evolve

ELSEVIER

YOU'VE JUST PURCHASED MORE THAN A TEXTBOOK!

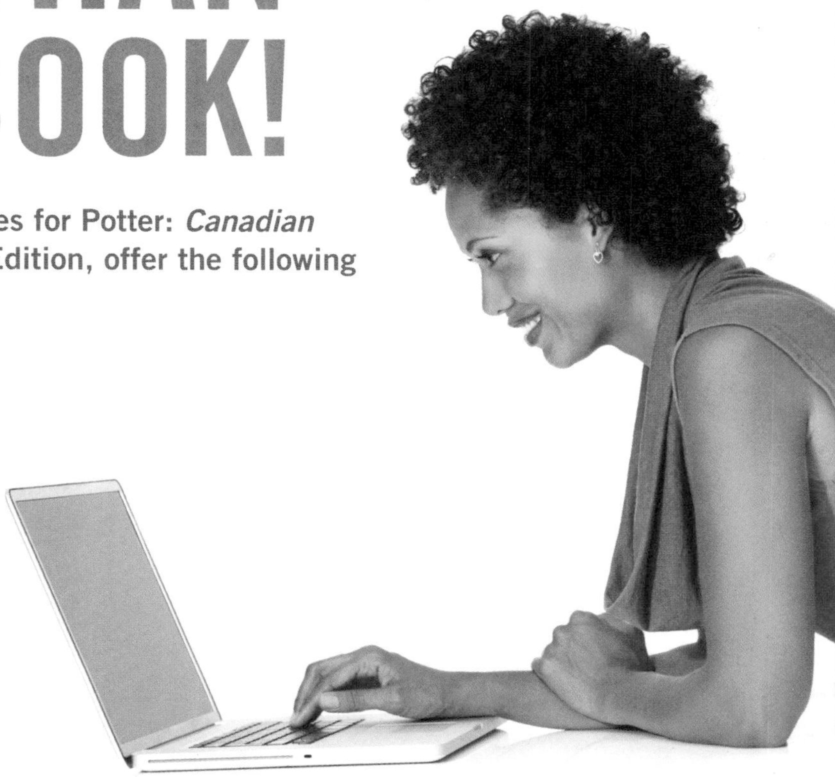

Evolve Student Learning Resources for Potter: *Canadian Fundamentals of Nursing*, Sixth Edition, offer the following features:

- Audio Glossary
- Case Studies
- Concept Map Creator
- Content Updates
- Examination Review Questions
- Key Points
- Skills Performance Checklists
- Tutorial – Calculations
- Tutorial – Fluids and Electrolytes
- Videos

Activate the complete learning experience that comes with each textbook purchase by registering at

http://evolve.elsevier.com/Canada/Potter/fundamentals/

REGISTER TODAY!

Canadian Fundamentals of Nursing

Sixth Edition

EDITORS

BARBARA J. ASTLE, RN, PhD
Associate Professor
Director, Centre for Equity & Global Engagement (CEGE)
School of Nursing
Trinity Western University
Langley, British Columbia

WENDY DUGGLEBY, RN, PhD
Professor
Associate Dean Research, and Nursing Research Chair, Aging and Quality of Life
Director Innovations in Seniors Care Research Unit
Faculty of Nursing
University of Alberta
Edmonton, Alberta

US NINTH EDITION EDITORS

Patricia A. Potter, RN, MSN, PhD, FAAN
Director of Research
Patient Care Services
Barnes-Jewish Hospital
St. Louis, Missouri

Anne Griffin Perry, RN, MSN, EdD, FAAN
Professor Emerita
School of Nursing
Southern Illinois University Edwardsville
Edwardsville, Illinois

Patricia A. Stockert, RN, BSN, MS, PhD
President, College of Nursing
Saint Francis Medical Center College of Nursing
Peoria, Illinois

Amy M. Hall, RN, BSN, MS, PhD, CNE
Chair and White Family Endowed Professor of Nursing
Dunigan Family Department of Nursing and Health Sciences
University of Evansville
Evansville, Indiana

ELSEVIER

ELSEVIER

CANADIAN FUNDAMENTALS OF NURSING, SIXTH EDITION **ISBN: 978-1-77172-113-4**

This adaptation of *Fundamentals of Nursing,* 9th edition, by Patricia A. Potter, Patricia Stockert, Anne Griffin Perry, and Amy Hall is published by arrangement with Elsevier Inc.

ISBN: 978-0-323-32740-4

Notice

Knowledge and best practice in this field are constantly changing. As new research and expertise broaden our knowledge, changes in practice, treatment, and drug therapy may become necessary.

Practitioners and researchers must always rely on their own experience and knowledge in evaluating and using any information, methods, compounds, or experiments described herein. In using such information or methods they should be mindful of their own safety and the safety of others, including parties for whom they have a professional responsibility.

With respect to any drug or pharmaceutical products identified, readers are advised to check the most current information provided (i) on procedures featured or (ii) by the manufacturer of each product to be administered, and to verify the recommended dose or formula, the method and duration of administration, and contraindications. It is the responsibility of practitioners, relying on their own experience and knowledge of their patients, to make diagnoses, to determine dosages and the best treatment for each individual patient, and to take all appropriate safety precautions.

To the fullest extent of the law, neither the Publisher nor the authors, contributors, or editors assume any liability for any injury and/or damage to persons or property as a matter of products liability, negligence or otherwise, or from any use or operation of any methods, products, instructions, or ideas contained in the material herein.

The Publisher

Library and Archives Canada Cataloguing in Publication

Potter, Patricia Ann, author
Canadian fundamentals of nursing / Patricia A. Potter, RN, MSN, PhD, FAAN, Director of Research, Patient Care Services, Barnes-Jewish Hospital, St. Louis, Missouri [and 3 others] ; Canadian editors: Barbara J. Astle, RN, PhD, Associate Professor, Director, Centre for Equity & Global Engagement (CEGE), School of Nursing, Trinity Western University, Langley, British Columbia, Wendy Duggleby, RN, PhD, Professor, Associate Dean Research, and Nursing Research Chair Aging and Quality of Life, Faculty of Nursing, University of Alberta, Edmonton, Alberta. – Sixth edition.

Includes index.
ISBN 978-1-77172-113-4 (hardcover)

1. Nursing–Textbooks. 2. Nursing–Canada–Textbooks. 3. Textbooks. I. Astle, Barbara J., 1957–, editor II. Duggleby, Wendy Diane, 1953-, editor III. Title.

RT41.P68 2018 610.73 C2017-905541-0

VP Medical and Canadian Education: Madelene J. Hyde
Content Strategist (Acquisitions): Roberta A. Spinosa-Millman
Content Development Manager: Lisa Newton
Content Development Specialist: Martina van de Velde
Book Production Manager: Jeff Patterson
Senior Production Managers: Mary Pohlman, Cindy Thoms
Book Designer: Paula Catalano
Copy Editor: Jerrolyn Hurlbutt
Cover Designer: Brett J. Miller, BJM Graphic Design and Communications
Cover Images: Itana/Shutterstock.com
Typesetting and Assembly: Toppan Best-set Premedia Limited
Printing and Binding: Transcontinental Printing

Elsevier Canada
420 Main Street East, Suite 636, Milton, ON, Canada L9T 5G3
Phone: 416-644-7053

2 3 4 5 6 22 21 20 19 18

Printed in Canada

Ebook ISBN: 978-1-77172-114-1

CONTENTS

UNIT II Foundations of Nursing Practice

UNIT VIII Basic Physiological Needs

PREFACE TO THE STUDENT

Canadian Fundamentals of Nursing provides you with all of the fundamental nursing concepts and skills you will need in a visually appealing, easy-to-use format. As you begin your nursing education, it is very important that you have a resource that includes all of the information required to prepare you for lectures, classroom activities, clinical assignments, and examinations. We've designed this text to meet all of those needs.

Check out the following special learning aids featured in *Canadian Fundamentals of Nursing*.

Learning Objectives begin each chapter to help you focus on the key information that follows.

Key Terms are listed at the beginning of each chapter and are boldfaced and defined in the text. Page numbers help you quickly find where each term is defined.

Media Resources detail what electronic resources are available to you for every chapter.

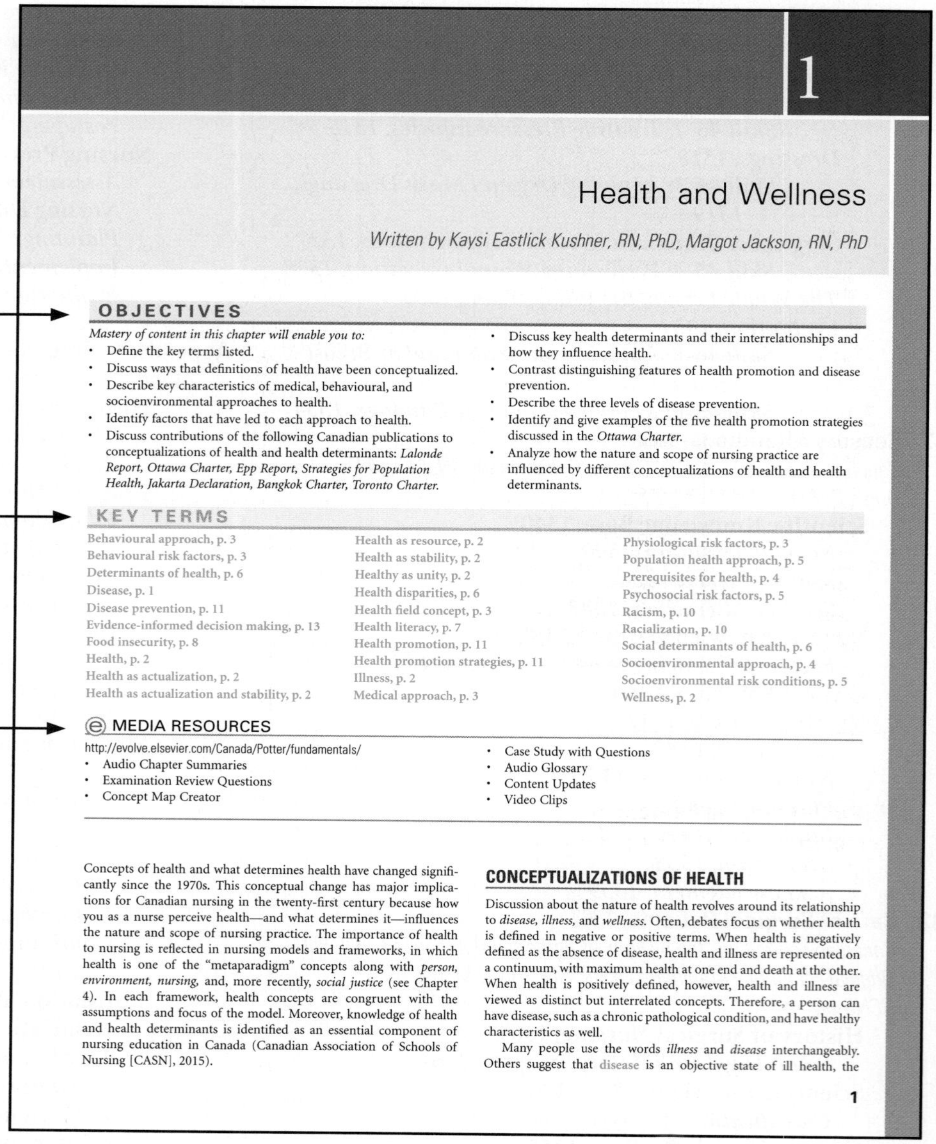
1

Health and Wellness

Written by Kaysi Eastlick Kushner, RN, PhD, Margot Jackson, RN, PhD

OBJECTIVES

Mastery of content in this chapter will enable you to:
- Define the key terms listed.
- Discuss ways that definitions of health have been conceptualized.
- Describe key characteristics of medical, behavioural, and socioenvironmental approaches to health.
- Identify factors that have led to each approach to health.
- Discuss contributions of the following Canadian publications to conceptualizations of health and health determinants: *Lalonde Report, Ottawa Charter, Epp Report, Strategies for Population Health, Jakarta Declaration, Bangkok Charter, Toronto Charter.*
- Discuss key health determinants and their interrelationships and how they influence health.
- Contrast distinguishing features of health promotion and disease prevention.
- Describe the three levels of disease prevention.
- Identify and give examples of the five health promotion strategies discussed in the *Ottawa Charter.*
- Analyze how the nature and scope of nursing practice are influenced by different conceptualizations of health and health determinants.

KEY TERMS

Behavioural approach, p. 3
Behavioural risk factors, p. 3
Determinants of health, p. 6
Disease, p. 1
Disease prevention, p. 11
Evidence-informed decision making, p. 13
Food insecurity, p. 8
Health, p. 2
Health as actualization, p. 2
Health as actualization and stability, p. 2
Health as resource, p. 2
Health as stability, p. 2
Healthy as unity, p. 2
Health disparities, p. 6
Health field concept, p. 3
Health literacy, p. 7
Health promotion, p. 11
Health promotion strategies, p. 11
Illness, p. 2
Medical approach, p. 3
Physiological risk factors, p. 3
Population health approach, p. 5
Prerequisites for health, p. 4
Psychosocial risk factors, p. 5
Racism, p. 10
Racialization, p. 10
Social determinants of health, p. 6
Socioenvironmental approach, p. 4
Socioenvironmental risk conditions, p. 5
Wellness, p. 2

MEDIA RESOURCES

http://evolve.elsevier.com/Canada/Potter/fundamentals/
- Audio Chapter Summaries
- Examination Review Questions
- Concept Map Creator
- Case Study with Questions
- Audio Glossary
- Content Updates
- Video Clips

Concepts of health and what determines health have changed significantly since the 1970s. This conceptual change has major implications for Canadian nursing in the twenty-first century because how you as a nurse perceive health—and what determines it—influences the nature and scope of nursing practice. The importance of health to nursing is reflected in nursing models and frameworks, in which health is one of the "metaparadigm" concepts along with *person, environment, nursing,* and, more recently, *social justice* (see Chapter 4). In each framework, health concepts are congruent with the assumptions and focus of the model. Moreover, knowledge of health and health determinants is identified as an essential component of nursing education in Canada (Canadian Association of Schools of Nursing [CASN], 2015).

CONCEPTUALIZATIONS OF HEALTH

Discussion about the nature of health revolves around its relationship to *disease, illness,* and *wellness.* Often, debates focus on whether health is defined in negative or positive terms. When health is negatively defined as the absence of disease, health and illness are represented on a continuum, with maximum health at one end and death at the other. When health is positively defined, however, health and illness are viewed as distinct but interrelated concepts. Therefore, a person can have disease, such as a chronic pathological condition, and have healthy characteristics as well.

Many people use the words *illness* and *disease* interchangeably. Others suggest that disease is an objective state of ill health, the

1

Key Concepts appear at the end of each chapter to help you review important content.

Review Questions at the end of each chapter help you review and evaluate what you have learned. Answers and rationales are provided at the back of the book.

Recommended Websites provide up-to-date online resources and are annotated to give you some information about each website.

Critical Thinking Exercises encourage you to think creatively and effectively to apply essential content.

BOX 7-7 FOCUS ON PRIMARY HEALTH CARE

How to Encourage Nurses Individually and Collectively to Work Toward Eliminating Social Inequities

- Utilize the principles of primary health care for the benefit of the public and patients receiving care.
- Understand that some groups in society are systemically disadvantaged, which leads to poorer health and diminished well-being. Nurses work to improve the quality of lives of people who are part of disadvantaged and vulnerable groups and communities, and they take action to overcome barriers to health care.
- Recognize and work to address organizational, social, economic, and political factors that influence health and well-being within the context of the nurse's role in the delivery of care.

information or seek assistance can be helpful strategies to address the issue causing moral distress. Even if formal or informal team discussions do not resolve ethical conflicts, discussions can be beneficial because they provide a way for nurses to have their concerns heard and legitimized. Nurse managers are also key team members for creating safe places where team discussions of challenging ethical issues can occur. The manager plays an essential role in offering support and the opportunity for the resolution of conflict to occur. Having the manager involved can help to reduce more distress.

KEY CONCEPTS

- Values clarification helps nurses explore personal values and feelings and to decide how to act on personal beliefs. It also facilitates nurse–patient communication.
- Ethics is the study of philosophical ideals of what is beneficial or valuable for all.
- A code of ethics provides a foundation for professional nursing. Such a code promotes accountability, responsibility, and advocacy.
- Theories of bioethics refer to ethical issues specific to the delivery of health care. They are based on the principles of autonomy, beneficence, nonmaleficence, and justice.
- Relational ethics theory encompasses more than bioethics; it addresses the role of relationships in the ethical delivery of health care. It maintains that the nurse–patient relationship is the foundation of nursing ethics.
- Ethical problems arise from differences in values, from technological advances, from end-of-life experiences, and from changes in work environments.
- A standard process for thinking through ethical dilemmas, including critical thinking skills, helps health care providers resolve conflict or uncertainty about correct actions.

CRITICAL THINKING EXERCISES

1. Complete the values clarification exercise (Box 7-1) with your classmates or others. Compare the answers and discuss the differences.
2. You are a clinic nurse in a small community clinic. A 17-year-old female patient has been coming to the clinic for treatment for and support with a sexually transmitted infection. During recent months, she has lost her support from a close friend. In addition, her parents are divorced, and she has little contact with them. Her health and well-being are of concern. Her appearance is unkempt, her nutritional status is not balanced, and she has admitted to being depressed. She asks for your help in planning her suicide. Discuss your response to her request. Begin by acknowledging the laws related to assisted suicide in Canada. Examine your personal feelings about suicide. Include a discussion about your understanding of sexually transmitted infections: Where do they come from? Who gets these infections? Why do people get these infections? What are your feelings and opinions about people with sexually transmitted infections? Construct your response, keeping in mind the theory of relational ethics. Discuss your role in this situation. What are your possible courses of action?
3. You have been assigned the care of a 98-year-old woman who was recently admitted with a diagnosis of pneumonia. She has a history of cardiac disease and takes a number of medications. She had been fairly active until the past few days, when her cough worsened and a fever developed. You note that her pulse has become weak and threadlike and that her respirations are increasingly laboured. The patient is now too weak to respond to you. When you mention to the family that you may need to call the physician and even take heroic life-saving measures, the patient's son and daughter become distraught, saying that they do not want their mother to be kept alive on "machines." They report that they have discussed this situation with their mother. You find that her wishes have not been documented in her chart. The family members have not discussed this situation with the patient's primary physician. What actions would you consider taking at this moment? Take into account the ethical principles of autonomy and beneficence and the idea of futile care. What are your personal values about interventions at the end of life?

REVIEW QUESTIONS

1. The nurse knows that values clarification plays a major role in
   1. Creating a set of rules for conduct
   2. Identifying values that should be accepted by all
   3. Resolving issues of "value conflict"
   4. Developing a code of ethics
2. In Canada, equitable access to health care means that all citizens have equal access to medically necessary services. Which ethical principle would reflect equal access to health care?
   1. Accountability
   2. Autonomy
   3. Relational ethics
   4. Justice
3. It may seem redundant when health care providers, including professional nurses, agree to "do no harm" to their patients. The point of this agreement is to reassure the public that in all ways, not only will the health care team work to heal patients but they also agree to do this in the least painful and harmful way possible. Which principle describes this agreement?
   1. Beneficence
   2. Accountability
   3. Nonmaleficence
   4. Respect for autonomy
4. A patient is admitted to a medical unit. The patient is fearful of hospitals. The nurse carefully assesses the patient to determine the exact fears and then establishes interventions designed to reduce

3. Assess the patient's point of view and prepare to articulate this point of view
4. Document all clinical changes in the medical record in a timely manner

8. Which action is *not* part of the nurse's role as patient advocate?
   1. Intervening if other people fail to respect the patient's dignity
   2. Protecting the patient's right to confidentiality and privacy
   3. Making nursing care decisions for the patient
   4. Advocating for appropriate use of interventions to minimize suffering
9. Mrs. Bruce, 68 years old, has been waiting to be seen in the outpatient symptom control clinic for the last 4 hours. Her daughter is becoming extremely anxious for her mother, and she approaches the triage desk. Which nursing action best reflects a relational ethics approach?
   1. In an assertive voice, the triage nurse comments that the clinic policy is to see people in order of medical priority, not waiting time.
   2. The nurse can sense that the daughter is becoming concerned regarding the time her mother has waited to be seen by the clinic nurse practitioner or oncologist, and without further discussion, the triage nurse assures her that everything will be just fine.
   3. As the daughter shares her narrative of needing to be seen, the nurse interjects to assure the daughter that the best effort will be made to get her mother seen in a timely manner.
   4. The nurse senses the daughter's angst. From behind the counter the nurse moves toward the daughter to listen. The nurse respectfully shares that at the present time there is not a room available, but the clinic team is working on moving a particular patient to an inpatient unit. The nurse explains further that, although she cannot predict the time, she will do her best to keep her informed.
10. Ethical dilemmas often arise over a conflict of opinion. Once the nurse has determined that the dilemma is ethical, which action should the nurse take first in negotiating the difference of opinion?

1. Consult a professional ethicist to ensure that the steps of the process occur in full
2. Gather all relevant information regarding the dilemma
3. List the ethical principles that inform the dilemma so that negotiations agree on the language of the discussion
4. Ensure that the attending physician has written an order for an ethics consultation to support the ethics process

Answers: 1. 3; 2. 4; 3. 3; 4. 4; 5. 4; 6. 2; 7. 3; 8. 3; 9. 4; 10. 2

Rationales for the Review Questions appear at the end of the book.

RECOMMENDED WEBSITES

Canadian Bioethics Society: http://www.bioethics.ca.
Founded in 1988 through the amalgamation of the Canadian Society of Bioethics and the Canadian Society for Medical Bioethics. Members include health care administrators, lawyers, nurses, philosophers, physicians, theologians, and other professionals concerned with the ethical and humane dimensions of health care. The website offers information about the annual CBS conference, national and international ethics organization links, and relevant ethics journals from a variety of disciplines.

W. Maurice Young Centre for Applied Ethics: http://www.ethics.ubc.ca.
Established by the University of British Columbia in 1993; primarily an interdisciplinary research centre in which a variety of ethics topics are studied. The website has links to other ethics organizations and ethics resources. The centre's newsletter is also available on the website.

John Dossetor Health Ethics Centre at the University of Alberta: http://www.bioethics.ualberta.ca.
The John Dossetor Health Ethics Centre is the only interdisciplinary, academic health ethics centre in Alberta and one of the first in Canada. The Centre is involved in health ethics education, research, and community engagement at the University of Alberta.

REFERENCES

Amjad, H., Towle, V., & Fried, T. (2014). Association of experience with illness and end-of-life care with advance care planning in older adults. *Journal of the American Geriatrics Society*, *62*(7), 1304–1309. doi:10.11111/jgs.12894.

Austin, W. (2007). The ethics of everyday practice: Healthcare environments as moral communities. *Advances in Nursing Science*, *30*(1), 81–88.

Beauchamp, T., & Childress, J. (2012). *Principles of biomedical ethics* (7th ed.). New York: Oxford University Press.

Bennett Jacobs, B., & Taylor, C. (2005). Medical futility in the natural attitude. *ANS. Advances in Nursing Science*, *28*, 288–305.

Bergum, V. (2013). Relational ethics in nursing. In J. Storch, P. Rodney, & R. Starzomski (Eds.), *Toward a moral horizon: Nursing ethics for leadership and practice*. Toronto: Pearson Education.

Bergum, V., & Dossetor, J. (2005). *Relational ethics: The full meaning of respect*. Hagerstown, MD: University Publishing Group.

Bilsen, J., Vander Stichele, R., Mortier, F., et al. (2004). Involvement of nurses in physician assisted dying. *Journal of Advanced Nursing*, *47*(6), 583–591. doi:10.1111/j.1365-2648.2004.02982.x.

Blondeau, D., Lavoie, M., Valois, P., et al. (2000). The attitude of Canadian nurses towards advance directives. *Nursing Ethics*, *7*(5), 399–411.

Boutain, D. (2005). Social justice in nursing: A review of the literature. In M. de Chesney (Ed.), *Caring for the vulnerable: Perspectives in nursing theory, practice, research*. Mississauga, ON: Jones & Barlett Publications.

Browne, A. (2000). When patients demand too much. *Health Ethics Today*, *11*(1), 2–3.

Canadian Association Schools of Nursing/Association Canadienne des Écoles de Sciences Infirmières [CASN/ACESI]. (2015). *National nursing education framework: Final report*. Ottawa: Author.

Canadian Health Services Research Foundation. (2006). *What's ailing our nurses? A discussion of the major issues affecting nursing human resources in Canada*. Ottawa: Author.

Canadian Nurses Association (CNA). (2012). *When private becomes public: The ethical challenges of and opportunities of social media*. Ottawa: Author.

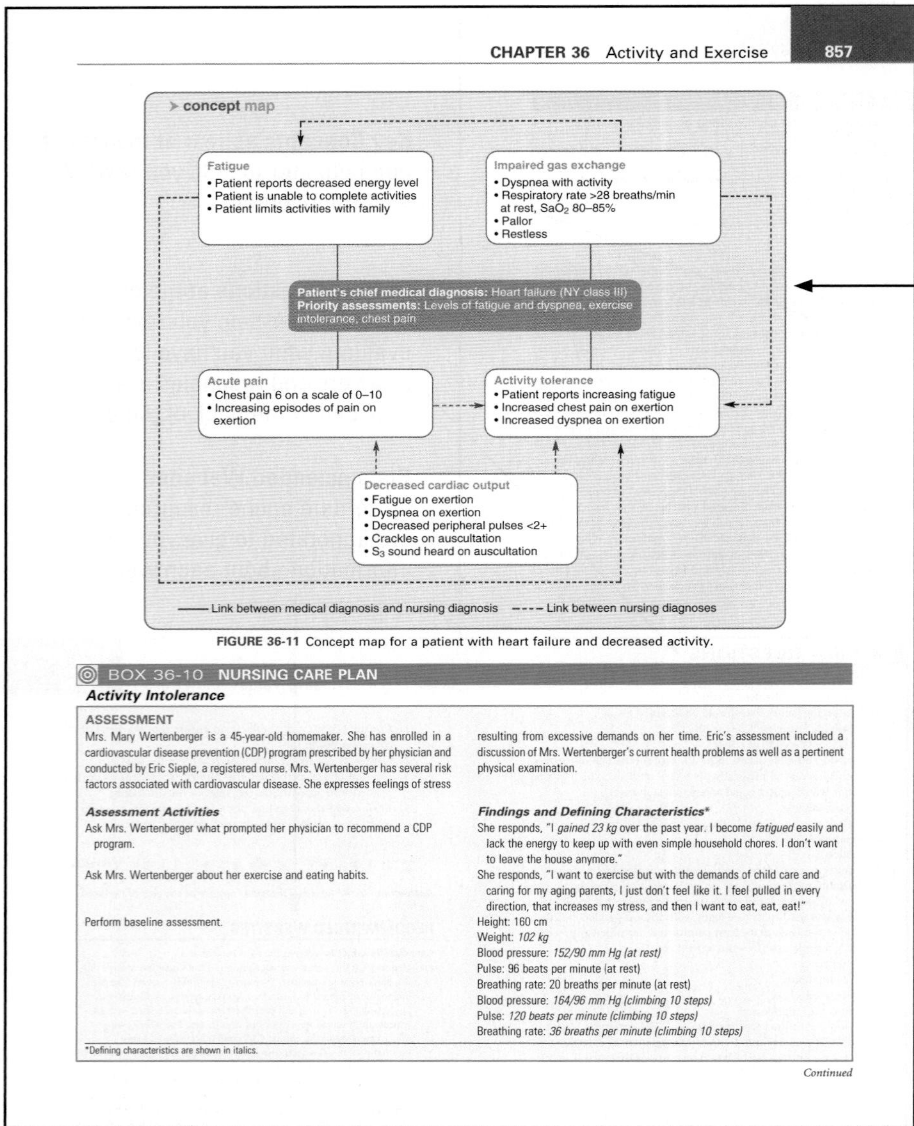

CHAPTER 36 Activity and Exercise 857

> concept map

Fatigue
• Patient reports decreased energy level
• Patient is unable to complete activities
• Patient limits activities with family

Impaired gas exchange
• Dyspnea with activity
• Respiratory rate >28 breaths/min at rest, SaO_2 80–85%
• Pallor
• Restless

Patient's chief medical diagnosis: Heart failure (NY class III)
Priority assessments: Levels of fatigue and dyspnea, exercise intolerance, chest pain

Acute pain
• Chest pain 6 on a scale of 0–10
• Increasing episodes of pain on exertion

Activity tolerance
• Patient reports increasing fatigue
• Increased chest pain on exertion
• Increased dyspnea on exertion

Decreased cardiac output
• Fatigue on exertion
• Dyspnea on exertion
• Decreased peripheral pulses <2+
• Crackles on auscultation
• S_3 sound heard on auscultation

—— Link between medical diagnosis and nursing diagnosis ---- Link between nursing diagnoses

FIGURE 36-11 Concept map for a patient with heart failure and decreased activity.

BOX 36-10 NURSING CARE PLAN

Activity Intolerance

ASSESSMENT

Mrs. Mary Wertenberger is a 45-year-old homemaker. She has enrolled in a cardiovascular disease prevention (CDP) program prescribed by her physician and conducted by Eric Sieple, a registered nurse. Mrs. Wertenberger has several risk factors associated with cardiovascular disease. She expresses feelings of stress resulting from excessive demands on her time. Eric's assessment included a discussion of Mrs. Wertenberger's current health problems as well as a pertinent physical examination.

Assessment Activities	***Findings and Defining Characteristics****
Ask Mrs. Wertenberger what prompted her physician to recommend a CDP program.	She responds, "I *gained 23 kg* over the past year. I become *fatigued* easily and lack the energy to keep up with even simple household chores. I don't want to leave the house anymore."
Ask Mrs. Wertenberger about her exercise and eating habits.	She responds, "I want to exercise but with the demands of child care and caring for my aging parents, I just don't feel like it. I feel pulled in every direction, that increases my stress, and then I want to eat, eat, eat!"
Perform baseline assessment.	Height: 160 cm Weight: *102 kg* Blood pressure: *152/90 mm Hg (at rest)* Pulse: 96 beats per minute (at rest) Breathing rate: 20 breaths per minute (at rest) Blood pressure: *164/96 mm Hg (climbing 10 steps)* Pulse: *120 beats per minute (climbing 10 steps)* Breathing rate: *36 breaths per minute (climbing 10 steps)*

*Defining characteristics are shown in italics.

Continued

Concept Maps show you the association among multiple nursing diagnoses and their relationship to medical diagnoses.

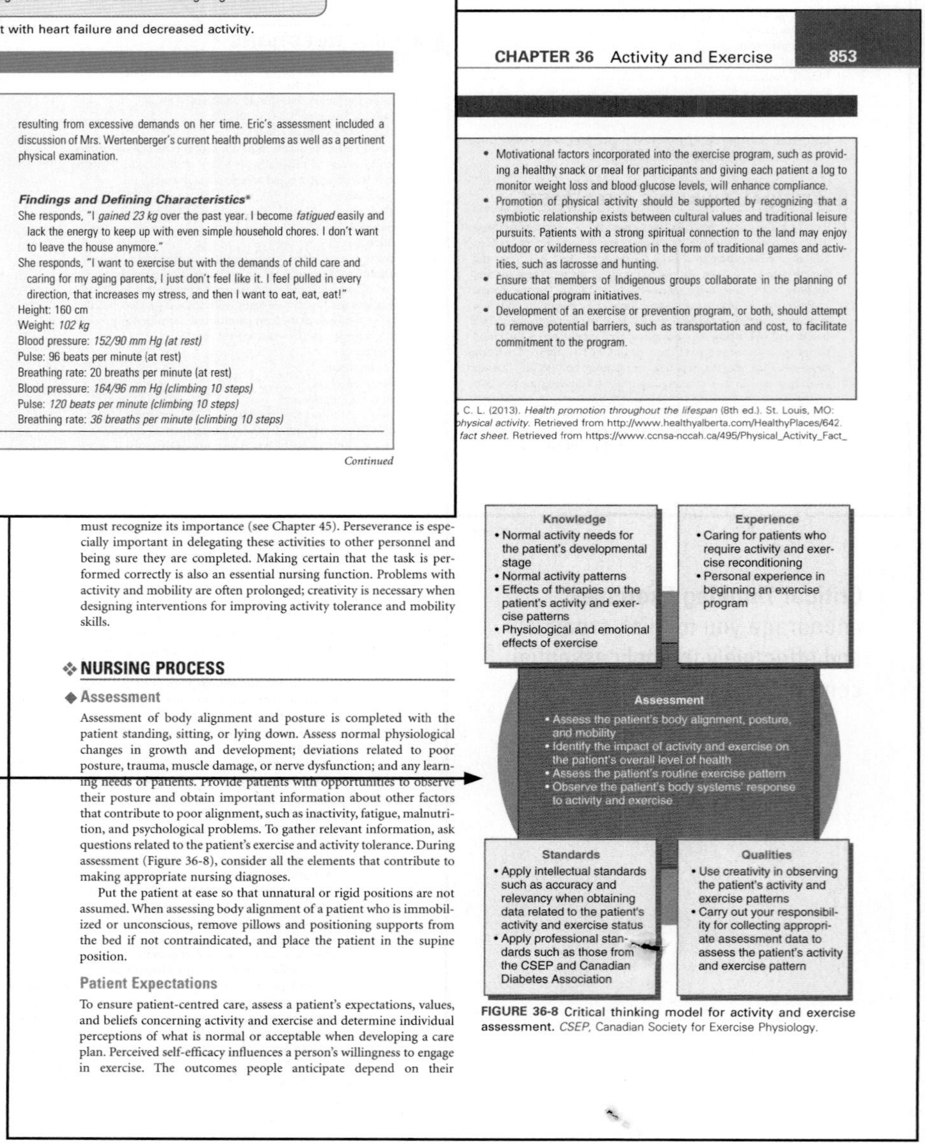

CHAPTER 36 Activity and Exercise 853

• Motivational factors incorporated into the exercise program, such as providing a healthy snack or meal for participants and giving each patient a log to monitor weight loss and blood glucose levels, will enhance compliance.
• Promotion of physical activity should be supported by recognizing that a symbiotic relationship exists between cultural values and traditional leisure pursuits. Patients with a strong spiritual connection to the land may enjoy outdoor or wilderness recreation in the form of traditional games and activities, such as lacrosse and hunting.
• Ensure that members of Indigenous groups collaborate in the planning of educational program initiatives.
• Development of an exercise or prevention program, or both, should attempt to remove potential barriers, such as transportation and cost, to facilitate commitment to the program.

, C. L. (2013). *Health promotion throughout the lifespan* (8th ed.). St. Louis, MO:
physical activity. Retrieved from http://www.healthyalberta.com/HealthyPlaces/642.
fact sheet. Retrieved from https://www.ccnsa-nccah.ca/495/Physical_Activity_Fact_

must recognize its importance (see Chapter 45). Perseverance is especially important in delegating these activities to other personnel and being sure they are completed. Making certain that the task is performed correctly is also an essential nursing function. Problems with activity and mobility are often prolonged; creativity is necessary when designing interventions for improving activity tolerance and mobility skills.

NURSING PROCESS

Assessment

Assessment of body alignment and posture is completed with the patient standing, sitting, or lying down. Assess normal physiological changes in growth and development; deviations related to poor posture, trauma, muscle damage, or nerve dysfunction; and any learning needs of patients. Provide patients with opportunities to observe their posture and obtain important information about other factors that contribute to poor alignment, such as inactivity, fatigue, malnutrition, and psychological problems. To gather relevant information, ask questions related to the patient's exercise and activity tolerance. During assessment (Figure 36-8), consider all the elements that contribute to making appropriate nursing diagnoses.

Put the patient at ease so that unnatural or rigid positions are not assumed. When assessing body alignment of a patient who is immobilized or unconscious, remove pillows and positioning supports from the bed if not contraindicated, and place the patient in the supine position.

Patient Expectations

To ensure patient-centred care, assess a patient's expectations, values, and beliefs concerning activity and exercise and determine individual perceptions of what is normal or acceptable when developing a care plan. Perceived self-efficacy influences a person's willingness to engage in exercise. The outcomes people anticipate depend on their

Knowledge
• Normal activity needs for the patient's developmental stage
• Normal activity patterns
• Effects of therapies on the patient's activity and exercise patterns
• Physiological and emotional effects of exercise

Experience
• Caring for patients who require activity and exercise reconditioning
• Personal experience in beginning an exercise program

Assessment
• Assess the patient's body alignment, posture, and mobility
• Identify the impact of activity and exercise on the patient's overall level of health
• Assess the patient's routine exercise pattern
• Observe the patient's body systems' response to activity and exercise

Standards
• Apply intellectual standards such as accuracy and relevancy when obtaining data related to the patient's activity and exercise status
• Apply professional standards such as those from the CSEP and Canadian Diabetes Association

Qualities
• Use creativity in observing the patient's activity and exercise patterns
• Carry out your responsibility for collecting appropriate assessment data to assess the patient's activity and exercise pattern

FIGURE 36-8 Critical thinking model for activity and exercise assessment. *CSEP,* Canadian Society for Exercise Physiology.

The unique **Critical Thinking Model** shows clearly how the nursing process and critical thinking come together to help you provide the best care for your patients.

The five-step **Nursing Process** provides a consistent framework for presentation of content in clinical chapters.

Research Highlight boxes provide abstracts of current nursing research studies and explain the implications for your daily practice.

physical limitations, which may affect their ability to manage their medications properly.

Once a medication has been given, careful monitoring of the effectiveness of the medication, its adverse effects, and signs of adverse reactions and/or drug interactions is necessary. If the medication has not achieved its desired effect, additional follow-up is needed. Within a collaborative model of care, nurses should be working closely with pharmacists and physicians if further follow-up or assessments are necessary (MacDonald, 2010).

Risk Management: Agency Policy and Procedure. Most institutions have nursing policy and procedure manuals to guide nursing practice. These manuals are updated annually on the basis of current evidence-informed practice literature. Policy and procedure manuals contain vital information for medication administration, including the types of medications nurses are permitted to administer, the preparation of medications, the administration of medications, and guidelines for evaluating patients' response to medications. For example, some agencies require nurses to complete specialized training to qualify them to safely administer IV chemotherapeutic agents. Furthermore, the administration of certain medications (e.g., IV inotropic medications for regulating a patient's blood pressure) are prohibited on general medicine and surgery units and permitted only in critical care areas where the patient is continuously monitored for responses to medication therapy.

Maintaining Patients' Rights. Because of the potential risks related to medication administration, patients have the right to the following:

- To be informed of the medication's name, purpose, action, and potential undesired effects
- To refuse a medication regardless of the consequences
- To have qualified nurses or physicians assess their medication history, including allergies and use of herbal therapies (Box 34-11)
- To be properly advised of the experimental nature of medication therapy and to give written consent for its use
- To receive labelled medications safely without discomfort in accordance with the rights of medication administration
- To receive appropriate supportive therapy in relation to medication therapy
- To not receive unnecessary medications
- To be informed whether medications are part of a research study

Nurses need to be aware of these rights and handle all inquiries by patients and their families courteously and professionally.

BOX 34-11 Nursing Assessment Questions

- What prescription and nonprescription medications do you take, when do you take them, and how do you take them? Do you have a list of medications from your pharmacy or your health care provider?
- What are your medications for?
- What adverse effects have you experienced?
- Have you ever stopped taking your medications? If so, why did you stop taking them?
- How do you help yourself to remember to take your medications?
- Do you have any allergies to medications or foods? If so, describe what happens when you take the medication or eat the food.
- Describe your normal eating patterns. What foods do you eat, and at what times do you normally eat?
- How do your religious or cultural beliefs influence your beliefs about your medications?
- How do you pay for your medications? Do you have additional insurance through your employer or pension plan to help cover the costs of your medication? Do you live close to a pharmacy? How do you access prescription medications in your community?
- What questions do you have about your medications?

NURSING PROCESS AND MEDICATION ADMINISTRATION

Assessment

To determine the need for and potential response to medication therapy, nurses assess many factors. To ensure safe medication administration, nurses must perform thorough physical assessments of all patients before administering medications.

History. Before administering medications, the nurse needs to obtain or review the patient's medical history. A patient's medical history provides indications or contraindications for medication therapy. A patient who has disease or illness is at risk for adverse medication effects. For example, if a patient has a gastric ulcer, compounds containing aspirin will increase the likelihood of bleeding. If a patient has a long-term health condition, such as diabetes or arthritis, the patient requires medications to treat these conditions. A patient's surgical history may also indicate the use of medications. For example, after a thyroidectomy, a patient may require hormone replacement.

History of Allergies. If the patient has a history of contact allergies or allergies to medication or food, the nurse needs to inform the other members of the health care team. Food allergies should be carefully documented because many medications include ingredients also found in food sources. For example, a patient who is allergic to shellfish may also be sensitive to any product containing iodine, such as Betadine or dyes used in radiological testing. To ensure patient safety, when patients are admitted to a hospital, they are issued an identification band that lists the medications they are allergic to. All allergies must be noted on the nurse's admission notes, the medication records, and the phy-

BOX 39-13 RESEARCH HIGHLIGHT

A Qualitative Systematic Review of Influences on Attendance at Cardiac Rehabilitation Programs After Referral

Research Focus

Attendance at cardiac rehabilitation and secondary prevention programs is instrumental in the prevention of heart disease in high-risk populations (Clark, King-Shier, Thompson, et al., 2012, p. 835). Up to half of all patients who are referred to these programs do not participate (Clark et al., 2012, p. 835). There has been little research done to examine strategies for increasing attendance and to identify what influences attendance after referral (Clark et al., 2012, p. 835). Identifying factors that influence patient decisions to attend cardiac rehabilitation and secondary prevention programs would inform potential interventions to increase access for those requiring cardiac health services (Clark et al., 2012, p. 836).

Research Abstract

The purpose of a study by Clark and colleagues (2012) was to examine the factors and processes that influence the decisions that patients make to attend cardiac rehabilitation and secondary prevention services. A systematic review using qualitative meta-analysis was the method employed to gather data. Relevant qualitative studies that met specific identified criteria were gathered from numerous databases and a meta-ethnographic approach was used to synthesize the results. For the purpose of this study, Clark and colleagues (2012) defined the term *attendance* as "whether eligible patients participate in a secondary prevention service after referral from a health professional" (p. 836). There were 90 studies that informed the results of this study (2010 patients, 120 caregivers, 312 professionals).

Evidence-Informed Practice

- There were both personal and contextual barriers and facilitators that influenced patients' decisions to attend cardiac rehabilitation and secondary prevention services (Clark et al., 2012, p. 840).
- The personal barriers to attendance were related to knowledge of programs, perceived beliefs about heart disease, patient identity, as well as financial and occupational constraints. An increased sense of control over heart disease and the benefits of services facilitated attendance (Clark et al., 2012, p. 838).
- The contextual barriers of attendance were related to long-distance travel to programs and a lack of support from family members. Interestingly, families and health care providers were considered influential in patient attendance (Clark et al., 2012, p. 840).
- Interventions that may promote patient attendance at cardiac rehabilitation and secondary preventions services include the following (Clark et al., 2012, p. 840):
  - Providing personalized feedback to patients on the "suitability" of services (p. 840)
  - Facilitating patients' sense of control over their cardiovascular health
  - With the assistance of members from the interdisciplinary team, engaging in conversations with both the patients and their families regarding their beliefs and perceptions related to heart disease and rehabilitation services
  - Using face-to-face or web-based mechanisms to facilitate required support.

Clark, A. M., King-Shier, K. M., Thompson, D. R., Spaling, M. A., Duncan, A. S., Stone, J. A., et al. (2012). A qualitative systematic review of influences on attendance at cardiac rehabilitation programs after referral. *American Heart Journal, 164*(6), 835–845. doi:10.1016/j.ahj.2012.08.020.

such as long-term care facilities, and patients over the age of 65 years (CDC, 2017b).

Healthy Lifestyle Behaviour. Identification and elimination of risk factors for cardiopulmonary disease is an important part of primary health care. Nurses need to encourage patients to eat a healthy, low-fat, high-fibre diet; to monitor their cholesterol, triglyceride, high-density lipoprotein (HDL), and low-density lipoprotein (LDL) levels and reduce stress; to exercise; and to maintain a body weight in proportion to their height.

Elimination of use of cigarettes and other tobacco products, reduction in exposure to pollutants, monitoring of air quality, and adequate hydration are additional behaviours that promote health. Patients should be encouraged to examine their habits and to make changes to achieve their goals.

Exercise is a key factor in maintaining a healthy heart and lungs. Patients should be encouraged to exercise three to four times a week for 20 to 30 minutes. Aerobic exercise is necessary to improve lung function, strengthen muscles, and achieve better health. Walking is one of the most efficient ways of getting a good aerobic workout. Many shopping malls have programs that allow people to enter the mall before shops open and to use the enclosed area for walking. Some have measured and posted the distances to help people plan their activity and measure their progress. Patients should be taught how to take their pulse and pace themselves; it is better to walk 15 minutes every day than to walk to exhaustion to achieve a goal. Patients should plan a time interval and walk for the designated time. Gradually, they will notice that the distance increases as their endurance and fitness improve.

Patients with cardiopulmonary alterations need to minimize their risk for infection, especially during the winter months. Nurses need to teach patients to avoid large, crowded places; to keep their mouth and nose covered; and to be sure to dress warmly, including a scarf, hat, and gloves. This is especially important during the peak of the influenza season.

Patients with known cardiac disease and those with multiple risk factors should be cautioned to avoid exertion in cold weather. Shovelling snow is especially risky and in many patients can precipitate a cardiac event. Other activities, such as hanging holiday lights and decorations in the extreme cold, can precipitate chest pain and bronchospasm. Patients should be advised to avoid drinking alcohol before going out into cold weather because it blunts the respiratory drive when used in excess and may contribute to exposure to the cold by making the patient feel warm when the patient is really not protected from the cold.

Patients should also be taught to plan for the hot summer months. Activities should be limited to early in the day or late in the evening, when temperatures are lower. Patients should take care to maintain adequate hydration and sodium intake; this is especially true for those patients taking diuretics. Caffeinated and alcoholic beverages should be limited or avoided completely, because they act as diuretics and can contribute to dehydration.

Environmental Pollutants. Avoiding exposure to second-hand smoke is essential to maintaining optimal cardiopulmonary function. Most businesses and restaurants now ban smoking or have separate areas designated as smoking areas. If patients are exposed to second-hand smoke in their home environment, counselling and

Nursing Care Plans feature a format that helps you understand the process of assessment, the relationship between assessment findings and nursing diagnoses, the identification of goals and outcomes, the selection of interventions, and the process for evaluating care.

Rationales for each of the interventions in the care plans help you to understand why a specific step or set of steps is performed.

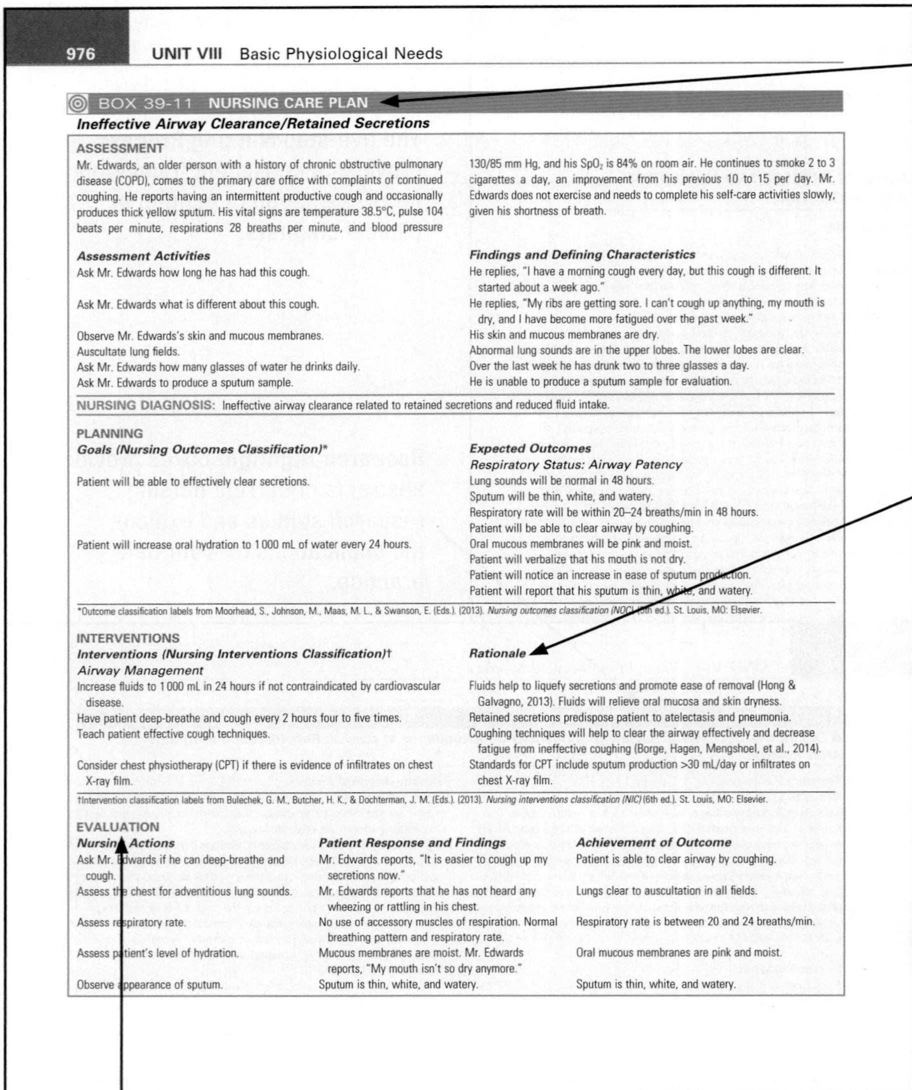

976 UNIT VIII Basic Physiological Needs

BOX 39-11 NURSING CARE PLAN

Ineffective Airway Clearance/Retained Secretions

ASSESSMENT

Mr. Edwards, an older person with a history of chronic obstructive pulmonary disease (COPD), comes to the primary care office with complaints of continued coughing. He reports having an intermittent productive cough and occasionally produces thick yellow sputum. His vital signs are temperature 38.5°C, pulse 104 beats per minute, respirations 28 breaths per minute, and blood pressure 130/85 mm Hg, and his SpO_2 is 84% on room air. He continues to smoke 2 to 3 cigarettes a day, an improvement from his previous 10 to 15 per day. Mr. Edwards does not exercise and needs to complete his self-care activities slowly, given his shortness of breath.

Assessment Activities	*Findings and Defining Characteristics*
Ask Mr. Edwards how long he has had this cough.	He replies, "I have a morning cough every day, but this cough is different. It started about a week ago."
Ask Mr. Edwards what is different about this cough.	He replies, "My ribs are getting sore. I can't cough up anything, my mouth is dry, and I have become more fatigued over the past week."
Observe Mr. Edwards's skin and mucous membranes.	His skin and mucous membranes are dry.
Auscultate lung fields.	Abnormal lung sounds are in the upper lobes. The lower lobes are clear.
Ask Mr. Edwards how many glasses of water he drinks daily.	Over the last week he has drunk two to three glasses a day.
Ask Mr. Edwards to produce a sputum sample.	He is unable to produce a sputum sample for evaluation.

NURSING DIAGNOSIS: Ineffective airway clearance related to retained secretions and reduced fluid intake.

PLANNING

*Goals (Nursing Outcomes Classification)**	*Expected Outcomes*
	Respiratory Status: Airway Patency
Patient will be able to effectively clear secretions.	Lung sounds will be normal in 48 hours. Sputum will be thin, white, and watery. Respiratory rate will be within 20–24 breaths/min in 48 hours. Patient will be able to clear airway by coughing.
Patient will increase oral hydration to 1 000 mL of water every 24 hours.	Oral mucous membranes will be pink and moist. Patient will verbalize that his mouth is not dry. Patient will notice an increase in ease of sputum production. Patient will report that his sputum is thin, white, and watery.

*Outcome classification labels from Moorhead, S., Johnson, M., Maas, M. L., & Swanson, E. (Eds.). (2013). *Nursing outcomes classification (NOC)* (5th ed.). St. Louis, MO: Elsevier.

INTERVENTIONS

Interventions (Nursing Interventions Classification)†	*Rationale*
Airway Management	
Increase fluids to 1 000 mL in 24 hours if not contraindicated by cardiovascular disease.	Fluids help to liquefy secretions and promote ease of removal (Hong & Galvagno, 2013). Fluids will relieve oral mucosa and skin dryness.
Have patient deep-breathe and cough every 2 hours four to five times.	Retained secretions predispose patient to atelectasis and pneumonia.
Teach patient effective cough techniques.	Coughing techniques will help to clear the airway effectively and decrease fatigue from ineffective coughing (Borge, Hagen, Mengshoel, et al., 2014).
Consider chest physiotherapy (CPT) if there is evidence of infiltrates on chest X-ray film.	Standards for CPT include sputum production >30 mL/day or infiltrates on chest X-ray film.

†Intervention classification labels from Bulechek, G. M., Butcher, H. K., & Dochterman, J. M. (Eds.). (2013). *Nursing interventions classification (NIC)* (6th ed.). St. Louis, MO: Elsevier.

EVALUATION

Nursing Actions	*Patient Response and Findings*	*Achievement of Outcome*
Ask Mr. Edwards if he can deep-breathe and cough.	Mr. Edwards reports, "It is easier to cough up my secretions now."	Patient is able to clear airway by coughing.
Assess the chest for adventitious lung sounds.	Mr. Edwards reports that he has not heard any wheezing or rattling in his chest.	Lungs clear to auscultation in all fields.
Assess respiratory rate.	No use of accessory muscles of respiration. Normal breathing pattern and respiratory rate.	Respiratory rate is between 20 and 24 breaths/min.
Assess patient's level of hydration.	Mucous membranes are moist. Mr. Edwards reports, "My mouth isn't so dry anymore."	Oral mucous membranes are pink and moist.
Observe appearance of sputum.	Sputum is thin, white, and watery.	Sputum is thin, white, and watery.

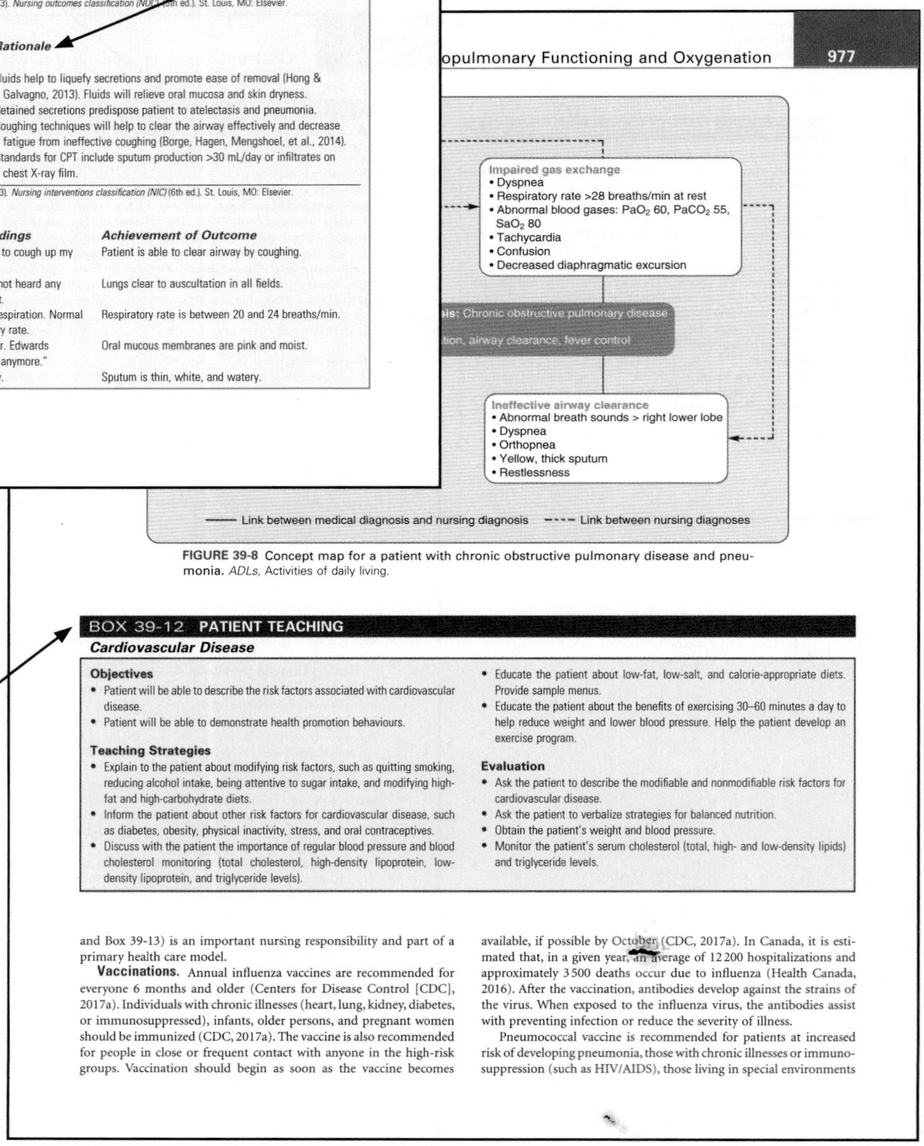

opulmonary Functioning and Oxygenation 977

FIGURE 39-8 Concept map for a patient with chronic obstructive pulmonary disease and pneumonia. *ADLs,* Activities of daily living.

BOX 39-12 PATIENT TEACHING

Cardiovascular Disease

Objectives
- Patient will be able to describe the risk factors associated with cardiovascular disease.
- Patient will be able to demonstrate health promotion behaviours.

Teaching Strategies
- Explain to the patient about modifying risk factors, such as quitting smoking, reducing alcohol intake, being attentive to sugar intake, and modifying high-fat and high-carbohydrate diets.
- Inform the patient about other risk factors for cardiovascular disease, such as diabetes, obesity, physical inactivity, stress, and oral contraceptives.
- Discuss with the patient the importance of regular blood pressure and blood cholesterol monitoring (total cholesterol, high-density lipoprotein, low-density lipoprotein, and triglyceride levels).
- Educate the patient about low-fat, low-salt, and calorie-appropriate diets. Provide sample menus.
- Educate the patient about the benefits of exercising 30–60 minutes a day to help reduce weight and lower blood pressure. Help the patient develop an exercise program.

Evaluation
- Ask the patient to describe the modifiable and nonmodifiable risk factors for cardiovascular disease.
- Ask the patient to verbalize strategies for balanced nutrition.
- Obtain the patient's weight and blood pressure.
- Monitor the patient's serum cholesterol (total, high- and low-density lipids) and triglyceride levels.

and Box 39-13) is an important nursing responsibility and part of a primary health care model.

Vaccinations. Annual influenza vaccines are recommended for everyone 6 months and older (Centers for Disease Control [CDC], 2017a). Individuals with chronic illnesses (heart, lung, kidney, diabetes, or immunosuppressed), infants, older persons, and pregnant women should be immunized (CDC, 2017a). The vaccine is also recommended for people in close or frequent contact with anyone in the high-risk groups. Vaccination should begin as soon as the vaccine becomes available, if possible by October (CDC, 2017a). In Canada, it is estimated that, in a given year, an average of 12 200 hospitalizations and approximately 3 500 deaths occur due to influenza (Health Canada, 2016). After the vaccination, antibodies develop against the strains of the virus. When exposed to the influenza virus, the antibodies assist with preventing infection or reduce the severity of illness.

Pneumococcal vaccine is recommended for patients at increased risk of developing pneumonia, those with chronic illnesses or immunosuppression (such as HIV/AIDS), those living in special environments

Evaluation sections explain how to evaluate and determine whether the outcomes have been achieved.

Patient Teaching boxes highlight what and how to teach patients and how to evaluate learning.

Evidence-Informed Practice boxes provide examples of recent state-of-the-science guidelines for nursing practice.

BOX 40-4 EVIDENCE-INFORMED PRACTICE

Preventing and Responding to Dehydration* in Older Persons

Evidence Summary

- Older persons are at increased risk of illness and death from dehydration, overhydration, and salt overload.
- Reduced thirst sensation and diminished appetite contribute to dehydration in older persons. Older people also have diminished capacity to correct volume losses.
- Chronic dehydration contributes to constipation in older persons.
- Adequate hydration in older persons is recommended for the prevention of falls, possibly related to hypotension or postural hypotension.
- Dehydration is a risk factor for delirium. The risk for delirium can be reduced as much as 33% with each additional glass of water consumed (El-Sharkawy et al., 2015).
- Signs and symptoms of dehydration can be easily confused with normal aging processes; therefore, assessment requires knowledge, skill, and commitment to acting on signs and symptoms.

Nursing Practice Guidelines

- Calculating fluid requirements should take into consideration individual characteristics including weight, gender, environmental factors, physical activity, and comorbidities, such as renal and cardiac disease.
- Identify risk factors for each older person from the following: age over 70 years, female, high or low body mass index, recent hospitalization, new admission to residential care, situations causing increased insensible loss (pyrexia), decreased access or ability to request fluids, and situations causing decreased intake, such as swallowing disorder (dysphagia), physical frailty, and decreased sentience. Diarrhea and vomiting are key causes of dehydration in older persons. Previous malnutrition, dehydration, polypharmacy, and having more than three medical conditions are significant risk factors.
- Establish an assessment, monitoring, and evaluation tool for identifying risk factors for older persons when initiating a caregiving relationship (e.g., on admission to residential care; with home assessment of older persons; routine health care visits)
- Assessment of hydration status should include physiological measures (urine specific gravity, urine colour, blood pressure, pulse, and respiration), as well as observed intake patterns and treatments. Recommend blood testing to determine cause and severity in suspected dehydration.
- Maintain fluid intake through documented planning using the nursing process in home, residential care, and hospital settings.
- Educate older persons and their family and friends on the importance of hydration.
- Evaluate acute losses such as diarrhea and vomiting.
- Attend more diligently to fluid balance in the context of medical issues such as diabetes, with the use of diuretics, with decreased cognitive level or functional status, and with reduced level of consciousness.
- Ensure availability of adequate fluids, including water, tea, coffee, milk, and other beverages, throughout the day and assist persons who are unable to access their own fluids. Replenish and refresh fluids through the day.
- Advocate for adequate staffing levels in residential and acute care, as inadequate staffing is closely linked to increased mortality (Shepherd, 2013).
- Promote audits of hydration practices and barriers or obstacles in health care settings and identify benchmarks for improved practice.
- Ongoing management consists of daily fluid goals, comparing current intake with physiological needs, and monitoring actual consumption of fluids and fluid-rich foods.
- Incorporate the offer of fluids, hot or cold, into regular rounds, socializing, and aspects of care using the "little and often" approach. Offer assistive devices, such as drinking straws or feeder cups, as necessary.
- Fluid status documentation should include hydration, eating habits, weight, vital signs, and fluid preferences.

*Dehydration is defined variably. Shepherd (2013) defines dehydration as equal to or greater than 1% loss of body mass through fluid loss. See text and Tables 40-3 and 40-4 for exploration of dehydration and tonicity.

fluids are also lost as burn exudate. Water vapour and heat are lost in proportion to the amount of skin that is burned away, increasing insensible losses. Blood leaks from damaged capillaries, adding to the loss of intravascular fluid volume. Sodium and water shift into the cells, further compromising ECF volume (Paul et al., 2016, p. 1844). Cell damage is accompanied by a loss of serum proteins, and a release of potassium into the intravascular fluid.

Respiratory disorders. Many alterations in respiratory function predispose the patient to respiratory acidosis. For example, pneumonia or sedative overdose interferes with the elimination of carbon dioxide due to hypoventilation. As the carbon dioxide continues to build up in the bloodstream, the body's compensatory mechanisms can no longer adapt, and the pH decreases. Likewise, hyperventilation that occurs with conditions such as fever or anxiety can cause respiratory alkalosis when too much carbon dioxide is expelled with the increased respiratory rate.

Gastrointestinal disturbances. Gastroenteritis and nasogastric suctioning result in a loss of fluid, potassium, and chloride ions. Hydrogen ions are also lost, resulting in metabolic alkalosis. In contrast, loss of bicarbonate-rich intestinal or pancreatic fluids (diarrhea, fistulas) can cause metabolic acidosis and also hypokalemia. Timely education of infant and child caregivers is necessary to prevent clinical dehydration when the infant or child is experiencing diarrhea.

NURSING KNOWLEDGE BASE

Developmental Factors

According to the Canadian Association of Schools of Nursing (CASN, 2015), foundational knowledge of human development expanding over the lifespan is an essential domain to consider when developing a plan of care. The developmental stage of the patient and the normal aging process can affect tissue oxygenation.

Infants and Toddlers. Infants and toddlers are at risk for upper respiratory tract infections as a result of frequent exposure to other children and exposure to second-hand smoke. In addition, during the teething process, some infants develop nasal congestion, which encourages bacterial growth and increases the potential for respiratory tract infection. Upper respiratory tract infections are usually not dangerous, and infants or toddlers recover with little difficulty.

School-Aged Children and Adolescents. School-aged children and adolescents are exposed to respiratory infections and respiratory risk factors such as second-hand smoke and cigarette smoking. A healthy child usually does not have adverse pulmonary effects from respiratory infections. A person who starts smoking in adolescence and continues to smoke into middle age, however, has an increased risk for cardiopulmonary disease and lung cancer.

Young and Middle-Aged Adults. Young and middle-aged adults are exposed to multiple cardiopulmonary risk factors: an unhealthy diet, lack of exercise, stress, over-the-counter and prescription drugs not used as intended, illegal drugs, and smoking. By reducing these modifiable factors patients may decrease their risk for cardiac or pulmonary diseases. During youth and middle age, lifelong habits and lifestyles are established. It is thus important to help these patients make good choices and informed decisions about the rest of their lives and their health care practices.

Older Persons. The cardiac and respiratory systems undergo changes throughout the aging process (Box 39-4). The changes are associated with calcification of the heart valves, SA node, and costal cartilages. The arterial system develops atherosclerotic plaques. Osteoporosis leads to changes in the size and shape of the thorax.

The trachea and large bronchi become enlarged from calcification of the airways. The alveoli enlarge, decreasing the surface area available for gas exchange. The number of functional cilia is reduced, causing a decrease in the effectiveness of the cough mechanism, putting the older person at increased risk for respiratory infections (Touhy & Jett, 2014). Ventilation and transfer of respiratory gases decline with age because the lungs are unable to expand fully, leading to lower oxygenation levels.

Lifestyle Risk Factors

Lifestyle modifications that influence cardiopulmonary functioning are frequently difficult because a patient is being asked to change a

Focus on Older Persons boxes prepare you to address the special needs of older persons.

BOX 39-4 FOCUS ON OLDER PERSONS

Changes to Cardiac and Respiratory Systems

- The tuberculin skin test is an unreliable indicator of tuberculosis in older persons. They frequently display false-positive or false-negative skin test reactions.
- Older persons are at an increased risk for reactivation of dormant organisms that have been present for decades, as a result of age-related changes in the immune system.
- The standard 5-TU Mantoux test is given and repeated or repeated with the 250-TU strength to create a booster effect.
- If the older person has a positive reaction, a complete history is necessary to determine any risk factors.
- Cardiac problems differ from other chronic conditions in that, when they become acute, symptoms worsen rapidly and necessitate hospitalization, whereas other chronic conditions can be managed in the home (Touhy & Jett, 2014).
- Regulating blood pressure in the older person results in 30% fewer strokes, 64% fewer cases of heart failure, 23% fewer fatal cardiac events, and 21% fewer cardiac-related deaths (Touhy & Jett, 2014).
- Mental status changes are often the first signs of respiratory problems and may include forgetfulness and irritability.
- Older persons may not complain of dyspnea until it affects the activities of daily living that are important to them.
- Changes in the older person's cough mechanism may lead to retention of pulmonary secretions, airway plugging, and atelectasis, if cough suppressants are not used with caution.
- Age-related changes in immune function lead to a decrease in cell-mediated and humoral immunity, causing an increased risk of respiratory infections (McCance & Huether, 2014).
- Alterations in the thorax that occur from ossification of costal cartilage, decreased space between vertebrae, and diminished respiratory muscle strength lead to impairment of chest expansion and oxygenation (Touhy & Jett, 2014).

Focus on Primary Health Care boxes draw attention to principles of primary health care and their application.

BOX 39-5 FOCUS ON PRIMARY HEALTH CARE

Positive Lifestyle Practices for Cardiopulmonary Health Promotion

As part of a primary health care focus, it is important to educate young to older persons about the following lifestyle practices that promote cardiopulmonary health:

- Maintain ideal body weight.
- Eat a low-fat, low-salt, calorie-appropriate diet.
- Engage in regular aerobic exercise 30 to 60 minutes daily.
- Use a filter mask when exposed to occupational hazards.
- Use stress-reduction techniques.
- Reduce exposure to secondary infections.
- Do not smoke.
- Avoid second-hand smoke and other pollutants.
- Have annual visits with a health care provider.
- Monitor blood pressure.
- Monitor cholesterol and triglyceride levels.
- Request an annual influenza vaccine, especially if at risk for the development of influenza.
- Request a pneumococcal vaccine, if appropriate.

Nursing Skills are presented in a clear, two-column format that includes Steps and Rationales to help you learn how and why a skill is performed.

Delegation Considerations guide you in delegating tasks to assistive personnel.

Critical Decision Points alert you to critical steps within a skill to ensure safe and effective client care.

CHAPTER 39 Cardiopulmonary Functioning and Oxygenation 983

SKILL 39-1 SUCTIONING

Delegation Considerations

If the patient has been assessed and determined to be stable, the skill of performing suctioning of an established tracheostomy can be delegated to an unregulated care provider (UCP) when the patient has a permanent tracheostomy tube or is receiving oropharyngeal suctioning. Before delegating this skill, do the following:

- Discuss with the UCP any unique modifications of the skill, such as the need to reapply any supplemental oxygen equipment following the procedure.
- Discuss appropriate suction limits.
- Instruct the UCP to report any change in the patient's respiratory status, signs and symptoms of hypoxemia, secretion colour or volume, or unresolved coughing or gagging.
- Instruct the UCP to report any change in the patient's colour, vital signs, or pain level.

Equipment

- Appropriate-size suction catheter (smallest diameter that will remove secretions effectively) or Yankauer catheter (oral suction)
- Nasal or oral airway (if indicated)
- Two sterile gloves or one sterile and one clean disposable glove (refer to technique)
- Clean towel or paper drape
- Portable or wall suction
- Mask, goggles, or face shield
- Connecting tube (1.8 metres)
- Pulse oximeter and stethoscope

Equipment for procedure without closed-suction catheter

- Small Y adapter (if catheter does not have a suction-control port)
- Water-soluble lubricant
- Sterile basin
- Sterile normal saline solution or water (approximately 100 mL)

PROCEDURE

STEPS	RATIONALE
1. Assess for signs and symptoms of upper and lower airway obstruction requiring nasotracheal or orotracheal suctioning, abnormal respiratory rate, adventitious sounds, nasal secretions, gurgling, drooling, restlessness, gastric secretions, or vomitus in mouth, and coughing without clearing secretions from airway.	• Physical signs and symptoms result from decreased oxygen to tissues, as well as pooling of secretions in upper and lower airways. A complete assessment is required before and after suction procedure (American Association of Respiratory Care [AARC], 2004).
2. Assess signs and symptoms associated with hypoxia and hypercapnia: decreased SpO_2, increased pulse and blood pressure, increased respiratory rate, apprehension, anxiety, decreased ability to concentrate, lethargy, decreased level of consciousness (especially acute), increased fatigue, dizziness, behavioural changes (especially irritability), dysrhythmias, pallor, and cyanosis.	• Physical signs and symptoms resulting from decreased oxygen to tissues indicate need for suctioning. Anxiety and pain consume oxygen and, in turn, worsen the signs of hypoxia.
3. Determine factors that normally influence upper or lower airway functioning:	
• Fluid status	
• Lack of humidity	
• Pulmonary disease, chronic obstructive pulmonary disorder, pulmonary infection	
• Anatomy	
• Changes in level of consciousness	
• Decreased cough or gag reflex, dysphagia, presence of a feeding tube	
• Allergies, sinus drainage	
4. Identify contraindications to nasotracheal suctioning: occluded nasal passages; nasal bleeding, epiglottitis, or croup; acute head, facial, or neck injury or surgery, coagulopathy, or bleeding disorder; irritable airway or laryngospasm or bronchospasm; gastric surgery with high anastomosis; myocardial infarction (AARC, 2004).	

CHAPTER 39 Cardiopulmonary Functioning and Oxygenation 985

STEPS	RATIONALE
(2) Attach Yankauer to connecting tubing. Check that equipment is functioning properly by suctioning a small amount of water or normal saline from the cup or basin.	
(3) Remove oxygen mask if present. Keep oxygen mask near patient's face. Nasal cannula may remain in place (if present).	• Allows access to patient's mouth. Reduces chances of hypoxia.

CRITICAL DECISION POINT: *Be prepared to quickly reapply oxygen mask if SpO_2 falls or respiratory distress develops during or at the end of suctioning.*

STEPS	RATIONALE
(4) Insert Yankauer into the patient's mouth. With suction applied, move catheter around mouth, including pharynx and gum line, until secretions are cleared.	• Movement of catheter prevents suction tip from invaginating oral mucosal surfaces, thus potentially causing trauma.
(5) Encourage patient to cough, and repeat suctioning if needed. Replace oxygen mask if used.	• Coughing moves secretions from lower to upper airways into mouth.
(6) Suction water from basin through catheter until catheter is cleared of secretions. Turn off suction.	• Clearing secretions before they dry reduces the probability of transmission of microorganisms and enhances delivery of preset suction pressures.
(7) Place catheter in a clean, dry area for reuse.	• Facilitates prompt removal of airway secretions when suctioning is needed in the future. Moist environment encourages microorganism growth.

CRITICAL DECISION POINT: *Do not store the catheter where it will come in contact with secretions or excretions, which promote bacterial growth. If the patient is capable of self-oral suctioning, place the catheter within reach.*

STEPS	RATIONALE
B. Nasopharyngeal and nasotracheal suctioning	
(1) Open lubricant. Squeeze small amount onto open sterile catheter package without touching package. Lubricant is *not* necessary for artificial airway suctioning.	• Prepares lubricant while maintaining sterility. Water-soluble lubricant is used to avoid lipoid aspiration pneumonia. Excessive lubricant can occlude the catheter.
(2) Apply sterile glove to each hand, or apply nonsterile glove to nondominant hand and sterile glove to dominant hand.	• Reduces transmission of microorganisms and allows nurse to maintain sterility of suction catheter.
(3) Pick up suction catheter with dominant hand without touching nonsterile surfaces. Pick up connecting tubing with nondominant hand. Secure catheter to tubing (see Step 17B(3) illustration).	• Maintains catheter sterility. Connects catheter to suction.

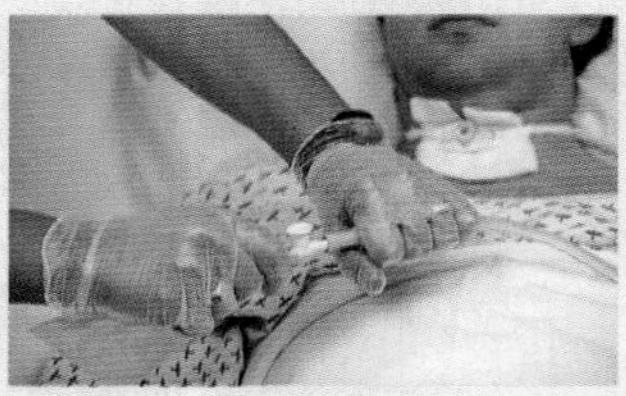

STEP 17B(3) Attaching catheter to suction.

STEPS	RATIONALE
(4) Check that the equipment is functioning properly by suctioning a small amount of normal saline solution from the basin.	• Ensures equipment function; lubricates catheter and tubing.
(5) Lightly coat distal 6–8 cm (2–3 inches) of catheter with water-soluble lubricant.	• Lubricates catheter for easier insertion.
(6) Remove oxygen delivery device, if applicable, with nondominant hand. *Without applying suction* and using dominant thumb and forefinger, gently insert catheter into naris during inhalation. ***Never apply suction during insertion.***	• Application of suction pressure while introducing catheter into nasopharyngeal tissues increases risk of damage to mucosa. When advanced into trachea, suction could damage mucosa and increase risk of hypoxia.
(7) *Nasopharyngeal:* As the patient takes a deep breath, insert catheter following natural course of naris; slightly slant catheter downward and advance to back of pharynx. Do not force through naris. In adults, insert catheter about 20 cm (6–8 inches); in older children, 16–20 cm (6–8 inches); in infants and young children, 4–14 cm (3–5½ inches) into trachea until resistance is met or patient coughs; then pull back 1–2 cm (1/2 inch).	• Proper placement ensures removal of pharyngeal secretions. Pulling back on catheter before initiating suctioning prevents invagination of the tracheal membrane (AARC, 2010).

Continued

STEPS	RATIONALE
14. The patient may assist by brushing. Hold toothbrush bristles at a 45-degree angle to gum line (see Step 14 illustration, part A). Be sure tips of bristles rest against and penetrate under gum line. Brush inner and outer surfaces of upper and lower teeth by brushing from gum to crown of each tooth. Clean biting surfaces of teeth by holding top of bristles parallel with teeth and brushing gently back and forth (see Step 14 illustration, part B). Brush sides of teeth by moving bristles back and forth (see Step 14 illustration, part C).	• Angle allows brush to reach all tooth surfaces and to clean under gum line where plaque and bacteria accumulate. Back-and-forth motion dislodges food particles caught between teeth and along chewing surfaces.
15. Have patient hold brush at a 45-degree angle and lightly brush over surface and sides of tongue (see Step 15 illustration). Avoid initiating gag reflex.	• Microorganisms collect and grow on the tongue's surface and contribute to bad breath. Gagging may cause aspiration of toothpaste. Evaluates patient's ability to use correct technique.

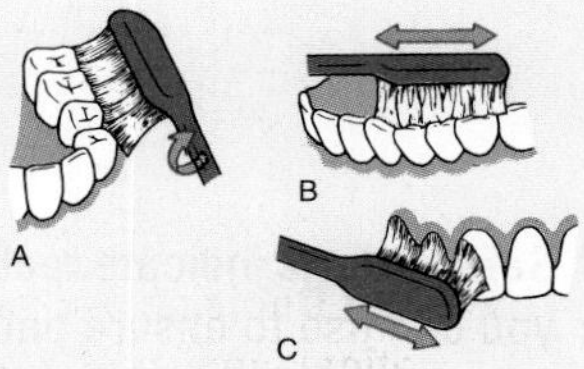

STEP 14 Directions for toothbrush placement. **A,** Gum line is brushed at a 45-degree angle. **B,** Parallel position is used for brushing biting surfaces. **C,** Lateral position is used for brushing sides of teeth.

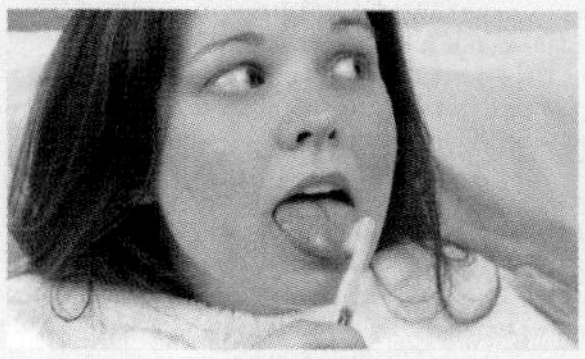

STEP 15 Assisting patient with brushing tongue.

Clear, close-up **photos** and **illustrations** show you how to perform important nursing techniques.

STEPS	RATIONALE
16. Allow patient to rinse mouth thoroughly: taking several sips of water, swishing water across all tooth surfaces, and spitting into the emesis basin.	• Irrigation removes food particles.
17. Allow patient to gargle and rinse mouth with mouthwash as desired.	• Mouthwash can be effective in reducing plaque and gingivitis (Canadian Dental Association, 2017).
18. Assist in wiping patient's mouth.	• Promotes sense of comfort.
19. Allow patient to floss.	
20. Allow patient to rinse mouth thoroughly with cool water and spit into emesis basin. Assist in wiping patient's mouth.	
21. Ask patient whether any area of oral cavity feels uncomfortable or irritated. Inspect the oral cavity.	
22. Assist patient to comfortable position, remove emesis basin and bedside table, raise side rail, and lower bed to the original position.	
23. Wipe off overbed table, discard soiled linen and paper towels in appropriate containers, remove soiled gloves, and return equipment to the proper place.	
24. Remove gloves, and perform hand hygiene.	
25. Ask patient to describe proper hygiene techniques.	

UNEXPECTED OUTCOMES

Dryness and inflammation of oral mucosa

Retraction of gum margins from teeth, localized areas of inflammation, and bleeding around gum margins

Signs of dental caries

RECORDING AND REPORTING

- Record all procedures on a flow sheet provided by your agency or facility. Note th
- Report any bleeding or the presence of lesions to the person in charge or the phy

HOME CARE CONSIDERATIONS

- Teach the patient and caregiver to assess the oral cavity daily to determine any

STEPS	RATIONALE
Unable to pass suction catheter through first naris attempted	• Try other naris or oral route. • Insert nasal airway, especially if suctioning through patient naris frequently. • Guide catheter along naris floor to avoid turbinates. • If obstruction is mucus, apply suction to relieve obstruction, but do not apply suction to mucosa. If obstruction is thought to be a blood clot, consult physician. • Increase lubrication of catheter.
Paroxysms of coughing	• Administer supplemental oxygen. • Allow patient to rest between passes of suction catheter. • Consult health care provider regarding need for inhaled bronchodilators or topical anaesthetics.
No secretions obtained	• Evaluate patient's fluid status. • Assess for signs of infection. • Determine need for chest physiotherapy. • Assess adequacy of humidification on oxygen delivery device.

RECORDING AND REPORTING

- Record the amount, consistency, colour, and odour of secretions and patient's response to procedure; document patient's pre-suctioning and post-suctioning cardiopulmonary status.

HOME CARE CONSIDERATIONS

- Nurses need to adhere to best practices for infection control while weighing cost-effectiveness in the setting of a chronic situation. If the patient has an established tracheostomy or requires long-term nasotracheal suctioning and infection is not present, clean suction technique is appropriate.
- Instruct the patient and family in infection-control measures for emptying the secretion jar. These secretions should be emptied in the toilet but they have a splash risk. Instruct the caregiver to apply a mask (shield if available) and gloves and bring the secretion jar as close to the toilet bowel as possible to decrease the risk of splash.

the time of suctioning. Sterile gloves are worn to perform the suction procedure. Closed suctioning involves a multiple-use suction catheter encased in a plastic sheath (Figure 39-11). Closed suctioning is most often used on patients who require mechanical ventilation to support their respiratory efforts, because it permits continuous delivery of oxygen while suction is performed, thus reducing the risk of oxygen desaturation. Although sterile gloves are not required in this procedure, at least nonsterile (i.e., disposable) gloves are recommended to prevent contact with splashes from body fluids.

Artificial Airways. An artificial airway is indicated for patients with a decreased level of consciousness or an airway obstruction and to aid in the removal of tracheobronchial secretions.

Oral Airway. The oral airway, the simplest type of artificial airway, prevents obstruction of the trachea by displacement of the tongue into the oropharynx (Figure 39-12). The oral airway extends from the teeth to the oropharynx, maintaining the tongue in the normal position. The correct-size airway must be used. Proper oral airway size is determined by measuring the distance from the corner of the mouth to the angle of the jaw just below the ear. The length is equal to the distance from the flange of the airway to the tip. If the airway is too small, the tongue is not held in the anterior portion of the mouth; if the airway is too large, it may force the tongue toward the epiglottis and obstruct the airway.

The airway is inserted by turning the curve of the airway toward the cheek and placing it over the tongue. When the airway is in the

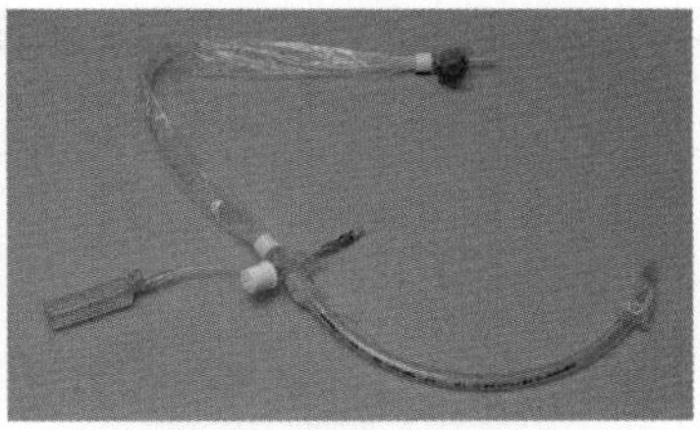

FIGURE 39-11 Ballard tracheal care, closed suction.

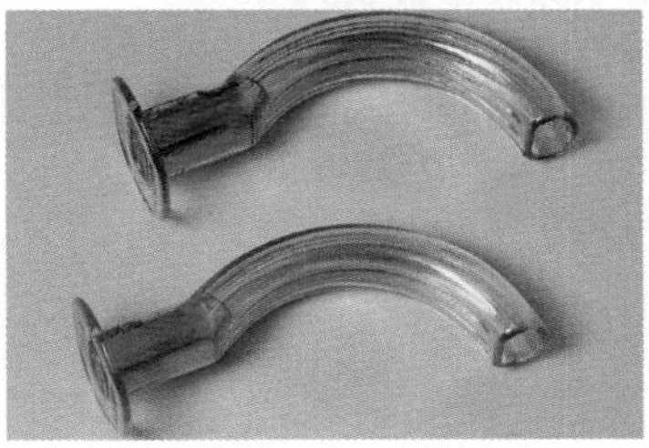

FIGURE 39-12 Artificial oral airways.

Recording and Reporting sections provide guidelines for what to chart and report with each skill.

Home Care Considerations explain how to adapt skills for the home setting.

1052 UNIT VIII Basic Physiological Needs

up to 5 to 7 days. No dressing is required for an STC once the wound has healed, unless the patient prefers one (Green, 2008, p. 45).

The external catheter should be measured and results documented daily to ensure that the catheter remains in the correct placement. The insertion site should be inspected daily for tenderness, signs of infection, erythema, warmth, and edema, and assessment should include palpation. The chest and neck should be assessed for engorged veins and for difficulty with movement. The nurse should also assess the patient for signs of systemic infection, such as fever, chills, and hypotension (Casey & Elliot, 2010, p. 78; Scales, 2011).

Prior to accessing a CVAD, the nurse conducts a 15-second rub with 70% isopropyl alcohol, povidone-iodine, or >0.5% chlorhexidine in alcohol solution (INS, 2016). New antimicrobial devices and approaches to preventing CR-BSI are being developed and include antimicrobial catheters, needleless access devices, dressings, and lock solutions (Casey & Elliot, 2010, p. 84). To prevent occlusion of the CVAD, the device is flushed and assessed for patency according to institutional policy. The use of heparin for flushing and locking is currently an area for further study and future recommendations (e.g., Mitchell, Anderson, Williams, et al., 2009; RNAO, 2008). Totally implanted ports, used for long-term treatment such as chemotherapy, are inserted surgically and are accessed by inserting a needle through the skin into the device. They can be used up to 2 000 times (Kelly, 2009, p. s11) and have the lowest incidence of infection (Casey & Elliot, 2010, p. 80).

Patient and family education is required for all patients with a CVAD. This should include care requirements and patient restrictions.

Administration of Intravenous Therapy

Types of solutions. Many prepared intravenous solutions are available for use (Table 40-9). Solutions are classified as hypertonic, isotonic, or hypotonic (see Figure 40-10, earlier in chapter). Osmolarity, reflecting the osmolar concentration in 1 L of solution (mOsm/L), is most often used to describe fluids outside the body (Hannon, Pooler, & Porth, 2010). A solution with the same osmolarity as blood plasma is called *isotonic*. A hypertonic solution, with a higher osmotic pressure, such as 3% sodium chloride, pulls fluid from cells, causing them to shrink. An isotonic solution, with the same osmotic pressure as plasma, such as 0.9% sodium chloride, expands the body's fluid volume without causing a fluid shift from one compartment to another. A hypotonic solution, with an osmotic pressure lower than plasma, such as 0.45% sodium chloride, moves fluid into the cells, causing them to enlarge. Each of these actions occurs through osmosis.

In general, isotonic fluids are used most commonly for extracellular volume replacement (e.g., FVD after prolonged vomiting). The decision to use a hypotonic or hypertonic solution is based on the specific fluid and electrolyte imbalances. For example, the patient with a hypertonic fluid imbalance will in general receive a hypotonic intravenous solution to dilute the ECF and rehydrate the cells. All intravenous fluids should be given carefully, especially hypertonic solutions, because these pull fluid into the vascular space by osmosis, resulting in an increased vascular volume that can lead to pulmonary edema, particularly in patients with heart or renal failure. Certain additives, most commonly vitamins and potassium chloride, are frequently added to intravenous solutions.

Safety Alert Under no circumstances should potassium chloride (KCl) be given by intravenous push. Direct intravenous infusion of KCl may cause death. If an intravenous fluid requires additives, a prescriber's order must specify the required additives—for example, "1 000 mL D51/2 NS with 20 mmol/L KCl at 125 mL/hour."

Patients with normal renal function who are receiving nothing by mouth should have potassium added to intravenous solutions. The body cannot conserve potassium, and even when the serum level falls, the kidneys continue to excrete potassium. Without oral or parenteral potassium intake, hypokalemia can develop quickly. Conversely, the nurse should verify that the patient has adequate renal function before administering an intravenous solution containing potassium, because hyperkalemia can develop quickly.

Equipment. Correct selection and preparation of intravenous equipment are necessary for safe and quick placement of an intravenous line (Figure 40-16). Because fluids are instilled into the bloodstream, sterile technique is necessary; the nurse should have all equipment organized for efficient insertion (see Skill 40-1). Intravenous cannulas are available in a variety of gauges. The larger the gauge, the smaller the diameter of the cannula. These cannulas are plastic tubing threaded over a needle. Once the cannula is inserted into the vein, the needle is withdrawn, leaving the cannula in place. Intravenous tubing or an intermittent infusion device, such as a needleless port, is then connected.

Safety Alert Intravenous pumps or volume-control (flow-control) devices ensure a prescribed rate of infusion. A prescribed rate of infusion is vital for children, patients with renal or cardiac failure, and critically ill patients. Electronic infusion devices must be used for medications that require precise rates of administration.

Safety Alerts indicate techniques you can use to ensure patient and nurse safety.

Initiating an intravenous line. A venipuncture is a technique in which a vein is punctured through the skin by a sharp, rigid stylet (e.g., butterfly needle or metal needle), a partially covered plastic catheter (over-the-needle catheter), or a needle attached to a syringe. When veins are fragile or collapse, venipuncture may become extremely

CHAPTER 40 Fluid, Electrolyte, and Acid–Base Balances 1065

people must receive only Rh-negative blood, whereas Rh-positive people can receive either Rh-negative or Rh-positive blood.

If incompatible or mismatched blood is transfused, a transfusion reactions occurs. The patient's, or recipient's, antibodies trigger RBC destruction. This response ranges from a mild response (e.g., faintness, dizziness) to severe anaphylactic shock or acute intravascular hemolysis, both of which can be life-threatening. Prompt intervention is required, including immediately stopping the transfusion, removing the tubing, and replacing the line with a normal saline infusion to maintain intravenous access.

Autologous Transfusion. Autologous transfusion, or autotransfusion, is the collection of a patient's own blood. The blood for an autologous transfusion can be obtained by preoperative donation up to 5 weeks before the planned surgery (e.g., heart, orthopedic, plastic, or gynecological). Patients can donate several units of their own blood, depending on the type of surgery and the ability of the patient to maintain an acceptable hematocrit. Another way to collect blood for an autologous transfusion is during perioperative blood salvage (e.g., during vascular and orthopedic surgery, organ transplant surgery, and traumatic injuries). The blood that has been salvaged is then reinfused during the surgery. Blood can also be salvaged postoperatively from mediastinal and chest tube drainage and after joint and spinal surgery. Autologous transfusions decrease the risk of complications such as mismatched blood and exposure to bloodborne infectious agents (Alexander, Corrigan, Gorski, et al., 2014).

TABLE 40-12 ABO Compatibilities for Transfusion Therapy

Component	Compatibilities	
Whole Blood	**Give Type-Specific Blood Only**	
Packed red cells (stored, washed, or frozen/washed)	***Donor***	***Recipient***
	0	0, A, B, AB
	A	A, AB
	B	B, AB
	AB	AB
Fresh-frozen plasma	***Donor***	***Recipient***
	0	0
	A	A, 0
	B	B, 0
	AB	AB, B, A, 0
Platelets	RBC: ABO and Rh compatible *preferred*	
	Donor	***Recipient***
	0	0, A, B, AB
	A	A, AB
	B	B, AB
	AB	AB

ABO, Blood group consisting of groups A, AB, B, and O.
Data from Alexander, M., Corrigan, A. M., Gorski, L. A., et al. (2014). *Core curriculum for infusion nursing* (4th ed.). Philadelphia: Lippincott.

Blood Transfusions. When transfusing blood or blood components, assessment is required before, during, and after the transfusion and for regulation of the transfusion, because of the risk of reactions and complications. Prior to transfusion the primary health care provider must obtain consent for transfusion, except in emergencies. The nurse then verifies that consent has been obtained, that it is current, and that the patient understands the reason for the blood transfusion. Patients with certain cultural backgrounds may abstain from blood transfusions (Box 40-13). The nurse should ask the patient if he or she has had a previous transfusion or a transfusion reaction. Before giving a transfusion, the nurse needs to explain the procedure and instruct the patient to report any side effects (e.g., chills, dizziness, or fever) once the transfusion begins. The nurse checks that the patient is properly identified, based on agency policy. This is critical to ensure that the patient is given the correct blood component, based on blood typing. Certain diagnostic tests are used to determine the need for blood component and the effectiveness of treatment, such as hemoglobin, platelet count, or tests related to clotting.

Infusion of blood components or blood products requires an order from the primary health care provider. The nurse checks patient identification, component or product to be administered, the amount or volume, the rate of administration, and any other requirements, such as premedication (e.g., intravenous diuretic). If the patient has an intravenous line in place, the nurse needs to assess the venipuncture site and determine the appropriate gauge of the intravenous catheter. A large catheter, such as 18 to 22 gauge, is recommended for adults unless rapid infusion is required (16–18 gauge). Blood administration tubing with a 70- to 260-micron filter is used, and the nurse needs to determine if the tubing is appropriate for the EID when using one. When priming blood administration tubing, 0.9% normal saline must be used to prevent hemolysis, or breakdown of RBCs. Timing of blood transfusion is extremely important. The infusion is begun within 30 minutes of accessing the blood component from the transfusion medical laboratory (TML) and is stopped after 4 hours. Bags and tubing are discarded in the biohazardous waste, according to agency policy.

Because of the danger of transfusion reactions, it is very important to use specific precautions and the ten rights of medication administration (see Chapter 34) in administering blood or blood products.

Cultural Aspects of Care boxes prepare you to care for patients of diverse populations and suggest actions needed to meet different cultural needs and preferences.

BOX 40-13 CULTURAL ASPECTS OF CARE

Preinfusion Assessments

When a patient's natural skin contains more melanin, it becomes more difficult to identify colour changes. Intravenous complications such as phlebitis and infiltration may not be easily detected. Patients from some cultural backgrounds experience fear related to the donor process for blood. Patients with certain religious (e.g., Jehovah's Witness) or personal beliefs may abstain from receiving blood transfusions or medications.

Implications for Practice

- Establish communication. Understand the values of family elders and know whom to speak with about intravenous procedures.
- Assess patients individually to determine their acceptance of or abstinence from therapeutic regimens.
- Appreciate patients' choice related to their therapy.
- Although some patients will abstain from receiving whole blood or packed red blood cells, they will accept other blood products or alternatives.

Adapted from Rudnicke, C. (2003). Transfusion alternatives. *Journal of Infusion Nursing, 26*(3), 29.

Procedural Guideline boxes provide streamlined, step-by-step instructions for performing basic skills.

BOX 38-12 PROCEDURAL GUIDELINE

Care of Dentures

Delegation Considerations

The skill of denture care can be delegated to an unregulated care provider (UCP). It is important to discuss the following with the UCP:

- To report any cracks found in the dentures
- To report any patient complaints of oral discomfort
- To report any signs of irritation, inflammation, or lesions

Equipment

- Soft-bristled toothbrush or denture toothbrush
- Denture cleaning agent or toothpaste
- Denture adhesive (optional)
- Glass of water
- Emesis basin or sink
- Washcloth
- Disposable gloves
- Denture cup (if dentures are to be stored after cleaning)

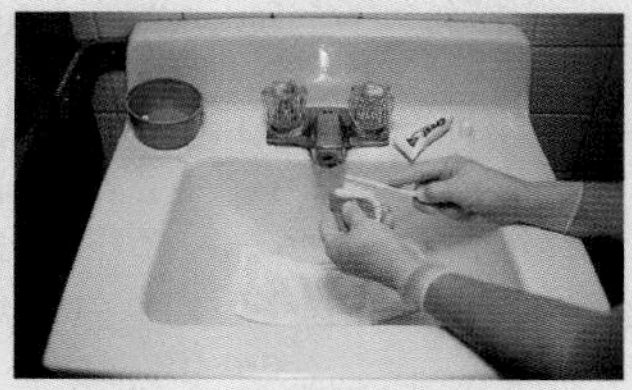

STEP 5 Brushing dentures.

Procedure

1. Ask patient whether dentures fit and whether the gums or mucous membranes are tender or irritated.
2. Ask patient about preferences for denture care and products used. If patient is unable to care for own dentures, you must provide this care. Clean dentures for the patient during routine mouth care.
3. Fill emesis basin with tepid water or, if using sink, place washcloth in bottom of sink and fill sink with 2.5 cm of water.
4. Remove dentures. If patient is unable to do this independently, perform hand hygiene and put on gloves, grasp upper plate at front with thumb and index finger wrapped in gauze, and pull downward. Gently lift lower denture from jaw, and rotate one side downward to remove from patient's mouth. Place dentures in emesis basin or sink.
5. Apply cleaning agent to brush and brush surfaces of dentures (see Step 5 illustration). Hold dentures close to water. Hold the brush horizontally, and use a back-and-forth motion to clean biting surfaces. Use short strokes from the top of the denture to biting surfaces to clean outer and inner teeth surfaces. Hold the brush vertically, and use short strokes to clean inner tooth surfaces. Hold the brush horizontally, and use a back-and-forth motion to clean the undersurface of dentures.
6. Rinse thoroughly in tepid water.
7. Some patients use an adhesive to seal dentures in place. If so, apply a thin layer to the undersurface before inserting.
8. If patient needs assistance with the insertion of dentures, moisten the upper denture and press firmly to seal it in place. Then insert moistened lower denture. Ask whether dentures feel comfortable.
9. Dentures should be removed at night and the gums cleaned gently. Dentures should be stored in a denture container that is labelled with the patient's name and placed in the bedside table to prevent loss.
10. Remove and discard gloves and perform hand hygiene.

Brushing and Combing. Frequent brushing and combing helps to keep hair clean and distributes oil evenly along hair shafts and prevents hair from tangling. Patients should be encouraged to maintain routine hair care. However, patients with limited mobility or weakness and those who are confused require assistance. Patients in a hospital or long-term care facility appreciate the opportunity to have their hair brushed and combed before being seen by others.

When caring for patients from different cultures, it is important to learn as much as possible from them or their family about their preferred hair care practices. Cultural preferences affect how hair is combed and styled. Nurses should never trim or cut a patient's hair without the patient's consent.

Long hair can easily become matted when patients are confined to bed, even for a short period. When lacerations or incisions involve the scalp, blood and topical medications can also cause tangling. Frequent brushing and combing keeps long hair neatly groomed. Braiding can help to avoid repeated tangles; however, braids should be unbraided periodically and the hair combed to ensure good hygiene. Braids made too tightly can result in bald patches. Nurses must always obtain permission from patients, if conscious, before braiding their hair.

To brush the hair, part it into two sections and separate each into two more sections. It is easier to brush smaller sections of hair. Brushing from the scalp toward the hair ends minimizes pulling. Moistening the hair with water frees tangles for easier combing.

Case Study boxes tell a real-life story concerning one or more topics in the chapter.

BOX 39-9 CASE STUDY

Understanding Cardiac Rehabilitation: A Personal Story and Case Study

During my evening shift Mr. Evans (a pseudonym), a 48-year-old male was admitted to the cardiac medical unit with a late-presenting myocardial infarction (MI). He presented to the emergency department with mid-scapular pain. Mr. Evans did not relate the symptoms to a cardiac event. One of our initial conversations indicated he was anticipating returning to work upon discharge from the hospital. I met his wife soon afterward, who shared with me her sense of being overwhelmed with the dietary changes, new medications, and her husband's "denial" of the current diagnosis. Toward the later part of my shift I took the opportunity to inquire about their understanding of the cardiac rehabilitation program and their intention to use the resource. I used this opportunity to teach Mr. Evans and his wife about cardiac rehabilitation. They developed an understanding of this resource and began to recognize that it was more than just an exercise program. Mr. Evans and his wife understood that cardiac rehabilitation encompassed a holistic approach to wellness with members of an interdisciplinary team who have expertise in different areas of clinical practice. Cardiac rehabilitation offered this couple ongoing support and strategies for lifestyle changes to promote wellness.

1. How do nurses assess patients' and families' readiness to learn?
2. What pertinent members of the interdisciplinary team support patients and families during cardiac rehabilitation? What are key elements of the conversation with patients and families regarding cardiac rehabilitation?
3. In addition to patients who have been diagnosed with an MI, what other patients might also benefit from cardiac rehabilitation?

BOX 39-10 NURSING DIAGNOSTIC PROCESS

Assessment Activities	Defining Characteristics	Nursing Diagnosis
Ask patient or family about patient's mood, attentiveness, memory, and activity level.	Confusion Decreased activity Fatigue Irritability Restlessness Sleepiness	*Impaired gas exchange related to decreased lung expansion*
Observe patient's respirations.	Dyspnea Impaired gas exchange related to collapsed alveoli Nasal flaring Tachypnea Use of accessory muscles	
Inspect skin and mucous membranes.	Diaphoresis Pallor Moist skin	
Auscultate chest.	Decreased respiratory excursion Abnormal, distant lung sounds	

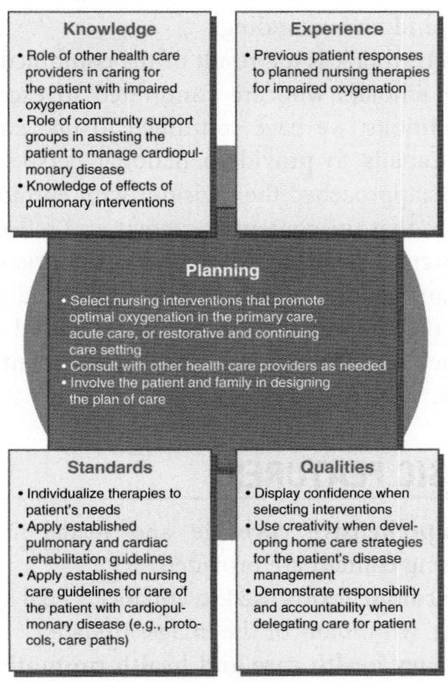

FIGURE 39-7 Critical thinking model for oxygenation planning.

lung conditions and is an essential component of primary health care. These professionals work with the patient and the community to optimize resources to assist the patient in attaining the highest level of wellness. In addition, professionals can help to identify community resources and support systems for both the patient and family in preventing and managing symptoms related to cardiopulmonary diseases.

◆ Implementation

Nursing interventions for promoting and maintaining adequate oxygenation include independent nursing actions such as health-promotion and disease-prevention behaviours, positioning, and coughing techniques. Interdependent or dependent interventions include oxygen therapy, lung inflation techniques, hydration, medication administration, and chest physiotherapy (CPT).

Health Promotion

Maintaining the patient's optimal level of health is important in reducing the number and severity of respiratory symptoms. Prevention of respiratory infections is foremost in maintaining optimal health. Providing cardiopulmonary-related health information (Box 39-12

REF[redacted]

The future of nursing in Canada in a globalized world is dynamic and ever-changing. It is imperative that our student nurses are prepared to have the necessary foundational knowledge of nursing and skills relevant to professional nursing practice. The nurses of tomorrow will continue to need to provide evidence-informed nursing practice in order to address the myriad of global health challenges to maintain and improve the health of Canadians. Professional nursing practice requires (a) critical thinking and critical reasoning, (b) the ability to collaborate and communicate with diverse clients and the interprofessional team, (c) patient/client advocacy, (d) excellence in clinical decision making, and (e) client/patient/community teaching within a broad spectrum of health services. Moreover, nursing practice will involve engaging in knowledge translation and leadership development and advocating for health policy change at the local, national, and global levels. *Canadian Fundamentals of Nursing* is specifically designed for students at all levels of undergraduate nursing programs. The text provides comprehensive coverage of fundamental nursing concepts, knowledge, research, and skills that are essential to informing nursing practice.

The sixth edition of *Canadian Fundamentals of Nursing* has been extensively revised, updated, and thoroughly edited to include the most current evidence, issues, and future directions for nursing in Canada. All chapters have been written or revised so that they reflect Canadian standards, traditions, research, and practice. *Canadian Fundamentals of Nursing* includes content covering the entire scope of primary, secondary, tertiary, rehabilitation, and end-of-life care. The focus is on the central role of primary health care in all areas of nursing practice. Emphasis is also placed on evidence-informed practice in skills and care plans to foster understanding of how research findings should guide clinical decision making. First-person accounts, in the form of case studies, of issues that have arisen in nursing practice are designed to engage the nursing student's attention and encourage more detailed reading and understanding.

This textbook is the result of the combined efforts of many expert nursing scholars who are committed to excellence. As in our previous editions, we have continued to use expert contributors from across Canada to provide a national perspective. All of these contributors approached the revisions with enthusiasm and worked hard to ensure that the content is current and reflects the Canadian health care system, Canadian health and social organizations, and uniquely Canadian health care issues in a globalized world. Reviewers scrutinized the chapters and made many helpful suggestions. We appreciate the conscientiousness and commitment of all these dedicated scholars.

CLASSIC FEATURES

- **Comprehensive** coverage and readability of all fundamental nursing content are provided.
- **Full-colour** text is used to enhance visual appeal and instructional value, with many of the images updated.
- **Primary health care and health promotion** issues are discussed throughout the text.
- **Chronic Illness** boxes pertain uniquely to the Canadian health care system.
- **Research Highlight** boxes are integrated throughout the text to provide current and applicable nursing research studies and explain the implications for daily nursing practice.
- **Patient/client education** is highlighted in boxes that list teaching objectives, strategies, and evaluation for clinical topics throughout the text.
- **Evidence-informed practice** is discussed throughout the text.
- **Evidence-Informed Practice** boxes provide examples of recent state-of-the-science guidelines for nursing practice.
- **Nursing** principles specific to older persons are addressed throughout the text.
- **Case Study** boxes present first-person accounts of issues in relation to chapter content.
- **Nursing Care Plans** guide students in how to conduct an assessment and analyze the defining characteristics that indicate nursing diagnoses. The plans include Nursing Interventions Classification (NIC) and Nursing Outcomes Classification (NOC) labels to familiarize students with this important nomenclature. The evaluation sections of the plans show students how to determine the expected outcomes and evaluate the results of care.
- **Concept Maps** demonstrate the relationships among nursing assessment, diagnosis, planning, intervention, and evaluation.
- **Procedural Guideline** boxes provide step-by-step instructions and photos about how to perform basic skills.
- **Video icons** indicate video clips associated with specific skills that are available in the Evolve Student Learning Resources.
- **End-of-chapter NCLEX review questions** assist students in critically reviewing what they have learned. Answers and rationales are provided at the end of this textbook.
- The annotated **Recommended Websites** section at the end of each chapter directs the student to current resources.
- A fully updated **Practical Nursing in Canada** appendix (Appendix A) provides important information on this nursing role in Canada.
- The **Laboratory Values** appendix (Appendix B) is a concise, up-to-date source of current laboratory values for use in clinical practice.
- **Media Resources** listed at the beginning of each chapter detail the available Evolve resources.
- Expert contributors and reviewers from across Canada have provided a national perspective.

NEW FEATURES

- A NEW chapter (Chapter 10) specifically addresses INDIGENOUS HEALTH, with particular reference made to the ***Truth and Reconciliation Commission (TRC) Report.***
- A NEW chapter (Chapter 18) addresses INTERPROFESSIONAL COLLABORATION, with a focus on patient-centred care, and there is greater emphasis on and integration of interprofessional collaboration in other chapters.
- Expanded content on THE DEVELOPMENT OF NURSING IN CANADA (Chapter 3), with addition of the history of the development of nursing education in Canada with baccalaureate, masters, nurse practitioners, and doctorate programs.
- A revised and updated chapter on EVIDENCE-INFORMED PRACTICE (Chapter 6), which includes the concept of **research literacy** as it applies to evidence-informed practice, and a discussion of **quality improvement (QI)**.
- Expanded content on NURSING VALUES AND ETHICS (Chapter 7), with emphasis on advance care planning, **medical assistance in dying (MAID)**, and the **revised CNA *Code of Ethics*.**

- Expanded content regarding LEGAL IMPLICATIONS IN NURSING PRACTICE (Chapter 8), with emphasis on medical assistance in dying (MAID) and updated information about the forthcoming changes in 2018 to laws governing the use of cannabis in Canada.
- Expanded content on GLOBAL HEALTH (Chapter 9), with emphasis on sustainable development goals (SDGs), environmental sustainability, planetary health, intersectoral action for health, health systems, intersectionality, culture in context, global violence, interprofessional collaboration, and competencies in global health.
- Inclusion of the concept of **clinical reasoning** in Chapter 12, CRITICAL THINKING IN NURSING PRACTICE, and integration of this concept into other chapters.
- Expanded and updated content on NURSING INFORMATICS AND CANADIAN NURSING PRACTICE (Chapter 16), with emphasis on eHealth and mHealth, the evolution of nursing informatics definitions, Canadian Organization for Advancement of Computers in Health (COACH) Health Information Professional (HIP) Competency Framework, Canada Health Infoway, International Classification for Nursing Practice (ICNP), and the *Nursing Informatics: Entry-to-Practice Competencies for Registered Nurses* from the Canadian Association of Schools of Nursing.
- Use of the term *older persons* instead of *older adults* throughout the text.
- A revised chapter on OLDER PERSONS (Chapter 24), including a palliative care approach.
- Expanded content on COMPLEMENTARY AND ALTERNATIVE APPROACHES IN HEALTH CARE (Chapter 35), with emphasis on other approaches for the treatment of chronic pain, health concerns, and health promotion.
- The updated chapter QUALITY AND PATIENT SAFETY (Chapter 37) includes new information on the importance of regulations for maintaining the workplace environment.
- Information about the 2017 **updated CNA *Code of Ethics*** has been integrated into many of the chapters.
- The Canadian **Medical Assistance in Dying (MAID)** legislation has been integrated into many of the chapters.
- Inclusion of the 2015 *National Nursing Education Framework Domains and Competencies* for baccalaureate nursing students from the Canadian Association of Schools of Nursing (CASN).
- Inclusion of the 2014 *Entry-to-Practice Public Health Nursing Competencies* for undergraduate nursing education from the Canadian Association of Schools of Nursing (CASN).
- Integration of the concept of **health literacy** into many of the chapters as it relates to learning new information.
- **References** have been updated throughout to include Canadian research and practice standards, such as the best nursing practice guidelines of Health Canada, Statistics Canada, the Canadian Nurses Association (CNA), and the Registered Nurses' Association of Ontario (RNAO). References have been organized by chapter and compiled at the end of each chapter.

LEARNING SUPPLEMENTS FOR STUDENTS

- The **Evolve Student Resources** are available online at http://evolve.elsevier.com/Canada/Potter/fundamentals/ and include the following valuable learning aids, organized by asset:
  - Audio Glossary
  - Case Studies
  - Concept Map Creator
  - Content Updates
  - Examination Review Questions
  - Key Points
  - Skills Performance Checklists
  - Tutorial – Calculations
  - Tutorial – Fluids and Electrolytes
  - Videos
- A thorough ***Study Guide With Skills Performance Checklists*** provides an ideal supplement to help students understand and apply the content of the text. Each chapter includes multiple sections:
  - Preliminary Reading includes a chapter assignment from the text.
  - Comprehensive Understanding provides a variety of activities to reinforce the topics and main ideas from the text.
  - Review Questions are multiple choice, requiring students to provide rationales for their answers. Answers and rationales are provided on the accompanying Evolve website.
  - Clinical chapters include critical thinking models that expand the case study from the chapter's care plan. Students are asked to develop a step in the model on the basis of the actions of the nurse and patient in the scenario. This helps students learn to apply both content learned and the critical thinking synthesis model.
  - Skills Performance Checklists are included so that students can evaluate skill competency.
- The handy ***Clinical Companion: Just the Facts*** complements, rather than abbreviates, the textbook. Content is presented in tabular, list, and outline formats that equip your students with a concise, portable guide to all of the facts and figures they'll need to know in their early clinical experiences.
- ***Virtual Clinical Excursions*** is an exciting workbook and CD-ROM package that brings learning to life in a virtual hospital setting. The workbook guides students as they care for patients, providing ongoing challenges and learning opportunities. Each lesson in *Virtual Clinical Excursions* complements the textbook content and provides an environment for students to practise what they are learning. This CD/workbook is available separately or packaged at a special price with the textbook.

TEACHING SUPPLEMENTS FOR INSTRUCTORS

- The **Evolve Instructor Resources** (available online at http://evolve.elsevier.com/Canada/Potter/fundamentals/) are a comprehensive collection of the most important tools instructors need, including the following:
  - **TEACH for Nurses** ties together every chapter resource you need for the most effective class presentations, with sections dedicated to objectives, teaching focus, instructor chapter resources, answers to chapter questions, and an in-class case study discussion. Teaching strategies include content highlights, student activities, online activities, and large-group activities.
  - The revised **Test Bank** contains more than 1300 multiple-choice questions with text page references and answers coded for NCLEX competencies and cognitive level. The ExamView software allows instructors to create new tests; edit, add, and delete test questions; sort questions by category, cognitive level, and question type; and administer and grade online tests.
  - Revised **PowerPoint Presentations** include over 1 500 slides for use in lectures.
  - The **Image Collection** contains more than 1 100 illustrations from the text for use in lectures.
  - **Simulation Learning System** is an online toolkit that helps instructors and facilitators effectively incorporate medium- to high-fidelity simulation into their nursing curriculum. Detailed

patient scenarios promote and enhance the clinical decision-making skills of students at all levels. The system provides detailed instructions for preparation and implementation of the simulation experience, debriefing questions that encourage critical thinking, and learning resources to reinforce student comprehension. Each scenario in the Simulation Learning System complements the textbook content and helps bridge the gap between lectures and clinicals. This system provides the perfect environment for students to practise what they are learning in the text for a true-to-life, hands-on learning experience.

MULTIMEDIA SUPPLEMENTS FOR INSTRUCTORS AND STUDENTS

- **Nursing Skills Online 4.0** contains 19 modules rich with animations, videos, interactive activities, and exercises to help students prepare for their clinical lab experience. The instructionally designed lessons focus on topics that are difficult to master and pose a high risk to the patient if done incorrectly. Lesson quizzes allow students to check their learning curve and review as needed, and the module exams feed out to an instructor grade book. Modules cover Airway Management, Blood Therapy, Bowel Elimination/Ostomy Care, Chest Tubes, Enteral Nutrition, Infection Control, Injections, IV Fluid Administration, IV Fluid Therapy Management, IV Medication Administration, Nonparenteral Medication Administration, Safe Medication Administration, Safety, Specimen Collection, Urinary Catheterization, Vascular Access, Vital Signs, and Wound Care. It is available alone or packaged with the text.
- **Clinical Skills: Essentials Collection** covers 144 of the most important nursing skills within fundamentals and health assessment. Each skill in this collection features a consistent seven-part framework to guide students through all aspects of the skill. From high-definition videos that demonstrate each step of the skill to an interactive supply list that visually familiarizes students with related equipment, your students will walk away with a firm understanding of how to properly perform each skill before they ever step foot in the clinical environment. Best of all, this remarkable training product includes competency checklists and interactive quizzes for each skill to help you easily keep tabs on your students' progress.

In this sixth edition of *Canadian Fundamentals of Nursing* we would like to acknowledge the expertise of our nursing scholars from across Canada, who ensured that the most up-to-date information was included so that our student nurses would have a fundamental textbook to meet their learning needs throughout their undergraduate nursing program. In addition, it was very important for us that the information provided prepared the student nurse to care for clients in local, national, and global contexts.

The task of updating a textbook of this magnitude is certainly an enormous undertaking that could only be accomplished through the collaborative efforts and commitment of the contributors, educator reviewers, editorial and production professionals, and our professional colleagues. We are so grateful for having the opportunity to collaborate with so many dedicated and committed individuals. We would like to acknowledge the following professionals from Elsevier:

- Martina van de Velde, Freelance Content Development Specialist, who provided outstanding leadership and capable organization of all parts of the developmental process and has been extremely supportive of all the contributors and editors. We were so grateful that we could work with Martina again, as this familiarity with each other fostered a sense of respect and collegiality that created a high-quality textbook.
- Mary Pohlman, Project Manager in the United States, for her dedication to the production of this edition.
- Roberta A. Spinosa-Millman, Content Strategist (Acquisitions) for Elsevier Canada, who oversaw the entire publication of this edition.
- Joyce Engel and Kerry Shoalts, who did an exemplary job in completing the *Study Guide* that accompanies this text.
- Daniela Freitas, Office Manager for Elsevier Canada, who ensured that the contracts and queries related to these matters were always attended to.
- Brenda Kirkconnell, Director, Educational Sales, Elsevier Canada, who has been actively involved in the promotion of the textbook.
- Ann Millar, former Director of International Content/Vice President, Publishing for Elsevier Canada, for her support of previous editions of this book.

We are very excited about this sixth edition of *Canadian Fundamentals of Nursing,* as it addresses many of the trends and issues that are so important for our student nurses to provide exemplary professional nursing practice in Canada and beyond.

Barbara J. Astle
Wendy Duggleby

CONTRIBUTORS

CANADIAN EDITORS

Barbara J. Astle, RN, PhD
Associate Professor
Director, Centre for Equity & Global Engagement (CEGE)
School of Nursing
Trinity Western University
Langley, British Columbia

Wendy Duggleby, RN, PhD
Professor, Associate Dean Research, and
Nursing Research Chair, Aging and Quality of Life
Faculty of Nursing
University of Alberta
Edmonton, Alberta

CANADIAN CONTRIBUTORS

Mary Ellen Andrews, RN(NP), PhD
Director of Nurse Practitioner Programs
Assistant Professor and Nurse Practitioner
College of Nursing
University of Saskatchewan
Saskatoon, Saskatchewan

Barbara J. Astle, RN, PhD
Associate Professor
Director, Centre for Equity & Global Engagement (CEGE)
School of Nursing
Trinity Western University
Langley, British Columbia

Colleen M. Astle, RN, BScN, MN, C Neph(C)
Nurse Practitioner
Dialysis Access, NARP
St. Marguerite Health Services Centre
Edmonton, Alberta

Chantal Backman, RN, MHA, PhD
Assistant Professor
Faculty of Health Sciences
School of Nursing
University of Ottawa
Ottawa, Ontario

Maureen A. Barry, RN, MScN
Associate Professor, Teaching Stream
Lawrence S. Bloomberg Faculty of Nursing
University of Toronto
Toronto, Ontario

Sylvia S. Barton, RN, PhD
Chair and Associate Professor
School of Nursing
University of Northern British Columbia
Prince George, British Columbia

Shelley Raffin Bouchal, RN, PhD
Associate Dean (Graduate Programs), Associate Professor
Faculty of Nursing
University of Calgary
Calgary, Alberta

Sherry Dahlke, PhD, RN, GCN(c)
Assistant Professor
Faculty of Nursing
University of Alberta
Edmonton, Alberta

Wendy Duggleby, RN, PhD
Professor, Associate Dean Research, and
Nursing Research Chair, Aging and Quality of Life
Faculty of Nursing
University of Alberta
Edmonton, Alberta

Susan M. Duncan, RN, PhD
Professor and Director
School of Nursing
University of Victoria
Victoria, British Columbia

Nancy A. Edgecombe, RN, BN, MN, PHD
Program Manager, Nursing and Health Sciences
Nunavut Arctic College
Iqaluit, Nunavut

Joyce Engel, RN, PhD
Associate Professor
Chair, Department of Nursing
Brock University
St. Catharines, Ontario

Caroline Foster-Boucher, RN, MN
Faculty Lecturer and Indigenous Nursing Coordinator
Faculty of Nursing
University of Alberta
Edmonton, Alberta

Frances Fothergill-Bourbonnais, RN, PhD
Professor Emeritus
School of Nursing, Faculty of Health Sciences
University of Ottawa
Ottawa, Ontario

Deborah Gibson, RN, MSN
Assistant Professor
School of Nursing
Trinity Western University
Langley, British Columbia

Jennifer Girvin, RN, MN
Nursing Faculty
Bachelor of Science in Nursing Program
College of the Rockies
Cranbrook, British Columbia

Sonya Grypma, RN, PhD
Dean and Professor
School of Nursing
Trinity Western University
Langley, British Columbia

Kathryn J. Hannah, C.M., RN, PhD
Professor (ADJ)
School of Nursing
University of Victoria
National Executive Lead
C-HOBIC Phase 2
Health Informatics Advisor
Canadian Nurses Association

Giuliana Harvey, RN, MN
Associate Professor
School of Nursing
Mount Royal University
Calgary, Alberta

Pamela G. Hawranik, RN, MN, PhD
Dean of Graduate Studies
Athabasca University
Athabasca, Alberta

Deborah Hobbs, RN, BScN, CIC
Infection Control Professional
University of Alberta Hospital
Edmonton, Alberta

Jim Hunter, RN, MSN
Program Head, Years 3, 4, and 5
British Columbia Institute of Technology
Burnaby, British Columbia

Kathleen F. Hunter, RN, NP, PhD, GNC(C), NCA
Professor
Faculty of Nursing
University of Alberta
Nurse Practitioner
Glenrose Hospital
Edmonton, Alberta

Margot Jackson, RN, PhD
Assistant Professor
Faculty of Nursing
University of Alberta
Edmonton, Alberta

Sonya L. Jakubec, RN, BHScN, MN, PhD
Associate Professor
School of Nursing
Mount Royal University
Calgary, Alberta

Darlaine Jantzen, RN, MA, PhD
Nursing Faculty
Camosun College
Victoria, British Columbia

Leanne Johnson, RN, MN
Nursing Instructor
Faculty of Nursing
University of Alberta
Edmonton, Alberta

Sharon Kaasalainen, RN, PhD
Associate Professor
School of Nursing
Research Fellow, HSFO/Michael G. Degroote Chair in Cardiovascular Nursing Research
Faculty of Health Sciences
McMaster University
Hamilton, Ontario

Margaret Ann Kennedy, RN, PhD, CPHIMS-CA
Chief Nursing Informatics Officer and Managing Partner, Clinical Informatics
Gevity Consulting Inc.
Halifax, Nova Scotia

Marnie L. Kramer, RN, PhD
Nursing Faculty
Bachelor of Science in Nursing Program
College of the Rockies
Cranbrook, British Columbia

Rosemary Kohr, RN, BA, BScN, MScN, PhD, Tertiary Care Nurse Practitioner Certificate (UWO, 1998)
Corporate Program Lead, Wound/Ostomy/Continence
Saint Elizabeth Health Care
Assistant Professor (Clinical Adjunct)
Faculty of Health Sciences
University of Western Ontario
London, Ontario

Kaysi Eastlick Kushner, RN, PhD
Professor Emeritus
Faculty of Nursing
University of Alberta
Edmonton, Alberta

Nicole Letourneau, RN, PhD, FCAHS
ACHF chair in Parent-Infant Mental Health
RESOLVE Alberta Director and Principal Investigator, CHILD Studies Program
Professor, Faculty of Nursing
Research Professor, Cumming School of Medicine
University of Calgary
Calgary, Alberta

Janet Luimes, RN(NP), MScN
Assistant Professor
College of Nursing
University of Saskatchewan
Saskatoon, Saskatchewan

Heather MacLean, RN, MN
Associate Professor
School of Nursing & Midwifery
Mount Royal University
Calgary, Alberta

Brenda L. Martelli, RN(EC), MEd
Pediatric Nurse Practitioner
Acute Pain Services
Children's Hospital of Eastern Ontario
Ottawa, Ontario

Judy Mill, RN, PhD
Professor Emeritus
Faculty of Nursing
University of Alberta
Edmonton, Alberta

Cynthia Murray, BN, MN, PhD
Associate Professor
School of Nursing
Memorial University
St. John's, Newfoundland

Judee E. Onyskiw, RN, BScN, MN, PhD
Associate Professor
Faculty of Nursing
MacEwan University
Edmonton, Alberta

Carole Orchard, BSN, MEd, EdD
Professor
Arthur Labatt Family School of Nursing
Western University
London, Ontario

Tanya Park, RN, PhD
Assistant Professor
Faculty of Nursing
University of Alberta
Edmonton, Alberta

Barbara Pesut, RN, PhD
Professor
Canada Research Chair, Health, Ethics and Diversity
School of Nursing
University of British Columbia, Okanagan
Kelowna, British Columbia

Pammla Lusenga Petrucka, RN, PhD
Professor
College of Nursing
University of Saskatchewan (Regina Site)
Regina, Saskatchewan

J. Craig Phillips, RN, PhD, LLM, ACRN, FAAN
Associate Professor
School of Nursing
University of Ottawa
Ottawa, Ontario

Donna M. Romyn, RN, PhD
Associate Vice President Research and Associate Professor
Faculty of Health Disciplines
Athabasca University
Athabasca, Alberta

Shawna M. Ryan, RN, MN
Nursing Faculty
Bachelor of Science in Nursing Program
College of the Rockies
Cranbrook, British Columbia

Monakshi Sawhney, RN(EC), PhD
Assistant Professor
School of Nursing
Queen's University
Kingston, Ontario

Carla Shapiro, RN, MN
Senior Instructor
College of Nursing
Rady Faculty of Health Sciences
University of Manitoba
Winnipeg, Manitoba

Jennifer Skelly, RN, PhD
Associate Professor
School of Nursing
McMaster University
Hamilton, Ontario

Candis Spiers, RN, MN
Nursing Faculty
College of the Rockies
Cranbrook, British Columbia

Tracy Stephen, RN, MN
Assistant Professor
School of Nursing
Trinity Western University
Langley, British Columbia

Claudette Taylor, PhD, RN, NP adult
Associate Professor
Cape Breton University
Sydney, Nova Scotia

Sally Thorne, RN, PhD
Professor, School of Nursing
Associate Dean, Faculty of Applied Science
University of British Columbia
Vancouver, British Columbia

Jill Vihos, RN, BScN, MN, PhD
Sessional Lecturer
Faculty of Nursing
University of Alberta
Edmonton, Alberta

Jeanette Vinek, RN, RScP, BScN, MHScN
Instructor 1
School of Nursing
University of British Columbia, Okanagan Campus
Kelowna, British Columbia

Kathryn Weaver, RN, PhD
Professor
Faculty of Nursing
University of New Brunswick
Fredericton, New Brunswick

Christina West, RN, PhD
Assistant Professor
College of Nursing
Rady Faculty of Health Sciences
University of Manitoba
Winnipeg, Manitoba

Jason Woytas, RN, MN, BSN
Faculty Lecturer
Faculty of Nursing
University of Alberta
Edmonton, Alberta

US CONTRIBUTORS

Michelle Aebersold, RN, PhD
Clinical Associate Professor
Director—Clinical Learning Center
School of Nursing
University of Michigan
Ann Arbor, Michigan

Katherine N. Ayzengart, MSN, RN
Associate Faculty
Nursing
MiraCosta College
Oceanside, California

Janice C. Colwell, RN, MS, CWOCN, FAAN
Advanced Practice Nurse
Surgery
University of Chicago Medicine
Chicago, Illinois

Maureen F. Cooney, DNP, FNP-BC
Adjunct Associate Professor of Nursing
FNP Program
Lienhard School of Nursing
College of Health Professions
Pace University
Pleasantville, New York;
Nurse Practitioner
Pain Medicine
Westchester Medical Center
Valhalla, New York

Margaret Ecker, RN, MS
Director of Nursing Quality (Retired)
Kaiser Permanente Los Angeles Medical Center
Los Angeles, California

Antoinette Falker, DNP, RN, CMSRN, CBN, GCNS-BC
Adjunct Faculty
Nursing Department
Webster University
Webster Groves, Missouri;
Clinical Nurse Specialist
Trauma, Geriatric Trauma, Acute Care Surgery, Bariatric Services
Barnes-Jewish Hospital
St. Louis, Missouri

Jane Fellows, MSN, CWOCN
Wound/Ostomy CNS
Advanced Clinical Practice
Duke University Health System
Durham, North Carolina

Linda Felver, RN, PhD
Associate Professor
School of Nursing
Oregon Health and Sciences University
Portland, Oregon

Victoria N. Folse, APN, PMHCNS-BC, LCPC, PhD
Director and Professor
Caroline F. Rupert Endowed Chair of Nursing
School of Nursing
Illinois Wesleyan University
Bloomington, Illinois

Lorri A. Graham, RN
Assistant Professor
Nursing
Saint Francis Medical Center College of Nursing
Peoria, Illinois

Amy M. Hall, RN, BSN, MS, PhD, CNE
Chair and White Family Endowed Professor of Nursing
Dunigan Family Department of Nursing and Health Sciences
University of Evansville
Evansville, Indiana

Tara Hulsey, PhD, RN, CNE, FAAN
Dean and E. Jane Martin Professor
School of Nursing
West Virginia University
Morgantown, West Virginia

Nöel Kerr, RN, PhD, CMSRN
Assistant Professor
School of Nursing
Illinois Wesleyan University
Bloomington, Illinois

Gayle L. Kruse, RN, ACHPN, GCNS-BC
APN Instructor
Graduate Department
Saint Anthony College of Nursing
Rockford, Illinois

Jerrilee LaMar, PhD, RN, CNE
Associate Professor of Nursing
Dunigan Family Department of Nursing and Health Sciences
University of Evansville
Evansville, Indiana

Kathy Lever, MSN, WHNP-BC
Associate Professor of Nursing
College of Education and Health Sciences
University of Evansville
Evansville, Indiana

Erin H. McCalley, RN, BSN, MS, CCRN, CCNS
Clinical Nurse Specialist
Nursing Education and Practice
Stanford Health Care
Stanford, California

Emily L. McClung, MSN, RN, PhD(c)
Nursing Instructor
Hiram College
Hiram, Ohio

Judith A. McCutchan, RN, ASN, BSN, MSN, PhD
Adjunct Nursing Faculty
Dunigan Family Department of Nursing and Health Sciences
University of Evansville
Evansville, Indiana

Patricia A. O'Connor, RN, MSN, CNE
Assistant Professor
College of Nursing
Saint Francis Medical Center College of Nursing
Peoria, Illinois

Wendy R. Ostendorf, RN, MS, EdD, CNE
Professor of Nursing
Neumann University
Aston, Pennsylvania

Jill Parsons, RN, PhD
Associate Professor of Nursing
MacMurray College
Jacksonville, Illinois

Kristine Rose, BSN, MSN
Assistant Professor
Nursing Education
Saint Francis Medical Center College of Nursing
Peoria, Illinois

Patsy L. Ruchala, RN, DNSc
Professor and Director
Orvis School of Nursing
University of Nevada Reno
Reno, Nevada

Matthew R. Sorenson, PhD, APN, ANP-C
Associate Professor/Associate Director
School of Nursing
DePaul University
Chicago, Illinois;
Clinical Scholar
Physical Medicine and Rehabilitation
Northwestern University Feinberg School of Medicine
Chicago, Illinois

Donna L. Thompson, MSN, CRNP, RNP-BC, CCCN-AP
Continence Nurse Practitioner
Division of Urogynecology
University of Pennsylvania Medical Center
Philadelphia, Pennsylvania;
Continence Nurse Practitioner
Urology Health Specialist
Drexel Hill, Pennsylvania;
Continence Consultant/Owner
Continence Solutions, LLC
Media, Pennsylvania

Leanne Armstrong, RN, BA, MHS, MN
Professor, School of Baccalaureate Nursing Tri-Campus
St. Lawrence College
Brockville, Ontario

Dr. Sherry Arvidson, RN, MN, EdD
Faculty of Nursing
University of Regina
Regina, Saskatchewan

Jasmine Balakumaran, RN, BScN, MScN
Nursing Faculty
Centennial College
Toronto, Ontario

Mona Burrows, RN(EC), BScN, MScN, PHC-NP
Professor, Collaborative BScN program
St. Lawrence College
Cornwall, Ontario

Erica Cambly, RN, MN
Assistant Professor, Teaching Stream
Lawrence S. Bloomberg Faculty of Nursing
University of Toronto
Toronto, Ontario

Seanna Chesney-Chauvet, RN, MN
Faculty Lecturer, Faculty of Nursing
University of Alberta
Edmonton, Alberta

Vanessa Corbett, LPN, MEd
School of Health and Wellness
Bow Valley College
Calgary, Alberta

Edward Venzon Cruz, RN, BN, MScN, PhD(Japan)
School of Community and Health Studies
Centennial College
Toronto, Ontario

Jan-Marie Graham, RN, MN
Assistant Professor, Faculty of Health Studies
Brandon University
Brandon, Manitoba

Shona Hommy, RN, BN, MHS GNC(c)
Health Careers Coordinator
Northern Lakes College
Slave Lake, Alberta

Coleen Karr, RN, BScN, MScN
Nursing Professor
Centennial College
Toronto, Ontario

Lori Kelly, RN DOHN, CCN(c)
Faculty, Allied Health Department
New Brunswick Community College
Saint John, New Brunswick

Shannon Lanctot-Shah, RN, MSN, DHSc, PhD(c)
Nursing Instructor
Selkirk College
Castlegar, British Columbia

Claudette McDonald, RN, MN
Practical Nursing Faculty
Nova Scotia Community College, Truro Campus
Truro, Nova Scotia

Andrea Miller
Professor, Nursing
Conestoga College
Kitchener, Ontario

Christina Murray, BA, BScN, RN, MN, PhD
Assistant Professor, School of Nursing
University of Prince Edward Island
Charlottetown, Prince Edward Island

Tia Louise Nymark, RN, BScN
Nursing Faculty
John Abbott College
Ste. Anne de Bellevue, Quebec

Holldrid Odreman, RN, MScN-Ed, PhD
Professor of Nursing, Program Coordinator, and Certified Simulationist
Niagara College
Welland, Ontario

Kathlyn Palafox, BSN, BCPID
Secondary Senior Educational Administrator
Canadian Health Care Academy
Surrey, British Columbia

Eva Hava Peisachovich, RN, PhD
Assistant Professor
School of Nursing, Faculty of Health
York University
Toronto, Ontario

Barbara Thompson, RN, BScN, MScN
Professor of Nursing, Health Programs
Sault College
Sault Ste. Marie, Ontario

1

Health and Wellness

Written by Kaysi Eastlick Kushner, RN, PhD, Margot Jackson, RN, PhD

OBJECTIVES

Mastery of content in this chapter will enable you to:

- Define the key terms listed.
- Discuss ways that definitions of health have been conceptualized.
- Describe key characteristics of medical, behavioural, and socioenvironmental approaches to health.
- Identify factors that have led to each approach to health.
- Discuss contributions of the following Canadian publications to conceptualizations of health and health determinants: *Lalonde Report, Ottawa Charter, Epp Report, Strategies for Population Health, Jakarta Declaration, Bangkok Charter, Toronto Charter.*
- Discuss key health determinants and their interrelationships and how they influence health.
- Contrast distinguishing features of health promotion and disease prevention.
- Describe the three levels of disease prevention.
- Identify and give examples of the five health promotion strategies discussed in the *Ottawa Charter.*
- Analyze how the nature and scope of nursing practice are influenced by different conceptualizations of health and health determinants.

KEY TERMS

Behavioural approach, p. 3
Behavioural risk factors, p. 3
Determinants of health, p. 6
Disease, p. 1
Disease prevention, p. 11
Evidence-informed decision making, p. 13
Food insecurity, p. 8
Health, p. 2
Health as actualization, p. 2
Health as actualization and stability, p. 2
Health as resource, p. 2
Health as stability, p. 2
Healthy as unity, p. 2
Health disparities, p. 6
Health field concept, p. 3
Health literacy, p. 7
Health promotion, p. 11
Health promotion strategies, p. 11
Illness, p. 2
Medical approach, p. 3
Physiological risk factors, p. 3
Population health approach, p. 5
Prerequisites for health, p. 4
Psychosocial risk factors, p. 5
Racism, p. 10
Racialization, p. 10
Social determinants of health, p. 6
Socioenvironmental approach, p. 4
Socioenvironmental risk conditions, p. 5
Wellness, p. 2

MEDIA RESOURCES

http://evolve.elsevier.com/Canada/Potter/fundamentals/

- Audio Chapter Summaries
- Examination Review Questions
- Concept Map Creator
- Case Study with Questions
- Audio Glossary
- Content Updates
- Video Clips

Concepts of health and what determines health have changed significantly since the 1970s. This conceptual change has major implications for Canadian nursing in the twenty-first century because how you as a nurse perceive health—and what determines it—influences the nature and scope of nursing practice. The importance of health to nursing is reflected in nursing models and frameworks, in which health is one of the "metaparadigm" concepts along with *person, environment, nursing,* and, more recently, *social justice* (see Chapter 4). In each framework, health concepts are congruent with the assumptions and focus of the model. Moreover, knowledge of health and health determinants is identified as an essential component of nursing education in Canada (Canadian Association of Schools of Nursing [CASN], 2015).

CONCEPTUALIZATIONS OF HEALTH

Discussion about the nature of health revolves around its relationship to *disease, illness,* and *wellness.* Often, debates focus on whether health is defined in negative or positive terms. When health is negatively defined as the absence of disease, health and illness are represented on a continuum, with maximum health at one end and death at the other. When health is positively defined, however, health and illness are viewed as distinct but interrelated concepts. Therefore, a person can have disease, such as a chronic pathological condition, and have healthy characteristics as well.

Many people use the words *illness* and *disease* interchangeably. Others suggest that disease is an objective state of ill health, the

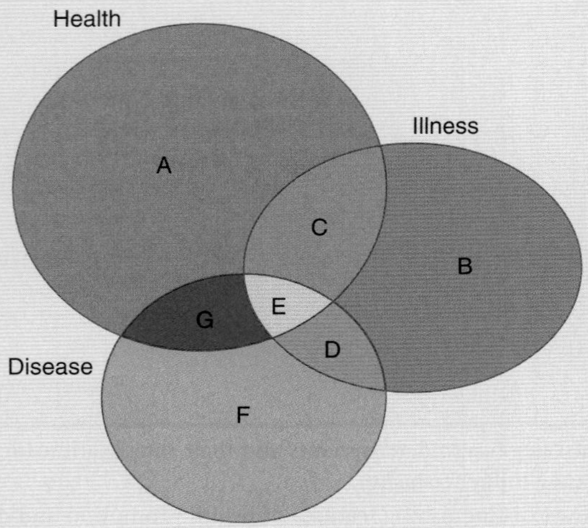

Legend

Circle A represents health or wellness, the clear area being experiences such as feeling vital, enjoying good social relationships, having a sense of purpose in life, and experiencing a connectedness to "community."

Circle B represents experiences of illness, the clear area representing illness that cannot be explained by conventional biomedical concepts and research.

Shaded area C is feeling "so-so," where little is required to tip one into wellness or illness.

Shaded area D is where a diagnosed pathology objectively validates and explains the subjective experience of illness.

Shaded area E represents feeling "so-so," being diagnosed with a pathology, and becoming sick.

Circle F represents diagnosed pathology, the clear area being undiagnosed or silent pathology, such as hypertension, CVD, congenital diseases, or cancers.

Shaded area G represents being diagnosed with a pathology, but still reporting oneself as feeling well or healthy.

FIGURE 1-1 Health, illness, and disease. CVD, cardiovascular disease. (From Labonte, R. [1993]. *Issues in health promotion series. 3. Health promotion and empowerment: Practice frameworks* [p. 18]. Toronto: Centre for Health Promotion, University of Toronto, & ParticipACTION.)

pathological process of which can be detected by medical science, whereas **illness** is a subjective experience of loss of health (Jensen & Allen, 1993; Labonte, 1993). Figure 1-1 shows the relationships among health, illness, and disease.

Definitions of health beyond the absence of disease usually have multidimensional components, including physical, mental, social, and spiritual health. Some scholars have considered this broad definition of health to be synonymous with wellness (Labonte, 1993; Pender, Murdaugh, & Parsons, 2015). Others have argued that **health** is an objective process characterized by functional stability, balance, and integrity, whereas **wellness** is a subjective experience (see discussion by Mackey, 2009). The word *health* is derived from the Old English word *hoelth*, meaning whole of body. Historically, physical wholeness was important for social acceptance, and people with contagious or disfiguring diseases were often ostracized. Good health was considered natural, whereas disease was considered unnatural. As science progressed, disease was regarded less negatively because it could be countered by scientific medicine. After World War II, the World Health Organization (WHO) (1947), in its constitution, defined health as "a state of complete physical, mental and social well-being, and not merely the absence of disease or infirmity." This is still the most commonly cited definition of health.

Classifications of Health Conceptualizations

Conceptualizations of individual health have been classified in a variety of ways. One way to organize conceptualizations is by dimensions that comprise the whole of a person's life or, alternatively, by the whole as a unitary life (i.e., not separable into dimensions):

- **Health as stability.** Health is defined as the maintenance of physiological, functional, and social norms, and encompasses views of health as a state, as a process, as adaptation and as homeostasis (Pender et al., 2015; Thorne, Canam, Dahinten, et al., 1998).
- **Health as actualization.** Health is defined as the actualization of human potential (Pender et al., 2015). Scholars and researchers who adhere to this definition often use the terms *health* and *wellness* interchangeably.
- **Health as actualization and stability.** Both actualization and stability concepts are incorporated in the definition of health as "the realization of human potential through goal-directed behaviour, competent self-care, and satisfying relationships with others, while adapting to meet the demands of everyday life and maintain harmony with the social and physical environments" (Pender et al., 2015, p. 13).
- **Health as resource.** The definition of health as a resource or asset emerged in the *Ottawa Charter for Health Promotion* (WHO, 1986) and includes capacities to fulfill roles, meet demands, and engage in the activities of everyday living (Pender et al., 2015; Williamson & Carr, 2009).
- **Health as unity.** Health is defined as "reflecting the whole person as process and is synonymous with self-transcendence" (Thorne et al., 1998, p. 1261) or actualization.

Most contemporary nursing theorists have conceptualized health as stability and/or actualization, although some have advanced the conceptualization of health as unity. Interestingly, Nightingale's definition of health reflects both the stability and actualization dimensions (Thorne et al., 1998).

In 1984, the WHO updated its conceptualization of health as:

> *the extent to which an individual or group is able, on the one hand, to realize aspirations and satisfy needs; and, on the other hand, to change or cope with the environment. Health is, therefore, seen as a resource for everyday life, not the objective of living; it is a positive concept emphasizing social and personal resources, as well as physical capacities. (p. 3)*

Rather than viewing health as an ideal state of well-being (as in the 1947 WHO definition), this definition, incorporating both actualization and stability dimensions, suggests that people in a variety of situations—even those with physical disease or nearing death—could be considered healthy.

Labonte (1993) developed a multidimensional conceptualization of health that reflects both actualization and stability perspectives. Aspects include the following qualities:

- Feeling vitalized and full of energy
- Having satisfying social relationships
- Having a feeling of control over one's life and living conditions

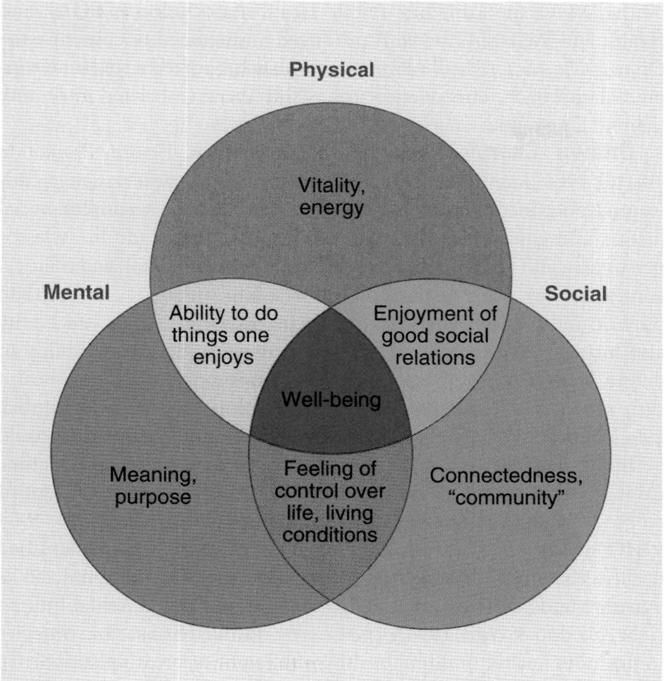

FIGURE 1-2 Dimensions of health and well-being. (From Labonte, R. [1993]. *Issues in health promotion series. 3. Health promotion and empowerment: Practice frameworks* [p. 20]. Toronto: Centre for Health Promotion, University of Toronto, & ParticipACTION.)

- Being able to do things that one enjoys
- Having a sense of purpose
- Feeling connected to community

Using the WHO dimensions of physical, mental, and social well-being, Labonte (1993) categorized these characteristics using a Venn diagram (Figure 1-2). The diagram clearly depicts the concept of holism, whereby health is more than the sum of the component parts in that the interrelationships between and among different components result in different aspects of health.

Nurse scholars conceptualize health in different ways (see Chapter 5 for further information on health). For example, the McGill Model of Nursing concept of health as coping and development is very congruent with the WHO (1984) definition (Gottlieb & Gottlieb, 2007). Jones and Meleis (1993) articulated health as empowerment: "Health is being empowered to define, seek, and find conditions, resources, and processes to be an effective agent in meeting the significant needs perceived by individuals" (p. 12). This conceptualization is congruent with Labonte's (1993) focus and reflects the essence of health promotion, to be discussed later. In a review of the concept of health, Rootman and O'Neill (2012) suggested that in view of current realities of the twenty-first century, a definition of health needs to be positive (not based on pathology or deficit), comprehensive (with a broad set of determinants), particularly attentive to the mental health dimension, and inclusive of quality of life and spirituality.

HISTORICAL APPROACHES TO HEALTH IN CANADA

In modern times, the three major approaches to health have been medical, behavioural, and socioenvironmental (Labonte, 1993). These approaches offer a useful framework for examining the evolution of health orientations in Canada.

Medical Approach

The **medical approach**, which represents a stability orientation to health, dominated Western thinking for most of the twentieth century. It emphasizes that medical intervention restores health. Health problems are defined primarily as **physiological risk factors**—physiologically defined characteristics that are precursors to or risk factors for disease. Examples include hypertension, hypercholesterolemia, genetic predispositions, and obesity. The biopsychosocial view of health (Engel, 1977) includes psychological and social elements; however, in practice, a medical focus on pathology was retained (Antonovsky, 1987). In the medical approach, the health care system is paramount to ensuring that populations remain healthy.

Focusing on treatment of disease was strongly supported after World War II, when new technological and scientific medical advances facilitated the medical approach. In Canada, postwar economic growth increased funding to build new hospitals. National health insurance was created to remove financial barriers to care. Many people believed that scientific medicine could solve most health problems and that accessible and quality health care (or, more correctly, illness care) would improve the health of Canadians. Within this approach, less emphasis was given to health promotion and disease prevention.

Behavioural Approach

By the early 1970s, increasingly large amounts of money were spent on health care, but the health status of the population did not improve proportionately. To better understand what contributed to illness and death, the Minister of Health and Welfare, Marc Lalonde, commissioned a study that resulted in the 1974 report *A New Perspective on the Health of Canadians.* This so-called *Lalonde Report* shifted emphasis from a medical to a **behavioural approach** to health. The report concluded that the traditional medical approach to health care was inadequate and that "further improvements in the environment, reductions in self-imposed risks, and a greater knowledge of human biology" were necessary to improve the health status of Canadians (p. 6). The *Lalonde Report* was the first modern government document in the Western world to acknowledge the inadequacy of a strictly biomedical health care system.

The *Lalonde Report* broadly defined health determinants as *lifestyle, environment, human biology,* and the *organization of health care.* This **health field concept** was widely used, modified, and expanded by other countries, and its release was a turning point in broadening Canadians' attitudes about factors that contribute to health, along with the role of government in promoting health (Health Canada, 1998). Of the four determinants, lifestyle received the most attention, perhaps because lifestyle behaviours contributed to chronic diseases (such as cancer and heart disease) and to injuries—both of which are the leading causes of morbidity and mortality in Canada (Labonte, 1993). In addition, greater understanding of behavioural social psychology revealed factors that motivated individuals to engage in healthy or unhealthy behaviours. In 1978, the Canadian government established the Health Promotion Directorate in the Department of National Health and Welfare, the first official health promotion undertaking of its kind. Its aim was to decrease **behavioural risk factors** such as smoking, substance abuse, lack of exercise, and an unhealthy diet. Public health programs such as Operation Lifestyle and ParticipACTION were developed through this department.

The behavioural approach places responsibility for health on the individual, thereby favouring health promotion strategies such as education and social marketing. Strategies are often based on the assumption that if people know the risk factors for disease, then they will engage in healthy behaviours. Indeed, health-enhancing practices among Canadians increased during this time. With the ParticipACTION initiative, for instance, many people increased their physical activity. Antismoking campaigns led to a substantial decrease in tobacco use.

Socioenvironmental Approach

By the mid-1980s, however, the behavioural approach to health and illness prevention was challenged. Studies showed that lifestyle improvements were made primarily by well-educated, well-employed, and higher-income Canadians. The *Lalonde Report* was criticized for deflecting attention from the environment and for how environment and lifestyle were defined. Lifestyle was viewed as being within an individual's control, with health risks as "self-imposed" behaviours. This supported "victim-blaming" and views that health was largely an individual responsibility. Critics suggested that health-related behaviours could not be separated from the social contexts (environments) in which they occurred. For example, living and working conditions were perceived as barriers to engaging in healthy behaviours (Labonte, 1993).

In the **socioenvironmental approach**, health is closely tied to social structures. For example, poverty and unhealthy physical and social environments, such as air pollution, poor water quality, and workplace hazards, are recognized as influencing health directly. Thus, Canadian public health providers expanded Lalonde's (1974) health field concept to emphasize the social context of health and the relationship between personal health behaviours and social and physical environments (Hancock & Perkins, 1985).

Internationally, more attention also was given to the social context of health. The WHO Regional Conference in Europe produced a discussion paper identifying the social conditions that influence health (WHO, 1984). Just as Canada led the behavioural approach to health with the *Lalonde Report,* it was now instrumental in focusing on social and environmental conditions. In 1986, the First International Conference on Health Promotion was held in Ottawa, sponsored by the WHO, the Canadian Public Health Association (CPHA), and Health and Welfare Canada. It produced a watershed document—the *Ottawa Charter for Health Promotion*—that supported a socioenvironmental approach. This document has since been translated into more than 40 languages.

Ottawa Charter. The *Ottawa Charter for Health Promotion* (WHO, 1986) identified **prerequisites for health** as peace, shelter, education, food, income, a stable ecosystem, sustainable resources, social justice, and equity. These prerequisites clearly go beyond lifestyles or personal health practices to include social, environmental, and political contexts. They place responsibility for health on society rather than only on individuals. The *Charter*'s focus on social justice and equity also incorporated the concept of *empowerment*—a person's ability to define, analyze, and solve problems—as an important goal for health care providers (Registered Nurses Association of British Columbia, 1994). Indeed, Wallerstein (1992) contended that powerlessness could be the underlying health determinant influencing other risk factors. Consequently, health promotion literature emphasizes the concept of empowerment. The *Ottawa Charter* incorporated the then-new 1984 WHO definition of health (discussed previously), which identified health as having both social and individual dimensions, emphasized its dynamic and positive nature, and viewed it as a fundamental human right (Naidoo & Wills, 1994). The *Charter* outlined five major strategies to promote health: building healthy public policy, creating supportive environments, strengthening community action, developing personal skills, and reorienting health services (detailed later in this chapter).

Achieving Health for All. Concepts from the *Ottawa Charter* were incorporated into another important Canadian document, *Achieving Health for All: A Framework for Health Promotion* (Epp, 1986). This report, developed under the leadership of Jake Epp, Minister of National Health and Welfare from 1984 to 1989, became Canada's blueprint for achieving the WHO goal of "Health for All 2000" (Figure 1-3).

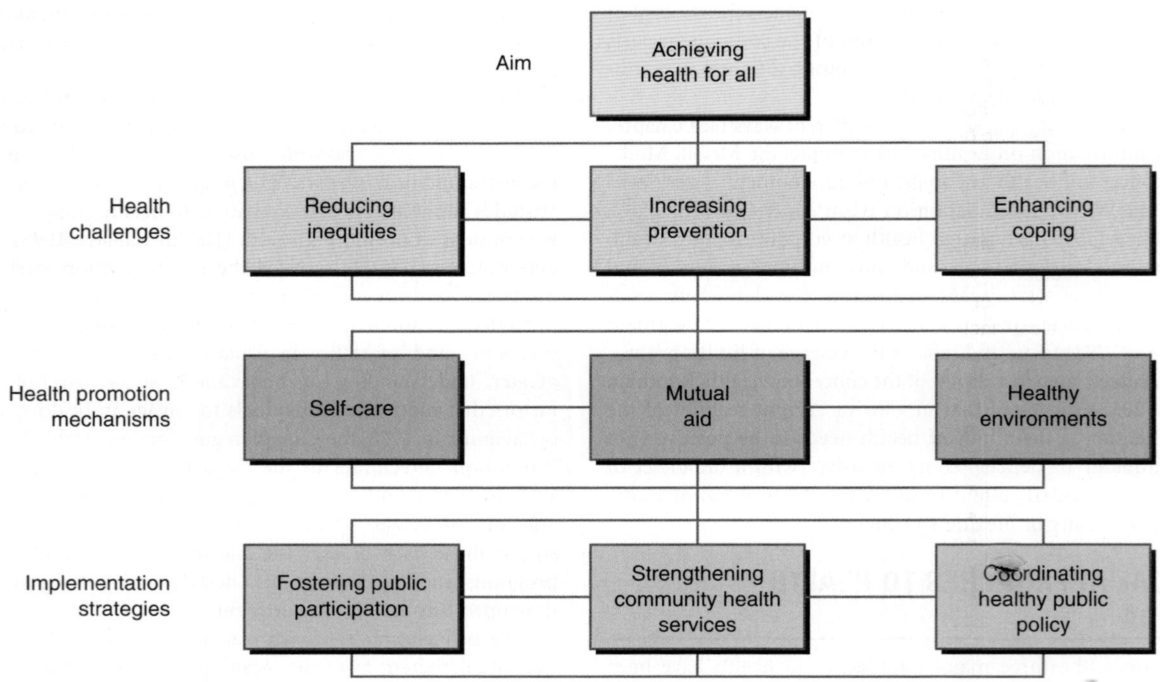

FIGURE 1-3 Achieving health for all: A framework for health promotion. (From Epp, J. [1986]. *Achieving health for all: A framework for health promotion* [p. 8]. Ottawa: Health and Welfare Canada. Reproduced with the permission of the Minister of Public Works and Government Services Canada, 2012.)

Epp's (1986) report identified three major health challenges: reducing inequities, increasing prevention, and enhancing coping mechanisms. The report acknowledged disparities in health, particularly between low- and high-income people, and that living and working conditions were critical determinants of health. The need for effective ways to prevent injuries, illnesses, chronic conditions, and disabilities was emphasized. The health challenge of enhancing people's ability to cope reflected an acknowledgement that the dominant diseases in Canada were chronic conditions that could not be cured. Thus people needed to be assisted in managing and coping with chronic conditions in order that they might live meaningful and productive lives. The *Epp Report* emphasized society's responsibility for providing supports for people experiencing chronic medical conditions, stress, mental illness, and problems associated with aging, as well as the need for supports for caregivers. The report identified self-care, mutual aid, and promotion of healthy environments as ways to address the three major health challenges, reflecting both personal and social responsibility. Specific strategies included fostering public participation, strengthening community health services, and coordinating healthy public policy.

The *Ottawa Charter* and the *Epp Report* each reflect a socioenvironmental approach in which health is seen as more than the absence of disease and engaging in healthy behaviours; rather, this approach emphasizes connectedness, as well as self-efficacy and the capacity to engage in meaningful activities (see Figure 1-2).

Risk Factors and Risk Conditions. Labonte (1993) categorized the major determinants of health in a socioenvironmental approach as psychosocial risk factors and socioenvironmental risk conditions:

- **Psychosocial risk factors** are complex psychological experiences resulting from social circumstances that include isolation, lack of social support, limited social networks, low self-esteem, self-blame, and low perceived power.
- **Socioenvironmental risk conditions** are social and environmental living conditions that include poverty, low educational or occupational status, dangerous or stressful work, dangerous physical environments, pollution, discrimination, relative political or economic powerlessness, and inequalities of income or power.

According to a socioenvironmental approach to health, political, social, and cultural forces affect health and well-being both directly and indirectly through their influence on personal health behaviours. Socioenvironmental risk conditions can contribute to psychosocial risk factors, which can then result in unhealthy behaviours (Figure 1-4). This means that health care providers should recognize the influence of environment on personal behaviours and that "health-inhibiting" behaviours could be coping strategies for managing the stress created by living and working conditions that decrease access to resources. In other words, "to change behaviour it may be necessary to change more than behaviour" (Wilkinson, 1996, p. 64). For example, in addition to working "downstream" to assist people who are experiencing the negative health effects of socioenvironmental conditions, nurses need to work "upstream" by advocating for policies that ensure affordable housing, financial support to patients with low incomes, and safe, fulfilling work environments.

Strategies for Population Health. In Canada, the determinants of health have been further emphasized through the **population health approach** (Public Health Agency of Canada, 2013). This approach, initiated by the Canadian Institute for Advanced Research, was officially endorsed by the federal, provincial, and territorial ministers of health in the report titled *Strategies for Population Health: Investing in the Health of Canadians* (Federal, Provincial, and Territorial Advisory Committee on Population Health [ACPH], 1994). In a population health approach, "the entire range of known individual and collective factors and conditions that determine population health status, and the interactions among them, are taken into account in planning action

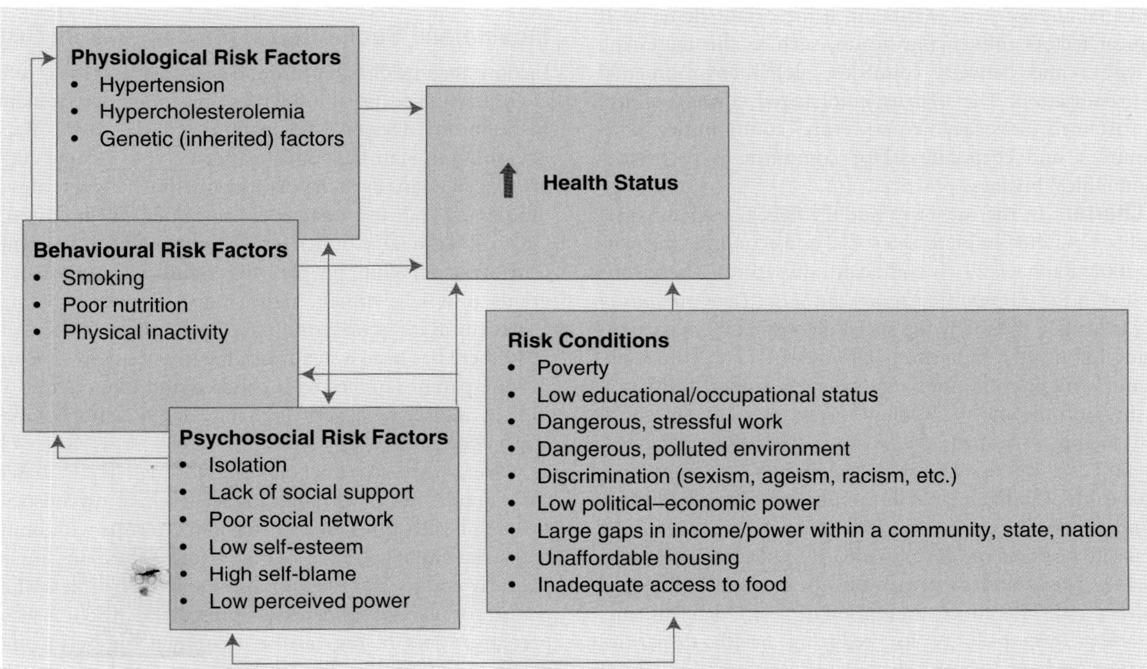

FIGURE 1-4 Socioenvironmental approach to health. (From Labonte, R. [1993]. *Issues in health promotion series. 3. Health promotion and empowerment: Practice frameworks* [p. 11]. Toronto: Centre for Health Promotion, University of Toronto, & ParticipACTION.)

to improve health" (Health Canada, 1998). The population health approach emphasizes the use of epidemiological data to determine the etiology of health and disease.

The key health determinants identified in the *Strategies for Population Health* report are as follows:

- Income and social status
- Social support networks
- Education
- Employment and working conditions
- Physical environments
- Biology and genetic endowment
- Personal health practices and coping skills
- Healthy child development
- Health services

In 1996, Health Canada added *gender, culture,* and *social environments* to this list. Note that the list includes determinants at the individual level (personal health practices and coping skills; biology and genetic endowment) and at the population level (education, employment, and income distribution).

Jakarta Declaration. The *Jakarta Declaration on Health Promotion Into the 21st Century* (WHO, 1997) emerged from the 4th International Conference on Health Promotion, the first to be held in a developing country and to involve the private sector. The *Jakarta Declaration* affirmed the *Ottawa Charter* prerequisites for health; added four other prerequisites (*empowerment of women, social security, respect for human rights,* and *social relations*); and declared poverty to be the greatest threat to health. The *Declaration* identified the following priorities for action: promoting social responsibility for health in public and private sectors; increasing investments for health in all sectors; consolidating and expanding partnerships for health to all levels of government and the private sector; increasing community capacity and empowering the individual; and securing adequate infrastructure for health promotion.

Bangkok Charter. The *Bangkok Charter for Health Promotion in a Globalized World* (WHO, 2005) affirmed health as a human right and emphasized mental and spiritual well-being as important elements. It identified critical factors influencing health, such as the increasing inequalities within and between countries, global environmental change, and urbanization. The *Charter* emphasized strong political action and sustained advocacy, empowering communities with adequate resources, and corporate sector commitment to healthy workplaces and ethical business practices.

Toronto Charter. In the early to middle 1990s, Canadian social and health policies resulted in increased social and economic inequalities (Bryant, 2002; Raphael, 2016) and health disparities. These concerns culminated in the *Toronto Charter on the Social Determinants of Health,* which identified the following social determinants as particularly important for health: Indigenous status, early life, education, employment and working conditions, food security, gender, health care services, housing, income and its distribution, social safety net, social exclusion, and unemployment and employment security. **Social determinants of health** can be defined as "the *economic and social conditions* that shape the health of individuals, communities, and jurisdictions as a whole ... [and] determine the extent to which a person possesses the physical, social, and personal resources to identify and achieve personal aspirations, satisfy needs, and cope with the environment" (Raphael, 2016, p. 3; italics ours). This conceptualization of health determinants emphasizes *societal* responsibility for reducing health disparities because it focuses on how a society distributes economic and social resources through its economic and social policies. A social determinants of health perspective calls attention to the political, economic, and social forces that shape policy decisions, thereby reflecting a critical/structural approach to health (Bryant, 2016). The social determinants of health identified in the *Toronto Charter* were chosen because they (a) are important to the health of Canadians, (b) are understandable to Canadians, (c) have clear policy relevance to decision makers and citizens, and (d) are especially timely and relevant (Raphael, 2016).

Concern about **health disparities** (i.e., differences in health status among different population groups) has been raised worldwide. The WHO Commission on Social Determinants of Health (WHO, 2008a) was charged with developing strategies to narrow health disparities through action on the social determinants of health. Nationally, the Health Disparities Task Group (2005), commissioned by the Public Health Agency of Canada (PHAC), identified socioeconomic status, Indigenous identity, gender, and geographic location as the most important factors contributing to health disparities. In 2007, the Senate Subcommittee on Population Health was established to examine the impact of social determinants of health on disparities and inequities in health (Senate Subcommittee on Population Health, 2009). The *Report on the State of Public Health in Canada* (PHAC, 2008), by Canada's first chief public health officer, also underscored health inequalities.

Health disparities are associated with inequitable access (unfair or unjust lack of access) to health determinants resulting from economic and social policies; therefore, the term *health inequities* (rather than *health inequalities* or *disparities*) may more accurately reflect the source and nature of health differences (Reutter & Kushner, 2010b).

DETERMINANTS OF HEALTH AND SOCIAL DETERMINANTS OF HEALTH

The following section introduces you to some of the major **determinants of health** affecting Canadians (Health Canada, 1996), with attention to the social determinants of health (Raphael, 2016). Although each determinant on its own contributes to health, the determinants are also interrelated and influence each other.

Income and Social Status (Income and Its Distribution)

Income, income distribution, and social status is the greatest determinant of health because it influences most other determinants (Canadian Institute for Health Information [CIHI], 2004; Raphael, 2016). According to Statistics Canada after-tax low-income cut-offs in 2008, 9% of Canadians lived in poverty, with much higher rates among single mothers (21%) and unattached nonelderly women (36%) and men (28%) (National Council of Welfare, 2008). Indigenous peoples, Canadians of colour, people with disabilities, and recent urban immigrants also have much higher rates of poverty compared to the Canadian average (see summary by Raphael, 2006). Although since 1980 there has been a steady decline in rates of low income, one-third of lone-parent families with children and one-quarter of unattached individuals seems a very high rate for a nation of relative wealth (Curry-Stevens, 2016).

Poverty exerts its effect on health through lack of material resources that support health, through higher levels of psychosocial stress, and through health-threatening behaviours to cope with limited resources and stress (Raphael, 2016). Low-income Canadians are more likely to die early and to suffer from most diseases, regardless of age, sex, race, culture, or place of residence (Phipps, 2003). About 20% of Canadians' premature loss of life can be accounted for by income differences (Raphael, 2016). People with lower incomes are more likely to have chronic health problems, particularly cardiovascular disease and type 2 diabetes (Raphael, Anstice, & Raine, 2003; Raphael & Farrell, 2002; Wilkins, Berthelot, & Ng, 2002); lower self-esteem, lower sense of mastery and coherence; and higher levels of depression (Federal, Provincial, and Territorial ACPH, 1999). With each step up the economic ladder, Canadians' health status improves, suggesting that this "social gradient" of health is related to more than absolute material deprivation (Raphael, 2016).

Low birth weight, an important marker for subsequent poor child and adult health, has a 43% higher incidence in poor neighbourhoods than in higher-income neighbourhoods (Wilkins et al., 2002). Children living in poverty are more likely to have chronic diseases such as asthma and type 2 diabetes, to suffer from malnutrition, to use emergency department services, and to die from injuries (Canadian Institute of Child Health, 2000; Shimmin, 2015). They are also at greater risk for cognitive difficulties, delayed vocabulary development, and behavioural problems (CIHI, 2004).

Income inequality (i.e., the increasing gap between the rich and the poor [Curry-Stevens, 2016]) also influences population health. Countries with greater economic inequality have lower overall health and life expectancies (Wilkinson & Picket, 2009). Although the mechanisms responsible for this association are complex and still being explored, one explanation suggests that income inequality may result in less public investment in sectors that affect health, such as education, health services, transportation, and housing (Auger & Alix, 2016).

Social Support Networks

Social support affects health, health behaviours, and health care utilization (Carpiano, 2007; Mikkonen & Raphael, 2010) through practical, emotional, informational, and affirmational support (House, 1981). Indeed, some experts believe that relationships may be as important to health as established risk factors such as obesity, smoking, and high blood pressure (Federal, Provincial, and Territorial ACPH, 1999). A strong body of research links social support with positive health outcomes (Carpiano, 2007; Richmond, Ross, & Egeland, 2007; Tomaka, Thompson, & Palacios, 2006), whereas social isolation, exclusion, and lack of supportive relationships increase stress and vulnerability to disease directly, and indirectly through increased risk behaviours such as smoking, substance abuse, and overeating (Mikkonen & Raphael, 2010).

In general, Canadians have reported high levels of support (Federal, Provincial, and Territorial ACPH, 1999). Four of five Canadians reported that they had someone to confide in, whom they could count on in a crisis or for advice, and who made them feel loved and cared for. Nevertheless, men, lone-parent families, and lower-income Canadians generally reported less support than did their respective counterparts. Support from families and friends and from informal and formal groups can provide practical aid during times of crisis and emotional support in times of distress and change. Social support assists in coping and making behavioural changes and can help individuals solve problems and maintain a sense of mastery and control over their lives. A Canadian population-based study found that higher levels of support and mastery were associated with lower psychological distress for men and women (Gadalla, 2009). A survey of young parents in Alberta identified spouses, family, and friends as major sources of support in encouraging healthy behaviours (exercise, diet) by providing emotional, affirmational, and practical support, including child care and financial assistance (Reutter, Dennis, & Wilson, 2001). Support interventions helped mothers of very preterm infants gain confidence in their parenting skills (Preyde, 2007), helped low-income women reduce or quit smoking (Stewart, Kushner, Greaves, et al., 2010), and enhanced support-seeking skills and reduced loneliness and parenting stress among Sudanese and Somali refugee new parents (Stewart, Makwarimba, Letourneau, et al., 2015). It is important to address social support in relation to not only individual behaviours but also the broader social, political, and economic context that shapes community norms, values, and behaviours (Richmond, 2007; Richmond & Ross, 2009).

Education and Literacy

Education and literacy are important influences on health status because they affect many other health determinants. Literacy can influence health both directly (e.g., reading medication prescriptions, safety instructions in workplaces) and indirectly through use of services, personal health practices, income, work environments, and stress levels. For example, people with low literacy skills are more likely to be unemployed, receive income support, earn minimum wages in unskilled jobs, have higher stress levels, and make less use of preventive services (Ronson McNicol & Rootman, 2016). Education increases job opportunities and income security, which provide knowledge and skills to solve problems and gain a sense of control (PHAC, 2004). People with higher education levels tend to smoke less, be more physically active, and have access to healthier foods and physical environments (Federal, Provincial, and Territorial ACPH, 1999).

Health literacy is a related but distinct concept that has evolved from an initial focus on functional literacy reading and math ability needed in everyday life to an expanded focus that includes interactive and critical literacy. As a progression from functional literacy, *interactive literacy* reflects advanced ability to apply new information to changing circumstances. *Critical literacy* reflects further advanced ability to "critically analyze information, and to apply this information to exert greater control over life events and situations" (Nutbeam, 2008, p. 2075).

Employment and Working Conditions (Unemployment and Employment Security)

(Un)employment, working conditions, and employment security significantly affect physical, mental, and social health. Paid work provides financial resources, a sense of identity and purpose, social contacts, and opportunities for personal growth (Smith & Polanyi, 2016). Unemployment is linked to material and social deprivation, adoption of health-threatening coping behaviours, psychological stress, and physical and mental health problems (Mikkonen & Raphael, 2010).

Working conditions can support health or pose health hazards. Smith and Polanyi (2016) identified qualities of available, adequate, appropriate, and appreciative work as pillars of workplace health. Healthy workplaces include job and employment security, safe physical conditions, reasonable work pace, low stress, opportunities for self-expression and individual development, participation, and work–life balance (Jackson & Rao, 2016). Temporary employees, part-time workers, and people working in low-wage jobs have high levels of job insecurity and frequent periods of unemployment. Often such jobs do not provide benefits or pensions, which can lead to uncertainty and stress (Menendez, Benach, Muntaner, et al., 2007; Tompa, Scott-Marshall, Dolinschi, et al., 2007). In 2000, more than one in four Canadian workers believed that their place of work was not healthy (Canadian Policy Research Networks, 2008). One third of Canadian workers in 2003 reported high stress at work, with even higher rates (45%) for health care workers (Wilkins, 2007). Indeed, the concern regarding negative workplace conditions in the health sector is considerable; nurses have had the highest or second-highest rates of absenteeism of all workers in Canada since the early 1990s (Villeneuve & MacDonald, 2006). Workplace stress is linked to increased risk of physical injuries, high blood pressure, cardiovascular disease, depression, and increases in tobacco and alcohol use (Jackson & Rao, 2016). In 2003, almost 10% of Canadian workers in trades, transport, and equipment operation sustained on-the-job injuries, which is more than four times the rate among workers in the "white-collar" sector (Wilkins & Mackenzie, 2007).

Physical Environments (Geography, Housing, Food Security)

The physical environment, an important determinant of health, includes factors in the built environment such as housing, food security, and community planning, as well as factors in the natural environment such as geography, environment quality, and climate change.

Lack of affordable, suitable, and adequate housing is a concern, as inadequate and insecure housing can affect health *directly* (e.g., presence of lead, asbestos, poor heating systems, overcrowding, dampness) and *indirectly* through its influence on other determinants (Bryant, 2009). Spending a disproportionate amount of income on rent, for example, reduces the amount of money that families can spend on food, clothing, recreation, and health care. Homelessness in Canada is increasing, in part because of reduced government funding of social housing and a lack of affordable rental accommodations (Bryant, 2009; Gaetz, Dej, Richter, et al., 2016; Khandor & Mason, 2007). Whereas historically, homelessness in Canada was experienced primarily by older single men, the current homelessness crisis involves substantial numbers of women, youth, and families, as well as veterans and Indigenous peoples (Gaetz et al., 2016). Homeless populations are at greater risk for a variety of health problems, including mental illness, substance abuse, suicide, tuberculosis, injuries and assaults, chronic medical conditions (e.g., respiratory and musculoskeletal), and poor oral and dental health, and for early death (Frankish, Hwang, & Quantz, 2005; Khandor & Mason, 2007).

Food insecurity (the limited or uncertain availability of nutritious foods) is a growing problem in Canada. In 2004, more than 40% of households with low or lower middle incomes reported food insecurity (Ledrou & Gervais, 2005); those receiving social assistance were particularly vulnerable. In March 2010, over 800,000 Canadians were assisted by food banks, a 9% increase over 2009 and the highest level on record. Over half (51%) of these users were social assistance recipients, and 51% were families with children, half of whom were two-parent families (Food Banks Canada, 2010). Food insecurity is significantly associated with multiple chronic conditions, distress, and depression (Tarasuk, 2016).

Municipalities throughout Canada have incorporated smoking bans in public places (and, in several jurisdictions, smoking bans in private cars when children are present) to limit involuntary exposure to tobacco smoke (second-hand smoke). There is no safe level of exposure to second-hand tobacco smoke (WHO, 2009). It can increase children's risk for sudden unexpected infant death (SUID), acute respiratory infections, ear problems, and reduced lung development and can increase adults' risk for coronary heart disease and lung cancer (US Department of Health and Human Services, 2006).

The determinant of physical environment also includes geographic conditions that may contribute to isolation and limit access to health care (McGibbon, 2016), as well as environmental quality; contaminants in air, water, food, and soil can adversely affect health, sometimes contributing to cancer, birth defects, respiratory illness, and gastrointestinal ailments. Children from low-income families, who often live in neighbourhoods located near highways and industrial areas, are particularly likely to be exposed to these contaminants (Center for Quality Growth and Regional Development, 2006).

Additionally, the effects of climate change on the health of populations and the planet itself have increased in magnitude. The Canadian Nurses Association (CNA) has produced several documents related to nursing's role in addressing climate change (CNA, 2008, 2009), including an excellent video and educational module available on its website. The need for sustainable ecosystems, a prerequisite for health first identified in the *Ottawa Charter,* is clearly becoming more critical; however, the relationship between human and environmental health is a relatively recent focus for nursing (Hansen-Ketchum, Marck, & Reutter, 2009).

Biological and Genetic Endowment

Heredity is strongly influenced by social and physical environments, and considerable effort has been expended to prevent congenital defects through monitoring and improved preconception and prenatal care (Federal, Provincial, and Territorial ACPH, 1999). This effort has led to substantial decreases in anomalies at birth. Yet, there is also increasing recognition that nature and nurture are not dichotomous influences on health but that "the social environment has a profound impact upon the function of one's genes, providing the context and stimulus for the variable expression of an inherited code" (Denburg & Daneman, 2010, p. 28).

Age is also a strong determinant of health. Many older people develop chronic diseases, although disability can be reduced with healthy aging (Healthy Aging and Wellness Working Group, 2006). Indeed, 70% of older people in Canada report good overall health, including good functional health and independence in activities of daily living (Shields & Martel, 2006). Nurses need to consider how much of the decline associated with aging is related to biological aging versus other determinants such as socioeconomic status, social support, and individual health practices.

Individual Health Practices and Coping Skills

Effective coping skills help people face challenges without resorting to risk behaviours such as substance misuse. Many so-called risk behaviours may, in fact, be coping strategies for stress and strain caused by living circumstances. For example, considerable evidence indicates that low-income women use smoking as a coping strategy (Stewart, Greaves, Kushner, et al., 2011). Three risk behaviours with major detrimental health consequences are physical inactivity, poor nutrition, and tobacco use.

Physical inactivity is a major risk factor for some types of cancer, diabetes, cardiovascular disease, osteoporosis, obesity, hypertension, depression, stress, and anxiety. In 2004, just over half (52%) of Canadians aged 12 and older were at least moderately active during their leisure time (equivalent to walking at least 30 to 60 minutes a day). Those who were active were more likely to rate their health as excellent or very good and to report lower levels of stress and were less likely to be overweight, obese, or hypertensive (Gilmour, 2007). However, actual physical measures of activity using accelerometer technique revealed that only 15% of Canadian adults meet the recommendation of 150 minutes of moderate-to-vigorous physical activity (MVPA) weekly (Colley, Garriguet, Janssen, et al., 2011a), and only 7% of children achieve the recommendation of 60 minutes of MVPA at least 6 days per week (Colley, Garriguet, Janssen, et al., 2011b).

Poor nutrition, particularly overconsumption of fats, sugars, and salt, is linked to such diseases as some cancers, cardiovascular diseases, type 2 diabetes, hypertension, osteoarthritis, and gallbladder disease and to functional limitations and disabilities (Tjepkema, 2006). Obesity is considered to be a major public health threat, and in 2010, the federal government launched a country-wide intersectoral initiative to curb child obesity (PHAC, 2010). The 2004 Canadian Community Health Survey (CCHS) revealed that 23% of adult Canadians were obese (body mass index [BMI] of 30 or more) and 36% were overweight (Shields, 2006); as BMI increased, so did the likelihood of reporting high blood pressure, diabetes, and heart disease. About 26% of children (aged 2–17 years) were overweight or obese (Shields, 2006). The 2004

CCHS (Nutrition section) indicated that 70% of children aged 4–8 years ate fewer than the minimum five servings of vegetables and fruit daily. Moreover, 25% of Canadians overall (and one-third of teenagers aged 14–18) had eaten at fast-food outlets the previous day (Garriguet, 2007), which feature foods high in fats and salt. Several factors influence food consumption patterns, including household income, food advertising, and availability of nutritious choices.

Tobacco use remains the leading preventable cause of death and disease in Canada (Makamowski Illing & Kaiserman, 2004). It is the only legal consumer product that can harm everyone exposed to it—and it kills up to half of those who use it as intended (WHO, 2008b). For every person who dies from smoking, another 20 continue to suffer with at least one serious tobacco-related illness, such as coronary heart disease, lung diseases, and cancers (US Department of Health and Human Services, 2010). The smoking rate in Canada in 2009 was 18% (Health Canada, 2013), but this burden is over-represented in more vulnerable populations, including those living in poverty (Physicians for a Smoke-free Canada, 2005) and Indigenous people (Health Canada, 2016). Half of all people with mental illness smoke, of whom 40% smoke more than 25 to 30 cigarettes per day, compared with 15% in the general population (de Leon & Diaz, 2005).

Clearly, many factors influence individual health behaviours (e.g., income, education, culture, and social support). Developing and maintaining health-enhancing behaviours requires not only health education but also social policies related to income security, product marketing, and supportive environments that make healthy choices the "easy" choices. In short, education is a necessary but not sufficient strategy.

Healthy Child Development (Early Life)

All health determinants influence child development, but healthy child development is a separate determinant because of its importance to lifelong health. The early life, which constitutes the period through adolescence, is critical for biological and brain development that shapes learning, behaviour, and health over the life course (McCain, Mustard, & Shanker, 2007; Provencal & Binder, 2015). During this stage of development, the brain is greatly responsive to environmental cues and undergoes dramatic changes. Healthy child development can be disrupted by excessive or prolonged activation of stress response systems in the body and brain, often referred to as *toxic stress*. Toxic stress has the potential to negatively affect the architecture of the developing brain (Centre for the Developing Child, 2014) and can often be linked to the determinants of health. Maternal and/or childhood exposure to environmental stressors such as poverty, violence, conflict, neglect, and food insecurity have been associated with many lifelong health concerns, including cognitive deficits, mental health and behavioural disorders, substance misuse, hypertension, type 2 diabetes, and coronary heart disease (Konrad, Herpertz, & Herpertz-Dahlmann, 2016; McCain et al., 2007; Provencal & Binder, 2015). Schools also play a role in healthy child development as they can provide an environment in which students feel secure, respected, challenged, and cared for, helping to ensure that children succeed academically. Community support is also important (McCain et al., 2007).

Quality early childhood education and care are particularly important in early child development, so much so that they have been singled out by some researchers as a combined social determinant of health (Friendly, 2016). High-quality programs promote cognitive development and social competence and support parents in education and employment. Canada has acknowledged the importance of early childhood intervention through its Early Childhood Development Initiative (Health Council of Canada, 2006); however, Canada lacks a national child care program.

Health Services (Health Care Services)

Approximately 25% of a population's health status is attributed to the health care services (Senate Subcommittee on Population Health, 2009). Quality and accessible primary care, hospital care, long-term care, home care, and public health services are therefore important to health. Prenatal care, well-child and immunization clinics, education services about health practices, and services that maintain older persons' health and independence are good examples of preventive and primary health care services (discussed further in Chapters 2 and 4). Principles of the *Canada Health Act*—universality, portability, accessibility, comprehensiveness, and public administration—apply to hospital and physician services, which cover only 70% of total health care costs. Medicare does not cover drug costs or dental care, and home care coverage varies across provinces (Mikkonen & Raphael, 2010), contributing to inequitable access. Increasingly, the trends in health care service provision are from institutionalized care to community-based care, toward decision making that is based on the best available evidence, and toward more regional administration. Considerable monies have been invested in initiatives that incorporate principles of primary health care; however, the progress in this regard has been relatively slow (Health Council of Canada, 2011).

Gender

Gender is "the array of society-determined roles, personality traits, attitudes, behaviours, values, relative power, and influence that society ascribes to the two sexes on a differential basis" (PHAC, 2004). When considering gender, one must examine men's as well as women's experiences (Bates, Hankivsky, & Springer, 2009). Many health issues are a function of gender-based social roles, and gender can influence health status, behaviours, and care (Armstrong, 2016; Bates et al., 2009; Spitzer, 2005); gender also influences all other health determinants (Armstrong, 2016). In Canada, men are more likely than women to experience extreme forms of social exclusion and to die prematurely, largely as a result of heart disease, unintentional fatal injuries, cancer, and suicide. Women, however, are more likely to suffer from depression, stress (often resulting from efforts to manage both paid and family work), chronic conditions such as arthritis and allergies, and injuries and death from family violence (Federal, Provincial, and Territorial ACPH, 1999; Mikkonen & Raphael, 2010). Moreover, gender plays a role in men's and women's experiences of sex-specific health concerns (e.g., pregnancy, prostate cancer, presentation of cardiovascular signs and symptoms), exposure to potential risk conditions (e.g., caregiving demands as traditionally women's responsibility), and interactions with health care providers (e.g., gender stereotypes, medicalization of health experience) (Pederson & Raphael, 2006).

Culture (Immigrant Status, Race, Indigenous Ancestry)

Cultural and ethnic factors influence people's interactions with a health care system, their participation in prevention and health promotion programs, their access to health information, their health-related lifestyle choices, and their understanding of health and illness (Health Canada, 1996). Cultural factors also influence whether and how health determinants are met (see Chapter 9 for further information about how culture is contextual). Language differences can lead to isolation and decreased social support networks. Among immigrants and refugees, health is negatively affected by unmet expectations; challenges to successful social integration; and difficulties arising from underemployment or unemployment, low income, and food and housing insecurity (Anderson, Reimer, Khan, et al., 2010; Dean & Wilson, 2009; Mikkonen & Raphael, 2010; Stewart, Makwarimba, Beiser, et al., 2010). The health of immigrants and refugees is also affected by experiences in their country of origin, such as exposure to violence, armed conflict, economic challenges, and patterns of migration (Ottersen, Dasgupta, Blouin, et al., 2014). These examples represent the complex political influences on the determinants of health that contribute to health inequity as introduced by the Oslo Commission on Global Governance for Health in 2014.

Racial disparities in health have been identified in Canada and are often attributed to bias, discrimination, and stereotyping in health care delivery (Nestel, 2012). The most basic cause for racialized health inequities is racism (Levy, Ansara, & Stover, 2013). **Racism** is defined as "an ideology that either directly or indirectly asserts that one group is inherently superior to others" (Levy et al., 2013, p. 5). **Racialization** is the "process by which societies construct races as real, different and unequal in ways that matter to economic, political and social life" (Levy et al., 2013, p. 5). Racialized individuals in Canada, particularly those who are visible minorities, are more likely to be unemployed, employed in hazardous work environments, have limited social benefits, and experience job insecurity than are nonracialized Canadians (Hyman, 2009). Racialization and racism adversely affect health in that they are linked to limited access to health resources, fewer socioeconomic opportunities, and fostering of unhealthy coping behaviours. As well, experiencing racism can cause significant stress, triggering negative psychological states such as anxiety and depression, which in turn initiate harmful physiological and biological processes in the cardiovascular, immune, and endocrine systems (Chae, Nuru-Jeter, Lincoln, et al., 2011; Clark, Anderson, Clark, et al., 1999; Harrell, Burford, Cage, et al., 2011; Hyman, 2009; Levy et al., 2013; Paradies, 2006; Pascoe & Richman, 2009).

Indigenous peoples of Canada are more likely to experience health inequities due to racism and the historical and contemporary discrimination experienced as a result of colonization (Levy et al., 2013). The forced placement of over 150 000 Indigenous children into government-funded residential schools from the 1870s until the late 1990s (Box 1-1) was established to eliminate parental involvement in the intellectual, cultural, and spiritual development of Indigenous children (Truth and Reconciliation Commission of Canada [TRC], 2015a). The impact of these injustices has been felt for generations and continues to affect the overall health and well-being of Canada's Indigenous populations. Indigenous peoples are much more likely to suffer acute and chronic diseases and to experience higher infant mortality and shorter life expectancy than the general Canadian population (Mikkonen & Raphael, 2010). For example, Indigenous youth living on reserve who are between the ages of 10 and 29 years are five to six times more likely to die by suicide than are non-Indigenous youth; 40% of deaths among Inuit youth are a result of suicide, compared to 8% in the rest of the population (TRC, 2015b). The link between the social health determinants (i.e., culture, social support, employment, income, and early childhood development) and the experiences of many of Canada's Indigenous people highlights the importance of culture in health outcomes, as well as the detrimental effects of racism and racialization on health. (See Chapter 10 for further information on Indigenous Health.)

Social Environments (Social Safety Net, Social Exclusion, Disability)

Social environments are defined as "the array of values and norms of a society [that] influence in varying ways the health and well-being of populations. In addition, social stability, recognition of diversity, safety, good working relationships, and cohesive communities provide a supportive society that reduces or avoids many potential risks to good health" (PHAC, 2004). The social environment is clearly related to other factors and expands on the social support determinant by incorporating broader community characteristics, norms, and values. Healthy social environments include freedom from discrimination and prejudice. The determinant of social environment is also evident in the *Jakarta Declaration*'s prerequisites of human rights, social security, and social relations (WHO, 1997). These prerequisites relate to social exclusion—the process by which people are denied opportunities to participate in many aspects of cultural, economic, social, and political life (Galabuzi, 2016). People most likely to be excluded are poor citizens, Indigenous people, new Canadians, and members of racialized or nonwhite groups; however, marginalization is also experienced by people on the basis of income, age, gender, activity and/or ability limitation, ethnicity, and sexual orientation. Social exclusion limits people's access to the resources that support health and their participation in community life (Stewart, Reutter, Makwarimba, et al., 2008). As well, a sense of community belonging has been linked to better self-rated general health and mental health (Shields, 2008). For example, Canadian youth who identify as lesbian, gay, bisexual, transgender, or queer (LGBTQ) experience disparities in their health and social outcomes compared to outcomes in their heterosexual peers (Knight et al., 2014). Health and social issues that this group of

BOX 1-1 CASE STUDY

The Truth and Reconciliation Commission of Canada (TRC)

During the 1870s, the Canadian government began to separate Indigenous children from their families and communities and place them into residential schools. This action was implemented as part of the greater colonization effort occurring in Canada. The objective of residential schools was to assimilate Indigenous children into the dominant culture by removing and isolating them from their home, family, and heritage. Children were taken from their homes primarily against their will and the will of their family. It was often stated that the residential schools were established to "kill the Indian" in the child (Truth and Reconciliation Commission [TRC], 2015a, p. 137).

For over 150 years, residential schools operated in Canada. Over 150 000 Indigenous children attended these schools. Many never returned. Often underfunded and overcrowded, these schools were used as a tool of assimilation by the Canadian state and churches. Thousands of students suffered physical and sexual abuse. All suffered from loneliness and a longing to be home with their families. The damages inflicted by these schools continue to this day (TRC, 2015b).

On June 11, 2008, Canada's Prime Minister, Stephen Harper, issued a statement of apology to all former students of Indian residential schools on behalf of the Government of Canada. In this statement, Harper apologized for the legacy and impact of the Indian residential schools on generations of Canada's Indigenous people and supported the Indian Residential Schools Settlement Agreement, which began September, 2007. A key foundational piece of this agreement was the Indian Residential Schools Truth and Reconciliation Commission. In 2009, the TRC began a multi-year process to listen to survivors, communities, and others affected by the residential school system. As a result of the TRC findings, and in efforts to make amends for the legacy of residential schools, the TRC made 94 *Calls to Action* to change governmental policies and programs in the areas of child welfare, education, language and culture, health, and justice (TRC, 2015c).

individuals face may include depression, anxiety, suicide ideation and/or attempts, homelessness, fear of family rejection, fear of violence, eating disorders, and physical abuse (Ylioja & Craig, 2014). A strong public health drive to address the inequities in health and social outcomes experienced by LGBTQ youth has led to some school boards in Canada establishing gay-straight alliances in schools to provide community and peer support to LGBTQ youth (Knight, Shoveller, Carson, et al., 2014).

Another important aspect of the social environment is the absence of violence, both in the home (child abuse, intimate partner violence, older person abuse) and in the community (youth violence, bullying, assault by strangers, violence due to property crimes, violence in the workplace). In 2009, 6% of the 19 million Canadians who had a current or former spouse reported being physically or sexually victimized by their partner in the past 5 years. Nearly 55 000 Canadian children and youth were the victims of sexual or physical assault, with 3 out of 10 assaults being perpetrated by a family member. More recently, police reported 2 400 Canadian seniors age 65 years and older as being victims of a violent crime by a family member (Statistics Canada, 2015). The health effects of family violence are devastating—for those experiencing or exposed to violence and for the perpetrators—and include negative psychological, physical, behavioural, academic, sexual, interpersonal, self-perceptual, or spiritual consequences, which may appear immediately or over time (Department of Justice Canada, 2009).

STRATEGIES TO INFLUENCE HEALTH DETERMINANTS

Health Promotion and Disease Prevention

The understanding that health is qualitatively different from disease has led to a differentiation of the concepts of health promotion and disease prevention, although they are interrelated. Pender and colleagues (2015) differentiated between health promotion and disease prevention as follows: **health promotion** is "directed toward increasing the level of well-being and self-actualization" (p. 27); **disease prevention** (specifically primary prevention) is "action to avoid or forestall illness/disease" (p. 26). On the other hand, Leavell and Clark's (1965) initial conceptualization of levels of prevention considered health promotion as one aspect of primary prevention and not necessarily disease specific. In contrast, the *Ottawa Charter* views health promotion as the overarching concept, defined as "the process of enabling people to increase control over, and improve, their health" (WHO, 1986). The following, more comprehensive, definition was offered by Nutbeam (1998):

> *Health promotion represents a comprehensive social and political process, it not only embraces actions directed at strengthening the skills and capabilities of individuals, but also action directed towards changing social, environmental and economic conditions so as to alleviate their impact on public and individual health. Health promotion is the process of enabling people to increase control over the determinants of health and thereby improve their health. Participation is essential to sustain health promotion action. (p. 351)*

Three levels of disease prevention correspond to the natural history of disease:

- *Primary prevention* activities protect against a disease before signs and symptoms occur (prepathogenesis stage of disease). Examples include immunization (to prevent infectious diseases) and reduction of risk factors (such as inactivity, smoking, and exposure to air pollution).
- *Secondary prevention* activities promote early detection of disease once pathogenesis has occurred, so that prompt treatment can be initiated to halt disease and limit disability. Examples include preventive screening for cancer (e.g., Pap test, testicular self-examination), blood pressure screening to detect hypertension, and blood glucose screening to detect diabetes.
- *Tertiary prevention* activities are initiated in the convalescence stage of disease and are directed toward minimizing residual disability and helping people to live productively with limitations. An example is a cardiac rehabilitation program after a myocardial infarction.

Nursing strategies guided by a prevention framework focus on assessment and alleviation of risk factors for disease. Health promotion, by contrast, may be viewed more broadly than disease prevention inasmuch as it emphasizes participation, empowerment, and equity and goes beyond individual health education to a broader ecological approach that incorporates community development and policy advocacy. Health promotion strategies, therefore, are often political because they emphasize addressing structural and systemic inequities and have a strong philosophy of social justice. Health promotion is guided by the following principles (CPHA, 1996):

- Health promotion addresses health issues in context.
- Health promotion supports a holistic approach.
- Health promotion requires a long-term perspective.
- Health promotion is multisectoral.
- Health promotion draws on knowledge from social, economic, political, environmental, medical, and nursing sciences, as well as from first-hand experiences.

HEALTH PROMOTION STRATEGIES

The *Ottawa Charter* identified five broad strategies to enhance health. The following is a brief introduction to each of these **health promotion strategies**. For further examples of each of these strategies see Reutter and Kushner (2010a).

1. Build Healthy Public Policy. Advocating healthy public policies is a priority strategy for health promotion in Canada. Indeed, some academics have suggested that this strategy is the foundation of all others because policies shape how money, power, and material resources are distributed to society (CPHA, 1996). Advocating healthy public policy means focusing on policies that create healthy living conditions. Because the determinants of health are broad, healthy public policy necessarily extends beyond traditional health agencies and government health departments to other sectors such as agriculture, education, transportation, labour, social services, energy, and housing. Therefore, policymakers in all government sectors and organizations should ensure that their policies have positive health consequences. This emphasis is reflected in national and international documents, including the recent *Adelaide Statement on Health in All Policies* (WHO, 2010). Advocating healthy public policy is best addressed through intersectoral collaboration. As a nurse, you might work with others to develop policy options, encourage public dialogue, persuade decision makers to adopt the healthiest option, and follow up to make sure the policy is implemented (CPHA, 1996). Cathy Crowe, a Toronto "street nurse," is an excellent example of a nurse who advocates for healthy public policy to reduce homelessness (Box 1-2).

Increasingly, policy advocacy is incorporated into nursing role statements (e.g., CPHA, 2010; International Council of Nurses, 2001) and nursing education curricula (Rains & Barton-Kriese, 2001; Reutter & Duncan, 2002; Reutter & Kushner, 2010b; Reutter & Williamson,

BOX 1-2 CASE STUDY

Cathy Crowe: Advocating Healthy Public Policy

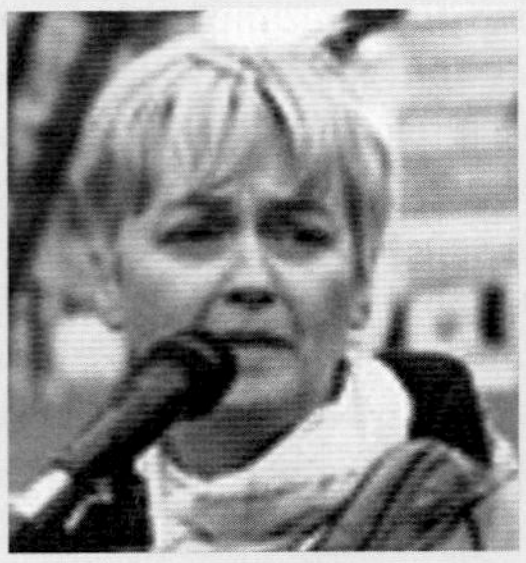

Cathy Crowe is a Toronto street nurse who has advocated for policies related to a variety of social determinants. Her work as an outreach street nurse in Toronto since the 1980s exemplifies nursing's role not only in attending to immediate health needs of people who are homeless but also advocating for policies that will provide more adequate and affordable housing to alleviate the root causes of these health problems. Crowe co-founded the Toronto Disaster Relief Committee (TDRC) in 1998, which declared homelessness a national disaster in Canada. The committee advocated a "1% solution," calling on the federal, provincial, and territorial governments to allocate an additional 1% of their budget to fully fund a national affordable housing program. The efforts of the TDRC increased awareness, both in large cities in Canada and at the United Nations, of Canada's housing problem. This awareness led to the appointment of a federal minister responsible for homelessness and federal emergency relief monies (e.g., for shelter beds, food banks, programs for homeless youth). Although monies were also made available to provide housing, the goal of a fully funded national housing strategy has not yet been realized, and homelessness continues to increase across Canada.

Crowe has fostered numerous coalitions and advocacy initiatives, working with homeless people and other organizations. The TDRC was involved in fighting the evictions of Toronto's Tent City in 2002 and succeeded in eventually securing housing for many residents. Crowe is currently on the board of directors of a nonprofit organization that is building affordable housing in Toronto. To raise awareness about children who are homeless, she co-produced the film *Home Safe,* set in several Canadian cities. As part of this initiative, a children's forum on homelessness was organized to provide children the opportunity to voice their concerns to the United Nations Special Rapporteur on Adequate Housing when he visited Canada. Crowe has also written a book, *Dying for a Home,* co-authored with activists who are homeless themselves.

Crowe has received numerous awards for her advocacy work. She sees advocacy as a critical nursing role and responsibility. You are encouraged to view her many speeches and activities on her website, at http://cathycrowe.ca. (Photo courtesy http://cathycrowe.ca/.)

2000). In your nursing care, it is important to think about what policies have contributed to the health situations of your patients, what policies would help alleviate health problems, and how you can champion public policies. For example, how do current welfare incomes, which are lower than poverty "lines" (low-income cut-offs), influence recipients' abilities to obtain adequate food and shelter and participate meaningfully in Canadian society? An informative resource on policy implications arising from social determinants of health is *Social Determinants of Health: The Canadian Facts* (see website at the end of the chapter). Reutter and Kushner (2010b) provide suggestions for the nursing role in policy advocacy, while Cohen and Reutter (2007) outline ways that nurses can engage in policy advocacy specifically related to child and family poverty.

2. Create Supportive Environments. The *Ottawa Charter* (WHO, 1986) states that "the overall guiding principle … is the need to encourage reciprocal maintenance, to take care of each other, our communities and our natural environment" (p. 2). This strategy helps ensure that physical environments are healthy and safe and that living and working conditions are stimulating and satisfying. Creating supportive environments also means protecting the natural environment and conserving natural resources (WHO, 1986).

An excellent example of an initiative that helps create supportive environments is the Comprehensive School Health Initiative, which focuses on improving school environments by providing health instruction, social support, support services, and positive physical environments (Mitchell & Laforet-Fliesser, 2003). Other examples of supportive environments include flexible workplace policies, quality child care programs that support early child development and parental employment, and baby- and senior-friendly community initiatives.

3. Strengthen Community Action. Strengthening communities is a requisite for successful health promotion and for community health nursing practices in Canada (CPHA, 2010). In this strategy, often referred to as *community development,* communities identify issues and work together to make changes that will enhance health. In a community development approach, health providers help community groups identify important issues and organize and implement plans and strategies to resolve these issues, often partnering with other community organizations (see Chapter 4). Public participation in all phases of community programming is key to community development. Examples of community development projects are community gardens and collective kitchens targeted to enhancing food security.

4. Develop Personal Skills. This strategy, which is probably most familiar to nurses, helps clients develop personal skills, enhance coping strategies, and gain control over their health and environments so that they can make healthy lifestyle choices. Personal skills development includes health education, but it also emphasizes adequate support and resources. Some examples of interventions to enhance personal skills include early intervention programs for children, home visiting by public health nurses, parenting classes, and falls reduction programs for seniors. On a broader level, examples include province-wide health communication initiatives aimed at improving nutrition and physical activity (e.g., *Healthy U* [Alberta], *Act Now* [B.C.]).

5. Reorient Health Services. Health system reform has two objectives: to shift emphasis from treating disease to improving health, and to make the health care system more efficient and effective (CPHA, 1996). A proactive approach to health requires improved access to primary health care services, increased community development, improved community-based care services, increased family-based care, and public participation. In Canada, there is considerable emphasis on developing the primary health care model, which nursing associations have advocated for many years (Reutter & Ogilvie, 2011; see also Chapters 2 and 4). Several Canadian documents have reiterated the urgency for the health sector to reorient its focus beyond provision of health care to reducing health inequities through action on the social determinants of health (e.g., Health Council of Canada, 2010; Health Disparities Task Group, 2005).

POPULATION HEALTH PROMOTION MODEL: PUTTING IT ALL TOGETHER

This chapter has presented two major approaches to health: health promotion and population health. Hamilton and Bhatti (1996)

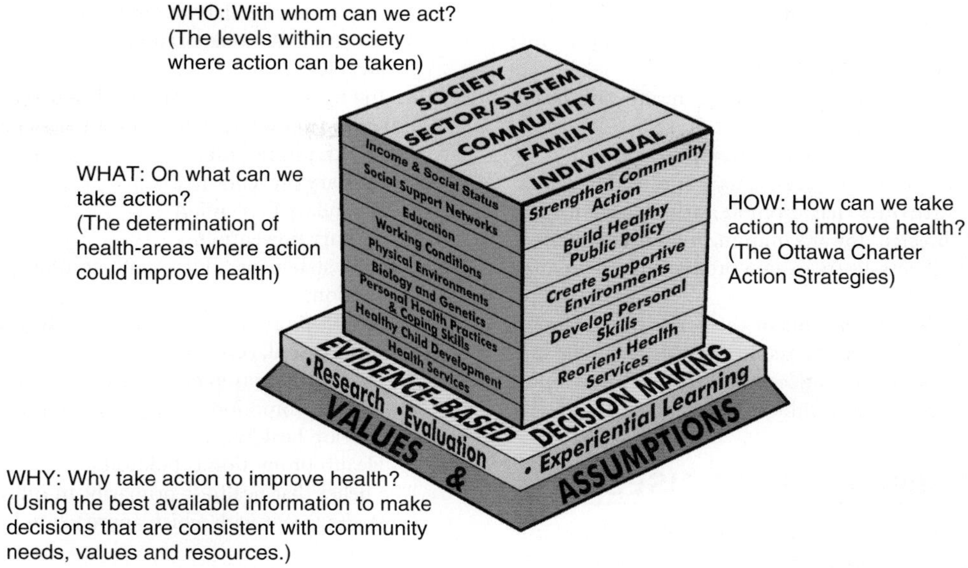

FIGURE 1-5 Population health promotion model. (From Hamilton, N., & Bhatti, T. [1996]. *Population health promotion: An integrated model of population health and health promotion.* Ottawa: Health Promotion Development Division, Health Canada. Copyright 1996 by Minister of Public Works and Government Services Canada.)

integrated these two concepts into one model that shows their relationship to each other (Figure 1-5). Aimed at developing actions to improve health, the model explores four major questions: "On *what* can we take action?"; "*How* can we take action?"; "With *whom* can we act?"; and "*Why* take action?" (Saskatchewan Health, Population Health Branch, 2002).

The document *Strategies for Population Health* (Federal, Provincial, and Territorial ACPH, 1994) indicates health determinant actions that could be taken (the "what"). The *Ottawa Charter* provides a comprehensive set of five strategies to enhance health (the "how"). Together, these documents suggest that, to enhance population health, action must be taken on a variety of levels (the "who"). Clearly, nurses must direct these strategies toward individuals and families, communities, individual sectors of society (such as health or environmental sectors), and society as a whole. For example, as a nurse, to promote the health of lower-income patients you can help them access resources and supports that will enhance their personal skills. Community programs such as school lunch programs, recreational activities, collective kitchens, and support groups can be provided. You can lobby government sectors responsible for housing and employment to implement healthy public policies pertaining to affordable housing, job creation, child care, income security, and financially accessible health services. On a societal level, nurses can raise awareness about the negative effects of poverty on health and well-being and can advocate for policies that will decrease poverty. The population health promotion model shows how **evidence-informed decision making** is a foundation to ensure that policies and programs focus on the right issues, take effective action, and produce successful results (Hamilton & Bhatti, 1996), the "why" of action (Saskatchewan Health, Population Health Branch, 2002). Evidence is informed by research, experiential learning, and evaluation of programs, policies, and projects. Values and assumptions that are the foundation of the model include the following:

- Stakeholders representing the various determinants must collaborate to address health determinants.
- Society is responsible for its members' health status.
- Health status is a result of people's health practices and their social and physical environments.
- Opportunities for healthy living are based on social justice, equity, and relationships of mutual trust and caring, rather than on power and status.
- Health care, health protection, and disease prevention complement health promotion.
- Active participation in policies and programs is essential.

SUMMARY

This chapter has introduced you to different ways of viewing health and health determinants, including the historical development of these concepts within the Canadian context. The content of the chapter challenges you to approach health situations broadly by identifying the myriad determinants that influence health. An increased understanding of health determinants should enable you to provide more sensitive care at the individual level and to consider strategies at the community and policy levels that will address the root causes of health situations.

KEY CONCEPTS

- Health conceptualizations and determinants influence the nature and scope of professional practice.
- Definitions of health can be classified in several ways; recent definitions reflect a multidimensional perspective and a positive orientation.
- Three recent approaches to health are medical, behavioural, and socioenvironmental.
- Behavioural approaches focus primarily on health practices.
- Socioenvironmental approaches emphasize psychosocial factors and socioenvironmental conditions.
- Health determinants are interrelated.

- Health literacy involves functional, interactive, and critical abilities needed to exert control over life events and circumstances that influence health experience and health status.
- Canada is a leader in ever-changing views of health and health determinants.
- Health promotion differs from disease prevention.
- Three levels of disease prevention are primary (protection against disease), secondary (activities that promote early detection), and tertiary (activities directed toward minimizing disability from disease and helping clients learn to live productively with their limitations).
- The *Ottawa Charter* identifies five major categories of health promotion strategies: building healthy public policies; creating supportive environments; strengthening community action; developing personal skills; and reorienting health care services.

CRITICAL THINKING EXERCISES

1. Describe your current level of health. What criteria did you use? Which definition of health discussed in this chapter best matches your understanding of health? Consider another definition of health discussed in this chapter. Does your current level of health change on the basis of this definition? How might your nursing practice differ depending on which conceptualization of health you choose to guide your practice? How might your definition of health change as you experience different life transitions (e.g., aging, parenthood)?
2. What do you consider to be the three most important health problems facing Canadians today? What are the major determinants of these problems? Which health promotion strategies would you consider the most appropriate to address them?
3. Imagine you are a community health nurse working in an area where many low-income women smoke. In a socioenvironmental approach to health, what questions would you need to address to decrease smoking behaviour in your area? How would your approach differ if you were using a behavioural approach to health?

REVIEW QUESTIONS

1. The *Lalonde Report* is significant in that it was the first to emphasize what?
   1. A behavioural approach to health
   2. A medical approach to health
   3. A socioenvironmental approach to health
   4. Physiological risk factors
2. What is the "watershed" document that marked the shift from a lifestyle to a socioenvironmental approach to health?
   1. *Lalonde Report*
   2. *Adelaide Statement on Health in All Policies*
   3. *Toronto Charter*
   4. *Ottawa Charter*
3. From a socioenvironmental perspective, what are the major determinants of health?
   1. Psychosocial risk factors and socioenvironmental risk conditions
   2. Physiological risk factors and behavioural risk factors
   3. Behavioural and psychosocial risk factors
   4. Behavioural and socioenvironmental risk factors
4. What is the main reason that intersectoral collaboration is a necessary strategy to reach the goal of "Health for All"?
   1. The determinants of health are broad.
   2. Intersectoral collaboration is cost-effective.
   3. Intersectoral collaboration encourages problem solving at a local level.
   4. Intersectoral collaboration is less likely to result in conflict.
5. Providing immunizations against measles is an example of what?
   1. Health promotion
   2. Primary prevention
   3. Secondary prevention
   4. Tertiary prevention
6. Which statement does *not* accurately characterize health promotion?
   1. Health promotion addresses health issues within the context of the social, economic, and political environment.
   2. Health promotion emphasizes empowerment.
   3. Health promotion strategies focus primarily on helping people develop healthy behaviours.
   4. Health promotion is political.
7. The belief that health is primarily an individual responsibility is most congruent with which approach to health?
   1. Medical
   2. Behavioural
   3. Socioenvironmental
   4. Critical/structural
8. Which statement does not accurately describe the Population Health Promotion Model?
   1. The model suggests that action can address the full range of health determinants.
   2. The model incorporates the health promotion strategies of the *Ottawa Charter.*
   3. The model focuses primarily on interventions at the societal level.
   4. The model attempts to integrate population health and health promotion concepts.
9. What is the most influential health determinant?
   1. Personal health practices
   2. Income and social status
   3. Health care services
   4. Physical environment
10. At what are health promotion activities aimed?
    1. Providing protection against disease
    2. Increasing the level of well-being
    3. Avoiding injury or illness
    4. Teaching clients to learn to live with their limitations

Answers: 1. 1; **2.** 4; **3.** 1; **4.** 1; **5.** 2; **6.** 3; **7.** 2; **8.** 3; **9.** 2; **10.** 2

Rationales for the Review Questions appear at the end of the book.

RECOMMENDED WEBSITES

Canadian Institute for Health Information (CIHI): https://www.cihi.ca/en

The CIHI is a not-for-profit Canadian organization working to improve the health of Canadians and the health care system. One of its goals is to generate public awareness about factors affecting good health. This website offers current information and numerous links to government health reports.

Public Health Agency of Canada: http://www.phac-aspc.gc.ca

The website of the Public Health Agency of Canada provides excellent information on many aspects of public health, including the population health approach and the determinants of health.

World Health Organization publications: http://www.who.int/pub/en/
This website provides links to the publications of the World Health Organization, including the *World Health Report.*

WHO Commission on Social Determinants of Health: http://www.who.int/social_determinants/en/
This web page provides many excellent papers pertaining to several determinants of health and provides a global perspective.

Social Determinants of Health: The Canadian Facts: http://www.thecanadianfacts.org/The_Canadian_Facts.pdf
This document summarizes the social determinants of health in the Canadian context and includes policy implications, references, and resources.

Social Determinants of Health e-Learning Course: https://www.cna-aiic.ca/en/on-the-issues/better-health/social-determinants-of-health/social-determinants-of-health-e-learning-course
This web site from the Canadian Nurses Association (CNA) provides on-line modules about how to integrate a social determinants lens into nursing practice.

REFERENCES

Anderson, J. M., Reimer, J., Khan, K., et al. (2010). Narratives of "dissonance" and "repositioning" through the lens of critical humanism: Exploring the influences on immigrants' and refugees' health and well-being. *Advances in Nursing Science, 33*(2), 101–112.

Antonovsky, A. (1987). *Unraveling the mystery of health: How people manage stress and stay well.* San Francisco: Jossey-Bass.

Armstrong, P. (2016). Public policy, gender, and health. In D. Raphael (Ed.), *Social determinants of health* (3rd ed., pp. 544–560). Toronto: Canadian Scholars' Press.

Auger, N., & Alix, C. (2016). Income, income distribution, and health in Canada. In D. Raphael (Ed.), *Social determinants of health: Canadian perspectives* (3rd ed., pp. 90–109). Toronto: Canadian Scholars' Press.

Bates, L. M., Hankivsky, O., & Springer, K. (2009). Gender and health inequities: A comment on the Final Report of the WHO Commission on the Social Determinants of Health. *Social Science & Medicine, 69*(7), 1002–1004.

Bryant, T. (2002). The role of knowledge in public health and health promotion policy change. *Health Promotion International, 17*(1), 89–98. doi:10.1093/heapro/17.1.89.

Bryant, T. (2009). *An introduction to health policy.* Toronto: Canadian Scholars' Press.

Bryant, T. (2016). Housing and health: More than bricks and mortar. In D. Raphael (Ed.), *Social determinants of health* (3rd ed., pp. 360–383). Toronto: Canadian Scholars' Press.

Canadian Association of Schools of Nursing/Association Canadienne des Écoles de Sciences Infirmières [CASN/ACESI] (2015). *National nursing education framework: Final report.* Ottawa: Author.

Canadian Institute for Health Information (CIHI) (2004). *Improving the health of Canadians.* Ottawa: Author.

Canadian Institute of Child Health (2000). *Low birth weight. Fact sheet.* In *The health of Canada's children: A CICH profile* (3rd ed.). Retrieved from http://www.cich.ca/PDFFiles/ProfileFactSheets/English/LBWEng.pdf.

Canadian Nurses Association (CNA) (2008). *The role of nurses in addressing climate change.* Ottawa: Author. Retrieved from https://cna-aiic.ca/~/media/cna/page-content/pdf-en/climate_change_2008_e.pdf.

Canadian Nurses Association (CNA) (2009). *Position statement: Climate change and health.* Ottawa: Author. Retrieved from https://www.cna-aiic.ca/~/media/cna/page-content/pdf-en/ps100_climate_change_e.pdf.

Canadian Policy Research Networks (2008). *Workplace health.* Retrieved from http://www.jobquality.ca/indicators/environment/phy1.shtml.

Canadian Public Health Association (CPHA) (1996). *Action statement for health promotion in Canada.* Ottawa: Author.

Canadian Public Health Association (CPHA) (2010). *Public health-community health nursing practice in Canada: Roles and activities* (4th ed.). Ottawa: Author. Retrieved from http://resources.cpha.ca/CPHA/Conf/Data/2010/A10-376e.pdf.

Carpiano, R. M. (2007). Neighborhood social capital and adult health: An empirical test of a Bourdieu-based model. *Health and Place, 13*(3), 639–655. doi:10.1016/j.healthplace.2006.09.001.

Center for Quality Growth and Regional Development (2006). *Healthy housing: Forging the economic and empirical foundation.* Atlanta, GA: Georgia Institute of Technology.

Centre for the Developing Child (2014). *Excessive stress disrupts the architecture of the developing brain (Working Paper 3)* (pp. 1–9). Boston, MA: National Scientific Council on the Developing Child Harvard University. Retrieved from http://developingchild.harvard.edu/wp-content/uploads/2005/05/Stress_Disrupts_Architecture_Developing_Brain-1.pdf.

Chae, D. H., Nuru-Jeter, A. M., Lincoln, K. D., et al. (2011). Conceptualizing racial disparities in health: Advancement of a socio-psychobiological approach. *Du Bois Review, 8*(1), 63–77. doi:10.1017/S1742058X11000166.

Clark, R., Anderson, N. B., Clark, V. R., et al. (1999). Racism as a stressor for African Americans: A biopsychosocial model. *American Psychologist, 54*(10), 805–816.

Cohen, B., & Reutter, L. (2007). Development of the role of public health nurses in addressing child and family poverty: A framework for action. *Journal of Advanced Nursing, 60*(1), 96–107. doi:10.1111/j.1365-2648.2006.04154.x.

Colley, R., Garriguet, D., Janssen, I., et al. (2011a). Physical activity of Canadian adults: Accelerometer results from the 2007 to 2009 Canadian Health Measures Survey. *Health Reports, 22*(1), 7–14.

Colley, R., Garriguet, D., Janssen, I., et al. (2011b). Physical activity of Canadian children and youth: Accelerometer results from the 2007 to 2009 Canadian Health Measures Survey. *Health Reports, 22*(1), 15–23.

Curry-Stevens, A. (2016). Precarious changes: A generational exploration of Canadian incomes and wealth. In D. Raphael (Ed.), *Social determinants of health* (3rd ed., pp. 60–89). Toronto: Canadian Scholars' Press.

Dean, J. A., & Wilson, K. (2009). 'Education? It is irrelevant to my job now. It makes me very depressed…': Exploring the health impacts of under/unemployment among highly skilled recent immigrants in Canada. *Ethnicity & Health, 14*(2), 185–204. doi:10.1080/13557850802227049.

de Leon, J., & Diaz, F. J. (2005). A meta-analysis of worldwide studies demonstrates an association between schizophrenia and tobacco smoking behaviors. *Schizophrenia Research, 76*(2–3), 135–157. doi:10.1016/j.schres.2005.02.010.

Denburg, A., & Daneman, D. (2010). The link between social inequality and child health outcomes. *Health Care Quarterly, 14*(Special Issue), 21–31. doi:10.12927/hcq.2010.21980.

Department of Justice Canada (2009). *What are the consequences of family violence? Family violence: Department of Justice Canada Overview Paper.* Retrieved from http://www.justice.gc.ca/eng/pi/fv-vf/facts-info/fv-vf/fv2-vf2.html#consequences.

Engel, G. L. (1977). The need for a new medical model: A challenge for biomedicine. *Science, 196*(4286), 129–136.

Epp, J. (1986). *Achieving health for all: A framework for health promotion.* Ottawa: Health and Welfare Canada.

Federal, Provincial, and Territorial Advisory Committee on Population Health (1994). *Strategies for population health: Investing in the health of Canadians.* Ottawa: Minister of Supply and Services Canada.

Federal, Provincial, and Territorial Advisory Committee on Population Health (1999). *Toward a healthy future: Second report on the health of Canadians.* Ottawa: Minister of Public Works and Government Services Canada.

Food Banks Canada (2010). *HungerCount 2010.* Retrieved from https://www.foodbankscanada.ca/getmedia/12a3e485-4a4e-47d9-9b90-ff8eff0ef89d/hunger-count-2010.pdf.aspx?ext=.pdf.

Frankish, C. J., Hwang, S., & Quantz, D. (2005). Homelessness and health in Canada. *Canadian Journal of Public Health, 96*(Suppl. 2), S23–S29.

Friendly, M. (2016). Early childhood education and care as a social determinant of health. In D. Raphael (Ed.), *Social determinants of health: Canadian perspectives* (3rd ed., pp. 192–217). Toronto: Canadian Scholars' Press.

Gadalla, T. (2009). Determinants, correlates and mediators of psychological distress: A longitudinal study. *Social Science & Medicine, 68*(12), 2199–2205. doi:10.1016/j.socscimed.2009.03.040.

Gaetz, S., Dej, E., Richter, T., et al. (2016). *The state of homelessness in Canada, 2016.* Toronto: Canadian Observatory on Homelessness.

Galabuzi, G. (2016). Social exclusion. In D. Raphael (Ed.), *Social determinants of health: Canadian perspectives* (3rd ed., pp. 388–418). Toronto: Canadian Scholars' Press.

Garriguet, D. (2007). Canadians' eating habits. *Health Reports, 18*(2), 17–32.

Gilmour, H. (2007). Physically active Canadians. *Health Reports, 18*(3), 45–65.

Gottlieb, L., & Gottlieb, B. (2007). The developmental/health framework within the McGill Model of Nursing. *Advances in Nursing Science, 30*(1), E43–E57.

Hamilton, N., & Bhatti, T. (1996). *Population health promotion: An integrated model of population health and health promotion.* Ottawa: Health Promotion Development Division, Health Canada.

Hancock, T., & Perkins, F. (1985). The mandala of health: A conceptual model and teaching tool. *Health Education, 24*(1), 8–10.

Hansen-Ketchum, P., Marck, P., & Reutter, L. (2009). Engaging with nature to promote health: New directions for nursing research. *Journal of Advanced Nursing, 65*(7), 1527–1538. doi:10.1111/j.1365-2648.2009.04989.x.

Harrell, C. J., Burford, T. I., Cage, B. N., et al. (2011). Multiple pathways linking racism to health outcomes. *Du Bois Review, 8*(1), 143–157. doi:10.1017/S1742058X11000178.

Health Canada (1996). *Towards a common understanding: Clarifying the concepts of population health.* Ottawa: Author.

Health Canada (1998). *Taking action on population health: A position paper for health promotion and programs branch staff.* Ottawa: Author.

Health Canada (2013). *Smoking prevalence. Canadian Tobacco Use Monitoring Survey.* Retrieved from http://hc-sc.gc.ca/hc-ps/tobac-tabac/research-recherche/stat/_ctums-esutc_prevalence/prevalence-eng.php.

Health Canada (2016). *First Nations, Inuit, and Aboriginal health: Tobacco.* Retrieved from http://www.hc-sc.gc.ca/fniah-spnia/substan/tobac-tabac/index-eng.php.

Health Council of Canada (2006). *Their future is now: Healthy choices for Canada's children and youth.* Toronto: Author.

Health Council of Canada (2010). *Stepping it up: Moving the focus from health care in Canada to a healthier Canada.* Retrieved from http://healthcouncilcanada.ca/en/index.php?page=shop.product_details&flypage=shop.flypage&product_id=134&category_id=16&manufacturer_id=0&option=com_virtuemart&Itemid=170.

Health Council of Canada (2011). *Taking the pulse. Health Council of Canada Review of the 10-year plan to strengthen health care.* Report to the Standing Senate Committee on Social Affairs, Science and Technology. Retrieved from http://www.healthcouncilcanada.ca/docs/speeches/2011/Senate_WrittenSubmission_EN.pdf.

Health Disparities Task Group of the Federal/Provincial/Territorial Advisory Committee on Population Health and Health Security (2005). *Reducing health disparities—Roles of the health sector: Discussion paper.* Retrieved from http://www.phac-aspc.gc.ca/ph-sp/disparities/pdf06/disparities_discussion_paper_e.pdf.

Healthy Aging and Wellness Working Group (2006). *Healthy aging in Canada: A new vision, a vital investment. From evidence to action. A background paper prepared for the Federal, Provincial and Territorial Committee of Officials (Seniors).* Retrieved from http://www.health.gov.bc.ca/library/publications/year/2006/Healthy_Aging_A_Vital_latest_copy_October_2006.pdf.

House, J. (1981). *Work, stress, and social support.* Menlo Park, CA: Addison-Wesley.

Hyman, I. (2009). *Racism as a determinant of immigrant health.* Retrieved from http://canada.metropolis.net/pdfs/racism_policy_brief_e.pdf.

International Council of Nurses (2001). *Guidelines on shaping effective health policy.* Geneva, Switzerland: Author.

Jackson, A., & Rao, G. (2016). The unhealthy Canadian workplace. In D. Raphael (Ed.), *Social determinants of health: Canadian perspectives* (3rd ed., pp. 150–170). Toronto: Canadian Scholars' Press.

Jensen, L., & Allen, M. (1993). Wellness: The dialectic of illness. *Image–the Journal of Nursing Scholarship, 25*(3), 220–224.

Jones, P., & Meleis, A. (1993). Health is empowerment. *Advances in Nursing Science, 15*(3), 1–14.

Khandor, E., & Mason, K. (2007). *The street health report 2007.* Retrieved from http://www.streethealth.ca/downloads/the-street-health-report-2007.pdf.

Knight, R. E., Shoveller, J. A., Carson, A. M., et al. (2014). Examining clinicians' experiences providing sexual health services for LGBTQ youth: Considering social and structural determinants of health in clinical practice. *Health Education Research, 29*(4), 662–670. doi:10.1093/her/cyt116.

Konrad, K., Herpertz, S. C., & Herpertz-Dahlmann, B. (2016). Early trauma: Long lasting, difficult to treat and transmitted to the next generation. *Journal of Neural Transmission, 123*(9), 1033–1035. doi:10.1007/s00702-016-1509-6.

Labonte, R. (1993). *Issues in health promotion series. 3. Health promotion and empowerment: Practice frameworks.* Toronto: Centre for Health Promotion, University of Toronto, & ParticipACTION.

Lalonde, M. (1974). *A new perspective on the health of Canadians.* Ottawa: Government of Canada.

Leavell, H., & Clark, A. (1965). *Preventive medicine for doctors in the community* (3rd ed.). New York: McGraw-Hill.

Ledrou, I., & Gervais, J. (2005). Food insecurity. *Health Reports, 16*(3), 47–51.

Levy, J., Ansara, D., & Stover, A. (2013). *Racialization and health inequities in Toronto.* Toronto: Toronto Public Health. Retrieved from http://www.toronto.ca/legdocs/mmis/2013/hl/bgrd/backgroundfile-62904.pdf.

Mackey, S. (2009). Towards an ontological theory of wellness: A discussion of conceptual foundations and implications for nursing. *Nursing Philosophy, 10*(2), 103–112. doi:10.1111/j.1466-769X.2008.00390.x.

Makamowski Illing, E., & Kaiserman, M. (2004). Mortality attributable to tobacco use in Canada and its regions, 1998. *Canadian Journal of Public Health, 95*(1), 38–44.

McCain, M. N., Mustard, J. F., & Shanker, S. (2007). *Early years study 2: Putting science into action.* Toronto: Council for Early Child Development.

McGibbon, E. (2016). Oppressions and access to health care: Deepening the conversation. In D. Raphael (Ed.), *Social determinants of health: Canadian perspectives* (3rd ed., pp. 491–520). Toronto: Canadian Scholars' Press.

Menendez, M., Benach, J., Muntaner, C., et al. (2007). Is precarious employment more damaging to women's health than men's? *Social Science & Medicine, 64*(4), 776–781. doi:10.1016/j.socscimed.2006.10.035.

Mikkonen, J., & Raphael, D. (2010). *Social determinants of health: The Canadian facts.* Retrieved from http://www.thecanadianfacts.org/The_Canadian_Facts.pdf.

Mitchell, I., & Laforet-Fliesser, Y. (2003). Promoting healthy school communities. *Canadian Nurse, 99*(8), 21–24.

Naidoo, J., & Wills, J. (1994). *Health promotion: Foundations for practice.* London, UK: Bailliere-Tindall.

National Council of Welfare (2008). *Poverty rates.* Retrieved from http://www.ncw.gc.ca/d.1tas.2t1@-eng.jsp?chrtid=3.

Nestel, S. (2012). *Colour coded health care: The impact of race and racism on Canadians' health.* Toronto: Wellesley Institute. Retrieved from http://www.wellesleyinstitute.com/wp-content/uploads/2012/02/Colour-Coded-Health-Care-Sheryl-Nestel.pdf.

Nutbeam, D. (1998). Health promotion glossary. *Health Promotion International, 13*(4), 349–364.

Nutbeam, D. (2008). The evolving concept of health literacy. *Social Science & Medicine, 67*(12), 2072–2078. doi:10.1016/j.socscimed.2008.09.050.

Ottersen, O. P., Dasgupta, J., Blouin, C., et al. (2014). The political origins of health inequity: Prospects for change. *Lancet, 383*(9917), 630–667. doi:10.1016/S0140-6736(13)62407-1. Retrieved from http://www.thelancet.com/pdfs/journals/lancet/PIIS0140-6736(13)62407-1.pdf.

Paradies, Y. (2006). A systematic review of empirical research on self-reported racism and health. *International Journal of Epidemiology, 35*(4), 888–901. doi:10.1093/ije/dyl056.

Pascoe, E. A., & Richman, L. S. (2009). Perceived discrimination and health: A meta-analytic review. *Psychological Bulletin, 135*(4), 531–554. doi:10.1037/a0016059.

Pederson, A., & Raphael, D. (2006). Gender, race, and health inequalities. In D. Raphael, T. Bryant, & M. Rioux (Eds.), *Staying alive: Critical perspectives on health, illness, and health care* (pp. 159–191). Toronto: Canadian Scholars' Press.

Pender, N., Murdaugh, C., & Parsons, M. (2015). *Health promotion in nursing practice* (7th ed.). Upper Saddle River, NJ: Pearson Prentice Hall.

Phipps, S. (2003). *The impact of poverty on health: A scan of research literature.* Ottawa: Canadian Institute for Health Information and Canadian Population Health Initiative. Retrieved from https://secure.cihi.ca/free_products/CPHIImpactonPoverty_e.pdf.

Physicians for a Smoke-Free Canada (2005). *Smoking in Canada: A statistical snapshot of Canadian smokers.* Retrieved from http://www.smoke-free.ca/pdf_1/SmokinginCanada-2005.pdf.

Preyde, M. (2007). Mothers of very preterm infants: Perspectives on their situation and a culturally sensitive intervention. *Social Work in Health Care, 44*(4), 65–83. doi:10.1300/J010v44n04_05.

Provencal, N., & Binder, E. B. (2015). The effects of early life stress on the epigenome: From the womb to adulthood and even before. *Experimental Neurology, 268*, 10–20. doi:10.1016/j.expneurol.2014.09.001.

Public Health Agency of Canada (2004). *What makes Canadians healthy or unhealthy?* Retrieved from http://www.phac-aspc.gc.ca/ph-sp/determinants/determinants-eng.php#income.

Public Health Agency of Canada (2008). *Report on the state of public health in Canada 2008: Addressing health inequalities.* Retrieved from http://www.phac-aspc.gc.ca/cphorsphc-respcacsp/2008/fr-rc/pdf/CPHO-Report-e.pdf.

Public Health Agency of Canada (2010). *Curbing childhood obesity.* Retrieved from http://www.phac-aspc.gc.ca/hp-ps/hl-mvs/framework-cadre/pdf/ccofw-eng.pdf.

Public Health Agency of Canada (2013). *What is the population health approach?* Retrieved from http://www.phac-aspc.gc.ca/ph-sp/approach-approche/appr-eng.php.

Rains, J., & Barton-Kriese, P. (2001). Developing political competence: A comparative study across disciplines. *Public Health Nursing, 18*(4), 219–224.

Raphael, D. (2006). *Poverty and policy in Canada.* Toronto: Canadian Scholars' Press.

Raphael, D. (2016). Social determinants of health: Key issues and themes. In D. Raphael (Ed.), *Social determinants of health: Canadian perspectives* (3rd ed., pp. 3–31). Toronto: Canadian Scholars' Press.

Raphael, D., Anstice, S., & Raine, K. (2003). The social determinants of the incidence and management of type II diabetes mellitus: Are we prepared to rethink our questions and redirect our research activities? *Leadership in Health Services, 16*(3), 10–20.

Raphael, D., & Farrell, E. (2002). Beyond medicine and lifestyle: Addressing the societal determinants of cardiovascular disease in North America. *Leadership in Health Services, 15*(4), 1–5.

Registered Nurses Association of British Columbia (1994). *Creating the new health care: A nursing perspective.* Vancouver: Author.

Reutter, L., Dennis, D., & Wilson, D. (2001). Young parents' understanding and actions related to the determinants of health. *Canadian Journal of Public Health, 92*(5), 335–339.

Reutter, L., & Duncan, S. (2002). Preparing nurses to promote health-enhancing public policies. *Policy, Politics and Nursing Practice, 3*(4), 294–305.

Reutter, L., & Kushner, K. (2010a). Health equity through action on the social determinants of health: Taking up the challenge in nursing. *Nursing Inquiry, 17*(3), 269–280. doi:10.1111/j.1440-1800.2010.00500.x.

Reutter, L., & Kushner, K. (2010b). The broad scope of health promotion in health assessment. In T. Stephen, D. L. Skillen, R. Day, et al. (Eds.), *Canadian Bates' guide to health assessment for nurses* (pp. 3–25). Philadelphia: Lippincott Williams & Wilkins.

Reutter, L., & Ogilvie, L. (2011). Primary health care: Challenges and opportunities for the nursing profession. In J. Ross-Kerr & M. Wood (Eds.), *Canadian nursing: Issues and perspectives* (5th ed., pp. 185–208). Toronto: Elsevier Canada.

Reutter, L., & Williamson, D. (2000). Advocating healthy public policy: Implications for baccalaureate nursing education. *Journal of Nursing Education, 39*(1), 21–26.

Richmond, C. (2007). Narratives of social support and health in Aboriginal communities. *Canadian Journal of Public Health, 98*(4), 347–351.

Richmond, C., & Ross, N. (2009). The determinants of First Nation and Inuit health: A critical population health approach. *Health and Place, 15*(2), 403–411. doi:10.1016/j.healthplace.2008.07.004.

Richmond, C., Ross, N., & Egeland, G. M. (2007). Social support and thriving health: A new approach to understanding the health of Indigenous Canadians. *American Journal of Public Health, 97*(10), 1827–1833. doi:10.2105/AJPH.2006.096917.

Ronson McNicol, B., & Rootman, I. (2016). Literacy and health literacy: New understandings about their impact on health. In D. Raphael (Ed.), *Social determinants of health: Canadian perspectives* (3rd ed., pp. 261–290). Toronto: Canadian Scholars' Press.

Rootman, I., & O'Neill, M. (2012). Key concepts in health promotion. In I. Rootman, S. Dupéré, A. Pederson, et al. (Eds.), *Health promotion in Canada: Critical perspectives* (3rd ed., pp. 18–32). Toronto: Canadian Scholars' Press.

Saskatchewan Health, Population Health Branch (2002). *A population health promotion framework for Saskatchewan Regional Health Authorities.* Saskatoon: Saskatchewan Health.

Senate Subcommittee on Population Health (2009). *A healthy, productive Canada: A determinant of health approach.* Retrieved from http://www.parl.gc.ca/Content/SEN/Committee/402/popu/rep/rephealth1jun09-e.pdf.

Shields, M. (2006). Overweight and obesity among children and youth. *Health Reports, 17*(3), 27–42.

Shields, M. (2008). Community belonging and self-perceived health. *Health Reports, 19*(2), 1–10.

Shields, M., & Martel, L. (2006). Healthy living among seniors. *Health Reports, 16*(Suppl.), 7–20.

Shimmin, C. (2015). *Backgrounder: The impact of poverty on health.* Retrieved from http://www.evidencenetwork.ca/archives/24642.

Smith, P., & Polanyi, M. (2016). Understanding and improving the health of work. In D. Raphael (Ed.), *Social determinants of health: Canadian perspectives* (3rd ed., pp. 171–191). Toronto: Canadian Scholars' Press.

Spitzer, D. (2005). Engendering health disparities. *Canadian Journal of Public Health, 96*(Suppl. 2), S78–S95.

Statistics Canada (2015). *Highlights: Family violence in Canada—A statistical profile.* Retrieved from http://www.statcan.gc.ca/pub/85-224-x/2010000/aftertoc-aprestdm2-eng.htm.

Stewart, M., Greaves, L., Kushner, K. E., et al. (2011). Where there is smoke there is stress: Low-income women identify support needs and preferences for smoking reduction. *Health Care for Women International, 32*(5), 359–383. doi:10.1080/07399332.2010.530724.

Stewart, M., Kushner, K. E., Greaves, L., et al. (2010). The impacts of a support intervention for low-income women who smoke. *Social Science & Medicine, 71*(11), 1901–1909. doi:10.1016/socscimed.2010.08.023.

Stewart, M., Makwarimba, E., Beiser, M., et al. (2010). Social support and health: Immigrants' and refugees' perspectives. *Diversity in Health, 7*(2), 91–103.

Stewart, M., Makwarimba, E., Letourneau, N., et al. (2015). Impacts of a support intervention for Zimbabwean and Sudanese refugee parents: "I am not alone". *Canadian Journal of Nursing Research, 47*(4), 113–140.

Stewart, M., Reutter, L., Makwarimba, E., et al. (2008). Left out: Perspectives on social exclusion and inclusion across income groups. *Health Sociology Review, 17*(1), 78–94. doi:10.5172/hesr.451.17.1.78.

Tarasuk, V. (2016). Health implications of food insecurity. In D. Raphael (Ed.), *Social determinants of health* (3rd ed., pp. 321–342). Toronto: Canadian Scholars' Press.

Thorne, S., Canam, C., Dahinten, S., et al. (1998). Nursing's metaparadigm concepts: Disimpacting the debates. *Journal of Advanced Nursing, 27*(6), 1257–1268.

Tjepkema, M. (2006). Adult obesity. *Health Reports, 17*(3), 9–25.

Tomaka, J., Thompson, S., & Palacios, R. (2006). The relation of social isolation, loneliness, and social support to disease outcomes among the elderly. *Journal of Aging and Health, 18*(3), 359–383. doi:10.1177/0898264305280993.

Tompa, E., Scott-Marshall, H., Dolinschi, R., et al. (2007). Precarious employment experiences and their health consequences: Towards a theoretical framework. *Work: A Journal of Prevention, Assessment, and Rehabilitation, 28*(3), 209–224.

Truth and Reconciliation Commission of Canada (2015a). *Canada's residential schools: The legacy.* Retrieved from http://www.myrobust.com/websites/trcinstitution/File/Reports/Volume_5_Legacy_English_Web.pdf.

Truth and Reconciliation Commission of Canada (2015b). *Honouring the truth, reconciling for the future.* Retrieved from http://www.trc.ca/websites/trcinstitution/File/2015/Honouring_the_Truth_Reconciling_for_the_Future_July_23_2015.pdf.

Truth and Reconciliation Commission of Canada (2015c). *Truth and reconciliation commission of Canada: Calls to action.* Retrieved from http://nctr.ca/assets/reports/Calls_to_Action_English2.pdf.

US Department of Health and Human Services (2006). *The health consequences of involuntary exposure to tobacco smoke: A report of the surgeon general—Executive summary.* A. Rockville, MD: Public Health Service, Office of the Surgeon General, Centers for Disease Control and Prevention.

US Department of Health and Human Services (2010). *How tobacco smoke causes disease: The biology and behavioral basis for smoking-attributable disease.* Atlanta, GA: US Department of Health and Human Services, Centers for Disease Control and Prevention, National Center for Chronic Disease Prevention and Promotion, Office on Smoking and Health.

Villeneuve, M., & MacDonald, J. (2006). *Toward 2020: Visions for nursing.* Ottawa: Canadian Nurses Association.

Wallerstein, N. (1992). Powerlessness, empowerment, and health: Implications for health promotion programs. *American Journal of Health Promotion, 6*(3), 197–205.

Wilkins, K. (2007). Work stress among health care providers. *Health Reports, 18*(4), 33–36.

Wilkins, K., & Mackenzie, S. (2007). Work injuries. *Health Reports, 18*(3), 1–17.

Wilkins, R., Berthelot, J., & Ng, E. (2002). Trends in mortality by neighbourhood income in urban Canada from 1971 to 1996. *Health Reports, 13*(Suppl.), 1–28.

Wilkinson, R. (1996). *Unhealthy societies: The afflictions of inequality.* London: Routledge.

Wilkinson, R., & Picket, K. (2009). *The spirit level: Why more equal societies almost always do better.* Toronto: Penguin Group.

Williamson, D. L., & Carr, J. (2009). Health as a resource for everyday living: Advancing the conceptualization. *Critical Public Health, 19*(1), 107–122. doi:10.1080/09581590802376234.

World Health Organization (1947). *World Health Organization Act 1947. Constitution of the World Health Organization. Section 3.* Retrieved from http://www.austlii.edu.au/au/legis/cth/consol_act/whoa1947273/sch1.html.

World Health Organization (1984). *A discussion document on the concept and principles of health promotion.* Copenhagen, Denmark: European Office of the World Health Organization.

World Health Organization (1986). *Ottawa charter for health promotion.* Ottawa: Canadian Public Health Association.

World Health Organization (1997). *The Jakarta declaration on health promotion into the 21st century.* Retrieved from http://www.who.int/healthpromotion/conferences/previous/jakarta/declaration/en/.

World Health Organization (2005). *The Bangkok charter for health promotion in a globalized world.* Retrieved from http://www.who.int/healthpromotion/conferences/6gchp/hpr_050829_%20BCHP.pdf.

World Health Organization (2008a). *Closing the gap in a generation: Health equity through action on the social determinants of health. Commission on Social Determinants of Health. Final Report. Executive Summary.* Retrieved from http://whqlibdoc.who.int/hq/2008/WHO_IER_CSDH_08.1_eng.pdf.

World Health Organization (2008b). *WHO Report on the Global Tobacco Epidemic, 2008: The MPOWER package.* Geneva, Switzerland: Author.

World Health Organization (2009). *WHO Report on the Global Tobacco Epidemic, 2009: Implementing Smoke-free Environments.* Geneva, Switzerland: Author.

World Health Organization (2010). *Adelaide statement on health in all policies. Adelaide, Australia: Government of South Australia.* Retrieved from http://www.who.int/social_determinants/hiap_statement_who_sa_final.pdf.

Ylioja, T., & Craig, S. L. (2014). Exclusionary health policy: Responding to the risk of poor health among sexual minority youth in Canada. *Social Work in Public Health, 29*(1), 81–86. doi:10.1080/19371918.2011.619936.

2

The Canadian Health Care Delivery System

Written by Pammla Lusenga Petrucka, RN, PhD

OBJECTIVES

Mastery of content in this chapter will enable you to:

- Define the key terms listed.
- Discuss the evolution of Canada's social safety net and Medicare.
- Identify and define the principles of the *Canada Health Act* and significant legislation related to the Canadian health care system.
- Discuss principal factors influencing ongoing health care reform and the current health care delivery system.
- Discuss patients' rights to health care.
- Discuss specific issues and opportunities within the health care delivery system related to Indigenous peoples' health.
- Discuss multiple roles and challenges for all categories of regulated nurses in different health care settings.
- Describe five levels of health care and associated types of services.
- Identify various settings and models of care delivery in the Canadian health care system.
- Identify challenges and initiatives related to enhancing the quality of the Canadian health care delivery system.

KEY TERMS

Accessibility, p. 20
Acute care, p. 26
Adult day support programs, p. 27
Assisted-living facilities, p. 27
Comprehensiveness, p. 20
Continuity of care, p. 23
eHealth, p. 29
Electronic health record (EHR), p. 29
Evidence-informed practice, p. 29
Health promotion, p. 28
Home care, p. 27
Hospice, p. 28
Inpatient, p. 26
Insured residents, p. 20
Levels of health care, p. 28
Medicare, p. 19
mHealth, p. 29
Nursing informatics, p. 29
Outpatients, p. 26
Palliative care, p. 28
Parish nursing, p. 28
Portability, p. 20
Primary care (PC), p. 24
Primary health care (PHC), p. 21
Public administration, p. 20
Quality care, p. 29
Recentralization, p. 22
Regional health authorities, p. 22
Rehabilitation, p. 22
Remote monitoring, p. 29
Respite care, p. 29
Secondary care, p. 25
Self-care, p. 29
Social safety net, p. 19
Supportive care, p. 29
Sustainability, p. 20
Tertiary care, p. 25
Truth and Reconciliation Commission (TRC), p. 21
Universality, p. 20
Voluntary agencies, p. 27

MEDIA RESOURCES

http://evolve.elsevier.com/Canada/Potter/fundamentals/

- Audio Chapter Summaries
- Examination Review Questions
- Concept Map Creator
- Case Study with Questions
- Audio Glossary
- Content Updates
- Video Clips

Nurses are an essential part of the Canadian health care delivery system, constituting the largest group of human health resources and recognized as invaluable to the health of Canadians. Nursing services are necessary for virtually every patient seeking care. Between 2006 and 2015, the number of regulated nurses (employed and unemployed) in Canada grew by 18.5% (351 048 to 415 864) (Canadian Institute for Health Information [CIHI], 2016a). In 2015, there were 283 575 registered nurses (RNs), including 4090 nurse practitioners (NPs), in Canada (72.46% of the regulated nursing workforce), 101 319 (25.9%) licensed practical nurses (LPNs), and 5465 (1.4%) registered psychiatric nurses (RPNs) (CIHI, 2016a) (Box 2-1).

Since the late 1990s, the size of the Canadian nursing workforce has remained relatively stable. Building the Future (Kephart, Maaten, O'Brien-Pallas, et al., 2004) was the first national study endorsed by stakeholder groups to outline a long-term strategy to ensure adequate Canadian nursing human resources. The Canadian National Expert Commission (Canadian Health Services Research Foundation [CHSRF], 2012a, 2012b) sought input into the future of nursing in achieving "Better Health. Better Care. Better Value. Best Nursing," considering strategies and policies to enable more effective use of existing health care providers throughout the health system. In recent years, the nursing workforce has been challenged by aging of workers, high

BOX 2-1 Facts About Nursing in Canada, 2016

- For RNs, 63.3% practised in the hospital sector; 8.1% in long-term care; 15.7% in community and home care; and 13% in other settings.
- For LPNs, 47.2% practised in hospitals; 12.8% in the community; 31.9% in long-term care; and 8.1% in other settings.
- For RPNs, 44.7% worked in the hospital; 30.7% in the community; and 13.5% in nursing homes and long-term care.
- For RNs, in 2015, 48% were degree prepared.
- Foreign-graduate representation in the regulated nursing work force included 8.9% of RNs, 5.1% of LPNs, and 7.2% of RPNs.
- 17 947 RNs obtained CNA certification in 1 of 20 specialty areas.
- In 2015, the ratio of regulated nurses employed in Canada was one RN for every 119 persons and one LPN for every 347 persons.
- The ratio of NPs employed in Canada was one NP for every 1 020 433 persons (9.8 per 100 000).
- By gender, for RNs and NPs, 92.4% were female and 7.6% were male; for LPNs, 91% were female and 9% were male.
- Average age of RNs was 44.6 years; for LPNs it was 41, and for RPNs it was 46.
- For RNs, 25.5% were aged 55 years or older, 13.5% were aged 60 years or older, and 1.2% were aged 65 years or older. For LPNs, 17.1% were aged 55 or older, and 7.9% were aged 60 or older.
- 9 out of 10 Canadian graduates either remain in or return to the jurisdiction of graduation to practise, a continuous pattern since 2006.

Canadian Institute for Health Information. (2016). *Regulated nurses: Canada and jurisdictional highlights.* Ottawa, ON: Author; Maier, C. B., Barnes, H., Aiken, L. H., & Busse, R. (2016). Descriptive, cross-country analysis of the nurse practitioner workforce in six countries: Size, growth, physician substitution. *BMJ Open, 6*(9), e011901. doi:10.1136/bmjopen-2016-011901corr1.

BOX 2-2 Moments in Canadian Nursing History*

Throughout Canada's history, nurses have met the health care needs of individuals, families, and communities. As nurses encountered changing practice environments, such as world wars or the Great Depression, they transformed their practices and skills to each new situation. During English–French hostilities from 1756 to 1760, the Grey Nuns cared for sick and wounded soldiers, including British prisoners of war. This order was known for its excellent hospitals, offering care regardless of race, colour, creed, or financial status. By the middle of the twentieth century, nursing transformed from a predominately spiritual vocation to a secular profession (Mansell, 2004). Most nurses worked in hospitals and communities, although some were present in nursing and health care organizations such as the Red Cross, the Victorian Order of Nurses (VON), military or navy service, tuberculosis sanatoria, professional nursing associations, and nursing unions. Although "the practice of nursing is perceived as an integral part of health care services in Canada" (Mansell, 2004, p. 204), the struggle for professionalism and recognition has not been an easy one.

*Section contributor: S. L. Bassendowski, RN, EdD.

retirement rates, ethical international recruitment, and lack of full-time positions.

Nursing is integral to the health care delivery system, so understanding this system and how care is provided is imperative. As a practising nurse, you need to appreciate the complexities of a health care delivery system replete with human and fiscal resource challenges and imperatives for quality patient- and family-centred services. Financial pressures have challenged hospitals and other institutions to shift priorities and to control costs by changing the faces of the workforce, often using alternative staff and support services mixes. Nurses must participate in restructuring delivery systems and achieving excellence in health care through leadership, advocacy, and reinforcement of the values of safe, quality, ethical, patient- and family-centred, and evidence-informed patient care.

EVOLUTION OF THE CANADIAN HEALTH CARE SYSTEM

Despite significant changes since the 1960s, a network of national, provincial, and territorial social programs, referred to as the **social safety net**, remains in place to protect the most vulnerable members of Canadian society. Most programs target specific populations (e.g., older persons, children), while a few are universally accessible. For example, provincial social assistance programs provide income support to individuals who are unemployed or underemployed for long periods of time; the federal employment insurance program provides income support for short-term employment interruption. A key component of Canada's social safety net is provision of hospital and medical insurance, known as **Medicare**, which is funded by general taxation. Although referred to as a "national" program, Medicare is, in fact, an interlocking set of 10 provincial and 3 territorial insurance schemes that provide reasonable "prepaid access to medically necessary hospital and physician services for all citizens and permanent residents" (Health Canada, 2016a).

Medicare is a source of national pride and solidarity as a commitment to the well-being of Canada's citizens. It is also a source of national debate regarding costs, effectiveness, and sustainability. Sustainability requires long-term maintenance and invokes creation of "standards of health human resources, infrastructure, clinical outcomes and fiscal capacity" for the health system (Kondro, 2010).

Early Health Care in Canada

Europeans arriving in Canada in the fifteenth century brought infectious diseases that flourished under conditions of poor sanitation. Settlements enacted public health laws to control the spread of diseases. For years, government care was limited to essential services (e.g., care of insane persons, epidemics). Permanent boards of health did not exist; hence, families, churches, and local communities were expected to manage medical and social problems. The stories and efforts of the first Canadian nurses were legendary (Box 2-2).

Canada became a self-governing colony with the passage of the *British North America Act* (also known as the *Constitution Act*) in 1867, which united three colonies into the original four provinces of Ontario, Quebec, Nova Scotia, and New Brunswick. This Act accorded certain powers to the national (federal) and provincial governments. Responsibility for public health (including regulation of hospitals, education, and social services) fell to the provinces, whereas the federal government retained jurisdiction over public policy components such

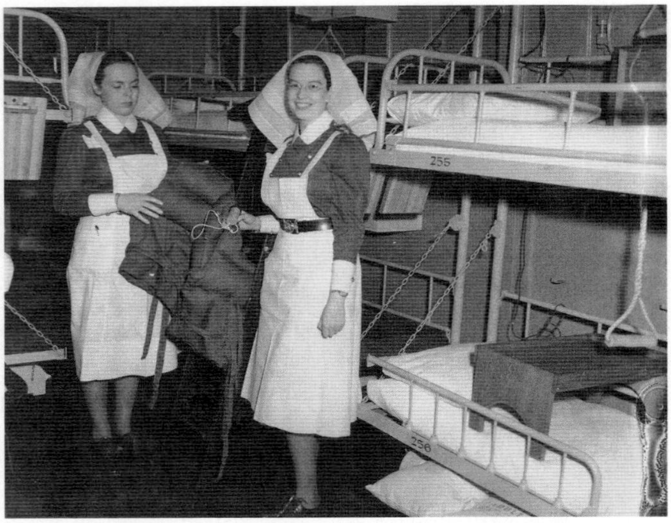

FIGURE 2-1 Military nurses. (Photo courtesy W. J. R. Bateman.)

as health care for Indigenous peoples and pharmaceutical safety (Storch, 2006).

As Canada's population grew and became urbanized and industrialized so, too, did substandard living conditions and sanitation, leading to more disease. Provinces enacted public health acts to establish local boards of health to hire medical health officers and sanitation inspectors, while nurses (ultimately the first public health nurses) continued working with the community and the poor.

By 1920, health and social programs had expanded, and voluntary agencies formed; the latter included the Children's Aid Society (in 1891), the Red Cross (in 1896), the Victorian Order of Nurses (in 1897), and the Canadian Mental Health Association (in 1918). Municipalities organized services for the poor and established hospitals. Patients who could not pay depended on charity (Figure 2-1). Fraternal societies (e.g., Knights of Columbus) and unions created trusts that members could access when ill, injured at work, or unemployed, becoming the precursors of modern employment insurance.

As urbanization continued, rural communities experienced difficulty attracting and paying physicians. The federal *Municipality Act* of 1916 gave communities the power to levy taxes to pay for physicians. But with the Great Depression, many people could not pay their medical bills and hospital stays caused financial ruin. With increasing needs, it became apparent that many provinces did not have the tax base to fund and ensure parallel services across the country.

These hardships inspired the Canadian provincial governments to create a prepaid medical and hospitalization insurance plan. In 1947, Premier Tommy Douglas of Saskatchewan introduced a public, universal hospital insurance plan, the basis of the first major federal initiative for national hospital insurance which led to the *Hospital Insurance and Diagnostic Services Act* (*HIDSA*) of 1957. For provinces establishing universal hospital insurance, *HIDSA* provided federal funds covering approximately half of service costs. By 1961, all provinces and territories were providing coverage for inpatient hospital care.

To ensure medical services outside of hospitals, Saskatchewan again took the lead. With federal government funding for half of the hospital insurance, Saskatchewan could afford to provide medical insurance and, in 1962, passed the *Medical Care Insurance Act*. The legislation was opposed by the province's physicians, who went on a 23-day strike, later reaching a compromise in which the physicians' autonomy to practise was preserved in exchange for agreeing to a single-payer insurance system to fund their services.

In 1964, the Royal Commission on Health Services (RCHS) was appointed to study provision of hospital and medical care to all Canadians and concluded that "strong federal government leadership and financial support for medical care" was needed (Wilson, 1995). The *Hall Commission Report* called for national expansion of the Saskatchewan model on a cost-shared basis similar to *HIDSA* (RCHS, 1965).

These recommendations led to the federal *Medical Care Act* of 1966. Federal grants were awarded on a cost-sharing basis with the provinces for programs meeting coverage criteria for hospital and physician services. Federal, provincial, and territorial governments agreed to share health care expenses equally. By 1972, all provincial and territorial insurance plans extended coverage to include medical services provided outside hospitals. Thus began modern Medicare, with all Canadians enjoying free access to hospital and medical care, regardless of ability to pay.

Although programs prospered, cost-sharing did not last. In 1977, the federal government enacted the *Federal Provincial Fiscal Arrangements and Established Programs Financing Act* to replace cost-sharing with block transfers of funds and a complicated formula of transferring tax points. These block transfers decreased federal contributions, which led some provinces to allow extra billing of patients by hospitals and providers above Medicare coverage.

The federal government's response was to enact the *Canada Health Act* in 1984, which amalgamated the *HIDSA* and *Medical Care Act*, effectively banning extra billing and user fees. The *Canada Health Act* added the principle of **accessibility** to the principles of **public administration**, **comprehensiveness**, **universality**, and **portability** (Table 2-1). Recently, a sixth principle—**sustainability**—has been debated. These principles apply to all **insured residents** (i.e., eligible residents) but exclude members of the Canadian Forces, Royal Canadian Mounted Police (RCMP), eligible veterans, inmates of federal penitentiaries, and some refugee claimants (Health Canada, 2016a). First Nations and Inuit health services receive special considerations, discussed later in this chapter. Under previous Acts, access to services was through physician gatekeepers, but the *Canada Health Act* allowed multiple points of access and insurance through additional care providers. Despite some opposition, by 1987 all provinces and territories were following *Canada Health Act* principles, "to protect, promote and restore the physical and mental well-being of residents of Canada and to facilitate reasonable access to health services without financial or other barriers" (Health Canada, 2011).

Along with the *Canada Health Act,* other federal legislation (Table 2-2) has influenced health and health services for Canadians in areas such as tobacco use, environmental health, and health research.

Indigenous Health Care

The *Indian Act* of 1985 (see http://laws-lois.justice.gc.ca/eng/acts/i-5/) identified the federal government's role in providing health care services to First Nations and Inuit (herein referred to as Indigenous) people. First Nations and Inuit Health Branch shares responsibility with communities, other federal government departments, and provincial/territorial partners in supporting optimal health outcomes for Canada's Indigenous people (Health Canada, 2016b). Since 1701, treaties with First Nations bands were signed—before confederation with the British government and after confederation with the Government of Canada—including a number of modern treaties (known as comprehensive land claims, such as the James Bay Claim) (Government of Canada [GOC], 2010). These treaties outlined agreements regarding land, services, and relationships; some (i.e., Treaty 6) included a health care services provision, often referred to as the "medicine chest" clause (GOC, 2010). Treaties enable direct delivery of services to Indigenous

TABLE 2-1 Principles of the *Canada Health Act* of 1984

Principle	Mandate	Actions/Exceptions
Public administration	Provincial and territorial plans operate on a nonprofit basis through a public authority	Regional authorities and some agencies (i.e., Cancer Agencies) are entrusted with delivery of programs and services.
Comprehensiveness	Cover medically necessary services; includes hospital and physician services. Determine medically necessary services (not defined in the Act), so differs in each province or territory	Access to surgical or medical hospital-based care with no out-of-pocket charges is ensured. Charges exist for extraordinary supplies or nonessential care elements (e.g., private duty nursing). Seeing a physician is without direct cost, but certain in-office procedures (e.g., wart removal, completion of medical forms) may involve patient payment. Coverage for programs such as long-term care and home care is not included.
Universality	Free of discrimination based on race, gender, income, ethnicity, or religion	Canadians are entitled to receive care that is respectful and embraces diversity. There remain challenges in achieving equity and equality under Medicare.
Portability	Enable insured residents access to health care services in another province or territory without cost or penalty. Provide continuous coverage for 3 months upon relocation in Canada to secure registration and coverage. Personal coverage required when moving or travelling outside of Canada.	Mobility across the country for purposes of travel, work, relocation, etc. is covered, but seeking care in another province/territory is only via prior approval through the jurisdiction where the individual holds a health card.
Accessibility	Provide insured residents reasonable access to health care facilities and providers, based on medical need regardless of ability to pay	Reasonable access is difficult to assess and measure. Varying levels of access to services exist for rural or remote people and urban people, often related to distance, health human resource availability, and facility capacities. Some individuals experience significant costs related to transportation (personal or ambulance), arguably a deterrent to access.

Adapted from Health Canada. (2016b). *Canada's health care system (Canada Health Act)*. Retrieved from https://www.canada.ca/en/health-canada/services/canada-health-caresystem.html; Romanow, R. (2002). *Building on values: The future of health care in Canada: Final report.* Ottawa: Commission on the Future of Health Care in Canada.

TABLE 2-2 Relevant Health-Related Legislation*

Legislation and Date Passed	Purpose
Canadian Environmental Protection Act, 1999 http://www.ec.gc.ca/lcpe-cepa	Regulates pollution prevention; promotes environmental protection and human health for sustainable development
Canadian Institutes of Health Research Act, 2000 http://www.cihr-irsc.gc.ca/e/9466.html	Strategizes and funds health-related research through 13 virtual institutes
Controlled Drugs and Substances Act, 1996 http://laws-lois.justice.gc.ca/eng/acts/C-38.8/	Controls certain drugs, precursors, and related substances
Emergency Management Act, 2007 http://laws-lois.justice.gc.ca/eng/acts/E-4.56	Develops and implements civil emergency plans; facilitates and coordinates across government levels and institutions, foreign governments, and international organizations
Food and Drugs Act, 1985 http://laws-lois.justice.gc.ca/eng/acts/F-27/	Regulates food, drugs, cosmetics, and therapeutic devices
Quarantine Act, 2005 http://laws.justice.gc.ca/eng/acts/Q-1.1/	Controls introduction and spread of infectious or contagious diseases
Tobacco Act, 1997 http://laws.justice.gc.ca/eng/acts/T-11.5/	Regulates manufacture, sale, labelling, and promotion of tobacco products

*Section contributor: T. McIntosh, PhD.

people, regardless of where they live in Canada, including **primary health care (PHC)** and emergency services on remote and isolated reserves where provincial or territorial services are not readily available; community-based health programs both on reserves and in Inuit communities; and noninsured health benefits programs (e.g., pharmaceuticals, dental, and medical transportation). All four levels of government (federal, provincial and territorial, and Indigenous) work collaboratively to improve and integrate responsive and appropriate health service delivery, with anticipated allocations for 2017–18 of $1.988 billion provided by an estimated 1 436 full-time-equivalent workforce (GOC, 2016).

The **Truth and Reconciliation Commission (TRC)** considered and brought attention to the events and impacts of Indian residential schools. Throughout its 5-year mandate, the TRC merged both truth (through over 6 500 stories, testimonials, document reviews, and other information seeking) and reconciliation as a means to rebuild and renew relationships between Canada's Indigenous and non-Indigenous peoples. The TRC (2015) released a six-volume final report with 94 calls to action, including seven directed at health, including increased sustainable funding for healing, embedding of cultural healing practices, cultural competency and safety training for all health care providers, and Indigenous professionals in health care (see Chapter 10 for further information regarding Indigenous health).

Indigenous self-governance is enabled through the "inherent right of self-government" under Section 35 of the *Canadian Constitution Act* of 1982. As self-governance models emerge, there will be challenges to health care providers to be "responsive to [Indigenous] political, economic, legal, historical, cultural and social circumstances" (Indian and Northern Affairs Canada, 2015).

ORGANIZATION AND GOVERNANCE OF HEALTH CARE

Under the *Canadian Constitution Act*, administration and delivery of health care services are primarily provincial or territorial responsibilities. The federal government has a role in health care financing, enforcement of the *Canada Health Act*, delivery of services to previously described targeted groups, and setting national agendas relating to public health and safety, pharmaceuticals, and biomedical/health services research.

Federal Jurisdiction

The federal government is charged to:

- Set and administer *Canada Health Act* principles.
- Assist in financing provincial and territorial health care services through transfer payments in alignment with *Canada Health Act* principles.
- Deliver or co-deliver health services for targeted groups.
- Provide national policy and programming to promote health and prevent disease, such as healthy environment, consumer safety, health product regulation, and public health programs.

Provincial and Territorial Jurisdiction

Each provincial and territorial government is charged to:

- Develop and administer its own health care insurance plan.
- Manage, finance, and plan insurable health care services and delivery, in compliance with *Canada Health Act* principles (see Table 2-1).
- Determine organization and location of health care facilities, mix of health provider workforce, and fiscal allocations for health care services.
- Reimburse physician and hospital expenses and provide co-payment with users for select rehabilitation and long-term care services.

Each provincial and territorial plan is unique in coverage, such as for drugs taken outside of hospitals, ambulance services, and home care. Health Canada (2011) provides general information on the eligibility and availability for programs and services on its website. To offset costs for services not covered by provincial or territorial insurance, Canadians can buy private health insurance or participate in employer-offered plans.

Professional Jurisdiction

Most health professions (i.e., medicine, nursing, pharmacology) in Canada are self-regulated, allowing them to determine, monitor, and manage standards, competencies, codes of ethics, and disciplinary actions for their respective members. Some professions are regulated through governments (e.g., emergency medical technicians in Ontario) or other regulatory mechanisms (e.g., osteopathic physicians in British Columbia). In some cases, so-called omnibus legislation regulates several professions simultaneously (e.g., Alberta's *Health Disciplines Act* of 2000).

HEALTH CARE SPENDING

"Canadians pay, directly or indirectly, for every aspect of our health care system through a combination of taxes, payments to government, private insurance premiums, and direct out-of-pocket fees of varying types and amounts" (Romanow, 2002, p. 24). In 2016, total health care spending reached approximately $228 billion (70% public spending; 14.6% out of pocket; 12.2% private insurance; 3.2% other), representing a 2.7% increase from 2015 while maintaining a relatively stable 70–30 split (CIHI, 2016b). According to the CIHI (2016b, 2016c), hospital and health care institutions (29.5%), drug sales (16%), and physician services (15.3%) account for more than 60% of health care spending. In 2016, $6 299 per person was spent on health care, in comparison with $5 614 in 2010 and $4 548 in 2006 (CIHI, 2016b). In 2014, trends showed higher per capita spending for infants (at $10 800) and older persons (ranging from $6 424 [age 65–69] to $21 150 [over 80]) than for younger adults (CIHI, 2016b). Although older persons constitute less than 16% of the population, they account for 44.6% of government health care spending (CIHI, 2016b).

Canada was ranked fifth ($5 543 per person) for health care spending, lower than first-ranking United States spending at $11 126, but above the average spending of member countries of the Organization of Economic Co-operation and Development (OECD) at $4 463 (OECD, 2016a). Canada continues to rank in the mid-range of OECD countries on quality indicators such as life expectancy, self-reported health status, and disease-specific mortality rates (OECD, 2016a).

TRENDS AND REFORMS IN CANADA'S HEALTH CARE SYSTEM

Since the 1980s, rapid changes in health care delivery, technologies, and public expectations have challenged all levels of government to reconstruct a health care system that balances current and future political, legal, economic, and social realities. Two influential national reports on Canada's health care system reforms are *The Kirby Report* (Kirby, 2002) and the report from Romanow's Commission on the Future of Health Care in Canada (CFHC) (Romanow, 2002).

In most provinces, restructuring and health reform became entrusted to regional health authorities, led by appointed or elected community representatives whose mandates, roles, and responsibilities are provincially legislated (Lewis & Kouri, 2004). Regionalization was intended to streamline health services, reduce fragmentation, respond to local needs, improve public participation, and address the continuum of health care services (McIntosh, Ducie, Burka-Charles, et al., 2010). Although these principles were initially promising, the process has not lived up to its potential, becoming primarily a fiscal exercise rather than a philosophical or health-motivated reform (McIntosh et al., 2010).

Framed within the determinants of health, reforms were intended to deliver better-quality and appropriate care at lower cost by adopting sound business and managerial strategies. To date, reforms have resulted in incomplete devolution to the regional boards and government's persistent control of key elements that might have enabled true regionalization to occur (Collier, 2010a).

Currently, there is a trend toward recentralization of health authorities. In 2005, Prince Edward Island dissolved its long-standing health boards and transferred the responsibility to the Department of Health, which has since morphed to become Health PEI (an arm's-length Crown Corporation) (Institute of Public Administration in Canada [IPAC], 2013). In 2008, Alberta went from nine regional health authorities to one province-wide health authority (known as Alberta Health Services), with the stated rationales of improving governance/accountability, management, health care levels, and standardized services to all Albertans (Healthy Debate, 2013). British Columbia also restructured its health authorities, going from 20 regional boards to 5 regional authorities and 1 provincial authority (IPAC, 2013), and recently, Saskatchewan announced a further reduction, from an initial 32 provincial health boards to one (Abrametz, Bragg, & Kendall, 2016).

Policy reform (such as regionalization) is only one means to change health care delivery; other catalysts include emerging medical technology, such as a new diagnostic approach (i.e., point-of-care testing in lieu of laboratory drawn tests) or robotics (i.e., remote presence nursing), and information and communication technologies (i.e., wireless devices) (Lazar, Lavis, Forest, et al., 2013).

In 2004, the federal government initiated a transfer scheme (i.e., *10-Year Plan to Strengthen Health Care*) to increase efficiency and sustainability of the Canadian health care system (Health Canada, 2006). This plan furthered the dialogue on shared values such as person-centred, accountable, efficient, and equitable health care but remained silent on shared and sustainable solutions directions (CHSRF, 2011).

For 2017–18, a new federal funding model was introduced, whereby the provinces and territories will receive $72.8 billion in transfer payments, of which $37.15 billion are Canada Health Transfer (CHT) payments (GOC, 2017). Payments are aligned with mandatory requirements per the *Canada Health Act*. In the past, CHT was adjusted to address tax bases in each province/territory, but the new model is on a per capita basis. Since 2004, the CHT grew by 6% per year; however, in 2017, this amount fell to 3.5%. Some groups estimated a $31 to $43.5 billion loss to the provinces over a 10-year period (Council of Canadians, 2016). The 2017 federal budget committed $6 billion over 10 years for home care (including support for home, community, and palliative services as well as informal caregivers) and $5 billion for mental health initiatives (GOC, 2017). Five-year targeted federal funding will invest in access to affordable and appropriate medications ($140.3 million); technologically mediated health initiatives ($300 million), such as e-prescribing, virtual care, and e-health records; and evidence-informed decision making and improved data uptake for health system enhancements ($53 million) (GOC, 2017). An additional $17 million per year for 3 years will be directed to health care innovations and improvements (GOC, 2017).

Role of Nurses in Health Care Policy

Individually and collectively, nurses are integral to policy advocacy, development, and implementation (Falk-Raphael & Betker, 2012). Health care needs a coordinated, integrated approach by nurses if they are to inform policy decisions and help shape the country's health care systems (Villeneuve, 2017; Villeneuve & MacDonald, 2006). Almost continually since the late 1950s, the federal government position of a senior or chief nurse has existed (i.e., Office of Nursing Policy), and many provincial governments host similar positions. The Office of Nursing Policy is charged with health policy and program development through evidence-informed nursing perspectives (Health Canada, 2009). These nurses contribute to health policy decisions, present government perspectives to nurses and patients, and articulate the potential impact of policy decisions to stakeholders.

RIGHT TO HEALTH CARE

The consensus in Canada is that everyone has a right to health care; however, neither the *Canadian Charter of Rights and Freedoms* of 1982 nor the *Canada Health Act* explicitly include health care as a right. Therefore, federal and provincial legislation must embed legal entitlement. (Only Quebec has health care rights in its legislation.)

Rights Within the Health Care System

Calls from various sources have arisen for a health covenant (Romanow, 2002), health guarantee (Kirby, 2002), or a patient-centred charter (Collier, 2010b) to specify the rights, obligations, and expectations of governments, citizens, and health care providers. A key recommendation of Saskatchewan's independent *Patient First Review* was to "make patient- and family-centred care the foundation and principal aim of the Saskatchewan health system…as an overarching guide for health care organizations, professional groups and others to make the Patient First philosophy a reality in all work places" (Dagnone, 2009).

Although, in practice, no statutory requirement exists in Canada to include patient advocacy groups in the policymaking process, a number of national groups (e.g., Canadian Cancer Society), as well as disease-specific patient groups, are involved. These groups in variably come together to share information, endorse, report on, advocate, or critique health care policy decisions from the consumer's perspective (Consumer Association of Canada, 2017).

As for Canadian health care worker rights, there are expectations: the right to reasonable working conditions, including safety; absence of discrimination, abuse, and harassment of any type; and the right to refuse dangerous work, and access to proactive measures (such as personal protective equipment) (Nordal, 2010). Professional associations and unions work to establish and protect the rights of health care workers.

PRIMARY HEALTH CARE

Primary health care (PHC) is a foundation of Canada's health care system, providing an entry point of contact into the health care system as well as being the vehicle for continuity of care (Health Council of Canada [HCC], 2008). (See Chapter 17 for more on continuity of care.) Health systems based on PHC are more effective and efficient than those centred on specialty and tertiary care (Starfield, Shi, & Macinko, 2005). Initially, PHC was envisioned as addressing nonmedical determinants of health to improve health (HCC, 2008) by connecting health status and social determinants of health (i.e., employment, poverty, lifestyle, environment, and genetic endowment). Other documents, such as the *Alma-Ata Declaration on PHC* (World Health Organization [WHO], 1978) and the *Ottawa Charter for Health Promotion (Charter)* (Lalonde, 1986), informed population health and health promotion approaches globally. The Canadian federal, provincial, and territorial health departments have all established units that focus on, promote, and fund PHC-based programs and services.

PHC is a philosophy and model for improving health that supports essential health care services, with a strong emphasis on the principles of health promotion and disease prevention. In PHC, the importance of determinants of health and strategies to advance individual and population health is recognized (HCC, 2008). According to the WHO (2017), the goal of PHC is to achieve better health for all by:

- Addressing equity issues for health
- Providing patient- and community-relevant and accessible health services and programs
- Situating health intersectorally
- Building collaborative models for program and policy dialogues
- Embedding patient, stakeholder, and partner participation

As an integrated approach, PHC involves building a related spectrum of programs and services (i.e., housing, education) beyond the traditional health care system. The PHC model (Figure 2-2) focuses on

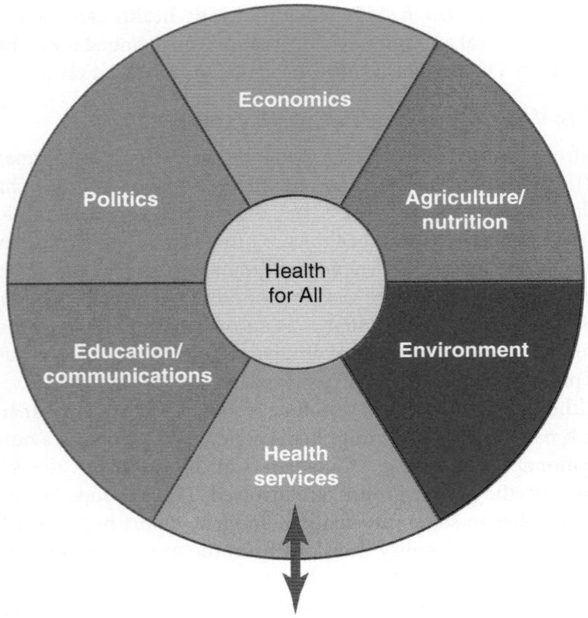

FIGURE 2-2 Primary health care model: A multisectoral or intersectoral approach. (From Shoultz, J., & Hatcher, P. A. [1997]. Looking beyond primary health care: An approach to community-based action. *Nursing Outlook, 45*[1], 24. © 1996 by P. Hatcher, J. Shoultz, and W. Patrick.)

intersectoral collaboration among health professionals, community members, and others, emphasizing health promotion, development of health policies, and prevention of diseases for all. PHC may and often does look different in each community, as it is derived from the needs of consumers and patients, access to health professionals, assets of specific communities (i.e., water supply, school, air quality), and proximity or transport to health care services.

According to Health Canada (2012), PHC services may include the following:

- Prevention and treatment of disease, illness, and injury
- Essential emergency services
- Care including primary mental health, maternity, rehabilitation, and palliative and end-of-life care
- Health promotion
- Inter-agency and inter-program referrals and coordination

From 2000 to 2006, the PHC Transition Fund provided opportunities to move PHC forward as integral to health care renewal. Support was provided for pan-Canadian, provincial/territorial, and multijurisdictional efforts and for Indigenous and minority language projects (GOC, 2007a) aimed at increasing access and coordination of PHC programs, services, and multidisciplinary teams on a 24/7 basis. One national initiative was "Getting a Grip on Arthritis," which undertook capacity building among PHC providers and people living with arthritis to improve prevention, advance early detection, emphasize comprehensiveness of care, and increase access to timely specialty care and self-management (GOC, 2007b). The training model for health professionals is transferable to other chronic diseases and patient groups. At a provincial level, Newfoundland and Labrador undertook an initiative to promote interdisciplinary team approaches to PHC, using key strategies including community-based advisory bodies, a provincial nurse-managed phone line, and establishment and capacity building of a core set of PHC teams supplemented by fiscal, technical, and relational supports (GOC, 2007c). The learnings reflected improvements in teamwork and enhanced information sharing, professional education, and extension of the interprofessional team models.

Throughout this book, "Focus on Primary Health Care" boxes highlight the vital role that nurses play in providing PHC. Box 2-3 links health care situations to PHC principles. Knowledge of primary health care is identified as an essential component of nursing education in Canada (Canadian Association of Schools of Nursing [CASN], 2015).

Barriers to Primary Health Care

The meaning of PHC has caused confusion among health care consumers and even health care providers. The distinction between PHC and **primary care (PC)** is difficult. PC focuses on personal health services, whereas PHC extends beyond PC to include health education, nutrition, maternal and child health care, family planning, immunizations, and control of locally endemic diseases. PHC affords patients the opportunity to be active and engaged, to "work the system" to their advantage, and to be a member of their care team (Nelson, Torchia, MacTavish, et al., 2014).

Interprofessional primary care (IPC) teams are not homogeneous groups, varying according to funding, purpose, governance, and maturity (i.e., length of team's existence) (Canadian Alliance for Sustainable Health Care [CASHC], 2012). Barriers to improving PHC collaboration fall into three distinct levels—individuals, practice, and system (CASHC, 2012). *Individual-level barriers,* such as lack of role clarity and trust, are often attributed to limited knowledge of other team members' knowledge, skills, and scopes of practice. To alleviate this barrier, a number of providers' scopes of practice may provide education for pain management, emphasizing the need for coordination and negotiation in order to remain focused on patient outcomes and quality of care (Canadian Medical Association, 2015). *Practice-level barriers,* according to the CASHC (2012), are closely linked to hierarchical issues at the level of governance and leadership, as well as to strategic team attributes and skills (i.e., skill mix, communications). Thus leadership is now necessarily shared with a more transformative management style found to be more appropriate in PHC teams (Canadian Interprofessional Health Collaborative [CIHC], 2010). Although there is no specific formula for composition of an IPC team, this factor seems to be contextual depending on patient attributes (including culture), location, health services availability, and scope of team members (Oelke, Thurston, & Arthur, 2013). For example, an Indigenous chronic renal insufficiency patient seeing the nephrologist, traditional healer, clinical nurse specialist, home care nurse, pharmacist, nutritionist, and occupational therapist in a single visit is more likely to experience a "whole-system" approach, maximizing scopes of practice of all team members. Given the imperative for collaboration and communication, issues of time (i.e., availability) and space (i.e., co-location) (Oandasan, Gotlib, Conn, et al., 2009) are often cited as barriers. Lack of interprofessional education, appropriate funding, and monitoring and evaluation are *system-level barriers* according to the CASHC (2012). Ineffective interprofessional collaboration is often attributed to members' lack of education and training related to interprofessional practice, collaboration, and team function (Drummond, Abbott, Williamson, et al., 2012). Remuneration and incentive strategies also challenge IPC, given the differing compensation arrangements for team members and payment schedules often tied to physician-initiated activities (i.e., referrals, testing) (Bainbridge, 2010). The Canadian Interprofessional Health Collaborative (2010) advocates and promotes six core competencies (i.e., interprofessional communication; patient-, client-, family-, and community-centred care; role clarification; team functioning; collaborative leadership; and interprofessional conflict resolution) as bringing clarity to future areas of

BOX 2-3 FOCUS ON PRIMARY HEALTH CARE

The Four Pillars of Primary Health Care*

PHC models describe the four pillars of teams, access, information, and healthy living.

Teams

In a 2016 report, 49% of respondents indicated seeing one to two providers in addition to their physician, while another 14% indicated seeing three to five additional providers (Canada Health Infoway, 2016). PHC interdisciplinary teams or networks deliver patient-centred care, which improves access through collaboration, coordination, continuity, and quality (Primaryhealthcareteams.ca, 2014). It has remained difficult to capture and determine the full impact of PHC teams, and only 39% of Canadians indicated having access to such teams (Health Canada, 2015). The CIHI has created and measured a series of indicators to determine effectiveness of PHC (i.e., access to a family medicine physician or NP/RN) (CIHI, 2016d).

West Winds Primary Health Centre (WWPHC) in Saskatoon is a PHC centre addressing the health care needs of men, pregnant and nonpregnant women, adolescents, children, newcomers, Indigenous peoples, and older persons. Through transdisciplinary and intersectoral collaboration, WWPHC provides a full range of services that include but are not limited to health promotion, chronic disease prevention and management (i.e., diabetes education), mental health (including maternal) and addiction services, public health, foundational programs (Healthy Mother-Healthy Baby, Food for Thought), and dental clinics. The staff includes physicians, nutritionists, psychologists, nurses, NPs, therapists (i.e., occupational, physical), speech-language pathologists, pharmacists, social workers, and clinical researchers. A community participation working group and a collaborative practice resource group provide direction and support development of evidence-informed programs.

Access

Although over 80% of Canadians reported having access to a regular family doctor, slightly more than half report having difficulties accessing after-hours PHC services (CIHI, 2016d).

In urban settings, interprofessional teams often work to bring PHC to the streets. They work with vulnerable groups—those in poor health (often with addictions, HIV/AIDS, hepatitis C) or who are homeless, malnourished, and/or lacking support—to assess and monitor health status and provide care "in place." Nurses on "PHC street teams" care for individuals and communities in need; for example, one nurse runs a community program called "Having Healthy Babies" for young, vulnerable women, co-located at a centre near the train tracks, thereby increasing accessibility, and advocates for a "chili lunch" program through local church and business communities for "on-the-street" youth.

Information

Less than a decade ago, 17.1% of people reported difficulty in accessing health information on a continuous basis (CIHI, 2009), but ubiquity of the Internet has the potential to transform the health care environment. Using technology to improve efficiency and quality is a critical part of health care renewal (Health Council of Canada, 2008), with 80% of information seekers reporting convenience, easy access to recent health information, and anonymity as the primary reasons for online access (Vance, Howe, & Dellavalle, 2009). Tools (e.g., electronic health record [EHR], diagnostic equipment) and skills (e.g., telehealth) facilitate quality, access, and coordination of information.

Canada Health Infoway (CHI) is a federally funded, independent, not-for-profit organization with federal, provincial, and territorial representation (2011). CHI fosters and accelerates the development and adoption of electronic health (e-health) information systems on a pan-Canadian level. CHI envisions a high-quality, sustainable, and effective info-structure to provide Canadians and health professionals with timely, appropriate, and secure access to information, such as supporting triage nurses to monitor patient kiosks at the Scarborough Hospital (CHI, 2011). According to CHI (2016), 74% of Canadians believed digital health had potentially positive impacts, and they believed that digital technologies enhanced comprehensive patient histories (85%) and coordination of care (86%). Most Canadians indicated that digital health improves knowledge of their health (77%), increases confidence in health self-management (69%), and informs discussions with their doctor (74%) (CHI 2016).

Healthy Living

Practitioners within PHC embrace strategies of prevention, chronic illness management, and self-care while recognizing that factors outside the health care system (e.g., social, economic, environmental) influence individual and community health.

An example is a public health nurse in southern Ontario running a program that educated low-income mothers about nutrition, child development, and community action. The women shared strategies to meet their families' nutritional requirements on tight budgets. Upon learning that a national bakery was closing its local day-old-bread outlet, the nurse coached the women to call a local newspaper reporter who, in turn, contacted the bakery's president and persuaded the owner to keep the outlet open, thereby benefitting the entire community.

*Section contributor: V. R. Ramsden, RN, PhD.
Canadian Nurses Association. (2003). Primary health care—The time has come. *Nursing Now,* 16, 1–4.

training and development (see Chapter 18 for further information about interprofessional collaboration).

Challenging the adoption of PHC is an underlying concern as "many Canadians see the health system as an 'illness care' system that will be there when they need it" (Canadian Nurses Association [CNA], 2003). Some fear that if monies are dedicated to PHC priorities and implementation, benefits will be limited, at least in the near term. PHC is a sensible approach to health care that is cost-effective and benefits most people. For example, by attending a community health program on infant and child care, parents learn the importance of recognizing signs and symptoms of urinary tract infection (UTI) in children and the importance of seeking medical treatment. With this knowledge comes prevention of long-term serious complications of untreated UTIs, such as potential kidney damage, and future reduced health care costs.

FUTURE OF PRIMARY HEALTH CARE

Strengthening PHC will address Canadians' needs for consistent access to comprehensive evidence-informed services, a range of providers, patient-centred approaches, and, ultimately, more equitable and inclusive programs and services (Sodani & Sharma, 2012). For example, trauma programs will have health promotion activities (road safety education), preventive programming (helmet legislation), secondary care and tertiary care (emergency transportation), and rehabilitation (head injury–related recovery programs). Programs will cover multiple sites, may be defined by a particular disease or population group (e.g., children), and will comprise multiple disciplines and sectors of society (e.g., health care, education, justice systems).

Because of its integrated approach, PHC may hold the key to Canada's looming health care crisis. By integrating and investing in

BOX 2-4 CASE STUDY

Primary Health Care

During a community meeting in a core area of a small city, parents, educators, health care providers, and volunteers agree to pilot an integrated program to reduce obesity in children. Social services staff and volunteers run a breakfast program. Fruits and vegetables for twice-daily snacks are donated by a local grocery store. Nutritionists and kinesiologists educate teachers to integrate nutrition and physical fitness into the curriculum. Schools commit to having students and teachers participate in activities for at least 30 minutes every day and establish rules for school lunches (e.g., no soft drinks). Nurse practitioners arrange visits with the parents of children identified as being overweight or at risk. If only 10% of the children in the program develop a healthier lifestyle, future savings to the health care system will pay for program costs.

health care, education, social services, and voluntary sectors, competition for government monies may decline and each sector will articulate beyond their own boundaries (Box 2-4).

SETTINGS FOR HEALTH CARE DELIVERY

Although health care delivery varies across Canada, three types of delivery agencies are comparable: institutional, community and voluntary, and private-sector agencies.

Institutional Sector

Institutional agencies, including hospitals, long-term care facilities, psychiatric facilities, and rehabilitation centres, offer health care services to **inpatients** (who stay at an institution for diagnosis, treatment, or rehabilitation). Most offer services to **outpatients** (who visit an institution for select services).

Hospitals. Hospitals have traditionally been considered major health care agencies, most specializing in acute care services. **Acute care** is health care delivered for a short time (usually days to weeks, typically less than 3 months) in which an immediate health problem is diagnosed, treated, or both. Hospital services may include emergency and diagnostic, inpatient, surgical intervention, intensive care, outpatient, and rehabilitation services. The numbers of hospitals, hospital beds, and admissions in Canada have decreased significantly since the 1990s, creating pressures in dealing with the patients who have more acute and specialized needs. In 2013, Canada had 2.68 acute beds per 1 000 population, mirroring the United States (2.93), but significantly lower than Australia's 3.75 beds and Japan's 13.32 beds (OECD, 2016b). Hospitals strive to provide quality care with the newest treatments and technologies and to facilitate appropriate, safe, and timely patient discharge to the appropriate environment in which to manage residual needs.

Hospitals are distinguished by their size (e.g., community hospitals), service provision (e.g., cancer care hospitals, children's hospitals), and connection to academic institutions (e.g., university health science centres), as well as by public or private status. Public hospitals are financed and operated by a local, provincial, or national government entity, whereas private hospitals are owned and operated by groups such as churches, corporations, and charitable organizations. Military hospitals, although limited in Canada, provide medical services to members of the military and their families. Veterans' hospitals provide residential care, extended care, and rehabilitation to aging, injured, and disabled military veterans.

Roles and functions of hospitals and hospital-based nurses have evolved in this era of health care reform. Hospital nurses use critical thinking skills (see Chapter 12 for further information about critical thinking and critical reasoning), apply the nursing process, coordinate and delegate care (see Chapter 11 for further information about collaborative practice), invoke evidence-informed practices, and stress patient teaching and post-discharge self-care (see Chapter 20 for further information about patient education). Nurses participate in clinical care rounds and discharge planning as a critical interdisciplinary strategy for continuity of care, facilitating safe transitions of patients between levels of care and the community. Many hospital nurses specialize as clinical nurse specialists, caring for patients with specific needs (e.g., palliative) or specific diseases (e.g., cardiovascular). Other hospital roles include nurse manager, infection control coordinator, clinical educator, and clinical nurse researcher.

Long-Term Care (LTC) Facilities. LTC (extended care) facilities provide accommodations and 24-hour intermediate and custodial care (e.g., nursing, rehabilitation, dietary, recreational, social, and spiritual services) for residents of any age with chronic or debilitating illnesses or disabilities. Most residents are frail, older persons with multiple health issues (see Chapter 24 for further information about caring for older persons). Some are younger adults with severe, chronic health conditions (see Chapter 23 for further information about chronic conditions with younger adults). LTC facilities function as the resident's temporary or permanent home; therefore, the surroundings are as homelike as possible. The philosophy of care is to provide a planned, systematic, and interdisciplinary approach that helps residents reach and maintain their highest level of function. LTC facilities are not part of the insured services bundle within the *Canada Health Act*, although many provincial and territorial plans do provide some coverage. In these settings, nurses plan and coordinate resident care, manage chronic illnesses, and conduct rehabilitation programs and assume roles in education (see Chapter 20 for further information about patient education), communication (see Chapter 17 for further information about relational communication), administration, and family-related interventions (see Chapter 19 for further information about family assessments).

Psychiatric Facilities. Located in hospitals, independent outpatient clinics, or mental health clinics, psychiatric facilities offer inpatient and outpatient services. Mental health is often seen as one of the "orphan children of Medicare," never being fully integrated into the health care system (Romanow, 2002). Nurses in these facilities collaborate with doctors, psychologists, social workers, and therapists to make plans that enable a patient to return to the community. At discharge from inpatient facilities, patients are usually referred for follow-up to community-based agencies. Nurses working in these settings are especially skillful in communication skills (see Chapter 17), case management, and patient safety (see Chapter 37).

Rehabilitation Centres. A *rehabilitation centre* is a residential institution providing therapy and restorative training to decrease patients' dependence on care. Many centres offer programs to teach the patient, patient's family, or both to achieve optimal function after a stroke, head or spinal cord injury, or other impairment. Substance rehabilitation centres help patients withdraw from alcohol and drug dependence and return to the community. Nurses in rehabilitation centres collaborate closely with physical and occupational therapists, psychologists, and social workers, working with patients experiencing stress and adapting to challenges to mobility and/or safety.

Community Sector

Community services are directed at primary and secondary care, described later in this chapter, and should be accessible to patients in locations where they live, work, play, and engage. The focus is on empowerment and community development opportunities that effect change at the broadest social level by reducing inequities in access to health services by identifying and removing barriers (Mikkonen & Raphael, 2013). Community health nurses (CHNs) oversee and participate in outreach programs that provide services and locate patients who might not seek care at traditional health care centres. According to the Community Health Nurses of Canada (CHNC) (2013), CHNs work in diverse rural and urban settings such as public health units, family practices, workplace, outpost stations, the street, faith organizations, schools, and correctional institutions. CHNs' primary role is to "promote, protect, and preserve the health of individuals, families, groups, communities, and populations in the settings where they live, work, learn, worship and play in an ongoing and/or episodic process" (CHNC, 2013). Nurses practising in the community sector are involved in community-based nursing (see Chapter 4) and caring throughout the lifespan (see Unit V).

Public Health. Public health is committed to ensuring conditions and circumstances in which people can be healthy through appropriate screening, assessment, development, monitoring, and support (i.e., public policy). Public health differs from many clinical practice settings in its focus on entire populations or subsets of populations rather than on individual patients.

Activities related to pandemic planning, One Health (i.e., interdisciplinary consideration of animal-human-environment health-related challenges and care), and global surveillance have put public health in the forefront (Kahn, 2017) with regard to protection and promotion efforts. Public health nurses work closely with a range of health care providers, including medical health officers, therapists, psychologists, nutritionists, and environmental and public health inspectors. Nurses are the primary professionals in public health clinics offering well-baby clinics, school health programs, sexually transmitted infections surveillance, and screening programs, as well as health promotion (e.g., tobacco reduction) and disease prevention programs.

Physician Offices. Physician offices offer PC focusing on diagnosis and treatment of specific illnesses rather than on health promotion. The majority of Canadian physicians function as private contractors within the publicly funded health care system, working on a fee-for-service basis. In this setting, nurses record vital signs, prepare patients for examination, and collaborate with physicians to conduct physical examinations, document histories, offer health education, and recommend therapies. Nurse practitioners often partner in these settings focusing on wellness care, minor emergencies, chronic disease screening and monitoring, ordering and interpreting diagnostic tests, and prescribing medications (Canadian Medical Protective Association, 2014).

Community Health Centres (CHCs) and Clinics. CHC teams plan, manage, and deliver comprehensive services to designated geographic areas or specific at-risk populations. According to the Canadian Association of Community Health Centres (2017), CHCs are the first point of contact offering a range of primary health, social, rehabilitation, and other noninstitutional services delivering integrated, locally relevant patient-centred services and programs.

Increasingly, NPs and nurses are managing CHCs, with the intention of enabling patients to assume more responsibility for their health. NPs have become CHC team members focused on prevention and supportive services rather than on traditional practitioner–driven curative and rehabilitative care.

Assisted Living. Assisted-living facilities are community-based residential facilities where adults live and receive a range of support services, including personalized assistance in achieving optimal independence. These facilities usually combine professional and nonprofessional staff on an around-the-clock basis. Personal assistance services promote maximum dignity and independence through meal preparation, personal hygiene practice, mobility, and socialization.

Home Care. Canadian health care is shifting from an institution-based system to one in which community care is playing a greater role (see Chapter 4). Home care is the provision of health care services (i.e., short-term postoperative recovery, end-of-life [EOL] care) and equipment to patients and families in their homes, residential settings, hospitals, and ambulatory clinics (CIHI, 2017). Home care is an uninsured extended health service (Canadian Home Care Association [CHCA], 2013). All provinces and territories fund assessment and case management, nursing care, and support services for eligible patients, while patients may pay for extra professional or support services through insurance or pay-for-service arrangements. The federal government delivers home care services to First Nations people on reserves and Inuit people in designated communities, members of the armed forces and the RCMP, federal inmates, and eligible veterans.

Home care involves primarily nursing care plus adjunct professional and nonprofessional services (i.e., physiotherapy, social work, speech therapy). Support services are nonmedical services and include personal care, assistance with activities of daily living, and assistance with home management.

Nurses working in home care experience all levels of care within the home setting (see "Levels of Care") as well as complex caseloads. The CHCA (2012) states that home care is a cost-effective alternative to acute care, maintaining patients at optimal levels of functioning, delaying institutionalization, and providing a viable substitution for health services (e.g., wound care comprises 50% of care delivered by home care providers). The CHCA's (2014) Vision 2020 describes an integrated system providing appropriate and accessible services that support individuals and families to remain independent in their own homes while preserving dignity, safety, and quality of life.

Adult Day Support Programs (ADSPs). As an alternative to hospitalization, adult day support programs may be associated with a hospital or LTC facility or exist independently and provide continuous health care services for specific patients (e.g., those with dementia, those needing physical rehabilitation or counselling). Nearly 45% of Canadians indicated that they had provided care to a family member or friend with a long-term health condition, disability, or age-related need (Vanier Institute of the Family, 2017). ADSPs play a critical role in enabling a caregiver's participation in care while continuing to work. Nurses in ADSPs provide continuity between the care delivered at home and ADSPs. For instance, nurses administer treatments, encourage patients to adhere to prescribed medication regimens (see Chapter 34), link patients with community resources (see Chapter 4), and provide counselling services (see Chapter 19).

Community and Voluntary Agencies. National, provincial, and regional voluntary agencies (e.g., Cystic Fibrosis Canada, Diabetes Canada) meet needs for target populations, circumstances (i.e., shut-ins) or conditions (i.e., disease-specific). Most voluntary agencies offer programs to educate about, prevent, and detect specific conditions rather than treat them. Voluntary agencies depend on the help of professional volunteers (e.g., VON [Victorian Order of Nurses]) and lay volunteers (e.g., Meals on Wheels). Many offer financial support or scholarships for training health care providers and students through fundraising and donations.

Occupational Health. More than 2 000 members of the Canadian Occupational Health Nurses Association (2011) deliver integrated occupational health and safety services to individual and communities of workers. RNs certified in occupational health have met specific eligibility requirements, passed a written examination, and achieved a national standard of competency.

Hospice and Palliative Care. Palliative care is an interdisciplinary EOL approach to care which manages life-threatening or serious illnesses, regardless of age or condition, with the intent of improving quality of life, addressing physical and psychological symptoms, and facilitating a dignified death. It includes caregiver support during and beyond the palliative care involvement. Palliative care, recognizing diverse needs, capacities, and cultural practices, is available in hospitals, homes, shelters, LTC facilities, and hospices.

A hospice is a family-centred care system that enables a person to live in comfort, with independence and dignity, while living with a life-ending illness. Hospice care is palliative, not curative (see Chapter 25). Its multidisciplinary approach involving physicians, nurses, social workers, pharmacists, and pastoral care staff is crucial. Hospice nurses work in hospitals, free-standing hospices, or the home, caring for the patient and family during the terminal phase of illness and at the time of death, and through the bereavement phase they provide counselling for the family and can assist in finding a support network (see Canadian Virtual Hospice at http://www.virtualhospice.ca/en_US/Main+Site+Navigation/Home.aspx).

With Canada's current aging population and increasing chronicity levels, there is an imperative for a well-constructed and responsive integrated EOL care system. In 2015, Canada ranked 11th out of 80 countries on the international "Quality of Death" index, which considers hospice and palliative care environments as well as other EOL care factors (Economist Intelligence Unit, 2015).

Currently, palliative and hospice care is inconsistently offered across Canada, reflecting the lack of policies, training, and funding related to EOL care as well as variances in delivery based on location and program criteria. Program offerings, such as palliative drug coverage, nursing/personal care services, and hospice care, are nonstandardized despite savings of nearly $8 000 per person when palliative care replaces hospital-based care (Hodgson, 2012). As a result, families and charitable entities frequently bear significant costs.

EOL care is complex and replete with contradictions. Although most Canadians express a desire to die on their own terms in the presence of loved ones, over 60% of deaths occur in a hospital (Statistics Canada, 2013). Most Canadians (73%) feel that the government places too little emphasis on EOL care, but less than half had spoken with family or friends regarding their EOL desires, and only 9% reported ever speaking with their health team about EOL care wishes (Canadian Hospice Palliative Care Association [CHPCA], 2013).

Health care providers and politicians must engage in dialogues related to advance care planning (where a capable adult indicates personal health care decisions in the event of incapacitation) (CHPCA, 2013) and medical assistance in dying (Bill C-14) to ensure the Canadian public comprehends and engages in EOL planning (Quality End-of-Life Care Coalition of Canada [QEoLCC], 2010).

Between 2011 and 2014, the QEoLCC developed a framework for integration of the palliative care model (i.e., The Way Forward Initiative). In 2016, the federal government announced an additional $3 billion in funding to home care, from which funding for palliative care would be drawn (GOC, 2017).

Parish Nursing. Parish nursing (or faith community nursing) is becoming more popular as faith-based communities promote and maintain members' health. According to the Canadian Association for Parish Nursing Ministry [CAPNM] (2017), a parish nurse is an RN with specialized knowledge who is called to the ministry and affirmed by a faith-based community to promote health, healing, and wholeness through advocacy, counselling, education, and intersectoral referrals (CAPNM, 2017).

LEVELS OF CARE

Five levels of health care exist: promotive, preventive, curative (diagnosis and treatment), rehabilitative, and supportive (including home care, LTC, and palliative care) (CNA Now, 2015).

Level 1: Health Promotion

The first level of health care, health promotion, focuses on "enabling people to increase control over, and to improve their health" (WHO, 1986) across a range of settings. Although rooted in health education (McManus, 2013), health promotion takes an interdisciplinary approach to provision of wellness services, such as antismoking education, promotion of self-esteem in children and adolescents, and advocacy for healthy public policy.

The *Ottawa Charter for Health Promotion* (the *Charter*) (Lalonde, 1986) lists five action strategies for health promotion: building healthy public policy, creating supportive environments, strengthening community action, developing personal skills, and reorienting health care services. Furthermore, the foundation of health promotion consists of "the fundamental conditions and resources for health, [which] are peace, shelter, education, food, income, a stable ecosystem, sustainable resources, social justice, and equity" (Lalonde, 1986) (see Chapter 1). The *Charter* details how health care providers enable patients to make decisions that affect their health.

Level 2: Disease and Injury Prevention

The second level includes illness prevention services to help patients, families, and communities reduce risk factors for disease and injury (see Chapter 4). Prevention strategies include clinical actions (immunizing), behavioural aspects (support groups), and environmental actions (climate control activism) (see Chapter 1).

Level 3: Diagnosis and Treatment

Diagnosis and treatment focus on recognizing and managing individual patients' existing health problems at three sublevels: primary, secondary, and tertiary.

- *Primary care* (PC) is the first contact of a patient with the health care system that leads to a decision regarding a course of action to resolve any actual or potential health problem. PC providers include physicians and NPs in practice settings such as physicians' offices, nurse-managed clinics, community health centres, and schools. The focus is on early detection, routine care, and education to prevent recurrences. (Recall and note differences from PHC.)
- *Secondary care* usually occurs in hospital or home settings and involves specialized medical service by a physician specialist or a hospital on referral from a PC practitioner. Secondary care considers definitive or extended diagnosis.
- *Tertiary care* is specialized technical care in diagnosing and treating complicated health problems. Tertiary care occurs in regional, teaching, university, or specialized hospitals that house sophisticated diagnostic equipment.

Level 4: Rehabilitation

The aim of rehabilitation nursing is to improve the health and quality of life of those facing life-altering conditions, regardless of age or circumstances, by promoting and advancing "the art, science, and practice of professional rehabilitation nursing practice through education, advocacy, collaboration, and research" (Canadian Association of Rehabilitation Nurses, 2017). Rehabilitation occurs after a physical or mental health illness, injury, or chemical addiction or is related to chronic illness, disability, frailty, and aging. Ideally, rehabilitation begins the moment a patient enters a health care setting for treatment as part of an interdisciplinary effort (i.e., therapists [physical, occupational, respiratory], nurses). As a condition stabilizes, rehabilitation assists patients in returning to their previous level of function or reaching an optimal level of function, thereby enhancing quality of life while promoting independence and self-care. For example, some patients undergo physiotherapy before major joint repair to enhance their recovery (see Chapter 36). Nurses have a key role in the continuity-of-care aspects of rehabilitation across agencies and settings.

Level 5: Supportive Care

Patients of all ages with illnesses or disabilities that are chronic (i.e., are long term) or progressive (i.e., worsen over time) may require supportive care. Supportive care consists of health, personal, and social services provided over a prolonged period to people who are disabled, who do not function independently, or who have a terminal disease. With increasing lifespans, escalating chronic conditions, and diverse care settings (i.e., institutional, community, and home), demand for supportive care will continue to grow. Two examples of supportive care include the following:

Palliative care serves people living with progressive, life-threatening illnesses or conditions. Palliative care, whether provided in the hospital, hospice, or home, addresses physical, emotional, social, and spiritual needs of the patient and family. (Please refer to previous description in Hospice and Palliative Care section.)

Respite care provides short-term relief or time off for family caregivers by health care providers and/or trained volunteers in either institutional (i.e., ADSP) or home settings.

CHALLENGES TO THE HEALTH CARE SYSTEM

Canada's health care system is challenged with a range of cost accelerators in pursuit of achieving equity in care and access for all. Nursing education programs must consider and build awareness of these issues through increasing knowledge of "professional and organizational structures" of graduates, who will need to have greater understanding of nursing's embeddedness in sociopolitical, historical, and economic contexts (CASN, 2015, p.10).

Cost Accelerators

Digital Health Technologies. New technologies, such as new-generation antibiotics or diagnostic imaging equipment, have become integral in the palette of care modalities. Their effectiveness has reduced mortality and morbidity rates while, at times, having an impact on health care costs.

As an essential element of future health care delivery, eHealth (see Chapter 16) is embedded in a number of health applications from administrative to direct care. There is an emphasis on developing a national health info-structure to support direct care, telehealth, mHealth (mobile applications), remote monitoring, remote presence (robotics), and maintenance of electronic health records (EHRs). (See Chapter 15 for more on EHRs.) Remote monitoring supports information-based, near real-time health care linking medical providers to patients who are not co-located. Robots are becoming a part of the care team complement, assisting with supporting patients, students, and health care providers. Nursing informatics is an emerging area that "integrates nursing, its information and knowledge and their management with information and communications technologies to improve the health of people, families, and communities worldwide" (Canadian Nursing Informatics Association, 2011).

Demographics. According to Statistics Canada (2017), Canada's population exceeds 35 million individuals, of which 5.4 million (15.3% of the population) are seniors (persons aged 65 years and over) (Statistics Canada, 2015). As the population ages, chronic and age-related diseases are increasing in frequency, further challenging the health care system.

Consumer Involvement and Personalized Medicine. Canadians are better informed than ever about their health care options and demand a high level of quality care. For example, patients might request an expensive diagnostic test such as magnetic resonance imaging (MRI), whereas previously an X-ray would have sufficed. There is a growing presence of and demand for self-care activities to enhance health, prevent disease, evaluate symptoms, and restore health either independently or in collaboration with health care providers (Consumer Health Products–Canada, 2009). Another aspect is in the awareness and demand for increasingly customized and personalized approaches to care using screening and genetic profiling for precise diagnosis and customizing therapeutics.

Equality and Quality

The aim of the Canadian health care system is to provide quality care and access to care for all.

Cultural Competence, Safety, and Humility. Canada is a country of diversity, creating an imperative for a health care system and for providers to be responsive and respectful (see Chapter 9). The emerging models for care must embrace a range of skills, competencies, and approaches that demonstrate genuine presence, caring, and understanding as well as reflective practice.

As discussed earlier, the federal government has a key role in the provision of health care services to Indigenous people. The shift in the health structures and PHC seem to hold the promise of aligning with Indigenous peoples' beliefs, especially with regard to holism and integration. Many policy and research approaches are increasingly calling for "Two-Eyed Seeing" as a framework for innovatively moving forward with Indigenous health (Martin, 2012).

Immigration has shaped Canada's population historically. According to Statistics Canada (2017), there were 437 815 more people living in Canada than in the previous year. The proportion of immigrants could reach 30% by 2036, nearly a 105% increase from the 2011 profile (Canadian Press, 2017). Newcomer health status varies, based on their reasons for immigration, place or circumstances of origin, and social supports (Wayland, 2006). Issues of income, psychological well-being, religion, and ethnic support are important aspects of adjustment and risk reduction (Wayland, 2006).

Evidence-Informed Practice (EIP). Evidence-informed practice and decision making is a critical approach to improving care delivery and potentiating optimal patient outcomes (Ciliska, 2013) (see Chapter 6 for further information about the research process). A range of EIP resources are available on CNA's portal called NurseONE (http://www.nurseone.ca/). The Canadian Institutes of Health Research (2016) Evidence-Informed Health Care Renewal initiative has contributed to the practice and policy knowledge base as well as knowledge transfer on strengthening and sustaining the Canadian health care system.

Quality and Patient Safety. The Canadian Patient Safety Institute (CPSI) (2016) focuses on four areas of patient safety: medication (incidents, management), surgical care (postoperative infections, retained objects), infection prevention and control (antibiotic resistance, hand hygiene), and home care safety (falls, abuse). In 2014–15, nearly 140 000 hospitalizations (5.6% of hospitalizations) resulted in preventable incidents, with 20% of these individuals experiencing multiple harmful events (CIHI, 2016e). About two-thirds of the events were either care or medication related (e.g., medication misadministration, infections), and the remainder were either procedure-related (e.g., incorrect procedure) or patient accidents (e.g., falls) (CIHI, 2016f).

Quality Workplaces. Health care is delivered in a diverse range of environments, a situation that challenges quality issues and affects recruitment and retention. Sustainable and quality workforces, organizational efficiency, and improved patient care are related to improved work environments; efforts toward these goals catalyzed the formation of the Federal/Provincial/Territorial Committee on Health Workforce (Health Canada, 2016c).

Privatization of Services. Governments are struggling to maintain the principle of universality against the benefits and challenges of privatization. At present, not all health care services are available and accessible to all Canadians. For example, infertility treatment procedures are performed in private offices, available to patients who can afford them.

Health Care Human Resources. In 2012, more than 1.7 million people (about 11.2% of the total workforce) in Canada worked directly in health-related occupations, making this the second largest employment sector (CIHI, 2015). Despite these numbers, accessibility to health care services is compromised by shortages of physicians, nurses, and other health care providers in targeted areas (such as rural or remote locations and specialty areas). Health Canada (2016c) states that health human resources planning must occur within the broader health care system, recognizing systemic challenges of wait times, patient safety, and bed closures. In addition, efforts to address underrepresentation of Indigenous people in the health workforce are subsumed within the Pan-Canadian strategy (Health Canada, 2016c). Five key strategic actions proposed for achieving a representative and culturally competent human resource cadre are integration of Indigenous ways of knowing, reduction of institutional barriers, increased recruitment and retention for education, increased recruitment and retention for practicing nurses, and building leadership and advocacy capacities (CNA, 2014).

Improved Patient Outcome Metrics. Patient outcomes need to be developed, captured, and visualized in order to address increased accountability and the sense of urgency to determine performance in health care. As reform of the Canadian health system continues, there will be increasing expectations for efficiency and effectiveness measures to reflect improvements. Coupled with these measures it will be necessary ensure appropriate data visualization and knowledge translation of findings across sectors and stakeholder groups and, importantly, to consumers.

NURSING'S FUTURE IN THE EMERGING HEALTH CARE SYSTEM

This chapter provided extensive discussion about the restructuring and challenges within the Canadian health care system. In this context of restructuring and complexity in the Canadian system, nursing roles continue to evolve and diversify. In the future, nurses will increasingly be regarded as critical stakeholders, partners, and providers within the emerging health care system. Nursing's contributions to health and health care in Canada range from direct care to active participation in the reformation processes as well as maintaining a continuous presence in the pursuit of equality in access for all patient groups. Nursing has been instrumental in the advancement of advanced nursing practice, interdisciplinary practices, and collaborative efforts for the betterment of society (Seenandan-Sookdeo, 2012). At the same time, nursing is conspicuous in its absence in the executive and decision-making levels of health care agencies; thus the "policy impact of the nursing voice, knowledge and experience is minimal and we must turn the reality around" (Shamian, 2014). A critical role of nursing in health policy is to peel back the layers of policy complexity in the effort to reduce and eliminate health disparities. As nurses strive to reduce health inequities and address the social determinants of health, there is a need to strengthen their policy presence through understanding, critical analysis, and voice (advocacy) (Reutter & Kushner, 2010).

KEY CONCEPTS

- Medicare is a key component of Canada's social safety net.
- All levels of government play a major role in co-funding national health insurance and setting health care policy in accordance with the *Canada Health Act.*
- The *Canada Health Act* forbids extra billing and user fees, while articulating the five principles of public administration, comprehensiveness, universality, portability, and accessibility.
- Health care services are provided in institutional, community, and home settings; across all age groups; and for individual, family, group, and community populations.
- Five levels of health care are promotive, preventive, curative, rehabilitative, and supportive.
- Escalating costs, technological innovations, and consumer expectations challenge the health care system in efforts to deliver innovative, efficient, and quality care.
- Equality, equity, access, interdisciplinary approaches, communication, and continuity of care challenge the health care system.
- The primacy of PHC and home care align with the reforming health care environment and cost-effectiveness.
- Successful health promotion and disease prevention programs help patients acquire healthier lifestyles and achieve an optimal quality of life.
- Sufficient, diverse, and qualified human health resources are essential for a culturally competent workforce attending to a culturally safe Canadian health care system.
- Enhancing the health of Canada's Indigenous peoples is a significant challenge to society and to the health care system.
- Nurses must continually seek out information and evidence to remain responsive to providing quality, culturally competent, and safe care.

CRITICAL THINKING EXERCISES

1. Debate the following challenges facing the Canadian health care system: escalating costs, privatization, continuity of care, regionalization/centralization, and digital health.
2. Consider and describe how the economy and technology have changed the Canadian health care system. What are the implications for nursing? For patients and families?
3. Mr. W., a 68-year-old widower with no immediate family support, is scheduled to have major surgery to replace the joint in his hip. He is generally in good health and lives in a seniors-only apartment complex in a small town. Describe the types of health care services, safety issues, interprofessional competencies, and technological supports that might play a part in his postsurgical care.

REVIEW QUESTIONS

1. A nurse working in a new position in policy development has been asked to identify agencies in Canada that have undertaken an effort to reduce wait times, reduce duplication of tests, and support coordination of care. Which of the following agencies would you expect to be on the list? *(Select all that apply.)*
   1. Canada eHealth
   2. Canadian Institute for Health Information
   3. Canada Health Infoway
   4. Canadian Institutes for Health Research
   5. Consumer Association of Canada
2. Which of the following people fall outside the *Canada Health Act*? *(Select all that apply.)*
   1. Indigenous peoples
   2. RCMP members
   3. Recently arrived newcomers
   4. Members of military services
   5. Persons in transit between provinces
3. A nursing student is discussing public health with her preceptor and asks about the main focus of public health. The mentor responds that public health primarily focuses on:
   1. Reporting
   2. Promotion
   3. Intervention
   4. Institutionalization
   5. Immunization
4. The *Canada Health Act* embraces which of the following five principles:
   1. Social justice, equity, acceptability, efficiency, effectiveness
   2. Accountability, equality, economy, collaboration, coordination
   3. Insured health services, provider compensation, hospital services, community care, and pharmaceuticals
   4. Public administration, comprehensiveness, universality, portability, accessibility
5. At the clinic, the nurse sees a middle-aged woman who is nearing exhaustion caring for her aging mother, who is experiencing dementia. As the nurse opens the dialogue on potential placements for her mother, it is obvious that there is a lack of understanding about the existence of community agencies such as ____________________, which might provide an alternative for this family.
   1. Home care
   2. Palliative care
   3. Hospital care
   4. Ambulatory care
   5. Adult day support
6. A nurse practitioner is establishing an interprofessional team to work with pregnant newcomer women, focusing on nutrition. In addition to the nurse, the three most critical members of the team at this early stage will include: *(Select all that apply.)*
   1. Obstetrics specialist
   2. Dietitian
   3. Pharmacist
   4. Social worker
   5. Translator
7. A nurse practitioner who is working in a northern remote community notes a trend toward depression and anxiety among a subset of the population in the 40–60 age group who were residential school survivors. A culturally competent strategy to work with this group might be to:
   1. Provide individual counselling on a case-by-case basis to protect confidentiality.
   2. Offer a weekly peer support program.
   3. Work with the elder and chief of the community to determine a way forward.
   4. Consult with a psychologist or psychiatrist before undertaking any programming to affirm risks and potential barriers.
8. Management has requested a brief report from the nurse manager on a human resources plan for the next 5 years. Which of the following statements best represents the factors that should be mentioned?
   1. We should be working with our aging nurses to transition out of full-time work and let younger nurses be mentored into their vacated positions.
   2. With all the workplace injuries, we should be hiring an occupational therapist or there will soon be no nurses working.
   3. We will soon be able to replace nurses with robots and technology, so that is where we should be investing.
   4. We are not educating enough nurses, so we may have to recruit from international pools to fill positions.
   5. There are too many variables to be able to predict what will be needed in 5 years, so the best we can do is try to keep the nurses we have.
9. A nurse organizes a blood pressure screening program as a ______________ strategy.
   1. Primary level
   2. Secondary level
   3. Tertiary level
   4. Rehabilitative level
10. Primary care can only be provided by a physician or in a hospital setting.
    1. True
    2. False

Answers: 1. 2, 3, 4; **2.** 1, 2; **3.** 2; **4.** 4; **5.** 5; **6.** 2, 4, 5; **7.** 3; **8.** 1; **9.** 2; **10.** 2

Rationales for the Review Questions appear at the end of the book.

RECOMMENDED WEBSITES

Canadian Foundation for Healthcare Improvement: http://www.cfhi-fcass.ca/Home.aspx
This site addresses initiatives of the Foundation to advance promising innovations across health care organizations to improve patient care, health outcomes, and efficiencies.

Canada Health Infoway: https://www.infoway-inforoute.ca/
A not-for-profit corporation created by Canada's First Ministers to foster and accelerate development and adoption of digital health innovations across all groups.

Canadian Institute of Health Information: https://www.cihi.ca
A not-for-profit organization seeking to improve the health care system and the health of Canadians by providing timely and essential health information.

Canadian Public Health Association: http://www.cpha.ca
A national, not-for-profit association seeking excellence in public health nationally and internationally and seeking universal and equitable access to basic health-sustaining conditions.

Health Canada: http://www.hc-sc.gc.ca
This site provides links to information about the Canadian health care system, such as the *Canada Health Act* legislation, budget information, and federal reports.

Canadian Patient Safety Institute: http://www.patientsafetyinstitute.ca
This institute was established to build and advance a safer health care system for Canadians. It reports on activities in leadership across health sectors and health care systems, highlights promising practices, and raises awareness with stakeholders and the public about patient safety.

REFERENCES

Abrametz, B., Bragg, T., & Kendel, D. (2016). *Optimizing and integrating patient centred care: Saskatchewan Advisory Panel on Health System Structure report.* Retrieved from https://www.saskatchewan.ca/~/media/news%20release%20backgrounders/2017/jan/saskatchewan%20advisory%20panel%20on%20health%20system%20structure%20report.pdf.

Bainbridge, I. (2010). Interprofessional education for interprofessional practice. Will future health care providers embrace collaboration as one answer to improved quality of care? *UBCMJ, 2*(1), 9–10.

Canada Health Infoway (CHI). (2011). Involving patients in healthcare through IT. *E-HEALTH: The enterprise of healthcare.* Retrieved from http://ehealth.eletsonline.com/2011/04/world-8/.

Canada Health Infoway (CHI) (2016). *Connecting patients for better health.* Ottawa, ON: Author.

Canadian Alliance for Sustainable Health Care (CASHC). (2012). *Improving primary health care through collaboration.* Ottawa: The Conference Board of Canada. Retrieved from www.wrha.mb.ca/professionals/collaborativecare/files/IPHCTC-Briefing2.pdf.

Canadian Association for Parish Nursing Ministry (CAPNM). (2017). *Parish nursing fact sheet.* Retrieved from http://www.capnm.ca/fact_sheet.htm.

Canadian Association of Community Health Centres (CASHC). (2017). *About community health centres.* Retrieved from www.cachc.ca/about-chcs/.

Canadian Association of Rehabilitation Nurses. (2017). *Mission.* Retrieved from http://carn.ca/about/.

Canadian Association of Schools of Nursing (CASN). (2015). *National nursing education framework final report.* Ottawa: CASN/ACESI.

Canadian Health Services Research Foundation (CHSRF). (2011). *Provincial and territorial health system priorities: An environmental scan.* Retrieved from www.cfhi-fcass.ca/Libraries/Commissioned_Research_Reports/EScanPTHealthSysPriorities-EN.sflb.ashx.

Canadian Health Services Research Foundation (CHSRF). (2012a). *Better health.* Ottawa, ON: CNA/CHRSF.

Canadian Health Services Research Foundation (CHSRF). (2012b). *Better care.* Ottawa, ON: CNA/CHRSF.

Canadian Home Care Association (CHCA). (2012). *CHCA on the issues: Wound care.* Retrieved from http://www.cdnhomecare.ca/content.php?doc=263.

Canadian Home Care Association (CHCA). (2013). *Portraits of home care in Canada. Executive precis.* Retrieved from http://www.cdnhomecare.ca/media.php?mid=3394.

Canadian Home Care Association (CHCA). (2014). *Advocacy: Vision of home care 2020.* Retrieved from http://www.cdnhomecare.ca/content.php?doc=243.

Canadian Hospice Palliative Care Association (CHPCA). (2013). *What Canadians say: The Way Forward survey report.* Retrieved from http://www.hpcintegration.ca/media/51032/The%20Way%20Forward%20-%20What%20Canadians%20Say%20-%20Survey%20Report%20Final%20Dec%202013.pdf.

Canadian Institutes for Health Information (CIHI) (2009). *Primary health care (PHC) indicators chartbook: An illustrative example of using PHC data for indicator reporting.* Ottawa: Author.

Canadian Institutes for Health Information (CIHI). (2015). *Canada's health care systems and health workforce by the numbers.* Retrieved from http://www.royalcollege.ca/rcsite/documents/health-policy/2015-canada-health-care-systems-by-numbers-diverty.pdf.

Canadian Institutes for Health Information (CIHI). (2016a). *Regulated nurses: Canada and jurisdictional highlights.* Ottawa, ON: CIHI.

Canadian Institutes for Health Information (CIHI). (2016b). *National health expenditure trends: 1975–2016.* Ottawa, ON: CIHI.

Canadian Institutes for Health Information (CIHI). (2016c). *Prescribed drug spending in Canada.* Ottawa, ON: CIHI.

Canadian Institutes for Health Information (CIHI). (2016d). *Primary health care in Canada: A chartbook of selected indicator results.* Ottawa, ON: CIHI.

Canadian Institutes for Health Information (CIHI). (2016e). *Measuring patient harm in Canadian hospitals.* Retrieved from https://www.cihi.ca/sites/default/files/document/hospital_harm_summary_en.pdf.

Canadian Institutes for Health Information. (2016f). *Patient harm in Canadian hospitals? It does happen.* Retrieved from https://www.cihi.ca/en/patient-harm-in-canadian-hospitals-it-does-happen-infographic.

Canadian Institutes for Health Information (CIHI). (2017). *Home care.* Retrieved from https://www.cihi.ca/en/home-care.

Canadian Institutes of Health Research (CIHR). (2016). *EIHR Portal.* Retrieved from http://www.cihr-irsc.gc.ca/e/43628.html.

Canadian Interprofessional Health Collaborative (CIHC). (2010). *A national interprofessional competency framework.* Retrieved from http://www.cihc.ca/files/CIHC_IPCompetencies_Feb1210.pdf.

Canadian Medical Association (2015). *Best practices and federal barriers: Practice and training of health professionals.* Ottawa: Author.

Canadian Medical Protective Association. (2014). *Physicians and nurse practitioners: Working collaboratively as independent health professionals.* Retrieved from https://www.cmpa-acpm.ca/-/physicians-and-nurse-practitioners-working-collaboratively-as-independent-health-professionals.

Canadian Nurses Association. (2003). Primary health care—The time has come. *Nursing Now, 16,* 1–4.

Canadian Nurses Association (CNA). (2014). *Aboriginal health nursing and Aboriginal health.* Retrieved from https://www.cna-aiic.ca/~/media/cna/page-content/pdf-en/aboriginal-health-nursing-and-aboriginal-health_charting-policy-direction-for-nursing-in-canada.pdf?la=en.

Canadian Nursing Informatics Association. (2011). *Introduction: Nursing informatics.* Retrieved from http://cnia.ca.

Canadian Occupational Health Nurses Association. (2011). *Improving the health and safety of workers by speaking with a national Canadian voice.* Retrieved from http://www.cohna-aciist.ca.

Canadian Patient Safety Institute (CPSI). (2016). *Topics.* Retrieved from http://www.patientsafetyinstitute.ca/en/topic/Pages/default.aspx.

Canadian Press. (2017). Immigrants could make up one-third of Canada's population by 2036: Stats Can. *The Star.* January 25, 2017.

Ciliska, D. (2013). *Evidence informed decision making.* Retrieved from http://ccebn.mcmaster.ca/documents/2013_%20Introduction-to-EIDM.pdf.

Now, C. N. A. (2015). *Primary care, primary health care.* Retrieved from https://canadian-nurse.com/articles/issues/2015/june-2015/cna-now?page=8.

Collier, R. (2010a). Is regionalization working? *Canadian Medical Association Journal, 182*(4), 331–332. doi:10.1503/cmaj.109-3167.

Collier, R. (2010b). Accountability key for patient charter. *Canadian Medical Association Journal, 182*(6), doi:10.1503/cmaj.109-3192.

Community Health Nurses of Canada (CHNC). (2013). *Canadian community health nursing professional practice model.* Retrieved from http://www.cna-aiic.ca/sitecore%20modules/web/~/media/cna/page-content/pdf-en/canadian_community_health_nursing_e.pdf.

Consumer Association of Canada. (2017). *Mandate and mission.* Retrieved from http://www.consumer.ca/en/mandate-and-mission/.

Consumer Health Products–Canada. (2009). *Formal recognition of self-care.* Retrieved from http://www.chpcanada.ca/en/advocacy-action/formal-recognition-self-care.

Council of Canadians. (2016). *Health care transfer payments to be discussed at federal-provincial summit.* Retrieved from https://canadians.org/blog/health-care-transfer-payments-be-discussed-federal-provincial-summit.

Dagnone, T. (2009). *For patients' sake: Patient First Commissioner report to the Saskatchewan Minister of Health.* Regina: Government of Saskatchewan, Ministry of Health.

Drummond, N., Abbott, K., Williamson, T., et al. (2012). Interprofessional primary care in academic family medicine clinics. *Canadian Family Physician, 58*(8), e450–e458.

Economist Intelligence Unit. (2015). *The 2015 Quality of Death Index ranking palliative care across the world.* Retrieved from https://www.eiuperspectives.economist.com/sites/default/files/2015%20EIU%20Quality%20of%20Death%20Index%20Oct%2029%20FINAL.pdf.

Falk-Raphael, A., & Betker, R. (2012). Witnessing social injustice downstream and advocating for health equity upstream: The trombone slide of nursing. *Advances in Nursing Science, 35*(2), 98–112. doi:10.1097/ANS.0b013e31824fe70f.

Government of Canada. (2007a). *Primary health care transition fund.* Retrieved from https://www.canada.ca/en/health-canada/services/primary-health-care/primary-health-care-transition-fund.html#a1.

Government of Canada. (2007b). *Primary health care transition fund—Funded initiatives.* Retrieved from http://www.apps.hc-sc.gc.ca/hcs-sss/phctf-fassp.nsf/WEB?ReadForm&lang=eng&.

Government of Canada. (2007c). *Newfoundland and Labrador.* Retrieved from http://www.apps.hc-sc.gc.ca/hcs-sss/phctf-fassp.nsf/WebProject/0005?OpenDocument&lang=eng&.

Government of Canada. (2010). *Indigenous and Northern Affairs Canada: Treaties with Aboriginal people in Canada.* Retrieved from https://www.aadnc-aandc.gc.ca/eng/1100100032291/1100100032292.

Government of Canada. (2016). *Corporate management reporting—health.* Retrieved from http://www.canada.ca/en/health-canada/corporate/transparency/corporate-management-reporting/report-plans-priorities.html.

Government of Canada. (2017). *Budget plan. Chapter 3—A strong Canada at home and in the world.* Retrieved from http://www.budget.gc.ca/2017/docs/plan/chap-03-en.html.

Health Canada. (2006). *Health care system—A 10-year plan to strengthen health care.* Retrieved from https://www.canada.ca/en/health-canada/services/health-care-system/health-care-system-delivery/federal-provincial-territorial-collaboration/first-ministers-meeting-year-plan-2004/10-year-plan-strengthen-health-care-backgrounders.html.

Health Canada. (2009). *Office of Nursing Policy.* Retrieved from https://www.canada.ca/en/health-canada/corporate/about-health-canada/branches-agencies/strategic-policy-branch/office-nursing-policy.html.

Health Canada. (2011). *Canada Health Act—Frequently asked questions.* Retrieved from https://www.canada.ca/en/health-canada/services/health-care-system/canada-health-care-system-medicare/canada-health-act-frequently-asked-questions.html.

Health Canada. (2012). *What is primary health care?* Retrieved from https://www.canada.ca/en/health-canada/services/primary-health-care/about-primary-health-care.html.

Health Canada. (2015). Health Canada, *Primary health care.* Retrieved from http://www.hc-sc.gc.ca/hcs-sss/prim/index-eng.php.

Health Canada. (2016a). *Canada's health care system.* Retrieved from https://www.canada.ca/en/health-canada/services/canada-health-care-system.html.

Health Canada. (2016b). *First Nations and Inuit health.* Retrieved from https://www.canada.ca/en/health-canada/services/first-nations-inuit-health.html.

Health Canada. (2016c). *Health care system—Committee on Health Workforce.* Retrieved from https://www.canada.ca/en/health-canada/services/health-care-system/health-human-resources/committee-health-workforce.html.

Health Council of Canada. (2008). *Fixing the foundation: An update on primary health care and home care renewal in Canada.* Ottawa: Author.

Healthy Debate. (2013). *Restructuring Alberta's health system.* Retrieved from http://healthydebate.ca/2013/10/topic/politics-of-health-care/restructuring-alberta-health.

Hodgson, C. (2012). *Cost-effectiveness of palliative care: A review of the literature.* Ottawa, ON: CHPCA.

Indian and Northern Affairs Canada. (2015). *Fact sheet: Aboriginal self-government.* Ottawa: Author. Retrieved from http://www.ainc-inac.gc.ca/ai/mr/is/abgov-eng.asp.

Institute of Public Administration in Canada. (2013). *Health governance models in Canada: A provincial perspective.* Toronto: Author.

Kahn, L. (2017). The one health way. *Springer Nature, 543,* S47.

Kephart, G., Maaten, S., O'Brien-Pallas, L., et al. (2004). *Building the future: An integrated strategy for nursing human resources in Canada—Research synthesis report.* Ottawa: The Nursing Sector Study Corporation. Retrieved from https://www.cna-aiic.ca/~/media/cna/page-content/pdf-fr/simulation_analysis_report_e.pdf?la=en.

Kirby, M. J. L. (2002). *The health of Canadians—The federal role. Vol. 6: Recommendations for reform.* Ottawa: Standing Senate Committee on Social Affairs, Science and Technology. Retrieved from http://www.parl.gc.ca/37/2/parlbus/commbus/senate/com-e/soci-e/rep-e/repoct02vol6-e.htm.

Kondro, W. (2010). Nation's physicians urge re-opening of Canada Health Act. *Canadian Medical Association Journal, 182*(13), doi:10.1503/cmaj.109-3352.

Lalonde, M. (1986). *Ottawa charter for health promotion: An international conference on health promotion.* Ottawa: Author.

Lazar, H., Lavis, J. M., Forest, P.-G., et al. (2013). *Paradigm freeze: Why is it so hard to reform health-care policy in Canada?* Kingston, ON: Queen's University, School of Policy Studies.

Lewis, S., & Kouri, D. (2004). Regionalization: Making sense of the Canadian experience. *Healthcare Papers, 5*(1), 12–31.

Mansell, D. (2004). *Forging the future: A history of nursing in Canada.* Ann Arbor, MI: Thomas Press.

Martin, D. H. (2012). Two-eyed seeing: a framework for understanding indigenous and non-indigenous approaches to indigenous health research. *Canadian Journal of Nursing Research, 44*(2), 20–42.

McIntosh, T., Ducie, M., Burka-Charles, M., et al. (2010). Population health and health system reform: Needs-based funding for health services in five provinces. *Canadian Political Science Review, 4*(1), 42–61.

McManus, A. (2013). Health promotion innovation in primary health care. *Australasian Medical Journal, 6*(1), 15–18. doi:10.4066/AMJ.2013.1578.

Mikkonen, J., & Raphael, D. (2013). *Social determinants of health: The Canadian facts.* Toronto: York University School of Health Policy and Management.

Nelson, M., Torchia, M. G., Mactavish, J. B., et al. (2014). Working the system: The experience of being a primary care patient. *Patient Experience Journal, 1*(1), 37–42.

Nordal, R. (2010). Workplace violence. *CBA National Administrative Law, Labour & Employment Law and Privacy & Access Law Conference.* November 26–27, 2010.

Oandasan, I. F., Gotlib, L., Conn, L., et al. (2009). The impact of space and time on interprofessional teamwork in Canadian primary health care settings: Implications for health care reform. *Primary Health Care Research and Development, 10*(2), 151–162.

Oelke, N. D., Thurston, W. E., & Arthur, N. (2013). Intersections between interprofessional practice, cultural competency, and primary healthcare. *Journal of Interprofessional Care, 27*(5), 365–372. doi:10.3109/13561820.2013.785502.

Organization of Economic Co-operation and Development (OECD). (2016a). *OECD health statistics—2014.* Retrieved from http://www.oecd.org/health/healthdata.

Organization of Economic Co-operation and Development (OECD). (2016b). *Health at a Glance 2015: OECD Indicators—Hospital beds per 1 000 population, 2000 and 2013 (or nearest year). doi:10.1787/health_glance-2015-graph75-en.*

Primaryhealthcareteams.ca. (2014). *Interdisciplinary primary care teams.* Retrieved from http://www.primaryhealthcareteams.ca.

Quality End-of-Life Care Coalition of Canada (2010). *Blueprint for action 2010 to 2020.* Ottawa: Author.

Reutter, L., & Kushner, K. (2010). Health equity through action on the social determinants of health: Taking up the challenge in nursing. *Nursing Inquiry, 17*(3), 269–280. doi:10.1111/j.1440-1800.2010.00500.x.

Romanow, R. J. (2002). *Building on values: The future of health care in Canada—Final report.* Ottawa: Commission on the Future of Health Care in Canada.

Royal Commission on Health Services (RCHS) (1965). *Hall commission report (Vol. 2).* Ottawa: Author.

Seenandan-Sookdeo, K. I. (2012). The influence of power in the Canadian healthcare system. *Clinical Nurse Specialist,* 107–112. doi:10.1097/NUR.0b013e31824590ba.

Shamian, J. (2014). The role of nursing in health care. *Revista Brasileria Enfermagem, 67*(6), 867–868.

Sodani, P. R., & Sharma, K. (2012). Strengthening primary level health service delivery: Lessons from a state in India. *Journal of Family Medicine and Primary Care, 1*(2), 127–131.

Starfield, B., Shi, L., & Macinko, J. (2005). Contribution of primary care to health systems and health. *Milbank Quarterly, 83*(3), 457–502.

Statistics Canada. (2013). *Deaths in hospital and elsewhere, Canada, provinces and territories, annual.* Retrieved from http://www5.statcan.gc.ca/cansim/a26?lang=eng&id=1020509&p2=33.

Statistics Canada. (2015). *Growth of Canadian population from 2013 to 2063.* Retrieved from http://www.statcan.gc.ca/pub/91-520-x/2014001/section02-eng.htm.

Statistics Canada. (2017). *Population, by year, by province by territory.* Retrieved from http://www.statcan.gc.ca/tables-tableaux/sum-som/l01/cst01/demo02a-eng.htm.

Storch, J. (2006). Canadian health care system. In M. McIntyre, E. Thomlinson, & C. McDonald (Eds.), *Realities of Canadian nursing: Professional, practice, and power issues* (pp. 29–53). Philadelphia: Lippincott Williams & Wilkins.

Truth and Reconciliation Commission (TRC). (2015). *Calls to action.* Retrieved from http://www.trc.ca/websites/trcinstitution/File/2015/Findings/Calls_to_Action_English2.pdf.

Vance, K., Howe, W., & Dellavalle, R. P. (2009). Social internet sites as a source of public health information. *Dermatology Clinics, 27,* 133–136.

Vanier Institute of the Family. (2017). *Family caregiving in Canada: A fact of life and a human right.* Retrieved from http://www.vanierinstitute.ca/family-caregiving-in-canada/.

Villeneuve, M. J. (2017). *Public policy and Canadian nursing: Lessons from the field.* Toronto, ON: Canadian Scholars.

Villeneuve, M., & MacDonald, J. (2006). *Towards 2020: Visions for nursing.* Ottawa: Canadian Nurses Association.

Wayland, S. V. (2006). *Unsettled: Legal and policy barriers for newcomers to Canada.* Retrieved from http://www.canada.metropolis.net/publications/pf_9_ENG_Immigration.pdf.

Wilson, D. M. (1995). *The Canadian health care system.* Edmonton: Health Canada.

World Health Organization. (1978). *Declaration of Alma-Ata: International conference on primary health care,* Alma-Ata, USSR, 6–12 September 1978. Geneva, Switzerland: Author.

World Health Organization. (1986). *The Ottawa Charter for Health Promotion: 1st International Conference on Health Promotion.* Ottawa, ON, 17–21 November.

World Health Organization. (2017). *Primary health care.* Retrieved from http://www.who.int/topics/primary_health_care/en/.

3

The Development of Nursing in Canada

Written by Sonya Grypma, PhD, RN

According to present indications there will be proportionately fewer acute cases to care for and more chronic, fewer physical and more mental breakdowns, fewer sick-a-bed patients and more sick on their feet.

—Isabel Maitland Stewart, The Education of Nurses, 1945

To answer the question of what nurses should know, we must first answer the question of what nurses should do/be doing in the next 10 years.

—Canadian Nurses Association, A Course for the Future, 1966

OBJECTIVES

Mastery of content in this chapter will enable you to:

- Define the key terms listed.
- Discuss the historical development of professional nursing.
- Discuss the historical development of nursing education in Canada.
- Discuss the historical development of nursing practice in Canada.

KEY TERMS

Baccalaureate as entry-to-practice, p. 41
Canadian Nurses Association (CNA), p. 40
Code of ethics, p. 41
Education reform, p. 41
International Council of Nurses (ICN), p. 39
Victorian Order of Nurses (VON), p. 39

MEDIA RESOURCES

http://evolve.elsevier.com/Canada/Potter/fundamentals/

- Audio Chapter Summaries
- Examination Review Questions
- Concept Map Creator
- Case Study with Questions
- Audio Glossary
- Content Updates
- Video Clips

When nursing leader Isabel Maitland Stewart made her prediction in 1945 on the future of nursing, she wrote with the belief that nursing educators should prepare nurses not for only what *is*, but also what *might be*. Anticipating what nursing practice will look like when current students graduate is an important and challenging aspect of nursing education. One way to anticipate the future of nursing is to track changing social and political trends and related health care policies—something that provincial and national nursing associations do well (see Chapter 2 for further information about health care policies). Another is to stay abreast of cutting edge research—something that nursing and health care researchers do well (see Chapter 6 for further information about research). A third way is to study nursing's past. By identifying key persons, issues, and events in nursing and how these have changed over time, this chapter intends to help readers envision nursing's future and their role in shaping it.

WHY NURSING HISTORY MATTERS

Early nurse leaders made nursing history a core component of nurses' education (Toman & Thifault, 2012). During the first wave of nursing history (1870–1970), comprehensive works like Nutting and Dock's four-volume *History of Nursing* (1907–12) were required reading in nursing programs worldwide. By the 1970s, nursing history was set aside to make way for the emerging field of nursing theory. The field sat dormant until the 1990s, when women's historians "discovered" nursing and began to reintroduce nurses to themselves. If the first wave focused on nursing leaders who established associations (Bates, Dodd, & Rousseau, 2005), the second wave of nursing history (1990 to present) includes the lives and experiences of ordinary nurses and the events and social structures that helped shape nursing into what it is today. Despite the increase in superb historical studies, nursing history had all but disappeared from the curriculum by the end of the twentieth century (Toman & Thifault, 2012). In Canada and elsewhere, small groups of historians are working actively to reintroduce history into nursing curricula (Toman & Thifault, 2012).

According to Nelson (2009), historical amnesia is dangerous. As this chapter will demonstrate, nursing history provides context, explains the present, and provides a way to look forward (Grypma, 2017). History is the basis for an informed and critical understanding of our society (Tosh, 2008). It serves as an overarching conceptual framework that allows us to more fully understand the various meanings of nursing and the different experiences of nurses (D'Antonio, 2003). Historical perspectives facilitate sharper reflection on the current system and clearer understanding of key stakeholders within and beyond it (Davey, 2012). History explains the present by recognizing that what happens in the present is not an accident; it has a past (Lynaugh, in D'Antonio & Fairman, 2010). The relationship between nursing's past and present is experienced by nurses who research history: reading historical archives can bring a profound sense of déjà-vu (Nelson, 2009). "Memory is necessary," Nelson notes. "We need to know who we are if we have any hope of knowing where we are going" (p. 787).

In 2008, the Canadian Nurses Association (CNA) developed a position statement on promoting nursing history, noting that learning from the lessons of history is "critical to advancing the profession in the interests of the Canadian public" (CNA, 2007). This statement outlined the responsibilities of nurses across the whole gamut of roles and settings to promote nursing history. The Canadian Association for Schools of Nursing (CASN) also considers nursing history an essential component of nursing education, emphasizing in the *CASN National Nursing Education Framework* (2015) that nursing programs must prepare students to demonstrate "foundational knowledge of nursing including nursing history, nursing theories, and other theories relevant to nursing practice" (p. 10). This chapter introduces readers to key nursing events and persons in Canadian nursing history, with an emphasis on the twentieth century.

CARE OF STRANGERS: THE EARLY HISTORY OF NURSING

Historians generally point to 1639 as the starting point of nursing in Canada. This is the year that the Hôtel-Dieu de Québec first opened. Hôtel-Dieu is Canada's first hospital and was the only hospital in North America at that time, other than one located in the Dominican Republic (CNA, 2013). In that sense, the roots of nursing and health care in North America may be found in the values and ideals of the European settlers in New France. At a time when knowledge of disease was primitive, technology was virtually nonexistent, and a few herbal remedies were the only medicines available, the practice of nursing developed as an integral part of the emerging health care system. Nursing care was often the sole weapon in fighting infectious disease. Its importance is underscored in accounts of the devastating epidemics of smallpox, diphtheria, cholera, typhus, trachoma, scarlet fever, and other infectious diseases that ravaged the population in continuing episodes (Paul & Ross-Kerr, 2011).

A long-established Indigenous society existed in North America before the arrival of the first settlers. At the time of the first sustained contact with European people, the estimated number of Indigenous people in North America was about 500 000 (Royal Commission on Aboriginal Peoples, 1996). Indigenous peoples also had health care knowledge of their own, including the use of herbal remedies to relieve symptoms of some diseases. Even after municipalities began to build hospitals and the number of doctors and nurses in Western Canada grew after 1890, acquiring such services remained prohibitive due to cost and distance. Thus, during the late nineteenth and early twentieth centuries, Indigenous women played essential roles within their own and newcomer communities as midwives, nurses, and caregivers. They used Indigenous knowledge to care for many White settlers in Western Canada (Burnett, 2008). In this way, Indigenous and settler groups had formalized social structures for the care of ill, injured, birthing, and dying persons long before hospitals were built and "modern" nursing was established.

The First Nurses and Hospitals in New France

From the outset of the settlement in New France, it was nurses rather than physicians who both provided and administered health care for Indigenous peoples and settlers. In 1608, Samuel de Champlain selected Quebec ("New France") as the site for a colony of settlers to support the growing fur trade. The first laywoman to provide nursing care in New France was Marie Rollet Hébert. She and her husband emigrated at the request of Champlain in 1617. Mme Hébert is known for confronting the popular notion (at that time) that Indigenous people needed to be "saved" by Europeans (CNA, 2013). Although she was a layperson, Mme Hébert extended care to Indigenous peoples and settlers who were ill, just as she would for ill family members.

The first nurses to tend the sick in a type of health care centre were male attendants at a "sick bay" established at the French garrison in Port Royal in Acadia in 1629 (Gibbon & Mathewson, 1947). The Jesuit priests, who were missionary immigrants to New France, also served as nurses. Their care for the sick aided their mission to convert Indigenous people to Christianity. Their call for assistance led to the missionary efforts of religious orders and lay persons, all of whom came to New France voluntarily to assist the Jesuits.

The first nursing mission was established in 1639 at Sillery, outside the citadel of Quebec, by three Augustinian nuns who were Hospitalières de la Miséricorde de Jésus. No sooner had they arrived when they found themselves overwhelmed with patients from the raging smallpox epidemic. As the population grew, they had enough new recruits that they no longer needed to ask for nuns to come from France to assist them. This mission later became known as Hôtel-Dieu, Quebec's first hospital. As a result of the Iroquois wars, the nuns abandoned this mission at Sillery in 1644 and moved it inside the citadel. An indication of the quality of the care provided by the nuns is the fact that 93% of the patients admitted to the Hôtel-Dieu de Québec survived (Hamelin, 1981; Rousseau, 1977).

In 1641, Jeanne Mance came to New France to found a hospital in the yet unsettled region of Ville Marie (later Montreal). Her intentions to care for the sick were viewed with suspicion by the settlers at Quebec, where they spent the winter. When she arrived at Ville Marie in 1642, Mance was the only person with health care knowledge in the new settlement. She was a leader in the community and became an inspiration for later generations of nurses (Box 3-1).

The Birth of Home Visiting

A uniquely Canadian order of nuns, the Sisters of Charity of Montreal ("Grey Nuns") was formed in 1738 by Marguerite d'Youville. They were a noncloistered order, beginning as a small group of women with charitable intentions who "agreed to combine their possessions in a house of refuge chiefly for the poor" (Gibbon & Mathewson, 1947, p. 45). They engaged in many activities in order to subsist, such as admitting wealthy paying guests to hospital as well as patients who required care. They also made military garments and tents, started a brewery and a tobacco plant, and operated a freight and cartage business (Ross-Kerr, 2011). Because what they were doing was highly unusual they were called "les soeurs grises," a derogatory term with a double meaning—the "grey nuns" and the "tipsy nuns." Still, they were respected for their work and were given a charter to take over the General Hospital of Montreal.

Health Care in the West and the Grey Nuns

In 1844, four Grey Nuns embarked on a perilous canoe journey from Montreal to St. Boniface, Manitoba, where their mission was to care for the sick. Soon after their arrival, a series of epidemics began. The nuns visited the sick at home, where they cared for people with measles,

BOX 3-1 **Milestones in Canadian Nursing History**

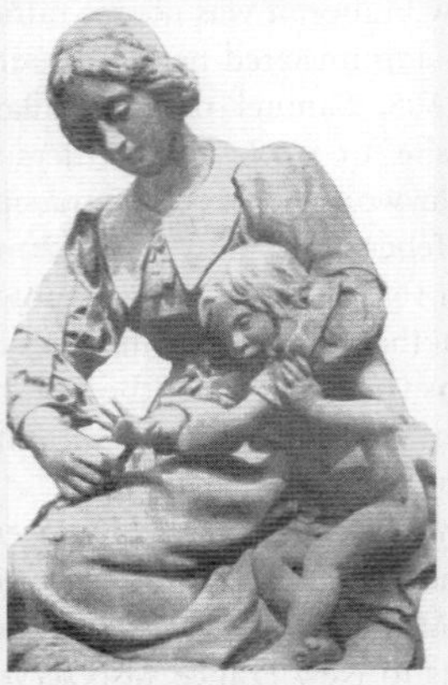

Jeanne Mance, 1606–1673

Jeanne Mance was born to a wealthy family in Langres, France, in 1606. She was the daughter of a wealthy legal advisor to the court of the King of France and decided early on to devote her life to God. She learned about New France from a cousin, a Récollet priest who had served there. She gained nursing knowledge and skills in Langres, where an epidemic of plague occurred and many people were wounded in the Thirty Years' War. Supported by a wealthy widow who wanted to finance a hospital at Ville Marie, Jeanne Mance sailed to New France with Paul de Chomédey, Sieur de Maisonneuve, and his band of 40. Maisonneuve's mission was to establish a settlement at Ville Marie, but arriving in Quebec after a 2-month voyage, the settlers learned that the governor was suspicious of their mission, and he tried to dissuade them from it.

They decided that it was too late in the summer to try to build the colony, so they remained in Quebec, involving themselves in the community. Mance spent time learning about nursing and health care in New France from the Augustinian nuns in their hospital.

In the spring, the settlers set out for Ville Marie in three boats and immediately began building houses and the Hôtel-Dieu. The next year, during an attack by the Iroquois, several settlers were killed, and others were taken hostage. The remaining settlers managed to finish the hospital and build a stockade around their colony. However, the attacks increased, and Mance was kept busy caring for both wounded settlers and Indigenous people. By 1649, the settlers' funds were low, and the colony was close to having to disband. Mance sailed to Paris, where she raised money and recruited settlers. Over the next few years, relations with the Iroquois continued to be poor. A guard was placed at the hospital and Mance slept within the fort. In 1650, the Iroquois killed 30 of 70 settlers.

Maisonneuve went to France in 1651 to gain further support and did not return for 2 years. This period was difficult, but Mance held the colony together during his absence. After a truce was reached between the French and the Iroquois in 1654, Mance was able to move back to the Hôtel-Dieu. In 1657, Mance fell on the ice, fractured her right arm in two places, and dislocated her wrist; as a result, she experienced continuing disability. She decided to make another trip to France to ask the order of nuns at La Flèche to come and help her in the hospital. While in Paris, during prayer at the Seminary of Saint Sulpice, she discovered she could move her arm without pain, and it healed miraculously. She returned to the colony, then made her last trip to France in 1663, again to solicit funding for the colony because it was, again, close to bankruptcy. En route back, she contracted typhus and nearly died. She was shocked to find upon her return that Maisonneuve had been replaced as governor. In declining health, Mance was less able to help at the hospital. She died peacefully in her sleep in 1673.

As well as founding and managing the Hôtel-Dieu, Mance assisted Maisonneuve in running the colony as confidant, advisor, and accountant. She is hailed as a founder of the city of Montreal. Today, the Canadian Nurses Association awards its highest honour in her name.

dysentery, and smallpox, and treated them with medicines and local herbs.

In 1859, another group of Grey Nuns travelled from Montreal by rail through the United States and then North to St. Boniface. They set off by ox cart over rough terrain to arrive in what is now Alberta to establish their first mission in Lac Ste. Anne. Arriving before most of the settlers, the nuns established systems of health care to care for the sick, eventually including a separate hospital building. They also established small missions in what is now northern Saskatchewan and the Northwest Territories to provide health care in Indigenous settlements. In 1895, they were asked to construct a hospital in Edmonton (the General Hospital) because settlement was burgeoning there.

During the Northwest Rebellion of 1885, nurses and physicians were called to duty to care for those wounded in the rebellion of Métis and First Nations people against the governing authority of the Dominion of Canada. Among those who responded to the call for "trained" nurses were six Sisters of St. John the Divine, under the leadership of Mother Hannah Grier Coombs. Established in Toronto only a year earlier as the first Canadian Anglican Sisterhood, the group arrived at the base hospital in Moose Jaw after a 6-week journey from Toronto. Two months after Louis Riel's surrender, the nuns returned to Toronto, where they established the first surgical hospital for women (Domm, 2010).

The Lady With the Lamp: Florence Nightingale

The movement to improve standards of nursing care in the mid-nineteenth century was spearheaded by Florence Nightingale, who is considered the founder of modern nursing. Nightingale was first brought to public attention in 1854, shortly after she was appointed superintendent of English nurses in Turkey during the Crimean War (1853–56). Nightingale was among those in London who were horrified by newspaper stories from Crimea. The detailed coverage and immediacy of the news "shattered the façade of a competent army high command and ignited a storm of outrage" (Dossey, 1998, p. 109). When a *London Times* correspondent drew attention to the lack of British nurses, Nightingale readily agreed to take a team of nurses to the war (McDonald, 2001). After arriving at Scutari, Nightingale was revolted by the filth, disease, and mortality. Through her reforms, the soldier mortality rate was reduced from 42% to just 2.2% in 6 months. War correspondents were enamored by Miss Nightingale. *The Times* described her as a "ministering angel without any exaggeration in these hospitals, and as her slender form glides quietly along each corridor, every poor fellow's face softens with gratitude at the sight of her" (cited in Dossey, 1998, p. 112).

Critical public acclaim for her work in the Crimea, in which the lives of thousands of wounded British soldiers were saved through good nursing, riveted public attention on the need for change. In 1855, while Nightingale was still in the Crimea, the English government established a "Nightingale Fund" that would be used to promote nurses' training in England. By the time Nightingale returned to England, in 1856, she was a national heroine. A flattering poem published by American poet H. W. Longfellow in 1857 solidified her reputation as the Lady with the Lamp, whose presence transformed the lives of miserable, hospitalized soldiers. It reads, in part:

> *Lo! In that house of misery/ a lady with a lamp I see/ pass through the glimmering doom/ and flit from room to room/ and slow, as in a dream of bliss/ the speechless sufferer turns to kiss/ her shadow, as it falls/ upon the darkening walls.*
>
> ***(Longfellow, 1857, in Grypma, 2005a, p. 25)***

The Nightingale Fund was used to establish the first Nightingale School of Nursing, at St. Thomas' Hospital London, in 1860. Nightingale did not work in the school herself; it followed an administrative model she created. The Nightingale system of education ("Nightingale model") became the standard for nursing in England, and around the world, for the next century. The Nightingale model was a hospital-based model overseen by a trained superintendent, trained staff members who also acted as instructors, and a cadre of nursing students who provided the bulk of the care.

In 1860 Nightingale also published her book *Notes on Nursing.* Its first edition sold out within a month (Dossey, 1998). Focused more on health than illness care, it was designed for use in the home by lay women and nurses. In it, Nightingale stressed the need for good environmental conditions, like clean air and water, that would allow nature to cure naturally. The nurses' role was to put the patients in the best position for nature to act upon them. This was the formula she had used to such good effect in the Crimea.

Brought up in a wealthy family, Nightingale railed against the customs of her time that did not allow middle- and upper-class women to work outside the home: "Why have women passion, intellect, moral activity—these three— and a place in society where no one of the three can be exercised?" (Nightingale, 1872/1979, p. 25). She was well educated and, against the wishes of her family, sought to prepare herself for nursing in 1850 by travelling to Kaiserwerth, Germany, where she worked with the German deaconesses under Pastor Fliedner. In 1853, she accepted the post of superintendent at Harley Street Hospital in London. Soon after, reports reached London of the appalling conditions for British wounded soldiers. It was Sidney Herbert, British Secretary of State at War and a personal friend of Nightingale, who asked her to organize a group of nurses to go to the Crimea in 1854.

Nightingale's success in the Crimea and following work triggered a remarkable shift in public attitudes toward the acceptability of women doing nursing outside the home. At the same time, advances in health care and the expansion in the number and importance of hospitals created a need for nurses, and the nursing profession became one of the most significant avenues of work for women. Nursing became an instrument of women's emancipation against the prevailing middle-class restrictions on women working outside the home.

After her service during the Crimean War, Nightingale became an advocate for the health of people, health care reform, and educational preparation for nursing. She made her views known through voluminous writings and lobbied members of parliament to act on her views. She drew her conclusions from health data that she collected and analyzed, and she became the first female statistician. The 16-volume *Collected Works of Florence Nightingale* (2001–2012) by Lynn McDonald makes available the full range of Nightingale's written work. Nightingale responded viscerally to situations that frustrated and angered her, including the lack of an active role for women in Victorian society and the lack of social action by religious men and women in general. Nurses can learn from her intellectual mischief, unquenchable curiosity, and stubborn resistance to the status quo (Grypma, 2005b).

GLOBALIZATION AND THE EMERGENCE OF MODERN NURSING

The history of modern nursing, at its heart, is a story of globalization. Nursing history is strewn with examples of nurses travelling across geographic and national boundaries to bring nursing service and training to communities in need (Grypma & Wu, 2012). In 1639 the first Catholic *religieuses hospitalières* sailed to New France to work at the Hôtel-Dieu de Québec (Violette, 2005). In 1819 France sent the Sisters of St. Joseph of Cluny to West Africa to engage in medical missions in Senegal (Grundmann, 2005). In 1844 the Grey Nuns travelled from Montreal to remote settlements in Canada's west and north where, in some regions, their influence has continued until the present day (Canadian Broadcasting Corporation, 2010). Indeed, Catholic religious orders were instrumental in the development of hospitals and nursing services in the United States, Canada, and Australia (Nelson, 2001; Paul, 2005). At the same time that Florence Nightingale's formal, standardized method of hospital-based nurses' training and practice was gaining popularity, a unique set of sociopolitical factors converged to set the stage for a new Anglo-Protestant brand of missionary nursing—and the birth of Canada's overseas missionary nursing movement.

Missionary Nursing

The importance of Christian missions to three centuries of Canadian nursing peaked with the missionary movement that started in China in the late 1880s and spread across the globe. In the late 1880s, China's defeat in the Opium Wars, the women's suffrage movement, the establishment of professional nursing education, advances in transportation, and the evangelistic student missionary movement converged to provide an unprecedented opportunity for unmarried, ambitious, and intelligent women looking for a way to express their religion in practical terms—as missionary nurses (Grypma & Wu, 2012). When the Presbyterian Church in Canada commissioned its first missionary nurse, Harriet Sutherland, to China in 1888, it initiated a wave of an estimated 100 Canadian missionary nurses to China (Figure 3-1). Before Mao Zedong's expulsion of foreigners from China in 1949, these Canadian nurses helped to establish hospitals and training schools in at least five provinces of China. They were among the cadre of Western missionaries credited with the birth and growth of modern nursing in China (Grypma, 2008). Although Canadian missionary nursing would continue in other regions, after the closure of the China field in 1949, missionary nursing moved from the centre to the margins of Canadian nursing practice (Grypma, 2007), largely ending the missionary era of nursing.

Canadian nurses' interest in international work continued past the missionary era, with the movement of Canadian nurses into postwar organizations such as the World Health Organization (WHO), which was established in 1948. Lyle Creelman, for example, was one among a number of Canadian nurses who worked with the United Nations Relief and Rehabilitation Administration (UNRRA), an international

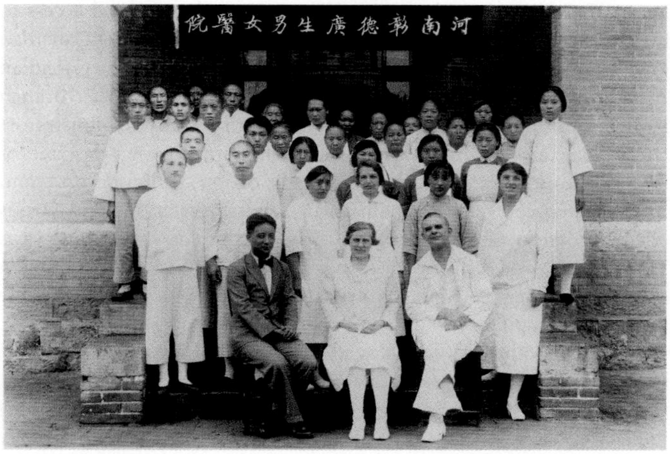

FIGURE 3-1 Canadian missionary nurses in Huaiqing, China, during the 1930s. (United Church of Canada Archives, Toronto. Access #1999.001P-1657.)

relief agency that operated between 1943 and 1947. UNRRA's mandate was to administer relief for victims of war through provision of essential services, including medical services. Its functions were later transferred to the WHO. Canadian nurse Margaret Jackson was employed by the WHO in Iran from 1954 to 1956 (Wytenbroek, 2015). Lyle Creelman became the chief nursing officer of the WHO from 1954 to 1968 (Armstrong-Reid, 2014).

Nursing in Remote Regions and Indigenous Communities

Remote nursing is a distinguishing feature of Canadian nursing. Outpost and outport nursing stations provided care for northern, newcomer, and Indigenous communities dispersed across Canada's vast landscape before physicians and other health care providers arrived in these areas. Since the early twentieth century, people living in regions considered too small or too remote for hospitals or physician care have depended on nurses for their health care needs. Nursing work in remote regions was crucial and all-encompassing. In the absence of physicians, nurses in outpost and outport nursing stations have provided public health, diagnostic, and emergency medical services. Nurses have learned and practised medical skills independently through necessity. Having experienced high levels of independence, northern nurses have resented and resisted situations that call for subservience to physicians or other "southern" authorities keen to restrict their care (Rutherdale, 2010).

The Grenfell Mission relied heavily on nurses in its efforts to provide health care for people living along hundreds of miles of coastline in Newfoundland and Labrador between 1894 and 1981. In addition to standard nursing duties, the station nurse's responsibilities involved operating the dispensary, midwifery, public health, first aid, and dentistry (Coombs-Thorne, 2010). Similarly, nurses working at Red Cross outpost stations in Ontario between 1922 and 1984 acquired diverse skills considered more in the purview of physicians, including suturing wounds, administering anaesthesia, taking X-rays, and diagnosing illnesses (Elliott, 2010) (Figure 3-2).

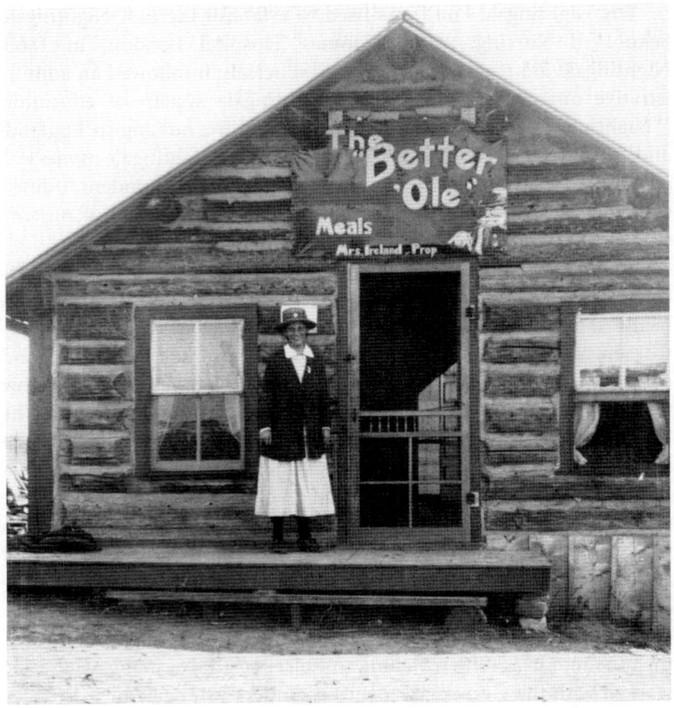

FIGURE 3-2 Red Cross nurse stopping for lunch, Pouce Coupe, British Columbia, circa 1920s. (Glenbow Archives, NA-2903-67.)

Prior to World War II, living conditions for northern populations—primarily Indigenous—were appalling. Most Western health care to the Arctic was provided under the auspices of Anglican and Roman Catholic churches, as "home" missions. In northern Saskatchewan there was an almost complete absence of government-run services. The end of World War II brought an onset of resource development in northern regions of Canada. As a result of the federal 1957 *Hospital Insurance and Diagnostic Services Act* and subsequent provincial legislation, Canadians have come to expect universal and equal access to hospitals and health care services (Meijer-Drees, 2013). The Canadian government increased its efforts to provide health care in the Canadian Arctic and, by 1963, the "Indian and Northern Health Services" branch had a staff of 2 500 nurses, doctors, dentists, and administrators (Rutherdale, 2010). In northern Saskatchewan, nursing was one of many institutions introduced into the region to modernize and improve people's lives (McBain, 2010). Nursing stations and nurses played a vital role in providing much-needed professional health care. Those who worked in these settings had the opportunity to develop skills, confidence, and independence not typical of—or transferrable to—urban hospital settings.

It is important to note that while Canada's publicly funded universal health care system represents an "almost sacred hallmark of what we collectively believe defines Canadian society," social history of medical services reveals a clear difference in the substance and delivery of health care to Indigenous and non-Indigenous populations (Meijer-Drees, 2013, XVII). Between the 1940s and 1970s, Canada's federal government offered Indigenous peoples separate health care services from that available to non-Indigenous Canadian citizens. One of the key objectives of the Canadian Indigenous Nurses Association (2010) is to engage in and conduct research on Indigenous health nursing and Indigenous peoples' access to health care. Emerging historical research into the human side of Indigenous health care—that is, based on the voices and stories of the people who experienced Canada's Indian Health Services (Meijer-Drees, 2013)—will help nurses to more fully understand, and respond appropriately to, the health care needs of Indigenous peoples.

Gender and Diversity in Nursing

For much of its early history, nursing in Canada was considered a suitable profession for young, unmarried, White, Christian women (Grypma, 2008). In the early twentieth century there was an unwritten rule that Canadian nursing schools would not admit non-White or non-English-speaking students; nor would they admit men. In 1931, less than 1% of graduate nurses listed themselves as being of Indian, Japanese, or Chinese origin; 94% were of British or French ancestry (Kulig & Grypma, 2006). When Chinese and Japanese-Canadian women were admitted to Vancouver General Hospital in the 1930s, it was on the assumption that they would work in "their own" communities (McPherson, in Kulig & Grypma, 2006, p. 14). Black Canadian nurses who entered nursing in the 1950s had been subjected to legal ordinances as children that created separate facilities for Blacks and Whites. The few who were allowed into nursing programs were placed in segregated residences (Flynn, 2009). Such exclusionary practices were common. Even patients were segregated on the basis of culture and ethnicity. For example, in early twentieth-century British Columbia (prior to 1920), Chinese and Japanese communities organized and financed private hospitals to serve their local communities, for both humanitarian and political ends (Vandenberg, 2015). In the 1930s the Vancouver General Hospital had a "foreign ward" for Chinese, Hindu, Mexican, and Japanese patients (Grypma, 2008).

Since the 1960s and 1970s, the profession has become increasingly aware of the need for gender balance and social diversity in nursing. As a profession, nursing is in transition from one that has been predominantly female in character to one that is gender balanced. Traditional societal values that negate nurturing roles for men have been changing. However, even though the number of men employed in nursing in Canada has increased, the most recent statistics show the proportion of male nurses as only 6.4% of the total nurse population, a slight increase over the 4.7% it represented in 2000 (CNA, 2012). Meadus and Twomey (2011) note that while women have been moving into previously male-dominated health professions such as medicine and pharmacy, the movement of men into nursing is slow. They argue that nursing education could be more proactive in promoting an appropriate learning environment for male students. For example, male students would benefit from clinical placements with male registered nurses, placement in clinical groups with at least one other man, and assignment of female and male patients (Meadus & Twomey, 2011). Still, although many factors have deterred men from pursuing careers in nursing, some of the negative influences are slowly beginning to change.

Canadian society has also become more multicultural. The increase in racial, ethnic, and cultural diversity has meant that individuals of different races, ethnic descent, and cultural backgrounds are present in every major population and occupational group. The benefit to Canada of this diversity is inestimable and provides a far richer background for local, national, and global relationships. Some groups have historically been underrepresented in certain professions, including nursing, in comparison with their representation in the population. Recognition of the contributions of different ethnic and cultural groups, including Indigenous groups, to the cultural mosaic in Canadian society has been slow in coming but is gaining traction.

In 2003, Villeneuve (2002–2003) decried the fact that the majority of nurses in Canada remained White and female. There has since been pressure for the profession to address the need for cultural diversity and to create a truly integrated health care workforce that embraces all types of diversity (Registered Nurses Association of Ontario [RNAO], 2007). This includes diversity based on culture, religion, ethnicity, gender, ability, and sexual orientation, with growing awareness of a need to reflect and address lesbian, gay, bisexual, transgendered, intersexed, and queer (LGBTQ+) patient health needs (Dysart-Gale, 2010).

NURSING EDUCATION IN CANADA

In 1860, Florence Nightingale established a financially independent school of nursing in association with St. Thomas's Hospital in London, England, with funds from the Nightingale Fund, a large sum of money from unsolicited donations to Nightingale in appreciation for her work in the Crimea. However, the educational model of the Nightingale school was missing from the new hospital schools in Canada. This was largely because the new schools had no financing and required students to provide nursing service to the hospital in return for their education and living expenses, which enabled hospitals to provide nursing services at minimal cost. The race to establish hospitals in the early 1890s was undoubtedly spurred on by the financial benefits of establishing associated schools of nursing. The financial advantage to the hospital of operating a school of nursing was clear, and this led to the need for hospitals to establish schools of nursing to give them a competitive edge relative to other institutions to which paying patients might turn for care. Operating a training school also provided security against incurring a financial loss if the number of paying patients dropped at any point. Therefore, the education of nurses became closely associated with hospitals as Canada established both hospitals and schools of nursing. A training school attached to a hospital ensured a higher standard of care than one without a school (Young, 1994).

The First Canadian Nursing Schools

The first hospital diploma school in Canada, the St. Catharines Training School, opened in 1874 at the St. Catharines General and Marine Hospital. Admission standards were "plain English education, good character, and Christian motives" (*St. Catharines Annual Report*, cited by Healey, 1990). Students learned chemistry, sanitary science, physiology, anatomy, and hygiene. They were taught to observe patients for changes in temperature, skin condition, pulse, respirations, and functions of organs and to report "faithfully" to the attending physician (Healey, 1990).

The School for Nurses at the Toronto General Hospital was established in 1881; Mary Agnes Snively was appointed superintendent in 1884 (Box 3-2). Although work and living conditions were poor, Snively worked hard to improve the program. In 1896, she introduced a 3-year course with 84 hours of practical nursing and 119 hours of instruction by the medical staff (Gibbon & Mathewson, 1947).

The move to establish hospital schools of nursing swept the country. In 1887 the Winnipeg General Hospital initiated the first Training School for Nurses in Western Canada. A measure of its success was that 134 of its graduates served as nurses in World War I (Gibbon & Mathewson, 1947). By 1890, hospitals in Montreal, Fredericton, Saint John, Halifax, and Charlottetown had opened schools. Vancouver General Hospital began a school in 1891, and in Alberta, a school was opened in Medicine Hat in 1894. By 1930, there were approximately 330 schools of nursing in Canada (CNA, 1968).

The Impact of Nursing Organizations on Nursing Education

The Victorian Order of Nurses. At the same time that hospital training schools for nurses were being established, nurses began to advocate for improved educational standards and passage of legislation for their profession. Women's associations were instrumental in the public health care crusade in Canada and in the rise of nursing organizations. The National Council of Women, under the presidency of Lady Ishbel Aberdeen, wife of the governor general of Canada, approved the formation of the Victorian Order of Nurses (VON) in 1898. Lady Aberdeen had conceived the idea of establishing the VON after she discovered the plight of women in Western Canada who had to give birth in remote locations with no assistance. The formation of the VON signified a professional standard of education for Canadian nurses that recognized the need not only for altruism and compassion but also for nursing knowledge (Figure 3-3).

The International Council of Nurses. The International Council of Nurses (ICN) started out as a small organization in the broader context of the women's movement (Boschma, 2014). The organization was founded in 1899 as the initiative of British nurse and suffragist Ethel Gordon Manson (later Mrs. Bedford Fenwick), a prominent leader in the British Nurses Association. The goals for the founders of the ICN were the professional welfare of nurses, the interests of women, and the improvement of the people's health. The founding members were part of a growing number of women who were active in social and health care reform and who simultaneously sought to improve women's social position, including the right to vote (Boschma, 2014, p. 115).

In 1899, Bedford Fenwick founded the ICN, with Britain, Germany, and the United States as member organizations. Nations without national nursing organizations could not become members. Although Canada did not yet have a national nursing organization, Mary Agnes

BOX 3-2 Milestones in Canadian Nursing History

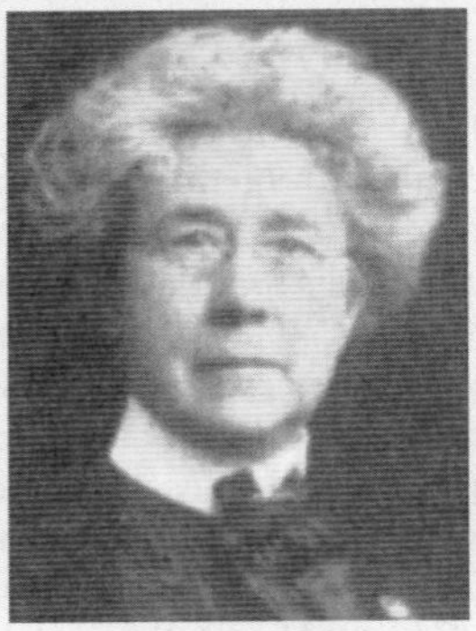

Mary Agnes Snively, 1847–1933

Born in St. Catharines, Ontario, Mary Agnes Snively was a teacher before she was a nurse. Upon graduation from the school of nursing at Bellevue Hospital, New York, in 1894, she was appointed Lady Superintendent of Nurses at Toronto General Hospital and director of the school of nursing. The school, founded along with the hospital 3 years earlier, was in a state of disorganization.

Students provided most of the nursing care at Toronto General Hospital, at little cost to the hospital. Snively found no organized plan for classes or clinical experience, nor was there a residence (students were housed in various locations in the hospital). Written records of nursing care, medical orders, and client histories were also lacking. Recruiting desirable applicants was difficult because students in the school faced so many hardships that parents were reluctant to allow their daughters to seek admission.

Snively rectified all of these deficiencies. A residence was soon built; she developed a curriculum plan, including nursing theory and practice; and she lengthened the education period to 3 years. By the end of her tenure in 1910, the Toronto General Hospital school was thriving as the largest school of nursing in Canada with hundreds of graduates, a full complement of students, and many more seeking admission. All parental skepticism had been overcome, and Toronto General Hospital served as a model for others across the country.

Snively achieved acclaim for her organizational work. She helped found the first nurses' alumnae association in Canada at Toronto General Hospital in 1894. She also attended the historic 1899 founding meeting of the International Council of Nurses (ICN) in London, England, and was elected first honorary treasurer of the ICN, even though Canada did not have the necessary national nursing association to become an ICN member at the time. In 1907, Snively established the Canadian Society of Superintendents of Training Schools of Nursing, and, recognizing that an organization that would include all nurses would be needed for Canada to become a member of the ICN, she was the driving force behind the 1908 founding of the Provisional Organization of the Canadian National Association of Trained Nurses (later the CNA), becoming its first president. She shepherded the entry of the fledgling Canadian organization to membership in the ICN and served later as ICN vice president.

Gibbon, J. M., & Mathewson, M. S. (1947). *Three centuries of Canadian nursing.* Toronto, ON: Macmillan; and Riegler, N. (1997). *Jean I. Gunn, nursing leader.* Markham, ON: Associated Medical Services with Fitzhenry and Whiteside.

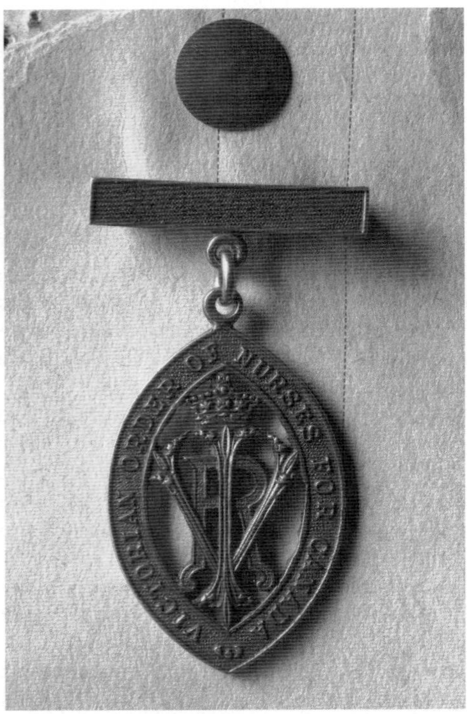

FIGURE 3-3 **Victorian Order of Nurses badge, Edmonton, Alberta, 1927.** (Glenbow Archives, NC-6-12085.)

Snively was elected the first treasurer of the ICN until 1904 (CNA, 2013). The formation of the ICN was a catalyst in organizing Canadian nurses. The *Canadian Nurse* journal was established in 1905. Initially envisioned as a way to connect the alumnae of nursing schools, it became a national nurse's journal "to aid in uniting and uplifting the profession and in keeping alive that esprit de corps and desire to grow better and wiser in work and life" (CNA, 2013, p. 16). While others focused on establishing a national journal, Snively focused on organizing superintendents of nursing schools. In 1907 she was named the first president of the Canadian Society of Superintendents of Training Schools for Nurses (CSSTN). In 1908, the new Canadian Association of Trained Nurses (CNATN, later CNA) was established, with Snively as its first president. In 1909, the CNATN was officially welcomed into the ICN. For almost a century the ICN has sustained its place as the key organization for uniting nurses around the globe (Boschma, 2014, p. 115). In 2013, Judith Shamian became the third Canadian nurse to serve as ICN president (Alice Girard was the first Canadian resident elected to presidency, in 1965; Euphemia Jane Taylor was born in Canada but had immigrated to the United States at the time of her presidency in 1937) (CNA, 2013, p. 230).

The Origins of the Canadian Nurses Association and Provincial Nursing Associations

After becoming a full-fledged member of the ICN in 1909, the CNATN streamlined its organization when registration of nurses was established through legislation in each province. Its name was changed to the **Canadian Nurses Association (CNA)** in 1924, and it became a federation of provincial associations in 1930 (CNA, 1968).

The struggle for women's rights helped nurses to secure laws to regulate their profession. Nurses formed provincial nurses' associations and sought legislation that would set educational standards and improve nursing care. The first province to gain legislation was Nova Scotia, where a voluntary registration act was passed in 1910. It also allowed nongraduate nurses to register. Initial acts passed in other provinces contained more restrictive standards. Admission criteria and curricula were set for nursing schools, as were rules governing the registration and discipline of practising nurses.

Provincial or territorial legislation and regulations are used to grant qualified nurses the legal authority to use the title "registered nurse" or "RN" (CNA, 2015). The distinguishing feature of mandatory rather than permissive legislation is a statute containing a definition of the scope of nursing practice, as well as protecting the use of the title of *registered nurse.* Permissive legislation only protects the title of *registered nurse* (Wood, 2011). Licensure laws are designed to protect the public against unqualified and incompetent practitioners.

In 1979 Sister Simone Roach was appointed by the CNA to develop a new code of ethics for Canadian nurses (Meyers, 2013). Roach identified two underlying values: "(1) Caring as a unique focus of nursing and (2) Respect for persons, and its related principle, the sanctity of human life" (Meyers, 2013, p. 238). Approved by the CNA Board of Directors in 1980, the code intended to provide meaningful guidelines for nurses experiencing ethical conflicts in daily practice. Through its various iterations since then, the *CNA Code of Ethics for Registered Nurses* (2017) has remained a value-based, rather than a rule-based, code for Canadian nurses (Storch, in Meyers, 2013).

The First University Programs

The devastating consequences of World War I and the influenza pandemic of 1918 led to support for public health programs and new patterns of health care delivery. Community health care was promoted, and nurses were seen as central participants who needed university-level education. To this end, the Canadian Red Cross Society awarded grants to a number of Canadian universities to develop postgraduate courses in public health nursing: University of Toronto, McGill University, University of British Columbia, University of Alberta, Dalhousie University, and University of Western Ontario (Canadian Red Cross Society, 1962).

The first Canadian undergraduate nursing degree program was established at the University of British Columbia in 1919, with Ethel Johns as director. The operating costs of the new department were to be borne by the hospital, an incentive for the university to support the program. The program was nonintegrated—that is, "the university assumed no responsibility for the two or three years of nursing preparation in a hospital school of nursing" (Bonin, 1976, p. 7).

Several new 5-year, nonintegrated degree programs began at Canadian universities in the 1920s and 1930s: University of Western Ontario, University of Alberta, l'Institut Marguerite d'Youville, University of Ottawa, and St. Francis Xavier University. The University of Toronto was the first in Canada to approve a degree in nursing, in 1942.

HEALTH CARE AND EDUCATIONAL REFORM

The Weir Report

Between 1874, when the first Canadian nursing school was opened, and the 1930s, when Canada boasted 330 hospital training schools (Paul & Ross-Kerr, 2011), nursing education remained virtually unchanged; hospitals used an apprenticeship-style training (Pijl-Zieber, Grypma, & Barton, 2014). Nursing students were the primary means of staffing hospitals. Hospitals provided a low-cost education; students provided a low-cost service. Growing concern about the quality of nursing education and exploitation of nursing students led to a nationwide study on nursing education, jointly funded by the CNA and the Canadian Medical Association (CMA). The resultant Survey of Nursing Education in Canada (Weir, 1932) confirmed widespread insufficient classroom instruction and lack of variety in clinical experience. The report recommended that nurse preparation be transferred from hospitals to the general education system, and that nurses receive adequate liberal arts as well as technical education at the degree level. Despite these recommendations, by the 1960s, 95% of Canadian nurses were still being trained in hospitals (Pijl-Zieber, Grypma, & Barton, 2014).

Education Reform

Preparing a sufficient number of graduate nurses became the rallying cry of the 1940s, both during the war and throughout the late 1940s and 1950s. In the expansionist years of the 1960s, nursing leaders called for nursing education reform: better-prepared faculty in schools, and high quality and standards as priorities in nursing education programs. Sparked by an interest in accreditation, the CNA sponsored a second nationwide survey of nursing education, conducted by Helen Mussallem. The resultant 1960 *Spotlight on Nursing Education* found that only 16% of schools met criteria for accreditation (Pijl-Zieber et al., 2014). Mussallem's recommendation that the CNA focus on upgrading nursing education led to a 1964 report, *A Path to Quality*, intended to prepare a plan to revise nursing education. The 1965 Royal Commission on Health Services, led by Justice Emmett Hall, called for separation of nursing education from hospital services (Baker, 2014). Both reports recommended a two-tiered education system with baccalaureate-prepared leaders and diploma-prepared bedside nurses (Baker, 2014; Pijl-Zieber et al., 2014). Hall's report successfully launched the demise of the hospital training schools and the addition of 10 baccalaureate nursing programs.

Baccalaureate as Entry-to-Practice

By the 1960s, a movement to separate nursing education programs from the authority of hospitals began in earnest. Two-year programs in nursing began to appear, and Ontario, Quebec, and Saskatchewan developed a system of diploma education based entirely in community colleges. This transfer of diploma programs to the general education system was in full swing when the Alberta Task Force on Nursing Education recommended in 1975 that all new graduates be prepared at the baccalaureate level before entering professional practice. The position was endorsed by the Alberta Association of Registered Nurses in 1976.

The reluctance of provincial governments over two decades to endorse the baccalaureate standard for entry to the practice of nursing reflected the fact that equality in education for women in nursing did not come easily.

In 1982, the CNA approved a resolution for baccalaureate as entry-to-practice (BETP) with a target date of the year 2000. The entry-to-practice position stipulated that all new graduates in nursing must be qualified at the baccalaureate level when they entered the professional practice of nursing. The year 2000 was initially set as a goal for implementation. Although this position originally was put forward by a government committee in Alberta in 1975, it became a highly valued goal of the nursing profession across the country in less than a decade. When nursing organizations put forward their statements supporting the position, they hoped that the position would become a reality by the expected date. At the same time, they recognized from the outset that achieving the position would be unlikely by the year 2000; it was simply a target date to assist with moving toward the goal. Contrary to what many believed, the position never had any kind of legal or political mandate.

By 1988, when the New Brunswick Association of Registered Nurses endorsed the position, all provincial associations had declared their support (CNA, 1991). The announcement by the premier of New Brunswick in 1992 that the baccalaureate degree should be a prerequisite to the practice of nursing was the first such endorsement by a first minister of a Canadian province (Nurses Association of New Brunswick, 1992). Implementation of the baccalaureate standard occurred first in Prince Edward Island in 1992 but would not have been the case without the strong support of its provincial government. Slowly but surely other provincial governments endorsed the position and made adjustments in the capacity of their provincial degree-granting nursing education programs to accommodate all students studying nursing at the undergraduate level. Between 2000 and 2010, BETP was realized throughout Canada, with the exception of Quebec (Baker, 2014).

INFLUENCE OF PERIODS OF SOCIAL UPHEAVAL ON NURSING

Public Health, Military Conflicts, and the Emergence of University Nursing Education

The struggle for social equality, which became a rallying cry for women in the first quarter of the twentieth century, also took hold on the prairies where the energies of women and men alike were required to work the land and to provide the services that were necessary in a frontier milieu. Women in Western Canada became seriously involved in commenting on needs in health and education and developed organizations to put forward their ideas. Five Alberta women—Nellie McClung, Emily Murphy, Henrietta Muir Edwards, Louise McKinney, and Irene Parlby—pressed forward with "the persons case," petitioning the Supreme Court of Canada and ultimately the Privy Council of Great Britain to declare that women were "persons" and, as such, could be elected to public office. Education had long been viewed by women as a means of surmounting perceived inequities in society. This was also true in nursing, as confirmed by Baumgart and Kirkwood (1990): "Nursing within the university metaphorically represents the struggle of women to have their experience and knowledge validated and legitimized, and their professional expertise recognized as a university discipline" (p. 510).

Canadian nurses who served in the military during World War I (1914–1918) left an extraordinary legacy (Toman, 2016). During that time, a small cadre of 2 845 women cared for over 750 000 patients in 135 medical units over the duration of the war. Serving mostly in France, England, and the Mediterranean, these nurses worked close to the front lines or along evacuation routes to military hospitals, adapting their nursing to extreme wartime conditions. Although recognized through public memorials, such as the CNA War Memorial in Canada's Parliament Buildings, it is only recently that their work has been a subject of serious study (Toman, 2016) (Figure 3-4).

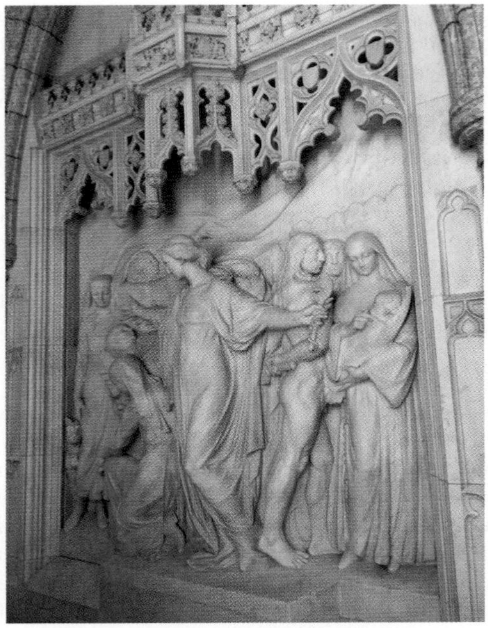

FIGURE 3-4 **Canadian Nurses Association (CNA) Memorial at the Parliament Buildings in Ottawa, Canada.** (Courtesy Sonya Grypma, RN, PhD.)

The devastating consequences of the war were compounded by the worldwide influenza epidemic of 1918 and 1919. Concerns over the "Spanish flu" led to support for public health programs and new patterns of health care delivery to prevent disease and improve the health and well-being of the Canadian populace. The impetus for the introduction of nursing programs to the university, then, was the perceived need for additional and highly capable nursing staff for public health work. In the aftermath of World War I, the impact of casualties and disability led to new value being placed on promoting and maintaining health. The health of mothers and children was seen as particularly critical to the nation because nurturing the health of the young was believed to raise the likelihood that the adult population of the future would be healthier than that of the past. In the new movement to promote health in the community, nurses were seen as central players with a need for additional, university-level preparation for their work.

Because of these issues, the Canadian Red Cross Society became a partner in establishing the League of Red Cross Societies and in planning an international program for peacetime activity in public health: "It was decided that there should be a great worldwide public health organization to help bring up the standards of physical and mental fitness of the world … the promotion of health, the prevention of disease and the mitigation of suffering throughout the world" (Gibbon & Mathewson, 1947, p. 342). This organization served as a catalyst for the development of university programs in nursing. A national committee was formed with representatives from the Canadian National Association of Trained Nurses, the Canadian Red Cross Society, and the St. John Ambulance Association and they endorsed resolutions on September 10, 1919 to approach the universities with a view to support the establishment of nursing departments (Canadian Red Cross Society, 1962). This was followed by 3-year grants from the Canadian Red Cross Society to six Canadian universities for the development of postgraduate courses in public health nursing. Funds for the provision of facilities for postgraduate instruction in public health nursing subsidized special courses for 3 years at the University of Toronto, McGill University, the Universities of British Columbia and Alberta, and Dalhousie University (Gibbon & Mathewson, 1947, p. 342).

When the first course in public health nursing was offered at the University of Alberta in 1918, shortly after the establishment of the Public Health Nursing Service, it became the first nursing program offered by a university in Canada (Department of Public Health Nursing, 1918). This course was of 2 months duration and began on April 1, 1918 (Stewart, 1979). A second course was held in 1919; a third in 1921. The *Public Health Nurses' Act*, passed in 1919, formalized the program and designated the University of Alberta as the institution offering the course, specifying that it would lead to a certificate or diploma, and authorized the graduate to "affix after her name the letters 'PH.'"

From the Depression to the Post–World War II Years

The Great Depression "brought unemployment and hardship to nurses" (Allemang, 1974, p. 172). Patients could no longer afford to employ private-duty nurses, which had been the most promising area of employment for graduate nurses (Gunn, 1933). During the Depression, Canadian universities faced reduced revenues, staff lay-offs, and difficult working conditions. The Depression was especially hard on McGill University, which depended on funds from private sources. During the Depression, raising private funds became next to impossible. Leaders of McGill's nursing school had fought unsuccessfully for years for a degree program. Once the university's finances began to deteriorate, the Board of Governors threatened to close the school altogether. The school's director gave up her salary, the faculty bought books for the library, and nursing alumnae groups all over the country raised funds to ensure the survival of the McGill nursing school (Tunis, 1966).

During World War II, health education again became a priority as doctors and nurses were needed to care for military personnel, as well as civilians. Nurses who held critical positions as administrators, supervisors, teachers, and public health nurses were recruited for military service and left their positions. A shortage of nurses soon developed. During and after the war, a new interest in nursing education led to increased external university funding, more scholarships and bursaries from private foundations, the growth of existing schools, and the founding of new programs between 1941 and 1949 (at Queen's, McMaster, Manitoba, Mount Saint Vincent, and Dalhousie). The new interest in nursing education led to exciting innovations. In 1942, the University of Toronto introduced an integrated basic degree program. Under the leadership of Edith Kathleen Russell (see Chapter 4), courses in arts and sciences were taught concurrently with nursing courses to enhance student development. Also, university instructors supervised student clinical practice in the health care agencies. At McGill, new funds flowed in, and in 1944, supporters of the school were rewarded with a 5-year nonintegrated degree program. In 1946, 4 years after the introduction of the University of Toronto basic degree program, a second basic degree program was developed at McMaster University under Gladys Sharpe's direction.

Emerging From Economic and Military Crises

In the 1960s, existing nursing degree programs expanded, and new programs emerged in other universities. The first master's degree program in nursing was established at the University of Western Ontario in 1959, followed in the 1960s and 1970s by similar programs in universities across the country. In 1962, the Canadian Nurses Foundation was established as an entity separate from the CNA, to provide scholarships, bursaries, and fellowships for graduate study in nursing.

Nursing schools' financial dependence left them at the mercy of hospital administrators. "The lack of nursing instructors and of other graduate nurses on patient care units meant that there were few role models for students for observation, questions and general discussion. In most cases senior students were left in charge of teaching junior students, and this with very limited supervision" (Paul, 1998, pp. 133–134). Many authorities have suggested that this was not a true apprenticeship model because it lacked the "master craftsman" (someone with highly developed skills) to guide the students (Chapman, 1969).

Nursing leaders called for better faculty preparation, more integrated programs, and more university-based opportunities for students, such as student placements and increased enrollments. The movement to separate nursing education programs from the authority of hospitals began in earnest, particularly after the studies on nursing education conducted in the early 1960s identified persistent problems.

Universities resisted introducing basic integrated degree programs because of the costs associated with the low student–teacher ratios required for clinical nursing. It was cheaper for them to let hospitals finance clinical education, but this meant that universities granted degrees for work over which they had no control. In 1964, the Royal Commission on Health Services castigated universities for this practice. By the late 1960s, the basic integrated degree program, modeled on the program at the University of Toronto, finally became the prototype for the establishment of integrated programs in nursing in universities across the nation.

In 1967, Dalhousie University offered the first education program for nurse practitioners (NPs) working in remote nursing stations (Worster, Sardo, Thrasher, et al., 2005). In 1973, the CNA and CMA released a joint statement, agreeing on the need for an expanded role for nurses (Canadian Nurse, 1973). That same year, a group of NP graduates from two newly established NP education programs at the University of Toronto and McMaster University established the Nurse Practitioners' Association of Ontario (NPAO, n.d.). However, these programs were closed in 1983 as a result of lack of both funding for positions and legislative support for the role. Despite this, approximately 250 NPs worked in Ontario through the 1980s and early 1990s, primarily in community health centres and northern nursing stations (Worster et al., 2005). In 1995, NP university programs were re-established. In 1997, Ontario passed the *Expanded Nursing Services for Patients Act*, which allowed registered nurses who hold an extended certificate to provide primary health care services (Legislative Assembly of Ontario, 1997).

Throughout the 1970s and 1980s, university faculties and schools of nursing developed research resources so that they could offer graduate programs first at the master's level and then at the doctoral level. The first doctoral nursing program was established at the University of Alberta Faculty of Nursing on January 1, 1991, and others quickly followed.

Nursing Education Today

With continuing expansion of health care knowledge and technology, beginning practitioners require a broad educational foundation. New curricula and collaborative baccalaureate programs across the country attest to the profession's commitment to maintaining high standards of health care and responding to society's changing health care needs. In collaborative programs, students may take part or all of their degree at a partner institution to the university that is granting the degree, such as a college in another region. The Internet, digital technology, electronic health records, computerized learning and testing programs, and online courses provide practising nurses with many options to complete degrees. The CNA's nursing portal, NurseOne, has made database information available to nurses across the country. Some universities have innovative programs at the baccalaureate level, including accelerated programs in which candidates hold a baccalaureate degree in other fields. Baccalaureate, master's, and doctorate programs are offered online, in all or in part.

Standards for nursing education are monitored by provincial regulators and associations and by the Canadian Association for Schools of Nursing (CASN) to ensure that educational programs are of appropriate quality and that they respond to changes in health care. On a national level, the CASN has developed the *National Nursing Education Framework*, a national, consensus-based framework describing expectations for baccalaureate, master's and doctoral programs in nursing education (CASN, 2015). As professionals, nurses must acquire, maintain, and continuously enhance the knowledge, skills, attitudes, and judgement necessary to meet patient needs in an evolving health care system. The responsibility for educational support for competent nursing practice is shared among individual nurses, professional nursing organizations, educational institutions, and governments (Wood, 2011).

The need for nurses with graduate degrees is rising, along with the need for research. A master's degree in nursing (typically a Master of Nursing [MN] or Master of Science in Nursing [MSN]) is necessary for nurses seeking positions as clinical nurse specialists, nurse administrators, or nurse educators. Most master's programs in Canada now offer streams in nursing leadership, education, and advanced practice. This provides advanced preparation in nursing science, theory, and

TABLE 3-1 Designations of Nursing in British Columbia—An Exemplar*

Title	Education	Licensing Exam	Registration Required	Regulatory Body	Professional Association
Licensed Practical Nurse (LPN)	Recently standardized as 2-year program	Canadian Practical Nurses Registration Exam (CPNRE)	Must be registered with CLPNBC	College of Licensed Practical Nurses of BC	Licensed Practical Nurses Association of BC
Registered Nurse (RN)	Baccalaureate degree: 4-year; Accelerated; Post-degree	National Council Licensure Examination for Registered Nurses (NCLEX-RN)	Must be registered with CRNBC	College of Registered Nurses of BC	Registered Nurses Association of BC
Registered Psychiatric Nurse (RPN)	Baccalaureate degree Diploma in Psychiatric Nursing Degree completion for RPNs	Registered Psychiatric Nurses of Canada Exam (RPNCE)	Must be registered with CRPNBC	College of Registered Psychiatric Nurses of BC	Association of Registered Nurses of BC
Nurse Practitioner	Masters of Nursing: MN-NP and MScN-FNP	Objective Structured Clinical Exam (OSCE); Written exams: Family, Adult or Pediatric stream	Must be registered with CRNBC	College of Registered Nurses of BC	BC Nurse Practitioner Association
Graduate Education for Advanced Practice, Leadership, Educator, and Researcher Roles					
Master's prepared RN	Masters in Nursing (MN) or Masters of Science in Nursing (MSN)	No provincial exam; must complete institutional requirements (e.g.; capstone project; thesis)	Must be registered with CRNBC to work as RN in BC	College of Registered Nurses of BC	Association of Registered Nurses of BC
Doctoral-prepared RN	PhD in Nursing	No provincial exam; must complete institutional requirements (e.g., comprehensive exam; dissertation)	Must be registered with CRNBC to work as RN in BC	College of Registered Nurses of BC	Association of Registered Nurses of BC

*The term *nurse* is used in Canada to refer to a number of different categories of nursing roles. Each category (or designation) has its own educational standards, regulatory bodies, and associations, which may vary from province to province. This table outlines the various nursing titles in the province of British Columbia. The Nurses and Nurse Practitioners of BC includes each of the professional associations listed in the table.

practice, with emphasis on evidence-informed clinical practice and knowledge translation.

For RNs who would like to become nurse practitioners, most NP programs in Canada are offered at the graduate level, but there is variation across provinces. In British Columbia, NPs were first legislated in 2005 (College of Registered Nurses of British Columbia [CRNBC], 2017). NPs in British Columbia work in many practice settings and across three "streams," or populations: family, adult, and pediatrics. NPs are not substitutes for physicians, but their roles complement one another to improve patient access. NPs bring the nursing focus of teaching, counselling, and support to the diagnostics and treatment they provide (CRNBC, 2017). The focus of NP education in British Columbia is on family practice, and three universities offer NP options, all within master's of nursing programs (MN-NP or MScN-FNP).

In comparison, Ontario has had primary health care NPs since the 1970s, although the role was first regulated in 1998 through the introduction of the "extended class" designation (Health Force Ontario, 2017). Adult and pediatric NPs (formerly known as acute care NPs) have worked in Ontario hospitals since the late 1980s. There are now four NP specialty certificates in the Extended Class: NP-Primary Health Care, NP-Pediatrics, NP-Adult, and NP-Anesthesia (Health Force Ontario). The only approved NP program in Ontario is the Ontario Primary Health Care Nurse Practitioner Program (OPHCNPP), a 12-month, post-baccalaureate certificate program offered through a consortium of nine universities, some as part of a master's degree (MN-PHCN) and others as a PHCN certificate (OPHCNPP, n.d.). In Ontario, NPs work in community health, long-term care, palliative care, Indigenous centres, community-based facilities, and ambulatory care centres as well as on family health teams (OPHCNPP, n.d.). Across Canada, while most NP programs exist at the graduate level, there continues to be diversity in entry to practice requirements for NPs (CASN, 2011a).

Canadian doctoral education in Canada is focused on PhD programs in nursing; there are no profession- or practice-based doctoral programs (CASN, 2011b). Nurses with doctorates can undertake research that advances knowledge and evidence-informed practice (see Chapter 6 for further information about research). This research enhances the quality of nursing care and improves Canadians' health outcomes. Table 3-1 lists the various designations of nursing in British Columbia as an example of the variations in nursing in Canada today.

CONCLUSION

Organized nursing has been a part of the social setting in Canada since the early days of the European settlement at Quebec, a period of almost four centuries. The first nurses who came to found hospitals and to provide care for Indigenous people and settlers were motivated by altruism and serve as excellent role models for nurses today. Altruism, a hallmark of any profession, remains an important characteristic of the nursing profession despite vast differences between the health care settings of the early days and those of today.

A fundamental and guiding principle of the French-Canadian hospitals that survived largely intact into the twentieth century was that care was available to all people regardless of their background, status in life, or ability to pay. This continues to be a principle for which nurses, through their professional organizations, have argued in national debates on the nature and continuing direction of Canada's national health care insurance program. In the presence of pressure to reshape Medicare, nurses have continued to strongly resist calls for privatization of more aspects of the health system. They have also repeatedly called for all health care providers to be remunerated on a salary or contract basis (Ross-Kerr, 2011).

Multidisciplinary and interprofessional teams are an integral component of the health care organization in the community. However, nurses are the primary health care providers both in home care and in community health settings. Thus, expanded and enhanced educational systems for nurses that incorporate knowledge and skills for community health and home care nursing are essential to meet the health needs of the populace today.

The transformation of the nursing profession and of the educational programs that support it since the nineteenth century has been truly remarkable. Nurses have demonstrated the value of their service, the integrity of their goals, the quality of their educational programs, and the strength of their commitment. It is certain that the nursing profession will continue to evolve in the interest of providing high-quality nursing care.

KEY CONCEPTS

- Nursing has responded to the health care needs of society, influenced over time by economic, social, and cultural factors.
- Nursing in Canada is rooted in the traditions of nursing that developed in New France.
- Florence Nightingale revolutionized nursing as an acceptable profession for women as lay nurses in the late 1800s and early 1900s.
- The development of a system of nursing education in Canada emerged from the early nursing sisterhoods and from schools of nursing associated with hospitals.
- Baccalaureate entry-to-practice was fully implemented in English-speaking Canada.
- Basic nursing education is acquired in college, collaborative college-university, or university programs.
- The ranks of the profession are moving toward gender balance and increased diversity that reflects the Canadian population.

CRITICAL THINKING EXERCISES

1. Explain the importance of Florence Nightingale's work to establish nursing as a profession.
2. Identify some of the enduring values that have emerged from the history of nursing in Canada.
3. Observe various levels of nursing practice, such as a staff nurse, nurse practitioner, and nurse educator. Identify similarities and differences in their roles and educational preparation.
4. Outline some career objectives for yourself after completing your nursing program. Think about what you want to do as a professional nurse, and then outline strategies for achieving these goals.

REVIEW QUESTIONS

1. The founder of modern nursing is
   1. Hippocrates
   2. Florence Nightingale
   3. Jeanne Mance
   4. Mary Agnes Snively
2. The earliest role of nurses involved
   1. Caring for the sick at home
   2. Using herbal remedies to relieve symptoms
   3. Caring for the sick in hospitals
   4. Supervising nursing students
3. The religious roots of nursing in Canada can be seen in the development of:
   1. The ICN
   2. The VON
   3. The code of ethics
   4. BETP
4. The following characteristic of nursing in Canada today can be traced back to Nightingale:
   1. The high percentage of men in nursing
   2. The apprenticeship model
   3. Public health education
   4. Nursing as a highly regarded profession
5. Minimum standards for nursing education are set by:
   1. The nursing school
   2. The provincial regulators and associations
   3. The Canadian Nurses Association
   4. The Canadian Nurses Federation

Answers: 1. 2; 2. 2; 3. 3; 4. 4; 5. 2

Rationales for the Review Questions appear at the end of the book.

RECOMMENDED WEBSITES

Canadian Association for the History of Nursing/Association canadienne pour l'histoire du nursing (CAHN-ACHN): https://cahn-achn.ca/
An affiliate group of the CNA, the CAHN offers information about Canadian nursing history and promotes historical research.

Canadian Association for Schools of Nursing/Association canadienne des ecoles de sciences infirmieres (CASN-ACESI): http://www.casn.ca/
CASN is the national voice for nursing education, research, and scholarship and represents baccalaureate and graduate nursing programs in Canada

Canadian Nurses Association (CNA): https://www.cna-aiic.ca/en
The CNA is the national professional voice of registered nurses in Canada, representing nearly 139 000 members.

Canadian Nursing Students' Association/L'Association de etudiant(e)s infirmier(eres) du Canada (CNSA-AEIC): http://cnsa.ca/
This is the national voice of Canadian nursing students.

Nurse Practitioner History in Ontario: http://www.npao.org/nurse-practitioners/history/
This site provides the history of nurse practitioners in Ontario, where NPs have worked since the early 1970s.

REFERENCES

Allemang, M. M. (1974). *Nursing education in the United States and Canada, 1873–1950: Leading figures, forces, views on education*. Unpublished doctoral dissertation, University of Washington, Seattle.

Armstrong-Reid, S. (2014). *Lyle Creelman: The frontiers of global nursing*. Toronto: University of Toronto Press.

Baker, C. (2014). Commentary. *Nursing Leadership, 27*(4), 35–39.

Bates, C., Dodd, D., & Rousseau, N. (2005). *On all frontiers: Four centuries of Canadian nursing*. Ottawa: University of Ottawa Press/Canadian Museum of Civilization.

Baumgart, A., & Kirkwood, R. (1990). Social reform versus education reform: University education in Canada, 1919–1960. *Journal of Advanced Nursing, 15*(5), 510–516.

Bonin, M. A. (1976). *Trends in integrated basic degree nursing programs in Canada: 1942–1972*. Unpublished doctoral dissertation, University of Ottawa, Ottawa, ON.

Boschma, G. (2014). International nursing history: The International Council of Nurses History Collective and beyond. *Nursing History Review, 22*, 114–118.

Burnett, K. (2008). The healing work of Aboriginal women in Indigenous and newcomer communities. In J. Elliott, M. Stuart, & C. Toman (Eds.), *Place and practice in Canadian nursing history*. Vancouver: University of British Columbia Press.

Canadian Association for Schools of Nursing (CASN). (2011a). *Nurse practitioner education in Canada*. Retrieved from http://casn.ca/wp-content/uploads/2014/12/EnvironmentalScanofNursePractitionerProgramsEn.pdf.

Canadian Association for Schools of Nursing (CASN). (2011b). *Position statement: Doctoral education in nursing in Canada*. Retrieved from http://casn.ca/wp-content/uploads/2014/10/DoctoralEducation2011.pdf.

Canadian Association for Schools of Nursing (CASN). (2015). *National nursing education framework: Final report*. Retrieved from http://www.casn.ca/wp-content/uploads/2014/12/Framwork-FINAL-SB-Nov-30-20151.pdf.

Canadian Broadcasting Corporation. (2010) *Grey Nuns leave NWT after 143 years*. Retrieved from http://www.cbc.ca/news/canada/north/grey-nuns-leave-n-w-t-after-143-years-1.920931.

Canadian Indigenous Nurses Association (CINA). (2010). *About C.I.N.A*. Retrieved from http://www.indigenousnurses.ca/About/AboutCINA.

Canadian Nurse. (1973). The expanded role of the nurse: A joint statement of CNA-CMA. *Canadian Nurse, 69*, 23–25.

Canadian Nurses Association (CNA). (1968). *The leaf and the lamp*. Ottawa, ON: Author.

Canadian Nurses Association (CNA). (1991). NB for BN: Province joins nurses' call for degree. *Edufacts, 1*(2), 1.

Canadian Nurses Association (CNA). (2007). *Position statement: The value of nursing history today*. Ottawa, ON: Author.

Canadian Nurses Association (CNA). (2012). *2010 workforce profile of registered nurses in Canada*. Retrieved from http://www.cna-aiic.ca/~/media/cna/page-content/pdf-en/2010_rn_snapshot_e.pdf.

Canadian Nurses Association (CNA). (2013). *One hundred years of service, 1908–2008*. Ottawa: Author.

Canadian Nurses Association (CNA). (2015). *Framework for the practice of registered nurses in Canada*. Retrieved from https://www.cna-aiic.ca/~/media/cna/page-content/pdf-en/framework-for-the-pracice-of-registered-nurses-in-canada.pdf?la=en.

Canadian Red Cross Society. (1962). *The role of one voluntary organization in Canada's health services: A brief presented to the Royal Commission on Health Services*. Toronto, ON: Author.

Chapman, M. E. (1969). *Nursing education and the movement for higher education for women: A study of interrelationship, 1870–1900*. Unpublished doctoral dissertation, Columbia University, New York.

College of Registered Nurses of BC (CRNBC). (2017). *Nurse practitioners*. Retrieved from https://www.crnbc.ca/QA/NP/Pages/Default.aspx.

Coombs-Thorne, H. (2010). Mrs. Tilly had a very hasty wedding! The class-based response to marriages in the Grenfell mission of Newfoundland and Labrador. *Canadian Bulletin of Medical History, 27*(1), 123–138.

D'Antonio, P. (2003). Editor's note. *Nursing History Review, 11*, 1.

D'Antonio, P., & Fairman, J. (2010). Guest editorial: History matters. *Nursing Outlook, 58*(2), 113–114.

Davey, E. (2012). New players through old lenses: Why history matters in engaging with Southern actors. *Humanitarian Policy Group Brief, 48*, 1–4. Retrieved from http://www.odi.org.uk/sites/odi.org.uk/files/odi-assets/publications-opinion-files/7726.pdf.

Department of Public Health Nursing. (1918). *Annual Report, 1918*. Edmonton: Provincial Archives of Alberta.

Domm, E. (2010). From the streets of Toronto to the Northwest Rebellion: Hannah Grier Coome's call to duty. In M. Rutherdale (Ed.), *Caregiving on the periphery: Historical perspectives on nursing and midwifery in Canada*. Montreal & Kingston: McGill-Queen's University Press.

Dossey, B. M. (1998). Florence Nightingale: A 19th century mystic. *Journal of Holistic Nursing, 16*(2), 112.

Dysart-Gale, D. (2010). Social justice and social determinants of health: Lesbian, gay, bisexual, transgendered, intersexed and queer youth in Canada. *Journal of Child and Adolescent Psychiatric Nursing, 23*(1), 23–28.

Elliott, J. (2010). A negotiated process: Outpost nursing under the Red Cross in Ontario, 1922–84. In M. Rutherdale (Ed.), *Caregiving on the periphery: Historical perspectives on nursing and midwifery in Canada*. Montreal & Kingston: McGill-Queen's University Press.

Flynn, K. (2009). Beyond the glass wall: Black Canadian nurses, 1940–1970. *Nursing History Review, 17*, 129–152.

Gibbon, J. M., & Mathewson, M. S. (1947). *Three centuries of Canadian nursing*. Toronto, ON: Macmillan.

Grundmann, C. H. (2005). *Sent to heal! Emergence and development of medical missions*. Lanham, MD: University Press of America.

Grypma, S. (2005a). Florence Nightingale's changing image, Part I: Nightingale the feminist, statistician and nurse. *Journal of Christian Nursing, 22*(3), 22–28.

Grypma, S. (2005b). Florence Nightingale's changing image, Part II: From saint to fiend to modern mystic. *Journal of Christian Nursing, 22*(4), 6–14.

Grypma, S. (2007). Withdrawal from Weihui: China missions and the silencing of missionary nursing, 1888–1947. *Nursing Inquiry, 14*(4), 306–319.

Grypma, S. (2008). *Healing Henan: Canadian nurses at the North China Mission, 1888–1947*. Vancouver: University of British Columbia Press.

Grypma, S. (2017). Historically-informed nursing: The untapped potential of history in nursing education. *Quality Advancement in Nursing Education/Avancees en formation infirmiere, 3*(1), Article 5.

Grypma, S., & Wu, N. (2012). China confidential: Methodological and ethical challenges in global nursing historiography. *Nursing History Review, 20*(1), 162–183. doi:10.1891/1062-8061.20.162.

Gunn, J. I. (1933). Educational adjustments recommended by the survey. *Canadian Nurse, 29*, 139–145.

Hamelin, J. (1981). *Histoire du Québec*. Montreal: Editions France/Amerique.

Healey, P. (1990). *The Mack training school for nurses*. Unpublished doctoral dissertation, University of Texas, Austin.

Health Force Ontario. (2017). *Nurse practitioners*. Retrieved from http://www.healthforceontario.ca/en/Home/Nurses/Training_%7C_Practising_In_Ontario/Nursing_Roles/Nurse_Practitioners.

Kulig, J., & Grypma, S. (2006). Honouring pioneer aboriginal nurses from the Blood reserve. *Alberta RN, 62*(8), 14–16.

Legislative Assembly of Ontario. (1997). 36:1 Bill 27, *Expanded Nursing Services for Patients Act*, 1997. Toronto: Author. Retrieved from http://www.ontla.on.ca/web/bills/bills_detail.do?locale=en&BillID=1349&isCurrent=false&BillStagePrintId=.

McBain, L. (2010). Caring, curing and socialization: The ambiguities of nursing in Northern Saskatchewan, 1944–57. In J. Elliott, M. Stuart, & C. Toman (Eds.), *Place and practice in Canadian nursing history*. Vancouver: University of British Columbia Press.

McDonald, L. (2001). *Florence Nightingale: An introduction to her life and family; Volume 1 of the collected works of Florence Nightingale*. Waterloo, ON: Wilfrid Laurier University Press.

Meadus, R. J., & Twomey, J. C. (2011). Men student nurses: The nursing education experience. *Nursing Forum, 46*(4), 269–279.

Meijer-Drees, L. (2013). *Healing histories: Stories from Canada's Indian hospitals*. Edmonton AB: University of Alberta Press.

Meyers, E. M. (2013). *Two roads diverged in a wood: The story of caring theorist Sister M. Simone Roach*. Unpublished PhD Dissertation. University of Alberta.

Nelson, S. (2001). *Say little, do much: Nursing, nuns, and hospitals in the nineteenth century*. Philadelphia: University of Pennsylvania Press.

Nelson, S. (2009). Historical amnesia and its consequences: The need to build histories of practice. *Texto Contexto Enferm, Florianópolis, 18*(4), 781–787.

Nightingale, F. (1979). *Cassandra*. New York: The Feminist Press of the City University of New York. (Original work published 1872).

Nurse Practitioners Association of Ontario (NPAO). (n.d.). *Men's health guidelines complimentary for practitioners*. Retrieved from http://www.npao.org/nurse-practitioner/history/history.

Nurses Association of New Brunswick. (1992). *Annual reports 1991–1992*. Fredericton: Author.

Nutting, M. A., & Dock, L. L. (1907–1912). *A history of nursing* (Vol. 1–4). New York: G.P. Putnam's Sons.

Ontario Primary Health Care Nurse Practitioner Program. (n.d.). *What is a nurse practitioner?* Retrieved from http://np-education.ca/?page_id=13373.

Paul, P. (1998). Nursing education becomes synonymous with nursing service: The development of training schools. In J. C. Ross-Kerr (Ed.), *Prepared to care: Nurses and nursing in Alberta* (pp. 133–134). Edmonton, AB: University of Alberta Press.

Paul, P. (2005). Religious nursing orders of Canada: A presence on all western frontiers. In C. Bates, D. Dodd, & N. Rousseau (Eds.), *On all frontiers: Four centuries of Canadian nursing* (pp. 125–139). Ottawa: University of Ottawa Press and Canadian Museum of Civilization.

Paul, P., & Ross-Kerr, J. (2011). Nursing in Canada, 1600 to the present: A brief account. In J. C. Ross-Kerr & M. J. Wood (Eds.), *Canadian nursing: Issues and perspectives* (5th ed., pp. 18–41). Toronto, ON: Elsevier Canada.

Pijl-Zieber, E., Grypma, S., & Barton, S. (2014). Baccalaureate nursing education: Has it delivered? A retrospective critique. *Nursing Leadership, 27*(2), 27–34.

Registered Nurses Association of Ontario (RNAO). (2007). *Health work environments best practice guidelines: Embracing cultural diversity in health care; developing cultural competence*. Toronto: Author.

Ross-Kerr, J. C. (2011). Issues of gender and diversity in nursing. In J. C. Ross-Kerr & M. J. Wood (Eds.), *Canadian nursing: Issues and perspectives* (5th ed.). Toronto: Elsevier Canada.

Rousseau, F. (1977). Hôpital et société en Nouvelle-France: L'Hôtel-Dieu de Québec à la fin du XVIIiéme siécle. *Revue de l'histoire de Amérique francaise, 31*(1), 29–47.

Royal Commission on Aboriginal Peoples. (1996). From time immemorial: A demographic profile. (Chap. 2). In *Report of the Royal Commission on Aboriginal Peoples: Vol. 1. Looking forward looking back.* Ottawa, ON: Indian and Northern Affairs Canada.

Rutherdale, M. (2010). *Caregiving on the periphery: Historical perspectives on nursing and midwifery in Canada.* Montreal & Kingston: McGill-Queen's University Press.

Stewart, I. (1979). *These were our yesterdays: A history of district nursing in Alberta.* Calgary: Friesen Printers.

Toman, C. (2016). *Sister soldiers of the Great War: The nurses of the Canadian Army Medical Corps.* Vancouver: University of British Columbia Press.

Toman, C., & Thifault, M. C. (2012). Historical thinking and the shaping of nursing identity. *Nursing History Review, 20,* 184–204.

Tosh, J. (2008). *Why history matters.* New York: Palgrave Macmillan.

Tunis, B. L. (1966). *In caps and gowns.* Montreal: McGill University Press.

Vandenberg, H. (2015). *Race, hospital development and the power of community: The history of Chinese and Japanese hospitals in British Columbia from 1880–1920.* Unpublished PhD dissertation. University of British Columbia School of Nursing.

Villeneuve, M. J. (2002–2003). Healthcare, race and diversity: Time to act. *Hospital Quarterly, 6*(2), 67–73.

Violette, B. (2005). Healing the body and saving the soul: Nursing sisters and the first Catholic hospitals in Quebec (1639–1880). In C. Bates, D. Dodd, & N. Rousseau (Eds.), *On all frontiers: Four centuries of Canadian nursing* (pp. 57–71). Ottawa: University of Ottawa Press and Canadian Museum of Civilization.

Weir, G. M. (1932). *Survey of nursing education in Canada.* Toronto, ON: University of Toronto Press.

Wood, M. J. (2011). Monitoring standards in nursing education. In J. C. Ross-Kerr & M. J. Wood (Eds.), *Canadian nursing: Issues and perspectives.* Toronto: Elsevier Science.

Worster, A., Sardo, A., Thrasher, C., et al. (2005). Understanding the role of nurse practitioners in Canada. *Canadian Journal of Rural Medicine, 10*(2), 89–94.

Wytenbroek, L. (2015). Negotiating relationships of power in a maternal and child health center: The experience of WHO Nurse Margaret Campbell Jackson in Iran, 1954–1956. *Nursing History Review, 23*(1), 87–122.

Young, S. L. (1994). *Standards in diploma nursing education: The involvement of the University of Alberta, 1920–1970.* Unpublished master's thesis, University of Alberta, Edmonton.

4

Community Health Nursing Practice

Written by Kaysi Eastlick Kushner, RN, PhD, Margot Jackson, RN, PhD

OBJECTIVES

Mastery of content in this chapter will enable you to:

- Define the key terms listed.
- Explain the relationship between community health nursing and primary health care.
- Discuss the roles and functions of the community health nurse.
- Differentiate between public health nursing and home health nursing.
- Explain the characteristics of clients who are structurally vulnerable.
- Describe the standards, competencies, roles, and activities important for success in community health nursing practice.
- Describe elements of a community assessment.

KEY TERMS

Community, p. 48
Community-based nursing, p. 53
Community health nursing, p. 50
Community health nursing practice, p. 49
Empowerment, p. 51
Harm reduction, p. 56
Home health nursing, p. 53
Population, p. 48
Population health, p. 52
Primary health care, p. 50
Public health, p. 51
Public health nursing, p. 51
Public health principles, p. 52
Social justice, p. 49
Vulnerable populations, p. 54

MEDIA RESOURCES

http://evolve.elsevier.com/Canada/Potter/fundamentals/

- Audio Chapter Summaries
- Examination Review Questions
- Concept Map Creator
- Case Study with Questions
- Audio Glossary
- Content Updates
- Video Clips

Today's health care climate is rapidly changing in response to economic pressures, technological and medical advances, and client participation in health care. As a result, many clients are receiving care in the community rather than in hospital. There is a growing need to deliver health care where people live, work, and learn (Community Health Nurses of Canada [CHNC], 2011). Community health nursing care focuses on health promotion and protection, disease and injury prevention, and restorative and palliative care. The goals of community health nursing are to keep individuals healthy, encourage client participation and choice in care, promote health-enhancing social and physical environments, and provide in-home care for ill or disabled clients.

Promoting individual and community health has always been key to the holistic practice of nursing. In the 1730s, the Grey Nuns were established as Canada's first community nursing order. More than a century later, in England, Florence Nightingale articulated a nursing philosophy grounded in knowledge of environmental conditions. By the end of the century, the Victorian Order of Nurses was providing in-home nursing, often in outpost and remote regions. After World War I, community nursing responsibilities "extended to screening programs to detect disease at early stages, to helping to maintain a healthy environment, and to providing nursing care" (Ross-Kerr, 2011, p. 25).

Canadians such as Kate Brighty Colley (Box 4-1) and Edith Kathleen Russell (Box 4-2) pioneered community and public health nursing in Canada. Today, nursing is leading the way in assessing, implementing, and evaluating public and community-based health services needed by patients. Community health nursing is essential for improving the health of the general public.

PROMOTING THE HEALTH OF POPULATIONS AND COMMUNITY GROUPS

Nurses practising in the community face many challenges in promoting the health of populations and community groups. A **population** is a collection of individuals who have in common one or more personal or environmental characteristics (Maurer & Smith, 2005). Examples of populations are Canadians inclusively and, more specifically, older persons or a cultural group such as Indigenous peoples. A healthy population is composed of healthy individuals, and the health status of individuals is considered an overall aggregate that reflects an average or general health status. To determine a population's health status, individual characteristics (such as occurrence of illness, disability, and death; lifespan; education; and living conditions) are considered. A **community** is a group of people who share a geographic (locational)

BOX 4-1 Milestones in Canadian Community Health Nursing History

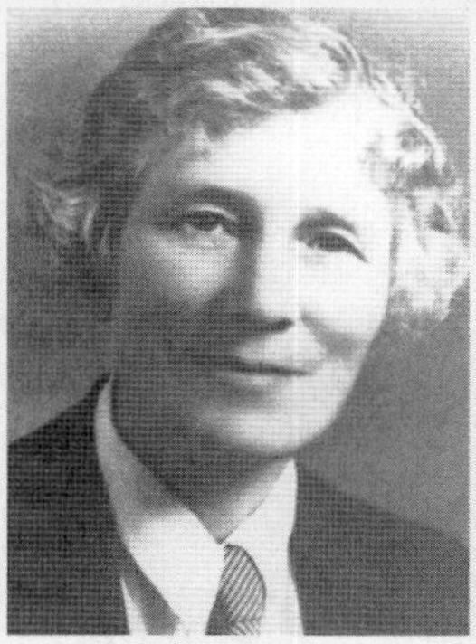

Kate Brighty Colley, 1883–1985

Born in England in 1883, Kate Brighty immigrated with her parents to Nova Scotia at the age of 3 years. She graduated from the Royal Alexandra Hospital School of Nursing in Edmonton in 1917, after which she enlisted with the Canadian Army Medical Corps in Calgary.

After completing a course in public health nursing at the University of Alberta in 1919, Brighty was one of the first nurses to be appointed to the staff of the new Alberta Department of Public Health.

In the same year, Brighty was appointed matron of the second municipal hospital in Alberta, the Mission Hospital at Onoway. Because there were no physicians in the region, she and her two employees staffed the hospital and visited rural patients on horseback. In 1923, she returned to the Department of Public Health to establish a district nursing centre at Buck Lake, southwest of Edmonton, an area that had no roads at the time, and then another centre, farther north at Wanham, near the Peace River. Here, she travelled by cutter to assist women in labour and those who were ill.

In 1925, Brighty took a postgraduate course in public health nursing at Columbia University, New York. Upon her return to Alberta in 1928, she was appointed director of the Department of Public Health Nursing. Brighty established a number of new district nursing centres. As a former district nurse, she understood the problems these nurses faced, and she travelled widely to visit staff. She expanded the health education program and gave radio talks on health, hygiene, nutrition, and child welfare. These broadcasts were important to residents of remote areas, where little formal health care was available.

After 24 years of service to the Department of Public Health Nursing, she retired in 1943, and in 1970, she published *While Rivers Flow: Stories of Early Alberta*, experiences and short stories based on her public health nursing practice.

Brighty, K. (1942). *Collection of facts for a history of nursing in Alberta: 1864–1942.* Edmonton: Alberta Association of Registered Nurses; and Brighty Colley, K. (1970). *While rivers flow: Stories of early Alberta.* Saskatoon: The Western Producer; and Stewart, I. (1979). *These were our yesterdays: A history of district nursing in Alberta.* Altona, MB: Friesen Printers.

BOX 4-2 Milestones in Canadian Community Health Nursing History

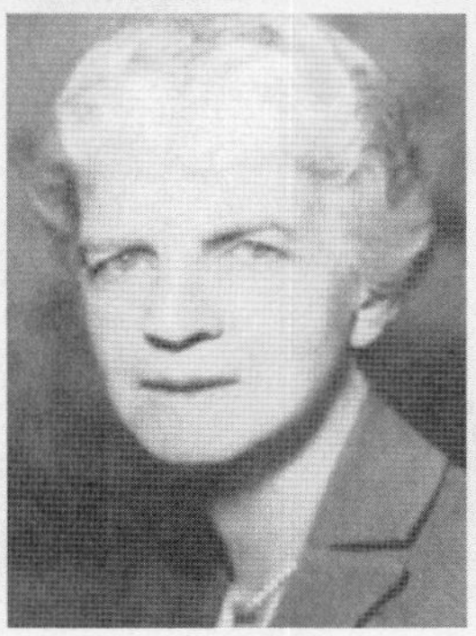

Edith Kathleen Russell, 1886–1964

Edith Kathleen Russell was born in Windsor, Nova Scotia, in 1886. She entered the Toronto General Hospital School of Nursing in 1915 and, after graduating, worked with the Department of Public Health in Toronto. In 1920, the Department of Public Health Nursing at the University of Toronto was established, and Russell was appointed its first director.

Russell recognized the great need for improved nursing education. At the time, the norm was an apprenticeship system in hospital schools, in which students, rather than graduate nurses, fulfilled nursing tasks. Russell gained the support of the University of Toronto and the Rockefeller Foundation for an experiment in basic nursing education and, in 1933, established a diploma program that prepared nurses for hospital and public health nursing. In 1942, her program evolved into an integrated basic degree program controlled by the university, in which clinical practice was obtained at affiliated hospitals under supervision of university instructors. This program was the first of its kind in Canada and was hailed throughout the world as an important new system of nursing education. Edith Kathleen Russell is widely recognized as the architect of the integrated degree nursing program.

Carpenter, H. (1982). *A divine discontent: Edith Kathleen Russell, reforming educator.* Toronto: University of Toronto Faculty of Nursing. Photo Credit: University of Toronto Archive (2010-40-2cMS). Reproduced by permission of Helen M. Carpenter (BS, MPH, EdD).

dimension and a social (relational) dimension (Diem & Moyer, 2015; Laverack, 2004). The social dimension—which comprises individual relationships, interactions among groups, and shared characteristics among members—distinguishes a community from a population. Examples of communities are geographic groupings (e.g., neighbourhoods) and shared-interest groups (e.g., women's health networks). A healthy community consists of healthy individuals engaged in collective relationships that create a supportive living environment. Both individual and community characteristics are used to determine community health status. Key characteristics of a healthy community include a collective capacity to solve problems; adequate living conditions; a safe environment; and sustainable resources such as employment, health care, and educational facilities.

COMMUNITY HEALTH NURSING PRACTICE

The scope of **community health nursing practice** includes population health promotion, protection, maintenance, and restoration; community, family, and individual health promotion; and individual rehabilitation or palliative care. Community health nurses "promote, protect, and preserve the health of individuals, families, groups, communities, and populations" (CHNC, 2013, p. 2). Practice involves coordinating care and planning services, programs, and policies by collaborating with individuals, caregivers, families, other disciplines, communities, and governments. Practice combines knowledge of nursing theory, including the metaparadigm concepts of person, health, nursing, environment, and social justice as a theoretical foundation, social sciences, and public health science (CHNC, 2013). Figure 4-1 depicts the multiple components of community health nursing practice. **Social justice** is rooted in notions of societal (social) responsibility and fairness (justice). "Social justice is the equitable, or fair, distribution of society's benefits, responsibilities and their consequences. It focuses on the relative position of social advantage of one individual or social group in relation to others in society as well as on the root causes of inequities and what can be done to eliminate them" (Canadian Nurses Association [CNA], 2010, p. 13). Social justice encompasses equity, human rights, democracy and civil rights, capacity building, just institutions, enabling environments,

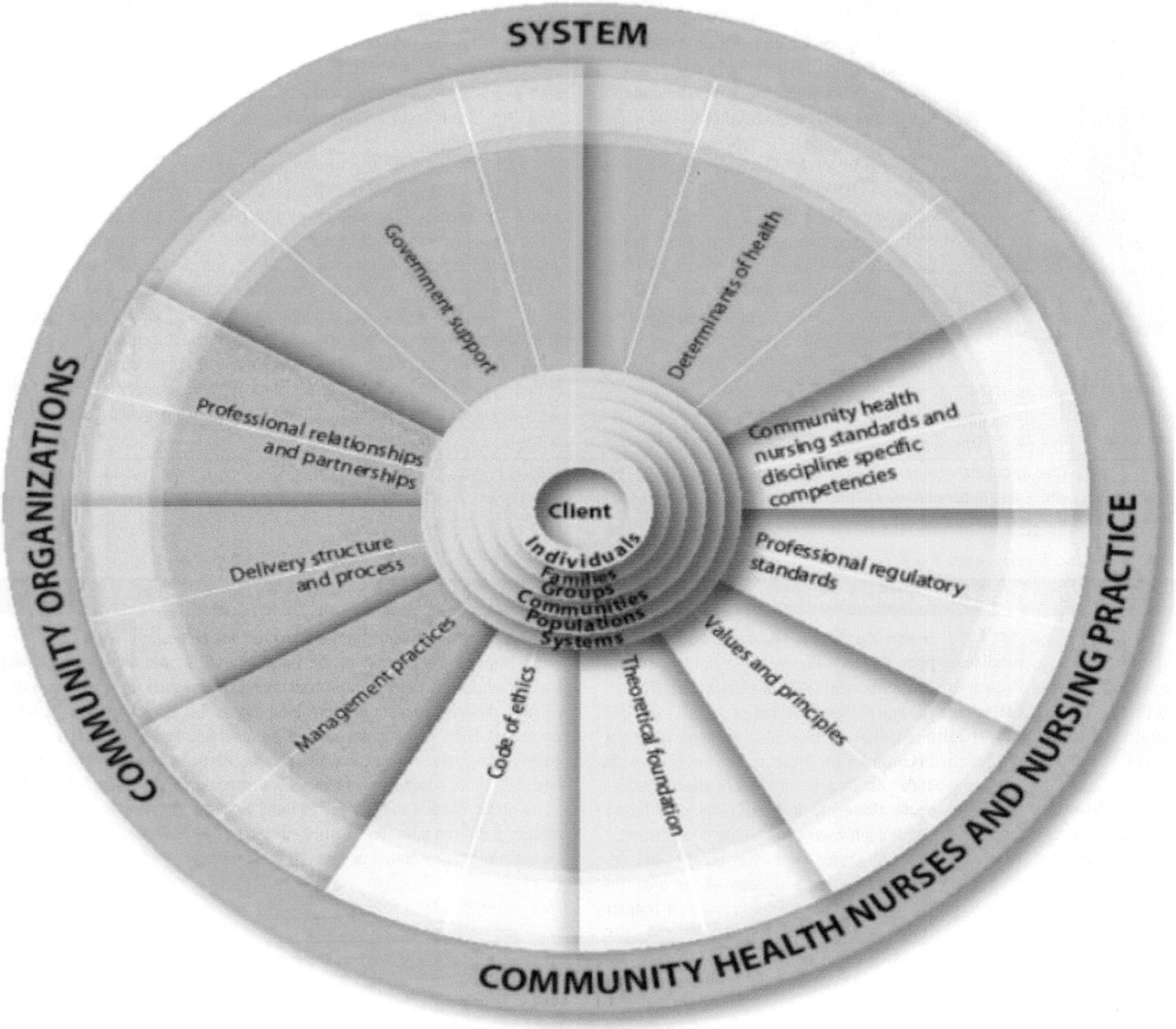

FIGURE 4-1 Canadian community health nursing professional practice model. (From Community Health Nurses of Canada. [2013]. *Canadian community health nursing professional practice model.* Retrieved from https://www.chnc.ca/upload/membership/document/2016-07/canadiancommunityhealthnursingprofessionalpracticecompoments-e_1.pdf.)

poverty reduction, ethical practice, advocacy, and partnerships (CNA, 2010).

Community health nursing includes public health nursing, home health (community-based) nursing, and community mental health nursing, as well as a variety of other specialties such as outpost nursing (Box 4-3), street health, and parish nursing (CHNC, 2011; see also Stamler & Yiu, 2016; and Stanhope, Lancaster, Jakubec, et al., 2017, for in-depth descriptions of community health nursing roles in Canada). Occupational health nursing has emerged as a distinctive specialized practice, although it is arguably within the inclusive focus of community health nursing.

The community health nursing focus is broad, emphasizing both the community's health and direct care to subpopulations within that community. By focusing on subpopulations, the community health nurse cares for the whole community and considers the individual to be one member of a group. The practice focus of different specialties within community health nursing varies: for example, home health nurses focus on individual clients, then broaden their view to consider family and community, whereas public health nurses more often shift from a broad view of populations to narrow their focus to specific vulnerable groups or families (CHNC, 2011).

Regardless of specific role, function, or setting, community health nursing practice is guided by values of caring, principles of primary health care, multiple ways of knowing, individual and community partnerships, empowerment, and social justice (CHNC, 2013). **Primary health care** focuses on education, rehabilitation, support services,

BOX 4-3 CASE STUDY

Outpost Nursing in Remote and Northern Communities

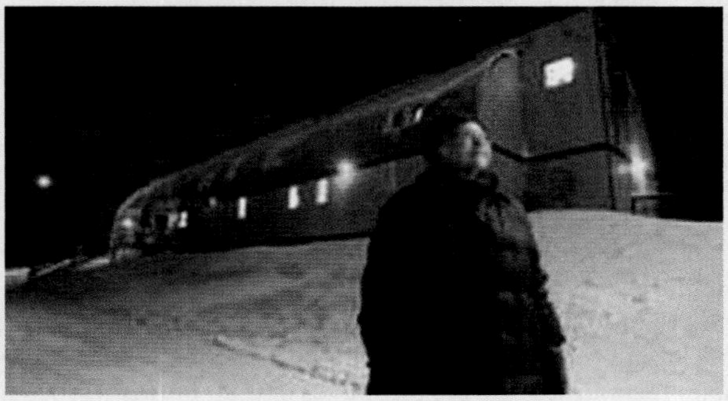

Providing health care services to Canada's remote and northern communities has been a challenge due to geographic location as well as Indigenous and northern cultural and linguistic barriers (Grypma, Wolfs, & Reimer-Kirkham, 2012; Tarlier, Johnson, & Whyte, 2016). Health care in these regions is most commonly provided by outpost nurses who assume the role of both primary care provider and primary health care provider. Tarlier and colleagues' (2016) qualitative study with experienced outpost nurses revealed the essential work of relationship and trust building within communities and the complex interrelations that exist among "autonomy, authority, power, ethics, responsibility, and the reciprocity of relationships" (p. 183).

Outpost nurses are responsible for incorporating disease prevention, health promotion, and population health and community development practices alongside providing illness management, treatment, and clinical assessment (Health Canada, 2016; Tarlier et al., 2016). Nurses working in these regions also take on the role of community health nurse by visiting new parents, helping with new baby care, and providing immunization. Provision of these services is often complex and challenging, as the health status of individuals within these communities tends to be poorer than in other regions of Canada (Tarlier et al., 2016). These regions tend to be populated primarily by Indigenous peoples who have faced a loss of cultural identity and traumatization due to colonization and the residential school system. Communities within the northern regions of Canada experience higher rates of death, suicide, alcohol and drug dependence, disease, and trauma (Tarlier et al., 2016). The contributors to these health challenges and issues are multifaceted and reflect the strong impact of the social determinants of health within these communities.

Nurse Cathy Rose stands outside the Resolute Bay Health Centre in Resolute, Nunavut, on November 21, 2013. Ms. Rose, originally from Kitchener, Ontario, has been working in the North for 28 years. Photo Credit: Peter Power/*The Globe and Mail.*

health promotion, and disease prevention. It involves multidisciplinary teams and collaboration with other sectors, as well as with secondary and tertiary care facilities (see Chapter 2). Primary health care principles guide community health nurses to use empowerment-based models of community practice (Chalmers & Bramadat, 1996; CHNC, 2011). **Empowerment** may be most simply described as a psychological, cultural, social, or political process by which people, individually and collectively in organizations and communities, exercise their ability to effect change to enhance control, quality of life, political effectiveness, and social justice (Canadian Public Health Association [CPHA], 2010). Empowerment is both an outcome and a process by which that outcome is achieved. Empowerment exists in dynamic power relations among people, which from a health promotion perspective are expressed as "power with" rather than "power over" relations (Labonte, 1993). Although empowerment is commonly conceptualized as a process continuum from personal to small group to community organization to partnership to social and political action (Laverack, 2004), Labonte's holosphere (Venn diagram) better depicts the interrelated and nonlinear dynamic of empowering processes in practice. Criticisms that empowerment is often misinterpreted as increasing individual responsibility but overlooking power and control (Cooke, 2002) highlight the importance of action to ensure that adequate resources are available for individuals and for groups and communities collectively. Such action would be grounded in ethical commitment to inclusion, diversity, participation, social justice, advocacy, and interdependence as a complementary foundation to the Canadian Nurses Association (CNA, 2017) Code of Ethics intended to guide all nursing practice (Racher, 2007).

Empowerment-based skills of patient advocacy, communication, and the design of new systems in cooperation with existing systems help make community health nursing practice effective. The Canadian Community Health Nursing Practice Model (CHNC, 2013) articulates how community health nursing care encompasses actions aimed at illness care; illness, disease, or injury prevention; and health promotion. Nursing actions are guided by approaches oriented to capacity building, participation, collaboration, inclusiveness, equity, social justice, and advocacy. These actions complement one another, even as their underlying aims, approaches to care, and perceptions of clients may differ.

Community health nursing practice requires a distinct set of skills and knowledge. The National Nursing Education Framework (Canadian Association of Schools of Nursing [CASN], 2015) identifies five domains essential to undergraduate nursing that include essential components relevant to preparation for community health nursing practice. For example, baccalaureate-educated nurses should have foundational skills in communication and collaboration, as well as in assessment, planning, and provision of care with diverse patients, along with foundational knowledge of population health, social justice, primary health care, health disparities, vulnerable populations, and determinants of health (CASN, 2015). Expert community health nurses understand the needs of a population or community through experiences with individuals, families, and groups. They think critically in applying a wide range of knowledge to find the best approaches for partnering with their patients. In 2006, the CNA introduced a community health nursing certification (CNA, 2006). Certification confirms practitioner competence in the specialty, recognizes nurses who meet the national standards of the specialty, and promotes excellence in nursing care for the Canadian population (see CHNC, 2013, and CNA, 2006, for standards and certification procedures).

Public Health Nursing

Public health nursing merges knowledge from public health science, social sciences, and primary health care with professional nursing theories to safeguard and improve the health of populations in the community (CHNC, 2011; CPHA, 2010). To understand public health nursing, it is necessary to know how public health works. The emphasis in **public health** is on the health of the entire population. Historically, government-funded agencies have supported public health programs that improve food and water safety and provide adequate sewage disposal. Public health policy has largely been responsible for the dramatic gain in life expectancy for North Americans during the past century (McKay, 2016; Shah, 2003). The goal of public health is to achieve a healthy environment for everyone. **Public health principles** of disease prevention, health promotion and protection, and healthy public policy (CPHA, 2010) can be applied to individuals, families, groups, or communities. Public health practice calls for competencies (i.e., knowledge, skills, attitudes) that cross the boundaries of specific disciplines and are independent of programs and roles (Canadian Association of Schools of Nursing [CASN], 2014; Public Health Agency of Canada [PHAC], 2007). These competencies include "public health sciences in nursing practice; population and community health assessment and analysis; population health planning, implementation, and evaluation; partnerships, collaboration and advocacy; and communication in public health nursing" (CASN, 2014, p. 3; see also CHNC, 2009; PHAC, 2007).

A public health focus requires understanding the needs of a population. Focus may be narrowed to vulnerable populations (e.g., low-income families, recent immigrants). Public health professionals must understand factors influencing the health promotion and health maintenance of groups, trends and patterns influencing disease or risk occurrence within populations, physical and social environmental factors contributing to health and illness, and political processes used to influence public policy (see Chapter 1, "Determinants of Health and Social Determinants of Health").

Population health is defined by the Public Health Agency of Canada (PHAC, 2016) as "an approach to health that aims to improve the health of the entire population and to reduce health inequities among population groups." The concept was introduced in 1989 by the Canadian Institute for Advanced Research, grounded in the recognition that determinants of health interact in complex ways to influence health. The population health promotion approach (Hamilton & Bhatti, 1996) provides a framework for thinking about health and taking action to improve the health of populations. Action is directed primarily at community levels. Strategies address the determinants of health in order to improve population health and reduce risks (see Chapter 1). Most health determinants involve other sectors of society, such as education, agriculture, business, and government. Multisectoral collaboration between the health sector and other sectors is essential, broadening the scope of nursing practice in the community. Population-based public health programs focus on disease prevention, health protection, and health promotion, which provide a foundation for health care services at all levels (see Chapter 2).

Using public health principles helps public health nurses to understand the environments in which clients live, the factors that influence client health, and the types of interventions supportive of client health. Public health nurses perceive value in their distinctive practice, which enables them to see "the big picture" as a result of their "broad health knowledge base, in-depth understanding of the community and community resources, and ... appreciation of individual–family–community interrelationships" (Reutter & Ford, 1996, p. 8). Figure 4-2 illustrates a framework for public health programs that provides a means of organizing program development in public health practice (Edwards & Moyer, 2000).

Successful public health nursing practice involves empowerment-based strategies initiated by building relationships with the community and being responsive to changes within it (Aston, Meagher-Stewart, Edwards, et al., 2009; Baisch, 2009; CPHA, 2010; CHNC, 2011). For example, when increasing numbers of grandparents are caring for their grandchildren in a community, nurses can collaborate with local schools and agencies to create a program that might include an opportunity for peer support and education about available resources. The public health nurse is responsive by being active in the community; knowing its members, needs, and resources; working collaboratively to establish health promotion and disease prevention programs; and

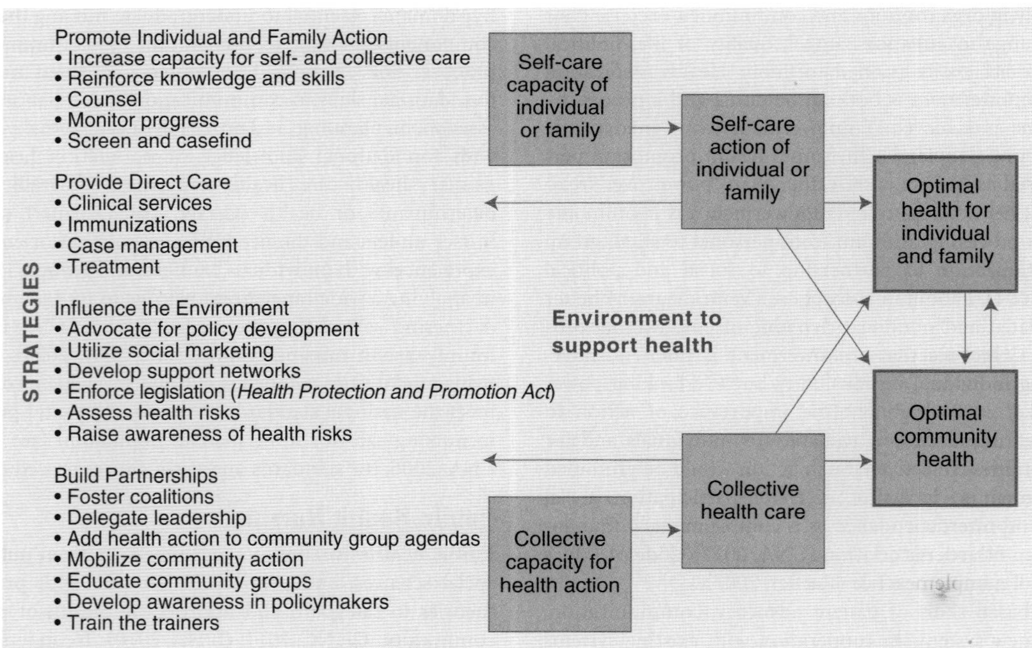

FIGURE 4-2 Framework for public health programs. (From N. Edwards et al. [1995]. *Building and sustaining collective health action: A framework for community health practitioners.* Ottawa: Community Health Research Unit, Pub. No. DP95-1, as cited by Edwards, N. C., & Moyer, A. [2000]. Community needs and capacity assessment: Critical component of program planning. In M. J. Stewart [Ed.], *Community nursing: Promoting Canadians' health* [2nd ed., p. 433], Toronto: W. B. Saunders.)

advocating for program and public policies that promote health and build capacity to identify and address health issues among individuals, families, communities, and service providers. This means developing and maintaining relationships with other professional systems and individuals and encouraging them to respond to a population's needs.

Home Health Nursing

Home health nursing, also known as **community-based nursing**, involves acute, chronic, and palliative care of individuals and their families that enhances their capacity for self-care and promotes autonomy in decision making (Hunt, 2013; CHNC, 2011). Nursing takes place in community settings such as the home, a long-term care facility, or a clinic. The nurse's competence is based on critical thinking and decision making at the level of the individual client: assessing health status, selecting nursing interventions, and evaluating care outcomes. Because they provide care where clients live, work, and play, home health nurses need to be individual- and family-oriented and also need to appreciate the community context (CHNC, 2010).

Components of home health nursing practice include self-care as a client and family responsibility, preventive care, care within the community context, continuity of care between home and health system services, and collaborative client care among health practitioners (CHNC, 2011). Nurses use their clinical expertise to provide direct care (e.g., a case manager monitors clients recovering from stroke and provides rehabilitation services). Nursing supports and improves clients' quality of life. Illness is seen as one aspect of clients' everyday lives. Nursing tends to be problem focused, addressing client needs for primary, secondary, and tertiary prevention (CHNC, 2011).

A strong theoretical foundation for home health nursing, and community health nursing broadly, is provided by the human ecological model, which conceptualizes human systems as open and interactive with the environment (Aston et al., 2009; Baisch, 2009; Chalmers, Bramadat, & Andrusyszyn, 1998). In an ecological model, the individual is viewed within the larger systems of family, social network, community, and society, which is commonly depicted as concentric circles: an innermost circle of the client and the immediate family, a second circle of people and settings that have frequent contact with the client and family, a third circle of the local community and its values and policies, and an outermost circle of larger social systems such as business and government. A home health nurse must understand the interaction of all systems while caring for clients and families in the home environment. Nurses typically become involved in the domain of the first three circles. For example, as a home health nurse, you work closely with a client recently diagnosed with diabetes and with the family to establish a care plan. You use observations of the client's lifestyle when considering an exercise schedule and meal routines. Knowing community resources (e.g., shops with glucose monitoring supplies, local diabetes support groups) enables you to provide comprehensive support.

Home health nursing is family-centred care (CHNC, 2010; Hunt, 2013). This care requires knowledge of family theory (see Chapter 19), global health (see Chapter 9), communication (see Chapter 17), and group dynamics. Empowerment-based strategies guide the nurse to work in partnership with clients and families (Toofany, 2007) in planning, decision making, implementation, and evaluation of health care approaches.

THE CHANGING FOCUS OF COMMUNITY HEALTH NURSING PRACTICE

Community health nursing practice has changed since the 1960s in response to social, economic, and political influences. Changes were documented by Chalmers and colleagues (1998), who interviewed community health nurse educators, administrators, and staff nurses who worked in public health agencies, home health services, and community health centres in Manitoba. The nurses noted shifts in practice focus from universal programs to programs directed toward high-risk or vulnerable groups, from generalized to specialized practice, and from delivery of traditional public health services to more community-based acute care. These shifts resulted in increasing demands on community health nurses to manage more complex care situations. In 2005, Meagher-Stewart, Aston, Edwards, et al. reported the practice challenges articulated by public health nurses and nurse administrators in Nova Scotia (Box 4-4), highlighting conditions that undercut their ability to work directly with patients, a highly valued aspect of their practice. The trends identified by Chalmers et al. remain relevant because they reflect continuing shifts and related challenges in community health nursing practice over a decade after they were publicized.

BOX 4-4 Challenges to Community Health Nursing Practice

- Pulled between documenting work and valued practice with clients
- Torn between prescribed programs and community partnership activities
- "Never enough time," especially for higher needs
- Increased task orientation, specialization, and working in silos
- Lack of evaluation of program effectiveness
- Increasing inequity of programs to rural, older-person, and low-income populations
- Feeling stretched related to shortage of nursing and administrative support staff
- Staying current on health information
- Loss of connection and visibility with the community

From Meagher-Stewart, D., Aston, M., Edwards, N., Smith, D., Young, L., Woodford, E., et al. (2005). *The study of public health nurses in primary health care. Fostering citizen participation and collaborative practice: Tapping the wisdom and voices of public health nurses in Nova Scotia.* Research report (p. 6). Halifax: Dalhousie University. Retrieved from http://preventionresearch.dal.ca/pdf/PHN_study_Nov25.pdf.

Although many changes are consistent with the principles of primary health care and health promotion, there is concern that some changes put universal accessibility of public health nursing services at risk (Meagher-Stewart et al., 2005). This concern has also emerged in home health practice, in which a policy agenda of increasing medicalization "potentially leads to further marginalization of the most vulnerable" (Duncan & Reutter, 2006, p. 242). Home health care case managers have expressed concern about limits on their practice arising from a conflict between professional discourse that guides practice and economic discourse that drives organizational priorities (Ceci, 2006). Underwood, Mowat, Meagher-Stewart, et al.'s (2009) examination of enablers to public health nursing practice identifies opportunities to enhance capacity to counter current system pressures. They concluded that "community nurses work well together, but need time, flexible funding and management support to strengthen relationships with their communities and clients and to build partnerships with other professionals" (p. I-10).

Vulnerable Populations: People Who Live in Vulnerable Circumstances

Community health nurses care for clients from diverse cultures and backgrounds and with various health conditions. However, because of changes in the health care delivery system, high-risk groups have become the nurses' principal clients.

Vulnerable populations of clients are those who are likely to develop health problems as a result of excessive risks, who experience barriers when trying to access health care services, or who are dependent on others for care. Vulnerability can be understood in relation to the determinants of health, particularly social determinants that compromise socioeconomic status, literacy, and social inclusion (see Chapter 1). People who live in poverty, people who are homeless, people who live in precarious circumstances (such as women in abusive interpersonal relationships), people with chronic conditions and disabilities, and people who engage in stigmatizing risk behaviours (including substance abuse and unsafe sexual practices), as well as Indigenous peoples and new immigrants and refugees, are examples of vulnerable populations (Beiser & Stewart, 2005). Individuals and their families often belong to more than one of these groups and may live in communities that can be characterized as vulnerable. Frequently, clients in vulnerable circumstances come from a variety of cultures, have beliefs and values different from the mainstream culture, face language barriers, and have few sources of social support (Chalmers et al., 1998; Mikkonen & Raphael, 2010). Their distinctive needs contribute to the challenges that community nurses face.

To provide competent care to people who live in vulnerable circumstances, nurses in community health care practice must be comfortable with diversity as valuable to individual and social well-being. Culture, ethnicity, ability, economic status, gender, and sexual orientation are all aspects of diversity in Canadian society. Comfort with diversity requires more than tolerance of difference, which implies that the dominant culture is the reference point. Chapter 9 addresses factors influencing individual differences within culture within context and the nurse's role in providing culturally competent and safe care. To provide culturally competent and safe care, the nurse must be able to understand clients' cultural beliefs, values, and practices within their context in order to work with them to determine their needs and the interventions most likely to improve their health. The nurse should not judge or evaluate a client's beliefs and values about health in terms of the nurse's own culture. Communication and caring practices are crucial for understanding clients' perceptions and for planning effective, culturally competent and safe health care. Thus nurses need to be aware of cultural and ethnic determinants of health, differing beliefs about health and medicine among ethnic communities, and barriers to accessing care that affect members of minority or marginalized populations.

People who live in vulnerable circumstances typically experience poorer health outcomes than people with ready access to resources and health care services (Beiser & Stewart, 2005; Raphael, 2016). Members of vulnerable groups frequently experience cumulative risk factors or combinations of risk conditions that make them more sensitive to adverse effects of individual risk factors that others might overcome (Raphael, 2016). Community health nurses must assess clients who are structurally vulnerable by considering multiple risk factors and the clients' strengths. Box 4-5 summarizes guidelines for assessing clients from vulnerable population groups.

BOX 4-5 Guidelines for Assessing People Who Live in Vulnerable Circumstances

Setting the Stage

- Create a comfortable, nonthreatening environment.
- Learn as much as you can about the culture of the clients you work with, to understand traditions and values that influence their health care practices.
- Provide culturally competent and safe assessment by understanding the meaning of language and nonverbal behaviour in the client's culture.
- Be aware that the individual or family may have priorities, such as financial or legal problems, that, within your scope as a nurse, you may need to help them deal with before specific health concerns can be addressed.
- Collaborate with others as appropriate; connect your client with someone who can help.

Nursing History of an Individual or a Family

- You may have only one opportunity to work with a person or family. Try to document a history that provides essential information you need to help on that day. Organize what you need to ask, and be prepared to explain why the information is necessary.
- Use a modified comprehensive assessment form to focus on the distinctive needs of the client. Be flexible. With some clients, it is impractical and unethical to ask all questions on the form.
- Include questions about social support, economic status, resources for health care, current health problems, medication, and how the person or family manages their health. Your goal is to obtain information that will enable you to provide family-centred care, work with strengths, and address concerns.

Physical Examination or Home Assessment

- Complete as thorough a physical examination (on an individual) or home assessment as you can. Collect only information you can use to work with the individual or family.
- Be alert for indications of mental or physical abuse, substance use, or differences from expected physical examination findings.
- Observe a family's living environment. Does the family have running water, functioning plumbing, electricity, and access to a telephone? Is paint peeling on the walls and ceilings? Are room ventilation and temperature adequate? Is the home next to a busy highway, exposing the family to high noise levels and automobile exhaust?

Adapted from Sebastian, J. G. (2006). Vulnerability and vulnerable populations: An overview. In M. Stanhope & J. Lancaster (Eds.), *Foundations of nursing in the community: Community-oriented practice* (pp. 403–417). St. Louis, MO: Mosby.

People Who Live in Poverty or Are Homeless. People who live in poverty are more likely to live in hazardous environments, work at high-risk jobs, eat less nutritious foods, and experience multiple stressors. They often face practical problems such as limited access to transportation, limited quality child care to support employment, and limited medication or dental coverage from supplementary health benefits. Low-income status is prevalent among lone-parent families, unattached older persons (mostly women), and Indigenous families (Canadian Population Health Initiative, 2004; Raphael, 2016). People who are homeless have even fewer resources than do people living on low incomes. Their vulnerability lies in their social condition, lifestyle, and environment, all of which diminish their ability to maintain or improve their health or access to health care. People who are homeless may live on the streets, in temporary accommodation such as shelters and boarding houses, or serially stay with friends (couch surf). They may distrust health and social services as bureaucratic and judgemental, using them only when their health has deteriorated (Pauly, 2014; Wen, Hudak, & Hwang, 2007). Chronic health problems worsen because of barriers to supportive self-care and medical care. People who are homeless have a high incidence of mental illness and substance abuse. Nurses can help people identify their capacities and resources, their eligibility for assistance, and interventions to help improve their health (Figure 4-3). For example, Cathy Crowe's work as a street nurse in Toronto includes direct care such as "dressing a wound under a highway overpass" and "treating frostbite" as well as advocacy such as "constantly seeking donations like Gatorade to counter dehydration"

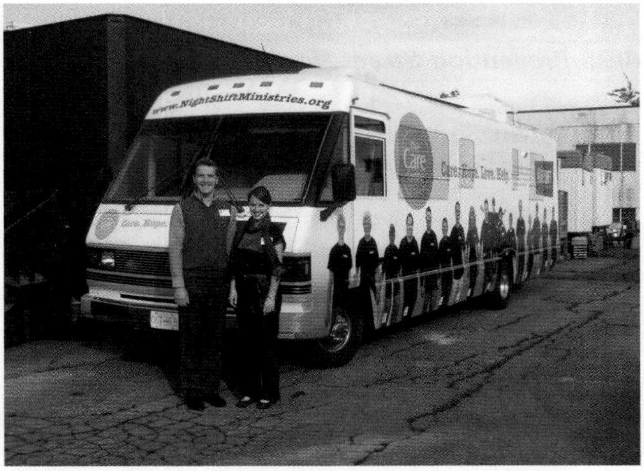

FIGURE 4-3 Nursing students working in a Care Bus to provide basic health care to the homeless population. (Courtesy Barbara J. Astle, RN, PhD.)

and "documenting police-inflicted injuries" (Crowe, 2007, p. 6) (see Box 1-2 in Chapter 1).

People in Precarious Circumstances. Women are at greater risk for problems related to low income, violence, and the stressors associated with unpaid caregiving. Such risks are further complicated for some women by living in geographically isolated settings that challenge women's capacities to maintain their health (Leipert & Reutter, 2005). Community health nurses' work is guided by their recognition of the need to listen to, respect, and communicate with women in their communities (Leipert, Regan, & Plunkett, 2015).

Physical, emotional, and sexual abuse and neglect are major public health problems, particularly affecting older persons, women, and children (CPHA, 2010; Sebastian, 2006). Abuse occurs in many settings, including the home, workplace, school, health care facility, and public areas, and is most often committed by an acquaintance of the victim (CPHA, 2010). When dealing with clients at risk for or who may have suffered abuse, nurses must seek to provide protection for them. Interviews with clients should occur in private when the individual suspected of being the perpetrator is not present. Clients who have been abused often fear retribution if they discuss their problems with a health care provider. Most regions have reporting agencies or hotlines for notification when an individual has been identified as being at risk, and nurses can work with clients to reflect on concerns, identify acceptable alternatives, and make decisions about their situation.

Unintentional injuries, unemployment, depression, and suicide are a concern among youth, particularly young men and those in Indigenous communities. As Gillis noted in 2000, "Community health nurses who are concerned with adolescent health promotion must consider the broad range of factors that affect adolescent health decisions and behaviours. Individual, family and environmental factors must be considered, together with many structural and societal factors" (p. 257). These considerations remain relevant for nurses working with youth today (Registered Nurses' Association of Ontario, 2010; YouThrive, 2017).

A focus on how the physical environment influences health has re-emerged as a priority for community health nurses, reflecting increasing public concerns about potential exposure to hazardous physical environments. These environments include natural and built environments. The quality of the built environment of daily life—dwellings, schools, workplaces, and community spaces—has an impact on individual and community health. Environmental racism, documented in "communities of colour" who experienced disproportionate exposure to hazardous waste facilities, landfills, and incinerators (Taylor, 2014), is a form of environmental injustice, encompassing racial and class-based discrimination that underpins such exposures in marginalized communities. An environmental justice perspective can support action to address inequitable distribution of health-promoting amenities, such as walkable neighbourhoods and park space, and of hazardous exposures, such as unsafe housing, toxic industrial sites, and polluted ground waters (Cutts, Darby, Boone, et al., 2009).

People Living With Chronic Conditions and Disabilities. "Chronic conditions are impairments in function, development, or disease states that are irreversible or have a cumulative effect" (Ogden Burke, Kauffmann, Wiskin, et al., 2000, p. 211). There are physical and emotional aspects of living with chronic conditions. Societal trends toward greater family mobility, maternal employment, smaller families, and female-headed, lone-parent, low-income families are challenges for families caring for children with chronic conditions (Woodgate, Edwards, Ripat, et al., 2015). Older persons experience more chronic conditions as they age (Denton & Spencer, 2010). The shift in health care service delivery from institutional to community-based care places demands on families, particularly women, to provide caregiving in the community. Nurses need to work with individuals, families, and communities to promote adequate support for family caregivers and access to resources and services.

For a client with a severe mental illness, multiple health and socioeconomic problems must be explored. Many such clients are homeless or marginally housed. Others are unable to work or provide self-care. They require medication therapy, counselling, housing, and vocational assistance. No longer hospitalized in long-term psychiatric institutions, clients with mental illness are offered resources within their community. However, many communities face continuing difficulties establishing comprehensive, coordinated, and accessible service networks (Dewa, Jacobson, Durbin, et al., 2010; Shah, 2003). Many clients who lack functional skills are left with fewer, more fragmented services.

Collaboration among community resources is key to helping people with mental illness obtain health care. For example, the interdisciplinary Psychiatric Outreach Team of the Royal Ottawa Hospital provides mobile services to shelters and drop-in centres to initiate mental health care, assist in linking clients to community resources, and provide education and assistance in connecting with mental health and addiction treatment (Farrell, Huff, MacDonald, et al., 2005).

With the increasing population of older persons, there is a corresponding increase in the number of patients with chronic disease and a greater demand for health care (Osborn, Moulds, Squires, et al., 2014). In providing health care to this population, nurses need to view health promotion from a broad perspective, by understanding what health means to older persons and ways they can maintain their own health. Individuals who feel empowered to control their own health may experience an enhanced engagement with health promotion efforts and a sense of health as a resource for everyday living (McWilliam, Vingilis, Ward-Griffin, et al., 2014). Through empowering patients to maintain their health, nurses can help improve the quality of life for older persons.

People Who Engage in Stigmatizing Risk Behaviours. Potentially stigmatizing risk behaviours include substance misuse and abuse and unsafe sexual practices. The social determinants of health provide a holistic perspective to address social and structural conditions that influence behaviour and to challenge the "unprecedented reliance on interventions that focus on addressing what is wrong with the individual" (Shoveller & Johnson, 2006, p. 56). *Substance misuse* is a general term for the use of illegal drugs, the abuse of alcohol, and the misuse or abuse of prescribed medications such as anti-anxiety drugs and narcotic analgesics. Clients who misuse substances also frequently have health and socioeconomic problems. A substantial proportion of adult HIV and AIDS cases have been attributed to injection drug use (Geduld & Gatali, 2003).

Substance misuse, particularly alcohol abuse, remains a serious problem among Canadian adolescents (Health Canada, 2007; Leatherdale & Ahmed, 2010). Socioeconomic problems often result from financial strain, employment loss, and family breakdown. The incidence of unsafe sexual practices and multiple risk-taking behaviours remains high among young people (Smylie, Medaglia, & Maticka-Tyndale, 2006). Unsafe sex creates serious health and social risks, including the risks of unplanned pregnancy and acquiring sexually transmitted infections (e.g., HIV infection and AIDS). Unplanned adolescent pregnancy is associated with risks for both mothers and infants, including pregnancy complications (Fleming, Tu, & Black, 2012), low income, low academic achievement, unemployment, violence (Oulman, Kim, Yunis, et al., 2015), and stigma (Fulford & Ford Gilboe, 2004).

Community health nurses can partner with clients to assess the circumstances that contribute to substance use, unsafe sexual practices, and other risk behaviours and identify strategies to address the often multiple and interrelated concerns. For example, Steenbeek (2004) identified strategies such as peer leader training and self-advocacy skill development within an empowering health promotion framework to prevent sexually transmitted infections among Indigenous youth. The AIDS Prevention Street Nurse Program (Box 4-6) and the Case Study (Box 4-7) illustrate **harm reduction**, an important but controversial approach to health promotion that is based on user input and demand, compassionate pragmatism, and commitment to offering alternatives to reduce risk behaviour consequences, to accept alternatives to abstinence, and to reduce barriers to treatment by providing user-friendly access (Hilton, Thompson, Moore-Dempsey, et al., 2001a; Pauly, Goldstone, McCall, et al., 2007; Shah, 2003).

BOX 4-6 RESEARCH HIGHLIGHT

AIDS Prevention Street Nurse Program

Research Focus

The AIDS Prevention Street Nurse Program in Vancouver provides outreach services for preventing HIV and sexually transmitted infection in vulnerable, high-risk clients (Hilton, Thompson, & Moore-Dempsey, 2009; Hilton, Thompson, Moore-Dempsey, et al., 2000, 2001b). The program was awarded the Provincial Health Officer's Award of Excellence in 2007 and acknowledged as symbolizing best nursing practices and organizational commitment. Community health nurses with the program use harm reduction and health promotion approaches in their work. Harm reduction includes needle exchange for injection drug use, education to promote safer drug use and sexual behaviour, and support to patients in addiction treatment programs. Nurses go where the clients are: clinics, drop-in centres, detoxification centres, jails, door-to-door in hotels, or on the street.

Research Abstract

The purpose of the program evaluation study was to describe the nurses' work and its impact on clients, the challenges that nurses faced, and the program fit with other services (Hilton et al., 2001b). Program nurses were interviewed, as were client of the program, including youths living on the streets, sex trade workers, and injection drug users. Challenges facing nurses include building trust with clients, providing needed care or resources, and involving other health care providers. Clients reported gaining knowledge, feeling better about themselves, being supported, and changing their behaviours to help themselves and others (Hilton et al., 2000, 2001b).

Evidence-Informed Practice

- Key strategies for reaching vulnerable populations include working with clients "at their location, on their own terms, and according to their own agenda" (Hilton et al., 2001b, p. 274) and encouraging and facilitating client participation and choice.
- Client empowerment can be promoted through nurses' nonjudgemental care, trust, and respect.
- Educating marginalized clients about health promotion and harm prevention increases their self-concept and encourages them to change their behaviour.

Hilton, B. A., Thompson, R., & Moore-Dempsey. L. (2009). Evaluation of the AIDS prevention street nurse program: One step at a time. *Canadian Journal of Nursing Research, 41*(1), 238–258; Hilton, A. B., Thompson, R., Moore-Dempsey, L., & Hutchinson, K. (2001). Urban outpost nursing: The nature of the nurses' work in the AIDS prevention street nurse program. *Public Health Nursing, 18*(4), 273–280; and Thompson, R., Hilton, A. B., Moore-Dempsey, L., & Hutchinson, K. (2000). AIDS prevention on the streets: Vancouver nurses are taking AIDS prevention to the streets. *Canadian Nurse, 96*(8), 24–28.

Standards, Competencies, Roles, and Activities in Community Health Nursing

Nurses in community health practice must have a broad base of knowledge and skills in order to work with clients to meet their health care needs and develop community relationships. Primary health care and health promotion approaches help nurses recognize the interplay between individual experience and social conditions, the value of diversity, and the importance of building capacity to promote health-enhancing change. The CHNC (2011) has identified seven standards of practice for community health nurses: health promotion; prevention and health protection; health maintenance, restoration, and palliation; professional relationships; capacity building; access and equity; and professional responsibility and accountability. These standards "define the scope and depth of community nursing practice; establish criteria and expectations for acceptable nursing practice and safe, ethical care; and inspire excellence in and commitment to community nursing practice" in nursing care, education, administration, and research (CHNC, 2011, p. 7). Nurses in community health nursing practice are responsible for meeting these professional nursing standards (CHNC, 2011). In addition, nurses in the specialty practice areas of public health or home health are responsible for meeting relevant competencies (i.e., having required knowledge, skills, and attitudes) (see CHNC, 2009, 2010; PHAC, 2007).

Community health nurses have multiple important roles in health promotion, disease and injury prevention, health protection, health surveillance, population health assessment, and emergency preparedness and response (CPHA, 2010). A summary of key activities engaged in by nurses in meeting responsibilities for these multiple roles was articulated in 1990 and updated in 2010 by the CPHA and is presented in the following sections.

Communication. *Communication* skills support all other activities in community health nursing practice. Skill as an effective communicator is closely related to the leadership and advocacy skills of the facilitator. Nurses may use negotiation and mediation to foster collaboration.

Facilitation. To *facilitate* is to promote. Community health nurses work within a participatory process to identify issues, develop goals for change, and implement strategies for action and evaluation of results. Leadership and advocacy skills are key to these activities.

Leadership. *Leadership* focuses on supporting processes that build capacity among participants, rather than on directing or controlling decision making. To develop proactive approaches to health and

BOX 4-7 CASE STUDY

Harm Reduction Nursing

Harm reduction initiatives exemplify community health nursing practice guided by primary health care, health promotion, empowerment, and ethical principles. The leadership, creativity, and dedication of nurses have contributed significantly to the development of these initiatives. Services may include health assessments, testing for sexually transmitted infections, screening, immunizations, minor treatments, emergency care, health education and counselling, advocacy, and support for natural helpers, in addition to needle exchange for people living in vulnerable circumstances. For example, Wood, Zettel, and Stewart (2003) successfully advocated for the establishment of a supervised injection site for injection drug users as part of the day program services provided by the Dr. Peter Centre in Vancouver's Downtown Eastside. Collaborating with local HIV and AIDS network members, researchers, and street nurses, they developed policies, procedures, and protocols to deliver harm reduction services to a highly vulnerable population in which stigmatizing risk behaviours were compounded by homelessness, precarious life circumstances, and chronic conditions and disabilities. In addition to the supervised injection site, nurses provide sterile drug injection supplies through a needle exchange program, teach about safer sex, offer condoms, talk with sex trade workers about safer ways of dealing with johns, counsel on addiction, support methadone maintenance regimens, and help when individuals are ready to enter detoxification programs or rehabilitation (Griffiths, 2002, p. 12). Serving the same population in Vancouver, Insite, North America's first dedicated legal supervised drug injection facility, opened in 2003 with diverse stakeholder engagement. Insite provides health care, counselling, education, and support from a multidisciplinary team that includes nurses (Small, Palepu, & Tyndall, 2006; Wood, Wood, Lai, et al., 2008). Since 1989, nurses with the Streetworks initiative in Edmonton have worked from several fixed daytime sites and from a mobile van for evening outreach to offer harm reduction strategies in partnership with agencies serving the inner-city community.

Nursing services have expanded from needle exchange to include a range of health services as well as special initiatives to support street-involved youth and pregnant women. Nurses' work in these initiatives illustrates many of the role dimensions needed for community health practice, including activities as communicator, facilitator, collaborator, coordinator, educator, care or service provider, community developer, policy formulator, and researcher. "Using professional practice to create change, the passion and leadership of a few nurses are resulting in an innovative approach. If such an approach were adopted across Canada, the number of human lives and health care dollars saved would be monumental" (Wood et al., 2003, p. 24). You are encouraged to reflect on these nursing roles and activities by reading more about these and similar programs in communities across the country.

Websites

Dr. Peter Centre: http://www.drpeter.org/dr-peter-centre/

Insite: http://www.vch.ca/public-health/harm-reduction/supervised-injection-sites

StreetWorks: http://www.streetworks.ca/pro/index.html

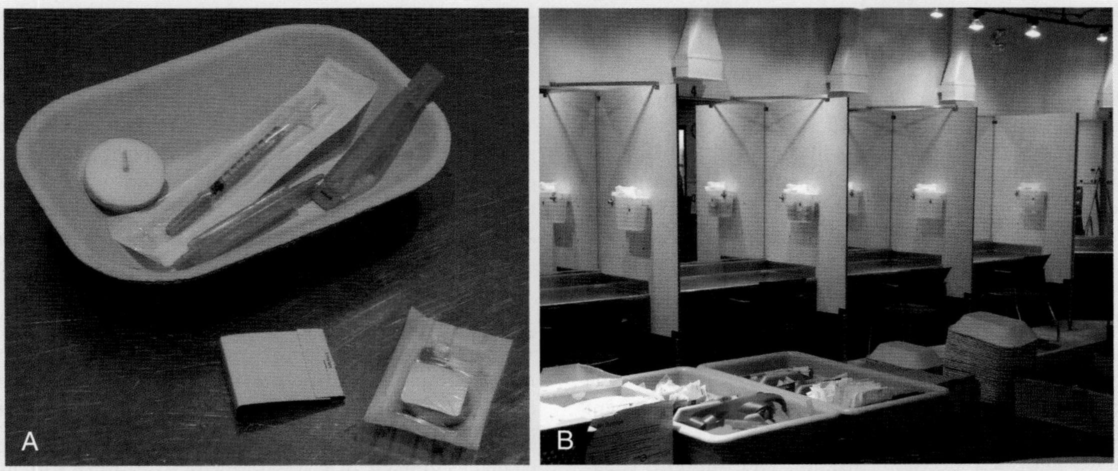

Harm reduction nursing practice at Vancouver's Insite showing an injection kit that contains sterile drug injection supplies (A), and the interior of the facility (B). (Vancouver Coastal Health: http://www.vch.ca/public-health/harm-reduction/supervised-injection-sites)

environmental issues, nurses need to apply knowledge of professional, community, and political issues and processes.

Advocacy. *Advocacy,* underpinned by commitment to equity and social justice, fosters attention and action to address social determinants of health and accessibility of care, especially among vulnerable populations. Community health nurses may help clients become aware of issues that influence their health, build capacity to speak for themselves, and access resources to address issues.

Consultation. Community health nurses *consult* with clients as well as with community members, health care providers, professionals from other disciplines, members of other sectors, policymakers, and government officials. Nurses respond to inquiries about and make referrals to community resources. By developing collaborative relationships, nurses support client access to these resources.

Team Building and Collaboration. *Team building and collaboration* is a way of working together, characterized by recognition of interdependence, collective responsibility, and negotiated equity in relationships (Gray, 1989; Labonte, 1993). Nurses may participate in a team or collective process as a collaborator with clients, community members, agencies, and sectors. This process is supported by developing honest relationships and mutual respect, recognizing many forms of expertise, valuing diversity, and being organized and committed.

Building Capacity. *Building individual and collective capacity* is a means to address health issues and overcome barriers to achieve enhanced quality-of-life outcomes (Labonte, Woodward, Chad, et al., 2002). Community health nurses may help community members understand their strengths and abilities, develop leadership, extend social networks, and work together. Group process skills are integral to supporting capacity-building activities.

Building Coalitions and Networks. Community health nurses also use capacity-building skills in situations where there is need for *building coalitions and networks* to support collective action on health issues. Nurses may work with community members to identify the type of coalition or network that best fits their intended purpose, to clarify leadership roles, to create links between the coalition or network and the community at large, and to provide requested support to the coalition or network.

Outreach. *Outreach* supports a holistic approach to community nursing practice and is particularly critical when working with vulnerable populations. Outreach often involves locating services in places that are considered safe or comfortable for potential users, using acceptable approaches to care, and working with clients "where they are at," including using harm reduction strategies.

Resource Management, Planning, Coordination. *Coordination*, often also involving resource management and planning, has long been associated with nursing practice. Nurses work with clients and diverse agencies to plan and coordinate activities, resources, access, and care to promote client health. These activities complement activities focused on education, care/counselling, and community development.

Case Management. *Case management* skills are closely linked with resource management, planning, and coordination skills and activities. Community health nurses' work will commonly involve case finding, including identification of potential clients who are structurally vulnerable, in addition to assessment as a basis for planning, implementing, and evaluating actions to address identified issues. Development of trusting relationships with clients, capacity building, and collaboration are central to effective case management.

Care/Counselling. Community health nurses provide *care/counselling* as they work with clients to promote and protect health and to prevent injury and illness. In many communities, home visiting remains integral to practice, as do services such as health assessment and immunization clinics. Nurses treat illness, monitor risk conditions, educate or guide informed decision making, and support client self-care.

Referral and Follow-Up. Community health nurses work with individuals and families to make decisions about appropriate *referral and follow-up* care, services, or resources. Nurses will need to develop and link with other providers, agencies, and networks to support effective and appropriate referral and follow-up.

Screening. *Screening* is intended to identify emerging, typically presymptomatic health problems for early treatment and improved health outcomes. Screening contributes to timely case finding. Nurses work to ensure that clients understand and consent to screening activities, that acceptable approaches are used to support culturally safe and competent care, and that appropriate referral and follow-up are completed.

Surveillance. *Surveillance* information is used to enhance understanding of health threats or problems, their natural course, and intervention effectiveness. Nurses may be involved in informal surveillance as well as formal or legally mandated protocols that contribute to documenting, interpreting, and sharing relevant surveillance information.

Health Threat Response. Community health nurses may be involved in *health threat response* procedures, such as when a natural disaster occurs in a community. Nurses must understand and follow established procedures that may include case investigation, provision of preventive care, and referral and follow-up for those needing treatment.

Health Education. Skillful and effective client education with individuals and groups requires a broad knowledge base, as well as communication and learning process skills. Nurses provide information to support community, family, and individual decision making. Nurses may participate in formal education sessions, such as prenatal classes, or in informal sessions, such as discussions with families during home visits.

Community Development. Community health nurses apply knowledge of *community assessment and development* to support community participation. Participation encourages open identification of issues, shared decision making, egalitarian relationships, and collective ownership of action (Labonte, 1993). Participation and empowerment are closely linked.

Policy Development and Implementation. Activities related to *policy development and implementation* include identifying the need for policy and program development; participating in program development, implementation, and evaluation; helping establish policies to support practice; and using political processes to promote health. Nurses need to support the collective voice of professional associations (e.g., CNA, CHNC) to advocate for health-enhancing public policy. Falk-Rafael (2005) contends that "nurses, who practice at the intersection of public policy and personal lives, are, therefore, ideally situated and morally obligated to include political advocacy and efforts to influence health public policy in their practice" (p. 212).

Research and Evaluation. *Research and evaluation* are used to generate information, identify issues, determine directions for action, consider strategies to promote change, and assess results. Nurses need to review research and apply knowledge to practice. Nurses may also engage in research and evaluation projects as a participant or investigator to support evidence-informed decisions about practice.

COMMUNITY ASSESSMENT

As a community health nurse, you need to assess the community, the environment in which people live and work. Without an understanding of that environment, any effort to promote health and to support change is unlikely to succeed, whether you work with an individual, a family, a group, or a community as client.

The community can be seen as having three components: the locale or structure, the social systems, and the people. A complete assessment involves studying each component to understand the health status of the people and the health determinants that influence their health as a basis on which to identify needs for health policy, health program development, and service provision. (For detailed descriptions of community assessment strategies, see community health nursing textbooks such as those by Diem & Moyer, 2015; Stamler & Yiu, 2016; Stanhope, Lancaster, Jakubec, et al., 2017; and Vollman, Anderson, & McFarlane, 2017.) To assess the locale or structure, you might travel around the community and observe the physical environment, the location of services, and the places where residents congregate (completing a windshield or walking survey). Information about social systems, such as schools, health care facilities, recreation, transportation, and government, may be acquired by visiting various sites and learning about their services (observing activities, interviewing key informants).

Community statistics from a local library or health department can help with assessing a population's demographics and health status (reviewing population data). Discussion with community members, including a social and environmental health history (interviewing key informants, holding focus groups), is also helpful to identify priority issues within the community. It is essential to identify community resources and capacities, as well as issues and problems (Diem & Moyer, 2015).

Recall the determinants of health as you consider the following scenario. As a community health nurse, you wish to familiarize yourself with the local area to help you begin to identify potential health concerns and available resources that will guide your work with the community. Your windshield and walking surveys reveal an older, high-density neighbourhood where pawn shops and bars outnumber grocery stores, schools, and community recreation facilities. You observe a culturally diverse population, including young families and older people who interact with each other at community events sponsored by faith-based groups and social agencies. Your observations are reinforced in discussions as you develop relationships with community leaders and health and social agency staff, whose perspectives are supported by census tract data and regional health statistics. You are alerted to tensions related to high unemployment and language barriers to services. Once you have a good understanding of the community, you may then perform individual or family client assessment against that background. For example, consider assessment of families in a low-income housing complex. Is lighting along walkways and entryways operational? Do they feel comfortable calling on their neighbours for assistance if necessary? Are health and social services easy to reach when needed? Do they feel a sense of belonging in the neighbourhood? No individual or family assessment should occur in isolation from the environment and conditions of the community setting. A collaborative approach to community assessment grounded in an empowerment process helps establish working relationships, identify shared concerns, recognize collective capacities, and develop effective strategies to enhance health.

PROMOTING CLIENTS' HEALTH

The challenge for nurses in community health practice is how to promote and protect the health of clients, whether within the context of their community or with the community as the focus. Community health nurses may bring together the resources necessary to improve the continuity of client care. In collaboration with clients, health care and social service providers, and other community members, nurses coordinate health care services, locate appropriate social services, and develop innovative approaches to address clients' health issues.

Perhaps the key to being an effective community health nurse is the ability to understand clients' everyday lives. The foundation for this understanding is the establishment of strong, caring relationships with clients (see Chapters 17 and 18) that support empowerment as an active process rooted in cultural, religious, and personal belief systems and awareness of links between personal lives, community experiences, and social political contexts (Falk-Rafael, 2001, 2005). The quasi-insider status of nurses in a community often enables them to identify local patterns and needs that can be addressed through programs, policies, and advocacy (Baisch, 2009; SmithBattle, Diekemper, & Leander, 2004) that are responsive, supportive, and effective. The day-to-day activities of family and community life and the cultural, economic, and political environment influence how they adapt nursing interventions. Once a nurse acquires an understanding of an individual's or family's life, interventions designed to promote health and prevent disease can be introduced. Similarly, understanding the relationships, activities, and concerns of groups and communities is central to health promotion practice. A continuing challenge for community health nurses is to take up their practice in ways that establish meaningful, respectful engagement with people in their communities and that promote individual, family, and collective empowerment, to enhance health in everyday life.

KEY CONCEPTS

- A successful community health nursing practice involves building relationships with the community members and being responsive to changes within the community.
- The principles of public health nursing practice support assisting individuals in acquiring a healthy environment in which to live.
- The public health nurse cares for the community as a whole and considers the individual or family to be one member of a population or potential group at risk.
- The home health nurse's competence is based on decision making at the level of the individual client.
- Within an ecological model of home health nursing, the individual is viewed within the larger systems of family, social network, community, and society.
- Vulnerable individuals and their families often belong to more than one vulnerable group.
- The distinctive needs of persons who are structurally vulnerable contribute to the challenges that nurses face in caring for these clients.
- Exacerbations of chronic health problems are common among homeless people because they have few resources.
- An important principle in dealing with clients at risk for or who may have suffered abuse is protection of the client.
- Clients who engage in risk behaviours such as substance misuse may respond to a harm reduction approach.
- In community health practice, it is important to understand what health means to clients and what they do to maintain their own health.
- A community health nurse must be competent in fulfilling a multidimensional role, including engaging in communication; facilitation; leadership; advocacy; consultation; team building and collaboration; building capacity; building coalitions and networks; outreach; resource management, planning, and coordination; case management; care/counselling; referral and follow-up; screening; surveillance; health threat response; health education; community development; policy development and implementation; and research and evaluation activities.
- Assessment of a community includes assessing population health status and relevant determinants of health in relation to three elements: locale or structure, the social systems, and the people.
- An important consideration in becoming an effective community health nurse is to strive to understand clients' lives.

CRITICAL THINKING EXERCISES

1. You are working with the family of a severely disabled child and learn that no respite services to provide parental support, and only limited educational resources, are available in your community. What activities or roles of the community health nurse would be important to establish a special education day care service, operated by volunteer educators?
2. Mr. Crowder is a 42-year-old man with diabetes mellitus and visual impairment. Your assessment reveals that he is homeless and spends nights in a local shelter. He is not able to buy medications or ensure

adequate diet to control his blood glucose. What factors might you consider to support Mr. Crowder's self-care?

3. Conduct a community assessment of an area that you have visited infrequently. Observe the community locale by driving or walking through the more populated area. Look for the following services: hospital, clinic, pharmacy, grocery store, schools, park or playground, and police and fire departments.

REVIEW QUESTIONS

1. What are the overall goals of a population health approach?
   1. Maintain and improve the population's health and eliminate health disparities
   2. Gather information on incidence rates of certain diseases and social problems
   3. Assess the health care needs of individuals, families, or communities
   4. Develop and implement public health policies and improve access to acute care
2. Public health nursing merges knowledge from professional nursing theories and what science?
   1. Population sciences
   2. Public health sciences
   3. Environmental sciences
   4. Social sciences
3. Home health nursing involves acute, chronic, and palliative care of clients and families to enhance their capacity for which activity?
   1. Nursing care that promotes autonomy in decision making
   2. Improving their health care and self-care
   3. Self-care and autonomy in decision making
   4. Learning about their illnesses
4. Persons who are structurally vulnerable are more likely to develop health problems as a result of which circumstances?
   1. Acute diseases, homelessness, and poverty
   2. Lack of transportation, dependence on others for care, and lack of initiative
   3. Poverty, lack of education, and mental illness
   4. Excess risks, barriers to health care services, and dependence on others for care
5. Which is not an aspect of competent care for persons who are structurally vulnerable?
   1. Providing culturally appropriate care
   2. Creating a comfortable, nonthreatening environment
   3. Assessing living conditions
   4. Offering financial or legal advice
6. What are major public health problems affecting older persons, women, and children?
   1. Prescribed medication abuse, poverty, sexual abuse
   2. Physical, emotional, and sexual abuse, as well as neglect
   3. Acute illnesses, neglect, substance abuse
   4. Financial strain, poverty, physical abuse
7. What does a successful community health nursing practice require?
   1. A graduate degree in health education or health promotion
   2. Building relationships with and responding to changes in the community
   3. Taking a passive role to allow the community to initiate change
   4. Subspecialty education in public health sciences
8. Teaching classes about infant care, cancer screening, and home safety adaptations for older people are examples of a nurse engaging in which activity?
   1. Consultation
   2. Collaboration
   3. Health education
   4. Facilitation
9. A community health nurse who is directing a client to community resources is an example of which activity?
   1. Consultation
   2. Collaboration
   3. Coordination
   4. Research
10. What three elements are included in a community assessment?
    1. Locale or structure, social systems, and people
    2. People, neighbourhoods, and social systems
    3. Health care systems, geographic boundaries, and people
    4. Environment, families, and social systems

Answers: 1. 1; **2.** 2; **3.** 3; **4.** 4; **5.** 4; **6.** 2; **7.** 2; **8.** 3; **9.** 1; **10.** 1

Rationales for the Review Questions appear at the end of the book.

RECOMMENDED WEBSITES

Canadian Public Health Association: http://www.cpha.ca
The Canadian Public Health Association (CPHA) is a national, independent, not-for-profit, voluntary association representing public health care in Canada.

Community Health Nurses of Canada: http://www.chnc.ca/
The CHNC is a national organization. It provides standards and information on community health nursing.

Fact Sheet: The Primary Health Care Approach: https://www.cna-aiic.ca/~/media/cna/page-content/pdf-en/fs02_primary_health_care_approach_june_2000_e.pdf?la=en
This Canadian Nurses Association publication defines and describes primary health care in Canada.

Public Health Agency of Canada: Health Promotion: http://www.phac-aspc.gc.ca/hp-ps/index-eng.php
This federal website provides links to many useful health promotion resources and guides that will aid health professionals and community leaders.

Victorian Order of Nurses: http://www.von.ca/
The Victorian Order of Nurses (VON) is Canada's leading charitable organization addressing community health and social needs.

REFERENCES

Aston, M., Meagher-Stewart, D., Edwards, N., et al. (2009). Public health nurses' primary health care practice: Strategies for fostering citizen participation. *Journal of Community Health Nursing, 26*(1), 24–34. doi:10.1080/07370010802605762.

Baisch, M. J. (2009). Community health: An evolutionary concept analysis. *Journal of Advanced Nursing, 65*(11), 2464–2476. doi:10.1111/j.1365-2648.2009.05068.x.

Beiser, M., & Stewart, M. (2005). Reducing health disparities. *Canadian Journal of Public Health, 96*(Suppl. 2), S4–S5.

Canadian Association of Schools of Nursing (CASN). (2014). *Entry-to-practice public health nursing competencies for undergraduate nursing education*. Ottawa: Author.

Canadian Association of Schools of Nursing (CASN). (2015). *National nursing education framework: Final report*. Ottawa: Author.

Canadian Nurses Association (CNA). (2006). *Community health nursing certification*. Ottawa: Author.

Canadian Nurses Association (CNA). (2010). *Social justice…a means to an end, an end in itself* (2nd ed.). Ottawa: Author.

Canadian Nurses Association (CNA). (2017). *Code of ethics for registered nurses*. Ottawa: Author.

Canadian Population Health Initiative. (2004). *Summary report: Improving the health of Canadians*. Ottawa: Canadian Institute for Health Information.

Canadian Public Health Association (CPHA). (2010). *Community health—Public health nursing in Canada: Preparation and practice*. Ottawa: Author.

Ceci, C. (2006). Impoverishment of practice: Analysis of effects of economic discourses in home care case-management practice. *Nursing Leadership, 19*(1), 56–68.

Chalmers, K. I., & Bramadat, I. J. (1996). Community development: Theoretical and practical issues for community health nursing in Canada. *Journal of Advanced Nursing, 24*(4), 719–726.

Chalmers, K. I., Bramadat, I. J., & Andrusyszyn, M. A. (1998). The changing environment of community health practice and education: Perceptions of staff nurses, administrators, and educators. *Journal of Nursing Education, 37*(3), 109–117.

Community Health Nurses of Canada (CHNC). (2009). *Public health nursing discipline specific competencies* (Version 1.0). Retrieved from http://phabc.org/wp-content/uploads/2015/07/Community-Health-Nurses-Public-Health-Core-Competencies.pdf.

Community Health Nurses of Canada (CHNC). (2010). *Home health nursing competencies* (Version 1.0). Retrieved from http://neltoolkit.rnao.ca/sites/default/files/Home%20Health%20Nursing%20Competencies_March%202010.pdf.

Community Health Nurses of Canada (CHNC). (2011, March). *Canadian community health nursing: Professional practice model and standards of practice*. Retrieved from http://www.chnig.org/wp-content/uploads/2016/02/chnc-standards.pdf.

Community Health Nurses of Canada (CHNC). (2013). *Canadian community health nursing professional practice model*. Retrieved from https://www.chnc.ca/upload/membership/document/2016-07/canadiancommunityhealthnursingprofessionalpracticecompoments-e_1.pdf.

Cooke, H. (2002). Empowerment. In G. Blakeley & V. Bryson (Eds.), *Contemporary political concepts* (pp. 162–178). London, UK: Pluto Press.

Crowe, C. (2007). *Dying for a home: Homeless activists speak out*. Toronto: Between the Lines.

Cutts, B., Darby, K., Boone, C., et al. (2009). City structure, obesity, and environmental justice: An integrated analysis of physical and social barriers to walkable streets and park access. *Social Science & Medicine, 69*(9), 1314–1322. doi:10.1016/j.socscimed.2009.08.020.

Denton, F., & Spencer, B. (2010). Chronic health conditions: Changing prevalence in an aging population and some implications for the delivery of health care services. *Canadian Journal of Aging, 29*(1), 11–21. doi:10.1017/S0714980809990390.

Dewa, C. S., Jacobson, N., Durbin, J., et al. (2010). Examining the effects of enhanced funding for specialized community mental health programs on continuity of care. *Canadian Journal of Community Mental Health, 29*(Special Issue Supplement), 23–40.

Diem, E., & Moyer, A. (2015). *Community and public health nursing: Learning to make a difference through teamwork* (2nd ed.). Toronto: Canadian Scholars' Press.

Duncan, S., & Reutter, L. (2006). A critical policy analysis of an emerging agenda for home care in one Canadian province. *Health and Social Care in the Community, 14*, 242–253. doi:10.1111/j.1365-2524.2006.00616.x.

Edwards, N. C., & Moyer, A. (2000). Community needs and capacity assessment: Critical component of program planning. In M. J. Stewart (Ed.), *Community nursing: Promoting Canadians' health* (2nd ed., pp. 420–442). Toronto: W. B. Saunders.

Falk-Rafael, A. (2001). Empowerment as a process of evolving consciousness: A model of empowering care [Electronic version]. *Advances in Nursing Science, 24*(1), 1–16.

Falk-Rafael, A. (2005). Speaking truth to power: Nursing's legacy and moral imperative. *Advances in Nursing Science, 28*(3), 212–223.

Farrell, S., Huff, J., MacDonald, S., et al. (2005). Taking it to the street: A psychiatric outreach service in Canada. *Community Mental Health Journal, 41*(6), 737–746. doi:10.1007/s10597-005-6430-7.

Fleming, N. A., Tu, X., & Black, A. Y. (2012). Improved obstetrical outcomes for adolescents in a community-based outreach program: A matched cohort study. *Journal of Obstetrics and Gynaecology Canada, 34*(12), 1134–1140.

Fulford, A., & Ford-Gilboe, M. (2004). An exploration of the relationships between health promotion practices, health work, and felt stigma in families headed by adolescent mothers. *Canadian Journal of Nursing Research, 36*(4), 47–72.

Geduld, J., & Gatali, M. (2003). Estimates of HIV prevalence and incidence in Canada, 2002 [Electronic version]. *Canada Communicable Disease Report, 29*, 197–207.

Gillis, A. J. (2000). Adolescent health promotion: An evolving opportunity for community health nurses. In M. J. Stewart (Ed.), *Community nursing: Promoting Canadians' health* (2nd ed., pp. 241–261). Toronto: W. B. Saunders.

Gray, B. (1989). *Collaborating: Finding common ground for multiparty problems*. San Francisco, CA: Jossey-Bass.

Griffiths, H. (2002). Dr. Peter Centre: Removing barriers to health care services. *Nursing BC, 34*(5), 10–14.

Grypma, S., Wolfs, D., & Reimer-Kirkham, S. (2012). Returning home: Historical influences on home healthcare in Canada. *Home Healthcare Nursing, 30*(8), 453–460. doi:10.1097/NHH.ob013e3182650142.

Hamilton, N., & Bhatti, T. (1996). *Population health promotion: An integrated model of population health and health promotion*. Ottawa: Health Promotion Development Division, Health Canada.

Health Canada. (2007). *Canadian addiction survey (CAS): A national survey of Canadians' use of alcohol and other drugs. Substance use by Canadian youth*. Ottawa: Minister of Health.

Health Canada. (2016). *First Nations and Inuit health: Health care services*. Retrieved from https://www.canada.ca/en/health-canada/services/first-nations-inuit-health.html.

Hilton, B. A., Thompson, R., Moore-Dempsey, L., et al. (2000). AIDS prevention on the streets. *Canadian Nurse, 96*(8), 24–28.

Hilton, B. A., Thompson, R., Moore-Dempsey, L., et al. (2001a). Harm reduction theories and strategies for control of human immunodeficiency virus: A review of the literature. *Journal of Advanced Nursing, 33*(3), 357–370.

Hilton, B. A., Thompson, R., Moore-Dempsey, L., et al. (2001b). Urban outpost nursing: The nature of nurses' work in the AIDS Prevention Street Nurse Program. *Public Health Nursing, 18*(4), 273–280.

Hilton, B. A., Thompson, R., & Moore-Dempsey, L. (2009). Evaluation of the AIDS Prevention Street Nurse Program: One step at a time. *Canadian Journal of Nursing Research, 41*(1), 238–258.

Hunt, R. (2013). *Introduction to community-based nursing* (5th ed.). New York: Wolters Kluwer/Lippincott Williams & Wilkins.

Labonte, R. (1993). *Health promotion and empowerment: Practice frameworks*. Toronto: Centre for Health Promotion, University of Toronto, & Participaction.

Labonte, R., Woodward, G., Chad, K., et al. (2002). Community capacity building: A parallel track for health promotion programs. *Canadian Journal of Public Health, 93*(3), 181–182.

Laverack, G. (2004). *Health promotion practice: Power and empowerment*. Thousand Oaks, CA: Sage.

Leatherdale, S., & Ahmed, R. (2010). Alcohol, marijuana, and tobacco use among Canadian youth: Do we need more multi-substance prevention programming? *Journal of Primary Prevention, 31*(3), 99–108. doi:10.1007/s10935-010-0211-y.

Leipert, B., Regan, S., & Plunkett, R. (2015). Working through and around: Exploring rural public health nursing practices and policies to promote rural women's health. *Online Journal of Rural Nursing and Health Care, 2015*(1), 74–99. doi:10.14574/ojrnhc.v15i1.342.

Leipert, B., & Reutter, L. I. (2005). Developing resilience: How women maintain their health in northern geographically isolated settings. *Qualitative Health Research, 15*(1), 49–65. doi:10.1177/1049732304269671.

Maurer, F. A., & Smith, C. M. (2005). *Community/public health nursing practice: Health for families and populations* (3rd ed.). St. Louis: Elsevier.

McKay, M. (2016). The history of community health nursing in Canada. In L. L. Stamler & L. Yiu (Eds.), *Community health nursing: A Canadian perspective* (4th ed., pp. 1–19). Toronto: Pearson Prentice Hall.

McWilliam, C. L., Vingilis, E., Ward-Griffin, C., et al., the South West Community Care Access Centre Collaborative Group, & the Champlain Community Care Access Centre Collaborative Group. (2014). An evaluation of the effectiveness of engaging Canadian clients as partners in in-home care. *Health and Social Care in the Community, 22*(2), 210–224. doi:10.1111/hsc.12082.

Meagher-Stewart, D., Aston, M., Edwards, N., et al. (2005). *The study of public health nurses primary health care practice. Fostering citizen participation and collaborative practice: Tapping the wisdom and voices of public health nurses in Nova Scotia*. Research Report, Dalhousie University, Halifax, NS.

Mikkonen, J., & Raphael, D. (2010). *Social determinants of health: The Canadian facts*. Retrieved from http://www.thecanadianfacts.org/The_Canadian_Facts.pdf.

Ogden Burke, S., Kauffmann, E., Wiskin, N. M. W., et al. (2000). Children with chronic conditions and their families in the community. In M. J. Stewart (Ed.), *Community nursing: Promoting Canadians' health* (2nd ed., pp. 211–240). Toronto: W. B. Saunders.

Osborn, R., Moulds, D., Squires, D., et al. (2014). International survey of older adults finds shortcomings in access, coordination, and patient-centered care. *Health Affairs, 12*, 2247–2255. doi:10.1377/hlthaff.2014.0947.

Oulman, E., Kim, T. H. M., Yunis, K., et al. (2015). Prevalence and predictors of unintended pregnancy among women: An analysis of the Canadian maternity experiences survey. *BMC Pregnancy and Childbirth, 15*(260), 1–8. doi:10.1186/s12884-015-0663-4.

Pauly, B. (2014). Close to the street: Nursing practice with people marginalized by homelessness and substance use. In S. W. Hwang, R. McNeil, & M. Guirguis-Younger (Eds.), *Homelessness & health in Canada* (pp. 211–232). Ottawa: University of Ottawa.

Pauly, B., Goldstone, I., McCall, J., et al. (2007). The ethical, legal and social context of harm reduction. *Canadian Nurse, 103*(8), 19–23.

Public Health Agency of Canada (PHAC). (2007). *Core competencies for public health in Canada Release 1.0*. Ottawa: Author.

Public Health Agency of Canada (PHAC). (2016). *What is the population health approach?* Retrieved from http://www.phac-aspc.gc.ca/ph-sp/approach-approche/appr-eng.php#history.

Racher, F. (2007). The evolution of ethics for community practice. *Journal of Community Health Nursing, 24*(1), 65–76.

Raphael, D. (2016). Social determinants of health: Key issues and themes. In D. Raphael (Ed.), *Social determinants of health: Canadian perspectives* (3rd ed., pp. 3–31). Toronto: Canadian Scholars' Press.

Registered Nurses' Association of Ontario. (2010). *Enhancing healthy adolescent development*. Toronto: Registered Nurses' Association of Ontario.

Reutter, L. I., & Ford, J. S. (1996). Perceptions of public health nursing: Views from the field. *Journal of Advanced Nursing, 24*(1), 7–15.

Ross-Kerr, J. C. (2011). Nursing in Canada, 1600 to the present: A brief account. In J. Ross-Kerr & M. J. Wood (Eds.), *Canadian nursing: Issues and perspectives* (5th ed., pp. 18–41). Toronto: Elsevier Canada.

Sebastian, J. G. (2006). Vulnerability and vulnerable populations: An introduction. In M. Stanhope & J. Lancaster (Eds.), *Foundations of nursing in the community: Community-oriented practice* (2nd ed., pp. 403–417). St. Louis: Mosby.

Shah, C. P. (2003). *Public health and preventive medicine in Canada* (3rd ed.). Toronto: Elsevier Canada.

Shoveller, J., & Johnson, J. (2006). Risky groups, risky behaviour, and risky persons: Dominating discourses on youth sexual health. *Critical Public Health, 16*(1), 47–60. doi:10.1080/09581590600680621.

Small, D., Palepu, A., & Tyndall, M. (2006). The establishment of North America's first state sanctioned supervised injection facility: A case study in culture change. *International Journal of Drug Policy, 17*(2), 73–82. doi:10.1016/jdrugpo.2005.08 .004.

SmithBattle, L., Diekemper, M., & Leander, S. (2004). Moving upstream: Becoming a public health nurse, part 2. *Public Health Nursing, 21*(2), 95–102.

Smylie, L., Medaglia, S., & Maticka-Tyndale, E. (2006). The effect of social capital and socio-demographics on adolescent risk and sexual health behaviours. *Canadian Journal of Human Sexuality, 15*(2), 95–112.

Stamler, L. L., & Yiu, L. (Eds.), (2016). *Community health nursing: A Canadian perspective* (4th ed.). Toronto, ON: Pearson Prentice Hall.

Stanhope, M., Lancaster, J., Jakubec, S. L., et al. (2017). *Community health nursing in Canada* (3rd ed.). Toronto: Elsevier Canada.

Steenbeek, A. (2004). Empowering health promotion: A holistic approach in preventing sexually transmitted infections among First Nations and Inuit adolescents in Canada. *Journal of Holistic Nursing, 22*(3), 254–266.

Tarlier, D. S., Johnson, J. L., & Whyte, N. B. (2016). Voices from the wilderness: An interpretive study describing the roles and practice of outpost nurses. *Canadian Journal of Public Health, 94*(3), 180–184.

Taylor, D. E. (2014). *Toxic communities: Environmental racism, industrial pollution, and residential mobility*. New York: NYU Press.

Toofany, S. (2007). Empowering older people. *Nursing Older People, 19*(2), 12–14.

Underwood, J., Mowat, D., Meagher-Stewart, D., et al. (2009). Building community and public health nursing capacity: A synthesis report of the national community health nursing study. *Canadian Journal of Public Health, 100*, I-1–I-11.

Vollman, A. R., Anderson, E. T., & McFarlane, J. (2017). *Canadian community as partner: Theory & multidisciplinary practice* (4th ed.). New York: Wolters Kluwer.

Wen, C. K., Hudak, P. L., & Hwang, S. W. (2007). Homeless people's perceptions of welcomeness and unwelcomeness in healthcare encounters. *Journal of General Internal Medicine, 22*(7), 1011–1017. doi:10.1007/si1606-007-0183-7.

Wood, R. A., Wood, E., Lai, C., et al. (2008). Nurse delivered safer injection education among a cohort of injection drug users: Evidence from the evaluation of Vancouver's supervised injection facility. *International Journal of Drug Policy, 19*(3), 183–188. doi:10.1016/j.drugpo.2008.01.003.

Wood, R. A., Zettel, P., & Stewart, W. (2003). The Dr. Peter Centre: Harm reduction nursing. *Canadian Nurse, 99*(5), 20–24.

Woodgate, R. L., Edwards, M., Ripat, J. D., et al. (2015). Intense parenting: A qualitative study detailing the experiences of parenting children with complex care needs. *BMC Pediatrics, 15*(197), 1–15. doi:10.1186/s12887-015-0514-5.

YouThrive. (2017). *Supporting communities to create places where all youth thrive*. Retrieved from http://www.youthrive.ca/node/3.

Theoretical Foundations of Nursing Practice

Written by Sally Thorne, RN, PhD

OBJECTIVES

Mastery of content in this chapter will enable you to:

- Define the key terms listed.
- Describe selected theories of nursing practice and differentiate between them.
- Describe challenges inherent in theorizing about nursing practice.
- Recognize selected conceptual frameworks associated with nursing practice.
- Appreciate the historical development of thought related to nursing practice.
- Interpret current debates surrounding various theories of nursing practice.
- Describe relationships between theorizing and other forms of nursing knowledge.
- Appreciate the role of "theorizing" about the essence of nursing.

KEY TERMS

Assumption, p. 63
Concept, p. 63
Conceptual framework, p. 64
Conceptualization, p. 63
Descriptive theory, p. 65
Grand theory, p. 65
Metaparadigm concepts, p. 66
Middle-range theory, p. 65
Models for nursing, p. 63
Nursing diagnosis, p. 65
Nursing process, p. 65
Nursing science, p. 63
Nursing theory, p. 63
Paradigms, p. 67
Philosophy of science, p. 64
Praxis, p. 71
Prescriptive theory, p. 65
Proposition, p. 63
Theoretical model, p. 64
Theory, p. 63
Ways of knowing, p. 67

MEDIA RESOURCES

http://evolve.elsevier.com/Canada/Potter/fundamentals/

- Audio Chapter Summaries
- Examination Review Questions
- Concept Map Creator
- Case Study with Questions
- Audio Glossary
- Content Updates
- Video Clips

Although many nursing tasks can be mastered by anyone trained to perform them, the hallmark of nursing practice is a unique body of knowledge combined with a set of principles that guide the systematic application of that knowledge in an expanding array of contexts. The aim of **nursing theory** is to organize knowledge about nursing to enable nurses to use it in a professional and accountable manner (Beckstrand, 1978).

A **theory** is a purposeful set of **assumptions** or **propositions** that identify the relationships between **concepts**. Theories are useful because they provide a systematic view for explaining, predicting, and prescribing phenomena. Although nursing theories are not generally propositional, they reflect a **conceptualization** of nursing for the purpose of describing, explaining, predicting, or prescribing care (Meleis, 2012). Theories constitute one aspect of disciplinary knowledge and create vital linkages to how inquiry is approached (Fawcett, Watson, Neuman, et al., 2001). Nursing theories provide nurses with a perspective from which to view client situations, a way to organize data, and a method of analyzing and interpreting information to bring about coherent and informed nursing practice.

EARLY NURSING PRACTICE AND THE EMERGENCE OF THEORY

Although nursing practices have been documented throughout history (Yura & Walsh, 1973), the advent of modern nursing practice, in which the knowledge and practice of nursing are formalized into a professional context, is often attributed to the work of Florence Nightingale, a visionary leader in Victorian England who created systems for nursing education and practice (see Chapter 3). Contemporary scholars now consider Nightingale's work as an early theoretical and conceptual **model for nursing**. Her descriptive theory provided nurses with a way to think about nursing practice in a frame of reference that focuses on patients and the environment.

Since Nightingale's era, the status of nursing practice has paralleled that of the authority of women in society. After World War II, major developments in science and technology had a powerful influence on health care, including nursing practice. **Nursing science** came into its own. No longer simply applying the knowledge of other disciplines, nurses now began to acquire a unique body of knowledge about the practice of nursing.

Since the 1960s, scientific knowledge has proliferated across all disciplines. In particular, knowledge about nursing has drawn from and contributed to developments in health sciences, basic physical sciences, social and biobehavioural sciences, social theory, ethical theory, and the **philosophy of science** (which will be further discussed under the section "Philosophy of Nursing Science" in this chapter). Each of these sources has relevance for the interpretation of nursing care and the synthesis of relevant facts and theories for application to practice.

A number of major developments in nursing theory occurred in the late 1960s (Meleis, 2012). The health care system was expanding and changing, influenced by scientific discoveries and technological applications. Disease intervention became more sophisticated and scientifically driven. The focus of society shifted from simply attending to sick and injured people toward the larger problem of curing and eradicating disease, which expanded the influence of physicians over the structure of health care delivery. For the first time, nurses realized the urgency of articulating exactly how their role differed from those of the other health care providers (Chinn & Kramer, 2011; Engebretson, 1997; Fawcett, 2004; Newman, 1972).

The drive for early theorizing about the practice of nursing was led by nurse educators, who noted that traditional ways of preparing professional nurses were rapidly becoming outdated. Until the 1960s, a nursing apprenticeship model, augmented by lectures offered by physicians, had seemed sufficient. Around this time, nursing educational leaders became inspired to theorize about nursing in order to structure and define what a curriculum oriented to nursing knowledge might contain (Dean, 1995; Orem & Parker, 1964; Torres, 1974). This meant grappling with large theoretical and philosophical questions, such as the following:

- What are the focus and scope of nursing?
- How is nursing unique and different from other health care professions?
- What should be the appropriate disciplinary knowledge for professional nursing practice?

To answer these questions, early theorists developed **conceptual frameworks**, in which they organized core nursing concepts and proposed relationships among these concepts. These conceptual frameworks were "mental maps" whose purpose was to make sense of the information and decisional processes that nurses needed to apply knowledge to nursing practice (Ellis, 1968; Johnson, 1974; McKay, 1969; Wald & Leonard, 1964). Expressing knowledge about nursing in scientific language created a context in which nursing science gained stature and flourished (Cull-Wilby & Peppin, 1987; Jones, 1997). However, these nursing theories were not the kind of scientific theories that could be confirmed or disproved with empirical evidence (Levine, 1995); rather, they represented ideas about how nurses might organize knowledge, as well as the processes by which they would apply that knowledge to unique practice situations. Table 5-1 defines some of the basic terms that are used in theorizing about scientific issues.

TABLE 5-1 The Terminology of Scientific Theorizing

Term	Description	Example
Concept	A mental formulation of objects or events, representing the basic way in which ideas are organized and communicated	Anxiety
Conceptualization	The process of formulating concepts	Framing behavioural patterns as anxiety related
Operational definition	A description of concepts, articulated in such a way that they can be applied to decision making in practice. It links concepts with other concepts and with theories, and it often includes the essential properties and distinguishing features of a concept.	Differentiation and measurement of state and trait anxiety
Theory	A purposeful set of assumptions or propositions about concepts; shows relationships between concepts and thereby provides a systematic view of phenomena so that they may be explained, predicted, or prescribed	Social determinants of illness
Assumption	A description of concepts or connection of two concepts that are accepted as factual or true; includes "taken for granted" ideas about the nature and purpose of concepts, as well as the structure of theory	"Nursing exists to serve a social mandate."
Proposition	A declarative assertion	"Clients who receive appropriate nursing care have better health outcomes."
Phenomenon	An aspect of reality that can be consciously sensed or experienced (Meleis, 2012); nursing concepts and theories represent the theoretical approach to making sense of aspects of reality of concern to nursing	Pain
Theoretical model	Mental representation of how things work. For example, an architect's plan for a house is not the house itself but rather the set of information necessary to understand how all of the building elements will be brought together to create that particular house.	Biopsychosocial model of health
Conceptual framework	The theoretical structure that links concepts together for a specific purpose. When its purpose is to show how something works, it can also be described as a theoretical model. Nursing conceptual frameworks link major nursing concepts and phenomena to direct nursing decisions (e.g., what to assess, how to make sense of data, what to plan, how to enact a plan, and how to evaluate whether the plan has had the intended outcome). Conceptual frameworks are also often referred to as nursing models or nursing theories (Meleis, 2012).	Orem's (1971) self-care model for nursing

NURSING PROCESS

Early nursing theorists sought to organize the knowledge about the practice of nursing that nurses draw upon to direct their approach to clinical encounters. However, theorists generally lacked ways of systematically explaining how nurses work with knowledge in new situations (Field, 1987). An important early step in the application of knowledge to nursing practice was Orlando's (1961) development of a problem-solving approach that came to be known as the **nursing process** (Yura & Walsh, 1973). This process originally involved four steps: assessment, planning, intervention, and evaluation, whereby each step represented a distinct way in which general nursing knowledge could be applied to unique and individual nurse–patient situations (Carnevali & Thomas, 1993; Henderson, 1966; Meleis, 2012; Torres, 1986):

- Assessment phase: Nurses would gather information, including biological, sociocultural, environmental, spiritual, and psychological data, to create an understanding of the patient's unique health or illness experience. Organizing the data would enable the nurses to interpret major issues and concerns (Barnum, 1998) and produce a **nursing diagnosis**: the nurse's perspective on the appropriate focus for the patient (Durand & Prince, 1966).
- Planning phase: Nurses would prioritize the issues raised during assessment in relation to the nursing diagnoses, identify which issues could be supported or assisted by nursing intervention, and create a plan of care.
- Intervention phase: The plan of care would be carried out.
- Evaluation phase: The plan's success or failure would be judged both against the plan itself and against the patient's overall health status; that is, it would be determined whether the intended outcomes had been achieved or whether the nursing intervention strategies required revision. The nursing process was intended as a sequence within which thoughtful interpretation always preceded action, and the effects of action were always evaluated in relation to the original situation.

The nursing process was widely accepted by nurses because it was a logical way to describe basic problem-solving processes in which knowledge was used effectively to guide nursing decisions (Henderson, 1982). Nurses quickly adopted the nursing process because it represented a continuous, rapid cycling of information through each of the phases. Although it was useful for organizing and applying knowledge to clinical practice (Meleis, 2012), some later theorists began to challenge the nursing process as being too linear and rigid for nursing's purposes (Varcoe, 1996).

In current practice, terms such as *clinical judgement* are used to refer to reasoning processes that rely on *critical thinking* and multiple ways of knowing; clinical judgement implies the systematic use of the nursing process to invoke the complex intuitive and conscious thinking strategies that are part of all clinical decision making in nursing (Alfaro-LeFevre, 2017; Benner & Tanner, 1987; Tanner, 1993).

CONCEPTUAL FRAMEWORKS

The conceptual framework builders of the late 1960s and after are usually referred to as the *nursing theorists.* All were fascinated with how effective nurses systematically organize general knowledge about nursing in order to understand an individual patient's situation and determine which of many available strategies would work best to restore health and ameliorate or prevent disease (Orem & Parker, 1964). This reasoning process was different from linear, cause-and-effect reasoning, and it was what the nursing theorists understood to be the hallmark of excellence in nursing practice (Barnum, 1998; Meleis, 2012). Indeed, when effective nurses made intelligent clinical decisions, it was often difficult to determine the precise dynamics that explained how those nurses applied that knowledge (Benner, Tanner, & Chesla, 2009).

The building of nursing models was an attempt to theorize how all nurses might be taught to organize and synthesize knowledge about nursing so that they would develop advanced clinical reasoning skills (Raudonis & Acton, 1997). Theorists who developed these frameworks and models sought to depict theoretical structures that would enable a nurse to grasp all aspects of a clinical situation within the larger context of available options for nursing care. Table 5-2 describes four types of theory: **grand theory**, **middle-range theory**, **descriptive theory**, and **prescriptive theory**.

METAPARADIGM CONCEPTS

Each conceptual framework was an attempt to define nursing by creating a theoretical definition for the substance and structure for

TABLE 5-2 Types of Theory

Type of Theory	Description
Grand theory	Global, conceptual framework that provides insight into abstract phenomena, such as human behaviour or nursing science. Grand theories are broad in scope and therefore require further application through research before the ideas they contain can be fully tested (Chinn & Kramer, 2011). They are intended not to provide guidance for specific nursing interventions but rather to provide the structural framework for broad, abstract ideas about nursing. They are sometimes called paradigms because they represent distinct world views about those phenomena and provide the structural framework within which narrower-range theories can be developed and tested.
Middle-range theory	Encompasses a more limited scope and is less abstract. Middle-range theories address specific phenomena or concepts and reflect practice (administration, clinical, or teaching). The phenomena or concepts tend to cross different nursing fields and reflect a variety of nursing care situations.
Descriptive theory	Describes phenomena (e.g., responding to illness through patterns of coping), speculates on why phenomena occur, and describes the consequences of phenomena. Descriptive theories have the ability to explain, relate, and, in some situations, predict phenomena of concern to nursing (Meleis, 2012). Descriptive nursing theories are designed not to direct specific nursing activities but rather to help explain client assessments and possibly guide future nursing research.
Prescriptive theory	Addresses nursing interventions and helps predict the consequences of a specific intervention. A prescriptive nursing theory should designate the prescription (i.e., nursing interventions), the conditions under which the prescription should occur, and the consequences (Meleis, 2012). Prescriptive theories are action oriented, which tests the validity and predictability of a nursing intervention. These theories guide nursing research to develop and test specific nursing interventions (Fawcett, 2004).

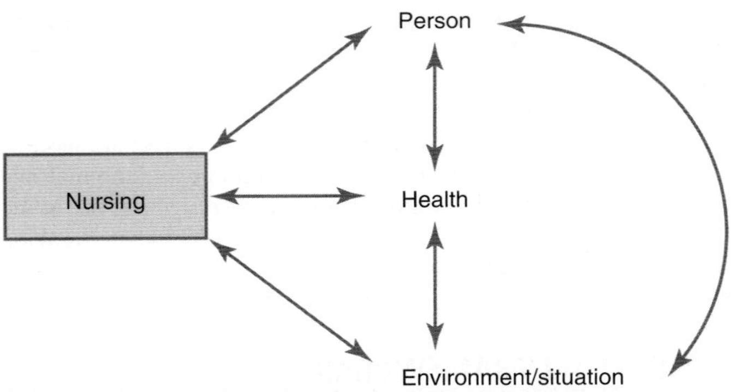

FIGURE 5-1 Nursing's metaparadigm concepts.

determining the key bodies of knowledge that would be needed to understand particular clinical situations (Figure 5-1). This collective body of knowledge was called the **metaparadigm concepts** and included the concepts of person, environment, health care, and nursing care (Fawcett, 1992).

Client and Person

By the 1960s, professional leaders recognized that nurses did much more than simply care for hospitalized patients. Because of this, nursing theorists started to use the term *client,* rather than *patient,* to refer to the person at the centre of any nursing process. The term signified a range of health states, including both sickness and wellness, and an explicitly interactive relationship between the nurse and the persons to whom care was directed. At the same time, nurses were becoming aware of their potential to deliver care beyond the individual—that is, to families, groups, and communities. Although theories to articulate the role of nursing care in families and communities also began to arise around this time, most early conceptual models focused on the individual.

To help nurses systematically organize and make sense of the vast amount of information that might be relevant to the care of any particular client, most early models clearly defined the concept of the person. Theorists variously understood a person as a system of interacting parts, a system of competing human needs, or an entity with biological, psychological, social, and spiritual dimensions. Each framework drew attention to multiple aspects of human experience so that the nurse could understand each instance of wellness and illness for its uniqueness within the context of that individual's body, feelings, and situation. Each model depicted a way of thinking about a whole individual, with the aim of helping nurses understand how the implications of any action or intervention could be systematically individualized toward the benefit of all facets of that individual.

Environment

Each conceptual framework reflected an understanding that the person is part of and interacts with a complex environmental system. This environment may involve the person's family and social ties, the community, the health care system, as well as the geopolitical issues that affect health. The early conceptual frameworks helped shape nurses' increasing appreciation of how to work within a larger context of every experience of wellness and illness. In so doing, these frameworks led to a future in which nurses would spearhead advances in social and health care policy, health promotion, and community development.

Health

Because nursing exists within a social mandate to improve the health of both the individual and society, the early theorists struggled to articulate the overarching goal that drives nursing practice. They defined health as much more than simply the absence of disease or injury but rather as an ideal state of optimal health or total well-being toward which all individuals could strive (see Chapter 1). This definition reflected a vision of nursing care that was relevant to both the individual and society, and applied to all clients, sick or well. It recognized that persons with chronic disease could strive for better health and that overall health could be compromised by psychosocial or spiritual challenges, even among the most physically fit individuals. Although perfect health was not necessarily achievable, this broad conceptualization guided nurses to help all clients reach outcomes that were productive and satisfying.

Nursing

Each early conceptual framework included a unique definition of nursing that linked a view of the client with an understanding of the person's environment, life, and health goals. Built on a distinct subset of knowledge, each conceptual framework presented a coherent and complete belief system about nursing practice, although each did so in different terms and with a different alignment of ideas. Because most nursing scholars of the era assumed that one model would eventually become dominant (Meleis, 2012), competition among the frameworks occurred. Over time, as enthusiasm for the idea of implementing theory-based practice grew, the application of the frameworks in practice became rigid and codified. Although the original focus had been on guiding nurses to think systematically, the implementation process caused the emphasis to shift toward such aspects as using language in particular ways and filling out assessment forms correctly. Many experienced nurses began to conclude that these frameworks actually inhibited their systematic thinking, and much debate ensued with regard to the utility of the models.

PHILOSOPHY OF NURSING SCIENCE

When nursing theorists began developing their frameworks and models, nurses understood the process of building a knowledge base as a matter of science and discovery. In that context, theories were considered logical propositions that could be rigorously tested for their capacity to answer (or not answer) the hypothetical questions posed by a discipline. However, while creating frameworks for the complex reasoning in nursing practice, these early theorists were applying traditional scientific ways of understanding how knowledge works without fully appreciating the limitations of science, especially in relation to complex problems. As thinkers in all disciplines began to move beyond their traditional boundaries, other possibilities for the development of knowledge about the practice of nursing began to emerge.

Scientific Revolutions

Thomas S. Kuhn, a philosopher of science, created a way of thinking about science and knowledge that expanded thought in many disciplines. First published in 1962, his book *The Structure of Scientific Revolutions* was popularized in the 1970s and 1980s as scholars began to realize the potential of its ideas to support new thinking about how knowledge is built. Kuhn challenged the traditional notion of science as a logical progression of discoveries, arguing that major scientific developments occurred only when scientists thought about problems in radically new ways. These ways of thinking departed from the traditional to such an extent that an entirely different world view, or "paradigm shift," developed. According to Kuhn, scientific advances happen when people think creatively and look beyond established norms. Such creative thinking could stimulate new understandings of problems that were once considered irresolvable (e.g., quantum physics introduced the idea that the behaviour of very small particles could explain atomic behaviour in ways that defied explanation through conventional Newtonian physics). This new way of thinking about the philosophy of science led nurses to consider their theoretical frameworks as not only theoretical propositions about logical relationships among concepts but also as actual world views, or **paradigms**, that might help them grasp the complexities of nursing (Fry, 1995).

Complexity Science

A second major shift in scientific thinking occurred with the introduction of chaos theory (Gleick, 1987). Originating from observations in physics that predictable patterns existed among factors that could not be predicted scientifically, this theory created a new way of approaching complex situations. In rejecting the simple cause-and-effect relationships used in traditional science, chaos theory led to what has been termed *complexity science.* In this kind of science, dynamic and interactive phenomena are reduced to the smallest properties that can be observed within their natural context so that their interactions can be interpreted with as little interference as possible from prior assumptions. For example, chaos theory explains how, in sensitive weather systems, minor variations in initial conditions (e.g., barometric pressure) might explain large-scale physical patterns over time (e.g., hurricanes). These ideas created a new language to apply to scientific thinking. Because experiences of health and illness are exceedingly difficult to understand out of their individual context, chaos theory offered a new way to approach nursing science (Coppa, 1993; Ray, 1998).

WAYS OF KNOWING IN NURSING PRACTICE

As ideas shifted, nursing theorists also realized that science was just one of several forms of knowledge necessary for their practice discipline. In 1978, Carper published an influential paper in which she used the expression **ways of knowing** to refer to patterns of knowledge application in nursing practice. Carper articulated a critical role in nursing practice not only for empirical science but also for ethical, personal, and aesthetic knowledge; this idea has become foundational to our understanding of the multiple lenses nursing uses to interpret complex phenomena (see Chapter 6 for further information about evidence-informed practice). Later theorists added sociopolitical knowledge (White, 1995), emancipatory knowing (Chinn & Kramer, 2011), and critical thinking (see Chapter 12 for further information about critical thinking) to the list of central ways of knowing that are essential to the highest quality of clinical nursing. These ideas contributed to discussions emerging in other social and life sciences around *how* nurses know what they know (Chinn & Kramer, 2011; Kikuchi & Simmons, 1999).

PARADIGM DEBATES WITHIN NURSING

With the new philosophical approach to scientific knowledge, nurses struggled with how to define their work as both an art and a science and as both applied and practical (Donaldson, 1995; Johnson, 1991; Rodgers, 1991; Sarter, 1990). Ideas about the theoretical foundations of nursing practice shifted. Some scholars began to question conceptual models as a valid form of theorizing (Holden, 1990). The frustration resulting from overly formal and rigid approaches to applying many of these models led to a period of what has been called *model bashing* (Engebretson, 1997). However, the question confronting the early theorists remained as follows: How does a nurse organize and make sense of all available knowledge and apply it intelligently to the challenges that arise in an individual clinical case?

In this context, many nurse scholars began to recognize that the original theories were better understood as philosophical statements than scientific prescriptions. However, one group of theorists, considering some of the original theories to be overly simplistic and insufficiently holistic, began to categorize various nursing models as reflective of two entirely different paradigms of thinking (Parse, 1987). Considering the majority of nursing models and frameworks to be old-fashioned and outdated, this group of theorists coined the term *totality paradigm frameworks* to describe them, contending that this kind of model reduced an understanding of the human person to fragmented parts out of context. They further proposed the term *simultaneity paradigm frameworks* to depict a set of conceptual frameworks they considered to be radically different and preferable by virtue of being both holistic and philosophically sophisticated (Parse, 1987). Some advocates of simultaneity theories continue to depict the diverse universe of theorizing about nursing as reflecting these two mutually exclusive groupings, positioning one set of conceptual frameworks as philosophically and morally superior to what they understand the other to represent (Cody, 1995; Nagle & Mitchell, 1991; Newman, 1992).

◆ NURSING DIAGNOSIS

Another discussion about nursing theory centred on nursing diagnosis. The scholars who devised conceptual frameworks focused on models to assess and interpret data about individual patient situations. However, the conceptual frameworks were less explicit about how to plan, implement, and evaluate nursing care. To fill this gap, nursing diagnosis emerged as an additional phase in that process. In making explicit the idea that nurses arrived at a clinical judgement relating to actual or potential health processes, it became a discrete focus of theorizing about nursing care.

In the 1970s, some scholars noted a need for precise language to categorize and document nursing diagnoses into a taxonomy (Warren & Hoskins, 1990). This resulted in the formation of the North American Nursing Diagnoses Association (NANDA) (see Chapter 13 for further information about NANDA), which held a series of consensus conferences to establish a list of the common patient problems addressed by practising nurses. The nursing diagnosis movement led to considerable general debate on the merits of using NANDA's fixed list of nursing diagnoses as compared to the theoretically infinite options for nursing care that had been intended by the conceptual models (Fitzpatrick, 1990; Roy, 1982). Although it is recognized as practical rather than theoretical (Fitzpatrick, 1990), NANDA's list has become a popular device for organizing nursing care in part because it enables efficient categorization into electronic databases and the subsequent standardization of nursing care plans (Warren & Hoskins, 1990). However, despite its popularity with health care administrators, NANDA's list is recognized by many nurses as a system that relies entirely upon an agreement about what constitutes average wellness and illness experiences. It can therefore create worrisome barriers to the individualized care of patients (Lee, Chan, & Phillips, 2006).

REFLECTIONS ON CONCEPTUALIZING NURSING

The scientific and philosophical aspects of today's nursing practice are built on the foundation of early theorizing about nursing. The history of "nursing theory" is the story of an enlightened attempt to articulate excellent clinical reasoning in nursing care. How effective nurses actually use knowledge within the complexity of their clinical reasoning is, however, still difficult to determine. In this context, theorizing about nursing is perhaps best understood as an extended philosophical struggle to make sense of how highly skilled nurses actually think. Instead of arguing the advantages of one nursing theory over another, nursing scholars of today appreciate the creativity of their predecessors within the constrained conceptual contexts in which they were expected to operate.

MAJOR THEORETICAL MODELS

Some of the major theoretical models are summarized briefly in Box 5-1 and Box 5-2; the similarities and differences among them are illustrated. Note, however, that because many nursing theorists based their models on complex combinations of theories from many disciplines, the categorization used here is somewhat oversimplistic. It may be helpful to view the conceptual frameworks in terms of larger theories upon which they have drawn, such as adaptation theory, systems theory, or human needs theory.

Practice-Based Theories

All conceptual models of nursing are designed to guide and shape practice. Although their theoretical inspiration is derived directly from the practice setting, many conceptual models do not capture all of what might be influencing that practice, such as societal and demographic changes, current health care belief models, and therapeutic strategies, as well as the political struggles inherent in health care delivery. The early practice theories, therefore, reflect the issues that were shaping the role and context of nursing during those specific time frames.

Florence Nightingale. Whereas most later theorists drew on social and psychological theories, Nightingale was directly inspired by nursing practice. Writing *Notes on Nursing* in 1859, she described conditions necessary to promote health and healing. Her observations during the Crimean War led to the first set of principles for nursing practice, acknowledging the particular importance of the environment, including clean living areas, fresh air, and the presence of light.

BOX 5-1 Milestones in the Development of Nursing Theory

1859	Florence Nightingale's *Notes on Nursing: What It Is and What It Is Not* was published (updated version published 1946).
1952	*Nursing Research* (the first peer-reviewed scientific journal about nursing care) was established.
1952	Hildegard Peplau's text *Interpersonal Relations in Nursing* was published.
1955	Virginia Henderson's definition of nursing was first published in the 5th edition of Harmer and Henderson's (1955) basic nursing text.
1961	Ida Orlando introduced the nursing process.
1970	Martha Rogers's model was first published.
1970	Callista Roy's model was first published.
1971	Dorothea Orem's model was first published.
1976	The North American Nursing Diagnosis Association (NANDA) list of nursing diagnoses was first published.
1976	The University of British Columbia model of nursing practice was first published (Campbell et al., 1976).
1978	Barbara Carper's paper on fundamental patterns of knowing in nursing practice was published.
1979	Evelyn Adam's model was first published (English version published 1980).
1981	Rosemarie Parse's model was first published.
1987	The McGill model of nursing was first published (Gottlieb & Rowat, 1987)
2000	The Prince Edward Island conceptual model for primary care nursing was published (Munro, Gallant, MacKinnon, et al., 2000).
2013	*Strengths-Based Nursing*, building on the McGill model, was published (Gottlieb, 2013).

BOX 5-2 Key Underpinnings and Major Premises of Nursing Theorists

Theorist	Key Underpinnings	Major Premises
Nightingale	Practice observations; epidemiology	Creating an environment conducive to healing
Peplau	Harry Stack Sullivan's theory of interpersonal relations	Nursing as an interpersonal process; understanding the behaviour of others
Henderson	Basic human needs	Assisting the individual, sick or well, to perform those activities that he or she would perform unaided given the strength, will, or knowledge
Travelbee	Existential philosophy	Preventing, coping with, and making meaning of illness and suffering
Rogers	Wasserman's energy fields	Focus on unitary or irreducible human being and environment as pan-dimensional energy fields
Roy	Helson's adaptation theory	Facilitating manas an adaptive system
Johnson	Chin's theory of behavioural systems	Maintaining stability and balance through adjustments and adaptation to the forces that impinge on them
Orem	Philosophy of human capability	Maintaining capacity for self-care
Neuman	Open system affected by intrapersonal, interpersonal, and extrapersonal stressors	Addressing variables affecting the client's response to stressors
UBC	von Bertalanffy's general systems theory and Lewin's field theory	Nurturing the person as a behavioural system during critical periods of the life cycle
Adam	Basic human needs with biological, physiological, and psychosociocultural dimensions	Nursing as a helping process of restoring independence to satisfy basic human needs
Parse	Dilthey's human science philosophy	Indivisible human beings and environment co-create health, structured around abiding themes of meaning, rhythmicity, and transcendence
McGill	Practice observations	Focus on health rather than illness; family as context
Watson	Phenomenal field/unitary consciousness	Nursing as caring; clinical caritas processes

The role of nursing care included ensuring that wounded soldiers were warm, comfortable, and adequately fed. Torres (1986) noted that Nightingale demonstrated how to think about patients and their environment. By shifting the focus from disease processes toward an environment conducive to healing, Nightingale's conceptualization clearly differentiated the role of nursing from that of medicine.

The McGill Model. Dr. Moyra Allen (Box 5-3) conceived the McGill model, and she and her colleagues developed it (Gottlieb & Rowat, 1987). Systematically studying actual nursing situations, Allen and her colleagues created a way of thinking about nursing that focused on promoting health. They recognized that many patients' health concerns were best approached through changes in lifestyle. The McGill scholars focused on the individual in the context of the family and, like Nightingale, viewed nursing as complementary to medicine. The main features of the McGill model were "a focus on health rather than illness and treatment, on all family members rather than the patient alone, on family goals rather than on the nurse's, and on family strengths rather than their deficits" (Gottlieb & Feeley, 1999, p. 194). Over time, the model has been further developed to demonstrate its application within a range of clinical contexts and settings (e.g., Feeley & Gerez-Lirette, 1992; Feeley & Gottlieb, 1998; Gottlieb, 2013).

Needs Theories

Many early theorists organized their thinking by conceptualizing the patient as representing a collection of needs. This reflected a common orientation to studying the nature of people, popularized in the 1960s, in which needs, drives, and competencies were thought to hold potential for explaining human behaviour. Of these theories, Maslow's (1954) hierarchy of needs was one of the best known and most influential. The idea that complex human behaviour can be best explained as a response to the competing demands of various basic needs is featured prominently in many nursing models.

Virginia Henderson. Henderson (Harmer & Henderson, 1955) conceptualized the patient as a compilation of 14 basic human needs: to breathe, eat and drink, eliminate waste products, move and maintain posture, rest and sleep, dress and undress, maintain body temperature, be clean, avoid danger, communicate, worship, work, play, and learn. Viewing the patient in this way clearly defined the nurse's role. Accordingly, Henderson defined nursing practice as assisting the individual, sick or well, in the performance of activities that contribute to health, recovery, or a peaceful death. Henderson's model has remained popular in practice because its language is familiar and easily comprehensible and because it explains how a person's biological, psychological, social, and spiritual components combine to influence the way illness is experienced and health can be regained.

Dorothea Orem. Orem's (1971) self-care theory, the origins of which lay in Henderson's work, was used widely in both nursing practice and research. Orem's theory addressed the ways in which people are responsible for meeting the following universal self-care requisites:

- Maintaining sufficient intake of air, water, and food
- Maintaining a balance between activity and rest, and between solitude and interaction
- Providing for elimination processes
- Preventing hazards to life, functioning, and well-being
- Promoting functioning and growth in social groups in accordance with human potential

Drawing on both human need and developmental theory, Orem's theory focused on the individual's role in maintaining health. This theory emerged at a time when the passive role of the patient was being questioned and the health care system was beginning to shift away from full responsibility for people's health. With increased understanding of illness patterns, Orem acknowledged the effects of multiple lifestyle factors such as smoking, diet, and exercise, reminding nurses that patients can look after their own health and that they must learn to care for themselves within their families and communities. Thus, the role of the nurse, according to Orem, was to act temporarily for the patient until the patient could resume a more independent role in self-care.

Interactionist Theories

Interactionist theories focused on the relationships between nurses and their clients. These theories defined more clearly the specific human communicative and behavioural patterns by which practitioners met their patients' needs. As the theorists reframed definitions of the nursing profession, they drew from the work of psychologists and psychoanalysts such as Harry Stack Sullivan, Abraham Maslow, and Sigmund Freud.

Hildegard Peplau. Peplau, a psychiatric specialist, defined the core of nursing care as the interpersonal relationship between the nurse and the patient. Building upon the ideas of psychoanalyst Harry Stack Sullivan, Peplau depicted the practice of nursing as an interactive and therapeutic relationship. Peplau felt that such relationships allowed nurses to challenge the practice of long-term stays in large inpatient psychiatric hospitals and to envision supporting patients to achieve independent living. "The kind of person each nurse becomes makes a substantial difference in what each patient will learn as he is nursed through his experience with illness" (Peplau, 1952, p. vii). According to Peplau, a nurse was "an investigator, prober, interpreter, and

BOX 5-3 Milestones in Canadian Nursing History

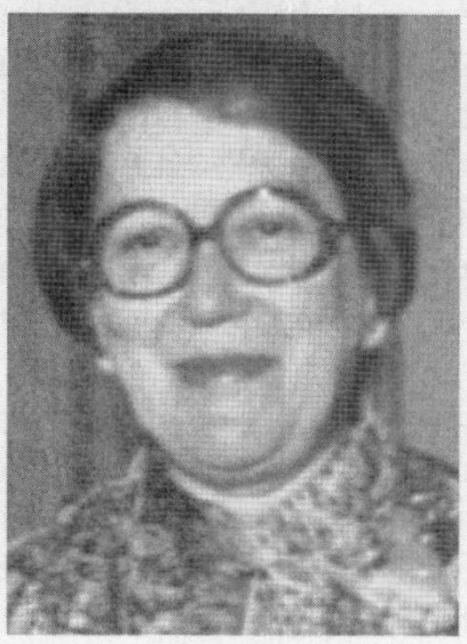

Moyra Allen, 1921–1996

A creative and independent thinker, Moyra Allen was one of the first Canadian nurses to earn a doctoral degree. She lobbied for collective bargaining rights for nurses and was the founding president of the United Nurses of Montreal. She was also the founder of *Nursing Papers,* later renamed the *Canadian Journal of Nursing Research.*

Allen was a founding member of the World Health Organization committee that developed the criteria for accreditation of nursing schools. She designed an evaluation model for nursing schools and evaluated schools in South America, India, and Ghana. She joined the faculty of the School of Nursing at McGill in 1954 and became professor emeritus in 1985 upon her retirement.

In demonstrating her model of nursing, now known as the McGill model, Dr. Allen established The Health Workshop in 1977, a community health facility, in which she put into practice a developmental concept of health and nursing as a prototype of primary health care. The workshop, viewed as complementary to existing services, was staffed with nurses, a community development officer, and a health librarian. The workshop's purpose was to demonstrate the validity of a local health resource managed by nurses that focused on long-term family health. It proved to be an innovative means of improving the health status of families coping with illness and other problems.

Allen received numerous awards, including the Jeanne Mance Award, which recognizes major contributions to the health of Canadians. In 1986, she was named an Officer of the Order of Canada for her outstanding contributions to Canadian nursing.

reporter, using the rich data she extracts from the patient concerning his life. She develops insights, his and hers, into the meaning of a patient's behaviour and helps the patient recognize and change patterns that obstruct achievement of his goals" (Barnum, 1994, p. 217). An early advocate of an orderly and systematic approach to care, Peplau created a way of thinking about nursing care that directed nurses toward preventing illness and maintaining health.

Joyce Travelbee. Writing in the late 1960s and early 1970s, Travelbee also viewed nursing care as an interpersonal process. In contrast to Peplau's more psychoanalytic orientation, Travelbee drew on a school of thought known as *existential philosophy* to guide her theorizing. Travelbee (1971) viewed the "client" as including not only the individual but also the individual's family and community, and she articulated the role of the nurse as assisting clients to "prevent or cope with the experience of illness and suffering and, if necessary, to find meaning in these experiences" (p. 7). Travelbee emphasized that nurses must recognize the humanity of their clients, suggesting that even the term *patient* should be regarded as a stereotypical categorization. Recognizing the reciprocity of human interaction, Travelbee focused attention on the communication that occurs between nurses and their clients as an important vehicle for finding meaning in illness.

Evelyn Adam. Influenced by Dorothy Johnson, as well as by earlier interactionist theorists (George, 1995), Canadian theorist Evelyn Adam (1979, 1980) articulated the essence of nursing as a helping process. From her perspective, the nurse played a complementary-supplementary role in supporting the patient's strength, knowledge, and will. Adam's model drew on Henderson's framework of basic human needs and extended it into a model that would explain not only how nurses conceptualized the patient but also how they applied that knowledge in the context of a helping relationship characterized by empathy, caring, and mutual respect.

Systems Theories

In the 1970s and 1980s, as conceptual models of nursing became more sophisticated and structured, several theorists drew on general systems theory (von Bertalanffy, 1968) for guidance in conceptualizing the complexity of human health. The main appeal of systems theory was that it accounted for the whole of an entity (the system) and its component parts (subsystems), as well as the complex interactions between the parts and the whole. In this way, systems theory allowed theorists to expand the conceptualization of nursing practice through both structure and process, whereby the individual was viewed as an open system in constant interaction with his or her environment. Being outside the system, the nurse became one of the many forces to have an effect on that system. Using this perspective, nurses were encouraged to appreciate the interactions of a system with its component parts and with its environment. Systems approaches helped nurses recognize that intervention in any one part of a system would produce consequent reactions in other parts, as well as in the system as a whole. Regardless of how each theorist depicted the nature of the system, these general principles common to all living systems were featured in each of the nursing systems models.

Dorothy Johnson. Johnson's theoretical work was popularized in the early 1960s through distribution of her class notes and speeches, but it remained unpublished until much later (Grubbs, 1980; Johnson, 1980). In her nursing model, Johnson identified the individual as a behavioural system with seven subsystems, each of which has a goal, a set of behaviours, and a choice. The notion of goals of the subsystems was based on the drives that were considered universal and applicable to all patients. However, the meanings attributed to each goal and the set of behaviours for achieving goals were seen as highly individual and unique to each patient. Together with the choices made by the patient in relation to meeting his or her behavioural system goals, each subsystem also had a function that could be considered analogous to the physiological function of a biological system (Meleis, 2012).

The University of British Columbia Model. The behavioural systems model developed at the University of British Columbia (UBC) School of Nursing was inspired by Johnson's model and developed by a committee led by Margaret Campbell that included several of Johnson's former students. Broadening the view of human experience on the basis of behavioural drives, the UBC model depicted the behavioural system as being composed of nine basic human needs, each of which is shaped by the psychological and sociocultural environment within which it is expressed (Campbell, Cruise, & Murakami, 1976). Whereas needs were considered universal and therefore fundamental to human experience, the specific goals toward which needs-related human behaviour were directed and the strategies for achieving those goals were recognized as unique to individuals and their particular physiological, psychological, or social circumstances (Thorne, Jillings, Ellis, et al., 1993). Thus, the UBC model provided a structure by which general knowledge about human health and illness could be combined with particular knowledge about each individual patient. In accordance with the tenets of general systems theory, the goal of nursing practice was balance of the behavioural system. The nurse's role was to foster, protect, sustain, and teach (Campbell, 1987) and thereby bring about not only system balance but also stability and optimal health.

Betty Neuman. Neuman's approach to theorizing about nursing differed from that of other systems theorists in that it did not rely on concepts concerning needs and drives, nor did it break the system into any component parts. Neuman understood the person to be a physiological, psychological, sociocultural, developmental, and spiritual being (Meleis, 2012) and oriented the attention of the nurse to the "client system" in a health care–oriented and holistic manner (Neuman, 1982). Neuman considered the client system to have innate factors consistent with being human, as well as unique factors that characterized each individual person. According to Neuman, each client had a unique set of response patterns determined and regulated by a core structure. Neuman believed that because the person was vulnerable to environmental stressors, the role of the nurse ought to focus on actual and potential stressors. In this way, Neuman's model focused on prevention.

Sister Callista Roy. In contrast to most other systems theorists, Roy considered the client not as a behavioural system but rather as an adaptive one. She viewed the person as a biopsychosocial being in constant interaction with a changing environment (Roy, 1984). Her model depicted four modes of adaptation: physiological needs, self-concept, role function, and interdependence (Roy, 1974). She conceptualized the person as an adaptive system with two major internal processes by which to adapt: the cognator and the regulator subsystems (Roy & Andrews, 1999). Roy used these mechanisms to describe and explain the interconnectedness of all aspects of human adaptation and to conceptualize the role of the nurse in managing the stimuli that influence that adaptation (Meleis, 2012).

Simultaneity Theories

The theorists who identified their work as belonging to the simultaneity paradigm considered their theories to be fundamentally distinct from the practice, needs, interactionist, and systems theories. Although simultaneity theories were first articulated long before the paradigm debate arose and before the terms *simultaneity* and *totality* were used to categorize the theories, the language of simultaneity has become prominent in distinguishing this group of nursing theories from others. A characteristic feature of these theories is what Rogers (1970) called the *unitary human being*. Previous theorists had sought to identify aspects of the individual that not only represented an abstract conceptualization of the whole but also provided a comprehensive understanding of the person in terms of his or her parts (such as problems, needs, or goals). In contrast, the simultaneity theorists viewed the individual as an entirely irreducible whole, inherently and "holographically" connected with the universal environment (Parse, 2004). Thus, these theories represented a distinctive approach to articulating an understanding of the client of nursing as well as nursing's role in relation to that client.

Martha Rogers. Martha Rogers's (1970) model was revolutionary in presenting the client not simply as a person but as an energy field in constant interaction with the environment, which itself was also an irreducible energy field, coextensive with the universe (Meleis, 2012). According to Rogers, who based her theory on her interpretations of evolving ideas in physics, the role of nursing was to focus on the life process of a human being along a time–space continuum (Rogers, 1970). An early proponent of pattern recognition, Rogers believed that pattern gave the energy field its identity and its distinguishing characteristics (Meleis, 2012). The objective of nursing practice became one of helping clients reach their maximum health potential in the context of constant change and to develop what Rogers referred to as homeodynamic unity within diversity.

Rosemarie Parse. Parse's (1981) theory of "man-living-health," later termed *human becoming* theory (Parse, 1997) and over time evolving into the *human becoming school of thought* (Parse, 2007), was another view of the individual as a unitary being who is "indivisible, unpredictable, and everchanging" and "a freely choosing being who can be recognized through paradoxical patterns co-created all-at-once in mutual process with the universe" (Parse, 2004, p. 293). According to Parse's perspective, the caring presence of nurses and their particular patterns of relating support individuals in the human "becoming" process. Within Parse's nursing theory, the goal of nursing is articulated not in traditional definitions of health but rather as the notion of people in a continuous process of making choices and changing health priorities. According to Parse's theory, nurses engage with people in their process of "becoming" through the application of three core processes referred to as explicating, dwelling with, and moving beyond (Parse, 1999).

Jean Watson. Watson (1979) considered the individual to be a totality who can be viewed as a transpersonal self. According to Watson, in contrast to depictions of the individual as a body and an ego, it is more useful to understand the individual as "an embodied spirit; a transpersonal transcendent evolving consciousness; unity of mind body spirit; person-nature-universe as oneness, connected" (Watson, 1999, p. 129). Watson therefore believed that nurses must do far more than deal with physical illness: they must attend to their primary function, which is caring. From Watson's perspective, caring infuses all aspects of a nurse's role and draws attention to nursing acts as embodying an aesthetic that facilitates both healing and growth.

Each of the models just described attracts continual analysis and implementation. In some instances, nurses draw on them holistically as a coherent approach to guide all of their practices. More often, nurses today consider themselves informed by the intellectual structure that any good framework provides, but typically expand their thinking beyond the limitations of a single model as their practice develops and progresses.

THEORIZING IN THE FUTURE

Theoretical knowledge leads us to reflect on "the basic values, guiding principles, elements, and phases of a conception of nursing" (Meleis, 2012). The goals of theoretical knowledge are to stimulate thinking and create a broad understanding of the science and practice of the nursing discipline (King & Fawcett, 1997). Although nurses today can appreciate the inherent complexity of these objectives, the creativity and vision modelled by these early theorists continue to inspire theorizing about the essence of nursing.

Nursing is solidly established as a distinct health care discipline with its own unique science. In addition, current theorists draw heavily from philosophy to resolve some of nursing's theoretical challenges. However, as Kikuchi (1999) pointed out, much of the theorizing about the purpose of nursing has confused rather than clarified thinking. As nursing scholarship evolves to include stronger philosophical and scientific inquiry, nursing practice must be conceptualized with increasing clarity (Silva, Sorrell, & Sorrell, 1995). Nurse philosophers, as well as scientists, are continuing to use new ways of tackling nursing's most complex theoretical feature, which is applying expanding, dynamic, and multiple sources of knowledge to a diverse range of client situations. This problem of understanding the general and applying it to the particular features in the work of many contemporary nursing scholars.

Meleis (1987), a scholar of nursing theory, challenged nurses to direct their theorizing away from the processes by which nurses use knowledge and toward the equally challenging issues associated with the substance of that knowledge. In accepting this challenge, many nursing scholars have shifted their theorizing about nursing to include both theoretical and substantive knowledge. Liaschenko (1997; Liaschenko & Fisher, 1999) oriented this theorizing into three levels of abstraction: knowing the case, knowing the patient, and knowing the person. Engebretson (1997) positioned nursing theory in relation not only to biomedicine but also to Eastern and holistic understandings of health and illness. Starzomski and Rodney (1997) worked toward articulating the link between definitions of health and more philosophical notions of the greater social good. Campbell and Bunting (1991) explored the possibilities of using critical social and feminist theories for emancipatory theorizing in nursing. Watson (1990; see also Brenwick & Webster, 2000) developed the idea of embedding "caring" as a moral component into nursing theory. Yeo (1989) considered the implications of ethical reasoning for nursing theory. In Canada, nurses at the Prince Edward Island School of Nursing developed a conceptual framework for nursing grounded in the social determinants of health (Munro, Gallant, MacKinnon, et al., 2000), and Gottlieb (2013) developed the McGill model into a comprehensive philosophy of care based on holism and a strengths-based orientation to engagement.

The capacity to provide a rationale for nursing actions and decisions based on theoretical knowledge is a recognized core competency for nursing practice in Canada (Canadian Association of Schools of Nursing, 2015). However, as this review of the history of theorizing in nursing illustrates, linking theory with practice requires a dynamic and evolving skill set. The inherent complexities underlying interrelationships between theory and practice are therefore of increasing interest to nursing scholars.

A dialogue representing the dynamic interaction between theorizing and clinical practice (often termed **praxis**) has started to emerge (Clarke, James, & Kelly, 1996; Mitchell, 1995; Reed, 1995; Reed & Ground, 1997; Thorne, 1997). This newer form of theorizing does not seek static truths about nursing practice, as it considers all truths to be potentially illusory. Rather, it seeks to create a coherent foundation upon which nurses can build, challenge, and integrate an infinite range of new ideas, new forms of knowledge, and new paths toward action. For some theorists, this notion of praxis represents a blend of what has been described as the art and science of nursing (Newman, 2002). For others, it reflects a call to engaging with knowledge in a reflexive manner that invokes emancipation and fuels action (Kagan, Smith, Cowling, et al., 2010).

As Levine once wrote, "Theory is the poetry of science" (1995, p. 14). In this manner, theorizing in nursing becomes the engine by which ideas about the discipline are advanced over time. It brings the old and familiar concepts of nursing together and shapes them into bold and exciting new configurations, rendering previously disconnected aspects of the human experience part of a greater whole. In so doing, it makes the intellectual excitement of the discipline come alive.

KEY CONCEPTS

- The hallmark of nursing practice is its unique body of knowledge and the way nurses use it.
- Nursing science has evolved within a historical and social context.
- Nursing theory represents the attempts by nursing scholars to articulate ways in which knowledge from multiple sources can be systematically applied in a wide variety of ways to guide professional, accountable, and defensible nursing practice.
- Much of the early theorizing about nursing practice was specifically designed to guide nursing curriculum development so that nursing education would be focused on the knowledge unique to nursing care.
- The nursing process is the fundamental problem-solving process by which new situations are assessed, plans are developed, and interventions are performed and evaluated.
- Nursing care requires the application of general knowledge to an infinite range of unique situations. Nursing process and nursing theory represent strategies to guide the application process.
- The major components of nursing theory, sometimes called the *metaparadigm concepts,* are person, environment, health, and nursing.
- Nurses' understanding of the role of science has changed as more complex forms of science have been articulated by philosophers of science; science is no longer limited to simple relationships such as cause and effect but instead provides strategies for understanding increasingly complex relationships and phenomena.
- Nursing knowledge derives from various sources in addition to science, including aesthetics, personal knowing, sociocultural understanding, and ethics.
- Nursing theorists based their conceptual frameworks on various ways of thinking about human behaviour and experience. Some framed their ideas within theories of human behaviour, such as needs, interaction, or systems, and others drew their primary inspiration from what they observed in excellent nursing practice.
- Nursing conceptual frameworks include those for understanding both the person as the nurse's client and the nurse's role in relation to that client.
- Although each framework may have attempted to organize nursing knowledge and systematic reasoning processes in a different way, each was aiming for a very similar ideal of excellent decision making in nursing practice.
- Although nursing theoretical frameworks are no longer considered useful as prescriptive models for practice, they provide a way of conceptualizing nursing's interests and of identifying researchable nursing problems.
- As the practice of theorizing about nursing care evolves, the role of philosophy in helping nurses understand their relationship to knowledge has become increasingly relevant.

CRITICAL THINKING EXERCISES

1. How do you think that different ways of conceptualizing the client might influence the kinds of decisions that nurses might make in their practice? Consider how understanding the person in terms of needs, system theory, or interaction might lead you to notice certain things and not others.
2. What sorts of gaps in information or misunderstandings might occur if nurses failed to use a systematic way of thinking about each individual in their care?
3. How do you think that conceptual frameworks and nursing theories might be used to generate research questions for developing knowledge for evidence-informed practice?
4. Why is it useful for nurses to question how they know what they think they know?

REVIEW QUESTIONS

1. A theory is best understood as a set of assumptions or propositions that becomes useful when it does which of the following?
   1. Helps people meet their self-care needs
   2. Isolates concepts
   3. Helps the nurse implement care
   4. Provides a systematic view of explaining, predicting, and prescribing phenomena
2. The enterprise of early theorizing about nursing practice was primarily driven by:
   1. Physicians
   2. Political leaders
   3. Nursing educators
   4. Policymakers
3. The nursing process in its original form involved which four basic steps?
   1. Assessment, planning, intervention, evaluation
   2. Assessment, nursing diagnosis, planning, intervention
   3. Nursing diagnosis, planning, intervention, evaluation
   4. Planning, assessment, intervention, evaluation
4. The metaparadigm concepts that formed the structure of concepts that nursing theories were concerned about included:
   1. The person, environment, health, and nursing
   2. Caring, health promotion, and supportive care
   3. Chaos theory and systems theory
   4. Existentialism, phenomenology, and metaphysics
5. The main question to which the early nursing theorists put their attention was to work out which of the following?
   1. How to differentiate between nursing theories and medical theories
   2. How to reconcile the generalizations of the North American Nursing Diagnoses Association with the unique situations of each client
   3. How to organize and make sense of general nursing knowledge and apply this knowledge to an individual clinical case
   4. Whether to use theories from other disciplines such as philosophy and to apply them to nursing
6. According to Kuhn, scientific advances are most likely to happen when creative individuals do which of the following?
   1. Approach a problem in a new way
   2. Use the cause-and-effect model to solve problems
   3. Use the work of other scientists to solve problems
   4. Use empirical evidence to solve problems

7. The central idea characterizing the McGill model for nursing is that it:
   1. Focuses on health rather than on illness or treatment
   2. Accounts for holistic aspects of the individual, rather than component parts
   3. Views the person as an energy field in constant interaction with the environment
   4. Considers the human experience to be based on behavioural drives
8. Building upon a psychoanalytic perspective, theorist Hildegard Peplau considered which of the following as fundamental aspects of nursing practice?
   1. Interacting in a therapeutic manner
   2. Developing the relationship between the nurse and patient
   3. Investigating the meaning of patient behaviour
   4. All of the above
9. The distinctive contribution that Canadian theorist Evelyn Adam added to nursing's thinking at the time was a conceptualization of the essence of nursing as:
   1. A collaboration with health care providers
   2. A helping process
   3. The management of patients and health care systems
   4. All of the above
10. The idea that nursing theorists drew specifically from systems theories was to consider the human being as:
    1. An irreducible whole
    2. A whole and component parts in intricate interaction with one another
    3. An embodiment of mind, body, and spirit
    4. All of the above
11. The most distinctive feature of Rosemarie Parse's theory is that it considers the individual as a unitary being who is engaged in which of the following?
    1. Seeking health
    2. Engaging in a continuing process of making choices
    3. Striving for homeostasis
    4. All of the above

Answers: 1. 4; **2.** 3; **3.** 1; **4.** 1; **5.** 3; **6.** 1; **7.** 1; **8.** 4; **9.** 2; **10.** 2; **11.** 2

Rationales for the Review Questions appear at the end of the book.

REFERENCES

Adam, E. (1979). *Être infirmière*. Montreal: Editions HRW Ltée.

Adam, E. (1980). *To be a nurse*. Philadelphia: W. B. Saunders.

Alfaro-LeFevre, R. (2017). *Critical thinking, clinical reasoning, and clinical judgment: A practical approach* (6th ed.). Philadelphia: W. B. Saunders.

Barnum, B. J. S. (1994). *Nursing theory: Analysis, application, evaluation* (4th ed.). Philadelphia: J. B. Lippincott.

Barnum, B. J. S. (1998). *Nursing theory: Analysis, application, evaluation* (5th ed.). Philadelphia: Lippincott Williams & Wilkins.

Beckstrand, J. (1978). The notion of a practice theory and the relationship of scientific and ethical knowledge to practice. *Research in Nursing & Health*, *1*(3), 131–136. doi:10.1002/nur.4770010306.

Benner, P., & Tanner, C. (1987). Clinical judgment: How expert nurses use intuition. *The American Journal of Nursing*, *87*(1), 23–31. doi:10.2307/3470396.

Benner, P., Tanner, C. A., & Chesla, C. A. (2009). *Expertise in nursing practice: Caring, clinical judgment, and ethics* (2nd ed.). New York: Springer.

Brenwick, J. M., & Webster, G. A. (2000). *Philosophy of nursing: A new vision for health care*. Albany, NY: State University of New York Press.

Campbell, J. C., & Bunting, S. (1991). Voices and paradigms: Perspectives on critical and feminist theory in nursing. *ANS. Advances in Nursing Science*, *13*(3), 1–15.

Campbell, M. A. (1987). *The UBC model for nursing: Directions for practice*. Vancouver: University of British Columbia School of Nursing.

Campbell, M. A., Cruise, M. J., & Murakami, T. R. (1976). A model for nursing: University of British Columbia School of Nursing. *Nursing Papers*, *8*(2), 5–9. Retrieved from http://cjnr.archive.mcgill.ca/article/view/588.

Canadian Association of Schools of Nursing. (2015). *National nursing education framework: Final report*. Ottawa: Author.

Carnevali, D. L., & Thomas, M. D. (1993). *Diagnostic reasoning and treatment decision making in nursing*. Philadelphia: Lippincott.

Carper, B. A. (1978). Fundamental patterns of knowing in nursing. *ANS. Advances in Nursing Science*, *1*(1), 13–23.

Chinn, P. L., & Kramer, M. K. (2011). *Integrated knowledge development in nursing* (8th ed.). St. Louis: Mosby.

Clarke, B., James, C., & Kelly, J. (1996). Reflective practice: Reviewing the issues and refocusing the debate. *International Journal of Nursing Studies*, *33*(2), 171–180. doi:10.1111/j.1741-2005.1938.tb04432.x.

Cody, W. K. (1995). About all those paradigms: Many in the universe, two in nursing. *Nursing Science Quarterly*, *8*, 144–147. doi:10.1177/089431849500800402.

Coppa, D. F. (1993). Chaos theory suggests a new paradigm for nursing science. *Journal of Advanced Nursing*, *18*(6), 985–991. doi:10.1046/j.1365-2648.1993.18060985.x.

Cull-Wilby, B. L., & Peppin, J. I. (1987). Towards a coexistence of paradigms in nursing knowledge development. *Journal of Advanced Nursing*, *12*(4), 515–521. doi:10.1111/j.1365-2648.1987.tb01361.x.

Dean, H. (1995). Science and practice: The nature of knowledge. In A. Omery, C. E. Kasper, & G. G. Page (Eds.), *In search of nursing science* (pp. 275–290). Thousand Oaks, CA: Sage.

Donaldson, S. K. (1995). Nursing science for nursing practice. In A. Omery, C. E. Kasper, & G. G. Page (Eds.), *In search of nursing science* (pp. 3–12). Thousand Oaks, CA: Sage.

Durand, M., & Prince, R. (1966). Nursing diagnosis: Process and decision. *Nursing Forum*, *5*(4), 50–64. doi:10.1111/j.1744-6198.1966.tb00348.x.

Ellis, R. (1968). Characteristics of significant theories. *Nursing Research*, *17*(3), 217–222. doi:10.1097/00006199-196805000-00009.

Engebretson, J. (1997). A multiparadigm approach to nursing. *ANS. Advances in Nursing Science*, *20*(1), 21–33.

Fawcett, J. (1992). Contemporary conceptualizations of nursing: Philosophy or science. In J. F. Kikuchi & H. Simmons (Eds.), *Philosophic inquiry in nursing* (pp. 55–63). Newbury Park, CA: Sage.

Fawcett, J. (2004). *Contemporary nursing knowledge: Analysis and evaluation of nursing models and theories* (2nd ed.). Philadelphia: F. A. Davis.

Fawcett, J., Watson, J., Neuman, B., et al. (2001). On nursing theories and evidence. *Journal of Nursing Scholarship*, *33*(2), 115–119. doi:10.1111/j.1547-5069.2001.00115.x.

Feeley, N., & Gerez-Lirette, T. (1992). Development of professional practice based on the McGill model of nursing in an ambulatory care setting. *Journal of Advanced Nursing*, *17*(7), 801–808. doi:10.1111/j.1365-2648.1992.tb02001.x.

Feeley, N., & Gottlieb, L. N. (1998). Classification systems for health concerns, nursing strategies, and client outcomes: Nursing practice with families who have a child with a chronic illness. *The Canadian Journal of Nursing Research*, *30*(1), 45–49. Retrieved from http://cjnr.archive.mcgill.ca/article/view/1424.

Field, P. A. (1987). The impact of nursing theory on the clinical decision-making process. *Journal of Advanced Nursing*, *12*(5), 563–571. doi:10.1111/j.1365-2648.1987.tb03046.x.

Fitzpatrick, J. J. (1990). Conceptual basis for the organization and advancement of nursing knowledge: Nursing diagnosis/taxonomy. *Nursing Diagnosis*, *1*(3), 102–106. doi:10.1111/j.1744-618X.1990.tb00251.x.

Fry, S. T. (1995). Science as problem solving. In A. Omery, C. E. Kasper, & G. G. Page (Eds.), *In search of nursing science* (pp. 72–80). Thousand Oaks, CA: Sage.

George, J. B. (Ed.), (1995). *Nursing theories: The base for professional nursing practice* (4th ed.). Norwalk, CT: Appleton Lange.

Gleick, J. (1987). *Chaos: Making a new science*. New York: Penguin.

Gottlieb, L. N. (2013). *Strengths-based nursing care: Health and healing for person and family*. New York: Springer.

Gottlieb, L. N., & Feeley, N. (1999). Nursing intervention studies: Issues related to change and timing in children and families. *The Canadian Journal of Nursing Research*, *30*(4), 193–212. Retrieved from http://cjnr.archive.mcgill.ca/article/view/1485.

Gottlieb, L. N., & Rowat, K. (1987). The McGill model of nursing: A practice-derived model. *ANS. Advances in Nursing Science*, *9*(4), 51–61.

Grubbs, J. (1980). An interpretation of the Johnson behavioral system model for nursing practice. In J. P. Riehl & C. Roy (Eds.), *Conceptual models for nursing practice* (2nd ed., pp. 217–254). New York: Appleton-Century-Crofts.

Harmer, B., & Henderson, V. (1955). *Textbook of the principles and practice of nursing* (5th ed.). New York: Macmillan.

Henderson, V. (1966). *The nature of nursing*. New York: Macmillan.

Henderson, V. (1982). The nursing process: Is the title right? *Journal of Advanced Nursing*, *7*(2), 103–109. doi:10.1111/j.1365-2648.1982.tb00217.x.

Holden, R. J. (1990). Models, muddles and medicine. *International Journal of Nursing Studies, 27*(3), 223–234. doi:10.1016/0020-7489(90)90037-J.

Johnson, D. E. (1974). Development of theory: A requisite for nursing as a primary health profession. *Nursing Research, 23*(5), 372–377.

Johnson, D. E. (1980). The behavioral system model for nursing. In J. P. Riehl & C. Roy (Eds.), *Conceptual models for nursing practice* (2nd ed., pp. 207–216). New York: Appleton-Century-Crofts.

Johnson, J. L. (1991). Nursing science: Basic, applied, or practical? Implications for the art of nursing. *ANS. Advances in Nursing Science, 14*(1), 7–16.

Jones, M. (1997). Thinking nursing. In S. E. Thorne & V. E. Hayes (Eds.), *Nursing praxis: Knowledge and action* (pp. 125–139). Thousand Oaks, CA: Sage.

Kagan, P. N., Smith, M. C., Cowling, W. R., et al. (2010). A nursing manifesto: An emancipatory call for knowledge development, conscience, and praxis. *Nursing Philosophy, 11*(1), 67–84. doi:10.1111/j.1466-769X.2009.00422.x.

Kikuchi, J. F. (1999). Clarifying the nature of conceptualizations about nursing. *The Canadian Journal of Nursing Research, 30*(4), 115–128. Retrieved from http://cjnr.archive.mcgill.ca/article/view/1478.

Kikuchi, J. F., & Simmons, H. (1999). *Scholarly Inquiry for Nursing Practice, 13*(1), 43–56.

King, I. M., & Fawcett, J. (1997). *The language of nursing theory and metatheory.* Indianapolis, IN: Sigma Theta Tau International Center Nursing Press.

Kuhn, T. S. (1962). *The structure of scientific revolutions.* Chicago: University of Chicago Press.

Lee, J., Chan, A. C., & Phillips, D. R. (2006). Diagnostic practice in nursing: A critical review of the literature. *Nursing and Health Sciences, 8*(1), 57–65. doi:10.1111/j.1442-2018.2006.00267.x.

Levine, M. E. (1995). The rhetoric of nursing theory. *Image–the Journal of Nursing Scholarship, 27*(1), 11–14. doi:10.1111/j.1547-5069.1995.tb00807.x.

Liaschenko, J. (1997). Knowing the patient? In S. E. Thorne & V. E. Hayes (Eds.), *Nursing praxis: Knowledge and action* (pp. 23–38). Thousand Oaks, CA: Sage.

Liaschenko, J., & Fisher, A. (1999). Theorizing the knowledge that nurses use in the conduct of their work. *Scholarly Inquiry for Nursing Practice, 13*(1), 29–42.

Maslow, A. H. (1954). *Motivation and personality.* New York: Harper & Row.

McKay, R. (1969). Theories, models, and systems for nursing. *Nursing Research, 18*(5), 393–400.

Meleis, A. I. (1987). ReVisions in knowledge development: A passion for substance. *Scholarly Inquiry for Nursing Practice, 1*(1), 5–19.

Meleis, A. I. (2012). *Theoretical nursing: Development and progress* (5th ed.). Philadelphia: Lippincott Williams & Wilkins.

Mitchell, G. J. (1995). Reflection: The key to breaking with tradition. *Nursing Science Quarterly, 8*(2), 57. doi:10.1177/089431849500800204.

Munro, M., Gallant, M., MacKinnon, M., et al. (2000). The Prince Edward Island Conceptual Model for Nursing: A nursing perspective of primary health care. *The Canadian Journal of Nursing Research, 32*(1), 39–55. Retrieved from http://cjnr.archive.mcgill.ca/article/view/1563.

Nagle, L. M., & Mitchell, G. J. (1991). Theoretic diversity: Evolving paradigmatic issues in research and practice. *ANS. Advances in Nursing Science, 14*(1), 17–25.

Neuman, B. M. (1982). *The Neuman systems model: Application to nursing education and practice.* Norwalk, CT: Appleton-Century-Crofts.

Newman, M. A. (1972). Nursing's theoretical evolution. *Nursing Outlook, 20*(7), 449–453.

Newman, M. A. (1992). Prevailing paradigms in nursing. *Nursing Outlook, 40*(1), 10–13, 32.

Newman, M. A. (2002). The pattern that connects. *ANS. Advances in Nursing Science, 24*(3), 1–7.

Nightingale, F. (1946). *Notes on nursing: What it is and what it is not.* Philadelphia: Lippincott. (Original work published 1859).

Orem, D. E. (1971). *Nursing: Concepts of practice.* New York: McGraw Hill.

Orem, D. E., & Parker, K. S. (1964). *Nursing content in preservice nursing curriculums.* Washington, DC: Catholic University of America Press.

Orlando, I. J. (1961). *The dynamic nurse–patient relationship: Function, process, and principles.* New York: G. P. Putnam's Sons.

Parse, R. R. (1981). *Man–living–health: A theory of nursing.* New York: Wiley.

Parse, R. R. (1987). *Nursing science: Major paradigms, theories, and critiques.* Philadelphia: W. B. Saunders.

Parse, R. R. (1997). The human becoming theory: The was, is, and will be. *Nursing Science Quarterly, 10*(1), 32–38. doi:10.1177/089431849701000111.

Parse, R. R. (1999). Nursing science: The transformation of practice. *Journal of Advanced Nursing, 30*(6), 1383–1387. doi:10.1046/j.1365-2648.1999.01234.x.

Parse, R. R. (2004). The many meanings of unitary: A plea for clarity. *Nursing Science Quarterly, 17*(4), 293. doi:10.1177/0894318404268810.

Parse, R. R. (2007). The human becoming school of thought in 2050. *Nursing Science Quarterly, 20*(4), 308–311.

Peplau, H. E. (1952). *Interpersonal relations in nursing.* New York: G. P. Putnam's Sons.

Raudonis, B. M., & Acton, G. J. (1997). Theory-based nursing practice. *Journal of Advanced Nursing, 26*(1), 138–145. doi:10.1046/j.1365-2648.1997.1997026138.x.

Ray, M. A. (1998). Complexity and nursing science. *Nursing Science Quarterly, 11*(3), 91–93. doi:10.1177/089431849801100302.

Reed, J., & Ground, I. (1997). *Philosophy for nursing.* London: Arnold.

Reed, P. G. (1995). A treatise on nursing knowledge development for the 21st century: Beyond postmodernism. *ANS. Advances in Nursing Science, 17*(3), 70–84.

Rodgers, B. L. (1991). Deconstructing the dogma in nursing knowledge and practice. *Image–the Journal of Nursing Scholarship, 23*(3), 177–181. doi:10.1111/j.1547-5069.1991.tb00665.x.

Rogers, M. E. (1970). *An introduction to the theoretical basis of nursing.* Philadelphia: F. A. Davis.

Roy, C. (1970). Adaptation: A conceptual framework for nursing. *Nursing Outlook, 18*(3), 42–45.

Roy, C. (1974). The Roy adaptation model. In J. P. Riehl & C. Roy (Eds.), *Conceptual models for nursing practice* (pp. 135–144). New York: Appleton-Century-Crofts.

Roy, C. (1982). Historical perspective of the theoretical framework for the classification of nursing diagnosis. In M. J. Kim & D. A. Moritz (Eds.), *Classification of nursing diagnoses: Proceedings of the third and fourth national conferences held in St. Louis, MO, in 1978 and 1980* (pp. 235–246). New York: McGraw-Hill.

Roy, C. (1984). *Introduction to nursing: An adaptation model* (2nd ed.). Englewood Cliffs, NJ: Prentice Hall.

Roy, C., & Andrews, H. A. (1999). *The Roy adaptation model: The definitive statement* (2nd ed.). East Norwalk, CT: Appleton & Lange.

Sarter, B. J. (1990). Philosophical foundations of nursing theory: A discipline emerges. In N. L. Chaska (Ed.), *The nursing profession: Turning points* (pp. 223–229). St. Louis: Mosby.

Silva, M. C., Sorrell, J. M., & Sorrell, S. C. (1995). From Carper's patterns of knowing to ways of being: An ontological philosophical shift in nursing. *ANS. Advances in Nursing Science, 18*(1), 1–13.

Starzomski, R., & Rodney, P. (1997). Nursing inquiry for the common good. In S. E. Thorne & V. E. Hayes (Eds.), *Nursing praxis: Knowledge and action* (pp. 219–236). Thousand Oaks, CA: Sage.

Tanner, C. A. (1993). Rethinking clinical judgment. In N. L. Diekelman & M. L. Rather (Eds.), *Transforming RN education: Dialogue and debate* (2nd ed., Publication No. 14-2511, pp. 15–41). New York: National League for Nursing.

Thorne, S. E. (1997). Introduction: Praxis in the context of nursing's developing inquiry. In S. E. Thorne & V. E. Hayes (Eds.), *Nursing praxis: Knowledge and action* (pp. xi–xxiii). Thousand Oaks, CA: Sage.

Thorne, S., Jillings, C., Ellis, D., et al. (1993). A nursing model in action: The University of British Columbia experience. *Journal of Advanced Nursing, 18*(8), 1259–1266. doi: 10.1046/j.1365-2648.1993.18081259.x.

Torres, G. (1974). Curriculum process and the integrated curriculum. In National League for Nursing (Ed.), *Unifying the curriculum: The integrated approach* (Publication No. 15-1522, pp. 15–31). New York: National League for Nursing.

Torres, G. (1986). *Theoretical foundations of nursing.* Norwalk, CT: Appleton-Century-Crofts.

Travelbee, J. (1971). *Interpersonal aspects of nursing.* Philadelphia, PA: F. A. Davis.

Varcoe, C. (1996). Disparagement of the nursing process: The new dogma? *Journal of Advanced Nursing, 23*(1), 120–125. doi:10.1111/j.1365-2648.1996.tb03144.x.

von Bertalanffy, L. (1968). *General systems theory: Foundations, development, application.* New York: George Braziller.

Wald, F. S., & Leonard, R. C. (1964). Toward development of nursing practice theory. *Nursing Research, 13*(4), 309–313.

Warren, J. J., & Hoskins, L. M. (1990). The development of NANDA's nursing diagnosis taxonomy. *Nursing Diagnosis, 1*(4), 162–168. doi:10.1111/j.1744-618X.1990.tb00434.x.

Watson, J. (1979). *Nursing: The philosophy and science of caring.* Boston: Little, Brown.

Watson, J. (1990). Caring knowledge and informed moral passion. *ANS. Advances in Nursing Science, 13*(1), 15–24.

Watson, J. (1999). *Postmodern nursing and beyond.* Edinburgh: Churchill Livingstone.

White, J. (1995). Patterns of knowing: Review, critique, and update. *ANS. Advances in Nursing Science, 17*(4), 73–86.

Yeo, M. (1989). Integration of nursing theory and nursing ethics. *ANS. Advances in Nursing Science, 11*(3), 33–42.

Yura, H., & Walsh, M. B. (1973). *The nursing process: Assessing, planning, implementing, evaluating* (2nd ed.). New York: Appleton-Century-Crofts.

6

Evidence-Informed Practice

Canadian content written by Wendy Duggleby, RN, PhD, Barbara J. Astle, RN, PhD

OBJECTIVES

Mastery of content in this chapter will enable you to:

- Define the key terms listed.
- Explain the need for evidence to inform nurses' decision making.
- Identify the steps of evidence-informed decision making.
- Discuss methods for developing new nursing knowledge.
- Explain how nursing research improves nursing practice.
- Discuss the steps of the research process.

KEY TERMS

Evidence-informed decision making, p. 75
Evidence-informed practice, p. 75
Informed consent, p. 83
Nursing research, p. 79
Qualitative nursing research, p. 83
Quantitative nursing research, p. 81
Research, p. 79
Research literacy, p. 78
Research process, p. 80

MEDIA RESOURCES

http://evolve.elsevier.com/Canada/Potter/fundamentals/

- Audio Chapter Summaries
- Examination Review Questions
- Concept Map Creator
- Case Study with Questions
- Audio Glossary
- Content Updates
- Video Clips

Natalie has been a nurse in the emergency department (ED) for more than 5 years. During that time, the nurses have followed a policy of restricting the presence of family members when patients experience critical events that necessitate resuscitation. The nurses have assumed that the experience of watching a family member undergoing resuscitation is too traumatic for family members. However, Natalie has noticed for some time that the families of resuscitated patients experience significant stress when they are unable to stay with their family member. Later, after the resuscitation, the families may express anger or resentment toward staff. Natalie raises a question with the other nurses in the department: "What if we allowed family presence during resuscitation? What would be the outcomes for the families? Is it possible that families can benefit?"

Natalie then began to look for evidence in the scientific literature to inform her practice and to change policy in the ED. In reading the literature, she found that when a person witnessed the resuscitation of their family member in the ED, their trust of the health care team increased and it assisted them in the grieving process if the patient did not survive (Leske, McAndrew, & Brasel, 2013). Other benefits were that the health care team viewed the patient more as a person and that having a family member present was of comfort for the patient. Studies recommended the development of a protocol for family-witnessed resuscitation in the ED and education sessions for staff (Lowry, 2012).

Most nurses like Natalie practise nursing according to what they learn in their nursing education, their experiences in practice, and the policies and procedures of their health care agency. In Natalie's case, the evidence from the scientific literature provided a basis for her and her colleagues to make evidence-informed decisions to provide the highest quality of care to their patients and families.

WHY EVIDENCE?

The Canadian Nurses Association's (CNA's) 2015 *Framework for Nursing Practice* states that nurses must use evidence-informed decision making. This means that scientific evidence is integrated into the decision making of every nurse. Additionally, knowledge of research, methodologies, critical inquiry, and evidence is acknowledged as a core domain to inform nursing practice (Canadian Association of Schools of Nursing, 2015). Multiple terms are used to describe the utilization of research by nurses in their practice, such as *research-based nursing practice, evidence-based practice, evidenced-based decision making,* **evidence-informed practice**, and *evidence-informed decision making. Evidence-based practice* refers to the use of evidence in the nurses' practice (Melnyk & Fineout-Overholt, 2015), whereas *evidence-informed decision making* refers to the use of evidence from research using a variety of methodologies within a framework of clinical judgement (Canadian Institutes of Health Research [CIHR], 2012). **Evidence-informed decision making** is defined by the CNA (2015) as "a continuous interactive process involving the explicit, conscientious and judicious consideration of the best available evidence to provide care. It is essential to optimize outcomes for individual clients, promote healthy communities and populations, improve clinical practice, achieve cost-effective nursing care and ensure accountability and transparency in decision-making within the health care system" (p. 27). As a result, evidence-informed decision making enables nurses to make accurate, timely, and appropriate clinical decisions. In this chapter, we will be using the term *evidence-informed decision making.*

Relationship Between Evidence-Informed Decision Making, Research, and Quality Improvement

Nurses conduct research in a variety of settings and with a variety of methods. Student nurses and practitioners participate in investigations of patient outcomes and nursing care specific to their place of practice, commonly called *quality assurance* or *improvement studies.* In these types of studies, data are collected to determine the influence of nurses on achievement of patient care objectives in a particular clinical setting. Because the results usually apply only to one facility, quality improvement (QI) studies are not considered research. However, such studies are important to the facility involved because they can demonstrate the contributions made by nurses to patient care and help the facility to improve processes, if necessary.

Evidence-informed decision making, research, and QI are closely interrelated. All three processes require nurses to use the best evidence to provide the highest quality of patient care. As a nurse, you should know the differences between these terms and know which process to select when you face clinical problems or you wish to improve patient care. Although you will use all of these in nursing practice, it is important to know the similarities and differences among them (see Table 6-1). When implementing evidence-informed decision making, it is important to first review evidence from appropriate research and QI data. This information can help you better understand the extent of a problem in practice and within your organization. QI data inform you about how processes work in an organization and thus offer information about how to make changes.

DEVELOPMENT OF NURSING KNOWLEDGE

Nursing knowledge must be expanded continuously to keep approaches to nursing care relevant and current; it is the foundation of the profession of nursing. Without new knowledge, nursing cannot improve therapies such as infant care, pain management, grief counselling, or patient education. The major source of new knowledge is research, which can provide a solid foundation for nursing practice. It is important to translate the best evidence into best practices at a patient's bedside. Nurses need a sound knowledge base to support practice, and research is essential for building that knowledge.

Professional nurses must stay informed about current evidence. This is not easy to do. Students may diligently read the assigned materials from texts and articles and assume they have the latest information. A good textbook incorporates evidence into the practice guidelines it describes. However, it takes about 2 years for a book to be written, published, and in print; therefore, the scientific literature used in the book can be outdated by the time the book is published. Articles, particularly scientific ones, are more likely to be current, but the findings may not be easily applied. They may be inconclusive, or the particular practice that would incorporate the research may not have been studied yet. Moreover, these articles are not readily available to staff nurses at the bedside. It is a distinct challenge to obtain the best, most current evidence when you need it for patient care.

The sources of information about evidence are well-designed, systematically conducted research studies, found in scientific journals.

TABLE 6-1 Similarities and Differences Among Evidence-Informed Decision Making, Research, and Quality Improvement

	Evidence-Informed Decision Making	Research	Quality Improvement
Purpose	Use of information from research, professional experts, personal experience, and patient preferences to determine safe and effective nursing care with the goal of improving patient care and outcomes	Systematic inquiry answers questions, solves problems, and contributes to the generalizable knowledge base of nursing; it may or may not improve patient care.	Improves local work processes to improve patient outcomes and efficiency of health systems; results usually not generalizable
Focus	Implementation of evidence already known into practice	Evidence is generated to find answers for questions that are not known about nursing practice.	Measures effects of practice and/or practice change on specific patient population
Data sources	Multiple research studies, expert opinion, personal experience, patients	Subjects or participants have predefined characteristics that include or exclude them from the study; the researcher collects and analyzes data from subjects.	Data from patient records or patients who are in a specific area, such as on a patient care unit or admitted to a particular hospital
Who conducts the activity?	Practising nurses and possibly other members of the health care team	Researchers who may or may not be employed by the health care agency and usually are not a part of the clinical health care team conduct it.	Employees of a health care agency, such as nurses, physicians, pharmacists
Is activity part of regular clinical practice?	Yes	No	Yes
Is approval needed from an institutional review board?	Sometimes	Yes	Sometimes
Funding sources	Internal, from health care agency	Funding is usually external, such as a grant	Internal, from health care agency

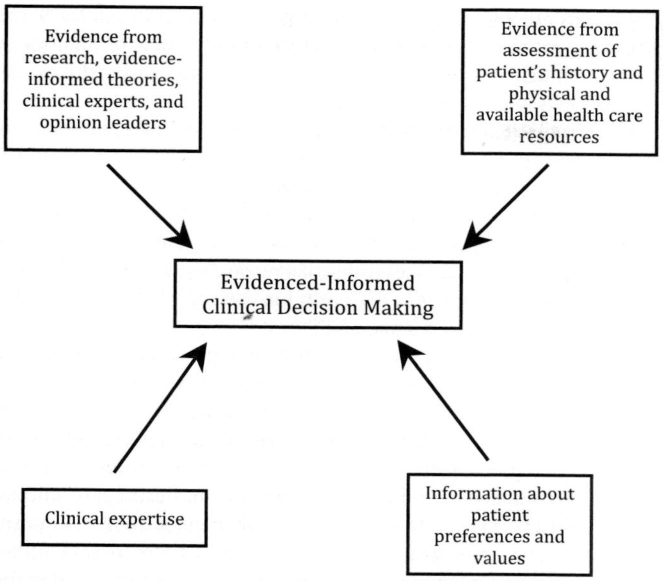

FIGURE 6-1 Processes involved in evidence-informed decision making.

Nurses need to have the ability to locate, understand, and critically evaluate evidence for application to practice. When no evidence is available, tradition prevails.

Nonresearch evidence is another source of information to support practice. This includes quality improvement and risk management data; international, national, and local standards; infection control data; chart reviews; and clinical expertise. These sources can be valuable, but their value never approaches that of research evidence.

A third source of evidence that must be incorporated into good clinical decisions consists of individual patients and their values, beliefs, and experience. No efficacious clinical decision can be made without consideration of the uniqueness of the patient. Figure 6-1 illustrates the process for evidence-informed decision making.

Steps to foster success in evidence-informed decision making are summarized in Box 6-1.

RESEARCHING THE EVIDENCE

Ask the Clinical Question

Clinical questions arise out of your nursing practice and represent problems that you wonder about or things that do not make sense to you. For example, while caring for an unconscious patient, you might wonder, "What is the best cleaner to use when I provide mouth care to this patient?" Or you might notice that there has been an increase in patient falls on your unit, leading you to ask, "How can I reduce falls on my unit?"

Clinical questions that arise from your nursing practice should first be addressed by looking to see if the answer is readily available. Important sources of this type of information can be found in practice guidelines available from professional associations. All professions have focused on ensuring that service professionals understand practice guidelines. "Best practices" are guiding principles leading to the most appropriate courses of action in certain standard practice situations. They are based on the accumulated research findings, as well as on evidence from practice. An example is the Best Practice Guidelines, developed by the Registered Nurses Association of Ontario (RNAO). The RNAO has 50 published guidelines, as well as a toolkit and educator's resource to implement these guidelines into practice.

BOX 6-1 Steps for Successful Evidence-Informed Practice

1. Ask a question that clearly presents the clinical problem.
2. Identify and gather the most relevant and best evidence.
3. Critically appraise the evidence.
4. Integrate all evidence with clinical expertise, patients' preferences, and patients' values to make a practice decision or change.
5. Evaluate the outcome of the practice decision or change.

From Melnyk, B. M., & Fineout-Overholt, E. (2015). *Evidence-based practice in nursing and health care. A guide to best practice* (3rd ed.). Philadelphia, PA: Lippincott Williams & Wilkins. Reprinted by permission of Lippincott Williams & Wilkins.

The questions you ask will eventually lead you to the evidence required for an answer. When you consult the empirical literature for an answer, you will want to read the most informative four to six articles that address your practice question specifically, not be mired in hundreds of articles that might have some relationship to your question. This means that your question must be well stated and focused on just the relevant components of the issue. Unfocused questions ("What is the best way to reduce wandering?" "What is the best way to measure blood pressure?") are too vague and will lead to many irrelevant sources of information. LoBondo-Wood, Haber, Cameron, and Singh (2017) suggested using a "PICOT" format to state your question. A PICOT question has five components:

P = Patient population of interest: What are the age, gender, ethnicity, and disease or health problem of the patients?
I = Intervention of interest: What is the best intervention (treatment, diagnostic test, prognostic factor)?
C = Comparison of interest: What is the usual standard of care or current intervention used now in practice?
O = Outcome: What result (e.g., change in patient behaviour, physical finding) do you want to achieve as a result of the intervention?
T = Time: What is the time frame in which you think the change will occur?

Do not be satisfied with clinical routines if they do not improve the patient's quality of life. Always ask questions and use critical thinking to consider better ways to provide patient care. The questions you raise by using a PICOT format help you identify knowledge gaps within a clinical situation and assist you in making sound clinical decisions for change.

Collect the Best Evidence

Once you have a clear and concise PICOT question, you are ready to search for evidence. You can find the evidence you need in a variety of sources: agency policy and procedure manuals, quality improvement data, existing clinical practice guidelines, or bibliographical databases. Always ask for help to find appropriate evidence. Nursing faculty are always a key resource, as are advanced practice nurses, staff educators, infection control nurses, and librarians.

When you go to the literature for evidence, a librarian can help you locate the appropriate databases. The databases contain published empirical studies, including peer-reviewed research. An article that has undergone peer review has been reviewed by a panel of experts before publication. The search process requires you to come up with keywords or phrases from your PICOT question that most accurately describe what you want from the search. The librarian can help you find the language that yields the most informative results. You usually need to adjust the wording of your search criteria until you get the results you want.

The best-known databases for nursing literature are MEDLINE and CINAHL. These are comprehensive databases containing articles from most nursing and health journals. These are usually available at no cost to students through the university or college library.

Research Literacy—Critique the Evidence

The most difficult step in the evidence-informed practice process is critiquing or evaluating the available evidence (Hines, Ramsbotham, & Coyer, 2015; Jakubec & Astle, 2017). **Research literacy** is an essential competency for evidence-informed practice; it is the ability to locate, understand, and critically evaluate empirical literature for application in practice (Jakubec & Astle, 2017). This term is different from the term *research capacity,* which is the ability to conduct research (Fitchett, Tartaglia, Dodd-McCure, et al., 2012; Williamson, 2007).

The critiquing of evidence involves determining its value, feasibility, and utility for changing practice. When you critique evidence, first evaluate the scientific merit and clinical applicability of each study's findings. Then, with a group of studies and expert opinion, determine what findings have a strong enough basis for use in practice. After critiquing the evidence, you will be able to answer the questions: Do the articles together offer evidence to explain or answer your PICOT question? Do the articles show that the evidence is true and reliable? Can you use the evidence in practice? Because you are a student and new to nursing, it will take time to acquire the skills to critique evidence like an expert. When you read an article from the literature, do not let the statistics or technical wording cause you to stop reading the article. Know the elements of an article, and use a careful approach when you review each one. Evidence-informed articles include the following elements:

- *Abstract:* An abstract is a brief summary of the article that quickly tells you whether the article is research or clinically based. An abstract summarizes the purpose of the study or clinical query, the major themes or findings, and the implications for nursing practice.
- *Introduction:* The introduction contains information about the purpose of the article and the importance of the topic for the audience who reads the article. Brief supporting evidence is usually presented as to why the topic is important from the author's point of view. Together, the abstract and introduction tell you whether you want to read the entire article. You will know if the topic of the article is similar to your PICOT question or related closely enough to provide you with useful information. Continue to read the next elements of the article.
- *Literature review or background:* A useful article has a detailed background of the existing level of science or clinical information about the topic of the article. Therefore, it offers an argument about what led the author to conduct a study or report on a clinical topic. This section of an article is valuable. Perhaps the article itself does not address your PICOT question in the way you desire, but it may lead you to other articles that are more useful. A literature review of a research article indicates how past research led to the researcher's question. For example, an article about a study designed to test an educational intervention for older-person family caregivers includes a review of the literature describing characteristics of caregivers, the type of factors influencing caregivers' ability to cope with stressors of caregiving, and any previous educational interventions used with families.
- *Manuscript narrative:* "Middle sections," or narratives, of articles differ according to the type of evidence-informed article they are (Melnyk & Fineout-Overholt, 2015). A clinical article describes a clinical topic and often includes a description of a patient population, the nature of a certain disease or health alteration, how patients are affected, and the appropriate nursing therapies. Some clinical articles explain how to use a therapy or new technology. A research article will contain several subsections within the narrative, including the following:
  - *Purpose statement:* A purpose statement explains the focus or intent of a study. It identifies what concepts were researched. This includes research questions or hypotheses—predictions made about the relationship or difference between study variables (concepts, characteristics, or traits that vary within or among subjects). An example of a research question is as follows: "What characteristics are common among older persons who have annual breast screening?"
  - *Methods or design:* The methods or design section explains how a research study is organized and conducted in order to answer the research question or to test the hypothesis. This explanation includes the type of study to be conducted (e.g., randomized control trial, case–control study, or qualitative study) and how many subjects or persons are in a study. In health care studies, "subjects" may include patients, family members, or health care staff. The language in the methods section is sometimes confusing because it contains details about how the researcher designs the study to minimize bias and thereby obtain the most accurate results possible. Consult with your instructor or other researchers as a resource to help interpret this section.
  - *Results or conclusions:* Clinical and research articles have a summary section. A clinical article explains the clinical implications for the topic presented, whereas a research article details the results of the study and explains whether a hypothesis is supported or how a research question is answered. For a qualitative study, the article presents a thorough summary of the descriptive themes and ideas that arise from the researcher's analysis of data. A quantitative study will present data using statistical analysis. Read carefully, and ask whether the researcher describes the results and whether the results were significant. Have a faculty member assist you in interpreting statistical results. A helpful results section also discusses any limitations to a study. This information on limitations is valuable in helping you decide whether you want to use the evidence with your patients.
- *Clinical implications:* A research article includes a section that explains whether the findings from the study have clinical implications. This section also explains how to apply findings in a practice setting for the type of subjects studied.

After you have critiqued each article for your PICOT question, synthesize or combine the findings from all of the articles to determine the state of the evidence. Use critical thinking to consider the scientific rigour of the evidence and how well it answers your area of interest. Consider the evidence in view of your patients' concerns and preferences. Your review of articles offers a snapshot conclusion that is based on combined evidence about one focused topical area. As a clinician, judge whether to use the evidence for a particular patient or group of patients, who usually have complex medical histories and patterns of responses (Melnyk & Fineout-Overholt, 2015). It is ethically important to consider evidence that benefits patients and does no harm. Decide whether the evidence is relevant, is easily applicable in your setting of practice, and has the potential for improving patient outcomes.

INTEGRATE THE EVIDENCE

Once you decide that the evidence is strong and applicable to your patients and clinical situation, incorporate the recommended evidence into practice. Your first step is to simply apply the research in your plan of care for a patient. Use the evidence you find as a rationale for an intervention you plan to try. For instance, you learned about an approach for bathing older persons who are restless, and you decide to use the technique during your next clinical assignment. You use the bathing technique with your own assigned patients, or you work with a group of other students or nurses in revising a policy and procedure or in developing a new clinical protocol. In another example, after being concerned about the rate of intravenous catheter dislodgement, you consult the evidence to compare the efficacy of gauze dressings with that of transparent dressings. The literature suggests that fewer catheter dislodgements occur with transparent dressings on peripheral intravenous sites than with gauze dressings, with no increase in phlebitis or infiltration rates (Melnyk & Fineout-Overholt, 2015). As a result of your findings, you meet with the policy and procedure committee of your institution to recommend the use of transparent dressings routinely. You then implement the use of transparent dressings in the routine care of peripheral intravenous catheters.

Evidence is useful in a variety of ways in formulating teaching tools, clinical practice guidelines, policies and procedures, and new assessment or documentation tools. Depending on the amount of change needed to apply evidence in practice, it becomes necessary to involve a number of staff from a given nursing unit. It is important to consider the setting in which you want to apply the evidence: Do all staff members support the change? Does the practice change fit with the scope of practice in the clinical setting? Are resources (time, administrative support, and staff) available to make a change? When evidence is not strong enough to apply in practice, your next option is to conduct a pilot study to investigate your PICOT question. A pilot study is a small-scale research study or a study that includes a quality or performance improvement project. As a nursing student integrating evidence, your study begins with searching for and applying the most useful evidence to improve the care you provide directly to your patients. The evidence available within nursing literature gives you almost unlimited access to innovative and effective nursing interventions. Using an evidence-informed practice approach helps you improve your skills and knowledge as a nurse and improve outcomes for your patients.

EVALUATE THE PRACTICE DESIGN OR CHANGE

After applying evidence in your practice, your next step is to evaluate its effect. How does the intervention work? How effective was the clinical decision for your patient or practice setting? Sometimes your evaluation is as simple as determining whether the expected outcomes you set for an intervention are met. For example, after the use of a transparent intravenous dressing, does the catheter dislodge, or does the complication of phlebitis develop? When you use a new approach to preoperative teaching, does the patient learn what to expect after surgery?

When an evidence-informed practice change occurs on a larger scale, an evaluation is more formal. For example, evidence of factors that contribute to pressure ulcers might lead a nursing unit to adopt a new skin care protocol. To evaluate the protocol, the nurses track the incidence of pressure ulcers over a course of time (e.g., 6 months to a year). In addition, the nurses collect data to describe both the patients who develop ulcers and those who do not. This comparative information is valuable for determining the effects of the protocol and whether modifications are necessary.

SUPPORT FOR EVIDENCE-INFORMED PRACTICE

Nursing practice is based on theory, professional values, and evidence. Nurses base decisions on these factors, as well on other influences such as individual values, ethics, legislation, patient choice, and practice environments. The CNA position statement on evidence-informed decision making specifies its importance in providing quality nursing care and in effecting change across the health care system. The evidence to be used in practice is derived through research and the scientific evaluation of practice. The CNA believes that individual nurses must read and critique evidence-informed literature in order to provide high-quality care to clients (CNA, 2010).

THE DEVELOPMENT OF RESEARCH IN NURSING

Research is the primary means by which new knowledge is discovered and brought into practice to improve the care that nurses provide to their patients. It is a systematic process in which questions that generate knowledge are asked and answered. This knowledge becomes part of the scientific basis for practice and may be used to validate interventions.

Nursing research is a systematic examination of phenomena important to the nursing discipline, as well as to nurses, their patients, and families. Its purpose is to expand the knowledge base for practice by answering nurses' questions. Nursing research addresses a range of issues related to actual and potential patient populations and to individual and family responses to health problems. Some research tests nursing theories; other research generates theory from findings. This "back-and-forth" relationship between theory and research is the way knowledge develops in any discipline (Polit & Beck, 2017). In the current health care environment, nursing research is frequently undertaken in multidisciplinary teams, in which nurses examine factors relevant to nursing in the context of the larger health care picture. The scientific knowledge needed for nursing practice is discovered, tested, and enhanced through nursing research. The multidisciplinary nature of nursing challenges nurses not only to keep up with nursing research but also to know the status of research in other health disciplines, as well as in the behavioural, social, and physical sciences.

The International Council of Nurses (ICN) is a staunch supporter of nursing research as a means to improve people's health and welfare. Research is a way to identify new knowledge, improve education and practice, and use resources effectively. In 1999, the ICN established the ICN Research Network. The network provides a means for sharing research ideas, results, and progress around the world. Network members communicate with one another through the ICN website, as well as at annual conferences. In 2015, the ICN Research Network developed a tool to increase the visibility of nursing research and to encourage nurses to use research (ICN, 2015). The tool is a visual representation of the research process (Figure 6-2).

Nursing research improves nursing practice, raising the profession's standards. Involvement in research takes many forms, including designing studies, being on a research team, collecting data, and using research findings to change clinical practice, improve patient outcomes, and contain health care costs. Promoting research and using it in practice increases the scientific knowledge base for nursing practice. Patients benefit from these improvements to practice, as is evident in the case study at the beginning of this chapter.

THE HISTORY OF NURSING RESEARCH IN CANADA

During the Crimean War, Florence Nightingale's detailed and systematic observation of nursing actions and outcomes resulted in major changes in nursing practice. Her work demonstrated the importance of systematic observational research to nursing practice.

In Canada, the establishment of university nursing courses starting in 1918, followed by master's degree programs in the 1950s and 1970s

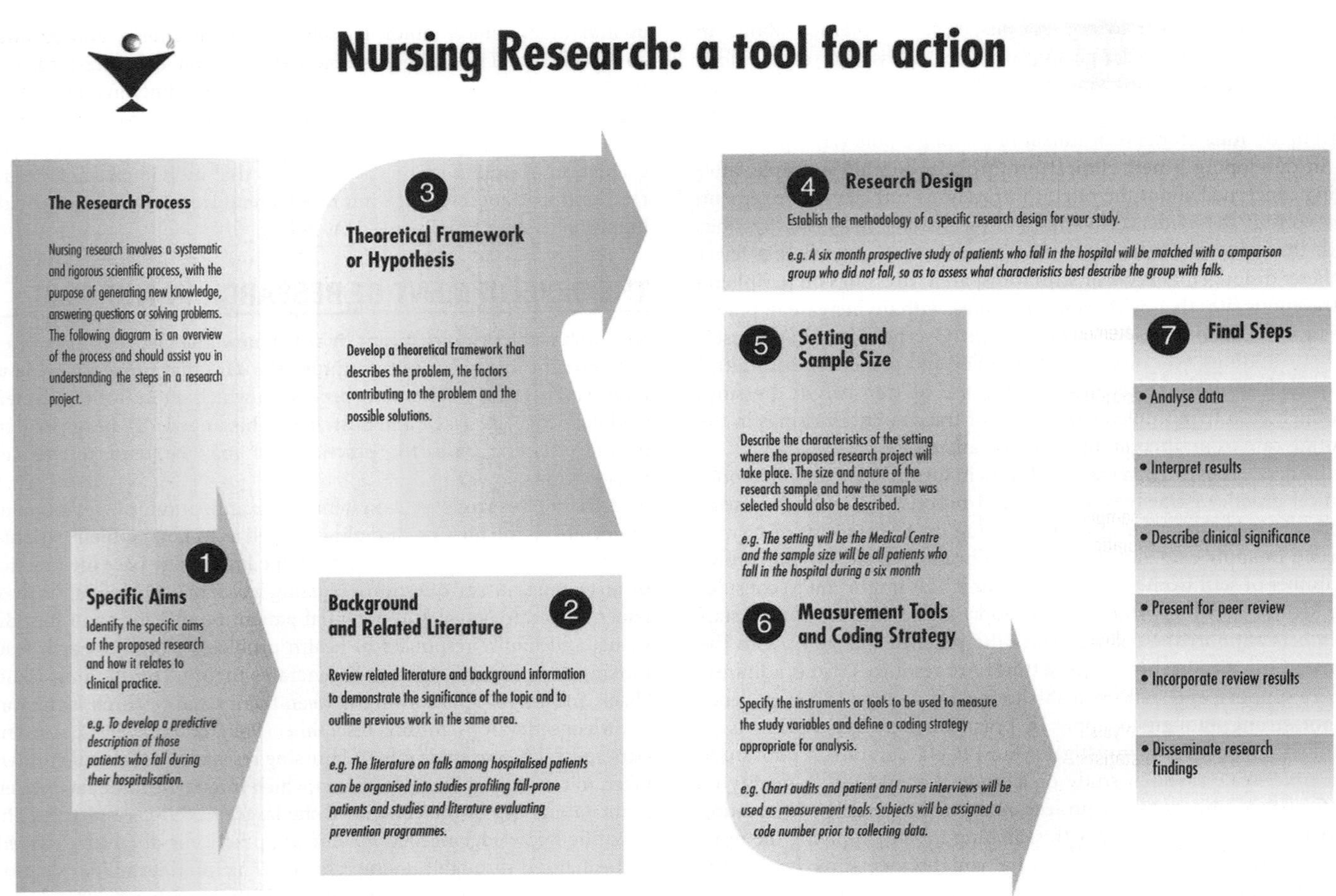

FIGURE 6-2 **A visual representation of the research process.** (International Council of Nurses. [2015]. *Nursing research: a tool for action.* Retrieved from http://www.icn.ch/networks/nursing-research-a-tool-for-action/.)

and by doctoral programs in the 1990s and 2000s, was crucial to the development of nursing research (see Chapter 3). The first master's degree program, established at the University of Western Ontario (now Western University) in 1959, highlighted the need for Canadian research capacity in nursing.

The first nursing research journal, *Nursing Research,* was launched in the United States in 1952. The first nursing research journal published in Canada, *Nursing Papers* (later the *Canadian Journal of Nursing Research*), was established at McGill University in 1969. Other journals were later established, and today, nurses publish their research, both within nursing and in interdisciplinary fields, in hundreds of journals.

Since the 1970s and 1980s, the two major factors in the development of nursing research have been the establishment of research training through doctoral programs and the establishment of funding to support nursing research. Throughout the 1970s and 1980s, university faculties and schools of nursing built their research resources so that they could establish doctoral programs. The first provincially approved doctoral nursing program was established at the University of Alberta Faculty of Nursing in 1991. Another was established at the University of British Columbia School of Nursing later that year, and programs at McGill University and the University of Toronto followed in 1993. Now there are many doctoral nursing programs in universities across Canada.

Growing awareness of the importance of nursing research gradually led to the availability of research funds. The year 1964 marked the first time that a federal granting agency funded nursing research in Canada (Good, 1969). In 1999, 14 years after the U.S. government had established funding for nursing research under the National Institutes of Health, the Canadian government established the Nursing Research Fund, budgeting $25 million for nursing research ($2.5 million over each of the following 10 years). The research areas targeted for support included nursing policies, management, human resources, and nursing care. Although this funding is no longer available, nurse researchers have been successful at obtaining Tri-Council funding nationally and international funding to support their programs of research. *Tri-Council* is a term referring to three federal research agencies: Canadian Institutes of Health Research, National Science and Engineering Research Council of Canada, and the Social Sciences and Humanities Research Council.

NURSING RESEARCH

There are several types of research that can inform nursing evidence-informed decision making. The type of research that is conducted depends on the research question or purpose.

Wood and Ross-Kerr (2011) describe the **research process** as follows: the process begins with a researchable question. If properly stated, the question guides the rest of the process; thus, asking the question is a crucial step. Three levels of questions exist, and the appropriate level is chosen based on how much is known about the research topic. Once an initial question has been formulated, the literature is searched to discover what is already known about the topic and to

TABLE 6-2 **Basic Steps in Planning Nursing Research**

Steps	Level I	Level II	Level III
Question	What?	What is the relationship?	Why?
Problem	Little known about topic	Conceptual base; variables have been studied before	Theoretical base
Purpose	Declarative statement	Question or hypothesis	Hypothesis
Design	Exploratory descriptive, Historical or Philosophical approaches	Descriptive survey, correlational or comparative	Nonexperimental or experimental
Sample	Convenience sample or total population	Convenience sample or total population	Convenience sample or total population
Methods	Qualitative, unstructured data; quantitative descriptive data	Quantitative data	Quantitative data
Analysis	Qualitative analysis; descriptive statistic	Correlation or tests of association; regression analysis	Differences between means test
Answer	Description of processes, meaning concepts, or population	Explanation of relationship among variables	Test of theory

Adapted from Wood, M., & Ross-Kerr, J. (2011). *Basic steps in planning nursing research: From question to proposal.* Sudbury, MA: Jones & Bartlett.

determine whether the question must be revised in light of prior knowledge. The level of the question determines the research design needed to answer it. Table 6-2 describes the basic steps in planning nursing research and corresponding types of research designs that might be used.

The research design provides the ground rules for data collection and analysis, ensuring that the research question will have a valid answer. The design steps are systematic and precise in order to control unwanted influences that might affect the answer. For example, in a study of the relationship between diet and heart disease, influences such as stress or smoking must be controlled because they are known to influence heart disease. The design also specifies the type of sample and sample selection techniques that will provide the most useful data for the study.

Data are gathered from the sample through measurement techniques that quantify the variables in the research question. Techniques include interviews, tests of knowledge, and physiological measures such as heart rate and blood pressure. When the evidence is analyzed, the result answers the original question and becomes the basis for discovering new knowledge.

RESEARCH DESIGNS

Nursing research approaches vary, depending on the specific problem to be studied. They are sometimes categorized as quantitative and qualitative. Neither is used exclusively in nursing research, and both approaches are now often combined (mixed-methods research). The research approach used is the one that is considered the best one to answer the research question. The next section describes some common research designs in these two categories.

Quantitative Nursing Research

Quantitative nursing research is the investigation of nursing phenomena that can be precisely measured and quantified. Examples are pain severity, rates of wound healing, and body temperature changes. The goal is to test theory and use numerical data, statistical analysis, and controls to eliminate bias (Polit & Beck, 2017).

Experimental Research. Experiments are appropriate designs for questions at level III (see Table 6-2), which concern why one variable causes a predictable change in another variable. In an experimental design, the conditions under which the variables are studied are tightly controlled to provide objective testing of hypotheses, which predict cause-and-effect relationships. Experimental research requires that the data be collected and quantified in a prescribed manner.

The requirements of an experimental design are as follows:

- The study usually includes at least one control or comparison group that does not receive the nursing treatment or intervention being investigated. The results for this group are compared with those of the experimental group, which is the group that receives the treatment or intervention. The subjects—people selected for the comparison and experimental groups—are randomly assigned to these groups, so that the groups are as similar as possible to each other before the intervention. Random assignment of subjects ensures that all subjects have the same chance to be in the control or experimental (treatment) group and that variables that could affect the outcome of the study are randomly distributed between the groups and therefore are no more likely to affect experimental subjects than to affect control subjects.
- An experimental variable must be manipulated by the researcher. For example, in a study of the effect of preoperative teaching on postoperative anxiety, the researcher manipulates preoperative teaching by providing it for the experimental group but not for the control group. The expectation is that the differences in postoperative anxiety measures between the two groups can be attributed to the effect of preoperative teaching because all other factors are under control. However, the researcher cannot control subjects' prior experiences, such as hearing other patients' stories about surgery. Psychological factors, which cannot be controlled, may influence a subject's level of anxiety. If subjects are randomly assigned to the two groups, however, those with negative prior experiences should be distributed equally between the two groups, and these experiences would affect both groups equally. Thus, differences between the groups in postoperative anxiety can still be attributed to the preoperative teaching intervention.
- The researcher proposes theory-based and statistically tested hypotheses about the action of the variables to answer the research question. For example, in a study of preoperative teaching, the hypothesis might be as follows: "Patients who receive interactive preoperative teaching will have significantly lower postoperative anxiety levels than will patients who receive other teaching methods." The researcher must explain why a lower anxiety level is expected, in a discussion of the theory behind the study.

A quasi-experimental research design is one in which groups are formed and the conditions are controlled, but the subjects are not randomly assigned to a control group or to treatment conditions. These designs also answer level III questions (Wood & Ross-Kerr, 2011). An example of a study using this design is given in Box 6-2. In

BOX 6-2 RESEARCH HIGHLIGHT

Evaluation of the Living With Hope Program for Rural Women Caregivers of Persons With Advanced Cancer

Research Focus

Duggleby, Williams, Cooper, et al. (2013) used a quasi-experimental design to collect both quantitative and qualitative data, to evaluate the effectiveness of a "Living with Hope Program," developed to support rural women caring for a person with advanced cancer in their home.

Research Abstract

Hope has been identified as a key psychosocial resource among family caregivers to manage and deal with the caregiver experience. The Living with Hope Program is a self-administered intervention that consists of watching an international award–winning *Living with Hope* film and participating in a 2-week hope activity ("Stories of the Present"). The purpose of this study was to examine the effects of the Living with Hope Program on self-efficacy (General Self-Efficacy Scale), loss and grief (Non-Death Revised Grief Experience Inventory), hope (Herth Hope Index), and quality of life (Short-Form 12 version 2 [SF-12v2]) in rural women caring for persons with advanced cancer and to model potential mechanisms through which changes occurred.

Methods

A time-series embedded mixed-method design was used, with quantitative baseline outcome measures repeated at day 7, day 14, and 3, 6, and 12 months. Qualitative data from the hope activity informed the quantitative data. Thirty-six participants agreed to participate, with 22 completing all data collection. General estimating equations were used to analyze the data.

Results

Herth Hope Index scores ($p = 0.05$) had increased significantly from baseline at day 7. General Self-Efficacy Scale scores were significantly higher than baseline at all data time points. In addition, as Herth Hope Index scores increased ($p < 0.001$) and Non-Death Revised Grief Experience Inventory scores decreased ($p = 0.01$), SF-12v2 mental health summary scores increased. Qualitative data suggested that through the hope activity ("Stories of the Present"), the participants were able to find hope in their experience.

Implications for Practice

- Family caregivers are essential in that persons with advanced cancer can remain in their communities.
- Hope is an important psychosocial resource for rural women who are caring for persons with advanced cancer.
- Nurses can use the Living with Hope Program to increase hope and improve quality of life for rural women caregivers of persons with advanced cancer. It also may decrease loss and grief, and increase their confidence in their ability to deal with difficult situations.

Duggleby, W., Williams, A., Cooper, D., Holtslander, L., Ghosh, S., Hallstrom, L., & Thomas R. (2013). Evaluation of the Living with Hope Program for rural women caregivers of persons with advanced cancer. *BMC Palliative Care, 12,* 36. doi:10.1186/1472-684X-12-36. Retrieved from http://www.biomedcentral.com/1472-684X/12/36.

many health care settings, assigning subjects randomly to experimental and control groups is not feasible. Quasi-experimental research is often carried out for practical reasons related to the subjects themselves. For example, to test the effect of a new intervention in the care of patients with Alzheimer's disease, carrying out two treatments on the unit at the same time might confuse the subjects. A quasi-experiment could entail the use of two care units: one as the experimental unit, in which all subjects receive the new intervention, and the second as the control group, in which subjects receive the usual care but not the new intervention. The two groups are compared before and after the intervention with regard to the outcome variable. The weakness in a quasi-experiment is that the researcher does not know whether the two groups were equivalent before the intervention. Unrecognized differences between the two units might exist that could influence the outcome of the study. For instance, subjects in one unit might have more cognitive impairment than do those in the other unit, and this difference could influence the outcome.

Descriptive Survey Designs. *Surveys* are designed to answer level II questions about relationships among variables. The research question that leads to a survey design begins with "What is the relationship between …?" and addresses two or more variables (Wood & Ross-Kerr, 2011)—for example, the relationship between ethnicity and suicide among university students.

In many types of research, investigators use surveys in which people in a group are compared with regard to two or more variables. The purpose is to discover relationships among variables in the population. In a survey design, the sample determines whether the survey yields informative or uninformative results. The sample should be representative of the population so that generalizations can be made on the basis of the sample data. Surveys contain three key elements. First, a random sample of the population must be drawn, from which inferences can be made about the population. Second, the population sampled should be large enough to keep sampling error to a minimum. Third, the measurement tools (e.g., questionnaires, interviews) must yield accurate measurements of the study variables.

Exploratory Descriptive Designs. Exploratory descriptive designs provide in-depth descriptions of populations or variables not previously studied. Level I (basic) questions are asked because not much is known about the topic. They typically begin with "what"; for example, "What are the health-promoting behaviours of older persons living in subsidized housing?" The results provide a detailed description of the variable or population. No relationships among variables are posited at this stage, although the results might indicate that relationships should be examined in subsequent research.

Data Analysis. All quantitative studies entail the use of statistical analysis. In experimental designs, researchers must discover whether the experimental and control groups are significantly different from each other after the intervention has been applied. Statistical tests that provide a test of group means, median, or modes are generally used for experiments.

Descriptive survey designs entail the use of statistical techniques to test for significant relationships among the variables. In general, these are correlational tests that indicate whether one subject's score on one variable (e.g., blood pressure) is related to the same subject's score on another variable (e.g., weight). The results of a correlational analysis of these two variables would reveal how much influence increased body weight has on blood pressure.

Exploratory descriptive studies entail the use of several techniques to analyze data, depending on the type collected. Unstructured data that do not lend themselves to numerical form are summarized verbally. If quantitative measures are used to collect the data, they can be described both numerically and verbally. Descriptions usually include

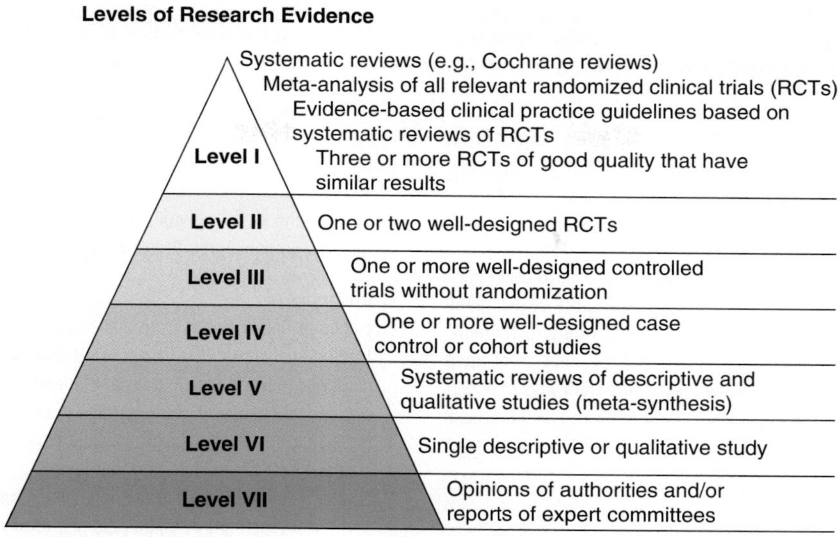

FIGURE 6-3 Hierarchy of evidence for quantitative research. (Melnyk, B. M., & Fineout-Overholt, E. [2015]. *Evidence-based practice in nursing and health care. A guide to best practice* [3rd ed.]. Philadelphia, PA: Lippincott Williams & Wilkins.)

measures of central tendency (mean, median, or mode) and dispersion (range, standard deviation).

The pyramid in Figure 6-3 represents the hierarchy of available quantitative evidence. At the top of the pyramid are systematic reviews and meta-analyses. These reviews have been conducted by experts in the clinical area, who review the evidence about a specific clinical question or issue and summarize the state of the science. Of primary importance in these reviews are the randomized controlled trials (RCTs) that have been conducted on the topic. On occasion, they include other types of research as well. Although the majority of nursing research is not at the level of the RCT, it is considered the "gold standard" in quantitative scientific research, in which the effect of a specific treatment or intervention is tested through the use of experimental and control groups. A systematic review of RCTs in which an intervention (such as computerized interactive patient teaching) is used would answer a PICOT question about the effectiveness of this intervention in managing the blood glucose levels of patients with newly diagnosed diabetes. However, this hierarchy does not apply to qualitative research, which has an important role in evidence-informed decision making (CIHR, 2012).

Qualitative Nursing Research

Qualitative nursing research poses questions about nursing phenomena that cannot be quantified and measured. To answer questions about these phenomena, researchers must understand the perspective of the person in the situation. Researchers using qualitative methods can choose one of many design strategies. The research question is the basis for the choice of design. Examples of qualitative designs that may be used in nursing research include ethnography, phenomenology, grounded theory, participatory action research, interpretive descriptive research, and narrative inquiry. In addition, each of the various qualitative methods has its own unique underlying philosophy as well as data collection and analysis approaches. For example, one qualitative approach that has been developed to specifically answer nursing practice questions is interpretive description (Thorne, 2016). Box 6-3 provides an example of a study using this methodological approach.

Transferability is an important concept to understand when using qualitative research findings in practice. It refers to the extent to which the findings of a qualitative study are thought to be meaningful and applicable to similar cases or other situations (Melnyk & Fineout-Overholt, 2015). You can assess transferability by asking the following questions:

1. Do the findings make sense with your own observations?
2. Were the study participants similar to those you care for?
3. Do the findings provide insights or make you think differently regarding your own experience?
4. Do the findings add new understandings to existing knowledge in the field? (Melnyk & Fineout-Overholt, 2015, p. 486)

Although there is not a hierarchy of evidence for qualitative research, there are systematic reviews and metasynthesis (combining of findings from several qualitative studies) that would help you determine if you wish to use the knowledge from qualitative studies in practice.

Conducting Nursing Research

Clinical nursing research should be undertaken by nurses educated to conduct scientific investigations (Figure 6-4). An experienced researcher is usually more qualified than a beginner to undertake a complex, long-term project. Nurses new to research may, however, assist with data collection, conduct replication studies (studies previously performed elsewhere), or conduct less complex studies.

ETHICAL ISSUES IN RESEARCH

Research must meet ethical standards in ways that respect the dignity and preserve the well-being of human research participants. In Canada, every health care facility and university receiving public funds for research must meet federal standards for protecting human research participants. The most recent standard is the *Tri-Council Policy Statement* (Canadian Institutes of Health Research et al., 2010), which requires that the institution have in place a research ethics board (REB) to review all research proposals to determine whether ethical principles are being upheld (Box 6-4). The REB focuses on informed consent and weighs benefits versus harms from the research. No research may be performed in a university or health care facility without the approval of the REB. All proposals are subject to review. However, if data collection processes (such as quality assurance studies) are a normal part of institutional business, performance reviews, or testing within

BOX 6-3 RESEARCH HIGHLIGHT

Discerning Success of Indigenous Health Students in Community-Based Programs

Research Focus

This study (Harder, Astle, Grypma, et al., 2016) was developed to explore how members of a community with a community-based program describe Indigenous health student success and factors that influence it.

Research Abstract

In recent years, public postsecondary educational institutions have been partnering with Indigenous educational societies to provide community-based health care programs in remote communities. The term *community* refers to students' geographical home region, the population of which may consist of both Indigenous and non-Indigenous peoples. The purpose of this study was to understand how people from one such community described the success of students who participated in those programs. The factors that influence the success of students were also explored.

Methods

This qualitative study used an inductive methodological approach called interpretive description and was informed by concepts from Indigenous decolonizing perspectives. With interpretive description, researchers are encouraged to uncover opportunities to deconstruct prior knowledge and to generate new insights that provide understanding of a specific context. It is considered to be a method of particular value to nursing research in that it is concerned with findings that are useful or applicable in nursing practice. Interviews were conducted with eight participants from a community in the northern part of a province in Western Canada. The participants included Indigenous students and community stakeholders.

Findings

The core theme of *courage* and three categorical themes of *nurturing the learning, owning the learning,* and *discerning success for learning* emerged from the data, which revealed the changes that students made in their lives as they moved through their educational journeys. Participants described that learning needed to be nurtured and that students achieved greater success when they took ownership for their learning. The participants also described success as being influenced by previous educational experiences, meeting community needs, and personal growth in the students.

Conclusions

Five conclusions emerged from this study:

1. Finding the courage to overcome fears and barriers was instrumental in students' educational journeys. Students often had to make life-changing choices that required great courage in order to advance in their education;
2. Receiving nurturing through a whole-person approach appeared to promote success in students' learning journeys;
3. Students following their educational paths were fostered through the support and encouragement of instructors and family members;
4. Students learning to believe in themselves was a key element of success; and
5. Student success was experienced as a collective community success.

Implications for Community-Based Education and Research

Nurses who are involved in community-based education may consider the following:

1. Promote ways in which Indigenous students can experience feelings of success in the early stages of their educational journeys;
2. Provide orientation sessions for nursing instructors hired to teach in community-based programs that discuss the importance of nurturing the Indigenous student learners; and
3. Discover Indigenous students' gifts prior to having them enter educational programs.

Harder, M., Astle, B., Grypma, S., & Voyageur, E. (2016)). Discerning success of Indigenous health students in community-based programs. *Quality Advancement in Nursing Education—Avancées en formation infirmière, 2*(2), Article 5, 1–19. doi:10.17483/2368-6669.1076.

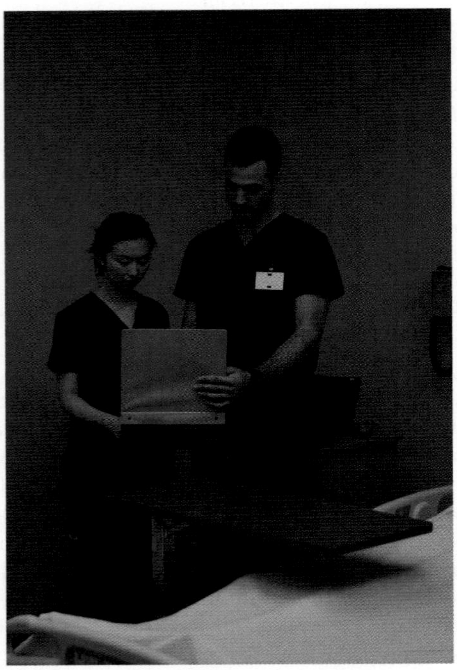

FIGURE 6-4 Nurses collaborating on research. (Courtesy Barbara J. Astle, RN, PhD.)

BOX 6-4 Guiding Ethical Principles for Research in Canada

1. *Respect for human dignity:* All research must be conducted in a manner that is sensitive to the inherent worth of human beings.
2. *Respect for persons*: Includes the obligation to respect autonomy of human research subjects and at the same time to protect those with developing, impaired, or diminished autonomy.
3. *Concern for welfare*: Researchers and ethics review boards should aim to protect the welfare of participants and, when possible, promote their welfare.
4. *Respect for privacy and confidentiality:* Standards of privacy and confidentiality protect the access, control, and dissemination of personal information and thus help protect mental or psychological integrity. These standards are consonant with values underlying privacy, confidentiality, and anonymity.
5. *Justice*: This principle reflects the importance of treating people fairly and equitably. This treatment includes ensuring that research participants are not unduly burdened by research or denied access to the benefits of research.

Adapted from Canadian Institutes of Health Research, the Natural Sciences and Engineering Research Council of Canada, & the Social Sciences and Humanities Research Council of Canada. (2014). *Tri-Council policy statement: Ethical conduct for research involving humans* (2nd ed.). Retrieved from http://www.pre.ethics.gc.ca/pdf/eng/tcps2/TCPS_2_FINAL_Web.pdf.

normal educational requirements and are not for research purposes, they are exempt from REB review.

To refine existing knowledge and develop new knowledge, investigators in clinical research sometimes use new procedures whose outcome is doubtful or unknown. This research may seem to conflict with the purpose of nursing practice, which is to meet specific patients' needs. In such cases, the investigator must structure the research to avoid or minimize harm to the subjects. Although not all undesirable effects can be anticipated, investigators are obligated to inform everyone involved about the known potential risks. Other basic human rights must also be observed. These principles are set forth by the CNA (2017). Procedures for obtaining informed consent must be outlined in the study protocol. The consent form must describe in lay language the purpose of the study, the role of the subjects, types of data that are to be obtained, how the data are obtained, the duration of the study, subject selection, procedures, risks to the subject (including financial risks), potential benefits (including the possibility of no benefit), alternatives to participation, and contact information concerning the principal investigator and local REB. The consent process gives subjects complete information regarding the study's risks, benefits, and costs so that they can make an informed decision.

The REB also determines whether the investigator has the necessary knowledge and skills to undertake the research, including familiarity with the clinical area in which the data will be collected and sufficient research training and experience. For example, a nurse planning a study of psychiatric patients should be familiar with psychiatric nursing principles and theory, as well as research procedures for data collection and analysis.

Rights of Other Research Participants

Student nurses and practising nurses may be asked to participate in research as data collectors or may be involved in the care of patients participating in a study. All participants, including health care providers, have the right to be fully informed about the study, its procedures (including the consent process and risk factors), and physical or emotional injuries that patients could experience as a result of participation. Often, the physical risks are more obvious than the emotional risks. For example, patients may be asked to give highly personal, intrusive information; some may find this experience stressful. The researcher should prepare all participants, including nurses delivering care, for this possibility and assist them in coping with the effects. Participants also have the right to see review forms from the REB that certify approval of the study. Participants can refuse to perform research procedures if they are concerned about ethical aspects.

APPLYING RESEARCH FINDINGS IN NURSING PRACTICE

Research evidence as a basis for scholarly, professional decision making in clinical practice is essential for providing competent, efficient, and state-of-the art nursing care (Melnyk & Fineout-Overholt, 2015). As a nurse, you can make links between research findings and nursing care by identifying appropriate clinical problems, reading peer-reviewed literature from numerous sources, and incorporating evidence-informed practice activities into the nursing practice of your nursing unit or agency.

In a policy statement, the CNA (2010) stated that evidence-informed decision making by registered nurses is key to quality nursing practice. Nurses need not only skills to access and appraise existing research but also scientific knowledge and skills to change practice settings and to promote evidence-informed decisions about patient care.

Evidence-informed nursing practice deemphasizes ritual, isolated, and unsystematic clinical experiences; ungrounded opinion; and tradition as bases for nursing practice. It stresses the use of research findings and, as appropriate, quality improvement data, other evaluation data, and the consensus of recognized experts and affirmed experience to support a specific practice (Melnyk & Fineout-Overholt, 2015). Many aspects of health care are not justly served by the research in only one discipline. The expertise of several disciplines must be brought to bear on complex health issues. Just as nurses play a vital role on the health care team, so, too, are they crucial to multidisciplinary health research. Policymakers in the broader arena of health care must account for nursing practice, which is so essential to patient care. Nurses need a sound knowledge base to support practice, and research is essential for building that knowledge.

KEY CONCEPTS

- Evidence-informed decision making includes knowledge from research, clinical expertise and patient preferences, and values.
- Development of nursing knowledge is essential to the profession of nursing.
- Research literacy is an essential competency for evidence-informed practice.
- Conducting research studies is critical to the development of evidence.
- How a study is conducted (study design) is dependent on the research question being asked.
- When human subjects participate in research, the researcher must obtain informed consent of study subjects, must maintain the confidentiality of subjects, and must protect subjects from undue risk or injury.
- When summarizing data reported in a research study, the nurse should note when, how, where, and by whom the investigation was conducted and who and what were studied.
- A researchable clinical nursing problem is one that is not satisfactorily resolved by current nursing interventions, occurs frequently in a particular group, can be measured or observed, and has a possible solution within the realm of nursing practice.
- To determine whether research findings can be used in nursing practice, the nurse considers the scientific worth of the study by substantiating evidence from other studies, the similarity of the research setting to the nurse's own clinical practice setting, the status of current nursing theory, and factors affecting the feasibility of application.

CRITICAL THINKING EXERCISES

1. A nurse is concerned about learning how to properly insert an intravenous catheter. Explain the benefits to the patient if the nurse learns how to do this by drawing from information in the research literature rather than from current practice.
2. The research literature reflects many different methods for inserting intravenous catheters. If you wished to determine the best method for doing this, use PICOT to clarify the findings.
3. If you wanted to design a study to answer a specific research question about the best way to insert intravenous catheters, how would you do this?

REVIEW QUESTIONS

1. Evidence-informed decision making is important because it:
   1. Is based on current nursing practice
   2. Has been found to improve patient care
   3. Includes information from the Internet
   4. Includes information only from randomized control trials
2. Which research method is quantitative?
   1. Grounded theory
   2. Phenomenology
   3. Ethnography
   4. Quasi-experimental research
3. Procedures for obtaining informed consent do *not* include:
   1. Describing the purpose of the study
   2. Describing the role of the subjects
   3. Giving the names of other participants in the study
   4. Describing the risks that the subject may incur
4. In a quasi-experimental research design, subjects are assigned to:
   1. An empirical group
   2. An ethnographic group
   3. Either a control group or a treatment condition, but not randomly
   4. An experimental group
5. Evidence-informed decision making:
   1. Enables the transfer of clinical practice techniques into policy
   2. Requires that evidence be always research based
   3. Is synonymous with research-based practice
   4. Entails the use of knowledge based on research studies and takes into account a nurse's clinical experience and patient preferences

Answers: 1. 2; 2. 4; 3. 3; 4. 3; 5. 4

Rationales for the Review Questions appear at the end of the book.

RECOMMENDED WEBSITES

Canadian Health Services Research Foundation: http://www.chsrf.ca
This website contains information about funding for health services research.

Canadian Institutes of Health Research (CHIR): http://www.cihr-irsc.gc.ca/e/193.html
This website contains information on evidence-based informed decision making, evidence-informed practice, and using research in practice (knowledge translation). It also contains pages for all 13 CIHR institutes.

Canadian Nurses Association: http://www.cna-aiic.ca/
This website contains information about policies and position statements for nursing research in Canada, as well as information about research funding.

Canadian Nurses Foundation: http://www.cnf-fiic.ca/
This website provides information about available research funding and about scholarships for students.

REFERENCES

Canadian Association of Schools of Nursing. (2015). *National nursing education framework: Final report*. Ottawa: Author.

Canadian Institutes of Health Research. (2012). *Introduction to evidence-informed decision making*. Retrieved from http://www.cihr-irsc.gc.ca/e/45245.html.

Canadian Institutes of Health Research, the Natural Sciences and Engineering Research Council of Canada, & the Social Sciences and Humanities Research Council of Canada. (2010). *Tri-Council policy statement: Ethical conduct for research involving humans*. Retrieved from http://www.pre.ethics.gc.ca/pdf/eng/tcps2/TCPS_2_FINAL_Web.pdf.

Canadian Nurses Association. (2010). *Policy statement: Evidence-informed decision-making and nursing practice*. Ottawa: Author. Retrieved from https://www.cna-aiic.ca/~/media/cna/page-content/pdf-en/ps113_evidence_informed_2010_e.pdf?la=en.

Canadian Nurses Association. (2015). *Framework for the practice of registered nurses in Canada* (2nd ed.). Ottawa: Author. Retrieved from https://www.cna-aiic.ca/~/media/cna/page-content/pdf-en/framework-for-the-practice-of-registered-nurses-in-canada.pdf?la=en.

Canadian Nurses Association. (2017). *Code of ethics for registered nurses*. Ottawa: Author.

Duggleby, W., Williams, A., Cooper, D., et al. (2013). Evaluation of the Living with Hope Program for rural women caregivers of persons with advanced cancer. *BMC Palliative Care, 12*, 36. doi:10.1186/1472-684X-12-36.

Fitchett, G., Tartaglia, A., Dodd-McCure, D., et al. (2012). Educating chaplains for research literacy: Results of a national survey of clinical pastoral education residency programs. *Journal of Pastoral Care & Counseling, 66*(1), 1–12. doi:10.1177/154230501206600103.

Good, S. R. (1969). *Submission to the study of support of research in universities for the Science Secretariat of the Privy Council*. Ottawa: Canadian Nurses Association and Canadian Nurses Foundation.

Harder, M., Astle, B., Grypma, S., et al. (2016). Discerning success of Indigenous health students in community-based programs. *Quality Advancement in Nursing Education, 2*(2), Article 5, 1–19. doi:10.17483/2368-6669.1076.

Hines, S., Ramsbotham, J., & Coyer, F. (2015). The effectiveness of interventions for improving the research literacy of nurses: A systematic review. *Worldviews Evidence Based Nursing, 12*(5), 265–272. doi:10.1111/wvn.12106.

International Council of Nurses. (2015). *Nursing research: a tool for action*. Retrieved from http://www.icn.ch/networks/nursing-research-a-tool-for-action/.

Jakubec, S. L., & Astle, B. J. (2017). *Research literacy for health and community practice* (1st ed.). Toronto: Canadian Scholars/Women's Press.

Leske, J. S., McAndrew, N. S., & Brasel, K. J. (2013). Experiences of families when present during resuscitation in the emergency department after trauma. *Journal of Trauma Nursing, 20*(2), 77–85. doi:10.1097/JTN.0b013e31829600a8.

LoBiondo-Wood, G., Haber, J., Cameron, C., et al. (2017). *Nursing research in Canada: Methods, critical appraisal, and utilization* (4th ed.). Toronto: Elsevier.

Lowry, E. (2012). "It's just what we do": A qualitative study of emergency nurses working with well-established family presence protocol. *JEN: Journal of Emergency Nursing, 38*(4), 329–334. doi:10.1016/j.jen.2010.12.016.

Melnyk, B. M., & Fineout-Overholt, E. (2015). *Evidence-based practice in nursing and health care. A guide to best practice* (3rd ed.). Philadelphia: Lippincott Williams & Wilkins.

Polit, D. F., & Beck, C. T. (2017). *Nursing research: Generating and assessing evidence for nursing practice* (10th ed.). Philadelphia: Wolters Kluwer.

Thorne, S. E. (2016). *Interpretive description: Qualitative research for applied practice*. New York: Routledge.

Williamson, G. R. (2007). *Making sense of research: An introduction for health and social care practitioners* (3rd ed.). Hoboken, NJ: Blackwell.

Wood, M., & Ross-Kerr, J. (2011). *Basic steps in planning nursing research, from question to proposal* (7th ed.). Sudbury, MA: Jones and Bartlett.

7

Nursing Values and Ethics

Written by Shelley Raffin Bouchal, RN, PhD, Barbara J. Astle, RN, PhD

OBJECTIVES

Mastery of content in this chapter will enable you to:

- Define the key terms listed.
- Discuss the role of values in the study of ethics.
- Examine and clarify personal values.
- Discuss how values influence patient care.
- Explain the relationship between ethics and professional nursing practice.
- Describe some basic ethical philosophies relevant to health care.
- Apply a method of ethical analysis to a clinical situation.
- Identify contemporary ethical issues in nursing practice.

KEY TERMS

Accountability, p. 89
Advance care planning (ACP), p. 96
Advocacy, p. 89
Answerability, p. 89
Applied ethics, p. 91
Autonomy, p. 91
Beneficence, p. 91
Bioethics, p. 91
Biomedical ethics, p. 91
Care theory, p. 92
Code of ethics, p. 87
Consequentialism, p. 91
Constrained moral agency, p. 90
Cultural values, p. 88
Deontology, p. 91
Descriptive moral theory, p. 90
Embodiment, p. 92
Engagement, p. 92
Environment, p. 92
Ethical dilemma, p. 92
Ethics, p. 87
Informed consent, p. 90
Justice, p. 92
Medical assistance in dying (MAID), p. 96
Medical futility, p. 95
Metaethics, p. 90
Moral distress, p. 97
Moral integrity, p. 97
Moral residue, p. 97
Mutuality, p. 92
Nonmaleficence, p. 91
Normative ethics, p. 90
Relational ethics, p. 92
Responsibility, p. 89
Social justice, p. 92
Teleology, p. 91
Utilitarianism, p. 91
Value, p. 87
Values clarification, p. 88

MEDIA RESOURCES

http://evolve.elsevier.com/Canada/Potter/fundamentals/

- Audio Chapter Summaries
- Examination Review Questions
- Concept Map Creator
- Case Study with Questions
- Audio Glossary
- Content Updates
- Video Clips

Values and ethics are inherent in all nursing acts. A **value** is a strong personal belief and an ideal that a person or group (such as nurses) believes to have merit. **Ethics** is the study of the philosophical ideals of right and wrong behaviour based on what one thinks one ought (or ought not) to do. The term also commonly refers to the values and standards that individuals and professions strive to uphold (e.g., health care ethics, nursing ethics). In other words, ethics are a reflection of what matters most to people or professions. Nurses and other health care providers agree to national codes of ethics that offer guidelines for responding to difficult situations that occur in practice and demonstrate to the public an overview of professional practice standards. For example, the Canadian Nurses Association (CNA, 2017a) publishes a **code of ethics** that outlines nurses' professional values and ethical commitments to their patients and the communities they serve. Revisions to the code of ethics normally occur every 5 to 7 years.

Because of their prominent and intimate role in the provision of health care, nurses continually make decisions about the correct course of action in different circumstances. In many situations, no answer or course of action is best. To manage such difficult situations, nurses need a keen awareness of their values and those of their patients, a good understanding of ethics, and a sound approach to ethical decision making. They also must be guided by a broader understanding of ethics through the application of philosophies, theories, and sets of principles. In addition, students should refer to the Canadian Association of Schools of Nursing (CASN) *National Nursing Education Framework* (2015) nursing ethics competencies, offered in domains such as *knowledge* 1.7, *nursing practice,* 3.1, and *professionalism,*

5.1, to create and maintain a growth and development competency portfolio.

VALUES

Values are at the heart of ethics. Values influence behaviour on the basis of the conviction that a certain action is correct in a certain situation. An individual's values reflect cultural and social influences, relationships, and personal needs. Values vary among people, and they develop and change over time. In the context of beliefs about morality, values generate rights and duties.

In nursing, value statements express broad ideals of nursing care and establish reasonable directions for practice. The CNA (2017a, pp. 8–17) *Code of Ethics for Registered Nurses* is organized around seven values that are central to ethical nursing practice. These values include providing safe, compassionate, competent, and ethical care; promoting health and well-being; promoting and respecting informed decision making; preserving dignity; maintaining privacy and confidentiality; promoting justice; and being accountable. Each provincial nursing association also has shared values, such as those held in position statements and practice standards. These standards reflect the values of the profession and clarify what is expected of you as a practising nurse.

Because of the intimacy of the nurse–patient relationship, you must be aware of your personal values, as well as the values of patients, physicians, employers, or other groups. To understand the values of others, it is important to understand your own values: what they are, where they came from, and how they relate to others' values.

Values Formation

People acquire values in many ways, beginning in early childhood. Throughout childhood and adolescence, people learn to distinguish right from wrong and to form values on which to base their actions. This is known as *moral development* (see Chapter 22). Family experiences strongly influence value formation.

Values are also learned outside the family. A person's culture, ethnic background, and religious community strongly influence that person's values, as do schools, peer groups, social media, and work environments. **Cultural values** are those adopted as a result of a social setting (see Chapter 9). A basic task of the young adult is to identify personal values within the context of the community. Over time, the person acquires values by choosing some values that are strongly upheld in the community and by discarding or transforming others. A person's experience as well as lack of experience also influences his or her values.

Values Clarification

Within the context of nursing, several layers of values inform the ethical questions and actions that you as a nurse will consider in your practice. Clarifying your values helps you articulate what matters most and what priorities are guiding your life and decision making. Values influence how you interpret confusing or conflicting information. Values change as you mature and experience new situations. As you become more aware and reflective about who you are, you may consider embracing or modifying your value set. As a result, you may modify your attitudes and behaviour. The willingness to change reflects a healthy attitude and an ability to adapt to new experiences.

To adopt new values, you must be aware of your existing values and how they affect behaviour. **Values clarification** is the process of appraising personal values (Box 7-1). It is not a set of rules, nor does it suggest that certain values should be accepted by all people; rather, it is a process of personal reflection. When you clarify your values, you make careful choices. The result of values clarification is greater self-awareness and personal insight.

BOX 7-1 Values Clarification Questions

Describe a situation in your personal or professional experience in which you felt uncomfortable, in which you believed that your beliefs and values were being challenged, or in which you believed your values were different from others'.

- As you record the situation, mention how you felt physically and emotionally at the time you experienced the situation.
- Write down your feelings as you remember the situation. Are your current reactions any different from those when you were actually in the situation?
- What personal values do you identify in the situation? Try to remember where and from whom you learned these values. Do you completely agree with the values, do you question some aspect of the values, or do you wonder about their validity?
- What values do you think were being expressed by others involved? Are they similar to or different from your own values?
- What do you think you reacted to in the situation?
- Can you remember having similar reactions in other situations? If you do, how were the situations similar or different?
- How do you feel about your response to the situation? If you could repeat the scenario, would you change something about it? Rewrite the scenario with the same changes. What might be the consequences of these same changes?
- How do you feel about the new scenario?
- What do you need to do to reinforce behaviours, ideals, beliefs, and qualities that you have identified as personal values in this situation? When and how can you do this?

From Burkhardt, M. A., & Nathaniel, A.K. (2014). *Ethics and issues in contemporary nursing* (4th ed.). Stamford CT: Cengage Learning. Inc. Reproduced by permission (www.cengage.com/permissions).

By understanding your personal values, you will become more sensitive to the values of others. In *values conflict,* personal values are at odds with those of a patient, a colleague, or an institution. Values clarification plays a major role in resolving these dilemmas. In addition, you can better advocate for a patient when you can identify your personal values and the values of the patient.

Relational communication can encourage the patient to examine personal thoughts and actions. When you make a clarifying response, it should be brief and nonjudgemental. For example, when talking with a patient who exercises only rarely, you might ask, "What is your understanding of the purpose of exercise?" A supportive clarifying response encourages the patient to think about personal values after the exchange is over and does not impose your own values onto the patient. In this way, you respect the patient's values and avoid inappropriately introducing personal values into the conversation.

ETHICS

Ethics is the study of good conduct, character, and motives. It is concerned with determining what is good or valuable for all people. Often the terms *ethics* and *morals,* or *morality,* are used interchangeably (Johnstone, 2015), inasmuch as both words are derived from an original meaning of "custom or habit." Johnstone suggested that it is not incorrect to use these terms interchangeably and that the choice is a matter of personal preference rather than of philosophical debate. The classic textbook definition of *ethics* is a "generic term for various ways of understanding and examining the moral life" (Beauchamp & Childress, 2012, p. 1). Essentially, ethics requires one to be critically reflective, exploring one's values, behaviours, actions, judgements, and justifications (Beauchamp & Childress, 2012, p. xii). In this chapter, the terms *ethics* and *morals* are used interchangeably.

Nursing and Ethics

Codes of Ethics. The code is a statement of the ethical values of nurses and of nurses' commitments to persons with health care needs and persons receiving care (CNA, 2017a, p. 2). It is intended for nurses in all contexts and domains of nursing practice (clinical practice, education, administration, research and policy; CNA 2015a)) and at all levels of decision making (CNA, 2017a, p. 2). In Canada, nursing is a self-regulating profession. As part of being self-regulatory, nurses are bound to a code of ethics to serve and protect the public. The code developed by nurses for nurses serves the profession with practical orientation supported by theoretical diversity. (CNA, 2017a).

As stated in the CNA (2017a) *Code of Ethics*, "the code provides guidance for ethical relationships, responsibilities, behaviours and decision-making and it is to be used in conjunction with professional standards, best practice, research, laws, and regulations that guide practice" (CNA, 2017a, p. 2). The code offers nurses guidance when they are working through ethical challenges that emerge from practice as nurses care for persons and working with interprofessional colleagues in healthcare.

The CNA (2017) and the International Council of Nurses (2012) have established widely accepted codes for nurses that reflect the principles of responsibility, accountability, and advocacy (Boxes 7-2 and 7-3).

Responsibility. Responsibility refers to the characteristics of reliability and dependability. It implies an ability to distinguish between right and wrong. In professional nursing, responsibility includes a duty to perform actions adequately and thoughtfully. When administering a medication, for example, you as a nurse are responsible for assessing the patient's need for the drug, for administering it safely and correctly, and for evaluating the patient's response to it. By agreeing to act responsibly, you gain trust from patients, colleagues, and society.

Nurses in all domains of practice uphold responsibilities related to all the values in the code of ethics. Nurses are responsible in their interactions with individual patients, families, groups, populations, communities, and society, as well as with students, nursing colleagues, and other health care colleagues. These responsibilities serve as the foundation for articulating nursing values to employers, other health care providers, and the public (CNA, 2017a).

Accountability. Accountability is grounded in the moral principles of fidelity (faithfulness) and respect for the dignity, worth, and self-determination of patients and others with whom nurses work. As accountable professionals, "nurses are honest and practise with integrity in all of their professional interactions" (CNA, 2017a, p. 16). Accountability means being able to accept responsibility or to account for one's actions and refers to being answerable to someone for something one has done. Answerability means being able to offer reasons and explanations to other people for aspects of nursing practice. When explanations are not readily available to patients, the nurse might seek advice of other health care providers or search for evidence that would support best practice. Nurses need to balance accountability to the patient, the profession, the employer, and society. For example, you may know that a patient who will be discharged soon is confused about how to self-administer insulin. The action that you take in response to this situation is guided by your sense of accountability. The patient, the institution, and society rely on your judgement and trust you to take action in response to this situation. You may request more hospitalization to provide further teaching, or you may arrange home care to continue teaching at home. The goal is the prevention of injury to the patient. Your sense of accountability guides actions that achieve this goal.

According to the CNA (2017a), nurses who are enacting professional accountability are (1) keeping up with professional standards, laws, and regulations; (2) ensuring that they have the competence to provide these practices; (3) maintaining their fitness to practise, ensuring that they have the necessary physical, mental, and emotional capacity to practise safely and competently; (4) sharing their knowledge with other nurses, nursing students, and other health-care providers through mentorship and giving feedback; and (5) advocating for comprehensive and equitable mental health care services.

Professional accountability is also the mandate of professional associations. Professional associations both check unethical practice in a profession and support conscientious professionals who may be under pressure to act unethically or to overlook unethical activity by colleagues. Professional nursing associations have the authority to register and discipline nurses. They also set and maintain professional standards of practice and communicate them to the public. These standards, developed by nursing clinical experts, provide a basic structure against which nursing care is objectively measured.

Advocacy. The ethical responsibility of advocacy means acting on behalf of another person, speaking for persons who cannot speak

BOX 7-2 Canadian Nurses Association Code of Ethics (2017)

Part I: Nursing Values and Ethical Responsibilities

There are seven primary values and responsibility statements related to each value:

A. Providing safe, compassionate, competent, and ethical care
B. Promoting health and well-being
C. Promoting and respecting informed decision making
D. Honouring dignity
E. Maintaining privacy and confidentiality
F. Promoting justice
G. Being accountable

Part II: Ethical Endeavours Related to Broad Societal Issues

Part two of the code describes activities that nurses enact to address social inequities. Ethical nursing practice involves striving towards addressing broader elements of social justice that relate to health and well-being.

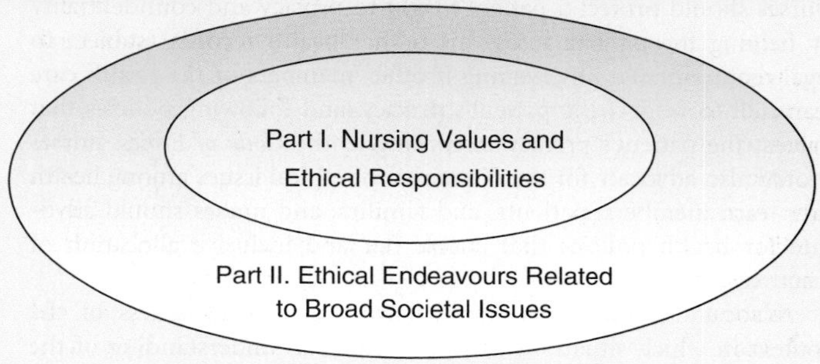

Canadian Nurses Association. (2017). *Code of ethics for registered nurses*. Ottawa: Author.

BOX 7-3 International Council of Nurses: The Code of Ethics for Nurses

Nurses have four fundamental responsibilities: to promote health, to prevent illness, to restore health, and to alleviate suffering. The need for nursing care is universal. Inherent in nursing care is respect for human rights, including cultural rights, the right to life and choice, the right to dignity, and the right to be treated with respect. Nursing care is respectful of and unrestricted by considerations of age, creed, culture, disability or illness, gender, sexual orientation, nationality, politics, race, economic status, or social status. Nurses render health services to the individual, the family, and the community, and they coordinate their services with those of related groups.

Nurses and People

The nurse's primary professional responsibility is to people who require nursing care. In providing care, the nurse promotes an environment in which the human rights, values, customs, and spiritual beliefs of the individual, family, and community are respected. The nurse ensures that the individual receives sufficient and timely information in a culturally appropriate manner on which to base consent for care and related treatment. The nurse holds in confidence personal information and uses judgement in sharing this information. The nurse shares with society the responsibility for initiating and supporting action to meet the health and social needs of the public, in particular those of vulnerable populations. The nurse advocates for equity and social justice in resource allocation, access to health care, and other social and economic services. The nurse demonstrates professional values such as respectfulness, responsiveness, compassion, trustworthiness, and integrity.

Nurses and Practice

The nurse carries personal responsibility and accountability for nursing practice and maintaining competence by continual learning. The nurse maintains a standard of personal health such that the ability to provide care is not compromised. The nurse uses judgement regarding individual competence when accepting and delegating responsibility. The nurse at all times maintains standards of personal conduct which reflect well on the profession and enhance its image and public confidence. The nurse, in providing care, ensures that the use of technology and scientific advances are compatible with the safety, dignity, and rights of people.

Nurses and the Profession

The nurse assumes the major role in determining and implementing acceptable standards of clinical nursing practice, management, research, and education. The nurse is active in developing a core of research-based professional knowledge that supports evidence-based practice. The nurse is active in developing and sustaining a core of professional values. The nurse, acting through the professional organization, participates in creating a positive practice environment and maintaining safe, equitable social and economic working conditions in nursing. The nurse practises to sustain and protect the natural environment and is aware of its consequences on health. The nurse contributes to an ethical organizational environment and challenges unethical practice settings.

Nurses and Co-Workers

The nurse sustains a collaborative and respectful relationship with co-workers in nursing and other fields. The nurse takes appropriate action to safeguard individuals, families, and communities when their health is endangered by a co-worker or any other person.

Adapted from International Council of Nurses. (2012). *ICN code of ethics for nurses.* Geneva, Switzerland: Author. Reprinted by permission of International Council of Nurses.

for themselves, or intervening to ensure that views are heard. Advocacy recognizes the need for improvement of systems and societal structures to create equity and better health for all (CNA, 2017a). Individually and collectively nurses advocate towards eliminating social inequities. This includes protecting the patient's right to choice by providing information, obtaining **informed consent** for all nursing care, and respecting patients' decisions. Nurses should protect patients' right to dignity by advocating for appropriate use of interventions in order to minimize suffering, intervening if other people fail to respect the dignity of the patient, and working to promote health and social conditions that allow patients to live and die with dignity. Nurses should protect a patient's right to privacy and confidentiality by helping the patient access his or her health records (subject to legal requirements), intervening if other members of the health care team fail to respect the patient's privacy, and following policies that protect the patient's privacy. According to the *Code of Ethics,* nurses should also advocate for the discussion of ethical issues among health care team members, patients, and families, and nurses should advocate for health policies that enable fair and inclusive allocation of resources.

Advocacy requires that nurses have a strong awareness of the context in which situations arise, as well as an understanding of the influence of power and politics on how they make decisions. If as a nurse you experience **constrained moral agency**—that is, if you feel powerless to act for what you think is right, or if you believe your actions will not effect change—then you will have difficulty being an effective advocate.

Ethical Theory

Ethics concern the examination of the moral basis for judgements, actions, duties, and obligations. For centuries, moral philosophers have tried to answer perplexing questions that help us understand the world. They structure this understanding in the form of philosophical theories. Different branches of philosophy answer different questions that people are grappling with. The field of ethics, also called moral philosophy, addresses questions like "What is the meaning of right and good, or ought and should?" **Descriptive moral theory** explains what people do or think about moral issues. For example, a descriptive theory might emerge from studies of how nurses make moral decisions. Such theory describes the rules, principles, and values that people apply when making moral decisions or judgements in different situations. Taking this one step further, philosophers ask, "Do we believe this is the right way to make moral decisions, just because many people do it this way?" Answering that question requires an understanding of what the "right" way would be. This understanding is called **metaethics**. A person studying metaethics might ask if "good" is socially related, an expression of emotion, or the will of a higher power, such as God. Is "good" out there to be discovered, or is it really socially constructed? Is there a true "right," and on what moral basis can moral judgements be assessed as being true or false?

Another branch of moral philosophy is **normative ethics**. A normative ethical theory is prescriptive, in that it tells us how we ought to think about moral questions. Normative ethical theory presents us with rules, values, and principles that allow us to judge the quality and the way we make and evaluate decisions, based on our obligations to others. Normative theories question or reveal our obligations as nurses. These are clearly stated in the CNA *Code of Ethics for Registered Nurses.*

In **applied ethics** (or practical ethics) we look at how decisions should be made in particular situations, asking questions about what moral belief and values should apply in specific contexts. Theories that address issues of right or ought in applied ethics move across disciplines. Applied ethics specific to nursing help us to examine our practice and how our behaviours are shaped by our practice as nurses. A nurse might reflect on how medical technology changes the way he or she communicates with family members regarding nutrition at the end of life. The following section introduces a variety of contemporary ethical theories. It is neither exclusive nor comprehensive.

Deontology. A traditional ethical theory, **deontology** is the system of ethics that is perhaps most familiar to practitioners in health care. Its foundations are often associated with the work of the eighteenth-century philosopher Immanuel Kant (1724–1804). In deontology, actions are defined as right or wrong on the basis of their right-making characteristics such as fidelity to promises, truthfulness, and justice (Beauchamp & Childress, 2012). The essence of right or wrong is located within deontological principles. Deontologists specifically do not look to consequences of actions to determine rightness or wrongness. Instead, they critically examine a situation for the existence of essential rightness or wrongness. Ethical principles such as justice, allowing free choice (autonomy), and doing the greatest good (beneficence) serve to define right or wrong. If an act is just, respects autonomy, and provides good, then the act is ethical. The process depends on a mutual understanding and acceptance of these principles.

Difficulty arises when one must choose among conflicting principles, which is often the case in ethical dilemmas concerning health care. For example, applying the principle of respect for autonomy can be confusing when dealing with the health care of children. The health care team may recommend a treatment, but a parent may disagree with or refuse the recommendation. In discussion of the dilemma, as the nurse you may refer to a guiding principle such as respect for autonomy. However, questions remain: Whose autonomy should receive the respect? That of the parents? Who should advocate for the child's best interest? Society often struggles to understand who should be ultimately responsible for the well-being of children. A commitment to respect autonomy does not guarantee that controversy can be avoided.

Utilitarianism. According to a utilitarian system of ethics, the value of something is determined by its usefulness. This philosophy, **utilitarianism**, may also be known as **consequentialism** because its main emphasis is on the outcome or consequence of action. A third term associated with this philosophy is **teleology** (from the Greek word *telos,* meaning "end"), which is the study of ends or final causes. Its philosophical foundations were first proposed by John Stuart Mill (1806–1873), a British philosopher and social commentator. The greatest good for the greatest number of people is the guiding principle for determining the correct action in this system. As with deontology, this theory relies on the application of a certain principle, namely measures of "good" and "greatest" (Beauchamp & Childress, 2012). The difference between utilitarianism and deontology is in the focus on consequences or outcomes. Utilitarianism concerns the effect that an act will have; deontology concerns the presence of principle, regardless of outcome.

Individuals or groups may have conflicting definitions of "greatest good." For example, research suggests that education regarding safer sex practices may reduce the spread of the human immunodeficiency virus. Some scholars argue, however, that education about sex should be provided by the family and that sex education in public schools diminishes the role and the value of the family. For them, the greater good is the preservation of family values and the protection of individual choices regarding sex education of children. For other scholars, however, the "greater good" is defined as educating the greatest number of people in the most effective way possible. The concepts of utilitarianism provide guidance, but they do not invariably provide for universal agreement.

Bioethics. In the 1970s, a group of ethics scholars concluded that then-current ethical theories were not sufficient for the health care field because they did not provide specific guidance for important moral questions that arose in the context of medicine. **Biomedical ethics** came to denote ethical reasoning for physicians, whereas **bioethics** became the general term for principled reasoning across health care professions. Bioethical theory is obligation-based, outcome-oriented, and based on reason (Oberle & Raffin Bouchal, 2009). The central idea of bioethics is that moral decision making in health care should be guided by four principles: autonomy, beneficence, nonmaleficence, and justice. According to this theory, health care providers should examine each situation, determine which of the principles has priority, and use that principle to guide action.

Autonomy. **Autonomy** refers to one's ability to make choices for oneself that should be based on full understanding, free of controlling influences (Beauchamp & Childress, 2012). Respect for another person's autonomy is fundamental to the practice of health care. It is the reason why patients should be included in all aspects of decision making regarding their care. The agreement to respect autonomy involves the recognition that patients are free to make choices and have the capacity to do so. Health care providers assess patient capacity and help to facilitate decision making. For example, the purpose of the preoperative consent that patients must read and sign before surgery is to ensure in writing that the health care team respects the patient's choice by obtaining permission to proceed. The consent process implies that a patient may refuse treatment, and in most cases, the health care team must agree to follow the patient's wishes. Health care providers agree to abide by a standard of respect for the patient's autonomy, which comes directly from Kant's ethics and his idea of respect for persons.

Beneficence. **Beneficence** means doing or promoting good for others. It speaks directly to the duty or obligation, as in deontological theories. Commitment to beneficence helps guide difficult decisions concerning whether the benefits of a treatment may be challenged by risks to the patient's well-being or dignity. For example, vaccination may cause temporary discomfort, but the benefits of protection from disease, both for the patient and for society, outweigh the patient's discomfort. The agreement to act with beneficence also requires that the best interests of the patient remain more important than self-interest. For example, as the nurse you do not simply follow medical orders; you act thoughtfully to understand patient needs and then work actively to meet those needs.

Nonmaleficence. *Maleficence* refers to harm or hurt; thus **nonmaleficence** is the avoidance of harm or hurt. The health care provider tries to balance the risks and benefits of a plan of care while striving to cause the least harm possible. This principle is often helpful in guiding discussions about new or controversial technologies. For example, a new bone marrow transplantation procedure may provide a chance for cure. The procedure, however, may entail long periods of pain and suffering. These discomforts should be considered in view of the suffering that the disease itself might cause and in view of the suffering that other treatments might cause. The commitment to provide least harmful interventions illustrates the term *nonmaleficence.* The standard of nonmaleficence promotes a continuing effort to consider the potential for harm even when it may be necessary to promote health.

Justice. Justice refers to fairness. The term is often used during discussions about resources: when competition for a scarce resource exists, justice mandates that decisions be fair and, to the greatest extent possible, unbiased. In decisions about which patient receives an available lung for transplantation, for example, it is understood that the lung will be allocated as fairly as possible. Understandings of fairness depend on community values. In Canadian society, community standards dictate that the decision should not depend on who has the higher intellect or larger salary; instead, the decision must be based on need alone. Of course, the definition of need can be debated, and when two people have equal need, nothing in the theory helps health care providers decide between them. These are ethical questions that require further exploration of values, principles, and priorities to guide decisions in resource allocation.

The literature also mentions other prevalent forms of justice that you need to understand, such as social justice. Social justice is often related to a concern for the equitable distribution of benefits and burdens in society (Boutain, 2005), with the view that broad social change is necessary to address the determinants of health and reduce inequalities of health (World Health Organization Commission on Social Determinants of Health, 2008) (refer to Chapters 1 and 9 for further information about social justice). Other scholars of bioethics, including Canadians Michael Yeo, Anne Moorhouse, Pamela Kahn, and Patricia Rodney (2010), who have written about nursing ethics, have incorporated a number of other principles such as fidelity (faithfulness), veracity (truth-telling), and confidentiality.

Feminist Ethics. Feminist ethicists consider their work a critique of conventional ethics, as well as a critique of social values. Their work focuses on the continuing inequalities between people (Lindemann, 2006). A feminist ethics approach embodies features of being attentive to issues of difference, power dynamics, and context and relatedness (Yeo et al., 2010). Feminist ethics is relevant for nurses in the deliberation of ethical issues as an expressive and collaborative process. Nurses hear the stories of patients and consider their social context in making ethical decisions.

Changes in attitudes toward women reflect new perspectives in women's relationships with family, work, science, and society (Sherwin, 1992). For example, until the early 1980s, moral development was thought to reach the highest stages more often in men than in women. According to this thinking, moral development occurred in predictable stages. The most complex stage involved a sense of justice, and young girls did not reach this stage as often as did young boys (Kohlberg, 1981). Findings of research in the early 1980s disputed this conclusion. Gilligan (1982) proposed that Kohlberg's tools to measure moral development were gender biased. Gilligan went on to build a revised theory of moral development from her findings. She attempted to accommodate gender differences. Specifically, she concluded that young girls tend to pay attention to community and to individual circumstances and that young boys tend to process dilemmas through ideals or principles determined abstractly.

Feminism proposes that gender makes a difference in the construction of roles and identities in society and, accordingly, in how individuals and groups are treated. Feminist ethicists hold the belief that society remains "patriarchal" in many ways (Yeo et al., 2010). Hilde Lindemann Nelson (2000), a prominent feminist scholar in the United States, provided a history of the development of feminist ethics and bioethics in which she notes that feminist attention to gender and gender-related issues gave rise to an important perspective called care theory. This theory is concerned with a type of virtue ethic that gives moral weight to caring for others. This was an important development in thinking about ethics because it moved attention away from the traditional masculine virtues toward those that had traditionally been considered more feminine.

Relational Ethics. It is becoming increasingly apparent that relationships are the basis of ethics in nursing. According to relational ethics theory, ethical understandings are formed in, and emerge from, a person's relationships with others, whether those others are patients, families, communities, or colleagues (Bergum, 2013; Bergum & Dossetor, 2005; Hartrick, Doane, & Varcoe, 2007; Wright & Brajtman, 2011). According to Bergum (2013), relational ethics is a way of "being," displayed in everyday interactions rather than a mode of decision making. It is how you as a nurse insert a needle, enter into conversation, show respect, or behave with other people.

Relational ethics focuses on the role of relational context or the experience of the relationships in shaping moral choices (Bergum, 2013; Wright & Brajtman, 2011). In research on relational ethics, Bergum (2013) identified four themes: environment, embodiment, mutual respect, and engagement. Environment concerns critical elements or characteristics of the health care system within which you work and how the nature of your relationships is affected by this system. Bergum encouraged nurses to consider the entire health care arena as a network or matrix in which each part is connected, either directly or indirectly, to the other. An awareness of this connectedness encourages you to look beyond the immediate situation and try to envision a broader context. It also makes you conscious of how power and politics affect your entire system of care (Oberle & Raffin Bouchal, 2009).

In relational ethics, embodiment means recognizing that the mind–body split is artificial and that healing for both patient and family cannot occur unless "scientific knowledge and human compassion are given equal weight [and it is recognized that] emotion and feeling are as important to human life as physical signs and symptoms" (Bergum, 2013, p. 132). Such recognition requires you to become truly aware of what other people may be experiencing. You must make this awareness a part of your own experience. The nurse–patient relationship requires that you value patients and treat them with respect. Within the nurse–patient relationship, you use nursing knowledge to enhance the patient's health and well-being. You always consider the unique needs of the patient as an individual. Mutual respect is created, with attention to both your and the patient's needs, wishes, expertise, and experience (Bergum & Dossetor, 2005). Mutuality, loosely defined as a relationship that benefits both you and the patient and harms neither, requires your and the patient's willingness to participate in a relationship that embraces the values and ideas of one another as a means of developing new understandings, rather than judging the other person's values and ideas.

Engagement means connecting with another person in an open, trusting, and responsive manner. Bergum (2013) suggested that it is through this connection that you develop a meaningful understanding of the other person's experience. Engagement takes skill and practice, inasmuch as it requires a commitment to keeping the relationship caring and respectful. Bergum asserted that engagement "does not ask for *selflessness* on the practitioner as both are recognized as *whole beings*" (p. 137). Engagement requires that you connect with the patient but, at the same time, set boundaries in such a way that the relationship remains on a professional level. Knowing how much to engage with another person is one of the greatest challenges in nursing.

ETHICAL ANALYSIS AND NURSING

An ethical dilemma is a conflict between two sets of human values, both of which are judged to be "good" but neither of which can be fully served. Ethical dilemmas can cause distress and confusion for patients and caregivers. As a nurse, you may well be faced with ethical questions that have not been examined previously and for which no practical wisdom exists. You must be able to examine issues and apply experience and wisdom in each situation. The CNA (2017a) *Code of Ethics* identifies the responsibility of nurses to maintain their "fitness to practise" as having the "necessary physical, mental or emotional capacity to practise safely and competently" (p. 17). Such fitness requires nurses to be knowledgeable and skillful as they engage in problem solving. Ethical issues must be analyzed carefully and deliberately. Ethical analysis involves descriptive, conceptual, and normative processes. Analysis of situations begins with acquiring knowledge to gain a sense of what is going on (descriptive analysis), as well as finding out about relevant policies, laws, relationships, and stakeholders. Conceptual analysis is clarifying the meaning of the situation, values, and assumptions of all individuals involved. Normative analysis focuses on what ought to be done, based on the people involved and the values of the people (Yeo et al., 2010).

Resolving an ethical dilemma requires deliberate, critical, and systematic thinking (Box 7-4). It also requires negotiation of differences (between beliefs, values, opinions, and so forth), incorporation of conflicting ideas, and an effort to respect differences of opinion. The process of negotiating ethical dilemmas may be in part the process of understanding ambiguities. Nurses need to be knowledgeable and adept in making logical, fair, and consistent decisions. Ethical decision-making models offer a variety of methods for reaching informed conclusions (Box 7-5).

Documentation of the ethical process can take a variety of forms. Whenever the process involves a family conference or results in a change in the plan of care, the process should be documented in the medical record. At some institutions, the ethics committee may use a formal consultation format whenever a request for discussion arises. If the ethical dilemma does not directly affect patient care, however, discussion may be documented by minutes from a meeting or in a memorandum to affected parties. In the following case study, the nursing concerns and the family conferences would be recorded in the medical record and in nursing flow sheets.

On your unit, a 35-year-old woman has been hospitalized in the final stages of brain cancer. She is a single mother with two young children. Although she has been treated by both conventional and experimental treatments, the tumour has continued to grow, and the medical team has agreed that further treatment would be futile. You have cared for this patient during past hospital admissions, and during an especially open discussion, she expressed wishes to explore "do not resuscitate" (DNR) orders. During the current admission, her primary physician is out of town. The attending physician does not know the patient personally, but he has spent time with her. He has reviewed the clinical data and agrees that the patient is entering the terminal stage of the disease. In his opinion, however, the patient is not ready to discuss end-of-life

BOX 7-4 How to Analyze an Ethical Dilemma

Step 1: Determine whether the issue is an ethical dilemma.
Step 2: Gather all the information relevant to the case.
Step 3: Examine and determine your own values on the issues.
Step 4: Verbalize the problem.
Step 5: Consider possible courses of action.
Step 6: Reflect on the outcome.
Step 7: Evaluate the action and the outcome.

BOX 7-5 Two Ethical Decision-Making Frameworks

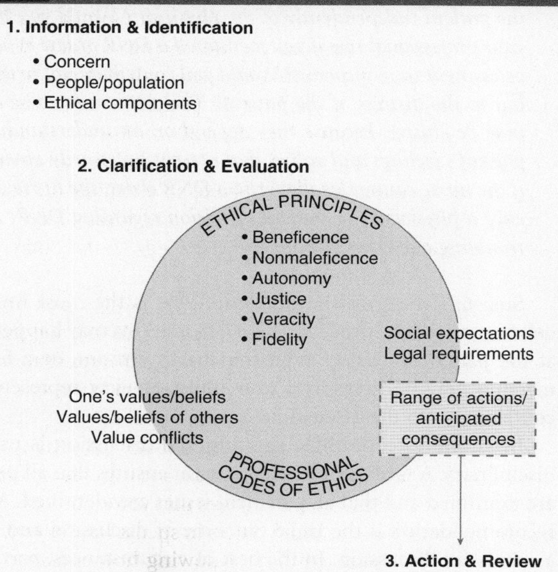

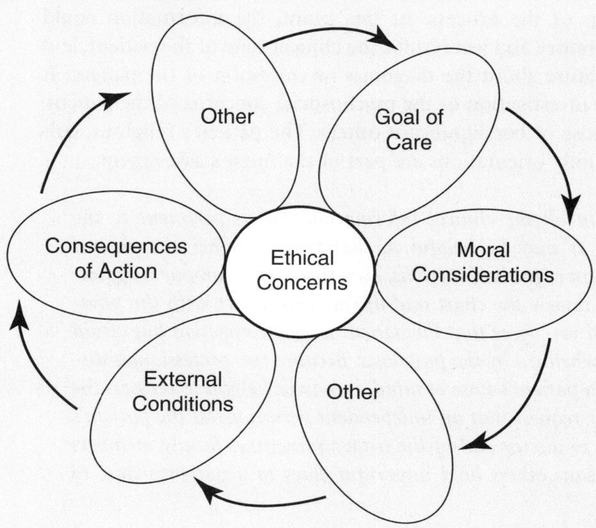

Diagram on left: From Storch, J. L. (2013). Model for ethical decision making for policy and practice. In J. Storch, P. Rodney, & R. Starzomski (Eds.), *Toward a moral horizon: Nursing ethics for leadership and practice* (p. 538). Toronto: Pearson Education. **Diagram on right:** From College and Association of Registered Nurses of Alberta. (2010). A model for questioning. In *Ethical decision-making for registered nurses in Alberta: Guidelines and recommendations* (p. 17). Edmonton: Author. Retrieved from http://www.nurses.ab.ca/content/dam/carna/pdfs/DocumentList/Guidelines/RN_EthicalDecisions_May2010.pdf#page=19. Reprinted by permission of College and Association of Registered Nurses of Alberta.

issues. He states that the patient has declined to discuss DNR orders with him. You ask the physician to convene a family conference about the issues. He refuses, stating that he believes the patient is not ready to participate.

Step 1: Is this an ethical dilemma? What may at first appear to be a question of ethics may be resolved by clarifying your knowledge about clinical facts. A review of policy and procedure, or of standards of care, may reveal legal obligations that determine a course of action, regardless of personal opinion. If the question remains perplexing, and the answer will be profoundly relevant to several areas of human concern, then an ethical dilemma may exist.

The single mother's situation meets the criteria for an ethical dilemma. Further review of scientific data will probably not contribute to a resolution of the dilemma, but it is important to review the data carefully to make this determination. The disagreement does not revolve around whether the patient is in a terminally ill state, so further clinical information will not change the basic question: Should the patient have an opportunity to discuss DNR orders at this time? The question is perplexing. Two professional team members disagree on an assessment of a patient's readiness to confront the difficult issues related to dying. The answer to the question "Is this patient ready to discuss end of life?" has important implications. If she is not ready, then raising the issue may cause anguish and fear in the patient and her family. If she is ready and the team avoids discussion, she may suffer unnecessarily in silence. If she is very close to death, then in the absence of a DNR order, cardiopulmonary resuscitation (CPR) will be performed in a futile situation. You know that CPR can cause pain. If applied in a situation in which the patient's life is unlikely to be extended or improved, CPR could prolong her suffering and reduce her dignity.

Step 2: Gather as much information as possible that is relevant to the case. Because resolution to dilemmas may arise from unlikely sources, it is important to incorporate as much knowledge as possible at every step of the process. At this point, the information could include laboratory and test results, the clinical state of the patient, and current literature about the diagnosis or condition of the patient. It may include investigation of the psychosocial concerns of the patient, as well as those of her significant others. The patient's religious, cultural, and family orientations are part of the nurse's assessment.

You obtain all the clinical information that is pertinent to the question. It may be helpful to determine whether the patient retains most cognitive functions, even though her tumour is aggressive. You review the chart and discuss this aspect with the physician, and you agree that the patient is fully competent but afraid and overwhelmed by the prognosis. Because two professionals disagree on a patient's state of mind, it may be helpful to reassess the patient or request that an independent person assess the patient's readiness to discuss end-of-life issues. Sometimes family members or significant others hold important clues to a patient's state of mind.

Step 3: Examine and determine your own values on the issues. This step is important for all participants in the discussion. At this stage, as the patient's nurse, you and the other participants practise values clarification, and you differentiate between your own values and the values of the patient and those of other health care team members. Essential parts of the goal are to form your own opinion and to respect others' opinions.

At this point, you stop to reflect on your own values. Your own religious practices may allow you to decide to forgo further treatment if you were in the patient's condition. You also may not yet have family members who rely on you, such as children or elderly parents. This patient's religious practices may be more strictly constructed than your own. Her religion discourages actions that diminish life in any way, and you realize that she may have come to see a DNR order as giving up, or as "acting like God." In addition, you understand that the attending physician has not had time to know this patient as her own physician has or as you have. You continue to believe that the patient would be capable of a discussion, despite her statements to the physician. In fact, you believe that she would benefit from a discussion, because perhaps the presence of an unfamiliar caretaker, combined with declining physical health, has silenced her, even though her fears and concerns persist.

Step 4: Verbalize the problem. Once all relevant information has been gathered, accurate definition of the problem may proceed. It is helpful to state the problem in a few sentences. By agreeing to a statement of the problem, the health care team, the patient, and the family can proceed with discussion in a focused way.

Here, the problem seems to be this: whether this patient should discuss DNR at this time. Determine the benefits and risks of a DNR order at this time. Other important questions relate to the patient's current state of mind: Is she afraid to speak? Is she feeling cut off from her normal network (a primary physician)? Are these feelings contributing to confusion about DNR decisions?

Step 5: Consider possible courses of action. What options are available within the context of the situation and the patient's values?

Once you have asked the basic question, other questions and possible courses of action arise. Should you initiate a discussion with the patient independently of the physician? Would you be outside your professional role if you facilitated a DNR order? What if your assessment were incorrect? Would you contribute not to the dignity but to the distress of the patient? The answers to these questions may be elusive, because they depend on an understanding of the patient's feelings and values that are not necessarily obvious. Even if the nurse cannot legally write a DNR order, the nurse can influence a physician's or patient's decision regarding DNR; therefore, troubling questions remain.

Step 6: Reflect on the outcome. This is the most important and delicate step of the process. These negotiations may happen informally at the patient's bedside or in the charting room, or a formal ethics meeting may be necessary. Your point of view represents a unique contribution to the discussion.

In an ethics committee meeting, the discussion is usually multidisciplinary. A facilitator or chairperson ensures that all points of view are examined and that all pertinent issues are identified. A decision or recommendation is the usual outcome of discussion and the result of a successful discussion. In the best of circumstances, participants discover a course of action that meets criteria for acceptance by all. On occasion, however, participants may leave the discussion disappointed or even opposed to the decision.

The discussion focuses on the disagreement between your assessment and the physician's regarding the patient's readiness to discuss end-of-life issues. The principles involved during the discussion include beneficence and nonmaleficence: Which plan would provide the most good for this patient—a DNR order or no order? A separate question addresses the patient's point of view: Would a discussion with the patient promote well-being or promote anguish? Furthermore, according to the principle of autonomy, a troublesome question remains: Does the patient want something different from the desire she is expressing?

With several members of the health care team present, the discussion proceeds. You present your point of view. You continue to sense that the patient is ready to discuss DNR orders but that she may be reluctant to trust the circumstances of this admission. You respect the attending physician and his analysis and continue to be concerned that the patient may have experienced a change of mind between the last admission and this one. In the end, the team proposes a formal meeting with the patient, in which you, the attending physician, and a supportive family member are present. You support this proposal because you sense that it will maximize the support of the patient's existing network. In addition, you recognize that in a trusting environment, the patient is more likely to express fears, insecurities, and wishes. Team members agree to keep the discussion open-ended and exploratory. You suggest that rather than asking whether the patient wants a DNR order, the team could wait for her to bring up the issue. In this way, the team could be assured of her consent and willingness to participate in the discussion.

Step 7: Evaluate the action and the outcome.

At the meeting, the patient in fact opens up. She expresses relief at the chance to explore her options and feelings. Pain management issues are clarified. She wants to discuss a DNR order but requests a visit from her priest before making a final decision.

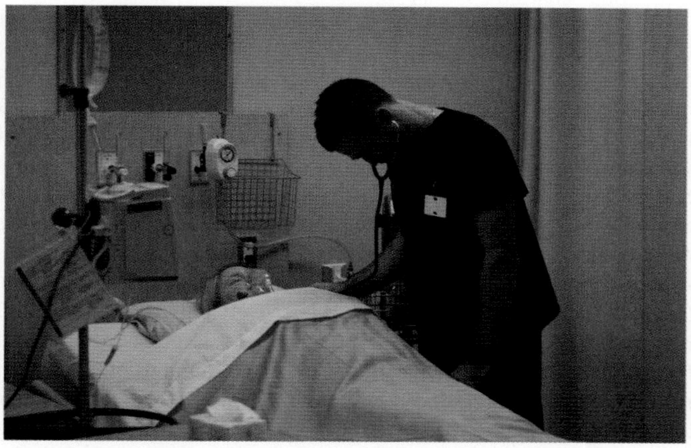

FIGURE 7-1 Nurses often struggle when patients are receiving care that they believe is prolonging their suffering and their life. (Courtesy Barbara J. Astle, RN, PhD.)

ETHICAL ISSUES IN NURSING PRACTICE

With increased professional responsibility and accountability, and with changes in the workplace and health care system, nurses are facing a myriad of ethical issues with greater frequency. They face ethical issues daily while caring for patients and families, while relating to other health care providers and institutions, and while dealing with global societal issues. The following section explores current issues in which ethical challenges arise. As a nurse, you have a unique understanding of ethical situations based on the context in which you practise. For example, a home care nurse may recognize moral dimensions of practice that are particular to that setting and have a way of thinking about ethical challenges that will help the patient and family know how best to act in a given situation. In other words, answers to moral problems must be negotiated in the context in which they arise; no two settings are alike.

Patient Care Issues

Futile Care. In the early 1980s, issues such as enhanced life-sustaining technologies, patients' rights movements, and growing concerns about using health care resources in a cost-effective and efficient manner led to academic discussions, debates, and practice policies on medical futility. Medical futility is defined as a medical treatment that is considered impossible or unlikely to achieve its therapeutic goal, or suggests that there is something problematic about the goal (Browne, 2000). Patients often worry, in the event of their becoming incapacitated and unable to express their wishes, that they will be "hooked up to machines" and receive treatment that they do not desire (Figure 7-1). At issue is whether clinicians are sufficiently objective to establish that a given intervention is futile, as determinations of futility are often laden with biases.

Although health care providers are best equipped to determine the physical benefits of treatment, only the patient or people who know the patient best can determine whether treatment is advancing the patient's overall well-being. Bennett Jacobs and Taylor (2005) identified this issue as "qualitative" futility or subjective determination, in which not just medical facts but also values lead the patient or the patient's surrogate decision makers to conclude that the treatment has no benefit according to those values (Ulrich, Taylor, Soeken, et al., 2010).

Achieving holistic outcomes of care must be based on an interplay of physical facts and subjective values. Taylor (1995) suggested the following four classifications of futility: (1) not futile: beneficial to both physical and overall well-being; (2) futile: nonbeneficial to either physical or overall well-being; (3) futile from the patient's perspective: medically indicated but not valued by the patient; and (4) futile from the clinicians' perspective and not medically indicated but valued by the patient (p. 301). It is evident that these classifications have objective and subjective dimensions, as well as quantitative and qualitative dimensions, and constitute a more complete way of viewing the complex notion of futility.

The issue of who has priority in health care decision making remains complex and often troublesome. The potential for futility conflicts is high in situations of critically and chronically ill patients. What, then, is the nurse's role? Taylor (1995) suggested that nurses play a leading role in working toward pursuing negotiated compromise between health care providers and patients equally, for the best possible outcome for the particular patient. She suggested that this may be accomplished "by identifying patients, families, and health care teams at risk of experiencing conflict about futile care, and then initiating dialogue that may prevent or resolve conflict" (p. 303). Rather than subscribing to categories of levels of futility to drive decision making, many health care agencies have now developed end-of-life guidelines that are tailored to patients' needs. These guidelines include a determination of levels of intervention or goals of care that range from fully acute to palliative/comfort care (Rocker & Dunbar, 2000). Levels of intervention are based on the premise that specific interventions may either be withheld or administered on the basis of individual patient needs and that supportive/palliative care ought to be integrated with all levels. Advance care planning is one way to address this problem.

Advance care planning (ACP) is a multidimensional process that involves health care providers in discussion with patients to ensure that they clearly understand their illness, its trajectory, and available treatment options. ACP includes the expression and comprehension of a patient's beliefs and values and the translation of these beliefs and values into medical decisions (Lum & Sudore, 2016; Lund, Richardson, & May, 2015). Families of patients are frequently included in these conversations (Lum & Sudore, 2016; Lund et al., 2015). During the ACP process, patients can also identify surrogate decision makers should they become unable to make their own health care decisions (Lum & Sudore, 2016; Lund et al., 2015). ACP, when utilized and implemented effectively, has the potential to improve patient and family experiences during end of life. The number of unwanted medical interventions is decreased, and health care providers are better able to deliver quality care that aligns with patients' wishes following ACP conversations (Lum & Sudore, 2016). ACP ensures that the patient's voice informs future care (Chrash, Mulich, & Patton, 2011). Yet, despite its benefits, ACP remains an underutilized tool in health care (Amjad, Towle & Fried, 2014).

Ideally, ACP should be facilitated by multiple health care providers (physicians, nurses, social workers, chaplains, and others). Nurses assume the role of educators and advocates for their patients. In these roles, they provide support and information regarding care decisions. Nurses encourage all individuals in their care (patients and families) "to reflect on, communicate and document their values (i.e., personal, cultural, religious and those that constitute a legacy for enduring and sustaining life), in addition to health and personal care wishes that include end-of-life care" (CNA, 2015b, p. 5). Nurses are involved in advocating for patients' rights, and nursing research has found that their presence is an important factor in helping patients to develop advance directives (living wills and identifying a surrogate decision maker) (Blondeau, Lavoie, Valois, et al., 2000; CNA, 2015a).

Medical Assistance in Dying (MAID). Canada's approach to choice regarding end-of-life care and decision making has undergone unprecedented change over the past few years. One of the most significant changes occurred on January 15, 2016, when the Supreme Court of Canada suspended the operation of its declaration in *Carter v. Canada,* permitting physician-assisted death (CNA, 2017b). The House of Commons and Senate responded by establishing a Special Joint Committee that produced a report entitled *Medical Assistance in Dying: A Patient-Centred Approach.* Several recommendations made by the committee included that the term **medical assistance in dying (MAID)** replace "physician-assisted death." On June 17, 2016, Bill C-14 received royal assent, making it possible to allow eligible persons to receive MAID in Canada under specific circumstances. This legislation revises the *Canadian Criminal Code* to include exemptions (legal protection in accordance with the law) for health care providers such as registered nurses who may help to provide MAID under the direction of a physician or nurse practitioner, and establishes safeguards for persons.

MAID is defined in the Act as (a) the administering by a medical practitioner or nurse practitioner of a substance to a person, at their request, that causes their death, or (b) the prescribing or providing by a medical practitioner or nurse practitioner of a substance to a person, at their request, so that they may self-administer the substance and in doing so cause their own death (Parliament of Canada, 2016). Each province, based on their shared responsibility for health care, may choose to develop additional legislation and/or policies to clarify the rules governing the everyday practice of MAID (CNA, 2017b). Health care providers who choose to participate in MAID must comply with those additions since, according to the MAID legislation, "medical assistance in dying must be provided with reasonable knowledge, care and skill and in accordance with any applicable provincial laws, rules or standards" (Parliament of Canada, 2016, c.3, s. 241.2 [1][7]).

Nursing regulatory bodies across the country have the legal mandate to protect the public by ensuring that nurses who practise are qualified and provide safe, competent, ethical care. They are responsible for setting standards and guidelines that apply to the scopes of practice (nurse practitioners, registered nurse, registered psychiatric nurse) established for nurses under provincial or territorial legislation (CNA, 2017b). Registered nurse and licensed practical nurse guidelines regarding MAID across the country are currently in different stages of development. The completed document from the College of Licensed Practical Nurses and Registered Nurses of Nova Scotia is one example. Common elements include (a) the role of nurses in end-of-life care and MAID; (b) what to do if a persons asks about medical assistance in dying (the nurse can explore reasons for the person's request, but this should be done in the context of a conversation about all other life options, including palliative care); (c) providing information on medical assistance in dying on the person's explicit request (nurses do not initiate a discussion on medical assistance in dying with persons because this could be interpreted as counselling a person to die or the person may feel pressured); (d) person eligibility (nurses are not permitted to determine the persons's eligibility as this is the role of the nurse practitioner or physician); (e) statutory safeguards (in section 241.2[3] in the *Criminal Code*); (f) administration of medication for assisted dying (nurses are not authorized to administer the medication); (g) privacy and confidentiality (respecting privacy of persons involved in MAID, including the person's wishes about communicating with family members); (h) documentation (nurses document according to agency policy); (i) witnessing a written request for MAID (nurses do not act as an independent witness; rather, the role of the witness is to confirm the identity of the person requesting medical assistance in dying, attest to the person's apparent understanding of the request being made, and, to the extent possible, affirm that the person is acting voluntarily, free of duress or coercion); and (j) conscientious objection (based on a nurse's moral beliefs and values, he or she may decline to participate in any aspect of person care connected with MAID; however, nurses must promptly inform their employer but not abandon persons until alternative care arrangements can be made to meet the person's needs) (College of Registered Nurses of Nova Scotia [CRNNS], 2016).

Nurses are intimately involved in end-of-life care processes, and in many cases "they play an important role in the development of these processes" (Gastmans, 2012, p. 603). Many studies have shown that registered nurses are the first caregivers to receive a request for MAID (Bilsen, Vander Stichele, Mortier, et al., 2004; CNA, 2017b; Inghelbrecht, Bilsen, Mortier, et al., 2009). The CNA (2017b) document *National Nursing Framework on Medical Assistance in Dying in Canada* will be a valuable resource for all nurses and students to gain a greater understanding of MAID as it unfolds in the Canadian context. In essence, nurses have a unique perspective and bring an important contribution to providing end-of-life care that includes medical assistance in dying (CNA, 2017b).

Issues of Safety and Ethics Related to the Work Environment

Social Networking and Safety. The online presence of social networks presents ethical challenges for nurses. On the one hand, social networks can be a supportive source of information about patient care or professional nursing activities. Social media can provide nurses with emotional support when encountering hardships at work with colleagues or patients. On the other hand, the risk to patient privacy is great. Even if a nurse posts an image of a patient without any obvious identifiers, the nature of shared media reposting can result in the image surfacing in a place where just the context of the image provides clues for friends or family to identify the patient.

Becoming friends with a patient in online chat rooms, on Facebook, or on other public sites interferes with a nurse's ability to maintain a therapeutic relationship. Friendship with a patient always comes with the risk of clouding your ability to remain objective in your clinical perceptions. The public nature of online relationships poses the additional risk that other patients may see and learn more than they should know about you and other patients. They may not trust you to remain impartial (i.e., available equally to each patient in your assignment).

Workplace policies will help to answer questions you have about when and where it is appropriate to engage in social media regarding workplace stories or issues. The CNA's (2012) *Ethics in Practice* paper on the challenges and opportunities of social media identifies the central concern as being patient confidentiality and privacy. This important document offers useful social media etiquette for nurses to maintain professional standards while using these technologies (CNA, 2012). The CNA cautions that the "use of social media is not considered in any way 'private' but is firmly within the public domain, with a potential audience of many thousands if not millions" (p. 2). Given the nonprivate nature of media platforms such as Facebook, the posting of information with well-intended goals, such as professional consulting purposes, could potentially lead to harm to both the nurse and the patient. A breach in private information can lead to serious legal and disciplinary actions.

Social media, when used sensibly, can also afford potential benefits to nurses. Networking with other nurses who have similar interests can lead to professional growth, learning opportunities, and knowledge transfer of key information to support continuing education. Social media can also be a way of sharing nursing knowledge as a way of offering the public a glimpse of the significance of the nursing role.

Working With a Health Care Team to Promote Safe Care. Nurses are responsible for providing safe, compassionate, competent, and ethical care (CNA, 2017a). In ensuring safety, care must be such that harm is minimized. Lack of control over important aspects of the environment can lead to ethically ambiguous situations (Austin, 2007). Complex life-and-death events, multiple role responsibilities, loyalties and expectations, reduced numbers of skilled health care providers, minimal clinical nursing leadership, interdisciplinary team conflict, and autocratic organizational decision making may all contribute to creating personal moral conflict for nurses (Austin, 2007; Canadian Health Services Research Foundation, 2006).

Causing harm to patients in the form of pain and suffering from continuing treatment is a source of **moral distress** for nurses that they often believe could be avoided. "Moral distress arises when nurses are unable to act according to their moral judgement" (Rodney, 2017, s-7). Sometimes nurses find it hard to care for a patient when other health care providers, usually physicians, make choices that nurses think are causing more harm than good. For example, the situation of a patient in intensive care who is comatose but seems to experience great pain when turned over can be very upsetting for nurses. They may experience moral distress if they feel that they are, in effect, torturing the patient each time they turn him or her over. Keeping patients safe from harm can be difficult, and sometimes it requires great ethical sensitivity to be aware of harms that are being caused. In these situations, nurses may lose their sense of **moral integrity** or "wholeness" when they are committed to certain values and beliefs that are not upheld because of situational constraints. If these situations continue and integrity is compromised, nurses may experience **moral residue**, when they seriously compromise themselves or allow themselves to be compromised (CNA, 2017a, p. 7). In such situations, relational ethics can help you know what the patient considers harm, and it is crucial to engage in discussions with your patients and colleagues.

In a multidisciplinary environment, all health care providers must take responsibility and work with colleagues at all levels of the system for the care that is provided (Boxes 7-6 and 7-7). Moral distress can be a very lonely experience, but meeting with co-workers to discuss the conflict, assess others' reactions to the situation, obtain additional

BOX 7-6 RESEARCH HIGHLIGHT

Ethics in Nursing Practice

Research Focus

Schick Makaroff, Storch, Pauly, et al. (2014) were interested in investigating how frontline nurses and formal nurse leaders envision ethical nursing leadership. The authors were curious about how two different (yet interrelated) populations of nurses, frontline nurses, and formal nurse leaders (FNLs) envisioned ethical nursing leadership.

Background and Research Design

Attention to ethical leadership in nursing has diminished over the past several decades. This Canadian study used meta-ethnography to guide the analysis and synthesis of four studies that explored the notion of ethical nursing leadership. These four original studies were conducted from 1999 to 2008 in Canada with a total of 601 participants. The analytic strategy of lines-of-argument (Noblit & Hare, 1988) was used to synthesize key themes.

Evidence-Informed Practice

Data synthesis and comparison of similarities and differences revealed the following themes:

- Ethical nursing leadership must be responsive to practitioners and to the contextual system in which they and FNLs work.
- Ethical nursing leadership requires receiving and providing support to increase the capacity to practise and discuss ethics in day-to-day situations.

The authors concluded that there is an urgent need to strengthen and make visible ethical leadership among FNLs. Ethical leadership is an important aspect of creating an ethical climate in which both nurse and patient outcomes are enhanced. FNLs, however, are often caught in the tension between enacting ethical obligations of the profession and working with the priorities and needs of their health care organizations and governments. Current contexts in health care organizations emphasize business and market values. The ability of nurse leaders to enact ethical leadership based on values related to compassionate and competent care can easily be dismissed and devalued. The FNLs require support and resources to enact their ethical commitments.

Schick Makaroff, K., Storch, J., Pauly, B., & Newton, L. (2014). Searching for ethical leadership in nursing. *Nursing Ethics, 21*(6), 642–658.

BOX 7-7 FOCUS ON PRIMARY HEALTH CARE

How to Encourage Nurses Individually and Collectively to Work Toward Eliminating Social Inequities

- Utilize the principles of primary health care for the benefit of the public and patients receiving care.
- Understand that some groups in society are systemically disadvantaged, which leads to poorer health and diminished well-being. Nurses work to improve the quality of lives of people who are part of disadvantaged and vulnerable groups and communities, and they take action to overcome barriers to health care.
- Recognize and work to address organizational, social, economic, and political factors that influence health and well-being within the context of the nurse's role in the delivery of care.

information or seek assistance can be helpful strategies to address the issue causing moral distress. Even if formal or informal team discussions do not resolve ethical conflicts, discussions can be beneficial because they provide a way for nurses to have their concerns heard and legitimized. Nurse managers are also key team members for creating safe places where team discussions of challenging ethical issues can occur. The manager plays an essential role in offering support and the opportunity for the resolution of conflict to occur. Having the manager involved can help to reduce more distress.

KEY CONCEPTS

- Values clarification helps nurses explore personal values and feelings and to decide how to act on personal beliefs. It also facilitates nurse–patient communication.
- Ethics is the study of philosophical ideals of what is beneficial or valuable for all.
- A code of ethics provides a foundation for professional nursing. Such a code promotes accountability, responsibility, and advocacy.
- Theories of bioethics refer to ethical issues specific to the delivery of health care. They are based on the principles of autonomy, beneficence, nonmaleficence, and justice.
- Relational ethics theory encompasses more than bioethics; it addresses the role of relationships in the ethical delivery of health care. It maintains that the nurse–patient relationship is the foundation of nursing ethics.
- Ethical problems arise from differences in values, from technological advances, from end-of-life experiences, and from changes in work environments.
- A standard process for thinking through ethical dilemmas, including critical thinking skills, helps health care providers resolve conflict or uncertainty about correct actions.

CRITICAL THINKING EXERCISES

1. Complete the values clarification exercise (Box 7-1) with your classmates or others. Compare the answers and discuss the differences.
2. You are a clinic nurse in a small community clinic. A 17-year-old female patient has been coming to the clinic for treatment for and support with a sexually transmitted infection. During recent months, she has lost her support from a close friend. In addition, her parents are divorced, and she has little contact with them. Her health and well-being are of concern. Her appearance is unkempt, her nutritional status is not balanced, and she has admitted to being depressed. She asks for your help in planning her suicide. Discuss your response to her request. Begin by acknowledging the laws related to assisted suicide in Canada. Examine your personal feelings about suicide. Include a discussion about your understanding of sexually transmitted infections: Where do they come from? Who gets these infections? Why do people get these infections? What are your feelings and opinions about people with sexually transmitted infections? Construct your response, keeping in mind the theory of relational ethics. Discuss your role in this situation. What are your possible courses of action?
3. You have been assigned the care of a 98-year-old woman who was recently admitted with a diagnosis of pneumonia. She has a history of cardiac disease and takes a number of medications. She had been fairly active until the past few days, when her cough worsened and a fever developed. You note that her pulse has become weak and threadlike and that her respirations are increasingly laboured. The patient is now too weak to respond to you. When you mention to the family that you may need to call the physician and even take heroic life-saving measures, the patient's son and daughter become distraught, saying that they do not want their mother to be kept alive on "machines." They report that they have discussed this situation with their mother. You find that her wishes have not been documented in her chart. The family members have not discussed this situation with the patient's primary physician. What actions would you consider taking at this moment? Take into account the ethical principles of autonomy and beneficence and the idea of futile care. What are your personal values about interventions at the end of life?

REVIEW QUESTIONS

1. The nurse knows that values clarification plays a major role in
   1. Creating a set of rules for conduct
   2. Identifying values that should be accepted by all
   3. Resolving issues of "value conflict"
   4. Developing a code of ethics
2. In Canada, equitable access to health care means that all citizens have equal access to medically necessary services. Which ethical principle would reflect equal access to health care?
   1. Accountability
   2. Autonomy
   3. Relational ethics
   4. Justice
3. It may seem redundant when health care providers, including professional nurses, agree to "do no harm" to their patients. The point of this agreement is to reassure the public that in all ways, not only will the health care team work to heal patients but they also agree to do this in the least painful and harmful way possible. Which principle describes this agreement?
   1. Beneficence
   2. Accountability
   3. Nonmaleficence
   4. Respect for autonomy
4. A patient is admitted to a medical unit. The patient is fearful of hospitals. The nurse carefully assesses the patient to determine the exact fears and then establishes interventions designed to reduce

these fears. In this setting, how is the nurse practising patient advocacy?
1. Seeking out the nurse supervisor to talk with the patient
2. Documenting patient fears in the medical record in a timely manner
3. Working to change the hospital environment
4. Assessing the patient's point of view and preparing to articulate it

5. If a nurse assesses a patient for pain and then offers a plan to manage the pain, the principle that encourages the nurse to monitor the patient's response to the plan is
   1. Beneficence
   2. Justice
   3. Nonmaleficence
   4. Respect for autonomy
6. Including patients in decision making regarding their care and respecting their choices of treatment demonstrate the principle of
   1. Beneficence
   2. Autonomy
   3. Justice
   4. Veracity
7. Nurses agree to be advocates for their patients. Which nursing action has the highest priority?
   1. Seek out a nursing supervisor in situations involving conflict
   2. Work to understand the law as it applies to the patient's clinical condition
   3. Assess the patient's point of view and prepare to articulate this point of view
   4. Document all clinical changes in the medical record in a timely manner
8. Which action is *not* part of the nurse's role as patient advocate?
   1. Intervening if other people fail to respect the patient's dignity
   2. Protecting the patient's right to confidentiality and privacy
   3. Making nursing care decisions for the patient
   4. Advocating for appropriate use of interventions to minimize suffering
9. Mrs. Bruce, 68 years old, has been waiting to be seen in the outpatient symptom control clinic for the last 4 hours. Her daughter is becoming extremely anxious for her mother, and she approaches the triage desk. Which nursing action best reflects a relational ethics approach?
   1. In an assertive voice, the triage nurse comments that the clinic policy is to see people in order of medical priority, not waiting time.
   2. The nurse can sense that the daughter is becoming concerned regarding the time her mother has waited to be seen by the clinic nurse practitioner or oncologist, and without further discussion, the triage nurse assures her that everything will be just fine.
   3. As the daughter shares her narrative of needing to be seen, the nurse interjects to assure the daughter that the best effort will be made to get her mother seen in a timely manner.
   4. The nurse senses the daughter's angst. From behind the counter the nurse moves toward the daughter to listen. The nurse respectfully shares that at the present time there is not a room available, but the clinic team is working on moving a particular patient to an inpatient unit. The nurse explains further that, although she cannot predict the time, she will do her best to keep her informed.
10. Ethical dilemmas often arise over a conflict of opinion. Once the nurse has determined that the dilemma is ethical, which action should the nurse take first in negotiating the difference of opinion?
    1. Consult a professional ethicist to ensure that the steps of the process occur in full
    2. Gather all relevant information regarding the dilemma
    3. List the ethical principles that inform the dilemma so that negotiations agree on the language of the discussion
    4. Ensure that the attending physician has written an order for an ethics consultation to support the ethics process

Answers: 1. 3; **2.** 4; **3.** 3; **4.** 4; **5.** 4; **6.** 2; **7.** 3; **8.** 3; **9.** 4; **10.** 2

Rationales for the Review Questions appear at the end of the book.

RECOMMENDED WEBSITES

Canadian Bioethics Society: http://www.bioethics.ca.

Founded in 1988 through the amalgamation of the Canadian Society of Bioethics and the Canadian Society for Medical Bioethics. Members include health care administrators, lawyers, nurses, philosophers, physicians, theologians, and other professionals concerned with the ethical and humane dimensions of health care. The website offers information about the annual CBS conference, national and international ethics organization links, and relevant ethics journals from a variety of disciplines.

W. Maurice Young Centre for Applied Ethics: http://www.ethics.ubc.ca.

Established by the University of British Columbia in 1993; primarily an interdisciplinary research centre in which a variety of ethics topics are studied. The website has links to other ethics organizations and ethics resources. The centre's newsletter is also available on the website.

John Dossetor Health Ethics Centre at the University of Alberta: http://www.bioethics.ualberta.ca.

The John Dossetor Health Ethics Centre is the only interdisciplinary, academic health ethics centre in Alberta and one of the first in Canada. The Centre is involved in health ethics education, research, and community engagement at the University of Alberta.

REFERENCES

Amjad, H., Towle, V., & Fried, T. (2014). Association of experience with illness and end-of-life care with advance care planning in older adults. *Journal of the American Geriatrics Society, 62*(7), 1304–1309. doi:10.1111/jgs.12894.

Austin, W. (2007). The ethics of everyday practice: Healthcare environments as moral communities. *Advances in Nursing Science, 30*(1), 81–88.

Beauchamp, T., & Childress, J. (2012). *Principles of biomedical ethics* (7th ed.). New York: Oxford University Press.

Bennett Jacobs, B., & Taylor, C. (2005). Medical futility in the natural attitude. *ANS. Advances in Nursing Science, 28*, 288–305.

Bergum, V. (2013). Relational ethics in nursing. In J. Storch, P. Rodney, & R. Starzomski (Eds.), *Toward a moral horizon: Nursing ethics for leadership and practice.* Toronto: Pearson Education.

Bergum, V., & Dossetor, J. (2005). *Relational ethics: The full meaning of respect.* Hagerstown, MD: University Publishing Group.

Bilsen, J., Vander Stichele, R., Mortier, F., et al. (2004). Involvement of nurses in physician assisted dying. *Journal of Advanced Nursing, 47*(6), 583–591. doi:10.1111/j.1365-2648.2004.02982.x.

Blondeau, D., Lavoie, M., Valois, P., et al. (2000). The attitude of Canadian nurses towards advance directives. *Nursing Ethics, 7*(5), 399–411.

Boutain, D. (2005). Social justice in nursing: A review of the literature. In M. de Chesney (Ed.), *Caring for the vulnerable: Perspectives in nursing theory, practice, research.* Mississauga, ON: Jones & Barlett Publications.

Browne, A. (2000). When patients demand too much. *Health Ethics Today, 11*(1), 2–3.

Canadian Association Schools of Nursing/Association Canadienne des Écoles de Sciences Infirmières [CASN/ACESI]. (2015). *National nursing education framework: Final report.* Ottawa: Author.

Canadian Health Services Research Foundation. (2006). *What's ailing our nurses? A discussion of the major issues affecting nursing human resources in Canada.* Ottawa: Author.

Canadian Nurses Association (CNA). (2012). *When private becomes public: The ethical challenges of and opportunities of social media.* Ottawa: Author.

Canadian Nurses Association (CNA). (2015a). *Framework for the practice of Registered Nurses in Canada*. Retrieved from https://www.cna-aiic.ca/~/media/cna/page-content/pdf-en/framework-for-the-practice-of-registered-nurses-in-canada.pdf?la=en.

Canadian Nurses Association (CNA). (2015b). *The palliative approach to care and the role of the nurse*. Ottawa: Author.

Canadian Nurses Association (CNA). (2017a). *Code of ethics for registered nurses*. Ottawa: Author.

Canadian Nurses Association (CNA). (2017b). *National nursing framework on medical assistance in dying in Canada*. Ottawa: Author.

Chrash, M., Mulich, B., & Patton, C. (2011). The APN role in holistic assessment and integration of spiritual assessment for advance care planning. *Journal of the American Academy of Nurse Practitioners*, *23*(10), 530–536. doi:10.1111/j.1745-7599.2011.00644.x.

College of Registered Nurses of Nova Scotia (CRNNS), & College of Licensed Practical Nurses of Nova Scotia. (2016). *Medical assistance in dying: A guideline for nurses*. Retrieved from http://eol.law.dal.ca/wp-content/uploads/2016/07/NS-Nurses-MAID-Guidelines.pdf.

Gastmans, C. (2012). Nursing ethics perspectives on end-of-life care. *Nursing Ethics*, *19*, 603–604. doi:10.1177/0969733012453234.

Gilligan, C. (1982). *In a different voice*. Cambridge, MA: Harvard University Press.

Hartrick Doane, G., & Varcoe, C. (2007). Relational practice and nursing obligations. *ANS. Advances in Nursing Science*, *30*, 192–205. doi:10.1097/01.ANS.0000286619.31398.fc.

Inghelbrecht, E., Bilsen, J., Mortier, F., et al. (2009). Attitudes of nurses towards euthanasia and towards their role in euthanasia: A nationwide study in Flanders, Belgium. *International Journal of Nursing Studies*, *46*(9), 1209–1218. doi:10.1016/j.ijnurstu.2009.02.009.

International Council of Nurses. (2012). *ICN code of ethics for nurses*. Geneva, Switzerland: Author.

Johnstone, M.-J. (2015). *Bioethics: A nursing perspective* (6th ed.). Melbourne, Australia: Elsevier.

Kohlberg, L. (1981). *Essays on moral development* (Vol. 1–3). San Francisco, CA: Harper & Row.

Lindemann, H. (2006). *An invitation to feminist ethics*. New York: McGraw-Hill.

Lindemann Nelson, H. L. (2000). Feminist bioethics: Where we've been, where we're going. *Metaphilosophy*, *31*, 492–508. doi:10.1111/1467-9973.00165.

Lum, H. D., & Sudore, R. (2016). Advance Care planning and goals of care communication in older adults with cardiovascular disease and multi-morbidity. *Clinics in Geriatric Medicine*, *32*(2), 247–260. doi:10.1016/j.cger.2016.01.011.

Lund, S., Richardson, A., & May, C. (2015). Barriers to advance care planning at the end of life: An exploratory systematic review of implementation studies. *PLoS ONE*, *10*(2). doi:10.1371/journal.pone.0116629.

Noblit, G. W., & Hare, R. D. (1988). *Meta-ethnography: Synthesizing qualitative studies*. Thousand Oaks, CA: Sage.

Oberle, K., & Raffin Bouchal, S. (2009). *Ethics in Canadian nursing practice*. Toronto: Pearson.

Parliament of Canada, Senate, Special Joint Committee on Physician-Assisted Death. (2016). *Medical assistance in dying: A patient-centred approach*. 42nd Parliament, 1st Session. Retrieved from http://www.parl.gc.ca/HousePublications/Publication.aspx?Language=e&Mode=1&Parl=42&Ses=1&DocId=8120006.

Rocker, G., & Dunbar, S. (2000). Withholding or withdrawal of life support: The Canadian Critical Care Society Position Paper. *Journal of Palliative Care*, *16*(Suppl.), S53–S62.

Rodney, P. A. (2017). What we know about moral distress. *American Journal of Nursing*, *117*(Suppl.), S7–S10. doi:10.1097/01.NAJ.0000512204.85973.04.

Schick Makaroff, K., Storch, J., Pauly, B., et al. (2014). Searching for ethical leadership in nursing. *Nursing Ethics*, *21*(6), 642–658. doi:10.1177/09697330135113213.

Sherwin, S. (1992). *No longer patient: Feminist ethics and health care*. Philadelphia, PA: Temple University Press.

Taylor, C. (1995). Medical futility and nursing. *Image: The Journal of Nursing Scholarship*, *27*, 301–306.

Ulrich, M., Taylor, C., Soeken, K., et al. (2010). Everyday ethics: Ethical issues and stress in nursing practice. *Journal of Advanced Nursing*, *66*(11), 2510–2519. doi:10.1111/j.1365-2648.2010.05425.x.

World Health Organization Commission on Social Determinants of Health. (2008). *Closing the gap in a generation: Health equity through action on the social determinants of health*. Geneva, Switzerland: Author.

Wright, D., & Brajtman, S. (2011). Relational and embodied knowing: Nursing ethics within the interprofessional team. *Nursing Ethics*, *18*(1), 20–30. doi:10.1177/0969733010386165.

Yeo, M., Moorhouse, A., Khan, P., et al. (2010). *Concepts and cases in nursing ethics* (3rd ed.). Peterborough, ON: Broadview Press.

8

Legal Implications in Nursing Practice

Written by Carla Shapiro, RN, MN

OBJECTIVES

Mastery of content in this chapter will enable you to:

- Define the key terms listed.
- Explain legal concepts that apply to nurses.
- Describe the legal responsibilities and obligations of nurses.
- List sources for standards of care for nurses.
- Define legal aspects of nurse–patient, nurse–physician, nurse–nurse, and nurse–employer relationships.
- List the elements needed to prove negligence.
- Give examples of legal issues that arise in nursing practice.

KEY TERMS

Advance directive, p. 110
Adverse occurrence report, p. 111
Assault, p. 103
Battery, p. 103
Civil law, p. 101
Common law, p. 101
Euthanasia, p. 109
Incident report, p. 111
Informed consent, p. 106
Intentional torts, p. 103
Living will, p. 110
Medical assistance in dying (MAID), p. 110
Negligence, p. 104
Nursing practice acts, p. 102
Risk management, p. 111
Standards of care, p. 102
Statute law, p. 102
Tort, p. 103

MEDIA RESOURCES

http://evolve.elsevier.com/Canada/Potter/fundamentals/

- Audio Chapter Summaries
- Examination Review Questions
- Concept Map Creator
- Case Study with Questions
- Audio Glossary
- Content Updates
- Video Clips

Safe nursing practice includes knowledge of the legal boundaries within which nurses must function. Nurses must understand the law to protect themselves from liability and to protect their patients' rights. Nurses need not fear the law; rather, they should view it as representing what society expects from them. Laws are continually changing to meet the needs of the people they are intended to protect. As technology has expanded the role of the nurse, the ethical dilemmas associated with patient care have increased and often become legal issues as well. As health care evolves, so do the legal implications for health care. Although federal laws apply to all provinces and territories, nurses must be aware that laws do vary across the country. It is important for nurses to know the laws in their province or territory that affect their practice. Being familiar with the law enhances nurses' ability to be patient advocates.

LEGAL LIMITS OF NURSING

Nurses have a fiduciary relationship with their patients. A *fiduciary relationship* is one in which a professional (the nurse) provides services that, by their nature, cause the recipient (the patient) to trust in the specialized knowledge and integrity of the professional. In the fiduciary relationship, nurses are obligated to provide knowledgeable, competent, and safe care and act in the best interests of their patients.

Although legal actions against nurses were once rare, the situation is changing. The public is better informed now than in the past about their rights to health care and are more likely to seek damages for professional negligence. The courts have upheld the concept that nurses must provide a reasonable standard of care. Thus, it is essential that nurses understand the legal limits influencing their daily practice.

Sources of Law

The Constitution of Canada is the primary source of Canadian law (*Constitution Act*, 1867). It divides areas of responsibility between the federal government and the provinces. The federal government has authority over such matters as unemployment insurance, the postal service, and criminal law. The federal law applies across the country. The Constitution gives the provinces authority over matters such as the management of hospitals, solemnization of marriage, and civil rights. In the constitutional context, civil rights have a very broad meaning and refer to private relationships between people, including contract rights, ownership of property, and negligence disputes. In Canada, there are two systems that deal with private law issues: **civil law** (based on Roman law) in Quebec and **common law** (based on British common law) in the rest of the country. The three Canadian territories exercise many of the same powers as the provinces, as a result of authority having been delegated to them by the federal government.

When either a civil or a criminal case goes to court, decisions are based on statute law and previous case rulings. How courts rule on the circumstances and facts surrounding the case is called a *precedent.* If legal rulings are made in a case, the court is bound to follow that decision in subsequent similar cases. Not every jurisdiction has case law on a given issue. For example, cases regarding a patient's right to refuse treatment are not found in every province. However, the cases from another province or territory are often consulted. In general, breaches of private law result in the payment of money to compensate the aggrieved party for damages incurred. Violations of some public law statutes such as the Criminal Code of Canada may result in a range of remedies, including fines or imprisonment.

Statute law is created by elective legislative bodies such as Parliament and provincial or territorial legislatures. Federal statutes apply throughout the country, and provincial and territorial statutes apply only in the province or territory in which they were created. Examples of provincial statutes are the *Regulated Health Professions Act* (1991) in Ontario and nursing practice acts throughout the country, which describe and define nursing practice within each province.

Examples of federal statutes are the Criminal Code of Canada (1985), the *Assisted Human Reproduction Act* (2004), the *Controlled Drugs and Substances Act* (1996), and the *Food and Drugs Act* (1985).

Professional Regulation

Like all self-governing professions in Canada, nursing is regulated at the provincial or territorial level. Each province and territory has legislation that grants authority to a nursing regulatory body. These regulatory bodies are accountable to the public for ensuring safe, competent, and ethical nursing care. Regulatory bodies are responsible for granting certificates of registration, offering practice support, ensuring continuing competence of their members, investigating complaints against members' conduct, and disciplining members when necessary. A registered nurse in Saskatchewan was found guilty of professional misconduct following a post she made on Facebook regarding the care that her grandfather received on a palliative care unit prior to his death (Dinh, 2016; Saskatchewan Registered Nurses Association & Strom, 2016). The nurse was disciplined, and a notice of Appeal was filed with the Court of Queen's Bench as of April 27, 2017 in regards to the decision of the Discipline Committee October 18, 2016 and April 4, 2017. Regulatory bodies are also responsible for developing codes of ethics, setting standards of practice, and approving nursing education programs (McIntyre & McDonald, 2010). The Canadian Association of Schools of Nursing (CASN) has developed a framework outlining the expectations for nursing education programs from baccalaureate to doctoral preparation. The framework consists of six domains, with guiding principles for each level of education and the essential components applying to each (CASN, 2015).

Separate regulatory bodies exist for registered nurses and practical nurses. Some provinces also have regulatory bodies for registered psychiatric nurses. These regulatory bodies are called either the *provincial association* or the *college of nursing* (e.g., the College and Association of Registered Nurses of Alberta, the College of Nurses of Ontario). The trend appears to favour the college model, with a stronger focus on regulation of practice and accountability to the public.

Nurses must be registered by the professional nursing association or college of the province or territory in which they practise. The requirements for registration (or licensure, as applicable) vary across the country, but most provinces and territories have minimum education requirements and require the nurse to pass an examination. All provinces and territories (except Quebec) use the NCLEX examination. Quebec has created its own professional examination (OIIQ). Registration (or licensure) enables people to practise nursing and use the applicable nursing title and initials: registered nurse (RN) or registered practical nurse (RPN). All nurses' credentials must be verified, either by the listing of their names on a register or by their holding a valid licence to practise.

Registration can be suspended or revoked by the regulatory body if a nurse's conduct violates provisions in the registration statute. For example, nurses who perform illegal acts, such as selling controlled substances, jeopardize their registration status. Due process must be followed before registration can be suspended or revoked. *Due process* means that nurses must be notified of the charges brought against them and have an opportunity to defend themselves against the charges in a hearing. Such hearings do not occur in courts but are usually conducted by the regulatory body. If a nurse loses his or her professional licence, or if the nurse's name is removed from the provincial or territorial register, and if the case involves civil or criminal wrongs, then further legal consequences may follow.

Regulation of Nurse Practitioners

Over the past number of years, the role, responsibilities, and use of nurse practitioners (NPs) has evolved in Canada. The utilization and regulation of NPs varies from jurisdiction to jurisdiction across the country. In some provinces or territories (e.g., Newfoundland, Northwest Territories, Nunavut), the title "nurse practitioner" is protected, and in others (e.g., Manitoba) these nurses are identified in other ways such as RN/EP (extended practice) or RN/NP (nurse practitioner). It is important that nurses communicate their regulated title to their patients, families, and other members of the health care team. The differences in regulatory approaches among jurisdictions can be confusing to consumers and can affect the mobility of nurses across the country as a result of this (McIntyre & McDonald, 2010).

Standards of Care

Standards of care are legal guidelines for nursing practice. Standards establish an expectation of nurses to provide safe and appropriate patient care. If nurses do not perform duties within accepted standards of care, they may place themselves in jeopardy of legal action and, more important, place their patients at risk for harm and injury. Nursing standards of care arise from a variety of sources, including statutes; case law; and the detailed regulations, practice standards, and codes of ethics that are generated by the professional associations. Nursing standards are also outlined in the written policies and procedures of employing institutions.

All provincial and territorial legislatures have passed health professions acts, **nursing practice acts**, or both that define the scope of nursing practice. These acts set educational requirements for nurses, distinguish between nursing and medical practice, and generally define nursing practice. The rules and regulations enacted by the provincial or territorial regulatory body help define the practice of nursing more specifically. For example, a nursing association may develop a rule regarding intravenous therapy. All nurses are responsible for knowing the provisions of the nursing practice or regulated health professions act for the province or territory in which they work, as well as the rules and regulations enacted by the regulatory bodies of their province or territory.

Professional organizations are another source for defining standards of care. The Canadian Nurses Association (CNA) has developed standards for nursing practice, policy statements, and similar resolutions. The standards delineate the scope, function, and role of the nurse in practice. Nursing specialty organizations also have standards of practice defined for certification of nurses who work in specific specialty areas, such as the operating room or the critical care unit. The same standards also serve as practice guidelines for defining safe and appropriate nursing care in specialty areas.

The Canadian Council on Health Services Accreditation requires that accredited health care institutions have nursing policies and procedures in writing that detail how nurses are to perform their duties. These internal standards of care are usually quite specific and are found in procedural manuals on most nursing units. For example, a procedure or policy that outlines the steps that should be taken when a dressing is changed or medication is administered gives specific information about how nurses are to perform these tasks. Nurses must know the policies and procedures of their employing institution because they all must follow that standard of care. Institutional policies and procedures must conform to laws and cannot conflict with legal guidelines that define acceptable standards of care.

In a negligence lawsuit, these standards are used to determine whether the nurse has acted as any reasonably prudent nurse in a similar setting with the same credentials would act. A nursing expert is called to testify about the standards of nursing care as applied to the facts of the case. The expert may be called to define and explain to the court what a reasonably prudent nurse would have been expected to do in view of the facts of the case in any similar setting and with similar credentials. It is recognized and understood that nursing practice differs according to the rural or urban nature of the institutional setting. In addition, home health care, occupational health nursing, and other community-based clinical settings require that the expert be familiar with the standards of care in these settings, as opposed to the traditional hospital or institutional setting. The expert must have the appropriate credentials, the appropriate experience, and an understanding of what the standard of care should have been in the specific case. The expert witness is distinguished from the fact witness. Staff nurses may testify in a court proceeding as fact witnesses if they have first-hand personal experience with the facts of the case. The expert witness evaluates the defendant's professional judgements and behaviour under the circumstances being reviewed.

General duty nurses are legally responsible for meeting the same standards as other general duty nurses in similar settings. However, specialized nurses, such as nurses in a Critical Care Unit or nurses who perform dialysis, are held to standards of care and skill that apply to all professionals in the same specialty. All nurses must know the standards of care that they are expected to meet within their specific specialty and work setting. Ignorance of the law or of standards of care is not a defence against negligence.

LEGAL LIABILITY ISSUES IN NURSING PRACTICE

Torts

A **tort** is a civil wrong committed against a person or property. Torts may be classified as intentional or unintentional. **Intentional torts** are willful acts that violate another person's rights (Keatings & Smith, 2010). Examples are assault, battery, invasion of privacy, and false imprisonment. Negligence is an example of an unintentional tort.

Intentional Torts

Assault. **Assault** is conduct (such as a physical or verbal threat) that creates in another person apprehension or fear of imminent harmful or offensive contact. No actual contact is necessary in order for damages for assault to be awarded (Fridman, 2003; Osborne, 2003). Threats by a nurse to give a patient an injection or to restrain a patient for an X-ray procedure when the patient has refused consent constitute assault. The key issues are whether the patient was afraid of being harmed in the situation and whether the patient consented to a procedure. In a lawsuit wherein the tort of assault is alleged, the patient's consent would negate the claim of assault against a nurse.

Battery. **Battery** is any intentional physical contact with a person without that person's consent. The contact can be harmful to the patient and cause an injury, or it can be merely offensive to the patient's personal dignity (Osborne, 2013). In the example of a nurse's threats to give a patient an injection without the patient's consent, if the nurse actually gives the injection, it is considered battery. Battery could even be life-saving, as in the Ontario case of *Malette v. Shulman* (1990). In that case, the plaintiff was unconscious and bleeding profusely. The physician determined that she needed a life-saving blood transfusion. Before the transfusion, a nurse found a signed card in the plaintiff's purse that identified the patient as a Jehovah's Witness and stated that under no circumstances was she to receive blood. Despite this, the physician chose to administer the blood to preserve the patient's life. The plaintiff survived, recovered from her injuries, and successfully sued the physician for battery (Irvine, Osborne, & Shariff, 2013).

In some situations, consent is implied. For example, if a patient gets into a wheelchair or transfers to a stretcher of his or her own volition after being advised that it is time to be taken for an X-ray procedure, the patient has given implied consent to the procedure. A patient has the right to revoke or withdraw consent at any time.

Invasion of Privacy. The tort of invasion of privacy protects the patient's right to be free from unwanted intrusion into his or her private affairs. Patients are entitled to confidential health care. Nursing standards for what constitutes confidential information are based on professional ethics, the common law, and privacy statutes. The ideals of privacy and sensitivity to the needs and rights of patients who may not choose to have nurses intrude on their lives but who depend on nurses for their care guide the nurse's judgement. The nurse's fiduciary duty requires that confidential information not be shared with anyone else except on a need-to-know basis.

One form of invasion of privacy is the release of a patient's medical information to an unauthorized person, such as a member of the press, the patient's employer, or through social media. The information that is contained in a patient's medical record is a confidential communication. It should only be shared with health care providers for the purpose of medical treatment.

A patient's medical record is confidential. The nurse should not disclose the patient's confidential medical information without the patient's consent. For example, a nurse should respect a wish not to inform the patient's family of a terminal illness. Similarly, a nurse should not assume that a patient's spouse or family members know all of the patient's history, particularly with regard to private issues such as mental illness, medications, pregnancy, abortion, birth control, or sexually transmitted infections.

Confidentiality is not an absolute value, however, and in certain circumstances, breaching confidentiality is justifiable. At times, a nurse may be required by law (statutory duty) to breach confidentiality and disclose information to a third party. For example, each province and territory has laws that require health care workers to report suspected child abuse to a local child protection agency. In some jurisdictions, statutes require the notification of the police when there has been a gunshot or a stab wound (*Gunshot and Stab Wounds Mandatory Reporting Act*, 2008). Nurses may also be required to release information about a patient when they receive a subpoena (a legal order) to testify in court.

Nurses are under no legal obligation to release confidential information to the police except in rare cases in which the life, safety, or health of the patient or an innocent third party is in jeopardy (such as when a patient tells a nurse that he or she intends to hurt or kill someone). Such a statement should first be reported to the employer's administration or legal counsel before releasing it to the police (Canadian Nurses Protective Society [CNPS], 2014). Other admissions made by a patient to a nurse about past or future criminal activity may not have to be disclosed unless the nurse is compelled to do so by a court of law. The conflict between confidentiality and risk of public harm is not always clear. When a nurse has serious concerns about the welfare of others (e.g., if a patient is infected with human immunodeficiency virus [HIV] and admits to having unsafe sex or donating blood), the nurse should first suggest and strongly encourage the patient to disclose this information. If the patient refuses, the nurse should seek consultation with professional colleagues and supervisors. The need for privacy and confidentiality of privileged communication and the need for public safety would need to be weighed carefully.

Computers and Confidentiality. Most health care facilities use computer systems to maintain patient records. "Computerization in health care raises major legal concerns related to confidentiality of health records because of the potential for unauthorized access and data sharing" (Tapp, 2003). Access to confidential patient information is generally controlled by means of a variety of technological safeguards, including magnetized cards and passwords. It is important that these security devices not be shared with other people and that access cards are used to retrieve files only when warranted. The improper use of a magnetized card and password to seek out confidential information could lead to legal repercussions or disciplinary action. Particular care must be taken to protect portable devices, such as laptop computers and flash drives containing health information, as there have been cases where such devices were stolen from offices and cars (CNPS, 2009a, 2013).

Social media and other forms of electronic communication such as blogs, Facebook, Twitter, and YouTube are used by many people to communicate and network. Nurses must be extremely cautious about what information or images they post online, as any information in electronic form can be easily distributed and make its way into the public domain. There is the mistaken belief that deleted information no longer exists, that privacy controls are totally secure, and that anonymous postings provide protection. Breaches of privacy legislation can lead to disciplinary action by the professional regulatory body or to civil lawsuits alleging breaches of privacy (CNPS, 2010). The best way to avoid the inadvertent disclosure of confidential or private information about patients is by maintaining professional boundaries, following employer policies, not posting or sharing any patient-related information online, and not making disparaging comments about employers or colleagues, as these may be viewed as defamatory (CNPS, 2003).

False Imprisonment. The tort of false imprisonment serves to protect a person's individual liberty and basic rights. Preventing a patient from leaving a health care facility voluntarily may constitute the tort of false imprisonment. The inappropriate or unjustified use of restraints (e.g., by confining a person to an area, or by using physical or chemical restraints) may also be viewed as false imprisonment. Nurses must be aware of their facility's policies and specific legislation in their jurisdiction (e.g., under the *Mental Health and Consequential Amendments Act*, 1998) relating to when and how restraints can be used (CNPS, 2004).

Unintentional Torts

Negligence. When nurses are sued, most often the proceedings against them are for the tort of negligence, also referred to as *malpractice* (Irvine et al., 2013). Negligence in nursing is conduct that does not meet a standard of care established by law. No intent is needed for negligence to occur. It is characterized chiefly by inadvertence, thoughtlessness, or inattention. Negligence may involve carelessness, such as not checking an identification bracelet, which results in administration of the wrong medication. However, carelessness is not always the cause of misconduct. If nurses perform a procedure for which they have not been educated and do so carefully but still harm the patient, a claim of negligence can be made. In general, courts define *nursing negligence* as the failure to use the degree of skill or learning ordinarily used under the same or similar circumstances by members of the nursing profession (Box 8-1).

Nurses can be found liable for negligence if the following criteria are established: (1) the nurse (defendant) owed a duty of care to the patient (plaintiff); (2) the nurse did not carry out that duty; (3) the patient was injured; and (4) the nurse's failure to carry out the duty caused the injury.

The ability to predict harm (i.e., the foreseeability of risk) is evaluated in negligence cases. The circumstances surrounding the injury are evaluated to determine whether it was likely that the injury or harm to the patient could have been expected from the care that was or was not provided. In other words, had it not been for what the nurse did or did not do, could an injury have been prevented?

The case of *Downey v. Rothwell* (1974) is an example of nursing negligence. This case involved a plaintiff who suffered a severe arm injury when she fell off an examining table while under the care of a nurse. The patient, who had a history of epilepsy, informed the nurse that she was about to have a seizure. The nurse left the patient unattended on an examining table while she left the room for a few moments. During this time, the patient had a seizure, fell onto the floor, and broke her arm. The nurse should have anticipated that the patient could have fallen during a seizure and ensured her safety either by moving her to the floor or by putting up guardrails on the examining table. This case involved an undertaking by the nurse to provide care, a reliance by the patient on this nurse, and a foreseeable risk. The nurse was found negligent in this case, and her employers were held vicariously liable. "Vicarious liability is a legal doctrine that applies in situations where the law holds the employer legally responsible for the acts of its employees that occur within the scope and course of their employment" (CNPS, 1998).

In the case of *Granger v. Ottawa General Hospital* (1996), two nurses (a staff nurse and her team leader) were found negligent in the care they provided to a woman in labour. During labour, the plaintiff's fetal heart monitor strip showed deep, persistent, variable decelerations. The staff nurse did not appreciate that these were a sign of fetal distress and did not immediately report these findings to other members of the obstetrical team. The ensuing delay in care resulted in severe and permanent brain injury in the baby, leaving her severely disabled. In

BOX 8-1 Common Negligent Acts

- Medication errors that result in injury to patients
- Intravenous therapy errors that result in infiltrations or phlebitis
- Burns caused by equipment, bathing, or spills of hot liquids and foods
- Falls resulting in injury to patients
- Failure to use aseptic technique as required
- Errors in sponge, instrument, or needle counts in surgical cases
- Failure to give a report, or giving an incomplete report, to an incoming shift of health care staff
- Failure to monitor a patient's condition adequately
- Failure to notify a physician of a significant change in a patient's status
- Failure to properly delegate or supervise

this case, the nurses breached their duty to exercise appropriate skill in making an assessment and to communicate the information to the physicians.

Preventing Negligence. The best way for nurses to avoid being negligent is to follow standards of care; give competent health care; insist on appropriate orientation, continuing education, and adequate staffing; communicate with other health care providers; develop a caring rapport with the patient; and document assessments, interventions, and evaluations fully.

The health care record, or "chart," is a permanent record of the nursing process. The courts consult the patient's chart for a chronological record of all aspects of care provided from admission to discharge. As a legal document, it is the most comprehensive record of the care provided. Careful, complete, and thorough documentation is one of the best defences against allegations of negligence or violations of nursing standards (see Chapter 15). The record can show that even in the event of an adverse patient outcome, the nursing care that was provided met the expected standards. An institution has a legal duty to maintain nursing records. Nursing notes contain substantial evidence needed in order to understand the care received by a patient. If records are lost or incomplete, the care is presumed to have been negligent and therefore the cause of the patient's injuries. In addition, incomplete or illegible records undermine the credibility of the health care provider.

In the classic case of *Kolesar v. Jeffries* (1976), the Supreme Court of Canada addressed the issue of poor record keeping. In that case, a patient underwent major spinal surgery and was transferred to a surgical unit, where he was nursed on a Stryker frame. The patient was found dead the following morning. No nursing notes were recorded from 2200 hours the previous evening until 0500 hours, when he was found dead. Although at trial several nurses and nursing assistants testified that they had tended to the patient multiple times throughout the night, the court inferred that "nothing was charted because nothing was done." One of the nurses was held negligent in this patient's death.

It is very important for documentation to be accomplished in a timely manner. Any significant changes in the patient's condition must be reported to the physician and documented in the chart (see Chapter 15). Recording nursing care notes in a notebook and then transferring them to the chart at the end of the shift can be a dangerous practice. If this practice is followed, other health care providers may administer medications or provide care to the patient without up-to-date information. Harm may come to a patient whose record is not accurate and current. Nurses must always follow the particular style of charting adopted by their employer (CNPS, 2007a).

Truthful documentation is also essential. If an error is made in the documentation, it is important to follow the policies and procedures of the institution to correct it. Obliterating or erasing errors may appear to be concealing misconduct and lead to charges of fraud. The credibility of a nurse who goes to court is negatively affected if it appears that the nurse's initial charting has been changed after an injury has occurred to a patient. This scenario is exemplified in the case of *Meyer v. Gordon* (1981). Nurses did not adequately monitor a woman in labour, and their notes were sloppy and vague. The fetus experienced severe distress, required resuscitation on delivery, and was transferred to another hospital. When a nurse realized that the documentation was deficient, she altered it. However, the original chart had already been photocopied and sent to the second hospital. At trial, it was obvious that the original document had been tampered with. The court held that the nursing staff had been negligent in several ways, and the judge severely condemned the nurse's tampering with the evidence. The court commented, "My criticism of the defendant hospital is not confined to the lack of care of its nursing staff. The hospital chart contains alterations and additions which compel me to view with suspicion the accuracy of many of the observations which are recorded."

Nurses should also be familiar with the current nursing literature in their areas of practice. They should know and follow the policies and procedures of the institution in which they work. Nurses should be sensitive to common sources of injury to patients, such as falls and medication errors. Nurses must communicate with the patient, explain the tests and treatment to be performed, document that specific explanations were provided to the patient, and listen to the patient's concerns about the treatment.

Nurse–patient relationships are very important not only in ensuring quality care but also in minimizing legal risks. Trust needs to develop between a nurse and patient. Patients who believe that the nurses performed their duties correctly and were concerned with their welfare are less likely to initiate a lawsuit against the nurses. Sincere caring for patients is an essential role of the nurse and is an effective risk-management tool. However, caring does not protect nurses completely if negligent practice occurs. When a patient is injured, the investigation into the incident may implicate the nurses even if the patient feels kindly toward them.

Criminal Liability

Although most nursing liability issues involve negligence claims, criminal law is also relevant. The Criminal Code has many offences that could potentially be committed by nurses. For example, Canadian nurses have been charged with criminal offences such as assault, administering a noxious substance, criminal negligence that causes death (a category of manslaughter), and first-degree murder (Dubinsky, 2017). Many of the acts that can give rise to a tort claim for damages may also give rise to a criminal charge. A nurse who assaulted a patient could potentially face a civil suit for damages brought by the patient and a criminal charge of assault laid by the police. Sometimes the difference between the tort and the criminal charge is one of degree. The tort of negligence involves the breach of duty of care expected of a reasonably competent practitioner, whereas the offence of criminal negligence involves actions that reach the level of "wanton or reckless disregard for the lives or safety of other persons" (Criminal Code, 1985, Part VIII, Section 219 [1]).

Consent

A signed consent form is required for all routine treatment, procedures such as surgery, some treatment programs such as chemotherapy, and research involving patients. A patient signs general consent forms when admitted to the hospital or other health care facility. The patient or the patient's representative must sign a special consent or treatment form before each specialized procedure or treatment. According to the CNA *Code of Ethics*, "if a person receiving care is clearly incapable of consent, the nurse respects the law on capacity assessment and substitute decision making in the nurse's jurisdiction" (CNA, 2017a, p. 12; see also CNPS, 2009b). Provincial and territorial laws describe what constitutes the legal ability to give consent to medical treatment. Nurses should know the law in their own jurisdiction and be familiar with the policies and procedures of their employing institution regarding consent.

In general, the following factors must be verified for consent to be legally valid:

- The patient must have the legal and mental capacity to make a treatment decision.
- The consent must be given voluntarily and without coercion.
- The patient must understand the risks and benefits of the procedure or treatment, the risks of not undergoing the procedure

or treatment, and any available alternatives to the procedure or treatment.

If a patient is deaf, is illiterate, or does not speak the language of the health care providers an official interpreter must be available to explain the terms of consent. A family member or acquaintance who can speak a patient's language should not be used to interpret health information except as a last resort. A patient experiencing the effects of a sedative is not able to clearly understand the implications of an invasive procedure. Every effort should be made to assist the patient in making an informed choice.

Nurses must be sensitive to the cultural issues of consent. The nurse must understand the way in which patients and their families communicate and make important decisions. It is essential for nurses to understand the various cultures with which they interact. The cultural beliefs and values of the patient may be very different from those of the nurse. It is important for nurses not to impose their own cultural values on the patient (see Chapter 9).

Informed Consent

> *Nurses ensure that nursing care is provided with the person's informed consent. Nurses recognize and support a capable person's right to refuse or withdraw consent for care or treatment at any time.*
>
> ***[College of Registered Nurses of British Columbia, CRNBC; CNA, 2017, p. 11]***

Informed consent is a person's agreement to allow a medical action to happen, such as surgery or an invasive procedure, based on a full disclosure of the likely risks and benefits of the action, alternatives to the action, and the consequences of refusal (Garner & Black, 2009; Osborne, 2013). Informed consent creates a legal duty for the physician or other health care provider to disclose material facts in terms that the patient can reasonably understand in order to make an informed choice. The explanation should also describe treatment alternatives, as well as the risks involved in all treatment options. Failure to obtain consent in situations other than emergencies may result in a claim of battery. In the absence of informed consent, a patient may bring a lawsuit against the health care provider for negligence, even if the procedure was performed competently. Informed consent requires the provision of adequate information for the patient to form a decision and the documentation of that decision.

The following materials are required for informed consent (Osborne, 2013):

- A brief, complete explanation of the procedure or treatment
- Names and qualifications of people performing and assisting in the procedure
- A description of any possible harm, including permanent damage or death, that may occur because of the procedure
- An explanation of therapeutic alternatives to the proposed procedure or treatment, as well as the risks of doing nothing. Patients also need to be informed of their right to refuse the procedure or treatment without discontinuing other supportive care and of their right to withdraw their consent even after the procedure has begun.

Informed consent is part of the physician–patient relationship. Because nurses do not perform surgery or direct medical procedures, obtaining patients' informed consent is not *usually* one of nurses' duties. However, given the expanded role of nurse practitioners, obtaining a patient's informed consent to treatment or procedures is vital. Even though a nurse may assume the responsibility for witnessing the patient's signature on the consent form, the nurse does not legally assume the duty of obtaining informed consent. The nurse's signature for witnessing the consent does not mean that the nurse has provided information about risks and alternatives of a particular procedure, only that the patient voluntarily gave consent, that the patient's signature is authentic, and that the patient appears to be competent to give consent (Irvine et al., 2013). When nurses provide consent forms for patients to sign, the patients should be asked whether they understand the procedures to which they are consenting. If they deny understanding or if the nurse suspects that they do not understand, the nurse must notify the physician or nursing supervisor. Some consent forms also have a line for the physician to sign after explaining the risks and alternatives to a patient. Such a form is helpful in a court case when a patient alleges that consent was not informed. If a patient refuses treatment, this rejection should also be written, signed, and witnessed.

If a patient participates in an experimental treatment program or submits to use of experimental drugs or treatments, the informed consent form must be even more detailed and stringently regulated. An organization's institutional review board should review the information in the consent form for research involving human subjects. The patient may withdraw from the experiment at any time (see Chapter 7).

Many procedures that nurses perform (e.g., insertion of intravenous or nasogastric tubes) do not require formal written consent; nonetheless, patients' rights to give or refuse consent to treatment must be protected. Implied consent to treatment is often involved in nursing procedures. For example, when the nurse approaches the patient with a syringe in hand and the patient rolls over to expose the injection site, consent is implied. If the patient resists the injection either verbally or through actions, the nurse must not proceed with the injection. Forcing or otherwise treating a patient without consent could result in criminal or civil charges of assault and battery. Many advanced practice nurses are now autonomously treating patients. It is therefore likely that formal written consent for nursing procedures will also be expected for the treatment received from advanced practice nurse specialists.

Parents are usually the legal guardians of pediatric patients, and, therefore, consent forms for treatment must be signed by parents. If the parents are divorced, the form must be signed by the parent with legal custody. On occasion, a parent or guardian will refuse treatment for a child. In those cases, the court may intervene on the child's behalf. The practice of making the child a ward of the court and administering necessary treatment is relatively common in such cases.

The example of 13-year-old Tyrell Dueck from Saskatchewan illustrates such a case. The teenager received a diagnosis of cancer in 1998. He had completed part of the chemotherapy treatment when he decided that he did not want more treatment or the recommended amputation of his leg, believing that he had been "cured by God" and that further treatment was unnecessary. His statements were consistent with his family's Christian value system. Following his parents' advice, the boy wished to undergo alternative therapy at a clinic in Mexico. The treating physicians maintained that without further conventional treatment, Tyrell would die within a year. A judge concluded that Tyrell had been given inaccurate information by his father about the benefits and risks of the proposed alternative therapy and, therefore, was unable to make an informed consent or refusal. Thus, the family's wishes to forgo conventional treatment were legally overruled, and the boy's grandparents were to take him for treatments. Before the enforced treatment could be started, however, tests revealed that the cancer had already spread and the treatment would no longer be helpful. The teenager was returned to the care of his parents, and he died a short time later.

In some instances, obtaining informed consent is difficult or simply not possible. If, for example, the patient is unconscious, consent must be obtained from a person legally authorized to give consent on the patient's behalf. Other surrogate decision makers may have legally been delegated this authority through proxy directives or court guardianship procedures. In emergency situations, if it is impossible to obtain consent from the patient or an authorized person, the procedure required to benefit the patient or save the patient's life may be undertaken without liability for failure to obtain consent. In such cases, the law assumes that the patient would wish to be treated. This is referred to as the emergency doctrine.

Patients with mental health problems and frail older persons must also be given the opportunity to give consent. They retain the right to refuse treatment unless a court has legally determined that they are incompetent to decide for themselves.

Nursing Students and Legal Liability

Nursing students must know their own capabilities and competencies and must not perform nursing actions unless competent to do so. "However, if a student nurse performs a nursing action which is one an RN would perform (e.g., administration of an I.M. [intramuscular] injection), that student will be held to the standard of an RN. Student nurses, like all other nurses, are accountable for their own actions" (Phillips, 2002). In a few reported cases in Canada, nursing students were sued for negligence in their care of patients. A nursing student in Nova Scotia who caused permanent injury in a patient through an improperly administered intramuscular injection was found negligent, and the hospital was found vicariously liable for the student's actions (CNPS, 2007b; *Roberts v. Cape Breton Regional Hospital*, 1997). Thus, nursing students are liable if their actions cause harm to patients. However, if a patient is harmed as a direct result of a nursing student's actions or lack of action, the liability is generally shared by the student, the instructor, the hospital or health care facility, and the university or educational institution. Nursing students should never be assigned to perform tasks for which they are unprepared, and they should be carefully supervised by instructors as they learn new skills. Although nursing students are not considered employees of the hospital, the institution has a responsibility to monitor their acts. Nursing students are expected to ensure that their student status is known to patients and to perform as professional nurses would in providing safe patient care. Faculty members are usually responsible for instructing and observing students, but in some situations, staff nurses serving as preceptors may share these responsibilities. Every nursing school should provide clear definitions of student responsibility, preceptor responsibility, and faculty responsibility (CNPS, 2012).

When students are employed as nursing assistants or nurses' aides when not attending classes, they should not perform tasks that do not appear in a job description for a nurses' aide or assistant. For example, even if a student has learned to administer intramuscular medications in class, this task may not be performed by a nurses' aide. If a staff nurse overseeing the nursing assistant or aide knowingly assigns work without regard for the person's ability to safely conduct the task as defined in the job description, that staff nurse is also liable. If students employed as nurse's aides are requested to perform tasks that they are not prepared to complete safely, this information should be brought to the nursing supervisor's attention so that the needed help can be obtained.

The website of the CNPS (http://www.cnps.ca/ through its members-only section) is an excellent resource available to nursing students, providing information about legal risks nurses face in practice. However, nursing students are not entitled to receive legal consultation services or financial assistance from the CNPS; these services are provided only for the benefit of eligible registered nurses.

Professional Liability Protection

Most nurses in Canada are employed by publicly funded health care facilities that carry malpractice insurance. These facilities are considered employers and thus are vicariously liable for negligent acts of their employees, provided the employees were working within the normal scope and course of practice (Keatings & Smith, 2010).

Because of this legal principle, an employer will generally be liable to those who may have suffered damages as a result of the negligence of an employee. Consequently, a patient who considers himself or herself to have been injured by the actions of an employee will often look to the employer for compensation (CNPS, 1998). This legal principle does not apply when the employee is working outside the normal scope of his or her employment. Accordingly, a nurse who is self-employed or engages in activities that are not related to his or her employment (even if they are undertaken on the employer's premises) is solely liable for his or her own negligence. All nurses should be aware of their employment status as well as the availability and extent of their professional liability coverage.

The Canadian Nurses Protective Society is a nonprofit society established in 1988 to provide legal support and liability protection to nurses. The services of CNPS are available to registered nurses and nurse practitioners as a benefit of membership in a subscribing provincial or territorial professional association or college, with CNA membership, or by becoming a CNPS individual beneficiary. Eligible nurses can obtain confidential assistance from a nurse lawyer by contacting the CNPS toll-free by telephone, Monday to Friday from 0830 to 1630 Eastern Standard Time or Eastern Daylight Time at 1-800-267-3390.

A nurse providing emergency assistance at an accident scene may not be covered by an employer's insurance policy because the care given would not fall within the scope of employment. However, some provinces have adopted "Good Samaritan" laws (e.g., Alberta's *Emergency Medical Aid Act*, 2000) that prevent voluntary rescuers from being liable for negligent care provided during a rescue unless it can be proved that they displayed gross negligence. Nurses must be familiar with these laws in their own province or territory.

Abandonment, Assignment, and Contract Issues

Short Staffing. During nursing shortages or periods of staff downsizing, the issue of inadequate staffing may arise. Legal problems may result if the number of nurses is insufficient or if an appropriate mix of staff to provide competent care is lacking. If assigned to care for more patients than is reasonable, nurses should bring this information to the attention of the nursing supervisor. In addition, a written protest such as a workload or staffing report form should be completed to document the nurse's concerns about patient safety. Most provinces and territories have some reporting mechanism in place to document heavy workload or staffing situations. Although such a protest may not relieve nurses of responsibility if a patient suffers injury because of inattention, it would show that they were attempting to act reasonably. Whenever a written protest is made, nurses should keep a copy of this document in their personal files. Most administrators recognize that knowledge of a potential problem shifts some of the responsibility to the institution.

Nurses should not walk out when staffing is inadequate, because charges of abandonment could be made. A nurse who refuses to accept an assignment may be considered insubordinate, and patients would not benefit from having even fewer staff available. Delegation of appropriate tasks to other health care workers may be necessary and of value in some circumstances. The registered nurse is responsible to ensure the competence of the care provider and provide ongoing supervision (CNPS, 2000). It is important to know the institution's policies and procedures and the nursing union's collective agreement on how to handle such circumstances before they arise.

Floating. Nurses are sometimes required to "float" from the area in which they normally practise to other nursing units. Nurses must practise within their level of competence. Nurses should not be floated to areas where they have not been adequately cross-trained. Nurses who float should inform the nursing supervisor of any lack of experience in caring for the type of patients on the nursing unit. They should also request and be given orientation to the unit. A nursing supervisor can be held liable if a staff nurse is given an assignment he or she cannot safely perform. In one case (*Dessauer v. Memorial General Hospital,* 1981), a nurse in obstetrics was assigned to an emergency room. A patient entered the emergency room, complaining of chest pain. The obstetrical nurse gave the patient too high a dosage of lidocaine, and the patient died after suffering irreversible brain damage and cardiac arrest. The nurse lost the negligence lawsuit.

Prescriber's Orders. The physician is responsible for directing medical treatment. Nurses are obligated to follow physicians' orders unless they believe the orders are in error, violate hospital policy, or would harm patients. Therefore, all orders must be assessed, and if an order is found to be erroneous or harmful, further clarification from the physician is necessary. If the physician confirms the order and the nurse still believes it is inappropriate, the supervising nurse should be informed. A nurse should not proceed to perform a prescriber's order if harm to the patient is foreseeable. The nursing supervisor should be informed of and given a written memorandum detailing the events in chronological order; the nurse's reasons for refusing to carry out the order should also be written, to protect the nurse from disciplinary action. The supervising nurse should help resolve the questionable order. A medical or pharmacy consultant may be called in to help clarify the appropriateness or inappropriateness of the order. A nurse carrying out an inaccurate or inappropriate order may be legally responsible for any harm suffered by the patient.

In a negligence lawsuit against a physician and a hospital, one of the most frequently litigated issues is whether the nurse kept the physician informed of the patient's condition. To inform a physician properly, nurses must perform a competent nursing assessment of the patient to determine the signs and symptoms that are significant in relation to the attending physician's tasks of diagnosis and treatment. Nurses must be certain to document that the physician was notified and to document his or her response, the nurse's follow-up, and the patient's response. For example, nurses noticed that a patient with a cast on his leg was experiencing poor circulation in his foot. The nurses recorded these changes but did not notify the physician. Gangrene subsequently developed in the patient, and an amputation was required. The hospital, physician, and nursing staff were all charged with negligence.

The physician should write all orders, including "do not resuscitate" (DNR) orders, which some physicians may be reluctant to write out because they fear legal repercussions for criminal neglect or failure to act. The nurse must make sure that orders are transcribed correctly. Verbal orders are not recommended because they increase the possibilities for error. If a verbal order is necessary (e.g., during an emergency), it should be written and signed by the physician as soon as possible, usually within 24 hours. The nurse should be familiar with the institution's policy and procedures regarding verbal orders.

Dispensing Advice Over the Phone. Providing advice over the telephone is a high-risk activity because diagnosing over the phone is extremely difficult. The nurse is legally accountable for advice given over the phone. The most common allegations of negligence in this area are provision of inadequate advice, improper referrals, and failure to refer (CNPS, 2009c). It is essential that nurses precisely follow institutional guidelines and policies and thoroughly document each call to avoid serious repercussions for all parties.

Contracts and Employment Agreements. In Canada, most nurses belong to unions or associations that engage in collective bargaining on behalf of a group. The collective agreements between employers and union members are written contracts that set out the conditions of employment (e.g., salary, hours of work, benefits, layoffs, and termination). Many laws, including labour laws, apply to nurses. For example, laws outline eligibility for and details of workers' compensation and maternity benefits. It is important for nurses to understand the employment laws in the province or territory where they work.

By accepting a job, a nurse enters into an agreement with an employer. The nurse is expected to perform professional duties competently, adhering to the policies and procedures of the institution. In return, the employer pays for the nursing services and ensures that facilities and equipment are adequate for safe care.

LEGAL ISSUES IN NURSING PRACTICE

Abortion

In the 1988 case of *R. v. Morgentaler,* the Supreme Court of Canada ruled that the Criminal Code (1985) regulations on legal access to abortion were unconstitutional. The Criminal Code had required a woman seeking abortion to secure the approval of a hospital-based committee before the procedure could be performed. By rejecting the Criminal Code provisions, the Supreme Court in effect referred the abortion issue to Parliament, but Parliament has not rewritten a criminal law policy on abortion. Abortion is thus unregulated by law, which is tantamount to its legalization. However, the legal entitlement to abortion does not mean abortion services are readily available. Because health care facilities are not obliged to offer abortions, many do not do so. Thus, access remains a continuing issue.

Drug Regulations and Nurses

Canadian law closely regulates the administration of drugs. Two federal acts control the manufacture, distribution, and sale of food, drugs, cosmetics, and therapeutic devices in Canada: the *Food and Drugs Act* (1985) and the *Controlled Drugs and Substances Act* (1996). The *Food and Drugs Act* lists the drugs that can be sold only by prescription (e.g., antibiotics) and drugs that are subject to stringent controls (e.g., barbiturates, amphetamines). The distribution of these drugs requires specific handling and record keeping. The *Controlled Drugs and Substances Act* controls the manufacture, distribution, and sale of narcotics (e.g., morphine, codeine). However, it also regulates other drugs that are controlled in the same manner as narcotics, such as cocaine. Most institutions have policies about medication administration and record keeping, especially for controlled drugs and narcotics. Nurses must be aware of their employer's policies.

Nurses are not legally entitled to prescribe drugs. However, in several jurisdictions, nurse practitioners can prescribe certain non-narcotic or narcotic drugs specific to their area of practice. Which controlled substances NPs are authorized to prescribe, and what additional education is required for practising NPs to prescribe them, differs by province/territory (Canadian Nurse, 2013; CASN, 2016).

The administration of medications in accordance with a physician's prescription is a basic nursing responsibility. A competent nurse is expected to know the purpose and effect of any drug administered, as well as potential adverse effects and contraindications. It is also a nurse's responsibility to question any physician's orders that may be incorrect or unsafe. A nurse who follows a prescriber's order that is unclear or incorrect may be found negligent, disciplined, or dismissed by the employer, or investigated by the professional regulatory body (CNPS, 2007a).

Cannabis. The laws regarding the legalization and regulation of marijuana for both medical and recreational purposes are currently evolving in Canada. Since August 2016, the use of cannabis for medical purposes is governed by the *Access to Cannabis for Medical Purposes Regulations* (ACMPR). As use of cannabis grows, it is essential that nurses educate themselves on the federal, provincial, and territorial legislation that governs its use and consult current available evidence about potential health benefits and risks of cannabinoids (CNPS, 2017). Cannabis use in Canada will become legal in 2018 (Government of Canada, 2017). This may have further implications for health care providers.

Communicable Diseases

The care of people with communicable conditions such as HIV infection, hepatitis, or severe acute respiratory syndrome (SARS) or during a possible influenza pandemic has legal implications for nurses. Health care workers are at risk for exposure to communicable diseases because of the nature of their work. Despite the best attempts to protect oneself against communicable diseases through the proper and consistent use of protective gear (e.g., latex gloves or masks), accidental needle-stick injuries or life-threatening illnesses such as SARS and Ebola can occur. Nurses have an ethical and legal obligation to provide care to all assigned patients, and employers have an obligation to provide their employees with necessary protective gear. However, there may be "some circumstances in which it is acceptable for a nurse to withdraw from care provision or to refuse to provide care" (College of Registered Nurses of British Columbia (CRNBC, 2017, p. 1). "Unreasonable burden" is a concept raised in relation to duty to provide care and withdrawing from providing or refusing to provide care. "An unreasonable burden exists when your ability to provide safe care and meet the standards of practice is compromised by unreasonable expectations, lack of resources, or ongoing threats to personal well-being" (CRNBC, 2017, p. 1).

In all cases involving privacy, confidentiality, and disclosure, the rights of patients with a communicable disease must be balanced with the rights of the public or of health care providers. Both civil and criminal liability can result if private information is disclosed without authorization. Nurses must understand the reporting laws in the province or territory in which they practise. Courts can order disclosure of the records of patients with AIDS in situations that are not addressed by a statute, even without the patient's consent. Whenever information about a patient is requested by any third parties, including insurance companies or employers, nurses must obtain a signed release from the patient before releasing confidential information. Not every health care provider who comes in contact with a patient has a need to know the patient's disease status. Confidential information must be protected.

The courts have upheld the employer's right to fire a nurse who refuses to care for a patient with AIDS. Nurses who flatly refuse to care for HIV-infected patients or possibly a patient with SARS or Ebola may be reprimanded or fired for insubordination. According to the CNA's (2017a) *Code of Ethics for Registered Nurses,* nurses must not discriminate on the basis of a person's race, ethnicity, culture, political and spiritual beliefs, social or marital status, gender, gender identity, gender expression, sexual orientation, age, health status, place of origin, lifestyle, mental or physical ability, socio-economic status, or any other attributes (p. 15). One limitation outlined in the Code regarding a nurse's right to refuse care to a patient is that nurses are not obligated to comply with a patient's wishes when those wishes are contrary to the law. If care requested is contrary to the nurse's personal values, such as assisting with an abortion or medical assistance in dying (MAID), the nurse must provide appropriate care until alternative care arrangements are made.

Nurses must be concerned with balancing the right to protect themselves with protection of the patient's rights. Both are afforded protection against discrimination and protection of privacy by human rights legislation. Most current legal cases involving nurses and communicable diseases are related to the protection needed for nurses as employees. Strict compliance with standard precautions and routine practices and the use of transmission-based precautions (e.g., against airborne or droplet transmission) for patients known or suspected of having other serious illnesses is the nurse's wisest strategy (see Chapter 33).

End-of-Life Issues

Many legal issues surround the event of death, including a basic definition of when a person is considered dead. There is no federal legislation in Canada that defines death. The provinces of Manitoba, Newfoundland, and Prince Edward Island have legislatively defined death as "the irreversible cessation of all brain function" under respective vital statistics acts or included in organ/tissue donation legislation (Shariff, 2013). However, this "brain death" definition has become standard medical practice across Canada. Until the 1960s, death was defined as the irreversible cessation of cardiopulmonary function. However, two developments at that time necessitated a shift to consideration of the brain: (1) the emergence of artificial life-support devices that could maintain cardiopulmonary functioning in a brain-dead person, and (2) the emergence of organ transplantation. Death had to be redefined so that organs could be donated.

Homicide or Natural Death? The law draws a distinction between "killing" (an act of homicide) and "letting die." Withholding or withdrawing life-prolonging treatment is considered "letting die." The disease process causes the patient to die a natural death. Thus, a mentally competent patient has the legal right to refuse life-prolonging treatment. If, for example, such a patient requests that a ventilator be disconnected, understanding that she will die as a result, her wishes must be honoured in accordance with the principle of "no treatment without consent."

In the case of *Nancy B. v. Hôtel-Dieu de Québec* (1992), a young, mentally competent patient who was totally and permanently paralyzed by a neurological disease had twice asked that her ventilator be disconnected. After the second refusal, she sought a court order to enforce her will. The order was granted by the Quebec Superior Court, which ruled that as a mentally competent patient, she could not be treated without consent. Also, even if a patient has not asked for the termination of life-prolonging treatment (either directly or by way of an advance directive), physicians are still allowed, after consultation with family members, to terminate such treatment when it no longer offers any reasonable hope of benefit to the person. When patients reject life-prolonging treatment, the nurse focuses on the goal of caring versus curing.

Ethical and legal questions are raised by the related issues of euthanasia and assisted suicide. **Euthanasia** is an act undertaken by one person with the motive of relieving another person's suffering and the knowledge that the act will end the life of that person (Downie, 2004). Up until June 17, 2016, s.14 of the Criminal Code of Canada prevented an individual from obtaining the assistance of a doctor to end his or her life.

The prohibition on obtaining assistance in dying was challenged in Canada for the first time in 1993, when the Supreme Court of Canada ruled 5 to 4 against giving Sue Rodriguez the right to die by assisted suicide. The Victoria woman, who had amyotrophic lateral sclerosis

(ALS), later ended her life by suicide. On November 14, 2011, the Supreme Court of British Columbia began hearing arguments in a constitutional challenge to the Criminal Code sanctions against physician-assisted suicide. The trial, known as *Carter v. Attorney General of Canada*, was brought forward by the B. C. Civil Liberties Association and a group of individuals, including Gloria Taylor, who, like Sue Rodriguez, was afflicted with ALS (*Carter v. Canada* [Attorney General], 2011 BCSC 1371; Edwards, 2016).

In February 2015, a unanimous Supreme Court of Canada ruled in *Carter v. Canada* that sections of the Criminal Code violated the right to life, liberty, and security of the person, protected by s.7 of the *Canadian Charter of Rights and Freedoms* because the sections prohibited mentally competent adults from obtaining medical assistance to end their lives. This led to Bill C-14, an Act to amend the Criminal Code that now allows eligible individuals to request **medical assistance in dying (MAID)**. This legislation came into effect June 17, 2016, making it legally permissible for mentally competent adults who are suffering from a "grievous and irremediable medical illness, disease, or disability" in an advanced state causing intolerable suffering, to request MAID (Box 8-2). Only physicians or nurse practitioners can provide a person with MAID, either by administering a substance that causes death (euthanasia) or prescribing a substance (assisted suicide). Nurses, however, can assist by participating in discussions with individuals and family members, advocating for aggressive symptom management, and continuing to provide routine care. Nurses are not required to participate in the provision of MAID should they be morally opposed; however, the right to conscientious objection must be communicated with their supervisor as soon as they anticipate such a conflict arising.

It is essential that all health care providers have a thorough understanding of the law and of any related institutional processes and responsibilities (CNA, 2017b, 2017c; CNPS, 2016; Edwards, 2016).

BOX 8-2 Eligibility Criteria for Medical Assistance in Dying (MAID)

In order to be eligible for medical assistance in dying (MAID), a person must meet *ALL* of the following criteria:

- The person is eligible for publicly funded health services in Canada.
- The person is at least 18 years of age and capable of making health care decisions.
- The person has a GRIEVOUS and IRREMEDIABLE MEDICAL condition.
- The patient makes a voluntary request (no coercion) in writing (or by proxy, if the patient is unable to write), signed and dated in the presence of two independent witnesses.
- The patient must provide informed consent after being informed of all therapeutic options to relieve their suffering.

The definition of a GRIEVOUS and IRREMEDIABLE MEDICAL condition must meet *ALL* of the following criteria:

- The person has a serious and incurable illness, disease, or disability.
- The person is in an advanced state of irreversible decline in capacity.
- The illness, disease or disability OR the state of decline causes the patient enduring physical or psychological suffering that is intolerable and cannot be relieved under conditions considered acceptable to the patient.
- Natural death must be reasonably foreseeable, taking into account all of the person's medical circumstances.

Government of Canada. (2016). *An Act to amend the Criminal Code and to make related amendments to other Acts (medical assistance in dying).* S.C. 2016, c.3. Retrieved from http://laws-lois.justice.gc.ca/eng/AnnualStatutes/2016_3/FullText.html.

Advance Directives and Health Care Surrogates

The **advance directive** is a mechanism enabling a mentally competent person to plan for a time when he or she may lack the mental capacity to make medical treatment decisions. It takes effect only when the person becomes incompetent to speak for himself or herself. The advance directive is a more sophisticated concept than that of the living will, although the two terms are often confused. A **living will** is a document in which the person makes an anticipatory refusal of life-prolonging measures during a future state of mental incompetence. An advance directive, in contrast, is not restricted to the rejection of life-support measures; its focus is on treatment preferences, which may include both requests for and refusals of treatment. One caveat, at this time, is that a person cannot request MAID should they no longer be deemed mentally competent (http://laws-lois.justice.gc.ca/eng/AnnualStatutes/2016_3/FullText.html). The advance directive assumes two forms: the *instructional directive* (in which the maker of the document spells out specific directions for governing care, in more detail than is generally found in the living will), and the *proxy directive* (in which the person appoints someone as a health care agent to make treatment decisions on his or her behalf). Legislation in British Columbia, Alberta, Saskatchewan, Manitoba, Ontario, Prince Edward Island, Newfoundland and Labrador, and the Northwest Territories gives full legal effect to both kinds of directives; the proxy directive is also recognized in Quebec and the Yukon. Even in provinces and territories that do not recognize an instructional directive, nothing prohibits a physician from following a directive.

If nurses know about the existence of a health care directive, they are required to follow it. Nurses are also required to follow the wishes of a validly appointed proxy (assuming these instructions are legal). A proxy has the right to receive all medical information concerning the patient's condition and proposed plan of care. Failure to comply with a proxy's directions could result in charges of battery.

If a physician ignores the advance directive, the nurse must bring the advance directive to the physician's attention and document that he or she did so, along with the physician's response to this information. The nurse should also notify the nursing supervisor, who can then give direction regarding institutional policies and guidelines for such circumstances.

The *psychiatric advance directive* is a new type of advance directive. An individual with mental health problems completes this type of directive during periods of mental stability and competence. The directive outlines how the patient wishes to be treated in the future if the underlying mental illness causes him or her to lose decision-making capacity. For example, it may specify preferences for and against certain interventions (e.g., electroconvulsive therapy) or medications. The psychiatric advance directive can also designate a surrogate decision maker to act on the person's behalf in the event of an incapacitating mental health crisis.

Organ Donation

Legally competent people are free to donate their bodies or organs for medical use. Every province and territory has human tissue legislation that provides for both the *inter vivos* (live donor) and postmortem (cadaveric) donation of tissues and organs. For example, a mentally competent adult can donate a kidney, a lobe of the liver, or bone marrow. Statutes provide that adults may consent to organ donation after death. If the deceased has left no direction for postmortem donation, consent may be obtained from the person's family. In some provinces—Manitoba and Nova Scotia—the statutes contain "required request" provisions that take effect when a deceased person did not consent to organ removal but is considered a good donor candidate. In such an event, the physician is legally obliged to seek permission from the family. In many hospitals, a nurse transplantation coordinator performs this function. Since organs cannot be procured for transplant until death has been pronounced, and because of the critical shortage of organs available for transplant, national guidelines for pronouncing cardiac death for organ donation have been developed. Some provinces (e.g., Manitoba, New Brunswick, and Saskatchewan) do not accept cardiac death and rely strictly on brain death criteria. Despite the national guidelines, individual hospitals can determine whether to recognize cardiac death or not. Given variation across the country, it is essential that nurses be familiar with both provincial/territorial laws as well as institutional regulations (Library of Parliament, 2014).

Mental Health Issues

Treating patients with mental health problems raises legal and ethical issues. Provincial mental health legislation such as the *Mental Health and Consequential Amendments Act* (1998) provides direction for health care providers, protects patient autonomy, and recognizes that some individuals with severe mental health problems may lack the ability to appreciate the consequences of their health condition.

A patient can be admitted to a psychiatric unit involuntarily or on a voluntary basis. Patients admitted on a voluntary basis should be treated no differently than any other patient. They have the right to refuse treatment and the right to discharge themselves from the hospital. However, provincial or territorial mental health legislation provides that if the patient may cause harm to self or others, police officers (or other authorized parties) may bring the patient to a health care facility for examination and treatment without the patient's consent (Carver, 2013).

Potentially suicidal patients may be admitted to psychiatric units. If the patient's history and medical records indicate suicidal tendencies, the patient may be kept under supervision. A lawsuit may result if a patient attempts suicide within the hospital. The allegations in the lawsuits would be that the institution failed to provide adequate supervision or safeguard the facilities. Documentation of precautions against suicide is essential.

Public Health Issues

It is important that nurses, especially those employed in community health settings, understand the public health laws. Public health acts, which have been enacted in all provinces and territories, are directed toward the prevention, treatment, and suppression of communicable disease (Schulz, 2013). Community health nurses have the legal responsibility to follow the laws enacted to protect public health. These laws may include reporting suspected abuse and neglect, such as child abuse, elder abuse, or domestic violence; reporting communicable diseases; and reporting of other health-related issues to protect the public's health.

Some provinces (e.g., Ontario and New Brunswick) have legislation that requires proof of immunization for school entry. In these provinces, however, exceptions are permitted on medical or religious grounds and for reasons of conscience (Health Canada, 1997). Although a signed consent form is not required for an immunization, nurses are advised to obtain some documentation (evidence) that they discussed the risks and benefits with the parent or legal guardian. Nurses should be aware of their employer guidelines for documentation.

Every province and territory has child abuse legislation that requires health care providers, such as nurses, to report witnessed or suspected child abuse or neglect directly to child protection agencies. To encourage reports of suspected cases, the laws offer legal immunity for the reporter if the report is made in good faith. Health care providers who do not report suspected child abuse or neglect may be held liable for civil or criminal action. Several provinces and territories also have laws that require health care workers to report witnessed or suspected abuse of patients within facilities (e.g., *Protection of Persons in Care Act*, 2000, in Manitoba). These reports must be made directly to a public authority. Even if public reporting is not required, nurses should report all suspicions of patient abuse to their nursing supervisors. It is essential for nurses to know their provincial or territorial laws and employer policies regarding the reporting of abuse.

RISK MANAGEMENT

Risk management is a system of ensuring appropriate nursing care by identifying potential hazards and preventing harm from occurring (Guido, 2014). The steps involved in risk management include identifying possible risks, analyzing them, acting to reduce them, and evaluating the steps taken.

One tool used in risk management is the **incident report**, or **adverse occurrence report**. When a patient is harmed or endangered by incorrect care, such as a drug error, a nurse completes an incident report (see Chapter 15). Such reports are analyzed to determine how future problems can be avoided. For example, if incident reports show that drug errors commonly involve a new intravenous pump, the risk manager must ensure that staff members have been properly trained in its use. In-service education may be all that is necessary to prevent future errors.

The underlying rationale for quality assurance in risk-management programs is the highest possible quality of care. Some insurance companies and medical and nursing organizations require the use of quality assurance and risk-management procedures. Quality care is the responsibility of both the employer and the individual provider.

Risk management requires sufficient documentation. The nurse's documentation can be the evidence of what was done for a patient and can serve as proof that the nurse acted reasonably and safely. Documentation should be thorough, accurate, and performed in a timely manner. When a lawsuit is being evaluated, the nurse's notes are very often the first record to be reviewed by the plaintiff's counsel. If the nurse's credibility is questioned because of these documents, the risk of greater liability exists for the nurse. The nurse's notes are risk-management and quality assurance tools for the employer and the individual nurse.

Professional Involvement

Nurses must be involved in their professional organizations and on committees that define the standards of care for nursing practice. If current laws, rules and regulations, or policies under which nurses must practise do not reflect reality, nurses must become involved as advocates to see that the scope of nursing practice is accurately defined. Nurses must be willing to represent the nursing profession's perspective, as well as the patient's perspective in the community. Nurses can be powerful and effective when the organizing focus is the protection and welfare of the public entrusted to their care.

KEY CONCEPTS

- With increased emphasis on patient rights, nurses in practice today must understand their legal obligations and responsibilities to patients.
- The civil law system is concerned with the protection of a person's private rights, and the criminal law system deals with the rights of individuals and society.
- A nurse can be found liable for negligence if the following criteria are established: the nurse (defendant) owed a duty of care to the patient (plaintiff), the nurse did not carry out that duty, the patient was injured, and the nurse's failure to carry out the duty caused the patient's injury.
- Patients are entitled to confidential health care and freedom from unauthorized release of information.
- Under the law, practising nurses must follow standards of care, which originate in nursing practice acts and regulations, the guidelines of professional organizations, and the written policies and procedures of employing institutions.
- Nurses are responsible for confirming that the patient has given informed consent to any surgery or other medical procedure before the procedure is performed.
- Nurses are responsible for performing all procedures correctly and exercising professional judgement as they carry out prescriber's orders.
- Nurses are obligated to follow prescriber's orders unless they believe the orders are in error or could be detrimental to patients.
- Staffing standards determine the ratio of nurses to patients, and if the nurse is required to care for more patients than is reasonable, a formal protest should be made to the nursing administration.
- Mentally competent adults suffering from a "grievous and irremediable medical illness, disease or disability" in an advanced state may request medical assistance in dying.
- A competent adult can legally give consent to donate specific organs, and nurses may serve as witnesses to this decision.
- All nurses should know the laws that apply to their area of practice.
- Depending on provincial statutes, nurses are required to report suspected child abuse and certain communicable diseases.
- Nurses are patient advocates and ensure quality of care through risk management and lobbying for safe nursing practice standards.
- Nurses must file incident or adverse occurrence reports in all situations when someone could or did get hurt.

CRITICAL THINKING EXERCISES

1. Nurse Rossi and Nurse Kao are getting on an elevator to go down to the cafeteria. Several visitors are present in the elevator, as are hospital personnel. Nurse Rossi and Nurse Kao are talking about a patient who is in the Critical Care Unit who has just tested positive for HIV infection. They identify the patient as "the man in Room 14B." One of the visitors on the elevator who overhears this information is a woman who is engaged to the patient in Room 14B.
   a. Have Nurse Rossi and Nurse Kao breached a patient's right to confidential health care?
   b. Would the patient in Room 14B have any legal cause of action against the nurses?
   c. Even though the patient's fiancée may have a right to know the HIV status of her future husband, do the nurses have any duty to disclose confidential information to the fiancée?
2. While transporting a patient down the hall on a stretcher, Nurse Reyes stops to chat with an orderly. The side rails on the stretcher are down, and while Nurse Reyes has her back to the stretcher, the patient rolls over, falls off the stretcher, and fractures his hip. In a lawsuit by the patient against Nurse Reyes, what must the patient establish to prove negligence against the nurse?

REVIEW QUESTIONS

1. The nursing practice acts are an example of:
   1. Statute law
   2. Common law
   3. Public law
   4. Criminal law
2. Treating a patient without his or her consent is considered:
   1. Battery
   2. Negligence
   3. Implied consent
   4. Expressed consent
3. A nurse is sued for negligence for failure to properly monitor a patient after surgery. Which of the following statements are correct? *(Select all that apply.)*
   1. The nurse does not need any representation.
   2. The patient must prove that harm or injury occurred.
   3. The patient must show the nurse provided substandard care.
   4. The patient must show the nurse's actions or inactions caused the injury.
   5. The burden of proof is always the responsibility of the nurse.
4. A confused patient falling out of bed because side rails were not used when they were ordered is an example of which type of liability?
   1. False imprisonment
   2. Assault
   3. Battery
   4. Negligence
5. What should you do if you think the patient does not understand the procedure for which he or she is being asked to give consent?
   1. Do not be concerned if the consent is already signed.
   2. Notify the physician or nursing supervisor.
   3. Send the patient for the procedure and discuss it afterward.
   4. Ask a family member to give consent.
6. When a patient is harmed because of a nursing student's actions or lack of action, the liability is generally held by the:
   1. student
   2. student's instructor or preceptor
   3. hospital or health care facility
   4. All of the above
7. A nurse stops to help in an emergency at the scene of an accident. If the injured party files suit and the nurse's employing institution's insurance does not cover the nurse, the nurse would probably be covered by the:
   1. nurse's automobile insurance
   2. nurse's homeowner's insurance
   3. *National Care Act*, which may grant immunity from suit if the injured party consents
   4. Good Samaritan laws, which grant immunity from suit if no gross negligence is involved
8. The nurse is obligated to follow a prescriber's order unless
   1. The order is a verbal order
   2. The prescriber's order is illegible
   3. The order has not been transcribed
   4. The order is in error, violates hospital policy, or would be detrimental to the patient

9. When is it acceptable for a nurse to post information about a patient on a social networking site?
    1. If the patient's name is not provided
    2. If the posting is done anonymously
    3. If the site has privacy controls
    4. It is inappropriate to post patient information online

Answers: 1. 1; **2.** 1; **3.** 2, 3, 4; **4.** 4; **5.** 2; **6.** 4; **7.** 4; **8.** 4; **9.** 4

Rationales for the Review Questions appear at the end of the book.

RECOMMENDED WEBSITES

Canadian Nurses Association—Provincial/Territorial Members: https://www.cna-aiic.ca/en.

This CNA site offers up-to-date weblinks and contact information for all provincial and territorial nursing colleges and associations.

The Canadian Nurses Protective Society: http://www.cnps.ca.

The Canadian Nurses Protective Society (CNPS) helps nurses manage their professional legal risks by offering legal support and liability protection. The members-only section of the website provides information on a variety of legal topics affecting Canadian nursing practice.

Department of Justice Canada: www.justice.gc.ca.

This site provides links to consolidated statutes, including the Criminal Code (1985) of Canada.

The Health Law Institute of Dalhousie University: End-of-Life Law & Policy in Canada: http://eol.law.dal.ca/?page_id=221.

This site contains information about the Canadian law pertaining to various aspects of end-of-life care, including advance directives and withholding of life-sustaining treatment.

REFERENCES

Assisted Human Reproduction Act, S.C., c.2 (2004).

Canadian Association of Schools of Nursing (CASN). (2015). *National nursing education framework: Final report.* Retrieved from http://www.casn.ca/wp-content/uploads/2014/12/Framwork-FINAL-SB-Nov-30-20151.pdf.

Canadian Association of Schools of Nursing (CASN). (2016). *Nurse practitioner education competencies for prescribing controlled drugs and substances.* Retrieved from http://www.casn.ca/wp-content/uploads/2016/02/NP-Prescribing-Final-for-web.pdf.

Canadian Nurse (2013). *Expanding prescribing authority.* Ottawa: Author. Retrieved from https://www.canadian-nurse.com/articles/issues/2013/january-2013/expanded-prescribing-authority.

Canadian Nurses Association (CNA) (2017a). *Code of ethics for registered nurses.* Ottawa: Author.

Canadian Nurses Association (CNA) (2017b). *National nursing framework on medical assistance in dying in Canada.* Ottawa: Author.

Canadian Nurses Association (CNA) (2017c). *National nursing framework on medical assistance in dying in Canada.* Ottawa: Author. Retrieved from https://www.cna-aiic.ca/en/~/media/cna/page-content/pdf-en/cna-national-nursing-framework-on-maid.

Canadian Nurses Protective Society (CNPS). (1998, April). *Vicarious liability. infoLAW Bulletin, 7(1).*

Canadian Nurses Protective Society (CNPS). (2000, December). *Delegation to other health care workers. infoLaw Bulletin, 9(2).*

Canadian Nurses Protective Society (CNPS). (2003). *Defamation. infoLAW Bulletin, 12(3).*

Canadian Nurses Protective Society (CNPS). (2004, May). *Patient restraints. infoLAW Bulletin, 13(2).*

Canadian Nurses Protective Society (CNPS). (2007a, December). *Medication Errors. infoLAW Bulletin, 7(1).*

Canadian Nurses Protective Society (CNPS). (2007b, February). *Nursing students' FAQ.* Available to members only at http://www.cnps.ca/.

Canadian Nurses Protective Society (CNPS). (2009a, December). *Privacy and electronic medical records. infoLAW Bulletin, 18(1).*

Canadian Nurses Protective Society (CNPS). (2009b, December). *Telephone advice. infoLAW Bulletin, 6(1).*

Canadian Nurses Protective Society. (CNPS). (2009c, December). *Consent for the incapable adult. infoLAW Bulletin, 13(3).*

Canadian Nurses Protective Society (CNPS). (2010, December). *Social media. infoLAW Bulletin, 19(3).*

Canadian Nurses Protective Society (CNPS). (2012, February). *Supervision. infoLAW Bulletin, 20(1).*

Canadian Nurses Protective Society. (CNPS). (2013, November). *Mobile Devices in the Workplace. infoLAW Bulletin, 21(1).*

Canadian Nurses Protective Society. (CNPS). (2014, November). *Communicating with the Police. infoLAW Bulletin, 22(1).*

Canadian Nurses Protective Society (CNPS). (2016). *Medical assistance in dying: What every nurse should know.* Retrieved from http://www.cnps.ca/MAID.

Canadian Nurses Protective Society (CNPS). (2017). Cannabis for medical purposes: Legal implications for nurses. *The Canadian Nurse, 113*(1), 30–31.

Carter v. Canada (Attorney General), 2011 *BCSC 1371.*

Carver, P. (2013). Law and mental illness in Canada. In J. Irvine, P. Osborne, & M. Shariff (Eds.), *Canadian medical law* (4th ed.). Toronto: Carswell.

College of Registered Nurses of British Columbia (CRNBC) (2017). *Practice standard: Duty to provide care.* Vancouver: Author. Retrieved from: https://www.crnbc.ca/Standards/PracticeStandards/Pages/consent.aspx.

Constitution Act, 1867. Retrieved from http://laws-lois.justice.gc.ca/eng/Const/page-1.html.

Controlled Drugs and Substances Act, *S.C., c. 19* (1996).

Criminal Code of Canada, *R.S.C., c. C-46* (1985).

Dessauer v. Memorial General Hospital and Glorious Bourque, 96 N.M. 92; 628 P.2d 337; N.M (1981).

Dinh, V. (2016). *Facebook post leaves Prince Albert, Sask., nurse charged with professional misconduct. CBC News.* Retrieved from http://www.cbc.ca/news/canada/saskatoon/facebook-post-prince-albert-nurse-charged-professional-misconduct-1.3400676.

Downey v. Rothwell, *5 W.W.R. 311, 49 D.L.R. (3d) 82 (Alta. S.C. 1974).*

Downie, J. (2004). *Dying justice: A case for decriminalizing euthanasia and assisted suicide in Canada.* Toronto: University of Toronto Press.

Dubinsky, Z. (2017). *Nurse accused in seniors' deaths stated 'it wasn't accidental,' childhood friend says. CBC News.* Retrieved from http://www.cbc.ca/news/canada/elizabeth-wettlaufer-messages-glen-hart-1.4039077.

Edwards, M. (2016). Changing laws on medical assistance in dying: Implications for critical care nurses. *Canadian Journal of Critical Care Nursing, 27*(3), 18–23.

Emergency Medical Aid Act, R.S.N.W.T., c.E-4 (2000).

Food and Drugs Act, R.S.C., c. F-27 (1985).

Fridman, G. H. L. (2003). *Introduction to the Canadian law of torts* (2nd ed.). Markham, ON: LexisNexis.

Garner, B., & Black, H. (2009). *Black's law dictionary* (9th ed.). St. Paul, MN: West Publishing.

Government of Canada (2017). *Legalization and regulation of cannabis.* https://www.canada.ca/en/services/policing/justice/legalization-regulation-marijuana.html.

Granger v. Ottawa General Hospital, O.J. No. 2129 (Gen. Div. 1996).

Guido, G. (2014). *Legal and ethical issues in nursing* (6th ed.). Upper Saddle River, NJ: Prentice Hall.

Gunshot and Stab Wounds Mandatory Reporting Act (S.M. 2008, c.21). Retrieved from http://web2.gov.mb.ca/laws/statutes/ccsm/_pdf.php?cap=g125.

Health Canada. (1997, May). *Canadian national report on immunization, 1996.* Canada Communicable Disease Report (Suppl., Vol. 23, S4). Ottawa: Public Health Agency of Canada.

Irvine, J., Osborne, P., & Sharif, M. (Eds.) (2013). *Canadian medical law: An introduction for physicians, nurses and other health care professionals.* Toronto: Carswell.

Keatings, M., & Smith, O. (2010). *Ethical and legal issues in Canadian nursing* (3rd ed.). Toronto: Elsevier Canada.

Kolesar v. Jeffries, *9 O.R. (2d) 41, 59 D.L.R. (3d) 367 (S.C.C).* 1976.

Library of Parliament (2014). *Organ donation and transplantation in Canada.* Ottawa: Canada. Retrieved from: https://lop.parl.ca/content/lop/ResearchPublications/2011-113-e.pdf.

Malette v. Shulman, *CarswellOnt 642, 2 C.C.L.T. (2d), 1, 72 O.R. (2d),* (1990).

McIntyre, M., & McDonald, C. (2010). *Realities of Canadian nursing: Professional, practice, and power issues* (3rd ed.). Philadelphia, PA: Lippincott Williams & Wilkins.

Mental Health and Consequential Amendments Act, S.M., c. 36 (1998).

Meyer v. Gordon, *17 C.C.L.T. 1 (B.C. S.C).* 1981.

Nancy B. v. Hôtel-Dieu de Québec, *R.J.Q. 361, 86 D.L.R. (4th) 385, 69 C.C.C. (3d) 450 (S.C. 1992).*

Osborne, P. H. (2003). *Essentials of Canadian law: The law of torts* (2nd ed.). Toronto: Irwin Law.

Osborne, P. (2013). Consent to treatment. In J. Irvine, P. Osborne, & M. Shariff (Eds.), *Canadian medical law: An introduction for physicians, nurses and other health care professionals* (pp. 19–34). Toronto: Carswell.

Phillips, E. (2002). Managing legal risks in preceptorships. *Canadian Nurse, 98*(9), 25–26.

Protection of Persons in Care Act, *C.C.S.M. c. P144* (2000). Retrieved from http://web2.gov.mb.ca/laws/statutes/ccsm/p144e.php.

R. v. Morgentaler, *37 C.C.C. (3d) 449 (S.C.C. 1988).*

Regulated Health Professions Act, *1991, S.O., c. 18* (1991). Retrieved from http://www.e-laws.gov.on.ca/html/statutes/english/elaws_statutes_91r18_e.htm.

Roberts v. Cape Breton Regional Hospital, *162 N.S.R. (2d) 342 (S.C.)* (1997).

Saskatchewan Registered Nurses Association, & Strom, C. M. (2016). *Decision of the Discipline Committee.* Retrieved from http://www.srna.org/images/stories/RN_Competence/Comp_Assurance_Hearings/SRNA_Discipline_Decision_Strom_Redacted_Oct_27_2016.pdf.

Schulz, J. (2013). Public health law. In J. Irvine, P. Osborne, & M. Shariff (Eds.), *Canadian medical law* (4th ed.). Toronto: Carswell.

Shariff, M. (2013). Defining Death in Law and Medicine. In J. Irvine, P. Osborne, & M. Shariff (Eds.), *Canadian medical law: An introduction for physicians, nurses and other health care professionals* (4th ed.). Toronto: Carswell.

Tapp, A. (2003). New developments in privacy law. *The Canadian Nurse, 99*(3), 32.

9

Global Health

Written by Barbara J. Astle, RN, PhD, Sylvia S. Barton, RN, PhD, Leanne Johnson, RN, MN, Judy Mill, RN, PhD

OBJECTIVES

Mastery of content in this chapter will enable you to:

- Differentiate between global health, international health, and public health in the context of professional nursing.
- Describe factors and practices that contribute to environmental sustainability.
- Recognize and analyze epidemiological trends and patterns in the global burden of disease (GBD) and their relationship to population health.
- Describe the key challenges in the prevention and control of noncommunicable diseases (NCDs) and neglected tropical diseases (NTDs).
- Describe the United Nations (UN) Sustainable Development Goals (SDGs).
- Explain the potential positive health outcomes of the SDGs for groups, communities, and populations.
- Explain the phenomenon of global violence and its influence on the health of families, communities, and societies.
- Define the concept of intersectionality and its relevance to global health nursing.
- Describe the concepts of global citizenship and the professional roles of nursing in a global world.
- Describe the diversity of the Canadian population.
- Define key concepts related to health, illness, and diversity.
- Describe the historical development of the concept of culture, cultural competence, cultural safety, and cultural humility in relation to nursing practice.
- Analyze components of cultural assessment critical to understanding the values, beliefs, and practices of people experiencing cultural transitions.
- Apply research findings to the provision of culturally competent care that incorporates cultural safety and relational practice.
- Describe the role of nurses in responding to social and health challenges on a global scale.

KEY TERMS

MEDIA RESOURCES

http://evolve.elsevier.com/Canada/Potter/fundamentals/

- Audio Chapter Summaries
- Examination Review Questions
- Concept Map Creator
- Case Study with Questions
- Audio Glossary
- Content Updates
- Video Clips

GLOBAL HEALTH

As we progress through the twenty-first century, nurses have a key role to play in examining global health issues, developing solutions, and implementing change at both the local and global levels. It is imperative that such activities are informed by an understanding of health equity and social justice concepts, in order to respond to the pressing health and social challenges experienced by diverse populations worldwide (Canadian Association of Schools of Nursing [CASN], 2015; International Council of Nurses [ICN], 2014; Shamian & Ellen, 2016). As Ban Ki-Moon (2017) reminds us, "Saving our planet, lifting people out of poverty, advancing economic growth...these are one and the same fight. We must connect the dots between climate change, water scarcity, energy shortages, global health, food security and women's empowerment. Solutions to one problem must be solutions for all" (Brainy quotes, para. 1). Nursing's responsibility for global health is consistent with our history in advocating for social justice and is critical to ensure that global health inequities are minimized or eliminated. Thus, nurses need to have knowledge of key concepts related to the myriad of global health issues (CASN, 2015).

Global health refers to "the optimal well-being of all humans from the individual and collective perspective and is considered a fundamental human right, which should be accessible to all" (Canadian Nurses Association [CNA], 2009, p. 1). According to Koplan, Bond, Merson, et al. (2009), global health encompasses prevention, treatment, and care while focusing on the improvement of health for all and health equity. These authors argue that in addition to transnational health issues, global health is concerned with domestic health disparities. In addition they suggest that "the *global* in global health refers to the scope of problems, not their location" (p. 1994). For instance, poverty in inner-city neighbourhoods, limited access to health care in rural communities, and high rates of malaria among sub-Saharan African children are all examples of global health issues. In order to achieve global health, interdisciplinary collaboration and authentic partnerships between high-income and low- or middle-income countries are required to develop effective solutions for complex health issues (Koplan et al., 2009). Additionally, in order to strengthen health care systems, there is a need for a collaborative practice-ready workforce (Health Professions Networks Nursing and Midwifery, Human Resources for Health, 2010).

Koplan et al. (2009) suggest that global health overlaps with concepts derived from the disciplines of **public health**, global health, and **international health**. Each of these domains shares several common characteristics: a population-based and preventative focus, work with marginalized populations, a focus on multidisciplinary and interdisciplinary approaches, acknowledgement that health is a public good, an emphasis on systems and structures, and participation with key stakeholders. Table 9-1 compares the similarities and differences of each of the three domains.

Environmental Sustainability

Global **environmental sustainability** is defined as having an intact and healthy ecosystem (Government of Canada, 2017a). It has become increasingly apparent that having a healthy environment prevents disease (World Health Organization [WHO], 2016a). The WHO (2016a) estimated in 2012 that 12.6 million people died as a result of living or working in an unhealthy environment. Environmental risk factors, such as climate change; ultraviolet radiation; air, water, and soil pollution; and chemical exposures, contribute to more than 100 diseases and injuries. As a result, nurses have a role "to promote and support actions to optimize the health of the environment because of the link to human health" (CNA, 2017a, para 1). In addition, the focus on environmental sustainability has led to increased attention on the interdependence of humans, plants, and animals. This relationship has been referred to as **One Health**, which "recognizes that the health of people is connected to the health of animals and the environment" (Centers for Disease Control [CDC], 2017, para. 1). The primary goal of the One Health initiative is to foster collaboration between many disciplines working locally, nationally, and globally to achieve the best health for all people (CDC, 2017).

A related concept has been referred to as planetary health (Horton & Lo, 2015). In 2014, the Rockefeller Foundation Lancet Commission on Planetary Health met in Bellagio, Italy, and defined **planetary health** as "the achievement of the highest attainable standard of health, well-being, and equity worldwide through judicious attention to the human systems—political, economic, and social—that shape the future of humanity and the Earth's natural systems that define the safe environmental limits within which humanity can flourish. Put simply, planetary health is the health of human civilization and the state of the natural systems on which it depends" (Whitmee, Haines, Beyrer, et al.,

TABLE 9-1 Comparison of Global, International, and Public Health

	Global Health	International Health	Public Health
Geographical reach	Focuses on issues that directly or indirectly affect health but that can transcend national boundaries	Focuses on health issues of countries other than one's own, especially those of low and middle income	Focuses on issues that affect the health of the population of a particular community or country
Level of cooperation	Development and implementation of solutions often requires global cooperation	Development and implementation of solutions often requires bi-national cooperation	Development and implementation of solutions does not usually require global cooperation
Individuals or populations	Embraces both prevention in populations and clinical care of individuals	Embraces both prevention in populations and clinical care of individuals	Mainly focuses on prevention programs for populations
Access to health	Heath equity among nations and for all people is a major objective	Seeks to help people of other nations	Health equity within a nation or community is a major objective
Range of disciplines	Highly interdisciplinary and multidisciplinary within and beyond health sciences	Embraces a few disciplines but has not emphasized multidisciplinarity	Encourages multidisciplinary approaches, particularly within health sciences and with social sciences

From Koplan, J. P., Bond, T. C., Merson, M. H., Reddy, K. S., Rodriguez, M. H., Sewankambo, N. K., & Wasserheit, J. N. (2009). Towards a common definition of global health. *Lancet, 373*(9679), 1993–1995. doi:10.1016/S0140-6736(09)60332-9

2015). For example, as a result of deforestation, people and wildlife are in closer contact with one another, which can promote risks of various zoonotic diseases. In 2016, Prüss-Ustün, Wolf, Corvalán, and colleagues completed a comprehensive assessment of the burden of disease and reported that premature deaths and disease could be prevented through healthier environments. As a result, knowledge of the influences that environmental hazards and risks have on global health is important for nurses to critique and understand if they are to assist in the promotion of healthier environments.

It has become increasingly apparent that as the environment is affected by a host of other factors, such as climate change and natural disasters; the health of a population will be drastically altered. CNA believes that nurses have a key role "to promote climate change adaptation (that is, responding to the effects of climate change) and mitigation (taking action to reduce it)" (CNA, 2017b, para 3). With climate change, the danger of greenhouse gas emissions is one example in Canada that receives attention regarding environmental sustainability, resulting in some action within the portfolio of international development (Government of Canada, 2017). As a result, nurses can be instrumental in promoting behavioural changes in a population to reduce greenhouse gas (GHG) emissions. For example, nurses can educate persons about choices they can make for decreasing emissions from using their cars and using other forms of transportation, such as, riding a bike or walking (CNA, 2017b). As Thomas (2017) explains, an understanding of climate change and natural disasters is needed to transform economies and policies for a sustainable future. Natural disasters are a rising threat in response to the influence of global warming—there is a growing incidence of storms, floods, and droughts across the globe. The need for action in the form of sustainability requires a key understanding that the desires of the present must not lead to environmental destruction in the future.

Health Equity

Health equity is a concept that is fundamental to understanding and achieving global health for a population (see Chapter 4 for further information on population health). **Health disparities** are defined as "a particular type of health difference that is linked with social, economic, and/or environmental disadvantage. Health disparities adversely affect groups of people who have systematically experienced greater obstacles to health based on their racial or ethnic group; religion; socioeconomic status; gender; age; mental health; cognitive, sensory, or physical disability; sexual orientation or gender identity; geographic location; or other characteristics historically linked to discrimination or exclusion" (HealthyPeople.gov, 2014, para. 5). **Health inequities**, in contrast, refer to "those inequalities in health that are deemed to be unfair or stemming from some form of injustice. On one account, most of the health inequalities across social groups (such as class and race) are unjust because they reflect an unfair distribution of the underlying **social determinants of health (SDOH)** (for example, access to educational opportunities, safe jobs, health care, and social self-respect)" (Raphael, 2012, p. 2) (see Chapter 1 for further information on the social determinants of health). Through an understanding of politics and economics, Raphael helps us to understand how institutions and social structures shape the distribution of social, political, and economic resources that affect health inequities and disparities among the population. Thus, "an examination of how governing authorities come to either confront or ignore these health inequalities and the conditions that create them" becomes integral to the evolution of democratic societies (Raphael, 2012, p. 2; Raphael, 2016). Braveman and Gruskin (2003) suggest that **health equity** refers to the "absence of systematic disparities in health (and its key social determinants) that are systematically associated with social advantage/disadvantage" (p. 256). Health inequity puts disadvantaged groups at further disadvantage, with poverty often being the root cause. The inability of all persons living with human immunodeficiency virus (HIV) in sub-Saharan Africa to access care and treatment is an example of a health equity issue.

Braveman and colleagues (2011) caution that health inequity implies a judgement about the causality of differences and suggest that measuring health inequities relies on quantifying health disparities. The term *health equity* is a normative concept that reflects the value of social justice (Braveman, 2014; Braveman et al., 2011; Reutter & Kushner, 2010) (see Chapter 4 for further information on social justice). Thus, health equity is a critical and necessary element to achieve health for all, because of the underlying value that health is a human right. Reutter and Kushner (2010) argue that nursing has a strong and clear mandate to reduce health inequities among individuals, families, and communities, as well as to take action on the social conditions that contribute to health inequities. These authors suggest that nursing must provide sensitive, empowering care to individuals experiencing health inequities and, at the same time, participate in policy analysis and advocacy to reduce inequities.

Global Burden of Disease (GBD)

In order for nurses to address and understand some of the key issues in global health, it is imperative that they have access to reliable data and evidence. The **global burden of disease (GBD)** is an example of a metric that quantifies the health of populations at the regional, country, and other subnational levels (Skolnik, 2016). The GBD provides estimates of morbidity and mortality by cause, sex, age, and country for the period 1990 to the most recent year (GBD 2015 SDG Collaborators, 2016). In global health work, the composite indicator of health status that is most commonly used is called the *disability-adjusted life year,* or DALY. This indicator is consistently used in GBD studies. The DALY is the sum of years lost due to premature death (YLLs) and years lived with disability (YLDs). For example, for a man in Denmark who dies at age 50 with hypertension, he would have 25 years lost (YLLs), assuming the highest life expectancy for males in Denmark is 75 years. If this same Danish man lived with this disease for 10 years, and hypertension was assigned a burden of 0.5, then he would have lived with this disability for $10 \times 0.5 = 5$ YLDs. The DALY for this individual would be $25 + 5 = 30$ years.

Millennium Development Goals (MDGs) and Sustainable Development Goals (SDGs)

In 2000, the United Nations (UN) General Assembly established eight **Millennium Development Goals (MDGs)** to address key health and development issues affecting the global community (UN, 2015). A target date of 2015 was established to meet these goals. The MDGs were instrumental in creating a global partnership between all countries of the world and development institutions (WHO, 2015). While many achievements were made to meet the MDG targets, including reduction in poverty, educational improvements, reduction in child and maternal mortality, and improvements in lowering incidence of HIV, tuberculosis, and malaria, gaps between and within countries continue to exist, with vulnerable populations being most at risk.

In September 2015, to build on the MDGs, the UN General Assembly adopted the **Sustainable Development Goals (SDGs)**. The SDGs include 17 universal goals (Box 9-1) and 169 targets planned for the next 15 years and address the health and well-being of persons of all ages, including newborns, children, adolescents, and middle-age and older persons (UN, 2017a). The uniqueness of the SDGs is the importance for all countries to promote prosperity while providing protection to the planet. While the SDGs are not legally binding, there

BOX 9-1 The 17 Sustainable Development Goals Adopted by the UN General Assembly

1. End poverty in all its forms everywhere.
2. End hunger, achieve food security and improved nutrition, and promote sustainable agriculture.
3. Ensure healthy lives and promote well-being for all at all ages.
4. Ensure inclusive and equitable quality education and promote lifelong learning opportunities for all.
5. Achieve gender equality and empower all women and girls.
6. Ensure availability and sustainable management of water and sanitation for all.
7. Ensure access to affordable, reliable, sustainable, and modern energy for all.
8. Promote sustained, inclusive, and sustainable economic growth, full and productive employment, and decent work for all.
9. Build resilient infrastructure, promote inclusive and sustainable industrialization, and foster innovation.
10. Reduce inequality within and among countries.
11. Make cities and human settlements inclusive, safe, resilient, and sustainable.
12. Ensure sustainable consumption and production patterns.
13. Take urgent action to combat climate change and its impacts.
14. Conserve and sustainably use the oceans, seas, and marine resources for sustainable development.
15. Protect, restore, and promote sustainable use of terrestrial ecosystems, sustainably manage forests, combat desertification, and halt and reverse land degradation and halt biodiversity loss.
16. Promote peaceful and inclusive societies for sustainable development, provide access to justice for all, and build effective, accountable, and inclusive institutions at all levels.
17. Strengthen the means of implementation and revitalize the global partnership for sustainable development.

From United Nations (2017). *Sustainable development goals*. Retrieved from https://sustainabledevelopment.un.org/sdgs.

BOX 9-2 CHRONIC ILLNESS

Noncommunicable Disease—Diabetes Mellitus

What can nurses do to reduce the global incidence of diabetes mellitus (DM)?

- DM affects 422 million people globally, with the number of new cases increasing in low-income countries.
- Risk of heart attacks and strokes is 2–3 times higher in individuals with DM.
- DM may cause diminished blood flow, resulting in blindness, neuropathy, amputation, and kidney failure.

Nurse's Role

- Educate individuals about the importance of eating a healthy diet, being physically active, maintaining a healthy body weight, and abstaining from using tobacco to reduce the risk of developing DM.
- Discuss with individuals who are diagnosed with DM how to self-manage their disease, including how to access medications. (DM medications can be quite expensive. For example, the WHO reports that for persons living with DM in low- and middle-income countries, DM medications are only available in 65% of private and 49% of public health care facilities, respectively.)

Questions for Discussion

- When caring for patients with DM, what have you found to be effective in motivating behaviour change? What are the challenges?
- For patients diagnosed with DM, what do you think can be done about the high cost of diabetes medications and access to those medications?

From World Health Organization [WHO]. (2016). *Global report on diabetes*. Retrieved from http://apps.who.int/iris/bitstream/10665/204871/1/9789241565257_eng.pdf?ua=1; World Health Organization [WHO]. (2017). *Diabetes fact sheet*. Retrieved from http://www.who.int/mediacentre/factsheets/fs312/en/.

is an expectation that governments globally will assume ownership and establish national frameworks for achievement of the 17 goals (UN, 2017b). SDG number three specifically targets health directly, with five other goals focusing on environmental concerns. This approach aligns with a planetary perspective on health. The goals are primarily focused on ending poverty, protecting the planet, and ensuring prosperity (WHO, 2015). The UN General Assembly will closely monitor the progress over the subsequent 15 years (WHO, 2015). Nurses have a role in attaining the SDGs; the International Council of Nurses (2017) has stated that "nurses, as the primary providers of healthcare to all communities in all settings, are key to the achievement of the SDGs" (p. 3).

Noncommunicable Diseases

Noncommunicable diseases (NCDs), also known as chronic diseases, are not contagious, meaning they are not passed from individual to individual. There are four main types of noncommunicable diseases: cardiovascular diseases, chronic respiratory diseases, cancers, and diabetes (WHO, 2016b). The WHO stresses the importance of taking action to meet global targets to reduce the burden of NCDs, in order to prevent 16 million people dying prematurely (before the age of 70). It is acknowledged that many of these premature NCD deaths are preventable (WHO, 2014). Diabetes is one of the main NCDs that requires close attention from nurses (Box 9-2).

Neglected Tropical Diseases

Neglected tropical diseases (NTDs) are a diverse group of communicable diseases that predominate in tropical and subtropical conditions, affect more than one billion people, cost developing economies billions of dollars yearly, and occur in approximately 149 countries (WHO 2016c). NTDs are a group of chronic disabling conditions that primarily affect people who live in poverty, are without adequate sanitation, and are in close contact with infectious vectors and domestic livestock and other animals. Examples of some of the 17 major NTDs recognized by the WHO (2016c) are leprosy (Hansen's disease), dracunculiasis (guinea-worm disease), onchocerciasis (river blindness), and dengue and chikungunya.

Global Violence

It is imperative that nurses understand the relationship between violence and health. To gain perspective at the international level, nurses can consult varied resources by the WHO and UN on global violence. These organizations paint a dismal picture: globally about 1.6 million deaths occur every year as a result of violence, and at least 90% of those deaths take place in low- and middle-income countries (WHO, 2010). Worldwide, global violence is a leading cause of death for persons between 15 and 44 years of age (WHO, 2010). Violence against children is intolerable but, unfortunately, exists.

The *Global Status Report on Violence Prevention* (WHO, UN Development Program [UNDP], & UN Office on Drugs and Crime [UNODC], 2014) provides data retrieved from 133 countries and addresses different forms of violence—interpersonal violence, youth violence, elder abuse, intimate partner violence, and sexual violence. The report indicated that women, children, and older adults disproportionately experience nonfatal physical, psychological, and sexual abuse. Further, the data showed that about 25% of adults experienced physical abuse as children, 15% of women recalled sexual abuse as children, 33% of women described sexual and physical intimate partner violence, and 6% of older adults recounted abuse that had occurred in the past month (WHO, UNDP, & UNODC, 2014). Violence contributes to lifelong illnesses and premature death, particularly for women and children. Children who experience physical, emotional, and sexual violence are at greater risk for chronic diseases, HIV, severe mental health problems, crime, and drug abuse (WHO, UNDP, & UNODC, 2014). Many leading causes of death such as heart disease, stroke, cancer, and HIV are increased among people who have experienced violence, as such individuals may adopt harmful behaviours, such as smoking, alcohol and drug misuse, and unsafe sex, to mitigate the psychological impact of violence (WHO, UNDP, & UNODC, 2014).

Violence also places a heavy strain on health and criminal justice systems, social and welfare services, and the economic fabric of communities (WHO, UNDP, & UNODC, 2014). One of the challenges facing communities in responding to violence is to recognize that essential data on violence are often lacking. About 60% of countries do not have usable data on homicide from civil or vital registration sources (WHO, UNDP, & UNODC, 2014). For many of the countries where these data do exist, they often lack specificity, such as the sex and age of the victim, the relationship of victim to perpetrator, and the means of homicide—all of which are needed to design and monitor prevention efforts (WHO, UNDP, & UNODC, 2014). More disconcerting is the fact that most instances of violence against women, children, and adults do not come to the attention of authorities or service providers. Thus population-based surveys are a critical source of information to document the nature and extent of these problems. A growing number of scientific studies demonstrate that violence is preventable, yet there is great need for the international community to recognize interpersonal violence as an important health, criminal justice, development, and gender issue (WHO, UNDP, & UNODC, 2014).

Reports such as the *Global Status Report on Violence Prevention* have one directive in common: the need to scale up violence prevention programs, to enhance services for people experiencing violence, to better enforce laws, and to enact stronger legislation to protect vulnerable populations (WHO, UNDP, & UNODC, 2014). Much work needs to be done to create violence-free societies. Many organizations, including the Centers for Disease Control (CDC) in Atlanta, Georgia, United States, are committed to studying violence. As the knowledge grows and understanding increases, so will the effectiveness of violence prevention strategies that are implemented. Research on the interpersonal and social factors that are implicated in causing physical and psychological harm is needed by agencies and governments across nations in order to respond with science-informed prevention programs that can reduce injury and death caused by violence (WHO, 2010).

In every local context, knowledge of the availability of health care and of legal and social services for people experiencing violence can be delivered by nurses to clients and patients who are in need of it. Across every nation, nurses are in a key position to identify gaps and take team and community action to address violence that is all too prevalent in society (WHO, UNDP, & UNODC, 2014).

Gender Equality

Gender equality is the view that all people, regardless of gender, should be given equal treatment and not be discriminated against as a result of their gender. The United Nations Universal Declaration of Human Rights lists gender equality as one of its objectives, seeking to create equality in social situations, law, democratic activities, politics, the workplace, or any policy-designated realm (Gender equality, United Nations, 2017c). Gender inequality is viewed as a major obstacle to human development. Although progress in this area has occurred since 1990, girls and women throughout the world have not yet obtained gender equality. Discrimination related to education, health, political participation, employment, and the labour market that is experienced by women and girls results in negative developmental outcomes, reduced life opportunities, and compromised freedom of choice. The UN, along with other global agencies, has accepted several conventions focused on the promotion of gender equality (Gender Inequality Index [GII], 2016).

INTERSECTIONALITY

Intersectionality is a theoretical perspective regarding the influence of different social characteristics—race, ethnicity, gender, class, and socioeconomic status—on a particular phenomenon, such as the experience of health and its outcomes. For instance, by examining the interconnections between social relationships, dominance, and oppression, deeper insights may be revealed about a person's mental health status (Hankivsky, Reid, Cormier, et al., 2010).

An understanding of intersectionality is useful to nursing and offers a way to think about the complexities of human experience as well as making sense of them. Intersectionality arose from social, feminist, and postcolonial theories. In 1989, Black feminist scholar Crenshaw wrote on the influences of gender, ethnicity, cultural discrimination, geography, and immigration on health experiences and outcomes (Hankivsky, 2012). Crenshaw was particularly interested in Black feminism in the United States, Indigenous feminism, and Third World feminism. Her goal in the development of intersectionality theory was to describe the exclusion of Black women from the discourse that was focused on White feminism and antiracism (Hankivsky & Cormier, 2009). As a result, an intersectionality perspective was created that "moves beyond single or typically favoured categories of analysis (e.g., gender, race, and class) to consider simultaneous interactions between different aspects of social identity...as well as the impact of systems and processes of oppression and domination" (Hankivsky & Cormier, 2009, p. 3). Thus, an intersectionality perspective helps us to extend analytical boundaries of what we think we know about the health context of the human condition, to recognize that "these [multiple dimensions of social identity] come together in distinct ways and lead to distinct health outcomes for individuals [and] groups, providing context to health experiences and drawing attention to the dynamic interplay between different system levels" (Van Herk, Smith, & Andrew, 2011, p. 30).

Intersectionality theory is useful to building nursing knowledge. Nursing as a professional discipline includes attention to the needs of underserved or disadvantaged people across the lifespan. An intersectionality perspective offers a way to challenge the status quo and to generate knowledge and action focused on improving the welfare of marginalized and at-risk groups. A deeper understanding of poverty, marginalization, subordination, social exclusion, and social injustice will aid in directing attention toward reducing and eventually eliminating these conditions. Critical reflection related to the health of women, children, and family, and solutions to challenges arising from the complexities of gender and its interactions are needed (Hankivsky, 2012; Hankivsky & Cormier, 2009).

Nurses are well positioned to influence multilevel root causes of health disparities that deny people access to health services. Iyer, Sen, and Östlin (2008) conducted a literature review of class and gender and argued that a deeper understanding of the intersection of these two concepts was required. Specifically, the review revealed that the interactions of class and gender played a significant role in the health of women and their access to health services in high- and low-income countries (Iyer et al., 2008). Thus, intersectionality theory assisted the researchers to consider multiple factors that explained the health outcomes and to understand the interrelationships between these factors.

Intersectoral Action for Health (IAH)

The health and quality of life of populations in varying contexts are determined by many complex interrelated factors, many associated with the social determinants of health, such as education, transportation, and employment (all with social, environmental, and economic features) (Marmot & Allen, 2014). The health care sector alone cannot meet all the requirements for the health and well-being of a population. As a result, it is important that an **intersectoral action for health (IAH)** perspective be considered. This perspective refers to "the inclusion of several sectors in addition to the health sector when designing and implementing public policies to improve quality of life" (WHO, 2016d, para. 2). For example, local governments can assume a pivotal role in intersectoral action for health as they have influence over many health determinants related to education and transportation.

As explained by de Leeuw and Simos (2017), the term *intersectoral action for health* has been part of the terminology of health promotion and public health since the mid-1970s. The term achieved credence through the WHO, the Ottawa Charter, and the Alma Ata Declaration. Although there are various ideas related to the interpretation of this term, this focus of health promotion and public health hinges on working together for health, leveraging networks, and exercising action. Successful intersectoral action inspires people, groups, organizations, and communities to come together to jointly act on determinants of health and health concerns. For instance, to take action on human health affected by toxic and polluted environments, policies to reduce lead levels in paints and gasoline in some African nations are considered industrial and economic in nature. Such a population health concern clearly requires commitments from industry, but also deep involvement of other sectors, such as government (de Leeuw & Simos, 2017).

Global Citizenship

Global citizenship is a concept that has been discussed for many years and has been advocated by a variety of disciplines, including education, law, community health, epidemiology (Landorf & Feldman, 2015) and increasingly in nursing (Burgess, Reimer-Kirkham, & Astle, 2014; Mill, Astle, Ogilvie, et al., 2010; Chavez, Peter, & Gastaldo, 2008; Simpson, Jakubec, Zawaduk, et al., 2015). Mill and colleagues (2010) argue that it is necessary for professional nurses to examine their role and responsibilities in relation to global citizenship. As a framework, global citizenship is necessary to shift the perspectives of nursing students toward a more critical inquiry of global issues (Burgess et al., 2014). A **global citizen** incorporates not only an *inward* personal awareness and commitment to global issues but also *outward* actions on local or global issues (Hanson, 2010). Byers (2005) suggests that "global citizenship empowers individuals to participate in the decisions concerning their lives, including the political, economic, social, cultural and environmental conditions in which they live" (p. 37). The common thread in global citizenship is our *interconnectedness* and the acknowledgement that the local and global are intertwined, with one perspective not privileged over the other (Mill et al., 2010). According to Oxfam (2015), the characteristics of a global citizen include, but are not limited to, awareness of the wider world; respecting and valuing diversity; contributing to the community at a local and global level; striving toward sustainability in the world; taking responsibility for our own actions; and acting on social injustice. The roots of social responsibility in nursing can be traced to pioneers such as Florence Nightingale, Margaret Sanger, Lavinia Dock, and Lillian Wald (Kelley, Connor, Kun, et al., 2008). Nurses have an extensive history of working with the marginalized in society and continue to do so into the present, advocating for social justice across low- and high-resourced nations worldwide (CNA, 2010a).

CULTURAL DIVERSITY

Canada has always been a multicultural nation. **Multiculturalism** is a process whereby "many cultures co-exist in society and maintain their cultural differences. Multiculturalism also refers to the public policy of managing cultural diversity in a multiethnic society, emphasizing tolerance and respect for cultural diversity" (Srivastava, 2007a, p. 323). In Canada, multiculturalism is viewed as a fundamental belief that all citizens are equal. In 1971, Canada became the first country in the world to officially adopt a multiculturalism policy (Government of Canada, 2017b). Since then, various laws have been passed to protect and promote the rights of minorities in Canada (Box 9-3). As expressed in the spirit of the multicultural policy, citizens are able to retain their unique ethnocultural traditions within a Canadian context.

At the time of Confederation, more than 50 Indigenous groups—each with its own language and culture—lived in Canada, in addition to the founding British and French settlers and other settlers migrating primarily from European countries. Canada is well known as a country that embraces diversity, relying heavily on immigration for population

BOX 9-3 Legislation Recognizing Diversity in Canada

***Official Languages Act* (1969; Updated 1988)**
This Act recognizes English and French equally as Canada's official languages. The 1988 amendment to this Act outlines the obligations of Canadian federal institutions to be committed to promoting full recognition and use of both English and French in Canadian society, as well as supporting the development of the anglophone and francophone communities across the country.

***Canadian Constitution Act* (1982)**
This Act replaced the *British North America Act* as Canada's Constitution, outlining how Canada governs and structures its society. It also recognizes the Aboriginal peoples of Canada as Indians (Status and Non-Status), Inuit, and Métis.

Canadian Charter of Rights and Freedoms (1982)
Written into the *Canadian Constitution* in 1982, this charter is a statement of the basic human rights and freedoms of all Canadians.

***Canadian Multiculturalism Act* (1988)**
In recognition of Canada's cultural diversity, this Act enshrines the enhancement and preservation of multiculturalism in Canada.

growth. As a result, the societal landscape changes continuously, integrating people from many ethnic groups who have migrated to this country and formed a cultural mosaic that is uniquely Canadian.

The ethnocultural profile of Canada is continually evolving (Statistics Canada, 2017a). More than 250 ethnic origins or ancesteries were reported by the Canadian population in the 2016 census (Statistics Canada, 2017a). After Canadian, the other most frequently reported origins in 2016, either alone or with other origins, were English, French, Scottish, Irish, German, Italian, Chinese, Indigenous (see Chapter 10 for further information on Indigenous peoples), Ukrainian, East Indian, Filipino, Dutch, and Polish. According to the 2016 Canadian census, visible minorities accounted for 30% of Canada's total population, and of these 30% were born in Canada and 65.1% were born outside the country (Statistics Canada, 2017a). The *Employment Equity Act* defines visible minorities as persons, other than Indigenous groups, who are non-Caucasian in race or nonwhite in colour (Statistics Canada, 2013a).

The three largest visible minority groups in Canada are South Asians, Chinese, and Blacks. South Asians surpassed Chinese as the largest visible minority group in 2006 (Statistics Canada, 2013a). In 2016, South Asians represented 25.1% of all visible minorities and 4.8% of the total population, Chinese accounted for about 20.5% of the visible minority population and 4% of the total population, and Blacks accounted for 15.6% of the visible minority population and represented 22.3% of the population (Statistics Canada, 2017b).

Immigration and Migration

Canada's valuing of multiculturalism is reflected within the ethnocultural diversity of its population: approximately 20% of the total population are immigrants. According to the 2016 census, approximately one in five people of Canada's total population were born outside the country (Statistics Canada, 2017c). A *foreign-born population* is also known as an *immigrant population* and is defined as persons who are, or who have been, landed immigrants/permanent residents in Canada (Statistics Canada, 2013a). Canada ranks second only to Australia as the country with the highest proportion of foreign-born citizens. The largest groups of immigrants to Canada are from Asian and Middle Eastern countries; this fact has remained virtually unchanged since the 2001 census. In contrast, during 1971, only 12.1% of immigrants to Canada were born in Asian and Middle Eastern countries, and 61.6% were born in Europe. By 2011, 56.9% of recent immigrants were Asian and only 13.7% were European born (Statistics Canada, 2013a). By 2006, immigration had outpaced the natural birth rate of the country (Statistics Canada, 2013a). Thus, immigrants and refugees come to Canada from many places and are part of more than 200 ethnocultural groups across the country (Statistics Canada, 2017c). **Refugees** are individuals who are forced to flee from persecution in their home country. In 2016, the top five source countries from which refugees came to Canada were Nigeria, Hungary, China, Iraq, and Pakistan (Immigration Watch Canada, 2017). Asylum seekers are individuals who have fled their country and have sought international protection (United Nations High Commissioner of Refugees [UNHCR], 2017). Internally **displaced persons** are individuals who are forced to leave their homes because of conflict, violations of human rights, or environmental disasters, yet remain in their home country (UNHCR, 2017).

People immigrate to another country for various reasons and have different motivations for doing so. Refugees may be relocated without having chosen their new location, in contrast to immigrants, who are able to choose where they live. Refugees tend to experience greater dislocation and deprivation than do immigrants who enter Canada with specialized skills and education and who have the option to return to their homeland. Although acculturation and length of residence in the new country are related, outcomes may be affected by other factors, such as education, racial characteristics, and familiarity with language and religion.

As a nurse, you may ask patients about the circumstances that brought them to Canada and how they believe they are adjusting. It is important to understand any problems that the patient may have (such as becoming comfortable with routines or with the language used to arrange medical appointments) in order to make reasonable and appropriate adjustments to care (Box 9-4). Nurses should also be aware that newly arrived immigrants and refugees, depending on the geographic location from which they came, are vulnerable to a variety of health conditions, including tuberculosis, hepatitis B, anemia, dental caries, intestinal parasites, nutritional deficiencies, incomplete immunization, and mental and emotional concerns such as depression and post-traumatic stress disorder. New immigrants and refugees also

BOX 9-4 Use of an Interpreter

Health care providers and patients must communicate clearly and effectively to ensure safe, patient-centred, high-quality care (Access Alliance, 2009). Canadians who do not speak the two official languages, English or French, may have difficulty accessing health care services and may experience health inequities (Access Alliance, 2009). To improve access and address language barriers, professional interpreters can be utilized. Interpreters may be available through the hospital, health care centre, local community organizations, or a language telephone line. It is important that an interpreter be used consistently and appropriately to meet the needs of patients.

Appropriate use of an interpreter:
- Ask if a male or female interpreter is preferred.
- Allot extra time for the visit.

Before the appointment:
- Be respectful of the interpreter's time.
- Discuss goals of the visit with the interpreter, and emphasize that the patients must make all medical decisions themselves.

During the appointment:
- Sit in a triangular arrangement so that everyone can see nonverbal cues.
- Introduce the interpreter and patient. Clarify how much of the discussion the patient wants to have interpreted, as he or she may have some understanding of English or French.
- Look at patients directly when speaking and while the interpreter is speaking. Use "I" and "You."
- Speak slowly and clearly; use short sentences and pause frequently.
- Avoid medical jargon and repeat important information to reinforce key messages.

After the appointment:
- Debrief with the interpreter to find out if there is anything observed that the health care provider should be aware of.
- If available, provide written material in the patient's primary language.
- The interpreter can arrange any follow-up appointments with the patient.

From Access Alliance. (2009). *Literature review: Costs of not providing interpretation in health care* (Access Alliance publication LR0004). Toronto, Canada: Author. Retrieved from http://accessalliance.ca/wp-content/uploads/2015/03/Lit_Review_Cost_of_Not_Providing_Interpretation.pdf; Hilliard, R. (Ed.). (2016). *Using interpreters in health care settings.* Retrieved from http://www.kidsnewtocanada.ca/care/interpreters#using-an-interpreter-appropriately.

BOX 9-5 RESEARCH HIGHLIGHT

A Study of Iranian Immigrants' Experiences of Accessing Canadian Health Care Services: A Grounded Theory

Research Focus

The aim of this study by Dasjerdi, Olson, and Ogilvie (2012) was to explore and understand the experiences of Iranian immigrants who had accessed Canadian health care services.

Research Abstract

Canada is a multicultural society with a diverse population. Foreign-born individuals account for approximately 20% of the total population, and the health service needs of immigrants may differ from those born in Canada. Therefore, it is important to learn about the strategies that newcomers develop to access health care systems. The research question in this study was "What are the processes by which Iranian immigrants learn to access health care services in Canada?"

Methods

A constructivist grounded theory approach was utilized to answer the research question. Researchers who use grounded theory link concepts, events, and situations described by the research participants to generate a theory that shows the relationship among the elements. The participants included both refugees and those who came to Canada independently. Unstructured interviews were conducted to address the research question.

Findings

The core category that emerged from the research was *Tackling the Stumbling Blocks of Access,* and the basic social process (BSP) that was explored was *Becoming Self-Sufficient.* There are five stages to this BSP: becoming a stranger, feeling helpless, navigating/seeking information, employing strategies, and becoming integrated and self-sufficient. This process provided insight into why some Iranian immigrants were able to access Canadian health care effectively whereas others were not. Iranian immigrants in this study experienced many challenges in accessing health care services in Canada, and while some immigrants overcame these challenges, others continued to experience barriers.

Conclusions

Many elements influence Iranian immigrants' ability to access the health care system effectively and appropriately, including language proficiency, cultural differences, education, previous experiences, financial status, age, knowledge of the host country's health care services, and insider and outside resources.

Clinical Implications

- The findings highlight the need for a culturally competent health care system and for health care providers to be culturally aware and engage with clients from diverse backgrounds.
- Health care institutions may want to consider hiring health care providers who are immigrants themselves, in order to help culturally diverse populations gain trust in and access to the health care system.
- Medical interpreters and cultural brokers should be utilized during health care interactions.
- Nursing education programs should integrate culture and its effect on health into the curriculum and seek opportunities for students to work with the immigrant population.

Dasjerdi, M., Olson, K., & Ogilvie, L. (2012). A study of Iranian immigrants' experiences of accessing Canadian health care services: A grounded theory. *International Journal for Equity in Health, 11,* 55. doi:10.1186/1475-9276-11-55. Retrieved from http://www.equityhealthj.com/content/11/1/55.

frequently experience language barriers, social isolation, separation from family, loss and grief, and a lack of information about available resources. It is important that nurses explore the historical and sociopolitical background of a patient with regard to the specific immigrant community; this knowledge can assist nurses in formulating a plan of care (Lo & Pottinger, 2007). Nurses should be aware of, and advocate for, primary health care programs in the community that are specific to immigrants and refugees (Box 9-5).

Two other significant groups in Canada's cultural mosaic are Indigenous peoples and the population of French ancestry. In the 2016 census, there were more than 1.6 million people who identified themselves as Metis, First Nations or Inuit, representing 4.9% of the total Canadian population (Statistics Canada, 2017). (see Chapter 10 for further discussion about Indigenous health). Citizens who spoke only French totaled more than 7.1 million (20.6%) people, of more than 34 million Canadians, with the vast majority residing in Quebec (Statistics Canada, 2017). Nurses require an understanding of cultural differences in order to critically perceive the diversity influences that shape healing, well-being, and patterns of caring (Racher & Annis, 2012).

UNDERSTANDING CULTURAL CONCEPTS

Clarification of key concepts related to culture and ethnicity are crucial to understanding their complexity. The Canadian Nurses Association (2010b) describes **culture** broadly as shared patterns of learned values and behaviours that are transmitted over time and that distinguish the members of one group from another. Culture can include language, ethnicity, spiritual and religious beliefs, socioeconomic class, gender, sexual orientation, age, group history, geographic origin, and education, as well as childhood and life experiences. According to CNA's (2017c) *Code of Ethics,* When providing care, "nurses do not discriminate on the basis of a person's race, ethnicity, culture, political and spiritual beliefs, social or marital status, gender, gender identity, gender expression, sexual orientation, age, health status, place of origin, lifestyle, mental or physical ability or socioeconomic status or any other attribute" (p. 15). More recently, Hartrick Doane and Varcoe (2015) defined culture "as a dynamic relational process of selectively responding to and integrating particular historical, social, political, economic, physical, and linguistic structures and processes. That is, culture is relationally determined and contextual" (p. 139). This definition of culture allows nurses to avoid making incorrect assumptions, omitting other important influences, and stereotyping. As well, a relational definition of culture encourages nurses to explore the contextually mediated influences shaping one's life and health rather than basing their care on ethnicity, race, or nationality. In sum, "cultural difference is not limited to difference based on membership in an ethnic or racial group, but rather encompasses differences in experience, meaning, and what is significant to particular individuals and families" (Hartrick Doane & Varcoe, 2015, p. 139–140).

Ethnicity refers to groups whose members share a social and cultural heritage. In Canada, the prevalent cultures are anglophones and francophones with origins from Western Europe. **Subcultures** (e.g., Ukrainian and Acadian) represent various ethnic, religious, and other groups with distinct characteristics. Members of ethnic groups, for example, may share common values, language, history, physical characteristics, and geographical space. The most important characteristic of an ethnic group is that its members feel a sense of common identity. For example, people may declare their ethnic identity as Scottish, Vietnamese, or Colombian. A term that is usually contrasted with ethnicity is race, which is limited to the common biological attributes, such as skin colour, shared by a group (Spector, 2012).

Cultural pluralism is a perspective that "promotes respect for the right of others to have different beliefs, values, behaviours, and ways of life" (Racher & Annis, 2012, p. 159). Cultural relativism "fosters awareness and appreciation of cultural differences, rejects assumptions of superiority of one's culture and averts ethnocentrism" (Racher & Annis, 2012, p. 159). In any intercultural encounter, nurses "are challenged to be open and responsive to cultural differences, while respecting, protecting, and promoting the rights and well-being of those people and groups with whom they work" (Racher & Annis, 2012, p. 160). Because Canada is a major immigrant-receiving country, it is important for nurses to be able to provide care that is responsive to cultural differences. As Ogilvie (2011) suggests, such diversity requires nurses to seek out knowledge on what cultural competence is, what cultural safety is, and what the connection is between the two. Community health nurses, for example, may need to be knowledgeable about parenting in newcomer families in order to develop a portrait of the health and well-being of these families (Wilkinson, Anchan, Arthur, et al., 2010).

The processes of enculturation and acculturation facilitate cultural learning. Socialization into one's primary culture during childhood is known as enculturation. The process of adapting to and adopting characteristics of a new culture is acculturation (Cowan & Norman, 2006). Acculturation outcomes may result in varying degrees of affiliation with the mainstream culture (Spector, 2012). Assimilation is a process whereby a minority group gradually adopts the attitudes and customs of the mainstream culture (Srivastava, 2007b). In relation to acculturation, the notion of integration may be viewed as an example of an adaptive process of acculturation. *Multiculturalism,* by contrast, describes the situation when cultures coexist and maintain their cultural differences.

Cultural Conflicts

Culture provides the context for valuing, evaluating, and categorizing life experiences. As values, morals, and norms are transmitted from one generation to another, members of ethnic groups may display ethnocentrism, a tendency to view their own way of life as more valuable than others'. Health care providers who do not understand cultural differences often resort to cultural imposition, in which they use their own values and beliefs as the absolute guide to interpreting patients' behaviours and providing services. Hence, if a nurse believes that pain is to be borne quietly as a demonstration of strong moral character, that nurse may be annoyed by a patient's insistence on being given pain medication and, in denying the patient's discomfort, may exacerbate the patient's pain.

Ethnocentrism is the root of stereotypes, biases, and prejudices against other people perceived to be different from the valued group. Stereotypes are generalizations about any particular group that prevent further assessment of unique characteristics. When a person acts on his or her prejudices, discrimination may occur. Discrimination refers to treating people unfairly on the basis of their group membership. Racism involves specific actions and an attitude whereby one group exerts power over others on the basis of either skin colour or racial heritage; its effects are to marginalize and oppress some people and to endow others with privileges (Srivastava, 2007b). Often, people do not realize that they are displaying prejudice or discrimination; such displays may be simply negative or fearful reactions to cultural differences.

HISTORICAL DEVELOPMENT OF THE CONCEPT OF CULTURE

It is important for nurses to understand the historical development of the concept of culture and shifts in thinking about the provision of culturally competent care. Framed primarily within the Canadian context, this history is also best discussed in terms of culturally appropriate nursing practice and education. The importance of being culturally sensitive and aware of a diverse society has been acknowledged by nurses and continues to evolve. Nurses became aware of the conceptual limitations of culture, partly by studying the complexities of race (Ramsden, 2002). Through a critical cultural analysis of the significance of power relations and structural constraints on health and health care, nurses are conceptualizing new ways to provide culturally competent and culturally safe care (Anderson, Perry, Blue, et al., 2003; Baker, 2007; Browne, Varcoe, Smye, et al., 2009; Gustafson, 2007; Hartrick Doane & Varcoe, 2015; Racine, 2009; Ramsden, 2002; Smith, Edwards, Varcoe, et al., 2006).

A critical historical view of transcultural nursing, cultural competence, and cultural safety is important for understanding the strengths and limitations of these approaches in nursing practice and education (Gustafson, 2005; Hartrick Doane & Varcoe, 2015). Increasingly, nurse scholars are questioning whether the health needs of ethnocultural groups are being equitably met (Hartrick Doane & Varcoe, 2015). Health equity may be considered one of the prerequisites and conditions for health. Ogilvie, Astle, Mill, et al. (2005) explained that "nurses can play a pivotal role by becoming informed advocates, challenging their organizations to incorporate a global health mandate and exercising their rights as citizens to influence policy" (p. 25).

The discipline of anthropology and the seminal work by Leininger (2002a) relative to culture have provided the theoretical foundation for transcultural nursing (Glittenberg, 2004). Leininger (2002a) defined transcultural nursing as a comparative study of cultures, an understanding of similarities (culture universal) and differences (culture specific) across human groups in order to provide meaningful and beneficial delivery of health care. According to Leininger, the goals of transcultural nursing are to provide *culturally congruent* and *culturally competent care.*

Culturally congruent care is "the use of sensitive, creative, and meaningful care practices to fit with the general values, beliefs, and lifeways of clients" (Leininger & McFarland, 2002, p. 12). In other words, nurses must provide care that does not conflict with patients' valued life patterns and sets of meanings, which may be distinct from their own (Leininger, 2002b).

Leininger and McFarland (2002) defined culturally competent care as "the explicit use of culturally based care and health knowledge in sensitive, creative, and meaningful ways to fit the general lifeways and needs of individuals or groups for beneficial and meaningful health and well-being or to help them face illness, disabilities, or death" (p. 84). To provide culturally competent care, nurses must bridge cultural gaps in care, work with cultural differences, and enable patients and families to receive meaningful care. Nurses need to exhibit specific ability, knowledge, sensitivity, openness, and flexibility toward the appreciation of cultural difference. They are then able to develop effective and meaningful interventions that promote optimal health for patients, families, and communities.

Leininger's Sunrise Model (2002a) has been the prevailing model used in nursing to promote culturally competent care with people from diverse cultures. It has been used as a guide in nursing curricula and practice policies in North America for several decades. In addition, other scholars have developed models of cultural competency in which they have expanded Leininger's work. Davidhizar and Giger (1998;

Giger, 2013) developed a transcultural assessment model with a focus on cultural competency that is also used in nursing practice. The underlying premise of their model is that each person is culturally unique and should be assessed according to six cultural phenomena: communication, space, social organization, time, environmental control, and biological variations. This model suggests that these phenomena are apparent in all cultural groups, but their application to practice settings varies. Giger and Davidhizar's (2002) transcultural assessment model offers a means for nurses to assess patients' unique health care needs, including their specific cultural health practices.

Campinha-Bacote (2002) defined *cultural competence* as an ongoing process, whereby nurses continuously strive to work within the patient's cultural context. As a result, nurses develop cultural competence rather than possess it. This ongoing process involves integrating cultural awareness, knowledge, skill, encounters, and desire. *Cultural awareness* involves an in-depth self-examination to recognize biases, prejudices, and assumptions about other people in order to develop insight into one's own background. *Cultural knowledge* refers to knowing about the patient's culture. It involves learning about the values, health beliefs, care practices, and world views of diverse groups. The development of *cultural skills* involves the assessment of social, cultural, and biophysical factors that influence patient care. *Cultural encounters* involve engaging in cross-cultural interactions that can teach about other cultures. *Cultural desire* is the motivation and commitment to learn from other people, to accept the role as learner, to be accepting of cultural differences, and to build relationships based on cultural similarities.

Narayanasamy (2002), a nurse scholar in Britain, also developed a framework to foster the development of cultural competence. This framework is referred to as the ACCESS model (**a**ssessment; **c**ommunication; **c**ultural negotiation and compromise; **e**stablishing respect and rapport; **s**ensitivity; and **s**afety). The focus of this model is on developing cross-cultural communication, cultural negotiations, diversity, and celebrations, and on fostering cultural safety (Narayanasamy & White, 2005).

In Canada, CNA (2010b) advocates in its position statement that culturally competent care can and should be practised in all clinical settings. Cultural competence is viewed as a key concept in the application of knowledge, skill, attitudes, and personal attributes by nurses in the provision of appropriate care and services in relation to the cultural characteristics of patients. A nurse practising in this way, for instance, values diversity, is interested in and seeks out knowledge about cultural mores and traditions from diverse patients, and is sensitive to these traditions while caring for culturally diverse persons. Although nurses are responsible for providing culturally competent care, nursing regulatory bodies, professional associations, educational institutions, governments, health service agencies, and accreditation organizations share responsibility in supporting culturally competent care. Nurses are in a position to build partnerships with other health care providers, patients, and funding agencies to establish culturally diverse practices that optimize patients' health outcomes.

Cultural Safety and Humility

The provision of culturally competent care has been promoted since the 1960s. Since 2000, however, Canadian nurse scholars have begun to question the limitations of such an approach (Anderson et al., 2003; Kirkham, 2003) and to explore the concept of cultural safety as another approach to providing care to diverse groups. This approach is in contrast to the notion of transcultural nursing (Ramsden, 2002). The College of Registered Nurses of British Columbia's (2014) profile of newly graduated registered nurse practice focuses on the therapeutic caring and culturally safe relationships between patients and health care team members. The cultural safety literature is positioned within a critical social theory and postcolonial framework. The concept of cultural safety evolved over a number of years in New Zealand as nurses tried to identify a way in which health care providers could more effectively address the inequity in the health status of Maori people. This was combined with an analysis of the historical, political, social, and economic situations influencing the health of Maori people (Ramsden, 2002). Cultural safety involves considering the redistribution of power and resources in a relationship. The notion "is based on the premise that the term 'culture' is used in its broadest sense to apply to any person or group of people who may differ from the nurse/midwife because of socio-economic status, age, gender, sexual orientation, ethnic origin, migrant/refugee status, religious belief or disability" (Ramsden, 2002, Chapter 8, p. 3). In contrast to transcultural nursing, the term *culture* refers to ethnicity. As a result, the philosophy of cultural care has shifted from a notion of cultural sensitivity underpinning the provisions of care irrespective of culture to one of cultural safety with the recognition of power imbalances, an understanding of the nature of interpersonal relationships, and awareness of institutional discrimination (Aboriginal Nurses Association of Canada [ANAC], CASN, & CNA, 2009; Browne et al., 2009; CNA, 2010a; Racine, 2009). Thus, understanding and providing culturally competent and safe care has the potential to make a difference to the health of all culturally diverse groups.

Ramsden (2002) articulated that *cultural awareness* and *cultural sensitivity* are separate concepts and that those terms are not interchangeable with *cultural safety.* Achieving cultural safety is a step-wise progression from cultural awareness through cultural sensitivity to cultural safety (Figure 9-1). The outcome of cultural safety is that safe care, defined as such by patients who receive the care, is provided. According to Ramsden (2002), cultural sensitivity "alerts students to the legitimacy of difference and begins a process of self-exploration as the powerful bearers of their own life experience and realities which can have an impact on others" (Ramsden, 2002, Chapter 8, p. 4). Cultural awareness "is a beginning step toward understanding that

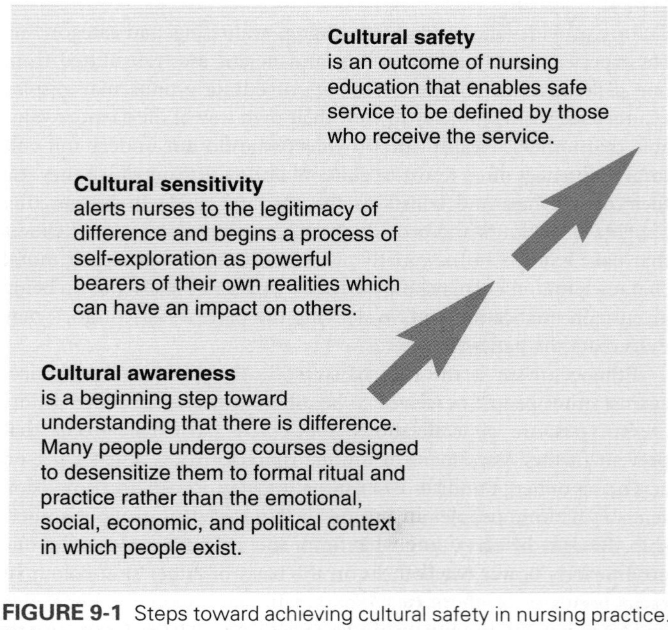

FIGURE 9-1 Steps toward achieving cultural safety in nursing practice. (Adapted from Ramsden, I. M. [2002]. *Cultural safety and nursing education in Aotearoa and TeWaipounamu* [unpublished PhD thesis]. Wellington, New Zealand: Victoria University of Wellington. Retrieved from http://culturalsafety.massey.ac.nz.)

BOX 9-6 Questions for Reflection and Building Awareness in Nursing

Personal Self-Awareness

What is my ethnic background? How does my knowledge of my ethnicity affect my identity? What meaning do I ascribe to my ethnic origins? How have they shaped who I am today? What cultural groups do I belong to? What are the rules, customs, and rituals that have been passed on to me and that I will pass on to the next generation of my family? How were these passed on to me, and what meaning do I give to them now? How do the rules and customs passed on to me inform how I engage with others?

Professional Self-Awareness

In my work, how do I relate to others of different cultures? What taken-for-granted assumptions am I prepared to make in the name of efficiency and time constraints? What stereotypes do I hold? How do these beliefs influence my practice? How do I maintain an attitude of cultural attunement in my work with groups and organizations? How do I bridge the differences between ethnic backgrounds in my work? What action might I take to improve my cultural attunement?

Organizational Awareness

What are the values and principles of my organization for working cross-culturally? How does my organization reflect behaviours, attitudes, policies, and structures when working cross-culturally? How does my organization value diversity, manage the dynamics of difference, acquire and institutionalize cultural knowledge, and adapt to diversity and the cultural contexts of the communities it serves?

Community Awareness

How do the dynamics of the community, such as racial tensions, enter into my work with community groups and organizations? When does difference make a difference? How does this community influence feelings of belonging among its residents? What actions do we take to be inclusive? How do we celebrate and honour cultural diversity? What do we need to do differently to be more inclusive and generate feelings of belonging among residents from all cultures?

Adapted from Hoskins, M. L. (1999). Worlds apart and lives together: Developing cultural attunement. *Child and Youth Care Forum, 28*(2), 73–85; Kirkham, S. (2003). The politics of belonging and intercultural health care. *Western Journal of Nursing Research, 25*(7), 762–780; Goode, T. (2004). *Cultural competence principles and continuum.* Washington, DC: National Center for Cultural Competence. Retrieved from https://ok.gov/odmhsas/documents/2)%20CC%20Principles%20-%20OK%20Increasing%20CC%20to%20Reduce%20BH%20Disparities%2010-29-15.pdf; and Racher, F. E., & Annis, R. C. (12). Honouring culture and diversity in community practice. In A. R. Vollman, E. T. Anderson, & J. McFarlane (Eds.), *Canadian community as partner: Theory & multidisciplinary practice* (3rd ed., p. 172). Philadelphia, PA: Lippincott Williams & Wilkins.

BOX 9-7 An Exemplary Relational Practitioner

1. *Identify* someone whom you would say is "good at relationships." Why did you identify that person? What qualities or characteristics stand out?
2. Now *identify* someone who is a nurse and is good at relationships. Think of someone with whom you have worked—perhaps a fellow student, a colleague, an instructor. What makes this person good at relationships? How is this person perceived by his or her colleagues?
3. *Compare notes* with someone else. Talk to someone who has thought about this question, or talk to someone who knows the person or people you have identified. Do you both value similar attributes and qualities?

From Doane, G. H., & Varcoe, C. (2005). *Family nursing as relational inquiry: Developing health-promoting practice* (p. 192). Philadelphia, PA: Lippincott Williams & Wilkins.

there is difference. Many people undergo courses designed to sensitize them to formal ritual and practice rather than the emotional, social, economic and political context in which people exist" (Ramsden, 2002, Chapter 8, p. 4). A strategy for achieving cultural awareness is to conduct a self-assessment in order to reflect on our biases and feelings. A set of questions for personal reflection is suggested for this purpose in Box 9-6. Another strategy is to observe nurses who are considered to be exemplary relational practitioners and to notice the particular qualities or characteristics they display when handling the cultural aspects of relationships (Box 9-7).

With regard to achieving cultural safety in nursing practice, Ramsden stated that "the skill for nurses does not lie in knowing the customs or even the health-related beliefs of ethno-specific groups. The step before that lies in professional acquisition of trust. Rather than the nurse determining what is culturally safe, it is consumers or patients who decide whether they feel safe with the care that has been given, that trust has been established, and that difference between the patient, the nurse and the institutions that underpin them can then be identified and negotiated" (Ramsden, 2002, Chapter 8, p. 4), as depicted in Figure 9-1. (See Chapter 10 for further information on cultural safety applied to the nursing care of Indigenous peoples.)

BOX 9-8 Using the Ideas of Cultural Safety

Start with the organization to inquire at the level of context:

- How are organizational practices supporting the health of nondominant groups?
- What policies or organizational practices diminish, demean, or disempower the cultural identity and well-being of any individual or group? How do such policies or practices support discrimination?
- What policies or organizational practices would recognize, respect, and nurture the unique cultural identities of people and families and safely meet their needs, expectations, and rights?

Examine nursing practices to inquire interpersonally:

- What is the unique identity of this person or family? What are this person's or family's needs and expectations?
- How can I practise to recognize, respect, and nurture that identity and meet those needs and expectations?

Use reflexivity to inquire intrapersonally:

- How do my own personal and cultural history, values, and beliefs influence my practice?
- How do my own economic, political, social, and historical location shape my practice?

From Hartrick Doane, G. & Varcoe, C. (2015). *How to nurse: Relational inquiry with individuals and families in changing health and health care contexts* (p. 180). Philadelphia, PA: Lippincott Williams & Wilkins.

As well, Hartrick Doane and Varcoe (2015) state that the "ideas of cultural safety are harmonious with a relational approach" (p. 179). The authors emphasize an "understanding of context and culture as inseparable, developing a relational consciousness, and inquiring at all levels" (p. 179). For nurses to integrate cultural safety in their practice, they suggest there are certain questions that are helpful to ask (Box 9-8).

In nursing, and in a wide variety of other disciplines, cultural humility is now viewed as important (Foronda, Baptiste, Reinholdt, et al., 2016). Cultural humility includes a variety of core features and consolidating definitions. Worthington, Davis, and Hook (2017) describe cultural humility as a lifelong learning experience, value, or virtue that shapes character traits across the lifespan. In addition, *cultural humility* refers to actions that demonstrate interpersonal respect and interpersonal reflection of one's cultural assumptions and biases. The focus of cultural humility offers something new as we continue to think about and apply cultural competence and safety frameworks. It is especially important to nursing as a profession that involves cross-cultural engagement, with applications across a wide variety of nursing domains (Worthington et al., 2017).

CULTURAL ASSESSMENT

A comprehensive cultural assessment is the basis for providing culturally competent care. A cultural assessment, combined with critical thinking skills, provides the knowledge necessary for transcultural nursing care (Andrews & Boyle, 2012). Cultural assessment is a systematic and comprehensive examination of the cultural care values, beliefs, and practices of individuals, families, and communities. The goal of cultural assessment is to generate from the patients themselves significant information that enables culturally congruent care (Leininger & McFarland, 2002). Several models of cultural assessment exist, each involving different levels of skill and knowledge. Leininger's Sunrise Model (Leininger & McFarland, 2002) demonstrates the inclusiveness of culture in everyday life and helps explain why cultural assessment must be comprehensive. According to the Sunrise Model, cultural care values, beliefs, and practices are embedded in the cultural and social structural dimensions of society, which include environmental contexts, language, and ethnohistory (i.e., significant historical experiences of a particular group). For older persons, for example, the experience of the Great Depression has sometimes resulted in a tendency to be frugal. Nurses must encourage patients to share stories about their lives that reveal how they think and the cultural lifestyle they embrace. Leininger's model differentiates folk care, which is caring as defined by the people, from the professional care, which is based on the scientific, biomedical system of care.

Whichever assessment model is used, the nurse can begin an assessment by knowing population demographic changes in the practice setting. In addition, background knowledge about a culture may assist the nurse in conducting a focused assessment when time is limited. Demographic information can be gathered from the local and regional census data, as well as from patients themselves. Demographic information might include the distribution of ethnic groups, education, occupations, and incidence of the most common illnesses. Comprehensive cultural assessment requires skill and time; hence, preparation and anticipation of needs are important.

A challenge in cultural assessment is the lack of ability to assess the multiple perspectives of patients and to interpret the information elicited. It helps to use open-ended questions (e.g., "What do you think caused your illness?"), focused questions (e.g., "Have you had this problem before?"), and contrast questions (e.g., "How different is this problem from the one you had previously?"). The aim is to encourage patients to describe values, beliefs, and practices that are significant to their care, which may be taken for granted unless otherwise revealed. Culturally oriented questions are by nature broad and require a lot of description. Table 9-2 provides a list of possible guiding questions (a cultural assessment guide) that focus on social and cultural dimensions of assessment.

Selected Components of Cultural Assessment

Cultural assessment is important in the total care of any patient. Over time, you will learn various skills needed to gather an accurate and comprehensive assessment. The following sections describe certain components of cultural assessment that provide information that can be useful in planning and providing nursing care. You may use the following information as a starting point to assess the similarities and differences of patients and families. However, it is best not to assume that because any two patients come from the same region or country they share similar values, beliefs, attitudes, and experiences. Other elements to consider are the social determinants of health, including early childhood development, education, employment and working conditions, food security, health care services, housing shortages, income, social safety nets, social exclusion, and unemployment and employment security (Commission on Social Determinants of Health, 2008; Hartrick Doane & Varcoe, 2015; Raphael, 2016).

Ethnohistory. Knowledge of a patient's country of origin and its history and ecological contexts is significant to the provision of health care. Haitian immigrants, for example, have linguistic and communication patterns distinct from those of Jamaicans, even though both groups come from the Caribbean region and may have a common history of oppression. Differences can be traced to their colonial history and intermingling with the local Indigenous people.

Social Organization. Cultural groups consist of units of organization delineated by kinship, status hierarchy, and roles for their members. Nurses need to consider all options when determining a patient's next of kin. This is especially relevant to new immigrants and refugees, who may have relocated without intact families. The status of a patient within the social hierarchy is generally linked with attributes such as age and gender, as well as with achievements such as education and position. The mainstream culture in Canada emphasizes achievement as the determinant of status, whereas other cultures may give higher priority to age and gender. In many Asian and African cultures, for instance, the eldest son is next in line after his father with regard to authority.

Socioeconomic Status, Biocultural Ecology, and Health Risks. The identification of health risks related to the environment should be assessed on admission of patients. Distinct health risks can be attributed to the ecological context of the environment. Immigrants from parts of Africa, Asia, and South America, for example, may have a higher incidence of parasitic infestations endemic to their country of origin.

Language and Communication. Linguistic and communication patterns are associated with different cultural groups. These patterns reflect the core cultural values of a society. In Western cultures that uphold individualism, assertive communication is valued because it demonstrates autonomy and self-determination. People are expected to say what they mean and to mean what they say. In collectivistic cultures, communication is shaped by the context of relationships among participants. Group harmony is the priority, so that participants interact on the basis of their expected positions and relationships within the social hierarchy. People are more likely to remain respectful and show deference to older persons or family leaders, even though they may disagree on an issue.

In cultural groups with distinct linear hierarchy, conflict is negotiated between people with the same level of position or authority. Identifying and working with family members at the appropriate hierarchy may prevent miscommunication. Nonverbal communication may also be shaped by culture. Culture influences the distance between participants in an interaction, the extent of touching, the degree of eye contact, and how much private information the patient shares. Patients use less distance when speaking to trusted affiliates and persons of the same gender, age, and social position. To minimize the distance when communicating with patients, nurses must consider taking up a relational approach to cultural nursing that greatly enhances the

TABLE 9-2 Cultural Assessment Guide

Subject	Suggested Questions
Cultural identity/ ancestry/heritage	Where were you born? Where were your parents born?
Ethnohistory	How long have you or your parents resided in this country? What is your ethnic background or ancestry? How strongly are you influenced by your culture? Why did you leave your homeland?
Social organization	Who lives with you? Whom do you consider members of your family? Where do you live? Where do other members of your family live? How do you contact them? How often do you have contact with your family members? Who makes the decisions for you or your family? Whom do you go to outside your family for support? What do you expect your family members to do for you? How different are your expectations of them now from your expectations at other times? What expectations do you have of your family members who are male, female, old, or young?
Socioeconomic status	What do you do for a living? What did you do back in your homeland? Where did you go to school? What level did you finish in school? How different is your life here from your life back in your homeland? Do you have a primary health care provider? What other health care providers have you seen?
Biocultural ecology and health risks	What is your purpose for coming here? What caused your problem? Have you had this problem before? Does this problem affect your life and your family? How? Do other members of your family have this kind of problem? How do you treat this problem at home? Whom do you go to for this kind of problem? What other plans do you have for dealing with this problem? What do you think we should do for you? What other problems do you have? Have these problems occurred with any other member of your family?
Language and communication	What language(s) do you speak at home? What language(s) are you most comfortable speaking? In what language(s) can you read and write? How do you want us to talk to you? How should we address you, or what should we call you? What kinds of communication upset or offend you? What words would you use to describe how you feel? Do you need an interpreter? Would you prefer a female or male interpreter?
Religion/ spirituality	Do you practice any religion? Who is your religious or spiritual leader? Do you want to be in touch with your religious leader? How do we contact your spiritual leader? What are some of the things we need to do within your religion? How do you practise your religion? Do you follow specific dietary practices?
Caring beliefs and practices	What do you do to keep yourself well? What do you do to show someone you care? How does your family or you take care of sick family members? Which caregivers do you seek when you are sick? How do you decide when to go to a caregiver and which one to go to? How different is what we do from what your family does for you when you are sick? Are we doing what you think we should be doing for you? How should we give you care?
Experience with professional health care	Since you came to this country, have you had contact with doctors or hospitals? How do you compare your past health care experiences with those of the present? What were some of the problems that you encountered? How were they resolved? What were the positive experiences you had? What type of health care provider do you prefer? Why? If you have a choice, what changes do you wish to see?

ability to know and respond to people (Hartrick Doane & Varcoe, 2005). A relational approach to nursing allows you not only to connect across differences but also to recognize more subtle cultural similarities and differences. Such an approach provides opportunities "to attend to issues of meaning, experience, race, history, culture, health, and sociopolitical systems. In addition, as we relationally honour and attend to such differences the potential for growth, change, and knowledge development is enhanced" (Hartrick Doane & Varcoe, 2005, p. 9).

Religion and Spirituality. Religious and spiritual beliefs may have a major influence on a person's attitudes toward health and illness, pain and suffering, and life and death. It is advisable for nurses to understand the various perspectives of patients. (see Chapter 28 for further information about religion and spirituality).

Caring Beliefs and Practices. Caring beliefs and practices incorporate a patient's perception of his or her ability to control circumstances or factors in the environment. Specifically, it may refer to a patient's perception of how he or she can influence causes of illness and use cultural healing modalities and healers. During cultural assessment, you should identify the health practices of the patient and respect them (Box 9-9).

Experience With Professional Health Care. All cultures have concepts of past, present, and future dimensions of time. An aspect of a patient's experience with professional health care, for instance, may

BOX 9-9 CASE STUDY

Identifying the Patient's Health Care Practices

A Chinese immigrant who recently arrived in Canada has given birth to her first child in the hospital. Once the newborn has been cared for and is resting, you ask the new mother if she would like to take a shower. The mother refuses politely. Her belief is that if she takes a shower, she could contract rheumatism in old age. Then the mother's food tray arrives, and she does not touch or eat anything. For this newcomer to Canada, the hospital food may seem different and served in an unfamiliar manner. Her family brings plain rice and salted pork into the hospital. They also bring two different soups, which are thought to bring heat, the "yang," into her body, thereby removing the impurities from her system.

In traditional Chinese culture, good health means achieving a balance between yin and yang. The belief is that all body systems interact with each other and with the environment to produce a balanced state of wellness. In consultation with the mother, you are able to assess and understand why she is refusing to shower and eat the hospital food. With this increased understanding, you are able to mutually negotiate with the mother some alternatives for her care to accommodate her needs, without jeopardizing her care or causing her distress. You appropriately assess that, rather than showering, the mother would prefer a basin of water and a cloth that she could use to clean herself. With regard to her dietary requests, you determine that she can eat the food from home as long as it does not interfere with or jeopardize her health status. As a result, your sensitivity and respect for the new mother's cultural beliefs enable her to relax and recover in a culturally safe environment. You were open to learning about the cultural beliefs of the new mother and then collaborating with her on decisions about care.

be your understanding of the patient's orientation of time. This information can be useful in planning care, arranging appointments for procedures, and helping a patient plan self-care activities at home.

GLOBAL HEALTH NURSING

Increasingly, there is an awareness of the importance of global health and its relevance for nursing education, practice, and research (Breakey, Corless, Meedzan, et al., 2015). Moreover, there is an acknowledgement that global is local, and local is global. This approach underscores the importance of nurses and other health professionals worldwide working collaboratively in order to address health inequities. International Council of Nursing (ICN) and WHO strongly advocates that every nurse can have a direct impact on health and is key to achieving the Sustainable Development Goals (SDGs) (Hughes, 2017; WHO 2018). In working in partnership with other professionals possessing the skills and expertise to address these inequities, health systems and equity in health can be strengthened (Astle, 2008; CNA, 2011a; Upval & Leffers, 2014).

Interprofessional Education and Collaborative Practice

Many health care systems in the world are struggling to oversee unmet health needs. Future health care providers will shoulder increasing responsibility for providing health services for some very complex health issues (Frenk, Chen, Bhutta, et al., 2010; WHO 2016c). As well, in nursing and other health care professions, globally there is a significant health care workforce shortage (Shaffer, 2014). In Canada, for example, there is a shortage of health care providers, predominantly in the rural and northern regions. Similarly, in sub-Saharan Africa, there is a critical shortage of health care providers, owing to migration among other reasons (Oglivie, Mill, Astle et al., 2007).

In response to the global health workforce shortage, in 2010, the WHO developed the "Framework for Action on Interprofessional Education and Collaborative Practice" as a guide for policymakers to implement interprofessional education and collaborative practice within their specific context (Health Professions Networks Nursing and Midwifery, 2010). **Interprofessional education** occurs "when students from two or more professions learn about, from and with each other to enable effective collaboration and improve health outcomes" (Health Professions Networks Nursing and Midwifery, 2010, p. 10). Interprofessional education is critical to ensuring that health care workers are able to address the complex health needs of their patients and clients in collaboration with other members of the health care team (CNA, 2011b). A **collaborative practice-ready workforce** "is a specific way of describing health workers who have received effective training in interprofessional education (Health Professions Networks Nursing and Midwifery, 2010, p. 10). Nurse educators have an important role to play in global health nursing to ensure that interprofessional education and collaborative practice opportunities are offered to students before entering the workplace. Ensuring that nursing students understand what it's like to work within interprofessional health care teams will help them understand "how to optimize the skills of their members, share case management and provide better health-services to patients and the community" (Health Professions Networks Nursing and Midwifery, 2010, p. 10).

Global Health Education/Global Health Competencies for Nursing

Over the past decade, there has been a growing interest in global health issues and a rapid increase in the development of global health and global health programs at the undergraduate and graduate levels (Jogerst, Callender, Adams et al., 2015). To address this increased interest, many Canadian nursing programs have integrated global health concepts and developed curricula with courses focusing specifically on global health. The University of Alberta, Trinity Western University, University of Toronto, McMaster University, and McGill University are just some of the universities making this shift in curricula. As well, the CASN (2015) as part of its educational framework at the undergraduate level emphasizes the importance for students to demonstrate knowledge of social justice, population health, environmental, and global health issues.

Curriculum development has accompanied the increase in global health programming, and initiatives have been undertaken to identify discipline-specific global health competencies in nursing (Astle, Redmond, & Reimer-Kirkham, in press; Wilson, Harper, Tami-Maury, et al., 2012), interprofessional competencies (Consortium of Universities for Global Health [CUGH], 2017; Jogerst et al., 2015), and understanding of host perspectives (Cherniak, Latham, Astle, et al., 2017a, 2017b). **Global health competencies** refers to the knowledge and skills that a nurse would possess when working in the area of global health. Research continues in nursing and other disciplines, which are working collaboratively toward implementation and evaluation of global health competencies, to better prepare health care providers to be global citizens.

National and International Organizations for Global Health

There are a number of national and international organizations that promote interprofessional collaboration and collaboration within nursing to advance global health (Box 9-10).

BOX 9-10 National and International Organizations for Global Health

Canadian Coalition for Global Health Researchers (CCGHR) http://www.ccghr.ca/
Canadian Nurses Association (CNA) https://www.cna-aiic.ca/en
Canadian Red Cross: http://www.redcross.ca/
Canadian Society for International Health (CSIH): http://www.csih.org
Consortium of Universities for Global Health (CUGH): https://www.cugh.org/
Global Advisory Panel on the Future of Nursing & Midwifery (GAPFON) (established 2013): Bridging the gaps for health: http://www.gapfon.org/
Global Nursing Caucus: Engaging nurses to advance global health: http://www.globalnursingcaucus.org/
Immigration, Refugees, and Citizenship Canada: http://www.cic.gc.ca/english/department/
International Council of Nurses (ICN): http://www.icn.ch/
Médecins sans Frontières (Doctors Without Borders Canada): http://www.msf.ca/
Nursing Now Campaign (2018). http://www.who.int/hrh/news/2018/nursing_now_campaign/en/
United Nations: http://www.un.org/en/index.html
World Health Organization (WHO): Health topics: Nursing: http://www.who.int/topics/nursing/en/

Implications for Nursing

In an increasingly globalized world, nursing has acknowledged the important role that nurses have in addressing some of the critical issues in the field of global health practice, education, and research. In order to be better prepared for caring for patients at the local and global levels, nurses must possess a foundational understanding of global health concepts and the complexities of culture; provide care using a relational approach in a culturally safe manner; work collaboratively and interprofessionally; and work in partnership with host institutions and countries. Areas that require further research include global health education, global citizenship, global health competencies, interprofessional collaboration, and global health partnerships. To achieve health equity, social justice, and human rights for all, it is essential that nurses acquire the necessary knowledge to provide competent and culturally safe care in their practice worldwide.

KEY CONCEPTS

- Global health is concerned with the health needs of people worldwide.
- Global citizenship is the active engagement of nurses in global health issues. As global citizens, nurses identify and act on health inequities in the population they work with at the local, national, and international levels.
- Global environmental sustainability is reliant on intact and healthy ecosystems.
- Sustainable Development Goals (SDGs) address the well-being of persons worldwide, which aligns with a planetary perspective on health.
- A relational definition of culture encourages nurses to explore the contextually mediated influences shaping one's life and health rather than basing their care on ethnicity, race, or nationality.
- Transcultural nursing is a comparative study and understanding of cultures to identify culture-specific and culture-universal caring constructs across ethnic groups.
- Culturally congruent care is meaningful, supportive, and facilitative because it conforms to valued life patterns of patients; it is achieved through cultural assessment.
- Culturally competent care requires knowledge, attitudes, and skills supportive of implementation of culturally congruent care.
- Cultural safety involves challenging stereotypes and assumptions to inquire into providing care to patients as defined by them.
- Cultural humility is a process that requires persons to acknowledge their own biases when engaging with others, which then provides a place to begin a relationship in an open and honest space.
- Nurses require education in global health issues and global health competencies in order to provide competent and culturally safe care worldwide.

CRITICAL THINKING EXERCISES

1. You are about to begin giving a male patient who is a practising Muslim his morning care when he states, "I don't want a bath now." He becomes annoyed when you try to explain that you must give him a bath at this time. Before you leave the room, he asks you to leave a basin of water and towel by his bedside. He also asks you to get his prayer rug from his closet.
   a. How should you respond to the patient?
2. A 50-year-old Chinese woman is hospitalized with a respiratory condition. She insists that you give her warm water and rub her back with Tiger Balm ointment. When she receives her lunch, consisting of a turkey sandwich, tossed salad, and milk, she keeps the turkey sandwich and tossed salad but asks that you take the milk away.
   a. How should you respond to the patient's requests?
   b. What is the significance of her requests?
   c. Why does she refuse her milk?

REVIEW QUESTIONS

1. Which of the following are environmental risk factors that nurses should know contribute to diseases and injuries to people worldwide? *(Select all that apply)*
   1. Chemical exposure
   2. Climate change
   3. Air, water, and soil pollution
   4. Ultraviolet radiation
2. The nurse assesses the health status of a population by analyzing the global burden of disease (GBD) of a country. The nurse's next step is to:
   1. Document the health status data
   2. Analyze the DALY indicator
   3. Validate the data with the country
   4. Assign the DALY indicator with a number
3. Which of the following are defining characteristics for the Sustainable Development Goals (SDGs)? *(Select all that apply.)*
   1. Align with a planetary perspective on health
   2. Focus on ending poverty
   3. Address the health of persons of all ages
   4. Target health risks of prosperous countries
4. The best definition for the term *multiculturalism* is:
   1. An experience with a new or different culture that is extremely negative
   2. A person who maintains his or her culture and interacts peacefully with people of other cultures
   3. A person who gives up his or her ethnic identity in favour of the dominant culture
   4. A person who adapts to and adopts a new culture

5. Cultural awareness involves in-depth self-examination that requires:
    1. Acknowledgement of one's background, and recognizing biases and prejudices
    2. Recognizing social, cultural, and biophysical factors
    3. Engagement in culturally safe interactions
    4. Motivation and commitment to caring
6. Nurses are responsible to provide culturally safe care for their patients. It is very important for the nurse to:
    1. Learn about vast cultures
    2. Deliver care that is based on knowledge of the patient's values, beliefs, and attitudes
    3. Influence treatment and care of patients
    4. Review cultural assessment models
7. Which of the following is the best definition of *ethnocentrism*:
    1. Stereotypes, biases, and prejudices
    2. Meanings by which people make sense of their experiences
    3. Cultural beliefs
    4. Individualism and self-reliance in achieving and maintaining health
8. The disparities in health outcomes between rich and poor patients is an example of:
    1. An attribution of illness to natural, impersonal, and biological forces
    2. Biological and sociocultural health risks
    3. An influence of socioeconomic factors in morbidity and mortality
    4. A combination of naturalistic, religious, and supernatural modalities
9. The concept of global health is best defined as:
    1. Issues that affect the health of the population of a particular community or country
    2. Prevention programs for populations
    3. Issues that directly or indirectly affect health that can transcend national boundaries
    4. Issues that affect the health of a few disciplines

Answers: 1. 1, 2, 3, 4; **2.** 2; **3.** 1, 2, 3; **4.** 2; **5.** 1; **6.** 2; **7.** 1; **8.** 3; **9.** 3.

Rationales for the Review Questions appear at the end of the book.

RECOMMENDED WEBSITES

Public Health Agency of Canada: https://www.canada.ca/en/public-health.html.

This website provides information on the prevention of diseases and injuries; the promotion of good physical and mental health; and information to support informed decision making.

United Nations (UN): http://www.un.org/en/index.html.

This website provides updates on maintaining peace and security, and the promotion and protection of human rights globally, as well as publications related to the Sustainable Development Goals (SDGs).

World Health Organization (WHO): http://www.who.int/en/.

This website provides links to publications on a variety of areas related to population health.

WHO Commission on Social Determinants of Health: http://www.who.int/social_determinants/thecommission/finalreport/en/.

This website provides publications related to the social determinants of Health (SDH).

REFERENCES

Aboriginal Nurses Association of Canada (ANAC), Canadian Association of Schools of Nursing (CASN), & Canadian Nurses Association (CNA) (2009). *Cultural competence and cultural safety in nursing education*. Ottawa, ON: ANAC.

Access Alliance (2009). *Literature review: costs of not providing interpretation in health care* (Access Alliance publication LR0004). Canada: Author. Retrieved from http://accessalliance.ca/wp-content/uploads/2015/03/Lit_Review_Cost_of_Not_Providing_Interpretation.pdf.

Anderson, J., Perry, J., Blue, C., et al. (2003). "Rewriting" cultural safety within the postcolonial and postnational feminist project: Toward new epistemologies of healing. *ANS. Advances in Nursing Science*, *26*, 196–214.

Andrews, M. M., & Boyle, J. S. (2012). *Transcultural concepts in nursing care* (6th ed.). Philadelphia, PA: Lippincott Williams & Wilkins.

Astle, B. J. (2008). *Building and sustaining international partnerships in higher education in nursing*. Doctoral Dissertation. Edmonton, AB: University of Alberta.

Astle, B., Redmond, A., & Reimer-Kirkham, S. (2017). Global health competencies to promote global citizenship in the baccalaureate nursing student: An interpretive description approach. *International Journal of Nursing Studies*, in press.

Baker, C. (2007). Globalization and the cultural safety of an immigrant Muslim community. *Journal of Advanced Nursing*, *57*(3), 296–305. doi:10.1111/j.1365-2648.2006.04104.x.

Brainy quote. (2017). *Ban Ki-moon quotes*. Retrieved from: https://www.brainyquote.com/authors/ban_kimoon.

Braveman, P. (2014). What is health equity and how does a life-course approach take us further toward it? *Maternal Child Health Journal*, *18*(2), 366–372.

Braveman, P., & Gruskin, S. (2003). Defining equity in health. *Journal of Epidemiology in Community Health*, *57*(4), 254–258. doi:10.1136/jech.57.4.254.

Braveman, P., Kumanyika, S., Fielding, J., et al. (2011). Health disparities and health equity: The issue is justice. *American Journal of Public Health*, *101*(Suppl. 1), S149–S155. doi:10.2105/AJPH.2010.300062.

Breakey, S., Corless, I. B., Meedzan, N. L., et al. (2015). *Global health nursing in the 21st century*. New York, NY: Springer.

Browne, A. J., Varcoe, C., Smye, V., et al. (2009). Cultural safety and the challenges of translating critically oriented knowledge in practice. *Nursing Philosophy*, *10*(3), 167–179. doi:10.1111/j.1466-769X.2009.00406x.

Burgess, C. A., Reimer-Kirkham, S., & Astle, B. (2014). Motivation and international clinical placements: shifting nursing students to a global citizenship perspective. *International Journal of Nursing Education Scholarship*, *11*(1), 1–8. doi:10.1515/ijnes-2013-0056.

Byers, M. (2005). Are you a global citizen? *The Tyee*, *5*, 35–37.

Campinha-Bacote, J. (2002). The process of cultural competence in the delivery of healthcare services: A model of care. *Journal of Transcultural Nursing*, *13*(3), 181–184. doi:10.1177/10459602013003003.

Canadian Association of Schools of Nursing/Association Canadienne des Écoles de Sciences Infirmières [CASN/ACESI] (2015). *National nursing education framework: Final report*. Ottawa: Author.

Canadian Nurses Association (2009). *Position statement: Global health and equity*. Ottawa: Author. Retrieved from https://www.cna-aiic.ca/~/media/cna/page-content/pdf-en/ps106_global_health_equity_aug_2009_e.pdf?la=en.

Canadian Nurses Association (2010a). *Social justice: A means to an end, an end in itself* (2nd ed.). Ottawa: Author. Retrieved from https://www.cna-aiic.ca/~/media/cna/page-content/pdf-en/social_justice_2010_e.pdf.

Canadian Nurses Association (2010b). *Position statement: Promoting cultural competence in nursing*. Ottawa: Author. Retrieved from https://www.cna-aiic.ca/~/media/cna/page-content/pdf-en/ps114_cultural_competence_2010_e.pdf?la=en.

Canadian Nurses Association (2011a). *Position statement: Global health partnerships*. Ottawa: Author. Retrieved from https://www.cna-aiic.ca/~/media/cna/page-content/pdf-en/ps115_global_health_partnerships_2011_e.pdf?la=en.

Canadian Nurses Association (2011b). *Position statement: Interprofessional collaboration*. Ottawa: Author. Retrieved from https://www.cna-aiic.ca/~/media/cna/page-content/pdf-en/interproffessional-collaboration_position-statement.pdf?la=en.

Canadian Nurses Association (2017a). *Position statement: Nurses and environmental health*. Ottawa: Author. Retrieved from https://www.cna-aiic.ca/en/~/media/cna/page-content/pdf-en/climate-change-and-health-position-statement.

Canadian Nurses Association (2017b). *Position statement: Climate change and health*. Ottawa: Author. Retrieved from https://www.cna-aiic.ca/en/~/media/cna/page-content/pdf-en/climate-change-and-health-position-statement.

Canadian Nurses Association (2017c). *Code of ethics for registered nurses*. Ottawa: Author. Retrieved from https://www.cna-aiic.ca/en/on-the-issues/best-nursing/nursing-ethics.

Centers for Disease Control and Prevention (CDC). (2017). *One Health*. Retrieved from https://www.cdc.gov/onehealth/.

Chavez, R. S., Peter, E., & Gastaldo, D. (2008). Nurses as global citizens: A global health curriculum at the University of Toronto, Canada. In V. Tschudin & A. J. Davis (Eds.), *The Globalization of Nursing* (pp. 175–186). Oxon, UK: Radcliffe.

Cherniak, W., Latham, E., Astle, B., et al. (2017a). Host perspectives on short-term experiences in global health: A survey [Abstract]. *Lancet Global Health*, *5*(S9), doi:10.1016/S2214-109X(17)30116-X.

Cherniak, W., Latham, E., Astle, B., et al. (2017b). Visiting trainees in global settings: Host and partner perspectives on desirable competencies. *Annals of Global Health*, *83*(2), 359–368. doi:10.1016/j.aogh.2017.04.007.

College of Registered Nurses of British Columbia (2014). *Competencies in the context of entry-level registered nurse practice in British Columbia.* (Publication No. 375-1). Vancouver: Author.

Commission on Social Determinants of Health (2008). *Closing the gap in a generation: Health equity through action on the social determinants of health (Final Report).* Geneva: World Health Organization (WHO). Retrieved from http://apps.who.int/iris/bitstream/10665/43943/1/9789241563703_eng.pdf.

Consortium of Universities for Global Health (CUGH). (2017). *Global health education competencies toolkit.* Retrieved from: http://cugh.org/resources/2063.

Cowan, D. T., & Norman, J. (2006). Cultural competence in nursing: New meanings. *Journal of Transcultural Nursing, 17*(1), 82–88. doi:10.1177/1043659605281976.

Dasjerdi, M., Olson, K., & Ogilvie, L. (2012). A study of Iranian immigrants' experiences of accessing Canadian health care services: A grounded theory. *International Journal for Equity in Health, 11*, 55. doi:10.1186/1475-9276-11-55. Retrieved from http://www.equityhealthj.com/content/11/1/55.

Davidhizar, R. E., & Giger, J. N. (Eds.), (1998). *Canadian transcultural nursing: Assessment and intervention.* St. Louis, MO: Mosby.

de Leeuw, E., & Simos, J. (2017). *Healthy cities: The theory, policy, and practice of value-based urban planning.* New York, NY: Springer Science.

Foronda, C., Baptiste, D., Reinholdt, M. M., et al. (2016). Cultural humility: A concept analysis. *Journal of Transcultural Nursing, 27*(3), 210–217. doi:10.1177/1043659615592677.

Frenk, J., Chen, L., Bhutta, Z. A., et al. (2010). Health professionals for a new century: Transforming education to strengthen health systems in an interdependent world. *Lancet, 376*, 1923–1958.

GBD 2015 SDG Collaborators. (2016). Measuring the health-related Sustainable Development Goals in 188 countries: A baseline analysis from the Global Burden of Disease Study 2015. *Lancet, 388*(10053), 1813–1850. doi:10.1016/S0140-6376(16)31467-2.

Gender equality. (2017, August 24). *Wikipedia, the Free Encyclopedia.* Retrieved from https://en.wikipedia.org/wiki/Gender_equality.

Gender Inequality Index (GII). (2016). *Human Development Reports.* Retrieved December 11, 2016 from http://hdr.undp.org/en/content/gender-inequality-index-gii.

Giger, J. N. (2013). *Transcultural nursing: Assessment and intervention* (6th ed.). St. Louis, MO: Mosby.

Giger, J., & Davidhizar, R. (2002). The Giger and Davidhizar transcultural assessment model. *Journal of Transcultural Nursing, 13*(3), 185–188.

Glittenberg, J. (2004). A transdisciplinary, transcultural model for health care. *Journal of Transcultural Nursing, 15*(1), 6–10. doi:10.1177/1043659603260037.

Government of Canada. (2017a). *Environmental sustainability.* Retrieved from http://www.international.gc.ca/development-developpement/priorities-priorites/enviro/index.aspx?lang=eng.

Government of Canada. (2017b). *Canadian multiculturalism act.* Retrieved from http://laws-lois.justice.gc.ca/eng/acts/C-18.7/page-1.html.

Gustafson, D. L. (2005). Transcultural nursing theory from a critical cultural perspective. *ANS. Advances in Nursing Science, 28*, 2–16.

Gustafson, D. L. (2007). White on whiteness: Becoming racialized about race. *Nursing Inquiry, 14*(2), 153–161. doi:10.1111/j.1440-1800.2007.00365.x.

Hankivsky, O. (2012). Women's health, men's health, and gender and health: Implications of intersectionality. *Social Science & Medicine, 74*(11), 1712–1720.

Hankivsky, O., & Cormier, R. (2009). *Intersectionality: Moving women's health research and policy forward.* Vancouver: Women's Health Research Network.

Hankivsky, O., Reid, C., Cormier, R., et al. (2010). Exploring the promises of intersectionality for advancing women's health research. *International Journal for Equity in Health, 9*, 5. doi:10.1186/1475-9276-9-5.

Hanson, L. (2010). Global citizenship, global health and the internationalization of the curriculum. *Journal of Studies in International Education, 14*(1), 70–88. doi:10.1177/1028315308323207.

Hartrick Doane, G., & Varcoe, C. (2005). *Family nursing as relational inquiry: Developing health-promoting practice.* Philadelphia, PA: Lippincott Williams & Wilkins.

Hartrick Doane, G., & Varcoe, C. (2015). *How to nurse: Relational inquiry with individuals and families in changing health and health care contexts.* Philadelphia, PA: Wolters Kluwer.

HealthyPeople.gov. (2014). *Disparities.* Retrieved from https://www.healthypeople.gov/2020/about/foundation-health-measures/Disparities.

Health Professions Networks Nursing and Midwifery, Human Resources for Health (2010). *Framework for action on interprofessional education & collaborative practice.* Geneva: World Health Organization. Retrieved from http://apps.who.int/iris/bitstream/10665/70185/1/WHO_HRH_HPN_10.3_eng.pdf?ua=1.

Horton, R., & Lo, S. (2015). Planetary health: a new science for exceptional action. *Lancet, 386*(10007), 1921–1922. doi:10.1016/S0140-6736(15)61038-8.

Hughes, F. (2017). Nurses: A voice to lead – achieving the Sustainable Development Goals. *International Nursing Review, 16*(1), 4. doi:10:1111/inr.12354.

Immigration Watch Canada [IMC] (2017). *Refugees Top 10 Source Countries 2011-2016.* Retrieved from http://immigrationwatchcanada.org/2017/03/13/refugees-top-10-source-countries-2011-2016/.

International Council of Nurses (ICN) (2014). *Nurses: A force for change, a vital resource for health.* Geneva, Switzerland: Author.

International Council of Nurses (ICN) (2017). *Nurses: A voice to lead: Achieving the SDGs.* Geneva, Switzerland: Author.

Iyer, A., Sen, G., & Östlin, P. (2008). The intersections of gender and class in health status and health care. *Global Public Health, 3*(Suppl. 1), 13–24. doi:10.1080/17441690801892174.

Jogerst, K., Callender, B., Adams, V., et al. (2015). Identifying interprofessional global health competencies for 21st-century health professionals. *Annals of Global Health, 81*(2), 240-247. doi:10.1016/j.aogh.2015.03.006.

Kelley, M. A., Connor, A., Kun, K. E., et al. (2008). Social responsibility: Conceptualization and embodiment in a school of nursing. *International Journal of Nursing Education Scholarship, 5*(1), 1–16.

Ki-Moon, B. (2017). *Quotes.* Author. Retrieved from https://www.brainyquote.com/quotes/authors/b/ban_kimoon.html.

Kirkham, S. (2003). The politics of belonging and intercultural health care. *Western Journal of Nursing Research, 25*, 762–780. doi:10.1177/0193945903256709.

Koplan, J. P., Bond, T. C., Merson, M. H., et al. (2009). Towards a common definition of global health. *Lancet, 373*(9679), 1993–1995. doi:10.1016/S0140-6736(09)60332-9.

Landorf, H., & Feldman, E. (2015). Global perspectives on global citizenship. In R. Reynolds, D. Bradbery, J. Brown, et al. (Eds.), *Contesting and constructing international perspectives in global education* (pp. 43–52). Rotterdam, Netherlands: Springer.

Leininger, M. (2002a). Culture care theory: A major contribution to advance transcultural nursing knowledge and practices. *Journal of Transcultural Nursing, 13*, 189–192. doi:10.1177/10459602013003005.

Leininger, M. (2002b). Essential transcultural nursing care concepts, principles, examples and policy statements. In M. Leininger & M. R. McFarland (Eds.), *Transcultural nursing: Concepts, theories, research and practice* (3rd ed., pp. 45–69). New York: McGraw-Hill.

Leininger, M., & McFarland, M. R. (2002). *Transcultural nursing: Concepts, theories, research and practice* (3rd ed.). New York: McGraw-Hill.

Lo, H., & Pottinger, A. (2007). Mental health practice. In R. H. Srivastava (Ed.), *The healthcare professional's guide to clinical cultural competence* (pp. 247–263). Toronto: Elsevier Canada.

Marmot, M., & Allen, J. J. (2014). Social determinants of health equity. *American Journal of Public Health, 104*(Suppl. 4), S517–S519. doi:10.2105/AJPH.2014.302200.

Mill, J., Astle, B., Ogilvie, L., et al. (2010). Linking global citizenship, undergraduate nursing education, and professional nursing: Curricular innovation in the 21st century. *Advances in Nursing Science, 33*(3), E1–E11.

Narayanasamy, A. (2002). The ACCESS model: A transcultural nursing practice framework. *British Journal of Nursing, 11*(9), 643–650.

Narayanasamy, A., & White, E. (2005). A review of transcultural nursing. *Nurse Education Today, 25*(2), 102–111. doi:10.1016/j.nedt.2004.09.011.

Nursing Now. (2018). http://www.nursingnow.org/launch/

Ogilvie, L. (2011). Health equity in newcomer health research: Setting the context for immigrant community health nursing research in Canada. *ICCHNR Symposium*, May 5, 2011, Edmonton. (Unpublished paper).

Ogilvie, L., Astle, B., Mill, J., et al. (2005). Global health and equity. Part II: Exploring solutions. *The Canadian Nurse, 101*(6), 25–28.

Ogilvie, L., Mill, J. E., Astle, B., et al. (2007). The exodus of health professionals from sub-Saharan Africa: Balancing human rights and societal needs in the twenty-first century. *Nursing Inquiry, 14*(2), 114–124. doi:10.1111/j.1440-1800.2007.00358.x.

Oxfam (2015). *Education for global citizenship: A guide for schools.* Author.

Prüss-Ustün, A., Wolf, J., Corvalán, C., et al. (2016). *Preventing disease through health environments: A global assessment of the burden of disease from environmental risks.* Geneva: World Health Organization (WHO). Retrieved from http://apps.who.int/iris/bitstream/10665/204585/1/9789241565196_eng.pdf.

Racher, F. E., & Annis, R. C. (2012). Honouring culture and diversity in community practice. In A. R. Vollmann, E. T. Anderson, & J. McFarlane (Eds.), *Canadian community as partner: Theory & multidisciplinary practice* (3rd ed., pp. 154–176). Philadelphia, PA: Lippincott Williams & Wilkins.

Racine, L. (2009). Examining the conflation of multiculturalism, sexism, and religious fundamentalism through Taylor and Bakhtin: Expanding post-colonial feminist epistemology. *Nursing Philosophy, 10*(1), 14–25. doi:10.1111/j.1466-76X.2008.00378.x.

Ramsden, I. M. (2002). *Cultural safety and nursing education in Aotearoa and Te Waipounamu.* Unpublished doctoral dissertation, Victoria University of Wellington, New Zealand.

Raphael, D. (2012). *Tackling health inequalities: Lessons from international experiences.* Toronto, ON: Canadian Scholars' Press.

Raphael, D. (Ed.), (2016). *Social determinants of health: Canadian perspectives* (3rd ed.). Toronto, ON: Canadian Scholars' Press.

Reutter, L., & Kushner, K. (2010). "Health equity through action on the social determinants of health": Taking up the challenge in nursing. *Nursing Inquiry, 17*(3), 269–280. doi:10.111/j.1440-1800.2010.00500.x.

Shaffer, F. A. (2014). Ensuring a global workforce: A challenge and opportunity. *Nursing Outlook, 62*(1), 1–4. doi:10.1016/j.outlook.2013.08.001.

Shamian, J., & Ellen, M. E. (2016). The role of nurses and nurse leaders on realizing the clinical, social, and economic return on investment in nursing care. *Healthcare Management Forum, 29*(2), 99–103. doi:10.1177/0840470416629163.

Simpson, D., Jakubec, S., Zawaduk, C., et al. (2015). Integrating global citizenship through local teaching practices. *Quality Advancement in Nursing Education, 1*(2), doi:10.17483/2368-6669.1031.

Skolnik, R. (2016). *Global health 101* (3rd ed.). Burlington, MA: Jones & Bartlett Learning.

Smith, D., Edwards, N., Varcoe, C., et al. (2006). Bringing safety and responsiveness into the forefront of care for pregnant and parenting aboriginal people. *ANS. Advances in Nursing Science, 29*, E27–E44.

Spector, R. E. (2012). *Cultural diversity in health and illness* (8th ed.). Upper Saddle River, NJ: Prentice Hall Health.

Srivastava, R. H. (Ed.), (2007a). *The healthcare professional's guide to clinical cultural competence*. Toronto: Elsevier Canada.

Srivastava, R. H. (2007b). Culture: Perspectives, myths, and misconceptions. In R. H. Srivastava (Ed.), *The healthcare professional's guide to clinical cultural competence* (pp. 28–52). Toronto: Elsevier Canada.

Statistics Canada (2013a). *Immigration and ethnocultural diversity in Canada. National household survey, 2011*. (Statistics Canada Catalogue No. 99-010-X2011001). Ottawa: Author. Retrieved from http://www12.statcan.gc.ca/nhs-enm/2011/as-sa/99-010-x/99-010-x2011001-eng.pdf.

Statistics Canada (2013b). *Aboriginal Peoples in Canada: First Nations People, Métis and Inuit. National Household Survey, 2011*. (Statistics Canada Catalogue no, 99-011-X2011001). Ottawa: Author. Retrieved from http://www12.statcan.gc.ca/nhs-enm/2011/as-sa/99-011-x/99-011-x2011001-eng.pdf.

Statistics Canada. (2017a). *Ethnic and cultural origins of Canadians: Portrait of a rich heritage*. http://www12.statcan.gc.ca/census-recensement/2016/as-sa/98-200-x/2016016/98-200-x2016016-eng.cfm.

Statistics Canada. (2017b). *Data Tables 2016*. http://www12.statcan.gc.ca/census-recensement/2016/dp-pd/dt-td/Rp-eng.cfm?LANG=E&APATH=3&DETAIL=0&DIM=0&FL=A&FREE=0&GC=0&GID=0&GK=0&GRP=1&PID=110531&PRID=10&PTYPE=109445&S=0&SHOWALL=0&SUB=0&Temporal=2017&THEME=120&VID=0&VNAMEE=&VNAMEF=.

Statistics Canada. (2017c). *Immigrant populations in Canada, 2016 Census in Population*. http://www.statcan.gc.ca/pub/11-627-m/11-627-m2017028-eng.htm.

Statistics Canada. (2017d). *Aboriginal peoples in Canada: Key results from the 2016 Censeu*. quotidien/171025/dq171025a-eng.htm.

Statistics Canada. (2017e). *English, French and official language minorities in Canada*. Retrieved from http://www12.statcan.gc.ca/census-recensement/2016/as-sa/98-200-x/2016011/98-200-x2016011-eng.cfm.

Thomas, V. (2017). *Climate change and natural disasters: Transforming economies and policies for a sustainable future*. NB: Transaction.

United Nations (2015). *The Millennium Development Goals report 2015*. New York: Author. Retrieved from http://www.un.org/millenniumgoals/2015_MDG_Report/pdf/MDG%202015%20rev%20(July%201).pdf.

United Nations (2017a). *Sustainable Development Goals Report 2017*. Retrieved from https://unstats.un.org/sdgs/files/report/2017/TheSustainableDevelopmentGoalsReport2017.pdf.

United Nations (2017b). *Sustainable development agenda*. Retrieved from http://www.un.org/sustainabledevelopment/development-agenda/.

United Nations. (2017c). *The universal declaration of human rights*. http://www.un.org/en/universal-declaration-human-rights/.

United Nations High Commissioner of Refugees (UNHCR). (2017). *Population statistics database*. Retrieved from http://popstats.unhcr.org/en/overview#_ga=1.230279774.352162355.1489117085.

Upval, M. J., & Leffers, J. M. (2014). *Global health nursing: Building and sustaining partnerships*. New York, NY: Springer.

Van Herk, K. A., Smith, D., & Andrew, C. (2011). Examining our privileges and oppressions: incorporating an intersectionality paradigm into nursing. *Nursing Inquiry, 18*(1), 29–39. doi:10.1111/j.1440-1800.2011.00539.x.

Whitmee, S., Haines, A., Beyrer, C., et al. (2015). Safeguarding human health in the Anthropocene epoch: Report of The Rockefeller Foundation-Lancet Commission on planetary health. *Lancet, 386*(10007), 1973–2028. doi:10.1016/S0140-6736(15)60901-1.

Wilkinson, L., Anchan, J., Arthur, N., et al. (2010). A portrait of the health and well-being of newcomer children and youth in the prairies. *Prairie Metropolis Centre Working Paper Series*. Published online at https://books.google.es/books/about/A_Portrait_of_the_Health_and_Well_being.html?id=1qi4nQAACAAJ&redir_esc=y.

Wilson, L., Harper, D. C., Tami-Maury, I., et al. (2012). Global health competencies for nurses in the Americas. *Journal of Professional Nursing, 28*(4), 213–222. doi:10.1016/j.profnurs.2011.11.021.

World Health Organization (WHO) (2010). *Injuries and violence: the facts*. Geneva: World Health Organization.

World Health Organization (WHO) (2014). *Global status report on noncommunicable diseases 2014*. Geneva: Author. Retrieved from http://www.who.int/nmh/publications/ncd-status-report-2014/en/.

World Health Organization (WHO). (2015). *Health in 2015 from MDGs Millennium goals to SDGs Sustainable development goals*. Retrieved from http://www.who.int/gho/publications/mdgs-sdgs/en/.

World Health Organization (WHO). (2016a). *Preventing disease through healthy environments: A global assessment of the burden of disease from environment risks*. http://www.who.int/healthsystems/about/en/.

World Health Organization (WHO). (2016b). *Noncommunicable diseases*. Retrieved from http://www.who.int/mediacentre/factsheets/fs355/en/.

World Health Organization (WHO). (2016c). *Neglected tropical diseases*. Retrieved from http://www.who.int/neglected_diseases/diseases/en.

World Health Organization (WHO). (2016d). *Intersectoral action for health*. Retrieved from http://www.who.int/kobe_centre/interventions/intersectorial_action/en/.

World Health Organization (WHO), the United Nations Development Programme (UNDP), & the United Nations Office on Drugs and Crime (UNODC). (2014) *Global status report on violence prevention 2014*. Retrieved December 3, 2016 from http://www.who.int/violence_injury_prCevention/violence/status_report/2014/en.

World Health Organization (WHO). (2018.) Nursing Now Campaign. http://www.who.int/hrh/news/2018/nursing_now_campaign/en/

Worthington, E. L., Jr., Davis, D. E., & Hook, J. N. (Eds.), (2017). *Handbook of humility: Theory, research, and applications*. New York, NY: Taylor and Francis.

10

Indigenous Health

Written by Sylvia S. Barton, RN, PhD, Caroline Foster-Boucher, RN, MN

OBJECTIVES

Mastery of content in this chapter will enable you to:

- Describe the Indigenous diversity of the Canadian population.
- Examine the Canadian history of colonization that includes pre-European and post-European contact.
- Differentiate between the historical timeline of key Indigenous events and legislation in Canada.
- Analyze components of colonialism to understand the complexities of the relationship that evolved between Indigenous peoples and Europeans.
- Examine the legacy of residential schools, which has had devastating consequences for Indigenous communities across Canada.
- Describe the concepts of structural racism, child welfare, poverty, and the justice system in relation to nursing practice.
- Differentiate between respect, trust, and spirituality in the context of caring for Indigenous people.
- Describe components of Indigenous cultural orientations in relation to nursing practice.
- Examine selected chronic illness experiences relevant to the Indigenous peoples of Canada.
- Apply research findings to the provision of nursing care of Indigenous peoples in Canada, with consideration of assessment and intervention underpinned by cultural safety, health equity, and social justice.
- Differentiate between Indigenous health from a global perspective and Indigenous health from a Canadian perspective.

KEY TERMS

Colonialism, p. 136
Cultural genocide, p. 138
Determinants of health, p. 144
Historical trauma, p. 136
Holistic view, p. 136
Indian Act, p. 134
Indigenous health, p. 141
Indigenous peoples, p. 133
Indigenous world view, p. 141
Intergenerational trauma, p. 137
Pre-European contact, p. 134
Post-European contact, p. 137
Residential schools, p. 137
Sixties Scoop, p. 139
Structural racism, p. 138
Theories of Indigenous health, p. 141
Truth and Reconciliation Commission, p. 138
Two-spirited, p. 147

MEDIA RESOURCES

http://evolve.elsevier.com/Canada/Potter/fundamentals/

- Audio Chapter Summaries
- Examination Review Questions
- Concept Map Creator
- Case Study with Questions
- Audio Glossary
- Content Updates
- Video Clips

INDIGENOUS DIVERSITY—THE CANADIAN PERSPECTIVE

Recognizing the diversity of Indigenous peoples of Canada requires an understanding of specific cultural groups in order to appreciate their contemporary health issues (Canadian Association of Schools of Nursing, 2015). **Indigenous peoples** represent an important and growing group within Canada. In 2011, the number of people who identified themselves as Indigenous (First Nations, Métis, and Inuit) surpassed 1.4 million (Statistics Canada, 2013a). Since the mid-1990s, the Indigenous population has increased significantly. Between 2006 and 2011, it grew by 20.1%, nearly four times faster than the 5.2% increase for the non-Indigenous population (Statistics Canada, 2013a). In 2011, Indigenous peoples accounted for 4.3% of the total population of Canada (Statistics Canada, 2013a). Of the three Indigenous groups, the First Nations population increased most between 2006 and 2011. Indigenous peoples in Canada also increasingly live in urban centres. In 2011, 56% lived in urban areas (including large cities or census metropolitan areas and smaller urban centres); this proportion increased from 49% in 1996 (Indigenous and Northern Affairs Canada [INAC], 2013a, 2016a). Furthermore, the Indigenous population is, on average, younger than the non-Indigenous population. Almost half (46%) of Indigenous peoples consist of children and youth aged 24 and younger, in comparison to 29% of the non-Indigenous population (INAC, 2013b).

The three Indigenous groups—First Nations, Métis, and Inuit—have their own unique languages, heritages, cultural practices, and spiritual beliefs (INAC, 2016b). These groups contain many subgroups, each with its own unique culture. The legal term *Indian* describes all the Indigenous peoples in Canada who are not Inuit. This includes the nations or groups of people who were originally living in Canada before the European explorers began to arrive in the 1600s (pre-contact), and the Métis, who are a specific cultural entity formed after contact with Europeans (post-contact) and before colonization. Legal definitions used to describe Indians in Canada include Status, non-Status, and Treaty Indians. *Status* Indians are registered under the **Indian Act** (INAC, 2013c), which regulates the management of reserves and sets out certain federal obligations. A *Treaty* Indian is a Status Indian who belongs to a First Nation that signed a treaty with the Crown (INAC, 2013c). Until recently, non-Status Indians and Métis peoples were not included as Indians under Section 91(24) of the *Constitution Act*. However, in 1999, four claimants brought action against the Canadian federal government, seeking a declaration that Métis and non-Status Indians fall within federal jurisdiction. In addition, their actions declared that Métis and non-Status Indians have the right to be consulted by, and to negotiate with, the federal government over needs, rights, and interests as Indigenous peoples. In what is now known as the "Daniels Decision" (*Daniels v. Canada* [Indian Affairs and Northern Development]), in 2016 the Supreme Court sided in favour of non-Status Indians and Métis as being "Indian" under S.91(24) of the *Constitution Act*. Currently, the federal government is closely examining this ruling to determine its meaning in terms of legislative authority (INAC, 2016c; Supreme Court of Canada, 2016).

Approximately 53 Indigenous languages in 12 different language families exist in Canada, with Algonquian being the largest and most widespread language family (Statistics Canada, 2015). Many Indigenous languages have identifiable dialects; however, some are in decline, owing to the history of assimilation policies carried out by the Canadian government, such as residential schooling. Interpreters who translate for Indigenous patients not only understand and translate the language but also make concepts relevant within the cultural realm, interpreting the culture for the health care provider. Accurately and culturally appropriate translated health care information can lead to patient empowerment and better health choices (Eggertson, 2014).

The Indigenous peoples of Canada are exceptionally diverse—culturally, linguistically, socially, economically, and historically—as well as in many other ways. There are distinct cultural differences between the Indigenous groups, derived from history and geographic influences on day-to-day life. The diversity of Indigenous peoples exists within Indian bands or First Nations across Canada (Assembly of First Nations, n.d.), within at least two distinct cultures of the Métis, and where differences emanate from particular historical experiences and geographic locations of the Inuit. Connecting diversity to Indigenous health, Waldram, Herring, and Young (2006) state:

> *The recognition and acceptance of such diversity is essential to an appreciation of developments in the healthcare field and to an appreciation of the myriad processes that have affected the health status of Indigenous people in both the pre-contact and post-contact periods. (p. 23)*

INDIGENOUS HISTORY IN CANADA

An appreciation of Indigenous history requires an understanding of the history of colonization that includes pre-European and post-European contact (see Table 10-1 for a historical timeline of key Indigenous events and legislation in Canada). **Pre-European contact** refers to the history of Indigenous peoples before exploration and settlement of the Americas by Europeans. During that period, Indigenous peoples were composed of distinct cultures from the Arctic, Western Subarctic, Eastern Subarctic, Northeastern Woodlands, Plains, Plateau, and Northwest Coast.

The Inuit have inhabited northern Canada for over 5 000 years. In 2011, there were 59 445 Inuit, which comprise 4.2% of the Indigenous population and 0.2% of the Canadian population (Statistics Canada, 2013a). Almost three-quarters of Inuit live in the northern part of Canada, in four territories (Inuit Nunangat) that were negotiated in land claim agreements with the federal government (Penny, O'Sullivan, & Senecal, 2012; Statistics Canada, 2013a). The four areas of Inuit Nunangat include Nunatsiavut (Northern Labrador), Nunavik (Northern Quebec), the Territory of Nunavut, and the Inuvialuit Settlement Region (Northwest Territories) (Penny et al., 2012). Each of the four regions has its own flag and history, as well as distinct geography and regional experiences of the people (Inuit Tapiriit Kanatami, 2017).

The Métis have been noted as a distinct Indigenous group in Canada, born from the union of Indigenous women and European men during the fur trade era, post-contact but precolonially. There are a variety of theories about who is Métis and how being Métis is defined. It is hard to pin down an unambiguous definition of Métis identity, although a number of definitions have been put forth by scholars and others (Andersen, 2016; Métis Nation of Alberta, 2017; Province of Alberta, 2015). There is disagreement, however, about whether a person's "mixedness" leads to a Métis identity, or whether a historical familial connection is what is necessary to be Métis. As to their exact genesis in time or place, literature offers a variety of theories, including a focus on the Red River settlements of what is now Winnipeg, and also in the Great Lakes Region, as well as a questioning of whether or not there is more diversity within the Métis community than currently noted. There is also disagreement about what propelled the Métis to establish nationhood—whether it was based on class structure, spirituality, occupation niches in the fur trading companies, political pressures, language, location, or a combination of factors (O'Toole, 2013).

Currently over 4 800 Métis live on eight provincial constitutionally protected settlements in Alberta, which are the only lands set aside for the Métis (Government of Alberta, 1990; Métis Settlements General Council, n.d.). In 2016, The Manitoba Métis Federation signed an agreement with the federal government to negotiate a land claim based on the 1870 *Manitoba Act* in which the Métis were promised land never received (Malone, 2016). Historically, the Métis have suffered great inequity and social exclusion from Canadian society. Currently, accurate statistics about the health of the Métis are minimal, owing to issues related to identity and misunderstood identity, interpretation of statistics, and other political pressures that influence defining who is Métis and how the data are gathered and interpreted (Andersen, 2016).

The term *First Nations* is derived from *Indian*, a legal term used in the *Indian Act* to refer to a Status Indian. The *Indian Act* was first passed in 1876 and has been amended a number of times since (see Box 10-1 for specific amendments). Its main purpose was to assimilate First Nations people into Canadian society. It sets out federal obligations toward "Indians" and regulates the management of reserves, money, and other resources for "Indians." The term *Indian* is generally not preferred by Indigenous people. A preferred term is *First Nation/s*, which can refer to a person or a group of First Nations people legally known as an Indian band (INAC, 2013c). Currently there are 634 First Nations or Indian bands in Canada.

A *reserve* is a piece of land that has been set aside by the federal government for the exclusive use of an Indian band or First Nation. Each First Nation may have one or more reserves based on treaty agreement and population. First Nations have a Chief and Council governance structure that was imposed on them through the *Indian Act*. Traditionally, this was not the way Indigenous peoples self-governed

TABLE 10-1 Indigenous Timeline: Key Events and Legislation

1500s and 1600s	**Early contact** between Indigenous peoples and Europeans. Relationship consisted of trading, mutual curiosity, and intermarriage. French settlement developed in Acadia.
1613	**Two Row Wampum Treaty** between Haudenosaunee and the Dutch in upstate New York—belts said to be created in order to record the agreement with two rows of purple shells symbolizing two boats (one Indigenous, one European) travelling side by side on the River of Life (Parmenter, 2013).
1664	Two Row Wampum Treaty between Haudenosaunee and the British Crown in Albany (Mohawks of the Bay of Quinte, n.d.; Parmenter, 2013).
1670	**Hudson's Bay Company** incorporated by the English Royal Charter. Headquarters at York Factory on Hudson's Bay, controlled fur trade in North America for two centuries (Hudson's Bay Company History Foundation, 2016a, 2016b).
1754–1763	**French and Indian War/Seven Years' War**—French and British colonies and their Indigenous allies were pitted against each other; it ended in Treaty of Paris; Britain gained control of French Canada and Acadia (Dickason & Newbigging, 2015).
1763	**Royal Proclamation of 1763**—issued by King George III to protect the land rights of Indigenous peoples by prohibiting purchase of or settling on Indigenous lands.
1834	**Mohawk Indian Residential School opens in Brantford Ontario** (TRC, 2015b).
1857	***British North America Act***—created Dominion of Canada and gave Canada jurisdiction over "Indians" and over lands reserved for "Indians" (Dickason & Newbigging, 2015).
1867	***Gradual Civilization Act***—introduced idea of enfranchisement for Indigenous peoples. Males age 21 and up, literate in English or French, with minimal education and "good moral character and free from debt" were eligible. If accepted, they would receive 20 hectares of land, and they would relinquish their treaty rights voluntarily. The government saw it as an honour that would be sought after; however, it was rejected by Indigenous peoples, with only a single candidate enfranchised by 1867 (Robinson, 2016).
1871–1921	Federal government of Canada entered into 11 numbered **treaties** with Indigenous peoples (Dickason & Newbigging, 2015).
1876	***Indian Act*** passed—introduced in 1876 as a consolidation of previous legislation which focused on assimilation of Indigenous peoples into Canadian society. Gave the government of Canada vast powers over First Nations people with regard to identity, political structures, cultural practices, governance, and education. It was amended several times, notably in 1951 and 1985 (Henderson & Parrott, 2016). (See Box 10-1 for amendments to *Indian Act* up to 1950.)
1880	**Department of Indian Affairs** is created by the government of Canada—has gone through numerous organizational and name changes since. Currently it is Indigenous and Northern Affairs Canada (Derworiz & Albers, 2015).
1883	Creation of Canada's **formal Indian residential school system**—three industrial schools opened in Western Canada by the Canadian government in partnership with Catholic and Anglican churches (TRC, 2015a).
1884	**Attendance at Indian residential schools compulsory** for Indigenous children between 7 and 16 years of age (TRC, 2015b).
1885	**Northwest Rebellion**—Uprising by Métis led by Louis Riel in what is now Manitoba against the government of Canada, with the grievance that Canada had failed to protect Métis rights, land, and survival as a distinct people. Riel and Métis surrendered; Riel was found guilty of treason and hanged (Beal, MacLeod, & Foot, 2015).
1948	**Compulsory attendance ends** at Indian residential schools (Canadian Baptists of Western Canada Justice and Mercy Network, 2013).
1951	**Changes to *Indian Act***—bans of traditional practices and ceremonies lifted; women included in band democracy (Dickason & Newbigging, 2015).
1960	**Indigenous people given right to vote** (Moss & Gardner-O'Toole, 1991).
1969	**White Paper** issued by the federal government proposing the *Indian Act* be repealed; abolishment of Department of Indian Affairs and provincial responsibility over Indigenous people, in order to assimilate Indigenous peoples into mainstream Canada. Indigenous peoples strongly resisted and put forth "Citizens Plus" (Red Paper), in which they insisted treaty and inherent rights be respected. The White Paper was retracted (Dickason & Newbigging, 2015).
1973	**Calder Case** ruling by the Supreme Court of Canada: legal assertion of Indigenous land rights, which led to comprehensive land claims policy to address Indigenous title claims (Cruickshank, 2017). **Indian Control of Indian Education paper** issued by the National Indian Brotherhood—policy adopted by the federal government (AFN, 2010).
1975	**James Bay Agreement** between Quebec, Cree, and Inuit communities (Dickason & Newbigging, 2015).
1982	**Constitutional recognition** of Indigenous and treaty rights, and *Aboriginal* peoples defined as Indian, Métis, and Inuit (Dickason & Newbigging, 2015).
1984	***Inuvialuit Claims Settlement Act*** (Dickason & Newbigging, 2015).
1985	***Indian Act* changes**—Métis and non-Status defined as Indian; **Bill C-31** allows women who lost their Indian status (due to marriage, widowing, or abandonment) to regain it (Dickason & Newbigging, 2015).
1990	**Oka crisis**—ignited by the town of Oka's plans for a golf course to be built on Mohawk burial grounds in Quebec; crisis lasted for 6 months (Dickason & Newbigging, 2015). **Meech Lake Accord** defeated in part by Elijah Harper in Manitoba Legislature (Dickason & Newbigging, 2015).

Continued

TABLE 10-1 Indigenous Timeline: Key Events and Legislation—cont'd

1991-1996	**Royal Commission on Aboriginal Peoples**; report released in 1996—most in-depth study of Indigenous issues up to this date (TRC, 2015d)
1992	Parliament passes motion citing **Louis Riel as the founder of Manitoba** (Parliament of Canada, 1992).
1996	**Last Indian residential school in Canada closes** (Gordon Indian Residential School, Punnichy, Saskatchewan).
1997	***Delgamuukw v. British Columbia***—Supreme Court decision regarding principles of Indigenous title, including property rights entitling the holders to exclusive possession and use of land and its resources (Dickason & Newbigging, 2015).
1999	**Nunavut created** (Dickason & Newbigging, 2015).
2000	**Nisaga'a Treaty approved** (Dickason & Newbigging, 2015).
2008	**Formal apology** for residential schools from Prime Minister Stephen Harper (TRC, 2015b). **Truth and Reconciliation Commission** officially launched (TRC, 2015d).
2012	**Idle No More** forms in response to alleged legislative abuses of Indigenous treaty rights by the federal government of Canada, specifically Bill C-45, an omnibus bill which produced sweeping legislative changes, including removal of protections for forests and waterways (Marshall, 2015).
2016	Canada removes objector status and officially adopts **United Declaration on the Rights of Indigenous Peoples** (Fontaine, 2016). **Truth and Reconciliation Commission of Canada** releases their final report with 94 calls to action (TRC, 2015d). Government of Canada launches an official inquiry into the missing and murdered Indigenous women in Canada (Government of Canada, 2016; Kirkup, 2016).

BOX 10-1 Amendments to the *Indian Act*, 1876–1950

Between 1876 and 1950, the purpose of the amendments to the *Indian Act* was to strengthen the philosophy of civilization and assimilation underlying the initial Act. Moreover, many of the changes to the Act granted the government greater powers to move Indigenous peoples and expropriate their lands for the purpose of non-Indigenous use.

Key amendments to the *Indian Act* during this period include the following:

- 1885: Prohibition of several traditional Indigenous ceremonies, such as potlatches.
- 1894: Removal of band control over non-Indigenous people living on reserves. This power was transferred to the Superintendent General of Indian Affairs.
- 1905: Power to remove Indigenous peoples from reserves near towns with more than 8 000 people.
- 1911: Power to expropriate portions of reserves for roads, railways, and other public works, as well as to move an entire reserve away from a municipality if it was deemed expedient.
- 1914: Requirement that western Indigenous people seek official permission before appearing in Indigenous "costume" in any public dance, show, exhibition, stampede, or pageant.
- 1918: Power to lease out uncultivated reserve lands to non-Indigenous people if the new leaseholder would use it for farming or pasture.
- 1927: Prohibition of anyone (Indigenous or otherwise) from soliciting funds for Indigenous legal claims without special licence from the Superintendent General. This amendment granted the government control over the ability of Indigenous people to pursue land claims.
- 1930: Prohibition of pool hall owners from allowing entrance of an Indigenous person who "by inordinate frequenting of a pool room either on or off an Indian reserve misspends or wastes his time or means to the detriment of himself, his family or household."

Adapted from Makarenko, J. (2008). *The Indian Act: Historical overview.* Retrieved from http://www.mapleleafweb.com/features/the-indian-act-historical-overview.html.

(St. Germain & Dyck, 2010), as many Indigenous groups are traditionally matriarchal (Allan & Smylie, 2015).

Historical knowledge of Indigenous history in Canada is foundational to understanding how Indigenous people currently view health. Such a vantage point includes an appreciation of health from a traditional Indigenous view, a Western biomedical view, and a combination view. Historically, Indigenous communities experienced healing and well-being through a **holistic view** of health, in which illness and treatment consisted of physical, emotional, mental, and spiritual dimensions. Traditional shamans, herbalists, and specialized healers worked within a holistic framework in order to heal afflicted persons (Earle, 2011; Waldram et al., 2006). Research provides evidence that Indigenous peoples were generally healthy and well nourished before contact, with death coming via injury, accidents, or wounds sustained in warfare. Diseases were likely minimal, and there is no evidence to date of widespread diffusion of disease pre-contact (Douglas, 2013).

Colonialism

What we refer to as colonialism is actually a theoretical framework for understanding the complexities of the relationship that evolved between Indigenous peoples and Europeans as they came into contact and as they later sustained those initial relationships in building a new reality in North America. Specifically, **colonialism** is the development of institutions and policies by European imperial and Euro-American settler governments toward Indigenous peoples (Truth and Reconciliation Commission [TRC], 2015b, p. 43-50). Nelson (2012) notes the importance of being aware of this history and to embrace an Indigenous healing journey. There is strong agreement that the experiences of colonialism resulted in much **historical trauma** (the nature of trauma as experienced over many years) for Indigenous people. Responding to many of the mental health challenges that Indigenous people experience in their lives requires a deep understanding of the historical, social, and economic contexts in which Indigenous families and communities are situated.

European contact began in the Eastern Arctic, where Norse made contact initially with Inuit starting in 1000 BC and continuing throughout the centuries. French explorers and fur traders settled on the lower east coast and introduced diseases such as smallpox, tuberculosis (TB), and measles, which killed thousands of Indigenous people. Scarce resources diminished Indigenous livelihoods, and malnutrition, starvation, and alcohol consumption made circumstances worse (Dickason & Newbigging, 2015; Waldram et al., 2006).

During post-European contact, Europeans established relationships with Indigenous people and colonization influenced Indigenous systems of government, trade, and health care. Over the years, the Canadian government displaced Indigenous people from their traditional lands and developed policies to isolate and assimilate them into Canadian society, which resulted in the destruction of Indigenous cultures. These oppressive and suppressive policies and the acts that followed had extensive negative effects on Indigenous cultural identities and governance structures (TRC, 2015c, p. 3-4). The Indian residential school system, for example, which no longer exists in Canada, left a legacy over several generations resulting in physical and psychological abuse that "is reflected in the significant educational, income, health and social disparities between Aboriginal people and other Canadians" (TRC, 2015b, p. 135).

Residential Schools

Residential schools and associated policies were a central element in colonial practices in Canada, wherein Indigenous children as young as 5 years old were separated from their parents, in many cases forcibly. The children were sent to residential schools to board year-round, in order to sever the link between identity and culture. This was part of a policy to eliminate Indigenous people as a distinct group and to assimilate them into mainstream Canadian society. The ulterior motive was to avoid the legal and financial obligations that the federal government had with Indigenous people, as well as to gain control over their lands and resources, thereby eliminating treaties, reserves, and Indigenous rights (TRC, 2015b, p. 3).

The government of Canada funded churches that included Roman Catholic, Anglican, United, Methodist, and Presbyterian to operate at least 139 residential schools beginning in the 1880s, the last one closing in 1996 (TRC, 2015b, p. 3) At least 150 000 Indigenous children attended these schools over approximately 130 years, in poorly built and maintained buildings, with limited numbers of inadequately trained staff. There was minimal regulation, and the few regulations that were in place were weakly enforced. The children were harshly disciplined and were forbidden to speak their language or practise any part of their own culture, including spirituality. They received a rudimentary education and were often forced to engage in chores to maintain the schools' operations. It is estimated that at least 3 200 children died from malnourishment, diseases such as TB, and abuse; this number includes those who ran away and those who froze to death. The number of children who died could be 5 to 10 times higher; however, given poor record-keeping, the full number may never be known (Mas, 2015; TRC, 2015a). In many cases, the schools did not record the name or gender of the children who died and generally did not send the child's body back to their home community to be buried (TRC, 2016a, p. 118, TRC, 2015b, p. 100). Physical and sexual abuse were rampant throughout the schools (TRC, 2015b, p. 105-110) and usually went unreported. If abuse was reported, little was done other than moving the perpetrator to another school or having the person resign. Few police investigations occurred, and prosecutions were rare.

The legacy of residential schools, one of the most long-lasting effects of colonialism, has had devastating consequences for Indigenous communities across Canada. Students who stayed at residential schools became institutionalized and had no experience in being parented. Because of their institutional upbringing, they were unable to learn how to parent; no such lessons were taught, and no such family interactions existed. The children and grandchildren of residential school survivors tell of growing up in abusive homes, with minimal affection and severe strictness and discipline—experiences similar to what the survivors experienced in residential school (Elias, Mignone, Hall, et al., 2012; TRC, 2015c p. 11-12, 32-33). This is now understood as intergenerational trauma. Intergenerational trauma is defined as the pathways by which the nature of trauma is understood and experienced by "Aboriginal survivors of the residential school system and their descendants" as well as "the pathways by which this trauma is transmitted from one generation to the next" (Aguiar & Halseth, 2015, p. 23). Suicide rates are much higher among children and grandchildren of survivors than for survivors themselves. The reasons for this are unclear, and the health issue requires further study. Some survivors turned to alcohol and other substances to cope with post-traumatic stress disorder; the effects of addiction have had a stronghold on some families and communities for decades. Diets have been poor as a result of minimal knowledge of nutrition and of food pattern issues derived from residential schools. Sexual abuse is rampant in some communities, as evidenced by recent reports (Elias et al., 2012; Kirkup & Ubelacker, 2016; TRC, 2015c, p. 70).

The government of Canada has failed in its assimilation goal, with Indigenous people surviving the atrocities of residential schools. However, the legacy of residential schools is still reflected in the significant health, educational, and income disparities between Indigenous people and other Canadians. Furthermore, intergenerational trauma is rampant, with some children who were abused becoming abusers, developing addictions as a way of coping, and being unable to parent their own children because of lack of experience of being parented.

Truth and Reconciliation

In the 1960s, with the onset of the assertion of Indigenous rights globally, the Civil Rights Movement in the United States, and the Catholic social justice movement that came to be known as liberation theology, churches began to examine their relationship with Indigenous peoples in Canada (TRC, 2015d). A number of churches apologized in the 1970s, 80s, and 90s for their treatment of, and the impact of their work on, Indigenous peoples in Canada (TRC, 2015d).

From the 1970s through to the 90s, residential school survivors wrote memoirs, accounts, and histories of their experiences. During this time, the Royal Commission on Aboriginal Peoples (RCAP) was established to study the evolution of the relationship among Aboriginal peoples, the government of Canada, and Canadian society as a whole. The final report was released in 1996, in which a full chapter was dedicated to residential schools. In response to RCAP, the federal government issued an action plan that included an apology and a healing fund entitled the *Aboriginal Healing Foundation* (AHF) (TRC, 2015d, p. 521-579).

Residential school survivors, however, organized into associations and turned to the courts through the 1980s and 90s. By 2005, more than 18 000 residential school survivors had filed lawsuits against the churches, the federal government, and other organizations involved as well as individuals who had committed the abuses. As a result of the staggering number of civil court cases and complex litigation, increasing costs, and the crippling effect on churches, the federal government created the Office of Indian Residential Schools Resolution (OIRSR). The OIRSR negotiated with churches and eventually launched the National Resolution Framework, of which a central element was the alternative dispute resolution process. However, this was met with much criticism and was eventually dropped. In the early 2000s, over 20 class action lawsuits were filed against the federal government. Eventually Indigenous organizations, church organizations, and the federal government began talks that would lead to the Indian Residential Schools Settlement Agreement (TRC, 2015d).

There were five main components of Truth and Reconciliation, of which the Truth and Reconciliation Commission (TRC) was one. These included the Common Experience Payment (CEP), in which all who had resided at a residential school would be eligible for a $10 000 CEP, plus an additional $3 000 for each year or partial year they attended (TRC, 2015d). There was also an independent assessment process available for those who had suffered abuse or neglect. This process used a points system in which a number of points were assigned to each claim, based on the type and frequency of assaults, as well as the consequences of the abuse. The number of points determined the claimant's award: the maximum amount was $275 000 dollars, plus an additional amount up to another $275 000 to be awarded in complex cases; 15% of each award would be paid to the survivor's counsel; $20 million was set aside for commemoration initiatives; and $125 million was set aside for the AHF to address the healing needs of Aboriginal people affected. The Anglican, Presbyterian, United, and Catholic churches all contributed funds (TRC, 2015d).

This agreement only covered Aboriginal people within the series of lawsuits, and the list of schools was limited to those with a residential component. It did not address the claims of Métis students, or a number of other situations and places, such as day schools (TRC, 2015d). There continue to be issues still being dealt with today. For instance, there is a class action lawsuit for First Nations people who attended residential schools during the day as day students (Canadian Broadcasting Company [CBC], 2016; Munson, 2016) and one for those who were in hospital but attended school during the day. These students were denied the CEP payout. The lawsuit is also seeking compensation for descendants of survivors and for First Nations bands that resided close to the schools.

In 2008, Prime Minister Stephen Harper issued a national apology in Parliament to Indigenous peoples in Canada. After Harper's statement, government opposition party leaders issued their own apologies. Then Indigenous leaders such as National Chief Phil Fontaine, Mary Simon, President of the Inuit Tapiriit Kanatami, and various others responded to the apologies (TRC, 2015d).

The TRC issued its final report in 2015. It comprises 10 books, or volumes, of information covering the full history, from early European imperialism to the year 2000; the final report includes survivors' stories and documentation of Inuit and Métis experiences, missing children and unmarked burials, and the legacy of residential schools. The TRC found that many of the 150 000 children who attended residential school were abused sexually, physically, emotionally, and spiritually. The TRC also stated that Canada was guilty of cultural genocide with respect to Indigenous people in Canada, which is the "destruction of those structures and practices that allow the group to continue as a group" (TRC, 2015a, p. 3). Instances of destruction of practices and structures included occupying and seizing land; forcing relocation of Indigenous peoples; confining them to reserves; disempowering them through replacement of existing forms of Indigenous government; and denying them basic rights, such as the right to practise their faith, the right to assemble, and the right to legal counsel.

The TRC released 94 calls to action to address the ongoing legacy of residential schools in Canada for Indigenous peoples. These calls to action address policy as well as institutional and governmental structures within Canada, such as child welfare, justice, education, language rights, government Indigenous funding programs, and health care. To help enact such actions, the TRC encouraged citizens to become a settler ally—teachers and learners who question how non-Indigenous people can change, as opposed to just Indigenous people changing (Box 10-2). In addition, calls to action were directed at the government to take steps to improve its policies and funding practices for a variety of aspects within the Indigenous realm, such as commencement of the inquiry into missing and murdered Indigenous women in Canada and adoption of the United Nations *Declaration on the Rights of Indigenous Peoples* (TRC, 2015c). Call to Action #24 is specifically directed at medical and nursing schools:

> *We call upon medical and nursing schools in Canada to require all students to take a course dealing with Aboriginal health issues, including the history and legacy of residential schools, the United Nations Declaration on the Rights of Indigenous Peoples, Treaties and Aboriginal rights, and Indigenous teachings and practices. This will require skills-based training in intercultural competency, conflict resolution, human rights, and anti-racism. (TRC, 2015c, p. 181)*

Structural Racism

Structural racism is the legitimized and normalized spectrum of attitudes, practices, and policies that consistently result in chronic and continuous substandard outcomes for Indigenous peoples. An example of structural racism within Indigenous communities involves the delays in service for on-reserve status First Nations children because of complex funding systems and delivery of services in health care as well as jurisdictional issues. Other children's health care is funded provincially or territorially. Health care services of on-reserve First Nations children, by contrast, are funded through the federal government but regulated through provincial/territorial systems and policies. Given the complexity of this process, services are often denied, delayed, or disrupted, which can lead to severe health consequences. Jordan's Principle was established in response to the death of a 5-year-old child, Jordan River Anderson, from Norway House First Nation, who died in hospital having never lived in a family home (despite having received medical approval to go home 2 years earlier) because of jurisdictional funding disputes by provincial and federal government agencies (Jordan's Principle Working Group, 2015). Jordan's Principle states that the agency that has first contact with the child and family must pay for services without delay and must sort out financial agreements with other agencies after the child has received services. This action was included in the TRCs 94 calls to action (Jordan's Principle Working Group, 2015).

Another example of greater harm resulting from structural racism involves assault of Indigenous women. According to the 2009 General Social Survey, approximately 67 000 Indigenous women aged 15 or older across the provinces self-reported that they had experienced one or more crimes of a violent nature such as sexual assault, robbery, and physical assault in the 12 months prior to the survey. This rate is almost three times higher than the rate reported by non-Aboriginal women and represents about two-thirds (63%) of Indigenous females aged 15 to 34 (Statistics Canada, 2013b). In recent years, it has become evident that a large number of Indigenous women in Canada have gone missing and been murdered. Estimates vary widely; the Royal Canadian Mounted Police (RCMP) has reported a total of nearly 1 200 missing and/or murdered Indigenous women (RCMP, 2015). Government ministers have indicated that the number is "way, way higher" than the RCMP estimates and could be as high as 4 000 women (Tasker, 2016). The RCMP found that 16% of all female homicide victims in Canada are Indigenous, despite Indigenous people making up only 4.3% of the total Canadian population, and that between 2001 and 2014, the average rate of homicide of Indigenous females was four times higher than that of other female victims in Canada (RCMP, 2015). The government of Canada launched the National Inquiry into Missing and Murdered Indigenous Women and Girls in December 2015 after much

BOX 10-2 A Set of Questions for Personal Reflection—Steps to Becoming a Settler Ally

What Is a Settler Ally?

A *settler ally* is someone who collectively considers how steps taken can advance the Truth and Reconciliation process (94 calls to action). All Canadians have been invited by the Truth and Reconciliation Commission of Canada to become a settler ally—teachers and learners who want to be informed of Indigenous–non-Indigenous historical relations; of Indigenous world views related to treaties, economic development, environment, community, and negotiations; and of instructional holistic approaches that are inclusive and safe, such as smudge ceremonies, talking circles, and Indigenous teachings.

Why Do Non-Indigenous Canadians Need to Share the Burden of the Residential School System?

> *If you have come to help me, you are wasting your time; but if you are here because your liberation is bound up with mine, then let us work together.* —Lilla Watson, Aboriginal Elder, activist, educator (Australia)

Steps to Becoming a Settler Ally

1. Self-awareness
   - Note circumstances throughout your life which have placed you where you are now—education, social support, family financial situation, and environment. Examine them for aspects that have matched dominant societal expectations—ethnicity, financial situation, dwelling, ability to go to school, clothing, transportation, social support.
   - Consider the history of your family in Canada. Are you settlers from generations back, or more recent settlers? What part did your family play in society during key times during the last 150 years in Canada? Were they settlers buying land, building a farm, or building a business, or were they newcomers that arrived in the last 20 years? Learn about your ancestry and the cultural history of your family.
   - What are your assumptions about what a good life is and how to attain it? What are your assumptions about right and wrong, about what causes the ills in society? Examine your assumptions and how they were formed. Did you gain them through discussion with family and friends? Through the media? Through school? What alternative viewpoints might there be?
2. Self-education
   - Access resources to find out about the history of Indigenous peoples in Canada.
   - Read about residential school, about treaties, about racism.
   - Watch videos, look at blogs, attend lectures and film screenings.
   - Discuss with Indigenous community members.
   - Discuss with settlers.
3. Create an open and supportive environment
   - Acknowledge and appreciate the similarities and differences among individuals and within groups.
   - Encourage an atmosphere of respect and trust.
   - Be open to feedback regarding yourself, organization, workplace, and community. Create safe spaces and opportunities to receive feedback.
   - Listen carefully and reflect on feedback.
   - Take action to move forward using feedback as a guide.
   - Recognize that mistakes will be made and sometimes that is how we learn.
   - Speak for yourself, not for others. Do things for others only if asked to.
4. Action
   - Recognize that identity as an ally comes from the community, not from oneself.
   - Share knowledge with those around you; help others understand privilege and oppression, colonization and decolonization.
   - Build partnerships with others and develop plans to promote structural change.
   - Stand up against and challenge oppression, racism, and colonization.
   - Stand with Indigenous peoples, do not lead them, do not speak for them. Follow them rather than lead. Be supportive and offer assistance in whatever way is needed. Recognize that there may be politics and processes that you may not be aware of in the Indigenous arena.

From Gehl, L. (2014). *A colonized ally meets a decolonized ally: This is what they learn.* Retrieved from http://www.lynngehl.com/black-face-blogging/a-colonized-ally-meets-a-decolonized-ally-this-is-what-they-learn; Pinch, S. (2014). *Revolution 101: How to be a settler ally.* Retrieved from http://rabble.ca/blogs/bloggers/activist-toolkit/2014/05/revolution-101-how-to-be-settler-ally; Theatre Communications Group. (n.d.). *Leadership development in interethnic relations: 4 steps to becoming an ally.* Retrieved from https://www.tcg.org/pdfs/events/fallforum/4_Steps_to_Becoming_an_Ally.pdf; *Unsettling America: Decolonization in theory and practice.* (n.d.). Retrieved from https://unsettlingamerica.wordpress.com/.

public pressure (Government of Canada, 2016; Native Women's Association of Canada, 2010).

Child Welfare. In 1955, fewer than 1% of Indigenous children were in government care in British Columbia. By 1964, 30% of the children in care in BC were Indigenous, suggesting a dramatic increase of Indigenous children in care. This pattern was similar to that in other parts of Canada and was initially referred to by an employee of the Ministry of Human Resources in BC as the **Sixties Scoop**, a term still used today to describe a phenomenon that continued into the 1990s. This phenomenon involved a situation in which children were apprehended from reservations and Indigenous families "on the slightest pretext" (Johnston, 1983, p. 23) in order to "save them from the effects of crushing poverty, unsanitary health conditions, poor housing and malnutrition" (Johnston, 1983, p. 23). Often these children were placed in non-Indigenous homes. The effects of removal from family and culture, however, were not considered. Some First Nations lost almost an entire generation of children in this way (Johnston, 1983).

Current discourse has placed the blame for the Sixties Scoop not on the compassion of social workers but instead on a continuation of the assimilation process and devaluation of the cultures of a colonized people. While residential schools were being phased out as the institutional agent of colonization, the child welfare system was still able to remove Indigenous children from families "in the best interest of the child" (Johnston, 1983, p. 24).

Research has found that many of the children who were removed and placed with non-Indigenous families did not fare well. In many cases, children were abused and suffered neglect, and they eventually left their adopted families. They were also affected by racialized power dynamics as well as loss of culture and identity (McKenzie, Varcoe, Browne, et al., 2016; Sinclair, 2007). These children struggled with identity and low self-esteem issues. Self-harm and suicide have occurred as a result in some cases (Carriere, 2005; MacDonald & MacDonald, 2007; Petrow, 2016; Sinclair, 2007). Currently in Canada, Sixties Scoop survivors are suing the federal government in class action lawsuits (Gallant, 2016). Johnston (1983) states:

> *In retrospect, the wholesale apprehension of Native children during the Sixties Scoop appears to have been a terrible mistake. While some individual children may have benefitted, many did not, nor did their families. And Native culture suffered one of many severe blows. (p. 62)*

The child welfare system in general offers services aimed at protecting children and encouraging family stability (Canadian Child Welfare Research Portal, n.d.). Across Canada, however, Indigenous children are over-represented in the child welfare system. In some provinces, the rate of out-of-home care for Indigenous children is over 10 times that of non-Indigenous children (Sinha, Trocmé, Fallon, et al., 2011). Prior to colonization, Indigenous families cared for their children according to their own belief systems and community values, laws, and traditions.

In the 1980s, due to concern from First Nations about the vast numbers of children in the child welfare system, the First Nations child and family service agencies emerged. By 2008, there were 125 of these agencies across Canada. Many of them developed culturally appropriate, community-based programs and approaches which focus on preventative strategies. The proportion of Indigenous children in out-of-home care, however, remains high; Indigenous children are still being removed from their families in record numbers by child welfare agencies. Adoptive families require assistance with complex needs and issues that have been shaped by colonial historical practices and intergenerational trauma (Sinha et al., 2011).

Poverty. Indigenous child poverty overall is at about 18% across Canada, which ranks Canada at 27th out of 34 countries in the Organization for Economic Cooperation and Development (Macdonald & Wilson, 2016). Indigenous children have much higher rates of child poverty than their non-Indigenous counterparts. In 2010, 60% of Indigenous on-reserve children lived in poverty, up from 56% in 2005. Thirty percent of non-Status First Nations children also live in poverty, as do 25% of Inuit children and 23% of Métis children. In contrast, 17% of non-Indigenous children in Canada live in poverty (Macdonald & Wilson, 2016). Manitoba and Saskatchewan have the highest rates of on-reserve status First Nations child poverty, at 76% and 69%, respectively (Macdonald & Wilson, 2016). These numbers only measure income; they do not give a picture of the other barriers that Indigenous children face, especially on reserves with poor housing, an underfunded education system, and other systemic structural issues that exacerbate the influence of low income. Currently, there are high levels of violence in some Indigenous communities, severe addiction issues, alarming health statistics, and poor living conditions such as derelict housing and a lack of potable water (TRC, 2015c).

The Justice System. The Canadian justice system has incarcerated a disproportionate number of Indigenous people and is thought to have an inadequate response to the criminal victimization of Indigenous people (TRC, 2015c, p. 186). Despite comprising only 4% of the Canadian population, 28% of all those admitted to sentenced custody across Canada are Indigenous. For Indigenous women, 43% of all women incarcerated in Canada are Indigenous (TRC, 2015c, p. 219).

Given the long history of inequity in justice, Indigenous people have viewed the justice system, including the police, the court, and the prison system, with fear and mistrust (TRC, 2015c). Historically, Indigenous people in Canada have been denied access to legal counsel. During the years of residential schools, despite complaints being made, there were few investigations into allegations of abuse and unexplained deaths of children (TRC, 2015c). Furthermore, the police were instrumental in enforcing attendance at residential schools. As more information about residential school abuse and deaths became known, police forces were involved in investigating allegations. However, few allegations resulted in charges being laid and justice being enacted.

Imprisonment of Indigenous persons removes them from their families and communities in a way that is similar to the role residential schools played. Prisons are violent and can be gateways to gang life, especially for youth. Significant issues in prison include racism and a lack of cultural programming. Because of intergenerational trauma, youth and young adults are affected in negative ways, which can lead to criminal behaviour resulting in prison time. Intergenerational trauma has severe effects on the children and grandchildren of residential school survivors (Box 10-3). The impacts of residential school, as mentioned earlier, include poverty, addiction, physical and emotional abuse, racism, family violence, child welfare involvement, and a lack of parenting skills, as well as a lack of cultural knowledge. Cultural

BOX 10-3 RESEARCH HIGHLIGHT

Indigenous Peoples and Historic Trauma: The Processes of Intergenerational Transmission

Within Western psychological frameworks, the understanding of the constellation of symptoms resulting from prolonged and repeated psychological and social trauma post in the diagnosis of post-traumatic stress disorder (PTSD). However, this diagnosis is seen as being too narrow for Indigenous people regarding the historic and intergenerational trauma experienced through colonialism and residential school over the past five generations. Experts in this area state that a PTSD diagnosis disregards community trauma and racism, as well as ignoring the impact of culture and broader systemic conditions which exacerbate and perpetuate the experiences of Indigenous people.

Several frameworks have been developed to describe long-term trauma. In the research conducted by Aguiar and Halseth (2015), the framework of historical trauma is described as having four key features, which distinguish it from PTSD: (1) increased complexity in the antecedents, evolution, and outcomes; (2) a phenomenon that is collective rather than individual and experienced over generations; (3) a phenomenon that is cumulative in its impacts over time; and (4) descendants being more susceptible to pathological dysfunction.

For Indigenous people, the term *colonial trauma response* is applied to the interaction between historical trauma and current trauma. The characteristics and patterns of behaviour found in trauma survivors can contribute to the intergenerational transmission of trauma. These characteristics and patterns include shame, which manifests itself in behaviours such as controlling acts, demanding perfection, blaming behaviours, denying feelings, and lacking ability to trust in relationships and to engage in open communication regarding shameful or compulsive behaviours. These behaviours may also include denying, disguising, or disqualifying behaviour that is disrespectful, abusive, or shameful. From these patterns of behaviour, other behaviours develop in adults who have been exposed to these as children. They include learned helplessness, anxiety, depression, and high-risk behaviours, among others.

The high rates of family violence in Indigenous families and communities is a profound manifestation of historic trauma, as are high levels of anxiety, hypervigilance, and depression. The pathways through which trauma is transmitted generationally include physiological, social, and psychological processes, all of which are complex and challenging to disrupt. Understanding these pathways, however, is critical to devising effective strategies to address the health and well-being of Indigenous people and of communities as a whole. A rebuilding and healing of communities, families, and individuals will require the re-establishment of pride and reconstruction of a positive sense of individual and collective identity.

Aguiar, W., & Halseth, R. (2015). *Aboriginal peoples and historic trauma: The processes of intergenerational transmission.* Prince George, BC: National Collaborating Centre for Aboriginal Health.

knowledge and the use of cultural knowledge systems have been shown to be stabilizing factors for Indigenous people (McIntosh, Moniz, Craft, et al., 2014; TRC, 2015c, p. 247; Wexler, White, & Trainor, 2015).

Fetal alcohol spectrum disorder (FASD) plays a role in the increasing incarceration rates of Indigenous people. It is estimated that 10 to 25% of all Canadians who are incarcerated suffer from FASD. For Indigenous people, there is often a connection between residential school experience, addiction, and FASD (TRC, 2015c, p. 222).

Another aspect of the justice system that has had an effect on some Indigenous people is what is known as the Gladue report. In 1999, the Supreme Court of Canada dismissed the appeal of a young Indigenous woman who had stabbed her boyfriend to death in 1995. In their decision they stated:

> *The fact that the reference to Aboriginal offenders is contained in section 718.2(e), in particular, dealing with restraint in the use of imprisonment, suggests that there is something different about Aboriginal offenders which may specifically make imprisonment a less appropriate or less useful sanction. (TRC, 2015c, p. 236)*

Since then, a number of jurisdictions have implemented a process in which an Indigenous offender can have a Gladue report written prior to sentencing, which details contextual information about the offender's life. This information is then taken into account when the offender is sentenced. While Gladue reports are insufficiently used, this approach recognizes that a one-size-fits-all type of sentencing is discriminatory toward Indigenous offenders and that the impact of colonization has caused extreme harm to Indigenous communities and families that is ongoing.

Other factors in the justice system that affect Indigenous offenders include possible community sentencing structures and policies; the impact of cultural programs in prisons, which are thought to decrease recidivism; and the over-representation of Indigenous youth among those incarcerated. Further, there is a blurring in communities of victims and offenders—previous victims of violence or abuse themselves may become offenders, committing those same acts (TRC 2015c, p. 272). One recommendation for the way forward is for Indigenous peoples to organize their own justice systems to be culturally appropriate and to practise restorative justice, which focuses on rehabilitation of offenders and reconciliation with the community at large (TRC, 2015c, p. 273).

CULTURAL ORIENTATIONS

Globally, Indigenous peoples have much in common in terms of **Indigenous world views** that include a strong connection to the land; millennia-old knowledge of the land and its uses; collective cultures focused on the good of the people, not the individual; and an elastic sense of time focused on seasons rather than hours (McCabe, 2008). In Canada, while there is a wide diversity of values, lifestyles, and perspectives within Indigenous communities, there are also commonalities (Kirmayer, Tait, & Simpson, 2008). Indigenous people view everything as being connected physically and spiritually, including knowledge, which is seen as holistic—there is trust for inherited wisdom and respect for all living things. Knowledge is passed down orally and spirituality is interwoven into daily life (Barnhardt & Kawagley, 2005). Many cultures are matriarchal (Goettner-Habendroth, 2012) and the view of the world is relational—everything is related and interconnected. Humans are related to the world around them, including with plants, rocks, animals, and spirits; humans are not viewed as the most important component. Reality is defined in a relational manner to ancestors, spirits, animals, plants, and rocks (Roy, 2014). By contrast, in Western tradition, human development and other theories often have linear trajectories, moving from lower to higher levels. This is not the case in the Indigenous world view. Views of health and other aspects of life are based on a circular view, in which the past, present, and future generations are connected.

In Canada, there are several ways of viewing health and healing. The Medicine Wheel Teachings and the Seven Grandfathers Teachings (or Seven Sacred Values)—**theories of Indigenous Health**—can be used as a framework when contemplating health and healing strategies (Kotalik, & Martin, 2016; Wenger-Nabigon, 2010). These frameworks do not fully integrate Eurocentric concepts. However, they can be used alongside Eurocentric views in order to deepen our understanding of parallel ways of seeing health and healing.

The circle is an important symbol in Indigenous healing that represents the interconnectedness of all beings. The Medicine Wheel, otherwise known as the Wheel of Life, the Circle of Life, the Hoop, or the Pimaatisiwin Circle (McCabe, 2008; Moodley & West, 2005; Wenger-Nabigon, 2010), is a symbolic, circular representation of the interconnectedness of life that denotes a philosophical foundation of a world view. It is used and presented in a range of ways, depending on who is using and presenting it. Often divided into four realms, it can be used to demonstrate the importance of balance or harmony among the four areas (discussed next) in order to achieve wellness. It surrounds the core, which is viewed as the person requiring healing. The Medicine Wheel can be used for teaching and for demonstrating the continuation and phases of the life cycle, as well as the four directions. It has been used in areas such as natural childbirth, mental illness, diabetes, cancer, and other illnesses (Wenger-Nabigon, 2010).

Central to the use of Medicine Wheel teachings is the core belief of sacredness, which is a fundamental principle integral to understanding Indigenous theories of healing and wellness. In different Indigenous cultures, a variety of colours are ascribed to specific parts of the circle. This includes the four directions, viewed as sacred. They form an important aspect in the teachings in that they are paired with aspects of the person as well as parts of nature, the seasons, and other elements. **Indigenous health** is understood in traditional Indigenous knowledge to be a balance among four components within a human: emotional, physical, spiritual, and mental. Poor health results from disharmony or imbalance between the four components (Marshall, Marshall, & Bartlett, 2015). If any of these dimensions is seen to be out of balance, the treatment prescribed attends to the imbalance of that dimension (Nabigon & Wenger-Nabigon, 2012). The traditional Indigenous health systems encompass a variety of modes of treatment including ceremonial, herbal and medicinal, and storytelling.

The person who prescribes may be a traditional healer, a medicine person, or an Elder who specializes in that area. Elders are not necessarily older adults; they are people upon whom the title is bestowed by the community as they become known for their extensive knowledge in an area of specialty, whether medicines, a knowledge of history, or other wisdoms. Elders are given high respect by the community.

Values are passed down through ceremony, teachings, and role-modelling by Elders and other community members. Depending on the Indigenous nation, these values may include kindness, sharing, noncompetitiveness, noninterference, and accepting responsibility for one's actions. In the Teachings of the Seven Grandfathers—a story from Ojibwe oral tradition—a baby is given gifts or teachings from powerful spirits known as the Seven Grandfathers. These teachings include learning about wisdom, love, respect, bravery, honesty, humility, and truth. In the teachings, the boy learns that there is an opposite of each gift or teaching. These teachings have been used in a variety of fields including social work, bioethics, and mental health and addictions (Kotalik & Martin, 2016).

In Canada, pre-contact Indigenous peoples had their own medicine systems and used ceremonies and a variety of healing methods to maintain health. Colonialism brought about overwhelming alterations in economic, political, and social structures, as well as in disease patterns and general health for Indigenous peoples. All aspects of life for Indigenous peoples were attacked or destroyed, including the ability to find food, their connection to the land, spirituality, languages, cultural behaviours and rituals, family connections and relationships, medicine ways, and the governing structures within groups. Indigenous identity was thoroughly attacked through colonial practices and policies, including placing Indigenous children in residential schools, where they were stripped of their names and given numbers instead. These children grew up with a diminished identity as an Indigenous person with a culture and language, rituals, ceremonies, and spirituality—aspects of life that are a part of every person's identity construction.

Indigenous identity has also been attacked through systemic devaluing and essentialism within institutions and government structures. In popular media negative stereotypes of Indigenous identity have appeared, such as "the drunken Indian" and "savage." In recent years, however, there has been a push toward reclaiming Indigenous identity through learning about cultures, traditions, traditional knowledge, languages, and medicine ways.

Identity is closely connected to health (Public Health Agency of Canada [PHAC], 2013a); research has shown a direct correlation between a decrease in Indigenous suicide rates and an increase in identity-preserving practices in Indigenous communities (Chandler & Lalonde, 2008). However, notions of identity involve intersections between historical, cultural, linguistic, geographic, and political dimensions, and not just traditional ways. Indigenous identity is also linked to phenotypes (braids, brown skin) and behavioural attributes; these are shaped by cultural scripts. Indigenous identity is a social construction that can unite or marginalize (Forte, 2013; Kirmayer et al., 2008). Those who are identified as being more "authentic" in terms of having an ideal ethnic image are privileged, while those who fail to embody the ideal ethnic image are marginalized. Ethnic identity is a factor in coping psychologically, in social interaction, and in community organization. All of these forms of identity contribute to Indigenous mental health.

The Sixties Scoop (Hanson, 2009), during which children were removed from their Indigenous families and placed in the welfare system to be fostered and adopted by non-Indigenous families, has led to generations of people struggling with identity. Many were raised in middle-class White families, and their first point of contact with the Indigenous world was through street services and addiction agencies, where they learned that they were a part of the most marginalized and oppressed group in Canada (Sinclair, 2007). As a result, Indigenous youth who were adopted have shown extremely poor self-esteem and high rates of suicidal ideation as they struggle with reconfiguring their identity.

Many Indigenous people have found it therapeutic to be reconnected to cultural teachings and ways of healing. Indigenous healing addresses issues of the spiritual, mental, physical, and emotional aspects, and so is well suited to helping Indigenous people and communities work toward wellness. It is important that health care providers recognize this and work with Indigenous people in using traditional ways to heal (Box 10-4).

As mentioned, notions of healing and well-being incorporate the four aspects of a person as seen in traditional Indigenous views—emotional, mental, physical, and spiritual. When these four components are in balance or in harmony, a person is seen as being healthy or well. However, beyond this, health is also connected to place. For the Inuit, place is described in terms of flora and fauna, snowdrift patterns, and animal trails. Relationships are built with the land and with all aspects of the land (Tagalik, 2015). When this holistic perspective is lost, the Inuit relate that they become disoriented and disconnected, with a lesser sense of belonging and wellness. It is felt that well-being comes through feeling the sense of peace on the land, and once felt, this feeling of peace will always be sought (Tagalik, 2015).

Environmental dispossession has added to a lack of wellness among Indigenous people in Canada. Traditionally, Indigenous people's teachings include having strong moral responsibility as protectors of the land. Struggles with the mining of resources and pollution of land and

BOX 10-4 RESEARCH HIGHLIGHT

Restoring the Blessings of the Morning Star: Childbirth and Maternal-Infant Health for First Nations Near Edmonton, Alberta

Disparities exist between Indigenous and non-Indigenous people in Canada regarding maternal-infant health, despite universal health care access and proximity to urban centres. Since the 1960s, a policy of evacuation was implemented, especially for remote communities in northern Canada, where Indigenous women were sent to tertiary care facilities in urban centres in southern Canada to await childbirth, sometimes weeks before their due date. However, research has demonstrated the importance of cultural safety in care; use of Indigenous beliefs, values and practices; and community-based approaches in midwifery and birthing. In the community-based, participatory, descriptive qualitative research study by Wiebe, Barton, Auger, et al. (2015), narratives from 75 Indigenous women were gathered as they spoke about the loss and separation inherent in birthing and maternity care that had moved them out of their community and into the hospital.

The need to reintegrate culturally based community support and Indigenous health perspectives into the childbirth experience was highlighted by participants. Five main themes were elicited: excluding the traditional Elders, moving childbirth out of the community, recalling the traditional teachings about childbirth, connecting spirituality with childbirth, and limited cultural safety in the health care system.

Recommendations included using a combination of Western medicine and a holistic, family-centred approach of traditional Indigenous communities' ways of knowing and doing in the health care system. This approach also encompasses the inclusion of Elders, Grandmothers, and other key female relatives into the circle surrounding pregnancy and birthing women in hospitals to provide traditional wisdom and guidance. It was also recommended that these traditional teachings and practices be available to those who request them. Another recommendation for an integrated health care program included having trained Indigenous doulas and/or midwives in a community-based role; they could accompany pregnant women through the entire process of pregnancy and labour and provide liaison support. The final recommendation was to have culturally safe health care providers caring for the women in order to prevent discrimination and prejudice and to help implement culturally relevant and safe health care practices that meet the needs of clients in a holistic manner.

Wiebe, A. D., Barton, S., Auger, L., Pijl-Zieber, E., & Foster-Boucher, C. (2015). Restoring the blessings of the Morning Star: Childbirth and maternal-infant health for First Nations near Edmonton, Alberta. *Aboriginal Policy Studies 5*(1), 47–68. doi:10.5663/aps.v5i1.23823

water have caused disruption to the health of Indigenous people. Land is seen as a place to heal and gain well-being. Water is seen as a healer, with cleansing properties. Notions of well-being are bound with the types of food one eats from the land, the land to which one is connected, and living on the land in harmony with family and community. Well-being comes from the spiritual relations one has with the land and food, and medicines from the land, as well as the social relationships one has with family and community (Richmond, 2015). Other key aspects in Indigenous conceptions of healing include Indigenous philosophies, cosmologies, ceremonies, identity, knowledge, lands and medicines, and environmental health (Steinhauer & Lamouche, 2015).

NURSING CONSIDERATIONS AND INDIGENOUS HEALTH

Respect is a fundamental aspect of nursing practice and is seen as a human value that addresses dignity and justice. Respect in nursing means acknowledging and appreciating the intrinsic value of others in an active and authentic way (Gallagher, 2007). In a study focused on First Nations people's meaning of respect, respect was seen as a process that is reciprocal and as being able to see and treat people as inherently worthy and equal in principle. Also, First Nations participants felt that respect was demonstrated by a willingness to be accepting and to listen actively, as well as genuinely trying to understand the situations patients found themselves in. Respect was shown through sincerity and explaining things in a way that a patient would be able to understand, thereby increasing patient autonomy. Lack of respect was shown through not ensuring privacy for patients, negative nonverbal behaviours, and behaviours that demonstrated discriminatory attitudes (Browne, 1995).

Trust has been described as an essential element of all nurse–patient relationships (Dinc & Gastmans, 2012). It involves vulnerability, dependency, and risk taking by the person exhibiting trusting behaviour. It also requires that nurses understand the unequal power relationship between themselves and their patient, as well as the vulnerable and dependent state of the patient (Dinc & Gastmans, 2012). Indigenous people have been described as a vulnerable population owing to the colonialism and racism that has affected every aspect of their lives over generations. Therefore, it is imperative that focus be placed on trust in the relationship between an Indigenous patient, family, or community and the health care provider. In order to build trusting relationships, nurses need to listen to their patients to find out who they are and what their needs are, as well as to show a willingness to adapt to the patient's, family's, or community's ways of being (Zeidler, 2011). Learning about the past history of Indigenous people and understanding how it might affect the behaviours and attitudes of Indigenous patients or families will help shape this relationship. Time is important in health care settings, and nurses are taught to be efficient. However, within Indigenous communities, relationships come before business. It is important to tend to the relationship first, in order to have sufficient trust to work toward the clinical aspects of caring for the patient and family. It is also important to understand how the concept of holism works in an Indigenous community and how a patient is connected to family, community, and a way of life (Zeidler, 2011). When treating a patient, these other aspects must be taken into consideration. For instance, ensuring that the family understands what is happening and that there is space provided for community members who come to visit is helpful and will shape the relationship further. Other aspects that contribute to a trusting relationship are keeping one's word, maintaining confidentiality, being reliable, and being kind and nonjudgemental (Zeidler, 2011).

Spirituality is important in many Indigenous people's lives. Traditional Indigenous faiths are believed to heal. In the holistic view of health for Indigenous people, spirituality is one of the four aspects within a person that must be in balance in order to be healthy. Therefore, it is important that efforts be made to ensure that Indigenous patients and families can practise their spirituality as completely as possible in a health care setting. This may involve finding out where they can hold ceremonies or ensuring that they can use sweet grass or other medicines which are burned, the smoke being used as a cleansing activity. It may mean locating the Indigenous helper or Elder in the health care setting who can assist the family or patient in tending to their spiritual needs. Items placed in the bed or on the wall or pinned to the patient's gown must not be moved without permission, as these items may hold spiritual and healing significance for the patient and family. Nurses should also know that not all Indigenous people follow traditional Indigenous faiths. Other faiths used by Indigenous people across Canada include Roman Catholicism, Protestantism, Pentecostalism, and others. The nurse needs to assess carefully to find out what the patient's spiritual needs are and to act accordingly (North American Indigenous Ministries, 2017; Public Safety and Emergency Preparedness Canada, 2006; Todd, 2016; Vancouver Native Pentecostal Church, n.d.).

It is important to recognize that while there may be many similarities, different Indigenous groups have their own interpretations and emphasis on various aspects of belief, Indigenous world views, and theories of Indigenous health. Further, not all Indigenous people believe in or seek out traditional healing. Because of colonization, many Indigenous people have lost their cultural knowledge or have not been taught about traditional healing practices. It is important to carefully assess where a person is on the continuum of what he or she believes in and the person's notions of healing and well-being in the context of cultural orientations. In caring for the Indigenous population, nurses must work cooperatively and in balance with Indigenous ways of knowing. These ways of knowing have developed over tens of thousands of years, and their use and sustenance are vital to the well-being of Indigenous people (Wenger-Nabigon, 2010).

ILLNESS EXPERIENCES—CHRONIC DISEASES

Implications for Nursing

The importance of cultural competency, safety, and humility for health care administrators, practitioners, and educators has been recognized by the Canadian Indigenous Nurses Association (CINA) and National Aboriginal Health Organization (NAHO). NAHOs (2012) document describes the origins of cultural competency and safety; a theoretical and methodological approach to cultural safety, an approach that originated with Aboriginal peoples; and the importance of its application to health care (refer to Chapter 9 for information on cultural safety).

Nursing and interdisciplinary scholars continue to research the health challenges faced by Aboriginal peoples, providing an analysis of health policy (Lavoie, Browne, Varcoe, et al., 2015) (Box 10-5). The exploration of cultural safety is also being taken up by other disciplines. From a sociological perspective, Brascoupé and Waters (2009) note how cultural safety "differs from cultural competence or trans-cultural training and practices" and indicate "why it's important to move from the concept of cultural safety to the outcome of cultural safety, namely the success of an interaction; [this] explores the idea of a shift from cultural safety for individuals to cultural safety at institutional and policy levels" (p. 6).

With regard to the success of an interaction, Harrowing, Mill, Spiers, et al. (2010) emphasize that such an outcome begins with

BOX 10-5 Indigenous Nursing Leader—Madeleine Kétéskwew Dion Stout

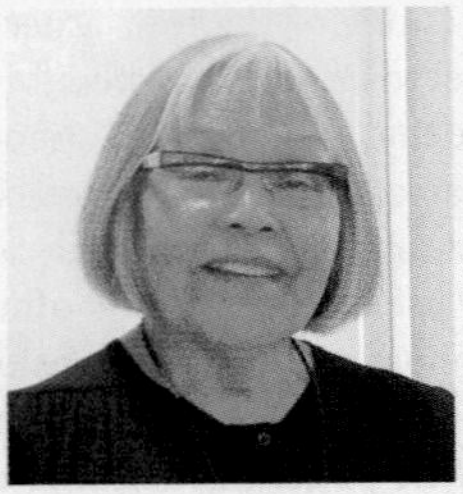

(Courtesy CARNE. Photograph by vsaranphoto.com.)

Madeleine Kétéskwew Dion Stout, a Cree speaker, was born and raised on the Kehewin First Nation in Alberta. After graduating from the Edmonton General Hospital as a registered nurse, she earned a bachelor's degree in nursing, with distinction, from the University of Lethbridge and a master's degree in international affairs from the Norman Paterson School of International Affairs at Carleton University. She serves on several Indigenous and non-Indigenous boards and committees, including the National Collaborating Centre for Aboriginal Health and, until recently, the First Nations Health Authority Board in British Columbia. In August 2007, she was appointed to the Mental Health Commission of Canada as an inaugural vice-chair of the Board of Directors. Madeleine is a past president of the Aboriginal Nurses Association of Canada and appointee to the National Forum on Health. She was a professor in Canadian Studies and founding director of the Centre for Aboriginal Education, Research and Culture at Carleton University in Ottawa. Now self-employed as the president of Dion Stout Reflections Inc., she adopts a Cree lens in her research, writing, and lectures on First Nations health. Her active involvement in several research projects funded by the Canadian Institutes of Health Research (CIHR) has her shaping the way social, health, and health care equity is best encouraged, cultivated, and disciplined for Indigenous people. She is the recipient of the Assiniwikamik Award from the Aboriginal Nurses Association of Canada; a Distinguished Alumnus Award from the University of Lethbridge, and an Honorary Doctor of Laws from the University of British Columbia, the University of Ottawa, and Carleton University. In November 2008, the Canadian Nurses Association of Canada selected Madeleine for the Centennial Award, given to 100 outstanding Canadian nurses. In March 2010 she won the National Aboriginal Achievement Award in the health category. Madeleine received the Order of Canada in 2015. She served as the Champion for the College and Association of Registered Nurses of Alberta (CARNA) during their centennial year in 2016. Madeleine is featured in the 2011 and 2012 editions of the *Canadian Who's Who*.

Personal communication with Caroline Foster-Boucher, March 29, 2017; Delta Optimist (2015). *Local nurse Madeleine Dion Stout appointed to the Order of Canada.* Retrieved from http://www.delta-optimist.com/news/local-nurse-madeleine-dion-stout-appointed-to-the-order-of-canada-1.1996258; Thunderbird Partnership Foundation. (2017). *Madeleine Dion Stout.* Retrieved from http://nnapf.com/events/hos2014-national-conference/madeleine-dion-stout-2/.

awareness of "the nurse's reflection on his or her personal and cultural history, values, and beliefs and continues with the situating of those understandings within a framework of power imbalances, institutional discrimination, and colonizer-colonized relationships" (p. 246). These interactional outcomes are also illustrated in the work of Smith, Edwards, Varcoe, et al. (2006), which focus on establishing safety and responsiveness as a mainstay of care for pregnant and parenting Aboriginal people. Their findings revealed that "safety and health care relationships and settings, and responsiveness to individuals' and families' experiences and capacities must be brought into the forefront of care. [These] results suggest that the intention of care must be situated in a broader view of colonizing relations to improve early access to, and relevance of, care during pregnancy and parenting for Aboriginal people" (p. E27). In situating the professional discipline of nursing in a broader view of colonizing relations, McGibbon, Mulaudzi, Didham, et al. (2013) emphasize that nursing must also look toward decolonizing itself, which includes understanding the colonization of nursing and strategies for increasing the counternarrative.

Clearly, major health disparities are found among Indigenous peoples in Canada. Causes of such disparities include impaired access to appropriate and adequate housing, income, education, and health care. As emphasized in this chapter, health inequities are largely due to historical colonialism and current-day postcolonial institutional racism, demonstrated in the policies and procedures of a variety of governmental institutions that influence Indigenous peoples negatively.

It is imperative that nurses understand the social determinants of health (SDOH) through an Indigenous lens, which helps to explain the underlying economic and social conditions that shape health. A **determinant of health** is a complex set of influences or circumstances that determine the level of health for people. Loppie Reading and Wien (2009) have organized SDOH as they relate to Indigenous people's health into three categories. *Proximal determinants of health* have a direct influence on health and include healthy behaviours (such as eating nutritious meals and exercising daily) and considerations of the physical and social environment. *Intermediate determinants of health* can be seen as the origin of proximal SDOH and include community infrastructure, resources, and systems (such as access to sidewalks, parks, and walking trails). *Distal determinants of health* have the most influence on a population's health and encompass the historical, political, social, and economic contexts from which intermediate and proximal SDOH are constructed (such as stable governance structures, competent leadership, and effective policing services).

Important proximal determinants of health that influence chronic diseases include health behaviours such as substance abuse, smoking, physical activity, and diet. These, however, must be considered in light of the sociopolitical context of Indigenous peoples, such as the influence of residential schools, other colonial policies, and racism in Canada. Intermediate determinants of health that influence Indigenous people include health care systems. Political, physical, and social access to these systems is limited and sometimes lacking for Indigenous peoples because of their physical location; lack of accounting for language and culture; governmental funding policies that result in inadequate, underfunded programs and personnel on reserve; and underlying racist attitudes and behaviours of health care providers that lead to poor and culturally unsafe care.

Education systems as an intermediate determinant of health, for example, are also inadequate for Indigenous peoples. Chronic underfunding of First Nations schools has resulted in lower education levels, lower income levels, and poorer living conditions. The Indigenous education system has always been designed with Indigenous perspectives and historical injustices in mind (McCorckle, 2015). Since the TRC Report, Canadian education systems have been working on ways to incorporate Indigenous knowledge and history of residential schools and colonialism into the current-day curriculum (Aboriginal Education Directorate Manitoba Education and Advanced Learning, 2016; Alberta Education, 2017; Alberta Teachers Association, 2015; First Nations Education Steering Committee & First Nations School Association, 2015; Gillmore, 2016; Murray, 2015; Ontario Ministry of Education, 2017; Reith & Stewart, 2015).

Community infrastructure, another intermediate determinant of health with associated opportunities in Indigenous communities, has been limited, contributing to economic insecurity and marginalization. Insufficient social resources, such as people who are able to develop or implement programs, have also led to decreased access to funding (Loppie Reading & Wien, 2009). Poor environmental stewardship, disempowerment, and contamination of wildlife, vegetation, and water have contributed to health problems (Parkes, 2010).

Addressing chronic disease requires appropriate skills and knowledge to create culturally safe chronic disease management programs in partnership with Indigenous communities. As well, advocating for improvements in the SDOH across sectors can help address chronic disease in the Indigenous population in Canada (Tobe, Maar, Roy, et al., 2015).

Current research evidence indicates that there is a propensity within the health care system to locate problems with the patient rather than with the health care provider when there are problems with care. For instance, when a patient does not show up to an appointment on time, the focus is on the deficit of the patient instead of asking why the system is set up in such a way that it does not work for this patient (Thurston et al., 2014). This deficit model leads to stereotyping of patients and to reinforcing apathy and neglect among health care providers. It is now acknowledged that Indigenous people would be better served by a system that is more culturally safe than by an historical expectation of change that is uncritically situated within the Indigenous population (Thurston, Coupal, Jones, et al., 2014).

Distal determinants of health affecting Indigenous health care require an understanding of colonialism, racism, social exclusion, and repression of self-determination for Indigenous people. As mentioned previously, colonial actions have resulted in Indigenous peoples being displaced from and dispossessed of traditional lands. Assimilation techniques, such as residential schools' destruction of culture, family ties, and language for Indigenous people, are examples of distal determinants of health. The influence of residential schools continues today, as exhibited in the lack of parenting knowledge and in other effects related to experiences of intergenerational trauma.

Racism and exclusion are demonstrated in inequities related to employment, education, and economic participation, alongside the unfair and hierarchical distribution of power and resources. The loss of self-determination for Indigenous peoples has been shown to be most influential, with secondary influences resulting from the interdependence of other SDOH.

The implications of all of these SODH for nursing among Indigenous people can be summed up by Reutter and Kushner's (2010) statement that "nursing has a clear mandate to ensure access to health and health-care by providing sensitive empowering care to those experiencing inequities and working to change underlying social conditions that result in and perpetuate health inequities" (p. 269). One reason why people become nurses is that they want to "act in ways that are respectful, compassionate, and equitable and that leave [them] feeling that [they] have somehow [contributed to the greater] good" (Hartrick Doane & Varcoe, 2005, p. 16). A relational approach to nursing shapes the places of inquiry and practice that determine how to find one's way through relationships, culture, safety, ethics, diversity, power, economics, communication, and history. A deep consideration of relational practice and nursing obligations offers an understanding of experience by which to imagine how one might incorporate reflexivity, intentionality, and openness into practice, education, and research. It is from such a position of nursing inquiry that nurses are better able to interpret personal life threads, eliciting from enmeshed personal and professional life stories the insight and wisdom that guide people in becoming better human beings. (Refer to Chapter 9 for information on implementing relational practice and to Chapter 18 for more information on patient-centred care.)

In critically analyzing nursing practice—as clinicians, educators, researchers, and administrators—it is essential that nurses, individually and collectively, enact and refine the role of the nurse in the provision of care with Indigenous peoples, as well as contribute to change. Wright (2015) states:

> *The nurse has a significant role to play in promoting a sense of respect for Aboriginal people in Canada, and improving the provision of culturally safe care. Nurses can also promote Aboriginal people to pursue careers in health care, and promote appropriate research strategies for researchers involved with Aboriginal people. It would seem that birthing in the north is progressing in the right direction, with return of birthing services to northern communities. Nurses can continue to advocate for Aboriginal people to gain self-governance for all of their healthcare services. (p. 6)*

It is in this spirit that the nursing profession will continue to develop the ability to adapt nursing practice to an Indigenous context, preserve the perspective of Indigenous peoples, sustain the holistic nature of responding to social and health challenges, and value new forms of partnership in respectful ways.

Diabetes Mellitus

Diabetes mellitus (type 2 diabetes) was a condition previously unknown prior to the 1940s but has been viewed as an epidemic in progress since the 1970s for Canadian Indigenous peoples (Howard, 2014; Kue Young, Reading, Elias, et al., 2000). Diabetes has a prevalence (dependent on location) that is three to five times higher in this population compared to non-Aboriginal Canadians (PHAC, 2011). Research has found that the lifetime risk of diabetes at 20 years old is 75.6% for First Nations men and 87.3% for First Nations women, compared to 55.6% and 46.5 % for non-Indigenous Canadians, respectively (Turin, Saad, Jun, et al., 2016). First Nations men and women reach a greater risk of diabetes at a much younger age than non–First Nations people, and First Nations people living rurally have a higher rate of diabetes than those living in an urban setting (Turin et al., 2016).

Contributing factors associated with these high rates are based on research involving an integrated understanding of genetic susceptibility, changes associated with transitioning from a physically active lifestyle to a sedentary lifestyle, and the intake of a diet that is high in sugar, fats, and salt. Other aspects that contribute include inequities in the social, political, and economic determinants of health, insufficient access to nutritious food, and barriers to appropriate health care, such as lack of comprehensive primary care and lack of specialized care within a reasonable distance (Rice, Te Hiwi, Zwarenstein, et al., 2016; Turin et al., 2016) (Box 10-6).

Type 2 diabetes is diagnosed with increasing frequency in Indigenous children (Dyck, Jiang, & Osgood, 2014; PHAC, 2011). Earlier onset of the disease leads to an earlier onset of complications, as well as excessive mortality rates among young and middle-aged adults. In Inuit communities, the rate of type 2 diabetes is still relatively low, but concerns have been raised that this may change if the Inuit alter their traditional eating patterns and lifestyle (Sefidbakht, Johnson-Down, Young, et al., 2015).

Indigenous Perspective. In considering diabetes in the Indigenous population, it is necessary to view this epidemic through a lens highlighting the impact of colonization and intergenerational trauma on determinants of health, such as personal coping habits and patterns of food use (Boxes 10-7 and 10-8). Howard (2014) has noted the impact of residential school experience on the eating habits of residential school survivors, who associated eating with abuse, trauma, and powerlessness. Wild animal meat and other Indigenous foods were denigrated and were replaced with food that was less nutritious (Howard, 2014).

BOX 10-6 RESEARCH HIGHLIGHT

Health Care Experiences of Indigenous People Living With Type 2 Diabetes in Canada

A recent study explored Indigenous perspectives on diabetes care. Findings indicated that study participants' experience of diabetes improved when they were able to engage in equitable and positive interactions with care providers and organizations. Participants cited negative experiences, such as being dismissed and lecturing by physicians. They also indicated that negative caregiver actions and attitudes triggered their residential school memories. These issues and lack of access to care were viewed as affecting how often they sought care and how willing they were to share all of their symptoms, regardless of their willingness to accept suggested treatments (Jacklin, Henderson, Green, et al., 2017). Recommendations for improved health care encounters included ensuring a positive relationship with Indigenous patients by tending to power differentials, incorporating a holistic view of health and treatment, and recognizing how important a trustful therapeutic relationship is between patient and health care provider in mitigating historical trauma and colonial history.

Jacklin, K. M., Henderson, R. I., Green, M. E., Walker, L. M., Calam, B., & Crowshoe, L. J. (2017). Health care experiences of Indigenous people living with type 2 diabetes in Canada. *Canadian Medical Association Journal, 189*(3), 106–112. doi:10.1503/cmaj.161098

BOX 10-7 The National Aboriginal Diabetes Association

As a result of the alarming increase in rates of diabetes among Indigenous people, in 1996 the National Aboriginal Diabetes Association (NADA) was formed (NADA, 2016a). In 1997, Health Canada initiated consultations with Indigenous organizations to develop a national Indigenous diabetes strategy. NADA provides diabetes resources and information for Indigenous people in Canada and hosts national conferences to raise awareness and share successes. They also partner with other groups in order to support projects focused on reducing complications from diabetes (NADA, 2016a). NADA receives funding through an annual contribution agreement instead of through multiyear funding agreements, which tend to increase stability of programming for such organizations. Despite this challenge in funding and increasing costs, NADA has focused their strategic plan on a 5-year cycle, from 2016 to 2021, with hopes of increased funding, multiyear funding agreements, and increased partnerships to assist with funding in order to strengthen programs.

HIV and AIDS

Human immunodeficiency virus (HIV) infections and cases of acquired immune deficiency syndrome (AIDS) among Canadian Indigenous peoples have increased steadily since the 1990s, whereas the annual number of AIDS cases has levelled off in the rest of the population. Indigenous people are over-represented among HIV and AIDS cases in Canada; although Indigenous persons make up about 4.3% of the Canadian population, it is estimated that they represent about 8.9% of all those living with HIV and AIDS, an increase of 17.3% from 2008 (PHAC, 2014). In addition, the HIV infection rate is about 3.5 times higher among Indigenous persons than non-Indigenous persons. Compared to their non-Indigenous counterparts, Indigenous persons diagnosed with HIV are more likely to be younger (31.6 vs 22.2% between 15 and 29 years old), female (47.3 vs 20.1%), and infected through intravenous drug use (58.1 vs 13.7%) (PHAC, 2014). In 2001, at the United Nations General Assembly, leaders from 189 member states committed to targets that would have halved HIV cases and thus would have reversed the global HIV/AIDS epidemic by 2015 (Box 10-9).

Indigenous Perspective. Indigenous people diagnosed with HIV/AIDS state that they have been devastated by the diagnosis, a similar reaction found in other diagnosed groups (Cain, Jackson, Prentice, et al., 2013). The differences, however, include the layering of trauma in their lives into which the diagnosis is situated, including intergenerational trauma, a history of familial violence, lack of being parented, loneliness, and lack of affection from parents. For many individuals the diagnosis either triggered a descent into depression or

BOX 10-8 The Aboriginal Diabetes Initiative

In 1999, First Nation and Inuit Health Branch launched the Aboriginal Diabetes Initiative (ADI) in order to provide funding to Indigenous communities that focus on health promotion, disease prevention, and screening and treatment services in more than 600 Indigenous communities in Canada (Health Canada, 2011, 2013). In 2015, the government of Canada announced that it would make the ADI a permanent program, to reduce "the health gap between Aboriginal and non-Aboriginal Canadians." Further, they stated, "This investment will help to create stable and predictable ongoing funding for health promotion, disease prevention and capacity building in First Nations, Inuit and Métis communities and supports Canada's vision of healthy individuals, families and communities" (Government of Canada, 2015b).

The renewed ADI features several areas of enhanced focus:

- Initiatives for children, youth, parents, and families
- Diabetes in childbearing women and pregnant women
- Community-led food security planning to improve access to healthy foods, including traditional and market foods
- Enhanced training for health provider's on clinical practice guidelines and chronic disease management strategies

Using local knowledge, First Nations and Inuit communities are encouraged to develop innovative, culturally relevant approaches aimed at increasing community wellness and ultimately reducing the burden of type 2 diabetes. Community activities funded through the ADI vary from one community to another and may include walking clubs, weight loss groups, diabetes workshops, fitness classes, community kitchens, community gardens, and healthy school food policies. The ADI also supports traditional activities, such as traditional food harvesting and preparation, canoeing, drumming, dancing, and traditional games (Health Canada, 2013).

BOX 10-9 Policy Highlight: Implications for Indigenous Health—HIV/AIDS

Globally, the Joint United Nations Program on HIV and AIDS (UNAIDS) is the main advocate for comprehensive and coordinated global action on the HIV/AIDS epidemic (UNAIDS, 2006). In Canada, the government supports the UNAIDS 90-90-90 treatment targets which focus on ensuring that 90% of HIV-positive people will know their status, 90% of people who know their status will be treated, and 90% of those treated will have their viral loads suppressed (Canadian AIDS Society, 2016a). There is also a focus on HIV/AIDS research that is community based specifically in Indigenous communities. However, there have been recent government funding cutbacks to HIV/AIDS organizations across Canada, which may influence the UNAIDS treatment targets in Canada. This is especially relevant for Indigenous people, for whom this may have far-reaching consequences (Canadian AIDS Society, 2016b).

increased already present depression, which was accompanied by increased self-abusive behaviours. For some Indigenous clients, the diagnosis triggered an evaluation of life, a searching and renewal of culture, and healing from trauma (Cain et al., 2013).

While research shows that intravenous drug abuse is a more common method of transmission of HIV for Indigenous people, there are currently no data or statistics on the effect of HIV/AIDS on two-spirited people (a term used by Indigenous people to identify a range of roles and identities that include gender, sex, and sexual identity). Historically, Indigenous people had a fluid view of gender and sexuality, which was deeply affected by colonization, including by residential schools (Hunt, 2016). However, HIV/AIDS has caused Indigenous communities to organize and become active, resulting in culturally safe programming and education initiatives that resonate for Indigenous youth, including two-spirited youth (Hunt, 2016) (Box 10-10).

Cancer

Cancer was relatively unknown among Indigenous peoples in Canada a few generations ago. However, studies have found dramatic increases in cancer rates among Indigenous Canadians in recent years, and it is now becoming one of the top three causes of death for First Nations people (Beben & Muirhead, 2016). Using statistics from 1991 to 2009, Withrow, Pole, Nishri, et al. (2017) found that First Nations people had poorer survival for 14 out of 15 common types of cancers than non-Indigenous people in Canada. This difference could not be explained away by income or location.

For the Métis, bronchus/lung cancer is the leading cause of death, with much higher rates among Métis men than among non-Métis men (Sanchez-Ramirez, Colquhoun, Parker, et al., 2016). Rates of incidence for other types of cancer were not particularly different between the Métis and other Canadians (Sanchez-Ramirez et al., 2016). The circumpolar Inuit population has the highest rate of lung cancer in the world, and the overall rate of cancer has increased especially for lung, colorectal, and female breast cancers. They are also at extremely high risk for the rare nasopharyngeal cancer (Kue Young, Kelly, Friborg, et al., 2016). The Inuit have a high prevalence of smoking; almost 63% of Canadian Inuit are daily smokers (Kue Young et al., 2016). The effects of colonization, residential schools, diet changes, and alterations in lifestyle have all been cited as factors in the increase of cancers among Indigenous people in Canada (Wakewich, Wood, Davey, et al., 2016).

Indigenous Perspective. There is a dearth of research about cancer from a Canadian Indigenous perspective. In one study that assessed Indigenous viewpoints of cancer that were from Australia, New Zealand, and Canada, researchers found that, in general, Indigenous people are fearful of a diagnosis of cancer. Some believe that because there are no words in certain Indigenous languages for cancer, there is minimal occurrence of cancer in the Indigenous population. Much of the information in this study, however, was from Australian, Polynesian, and New Zealand literature. In studies focusing on cervical cancer screening, Canadian Indigenous women discussed feeling fearful of being screened, owing to factors stemming from colonial history such as residential school. However, they felt great responsibility to take care of their health given their role as family caretakers. Other women spoke of being so busy with their caretaking activities and employment that they had no time for screening. Barriers to screening included a lack of female physicians—many Indigenous women feel uncomfortable with male physicians performing cervical screening—lack of transportation, employment factors, lack of health literacy, and a general mistrust of the health care system (Maar, Burchell, Little, et al., 2013).

Tuberculosis

Although the overall incidence of tuberculosis (TB) has dropped steadily since the 1960s, in 2011, the incidence rate of active TB disease reported for the Canadian-born Indigenous population was 34 times higher than for the Canadian-born non-Indigenous population. Further, the overall rate of TB disease and infection was almost six times greater than for the average Canadian population. Factors contributing to such a high rate include the historical context of colonialism, insufficient housing leading to overcrowded and often poorly ventilated living conditions, and environmental conditions. Challenges related to the health care system include complexities related to poor access to diagnosis and treatment in remote communities (Alvares, Orr, Wobeser, et al., 2014; PHAC, 2013b).

Indigenous Perspective. Even though historically TB has been devastating in Indigenous communities, many current patients have little knowledge of the specifics of historical TB in their families, according to a study conducted in Montreal, Quebec (MacDonald, Rigillo, & Brassard, 2010). Participants stated that details were not shared when parents and other family members went away to sanatoriums. Participants with TB also had some knowledge of TB as a lung disease that was serious, contagious, and potentially fatal. They gained their information generally from health care workers, television, and pamphlets. The TB treatment regimen was seen as a heavy burden that was exacerbated by language difficulties, lack of social support, racism, and mistrust of the health care system. There was also fear of getting a positive result when being screened for TB (MacDonald et al., 2010).

Chronic Obstructive Pulmonary Disease and Asthma

Statistics for rates of chronic obstructive pulmonary disease (COPD) among Indigenous peoples in Canada are higher than those for other

BOX 10-10 CASE STUDY

An Indigenous Man With HIV

James is a 50-year-old two-spirited man from the Muskoday First Nation in northern Saskatchewan. He recently saw his family doctor in Prince Albert for an HIV test. When he returned to see the doctor for his results, he was shocked to learn that his test was positive. James had lived with his partner Sam for more than 10 years; however, they had separated about 7 months ago. James is unsure of Sam's HIV status.

James has been referred to one of the nurses working in the sexually transmitted infections clinic for an assessment. During his first visit, James is very quiet and withdrawn, and it is difficult to engage him in a conversation. James would like to return to his home community to live, but he is hesitant to do so because he is afraid he will not be accepted. He receives his medical care on the basis of his First Nations status; however, he is worried that care for his HIV illness will not be covered.

1. What needs to be demonstrated during compassionate, culturally safe, and relationship-centred care with this patient?
2. How could the nurse demonstrate effective and culturally safe communication with this patient?

Canadians, with the epidemiology for Indigenous peoples resembling that of people in low- to middle-income countries. Inuit and First Nations people have higher rates of COPD than those for Métis people. Indigenous peoples, on average, have two times the rate of smoking for non-Indigenous people in Canada. Other factors include exposure to environmental contaminants, housing conditions such as mould and poor ventilation, and lower levels of education. In addition, poor nutrition, poverty, remote locations, and childhood exposure to cigarette smoke are further contributing factors (Gershon, Khan, Klein-Geltink, et al., 2014; Ospina, Voaklander, Senthilselvan, et al., 2015; Pahwa, Abonyi, Karunanayake, et al., 2015). Insufficient data were found to provide an Indigenous perspective.

Asthma is a significant respiratory disease among Indigenous children, affecting at least 10% (Castleden, Watson, Bennett, et al., 2016). Even though the rates are similar to those for other Canadian children, it is thought that Indigenous children receive fewer health care services related to treatment for asthma as a result of decreased access to health care services overall. Factors linked to incidence and severity of asthma in Indigenous communities include overcrowded or poorly ventilated housing, mould, tobacco and ceremonial smoke indoors, use of wood-burning stoves, lack of financial resources, and stressful home environments (Castleden et al., 2016; Senthilselvan, Selvanayagam, King, et al., 2015).

Furthermore, in many Indigenous communities, asthma is often underdiagnosed and undertreated because of under-reporting by families, for a variety of reasons. These include a lack of knowledge about asthma within Indigenous communities (including for health care providers), lack of funding for health promotion related to asthma, and issues for families and patients with asthma in obtaining appropriate and culturally safe care (Castleden et al., 2016). Asthma among Indigenous children is also associated with having frequent inner ear infections and low birth weight and allergies (Senthilselvan et al., 2015). Studies have shown that breastfeeding is protective for asthma in Indigenous children and thus should be promoted (Ming, Mandhane, & Senthilselvan, 2012).

Indigenous Perspective. In a study completed in five Mi'kmaq communities in Nova Scotia, few Indigenous children self-identified in school as having asthma diagnosed, owing to fear of stigma, exclusion, and isolation (Castleden et al., 2016). Children noted that they received support from their families as well as from their peers. Families also said that they needed better asthma care in the on-reserve health care centres and were reluctant to seek out medical intervention off reserve because of previous racism encountered in the health care system, the complexity of the funding for Indigenous health, and the lack of consistency found in information from health care providers (Castleden et al., 2016).

Cardiovascular Disease

Indigenous people in Canada have more than 10 times the rate of cardiovascular disease for other Canadians. This includes myocardial infarctions, strokes, coronary artery disease, and angina (Foulds, Bredin, & Warburton, 2016). The high rate is attributed to a higher prevalence of diabetes, hypertension, smoking, dyslipidemia, and dysglycemia (Tobe et al., 2015).

Indigenous Perspective. In a study examining contextual factors and health behaviours on the Six Nations reserve in Ontario, participants felt that the walkability score of the reserve was low in terms of lack of street connectivity, aesthetics, and safety (Joseph, Davis, Miller, et al., 2012). Further, participants identified high levels of cigarette smoking as being a problem on reserve. Food was bought outside the reserve, and participants spent more on food than non-Indigenous Canadians do in general (Joseph et al., 2012).

Indigenous women have been identified as having the highest levels of cardiovascular disease in the Indigenous population. Common themes among Indigenous women interviewed about cardiovascular disease (Medved, Brockmeier, Morach, et al., 2013) included disability and loss of life associated with family heart disease, a willingness to use Western medicine for treatment, and a lack of awareness of their own risk factors for heart disease due to being the family caregiver, often in chaotic and busy circumstances and often with insufficient support from the men in the family and community. They also expressed resentment at being told what to do for implementing lifestyle changes, an effect related to the impact of residential school on participants. Despite this resentment, many had in fact tried to change some of their lifestyle habits, even in the face of the economic challenges they encountered. Indigenous women, in general, did not place their heart condition as a top priority in their lives; they considered their families and caregiving responsibilities to be the major priority (Medved et al., 2013).

Otitis Media

It has been postulated that Indigenous populations did not experience otitis media (OM) prior to colonization and that colonization and the introduction of new pathogens have played a role in the increased incidence of OM among Indigenous populations (Bhutta, 2015). OM has generally been reported to be higher in incidence among Indigenous children than other Canadians (Bowd, 2005). One study, however, found that a cohort of First Nations children had a lower incidence than that for non-Indigenous children (Karunanayake, Albritton, Rennie, et al., 2016).

Accurate information about OM rates among the Indigenous population has been limited and variable owing to different definitions of OM and the inclusion of children of varying ages. Lack of access to health care, inconsistency in obtaining a diagnosis, and remote locations of First Nations communities are all contributing factors to these rates. Other factors found to increase the risk of OM include gender (male more than female), lower socioeconomic status, exposure to cigarette smoking, inadequate housing conditions, low birth weight, and daycare attendance.

Consequences of OM include hearing loss, which has been reported at rates as high as 44% for adult Inuit and 39% for adult First Nations people. Inuit appear to be more at risk, with contributing factors being exposure to wind, diet, activity in the winter, and increased rates of smoking (Bowd, 2005). As with other chronic illnesses, another factor contributing to the greater impact of OM is decreased access to appropriate medical care for children in remote communities. Recommendations for decreasing the incidence of OM include encouraging breastfeeding, having culturally safe and community-driven education health promotion programs about OM, taking antibiotics as prescribed, immunizing programs, and decreasing infant exposure to cigarette smoke (Bowd, 2005). Insufficient data were found to provide an Indigenous perspective on OM.

Rheumatic Disease

Rheumatic disease rates are higher in the Indigenous population in Canada than among non-Indigenous Canadians. This includes lupus, rheumatoid arthritis, osteoarthritis, and other connective tissue disorders such as spondyloarthropathies (Barnabe, Jones, Bernatsky, et al., 2017; Levy, Peschken, Tucker, et al., 2013; McDougall, Hurd, & Barnabe, 2017). Osteoarthritis rates range from 6 to 16% as opposed to 3.4 to 7.4% in the non-Indigenous population (McDougall et al., 2017). Lupus rates have been reported to be twice as high in the Canadian Indigenous populations as in the non-Indigenous Canadian population (McDougall et al., 2017). Arthritis is the most common chronic disease among Indigenous Canadians, with estimates of 1.3 to 1.6 times the rate of occurrence for non-Indigenous Canadians; high rates of disability have also been noted (Thurston et al., 2014). Smoking and indoor air pollution have been found to be associated with an increased risk of rheumatic diseases for the Canadian Indigenous population (McDougall et al., 2017).

Indigenous Perspective. Indigenous people with arthritis have described feelings of anger, frustration, and depression as a result of their experiences with arthritis. However, utilization of health care services is less than that of non-Indigenous people with arthritis, for a variety of reasons. These include coping behaviours described as "toughing it out," whereby arthritis is normalized because it is seen as a common affliction. Racism encountered within the health care system and challenges related to attending appointments are other complicating factors (Thurston et al., 2014).

Addictions

Addressing addictions through a chronic illness and traditional Indigenous health view lens (hybrid traditional Indigenous/Western health view) requires an understanding of a holistic perspective (emotional, mental, spiritual, and physical dimensions) situated within place, family, and community. When addressing addiction, traditional approaches may include using Indigenous values, perspectives, and knowledge as well as community involvement in program design. Promoting nonaddictive health may also include information on traditional diet, traditional Indigenous activities, and healing practices. Interventions may be diverse depending on the community and its particular values, customs, and history. Examples of effective approaches include storytelling; physical activities such as trapping and hunting; learning how to grow, harvest, and prepare traditional foods; bringing community members together for ceremonies; and having the community teach each other traditional crafting and other activities that focus on culture, self-determination, truth, and reconciliation. Social and rehabilitative interventions that increase individual and collective ownership and control, capacity, and empowerment are recognized as being important for reducing disparities, of which understanding the complexity of addictive behaviour are a part (Earle, 2011).

While it is difficult to collect accurate relevant data, the abuse of alcohol and other substances is perceived to be common in some Aboriginal communities (Firestone, Tyndall, & Fischer, 2015). Alcohol and substance abuse can be viewed as part of a set of complex issues affecting the social and physical well-being of the patient, family, and community. The National Native Alcohol and Drug Abuse Program was established to assist First Nations and Inuit community members in instituting and operating programs aimed at reducing and preventing alcohol, drug, and solvent abuse in Indigenous communities. The program emphasizes First Nations ownership of the prevention and treatment services. Together with the National Youth Solvent Abuse Program, a network of programming exists that focuses on prevention, early identification and intervention, screening, assessment and referral, treatment, discharge planning and aftercare, and performance measurement, research, and knowledge exchange (Government of Canada, 2015a).

Chronic addictive social and health challenges sometimes result in suicide. Suicide rates in Inuit and First Nations communities are variable, ranging from five times higher for Indigenous male youth compared to rates for non-Indigenous male youth to seven times higher for Indigenous females compared to rates for females of other ethnicities. They can also be up to 11 times higher for Inuit youth compared to rates for other Canadian youth (Bellamy & Hardy, 2015; Centre for Suicide Prevention, 2013). Possible factors that contribute to high suicide rates include psychobiological factors (pre-existing mental illness, personality disorders, dysfunctional cognitive style); intergenerational trauma resulting from colonial practices imposed on Indigenous peoples in Canada, such as residential school; socioeconomic conditions (poverty, unemployment); and cultural stress (loss of culture, language, and traditional coping mechanisms) (Centre for Suicide Prevention, 2013; TRC, 2015c, p. 151-153).

INDIGENOUS HEALTH—THE GLOBAL PERSPECTIVE

An Indigenous health global perspective takes into account an estimated 400 million Indigenous people who reside in countries on every continent around the world (Gracey & King, 2009; United Nations, 2015). Present trends reported by the United Nations (2009) indicate that Indigenous peoples represent approximately 15% of the poorest people globally yet make up only about 5% of the population worldwide. Poverty within Indigenous groups needs to be eradicated as poverty contributes to poor health associated with malnutrition, prevalent infections, environmental contamination, overcrowding, and inadequate hygiene. In addition, as King, Smith, and Gracey (2009) and the United Nations (2015) point out, Indigenous peoples have experienced entrenched discrimination and isolation due to their unique histories, traditions, cultures, languages, and geographic locations.

Indigenous peoples continue to suffer abuse and denial of human rights, including their right to health and right to land. Effects of colonization, powerful structural racism, and the burden of disease have resulted in long-standing societal and government denial of the complex and serious problems faced by Indigenous peoples. An understanding of Indigenous health requires an understanding of colonization and its effect on Indigenous people's existence (Gracey & King, 2009). Recognizing the burden of disease for Indigenous groups, thought to have resulted from transitioning from traditional to modern lifestyles, requires an understanding of obesity; type 2 diabetes; cardiovascular disease; and mental, social, and physical ailments linked to alcohol and substance misuse (Gracey & King, 2009). Postcolonial theoretical perspectives, social theory, and the work of Indigenous scholars are commonly used to guide thinking that can result in appreciating the detail and intricacies within Indigenous ways of viewing the world and thus a better understanding of their world. Topics of Indigenous health involve ethical issues relating to cultural pluralism and the development of culturally competent and culturally safe knowledge.

Common health disparities and inequities of Indigenous peoples are many. For example, the infant mortality rate in Latin America is 70% higher than it is for the non-Indigenous population (United Nations, 2009). In Australia, Indigenous children have a shorter life expectancy and higher burden of poor health compared to the non-Indigenous child population (United Nations, 2009). Connections between determinants of health and illness patterns and major health concerns such as obesity, type 2 diabetes, and TB as well as substance misuse are more common among Indigenous groups than for non-Indigenous populations (United Nations, 2009). Major health problems of Indigenous peoples are thought to be better understood as illness experiences that vary according to local culture and linguistic membership, geographic placement, and the extent of isolated living circumstances.

The Indigenous health crisis can be characterized by life expectancies that are lower than those for the general populations living in the same country. Along with hunger, inadequate food and dietary energy and nutrient deficiencies such as iron (due to intestinal parasites, blood loss, hypothyroidism, malaria, vitamin deficiencies, heavy metals such

BOX 10-11 Past Indigenous Nursing Leader: Jean Cuthand Goodwill (1928–1997)

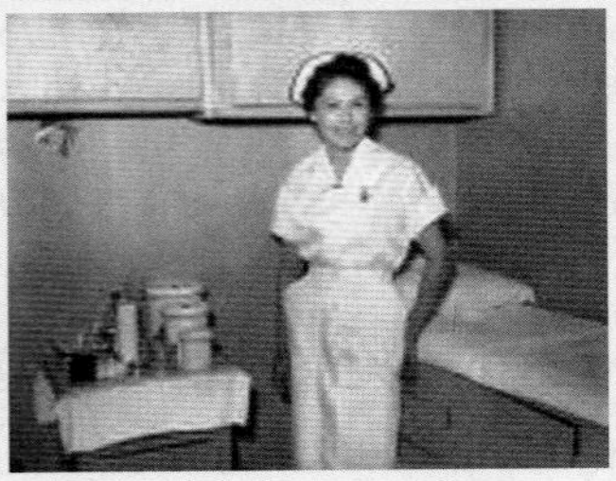
(Photo credit: Saskatchewan Archives Board, R-B6805)

Born on Little Pine First Nation, Saskatchewan, Jean studied nursing at the Holy Family Hospital in Prince Albert, Saskatchewan. She became the first Indigenous woman to finish a nursing program in Saskatchewan. Jean was influenced by spending time as a patient in a tuberculosis (TB) sanatorium in Prince Albert in her teen years, and also by watching her aunt Harriet Cuthand, who was a midwife and a medicine woman.

Jean became the first Indigenous head nurse at the La Ronge nursing station in northern Saskatchewan. In 1962, she became the executive director of the Indian and Métis Friendship Centre in Winnipeg. After marrying, adopting two children, being co-editor of *Indian News*, and helping develop *Tawwow* (a First Nations magazine), she co-founded the Indian and Inuit Nurses of Canada in 1974 (now the Canadian Indigenous Nurses Association). She served as president from 1983 to 1990. Jean became the first Indigenous woman in the federal public service to be appointed as special advisor to the Minister of National Health and Welfare, Monique Begin. After retirement from working in the Department of Indian Affairs and Northern Development, she became department head of Indian Health Studies at the Saskatchewan Indian Federated College of the University of Regina (now the First Nations University of Canada). She was on the Board of Directors for the Canadian Public Health Association, a founding member and past president of the Indigenous Nurses Association of Canada, and president of the Canadian Society for Circumpolar Health. Jean helped develop the National Native Access to Nursing Program at the University of Saskatchewan and the Indian Health Studies Department at the Saskatchewan Indian Federated College at the University of Regina. She received an Honorary Doctorate of Law from Queen's University in 1986 and the Order of Canada in 1992, as well as a National Excellence Award from the National Aboriginal Achievement Foundation in 1994. Jean Goodwill died in Regina on August 25, 1997, at the age of 69 from TB and leukemia. She was honoured posthumously by the Canadian Public Health Association by being named the recipient of the Ron Draper Health Promotion Award as well as having scholarships named in her honour by the Aboriginal Nurses Association of Canada (Indigenous Nurses of Canada Association) and Baxter Corporation.

From Cuthand, D. (n.d.). *Goodwill, Jean Cuthand (1928–97)*. Retrieved from http://esask.uregina.ca/entry/goodwill_jean_cuthand_1928-97.html; Petten, C. (1997). *Jean Goodwill: Footprints*. Retrieved from http://www.ammsa.com/content/jean-goodwill-footprints.

as zinc) are examples of nutritional deficiencies affecting Indigenous peoples (Gracey & King, 2009). Thus, nutritional deficiencies, diseases associated with cigarette smoking, accidents, poisonings, interpersonal violence, homicide, and suicide present similarities in health and illness experiences and their determinants across the great diversity of Indigenous groups (Gracey & King, 2009).

The United Nations (2009) indicates that the life expectancy of Indigenous peoples in Nepal is approximately 20 years lower than the non-Indigenous population, and for the Maori in New Zealand it is nearly 10 years lower than for non-Maori. These findings are important for several reasons. First, when considering Indigenous health worldwide, it is complex, and the variation in high rates among different Indigenous populations requires more attention and research. Second, as studies continue to present the epidemiological features of great disparities in health and disease statistics, advocacy related to the provision of health and social services that benefit Indigenous people is even more urgently required. Third, much of the empirical evidence is still replete with examples of the limited effectiveness of specific Indigenous health approaches that have been adapted to meet the needs of diverse Indigenous peoples globally.

Although global achievements directed at improving population health have been reached, the overall health of Indigenous populations lags far behind that of other populations (Pulver, Haswell, Ring, et al., 2010). In recent years, the health of some Indigenous groups has been considered improved, but access to holistic and culturally appropriate health services remains challenging, as does a deepening response to health problems related to the health of mothers and children, infectious diseases, and diseases related to urbanization and lifestyle (Gracey & King, 2009; United Nations, 2015). To make progress in the twenty-first century toward improving Indigenous health, nurses will need to play key roles in examining Indigenous health challenges, developing appropriate responses, and implementing knowledge and action through understanding. In responding to Indigenous health, nurses have participated in huge numbers and will continue to do so, continuing a history of advocacy related to health inequities and social injustices (Box 10-11). However, as Gracey and King (2009) emphasize, from a politics, policy, and future-directions perspective, assisting Indigenous peoples to build capacity in order to orchestrate effective services and programs and work closely with systems of health care will be part of the next wave of radical reorientation that is urgently needed.

KEY CONCEPTS

- The three Indigenous Canadian groups—First Nations, Métis, and Inuit—have their own unique languages, heritages, cultural practices, and spiritual beliefs.
- Colonialism is a theoretical framework for understanding the complexities of past relationships between Indigenous peoples and Europeans and as they later sustained those initial relationships in building a new reality in North America.
- The experiences of colonialism resulted in much historical trauma for Indigenous people.
- All Canadians have been invited by the Truth and Reconciliation Commission of Canada to become a settler ally—teachers and learners that question how non-Indigenous people can change, as opposed to just Indigenous people changing.
- Cultural orientations include theories of Indigenous health, the symbol of the circle, the Medicine Wheel, traditional healers, ceremony, teachings, and role-modelling of the elders.
- Nurses need to develop the ability to adapt nursing practice for use in an Indigenous context, to preserve the perspectives of Indigenous peoples, sustain the holistic nature of responding to social and health challenges, and value new forms of partnership in respectful ways.
- Addressing chronic disease requires appropriate knowledge and skills to create culturally safe chronic disease management programs in collaboration with Indigenous communities.
- Nurses' advocacy can improve the social determinants of health across sectors and help in treating and reducing chronic diseases in the Indigenous population in Canada.
- Almost 400 million Indigenous peoples reside in countries on every continent around the world.

- Structural racism is the legitimized and normalized spectrum of attitudes, practices, and policies that consistently result in chronic and continuous substandard outcomes for Indigenous peoples.

CRITICAL THINKING EXERCISES

1. You are a staff nurse at the hospital and involved in the education committee for the medical/surgical units. The person in charge of the education committee, another staff nurse, would like to have a multicultural day, as Heritage Days are coming up soon. The committee divides into teams to come up with ideas to highlight several cultures. At the meeting when you are all presenting your final ideas to the group, the team responsible for Indigenous people in America and Canada presents several ideas. One is for participants to paint their own "eagle" feather. Another involves making dreamcatchers out of kits from the dollar store. The last one is to make a smudging kit with sage that was bought from a gift shop. You recognize that there is a problem with all of these ideas. The team gets upset and leaves when you state your objections. You are then tasked with coming up with three ideas in order to showcase Indigenous people at the multicultural day.
   a. What objections do you voice to the team?
   b. What are some ideas that you might come up with that would be culturally safe?
2. You are the coordinator for a liver transplant team. A new patient comes in to see you for his pre-evaluation. He is an Indigenous patient with liver cancer who lives on a reserve near Edmonton. Over the course of the next few months, you meet with him three times to explain the process for a liver transplant and answer any questions. He shows up to all the appointments and seems to understand all that you have explained to him. On the day of a procedure to place radiation beads into his liver to combat his liver cancer, he does not show up and you cannot reach him. You call his niece, who also is unable to reach him. After 2 weeks have passed, he eventually calls you. He tells you he was too scared to go for the procedure.
   a. What can you do to help him?
   b. How might colonialism have impacted his life in such a way that his fear was triggered?
3. You are eventually able to encourage him to go for the procedure. His niece calls you a week later. She tells you that he is a spiritual leader in the community and that this was not taken into account when you did your teachings with him. She offers to meet with you to further discuss this so that future Indigenous patients will not have to go for treatment without their culture and spirituality being taken into account.
   a. Thinking about hospital policies and procedures, staff knowledge and community connections that the hospital may need to have to improve their care for Indigenous patients, what ideas do you have that could be helpful in tackling any or all of these areas?
   b. Where might you gather more information?
   c. Find an article or two from the nursing literature that might help you to make suggestions to the liver transplant unit and the clinical nurse educators in the hospital. Could this information improve policies, procedures, and knowledge of hospital staff relative to the care of Indigenous patients?
4. You are working at the community health centre and your next appointment is with a family of a single mother and her five children. You go out into the waiting area to see if they have arrived. The staff person at the desk says, "Oh, don't worry—they'll be late. They always are. They don't care. I don't even know why they bother coming in. It's so ridiculous. We end up having to reschedule them every time because they are always late. And she doesn't even have their immunization cards, she doesn't know when they were immunized last. And last time the kids had lice, so be careful going near them. Aboriginal families. You know what they're like!" You know that the policy is to reschedule patients who are over 15 minutes late for their appointment. Twenty-five minutes after their appointment time, the mother comes in with her five children aged 6 months to 10 years old. When you look at their chart, you realize the children are behind on their immunizations. You decide to speak with her in the waiting room. She tells you that they were immunized the summer previously on reserve, and that she has told the staff this. She also says she had trouble getting a ride to the clinic and the bus was late. She looks exhausted, and the baby has a cough. The staff tells you that they have to reschedule her, but you disagree.
   a. What do you do about her late appointment?
   b. How have social determinants of health impacted this woman and her family?
   c. How can you best help this woman and her family?
   d. What will you do about the staff member's statements about the woman and her family?

REVIEW QUESTIONS

1. An Indigenous patient tells the nurse that she has problems with being affectionate with her children and is worried that too much affection will spoil them. She says she never had affection from her parents and can't understand why people feel she should show more emotion to her children. This might be an example of which of the following?
   1. Historical trauma
   2. Colonialism
   3. Cultural trauma
   4. Cultural genocide
2. A patient states that he cannot get his health care equipment and medical supplies for home peritoneal dialysis paid for by the federal government when he is in his community. He lives on a reserve just outside the city. He says that in order to get the equipment paid for, he must live in the city where the provincial government will pay for it. What is this an example of?
   1. Institutionalism
   2. Colonialism
   3. Cultural genocide
   4. Personal racism
3. A hospitalized patient is a Cree man who has just been diagnosed with diabetes. He has asked the nurse for a sweet grass ceremony and to see the hospital Indigenous Elder. The nurse understands that in order to treat the man's diabetes she will have to take different cultural aspects into consideration. Which of the following aspects will the nurse have to take into consideration in writing a care plan for him?
   1. Historical trauma and spiritual genocide
   2. The patient's individualism and self-determination
   3. A holistic view of health, which includes spirituality
   4. A circular view of health, which includes individualism
4. A community health nurse is attending a cultural safety course where a co-worker tells the nurse that he knows all about Indigenous patients. He tells her that they have traditional beliefs

that she must understand, that she should attend their sweet grass ceremonies, and that they all went to residential school. The nurse knows that the co-worker needs more information in order to give culturally safe care. What else does he need to know?
   1. One should not attend their sweet grass ceremonies.
   2. Indigenous patients do not all have traditional beliefs.
   3. In order to understand their traditional beliefs, one must know what the Medicine Wheel is.
   4. Most Indigenous people who attended residential school have already passed away.
5. The incidence of COPD and asthma is higher for Indigenous people than it is for other Canadians. Which of the following are social determinants of health that contribute to these higher rates?
   1. Personal health practices and coping skills, physical environments, and education
   2. Gender, diet, and personal health practices
   3. Genetics, biology, and social status
   4. Family health practices, work environment, and colonialism
6. Asthma is under-reported in many Indigenous communities. What are some factors that contribute to this under-reporting?
   1. Medical personnel do not report it because of their racism.
   2. Indigenous families have decreased access to health care.
   3. No treatment is available for asthma.
   4. Indigenous medicine is effective for asthma.
7. Suicide rates are much higher in some Indigenous communities than in non-Indigenous communities. Which of the following has been shown to be an effective deterrent to suicide in Indigenous communities?
   1. Teaching youth how to make traditional Indigenous art.
   2. Ensuring there is a suicide prevention team flown into the community.
   3. Having information nights about suicide as well as information posters in the community.
   4. Having discussions with Indigenous youth about their suicidal thoughts.
8. The community health nurse on reserve has a free afternoon to plan a health promotion activity. Which of the following would be the best use of the nurse's time?
   1. Planning a smoking cessation program on reserve, which includes posters and a weekly meeting.
   2. Agreeing to help the band council plan an Indigenous-language program for the First Nation.
   3. Ensuring information is made available to all families about good nutrition for children.
   4. Buying a weight set for the recreation room in the community hall.
9. Which of these would be an example of cultural safety?
   1. Giving an Indigenous patient a braid of sweet grass
   2. Asking an Indigenous patient which residential school she attended
   3. Asking an Indigenous patient which First Nation he is from
   4. Calling the Indigenous Elder to come to the unit to help with the admission of an Indigenous patient
10. An Indigenous patient is on a strict diet because of heart failure. The nurse enters her room and catches her drinking out of a bottle that a family member brought in for her. She says it is traditional medicine. What is the most appropriate response?
   1. The nurse asks if she can give it to him so the nurse can send it to the lab for testing to assess if it is safe for her to drink.
   2. The nurse reiterates that she is not to eat or drink anything that is not on her diet and asks her to hand it over.
   3. The nurse is worried it might be alcohol and decides to discuss it with the charge nurse so that the doctor can be notified,
   4. The nurse asks the patient if she could tell him more about what the medicine is and explains that he is concerned about interactions with the medicines the patient is taking from the hospital.
11. A nursing instructor is teaching a cultural safety session to staff at the clinic. One nurse asks the instructor, "Who is a Métis person?" What is the instructor's best response?
   1. A Métis person is someone with mixed Indigenous ethnicity and other ethnicity.
   2. A Métis person is someone who is half Indigenous and half French.
   3. A Métis person is someone who self-identifies as Métis and lives in a Métis community.
   4. A Métis person is someone who self-identifies as Métis and has Indigenous ancestry from several generations ago.

Answers: 1. 1; **2.** 2; **3.** 3; **4.** 2; **5.** 1; **6.** 2; **7.** 1; **8.** 2; **9.** 3; **10.** 4; **11.** 3.

Rationales for the Review Questions appear at the end of the book.

RECOMMENDED WEBSITES

Canadian Foundation for Healthcare Improvement: Canadian Northern and Remote Healthcare Network: http://www.cfhi-fcass.ca/WhatWeDo/northern-remote-collaboration.

The aim of this network is to improve the health status of people living in northern and remote regions of Canada by providing opportunities for practitioners, leaders, and policymakers to network in order to build leadership and improve capacity.

Canadian Indigenous Nurses Association of Canada (CINA): http://www.indigenousnurses.ca.

The CINA works to improve the health of Indigenous people by supporting Indigenous nurses and promoting the development and practice of Indigenous nursing. Key objectives include, among others, working with communities, health provider's, and government institutions on addressing Canadian health system elements that address issues and concerns in Indigenous communities; engaging and conducting research on Indigenous health nursing; and promoting awareness nationally and internationally of the health needs of Canadian Indigenous people.

First Nations Child and Family Caring Society of Canada: https://fncaringsociety.com/who-we-are.

First Nations Child and Family Caring Society of Canada is a non-profit organization that provides resources to support the First Nations community to empower Indigenous children, youth, and families and works with national and international partners to promote the rights of Indigenous children, youth, and families.

Nasivvik: Centre for Inuit Health and Changing Environments: http://www.nasivvik.ca/research/funded-research/.

Funded by the Canadian Institutes of Health Research–Institute of Aboriginal Peoples' Health and based at Laval and Trent Universities, the Nasivvik Centre is a multidisciplinary research and training centre that focuses on building Inuit health research in key environmental health areas of importance to Inuit communities. Nasivvik is an Inuktitut word that means vantage point. It can be a height of land, a hummock of ice, or any place of elevation that affords an observer a clear view of their surroundings to make good observations (Zebedee Nungak).

National Collaborating Centre for Aboriginal Health: http://www.nccah-ccnsa.ca/en/.

The National Collaborating Centre for Aboriginal Health supports First Nations, Inuit, and Métis health equity and renewal through knowledge translation and exchange. It was established by the government of

Canada in 2005, is funded through the Public Health Agency of Canada, and is hosted by the University of Northern British Columbia.

Native Women's Association of Canada: https://www.nwac.ca/.

The Native Women's Association of Canada is an aggregate of 13 Canadian Indigenous women's organizations whose goal is to "enhance, promote and foster the social, economic, cultural and political well-being of First Nations and Métis women within First Nation, Métis, and Canadian societies" while respecting, promoting, defending, and enhancing Indigenous languages, traditions, beliefs, and ancestral laws.

Walking in Her Moccasins: http://walkinginhermoccasins.org/.

An experimental violence prevention resource for Indigenous men and boys officially launched Nationally in Canada in December 2017.

REFERENCES

Aboriginal Education Directorate Manitoba Education and Advanced Learning. (2016). *First Nation, Métis and Inuit Education Policy Framework: Transforming educational experiences through the five Rs: recognition, revitalization, relevance, relationships and reconciliation.* Retrieved from http://www.edu.gov.mb.ca/aed/fnmi_framework/document.pdf.

Aguiar, W., & Halseth, R. (2015). *Aboriginal peoples and historic trauma: The processes of intergenerational transmission.* Prince George, BC: National Collaborating. Retrieved from http://www.nccah-ccnsa.ca/Publications/Lists/Publications/Attachments/142/2015-04-28-AguiarHalseth-RPT-IntergenTraumaHistory-EN-Web.pdf.

Alberta Education. (2017). *Education for reconciliation—First Nations, Métis and Inuit curriculum. Overview.* Retrieved from https://education.alberta.ca/education-for-reconciliation/first-nations-m%C3%a9tis-inuit-curriculum/.

Alberta Teachers Association. (2015). *Truth and Reconciliation Commission's final report.* Retrieved from https://www.teachers.ab.ca/News%20Room/WebExtras/Pages/Truth-and-Reconciliation-Commission%E2%80%99s-Final-Report.aspx.

Allan, B., & Smylie, J. (2015). *First peoples, second class treatment: The role of racism in the health and well-being of Indigenous peoples in Canada.* Toronto, ON: The Wellesley Institute. Retrieved from http://www.wellesleyinstitute.com/wp-content/uploads/2015/02/Summary-First-Peoples-Second-Class-Treatment-Final.pdf.

Alvares, G. G., Orr, P., Wobeser, W. L., et al. (2014). Chapter 14: Tuberculosis prevention and care in First Nations, Inuit, and Metis people. In *Tuberculosis Standards* (7th ed.). Ottawa: Public Health Agency of Canada. Retrieved from http://www.respiratoryguidelines.ca/sites/all/files/Canadian_TB_Standards_7th_Edition_ENG.pdf.

Andersen, C. (2016). The colonialism of Canada's Métis health population dynamics: Caught between bad data and no data at all. *Journal of Population Research, 33*(1), 67–82. doi:10.1007/s12546-016-9161-4.

Assembly of First Nations (AFN). (n.d.). *Description of the AFN.* Retrieved from: http://www.afn.ca/en/about-afn/description-of-the-afn.

Assembly of First Nations (AFN). (2010). *First Nations control of First Nations education.* Retrieved from http://www.afn.ca/uploads/files/education/3._2010_july_afn_first_nations_control_of_first_nations_education_final_eng.pdf.

Barnabe, C., Jones, C. A., Bernatsky, S., et al. (2017). Inflammatory arthritis prevalence and health services use in the First Nations and non-First Nations populations of Alberta, Canada. *Arthritis Care and Research, 69*(4), 467–474. doi:10.1002/acr.22959.

Barnhardt, R., & Kawagley, A. O. (2005). Indigenous knowledge systems and Alaska Native ways of knowing. *Anthropology and Education Quarterly, 36*(1), 8–23.

Beal, B., MacLeod, R., & Foot, R. (2015). *Northwest rebellion.* Retrieved from http://www.thecanadianencyclopedia.ca/en/article/north-west-rebellion/.

Beben, N., & Muirhead, A. (2016). Improving cancer control in First Nations, Inuit and Métis communities in Canada. *European Journal of Cancer Care, 25*(2), 219–221. doi:10.1111/ecc.12479.

Bellamy, S., & Hardy, C. (2015). *Understanding depression in Aboriginal communities and families.* Prince George, BC: National Collaborating Centre for Health. Retrieved from http://www.nccah-ccnsa.ca/Publications/Lists/Publications/Attachments/150/2015-10-07-RPT-MentalHealth03-Depression-BellamyHardy-EN-Web.pdf.

Bhutta, M. (2015). Evolution and otitis media: A review, and a model to explain high prevalence in Indigenous populations. *Human Biology, 87*(2), 92–108. doi:10.11310/humanbiology.87.2.0092.

Bowd, A. D. (2005). Otitis media: Health and social consequences for Aboriginal youth in Canada's north. *International Journal of Circumpolar Health, 64*(1), 5–15. doi:10.3402/ijch.v64i1.17949.

Brascoupé, S., & Waters, C. (2009). Cultural safety: Exploring the concept of cultural safety to Aboriginal health and community wellness. *Journal of Aboriginal Health, November,* 6–41.

Browne, A. J. (1995). The meaning of respect: A First Nations perspective. *Canadian Journal of Nursing Research, 27*(4), 95–109.

Cain, R., Jackson, R., Prentice, T., et al. (2013). The experience of HIV diagnosis among Aboriginal people living with HIV/AIDS and depression. *Qualitative Health Research, 23*(6), 815–824. doi:10.1177/1049732313482525.

Canadian AIDS Society. (2016a). *Position statement: Treatment as prevention.* Retrieved from http://www.cdnaids.ca/position-statement-treatment-as-prevention/.

Canadian AIDS Society. (2016b). *Public Health Agency of Canada cutting funding to Canadian AIDS service organizations.* Retrieved from http://www.newswire.ca/news-releases/public-health-agency-of-canada-cutting-funding-to-Canadian-aids-service-organizations-596863811.html.

Canadian Association of Schools of Nursing/Association Canadienne des Écoles de Sciences Infirmières [CASN/ACESI] (2015). *National nursing education framework: Final report.* Ottawa: Author.

Canadian Baptists of Western Canada. (2013). *Aboriginal issues resources for the churches of the Canadian Baptists of Western Canada.* Retrieved from: http://cbwc.ca/wp-content/uploads/2017/04/CBWC-Aboriginal-Issues-Resources.pdf.

Canadian Broadcasting Company (CBC). (2016). *Deadline looms for bands to enter day scholar residential school suit.* Retrieved from http://www.cbc.ca/news/canada/north/deadline-looms-day-students-1.3407833.

Canadian Child Welfare Research Portal. (n.d.). *Frequently asked questions (FAQs).* Retrieved from http://cwrp.ca/faqs.

Carriere, J. (2005). Connectedness and health for First Nation adoptees. *Pediatric Child Health, 10*(9), 545–548. Retrieved from https://www.ncbi.nlm.nih.gov/pmc/articles/PMC2722640/.

Castleden, H., Watson, R. C., Bennett, E., et al. (2016). Asthma prevention and management for Aboriginal people: Lessons from Mi'kmaq communities, Unama'ki, Canada, 2012. *Preventing Chronic Disease, 13,* 1–9. doi:10.5888/pcd13.150244.

Centre for Suicide Prevention. (2013). *Aboriginal suicide prevention resource toolkit.* Retrieved from https://suicideinfo.ca/LinkClick.aspx?fileticket=MVIyGo2V4YY%3D&tabid=563.

Chandler, M. J., & Lalonde, C. E. (2008). Cultural continuity as a moderator of suicide risk among Canada's First Nations. In L. Kirmayer & G. Valaskakis (Eds.), *Healing traditions: The mental health of Aboriginal peoples in Canada* (pp. 221–248). Vancouver: University of British Columbia Press.

Cruickshank, D. A. (2017). *Calder case.* Retrieved from http://www.thecanadianencyclopedia.ca/en/article/calder-case/.

Derworiz, C. E., & Albers, G. (2015). *Indigenous and Northern Affairs Canada.* Retrieved from http://www.thecanadianencyclopedia.ca/en/article/aboriginal-affairs-and-northern-development-canada/.

Dickason, O. P., & Newbigging, W. (2015). *A concise history of Canada's First Nations* (3rd ed.). Don Mills, ON: Oxford University Press.

Dinc, L., & Gastmans, C. (2012). Trust and trustworthiness in nursing: An argument-based literature review. *Nursing Inquiry, 19*(3), 223–237. doi:10.1111/j.1440-1800.2011.00582.x.

Douglas, V. (2013). *Introduction to Aboriginal health and healthcare in Canada: Bridging health and healing.* New York, NY: Springer Publishing Company, LLC.

Dyck, R. F., Jiang, Y., & Osgood, N. D. (2014). The long term risks of end stage renal disease and mortality among First Nations and non-First Nations people with youth-onset diabetes. *Canadian Journal of Diabetes, 38*(4), 237–243. doi:10.1016/j.jcjd.2014.o3.005.

Earle, L. (2011). *Understanding chronic disease and the role for traditional approaches in Aboriginal communities.* Prince George: National Collaborating Centre for Aboriginal Health. Retrieved from http://www.nccah-ccnsa.ca/Publications/Lists/Publications/Attachments/45/chronic_disease_EN_web.pdf.

Eggertson, L. (2014). News: Health course helps Inuit interpreters tackle tough jobs. *Canadian Medical Association Journal, 186*(2), doi:10.1503/cmaj.109-4677.

Elias, B., Mignone, J., Hall, M., et al. (2012). Trauma and suicide behaviour histories among a Canadian Indigenous population: An empirical exploration of the potential role of Canada's residential school system. *Social Science and Medicine, 74*(10), 1560–1569. doi:10.1016/j.socscimed.2012.01.026.

Firestone, M., Tyndall, M., & Fischer, B. (2015). Substance use and related harms among Aboriginal people in Canada: A comprehensive review. *Journal of Healthcare for the Poor and Underserved, 26*(4), 1110–1131. doi:10.1353/hpu.2015.0108.

First Nations Education Steering Committee, & First Nations Schools Association. (2015). *Indian residential schools and reconciliation: Teacher resource guide.* Retrieved from http://www.fnesc.ca/wp/wp-content/uploads/2015/07/PUB-LFP-IRSR-10-2015-07-WEB.pdf.

Fontaine, T. (2016). *Canada officially adopts UN declaration on rights of Indigenous peoples.* Retrieved from http://www.cbc.ca/news/indigenous/canada-adopting-implementing-un-rights-declaration-1.3575272.

Forte, M. C. (2013). Introduction - "Who is an Indian": The cultural politics of a bad question. In M. C. Forte (Ed.), *Who is an Indian: Race, place and the politics of Indigeneity in the Americas* (pp. 3–51). Toronto: University of Toronto Press.

Foulds, H. J. A., Bredin, S. S. D., & Warburton, D. E. R. (2016). The vascular health status of a population of adult Canadian Indigenous peoples from British Columbia. *Journal of Human Hypertension, 4*(30), 278–284. doi:10.1038/jhh.2015.51.

Gallagher, A. (2007). The respectful nurse. *Nursing Ethics, 14*(30), 360–371.

Gallant, J. (2016). *Federal government asks judge to toss Sixties Scoop lawsuit. thestar.com.* Retrieved from https://www.thestar.com/news/gta/2016/11/29/federal-government-asks-judge-to-toss-sixties-scoop-lawsuit.html.

Gershon, A. S., Khan, S., Klein-Geltink, J., et al. (2014). Asthma and chronic obstructive pulmonary disease (COPD) prevalence and Health services use in Ontario Métis: A population-based cohort study. *PLoS ONE, 9*(4), e95899. doi:10.1371/journal.pone.0095899.

Gillmore, K. (2016). Teaching truth and reconciliation: Exploring residential schools in Canada. *Teach: Education For Today and Tomorrow*. Retrieved from http://www.teachmag.com/archives/8934.

Goettner-Habendroth, H. (2012). *Matriarchal societies: Studies on indigenous cultures across the globe*. New York, NY: Peter Lang AG.

Government of Alberta. (1990). *Constitution of Alberta Amendment Act, 1990 Chapter C-24*. Retrieved from http://www.qp.alberta.ca/documents/Acts/C24.pdf.

Government of Canada. (2015a). *Government of Canada commits to ongoing funding for Aboriginal programs*. Retrieved from http://www.newswire.ca/news-releases/government-of-canada-commits-to-ongoing-funding-for-aboriginal-health-programs-520293841.html.

Government of Canada. (2015b). *National Native alcohol and drug abuse program*. Retrieved from http://healthycanadians.gc.ca/anti-drug-antidrogue/funding-financement/hc-sc-nnadap-pnlaada-eng.php.

Government of Canada. (2016). *National inquiry into missing and murdered Indigenous women and girls*. Retrieved from https://www.aadnc-aandc.gc.ca/eng/1448633299414/1448633350146.

Gracey, M., & King, M. (2009). Indigenous health part 1: determinants and disease patterns. *Lancet, 374*, 65–75.

Hanson, E. (2009). *The Sixties Scoop and Aboriginal child welfare*. Retrieved from: http://alieastolot.weebly.com/uploads/5/0/3/4/50341847/sixties_scoop.pdf.

Harrowing, J. N., Mill, J., Spiers, J., et al. (2010). Critical ethnography, cultural safety, and international health research. *International Journal of Qualitative Methods, 9*, 240–251.

Hartrick Doane, G., & Varcoe, C. (2005). *Family nursing as relational inquiry: Developing health-promoting practice*. Philadelphia, PA: Lippincott Williams & Wilkins.

Health Canada. (2011). *Communities in action: Aboriginal diabetes initiative*. Retrieved from: https://www.canada.ca/en/health-canada/services/first-nations-inuit-health/reports-publications/diseases-health-conditions/communities-action-aboriginal-diabetes-initiative-health-canada-2011.html.

Health Canada. (2013). First Nations and Inuit health. *Diabetes*. Retrieved from https://www.canada.ca/en/health-canada/services/first-nations-inuit-health/diseases-health-conditions/diabetes.html.

Henderson, W. B., & Parrott, Z. (2016). *Indian Act*. Retrieved from http://www.thecanadianencyclopedia.ca/en/article/indian-act/.

Howard, H. A. (2014). Canadian residential schools and urban Indigenous knowledge production about diabetes. *Medical Anthropology, 33*(6), 529–545. doi:10.1080/01459740.2013.828722.

Hudson's Bay Company History Foundation. (2016a). *Hudson's Bay Company timeline: 1670*. Retrieved from http://www.hbcheritage.ca/classroom/timeline.

Hudson's Bay Company History Foundation. (2016b). *York Factory*. Retrieved from http://www.hbcheritage.ca/places/forts-posts/york-factory.

Hunt, S. (2016). *An Introduction to the health of two-spirit people: Historical, contemporary and emergent issues*. Prince George, BC: National Collaborating Centre for Aboriginal Health. Retrieved from http://www.nccah-ccnsa.ca/Publications/Lists/Publications/Attachments/156/2016-05-10-RPT-HealthTwoSpirit-Hunt-EN-Web.pdf.

Indigenous and Northern Affairs Canada (INAC). (2013a). *Fact sheet-2011 National Household Survey Aboriginal demographics, educational attainment and labour market outcomes*. Retrieved from https://www.aadnc-aandc.gc.ca/eng/1376329205785/1376329233875.

Indigenous and Northern Affairs Canada (INAC). (2013b). *Aboriginal demographics from the 2011 National Household Survey*. Retrieved from https://www.aadnc-aandc.gc.ca/eng/1370438978311/1370439050610.

Indigenous and Northern Affairs Canada (INAC). (2013c). *Common terminology*. Retrieved from https://www.aadnc-aandc.gc.ca/eng/1358879361384/1358879407462.

Indigenous and Northern Affairs Canada (INAC). (2015). *Timeline – Indian Residential Schools*. Retrieved from https://www.aadnc-aandc.gc.ca/eng/1332939430258/1332939552554.

Indigenous and Northern Affairs Canada (INAC). (2016a). *Urban Indigenous peoples*. Retrieved from https://www.aadnc-aandc.gc.ca/eng/1100100014265/1369225120949.

Indigenous and Northern Affairs Canada (INAC). (2016b). *Indigenous peoples and communities*. Retrieved from https://www.aadnc-aandc.gc.ca/eng/1100100013785/1304467449155.

Indigenous and Northern Affairs Canada (INAC). (2016c). *Indian status*. Retrieved from https://www.aadnc-aandc.gc.ca/eng/1100100032374/1100100032378.

Inuit Tapiriit Kanatami. (2017). *About Canadian Inuit*. Retrieved from https://www.itk.ca/about-canadian-inuit/.

Jacklin, K. M., Henderson, R. I., Green, M. E., et al. (2017). Health care experiences of Indigenous people living with type 2 diabetes in Canada. *Canadian Medical Association Journal, 189*(3), 106–112. doi:10.1503/cmaj.161098.

Johnston, P. (1983). *Native children and the child welfare system*. Ottawa, ON: The Canadian Council on Social Development. Retrieved from http://www.deslibris.ca/ID/413616.

Jordan's Principle Working Group (2015). *Without denial, delay or disruption: Ensuring First Nations children's access to equitable services through Jordan's Principle*. Ottawa, ON: Assembly of First Nations. Retrieved from http://cwrp.ca/sites/default/files/publications/en/jpreport_final_en.pdf.

Joseph, P., Davis, A. D., Miller, R., et al. (2012). Contextual determinants of health behaviours in an Aboriginal community in Canada: Pilot project. *BMC Public Health, 12*(1), 1–8.

Karunanayake, C. P., Albritton, W., Rennie, D. C., et al. & The Saskatchewan Rural Health Study Team. (2016). Ear infection and its associated risk factors in First Nations and rural school -aged Canadian children. *International Journal of Pediatrics*, 2016: 1523897. doi:10.1155/2016/1523897.

King, M., Smith, S., & Gracey, M. (2009). Indigenous health part 2: The underlying causes of the health gap. *Lancet, 374*, 76–85.

Kirkup, K. (2016). *Ottawa launches long-awaited inquiry into missing, murdered Indigenous women*. Global News. Retrieved from http://globalnews.ca/news/2862129/ottawa-set-to-launch-inquiry-into-missing-murdered-indigenous-women/.

Kirkup, K., & Ubelacker, S. (2016). *Solving the legacy of Indigenous sexual abuse: think globally, act nationally*. CBC News. Retrieved from http://www.cbc.ca/news/canada/manitoba/solving-the-legacy-of-indigenous-sexual-abuse-think-globally-act-nationally-1.3880907.

Kirmayer, L. F., Tait, C. L., & Simpson, C. (2008). The mental health of Aboriginal peoples in Canada: Transformations of identity and community. In L. Kirmayer & G. Valaskakis (Eds.), *Healing traditions: The mental health of Aboriginal peoples in Canada* (pp. 3–35). Vancouver, Canada: University of British Columbia Press.

Kotalik, J., & Martin, G. (2016). Aboriginal health care and bioethics: A reflection on the teaching of the seven grandfathers. *The American Journal of Bioethics, 16*(5), 38–43. doi:10.1080/15265161.2016.1159749.

Kue Young, T., Kelly, J. J., Friborg, J., et al. (2016). Cancer among circumpolar populations: An emerging public health concern. *International Journal of Circumpolar Health, 75*, doi:10.3402/ijch.v75.29787.

Kue Young, T., Reading, J., Elias, B., et al. (2000). Type 2 diabetes mellitus in Canada's First Nations: Status of an epidemic in progress. *Canadian Medical Association Journal, 163*(5), 561–566.

Lavoie, J., Browne, A. J., Varcoe, C., et al. (2015). Missing pathways to self-governance: Aboriginal health policy in British Columbia. *International Indigenous Policy Journal, 6*(1). Retrieved from http://ir.lib.uwo.ca/iipj/vol6/iss1/2.

Levy, D. M., Peschken, C. A., Tucker, L. B., et al. (2013). Influence of ethnicity on childhood-onset systemic lupus erythematosus: Results from a multiethnic multicenter Canadian cohort. *Arthritis Care and Research, 65*(1), 152–160. doi:10.1002/acr.21779.

Loppie Reading, C., & Wien, F. (2009). *Health inequalities and social determinants of Aboriginal peoples' health*. Retrieved from http://www.nccah-ccnsa.ca/docs/social%20determinates/nccah-loppie-wien_report.pdf.

Maar, M., Burchell, A., Little, J., et al. (2013). A qualitative study of provider perspectives of structural barriers to cervical cancer screening among First Nations women. *Women's Health Issues, 23*(5), e319–e325. doi:10.1016/j.whi.2013.06.005.

Macdonald, D., & Wilson, D. (2016). *Shameful neglect: Indigenous child poverty across Canada*. Ottawa, ON: Canadian Centre for Policy Alternatives. Retrieved from http://cwrp.ca/sites/default/files/publications/en/indigenous_child_poverty_2016.pdf.

MacDonald, M. E., Rigillo, N., & Brassard, P. (2010). Urban Aboriginal understandings and experiences of tuberculosis in Montreal, Quebec, Canada. *Qualitative Health Research, 20*(4), 506–523. doi:10.1177/1049732309360538.

MacDonald, N., & MacDonald, J. (2007). Reflections of a Mi'kmaq social worker on a quarter of a century work in First Nations child welfare. *First Peoples Child & Family Review, 3*(1), 34–45.

Malone, K. (2016). *Métis Nation 'finding ourselves in Confederation' with land claim negotiations, President of MMF says*. CBC News. Retrieved from http://www.cbc.ca/news/canada/manitoba/m%C3%A9tis-confederation-land-claim-negotiations-mmf-1.3854022.

Marshall, M., Marshall, A., & Bartlett, C. (2015). Two-eyed seeing in medicine. In M. Greenwood, S. De Leeuw, N. M. Lindsay, et al. (Eds.), *Determinants of Indigenous peoples' health in Canada* (pp. 16–24). Toronto: Canadian Scholars Press Inc.

Marshall, T. (2015). *Idle no more*. Retrieved from http://www.thecanadianencyclopedia.ca/en/article/idle-no-more/.

Mas, S. (2015). *Truth and Reconciliation Commission final report points to 'growing crisis' for Indigenous youth: Indigenous youth are overrepresented in Canada's prisons and child-welfare system*. CBC News. Retrieved from http://www.cbc.ca/news/politics/truth-and-reconciliation-final-report-1.3361148.

McCabe, G. (2008). Mind, body, emotions and spirit: Reaching to the ancestors for healing. *Counseling Psychology Quarterly, 21*(2), 143–152. doi:10.1080/09515070802066847.

McCorckle, K. (2015). A different kind of choice: Weighing the pitfalls and profits of education outside the First Nation. *Canada Education, 56*(2).

McDougall, C., Hurd, K., & Barnabe, C. (2017). Systematic review of rheumatic disease epidemiology in the indigenous populations of Canada, the United States, Australia, and New Zealand. *Seminars in Arthritis and Rheumatism, 37*(4), 503–521. doi:10.1016/j.semarthrit.2016.10.010.

McGibbon, E., Mulaudzi, F. M., Didham, P., et al. (2013). Toward decolonizing nursing: the colonization of nursing and strategies for increasing the counter-narrative. *Nursing Inquiry, 21*(3), 179–191. doi:10.1111/nin.12042.

McIntosh, K., Moniz, C., Craft, C. B., et al. (2014). Implementing school-wide positive behavioural interventions and supports to better meet the needs of Indigenous students. *Canadian Journal of School Psychology, 29*(3), 236–257.

McKenzie, H. A., Varcoe, C., Browne, A. J., et al. (2016). Disrupting the continuities among residential schools, the Sixties Scoop and child welfare: An analysis of colonial and neocolonial discourses. *International Indigenous Policy Journal, 7*(2), 1–24. doi:10.18584/iipj.2016.7.2.4.

Medved, M. I., Brockmeier, J., Morach, J., et al. (2013). Broken heart stories: Understanding Aboriginal women's cardiac problems. *Qualitative Health Research, 23*(12), doi:10.1177/1049732313509407.

Métis Nation of Alberta. (2017). *Definition of Métis.* Retrieved from http://albertametis.com/registry/registry/definition-of-metis/.

Métis Settlements General Council. (n.d.). *History in brief.* Retrieved from https://metissettlements.com/history/.

Ming, Y., Mandhane, P. J., & Senthilselvan, A. (2012). Association of breastfeeding with asthma in young Aboriginal children in Canada. *Canadian Respiratory Journal, 19*(6), 361–366. doi:10.1155/2012/402765.

Mohawks of the Bay of Quinte. (n.d.). *Culture: Two Row Wampum.* Retrieved from http://www.mbq-tmt.org/community/culture.

Moodley, R., & West, W. (Eds.), (2005). *Integrating traditional healing practices into counseling and psychotherapy.* Thousand Oaks, CA: Sage.

Moss, W., & Gardner-O'Toole, E. (1991). *Aboriginal people: History of discriminatory laws.* Retrieved from http://publications.gc.ca/Collection-R/LoPBdP/BP/bp175-e.htm.

Munson, J. (2016). *Dozens of bands join residential school day student lawsuit.* Retrieved from http://ipolitics.ca/2016/02/24/dozens-of-bands-join-residential-school-day-student-lawsuit/.

Murray, J. J. (2015). Revisioning science education in Canada: A new polar identity and purpose. *Canada Education, 55*(4).

Nabigon, H. C., & Wenger-Nabigon, A. (2012). 'Wise practices': Integrating traditional teachings with mainstream treatment approaches. *Native Social Work Journal: Indigenous Social Work Practices and theories, 8*, 43–55. Retrieved from https://zone.biblio.laurentian.ca/bitstream/10219/1981/1/NSWJournalV8_article2.pdf.

National Aboriginal Diabetes Association (NADA). (2016a). *History.* Retrieved from http://nada.ca/?page_id=287.

National Aboriginal Health Organization (NAHO). (2012). *Publications: Terminology.* Retrieved from http://www.naho.ca/publications/topics/terminology/.

Native Women's Association of Canada [NWAC]. (2010). *Fact sheet: Missing and murdered Aboriginal women and girls.* Retrieved from http://www.nwac.ca/wp-content/uploads/2015/05/Fact_Sheet_Missing_and_Murdered_Aboriginal_Women_and_Girls.pdf.

Nelson, S. (2012). *Challenging hidden assumptions: Colonial norms as determinants of Aboriginal mental health.* Prince George, BC: National Collaborating Centre for Aboriginal Health. Retrieved from http://www.nccah-ccnsa.ca/Publications/Lists/Publications/Attachments/70/colonial_norms_EN_web.pdf.

North American Indigenous Ministries. (2017). *About us.* Retrieved from: https://www.naim.ca/about/what-we-believe/.

Ontario Ministry of Education. (2017). *Indigenous education in Ontario.* Retrieved from http://www.edu.gov.on.ca/eng/aboriginal/supporting.html.

Ospina, M. B., Voaklander, D., Senthilselvan, A., et al. (2015). Incidence and prevalence of chronic obstructive pulmonary disease among Aboriginal peoples in Alberta, Canada. *PLoS ONE, 10*(4), doi:10.1371/journal.pone.0123204.

O'Toole, D. (2013). From entity, to identity to nation. In C. Adams, G. Dahl, & I. Peach (Eds.), *Métis in Canada: History, identity, law and politics* (pp. 143–203). Edmonton, AB: University of Alberta Press.

Pahwa, P., Abonyi, S., Karunanayake, C., et al. (2015). A community-based participatory research methodology to address, redress, and reassess disparities in respiratory health among First Nations. *BMC Research Notes, 8*, 199–210. doi:10.1186/s13104-015-1137-5.

Parkes, M. (2010). *Ecohealth and Aboriginal health: A review of common ground.* Retrieved from http://www.nccah-ccnsa.ca/docs/Ecohealth_Margot%20Parkes%202011%20-%20EN.pdf.

Parliament of Canada. (1992). 1st Session, 36th Parliament, 46-47-48 Elizabeth II, 1997-98-99. *The House of Commons of Canada Bill C-417 Louis Riel Act.* Retrieved from http://www.parl.gc.ca/HousePublications/Publication.aspx?DocId=2330320&Mode=1&Language=E&File=16.

Parmenter, J. (2013). The meaning of Kaswethan and the Two Row Wampum Belt in Haudenosaunee (Iroquois) history: Can Indigenous oral tradition be reconciled with the documentary record? *Journal of Early American History, 3*, 82–109. doi:10.1163/18770703-00301005.

Penny, C., O'Sullivan, E., & Senecal, S. (2012). *The Community Well-Being Index (CWB): Examining well-being in Inuit communities.* Unpublished report. Aboriginal Affairs and Northern Development Canada. Retrieved from http://assembly.nu.ca/library/Edocs/2012/000818-e.pdf.

Petrow, E. (2016). *A culture lost: Two stories of the Sixties Scoop.* Saskatoon Star Phoenix. Retrieved from http://thestarphoenix.com/news/saskatchewan/a-culture-lost-two-stories-from-the-sixties-scoop.

Province of Alberta (2015). *Metis Settlements Act. Revised Statutes of Alberta 2000 Chapter M-14.* Edmonton, AB: Alberta Queen's Printer. Retrieved from http://www.qp.alberta.ca/1266.cfm?page=m14.cfm&leg_type=Acts&isbncln=9780779786541.

Public Health Agency of Canada (PHAC) (2011). *Diabetes in Canada: Facts and figures from a public health perspective.* Ottawa: Author. Retrieved from http://www.phac-aspc.gc.ca/cd-mc/publications/diabetes-diabete/facts-figures-faits-chiffres-2011/pdf/facts-figures-faits-chiffres-eng.pdf.

Public Health Agency of Canada (PHAC). (2013a). *Aboriginal children: The healing power of cultural identity.* Retrieved from https://www.canada.ca/en/public-health/services/health-promotion/childhood-adolescence/programs-initiatives/aboriginal-head-start-urban-northern-communities-ahsunc/aboriginal-children-healing-power-cultural-identity.html.

Public Health Agency of Canada (PHAC). (2013b). *The Chief Public Health Officer's report on the state of public health in Canada, 2013 infectious disease—The never-ending threat.* Retrieved from https://www.canada.ca/en/public-health/corporate/publications/chief-public-health-officer-reports-state-public-health-canada/chief-public-health-officer-report-on-state-public-health-canada-2013-infectious-disease-never-ending-threat.html.

Public Health Agency of Canada (PHAC) (2014). *HIV/AIDS Epi updates. Chapter 8: HIV/AIDS among Aboriginal people in Canada.* Ottawa: Author. Retrieved from http://www.phac-aspc.gc.ca/aids-sida/publication/epi/2010/pdf/ch8-eng.pdf.

Public Safety and Emergency Preparedness Canada. (2006). *A matter of faith: A gathering of Aboriginal Christians, APC 24 CA. (Cat. No.: PS4-32/2006E.)* Retrieved from https://www.publicsafety.gc.ca/cnt/rsrcs/pblctns/mttr-fth-2006/mttr-fth-2006-eng.pdf.

Pulver, L. J., Haswell, M. R., Ring, I., et al. (2010). *Indigenous Health – Australia, Canada, Aotearoa, New Zealand and the United States—Laying claim to a future that embraces health for us all. World Health Report Background Paper 33.* Geneva: World Health Organization. Retrieved from http://www.who.int/healthsystems/topics/financing/healthreport/IHNo33.pdf.

Reith, T., & Stewart, B. (2015). *Canada's residential school story to be taught in schools this fall.* CBC News. Retrieved from http://www.cbc.ca/news/canada/edmonton/canada-s-residential-school-story-to-be-taught-in-classrooms-this-fall-1.3216399.

Reutter, L., & Kushner, K. (2010). "Health equity through action on the social determinants of health": Taking up the challenge in nursing. *Nursing Inquiry, 17*(3), 269–280. doi:10.111/j.1440-1800.2010.00500.x.

Rice, K., Te Hiwi, B., Zwarenstein, M., et al. (2016). Best practices for the prevention and management of diabetes and obesity-related chronic disease among Indigenous peoples in Canada: A review. *Canadian Journal of Diabetes, 40*(3), 216–225. doi:10.106/j.jcjd.2015.10.007.

Richmond, C. (2015). The relatedness of people, land and health. In M. Greenwood, S. De Leeuw, N. M. Lindsay, et al. (Eds.), *Determinants of Indigenous peoples' health in Canada* (pp. 47–63). Toronto: Canadian Scholars Press Inc.

Robinson, A. (2016). *Gradual Civilization Act.* Retrieved from http://www.thecanadianencyclopedia.ca/en/article/gradual-civilization-act/.

Roy, A. (2014). Aboriginal worldviews and epidemiological surveys: Overcoming incongruence. *International Journal of Multiple Research Approaches, 8*(1), 117–128.

Royal Canadian Mounted Police (RCMP). (2015). *Missing and murdered Aboriginal women: 2015 update to the national operational overview.* Retrieved from http://www.rcmp-grc.gc.ca/en/missing-and-murdered-aboriginal-women-2015-update-national-operational-overview.

Sanchez-Ramirez, D. C., Colquhoun, A., Parker, S., et al. (2016). Cancer incidence and mortality among the Métis population of Alberta, Canada. *International Journal of Circumpolar Health, 75*, doi:10.3402/ijch.v75.30059.

Sefidbakht, S., Johnson-Down, L., Young, T. K., et al. (2015). High protein and cholesterol intakes associated with emergence of glucose intolerance in a low-risk Canadian Inuit population. *Public Health Nutrition, 19*(10), 1804–1811. doi:10.1017/S1368980015003080.

Senthilselvan, A., Selvanayagam, J. N., King, M., et al. (2015). Prevalence and risk factors of asthma in First Nations children living on reserves in Canada. *Journal of Public Health, 106*(8), e483–e488. doi:10.17269/CJPH.106.5147.

Sinclair, R. (2007). Identity lost and found: Lessons from the Sixties Scoop. *First Peoples Family and Child Review, 3*(1), 65–82.

Sinha, V., Trocmé, N., Fallon, B., et al. (2011). *Kiskisik awasisak: Remember the children. Understanding the overrepresentation of First Nations children in the child welfare system.* Ottawa, ON: Assembly of First Nations. Retrieved from http://cwrp.ca/sites/default/files/publications/en/FNCIS-2008_March2012_RevisedFinal.pdf.

Smith, D., Edwards, N., Varcoe, C., et al. (2006). Bringing safety and responsiveness into the forefront of care for pregnant and parenting aboriginal people. *ANS. Advances in Nursing Science, 29*, E27–E44.

Statistics Canada (2013a). *Aboriginal peoples in Canada: First Nations people, Métis and Inuit. National Household Survey, 2011 (Catalogue no. 99-011-X2011001).* Ottawa: Author. Retrieved from http://www12.statcan.gc.ca/nhs-enm/2011/as-sa/99-011-x/99-011-x2011001-eng.pdf.

Statistics Canada (2013b). *Measuring violence against women: Statistical trends (Catalogue No. 85-002-x Juristat.).* Ottawa: Author. Retrieved from http://www.statcan.gc.ca/pub/85-002-x/2013001/article/11766-eng.pdf.

Statistics Canada (2015). *Aboriginal languages in Canada.* Ottawa, ON: Author. Retrieved from https://www12.statcan.gc.ca/census-recensement/2011/as-sa/98-314-x/98-314-x2011003_3-eng.cfm.

Steinhauer, D., & Lamouche, J. (2015). Miyo-pimatisiwin "A good path": Indigenous knowledges, languages, and traditions in education and health. In M. Greenwood, S. De Leeuw, N. M. Lindsay, et al. (Eds.), *Determinants of Indigenous peoples' health in Canada* (pp. 16–24). Toronto: Canadian Scholars Press Inc.

St. Germain, G., & Dyck, L. E. (2010). *First Nations elections: The choice is inherently theirs. Report of the Standing Senate Committee on Aboriginal Peoples.* Retrieved from http://www.parl.gc.ca/Content/SEN/Committee/403/abor/rep/rep03may10-e.pdf.

Supreme Court of Canada. (2016). *Daniels v. Canada (Indian Affairs and Northern Development).* Retrieved from https://scc-csc.lexum.com/scc-csc/scc-csc/en/item/15858/index.do.

Tagalik, S. (2015). Inuit knowledge systems, Elders and determinants of health. In M. Greenwood, S. De Leeuw, N. M. Lindsay, et al. (Eds.), *Determinants of Indigenous peoples' health in Canada* (pp. 25–32). Toronto: Canadian Scholars Press Inc.

Tasker, J. P. (2016). *Confusion reigns over number of missing and murdered Indigenous women.* CBC News. Retrieved from http://www.cbc.ca/news/politics/mmiw-4000-hajdu-1.3450237.

Thunderbird Partnership Foundation. (2017). *Madeleine Dion Stout.* Retrieved from http://nnapf.com/events/hos2014-national-conference/madeleine-dion-stout-2/.

Thurston, W. E., Coupal, S., Jones, C. A., et al. (2014). Discordant indigenous and provider frames explain challenges in improving access to arthritis care: A qualitative study using constructivist grounded theory. *International Journal for Equity in Health, 13*(1), 1–19. doi:10.1186/1475-9276-13-46.

Tobe, S. W., Maar, M., Roy, M. A., et al. (2015). Preventing cardiovascular and renal disease in Canada's Aboriginal populations. *Canadian Journal of Cardiology, 31*(9), 1124–1149. doi:10.1016/j.cjca.2015.05.024.

Todd, D. (2016). Canadian Aboriginals joining Christian clergy despite residential-school legacy. *Vancouver Sun.* Retrieved from http://www.vancouversun.com/life/douglas+todd+canadian+aboriginals+joining+christian+clergy+despite+residential+school+legacy/11700642/story.html.

Truth and Reconciliation Commission of Canada (2015a). *Canada's residential schools: The history, Part 1 Origins to 1939. The final report of the Truth and Reconciliation Commission of Canada* (Vol. 1). Montreal, Canada: McGill-Queen's University Press.

Truth and Reconciliation Commission of Canada. (2015b). *Honouring the truth, reconciling for the future. Summary of the final report of the Truth and Reconciliation Commission of Canada.* Retrieved from http://nctr.ca/assets/reports/Final%20Reports/Executive_Summary_English_Web.pdf.

Truth and Reconciliation Commission of Canada (2015c). *Canada's residential schools: The legacy. The final report of the Truth and Reconciliation Commission of Canada* (Vol. 5). Montreal & Kingston, Canada: McGill Queen's University Press. Retrieved from http://nctr.ca/assets/reports/Final%20Reports/Volume_5_Legacy_English_Web.pdf.

Truth and Reconciliation Commission of Canada (2015d). *Canada's residential schools: The history, Part 2 1939-2000* (Vol. 1). Montreal, Canada: McGill-Queen's University Press.

Truth and Reconciliation Commission of Canada. (2016a). *Canada's residential schools: Missing children and unmarked burials. The final report of the Truth and Reconciliation Commission of Canada, Volume 4.* Retrieved from http://nctr.ca/assets/reports/Final%20Reports/Volume_4_Missing_Children_English_Web.pdf.

Turin, T. C., Saad, N., Jun, M., et al. (2016). Lifetime risk of diabetes among First Nations people and non-First Nations people. *Canadian Medical Association Journal, 188*(16), 1147–1153. doi:10.1503/cmaj.150787.

UNAIDS. (2006). *Report on the global AIDS epidemic: Executive summary. A UNAIDS 10th anniversary special edition.* Retrieved from http://data.unaids.org/pub/GlobalReport/2006/2006_GR-ExecutiveSummary_en.pdf.

United Nations. (2009). *State of the world's indigenous peoples (Volume 1).* Retrieved from http://www.un.org/esa/socdev/unpfii/documents/SOWIP/en/SOWIP_web.pdf.

United Nations. (2015). *State of the world's indigenous peoples (Volume 2): Indigenous Peoples' access to health services.* Retrieved from http://www.un.org/esa/socdev/unpfii/documents/2015/sowip2volume-ac.pdf.

Vancouver Native Pentecostal Church. (n.d.). *About us.* Retrieved from http://www.vnpc.ca/about.html.

Wakewich, P., Wood, B., Davey, C., et al. & on behalf of the ACCSS Group. (2016). Colonial legacy and the experience of First Nations women in cervical cancer screening: A Canadian multi-community study. *Critical Public Health, 26*(4), 368–380. doi:10.1080/09581596.2015.1067671.

Waldram, J. B., Herring, A., & Young, T. K. (2006). *Aboriginal health in Canada: Historical, cultural, and epidemiological perspectives* (2nd ed.). Toronto: University of Toronto Press.

Wenger-Nabigon, A. (2010). The Cree medicine wheel as an organizing paradigm of theories of human development. *Native Social Work Journal: Indigenous Social Work Practices and Theories, 7*, 139–161. Retrieved from https://zone.biblio.laurentian.ca/bitstream/10219/387/1/NSWJ-V7-art6-p139-161.pdf.

Wexler, L., White, J., & Trainor, B. (2015). Why an alternative to suicide prevention gatekeeper training is needed for rural Indigenous communities: Presenting an empowering community storytelling approach. *Critical Public Health, 25*(2), 205–217. doi:10.1080/09581596.2014.904039.

Wiebe, A., Barton, S., Auger, L., et al. (2015). Restoring the blessings of the morning star: childbirth and maternal-infant health for women from First Nations near Edmonton, Alberta. *Aboriginal Policy Studies, 5*(1), 47–68. doi:10.5663/apsv5i123823.

Withrow, D. R., Pole, J. D., Nishri, E. D., et al. (2017). Cancer survival disparities between First Nation and non-aboriginal adults in Canada: Follow-up of the 1991 Census Mortality Cohort. *Cancer Epidemiology, Biomarkers & Prevention, 26*(1), 145–151. doi:10.1158/1055-9965.EPI-16-0706.

Wright, A. (2015). Role of the nurse in returning birth to the north. *Rural and Remote Health, 15*(3109), 1–6.

Zeidler, D. (2011). Building a relationship: Perspectives from one First Nations community. *Canadian Journal of Speech-Language Pathology and Audiology, 35*(2), 136–143.

11

Nursing Leadership, Management, and Collaborative Practice

Written by Susan M. Duncan, RN, PhD

OBJECTIVES

Mastery of content in this chapter will enable you to:

- Define the key terms listed.
- Describe entry-level professional nurse competencies related to leadership, management, and collaborative practice.
- Describe the relationships between nursing leadership and healthy practice environments, patient safety, and quality patient care outcomes.
- Describe theories of leadership and how they are evolving.
- Discuss how a nurse leader can contribute to collaborative practice and best practices implementation.
- Describe levels of management.
- Discuss ways to apply skills of clinical care coordination in nursing practice.
- Discuss principles for the appropriate delegation of patient care activities.
- Describe the purpose, elements, and models for quality practice environments and patient safety.
- Identify strategies for developing entry-level competencies related to management and leadership in nursing.

KEY TERMS

MEDIA RESOURCES

http://evolve.elsevier.com/Canada/Potter/fundamentals/

- Audio Chapter Summaries
- Examination Review Questions
- Concept Map Creator
- Case Study with Questions
- Audio Glossary
- Content Updates
- Video Clips

In this chapter, you will explore what it means to be a nurse leader in Canada and the world today. Nurses provide leadership for quality patient care and in promoting health in many roles and settings—from the point of care to organizational positions, including government. Nurses also enact leadership by engaging with the profession through its organizations, leading the future of nursing as it stands on the cusp of societal change (Whyte & Duncan, 2016). The Canadian Nursing Students' Association plays a leadership role by taking an informed stand on many issues shaping nursing education and practice today. Trends in nursing practice and health care set the dynamic context of leadership today—shifting scopes of practice, collaborative models of care, emerging roles in community health and primary care, medical assistance in dying (MAID) (see Chapters 7 and 8 for more information about MAID), increasing use of technology in care and information, and the Truth and Reconciliation Commission of Canada (2015) calls to action. In contemplating these trends, it is important to consider how you will learn about and influence these trends in ways that promote health.

The Canadian Association of Schools of Nursing (CASN) *National Nursing Education Framework* (CASN, 2015) identifies leadership as an essential component of baccalaureate education that prepares the student to coordinate nursing care and influence and advocate for change in nursing and health programs for health equity and social justice. As a nursing student, you will have opportunities to develop insights and awareness for change and influence that will lead to more just and equitable nursing programs and health outcomes. Nursing students have opportunities to provide leadership for practice and within their educational settings by bringing their vision and values for changes that are needed. See Box 11-1 for a case study that demonstrates how nursing students are making a difference in how a school

BOX 11-1 CASE STUDY

Nursing Students Leading the Way to Truth and Reconciliation in a University Setting

Students at Thompson Rivers University School of Nursing joined with their faculty members to form the Indigenous Health and Nursing Committee with the goal of leading the way to enacting the recommendations of the Truth and Reconciliation Commission of Canada (TRC) calls to action (TRC, 2015). The students from all years of their undergraduate program voluntarily joined the committee to provide leadership among students and across the university to begin the journey of reconciliation. The Commission (TRC, 2015) called for nursing education programs to graduate nurses with a deep awareness of "Aboriginal rights and Indigenous teachings, inter-cultural competencies, conflict resolution, human rights, and anti-racism" (p. 3). The students recognized that, as agents of change, they had the opportunity to promote awareness of the meaning and opportunities for meaningful reconciliation, and for culturally safe nursing practice, and health care delivery with Indigenous peoples. Students initiated activities such as workshops for understanding the colonial past and its impact on the health of Indigenous communities, surveyed the student body about their understandings of culturally safe practice, and made recommendations to the School of Nursing Council for curriculum change. They were also involved in community consultations to develop an Indigenous health and nursing elective.

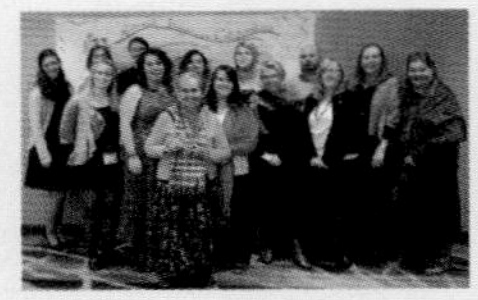
(Courtesy Star Mahara, RN, MN)

Subsequently, they attended and presented their experience of change and recommendations for the future at the 2015 national conference of the Aboriginal Nurses of Canada (now Canadian Indigenous Nurses Association [CINA]). Through their leadership, these students recognized the importance of collaborating with others, advocating for a vision of culturally safe practice, and engaging students in the process of enacting a vision of reconciliation and social justice. These students were developing essential leadership competencies in promoting change for social justice and optimal health.

BOX 11-2 Selected Entry-Level Staff Nurse Competencies Related to Leadership and Management

- Is accountable and accepts responsibility for own actions and decisions, and professional conduct
- Articulates the role and responsibilities of a registered nurse as a member of the nursing and health care team
- Demonstrates leadership in providing patient care by promoting healthy and culturally safe practice environments
- Displays initiative, a beginning confidence, and self-awareness in collaborative interactions within the health care team
- Organizes own workload and develops time-management skills for meeting responsibilities
- Supports the integration of quality improvement initiatives in nursing practice
- Demonstrates leadership in the coordination of care by
  - assigning client care;
  - delegating nursing activities to selected health care team members while ensuring that the delegated nursing activities are safely and competently performed; and
  - facilitating continuity of care
- Uses resources under one's control in a fiscally responsible manner to provide safe, appropriate, and ethical care
- Advocates for and supports healthy public policy and principles of social justice
- Engages in relational practice and uses ethical principles with the health care team to maximize collaborative client care

Adapted from College of Registered Nurses of British Columbia. (2015). *Competencies in the context of entry-level registered nurse practice in British Columbia. Leadership and management practices for healthy work environments.* Vancouver: Author. Retrieved from https://www.crnbc.ca/Registration/Lists/RegistrationResources/375CompetenciesEntrylevelRN.pdf.

of nursing and university take up the Truth and Reconciliation Commission's calls to action (2015).

You will develop your knowledge and practice of leadership and management roles in nursing early in your educational program, including relational aspects of addressing constant change in life and work environments and addressing conflict situations as opportunities for growth. As you develop the knowledge and skills to enter the nursing workforce, you will also learn how to become a leader among colleagues at the point of care in many health care settings. Phrases such as "from the bedside to the boardroom" (Institute of Medicine [IOM], 2011) and "leadership in every moment of practice" (Doane & Varcoe, 2015, p. 421) indicate the centrality of leadership in all nursing practice settings and roles.

From the list of competencies required of entry-level nurses in Box 11-2 it is apparent that leadership begins with a strong professional identity and accountability and is rooted in relational and ethical practice. For optimal nursing care, managers and leaders are needed to ensure both the vision for quality care and the management skills required for best practices and quality care (Hibberd, Smith, & Wylie, 2006). Whereas *leadership* refers to a shared vision, values, organizational strategy, and relationships, *management* most often refers to the competencies required to ensure the day-to-day delivery of nursing care according to available resources and standards of professional practice. To be effective in promoting a healthy work environment and a healthy society, nurses must demonstrate leadership practices that honour the importance of relationships, values, and ethics and in understanding better how we think about health and health systems (Doane & Varcoe, 2015; IOM, 2011; Wong, 2015). Nursing leadership is needed at every level, and nurses must be full partners in changing health systems with physicians and other providers and sectors of society (IOM, 2011). Figure 11-1 provides a conceptual model of leadership that has been identified as contributing to health outcomes.

In the current context of health care, in which qualified care providers are in short supply, competencies associated with leadership in nursing relate to creating environments for healthy working relationships and teamwork. A healthy work environment is most likely to retain nurses in practice settings in which they are both satisfied and able to provide high-quality care. Researchers note that transformational and relational models of leadership best contribute to healthy work environments for nurses, including nurse retention and recruitment needed for quality patient care (Cummings, MacGregor, Davey, et al., 2010; Wong & Laschinger, 2013). At the staff and patient level, this translates, for instance, into registered nurses working collaboratively with other members of the nursing team, as well as with providers from other disciplines and with patients and families.

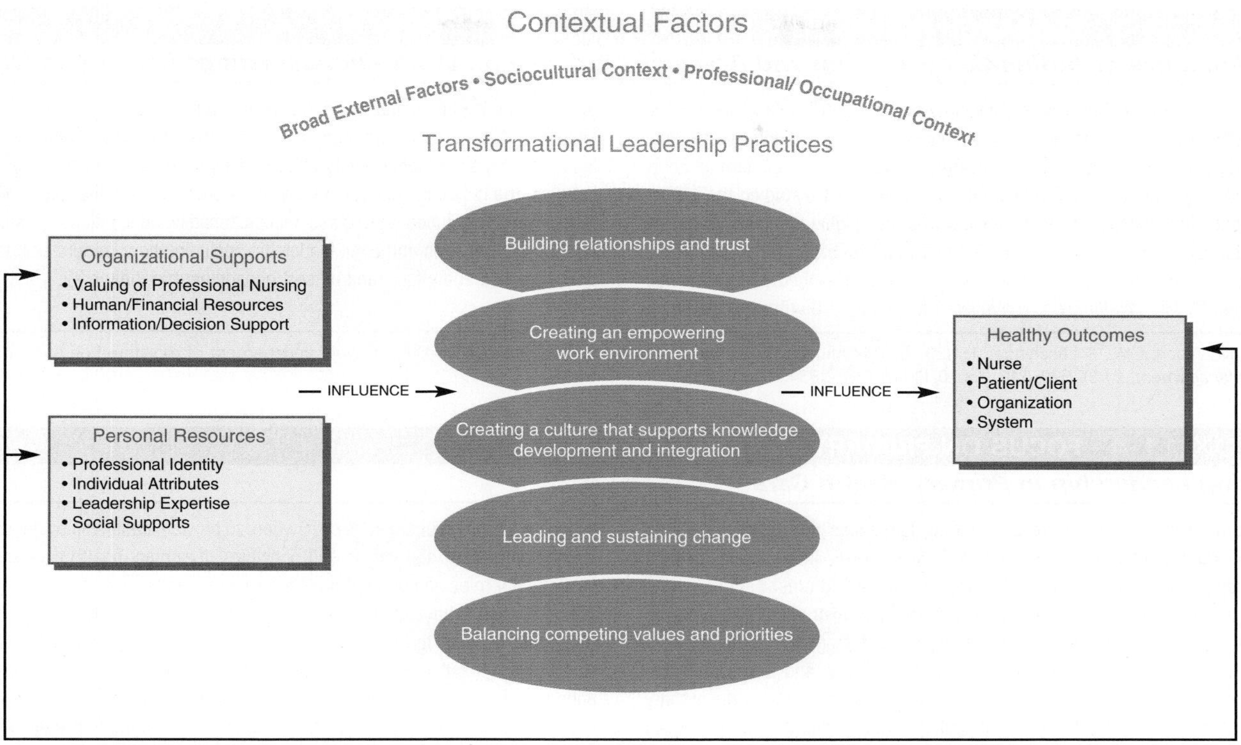

FIGURE 11-1 Conceptual model for developing and sustaining leadership. This model organizes and guides the discussion of the Registered Nurses' Association of Ontario (RNAO) recommendations. It provides a framework for understanding the leadership practices needed to achieve healthy work environments and the organizational supports and personal resources that enable effective leadership practices. (From Registered Nurses' Association of Ontario. [2013]. *The healthy work environments quick reference guide for nurses* [p. 23]. Toronto: Author.)

The importance of such work is most often discussed as collaborative practice, defined as working together toward mutually identified goals while valuing different perspectives and accountabilities of individual team members (Health Professions Network Nursing and Midwifery Office, 2010). This chapter therefore focuses on current thinking on nursing leadership and management, including definitions, roles and relationships, shifts to collaborative practice models, and the role of leaders in ensuring healthy practice environments and relational practice (Doane & Varcoe, 2015). The ideas and examples included in this chapter apply to the different practice settings in which nurses work: in homes, in institutions, and in communities.

LEADERSHIP THEORIES

Nurses draw on multiple views and theories of leadership that come from a variety of disciplines, including sociology, psychology, and management science. There is also an emerging body of research in nursing leadership and management that illuminates critical issues for nursing and nurses (Cummings et al., 2010; Wong, Cummings, & Ducharme, 2013). Theoretical perspectives on leadership inform how a nurse enacts leadership and defines her or his leadership style. Students may become familiar with one or more leadership theories and reflect on how these theories resonate with their own values and aspirations to make a difference through leadership.

One theory that has resonated with nurses is transformational leadership, which emphasizes how a leader with vision and values can inspire others in a given direction (Kouzes & Posner, 2017). Closely related to transformational theory is the idea of emotional intelligence of leaders who "lead with their heart" and engage in self-reflection and supportive and collaborative relationships while sharing power with those in their organization (Smith, Profetto-McGrath, & Cummings, 2009). Another theoretical perspective draws on the notion of servant leadership, in which leaders are motivated to serve others through their leadership while sharing their power with those at all levels of the organization (Greenleaf, 1977). Building on the ideas of sharing power and serving others through leadership, emergent theories of appreciative inquiry (Knibbs, Underwood, MacDonald, et al., 2010) and strengths-based leadership (Gottlieb, Gottlieb, & Shamian, 2012) describe how relational leaders can inspire others by building on what is working well and on the strengths and identities of nurses instead of focusing on issues and problems. Nursing and health care theorist Tim Porter-O'Grady is a noted author and speaker on the topic of "quantum leadership," which extends thinking about leadership into the dynamic context of the twenty-first century. Porter-O'Grady and Malloch (2015) describe the leadership styles and traits needed to transform nursing and health care in a society that is moving from the industrial age to the digital age of technology and knowledge-based economies. Leading change in this era will require leaders to develop competencies that are closely aligned with the relational and ethical values of nursing, as well as the ability to think at a systems level, inspire innovation, and collaborate for shared power.

In contemplating the impact of various leadership perspectives on nurses and patients in health care organizations, it is also important to consider where leadership is needed. Typically, organizations have senior leaders at the board of governors and executive levels of

BOX 11-3 RESEARCH HIGHLIGHT

The Influence of Authentic Leadership and Areas of Work Life on Work Engagement of Registered Nurses

Canadian nurse researchers are studying how leadership perspectives and styles contribute to nurses' experiences of engagement in their work, healthy and satisfying work environments, and ultimately high-quality patient care and outcomes. Researchers Bamford, Wong, and Laschinger (2013) studied the impact of authentic leadership, defined as leaders who are "highly reflective, transparent and instill trust and respect in their employees" (p. 530). "Relational transparency ... the presentation of one's genuine self" is embodied in authentic leadership (Avolio, Walumbwa, & Weber, 2009, cited in Bamford et al., 2013, p. 530). Drawing on an analysis of a survey of 600 nurses working in acute care hospitals, these researchers found that managers who demonstrated authentic leadership inspired higher levels of engagement and a stronger overall match between the nurse and his or her work in six areas of work life (Bamford et al., 2013). They concluded that nurse researchers should continue to study the relationship between authentic leadership, including how leaders embody relational practice and ethics, and nurses' engagement in their work.

Bamford, M, Wong, C.A., & Laschinger, H. (2013). The influence of authentic leadership and areas of worklife on work engagement of registered nurses. *Journal of Nursing Management, 21*(3), 529–540. doi:10.1111/j.1365-2834.2012.01399.x

BOX 11-4 FOCUS ON PRIMARY HEALTH CARE

Nursing Leadership in Primary Health Care

Nursing as a profession has taken a strong leadership role in implementing primary health care throughout the world. Since 1978, International Council of Nurses (ICN), Canadian Nurses Association (CNA), and other national, provincial, and territorial nursing associations have been instrumental in lobbying for inclusion of primary health care principles and programs in health care professional education, in service planning and delivery, and in research and evaluation. CNA (2009b) actively promotes initiatives to incorporate primary health care into nursing practice and policy. Primary health care principles enshrined in policy is the way to promote health for all people and is based on a social justice model and related values (Reutter & Ogilvie, 2011). Nursing advocacy for primary health care as the foundation of health care is required of leaders at all levels of practice and organizations (ICN, 2008; Reutter & Kushner, 2010).

There is reason to believe that nurses must play an even larger role in primary health care in the future (National Expert Commission, 2012; World Health Organization [WHO], 2008), to provide leadership necessary for transformational change in health systems worldwide. The WHO (2008) calls for a greater emphasis on primary health care to reform health systems worldwide, a process of change that will require nurses everywhere to provide leadership by demonstrating commitment to the values and principles of primary health care and envisioning new roles and opportunities to promote health.

If nurses are to have the influence that is needed to transform health systems, they must develop the vision, knowledge, and skills for primary health care. Nurses learn to influence systems through their work in organizations and, most importantly, by working collectively in nursing and other types of associations. Nursing associations have a pivotal role to play in ensuring that their voice and influence is expressed and represented as the largest group of health professionals worldwide:

> *The ICN and its member national nurses associations (NNAs) promote and support all efforts to improve the preparation of nurses for management, leadership and policy development. The preparation should be broad and must include the development of knowledge and skills for influencing change, engaging in the political process, social marketing, forming coalitions, working with the media and other means of exerting influence.*
>
> ***(ICN, 2008)***

organizations, mid-organizational-level leaders such as program and clinical managers, and leaders who are at the point of care. Recent analyses of nursing systems indicate that nurses are needed at all organizational levels, and more attention needs to be paid to leadership that inspires and supports nurses and nursing at the point of care. Therefore, nurses who are in formal leadership positions, such as at executive and managerial levels, must provide resources to develop leadership for practice at the point of care (Duncan, Rodney, & Thorne, 2014). The impact of leadership on nursing and patient outcomes at the point of care is a research priority in nursing (Box 11-3).

MANAGEMENT AND LEADERSHIP ROLES FOR NURSES

Nurses assume a wide variety of management and leadership roles in health care organizations with the aim of ensuring that patients receive safe and high-quality care. Research has shown that nurses must provide leadership to ensure that nursing care takes place in quality practice environments (Aiken, 2008; Aiken, Sloane, Bruyneel, et al., 2014; Health Canada, 2002) and that these work environments are essential for health, high-quality patient care, and patient safety (Aiken et al., 2014; Duncan et al., 2014; Estabrooks, Midodzi, Cummings, et al., 2005; Wong et al., 2013). A high-quality practice environment is also a healthy work environment, defined as "where nurses respect and are involved in decision-making" (Canadian Nurses Association [CNA] & Canadian Federation of Nursing Unions [CFNU], 2015, p. 1).

A **healthy practice environment** begins with the senior nurse leader in the organization, who most often holds the title of Chief Nurse Executive, Chief Nursing Officer, or Director or Vice-President of Nursing or of Patient Care (Health Canada, 2002). In 1999, the government of Canada instituted the first Office of Nursing Policy with Dr. Judith Shamian, RN, Executive Director, hired to provide leadership to ensure that attention was paid in government to the nursing perspective on programs and policies (Health Canada, 2009). These positions are key to ensuring that nurses influence the policy directions that governments take to provide high-quality nursing services for Canadians. In policy roles, nurses act as policy advocates and, as such, have made a difference throughout history; they continue to advocate for progressive public policy in primary health care and to achieve health equity (Reutter & Kushner, 2010) (see Chapter 1). As a student, you will learn the skills involved in nursing advocacy and assume the role of advocate to promote the health of people. Nurses today "stand on the shoulders of giants"; the nurse leaders of the past held a powerful vision for the development of nursing as a profession and advocated tirelessly to bring this vision to fruition ("A century of progress," 2005) (Box 11-4). An example of a Canadian nurse leader is Dr. Judith Shamian (Box 11-5).

Nursing Care Delivery Models, Collaborative Practice, and Nursing Teams

As in the past, a strong nurse leader at the senior level of the organization unites the strategic direction of the organization with the values and goals of nursing. Nurse executives must also build teams of leaders who work across the organization to implement best practices and develop high-quality work environments in which nursing practice can flourish. Although it takes a strong senior nursing leader to inspire a healthy work environment, the role and responsibility of every nurse is to provide leadership to make a difference by displaying attributes such as articulating a vision, enabling others to act, encouraging others, and taking initiative (CNA, 2009a). The leader and nursing staff must share a philosophy of care that integrates purpose, best practices, and concern for relationships, including how staff will work together and with patients and families (Box 11-6).

Integral to the philosophy of care is the selection of a nursing care delivery model and a management structure that support professional nursing practice. A *nursing care delivery model* is a system for organizing and delivering nursing care to patients and their families, and it represents structural and contextual elements of nursing practice (Fowler, Hardy, & Howarth, 2006, cited in CNA, Canadian Council for Practical Nurse Regulators, & Registered Psychiatric Nurses of Canada, 2012). Key factors contributing to success are strong nursing leadership, decision-making authority for nurses who provide direct care, and effective respectful communications with colleagues, physicians, and other health care providers (Health Canada, 2002; Canadian Patient Safety Institute, 2009).

Nursing care delivery models are designs that determine how nurses provide care. The choice of a nursing care delivery model is influenced by patient, provider, and organizational factors (Harris & McGillis Hall, 2012). Continuity of care is an extremely important concept in determining the choice of a nursing care delivery model. **Continuity of care** is defined as "a seamless continuous implementation of a plan of care that is reviewed and revised to meet the changing needs of the client" (Registered Nurses' Association of Ontario [RNAO], 2010, p. 61)—whether the client is a person, family, or population. It refers to continuity of information or knowledge, continuity of relationships between a patient and one or more health care providers over time, and continuity of management of care across organizational boundaries (Smith, Smith, Boechler, et al., 2006). In the choice of nursing care delivery models, it is important to consider how nurses ensure that a patient's plan of care is as consistent as possible. For instance, evidence shows that the presence and knowledge of the registered nurse is a key factor in determining quality patient care outcomes (Aiken et al, 2014; Wong, 2015). As change occurs in health care delivery and nursing practice, new care delivery models are evolving. In the current context, a patient care model known as the *collaborative practice model* is emerging. This model depends on strong professional identities and working relationships between nurses at all levels and with patients, other health care providers, and community members.

Nursing care delivery models of today entail higher staff ratios of unregulated care providers (UCPs) in many settings of practice,

BOX 11-5 Canadian Nurse Leader: Judith Shamian, President of the International Council of Nurses (2013–2017)

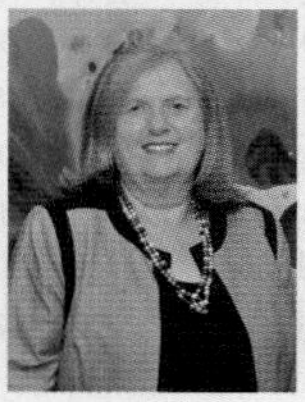

One dimension of nursing leadership is to engage politically and advocate for nursing and health in organizational and political arenas. Dr. Judith Shamian is a Canadian nurse who brings the political and global dimensions of nurse leadership to life. She is only the second Canadian nurse to be elected as president of International Council of Nurses (ICN). Upon her election in 2013, to serve a 4-year term, Dr. Shamian chose the word "impact" to guide her vision and mission during her term as president, citing how she sees the "power of nursing and the impact nurses have on the health of the global population" (ICN, 2013). As an international leader, she works to bring the voice of nurses and nursing to the most pressing health issues of our time. When asked in a recent interview about her goals, she responded that she wanted to "elevate the value of nursing on the world stage and in particular—engage nurses to assume influential positions in global organizations and politics" (Nagle, 2014, p. 30).

International Council of Nurses (ICN). (2013). Judith Shamian elected as new ICN President [International Perspectives], *International Nursing Review,* 60(1), 283-290. doi: 10.111/inr.12053.

BOX 11-6 Developing a Vision for a Nursing Unit or Program

What Is the Nursing Unit's Purpose or Mission?
- Articulating why it exists
- Ensuring that nursing services are based on primary health care principles
- Knowing the background of health needs and perspectives of patients and population (internal and external)
- Knowing the background of its collaborative team members: their professional preparation, identity, and unique contributions
- Demonstrating how it accomplishes organizational goals or vision

How Will Staff Work With Patients and Families?
- By placing a patient's and family's needs first with a patient-focused approach
- By involving patients and families as members of a collaborative practice team
- By making effective communication a priority

What Are the Standards of the Work Unit?
- Staff members adhere to professional accountability practice according to standards of practice and codes of ethics
- Staff members practise within a culture of safety
- The work unit integrates evidence-informed best practices
- Staff members work collaboratively with all members of the health care team

What Are the Key Values?
- Creating and maintaining a healthy practice environment
- Enacting the principles of primary health care
- Recognizing social justice issues
- Providing culturally safe care and responding to the Truth and Reconciliation Commission (TRC) calls to action
- Supporting relational practice and the upholding of the CNA *Code of Ethics*
- Being self-aware, motivated, and accountable
- Supporting a learning environment

including home care, institutional acute care, and residential long-term care. The title of the UCP typifies the role of providing front-line personal and delegated care to increasing numbers of patients across different health care settings in Canada. UCP practice is not defined by qualifications or established standards. The title of the role differs from province to province, as does its requirement for training or educational programs. In British Columbia, for example, UCPs are referred to as *health care assistants* (HCAs), and they are required to take a preparatory 6- to 8-month certification program offered in public and private postsecondary educational institutions.

Traditional Models of Care

Terms that describe **models of care** that have been present over the past century include *functional nursing*, *team nursing*, and *primary care*. These models have existed primarily in institutional settings, and elements of them may be seen in practice today. Functional nursing became popular during World War II in response to a nursing shortage, where nurses focused on tasks instead of assuming responsibilities for a group of patients. The disadvantages of functional nursing are problems with continuity of care, absence of a holistic view of patients, and the possibility that care will become mechanical and fragmented (Sportsman & MacMillan, 2015). Despite the critique of functional nursing, aspects of this model are still in practice today—for example, when a nurse assumes sole responsibility for all patient medications in a long-term care setting.

Team nursing developed in response to the nursing shortage after World War II (Sportsman & MacMillan, 2015). It involves the coordinated delivery of nursing care by various staff members. A registered nurse (RN) leads a team of other RNs, registered psychiatric nurses (RPNs), licensed practical nurses (LPNs), UCPs, or a combination of these professionals. The task orientation of the model in the past and the fact that nurses do not always interact with the same patients each day can result in a lack of continuity of care. An advantage of team nursing is the collaborative style that encourages each member of the team to help the other members. Elements of this former team nursing model may be present in emerging models of collaborative practice with the evolution to more patient care focused on participatory relationships with other members of the intraprofessional nursing team.

The **primary nursing** model aimed to place RNs at patients' bedsides and improve nursing accountability for patient outcomes and relationships among staff (Sportsman & MacMillan, 2015). Primary nursing supports a philosophy of strong nurse–patient relationships. Primary nursing maintains continuity of care across shifts, days, or visits. It can be applied in any health care setting. When a primary nurse is off duty, other team members, including RPNs, LPNs, or other RNs, follow the care plan. If differences in opinion occur, associate and primary nurses collaborate to redefine the plan as necessary. The strengths of this model may also be realized in new models of care that extend primary care models to fit the current health care delivery system and emphasize collaborative relationships, evidence-informed practice, and continuity of care (Jost, Bonnell, Chacko, et al., 2010; LeClerc, Doyon, Gravelle, et al., 2008).

The **case management** model is one that emphasizes the coordination of an array of health services and links them to patients and their families while streamlining costs and maintaining quality (Dadich, 2003). The term *case manager* has been criticized because patients and families are not "cases" to be managed (Smith et al., 2006). Case management, as it has evolved, is "a collaborative process which assesses, plans, implements, coordinates, monitors, and evaluates the options and services required to meet an individual's health needs, using communications and available resources to promote quality, cost-effective outcomes" (Case Management Society of America, 2016). Clinicians, as individuals or in teams, care for patients with specific conditions and associated care needs (e.g., patients with complex nursing and medical problems) and are usually held accountable for quality and cost management. Many case managers use critical pathways, or "care maps," which are multidisciplinary treatment plans for patients with specific case types (see Chapter 13). The plans help in the delivery of timely, coordinated care.

Roles of case managers vary across health care settings, including long-term care, home care, community mental health, and acute care institutions, and these professionals increasingly coordinate and integrate care across settings. Roles and responsibilities of case managers across settings include clinical expert, advocate, educator, facilitator, negotiator, manager, and researcher (Smith et al., 2006).

Collaborative Models of Care. Emerging models of care emphasize the role of the RN in providing continuity of care to patients across settings. Another goal of emerging models of care is to emphasize and acknowledge that the skill and knowledge of the RN are needed at the point of care, as well as providing coordination and management of teams.

The collaborative practice model is increasingly used by **intra-professional teams** (teams whose members provide nursing care) and by other health care providers who are members of the **interprofessional team**. All health professional education programs, including nursing, are called upon to prepare graduates to practise and lead collaborative team approaches to care (Health Professions Network Nursing and Midwifery Office, 2010). A call for collaborative practice development has been sounded across Canada because this model is viewed as the way to ensure that all professionals and providers can practise to the full potential of their role and competencies. Collaborative practice is therefore also the best way to ensure that health human resources are used most effectively during a time of shortage in the achievement of quality care and population health outcomes. It is important for students in nursing and other professional health care programs to learn the competencies associated with collaborative practice during their educational programs by focusing on relationships with nurses and others in diverse settings of care. Students and entry-level nurses need to acquire competencies that promote collaboration among teams of nurses and others to ensure that optimal care is provided. As a student nurse, you are an integral member of both nursing and interprofessional teams that cross health care settings, including acute care, mental health care, community and home care, and public and population health care. One of the first and most important responsibilities is to articulate the role and contribution of nurses to care, and then to be able to learn about and relate to the roles and responsibilities of other team members. Central to the collaborative practice model are the patient, family, and population as full participants in care or service delivery.

The RNAO has developed evidence-informed **Best Practice Guidelines** for intra-professional collaborative practice among nurses (RNAO, 2016) and interprofessional health teams among health professionals (RNAO, 2013). These guidelines show how teamwork and collaborative practice can be supported at individual, team, organizational, and system levels of nursing practice. The guidelines are comprehensive and indicate the need for transformational leadership to support a culture of teamwork and collaboration. One best practice guideline for supporting collaborative practice is the ability to share power, as identified in Box 11-7 (RNAO, 2013).

Nurses are well situated to provide leadership for collaborative practice in many health care settings. One example may be found in the home care setting, in which nurses work closely with UCPs, who provide a large amount of the continuous day-to-day care for patients

BOX 11-7 RNAO (2013) Recommendation 12: Power and Hierarchy in Teams

12.1: Team members demonstrate their willingness to share power by:

a. Building a collaborative environment through recognizing and understanding power and its influence on everyone involved;
b. Creating balanced power relationships through shared leadership, decision making; authority, and responsibility;
c. Including diverse voices in decision making;
d. Sharing knowledge openly; and
e. Working collaboratively with patients/clients and their families to plan and deliver care.

From Registered Nurses' Association of Ontario (RNAO). (2013). *Best Practice Guidelines: Developing and Sustaining Interprofessional Health Care. Optimizing patient, organizational and system outcomes* (p. 44). Toronto: Author.

who have been discharged from hospitals after undergoing surgery or who have chronic illnesses and disabilities. UCPs must have opportunities to meet and communicate regularly with the nurses and other professionals involved in the care of these patients, to ensure that they understand the patient situation and receive support for the challenges they face in providing care. Nurses can also aid UCPs by providing education and other supports so that they are able to contribute to best practices in important areas such as safety, emotional support, and wound healing. In this way, UCPs are recognized and valued for their role, and the continuity of care to a single patient or family is supported by UCPs, nurses, and other health care providers. Nurses who are employed in long-term or residential care settings may also provide leadership for collaborative practice by ensuring opportunities for communication and learning among professionals involved in teams or systems of care.

Home care delivery also often includes social workers, physicians, nutritionists, physiotherapists, and other health care providers, as well as nurses and UCPs, a situation requiring even more collaborative practice. According to the Health Professions Network Nursing and Midwifery Office (2010), "Collaborative practice in health-care occurs when multiple health workers from different professional backgrounds provide comprehensive services by working with patients, families, carers and communities to deliver the highest quality of care across settings" (p. 13). Implementing collaborative practice among professionals requires that no one professional group dominates, leadership is shared, and differences in knowledge and contributions are understood and respected. Educators and practice leaders in the health professions are working to envision and develop education strategies to prepare students to graduate with interprofessional competencies in order to carry out collaborative practice. iPANEL is an example of an initiative where nurse researchers work collaboratively with nurses in practice, patients and families, and other care providers to bring evidence that addresses the most pressing challenges of palliative care (Box 11-8).

Health care in the twenty-first century will require nurses to work with other members of the health care team and collaborate with other community members, agencies, and organizations outside the health sector. Intersectoral collaboration is a principle of primary health care, requiring nurses and others to develop skills in engaging with others to influence health in the broadest way possible. This ability to collaborate across professions and organizations requires the development of competencies in communication and conflict resolution, team functioning, and collaborative leadership that starts with a deep understanding of one's own professional role and contribution, as well as the appreciation of others' contributions (Canadian Interprofessional Health Collaborative [CIHC], 2010) (see Chapter 18 for further information about interprofessional practice).

BOX 11-8 Initiative for a Palliative Approach in Nursing: Evidence and Leadership (iPANEL)

iPANEL is an example of strong leadership and collaboration among nurse researchers, practising nurses, and other professionals with the goal of providing research and evidence to promote the best care for people with chronic and life-limiting illnesses. Palliative care is vital to promoting a quality of life during illnesses that are life limiting. Nurses are on the forefront of providing palliative care, and they require the most up-to-date knowledge to direct all aspects of their care.

iPANEL is a unique collaboration because it values and answers the kinds of questions and challenges that nurses face in their everyday practice, including:

- "What should I say?"
- "Can't we do better when she is so short of breath?"
- "What does she want for her future care? Is it my role to talk with her about this?"

Based on iPANEL.ca. (2012). *About us.* Retrieved from www.iPANEL.ca.

Decision Making

One of the most important recommendations for achieving healthy practice environments is that staff at all levels be involved in decision making about nursing practice. It is of utmost importance that the voice and decisions of nurses who are providing care are valued and acted upon. Of equal importance is that the most senior nurse in the organization be included in the executive decision-making level of the organizations and agencies, including those responsible for the delivery of home care, mental health care, public health care, or hospital care. The nurse executive supports managers and staff by creating a management structure that helps achieve organizational goals and provides support for participatory decision making and collaborative practice models. With a vision for nursing established, the manager helps staff realize that vision.

Decentralized or participatory management, in which decision making occurs at the staff level, is a vital part of a healthy work environment and effective health care organization; however, it has not been achieved to the extent needed. The advantage of this structure is that managers and staff are actively involved in shaping an organization's identity and determining success. Decentralized management requires workers to be empowered to accept greater responsibility for the quality of patient care (Mancini & Wong, 2015). A decentralized structure has the best potential to lead to positive outcomes, such as increased collaboration among staff, best practice implementation, and patient satisfaction (Table 11-1).

The nurse manager is crucial for the successful functioning of nursing units and systems. Figure 11-2 illustrates the responsibilities and competencies of nurse managers, including supervising, planning, scheduling, and staffing, as situated within a framework of leadership competencies.

Nurse leaders must enable decision making by the professionals who are most involved in patient care and must encourage inclusion rather than exclusion of staff (RNs, RPNs, LPNs, UCPs, unit administrators, and secretaries). Leaders of today are making crucial decisions about the nursing care delivery models and staff mix that will best meet patient needs and promote optimum health outcomes. Three national

TABLE 11-1 Examples of Management Structures

Structural Approach	Characteristics
Centralized management	A single administrator leads the organization, and directors oversee departments or programs. Decisions are made by the leader and directors, with little staff input. Managers have minimal responsibility or accountability for operation of the nursing unit. Staff do not feel involved in care processes, and collaborative practice is not supported.
Decentralized/participatory management	Staff members with the most knowledge about an issue participate in decision making. Structures such as professional practice councils exist to promote collaboration and decision making. Managers responsible for nursing care units or community programs often have accountability and responsibility for staffing decisions, budget, and day-to-day management of the work unit.
Matrix	Traditional units are reorganized into business units. Staff may report to several managers—such as one with responsibility for professional practice (e.g., nursing) and another with responsibility for a specific program (e.g., child and family health)—who may be from a variety of professional practice backgrounds.

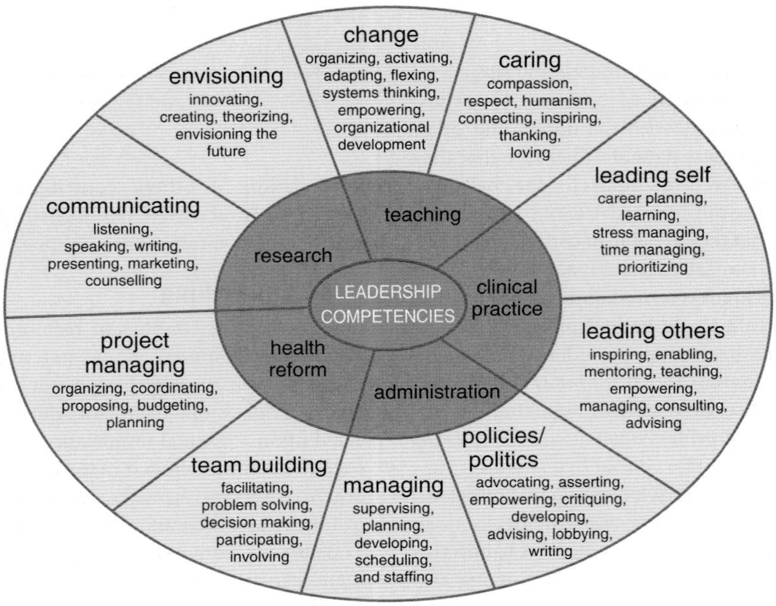

FIGURE 11-2 Management and leadership competencies. (From Canadian Nurses Association. [2005]. *Nursing leadership and development in Canada* [p. 28]. Ottawa: Author. Retrieved from https://www.cna-aiic.ca/~/media/cna/page-content/pdf-fr/nursing_leadership_development_canada_e.pdf?la=en.)

nursing groups representing RNs, LPNs, and RPNs have worked with leading nurse researchers, including Dr. Linda McGillis Hall, to identify evidence-informed guiding principles for making staff mix decisions for quality care (Box 11-9). These principles can only be realized through collaborative nursing leadership, with values of inclusiveness and evidence-informed decisions about nursing care delivery models.

Nurses must develop skills and knowledge to exercise responsibility, autonomy, authority, and accountability in order to participate fully in organizational decision making and collaborative practice (Anders & Hawkins, 2006).

Responsibility refers to the duties and activities that an individual is employed to perform. A professional nurse's responsibilities in a given role are outlined in a position description of the nurse's duties in patient care and of participation as a member of the nursing team. Managers must be sure that staff members understand their responsibilities, particularly during change. For example, when hospitals restructure and patient care delivery models change, the manager must clearly define the nurse's role within the new care delivery model. If decentralized decision making is in place, professional staff can help shape

BOX 11-9 Five Guiding Principles for Staff Mix Decision Making

- Decisions concerning staff mix respond to clients' health care needs and enable the delivery of safe, competent, ethical, quality, evidence-informed care in the context of professional standards and staff competencies.
- Decision making regarding staff mix is guided by nursing care delivery models based on the best evidence related to (1) client, staff, and organizational factors influencing quality care and work environments, and (2) client, staff, and organizational outcomes.
- Staff mix decision making is supported by the organizational structure, mission, and vision and by all levels of leadership in the organization.
- Direct care nursing staff and nursing management are engaged in decision making about the staff mix.
- Information and knowledge management systems support effective staff mix decision making.

From Canadian Nurses Association. (March, 2012). *Staff mix decision-making framework for quality nursing care.* Ottawa: Author.

the new nurse role. All nurses are responsible for knowing their role in developing competencies.

Innovation by nurses, increased productivity, higher employer retention of nurses, and greater patient satisfaction are results of autonomy in nursing practice (Keeley, Cashavelly, Cronin, et al., 2015).

Authority to act is the right to act in areas in which a nurse has been given and accepts responsibility according to legislation, standards, and the code of ethics governing the professional practice of nursing. Nurses have authority to act and to question actions concerning the practice of other professionals in relation to this scope of responsibility. For example, a nurse who as a case manager finds that the nursing team did not follow a discharge teaching plan for an assigned patient has the authority to consult with other nurses to learn why the plan was not followed. The nurse as case manager has accepted responsibility for the care of a group of patients and therefore has the final authority in selecting the best course of action for the patient's care, while collaborating with others to ensure quality outcomes.

Accountability means being answerable for one's actions. It means that as a nurse, you accept the commitment to provide excellent patient care and the responsibility for the outcomes of actions in providing that care (Anders & Hawkins, 2006). A nurse is accountable for patients' outcomes. In the example just described, the nurse as case manager is accountable for the patient's health outcomes by ensuring a continuity of care across hospitalization and home care.

A successful decentralized nursing unit exercises the four elements of decision making: responsibility, autonomy, authority, and accountability. The staff must meet routinely to discuss how to maintain equality and balance in these elements. Individuals should be comfortable in expressing differences of opinion and challenging the status quo, while understanding their own responsibility, autonomy, authority, and accountability.

Supporting Staff Involvement. In decentralized decision-making structures, all staff members actively participate in unit or agency activities (Figure 11-3). Staff members benefit from the knowledge and skills of the entire team. If the staff members value knowledge and their colleagues' contributions, patient care improves. The nursing manager supports staff involvement through the following approaches.

Establishment of Nursing Practice or Professional Shared Governance Councils. Chaired by senior clinical staff, these councils are empowered to maintain care standards for nursing practice (Gokenbach, 2007). The councils review and establish standards of care, develop policy and procedures, resolve patient satisfaction issues,

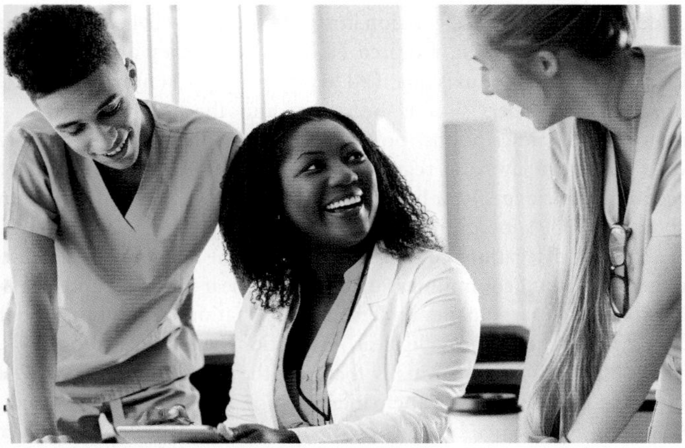

FIGURE 11-3 Students in nursing and other health care provider programs learning about their roles and contributions to collaborative practice. (Copyright © Steve Debenport/iStockphoto.)

or develop new documentation tools. Mechanisms are established to empower all staff to contribute input on practice issues. Managers might not sit on the council, but they receive progress reports. The types of work in the nursing unit are what determine council membership. Professionals from other disciplines (e.g., pharmacy, respiratory therapy, social work, medicine, or clinical nutrition) might participate in these councils. Professional practice councils can advocate for resources and conditions necessary for healthy practice environments and safety.

Interprofessional Collaboration. As previously described, collaborative practice among professionals from different disciplines is essential to ensuring that health human resources are used in the best possible way (CIHC, 2010) (see Chapter 18 for further information about interprofessional collaboration). Whenever systems or programs are redesigned, interprofessional involvement is crucial because most health care processes involve more than one discipline. Nurses must recognize the importance of prompt referrals and timely communication with other care providers. Inclusion of professionals from various disciplines in practice projects, in-service programs, conferences, and staff meetings fosters improvement in health outcomes. Learning the skills and knowledge for interprofessional practice begins in nursing education, thus student nurses are encouraged to seek practicum and other opportunities that allow them to work with other professionals and providers and articulate nursing's unique role and contribution to practice.

Communication and Information Technology. Communication is one of the leader's greatest challenges, especially in a large work group in which change is constant. It is difficult to ensure that all staff members and partners receive the correct messages. In the current health care environment, staff quickly become uneasy and distrusting if they fail to hear about planned changes in their work unit that often include the introduction of new information technology such as electronic health records and standardized nomenclatures for patient care (CASN, 2012) (see Chapter 15 for more information about documentation). A manager cannot be responsible for all communication but can use several approaches to communicate quickly and accurately with all staff, such as increasing presence on work units and using the new capacity of social media. Social media has radically altered patterns of communications in the workplace, resulting in the need for nurses to develop new competencies and ethical awareness of privacy and confidentiality considerations. As technology continues to evolve as a dominant mode of communication, nurse leaders must find ways to maintain the relational aspects of the workplace and provide opportunities for nursing presence and meaningful dialogue within organizations.

Developing a Learning Organization. Constant change is a reality of our time, and organizations and leaders must understand and embrace all that is new and provide a vision for new realities and directions (Porter-O'Grady & Malloch, 2015). In this era of unprecedented change, leaders and managers are challenged to develop the conditions for learning to flourish in what has been described as a *learning organization* (Senge, 2006). In learning organizations, many forms of knowledge are shared. Leadership strategies are needed to help nurses incorporate evidence-informed best practice guidelines into their nursing practice. These strategies include "support, role-modelling commitment to best practices, and reinforcing organizational policies and goals consistent with evidence-based care" (Gifford, Davies, Edwards, et al., 2006, p. 73). Technology such as web-based applications and social media will continue to transform how we learn and communicate in organizations, requiring attention to ethical issues such as privacy and confidentiality, as well as the power of the media to influence change in systems (Risling, 2016). These influences will require both vigilance and ethical consideration of managers and leaders.

Clinical Care Coordination

As a nursing student, you develop the skills necessary to ensure timely and effective patient care. At first, you may have only one patient, but eventually you will coordinate the care of groups of patients. Clinical care coordination includes decision making, priority setting, use of organizational skills and resources, time management, and evaluation.

Clinical Decisions. Leadership and decision-making skills are required as the nurse engages in the complex interactions—collaboration, negotiation, conflict resolution, and delegation—necessary to elicit the involvement of other people. Nursing students learn to value and practise patient centredness in every interaction. They also learn to adopt a critical thinking approach, applying understanding of patients' perspectives, one's knowledge, evidence-informed best practice guidelines, and experience to the decision-making process (see Chapter 12 for more information about critical thinking and clinical reasoning).

Priority Setting. Nurses must establish priorities of care as these relate to actions taken to meet patients' needs. This is particularly important in caring for groups of patients with health challenges involving immediate needs and actions to be taken.

Any patients can have priorities, which requires the nurse to use careful judgement in choosing a course of action. Priorities of care relate to nursing standards of practice as the benchmark of nurses' provision of care to persons, families, and communities. First-priority needs require immediate attention and most often relate to life-threatening or pain-related issues. Setting priorities also requires nurses to know the priority needs of each patient; assess each patient's needs as soon as possible, including the patient's and family's determination of priorities; and address needs in a timely manner through teamwork. Nurses must be constantly aware of resources needed to ensure that they are able to respond to priorities.

Time Management. Changes in health care delivery and increasing complexity in all settings of care can create time management challenges for nurses as they work to meet patients' needs (Harris & McGillis Hall, 2012). Time management skills can help nurses manage stress. These skills include reflecting on how one uses time, planning effectively, and being aware of competing priorities. Because of the complexity of practice, nurses are often required to juggle priorities and respond to multiple demands on their time. It is therefore most important to track these demands and ensure that resources are in place that allow the nurse to focus on priorities in a timely manner. Technology such as email correspondence has increased demands on nurses' time and often requires an immediate response. It is therefore important for nurses to realize and reflect on the impact of technology and other forces and to acquire the ability to set limits and refuse demands that are unreasonable.

Evaluation. Evaluation is one of the most important aspects of clinical care coordination. Evaluation is an ongoing process that provides focus and direction for each phase of nursing care. As a nurse, once you begin to provide care, you should also learn to immediately evaluate its effectiveness and the patient's response. In the evaluation process, you need to compare expected patient outcomes with actual outcomes. For example, a clinic nurse assesses a diabetic patient's foot ulcer to determine whether healing is progressing and expected outcomes are met. Upon evaluation, the nurse realizes the need to revise approaches to care and to introduce new therapies. Focusing on evaluation of a patient's progress and outcomes, rather than on tasks, lessens the chance of distraction. The nurse learns to keep the patient at the centre of the care by asking the patient for his or her ideas and evaluation of how he or she is experiencing the care plan.

Delegation. Changes in staff mix have resulted in more UCPs delivering care to patients (Harris & McGillis Hall, 2012). In the new working environment, a nurse must understand the evolving role of nursing and delegated care responsibilities in order to ensure the safety and quality of nursing care delivery. **Delegation** is "transferring the responsibility to perform a function or intervention to someone who would not otherwise have the authority to perform it (i.e., the function or intervention is not within the scope of practice or scope of employment of the care provider to whom the care is being delegated) (College of Registered Nurses of Nova Scotia [CRNNS] & College of Licensed Practical Nurses of Nova Scotia [CLPNNS], 2012). An important point here is that the person delegating the function remains accountable for the practice, while the delegate is responsible for performing it safely (CRNNS & CLPNNS, 2012; College of Registered Nurses of Ontario, 2013).

As a student, you will work with teams of nurses and UCPs during your practica in many health care settings, including home care, residential care, community health care, and acute care settings. As you develop in your role, it is important to learn about the roles and scopes of practice of UCPs in different practice settings. You will learn about how your role relates to that of the UCP and how the principles of delegation are applied in practice. Students and nurses also have access to valuable resources such as nursing practice consultants and practice guidelines to assist them in making complex decisions about delegation. The nurse may assume responsibility for the education, supervision, and support of UCPs as they perform delegated nursing activities.

Provincial regulations define the scope of an RN's practice, including activities that only RNs can perform (e.g., patient assessment and planning care). Although most provinces identify the delegation and supervision of work as an RN's responsibility, each province addresses the specifics of delegation differently. In Ontario, British Columbia, and Alberta, for example, legislation that applies to all regulated health care providers identifies specific tasks or activities that can be performed by only certain providers. In British Columbia, these authorized tasks are known as *reserved acts;* in Ontario, they are called *controlled acts;* and in Alberta, they are known as *restricted activities.* UCPs are not allowed to perform actions authorized for RNs unless those actions have been properly delegated by an RN and only if they are within the UCP's job description and employer policy.

An institution's policies, procedures, and job descriptions for UCPs provide specific guidelines regarding which tasks or activities can be delegated. The job description should specify any required education and the types of tasks UCPs can perform, either independently or under an RN's direct supervision. Institutional policy helps in defining the amount of training required of UCPs while they are employed. Procedures specify who is qualified to perform a given nursing procedure, whether supervision is necessary, and the type of reporting required. Job descriptions, policies, and procedures should comply with provincial laws and regulations. Nurses should have a means of accessing policies easily or have supervisory staff who can inform them about the UCP's job duties.

Effective delegation requires trust between the RN and UCPs. It also requires constant communication—sending clear messages and listening so that all participants understand expectations regarding patient care. An RN should provide clear instructions when delegating tasks. These instructions may initially focus on the procedure itself, as well as on the unique needs of the patient. As the RN becomes more familiar with a staff member's scope of practice, trust builds and fewer instructions may be needed, but clarification of patients' specific needs is always necessary.

A key step in delegation is evaluation of the staff member's performance and the patient's outcomes. When UCPs do a good job, it is

BOX 11-10 Summary of Points to Consider in Assignment and Delegation

Assignment = client and/or interventions—**within** individual scope of practice
Delegation = client interventions—**outside** individual scope of practice

Communication and collaboration are key components for successful assignment or delegation outcomes.

1. **Planning**
   - Has the client population been identified?
   - Is the model of care understandable and the role descriptions clear/available?
   - Are agency policies/procedures in place to support assignment/delegation?
   - Are the necessary supports/resources available to enable appropriate assignment or delegation?

2. **Assessment**
   a. Client Health Status and Care Needs
      - Is there a low risk associated with assignment or delegation?
      - Is the care requirement an ADL/IADL or does the client have complex needs?

   b. Right Context (Care Environment and Resources)
      - Is there a low risk associated with the assignment or delegation?
      - Is the decision based on sound nursing judgement?
      - Are the necessary agency supports in place and available; i.e., education, policies and procedures, appropriateness to delegatee's job description?
      - Is the assignment or delegation supported by the *RN Act, LPN Act* or other relevant legislation?
      - Has education been provided where necessary (especially for delegation)?
      - Are ongoing nursing assessment, care planning, and evaluation available?

   c. Right Intervention
      - Is the intervention in the client's best interest?
      - Are the results of the intervention reasonably predictable?
      - Is the intervention within the scope of practice of the assignee?
      - Do the *Standards of Practice for Registered Nurses* and *Code of Ethics* support the assignment or delegation?
      - Do the *Scope of Practice, Standards of Practice,* and *Code of Ethics* for LPNs support the assignment or delegation?
      - Is the intervention appropriate for assigning (within scope of practice) or delegating (outside scope of practice) within the context of practice?

   d. Right Person (determining the most appropriate competent health care provider)
      - Does the assignor/delegator have the competence and/or the authority to assign or delegate?
      - Does the assignee/delegatee have the necessary competence to accept the assignment or delegation so that client safety and well-being are not compromised?

3. **Supervision**
   - Is supervision required?
   - What type of supervision is required?
   - Is appropriate supervision available when necessary?

4. **Evaluation and Documentation**
   - Has the assignment or delegation been followed up with the appropriate documentation in the health record?
   - Is there a process for communicating the results/outcomes of the process and/or intervention?
   - Has the plan of care informed the decision to assign or delegate been evaluated?

5. **Adjustments to Nursing Care Plan/Plan of Care**
   - Are adjustments to the nursing care plan/plan of care required?

From College of Registered Nurses of Nova Scotia & College of Licensed Practical Nurses of Nova Scotia. (2012). *Assignment and delegation guidelines for registered nurses and licensed practical nurses* (p. 10). Halifax, NS: Author. Retrieved from https://crnns.ca/wp-content/uploads/2015/02/AssignmentandDelegationGuidelines.pdf.

important to provide praise and recognition. If the staff member's performance is unsatisfactory, the RN must give constructive feedback, specifically discussing mistakes and how they could have been avoided. Giving feedback in private in a professional manner preserves the staff member's dignity. A UCP may fail to meet expectations because of inadequate training or assignment of too many tasks. The RN may need to review or demonstrate a procedure with staff or schedule additional training with the education department. The delegation of too many tasks might be a nursing practice issue. All staff should discuss delegation on their unit because UCPs may need help in learning how to prioritize and RNs may need to ensure that they are not over-delegating. The College of Registered Nurses of Nova Scotia (CRNNS & CLPNNS, 2012) has developed guidelines for what a nurse must consider and do when assigning or delegating care (Box 11-10).

QUALITY CARE AND PATIENT SAFETY

As discussed throughout this chapter, safe and high-quality care is delivered when leadership, staffing models, and collaborative practice are in place to support it. Studies show that high-quality practice environments produce better patient outcomes and more satisfied patients and staff (Aiken et al., 2014; CNA, 2008).

Accreditation Canada (2017) engages at an organizational level "to improve client outcomes and health system performance" (see https://www.accreditation.ca). The organization engages people at all levels of the organization and the public to determine if organizations meet standards. Accredited organizations have achieved a standard of safety and quality in all aspects of the care provided including leadership, infection control, safe medication management, and other areas. Influential nurse leaders, including CNA's past president, Dr. Karima Velji, who is a vice-chair of the Board of Directors at Accreditation Canada, have influence on setting the highest standards for safety and quality care.

Quality in Nursing Practice

Quality Defined. Standards or guidelines define the meaning of quality. For example, to judge whether rehabilitation has been delayed, a standard of when rehabilitation should begin must exist. Quality of care in nursing practice is not arbitrarily defined. A definition of quality begins with the mission, vision, philosophy, and values of the nursing department. These statements define how all nurses within an organization are to perform and which services must be provided. Written values give direction for professional standards and care guidelines that lead to positive patient outcomes.

Professional Standards. Professional standards are authoritative statements used by the profession in describing the responsibilities for which its practitioners are accountable (Peters, 1995). They include the policies and position descriptions that identify performance expectations within an organization. Standards are an organization's interpretation of the professional's competency. The adherence to professional standards is measured through professional outcomes.

Care and Best Practice Guidelines. Best Practice Guidelines are evidence-informed resources to assist nurses in providing the best care possible (Folse & Wong, 2015). Guidelines can be developed by single disciplines or can be multidisciplinary in focus. Examples of nursing practice guidelines are found in the literature encompassing some of the examples referred to in this chapter, including wound care and prevention of falls. The effectiveness of nursing practice is measured through patient outcomes and the accumulation of evidence (Graham & Harrison, 2008).

Nurse-Sensitive Outcomes. *Outcomes* are conditions to be achieved as a result of care. It is important that the outcomes selected to measure the effectiveness of nursing care are related to the work that nurses do. A nurse-sensitive outcome reveals whether interventions are effective, whether patients progress, how well standards are being met, and whether changes are necessary. Examples of outcomes related to the implementation of Best Practice Guidelines may include incidence of pressure sores, falls in elderly patients, and hypertension control measures.

To judge whether standards of care are met, processes and outcomes are measured. For example, a staff team measures its success in implementing a new process of diabetes instruction and also measures the outcome: Can patients administer insulin correctly? When selecting quality indicators, teams should consider processes and related outcomes that are most likely to improve nursing practice. Processes to improve may include the following:

- A weak process that is causing problems (e.g., poor pain management for patients with cancer who are at home)
- A stable process that is adequate but can be improved (e.g., access to education and support for people with diabetes in rural communities)
- A process linked to negative outcomes (e.g., care of intravenous access sites with the occurrence of phlebitis)

Building a Culture of Safety

Patient safety has been recognized as a crucial component of health care delivery. The Canadian Patient Safety Institute (2009) has defined patient safety as "the reduction and mitigation of unsafe acts within the health care system, as well as through the use of best practices shown to lead to optimal patient safety." Issues such as staff shortages, new technology, and other demands on health care systems have prompted a re-examination of how errors and adverse events for patients can be prevented. Increasingly, the emphasis is on enabling health care providers to communicate effectively and to acknowledge and receive timely assistance for errors. This assistance includes the education of nursing and other health care students to view mistakes as learning, to know and prevent conditions that lead to unsafe practices, and to develop the competencies for safe practice (CASN, 2006; Davidson, Weisbrod, Gregory, et al., 2006). The Canadian Patient Safety Institute (2009) identified seven core domains of abilities for all health care providers, including their contributions to developing a culture of patient safety as a most important foundation (Box 11-11).

Coming Full Circle: Leadership for a High-Quality Work Life and High-Quality Health Care. Leaders and managers at all levels of health care organizations must do what they can to improve the quality of work life in health care in order to ensure patient safety and quality health care; evidence and awareness of this need are growing. For example, nurse fatigue has been identified as a current factor in patient safety requiring the attention of governments, organizations, and individual nurses (CNA & RNAO, 2010). Recommended solutions to the problem based on research include the role of nurse managers in instituting fatigue management policies and programs. These measures require significant changes in the workplace and collaboration with nursing unions and nursing education programs. Measures to be considered include rest and sleep policies, as well as reform of scheduling practices (CNA & RNAO, 2010). Nurse managers have significant responsibilities in implementing these solutions, and they provide leadership in this area to make a difference to both the quality of nurses' work lives and patient safety outcomes.

BOX 11-11 The Safety Competencies

Domain 1: Contribute to a Culture of Patient Safety

Health care professionals must be enabled to contribute to health care organizations, large or small, in ways that promote patient safety in their structure and function. Content in this domain could include but is not limited to the following aspects:

- Understanding of patient safety concepts, epidemiology, and basic theories
- Awareness of health care error
- Promotion of a systems approach to care and safety
- Promotion of staff empowerment to resolve unsafe situations
- Role modelling and demonstration of a commitment to leadership in safe practice
- Ensuring feedback on safety issues
- Integration of safe practices into daily activities
- Commitment to communication, teamwork, and quality
- Reporting of adverse events
- Commitment to a just, nonpunitive culture

Canadian Patient Safety Institute. (2009). *The safety competencies.* Ottawa: Author. Retrieved from http://www.patientsafetyinstitute.ca/en/toolsResources/safetyCompetencies/Documents/Safety%20Competencies.pdf#search=Domain%201%3A%20Creating%20a%20Culture%20of%20Patient%20Safety.

LEADERSHIP SKILLS FOR NURSING STUDENTS

Nursing students prepare for leadership roles. This does not mean that you as a student must quickly learn how to lead a nursing team; rather, you first learn to become an accountable and competent health care provider. Leadership development is ongoing throughout a career, and individual leadership styles are influenced from a variety of sources, including theories, best practices, mentors, role models, and experiences. You learn leadership by making clinical decisions, advocating for public health and quality care, learning from mistakes, seeking guidance, engaging in collaborative practice with nursing teams and other professionals, seeking mentors, and striving to improve during each patient interaction. Recent research in Canada has indicated that mentorship components of new graduate transition programs are key to helping new graduate nurses become part of the nursing workforce (Baumann, Hunsberger, & Crea-Arsenio, 2011; Brewer, Flavell, Trede, et al., 2016). Your nursing education program provides you with the opportunity to develop leadership competencies: advocacy, conflict management, collaborative practice, patient centredness, delegation, and evidence-informed decision making.

Career Development and Mentoring for Nursing Students

Nursing students have the opportunity to begin to envision their preferred career path early in their nursing education program. In fact, it is likely that students who do begin to plan their careers or "course of life work" are more likely to achieve their goals and develop personal and professional strengths that enable their future career satisfaction and success (Waddell, Donner, & Wheeler, 2009). As you develop a career vision, you may identify opportunities that can further your **career development** as a nurse leader, such as attending meetings of professional associations, presenting your work at student conferences, and finding a career coach or mentor (Cooper & Wheeler, 2010; Mata, Latham, & Ransome, 2010). Waddell et al. (2009) have developed the Career Planning and Development Model for students to use during their nursing education program (Figure 11-4). The model includes stages of planning that engage the student in learning about nursing realities and trends, developing a self-assessment, and creating a career vision and marketing approach. These authors contend that having a career vision is "perhaps the most forceful motivator for using your nursing practice placement and classroom experiences and your summer and part-time work opportunities to the fullest" (2009, p. 7).

Nursing leadership, including the concepts and competencies discussed in this chapter, is needed to shift the current culture of health care to achieve the vision of health care providers delivering high-quality health care, adopted by the collaborative. This means that nurses and other professionals working directly with patients and the mid-level managers have key roles to play in leading change. They must be inspired and supported through **mentoring** and by the implementation of leadership best practices guidelines and collaborative practice. Senior leaders must ensure adequate staffing and support for the culture of a healthy workplace. The way forward is to inspire lifelong learning at all levels of the organization and provide access and resources to education that enables staff to work with the patient and the patient's family at the centre of health care delivery and decision making.

Nurses working at all levels of organizations can contribute by making a commitment to this vision and being part of the change that is required to transform Canadian health care. Indeed, CNA in its centenary year inspired the theme of leadership for a transformed Canadian health care system and has called for Canadian nurses to "be the change" required to sustain quality health care for all. As a student and as a qualified nurse, you have the opportunity and the challenge to effect positive change in nursing practice and Canadian health care (Box 11-12).

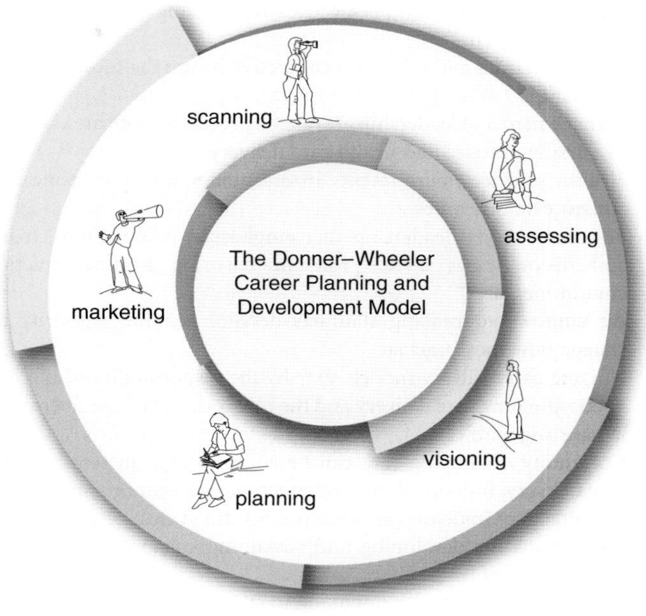

FIGURE 11-4 The Donner–Wheeler career planning and development model. (From Waddell, J., Donner, G. J., & Wheeler, M. M. [2009]. *Building your nursing career: A guide for students* [3rd ed., p. 2]. Toronto: Elsevier Canada.)

BOX 11-12 CASE STUDY

Leadership for Best Practices in Falls Prevention

Kaley Hart is a recently graduated registered nurse (RN) working in a residential care facility. Ann Best, the nurse manager of the facility, is aware of Kaley's interest in leadership for best practices. As a fourth-year student, Kaley had completed a special project on falls prevention in the facility, using local statistics on falls and evidence-informed practice guidelines. Ann wishes to enroll the long-term care facility in the National Collaborative on Falls in Long-Term Care (Registered Nurses' Association of Ontario [RNAO], 2007). This program requires the commitment of an improvement team consisting of five to seven staff members. Ann's vision is that the improvement team would be supported by the educational and research resources of this national program and by access to national experts in falls prevention. She sees this as an excellent opportunity for Kaley to be involved and to continue to develop her leadership skills in the areas of collaborative practice and best practices implementation.

At Ann's invitation, Kaley becomes involved with the quality improvement team, which also includes a nurse researcher from the university. Kaley begins her work by inspiring other nurses to become involved with the initiative, and she advocates for unregulated care providers (UCPs) and other professionals to become members of the team in order to achieve a broad perspective on the changes required to prevent falls. She refers to the Canadian statistic that falls are the leading cause of overall injury costs in Canada (SMARTRISK, 2009) and how they continue to increase among older persons in residential care settings (Public Health Agency of Canada, 2014). Kaley inspires a vision of changes to be made in the interest of preventing falls and achieving the best possible health outcomes for the residents in the facility. She advocates for residents' and their families' involvement in the initiative and seeks input from all patients and professionals as to how the learning sessions should take place in order to promote engagement as a learning community.

As a member of the team, Kaley contributes her knowledge of the RNAO (2007) *Falls Prevention Best Practices Guidelines and Supplement* (RNAO, 2010) and helps develop a practical approach to identifying residents who are at risk for falls. Drawing on her knowledge of collaborative practice, Kaley ensures that other members, including the physiotherapist, UCP, recreation therapist, nutritionist, and housekeeping manager, are able to contribute their experiences and ideas about risk management and participate in the learning sessions. Kaley takes the opportunity to praise the contributions of diverse team members and to facilitate input and participation from the residents.

An evaluation of the quality improvement team reveals high levels of participation and interest within the facility. The experience of being involved in a national initiative has contributed to the capacity for best practices implementation and evidence-informed practice. Kaley is inspired by the experience and has further developed her management and leadership competencies in the areas of inspiring a vision, leading change, facilitating collaborative practice, and developing respectful and supportive relationships among team members. She has worked with the nurse researcher at the local university to develop the plan for studying the impact of the changes on the incidence of falls over time. Of most importance is that Kaley looks forward to the next opportunity to make a difference in the health outcomes of the residents through the exercise of progressive management and leadership initiatives.

KEY CONCEPTS

- A leader must set a vision or philosophy for a work unit, ensure appropriate staffing, mobilize staff and institutional resources to achieve objectives, motivate staff members to carry out their work, set standards of performance, and make the right decisions to achieve objectives.
- Leadership theories and perspectives are evolving and informed by nursing research.
- Nursing's ethics and relational competencies are the foundation of leadership.
- Management and leadership are related processes; both are essential to nursing practice and health care delivery.
- Healthy practice environments are essential to quality nursing and patient care outcomes.
- Transformational leadership that emphasizes relationships, trust, and vision plays a key role in ensuring healthy practice environments.
- An empowered nursing staff has decision-making authority to change how they practise.
- Nursing care delivery models vary by the responsibility of the RN in coordinating care delivery and the roles other staff members play in assisting with care.
- Continuity of nursing care can be compromised in total patient care delivery, functional nursing practice, and team nursing.
- Best Practice Guidelines are evidence informed and contain recommendations for developing and sustaining collaborative practice models and leadership.
- For decentralized decision making to succeed, staff members must be aware that they have the responsibility, authority, autonomy, and accountability for the care they give and the decisions they make.
- A nurse manager can foster decentralized decision making by establishing nursing practice committees, supporting collaborative practice, implementing quality improvement plans, and maintaining timely staff communication.
- Clinical care coordination involves accurate clinical decision making, establishing priorities, efficient organizational skills, appropriate use of resources and time management skills, and an ongoing evaluation of care activities.
- To promote an enriching professional environment, each member of a nursing work team is responsible for open, professional communication.
- Delegation involves transferring responsibility for performing an activity while retaining accountability for the outcome.
- When accomplished correctly, delegation can improve job efficiency and job enrichment.
- An important responsibility for the nurse who delegates nursing care is evaluation of the staff member's performance and patient outcomes.
- In a quality improvement–oriented environment, every staff member becomes involved in finding ways to improve or change work processes so as to promote patient safety and quality care outcomes.
- Nurses' career development involves planning and opportunities for mentorship.

CRITICAL THINKING EXERCISES

1. John, an RN, is working with Tammy, a UCP, to manage care for five patients. John has completed morning assessments and rounds on the assigned patients and is giving Tammy directions for what she needs to do in the next hour. John says to Tammy, "Why don't you go to Room 415 and see what Mr. Thomas needs, and go to Room 418 to check if Mrs. Landry is doing all right." Based on what you know about delegation, were these appropriate or inappropriate delegations to Tammy? Provide a rationale for your answer.
2. You are a recently graduated RN working in a home care setting. The manager of the nursing program asks you to assist with the implementation of a collaborative practice model. She asks you to help her set the agenda for the first meeting to discuss the concept and principles of collaborative practice. What ideas and resources would you contribute to the agenda?
3. You have just received morning shift reports on your patients. You have been assigned the following patients:
   - A 52-year-old man who was admitted yesterday with a diagnosis of angina. He is scheduled for a cardiac stress test at 0900.
   - A 60-year-old woman who was transferred out of intensive care at 0630 today. She underwent uncomplicated coronary bypass surgery yesterday.
   - A 45-year-old man who experienced a myocardial infarction 3 days ago and is complaining of chest pain, which he rates as 5 on a scale of 0 to 10.
   - A 76-year-old woman who had a permanent pacemaker inserted yesterday and is complaining of incision pain, which she rates as 7 on a scale of 0 to 10.

   Which one of these patients do you need to see first? Explain your answer.

REVIEW QUESTIONS

1. Transformation leadership most fundamentally involves *(Select all that apply)*:
   1. Developing charismatic and highly influential leaders
   2. Envisioning new systems of care to get work done
   3. Developing relationships and involving others in change
   4. Introducing research and innovation
2. Collaborative practice models most fundamentally aim to
   1. Improve delegation between staff
   2. Improve communication between staff
   3. Place the patient at the centre of care delivery
   4. Ensure that health care providers can cover for one another
3. Delegation by nurses involves the following *(Select all that apply)*:
   1. Communication of the plan of care to the LPN
   2. Transferring accountability to another care provider
   3. Ensuring that the delegate has the skills and knowledge to perform the function
   4. Understanding team members' scopes of practice
4. The type of management structure that has a potential for greater collaborative effort, increased competency of staff, and ultimately a greater sense of professional accomplishment and satisfaction is
   1. Empowerment
   2. Primary nursing
   3. Total patient care
   4. Decentralized
5. While administering medications, the nurse realizes she has given the wrong dose of medication to a patient. The nurse acts by completing an incident report and notifying the patient's physician. The nurse is exercising
   1. Authority
   2. Responsibility
   3. Accountability
   4. Decision making

6. A manager who wishes to promote patient safety in the health care organization should focus on *(Select all that apply)*:
   1. Viewing mistakes as opportunities for learning
   2. Staffing models and ratios
   3. Systems for detecting mistakes
   4. Ensuring shared vision and values of quality and safety in care
7. A home care nurse is working with three UCPs who were recently hired and are new to their roles. For the first 2 weeks of their employment, the UCPs have been providing care for patients at home with complex wounds and caring for families in palliative care situations. The nurse believes in the principles of collaborative practice and wishes to support the UCPs in their development. An important first step would be to
   1. Provide an opportunity for the UCPs to talk about their experiences, questions, and roles
   2. Provide an educational session on palliative care
   3. Set up a mentoring system among the UCPs
   4. Discuss the role of the RN in home care
8. Leadership for the promotion of primary health care involves *(Select all that apply)*:
   1. Political action and advocacy
   2. Understanding how communities access care
   3. Implementing collaborative practice models
   4. Promoting the goal of health equity
9. The nurse checks on a patient who was admitted to the hospital with pneumonia. He has been coughing profusely and has required nasotracheal suctioning. He has an intravenous infusion of antibiotics. He is febrile. The patient asks the nurse whether he can have a bath because he has been perspiring profusely. The nurse may delegate to the UCP working with her today the task of
   1. Assessing vital signs
   2. Changing intravenous dressing
   3. Nasotracheal suctioning
   4. Administering a bed bath
10. An example of a nurse-sensitive outcome based on Best Practice Guidelines is *(Select all that apply)*:
    1. Rates of wound infection
    2. Percentage of time it takes to count narcotics by nursing staff every shift
    3. Number of falls among residents in a long-term care setting
    4. Time it takes for a patient to be transported from the emergency department to an inpatient nursing unit

Answers: 1. 2, 3, 4; **2.** 3; **3.** 3, 4; **4.** 4; **5.** 3; **6.** 1, 2, 4; **7.** 1; **8.** 1, 2, 3, 4; **9.** 4; **10.** 1, 3.

Rationales for the Review Questions appear at the end of the book.

RECOMMENDED WEBSITES

Academy of Canadian Executive Nurses (ACEN): http://www.acen.ca.
This is an association of nurses in leadership positions across the spectrum of health services. ACEN activities support leadership, advocacy and policy initiatives, and mentorship for emerging nurse leaders and executives.

Accreditation Canada: https://www.accreditation.ca/en/.
Accreditation Canada, formerly known as the Canadian Council on Health Services Accreditation, is a national, nonprofit, independent organization whose role is to help health services organizations, across Canada and internationally, examine and improve the quality of care and service they provide to their patients.

Canadian Association of Schools of Nursing (CASN): http://www.casn.ca.
The CASN is the national voice for nursing education, research, and scholarship and represents baccalaureate and graduate nursing programs across Canada.

Canadian Foundation for Healthcare Improvement: http://www.cfhi-fcass.ca/.
The website of the Canadian Foundation for Healthcare Improvement contains research resources for policymakers and for health system leaders and managers pertaining to staffing models, high-quality health work life, and high-quality health care.

Canadian Interprofessional Health Collaborative (CICH): http://www.cihc.ca.
The CICH is made up of health organizations, health educators, researchers, health professionals, and students across Canada. This collaborative shares best practices and advances knowledge in interprofessional practice and collaborative practice.

Canadian Nurses Association (CNA): https://www.cna-aiic.ca/en.
CNA is a federation of 11 provincial and territorial nursing associations representing more than 120,000 RNs. CNA's mission is to advance the quality of nursing in the interest of the public.

Canadian Nursing Students Association (CNSA): http://www.cnsa.ca/.
CNSA is the national voice of nursing students in Canada. For more than 30 years, the CNSA has represented the interests of nursing students to federal, provincial, and international governments and to other nursing and health care organizations.

Canadian Patient Safety Institute (CPSI): http://www.patientsafetyinstitute.ca/.
The CPSI is an independent not-for-profit corporation, operating collaboratively with health providers and organizations and with regulatory governments and bodies to build and advance a safer health care system for Canadians.

Donnerwheeler: http://www.donnerwheeler.com.
This website includes information and resources for career development and mentoring, developed by Canadian nurse leaders Gail Donner and Mary Wheeler.

International Council of Nurses (ICN): http://www.icn.ch/.
ICN is a federation of national nurses' associations, representing nurses in more than 120 countries. Operated by nurses for nurses, ICN works to ensure quality nursing care for all patients, sound health policies globally, and the advancement of nursing knowledge.

Registered Nurses' Association of Ontario (RNAO): http://www.rnao.org.
This website offers a complete and up-to-date inventory of Best Practice Guidelines, including implementation and evaluation.

Truth and Reconciliation Commission of Canada: www.trc.ca.
This website includes all of the archived and up-to-date proceedings of the Truth and Reconciliation Commission, including the document containing all of the calls to action. This resource is essential for nurses to provide leadership for understanding the meaning, shared responsibilities, and opportunities inherent in reconciliation.

REFERENCES

Accreditation Canada. (2017). *Corporate overview*. Ottawa: Author. Retrieved from https://www.accreditation.ca/corporate-overview.

A century of progress—Overview of significant themes and issues. (2005). *Canadian Nurse (Centennial Edition)*, *101*(7), 22–28.

Aiken, L. (2008). Economics of nursing. *Policy, Politics and Nursing Practice*, *9*(2), 73–79.

Aiken, L. H., Sloane, D. M., Bruyneel, L., et al. (2014). Nurse staffing and education and hospital mortality in nine European countries: a retrospective observational study. *Lancet*, *383*(9931), 1824–1830.

Anders, R. L., & Hawkins, J. A. (2006). *Mosby's nursing leadership and management online*. St. Louis: Mosby.

Avolio, B. J., Walumbwa, F. O., & Weber, T. J. (2009). Leadership: Current theories, research, and future directions. *Annual Review of Psychology*, *60*, 421–449.

Bamford, M., Wong, C. A., & Laschinger, H. (2013). The influence of authentic leadership and areas of worklife on work engagement of registered nurses. *Journal of Nursing Management*, *21*(3), 529–540. doi:10.1111/j.1365-2834.2012.01399.x.

Baumann, A., Hunsberger, M., & Crea-Arsenio, M. (2011). Workforce integration of new graduate nurses: Evaluation of a health human resources employment policy. *Healthcare Policy*, *7*(2), 47–59.

Brewer, M. L., Flavell, H. L., Trede, F., et al. (2016). A scoping review to understand "leadership" in interprofessional practice and education. *Journal of Interprofessional Care*, *30*(4), 408–415. doi:10.3109/13561820.2016.1150260.

Canadian Association of Schools of Nursing. (2006). *Position statement: Patient safety and nursing education.* Ottawa: Author.

Canadian Association of Schools of Nursing. (2012). *Nursing informatics entry-to-practice competencies for registered nurses.* Ottawa: Author.

Canadian Association of Schools of Nursing. (2015). *National nursing education framework: Final report.* Ottawa: Author.

Canadian Interprofessional Health Collaborative. (2010). *A national interprofessional competency framework.* Retrieved from https://www.cihc.ca/files/CIHC_IPCompetencies_Feb1210.pdf.

Canadian Nurses Association. (2008). *Unregulated health workers: A Canadian and global perspective.* Retrieved from https://www.cna-aiic.ca/~/media/cna/page-content/pdf-en/18%20-%20unregulated_health_workers_04_2008_e.pdf?la=en.

Canadian Nurses Association. (2009a). *Nursing leadership—Position statement.* Ottawa: Author.

Canadian Nurses Association. (2009b). *The next decade: CNA's vision for nursing and health.* Ottawa: Author.

Canadian Nurses Association, Canadian Council for Practical Nurse Regulators, & Registered Psychiatric Nurses of Canada. (2012). *Staff mix decision-making framework for quality nursing care.* Ottawa: Canadian Nurses Association.

Canadian Nurses Association & Canadian Federation of Nursing Unions. (2015). *Joint position statement: Practice environments: Maximizing outcomes for clients, nurses and organizations.* Ottawa: Author.

Canadian Nurses Association & Registered Nurses Association of Ontario. (2010). *Nurse fatigue and patient safety: Research report Executive Summary.* Ottawa: Author.

Canadian Patient Safety Institute. (2009). *The safety competencies—Enhancing patient safety across the health professions.* Retrieved from http://www.patientsafetyinstitute.ca/en/toolsResources/safetyCompetencies/Documents/Safety%20Competencies.pdf.

Case Management Society of America. (2016). *Member benefits: Why join?* Retrieved from http://www.cmsa.org/Individual/Membership/WhyJoin/tabid/166/Default.aspx.

College of Registered Nurses of British Columbia. (2015). *Competencies in the context of entry-level registered nurse practice in British Columbia.* Vancouver: Author.

College of Registered Nurses of Nova Scotia (CRNNS) & College of Licensed Practical Nurses of Nova Scotia (CLPNNS). (2012). *Assignment and delegation guidelines for registered nurses and licensed practical nurses.* Halifax: Authors.

College of Registered Nurses of Ontario. (2013). *Working with unregulated care providers.* Toronto: Author.

Cooper, M., & Wheeler, M. M. (2010). Career Talk. Building successful mentoring relationships. *Canadian Nurse, 106*(7), 34–35.

Cummings, G. G., MacGregor, T., Davey, M., et al. (2010). Leadership styles and outcome patterns for the nursing workforce and work environment: A systematic review. *International Journal of Nursing Studies, 47*, 363–385.

Dadich, K. A. (2003). Care delivery strategies. In P. S. Yoder-Wise (Ed.), *Leading and managing in nursing* (3rd ed., pp. 253–274). St. Louis: Mosby.

Davidson, D., Weisbrod, L., Gregory, D., et al. (2006). Case study: On the leading edge of new curricula concepts: Systems and safety in nursing education. *Canadian Journal of Nursing Leadership, 19*, 34–42.

Doane, G. H., & Varcoe, C. (2015). *How to nurse: Relational inquiry with individuals and families in changing health and health care contexts.* Philadelphia: Walters Kluwer.

Duncan, S., Rodney, P. A., & Thorne, S. (2014). Forging a strong nursing future: Insights from the Canadian context. *The Journal of Research in Nursing, 19*(7–8), 621–633. doi:10.1177/1744987114559063.

Estabrooks, C., Midodzi, W., Cummings, G., et al. (2005). The impact of hospital nursing characteristics on 30-day mortality. *Nursing Research, 54*(2), 74–84.

Folse, V. N., & Wong, C. A. (2015). Managing Quality and Risk. In P. S. Yoder-Wise & L. G. Grant (Eds.), *Leading and managing in Canadian nursing* (pp. 391–410). Toronto: Elsevier Canada.

Fowler, J., Hardy, J., & Howarth, T. (2006). Trialing collaborative nursing models of care: The impact of change. *The Australian Journal of Advanced Nursing, 23*(4), 40–46.

Gifford, W. A., Davies, B., Edwards, N., et al. (2006). Leadership strategies to influence the use of clinical practice guidelines. *Canadian Journal of Nursing Leadership, 19*, 72–88.

Gokenbach, V. (2007). Professional nurse councils: A new model to create excitement and improve value and productivity. *The Journal of Nursing Administration, 37*, 440–443.

Gottlieb, L. N., Gottlieb, B., & Shamian, J. (2012). Principles of strengths-based nursing leadership for strengths-based nursing care: A new paradigm for nursing and healthcare for the 21st century. *Nursing Leadership, 25*(2), 38–50. doi:10.12927/cjnl.2012.22960.

Graham, I. D., & Harrison, M. B. (2008). Appraising and adapting clinical practice guidelines. In N. Cullum, D. Ciliska, R. B. Haynes, et al. (Eds.), *Evidence-based nursing* (pp. 219–230). Oxford, UK: Blackwell.

Greenleaf, R. K. (1977). *Servant leadership: A journey to the nature of legitimate power and greatness.* New York: Paulist Press.

Harris, A., & McGillis Hall, L. (2012). *Evidence to inform staff mix decision-making: A focused literature review prepared for the Canadian Nurses Association.* Ottawa: CNA.

Health Canada. (2002). *Our health, our future: Creating quality workplaces for Canadian nursing.* Final report of the Canadian Nursing Advisory Committee. Ottawa: Author. Retrieved from https://www.canada.ca/en/health-canada/services/health-care-system/reports-publications/nursing/health-future-creating-quality-workplaces-canadian-nurses-final-report-canadian-nursing.html.

Health Canada. (2009). *Office of nursing policy (ONP).* Ottawa: Author. Retrieved from https://www.canada.ca/en/health-canada/corporate/about-health-canada/branches-agencies/strategic-policy-branch/office-nursing-policy.html.

Health Professions Network Nursing and Midwifery Office, Department of Human Resources for Health. (2010). *Framework for action on interprofessional education and collaborative practice.* Geneva: Author. Retrieved from http://apps.who.int/iris/bitstream/10665/70185/1/WHO_HRH_HPN_10.3_eng.pdf?ua=1.

Hibberd, J. M., Smith, D. L., & Wylie, D. M. (2006). Leadership and leaders. In J. M. Hibberd & D. L. Smith (Eds.), *Nursing leadership and management in Canada* (3rd ed., pp. 369–394). Toronto: Elsevier Canada.

Institute of Medicine (IOM). (2011). *The future of nursing: Leading change, advancing health.* Washington, DC: National Academies Press.

International Council of Nurses (ICN). (2008). *Participation of nurses in health services decision making and policy development position statement.* Geneva: Author. Retrieved from http://www.icn.ch/images/stories/documents/publications/position_statements/D04_Participation_Decision_Making_Policy_Development.pdf.

International Council of Nurses (ICN). (2013). Judith Shamian elected as new ICN President [International Perspectives]. *International Nursing Review, 60*(1), 283–290. doi:10.111/inr.12053.

Jost, S. G., Bonnell, M., Chacko, S., et al. (2010). Integrated primary nursing: A care delivery model for the 21st century knowledge worker. *Nursing Administration Quarterly, 34*(3), 208–216. doi:10.1097/NAQ.0b013e3181e7032c.

Keeley, A., Cashavelly, B., Cronin, J., et al. (2015). Exemplars of innovation in practice: Implications of the AONE-CIT and CMS innovation advisors projects within the Massachusetts General Hospital. *Nursing Administration Quarterly, 39*(4), 325–332. doi:10.1097/NAQ.0000000000000131.

Knibbs, K., Underwood, J., MacDonald, M., et al. (2010). Appreciative inquiry: A strengths-based research approach to building Canadian public health nursing capacity. *The Journal of Research in Nursing, 17*(5), 484–494. doi:10.1177/1744987110387472.

Kouzes, J. M., & Posner, B. Z. (2017). *The leadership challenge: How to make extraordinary things happen* (6th ed.). San Francisco: Jossey-Bass.

LeClerc, C. M., Doyon, J., Gravelle, D., et al. (2008). The autonomous-collaborative care model: Meeting the future head on. *Nursing Leadership, 21*(2), 63–75.

Mancini, M., & Wong, C. A. (2015). Understanding and designing organizational structures. In P. S. Yoder-Wise & L. G. Grant (Eds.), *Leading and managing in Canadian nursing* (pp. 149–169). Toronto: Elsevier Canada.

Mata, H., Latham, T. P., & Ransome, Y. (2010). Benefits of professional organization membership and participation in national conferences: Considerations for students and new professionals. *Health Promotion Practice, 11*(4), 450–453. doi:10.1177/1524839910370427.

Nagle, L. (2014). An interview with Dr. Judith Shamian, President, International Council of Nurses. *Nursing Leadership, 27*(1), 26–30.

National Expert Commission. (2012). *A nursing call to action: The health of our nation, the future of our health system.* Ottawa: CNA.

Peters, D. A. (1995). Outcomes: The mainstay of a framework for quality care. *Journal of Nursing Care Quality, 10*(1), 61–69.

Porter-O'Grady, T., & Malloch, K. (2015). *Quantum leadership* (4th ed.). Burlington, MA: Jones & Bartlett Learning.

Public Health Agency of Canada. (2014). *Seniors' falls—Second report.* Ottawa: Author.

Registered Nurses' Association of Ontario (RNAO). (2007, January). *Falls prevention—Building the foundations for patient safety. Self-learning package.* Toronto: Author. Retrieved from http://rnao.ca/sites/rnao-ca/files/Falls_Prevention_-_Building_the_Foundations_for_Patient_Safety._A_Self_Learning_Package.pdf.

Registered Nurses' Association of Ontario (RNAO). (2010, August). *Pilot evaluation of implementation and update of healthy work environment best practice guidelines: Final report.* Toronto: Author.

Registered Nurses' Association of Ontario (RNAO). (2013). *Best practice guidelines: Developing and sustaining interprofessional health care: Optimizing patient, organizational and system outcomes.* Toronto: Author.

Registered Nurses' Association of Ontario (RNAO). (2016). *Intra-professional collaboration among nurses.* Toronto: Author.

Reutter, L., & Kushner, K. E. (2010). Health equity through action on the social determinants of health: Taking up the challenge in nursing. *Nursing Inquiry, 17*(3), 269–280. doi:10.1111/j.1440-1800.2020.00500.x.

Reutter, L., & Ogilvie, L. (2011). Primary health care: Challenges and opportunities for the nursing profession. In J. C. Ross-Kerr & M. J. Wood (Eds.), *Canadian nursing: Issues and perspectives* (5th ed., pp. 185–208). Toronto: Elsevier Canada.

Risling, T. (2016). Social media and nursing leadership: Unifying professional voice and presence. *Nursing Leadership, 28*(4), 48–57. doi:10.12927/cjnl.2016.24561.

Senge, P. (2006). *The fifth discipline: The art and practice of the learning organization*. New York: Doubleday.
SMARTRISK. (2009). *The economic burden of injury in Canada*. Toronto: Parachute Canada. Retrieved from http://www.parachutecanada.org/downloads/research/reports/EBI2009-Eng-Final.pdf.
Smith, D. L., Smith, J. E., Boechler, V., et al. (2006). Structure and organization of nurses' work. In J. M. Hibberd & D. L. Smith (Eds.), *Nursing leadership and management in Canada* (3rd ed., pp. 199–237). Toronto: Elsevier Canada.
Smith, K. B., Profetto-McGrath, J., & Cummings, G. G. (2009). Emotional intelligence and nursing: An integrative literature review. *International Journal of Nursing Studies, 46*(12), 1624–1636. doi:10.1016/j.ijnurstu.2009.05.024.
Sportsman, S., & MacMillan, H. (2015). Care delivery strategies. In P. S. Yoder-Wise & L. G. Grant (Eds.), *Leading and managing in Canadian nursing* (pp. 256–278). Toronto: Elsevier Canada.
Truth and Reconciliation Commission of Canada (TRC). (2015). *Honoring the truth, Reconciling for the future: Summary of the final report of the TRC of Canada*. Ottawa: Author. Retrieved from http://www.myrobust.com/websites/trcinstitution/File/Reports/Executive_Summary_English_Web.pdf.
Waddell, J., Donner, G. J., & Wheeler, M. (2009). *Building your nursing career: A guide for students* (3rd ed.). Toronto: Elsevier Canada.
Whyte, N. B., & Duncan, S. M. (2016). Engaging nursing voice and presence during the federal election 2015. *Nursing Leadership, 29*(4), 19–34.
Wong, C. A. (2015). Editorial: Connecting nursing leadership and patient outcomes. *Journal of Nursing Management, 23*(3), 275–278. doi:10.1111/jonm.12307.
Wong, C. A., Cummings, G. G., & Ducharme, L. (2013). The relationship between nursing leadership and patient outcomes: A systematic review update. *Journal of Nursing Management, 21*(5), 709–724.
Wong, C. A., & Laschinger, H. K. S. (2013). Authentic leadership, performance, and job satisfaction: The mediating role of empowerment. *Journal of Advanced Nursing, 69*(4), 947–959. doi:10.1111/j.1365-2648.2102.06089.x.
World Health Organization (WHO). (2008). *Primary health care now more than ever*. Geneva: Author.

12

Critical Thinking in Nursing Practice

Canadian content written by Donna M. Romyn, RN, PhD
Original chapter by Patricia A. Potter, RN, MSN, PhD, FAAN

OBJECTIVES

Mastery of content in this chapter will enable you to:

- Define the key terms listed.
- Describe characteristics of a critical thinker.
- Consider the relationship between critical thinking and patient-centred care.
- Describe the components of a critical thinking model for clinical decision making.
- Explain the relationship between clinical experience and critical thinking.
- Discuss critical thinking competencies used in nursing practice.
- Discuss the nurse's responsibility in making clinical decisions.
- Discuss the relationship of the nursing process to critical thinking.
- Discuss the critical thinking attitudes used in clinical decision making.
- Explain how professional standards influence a nurse's clinical decisions.
- Describe how case-based learning fosters critical thinking.
- Describe how reflective writing promotes critical thinking.
- Discuss how concept maps can improve a nurse's ability to think critically.

KEY TERMS

Case-based learning, p. 182
Clinical decision-making process, p. 176
Clinical inference, p. 179
Clinical reasoning, p. 180
Concept map, p. 182
Critical thinking, p. 174
Decision making, p. 179
Diagnostic reasoning, p. 179
Evidence-informed knowledge, p. 175
Information literacy skills, p. 178
Nursing process, p. 176
Patient-centred care, p. 174
Problem solving, p. 179
Reflection, p. 182
Reflective writing, p. 182
Scientific method, p. 178

MEDIA RESOURCES

http://evolve.elsevier.com/Canada/Potter/fundamentals/

- Audio Chapter Summaries
- Examination Review Questions
- Concept Map Creator
- Case Study with Questions
- Audio Glossary
- Content Updates
- Video Clips

As a nurse, you will face many complex situations involving patients, family members, and other health care workers. To deal with these experiences effectively, you need to develop sound critical thinking skills so that you can approach each new problem with open-mindedness, creativity, confidence, and wisdom. When a patient develops a new set of symptoms, asks you to provide comfort measures, or requires a procedure, it is important to think critically and make prudent clinical judgements so that the patient receives the best nursing care possible. Critical thinking is not a simple, step-by-step linear process that you can learn overnight. Your ability to think critically will increase as you gain experience and progress from novice to expert nurse (Benner, 1984). Critical thinking is central to professional nursing practice because it allows you to test and refine nursing approaches, learn from successes and failures, apply nursing research findings, and ensure holistic patient-centred care.

CRITICAL THINKING DEFINED

Critical thinking is a complex phenomenon that can be defined as a process and as a set of skills. Definitions of critical thinking emphasize the use of knowledge and reasoning to make accurate clinical judgements and decisions. Accordingly, nurses recognize that an issue (e.g., patient problem or health-related concern) exists, analyze information about the issue (e.g., clinical data about the patient), evaluate information (e.g., review assumptions and evidence), and draw conclusions (e.g., decide how to proceed). In consultation with patients, nurses consider what is important in a situation, explore alternative solutions, consider ethical principles, and then make informed decisions about how to proceed. Consider the following case example:

Mr. Jacobs is a 58-year-old patient who had a radical prostatectomy for prostate cancer yesterday. His nurse, Tonya, finds him lying supine in bed with his arms extended along his sides and his hands clenched. When Tonya checks his surgical wound and drainage device, she notes that he winces when she gently palpates over the incisional area. She asks Mr. Jacobs when he last turned onto his side, and he responds, "Not since sometime last night." Tonya asks Mr. Jacobs if he is having incisional pain and he nods, saying, "It hurts too much to move." Tonya considers her observations and the information she has learned from the patient to determine that his pain is severe and his mobility is reduced because of it. Together, she and Mr. Jacobs decide to take action to relieve his pain so he can turn more frequently and begin to get out of bed to aid his recovery.

Critical thinking requires purposeful and reflective reasoning to examine ideas, assumptions and beliefs, principles, conclusions, and actions within the context of the situation. When you care for a patient, you begin to think critically by asking questions such as "What do I know about the patient's situation? How do I know it?" "What is the patient's situation now? How might it change?" "What is the patient's perspective on the situation?" "What else do I need to know to understand this situation better or improve it? How can I obtain that information?" "In what way will a specific therapy affect the patient?" "Are other options available?" "What health outcomes are important to the patient?" "How can I work with the patient to attain those outcomes?" By answering these questions, you are able to identify alternative solutions to address the patient's health-related concerns and to involve the patient in making decisions about the care provided. (Box 12-1 illustrates how strategies designed to foster critical thinking can promote patient-centred care.)

As you gain experience in nursing, avoid letting your thinking become routine or standardized. Instead, learn to look beyond the obvious in any clinical situation, explore the patient's unique responses to actual or potential health alterations, and recognize what actions are needed to benefit the patient. Over time, your experience with many patients will help you recognize patterns of behaviour (Tanner, 2006), see commonalities in signs and symptoms, and anticipate reactions to nursing interventions. Reflecting on your experiences will help you determine how the knowledge you gained working with one patient may be applicable to another patient's situation.

In Tonya's case, she knows that the patient is likely to have pain because the surgery was extensive. Her review of her observations and the patient's report of pain confirm that pain is a problem. Her options include giving Mr. Jacobs an analgesic and then waiting until it takes effect so that she can help him find a more comfortable position. Once his pain is less acute, Tonya might also ask Mr. Jacobs whether he would like to try some relaxation exercises and mobilization techniques she learned while caring for another postoperative patient that may be effective in increasing his mobility.

You can begin to learn to think critically early in your practice and use relevant information, knowledge, and communication technologies to support evidence-informed nursing practice (Canadian Association of Schools of Nursing [CASN], 2015a, p. 12). For example, as you learn about administering bed baths and other hygiene measures to your patients, take time to read the nursing literature about the concept of comfort. What are the criteria for comfort? How do patients from other cultures perceive comfort? What are the many factors that promote comfort? The use of **evidence-informed knowledge**—knowledge based on research or clinical expertise—makes you an informed critical thinker and improves patient outcomes.

Critical thinking requires not only cognitive skills, such as interpretation, analysis, inference, evaluation, explanation, and self-regulation, but also a nurse's habit (disposition) to ask questions, to be well informed, to be honest in facing personal biases, and to always be willing to reconsider and think differently about issues. Without these dispositions, sound critical thinking is unlikely to occur (Facione, 1990; Facione & Facione, 1996; Meherali, Profetto-McGrath, & Paul, 2015). When applied to nursing, these core critical thinking skills and critical thinking dispositions reveal the complex nature of

BOX 12-1 RESEARCH HIGHLIGHT

Putting the "Patient" Back Into Patient-Centred Care: An Education Perspective

Focus

The ethos of patient-centred care infers that care provided to patients is tailored to the specific needs of individual patients and that patients are engaged in making decisions about their care to the extent desired. Underlying this research study (Ferguson, Ward, Card, et al., 2013) was the question, "How do patients describe their experiences and roles in the interprofessional teams that provide their health care in an acute care medical inpatient unit?"

Abstract

Face-to-face interviews were conducted with 18 inpatients (10 men and 8 women) on an acute medical inpatient unit in a large Canadian hospital. In some cases, their family members participated in the interviews to add their perspectives or illuminate patient perspectives. The interview data were analyzed using an interpretive descriptive approach (Thorne, 2008). Five themes emerged related to patient expectations of and satisfaction with the quality of and their involvement in their care: (1) patients wanted to feel valued and respected by health care providers; (2) trust between patients and health care providers was essential to an effective relationship; (3) communication of relevant information was extremely important to patients; (4) patient perceptions of team relationships existed primarily with physicians, although other professionals were acknowledged; and (5) patients generally expressed satisfaction with care.

Evidence-Informed Practice

Patient-centred care is addressed in the education of all health care providers; however, the findings of this research indicate a need to emphasize the concept more extensively or differently. Suggested strategies included using case approaches, problem-based learning, and simulation experiences that emphasize the psychosocial aspects of patients' experiences of illness; engagement of patients and families in classroom discussions; academic assignments that involve students in the exploration of patients' experiences; concept maps that involve pathophysiological, psychological, social, emotional, and cultural factors; use of text and online resources that explore patient experiences; and patient- and family-focused rounds. Increasing the emphasis on patient-centred care in the education of health care providers was deemed by the researchers to be critical to patients in their experience of illness, both in acute care facilities and in the community.

Reference: Ferguson, L. M., Ward, H., Card, S., Sheppard, S., & McMurtry, J. (2013). Putting the 'patient' back into patient-centred care: An education perspective. *Nurse Education in Practice, 13*(4), 283-287. doi:10.1016/j.nepr.2013.03.016

TABLE 12-1 Critical Thinking Skills and Dispositions

Elements of Decision-Making Process	Critical Thinking Behaviour
Skill	
Interpretation	Be orderly in data collection. Look for patterns to categorize data (e.g., formulate nursing diagnoses [see Chapter 13]). Clarify any data about which you are uncertain.
Analysis	Be open-minded as you look at information about a patient. Avoid making careless assumptions. Ask whether the data reveal what you believe is true or whether other scenarios are possible.
Inference	Examine meanings and relationships in the data. Form reasonable hypotheses and conclusions on the basis of the patterns observed.
Evaluation	Assess all situations objectively. Use criteria (e.g., expected outcomes) to determine the effectiveness of nursing actions. Identify required changes. Reflect on your own behaviour.
Explanation	Support your findings and conclusions. Use knowledge and experience to select the strategies you use in the care of patients.
Self-regulation	Reflect on your experiences. Adhere to standards of practice. Apply ethical principles in your nursing practice. Identify in what way you can improve your own performance.
Dispositions or Habits	
Truth-seeking	Learn what is actually happening in a situation. Consider scientific principles and evidence, even if they do not support your preconceptions or personal beliefs.
Open-mindedness	Be receptive to new ideas and tolerant of other points of view. Respect the right of other people to hold different opinions. Be aware of your own prejudices.
Analyticity	Determine the significance of a situation. Interpret meaning. Anticipate possible results or consequences. Use evidence-informed knowledge in your nursing practice.
Systematicity	Be organized and focused in data collection. Use an organized approach to problem solving and decision making.
Self-confidence	Trust your own reasoning processes. Seek confirmation from experts when uncertain.
Inquisitiveness	Actively seek new knowledge.
Maturity	Accept that multiple solutions are possible. Reflect on your own judgements; be willing to consider other explanations. Use prudence in making, suspending, or revising judgements.

Adapted from Facione, P. (1990). *Critical thinking: A statement of expert consensus for purposes of educational assessment and instruction. The Delphi report: Research findings and recommendations prepared for the American Philosophical Association* (ERIC Doc No. ED 315-423). Washington, DC: Educational Resources Information Center (ERIC).

the clinical decision-making process (Table 12-1). Learning to apply these skills and establish critical thinking habits takes time and practice. Being open-minded, inquisitive, and systematic in thinking about practice situations will help you incorporate research findings in your clinical decision making.

Nurses who apply critical thinking in their work consider all aspects of a situation and make well-reasoned judgements about a variety of possible alternative actions rather than hastily and carelessly implementing solutions (Kataoka-Yahiro & Saylor, 1994). For example, nurses who work in crisis situations such as child abuse and suicide prevention programs act quickly when patient problems develop. These nurses must, however, exercise discipline in decision making to avoid premature and inappropriate decisions. Learning to think critically helps you to care for patients as their advocate and to make better informed choices about their care. Critical thinking is more than just problem solving; it is an attempt to continually improve how you apply knowledge when faced with problems in patient care.

A CRITICAL THINKING MODEL FOR CLINICAL DECISION MAKING

Thinking critically is a benchmark or standard for professional nursing competence. Kataoka-Yahiro and Saylor (1994) developed a model of critical thinking for nursing judgement based in part on previous work by Paul (1993), Glaser (1941), Perry (1979), and Miller and Malcolm (1990) (Figure 12-1). The model helps explain what is involved as you make clinical decisions and judgements about your patients. It also defines the outcome of critical thinking: nursing judgement that is relevant to nursing problems in a variety of settings.

Throughout this text, this model is used for applying critical thinking during the nursing process (see Chapter 5). Each clinical chapter of the text (Chapters 31 to 48) is organized by the steps of the nursing process and includes both scientific and nursing knowledge. It is your knowledge base (the first critical thinking component) that prepares you to make clinical judgements as a nurse. Figure 12-1 demonstrates how to apply elements of critical thinking in assessing patients, in planning the interventions you provide, and in evaluating the outcomes.

LEVELS OF CRITICAL THINKING IN NURSING

Your ability to think critically grows as you gain new knowledge and experience in nursing practice. Three levels of critical thinking in nursing—basic, complex, and commitment—are incorporated in the critical thinking model developed by Kataoka-Yahiro and Saylor (1994). As a beginning nursing student, you will apply the critical thinking model at the basic level. As you advance in practice, you will adopt complex critical thinking and commitment.

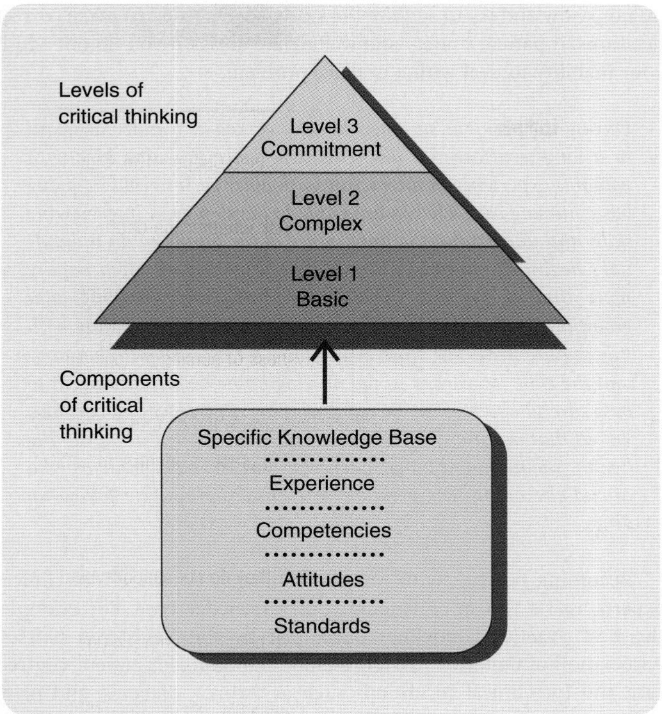

FIGURE 12-1 **Critical thinking model for nursing judgement.** (Redrawn from Kataoka-Yahiro, M., & Saylor, C. [1994]. A critical thinking model for nursing judgment. *Journal of Nursing Education, 33*[8], 351. Adapted from Glaser, E. [1941]. *An experiment in the development of critical thinking.* New York: Bureau of Publications, Teachers College, Columbia University; Miller, M., & Malcolm, N. [1990]. Critical thinking in the nursing curriculum. *Nursing & Health Care, 11*, 67; Paul, R. W. [1993]. The art of redesigning instruction. In J. Willsen & A. J. A. Blinker [Eds.], *Critical thinking: How to prepare students for a rapidly changing world.* Santa Rosa, CA: Foundation for Critical Thinking; and Perry, W. [1979]. *Forms of intellectual and ethical development in the college years: A scheme.* New York: Holt, Rinehart, & Winston.)

Basic Critical Thinking

At the basic level of critical thinking, thinking is concrete and based on a set of rules or principles. For example, as a student nurse, you use a hospital's procedure manual to confirm how to insert a Foley catheter. In completing this procedure for the first time, you will probably follow the procedure step by step without adjusting the procedure to meet a patient's unique needs (e.g., positioning to minimize the patient's pain or mobility restrictions) because you do not have enough experience to know how to individualize the procedure. At this level, answers to complex problems are seen to be either right or wrong (e.g., the Foley catheter balloon contains too much or not enough sterile water), and you may believe that one right answer exists for each problem. As you gain more experience in nursing, you will begin to explore the diverse opinions of expert others (e.g., instructors and staff nurse role models) and engage in more complex critical thinking.

Complex Critical Thinking

When you engage in complex critical thinking, you begin to separate your thinking processes from those of expert others and to analyze and examine choices more independently. Your thinking abilities and initiative to look beyond expert opinion begin to change as you realize that alternative, and perhaps conflicting, solutions to a problem or issue exist.

Consider the following case study:

Mr. Rosen is a 36-year-old man who injured his back in a skiing accident. He suffers from chronic pain but is refusing to take a prescribed analgesic. While discussing the importance of rehabilitation with Mr. Rosen, the nurse, Edwina, learns that Mr. Rosen practises meditation at home. In complex critical thinking, Edwina recognizes that for pain relief, the patient has options other than accepting analgesics. Edwina decides to also discuss other nonpharmacological interventions with Mr. Rosen and his other health care providers even though not all may agree about their potential efficacy in controlling his pain.

In complex critical thinking, you are willing to consider other options, including patient preferences regarding care, in addition to routine procedures, when complex situations develop. As a nurse, you learn to weigh the benefits and risks of each potential solution before making a final decision. Thinking becomes more creative, innovative, and patient-centred as you explore a broad range of perspectives and alternative solutions.

Commitment

The third level of critical thinking is commitment. You anticipate the need to make choices without assistance from other professionals, and then you assume responsibility and accountability for those choices. As a nurse, you do more than just consider the complex alternative solutions that a problem poses. At the commitment level, you choose an action or belief on the basis of the viability of the alternative solutions available, and you stand by your choice. Sometimes an action is to not take action, or you may choose to delay taking action as a result of your experience and knowledge. Because you take responsibility for the decision, you evaluate the results of the decision and determine whether it was appropriate or if a different approach is required.

COMPONENTS OF CRITICAL THINKING IN NURSING

Critical thinking consists of five components: knowledge base, experience, competencies, attitudes, and standards. These elements explain how nurses make clinical judgements that are necessary for safe, competent, and ethical nursing care. (Box 12-2 highlights the components of critical thinking in nursing.)

Specific Knowledge Base

Nurses must possess a sound knowledge base to think critically, formulate accurate clinical judgements and decisions, and improve clinical practice. Your knowledge base includes information and theory from the basic sciences, humanities, behavioural sciences, and nursing. The *Framework for the Practice of Registered Nurses in Canada* describes how nurses use their knowledge base in a different way than other health care providers and think holistically about patient problems and health-related matters (Canadian Nurses Association [CNA], 2015). For example, a nurse's broad knowledge base offers a physical, psychological, social, moral, ethical, legal, and cultural view of patients and their health concerns. The breadth and depth of your knowledge influence your ability to integrate and apply different kinds of knowledge and to think critically about nursing problems in a range of practice settings. Consider this scenario:

Robert Perez previously earned a bachelor's degree in education and taught high school for 1 year. He has successfully completed the required human and biological science courses in his nursing

BOX 12-2 Components of Critical Thinking in Nursing

I. Specific knowledge base
II. Experience in nursing
III. Critical thinking competencies
  A. General critical thinking competencies (scientific method, problem solving, and decision making)
  B. Specific critical thinking competencies in clinical situations (diagnostic reasoning, clinical inference, and clinical decision making)
  C. Specific critical thinking competency in nursing (use of nursing process)
IV. Attitudes for critical thinking
V. Standards for critical thinking
  A. Intellectual standards
  B. Professional standards
    1. Ethical criteria for nursing judgement
    2. Criteria for evaluation
    3. Professional responsibility

Adapted from Kataoka-Yahiro, M., & Saylor, C. (1994). A critical thinking model for nursing judgment. *Journal of Nursing Education, 33*(8), 351. Data from Paul, R. W. (1993). The art of redesigning instruction. In J. Willsen & J. A. A. Blinker (Eds.), *Critical thinking: How to prepare students for a rapidly changing world.* Santa Rosa, CA: Foundation for Critical Thinking.

program as well as those related to health ethics, fundamental nursing concepts, and communication principles. His first clinical course focuses on health promotion, with a clinical assignment in an outpatient primary care clinic. Although he is still new to nursing, his experience as a teacher and his preparation and knowledge base in nursing will help him know how to begin to make clinical decisions about patients' self-care and health promotion practices.

The proliferation of digital technologies influences how knowledge is documented, acquired, utilized, and shared in clinical practice. Building a sound knowledge base demands that you develop strong **information literacy skills**, which includes proficiency in knowing when information is needed and how to effectively find, retrieve, evaluate, and apply research findings (LoBiondo-Wood, Haber, Cameron, et al., 2017). Critical thinking dispositions, such as truth-seeking, being systematic, analytical, open-minded, and inquisitive, will allow you to become an informed consumer of information found in print, through social media, and on the Internet.

Experience

Nursing is a practice discipline and clinical nursing experiences are necessary for you to acquire clinical decision-making skills. In clinical situations, you learn from observing, sensing, talking with patients and families, and reflecting actively on your experiences. Clinical experience is the laboratory for evaluating nursing knowledge. You learn that "textbook" approaches form the basis for nursing practice, but you make safe adaptations or revisions in approaches to accommodate the setting, unique characteristics and desires of the patient, and the experience you gained from caring for previous patients. With experience, you begin to understand clinical situations, recognize cues of patients' health patterns, and interpret cues as relevant or irrelevant (Tanner, 2006). As a result, your critical thinking skills advance beyond the basic level. You also learn to seek new knowledge as needed, act quickly when events change, and make quality decisions that promote the patient's health and well-being. Critical thinkers admit what they do not know and try to acquire the knowledge needed to make correct decisions. A patient's safety and welfare are at risk if you do not admit your inability to deal with a practice problem.

During the previous summer, Robert worked as a nurse assistant in a long-term care facility. This experience provided him with valuable experience in interacting with older persons and in giving basic nursing care. He has been able to develop good interviewing skills and understand the importance of the family in an individual's health. He has also learned that older persons often require more time to perform activities such as eating, bathing, and grooming, and so he has adapted skill techniques for dealing with this requirement. His time in the physical assessment laboratory and the time he worked in the nursing home helped him begin to be a careful observer. As he reflects on his experiences, Robert also knows that much of what he learned can be applied in promoting health, wellness, and independence among the older patients who attend the outpatient primary care clinic for routine follow-up visits.

Becoming familiar with practice standards developed by clinical experts assists you in enhancing your knowledge base. For example, the Best Practice Guidelines developed by the Registered Nurses' Association of Ontario (RNAO) include standards for patient-centred care and for clinical conditions such as asthma, diabetes, and pain. Others focus on nursing practice issues such as cultural competence, end-of-life care, and woman abuse. The aim of Best Practice Guidelines is to incorporate research into practice, increase consistency of care, eliminate interventions that are of questionable value, and improve health outcomes. Visit the RNAO's website (http://www.rnao.org/bestpractices/) and those of other Canadian professional nursing associations to learn more about the range of practice guidelines that are available to help you develop a sound knowledge base for your nursing practice.

CRITICAL THINKING COMPETENCIES

Kataoka-Yahiro and Saylor (1994) described critical thinking competencies as the cognitive processes that a nurse uses to make judgements about the clinical care of patients. They include general critical thinking, specific critical thinking in clinical situations, and specific critical thinking in nursing.

General Critical Thinking Competencies

General critical thinking competencies are not unique to nursing. They include the scientific method, problem solving, and decision making.

Scientific Method. The **scientific method** is a systematic, ordered approach to gathering data and solving problems that is used in nursing, medicine, and various other disciplines. Nurse researchers use the scientific method to verify that a set of facts is true when testing research questions in nursing practice. Research incorporating the scientific method contributes to evidence-informed nursing practice and the development of Best Practice Guidelines.

The scientific method has five steps:

1. Identification of the problem
2. Collection of data
3. Formulation of a research question or hypothesis
4. Testing of the question or hypothesis
5. Evaluation of the results of the test or study

Consider the following example of the scientific method in nursing practice:

A nurse caring for patients who receive large doses of chemotherapy for ovarian cancer detects a pattern whereby these patients develop severe inflammation of the mouth (mucositis) (identifies the problem). The nurse reads research articles (collects data) about mucositis and learns about evidence that cryotherapy, in which patients keep ice in their mouths during the chemotherapy infusion, reduces the severity of the mucositis after treatment. The nurse asks (forms research question), "Can patients with ovarian cancer who receive chemotherapy have less severe mucositis when given cryotherapy instead of standard mouth rinse in the oral cavity?" The nurse then designs a study that compares the incidence and severity of mucositis in a group of patients who use cryotherapy with those in patients who use traditional mouth rinse (tests the question). The nurse hopes that the results from the study will give oncology nurses a better approach for reducing the frequency and severity of mucositis in cancer patients. A nurse in another oncology setting critically analyzes the study before implementing its recommendations for patient care (evaluates the results of the study).

Problem Solving. Everyone faces problems every day. When a problem arises, people obtain information and then use the information, in addition to what they already know, to find a solution. Patients routinely present problems in nursing practice. For example, a home care nurse visits a patient and learns that the patient cannot describe what medications she has taken for the past 3 days. The nurse must solve the problem of why the patient is not adhering to her medication schedule. The nurse knows the patient was recently discharged from the hospital and five medications were prescribed. When the nurse asks the patient to show the medications that she takes in the morning, the nurse notices that the patient is anxious and has difficulty reading the medication labels. The patient is able to tell the nurse the names of the medications she is to take but is uncertain about the times of administration. The nurse recommends having the patient's pharmacy relabel the medications in larger lettering. In addition, the nurse shows the patient examples of pill organizers that will help her sort her medications by time of day for a period of 7 days.

Effective problem solving also involves evaluating the solution over time to be sure that it is still effective. It becomes necessary to try different options if a problem recurs. As a continuation of the example just described, the nurse finds during a follow-up visit that the patient has organized her medications correctly and is able to read the labels without difficulty. The patient confirms that she is now more confident about her ability to follow her medication regimen. The nurse obtained information that correctly clarified the cause of the patient's problem, and the nurse tested a solution that proved successful. Having solved a problem in one situation adds to the nurse's experience in practice and enables the nurse to apply that knowledge in future situations with patients.

Decision Making. When you face a problem or situation and need to choose a course of action from several options, you are making a decision. Decision making is a product of critical thinking that focuses on problem resolution. Following a set of criteria helps you make a well-reasoned decision. For example, decision making occurs when a new parent chooses an infant car seat. To make a decision, the parent needs to recognize and define the problem (need to protect the infant) and assess all options (consider available models). The parent has to weigh each option against a set of criteria (e.g., safety rating; cost; ease of installation and use), test possible options (e.g., search Health Canada website for recall notices; seek advice from other parents), consider the consequences of the decision (safety of infant; risk of injury), and then make a final decision. Although the criteria follow a sequence of steps, decision making involves moving back and forth between steps when all criteria are considered. Decision making leads to informed conclusions that are supported by evidence and reason. Other examples of decision making include deciding on the specific dressing to be used for a patient with a surgical wound or selecting the best approach for teaching a family how to assist a patient who is returning home after a stroke. You learn to make sound decisions by approaching each clinical situation thoughtfully and by applying each component of the decision-making process described previously.

Specific Critical Thinking Competencies in Clinical Situations

Specific critical thinking competencies in clinical situations include diagnostic reasoning, clinical inference, and clinical decision making.

Diagnostic Reasoning and Clinical Inference. As soon as you receive information about a patient in a clinical situation, you begin diagnostic reasoning, a process of determining a patient's health status after you make physical and behavioural observations and after you assign meaning to the behaviours, physical signs, and symptoms exhibited by the patient. The information that you collect and analyze leads to a diagnosis of the patient's condition. An expert nurse sees the context of a patient situation (e.g., recognizes that a patient who is feeling lightheaded, has blurred vision, and has a history of diabetes is experiencing a problem with blood glucose levels), observes patterns and themes (e.g., symptoms including weakness, headache, hunger, and visual disturbances that suggest hypoglycemia), and chooses an appropriate intervention quickly (e.g., offers a food source containing glucose). Considering the context of the situation enhances the nurse's analytical skills (Ironside, 2005) and results in a more accurate diagnosis.

Part of diagnostic reasoning is clinical inference: the process of drawing conclusions from related pieces of evidence. An inference involves forming patterns of information from data before making a diagnosis. Seeing that a patient has lost his appetite and experienced a loss of weight over the past month, the nurse infers that the patient has a nutritional problem. An example of diagnostic reasoning is forming a nursing diagnosis such as imbalanced nutrition, less than body requirements (see Chapter 42).

Often you cannot make a precise nursing diagnosis during your first meeting with a patient. You will sometimes sense that a problem or health concern exists, but you do not have sufficient data to make a specific diagnosis. Some patients' physical conditions limit their ability to tell you about their symptoms. Other patients may choose not to share sensitive and important information during your initial assessment. For example, patients who live with mental illness or human immunodeficiency virus (HIV) may fear discrimination if they reveal their diagnosis. Other patients' behaviours and physical responses, such as those related to post-traumatic stress disorder (PTSD), may become observable only under certain conditions not present during your initial assessment. When you are uncertain of a diagnosis, continue data collection until you are able to determine the patient's unique situation.

In diagnostic reasoning, use patient data that you gather to logically explain a clinical judgement. For example, after turning a patient over in bed, you see an area of redness and a small blister on his right hip. You palpate the area and note that it is warm to the touch, and the patient complains of tenderness there. You push on the area with your finger, and, after you release pressure, the area does not blanch or turn white. You think about what you know about normal skin integrity and the effects of pressure. You form the conclusion the patient has a stage I pressure injury. As a new student, confirm your judgement with experienced nurses. At times, your clinical judgement may be incorrect (e.g., a blistered area is indicative of a stage II pressure injury [RNAO, 2016a]); however, nurse experts will give you feedback to build on in future clinical situations.

Nurses do not make medical diagnoses, but they do assess and monitor patients closely and compare the patient's signs and symptoms with those that are common to a medical diagnosis. This type of diagnostic reasoning helps nurses and other health care providers pinpoint the nature of a problem more quickly and select proper interventions. Similarities and differences between medical and nursing diagnoses are described in more detail in Chapter 13.

Clinical reasoning is a term that is also used to describe the cognitive process of thinking about patient issues, making inferences, and deciding on the actions to be implemented in a particular situation. Engaging in clinical reasoning involves collecting cues, processing information, coming to understand the patient problem or situation, planning and implementing interventions, evaluating outcomes, and reflecting on and learning from the process. As you gain experience in nursing, your ability to identify the salient aspects of patient situations and to differentiate between clinical problems that require immediate attention (difficulty breathing due to an adverse medication reaction) and those that are less acute (shortness of breath related to chronic pulmonary disease) will increase. As a result, you will be able to accurately identify patients who are at greatest risk of complications, make sound clinical judgements about how to intervene, and manage complex clinical situations effectively (Levett-Jones, Hoffman, Dempsey, et al., 2010).

Strategies such as "thinking-out-loud" (verbalizing your thinking) as you work through a simulated patient care scenario can be useful in honing your clinical reasoning skills (Forsberg, Ziegert, Hult, et al., 2014; Tanner, 2006). Using clinical reasoning, nursing knowledge, and other evidence to inform decision making in diverse practice situations enables you to provide safe, competent, compassionate, ethical, and culturally safe care to patients and families (CASN, 2015a, p. 13). Clinical reasoning incorporates critical thinking and is essential to sound clinical decision making.

Clinical Decision Making. Clinical decision making focuses on defining patient problems and selecting appropriate interventions. When you approach a clinical problem, such as a patient who is experiencing difficulty walking, you make a decision that identifies the problem (e.g., right-sided weakness) and choose nursing interventions (e.g., teach the use of appropriate assistive devices) for that patient. Use of clinical decision making distinguishes professional nurses from technical personnel. It is the professional nurse, for example, who takes immediate action when a patient's clinical condition deteriorates, decides whether a patient is experiencing complications that call for notification of a physician, or decides whether a teaching plan for a patient is ineffective and needs revision. Benner (1984) described clinical decision making as judgement that includes critical and reflective thinking and action and the application of scientific and practical knowledge.

Clinical judgement requires that you recognize the salient aspects of a clinical situation, interpret their meanings, and respond appropriately. It includes four components: noticing or grasping the situation; interpreting or developing a sufficient understanding of the situation to respond; responding or deciding on a course of action; and reflecting on or reviewing the actions taken and their outcomes. In making a clinical judgement, you consider the context of the situation and rely on analytical processes, intuition, and narrative thinking (i.e., thinking that occurs as a result of telling and interpreting stories). As you reflect on actions taken, you acquire clinical learning, which contributes to future clinical judgements (Tanner, 2006).

Nurses regularly encounter practice situations in which little is straightforward (Hartrick Doane & Brown, 2011). Each patient's problems are unique and products of many factors, including the patient's physical health, lifestyle, culture, relationship with family and friends, living environment, and experiences. Clinical decision making requires careful reasoning so that you choose the options for the best patient outcomes on the basis of the patient's condition, the priority of the problem, or health concern.

You improve your clinical decision making by knowing your patients. For example, an expert nurse who has worked on a general surgery unit for many years is more likely to detect signs of internal hemorrhage (e.g., fall in blood pressure, rapid pulse, change in consciousness) than is a new nurse. Over time, a combination of knowledge, experience, time spent in a specific clinical area, and the quality of relationships formed with patients allow expert nurses to know clinical situations and quickly anticipate and select the right course of action (Tanner, Benner, Chesla, et al., 1993). Spending more time during initial patient assessments to both observe patient behaviour and measure physical findings is a way to better know your patients. Accounts of patients' health challenges can help you learn about their experiences through their eyes and foster empathy. Consistently monitoring patients as problems occur helps you see how clinical changes develop over time. The selection of nursing actions is built on both clinical knowledge and patient data, including the following:

- The identified status and situation of the patient
- Knowledge about the clinical variables (e.g., patient's age, seriousness of the problem, pathological process of the problem, patient's pre-existing disease conditions) involved in the situation and how the variables are related
- Knowledge about the usual patterns of any diagnosed problem or prognosis and a judgement about the likely course of events and outcomes of the diagnosed problem, in view of any coexisting health risks the patient also possesses
- Additional relevant information about the patient's daily living situation, functional capacity, and social resources
- Knowledge about the nursing interventions available and the way in which specific actions will predictably affect the patient's situation
- Knowledge about the patient's desired health outcomes

After determining a patient's nursing care priorities, you select actions most likely to relieve each problem or to promote health, wellness, and quality of life. A wide range of choices is often available, from nurse-administered to patient self-care strategies. You collaborate with the patient and then select, test, and evaluate the chosen approaches. Making an accurate clinical decision enables you to set priorities for nursing action. Because each situation involves different patients and different variables, a certain activity is sometimes more of a priority in one situation and less of a priority in another. For example, if a home care patient is physically dependent, unable to eat, and incontinent of urine, skin integrity is of higher priority than if the patient were immobile but continent of urine and able to eat a normal diet. Do not assume that certain health situations produce automatic priorities. For example, an adolescent who has embarked on a smoking cessation program is expected to experience some withdrawal symptoms, which often become a priority of care. However, if the patient is experiencing anxiety about potential weight gain that decreases his ability to participate fully in the program, it becomes necessary for you to focus on ways to relieve the anxiety before the smoking cessation measures will be effective.

Nurses make decisions about individual patients and about groups of patients. You need to use criteria such as the clinical condition of the patients, their specific needs, risks involved in treatment delays, and patients' expectations of care to determine which patients have the most urgent priorities for care. For example, a patient in a community care centre who is experiencing a sudden drop in blood pressure along with a change in consciousness requires your attention immediately, in contrast to a small child who requires a routine immunization or a group of expectant parents attending a prenatal class. In order for you to manage the wide variety of problems associated with groups of patients, skillful, prioritized decision making is crucial. Learning to set priorities effectively takes time and experience. Consulting with more experienced nurses and being aware that priorities may change rapidly can help you identify and deal with unexpected events (Box 12-3).

Nursing Process as a Critical Thinking Competency

Nurses apply the nursing process as a critical thinking competency when delivering patient care. The nursing process is a five-step clinical decision-making approach that consists of assessment, diagnosis, planning, implementation, and evaluation (see Chapters 13 to 14). The purpose of the nursing process is to assist nurses in identifying and treating patients' health-related concerns and help patients attain agreed-upon health outcomes (Figure 12-2). The nursing process incorporates general (e.g., scientific method, problem solving, and decision making) and specific critical thinking competencies (e.g., diagnostic reasoning, inference, and clinical decision making), described earlier in this chapter, in a manner that focuses on a particular patient's unique needs. The format of the nursing process is unique to the discipline of nursing and provides a common language and process for nurses to "think through" patients' clinical problems (Kataoka-Yahiro & Saylor, 1994). Chapter 13 describes the nursing process in more detail.

The nursing process is often called a blueprint or plan for care. When you use the nursing process, you identify a patient's health-related concerns, clearly define a nursing diagnosis or collaborative problem, determine priorities of care, and set goals and expected outcomes of care. Then you develop and communicate a plan of care, perform nursing interventions, and evaluate the effects of your care. Involving your patient in each step of the nursing process helps ensure that care is patient-centred. As you become more competent in using the nursing process, you will be able to focus on multiple problems or diagnoses and move back and forth between steps when considering all the information available to you about a patient's concerns.

Attitudes for Critical Thinking

The fourth component of the critical thinking model incorporates the attitudes needed to think critically. An important part of critical thinking is interpreting, evaluating, and making judgements about the adequacy of various arguments and available data. Attitudes determine how a successful critical thinker approaches a problem or a situation that necessitates decision making. For example, when a patient complains of anxiety before undergoing a diagnostic procedure, the curious nurse explores possible reasons for the patient's concerns. The nurse also exhibits discipline and perseverance in taking responsibility to complete a thorough assessment to find the sources of the patient's anxiety. Knowing when you need more information, knowing when information is misleading, and recognizing your own knowledge limits and personal biases are examples of how critical thinking attitudes play a key role in decision making.

Standards for Critical Thinking

The fifth component of the critical thinking model includes intellectual and professional standards (Kataoka-Yahiro & Saylor, 1994).

Intellectual Standards. An *intellectual standard* is a guideline or principle for rational thought. You apply such standards when you conduct the nursing process. When you consider a patient problem, apply intellectual standards such as thoroughness, precision, accuracy, and consistency to make sure that all clinical decisions are sound. Efficacious use of the intellectual standards in clinical practice ensures that you do not perform critical thinking haphazardly.

Professional Standards. *Professional standards* for critical thinking refer to ethical criteria for nursing judgements, evidence-informed criteria for evaluation, and criteria for professional responsibility. Professional standards promote the highest level of quality nursing care for individuals and groups in institutional and community-based settings.

Ethical Criteria for Nursing Judgement. Effective nursing practice reflects sound ethical principles. Being able to focus on a patient's values and beliefs helps you make clinical decisions that are just, faithful to the patient's choices, and beneficial to the patient's health and well-being. *The Code of Ethics for Registered Nurses* (CNA, 2017) is based on core values that serve as a guide to ethical decision making

BOX 12-3 Clinical Decision Making for Groups of Patients

- Identify the nursing diagnosis and collaborative problems of each patient.
- Analyze patients' diagnoses or problems and decide which are most urgent in light of the patient's basic needs, changing or unstable status, and problem complexity.
- Consider the resources available for managing each problem, including unregulated care providers assigned to work with you and the patients' family members.
- Consider how to involve the patients as decision makers and participants in care.
- Decide how to combine activities to resolve more than one patient problem at a time.
- Decide what, if any, nursing care procedures to delegate to unregulated care providers so that you are able to spend your time on activities requiring professional nursing knowledge.

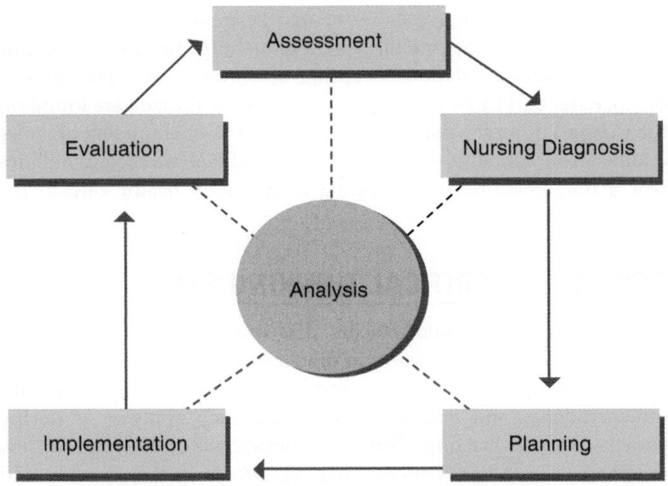

FIGURE 12-2 Five-step nursing process model.

in nursing practice. Among these values and ethical responsibilities are providing safe, compassionate, competent, and ethical care; promoting health and well-being; promoting and respecting informed decision making; preserving dignity; maintaining privacy and confidentiality; promoting justice; and being accountable. Critical thinkers maintain a sense of self-awareness through conscious awareness of their own values, beliefs, and feelings and of the multiple perspectives of patients, family members, staff, and peers in clinical situations. Chapter 7 summarizes ethical standards to use when you are faced with ethical dilemmas or problems.

One of the patients in a community health clinic is a young man who has signs and symptoms of chlamydia, a sexually transmitted infection. The patient has had the symptoms for more than 3 weeks and voices concern about what it will mean to have the infection. Richard, a nurse, examines the young man and finds that the patient has redness and itching on his penis, with a yellowish discharge. Richard checks further and asks whether the patient has pain on urination. He also assesses the patient for fever. Richard has limited knowledge about chlamydia, and so he consults with the clinic nurse practitioner, who explains the nature of the infection, the risks it poses to the patient, the usual course of treatment, and some of the legal and ethical guidelines that govern nurses' actions when working with patients with sexually transmitted infections. Richard returns to the patient and speaks confidently with him about chlamydia, the reason for his symptoms, the need to tell sex partners about the infection, and the importance of wearing a condom.

Criteria for Evaluation. Nurses routinely use evidence-informed criteria to assess patients' conditions, determine a course of action, and evaluate the efficacy of nursing interventions. For example, accurate assessment of symptoms such as pain or shortness of breath requires use of assessment criteria such as the duration, severity, location, aggravating or relieving factors, and effects on daily lifestyle (see Chapter 31). Assessment criteria enable you to accurately determine the nature of a patient's symptoms, select appropriate interventions, and later evaluate whether the interventions are effective. Another example is the use of the criteria incorporated in Best Practice Guidelines to differentiate between delirium, dementia, and depression in older persons in order to make prudent decisions about the care and services needed by patients and their caregivers to optimize clinical outcomes and reduce caregiver burden (RNAO, 2016b).

Professional Responsibility. The standards of professional responsibility that a nurse strives to achieve are the standards cited in institutional practice guidelines, professional organizations' standards of practice, and legislation governing nursing practice. The nursing practice standards that govern nurses' actions in Canada are found on the websites of provincial and territorial professional nursing organizations. These standards outline the responsibilities and accountabilities that a nurse assumes in providing high-quality health care to the public.

DEVELOPING CRITICAL THINKING SKILLS

To develop critical thinking skills, it is important to learn how to connect knowledge and theory in practice. Making sense of what you learn in the classroom, from reading, or from dialogue with patients, other students, and health providers and then applying it during patient care is challenging. Using strategies such as case-based learning, reflective writing, and concept mapping will help you develop and refine your critical thinking skills.

Case-Based Learning

Case-based learning is a strategy that helps you to explore complex problems and engage in decision making without the risk of harming a patient. It includes approaches such as case studies, problem-based learning, simulation, and virtual reality. Simulation and virtual reality can be used to practise psychomotor skills to enhance your knowledge base, respond to unanticipated events in a controlled environment, and receive immediate feedback on your performance. Using these technologies you can identify knowledge gaps, learn from your mistakes in a safe environment, and enhance your ability to solve problems and make clinical judgements in increasingly complex scenarios. Case-based strategies prepare you to apply diagnostic reasoning, inference, and clinical decision making in real-life situations and are a valuable complement to your clinical practice experiences (CASN, 2015b).

Reflective Writing

Reflective writing is a tool for developing critical thought that uses the process of **reflection** to purposefully recall a situation in order to discover its purpose or meaning. Reflective writing gives you the opportunity to describe a clinical experience in your own words, explore your perceptions and understanding of the experience, and become more aware of how you use clinical decision-making skills. It invites to you to consider questions such as "What have I learned from this experience?" and "What could I have done differently?" Reflection promotes knowledge transfer by enabling you to identify how previously acquired knowledge can be applied in another situation. Reflecting on your experiences is also an important component of monitoring your competence in nursing practice.

Reflective writing can also help you learn to know your patients better, even though you may not have had similar experiences. Instead of becoming a source of fear, diversity and difference can become an opportunity for you to come to understand their experience. Reflection allows you to examine your assumptions about what it means to be of a different age, race, or sexual orientation or to suffer from a mental illness. Similarly, reflecting on visual images, narratives, poetry, music, or drama offers you opportunities to examine multiple perspectives, challenge your assumptions, and develop self-awareness and empathy (Lapum & St-Amant, 2016). Box 12-4 reports on a research study in which photovoice was used as a tool in getting to know patients and their experiences.

Concept Mapping

As a nurse, you care for patients who have multiple nursing diagnoses. A **concept map** is a visual representation of patient problems and interventions that depicts their relationships to one another. Drawing a concept map can help you synthesize relevant data about a patient, including assessment data, health needs, nursing diagnoses, nursing interventions, and evaluation measures. It also helps you move beyond memorizing, recalling facts, and focusing on tasks that need to be done to organizing or linking information in a unique way so that the diverse information you have about a patient begins to connect to form meaningful patterns and concepts. When you see the relationship between the various patient diagnoses and the assessment data that support them, you gain a holistic understanding of a patient's clinical situation.

Concept maps take many visual forms (see Chapters 39 and 41 for examples). Select a format that allows the concept map to become a "living" document that can change as you develop and document your plan of care for the patient over time. The final map gives you a broader and more complex understanding of your patient's health care needs and demonstrates your integration of theory into practice. Save the

BOX 12-4 RESEARCH HIGHLIGHT

In Her Own Eyes: Photovoice As an Innovative Methodology to Reach Disadvantaged Single Mothers

Focus

Photovoice enables research participants to use cameras to capture issues central to their lives. In this study (Valiquette-Tessier, Vandette, & Gosselin, 2015), researchers explored how disadvantaged mothers experienced photovoice and how its use affected their participation in a community-based program, Toward Success, which aimed to enhance their social inclusion, parenting, and coping skills.

Abstract

Six disadvantaged single mothers were provided with a digital camera and were trained in the ethics of taking photographs and the mechanical use of the camera. Over a 2-week period, they took photographs and documented each photograph in a logbook. Each mother subsequently chose six photographs that were most significant in representing her reality. This same process was repeated over the next 2 weeks, following which each mother created and presented a poster showing her work, and all participants engaged in a group discussion about the themes emerging from the pictures selected. The photographs in the posters as well as the logbooks, transcripts from the poster presentations, group discussions, and semi-structured interviews were analyzed to identify emerging themes. Among the themes were a sense of accomplishment, a deeper understanding of self and their own reality, increased optimism, a sense of being unburdened, an increased sense of agency, a feeling of being experts in their own lives, and solidarity among participants.

Evidence-Informed Practice

On the basis of this study, the authors concluded that innovative methodologies, such as photovoice, can support community empowerment by focusing on participants' strengths, as well as their challenges, and by helping communities find adaptive and relevant solutions to their own difficulties.

Reference: Valiquette-Tessier, S-C., Vandette, M-P., & Gosselin, J. (2015). In her own eyes: Photovoice as an innovative methodology to reach disadvantaged single mothers. *Canadian Journal of Community Mental Health, 34*(1), 1–16. doi:10.7870/cjcmh-2014-022

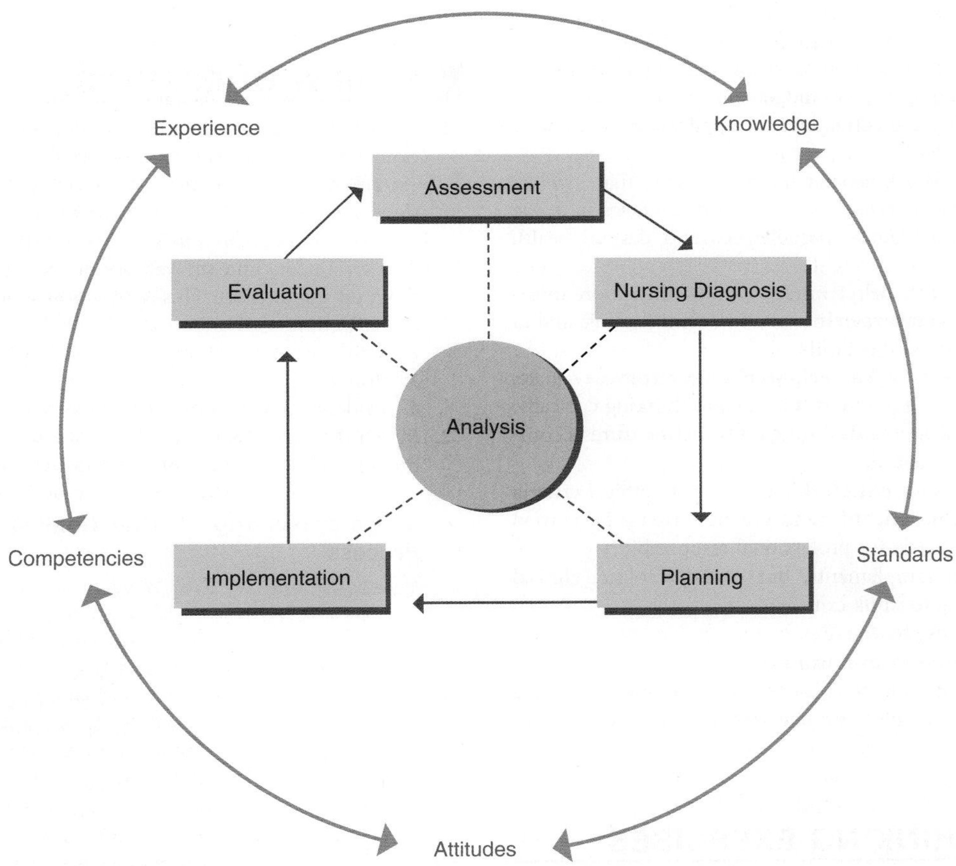

FIGURE 12-3 Synthesis of critical thinking with the nursing process competency.

concept maps you create and use them as a reference as you care for other patients with similar health concerns.

CRITICAL THINKING SYNTHESIS

Critical thinking is a reasoning process by which you use knowledge, reflect on previous experience, and integrate professional practice standards to provide competent and ethical nursing care to patients (Figure 12-3). Thinking critically requires dedication and a desire to grow intellectually. For novice nurses, it is important to learn the steps of the nursing process and to incorporate the elements of the critical thinking model in your practice. The two processes are intertwined in making quality decisions about patient care. The key components of critical thinking are integrated into other chapters in this text to help you better understand its relationship to the nursing process and make quality judgements and decisions about patient care.

KEY CONCEPTS

- Critical thinking is a process acquired through learning and experience.
- Nurses who apply critical thinking in their work focus on options for solving problems and making decisions, rather than rapidly and carelessly adopting solutions.
- Following a procedure step by step without adjusting to a patient's unique needs is an example of basic critical thinking.
- In complex critical thinking, a nurse learns that alternative and perhaps conflicting solutions to problems exist.
- The critical thinking model combines a nurse's knowledge base, experience, competence in nursing process, attitudes, and standards to explain how nurses make clinical judgements that are necessary for safe, effective nursing care.
- In diagnostic reasoning, you collect patient data and then logically develop a clinical judgement, such as a nursing diagnosis.
- When you face a clinical problem or situation and choose a course of action from several options, you are making a clinical decision.
- Clinical learning experiences are necessary for you to acquire clinical decision-making skills.
- You improve your clinical decision making by knowing your patients and including them in the decision-making process.
- Clinical decision making involves judgement that includes critical and reflective thinking and action and the application of scientific and practical knowledge.
- The nursing process is a blueprint for patient care that involves both general and specific critical thinking competencies in a way that focuses on the patient's unique needs and desired health outcomes.
- Critical thinking attitudes help a nurse to know when more information is needed, to know when information is misleading, and to recognize personal knowledge limits.
- Sound information literacy skills help you locate, retrieve, evaluate, and apply research findings and are essential to thinking critically.
- The use of intellectual standards during assessment ensures a complete database of information.
- Professional standards for critical thinking refer to ethical criteria for nursing judgements, scientific and practice criteria to be used for evaluation, and criteria for professional responsibility.
- Case-based learning complements, but cannot replace, clinical experience in learning to think critically.
- Reflective writing gives you the opportunity to define and express clinical experiences in your own words.
- Drawing a concept map enables you to gain a broader and more complex understanding of your patient's complex health care needs.

CRITICAL THINKING EXERCISES

1. You are meeting with an obese patient for the first time. She states that she has been successful in losing weight but is frustrated by her inability to maintain her weight loss. She reports having tried "virtually every fad diet" and "multiple exercise programs." She admits that as her weight increases, she tends to be become less active. She has become increasingly reluctant to leave her home because of the negative reactions of other people. In listening to her story, you attempt to imagine what it would be like to be in her situation and begin to examine your biases and assumptions about people who are obese. Your goal is to begin to discuss potential options with her for dealing with her situation. Describe the level of critical thinking that is necessary in this scenario and how it will assist you in helping this patient develop an effective plan of action.
2. Mr. Yousif is a terminally ill patient receiving home care. His wife and son are asking you about his pain control. Mrs. Yousif is requesting that her husband's medication be increased, even if it means he will be less responsive. She does not want her husband to suffer. The son is vehemently opposed to too much narcotic and feels that his father is still able to make decisions for himself. Mr. Yousif remains alert much of the time and is able to talk with you about his pain, his feelings regarding death. and his desire to die at home. How might you use critical thinking to help the family resolve this complex problem?
3. Reflect on a situation in which you needed to provide care to someone from a distinctly different culture. Construct a concept map that illustrates your approach to this situation. What were the key health challenges of concern to the patient? How were they related to each other? How did you approach knowing the patient? How did your beliefs and assumptions about the patient's culture change over time? What factors contributed to this change? Try to incorporate these factors into your concept map.

REVIEW QUESTIONS

1. You are scheduled to begin a clinical placement in an immunization clinic and are aware that some parents in the community are extremely concerned about the safety of childhood immunizations. Prior to your first day in the clinic, you conduct a comprehensive Internet search to learn more about the potential sources of their anxiety and the validity of the information available to them on the Internet. This is an example of:
   1. Reflection
   2. Truth-seeking
   3. Problem solving
   4. Evidence-informed decision making
2. Match the questions on the left with the appropriate step in the nursing process on the right.

Stage of Nursing Process	Question
1. Assessment	a. What actions will help the patient achieve his or her desired outcomes?
2. Nursing diagnosis	b. How will I know if the patient has achieved his or her desired outcomes?
3. Planning	c. How can I help the patient achieve his or her desired outcomes?
4. Implementation	d. What is the patient's health-related concern?
5. Evaluation	e. What are the patient's desired health outcomes?

3. A nurse uses an institution's procedure manual to confirm how to change a patient's nasogastric tubing. The level of critical thinking the nurse is using is
   1. Commitment
   2. Scientific method
   3. Basic critical thinking
   4. Complex critical thinking

4. A patient had hip surgery 24 hours ago. The nurse refers to the written plan of care, noting that the patient has a device collecting wound drainage. The physician is to be notified when the accumulation in the device exceeds 100 mL for the day. When the nurse enters the room, the nurse looks at the device and carefully notes the amount of drainage currently in the device. This is an example of
   1. Planning
   2. Assessment
   3. Intervention
   4. Nursing diagnosis
5. The nurse asks a patient how she feels about her impending surgery for breast cancer. Before the discussion, the nurse reviewed the description in his textbook of loss and grief in addition to therapeutic communication principles. The critical thinking component involved in the nurse's review of the literature is
   1. Experience
   2. Problem solving
   3. Knowledge application
   4. Clinical decision making
6. As the nurse enters a patient's room, she observes that the intravenous line is not infusing at the ordered rate. The nurse checks the flow regulator on the tubing, looks to see whether the patient is lying on the tubing, checks the connection between the tubing and the intravenous catheter, and then checks the condition of the site where the intravenous catheter enters the patient's skin. She readjusts the flow rate, and the infusion begins at the correct rate. This is an example of
   1. Inference
   2. Reflection
   3. Problem solving
   4. Evidence-informed decision making
7. In observing a new mother breastfeeding her baby, the public health nurse observes that the baby is fussy and is not sucking effectively. The nurse reviews the baby's record and finds that he has lost a considerable amount of weight since birth. The nurse conducts an assessment and notes that the baby has poor skin turgor. The mother reports that he urinates infrequently and sleeps only for very short periods of time between feedings. The nurse concludes that the baby is dehydrated and is at risk of becoming malnourished. This is an example of
   1. Inference
   2. Problem solving
   3. Diagnostic reasoning
   4. Applying nursing practice standards
8. Paul participates in a standardized patient simulation exercise designed to enhance therapeutic communication skills when working with clients experiencing mental health challenges. Later he asks, "What did I learn about myself that could hinder my therapeutic engagement with mental health clients? And, how can I rephrase my responses so that they do not have an unintended, detrimental effect on my nurse–patient relationships?" This is an example of
   1. Reflection
   2. Problem solving
   3. Knowing the patient
   4. Evidence-informed practice
9. Your community is engaged in a contested debate about whether or not it should open a needle-exchange program and a safe injection site for intravenous drug users. Some citizens believe that doing so condones drug abuse; others believe that such actions will reduce harm and save lives. You can appreciate both arguments but have not yet formulated your own position. Which of the following should you do in thinking critically about this complex question? *(Select all that apply)*
   1. Listen carefully to both points of view.
   2. Challenge your own beliefs about drug addiction.
   3. Examine the scientific arguments both for and against such initiatives.
   4. Support the communities that are reluctant to have the clinic in their neighbourhood.
   5. Assume that the people in authority who are speaking about the issue are well informed.
10. Match the clinical thinking skills and dispositions (habits) on the left with the corresponding critical thinking behaviour on the right.

Critical Thinking Skills and Dispositions	Critical Thinking Behaviour
1. Inference	a. Observe patterns and formulate conclusions
2. Evaluation	b. Ask how you can improve your clinical performance
3. Explanation	c. Consider opposing points of view
4. Self-regulation	d. Select criteria to assess the effectiveness of nursing interventions
5. Open-mindedness	e. Defend your conclusions

11. The nurse sits down to talk with her patient, whose sister died 2 weeks ago. The patient reports that she is unable to sleep, feels very fatigued during the day, and is having trouble at work. The nurse asks her to clarify the type of trouble, and the patient explains that she cannot concentrate or even solve simple problems. The nurse records the results of her assessment, describing the patient's problem as ineffective coping. This conclusion reflects the nurse's use of
   1. Inference
   2. Nursing process
   3. Evaluation criteria
   4. General critical thinking competencies

Answers 1. 2; **2.** 1(e); 2(d); 3(a); 4(c); 5(b); **3.** 3; **4.** 2; **5.** 3; **6.** 3; **7.** 3; **8.** 1; **9.** 1, 2, 3; **10.** 1(a); 2(d); 3(e); 4(b); 5(c); **11.** 1

Rationales for the Review Questions appear at the end of the book.

RECOMMENDED WEBSITES

Canadian Nurses Association: https://www.cna-aiic.ca/en.

A wide range of valuable resources, including the *Code of Ethics for Registered Nurses* (CNA, 2017), can be found on this website, as well as links to those of each of the provincial and territorial professional nursing associations in Canada. The position papers and other documents found on these websites demonstrate how Canadian nurse leaders have used critical thinking to explore important issues in nursing and nursing practice.

Concept Mapping Tools: https://uwaterloo.ca/centre-for-teaching-excellence/teaching-resources/teaching-tips/educational-technologies/all/concept-mapping-tools.

This site, created by the Centre for Teaching Excellence at the University of Waterloo, provides an overview of the strengths and limitations of several concept mapping tools. Other tools, including examples of nursing-related concept maps, can be accessed via the Internet.

Critical Thinking Community: http://www.criticalthinking.org.
The section of this website titled "Begin Here" includes links to a number of short articles specifically related to critical thinking in nursing and in health care. Explore the remainder of the website to locate yet other resources that may be of value to you in developing your critical thinking skills.

REFERENCES

Benner, P. (1984). *From novice to expert: Excellence and power in clinical nursing practice.* Menlo Park, CA: Addison-Wesley.

Canadian Association of Schools of Nursing/Association Canadienne des Écoles de Sciences Infirmières [CASN/ACESI]. (2015a). *National nursing education framework: Final report.* Ottawa: Author. Retrieved from http://www.casn.ca/wp-content/uploads/2014/12/Framwork-FINAL-SB-Nov-30-20151.pdf.

Canadian Association of Schools of Nursing. (2015b). *Practice domain for baccalaureate nursing education: Guidelines for clinical placements and simulation.* Ottawa: Author. Retrieved from http://www.casn.ca/wp-content/uploads/2015/11/Draft-clinical-sim-2015.pdf.

Canadian Nurses Association. (2015). *Framework for the practice of registered nurses in Canada.* Ottawa: Author. Retrieved from https://www.cna-aiic.ca/~/media/cna/page-content/pdf-en/framework-for-the-pracice-of-registered-nurses-in-canada.pdf?la=en.

Canadian Nurses Association. (2017). *Code of ethics for registered nurses.* Ottawa: Author. Retrieved from https://cna-aiic.ca/en/on-the-issues/best-nursing/nursing-ethics.

Facione, P. (1990). *Critical thinking: A statement of expert consensus for purposes of educational assessment and instruction. The Delphi report: Research findings and recommendations prepared for the American Philosophical Association.* ERIC Doc No. ED 315-423. Washington, DC: Educational Resources Information Center (ERIC).

Facione, N., & Facione, P. (1996). Externalizing the critical thinking in knowledge development and clinical judgement. *Nursing Outlook, 44,* 129–136.

Ferguson, L. M., Ward, H., Card, S., et al. (2013). Putting the 'patient' back into patient-centred care: An education perspective. *Nurse Education in Practice, 13*(4), 283–287. doi:10.1016/j.nepr.2013.03.016.

Forsberg, E., Ziegert, K., Hult, H., et al. (2014). Clinical reasoning in nursing, a think-aloud study using virtual patients—A base for an innovative assessment. *Nurse Education Today, 34,* 538–542. doi:10.1016/j.nedt.2013.07.010.

Glaser, E. (1941). *An experiment in the development of critical thinking.* New York: Bureau of Publications, Teachers College, Columbia University.

Hartrick Doane, G., & Brown, H. (2011). Recontextualizing learning in nursing education: Taking an ontological turn. *Journal of Nursing Education, 50,* 21–26. doi:10.3928/01484834-20101130-01.

Ironside, P. M. (2005). Teaching thinking and reaching the limits of memorization: Enacting new pedagogies. *Journal of Nursing Education, 44,* 441–449.

Kataoka-Yahiro, M., & Saylor, C. (1994). A critical thinking model for nursing judgment. *Journal of Nursing Education, 33*(8), 351–356.

Lapum, J. L., & St-Amant, O. (2016). Visual images in undergraduate nursing education. *Nurse Educator, 41*(3), 112–114. doi:10.1097/NNE.0000000000000214.

Levett-Jones, T., Hoffman, K., Dempsey, J., et al. (2010). The 'five rights' of clinical reasoning: An educational model to enhance nursing students' ability to identify and manage clinically 'at risk' patients. *Nurse Education Today, 30,* 515–520. doi:10.1016/j.nedt.2009.10.020.

LoBiondo-Wood, G., Haber, J., Cameron, C., et al. (2017). *Nursing research in Canada: Methods, critical appraisal, and utilization* (4th ed.). Toronto: Elsevier Canada.

Meherali, S. M., Profetto-McGrath, J., & Paul, P. (2015). Nursing students clinical thinking and research utilization. *Quality Advancement in Nursing Education/Avancées en formation infirmière, 1*(3), doi:10.17483/2368-6669.1052. Article 3.

Miller, M. A., & Malcolm, N. S. (1990). Critical thinking in the nursing curriculum. *Nursing and Health Care, 11,* 66–73.

Paul, R. W. (1993). The art of redesigning instruction. In J. Willsen & A. J. A. Blinker (Eds.), *Critical thinking: How to prepare students for a rapidly changing world.* Santa Rosa, CA: Foundation for Critical Thinking.

Perry, W. (1979). *Forms of intellectual and ethical development in the college years: A scheme.* New York: Holt, Rinehart, & Winston.

Registered Nurses' Association of Ontario (RNAO). (2016a). *Assessment and management of pressure injuries for the interprofessional team* (3rd ed.). Toronto: Author. Retrieved from http://rnao.ca/bpg/guidelines/pressure-injuries.

Registered Nurses' Association of Ontario (RNAO). (2016b). *Delirium, dementia, and depression in older adults: Assessment and care.* Toronto: Author. Retrieved from http://rnao.ca/sites/rnao-ca/files/DDD_BPG.pdf.

Tanner, C. (2006). Thinking like a nurse: A research-based model of clinical judgment in nursing. *Journal of Nursing Education, 45,* 204–211.

Tanner, C. A., Benner, P., Chesla, C., et al. (1993). The phenomenology of knowing the patient. *Image: Journal of Nursing Scholarship, 25,* 273–280.

Thorne, S. (2008). *Interpretive description.* Walnut Creek, CA: Left Coast Press.

Valiquette-Tessier, S.-C., Vandette, M.-P., & Gosselin, J. (2015). In her own eyes: Photovoice as an innovative methodology to reach disadvantaged single mothers. *Canadian Journal of Community Mental Health, 34*(1), 1–16. doi:10.7870/cjcmh-2014-022.

13

Nursing Assessment, Diagnosis, and Planning

Canadian content written by Marnie L. Kramer, RN, PhD, Shawna M. Ryan, RN, MN
Original chapter by Patricia A. Potter, RN, MSN, PhD, FAAN

OBJECTIVES

Mastery of content in this chapter will enable you to:

- Define the key terms listed.
- Identify and discuss the steps of nursing assessment.
- Explain the relationship of critical thinking to assessment, diagnosis, and planning.
- Differentiate between subjective and objective data.
- Discuss the purposes of a client interview and the use of interview techniques in obtaining a health history.
- Describe the components of a nursing history.
- Describe the relationship between data collection and data analysis.
- Explain the relationship between data interpretation, validation, and clustering.
- Differentiate between a nursing diagnosis, medical diagnosis, and collaborative problem.
- Describe the steps of the nursing diagnostic process.
- Explain the benefit of using the NANDA International nursing diagnoses in practice.
- Describe sources of diagnostic errors.
- Identify nursing diagnoses from a nursing assessment.
- Discuss criteria used in a priority setting.
- Describe goal setting and discuss the difference between a goal and an expected outcome.
- Develop a plan of care from a nursing assessment.

KEY TERMS

Actual nursing diagnosis, p. 199
Assessment, p. 188
Client-centred goal, p. 205
Client-centred plan of care, p. 200
Clinical criteria, p. 198
Closed-ended questions, p. 193
Collaborative problem, p. 196
Concept map, p. 195
Consultation, p. 207
Critical pathways, p. 207
Cue, p. 189
Data analysis, p. 195
Database, p. 189
Defining characteristics, p. 197
Diagnosis, p. 188
Diagnostic label, p. 199
Etiology, p. 199
Evaluation, p. 188
Expected outcomes, p. 204
Goals, p. 204
Health promotion nursing diagnosis, p. 199
Implementation, p. 188
Inference, p. 191
Interview, p. 192
Kardex, p. 207
Long-term goal, p. 205
Medical diagnosis, p. 196
NANDA International, p. 198
Nursing care plan, p. 206
Nursing diagnosis, p. 196
Nursing health history, p. 189
Nursing process, p. 188
Nursing-sensitive client outcome, p. 206
Objective data, p. 191
Open-ended questions, p. 193
Planning, p. 188
Priority setting, p. 203
Related factor, p. 199
Review of systems, p. 190
Risk nursing diagnosis, p. 199
Short-term goal, p. 205
Standard, p. 188
Subjective data, p. 191
Validation, p. 194
Wellness nursing diagnosis, p. 199

ⓔ MEDIA RESOURCES

http://evolve.elsevier.com/Canada/Potter/fundamentals/

- Audio Chapter Summaries
- Examination Review Questions
- Concept Map Creator
- Case Study with Questions
- Audio Glossary
- Content Updates
- Video Clips

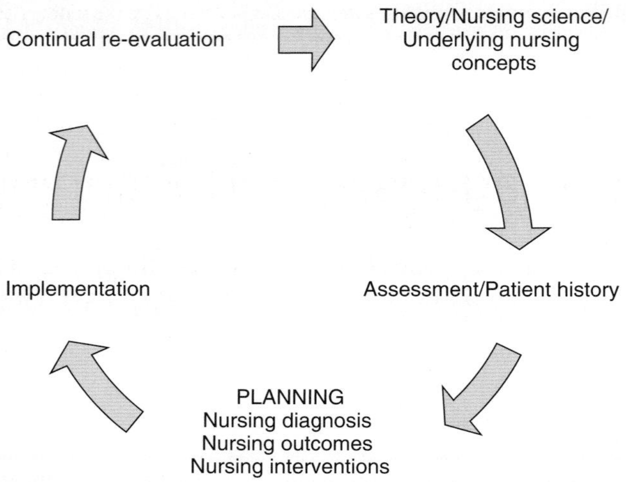

FIGURE 13-1 The modified nursing process. (From NANDA International. [2018]. *Nursing diagnoses: Definitions and classification, 2018–2020* [11th edition]. New York: Thieme [p. 36, Fig 5.2].)

When providing nursing care, nurses engage in an intellectual process of reasoning—the **nursing process** (University of British Columbia, n.d.). It is a cognitive framework through which one aims to identify, diagnose, and treat actual and potential health issues and challenges of clients from a holistic perspective. As a nursing student, you will begin by learning the steps of the nursing process: assessment, diagnosis, planning, implementation, and evaluation. As you gain familiarity with the nursing process, you will learn that it is not a linear approach; rather, the steps of the nursing process are unified and continuously relate to each other (Zamanzadeh, Valizadeh, Tabrizi, et al., 2015) (Figure 13-1). The nursing process guides clinical judgement, decision making, and reflective nursing practice when used in a manner that encourages critical thinking in each of the steps (Alfaro-Lefevre, 2012; Ofi & Sowunmi, 2012).

The nursing process begins with the first step, **assessment**, which is the collection of pertinent data to the client's health status or situation. While the client may come to the nurse with one problem in mind, the nurse spends time collecting a variety of different types of data in order to fully understand the client's priority needs. It is imperative to complete "holistic and comprehensive assessment of diverse clients, to plan and provide competent, ethical, safe compassionate nursing care" (Canadian Association of Schools of Nursing [CASN], 2015, Competency 3.1). In the next step, **diagnosis**, the nurse analyzes the assessment data in order to determine key issues and make clinical judgements in the form of a *nursing diagnosis.* This step is important because it directs the plan of care for the client. In this process, the nurse will *identify outcomes* for the client that are individualized to the client and his or her current situation. The next step is **planning**, which involves the creation of a formal plan that prescribes strategies and alternatives to attain the expected outcomes. The nurse then carries out **implementation** of the plan. This may occur by coordinating care delivery, providing health teaching and health promotion activities to the client, consulting with other health care providers, or providing medications or other therapies within the scope of practice of the registered nurse. Finally, the nurse conducts an **evaluation** of the client's response to the selected interventions and determines whether the interventions were effective.

Consider the following scenario:

Mr. Fletcher is a 56-year-old client who has been experiencing headaches and dizziness for the past 2 months. He lives in a rural community and works 12-hour shifts as a haul truck operator in an open pit coal mine. Mr. Fletcher is 23 kg overweight and has a sedentary lifestyle. He has been married for 25 years and has two grown children who no longer live at home. Mr. Fletcher recently attended a blood pressure clinic where he was told he had "high blood pressure". He has been referred to his local general practitioner for follow-up and the primary health care nurse is preparing to complete his initial health history and assessment. Mr. Fletcher has brought his wife with him for his clinic visit.

CRITICAL THINKING APPROACH TO ASSESSMENT

Assessment is the deliberate and systematic collection of data to determine a client's current and past health and functional status and to determine the client's present and past coping patterns (Carpenito, 2013). Nursing assessment consists of the following:

- Collection and verification of data from a primary source (the client) and secondary sources (e.g., family, health providers, and client record)
- The analysis of all data as a basis for developing nursing diagnoses, identifying collaborative problems, and developing a plan of individualized care

The purpose of assessment is to establish an individualized database about the client's health status to include his or her perceived needs, health challenges, and problems and to respond to these challenges or problems (Carpenito, 2013).

Nurses observe each client's behaviour, ask questions about the nature of the problem, listen to the cues that the client provides, and conduct a physical examination (see Chapter 32 for further information about conducting a health assessment). Sometimes they also interview family members who are familiar with the client's health problem and review any existing medical record data. It is important that nurses understand that the "coordination of client care in collaboration with individuals, families and other members of the health care team" is completed in all phases of the nursing process (CASN, 2015, Competency 3.10). All of the data collected form different sets or patterns of information that point to a diagnostic conclusion. Similarly, once a nurse understands the nature and source of a client's health problems, the nurse is able to provide client-focused interventions that will restore, maintain, or improve the client's health.

Critical thinking is foundational to a comprehensive and accurate nursing assessment (see Chapter 12 for further information about critical thinking). Critical thinking enables the nurse to have a broader perspective from which to form conclusions and make decisions about a client's health condition. While gathering data about a client, the nurse synthesizes relevant knowledge, recalls prior clinical experiences, applies critical thinking **standards** and available evidence, and uses standards of practice directing assessment in a meaningful and purposeful way (Figure 13-2). A nurse's knowledge of the physical, biological, and social sciences enables the nurse to ask relevant questions and collect history and physical assessment data relevant to the client's presenting health care needs. By using good communication skills and critical thinking intellectual standards, nurses collect complete, accurate, and relevant data.

Figure 13-2 highlights how critical thinking impacts the assessment process. Assessment is more than collecting data on a client; it also involves collecting the right data in a way that elicits openness from the client and integrates the nurse's knowledge base and experience. Nurses use provincial and national standards to guide their care and ensure best practice during this process. Most importantly, nurses who have strong assessment skills demonstrate an ability to be focused, detailed, and creative in their approach to assessment.

◆ ASSESSMENT

Nurses begin their assessment by documenting a comprehensive **nursing health history**, a detailed **database** that allows them to plan and carry out nursing care to meet clients' needs. Box 13-1 presents guidelines for documenting a comprehensive history. The goal of the health history is to focus on the client's strengths and available supports while also highlighting pressing or potential health challenges. As a nurse begins client assessment, he or she needs to think critically about what to assess. On the basis of the nurse's clinical knowledge and experience and the client's health history and responses, the nurse will determine what questions or measurements are appropriate. When a nurse first meets a client, the nurse makes a quick observational overview or screening. Usually an overview is based on a treatment situation. For example, a community health nurse assesses the neighbourhood and the community of the client; an emergency room nurse uses the circulation-airway-breathing (CAB) sequence; and an oncology nurse focuses on the client's symptoms from disease and treatment and on the grief response (Heart and Stroke Foundation of Canada, 2015).

Nurses learn to differentiate important data from the total data collected (Sullivan, 2012). A **cue** is information that a nurse obtains

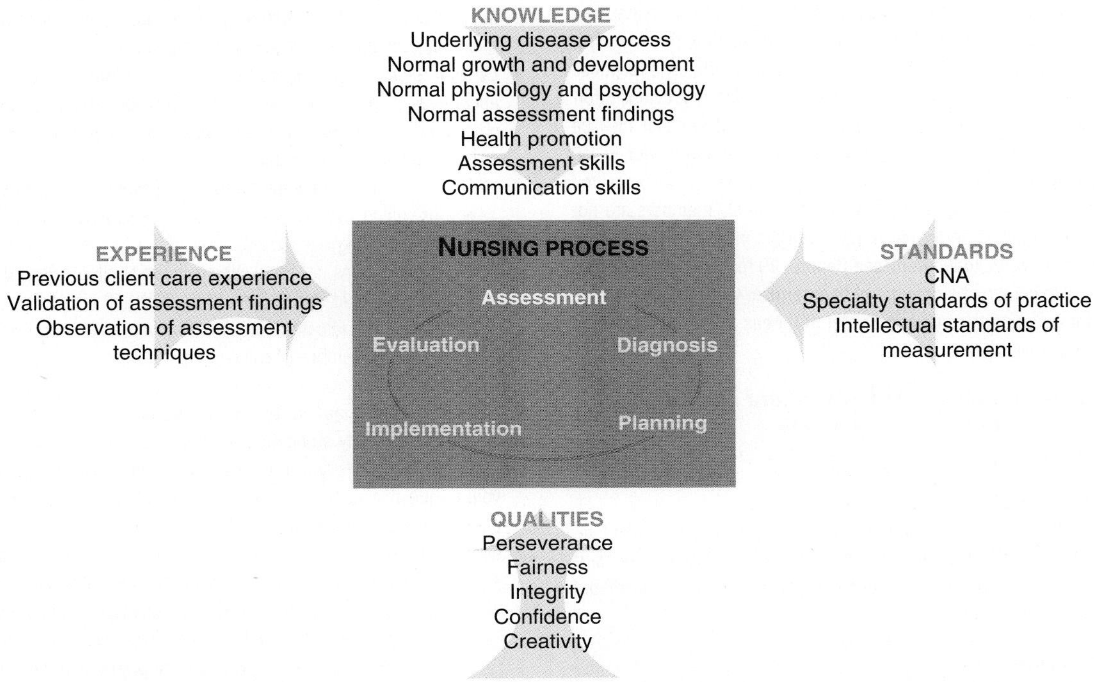

FIGURE 13-2 Critical thinking and the assessment process. *CNA,* Canadian Nurses Association.

BOX 13-1 Guidelines for Documenting a Comprehensive Nursing Health History

A. Identifying Data
- Name, age, sex, date, and place of birth

B. Source of History
- Relationship to client, any special circumstances, such as use of interpreter

C. Reason for Health History Interview
- Explain why you are interviewing the client at the present time (e.g., the client has just been admitted to an inpatient unit or clinic).

D. Current State of Health
- General state of physical, mental, social, and spiritual health, and health goals. If an illness is present, gather data about the nature of the illness by conducting a symptom analysis (see Chapter 32).

E. Developmental Variables
- Relationship status: single, married, partner, separated, widowed, divorced
- Number of children
- Developmental stage (see Chapter 21)
- Current occupation
- Significant life experiences (e.g., education, previous occupations, financial situations, retirement, coping or stress tolerance, and measures normally used to reduce stress)
- Safety hazards (e.g., biological, chemical, ergonomic, physical, psychosocial, reproductive)
- Housing, environmental hazards (e.g., type of housing, location, living arrangements; specific hazards in the home or community)
- Safety measures (e.g., use of seat belts, helmets, presence of smoke detectors and fire extinguishers, and other measures related to specific hazards of work, community, and home)

F. Psychological Variables
- Mental processes, relationships, support systems, statements regarding client's feelings about self

Continued

BOX 13-1 Guidelines for Documenting a Comprehensive Nursing Health History—cont'd

G. Spiritual Variables (see Chapter 28 for further information about spiritual health)

- Rituals, religious practices, beliefs about life, client's source of guidance in acting on beliefs, and the relationship with family in exercising faith

H. Sociocultural Variables

- Culture: values, beliefs and practices related to health and illness (see Chapter 9)
- Primary language and other languages spoken
- Recreation (exercise, hobbies, socializing, use of leisure time)
- Family and significant others, such as authorized representative, i.e., enduring power of attorney. Include family composition, relationships, special problems experienced by family, client's and family's response to stress, roles, and support systems. The family history provides information about family structure, interaction, and function that may be useful in planning care. For example, a cohesive, supportive family can help a client adjust to an illness or disability and should be incorporated into the plan of care. However, if the client's family members are not supportive, it may be better not to involve them in care.
- Outline a family tree (genogram; see Chapter 19 for further information about how to construct a genogram) to determine whether the client is at risk for genetic illnesses and to identify areas of health promotion and illness prevention.

I. Physiological Variables (Body Structure and Function)

History of Past Illnesses and Injuries

- Include dates

Current Medications

- Prescribed, over-the-counter, or illicit drugs. Include name, dosage, schedule, duration of and reason for use, and expected effects and adverse effects; if illicit drug, include type, amount, response, adverse reaction, drug-related accidents or arrests, attempts to quit

Review of Systems

The **review of systems** is a systematic method for collecting data on all body systems. Not all questions in each system may be covered in every history. Nevertheless, some questions about each system are included, particularly when a client mentions a symptom or sign. The nurse begins with questions about the usual functioning of each body system and any noted changes and follows with specific questions, such as the ones noted as follows for each system. Nurses also focus on measures taken by the client to promote and maintain health and those to prevent illness or injury. Therefore, after a set of questions is asked, the nurse will always follow up with a review of health promotion activities. The following are included in the review of systems:

- *General overall health state:* Ask how the client feels overall ("Have you experienced any recent health changes or symptoms?"), fever, chills, malaise, pain, sleep patterns and disturbances, fatigue, recent alterations in weight
- *Integumentary:* itching, colour or texture change, lesions, dryness and use of creams or lotions, changes in hair or nails
- *Ocular:* visual acuity, blurring, eye pain, recent change in vision, discharge, excessive tearing, date of last examination
- *Auditory:* hearing loss, pain, discharge, dizziness, perception of ringing in ears, wax
- *Upper respiratory:* nosebleeds, nasal discharge, nasal allergies, sinus problems, frequency of colds and usual method of treatment, sore throat and usual type of home remedy, hoarseness or voice changes
- *Lower respiratory:* use of tobacco (amount and number of years of smoking; exposure to tobacco smoke; if smoker, attempts to stop smoking), exposure to airborne pollutants, cough, sputum, wheezing, shortness of breath, tuberculosis test and results, date of last chest X-ray examination
- *Breasts and axillae:* rashes, lumps, discharge, pain, breast self-examination practices
- *Lymphatic:* pain, swelling
- *Cardiovascular:* chest pain or distress, precipitating causes, timing and duration, relieving factors, dyspnea, orthopnea, edema, hypertension, exercise tolerance, circulatory problems, varicose veins
- *Gastrointestinal:* appetite, digestion, food intolerance, dysphagia, heartburn, abdominal pain, nausea or vomiting, bowel regularity, use of laxatives, change in stool colour or contents, constipation or diarrhea, flatulence, hemorrhoids, rectal examinations
  - *Dietary pattern:* calculate number of servings per day of each of the food groups, using *Canada's Food Guide to Healthy Eating* (Health Canada, 2011) for serving size (see Chapter 42 for further information about nutrition); restrictions to food choice; special diets; use of salt; calculate adequacy of fluid intake (should be 30 to 40 mL of fluid per kilogram of body weight); indicate sources of calcium and amounts per day; alcohol use (average number of ounces per week, recent changes in pattern of consumption)
- *Urinary:* painful urination; blood, stones, or pus in urine; bladder or kidney infections; difficulty stopping urinary stream; dribbling or hesitancy; sudden feeling of need to urinate; frequent urination; nocturia (having to get up to void during the night); incontinence (see Chapter 43 for further information about urinary elimination)
- *Genital and reproductive:*
  - *Male:* puberty onset, difficulty with erections, emissions, testicular pain, libido, infertility, urethral discharge, genital lesions, exposure to and history of sexually transmitted infections, testicular self-examinations, testicular lump or pain, hernias, sexual preference, birth control method, safer sex practices used
  - *Female:* menses (onset, duration, regularity, flow, discomfort, date of most recent menstrual period), age at menopause (occurrence of hot flashes, night sweats, vaginal discharge), date of last Pap smear, pregnancies (number, miscarriages, abortions), exposure to and history of sexually transmitted infections, sexual preference, birth control method, safer sex practices used
- *Musculoskeletal:* pain, joint stiffness or swelling, restricted motion, muscle wasting, weakness, general mobility, use of mobility aids, ability to perform activities of daily living
- *Neurological:* injury, headaches, dizziness, fainting, abnormalities of sensation or coordination, tremors, seizures
- *Endocrine:* excessive sweating, thirst, hunger, or urination; intolerance of heat or cold; changes in distribution of facial hair; thyroid enlargement or tenderness; unexplained weight change; change in glove or shoe size
- *Hematological:* anemia, bruise or bleed easily, transfusions
- *Psychiatric:* depression, mood changes, difficulty concentrating, nervousness, anxiety, suicidal thoughts, irritability
- *Immunological:* communicable diseases (indicate disease and age at or year of onset), immunization status (indicate year of most recent immunization), allergies (known allergens and reactions; MedicAlert identification worn)

Adapted from Jarvis, C., Browne, A. J., MacDonald-Jenkins, J., Luctkar-Flude, M. (2014). *Physical examination & health assessment* (2nd Canadian ed., pp. 69–72). Toronto: Elsevier.

through use of the senses. An **inference** is one's judgement or interpretation of those cues. For example, a client's crying is a cue that can imply fear or sadness. The nurse asks the client about any concerns and makes known any nonverbal expressions noticed in an effort to direct the client to share his or her feelings. It is possible to miss important cues when a nurse conducts an initial overview. However, with creativity, flexibility, inquisitiveness, intuition, and open-mindedness the nurse can become aware of unusual or unexpected cues (Lunney, 2009).

As nurses collect data, they begin to categorize cues, make inferences, and identify emerging patterns, potential problem areas, and solutions. To do this well, nurses critically anticipate patterns, problems, and solutions, staying a step ahead in their assessment. Once the nurse asks a client a question or makes an observation, the information "branches" to an additional series of questions or observations (Figure 13-3). It is key that nurses anticipate assessment questions or the

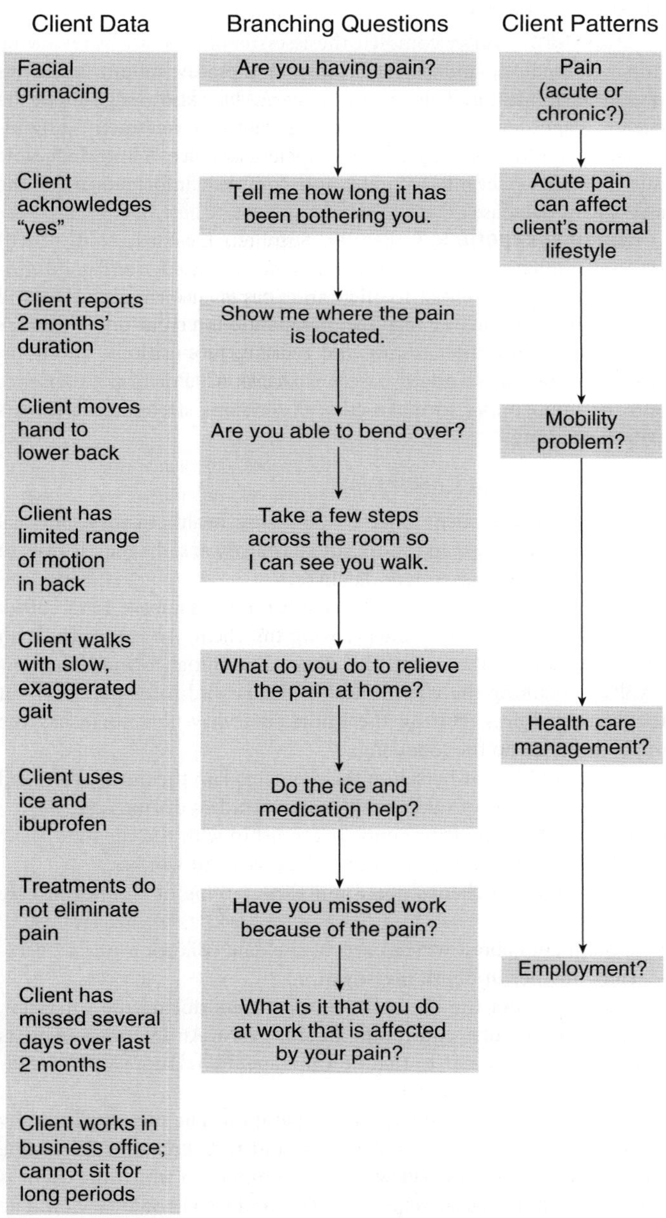

FIGURE 13-3 Example of branching logic for selecting assessment questions.

overall assessment may be incomplete or the nurse may miss relevant problem areas. Nurses learn to hone these skills and anticipate which questions to ask as they become more experienced in their practice.

Types of Data

Client data can be categorized in two ways: subjective and objective. **Subjective data** are clients' verbal descriptions of their health concerns. Subjective data are obtained through the health history and the nurse's questions and the explanation the client provides (Jarvis, Browne, MacDonald-Jenkins, et al., 2014). Only clients provide subjective data. Subjective data usually include feelings, perceptions, and self-report of symptoms. Although only clients provide subjective data relevant to their health condition, the data sometimes reflect physiological changes, which nurses further explore through objective data collection. For example, a client may state she feels nauseous. The nurse will then collect further data to support this symptom.

Objective data are observations or measurements of a client's health status. Inspection of the condition of a wound, description of an observed behaviour, and measurement of blood pressure are examples of objective data. The measurement of objective data is based on an accepted standard, such as the Celsius measure on a thermometer, centimetres on a measuring tape, or known characteristics of behaviours (e.g., anxiety or fear). Objective data may be considered a normal or abnormal finding. When nurses collect objective data, they apply critical thinking standards (e.g., whether the data are clear, precise, and consistent) to help interpret their findings. In the previous example of the subjective symptom of nausea, vomiting (emesis) would be a piece of objective data that would support this symptom.

Sources of Data

Nurses obtain data from a variety of sources. Each source of data provides information about the client's level of wellness, strengths, anticipated prognosis, risk factors, health practices and goals, and patterns of health and illness. Sources of data include primary, secondary, and tertiary sources (Nugent & Vitale, 2015, p. 70) (Box 13-2). The only *primary source* of data is the client. While *secondary sources* include information from someplace other than the client, this may include family members and the client's medical records. *Tertiary*

BOX 13-2 Sources of Data

Primary Sources

- Client
  Example: Client's description of the presenting problem and medical history, narratives of health experiences

Secondary Sources

Sources Outside the Client

- Client chart
  Examples: nursing notes/charting, physician progress notes, medication administration record, diagnostic and laboratory tests, interdisciplinary team notes. It is important to note that the client is dynamic and changing—chart data show the client's history and may not reflect the current health status of the client
- Family members/significant others

Tertiary Sources

Provide information to client's frame of reference (e.g., illness conditions)

- Relevant literature
- Nurse's experience (e.g. accepted commonalities among clients with similar physical and emotional responses) (Nugent & Vitale, 2015)

sources provide information outside the specific client's frame of reference and are a result of the nurse's or other health care team member's response to care. Sources include textbooks, a nurse's experience, and patterns noticed in other clients with similar presentations and conditions (p. 70).

Primary Sources

Client. A client is usually the nurse's best source of information. Clients who are conscious, alert, and able to answer questions correctly provide the most accurate information about their health care needs, lifestyle patterns, current and past illnesses, perception of symptoms, and changes in activities of daily living. Nurses always need to consider the setting for their assessment. It is important that the client has privacy and feels safe in disclosing health information. The nurse must also take the current situation into account when taking a health history. For example, a client experiencing acute symptoms in an emergency department will not offer as much information as one who comes to an outpatient clinic for a routine check-up. It is imperative that the nurse demonstrate a caring presence with the client by actively listening to the client's concerns and engaging in caring behaviours while completing an assessment (see Chapter 17 for further information about communication skills). In some instances, the use of a translator may be indicated when gathering primary data from the client. It is important to ensure that the nurse completes an accurate history and attends when a translator is being utilized for the client.

Secondary Sources

Family and Significant Others. Family members and significant others can be the most knowledgeable sources of information for infants or children, critically ill adults, and mentally challenged, disoriented, or unconscious clients. In cases of severe illness or emergency situations, families are sometimes the only available sources of information for nurses and the clients' health care providers. The family and significant others are important secondary sources of information. They confirm findings that a client provides (e.g., whether a client takes medications regularly at home or how well the client sleeps or eats). In cases where a language barrier exists, families can often assist in gathering information from the client in immediate situations. However, it is important to note that the nurse includes the family only when appropriate. A client may not always want the nurse to question the family or may not wish to reveal certain information in front of family members. It is important for the nurse to ask the client privately if he or she would like the family present during a health history and to always ask permission to have family or other health providers in the room while conducting a physical assessment.

Spouses or close friends often sit in during an assessment and provide their view of the client's health problems or needs. They not only supply information about the client's current health status but are able to tell when changes in the client's status occurred. Family members are often well informed because of their experiences living with the client and observing how health problems affect daily living activities. Family and friends make important observations about the client's needs that can affect the way care is delivered (e.g., how a client eats a meal or how a client makes choices). It is important to note the difference between using the family as a source of data and family nursing. *Family nursing* is a comprehensive primary care approach to the health of the entire family (see Chapter 19) that extends beyond collecting additional data about the client.

Health Care Team. Nurses frequently communicate with other health care team members in gathering information about clients. In the acute care setting, the change-of-shift report is a way for nurses from one shift to communicate information to nurses on the next shift (see Chapter 15 for further information about documentation). When nurses, physicians, physiotherapists, social workers, or other staff consult about a client's condition, they typically have information about the client. This information may include how the client is interacting within the health care environment, the client's physical or emotional reactions to treatment, the result of diagnostic procedures or therapies, and how the client responds to visitors. Every member of the team is a source of information for identifying and verifying information about the client.

Medical Records. The medical record is a source of the client's medical history, laboratory and diagnostic test results, current physical findings, and the medical treatment plan. Data in the records offer baseline and ongoing information about the client's response to illness and progress to date. Information in a client's record is confidential. The medical record is a valuable tool for checking the consistency and similarities of personal observations.

Tertiary Sources

Literature. Nurses complete the assessment database by reviewing nursing, medical, and pharmacological literature about a client's present health status. This review increases their knowledge about the client's diagnosed problems, expected symptoms, treatment, prognosis, and established standards of therapeutic practice. A knowledgeable nurse obtains relevant, accurate, and complete information for the assessment database.

Nurse's Experience. Benner, Sutphen, Leonard, et al. (2010) assert that integration of evidence-informed knowledge and good clinical reasoning is essential to elicit and process information that will lead the nurse to deliver relevant therapeutic interventions. A nurse's expertise develops after testing and refining propositions, questions, and principle- or standard-based expectations. Practical experience and the opportunity to make clinical decisions strengthen a nurse's critical thinking.

Methods of Data Collection

Nurses utilize the client interview, nursing health history, physical examination findings, and results of laboratory and diagnostic tests to establish a client's assessment database.

Interview. The first step in establishing a database is to collect subjective information by interviewing the client. An **interview** is an organized conversation with the client. The initial formal interview involves obtaining the client's health history and information about the current illness. During the initial interview, the nurse has the opportunity to do the following:

- Introduce him- or herself to the client, explain the nurse's role, and explain the role of other health care providers during care.
- Establish a caring therapeutic relationship with the client.
- Obtain insight about the client's concerns and worries.
- Determine the client's goals and expectations of the health care system.
- Obtain cues about which parts of the data collection phase necessitate further in-depth investigation.

The nurse and the client become partners during the interview, rather than the nurse controlling the interview. An interview consists of three phases, similar to that of a therapeutic relationship: orientation, working, and termination.

A successful interview requires preparation. The nurse collects any available information about the client and then creates a favourable environment for the interview. An environment in which the client is comfortable and relaxed helps the nurse conduct a good interview. The nurse must ask the client if he or she would like to conduct the interview alone or if the client would like to include family members.

Finally, the nurse selects a place private enough to enable the client to be comfortable when providing personal information.

Orientation Phase. During the orientation phase of the interview, the nurse introduces him- or herself, describes the nurse's position, and explains the purpose of the interview. It is imperative that nurses explain to clients why they are collecting data (e.g., for a nursing history or for a focused assessment) and assure them that any information obtained will remain confidential and will be used only by health care providers.

Working Phase. In the working phase of the interview, nurses gather information about the client's health status. The nurse does this by focused questioning and other communication strategies such as active listening, paraphrasing, and summarizing to promote a clear interaction (see Chapter 17 for further information about communicating). The use of open-ended questions encourages clients to describe their health histories in detail.

Nurses use **open-ended questions** whenever they want to explore broader issues and have clients describe their history in their own words. Open-ended questions can help to determine the client's priorities and primary concerns, because sometimes these can be different from what the nurse initially thinks the concern is. **Closed-ended questions** can all be answered by "yes" or "no" (or a choice of answers that the nurse provides); these should be limited to issues in which the nurse does not need additional information from the client (Box 13-3). Both types of questioning can help advance client care. While open-ended questions can elicit more information about a client's histories and perceptions of his or her health, closed-ended questions can help a client who is in acute pain or distress identify his or her emergent or priority needs.

During the working phase, the nurse obtains a nursing health history by exploring the client's current illness, health history, and expectations of care. The objective for collecting a health history is to identify patterns of health and illness, risk factors for physical and behavioural health problems, changes from normal function, and available resources for adaptation. The initial interview is normally the most extensive. Ongoing interviews, which occur each time a nurse interacts with the client, do not need to be as extensive; their purpose is to update the client's status and focus more on changes in previously identified problems and to identify new problems.

Termination Phase. As in the other phases of the interview, termination requires skill on the part of the interviewer. The nurse provides the client clues that the interview is coming to an end. For example, the nurse may say, "I want to ask just two more questions" or "We'll be finished in about 2 minutes." This helps the client maintain direct attention without being distracted by wondering when the interview will end. This approach also gives the client an opportunity to ask questions. When concluding an interview, the nurse summarizes the important points and asks the client whether the summary was accurate. The interview should end in a friendly manner, such as the nurse telling the client when the nurse will return to provide care.

A skillful interviewer adapts interview strategies on the basis of the client's responses. Nurses successfully gather relevant health data when they are prepared for the interview and able to carry out each interview phase with minimal interruption.

BOX 13-3 Examples of Open- and Closed-Ended Questions

Open-Ended Questions

Tell me how you are feeling.
Your discomfort affects your ability to get around in what way?
Describe how your spouse or partner has been helping you.
Give me an example of how you get relief from your pain at home.

Closed-Ended Questions

Do you feel as if the medication is helping you?
Who is the person who helps you at home?
Do you understand why you are having the X-ray examination?
Has the warm compress given you relief from your back pain?
Are you having pain now?
On a scale of 0 to 10, with 0 being no pain at all and 10 being the worse possible pain, how would you rate your pain?

Cultural Considerations in Assessment

Cultural assessments, combined with critical thinking skills, provide the knowledge necessary for nursing care. As a nurse, it is important to conduct any assessment with cultural competence and cultural safety (see Chapter 9 for further information on conducting a cultural assessment within a cultural context). This involves a conscientious understanding of your client's culture so that you can offer better care within differing value systems and act with respect and understanding without imposition of your own attitudes and beliefs (Seidel, Ball, Dains, et al., 2011). Good communication techniques are important when assessing a client whose culture is different from your own. Communication and culture are interrelated in the way feelings are expressed verbally and nonverbally.

When nurses interact to assess any specific client, they must first know their own cultural self. Cultural awareness can be achieved by engaging in self-reflection of biases and feelings (see Chapter 9 for more information about cultural awareness). Nurses need to avoid forming a sense of a client on the basis of prior information about the client's culture because this may not only affect the quality of client care but also cause harm to the client if the person is stereotyped or if assumptions are made about his or her health practices. The nurse needs to ask questions in a constructive and probing way to enable a full understanding of the client with regard to the client's priorities, beliefs about health, and health concerns.

Approaches to Indigenous Health Assessment

Nurses require skills-based training in intercultural competency, conflict resolution, human rights, and anti-racism (Truth and Reconciliation Commission of Canada [TRC], 2015, Call to Action 24) in order to provide safe and culturally competent care to Indigenous clients. This includes taking courses dealing with Indigenous health issues, including the history and legacy of residential schools, the *United Nations Declaration on the Rights of Indigenous Peoples* (United Nations, 2007), treaties and Aboriginal rights, and Indigenous teaching and practices (TRC, 2015, Call to Action 24). It is important that nurses also advocate, in consultation with Indigenous communities, to the federal Canadian government to publish annual progress reports and assess long-term trends impacting the health of Indigenous communities in Canada. Furthermore, nurses need to understand the value of Indigenous healing practices, assess clients for the use of these practices, and utilize them for the treatment of Indigenous clients in collaboration with Indigenous healers and Elders, when requested (TRC, 2015, Call to Action 22). Significant repercussions from the residential schooling system persist that may affect the health of Indigenous survivors of this system, their families, and future generations. However, it is imperative that nurses remember that assessing for any type of transgenerational or collective trauma should be conducted by nurses with expertise in this area of assessment. Beginning nurses should focus their efforts on general health assessment and building trusting and therapeutic relationships with their clients in order to come to know them as individuals, their experiences, and primary health concerns (see Chapter 10 for further information about assessing Indigenous health).

Nursing Health History

Nurses conduct a nursing health history during either their initial contact or an early contact with a client. The history is a major component of assessment. Although many health history forms are structured, nurses learn to use the questions as starting points. A good assessor learns to refine and broaden questions as needed in order to correctly assess the client's unique needs. Time and client priorities determine how complete a history is. The nurse can identify patterns of information about a client's health and illness by collecting data about all health dimensions (see Box 13-1). By incorporating data from all dimensions, the nurse can develop a complete plan of care.

Family History

The purpose of collecting the family history is to obtain data about immediate and blood relatives. The objectives are to determine whether the client is at risk for illnesses of a genetic or familial nature and to identify areas of health promotion and illness prevention (see Chapter 20 for further information about patient education). The family history also provides information about family structure, interaction, and function that is often useful in planning care (see Chapter 19 for further information about assessing the family). For example, a close, supportive family will help a client adjust to an illness or disability. If the client's family is not supportive, it is better to not involve family members in care. Stressful family relationships are sometimes a significant barrier when nurses try to help clients with problems involving loss, self-concept, spiritual health, and personal relationships.

Documentation of History Findings

As nurses conduct the nursing health history, they need to record their assessment in a clear, concise manner, using appropriate terminology. Standardized forms make it easy to enter data as the client responds to questions. In settings that have computerized documentation, entry of assessment data is easy. A clear, concise record is necessary for use by other health care providers (see Chapter 15 for further information about documentation). Regardless of the model used in a documentation system, nurses provide a thorough database inclusive of historical and current information about the client's health. This information then becomes the baseline against which nurses and the health care team evaluate any future changes.

Physical Examination

A *physical examination* is an investigation of the body to determine its state of health. A physical examination involves use of the techniques of inspection, palpation, percussion, auscultation, and smell (see Chapter 32 for further information about conducting a health assessment). A complete examination includes measurements of a client's height, weight, and vital signs and a head-to-toe examination of all body systems. By performing actual hands-on physical assessment, nurses gather valuable objective information that helps in forming accurate diagnostic conclusions. It is important for the nurse to conduct an examination with sensitivity and competence to prevent the client from becoming anxious.

Observation of Client Behaviour. Throughout an interview and physical examination, it is important for nurses to observe a client's verbal and nonverbal behaviours closely in order to enhance their objective database. Nurses learn to determine whether data obtained by observation matches what the client verbally communicates. For example, if a client expresses no concern about an upcoming diagnostic test but shows poor eye contact, shakiness, and restlessness, all suggestive of anxiety, then verbal and nonverbal data conflict. Observations direct the nurse to gather additional objective information to form accurate conclusions about the client's condition. An important aspect of observation includes a client's level of function: the physical, developmental, psychological, and social aspects of everyday living. Observation of the level of function differs from observations made during an interview. Observation of level of function involves watching what a client does, such as eating or decision making about preparing a medication, rather than what the client tells the nurse what he or she can do. Observation of function can occur in the home or in a health care setting during a return visit.

Diagnostic and Laboratory Data. The results of diagnostic and laboratory tests reveal or clarify alterations questioned or identified during the nursing health history and physical examination. For example, during the history documentation, the client reports having had a bad cold for 6 days and currently has a productive cough with brown sputum and mild shortness of breath. On physical examination, the nurse notices an elevated temperature, increased respirations, and decreased breath sounds in the right lower lobe. The nurse reviews the results of a complete blood cell count and notes that the white blood cell count is elevated (indicating an infection). In addition, the radiologist's report of a chest X-ray examination shows the presence of a right lower lobe infiltrate. Such findings combined are suggestive of the medical diagnosis of pneumonia and the associated nursing diagnosis of *impaired gas exchange.*

Some clients collect and monitor laboratory data in the home. For example, clients with diabetes mellitus often perform daily blood glucose monitoring. The nurse would then ask clients about their routine results to determine their responses to illness and elicit information about the effects of treatment measures. The nurse also compares laboratory data with the established norms for a particular test result, age group, and gender.

Interpreting Assessment Data and Making Nursing Judgements. The successful analysis and interpretation of assessment data requires critical thinking. When nurses correctly analyze data, they recognize patterns that lead them to make necessary clinical decisions about their client's care. These decisions are in the form of either nursing diagnoses or collaborative problems that require treatment from several disciplines (Carpenito, 2013). When nurses critically think about interpreting assessment information, they determine the presence of abnormal findings, what further observations they need in order to clarify information, and the client's health problems.

Data Validation. Before nurses begin analyzing and interpreting data, they need to validate the collected information they have, to avoid making incorrect inferences (Carpenito, 2013). **Validation** of assessment data is the comparison of data with another source to determine data accuracy. For example, a nurse observes a client crying and logically infers that this is related to hospitalization or a medical diagnosis. Making such an initial inference is not wrong, but problems can result if the nurse does not validate the inference with the client. In this case, the nurse may state, "I notice that you have been crying. Can you tell me about it?" By questioning the client, the nurse will discover the real reason for the crying behaviour. To validate the information obtained during an interview and history the nurse relies on the client to confirm it. The nurse also validates findings from the physical examination and observation of client behaviour, by comparing data in the medical record and by consulting with other nurses or health care team members. Often family or friends are able to validate assessment information. Validation opens the door for gathering more assessment data because it involves clarifying vague or unclear data. On occasion, the nurse may reassess previously covered areas of the nursing history or gather further physical examination data. It is important to continually analyze and think about a client's database in order to make concise, accurate, and meaningful interpretations. Critical thinking applied to assessment enables the nurse to fully understand the client's problems, to judge the extent of the problems carefully, and to discover possible relationships between the problems.

Analysis and Interpretation. After the nurse collects extensive information about a client, the nurse analyzes and interprets the data. The nurse begins analysis by organizing the information into meaningful and usable clusters, keeping in mind the client's response to illness. A *data cluster* is a set of signs or symptoms that are grouped together in a logical way. During data clustering, the nurse will organize data and focus attention on client functions to determine which support or assistance for recovery is needed. Data analysis involves recognizing patterns or trends in the clustered data, comparing them with standards, and then establishing a reasoned conclusion about the client's responses to a health problem. Patterns of meaning begin to form, enabling the nurse to make inferences about client problems.

Through reasoning and judgement, the nurse decides what information explains the client's health status. At times, additional information is required to clarify the nurse's interpretation. The ability to cluster or group data during analysis will help the nurse at becoming proficient in identifying individualized nursing diagnoses and identifying collaborative problems (see Figure 13-6).

During clustering, a cue or an individual sign, symptom, or finding will alert the nurse more than others do. Such cues are especially helpful in identifying nursing diagnoses.

Data Documentation

Data documentation is the last part of a complete assessment. The timely, thorough, and accurate documentation of facts is necessary when clients' data are recorded. Not only does documentation guide client care, it is also a legal and professional responsibility to record the client's status. If the nurse does not record an assessment finding or problem interpretation, that information is lost and unavailable to anyone else caring for the client. If the nurse does not record detailed and specific data, the person reading the report is left with only general impressions. The basic rule is to record all observations. Anything heard, seen, felt, or smelled should be reported exactly. It is important to record objective information in accurate terminology (e.g., "weighs 77.3 kg," "abdomen is soft and nontender to palpation"). Subjective information from a client is recorded in quotation marks. When entering data, the nurse should not generalize or form judgements through written communication. Conclusions about such data become nursing diagnoses and must be accurate. As nurses become more proficient at identifying data clusters and patterns of signs and symptoms, they are better able to conclude the existence of a correct problem. (Review Chapter 15 for details on documentation.)

Concept Mapping

A concept map is a visual representation that show the connections between a client's health problems. It fosters a holistic view of the client and identifies linkages between the multiple variables affecting the client's health. Constructing concept maps demonstrates and promotes critical thinking through the use of reflection, creativity, and insight (Harrison & Gibbons, 2013). The visual image of clients as holistic, multidimensional, and complex serves as a starting point for the development of a comprehensive, individualized care plan (Taylor & Wros, 2007). Figure 13-4 summarizes the primary assessment findings from Mr. Fletcher's scenario, introduced at the start of this chapter. Review these findings and write out any additional questions you may have about these findings or any additional questions you would ask the client at this time. It is helpful to address this scenario as a large group as an in-class exercise. In order to demonstrate how critical thinking is integrated into assessment, Figure 13-2 is applied here to this scenario:

Irene is the local primary health nurse assessing Mr. Fletcher. Irene has practised as a registered nurse for 25 years in this small, mountain community. She is familiar with the daily routines and stresses of a haul truck operator because her husband also works at the coal mine as a heavy-duty mechanic. Irene's practice experience has been in acute care and community health.

Knowledge: *Irene is concerned about Mr. Fletcher's high blood pressure and his identification of subjective symptoms such as headache and blurred vision because these are symptoms of advanced disease. She is aware that Mr. Fletcher may have had high blood pressure for years and may not have been aware of it because high blood pressure can be hidden in a client who does not take his own blood pressure regularly. She is concerned because prolonged hypertension can cause kidney failure, loss of vision, and cardiovascular and peripheral vascular disease. Irene also notes on his lab results that Mr. Fletcher has hyperlipidemia; this can worsen vascular disease when paired with uncontrolled hypertension. Irene suspects that Mr. Fletcher is also experiencing peripheral arterial disease due to his poor circulation in his feet, hair loss on his lower legs, and pain in his calf muscles when walking. Mr. Fletcher has a positive family history for heart disease, vascular disorders, and diabetes—all of these conditions can be genetically linked to future occurrences. She suspects that Mr. Fletcher may be smoking more than five cigarettes per day as he has hypertension, symptoms of vascular disease, a strong odour on his clothing, and stained fingers. However, there may be a reason why he is not disclosing this to her, and Irene has decided to build a trusting rapport with him before further questioning him about his smoking patterns. At this time, Irene is focused on gathering more information on Mr. Fletcher's key areas related to his hypertension, high lipid levels, and symptoms of vascular disease.*

Standards: *Irene draws from various resources to help guide her assessment and questioning. For example, Hypertension Canada (2016) has outlined the standards for the diagnosis and clinical pathways for the diagnosis of hypertension, and the Heart and Stroke Foundation of Ontario and Registered Nurses' Association of Ontario (2005) has a Best Practice Guideline for the treatment of hypertension that addresses both medical and nursing management. Irene is using both medical (e.g., pathophysiology, pharmacology, disease management) and nursing knowledge to guide her questioning; she is aware of her scope of practice as a registered nurse.*

Qualities: *Irene reflects on the assessment interview, her rapport with Mr. Fletcher, and her creativity in collecting information. She listens in the interview process to both what is being said and information that is not pointed out or is being avoided in the conversation. She conducts her interview in a therapeutic manner, ensuring that she is treating Mr. Fletcher fairly and with respect. She does not comment directly on his health practices at this time. Rather, she assesses his understanding, reasoning, and approaches to his health.*

Experience: *Irene's experience as a nurse in this region informs her approaches to her assessment and the questions she asks the client. Irene is familiar with the position of a haul truck operator. She is aware that they work long shifts, often have sleep issues due to shift work, and that the job is stationary (involves sitting for long periods). She is also familiar with risk factors for hypertension and vascular disease. Therefore, she knows what type of direct questions to ask and what to look for in her assessment. She is confident and proficient in her assessment techniques and knows how to cluster data in order to gain an understanding of emerging issues.*

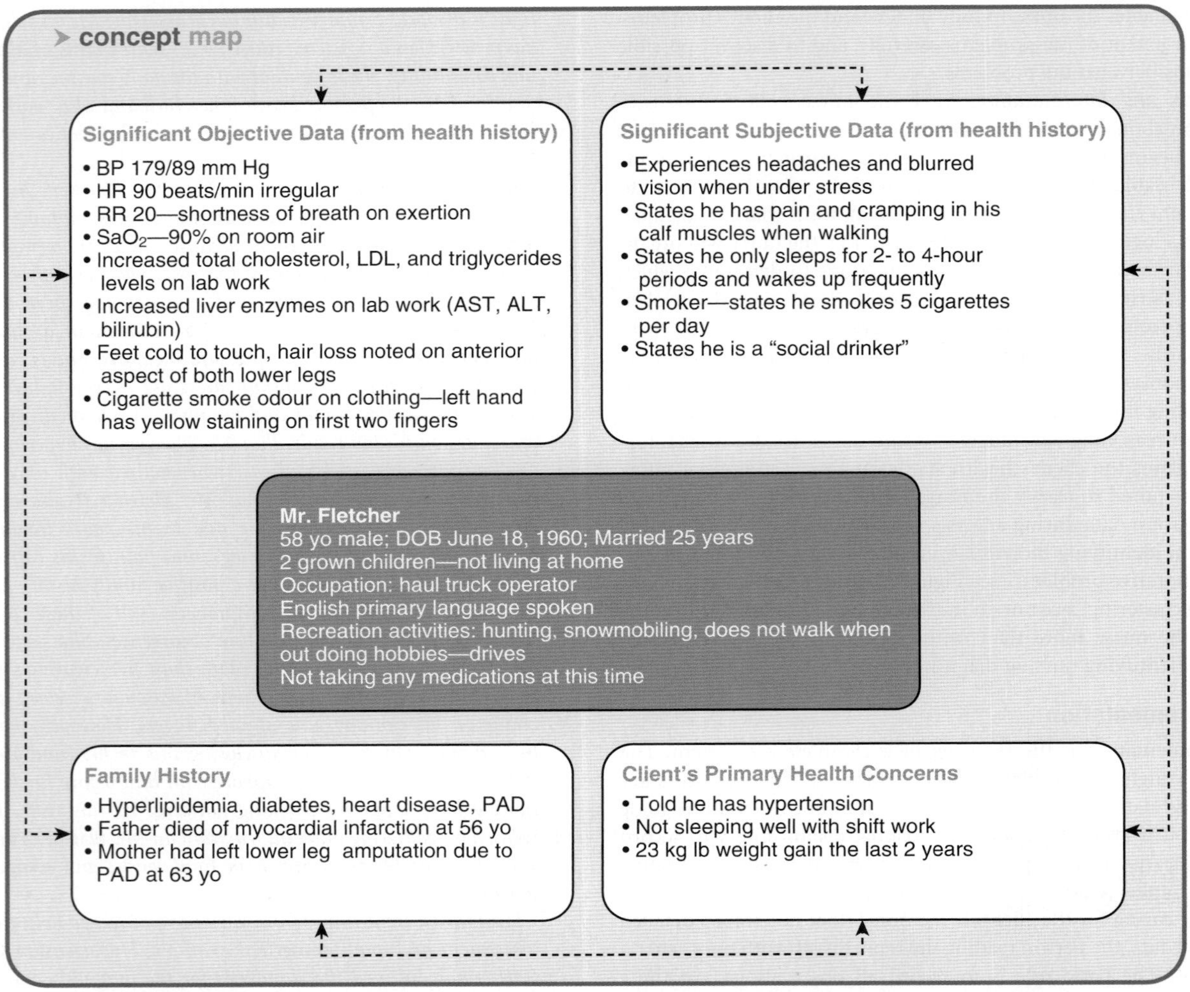

FIGURE 13-4 Concept map for Mr. Fletcher's assessment findings. *ALT,* Alanine aminotransferase; *AST,* aspartate aminotransferase; *BP,* blood pressure; *DOB,* date of birth; *HR,* heart rate; *LDL,* low-density lipoprotein; *PAD,* peripheral arterial disease; *RR,* respiratory rate; *SaO_2,* oxygen saturation; *yo,* years old.

◆ NURSING DIAGNOSIS

After a client is assessed thoroughly to compile a database, the next step of the nursing process is to form diagnostic conclusions that determine the nursing care that a client receives (Figure 13-5). Figure 13-6 outlines these specific steps to a nursing diagnosis and summarizes key phases of assessment. Some of the conclusions lead to nursing diagnoses whereas others do not. Diagnostic conclusions include problems treated primarily by nurses (nursing diagnoses) and problems necessitating treatment by several disciplines (collaborative problems).

When physicians refer to commonly accepted medical diagnoses, such as myocardial infarction, diabetes mellitus, or osteoarthritis, they all know the meaning of these diagnoses and the standard approaches to treatment. A **medical diagnosis** is the identification of a disease condition on the basis of a specific evaluation of physical signs, symptoms, the client's medical history, and the results of diagnostic tests and procedures. Physicians are licensed to treat diseases or pathological processes described in medical diagnostic statements. Nurses have a similar diagnostic language. **Nursing diagnosis**, the second step of the nursing process, determines health problems within the domain of nursing. The term *diagnose* means "distinguish" or "know." A nursing diagnosis is a clinical judgement about individual, family, or community responses to actual and potential health problems or life processes that is within the domain of nursing (NANDA International, 2018). Box 13-4 shows examples of nursing diagnoses.

A **collaborative problem** is an actual or potential physiological complication that nurses monitor to detect the onset of changes in a client's status (Carpenito, 2013). When collaborative problems develop, nurses intervene in collaboration with personnel from other health care disciplines. Nurses manage collaborative problems such as hemorrhage, infection, and cardiac dysrhythmia by using both physician-prescribed and nursing-prescribed interventions to minimize complications. For example, a client who has a surgical wound is at risk for developing an infection, and so a physician prescribes antibiotics. The nurse monitors the client for fever and other signs of infection and implements appropriate wound care measures.

Nursing diagnoses provide the basis for selection of nursing interventions to achieve outcomes for which nurses are accountable

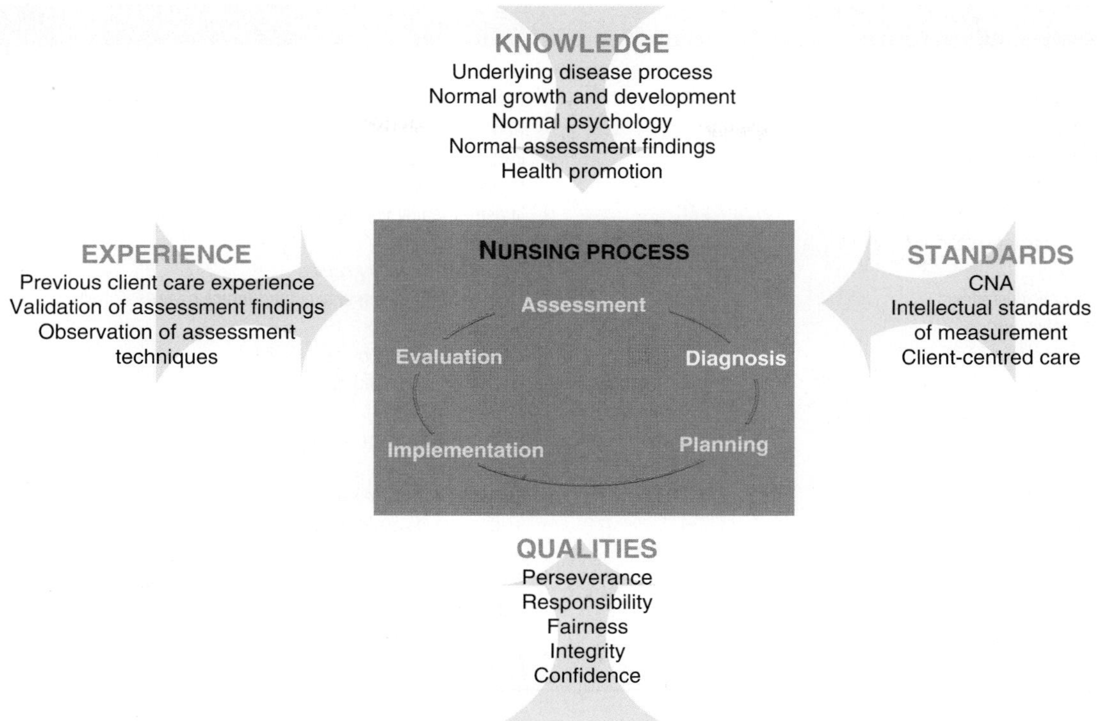

FIGURE 13-5 Critical thinking and the nursing diagnostic process. *CNA,* Canadian Nurses Association.

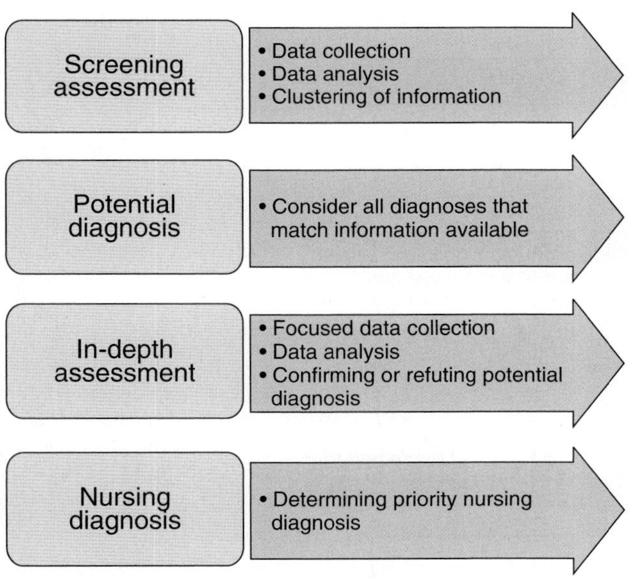

FIGURE 13-6 Steps in moving from assessment to diagnosis. (Adapted From NANDA International. [2018]. *Nursing diagnoses: Definitions and classification, 2018–2020* [11th edition]. New York: Thieme [p. 50, Fig 6.1]).

(NANDA International, 2018). A nursing diagnosis focuses on a client's actual or potential response to a health problem rather than on the physiological event, complication, or disease. In the case of the diagnosis *inadequate knowledge regarding postoperative routines,* collaborative problems occur or probably will occur in association with a specific disease, trauma, or treatment (Carpenito, 2013). Nurses require expert knowledge to assess a client's specific risk for these problems, to identify the problems early, and then to take preventive action (Figure 13-7). Critical thinking is necessary in identifying nursing diagnoses and collaborative problems so that nurses individualize care appropriately for their clients.

Nursing diagnosis is recognized in Canada as an innovative means of translating nursing observations and assessments into standard conclusions in a common nomenclature. Although nursing diagnosis is part of basic nursing preparation in Canada, it has not yet been incorporated into provincial and territorial nursing practice standards or legislation.

The use of standard formal nursing diagnostic statements (see Box 13-4) serves several purposes:

1. They provide a precise definition that gives all members of the health care team a common language for understanding the client's needs.
2. They enable nurses to communicate their actions among themselves, to other health care providers, and to the public.
3. They distinguish the nurse's role from that of the physician or other health care providers.
4. They help nurses focus on the scope of nursing practice.
5. They foster the development of nursing knowledge.

CRITICAL THINKING AND NURSING DIAGNOSTIC PROCESS

Diagnostic reasoning is a process of using assessment data about a client to logically explain a clinical judgement—in this case, a nursing diagnosis. The diagnostic process flows from the assessment process and includes decision-making steps. These steps include data clustering, identifying client needs, and formulating the diagnosis or problem.

Clusters and patterns of data often contain **defining characteristics**—the clinical criteria or assessment findings that help confirm an

BOX 13-4 Examples of Nursing Diagnoses

Reduced stamina
Risk for *reduced* stamina
Reduced *airway* clearance
Hypersensitivity reaction
Anxiety
Potential for *aspiration*
Potential for impaired parent–child *attachment*
Autonomic dysreflexia
Potential for *autonomic* dysreflexia
Risk-prone health *behaviour*
Potential for altered *body* image
Potential for imbalanced *body* temperature
Bowel incontinence
Inadequate *breastfeeding*
Interrupted *breastfeeding*
Reduced *breathing* pattern
Decreased *cardiac* output
Caregiver role strain
Potential for *caregiver* role strain
Inadequate verbal *communication*
Conflict (decisional, parental role)
Potential for *confusion*
Constipation
Potential for *constipation*
Contamination
Potential for *contamination*
Defensive *coping*
Impaired family *coping*
Impaired *coping*
Impaired community *coping*
Potential for sudden unexpected infant *death*
Impaired *denial*
Ineffective *dentition*
Potential for delayed *development*
Diarrhea
Potential for compromised human *dignity*
Moral *distress*
Potential for *disuse* syndrome
Inadequate *diversional* activity
Altered *energy* field
Altered *environmental* interpretation syndrome
Adult *failure* to thrive
Potential for *falls*
Dysfunctional *family* processes: alcoholism

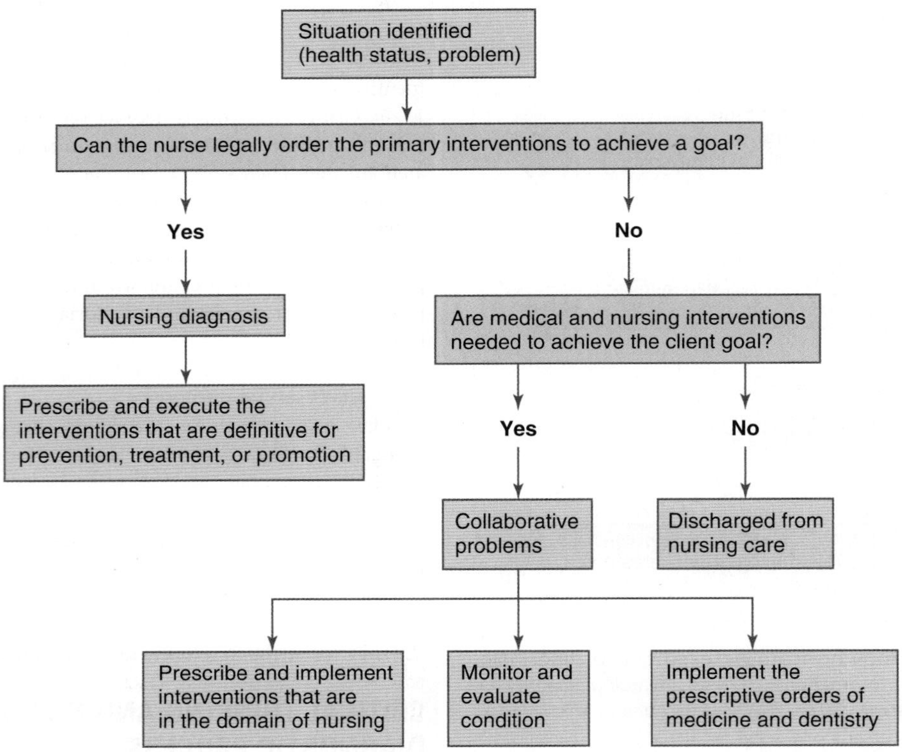

FIGURE 13-7 Differentiating nursing diagnoses from collaborative problems. (Copyright © 1990, 1988, 1985, by Lynda Juall Carpenito. Redrawn from Carpenito, L. J. [1995]. *Nursing diagnosis: Application to clinical practice* [6th ed.]. Philadelphia, PA: J. B. Lippincott.)

actual nursing diagnosis. Clinical criteria are objective or subjective signs and symptoms, clusters of signs and symptoms, or risk factors that lead to a diagnostic conclusion. A specific set of defining characteristics helps confirm identification of each NANDA International–approved nursing diagnosis (NANDA International, 2018). Nurses learn to recognize patterns of defining characteristics and then readily select the corresponding diagnosis.

Table 13-1 shows two examples of possible nursing diagnoses and their associated defining characteristics. As nurses analyze clusters of data, they begin to consider various diagnoses that might apply to the

TABLE 13-1 Examples of Nursing Diagnoses With Defining Characteristics

Diagnosis: Inadequate Gas Exchange	Diagnosis: Inadequate Breathing Pattern
Defining Characteristics	
Dyspnea	Dyspnea
Abnormal rate, rhythm, depth of breathing	Bradypnea
Abnormal arterial pH	Decreased vital capacity
Abnormal skin colour (pale, dusky)	Orthopnea
Hypoxemia	Altered chest excursion
Hypercarbia	Use of accessory muscles to breathe
Hypoxia	Tachypnea
Confusion	Pursed-lip breathing
Related Factors	
Ventilation-perfusion	Hyperventilation
Alveolar–capillary membrane changes	Pain
	Chest wall deformity
	Anxiety
	Musculoskeletal impairment
	Body position

client. For example, the diagnoses of *inadequate gas exchange* and *inadequate breathing pattern* have similar defining characteristics, including dyspnea, abnormal respiratory rate, and abnormal depth of breathing. As the nurse determines a diagnosis it is important to remember that the absence of certain defining characteristics suggests the rejection of a diagnosis under consideration. Thus, in the same example, if a client uses accessory muscles to breathe and demonstrates pursed-lip breathing, the correct diagnosis is not *inadequate gas exchange* but *inadequate breathing pattern.* It is important to examine the defining characteristics in the database carefully to confirm or eliminate a nursing diagnosis. To be more accurate, review all characteristics, eliminate irrelevant ones, and confirm the relevant ones.

While focusing on patterns of defining characteristics, the nurse compares a client's pattern of data with data that are consistent with normal, healthy patterns. The nurse uses accepted norms as the basis for comparison and judgement. These norms include laboratory and diagnostic test values, professional standards, and normal anatomical or physiological limits. When comparing patterns, the nurse judges whether the grouped signs and symptoms are normal for the client and whether they are within the range of healthy responses and isolates any defining characteristics not within healthy norms in order to identify a problem.

Before finalizing a nursing diagnosis, the nurse needs to review the client's general health care needs or problems. Identifying client needs enables the nurse to individualize nursing diagnoses by considering all assessment data and focusing on the more relevant data. NANDA International (2018) has two nursing diagnoses that apply to knowledge: *insufficient knowledge* and *potential for enhanced knowledge.* It is crucial to select the correct diagnostic label for a client's need. Usually from assessment to diagnosis, the information gathered progresses from general to specific. It helps to think of the problem identification phase in terms of the general health care problem and to think of the formulation of the nursing diagnosis in terms of the specific health problem.

Formulation of the Nursing Diagnosis

NANDA International (2018) identifies four types of nursing diagnoses: actual diagnoses, risk diagnoses, health promotion diagnoses, and wellness diagnoses. An **actual nursing diagnosis** describes responses to health conditions or life processes that exist in an individual, family, or community. Defining characteristics (manifestations, signs, and symptoms) that cluster in patterns of related cues or inferences support this diagnostic judgement (NANDA International, 2018). The selection of an actual diagnosis indicates that sufficient assessment data are available to establish the nursing diagnosis. *Acute pain* is an actual nursing diagnosis. Prioritizing established nursing diagnosis is an important component of the nursing process.

A **risk nursing diagnosis** describes human responses to health conditions or life processes that will possibly develop in a vulnerable individual, family, or community (NANDA International, 2018). Such data include physiological, psychosocial, familial, lifestyle, and environmental factors that increase the client's vulnerability to, or likelihood of, developing the condition.

A **health promotion nursing diagnosis** is a clinical judgement of a person's, family's, or community's motivation and desire to increase well-being and actualize human health potential, as expressed in their readiness to enhance specific health behaviours, such as those related to nutrition and exercise. Health promotion diagnoses can be used in any health state; they do not reflect current levels of wellness (NANDA International, 2018).

A **wellness nursing diagnosis** describes levels of wellness in an individual, family, or community that can be enhanced (NANDA International, 2018). It is a clinical judgement about an individual, group, or community in transition from a specific level of wellness to a higher level of wellness. Nurses select this type of diagnosis when the client wishes to or has achieved an optimal level of health. For example, *readiness for enhanced coping related to successful cancer treatment* is a wellness diagnosis, and the nurse and the family unit work together to adapt to the stressors associated with cancer survivorship. In doing so, the nurse incorporates the client's strengths and resources into a plan of care, with the outcome directed at improving the level of coping.

Components of a Nursing Diagnosis

The nursing diagnosis results from the assessment and diagnostic process. Throughout this text, nursing diagnoses are in a two-part format: the diagnostic label followed by a statement of a related factor. It is this two-part format that provides a diagnosis meaning and relevance for a particular client. In addition, all NANDA International–approved diagnoses have a definition. Risk factors are a component of all risk nursing diagnoses.

Diagnostic Label. The **diagnostic label** is the name of the nursing diagnosis as approved by NANDA International (2018). It describes the essence of a client's response to health conditions in as few words as possible. Diagnostic labels include descriptors used to give additional meaning to the diagnosis. For example, the diagnosis *impaired physical mobility* includes the descriptor *impaired* to describe the nature or change in mobility that best describes the client's response (Table 13-2). Examples of other descriptors are *compromised, decreased, deficient, delayed, effective, imbalanced, impaired,* and *increased.*

Related Factors. The **related factor** is a condition or **etiology** identified from the client's assessment data. It is associated with the client's actual or potential response to the health problem and can be changed through the use of nursing interventions. The inclusion of the "related to" phrase requires the nurse to use critical thinking skills to individualize the nursing diagnosis and then select nursing

TABLE 13-2 Comparison of Interventions for Nursing Diagnoses With Different Etiologies

Nursing Diagnoses	Interventions
Client A	
Anxiety related to uncertainty over surgery	Provide detailed instructions about the surgical procedure, recovery process, and postoperative care activities Plan formal time for client to ask questions
Deficient physical mobility related to acute pain	Administer analgesics 30 minutes before planned exercise Instruct client in technique to splint painful site during activity
Client B	
Anxiety related to loss of job	Consult with social work to arrange for job consulting Encourage client to continue health promotion activities (e.g., exercise, routine social activities)
Deficient physical mobility related to musculoskeletal injury	Have client perform active range-of-motion exercises to affected extremity every 2 hours Instruct client on use of three-point crutch gait

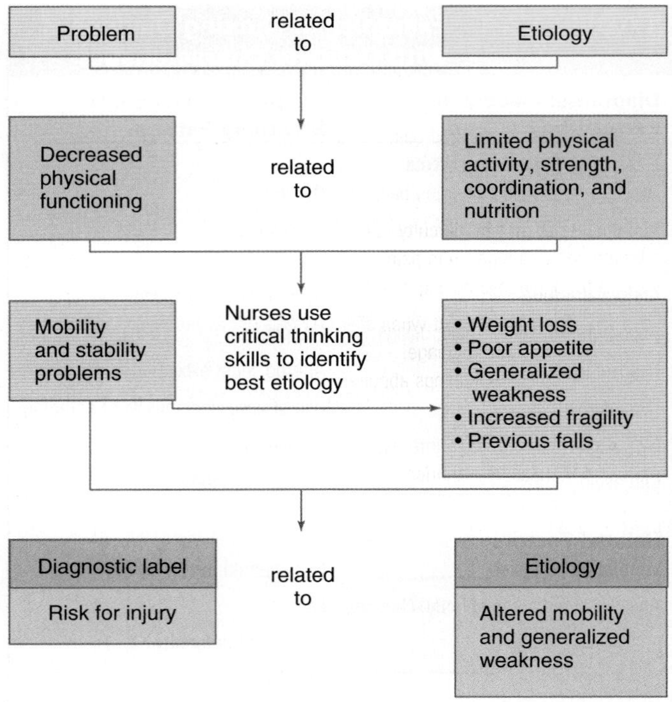

FIGURE 13-8 Relationship between a diagnostic label and an etiology (related factor). (Redrawn from Hickey, P. [1990]. *Nursing process handbook.* St. Louis, MO: Mosby.)

interventions (Figure 13-8). The origin or cause of the nursing diagnosis is always within the domain of nursing practice and a condition that responds to nursing interventions.

Sometimes health care providers record medical diagnoses as the etiology in the nursing diagnosis. This is incorrect. Nursing interventions do not change a medical diagnosis. However, nurses direct nursing interventions at behaviours or conditions that nurses are able to treat or manage. For example, the nursing diagnosis *acute pain related to herniated disc* is incorrect; nursing actions do not affect the medical diagnosis of a herniated disc. Instead, a diagnosis of *acute pain related to pressure on spinal nerves* results in nursing interventions directed at reducing stress on the vertebrae, improving body alignment, and offering nonpharmacological comfort measures.

Table 13-3 displays the association between a nurse's assessment of a client, the clustering of defining characteristics, and formulation of nursing diagnoses. The diagnostic process results in the formation of a total diagnostic label that enables a nurse to develop an appropriate client-centred plan of care. The defining characteristics and relevant etiologies are from NANDA International (2018).

Definition. NANDA International (2018) approved a definition for each diagnosis that follows clinical use and testing. The definition describes the characteristics of the human response identified. For example, the definition of the diagnostic label *deficient physical mobility* is the "limitation in independent, purposeful physical movement of the body or of one or more extremities" (NANDA International, 2018). Nurses refer to definitions of nursing diagnoses to assist in identifying a client's correct diagnosis.

Risk Factors. *Risk factors* are environmental, physiological, psychological, genetic, or chemical elements that increase the vulnerability of an individual, family, or community to an unhealthful event (NANDA International, 2018). They are a component of all risk nursing diagnoses. The risk factors are cues to indicate that a risk nursing diagnosis is applicable to a client's condition. Examples of risk factors for the nursing diagnosis *risk for infection* include invasive procedures, trauma, malnutrition, immunosuppression, and insufficient knowledge to avoid exposure to pathogens. The risk factors help nurses select the correct risk diagnosis, similar to the manner in which defining characteristics help nurses formulate actual nursing diagnoses. In addition, risk factors are valuable in planning preventive nursing interventions.

Support of the Diagnostic Statement. Nursing assessment data must support the diagnostic label, and the related factors must be included in these data. To collect complete, relevant, and correct assessment data, it helps to identify assessment activities that produce specific kinds of data. For example, asking the client about the quality and perception of pain elicits subjective data. However, if palpating an area elicits a facial grimace, that grimace is objective information. Likewise, asking a client to describe the perception of an irregular heartbeat elicits subjective information, and using auscultation to obtain a pulse elicits an objective measurement of heart rate and rhythm. As nurses review assessment data, they look for clusters of defining characteristics and consider whether they have probed and assessed the client accurately and thoroughly to gather a complete database.

CONCEPT MAPPING FOR NURSING DIAGNOSES

Figure 13-9 demonstrates a method for concept mapping a client's nursing diagnosis using the case study presented at the start of this chapter. While this specific concept map demonstrates nursing

TABLE 13-3 **Defining Characteristics and Etiologies to Confirm Nursing Diagnoses**

Assessment Activities	Defining Characteristics (Clustering Cues)	Nursing Diagnoses	Etiologies ("Related to")
Ask client to rate severity of pain on a scale from 0 to 10. Observe client's positioning in bed.	Client verbally reports pain at a level of 8 or 9 when it becomes sharp. Client bends knees while on back to lessen pain.	Acute pain	Physical pressure on spinal nerves
Ask whether client has difficulty falling asleep or awakens during night from pain. Observe for any nonverbal signs of discomfort.	Client reports feeling tired, awakens easily. Client moans and sighs when attempting to find comfortable position in bed.	Acute pain	Physical pressure on spinal nerves
Observe client's eye contact when client is talking. Observe client's body language. Ask client to describe feelings about surgery.	Client has poor eye contact when discussing surgery. Client is restless. Client is uncertain about what to expect after surgery and the outcome of surgery.	Anxiety	Threat to health status as a result of surgery
Give instruction in topic of interest, and return in 15 minutes to measure retention.	Client forgets details of explanation.	Anxiety	Threat to health status as a result of surgery

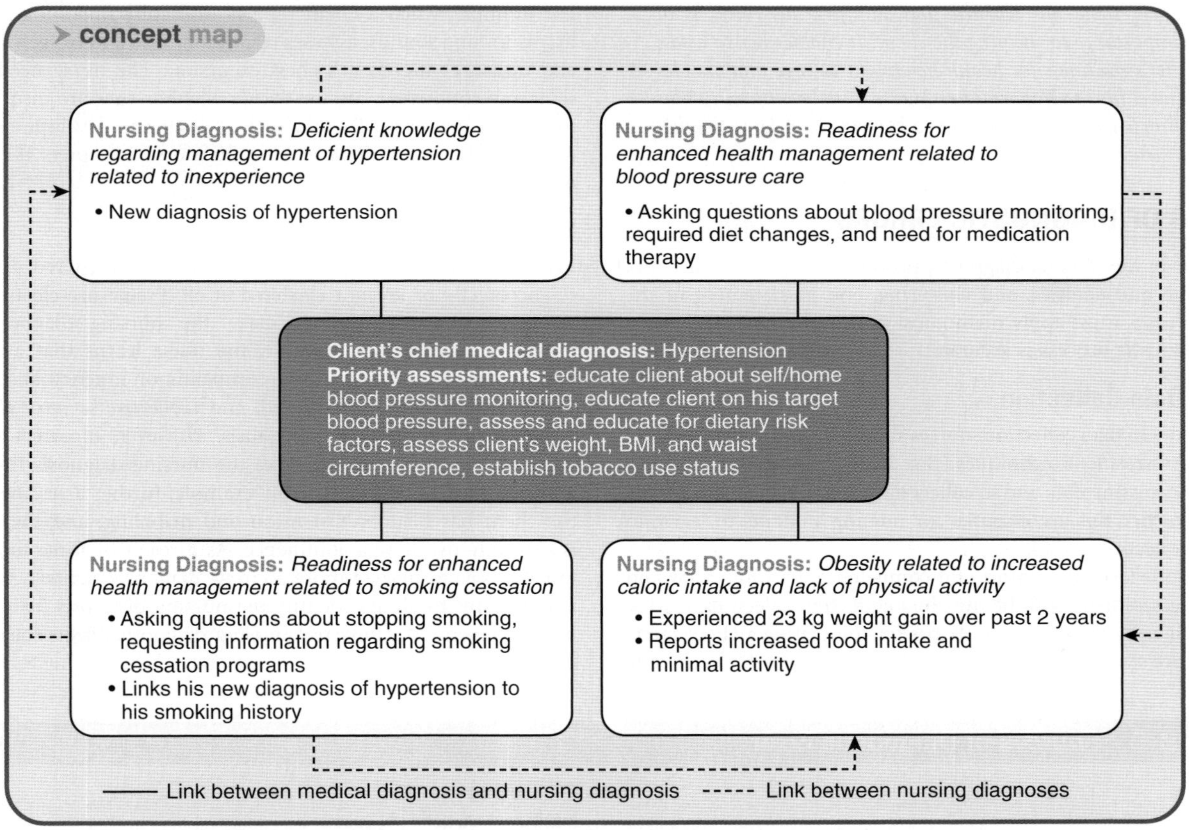

FIGURE 13-9 Concept map for Mr. Fletcher's nursing diagnoses. *BMI,* Body mass index.

diagnosis, it is also important to review other medical and collaborative problems that may influence client care. Laboratory values and diagnostic testing for client care may support both medical and nursing diagnosis that will be used in care planning. In the following example of how nurses engage critical thinking in the diagnostic process, Figure 13-5 is used as a template:

After assessing Mr. Fletcher, Irene, the registered nurse, recognizes that there are several areas for diagnosis coming forward for the client within both collaborative and nursing diagnostic frameworks. At this time, Irene decides to defer the potential signs of peripheral arterial disease to the physician or nurse practitioner and notes it as a collaborative concern on the client record. She turns her attention to nursing diagnosis related to Mr. Fletcher's primary concern of hypertension.

Knowledge: *Mr. Fletcher's blood pressure is considered high according to clinical guidelines. While is it not in Irene's scope of practice to prescribe medications for the management of* *hypertension (she notes this as a priority for the physician or nurse practitioner), she continues her assessment to further outline how Mr. Fletcher's lifestyle, weight, diet, exercise, alcohol intake, smoking, and stress may be leading to his hypertension.*

Standards: *Irene accesses the Registered Nurses' Association of Ontario (RNAO) (2005) Nursing Management of Hypertension to guide her assessment and formulation of nursing diagnosis. The Summary of Recommendations for this Best Practice Guideline is a useful tool for guiding her questioning and in helping direct her plan of nursing care. She also realizes that it would be helpful to follow a self-management framework with Mr. Fletcher because hypertension is considered a chronic health condition.*

Qualities: *Irene uses therapeutic techniques to ascertain more assessment information from Mr. Fletcher. She actively listens to his responses and focuses her questions on areas that require more information. She does not judge Mr. Fletcher for his weight gain or smoking, rather she assists him in linking these behaviours to his hypertension and seeks to understand how other social determinants of health or coping practices may be influencing these specific behaviours.*

Experience: *Irene has learned that this first interview is of primary importance for helping the client. It enables her to assess Mr. Fletcher's readiness for health behaviour change and enables her to connect him to important resources in the community that will help him learn more about his hypertension in order to develop successful strategies for self-care.*

SOURCES OF DIAGNOSTIC ERRORS

Errors occur in the nursing diagnostic process during data collection, interpretation and analysis, and clustering, and in statement of the diagnosis. Nurses must apply methodical critical thinking so that the nursing diagnostic process is accurate.

Errors in Data Collection

To avoid errors in data collection, nurses should be knowledgeable and skilled in all assessment techniques (Box 13-5). It is vital to check for inaccurate or missing data and to collect data in an organized way. The following practice tips are essential for nursing students to learn, to avoid data collection errors:

- Review your level of comfort and competence with interview and physical assessment skills before you begin data collection.
- Approach assessment in steps. Focus on completing a client interview before starting a physical examination. Perhaps focus on only one body system in order to learn how to gather a complete assessment. Then move to a more complex head-to-toe examination.
- Review your clinical assessments in clinical or classroom settings. They will provide you with a constructive learning opportunity to determine how to revise an assessment or to gather additional information.
- Determine the accuracy of your data. For example, when you auscultate abnormal lung sounds for the first time, be sure of what you hear through the stethoscope. To minimize the risk of inaccuracy, have a more experienced co-worker validate your findings or explain why they are incorrect. Validate your assessment data by double-checking and verifying them.
- Be organized in any examination. Have the appropriate forms and examination equipment ready to use. Be sure the environment is private, quiet, and comfortable for the client.

Errors in Interpretation and Analysis of Data

After data collection, nurses will review the database to decide whether it is accurate and complete. Data are reviewed to confirm that measurable, objective physical findings support subjective data. For example, when a client reports "difficulty breathing," the nurse listens to lung sounds, assesses respiratory rate and oxygen saturation, and measures the client's chest excursion. The nurse needs to consider any conflicting cues or decide whether cues are insufficient for forming a diagnosis. Factors such as a client's developmental stage, for example, may influence how the nurse interprets the meaning of cues.

Errors in Data Clustering

Errors in data clustering occur when data are clustered prematurely or incorrectly or are not clustered at all. Premature closure of clustering occurs when nurses make the nursing diagnosis before grouping all data. For example, the nurse learns that a client has had urinary incontinence and complains of urgency and nocturia. The available data are clustered, and *ineffective urinary elimination* is considered a probable diagnosis. However, incorrect clustering occurs when nurses try to make the nursing diagnosis fit the signs and symptoms obtained. In this example, further assessment reveals the client has bladder distension and dribbling, and the condition is probably overflow incontinence. As a result of these findings, the nurse is able to make a more accurate diagnosis: *urinary retention.* It is important to always identify the nursing diagnosis from the data, not the reverse. An incorrect nursing diagnosis affects the quality of client care.

BOX 13-5 Sources of Diagnostic Error

Collecting
Lack of knowledge or skill
Inaccurate data
Missing data
Disorganization
Stereotyping of clients or making assumptions that lead to collection of selective data

Interpreting
Inaccurate interpretation of cues
Failure to consider conflicting cues
Using an insufficient number of cues
Using unreliable or invalid cues
Failure to consider cultural influences or developmental stage

Clustering
Insufficient clustering of cues
Premature or early closure of clustering
Incorrect clustering

Labelling
Wrong diagnostic label selected
Existence of evidence that another diagnosis is more likely
Condition incorrectly overlooked as a collaborative problem
Failure to validate nursing diagnosis with client
Failure to seek guidance

Errors in the Diagnostic Statement

Inaccurately interpreting the nursing diagnosis may result in developing and delivering inappropriate interventions leading to undesirable outcomes (Lunney, 2009). To reduce errors, the diagnostic statement should be worded in appropriate, concise, and precise language. Nurses need to use correct terminology that reflects the client's response to the illness or condition. Use of standardized nursing language from NANDA International (2018) helps ensure accuracy. A diagnostic statement such as "unhappy and worried about health" is not a scientifically based diagnosis and it will lead to errors. The language needs to be more precise and appropriate, such as *impaired coping related to fear of medical diagnosis.* The problem and etiological portions of the diagnostic statement need to be within the scope of nursing in order to be diagnosed and treated.

Documentation

After the nurse has identified a client's nursing diagnoses, they are listed on the written plan of care. Within clinical facilities, nursing diagnoses are chronologically listed as they are identified, with the highest level diagnosis listed first.

◆ NURSING DIAGNOSES: APPLICATION TO CARE PLANNING

Nursing diagnosis is a mechanism for identifying the nursing care necessary for clients. Diagnoses provide direction for the planning process and the selection of nursing interventions to achieve desired outcomes for clients. Just as the medical diagnosis of diabetes guides a physician to prescribe a low-carbohydrate diet and medication for blood glucose control, the nursing diagnosis of *reduced skin integrity* directs a nurse to apply certain support surfaces to a client's bed and to initiate a turning schedule. In the next section, focused on the planning phase of the nursing process, you will learn how to unify the language of NANDA International with the Nursing Interventions Classification (NIC) and Nursing Outcomes Classification (NOC) to help facilitate the process of matching nursing diagnoses with accurate and appropriate interventions and outcomes. The care plan is a map for nursing care and demonstrates the nurse's accountability for client care. Accurate nursing diagnosis will assist in communicating to other health providers the client's health care issues and will help to guide the planning of relevant and appropriate nursing interventions.

◆ PLANNING

After a nurse identifies a client's nursing diagnoses and strengths, he or she will begin planning nursing care. Planning is a category of nursing behaviour in which a nurse sets client-centred goals, outlines expected outcomes, plans nursing interventions, and prioritizes and selects interventions that will resolve the client's problems and achieve the goals and outcomes. Planning requires critical thinking, applied through deliberate decision making and problem solving, to set priorities for a client. Many clients have multiple diagnoses and a number of health concerns. Successful planning requires the nurse to collaborate with the client and family, consult with other members of the health care team, and review related literature. This literature includes available evidence related to the client's health problems and concerns. A plan of care is dynamic and will change once the client's needs are met or new needs are identified.

ESTABLISHING PRIORITIES

Priority setting is the ranking of nursing diagnoses or client problems, through the use of principles such as urgency or importance, to establish a preferential order for nursing actions (Hendry & Walker, 2004; Figure 13-10). By ranking nursing diagnoses in order of importance, nurses attend to the client's most important needs first. Priorities help the nurse to anticipate and sequence nursing interventions for a client who has multiple nursing diagnoses and health problems. When feasible, nurses and clients select mutually agreed-upon priorities on the bases of the urgency of the problems, safety, the nature of the treatment indicated, and the relationship among the diagnoses.

Establishing priorities or determining urgency of the identified health problems is done on the basis of their severity or physiological importance (Lewis, Heitkemper, Dirksen, et al., 2014). Nursing diagnoses of conditions that, if untreated, result in harm to the client or others have the highest priorities. For example, *risk for other directed violence, impaired gas exchange,* and *decreased cardiac output* are typically high-priority nursing diagnoses that raise issues of safety, adequate oxygenation, and adequate circulation. *High priorities* are sometimes both physiological and psychological and may address other basic human needs. *Intermediate priority* nursing diagnoses involve the nonemergency, non–life-threatening needs of the client. *Low-priority* nursing diagnoses are not always directly related to a specific illness or prognosis but affect the client's future well-being. Many low-priority diagnoses focus on the client's long-term health care needs. The order of priorities changes as a client's condition changes, sometimes within a matter of minutes. Ongoing client assessment is essential for determining the priority of the client's nursing diagnoses.

In considering time as a factor in setting priorities, White (2003) explained that the planning of nursing care occurs in three phases: initial, ongoing, and discharge. *Initial planning* involves development of a preliminary plan of care after admission assessment and initial selection of nursing diagnoses. Because of progressively shorter lengths of hospitalization, initial planning is important in addressing nursing diagnoses and collaborative problems in order to hasten problem

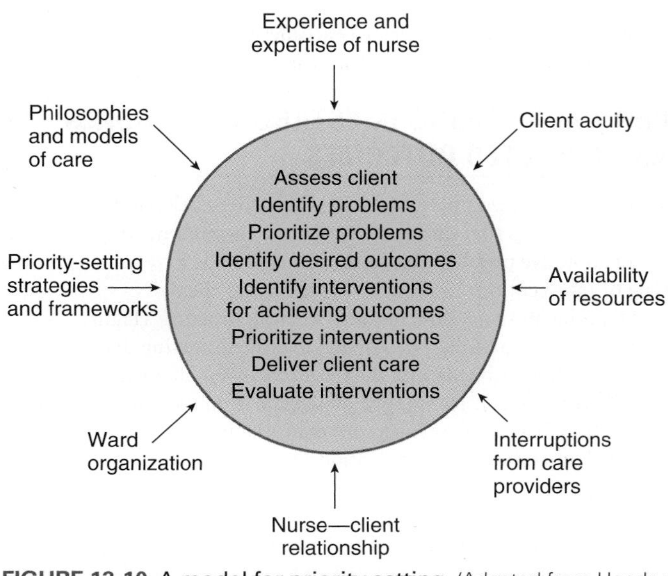

FIGURE 13-10 A model for priority setting. (Adapted from Hendry, C., & Walker, A. [2004]. Priority setting in clinical nursing practice. *Journal of Advanced Nursing, 47*[4], 427–436.)

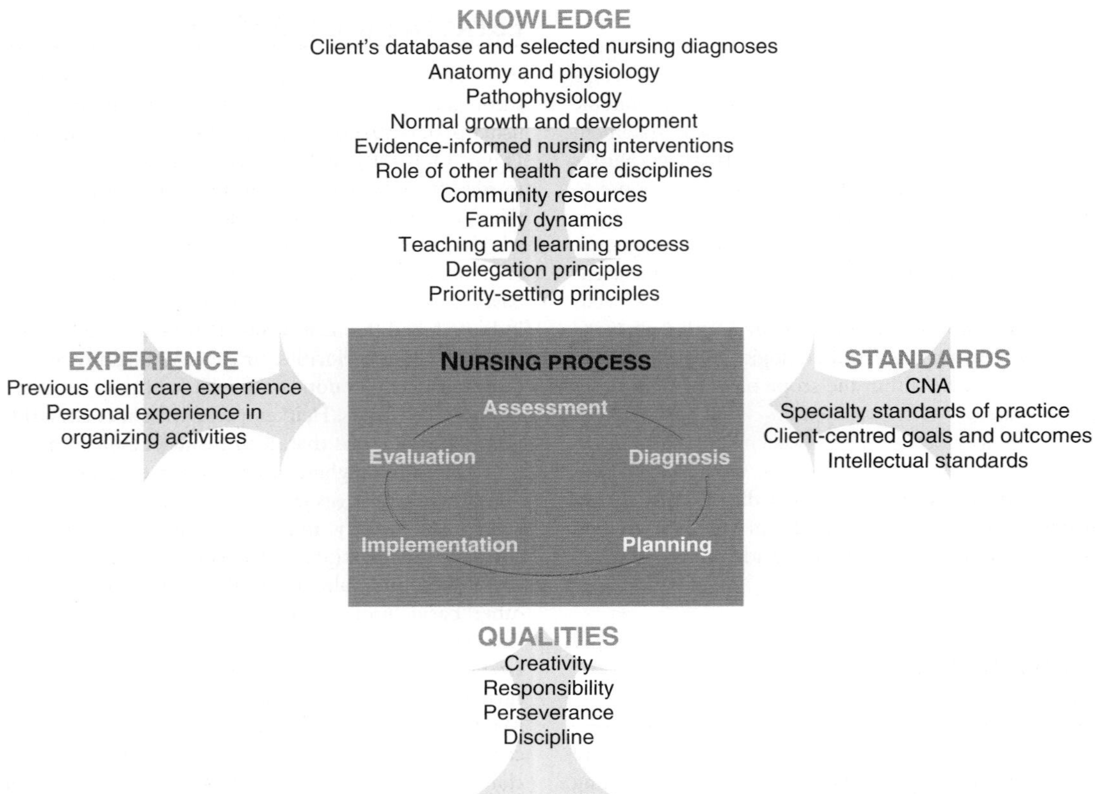

FIGURE 13-11 Critical thinking and the process of planning care. *CNA,* Canadian Nurses Association.

resolution. *Ongoing planning* involves continuous updating of the client's plan of care. As the client's condition changes, the nurse assesses new information about the client and evaluates the client's status. *Discharge planning* involves the anticipation and preparation for meeting the client's needs after discharge. This is a vital phase of planning that should begin upon admission or when care begins. It continues throughout the period of care.

Nurses prioritize the specific interventions or strategies used in order to help a client achieve desired goals and outcomes. It is important to involve the client in priority setting whenever possible; in some situations, the nurse and the client have different priorities.

CRITICAL THINKING IN ESTABLISHING GOALS AND EXPECTED OUTCOMES

Goals and **expected outcomes** are specific client behaviour or physiological responses that nurses set to achieve through nursing diagnosis or collaborative problem resolution. They provide a clear focus for the type of interventions necessary to care for the client.

Planning nursing care requires critical thinking (Figure 13-11). Nurses need to carefully evaluate the identified nursing diagnoses, the urgency of the problems, and the resources of the client and the health care delivery system. They apply knowledge from the nursing, medical, and sociobehavioural sciences to plan client care. To select goals, expected outcomes, and interventions, nurses must consider their previous experience with similar client problems, as well as any established standards for nursing practice.

The diagram in Figure 13-12 illustrates the relationships between nursing diagnoses, goals, expected outcomes, and nursing interventions. In order to help you to understand the role of critical thinking in establishing goals and expected outcomes, we return to Mr. Fletcher's case scenario and outline how the nurse uses this process in the planning of care:

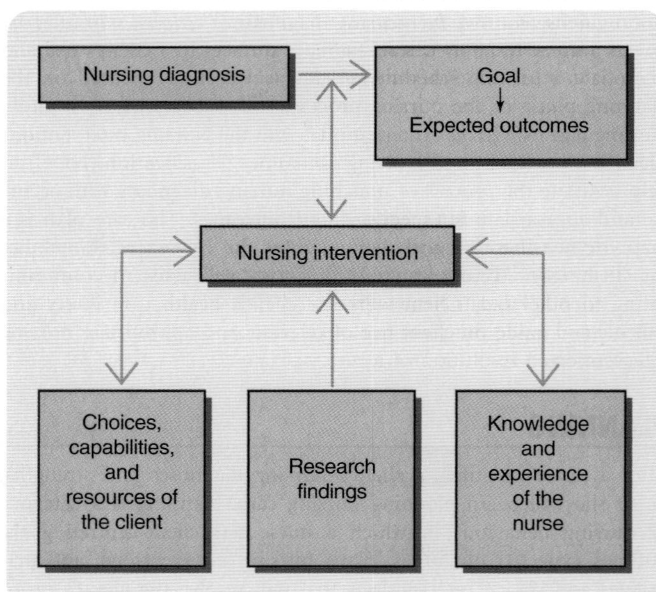

FIGURE 13-12 From diagnosis to outcome. (Revised and redrawn from Gordon, M. [1994]. *Nursing diagnosis: Process and application* [3rd ed.]. St. Louis, MO: Mosby.)

Irene begins planning with Mr. Fletcher in order to control and improve his hypertension. Knowing that hypertension is a chronic disease condition, Irene recognizes that Mr. Fletcher will need to be involved in his care and that he needs to help to set the expected outcomes for his care.

Knowledge: *Irene needs to educate Mr. Fletcher on the key aspects related to his hypertension: (1) how to recognize hypertension using clinical parameters, (2) how to monitor his blood pressure, (3) how to identify potential modifiable risk factors, and (4) how to recognize complications. Irene is aware that Mr. Fletcher is dealing with a new diagnosis and that she will need to prioritize and simplify the information given to him. It is likely that the physician or nurse practitioner will prescribe antihypertensive medication to Mr. Fletcher. In this case, Irene will work collaboratively to set goals for client outcomes resulting from medication therapy.*

Standards: *Irene uses the RNAO's (2005) Nursing Management of Hypertension guidelines to help formulate her teaching plan. She decides to focus on educating Mr. Fletcher about self and home blood pressure monitoring techniques and the appropriate equipment to use to assist in monitoring his hypertension. She will also use these guidelines to plan her educational strategies to guide Mr. Fletcher in optimizing a target blood pressure. She will work with him to identify lifestyle factors that may be contributing to his hypertension.*

Qualities: *Irene takes a client-centred approach in planning nursing care. She has developed a therapeutic relationship with Mr. Fletcher and will use both direct and indirect nursing interventions, accessing collaborative supports as required in her care planning.*

Experience: *For previous clients with newly diagnosed hypertension, Irene has found it helpful to teach them to take their blood pressure at home and to keep a log. This enables clients to see trends in their blood pressure throughout the day and to keep track of any symptoms that may be occurring for them. Irene has also found that including the client's partner or spouse and/or family in this education has led to increased understanding and practice of proposed strategies. Irene will set client-centred goals that are both short and long term.*

Goals of Care

A **client-centred goal** is a specific and measurable behavioural response that reflects a client's highest possible level of wellness and independence in function. Examples are "Client will perform self-care hygiene independently" and "Client will remain free of infection." A goal is realistic and based on client needs and resources. A client goal represents predicted resolution of a nursing diagnosis or health problem, proof of progress toward resolution, enhanced improved health status, or continued maintenance of optimal health (Carpenito, 2013). A goal involves only one behaviour or response. The example of "Client will administer a self-injection and demonstrate infection control measures" is incorrect because the statement includes two different behaviours: "administer" and "demonstrate." Instead, the goal should be worded as follows: "Client will administer a self-injection." The specific criteria you use to measure success of the goal are the expected outcomes: for example, "Client will prepare medication dose correctly" and "Client uses aseptic technique when preparing injection site." Each goal is time-limited so that the health care team has a common time frame for problem resolution. The time frame depends on the nature of the problem, etiology, overall condition of the client, and treatment setting.

A **short-term goal** is an objective behaviour or response that a client is expected to achieve in a short time, usually less than a week. In an acute care setting, goals are set for over a course of just a few hours. A **long-term goal** is an objective behaviour or response that a client is expected to achieve over a longer period, usually over several days, weeks, or months: for example, "Client will be tobacco-free within 60 days." Goal setting establishes the framework for the nursing care plan (Table 13-4).

Role of the Client in Goal Setting. It is important to work closely with clients in setting goals. Mutual goal setting is an activity that includes clients and families in prioritizing goals of care and in developing plans for action (Bulechek, Butcher, Dochterman, et al., 2013). Clients need to be able to engage in problem solving and decision making in order to participate effectively in goal setting. Goals that are determined with the client and have a clear action plan are more likely to be successful.

Expected Outcomes

An *expected outcome* is a specific measurable change in a client's status that is expected in response to nursing care. Expected outcomes provide a focus or direction for nursing care because they are the desired physiological, psychological, social, developmental, or spiritual responses that indicate resolution of clients' health problems. Derived from both short- and long-term goals, outcomes determine when a specific client-centred goal has been met.

Usually several expected outcomes for each nursing diagnosis and goal are listed. The reason for the multiple expected outcomes is that sometimes one nursing action is not enough to resolve a specific problem. In addition, the listing of the step-by-step expected outcomes assists in planning interventions. The nurse should write

TABLE 13-4 Examples of Goal Setting With Expected Outcomes

Nursing Diagnoses	Goals	Expected Outcomes
Acute pain related to pressure on spinal nerves	Client's level of comfort will improve before surgery.	Client will be able to turn without reported discomfort in 2 hours. Client's self-report of pain will be 3 or less on a scale of 0 to 10 by the time of scheduled surgery.
Anxiety related to uncertainty over surgery	Client will accept plan for surgical care before scheduled surgery.	Client will express less uneasiness about surgical experience in next 4 hours.
Deficient knowledge regarding postoperative activities related to inexperience	Client will understand treatment procedures planned postoperatively within 4 hours.	Client will describe purpose of postoperative exercises prior to scheduled surgery. Client will demonstrate use of incentive spirometer and deep breathing and coughing prior to scheduled surgery. Client will explain purpose of postoperative nursing care prior to scheduled surgery.
Impaired physical mobility related to acute back pain	Client will move independently in bed before surgery.	Client will initiate turning without additional discomfort within 2 hours. Client will position self for care procedures within 2 hours.

TABLE 13-5 Examples of NANDA International Nursing Diagnoses and Suggested NOC Linkages

Nursing Diagnosis	Suggested NOC-Based Outcomes (Examples)	Outcome Indicators (Examples)
Deficient knowledge	Knowledge: treatment procedures	Description of treatment procedure Description of steps in procedure
	Client satisfaction: teaching	Explanations provided in understandable terms Explanation of activity restrictions
Activity intolerance	Activity tolerance	Oxygen saturation with activity Pulse rate with activity Respiratory rate with activity
	Self-care status	Bathes self Dresses self Prepares food and fluid for eating

NOC, Nursing Outcomes Classification.

expected outcomes sequentially, specifying time frames for each. Time frames provide progressive steps to recovery and assist in ranking nursing interventions. In addition, time frames set limits for problem resolution.

The nurse should also write expected outcome statements in measurable terms. This enables the nurse to note the specific behaviour or physiological response expected for resolution of the problem. For example, "Client will have less pain" is an inaccurate outcome statement because the phrase "less pain" is nonspecific. The statement "Client will report pain acuity of less than 3 on a scale of 0 to 10" is accurate.

Nursing Outcomes Classification. In the current health care environment, considerable attention is paid to measuring outcomes sensitive to nursing interventions. Many health care administrators focus on outcomes in determining staffing and other resources in health care settings. The Iowa Intervention Project published the Nursing Outcomes Classification (NOC) and has linked the outcomes to NANDA International (2018) nursing diagnoses (University of Iowa College of Nursing, 2008). The Iowa researchers defined a **nursing-sensitive client outcome** as an individual, family, or community behaviour or perception that is measurable along a continuum in response to a nursing intervention. For any given NANDA International nursing diagnosis, multiple outcomes are suggested in NOC. These outcomes provide descriptions of the focus of nursing care and include indicators for measuring success with interventions (Table 13-5).

Combining Goals and Outcome Statements

Nurses within health care settings may refer to the terms, goals, and outcomes interchangeably. This is acceptable, as long as the criteria for writing goals and outcomes are met. For example, the statement "Client will achieve pain control as evidenced by reporting pain acuity of less than 3 on a scale of 0 to 10 within 24 hours" is an acceptable statement. The goal portion of the statement broadly describes the desired client status ("achieve pain control"), and the outcome portion of the statement contains the observable criterion ("3 on a [pain] scale") needed to measure success.

Guidelines for Writing Goals and Expected Outcomes

There are seven guidelines for writing goals and expected outcomes: client-centred, singular, observable, measurable, time-limited, mutual, and realistic.

Client Goal or Outcome. Outcomes and goals reflect client responses that are expected after nursing interventions. The nurse should write a goal to reflect client behaviour, not to reflect the nurse's goals or interventions. A correct outcome statement is "Client will ambulate in the hall three times a day." A common error is to write "Ambulate client in the hall three times a day."

Singular Goal or Outcome. The nurse should be precise in evaluating a client response to a nursing action. Each goal and outcome addresses only one behaviour or response.

Observable Goal or Outcome. Nurses need to be able to observe whether change in a client's status occurs. Changes in physiological findings and in the client's knowledge, perceptions, and behaviour are observable. Nurses observe outcomes by directly asking clients about their condition and by using assessment skills. For the outcome "Chest sounds will be clear on auscultation by 8/31," the nurse would auscultate the client's chest routinely after therapy (e.g., inhalation, percussion). The outcome statement "Client will appear less anxious" is not a correct statement because no specific behaviour for "will appear" is observable.

Measurable Goal or Outcome. It is imperative to learn to write goals and expected outcomes that set standards against which to measure the client's response to nursing care. Examples such as "Body temperature will remain between the normal range of 36.5 and 37.5°C" and "Apical pulse will remain between 60 and 100 beats per minute" enable the nurse to objectively measure changes in the client's status.

Time-Limited Goal or Outcome. The time frame for each goal and expected outcome indicates when the expected response should occur. Time frames assist in determining progress toward goals and outcomes.

Mutual Goal or Outcome. Mutually set goals and expected outcomes ensure that the client and nurse agree on the direction and time limits of care. Mutual goal setting increases clients' motivation and cooperation.

Realistic Goal or Outcome. It is important to set goals and expected outcomes that are achievable. Clients are then more likely to have a sense of empowerment that increases motivation and cooperation. In order to establish realistic goals, the nurse needs to assess the resources of the client, the family, the health care facility, and the community. The nurse should also be aware of the client's physiological, emotional, cognitive, and sociocultural influences and take into consideration the client's determinants of health.

WRITTEN PLANS OF CARE

In any health care setting, a nurse is responsible for developing a written plan of care for clients. The written plan of care may take several forms (e.g., a nursing card-filing system, standardized care plans, or computerized plans). In general, a written **nursing care plan** includes nursing diagnoses; goals, expected outcomes, or both; and specific nursing interventions, so that any nurse is able to quickly identify a client's clinical needs and situation. In hospitals and community-based settings, the client often receives care from more than one nurse, physician, or allied health provider. A written nursing care plan makes possible continuity and coordination of nursing care and consultation by a number of health providers.

Written care plans organize information exchanged by nurses in change-of-shift reports (see Chapter 16 for further information about nursing informatics). Nurses learn to focus their reports on the nursing care, treatments, and expected outcomes documented in their care plans, and the end-of-shift report allows for discussion of care plans and the overall progress with the next caregiver.

Institutional Care Plans

Institutional care plans become part of a client's legal medical record. Many hospitals still use a written Kardex nursing care plan. The Kardex card-filing system allows quick reference to the needs of the client for certain aspects of nursing care (see Chapter 15 for documentation). The care plan section of a Kardex system varies by agency and focuses on planned interventions to meet the needs of the client and family and to prepare the client for discharge from the hospital. The focus of a nursing care plan differs by setting and the evolving client situation. For example, nursing care plans developed for clients returning home are usually based solely on long-term health needs. Nursing care plans for same-day surgeries are usually focused on clients' short-term needs (e.g., immediate recovery from surgery and instructions for self-care at home). In a long-term care facility, plans of care focus on clients' long-term rehabilitation needs.

Computerized Care Plans. A majority of health care facilities now have some type of electronic health record (EHR) and documentation system (Health Canada, 2009). Software programs are available for nursing care plans. In many facilities, the format is for standardized care plans that list generalized nursing diagnoses, goals, outcome criteria, and interventions for specific clients. The nurse adds or deletes information by making selections from menus on the standardized form to individualize it for a client's needs. Computerized and standardized nursing care plans organize and enhance care planning. Their design incorporates current evidence-informed practice guidelines to achieve the desired client outcomes for a specific group of clients.

Care Plans for Community-Based Settings. Planning care for clients in community-based settings—for example, clinics, community centres, or clients' homes—involves using the same principles of nursing practice. In these settings, however, nurses need to complete a more comprehensive community, home, and family assessment. The client or family unit must be able to provide the majority of health care independently or with external resources provided to meet care demands (see Chapter 4 for further information about community health).

Critical Pathways. Critical pathways are multidisciplinary treatment plans that outline treatments or interventions that clients may require for treatment of a condition. Most pathways are based on medical rather than nursing diagnoses, but they incorporate related nursing diagnoses and associated nursing interventions. A critical pathway maps out, day to day or even hour to hour, the recommended interventions and expected outcomes. For example, a pathway for a surgical procedure such as a bowel resection will recommend on a day-by-day basis the client's activities, procedures, and discharge planning activities. A critical pathway improves continuity of care because it clearly maps out the responsibility of each health discipline and can be used to monitor a client's progress. Well-developed pathways incorporate current evidence in caring for clients with a specific condition. When critical pathways are used to plan care, some forms of documentation are eliminated (e.g., the nursing care plan, flow sheets, and nurses' notes) because all of the pertinent components are included in the pathway.

CONSULTING OTHER HEALTH CARE PROVIDERS

Planning involves consultation with members of the health team. Although consultation can occur at any step in the nursing process, it occurs most often during planning and implementation, when problems necessitating additional knowledge, skills, or resources arise. Consulting involves seeking the expertise of a specialist, such as a nurse educator, registered nurse, or clinical nurse specialist, to identify ways of approaching and managing the planning and implementation of therapies.

Nurse consultants frequently offer advice about difficult clinical problems. For example, a nursing student will consult with the registered nurse assigned to the same client about ways to individualize interventions, with a clinical specialist for wound care techniques, or with an educator for useful teaching resources. Nurses are consulted for their clinical expertise, client education skills, or staff education skills. Nurses also consult with other members of the health care team, such as physiotherapists, nutritionists, and social workers.

CONCLUSION

This chapter has outlined how the nurse approaches assessment, diagnosis, and planning within the nursing process. It is important to remember that nursing practice is complex, dynamic, and at times unpredictable; nurses must be able to prioritize, predict changes in health status, and adapt to new situations as necessary. While nurses utilize models of care, such as the nursing process, as a beginning structure for approaching, organizing, implementing and evaluating care, it is their critical thinking and holistic approaches to client care that help to provide safe, informed, and comprehensive client care. The next chapter approaches care planning in more detail and discusses the intervention and evaluation stages of the nursing process.

USING THE NURSING PROCESS TO ANSWER MULTIPLE-CHOICE AND MULTIPLE-RESPONSE EXAM QUESTIONS

The nursing process is an essential model for helping nursing students understand how nursing care unfolds. It is also a valuable tool to use when learning how to study for and take nursing exams. By understanding the nursing process in full, a nursing student can quickly determine what an exam question is asking and what the most logical answer or next step will be. It is important to speak to the role of the nursing process in exam taking because nursing students will be evaluated in their nursing programs through exams and on graduation by writing a registration exam for nursing licensure. This section addresses the basics of multiple-choice questions/multiple-response questions and the different taxonomies (or levels) of thinking that are used to underpin this form of evaluation (please note that the taxonomic levels identified are used in varying ways in education, but for the purpose of discussion are focused on multiple-choice/multiple-response exam-type questions). The role of the nursing process as it relates to assessment, diagnosis, and planning will also be discussed here for approaching and answering exam questions in these areas of focus.

To begin with, multiple-choice questions have varying level of difficulty, depending on what they are testing. *Knowledge/Comprehension*-level questions are the easiest because they test basic information or content that can be memorized. Here is an example of a knowledge-level question based on the content from this chapter:

The purpose of nursing assessment is to:

1. Make a diagnostic conclusion
2. Delegate nursing responsibility
3. Teach the client about his or her health
4. Establish a database concerning the client

This question is asking you to recall the purpose of an assessment, which is to establish a database concerning the client (answer 4). By memorizing the basic definition of an assessment, you are able to answer this question. While gathering basic knowledge through memorization is a step in acquiring your future knowledge base, it is important that you learn to extend your study strategies to include other forms of learning outside of memorization (e.g., flashcards, writing down notes and studying them). As your nursing program progresses, there will be fewer knowledge/comprehension-type questions on your exams and you will need to develop study strategies to help you apply and critically think about the information you are learning. (See Chapter 14 for an example of these exercises.)

The next level of questioning in multiple-choice/multiple-response testing is an *application question*. These questions ask you to apply information/knowledge to a new situation. An example of this type of question is as follows:

Casey is reviewing a client's list of nursing diagnoses in the medical record. The most recent nursing diagnosis is *constipation related to intestinal blockage*. Why is this nursing diagnostic statement incorrectly worded?

1. Identifying the clinical sign instead of an etiology
2. Identifying a diagnosis on the basis of prejudicial judgement
3. Identifying the diagnostic study rather than a problem caused by the diagnostic study
4. Identifying the medical diagnosis instead of the client's related factors to the diagnosis

This is a more difficult question than the previous one. In this question, you must understand what a nursing diagnosis is and how it is constructed. This question has given you an inaccurate nursing diagnosis: *constipation related to intestinal blockage*, and is asking you why it is wrong. The first part of the diagnosis is correct. Constipation is an approved NANDA diagnostic label (diagnosis code 00011); it is the second part of the diagnosis that is incorrect. In a nursing diagnosis, the second part is the etiology of the problem (factors that support the diagnosis), which must be within nursing terms and not described as a medical diagnosis (in this case, an intestinal blockage). Remember, nursing diagnoses are built to guide and direct nursing care. For example, if the constipation is due to the client having decreased fluid intake and being on bed rest, these would be the related factors in the nursing diagnosis. Therefore, the correct nursing diagnosis should read *constipation related to decreased fluid intake and immobility.* This nursing diagnosis allows for the development of a nursing care plan aimed at treating and preventing further constipation. In order to get this question correct you had to be successful in:

1. Remembering what the components of a nursing diagnosis were (diagnostic label and etiology [related factors])
2. Being able to apply this to a clinical context and demonstrate your understanding of the scope of a nursing diagnosis and how it differs from a medical diagnosis.

The last type of questions are *critical thinking or analysis*-level questions. These are often the most challenging types of questions because you are applying multiple sources of information, integrating foundational nursing knowledge, or being asked to prioritize between answers that are all correct, but you must choose the most immediate or best answer. An example of this type of question is as follows:

The nurse gathers the following assessment data. Which of the following cues form a pattern? (*Select all that apply.*)

1. The client is restless.
2. Fluid intake for 8 hours is 800 mL.
3. The client complains of feeling short of breath.
4. The client has drainage from a surgical wound.
5. Respirations are 24 per minute and irregular.
6. Client reports loss of appetite for more than 2 weeks.

To answer this question you begin by remembering what a "cue" is. Cues are client responses that enable the nurse to form patterns in order to formulate or support a diagnosis. In this case, there are several cues identified in the question. The most notable commonality in cues pertains to respiratory assessment: the client complains of feeling short of breath and the respirations are 24 per minute and irregular. In order to correctly answer this question, you also need to consider that the client is restless—this is associated with respiratory distress and is the final cue to establishing a pattern pertaining to respiratory distress in this client. Finally, you need the foundational knowledge of normal respirations and a recognition that 24 respirations per minute is considered tachypneic. To arrive at this correct answer, you needed to define a term, look for patterns, and then determine if the cues presented were considered normal or abnormal findings.

It is also helpful to reflect on common words, listed by Nugent and Vitale (2015), that are often present in the stem of the question when asking about the differing parts of the nursing process. This will help you understand exactly which part of the nursing process (assessment, diagnosis, planning, intervention, or evaluation) the question is speaking to (Table 13-6). When you approach an exam question, engage in the following steps (Kramer-Kile, 2015):

Step 1: Identify which phase of the nursing process is being addressed in the question stem. You can do this by isolating the verbs in the question stem and determining what the question is asking the nurse to do (see Table 13-6).

Step 2: Determine what the question is asking. Are you being asked to explore a part of the nursing process or to go to the next step? Are you supposed to prioritize among answers that are all correct? Or are you choosing the best answer, knowing that other answers may be incorrect?

Step 3: Link the potential answers back to the question stem and information provided.

Example:

The nurse assesses a 70-year-old male's laboratory results during a routine clinic visit. Which result would indicate a need for information and education? Please select your answer.

__RBC 5×10^{12}/L (5.0 million/mm^3)

__Serum albumin 25 g/L (2.5 g/dL)

__LDL cholesterol 3.37 mmol/L (130 mg/dL)

__Serum glucose 5 mmol/L (90 mg/dL)

(NCSBN Learning Extension question of the week. Retrieved from http://learningext.com.)

Step 1: This question is in the assessment phase of the nursing process, where the nurse is being asked to conduct *data analysis* in order to determine his or her priority nursing interventions.

Step 2: The question is asking you to first determine which lab values are normal and which are abnormal. The RBC (red blood cells), LDL (low-density lipoprotein) cholesterol, and serum glucose levels are all in the normal range. *(Please note that while you are learning about laboratory values in clinical practice, you will be given the reference ranges next to the client result in the lab report. It is common in nursing examination settings (particularly with registration exams) that you will be expected to note an abnormal laboratory value*

TABLE 13-6 Using the Nursing Process to Help Answer Exam Questions

Nursing Process	Questions in This Stage of the Nursing Process Often Ask You to:	Common Words in the Question Stem Identifying This Area
Assessment	• Perform an assessment technique • Obtain vital signs • Recognize normal and abnormal findings or values • Take a health history • Explore client feelings • Review diagnostic tests • Review or access a consultation from another health care provider	Inspect, identify, verify, observe, determine, notify, check, inform, question, communicate, verbal and nonverbal, signs and symptoms, stressors, adaptations, sources, perceptions, and assess
Analysis	• Clustering data • Determine priorities in data collection • Identifying further data that need to be examined • Interpreting data in the context of illness	Organize, categorize, re-examine, pattern, formulate, nursing diagnosis, reflect, relate, problem, interpret, contribute, related, decision, significant, deduction, statement, analysis
Planning	• Involve the client in the planning process • Set goals • Establish expected outcomes against which results of care can be compared for the purpose of evaluation • Plan appropriate interventions based on their effects • Establish priorities of nursing interventions • Anticipate client needs • Collaborate with others • Coordinate planned care with other disciplines • Recognize that plans must be flexible and modified on the basis of changing client needs	Achieve, desired, plan, effective, desired result, goal, priority, develop, formulate, establish, design, prevent, strategy, select, determine, anticipate, modify, collaborate, arrange, coordinate, expect, outcome

Source: Kramer-Kile, M.L. (2016). *Transitioning to the NCLEX-RN®: A Study Guide for Canadian-educated graduates* (2nd ed.). Kimberley, BC: Kramer-Kile Nurse Education Consultants Ltd. Registration No. 1122832. Retrieved from rnstudyguides.ca. Reprinted with permission.

without having the reference range provided—keep this in mind as you progress through your studies.)

Step 3: The question asks which result would indicate a need for more information and education. In this case, it is the low albumin level because it may indicate liver failure or malnutrition.

This question is challenging because you are applying the nursing process and recalling complex information at the same time. In order to answer this question, you were required to know what each of these laboratory tests were and their normal values. This is information that you will gain as you progress in your nursing program. This question was selected to show you that the information required to answer nursing exam questions becomes more complex. However, if you have strong skills in understanding foundational concepts such as the nursing process it will become easier to decipher the correct answer when you may not know the answer. This last example will demonstrate how to do this (Kramer-Kile, 2015):

A client's heart rate on initial assessment was 48 beats per minute. At the time, the nurse took a radial pulse and had difficulty palpating it. What is an appropriate next step for the nurse to take in this situation?

1. Call the physician immediately.
2. Take a blood pressure.
3. Auscultate the apical pulse.
4. Determine if the client is on beta-blocker therapy.

The answer is 3. In this question the nurse is in the assessment phase of the nursing process. The nurse has collected data and is now moving toward the next step of data verification. In order to verify that the low radial pulse is actually at 48 beats/minute the nurse takes an apical pulse to verify the rate. Calling the physician at this time is not appropriate because he or she would ask the nurse to verify the data. Determining if the client is on beta-blocker therapy would help the nurse to interpret potential assessment findings, but again, the question states that the pulse was collected using the radial site and it was difficult to palpate. Again, the client's heart rate needs to be verified.

Practice questions are a helpful resource that will assist you in learning to apply the nursing process. However, it is important that you answer practice questions after studying your nursing content. It is also helpful to try to construct your own practice questions after you have read a chapter in your textbook. This will help you to decipher and think through the content you have reviewed.

KEY CONCEPTS

- The nursing process employs critical thinking to identify, diagnose, and treat clients' responses to health and illness.
- Nursing assessment involves the collection and verification of data and the analysis of all data to establish a database about a client's perceived needs, health problems, and responses to those problems.
- By interpreting the meaning of cues, the nurse forms an inference, which then enables the nurse to identify meaningful clusters of information.
- To conduct a comprehensive assessment, nurses use a structured database format or a problem-oriented approach.
- The interview is an organized conversation with a client that begins by establishing a therapeutic relationship with the client and that aids in the investigation and discussion of the client's health care needs.
- Open-ended questions encourage clients to describe their health histories in detail, whereas closed-ended questions present a list of possible choices for the client.

- An interview includes three phases: orientation, working, and termination.
- Once a client provides subjective data, the nurse considers exploring the findings further by collecting objective data.
- During assessment, nurses critically anticipate and use an appropriate branching set of questions or observations to collect data, and cues of assessment information are clustered to identify emerging patterns and problems.
- Written data statements are descriptive, to the point, and complete and do not include inferences or interpretative statements.
- Family members and friends sometimes offer observations about the client's needs; these observations will affect the way the nurse delivers care.
- During assessment, nurses encourage clients to describe their histories of illnesses or health care problems.
- To form a nursing judgement, nurses critically assess a client, validate the data, interpret the information gathered, and look for diagnostic cues that will lead them to identify the client's problems.
- NANDA International has developed a common language that enables all members of the health care team to understand a client's needs.
- The analysis and interpretation of data require nurses to validate data, recognize patterns or trends, compare data with healthful standards, and then form diagnostic conclusions.
- The absence of defining characteristics suggests that the nurse reject a proposed diagnosis.
- Four types of nursing diagnoses exist: actual, at risk, wellness diagnoses, and health promotion.
- A nursing diagnosis is written in a two-part format, including a diagnostic label and an etiological or related factor.
- The "related to" factor of the diagnostic statement assists nurses in individualizing a client's nursing diagnoses and provides direction for their selection of appropriate interventions.
- Risk factors serve as cues to indicate that a risk nursing diagnosis applies to a client's condition.
- Concept mapping is a visual representation of a client's nursing diagnoses and their relationship with one another.
- Nursing diagnostic errors occur through errors in data collection, in interpretation and analysis of data, in clustering of data, or in the diagnostic statement.
- Nursing diagnoses improve communication between nurses and other health care providers.
- During planning, nurses determine client-centred goals, set priorities, develop expected outcomes of nursing care, and develop a nursing care plan.
- Priority setting helps nurses anticipate and sequence nursing interventions when a client has multiple nursing diagnoses and collaborative problems.
- Multiple factors in the nursing care environment influence priority setting.
- Goals and expected outcomes provide clear direction for the selection and use of nursing interventions and provide focus for evaluation of the effectiveness of the interventions.
- In setting goals, the time frame depends on the nature of the problem, etiology, overall condition of the client, and treatment setting.
- A client-centred goal is singular, observable, measurable, time limited, mutual, and realistic.
- An expected outcome is an objective criterion for goal achievement.
- Care plans and critical pathways increase communication among nurses and facilitate the continuity of care from one nurse to another and from one health care setting to another.

REVIEW QUESTIONS

1. The nurse completes a nursing health history with her client. In order to avoid incorrect inferences and ensure that the data are accurate, the nurse's next step is to:
   1. Analyze and interpret the data
   2. Document the data
   3. Validate data with the client
   4. Share the data with other health care providers
2. During data clustering, a nurse:
   1. Provides documentation of nursing care
   2. Reviews data with other health care providers
   3. Makes inferences about patterns of information
   4. Organizes cues into patterns that enable the nurse to identify nursing diagnoses
3. A nursing diagnosis is:
   1. The diagnosis and treatment of human responses to health and illness
   2. The advancement of the development, testing, and refinement of a common nursing language
   3. A clinical judgement about individual, family, or community responses to actual and potential health problems or life processes
   4. The identification of a disease condition on the basis of a specific evaluation of physical signs, symptoms, the client's medical history, and the results of diagnostic tests
4. One of the purposes of the use of standard formal nursing diagnostic statements is to:
   1. Evaluate nursing care
   2. Gather information on client data
   3. Help nurses to focus on the role of nursing in client care
   4. Facilitate understanding of client problems among health care providers
5. The nursing diagnosis *readiness for enhanced communication* is an example of:
   1. A risk nursing diagnosis
   2. An actual nursing diagnosis
   3. A potential nursing diagnosis
   4. A wellness nursing diagnosis
6. The nursing diagnosis *hypothermia* is an example of:
   1. A risk nursing diagnosis
   2. An actual nursing diagnosis
   3. A potential nursing diagnosis
   4. A wellness nursing diagnosis
7. The word *impaired* in the diagnosis *impaired physical mobility* is an example of:
   1. A descriptor
   2. A risk factor
   3. A related factor
   4. A nursing diagnosis
8. Nurses use a variety of assessment techniques for data collection. The nurse knows that the first appropriate assessment technique for data collection is to:
   1. Review client's medical record
   2. Interview client
   3. Consult health care team
   4. Review literature
9. Which of the following are defining characteristics for the nursing diagnosis *impaired urinary elimination*? (*Select all that apply.*)
   1. Nocturia
   2. Frequency
   3. Urine retention

4. Inadequate urinary output
5. Treatment with intravenous fluids
6. Sensation of bladder fullness

Answers: 1. 3; **2.** 4; **3.** 3; **4.** 4; **5.** 4; **6.** 2; **7.** 1; **8.** 2; **9.** 1, 2

Rationales for the Review Questions appear at the end of the book.

RECOMMENDED WEBSITES

Center for Nursing Classification and Clinical Effectiveness: https://nursing.uiowa.edu/center-for-nursing-classification-and-clinical-effectiveness

The University of Iowa's Center for Nursing Classification & Clinical Effectiveness was established to facilitate ongoing research of the Nursing Interventions Classification (NIC) and Nursing Outcomes Classification (NOC). This site provides an overview of the NIC and NOC and offers information about new classification material and publications.

NANDA International: http://www.nanda.org/

Through this website, NANDA International (formerly the North American Nursing Diagnosis Association) provides current information on nursing diagnosis research, publications, links, and Internet resources.

National Council of State Boards of Nursing (NCSBN): NCLEX-RN Test Plans: https://www.ncsbn.org/testplans.htm

This website outlines the current NCLEX-RN Test Plan. Currently, this is the registration exam used by the Canadian Council of Registered Nurse Regulators (CCRNR) and provincial regulatory bodies for registration in all the provinces and territories, except Quebec, as of January 2015.

Registered Nurses' Association of Ontario (RNAO): Nursing Best Practice Guidelines: http://www.rnao.org/bestpractices/

The RNAO has developed an extensive process to develop Best Practices Guidelines in a variety of areas of clinical nursing. They have received federal and provincial funding for this process, and their work has been made available to all Canadian nurses through this website, which lists all current guidelines that have been developed.

REFERENCES

Alfaro-Lefevre, R. (2012). Nursing process and clinical reasoning. *Nursing Education Perspectives, 33*(1), 7.

Benner, P., Sutphen, M., Leonard, V., et al. (2010). *Educating nurses: A call for radical transformation*. San Francisco: Jossey-Bass.

Bulechek, G. M., Butcher, H. K., Dochterman, J. M., et al. (2013). *Nursing interventions classification (NIC)* (6th ed.). St. Louis: Mosby.

Canadian Association of Schools of Nursing/Association Canadienne des Écoles de Sciences Infirmières (CASN/ACESI) (2015). *National nursing education framework: Final report*. Ottawa: Author. Retrieved from http://www.casn.ca/wp-content/uploads/2014/12/Framwork-FINAL-SB-Nov-30-20151.pdf.

Carpenito, L. J. (2013). *Nursing diagnosis: Application to clinical practice* (14th ed.). Philadelphia: Lippincott Williams & Wilkins.

Harrison, S., & Gibbons, C. (2013). Nursing student perceptions of concept maps: From theory to practice. *Nurse Education Perspectives, 34*(6), 395–399.

Health Canada (2009). *Government of Canada supports electronic health record system that will save time and lives*. Ottawa: Author. Retrieved from http://www.marketwired.com/press-release/government-canada-supports-electronic-health-record-system-that-will-save-time-lives-948454.htm. February 11.

Health Canada (2011). *Eating well with Canada's food guide*. Ottawa: Author. Retrieved from http://www.hc-sc.gc.ca/fn-an/alt_formats/hpfb-dgpsa/pdf/food-guide-aliment/view_eatwell_vue_bienmang-eng.pdf.

Heart and Stroke Foundation of Canada. (2015). *The 2015 guidelines for CPR and emergency cardiovascular care*. Retrieved from https://www.heartandstroke.ca/-/media/pdf-files/canada/cpr-2017/ecc-highlights-of-2015-guidelines-update-for-cpr-ecclr.ashx.

Heart and Stroke Foundation of Ontario & Registered Nurses' Association of Ontario (RNAO) (2005). *Nursing management of hypertension*. Toronto: Author. Retrieved from http://rnao.ca/bpg/guidelines/nursing-management-hypertension.

Hendry, C., & Walker, A. (2004). Priority setting in clinical nursing practice: Literature review. *Journal of Advanced Nursing, 47*, 427–436.

Hypertension Canada. (2016). II. *Criteria for diagnosis of hypertension and recommendations for follow-up*. Retrieved from http://guidelines.hypertension.ca/wp-content/docs/DAII_Criteria_for_Diagnosis_of_Hypertension_and_Recommendations_for_Follow-up.pdf.

Jarvis, C., Browne, A. J., MacDonald-Jenkins, J., et al. (2014). *Physical examination & health assessment* (2nd Canadian ed.). Toronto: Elsevier.

Kramer-Kile, M. L. (2015). *Transitioning to the NCLEX-RN®: A study guide for Canadian-educated graduates* (1st ed.). Kimberley, BC: Kramer-Kile Nurse Education Consultants Ltd. Retrieved from rnstudyguides.ca. Registration No. 1122832.

Lewis, S., Heitkemper, M., Dirksen, S., et al. (2014). *Medical-surgical nursing in Canada: Assessment and management of clinical problems* (3rd ed.). Toronto: Elsevier.

Lunney, M. (2009). *NANDA International: Critical thinking to achieve positive outcomes: Nursing case studies and analyses*. Indianapolis, IN: Wiley-Blackwell.

NANDA International. (2018). *Nursing diagnoses: Definitions and classification, 2018–2020* (11th ed.). New York: Thieme.

Nugent, P. M., & Vitale, B. A. (2015). *Test success: Test-taking techniques for beginning nursing students* (7th ed.). Philadelphia: F. A. Davis.

Ofi, B., & Sowunmi, O. (2012). Nursing documentation: Experience of the use of the nursing process model in selected hospitals in Ibadan, Oyo State, Nigeria. *International Journal of Nursing Practice, 18*(4), 354–362.

Registered Nurses' Association of of Ontario (RNAO). (2005) *Nursing management of hypertension: Summary of recommendations*. Retrieved from http://rnao.ca/sites/rnao-ca/files/storage/related/608_BPG_Hypertension_summary.pdf.

Seidel, H. M., Ball, J. W., Dains, J. E., et al. (2011). *Mosby's guide to physical examination* (7th ed.). St. Louis: Mosby.

Sullivan, E. A. (2012). Critical thinking in clinical nurse education: Application of Paul's model of critical thinking. *Nursing Education in Practice, 12*(6), 322–327. doi:10.1016/j.nepr.2012.03.005.

Taylor, J., & Wros, P. (2007). Concept mapping: A nursing model for care planning. *Journal of Nursing Education, 46*(5), 211–216.

Truth and Reconciliation Commission of Canada (2015). *Calls to action*. Winnipeg: Author. Retrieved from http://www.trc.ca/websites/trcinstitution/File/2015/Findings/Calls_to_Action_English2.pdf.

United Nations (2007). *United Nations declaration on the rights of Indigenous peoples*. Geneva: Author. Retrieved from http://www.un.org/esa/socdev/unpfii/documents/DRIPS_en.pdf.

University of British Columbia. (n.d.). *Assessment framework for nursing practice*. Retrieved from https://nursing.ubc.ca/files/documents/policies/Assessment%2520Framework%25202004_1.pdf.

University of Iowa College of Nursing. (2008). *CNC—Nursing outcomes classification (NOC)*. Retrieved from https://nursing.uiowa.edu/cncce/nursing-outcomes-classification-overview.

White, L. (2003). *Documentation and the nursing process*. Clifton Park, NY: Delmar Learning.

Zamanzadeh, V., Valizadeh, L., Tabrizi, F. J., et al. (2015). Challenges associated with the implementation of the nursing process: A systematic review. *Iranian Journal of Nursing and Midwifery Research, 20*(4), 411–419.

14

Implementing and Evaluating Nursing Care

Canadian content written by Jennifer Girvin, RN, MN, Candis Spiers, RN, MN, Marnie L. Kramer, RN, PhD
Original chapter by Patricia A. Potter, RN, MSN, PhD, FAAN

OBJECTIVES

Mastery of content in this chapter will enable you to:

- Discuss the differences between nurse-initiated, physician-initiated, and collaborative interventions.
- Discuss the process of selecting nursing interventions.
- Describe the purposes of a written nursing care plan.
- Explain the relationship of implementation to the nursing diagnostic process.
- Discuss the differences between protocols and medical directives or standing orders.
- Describe the association between critical thinking and selecting nursing interventions.
- Discuss steps taken to revise a plan of care before performing implementation.
- Describe and compare direct and indirect nursing interventions.
- Select appropriate interventions for an assigned client.
- Discuss the relationship between critical thinking and evaluation.
- Identify the five elements of the evaluation process.
- Explain the relationship between goals of care, expected outcomes, and evaluative measures in evaluating nursing care.
- Give an example of evaluative measures for determining clients' progress toward an outcome.
- Describe how evaluation leads to discontinuation, review, or modifying a plan of care.

KEY TERMS

Activities of daily living (ADLs), p. 221
Adverse reaction, p. 221
Client-centred goal, p. 222
Collaborative interventions, p. 214
Consultation, p. 214
Counselling, p. 221
Dependent nursing interventions, p. 214
Direct care, p. 214
Evaluative measures, p. 225
Independent nursing interventions, p. 214
Instrumental activities of daily living (IADLs), p. 221
Life-saving measure, p. 221
Medical directive, p. 218
Nursing intervention, p. 214
Outcome, p. 225
Preventive nursing actions, p. 222
Scientific rationale, p. 220
Standard of care, p. 224
Standing order, p. 218

MEDIA RESOURCES

http://evolve.elsevier.com/Canada/Potter/fundamentals/

- Audio Chapter Summaries
- Examination Review Questions
- Concept Map Creator
- Case Study with Questions
- Audio Glossary
- Content Updates
- Video Clips

INTRODUCTION

The previous chapter explored how assessment, diagnosis, and planning inform the nursing process. In this chapter the last two steps of the nursing process, implementation and evaluation, will be discussed. The following scenario, introduced in the previous chapter, will be used as an example to discuss concepts related to implementation and evaluation in the nursing process. Box 14-1 provides an example of the nurse's care planning for Mr. Fletcher:

Mr. Fletcher is a 56-year-old client who has been experiencing headaches and dizziness for the past 2 months. He lives in a rural community and works 12-hour shifts as a haul truck operator in an open-pit coal mine. Mr. Fletcher is 23 kg overweight and has a sedentary lifestyle. He has been married for 25 years and has two grown children who no longer live at home. Mr. Fletcher recently attended a blood pressure clinic where he was told he had "high blood pressure." He has been referred to his local general practitioner for follow-up and the primary health care nurse is preparing to complete his initial health history and assessment. Mr. Fletcher has brought his wife with him for his clinic visit.

Irene is the primary nurse completing care planning for Mr. Fletcher. Irene has engaged the assessment, diagnosis, and

BOX 14-1 NURSING CARE PLAN

Hypertension

ASSESSMENT

Mr. Fletcher is a 56-year-old man who presented to the clinic with headaches and dizziness over the last 2 months. His current blood pressure is 179/89 mm Hg, HR 90 beats per minute, and respirations 20 breaths per minute.

It is noted on his lab work that he has increased total cholesterol, low-density lipoprotein (LDL), and triglyceride levels. The nurse notes cigarette smoke odour on his clothing and he has yellow staining on his first two fingers.

Assessment Activities	*Finding and Defining Characteristics*
Assess client's weight, body mass index (BMI), and waist circumference	Client weighs 115 kg, 183 cm tall. BMI is 33.9. BMI of 30 or greater is considered a clinical indicator of obesity. Waist circumference of 102 cm (40 inches) is considered a clinical indicator of obesity.
Assess client's current activity level	Client states he hunts, rides snowmobile, does not walk far when out doing hobbies. Watches 4 hours of television per day.
Establish client's tobacco use status	Client states he smokes one pack of cigarettes per day
Assess client's dietary patterns and average daily caloric intake	Client states that he eats what he feels like and snacks often at work. Wife cooks all the meals in the home.

NURSING DIAGNOSIS: Deficient knowledge regarding management of hypertension related to inexperience

PLANNING

*Goal (Nursing Outcomes Classification)**	*Expected Outcomes*
Management of Hypertension	*Knowledge of Hypertension Risk Factors*
Client will identify lifestyle risk factors associated with the development of hypertension	Client will identify the target range for his blood pressure Client will link diet to the development of hypertension Client will increase physical activity Client will decrease tobacco consumption and work toward cessation

*Outcome classification labels from Moorhead, S., Johnson, M., Maas, M. L., & Swanson, E. (Eds.). (2013). *Nursing outcomes classification (NOC),* (5th ed.). St. Louis, MO: Elsevier.

INTERVENTIONS (NURSING INTERVENTIONS CLASSIFICATION)†

Self-Care Facilitation	*Rationale*
Work with client in achieving a collaborative goal regarding smoking cessation from a self-care model	Smoking cessation provides an opportunity for the client to work toward a goal within a self-care framework. The nurse is supportive in this process but the client directs his efforts aimed at stopping smoking.
Activity and Exercise Management Client implements plan to walk for 30 minutes four times a week	Begin the activity plan with a simple activity. Walking 30 minutes four times a week will help the client to start a pattern of physical activity that can be modified in the future. Intensity dynamic exercise for 30–60 minutes will help to treat hypertension.
Nutrition Support Client implements the DASH diet (Dietary Approaches to Stop Hypertension) in collaboration with dietitians and other members of the health care team	The DASH diet will aid the client in managing his hypertension and introduce him to the basic nutritional principles behind the management of hypertension.

†Intervention classification labels from Bulechek, G. M., Butcher, H. K., & Dochterman, J. M. (Eds.). (2013). *Nursing interventions classification (NIC)* (6th ed.). St Louis, MO: Elsevier.

EVALUATION

Nursing Actions	*Client Response and Finding*	*Achievement of Outcome*
Ask client to state three ways to help lower his hypertension	Mr. Fletcher identifies that his smoking is increasing his blood pressure. He states he will start by smoking only ½ a pack per day.	Role of smoking in hypertension is recognized as a contributing factor. Client is working toward a plan to stop smoking.
	Client states he is enjoying walking 30 minutes four times per week and his wife has also joined him.	Client has initiated an activity plan and his wife has joined him, leading to increased opportunities for success in the intervention.
	Client identifies that high-salt, high-calorie diets have an impact on increasing his BMI and hypertension.	Client recognizes the role of diet in the management of hypertension and is taking beginning steps to change and monitor his diet plan.

planning phases. She is now determining which nursing interventions to implement and outlining how she will evaluate his care. (Box 14-1 outlines the care plan she has constructed.)

This chapter will outline important considerations nurses make when implementing and evaluating nursing care.

IMPLEMENTATION

The *implementation* step of the nursing process initiates or completes planned actions or nursing interventions. This may include organizing and managing planned care, aiding with activities of daily living (ADLs), counselling or teaching the client and family, providing care, or the delegation of care to others (Nugent & Vitale, 2015, p. 82). The nurse aims to implement safe client care designed to achieve planned goals and expected outcomes (p. 82). There are a variety of differing interventions that may be initiated to ensure comprehensive client care. With a care plan based on clear and relevant nursing diagnoses, the nurse initiates interventions that are most likely to achieve goals and expected outcomes needed to support or improve the client's health status. A **nursing intervention** is any treatment, based on clinical judgement and knowledge, to enhance client outcomes (Bulechek, Butcher, & Dochterman, 2013). Ideally, interventions are evidence informed (see Chapter 6 for further information about research), providing the most current, up-to-date, and effective approaches addressing client problems, and include both direct and indirect care measures.

Direct care interventions are treatments performed through interactions with clients. For example, a client receives direct intervention in the form of medication administration, insertion of an intravenous infusion, or counselling during a time of grief. *Indirect care* interventions are treatments performed away from the client but on behalf of the client or group of clients (Bulechek et al., 2013). Indirect care measures include actions for managing the client's environment (e.g., safety and infection control), documentation, and interdisciplinary collaboration. Both direct and indirect care measures can be nurse-initiated, physician-initiated, and collaborative interventions. For example, client teaching is a direct, nurse-initiated intervention. The indirect intervention of **consultation** is a collaborative intervention.

Each intervention is rendered within the context of a client's unique situation. This may include the client's particular situation, how the client perceives the proposed interventions, and how the nurse can best support the client as they intervene.

TYPES OF NURSING INTERVENTIONS

Nursing interventions belong to three categories: nurse-initiated, physician-initiated, and collaborative. Interventions are based on client needs. Some clients require all three categories of interventions, whereas others need only nurse- and physician-initiated interventions.

Nurse-initiated interventions are **independent nursing interventions** (Nugent & Vitale, 2015). These do not require direction or orders from other health care providers. As a nurse, you act independently for clients. Nurses' actions are grounded in evidence-informed decision making. Examples include elevating an edematous extremity, instructing clients about adverse effects of medications, or directing a client how to splint an incision during coughing.

Physician-initiated interventions are **dependent nursing interventions**, or actions that require orders or directions from physicians (Nugent & Vitale, 2015). The interventions are directed toward treating or managing a medical diagnosis. Nurse practitioners working under collaborative agreements with physicians or who are licensed through provincial or territorial nursing legislation are also able to provide such orders or directions for care. Nurses intervene by carrying out these written orders or verbal orders in the case of emergency situations. Administering a medication and changing a dressing are examples of written physician-initiated interventions.

Each physician-initiated intervention requires specific nursing responsibilities that are based on nursing knowledge. For example, when administering medications, you are responsible for knowing the classification of the drug, its physiological action, the normal dosage, adverse effects, and nursing interventions related to its action or adverse effects (see Chapter 34 for further information about medications).

Interdependent nursing interventions, or **collaborative interventions**, are therapies that require the combined knowledge, skill, and expertise of numerous health care providers. Typically, when a nurse plans care for a client, the nurse reviews the necessary interventions and determines whether the collaboration is necessary. An interdisciplinary health care team conference about a client's care is useful in determining interdependent nursing interventions.

Nurses are required to have the appropriate and specific knowledge base, skills, and abilities that are evidence informed, to be able to recognize and question errors and thus competently care for assigned client populations (Table 14-1). The ability to recognize incorrect orders or therapies is the responsibility of the nurse before implementation of any order or therapy. Errors may occur in writing or transcribing orders. Clarifying an order is competent nursing practice and protects clients from harm. When nurses carry out an incorrect or inappropriate intervention, they are responsible for an error in judgement and are legally responsible for any complications resulting from the error (see Chapter 8 for further information about legal implications).

TABLE 14-1 Frequent Errors in Writing Nursing Interventions

Type of Error	Incorrectly Stated Nursing Intervention	Correctly Stated Nursing Intervention
Failure to precisely or completely indicate nursing actions	Turn client every 2 hours	Turn client every 2 hours, using the following schedule: 0800: supine 1000: left side 1200: prone 1400: right side (repeat this routine beginning at 1600 and 2400)
Failure to indicate frequency	Perform blood glucose measurements	Measure blood glucose before each meal: 0700, 1100, and 1600
Failure to indicate quantity	Irrigate wound once a shift: 0800, 1600, and 2400	Irrigate wound with 100 mL normal saline until clear: 0800, 1600, and 2400
Failure to indicate method	Change client's dressing once a shift: 0800, 1600, and 2400	Replace client's dressing with Neosporin ointment to wound and two dry 4×4 dressings secured with hypoallergenic tape, once a shift: 0800, 1600, and 2400

BOX 14-2 Choosing Nursing Interventions

Characteristics of the Nursing Diagnosis

Interventions should alter the etiological ("related to") factor or signs and symptoms associated with the diagnostic label.

- When an etiological factor cannot change, direct the interventions toward treating the signs and symptoms (e.g., NANDA International [2018] defining characteristics).
- For potential or high-risk diagnoses, direct interventions at altering or eliminating risk factors for the diagnosis.

Expected Outcomes

Because nurses state outcomes in terms used to evaluate the effect of an intervention, this language assists in selecting the intervention. NIC is designed to show the link to NOC (University of Iowa College of Nursing, 2008).

Evidence Base

Research evidence in support of a nursing intervention indicates the effectiveness of the intervention in certain types of clients.

- Refer to the evidence (e.g., research articles, evidence-informed decision making, or evidence-informed nursing practice protocols that describe the use of the evidence in similar clinical situations and settings).
- When research is not available, use scientific principles (e.g., infection control) or consult a clinical expert about your client population.

Feasibility

A specific intervention has the potential for interacting with other interventions.

- Be knowledgeable about the total plan of care.
- Consider cost: Is the intervention clinically effective and cost efficient?
- Consider time: Are time and personnel resources available?

Acceptability to the Client

A treatment plan needs to be acceptable to the client and/or family and must match the client's goals, health care values, and culture.

- Promote informed choice; help a client know how to participate in and anticipate the effect of interventions.

Capability of the Nurse

The nurse needs to have current knowledge of the intervention, its scientific basis, and considerations for implementation.

- Be prepared to carry out the intervention.
- Know the scientific rationale for the intervention.
- Have the necessary psychosocial and psychomotor skills to complete the intervention.
- Function within the specific setting and use health care resources effectively and efficiently.

Adapted from Bulechek, G. M., Butcher, H. K., & Dochterman, J. M. (2013). *Nursing interventions classification (NIC)* (6th ed.). St. Louis, MO: Mosby.

BOX 14-3 Purposes of the Nursing Interventions Classification (NIC)

1. Standardization of the nomenclature (e.g., labelling, describing) of nursing interventions. Standardizes the language nurses use to describe sets of actions in delivering client care.
2. Expansion of nursing knowledge about connections between nursing diagnoses, treatments, and outcomes. These connections will be determined through the study of actual client care through the use of a database that the classification will generate.
3. Development of nursing and health care information systems.
4. Teaching decision making to nursing students. Defining and classifying nursing interventions help teach beginning nurses how to determine a client's need for care and to respond appropriately.
5. Determination of the cost of services provided by nurses.
6. Planning for resources needed in all types of nursing practice settings.
7. Language to communicate the unique functions of nursing.
8. Link with the classification systems of other health care providers.

Adapted from Bulechek, G. M., Butcher, H. K., & Dochterman, J. M. (2013). *Nursing interventions classification (NIC)* (6th ed.). St. Louis, MO: Mosby.

SELECTION OF INTERVENTIONS

Interventions are not selected randomly. Clients with the diagnosis of *anxiety,* for example, may require a variety of interventions. Nurses treat anxiety related to the uncertainty of impending surgery very differently than anxiety related to a possible loss of family role function. When choosing interventions, the nurse considers six factors: (1) the nursing diagnosis, (2) goals and expected outcomes, (3) the evidence base (e.g., research or proven practice guidelines), (4) feasibility, (5) acceptability to the client, and (6) the nurse's competence (Bulechek et al., 2013) (Box 14-2). During deliberation, resources are reviewed, such as the nursing literature, standard protocols or guidelines, the Nursing Interventions Classification (NIC), critical pathways, policy or procedure manuals, and textbooks. For the nurse to have the best potential for achieving expected outcomes, it is important to collaborate with other professionals, review client's needs and priorities, and allow for previous experiences to aid in selecting nursing interventions for expected outcomes.

Nursing Interventions Classification (NIC)

The Iowa Intervention Project (1993) developed a set of nursing interventions that provide a level of standardization, which enhance communication of nursing care across all health care settings and enable health care providers to compare outcomes (Bulechek et al., 2013). The purpose of the Nursing Intervention Classification (NIC) model is outlined in Box 14-3. The NIC model has three levels: domains, classes, and interventions for ease of use. The domains are the highest level (Level 1) of the model, worded in broad terms (e.g., "safety" and "physiological: basic") to organize the more specific classes and interventions (Table 14-2). The second level of the model includes 30 classes, which offer useful clinical categories for reference in selecting interventions. The third level of the model includes the 514 interventions, defined as any treatment based on clinical judgement and knowledge, that a nurse performs to enhance the condition of a client who presents an alteration within the class (Bulechek et al., 2013). Each intervention can be performed with a variety of nursing activities (Box 14-4). Nursing activities are those commonly used in a plan of care. NIC-based interventions are also linked with NANDA International (2018) nursing diagnoses for ease of use. For example, if a client has a nursing diagnosis of *acute pain,* 21 recommended interventions, including pain management, cutaneous stimulation, and anxiety reduction, may be used. A variety of nursing care activities are presented with each of the recommended interventions.

TABLE 14-2 Nursing Interventions Classification (NIC) Taxonomy

Domain 1	Domain 2	Domain 3	Domain 4	Domain 5	Domain 6	Domain 7
Level 1 Domains						
1. Physiological: Basic Care that supports physical functioning	2. Physiological: Complex Care that supports homeostatic regulation	3. Behavioural Care that supports psychosocial functioning and facilitates lifestyle changes	4. Safety Care that supports protection against harm	5. Family Care that supports the family	6. Health System Care that supports effective use of the health care delivery system	7. Community Care that supports the health of the community
Level 2 Classes						
A. *Activity and Exercise Management:* Interventions to organize or assist with physical activity and energy conservation and expenditure	G. *Electrolyte and Acid–Base Management:* Interventions to regulate electrolyte/acid–base balance and prevent complications	O. *Behaviour Therapy:* Interventions to reinforce or promote desirable behaviours or alter undesirable behaviours	U. *Crisis Management:* Interventions to provide immediate short-term help in both psychological and physiological crises	W. *Childbearing Care:* Interventions to assist in understanding and coping with the psychological and physiological changes during the childbearing period	Y. *Health System Mediation:* Interventions to facilitate the interface between client/family and the health care system	c. *Community Health Promotion:* Interventions that promote the health of the whole community
B. *Elimination Management:* Interventions to establish and maintain regular bowel and urinary elimination patterns and manage complications due to altered patterns	H. *Drug Management:* Interventions to facilitate desired effects of pharmacological agents	P. *Cognitive Therapy:* Interventions to reinforce or promote desirable cognitive functioning or alter undesirable cognitive functioning	V. *Risk Management:* Interventions to initiate risk-reduction activities and continue monitoring risks over time	Z. *Childrearing Care:* Interventions to assist in rearing children	a. *Health System Management:* Interventions to provide and enhance support services for the delivery of care	d. *Community Risk Management:* Interventions that assist in detecting or preventing health risks to the whole community
C. *Immobility Management:* Interventions to manage restricted body movement and the sequelae	I. *Neurological Management:* Interventions to optimize neurological functions	Q. *Communication Enhancement:* Interventions to facilitate delivering and receiving verbal and nonverbal messages		X. *Lifespan Care:* Interventions to facilitate family unit functioning and promote the health and welfare of family members throughout the lifespan	b. *Information Management:* Interventions to facilitate communication among health care providers	
D. *Nutrition Support:* Interventions to modify or maintain nutritional status	J. *Perioperative Care:* Interventions to provide care before, during, and after surgery	R. *Coping Assistance:* Interventions to assist another to build on own strength, to adapt to a change in function, or to achieve a higher level of function				
E. *Physical Comfort Promotion:* Interventions to promote comfort using physical techniques	K. *Respiratory Management:* Interventions to provide care before, during, and immediately after surgery	S. *Client Education:* Interventions to facilitate learning				

TABLE 14-2 Nursing Interventions Classification (NIC) Taxonomy—cont'd

Domain 1	Domain 2	Domain 3	Domain 4	Domain 5	Domain 6	Domain 7
F. *Self-Care Facilitation:* Interventions to provide or assist with routine activities of daily living	L. *Skin/Wound Management:* Interventions to maintain or restore tissue integrity	T. *Psychological Comfort Promotion:* Interventions to promote comfort using psychological techniques				
	M. *Thermoregulation:* Interventions to maintain body temperature within a normal range					
	N. *Tissue Perfusion Management:* Interventions to optimize circulation of blood and fluids to the tissue					

From Bulechek, G. M., Butcher, H. K., & Dochterman, J. M. (2013). *Nursing interventions classification (NIC)* (6th ed.). St. Louis, MO: Mosby.

BOX 14-4 Example of Interventions and Associated Nursing Activities

Class: Physical Comfort Promotion Intervention–Environmental Management

Examples of Activities

- Create a safe environment for client
- Provide a clean, comfortable bed and environment
- Avoid unnecessary exposure, drafts, overheating, or chilling
- Provide music of choice
- Limit visitors
- Manipulate lighting for therapeutic benefit
- Bring familiar objects from home
- Allow family/significant other to stay with client

From Bulechek, G. M., Butcher, H. K., & Dochterman, J. M. (2013). *Nursing interventions classification (NIC)* (6th ed.). St. Louis, MO: Mosby.

CRITICAL THINKING IN IMPLEMENTATION

The selection of nursing interventions involves complex decision making and is based on critical thinking to ensure that an intervention is correct and appropriate for the clinical situation. Even when nurses have planned interventions for a client, good judgement, decision making, and reassessment are needed before each intervention is performed, understanding that clients' conditions sometimes change rapidly. Some points to consider when working with clients to meet their needs are as follows:

- Review the set of all possible nursing interventions for the client's problem.
- Review all possible consequences associated with each possible nursing action.
- Determine the probability of all possible consequences.
- Determine the effect of the intervention on the client.

The selection and performance of nursing interventions for a client is part of clinical decision making. The critical thinking model described in Chapter 12 provides a framework for making decisions about nursing care. As you proceed with an intervention, you should consider the purpose of the intervention, the steps in performing the intervention correctly, and the client's health status (Figure 14-1). It is essential to know the clinical standards of practice of each agency because procedures and standards of practice vary considerably. The standards of practice are guidelines for nursing practice and sanction principles to provide safe and competent care. To demonstrate the process of critical thinking in the implementation stage (Figure 14-2) for nursing diagnosis and interventions, we return to Mr. Fletcher's case study:

Irene, the nurse, has decided to focus on education as a primary direct nursing intervention for Mr. Fletcher. She will be focusing her efforts on a self-care framework to empower Mr. Fletcher to learn how to manage his hypertension.

Knowledge: *Irene approaches smoking cessation, exercise, and nutrition support as her direct nursing interventions for the management of hypertension. She also knows that she will need to teach Mr. Fletcher how to monitor his blood pressure at home. These are areas for education which she can address within her nursing scope of practice. If the physician or nurse practitioner orders antihypertensive medications for Mr. Fletcher, she will add this area of teaching into her care plan. Irene will be assessing Mr. Fletcher's readiness to learn and his learning styles in order to best support his learning.*

Standards: *Irene will aim to help Mr. Fletcher decrease his blood pressure below 140/80 mm Hg as per Best Practice Guidelines. She will help Mr. Fletcher to determine a target range for his blood pressure and determine strategies to assist him in recognizing the links between diet, exercise, and smoking in the development of hypertension. Irene understands that diet and lifestyle modification is a first step; if this is unsuccessful in*

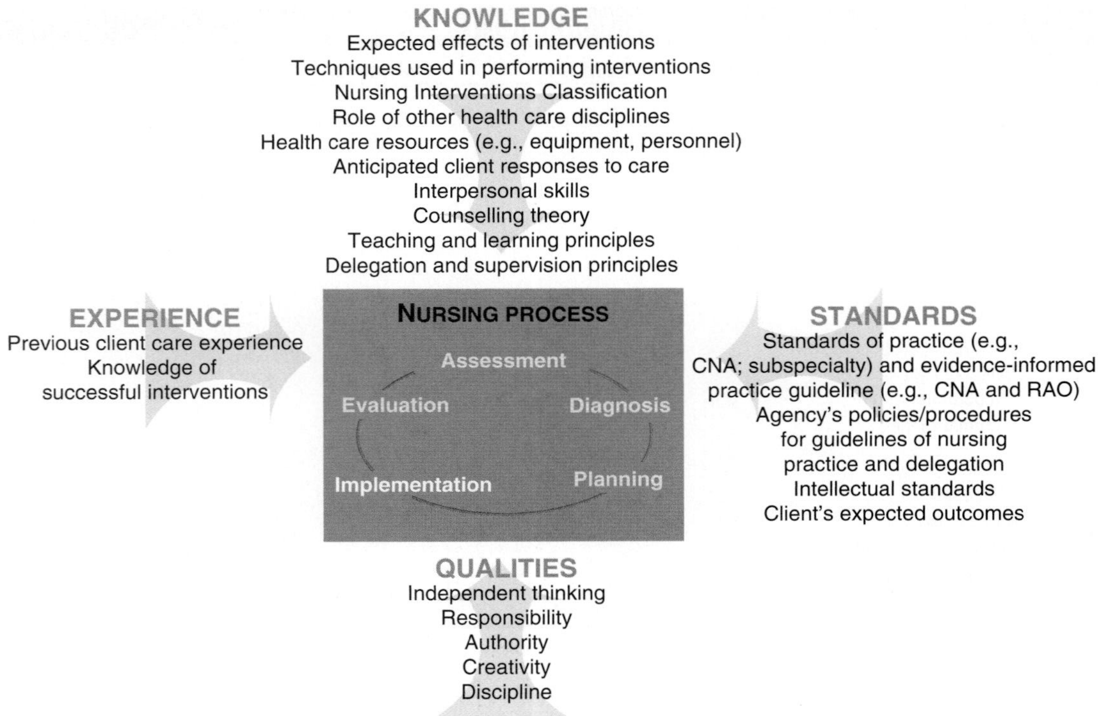

FIGURE 14-1 **Critical thinking and the process of implementing care.** CNA, Canadian Nurses Association; RNAO, Registered Nurses' Association of Ontario.

lowering his blood pressure, Mr. Fletcher may require medication therapy.

Qualities: *Irene recognizes that health behaviour change is challenging. Therefore, she sets reasonable short-term goals that will help to build Mr. Fletcher's confidence in managing his condition. She starts by helping him gain access to a home blood pressure monitor and teaches him and his wife to take their blood pressures at breakfast and before bed. She also finds two apps to download on his smartphone to help him keep track of his diet and cigarette consumption.*

Experience: *In the past, Irene has found that it is helpful for clients to log their blood pressure and to have an organized structure to approaching health behaviour modifications. Once Mr. Fletcher has learned to take his blood pressure, Irene will let him decide if he would like to approach diet change, exercise, or smoking cessation first. This will help him to stay focused on one task and not be overwhelmed by too many changes at once. Irene has found with smoking cessation that is it helpful to access support from the physician or nurse practitioner and to slowly cut back on cigarettes while establishing new habits in their place.*

STANDARD NURSING INTERVENTIONS

To facilitate good care planning, systems of standard nursing interventions are available to help the nurse. These are based on common health care problems for which standard interventions can serve as a reference point in determining what is necessary. Of more importance, if the standards are informed by evidence, interventions are more likely to improve client outcomes (see Chapter 6). Standard interventions, both nurse initiated and physician initiated, are available in the form of clinical guidelines or protocols, preprinted medical directives or standing orders, and NIC-based interventions.

Clinical Practice Guidelines and Protocols

A clinical guideline or protocol is a document that guides decisions and interventions for specific health care problems. The guideline or protocol is developed on the basis of an authoritative examination of current scientific evidence and assists nurses, physicians, and other health care providers in making decisions about appropriate health care for specific clinical circumstances. Clinicians within a health care agency sometimes choose to review the scientific literature and their own standard of practice to develop guidelines and protocols in an effort to improve their standard of care. For example, a hospital develops a rapid assessment protocol to improve the identification and early treatment of clients suspected of having a stroke. Clinical practice guidelines can also assist you in providing the best possible care. The *Best Practice Guidelines*, developed by the Registered Nurses' Association of Ontario (RNAO) (http://rnao.ca/bpg), is an excellent example of these. At times, Best Practice Guidelines are critiqued for being difficult to implement into nursing practice. In response, the RNAO recently created *Nursing Order Sets*, designed to make it easier to translate evidence into nursing practice by providing clear, concise, and actionable evidence-informed intervention statements. Examples of these Nursing Order Sets are available at the following website: http://rnao.ca/ehealth/nursingordersets.

Medical Directives or Standing Orders

A **medical directive** or **standing order** is a statement of orders for the conduct of routine therapies, monitoring guidelines, or diagnostic procedures, or a combination of these, for specific clients with identified clinical problems. These statements direct client care in various clinical settings and must be approved and signed by the prescribing physician, nurse practitioner, or health care provider. Medical directives or standing orders are common in critical care settings and other specialized practice settings in which clients' needs change rapidly and require

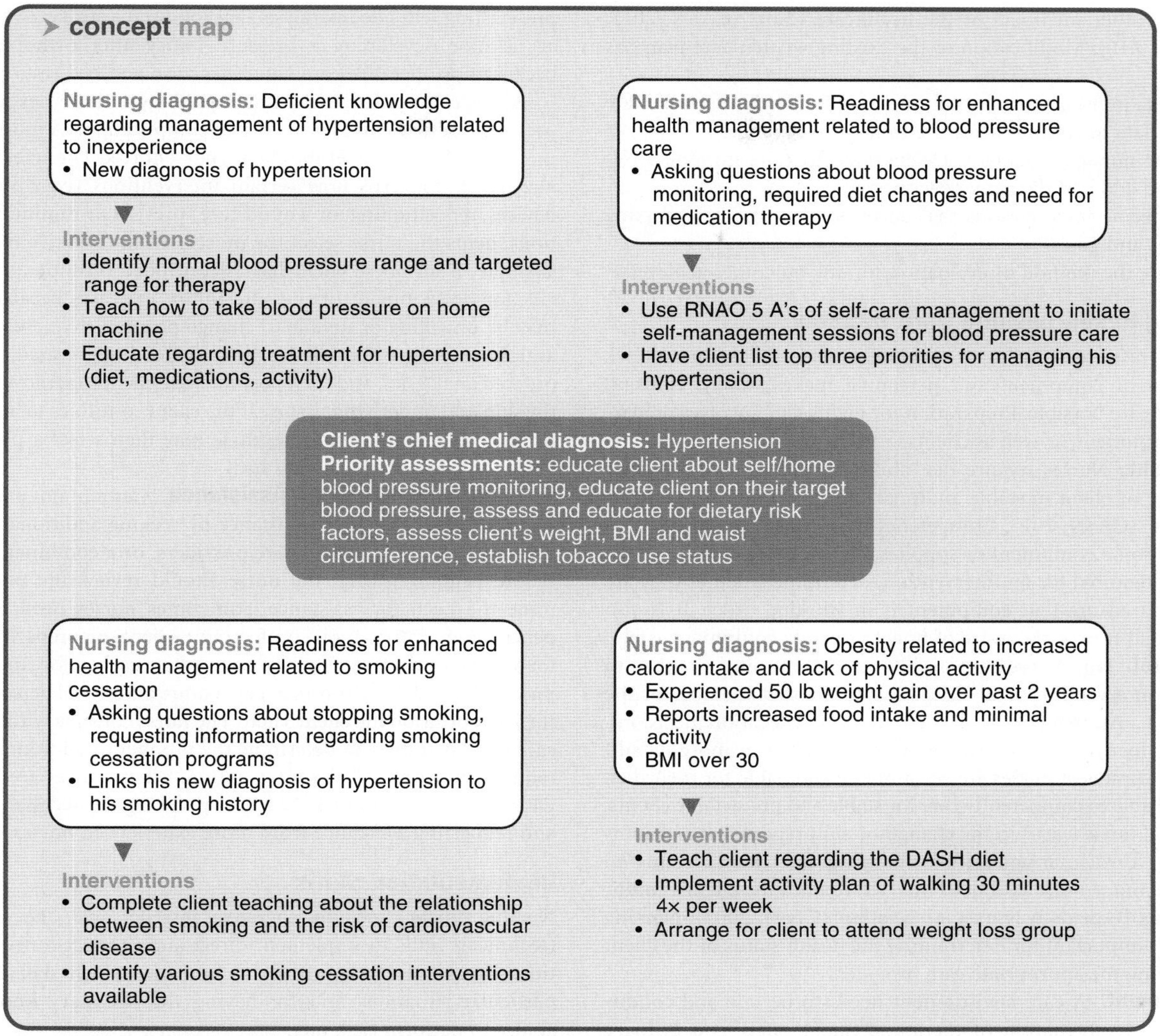

FIGURE 14-2 Concept map for planning Mr. Fletcher's nursing care. *BMI,* Body mass index; *RNAO,* Registered Nurses' Association of Ontario.

immediate attention. Examples include those for preoperative blood tests, those for postoperative exercises and positioning, and those for certain medications (such as heparin) for blood coagulation. When these statements are in place, the critical care nurse may administer the specified medication or conduct the specified action without first notifying the physician. Medical directives or standing orders are also common in community health settings in which physicians are not immediately available for consultation. Medical directives, standing orders, and clinical protocols give the nurse legal protection to intervene appropriately in the client's best interest.

◆ IMPLEMENTATION PROCESS

Preparation for implementation ensures efficient, safe, and effective nursing care. Preparatory activities include reassessing the client, reviewing and revising the existing nursing care plan, organizing resources and care delivery, anticipating and preventing complications, and implementing nursing interventions.

Reassessing the Client

Assessment is a continuous process that occurs each time the nurse interacts with a client. As new data are collected and client needs change or resolve, nurses modify the plan of care. During the initial phase of planning nursing care, the preliminary assessment may focus on one dimension of the client, such as level of comfort, or on one system, such as the cardiovascular system. Reassessment helps the nurse decide whether the proposed nursing action continues to be appropriate for the client's level of wellness. As outlined by the Canadian Association of Schools of Nursing's (CASN) *National Nursing Education Framework: Final Report,* "holistic and comprehensive assessment of diverse clients, to plan and provide competent, ethical and safe, and compassionate care" is essential in any assessment framework (CASN, 2015, Competency 3.1).

Reviewing and Revising the Existing Nursing Care Plan

After reassessing a client, the nurse reviews the care plan, compares assessment data in order to validate the nursing diagnoses, and determines whether the nursing interventions remain the most appropriate ones for the client's situation. If the client's status has changed and the nursing diagnosis and related nursing interventions are no longer appropriate, the nursing care plan is modified. An outdated or incorrect care plan compromises quality of nursing care. Most importantly, it is essential that any revision or review of the client care plan is done in "collaboration with individuals, families and other members of the healthcare team" (CASN, 2015, Competency 3.10). Modification of the existing written care plan has four steps:

1. Revise data in the assessment column to reflect current status. Date any new data to communicate the time of the change.
2. Revise the nursing diagnoses. Delete those that are no longer relevant, and add and date any new ones.
3. Revise specific interventions that correspond to the new nursing diagnoses and goals.
4. Determine the method of evaluation for any outcomes achieved.

Organizing Resources and Care Delivery

A facility's resources include equipment and skilled personnel. Organization of equipment and personnel makes timely, efficient, skilled client care possible. Preparation for giving care involves preparing the environment, as well as clients.

Equipment. Nurses require the "ability to monitor and manage complex care of client in stable and unstable contexts using multiple technologies" (CASN, 2015, Competency 3.5). Most nursing procedures require some equipment or supplies. Nurses must identify which supplies are required for an intervention, determine whether they are available, and ensure that equipment is in working order. It is also imperative that nurses are aware of how to operate equipment safely.

Personnel. Nurses are responsible for determining whether to perform an intervention or to delegate it to another member of the nursing team. Assessment of a client directs delegation decisions. (Chapter 11 focuses on the principles of delegation in more detail.) For example, practical nurses are accountable and liable for their own practice and able to competently care for stable and predictable clients. If a registered nurse learns in the change-of-shift report that a client is experiencing cardiac irregularities, changing the client's status to unstable, the nurse must assume primary care until the client's condition stabilizes (Canadian Nurses Association [CNA], 2003). Nursing judgement is important for determining the health status of the client and identifying the appropriate care provider.

Environment. A care environment needs to be safe and conducive to the implementation of therapies. Client safety is a primary concern. Nurses must anticipate circumstances that place clients at risk and must create a culture of client safety (Canadian Client Safety Initiative, 2009). If the client has sensory deficits, a physical disability, or an alteration in level of consciousness, it is important to arrange the environment to prevent injury. Privacy should be ensured during procedures that may require some body exposure. Also, lighting should be adequate for performing procedures correctly (see Chapter 37).

Client. Before providing care, the nurse needs to ensure that the client is as physically and psychologically comfortable as possible. The client needs to be comfortable during interventions. The nurse should control environmental factors at the outset, taking care of physical needs (e.g., elimination), minimizing the potential for interruptions, and positioning the client correctly. The client's strength and endurance need to be considered, and the nurse should plan only the level of activity that the client is able to tolerate comfortably. Awareness of the client's psychosocial needs helps the nurse create a favourable emotional climate. Some clients feel reassured by having a significant other present for encouragement and moral support.

Anticipating and Preventing Complications

Risks to clients arise from both illness and treatment. It is important for nurses to be alert for and recognize these risks, adapt interventions to the situation, evaluate the benefit of the treatment in relation to risk, and, finally, initiate risk-prevention measures. Many conditions heighten the risk for complications. For example, the client with pre-existing left-sided paralysis that followed a stroke 2 years earlier is at risk for developing a pressure injury after orthopedic surgery because postoperative care entails traction and bed rest.

A nurses' knowledge of pathophysiology and their experience with previous clients helps identify risk of complications. A thorough assessment reveals the level of the client's current risk. The scientific rationale, which concerns how certain interventions (e.g., pressure-relief devices, repositioning, or wound care) prevent or minimize complications, helps the nurse select the most useful preventive measures. For example, if an obese client has uncontrolled postoperative pain, the risk for development of pressure injury increases because the client may be unwilling or unable to change position frequently. The nurse anticipates when the client's pain will be aggravated, administers ordered analgesics, and then positions the client to remove pressure on the skin and underlying tissues. If the client continues to have difficulty turning or repositioning, the nurse may then select a pressure-relief device to place on the client's bed.

Identifying Areas of Assistance. Certain nursing situations require nurses to obtain assistance by seeking additional knowledge, nursing skills, unregulated care providers, or a combination of these. Before beginning care, the nurse should review the plan to determine the need for assistance. Sometimes nurses need assistance in performing a procedure, comforting a client, or preparing the client for a diagnostic test. For example, when caring for an overweight, immobilized client, the nurse may require additional personnel to help turn and position the client safely. The nurse consults with other health care team members to determine the number of additional personnel required to carry out the intervention. When nurses are less familiar with a situation, they prepare for it by seeking the necessary knowledge and requesting assistance from more experienced nurses.

Implementation Skills

Nursing practice includes cognitive, interpersonal, and psychomotor (technical) skills to implement direct and indirect nursing interventions. Nurses are responsible for knowing which skill is needed in particular situations and for having the necessary knowledge and ability to perform each one.

Cognitive Skills. Cognitive skills involve the application of critical thinking in the nursing process. To perform any intervention, nurses use good judgement and make sound clinical decisions. No nursing intervention is automatic or routine. Nurses critically think and anticipate in order to individualize care for clients and to ensure safety in their care.

Interpersonal Skills. Interpersonal skills are essential for effective nursing action. The nurse needs to develop a trusting relationship, express a caring attitude, and communicate clearly with the client and family (see Chapter 17 for further information about relational communication). Good interpersonal communication is crucial for keeping clients informed, providing individualized client teaching, and effectively supporting clients with challenging emotional needs.

Psychomotor Skills. Psychomotor skills require the integration of cognitive and motor activities. For example, when giving an injection, nurses need to understand anatomy, physiology, and pharmacology (cognitive skills) and use good coordination and precision to administer the injection correctly (motor skills). They are responsible for acquiring necessary psychomotor skills, through their experience in the nursing laboratory during their nursing education, and in practice while learning a new skill, through the use of interactive instructional technology, or through actual hands-on care of clients. Before performing a new skill, nurses always assess their level of competency and obtain the necessary resources to ensure that the client receives safe treatment.

DIRECT CARE

Nurses provide a wide variety of direct care measures. How a nurse interacts affects the success of any direct care activity, and a caring approach is essential. Nurses need to be sensitive at all times to a client's clinical condition, values and beliefs, expectations, and cultural views. All direct care measures require safe and competent practice. It is import to note that there are similar direct care activities within the scope of practice of registered nurses (RNs) and licensed practical nurses (LPNs)/registered practical nurses (RPNs). In these cases, team work and delegation of direct care activities is essential for the implementation of comprehensive nursing care. However, while scope of practice may overlap at times between RNs, LPNs, and RPNs, there may also be indications where the RN and LPN/RPN roles differ in approach. For example, a client who is newly diagnosed with a chronic disease condition may require extensive client teaching from the RN, while the LPN/RPN may focus on completing teaching from an established care plan for a client who is being discharged. This section will outline differing types of direct care measures from a general perspective that affects all nurses.

Activities of Daily Living

Activities of daily living (ADLs) are activities usually performed in the course of a normal day, including ambulation, eating, dressing, bathing, brushing the teeth, and grooming (see Chapter 38 for further information about hygiene). A client's need for assistance with ADLs is temporary, permanent, or rehabilitative. A client with impaired mobility because of bilateral arm casts has a temporary need for assistance. A client with an irreversible injury to the cervical spinal cord is paralyzed and thus has a permanent need for assistance. Occupational therapists and physiotherapists play key roles in rehabilitation to restore ADL function.

When an assessment reveals that a client is experiencing fatigue, a limitation in mobility, confusion, and pain, the client needs assistance with ADLs. For example, a client who experiences shortness of breath avoids eating because of the associated fatigue. The nurse assists the client by setting up meals, offering to cut up food, and planning for small and frequent meals to maintain nutrition. It is important to determine the client's preferences when assisting with ADLs and to let the client participate as much as possible. Involving the client in planning the timing and types of interventions enhances the client's self-esteem and willingness to assume more independence.

Instrumental Activities of Daily Living

Illness or disability sometimes alters a client's ability to be independent in society. Instrumental activities of daily living (IADLs) include such skills as shopping, preparing meals, writing cheques, and taking medications. Nurses within the home care and community health care settings frequently assist clients in finding ways to accomplish IADLs. Often, family and friends are excellent resources for assisting clients. In acute care, it is important to anticipate how illness will affect the client's ability to perform IADLs and to involve other health providers such as occupational therapists or social workers.

Physical Care Techniques

Nurses routinely perform a variety of physical care techniques when caring for a client. Examples include turning and positioning, changing dressings, administering medications, and providing comfort measures. Considerations in providing physical care include protecting the nurse and the client from injury, using infection control practices, following applicable practice guidelines, and staying organized. To carry out a procedure, nurses need to be knowledgeable about the procedure and how to perform it and about the expected outcomes.

Controlling for Adverse Reactions

An adverse reaction is a harmful effect of a medication, diagnostic test, or therapeutic intervention. Nurses are responsible for knowing the potential adverse reactions associated with nursing interventions as they provide client care.

Nursing actions that control for adverse reactions reduce or counteract the reaction. For example, when applying a moist heat compress, a nurse must take steps to prevent burning the client's skin. First, the nurse assesses the area where the compress is to be applied. Then the nurse inspects the area every 5 minutes for any adverse reaction, such as excessive reddening of the skin from the heat or skin maceration from the moisture of the compress. When completing a physician-initiated intervention, such as medication administration, nurses need to know about the potential adverse effects and reactions of the medication. After administration of the medication, the nurse evaluates the client for the expected outcomes and any adverse effects or reactions.

Nurses need to be knowledgeable about medications that counteract the adverse effects or have adverse reactions. For example, a client has an unknown hypersensitivity to penicillin, and hives develop after three doses. The nurse records the reaction, stops further administration of penicillin, and consults with the physician. Part of this process also includes anticipating an order for diphenhydramine (Benadryl), an antihistamine and antipruritic medication, to reduce the adverse reaction or allergic response and to relieve the itching. The nurse recalls how to access and administer this information in advance to help ensure client safety during this acute event.

Life-Saving Measures

A life-saving measure is a physical care technique performed when a client's physiological or psychological state is threatened (see Chapter 39 for further information about cardiopulmonary functioning). The purpose of life-saving measures is to restore physiological or psychological equilibrium. Such measures include administering emergency medications, instituting cardiopulmonary resuscitation, intervening to protect a confused or violent client, and providing a safe environment for a client experiencing a mental health crisis.

Counselling

Counselling is a direct care method that helps the client use a problem-solving process to recognize and manage stress and to facilitate interpersonal relationships. Nurses may engage in emotional, intellectual, spiritual, and psychological support for the client. "The ability to counsel and educate clients to promote health, symptom and disease management" is an essential skill of the nurse (CASN, 2015, Competency 3.9). A client and family who need nursing counselling may be upset or frustrated, but they are not necessarily disabled psychologically. Family caregivers need assistance in adjusting to the physical and emotional demands of caregiving. Likewise, the recipient of care also needs assistance in adjusting to the disability. Clients with psychiatric diagnoses require therapy provided by psychiatric nurses or by social workers, psychiatrists, or psychologists.

Many counselling techniques foster cognitive, behavioural, developmental, experiential, and emotional growth in clients. Counselling can be used to encourage individuals to examine available alternatives and decide which choices are useful and appropriate.

Teaching

Teaching is an important nursing responsibility and is related to counselling. Both involve using communication skills to create a change in the client. However, in counselling, the focus is on the development of new attitudes and feelings, whereas in teaching, the focus is on intellectual growth or the acquisition of new knowledge or psychomotor skills (Redman, 2007).

The purpose of health teaching is to help clients learn about their health status, ways of promoting health, and ways of caring for themselves. Some common examples of teaching by nurses are related to medication administration, activity restrictions, health promotion activities (e.g., diet, exercise, or smoking cessation), and knowledge about disease and related implications. The nurse's role includes assessment of clients' learning needs and readiness to learn. It is important to know the client and to be aware of cultural and social factors that influence a client's willingness and ability to learn. It is also important to know the client's health literacy levels, that is, whether the client can read directions or make calculations that sometimes are necessary with self-care skills. The teaching–learning process is an interaction between the nurse and the client in which specific learning objectives are addressed (see Chapter 20 for further information about patient education).

Preventive Measures

Preventive nursing actions promote health and prevent illness in order to avoid the need for acute or rehabilitative health care. Prevention includes assessment and promotion of the client's health potential, carrying out prescribed measures (e.g., immunizations), health teaching, and identification of risk factors for illness, trauma, or both (see Chapter 1 for further information about health promotion).

INDIRECT CARE

Indirect care measures are actions that support the effectiveness of direct care interventions (Bulechek et al., 2013). Nurses spend a good amount of time in indirect care activities (Box 14-5). Communication of information about clients (e.g., change-of-shift report and consultation) is essential to ensure that direct care activities are planned, coordinated, and performed with the proper resources.

Communicating Nursing Interventions

Any intervention provided for a client will be communicated in a written or oral format, or both. Written interventions are part of both the nursing care plan and the permanent medical record. In a nursing care plan, there are collaborative interventions that represent the contributions of all disciplines involved in caring for a client.

After completing nursing interventions, the nurse documents the treatment and client's response in the appropriate record (see Chapter 15 for further information about documentation). The entry usually includes a brief description of pertinent assessment findings, the specific procedure, the time and details of the procedure, and the client's response. The nurse also communicates nursing interventions verbally to other health care providers. Unless communication is clear, concise, accurate, and timely, caregivers can be uninformed, interventions may be needlessly duplicated, procedures may be delayed, or tasks may be left undone.

BOX 14-5 Examples of Indirect Care Activities

- Documentation
- Delegation of care activities to unregulated care providers
- Medical order transcription
- Infection control (e.g., proper handling and storage of supplies, use of protective isolation)
- Environmental safety management (e.g., make client rooms safe, strategically assigning clients in a geographic proximity to a single nurse)
- Computer data entry
- Telephone consultations with physicians and other health care providers
- Change-of-shift report
- Collecting, labelling, and transporting laboratory specimens
- Transporting clients to procedural areas and other nursing units

Adapted from Bulechek, G. M., Butcher, H. K., & Dochterman, J. M. (2013). *Nursing interventions classification (NIC)* (6th ed.). St. Louis, MO: Mosby.

Delegating, Supervising, and Evaluating the Work of Other Staff Members

Depending on the staffing system, not all of the nursing interventions may be performed by the nurse who develops the care plan. Some activities are delegated to other members of the health care team. Interventions such as skin care, ambulation, grooming, measuring vital signs in stable clients, and hygiene measures are examples of care activities that may be assigned to unregulated care providers. When a nurse delegates aspects of a client's care to another staff member, the nurse assigning tasks is responsible for ensuring that each task is appropriately assigned and completed.

ACHIEVING CLIENT-CENTRED GOALS

Nursing care is implemented to meet **client-centred goals** and outcomes. In most clinical situations, multiple interventions are necessary to achieve selected outcomes. Because clients' conditions may change rapidly, it is important to apply principles of care coordination, such as good time management, organizational skills, and appropriate use of resources, to ensure that nurses deliver interventions effectively and that clients achieve desired outcomes. Therefore, the nurse must demonstrate an ability to "recognize and respond safely, competently and ethically to rapidly changing client conditions and contexts" (CASN, 2015, Competency 3.4). Priority setting is also crucial in successful implementation because it helps the nurse to anticipate and sequence nursing interventions when a client has multiple nursing diagnoses and collaborative problems. Another way to achieve client-centred goals is to encourage and assist clients to follow their treatment plan. Consultation and collaboration are critical to achieving the client's goals and expected outcomes.

Effective discharge planning and teaching for clients and families require individualized care that is consistent with culture and health beliefs. The process should be initiated at the outset of care. Adequate and timely discharge planning and education of the client and family are the first steps in promoting a smooth transition from one health care setting to another or to home. To be effective with discharge planning and education, the nurse needs to individualize care and take into consideration the various factors that influence a client's health beliefs.

◆ EVALUATION

Evaluation is the final step of the nursing process. Evaluation involves two components: (1) an examination of a condition or situation and (2) a judgement as to whether change has occurred. Ideally, after an intervention takes place, evaluation will reveal an improvement. The nurse utilizes critical thinking skills throughout the nursing process, from gathering client data, to forming nursing diagnoses, to developing and implementing a plan of care. At the end of this process, during evaluation, the nurse reviews the expected outcomes for the client and judges whether or not the planned goals have been successful. Evaluation ensures that nursing care helped the client; if it did not, the nurse re-enters into the nursing process in order to continue to work toward improving the client's condition or well-being.

CRITICAL THINKING AND EVALUATION

Evaluation is an ongoing process whenever a nurse has contact with a client. Collaboration is a key component of the evaluation process and is found to be an overarching theme in client-centred care, according to Kitson, Marshall, Bassett, et al. (2012), who found that the relationship between the client and the health provider is one of three top themes in client-centred care. Nurses gather subjective data from the client as well as objective data from the family and health care team members prior to and following an intervention; this process ensures that all facets of the client's health are considered. Nurses also review knowledge regarding the client's current condition, treatment, resources available for recovery, and expected outcomes. In referring to previous experiences caring for similar clients, nurses are in a better position to know how to evaluate their client's needs. As in all steps of the nursing process, critical thinking remains a key component in the evaluative process. Critical thinking involves a purposeful, disciplined and systematic process of continual questioning, logical reasoning and reflecting through the use of interpretation, inference, analysis, synthesis and evaluation to achieve a desired outcome (College of Registered Nurses of British Columbia [CRNBC], 2012, p. 21). It also involves using standards to determine whether expected outcomes of care are achieved. Critical thinking fosters analysis of the findings in an evaluation to ensure that a client's health needs or goals have been met or that the client is able to improve or meet his or her health goals in a reasonable amount of time. Critical thinking also enables the identification of internal or external factors that may prevent recovery or the meeting of health goals.

During evaluation, nurses make clinical decisions and continually redirect nursing care. This involves the nurse's ability to "synthesize findings to develop or modify a person-centred plan of care" (CASN, 2015, Competency 3.3). Positive evaluations occur when desired outcomes are met. Unmet or undesirable outcomes, such as the continuation of severe pain, indicate that interventions are not effective in minimizing or resolving the actual problem or in avoiding the risk of a problem. Outcomes need to be realistic and adjusted on the basis of the client's prognosis, health goals, and nursing diagnoses. An unmet outcome indicates that the client has not responded to interventions as planned. As a result, the nurse needs to change the plan of care by trying different healing initiatives or changing the frequency or approach of existing healing initiatives. As a nurse, reflecting on the success or failure of previous interventions will enhance your clinical expertise when choosing relevant evidence-informed options for future clients.

This sequence of critically evaluating and revising therapies continues until the nurse and the client successfully and appropriately resolve the health issues, as defined by nursing diagnoses and client's goals. Remember that evaluation is dynamic and ever-changing, depending on the client's nursing diagnoses, health goals, and condition. As problems change, so will expectations of outcomes. A client whose health status continuously changes requires more frequent evaluation. In addition, nurses evaluate high-priority diagnoses first; in client centred-care, the priority will be that set by the client in collaboration with the nurse.

To highlight the role of critical thinking in evaluation (Figure 14-3), we return to the case scenario presented throughout this chapter. Irene is preparing to evaluate her implemented nursing activities for Mr.

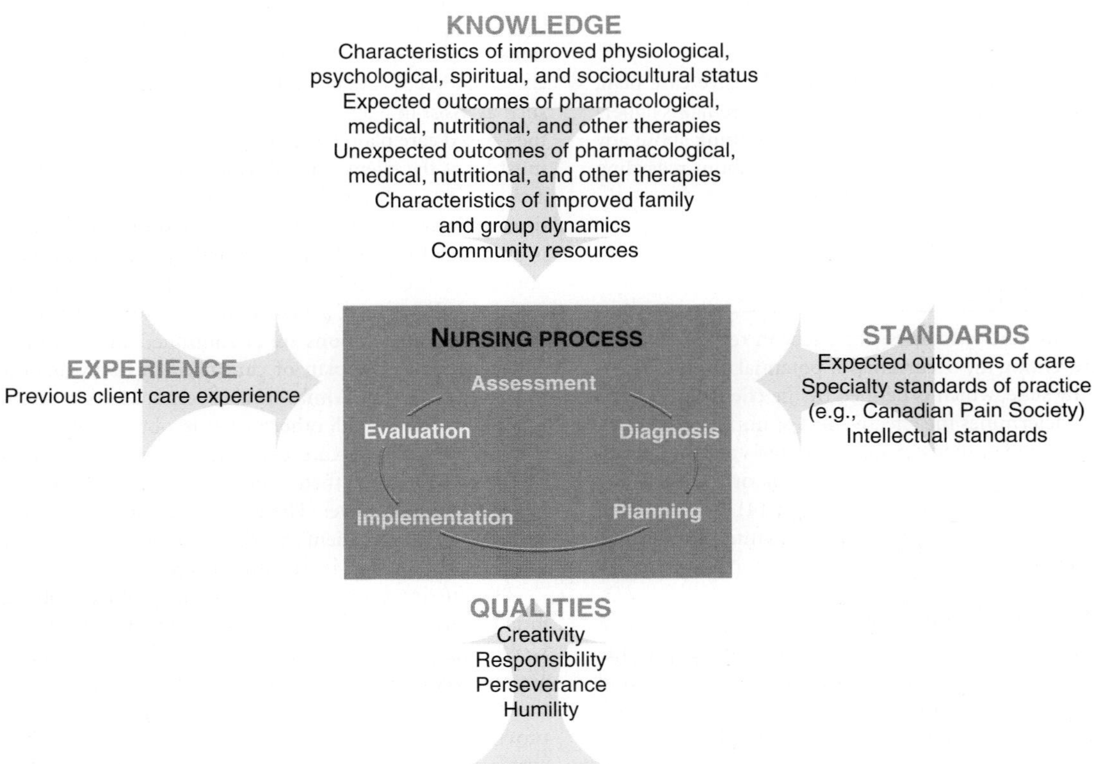

FIGURE 14-3 Critical thinking and evaluation.

Fletcher. She is using a critical thinking approach to frame her evaluative process (see Figure 14-3). She revisits her care plan in order to engage in the evaluation process (see Box 14-1).

Knowledge: *Irene meets with Mr. Fletcher and he identifies that his smoking influences his blood pressure. While keeping his blood pressure log, he developed an interest in taking his blood pressure before and after having a cigarette. He has decided to decrease his cigarette intake and try to stop smoking. He has also started walking 30 minutes per day with his wife. Irene knows that having outside support will help him to maintain this practice. His wife has also changed her cooking to include low-salt, low-fat foods and a lower daily caloric intake. Irene plans to seek collaborative support from the nurse practitioner because Mr. Fletcher's blood pressure is still 150/99 mm Hg despite his recent lifestyle changes. He will most likely require an antihypertensive medication to help support his lifestyle modification and to help decrease his cardiac risk.*

Standards: *Mr. Fletcher's blood pressure is still high according to clinical guidelines. While he is making significant strides in adopting a self-care approach, he may require extra support or new goals in order to decrease his overall blood pressure and to prevent complications.*

Qualities: *Irene takes a supportive approach, commending Mr. Fletcher on his changes in health behaviour. She helps him to interpret the data he has been collecting and talks about what is working and what he is still having difficulty with. She continues to work alongside him to manage his hypertension.*

Experience: *Irene notes that Mr. Fletcher is making a significant effort to improve his health. His self-care management may become more complicated as he integrates these new behaviours into different social settings. The next step in his care will include the introduction of collaborative approaches to the management of hypertension, including referral to a dietician to help further his education on healthy eating.*

The nurse in this scenario developed a comprehensive care plan, but her outcomes were only partially met and the client remains hypertensive. In order to understand the evaluation process, think about any additional evaluative data that you would like to ask about regarding this case as you read through the remaining sections.

◆ EVALUATION PROCESS

The purpose of nursing care is to assist the client in resolving actual health problems, preventing the occurrence of potential problems, and maintaining a healthy state, which is defined by the client. The evaluation process, which determines the effectiveness of nursing care, consists of five elements: (1) identifying evaluative criteria and standards; (2) collecting data to determine whether the criteria or standards are met; (3) interpreting and summarizing findings; (4) documenting findings and any clinical judgement; and (5) terminating, continuing, or revising the care plan.

Identifying Criteria and Standards

Nursing care is evaluated by critically analyzing the attainment of the client's identified goals and expected outcomes. A client's goals and expected outcomes are the objective criteria by which to judge a client's response to care. This client-centred approach to care plans falls directly in line with the CNA *Code of Ethics*, which states, "In health-care decision-making, in treatment and in care, nurses work with persons receiving care to take into account their values, customs and spiritual beliefs, as well as their social and economic circumstances without judgement or bias." (CNA, 2017, p. 12).

Goals. A *goal* is the expected behaviour or response that indicates resolution of a nursing diagnosis or maintenance of a healthy state. It is a summary statement of what will be accomplished when the client has met all expected outcomes. Successful achievement of this goal depends on the success of interventions, chosen from the Nursing Interventions Classification (NIC), which states that "the classification includes the interventions that nurses do on behalf of clients, both independent and collaborative interventions, both direct and indirect care" (Bulechek et al., 2013, p. 2). Goals are also often based on standards of care or guidelines established for minimal safe practice.

The evaluation of interventions concerns two factors: the appropriateness of the interventions selected and the correct application of the intervention. The appropriateness of an intervention is based on the standard of care for a client's health problem. A **standard of care** is the minimum level of care acceptable to ensure high quality of care. Standards of care define the types of therapies typically administered to clients with defined problems or needs. If a client who is receiving chemotherapy for leukemia has a specific nursing diagnosis, such as *nausea related to pharyngeal irritation,* the standard of care established by a nursing department for this problem includes pain control measures for pharyngeal irritation, mouth care guidelines, and diet therapy. The nurse reviews the standard of care to determine whether the right interventions have been chosen or whether additional ones are required. Increasing or decreasing the frequency of interventions is another approach for ensuring appropriate application of an intervention. Nurses adjust interventions on the basis of the client's actual response to therapy as well as previous experience with similar clients. For example, if a client continues to have congested lung sounds, the nurse counsels the client to increase the frequency of coughing and deep breathing exercises to remove secretions.

During evaluation, it is often found that some planned interventions are designed for an inappropriate level of nursing care. In this case, the level of care is changed by substituting a different action verb, such as *assist* in place of *provide* or *demonstrate* in place of *instruct,* in the revised care plan. For example, to assist a client in walking, a nurse must be at the client's side during ambulation, whereas providing an assistive device helps the client ambulate more independently. Also, demonstrating a skill requires that the nurse show a client how a skill is performed rather than simply telling the client how to perform it. Sometimes the level of care is appropriate but the interventions are unsuitable because of a change in the expected outcome. In this case, the current interventions are discontinued and new ones are planned. Any changes in the plan of care need to be made according to the nature of the client's unfavourable response. As a beginning nurse, it is good to consult with other nurses to obtain suggestions for improving the approach to care delivery. Senior nurses are often excellent resources because of their experience. Simply changing the care plan is not enough, however. The nurse needs to implement the new plan and re-evaluate the client's response to the nursing actions, keeping in mind that evaluation is a continuous process.

The nursing process is a systematic, problem-solving approach to individualized client care, but many factors affect each client with health care problems. Clients who have the same health care problem are not necessarily treated the same way. As a result, nurses will sometimes make errors in judgement. The systematic use of evaluation provides a way to catch these errors. By consistently incorporating evaluation into practice, it will minimize errors and ensure that the client's plan of care is appropriate and relevant.

Expected Outcomes. Outcomes have been broadly defined in the health care literature. *Outcomes* refer to the changes that have occurred as a result of nursing care (Harris & McGillis Hall, 2012). As indicated by Doenges, Moorhouse, and Murr (2016), when a client enters the health care system, regardless of physical environment, and enters into a relationship with a nurse, the nursing process steps are set in motion. In collaboration with the client, the nurse collects data, identifies client needs, establishes goals, creates measurable outcomes, and selects nursing interventions to assist the client in achieving these outcomes and health-related goals (Doenges et al., 2016). Examples of nursing-sensitive outcomes are reductions in pain severity, in incidence of pressure injuries, in nosocomial infections (e.g., *Clostridium difficile*), and in incidence of falls. In comparison, outcomes influenced largely by medical interventions include client mortality, hospital readmissions, and length of stay. **Outcomes** are statements of progressive, step-by-step responses or behaviours that must be achieved in order to accomplish the goals of care. An outcome defines the effectiveness, efficiency, and measurement of the results of nursing interventions. When client outcomes are achieved, the related factors for a nursing diagnosis usually no longer exist. During the planning phase (see Chapter 13 for further information about the planning process), it is important for the nurse to select an observable client state, behaviour, or self-reported perception that will reflect goal achievement.

TABLE 14-3 Linkages Between Nursing Outcomes Classification and Nursing Diagnoses

Nursing Diagnosis	Suggested Outcomes	Indicators (Examples)
Pain	Comfort level	Reported physical well-being Reported satisfaction with symptom control Expressed satisfaction with pain control
	Pain control	Recognition of pain onset Appropriate use of analgesics Control of reported pain
	Pain level	Reported pain severity Frequency of pain Muscle tension
Deficient knowledge	Knowledge: treatment procedures	Description of treatment procedures
	Knowledge: illness care	Description of disease process Description of prescribed activity

Adapted from Moorhead, S., Johnson, M., Maas, M., & Swanson, E. (2013). *Nursing outcomes classification (NOC)* (5th ed.) St. Louis, MO: Mosby.

Nursing-sensitive outcomes (Nursing Outcomes Classification [NOC]) were developed after NICs once nurses realized that NOCs also needed a classification system to aid in documenting in a nurse–client encounter. NOCs are designed to provide the language for the evaluation step of the nursing process. The purposes of NOC are (1) to identify, label, validate, and classify nursing-sensitive client outcomes; (2) to field test and validate the classification; and (3) to define and test measurement procedures for the outcomes and indicators using clinical data. The NOC system offers nursing-sensitive outcomes for NANDA International nursing diagnoses (Table 14-3). For each outcome, the NOC system specifies recommended evaluation indicators: the client behaviours or responses that are measures of outcome achievement. These nursing diagnoses are applied in a meaningful way to make informed, client-centred care (NANDA International, 2018).

Collecting Evaluative Data

Proper evaluation enables the nurse to determine the client's response to nursing care and whether the therapy was effective in improving the client's physical or emotional health. It is important to evaluate whether each client reaches a level of wellness or recovery that the health care team and client established in the goals of care. In addition, the nurse must determine whether he or she met the client's expectations of care. Nurses will ask clients questions about their perceptions of care, such as "Did your pain score out of 10, with 10 being the worst pain you have ever experienced to 0 being no pain, improve after the analgesic was administered?" and "Do you feel that your pain will be appropriately managed when you are discharged from the hospital today?" This level of evaluation is important for determining the client's satisfaction with care and for strengthening the partnering between the nurse and the client. Evaluating a client's response to nursing care requires the use of **evaluative measures**, which are simply assessment skills and techniques (e.g., auscultation of lung sounds, observation of a client's skill performance, discussion of the client's feelings, and inspection of the skin) (Figure 14-4). In fact, evaluative measures are the same as assessment measures, but nurses perform them when making decisions about the client's status and progress.

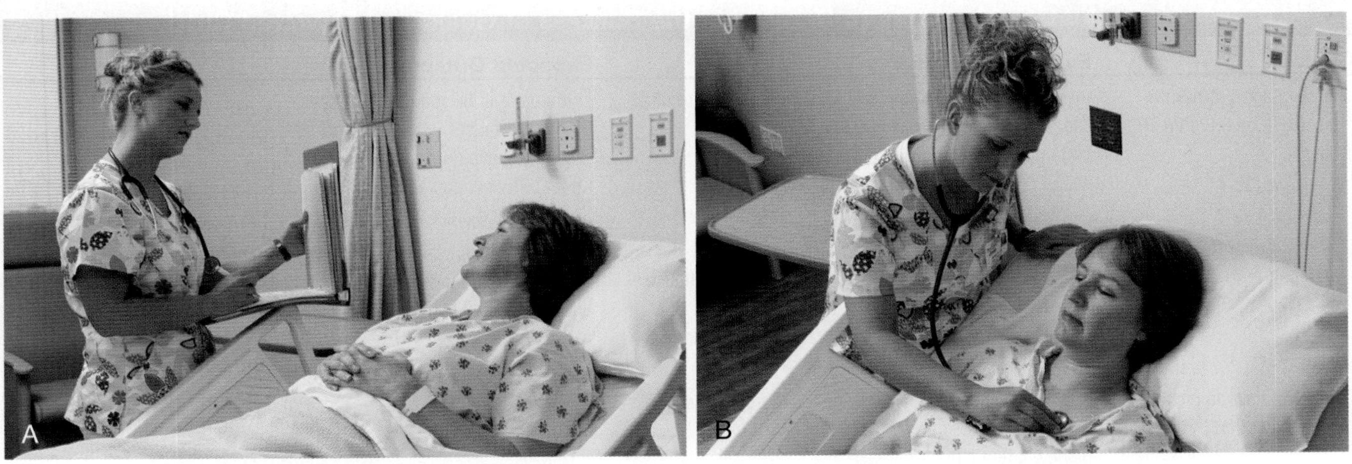

FIGURE 14-4 Evaluative measures. **A,** Nurse confirms client's medical history. **B,** Nurse evaluates client's lung sounds.

The intent of assessment is to identify any problems that exist. The intent of evaluation is to determine whether the known problems have remained the same, improved, worsened, or otherwise changed. In many clinical situations, it is important to collect evaluative measures over a period of time to determine whether a pattern of improvement or change exists. A one-time observation of a pressure injury is insufficient to determine that the injury is healing. It is important to note a consistency in change. For example, over a period of 2 days, you can observe whether the pressure injury is gradually decreasing in size, whether the amount of drainage is declining, and whether the redness of inflammation is resolving. Recognizing a pattern of improvement or deterioration enables the nurse to reason and decide whether the client's problems are resolved. The primary source of data for evaluation is the client. However, nurses also use input from the family and other caregivers; nursing colleagues can also serve as a source of evaluation when they are consulted regarding how a client responded to a nursing intervention during a previous shift.

Interpreting and Summarizing Findings

During an acute illness, a client's clinical condition changes, often minute by minute. In contrast, chronic illness results in slow, subtle changes. When nurses evaluate the effect of interventions, they are essentially performing another nursing assessment whereby they learn to recognize relevant evidence about a client's condition, even evidence that sometimes does not match clinical expectations. By applying clinical knowledge and life experiences, nurses learn to recognize complications or adverse responses to illness and treatment in addition to expected outcomes. Using evidence, they make judgements about a client's condition. To develop clinical judgement, nurses learn to match the results of evaluative measures with expected outcomes to determine whether a client's status is improving. When interpreting findings, the nurse, in conjunction with the client, compares the client's behavioural responses and the physiological signs and symptoms expected with the client's condition. By comparing expected and actual findings, the nurse can interpret and judge the client's condition and whether predicted changes have occurred (Table 14-4).

To objectively evaluate the degree of success in achieving outcomes of care, use the following steps:

1. Examine the outcome criteria to identify the exact desired client behaviour or response.
2. Assess the client's actual behaviour or response.
3. Compare the established outcome criteria with the actual behaviour or response.
4. Judge the degree of agreement between outcome criteria and the actual behaviour or response.
5. If the outcome criteria are not in agreement or are in only partial agreement with the actual behaviour or response, what are the barriers to agreement? Why was agreement not complete?

Evaluation is easier to perform after a nurse has cared for a client over a long period. The nurse is then able to make subtle comparisons of client responses and behaviours. When nurses have not had the chance to care for a client over an extended time, they improve evaluation by referring to previous experiences or asking colleagues who are familiar with the client to confirm evaluation findings. In short-term stay settings, a plan of care with clearly defined short- and long-term goals provides a framework to guide future care. The accuracy of any evaluation improves when nurses are familiar with the client's behaviour and physiological status or have cared for more than one client with a similar problem.

A central part of evaluation is to determine if each expected outcome was achieved and its place in the sequence of care. This aids the nurse in revising and redirecting the plan of care if outcomes are not met. Once a client achieves an outcome the nurse either continues the plan of care to reinforce the continuation of the outcome or discontinues the interventions because the goal is met. If the expected outcome was only partially achieved or not achieved at all, the care plan is reassessed and revised. It is important to note that if progress is not made, the goal or outcome is not met. At any time during treatment the client may withdraw treatment and/or goals can change regardless of being met or not depending on the client's desires (Table 14-5).

Documenting Findings

Documentation and reporting are an important part of evaluation and a legal necessity for nurses to complete. For nurses to make ongoing clinical decisions, a client's medical record must contain accurate information. Therefore, when documenting a client's response to interventions the nurse should always describe the same evaluative measures. For example, "the client was given 2.5 mg of IV [intravenous] morphine for 8/10 chest pain, after administration the pain level was 0/10." The aim is to present a clear description, informed by the evaluative data, of a client's progress or lack of progress. Written nursing progress notes, assessment flow sheets, clinical pathways, care

TABLE 14-4 Evaluative Measures to Determine the Success of Goals and Expected Outcomes

Goals	Evaluative Measures	Expected Outcomes
Client's stage 2 pressure ulcer will heal within 10 days	Inspect colour, condition, and location of pressure ulcer Measure diameter of ulcer daily Note odour and colour of drainage from ulcer	Erythema will be reduced in 2 days Diameter of ulcer will decrease in 5 days Ulcer will have no drainage in 2 days Client will have increased protein intake for wound healing Skin overlying ulcer will be closed in 7 days
Client will tolerate ambulation to end of hall by 11/20	Palpate client's radial pulse before exercise Palpate client's radial pulse 10 minutes after exercise Assess respiratory rate during exercise Observe client for dyspnea or breathlessness during exercise	Pulse will remain below 110 beats per minute during exercise Respiratory rate will remain within two breaths of client's baseline rate Client will deny feeling of breathlessness
Client will have improved grief resolution by 1/15	Ask client about frequency of periods of crying, sadness Review client's sleeping log Review client's dietary intake	Client reports decreased frequency of crying and sadness in 2 months Client has periods of 6 to 7 hours of sleep without interruption within 10 days Client has no weight loss in 1 month

TABLE 14-5 Examples of Objective Evaluation of Goal Achievement

Goals	Outcome Criteria	Client Response	Evaluation Findings
Client will self-administer insulin by 12/18	Client prepares insulin dosage in syringe by 12/17 Client demonstrates self-injection by 12/18	Client prepared accurate dosage in syringe on 12/17 Client administered morning insulin dosage and performed self-injection correctly on 12/18	Client has progressed and achieved desired behaviour
Client's lungs will be free of secretions by 11/30	Coughing will be nonproductive by 11/29 Lungs will be clear to auscultation by 11/30 Respirations will be 20 per minute by 11/30	Client coughed frequently and productively on 11/29 Lungs were clear to auscultation on 11/30 Respirations were 18 per minute on 11/29	Client will require continued therapy Condition is improving
Client will be able to perform self-care measures without discomfort in 2 days	Client will rate pain as 3 on a scale of 0–10 within 2 days Client will initiate bathing within 2 days	Client rates severe right-sided abdominal pain as 5 on a scale of 0–10 while attempting bathing on day 2	Client's condition still indicates a problem Client requires continued therapy with possibly new care measures

maps, and information shared between nurses during change-of-shift reports (see Chapter 15 for further information about documentation) communicate a client's progress toward meeting expected outcomes and goals for the nursing plan of care.

Care Plan Revision

Nurses evaluate expected outcomes and determine whether the goals of care have been met. They then decide whether the plan of care needs to be adjusted. If goals are successfully met, that portion of the care plan can be discontinued. If goals are unmet or partially met, the intervention continues. After the nurse evaluates a client, the nurse may want to modify or add nursing diagnoses with appropriate goals and expected outcomes and establish interventions. It is also important to redefine priorities. This is an important step in critical thinking: knowing how the client is progressing and how problems either resolve or worsen. With chronic conditions care plans are still used and require revisions based on the progression of the chronic health issue. Care plans help clients with chronic health issues become more proactive in responding to their health needs (Jansen, Heijmans, & Rijken, 2015).

Careful monitoring and early detection of problems are a client's first line of defence. Nurses must make nursing judgements pertaining to observations of what is occurring with a specific client and not merely of what happens to clients in general. Frequently, changes are not obvious. Evaluations are client specific, based on a close familiarity with each client's behaviour, physical status, and reaction to caregivers. Critical thinking skills and life experiences enhance accurate evaluation, which enables appropriate revision of ineffective care plans and discontinuation of therapy that has successfully resolved a problem.

Discontinuing a Care Plan

After a nurse determines that expected outcomes and goals have been met, he or she confirms this finding with the client, when possible. If the nurse and the client agree, that portion of the care plan is discontinued. Documentation of a discontinued plan ensures that other nurses will not unnecessarily continue interventions for that portion of the plan of care. Continuity of care ensures that care provided to clients is relevant and timely. In situations of chronic illness, care plans are still used and beneficial; expected outcomes in chronic conditions should aim to improve the quality of the chronic illness. This in turn leads to a better quality of life for clients, improved health outcomes, and decreased health care utilization (Jansen et al., 2015).

Modifying a Care Plan

When goals are not met, nurses identify the factors that interfere with goal achievement. A change in the client's condition, needs, or abilities usually necessitates alteration of the care plan. For example, when teaching self-administration of insulin, a nurse discovers that the client has developed a new problem, a tremor associated with an adverse effect of a medication. The client is unable to draw medication from a syringe or inject the needle safely. As a result, the original outcomes "Client will correctly prepare insulin in a syringe" and "Client will administer insulin injection independently" cannot be met. The nurse introduces new interventions (instructing a family member in insulin preparation and administration or introducing an alternative method of insulin administration, such as an insulin pen) and revises outcomes to meet the goal of care.

At times a lack of goal achievement results from an error in nursing judgement or failure to follow each step of the nursing process. Clients often have multiple and complex problems. When a goal is not achieved, no matter what the reason, the entire nursing process sequence should be repeated for that nursing diagnosis, to discover which changes in the plan are needed. The client is then reassessed, the accuracy of the nursing diagnosis is determined, new goals and expected outcomes are established, and new interventions are selected while adhering to national and provincial nursing standards.

A complete reassessment of all client factors relating to the nursing diagnosis and etiology is necessary when nurses modify a plan. Reassessment requires critical thinking as new data are compared with previously assessed information.

Knowledge from previous experiences helps to direct the reassessment process. Caring for clients and families who have had similar health problems gives the nurse a strong background of knowledge to use for anticipating client needs and knowing what to assess. As a nurse's experience increases so does his or her knowledge base to draw from. Reassessment reveals "missing links" (i.e., critical pieces of new information that were overlooked, which thus interfered with goal achievement). Nurses sort, validate, and cluster all new data to analyze and interpret differences from the original database. They also document reassessment data to alert other nursing staff to the client's status and communicate them to the client. After reassessment, the nurse determines what nursing diagnoses are accurate for the situation and the problem list is revised to reflect the client's changed status and/or goals.

Sometimes a new diagnosis is formed. As the client's condition changes, the diagnoses also change. For example, the nursing diagnosis *deficient knowledge related to inexperience* for a client with newly diagnosed diabetes was previously used in the care plan. The original plan was to instruct the client in how to self-administer insulin. After finding that the client has difficulty self-administering insulin because of a tremor associated with an adverse effect of a medication, the nurse reassesses the situation and finds that a family member is available as a resource. To develop a plan designed to educate a caregiver about the administration of insulin, the nurse then establishes a new diagnosis: *ineffective health maintenance related to impaired dexterity.*

Goals and Expected Outcomes

When revising care plans, it is imperative to collaboratively review with the client the goals and expected outcomes for needed changes. Nurses also need to examine the appropriateness of goals for unchanged nursing diagnoses, because a change in one problem sometimes affects other problems. Determining that each goal and expected outcome is realistic for the problem, etiology, and time frame is particularly important. Unrealistic expected outcomes and time frames hamper goal achievement. It is important to clearly document goals and expected outcomes for new or revised nursing diagnoses so that all team members are aware of the revised care plan. When the goal is still appropriate but has not yet been met, the nurse can try changing the evaluation data to allow more time. The nurse may also decide to change interventions. For example, when a client's pressure ulcer does not show signs of healing, the nurse chooses to use a different support surface or a different type of wound cleanser. All goals and expected outcomes are client centred, with realistic expectations for client achievement.

CONCLUSION

The evaluation of nursing care is a professional responsibility, and it is a crucial component of nursing care. Evaluation that focuses on a single client's plan of care enables the nurse to know the effectiveness of interventions and whether expected outcomes are met. At a system or institutional level, evaluation involves quality improvement and performance improvement activities that focus on the delivery of care provided by an agency or a specific nursing division within an agency. Through the continuous evaluation of care, nurses play a key role in the ongoing improvement of client care.

USING THE NURSING PROCESS AS A GUIDE FOR EXAM PREPARATION FOR TEST-TAKING STRATEGIES

The nursing process is a useful model for guiding the development of your future nursing practice. It is also an essential tool that will aid in organizing the vast amount of information you will be exposed to in your nursing program. If used in the right way, it can be an excellent tool to help you to frame your preparation for the NCLEX-RN, which is the registration exam you will write upon graduation in order to register with your provincial or territorial regulatory body. In Chapter 13, the use of the nursing process for test-taking was introduced. The remainder of this chapter will address how to identify questions focused on the implementation or evaluation stage of the nursing process (Table 14-6), and a study strategy using the nursing process as an organizational framework for approaching disease management will be discussed.

It is helpful to reflect on common words, listed by Nugent and Vitale (2015), that are often present in the stem of the question when asking about the different parts of the nursing process. This will help you to understand exactly which part of the nursing process (assessment, diagnosis, planning, intervention, or evaluation) that the question is speaking to (see if you can pick out words that would refer directly to the teaching process, as the terms listed can describe a variety of nursing actions in differing contexts). The following section will speak to components and content in each of the nursing process areas and provide examples of common words used to help identify each stage.

Step 1: Identify which phase of the nursing process is being addressed in the question stem. You will do this by isolating the verbs in the question stem and determining what the question is asking the nurse to do. The question step is the first part of a multiple choice or multiple response (select all that apply question) that contains the information and the question itself.

Step 2: Determine what the question is asking. Which content is being tested? Are you supposed to prioritize among answers that are all correct? Or are you choosing the best answer, knowing that other answers may be incorrect? Table 14-6 describes common themes and terminology in each phase of the nursing process that may be used in an exam question. Decide if you are being asked to find an answer that is compatible with that stage or if you are now moving to the next stage.

Step 3: Link the potential answers provided back to the question stem and information provided. Are they appropriate with respect to the information that you have been provided? Are they compatible with

TABLE 14-6 Using the Nursing Process to Help Answer Exam Questions

Nursing Process	Questions in This Stage of the Nursing Process Often Ask You to:	Common Words in the Question Stem Identifying This Area
Implementation	• Complete nursing actions based on goals established • Prioritize care • Delegate care as appropriate • Advocate for the client • Document all nursing interventions to therapeutic modalities	Change, assist, counsel, teach, give, supervise, perform, method, procedure, treatment, instruct, strategy, facilitate, provide, inform, refer, technique, motivate, delegate, implement
Evaluation	• Compare actual outcomes with expected outcomes • Communicate findings to health care team • Document and measure goal attainment • Review and modify nursing care plan • Reprioritize care plan based on evaluation	Expected, met, desired, compared, succeeded, failed, achieved, modified, reassess, ineffective, effective, response and evaluate

From Kramer-Kile, M. L. (2016). *Transitioning to the NCLEX-RN®: A study guide for Canadian-educated graduates* (2nd ed.). Kimberley, BC: Kramer-Kile Nurse Education Consultants Ltd. Registration No. 1122832. Retrieved from http://rnstudyguides.ca. Reprinted with permission.

the stage of the nursing process that you have identified? For example, if you have determined that you are in the implementation stage of the nursing process, you are looking for an action the nurse performs. If you are in the evaluation stage, you are looking for an outcome related to care.

It is useful to work with the following sample question to help understand how the nursing process can be applied to an exam question:

A client describes having severe abdominal discomfort. On assessment, it is found that the client's abdomen is distended and he has not passed flatus since his bowel resection surgery 24 hours earlier. Which of the following is a priority nursing action at this time?

1. Insert a nasogastric tube per health care provider order.
2. Offer the client ice chips.
3. Gather more assessment data.
4. Reassess the client in 15 minutes to see if the discomfort resolves.

In this question, it is made clear that the client is having abdominal discomfort due to decreased peristalsis of the bowel after a surgical procedure. This can turn into an emergent situation if it is not addressed immediately. Assessment data provided are that the client had surgery 24 hours earlier and that he has not passed flatus. The question asks, "Which of the following is a priority nursing action at this time?" The term *action* is associated with the implementation stage of the nursing process—it is focused on what the nurse can do within his or her scope of practice. The first step in answering this question is to focus on answers that are clearly nursing interventions set to resolve the identified problem.

Answer 1 (Correct): This is clearly a nursing action focused on alleviating the buildup of gas in the bowel. The insertion of a nasogastric tube is within a nurse's scope of practice; however, it must be under a health care provider's order or directive.

Answer 2 (Incorrect): Offering the client ice chips will not help to relieve the discomfort and may make the discomfort in the client's abdomen worse.

Answer 3 (Incorrect): Gathering more assessment data is not an appropriate action at this time. The question stem has provided enough information to determine that this client is at risk. The nurse needs to move from the assessment phase to the implementation phase of the nursing process.

Answer 4 (Incorrect): This is clearly within the evaluation phase of the nursing process. However, what is the nurse evaluating if he or she has not performed any nursing interventions?

❖ THE NURSING PROCESS AND STUDYING DISEASE MANAGEMENT

While there are many facets to nursing practice, including individual, community, and population approaches to health (which require more complex approaches to care), the nursing process is most easily applied to disease management frameworks. Clients may be living with a variety of disease conditions within acute, chronic, or palliative contexts. The nursing process can be used to map out what a plan of care would look like in these instances. For example, if a client has been diagnosed with a condition such as acute glomerulonephritis, the nurse would need to know what to assess with this condition, how it is diagnosed and related nursing diagnosis, how to plan care, the selected nursing and medical interventions for the client, and how to evaluate if these interventions have been successful. Students can begin "mapping" out different disease conditions early in their nursing programs in order to organize this information and provide a framework for study for in-class exams and the NCLEX-RN (Kramer-Kile, 2016). A key to understanding disease management is demonstrating knowledge in pathophysiology (what is happening in the body during the disease process). This can be linked with symptoms of disease that will direct the nursing in the assessment process.

The framework provided in Figure 14-5 can be used to help you understand the path and goal of care for disease management. The

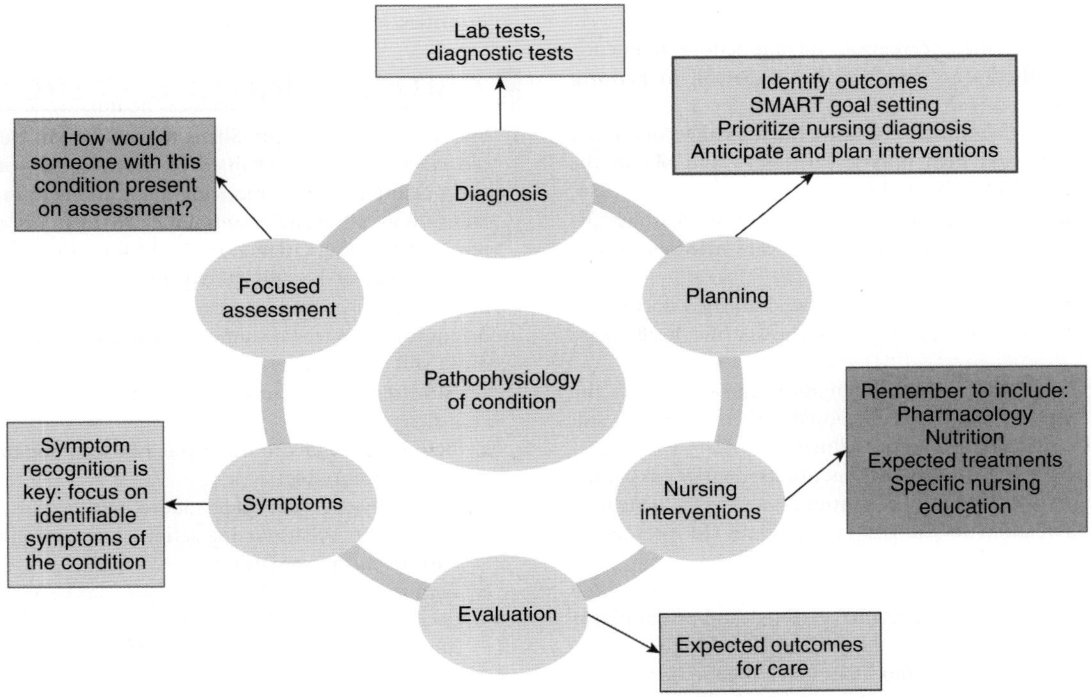

FIGURE 14-5 Using the nursing process to study disease and illness conditions. (From Kramer-Kile, M. L. [2016]. *Transitioning to the NCLEX-RN®: A study guide for Canadian-educated graduates* [2nd ed.]. Kimberley, BC: Kramer-Kile Nurse Education Consultants Ltd. Registration No. 1122832. Reprinted with permission.)

exercise outlined there would be useful to start during your pathophysiology course. Continue creating these study maps as you advance through your nursing program. It is recommended that you build these study maps while taking your pathophysiology course and moving into acute care practice. While these maps are excellent tools for your clinical practice and for studying, it is important to remember that real clients who are living with these conditions are individuals who may experience their symptoms, understanding, and acceptance of these conditions in differing ways that may directly impact their care. Therefore, the nursing process involves more than listing which activities should be directed through nursing care—it becomes a tool for learning how to critically think about the provision of holistic and comprehensive nursing care that treats more than the disease process; it is a recognition of the client and his or her role in managing the client's health.

It is often helpful to think of these maps as a guide for basic content. As you become more comfortable with the topic area you can begin to add to them. For example, it is helpful to attach relevant drug cards to the maps to help you learn the pharmacological treatment of a disease process. Some students also write case studies related to the disease condition on the back of their maps. This helps them to process the information they have learned. These maps are extremely useful when you are studying for the NCLEX-RN. If you build the maps through the program and save them when it comes time to study, instead of simply reading through your textbooks, you have already organized your study approach so you can study in the detail needed for the exam. It is also helpful to form study groups and to complete the maps together. A list of common diseases to map and a detailed description of the study mapping exercises is provided on the Potter Evolve website.

KEY CONCEPTS

- The Nursing Interventions Classification (NIC) taxonomy provides a standardization to assist nurses in selecting suitable interventions for clients' problems
- Correctly written nursing interventions include actions, frequency, quantity, and method, and they specify the person to perform them.
- Consultation and collaboration increase a nurse's knowledge about a client's problem and help nurses learn skills and obtain the resources needed to solve the problem.
- Implementation is the step of the nursing process in which the nurse provides direct and indirect nursing care interventions to clients.
- Clinical guidelines or protocols are evidence-informed documents that guide decisions and interventions for specific health care problems.
- During the initial phase of implementation, nurses reassess the client to determine whether the proposed nursing action is still appropriate for the client's level of wellness.
- To anticipate and prevent complications, nurses identify risks to the client, adapt interventions to the situation, evaluate the benefit of a treatment in relation to the risk, and initiate risk-prevention measures to create a culture of client safety.
- Successful implementation of nursing interventions requires the nurse to use appropriate cognitive, interpersonal, and psychomotor skills.
- Counselling is a direct care method that helps clients use problem solving to recognize and manage stress and to facilitate interpersonal relationships.
- Preventive nursing actions include assessment and promotion of the client's health potential, application of prescribed measures (e.g., immunizations), health teaching, and identification of risk factors for illness, trauma, or both.
- A concept map provides a visually graphic way to understand the relationship between a client's nursing diagnoses and interventions.
- Evaluation is a step of the nursing process that allows nurses to determine whether nursing interventions are successful in improving a client's condition or well-being.
- During evaluation, the appropriateness of the intervention should be assessed, as should the outcome.
- Evaluation involves two components: an examination of a condition or situation and a judgement as to whether change has occurred.
- During evaluation, nurses apply critical thinking to make nursing decisions and redirect nursing care to best meet clients' needs.
- Evaluation findings are positive when desired outcomes are met; this enables nurses to conclude that their interventions were effective.
- When the client's actual response (e.g., behaviours and physiological signs and symptoms) to nursing interventions are compared with expected outcomes established during planning, the nurse determines whether goals of care are met. At this time, the nurse should also determine whether the goals, outcomes, or both were realistic.
- Evaluative measures are assessment skills or techniques that nurses use to collect data for evaluation.
- It sometimes becomes necessary to collect evaluative measures over time to determine whether a pattern of change exists.
- To interpret evaluative findings, the nurse needs to examine the outcome criteria, assess the client's actual behaviour or response, compare the outcome criteria with the actual behaviour or response, and judge the degree of agreement.
- Through documentation of evaluative findings, all members of the health care team can know whether a client is progressing.
- The evaluative process may change a client's nursing diagnoses, priorities, and interventions.

CRITICAL THINKING EXERCISES

1. Sue is a nursing student. She is to care for Mr. Nelson, a 63-year-old client who was admitted to the hospital with heart failure and pneumonia. He is receiving medications to improve his heart failure and intravenous antibiotics to treat his pneumonia. He reports becoming fatigued easily during care activities and states, "I feel short of breath if I try to do too much." Sue notes he has 3+ edema in his lower extremities. Sue has identified nursing diagnoses of *decreased cardiac output* and *activity intolerance.* Sue must still perform hygiene measures, change the client's intravenous dressing, get him up into a chair, and measure noontime vital signs.
   a. Before she begins to intervene, how can Sue make Mr. Nelson more comfortable?
   b. What objective data does Sue obtain as part of her nursing assessment? What nursing actions may be implemented on the basis of this information?
   c. Because Sue thinks that Mr. Nelson may be at risk of falling, she decides to get assistance from a colleague before trying to get him into a chair. This is an example of what type of implementation skill?
   d. When changing Mr. Nelson's intravenous dressing, Sue cleans the insertion site in accordance with clinical practice guidelines and checks the site for signs of phlebitis. These steps are examples of what type of direct care measure?

2. Mr. Vicar has been visiting the clinic for more than a month. He visits weekly for follow-up care for a chronic venous stasis ulcer of the left leg. The nurse's note at the time of his first visit contained the following information: "Ulcer with irregular margins, 4 cm wide by 5 cm long, approximately 0.5 cm deep, draining foul-smelling purulent yellowish drainage. Subcutaneous tissue visible. Skin around ulcer, brownish rust in colour. Zinc oxide and calamine gauze applied to ulcer; elastic wrap bandage applied to gauze. Client instructed to return in 1 week." The stated goal is "Wound will demonstrate healing within 4 weeks." As the nurse who is caring for the client on the follow-up visit, what expected outcomes would you anticipate for this goal? What evaluative measures would you use to determine whether the wound is healing?

REVIEW QUESTIONS

1. The client signals the nurse to the room with the call light. The nurse enters the room and finds that the drainage tube to the abdominal wound is disconnected, the intravenous line has 100 mL of fluid remaining, and the client has asked to be turned. Which of the following should the nurse perform first?
   1. Reconnect the drainage tubing.
   2. Inspect the condition of the intravenous dressing.
   3. Improve the client's comfort and turn her onto her side.
   4. Go to the medication room and obtain the next intravenous fluid bag.
2. Which of the following expected outcomes are written correctly? (*Select all that apply.*)
   1. Client will remain afebrile until discharge
   2. Intravenous site will be without phlebitis by the third post-operative day
   3. Provide incentive spirometry for deep breathing every 2 hours
   4. Client will report pain and turn more freely by the first post-operative day
3. The nurse writes an expected outcome statement in measurable terms. An example is:
   1. Client will be pain free
   2. Client will have less pain
   3. Client will take pain medication every 4 hours
   4. Client will report pain acuity less than 4 on a scale of 0 to 10
4. Collaborative interventions are therapies that require:
   1. Nurse and client intervention
   2. Physician and nurse intervention
   3. Client and physician intervention
   4. Multiple health care providers
5. Nurses are responsible for an individualized written plan of care for clients. It is most important for the nurse to:
   1. Use a critical pathway to provide a strict plan of care
   2. Complete a concept map to comprehensively manage one problem at a time
   3. Collaborate with the client and family in the development of the plan
   4. Understand that nursing care plans are the same despite different settings and client situations
6. A number of different types of nursing interventions may be incorporated into the plan of care. Which of the following interventions is an example of a specific life-saving measure that the nurse may implement?
   1. Administering analgesics
   2. Performing cardiopulmonary resuscitation on an unconscious client
   3. Initiating stress-reduction therapy
   4. Teaching the client how to take his or her pulse
7. A nurse guides a client with pneumonia to complete deep breathing and coughing exercises. Which of the following actions would the nurse use to evaluate this intervention?
   1. Suctioning the airway
   2. Sitting client up in bed
   3. Auscultating lung sounds
   4. Asking client to describe type of discomfort
8. The evaluation of nursing care is a professional responsibility and crucial to determining whether, after application of the nursing process, the client's condition or well-being improves. One of the five elements of the evaluation process is "identifying evaluative criteria and standards." On what objective criteria does the nurse base judgement of a client's response to care?
   1. Goals and expected outcomes
   2. Client states "I am feeling better."
   3. Nursing diagnosis
   4. Effective communication by the client
9. Mr. Gunderson returns to the walk-in clinic after taking a 7-day course of antibiotic therapy and is still exhibiting signs of pneumonia. What should be the nurse's initial action?
   1. Arrange for the physician to order a different antibiotic.
   2. Obtain another sputum specimen for a culture and sensitivity.
   3. Determine if Mr. Gunderson took the medication as prescribed.
   4. Make an appointment for Mr. Gunderson to be seen by the physician.

Answers 1. 1; **2.** 1, 2; **3.** 4; **4.** 4; **5.** 3; **6.** 2; **7.** 3; **8.** 1; **9.** 3.

Rationales for the Review Questions appear at the end of the book.

RECOMMENDED WEBSITES

Canadian Nurses Association (CNA): https://www.cna-aiic.ca/en
This expansive nursing website provides comprehensive information regarding many nursing issues such as nursing care delivery models and standards and best practices. The CNA's *Code of Ethics for Registered Nurses* is an example of the type of documents available on this site.

Center for Nursing Classification & Clinical Effectiveness: https://nursing.uiowa.edu/center-for-nursing-classification-and-clinical-effectiveness
The University of Iowa's Center for Nursing Classification & Clinical Effectiveness was established to facilitate ongoing research of the Nursing Interventions Classification (NIC) and Nursing Outcomes Classification (NOC). This website provides an overview of the NIC and NOC and offers information about new classification material and publications.

NANDA International: http://www.nanda.org/
Through this website, NANDA International provides current information on nursing diagnosis research, publications, support resources, and Internet resources.

Registered Nurses' Association of Ontario (RNAO): Best Practices Guidelines: http://rnao.ca/bpg
The RNAO has an extensive process for developing Best Practices Guidelines in a variety of areas of clinical nursing. They have received federal and provincial funding for this process, and the results of their work have been made available to all Canadian nurses through this website, which lists all current guidelines that have been developed.

REFERENCES

Bulechek, G. M., Butcher, H. K., & Dochterman, J. M. (2013). *Nursing interventions classification (NIC)* (6th ed.). St Louis, MO: Mosby.

Canadian Association of Schools of Nursing/Association Canadienne des Écoles de Sciences Infirmières [CASN/ACESI] (2015). *National nursing education framework: Final report*. Ottawa: Author. Retrieved from http://www.casn.ca/wp-content/uploads/2014/12/Framwork-FINAL-SB-Nov-30-20151.pdf.

Canadian Client Safety Initiative. (2009). *Safety competencies framework*. Retrieved from http://www.patientsafetyinstitute.ca/en/toolsResources/safetyCompetencies/Documents/Safety%20Competencies.pdf.

Canadian Nursing Association (CNA) (2003). *Position statement: Staffing decisions for the delivery of safe nursing care*. Ottawa: Author. Retrieved from http://www.cna-aiic.ca/~/media/cna/page-content/pdf-en/ps67_staffing_decisions_delivery_safe_nursing_care_june_2003_e.pdf.

Canadian Nurses Association (CNA) (2017). *Code of Ethics for Registered Nurses*. Ottawa: Author.

College of Registered Nurses of British Columbia (CRNBC). (2012). *Professional standards for registered nurses and nurse practitioners*. Vancouver, BC. Retrieved from https://crnbc.ca/Standards/Lists/StandardResources/128ProfessionalStandards.pdf.

Doenges, M., Moorhouse, M., & Murr, A. (2016). *Nursing diagnosis manual: Planning, individualizing and documenting client care* (5th ed.). Philadelphia: F.A. Davis.

Harris, A., & McGillis Hall, L. (2012). *Evidence to inform staff mix decision-making: A focused literature review*. Ottawa: Canadian Nurses Association. Retrieved from https://www.cna-aiic.ca/~/media/cna/page-content/pdf-en/staff_mix_literature_review_e.pdf.

Iowa Intervention Project. (1993). The NIC taxonomy structure. *Image–the Journal of Nursing Scholarship, 25*(3), 187–192.

Jansen, D., Heijmans, M., & Rijken, M. (2015). *Individual care plans for chronically ill clients within primary care in the Netherlands: dissemination and associations with client characteristics and clients-perceived quality of care*. Den Haag, Netherlands: NIVEL—The Netherlands Institute for Health Services Research. Retrieved from http://www.narcis.nl/publication/RecordID/publicat%3A5183.

Kitson, A., Marshall, A., Bassett, K., et al. (2012). What are the core elements of client-centered care? A narrative and synthesis of the literature from health policy. *Journal of Advanced Nursing, 69*(1), 4–15. doi:10.1111/j.1365-2648.2012.06064.x.

Kramer-Kile, M. L. (2016). *Transitioning to the NCLEX-RN®: A study guide for Canadian-educated graduates* (2nd ed.). Kimberley, BC: Kramer-Kile Nurse Education Consultants Ltd. Registration No. 1122832.

NANDA International. (2018). *Nursing diagnoses: Definitions and classification 2018–2020* (11th ed.). New York: Thieme.

Nugent, P. M., & Vitale, B. A. (2015). *Test success: Test-taking techniques for beginning nursing students* (7th ed.). Philadelphia: F.A. Davies.

Redman, B. K. (2007). *The practice of client education* (10th ed.). St. Louis, MO: Mosby.

University of Iowa College of Nursing. (2008). *Nursing outcomes classification*. Retrieved from https://nursing.uiowa.edu/cncce/nursing-outcomes-classification-overview.

15

Documenting and Reporting

Canadian content written by Maureen A. Barry, RN, MScN
Original chapter by Noël Kerr, RN, PhD, CMSRN

OBJECTIVES

Mastery of content in this chapter will enable you to:

- Identify purposes of a health care record.
- Discuss legal guidelines for documentation.
- Identify ways to maintain confidentiality of electronic and written records.
- Describe six quality guidelines for documentation and reporting.
- Describe the different methods used in record keeping.
- Discuss the advantages of standardized documentation forms.
- Identify elements to include when documenting a patient discharge plan.
- Describe the role of critical pathways in interdisciplinary documentation.
- Identify the important aspects of home care and long-term care documentation.
- Explain how to verify telephone orders.
- Describe the purpose and content of a change-of-shift report.
- Discuss the use of electronic health records in documentation.
- Describe the advantages of clinical information systems.

KEY TERMS

Acuity ratings, p. 245
Case management, p. 243
Change-of-shift report, p. 246
Charting by exception (CBE), p. 242
Clinical decision support system (CDSS), p. 249
Clinical information system (CIS), p. 249
Computerized provider order entry (CPOE), p. 249
Consultation, p. 238
Critical pathways, p. 243
Data–action–response (DAR) notes, p. 242
Documentation, p. 233
Electronic health record (EHR), p. 236
Electronic medical record (EMR), p. 236
Firewall, p. 237
Flow sheets, p. 244
Focus charting, p. 242
Health informatics, p. 249
Identification–situation–background–assessment–recommendation–read back (I-SBAR-R) technique, p. 248
Incident (occurrence) report, p. 248
Information technology (IT), p. 249
Kardex, p. 244
Nursing clinical information system (NCIS), p. 250
Personal Information Protection and Electronic Documents Act (PIPEDA), p. 237
Problem–intervention–evaluation (PIE), p. 242
Problem-oriented medical record (POMR), p. 242
Records, p. 238
Reports, p. 238
Referrals, p. 238
Situation–background–assessment–recommendation (SBAR) technique, p. 248
Source record, p. 242
Standardized care plans, p. 244
Subjective–objective–assessment–plan (SOAP), p. 242
Subjective–objective–assessment–plan–intervention–evaluation (SOAPIE), p. 242
Transfer of accountability (TOA), p. 247
Transfer report, p. 248
Variance, p. 243

MEDIA RESOURCES

http://evolve.elsevier.com/Canada/Potter/fundamentals/

- Audio Chapter Summaries
- Examination Review Questions
- Concept Map Creator
- Case Study with Questions
- Audio Glossary
- Content Updates
- Video Clips

Documentation is a nursing action that produces a written account of pertinent patient data, nursing clinical decisions and interventions, and patient responses in a health record (O'Toole, 2013). Documentation within a patient health care record is a vital aspect of nursing practice. According to Philipsen, Carruthers, Chi, et al. (2014), approximately 21.5% of nursing practice time is concerned with documentation. Nursing documentation needs to be accurate and comprehensive. Nursing documentation systems need to be flexible enough to retrieve clinical data, facilitate continuity of care, track patient outcomes, and reflect current standards of nursing practice.

Information in a patient's record provides a detailed account of the level of quality of care delivered. The quality of care, the standards of regulatory agencies and nursing practice, and legal guidelines make documentation and reporting an extremely important nursing responsibility.

Effective documentation can positively affect the quality of life and health outcomes for patients and minimize the risk of errors. Accrediting agencies such as Accreditation Canada offer guidelines for documentation. However, documentation and reporting practices differ among institutions and jurisdictions and are influenced by ethical, legal, medical, and agency guidelines.

As a member of the health care team, the nurse needs to communicate information about patients accurately and in a timely, effective manner. The quality of patient care depends largely on the ability of health care providers to communicate with one another. All care providers require accurate information about patients in order to devise an organized, comprehensive care plan. If the care plan is not communicated to all members of the health care team, care can be fragmented, tasks repeated, and therapies delayed or omitted. Data recorded, reported, or communicated to other health care providers are confidential, and the confidentiality of these data must be protected.

PURPOSES OF MEDICAL RECORDS

A patient's medical record is a valuable source of data for all members of the health care team. Data entered into the medical record facilitates interdisciplinary communication and care planning; provides a legal record of care provided; facilitates funding and resource management; and allows for auditing, monitoring, and evaluation of care provided. Medical records also serve as sources of research data and as learning resources for nursing and health care education.

Communication and Care Planning

A patient's medical record is one way that health care team members communicate about patient needs and progress responses to care, individual therapies, content of conferences, patient education, and discharge planning. The plan of care needs to be clear to everyone reading the chart. The record should be the most current and accurate source of information about a patient's health care status.

In the medical record, as a nurse, always communicate the manner in which you conduct the nursing process with a patient. The admitting nursing history and physical assessment are comprehensive and provide baseline data about the patient's health status on admission to the facility. These data usually include biographical information (e.g., age and marital status), method of admission, reason for admission, a brief medical-surgical history (e.g., previous surgeries or illnesses), allergies, current medication (prescribed and over-the-counter), the patient's perceptions about illness or hospitalization, and a review of health risk factors. Results of a physical assessment of all body systems are either documented in the nursing history or included on a separate form (see Chapter 32 for further information about physical assessment).

The medical record provides data that you use to identify and support nursing diagnoses, establish expected outcomes of care, and plan and evaluate interventions. Information from the record adds to your observations and assessment. You do not need to collect information that is already available. If you have reason to believe that the information is inaccurate, information should be verified and appropriate changes made to the patient's record.

Legal Documentation

Accurate documentation is one of the best defenses against legal claims associated with nursing care (see Chapter 8 for further information about legal implications). From a legal perspective, the purpose of documentation is to provide proof of health care provided. Documentation should accurately and fully document patient care as well as the patient's response to that care. According to Cartwright-Vanzant (2010, p. 134), the medical record is vital evidence in negligent practice lawsuits and considered as important as the testimony of witnesses in the courtroom. To limit nursing liability, as the nurse you must clearly document that individualized, goal-directed nursing care, based on the nursing assessment, was provided to a patient and that you continue to monitor for, document, and report deterioration. The record must describe exactly what happened to a patient. Charting should be performed immediately after care is provided. Nursing care may have been excellent, but in a court of law, care not documented is care not provided (Bryden, 2016). When the chart is reviewed in court, it must show that the patient received the best and most appropriate care possible. In the health care record, you need to indicate all assessments, interventions, patient responses, instructions, and referrals. It is important to complete all documentation on appropriate forms and to be sure that patient-identifying information (patient's name and identification number) is on every page of documentation.

DeMilliano (2017) has identified eight common charting mistakes that can result in malpractice: (1) failing to record pertinent health or drug information, (2) failing to record nursing actions, (3) failing to record that medications have been given, (4) recording on the wrong chart, (5) failing to document a discontinued medication, (6) failing to record drug reactions or changes in the patient's condition, (7) transcribing orders improperly or transcribing improper orders, and (8) writing illegible or incomplete records. Table 15-1 provides guidelines for legally sound documentation.

Funding and Resource Management

The patient care record shows how health care agencies have used their financial resources. Various tools help monitor the timing and reasons for health team–patient interactions. These data are then compared with documented entries on the chart to demonstrate the need for and efficacy of health care resources. In some workload assignment systems, health care interactions and tasks are assigned specified points in relation to time spent with each patient.

Auditing and Monitoring

A regular review of information in patient records helps the nurse evaluate the quality and appropriateness of care. This audit may be either a review of care received by discharged patients or an evaluation of care currently being given. Most Canadian health care agencies have continuous quality improvement programs and teams to monitor and improve the delivery of health care services. These teams often contain members from across the organization, and they normally perform the self-assessment requirements of Accreditation Canada (see Chapter 11). Nurses or interdisciplinary members of a committee monitor or review records throughout the year to determine the degree to which quality improvement standards are met. Deficiencies are explained to the nursing staff so that corrections in policy or practice can be made.

Research

Statistical data relating to the frequency of clinical disorders, complications, use of specific medical and nursing therapies, recovery from illness, and deaths can be gathered from patient records. For example,

TABLE 15-1 Legal Guidelines for Documentation

Guidelines for Electronic and Written Documentation	Rationale	Correct Action
Do not document retaliatory or critical comments about a patient or care provided by another health care provider. Do not enter personal opinions.	Statements can be used as evidence for nonprofessional behaviour or poor quality of care.	Enter only objective and factual descriptions of a patient's behaviour or the actions of another health care provider. Quote all patient statements.
Correct all errors promptly.	Errors in recording can lead to errors in treatment or may imply an attempt to mislead or hide evidence.	Avoid rushing to complete documentation; be sure that information is accurate and complete.
Record all facts.	Record must be accurate, factual, and objective.	Be certain entry is factual and thorough. A person reading your documentation needs to be able to determine that a patient received adequate care.
Document as close as prudently possible to the time of the event.	Most accurate method of recalling details. Details can be lost and discrepancies can arise the longer the wait to the documentation of the event.	Document as soon after the event as possible to ensure accuracy.
If an order is questioned, record that clarification was sought.	If you perform an order known to be incorrect, you are just as liable for prosecution as the prescriber is.	Do not record, "physician made error"; instead, chart that "Dr. Wong was called to clarify order for analgesic." Include the date and time of phone call, whom you spoke with, and the outcome.
Document only for yourself.	You are accountable for information you enter into a patient's record.	Never enter documentation for someone else. Check agency policy for circumstances when a third party may document for another nurse (e.g., designated recorder for emergency situations).
Avoid using generalized, empty phrases such as "status unchanged" or "had good day."	This type of documentation is subjective and does not reflect patient assessment.	Use complete, concise descriptions of assessments and care so that documentation is objective and factual.
Begin each entry with the date and time and end with your signature and credentials.	Ensures that the correct sequence of events is recorded; signature documents who is accountable for care delivered.	Do not wait until end of shift to record important changes that occurred several hours earlier; sign each entry according to agency policy (e.g., Mei Lin, LPN).
Avoid "precharting" (documenting an entry before performing a treatment or an assessment or before giving a medication).	Invites error and thus endangers the health and safety of the patient; it is also illegal and can constitute falsification of health care records.	Document during or immediately after giving care or after administering a medication.
Protect the security of your password for computer documentation.	Maintains security and confidentiality.	Once logged into a computer, do not leave computer screen unattended. Log out when you leave the computer. Make sure the computer screen is not accessible for public viewing.
Guidelines Specific to Written Documentation	**Rationale**	**Correct Action**
Do not erase, apply correction fluid to, or scratch out errors made while recording.	Charting becomes illegible: It may appear as if you were attempting to hide information or deface record.	Draw a single line through error; write "error," above it, and sign your name or initials and date it. Then record note correctly.
Do not leave blank spaces or lines in a written nurse's progress notes.	Allows another person to add incorrect information in open space.	Chart consecutively, line by line; if space is left, draw a line horizontally through it and place your signature and credentials at the end.
Record all entries legibly and in black ink. Do not use felt-tip pens or erasable ink.	Illegible entries can be misinterpreted, thereby causing errors and lawsuits; ink from felt-tip pens can smudge or run when wet and may destroy documentation; erasures are not permitted in clinical documentation; black ink is more legible when records are photocopied or scanned.	Never use pencil to document in a written clinical record. Never erase entries or use correction fluid. To indicate an error in written documentation, place a single line through the inaccurate information and write your signature with credentials at the end of the text that has been crossed out.

as part of a quality improvement program for patients receiving intravenous therapy, a nurse manager reviews patients' records to investigate the incidence of infection in patients with a specific type of intravenous catheter. This review reveals that the infection rate is increased, and the nurse manager and staff nurses design a new method for intravenous catheter care. Once this new intervention is implemented, the manager again reviews patients' records to determine whether the infection rate decreases.

A nurse may use patients' records during a clinical research study to investigate a new nursing intervention. For example, a nurse wants to compare a new method of pain control with a standard pain protocol, by using two groups of patients. The patient records provide data on the two types of interventions: the new method and the standard pain control. The nurse researcher collects data from the patients' records that describe the types and doses of analgesic medications used, objective assessment data, and patients' subjective reports of pain relief. The researcher then compares the findings to determine whether the new method was more effective.

Some data collection activities may be part of the quality improvement practices at an agency, whereas other activities may be actual clinical research studies. Different types of permission must be secured before a researcher can review patient records for any type of research study or data analysis. The researcher must be sure that the data collection and analysis adhere to provincial, territorial, and agency policies.

Education

One way to learn the nature of an illness and an individual's response to it is to read a patient care record. A patient's record contains a variety of information, including diagnoses, signs and symptoms of disease, successful and unsuccessful therapies, diagnostic findings, and patient behaviours. No two patients have identical records, but in the course of clinical training nursing and other health care students review records of patients who have similar health problems to identify patterns of information and anticipate the type of care required for a patient.

THE SHIFT TO ELECTRONIC DOCUMENTATION

Traditionally health care providers documented on paper medical records. Paper records are episode oriented, with a separate record for each patient visit to a health care agency. Key information such as patient allergies, current medications, and complications from treatment are sometimes lost from one episode of care (e.g., hospitalization or clinic visit) to the next, jeopardizing a patient's safety (Hebda & Czar, 2013).

To enhance communication among health care providers and thus patient safety, Canadian Health Infoway had a mandate to partner with jurisdictions for the development and implementation of an electronic health record (EHR) to support effective health care delivery for Canadians. By December 2010, 49% (target was 50%) of Canadians had an EHR (Canada Health Infoway, 2011). According to Canada Health Infoway (2016), 73% of primary care physicians were using an electronic medical record (EMR) in 2015 (up from 24% in 2007), and there are more than 139 000 active EMR users in Canada in 2016 (p. 5).

Although the terms EHR and EMR frequently are used interchangeably in practice, there are differences between them. An *EHR* is a digital version of patient data that is found in traditional paper records. The term *EHR* is used increasingly to refer to a longitudinal (lifetime) record of all health care encounters for an individual patient (Hebda & Czar, 2013). An *EMR* is the legal record that describes a single encounter or visit created in hospitals and outpatient health care settings that is the source of data for the EHR (Hebda & Czar, 2013).

To meet agreed-on standards, EHRs are expected to have the following attributes or components (Hebda & Czar, 2013):

- Provide a longitudinal or lifetime patient record by linking all patient data from previous health care encounters
- Include a problem list indicating current clinical problems for each health care encounter, the number of occurrences associated with all past and current problems, and the current status of each problem
- Require the use of accepted, standardized measures to evaluate and record health status and functional levels
- Provide a method for documenting the clinical reasoning or rationale for diagnoses and conclusions that allows clinical decision making to be tracked by all providers who access the record
- Support confidentiality, privacy, and audit trails
- Provide continuous access to authorized users at any time
- Allow multiple health care providers access to customized views of patient data at the same time
- Support links to local or remote information resources such as databases using the Internet or intranet resources based within an organization
- Support the use of decision analysis tools
- Support direct entry of patient data by physicians
- Include mechanisms for measuring the cost and quality of care
- Support existing and evolving clinical needs by being flexible and expandable

The promise of the EHR is twofold: (1) making a positive impact on the quality of patient care through interprofessional collaboration with improved data availability and information synthesis, and (2) improving patient safety through the use of clinical decision support (Saleem, Flanagan, Wilck, et al., 2013). The EHR provides access to a patient's health record information at the time and place that clinicians need it. A unique feature of an EHR is its ability to integrate all patient information into one record, regardless of the number of times a patient enters a health care system. An EHR also includes results of diagnostic studies that may include diagnostic images (e.g., X-ray film or ultrasound images) and decision support software programs. Because an unlimited number of patient records potentially can be stored within an EHR system, health care providers can access clinical data to identify quality issues, link interventions with positive outcomes, and make evidence-informed decisions. Here is an example of how an EHR works: A patient with a complex medical history sees multiple specialists to manage his or her health, such as an endocrinologist to address diabetes, a pulmonologist to manage emphysema, and a cardiologist to manage heart failure and atrial fibrillation. Each of these providers is able to access patient data from the EMR at the same time.

Accurate documentation within an EHR facilitates interprofessional communication; helps to meet professional, regulatory, and legal requirements; and aids in quality improvement efforts and health care research (Blair & Smith, 2012). Members of the health care team use EHRs to improve continuity of health care from one episode of illness to another. A clinician accesses relevant and timely information about a patient and focuses on the priority problems to make timely, well-informed clinical decisions. An EHR includes tools to guide and critique medication administration (see Chapter 34) and basic decision-support tools such as physician order sets and interdisciplinary treatment plans. The key advantages of an EHR for nursing include a means for nurses to compare current clinical data about a patient with data from previous health care encounters and to maintain an ongoing record of health education provided to a patient and the patient's response to that information.

INTERPROFESSIONAL COMMUNICATION WITHIN THE MEDICAL RECORD

The quality of patient care depends on the nurse's ability to communicate with other members of the health care team. Regardless of whether documentation is entered electronically or on paper, each member of the health care team needs to document patient information in an accurate, timely, concise, and effective manner to develop and maintain an effective, organized, and comprehensive plan of care. When a plan is not communicated to all members of the health care team, care becomes fragmented, tasks are repeated, and delays or omissions in care often occur.

The health care environment creates many challenges for accurately documenting and reporting the care delivered to patients.

CONFIDENTIALITY

Whether the transfer of patient information occurs through verbal reports, written documents, or electronic transfer, nurses must follow certain principles to maintain confidentiality of information. Nurses are legally and ethically obligated to keep information about patients confidential. Under the domain of professionalism in the *National Nursing Education Framework*, the Canadian Association of Schools of Nursing (CASN, 2015) lists "the ability to ensure client confidentiality and privacy (including in the context of social media)" as an essential component of baccalaureate nursing education (p. 16). Only members of the health care team who are directly involved in a patient's care have legitimate access to the medical record. Thus, the nurse discusses a patient's diagnosis, treatment, assessment, and/or any personal conversations only with members of the health care team who are involved in a patient's care. The nurse must not share information with other patients or health care team members who are not caring for a patient. Patients have the right to request copies of their medical records and read the information. Each institution has policies that describe how medical records are shared with patients or other people who request them. In most situations, patients are required to give written permission for release of medical information.

Sometimes nurses use health care records for data gathering, research, or continuing education. As long as a nurse uses a record as specified and permission is granted, this is permitted. When you are a student in a clinical setting, confidentiality and compliance with *Personal Information Protection and Electronic Documents Act* (PIPEDA) are part of professional practice (see Chapter 16). You can review your patients' medical records only for information needed to provide safe and effective patient care. For example, when you are assigned to care for a patient, you need to review the patient's medical record and plan of care. You do not share this information with classmates (except for clinical conferences) and do not access the medical records of other patients on the unit. Access to EHRs is traceable through user log-in information. Not only is it unethical to view medical records of other patients, but breaches of confidentiality lead to disciplinary action by employers and dismissal from work or nursing school. To protect patient confidentiality, ensure that written or electronic materials used in your student clinical practice do not include patient identifiers (e.g., room number, date of birth, demographic information), and never print material from an EHR for personal use.

Before the beginning of clinical placements, students and instructors may be required to sign confidentiality agreements with the agencies in question. Students need to understand the practice standards and laws concerning confidentiality. A breach of confidentiality is often a careless rather than a deliberate act. Students need to make sure that patient-identifiable information (e.g., files, stickers, information in notebooks, worksheets) is not taken home and that it is disposed of correctly in a secure bin for shredding. Examples of breaches of confidentiality are accessing information not related to your duties, discussing patient information in an inappropriate area, such as in an elevator or on public transport, revealing to a caller confidential patient or co-worker details, emailing patient information through a public network such as the Internet, and leaving confidential material in a public area. Even after you are no longer on placement at an agency, you are obligated to maintain the confidentiality of patients and co-workers at that agency.

Privacy, Confidentiality, and Security Mechanisms

Electronic documentation has legal risks. It is possible for anyone to access a computer station within a health care agency and gain information about almost any patient. Therefore, protection of information and computer systems is a top priority. As described in Chapter 16, Canada has both provincial/territorial and national privacy legislation to protect personal health information in electronic or other forms. Under the *Personal Information Protection and Electronic Documents Act* (PIPEDA), ensuring appropriate access to and confidentiality of personal health information (PHI) is the responsibility of all people working in health care. PHI includes individually identifiable health information such as demographic data; facts that relate to an individual's past, present, or future physical or mental health condition; provision of care; and payment for the provision of care that identifies the individual (Hebda & Czar, 2013).

The ***Personal Information Protection and Electronic Documents Act* (PIPEDA)** is federal legislation that protects personal information, including health information. PIPEDA delineates how private-sector organizations may collect, use, or disclose personal information in the course of commercial activities. Individuals have the right to access and request correction of any personal information collected about them as well. PIPEDA applies to all organizations engaged in commercial activities unless the federal government exempts an organization or activity in a province with similar legislation. PIPEDA is discussed in more detail in Chapter 16.

Most security mechanisms for computerized information systems use a combination of logical and physical restrictions to protect information. For example, an automatic sign-off is a safety mechanism that logs a user off a computer system after a specified period of inactivity (Hebda & Czar, 2013). Other security measures include firewalls and the installation of antivirus and spyware-detection software. A **firewall** is a combination of hardware and software that protects private network resources (e.g., the information system of the hospital) from outside hackers, network damage, and theft or misuse of information.

Physical security measures include placing computers or file servers in restricted areas or using privacy filters for computer screens visible to visitors or others without access. This form of security has limited benefit, especially if an organization uses mobile wireless devices such as notebooks, tablets, personal computers (PCs), and smart phones. These devices are easily misplaced or lost, falling into the wrong hands. Some organizations use motion detectors or alarms with these devices to help prevent theft.

Access or log-in codes along with passwords are frequently used for authenticating authorized access to electronic records. A *password* is a collection of alphanumeric characters that a user types into a computer before accessing a program after the entry and acceptance of an access code or user name. Strong passwords use combinations of letters, numbers, and symbols that are difficult to guess. When using a health care agency computer system, it is essential that you do not share your computer password with anyone under any circumstances. A good system requires frequent, random changes in personal passwords to prevent unauthorized people from tampering with records. A password does not appear on the computer screen when it is typed, nor should it be known to anyone but the user and information system administrators (Hebda & Czar, 2013). In addition, most health care personnel are only given access to patients in their work area. Some staff (e.g., administrators or risk managers) have authority to access all patient records. To protect patient privacy, health care agencies track who accesses patient records and when they access them. Disciplinary action, including loss of employment, occurs when nurses or other health care personnel inappropriately access patient information.

Handling and Disposing of Information

Maintaining the confidentiality of medical records is an essential responsibility of all members of the health care team. It is equally important to safeguard any information that is printed from the record or extracted for report purposes. For example, you print a copy of a nursing activities work list to use as a day planner while providing patient care. You refer to information on the list and write notes to enter later into the computer. Information on the list is PHI; you do not leave it out for view by unauthorized people. Destroy (e.g., shred) anything that is printed when the information is no longer needed. Nursing students must write down patient data needed for clinical paperwork directly from a patient's medical record on the computer screen or the physical chart. When writing patient data onto forms or including it in papers written for nursing courses, you need to de-identify all patient data. Do not remove patient information that is printed out from a clinical agency. If you need to remove printed information from a clinical setting, de-identify all PHI, keep the documents secure, and destroy documents by shredding or disposing of them in a locked receptacle as soon as possible.

Historically the primary sources for inadvertent, unauthorized disclosure of PHI occurred when information was printed from a patient record and/or faxed to other health care providers. Thus, nurses need to destroy all papers containing PHI (e.g., social insurance number, date of birth or age, patient's name or address) immediately after using or faxing them. Most agencies have shredders or locked receptacles for shredding and incineration. Some nurses work in settings where they are responsible for erasing files from a computer hard drive that contain calendars, surgery or diagnostic procedure schedules, or other daily records that contain PHI (Hebda & Czar, 2013). It is important to know and follow the disposal policies for records in the institution where you work.

Health care facilities and departments have policies for the use of fax machines, which specify the types of information that can be faxed, allowable recipients of the information, where information is sent, and the process used to verify that information was sent to and received by the appropriate person(s). Nurses should fax only the amount of information that is requested or required for immediate clinical needs. The following are some steps to take to enhance fax security (Hebda & Czar, 2013):

- Confirm that fax numbers are correct before sending to be sure that you direct information properly.
- Use a cover sheet to eliminate the need for the recipient to read the information to determine who gets it. This is especially important if a fax machine serves a number of different users.
- Authenticate at both ends before data transmission to verify that source and destination are correct. Use the cover sheet to list intended recipient(s), the sender, and the phone and fax numbers. Verify the fax number on the transmittal confirmation sheet.
- Use programmed speed-dial keys to eliminate the chance of a dialing error and misdirected information.
- Use the encryption feature on the fax machine. Encoding transmissions makes it impossible to read confidential information without the encryption key.
- Place fax machines in a secure area and limit machine access to designated individuals.
- Log fax transmissions. This feature is often available electronically on the machine.

INTERPROFESSIONAL COMMUNICATION WITHIN THE HEALTH CARE TEAM

Patient care requires effective communication among members of the health care team. Communication takes place through the patient's record or chart and reports.

A patient's **record**, or *chart*, is a confidential, permanent legal document of information relevant to a patient's health care. Information about the patient's health care is recorded after each contact with the patient. The record is a continuing account of the patient's health care status and is available to all members of the health care team. All health records contain the following information:

- Patient identification and demographic data
- Informed consent for treatment and procedures
- Advance directives
- Admission nursing history
- Nursing diagnoses or problems and the nursing or interdisciplinary care plan
- Record of nursing care treatment and evaluation
- Medical history
- Medical diagnosis
- Therapeutic orders
- Progress notes for various health care providers
- Reports of physical examinations
- Reports of diagnostic studies
- Record of patient and family education
- Summary of operative procedures
- Discharge plan and summary

Reports are oral, written, or audiotaped exchanges of information between caregivers. Reports commonly compiled by nurses include change-of-shift reports, telephone reports, transfer reports, and incident or occurrence reports (discussed later in this chapter). A physician or nurse practitioner may call a nursing unit to receive a verbal report on a patient's condition and progress. A laboratory submits a written report about the results of diagnostic tests.

Team members communicate information through discussions or conferences (Figure 15-1). For example, a discharge planning conference often involves members of several disciplines (e.g., nursing, social work, dietary, medicine, and physiotherapy) who meet to discuss the patient's progress toward established discharge goals. **Consultations** are another form of discussion whereby one professional caregiver gives formal advice about the care of a patient to another caregiver. For example, a nurse caring for a patient with a chronic wound may need a consultation with a wound care specialist. **Referrals** (an arrangement for services by another care provider), consultations, and conferences must be documented in a patient's permanent record so that all caregivers can plan care accordingly.

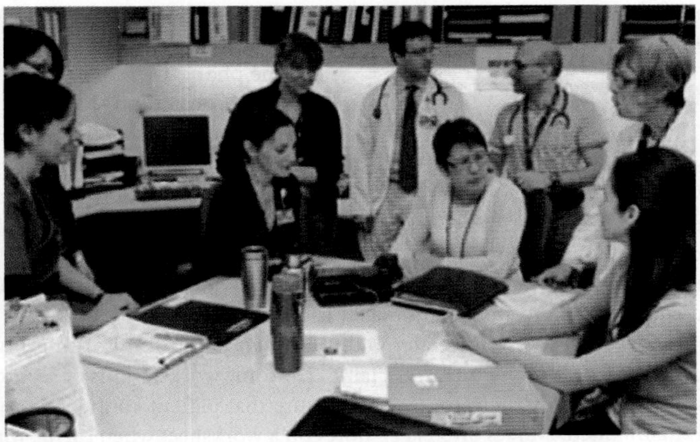

FIGURE 15-1 Staff communicate information about their patients during an interprofessional team conference. (From Registered Nurses' Association of Ontario [RNAO]. [2013]. *Developing and sustaining interprofessional health care: Optimizing patient, organizational and system outcomes.* Retrieved from http://rnao.ca/bpg/guidelines/interprofessional-team-work-healthcare.)

GUIDELINES FOR QUALITY DOCUMENTATION AND REPORTING

High-quality documentation enhances efficient, individualized patient care and has the potential to improve patient outcomes. According to Jefferies, Johnson, and Griffiths (2010), nursing documentation too often consists of a list of tasks performed, and the production of quality documentation can be a challenge for nurses. Quality documentation has six important characteristics: it is factual, accurate, complete, current, and organized, and it complies with standards set by Accreditation Canada and by provincial or territorial regulatory bodies. It is easier to maintain these characteristics if you continually seek to express ideas clearly and succinctly by (Beach & Oates, 2014):

- Sticking to the facts
- Writing in short sentences
- Using simple, short words
- Avoiding the use of jargon or abbreviations

Factual

A factual record contains descriptive, objective information about what a nurse sees, hears, feels, and smells. Avoid vague terms such as *appears*, *seems*, or *apparently*. These words suggest that you are stating an opinion; they do not communicate facts accurately and do not inform another caregiver of the details regarding the behaviours exhibited by the patient. Objective data are obtained through direct observation and measurement (e.g., "BP 80/50, patient diaphoretic, heart rate 102 and regular"). Objective documentation includes the observations of the patient's behaviours. The only subjective data that you include in the record is what the patient says. When recording subjective data, you document the patient's exact words within quotation marks wherever possible. Include objective data to support subjective data so your documentation is as descriptive as possible. For example, instead of documenting "the patient seems anxious," provide objective signs of anxiety and document the patient's statement about the feeling(s) experienced (e.g., "the patient's pulse rate is 110/beats/min, respiratory rate is slightly laboured at 22 breaths/min, and the patient states 'I feel very nervous'").

Accurate

The use of exact measurements establishes accuracy and helps the nurse determine if a patient's condition has changed in a positive or negative way. For example, a description such as "intake, 360 mL of water" is more accurate than "Patient drank an adequate amount of fluid." Documenting that an abdominal wound is "5 cm in length without redness, drainage, or edema" is more descriptive than "large wound healing well." Documentation of concise data should be clear and easy to understand. Avoid the use of unnecessary words and irrelevant detail. For example, the fact that the patient is watching TV is only necessary when this activity is significant to the patient's status and plan of care.

Most health care institutions develop a list of standard abbreviations, symbols, and acronyms to be used by all members of the health care team in documenting or communicating patient care and treatment. Approved abbreviations and acronyms vary, depending on the type of facility (i.e., long-term versus acute care facility). Use of an institution's accepted abbreviations, symbols, and system of measures (e.g., metric) ensures that all staff members use the same language in their reports and records. Always use abbreviations carefully to avoid misinterpretation. For example, "od" (every day) can be misinterpreted to mean "O.D." (right eye). If abbreviations are confusing, to minimize errors, you should spell terms out in their entirety.

The Institute for Safe Medication Practices (ISMP) (2015) has published an extensive list of error-prone abbreviations, symbols, and dose designations that health care institutions need to consider adding to their "Do Not Use" lists (see Chapter 34 for further information about abbreviations). Suggestions include writing "unit" instead of "U", always using a zero before a decimal point in a decimal fraction (e.g., "0.25 mg"), and not writing a zero alone after a decimal point (e.g., writing "5 mg," not "5.0 mg").

Correct spelling demonstrates a level of competency and attention to detail. Many terms can easily be misinterpreted (e.g., *dysphagia* and *dysphasia*). Some spelling errors can also result in serious treatment errors (e.g., the names of certain look alike–sound alike medications, such as *morphine* and *hydromorphone,* are similar). Transcribe medication names carefully to ensure that patients receive the correct medication.

Record entries must be dated, and a method for identifying the authors of entries must be in place. Each entry in a patient's record ends with the caregiver's full name or initials and credentials/title/role such as "Holly Lee, LPN." If initials are used in a signature, the full name and credentials/title/role of the individual need to be documented at least once in the medical record to allow others to readily identify the individual. As a nursing student, enter your full name and student nurse (SN) abbreviation, such as "Henri Gauthier, SN." The abbreviation for student nurse varies between SN/SPN for student nurse/student practical nurse or NS/PNS for nursing student/practical nursing student. Include your educational institution when required by agency policy.

Records must reflect accountability during the time frame of the entry. Accountability is best accomplished when you chart only your own observations and actions. Your signature holds you accountable for information recorded.

You should refer to agency policy before making late entries, correcting errors, or completing an omission. Late entries are often documented by writing the current date and time in the next available space as close to the late entry as possible and writing "late entry for [date and shift]." For adding information to an existing entry, using the current date and time in the next space and adding "addendum to note of [date and time of prior note]" is a good practice.

Complete

The information within a recorded entry or a report must be complete, containing appropriate and essential information. Criteria for thorough communication exist for certain health problems or nursing activities (Table 15-2). It is important to document all nursing interventions, such as education and psychosocial support, as this information and the outcomes of these interventions are not often recorded in nursing documentation (Jefferies et al., 2010). An example of a thorough nurse's note is as follows:

> *1915 hrs: Patient verbalizes sharp, throbbing pain localized along lateral side of right ankle, beginning approximately 15 minutes after twisting his foot on the stairs at 1700. Patient rates pain as 8 on a scale of 0–10. Pain increased with movement, slightly relieved with elevation. Pedal pulses equal bilaterally. Right ankle circumference 1 cm larger than left. Bilateral lower extremities warm, pale pink, skin intact, responds to tactile stimulation, capillary refill less than 3 seconds. Ice applied. Percocet 2 tabs (PO) given for pain. Patient states pain somewhat relieved with ice, rates pain as 6 on a scale of 0–10. Dr. P. Yoshida notified. Lee Turno, RN.*
>
> *1945 hrs: States pain was somewhat relieved with ice and now rates pain as a 3 on a scale of 0–10. States, "The pain medication really helped." Lee Turno, RN*

Frequently you will use flow sheets or graphic records to document routine activities such as daily hygiene care, vital signs, and pain assessments. Describe these data in greater detail when they are relevant, such as when a change in functional ability or status occurs. For example, if your patient's blood pressure, pulse, and respirations are elevated above expected values following a walk down the hall, document additional description about the patient's status and response to the walk in the appropriate place in the medical record (e.g., nurse's notes).

Current

Timely entries are essential to the patient's ongoing care. Documentation should occur during or as soon as possible after the incident or intervention, and events should be described chronologically to reflect a clear record of exactly what happened. To increase accuracy and decrease unnecessary duplication, many health care agencies keep records or computers near the patient's bedside to facilitate immediate documentation of information as it is collected.

Flow sheets (described later in this chapter) are a means of entering current information quickly. Portable electronic workstations or secure wall cabinets in patient rooms help ensure that patient confidentiality is maintained. Nurses often keep notes on a worksheet when caring for several patients, making notes as the care occurs to ensure that entries recorded later in the record are accurate. The following activities and findings should be communicated at the time of occurrence:

- Vital signs
- Pain assessment
- Administration of medications and treatments
- Preparation for diagnostic tests or surgery, including preoperative checklist
- Change in patient's status and who was notified (e.g., nurse practitioner, physician, manager, patient's family)
- Admission, transfer, discharge, or death of a patient
- Treatment for a sudden change in patient's status
- Patient's response to treatment or intervention

Most health care agencies use military time, a 24-hour system that avoids misinterpretation of "a.m." and "p.m." times (Figure 15-2). Instead of two 12-hour cycles in standard time, the military clock is one 24-hour time cycle. The military clock ends with midnight (2400)

TABLE 15-2 Examples of Criteria for Documentation and Reporting

Topic	Criteria to Report or Record
Subjective assessment data	Patient's description of episode in quotation marks; for example, "I feel as if I have an elephant sitting on my chest, and I can't catch my breath." Describe in patient's own words the onset, location, description of condition (severity, duration, frequency; precipitating, aggravating, and relieving factors) (e.g., "The pain in my left knee started last week after I knelt on the ground. Every time I bend my knee, I have a shooting pain on the inside of my knee.")
Objective assessment data (e.g., rash, tenderness, breath sounds or descriptions of patient behaviour [e.g., anxiety, confusion, hostility])	Onset, location, description of condition (e.g., 1100 hrs: 2 cm raised pale red area noted on back of left hand). Onset, precipitating factors, behaviours exhibited (e.g., pacing in room, avoiding eye contact with nurse), patient statements (e.g., repeatedly stating, "I have to go home now.")
Nursing interventions, treatments and evaluation (e.g., enema, bath, dressing change)	Time administered, equipment used (if appropriate), patient's response (objective and subjective changes) compared to previous treatment (e.g., denied incisional pain during abdominal dressing change, ambulated 100 metres in hallway without assistance).
Medication administration	At time of administration when using a computerized bar-code medication administration program (or immediately after administration), document time medication given, medication name, dose, route, preliminary assessment (e.g., pain level, vital signs), patient response, or effect of medication. For example: 1500 hrs: Reports "throbbing headache all over my head." Rates pain at 6 (scale 0 to 10). Tylenol 650 mg given PO. 1530 hrs: Patient reports pain level 2 (scale 0 to 10) and states, "the throbbing has stopped."
Patient and/or family teaching	Information presented; method of instruction (e.g., discussion, demonstration, videotape, booklet); and patient response, including questions and evidence of understanding such as return demonstration, or change in behaviour.
Discharge planning	Measurable patient goals or expected outcomes, progress toward goals, need for referrals.

and begins with 1 minute after midnight (0001). For example, 10:22 a.m. is 1022 military time; 1:00 p.m. is 1300 military time.

Organized

As a nurse, you want to communicate information in a logical order. For example, an organized note describes the patient's pain, the nurse's assessment and interventions, and the patient's response. To write notes about complex situations in an organized manner, think about the situation and make notes of what is to be included before you begin to write in the permanent legal record.

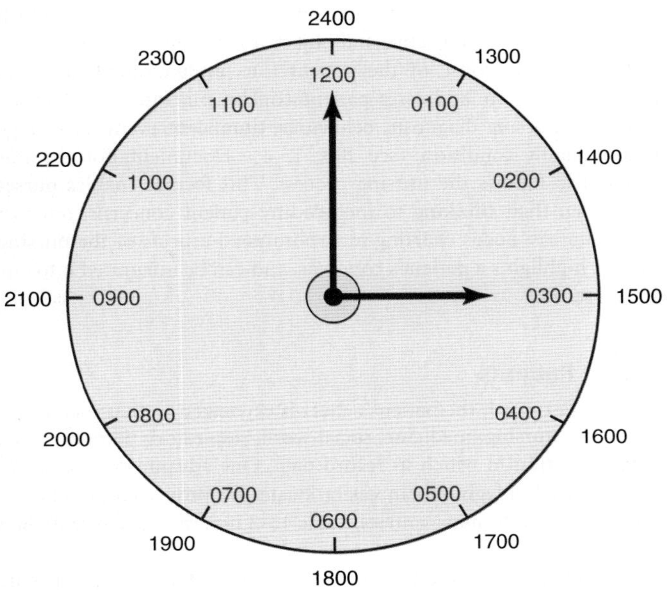

FIGURE 15-2 Comparison of 24 hours of military time with the hourly positions for civilian time on the clock face.

Compliant With Standards

Documentation needs to follow standards set by Accreditation Canada and by provincial or territorial regulatory bodies to maintain institutional accreditation and to decrease the risk of liability. Current standards require that all patients who are admitted to a health care institution undergo physical, psychosocial, environmental, and self-care assessments; receive patient education; and be provided discharge planning. In addition, criteria for standards stress the importance of evaluating patient outcomes, including the patient's response to treatments, teaching, or preventive care.

The nursing service department of each health care agency selects a method of documenting patient care. The method reflects the philosophy of the nursing department and incorporates the standards of care. Because the nursing process shapes a nurse's approach and direction of care, effective documentation also reflects the nursing process.

METHODS OF DOCUMENTATION

There are several documentation methods for recording patient assessment data and progress notes (Box 15-1). Regardless of whether documentation is entered electronically or on paper, each health care agency selects a documentation system that reflects its philosophy of nursing. The same system is used throughout a specific agency and is sometimes used throughout a health care system as well.

Narrative Documentation

Narrative documentation is the method traditionally used to record patient assessment and nursing care provided. It is simply the use of a storylike format to document information. In an electronic nursing information system, this is accomplished through use of free text entry or menu selections (Hebda & Czar, 2013). Narrative documentation tends to be time consuming and repetitious. It requires the reader to sort through a lot of information to locate desired data. However, some nurses believe that in certain situations, use of this method provides

BOX 15-1 Examples of a Nursing Progress Note Written in Different Formats

Narrative Note

Patient stated, "I'm worried about the surgery. Last time I had a lot of pain when I got out of bed." Discussed importance of postoperative ambulation and demonstrated turning, coughing, deep-breathing (TCDB) exercises. Patient set postoperative pain-rating goal at 4 on scale of 0 to 10. Discussed analgesic plan of care and reassured that analgesics will be offered around the clock as ordered. Encouraged to tell nursing staff as soon as possible if pain is not relieved. Provided with teaching booklet on postoperative care. Stated, "I feel less anxious about my pain now." Verbalized understanding of the importance of postoperative ambulation and confidence in the plan of care.

SOAP (Subjective—Objective—Assessment—Plan) Note

S: "I'm worried about the surgery. Last time I had a lot of pain when I got out of bed."
O: Asking multiple questions about how postoperative pain will be addressed.
A: Anxiety related to perceived threat of postoperative pain as evidenced by statement of prior experience with uncontrolled postoperative pain.
P: Explain routine postoperative analgesic plan of care. Encourage to inform nursing staff as soon as possible if pain is not relieved. Explain rationale for early postoperative ambulation and demonstrate TCDB exercises. Provide teaching booklet on postoperative nursing care.

PIE (Problem—Intervention—Evaluation) Note

P: Anxiety related to perceived threat of postoperative pain as evidenced by statement of prior experience with uncontrolled postoperative pain.
I: Explained importance of postoperative ambulation and demonstrated TCDB exercises. Described analgesic plan of care. Encouraged to inform nursing staff as soon as possible if pain is not relieved. Provided teaching booklet on postoperative nursing care.
E: Stated, "I feel less anxious about postoperative pain now" and performed return demonstration of TCDB exercises correctly.

Focus Charting DAR (Data—Action—Response) Note

D: Patient stated, "I'm worried about the surgery. Last time I had a lot of pain when I got out of bed." Asked frequent questions about postoperative pain management.
A: Discussed importance of postoperative ambulation and demonstrated TCDB exercises. Described postoperative analgesic plan of care that is in place. Provided teaching booklet on postoperative nursing care.
R: Demonstrated TCDB exercises correctly. States, "I feel better knowing how my pain will be treated."

better detail of individual patient assessment findings and/or complex patient situations (Kerr, 2013). Physicians and other health care providers review nursing documentation for details about changes in a patient's condition (Penoyer, Cortelyou-Ward, Noblin, et al., 2014). One of the limitations of electronic documentation is the limited use of narrative documentation. Some areas of the EMR are designed to use multiple checkboxes or drop-down lists, which some believe may not adequately convey the details of significant events that result in a change in patient condition (Kerr, 2013; Penoyer et al., 2014). EMRs that incorporate options for narrative descriptions in a format that is easily retrieved and reviewed may enhance clinician communication and interdisciplinary understanding for patient care.

Problem-Oriented Medical Records or Health Care Records

The problem-oriented medical record (POMR) is a system of organizing documentation to place the primary focus on patients' individual problems. Data are organized by problem or diagnosis. Ideally each member of the health care team contributes to a single list of identified patient problems. This assists in coordinating a common plan of care. The POMR has the following major sections: database, problem list, care plan, and progress notes.

Database. The database section contains all available assessment information pertaining to the patient (e.g., history and physical examination, nursing admission history and ongoing assessment, physiotherapist's assessment, laboratory reports, and radiological test results). The database provides the foundation for identifying patient problems and planning care. As new data become available, the database is revised. It accompanies patients through successive hospitalizations or clinic visits.

Problem List. After analyzing data, health care team members identify problems and make a single problem list. The problem list includes a patient's physiological, psychological, social, cultural, spiritual, developmental, and environmental needs. Team members list the problems in chronological order and file the list in the front of the patient's record to serve as an organizing guide for patient care. Team members add and date new problems as they arise. When a problem has been resolved, the text of that problem is highlighted, or lined out, and the date is recorded.

Care Plan. Disciplines involved in a patient's care develop a care plan or plan of care for each problem (see Chapter 13 for further information about the plan of care for patients). Nurses document the plan of care in a variety of formats; generally all of these formats include nursing diagnoses, expected outcomes, and interventions.

Progress Notes. Health care team members monitor and record the progress made toward resolving a patient's problems in progress notes. Health care providers write progress notes in one of several formats or structured notes within a POMR (see Box 15-1).

One method is the subjective–objective–assessment–plan (SOAP) note. The acronym SOAP stands for **S**ubjective data (verbalizations of the patient), **O**bjective data (that which is measured and observed), **A**ssessment (diagnosis based on the data), and **P**lan (what the caregiver plans to do). In some institutions, an "I" and an "E" are added (i.e., SOAPIE), for **I**ntervention and **E**valuation. The logic of the SOAPIE note format is similar to that of the nursing process. The nurse collects data about a patient's problems, draws conclusions, develops a plan of care, and then evaluates the outcome(s). Each SOAP note is numbered and titled according to the problem on the list that it addresses.

A second progress note method is the problem–intervention–evaluation (PIE) format (see Box 15-1). It is similar to SOAP charting in its problem-oriented nature. However, it differs from the SOAP method in that PIE charting originated in nursing practice, whereas SOAP charting originated from medical records. The PIE format simplifies documentation by unifying the care plan and progress notes. PIE notes differ from SOAP notes in that the narrative does not include assessment information. A nurse's daily assessment data appear on flow sheets, preventing duplication of data. The narrative note includes the problem, the intervention, and the evaluation. The PIE notes are numbered or labelled according to the patient's problems. Resolved problems are dropped from daily documentation after the nurse's review. Continuing problems are documented daily.

The third format used for notes within a POMR is focus charting. It involves the use of data–action–response (DAR) notes, which include **D**ata (both subjective and objective), **A**ction or nursing intervention, and **R**esponse of the patient (i.e., evaluation of effectiveness). A DAR note addresses patient concerns: a sign or symptom, condition, nursing diagnosis, behaviour, significant event, or change in a patient's condition (see Box 15-1). Documentation in this format also follows the nursing process. This format enables nurses to broaden their thinking to include any patient concerns, not just problem areas. Focus charting incorporates all aspects of the nursing process, highlights a patient's concerns, and can be integrated into any clinical setting.

Source Records

In a source record, the patient's chart is organized so that each discipline (e.g., nursing, medicine, social work, respiratory therapy) has a separate section in which to record data. One advantage of a source record is that caregivers can easily locate the proper section of the record in which to make entries. Table 15-3 lists the components of a source record.

A disadvantage of the source record is that details about a specific problem may be distributed throughout the record. For example, in the case of a patient with bowel obstruction, the nurse describes in the nurses' notes the character of abdominal pain and the use of relaxation therapy and analgesic medication. In a separate section of the record, the physician's notes describe the progress of the patient's condition and the plan for surgery. The findings of X-ray examinations that reveal the location of the bowel obstruction are in the test results section of the record.

The nursing notes or interdisciplinary progress notes section is where nurses enter a narrative description of nursing care and the patient's response (Box 15-2). It is also a section for documenting care that is provided by the physician or nurse practitioner in the nurse's presence. The nurse may record key diagnostic test results from other sections of the record in the nurses' notes if they are of major importance in the care of the patient.

Charting by Exception

The philosophy behind charting by exception (CBE) is that a patient meets all standards unless otherwise documented. The method was introduced in the early 1980s. Although the philosophy behind the method has consistently raised professional concern (Kerr, 2013), many computerized nursing documentation systems use a CBE design. Exception-based documentation systems incorporate standards of care, evidence-informed interventions, and clearly defined criteria for nursing assessment and documentation of "normal" findings. The predefined statements used to document nursing assessment of body systems are called *within defined limits (WDL)* or *within normal limits*

TABLE 15-3 Organization of Traditional Source Record

Sections	Contents
Admission sheet	Specific demographic data about patient: legal name, identification number, sex, age, birth date, marital status, occupation and employer, health card number, nearest relative to notify in an emergency, religious affiliation, name of attending physician, date and time of admission
Order sheet	Record of prescriber's orders for treatment and medications, with date, time, and physician's signature
Nurse's admission assessment	Summary of nursing history and physical examination
Graphic sheet and flow sheet	Record of repeated observations and measurements such as vital signs, daily weights, and intake and output
Medical history and examination	Results of initial examination performed by physician, including findings, family history, confirmed diagnoses, and medical plan of care
Medication administration record (MAR)	Accurate documentation of all medications administered to patient: date, time, dose, route, and nurse's signature
Progress notes	Ongoing record of patient's progress and response to therapy completed by all members of the health care team. Included in this section is a narrative record of the nursing process written by nurses: assessment, nursing diagnosis, planning, implementation, and evaluation of care
Health care disciplines' records	Entries made into record by all health care–related disciplines: radiology, social work, laboratories, physiotherapy, and so forth
Discharge summary	Summary of patient's condition, progress, prognosis, rehabilitation, and teaching needs at time of dismissal from hospital or health care agency

BOX 15-2 Sample Narrative Note

May 24, 2018

1100 hrs: Patient states, "I'm having a hard time catching my breath." R [Respirations], laboured at 32/min; P [pulse] 120; BP 112/70. Oxygen saturation 90% on room air. Patient alert and oriented. Patient using intercostal muscles during inspiration. Wheezes noted in both lower lobes. Chest excursion equal bilaterally. Elevated head of bed to Fowler's position. Obtained arterial blood gas (ABG) sample at 1045. O_2 (oxygen) started at 2 L/min per nasal prongs as ordered. Remained at bedside to calm patient.

Pam Haske, RN

1130 hrs: Results of ABGs reported to Dr Stein are pH 7.34; PCO_2 [partial pressure of carbon dioxide] 44 mm Hg; PO_2 [partial pressure of oxygen] 80 mm Hg. Patient states, "It is easier to breathe now." R 24/min; P 96; BP 110/72. Oxygen saturation 97% on O_2 at 2 L/min per nasal prongs, lips pale pink; capillary refill less than 3 seconds. Wheezing still audible on auscultation. Patient remains in high Fowler's position.

Pam Haske, RN

(WNL) definitions. They consist of written criteria for a "normal" assessment for each body system. Automated documentation within a computerized documentation system allows nurses to select a WDL statement or to choose other statements from a drop-down menu that allow description of any assessment findings that deviate from the WDL definition or that are unexpected (Hebda & Czar, 2013). The nurse writes a progress note only when a patient's assessment does not meet the standardized criteria for "normal" in one or more body systems. When changes in a patient's condition develop, the nurse needs to include a thorough and precise description of the effects of the change(s) on the patient and the actions taken to address the change(s) in the progress note.

Case Management and Use of Critical Pathways

The **case management** model of delivering care (see Chapter 11 for management models) incorporates an interdisciplinary approach to documenting patient care. In many organizations, the standardized plan of care is summarized into **critical pathways** for a specific disease or condition. Critical pathways (also known as clinical pathways, practice guidelines, or CareMap tools) are interprofessional care plans that identify patient problems, key interventions, and expected outcomes within an established time frame (American Health Consultants, 2015). The document facilitates the integration of care because all health care team members use the same critical pathway to monitor a patient's progress during each shift or, in the case of home care, every visit (Chan, Webster & Bowers, 2016). Many organizations summarize the standardized plan of care into critical pathways for a specific disease or condition. For example, in cancer care some pathways focus on malignancies that have a higher incidence, such as breast, colon, prostate, and lung cancers and certain types of blood cancers (DeMartino & Larsen, 2012). Evidence-informed critical pathways improve patient outcomes. For example, one critical pathway to manage pain caused by vascular-occlusive crisis in patients with sickle cell disease significantly improved the time interval between patient triage and administration of first analgesic dose and the likelihood of ketorolac administration in a pediatric emergency department (Ender, Krajewski, Babineau, et al., 2014).

Critical pathways eliminate the need for nurses' notes, flow sheets, and nursing care plans because the pathway document integrates all relevant information. Unexpected occurrences, unmet goals, and interventions not specified within the clinical pathway time frame are called *variances*. A **variance** is present when the activities on the clinical pathway are not completed as predicted or the patient does not meet the expected outcomes. An example of a negative variance is when a patient postoperatively develops pulmonary complications necessitating oxygen therapy and monitoring with pulse oximetry. An example

BOX 15-3 Example of Variance Documentation

You are using a critical pathway for "Routine Postoperative Care" for a 56-year-old man who had abdominal surgery yesterday. One of the expected outcomes for postoperative day 1 on the critical pathway document is "Afebrile with lungs clear bilaterally." This patient has an elevated temperature, his breath sounds are decreased bilaterally in the bases of both lungs, and he is slightly confused.

The following is an example of how you document this variance on the pathway:

"Breath sounds diminished bilaterally at the bases. T 37.8° C; P 92; R 28/min; oxygen saturation 84% on room air. Daughter states he is "confused" and did not recognize her when she arrived a few minutes ago. Oxygen started at 2 L/min via nasal prongs. Head of bed elevated. Oxygen saturation improved to 92% after 5 minutes. Dr. P. Yoshida notified of change in status. Daughter remains at bedside."

of a positive variance is when a patient progresses more rapidly than expected (e.g., use of a Foley catheter may be discontinued a day early). A variance analysis is necessary to review the data for trends and for developing and implementing an action plan to respond to the identified patient problems (Box 15-3). In addition, variances may result from changes in the patient's health or may occur as a result of other health complications not associated with the primary reason why the patient requires care. Once a variance has been identified, the nurse modifies the patient's care to meet the needs associated with the variance.

COMMON RECORD-KEEPING FORMS

Nurses use a variety of electronic or paper forms for the type of information routinely documented. The categories or data fields within a form are usually derived from institutional standards of practice or guidelines established by accrediting agencies.

Admission Nursing History Form

A nursing history form is completed when a patient is admitted to a nursing care unit. The history form guides the nurse through a complete assessment to identify relevant nursing diagnoses or problems (see Chapter 13). Data on history forms provide baselines that can be compared with changes in the patient's condition.

Flow Sheets and Graphic Records

Acute and critical care nurses commonly use flow sheets and graphic records to document physiological data and routine care. Within a computerized documentation system, these forms allow the nurse to quickly and easily enter assessment data about a patient, such as vital signs, admission and/or daily weights, and percentage of meals eaten. They also facilitate the documentation of the provision of routine, repetitive care, such as hygiene measures, ambulation, and safety and restraint checks. These documents provide current patient information accessible to all members of the health care team and help team members quickly see patient trends over time (Box 15-4). Any occurrence on a flow sheet that is unusual or represents a significant change in a patient's condition is explained in detail in a progress note. For example, if a patient's blood pressure becomes dangerously high, you first complete and record a focused assessment and then document the action taken in a progress note.

BOX 15-4 Benefits of Using a Flow Sheet

- Information is accessible to all members of the health care team.
- Time spent on writing a narrative note is decreased.
- Information is current.
- Errors resulting from transfer of information are decreased.
- Team members can quickly see trends over time.

Patient Care Summary or Kardex

Many agencies now have computerized systems that provide basic, summative information in the form of a patient care summary. This is printed out for each patient during each shift. This summary is continually updated and provides the nurse with a current detailed list of orders, treatment, and diagnostic testing. In some settings, a Kardex system, a portable "flip-over" file or binder, is kept at the nurses' station. Most Kardex forms have an activity and treatment section and a nursing care plan section that organize information for quick reference as nurses give change-of-shift reports or make walking rounds. An updated Kardex form eliminates the need for repeated referral to the chart or computer record for routine information throughout the day. Information commonly found on the patient care summary or Kardex form includes the following:

- Basic demographic data (e.g., age, sex, religious affiliation)
- Hospital identification number
- Physician's name
- Primary medical diagnosis
- Medical and surgical history
- Current prescriber's treatment orders to be carried out by the nurse (e.g., dressing changes, ambulation, glucose monitoring)
- Nursing care plan
- Nursing orders (e.g., education sessions, symptom relief measures, counselling)
- Scheduled tests and procedures
- Safety precautions to be used in the patient's care
- Factors related to activities of daily living
- Contact information about nearest relative or guardian or person to contact in an emergency
- Emergency code status
- Allergies

Standardized Care Plans

Some institutions use standardized care plans to make documentation easier for nurses. The plans, based on the institution's standards of nursing practice, are preprinted, established guidelines that are used to care for patients who have similar health problems. After a nursing assessment is completed, the staff nurse identifies the standard care plans that are appropriate for the patient. The care plans are placed in the patient's health care record. The standardized plans can be modified (and changes are noted in ink) to individualize the therapies. Most standardized care plans also allow the nurse to write in specific goals or desired outcomes of care and the dates by which these outcomes should be achieved.

One advantage of standardized care plans is establishment of clinically sound standards of care for similar groups of patients. These standards can be useful when quality improvement audits are conducted. These care plans can help nurses recognize the accepted requirements of care for patients and also improve continuity of care.

The use of standardized care plans is controversial. The major disadvantage is the risk that the standardized plans prevent nurses from providing unique, individualized therapies for patients.

Standardized care plans cannot replace the nurse's professional judgement and decision making. In addition, care plans need to be updated on a regular basis to ensure that content is current and appropriate.

Discharge Summary Forms

It is important to prepare patients for an efficient, timely discharge from a health care facility. A patient's discharge should also result in desirable outcomes. Multidisciplinary involvement in discharge planning helps ensure that a patient leaves the hospital in a timely manner with the necessary resources in place (Box 15-5).

Ideally, discharge planning begins at admission. The nurse needs to revise the care plan as the patient's condition changes. The patient and family members need to be involved in the discharge planning process so that they have the information needed to return the patient home. Discharge information and instructions should include data such as the following:

- Instruction about potential food–drug interactions, nutrition intervention, and modified diets
- Rehabilitation techniques to support adaptation to, or functional independence in, the environment, or both
- Access to available community resources
- Circumstances in which patients should obtain further treatment or follow-up care
- Methods of obtaining follow-up care
- The patient's and family's responsibilities in the patient's care
- Medication instructions, including the times and reasons to take each medication, the dose, the route, precautions, possible adverse reactions, and information about when and how to get prescriptions refilled

Furthermore, a common standard in nursing practice is to educate patients about the nature of their disease process, its likely progress, and the signs and symptoms of complications.

All of this information is included in a discharge summary that is printed out and given to the patient or family or to the home care, rehabilitation, or long-term care agency on discharge but remains in the EHR as a record of the discharge teaching that was provided (see Box 15-5). Discharge summary forms help make the summary concise and instructive. A summary form emphasizes previous learning by the patient and family and care that should be continued in any restorative care setting. When given directly to patients, the form may be attached to pamphlets or teaching brochures.

BOX 15-5 Discharge Summary Information

- Use clear, concise descriptions in the patient's own language.
- Provide step-by-step instructions for how to perform any procedure that the patient or family will be doing independently (e.g., emptying a urinary catheter or self-administration of an injectable medication). Reinforce explanation with printed instructions.
- Identify precautions to follow when performing self-care or administering medications.
- Review signs and symptoms of complications that a patient or family member needs to report to a health care practitioner.
- List names and phone numbers of health care providers and community resources that the patient or family member can contact.
- Identify any unresolved problem, including plans for follow-up and continuous treatment.
- List actual time of discharge, mode of transportation, and who accompanied the patient.

ACUITY RATING SYSTEMS

Nurses use **acuity ratings** to determine the hours of care and number of staff required for a given group of patients every shift or every 24 hours. A patient's acuity level, usually determined by assessment data entered into a computer program by a registered nurse, is based on the type and number of nursing interventions (e.g., intravenous [IV] therapy, wound care, or ambulation assistance) required by a patient over a 24-hour period. Although acuity ratings are not part of a patient's medical record, nursing documentation within the medical record provides evidence to support the assessment of an acuity rating for an individual patient.

The acuity level is a classification used to compare one or more patients to another group of patients. For example, an acuity system classifies bathing patients from 1 (independent in all but one or two aspects of care; almost ready for discharge) to 5 (totally dependent in all aspects of care; requiring intensive care). Using this system, for example, a patient returning from surgery requiring frequent monitoring and extensive care has an acuity level of 3 compared with another patient awaiting discharge after a successful recovery from surgery who has an acuity level of 1. Accurate acuity ratings justify the number and qualifications of staff needed to safely care for patients. The patient-to-staff ratios established for a unit depend on a composite gathering of 24-hour acuity data for all patients receiving care.

DOCUMENTATION IN THE HOME HEALTH CARE SETTING

As a result of shorter hospitalizations and larger numbers of older persons who require home care services, home health care is expanding. Because patients are leaving acute care settings earlier, increasing numbers of home care patients are presenting in the community setting with more acuity (i.e., sicker). The focus in home health care is on family-centred care and forming a partnership or collaboration with the patient and the family to help the patient regain health, to help the family take over the patient's care, or to help accomplish both. Documentation in the home health care system has different implications than in other areas of nursing. Two primary differences are that the majority of the care is performed by the patient and family and that the nurse is often teaching and helping the patient and family achieve greater independence. Nurses must have astute assessment skills to gather the needed information about changes in the patient's health care status. In addition, documentation systems need to provide the entire health care team with the information needed for them to work together effectively (Box 15-6).

BOX 15-6 Home Care Forms for Documentation

The usual forms used to document home care include the following:

- Assessment forms
- Referral source information or intake form
- Discipline-specific care plans
- Physician's plan of treatment
- Professional order form (e.g., MD, speech language pathologist, specialty nurses)
- Medication administration record
- Clinical progress notes
- Miscellaneous (case conference notes, professional communication forms, private billing forms, insurance company forms)
- Discharge summary

In the home care setting, the patient is the guardian of the health care record. A hard copy of the health care record is kept in the patient's home, and the patient is responsible for its safekeeping. Communication is crucial in home care because much of the interaction between health care providers is conducted virtually by phone or fax over password-protected voice mail or secure fax lines. With the increasing availability of smart phones and laptop computers or tablets, home health care records can be available in multiple locations, improving accessibility to information and facilitating interprofessional collaboration.

DOCUMENTATION IN THE LONG-TERM HEALTH CARE SETTING

An increasing number of older persons require care in long-term care or residential facilities. Many individuals live in this setting for the rest of their lives and are therefore referred to as *residents* rather than as *patients.* In long-term care settings, nursing personnel face challenges much different from those in acute care settings. Residents' health is often stable, and daily documentation can be completed on flow sheets. Assessments performed several times a day in acute care settings are required only weekly or monthly in long-term care settings.

Governmental agencies and provincial and territorial laws are instrumental in determining the standards and policies for documentation. Documentation is used to review the levels of care given to and needed by residents in long-term care facilities. Although most long-term care facilities have different documentation systems, these systems are based on the need for a concise, nonduplicating method of documentation and on the importance of nursing documentation in support of evidence-informed practice (Box 15-7).

DOCUMENTING COMMUNICATION WITH PROVIDERS AND UNIQUE EVENTS

Telephone Calls Made to a Health Care Provider

Document every phone call you make to a health care provider. Your documentation includes when the call was made, who made it (if you did not make the call), who was called, to whom information was given, what information was given, and what information was received. An example is as follows: "May 20, 2017 (2030 hrs): Called Dr. Morgan's office. Spoke with Sam Thomas, RN, who will inform Dr. Morgan that Mr. Wade's potassium level drawn at 2000 hrs was 5.9 mEq/dL. Informed that Dr. Morgan will call back after he is finished seeing his current patient. Carla Skala, RN."

Telephone and Verbal Orders

Telephone orders (often written "TO") occur when a health care provider gives therapeutic orders over the phone to a registered nurse. Verbal orders (often written "VO") occur when a health care provider gives therapeutic orders to a registered nurse while they are standing in close proximity to each other. TOs and VOs usually occur at night or during emergencies; they should be used only when absolutely necessary and not for the sake of convenience. In some situations, it is prudent to have a second person listen to TOs. Check agency policy. Box 15-8 provides guidelines that promote accuracy when receiving TOs or VOs.

The nurse receiving a TO or VO enters the complete order into the computer using the computerized provider order entry (CPOE) software or writes it out on a physician's order sheet for entry in the computer as soon as possible. After taking the order, the nurse reads it back using the "read-back" process and documents that he or she did this, to provide evidence that the information received (such as call-back instructions and/or therapeutic orders) was verified with the provider. An example follows: "*March 4, 2017 (0815 hrs) Change IV fluid to Lactated Ringer's with potassium 20 mEq per litre to run at 125 mL/hour. TO: Dr. Knight/J. Woods, RN, read back.*" The health care provider later verifies the TO or VO legally by signing it within a set time (e.g., 24 hours) as set by hospital policy.

Change-of-Shift Reports

At the end of each shift, nurses report information about their assigned patients to the nurses working on the next shift. While there is an increasing awareness that high-quality handover practices are critical to ensure patient safety and continuity of care among nurses, there is very little evidence for what constitutes best practice in change-of-shift reports (Riesenberg, Leisch, & Cunningham, 2010). Various terms are used to describe this exchange of information, such as *change-of-shift reports, patient care handover, transfer of accountability (TOA), handoffs, bedside reporting,* or *shift handover.*

Nurses give a **change-of-shift report** orally in person, by audiotape recording, by writing information on a summary report sheet, or by standing at the patient's bedside. Oral reports can be given in conference rooms, with staff members from both shifts participating, but this

BOX 15-7 Components of Documentation in Long-Term Care

Section 1: The Health Care Record
The health care record includes the resident's name and medical number; date and time of admission; change in resident's condition; informed consent; note or discharge summary; incident reporting; monthly summary charting; and type of therapy and treatment time.

Section 2: Resident Assessments and Related Documents
This section consists of the admission record; preadmission assessment; admission assessment; assessment of risk for falls; skin assessment; bowel and bladder assessment; physical restraint assessment; record of self-administration of medication; nutrition assessment; and activities, recreation, or leisure interests.

Section 3: Other Records
Other records include drug therapy records, medication or treatment records, flow sheets or other graphic records, laboratory and special reports, consent forms, acknowledgements and notices, advance directives, and discharge or transfer records.

BOX 15-8 Guidelines for Telephone Orders and Verbal Orders

- Clearly determine the patient's name, room number, and diagnosis.
- Repeat any prescribed orders back to the physician or health care provider.
- Use clarification questions to avoid misunderstandings.
- Write telephone order ("TO") or verbal order ("VO"), including date and time, name of patient, and the complete order; sign the names of the physician or other health care provider and nurse.
- Follow agency policies; some institutions require telephone (and verbal) orders to be reviewed and signed by two nurses.
- The physician must co-sign the order within the time frame required by the institution (usually 24 hours).

is no longer as common as it used to be. Oral reports most often take the form of one-to-one reports—for example, a report given by the night nurse to the day nurse (Figure 15-3). An advantage of oral reports is that they allow staff members to ask questions or clarify explanations. The nurses can see the patient together to perform needed assessments, evaluate progress, and discuss the interventions best suited to the patient's needs. An audiotape report is given by the nurse who has completed care for the patient; this type of report is left for the nurse on the next shift to review. However, it is essential to schedule an opportunity for the incoming nurses to ask questions for clarification after they listen to the taped report. According to Popovich (2011, p. 59), human factors such as "stress, distraction, and communication problems" make change-of-shift reports more prone to error. Several Canadian hospitals have implemented standardized bedside safe patient handoffs using transfer of accountability (TOA) practice guidelines developed by their institution. The process provides an opportunity for the outgoing night nurse and the incoming day nurse to engage in a verbal report and to complete a patient safety checklist at the bedside.

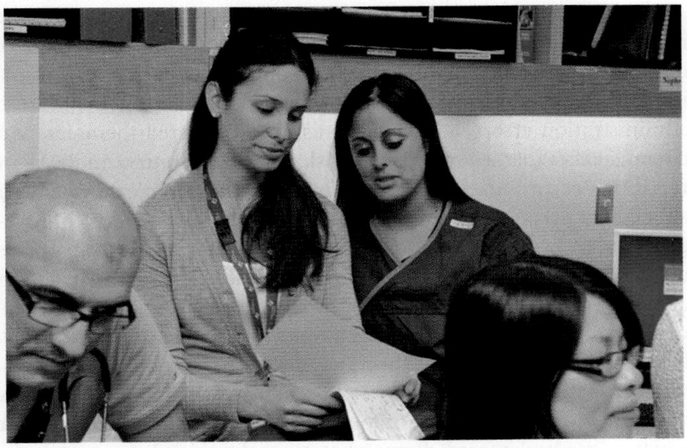

FIGURE 15-3 One-to-one change-of-shift report at nursing station. (From RNAO. [2013]. *Developing and sustaining interprofessional health care: Optimizing patient, organizational and system outcomes* [p. 8]. Retrieved from http://rnao.ca/bpg/guidelines/interprofessional-team-work-healthcare.)

Because nurses have many responsibilities, it is important to compile a change-of-shift report quickly and efficiently (Table 15-4). An effective report describes patients' health status and tells staff on the next shift exactly what kind of care the patients require. A change-of-shift report should *not* simply be a reading of documented information. Instead, significant facts about patients are reviewed (e.g., condition of wounds, episodes of chest pain) to provide a baseline for comparison during the next shift. Data about patients need to be objective, current, and concise.

An organized report follows a logical sequence. The following is an example of a change-of-shift report:

Background information: Cy Tolan in bed 4, a 32-year-old patient of Dr. Lang, is scheduled for a colon resection this morning at 0800 hrs. He has had ulcerative colitis for 2 years with recent bouts of frank bleeding in his stools. He was admitted at 0600 hrs this morning with slight abdominal discomfort. This is his first experience with surgery. He knows he may require a colostomy. He has been NPO (had nothing by mouth) since midnight at home.

Assessment: Mr. Tolan mentioned that he was unable to sleep last night. He had many questions about surgery on admission this morning.

Nursing diagnosis: His chief nursing care problems are anxiety related to inexperience with surgery and risk for body image disturbance.

Teaching plan: I talked to him about postoperative routines and answered all his questions. He attended the preoperative admission clinic 2 weeks ago, but he did not have as many concerns at that time. He stated that he felt less anxious now that he knows what to expect.

Treatments: I started an intravenous infusion of normal saline in his left arm at 0645 hrs and it is running at 125 mL/hr.

Family information: His wife came with him this morning and will wait in the surgical waiting room till his surgery is complete.

Discharge plan: Mr. Tolan is a very active person and participates in strenuous sports such as swimming. Mrs. Tolan is concerned about how he might react to a colostomy. I suggest making a referral to the enterostomal therapist early, if the colostomy is performed.

TABLE 15-4 Change-of-Shift Reports: Dos and Don'ts

Dos	Don'ts
Do provide only essential background information about patient (i.e., name, sex, age, physician's diagnosis, and medical history).	Don't review all routine care procedures or tasks (e.g., bathing, scheduled changes).
Do identify patient's nursing diagnoses or health care problems and their related causes.	Don't review all biographical information already available in written form.
Do describe objective measurements or observations about patient's condition and response to health problem, and emphasize recent changes.	Don't use critical comments about patient's behaviour, such as "Mrs. Wills is so demanding."
Do share significant information about family members as it relates to patient's problems.	Don't make assumptions about relationships between family members.
Do continuously review ongoing discharge plan (e.g., need for resources, patient's level of preparation to go home).	Don't wait until near discharge to discuss the plan.
Do relay to staff significant changes in the way therapies are given (e.g., different position for pain relief, new medication).	Don't describe basic steps of a procedure.
Do describe instructions given in teaching plan and patient's response.	Don't explain detailed content unless staff members ask for clarification.
Do evaluate results of nursing or medical care measures (e.g., effect of back rub or analgesic administration), and describe results specifically.	Don't simply describe results as "good" or "poor."
Do be clear about priorities to which incoming staff must attend.	Don't force incoming staff to guess what to do first.

Priority needs: Right now, Mr. Tolan is relaxing in his room. All preoperative procedures have been completed except for his preoperative antibiotic, due on call to the operating room.

A professional demeanour is essential when giving a report about patients or family members. It is often necessary to describe the interactions among patients, nurses, and family members in behavioural terms. Nurses must avoid using judgemental language such as *uncooperative, difficult,* or *bad* when describing such behaviours.

In many settings, unregulated care providers (UCPs) are involved in the change-of-shift report. UCPs are part of the health care team and can contribute more when they also know a patient's condition and the nursing team's priorities in care. The nurse can use the report to emphasize to UCPs the tasks that need to be accomplished.

Transfer Reports

Patients may transfer from one unit to another to receive different levels of care. For example, patients transfer from a Critical Care Unit or the recovery room to general nursing units when they no longer require intense monitoring. To promote continuity of care, the nurse may give transfer reports by phone or in person. When giving a transfer report, the nurse needs to include the following information:

- Patient's name, age, name of primary physician, and medical diagnosis
- Summary of progress up to the time of transfer
- Patient's current health status (physical and psychosocial)
- Patient's allergies
- Patient's emergency code status
- Patient's family support (e.g., spouse or partner, children, parents)
- Patient's current nursing diagnoses or problem and care plan
- Any critical assessments or interventions to be completed shortly after transfer (helps receiving nurse to establish priorities of care)
- Need for any special equipment, such as isolation equipment, suction equipment, or traction

After completion of the transfer report, the receiving nurse needs an opportunity to ask questions about the patient's status. In some cases, written documentation must include a record of information reported.

Using SBAR or I-SBAR-R for Communication

Nurses communicate information about patients so that all team members can make appropriate decisions about the care of patients. Any verbal report must be timely, accurate, and relevant. Many Canadian hospitals use the situation–background–assessment–recommendation (SBAR) technique or identification–situation–background–assessment–recommendation–read back (I-SBAR-R) technique (Box 15-9) to share important patient information in an effective and efficient way and to help standardize communication (Institute for Healthcare Improvement, 2017). The SBAR/I-SBAR-R technique is a situational briefing system that fosters a culture of patient safety. This technique (see Box 15-9) can be incorporated into a variety of ways of reporting (e.g., a nurse's report to a physician about a critically ill patient, change-of-shift reports about individual patients) and can be adapted for use with or by other health care providers.

Incident or Occurrence Reports

An *incident* or *occurrence* is any event that is not consistent with the routine, expected care of a patient or the standard procedures in place on a health care unit. Examples include patient falls, needle-stick injuries, a visit by someone who has symptoms of illness, medication administration errors, accidental omission of ordered therapies, and circumstances that led to injury or risk for patient injury. An incident report (or occurrence or safety learning report) is completed whenever an incident occurs. They are an important part of the quality improvement program of a unit (see Chapter 11). A *near miss* (or *close call*) is defined as "an event that could have resulted in unwanted consequences, but did not because either by chance or through timely intervention the event did not reach the patient" (ISMP, Canada, 2017). When an incident occurs, as the nurse, document an objective description of what happened; what you observed; and the follow-up actions taken, including notification of the patient's health care provider in the patient's medical record. Remember to evaluate and document the patient's response to the incident.

Incident or occurrence reports contain confidential information; distribution of the report is limited to those responsible for reviewing

BOX 15-9 The Identification-Situation–Background–Assessment–Recommendation-Repeat Back (I-SBAR-R) Technique

When calling the physician, follow the I-SBAR-R process as follows:

Identification: Who is calling and who are you calling about?

- Identify yourself and your role
- Identify the unit, the patient, and the room number

Situation: What is the situation you are calling about?

- Briefly state the problem: What it is, when it started, and the severity

Background: Provide background information as necessary related to the situation, including the following:

- The admitting diagnosis, date of admission, and pertinent medical history
- List of current medications, allergies, intravenous fluids, and laboratory tests
- Laboratory results (date and time each test was performed and results of previous tests for comparison)
- Other clinical information
- Code status

Assessment: What is your assessment of the situation?

Examples include the following:

- Most recent vital signs
- Changes in vital signs or assessment from previous assessments

Recommendations: What is your recommendation, or what do you think needs to be done?

Examples include the following:

- Patient to be admitted or transferred
- New medication or further tests
- Patient to be seen now
- Orders to be changed

Repeat Back:

- Repeat back orders that have been given
- Clarify any questions

Adapted from Joint Commission on Accreditation of Healthcare Organizations. (2005, February). The SBAR technique: Improves communication, enhances patient safety. *Joint Commission Perspectives on Patient Safety, 5*(2), 2; Enlow, M., Shanks, L., Guhde, J., & Perkins, M. (2010). Incorporating interprofessional communication skills (ISBARR) into an undergraduate nursing curriculum. *Nurse Educator, 35*(4), 176–180; and Grbach, W., Struth, D., & Vincent, I. (2008). *Reformulating SBAR to "I-SBAR-R."* Chapel Hill, NC: Quality and Safety Education for Nurses. Retrieved from http://qsen.org/reformulating-sbar-to-i-sbar-r/.

the forms. It is important to follow agency policy when making an incident report and file the report with the risk-management department of your agency. Analysis of incident reports helps identify trends in an organization that provide justification for changes in policies and procedures or for in-service programs. Do not include any reference to an incident in the medical record. A notation about an incident report in a patient's medical record makes it easier for a lawyer to argue that the reference makes the incident report part of the medical record and therefore subject to attorney review.

INFORMATION MANAGEMENT IN HEALTH CARE

Information technology (IT) refers to the management and processing of information, generally with the assistance of computers. **Health informatics** (see Chapter 16) is the "intersection of clinical, IM/IT [Information Management/Information Technology] and management practices to achieve better health" (Canadian Organization for Advancement of Computers in Health [COACH] 2012, p. 8). A health care information system (HIS) is a group of systems used within a health care organization to support and enhance health care. An HIS consists of two major types of information systems: clinical information systems and administrative information systems. Together the two systems operate to make the entry and communication of data and information more efficient. Any single health care agency uses one or several of these systems.

Nursing competence in health care informatics is becoming a priority as health care providers and facilities across Canada implement electronic documentation. Nurses need informatics competencies to deliver safer and more efficient care, to add to the nursing professional knowledge base, and to facilitate the growth of evidence-informed practice. Professional organizations recommend that all nurses acquire a minimal level of awareness and competence in informatics and use of IT. Under the domain of communication and collaboration in the National Nursing Education Framework (CASN, 2015), the CASN lists "the ability to communicate using information technologies to support engagement with patients/clients and the interprofessional team" as an essential component of baccalaureate nursing education (p. 15). The Nursing Informatics Entry-to-Practice Competencies for Registered Nurses (CASN, 2012) outlines three entry-to-practice competencies related to nursing informatics: (1) use of relevant information and knowledge to support the delivery of evidence-informed patient care; (2) use of information and communication technologies (ICTs) in accordance with professional and regulatory standards and workplace policies; and (3) use of ICTs in the delivery of patient/client care (pp. 6–10). These nursing informatics competencies are considered the minimum knowledge and skills that new graduate nurses require in order to practise.

Competence in informatics is not the same as computer competency. To become competent in informatics, nurses need to be able to use evolving methods of discovering, retrieving, and using information in practice (Hebda & Czar, 2013). This means that, as a nurse, you learn to recognize when information is needed and have the skills to find, evaluate, and use that information effectively. You also need to know how to use clinical databases within your institution and apply the information so you can deliver high-quality, appropriate patient care.

Clinical Information Systems

All members of the interprofessional health care team, including nurses, physicians, pharmacists, social workers, and therapists, use programs available on a **clinical information system (CIS)**. These programs include monitoring systems; order entry systems; and laboratory, radiology, and pharmacy systems. A monitoring system includes devices that automatically monitor and record biometric measurements (e.g., vital signs, oxygen saturation, cardiac index, and stroke volume) in acute care, critical care, and specialty areas. The devices electronically send measurements directly to the nursing documentation system.

Order-entry systems allow nurses to order supplies and services from another department. An example is a computer program that provides the ability to order sterile supplies from the central supply department. This eliminates the use of written order forms and expedites the delivery of needed supplies to a nursing unit. **Computerized provider order entry (CPOE)** systems allow health care providers to directly enter orders for patient care into the hospital information system. In advanced systems, CPOE has built-in reminders and alerts that help a health care provider select the most appropriate medication or diagnostic test. The direct entry of orders eliminates issues related to illegible handwriting and transcription errors. In addition, a CPOE system potentially speeds the implementation of ordered diagnostic tests and treatments, which improves staff productivity and saves money because the unit secretary no longer transcribes a written order onto a nursing order form (Hebda & Czar, 2013). Orders made through CPOE are integrated within the record and sent to the appropriate departments (e.g., pharmacy or radiology).

Clinical decision support systems (CDSS) are computerized programs used within the health care setting to aid and support clinical decision making. When used to support nursing decisions it is called a *nursing CDSS* (Figure 15-4). The knowledge base within a CDSS contains rules and logic statements that link information required for clinical decisions to generate tailored recommendations for individual patients, which are presented to nurses as alerts, warnings, or other information for consideration (Lee, 2013). For example, an effective CDSS notifies health care providers of patient allergies before ordering a medication, which enhances patient safety during the medication ordering process. CDSSs also improve nursing care. When patient assessment data are combined with patient care guidelines, nurses are

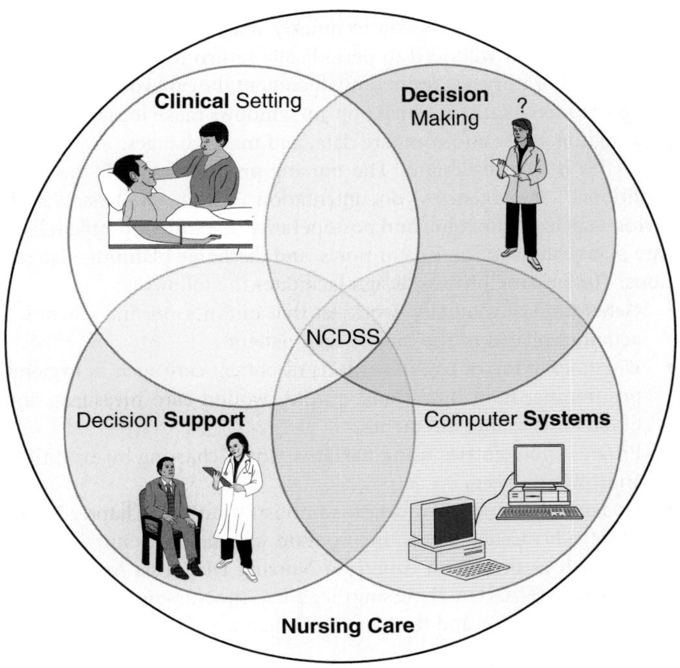

FIGURE 15-4 Model of a nursing clinical decision support system (NCDSS).

BOX 15-10 EVIDENCE-INFORMED PRACTICE

Effect of Clinical Decision Support Systems on Patient Outcomes

PICO Question: Do nurses who work at health care agencies that use clinical decision support systems (CDSSs) provide safer and more effective patient care when compared with nurses who work at agencies that do not use CDSSs?

Evidence Summary

Nurses who provide evidence-informed care at the bedside provide safe and effective care. However, one barrier to implementing evidence-informed practice is getting information to nurses at the bedside when they need it. Several studies investigated the effect of the CDSS on patient outcomes. Harrison, Stalker, Henderson, et al. (2013) examined the impact of a nursing CDSS integrated with the electronic heart record developed to facilitate adherence to guidelines for the management of hypoglycemia. Data were collected and reviewed 6 months before implementation, 6 months following implementation, and 7 to 12 months after implementation of the CDSS. The findings of this study demonstrated a statistically significant improvement in adherence to use of the clinical guideline. The study also showed that the protocol was almost three times as likely to be followed 7 to 12 months after implementation of the CDSS.

Current evidence also shows that use of CDSS improves adherence to implementation of evidence-informed sepsis care in Critical Care Units (Giuliano, Lecardo, & Staul, 2011) and completion of screening for osteoporosis in primary care settings (DeJesus, 2012). These studies show that CDSSs that provide automatic decision support at the time and place nurses need it enhance the quality and safety of patient care. CDSSs also help nurses initiate evidence-informed care faster and with more accuracy, improving patient outcomes.

Application to Nursing Practice

- CDSSs enhance the implementation of evidence-informed practice into nursing care because they remind nurses which interventions need to be implemented for specific patients at the time the care is needed.
- Nurses need to be involved in the design and selection of CDSSs to ensure that they provide clinical decision support effectively and efficiently.
- Nurses need to evaluate patient outcomes when CDSSs are used. They also need to be involved in developing solutions to improve the effectiveness of CDSSs when opportunities for improvement are identified.

better able to implement evidence-informed nursing care, resulting in improved patient outcomes (Box 15-10).

Nursing Clinical Information Systems

A well-designed nursing clinical information system (NCIS) incorporates the principles of nursing informatics to support the work that nurses do by facilitating documentation of nursing process activities and offering resources for managing nursing care delivery. As a nurse, you need to access a computer program easily, review a patient's medical history and health care provider's orders, and then go to the patient's bedside to conduct a comprehensive assessment. Once you complete an assessment, you will enter data into the computer terminal at the patient's bedside and develop a plan of care from the information gathered. This allows you to quickly share the plan of care with your patient. You will need to periodically return to the computer to check on laboratory test results and document the care you deliver. The computer screens and optional pop-up windows make it easy to locate information, enter and compare data, and make changes.

NCISs have two designs. The nursing process design is the most traditional. It organizes documentation within well-established formats such as admission and postoperative assessment problem lists, care plans, intervention lists or notes, and discharge planning instructions. The nursing process design facilitates the following:

- Generation of a nursing work list that outlines routine scheduled activities related to the care of each patient
- Documentation of routine aspects of patient care such as hygiene, positioning, fluid intake and output, wound care measures, and blood glucose measurements
- Progress note entries using narrative notes, charting by exception, and/or flow sheets
- Documentation of medication administration (see Chapter 34)

More advanced systems incorporate standardized nursing languages such as the North American Nursing Diagnosis Association–International (NANDA-I) nursing diagnoses, the Nursing Interventions Classification (NIC), and the Nursing Outcomes Classification (NOC) into the software.

The other model for an NCIS is the protocol or critical pathway design (Hebda & Czar, 2013). This design facilitates interdisciplinary management of information because all health care providers use evidenced-informed protocols or critical pathways to document the care they provide. The information system allows a user to select one or more appropriate protocols for a patient. An advanced system merges multiple protocols, using a master protocol or path to direct patient care activities. Standard health care provider order sets are included in the protocols and automatically processed. The system integrates appropriate information into the medication delivery process to enhance patient safety. In addition, the system identifies variances of the anticipated outcomes on the protocols as documentation is entered. This provides all caregivers the ability to analyze variances and offer an accurate clinical picture of a patient's progress.

Advantages of a Nursing Clinical Information System. Anecdotal reports and descriptive studies suggest that NCISs offer important advantages to nurses in practice. According to Hebda and Czar (2013), some specific advantages include the following:

- Better access to information
- Enhanced quality of documentation through prompts
- Reduced errors of omission
- Reduced hospital costs
- Increased nurse job satisfaction
- Compliance with requirements of accrediting agencies
- Development of a common clinical database
- Enhanced ability to track records

Many NCISs include content-importing technologies that allow the use of templates, macros, automated data points, and the ability to copy forward either parts of or entire nursing shift assessments that enable nurses to quickly document their assessment or the care they provided. These features have benefits and risks associated with their use. When allergy and current medication lists are automatically imported into nursing admission documentation from a previous hospital encounter, the nurse needs to meticulously review this information for accuracy and update it as needed to avoid documentation errors and patient safety concerns. When nursing shift assessment data are copied forward from a previous shift or day, the data must be updated so they accurately reflect a patient's current clinical status (Weis & Levy, 2014).

KEY CONCEPTS

- The electronic (or paper-based) medical record is a legal document and requires information describing the care delivered to a patient.
- All information contained in the medical record is confidential; access to patient records is limited to individuals involved in the care of the patient.
- Interdisciplinary communication arising among members of the health care team is essential, and the medical record is one tool that supports and facilitates that communication.
- Accurate record keeping requires an objective interpretation of data with precise measurements, correct spelling, and proper use of abbreviations.
- A nurse's electronic or handwritten signature on an entry in a record designates accountability for the contents of that entry.
- To keep medical records accurate, any change in a patient's condition warrants immediate documentation about the event and the action that was taken to address the change.
- Protection of the confidentiality of patients' health information and the security of computer systems are top priorities that include log-in processes, audit trails, firewalls, data-recovery processes, and policies about handling and disposing of data to protect patient information.
- Problem-oriented medical records (POMRs) are organized by the patient's health care problems.
- SOAP, SOAPIE, PIE, and DAR charting formats organize entries in the progress notes according to the nursing process.
- Home care documentation is accessible to a variety of caregivers in the home.
- Long-term care documentation is interdisciplinary. Assessments performed several times a day in the acute care setting are required only weekly or monthly in long-term care.
- Patient care information communicated to providers through telephone orders must always be verified by using and documenting use of the "read-back" process.
- Incident or occurrence reports objectively describe any event that is not consistent with the routine care of a patient.
- The major purpose of the change-of-shift report is to maintain continuity of care.
- A hospital information system consists of two major types of information systems: CIS and administrative information systems.
- Computerized information systems provide information about patients in an organized and easily accessible fashion.
- Protection of the confidentiality of patient health information and the security of computer systems should be a top priority.
- Nursing informatics facilitates the integration of data, information, and knowledge to support clinical decision making of nurses and other health care providers in all roles and settings.

CRITICAL THINKING EXERCISES

1. Joseph Vojnovic is an 80-year-old man admitted with a diagnosis of possible pneumonia. He complains of general malaise and a frequent productive cough, which produces thick, yellow sputum. Vital sign measurements are as follows: blood pressure, 150/90 mm Hg; pulse rate, 92 beats per minute; respiration rate, 22 breaths per minute; and temperature, 38.5°C. During your initial assessment, he coughs violently for 40 to 45 seconds without expectorating. He exhibits wheezes and coarse crackles at both bases of the lungs. He states, "It hurts in my chest when I cough." Differentiate between objective and subjective data in this case example.
2. The nurse positions Mr. Vojnovic in a semi-Fowler's position, encourages him to increase his fluid intake, and gives him acetaminophen (Tylenol), 650 mg PO, as ordered for fever. One hour later, his vital sign measurements are as follows: blood pressure, 130/86 mm Hg; pulse, 86 beats per minute; respiration rate, 22 breaths per minute; and temperature, 37.7°C. He states that he has been able to sleep. His fluid intake over the past hour has been 200 mL of water. Use the given information to write a nurse's progress note using the PIE format.
3. Near the end of your shift, you have identified *fluid volume deficit* as a nursing diagnosis for Mr. Vojnovic. Since his admission, he has had a fluid intake of about 600 mL, and his urine output was 300 mL of dark, concentrated urine. His temperature is back up to 38.4°C, his mucous membranes are dry, and he states that he feels very weak. List what should be included in the change-of-shift report.
4. Several days later, after treatment with intravenous antibiotics, Mr. Vojnovic is feeling much better and preparations are being made for discharge. He is to take cephalexin (Keflex) 500 mg every 6 hours, for the next 10 days; continue to drink extra fluids; and get extra rest. He lives alone. Although he is generally cooperative, he does not like drinking water or taking pills. He is to make an appointment with his physician for 1 week from today and should call the physician if symptoms recur. Write a discharge summary that is concise and instructive.

REVIEW QUESTIONS

1. A fellow nursing student is a patient in the hospital where a student nurse has a clinical placement. What should the student nurse do when he sees his ill classmate during a patient transfer to that unit?
   1. Keep the information private.
   2. Advise a few of the ill student's friends so that they can visit.
   3. Visit the ill student during lunch break.
   4. Access the ill student's EHR to see if the student is well enough for a visit.
2. A manager notes the following entry in the nurses' notes from a community patient's health care record, "Patient is difficult to care for. Refuses advice for improving appetite." Which of the following suggestions should the manager give to the community health nurse who entered the note?
   1. Avoid rushing when charting an entry.
   2. Use correction fluid to remove the entry.
   3. Draw a single line through the statement and initial it.
   4. Enter only objective and factual information about the patient.
3. A patient tells the nurse, "I have stomach cramps and feel nauseated." Which type of data is this?
   1. Objective
   2. Historical
   3. Subjective
   4. Assessment
4. During your visit to a patient's home, your patient says, "I do not know what is going on; I cannot get an explanation from my doctor about the results of my test. I want something done about this." Which of the following is the most appropriate documentation of the patient's emotional status?
   1. The patient has a defiant attitude and demands his test results.
   2. The patient appears to be upset with his physician about his test results.
   3. The patient is demanding and complains frequently.
   4. The patient states he is frustrated by the lack of information about his test results.

5. Patients frequently request copies of their health care records. Which of the following statements is true regarding patient access to health care records?
   1. Patients have the right to read those records.
   2. Patients are not allowed to read those records.
   3. Only the health care workers have access to the records.
   4. Only the families may read the records.
6. Accurate entries are an important characteristic of good documentation. Which of the following charting entries is most accurately written?
   1. Patient ambulated in hall with assistance, exercise well tolerated.
   2. Patient ambulated 15 m (50 feet) up and down hall, exercise well tolerated.
   3. Patient ambulated 15 m (50 feet) up and down hall with assistance from nurse. Spouse also accompanied patient during the walk.
   4. Patient ambulated 15 m (50 feet) with assistance from nurse. Pre-exercise HR 88; post-exercise HR 94.
7. What is the purpose of acuity ratings?
   1. To guide all nursing care
   2. To document the patient admission
   3. To determine hours of care needed
   4. To establish guidelines for patient care
8. Label each line of documentation with the appropriate SOAP category: (Subjective [S], Objective [O], Assessment [A], Plan [P]).

   1. ___ Repositioned patient on right side. Encouraged patient to use patient-controlled analgesia.
   2. ___ "The pain increases every time I try to turn on my left side."
   3. ___ Acute pain related to tissue injury from surgical incision.
   4. ___ Left lower abdominal surgical incision, 7.5 cm (3 inches) in length, closed, sutures intact, no drainage. Pain noted on mild palpation.

9. A nurse is documenting his telephone report to a registered nurse (RN) who is receiving his patient later in the day at another agency. The nurse begins by writing the date and time the report was given and the name of the RN taking the report. Which pieces of information does the nurse include in the telephone call documentation? *(Select all that apply.)*
   1. The patient's name, age, and admitting diagnoses
   2. The discussion of any patient allergies to food and medications
   3. That the nurse receiving the report was advised that the patient is "needy" and "on the call light all the time"
   4. That the patient's pain rating went from 8 to 2 on a scale of 0 to 10 after receiving Tylenol 650 mg
   5. Description of any unresolved problems and current interventions in place
10. A beginning nursing student is completing documentation of care under direct observation from her preceptor. Which of the following actions would require intervention as they are inappropriate? The nursing student: *(Select all that apply.)*
    1. Documents a medication given by another nursing student.
    2. Includes the date and time of the entry into the medical record.
    3. Enters assessment data into the electronic medical record using the computer mounted on the wall in the patient's room.
    4. Leaves a slip of paper with her user name and password in the patient's room.
    5. Starts to enter "Docusate sodium 100 mg ordered at 08:00 held. Patient declined to take dose stating, 'I had several loose stools yesterday, and I'm afraid if I take this dose the problem will get worse,'" as a narrative comment.
11. A group of nurses is discussing the advantages of using computerized provider order entry (CPOE). Which statement indicates that the nurses understand the major advantage of using CPOE?
    1. "CPOE reduces transcription errors."
    2. "CPOE reduces the time needed for health care providers to write orders."
    3. "CPOE eliminates verbal and telephone orders from health care providers."
    4. "CPOE reduces the time nurses use to communicate with health care providers."
12. The nurse enters the patient assessment data and information that the head of the patient's bed is elevated to 20 degrees and that he is receiving nasogastric tube feedings at 45 mL/hr. An alert appears on the computer screen warning that this patient is at a high risk for aspiration because the head of the bed is not elevated enough. This warning is known as which type of system?
    1. Electronic health record
    2. Clinical documentation
    3. Clinical decision support system
    4. Computerized physician order entry
13. What is the appropriate way for a nurse to dispose of information printed out from a patient's electronic health record?
    1. Rip the papers up into small pieces and place the pieces into a standard trash can.
    2. Place all papers in the flip-top binder designated for that patient that is located in the nurse's station on the patient care unit.
    3. Place papers with patient information in a secure bin marked for shredding.
    4. Ask one of the unit clerks to dispose of the papers at their convenience.

Answers: 1. 1; **2.** 4; **3.** 3; **4.** 4; **5.** 1; **6.** 4; **7.** 3; **8.** S = 2; O = 4; A = 3; P = 1; **9.** 1, 2, 4, 5; **10.** 1, 4; **11.** 1; **12.** 3; **13.** 3.

Rationales for the Review Questions appear at the end of the book.

RECOMMENDED WEBSITES

Accreditation Canada: http://www.accreditation.ca/

Accreditation Canada is a national, nonprofit, independent organization whose role is to help health and social service organizations, across Canada and internationally, examine and improve the quality of care and service they provide to their patients through a voluntary external peer review.

Canada Health Infoway: https://www.infoway-inforoute.ca

Canada Health Infoway (Infoway) is a federally funded, independent, not-for-profit organization. Members include the 14 federal, provincial, and territorial deputy ministers of health. Infoway has a mandate to foster and accelerate the development and adoption of electronic health information systems and EHRs across Canada.

Canadian Nurses Association: Provincial and Territorial Regulatory Bodies: http://www.cna-aiic.ca/en/becoming-an-rn/regulation-of-rns/regulatory-bodies/

This part of the website of the Canadian Nurses Association provides links to each provincial and territorial nursing association. Most associations provide information about documentation standards and requirements in their province or territory.

Canadian Nursing Informatics Association: https://cnia.ca/

The Canadian Nursing Informatics Association (CNIA) is affiliated with the Canadian Nurses Association and has been established as the voice for health informatics in Canada. *Nursing informatics* refers to the integration of nursing science, computer science, and information science to document and communicate data and knowledge in nursing practice.

***The Personal Information Protection and Electronic Documents Act* (PIPEDA):** https://www.priv.gc.ca/en/privacy-topics/privacy-laws-in-canada/the-personal-information-protection-and-electronic-documents-act-pipeda/

The *Personal Information Protection and Electronic Documents Act* (PIPEDA) is the federal privacy law for private-sector organizations. It sets out the ground rules for how agencies must handle personal information.

REFERENCES

American Health Consultants. (2015). They're back! Clinical pathways are in favor again. *Hospital Care Management, 23*(2), 13–15.

Beach, J., & Oates, J. (2014). Maintaining best practice in record-keeping and documentation. *Nursing Standard, 28*(36), 45–50.

Blair, W., & Smith, B. (2012). Nursing documentation: Frameworks and barriers. *Contemporary Nurse, 41*(2), 160–168. doi:10.5172/conu.2012.41.2.160.

Bryden, C. (2016). *Documentation and nursing: A legal perspective*. Presentation sponsored by the RNAO Legal Assistance Program. Retrieved from http://rnao.ca/sites/rnao-ca/files/Documentation_and_Nursing.pdf.

Canada Health Infoway. (2011). *Summary corporate plan 2011–2012*. Retrieved from https://www.infoway-inforoute.ca/en/component/edocman/resources/i-infoway-i-corporate/business-plans/11-summary-corporate-plan-2011-2012.

Canada Health Infoway. (2016). *A conversation about digital health: Canada Health Infoway Annual Report 2015–2016*. Retrieved from https://www.infoway-inforoute.ca/en/component/edocman/3098-annual-report-2015-2016/view-document.

Canadian Association of Schools of Nursing/Association Canadienne des Écoles de Sciences Infirmières (CASN/ACESI). (2012). *Nursing informatics: Entry-to-practice competencies for registered nurses*. Retrieved from http://www.casn.ca/wp-content/uploads/2014/12/Nursing-Informatics-Entry-to-Practice-Competencies-for-RNs_updated-June-4-2015.pdf.

Canadian Association of Schools of Nursing/Association Canadienne des Écoles de Sciences Infirmières (CASN/ACESI). (2015). *National nursing education framework—Final report*. Retrieved from http://www.casn.ca/wp-content/uploads/2014/12/Framwork-FINAL-SB-Nov-30-20151.pdf.

Canadian Organization for Advancement of Computers in Health (COACH). (2012). *Health informatics professional core competencies. Version 3.0*. Retrieved from http://1d2u096vz192r028wlywji1c.wpengine.netdna-cdn.com/wp-content/uploads/2017/03/Health-Informatics-Core-Competencies.pdf.

Cartwright-Vanzant, R. C. (2010). Medical record documentation: Legal aspects in neonatal nursing. *Nursing & Infant Nursing Reviews, 10*(3), 134–137. doi:10.1053/j.nainr.2010.06.008.

Chan, R. J., Webster, J., & Bowers, A. (2016). End-of-life care pathways for improving outcomes in caring for the dying. *The Cochrane Database of Systematic Reviews*, (12), CD008006. doi:10.1002/14651858.CD008006.pub4.

DeJesus, R. S. (2012). Use of clinical decision support system to increase osteoporosis screening. *Journal of Evaluation in Clinical Practice, 18*(4), 926. doi:10.1111/j.1365-2753.2012.01878.x.

DeMartino, J. K., & Larsen, J. K. (2012). Equity in cancer care: Pathways, protocols, and guidelines. *Journal of the National Comprehensive Cancer Network, 10*(Suppl. 1), S1–S9.

DeMilliano, M. (2017). *8 Common charting mistakes to avoid*. Hatboro, PA: Nurses Service Organization. Retrieved from http://www.nso.com/risk-education/individuals/articles/8-Common-Charting-Mistakes-To-Avoid.

Ender, K. L., Krajewski, J. A., Babineau, J., et al. (2014). Use of a clinical pathway to improve the acute management of vaso-occlusive crisis pain in pediatric sickle cell disease. *Pediatric Blood and Cancer, 61*(4), 693–696.

Giuliano, K. K., Lecardo, M., & Staul, L. (2011). Impact of protocol watch on compliance with the surviving sepsis campaign. *American Journal of Critical Care, 20*(4), 313–321. doi:10.4037/ajcc2011421.

Harrison, R. L., Stalker, S. L., Henderson, R., et al. (2013). Use of a clinical decision support system to improve hypoglycemia management. *MEDSURG Nursing Journal of Adult Health, 22*(4), 250–254, 263.

Hebda, T., & Czar, P. (2013). *Handbook of informatics for nurses & healthcare professionals* (5th ed.). Upper Saddle River, NJ: Pearson Education.

Institute for Healthcare Improvement (2017). *SBAR Toolkit*. Retrieved from http://www.ihi.org/resources/Pages/Tools/sbartoolkit.aspx.

Institute for Safe Medication Practices (ISMP). (2015). *ISMP's list of error-prone abbreviations, symbols, and dose designations, 8*(24). Retrieved from https://www.ismp.org/tools/errorproneabbreviations.pdf.

Institute for Safe Medication Practices (ISMP) Canada. (2017). *Definitions of terms*. Retrieved from https://www.ismp-canada.org/definitions.htm.

Jefferies, D., Johnson, M., & Griffiths, R. (2010). A meta-study of the essentials of quality nursing documentation. *International Journal of Nursing Practice, 16*(2), 112–114. doi:10.1111/j.1440-172X.2009.01815.x.

Kerr, N. (2013). 'Creating a protective picture': A grounded theory of RN decision-making when using a charting-by-exception documentation system. *MEDSURG Nursing Journal of Adult Health, 22*(2), 110–118.

Lee, S. (2013). Features of computerized clinical decision support systems supportive of nursing practice. *Computers, Informatics, Nursing, 31*(10), 477–495. doi:10.1097/01.NCN.0000432127.99644.25.

O'Toole, M. (Ed.), (2013). *Mosby's dictionary of medicine, nursing & health professions* (9th ed.). St. Louis: Elsevier.

Penoyer, D. A., Cortelyou-Ward, K. H., Noblin, A. M., et al. (2014). Use of electronic health record documentation by healthcare workers in an acute care hospital system. *Journal of Healthcare Management, 59*(2), 130–144.

Philipsen, N., Carruthers, W., Chi, G., et al. (2014). A mixed-methods assessment of time spent documenting by nurses using an electronic medical records system. *2014 Systems and Information Engineering Design Symposium (SIEDS)*, 118–123. doi:10.1109/SIEDS.2014.6829925.

Popovich, D. (2011). 30-second head-to-toe tool in pediatric nursing: Cultivating safety in handoff communication. *Pediatric Nursing, 37*(2), 55–60.

Riesenberg, L. A., Leisch, J., & Cunningham, J. M. (2010). Nursing handoffs: A systematic review of the literature. *American Journal of Nursing, 110*(4), 24–34. doi:10.1097/01.NAJ.0000370154.79857.09.

Saleem, J. J., Flanagan, M. E., Wilck, N. R., et al. (2013). The next-generation electronic health record: Perspectives of key leaders from the US Department of Veterans Affairs. *Journal of American Medical Informatics Association, 20*(e1), e175–e177. doi:10.1136/amiajnl-2013-001748.

Weis, J. M., & Levy, P. C. (2014). Copy, paste, and cloned notes in electronic health records. *Chest, 145*(3), 632–638. doi:10.1378/chest.13-0886.

16

Nursing Informatics and Canadian Nursing Practice

Written by Margaret Ann Kennedy, RN, PhD, CPHIMS-CA, Kathryn J. Hannah, C.M., RN, PhD

OBJECTIVES

Mastery of content in this chapter will enable you to:

- Define the key terms listed.
- Describe how nursing informatics differs from routine use of technologies in nursing practice.
- Identify key Canadian issues and challenges in managing nursing data.
- Compare Canadian strategies for identifying and documenting key nursing data.
- Discuss how health information data standards influence Canadian nursing practice.
- Discuss why using standardized nursing data is important for acknowledging the professional contributions of nursing to health outcomes of Canadians.
- Develop a beginning understanding of the scope of nursing informatics concepts and the ways in which nurses can be involved in nursing informatics.
- Discuss the relationship between national privacy legislation and nursing practice in the context of a digital practice environment.
- Discuss how the Canadian Nurses Association's national e-nursing strategy will influence current and future nursing practice.

KEY TERMS

MEDIA RESOURCES

http://evolve.elsevier.com/Canada/Potter/fundamentals/

- Audio Chapter Summaries
- Examination Review Questions
- Concept Map Creator
- Case Study with Questions
- Audio Glossary
- Content Updates
- Video Clips

As health care systems respond to an increasingly complex technological environment and the progression of location-independent health care available through digital technologies (or connected health care), long-standing routines and tools are being superseded by strategic, adaptive, and evidence-informed practices that demand high-quality, timely health information. In an era when complex health care is delivered by dynamic multidisciplinary teams in increasingly diverse locations, effective nursing documentation is critical to support clinical judgement and decision making, as well as to support aggregation with documentation from other nurses and clinical disciplines to support optimal patient outcomes. Current information needs in health care challenge nurses to identify the elements of their practice that are most critical for use in nursing decision making. Nursing informatics (NI), a specialty area of nursing practice dedicated to optimal use of information and communication technology to support professional nursing practice and enable optimal patient outcomes, has been developed to respond to this challenge and continues to support the progression of the effective use of information in nursing practice and documentation.

Hannah, Ball, and Edwards (2006) tracked the evolution of technology in health care, noting that since its introduction in the health care sector, nursing has recognized the value of information and communications technology (ICT) to inform effective practice and has fostered technological development in support of patient care. Well-established ICT applications in health care include patient scheduling and transfer, billing and financial management, diagnostic imaging, lab reporting, order entry applications, pharmacy, patient documentation systems, clinical support tools, remote consultation and triage, as well as resource management applications. Innovative and explosive development of digital tools supporting health information management for both clinicians and consumers have pushed the boundaries of traditional conceptualizations of health care, with terms such as eHealth (electronic health care) and mHealth (mobile health care) fully embedded into the daily language of clinicians and Canadians. The World Health Organization (WHO, 2017) defines eHealth as "the use of information and communication technologies (ICT) for health. Examples include treating patients, conducting research, educating the health workforce, tracking diseases and monitoring public health."

Developers of health care software solutions offer integrated suites of applications that incorporate multiple tools for health care facilities or regions, and many health care institutions customize software to meet specific needs. Efforts are underway in every Canadian province and territory to develop a jurisdictional electronic health record (EHR)—a longitudinal record of an individual's health status (including diagnosed morbid conditions), diagnostic tests, treatments, and results—that will be interoperable with a pan-Canadian EHR. This movement toward provincial and national EHRs requires that developers or vendors incorporate into their information systems the capacity for interoperability with other vendors' systems in order to provide the ability for patient information to be communicated along with the patients as they move across all sectors of the regional, provincial, or national health care delivery system.

However, in spite of the vast array of technologies currently available in health care, nurses must continue to contextualize technology within the scope of their professional practice. Leaders such as Porter-O'Grady (2014) have advocated that nursing practice must be value based, particularly in digital environments where real-time data can be provided to clinicians regarding the validity and impact of interventions. This requires that nurses and nurse leaders recognize that a future relying on digital health necessarily includes informatics competencies and a shift in practice to incorporate such competencies seamlessly across all practice domains (Hussey & Kennedy, 2016; Remus & Kennedy, 2012). The Canadian Nurses Association (CNA) and Canadian Nursing Informatics Association (CNIA) (2017) Joint Position Statement on NI extends this further and links practice to NI understanding, stating, "Just as ICT and digitally connected health are becoming integral to nursing practice, nursing informatics knowledge will be integral to evolving models of care…in digitally connected health environments that maintain the caring core of nursing" (p. 4).

NURSING INFORMATICS AND THE CANADIAN HEALTH CARE SYSTEM

As nurse leaders witnessed the technology explosion, pioneers in NI recognized that nursing needed to be strategic regarding the adoption of technology to support professional practice and assess how nurses could respond to the demands related to using such technology (Hannah, Ball, & Edwards, 1994). The term *nursing informatics* was introduced initially by Dr. Marion Ball at the 1983 International Medical Informatics Association (IMIA) Conference in Amsterdam (Hannah et al., 2006). In the 1980s, NI emerged as a new nursing specialty in health information management. Since the first text devoted to NI in 1984 by Ball and Hannah, journals and texts have proliferated across Canada and internationally, with both traditional and online resources reflecting discipline-specific informatics (e.g., nursing, medicine, health) and broader more collaborative topics in informatics and innovation.

Hannah and colleagues (2006) challenge that, despite the escalation of technology in health care and the recognition of NI, the persistent absence of universally accepted methods for defining and coding nursing contributions to health outcomes is a significant obstacle to the collection of nursing data and has spurred accelerated innovation. Initiatives in capturing, documenting, and sharing nursing contributions through tools such as C-HOBIC (Canadian Health Outcomes for Better Information and Care), nursing dashboards, and standardizing nursing data are evidence of a change in perspective regarding nursing data and a commitment to articulating how interventions impact patient outcomes. These initiatives will be discussed later throughout this chapter.

Defining Nursing Informatics

A variety of definitional perspectives evolved as NI pioneers and practitioners attempted to conceptualize and represent their practice to others. Early definitions of NI focused on technology and effective utilization in practice, while more recent definitions focus more on the role of information management and the role of the nurse as an information manager. Figure 16-1 presents the evolution of NI definitions from focusing on technology and its novel role to broader, more conceptual definitions, to role-based definitions, and, most recently, to integrated practice-based definitions that reflect the convergence of information management, information technology, and nursing practice in an internationally supported, integrated definition. At the 2009 Helsinki conference, the International Medical Informatics Association (IMIA) Nursing Informatics Special Interest Group (IMIA, 2009) declared, "Nursing informatics science and practice integrates nursing, its information and knowledge and their management with information and communication technologies to promote the health of people, families and communities world wide." It is worth noting that the preceding IMIA-NI definition has become the most widely accepted definition for NI, and the discipline has largely moved on from generating definitions of NI to the actual practice, research, and teaching of NI.

Evolution of Informatics in the Canadian Health Care System

The events occurring over the last 30 years have culminated in national attention regarding the need for timely, secure, and appropriate health information access. Multiple health care and standards development organizations operate to coordinate broad documentation of health information and monitoring of the Canadian health care system. It is essential that nurses have both an awareness and understanding of the roles and relevance of each of these entities in relation to nursing practice.

Health informatics encompasses all health care disciplines, and the unique application of informatics knowledge and skills reflects specialties such as medical informatics, nursing informatics, and dental informatics. Digital Health Canada (formerly the Canadian Organization for Advancement of Computers in Health, or COACH),

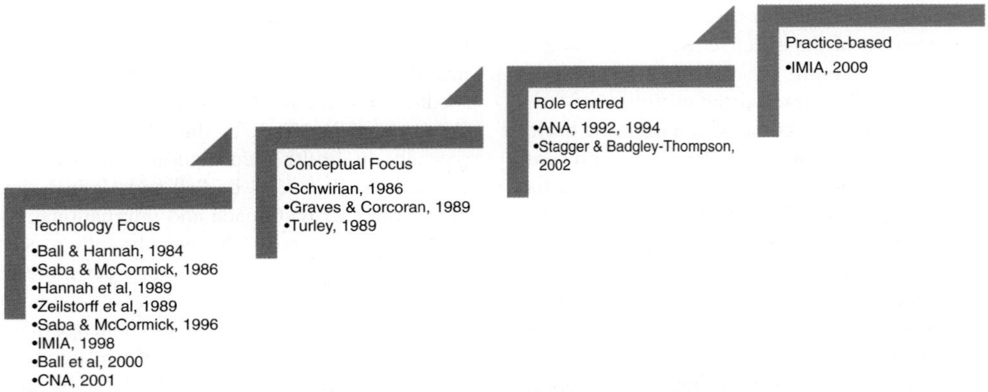

FIGURE 16-1 Evolution of nursing informatics definitions. *ANA,* American Nurses Association; *CNA,* Canadian Nurses Association; *IMIA,* International Medical Informatics Association.

Canada's health informatics association, defines "health informatics (HI) as the intersection of clinical, IM/IT (Information Management/ Information Technology) and management practices to achieve better health" (COACH, 2013, p. 8). The recognition and growth of health informatics occurred over many years as the result of dedicated efforts of many professionals and clearly recognizes the dependency on clinical expertise, as reflected in the Health Information Professional (HIP) Competency Framework illustrated in Figure 16-2. Although this chapter recognizes the existence of other types of informatics practice in the health sector, the focus will remain on NI.

From the mid-1980s onward, Canada's health information infrastructure experienced numerous evolutions and reconfigurations, all of which had significant implications for nursing and led to the establishment of sentinel health information organizations. The 1989 Canadian merger between the National Hospital Productivity Improvement Program and the Management Information System Project, which led to the Management Information System (MIS) Group, was an important event in Canadian health care information management (Hannah et al., 2006). The MIS Group, according to Hannah et al. (2006), developed guidelines on the collection of data for demographic, statistical, and resource utilization and consumption purposes. The problem with the MIS data is that, like hospital discharge summaries, this health information was restricted to physician-driven data and contained no clinical nursing data elements. Hannah et al. (2006, p. 89) made the point that "noteworthy, again, is the *total absence* of clinical nursing data."

The Wilk Report (National Task Force on Health Information, 1991) had a significant effect on Canadian health information, triggering the 1993 merger of the MIS Group, Hospital Medical Records Institute, portions of Statistics Canada, and portions of Health and Welfare Canada to create the Canadian Institute for Health Information (CIHI) (Hannah, 2005). CIHI is the national, independent, and not-for-profit body that records, analyzes, and disseminates essential data and analysis on Canada's health system and the health of Canadians (CIHI, 2017). Although not initially attentive to nursing data, this institution later became more important to several issues directly influencing nursing, including issues related to nursing workforce recruitment and retention.

In response to recommendations issued by the National Forum on Health for a pan-Canadian EHR, the federal government committed an initial $500 million to the development of eHealth, which included the EHR, telehealth, and Internet-based health information (CNA, 2006a; Hannah, 2005). Canada Health Infoway (Infoway), incorporated in 2001, was a key outcome of the federal, provincial, and territorial partnership (Canada Health Infoway, 2016a). Infoway has a national mandate to generate consensus on health information standards, to drive the national agenda of creating an EHR system, and to act as the liaison to international standards development organizations (Canada Health Infoway, 2016a). Infoway fulfills this mandate by partnering with jurisdictions as a "strategic investor" to share costs of implementing health information management projects and provides additional project benefits analysis. Since 2001, the federal government has allocated $2.1 billion to Infoway to support the development of EHRs in Canada (Canada Health Infoway, 2016a). In the 2017 budget, the federal government reconfirmed its commitment to improve the health of Canadians through digital health innovation by announcing an additional $300 million investment in Canada Health Infoway (Canada Health Infoway, 2017a).

Six core components make up an EHR (Canada Health Infoway, 2016a):

- Patient registry
- Provider registry
- Diagnostic images
- Laboratory results
- Drugs dispensed
- Clinical reports/immunization

Since its inception, Infoway has approved allocation of more than $2 billion, or 97.4% of its total funding, across all its program areas (Canada Health Infoway, 2016a, p. 33). To date, Infoway has committed more than $1.877 billion to various provincial and territorial projects and programs, resulting in more than 419 projects in various stages of evolution, ranging from planning to near completion (Canada Health Infoway, 2016a).

Infoway-funded projects vary in nature—telehealth, registries, picture archiving and communication systems (PACS), and lab and drug information systems—all enabling a faster response time between assessment and treatment. And while every province and territory in Canada is engaged in advancing the implementation of EHRs, with investment from Infoway, attention has shifted from getting projects started to quantifying value and benefits of these systems and projects. Infoway estimates that $200 million is saved annually through electronic health initiatives and projects, and that $16 billion has been saved since 2007 (Canada Health Infoway, 2016a). Figure 16-3 illustrates the benefits documented across Canada.

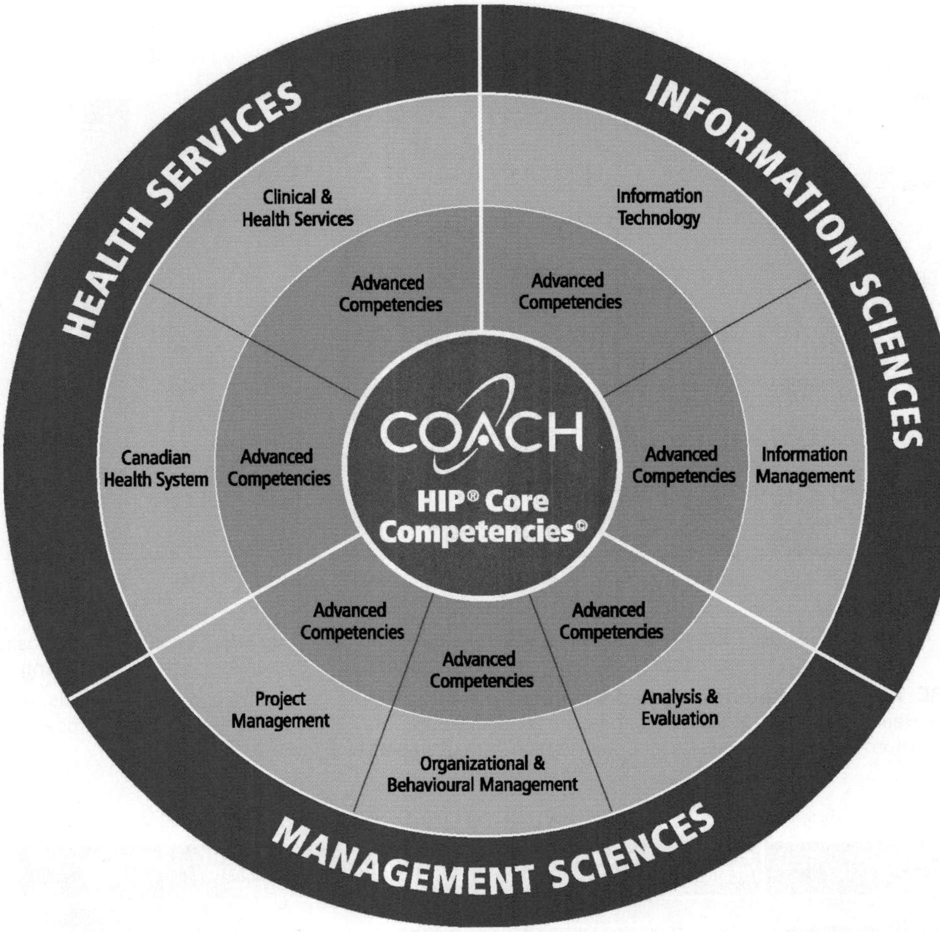

FIGURE 16-2 COACH HIP competency framework. (From COACH. [2012]. *Health informatics professional core competencies* [p. 11]. Toronto: Author. Retrieved from https://www.coachorg.com/en/resourcecentre/resources/Health-Informatics-Core-Competencies.pdf. Reprinted with permission from COACH: Canada's Health Informatics Association, copyright 2017. HIP is a registered trademark of COACH: Canada's Health Informatics Association. HIP Core Competencies is a copyright of COACH: Canada's Health Informatics Association.)

STANDARDS AND CLINICAL INTEROPERABILITY

Standards in health care data management refer to a nationally or internationally agreed-upon protocol for representing all types of health information, including types of care provided, location of care provision, pharmacy ordering and dispensing, and billing messages. Standards ensure that data are consistently represented and exchanged and thus consistently *understood* by clinicians and health information systems. This consistent understanding and interpretation of health data contribute to the provision of quality care as well as increasing patient safety.

Canada Health Infoway (2016a) has noted that standards ensure interoperability by supporting information exchange and identified standards as a critical foundation for the interoperable electronic health record (iEHR). Canada Health Infoway (2016a) demonstrates how "standards support integrated, patient-centric health records enabling a longitudinal view of an individual's key health history and care…and that this critical information can be updated, managed, shared and interpreted in a meaningful secure way, when and where required" (p. 5).

There are a number of ways in which standards play a role in shaping health care data. Standards support both *technical needs* regarding consistent communication or transmission of health data in system messages and *business needs* regarding actual clinical work processes and clinical content of messages. For example, a gap may be identified where clinicians need to consistently describe a particular condition or clinical situation and exchange patient data to deliver optimal care. Clinical terminology standards such as SNOMED CT® (Systematized NOmenclature of MEDicine Clinical Terms®), LOINC (Laboratory Observation Identifiers Names and Codes), and others influence how clinical practice is documented, while technical standards such as HL7 FHIR (Health Level 7 Fast Healthcare Interoperability Resources) support transmission and exchange across the health care system.

Infoway's commitment to standards development, formerly through structures such as the Standards Collaborative, helped develop and support Canadian adoption of relevant international health information standards, such as SNOMED CT, HL7, and numerous standards of the International Organization for Standardization (ISO). As of 2011, standards supporting all six key components of the Electronic

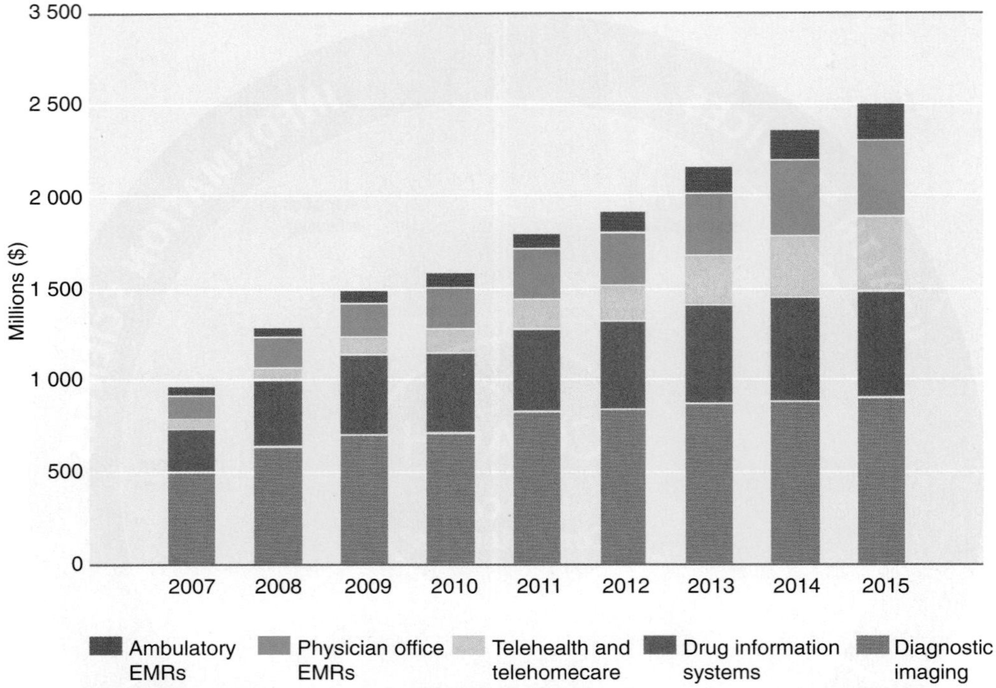

FIGURE 16-3 Estimated aggregated benefits (in millions). EMRs, electronic medical records. (From Canada Health Infoway. [2016]. *Annual report 2015–2016* [p. 14, Figure 6]. Retrieved from https://www.infoway-inforoute.ca/en/home/95-accountability/7064-annual-report-highlights-2015-2016.)

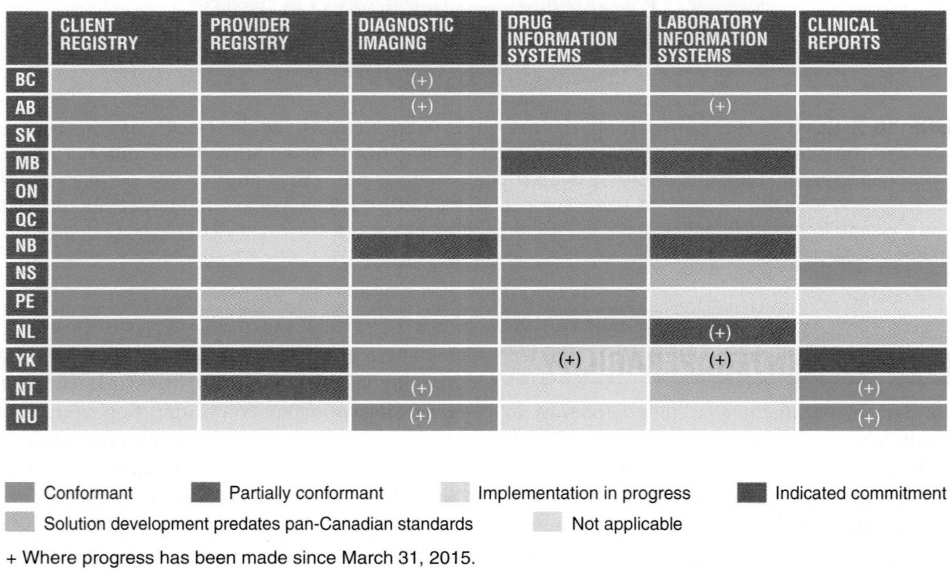

FIGURE 16-4 Standards conformance by jurisdiction, March 31, 2016. (From Canada Health Infoway. [2016]. *Annual report 2015–2016* [p. 15, Figure 7]. Retrieved from https://www.infoway-inforoute.ca/en/home/95-accountability/7064-annual-report-highlights-2015-2016.)

Health Record Solution (EHRS) and the EHRS Blueprint have been developed in Canada (Canada Health Infoway, 2016a). To date, all jurisdictions in Canada are at least partially conformant and/or have commitments to become conformant with pan-Canadian standards supporting the six components of the EHR, while two jurisdictions are completely conformant (Canada Health Infoway, 2016a). Figure 16-4 illustrates the progression of inclusion and conformance with pan-Canadian standards across all jurisdictions in Canada.

As standards development initiatives matured across Canada, Infoway's focus shifted from development to the practical use and implementation of standards. To this end, the issue of *clinical interoperability* became a central focus of Infoway communications and

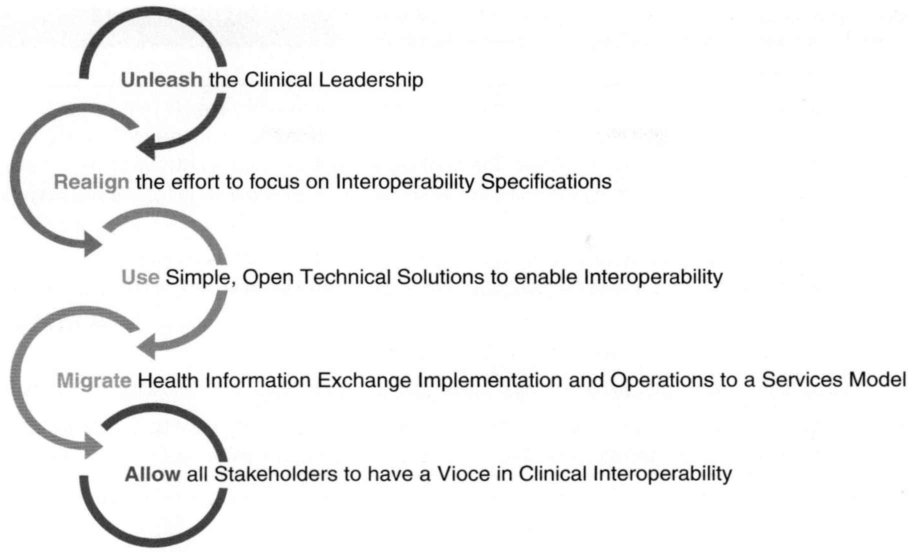

FIGURE 16-5 Infoway path to clinical interoperability. (From Canada Health Infoway. [2014]. *The Path Forward: Accelerating Clinical Interoperability in Canada—Strategy.* Retrieved from https://ic.infoway-inforoute.ca/en/resources/docs/cistratdocs/40-the-path-forward.)

effort (Canada Health Infoway, 2014, 2015, 2016b, 2016c). Figure 16-5 presents the component of the clinical interoperability strategy. As indicated, this approach is grounded in clinical engagement and stakeholder inclusivity, innovation, and using digital solutions to solve real-world clinical challenges (Canada Health Infoway, 2016b).

Standardizing Nursing Language

A long-standing perception among many nurses is that nursing, as a professional practice, is generally considered invisible in regard to formal and tangible recognition (Clark, 1999; Clark & Lang, 1992; CNA, 2000; Hannah et al., 2006; Marck, 1994; Norwood, 2001; Powers, 2001; Weyrauch, 2002). Clark (1999, p. 42) observed that, in spite of representing the largest group of health care clinicians, nursing was invisible in health policy decisions, in descriptions of health care, in contracts, and in service specifications.

Clark and Lang (1992, p. 109) famously declared in their assessment of the invisibility of nursing, "If we cannot name it, we cannot control it, finance it, teach it, research it, or put it into public policy." Numerous pioneering nurse informaticists supported this position, including Graves and Corcoran (1989), Werley (1988), Ball, Hannah, Newbold, et al. (2000), and others, arguing that in order to give nursing visibility, a standardized language is required to reflect what nursing is and what nursing does. In order to accomplish this, significant effort and numerous incremental initiatives would be necessary to distinguish specific components of nursing data and identify key concepts, data sets, and outcomes of care.

Health Information: Nursing Components

Before a standardized nursing language is adopted, it is necessary to identify the most important data elements required for effective nursing decision making and evaluation. The minimum number of essential nursing data elements is referred to as a *nursing minimum data set (NMDS)*. The Canadian NMDS was established in 1992 in a joint conference sponsored by the Alberta Association of Registered Nurses (AARN), the MIS Group and CNA (Giovannetti, Smith, & Broad, 1999). The nursing components of health information, the Canadian version of an NMDS, is known as **Health Information: Nursing Components (HI:NC)**. Since 1992, there has been consensus among Canadian nurses that HI:NC comprises five categories of elements: patient status, nursing interventions, patient outcomes, nursing resource intensity, and primary nurse identifier (AARN, 1994; CNA, 2000, 2001a). CNA describes HI:NC as the "most important pieces of data about the nursing care provided to the client during a health care episode" (2000, p. 5). Table 16-1 presents the HI:NC definitions.

In addition to the foundational work on HI:NC, ongoing effort went into articulating nursing requirements in the EHR. The Nursing Reference Group, hosted by Canada Health Infoway and co-chaired jointly by Infoway and CNA (2012), sponsored a working group that developed the *Pan-Canadian Nursing EHR Business and Functional Elements Supporting Clinical Practice* document. This reference document provides guidance on how nursing data should be incorporated into EHRs and covers such topics as privacy and security, safety, data sources, usability, clinical decision support, collaborative practice, communications, information use, and data access.

In 2016, the inaugural National Nursing Data Standards Symposium was held at the University of Toronto, with the sponsorship of CNA, CIHI, Canada Health Infoway, CNIA, and numerous health informatics industry vendors. Sixty nurse leaders, representatives from the host organizations, and industry vendors from across Canada met to collaborate on a national strategy to "represent, teach, capture, and report nursing practice in Canada" (Nagle & White, 2016). With focused streams of discussion on clinical, education, research, and policy, the outcomes of the symposium included a commitment to establishing a national taskforce that would ultimately develop and evaluate a framework for nursing data standards for use across Canada. This work continues, with an annual symposium to advance the objective of ensuring nursing is represented using standardized data within and across practice domains. In 2017 more than 100 nurse leaders, nurse informaticians, and vendors convened to further this activity.

TABLE 16-1 Health Information: Nursing Components

Nursing Component	Definition
Patient status	A label for the set of indicators that reflect the phenomena for which nurses provide care, relative to the health status of patients (McGee, 1993). Although patient status is similar to nursing diagnosis, the term *patient status* is preferred because it represents a broader spectrum of health and illness. The common label *patient status* is inclusive of input from all disciplines. The summative statements referring to the phenomena for which nurses provide care (i.e., nursing diagnosis) are merely one aspect of patient status at a point in time, in the same way as medical diagnosis.
Nursing interventions	Purposeful and deliberate health-affecting interventions (direct and indirect), based on assessment of patient status, which are designed to bring about results that benefit patients (Alberta Association of Registered Nurses [AARN], 1994).
Patient outcome	The "clients' status at a defined point(s) following health care [affecting] intervention" (Marek & Lang, 1993). It is influenced to varying degrees by the interventions of all care providers.
Nursing intensity	"Refers to the amount and type of nursing resource used to [provide] care" (O'Brien-Pallas & Giovannetti, 1993).
Primary Nurse Identifier	A single, unique, lifetime identification number for each individual nurse. This identifier is independent of geographic location (province or territory), practice sector (e.g., acute care, community care, public health), or employer.

From Hannah, K. J. (2005). Health informatics and nursing in Canada. *Healthcare Information Management and Communications, 19*(3), 49. Reprinted by permission of Healthcare Computing and Communications Canada, Inc.

BOX 16-1 RESEARCH HIGHLIGHT

Evaluating Standardized Nursing Terminology

Research Focus

Nursing data have not historically been included in national data repositories for a variety of reasons, including the lack of a single nursing terminology to describe the nursing contribution to patient/client care (i.e., nursing practice). Consequently, health care decisions have been made in the absence of valuable nursing data. The need for a standardized nursing language stimulated the development of the International Classification for Nursing Practice (ICNP). Testing was necessary to evaluate the representational capacity of this terminology for Canadian nursing practice. Kennedy (2005) examined the effectiveness of the ICNP in representing the contributions of nursing to health care outcomes in Canada. ICNP was used to code retrospective nursing data extracted from patient records originating in acute care, inpatient mental health, home health care, and long-term care practice settings. In spite of a wide variation in documentation practices, ICNP achieved matches with a significant majority of nursing data, thereby confirming the utility of ICNP for documenting nursing practice in Canada.

Representing Nursing Practice

ICNP represents Canadian nursing practice with high accuracy. Variations and gaps in nursing documentation practices are further evidence of the need for standardized terminology to ensure that at least minimum nursing data are recorded.

Kennedy, M. A. (2005). *Packaging nursing as politically potent: A critical reflexive cultural studies approach to nursing informatics.* Unpublished doctoral dissertation, University of South Australia, Adelaide, Australia; Kennedy, M. A., & Hannah, K. J. (2007). Representing nursing practice: Evaluating the effectiveness of a nursing classification system. *Canadian Journal of Nursing Research, 39*(7), 58–79.

An overview of computerized nursing documentation is provided in Chapter 15. Some clinical information systems incorporate the HI:NC and nursing functional requirements into the architecture or design of the nursing componenet of the clinical documentation system. This enables capture of the most significant data reflective of the nursing contribution to patient care. Many versions of computerized nursing documentation systems continue to evolve, relying on the underlying philosophy of documentation to support design. For example, many systems do not encourage narrative documentation but provide checklists of common activities and encourage exception charting. Please review Chapter 15 for additional discussion of this issue.

International Classification for Nursing Practice

The **International Classification for Nursing Practice® (ICNP®)** is a formal terminology developed by the **International Council of Nurses (ICN)** (ICN, 2015a) in response to concerns regarding the visibility of nursing contributions in health care and calls for standardization of nursing data for comparability and analysis, as well as evidence-informed practice (Box 16-1). ICN proposed the use of a single unified terminology to represent nursing practice. The goals were to capture nursing practice across practice settings, cultures or languages, and geographic settings, while simultaneously ensuring that professionals who used this new terminology could communicate with the numerous nursing terminologies already in use. Initially endorsed for development in 1989 by resolution at the ICN Nineteenth Quadrennial Conference, ICNP has evolved through multiple iterations and is currently updated and released biannually to coincide with the ICN Congress (ICN, 2015b).

ICNP is a standardized terminology for nursing practice and is built using the Web Ontology Language (OWL) (ICN, 2015a, 2015b). This enables ICNP to function both as a reference terminology (within the system) and an interface terminology (facing users in a system interface). ICNP has a seven-axis model, which includes Focus, Judgement, Action, Means, Location, Client, and Time (ICN, 2017a). In addition to viewing ICNP by the axes, users can also view the terminology by hierarchy or in a simple list (Figure 16-6). ICN also reports that as ICNP implementations have advanced, some users have experienced success with the seven-axis model; however, the dominant trend has been to use precoordinated concepts or expressions that are accessible through the Diagnosis and Outcome axis or the Intervention axis (ICN 2015b).

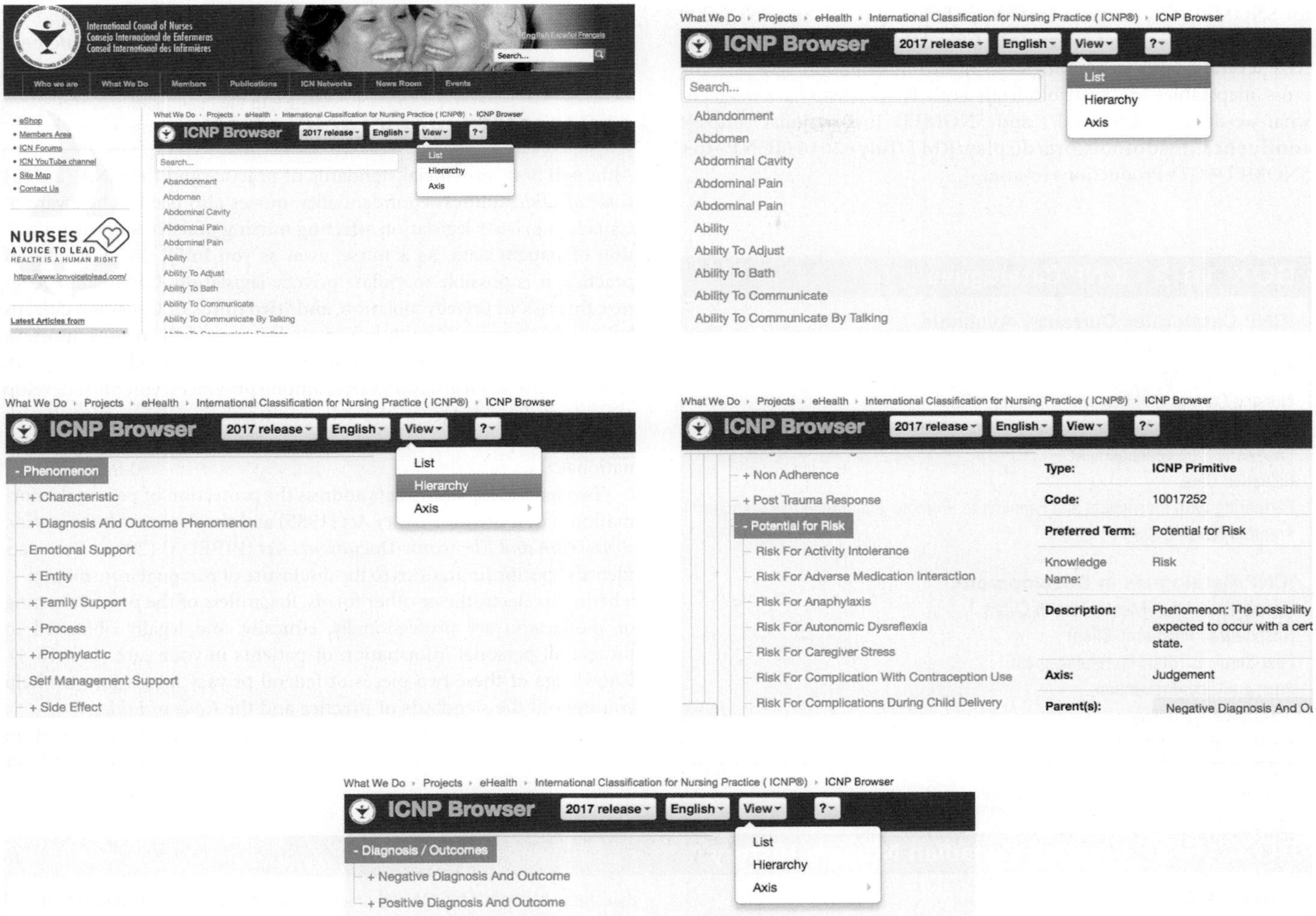

FIGURE 16-6 International Classification for Nursing Practice® (ICNP®) browser views. (International Council of Nurses. [2017]. ICNP browser. Retrieved from http://www.icn.ch/ICNP-Browser-NEW.html. Reprinted with permission.)

ICNP is used to generate statements of nursing diagnoses, nursing actions, and nursing outcomes, using terms arranged in a hierarchical order and in catalogues (or subsets) of precombined terms. ICNP provides "805 precoordinated terms for nursing diagnoses and outcome statements, and 1019 precoordinated intervention statements" (ICN, 2015b, p. 4). As of 2017, eight individual catalogues were available to users, with additional catalogues in development (2017b; Box 16-2). As development is ongoing internationally, these numbers will continue to grow over time.

Catalogues are made up of nursing data subsets of diagnoses, actions, and outcomes specific to various practice areas or specialties (such as wound care) and continue to be developed. To begin catalogue development, nurses select a health care topic based on the needs of patients. The organization of the catalogue content is determined by the nurses as ICNP diagnoses, outcomes, and interventions are identified. ICN (2015b) notes that catalogues can fill a practical need in building health information systems with all the benefits of being part of a unified nursing language.

In 2001, CNA endorsed the ICNP "for use in Canada as a foundational classification system for nursing practice in Canada" (CNA, 2001b). This endorsement was renewed in 2006 (CNA, 2006a). Although Canada Health Infoway, in consultation with various stakeholder groups, adopted SNOMED CT as the preferred terminology for the pan-Canadian EHR, ICNP remains the preferred terminology for nursing. ICN, which holds the intellectual property rights to ICNP, collaborated with SNOMED International (formerly known as the **International Health Terminology Standards Development Organization [IHTSDO]**), which holds the intellectual property rights for SNOMED CT, to create cross maps between ICNP and SNOMED CT, enabling users and systems, in Canada and elsewhere, to effectively leverage both terminologies in health information systems. The cross map tables are available from both ICNP (http://www.icn.ch/what-we-do/icnp-download/) and SNOMED International (https://confluence.ihtsdotools.org/display/RMT/July+2016+ICNP+to+SNOMED+CT+Production+release).

BOX 16-2 ICNP Catalogues

ICNP Catalogues Currently Available

Community Nursing
Disaster Nursing
Nursing Care of Children with HIV and AIDS
Nursing Outcome Indicators
Paediatric Pain Management
Palliative Care
Partnering with Individuals and Families to Promote Adherence to Treatment
Prenatal Nursing Care

ICNP Catalogues in Development

Hospitalized Adult Mental Health Client
Hospitalized Paediatric Client
Post-Surgical Total Hip Replacement
Pressure Ulcer Prevention
Special Care Nursery
Adult Pain Management

For discussion of CNA's use of ICNP to collect information on patient outcomes through the C-HOBIC (Canadian Health Outcomes for Better Information and Care) initiative, see Box 16-3.

CANADIAN PRIVACY LEGISLATION

Although both provincial standards of practice and the CNA (2017a) *Code of Ethics* address confidentiality, nurses also need to be aware of Canadian privacy legislation affecting nursing practice and the protection of patient data. As a nurse, even as you fulfill the standards of practice, it is possible to violate privacy legislation. Canadians recognize this risk of privacy violation, and "two thirds of Canadian citizens believe that personal health information is one of the most important areas in need of protection under privacy laws" (Roch, 2008, p. 8). Although privacy legislation varies among provinces, you must develop a working knowledge of the relevant legislation supporting health information protection (Gershon & Tu, 2008), both provincial and national.

Two federal legislative acts address the protection of personal information. These are the *Privacy Act* (1985) and the ***Personal Information Protection and Electronic Documents Act*** **(PIPEDA)** (2004). Both acts identify specific limitations to the disclosure of personal information—whether in electronic or other forms. Regardless of the practice setting or mode, you are professionally, ethically, and legally obligated to protect all personal information of patients in your care (Box 16-4). Knowledge of these two pieces of federal privacy legislation can help you uphold the standards of practice and the *Code of Ethics*.

According to the *Privacy Act*, Section 8.1, "Personal information under the control of a government institution shall not, without

BOX 16-3 Creating Canadian Nursing History

The C-HOBIC Initiative

In 2007, the Canadian Nurses Association (CNA) launched a multi-province project, with financial investment by Canada Health Infoway, focused on collecting information reflecting evidence-informed, nursing-sensitive patient outcomes (CNA, 2008). Drawing on the work of the original **Health Outcomes for Better Information and Care (HOBIC)** project, the **Canadian Health Outcomes for Better Information and Care (C-HOBIC)** project (http://c-hobic.cna-aiic.ca/about/default_e.aspx) is implementing a standardized nursing documentation approach for capturing, analyzing, and reporting nursing-sensitive outcomes for acute care, complex continuing care, long-term care, and home care.

The C-HOBIC project addresses gaps in health information related to nursing's contribution to patient outcomes and addresses the need for standardized nursing data for inclusion on patient admission and discharge summaries. The major components of this project are a systematic approach to gathering nursing content that is documented using a standardized clinical terminology and coded in a format suitable for inclusion in the electronic health records being developed or implemented by the participating provinces. This project uses a standardized clinical terminology, the International Classification for Nursing Practice (ICNP), and provides an opportunity for Canadian nurses to make substantive contributions to the ongoing development of ICNP.

Mapping challenges provided an immediate opportunity for Canadian nurses to contribute to the iterative development of ICNP by proposing multiple new terms and to a catalogue of precombined terms for inclusion in ICNP that are uniquely Canadian and reflect C-HOBIC concepts. The initial mapping to ICNP Version 1.0 was validated at a national forum (Kennedy, 2008; Kennedy, Hannah, & White, 2008) that included C-HOBIC partners, nursing informatics experts, nurse educators, nurse researchers, representatives from government ministries, policy institutions and practice environments, and two international ICNP experts. In total, 96 concepts were addressed in the mapping aspect of the C-HOBIC project: 58 HOBIC concepts were matched and validated as C-HOBIC terms, 13 HOBIC concepts were partially mapped to ICNP, and a new term was required in ICNP in order to fully communicate the original concept in C-HOBIC; 24 new C-HOBIC terms were proposed for inclusion in ICNP to represent concepts that did not match, and only one HOBIC concept ("Activity did not occur") could not be mapped to ICNP. In addition, two HOBIC ordinal scales were retained for use in C-HOBIC, including the pain scale and the number of falls. The final results of the C-HOBIC work were used to create the ICNP Nursing Outcomes Indicators Catalogue for use internationally (Figure 16-7). The ICNP Outcomes Catalogue and Canadian innovations generated through the C-HOBIC initiative are increasingly used internationally as other countries prioritize outcome documentation and analysis (ICN, 2011).

On January 11, 2012, Canada Health Infoway endorsed the C-HOBIC/ICNP Data Set as a Canadian Approved Standard (CAS) (Canadian Health Infoway, 2017b). This is the first nursing data standard approved as CAS, and Canada is the first country in the world to approve an ICNP Catalogue as a national standard.

The C-HOBIC work has continued to evolve and was used to create the Nursing Outcomes Indicators Catalogue in ICNP in 2013. Additionally, C-HOBIC has been mapped to SNOMED CT and validated through international consensus at SNOMED International (http://www.snomed.org). Critical next steps are to continue collaboration with the Canadian Institute of Health Information (CIHI) to ensure that C-HOBIC is included in the **Discharge Abstract Database (DAD)** (Figure 16-8), thereby consistently documenting these standardized outcomes measures for every hospital admission across Canada.

the consent of the individual to whom it relates, be disclosed by the institution" (Government of Canada, 2016). The PIPEDA is federal legislation governing the disclosure of personal health information in any electronic environment. This act extends the *Privacy Act* by addressing specific risks associated with electronic data collection, storage, retrieval, and communication. The purpose of PIPEDA, as updated in March 2006, is to "establish, in an era in which technology increasingly facilitates the circulation and exchange of information, rules to govern the collection, use and disclosure of personal information in a manner that recognizes the right of privacy of individuals with respect to their personal information and the need of organizations to collect, use, or disclose personal information for purposes that a reasonable person would consider appropriate in the circumstances" (Government of Canada, 2017; https://www.priv.gc.ca/en/privacy-topics/privacy-laws-in-canada/the-personal-information-protection-and-electronic-documents-act-pipeda/r_o_p/). Furthermore, PIPEDA restricts the disclosure of personal information under only the most stringent of conditions, such as law enforcement requirements (Government of Canada, 2017).

The PIPEDA was initially applicable only to personal information collected or used in commercial activities by private-sector entities regulated by the federal government. However, the Act has been extended over time to cover the retail sector, publishing companies, the service industry, manufacturers, and other provincially regulated organizations, as well as sector-specific data such as health information.

The PIPEDA applies to Canadian jurisdictions unless the federal government acknowledges an exemption based on provincial legislation that is substantially similar. As of 2011, British Columbia, Alberta, Quebec, and, most recently, Ontario are considered to have legislation substantially similar to PIPEDA (Office of the Privacy Commissioner, 2014). Despite provincial acts taking precedence within provinces, federal legislation continues to govern the transmission of personal information across and between provincial boundaries.

In addition to domestic legislation, other factors also affect the privacy of the EHR. Infoway's privacy mandate is to support private, secure, and protected information in the EHR. In the course of doing so, Infoway and their partners leverage applicable international standards (for example, from the ISO) that operate in alignment with Canadian legislation and further support the privacy and security of health data in electronic health care systems.

Despite the complex nature of privacy legislation and the standards that support privacy activities, as a nurse, you must exercise diligence in examining and applying these pieces of legislation to your professional nursing practice. The privacy legislation by province can be reviewed at: https://www.priv.gc.ca/en/privacy-topics/privacy-laws-in-canada/02_05_d_15/. Please refer to Chapter 15 to explore how PIPEDA relates to specific nursing documentation.

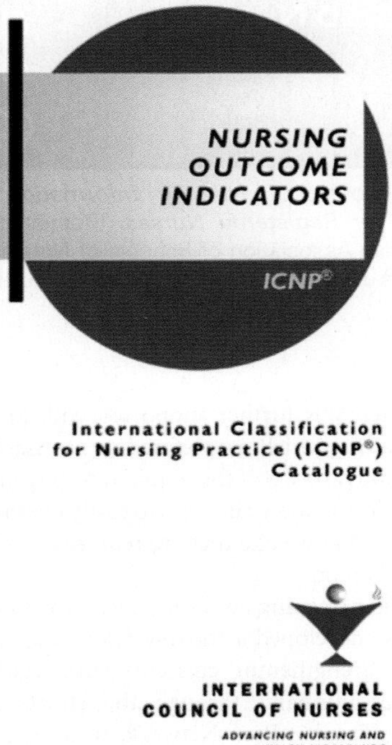

FIGURE 16-7 International Classification for Nursing Practice® (ICNP®) Nursing Outcome Indicators Catalogue. (From International Council of Nurses. Reprinted with permission from ICN, May 2017.)

BOX 16-4 Distinguishing Types of Protected Information

The *Personal Information Protection and Electronic Documents Act* (PIPEDA) distinguishes "personal information" from "personal health information" and provides specific definitions for both:

"*Personal health information,*" with respect to an individual, whether living or deceased, means

(a) information concerning the physical or mental health of the individual;
(b) information concerning any health service provided to the individual;
(c) information concerning the donation by the individual of any body part or any bodily substance of the individual or information derived from the testing or examination of a body part or bodily substance of the individual;
(d) information that is collected in the course of providing health services to the individual; or
(e) information that is collected incidentally to the provision of health services to the individual.

"*Personal information*" means information about an identifiable individual but does not include the name, title, or business address or telephone number of an employee of an organization.

Personal Information Protection and Electronic Documents Act, S.C. 2000, c. 5. Retrieved from http://laws-lois.justice.gc.ca/eng/acts/P-8.6/page-1.html#h-3.

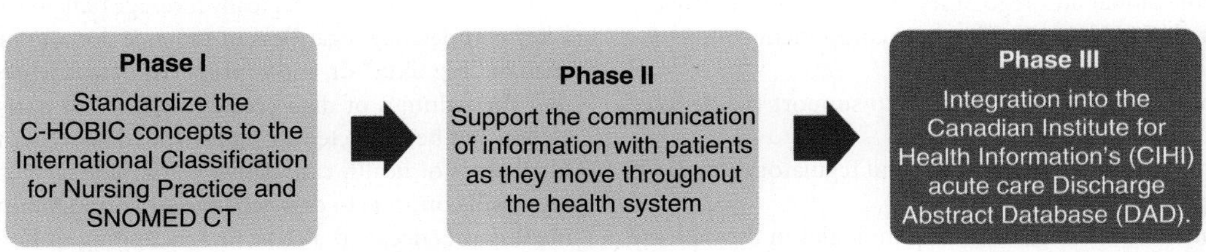

FIGURE 16-8 C-HOBIC project phases.

INFORMATICS COMPETENCIES AS A STRATEGIC DIRECTION

CNA (2006b) released the *e-Nursing Strategy for Canada* to direct the coordinated integration of technology into Canadian nursing practice. The strategy addresses both medium- and long-term targets, with the overall goal of improving both nursing practice and outcomes for patients and clients. This strategy is intended to completely integrate ICT in such a way that the "e" in *e-nursing* is no longer required. ICT will simply be another tool that nurses use in their practice (CNA, 2006b). CNA (2006b, p. 4) identified seven key outcomes that are projected to emerge from the *e-Nursing Strategy*:

1. Nurses will integrate ICT into their practice to achieve desirable patient outcomes.
2. Nurses will have the required information and knowledge to support their practice.
3. Human resources planning will be facilitated.
4. New models of nursing practice and health services delivery will be supported.
5. Nursing groups will be well connected.
6. ICT will improve the quality of nurses' work environments.
7. Canadian nurses will contribute to the global community of nursing.

Three fundamental directions for CNA's *e-Nursing Strategy* were developed among working groups and national feedback: access, competencies, and participation. *Access* to quality ICT in the practice environment is imperative if Canadian nurses are to realize the full benefits of technology in their practices. CNA (2008) noted that health care organizations have a responsibility to ensure that nurses have connectivity—tools such as computers and mobile technology (e.g., laptops, smart phones and mobile tablets, wireless technology), as well as resource databases and Internet resources—that will support professional practice. Surprisingly, access continues to be a challenge in many health care environments, and all nurses must continue to advocate for access to digital tools and databases to support patient outcomes and evidence-informed care. At the time of writing, CNA's *e-Nursing Strategy* is being reviewed and a revision should be published in 2019.

CNA (2008) encourages nurses to develop *competencies* in the application of ICT and has recommended that such competencies be part of both undergraduate and graduate-level nursing programs. As a nursing student, just as you have a responsibility to develop competencies in performing a variety of patient care tasks, such as assessments and treatments, it is also your responsibility to develop and maintain competencies in technological applications that support information management in professional practice.

In 2014, the Canadian Association of Schools of Nursing (CASN) convened several working groups to identify and establish entry-level informatics competencies for registered nurses (Figure 16-9). Through this initiative, CASN, with investment by Infoway, provided a clear path for faculty and nursing students with the knowledge, tools, and support they need to teach, learn, and practice in technology-enabled practice settings. Three primary competencies contribute to a single overarching competency that is identified as "uses information and communication technologies to support information synthesis in accordance with professional and regulatory standards in the delivery of patient/client care" (CASN, 2015). The three component competencies include the following:

1. Uses relevant information and knowledge to support the delivery of evidence-informed patient care
2. Uses ICTs in accordance with professional and regulatory standards and workplace policies
3. Uses information and communication technologies in the delivery of patient/client care

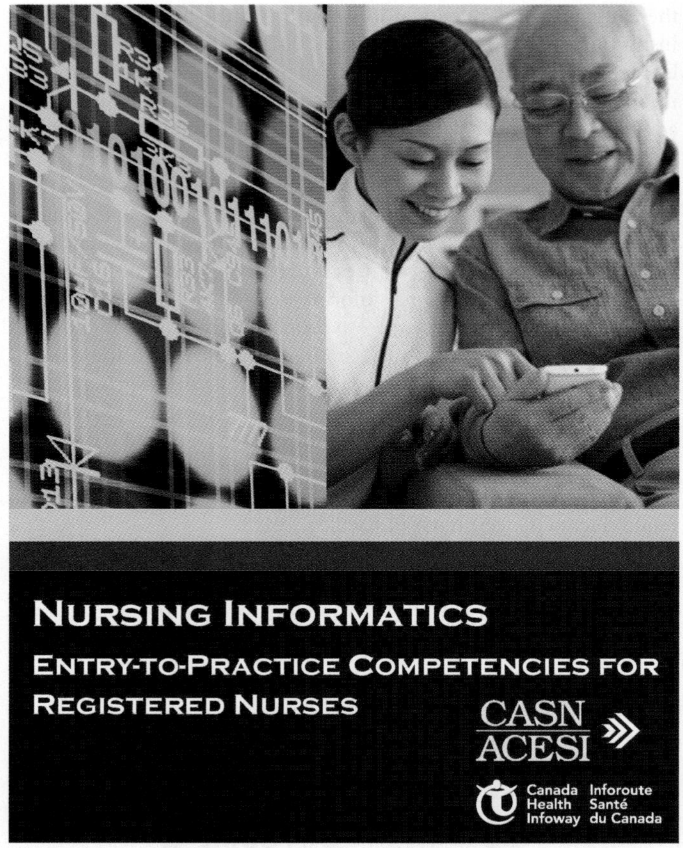

FIGURE 16-9 Cover of *Nursing Informatics Entry-to-Practice Competencies for Registered Nurses.* (Reprinted with permission from the Canadian Association of Schools of Nursing, copyright 2015. This illustration is used with permission of the Canadian Interprofessional Collaborative.)

Each competency is further supported with knowledge and performance indicators, which are defined as assessable and observable examples of various aspects of the required competency (CASN, 2015). This enables clinicians and evaluators to easily identify the specific type of behaviours and knowledge that are required to meet the respective competency statements.

As part of their ongoing commitment to nursing faculty development, CASN also developed a *Nursing Informatics Teaching Toolkit* to support faculty strengthening curricula with regard to teaching NI competencies. Additionally, through the efforts of CASN Digital Health Nursing Faculty Peer Network, a second faculty resource, *Consumer Health Solutions: A Teaching and Learning Resource for Nursing Education*, was developed, ensuring that faculty across Canada have access to key NI content to mentor nursing students. Furthermore, CASN has established peer support workshops for faculty to facilitate development of NI expertise among faculty.

Knowing how to strategically leverage data to make decisions is also a key competency regardless of practice domain or role. The prominence of "big data" or, more properly, data science, is the recognition that the volumes of data created daily in all parts of the health care system can be subjected to sophisticated analytics to inform decisions in all areas of health care delivery and management. This burgeoning topic will continue to drive change and opportunity in health care and nursing practice, and a clear understanding of how nurses can use all types of data to support practice and patient outcomes is imperative.

BOX 16-5 CASE STUDY

Role of an Electronic Community of Practice to Create Interest and Positive Attitude Toward Nursing Informatics: The BC Experience

By Elizabeth Borycki and Noreen Frisch

University of Victoria Schools of Health Information Science and Nursing; Co-Leaders of the InspireNet eHealth Action Team

Nurses in British Columbia are connecting! For the purpose of garnering interest in nursing health services research, the BC Nursing Research Initiative, through the Michael Smith Foundation for Health Research, has funded a BC Nursing Health Services Research Network, now renamed as InspireNet (**I**nnovative **N**ursing **S**ervices and **P**ractice **I**nformed by **R**esearch and **E**valuation). InspireNet's goals include creating collaborative advantages by bringing like-minded people together to foster research, knowledge translation, and practice readiness. Based on an understanding that connections between and among people who are geographically dispersed require virtual connections, InspireNet uses Web 2.0 and 3.0 technologies to conduct its work "virtually" through a website and by organizing its members into action teams that function as communities of practice. Wenger, McDermott, and Snyder (2002) describe *communities of practice* as groups of people who share a concern, a set of problems, or a passion about a topic, and who deepen their knowledge and expertise in the area of that topic by interacting on an ongoing basis. Electronic communities of practice (eCOPs) use social networking capabilities to support the establishment and work of groups of people.

After 18 months in operation, the InspireNet project had over 800 members connecting to each other through an e-newsletter, a password-protected database of members, a monthly blog prepared by members on current topics, and password-protected memberships in eCOPs called "InspireNet Action Teams." The Action Team eCOPs are formed around topics or areas of interest. Perhaps not surprisingly, nurses interested in all of the various aspects of informatics were early adopters of an eCOP, which they have labelled the *eHealth, eTechnologies and Informatics Action Team.*

In an area of nursing where nurses are covering new ground (like informatics), and where nurses who have an interest in the topic may be few and far between, the connections found in a virtual environment can be critical. The InspireNet eHealth eCOP has brought over 50 nurses together in a short period of time. They have tuned into web-based conferencing to learn about and discuss issues such as basic informatics, the need for education to address informatics, and the state of informatics work in their province. They have connected nurses who work in information technology units with nurses who work in professional practice offices. They have learned about membership in the Canadian Nursing Informatics Association (CNIA) and have had speakers from afar (from Canada) on topics such as C-HOBIC and (from Europe) on demonstrations of fully implemented electronic nursing documentation systems. They have established a journal club to learn about some of the latest work in nursing informatics. And they have accomplished all of these activities without leaving home!

We encourage you, as beginning students in nursing, to participate in exploring the role that networking can play in your professional development and support. For starters, we recommend exploring membership in nursing organizations (such as CNIA) for the purpose of finding those with interests similar to yours and seeking to establish connections with other nurses who wish to make a difference in Canadian nursing practice.

Networking may well be the future of social capital for nurses. Try it out for yourself.

Wenger, E., McDermott, R., & Snyder, W. (2002). *Cultivating communities of practice.* Boston: Harvard Business School Press. For further information, go to http://www.InspireNet.ca.

Exciting examples of innovative nursing practice incorporating information and communications technology are continually evident across Canada (Box 16-5). The French Canadian ICNP Research & Development Centre, located at the Université de Sherbrooke, is actively developing a health information system using ICNP for simulation training (Figure 16-10). This system is being used to support student understanding and experience using standardized nursing terminologies and documenting in digital environments.

Innovation in care provision has been occurring for quite some time across Canada (Table 16-2). For example, Goodwin, Matthews, Carr, et al. (2008) combined telemedicine and telemonitoring with patient education and peer supports in assisting chronically ill patients to stay at home in rural Ontario. Without this program, these patients would have had to travel for care provision and would have potentially experienced more frequent hospitalizations, loss of independence, and significantly less self-care. Tracey (2008) described how a standardized assessment approach is in pilot testing at two sites. This pilot format will ultimately replace six different assessment forms, contributing to more systematic data collection and greater capacity for data aggregation and analysis.

The third fundamental direction for CNA's *e-Nursing Strategy* (CNA, 2006b, p. 12) involves *participation,* which includes strategic partnerships with nurses in clinical practice; employers and administrators; federal, provincial, and territorial ministries; nursing organizations (professional associations, regulatory bodies, educational groups, and unions); and educators and researchers. The concept of partnership has far-reaching consequences: with effective partnerships, nurses can contribute to the selection and design of information technology applications and contribute to educational programs. For example, many health care institutions and agencies have clinical committees that collaborate with IT experts in the design and selection of electronic documentation systems. Especially as a novice nurse, you have both the knowledge and opportunity to contribute your insights about which information management systems are user friendly or present unexpected challenges. It is also helpful to have this type of clinician involvement when system revision or adaptation is required. Even small changes can sometimes have a significant impact on the capture of appropriate nursing data and how nurses view the system. Without partnerships, you, and all nurses, risk being excluded from decision making and and consequently using systems that are selected without valuable clinician contributions.

The CNA portal NurseONE is a key component of the *e-Nursing Strategy*. The portal was initially funded from a grant from the First Nations and Inuit Health Branch (FNIHB) of Health Canada (CNA, 2017b). NurseONE enables registered nurses and nursing students to register, create a personal profile, and customize use of the site's tools and resources. NurseONE provides such services as the following:

- Professional links (resources with clinical or professional orientation)
- Professional development (including resources for continuing competence, online and continuing education, and career development)
- Library (access to numerous articles and publications)
- NurseConnect (use of the portal to create discussion groups among individual subscribers)

Resources available to subscribers also include conducting self-assessments, creating individualized learning plans, and developing an

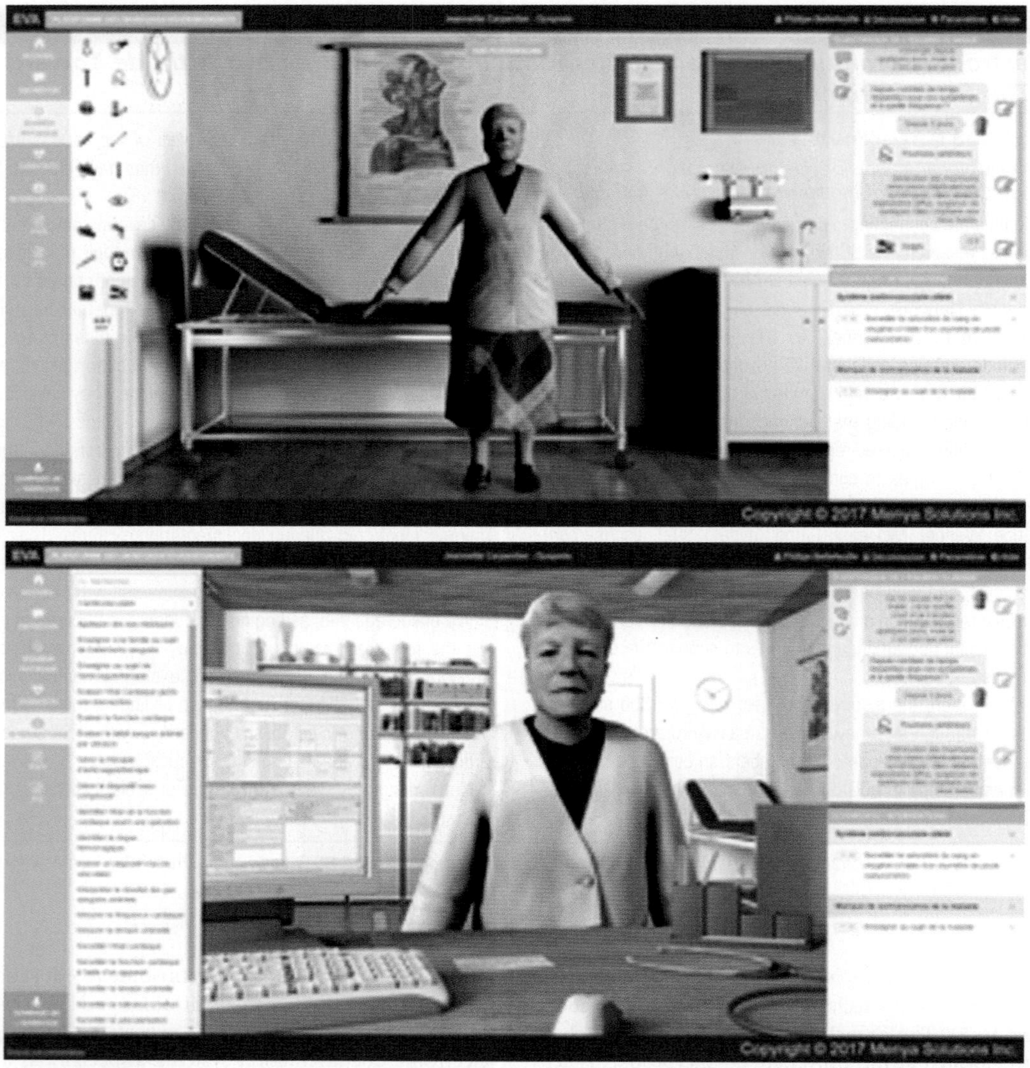

FIGURE 16-10 **Université de Sherbrooke Information System Simulation Tool.** (Reprinted with permission from Menya Solutions Inc., 2015.)

online professional portfolio. Users can also track current news and nursing information, receive updates and alerts on items of interest, access educational opportunities, and search for practice support on the NurseONE site. This site will continue to develop over time and provides a centralized professional nursing forum for Canadian nurses.

CLINICIAN ENGAGEMENT AND INFORMATICS COMMUNITIES

Many Canadian and international health informatics communities exist that offer exciting opportunities for participation in support, educational programs, and networking. Of most importance, these communities always welcome new members who are interested in advancing informatics. As noted throughout this chapter, involving clinicians in the selection, design, and revision of technology is critically important. As a professional, you have both an obligation and a right to be involved in issues that affect your professional practice and your work environment.

Many informatics organizations have specific strategies to foster clinician engagement or to encourage clinicians to become involved; despite historical scarcity, clinician engagement is increasingly recognized as essential to effective design, adoption, and evaluation. Mercer (2008) promoted involvement through five questions (the "5 Ws"): (1) What is it? (2) Who should be involved? (3) Why is it important? (4) Where does it fit? and (5) When should clinicians get involved? Mercer advocated immediate involvement in any clinical environment.

As the national professional body representing Canadian nurses, the CNA has a mandate to support professional nursing practice, which includes supporting the integration of NI in Canada. CNA has issued many position statements and professional guidelines to support all nurses as technology has become increasingly integrated into Canadian practice environments. CNA provides an excellent starting point from which you can explore NI in Canada.

The Canadian Nursing Informatics Association (CNIA) is the national special interest group dedicated to the advancement of NI in Canada (Box 16-6) and is designated as a group affiliated with the CNA. Also affiliated with Digital Health Canada (formerly COACH), the CNIA is the Canadian nursing representative to the International Medical Informatics Association–Special Interest Group in Nursing

TABLE 16-2 Snapshots of Informatics Progress Across Canada

Initiative	Overview	For More Information
North York General Hospital (NYGH) has achieved comprehensive informatics advancement and received the prestigious 2016 HIMSS Enterprise Davies Award	Among their achievements from interprofessional collaboration on implementing a number of informatics initiatives, NYGH reported: • Prevention and reduction of more than 11 000 medication errors as a direct result of implementing a closed-loop medication administration system. Manual entry of medications was eliminated. The system generates alerts to staff if medications about to be administered do not match the active orders on the electronic chart. • Venous thromboembolism occurrences were cut in half using computerized provider order entry (CPOE) and clinical decision support tools such as order sets and alerts. • Significant reductions in probability of in-hospital death due to medication errors, pneumonia, and exacerbation of chronic obstructive pulmonary disease (COPD) as a result of the safety and quality improvements gained from CPOE, clinical decision support, and medication reconciliation.	Canadian Healthcare Technology (2017a, 2017b): http://www.canhealth.com/blog/nygh-to-receive-prestigious-himss-award/ http://www.canhealth.com/wordpress/wp-content/uploads/2017/03/Canadian-Healthcare-Technology-2017-03.pdf
Vancouver Coastal Health (VCH), the Provincial Health Services Authority (PHSA) and Providence Health Care (PHC)	The Clinical & Systems Transformation (CST) project is one of the largest and most complex projects in Canada. It is designed to transform health care delivery systems and processes to improve the quality and consistency of the patient and caregiver experience. CST will establish common clinical and process standards, including workflows, order sets, clinical guidelines, integrated plans of care, and a common electronic health record, and enable clinicians to access client data where and when needed.	About CST: http://cstproject.ca/about-cst
VON Canada mobile solution	VON Canada has implemented a mobile app that has increased productivity by 25%, reduced mileage costs by 15%, and enables them to provide services to one additional client per day as a result. Staff can connect more efficiently with each other, document in real time, connect with clients, and reduce wait times for new clients.	Canadian Healthcare Technology (2017c): http://www.canhealth.com/wordpress/wp-content/uploads/2017/03/Canadian-Healthcare-Technology-2017-03.pdf
Island Health in BC has implemented a relief nurse shift scheduler	Island Health implemented Automatic Shift Callout (ASC) in combination with their existing workforce management system. As a result, schedulers have doubled the number of calls they make to potential relief nurses, are now able to provide 2–20 days' advance notice to relief nursing staff, and are reporting significant optimization of staff resourcing.	Canadian Healthcare Technology (2016): http://www.canhealth.com/blog/relief-nurse-scheduling-improved-using-vocantas/

Informatics (IMIA–NI) (IMIA, 1998). Originally functioning as a special-interest group within COACH, this group disbanded in 2000 and resumed as CNIA (CNIA, 2011). CNIA's mandate includes the following:

- To provide nursing leadership for the development of nursing and health informatics in Canada
- To establish national networking opportunities for nurse informaticians
- To facilitate informatics educational opportunities for all nurses in Canada
- To engage in international NI initiatives
- To act as a nursing advisory group in matters of nursing and health informatics

Since being founded, CNIA has hosted successful national NI conferences, provided educational offerings, and advocated for the advancement of NI in Canada. CNIA continues to evolve, producing an online newsletter and offering new initiatives that support nurses' continuing education opportunities.

As noted earlier in this chapter, Digital Health Canada (formerly COACH) is another organization dedicated to promoting health informatics within the Canadian health system, through education, information, networking, and communication. COACH was formed in 1975 by software developers and health care clinicians (COACH, 2017). Their original focus was to support effective use of information technology and systems among Canadian health institutions by sharing ideas and efforts. This focus has expanded to include the effective use of health information for decision making.

Digital Health Canada's multidisciplinary membership encompasses more than 1 300 individuals, including health care executives, physicians, nurses and allied health providers, researchers and educators, chief information officers, information managers, technical experts, consultants, and information technology vendors (COACH, 2017). Member organizations include health care service deliverers, government and nongovernment agencies, consulting firms, commercial providers of information and telecommunications technologies, and educational institutions.

In addition to the groups discussed here, you can contribute your clinician perspective to the various Communities of Practice and Working Groups sponsored by Infoway. In keeping with the priority on clinical interoperability, clinicians are welcomed and encouraged to participate and contribute their expertise on health care and informatics initiatives.

BOX 16-6 Getting to Know Your Canadian Nursing Informatics Association

The mission of the Canadian Nursing Informatics Association (CNIA) is to enable the improvement of nursing through the use of evidence-informed practice using nursing informatics, information technology, and information management.

The goals of this national organization include the following:

1. Influence and advance the use of nursing informatics and nursing data standards.
2. Connect nurses and health providers across the country for the purpose of improving best practice.
3. Support nurses in practice and education by providing resources for the advancement of nursing informatics competencies via training, tool kits, standards, and communities of practice.
4. Establish best practices in clinical information technology and information management.

Membership offers benefits such as access to a network of national nursing informatics experts and communication forums, valuable educational opportunities and conference events, and the ability to contribute to national discussions shaping the nursing informatics space. Find out more about CNIA at http://cnia.ca/.

Canadian Nursing Informatics Association. (2011). *2011 Strategic plan*. Toronto: Author.

Participating in these Communities and Working Groups not only supports your professional practice but also offers you an opportunity for professional development and mentoring. While many experienced nurses are currently involved in Infoway advisory groups, the Communities and Working Groups consistently need and solicit clinician engagement. The distinction between these two types of groups is that Working Groups typically focus on a specific challenge, whereas the Community may address multiple issues that support both specific and broader issues. The Working Groups can be accessed at: https://ic.infoway-inforoute.ca/en/collaboration/wg, and Communities at: https://ic.infoway-inforoute.ca/en/collaboration/communities.

You can also choose to participate in a variety of international informatics organizations. These include the American Medical Informatics Association (AMIA), the International Medical Informatics Association (IMIA), and the Health Informatics Society of Australia (HISA), all of which host special-interest groups in NI. You can be involved at every level of information management in health care. Your challenge and opportunity is to decide where your interest and energy can be best used.

In addition to the formal organizations that you may consider joining, numerous informal communities are devoted to NI and creating dialogue among nurses. You may decide to explore a variety of informal communities or social entities, including the following:

- *Blogs:* These are online diaries, generally sponsored by individuals, which are occasionally interactive but typically present only the thoughts and opinions of the blog's sponsor.
- *Wikis:* These are web pages that are interactive and allow subscribers to modify or contribute to the content. Subscribers are able to use any web browser. Wikis also allow users to incorporate hyperlinks and use a simplified language to create new pages and linkages rapidly.
- *Listservs and discussion groups:* These are email distribution lists. NI sites allow and encourage users to subscribe to the listserv or discussion groups so they can receive regular contact and updates regarding content, activities, or networking opportunities. These tools also allow participants to ask questions, post messages, and network with colleagues.
- *Social media:* Communities such as Facebook or Twitter allow subscribers to join or follow groups who are interested in shared interests and activities. These web-based communities include a variety of ways in which subscribers may communicate, such as chat, messaging, email, blogs, video, voice chat, file sharing, discussion groups, and message boards. Interest groups and organizations are regularly using these types of social media tools to create communities of practice and share experiences. Nurses who use these tools must do so in a fashion consistent with the ethical practice of nursing and privacy legislation.

The value of interest in informal networking cannot be underestimated; however, you should not depend solely on these types of forums for consistent, professional, and credible health informatics information. Some sites may offer highly professional informatics advice or information; unfortunately, no standards exist with regard to either content or process. Many sites offer only personal or anecdotal commentary and may provide misleading information, which can create liability if used in professional practice. Consequently, you must critically evaluate the content of these informal sites and groups to determine the validity of the content, the credibility of the organization or group, and the intent of the networking tool. The most effective way to obtain reliable and authoritative information is through formalized organizations that are committed to the professional advancement of informatics.

CRITICAL THINKING EXERCISES

1. You have been assigned to lead a team tasked with implementing a standardized nursing terminology for your hospital. What critical topics would you assign your team for review? What groups would you connect with to initiate discussions on best practices? What would be the top four activities necessary to proceed with this task?
2. During the course of documenting an admission assessment, you note that your patient has had a previous admission to a psychiatric unit. One of your colleagues is a neighbour of the patient and asks you to confirm whether this patient has a psychiatric history. Your colleague is not providing care to the patient. How do you respond to this inquiry? What pieces of legislation do you consider in helping you come to a decision?

REVIEW QUESTIONS

1. Changes that occurred in the health care system over the last few decades that have contributed to the recognition of nursing informatics include which of the following:
   1. Decreasing technology in health care and the evolution toward evidence-informed practice
   2. Requests for nursing informatics from administrators and national databases
   3. A recognition among nurses that specific nursing data must be documented consistently in order to create high-quality health data, support evidence-informed decision making, and represent nursing contributions
   4. Competition among professions to lead technology adoption
2. The factors behind the need for standardized nursing documentation include which of the following?
   1. To facilitate aggregation of nursing data and support data analysis

2. To enhance communication among nurses
3. To improve representation regarding nursing contributions
4. All of the above

3. Which of the following standardized nursing terminology is being used in Canada?
   1. interRAI
   2. ICNP
   3. SNOMED CT
   4. HOBIC
4. Which of the following privacy legislation influences nursing practice in Canada?
   1. PIPEDA and the *Privacy Act*
   2. PIPEDA and SCWGs
   3. Standards Collaborative Working Groups (SCWG) and Standards
   4. *Privacy Act* and *Code of Ethics*
5. How can you, as a nurse, enact the *e-Nursing Strategy*?
   1. Buy your own laptop, and design a nursing-related website
   2. Complete mandatory education on your hospital information system
   3. Support access to technology for all nurses, develop your technology competencies, and participate in advancing information and communication technology and nursing informatics
   4. Work at the Canadian Nurses Association
6. What nursing or health informatics communities are available to nurses?
   1. CNIA, IMIA-SIGNI
   2. CNA, CMA
   3. HOBIC, TTYL
   4. CSA, ICD-10

Answers: 1. 3; 2. 4; 3. 2; 4. 1; 5. 3; 6. 1

Rationales for the Review Questions appear at the end of the book.

RECOMMENDED WEBSITES

American Medical Informatics Association (AMIA): http://www.amia.org/.
AMIA is a national association in the United States that is dedicated to the adoption and advancement of technology in health care.

American Medical Informatics Association—Alliance for Nursing Informatics: http://www.amia.org/programs/alliance-nursing-informatics.
The American Medical Informatics Association—Nursing Informatics is a special-interest group within the American Medical Informatics Association. This group is focused on the advancement of informatics as it relates specifically to American professional nursing practice.

Canada Health Infoway: http://www.infoway-inforoute.ca/.
Canada Health Infoway is Canada's national not-for-profit body that generates consensus on health information standards, drives the national agenda of creating an EHR, and acts as the liaison to international standards development organizations.

Canadian Association of Schools of Nursing (CASN) Digital Health In Nursing Education: http://www.casn.ca/education/digital-healthnursing-informatics-casn-infoway-nurses-training-project/.
This inventory includes a variety of events and resources on integration of nursing informatics into nursing practice across Canada.

Canadian Nursing Informatics Association (CNIA): https://cnia.ca.
CNIA is Canada's national body with a mission to advance nursing informatics in Canada.

Canadian Organization for Advancement of Computers in Health (COACH): http://coachorgnew.com.
COACH is a Canadian not-for-profit association that is dedicated to the effective integration of technology in health care. This association is one of the largest informatics associations in Canada and includes members from all health care disciplines. COACH recently completed a rebranding initiative to better align and respond to industry needs and priorities around digital health. Moving forward, COACH will be known as Digital Health Canada (http://digitalhealthcanada.com/).

Health Informatics Society of Australia (HISA): http://www.hisa.org.au/.
HISA is the national not-for-profit association for advancing informatics in Australia.

International Medical Informatics Association (IMIA): http://imia-medinfo.org/wp/.
IMIA is an international not-for-profit association dedicated to the adoption and advancement of technology in health care.

International Medical Informatics Association—Nursing Informatics: http://imia-medinfo.org/wp/sig-ni-nursing-informatics/.
The International Medical Informatics Association—Nursing Informatics is a special-interest group within the International Medical Informatics Association. This group is focused on the advancement of nursing informatics with international implications.

Nursing Informatics Australia: https://www.hisa.org.au/nia/.
Nursing Informatics Australia is a special-interest group within the Health Informatics Society of Australia. This group is focused on the advancement of informatics as it relates specifically to professional nursing practice in Australia.

National Institute of Nursing Informatics: https://bloomberg.nursing.utoronto.ca/pd/professional-development/informatics.
This 3-day educational program for nurse educators, nurse leaders, or nurses interested in careers in nursing informatics is held in Toronto.

NurseONE: http://www.nurseone.ca/.
The NurseONE site is one of the outcomes of the Canadian Nurses Association *e-Nursing Strategy*. This site offers nurses a diverse array of educational tools, professional practice supports, and networking opportunities.

Office of the Privacy Commissioner of Canada: https://www.priv.gc.ca/en/.
This site provides access to a range of privacy-related materials, including the *Privacy Act* and *Personal Information Protection and Electronic Documents Act* (PIPEDA).

REFERENCES

Alberta Association of Registered Nurses (AARN) (1994). *Client status, nursing intervention, and client outcome taxonomies: A background paper*. Edmonton: Author.

Ball, M. J., & Hannah, K. J. (1984). *Using computers in nursing*. Reston, VA: Reston Publishing.

Ball, M. J., Hannah, K. J., Newbold, S. K., et al. (Eds.), (2000). *Nursing informatics: Where caring and technology meet* (3rd ed.). New York: Springer.

Canada Health Infoway. (2012). *Pan-Canadian nursing EHR business and functional elements supporting clinical practice*. Retrieved from https://www.infoway-inforoute.ca/en/component/edocman/resources/guides-workbooks/444-pan-canadian-nursing-ehr-business-and-functional-elements-supporting-clinical-practice.

Canada Health Infoway. (2014). *The path forward: Accelerating clinical interoperability in Canada—Strategy*. Retrieved from https://ic.infoway-inforoute.ca/en/resources/docs/cistratdocs/40-the-path-forward.

Canada Health Infoway. (2015). *Clinical interoperability action plan & notes*. Retrieved from: https://ic.infoway-inforoute.ca/en/resources/docs/cistratdocs/254-clinical-interoperability-action-plan-notes-may-2015/file.

Canada Health Infoway (2016a). *A conversation about digital health: Annual report 2015–2016*. Toronto: Author. Retrieved from https://www.infoway-inforoute.ca/en/component/edocman/resources/i-infoway-i-corporate/annual-reports/3098-annual-report-2015-2016.

Canada Health Infoway. (2016b). *National collaboration on clinical interoperability and digital health standards*. Retrieved from https://www.infoway-inforoute.ca/en/component/edocman/supporting-documents/partnership/3196-national-collaboration-on-clinical-interoperability-and-digital-health-standards.

Canada Health Infoway. (2016c). *Clinical peer leader networks support advanced clinical use and patient-centred digital health solutions*. Retrieved from https://www.infoway-inforoute.ca/en/what-we-do/news-events/newsroom/2016-news-releases/6739-clinical-peer-leader-networks-support-advanced-clinical-use-and-patient-centred-digital-health-solutions.

Canada Health Infoway (2017a). *Federal government announces new funding for Canada Health Infoway*. Toronto: Author. Retrieved from https://www.infoway-inforoute.ca/en/what-we-do/news-events/newsroom/2017-news-releases/7387-federal-government-announces-new-funding-for-canada-health-infoway.

Canada Health Infoway. (2017b). *Canadian outcomes for better information and care (C-HOBIC)*. Retrieved from https://ic.infoway-inforoute.ca/en/standards/inventory/c-hobic.

Canadian Association of Schools of Nursing (CASN). (2015). *Nursing informatics: Entry-to-practice competencies for registered nurses*. Retrieved from http://www.casn.ca/wp-content/uploads/2014/12/Nursing-Informatics-Entry-to-Practice-Competencies-for-RNs_updated-June-4-2015.pdf.

Canadian Healthcare Technology. (2016). *Island Health in BC has implemented a relief nurse shift scheduler. News blast February 17, 2016*. Retrieved from http://www.canhealth.com/blog/relief-nurse-scheduling-improved-using-vocantas/.

Canadian Healthcare Technology. (2017a). NYGH to receive prestigious HIMSS award. *Canadian Healthcare Technology*. Retrieved from http://www.canhealth.com/blog/nygh-to-receive-prestigious-himss-award/.

Canadian Healthcare Technology. (2017b). Innovative NYGH scoops up e-health award of excellence at HIMSS. *Canadian Healthcare Technology*, *22*(3), Retrieved from http://www.canhealth.com/wordpress/wp-content/uploads/2017/03/Canadian-Healthcare-Technology-2017-03.pdf.

Canadian Healthcare Technology. (2017c). VON Canada's mobile solution has increased productivity 25 percent. *Canadian Healthcare Technology*, *22*(3), 17. Retrieved from http://www.canhealth.com/wordpress/wp-content/uploads/2017/03/Canadian-Healthcare-Technology-2017-03.pdf.

Canadian Institute of Health Information (CIHI). (2017). *About CIHI*. Retrieved from https://www.cihi.ca/en/about-cihi.

Canadian Nurses Association (CNA) (2000). *Collecting data to reflect nursing impact: Discussion paper*. Ottawa: Author.

Canadian Nurses Association (CNA). (2001a). What is nursing informatics and why is it so important? *Nursing Now*, *11*.

Canadian Nurses Association (CNA) (2001b). *Position statement: Collecting data to reflect the impact of nursing practice*. Ottawa: Author.

Canadian Nurses Association (CNA) (2006a). *Position statement: Nursing information and knowledge management*. Ottawa: Author. Retrieved from https://www.cna-aiic.ca/~/media/cna/page-content/pdf-en/nursing-information-and-knowledge-management_position-statement-2006.pdf?la=en.

Canadian Nurses Association (CNA) (2006b). *E-nursing strategy for Canada*. Ottawa: Author. Retrieved from https://www.cna-aiic.ca/~/media/cna/page-content/pdf-en/e-nursing-strategy-for-canada.pdf?la=en.

Canadian Nurses Association (CNA) (2008). *Mapping Canadian clinical outcomes in ICNP*. Ottawa: Author.

Canadian Nurses Association (CNA) (2017a). *Code of ethics for registered nurses*. Ottawa: Author.

Canadian Nurses Association (CNA) (2017b). *NurseOne*. Ottawa: Author. Retrieved from https://www.nurseone.ca.

Canadian Nurses Association (CNA) & Canadian Nursing Informatics Association (CNIA) (2017). *Joint position statement: Nursing informatics*. Ottawa: Author. Retrieved from https://www.cna-aiic.ca/en/~/media/cna/page-content/pdf-fr/nursing-informatics-joint-position-statement.

Canadian Nursing Informatics Association (CNIA) (2011). *2011 Strategic plan*. Toronto: Author.

Canadian Organization for Advancement of Computers in Health (COACH). (2013). *HIP competencies, version 3.0: Equipping HI professionals for the future*. Retrieved from https://ams.coachorg.com/inventory/PurchaseDetails.aspx?Id=f1867f53-f22d-4705-a1b4-99db528cc574.

Canadian Organization for Advancement of Computers in Health (COACH). (2017). *COACH: Canada's health informatics association*. Retrieved from http://coachorgnew.com.

Clark, D. J. (1999). A language for nursing. *Nursing Standard*, *13*(31), 42.

Clark, J., & Lang, N. M. (1992). Nursing's next advance: An international classification system for nursing practice. *International Nursing Review*, *39*(4), 109–112, 128.

Gershon, A. S., & Tu, J. (2008). The effect of privacy legislation on observational research. *Canadian Medical Association Journal*, *178*(7), 871–873.

Giovannetti, P., Smith, D., & Broad, E. (1999). Structuring and managing health information. In J. Hibberd & D. Smith (Eds.), *Nursing management in Canada* (2nd ed., pp. 297–318). Toronto: Saunders.

Goodwin, S., Matthews, S., Carr, H., et al. (2008). Transforming home and community care. *The Canadian Nurse*, *104*(5), 30–31.

Government of Canada. (2016). Privacy Act. *Bill C-21. Ottawa: Department of Justice*. Retrieved from http://laws-lois.justice.gc.ca/eng/acts/P-21/.

Government of Canada. (2017). Personal Information Protection and Electronic Documents Act. *Bill C-6. Ottawa: Department of Justice*. Retrieved from http://laws-lois.justice.gc.ca/eng/acts/P-8.6/index.html.

Graves, J. R., & Corcoran, S. (1989). The study of nursing informatics. *Image: Journal of Nursing Scholarship*, *21*, 227–231.

Hannah, K. J. (2005). Health informatics and nursing in Canada. *HCIM&C*, *XIX*, *3*, 45–51.

Hannah, K. J., Ball, M. J., & Edwards, M. J. A. (1994). *Introduction to nursing informatics*. New York: Springer-Verlag.

Hannah, K. J., Ball, M., & Edwards, M. J. A. (2006). *Introduction to nursing informatics* (3rd ed.). New York: Springer-Verlag.

Hussey, P., & Kennedy, M. A. (2016). Instantiating informatics within nursing practice for integrated patient centered holistic models of care: A discussion paper. *Journal of Advanced Nursing*, *75*(5), 1030–1041. doi:10.1111/jan.12927.

International Council of Nurses (ICN) (2011). *Nursing outcome indicators: A shared project with the Canadian Nurses Association*. Geneva, Switzerland: Author.

International Council of Nurses (ICN). (2015a). *ICNP definition*. Retrieved from http://www.icn.ch/what-we-do/definition-a-elements-of-icnpr/.

International Council of Nurses (ICN). (2015b). *ICNP technical implementation guide*. Retrieved from http://www.icn.ch/images/stories/documents/publications/free_publications/ICNP_Technical_Implementation_Guide.pdf.

International Council of Nurses (ICN). (2017a). *ICNP browser*. Retrieved from http://www.icn.ch/ICNP-Browser-NEW.html.

International Council of Nurses (ICN). (2017b). *ICNP catalogues*. Retrieved from http://www.icn.ch/what-we-do/icnpr-catalogues/.

International Medical Informatics Association (IMIA). (1998). *Special interest group—Nursing informatics*. Retrieved from http://imia-medinfo.org/wp/sig-ni-nursing-informatics/.

International Medical Informatics Association (IMIA). (2009). *IMIA-NI definition of nursing informatics updated*. Retrieved from https://imianews.wordpress.com/2009/08/24/imia-ni-definition-of-nursing-informatics-updated/.

Kennedy, M. A. (2005). *Packaging nursing as politically potent: A critical reflexive cultural studies approach to nursing informatics*. Unpublished doctoral dissertation, University of South Australia, Adelaide, Australia.

Kennedy, M. A. (2008). *Mapping clinical outcomes in ICNP, Version 1.0: The C-HOBIC Project* (Final Report). Merigomish, NS: Kennedy Health Informatics Inc.

Kennedy, M. A., Hannah, K. J., & White, P. (2008). C-HOBIC: Mapping a path for Canada in nursing documentation. *Canadian Nurse*, *104*(5), 27–29.

Marck, P. (1994). The problem with good nursing care…it is often invisible. *Alberta Association of Registered Nurses Newsletter*, *50*(5), 10–11.

Marek, K., & Lang, N. (1993). Nursing sensitive outcomes. In Canadian Nurses Association (Ed.), *Papers from the Nursing Minimum Data Set Conference* (pp. 100–120). Ottawa: Canadian Nurses Association.

McGee, M. (1993). Response to V. Saba's paper on nursing diagnostic schemes. In Canadian Nurses Association (Ed.), *Papers from the Nursing Minimum Data Set Conference* (pp. 64–67). Ottawa: Canadian Nurses Association.

Mercer, C. (2008). The five Ws of clinical engagement. *Canadian Nurse*, *104*(5), 9–10.

Nagle, L., & White, P. (2016). *National nursing data standards symposium: Proceedings*. Toronto: Author.

National Task Force on Health Information (1991). Health information for Canada. In M. Wilk (Ed.), *Wilk report*. Ottawa: National Health Information Council, Health Canada.

Norwood, S. (2001). NP education: The invisibility of advanced practice nurses in popular magazines. *Journal of the American Academy of Nurse Practitioners*, *13*(3), 129–134.

O'Brien-Pallas, L., & Giovannetti, P. (1993). Nursing intensity. In Canadian Nurses Association (CNA) (Ed.), *Papers from the Nursing Minimum Data Set Conference* (pp. 68–76). Ottawa: Canadian Nurses Association.

Office of the Privacy Commissioner of Canada, Government of Canada. (2014). *Overview of privacy legislation in Canada*. Retrieved from https://www.priv.gc.ca/en/privacy-topics/privacy-laws-in-canada/02_05_d_15/.

Porter-O'Grady, T. (2014). Leading the revolution in nursing practice: Advancing health in the digital age. *Canadian Journal of Nursing Leadership*, *27*(2), 14–20.

Powers, P. (2001). The image of nursing in hospital promotional materials: A discourse analysis. *Scholarly Inquiry for Nursing Practice*, *15*(2), 91–107.

Remus, S., & Kennedy, M. A. (2012). Innovation in transformative nursing leadership: Nursing informatics competencies and roles. *Canadian Journal of Nursing Leadership*, *25*(4), 14–26. doi:10.12927/cjnl.2012.23260.

Roch, J. (2008). Protecting health information is of paramount importance. *Canadian Nurse*, *104*(5), 8.

Tracey, P. (2008). Integrating a standardized assessment into acute care settings: One LHIN's approach. *Canadian Nurse*, *104*(5), 25–26.

Wenger, E., McDermott, R., & Snyder, W. (2002). *Cultivating communities of practice*. Boston: Harvard Business School Press.

Werley, H. H. (1988). Introduction to the nursing minimum data set and its development. In H. H. Werley & N. M. Lang (Eds.), *Identification of the nursing minimum data set* (pp. 1–15). New York: Springer.

Weyrauch, B. (2002). President's message: DNA joins alliance to increase nursing's visibility. *Dermatology Nursing*, *14*(6), 356.

World Health Organization (WHO). (2017). *eHealth*. Retrieved from http://www.who.int/topics/ehealth/en/.

17

Communication and Relational Practice

Written by Sonya L. Jakubec, RN, BHScN, MN, PhD, Barbara J. Astle, RN, PhD

OBJECTIVES

Mastery of content in this chapter will enable you to:

- Define the key terms listed.
- Describe aspects of critical thinking that are important to the communication process.
- Describe the five levels of communication and their uses in nursing.
- Describe the basic elements of the communication process.
- Discuss the role of communication in relational practice.
- Identify the practices important for relational inquiry.
- Identify significant features and therapeutic outcomes of nurse–patient helping relationships.
- List nursing focus areas within the four phases of a nurse–patient helping relationship.
- Describe qualities, behaviours, and approaches that affect interprofessional communication.
- Discuss effective approaches to communicating with patients at various developmental levels.
- Identify patient health states and conditions that contribute to impaired communication.
- Discuss nursing care measures for patients with special communication needs.

KEY TERMS

Active listening, p. 282
Aphasia, p. 286
Assertive, p. 279
Authenticity, p. 272
Autonomy, p. 279
Channels, p. 274
Collaborative communication, p. 278
Communication, p. 271
Elderspeak, p. 280
Empathy, p. 282
Environment, p. 275
Expressive aphasia, p. 286
Feedback, p. 274
Global aphasia, p. 286
Initiative, p. 272
Intentionality, p. 282
Interpersonal communication, p. 273
Interpersonal variables, p. 275
Intrapersonal communication, p. 273
Message, p. 274
Metacommunication, p. 277
Mutuality, p. 272
Narrative interactions, p. 278
Nonverbal communication, p. 275
Perception, p. 272
Perceptual biases, p. 272
Public communication, p. 274
Questioning beyond the surface, p. 272
Receiver, p. 274
Receptive aphasia, p. 286
Referent, p. 274
Reflexivity, p. 273
Relational communication, p. 272
Relational inquiry, p. 280
Relational practice, p. 272
Seeking contextual knowledge, p. 273
Sender, p. 274
Small-group communication, p. 274
Spiritual inquiry, p. 273
Symbolic communication, p. 277
Sympathy, p. 285
Therapeutic communication techniques, p. 282
Transpersonal communication, p. 273
Verbal communication, p. 275

MEDIA RESOURCES

http://evolve.elsevier.com/Canada/Potter/fundamentals/

- Audio Chapter Summaries
- Examination Review Questions
- Concept Map Creator
- Case Study with Questions
- Audio Glossary
- Content Updates
- Video Clips

Communication is a lifelong learning process for the nurse. Nurses are intimately involved with patients and their families throughout the lifespan. Nurses must communicate effectively with people who are in some of the most stressful of life's circumstances. They function as patient advocates and as members of interprofessional teams where other members may have different priorities for patient-centred care. Nurses must also communicate their own needs to avoid burnout and to continue providing effective care (Balzer Riley, 2016). Despite the competing demands on nurses' time and increasing technological complexity, it is the intimate nurse–patient connection that makes the difference in the quality of care and in the meaning of the illness experience for both (Balzer Riley, 2016). Therefore, competency in a variety of communication techniques supports the nurses' ability to develop and maintain therapeutic relationships. The importance of communication and collaboration is identified as a key domain of nursing education in Canada (Canadian Association of Schools of Nursing, 2015). Effective communication promotes interprofessional collaboration (IPC) with others in the health care team, helps ensure that ethical and legal responsibilities and professional practice standards are met, and contributes to positive patient outcomes (Registered Nurses' Association of Ontario, 2013; Wagner, Liston, & Miller, 2011) (see Chapter 18 for further information on interprofessional practice). Ineffective communication may lead to poor patient outcomes, increases in adverse incidents, and decreases in professional credibility. The Conference Board of Canada considers communication and interpersonal relationship skills to be crucial for successful employment and the establishment of healthy work environments (Devito, Shimoni, & Clark, 2015).

The qualities, behaviours, and therapeutic communication techniques described in this chapter characterize professionalism in helping relationships. Although the term *patient* is often used, the same principles can be applied in communicating with any person, group, or population in any nursing situation.

COMMUNICATION AND INTERPERSONAL RELATIONSHIPS

At the core of nursing care are therapeutic interpersonal relationships based on caring, mutual respect, and dignity. Communication is the means to establishing these helping-healing relationships. As all behaviour communicates, and all communication influences behaviour, nurses must become experts in communication if they are to provide effective care.

Relational practice is "guided by conscious participation with clients using a number of relational skills including listening, questioning, empathy, mutuality, reciprocity, and self-observation, reflection, and a sensitivity to emotional contexts" (College of Nurses of Ontario, 2014, p. 13). The nurse's capacity to be in relation with other people—to take initiative in establishing and maintaining a relationship, to be authentic and responsive to the other person—is a crucial aspect of interpersonal communication. The will and active intention of nurses to join people where they are is what is meant by initiative in **relational communication**. Reaching out and listening are parts of taking **initiative**. Being spontaneous and genuine, aware of the in-the-moment experiences of the patient and one's self, are aspects of **authenticity**. Authenticity is often one of the characteristics of nurses that imbues the trust of the public. Hartrick Doane and Varcoe (2015) explain that "when a nurse has the initiative to be with another in an authentic way, she or he is able to respond to the other as they are in that moment" (p. 193). Effective interpersonal communication also requires a sense of **mutuality** and being in a mutual relation. Being "in synch" in this way is based on a belief that the nurse–patient relationship is a partnership and that both partners are equal participants. Mutuality requires that both participants respect each other's autonomy and value system and are committed to the patient's well-being (Arnold & Boggs, 2015). In their work, nurses honour the fact that people are complex and ambiguous beings. Often, more is communicated than is initially apparent, and patient responses are not always what you might expect. **Questioning beyond the surface** is an approach to inquiry that nurses employ that facilitates relational practice within complex circumstances of health and illness. Nurses are further able to engage with complexity and uncertainty and expand their capacity to communicate by focusing on their relational capacity and the following skills (Hartrick Doane & Varcoe, 2005):

- Letting be
- Listening
- Self-observation
- Questioning to look beyond the surface
- Intentionality
- Interrupting contextual constraints
- Reimagining

In addition, Hartrick Doane and Varcoe (2015) propose the importance of developing a relational inquiry approach in order to be consistent with the "realities of contemporary nursing situations" (p. 7) when they state that relational inquiry is an approach to competence in its fullest sense in nursing practice (see Chapter 9 for further information about a relational inquiry approach to nursing competence).

Therapeutic communication occurs within a healing environment between a nurse and a patient (Arnold & Boggs, 2015). Nurses know that attitudes and emotions are easily transmitted and can be communicated intentionally or unintentionally. Every nuance of posture, every small expression and gesture, every word chosen, every attitude held—all have the potential to hurt or heal. Because thought patterns (positive or negative), intention, and behaviour directly influence human energy fields and, therefore, health, nurses have a tremendous ethical responsibility to pay careful attention to their communication with patients.

Complementary perspectives of communication and relationships draw upon notions of balance (Hunter, Logan, Goulet, et al., 2006) and energy fields (Gueldner, Michel, Bramlett, et al., 2005) as aspects of communication that permeate and connect all beings. Although the use of energy and nature to heal is a relatively new concept in Western cultures, it has long existed in Indigenous and Eastern cultures. Most nurses embrace the profession's view of people as holistic beings and have experienced synergy in human interactions. All communication must be respected for its potential power and not carelessly misused to hurt, manipulate, or coerce patients. Good communication empowers patients and enables them to know themselves and make their own choices, which is an essential aspect of the healing process. Nurses have an opportunity to create positive outcomes for themselves, patients, and colleagues through therapeutic communication.

DEVELOPING COMMUNICATION SKILLS

Gaining expertise in communication requires an understanding of the communication process, commitment to an evolving capacity to be in relation to others, and in-depth reflection about personal communication experiences (Balzer Riley, 2016). In addition, the qualities of good critical thinking and problem solving are important to the communication process. Curiosity, perseverance, creativity, self-confidence, independence, fairness, integrity, and humility are useful in approaching a problem (see Chapter 12 for further information on critical thinking).

Interpersonal communication may be challenging because it is based on an individual's perception of received information and is therefore subject to misinterpretation. **Perception** is based on information acquired through the five senses of sight, hearing, taste, touch, and smell (Austin & Boyd, 2014). It is a process of mentally organizing and interpreting sensory information to arrive at a meaningful conclusion. An individual's culture, education, and personal background also influence perception (see Chapter 9). Critical thinking and self-reflection can help nurses overcome **perceptual biases**, which are human tendencies that interfere with accurately perceiving and interpreting messages from other people. People often assume that others would think, feel, act, react, and behave as they themselves would in similar circumstances. People tend to distort or ignore information that goes against their expectations, preconceptions, or stereotypes (Beebe, Beebe, Redmond, et al., 2014). By thinking critically about personal communication habits, you will gain awareness of these tendencies and become more responsive to your patients and your goals of therapeutic communication.

As communication skills develop, competence in the nursing process occurs. Integration of communication skills throughout the nursing process facilitates collaboration with patients and members of the interprofessional team (Box 17-1). Communication skills are used to gather, analyze, and transmit information and to accomplish the work of each step of the process. Assessment, diagnosis, planning, implementation, and evaluation all depend on effective communication among nurse, patient, family, and interprofessional colleagues. Although the nursing process is a reliable framework for patient-centred care, it does not work well unless you master the art of effective interpersonal communication and relational inquiry.

The nature of the communication process requires nurses to constantly make decisions about what, when, where, why, and how to convey messages to other people. Decision making is always contextual; unique features of any situation influence the nature of the decisions made. For example, the importance of following a prescribed diet will be explained differently to a patient with a newly diagnosed medical condition than to a patient who has repeatedly chosen not to follow diet restrictions. In nursing communication, **seeking contextual knowledge** is the building block to providing context-based and relevant care (Hartrick Doane & Varcoe, 2015). Effective communication skills such as "seeking contextual knowledge" are easy to learn, but their application is more difficult and nuanced. Deciding which approach is most responsive to each unique nursing situation is challenging and requires tremendous self-awareness and reflexivity. **Reflexivity** is being aware of your own patterns of communication and response to communication, as well as the responses you are evoking in others. When considering self-awareness, imagine how communication about specific diagnoses such as cancer or end-of-life conditions and dealing with patient and family emotions might be challenging to you. Certainly, some nurses struggle to cope with their own reactions and emotions when communicating difficult news to families and patients (Sheldon, Barrett, & Ellington, 2006).

Throughout this chapter, brief clinical examples will guide you in approaches for effective communication. Because the best way to acquire skill is through practice, it is useful for you to know yourself and your own habits, as well as typical responses to situations. Discussing and role-playing these scenarios before experiencing them at the point of care may be helpful (Wagner et al., 2011).

BOX 17-1 Communication Throughout the Nursing Process

Assessment
- Verbal interviewing and history taking
- Visual and intuitive observation of nonverbal behaviour
- Documentation of visual, tactile, and auditory data during physical examination
- Written medical records, diagnostic test results, and literature review

Nursing Diagnosis
- Intrapersonal analysis of assessment findings
- Validation of health care needs and priorities through verbal discussion with patient
- Handwritten or electronic documentation of nursing diagnosis

Planning
- Interpersonal or small-group planning sessions with health care team
- Interpersonal collaboration with patient and family to determine implementation methods
- Written documentation of expected outcomes
- Written or verbal referral to members of the health care team

Implementation
- Delegation and verbal discussion with health care team
- Verbal, visual, auditory, and tactile health teaching activities
- Provision of support through therapeutic communication techniques
- Contact with other health care resources and the interprofessional collaboration team
- Written documentation of patient's progress in medical record
- Communicating targeted, effective public and population health messages

Evaluation
- Acquisition of verbal and nonverbal feedback
- Comparison of actual and expected outcomes
- Identification of factors affecting outcomes
- Modification and update of care plan
- Verbal or written explanation, or both, of revisions of care plan to patient
- Receiving and responding to feedback about one's own nursing care

LEVELS OF COMMUNICATION

Nurses use different levels of communication in their professional role: intrapersonal, interpersonal, transpersonal, small group, and public.

Intrapersonal Communication

Intrapersonal communication, exemplified in one's thinking, is also known as *self-talk* or *inner thought.* It is a powerful form of communication that occurs *within* an individual (Beebe et al., 2014). Nurses and patients use intrapersonal communication to develop self-awareness and a positive self-concept that can facilitate self-expression and improve health and self-esteem by replacing negative thoughts with positive assertions.

Interpersonal Communication

Interpersonal communication is the one-to-one interaction between the nurse and patient that often occurs face to face. It is the level most frequently used in nursing practice. It takes place within a social context and includes all the symbols and cues used to give and receive meaning.

Sometimes messages are received differently than the messenger intended. Nurses work with people who have different opinions, experiences, values, and belief systems; therefore, meaning must be validated or mutually negotiated between participants.

Transpersonal Communication

Transpersonal communication occurs within a person's spiritual domain. Nurses communicate and relate to their patients within this domain (see Chapter 28). **Spiritual inquiry** is an approach to communication whereby nurses can join with their patients to create a road map of what is meaningful, significant, and important for the patient in their unique context. This inquiry illuminates the patient's contexts, understandings, experiences, and hopes. It is through such dialogue that nurses can communicate with patients in times of deeper, often complex, conflicted, and ambiguous situations (Hartrick Doane & Varcoe, 2015).

Small-Group Communication

Small-group communication is interaction that occurs when a small number of people meet together and share a common purpose. This type of communication is usually goal-directed and requires an understanding of group dynamics. When nurses work on committees, lead patient support groups, form research teams, or participate in patient-centred care conferences, they are using the small-group communication process. For small groups to function effectively, members must feel accepted, comfortable in sharing ideas and thoughts openly and honestly, and able to actively listen to other group members and consider possible alternative viewpoints (Arnold & Boggs, 2015).

Public Communication

Public communication is interaction with an audience. Nurses have opportunities to speak with groups of consumers about health-related topics, present scholarly work to colleagues at conferences, lead classroom discussions with peers or students, and engage in public advocacy or media activities. Public communication requires special adaptations in eye contact, gestures, and voice inflection and the use of media materials to communicate messages effectively. The purpose of public communication by nurses is to increase audience knowledge about health-related topics, health care issues, and other issues important to the nursing profession.

BASIC ELEMENTS OF THE COMMUNICATION PROCESS

Communication is an ongoing, dynamic, and multidimensional process. Its basic elements are illustrated in Figure 17-1 and described in the following paragraphs. This simple model represents what is, in practice, a very complex process. The model helps identify essential components of communication.

Referent

The referent motivates one person to communicate with another. In a health care setting, sights, sounds, odours, time schedules, messages, objects, emotions, sensations, perceptions, ideas, and other cues trigger communication. When a nurse knows the stimulus that triggered communication she or he can develop and organize messages for effective communication.

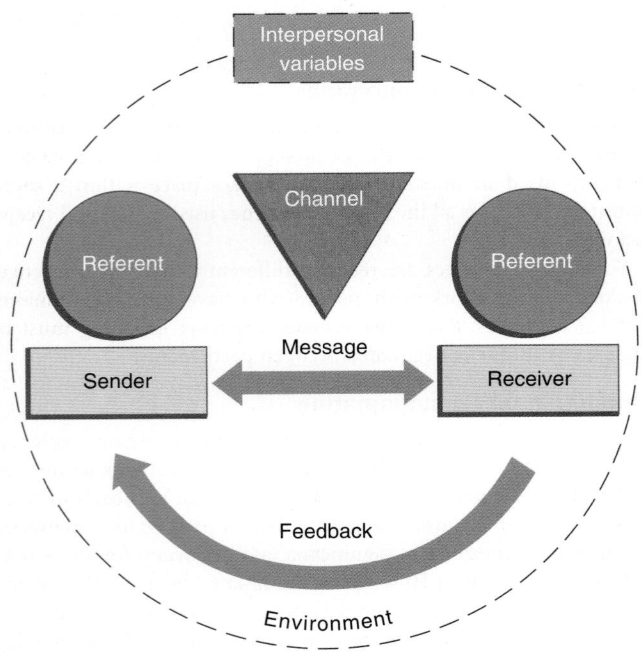

FIGURE 17-1 Communication is an active process between sender and receiver.

Sender and Receiver

The sender is the person who encodes and delivers the message, and the receiver is the person who receives and decodes the message. The sender puts ideas or feelings into a form that can be transmitted and is responsible for accuracy and emotional tone. The sender's message acts as a referent for the receiver, who is responsible for attending to, decoding, and responding to the sender's message. Sender and receiver roles are fluid and change back and forth as people interact; sometimes sending and receiving even occur simultaneously. The more the sender and receiver have in common and the closer their relationship, the more likely they will accurately perceive one another's meaning and respond accordingly.

Messages

The message is the content of the communication. It contains verbal, nonverbal, and symbolic expressions of thoughts or feelings that are transmitted from the sender to the receiver (Arnold & Boggs, 2015). Personal perceptions sometimes distort the receiver's interpretation of the message. Two nurses can provide the same information and yet convey very different messages according to their personal communication styles. One nurse can send the same message to two people and be understood differently by each. You can send effective messages by expressing yourself clearly, directly, and in a manner familiar to the receiver. By watching the listener for nonverbal cues that suggest confusion or misunderstanding, you can determine whether the message needs to be clarified. Communication can be difficult when participants have different levels of education and experience. "Your incision is well approximated without purulent drainage" means the same as "Your wound edges are together, with no signs of infection," but the latter is easier to understand. You must be sure patients can read before you send messages in writing.

Channels

Channels are means of conveying and receiving messages through visual, auditory, and tactile senses. Facial expressions send visual messages, spoken words travel through auditory channels, and touch crosses tactile channels. The more channels the sender uses to convey a message, the more clearly the message is usually understood. For example, when teaching about insulin self-injection, the nurse talks about and demonstrates the technique, gives the patient printed information, and encourages hands-on practice with the vial and syringe. Nurses use verbal, nonverbal, and mediated (technological) communication channels. They send and receive information in person; by informal or formal writing; over the telephone or pager; by audio and video recording; and through fax, email, and interactive electronic or social networking media.

Feedback

Feedback is the message returned by the receiver. It indicates whether the intended meaning of the sender's message was understood by the receiver. Senders need to seek verbal and nonverbal feedback to ensure that clear communication has occurred. To be effective, the sender and receiver must be sensitive and open to each other's messages, clarify the messages, and modify behaviour accordingly. In a social relationship, both participants assume equal responsibility for seeking openness and clarification, but in the nurse–patient relationship, this responsibility is primarily the nurse's.

Interpersonal Variables

Interpersonal variables are characteristics within both the sender and receiver that influence communication. People perceive events differently (Austin & Boyd, 2014). A nurse might say, "You have been very quiet since your family left. Is something on your mind?" One patient might perceive the nurse's question as showing caring and concern; another might perceive the nurse as being intrusive. It is the responsibility of the nurse to seek out the variables and contexts that will communicate sensitively and effectively. Other interpersonal variables include educational and developmental levels, sociocultural backgrounds, values and beliefs, emotions, gender, physical health status, and roles and relationships. Variables associated with illness, such as pain, anxiety, and medication effects, can also affect nurse–patient communication and should all be considered in communication choices (Feldman-Stewart, Brundage, & Tishelman, 2005).

Environment

The environment is the setting for sender–receiver interaction. For effective communication, the environment should meet nurse and patient needs for physical and emotional comfort and safety. Noise, temperature extremes, distractions, and lack of privacy or space create confusion, tension, and discomfort. Environmental distractions are common in health care settings and interfere with messages sent between people. Establishing as comfortable an environment as possible to create favourable conditions for effective communication is a role of the nurse.

FORMS OF COMMUNICATION

Messages are conveyed verbally, nonverbally, concretely, and symbolically. As people communicate, they express themselves through words, movements, voice inflection, facial expressions, and use of space. These elements work in harmony to enhance a message and can also conflict with one another to contradict or confuse the message.

Verbal Communication

Verbal communication entails the use of spoken or written words. Verbal language is a code that conveys specific meaning through a combination of words. The most important aspects of verbal communication are discussed next.

Vocabulary. Communication is unsuccessful if senders and receivers cannot decode each other's words and phrases. When a nurse cares for a patient who speaks another language, the services of an interpreter may be necessary. Even those who speak the same language use subcultural variations of certain words: *dinner* may mean a noon meal to one person and the last meal of the day to another. Medical jargon (technical terminology used by the interprofessional collaborative practice team) may sound like a foreign language to patients and should be used only with other IPC practitioners. Children have more limited vocabularies than do adults and may use special words to describe bodily functions or a favourite blanket or toy. Teenagers often use words in unique ways that are unfamiliar to adults.

Denotative and Connotative Meaning. A single word can have several meanings. Individuals who use a common language share the denotative meaning: *baseball* has the same meaning for everyone who speaks English, but *code* denotes cardiac arrest to health care providers. The connotative meaning is the interpretation of a word's meaning influenced by the thoughts, feelings, or ideas that people have about the word. Families who are told that a loved one is "in serious condition" may believe that death is near, but to the nurse *serious* may simply describe the nature of the condition. As a nurse you need to select words carefully, avoiding terms that can be easily misinterpreted, especially when explaining a patient's medical condition or therapy. Even a much-used phrase such as "I'm going to take your vital signs" can be unfamiliar to an adult or frightening to a child.

Pacing. Messages are conveyed more successfully when sent at an appropriate speed or pace. It is important to speak slowly enough to enunciate clearly. Talking rapidly, using awkward pauses, or speaking slowly and deliberately can convey an unintended message. Long pauses and rapid shifts to another topic may be unsettling for a patient. Pacing is improved by thinking before speaking and by developing awareness of the cadence of your speech.

Intonation. Tone of voice dramatically affects the meaning of a message. Depending on intonation, even a simple question or statement can express enthusiasm, anger, concern, or indifference. To avoid sending unintended messages, be aware of your tone of voice. For example, patients may interpret a nurse's tone of voice as condescending, and further communication may be inhibited. A patient's tone of voice is also highly relevant to communication and may provide information about his or her emotional state or energy level.

Clarity and Brevity. Effective communication is simple, brief, and direct. Fewer words result in less confusion. You can achieve clarity by speaking slowly, enunciating clearly, and using examples to make explanations easier to understand. Repeating important parts of a message also clarifies communication. Phrases such as "you know" or "okay?" at the end of every sentence detract from clarity, as well as professionalism. Brevity is achieved by using short sentences and words that express an idea simply and directly. "Where is your pain?" is much better than "I would like you to describe for me the location of your discomfort."

Timing and Relevance. Timing is critical in communication. Even though a message is clear, poor timing can limit its effectiveness. For example, you should not begin routine teaching when a patient is in severe pain, is in emotional distress, or is distracted by pressing matters. Often the best time for interaction is when a patient expresses an interest in communicating. If messages are relevant or important to the situation at hand, communication is more effective. For example, when a patient is facing emergency surgery, discussing the risks of smoking is less relevant than explaining preoperative procedures.

Nonverbal Communication

Nonverbal communication makes use of all five senses and refers to transmission of messages that do not involve the spoken or written word. Researchers have estimated that approximately 7% of meaning is transmitted by words, 38% by vocal cues, and 55% by nonverbal body cues. Nonverbal communication serves to accent, complement, contradict, regulate, repeat, or substitute for verbal messages (Devito et al., 2015). Nonverbal communication is unconsciously motivated and thus reflects a person's intended meaning more accurately than spoken words (Austin & Boyd, 2014). When verbal and nonverbal communication are incongruous, the receiver usually "hears" the nonverbal message as the true message.

All kinds of nonverbal communication are important, but interpreting them is often difficult. Sociocultural background is a major influence on the meaning of nonverbal behaviour. Nonverbal messages between people of different cultures are easily misinterpreted. Because the interpretation of nonverbal behaviour is subjective, it is important to check its perceived meaning (Adler et al., 2008). Assessing nonverbal messages is an important communication skill that is highly consequential to patient assessment and nursing care (Austin & Boyd, 2014).

Personal Appearance. Personal appearance includes physical characteristics, facial expression, manner of dress and grooming, and adornments. These factors help communicate physical well-being, personality, social status, occupation, religion, culture, and self-concept. First impressions are largely based on appearance. Nurses learn to develop a general impression of patient health and emotional status through appearance, and patients develop a general impression of the nurse's professionalism and caring in the same way.

Posture and Gait. Posture and gait are forms of self-expression. The ways that people sit, stand, and move reflect attitudes, emotions, self-concept, and health status. For example, an erect posture and a quick, purposeful gait communicate a sense of well-being and confidence. Leaning forward conveys attention. A slumped posture and a slow, shuffling gait may be indicative of depression, illness, discomfort, or fatigue.

Facial Expression. The face is the most expressive part of the body. Facial expressions convey emotions such as surprise, fear, anger, happiness, and sadness. Some people have an expressionless face, or flat affect, which reveals little about what they are thinking or feeling. An incongruent affect is a facial expression that does not match the content of a verbal message—for example, smiling when describing a sad situation. People are sometimes unaware of the messages their expressions convey. For example, a nurse may frown in concentration while doing a procedure and the patient may interpret this as anger or disapproval. Patients closely observe nurses. Consider the impact a nurse's facial expression might have on a person who asks, "Am I going to die?" The slightest change in the eyes, lips, or facial muscles will reveal the nurse's feelings. Although it is hard to control all facial expression, the nurse should try to avoid showing shock, disgust, dismay, or other distressing reactions in the patient's presence.

Eye Contact. People signal readiness to communicate through eye contact. Among many European and American people, maintaining eye contact during conversation shows respect and willingness to listen. Eye contact also allows people to closely observe one another. Lack of eye contact may indicate anxiety, defensiveness, discomfort, or lack of confidence in communicating. However, among some Asian and Aboriginal people, eye contact may be considered intrusive, threatening, or harmful. Eye movements can also communicate feelings and emotions. Standing above a person (looking downward) conveys authority, whereas interacting at the same eye level indicates equality in the relationship. Rising to the same eye level as an angry person communicates self-assertion.

Gestures. Gestures emphasize, punctuate, and clarify the spoken word, and they may communicate volumes when speech is not possible. Gestures alone carry specific meanings and create messages. A finger pointed toward a person may communicate several meanings, but when accompanied by a frown and stern voice, the gesture conveys an accusation or a threat. Pointing to an area of pain may be more accurate than verbally describing the location.

Sounds. Sounds such as sighs, moans, groans, or sobs also communicate feelings and thoughts. When combined with other nonverbal communication, sounds help send messages. Sounds can be interpreted in several ways: sighing often suggests boredom or anxiety, moaning may convey pleasure or suffering, and crying may communicate happiness, sadness, or anger. As a nurse you need to validate such nonverbal messages with the patient in order to interpret them accurately. Simply noticing the sound, such as stating, "I hear you sighing so strongly," can impart concern and listening to what is not spoken.

Personal Space. Personal space is the need to gain, maintain, and defend one's right to their space. Personal space is important because it provides people with a sense of identity, security, and control. Personal space can be distinguished and made visible to other people, as with a fence around a yard or a curtain around a bed in a hospital room. Personal space, however, is invisible and individual, connoting boundaries beyond the physical territory. Boundaries such as physical or emotional space can be defended just like another sort of fence or barrier. Some people choose when to open the gate of a fence, and others simply leave the boundary wide open, taking whatever comes through. When personal space becomes threatened, people respond defensively and communicate less effectively. Specific contexts may dictate whether the physical or emotional distance between nurse and patient is appropriate. Because of the nature of caregiving, nurses often must move into a patient's personal space, even entering a more vulnerable zone in that personal space. For instance, when conducting an in-depth patient assessment or performing an intervention such as wound care, there is necessarily close personal and emotional contact between nurse and patient. Before entering a patient's personal space, it is essential that you prepare both your patient and the environment. By explaining to your patient what you will do and preparing the environment for nursing interventions, your patient will recognize a shift toward the establishment of a therapeutic interaction. You need to convey confidence, gentleness, and respect for privacy, especially when your actions will require intimate contact or involve a patient's vulnerable zone. Box 17-2 provides examples of nursing actions within zones of personal space (Austin & Boyd, 2014) and zones of touch.

BOX 17-2 Zones of Personal Space and Touch

Zones of Personal Space

Intimate Zone (0 to 45 cm)

Holding a crying infant
Performing physical assessment
Bathing, grooming, dressing, feeding, and toileting a patient
Changing a patient's dressing

Personal Zone (45 cm to 1 m)

Sitting at a patient's bedside
Taking the patient's health history
Teaching an individual patient
Exchanging information with health care staff at change of shift

Social Zone (1 to 4 m)

Participating in patient-centred care rounds
Sitting at the head of a conference table
Teaching a class for patients with a specific disease
Conducting a family support group session

Public Zone (4 m and Greater)

Speaking at a community forum
Testifying at a legislative hearing
Lecturing to a class of students

Zones of Touch

Social Zone (Assess for Permission to Touch)

Hands, arms, shoulders, back

Consent Zone (Consent Needed)

Mouth, wrists, feet

Vulnerable Zone (Consent and Special Care Needed)

Face, neck, front of body

Intimate Zone (Consent and Great Sensitivity Needed)

Genitalia, rectum

Symbolic Communication

Good communication requires awareness of symbolic communication, the verbal and nonverbal symbolism used to convey meaning. Art and music are forms of symbolic communication that nurses use to enhance understanding and promote healing. Lane (2006, 2008) found that creative expressions such as art, music, and dance have a healing effect on patients. Patients reported decreased pain and greater joy and hope, and were often more open to communication when creative expressions were part of therapeutic communication.

Metacommunication

Metacommunication is a broad term that refers to all factors that influence how a message is perceived by other people (Arnold & Boggs, 2015). It is communication *about* communication (Devito et al., 2015) that reflects the relational aspects of messages (Adler, Procter, Towne, et al., 2008) and helps people better understand what has been communicated. For example, a nurse observes a young patient holding his body rigidly, and his voice is sharp as he says, "Going to surgery is no big deal." The nurse replies, "You say having surgery doesn't bother you, but you look and sound tense. I'd like to help." Awareness of the tone of the verbal response and the nonverbal behaviour may result in further exploration of the patient's feelings and concerns.

PROFESSIONAL NURSING RELATIONSHIPS

The nurse's application of knowledge, understanding of human behaviour and communication, and commitment to ethical behaviour all contribute to the formation of professional relationships. The intention to promote caring and respect for other people will help you be more successful in establishing professional relationships.

Nurse–Patient Helping Relationships

Helping relationships are the foundation of clinical nursing practice. In such relationships, the nurse assumes the role of professional helper and comes to know the patient as an individual who has unique health care needs, human responses, and patterns of living. The relationship is therapeutic, promoting a psychological climate that facilitates positive change and growth. Therapeutic communication allows patients to achieve their health care–related goals and attain optimal personal growth (Arnold & Boggs, 2015). It includes an explicit time frame and a goal-directed approach, and confidentiality is an expected feature. The nurse establishes, directs, and takes responsibility for the interaction, and the patient's needs take priority over the nurse's needs. The relationship is also characterized by the nurse's nonjudgemental acceptance of the patient. Acceptance conveys a willingness to hear a message or to acknowledge feelings. It does not mean you always agree with the patient or approve of the patient's decisions or actions. A helping relationship between nurse and patient does not just happen; you create it through care, skill, and the development of trust.

The nurse–patient helping relationship is characterized by a natural progression of four goal-directed phases: preinteraction, orientation, working, and termination phases (Box 17-3). These phases often begin before the nurse meets the patient and continue until the caregiving relationship ends. Even a brief interaction can exhibit an abbreviated version of these four phases. For example, the student nurse gathers patient information to prepare in advance for caregiving, meets the patient and establishes trust, accomplishes health care–related goals through use of the nursing care process, and says goodbye at the end of the shift or when the patient leaves the unit.

Socializing is an important initial component of interpersonal communication. It helps people get to know one another and relax. It is easy, superficial, and not deeply personal, whereas therapeutic interactions are often more difficult, intense, and uncomfortable. A nurse often uses social conversation to lay a foundation for a closer relationship, for example: "Hi, Mr. Simpson. I hear it's your birthday today. Happy birthday!" A friendly, informal, and warm communication style helps establish trust, but nurses must get beyond social conversation to talk about issues or concerns affecting the patient's health. During

BOX 17-3 Phases of the Helping Relationship

Preinteraction Phase

Before meeting the patient, the nurse accomplishes the following tasks:

- Reviews available data, including the medical and nursing history
- Talks to other caregivers who may have information about the patient
- Anticipates health care concerns or issues that may arise
- Identifies a location and setting that will foster comfortable, private interaction with the patient
- Plans enough time for the initial interaction

Orientation Phase

When the nurse and patient meet and get to know one another, the nurse accomplishes the following tasks:

- Sets the tone for the relationship by adopting a warm, empathetic, caring manner
- Recognizes that the initial relationship may be superficial, uncertain, and tentative
- Expects the patient to test the nurse's competence and commitment
- Closely observes the patient and expects to be closely observed by the patient
- Begins to make inferences and form judgements about patient messages and behaviours
- Assesses the patient's health status
- Prioritizes the patient's problems and identifies the patient's goals
- Clarifies the patient's and nurse's roles
- Negotiates a contract with the patient that specifies who will do what
- Lets the patient know when to expect the relationship to be terminated

Working Phase

When the nurse and patient work together to solve problems and achieve goals, the nurse accomplishes the following tasks:

- Encourages and helps the patient to express feelings about his or her health
- Encourages and helps the patient to explore own feelings and thoughts
- Provides information that the patient needs to understand and to change behaviour
- Encourages and helps the patient to set goals
- Takes actions to meet the goals set with the patient
- Uses therapeutic communication skills to facilitate successful interactions
- Uses appropriate self-disclosure and confrontation

Termination Phase

During the ending of the relationship, the nurse accomplishes the following tasks:

- Reminds the patient that relationship termination is near
- Evaluates goal achievement with the patient
- Reminisces about the relationship with the patient
- Separates from the patient by relinquishing responsibility for his or her care
- Facilitates a smooth transition for the patient to other caregivers as needed

BOX 17-4 EVIDENCE-INFORMED PRACTICE

Expanding Capacity for Positive Nurse–Patient Relationships Through Enhanced Communication Skills

Some students and nurses may claim: "I'm more technically inclined—communication and relationship skills are not really my strength." While we all have particular strengths and weaknesses in our nursing practice, research shows that, with skills, training, and practice, we can continue to enhance our capacity for communication with positive outcomes for our helping relationship and patient outcomes. Veronique Boscart, of the University of Toronto, conducted a study to evaluate the effect of a 3-hour communication skills training session on the quality of verbal interactions between nursing staff and patients in a chronic care facility. Before the training, which included a lecture, role playing, discussion, and reflection, the staff nurses in chronic care nursing practice were predominantly task oriented and their style of communication was largely authoritative and advice giving in nature. Findings of the study revealed that, even several months following the training, with practice and attention on skills such as inquiry, listening, and validation, the positive qualities of nurse–patient interactions were greatly enhanced. Boscart's study shows that effective communication is something we can learn, and that with practice we can continue to expand our capacity for relational practice (Hartrick-Doane & Varcoe, 2005).

Boscart, V. M. (2009). A communication intervention for nursing staff in chronic care. *Journal of Advanced Nursing, 65*(9), 1823–1832.

social conversation, patients may ask personal questions about the nurse's family, place of residence, and so forth. Students often wonder whether it is appropriate to reveal such information. The skillful nurse uses judgement about what to share and provides minimal information or deflects such questions with gentle humour and refocuses conversation back to the patient.

Creating a therapeutic environment depends on your ability to communicate, comfort, and help patients meet their needs. Comfort is crucial in the practice of nursing. Therapeutic interactions increase feelings of personal control by helping patients feel secure, informed, and valued. Optimizing personal control facilitates emotional comfort, which minimizes physical discomfort and promotes recovery. Creating an emotionally comfortable interaction is something that can be learned, as discussed in the evidence-informed practice guideline in Box 17-4 (Boscart, 2009).

In a therapeutic relationship, nurses often encourage patients to share personal stories, which are called **narrative interactions**. Through narrative interactions, such as reminiscing with patients, you begin to understand the context of patients' lives and learn what is meaningful from their perspective (Shattell & Hogan, 2005). For example, a nurse asked a patient to tell about a time in his life when he had to make a difficult decision. The patient related the following story:

> *"When I was a young man, I worked on the family farm. An uncle died and left me some money. All of a sudden, I could afford to go to university, but Dad didn't want me to go because he needed me there. I had to decide whether to stay or go, and it was real hard because at first I just wanted to get away. I talked to our preacher, and he said it was up to me, to pray about it and do what my heart told me to. So I stayed. Oh, I've thought from time to time what I might have made of myself, but I never regretted it. I had a good life in farming."*

From this brief story, the nurse understood that it was important to the patient to put his family's needs above his personal desires and that seeking spiritual guidance was an important component of his decision making. This same information may not have been revealed had the nurse used a standard history that usually elicits only short answers.

Collaboration between nurses and patients builds relationships and is based on principles of mutual gain and respect. It reflects a desire to satisfy the needs of both parties (Dubrin & Geerinck, 2014). **Collaborative communication** promotes personal responsibility, enables self-expression, and strengthens the patient's problem-solving ability. In addition to patient–nurse communication, nurses also communicate collaboratively with the interprofessional team. These skills are highly consequential to patient outcomes (Institute of Medicine, 2015).

Nurse–Family Relationships

Many nursing situations, especially those in the community, require the nurse to form helping relationships with entire families. The same principles that guide one-to-one helping relationships also apply when the patient is a family unit; however, communication within families requires additional understanding of the complexities of family dynamics, needs, and relationships (see Chapter 19).

Interprofessional Collaborative Practice (ICP) Relationships

Nurses function in roles that require interaction with interprofessional teams (see Chapter 18 for further information on interprofessional practice). Many elements of the nurse–patient helping relationship also apply to collegial relationships, which focus on accomplishing the work and goals at the point of care. Communication in such relationships may be geared toward team building, facilitating group process, collaboration, consultation, delegation, supervision, leadership, and management (see Chapter 11). Nurses need a variety of communication skills, including presentational speaking, persuasion, group problem solving, providing performance reviews, and writing business reports.

Social and therapeutic interactions are needed between the nurse and members of the interprofessional team to build morale and strengthen relationships within the work setting. Within the interprofessional team, all members need friendship, support, guidance, and encouragement from one another to cope with the many stressors imposed by the demands of the health care context (Gottlieb & Feeley, 2006).

Nurse–Community Relationships

Many nurses form relationships with community groups by participating in local organizations, volunteering for community service, or becoming politically active. In a community-based practice, nurses establish relationships with their community (Jakubec & Pike-MacDonald, 2016) (see Chapter 4 for more information about communication in community practice). Communication in the nurse–community relationship includes neighbourhood newsletters, public bulletin boards, newspapers, radio, television, electronic information sites, and social media, whereby community health information is shared.

ELEMENTS OF PROFESSIONAL COMMUNICATION

Professional appearance, demeanour, and behaviour are important in establishing your trustworthiness and competence. They communicate the impression that you have assumed the professional helping role, are clinically skilled, and are focused on the patient. Professional behaviour should communicate warmth, friendliness, confidence, skill, and competence. Professionals speak in a clear, well-modulated voice, use good grammar, listen to other people, help and support colleagues, and communicate effectively. Being punctual, organized, well prepared, and equipped for the responsibilities of the nursing role also communicate professionalism.

Courtesy

Common courtesy is part of professional communication. To practise courtesy, always greet and say goodbye to patients and knock on doors before entering. A courteous nurse will also state his or her purpose, address people by name, say "please" and "thank you" to members of the interprofessional team, and apologize for inadvertently causing distress. When a nurse is discourteous, he or she is perceived as rude or insensitive. Such behaviour sets up barriers between nurse and patient and causes friction among members of the interprofessional team.

Use of Names

Self-introduction is important. Failure to give a name, indicate status (e.g., student nurse, registered nurse, or licensed practical nurse), or acknowledge the patient creates uncertainty about the interaction and conveys a lack of commitment or caring. Making eye contact with and smiling at people communicates recognition. Addressing other people by name conveys respect for human dignity and uniqueness. Asking how to pronounce someone's name and taking the initiative to say the name correctly lays the groundwork for communication. Because using last names is respectful in most cultures, nurses usually use the patient's last name in the initial interaction, but they may use the first name in subsequent interactions at the patient's request. It is important to ask other people how they would like to be addressed and to honour their preferences. Using first names is appropriate for infants, young children, confused or unconscious patients, and close colleagues. Terms of endearment such as "honey," "dear," "Auntie," or "sweetheart" are inappropriate; they may be perceived as disrespectful and unprofessional. The use of plural pronouns such as "we" when referring to patients implies a loss of independence and may be interpreted as condescending. Referring to a patient by diagnosis, room number, or another attribute is demeaning and implies that you do not care enough to know the patient as an individual.

Trustworthiness

Trust entails relying on someone without doubt or question. Being trustworthy means following through on what you say you are going to do. To foster trust, you need to communicate warmth and demonstrate consistency, reliability, honesty, integrity, competence, and respect. Sometimes it is not easy for a patient to ask for help. Trusting another person involves risk and vulnerability, but it also fosters open, therapeutic communication and enhances the expression of feelings, thoughts, and needs. Without trust, a nurse–patient relationship rarely progresses beyond social interaction and superficial care. Knowingly withholding key information, lying, or distorting the truth violates both legal and ethical standards of practice. Maintaining confidentiality and protecting a patient's privacy are also important aspects of communicating a trustworthy professional relationship. Sharing personal information or gossiping about other people communicates the message that you cannot be trusted and damages interpersonal relationships.

Autonomy and Responsibility

Autonomy is the ability to be self-directed and independent in accomplishing goals and advocating for other people. Nurses make choices and accept responsibility for the outcomes of their actions (Halter, Pollard, Haase, et al., 2014). They take initiative in solving problems and communicate in a manner that reflects the importance and purpose of the therapeutic interaction (Arnold & Boggs, 2015). Recognizing the patient's autonomy is important to effective communication.

Assertiveness

Assertive communication allows individuals to act in their own best interests without infringing on or denying the rights of other people (Devito et al., 2015). Assertiveness conveys self-assurance and respect for other people (Austin & Boyd, 2014).

Nurses teach assertiveness skills to other people as a means of promoting personal health. Assertive people express feelings and emotions confidently, spontaneously, and honestly. They make decisions and control their lives more effectively than do nonassertive individuals. They can deal with criticism and manipulation by other people and learn to say no, set limits, and resist other people's efforts to impose guilt. For instance, a nurse, when being asked to complete multiple tasks, may set limits by stating: "I will be able to get to that task, but only later today. Will that still work for you?"

Assertive responses are characterized by feelings of security, competence, power, optimism, and professionalism. They are good tools for dealing with criticism, change, negative conditions in personal or professional life, and conflict or stress in relationships. Assertive responses often contain "I" messages, such as "I want," "I need," "I think," and "I feel."

❖ COMMUNICATION WITHIN THE NURSING PROCESS

In the following sections, the focus of the nursing process is on providing care for patients who need special assistance with communication. The section on implementation, to follow, contains examples of therapeutic communication techniques that are appropriate strategies for use in any interpersonal nursing situation.

◆ Assessment

Assessment of a patient's ability to communicate includes gathering data about the many contextual factors that influence communication. The word *context* refers to all the parts of a situation that help determine its meaning. A context includes all the environmental factors that influence the nature of communication and interpersonal relationships. This includes the participants' internal factors and characteristics, the nature of their relationship, the situation prompting communication, the environment, and the sociocultural elements present (Beebe et al., 2014). Box 17-5 lists the contextual factors that influence communication. Understanding these contextual factors helps you make sound decisions during the communication process.

Physical and Emotional Factors. Assessing the psychophysiological factors that influence communication is especially important. Many altered health states and human responses limit communication. People with hearing or visual impairments have fewer channels through which to receive messages (see Chapter 47). Facial trauma, laryngeal cancer, tracheostomy, or endotracheal intubation often

BOX 17-5 Contextual Factors That Influence Communication

Psychophysiological Context

This refers to the internal factors that influence communication:

- Physiological status (e.g., pain, hunger, weakness, dyspnea)
- Emotional status (e.g., anxiety, anger, hopelessness, euphoria)
- Growth and development status (e.g., age, developmental tasks)
- Unmet needs (e.g., safety or security; love or belonging)
- Attitudes, values, and beliefs (e.g., meaning of illness experience)
- Perceptions and personality (e.g., optimistic or pessimistic, introverted or extroverted)
- Self-concept and self-esteem (e.g., positive or negative)

Relational Context

This refers to the nature of the relationship between the participants:

- Social, helping, or working relationship
- Level of trust between participants
- Level of caring expressed
- Level of self-disclosure between participants
- Shared history of participants
- Balance of power and control

Situational Context

This refers to the reason for the communication:

- Information exchange
- Goal achievement
- Problem resolution
- Expression of feelings

Environmental Context

This refers to the physical surroundings in which communication takes place:

- Privacy level
- Noise level
- Comfort and safety level
- Distraction level

Cultural Context

This refers to the sociocultural elements that affect the interaction:

- Educational level of participants
- Language and self-expression patterns
- Customs and expectations
- Media influences

prevent movement of air past vocal cords or mobility of the tongue, which results in an inability to articulate words. An extremely breathless person must use oxygen to breathe rather than speak. People with aphasia after a stroke or in late-stage Alzheimer's disease often cannot understand or form words. People with delirium cannot focus attentively, and those with dementia often cannot make sense of what is being said. Certain mental illnesses such as psychoses or depression cause patients to demonstrate flight of ideas (words do not keep up to rapidly changing thoughts), constant verbalization of the same words or phrases, a loose association of ideas, or slowed speech pattern. People who are highly anxious are sometimes unable to perceive environmental stimuli or hear explanations. Unresponsive or heavily sedated people cannot send or respond to verbal messages.

Review of the patient's medical record helps provide relevant information about the patient's ability to communicate. Through the health history and physical examination, the nurse documents physical barriers to speech, neurological deficits, and pathophysiological conditions that affect hearing or vision. Reviewing the patient's medication record is also important. For example, opiates, antidepressants, neuroleptics, hypnotics, or sedatives may cause a patient to slur words or use incomplete sentences. The nursing progress notes may reveal other factors that contribute to communication difficulties, such as the absence of family members who could provide more information about a confused patient.

Assessment should include communicating directly with patients to provide information about their ability to attend to, interpret, and respond to stimuli. If patients have difficulty communicating, it is important to assess the effects of the problem. Patients who cannot communicate effectively will often have difficulty expressing their needs and responding appropriately to the environment. A patient who is unable to speak is at risk for injury unless the nurse identifies an alternative communication method. Assistive communication tools and devices may support the nurse in assessment and communication more generally. Some of these tools involve assistive technologies, whereas others may be more simplistic, for example, nonverbal techniques such as simple sign language, lip reading, and so on (Finke, Light, & Kitko, 2008). If barriers make it difficult to communicate directly with the patient, then family or friends become important sources of collateral information about the patient's communication patterns and abilities, as well as for general assessment.

Developmental Factors. Aspects of a patient's growth and development also influence nurse–patient communication. For example, an infant's self-expression is limited to crying, body movement, and facial expression, whereas most older children express their needs more directly, through speech and specific actions such as pointing. Nurses adapt communication techniques to the developmental needs of infants and children (see Chapters 21 and 22 for further discussion of communication with children). Communication with children and their parents requires special considerations. It is important to include the parents, child, or both as sources of information about the child's health, depending on the child's age.

Advancing age may also affect communication abilities. According to Statistics Canada, older persons represent the fasting-growing sector of the population, of which 6 to 12% will experience speech, language, or voice difficulties (Speech Language & Audiology Canada (SAS) (2017)). Although some older persons have varied communication barriers, nurses need to avoid the patronizing tone of what is referred to as "**elderspeak**," or condescending baby talk. Rather, nurses should communicate simply, clearly, and with respect to provide humanistic care for the unique needs of their older patients (Cunningham & Williams, 2007). Box 17-6 highlights tips for communicating with older persons who have communication needs and barriers. These tips can be applied to all patients with communication problems.

Sociocultural Factors. Culture, like communication more broadly, is a process that is experienced between people in a relationship. Awareness of the relational process of culture, beginning with an appreciation of one's own individual perspective, power, and privilege, can facilitate communication and understanding between nurses and their patients (see Chapter 9). Nurses can communicate in what is considered culturally safe **relational inquiry** (Hartrick Doane & Varcoe, 2015) by responding to their patients and families, following their lead, appreciating their unique contexts, acknowledging difference, and engaging with the relational capacities mentioned earlier.

Make a conscious effort to avoid interpreting messages from your own cultural perspective and to consider communication within the context of the patient's background.

BOX 17-6 FOCUS ON OLDER PERSONS

Tips for Improved Communication With Older Persons Who Have Communication Needs or Barriers

- Capture the patient's attention before speaking.
- Check for hearing aids and glasses.
- Introduce yourself.
- Choose a quiet, well-lit environment, and minimize visual and auditory distractions.
- Face the patient, and use facial expressions and gestures as needed.
- Amplify your voice if necessary, but do not shout because it distorts sound and your facial expression could be misinterpreted. Speak clearly at a moderate rate.
- Allow time for the patient to respond. Do not assume the patient is being uncooperative if the patient makes no response or a delayed response.
- Give patients time to ask questions and clarify responses.
- Whenever possible, ask a family member or caregiver to join you and the patient in the room. Such people are usually most familiar with the patient's communication patterns and can assist in the communication process.

Gender. Gender is another factor that influences how people think, act, feel, and communicate. Male and female communication patterns tend to differ, which can sometimes create barriers to effective communication (Beebe et al., 2014). Males tend to use less verbal communication but are more likely to initiate conversations and address issues directly. Females tend to disclose more personal information, use more active listening, and respond in ways that encourage continued conversation. A male nurse might say to his colleague, "Help me turn Jeremy." A female nurse might say, "Jeremy needs to be turned," expecting her colleague to understand the implied request for help.

To practise gender sensitivity in communication, recognize the differences in male and female communication patterns to avoid misinterpreting messages sent by someone of the opposite gender. Conversations with sexual overtones, gender-denigrating jokes, and male–female stereotyping communicate a lack of professionalism.

◆ Nursing Diagnosis

Most individuals experience difficulties with some aspect of communication. People who are free of illness or disability may lack skills in attending, listening, responding, and self-expression. Often, nurses will direct care toward individuals who experience more serious communication impairments, though support for everyone's communication regardless of abilities is part of the nursing process.

The primary nursing diagnostic label used to describe the patient with limited or no ability to communicate verbally is *impaired verbal communication.* This is the state in which the ability to receive, process, transmit, and use symbols is decreased or absent (Doenges, Moorhouse, & Murr, 2016). Defining characteristics include the inability to articulate words, inappropriate verbalization, difficulty forming words, and difficulty in comprehending, which the nurse clusters together to form the diagnosis. This diagnosis is useful for a wide variety of patients with special problems and needs related to communication, such as impaired perception, reception, and articulation. Although a patient's primary problem may be impaired verbal communication, the associated difficulty in self-expression or altered communication patterns may also contribute to other nursing diagnoses:

- Anxiety
- Social isolation
- Ineffective coping
- Compromised family coping
- Powerlessness
- Impaired social interaction

Contributing and contextual factors for a nursing diagnosis focus on the origins of the communication disorder. In the case of impaired verbal communication, these are physiological, mechanical, anatomical, psychological, social/cultural, or developmental in nature. Accuracy in the identification of related factors is necessary to selecting interventions that can effectively resolve the problem. For example, the diagnosis of *impaired verbal communication related to cultural diversity* would be managed very differently than the diagnosis of *impaired verbal communication related to deafness.*

◆ Planning

Once you have identified the origins and context of the patient's communication impairment, you must consider several factors as you design a responsive approach and nursing care plan. Motivation is a factor in improving communication; patients often must be encouraged to try different approaches. It is especially important to involve the patient and family in decisions about the plan of nursing care to determine whether suggested methods are acceptable. Patients and families must be patient with themselves and each other when learning new skills if communication is to be effective. When the focus is on practising communication, in some instances arranging for a quiet, private place that is free of distractions may be helpful. Communication aids, such as a writing board for a patient with a tracheostomy, an electronic communication device for a patient with autism, or a special call system for a patient with paralysis, may enhance communication.

Goals and Outcomes. The primary goal of nursing interventions is to facilitate the development of trust between the patient and members of the health care team. It is important to identify expected outcomes for all patients, particularly when impaired communication is a concern. Outcomes are specific and measurable and provide the means to determine whether the broader goal is met. For example, outcomes for the patient might be as follows:

- The patient initiates conversation about diagnosis or health care problem.
- The patient is able to attend to appropriate stimuli.
- The patient conveys clear and understandable messages with family members and members of the health care team.
- The patient expresses increased satisfaction with the communication process.

At times, you will care for well patients whose difficulty in sending, receiving, and interpreting messages interferes with healthy interpersonal relationships. In this case, impaired communication may be contributing to other nursing diagnoses such as *impaired social interaction* or *ineffective coping.* In such cases, you need to plan interventions to help your patients improve their communication skills. For example, you could model effective communication techniques and provide feedback regarding the patient's communication. Role playing helps patients rehearse situations in which they have difficulty communicating. Expected outcomes for a patient in this situation might include demonstrating the ability to appropriately express needs, feelings, and concerns; communicating thoughts and feelings more clearly; engaging in appropriate social conversation with peers and staff; and increasing feelings of autonomy and assertiveness.

Setting of Priorities. It is essential for the nurse to be available for communication with some immediacy so that the patient is able to express any pressing needs or problems. This may involve an intervention as simple as keeping a call light within reach for a patient restricted to bed or providing a communication augmentative device for the patient to use (e.g., message board, Braille keyboard). When you plan to have lengthy interactions with a patient, it is important to address physical care priorities (i.e., pain or elimination needs) first, so that the patient is comfortable and the discussion is uninterrupted.

Continuity of Care. To ensure an effective care plan, you may need to collaborate with other members of the interprofessional team who have expertise in communication strategies. Speech therapists help patients with aphasia; interpreters may be of use to communicate with patients who speak a diversity of languages; and psychiatric nurse specialists support communication with patients in crisis, or those who may be experiencing altered moods, behaviours, anxiety states, or disordered thoughts and perceptions (Austin & Boyd, 2014).

◆ Implementation

In carrying out any care plan, nurses use communication techniques that are appropriate for the patient's individual needs. Before learning how to adapt communication methods to help patients with serious communication impairments, it is necessary to learn the communication skills and approaches that serve as the foundation for professional communication. It is also important to understand approaches that create barriers to effective interaction (Devito et al., 2015).

Therapeutic Communication Techniques. Therapeutic communication techniques are specific responses that encourage the expression of feelings and ideas and convey acceptance and respect. By learning these techniques, you develop awareness of the variety of nursing responses available for use in different situations. Although some of the techniques seem artificial at first, skill and comfort in using them do increase with practice. Tremendous satisfaction will result from the development of therapeutic relationships and achievement of desired patient outcomes.

Active Listening. Active listening means being attentive to what the patient is saying both verbally and nonverbally. It enhances trust and facilitates patient communication because it demonstrates acceptance and respect for the patient. Several nonverbal skills facilitate active listening. They can be identified by the acronym *SOLER* (Townsend, 2013):

S: *Sit* facing the patient. This posture indicates that you are there to listen and are interested in what the patient is saying.

O: Keep an *open* posture (i.e., keep arms and legs uncrossed). This posture suggests that you are receptive ("open") to what the patient has to say. A "closed" position may convey a defensive attitude, possibly invoking a similar response in the patient.

L: *Lean* toward the patient. This posture indicates that you are involved and interested in the interaction.

E: Establish and maintain intermittent *eye contact*. This behaviour conveys your involvement in and willingness to listen to what the patient is saying. Absence of eye contact or shifting of the eyes indicates that you are not interested in what the patient is saying.

R: *Relax*. It is important to communicate a sense of being relaxed and comfortable with the patient. Restlessness communicates a lack of interest and also conveys a sense of discomfort that may extend to the patient.

Sharing Observations. Nurses make observations by commenting on how the patient looks, sounds, or acts. Stating observations often helps the patient communicate without the need for extensive questioning, focusing, or clarification. This technique helps start a conversation with quiet or withdrawn people. Do not state observations that might anger, embarrass, or upset the patient, such as telling someone "You look a mess!" Even if such an observation is made with humour, the patient may be offended or feel belittled.

Sharing observations differs from making assumptions, which means drawing unwarranted conclusions about the patient without validating them. Making assumptions puts the patient in the position of having to contradict the nurse. Examples might include the nurse interpreting fatigue as depression or assuming that untouched food indicates lack of interest in meeting nutritional goals. Making observations is a gentler approach of simply witnessing, without judgement about what might be happening: "You look tired" is very different from the attached judgement of "You look tired. Were you up all night?"; "You seem different today" is different from "You seem much better today" and simply stating "I see you are wearing lipstick today" conveys something quite distinct from "You look very beautiful."

Sharing Empathy. Empathy is the ability to emotionally and intellectually understand another person's reality, to accurately perceive unspoken feelings, and to communicate this understanding to the other person (Devito et al., 2015). Empathy is expressed when you seek to explore the perspective of another person. Cultivating an ability to empathize requires patience, a sense of curiosity, and a willingness to understand a patient's context and viewpoint. This requires a relational approach starting with a willingness to open the relational space and take action. Empathy can also be expressed in relational communication through strong intentionality, or a consciousness of the purpose and intention of one's communication, and *reflexivity*, which is an attention to one's responses and feelings as they influence communication and decision making (Hartrick Doane & Varcoe, 2007). Such empathic understanding requires you to be self-aware, sensitive, and imaginative, especially if you have not had similar experiences. Statements reflecting empathy are highly effective because they indicate you heard the emotional content, as well as the factual content, of the communication. Empathic statements are neutral and nonjudgemental and help to provide validation to the patient and establish a trusting relationship. For example, to an angry patient who has limited mobility after a stroke, you might say, "It must be very frustrating to know what you want to do and not be able to do it."

Sharing Hope. It is important to recognize that hope is essential for healing, thus nurses need to learn to communicate a "sense of possibility" to other people. Appropriate encouragement and positive feedback—without minimizing the reality of an illness situation or instilling false hope—are important in fostering hope and self-confidence. This can encourage people to take the steps necessary in order to reach their goals. As a nurse, you can instill hope by commenting on the positive aspects of the other person's behaviour, performance, or response. Sharing a vision of the future is a way of reimagining their situation, which can foster hopefulness and creativity through communication. Reminding patients of their internal resources and coping abilities also conveys a sense of hope as a way to establish action and build relationships. You can also reassure patients that many kinds of hope exist, and that meaning and personal growth can arise from illness experiences. For example, you might say to a patient discouraged about progressive changes in mobility: "I have seen your courage and creativity in the past and am curious about how you might be preparing for the changes in your abilities now."

Sharing Humour. Humour is an important but underused resource in nursing communication (Wilkins & Eisenbraun, 2009). Research suggests that a sense of humour is a useful coping strategy for patients, health care providers, and families and an essential communication tool for nurses, as it can strengthen the helping relationship (Wanzer,

Booth-Butterfield, & Booth-Butterfield, 2005). Humour has been shown to have positive effects on both a person's emotional and physiological state (Tse, Lo, Cheng, et al., 2010; Wilkins & Eisenbraun, 2009).

Humour is not without potential communication challenges. It is common for nurses to care for patients from diverse cultures. When nurses interact with patients who communicate in languages other than their own, it is important to acknowledge that nuances of jokes and humour can be misunderstood. Similarly, when either a nurse or a patient attempts to communicate humour while speaking in a language other than that most familiar to them, mistakes and misunderstandings may also occur. Regardless of culture or background, what is humorous to one person simply may not be funny to another.

Health care providers sometimes use negative humour to deal with extreme tension and stress in the workplace, but this can be problematic. What is referred to as "grey zone" humour constitutes behaviours like teasing, practical jokes, and sarcasm. "Gallows humour" speaks to the more grim or dark style of humour, often used in very difficult situations to relieve anxiety or release anger in order to transform negative feelings into something lighter in mood. This humour frequently includes topics such as body fluids, body parts, physical or slapstick humour, and so on (Buxman, 2008). This style of humour has a high potential to be perceived as tasteless and lacking in caring by people uninvolved in the situation. When nurses use this style of humour within earshot of patients or their loved ones, great emotional distress can result. When nurses use humour judiciously and carefully, however, in communication with patients, it can be a highly therapeutic strategy.

Sharing Feelings. Emotions are subjective feelings that result from thoughts and perceptions. Feelings are not right, wrong, good, or bad, although they may be experienced as pleasant or unpleasant. Even though withholding feelings can increase stress and exacerbate illness, people may do so in an attempt to ward off unpleasant feelings or adhere to expectations of others or societal norms. Nurses can gently help patients express their emotions by making observations, acknowledging feelings, encouraging communication, giving them permission to express "negative" feelings, and modelling healthy emotional self-expression. At times, patients direct anger or frustration prompted by their illness toward nurses, who should not take such expressions personally. Acknowledging patients' feelings demonstrates empathy and communicates that you have listened to and understood the emotional aspects of their situation.

When you care for patients, you must be aware of your own emotions because strong feelings may be difficult to hide. Students may wonder whether it is helpful for nurses to share their feelings with patients. Sharing emotion makes nurses seem more human and often brings people closer. It is appropriate to share feelings of caring, or even cry with other people, as long as you are in control of the expression of those feelings and do so in a way that does not burden the patient or break confidentiality. Patients are perceptive and can sense a nurse's emotions. It is usually inappropriate, and may interfere with assessing and caring for the patient, to discuss one's negative personal emotions, such as anger or sadness, with patients. A social support system of colleagues is helpful, as are strategies for supervision and debriefing; employee assistance programs, peer group meetings, and the use of interprofessional teams such as social work and pastoral care may provide avenues for nurses to safely express feelings away from patients.

Using Touch. Many patients experience feelings of isolation related to their personal and social contexts, as well as the increasing technological features of society more generally. Thus, nurses are required, more than ever, to communicate a human connection to their patients. Touch is an important element of communication that conveys many messages, such as affection, emotional support, encouragement, tenderness, and personal attention. People have unique perspectives on touch based on their past experiences and health conditions. For instance, patients in psychosis may misinterpret touch as threatening; patients who have experienced abusive or violent contact from others may be fearful of even well-intentioned touch from a nurse. Touch may also be misinterpreted by some patients as sexual or romantic (Gleeson & Higgins, 2009). In response to the patient's lead, holding a hand or offering a gentle touch on the shoulder may, however, be an expression of comfort, reassurance, and care for some, and may convey empathy in situations when words are insufficient (Arnold & Boggs, 2015) (Figure 17-2).

Students may initially find giving intimate care stressful, especially when caring for patients of the opposite gender. Students learn to cope with intimate contact by changing their perception of the situation. Because much of what nurses do involves touch, you must learn to be sensitive to people's reactions to touch and communicate effectively when touch is required. Touch should be as gentle or as firm as needed and delivered in a comforting, nonthreatening manner. In certain situations, you will need to withhold touch, for example, when interacting with highly suspicious or angry people who may respond negatively or even violently when touched.

Using Silence. It takes time and experience to become comfortable with silence. Most people have a natural tendency to fill silences with words, but sometimes silences serve the need for time for the nurse and patient to observe one another, to really *listen*, to sort out their feelings, think about how to say things, and consider what has been communicated. Silence is an important skill in the capacity to relate with curiosity, to live with *complexity and uncertainty,* and to relate with vulnerability (Hartrick Doane & Varcoe, 2015, p. 22). Silence may provide sufficient space for some patients to talk freely without the constraint of relying on particular patterns of question and answer. Silence allows patients to think and gain insight into their situation, which is crucial to *reimagining* and hope. In general, you should allow the patient to initiate when the silence is to be broken (Austin & Boyd, 2014).

Silence is particularly useful when people are confronted with decisions that require much thought. For example, silence may help a patient gain the confidence needed to share the decision to refuse medical treatment. Silence also allows the nurse to attend to nonverbal messages, such as worried expressions or loss of eye contact. Remaining silent demonstrates the nurse's patience and responsiveness to the patient who may be unable to reply quickly. Silence may be especially therapeutic during times of profound sadness or grief (Box 17-7).

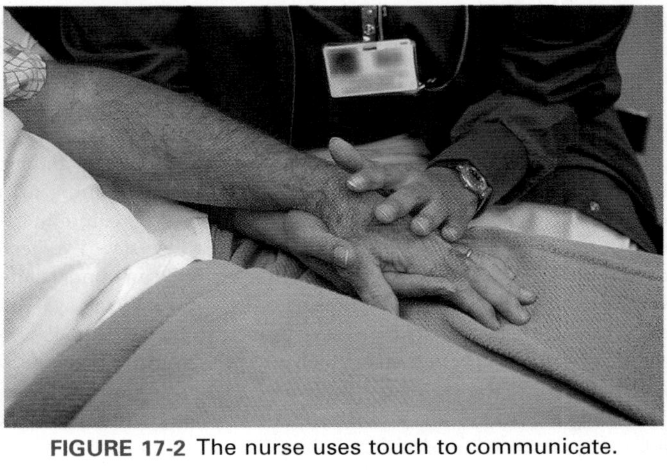

FIGURE 17-2 The nurse uses touch to communicate.

BOX 17-7 CASE STUDY

Communication With a Patient at End of Life

A young third-year nursing student who was assigned to care for a patient at the end of life came to me, as her nursing instructor, to discuss her assignment. The student nurse appeared to be anxious and distraught and was tearful. She requested a change of assignment and, when asked why she felt she needed to be moved, she stated: "I just don't know what I'm supposed to be *doing* with her. She is asking for her family, but they aren't there. She's dying and I just don't know what to do to *help* her." I asked the student what she was doing while she was in the room and she said: "I'm just sitting there holding her hand and listening to her when she's awake. She really isn't talking much, and she drifts off to sleep a lot, but she's afraid of being left alone, so I'm just holding her hand and letting her know I'm there, even when she's sleeping; that way she'll know she's not alone whenever she wakes up. I make sure she's comfortable but I don't know what else she needs. I'm just not *doing* anything." As I looked into her tear-filled eyes, I simply asked her, "So, what makes you think you aren't doing anything?" Communication involves so much more than dialogue. In this case, communication involved very little verbal interaction; it involved active listening, shared empathy, comfort care, gentle touch, silence, presence, and "being with," as the student compassionately accompanied the patient through her final stage of life and assisted with her transition into death.

Providing Information. Providing relevant information that the patient needs or wants to know empowers the patient to make informed decisions, experience less anxiety, and feel safe and secure. It is also an integral aspect of health teaching. Hiding information from patients is not usually helpful, particularly when they are seeking it. If a physician withholds information, you need to clarify the reason with the physician. Patients have a right to know about their health status and what is happening in their environment. Information of a distressing nature needs to be communicated with sensitivity, at a pace appropriate to what the patient can absorb, and in general terms at first—for example: "Majid, your heart sounds have changed from earlier today, and so has your blood pressure. I'll let your doctor know." It is important to provide information that enables patients and family members to understand what is happening and what to expect: "Mrs. Ghaed, Majid is getting an echocardiogram right now. This test uses painless sound waves to create a moving picture of his heart structures and valves and should tell us what is causing his murmur."

Clarifying. To check whether understanding is accurate, restate an unclear or ambiguous message to clarify the sender's meaning or ask the other person to rephrase it, explain further, or give an example of what he or she means. Without clarification, you may make invalid assumptions and miss valuable information. Despite efforts at paraphrasing, you sometimes will still not understand the patient's message and should let the patient know that this is the case—for example: "I'm not sure I understand what you mean by 'sicker than usual.' What is different now?"

Focusing. Focusing centres on key elements or concepts of a message. If conversation is vague or rambling or if patients begin to repeat themselves, focusing is a useful technique. Do not use focusing if it interrupts patients while they are discussing an important issue. Rather, use focusing to guide the direction of conversation to important areas: "We've talked a lot about your medications, but let's look more closely at the trouble you're having in taking them on time."

Paraphrasing. Paraphrasing is restating another person's message more briefly in your own words. Through paraphrasing, you let the patient know you are actively involved in the search for understanding. Practice is required to paraphrase accurately. If the meaning of a message is changed or distorted through paraphrasing, communication becomes ineffective. For example, a patient may say, "I've been overweight all my life and never had any problems. I can't understand why I need to be on a diet." Paraphrasing this statement by saying, "You don't care if you're overweight or not," is incorrect. It would be more accurate to say, "I hear you saying that you're not convinced you need a diet because you've stayed healthy."

Asking Relevant Questions. Nurses ask relevant questions to seek information needed for decision making. Nurses should ask only one question at a time and fully explore one topic before moving to another area. During patient assessment, questions should follow a logical sequence and proceed from general to more specific. Open-ended questions allow the patient to take the conversational lead and introduce pertinent information about a topic, for example, "What's your biggest concern now?" Focused questions are used when more specific information is needed in an area: "How has your pain affected your life at home?" Patients should be allowed to fully respond to an open-ended question before the nurse asks more focused questions. Closed-ended questions elicit yes, no, or one-word responses, such as the question "How many times a day are you taking pain medication?" Although closed-ended questions are helpful during assessment, they are generally less useful during therapeutic exchanges.

Asking too many questions is sometimes dehumanizing. Seeking primarily factual information does not allow you or your patient to establish a meaningful relationship or deal with important emotional issues. It is a way to ignore uncomfortable areas in favour of more comfortable, neutral topics. A useful exercise is to try conversing with another person without asking a single question. By giving general leads ("Tell me about it"), making observations, paraphrasing, focusing, providing information, and so forth, you may discover important information that would have remained hidden if communication were limited primarily to questions.

Summarizing. Summarizing is a concise review of key aspects of an interaction. Summarizing brings a sense of satisfaction and closure to an individual conversation and is especially helpful during the termination phase of a nurse–patient relationship. By reviewing a conversation, participants focus on key issues and add relevant information as needed. Beginning a new interaction by summarizing a previous one helps the patient recall topics discussed and shows the patient that the nurse has analyzed the communication. Summarizing also clarifies expectations, as in this example of a nurse manager who has been working with a dissatisfied employee: "You've told me a lot of reasons about why you don't like this job and how unhappy you've been. We've also come up with some possible ways to make the situation better, and you've agreed to try some and let me know if any of them help."

Self-Disclosure. Self-disclosures are subjectively true, personal experiences about the self that are intentionally revealed to another person. This is not therapy for the nurse; rather, it shows patients that the nurse understands and that their experiences are not unique. You may choose to share experiences or feelings similar to those of the patient and emphasize both the similarities and differences. This kind of self-disclosure is indicative of the closeness of the nurse–patient relationship and involves a particular kind of respect for the patient. It is offered as an expression of genuineness and honesty and is an aspect of empathy (Austin & Boyd, 2014). Self-disclosure should be relevant and appropriate and made to benefit the patient. Self-disclosure should be used sparingly so that the patient remains the focus of the interaction. For example, in response to a patient who has suffered a loss, the nurse might say, "That happened to me once, too. I was devastated … I went for counselling, and it really helped. What are your thoughts about seeing a counsellor?"

Confrontation. To confront someone in a therapeutic way, you help the other person become more aware of inconsistencies in his or her feelings, attitudes, beliefs, and behaviours (Austin & Boyd, 2014). Use of this technique improves patient self-awareness and helps the patient recognize growth and deal with important issues. Confrontation should be used only after you have established a trusting relationship with the patient, and it requires gentleness and sensitivity. For example, the nurse might say to a patient who has chronic pain and decided to forego surgery, "You say you've already decided what to do, but you're still talking a lot about your options."

Nontherapeutic Communication Techniques. Certain communication techniques hinder or damage professional relationships. These specific techniques are referred to as *nontherapeutic* or *blocking* and will often cause recipients to activate defences to avoid being hurt or negatively affected. Nontherapeutic techniques tend to discourage further expression of feelings and ideas and may engender negative responses or behaviours in other people.

Asking Personal Questions. Asking personal questions that are not relevant to the situation but simply to satisfy one's curiosity (e.g., "Why don't you and John get married?") is not appropriate professional communication. Such questions are invasive and unnecessary. If patients wish to share private information, they will. To learn more about the patient's interpersonal roles and relationships, ask a question such as "How would you describe your relationship with John?"

Giving Personal Opinions. When the nurse provides a personal opinion (e.g., "If I were you, I'd put your mother in a long-term care facility"), it takes decision making away from the patient. It inhibits spontaneity, stalls problem solving, and creates doubt. Personal opinions differ from professional advice. At times, patients need suggestions and help to make choices. Suggestions should be presented to patients as options because the final decision rests with the patient. Remember that the problem and its solution belong to the patient. A much better response is "Let's talk about what options are available for your mother's care."

Changing the Subject. When another person is trying to communicate something important, changing the subject (e.g., "Let's not talk about your problems with your job. It's time for your walk") is rude and shows a lack of empathy and mutuality. It tends to block further communication, and the sender then withholds important messages or fails to openly express feelings. Thoughts and spontaneity are interrupted, ideas become tangled, and information provided may be inadequate. In some instances, changing the subject serves as a face-saving manoeuvre. If this happens, reassure the patient that you will return to his or her concerns: "After your walk, let's talk some more about what's going on with your job."

Automatic Responses. Stereotypes (e.g., "Older persons are always confused" or "Administration doesn't care about the staff") and labels are generalized beliefs held about people. A cliché is a generalizing comment such as "You can't win them all" that tends to dismiss the other person's feelings and minimize the importance of his or her message. These automatic responses communicate that you are not taking concerns seriously or responding thoughtfully. Another kind of automatic response is parroting, repeating what the other person has said, word for word. Parroting is easily overused and is not as effective as paraphrasing. Automatic remarks about other people lead to assumptions and closed communication that reflects poor nursing judgement and may well threaten nurse–patient or nurse–team relationships. Nurses may get in the habit of these automatic responses as a defence mechanism or as a way to compartmentalize and organize their work. Observation of one's habitual techniques and approaches is key to self-awareness and communication with others (Austin & Boyd, 2014).

A nurse who is excessively task oriented automatically makes the task or procedure the central focus of interaction with patients, missing opportunities to communicate with patients as individuals and meet their needs. When you first perform technical tasks, you may have difficulty integrating therapeutic communication because of your need to focus on the procedure. In time, you will learn to integrate communication with high-visibility tasks and accomplish several goals—including relational inquiry—simultaneously.

False Reassurance. When a patient is seriously ill or distressed, you may be tempted to offer hope to the patient with statements such as "Don't worry, everything will be all right"; "You'll be fine"; or "You have nothing to worry about." When a patient is reaching for understanding, false reassurance discourages open communication. Offering reassurance not supported by facts or based in reality typically does more harm than good. Although you may be attempting to be kind, such reassurance has the secondary effect of helping you avoid the patient's distress, tends to block conversation, and discourages further expression of feelings. A more relational nursing response is "It must be difficult not to know what the surgeon will find. What might be helpful to you at this time?"

Sympathy. Sympathy is concern, sorrow, sadness, or pity felt for the patient generated by personal identification with the patient's needs (Grover, 2005). Sympathy is a subjective vision of another person's viewpoint that prevents a clear perspective of the issues confronting that person. If you overidentify with the patient (e.g., "I'm so sorry about your mastectomy; it must be terrible to lose a breast"), you will lose objectivity and be unable to effectively help the patient work through his or her situation (Arnold & Boggs, 2015). Although sympathy is a compassionate response to another's situation, it may not be as responsive and therapeutic as empathy. A more empathic approach is "The loss of a breast is a major change. How do you think it will affect your life?"

Asking for Explanations. You may be tempted to ask your patient to explain why he or she believes, feels, or has acted in a certain way (e.g., "Why are you so anxious?"). Patients frequently interpret "why" questions as accusations or think you already know the reason and are simply testing them. "Why" questions tend to interrupt patients' descriptions of their feelings and experience and cause them to refocus their energy into intellectual or defensive responses (Shattell & Hogan, 2005). Regardless of your motivation, "why" questions can cause resentment, insecurity, and mistrust. If you require additional information, it is best to phrase questions to avoid using "why"—for example, "You seem upset. What's on your mind?" or "Tell me about how you are feeling today compared to yesterday" is more likely to help the anxious patient to communicate.

Approval or Disapproval. It is important to not impose your personal attitudes, values, beliefs, and moral standards on other people while in the professional helping role (e.g., "You shouldn't even think about assisted suicide; it's not right"). Other people have the right to speak their minds and make their own decisions. Judgemental responses often contain terms such as *should, ought, good, bad, right,* and *wrong.* Agreeing or disagreeing conveys the subtle message that you are making value judgements about the patient's decisions. Approving implies that the behaviour being praised is the only acceptable one. Often the patient shares a decision not in an effort to seek approval but to provide a means to discuss feelings. On the other hand, disapproving implies that the patient needs to meet your expectations or standards. Instead, help patients explore their own beliefs and decisions. The nursing response "I'm surprised you're considering assisted suicide; tell me more" gives the patient a chance to express ideas or feelings without fear of being judged.

Defensive Responses. Becoming defensive in response to criticism (e.g., "No one here would intentionally lie to you") implies that the other person has no right to an opinion. The sender's concerns are ignored when you focus on the need for self-defence, defence of the health care team, or defence of other people. When patients express criticism, it is important to listen to what they have to say. Listening does not imply agreement. To discover reasons for a patient's anger or dissatisfaction, you must listen without defensiveness or judgement and criticism. By avoiding defensiveness, you can defuse anger and uncover deeper concerns: "It sounds as if you believe people have been dishonest with you. That must make it difficult for you to trust anyone."

Passive or Aggressive Responses. Passive responses (e.g., "Things are bad, and I can't do anything about it") serve to avoid conflict or sidestep issues. They reflect feelings of sadness, depression, anxiety, powerlessness, and hopelessness. Aggressive responses (e.g., "Things are bad, and it's all your fault") provoke confrontation at the other person's expense and reflect feelings of anger, frustration, resentment, and stress. When nurses lack assertiveness skills, they may also use triangulation, complaining to a third party rather than confronting the problem or expressing concerns directly to the source. This lowers team morale and draws other people into the conflict situation. Assertive communication establishes boundaries and expectations without the blame or judgement implied in passive and aggressive responses. An assertive approach imparts intention and action that will support the ongoing professional therapeutic relationship.

Arguing. Challenging or arguing against perceptions (e.g., "How can you say you didn't sleep a wink, when I heard you snoring all night long?") denies that they are real and valid to the other person. They imply that the other person is lying, misinformed, or uneducated. Skillful nurses give information or present reality in a way that avoids argument: "You feel as if you didn't get any rest at all last night, even though I thought you slept well because you seemed peaceful when I checked your room during the night."

Adapting Communication Techniques for the Patient With Special Needs. The temporary or permanent loss of the ability to speak is extremely traumatic to an individual. It is important to assess a patient's alternative communication method and whether it causes anxiety in the patient. Patients who have undergone laryngectomies often write notes, use communication boards or laptop computers, speak with mechanical vibrators, or use esophageal speech. Patients with endotracheal or tracheostomy tubes have a temporary loss of speech. Most use a notepad to write their questions and requests. However, the patient may become incapacitated and unable to write messages. You need to determine whether the patient has developed a sign language or system of symbols to communicate needs. If not, you may need to assist the patient in developing a meaningful method during a new or temporary loss of communication.

Interacting effectively with patients who have conditions that impair communication requires special thought, sensitivity, creativity, and responsiveness. Such patients benefit greatly when you adapt communication techniques to their unique circumstances or developmental level. For example, if you are caring for a patient with impaired verbal communication related to mechanical ventilation, you can provide a visual table or construct a coded hand signal to exchange necessary communication. You and the patient can use such tools to help communicate for assessment and interventions. Similar techniques can be used with patients suffering with aphasia or some dementias.

Patients with **aphasia** may be unable to produce or understand language. **Expressive aphasia**, a motor type of aphasia, is the inability to name common objects or to express simple ideas in words or writing. For example, a patient may understand a question but be unable to express an answer. Sensory or **receptive aphasia** is the inability to understand written or spoken language. The patient may be able to express words but is unable to understand the questions or comments of others. **Global aphasia** is the inability to understand language or communicate orally.

When caring for patients with special needs regarding communication, you need to direct nursing actions toward meeting the goals and expected outcomes identified in the plan of care, addressing both the communication impairment and its contributing factors. Box 17-8 lists many methods available to encourage, enhance, restore, or substitute for verbal communication. You must be sure that the patient is physically able to use the chosen method and that it does not cause frustration by being too complicated or difficult.

Effective communication involves adapting to any special needs resulting from sensory, motor, or cognitive impairments that are present. Box 17-9 addresses communication and relational practice in the Critical Care Unit.

◆ Evaluation

To determine whether the plan of care has been successful, both the nurse and patient evaluate the patient's communication outcomes. You need to evaluate nursing interventions to determine what strategies or interventions were effective and what changes in the patient's situation resulted because of the interventions. For example, if using pen and paper proves frustrating for a nonverbal patient whose handwriting is shaky, you need to revise the care plan to include use of a picture board instead. If expected outcomes are not met or progress is not satisfactory, you need to determine what factors influenced the outcomes and then modify the plan.

You can evaluate the effectiveness of your own communication by videotaping practice sessions with peers, making recordings, and analyzing written records of your verbal and nonverbal interactions with patients. Process recording analysis reveals faults in personal communication techniques, so that you can improve their effectiveness. Box 17-10 contains a sample communication analysis of such a record. Analyzing a process recording enables you to evaluate the following:

- Determine whether the nurse encouraged openness and allowed the patient to "tell his or her story," expressing both thoughts and feelings
- Identify any missed verbal or nonverbal cues or conversational themes
- Examine whether nursing responses blocked or facilitated the patient's efforts to communicate
- Determine whether nursing responses were positive and supportive or superficial and judgemental
- Examine the type and number of questions that were asked
- Determine the type and number of therapeutic communication techniques used
- Discover any missed opportunities to use humour, silence, or touch

Evaluation of the communication process helps you gain confidence and competence in interpersonal skills. Becoming an effective communicator greatly increases your professional satisfaction and success. No skill is more basic, and no tool more powerful, than communication.

BOX 17-8 Communicating With Patients Who Have Special Needs

Patients Who Cannot Speak Clearly (Aphasia, Dysarthria, Muteness)

- Listen attentively, be patient, and do not interrupt.
- Ask simple questions that require yes or no answers.
- Allow time for understanding and response.
- Use visual cues (e.g., words, pictures, and objects) when possible.
- Allow only one person to speak at a time.
- Do not shout or speak too loudly.
- Encourage the patient to converse.
- If you have not understood the patient, let him or her know.
- Collaborate with a speech therapist as needed.
- Use communication aids:
    - Pad and felt-tipped pen or Magic Slate
    - Communication board with commonly used words, letters, or pictures denoting basic needs
    - Call bells or alarms
    - Sign language
    - Use of eye blinks or movement of fingers for simple responses ("yes" or "no")

Patients Who Are Cognitively Impaired

- Reduce environmental distractions while conversing.
- Capture the patient's attention before you speak.
- Use simple sentences, and avoid long explanations.
- Ask one question at a time.
- Allow time for the patient to respond.
- Be an attentive listener.
- Include family and friends in conversations, especially in topics known to the patient.

Patients Who Are Hearing Impaired

- Check for the presence of hearing aids.
- Reduce environmental noise.
- Get the patient's attention before you speak.
- Face the patient so that your mouth is visible.
- Do not chew gum.
- Speak at normal volume; do not shout.
- Rephrase rather than repeat, if your message is misunderstood.
- Provide a sign language interpreter if this is indicated.

Patients Who Are Visually Impaired

- Check for use of glasses or contact lenses.
- Identify yourself when you enter the room, and notify the patient when you leave the room.
- Speak in a normal tone of voice.
- Do not rely on gestures or nonverbal communication to convey messages.
- Use indirect lighting, avoiding glare.
- Use an appropriate font size for the impairment (i.e., at least 14-point print).

Patients Who Are Unresponsive

- Call the patient by name during interactions.
- Communicate both verbally and by touch.
- Speak to the patient as though he or she can hear.
- Explain all procedures and expected sensations.
- Provide orientation to person, place, and time.
- Avoid talking about the patient to other people in his or her presence.
- Avoid saying things that the patient should not hear (e.g., gossip or speculations about patient's condition).
- Always assume that patients can hear and understand everything said at their bedside.

Patients Who Do Not Speak English

- Speak to the patient in a normal tone of voice (shouting may be interpreted as anger).
- Establish a method for the patient to signal a desire to communicate (call light or bell).
- Provide an interpreter (translator) as needed (for further information on working with an interpreter see Chapter 9).
- Develop communication board, pictures, or cards.
- Translate words from the English list into the patient's native language for the patient to make basic requests.
- Ensure that a dictionary (English-French, English-Blackfoot, and so forth) is available if the patient can read.

BOX 17-9 EVIDENCE-INFORMED PRACTICE

Communication and Relational Practice in the Critical Care Unit

People admitted to Critical Care Units (CCUs) during periods of critical illness may be intubated and on respirators and unable to speak. This, and the highly technological focus of care, can be a source of distress for patients; however, the nurse–patient communication in this setting is poorly understood. In a descriptive observational study of the noninterventional, routine care of patients in a medical and cardiothoracic surgical CCU, the authors attempted to describe communication interactions between nurses and nonspeaking critically ill patients in these settings. The study used video-recorded interactions between 10 randomly selected nurses and 30 critically ill adults. The patients, who were awake, responsive, and unable to speak because of respiratory tract intubation, were rated for frequency, success, quality, communication methods, and use of assistive communication techniques. Patients also self-rated ease of communication. The study found that nurses initiated most (86.2%) of the communication exchanges, with a mean of 2.62 exchanges per minute. The most common positive nurse act was making eye contact with the patient. Communication exchanges were generally (>70%) successful, but communications about pain were more than 37% unsuccessful. Patients rated 40% of the communication sessions with nurses as somewhat difficult to extremely difficult. Assistive communication strategies and materials (e.g., writing supplies, white boards, electronic tablets, etc.) were not well used. The study highlighted several areas for improvement in communication between nurses and nonspeaking CCU patients, specifically regarding listening, communication about pain, and the use of assistive communication strategies and materials.

Happ, M. B., Garrett, K., Thomas, D. D., et al. (2011). Nurse–patient communication interactions in the intensive care unit. *American Journal of Critical Care, 20*(2), e28–e40. doi:10.4037/ajcc2011433

BOX 17-10 Sample Communication Analysis

NURSE: Good morning, Mr. Simpson. [Smiles and approaches bed, holding clipboard]
- Acknowledging by name, social greeting to begin conversation

PATIENT: What's good about it? [Arms crossed over chest, frowning, with a direct stare]
- Nonverbal signs of anger

NURSE: You sound unhappy. [Pulls up chair and sits at bedside]
- Sharing observation, nonverbal communication of availability

PATIENT: You'd be unhappy, too, if nobody would answer your questions. [Angry tone of voice, challenging expression]
- Further expression of feelings, facilitated by nurse's accurate observation

NURSE: This hospital has a fine staff, Mr. Simpson. I'm sure no one would intentionally keep information from you.
- Feeling threatened and being defensive: a nontherapeutic technique

PATIENT: All right, then: Why wouldn't that girl tell me what my blood sugar was?

NURSE: I'm not sure. If I were you, I'd forget about it and get a fresh start.
- Giving advice and using cliché, which is nontherapeutic; would have been better to acknowledge that the patient had a right to know the information

NURSE: I'm going to test your blood sugar levels in a minute, and I'll tell you the results. [Performs test] Your blood sugar level was 20.
- Providing information, demonstrating trustworthiness

PATIENT: That's up pretty high, isn't it? [Worried facial expression]
- Feeling very concerned about test results

NURSE: [Nods; long pause]
- Nonverbal affirmation, use of silence to allow patient time to absorb information and gather thoughts

PATIENT: I'm so afraid complications will set in because my blood sugar is high. [Stares out window]
- Feeling free to express deeper concerns, which are hard to face

NURSE: What kinds of things are you worried about?
- Open-ended question to elicit information

PATIENT: I could lose a leg, as my mother did. Or go blind. Or have to live hooked up to a kidney machine for the rest of my life.

NURSE: You've been thinking about all kinds of things that could go wrong, and it adds to your worry not to be told what your blood sugar is.
- Summarizing to let patient "hear" what he has communicated

PATIENT: I always think the worst. [Shakes head in exasperation]
- Expressing insight into his "inner dialogue"

NURSE: I'll pass along to the technician that it's okay to tell you your blood sugar levels. And later this afternoon, I'd like us to talk more about some things you can do to help avoid these complications and set some goals for controlling your blood sugar. [Stands up, keeps looking at patient]
- Providing information, encouraging collaboration and goal setting; giving nonverbal cue that conversation is nearing end

PATIENT: Okay, I'll see you later.

KEY CONCEPTS

- Communication is a powerful therapeutic tool and an essential nursing skill used to influence other people and achieve positive health care outcomes.
- Relational inquiry depends on approaches to communication that enhance the nurse's capacity to be in relation to patients in often very uncertain and difficult circumstances.
- Communication involves the entire human being: body, mind, emotions, and spirit.
- Critical thinking facilitates communication through creative inquiry, focused self-awareness, reflexivity, empathy, and awareness of other people, as well as the intentionality of purposeful analysis, and control of perceptual biases.
- Nurses consider many contexts and factors influencing communication when making decisions about what, when, where, how, why, and with whom to communicate.
- Nurses use intrapersonal, interpersonal, transpersonal, small-group, and public interaction to achieve positive change and health goals.
- Communication is most effective when the receiver and sender accurately perceive the meaning of each other's messages.
- Message transmission is influenced by the sender's and receiver's physical and developmental status, perceptions, values, emotions, knowledge, sociocultural background, roles, and environment.
- Effective verbal communication requires appropriate vocabulary, intonation, clear and concise phrasing, proper pacing of statements, and proper timing and relevance of a message.
- Nonverbal communication often conveys the true meaning of a message more accurately than verbal communication.
- Helping relationships are strengthened when the nurse demonstrates caring by establishing trust, empathy, autonomy, confidentiality, and professional competence.
- Effective communication skills are facilitative and tend to encourage the other person to openly express ideas, feelings, or concerns.
- Ineffective communication techniques are inhibitive and tend to block the other person's willingness to openly express ideas, feelings, or concerns.
- The nurse must blend social and informational interactions with therapeutic communication skills so that other people can explore feelings and manage health issues.
- Older persons with sensory, motor, or cognitive impairments require the adaptation of communication techniques to compensate for their loss of function and special needs.
- Patients with impaired verbal communication require special consideration and alterations in communication techniques to facilitate the sending, receiving, and interpreting of messages.
- Desired outcomes for patients with impaired verbal communication include increased satisfaction with interpersonal interactions, the ability to send and receive clear messages, and attending to and accurately interpreting verbal and nonverbal cues.

CRITICAL THINKING EXERCISES

1. Ms. Louise George, an Indigenous Elder and a member of the Haida community of Atewaas, must learn how to manage her diabetes mellitus and self-administer insulin injections. Considering the elements of critical thinking for communication, what communication approaches and skills could you use to help her?

2. Jasmine, a nurse colleague of Siew Ping, is having difficulty interacting assertively with Dr. Fielding, a physician who has an abrupt, intimidating communication style. Jasmine frequently complains of tension headaches, pent-up anger, and crying easily. What can Siew Ping do to help Jasmine?
3. Mr. Hess, a patient with Parkinson's disease living at a long-term care facility, has a stiff, expressionless face from his disease. He sits slumped in a recliner chair all day and seems lost in his own world, rarely looking at or interacting with anyone. When he does talk, he mumbles in a soft voice, and his words are difficult to understand. What communication skills would support your relational inquiry with Mr. Hess?
4. Ms. Velma Eberhard, a member of a Hutterite colony in western Canada, is considering whether she should have her two young children immunized before they begin attending school. What communication skills could you use to help her decide, and what traps do you need to avoid in communication about information and decision making?
5. Ms. Esther Simons, a patient who is receiving palliative care, confides in you that she feels overwhelmed with the number of issues she must attend to, now that she's facing the possibility of death. She says, "My thoughts are all over the place. I don't know where to start." What communication skills, based on the critical thinking model, can you use to help her at this point?

REVIEW QUESTIONS

1. The statement that best explains how communication is not about the message that was intended, but rather the message that was received, is:
    1. Clear communication can ensure the patient will receive the message intended.
    2. Authenticity in communication is the responsibility of the sender and the receiver.
    3. Attention to personal space (physically and emotionally) can minimize misinterpretation of communication.
    4. Contextual factors, such as attitudes, values, beliefs, and self-concept, influence relational capacity and communication.
2. Nurses demonstrate active listening by:
    1. Agreeing with the patient
    2. Repeating everything the patient says to clarify
    3. Assuming a relaxed posture, establishing eye contact, and leaning toward the patient
    4. Smiling and nodding continuously throughout the interview
3. During the orientation phase of the helping relationship, a nurse
    1. Discusses the cards and flowers in the room
    2. Works together with the patient to establish goals
    3. Reviews the patient's history to identify possible health concerns
    4. Uses therapeutic communication to manage the patient's confusion
4. It would be most helpful for the nurse working with a patient who has expressive aphasia to:
    1. Ask open-ended questions
    2. Speak loudly and use simple sentences
    3. Allow extra time for the patient to respond
    4. Encourage a family member to answer for the patient
5. Communication for the patient's plan of care requires that the nurse:
    1. Collaborate with other interprofessional colleagues and the patient's family to provide combined expertise in planning care
    2. Consult the physician for direction in establishing goals for the patient
    3. Depend on the latest literature to complete an excellent plan of care for patients
    4. Work independently to plan and deliver care and not depend on other staff for assistance
6. "I'm not sure I understand what you mean by 'sicker than usual.' What is different now?" reflects the therapeutic technique of:
    1. Paraphrasing
    2. Providing information
    3. Clarifying
    4. Focusing
7. "We've talked a lot about your medications, but let's look more closely at the trouble you're having in taking them on time." This example demonstrates the therapeutic communication skill of:
    1. Paraphrasing
    2. Providing information
    3. Clarifying
    4. Focusing
8. Students who provide themselves with positive messages about their abilities demonstrate communication at the _______ level.
    1. Public
    2. Intrapersonal
    3. Interpersonal
    4. Transpersonal
9. A nurse working with older persons is advised to avoid:
    1. Touching the patient
    2. Shifting from subject to subject
    3. Allowing the patient to reminisce
    4. Asking the patient how he or she feels
10. The nurse completing a patient's health history should acknowledge the appropriate zone of personal space and touch as:
    1. 0 to 45 cm from the patient
    2. 45 cm to 1 m from the patient
    3. 1 to 4 m from the patient
    4. 4 m or farther from the patient

Answers: 1. 4; **2.** 3; **3.** 1; **4.** 3; **5.** 1; **6.** 3; **7.** 4; **8.** 2; **9.** 2; **10.** 2

Rationales for the Review Questions appear at the end of the book.

RECOMMENDED WEBSITES

American Sign Language Browser: http://www.commtechlab.msu.edu/sites/aslweb/browser.htm.

This website provides an English and manual alphabet and dictionary, a brief history of sign language, and links to other relevant websites.

Canadian Hearing Society: http://www.chs.ca/communication.

This website provides information about communication and interpreting support for those in Canada with hearing impairments.

Communicative Disorders Assistant Association of Canada: http://www.cdaac.ca/links.htm.

This website provides links to various Canadian and international resources for people with conditions that affect communication.

Establishing Therapeutic Relationships. Registered Nurses' Association of Ontario: Best Practice Guidelines.

- *e-Learning Program:* http://rnao.ca/bpg/guidelines/resources/elearning-program-establishing-therapeutic-relationships
- *Video:* http://old.rnao.org/TR_Video/index.html

Medscape: http://www.medscape.com/px/urlinfo.

Medscape is a resource for physicians and nurses that requires a one-time registration (free of charge) and offers links to current literature on numerous health care topics. Enter "Communication" in the search frame, and the site will list current articles on communication in health care.

REFERENCES

Adler, B., Procter, R. F., Towne, N., et al. (2008). *Looking out: Looking in* (3rd ed.). Scarborough, ON: Nelson Education, Ltd.

Arnold, E., & Boggs, K. (2015). *Interpersonal relationships: Professional communication skills for nurses* (7th ed.). St. Louis: Saunders.

Austin, W., & Boyd, M. A. (Eds.), (2014). *Psychiatric and mental health nursing for Canadian practice* (3rd ed.). Philadelphia: Lippincott Williams & Wilkins.

Balzer Riley, J. (2016). *Communication in nursing* (8th ed.). St. Louis, MO: Mosby.

Beebe, S. A., Beebe, S. J., Redmond, M. V., et al. (2014). *Interpersonal communication: Relating to others* (6th ed.). Toronto: Pearson Education.

Boscart, V. M. (2009). A communication intervention for nursing staff in chronic care. *Journal of Advanced Nursing, 65*(9), 1823–1832. doi:10.1111/j.1365-2648.2009.05035.x.

Buxman, K. (2008). Humor in the OR: A stitch in time. *Association of Operating Room Nurses Journal, 88*(1), 67–77. doi:10.1016/j.aorn.2008.01.004.

Canadian Association of Schools of Nursing/Association Canadienne des Écoles de Sciences Infirmières (CASN/ACESI). (2015). *National nursing education framework: Final report*. Ottawa: Author. Retrieved from http://www.casn.ca/wp-content/uploads/2014/12/Framwork-FINAL-SB-Nov-30-20151.pdf.

College of Nurses of Ontario. (2014). *Competencies for entry-level registered nurse practice*. Toronto: Author.

Cunningham, J., & Williams, K. N. (2007). A case study of resistiveness to care and elderspeak. *Research and Theory for Nursing Practice, 21*(1), 45–56. doi:10.1891/rtnpij-v21i1a006.

Devito, J., Shimoni, R., & Clark, D. (2015). *Messages: Building interpersonal communication skills* (5th ed.). Toronto: Pearson.

Doenges, M. E., Moorhouse, M. F., & Murr, A. C. (2016). *Nursing diagnosis manual: Planning, individualizing, and documenting client care* (5th ed.). Philadelphia: F. A. Davis.

Dubrin, J., & Geerinck, T. (2014). *Human relations: Interpersonal, job-oriented skills* (4th ed.). Toronto: Pearson.

Feldman-Stewart, D., Brundage, M., & Tishelman, C. (2005). A conceptual framework for patient–professional communication: An application to the cancer context. *Psycho-Oncology, 14*, 801–809. doi:10.1002/pon.950.

Finke, E. H., Light, J., & Kitko, L. (2008). A systematic review of the effectiveness of nurse communication with patients with complex communication needs, with a focus on the use of augmentative and alternative communication. *Journal of Clinical Nursing, 17*(16), 2102–2115. doi:10.1111/j.1365-2702.2008.02373.x.

Gleeson, M., & Higgins, A. (2009). Touch in mental health nursing: An exploratory study of nurses' views and perceptions. *Journal of Psychiatric Nursing, 16*, 382–389. doi: 10.1111/j.1365-2850.2009.01389.x.

Gottlieb, L. N., & Feeley, N. (2006). *The collaborative partnership approach to care: A delicate balance*. Toronto: Elsevier Canada.

Grover, S. M. (2005). Shaping effective communication skills and therapeutic relationships at work: The foundation of collaboration. *American Association of Occupational Health Nurses Journal, 53*, 177–182.

Gueldner, S. H., Michel, Y., Bramlett, M. H., et al. (2005). The Wellbeing Picture Scale: A revision of the index of field energy. *Nursing Science Quarterly, 18*(1), 43–50. doi:10.1177/0894318404272107.

Halter, M. J., Pollard, C., Haase, M., et al. (2014). *Varcarolis' Canadian psychiatric mental health nursing* (1st ed.). Toronto: Elsevier.

Hartrick Doane, G., & Varcoe, C. (2005). *Family nursing as relational inquiry: Developing health-promoting practice*. Philadelphia: Lippincott Williams & Wilkins.

Hartrick Doane, G. H., & Varcoe, C. (2007). Relational practice and nursing obligations. *Advances in Nursing Science, 30*(3), 192–205.

Hartrick Doane, G. H., & Varcoe, C. (2015). *How to nurse: Relational inquiry with individuals and families in changing health care contexts*. Philadelphia: Wolters Kluwer/Lippincott Williams & Wilkins.

Hunter, L. M., Logan, J., Goulet, J., et al. (2006). Aboriginal healing: Regaining balance and culture. *Journal of Transcultural Nursing, 17*(1), 13–22. doi:10.1177/1043659605278937.

Institute of Medicine. (2015). *Measuring the impact of interprofessional education (IPE) on collaborative practice and patient outcomes: A consensus study*. Washington, DC: National Academies Press.

Jakubec, S. L., & Pike-MacDonald, S. (2016). *Community health nursing in Canada* (3rd ed.). Toronto: Elsevier.

Lane, M. R. (2006). Arts in health care: A new paradigm for holistic nursing practice. *Journal of Holistic Nursing, 24*(1), 70–75. doi:10.1177/0898010105282465.

Lane, M. R. (2008). Spirit-body healing II: A nursing intervention model for spiritual/creative health. *Cancer Nursing, 31*(3), E24–E31. doi:10.1097/01.NCC.0000305719.90894.e9.

Registered Nurses' Association of Ontario (RNAO). (2013). *Developing and sustaining interprofessional health care: Optimizing patients/clients, organizational, and system outcomes*. Toronto: Author.

Shattell, M., & Hogan, B. (2005). Facilitating communication: How to truly understand what patients mean. *Journal of Psychosocial Nursing, 43*(10), 29–32.

Sheldon, L. K., Barrett, R., & Ellington, L. (2006). Difficult communication in nursing. *Journal of Nursing Scholarship, 38*, 141–147. doi:10.1111/j.1547-5069.2006.00091.x.

Speech-Language & Audiology Canada (SAC). (2017). *Seniors*. Retrieved from http://www.sac-oac.ca/public/seniors.

Townsend, M. (2013). *Essentials of psychiatric mental health nursing: Concepts of care in evidence-based practice* (7th ed.). Philadelphia, PA: F. A. Davis.

Tse, M. N., Lo, A. P., Cheng, T. L., et al. (2010). Humor therapy: Relieving chronic pain and enhancing happiness for older persons. *Journal of Aging Research, 2010*, 2090–2099. doi:10.4061/2010/343574.

Wagner, J., Liston, B., & Miller, J. (2011). Developing interprofessional communication skills. *Teaching and Learning in Nursing, 6*(3), 97–101.

Wanzer, M., Booth-Butterfield, M., & Booth-Butterfield, S. (2005). "If we didn't use humor, we'd cry": Humorous coping communication in health care settings. *Journal of Health Communication, 10*(2), 105–125. doi:10.1080/10810730590915092.

Wilkins, J., & Eisenbraun, A. J. (2009). Humor theories and the physiological benefits of laughter. *Holistic Nursing Practice, 23*(6), 349–354.

18

Patient-Centred Care: Interprofessional Collaborative Practice

Written by Carole Orchard, BSN, MEd, EdD

OBJECTIVES

Mastery of content in this chapter will enable you to:

- Define the key terms listed.
- Challenge your existing values and how these relate to nursing professional values.
- Explore how you gain and use your knowledge.
- Gain an understanding of how your own and professional ways of knowing will shape how you approach and provide nursing care.
- Explore how to integrate your growing nursing professional identity with that of an interprofessional identity.
- Explore your own ways of learning and how these can be integrated to support your learning of how to be a professional nurse and provide care to patients.
- Gain an understanding of the frameworks that provide guidance to what nursing professional practice entails.
- Gain beginning practice in how to develop patient-centred practice using a judgement framework within the context of a case scenario.
- Explore how as a beginning nurse professional you can work within interprofessional teams.
- Reflect on values, knowledge, skills, and judgements that have evolved through your learning in this chapter.

KEY TERMS

Action, p. 296
Aesthetic knowing, p. 297
Analytic interpreting, p. 297
Antecedents, p. 295
Assessment, p. 296
Behaviourism, p. 296
Clinical decision-making process, p. 293
Collaborative leadership, p. 303
Constructed knowing, p. 293
Context, p. 296
Empirical knowing, p. 293
Entry-to-practice competencies, p. 294
Ethical knowing, p. 293
Evaluation, p. 296
Feeling, p. 296
Interprofessional communication, p. 300
Interprofessional competencies, p. 295
Interprofessional conflict resolution, p. 303
Interprofessional patient-centred collaborative practice, p. 299
Intervention, p. 296
Intuitive interpreting, p. 297
Narrative interpreting, p. 297
Noticing, p. 296
Norms, p. 302
Nursing process, p. 295
Patient-centred care, p. 300
Patterns of knowing, p. 293
Perception, p. 295
Personal knowing, p. 293
Planning, p. 296
Procedural knowing, p. 292
Received knowing, p. 292
Reflection, p. 298
Reflection-in-action, p. 298
Reflection-on-action, p. 298
Responding, p. 298
Role clarification, p. 299
Silence, p. 292
Situation–background–assessment–recommendation (SBAR) technique, p. 301
Social contact theory, p. 295
Socialization, p. 298
Subjective knowing, p. 292
Team functioning, p. 302
Thought, p. 296
Values, p. 293
Ways of knowing, p. 292

MEDIA RESOURCES

http://evolve.elsevier.com/Canada/Potter/fundamentals/

- Audio Chapter Summaries
- Examination Review Questions
- Concept Map Creator
- Case Study with Questions
- Audio Glossary
- Content Updates
- Video Clips

It would be remiss for a chapter titled "Patient-Centred Care" not to begin with the story of a patient or client—in this case, Mrs. Black and her family. Nurses need to gain an understanding of the story concerning why a patient is seeking nursing help in their care. These stories must be rich enough for nurses to gain an appreciation for the complex health and social issues many patients are faced with. A failure to learn about their full story can interfere with effectiveness in nursing care and in patients' capacity to reach a health outcome that is realistic to their situation. Here you will meet Mrs. Black and her family. You may also access a video clip of this case by going to the case studies, at http://www.ipe.uwo.ca/Administration/case.html. Through her story, you will learn how to make your nursing care truly patient- and family-centred.

JANE BLACK'S STORY

Jane Black is a 32-year-old mother of three who has just been admitted into the hospital unit that you are working on today. Her diagnosis is diabetes and pregnancy. She is 22 weeks pregnant. She was found at home by her husband when she became drowsy and was having difficulty focusing. She has an intravenous line (IV) of D5W running and was given a loading dose of insulin. Since she is a newly diagnosed diabetic who is also dealing with her pregnancy, she has been hospitalized by Dr. Johansen. Mrs. Black's three children came in with her and her husband, as there was no one else at home to take care of them. They are two girls, 3 and 7 years of age, and a boy who is 5 years old. Mr. Black is a long-distance truck driver who is frequently on the road. He is next scheduled to leave in 2 days. Mrs. Black is a stay-at-home mother who is very devoted to her children.

They live in a three-bedroom apartment that they rent. In talking to Mr. Black, you find out that one of their daughters (the 7-year-old) has cystic fibrosis (CF) and requires a great deal of his wife's time to ensure her lungs remain as clear as possible. Mr. Black asks if there is anywhere he can smoke. You notice that he has tobacco-stained fingers. He also is somewhat overweight. Mr. Black comments to you that he is concerned about how he can manage the children with his wife in the hospital and wonders how quickly she can be discharged home. Mrs. Black also informs you that she has weakness in the right side of her body because of a previous "small stroke" she had about 5 years ago. She tells you she is worried about whether she has to take insulin by injection, because she is right-handed and does not have full use of her right hand since the stroke.

On further listening to Mrs. Black, you find out from her that she has experienced a great deal of thirst and has had frequency [having to void often] for a while but thought it was related to her pregnancy. She also tells you that her mother is a diabetic. Her mother has had a lot of problems with her eyesight, and recently her doctor told her that her kidneys were starting to fail.

(Adapted from Interprofessional Health Education and Research [IPHER]. [2014].* Case of Jane Black. *London, ON: University of Western Ontario. Retrieved from http://www.ipe.uwo.ca/Administration/CaseScenarios/Case%20of%20Jane%20Black.pdf. Reprinted with permission.)

In this case, you can see the complex interplay of the family and their social issues that are affected by the environmental factors around housing, finances, parenting, and child-rearing needs. By only focusing on the immediate needs of Mrs. Black, you would neglect the many other factors that are affecting this family because of her illness. Therefore, when nurses provide care that is patient centred, nurses must integrate a number of dimensions into their practice. As you move through this chapter you will explore how you can prepare yourself to be able to address stories such as Mrs. Black's. This story is woven through the chapter as a way of assisting you to understand how nursing care decisions are made to be patient centred.

KNOWING

As you move forward in shaping your nursing practice, you will all use both, your ways of knowing (Blenky et al, 1986), and also our professional patterns of knowing (Carper, 1978). Each of these terms is discussed in the next sections.

Ways of Knowing

Becoming a professional nurse requires that you first look deeply within yourself, because the values you bring with you into your nursing studies influence your future nursing practice. The way you "know" what you know is influenced by how you look at issues and address them. Blenky, Clinchy, Goldberger, et al. (1986) carried out a study of women's approaches to how they develop their self, voice, and mind. The authors discovered that there are five **ways of knowing**: silence, received knowing, subjective knowing, procedural knowing, and constructed knowing.

Through **silence**, people "feel passive, reactive, and dependent, they see authorities as being all-powerful, if not overpowering" (p. 27). For instance, if Mrs. Black used silence, she would listen to whatever you as her nurse told her and would do as you wished, but she would not question why because she would see you as an authority that she must obey. Therefore, it would be difficult for her to enter into a relationship with you that is patient centred, unless you could encourage her to participate in her care with you. In order for her care to be patient centred, a partnership would need to be established between you as her nurse in a way that you both learn from each other.

Nurses whose knowing relates to **received knowing** believe what they know on the basis of what they hear, and thus they learn through listening. For example, when you take notes in a class and only memorize these notes and then repeat the notes back in your reflections, you are practising received knowing. If you asked Mrs. Black to repeat the instruction you provided to her and she was able to do this but did not question why this was important to her care she might be using received knowing. Again, this would not be a true partnership that is needed for patient-centred care to occur. In order to establish a partnership, you would need to encourage her to share how her life situation will affect her being able to do what you are guiding her in.

However, if you, as a nurse, listen to what others say and then internalize it to assess its meaning to you, you are practising **subjective knowing**. For example, if Mrs. Black shared that she wondered how she might be able to care for herself at home, she might be demonstrating subjective knowing. Mrs. Black would therefore be more likely to be able to participate with you in making decisions about her care, allowing for a partnership to be created. When this internalization becomes a debate within yourself as to what its meaning is to you, you are beginning to use your **procedural knowing**. For example, if Mrs. Black then debated the importance of being at home to care for her daughter with CF, while also realizing that this new diagnosis of diabetes means she could not fulfill this role, leading her to explore who might be able to provide her daughter's care at home, she might be demonstrating procedural knowing. In this form of knowing, you are beginning to identify what your assumptions are and how these relate to your own values. If Mrs. Black was using procedural knowing, then a partnership between the two of you would be a likely way of working together.

And finally, when you are able to compare what you hear against your assumptions and challenge your own assumptions and those of others, you have moved into constructed knowing. If Mrs. Black uses constructed knowing, she might identify which aspects of her daughter's care different family members at home could provide, and then in her mind could develop a plan for discussing their individual roles to achieve the total care that needs to be provided while she is incapacitated. Again, a partnership between you both can be achieved without modifying your interaction with the patient. When the more active forms of knowing (received, procedural, and constructive) provide the means for a nurse–patient partnership to be established, this allows for patient-centred care to occur.

While nursing professional practice requires nurses to use their procedural and constructed knowing, it is important to remember that patients are not always operating at the same level. The success of nursing care with them requires nurses to explore with them the story that brought them into the hospital, to gain insight into how they arrived at the decision to seek help. This will allow you as a nurse to determine how you might develop a relationship with your patient and create a patient-centred partnership.

In summary, for all, knowing by receiving knowledge means deferring to an "authority figure" and accepting without debate what that person teaches you; knowing by procedural knowing means receiving knowledge from others but also considering how this knowledge relates to what you understand. Knowing by constructing knowledge means experiencing something and then considering its meaning not only to you but also to others; you also listen to others and consider their perspective and assess this in relation to yourself.

In applying these ways of knowing to your own nursing practice, questions to consider include the following:

- How do you currently know—by being silent, by receiving knowledge, by perceiving knowledge, or by constructing knowledge?
- What action might you need to take to move yourself into the next level of knowing?
- What way of knowing does Mrs. Black present in her story? What impact would it have on how you partnered with her?

Professional Patterns of Knowing

As you move forward and develop into the nurse you wish to be, you will expand your ways of knowing beyond those just identified. Carper (1978) identified four patterns of knowing that are essential to nursing knowledge development: empirical knowing, or "the science of nursing"; aesthetic knowing, or "the art of nursing"; personal knowing; and ethical knowing, or "moral knowledge in nursing" (p. 14).

Empirical Pattern of Knowing. As you learn about theories and findings from research studies that underpin nursing practice, your understanding about how you can implement patient-centred nursing practice will expand. When knowledge you apply to your practice arises from exploratory, descriptive, or inferential studies about key findings that influence aspects of practice, you will generate knowledge to guide your clinical decision-making process around one of your patterns of knowing referred to as empirical knowing.

However, as Carper and others remind us, this is but one pattern of knowing that nurses use. It does align with much of the research evidence applied in evidence-informed practice, but it also can be limited when it does not include the complex health and social aspects of families that influence how a patient can respond to such approaches. This does not mean empirical knowing is not a valuable asset to nursing practice, but it is only one aspect of nursing patterns of knowing.

Aesthetic Knowing. The way we begin to shape our approaches to care using empirical knowing allows us to reflect on our comfort levels. This is where our personalities and approaches to creating relationships with others come into play. Returning to Mrs. Black and her family, you might approach her daughter with CF who is visiting with her mother, squat down to her height, and ask her how she is doing and how her breathing is today. Then you might ask her what she has been able to do on her own to help with her breathing. You do this because you know from working with children that they like to participate in adult conversations and share what they are doing, rather than be told what to do. This scenario illustrates the integration of empirical knowledge about the impact of CF on her lung capacity coupled with an aesthetic pattern of knowing how to approach children. Another nurse might like to draw pictures and encourage the daughter to draw a picture of how she is feeling today. This action might result in different information being gained. Hence, there is no single way to use an aesthetic pattern of knowing. When you are able to use your own comfort level to develop relationships with your patients and their families, you are more likely to be seen by them as being genuine. Genuineness forms a basis for trust. Hence, your aesthetic pattern of knowing relates to how you, as a unique individual, choose to respond in a patient situation. It is a reflection of your personality and your creativity.

Personal Knowing. How we use our aesthetic pattern of knowing is also based on our pattern of personal knowing. Our personal pattern reflects the knowledge that we bring into our nursing understanding that has been accumulated from experiences in our lives to date. Our means of interacting with others, body movements, expressions of emotions, values that influence the way we view our nursing practice, and interactions with patients, families, and other health care providers create our personal pattern of knowing. Carper (1978) states that, in essence, personal knowing "involves interactions, relationships and transactions between the nurse and the patient-client" (p. 18). Whether practising at the procedural or constructed level of knowing, using empirical and aesthetic patterns of knowing, we are influenced by our personal pattern of knowing.

Ethical Knowing. How we select from our empirical, aesthetic, and personal patterns of knowing is also influenced by our pattern of ethical knowing, which is shaped initially by our own values. Values are ideals that have significant meaning or importance to you as a person, to your family, or to your community (Keatings & Smith, 2009, p. 16). They arise from a person's cultural, societal, or family norms and shape an individual's morality—that is, what one knows to be right or wrong. In the nursing profession, all members need to have a similar set of nursing professional values. These values form the basis of a profession's code of ethics. One of the characteristics of a profession is having a code of ethics. The Canadian Nurses Association's (CNA's) *Code of Ethics* (2017, p. 3) includes the following values:

- Providing safe, compassionate, competent and ethical care
- Promoting health and well-being
- Promoting and respecting informed decision making
- Honouring dignity
- Maintaining privacy and confidentiality
- Promoting justice
- Being accountable

You will need to integrate these values into your own personal values as you socialize yourself to being a professional nurse. These values begin to shape how you approach the care of your patients. If your own personal values are at odds with nursing professional values, then you will need to spend time trying to understand this disjuncture and how you will set aside your own contrary values to ensure that when you practise as a professional nurse you are not neglecting any of the nursing *Code of Ethics* values in caring for patients.

Now let's go back to our patient, Mrs. Black, and your initial "judgement" of the family and their situation. After considering your nursing values, have you changed any of your initial judgements about Mrs. Black and her family? If so, which of the nursing values does this shift in judgement relate to? How will you ensure that the judgement you initially made of Mrs. Black and her family will not interfere with your enactment of these professional nursing values?

The Canadian nursing *Code of Ethics* provides a foundation for how professional nurses practice in Canada. Provincial regulators then use the *Code of Ethics* in generating sets of practice standards that reflect the *nurses' act* in each province and territory. These standards of practice help nurses understand how they can integrate the various patterns of knowing into decision making and the enactment of care into their practice. Therefore, the standards of practice become the norms that nurses use in their professional practice.

Table 18-1 presents one set of nursing practice standards for nurses who practise in Ontario. Your provincial regulator of nursing practice will have its own set of nursing practice standards. You are encouraged to seek these out through your provincial regulator's website (many of which are listed in the "Recommended Websites" section at the end of this chapter).

These standards are designed to be applied across all settings and situations that nurses find themselves in. But they can be difficult to carry out fully as you are learning to become a professional nurse. Your program faculty will assist you in learning your nursing practice so that you will be able to implement the entry-to-practice competencies. The Canadian nursing **entry-to-practice competencies** (Figure 18-1) comprise a common framework of nursing competencies in Canada. All

TABLE 18-1 Nursing Practice Standards

Standard	Statement of Standard
1. Accountability	Each nurse is accountable to the public and responsible for ensuring that her or his practice and conduct meets legislative requirements and the standards of the profession.
2. Continuing competence	Each nurse maintains and continuously improves her or his competence by participating in the College of Nurses of Ontario's Quality Assurance (QA) program.
3. Ethics	Each nurse understands, upholds, and promotes the values and beliefs described in the Ethical Framework (1999).
4. Knowledge	Each nurse possesses, through basic education and continuing learning, knowledge relevant to her or his professional practice.
5. Knowledge application	Each nurse continually improves the application of professional knowledge.
6. Leadership	Each nurse demonstrates her or his leadership by providing, facilitating, and promoting the best possible care/service to the public.
7. Relationships Therapeutic nurse–client relationships Professional relationships	Each nurse establishes and maintains respectful, collaborative, therapeutic, and professional relationships.

From College of Nurses of Ontario: http://www.cno.org/docs/prac/41006_ProfStds.pdf.

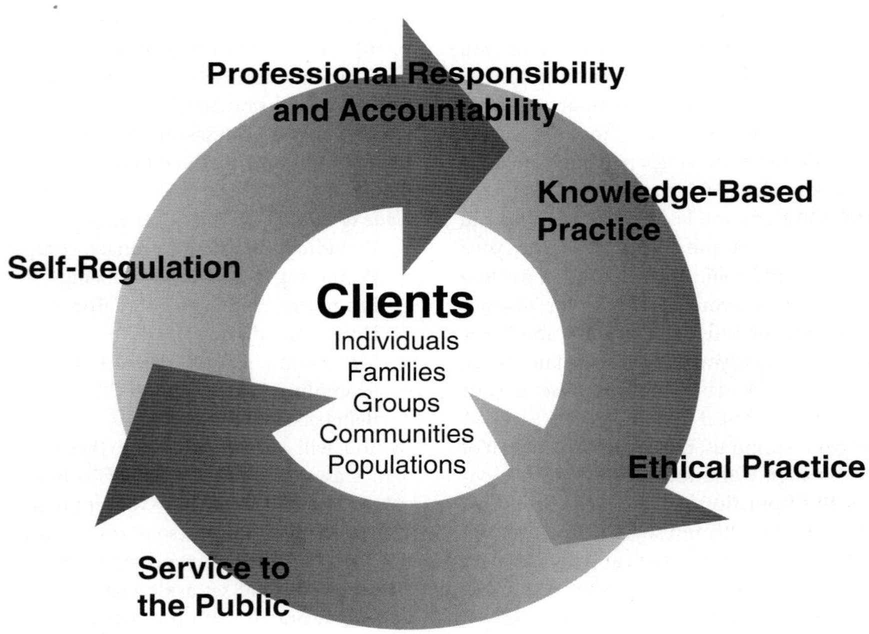

FIGURE 18-1 National framework for organizing practice competencies. (From Black, J., Allen, D., Redfern, L., et al. [2008]. Competencies in the context of entry-level registered nurse practice: a collaborative project in Canada. *International Nursing Review, 55*, 176 [Figure 2].)

TABLE 18-2 Knowledge-Based Practice

Category	Competency	What Competency Entails
Knowledge-based practice	Specialized body of knowledge	Has a knowledge base: From nursing which is informed by other disciplines concerning current health care issues About human growth, development, and role transitions for people of all ages and genders, especially how these impact various states of health and wellness In the health sciences including physiology, pathophysiology, pharmacology, microbiology, epidemiology, genetics, immunology, and nutrition About workplace health and safety including body mechanics, safe work practices, and prevention and management of aggressive or violent behaviour In social sciences, the humanities, and health-related research, (e.g., culture, power relations, spirituality, philosophical and ethical reasoning)
Competent application of knowledge	Ongoing holistic assessment	Engages clients in an assessment of the following: physical, emotional, spiritual, cognitive, developmental, environmental, social, and information or learning needs, along with their meaning of health Analyzes and interprets data obtained in client assessments to draw conclusions about client health status and make a nursing diagnosis where appropriate Engages clients in identifying their health needs, strengths, capacities, and goals Collaborates with other health care team members to identify actual and potential client health care needs, strengths, capacities, and goals

From College of Registered Nurses of Manitoba (2007). *Entry level competencies for registered nurses in Manitoba.* Winnipeg, MB: Author.

nursing programs are approved by their provincial regulators on the basis of how well their graduates are prepared to meet the competencies for entering practice.

These competencies are organized around professional responsibility and accountability, knowledge-based practice, ethical practice, service to the public, and self-regulation. Practice standards and competencies will assist both you (the aspiring nurse) and your learning facilitators to ensure that you learn the knowledge, skills, attitudes, and values necessary to practise nursing. A selected example of one of these competencies (knowledge-based practice) is listed in Table 18-2.

At the same time, learning only within the discipline of nursing creates difficulties when practising with other professionals; rarely will you be in practice situations where only a professional nurse is involved in a patient's care. Consider all the other health care providers who need to be involved (e.g., nurse, social worker, physician, physiotherapist, to name a few). You will already have a comfort level in using your developing nursing knowledge with other nurses, but in today's health care system, you also must interact with other health care providers. To help you begin to develop your interaction with health care providers working in a setting for your practice experience, we will explore some useful tips from **social contact theory**.

When groups (such as your nursing class) study together, they establish strong in-group cohesiveness and loyalty to the group. Consequently, all others outside the in-group (i.e., the other professionals) are seen as out-group members, and those in the in-group feel a level of distrust toward them regarding their understanding of the care needs of patients, such as Mrs. Black. This leads to problems of trust and compromises the ability to work collaboratively with other health care providers. It is helpful to be able to explain your role and your current level of competence in your nursing practice to the other health care providers involved in the patient's care, but in the context of a question you have or help you are seeking from them. Working with other health care providers will be discussed in the context of interprofessional collaborative practice later in this chapter.

The four patterns of knowing help to provide a supporting framework for your professional practice as a nurse, along with the *Code of Ethics*, standards of practice, entry-to-practice competencies, and **interprofessional competencies** (Figure 18-2). Now that we have explored all the various ways you develop and use your knowledge, we will address how your own way of knowing and evolving professional patterns of knowing can be used to create a plan of care for a patient like Mrs. Black.

THINKING

In the knowing section of this chapter we explored what can be termed the **antecedents** used to bring us to the point of being able to provide nursing care for Jane Black (the family in our case scenario). Now we will begin to look at how we can bring the knowledge you are learning in all of your nursing courses to create a plan of care. This is the type of thinking you use to gain insight into some means you want to share with Mrs. Black that might be of help to her.

There are two common approaches that can be used in this thinking process: the nursing process and the clinical judgement model. We will first briefly explore how the nursing process evolved and what it comprises, and then we will explore the clinical judgement model. To align with this chapter's focus on patient-centred collaborative process, the integration of Mrs. Black's case will use the latter approach.

NURSING PROCESS

In the mid-1970s, Orlando put forward her view that nursing would not receive its just rewards until there is "learning to understand what is happening between the nurse and the patient, the central core of the nurse's practice and the framework for the help the nurse gives the patient" (Schmieding, 1983, p. 75). She theorized that nursing is about patients coming to seek help from nurses, and the role of nurses is to find out what help patients need from nurses and then explore how nurses can meet their needs. To support this, Orlando's research focused on the process that nurses used to arrive at good outcomes for their patients. She called these good outcomes "deliberate formulations," which were later renamed as the "nursing process."

Orlando's work transformed the way nurses practised nursing into what was termed the **nursing process**. Within the nursing process, Orlando believed that nurses needed to use a sequence of the following steps: (1) **perception**—finding out how the person perceives using the

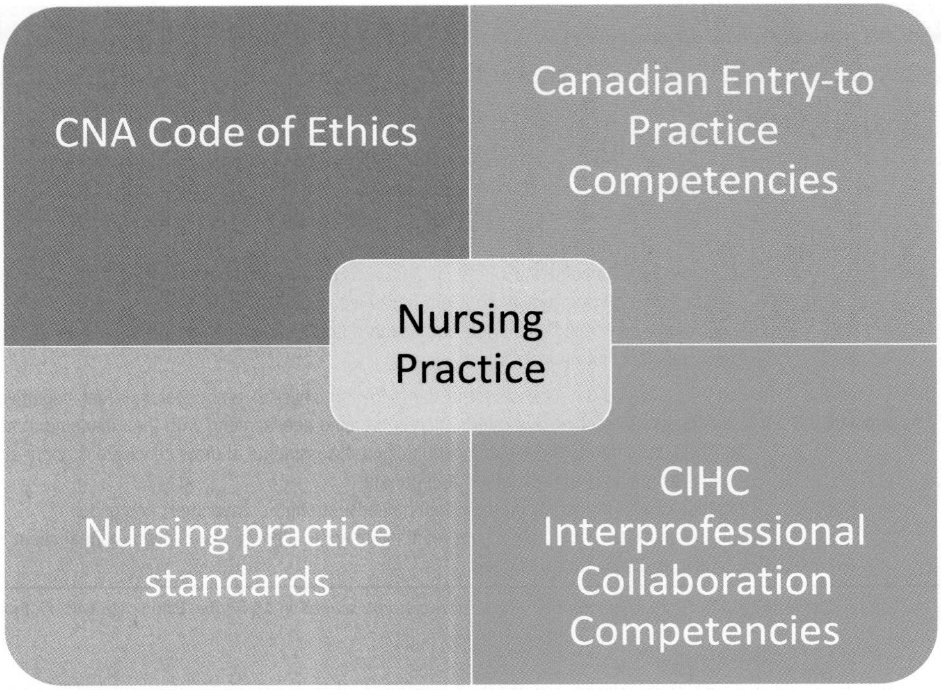

FIGURE 18-2 Foundation of nursing practice. CIHC, Canadian Interprofessional Health Collaborative; CNA, Canadian Nursing Association.

five senses; (2) **thought**—this perception stimulates automatic thinking; (3) **feeling**—thinking stimulates feelings; and (4) **action**—the person takes action. The processing of these four components within the nurse–patient encounter takes place through the nursing process. The process continues until all unmet needs are addressed, or the patient chooses to withdraw from the ongoing interaction with the nurse.

The introduction of the nursing process created a significant shift in nursing practice. This shift occurred at a time when society was continuing to adopt stimulus–response approaches to learning and action, also referred to as **behaviourism**. Previously, the measure of success in nursing care had been related to which changes in patient behaviours could be observed. The nursing profession adopted Orlando's concept of nursing process and institutionalized its application through a linear set of problem-solving stages: **assessment**, **planning**, **intervention**, and **evaluation**. In assessment, generally the nurse is provided with a set of guidelines as to what is to be assessed. Approaches vary depending on the health care agency—some develop their forms related to a specific nursing theory, whereas others may use a "head-to-toe" check system. The criticism of the current approaches relates to how well these assist in linking all the components of nursing care. Others suggest that the centrality of listening to the patient's story about why they are seeking help is often missed (Sahlsten, Larsson, Plos, et al., 2005). During planning, a set document is provided that generally provides the means to enter data collected against set goals for each identified problem or nursing diagnosis. The limitation of the nursing process is in its failure to allow for the thinking processes that shape nurses' decision making for patient care outcomes.

CLINICAL JUDGEMENT MODEL

Tanner (2006) provided an innovative model for pulling all learning together, which she calls the *model of clinical judgement* (Figure 18-3). In her model, she suggests there are four aspects needed to bring all the pieces of information—here, about the Black family—together: *noticing, interpreting, responding,* and *reflecting.*

All of these aspects are influenced by the **context**, or situation where the patient–nurse encounter occurs, the background of all persons involved, and the relationships that develop between the nurse and patient and family—in the case scenario, Mrs. Black and Mr. Black.

Noticing

Noticing equates to *assessment* in the traditional nursing process. In this process, as the nurse reading the case about the Black family you need to notice what key aspects are being presented to more fully understand how each relates to actual observable signs and statements from Mrs. Black. A patient's story is not always told in a clear, chronological order, and not all of the pieces fit nicely together as the story is first presented. Often, there are pieces in the story that are missing. These pieces are critical for you to gain a full picture of the situation that the Black family currently find themselves in. First, take the key points presented in the case. Then consider what more you need to learn in order to be able to fully understand the situation and how you might be able to develop a plan to address these needs for the family. In a real situation, you would go back and ask the family members for more information. A critical piece of information to ask any patient is what his or her goals are. This helps you to focus your further exploration around the patient's goals. As an aspiring registered nurse, you need to realize that time in practice is critical for being able to meet your future workload, so now is the time to create efficient ways to enact your role. Saving time by developing your planning around the patient's goals is an important means to achieving this efficiency in practice. Goals also help you to think within yourself about what nursing knowledge you need to help this family. Once you have completed the noticing phase, you are ready to move into interpreting.

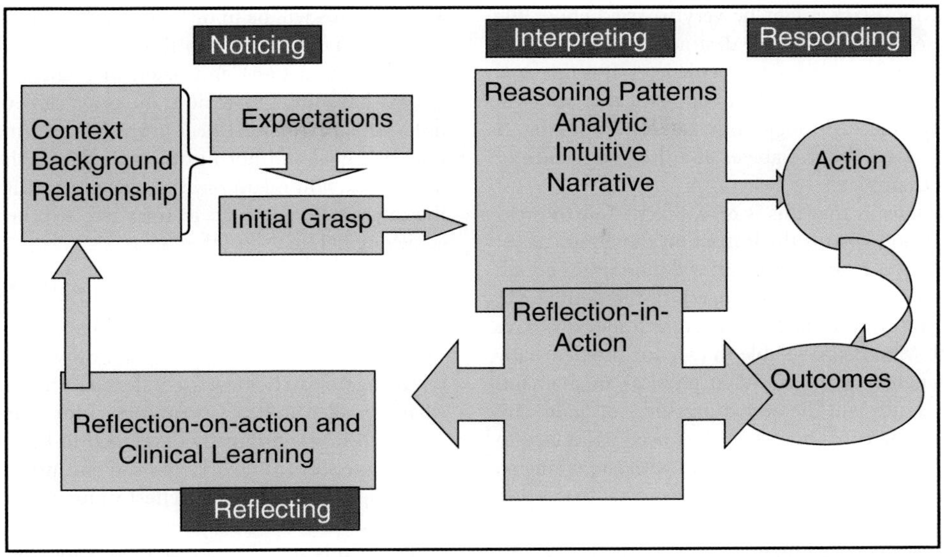

FIGURE 18-3 Tanner's model of clinical judgement. (From Tanner, C. [2006]. Clinical judgment model. *Journal of Nursing Education, 45*[6], p. 208.)

Interpreting

Interpreting means translating information gained in seeking information about a patient using knowledge and skills learned into meaningful actions. As you review the patient's set goal(s) as well as all the aspects identified in your noticing, you then identify evidence you have collected and interpret its meaning within your growing knowledge from theory learning, reading on your own, or previous experience.

To help you see how all aspects identified in your noticing are being addressed, take a piece of paper and draw four columns. Title the first column "Noticing" and the second column "Interpreting." Then, enter all of your noticing aspects into the first column and start thinking about how you can interpret the meaning of each aspect to Mrs. Black and her family in the second column.

Now consider what needs to be addressed in the context of Mrs. Black's presented goals. This is similar to the planning phase of the traditional nursing process. According to Tanner (2006), interpreting information is influenced by three types of reasoning patterns: analytic, intuitive, and narrative. In using **analytic interpreting** you can expand on your noticing aspects by focusing on one family member at a time: Jane Black, Mr. Black, the daughter with CF, and the other children. Then, based on the information you gained in noticing, decide what the health issues are for each person that you need to address. For Mr. Black, you could focus on his smoking and weight problem. For the daughter with CF, her care needs are to ensure that her breathing capacity is not impaired. These are the physical needs. In determining what you feel needs to be attended to, you need to shape this around the expressed goals, but you can also present alternatives related to those goals. You will use all the data you have obtained from the Black family and then add to this knowledge relating to physiology, anatomy, and pathophysiology that you have gained about diabetes, smoking, CF, obesity, and pregnancy. This is quite a list, but knowing about these elements is key to the analytic reasoning pattern you use in developing a plan of interaction with the Black family. Further considerations include the following: What would be the genetic impacts of diabetes on Mrs. Black and the children? What care will Mrs. Black require in order to manage herself postdelivery? What are the concerns of other family members about Mrs. Black and the new baby?

Tanner suggests that you consider which treatments and/or actions will be required to achieve the goals, and then explore with Mrs. Black which alternative approaches might also be possible for achieving these goals. In patient-centred care, you need to take your work on establishing goals to the patient and discuss these with him or her and adjust them on the basis of the patient's goal(s), not just your own, for successful outcomes. In an actual situation, you would combine the above information with actual clinical data, such as tests, blood work, and physical assessment data, to determine the likely achievement of the goals. This constitutes the analytic processes used in interpreting for a patient such as Mrs. Black and her family.

Tanner (2006) identifies another pattern of reasoning that nurses use: **intuitive interpreting**. She states, "intuition is characterized by immediate apprehension of a clinical situation and is a function of experience with similar situations" (p. 207). Depending on the nursing practice experience you have had up to this point, you will bring learning forward as you consider how you will approach the family and their care. McCurcheon and Pincombe (2001) suggest that intuition "is the result of a complex interaction of attributes, including experience, expertise, and knowledge, along with personality, environment, acceptance of intuition as a valid 'behaviour' and the presence of a nurse/client relationship" (p. 344). Even though you are just at the beginning of your nursing studies, you will also bring to it your own experiential learning (personal knowing) that was gained before you entered nursing. This experiential learning evolved from the environment you grew up in, your personality, and your evolving nursing knowledge and practice (**aesthetic knowing**). These components will help you shape how you develop your nurse–patient relationships in practice. For example, just the way in which Mrs. Black expresses her concerns will help you determine what is most important to her and what you will need to address in order to get past her concerns and work on one that you feel is equally important for her health.

Tanner (2006) notes that nurses add to their analytic and intuitive interpretation through use of **narrative interpreting**. She suggests that narrative thinking occurs during the nurse's interactions with a patient and family and "involves trying to understand the particular case and is viewed as human beings' primary way of making sense of experience, through an interpretation of human concerns, intents, and motives"

(p. 207). For example, Mrs. Black might be very worried about the diabetes diagnosis and feel that her life is destined to end in renal failure because of her mother's experience with diabetes. It is this type of information, shared because of unspoken concerns, that you will need to explore with Mrs. Black through your narrative thinking. It will allow you to provide facts about diabetes and the importance of blood sugar control, for example.

Another point to consider is that this is Mrs. Black's fourth pregnancy. Was it planned? If not, what is the impact on the family of yet another child? The family lives in an apartment: will it be large enough for the growing family? Is this an issue of concern to the family? Mr. Black is on the road a great deal of time. What impact does this have on Mrs. Black? How will Mrs. Black be able to care for the new baby while managing their daughter with CF? What physical, mental, and social costs to her own health will the added pressures of child care have on her? What about their income—will they need assistance to manage? How can you structure your relationship with the family so that it is both professional but at the same time allows trust to develop so that you can explore these questions with the family? How will you determine the right time to approach these issues with the Blacks? All of these alerts should come to your attention and will require you to use your narrative thinking to ensure that you gain an understanding of which of these issues is significant to Mrs. Black and her family. Knowing such information enables you to intervene with facts and supports. Each success in Mrs. Black's care is dependent on what is important as a goal or goals to her.

Consider what further knowledge you need to check on, what you feel you need to know to inform yourself about each of the points that is not known to you at this time. Then do your research on these missing pieces of needed knowledge. Consider what you feel confident in working on, related to the goals that Mrs. Black has agreed to. See which of these aspects may be out of your depth of understanding and may require you to request assistance from other health care providers.

Responding

Responding means developing actions and planning implementation to address a patient's identified health and social issues. Discuss with Mrs. Black what planned interventions you are proposing, and seek her agreement on which of these she can support. Then consider the evidence that is needed for Mrs. Black and you to determine if each goal has been reached.

As you can see, patient-centred care requires this ongoing interaction and negotiation with the patient, and may at times necessitate an adaptation of your plan so that it is acceptable to the patient. Furthermore, in this case you need to discuss with Mrs. Black how she and you will know when the goal has been reached. This is a key aspect for responding. Finally, you need to carry out the plan in consultation with Mrs. Black. Shaping your care plan around what Mrs. Black is able and willing to do to achieve her set goals is key to effective patient-centred care.

Reflecting

Reflection is a process that occurs at two levels: assessing a patient's responses during provision of care and then again following completion of a patient's care when evaluating your work. Good nursing care requires that nurses frequently reflect on what has occurred with their care. Citing the work of Schön, Tanner (2006) suggests that two types of reflection are required: **reflection-in-action** and **reflection-on-action**. In reflection-in-action, you consider how your planned interventions are having an impact on moving toward the outcome you are seeking and how the patient, in this case Mrs. Black, is responding to your actions. Coming to agreement about what the focus of achievements will be in order to reach goals helps to prepare you and the patient to reflect on how reaching the goal is progressing (reflection-in-action) and, later, to look back at what you and the patient have done to achieve the goals (reflection-on-action). This is not a straightforward, linear process. Sometimes there is movement in only one goal and not in others. If that is the case, in working with Mrs. Black, you might have to renegotiate with her to help her adjust the interventions, which in turn can help her move forward toward achieving her goals in other areas.

An Assessment Rubric for Tanner's Model

At this point you may be thinking, "Well, it's fine for the author to say that this will all come together, but how will I know if what I am doing is moving toward this level of understanding?" Lasater (2007) developed what she called an "assessment rubric" for Tanner's model (Table 18-3). Although it was originally developed to be used by faculty members to evaluate students' work, you can also use her criteria to judge your emerging ability to provide effective judgements in providing care for Mrs. Black and her family.

Frequently in nursing care there are many options available to us. When we ground our practice in a patient-centred philosophy, it is up to the patient and family to decide which of the goals they wish to work on. Therefore, until you interact with the patient and family, you will not be able to finalize any plan you wish to develop.

Going back to the earlier discussion about Orlando and others' conception of the nursing process, the nursing focus is the patient and what the patient wishes help with. This perspective clearly places the control of the interaction in the hands of the patient. But in the quest for professional respect, nursing has often veered toward defending professional expertise. This has created a power differential between the patient and the nurse. If we reconceptualize health care toward a patient-centred focus and away from a system-centred focus (as currently exists), then the expertise of patients, based on their lived experience with their health issues, becomes a critical focus of care. Patients are the experts in their management of illness. The nurse's role is very episodic, in that the nurse only encounters the patient and family at key points, when they desire nursing assistance. Hence, nurses need to see themselves as partners. Partnering with patients does not mean nurses are totally responsible for a patient's care. Today, because of the complexity of health and social issues that many patients experience, no one health care provider has sufficient knowledge, skills, and expertise to meet all the needs of patients. Hence, while nurses are held accountable for the nursing knowledge, skills, and expertise provided to their patients, this is but a part of the totality of care. Addressing the totality of care requires that you learn to practise within your developing professional role and also learn how you can then practise as a member of interprofessional patient-centred collaborative teams.

As you think back over all the issues that the Black family is facing, which other health care providers do you think may need to assist you and the family in addressing all of their health and social issues? How would you get their input in care planning in a health care institution? Does the health care institution use a team concept for meeting the complex care needs of patients and their families? If it does not, how can you suggest that other health care providers be consulted to ensure that the best care is provided?

As you learn about the role of a professional nurse, you will begin socialization into the profession. **Socialization** is the development of behaviours and attitudes deemed necessary to fit into a cultural group, in this case, the *nursing culture*. In reality, you started this socialization long before you began your nursing studies. Your socialization was shaped by people you talked to about nursing and by the media (both

TABLE 18-3 Assessing Critical Thinking Associated With Application of Tanner's (2006) Clinical Judgement Model

Assessing Effectiveness of Judgement Making	Questions to Consider
Noticing	• What did you observe? • What did you hear? • Did you gain a comprehensive understanding of how the patterns and relationships you identified in the case scenario would likely play out in a real situation with a patient? • Were there key assessment aspects that you failed to consider as being important to understanding Mrs. Black and her care needs? • Why did you fail to consider these? • When you considered the patterns that were emerging from all of the information you gained about Mrs. Black and her family, did you discover any new patterns following some research about each of the patterns? • Were the relationships you identified supported by your readings? • How will you connect relationships between patterns in actual patient encounters? • How will you identify any deviations from the expected patterns in an actual patient encounter? • What information did you need to find to support your full understanding of patterns and relationships in the Black family's care? • Did you find sufficient information to assist you in gaining confidence in moving ahead to interpret both the scenario and learned knowledge from the literature?
Interpreting	• How did you set priorities for care goals with the patient and family? • How well did you make sense of the interrelationship between your identified patterns and relationships, the data you learned from the literature search, and the data you collected from Mrs. Black and her family members?
Responding	• How well are you prepared to interact with the Blacks? • Will you be able to provide a calm environment and exude a confident manner? • How will you choose words that will convey clear communication? • How proficient are you in the skills you will need to implement for Mrs. Black?
Reflecting	• Did you consistently assess how well your planning for Mrs. Black's care fit with her goals and their achievement? • Were you able to connect each of your planned actions to specific goals? • Did you and Mrs. Black develop how you would both know when she was progressing toward her goal achievement? • How would you know when one of her goals was achieved?

textual and visual), leading you to believe certain things about what a nurse is and does. In order to make this career choice, you also explored what other health care providers do. Both sets of beliefs contain truths and myths. While your nursing program will help you to shape your professionalism, it will also cause you to cast off these myths about nursing that are based on information you learned before you came into your program. However, if you do not also attend to learning about the knowledge and roles of other health care providers, your internalized myths about other health professionals will persist well into your practice. This is a further component to address from an interprofessional perspective; it is referred to as **role clarification**. Role clarification requires that you be able to explain to another what a professional nurse's role is and what knowledge and skills you, as a nurse, bring to your patient-centred care (read the activity outlined in Box 18-1).

BOX 18-1 Learning Activity: Role Clarification

Reflect for a moment on what thoughts came to mind as you read the case about Mrs. Black and her family at the start of this chapter. Which values do you hold that influence the way you assessed the members of Mrs. Black's family and their current situation? Take a minute to write these down

Thinking back to your exploration of the nursing role, prepare a written presentation about how you will discuss your nursing role, knowledge, and skill with another student in a health care profession outside of nursing. Then try it out on a friend in another health-related professional program.

Being able to explain what a nurse's role is can help patients such as Mrs. Black, as well as other health care providers, appreciate how they can work with you in interprofessional team work.

INTERACTING

When nurses interact with other health care providers, the artistry that nurses use is often an interplay of balancing what they can provide to the care process while interfacing with the way others see the care needs of patients. Varying aesthetic patterns across disciplines can lead to perceived power disputes among professionals, as well as to disputes between professionals and patients. Interprofessional collaborative practice is about learning to respect the knowledge and skills that are brought into the care process and identifying who is the most appropriate professional to support patients' care needs at key times in their care. When power imbalances occur, these are counterproductive to both effective nursing and effective patient-centred care.

Being a member of such a team requires that the nurse understand how the nursing professional role fits in collaboration with the patient and the interprofessional team. **Interprofessional patient-centred collaborative practice** "involve[s] a partnership between a team of health [care] professionals and a client in a participatory, collaborative and coordinated approach to shared decision-making around health and social issues" (Orchard, Curran, & Kabene, 2005).

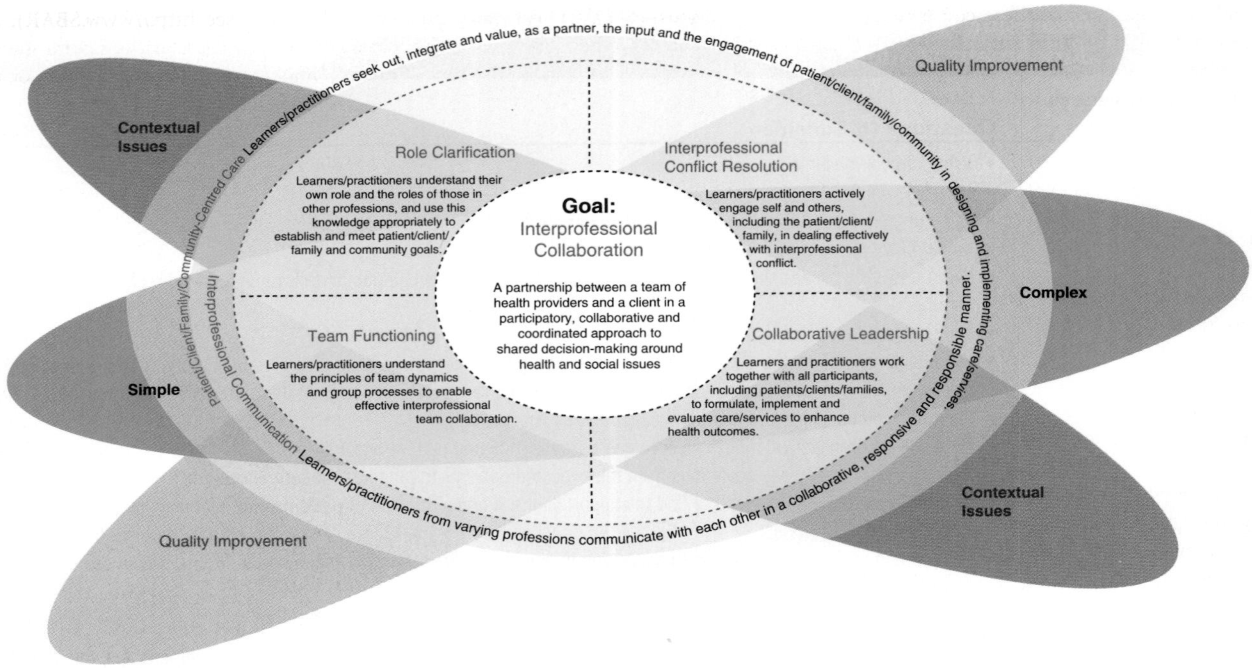

FIGURE 18-4 Canadian Interprofessional Health Collaborative (CIHC) National Interprofessional Competency Framework. (From Canadian Interprofessional Health Collaborative [CIHC]. [2010, February]. *A national interprofessional competency framework* (p. 17). Vancouver, BC: Author. Retrieved from https://www.cihc.ca/files/CIHC_IPCompetencies_Feb1210.pdf. Reprinted with permission from the Canadian Association of Schools of Nursing, Copyright 2015. This illustration is used with permission of the Canadian Interprofessional Collaborative.)

This definition has been chosen as the goal within the Canadian Interprofessional Health Collaborative (CIHC) Interprofessional Collaborative Competency Framework (Figure 18-4). This framework provides health care providers with a means to understand which competencies they need to enact in order to practise collaboratively within a patient's health care team.

In reality, *team* is an amorphous term. In health care, consistency in the composition of teams is often fragmentary, owing to the varying needs of patients. But the concepts within a team may be more important to focus on in order to gain an understanding of what it means to function within a team or group.

In health care, the composition of the health care team changes with each patient, and often team members come and go during the course of care. Hence, the approach nurses use to work within collaborative teams has to be adapted to address the realities of health care. The CIHC competency framework attempts to do just this. First, the framework focuses on how the team functions together—how the team achieves being an intact social unit with its "members" working together. In working together, the team members demonstrate sharing responsibilities and using their interdependencies in managing their relationships across the boundaries of each team member's professional competencies to provide care around agreed-upon shared goals. What, then, makes a team collaborative in their practice? Collaboration can be viewed as both an outcome of a team working together with a patient or as a process used by the team members with their patients in working together to make shared judgements about care to achieve the best outcomes for their patients. Hence, the CIHC competency framework focuses on the judgements made within a group of team members working interdependently with each other with a shared set of decisions to reach shared goals set in consultation with their patients.

Collaborative practice in health care teams is not a constant. Each experience can be unique, thus requiring ongoing reflection about the team's effectiveness in making judgements with its patients. The competencies are interdependent: they overlap and cannot be separated because all are needed to achieve this form of practice. Therefore, the competency framework is viewed as an oval that includes six competency domains. It begins with **patient-centred care**, as well as family- and community-centred care, which ensures that the focus of all care includes their participation in the care, no matter where they are located. Patient-centred care is achieved through **interprofessional communication**, which entails verbal and nonverbal interactions that occur between health care providers and include communicating with patients and family members during team-based meetings. Such communication is based on understanding each other's roles through *role clarification*, which allows team members to work together through a set of team norms to enact team functioning, using a collaborative leadership approach and addressing and resolving interprofessional conflicts or disagreements as they occur (see Figure 18-4).

We have already discussed the first competency domain, patient-, client-, family-, and community-centred care, throughout this chapter. It is described as care in which learners "seek out, integrate, and value ... the engagement of the patient/client/family/community in designing and implementing care/services" (CIHC, 2010, p. 13). Additional support for focusing on both communication and collaboration for nurses can be found in the Canadian Association of Schools of Nursing (CASN, 2015) *National Nursing Education Framework*, which emphasizes the importance of "the ability to communicate using information technologies to support engagement with patients/clients and the interprofessional team" (Domain 4: Communication and Collaboration; p. 15).

We will now take each of these competency domains and discuss some key aspects for you to focus on as you gain practice experiences in your program and learn how to work interprofessionally with others, including patients and their family members.

Interprofessional Communication

You have likely already studied communication in your program (and in Chapter 17). Now we will build on that learning by focusing on key aspects that are affected when you work with other health care providers.

When working with other health care providers, it is important to enter into *interactions* with others and create a shared understanding through an exchange of knowledge, skills, and expertise within a moral/ethical framework of practice (Hindmarsh, & Pilnick, 2002). In essence, when you come to work with other health care providers, you are using communication that consists of unique nursing language and/or meanings, nursing-specific communication patterns, and nursing professional ethical values. Thus, in trying to reach a shared meaning in the message you send to your non-nursing health provider colleagues, there is a greater likelihood of not being fully heard, understood, or both. Interestingly, Adler, Rolls, Proctor, et al. (2009) remind us that whenever we communicate with someone else, we focus on the content of our message, but in reality, our relationship with the other person is actually equally important. Within that relationship, four aspects will influence how the other person receives your message. These are affinity, immediacy, respect, and control, as outlined here:

- *Affinity*—How the person views you and knows about your competence will influence how well that person will listen to you and your message.
- *Immediacy*—How urgent is the message you are sending? For example, if one of your patient's vital signs is far outside the norms, then there is an immediate need to report and gain direction for what intervention should be provided. On the other hand, the patient may be asking when he or she is going to be discharged home. In this case, it is more routine to ask about this issue for your patient. You may decide this information is less urgent and choose to wait and ask at the next "bullet round" (interprofessional short sessions often provided in the morning for a team to discuss needed decisions to be made that day).
- *Respect*—Gaining respect from the team is always a difficult task when you are a student who comes into the unit, perhaps only one or two days a week, and when you are working under the guidance of the nurse who is responsible for your patient's care. If that nurse opens the communication with the team by asking you to pose the question, then this support can help the team listen to your message about that patient.
- *Control*—The openness of a team member in listening to you is often related to the control and power they hold over you. When a team member provides you with an opportunity to pose a question to the team about your patient, there is a greater likelihood that the team will also accept the information you convey.

Hence, the relationship a person has with the team determines how well the message being delivered by any means is actually received, interpreted, and responded to.

Situation, Background, Assessment, and Recommendation (SBAR). The key to effective interprofessional communication is creating a message that is well formulated and presented in a way that bypasses the problems that profession-specific words and approaches can pose. It is advocated that all health care providers use what is referred to as *SBAR* when providing communications. The **situation–background–assessment–recommendation (SBAR) technique** was developed by the U.S. military to improve communications, and it has also been adopted into health care (see http://www.SBAR). Studies have shown it to be effective in improving clarity of communications in teams (Andreoli, Fancott, Velji, et al., 2010; Enlow, Shanks, Guhde, et al., 2010; Marshall, Harrison, & Flanagan, 2009).

Why does it work so well? If we consider communication theory and how we process information, SBAR makes good sense for helping to create shared meanings in interprofessional care. Think about sending a message to a friend: If you want to find out if your friend wants to go to a movie with you tomorrow evening, how would you communicate this information? Let's try to formulate your SBAR message:

Communication Element	Message
Situation	Hi, John, have you heard about the movie *La La Land*? It's playing at the cinema in the local mall. The feedback on Facebook says it is really good.
Background	I remember that you love this kind of movie.
Assessment	I know you don't have a car, so I could pick you up if you like. I was thinking of going on Thursday, to the early show at 5 p.m., right after our last class that day.
Recommendations	So please let me know if you would like to come on Thursday, and if you would like me to drive you. If you want to come, I will go online and buy the tickets.

In this example, if John didn't know why you were texting him, he would not know what you want to contact him about, and he might choose to not respond right away. This is the same in professional communications with another health care provider, particularly if you need another health care provider's help to address something that concerns you about your patient. You first share the *situation*. This allows the person you are communicating with to be able to picture who the patient is and which issue needs his or her help. In the next component, *background*, you convey aspects about previous situations, or new changes that are different from the previous day, for example. The health care provider receiving your message is then able to compare the current situation with previous functioning of the patient, for example. Next, you share your *assessment* of the situation. This allows the health care provider receiving this information to connect what you have observed within the situation. Processing of information allows for connecting the situation and the background with what you assessed in the patient. Finally, you present to the health care provider what your *recommendation* is within your professional competence for practice. In this way, you have helped the other health care provider to process the information using a shared meaning of the situation, background, assessment, and recommendation.

As a student, when you communicate with a physician, it is likely that you will feel anxious about making the call. Preparing your communication using SBAR will help you to ensure that the physician can then ask you questions within the parameters of what you have shared. Such a package of information is welcomed, as the physician is likely having to address issues with several of his or her patients on the same day. The reminders provided through background help to shape the direction of information that you are likely to receive. And the physician will learn to respect you, even if you are a student nurse.

To help you create an SBAR communication, we will refer back to the case involving Mrs. Black. You check her glucometer reading at 11 a.m. and note that it is 10. You are concerned and discuss your worry with her assigned nurse. You both agree that the physician needs to be contacted. Try to create your own SBAR for Mrs. Black's physician managing her diabetes, using the following chart:

	Message to be communicated
S Situation	
B Background	
A Assessment	
R Recommendation	

Role Clarification. The role nurses enact within a team actually often constitutes roles. Earlier in this chapter we discussed the characteristics of a registered nurse and how your standards of practice and entry-to-practice competencies guide you in your practice as a professional nurse. This presentation of your professional role as a nurse is termed a "generic role"—that is, how you are being prepared to be able to practise in any setting. However, when you work with a patient such as Mrs. Black in a team environment, you adjust the knowledge, skills, and your expertise to the situation that Mrs. Black and her family present. Hence, nurses do not use all their nursing knowledge and skills with every patient. Within an interprofessional collaborative team, the nursing knowledge, skills, and expertise used with a specific patient, such as Mrs. Black, is referred to as the nurse's "focal role." It is a set of components from all the nurse's knowledge and skills that is needed at a specific time.

In addition, all team members need to understand how they can participate within their team. The role the nurse uses in the team is then termed a "functional role." We will discuss this role more fully next, under "Team Functioning."

Role clarification has been shown to be a critical element for working collaboratively in teams. This means you not only need to know and be able to articulate your nursing knowledge, skills, and expertise but also need to know that other members of your team can do this.

Most nursing programs in Canada now address this learning as part of the program. If this is not the case in your program, you can learn about other health care providers and their roles at Western University's Office of Interprofessional Health Education & Research (IPHER): http://www.ipe.uwo.ca.

A key area that is beginning to be studied is the role of the patient and family or chosen caregiver within the team. Their roles in the team are equally as important as the role of each health care provider. The IPHER website also provides a description of the patient and caregiver roles.

Team Functioning. In order for a team to function collaboratively, its members need to attend to developing some norms for consistency when they work together. **Norms** are standards that are created and shared by team members to set a tone for teamwork. These are often referred to as the dynamic of **team functioning**. Cohen and Bailey (1997) state that a team is "…a collection of individuals who are *interdependent* in their tasks, who *share responsibility* for outcomes, who see themselves and are seen by others as an *intact social entity* embedded in one or more larger social systems and who *manage their relationships* across organizational boundaries."

Therefore, norms for collaborative health care team functioning relate to *interdependencies* within a team, how the members *share responsibility* for the care outcomes of their patients, and how these members work together around a set of *shared goals* within the overall organization in which they work (Gittell, Godfrey, & Thistlethwaite, 2013; van Schaik, O'Brien, Almeida, et al., 2014). To appreciate team interdependencies, the sharing of knowledge, skills, and expertise can start the process of learning where specific areas of expertise exist and can be used. Also, knowing about each other's roles as professionals helps the health care team members learn where there are shared areas of knowledge and skills. In this process, there is a clarification of *role boundaries*. Knowing about shared areas relieves the potential problem of one health care provider trying to limit another's practice because they believe that they are the only health provider who can perform in a specific area of care.

Developing collaborative team functioning necessitates creating trust in the team. Trust is essential for effective collaborative practice. Research by McAllister (1995) and further developed by Costa (2003) has identified a two-phased process for developing trust of a team toward each member. First, a member's *competence* is assessed. This supports the importance of a member sharing outright his or her knowledge, skills, and expertise. This allows the other members to take this information and assess the key areas identified, rather than searching through all the first member's performance aspects to determine if they will trust that person. In the second phase, one's ability to work within the team is assessed. This consists of a member's willingness to *assume responsibility and accountability* for aspects of care that reflect his or her professional knowledge and skills, as well as assuming a role in the team to assist in its functioning (Costa, 2003).

One of the areas where a functioning role might be demonstrated is assuming one of the roles during team meetings. Team meetings need to have a structure and guidelines for attending to meeting processes. These need to be agreed to by the collaborative team and are part of a team's norms. The roles include chair, recorder, summarizer, and re-director. The *chair* can rotate within the team membership to ensure the same person is not always required to assume this role. The *summarizer* is the person who assists both the chair and the team to periodically remind team members about what they have discussed and agreed to. The *recorder* takes notes as the meeting progresses. Finally, the *re-director* helps the team if the discussion deviates away from the central discussion topic. Guidelines around the use of these roles should be set by the team. In an effective collaborative team, these guidelines are consistently applied to the team's work. To get acquainted with these roles, try assuming one in your next small-group learning session, to gain an appreciation for their value in moving discussion forward and reaching decisions for actions.

Guidelines are also needed to direct how collaborative team members will share information. The SBAR technique discussed earlier in the chapter is used to attend to *what* needs to be communicated (the content), but these additional communication guidelines relate to the *means* or mechanisms that will be used within the team (e.g., text messaging, email, paging, etc.). Guidelines are also needed to determine *when* (needed timing) communications are required and *who* needs to provide the communications. When these guidelines are created and used within a collaborative team, there is a greater likelihood that interdependencies and shared responsibilities within the team can be achieved. A dynamic team is then able to establish *complementary relationships* that result in a cohesive and shared plan of care with the patient and team members.

When a team is dynamic, it has a *cohesiveness* that reflects how its members are *committed to a common task* (in our case, patient care) and subsequently are *motivated to stay* in the team. Motivation to remain is dependent on the rewards that members see for this teamwork. Hence, it is important to ensure that rewards are not individually allocated but are team based for outcomes of teamwork. When equivalent reward structures are in place, members are more willing to contribute to the outcomes of the team's work.

TABLE 18-4 Comparison of Transformative Leadership Elements for a Leader and an Interprofessional Team

Leadership Element (Kouzes & Posner, 2006)	Role of a Transformative Leader	Interprofessional Client-Centred Collaborative Team
Inspire a shared vision	Helps the group to see a desired future	Members focus on client-specified goals and, when the team considers how to get there, help each other to bring their ideas together in an agreed-upon plan with the patient
Enable others to act	Seeks opportunities to innovate and take risks	Members help to guide the team in promoting respect for all members and in arriving at shared goals with patients and team members; encourage other members to take on the leadership role and support patients in their decision making with the team
Challenge the process	Seeks opportunities to innovate and take risks	Collaborative leader in the team carries out ongoing reflection on how the team is working together with the patient and, based on feedback, makes needed changes; thinks about their provider roles within an interprofessional patient-centred context
Encourage the heart	Recognizes contributions of others	Collaborative leader in the team recognizes the positive work of all team members, including the patient, toward meeting patient-set goals for care; helps team members with the patient, celebrates achievement of steps toward patient-set goals of care and well-being

From Orchard, C., & Rykhoff, M. (2015). Collaborative leadership within interprofessional practice. In D. Forman, M. Jones, & J. Thistlethwaite (Eds.), *Leadership and collaboration: Further developments for interprofessional education* (p. 83). Houndsmill, Basingstoke, Hampshire, UK: Palgrave Macmillan.

Think back to a positive team experience. Why was it so positive? Which of the norms discussed were present? Now consider a negative team experience. What was negative about it? Which of the norms discussed here were not present?

Collaborative Leadership. Collaborative leadership is a form of leadership in which all team members work together to achieve a common and agreed-upon set of goals. There is a leader or, as discussed earlier, the person in the chair role who assumes a coordinating function to ensure that the work agreed to by team members is moving ahead as planned in order to achieve the team's shared goals. This leader can also bring the group together in the event that some agreed-upon aspects of the work need to be renegotiated because of unanticipated factors. In collaborative leadership, the coordinator may move around the team so that everyone has the opportunity to learn to lead in the team. In collaborative leadership, all the team members hold the team responsible for meeting planned outcomes. Elements of a team that can demonstrate collaborative leadership include Kouzes and Posner's (2006) elements of leadership, adapted by Orchard and Rykhoff (2015) for this form of leadership (Table 18-4).

The next time you are in a group learning situation, try using these elements of collaborative leadership to see how they work.

Interprofessional Conflict Resolution. Conflict and its resolution is a component of interprofessional communication. However, distrust can occur when professionals from several disciplines are put together and expected to function collaboratively without attention to interprofessional collaborative team building. Thus, in practice, for example, it is not uncommon to hear nurses complain about another health care provider over coffee and behind that professional's back. This distrust can cause one to feel that only members of one's profession really understand the care that a patient needs. In reality, if we were in the other person's profession, a similar discussion would occur about nurses in their coffee conversations. Hence, overall, there needs to be a process for resolving such conflicts and stopping this destructive form of questioning others' competence. How can this be done? As with team functioning, the team needs to be in agreement on a process they can use to address any disagreements. The foundation for this process requires openness in realizing that each member of the team is presenting suggestions that have value regarding what is being discussed. It is important for each team member to listen to and consider each suggestion in relation to their own potential bias against the idea or the person providing it. An example of an interprofessional conflict resolution process with its elements is as follows (Orchard, 2016, p. 268):

- Create openness to hear others' views.
- Consider all views within your own perspective.
- Consider biases that might exist in your viewpoint.
- Consider justification for your biases and how you can come to terms with others' views.
- Weigh the alteration in your view, based on others' views in the context of the patient's safety.
- Share your thinking with the other team members.
- Hear each other's viewpoints.
- Come to a shared agreement.

KEY CONCEPTS

- Patient-centred care is at the heart of nursing professional practice.
- Interprofessional patient-centred collaborative practice begins by first gaining an understanding of one's own knowing within the context of ways of knowing.
- Five ways of knowing include silence, received knowing, subjective knowing, procedural knowing, and constructed knowing.
- Nursing professional patterns of knowing include empirical, aesthetic, personal, and ethical knowing.
- A nurse's knowing is then applied to how the nurse thinks about his or her reasoning process in nursing practice.
- Two approaches used in a nurse's thinking process are the nursing process and the judgement model.
- The nursing process involves perception, thought, feeling, and action.
- The clinical judgement model involves noticing, interpreting, responding, and reflecting.
- Tanner's judgement model of practice is useful for fitting nursing practice within both a nursing professional and interprofessional collaborative team.
- Identifying the nurse's role when working within interprofessional teams of health care providers can enhance competence in such teamwork.

CRITICAL THINKING EXERCISES

1. Challenge your existing values and how these relate to nursing professional values by considering the following case scenario:

   You are a student nurse working with a community health nurse and a social worker in a walk-in clinic in an inner-city area. This is the second week you have been in this placement as part of your initial community health practicum. Jonathan Brown is a 26-year-old male who comes in requesting to be tested for HIV. You notice that he is well groomed and wearing business apparel. He tells you that he is an accountant and has been working in a large accounting firm for the past 3 years. He has just completed his CGA certification and is excited to be joining the firm next month as a chartered accountant. However, he tells you he is concerned because he will have to go through a medical examination for life insurance as part of the firm's employment process. He tells you he is gay and in an active relationship with his boyfriend. He is hoping that the staff in the clinic can help him to determine what his HIV test might show and hopes it will be negative.

   a. What points did you notice in this case scenario?
   b. How are you interpreting what he is requesting be done?
      1. How did you analyze this request and determine what knowledge you already have and what you still need to learn?
      2. What feelings and intuitions emerged as you read over this case scenario? Which values were challenged within yourself that may have caused these feelings?
      3. What further information do you need to ask about from him and your preceptors (community health nurse and social worker) in order to fully understand his request and what services the walk-in clinic can provide?
   c. Determine how you would respond to this situation:
      1. What goals would you set with Jonathan to meet his needs?
      2. What interventions will be provided to meet the goals that have been set?
      3. What evidence will you identify to assess how well the goals are being achieved?
   d. During your reflection-on-action related to this case scenario what surprised you about yourself? Were the feelings and values that emerged unique to your personal values? And were they also consistent with the CNA *Code of Ethics*?
      1. Reflect on what thoughts came through your mind as you read the case scenario at the start of this chapter.
      2. Which values do you hold that influenced the way you judged the members of this family and their current situation?
      3. After considering your nursing values, have you changed any of your initial judgements?
2. To explore how you gain and use your knowledge, consider the following questions:
   a. What ways of knowing have you brought with you into your nursing development?
   b. When you reflect on recent experiences, what was the quality of your listening?
   c. Did you gain knowledge related to your plan of care?
   d. Did you gain an understanding of what is important to the patient about resolving health issues?
   e. Did you gain insight into how the patient wants to cope with the current health issues and how this will have an impact on accepted societal roles?
   f. In terms of clinical learning, what did you learn that you will use in future patient situations?
3. To gain an understanding of how your own and professional ways of knowing will shape how you approach and provide nursing care, consider the following questions:
   a. What ways of knowing do you usually use? Will your current ways of knowing help you to reason through the needs of your patients?
   b. Discuss how you will develop nursing ways of knowing.
   c. How will you ensure that all of Carper's patterns of knowing become part of your professional development shaping your practice?
4. Explore how to integrate your growing nursing professional identity with that of an interprofessional identity:
   a. Reflecting on the interprofessional competencies, how will you ensure that you develop the abilities required to demonstrate good judgements when working interprofessionally?
   b. What actions will you take to gain exposure to interprofessional learning with, from, and about other health providers?
   c. How will you enact your nursing code of ethics within practice situations to ensure that the patient's and family's voices are heard and part of their care planning?
   d. How will you gain both an understanding of and practice in developing collaborative teamwork skills?
   e. How will you identify and work through conflicts or disagreements that may arise during teamwork?
   f. How will you develop the ability to take responsibility for agreed-upon care interventions that reside within the nursing standards of practice and demonstrate accountability for completing assigned activities?
   g. How will you evaluate your own performance with the team and revise your future interactions based on your reflection?
   h. As a beginning nurse it is very important to be able to describe your roles, knowledge, and skills to other members of an interprofessional team. Prepare your own written presentation on how you would discuss your nursing role, knowledge, and skills to another student in a discipline other than nursing.
5. It is important to explore your own ways of learning and how these can be integrated to support your learning in how to be a professional nurse and provide care to patients. To gain understanding of the frameworks that provide guidance to what nursing professional practice entails, you can use concept mapping—specifically identifying patterns to inform nursing care for Mrs. Black from the chapter's case example.
   a. Ask yourself if there is a pattern among these health issues Mrs. Black finds herself in.
   b. Is her pregnancy the underlying issue to shape a pattern?
   c. Did the pregnancy cause an inadequate glycogen conversion in her islet cells of the pancreas?
   d. Or has an endocrine imbalance resulting from her pregnancy caused interference with the effective metabolism of sugars?
   e. What is the pattern?
   f. Perhaps there are several theorized patterns. As a nurse, does the theorized pattern really matter to the care you will provide?
   g. Is there also a relationship between pregnancy and hyperclotability in Mrs. Black?
   h. If so, is she at an increased risk of another stroke?
   i. How does this fit into your pattern of care for Mrs. Black?
   j. What genetic predisposition might be present considering that Mrs. Black already has one daughter with cystic fibrosis?
   k. Does this add to your evolving pattern for her care?
6. Use concept mapping to link patterns identified in Question 5 to forming relationships and how these would inform your nursing care for Mrs. Black.

a. Can the pattern you have begun to recognize now create interconnections to form relationships for your care planning?
b. What impact is her illness going to have on her level of worry about her children and particularly how her daughter with cystic fibrosis will receive the critical care she needs to keep her lungs clear?
c. What about her living accommodations?
d. How will she be able to care for two children needing intensive home care from her when she has continuing weakness in her hand and arm?
e. What impact will her diabetes have on her ability to care for herself and her family?

REVIEW QUESTIONS

1. Sally Jones is a second-year BScN student who was assigned to Mrs. Brandt. Mrs. Brandt, upon seeing Sally, started to cry. Sally was very confused as to what was going on. She asked Mrs. Brandt if something was wrong. Mrs. Brant told her she had just received a phone call from her granddaughter to tell her that she was expecting Mrs. Brandt's first great grandchild. The pattern of knowing that Sally Jones applied in this situation is an example of: *(Select all that apply.)*
   1. Personal knowing
   2. Aesthetic knowing
   3. Ethical knowing
   4. Empirical knowing
   5. Emancipatory knowing
2. Jordan Smith was in a community rotation and encountered a homeless youth on the street as he was walking toward his placement with a non-profit agency. The youth asked him for "change to buy a coffee." Jordan initially felt he should ignore the youth, but then recalled a discussion his class had that week about nursing's role in addressing socially unjust situations in practice. Jordan turned and called to the youth and asked if he would like to join him for a coffee and something to eat. The youth looked surprised by this response, but agreed. As the two sat over their coffees, Jordan started asking the youth about what situations caused him to end up on the street. As the youth explained his situation, Jordan began to fully appreciate how the city and its services were letting this youth down, who just wanted, as he said, "to have a life without being abused all the time." Which of the following ethical values are demonstrated in this situation? *(Select all that apply.)*
   1. Providing safe, compassionate, competent, and ethical care
   2. Promoting and respecting informed decision making
   3. Preserving dignity
   4. Promoting justice
   5. Being accountable
3. Refer back to the scenario presented for Jordan Smith in Question 2. Which of the following aspects of Tanner's judgement model are demonstrated in the scenario? *(Select all that apply.)*
   1. Noticing
   2. Interpreting
   3. Responding
   4. Reflection-in-action
   5. Reflection-on-action
4. As a soon-to-graduate registered nurse (RN), Jasmine Alam has learned to practise as a "real" nurse from her clinical and community experiences in her program. However, Jasmine is starting to worry about how she will be able to assume her RN role and interact with other health care providers who have so much more experience than she does. She recently participated in an interprofessional education workshop at her university that focused on communicating within teams. Yesterday she was in a practice setting and the physician, who was one of her patient's doctors, confronted her and challenged her regarding whether her patient had had her MRI (magnetic resonance imaging) scan yet, since it had been ordered for early yesterday morning. Jasmine was very taken aback by this confrontation with the physician, and she was speechless. She knew that her patient had not been for an MRI, but was worried about how the doctor would respond if she told him this. There was a very good reason for the patient not having received the MRI—the machine was not working and the unit staff had called to cancel all tests for that day. Communication consists of both content and relational aspects associated with how it is received. Which of the following relational aspects were at play in this scenario that likely resulted in Jasmine not being able to respond to the doctor? *(Select all that apply.)*
   1. Affinity
   2. Immediacy
   3. Respect
   4. Control

Answers: 1. 1, 2; **2.** 2, 3, 5; **3.** 2, 3, 4; **4.** 1, 3, 4

Rationales for the Review Questions appear at the end of the book.

RECOMMENDED WEBSITES

Association of Registered Nurses of Newfoundland & Labrador (ARNNL): https://www.arnnl.ca/standards-code-ethics.
This website provides another perspective on how a licensing organization sets nurses' standards of practice and codes of ethics for its members to enact.

Association of Registered Nurses of Prince Edward Island (ARNPEI): https://www.arnpei.ca/images/pdf/Standards%20for%20Nursing%20Practice%202016.pdf
This link opens to the standards of practice for nurses who are licensed to practise in Prince Edward Island.

Canadian Nurses Association (CNA) Code of Ethics for Registered Nurses: https://cna-aiic.ca/en/on-the-issues/best-nursing/nursing-ethics
This link provides a national orientation to the Code of Ethics and its values that all Canadian nurses adhere to. While it is a national code because of the provincial responsibility for health care and education based on the BNA Act, variations can be viewed by checking for the Code of Ethics set by each of the provincial licensing bodies for its nurses.

College & Association of Registered Nurses of Alberta (CARNA): http://www.nurses.ab.ca/content/dam/carna/SUFS/index.html
This link is a resource to the CARNA Practice Standards for Regulated Members.

College of Nurses of Manitoba: Entry Level Competencies for Registered Nurses: https://www.crnm.mb.ca/uploads/document/document_file_92.pdf/
In this link you will view a variance to the other province regulators. In Alberta they refer to their standards as competencies. They also integrate their Code of Ethics into their standard for Ethical Practice.

College of Nurses of Ontario: Practice Standard: http://www.cno.org/docs/prac/41006_ProfStds.pdf
The College of Nurses of Ontario again separate their practice standards and their Code of Ethics. These again are the requirements for nurses to practice within Ontario.

College of Nurses of Ontario: Professional Standards: http://www.cno.org/en/learn-about-standards-guidelines/educational-tools/learning-modules/ethics/ethical-values/
In this link the College of Nurses of Ontario provide a video to explain what is categorized as ethical practice for nurses in Ontario.

College of Registered Nurses of British Columbia (CRNBC): https://www.crnbc.ca/Standards/PracticeStandards/Pages/Default.aspx/

The College of Registered Nurses of British Columbia provide an additional menu within this link that allows you to click on each of their practice standards. Within this same link the B. C. nurses' scope of practice is also outlined.

College of Registered Nurses of Nova Scotia: Entry-Level Competencies: https://crnns.ca/wp-content/uploads/2015/02/RNStandards.pdf

This link provides you with a series of slides about the College of Registered Nurses of Nova Scotia's Standards of Practice. In Nova Scotia nurses follow the CNA Code of Ethics.

Interprofessional Health Education & Research (IPHER): Professions—Nursing: http://www.ipe.uwo.ca/Professionals/nurses.html

In this link is a description of what nurses do. This importance of our ability to describe our role is critical within interprofessional teams. This description still needs work but is one that seems to reflect some of the components of our practice.

Nurses Association of New Brunswick (NANB): http://www.nanb.nb.ca/practice/standards

This link provides access to both the Nurses Association of New Brunswick's Standards for Nursing Practice in New Brunswick as well as their Code of Ethics.

Ordre des infirmieres et infirmiers auxiliaires du Quebec: http://www.oiiaq.org/en/order/professional-system

This link provides access to the Quebec professional code which is applied to all professions.

PDA Cortex: http://www.pdacortex.com/

This is a link to the Journal of Mobile Informatics.

Registered Nurses Association of Northwest Territories & Nunavut: http://www.rnantnu.ca/sites/default/files/Entry%20Level%20Competencies%20%20Feb%202014%20PDF.pdf

This link provides a slide set about the Entry to Practice competencies expected of any nurses wishing to practise in the Northwest Territories & Nunavut.

Saskatchewan Registered Nurses Association (SRNA): https://www.srna.org/images/stories/Nursing_Practice/Resources/What_is_a_Registered_Nurse_2015_09_14.pdf

In this link the Saskatchewan Registered Nurses Association provides a comprehensive statement about what a nurse is and the scope of a nurse's practice.

Online Journal of Nursing Informatics: http://ojni.org/issues/?p=1706

This link takes you to the online journal of nursing informatics which can be a source to learning about various applications that you can use and upload into your smart phones for use in practice.

Free Apps for Nurses and Nursing Students: http://findnursingschools.com/blog/12-free-apps-for-nurses-and-nursing-students/

This link provides access to free apps to use on your smart phones and other devices. However, they are United States based.

Yukon Registered Nurses Association: http://yukonnurses.ca/images/YRNA/Documents/Standards2013.pdf

This link provides you with access to the Yukon Registered Nurses Association's Standards for Practice.

REFERENCES

Adler, R. B., Rolls, J. A., Proctor, R. F., III, et al. (2009). *Looking out/looking in: Brief Canadian edition*. Toronto: Nelson Education Ltd.

Andreoli, A., Fancott, C., Velji, K., et al. (2010). Using SBAR to communicate falls risk and management in inter-professional rehabilitation teams. *Healthcare Quarterly, 13*(13), 94–101.

Blenky, M. F., Clinchey, B. M., Goldberg, N. R., et al. (1986). *Women's ways of knowing: The development of self, voice, and mind*. New York: Basic Books.

Canadian Association Schools of Nursing (CASN). (2015). *National nursing education framework: Final report*. Retrieved from http://www.casn.ca/wp-content/uploads/2014/12/Framwork-FINAL-SB-Nov-30-20151.pdf.

Canadian Interprofessional Health Collaborative (CIHC). (2010). *National interprofessional competency framework*. Vancouver: Author. Retrieved from https://www.cihc.ca/files/CIHC_IPCompetencies_Feb1210.pdf.

Canadian Nurses Association (CNA) (2017). *Code of ethics for registered nurses*. Ottawa: Author.

Carper, B. A. (1978). Fundamental patterns of knowing in nursing. ANS/practice oriented theory, Part I. *Advances in Nursing Science, 1*(1), 13–23.

Cohen, S. G., & Bailey, D. E. (1997). What makes teams work? Group effectiveness research from the shop floor to the executive suite. *Journal of Management, 23*, 239–290.

Costa, A. C. (2003). Work team trust and effectiveness. *Personnel Review, 32*(5), 605–622. doi:10.1108/00483480310488360.

Enlow, M., Shanks, L., Guhde, J., et al. (2010). Incorporating interprofessional communication skills (ISBAR) into an undergraduate nursing curriculum. *Nurse Educator, 35*(4), 176–180. doi:10.1097/NNE.0b013e3181e339ac.

Gittell, J. H., Godfrey, M., & Thistlethwaite, J. (2013). Interprofessional collaborative practice and relational coordination: Improving healthcare through relationships. *Journal of Interprofessional Care, 27*(3), 210–213. doi:10.3109/13561820.2012.730564.

Hindmarsh, J., & Pilnick, A. (2002). The tacit order of teamwork: Collaboration and embodied conduct in anesthesia. *Sociological Quarterly, 43*(2), 139–164. doi:10.1111/j.1533-8525.2002.tb00044.x.

Keatings, M., & Smith, O. N. (2009). *Ethical and legal issues in Canadian nursing* (3rd ed.). Toronto: W.B. Saunders.

Kouzes, J. M., & Posner, B. Z. (2006). *Student leadership practices inventory: Facilitator's Guide* (2nd ed.). San Francisco: Jossey-Bass.

Lasater, K. (2007). Clinical judgment development: Using simulation to create an assessment rubric. *The Journal of Nursing Education, 45*(11), 496–503.

Marshall, S., Harrison, J., & Flanagan, B. (2009). The teaching of a structured tool improves the clarity and content of interprofessional clinical communication. *Quality and Safety in Health Care, 18*(2), 137–140. doi:10.1136/qshc.2007.025247.

McAllister, D. J. (1995). Affect- and cognition-based trust as foundations for interpersonal cooperation in organizations. *Academy of Management Journal, 38*, 24–59.

McCurcheon, J. J. I., & Pincombe, J. (2001). Intuition: An important tool in the practice of nursing. *Journal of Advanced Nursing, 35*(5), 342–348.

Orchard, C. (2016). The APN and interprofessional collaborative practice competence. In E. Staples, S. L. Ray, & R. A. Hannon (Eds.), *Canadian perspectives on advanced practice nursing* (pp. 254–273). Toronto: Canadian Scholars' Press.

Orchard, C., Curran, V., & Kabene, S. (2005). Creating a culture for interdisciplinary collaborative professional practice. *Medical Education Online [Electronic Resource], 10*(11), 1–13. doi:10.3402/meo.v10i.4387.

Orchard, C., & Rykhoff, M. (2015). Collaborative leadership within interprofessional practice. In D. Forman, M. Jones, & J. Thistlethwaite (Eds.), *Leadership and collaboration: Further developments for interprofessional education* (pp. 71–94). Houndsmill, Basingstoke. Hampshire, UK: Palgrave Macmillan.

Sahlsten, M. J. M., Larsson, I. E., Plos, K. A. E., et al. (2005). Hindrance for patient participation in nursing care. *Scandinavian Journal of Caring Sciences, 19*, 223–229. doi:10.1111/j.1471-6712.2005.00336.x.

Schmieding, N. J. (1983). The analysis of Orlando's nursing theory based on Kuhn's theory of science. In P. Chinn (Ed.), *Advances in nursing theory development* (pp. 63–87). Rockville, MD: Aspen Systems.

Tanner, C. (2006). Thinking like a nurse: A research-based model of clinical judgment in nursing. *The Journal of Nursing Education, 45*(6), 204–211.

van Schaik, S. M., O'Brien, B. C., Almeida, S. A., et al. (2014). Perceptions of interprofessional teamwork in low-acuity settings: A qualitative analysis. *Medical Education, 48*(6), 583–592. doi:10.1111/medu.12424.

19

Family Nursing

Written by Christina H. West, RN, PhD, Sonya L. Jakubec, RN, BHScN, MN, PhD

OBJECTIVES

Mastery of content in this chapter will enable you to:

- Define the key terms listed.
- Discuss how the term *family* can be defined.
- Examine current trends in the Canadian family.
- Discuss how family members influence one another's health.
- Compare family as context, family as patient, and family *in* context, explaining how these different perspectives influence nursing practice with families.
- State the three major categories of the Calgary Family Assessment Model (CFAM) and understand subcategories important to consider in a family assessment.
- Describe key concepts of the Calgary Family Intervention Model (CFIM).
- Discuss family nursing as relational inquiry.
- Describe key concepts and approaches to relational inquiry–based practices for family nursing.
- Ask assessment questions to learn relevant information about family functioning in the context of health or illness.
- Discuss the relational approaches and practices needed to conduct a family interview and effectively intervene with the family in nursing practice.

KEY TERMS

Alliances and coalitions, p. 318
Beliefs, p. 318
Calgary Family Assessment Model (CFAM), p. 313
Calgary Family Intervention Model (CFIM), p. 318
Circular communication, p. 317
Circular questions, p. 319
Commendation, p. 319
Context (families *as* context, families *in* context, families as patient), p. 311
Ecomap, p. 315
Emotional communication, p. 316
Family, p. 308
Family forms, p. 308
Family nursing, p. 308
Genogram, p. 315
Hardiness, p. 310
Illness narrative, p. 320
Influence, p. 317
Linear questions, p. 318
Nonverbal communication, p. 317
Problem solving, p. 317
Reciprocity, p. 320
Relational inquiry, p. 311
Resiliency, p. 310
Roles, p. 317
Verbal communication, p. 317

MEDIA RESOURCES

http://evolve.elsevier.com/Canada/Potter/fundamentals/

- Audio Chapter Summaries
- Examination Review Questions
- Concept Map Creator
- Case Study with Questions
- Audio Glossary
- Content Updates
- Video Clips

The role of the family in health care has evolved significantly in previous years. In the early twentieth century, visiting public health nurses and private duty nurses worked closely with family members, providing care in the patient's home. After World War II, with the development of a national health care system in Canada, the location of most nursing services shifted to hospital settings. With these historical changes in health care, families were largely excluded from their relatives' nursing care, while physicians and nurses came to be considered the experts in health care provision (Elliott, Stuart, & Toman, 2009). Although tensions between the role of professionals and family members in health care continue to persist (Coyne, 2013; Rankin, 2015), families and nurses have increasingly forged more collaborative relationships. Family nursing is a highly contextual, relational, and skill-based practice that is further complicated by the high intensity of the clinical contexts where it is practised.

Within family nursing practice, nurses need to simultaneously attend to the needs of multiple family members in the context of a complex health care environment (Registered Nurses' Association of Ontario [RNAO], 2015). An example of the complexity faced in contemporary nursing practice is palliative home care with patients and families who live in rural settings, several hundred kilometres from urban health services (Robinson, Pesut, & Bottorff, 2012). The location of a patient's care may create significant challenges for the family in relation to travel, employment, and finances. Other examples include frail older persons isolated from family and friends as they enter the health care system, or recently immigrated families who must face a child's serious illness in the context of significant language, cultural, and economic barriers.

It is within these diverse and challenging clinical and family contexts that nurses strive to provide *family-centred care,* an approach that is characterized by dignity and respect, information sharing, patient and family participation, and family–professional collaboration (RNAO, 2015). Despite the growing adoption of family-centred care within modern health care settings, implementation of this approach has been challenging (Coyne, 2013). Further, Rankin (2015) reported that patient- and family-centred care is "organized to be empty rhetoric" (p. 533), acting to socially organize nurses' work to meet the efficiency-based priorities of the health care system rather than the needs of family members. A lack of research, shared language, and collaborative practice approaches have posed significant challenges to the implementation of family-centred care (Clay & Parsh, 2016). Wright and Leahey (2013) argue that family-centred care can be responsibly and respectfully achieved only through the use of clearly articulated relational, family assessment, and family intervention frameworks.

Family nursing is based on the assumption that every person, regardless of age, is a member of some type of family form and carries family experiences that have profound influences on their lives and approaches to health care (Hartrick Doane & Varcoe, 2015). Also central is the assumption that individuals are best understood within the context of the family. A change in one family member, such as an illness or health condition, affects the other family members. Family nursing promotes, supports, and provides for the well-being and health of the family and individual family members (Wright & Leahey, 2013). Nurses need to understand the relational contexts as well as the particular strengths and needs of each family that they encounter in practice. It is also important that nurses work to understand the geo-social, economic, and political influences that shape each family's life experience. Through skilled relational inquiry (Hartrick Doane & Varcoe, 2015) and the use of family assessment and intervention frameworks, nurses can effectively collaborate with families to enhance the unique strengths and resources they possess (Gottlieb, 2013; Hartrick Doane & Varcoe, 2015; Wright & Leahey, 2013). Nurses are encouraged to move beyond understanding family as an entity and into the sensitive mediation of the nurse–family relationship as well as the relationships shared between family members. The goal of family nursing is to help the family and its individual members achieve and maintain optimal health throughout and beyond the illness experience.

WHAT IS A FAMILY?

Defining *family* within complex relational and clinical contexts is not a simple undertaking. Different definitions have resulted in heated debates among social scientists and legislators. Formal definitions have included understandings of family as a biological or legal entity and as social networks complete with personally or institutionally organized values and ideologies. To some patients, family may include only people who are related by marriage, birth, or adoption.

Other patients consider aunts, uncles, close friends, cohabiting people, and even pets as family. Families are as diverse as the individuals that compose them, and patients, as well as health care providers, hold deeply ingrained beliefs and values about family. It is important that nurses explore these values and beliefs within their nursing practice with families. Thus, **family** is defined as a set of relationships that each patient identifies as a network of individuals who influence each other's lives, regardless of whether actual biological or legal ties exist. In other words, each person has an individual definition of who or what constitutes family (RNAO, 2015).

As a nurse, your personal beliefs do not have to coincide with those of the patient, but to provide responsive, individualized, and compassionate care, it is important to have an awareness of your own history, values, and beliefs and an understanding that families are diverse in form and expression. Families are unique, each having their own strengths, resources, and challenges (Hartrick Doane & Varcoe, 2015; Wright & Bell, 2009; Wright & Leahey, 2013). Families nonetheless share some general characteristics that include future obligations and caregiving functions, such as protection, nourishment, and socialization of family members (McGoldrick, Garcia Preto & Carter, 2016).

CURRENT TRENDS IN THE CANADIAN FAMILY

Although the institution of the family remains strong, the family itself is changing. Nurses need to be aware of current trends and social factors that affect the structure and function of the family. The following information about current family trends is based on data from Statistics Canada's 2016 censuses (Statistics Canada, 2017a) and prior household survey data (Statistics Canada, 2012).

Family Forms

Family forms are patterns of people considered by family members to be included in the family (Box 19-1). Although all families have some common characteristics, each family form has unique challenges and strengths. It is important for nurses to maintain an open mind about what constitutes a family so that potential resources and concerns are not overlooked.

Divorce rates have increased dramatically since the 1950s, and although the rate seems to be dropping, it is now estimated that 41% of Canadian marriages will end in divorce. While the majority of children in lone-parent families live with a divorced or separated lone parent (56.2%), over one-third (37.4%) live with a lone parent who has never married (Statistics Canada, 2015). Many divorced adults do eventually remarry or form new family units, which results in blended families with complex sets of relationships among step-parents, stepchildren, half-brothers and half-sisters, and extended family members. When transitioning to a blended family, parents undergo difficult emotional challenges, while simultaneously managing the intense sadness, anger, and confusion experienced by children, extended family members, friends, and ex-spouses. Divorced and re-coupled families require an entirely new paradigm as they move forward in family life (McGoldrick et al., 2016).

Lesbian, gay, bisexual, and transgender individuals are connected to family through their membership in families of origin, as well as in the families they have chosen to create both within and outside the context of legal marriage (McGoldrick et al., 2016). These individuals and couples may face multiple challenges within the family life cycle, including those associated with identity development, the process of coming out, coupling, parenting, and transitions in later life.

There has been a significant decline in the number of parents staying at home, outside of the formal workforce, to care for children—from 1.5 million in 1976 to 0.5 million in 2015. While the vast majority of stay-at-home parents are women, men are increasingly taking on this role. In 2015, men represented 1 in 10 stay-at-home parents in Canada (Statistics Canada, 2016a). Grandparents have also increasingly taken responsibility for the raising of grandchildren. In 2011, close to 600 000 grandparents aged 45 and over lived with their grandchildren, accounting for 8% of all grandparents and for 4% of the overall population in this age group (Statistics Canada, 2015). Sharing a home with one's grandchildren is influenced by numerous factors,

BOX 19-1 Family Forms

Blended Family
Formed when both parents bring children from previous relationships into a new, joint living situation or when children from the current union and children from previous unions are living together

Extended Family
Includes the nuclear family and other relatives (perhaps grandparents, aunts, uncles, cousins)

Lone-Parent Family
Consists of one parent and one or more children. The lone-parent family is formed when one parent leaves the nuclear family because of death, divorce, or desertion or when a single person decides to have or adopt a child.

Step-Family
Formed when at least one child in a household is from a previous relationship of one of the parents

Traditional Nuclear Family
Consists of a mother and father (married or common-law) and their children

Family Forms—Increasing Diversity
Family forms and family relationships within Canada have become increasingly diverse. They include married and common-law couples without children, families in which grandparents provide care for their grandchildren, adults living alone, and same-sex couples (with or without children). The rates of traditional families (two married parents and children living together) in Canada is declining, while the proportion of common-law and lone-parent families is increasing. Today, the average Canadian household consists of 2.5 people, and for the first time in 2011, there were more one-person households (27.6%) (a number now totaling 28.2%, based on the 2016 Census [Statistics Canada, 2017b]). than couple households with children (26.5%) (Statistics Canada, 2017a). These changes hold significant societal implications. For instance, smaller families and more people living alone have led to an increasing need for affordable child care in Canada. Further, the care and support of young children or older Canadians is now spread among a decreasing number of family members.

including the ethnocultural, sociodemographic, and economic characteristics of the population (Statistics Canada, 2015).

Family Changes and Challenges: Understanding the Influence of Sociocultural Contexts

Sociocultural and economic changes are significantly increasing challenges to family health. Many families find themselves unable to respond effectively to complex family challenges (e.g., violence, addictions, illness, learning disabilities, cognitive decline and/or dementia). These family challenges can undermine existing relationships of care, leaving family members more vulnerable and socially isolated during times when support is most needed (Luxton, 2011; Reiter, 2015). Recognizing these changes and challenges is crucial within family nursing assessment and intervention.

Pregnancy for Teens and Older Moms

The rates of pregnancies of teen moms and women in their 20s has steadily decreased, while the pregnancy rate for older mothers aged 30–39 and 40–49 increased between 2009 and 2013 in Canada (Statistics Canada, 2016b). Nevertheless, adolescents who give birth are now more likely to raise their children as single parents or within the context of extended family units rather than placing their children for adoption. A teenage pregnancy often has significant health and social consequences for children and mothers, and can severely strain family relationships and family resources. In addition, these families are at increased risk for living in poverty related to disruptions in maternal education and limited career opportunities. These risks are of particular concern for Inuit (Moisan, Baril, Muckle, et al., 2016) and First Nations (Garner, Guimond, & Senécal, 2013) adolescents, who have higher rates of pregnancy than do non-Indigenous adolescents.

Domestic Roles

Domestic roles have become more complex, as families are increasingly made up of two wage earners or living in single-person households (Statistics Canada, 2016c). Balancing employment and domestic responsibilities creates a variety of challenges regarding child and elder care, as well as household work. Concerns that maternal employment is detrimental to children's development and well-being are limited and unsubstantiated (Brooks-Gunn, Han, & Waldfogel, 2010). However, finding high-quality child care and managing domestic tasks can be a major challenge. Management of domestic tasks and parenting responsibilities varies substantially from family to family. Many fathers are now expected and want to participate more fully in day-to-day parenting responsibilities. Additionally, cultural groups such as Indigenous, European, African, Asian, and South Asian communities have historically valued and maintain extended family involvement in family caregiving (Hsieh, Mercer, & Costa, 2017; Lindstrom, Choate, Bastien, et al., 2016; Luxton, 2011) (see Chapter 9 for further information on the diversity seen in the Canadian population).

Economic Status

In 2014, the median annual income of Canadian families was about \$75 700. The median annual income for lone-parent households was \$43 400 (Statistics Canada, 2016d). Distribution of wealth greatly affects the capacity to maintain health. Low educational preparation, poverty, and decreased amounts of support all magnify the impact of illness on the family and increase the amount of illness in the family. In Canada 4.5 million people, or 13.0% of the population, lived in low income in 2014 (Statistics Canada, 2016d). Dual-income families account for nearly 7 in 10 families with children at this time, a rate that has doubled over the past 40 years (Statistics Canada, 2016c).

Indigenous Families

Individual, family, and community impacts of social and health inequities and disparities in Canadian society are profound (Browne, Varcoe, Lavoie, et al., 2016) and require nursing attention. Indigenous peoples' families are the fastest-growing group with children younger than 24 years. Indigenous peoples' family structures tend to be larger, have younger family members, and contain greater diversity in family members than do non-Indigenous families (Hsieh et al., 2017). Each group of Indigenous peoples has its own traditions, rituals, relationships, and functions that need to be taken into account in nursing care. They are undergoing substantial changes while trying to maintain traditional culture, structure, and function. These families have multigenerational structures that often consist of a network of grandparents, parents, children, aunts, uncles, and cousins. Each member has obligations to the family. Traditionally, Indigenous children are held in high esteem and there is an expectation that they be treated gently and protected from harm (Muir & Bohr, 2014). Traditional Indigenous family values and intergenerational family and parenting patterns were lost, however, over decades of cultural disruption and trauma. Historical acts of forced assimilation were founded on the belief that Indigenous values were inferior to those of the dominant culture (Muir & Bohr, 2014). In the post–Truth and Reconciliation era, traditional values and Indigenous voices are being reclaimed and re-examined, including family values (Lindstrom et al., 2016). The Calgary Family Assessment and Intervention Models (Wright & Leahey, 2013), as well as Hartrick Doane and Varcoe's (2005, 2015) approach to relational inquiry with families, can assist nurses in creating sensitivity, cultural safety, and attentiveness to both the strengths of and challenges faced by the Indigenous families they encounter in practice.

Family Caregivers

Persons 80 years of age and older are Canada's fastest-growing age group. One out of every seven Canadians is an older person. Life expectancy is 84 years for women and 80 years for men (World Health Organization, 2016). The aging population has affected the family life cycle, especially the middle generation, as many family members serve as informal caregivers for older persons and other persons with disabilities. The majority of these caregivers are women, and they frequently provide 10 hours or more of unpaid assistance per week (Duxbury, Higgins, & Schroeder, 2009). Family caregiving involves the routine provision of services and personal-care activities for a family member by spouses, siblings, or children. Caregiving activities include personal care (bathing, feeding, or grooming), monitoring for complications or adverse effects of medications, instrumental activities of daily living (shopping or housekeeping), and ongoing emotional support. The respite needs of family caregivers are an important aspect of assessment and intervention given the changes occurring within the sociocultural and economic contexts of family health.

Although family caregivers often find that providing care has many rewards, this group frequently must balance caring for a family member with many other ongoing demands (e.g., raising children, working full-time, or dealing with personal problems or illness) and may suffer physical and emotional health challenges related to the competing demands (Duxbury et al., 2009; McGoldrick et al., 2016). Box 19-2 provides a list of family nursing gerontological concerns.

THE FAMILY AND HEALTH

The family is the primary context in which health promotion and disease prevention take place (Box 19-3). The health of the family is influenced by many factors such as biology, social status, economic resources, politics, violence, and geographic and environmental contexts. Each family's beliefs, values, and practices also strongly influence the health-promoting behaviours of its members (Hartrick Doane & Varcoe, 2005, 2006, 2015). The health status of each individual influences how the family unit functions and its ability to achieve its goals. When the family meets its goals, its members tend to feel positive about themselves and their family. Conversely, when they do not meet goals, families may view themselves as ineffective.

Attributes of Healthy Families

Researchers have focused on hardiness and resiliency as mediating factors for long-term health. Hill's (1958/2003) classic research attempted to explain the reactions of crisis-proof and crisis-prone families in order to foster strength. A crisis-proof, or effective, family can integrate the need for stability with the need for growth and change. This type of family has a flexible structure for task performances and is receptive to help from outside the family system while maintaining a sense of strength and stability. An effective family exerts influence on the immediate environment of home, neighbourhood, and school, whereas a crisis-prone family may lack, or believe it lacks, control over these environments.

Family **hardiness** has been defined as the internal strengths and durability of the family unit and is characterized by a sense of control over the outcome of life, perceiving change as beneficial and growth producing, and having active rather than passive approaches to stressful events (McCubbin, McCubbin, & Thompson, 1996). A hardy family can thus transcend inevitable lifestyle changes. Family **resiliency** is the ability to cope with expected and unexpected stressors: role changes, developmental milestones, and crises. The goal of the family is not only to survive the challenge but also to thrive and grow with knowledge acquired in the challenge.

Black and Lobo (2008) defined *family resiliency* as successful coping under conditions of stress and adversity that enables individuals and the family unit to flourish with support. Factors influencing family resiliency include positive outlook; spirituality; flexibility; cohesiveness; clear communication; financial management; shared family

BOX 19-2 FOCUS ON OLDER PERSONS

- Nurses need to carefully consider caregiver strain; caregivers are typically older persons whose own physical stamina may be declining, or middle-age children who often have other responsibilities.
- Older families have a different social network than younger families; friends and same-generation family members may have died or have been ill themselves. Nurses can look for social support within the community and within resources of the patient's religious affiliation.
- Physical health impairments increase the risk of depression in older persons.
- As in the other stages of life, members of older families need to work on developmental tasks (see Chapter 24 for further information about older persons).
- Abuse of older persons occurs across all social classes, with family members and family caregivers being the most frequent abusers (Ford-Gilboe, Varcoe, Wuest, et al., 2011). Unexplained bruises and skin trauma should not be ignored by health care providers.

BOX 19-3 FOCUS ON PRIMARY HEALTH CARE

Family nursing practice focuses on active collaboration with individual members and the family unit with the goal of supporting their efforts to reach optimal levels of health and well-being. Community health nurses meet families in a wide variety of primary health care settings and have many opportunities to implement holistic family nursing practices. Nursing practices in health promotion include, but are not limited to, neonatal assessments, bereavement visits, school health care, occupational health care, substance abuse programs, palliative care, infusion clinics, and home care. Research has shown that these nursing interventions have a positive impact on the health outcomes of families (MacMillan, Wathen, Jamieson, et al., 2009).

involvement in recreation, routines, and rituals; and support networks. Communication is particularly crucial to resilience and general family functioning. It enables individuals within a family unit to express needs, wants, and concerns to one another. Through communication, family members are able to resolve everyday challenges, promote health of all members, and develop resilience for extraordinary challenges (Black & Lobo, 2008).

Health promotion programs, psychosocial supports, and family counselling or therapy aimed at enhancing communication and other resiliency attributes are available for families and children in many communities. Nurses need to make themselves aware of family-oriented community resources so that families can be referred as needed.

FAMILY NURSING CARE

The Canadian Association for Schools of Nursing (2015) has developed a national nursing education framework that emphasizes family nursing in a number of key competency domains, including knowledge of relational practice to affect health outcomes of individuals, families and communities; collaborative practice with families; and family health promotion. This collaborative family nursing practice must be based on mutual respect and trust. Nurses should examine family patterns, relationships, and interactions when they consider how a health challenge or illness affects a family and, conversely, how a family affects a health challenge or illness (Wright & Leahey, 2013). A nurse's relationship with the family has a significant influence on patient and family functioning and health outcomes (MacMillan, Wathen, Jamieson, et al., 2009) (Figure 19-1).

Although health care systems in the past tended to emphasize the individual, a family focus is now needed in order to be able to safely discharge patients to the care of the family or community settings. There is also a pressing need to address within nursing practice the challenges faced by multiple family members, the patient, and the family unit. To begin your nursing practice with families, you must have scientific knowledge of family theory and family nursing. Family nursing care focuses on family as context, family as patient, and an understanding of families in context. The approaches used depend on the particular situation and the self-awareness and abilities of the nurse.

Family as Context

When considering the family as **context**, the focus is either on the individual patient within the context of his or her family or on the family with the individual as context (RNAO, 2015). The approach used relates to the clinical setting, clinical problem, and practical considerations. An example of the first approach is a situation in which a nurse interviews a man with heart disease, asking the man's wife about the family's diet and possible family stressors. The wife's ability to support her husband's efforts at changing eating patterns and use of stress management techniques are also assessed. The main focus is on the health of the patient within the environment of the family. An example of the second approach is a situation in which a community health nurse interviews the adult daughter of a woman with multiple sclerosis, discussing how she is coping with her mother's care. Family members may need direct support and nursing intervention themselves.

With both approaches, the nurse assesses the extent to which the family supports the individual's basic needs. Family members are considered valuable resources for assessment and intervention. They provide information about how they have been helping the patient maintain health and manage health problems. When patients are unable to communicate, families provide important information about the patient and indicate the patient's wishes. Nurses need to be competent at considering the family as context. Even if there is no opportunity to involve the family directly, the patient is still considered as a member of a family.

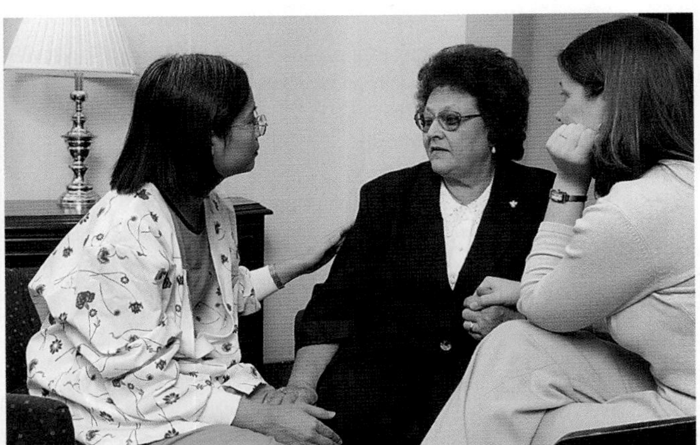

FIGURE 19-1 Nurse (*left*) and family members.

Family as Patient

When approaching the family as patient, the focus is on the entire family—its processes and relationships (e.g., parenting, impacts of the marital relationship, or family caregiving). Family patterns and interactions among family members are the focus, rather than individual characteristics. The nursing process concentrates on how these patterns and processes are consistent with achieving and maintaining family and individual health. Nursing practice that focuses on family as patient is also known as *family systems nursing* and requires in-depth knowledge of family dynamics and family systems theory (Wright & Leahey, 2013). Therefore, nurses who specialize in family systems nursing often have advanced skills and training. An interdisciplinary approach is helpful when dealing with complex family systems. In your own nursing practice, it is important that you are aware of the limits of nursing practice and make referrals when appropriate. Considering the family as the patient, you aim to support communication and healthy family functioning among family members (Wright & Leahey, 2013). Often you must support conflict resolution between family members so that each member can confront and resolve challenges in a healthy way. You also may link family members to external and internal resources as necessary. Ultimately, your aim is to help the family achieve optimal functioning.

Understanding Family in Context: Relational Inquiry With Individuals and Families

Family nursing as relational inquiry invites nurses to consider the ways in which families and nurses are embedded within diverse and complex life contexts. Hartrick Doane and Varcoe (2005, 2015) articulate the importance of critically attending to the social, political, economic, and geographic contexts that influence both family members and nurses who care for them. Nurses need to continually explore how personal and professional definitions of *health* and *family* may shape, and possibly constrain, their nursing practice with families (Hartrick Doane & Varcoe, 2005, p. 24). A nurse's perceptions, values, and beliefs about the meaning of family can greatly influence the quality of the therapeutic relationship, the health of patients and families, and the quality of work life experienced by nurses. In a **relational inquiry** approach, nurses seek to expand their contextual knowledge of families, developing a more in-depth and comprehensive consideration of the historical,

BOX 19-4 Relational Capacities

Key concepts of relational practice with families include the following:
- Self-awareness (in relationship with others)
- Context/culture
- Perception/personal meaning
- Relational capacity (approaches identified in detail below)

Relational capacities:
- Ways of being in relationship
  - Presence/mindfulness
  - Synchrony/mutuality
  - Capacity for ambiguity
  - Intentionality/congruence
  - Genuineness
  - Warmth
  - Respect
  - Attending/listening (including listening for difference)
  - Boundaries
- Understanding another's personal meaning
  - Empathy
  - Clarification/perception checking/verbalizing the implied
  - Validating
  - Question posing, focusing, and reflecting
  - Use of silence
  - Summarizing/placing events in a time sequence
- Expressing/sharing your own personal meaning
  - Constructive giving/receiving of feedback
  - Assertiveness
  - Conflict resolution
  - Sharing information

Adapted from Hartrick Doane, G., & Varcoe, C. (2005). *Family nursing as relational inquiry: Developing health-promoting practice* (p. 228; Box 7.1). Philadelphia: Lippincott Williams & Wilkins.

economic, political, social, environmental, and geographic influences at play when families encounter illness or other difficulties related to life transitions.

The nurse's awareness of his or her own values and beliefs, as well as a critical, reflective consideration of different understandings of health and family, will enhance the nurse's ability to hear the unique stories of family members' lives. Nurses must explore potential biases they may hold, how those biases may influence the questions they ask, and their ability or inability to listen for and to the experiences of family members.

This practice is guided by a number of relational capacities that have been described by Hartrick Doane and Varcoe (2005) (Box 19-4). These skills include listening, questioning, empathy, mutuality, reciprocity, self-observation, reflection, and a sensitivity to emotional contexts (also see Chapter 17 for further information about relational practice in communicating). This approach highlights working across differences and acknowledging that power and differences are important, often invisible, features of relationships. This practice begins by entering into relation, inquiring into the family health and healing experience, following the lead of families, and learning to let be (Box 19-5). Within your own practice, consider how you might look beyond the surface of patients and families, entering your practice with an approach of inquiry, while drawing on the assessment and intervention processes described in Box 19-5.

ASSESSING THE CHALLENGES, STRENGTHS, AND NEEDS OF THE FAMILY: THE CALGARY FAMILY ASSESSMENT MODEL

Family assessment skills are also essential in providing responsive, compassionate, and respectful family care and support. To help families adjust to acute and chronic illness, nurses need to understand the

BOX 19-5 Relational Inquiry: Assessing and Intervening Approaches

1. Entering into relation: Getting "in sync" with a family
   - Conscious participation—walking alongside the family
   - Stopping to look, listen, and hear
   - Unconditional positive regard
   - Being in sync
2. Being in collaborative relation: Staying "in sync"
   - Family and nurse working together to assess and intervene
3. Inquiring into the family health and healing experience
   - Inquiry into what is meaningful to the family
   - Keeping family at the centre of view
4. Following the lead of families
   - Taking cues from families
   - Taking a stance of curiosity, unknowing, and uncertainty
   - Using theoretical knowledge to enhance sensitivity to family experience
   - Scrutinizing theoretical and expert knowledge against family experience
5. Listening to and for
   - Listening through phenomenological, critical, spiritual, and socioenvironmental health-promotion lenses
6. Self-observation
   - Participating consciously and intentionally
   - Self-knowing
7. Letting be and change
   - Letting be to know who this family is and what is happening for them
   - Creating the opportunity for family to come to know more about their own experience, patterns, capacities, challenges, and contextual constraints
8. Collaborative knowledge development
   - Drawing on family knowledge (experiential, historical, sociocultural), and drawing on nursing knowledge (scientific, theoretical, biomedical, political, practical)
9. Pattern recognition
   - Identifying underlying patterns of experience and responses
   - Identifying patterns of capacity and capacity–adversity
10. Naming and supporting capacity
    - Seeing and recognizing strengths
    - Looking beyond the surface
    - Honouring the family's version of the story
    - Working with the family to enhance capacity and address adversity
11. Emancipatory action
    - Recognizing and naming inequities and structural conditions
    - Drawing on and sharing contextual knowledge
    - Introducing alternative discourses
    - Devoting energy to remedying structural inequities and creating coalitions

Adapted from Hartrick Doane, G., & Varcoe, C. (2005). *Family nursing as relational inquiry: Developing health-promoting practice* (p. 228; Box 7.1). Philadelphia: Lippincott Williams & Wilkins.

relationships that family members share, what the illness means to family members, how the illness has influenced family functioning, how the family has been affected by the illness, and the support that the family is most in need of (Wright & Leahey, 2013). Box 19-6 lists the particular features of families who should be considered for a family assessment. During an assessment, the nurse, patient, and family engage relationally and collaboratively in conversation to share information with each other and explore family members' experiences of illness, while simultaneously reflecting on issues important to the patient and family's well-being.

BOX 19-6 Features of Families Who Should Be Considered for a Family Assessment

Families who may benefit most from a family assessment include those who

- Are experiencing emotional, physical, or spiritual suffering or disruption caused by a family crisis (e.g., acute, chronic, or life-threatening illness, injury, death, addiction, and/or suspected family violence)
- Are experiencing emotional, physical, or spiritual suffering or disruption caused by a developmental milestone (e.g., birth, marriage, child leaving home)
- Define a problem or illness as a family issue (e.g., the impact of chronic illness on the family)
- Have a child or adolescent whom they identify as having difficulties (e.g., cyberbullying at school, fear of cancer treatment)
- Are experiencing issues that are serious enough to jeopardize family relationships (e.g., terminal illness, abuse, addictions)
- Have a family member who is about to be admitted to the hospital for psychiatric or mental health care
- Have a child admitted to the hospital

Adapted from Wright, L. M., & Leahey, M. (2013). *Nurses and families: A guide to family assessment and intervention* (6th ed., p. 5). Philadelphia: FA Davis.

The Calgary Family Assessment Model (CFAM) is a relational, strengths-focused practice model that guides nurses in the completion of comprehensive family assessment (Wright & Leahey, 2013). The CFAM has received international recognition and has been adopted by schools of nursing around the world. The CFAM focuses on three major categories of family life: structural, developmental, and functional dimensions. Each category has several subcategories; however, not all subcategories will be relevant to every family (Figure 19-2). Nurses must decide, on a family-by-family basis, which subcategories are most relevant. Using too many subcategories may result in an overwhelming amount of data and questions for family members; using too few may yield insufficient data, which can distort a family's strengths and/or challenges. The model can be consulted during discussions about family issues.

Structural Assessment

The structural dimension of the family assessment includes the following:

- *Internal structure:* the people who are included in the family and how they are relationally connected to one another
- *External structure:* the relationships the family shares with people and institutions outside the family unit
- *Context:* the whole situation or background relevant to the family

Internal Structure. The internal structure of the family—the composition and relationships shared by family members—can be further divided into six subcategories: family composition, gender, sexual orientation, rank order, subsystems, and boundaries.

Family Composition. *Family composition* refers to the individual members who form the family. The family composition is not limited

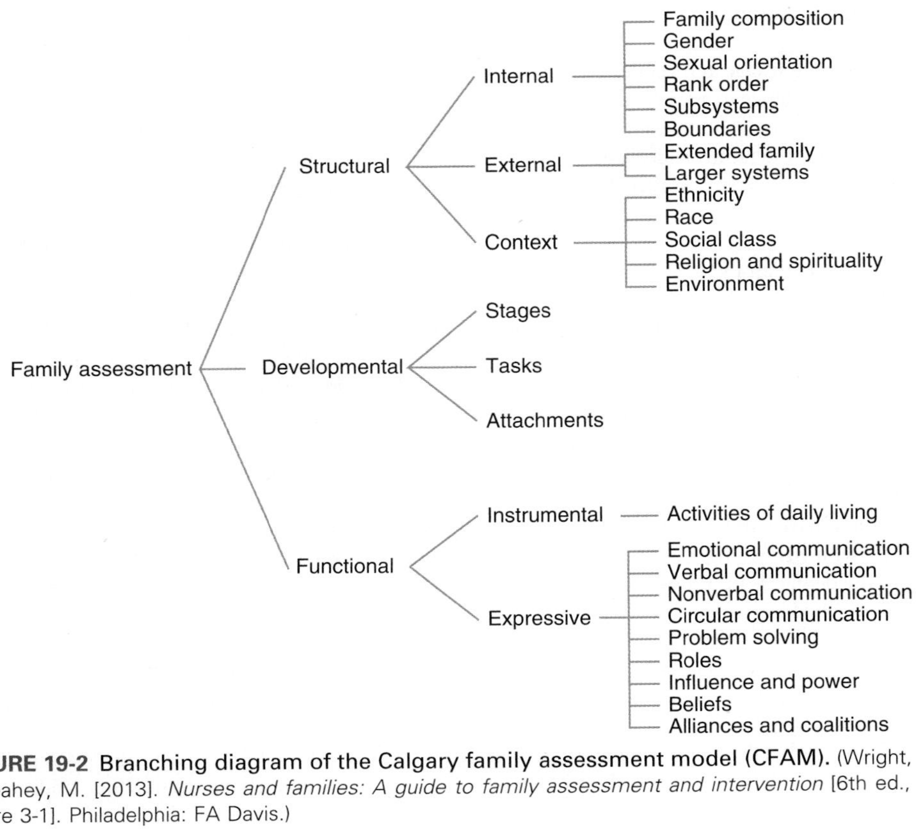

FIGURE 19-2 Branching diagram of the Calgary family assessment model (CFAM). (Wright, L. M., & Leahey, M. [2013]. *Nurses and families: A guide to family assessment and intervention* [6th ed., p. 52, Figure 3-1]. Philadelphia: FA Davis.)

to the traditional, nuclear family; it may include any of the various family forms, which were previously discussed (see Box 19-1). It is important to note whether any recent additions or losses in the family composition have occurred.

Questions to ask the family

- Who is in your family?
- Does anyone else live with you—for example, grandparents, boarders?
- Has anyone recently moved out of your household, married, or died?
- Can you think of anyone else who is like a family member but is not biologically related?

Gender. *Gender* is the set of beliefs about or expectations of masculine and feminine behaviours and experiences. These beliefs are fundamental to intimate relationships and are influenced by culture, religion, and family. It is useful to understand how male and female members of a particular family may view and experience the world differently.

Questions to ask the family

- How have your parents' ideas about masculinity and femininity affected your own? Have your ideas about gender been challenged in any way since you became parents?
- Do you have expectations of your children on the basis of their gender?
- Is the division of labour at home based on gender roles?

Sexual Orientation. *Sexual orientation* refers to heterosexual, gay, lesbian, bisexual, or transgendered orientation (see Chapter 27 for further information about sexual orientation). Heterosexism, a belief that male–female bonding is the only legitimate type of bonding, is a form of bias that can affect families and health care providers. Discrimination based on sexual orientation remains a problem. Unless relevant to the patient or family's presenting concern, you do not usually ask questions about sexual orientation, but avoid stereotyping or making assumptions when you ask general questions.

Rank Order. The order of children by age and gender is called *rank order.* The birth order, gender, and distance in age between siblings are important considerations because they may influence roles and behaviours. The child's characteristics and the family's idealized "program" for the child (going to school, college, university, work, getting married, and so forth) are also important.

Questions to ask the family

- How many children are in your family?
- What are the children's ages?
- Do you have distinct expectations for the oldest and younger children?

Subsystems. *Subsystems* are smaller groups of relationships (i.e., based on generation, interests, skills, or gender) within a family. For example, a family could have a sibling subsystem, a husband–wife subsystem, and a parent–child subsystem. Each family member usually belongs to several subsystems, and in each subsystem, they play a different role, use different skills, and have a different level of power (i.e., a teenager behaves differently with her younger sister than she does with her father). Adapting to the demands of different subsystems is a necessary skill for each family member.

Questions to ask the family

- What groups have you noticed in your family?
- Are there times when disagreements occur among and between the subgroups in your family?
- If your family had more or fewer subgroups, what effect do you think that might have? What might you most like to change about the subgroups in your family?

Boundaries. Boundaries define family subsystems and distinguish one subsystem from another. They influence how members participate in each subsystem. For example, a child in a parent–child subsystem may be given certain responsibilities and power but is not expected to be involved with family decision making. Boundaries can be weak, rigid, or flexible, and they change over time as family members age or are gained or lost.

Questions to ask the family

- Who do you talk with when you feel happy? Who do you talk to when you feel sad?
- Does the family have any "unwritten" rules about topics never to be discussed outside of the family?

External Structure. *External structure* refers to the connections that family members have to persons outside the family. Two subcategories of external structure exist: extended family and larger systems.

Extended Family. *Extended family* includes the family of origin, the current generation, and step-relatives. How each member sees himself or herself as an individual, yet also as part of the family, should be critically assessed. You should note whether family members make many references to the extended family during the interview and inquire about the nature of the relationships shared with extended family members.

Questions to ask the family

- Where do your parents live? How often do you have contact with them and your siblings?
- Which family members do you see or speak with regularly? Who in your extended family are you the closest to?
- Have members of your extended family been helpful to you during this time of illness? In what way?

Larger Systems. *Larger systems* are groups with whom the family has meaningful contact. Groups include health care organizations, work, religious affiliations, school, friends, and social agencies such as public welfare, child welfare, foster care, and courts. Usually, contact with such larger systems is helpful. However, some families have difficult relationships with individuals from these groups, which can create stress for the family.

Questions to ask the family

- How many health agencies regularly interact with you?
- What agency professionals are involved with your family? How have they been helpful or not helpful to your family? How are you hoping I might support you differently than other professionals involved in your family's care?

Context. *Context* refers to the situation or background relevant to the family. A family can be viewed in the context of ethnicity, race, social class, religion and spirituality, and environment.

Ethnicity. *Ethnicity,* which is the concept of a family's cultural, historical, geographic, linguistic, and ethnic heritage, can greatly influence family interaction. Ethnicity may influence a family's functioning, structure, perspectives, values, health beliefs, and philosophies (see Chapter 9 for further information about ethnicity). Cultural and ethnic heritage can affect, for example, religious practices, child-rearing practices, recreational activities, and nutrition. Individually focused assessment is important, as different members of an ethnic group may subscribe to differing beliefs, traditions, and restrictions, even within the same generation.

Questions to ask the family

- Do you think of your family as having a strong ethnic identity?
- Has your ethnic background influenced your health care?
- Could you tell me about ethnic traditions you practise? How are these traditions helpful to your family?

Race. *Race* (biological characteristics such as skin and hair colour) influences individual and group identification and is closely connected to ethnicity. Family members' interactions among themselves and with health care providers are influenced by racial attitudes, stereotypes, and discrimination. If ignored, these influences may constrain the nurse and family's relationship.

Question to ask the family

- If you and I were of the same race, would our conversation be different? How?

Social Class. *Social class* is shaped by education, income, and occupation. Each class has its own values, lifestyles, and behaviours that influence family interaction and health care practices.

Questions to ask the family

- What is your job? How many hours a week do you work? How does this affect family life?
- Does anyone in the family work shifts? How does that influence your family functioning?
- What level of education have you completed?
- Does your family have economic challenges at this time?

Religion and Spirituality. Family members' spiritual or religious beliefs, rituals, and practices can influence their ability to cope with or manage an illness or health concern (McLeod & Wright, 2008; Walsh, 2010a, 2010b; Wright, 2005, 2008; Wright & Bell, 2009). Spirituality is often an underused resource in family nursing (see Chapter 28 for further information about spiritual health). Increasingly, families choose to explore the spiritual beliefs and practices that best fit their multifaith lives, beliefs about spirituality, and relationships. Spiritual assessment and support will therefore be highly individualized within an inquiry-oriented approach (Hartrick Doane & Varcoe, 2006; Walsh, 2010a).

Questions to ask the family

- What spiritual practices does your family have? What priority do these practices hold in your family? Have your family's spiritual beliefs changed or been challenged in any way during this illness?
- Are you involved in a particular church, temple, mosque, synagogue, group, religious or spiritual community?
- Would you discuss a family problem with anyone from your place of worship?
- Do you consider your spiritual beliefs a resource? A source of stress?

Environment. The family *environment* refers to the larger community, neighbourhood, and home contexts. Environmental factors that may affect family functioning include availability or lack of adequate space and of access to schools, day care, recreation, and public transportation.

Questions to ask the family

- What are the advantages and disadvantages of living in your neighbourhood?
- What community services does your family use?
- What community services would you like to learn about?

Structural Assessment Tools. The CFAM encourages you to work with family members to create genograms and ecomaps to facilitate documentation and understanding of the family structure and its contact with outside individuals and organizations. A **genogram** is a sketch of the family structure and relevant information about family members (Figure 19-3). Some agencies have genogram forms, but genograms can also be sketched on other forms, such as admission forms and records. The genogram becomes part of the documentation about the patient and family. An **ecomap** is a sketch of the family's relationships with persons and groups outside the family (Figure 19-4). The family members who share the household are depicted in the

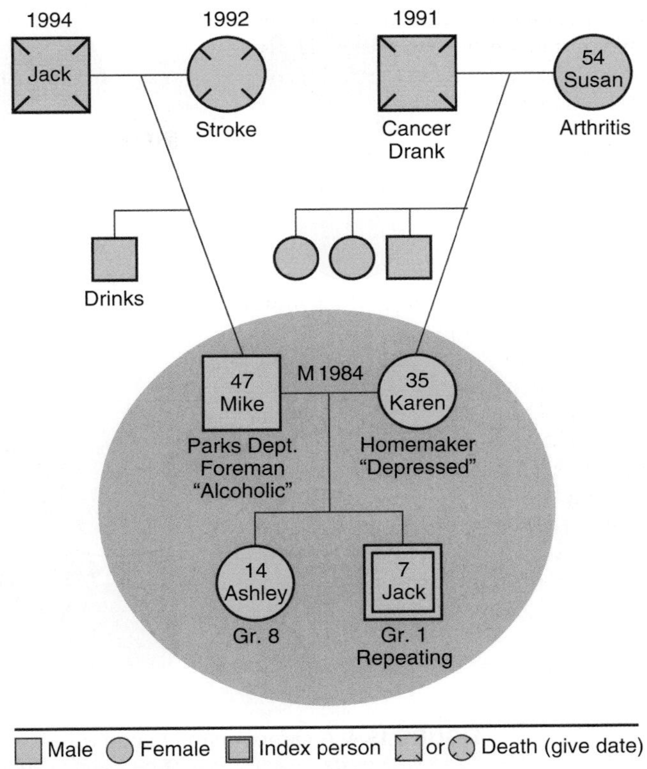

FIGURE 19-3 A sample family genogram. (Adapted from Wright, L. M., & Leahey, M. [2013]. *Nurses and families: A guide to family assessment and intervention* [6th ed., p. 79, Figure 3-4]. Philadelphia: FA Davis.)

centre of the ecomap, and various important extended family members or larger systems are sketched in to show their relationship to the family.

Nurses are encouraged to draw genograms and ecomaps for families with whom they will be involved for more than one day. Information for brief genograms and ecograms can be gleaned from family members during the initial assessment of the family structure. The most essential information for genograms includes data about ages, occupation or schooling, religion, ethnicity, and current health status of family members. For a brief genogram, the focus is only on information relevant to the family and the health problem. The shared creation of a genogram by a nurse and family can be an important time for the nurse to engage with the family, forming a relational connection between family members and the nurse. Engagement can be facilitated through the use of humour, curiosity, and invitations for family members to describe the strengths they see in one another. For example, the nurse might ask a child (8 years old), "What do you most like about your dad?"

Developmental Assessment

Families, like individuals, change and grow over time. Although each family is unique, all families tend to go through certain stages that require family members to adjust, adapt, and change roles. Each developmental stage presents challenges and includes tasks that need to be completed before the family can successfully move on to the next stage. Family development is more than the concurrent development of children and adults. It is the interaction between an individual's development and the phase of the family developmental life cycle that can be significant for family functioning. Therefore, in addition to

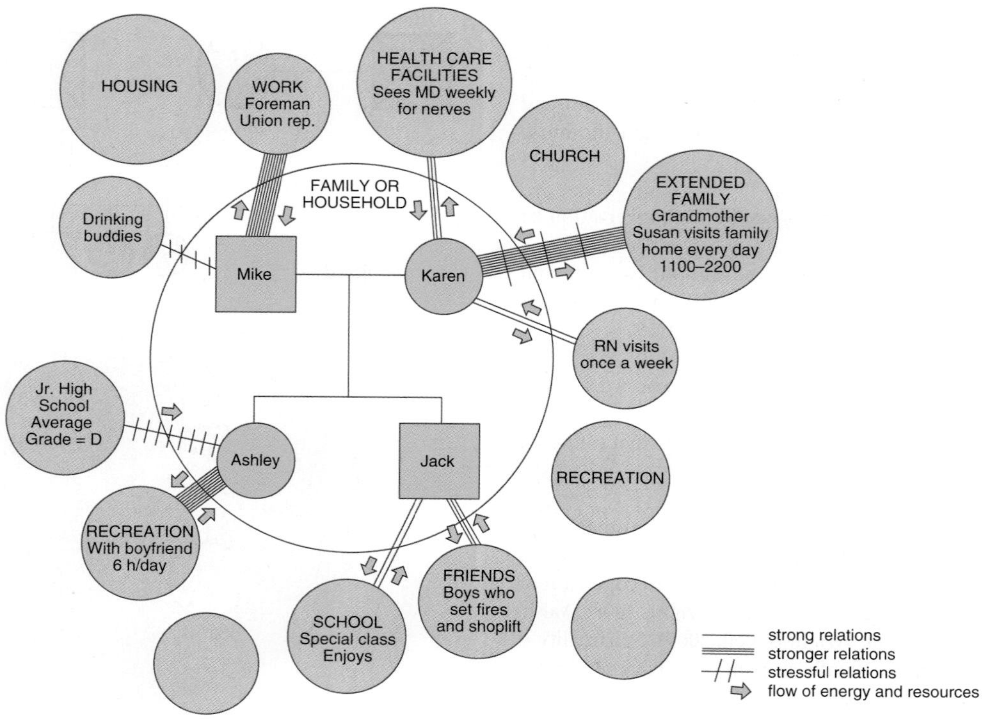

FIGURE 19-4 A sample family ecomap. (Adapted from Wright, L. M., & Leahey, M. [2013]. *Nurses and families: A guide to family assessment and intervention* [6th ed., p. 89, Figure 3-10]. Philadelphia: FA Davis.)

understanding family structure, nurses need to understand the developmental life cycle of each family.

In their articulation of the expanded family life cycle, McGoldrick and colleagues (2016) described the emotional process of life cycle transition, as well as the family development tasks for different stages. The family life cycle stages they describe include "Emerging Young Adults, Couple Formation: The Joining of Families, Families with Young Children, Families with Adolescents, Launching Children and Moving on at Midlife, Families in Late Middle Age, and Families Nearing the End of Life" (pp. 24-25). Additionally, the unique challenges faced by lone-parent, lesbian, gay, bisexual, and transgender families, as well as those facing transitions related to divorce, are discussed. Understanding family development theory can help nurses to promote health during expected family life cycle transitions and experiences of illness. For further information, please see *The Expanding Family Life Cycle: Individual, Family, and Social Perspectives* (5th ed.) (McGoldrick et al., 2016).

Functional Assessment

A *functional assessment* focuses on how family members interact and behave toward each other. Nurses assess family functioning by closely observing the interactions of family members in two subcategories: instrumental and expressive functioning.

Instrumental Functioning. *Instrumental functioning* refers to the normal activities of daily living, such as preparing meals, eating, sleeping, and attending to health needs. For families with health problems, these activities often become a challenge. Roles may change as family members cope with a relative's illness and disability. Within the context of illness, nurses and other health care providers play an important role in accessing practical and financial resources to support family members' instrumental needs (e.g., financial resources for medical supplies that parents need to care for an ill child at home).

Questions to ask the family

- Who is usually responsible for housekeeping and child care?
- Do other family members help with these tasks?
- Does anyone in the family require help with activities of daily living?
- Who will be primarily responsible for cleaning Mary's Broviac line (an intravenous access device for the administration of medications and blood tests) when she is discharged home?

Expressive Functioning. *Expressive functioning* refers to the ways in which people communicate. The significance of communication within the family cannot be emphasized enough, for it has a profound impact on a family's adjustment to illness and on their resiliency in the face of developmental and illness-related challenges. Illness and disability often challenge and alter expressive functioning within the family. A diagnosis may cause intense feelings of anxiety or grief, both within the person being diagnosed and within other family members. Nurses should encourage families to explore their understanding of illness and how it affects their lives. Nurses may need to assist family members with these difficult conversations, given the emotional intensity of this communication (Box 19-7). There are 10 subcategories of expressive functioning: emotional, verbal, nonverbal, and circular communication; problem solving; roles; influence and power; beliefs; and alliances and coalitions.

Emotional Communication. Emotional communication encompasses the range and types of feelings that are expressed by the family. Most families express a wide range of feelings. Families with problems may have rigid patterns and narrower ranges of emotional expression (e.g., a family coping with a father's cancer diagnosis may be anxious and unable to express optimism or hope for the future). Family roles and gender may affect emotional expression. For example, brothers and sisters who have a sibling with a life-threatening illness may not express their own experiences of suffering because they want

BOX 19-7 RESEARCH HIGHLIGHT

Therapeutic Conversations With Family Members Experiencing Childhood Cancer

Children with cancer, and their families, experience physical, emotional, spiritual, and relational illness distress. Families have described the sadness and fear they live with and the difficulty experienced in talking about cancer. Despite calls for comprehensive psychosocial intervention, childhood cancer research that examines family intervention has been limited. West, Bell, Woodgate, and Moules (2015) conducted a qualitative study that analyzed videotaped therapeutic conversations from the Family Nursing Unit, University of Calgary, as well as research interviews with family members (16) and nurse clinicians (3) following their participation in a family systems nursing clinical intervention. The philosophical hermeneutic research study explored the internalized questions that parents, ill children, brothers, and sisters ask themselves while living with childhood cancer, and how nurses could better attend to their suffering. Nursing interventions that were found to lessen illness suffering included bringing the family and nurse together for the purpose of a therapeutic conversation, and creating a therapeutic space where illness suffering was brought forward through the sharing of illness experiences with the nurse, as well as with other family members. West and colleagues (2015) found that when nurses invited family members into a reflective, listening stance, they were able to hear each other's illness experiences, which facilitated new interpretations of their suffering. Integral to this intervention process was the nurse's presence, described as a "holding" or "containing" of suffering, giving family members the experience of being heard, and opening families to new interpretations of their suffering through the offering of alternative illness beliefs. Questions and nursing responses that invited family members to externalize their inner dialogue were particularly helpful in lessening suffering. Sharing commendations with family members was another valuable nursing intervention that helped to enhance family strengths and lessen experiences of suffering.

An interview excerpt with Jason (12-year-old brother, research participant) highlights the profound importance of family nursing practices:

> *Jason: When Cameron was sick, I was like, "Oh, my parents don't love me ... they want to spend all the time with Cameron, I got no family." And then we went to the FNU [Family Nursing Unit], and we had fun, and I realized that my family was like any other ... we just went through ... a hard ... a traumatic situation ... otherwise, we're a normal family* (p. 279).

West, C. H., Bell, J. M., Woodgate, R. L., & Moules, N. J. (2015). Waiting to return to normal: An exploration of family systems intervention in childhood cancer. *Journal of Family Nursing, 21*(2), 261–294. doi:10.1177/1074840715576795

to protect their family from further distress and worry (Woodgate, 2006).

Questions to ask the family

- How can you tell when each member of your family is happy, sad, or under stress?
- How do you express happiness, sadness, or stress?
- Johnny, when you are sad or worried, who in the family do you most like to spend time with or talk to about that?

Verbal Communication. Nurses should observe a family's verbal communication, focusing on the meaning of the words in terms of the relationship. Is communication among family members clear and direct, or is it vague and indirect? It is useful to ask family members about how well the family communicates.

Questions to ask the family

- Which family member communicates most clearly?
- How might your family members communicate with each other more effectively?
- Families sometimes find it helpful to talk with one of the nurses about their life at home after learning about an illness. Do you think your family would find that helpful?

Nonverbal Communication. Nonverbal communication consists of messages conveyed without words, including body language, eye contact, gesturing, crying, and tone of voice. An example of a nonverbal communication is children's body language regarding each other or in response to their father's abuse of alcohol.

Questions to ask the family

- How do you think your daughter feels when your son rolls his eyes while she's talking?
- Who shows the most distress when talking about your dad's drinking? What are some of the nonverbal signals that indicate your daughter is distressed when talking about her dad's drinking?

Circular Communication. Circular communication refers to reciprocal communication between family members; that is, each person influences the behaviour of the other. Circular communication can be adaptive or maladaptive. For example, an adaptive communication pattern occurs when a parent comforts a child when the child cries. Because the parent responds to the child, the child feels safe and secure. An example of a maladaptive communication pattern is when a parent criticizes a teenager for not phoning home. The teenager is angry for being criticized and avoids the parent, and then the parent becomes angrier and criticizes more.

Questions to ask the family

- You mentioned that your teenager does not phone home. What do you do then?
- What do you think your daughter is thinking when you criticize her?

Problem Solving. Problem solving refers to how a family thinks about actions to take to resolve difficult situations.

Questions to ask the family

- Who first notices problems? How does your family tend to deal with problems?
- Is one member more proactive than others about solving problems?

Roles. Roles are established patterns of behaviour for family members, often developed through interactions with others. Formal roles include those of mother, husband, friend, and so forth. Informal roles can include, for example, those of "the softy," "the angel," or "the scapegoat." In the context of illness, family members often must take on new roles, such as medical caregiver.

Question to ask the family

- Who is the "good listener"... who is "the angel" in your family?

Influence. Influence refers to methods of affecting or controlling another person's behaviour. Influence may be instrumental (e.g., rewards for behaviour such as the promise of candy, computer time), psychological (communication to influence behaviour such as praise, admonishment), or corporal (the use of body contact, such as hugging, hitting).

Questions to ask the family

- What method does your mom use to get you to go to bed on time?

- How does your grandma get your brother to attend school when he refuses?

Beliefs. Beliefs are individual- and family-held fundamental ideas, values, opinions, and assumptions (Wright, Watson, & Bell, 1996). Understanding the core beliefs (Wright & Bell, 2009) of family members is central to understanding their suffering and to facilitating healing in the context of illness (Wright et al., 1996; Wright & Bell, 2009). Beliefs influence behaviour and how the family adapts to illness. For example, if a family believes that vaccinations may cause disabilities, the parents may decline vaccinating an infant. Beliefs may also influence how a family responds to another member's depression or chronic pain.

Questions to ask the family

- What do you believe causes your husband's depression?
- What do you believe would be the effect on your chronic pain if you chose to participate in that treatment?

Alliances and Coalitions. Alliances and coalitions involve the directionality, balance, and intensity of relationships among family members or between families and nurses.

Questions to ask the family

- If the children are playing well together, who would be most likely to get them to start fighting?
- Is there anything that you were hoping we would talk about today that we haven't spoken about?

TABLE 19-1 The ABCs of Engaging Families

A	B	C
Assume an active, confident approach.	Begin by providing structure to the meeting (time frame, orientation to the context).	Create a context of mutual trust.
Ask purposeful questions that draw forth family assessment data.	Behave in a curious manner, and take an equal interest in all family members, whether present or not.	Clarify expectations about your role with the family.
Address all who are present, including small children.	Build on family strengths by offering commendations to the family.	Collaborate in decision making, health promotion, and health management.
Adjust the conversation to children's developmental stages.	Bring relevant resources to the meeting (list of agencies, phone numbers, pamphlets).	Cultivate a context of racial and ethnic sensitivity. Commend family members.

Adapted from Levac, A. M. C., Wright, L. M., & Leahey, M. (2002). Children and families: Models for assessment and intervention. In J. A. Fox (Ed.), *Primary health care of infants, children, and adolescents* (2nd ed., p. 111). St. Louis: Mosby.

FAMILY INTERVENTION: THE CALGARY FAMILY INTERVENTION MODEL

After assessment, nurses intervene to help families meet their needs, face challenges, and appreciate their strengths. A range of family nursing interventions can be offered to families in the context of a therapeutic relationship. Some, such as parent education and caregiver support, are general; others are specific and require therapeutic communication and family interviewing skills. The ultimate goal is to help family members discover alternative solutions that may lessen or alleviate emotional, physical, and spiritual suffering. Whether caring for a patient with the family as context or directing care to the family as patient, the aim of nursing interventions is to enhance family members' abilities in certain areas, remove barriers to health care, and perform actions that the family cannot perform for itself. Nurses guide the family in problem solving, provide practical services, and convey a sense of acceptance and caring by listening carefully to family members' experiences, concerns, suggestions, and questions.

Interventions for each family must be individualized and focus on particular areas of family functioning (cognitive, affective, behavioural) (Wright & Leahey, 2013). Nurses can only *offer* interventions and must not instruct or insist on a particular kind of change or way of family functioning. Nurses need to sensitively attend to ideas or interventions that the family perceives as being most helpful (Wright & Leahey, 2013).

The Calgary Family Intervention Model (CFIM) is a companion to the CFAM and can be used as a guide for nursing intervention with the family (Wright & Leahey, 2013). The CFIM focuses on promoting and improving family functioning in three domains: cognitive, affective, and behavioural. Interventions may affect functioning in any or all of the three domains. For example, when a clinic nurse informs a wife that her husband, who has amyotrophic lateral sclerosis, is still capable of large gross motor movement, the nurse can suggest he help with chores in the house, such as bringing the laundry upstairs. This intervention may challenge the wife's thinking that her husband was incapable of work, influence her to feel less depressed over her husband's declining physical capacity, and lead her to change her behaviour by including her husband when performing other household chores.

The CFIM recommends many relational nursing practices that promote family health and functioning, including asking interventive questions, offering commendations, providing information, validating emotional responses, encouraging illness narratives, supporting family caregivers, and encouraging respite. Central to this interventional practice is the nurse's engagement with family members in a thoughtful, purposeful relation (Table 19-1). Within CFAM and CFIM, as well as in the Illness Beliefs Model (Wright & Bell, 2009; Wright et al., 1996), nurses are guided to continually attend to the cultivation of a relationship that is collaborative, responsive, and nonhierarchical. Within this relationship, there is a privileging of family expertise and a commitment to listening deeply to the concerns, suffering, and questions of family members.

The guidance provided by Hartrick Doane and Varcoe (2005, 2015) in their discussion of relational inquiry is another helpful resource for your relational engagement with the families you encounter in your practice.

Asking Interventive Questions

One of the most effective ways that nurses can help families is by engaging in therapeutic conversations with families and asking them questions. Questions lead the family to reflect on their situation, clarify opinions and ideas, and understand how they are affected by their family member's illness or condition. By hearing their own responses to questions, as well as the responses of others, family members can better understand themselves and each other and perhaps discover new possibilities for health and healing. Interventive questions also elicit information important to the nurse.

There are two types of interventive questions: linear and circular (Tomm, 1987, 1988). Linear questions elicit information about a

TABLE 19-2 Three Types of Circular Questions

	EXAMPLES TO ELICIT CHANGE		
Purpose of Question	**Cognitive Domain**	**Affective Domain**	**Behavioural Domain**
Difference Question			
Explores differences between people, relationships, time, ideas, or beliefs	What is the best advice given you about supporting your son with AIDS? What is the worst advice?	Who in the family is most worried about how AIDS is transmitted?	Which family member is best at getting your son to take his medication on time?
Behavioural Effect Question			
Explores connections between how one family member's behaviour affects other members	What do you know about the effect of life-threatening illness on children?	How does your son show that he is afraid of dying?	What could you do to show your son that you understand his fears?
Hypothetical/Future-Oriented Question			
Explores family options and alternative actions or meanings in the future	What do you think will happen if these skin grafts continue to be painful for Dan?	If Dan's skin grafts are not successful, what do you think his mood will be? Angry? Resigned?	When will your son engage in treatment for his contractures?

Adapted from Wright, L. M., & Leahey, M. (2013). *Nurses and families: A guide to family assessment and intervention* (6th ed., p. 156). Philadelphia: FA Davis.

patient or family. They explore a family member's descriptions or perceptions of an illness or life challenge. For example, linear questions may be used when exploring a couple's perceptions of their daughter's anorexia nervosa: "When did you notice that your daughter had changed her eating habits?" "Has she been hospitalized in the past for this problem?" These questions inform the nurse of the daughter's eating patterns and illuminate family perceptions or beliefs about eating patterns.

Circular questions help determine possible changes for a patient's or family's life. They help the nurse understand relationships between individuals, beliefs, and events and elicit valuable information to help create change. In this way, circular questions often help patients make new cognitive connections, paving the way for changes in family behaviours. For example, with the same family, the nurse could ask, "Who is most worried about Cheyenne's anorexia?" or "How does Ellen show that she's worrying the most?" Although linear questions may imply that you know what is best for the family, circular questions facilitate change by inviting the family to discover their own answers. Linear questions tend to target specific yes or no answers, thereby limiting options for the family; for example, "Have you tried time out to discipline your 3-year-old?" An alternative circular question might be "Which type of discipline seems to work best for your child?" Several types of circular questions exist; each can affect the cognitive, affective, and behavioural domains. These types include difference questions, behavioural effect questions, hypothetical or future-oriented questions, and triadic questions (Tomm, 1987, 1988; Wright & Leahey, 2013) (Table 19-2).

Offering Commendations

Families do not always view themselves as having inherent strength and resilience. As their nurse, you can help the family become aware of their unique strengths, thus increasing their potential and capabilities. A **commendation** is a conversational statement emphasizing family strengths and abilities. While spending time with the family, you may observe many instances in which the family displays strengths. It is important to acknowledge these with the family so that they can recognize and appreciate their capabilities. By commending a family's strengths and capacities, you can offer family members a new view of themselves, and this may invite a change in how they view their health challenges. Look for patterns of behaviour to commend, rather than a single occurrence. For example, you may say, "Your family has shown courage living with your wife's cancer for 5 years" or "I'm impressed with how the family worked together during the crisis." Families coping with chronic, life-threatening, or psychosocial problems frequently feel hopeless in their efforts to overcome or live with the illness. Therefore, you should offer as many truthful, genuine commendations as possible. In a qualitative research study exploring the practice of commendations, family members shared their belief that commendations were part of the "special, meaningful, and caring relationships that they developed with the therapists [nurses]. Commendations were not techniques... but *a way of being with people in the world*" (Hougher Limacher, 2008, p. 99).

Family strengths include clear communication, adaptability, healthy boundaries, support and nurturing among family members, and the use of crisis for growth. You can help the family focus on these strengths rather than on weaknesses.

Providing Information

Families need information from health care providers about developmental issues, health promotion, and illness management, especially if the illness is complex (Hartrick Doane & Varcoe, 2015). Accurate, timely information is essential for the family to make decisions and cope with difficult situations. Health education is a process by which information is exchanged between the nurse, patient, and family. Family and patient needs for information may be elicited through direct questioning but are often far more subtle. In this role of educator, you may recognize, for example, that a new father is fearful of cleaning his newborn's umbilical cord stump or that an older woman is not using her cane safely. Respectful communication is required. Nurses often share information subtly: "I notice you are trying to not touch the umbilical cord stump; I see that a lot with other new parents" or "You use the cane the way I did before I was shown a way to keep from falling or tripping over it; do you mind if I show you?" When you assume a humble, caring position instead of coming across as an authority on the subject, this attitude often decreases the patient's defences and invites the family to listen without feeling embarrassed.

Validating or Normalizing Emotional Responses

Validating intense emotions can alleviate a family's feelings of isolation and loneliness and help family members make the connection between a family member's illness and their own emotional response. For example, after a diagnosis of a life-shortening illness, families frequently feel powerless or frightened. It is important to validate these strong emotions as normal and reassure families that they will adjust and learn new ways to cope. You may do this by sharing experiences you have had with other families who have faced a similar situation.

Encouraging Illness Narratives

Too often, patients and family members are encouraged to talk only about the medical aspects of their illness rather than the emotional aspects. An **illness narrative** is the person's story of how the illness affects his or her whole being, including emotional, intellectual, social, and spiritual dimensions (Kleinman, 1988; Wright & Bell, 2009). Hearing the person's illness narrative will help you understand the person's/family's strengths and challenges, and the beliefs they hold about their illness experience. This information enables you to offer commendations to the family. Many people also find that telling their story helps them better understand themselves, their experience, and their family's experience. Families also benefit from listening to one another's illness narratives. Prior to meeting with their nurse, families may not have had the opportunity to hear and understand how other family members have suffered in living with illness (Boxes 19-7 and 19-8).

Communicating what it is like to live with individual, separate experiences, particularly the experience of illness, is a powerful human need (Wright, 2005). Frequently, nurses believe that listening entails an obligation to "fix" whatever concerns or problems are raised. However, showing compassion through deep listening and offering commendations are usually more therapeutic or helpful than offering solutions to problems (Hougher Limacher, 2008; Wright & Bell, 2009).

Encouraging Family Support

Family functioning is enhanced by encouraging and assisting family members to listen to each other's concerns and feelings. This assistance can be particularly useful if a family member is embracing some constraining beliefs when a loved one is dying or has died (RNAO, 2015; Wright & Nagy, 1993). For example, a family may believe that talking with the ill person about death and dying would hasten the person's death.

Supporting Family Caregivers

Family members are often afraid of becoming involved in the care of an ill member without a nurse's support. One way the nurse can best provide care is through supporting family caregivers. Without preparation and support, caregiving can be stressful, causing a decline in the health of the caregiver and care receiver or the development of abusive relationships.

Despite its demands, caregiving, whether one spouse caring for the other or a child caring for a parent, can be a positive and rewarding experience (Duxbury et al., 2009). The interpersonal dynamics between family members influence the ultimate quality of caregiving. Nurses can play a key role in helping family members develop better communication and problem-solving skills needed for caregiving.

Researchers have identified variables, such as caregiver and care recipient expectations, that influence caregiving quality. Carruth (1996) studied the concept of **reciprocity**, in which care recipients acknowledged the importance of the caregiver's help, and contributions to a caregiver's self-worth. When the caregiver knows that the care recipient appreciates his or her efforts and values the assistance provided, the caregiving relationship is healthier and more satisfying.

Encouraging Respite

Nurses should encourage respite for caregivers, who may feel guilty about or not even recognize their need to withdraw, even temporarily, from caregiving tasks. Sometimes an ill person may be encouraged to accept another person's temporary assistance so that family members can take a break. Whatever the situation, the nurse should remember that each family's need for respite varies.

Providing care and support for family caregivers often involves using available family and community resources for respite. Caregiving burden can be lessened by the use of a caregiving schedule when multiple family members are participating, the sharing of any financial burdens posed by caregiving, and communication of support from extended family members who live at a distance. However, it is important to understand the relationship between potential caregivers and care recipients. If the relationship is not a supportive one, community services may be a resource for both the patient and family.

Services that may be beneficial to families include caregiver respite, caregiver support groups, housing and transportation services, food and nutrition services, housecleaning, legal and financial services, home care, hospice, and mental health resources. Before referring a family to a community resource, it is crucial that nurses are aware of the community services themselves, understand the family's dynamics, and know whether such support is desired or welcomed. A family caregiver may resist help, feeling obligated to be the sole source of support to the care recipient. Nurses must be sensitive to family relationships and help normalize the demands of caregiving and the need for respite.

BOX 19-8 EVIDENCE-INFORMED PRACTICE

Lessons Learned From the Study of Therapeutic Conversations Between Nurses and Family Members Living With Childhood Cancer

- Nurses should offer families the opportunity to gather together in order to speak about the suffering they experience living with illness. Family members may be unable to speak directly with one another about intense emotions and illness suffering.
- The nurse's presence with family members for the purpose of a therapeutic conversation can facilitate sharing and a lessening of suffering. The nurse's ability to create a safe relational space where suffering is explored and contained or held by the nurse is particularly important.
- Careful relational engagement, eliciting the illness narrative, asking circular questions, offering commendations, as well as externalizing inner dialogue are particularly helpful interventions that may lessen suffering. The exploration of alternative illness beliefs within the therapeutic conversation opens possibilities for family healing and new ways of living with illness.
- When a family member shares his or her illness narrative with a nurse, other family members are able to adopt a listening, reflective stance, enabling the family to listen and understand each other's experiences differently.

West, C. H., Bell, J. M., Woodgate, R. L., & Moules, N. J. (2015). Waiting to return to normal: An exploration of family systems intervention in childhood cancer. *Journal of Family Nursing, 21*(2), 261–294. doi:10.1177/1074840715576795

INTERVIEWING THE FAMILY

With a clear conceptual framework for assessment and intervention, you can begin to learn the competencies and skills needed to conduct family interviews. Family interviews follow the same basic principles as any patient interview (see Chapter 13 for further information about interviewing patients). However, family interviews have the complexity of more people and multiple relationships. You must develop keen perceptual, conceptual, and executive skills. *Perceptual skills* refer to the ability to make relevant observations. In family interviewing, you must observe multiple interactions and relationships simultaneously. *Conceptual skills* constitute the ability to formulate observations of the entire family and give meaning to those observations. Remember that observations and subsequent judgements are subjective and not conclusive. *Executive skills* are the actual therapeutic interventions you offer in the context of a family interview. These therapeutic interventions elicit responses from family members and are the basis for further observations and conceptualizations.

During an interview, observe and listen for responses from a patient and family to formulate further therapeutic interventions. The type of intervention that you offer depends on your clinical expertise and experience in working with families, as well as the unique challenges and strengths of the family members you are working with. The four stages of a family interview are engagement, assessment, intervention, and termination. Each of these stages will include specific perceptual and executive skills. For more information on the skills and stages of conducting a family interview, see *Nurses and Families: A Guide to Family Assessment and Intervention* (Wright & Leahey, 2013). With these skills you can assess, explore, and identify strengths and problems in the familiar process of engagement, assessment, intervention, and termination (see Chapter 17 for further information about communication skills). You can also decide to intervene or to refer the family to another health provider. These skills should not necessarily be applied to all families. You should tailor the interview to each family's individual context.

It is important to realize that not all family interviews are formal, lengthy processes. Even if you do not have the time for a formal family interview, you can still engage the family in productive, therapeutic conversations. Every conversation between you and the patient or family members can improve communication and understanding. Therapeutic conversations can be as short as one sentence or as long as time allows. All therapeutic conversations, regardless of time, have the potential to unite the family (Wright & Leahey, 2013). Even brief interviews or conversations have tremendous healing potential because they offer families the opportunity to acknowledge and affirm their problems and seek solutions (Wright & Bell, 2009; Wright & Leahey, 2013).

The integration of task-oriented patient care with interactive, purposeful conversation distinguishes a time-effective interview (taking less than 15 minutes). Providing information and involving the family in decision making are integral parts of the therapeutic process. You should search for opportunities to engage in purposeful conversations with families, which may include the following:

- Routinely inviting families to accompany the patient to the unit, clinic, or hospital
- Routinely including families' participation in the admission procedure
- Routinely inviting families to ask questions
- Acknowledging the patient and family's expertise in managing the health problem at home
- Routinely consulting patients and families about their ideas regarding treatment and discharge

KEY CONCEPTS

- Family members influence one another's health beliefs, practices, and status.
- The concept of family is highly individual; thus, nurses should base care on the patient's definition of family rather than on an inflexible definition of family.
- Family nursing care requires that nurses continually examine the current trends in the Canadian family and their health care implications.
- A healthy, resilient family is able to integrate the need for stability with the need for growth and change. The family can be viewed as context, in which the nurse focuses either on the individual patient within the context of his or her family or on the family with the individual as context, or the family can be viewed as patient (family systems nursing), in which the nurse focuses on family interactions.
- The CFAM is a conceptual framework that guides nurses in assessing the structural, developmental, and functional aspects of the family.
- Genograms and ecomaps are structural assessment tools that provide a pictorial image of the family's structure and relation to outside influences.
- Family members as caregivers are often spouses who may be either older persons themselves or adult children trying to work full-time, care for aging parents, and enable children to move out of the home (launch children) successfully.
- Illness and disability often alter expressive functioning and communication within the family.
- Relational inquiry with families is concerned with understanding the family in context (interpersonal, social, geo-political, historical, environmental context).
- A number of relational capacities that support being in relation with families in a mode of inquiry that balances letting be and emancipator action are key components to family nursing as relational inquiry.
- The CFIM is a companion to the CFAM that guides nurses in implementing family interventions; it is focused on improving family functioning in three domains: cognitive (thinking), affective (feeling), and behavioural (doing).
- One of the simplest and most effective ways that nurses can help families is by asking them circular questions.
- Offering commendations is important because they encourage the family to recognize their strengths and competencies.
- Other nursing interventions to help the family include providing information, validating emotional responses, encouraging patients to provide illness narratives, supporting family caregivers, and encouraging respite for family caregivers.
- Family caregiving is an interactional process that occurs within the context of the relationships among its members.
- Family interviews require nurses to have perceptual, conceptual, and executive skills; interviews may be formal and lengthy or casual and brief.

CRITICAL THINKING EXERCISES

1. Kathy is a palliative care nurse working with a family of four: Melinda, a 45-year-old single mother; her adolescent sons, Etan and Matthew; and Heng, her 76-year-old mother, who is in the last stages of terminal breast cancer. The family has lived together for 10 years, ever since they immigrated to Canada from Hong Kong. Heng helped Melinda parent Etan and Matthew and supported

Melinda when her husband died 5 years ago. Melinda has decided to care for her mother in the family's home until Heng dies. Kathy will assist this family in achieving their goal. Kathy has just had in-service training in using CFAM.

a. What parts of the CFAM should Kathy use when assessing the family's needs?
b. How can Kathy help the family achieve their goal of caring for their aging family member at home?
c. How can Kathy determine this family's strengths, suffering, and resources?
d. What cultural aspects are important to consider for a family who has immigrated to Canada and is now facing the death of a loved one?
e. What self-awareness and reflection will support a relational inquiry approach to the assessment and interventions?

2. Dan and Kim divorced 7 years ago, and neither has remarried. They have three daughters, aged 10, 12, and 14. At the time of the divorce, Dan was HIV positive, and has remained so for 5 years. Kim has had repeated tests and remains HIV negative. Dan is responding to therapy slowly. Kim and Dan share parenting responsibilities and have a friendly relationship. They have decided it would be easier for the family to live together again so that Dan can actively participate in his children's lives without placing caregiver demands on Kim when the extended family visits overnight. Kim also wants to care for her former husband.
   a. What family development tasks are important to assess for this family as the members attempt to reunite?
   b. How should the nurse determine what support services the family needs?
   c. What assessment questions would be useful to ask in order to assess how the illness is affecting this family? Do family members have any signs of emotional, physical, or spiritual suffering?
3. Gilles Leduc and Xavier Bothe, both in their early 50s, are the youngest members of large families. They work full-time and have two teenage children. Both sets of their parents are in their 80s and have chronic health problems. All of their siblings live farther away.
   a. How can the nurse help Gilles and Xavier access resources to aid in caring for their parents and maintain the responsibilities of their own family unit?
   b. What developmental tasks does this family have?
   c. What kinds of questions can you ask to assess the family's emotional and verbal communication (found in CFAM's functional assessment category)?

REVIEW QUESTIONS

1. Who should a nurse consider as family?
   1. Parents and their children
   2. People related by marriage, birth, or adoption
   3. The nuclear family and aunts, uncles, grandparents, and cousins
   4. A set of relationships that the patient identifies as family
2. The patient is remarried, and her two children from a previous marriage live in the same household. Her husband's children visit on the weekend. This is an example of which form of family configuration?
   1. A nuclear family
   2. A blended family
   3. An extended family
   4. An alternative family
3. What is the primary social context in which health promotion and disease prevention take place?
   1. At educational institutions
   2. From friends and colleagues
   3. From physicians and nurses
   4. In the family
4. What are two factors that contribute to the long-term health of a family?
   1. Structure and function
   2. Caregiving and reciprocity
   3. Hardiness and resiliency
   4. Context and system
5. What does the nurse focus on when viewing the family as patient?
   1. Health and development of an individual member existing within a specific environment
   2. Family process and relationships
   3. Family relational and transactional concepts
   4. Family within a system
6. What does asking a patient "Who is in your family?" help the nurse assess?
   1. Internal structure
   2. External structure
   3. Context
   4. Instrumental functioning
7. What is a goal of approaching family from a relational inquiry perspective?
   1. Professional collaboration
   2. Systematic problem solving
   3. Inquiry to understand the family in context
   4. Circular questions
8. What are two of the components of relational inquiry?
   1. Using both open- and closed-ended questions
   2. Applying both a strict assessment format and corresponding interventions
   3. Incorporating both letting be and emancipatory action
   4. Assessing the presenting problem and history of the presenting problem
9. Emotional communication belongs to which CFAM subcategory?
   1. Instrumental functioning
   2. Development
   3. Internal structure
   4. Expressive functioning
10. "What do you think when your husband won't visit your son in the hospital?" is an example of a circular question. What can asking the family circular questions accomplish?
    1. Facilitating change by inviting the family to discover their own answers
    2. Encouraging family members to be caregivers
    3. Validating their emotional responses
    4. Targeting specific yes or no answers
11. Which intervention can the nurse accomplish during a family interview?
    1. Educate the family
    2. Enforce change
    3. Engage a family to assess, explore, and identify strengths and problems
    4. Establish roles

Answers: 1. 4; **2.** 2; **3.** 4; **4.** 3; **5.** 2; **6.** 1; **7.** 3; **8.** 3; **9.** 4; **10.** 1; **11.** 3

Rationales for the Review Questions appear at the end of the book.

RECOMMENDED WEBSITES

Family Nursing Resources: http://www.familynursingresources.com
Family nursing videos, books, DVDs, and family genographs are available on this website.

International Family Nursing Association: http://internationalfamilynursing.org
Resources for family nursing practice, education, and research. An online community that promotes connection with family nurses globally.

Journal of Family Nursing: http://jfn.sagepub.com
The *Journal of Family Nursing* (JFN) "is a peer-reviewed, quarterly journal of nursing research, practice, education, and policy issues, as well as empirical and theoretical analyses on the subject of family health. Its interdisciplinary, international, and collaborative perspectives examine cultural diversity and families across the life cycle" (Sage Journals, 2012, paragraph 1).

Vanier Institute of the Family: http://www.vanierinstitute.ca
The Vanier Institute of the Family aims to "create awareness of, and to provide leadership on, the importance and strengths of families in Canada and the challenges they face in their structural, demographic, economic, cultural and social diversity" (Vanier Institute, About Us, paragraph 1). This website highlights news articles, research, publications, policies, and networks that focus on the family.

REFERENCES

Black, K., & Lobo, M. (2008). A conceptual review of family resilience factors. *Journal of Family Nursing, 14*(1), 33–55. doi:10.1177/1074840707312237.

Brooks-Gunn, J., Han, W., & Waldfogel, J. (2010). First-year maternal employment and child development in the first 7 years. *Monographs of the Society for Research in Child Development, 75*(2), 59–69. doi:10.1111/j.1540-5834.2010.00562.x.

Browne, A. J., Varcoe, C., Lavoie, J., et al. (2016). Enhancing health care equity with indigenous populations: Evidence-based strategies from an ethnographic study. *BMC Health Services Research, 16*(1), 544. doi:10.1186/s12913-016-1707-9.

Canadian Association for Schools of Nursing/Association Canadienne des Écoles de Sciences Infirmières (CASN/ACESI). (2015). *National nursing education framework: Final report.* Retrieved from http://www.casn.ca/wp-content/uploads/2014/12/Framwork-FINAL-SB-Nov-30-20151.pdf.

Carruth, A. K. (1996). Development and testing of the Caregiver Reciprocity Scale. *Nursing Research, 45*(2), 92–97.

Clay, A. M., & Parsh, B. (2016). Patient- and family-centered care: It's not just for pediatrics anymore. *AMA Journal of Ethics, 18*(1), 40. doi:10.1001/journalofethics.2016.18.1.medu3-1601.

Coyne, I. (2013). Families and health-care professionals' perspectives and expectations of family-centred care: Hidden expectations and unclear roles. *Health Expectations, 18*(5), 796–808. doi:10.1111/hex.12104.

Duxbury, L., Higgins, C., & Schroeder, B. (2009). *Balancing paid work and family caregiving responsibilities: A closer look at family caregivers in Canada.* Ottawa: Human Resources and Skills Development Canada.

Elliott, J., Stuart, M., & Toman, C. (2009). *Place and practice in Canadian nursing history.* Vancouver: UBC Press.

Ford-Gilboe, M., Varcoe, C., Wuest, J., et al. (2011). Nursing practice in relation to family violence. In J. Humphreys & J. Campbell (Eds.), *Family violence and nursing practice.* (2nd ed.). New York: Springer.

Garner, R., Guimond, E., & Senécal, S. (2013). The socio-economic characteristics of First Nation teen mothers. *International Indigenous Policy Journal, 4*(1), doi:10.18584/iipj.2013.4.1.9. Retrieved from http://ir.lib.uwo.ca/iipj/vol4/iss1/9.

Gottlieb, L. N. (2013). *Strengths-based nursing care: Health and healing for person and family.* New York: Springer.

Hartrick Doane, G., & Varcoe, C. (2005). *Family nursing as relational inquiry. Developing health promoting practice.* Philadelphia, PA: Lippincott Williams & Wilkins.

Hartrick Doane, G., & Varcoe, C. (2006). The "hard spots" of family nursing: Connecting across difference and diversity. *Journal of Family Nursing, 12*(1), 7–21. doi:10.1177/1074840705284210.

Hartrick Doane, G. H., & Varcoe, C. (2015). *How to nurse: Relational inquiry with individuals and families in changing health care contexts.* Philadelphia, PA: Wolters Kluwer/Lippincott Williams & Wilkins.

Hill, R. (2003). Generic features of families under stress. In P. Boss & C. Milligan (Eds.), *Family stress: Classic and contemporary readings.* (pp. 177–190). Thousand Oaks, CA: Sage. (Original work published 1958).

Hougher Limacher, L. (2008). Locating relationships at the heart of commending practices. *Journal of Systemic Therapies, 27*(4), 90–105. doi:10.1521/jsyt.2008.27.4.90.

Hsieh, J. Y., Mercer, K. J., & Costa, S. A. (2017). Parenting a second time around: The strengths and challenges of Indigenous grandparent caregivers. *Grand Families: The Contemporary Journal of Research, Practice and Policy, 4*(1), Retrieved from http://scholarworks.wmich.edu/grandfamilies/vol4/iss1/8.

Kleinman, A. (1988). *The illness narratives: Suffering, healing, and the human condition.* New York: Basic Books.

Lindstrom, G., Choate, P., Bastien, L., et al. (2016). *Nistawatsimin: Exploring First Nations parenting: A literature review and expert consultation with Blackfoot Elders.* Calgary, AB: Mount Royal University.

Luxton, M. (2011). *Changing families, new understandings. Contemporary family trends.* Ottawa: Vanier Institute of the Family.

MacMillan, H. L., Wathen, C. N., Jamieson, E., et al. (2009). McMaster Violence Against Women Research Group. *Journal of American Medical Association, 302*(5), 493–501.

McCubbin, M. A., McCubbin, H. I., & Thompson, A. I. (1996). Family Hardiness Index (FHI). In H. I. McCubbin, A. I. Thompson, & M. S. McCubbin (Eds.), *Family assessment: Resiliency, coping, and adaptation, inventories for research and practice.* Madison, WI: University of Wisconsin Press.

McGoldrick, M., Garcia Preto, N., & Carter, B. (Eds.), (2016). *The expanding family life cycle: Individual, family, and social perspectives.* (5th ed.). Boston: MA: Pearson.

McLeod, D. L., & Wright, L. M. (2008). Living the as-yet unanswered: Spiritual care practices in family systems nursing. *Journal of Family Nursing, 14*(1), 118–141.

Moisan, C., Baril, C., Muckle, G., et al. (2016). Teen pregnancy in Inuit communities—gaps still needed to be filled. *International Journal of Circumpolar Health, 75*, 1–7. doi:10.3402/ijch.v75.31790.

Muir, N. M., & Bohr, Y. (2014). Contemporary practice of traditional Aboriginal child rearing: A review. *First Peoples Child & Family Review, 9*(1), Retrieved from http://journals.sfu.ca/fpcfr/index.php/FPCFR/article/view/231.

Rankin, J. M. (2015). The rhetoric of family centred care: An institutional ethnography into what actually happens. *Journal of Advanced Nursing, 71*(3), 526–534. doi:10.1111/jan.12575.

Registered Nurses' Association of Ontario (RNAO). (2015). *Person- and family-centred care.* Toronto, ON: Author.

Reiter, M. D. (2015). *Substance abuse and the family.* New York: Routledge.

Robinson, C. A., Pesut, B., & Bottorff, J. L. (2012). Supporting rural family palliative caregivers. *Journal of Family Nursing, 18*(4), 467–490. doi:10.1177/1074840712462065.

Statistics Canada. (2012). *Portrait of families and living arrangements in Canada, 2011 census of population* (Catalogue no. 98-312-X2011001). Ottawa: Minister of Industry.

Statistics Canada. (2015). *Portrait of families and living arrangements in Canada.* Retrieved from http://www12.statcan.gc.ca/census-recensement/2011/as-sa/98-312-x/98-312-x2011001-eng.cfm.

Statistics Canada. (2016a). *Canadian megatrends: The changing profile of stay-at-home parents.* Retrieved from http://www.statcan.gc.ca/daily-quotidien/160928/dq160928e-eng.htm.

Statistics Canada. (2016b). *Teen pregnancy: Pregnancy outcomes by age group.* Retrieved from http://www.statcan.gc.ca/eng/help/bb/info/teen.

Statistics Canada. (2016c). *Canadian megatrends: The rise of the dual-earner family with children.* Retrieved from http://statcan.gc.ca/daily-quotidien/160530/dq160530c-eng.htm.

Statistics Canada. (2016d). *Canadian income survey 2014.* Retrieved from http://www.statcan.gc.ca/daily-quotidien/160708/dq160708b-eng.htm.

Statistics Canada. (2017a). *The shift to smaller households over the past century.* Retrieved from http://www.statcan.gc.ca/pub/11-630-x/11-630-x2015008-eng.htm.

Statistics Canada (2017b). *2016 Census topic: Families, households and marital status.* Retrieved from http://www12.statcan.gc.ca/census-recensement/2016/rt-td/fam-eng.cfm

Tomm, K. (1987). Interventive interviewing: Part II. Reflexive questioning as a means to enable self-healing. *Family Process, 26*(2), 167–183.

Tomm, K. (1988). Interventive interviewing: Part III. Intending to ask lineal, circular, strategic or reflexive questions? *Family Process, 27*(1), 1–15.

Walsh, F. (2010a). Spiritual diversity: Multifaith perspectives in family therapy. *Family Process, 49*(3), 330–348. doi:10.1111/j.1545-5300.2010.01326.x.

Walsh, F. (2010b). *Spiritual resources in family therapy.* (2nd ed.). New York: Guilford Press.

West, C. H., Bell, J. M., Woodgate, R. L., et al. (2015). Waiting to return to normal: An exploration of family systems intervention in childhood cancer. *Journal of Family Nursing, 21*(2), 261–294. doi:10.1177/1074840715576795.

Woodgate, R. L. (2006). Siblings' experiences with childhood cancer: A different way of being in the family. *Cancer Nursing, 29*(5), 406–414.

World Health Organization. (2016). *World Health Statistics: Canada.* Retrieved from http://www.who.int/countries/can/en/.

Wright, L. M. (2005). *Spirituality, suffering, and illness: Ideas for healing.* Philadelphia, PA: F. A. Davis.

Wright, L. M. (2008). Softening suffering through spiritual care practices: One possibility for healing families. *Journal of Family Nursing, 14*(4), 394–411.

Wright, L. M., & Bell, J. M. (2009). *Beliefs and illness: A model for healing.* Calgary: 4th Floor Press.

Wright, L. M., & Leahey, M. (2013). *Nurses and families: A guide to family assessment and intervention.* (6th ed.). Philadelphia: F. A. Davis Company.

Wright, L. M., & Nagy, J. (1993). Death: The most troublesome family secret of all. In E. I. Black (Ed.), *Secrets in families and family therapy.* (pp. 121–137). New York: W. W. Norton.

Wright, L. M., Watson, W. L., & Bell, J. M. (1996). *Beliefs: The heart of healing in families and illness.* New York: Basic Books.

20

Patient Education

Canadian content written by Nancy A. Edgecombe, RN-NP, BN, MN, PhD
Original chapter by Katherine N. Ayzengart, MSN, RN

OBJECTIVES

Mastery of content in this chapter will enable you to:

- Define the key terms listed.
- Identify appropriate topics that address a patient's health education needs.
- Explain the role of the nurse in patient education.
- Describe the purposes of patient education.
- Determine appropriate communication principles when providing patient education.
- Describe the domains of learning.
- Identify basic learning principles.
- Discuss how to integrate health education into patient-centred care.
- Differentiate factors that determine readiness to learn from those that determine the ability to learn.
- Compare and contrast the nursing and teaching processes.
- Write learning objectives for a teaching plan.
- Establish an environment that promotes learning.
- Include patient teaching while performing routine nursing care.
- Use appropriate methods to evaluate learning.

KEY TERMS

Affective learning, p. 327
Analogies, p. 338
Cognitive learning, p. 327
Health literacy, p. 338
Learning, p. 327
Learning objectives, p. 331
Motivation, p. 330
Patient-centred approach, p. 324
Patient-centred care, p. 331
Psychomotor learning, p. 327
Reinforcement, p. 336
Return demonstration, p. 337
Social learning theory, p. 330
Teaching, p. 326

MEDIA RESOURCES

http://evolve.elsevier.com/Canada/Potter/fundamentals/

- Audio Chapter Summaries
- Examination Review Questions
- Concept Map Creator
- Case Study with Questions
- Audio Glossary
- Content Updates
- Video Clips

Patient education is one of the most important roles for nurses in any health care setting. Patients and family members need health education so that they can make informed decisions about their health care and lifestyle. With the current trend of shorter hospital stays, increased demands on nurses' time, and greater numbers of patients with acute conditions and of chronically ill patients, high-quality patient education has become even more important. Initial patient education often takes place in the hospital while patients are in the highly stressful acute stage of their illness, and education may not be completed at the time of discharge. Nurses, both in the hospital and the community, are not only the primary source of information for people adjusting to health problems but also often in the role of clarifying information provided by physicians and other health care providers (Bergh, Friberg, Persson, et al., 2015). In primary health care settings, nurses are often the main source of information about health promotion and illness prevention (see Chapter 4 for further information about health promotion). By taking a **patient-centred approach** to patient education, the nurse helps patients to be active participants in their education and is better able to self-manage their needs and care with health providers across health care settings (Box 20-1).

In order for nurses to be effective patient educators, they require knowledge and abilities that are considered essential domains of nursing education; these include knowledge, critical inquiry, communication and collaboration, professionalism, and leadership (Canadian Association of Schools of Nursing [CASN], 2015). Nurses use both the art and science of nursing to provide professional care to their patients, whether they are individuals, families, or groups. Providing patient education requires critical thinking and utilization of the best evidence available. Nurses regularly communicate and collaborate with other members of the health care team to provide patient-centred education to a diverse patient population. Their relationships with patients and their position within the health care team result in nurses often assuming a leadership role in health education.

Over the past couple of decades, the general public has become more assertive in seeking knowledge, understanding health, and finding resources available within the health care system. Nurses need

BOX 20-1 CHRONIC ILLNESS

Self-Management of Chronic Disease

The incidence of chronic illness is increasing with the growing older person population. The importance of self-management of chronic illness and disease includes a significant education component, focusing on knowledge of the chronic disease and on self-management skills.

The focus of self-management education is to provide patients and their families with information and knowledge necessary for them to understand their chronic disease as well as the skills for medical management and living with their chronic disease. This person-centred approach is based on the view that patient outcomes improve if patients not only understand their illness but also develop the knowledge and skills to "identify and address problems related to living with a chronic disease" (Stenburg, Haaland-Overby, Fredriksen, et al., 2016, p. 1760). While self-management patient education can be offered in a variety of settings and using a variety of methods, research has identified some common benefits and challenges: participants in patient self-management experienced improved awareness of their conditions, less symptom distress, and acquisition of self-management skills. Participants reported that peer and social support, mutual learning, and networking resulted in them feeling less isolated and that they learned from other people's experiences in living with their chronic disease.

By learning how others have been able to manage their chronic disease, participants expressed feeling hopeful about their future and their ability to live with their chronic illness. As patients learned to self-manage their illness, they had increased awareness of their disease and its management, and some reported improved quality of life, ability to manage their disease, and navigation of the health care system. Use of a person-centred approach in self-management education resulted in participants being able to move beyond learning about their illness to sharing experiences and learning how to cope with their illness.

By incorporating a person-centred approach to self-management patient education, nurses can facilitate patients' understanding of their chronic disease and how to live with their disease. This leads to patients' increased confidence in their ability to adapt their lives to their chronic disease and to navigate the health care system, which in turn leads to improved quality of life. Learning with and from other people with chronic disease at other stages provides peer and social supports that reduce isolation and identify real-life experiences on how to manage their chronic disease. This can result in patients' increased hope and optimism about their disease, improved quality of life, and enhanced ability to manage their illness and use the health care system.

Stenburg, U., Haaland-Overby, M., Fredriksen, K., Westermann, T. K., & Kvisvik, T. (2016). A scoping review of the literature on benefits and challenges of participating in patient education programs aimed at promoting self-management for people living with chronic illness. *Patient Education and Counseling, 99*(11), 1759–1771. doi:10.1016/j.pec/2016.07.027.

to assist patients in navigating all of the information available to them through all forms of media. The Internet and other forms of technology (telehealth, eHealth) provide nurses and patients with vast amounts of information, some reliable and some not. Patients need guidance regarding the selection of current and reliable resources. Nurses must be able to discuss with patients the criteria for evaluating sources for validity and reliability, educate patients on the use of social media and technology as a medium for providing health information, and facilitate self-management of individual health needs that is explored and used by nursing and other health providers. The teaching material provided by nurses must honour the copyright rules and must reference both written information and illustrations that are used to support patient learning.

As a nurse providing patient education, you will need to be mindful of the increasing emphasis on scientific evidence and the diminished focus on other kinds of evidence of the efficacy or effectiveness of therapeutic interventions. You should also have a broad perspective of what constitutes meaningful evidence to support the significance of testimonials, lived experiences, and other ways of knowing. Because critical thinking is essential in nursing care, you need to remember that knowledge is limited, beliefs change, and conclusions are temporary. Nonetheless, a well-designed, comprehensive teaching plan that meets a learner's needs can improve quality of care, help patients gain optimal wellness, increase their independence, and reduce health care costs (Bastable, 2017).

GOALS OF PATIENT EDUCATION

The goal of patient education is to assist individuals, families, or communities in achieving optimal health (Edelman, Kudzma, & Mandle, 2014). Education is an important component of primary health care. It helps individuals, families, and communities to develop the knowledge, understanding, and skills necessary to maintain, improve, and manage their health; reduces hardship; helps contains health care costs; and enables people to take control of and manage their own health (Bergh et al., 2015). Patient education has three main goals (Box 20-2):

- Maintaining and promoting health and preventing illness
- Restoring health
- Optimizing quality of life with impaired functioning

Maintaining and Promoting Health and Preventing Illness

In the home, clinic, or other community health care settings, nurses provide information and skills that people need to maintain, manage, and improve their health (see Box 20-2). For example, in prenatal classes, nurses teach expectant parents about fetal development and physical and psychological changes during pregnancy. They also teach about the importance of healthy food choices, exercise, and avoiding substances that might harm the fetus. Greater knowledge can result in better health. When patients become more health conscious, they are more likely to effectively manage their health and to seek early diagnosis of health problems (Zuniga, Kirk, Mier, et al., 2012). With the growth and development of Internet access and of health-related websites, patients have been able to access more health information and resources directly. The use of social media, interactive health information sites, and smartphone applications has the potential to enhance health education and patient self-management (Nimkar, 2016).

Restoring Health

Many patients seek information and skills that will help them manage, regain, or maintain their health (see Box 20-2). However, patients who find it difficult to adapt to illness may be more passive in their approach. As a student nurse, you will learn to identify barriers to learning, to recognize patients' willingness to learn, and to help motivate their interest in learning (London, 2016).

The family can be a vital part of a patient's return to health, and they may need to know as much as the patient about the patient's recovery. If the nurse excludes the family from a teaching plan, conflicts

BOX 20-2 Topics for Health Education

Health Maintenance and Promotion and Illness Prevention

Educate patients about the following:

- First aid
- Health resources (e.g., Internet)
- Avoidance of risk factors (e.g., smoking, alcoholism, obesity)
- Stress management
- Typical growth and development patterns
- Proper hygiene
- Immunizations (e.g., recommendations, risks and benefits)
- Prenatal care and normal child-bearing
- Nutrition
- Exercise
- Safety (in home and health care setting)
- Screening for common conditions (e.g., blood pressure, poor vision, cholesterol level)
- Behaviour modification to change risky behaviours (e.g., smoking cessation, treatment for substance abuse)

Restoration of Health

Educate patients about the following:

- Patient's disease or condition
- Anatomy and physiology of body system affected by disease or condition
- Cause of disease
- Origin of symptoms
- Expected effects on other body systems
- Prognosis
- Limitations on function
- Rationale for treatment
- Medications
- Alternative therapies (evidence regarding risks and benefits)
- Tests and therapies
- Nursing measures
- Surgical intervention
- Expected duration of care
- Hospital or clinic environment
- Hospital or clinic staff
- Long-term care implications
- Methods for patient's participation in care
- Limitations imposed by disease or surgery

Optimizing Quality of Life When Functions Are Impaired

Educate patients about the following:

- Home care
- Medications
- Intravenous therapy
- Diet
- Activity
- Self-help devices
- Rehabilitation of remaining function
- Allied health services (e.g., physiotherapy, occupational therapy, speech therapy)
- Prevention of complications
- Knowledge of risk factors
- Implications of noncompliance with therapy
- Environmental alterations
- Self-help and support groups

regarding the patient's care may arise. For example, if the family does not understand a patient's need to regain independent function, their efforts may encourage dependency and thus slow the patient's recovery. It is also important for the nurse to assess the patient–family relationship before involving the family in a teaching plan (see Chapter 19).

Coping With Impaired Functioning

Some patients must learn to cope with permanent health alterations. For example, a patient who loses the ability to speak after surgery of the larynx must learn new ways to communicate. A patient with severe heart disease must learn to modify risk factors that might cause further heart damage. After the patient's needs are identified and the family has displayed willingness to help, the nurse teaches family members to assist the patient with health care management (e.g., giving medications through gastric tubes and performing passive range-of-motion exercises).

TEACHING AND LEARNING

Teaching is an interactive process that promotes learning. Teaching and learning generally begin when a person identifies a need for knowing or acquiring an ability to do something. A nurse-teacher provides information that prompts the patient to engage in activities that lead to a desired change (Box 20-3). Teaching is most effective when it addresses the learner's needs, learning style, and capacity. The teacher assesses these needs by asking questions, observing the patient, and determining the patient's interests. With successful teaching, patients can learn new skills or change existing attitudes (Bastable, 2014).

Role of the Nurse in Teaching and Learning

The role of the nurse in patient education is multifaceted. It involves creating or adapting the environment to facilitate learning, using a patient-centred approach in assessing the learning needs of the patient, and using the most appropriate educational strategy (Registered Nurses' Association of Ontario [RNAO], 2012). Nurses have an ethical responsibility to teach their patients and enable them to self-manage their health (Redman, 2011). The Canadian Nurses Association's (2017) *Code of Ethics* states that patients have the right to make informed decisions about their care. The information that patients need to make such decisions must be accurate, complete, and relevant to their needs. Nurses should anticipate patients' needs for information on the basis of their overall condition (physical, mental, emotional, spiritual), identified risks, and interdisciplinary treatment plans. Nurses often clarify information provided by physicians and other health care providers and may become the patient's primary source of information for adjusting to health problems (Bastable, 2017).

Patients and their families often ask nurses for health information, and it is easy to identify the need for teaching when patients request information. However, in some cases, the need for information may be less apparent. Nurses need to observe and listen carefully to determine patients' needs for information and learning. When nurses value education and ensure that patients learn necessary information, patients are better prepared to assume health care responsibilities. To be an effective nurse educator, you must do more than just pass on facts; you must determine what patients need to know, find time when they are ready to learn, and evaluate the impact of patient education on patient outcomes (Bastable, 2014, 2017; London, 2016).

BOX 20-3 RESEARCH HIGHLIGHT

The Effectiveness of Combined Group and Individual Nurse-Directed Patient Education

Research Focus

This study focused on the effects of nurse-led education programs using a combination of group and individual education for patients with chronic inflammatory polyarthritis.

Research Abstract

Grønning, Rannestad, Skomsvoll, and colleagues (2013) wanted to know if a combination of group and individual education sessions would constitute a cost-effective method of patient education that can improve patient well-being and self-efficacy. The study was carried out through a randomized control trial. The control group received no structured patient education, and the intervention group received three structured nurse-led group education sessions followed by an individual education session. Group education sessions were delivered at 2-week intervals and lasted 45 minutes. The first group session addressed the process of arthritis, including symptoms, the cyclic nature of symptoms, and prognosis. The second group session focused on medical treatment of arthritis, including observing for adverse effects. In the third group session, health lifestyle, coping, and community resources were explored, including exercise, nutrition, problem solving, self-management, and living with arthritis. These three sessions were followed by an individual education session based on content identified by the patients, their recent experience of the disease, and related health goals. Evaluation of the intervention and control group members was done through survey and questionnaires, which measured utilization of health services, coping, self-efficacy, and health status.

Findings indicated that, at 12 months, the intervention group had a greater feeling of well-being, less reported disease activity, and better coping and health status scores compared to the control group. Use of the health care system and self-efficacy were not significantly different between the intervention and control groups. Findings indicated that a combined group and individual approach to patient education is beneficial. It enables efficient use of time to present information to patients and helps patients to explore their own educational needs. While this approach improved patients' experiences of their illness relating to some outcomes, it also demonstrated the need for ongoing health education interactions for other outcomes.

Research Highlights

- A combination of structured group followed by individual education sessions results in improved outcomes relating to feelings of well-being, disease activity, coping, and health status.
- Over time, some outcomes were not maintained and required reinforcement.
- Combined group and individual educational programs are cost-effective.

Grønning, K., Rannestad, T., Skomsvoll, J.F., Rygg, L.Ø., & Steinsbekk, A. (2013). Long-term effects of a nurse-led group and individual education programme for patients with chronic inflammatory polyarthritis—a randomised controlled trail. *Journal of Clinical Nursing, 23*(7-8), 1005–1017. doi: 10.1111/jocn/12353.

Teaching as Communication

Effective teaching depends on effective communication (see Chapter 17). To be a good teacher, you must listen empathetically, observe astutely, and speak clearly. Many intrapersonal variables—including attitudes, values, culture, emotions, and knowledge—influence both the nurse's and patient's styles and approaches. Both you and the patient are also affected by the patient's motivation and ability to learn, which depend on physical and psychological health, education, developmental stage, and previous knowledge.

DOMAINS OF LEARNING

Learning occurs in three domains: cognitive (understanding), affective (attitudes), and psychomotor (motor skills) (Bastable, 2014; Bloom, 1956). Any topic to be learned may involve one domain, all domains, or any combination of the three. For example, patients with diabetes must learn how diabetes affects the body and how to control blood glucose levels for better health (cognitive domain). They must also learn to accept the chronic nature of diabetes by learning positive coping mechanisms (affective domain). Finally, many patients with diabetes must learn to test their blood glucose levels at home. This requires learning how to use a glucose meter (psychomotor domain). By understanding each learning domain, nurses can select appropriate teaching methods (Box 20-4).

Cognitive Learning

Cognitive learning includes all intellectual behaviours and requires thinking (Krau, 2011). In the hierarchy of cognitive behaviours, the simplest behaviour is remembering, whereas the most complex is creating. Cognitive learning includes the following:

- Remembering: the ability to learn new information and to retrieve knowledge from long-term memory
- Understanding: the ability to construct the meaning of learned material
- Applying: the use of abstract, newly learned ideas in a practical situation
- Analyzing: the breaking down of information into organized parts and determining how the parts relate to one another
- Evaluating: making judgements based on criteria and standards
- Creating: combining elements to form a coherent and functional whole

Affective Learning

Affective learning concerns expressions of feelings and acceptance of attitudes, opinions, or values. Values clarification (see Chapter 7) is an example of affective learning. The simplest behaviour in the affective learning hierarchy is receiving, and the most complex is characterizing (Krau, 2011; Krathwohl, Bloom, & Masia, 1964).

- Receiving: the willingness to attend to another person's words
- Responding: active participation through listening and reacting verbally and nonverbally
- Valuing: attachment of worth to an object, concept, or behaviour, demonstrated by the learner's actions
- Organizing: development of a value system by identifying and organizing values and resolving conflicts
- Characterizing: action and response with a consistent value system

Psychomotor Learning

Psychomotor learning involves acquiring skills that require the integration of mental and muscular activity, such as the ability to walk or to use an eating utensil. The simplest behaviour in the hierarchy is perception and the most complex is origination (Krau, 2011).

- Perception: awareness of objects or qualities through the use of sense organs

BOX 20-4 Appropriate Teaching Methods Based on Domains of Learning

Cognitive

Discussion (One-on-One or Group)
May involve nurse and one patient or nurse with several patients
Promotes active participation and focuses on topics of interest to patient
Facilitates peer support
Enhances application and analysis of new information

Storytelling
Can involve individual or group
Facilitates cultural relevance and safety
Enhances application of new information to a familiar context

Lecture
Is more formal method of instruction because it is teacher controlled
Helps learner acquire new knowledge and gain comprehension

Question-and-Answer Session
Is designed specifically to address patient's concerns
Assists patient in applying knowledge

Role Play and Discovery
Encourages patient to actively apply knowledge in controlled situation
Promotes synthesis of information and problem solving

Independent Projects (e.g., Computer-Assisted Instruction) and Field Experience
Assists patient to assume responsibility for learning at own pace
Promotes analysis, synthesis, and evaluation of new information and skills

Affective

Role Play
Encourages expression of values, feelings, and attitudes

Discussion (Group)
Enables patient to acquire support from other people in group
Encourages patient to learn from other people's experiences
Promotes responding, valuing, and organizing

Discussion (One-on-One)
Facilitates discussion of personal, sensitive topics of interest or concern

Psychomotor

Demonstration
Provides presentation of procedures or skills by nurse
Encourages patient to model nurse's behaviour
Allows nurse to control questioning during demonstration

Practice
Enables patient to perform skills by using equipment in a controlled setting
Allows repetition

Return Demonstrations
Enables patient to perform skill as nurse observes
Provides excellent source of feedback and reinforcement

Independent Projects and Games
Require teaching method that promotes adaptation and initiation of psychomotor learning
Enable learner to use new skills

- Set: a readiness (mental, physical, or emotional) to take a particular action
- Guided response: the performance of an act under the guidance of an instructor, involving imitation of a demonstrated act
- Mechanism: a higher level of behaviour by which a person gains confidence and skill in performing a behaviour that is more complex or involves several more steps than does a guided response
- Complex overt response: the smooth and accurate performance of a motor skill that requires a complex movement pattern
- Adaptation: the ability to change motor response when unexpected problems occur
- Origination: use of existing psychomotor skills and abilities to perform a highly complex motor act that involves creating new movement patterns

BASIC LEARNING PRINCIPLES

Before nurses can teach, they must understand how people learn. Learning depends on the learning environment and on the individual's ability to learn, learning style, and motivation to learn. Learning takes place both in formal learning sessions, which involve planned learning activities, and in teachable moments, which allow nurses to spontaneously take advantage of teaching opportunities as they occur in day-to-day contact with patients.

Learning Environment

Patient education takes place in a variety of settings: the patient's home, community centres, classrooms, and hospital rooms. The ideal environment for learning is a well-lit, well-ventilated room with appropriate furniture and a comfortable temperature. A quiet setting with few distractions and interruptions can help a person to concentrate. Nurses can provide privacy even in a busy hospital by closing cubicle curtains or taking the patient to a quiet spot. In the home, a bedroom might separate the patient from household activities. If the patient desires, family members or significant others may share in discussions. However, some patients may be reluctant to discuss their illness when other people, even close family members, are in the room. An ideal environment is not always achievable, however, and rather than miss a teachable moment, nurses can adapt the environment as much as possible to provide privacy and minimize distractions.

Ability to Learn

The ability to learn depends on emotional, intellectual, and physical capabilities and on developmental stage. If a patient's learning ability is impaired, the nurse should modify or postpone teaching activities.

Emotional Capability. Emotions can aid or prevent learning. Mild anxiety may help a person focus. However, stronger levels of anxiety can be incapacitating, creating an inability to attend to anything other than to relieving the anxiety. The prospect of change makes many people anxious. Seriously ill people, who are faced with multiple

BOX 20-5 Teaching Methods Based on Patient's Developmental Capacity

Infant
Maintain consistent routines (e.g., feeding, bathing).
Hold infant firmly while smiling and speaking softly, to convey sense of trust.
Have infant touch different textures (e.g., soft fabric, hard plastic).

Toddler
Use play to teach procedure or activity (e.g., handling examination equipment, applying bandage to doll).
Offer picture books that describe a story of children in a hospital or clinic.
Use simple words such as "cut" instead of "laceration," to promote understanding.

Preschooler
Use role playing, imitation, and play to make learning fun.
Encourage questions and offer explanations; use simple explanations and demonstrations.
Encourage several children to learn together through pictures and short stories about how to perform hygiene.

School-Age Child
Teach necessary psychomotor skills. (Complicated skills, such as learning to use a syringe, may take considerable practice.)
Offer opportunities to discuss health problems and answer questions.

Adolescent
Help adolescent learn about feelings and need for self-expression.
Collaborate with adolescent on teaching activities.
Let adolescent make decisions about health and health promotion (safety, sex education, substance abuse).
Use problem solving to help adolescent make choices.

Young or Middle-Age Adult
Encourage participation in teaching plan by setting mutual goals.
Encourage independent learning.
Offer information so that adult can understand effects of health problem.

Older Person
Teach when patient is alert and rested.
Involve adult in discussion or activity.
Focus on wellness and the person's strength.
Use approaches that enhance sensorially impaired patients' reception of stimuli (see Chapter 47).
Keep teaching sessions short.

losses, may be extremely anxious and distressed. Nurses must be sensitive to a patient's level of anxiety. If a person is incapacitated by anxiety, the nurse needs to find a way to alleviate the anxiety. This may mean teaching relaxation techniques before attempting to teach a task or a procedure.

Intellectual Capability. Patients have different levels of intellectual ability. Nurses must assess a patient's knowledge and intellectual level before beginning a teaching plan. For example, measuring liquid or solid food portions requires the ability to perform mathematical calculations. Reading a medication label or discharge instructions requires reading and comprehension skills. Following directions when performing self-care in accordance with limitations requires comprehension and application skills.

Physical Capability. The ability to learn often depends on physical health. To learn psychomotor skills, a patient must possess the necessary strength, coordination, and sensory acuity. Nurses should not overestimate a patient's physical ability. The following physical attributes are necessary for learning psychomotor skills:

- Size (height and weight adequate for performing the task or using the equipment, such as crutch walking)
- Strength (ability of the patient to follow a strenuous exercise program)
- Coordination (dexterity needed for complicated motor skills, such as using utensils, changing a bandage, or opening a medication container)
- Sensory acuity (visual, auditory, tactile, gustatory, and olfactory resources needed to receive and respond to messages taught)

Any physical condition (e.g., pain, fatigue, hunger) that depletes energy also impairs the ability to learn. For example, a patient in a weakened state who has just spent hours undergoing diagnostic tests is likely to be too fatigued to learn. Nurses need to assess the patient's energy level by noting the patient's willingness to communicate, the degree of activity initiated, and the patient's responsiveness to questions. Teaching may be halted if the patient needs rest.

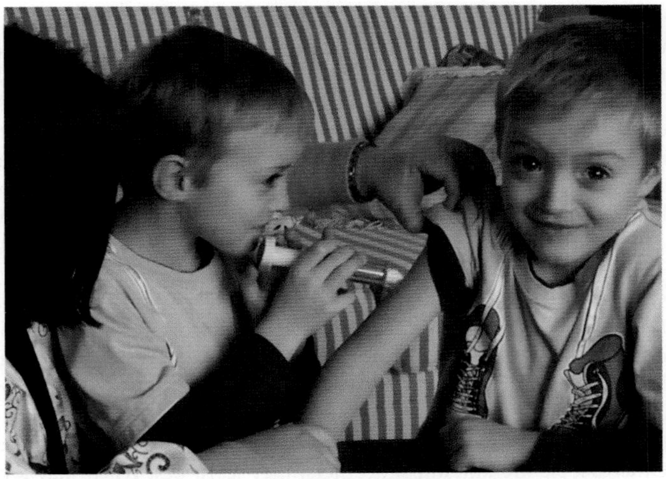

FIGURE 20-1 Teaching aids for children. The nurse uses a developmentally appropriate toy syringe to teach about immunization to school-aged children.

Developmental Stage. Age and stage of development affect the ability to learn (Box 20-5). Without proper biological, motor, language, and personal–social development, many types of learning cannot take place.

Learning in Children. As a child matures, intellectual growth progresses from concrete to abstract. Therefore, information should be understandable, and the expected outcomes should be realistic and based on the child's developmental stage. Developmentally appropriate teaching aids should also be used (Figure 20-1).

Adult Learning. Many adults are independent, self-directed learners. However, they may become dependent in new learning situations. Adults typically learn more successfully when they are encouraged to

BOX 20-6 CASE STUDY

"To Take or Not to Take"

In preparation for a trip to Vietnam and Cambodia, Mr. and Mrs. Bennet visited a travel clinic, which recommended that they update their immunization (diphtheria-pertussis-tetanus, hepatitis A, typhoid) and take antimalarial drugs for the Cambodia portion of the trip (atovaquone/proguanil [Malarone], one pill daily starting 1 day before stay and continuing during stay and 1 week after). When they came in for their immunizations, they expressed some concerns about taking the antimalarial drugs. They had been talking to friends who told them these antimalarial drugs had severe adverse effects and caused hallucinations. They had investigated several Internet sites that their friends had recommended; these sites indicated that antimalarial drugs were not required for where they were going. Mrs. Bennet emailed the Cambodian Consulate in Canada and was told that malaria was not a concern where they were going.

Assessment

- Concerned about health but received mixed messages about the need for antimalarial drugs
- Concerned about serious adverse effects of drugs
- Motivated to learn

Plan

- Discussed with Mr. and Mrs. Bennet criteria evaluating websites for health information (author, age, conflict of interest, whether evidence informed rather than opinion based)
- Provided list of reliable travel health sites (Health Canada, World Health Organization, US Centers for Disease Control and Prevention)
- Identified other measures to reduce risk of contracting malaria (using mosquito repellent, limiting time outside at night, staying in air-conditioned rooms or mosquito nets, wearing protective clothing)
- Discussed various drugs used for malaria and the incidence and type of adverse effects
- Explored the risk of not taking medication and implications of contracting malaria
- Identified other resources of information (travel agents, pharmacists)

Outcome

Mr. and Mrs. Bennet visited several reliable sources on the Internet and talked to their pharmacist. They identified several strategies to minimize exposure to mosquitoes on their travels. Mr. Bennet learned that the risk of adverse effects from the Malarone was minimal and decided to take the drug. Mrs. Bennet also recognized that the risk for adverse effects was minimal; however, because of her concern about those adverse effects, she decided not to take the Malarone. She was more comfortable taking the risk because she understood that if she developed a high fever and flu-like illness at any time up to a year after the trip, she had to seek immediate medical attention.

use past experiences to solve problems. When teaching adult patients, nurses need to collaborate with them on educational topics and goals. Needs or issues that are important to the adult should be addressed early in the teaching–learning process. Ultimately, adults must accept responsibility for changing their own behaviours. Assessing what the adult patient currently knows, teaching what the patient wants to know, and setting mutual goals will improve the outcomes of care and education (Bastable, 2014).

Learning Style and Preference

People have different learning styles. Everyone processes information differently by seeing and hearing, reflecting and acting, reasoning logically and intuitively, and analyzing and visualizing. Some people are visual learners; they learn best by watching. Audiovisual presentations and visual demonstrations often work best for this type of learner. Other people are kinesthetic learners; they learn best when they are able to manipulate tools and find out how they work. Some people learn by taking detailed notes; others prefer to only listen. Some people need to be engaged in activities and discussion in order to learn effectively. Others may be too shy to enjoy this type of learning and prefer to learn from an orderly, structured presentation.

Environmental, social, emotional, psychological, and physical stimuli affect people differently. Some people prefer complete silence in the learning environment, whereas others prefer background sounds. Some prefer to learn in a group; others, on their own. Different people prefer different times of the day for learning experiences.

When developing teaching plans, you should assess the favoured learning style and preferences of the patient. With groups, it may not be possible to address every patient's preferences. However, including a combination of approaches to meet multiple learning styles can ensure that most people's learning preferences are met (Bastable, 2017). When the patient is having difficulty with learning, you should consider a change to accommodate a different learning style.

Motivation to Learn

Motivation is a person's desire or willingness to learn, and it influences a person's behaviour (Pender, Murdaugh, & Parson, 2015; Box 20-6). If a person is not ready or does not want to learn, learning is unlikely to occur. The stimuli for motivation vary between individuals and may be social, task mastery, or physical in nature. *Social motives* reflect a need for connection, social approval, or self-esteem. For example, the motivation to exercise may be linked to the social aspects of the exercise activities (Stevinson, Wiltshire, & Hickson, 2015). *Task mastery motives* are driven by desire for achievement. For example, a high school student with diabetes begins to test blood glucose levels and determine insulin dosages before leaving home and establishing independence. The desire to live independently and manage the disease provides the motivation to master the task or skill. After succeeding at a task, a person is usually motivated to achieve more. *Physical motives* come from a desire to maintain and improve health. Patients motivated by the need to survive or overcome hardship are often more motivated than those who wish merely to improve their health (Pender et al., 2015). For example, a patient who has undergone a leg amputation may be extremely motivated to learn to use assistive devices, whereas a patient who is overweight but otherwise healthy may not be motivated to exercise.

Many people do not adopt new health behaviours or change unhealthy behaviours unless they perceive a disease as a threat, overcome barriers to changing health practices, and see the benefits of such changes (Pender et al., 2015). Thus, a patient with lung disease may continue to smoke. An obese patient may worsen a heart condition by refusing to follow a low-fat diet.

Motivation and Social Learning Theory. Health education often involves changing people's attitudes and values. Change can occur only when education plans and interventions are based on sound learning theories. A number of theories address the complex patient education process (Bastable, 2014). One of these is **social learning theory**, which helps educators understand learners and develop interventions that enhance motivation and learning (Bandura, 2001; Bastable, 2014; Stevinson et al., 2015).

When people believe that they can execute a particular behaviour, they are more likely to perform the behaviour consistently and correctly (Bandura, 1997). *Self-efficacy,* a social learning theory concept, is a person's perceived ability to successfully complete a task. Beliefs about self-efficacy arise from four sources: verbal persuasion, vicarious experiences, enactive mastery experiences, and physiological and affective states (Bandura, 1997). Understanding these sources enables nurses to develop appropriate interventions. For example, a nurse teaching a boy with asthma to use an inhaler expresses positive reinforcement (verbal persuasion) by encouraging him to use the inhaler himself. The nurse then demonstrates to the boy how to use the inhaler (vicarious experience). The boy successfully uses the inhaler by himself (enactive mastery experience). As the boy is able to control his asthma by using the inhaler, the nurse gives him positive feedback, which further enhances his confidence to use the inhaler (physiological and affective states). Interventions such as these enhance perceived self-efficacy, which in turn improves the achievement of desired outcomes.

Motivation and Transtheoretical Model of Change. Health education may involve changes in behaviour, and for many people, behavioural change is often challenging and difficult. It involves a process that occurs over time through a series of stages. By identifying a patient's stage of change and focusing learning activities to match the patient's stage, the nurse can facilitate the learner's motivation to change and his or her transition from one stage to the next.

Five stages involved in behaviour change have been identified; these have been used, for example, in smoking cessation activities (Prochaska & DiClemente, 1992; Robinson & Vail, 2012):

- Precontemplation: is unaware of need for change and has no intention of changing behaviour
- Contemplation: is aware of need for change and intends to change behaviour sometime in the future
- Preparation: alters behaviour in minor ways with the intention to make substantive changes in the immediate future
- Action: modifies behaviour and experiences in order to make sustainable change
- Maintenance: focuses on not reverting to previous behaviour and on solidifying new behaviours

A Patient-Centred Approach to Patient Education. Patient-centred care is a standard of care that positions the patient as the focus of care delivery and as a partner in the delivery of care (McCance, McCormack, & Dewing, 2011). To provide a patient-centred approach to patient education, nurses must use both social learning theory and the nursing process. The L.E.A.R.N.S. model, developed by the RNAO (2012), provides a nursing process framework incorporating social learning theory that facilitates a patient-centred approach. The L.E.A.R.N.S. model consists of the following (RNAO, 2012, p. 20):

- **Listen** to patient needs.
- **Establish** therapeutic partnership relationships.
- **Adopt** an intentional approach to every learning encounter.
- **Reinforce** health literacy.
- **Name** new knowledge via teach-back.
- **Strengthen** self-management via links to community resources.

Using this approach, the patient is involved as a partner in the learning process.

INTEGRATING THE NURSING AND TEACHING PROCESSES

The nursing and teaching processes are related and usually take place concurrently. Like the nursing process, the teaching process requires assessment, nursing diagnosis, planning, implementation, and evaluation. However, the processes are not exactly the same: the nursing process is broader. For example, determining a patient's health needs requires assessing all data sources. The teaching process is focused on data sources that reveal the patient's learning needs, willingness and ability to learn, and available teaching resources. The teaching process is especially useful for teaching large groups, where individual learning needs and styles may vary. Table 20-1 compares the teaching and nursing processes.

The teaching process requires assessment. The patient's ability to learn, motivation, and needs should be assessed and analyzed. A diagnostic statement specifies the information or skills that the patient requires. The nurse sets specific learning objectives (i.e., what the learner will be able to do after successful instruction) and implements the teaching plan by using teaching and learning principles to ensure that the patient acquires knowledge and skills. Finally, the teaching

TABLE 20-1 Comparison of the Nursing and Teaching Processes

Basic Steps	Nursing Process	Teaching Process
Assessment	Collect data about patient's physical, psychological, social, cultural, developmental, and spiritual needs from patient, family, diagnostic tests, medical record, health history, learning style, and literature.	Gather data about patient's learning needs, motivation, ability to learn, and teaching resources from patient, family, learning environment, medical record, health history, and literature.
Analysis	Identify appropriate health concern based on assessment findings, including deficits.	Identify patient's learning needs on the basis of three domains of learning.
Planning	Develop individualized care plan. Set diagnosis priorities on the basis of patient's immediate needs. Collaborate with patient on care plan.	Establish learning objectives, stated in behavioural terms. Identify priorities regarding learning needs. Collaborate with patient on teaching plan. Identify type of teaching method to use.
Implementation	Perform nursing care therapies. Include patient as active participant in care. Involve family or significant other in care as appropriate.	Implement teaching methods. Actively involve patient in learning activities. Include family or significant other in participation as appropriate.
Evaluation	Identify success in meeting desired outcomes and goals of nursing care. Alter interventions as indicated when goals are not met.	Determine outcomes of teaching–learning process. Measure patient's ability to achieve learning objectives. Reinforce information as needed.

process requires an evaluation of learning; this evaluation is based on learning objectives.

◆ Assessment

During assessment, the nurse works with the patient to determine the patient's health care needs (see Chapter 13). The patient may indicate a need for health care information, or the nurse may identify a need for education. Learning needs identified by both the patient and the nurse determine the content to be learned. By performing an effective assessment, nurses can individualize instruction for each patient. Nurses need to ask specific questions to assess a patient's unique learning needs (Box 20-7).

Learning Needs. Most patients can identify at least some of their own learning needs. Effective questioning and assessment tools help nurses determine a patient's perceived learning needs. By listening carefully and using open-ended and closed-ended questions (see Chapter 17), nurses can often find out what a patient's needs are. Because a patient's health status is dynamic, assessment is an ongoing activity. Nurses should assess for the following:

- Information or skills needed by the patient to perform self-care and to understand the implications of a health problem (Health care team members anticipate learning needs related to specific health problems—for example, teaching an adolescent boy to perform testicular self-examination.)
- Patients' experiences that influence the need to learn
- Information that family members or significant others require to support the patient's needs (The amount of information needed depends on the extent of the family's role in helping the patient.)

Ability to Learn. The ability to learn can be impaired by many factors, including body temperature, electrolyte levels, oxygenation status, and blood glucose level. Several factors may influence a patient at one time. The nurse assesses the patient's ability to learn by considering the following:

- Physical strength, movement, dexterity, and coordination (The nurse determines the patient's ability to perform skills.)
- Sensory deficits that may affect the ability to understand or follow instruction (see Chapter 47)
- Reading level (Reading level can be difficult to assess because functional illiteracy is often easy to conceal; one way to assess a patient's reading level and level of understanding is to ask the patient to read instructions from a teaching brochure and then explain its meaning.)
- Developmental level (developmental level influences teaching approaches [see Box 20-5])
- Cognitive function (Cognitive function includes memory, knowledge, association, and judgement.)

Motivation to Learn. To identify a patient's motivation level, nurses can ask questions that will help them determine whether a patient is prepared and willing to learn. The patient's motivation is assessed by studying the following:

- Behaviour (e.g., attention span, tendency to ask questions, memory, and ability to concentrate during the teaching session)
- Health beliefs and perception of a health problem and the benefits and barriers to treatment (e.g., ask a patient with coronary artery disease, "Explain how heart disease will affect you over time. What is the value of eating a low-fat diet?")
- Perceived ability to complete a required healthy behaviour
- Desire to learn
- Attitudes about health care providers (e.g., role of patient and nurse in making decisions, such as asking, "In what way can I best help you?")
- Knowledge of information to be learned (The patient must play an active role in seeking health-related information.)
- Pain, fatigue, anxiety, or other physical symptoms that can interfere with the ability to maintain attention and participate (In acute care settings, a patient's physical condition can easily detract from learning.)
- Sociocultural background (A patient's beliefs and values about health and various therapies may be influenced by sociocultural norms or tradition [see Chapter 9]; educational efforts can be especially challenging when patients and educators do not speak the same language.)
- Learning style preference (Patients who learn better by seeing and hearing may benefit from a video; patients who learn best by reasoning logically and intuitively may learn better if presented with written material that they can analyze and discuss with others.)

Teaching Environment. Nurses need to assess the following factors when choosing a teaching environment:

- Distractions or persistent noise (a quiet area should be set aside for teaching)
- Comfort of the room, including ventilation, temperature, lighting, and furniture
- Room facilities and available equipment

Resources for Learning. Assessment of resources includes a review of available teaching tools and guidelines (RNAO, n.d.). If a patient requires family support, the nurse should evaluate the readiness and ability of family and friends to learn to care for the patient and review resources in the home. The nurse needs to assess the following:

- The patient's willingness to have family members involved in the teaching plan and care (Information about the patient's health care is confidential unless the patient chooses to share it.)

BOX 20-7 Nursing Assessment Questions

Ask Patients

What do you want to know?

What do you know about your illness and your treatment plan?

How does (or will) your illness affect your current lifestyle?

What barriers currently exist that are preventing you from managing your illness the way you would like to manage it?

What cultural or spiritual beliefs do you have regarding your illness and the prescribed treatment?

What experiences have you had that are similar to what you are experiencing now?

Together we can choose the best way for you to learn about your disease. How can I best help you?

What role do you believe your health care provider should take in helping you manage your illness or maintain health?

When you learn new information, do you prefer to have the information given to you in pictures or written down in words?

When you give someone directions to your house, do you tell the person how to get there, write out the instructions, draw a map, or just give the person the address to enter in a smart phone for directions?

How involved do you want your family to be in the management of your illness?

Ask Family Members

When are you available to help, and how do you plan to help your loved one?

Your spouse needs some help. How do you feel about learning how to assist him or her?

- Family members' perceptions and understanding of the patient's illness and its implications (Family members and patients' perceptions should match; otherwise, conflicts may arise in the teaching plan.)
- Family's willingness and ability to participate in care (Family members must be responsible, willing, and able to assist in care activities, such as bathing or administering medications.)
- Resources in the home (These resources include health care equipment, access to technology, and a suitable rearrangement of rooms.)
- Teaching tools, including brochures, audiovisual materials, or posters. Printed material should present current and easy-to-understand information that matches the patient's reading level.

◆ Nursing Diagnosis

After assessing the patient's ability and need to learn, the nurse interprets data to form an accurate health focus. This focus ensures that teaching will be goal directed and individualized. If a patient has several learning needs, the nursing foci guide priority setting. By classifying diagnoses according to the three learning domains, the nurse can focus on subject matter and teaching methods. Examples of nursing foci that indicate a need for education include the following:

- Health maintenance
- Health-seeking behaviours
- Health self-management
- Mastery of health-related skill
- Deficient knowledge

When health care problems can be managed through education, the foci of patient education are *knowledge* and *skills.* For example, an older person may be unable to manage a medication regimen because of the number of medications that must be taken at different times of the day. Education may improve the patient's ability to schedule and take the medications.

Some nursing foci also indicate that teaching is inappropriate. You may identify conditions that hinder learning (e.g., nursing focus of pain or activity intolerance). In these cases, you should delay teaching until the nursing focus is resolved or the health problem is controlled.

◆ Planning

After identifying a patient's learning needs and identifying a nursing focus, the nurse develops a teaching plan, sets goals and expected outcomes, and works with the patient to select a teaching method (Box 20-8). Expected outcomes or learning objectives determine which teaching strategies and approaches are appropriate. Patient participation is essential.

Developing Learning Objectives. Learning objectives identify the expected outcome of instruction and establish learning priorities. Objectives help nurses manage time and resources.

Objectives are either for a short term or a long term. Short-term objectives meet the patient's immediate learning needs, such as needing knowledge about an upcoming test. Long-term objectives, which are often broader, help a patient adapt to a long-term challenge. Learning objectives, which will guide the teaching plan, include the same criteria as outcomes in a nursing care plan:

- Singular behaviours
- Observable or measurable content
- Timing or conditions under which the objective is measured
- Goals mutually set by the nurse and patient

Each objective focuses on a single behaviour that will determine the patient's ability to meet health care outcomes. A behavioural objective contains an active verb, describing what the learner will do after the objective is met (e.g., "*will administer* an injection"). Behavioural objectives are measurable and observable and indicate how learning will be evidenced (e.g., "will perform *three-point crutch gait*"). The objective describes precise behaviours and content. Nurses should avoid vague or nonspecific objectives that do not explain what the learner is to do.

An objective is more precise when it describes the conditions or timing under which the behaviour occurs. Conditions and time frames should be realistic and designed for the learner's needs (e.g., "will identify the side effects of medication by discharge"). It also helps to consider conditions under which the patient or family will perform the behaviour (e.g., "will walk from bedroom to bathroom, using crutches"). Nurses set criteria for acceptable performance on the basis of the desired level of accuracy, success, or satisfaction. For example, "a patient undergoing therapy for a fractured leg will walk on crutches to the end of the hall within three days." Criteria are more acceptable when the teacher and learner establish them mutually. However, the nurse serves as a resource in setting the minimum criteria for success.

After formulating objectives, the nurse and patient establish a teaching plan. It is the nurse's responsibility to integrate basic teaching principles and develop a well-timed, organized teaching plan.

Setting Priorities. The teaching plan is prioritized according to the patient's immediate needs, nursing diagnoses, learning objectives, main concerns, anxiety level, and the time available to teach.

Timing. When is the right time to teach? Before a patient is hospitalized? When a patient enters a clinic or a long-term care facility? At discharge? At home? All of these times are correct because patients continue to have learning needs and opportunities as long as they stay in the health care system. As the nurse, you should plan to teach when a patient is most attentive, receptive, and alert. However, timing can be difficult, particularly in an acute care setting, because the focus is on an early discharge. By the time the patient is ready to learn, discharge may already be scheduled. Therefore, you need to anticipate a patient's educational needs.

The length of teaching sessions also influences learning. Concentration decreases with prolonged sessions. You can assess a patient's level of concentration by observing nonverbal cues such as poor eye contact or slumped posture. Teaching sessions should be held often enough to document the patient's learning progress. The frequency of sessions depends on the learner's abilities and the complexity of the material. For example, a child in whom diabetes has been newly diagnosed will require more visits to an outpatient centre than will an older person who has been managing diabetes for 15 years. Intervals between teaching sessions should not be so long that the patient might forget information.

Organizing Teaching Material. An outline helps organize information into a logical sequence. Material should progress from simple to complex. A person needs to learn simple facts and concepts before learning associations or complex concepts.

Essential content should be taught first because people are more likely to remember information that is taught early. Repetition reinforces learning. Summarizing key points helps the learner remember important information (Bastable, 2014).

Maintaining Attention and Promoting Participation. Active participation is key to learning. People learn better when more than one of the body's senses is stimulated. Nurses should engage the patient's interest by changing the tone and intensity of their voice, making eye contact, using gestures, asking questions, and encouraging participation with activities such as role playing.

Building on Existing Knowledge. An effective teacher presents information that builds on a learner's existing knowledge. For example, a patient who has had multiple sclerosis must begin a new medication that is given subcutaneously. On assessment, the nurse asks the patient

BOX 20-8 NURSING CARE PLAN

Learning Needs

ASSESSMENT

Connie, a nurse in a surgeon's office, is preparing John for a colon resection, which is scheduled in 1 week. John, aged 75, has recently received a diagnosis of colorectal cancer. Connie's assessment focuses on John's readiness to learn, available resources, and factors that might affect his ability to understand the procedure and related postoperative care.

Assessment Activities	***Findings and Defining Characteristics***
Assess John's readiness to learn, and ask what the surgeon has already told him about the surgery.	John responds, "I can't remember what the doctor told me at my last appointment. My surgery is scheduled for next week."
Ask John to explain postoperative care, including performing a return demonstration of deep breathing and coughing.	John is unable to describe postoperative care or provide a return demonstration of deep breathing and coughing.
Assess John's visual acuity.	John says he has difficulty reading small print.

NURSING FOCUS: Lack of recall and exposure to information

PLANNING

Goals (Nursing Outcomes Classification)*	***Expected Outcomes**** ***Knowledge: Treatment Regimen***
John will describe preoperative and postoperative care to the nurse before surgery.	John will verbalize understanding of surgical procedure and related care on the day of surgery.
John will participate in postoperative care during hospitalization.	John will demonstrate deep breathing and coughing; he will advance his level of activity after his surgery.

*Outcome labels from Moorhead, S., Johnson, M., Maas, M. L., & Swanson, E. (Eds.). (2013). *Nursing outcomes classification (NOC)* (5th ed.). St. Louis, MO: Mosby.

INTERVENTIONS (NURSING INTERVENTIONS CLASSIFICATION)†

Learning Readiness Enhancement	***Rationale***
Determine readiness to learn and what the patient perceives as important to know.	Adult patients' learning is enhanced when they are ready to learn and the information is perceived as important (Bastable, 2014).
Learning Facilitation	
Give patient large-print brochure describing preoperative and postoperative care during educational session. Provide patient with Internet address associated with clinic to access patient information and instructional video clips.	Providing patients with educational methods that use multiple senses is effective in educating older persons. Large fonts with contrasting colours are easier for older persons to see (Sadowski, 2011).
Explain postoperative care, demonstrate deep breathing and coughing, and have patient perform return demonstration.	Improving self-efficacy by using role modelling and by having the patient perform behaviours enhances the successful adoption of healthy behaviours (Bandura, 1997).

†Intervention classification labels from Bulechek, G. M., Butcher, H. K., Dochterman, J. M., & Wagner, C. (Eds.). (2008). *Nursing interventions classification (NIC)* (6th ed.). St. Louis, MO: Mosby.

EVALUATION

Nursing Actions	***Patient Response and Finding***	***Achievement of Outcome***
Ask John what he can expect before and after surgery.	John is able to state understanding of preoperative and postoperative care.	John's anxiety level has decreased, and he reports that he is ready for surgery.
Observe patient as he demonstrates deep breathing and coughing and advances his activity postoperatively.	John is able to cough and breathe deeply postoperatively, but he is hesitant to advance his activity level after surgery.	Outcome of advancing activity postoperatively has not been totally achieved. Address and manage barriers inhibiting attainment of this outcome (e.g., pain), and continue to encourage and educate patient.

about experience with injections. The patient explains that she gave her father insulin injections for many years. The nurse can then individualize the teaching plan by building on the patient's previous knowledge and experience with insulin injections.

Selecting Teaching Methods. A teaching method is the way that the teacher delivers information. It is based on the patient's learning needs. More than one method may be used for instruction. For example, a patient who learns best in the psychomotor domain will benefit from demonstrations and supervised practice. The patient masters skills by manipulating equipment and practising manual skills. Discussions, question-and-answer sessions, and formal lectures can all be effective methods, depending on the patient's needs and learning style. When choosing appropriate teaching methods, nurses should encourage patients to offer suggestions (Box 20-9).

Selecting Resources. Nurses are responsible for ensuring that patients' educational needs are met. Sometimes patients' needs are highly complex. In these cases, nurses need to identify appropriate health education resources within the health care system or the community. Examples of resources for patient education are diabetes education clinics, cardiac rehabilitation programs, prenatal classes, and support groups. Nurses should obtain a referral if necessary, encourage patients to attend these sessions, and reinforce information taught.

BOX 20-9 PATIENT TEACHING

Teaching Strategies

- Establish trust with the patient before beginning the teaching–learning session.
- Limit teaching objectives.
- Use simple terminology to enhance the patient's understanding.
- Avoid medical jargon. If necessary, explain medical terms by using basic one- or two-syllable words.
- Schedule short teaching sessions at frequent intervals; minimize distractions during teaching sessions.
- Begin and end each teaching session with the most important information.
- Present information slowly, pacing to provide ample time for the patient to understand the material.
- Repeat important information.
- Provide many examples that have meaning to the patient; for example, relate new material to a previous life experience.
- Build on existing knowledge.
- Use visual cues and simple analogies when appropriate.
- Ask the patient for frequent feedback to determine whether the patient comprehends information.
- Demonstrate procedures such as measuring dosages; ask for return demonstrations (which provide opportunities to clarify instructions and time to review procedures).
- Provide teaching materials that reflect the reading level of the patient; use material that is written with short words and sentences, large type, and simple format (in general, information written on a Grade 5 reading level is recommended for adult learners).
- Provide teaching materials that reflect health literacy of the patient; use material that avoids jargon, acronyms, and unnecessary medical terminology and defines medical terms that are necessary.
- Model appropriate behaviour and use role playing to help patient learn how to ask questions and ask for help effectively.
- Pace the delivery of material so that patients can progress at their own speed.
- Include family members or other caregivers in the education process.

Data from Bastable, S. (2014). *Nurse as educator: Principles of teaching and learning for nursing practice* (4th ed.). Sudbury, MA: Jones & Bartlett; London, F. (2016). *No time to teach: The essence of patient and family education for health care providers* (2nd ed.). Atlanta, GA: Pritchett & Hall.

BOX 20-10 Example of Nursing Interventions Based on Patient's Learning Needs

Assessment Data

Mr. Kennedy, aged 67, has a 15-year history of type 2 diabetes. He is in the hospital because of an infected foot ulcer that necessitates frequent dressing changes. Mr. Kennedy used to take oral hypoglycemic agents to control his blood glucose levels. However, he now needs to start home insulin injections because of the infection and wound. He must also learn how to change his dressings. Mr. Kennedy is anxious about his discharge and requests information about a local diabetes support group and Internet resources. The case manager indicates that Mr. Kennedy will be discharged soon.

Cognitive Interventions

- Ask Mr. Kennedy about what he believes he needs to know before his discharge.
- Encourage Mr. Kennedy to help establish learning outcomes and goals.
- Provide Mr. Kennedy with teaching materials regarding insulin preparation and administration, and how to recognize and manage hypoglycemia and hyperglycemia.
- During teaching sessions, give Mr. Kennedy examples of what problems he might experience at home and ask him how he would respond to the situations (e.g., "If the wound's drainage increases and it looks like there is pus, what would you do?").
- Provide Mr. Kennedy with the URL for the Canadian Diabetes Association.

Affective Interventions

- Encourage Mr. Kennedy to attend a support group meeting, if possible, to facilitate learning from others' experiences.
- Encourage Mr. Kennedy to verbalize his feelings and fears about this change in his health status.
- Have Mr. Kennedy role play how he will respond to his friends when they ask him about his health status.
- As he acquires new skills and behaviours, provide Mr. Kennedy with feedback and positive reinforcement.

Psychomotor Interventions

- Demonstrate insulin preparation and injection techniques.
- Demonstrate use of blood glucose meter and recording of blood glucose measurements.
- Demonstrate dressing changes.
- Ask Mr. Kennedy to perform return demonstrations of insulin preparation and injection, blood glucose testing, and dressing changes.

Writing Teaching Plans. In all health care settings, nurses develop written teaching plans for use by colleagues. The nurse responsible for developing the teaching plan incorporates all pertinent information into the plan, including topics for instruction, resources (e.g., equipment, teaching booklets, and referrals to education programs), recommendations for involving family, and objectives of the teaching plan. A plan may be detailed or in outline form.

In an acute care setting, plans are concise and focused on the primary learning needs of the patient because time for teaching is limited. A home care teaching plan or outpatient clinic plan may be more comprehensive because nurses may have more time to instruct patients, and patients are often less anxious in outpatient settings.

A plan should provide continuity of instruction, particularly when several nurses are involved in a patient's care. The more specific the plan is, the easier it is to follow.

◆ Implementation

Implementing a teaching plan depends on a nurse's ability to analyze assessment data when identifying learning needs and developing the teaching plan (see Box 20-8). The nurse needs to evaluate the learning objectives and determine the best teaching and learning methods to help the patient to meet expected goals and outcomes. A diversified approach can be used to create an active learning environment (Box 20-10).

Teaching Approaches. A teaching approach is different from a method. Because a learner's needs and motives can change over time, nurses must be ready to modify teaching approaches.

Telling. The telling approach is useful when limited information must be taught (e.g., preparing a patient for an emergency diagnostic procedure). The nurse outlines the task to be done and the patient's role and gives instructions—for example, explaining the insertion of an intravenous line and the need for the patient to remain still. This method provides no opportunity for feedback.

Selling. The selling approach entails two-way communication. The nurse needs to pace instruction according to the patient's response. Specific feedback is given to the patient who learns successfully. For example, when the patient learns a step-by-step procedure for changing a dressing, first the patient learns to remove the old dressing, then to clean the wound, and finally to apply a new dressing.

Participating. Participating involves setting objectives and becoming involved in the learning process together. The patient helps decide content, and the nurse guides and counsels the patient with pertinent information. Opportunities are provided for discussion, feedback, mutual goal setting, and revision of the teaching plan. For example, a patient's request for information about improving physical fitness leads to a discussion with the patient in which the nurse identifies key areas of interest, such as weight loss and improving cardiovascular fitness. Together with the patient, the nurse identifies goals and learning strategies.

Entrusting. The entrusting approach provides the patient with the opportunity to manage self-care. The nurse observes the patient's progress and remains available to assist without introducing more new information. For example, a patient with metabolic syndrome has decided to make lifestyle changes (e.g., improve diet and exercise) to improve his health. The nurse provides resources and recommends other sources of information. The nurse then meets with the patient on a regular basis to check progress and provide additional information.

Reinforcing. Reinforcement is the use of a stimulus that increases the probability of a response. A person who receives positive reinforcement before or after learning a desired behaviour is likely to repeat the behaviour. People usually respond better to positive reinforcement (Bastable, 2014). The effects of negative reinforcement, such as criticizing, can decrease an undesired response but are less predictable and often undesirable. Feedback is a common form of reinforcement.

Three types of reinforcers are social, material, and activity. Most nurses use social reinforcers (e.g., encouraging words) to acknowledge a learned behaviour. Examples of material reinforcers are food, toys, and music. These reinforcers work best with young children. Activity reinforcers are based on the principle that people are motivated to engage in an activity if, after its completion, they are able to engage in a more desirable activity. For example, patients with dementia may be more willing to bathe if they can go for a walk with the nurse afterward. Activity reinforces work when a patient is self-motivated. Choosing an appropriate reinforcer requires attention to individual preferences. Observing behaviour often helps reveal the best reinforcer to use. Reinforcers should never be used as threats and are not effective with every patient.

Incorporating Teaching Into Nursing Care. Many nurses teach effectively while delivering nursing care. This is taking advantage of teachable moments (London, 2016). This activity becomes easier as you gain confidence in clinical skills. For example, while hanging a blood bag, you explain to the patient why the blood is needed, and you describe the symptoms of transfusion reactions that should be reported immediately. When you follow a teaching plan informally, the patient feels less pressure to perform, and learning becomes more of a shared activity. Teaching during routine care is efficient and cost-effective (Figure 20-2).

Implementing Teaching Methods. The nurse's choice of teaching methods depends on the patient's learning needs, the time available for teaching, the environment, the resources, and the nurse's own comfort level with teaching. Skilled teachers are flexible in altering teaching methods according to the learner's responses and in using teaching tools that work best with a particular method. Various teaching tools are detailed in Table 20-2.

One-on-One Discussion. In one-on-one discussion, you present information informally, providing the patient with the opportunity to ask questions or share concerns. During the discussion, you can use various teaching aids such as models or diagrams, depending on the patient's learning needs.

Group Instruction. Groups are an economical way to teach several patients at once. Patients interact and learn from other's experiences. Groups can also foster positive attitudes that help patients meet learning objectives (London, 2016).

Group instruction often involves lecture, activities, and discussion. Lectures are highly structured and help patients learn standard content. However, they do not encourage active thinking; thus, activities, discussion, and practice sessions are essential (London, 2016).

Preparatory Instruction. Patients are often anxious about unfamiliar tests or procedures. By providing information about procedures, nurses help patients anticipate what will happen. Guidelines for giving preparatory explanations are as follows:

- Describe physical sensations during the procedure, but do not evaluate them. For example, when you draw a blood specimen, explain to the patient that he or she will feel a sticking sensation as the needle punctures the skin.

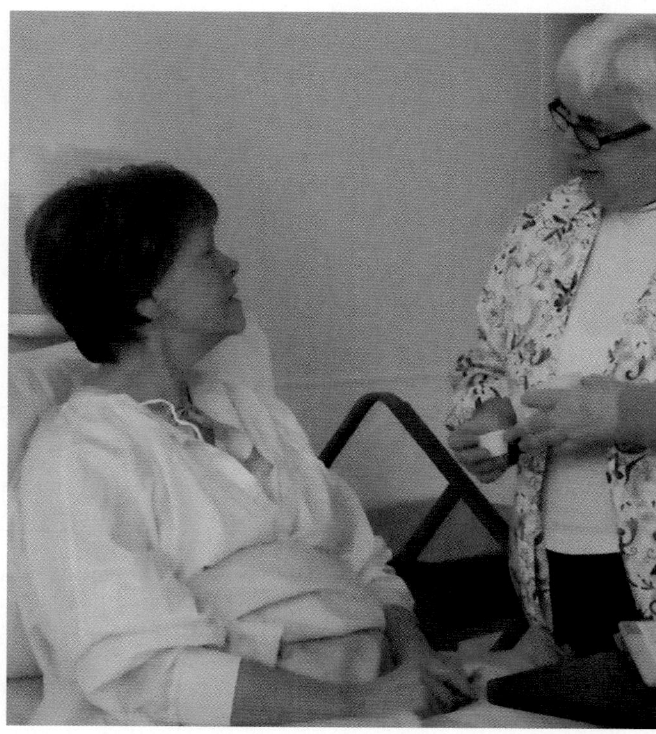

FIGURE 20-2 Teaching during routine care. The nurse uses administration of medication to assess a patient's knowledge about medications and provides additional information as needed.

TABLE 20-2 Teaching Tools for Instruction

Description of Tool	Implications for Learning
Printed Material	
Written teaching tools such as pamphlets, booklets, and brochures	Material must be easily readable for learner. Information must be accurate and current. Method is ideal for understanding complex concepts and relationships.
Programmed Instruction	
Written sequential presentation of learning steps requiring that learners answer questions and that teachers tell them whether their answers are right or wrong	Instruction is primarily verbal, but teacher may use pictures or diagrams. Method requires active learning, giving immediate feedback, correcting wrong answers, and reinforcing right answers. Learner works at own pace.
Computer Resources	
Computer Programs	
Programmed instruction format in which computers store response patterns for learners and select further lessons on basis of these patterns (programs can be individualized)	Method requires reading comprehension, psychomotor skills, and familiarity with computer.
Internet Resources	
Provides access to instructional resources that might not be available locally and that may be interactive and include demonstrations, video clips, self-directed modules, and web-based learning	Method requires access to the Internet, psychomotor skills, and familiarity with computer.
Audiovisual Materials	
Diagrams	
Illustrations that show interrelationships by means of lines and symbols	Method demonstrates key ideas and summarizes and clarifies key concept.
Graphs (Bar, Circle, or Line)	
Visual presentations of numerical data	Graphs help learner to grasp information quickly about single concept.
Charts	
Highly condensed visual summaries of ideas and facts that may highlight series of ideas, steps, or events	Charts demonstrate relationship of several ideas or concepts. Method helps learners know what to do.
Pictures	
Photographs or drawings used to teach concepts in which the third dimension of shape and space is not important	Photographs are more desirable than diagrams because they more accurately portray the details of the real item. Drawings are pertinent for removing the superfluous detail present in real objects.
Physical Objects	
Use of actual equipment, objects, models, or simulation to teach concepts or skills	Models are useful when real objects are too small, large, or complicated or are unavailable. Learners can manipulate objects that are to be used later in skill.
Other Audiovisual Materials	
Slides, audiotapes, television, and videotapes used with printed material or discussion	Materials are useful for patients with reading comprehension problems and visual deficits.

- Describe the cause of the sensation to prevent misinterpretation of the experience. For example, explain that a needle stick burns because the alcohol used to cleanse the skin enters the puncture site.
- Prepare patients only for aspects of the experience that are common to other patients. For example, explain that it is normal for a tight tourniquet to cause a person's hand to tingle and feel numb.

Demonstrations. Demonstrations are used to teach psychomotor skills, such as preparing a syringe, bathing an infant, walking with a crutch, or measuring a pulse. Patients need to observe a skill before practising it. Demonstrations are most effective when patients first observe the nurse doing the skill and then perform a **return demonstration** to practise the skill. A demonstration should be combined with discussion to clarify concepts and feelings. An effective demonstration requires advanced planning:

- Position the patient to provide a clear view of the demonstration.
- Review the rationale and steps of the procedure.
- Assemble and organize equipment. Make sure it works.
- Perform each step in sequence while analyzing the knowledge and skills involved.
- Determine when to give explanations, considering the patient's learning needs.
- Adjust speed and timing of the demonstration according to the patient's abilities and anxiety level.

The nurse should demonstrate the steps of a procedure in the same order in which the patient will perform them. The demonstration involves the following:

- Performing each step slowly and accurately
- Encouraging the patient to ask questions so that each step is understood
- Explaining the rationale for each step
- Allowing the patient to observe each step
- Providing the patient with the opportunity to handle equipment and practise the procedure under supervision

The patient demonstrates the procedure to ensure that learning has occurred. The demonstration should occur under the same conditions that will be experienced at home or in the place where the procedure is to be performed. For example, for a patient learning to walk with crutches, the nurse needs to simulate the home environment. If short, narrow steps lead to the patient's bedroom, the patient should learn to climb similar stairs in the hospital.

Analogies. Learning occurs when a teacher translates complex language or ideas into words or concepts that the patient understands. Analogies aid learning by supplementing verbal instruction with familiar images that make complex information simpler and understandable. For example, to explain arterial blood pressure, an analogy is the flow of water through a hose. To use analogies, follow these general principles:

- Be familiar with the concept.
- Know the patient's background, experience, and culture.
- Keep the analogy simple and clear.

Role Playing. Role playing can be used to teach new ideas and attitudes. During role playing, patients play themselves or someone else and rehearse a desired behaviour. For example, you can teach a parent to respond to a child's behaviour by pretending to be a child having a temper tantrum. This role playing provides the parent with the opportunity to practise responding in this situation. You then evaluate the parent's response and determine whether an alternative approach would be more appropriate. Role playing helps patients learn skills and feel confident in their ability to perform them independently.

Simulation. Simulation can be used to teach problem solving, application, and independent thinking. During individual or group discussion, a nurse poses a problem or situation for patients to solve. For example, patients with heart disease are asked to plan a low-fat meal. The nurse will then ask the patients to present their diet, providing an opportunity to identify mistakes and reinforce correct information.

Paying Attention to Learning Barriers. Many situations or conditions present a barrier to learning. For example, the patient may have a low reading level (functionally illiterate), a learning disability, a sensory alteration, or depression; may be suffering the effects of prescribed medications or adjusting to life changes or transitions; or may have a poor memory. Patients understand fewer medical words than health care providers predict. Unfortunately, health care providers often use medical terminology and jargon, which prevents patients from understanding the written health information they are given (Huff, 2011). Nurses should pay special attention to the learning needs of patients who have reading problems, learning disabilities, and sensory alterations and of those whose first language is not English or French.

Illiteracy and Learning Disabilities. A 2012 survey on literacy rates in Canada (Statistics Canada & Organization for Economic Cooperation and Development, 2016) indicated that about 11% of Canadian adults fall within the lowest level of literacy. These people have only rudimentary reading and writing skills; for example, they are not able to read and understand a label on a medicine container. An additional 27% of Canadians may read only material that is simple and familiar. Therefore, a substantial number of Canadians have problems with reading materials encountered in everyday life. To compound this problem, the readability of printed material ranges from elementary school level to college level. Researchers have found that printed educational material is consistently written above most patients' reading level (Ryan, Logsdon, McGill, et al., 2014). Health care providers need to screen materials for readability and clarity.

Some people have learning disabilities, which are disorders that may impair ability to acquire, organize, remember, understand, or apply information (Learning Disabilities Association of Canada, n.d.). The ability to learn or use oral or written language, mathematics, or both may be poor. Teaching strategies need to be adapted to accommodate their learning needs. For example, patients with attention deficit–hyperactivity disorder may have difficulty recalling information and staying focused during educational sessions; they may also have a low threshold of frustration (Bastable, 2014). Teaching activities should be kept short in an environment with minimal competing stimuli.

Health Literacy. Health literacy refers to a patient's ability to find, access, read, and understand reliable health information and to use that information to make informed decisions about their health. Many patients have difficulty accessing and understanding health information (RNAO, 2012; Stiles, 2011; Ward-Smith, 2012). Aspects of health literacy of note are the ability to identify, access, and use reliable information. Patients no longer depend solely on their health care provider. They are bombarded with health-related advertisements and may seek information on the Internet, some of which is incomplete or inaccurate. They can be either well informed about their health or misinformed about their health, depending on their health literacy. Patient information needs to be presented clearly, avoiding medical terminology, jargon, and acronyms that the patient may not be familiar with.

Sensory Alteration and Other Barriers. Some patients, including many older persons, have sensory deficits (see Chapter 47). Sensory changes such as visual and hearing deficits necessitate teaching methods that enhance functioning. For example, you need to face a patient with hearing problems and speak in a low tone of voice during discussions (lower tones are easier to hear than higher tones). Clearly written materials should be provided. Patients with visual problems can benefit from large-print materials. Patients with slower cognitive function and reduced short-term memory (as in some older persons and patients who have had strokes) learn and remember effectively if the learning is paced properly and the material is relevant to the learner's needs and abilities.

Language. The diverse backgrounds of Canadians can challenge nurses to provide culturally safe care (see Chapters 9 and 10 for further information about cultural safety). Patients may not understand instructions that are not in their native language (see Chapters 9 and 17 for further information about communication). As a nurse, you need to ascertain a patient's fluency in English or French before you choose teaching methods or tools. If possible, instruction should be done collaboratively with an interpreter (London, 2016).

Cultural Diversity. Nurses need to have knowledge of patients' cultural background, values, and beliefs (see Chapters 9 and 10 for further information about cultural diversity), as well as the patient's ability to understand both verbal and written material (Farahani, Sahragard, Carroll, et al., 2011). When educating patients of cultural groups different from your own, you need to be aware of the distinctive aspects of their cultures and develop teaching strategies that are respectful of cultural beliefs, values, and behaviours.

Needs of Patients With Severe Illness. Adapting to serious illness or disability is difficult for most people. Often, they need to grieve resulting losses. The grieving process gives them time to adapt psychologically to the emotional and physical implications of illness. People experience grief (see Chapter 25) at different rates and sequences, depending on their self-concept before illness, the severity of the illness, and the changes and losses caused by the illness. Sensitivity is required to educate patients while they are grieving and are adjusting to their illness.

Readiness to learn is related to the grieving stage (Table 20-3). Patients cannot learn when they are unwilling or unable to accept the reality of illness. However, properly timed teaching can help a patient to adjust to illness or disability. The nurse can identify the patient's stage of grieving on the basis of the patient's behaviours. When the patient enters the stage of acceptance, the stage compatible with learning, the nurse can then introduce a teaching plan. Continuous assessment of the patient's behaviours is used to determine the stages of grieving.

◆ Evaluation

Patient education is not complete until outcomes of the teaching–learning process have been evaluated (see Box 20-8). Nurses need to determine whether patients have learned the material. Evaluation reinforces correct behaviour, helps learners realize how they should change incorrect behaviour, and helps the nurse determine the adequacy of the teaching (Bastable, 2014). Success depends on the patient's ability to meet the established outcome and goals, and these in turn are the means by which the nurse can evaluate success. The following checklist helps in evaluating patient education:

- Were educational goals set mutually between the nurse and the patient?
- Were the patient's goals or outcomes realistic and observable?
- Is the patient able to demonstrate the behaviour or skill on multiple occasions?
- How well is the patient able to answer questions about the topic?
- Does the patient continue to have a difficulty in understanding the information or performing a skill? If so, what changes in interventions should be made to enhance skill attainment?

Measurement Methods. Under direct observation, the patient should demonstrate the behaviours described in the learning objectives. If the evaluation process indicates a deficit in knowledge or skill, the nurse must repeat or modify the teaching plan. By watching patients demonstrate behaviours, nurses can see whether correct techniques are being used. However, a patient may behave differently later. Therefore, observation works best in real-life situations.

Oral and written questioning are other useful evaluation methods. Questions are best used for behaviours that are not easily demonstrated. The nurse should phrase questions to ensure that the learner understands them and that objectives are truly measured.

Another form of evaluation includes self-reports (oral and written) and self-monitoring (written). An example is a patient's written log of the foods eaten in a specific time period, in comparison with a new diet. Nurses rely on patients' honesty and memory in self-reporting.

Patient Expectations. Evaluations of nursing care and teaching sessions help determine whether a patient's needs and expectations

TABLE 20-3 Relationship Between Learning and Psychosocial Adaptation to Illness

Stage	Patient's Behaviour	Nursing Activities	Rationale
Denial or disbelief	Patient avoids discussion of illness ("Nothing is wrong with me"), withdraws from others, and disregards physical restrictions. Patient suppresses and distorts information that has not been presented clearly.	Provide support, empathy, and careful explanations of all procedures while they are being done. Let patient know you are available for conversation. Explain situation to family or significant other if appropriate. Teach in present tense (e.g., explain what patient needs to know to be discharged).	Patient is not prepared to deal with problem; attempts to teach patient will result in further anger or withdrawal. Provide only information that patient pursues or requires.
Anger	Patient blames and complains and often directs anger toward nurse or others.	Do not argue with patient, but listen to concerns. Teach in present tense. Reassure family of the normality of patient's behaviour.	Patient needs opportunity to express feelings and anger. Patient is still not prepared to face future.
Bargaining	Patient offers to live better life in exchange for promise of better health (e.g., "If God lets me live, I promise to manage my disease better").	Continue to introduce only reality and teaching in present tense.	Patient is still unwilling to accept limitations.
Resolution	Patient begins to express emotions openly, realizes that illness has created changes, and begins to ask questions.	Encourage expression of feelings. Begin to share information needed for future, and set aside formal times for discussion.	Patient begins to perceive need for assistance and is ready to accept responsibility for learning.
Acceptance	Patient recognizes reality of condition, actively pursues information, and strives for independence.	Focus on future skills and knowledge required. Continue to teach in present tense. Involve family in planning and teaching for discharge.	Patient is more easily motivated to learn. Acceptance of illness reflects willingness to deal with its implications.

have been met. At the end of the session, the nurse asks the patient whether he or she has questions; in this way, the nurse can identify information that was missing and should have been covered. Patients may also fill out written evaluations of a teaching session or course. Anonymous written evaluations may be more truthful than face-to-face evaluations.

Evaluation may reveal new learning needs or new factors that are interfering with learning, in which case the nurse should try alternative teaching methods. When a patient has difficulty in an acute care setting, the nurse may make a referral to resources, such as home care or an outpatient clinic, for further education and evaluation.

Documentation. Because patient teaching often occurs informally, it is difficult to document it consistently. Nurses are legally responsible for providing accurate, timely information that promotes continuity of care; therefore, it is essential to document the outcomes of teaching. The following should be documented with regard to patient education:

- *Assessment data and reassessment of learning needs.* Such data and evaluation provide important information for when the teaching plan is developed.
- *Nursing analysis, patient needs, and educational priorities.* These provide support for goals and outcomes that are established.
- *Interventions planned.* A specific plan, including the methods to be used in instruction, enhances continuity of care. When planned interventions are provided, the nurse can determine what information needs to be provided to the patient.
- *Interventions provided.* Specifically describing the subject matter enables other nurses to follow up and reinforce teaching (e.g., "Explained side effects of Inderal" or "Demonstrated umbilical cord care"). Note the date, time, and specific patient or patients taught. Avoid generalizations (e.g., "medications taught"). Resources used, such as pamphlets or audiovisual materials, are documented in the patient's record.
- *Patient's response and outcomes of care.* In documenting evidence of learning (e.g., a return demonstration or the ability to verbalize the purpose and adverse effects of a medication), the nurse is informing staff about the patient's progress and identifying information that must still be taught.
- *Ability of patient, family, or both to manage needs after discharge.* An evaluation of remaining educational needs on discharge helps with identifying the need for outpatient or home health care follow-up. If referrals are appropriate, the patient, family, or both are often able to meet their needs.

KEY CONCEPTS

- The nurse ensures that patients, families, and communities receive information needed to maintain optimal health.
- Health education is aimed at the promotion, restoration, and maintenance of health.
- Teaching is most effective when it is responsive to the learner's needs.
- Teaching is a form of interpersonal communication, with the teacher and student actively involved in a process that increases the student's knowledge and skills.
- The ability to learn depends on a person's physical and cognitive attributes.
- The ability to attend to the learning process depends on physical comfort and anxiety levels and on the presence of environmental distraction.
- A person's health beliefs influence the willingness to gain knowledge and skills necessary to maintain health.
- Teaching must be timed to coincide with the patient's readiness to learn.
- Patients of different age groups require different teaching strategies as a result of developmental capabilities.
- The patient should be an active participant in a teaching plan: agreeing to the plan, helping choose instructional methods, and recommending times for instruction.
- Learning objectives describe what a person is to learn in behavioural terms.
- A combination of teaching methods improves the learner's attentiveness and involvement.
- A teacher is more effective when presenting information that builds on a learner's existing knowledge.
- Nurses should assess which learning materials, methods, and approaches will be most effective for each patient, on the basis of each patient's individual abilities and challenges.
- A nurse evaluates a patient's learning by observing performance of expected learning behaviours under desired conditions.
- Effective documentation describes the entire process of patient education, promotes continuity of care, and demonstrates that educational standards have been met.

CRITICAL THINKING EXERCISES

1. Mrs. S. has a 10-year history of hypertension and a 5-year history of diabetes. Recently, her hypertension has worsened and she has received a diagnosis of depression. Her medications, which have recently been changed, include 25 mg of captopril (Capoten) three times a day; 240 mg of diltiazem (Cardizem CD) every morning; 1500 mg of metformin (Glucophage XR) before the evening meal; and 100 mg of sertraline (Zoloft) by mouth at bed time. You identify the priority nursing focus *additional knowledge related to change in medications.* You want to develop a plan of care in which the three domains of learning are used. What are the patient's teaching priorities? Which learning needs would necessitate a cognitive method? Which needs would be more appropriate to satisfy through affective or psychomotor methods?
2. You are caring for a patient who is being discharged after an appendectomy. He takes medication to treat attention deficit–hyperactivity disorder. Which teaching strategies should you use when providing discharge information to this patient?
3. A 23-year-old man has recently sustained a spinal cord injury after being involved in a diving accident that has left him paralyzed from the waist down. He verbally abuses the staff and expresses anger toward his family and friends when they come to visit. He needs to begin learning transfer techniques. Which stage of grieving is this patient experiencing? What approach should you take in planning education for this patient?
4. A 65-year-old woman is taking her 72-year-old husband home after surgery. Which strategies should you use in helping this couple make the transition to home smoothly?

REVIEW QUESTONS

1. A patient must learn to use an inhaler. Acquisition of this skill will require learning in which domain?
   1. Cognitive
   2. Affective
   3. Psychomotor
   4. Attentional

2. The nurse is planning to teach a patient about the importance of exercise. What is the best time for teaching to occur?
   1. When visitors are in the room
   2. When the patient indicates being pain free
   3. Just before lunch, when the patient is most awake and alert
   4. When the patient is talking about current stressors in his or her life
3. A patient with newly diagnosed cervical cancer is going home. The patient is avoiding discussion of her illness and postoperative orders. In teaching the patient about discharge instructions, the nurse should:
   1. Teach the patient's spouse
   2. Focus on knowledge the patient will need in a few weeks
   3. Provide only the information the patient needs to go home
   4. Convince the patient that learning about her health is necessary
4. A community health nurse is about to teach a Grade 12 health class about nutrition. To achieve the best learning outcomes, the nurse should: *(Select all that apply.)*
   1. Provide information by using a lecture
   2. Use simple words to promote understanding
   3. Complete an extensive literature search focusing on eating disorders
   4. Develop topics that include activities and problem solving
   5. Explore with students their understanding of nutrition to determine educational needs
5. The nurse is organizing a disease prevention program for a specific cultural group. To effectively meet the needs of this group the nurse will: *(Select all that apply.)*
   1. Assess the needs of the community in general
   2. Involve those affected by the problem in the planning process.
   3. Use educational materials that are simplistic and have many pictures
   4. Assess commonly held health beliefs among the cultural group
   5. Educate the group about the Western concepts of health and illness
   6. Include cultural practices that are relevant to this community
6. A patient who is having chest pain is about to undergo an emergency cardiac catheterization. Which of the following is the most appropriate teaching approach in this situation?
   1. Telling
   2. Selling
   3. Entrusting
   4. Participating
7. The nurse teaching a parenting class to a group of pregnant adolescents has given the adolescents baby dolls to bathe and talk to. This is an example of:
   1. Simulation
   2. An analogy
   3. Role playing
   4. A demonstration
8. A patient with a learning disability is starting to take a new antihypertensive medication. In teaching the patient about the medication, the nurse should: *(Select all that apply.)*
   1. Demonstrate measuring dosages and ask for a return demonstration
   2. Provide only written material
   3. Present the information several times
   4. Expect the patient to understand the information quickly
9. A patient must learn how to administer a subcutaneous injection. The nurse knows the patient is ready to learn when the patient:
   1. Has been given written instructions
   2. Expresses the importance of learning the skill
   3. Can see and understand the markings on the syringe
   4. Has the dexterity needed to prepare and inject the medication
10. A patient who is hospitalized has just received a diagnosis of diabetes. He needs to learn how to give himself injections. The best teaching method(s) would be: *(Select all that apply.)*
    1. Demonstration
    2. Group instruction
    3. One-on-one discussion
    4. Simulation
    5. Step-by-step instructional video
11. A nurse needs to teach a young woman newly diagnosed with asthma how to manage her disease. Which of the following topics does the nurse teach first?
    1. How to use an inhaler during an asthma attack
    2. The need to avoid people who smoke, to prevent asthma attacks
    3. Where to purchase a medical alert bracelet that says she has asthma
    4. The importance of maintaining a healthy diet and exercising regularly
12. A nurse is teaching a 27-year-old man how to adjust his insulin dosages on the basis of his blood sugar results. This type of activity addresses learning in the cognitive domain at the level of ___________.

Answers: 1. 3; **2.** 2; **3.** 3; **4.** 4, 5; **5.** 2, 4, 6; **6.** 1; **7.** 3; **8.** 1, 3; **9.** 2; **10.** 1, 4, 5; **11.** 1; **12.** application

Rationales for the Review Questions appear at the end of the book.

RECOMMENDED WEBSITES

Canadian Public Health Association: http://www.cpha.ca.
This website provides both national and international information and resources on public health issues and services.

Health Canada: http://www.hc-sc.gc.ca.
This website provides many resources on a variety of health issues and topics to assist in patient education.

National Institutes of Health: https://health.nih.gov/.
Prepared by the National Institutes of Health in the United States, this website provides a great many resources for patient education.

Public Health Agency of Canada: https://www.canada.ca/en/public-health.html.
This website provides information and resources on a variety of public health issues and topics, including health promotion, healthy living, diseases, and injury prevention.

Registered Nurses' Association of Ontario (RNAO): http://rnao.ca/bpg/guidelines/facilating-client-centred-learning.
This website provides Best Practice Guidelines and other resources relating to patient education.

REFERENCES

Bandura, A. (1997). *Self-efficacy: The exercise of control.* New York: W. H. Freeman.

Bandura, A. (2001). Social cognitive theory: An agentic perspective. *Annual Review of Psychology, 52,* 1–26.

Bastable, S. (2014). *Nurse as educator: Principles of teaching and learning for nursing practice* (4th ed.). Sudbury, MA: Jones & Bartlett.

Bastable, S. (2017). *Essentials of patient education* (2nd ed.). Sudbury, MA: Jones & Bartlett.

Bergh, A., Friberg, F., Persson, E., et al. (2015). Registered nurses' patient education in everyday primary care practice: Managers' discourse. *Global Qualitative Nursing Research, 2,* doi:10.1177/2333393615599168.

Bloom, B. S. (Ed.), (1956). *Taxonomy of educational objectives: The classification of educational goals: Vol. 1. Cognitive domain.* New York: Longman.

Canadian Association of Schools of Nursing/Association Canadienne des Écoles de Sciences Infirmières (CASN/ACESI) (2015). *National nursing education framework*. Ottawa ON: Author. Retrieved from http://www.casn.ca/wp-content/uploads/2014/12/Framwork-FINAL-SB-Nov-30-20151.pdf.

Canadian Nurses Association (2017). *Code of ethics for registered nurses*. Ottawa: Author.

Edelman, C. L., Kudzma, E. C., & Mandle, C. L. (2014). *Health promotion throughout the life-span* (8th ed.). St. Louis, MO: Mosby.

Farahani, M. A., Sahragard, R., Carroll, J. K., et al. (2011). Communication barriers to patient education in cardiac inpatient care: A qualitative study of multiple perspectives. *International Journal of Nursing Practice, 17*(3), 322–328. doi:10.1111/j.1440-172X.2011.01940.x.

Huff, C. (2011). Does your patient really understand? *Hospitals and Health Networks, 85*(10), 34–35, 37–38, 2.

Krathwohl, D. R., Bloom, B. S., & Masia, B. B. (1964). *Taxonomy of educational objectives: The classification of educational goals: Handbook 2. Affective domain*. New York: David McKay.

Krau, S. (2011). Creating educational objectives for patient education using the new Bloom's taxonomy. *Nursing Clinics of North America, 46*(3), 299–312. doi:10.1016/j.cnur.2011.05.002.

Learning Disabilities Association of Canada. (n.d.). *Learning disabilities at a glance*. Retrieved from http://www.ldac-acta.ca/learn-more/ld-basics.

London, F. (2016). *No time to teach: The essence of patient and family education for health care providers* (2nd ed.). Atlanta, GA: Pritchett & Hall.

McCance, T., McCormack, B., & Dewing, J. (2011). An exploration of person-centredness in practice. *OJIN: The Online Journal of Issues in Nursing, 16*(2), Manuscript 1. doi:10.3912/OJIN.Vol16No02Man01.

Nimkar, S. (2016). Promoting individual health using information technology: Trends in the US health system. *Health Education Journal, 75*(6), 744–752. doi:10.1177/0017896916632790.

Pender, N. J., Murdaugh, C. L., & Parsons, M. A. (2015). *Health promotion in nursing practice* (7th ed.). Upper Saddle River, NJ: Prentice Hall.

Prochaska, J. C., & DiClemente, C. C. (1992). Stages of change in the modification of problem behaviors. In M. Hersen, R. M. Eisler, & P. M. Miller (Eds.), *Progress in behaviour modification* (pp. 184–218). Newbury Park, CA: Sage.

Redman, B. K. (2011). Ethics of patient education and how do we make it everyone's ethics. *Nursing Clinics of North America, 46*(3), 283–289. doi:10.1016/j.cnur.2011.05.001.

Registered Nurses' Association of Ontario (RNAO) (2012). *Facilitating client-centreed learning*. Toronto ON: Author. Retrieved from http://rnao.ca/sites/rnao-ca/files/BPG_CCL_2012_FA.pdf.

Registered Nurses' Association of Ontario (RNAO) (n.d.). *Guidelines*. Toronto ON: Author. Retrieved from http://rnao.ca/bpg/guidelines.

Robinson, L. M., & Vail, S. R. (2012). An integrative review of adolescent smoking cessation using the transtheoretical model of change. *Journal of Pediatric Health Care, 26*(5), 336–345. doi:10.1016/j.pedhc.2010.12.001.

Ryan, L., Logsdon, M. C., McGill, S., et al. (2014). Evaluation of printed health education materials for use by low education families. *Journal of Nursing Scholarship, 46*(4), 218–228. doi:10.1111/jnu.12076.

Sadowski, C. A. (2011). Providing health information to older adults. *Reviews in Clinical Gerontology, 21*(1), 55–66. doi:10.1017/S0959259810000316.

Statistics Canada & Organization for Economic Co-operation and Development (OECD) (2016). *Education indicators in Canada: An international perspective 2016*. Ottawa: Author. Retrieved from http://www.statcan.gc.ca/pub/81-604-x/2016001/toc-tdm-eng.htm.

Stevinson, C., Wiltshire, G., & Hickson, M. (2015). Facilitating participation in health-enhancing physical activity: A qualitative study of parkrun. *International Journal of Behavioral Medicine, 22*(2), 170–177. doi:10.1007/s12529-014-9431-5.

Stiles, E. (2011). Promoting health literacy in patients with diabetes. *Nursing Standard, 26*(8), 35–40.

Ward-Smith, P. (2012). Health literacy. *Urologic Nursing, 32*(3), 168–170, 167.

Zuniga, G. C., Kirk, S., Mier, N., et al. (2012). The impact of asthma health education for parents of children attending head start centers. *Journal of Community Health, 37*(6), 1296–1300. doi:10.1007/s10900-012-9571-y.

21

Developmental Theories

Canadian content written by Nicole Letourneau, RN, PhD, FCAHS
Original chapter by Tara Hulsey, PhD, RN, CNE, FAAN

OBJECTIVES

Mastery of content in this chapter will enable you to:

- Define the key terms listed.
- Identify basic principles of growth and development.
- Discuss factors influencing growth and development.
- Identify five major traditions that underlie modern developmental theories.
- Name and describe the major developmental theories associated with each tradition.
- Describe and compare the mechanisms that underlie the major developmental theories.
- Discuss nursing implications associated with the application of developmental principles to patient care.

KEY TERMS

Accommodation, p. 347
Assimilation, p. 347
Attachment, p. 352
Autonomous stage, p. 348
Biophysical developmental theories, p. 344
Bowlby's attachment and separation theory, p. 352
Bronfenbrenner's bioecological theory, p. 354
Cognitive developmental theories, p. 346
Contextual tradition, p. 354
Conventional stage, p. 348
Developmental health, p. 355
Dialectic tradition, p. 355
Differentiation, p. 346
Dynamic maturational model of attachment, p. 352
Ego, p. 350
Epigenesis, p. 352
Epigenetics, p. 355
Erikson's theory of eight stages of life, p. 350
Exosystem, p. 355
Freud's psychoanalytic model of personality development, p. 349
Havighurst's developmental tasks, p. 354
Id, p. 350
Individuation, p. 349
Kohlberg's theory of moral development, p. 348
Libido, p. 349
Macrosystem, p. 355
Maturation, p. 346
Mechanisms of development, p. 344
Mechanistic tradition, p. 354
Mesosystem, p. 355
Microsystem, p. 355
Moral developmental theories, p. 348
Organicism, p. 344
Piaget's theory of cognitive development, p. 347
Piaget's theory of moral development, p. 348
Population health approach, p. 355
Premoral stage, p. 348
Protective processes, p. 356
Psychoanalytic and psychosocial tradition, p. 349
Resilience, p. 356
Separation, p. 349
Superego, p. 350
Temperament, p. 346
Vulnerability processes, p. 356
Zone of proximal development, p. 355

MEDIA RESOURCES

http://evolve.elsevier.com/Canada/Potter/fundamentals/

- Audio Chapter Summaries
- Examination Review Questions
- Concept Map Creator
- Case Study with Questions
- Audio Glossary
- Content Updates
- Video Clips

All people progress through phases of growth and development, from the simple to the complex, at a highly individualized rate. Understanding typical growth and development helps nurses to predict, prevent, and detect any changes from patients' expected patterns and to develop approaches and programs that can further enhance the developmental well-being of individuals (Berk, 2008; Bukatko, 2012). Drawing on theories from the natural and biomedical sciences, as well as behavioural and social sciences, to explain the influence of early experience on lifespan development enables nurses in caring for patients (Green & Piel, 2016; McCain, Mustard, & Shanker, 2007) and provides a foundation for nurses' advocacy for appropriate developmental care for vulnerable children, adults, and families (Canadian Association for Schools of Nursing [CASN], 2015). Knowledge of human developmental processes is crucial to optimal nursing education (CASN, 2015) as it helps nurses in assessing and treating a patient's response to an illness and in planning appropriate individualized care for patients.

Historically, growth and development have been described as orderly, predictable processes beginning with conception and continuing until death, but this view is increasingly recognized as overlooking differences in gender, culture, and sexuality. Today, it is no longer assumed that all people progress through universal linear phases of growth and development. Human growth and development are now seen as processes in which sociocultural, biological, and psychological forces interact with the individual over time (Berk, 2008; Green & Piel, 2016). As a result, theorists have changed their focus from describing growth and development to explaining it: How do humans develop? What are the mechanisms, or explanatory components, that underlie human growth and development?

In this chapter, five broad traditions of human development are introduced, and the mechanisms of development espoused by key theorists are outlined. Examples of implications for the nursing process that follow from the mechanisms are offered (see Chapters 22, 23, and 24 for further information about descriptions of human development).

GROWTH AND DEVELOPMENT

Growth and development are synchronous processes that are interdependent in the healthy individual. Growth and development depend on a sequence of endocrine, genetic, constitutional, environmental, and nutritional influences (Edelman, Kudzma, & Mandle, 2013).

Physical Growth

Growth is the quantitative, or measurable, aspect of an individual's increase in physical measurements. Measurable growth indicators include changes in height, weight, teeth, skeletal structures, and sexual characteristics. For example, children generally double their birth weight by 5 months of age and their birth height by 36 months. Physical growth is not only genetic but also affected by other contextual factors, such as socioeconomic status.

Development

Development is a progressive and continuous process of change leading to increased skill and capacity to function. Development is the result of complex interactions between biological and environmental influences (Green & Piel, 2016). These changes are qualitative in nature and difficult to measure in exact units. Developmental changes have certain predictable characteristics: They proceed from simple to complex, from general to specific, from head to toe (cephalocaudal), and from the trunk to the extremities (proximodistal). For example, a child's progressions from rolling over to crawling to walking are developmental changes.

Factors Influencing Growth and Development

Three major categories of factors influence human growth and development: (1) genetic or natural forces within the person, (2) the environment in which the person lives, and (3) the interaction that takes place between these two factors (Table 21-1). Nurses apply knowledge of these factors when selecting approaches to promote typical growth and developmental progression. It is important, for example, that as part of planning for a patient's pregnancy, nurses consider the patient's genetic endowment, age, socioeconomic status, culture (Box 21-1), available support system, and preconception state of health.

BOX 21-1 CULTURAL ASPECTS OF CARE

Canadian Indigenous People

Nurses need to assess the cultural background of each patient and be prepared to change their practice so that it is congruent with the patient's beliefs and values concerning growth and development. For example, within many Indigenous cultures, the concept of a circle or cycle is a fundamental theme and can be applied to human development and health issues (Douglas, 2013; Greenwood, de Leeuw, Lindsay, et al., 2015). The human life cycle is symbolized by the Medicine Wheel, which has four sections, often depicted as a circle with four equal-sized sections. The four sections are linked to the stages of life—birth, youth, adulthood, and death, or the four aspects of human life—spiritual, emotional, intellectual, and physical, or even the four seasons. Its basic symbolism represents a holistic relationship between health, the community, and natural world, including plants, animals, and human lives over time (Douglas, 2013). All aspects of human development are viewed as being in harmony with the cycle of life in nature. As in nature, each part of the cycle needs to be balanced with the other parts. Roles and expectations related to developmental age reflect traditional values of respect, honour, balance, and harmony.

TRADITIONS OF DEVELOPMENTAL THEORIES

A *theory* is an organized, often observable, logical set of statements about a subject. Human developmental theories are models intended to account for how and why people develop as they do (Green & Piel, 2016). All of the theories of development discussed in this chapter make different contributions to our understanding of the developmental process.

To help you understand the various developmental theories, this chapter has been grouped into five traditions of (or ways of thinking about) theory development: organicism, psychoanalytic and psychosocial, mechanistic, contextualism, and dialecticism (see Chapters 20 and 28 for further information about learning and spiritual development, respectively).

Each tradition of developmental theory emphasizes different underlying developmental mechanisms. **Mechanisms of development** are the explanatory components of each theory, or the means by which the developmental tasks are achieved. They are the processes or factors that underlie the developmental process within each theory, and they enable developmental progression. These underlying mechanisms are proposed to be universal and to function across the lifespan (not just in childhood) and cultures. Although developmental theories are often presented within a framework of stage-like progressions, what the stages actually represent are the outcomes produced by these mechanisms at each specific age.

ORGANICISM

Organicism refers to a theoretical focus on the organism itself. According to theories in this tradition, development is a result of biologically driven behaviour and the person's adaptation to the environment. Biophysical and cognitive–moral theories of development are included in this tradition.

Biophysical Developmental Theories

Biophysical developmental theories describe and explain how the physical body grows and changes. The changes that occur as a person grows from fetus, to neonate, to child, and finally to adult can be quantified and compared against established norms; however, regional and cultural differences may exist, as may differences related to the availability of resources in the environment for adequate growth.

How does the physical body age? What are the triggers that change the body's physical characteristics from childhood through

TABLE 21-1 Major Factors That Influence Growth and Development

Categories	Implications
Genetic or Natural Factors	
Heredity	Genetic endowment determines sex, skin, hair and eye colour, physical growth, stature, and, to some extent, psychological uniqueness.
Temperament	Temperament is the characteristic psychological disposition with which the child is born, typically ranging from difficult to flexible. It influences interactions between an individual and the environment.
Environmental Factors	
Family	The purpose of family is to protect, teach, and nurture its members. The functions of family include means for survival, security, promotion of healthy emotional and social development, assistance with maintenance of relationships, instruction about society and world, and assistance in learning roles and behaviours. Family influences values, beliefs, customs, and specific patterns of interaction and communication.
Peer group	The peer group provides a new and different learning environment from the family, with different patterns and structures of interaction and communication, necessitating a different style of behaviour. The functions of the peer group include allowing the individual to learn about success and failure; to validate and challenge thoughts, feelings, and concepts; to receive acceptance, support, and rejection as a unique person apart from family; and to achieve group purposes by meeting demands, pressures, and expectations.
Health environment	The level of health affects an individual's responsiveness to the environment and responsiveness of others to the individual. It determines availability and accessibility of resources to support health.
Nutrition	Growth is regulated by dietary factors. Adequacy of nutrients influences whether and how physiological needs, as well as subsequent growth and development needs, are met. The availability of quality nutrients also affects growth.
Rest, sleep, and exercise	Balance between rest, sleep, and exercise is essential for rejuvenating the body, while disturbances diminish growth, and equilibrium reinforces physiological and psychological health.
Living environment	Factors affecting growth and development include season, climate, community life, socioeconomic status, and quality of the physical environment (air, water, land). An embryo may be exposed to teratogenic substances (e.g., alcohol, chemicals, or radiation) that cause abnormal development.
Political and policy environment	Municipal, provincial, and federal policies directly affect the health and well-being of individuals, families, and communities.
Interacting Factors	
Life experiences	Individuals develop by applying what has been learned through experience to their current situation. Experiences emerge from both biological and environmental sources. The individual deduces meaning from these experiences and bases further actions on them. The epigenome—genetic expression—changes in response to experience.
Prenatal health	Biological and maturational factors (genetics; maternal age; medical problems) and environmental factors (maternal health; stress, nutrition; use of tobacco, drugs, and alcohol; use of prenatal services) together affect fetal growth and development.
State of health	Health is a product of both intrinsic (biology) and extrinsic (quality of environment, availability of resources for health) factors. Changes to health status such as illness or injury may cause inability to cope with and respond to underlying processes and demands of development.

adolescence to adulthood? Biological influences on development include many factors, such as genetics and exposure to teratogens (e.g., maternal diseases, drugs, X-rays, or other hazardous substances that interfere with the normal development of the fetus). All biophysical developmental theories give some credence to the roles of nature (genetics) and nurture (caregiving environment and resources). However, the theories differ on how much influence individual and environmental forces have on development.

Gesell's Theory of Maturational Development. Arnold Gesell (1880–1961) was a psychologist who obtained his medical degree to help him explain the physiological processes he observed in the behaviour of children. Through extensive observations in the 1940s, he developed behavioural norms that serve as a primary source of information for childhood development today.

Fundamental to Gesell's theory of development is the notion that the pattern of growth and development is directed by the activity of genes, although at that time, the genetic mechanism was unknown to him. He believed that environmental factors can support, change, and modify the pattern but do not generate the progressions of development (Gesell, 1948). Gesell proposed that the pattern of maturation follows a fixed developmental sequence in all humans and that critical periods exist in which the presence or absence of particular experiences makes a biological system functional or nonfunctional (Weizmann & Harris, 2012). Gesell based some of his observations on the visual system (Gesell, Ilg, & Bullis, 1949). He noted that visual defects not identified until the start of school may be associated with underdeveloped brain pathways that will impair long-term vision. New research on child neglect shows a similar pattern—if a child is neglected physically and emotionally early in life, this affects the child's developing brain, with long-term reductions in brain volume compared to that in non-neglected peers (National Scientific Council on the Developing Child, 2012).

Sequential development is seen in fetuses; that is, the various organ systems develop in a specific order (Crandell, Crandell, & Vander Zanden, 2012). After birth, children grow according to their genetic blueprint and gain skills in an orderly manner, but at each individual's own pace. For example, most children learn first how to hold a cup with digital grasp at about 15 months of age and later how to lift, drink from, and replace the cup at 21 months of age. Gesell clarified that not every child develops those skills at exactly the same ages. He pointed out that the environment does play a part in the development of the child but that it does not have any part in the sequence of development. Gesell believed that children could not be pushed to develop faster than their own unique timetables permitted. He also proposed that the biological body determines behavioural development. Researchers continue to use Gesell's theories today, probing for gene–environment interactions in human development (Cicchetti & Rogosch, 2012).

Mechanisms of Maturational Development. Maturation is the biological internal regulatory mechanism that governs the emergence of all new skills and abilities that appear with advancing age (Crandell et al., 2012). Maturation involves an individual's biological ability, physiological condition, and desire to learn more mature behaviour. To mature, the individual may have to relinquish previous behaviour and learning, integrate new patterns into existing behaviour, or both. Maturation influences the sequence and timing of the changes associated with growth and development. For example, the child relinquishes crawling for walking because walking permits greater investigation of the environment and more learning. However, the child cannot walk until the biological ability and structures to perform the action (i.e., increased muscle cells and tone) have developed.

Differentiation is the process by which cells and structures become modified and refine their characteristics. Development of activities and functions progresses from simple to complex. Embryonic cells begin as vague and undifferentiated and develop into complex, highly diversified cells, tissues, and organs.

Nursing Implications of Maturational Development. As a nurse, you need to consider maturational development in your care planning when you help mothers sequence child play activities appropriate for learning of sitting, rolling, creeping, crawling, and walking. You must consider sequential development of fetuses and critical periods when you counsel expectant mothers about environmental teratogens during the first trimester of pregnancy. One way to support development during critical periods is to develop or implement early intervention programs for parents.

Chess and Thomas's Theory of Temperament Development. Temperament is a physical and emotional response style that affects a child's interactions with others (Hockenberry & Wilson, 2015). It is the way a person adjusts to life experiences, and it is thought to originate within the person's genetic makeup. A child's temperament influences how others respond to the child and to his or her needs. Knowledge of temperament helps parents to have a clearer perspective of their child and enables health care providers to guide them appropriately (Hockenberry & Wilson, 2015).

Psychiatrists Stella Chess (1914–2007) and Alexander Thomas (1915–2003) conducted a landmark 20-year longitudinal study of development that included children from a range of populations, including children of middle-income parents and intellectually disabled children of lower-income parents. The breadth of the data allowed them to look at the behaviour of people from childhood to early adulthood as they interacted with their environment. Their work defined the concept of temperament (Chess & Thomas, 1995), and they proposed that temperament is biologically derived.

Chess and Thomas (1995) described three common categories of temperament, although because of individual variation, approximately 30% of children cannot be classified in any of these groups:

- The *easy child* is easygoing and even-tempered, regular and predictable in his or her habits, and open-minded, flexible and adaptable to change. Mood expressions are mild to moderately intense and typically positive.
- The *difficult child* is highly active, irritable, and irregular in habits. Negativity in interactions and withdrawal from other people is typical, and the child requires a highly structured environment. He or she adapts slowly to new routines, new people, or new situations. Mood expressions are usually intense and primarily negative.
- The *slow-to-warm-up child* typically reacts negatively and with mild intensity to new stimuli. He or she adapts slowly with repeated contact unless pressured and responds with mild but passive resistance to novelty or changes in routine.

Mechanisms of Temperament Development. According to temperament theory, biologically derived temperament characteristics drive children's interaction with the environment. Chess and Thomas (1995) proposed that it is through "goodness of fit" between the individual and the immediate environment that human development is modulated. This places significant responsibility for child development outcomes within the family. For instance, the difficult child who has trouble making the transition from one activity or environment to a new one functions best in a family that maintains routines and has a slow, easy attitude toward the introduction of change. The same child in a family that has few routines has much more difficulty moving from one activity (such as play) to the next activity (such as sleep). The first scenario is an example of "goodness of fit" between the temperament of the child and the family environment. However, recent research has suggested that temperament may be a function of fetal exposures to, for example, excessive maternal stress hormones during pregnancy or birth complications (Laplante, Brunet, & King, 2016; O'Connor, Bergman, Sarkar, et al., 2013).

Nursing Implications of Temperament Development. Nurses can help families identify the unique characteristics of their infants and children. For instance, a parenting program called "Keys to Caregiving" (Nursing Child Assessment Satellite Training [NCAST], 1999; see Feeley, Zelkowitz, Westreich, et al., 2011 for example of use) that consists of professional self-educational videos and parent pamphlets, assists nurses in helping new parents identify their infants' usual behaviour and communication styles. In Keys to Caregiving, new parents are taught about infant cues and behaviours that signify needs (e.g., hunger, desire for playful attention), infant states and how to modulate infant states (e.g., helping soothe a fussy baby), and optimal parenting practices that promote sensitive, nurturant relationships between caregivers and infants. This information helps families adapt their habits and routines to match their children's temperaments. Nurses can also consider temperament styles when working with adults and families in teaching or support situations.

Cognitive Developmental Theories

Cognitive developmental theories focus on reasoning and thinking processes, including the changes in how people perform intellectual operations. These operations are related to the ways people learn to understand the world in which they live. Mental processes, including perceiving, reasoning, remembering, and believing, affect certain types of emotional behaviour. For example, a typical child will have a different emotional reaction to the death of a grandparent than to the death of an older sibling or a parent.

Unlike biophysical developmental theories, cognitive developmental theories emphasize that although the developmental process originates with the person, it is greatly influenced by interactions between the person and the environment. Therefore, theories of cognitive development emphasize the active role that the individual plays in the developmental process. Cognitive theories are considered to be within the organicism tradition because development is still viewed as originating within the organism.

Piaget's Theory of Cognitive Development. Jean Piaget (1896–1980), a Swiss biologist and philosopher, studied how people come to know their world. Piaget's theory of cognitive development addresses the development of children's intellectual organization and how they think, reason, perceive, and make meaning of the physical world. His theory includes four periods, each of which subsumes a number of stages (Table 21-2). He recognized that people move through these specific periods at different rates but in the same sequence or order (Piaget, 2000). Piaget also theorized that this would be true in all cultures. He acknowledged that biological maturation plays a role in this developmental theory but believed that rates of development depend on the intellectual stimulation and challenge in the environment of the person. Piaget found that children acquire knowledge through acting on the environment. In other words, the individual plays an active role in his or her development (Berk 2013; Green & Piel, 2016).

Mechanisms of Cognitive Development. Although it is helpful to be aware of the stages, the importance of Piaget's theory is that development is considered a spontaneous process in which individuals play an active role in their own development. Environmental challenges are internalized through the mechanisms of assimilation and accommodation. Assimilation is the process of making sense of new information in comparison with what is already known. Accommodation is the process of adapting ways of thinking to a new experience or new information. Together, these processes reflect

TABLE 21-2 Piaget's Theory of Cognitive Development

Stage	Description	Nursing Implications
Period 1: Sensorimotor (birth to 2 years of age)	The infant develops the schema or action pattern for dealing with the environment (Berk, 2013; Piaget, 2000). These schemas may include mouthing, looking, vocalizing, grasping, or hitting (Figure 21-1). Schemas become self-initiated activities; for example, the infant who learns that mouthing or sucking achieves a pleasing result generalizes the action to suck fingers, blanket, or clothing. Successful achievement leads to greater exploration. In the second year, children are able to form primitive mental images as they acquire object permanence. Before this, they do not realize that objects out of sight exist. When a 6-month-old is shown a toy before it is hidden, he or she will not search for it. At 18 months, the child can understand that even if it cannot be seen, it still exists and will search for it.	Educate parents about the need to promote infants' exploration of the environment. Such education supports development of action patterns that help the children achieve motor and cognitive skills. Observe parents during interactions with their infants. Reinforce parents' sensitivity and responsiveness to infant behaviours.
Period 2: Preoperational (2 to 7 years of age)	Children learn to think with the use of symbols and mental images. Still egocentric, the child sees objects and people from only one point of view: the child's own. Play is the initial method of nonlanguage use of symbols. This is a time of parallel play. Parallel play can be observed as children engage in activities side by side without a common goal. Imitation and make-believe play are ways to represent experience (Berk, 2013; Piaget, 2000). Later, language develops and broadens possibilities for thinking about the past or the future. Children can now communicate about events with others. As the language fits into a logical form, it mirrors the thinking process at the time.	Recognize the use of play as the way the child understands the events taking place. Parents can be assisted in the use of play materials such as toy thermometers and stethoscopes to encourage children to communicate feelings about health care procedures. Parents can also be encouraged to read and use rich language with their children to promote literacy and language development.
Period 3: Concrete operations (7 to 11 years of age)	Children achieve the ability to perform mental operations. For example, the child can think about an action that before was performed physically. At the earlier stage, the child could count to 10, but at this stage, he or she can count and understand what each number represents. Children can describe a process without actually performing it. At this stage, they are able to coordinate two perspectives. In other words, they can appreciate the difference between their perspective and that of a friend. Reversibility is the primary characteristic of concrete operational thought. Children can mentally reverse the direction of their thoughts. Children can mentally classify objects according to their quantitative dimensions, known as seriation. Another major accomplishment of this stage is conservation, or the ability to see objects or quantities as remaining the same despite a change in their physical appearance (Berk, 2013; Piaget, 2000). Children can begin to cooperate and share with new information about the acts they perform.	Encourage parents to guide the child to perform helpful activities within the home, such as doing chores in exchange for privileges (television or computer time, play with friends). Parents can encourage children to take another person's perspective or to plan ahead in school work deadlines.
Period 4: Formal operations (11 years to adulthood)	The individual's thinking moves to abstract and theoretical subjects. Thinking can venture into such subjects as achieving world peace, finding justice, and seeking meaning in life. Adolescents can organize their thoughts in their minds. They have the capacity to reason with regard to possibilities. New cognitive powers allow the adolescent to achieve more far-reaching problem solving. This thinking matures, and the depth of understanding increases with experience.	Include the adolescent in decision making about his or her own health care that is based on his or her ability to think abstractly.

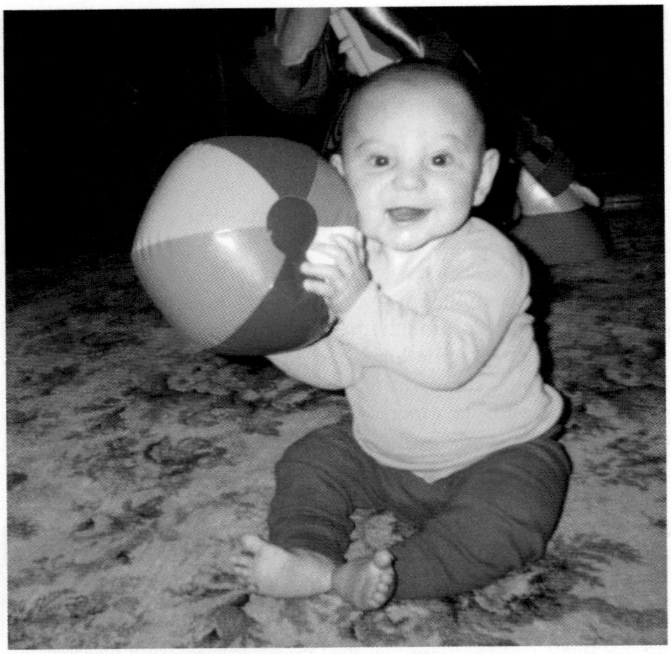

FIGURE 21-1 Piaget's theory of cognitive development, sensorimotor stage. Successfully achieving action patterns, such as grasping, leads to learning and more exploration.

adaptation to new information or experience (Feldman, 2017). In a health care situation, a person who has a headache can evaluate it as an everyday or usual experience. In this process, the person is assimilating it to what he or she knows already as the experience of his or her body; that is, the person occasionally has headaches. When headaches become extreme or constant, then the person needs to understand the headache pain differently in the experience of his or her body. For instance, the person may learn to see himself or herself as a person who has migraines or as a person with a brain tumour who requires surgery.

The mechanisms of cognitive development apply across the lifespan and to all patient situations. Thus, they also apply to the moral theories and theories of adult development that are described in the following sections.

Nursing Implications of Cognitive Development. Most patients need to know about new ways of adjusting or behaving with regard to their health. Assimilation and accommodation represent adaptation of the patient to new health challenges. Nurses need to support this process by providing information and support as patients come to terms with new health situations. Nurses must also offer positive feedback when patients successfully adapt to their challenges.

Moral Developmental Theories

Moral developmental theories are a subset of cognitive theory and describe the development of moral reasoning. *Moral reasoning* is how people think about the rules of ethical or moral conduct, but it does not predict what a person would actually do in a given situation. *Moral development* is the ability of an individual to distinguish right from wrong and to develop ethical values on which to base his or her actions (Berk, 2013). Although various theorists have addressed moral development, Piaget and Kohlberg proposed the most comprehensive theories of moral development. These theories are within the organicism tradition because they are grounded in cognitive development theory and development is seen as originating from within the individual. In the context of nursing interventions, the mechanisms of cognitive development also apply to the moral development theories because they both emerged from the original work of Piaget.

Piaget's Theory of Moral Development. Piaget believed that moral development goes through a series of successive stages, just as cognition and learning do. Piaget's theory of moral development presents three stages of morality: the premoral stage, the conventional stage, and the autonomous stage (Feldman, 2017; Green & Piel, 2016). In the premoral stage, the child feels no obligation to follow rules. In the conventional stage, children follow the rules set up by people in authority, such as their parents, teachers, clergy, or police. When a person reaches the stage of autonomous morality, moral judgements are based on mutual respect for the rules. A person also considers the consequences of a moral decision. In making moral judgements that involve others, the person at this stage starts to consider information related to the subjective intent (Patanella, 2011).

Piaget believed that children initially follow the rules without understanding them. Children see these rules as fixed and handed down by adults or by a higher authority (e.g., God) and therefore think they cannot change them. Young children base their moral decisions on the extent of the consequences to the action, not necessarily on the action itself. For example, a young child may refrain from eating a cookie before supper, not because the mother said not to but because the child is afraid of the punishment that would result if he or she did. Around 10 or 11 years of age, children's cognitive ability matures and the rules they follow are understood within the context of community life. Children understand that the rules can be modified "by legal channels" if everyone agrees to change the rules (Patanella, 2011). Moral maturity is the internalization of the principles—that is, the desire to weigh all of the relationships and circumstances before making a decision.

Kohlberg's Theory of Moral Development. Lawrence Kohlberg (1927–1987) expanded on Piaget's moral developmental theory. From a series of moral dilemmas presented to boys aged 10, 13, and 16 years, he identified six stages of moral development occurring at three levels (Kohlberg, 1981; Table 21-3). Kohlberg found a link between moral development and Piaget's cognitive development theory. He theorized that a child's moral development does not advance if the child's cognitive development does not also mature. In this way, Kohlberg's theory of moral development follows Piaget's cognitive developmental theory. According to Kohlberg, levels and stages do not occur at specific ages, and people attain different levels of moral development.

Kohlberg's Critics. Although Kohlberg is recognized as a leader in moral developmental theory, critics have questioned the applicability of his study beyond the study population of male adolescents of the Western philosophical tradition. Research attempting to support Kohlberg's (1981) theory with people raised in the Eastern philosophies found that those study participants never proceeded beyond stages 3 or 4 of Kohlberg's model. Does that mean that they have not reached as high a level of moral development as most of the adults raised in the Western traditions? Or is it that Kohlberg's research design did not allow a way to measure moral development in people raised within a different culture?

Kohlberg's (1981) study has also been criticized for age and gender biases. Carol Gilligan was one important critic. As Kohlberg's contemporary, she concentrated on how Kohlberg's findings may have been biased by a narrow focus on only boys. According to Gilligan (1993), all developmental theories are subject to gender bias, and only since the 1990s have scholars researched and recognized the differences between men and women in the way they think and how they have been raised to make decisions.

Gilligan's Theory. Carol Gilligan (1936–) proposed that Kohlberg's (1981) theory is biased in favour of men. She believed

TABLE 21-3 Kohlberg's Moral Development Theory

Level and Stage	Description	Nursing Implications
Level I: Preconventional level	The person reflects on moral reasoning based on personal gain. The person's moral reason for acting, the "why," relates to the consequences that the person believes will occur. These consequences can occur in the form of punishment or reward. Therefore, children may view illness as a punishment for fighting with their siblings or disobeying their parents.	Nurses should be aware of this thinking and reinforce teaching that the child cannot become ill because of wrongdoing.
Stage 1: Punishment and obedience orientation	Response to a moral dilemma is in terms of absolute obedience to authority and rules. Avoidance of punishment or the unquestioning deference to authority is characteristic behaviour. The child will do something because an authority figure tells him or her to do it.	
Stage 2: Instrumental relativist orientation	The person recognizes that more than one view may be correct. The decision to do something morally correct is based on satisfying one's own needs and occasionally the needs of others.	
Level II: Conventional level	The person sees moral reasoning based on his or her own personal internalization of societal and others' expectations. A person wants to fulfill the expectations of the family, group, or nation; develop loyalty to the dominant order; and actively maintain, support, and justify the order. Moral decision making at this level moves from "What's in it for me?" to "How will it affect my relationships with others?"	Nurses may observe this level of moral development when family members make end-of-life decisions for their loved ones. Grief support will involve an understanding of the level of moral decision making of each family member (see Chapter 25).
Stage 3: Good boy–nice girl orientation	The individual wants to please others and win approval by "being nice," which means having good motives, showing concern for others, and keeping mutual relationships through trust, loyalty, respect, and gratitude.	
Stage 4: Society-maintaining orientation	Focus expands from relationships with others to societal concerns. Correct behaviour is doing one's duty, showing respect for authority, and maintaining the social order. Adolescents in this stage may choose not to attend a party at which drugs will be used, not because they are afraid of getting caught but because they know that using drugs is not healthy.	
Level III: Postconventional level	The person finds a balance between basic human rights and obligations and societal rules and regulations. Individuals reject moral decisions based on authority or conformity to groups in favour of defining their own moral values and principles. Individuals at this stage start to envision an ideal society.	Focus not only on your individual practice but also on social determinants that affect the well-being of a community, such as poverty and homelessness.
Stage 5: Social contract orientation	An individual follows the laws but recognizes the possibility of changing the law to improve society. The individual also recognizes that different social groups may have different values but believe in basic rights, such as liberty and life.	
Stage 6: Universal ethical principle orientation	"Right" is defined by the decision of conscience in accord with self-chosen ethical principles. These principles, such as the Golden Rule, are abstract and appeal to logical comprehensiveness, universality, and consistency (Kohlberg, 1981). Whereas stage 5 emphasizes the basic rights and the democratic process, stage 6 defines the principles by which agreements will be most just.	

that men and women develop in parallel ways, with one not being superior to the other. Gilligan's argument is basically that the developmental difference between women and men is in relationships and issues of dependency (Gilligan, 1993). Separation and individuation are critically tied to male development. **Separation** refers to the boy's recognition of biological distinctness and is based on his emergence from a dependent relationship with his mother. This separation from the mother is essential for the boy in his development of masculinity. Girls do not need to separate from their mothers to achieve feminine identity; it is through this attachment to their mother that their identity is formed. In most developmental theories, the achievement of increasing separation is a developmental norm. When women are measured against this norm as it relates to their need to maintain relationships, they are seen as failures or as less evolved developmentally. **Individuation** is based on the child's awareness of differences in will, viewpoint, and needs. This process enables the individual to gradually assume a more independent role and identity.

Male moral development may focus on logic, justice, and social organization, whereas female moral development focuses on interpersonal relationships. Of interest is that in studies whose research design is based on Gilligan's critique, findings have been inconclusive. As a result, Gilligan's position remains controversial (Slote, 2016).

PSYCHOANALYTIC AND PSYCHOSOCIAL TRADITION

Theories in the **psychoanalytic and psychosocial tradition** describe the development of personality, thinking, behaviour, and emotions. This development is thought to occur with varying degrees of influence from internal biological forces and external societal and cultural forces.

Sigmund Freud

The first scholar to provide a formal, structured theory of personality development was Sigmund Freud (1856–1939). His goal was to promote successful participation in society through the development of balance between pleasure-seeking drives and societal pressures. In **Freud's psychoanalytic model of personality development**, he asserted that mature adults should have a strong sense of conscience that allows for the experience of pleasure within the boundaries of society. He believed that two internal biological forces essentially drive psychological change in the child: sexual (**libido**) and aggressive energies. The motivation for behaviour is to achieve pleasure and avoid pain created by these forces. These forces come into conflict with the reality of the world as maturational changes occur.

Freud's theory accounts for five psychosexual developmental stages, each associated with different pleasurable zones that serve as the foci for gratification and bodily pleasure (Berk, 2013; Feldman, 2017; Kliegman, Stanton, Geme, et al., 2016; Table 21-4). Freud's theory has been soundly criticized for gender and cultural biases and for an extreme focus on sexuality in development. Freud's critics contend that people are more influenced by their life experiences than by their sexual energies. Despite these criticisms, Freud provided a basis for observation of emotion, behaviour, and sexuality that has been very influential in the development of many other psychoanalytic theories. Indeed, many agree that development is an ongoing process of resolving conflict between issues of biological maturation and societal expectations.

Mechanisms of Freud's Theory. Components of personality emerge through Freud's developmental stages. The mechanisms of Freud's personality development theory are the id, the ego, and the superego. Freud believed that the functions of these mechanisms regulate behaviour. The **id**—basic instinctual impulses and drives to achieve pleasure—is the most primitive part of the personality and originates in the infant. The **ego** represents the reality mechanism mediating conflicts between the environment and the forces of the id. The ego helps us judge reality accurately, regulate impulses, and make good decisions. The third mechanism, the **superego**, performs regulating, restraining, and prohibiting actions. Often referred to as the *conscience*, the superego is influenced by the standards of outside social forces (parents, teachers).

Nursing Implications of Freud's Theory. The functions of the id, ego, and superego form the historical basis of many, if not all, subsequent theories of personality and social emotional development. It is important to remember that according to Freudian theory, mature human personality is the product of conflict between instinctual drives to achieve pleasure and the restraints of adaptive human society. When activities associated with basic pleasure (e.g., eating, sexual activity, and elimination) are altered by illness or disability, knowledgeable and empathetic nursing care is required.

Erikson's Theory of Eight Stages of Life

Erik Erikson (1902–1994) expanded Freud's psychoanalytic stages into a psychosocial model that covered the whole lifespan, not just childhood and adolescence (Erikson, 1993, 1997; Kliegman et al., 2016). He broadened the factors responsible for influencing development to include socialization.

According to **Erikson's theory of eight stages of life**, each person goes through eight stages of development (Table 21-5). In each stage, the person needs to accomplish a particular task before moving on to

TABLE 21-4 Freud's Five Stages of Psychosexual Development

Stage	Description	Nursing Implications
Stage 1: Oral (birth to age 12–18 months)	Initially, sucking and oral satisfaction is not only necessary for living but also extremely pleasurable in its own right. Late in this stage, the infant begins to realize that the mother or parent is something separate from self. Disruption in the physical or emotional availability of the parent (e.g., inadequate bonding or chronic illness) could have an impact on the infant's development.	For an infant, feeding and sucking produces pleasure and comfort and promotes self-regulation. Teach parents that feedings should be offered whenever the infant requires them. As well, encourage parents to help their infant self-soothe by making the infant's hands available for sucking.
Stage 2: Anal (ages 12–18 months to 3 years)	The focus of pleasure changes to the anal zone. Children become increasingly aware of the pleasurable sensations of this body region with interest in the products of their effort. Through the toilet-training process, the child is asked to delay gratification in order to meet parental and societal expectations.	Teach parents that toilet training should be as positive an experience as possible. Praise helps the child achieve a sense of control. Development is not always a smooth, uninterrupted process of moving forward to more advanced stages. Teach parents to understand that successes are often accompanied by failures in the normal progression of development.
Stage 3: Phallic or Oedipal (ages 3–6 years)	The genital organs become the focus of pleasure. The boy becomes interested in the penis; the girl becomes aware of the absence of the penis, known as *penis envy*. This is the time of exploration and imagination as the child fantasizes about the parent of the opposite sex as his or her first love interest, known as the *Oedipal complex* (in boys) or *Electra complex* (in girls). By the end of this stage, the child attempts to reduce this conflict by identifying with the parent of the same sex in a way to win recognition and acceptance.	Assure parents that a child's identifying with the parent of the same sex is a normal developmental phase.
Stage 4: Latency (ages 6–12 years)	Sexual urges from the earlier Oedipal stage are repressed and channelled into productive activities that are socially acceptable. Within the educational and social worlds of the child, much is to be learned and accomplished. The child places energy and effort into these worlds.	Encourage the child to pursue physical and intellectual challenges that will provide opportunities to explore and develop abilities and competencies.
Stage 5: Genital (puberty through adulthood)	This is a time of turbulence when earlier sexual urges reawaken and are directed toward an individual outside the family circle. Unresolved prior conflicts surface during adolescence. Once conflicts are resolved, the individual is then capable of having a mature adult sexual relationship.	Educate parents that the child needs to be encouraged to be independent and make his or her own decisions, within safe limits. Help parents to empathize and identify with their growing adolescent. As parent–child conflicts associated with increasing adolescent independence arise, empathy will help the parent to understand the adolescent's point of view.

TABLE 21-5 Erikson's Theory of Eight Stages of Life

Stage	Description	Nursing Implications
1. Trust versus mistrust (infancy: birth to age 1 year)	The infant learns to trust others. Trust is achieved when the infant will let the caregiver out of sight without undue distress. Key to this stage is consistent caregiving. The question answered at this stage is "Can I trust the world?"	The parent's struggle with building competence can be assisted by the nurse's use of anticipatory guidance and other educative interventions. The parent may need guidance to understand the importance of a safe, nurturing environment when meeting the child's needs.
2. Autonomy versus sense of shame and doubt (toddler years: ages 1–3 years)	The toddler learns to be independent and develops self-confidence. Not learning independence creates feelings of shame and self-doubt. Independence is accomplished through self-care activities, including walking, feeding, and toileting. Toddlers also develop autonomy by making choices. The question answered at this stage is "Can I control my own behaviour?"	Nurses can use empathetic guidance to offer support for and understanding of the challenges of this stage. Parents can be taught to use nonviolent disciplinary methods with their children that promote safety, yet discipline. Teach parents to offer children a limited number of choices, so as not to overwhelm, but to promote children's developing sense of self-efficacy and competence.
3. Initiative versus guilt (preschool years: ages 3–6 years)	The child learns to initiate his or her activities. Accomplishing this task teaches the child to seek challenges in later life. Children use fantasy and imagination to explore their environment. Conflicts often arise between the child's desire to explore and the limits placed on his or her behaviour. These conflicts may lead to feelings of frustration and guilt. The question answered during this stage is "Can I become independent of my parents and explore my limits?"	Teaching impulse control and cooperative behaviours to the child is necessary at this stage. Children can be shown appreciation for independent behaviours that demonstrate prosocial skills, such as sharing, kindness to others, and helping with household chores.
4. Industry versus inferiority (middle childhood: ages 6–11 years)	The child develops a sense of competence in physical, cognitive, and social areas. Not learning new skills may lead to a sense of inadequacy and inferiority. Successfully achieving this task leads to positive attitudes toward work in adulthood (Erikson, 1993). The question answered at this stage is "Can I master the skills necessary to survive and adapt?"	Encourage parents to offer the child many opportunities to pursue new interests and challenges in extracurricular activities, such as sports, music, and art.
5. Identity versus role confusion (adolescence: ages 12–18 years)	The task of adolescence is to try out several roles and form a unique identity. Dramatic physiological changes associated with sexual maturation also mark this stage. Acquiring a sense of identity is essential for making later adult decisions such as vocation or marriage partner. New social demands, opportunities, and conflicts arise in relation to the emergent identity and separation from family. The question answered at this stage is "Who am I, and what are my beliefs, feelings, and attitudes?"	Provide education and anticipatory guidance for the parent about the changes in and challenges to the adolescent. Also assist hospitalized adolescents in dealing with their illness by giving them enough information to allow them to make decisions about their treatment plan.
6. Intimacy versus isolation (young adulthood: ages 18–35 years)	The primary task of young adulthood is to form close, personal relationships. This is the time to become fully active in the community. If young adults have not achieved a sense of personal identity, they may be unable to form meaningful attachments, and they experience feelings of isolation. The question answered during this stage is "Can I give of myself fully to another?"	Understand that during hospitalization, young adults may benefit from the support of their partners or significant others because this support helps fulfill their need for intimacy.
7. Generativity versus self-absorption and stagnation (middle adulthood: ages 35–65 years)	The task of middle adulthood is to help younger people. The ability to expand one's personal and social involvement is crucial for this stage of development. Middle-aged adults should be able to see beyond their needs and accomplishments and view the needs of society. Dissatisfaction with one's achievements often leads to self-absorption and stagnation. The question answered during this stage is "What can I offer succeeding generations?"	Assist adults in choosing creative ways to foster social development. Middle-aged people may find a sense of fulfillment from volunteering some time in a local school, hospital, community centre, or place of worship.
8. Integrity versus despair (old age: age 65 years and older)	Older persons reflect on their life and feel satisfaction or disappointment. By suffering physical and social losses, such as those through retirement or illness, the person may also suffer loss of status and function. The person may also have internal struggles, such as the search for meaning in life. Meeting these challenges creates the potential for growth and wisdom (Figure 21-2). The question answered during this stage is "Has my life been worthwhile?"	Nurses can contribute to the valuing of people at all ages and stages in their communities. For example, by promoting older persons' involvement in volunteer activities, such as youth mentoring, you display value for the skills and experience of older people, and such mentoring helps the younger generation feel important.

Based on Erikson, E. (1993). *Childhood and society*. New York: W. W. Norton; Erikson, E. (1997). *The lifecycle completed*. New York: W. W. Norton.

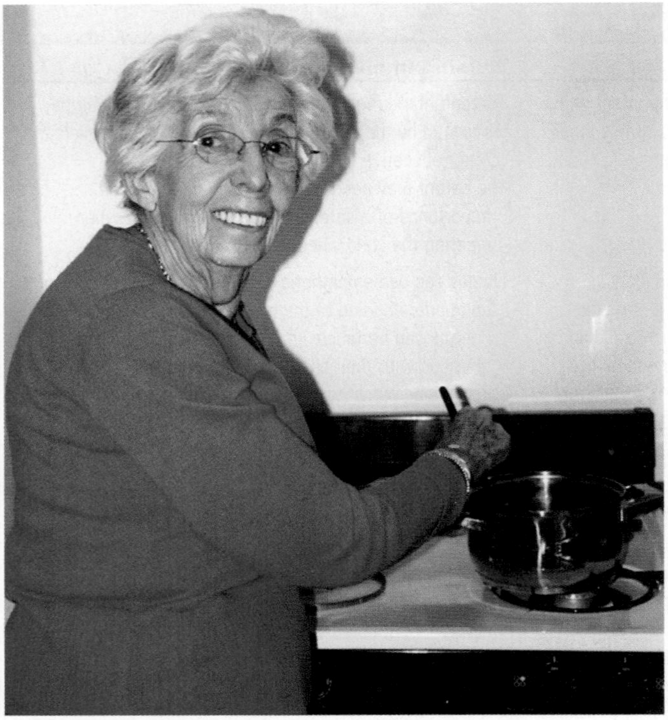

FIGURE 21-2 Maintaining independence is important to a person's self-esteem.

the next stage. Each task is framed with opposing conflicts that the person must balance. For example, an adolescent needs to develop a sense of personal identity despite many conflicting societal choices (stage 5, identity versus role confusion). Each stage builds upon the successful resolution of the previous developmental conflict. Readiness for the task is necessary for success. Once mastered, tasks are challenged and tested during new situations or at times of conflict (Hockenberry & Wilson, 2015). For example, the infant's trust is built through consistent, reliable caregiving, and the concept of trust is tested when an infant is hospitalized or after the birth of a new sibling.

Mechanisms of Erikson's Theory. *Maturation* and *ego* activity are the primary mechanisms of development in Erikson's theory of eight stages of life. The ego mediates the conflicts between the biological needs and societal norms, and maturation establishes the timeline of this mediation. The developmental result of these mechanisms is described as an epigenesis (successive gradual change). If the process is adaptive, then a person has successive positive outcomes.

Nursing Implications of Erikson's Theory. The theory of the eight stages of life implies that the quality of early developmental work is important. For instance, children who live in environments in which violence is common and trust has not been attained are at greater risk of experiencing poor intimate relationships. The mechanism of epigenesis implies that the original required trust elements cannot be retrieved; at best, such a person can learn only to live with the fear and anger associated with this mistrust. Nurses therefore need to practise within the health promotion model to build the familial, community, and societal supports necessary for supporting vulnerable children to achieve successful transitions at each stage (e.g., trust, autonomy, initiative).

John Bowlby

John Bowlby (1907–1990) was a child psychiatrist interested in children's mental health. According to Bowlby's attachment and separation theory, the conflict between attachment and separation needs to be resolved to produce healthy social and emotional developmental outcomes across the lifespan. Attachment refers to the tie or relationship between an individual and another person, such as a parent or caregiver. A basic premise of the theory is that the quality of attachment relationships stems from interactions between infants and caregivers. These interactions reflect the degree to which infants can rely on their caregivers to provide proximity and companionship, a safe haven in the presence of threat or anxiety, and a secure base from which to explore. Insecure attachment results in developmental challenges across the lifespan including difficulty in new relationships (including work, friendship, and intimate relationships) (Sroufe, 2005).

Mechanisms of Bowlby's Theory. Early in life, two complementary behavioural systems, attachment and caregiving, combine into a self-regulating system that supports people in their healthy attachments to and separations from others. The child's experiences within this self-regulating system cause the child to develop a cognitive working model (or "map") of self, other, and the relationship between them. The ability to regulate emotion and behaviour (Box 21-2) is influenced by this working model at each developmental stage throughout life.

Extensions to Bowlby's Theory of Attachment and Separation

Mary Ainsworth (1913–1999) was an American-Canadian psychologist who is known for operationalizing the measurement of attachment as conceptualized by Bowlby. Patricia Crittenden (1945–) was Ainsworth's student and was heavily influenced by the work of both Bowlby and Ainsworth (1979) in developing her dynamic maturational model of attachment (Crittenden, 2008; Crittenden & Claussen, 2003). In this model, behavioural and psychiatric developmental disorders are considered within the context of family attachment relationships. Early attachment patterns link to later health and development (Puig, Englund, Simpson, et al., 2013; Veríssimo, Santos, Fernandes, et al., 2014). Unlike the work of other attachment theorists, the model considers the impact of intimate relationships at different life stages including preschool, school-age, adolescence, and adulthood, in addition to infancy.

Mechanisms of the Dynamic Maturational Model of Attachment. The interaction between brain development and experiences with caregivers is central in the development of self-protective strategies that individuals use over their lifespan (Box 21-3). Attachment strategies are employed to promote safety and security in relationships (Crittenden & Claussen, 2003; Crittenden & Landini, 2011). Patterns of attachment are dominated by "cognitive" and "affective" strategies and may be categorized as types A and C, respectively. Ainworth described infants' attachment patterns (Ainsworth, 1979), and as suggested above, Crittenden extended the observations to include preschool, school-age, adolescent, and adult patterns. People with type A patterns tend to minimize awareness of negative feelings, compulsively perform what they expect will be reinforced, and avoid doing what will be punished (Crittenden & DiLalla, 1988). People with type C patterns rely on feelings as guides to behaviour because they lack confidence in what will happen next. When familial relationships fail to protect the child (or adult parent), type A and type C coping strategies become more extreme. For example, a child reared by an unresponsive caregiver may learn that "acting out" elicits a needed response from the caregiver. As the child grows and becomes an adult, he or she may seek attention with extreme emotional outbursts, acting coercively or aggressively in other adult relationships (type C) (Crittenden & Kulbotten, 2007). Another pattern, type B, is characterized by a tendency to use a balance of type A and type C strategies (Green & Piel, 2016).

BOX 21-2 CASE STUDY

Jonathan is 5 years old. His mother has brought him to the pediatrician at the advice of his kindergarten teacher. You are the clinic nurse, charged with taking Jonathan's history. His mother removes Jonathan's winter coat and collects his mittens. She takes time to locate crayons and paper for Jonathan during the office visit. However, Jonathan does not settle for long. As you begin your assessment, you observe Jonny, as she calls him, spend a minute with the crayons before breaking one and then moving on to examine the stethoscope and then the next item in the office that intrigues him more. Jonny rips the paper, and his mother makes no move to correct him. He smiles at you and seems content to move chaotically about in the office.

As you proceed through your assessment, you learn that Jonny accomplished typical milestones (walking, talking, toilet training) on time and had a few ear infections but no other physical health problems. His weight and height are normal. He gets along well with the other kids, except for the occasional skirmish over a toy. His mother notes that he does not sit still for very long, but, she says, Jonny loves to be read to and can curl up for half an hour easily during story time with her. The mother tells you that since her husband, who is in the military, was deployed 3 months ago, she rarely has individual time for Jonny or her other children. His dad could "make him mind," and so since his dad's deployment, she has given up on trying to make him sit still in church, leaving him instead in a supervised playroom. She adds that her kids miss their dad but Jonny's older siblings grew accustomed to his absences over time. As she begins to talk about Jonny's dad, Jonny climbs into his mother's lap and starts playing a shooting game with a car on the counter. Jonny's mom gently "shoos" him away. Jonny slides to the floor but returns with a book held out to his mother. She says, "Sorry, not now, Jonny," and tells you the teacher's concern about his activity level, inability to hold a pencil properly, and failure to pay attention to learning tasks in class. The mother relays the teacher's concern that he may have attention deficit–hyperactivity disorder. You wonder whether Jonny's activity level has anything to do with his father's deployment (separation from his dad) and the decreased time that Jonny's mother has for him (separation anxiety and lack of secure base). The mother wonders whether medication would help Jonny have an easier time in kindergarten, and she asks you for your opinion.

BOX 21-3 RESEARCH HIGHLIGHT

Toxic Stress and Development

In response to stressors such as difficult and challenging experiences, humans physiologically respond by increasing the capacity to think and act. Energy stores are mobilized and heart rate and blood pressure are increased to enable more attention, awareness, and responsiveness to the environment. When stress is controllable, short-lived, and predictable, it can help us learn to be adaptive and resilient. This is a good form of stress. Some forms of stress are tolerable even though they challenge our abilities to cope. The death of a loved one or moving to a new city are examples of inevitable forms of adverse events that are made tolerable by support from our social network and by the fact that many other people have faced similar experiences. But what if the challenges we face are uncontrollable, unpredictable, and pervasive? This is toxic stress.

Toxic stress is a form of stress that results in chronic activation of the biological stress response system with harmful consequences for child development. Experiences that are chronically disruptive, abusive, neglectful, or unpredictable flood the brain with chemicals that, in large persistent doses, impair neuronal growth and ultimately make it harder for the brain to form healthy connections. In this way, toxic stress leaves a lasting biological fingerprint of damage on brain structure and function.

For example, parents suffering from mental illness, addictions to substances of abuse, or domestic violence are less able to respond sensitively to their infants to meet their needs, placing the infants at risk for unpredictable, neglectful, or abusive parenting. As infants are completely reliant on their parents to have their basic needs met, these situations chronically activate infants' stress systems and produce changes to the structure and function of some brain regions.

Two major brain regions that are known to be affected by toxic stress are the hippocampus and the prefrontal cortex. These brain regions are particularly important to the development of memory and self-regulation—the foundations of school and social success. Over time, the effects of toxic stress on brain structure and function can lead to shifts in patterns of behaviour from more organized to more habitual with the result that children become more rigid and less capable of independent problem solving.

The effects of toxic stress are particularly worrisome in early childhood because the brain is exquisitely sensitive to experience during this phase of rapid brain development. As well, children's future brain development builds upon current and past brain development. Thus, changes in brain structure and function due to toxic stress produce cumulative changes—affecting not only current aspects of development for a given stage, but also the next stage that builds upon previous growth. To summarize, it seems that the common adage "what doesn't kill you will make you stronger" is true of good stress, but when it comes to toxic stress, "what doesn't kill you now may kill you later."

Letourneau, N. (2012). Toxic stress in early caregiving and child health. *Canadian Nurse, 108*(3), 48.

Nursing Implications of the Dynamic Maturational Model of Attachment. As a nurse, you will need to design approaches that address both the quality of the attachment system and the caregiving system. Crittenden (2008) asserted that recognizing patients' attachment strategies is crucial for providing helpful treatments and reducing the risk of inappropriate treatment. For instance, in the situation in which a young child is hospitalized, you would need to consider the security of the child and to provide high-quality substitute care, including making developmentally appropriate efforts to keep the child attached to his or her primary caregiver (e.g., using pictures, phone calls, liberal visiting hours, parent sleepovers). If you are working in mental health care, you need to recognize that patients' apparently maladaptive coping strategies (e.g., obsessive–compulsive disorder, anxiety) may be strategies developed to cope with adverse relationships with attachment figures. Alternatively, in working with parents in impoverished environments, you need to support the caregivers through the provision of material, social, and educational resources that will promote safety and security of both adults and children. Nurses need to advocate for appropriate support resources for families in which caregiving may be compromised as a result of stress associated with parental poverty, mental illness, or lack of education (Shonkoff, Garner, Siegel, et al., 2012).

Havighurst's Developmental Tasks

Robert Havighurst (1900–1991) was influenced by Erikson's work and observations of the developmental tasks crucial for healthy development. Havighurst defined a series of age-specific essential tasks, such as learning to walk, getting ready to read, learning social and gender roles, developing independence, selecting a mate, rearing children, and, finally, adjusting to decreasing physical strength and health. The essential tasks arise from predictable internal and external pressures, such as increasing physical maturity, cultural pressure of society, and the individual's personal goals and aspirations (Havighurst, 1972).

According to **Havighurst's developmental tasks**, several sources of pressure may be present at the same time. Increasing physical maturity is associated with the development of skills such as walking, talking, or eating. Cultural pressure creates the conditions necessary to learn social behaviours and ethical norms. An adolescent girl may be physically able to bear a child, but the preparation and timing for the onset of parenthood can also be considered from a perspective of pressure from both the youth and adult cultures (Havighurst, 1972).

Havighurst believed that at certain critical periods, the individual is most receptive to the learning necessary to achieve success in performing these tasks. Effective learning and achievement of tasks during one period lead to happiness and success with later tasks. Failure leads to unhappiness, disapproval by society, and difficulty with later tasks. An example is the struggle that adolescents might experience in preparing for a work career after having failed to develop fundamental skills in reading and math (Havighurst, 1972; Seiffge-Krenke & Gelhaar, 2008).

Havighurst's theory is limited in its cultural application, according to critics who believe that it describes developmental milestones from the perspective of middle-class norms within the United States. It would be difficult to fit all cultural or ethnic mores within this theoretical framework (Klaczynski, 1990).

Mechanisms and Nursing Implications of Havighurst's Theory. Havighurst's work built on that of Freud and Erikson. Therefore, the mechanisms and nursing implications from Freud and Erikson also apply to Havighurst's developmental tasks (Table 21-6).

MECHANISTIC TRADITION

According to the **mechanistic tradition**, the organism is similar to a machine. Development depends on the level of stimulation, the kind of stimulation, and the history of stimulation from the environment. The environment is considered to activate human development (Bornstein & Lamb, 2015), and behaviour is seen as responsive to environmental forces rather than driven only by internal causes such as maturation. Social learning theory follows from this tradition and is presented in Chapter 20.

CONTEXTUALISM

The way that human development is described and explained is increasingly tied to the understanding of environment and context. Developmental theories within the **contextual tradition** focus on the relationship between the individual and his or her social context. Within this tradition, the individual and the environment are viewed as mutually influential, acting on one another in dynamic interaction (Bornstein & Lamb, 2015). Human development is the process of continuously adapting to changing environments.

Bioecological Theory

Urie Bronfenbrenner (1917–2005), a developmental psychologist at Cornell University, developed a theory that stresses the importance of the interaction between the developing individual and his or her surrounding social environments. **Bronfenbrenner's bioecological theory** involves considering multiple "layers" of the environment:

TABLE 21-6 Developmental Theorists for Adult Stages

Adult Stages	Erikson's Description	Havighurst's Description
Early-early adult (ages 16–22 years)	Intimacy versus isolation	Early adulthood stage
Middle-early adult (ages 22–28 years)	Ability to form intimate relationships	Selecting a mate Learning to live with a marriage partner Starting a family Rearing children Getting started in an occupation Taking on civic responsibilities Finding a congenial social group
Early-middle adult (ages 28–45 years)	Generativity versus self-absorption and stagnation Ability to expand personal and social involvement	Middle age Assisting teenage children to become responsible adults Achieving adult social and civic responsibility Reaching and maintaining satisfactory performance in one's occupation Developing adult leisure-time activities Relating to one's spouse as a person Accepting and adjusting to the physiological changes of middle age Adjusting to aging of parents
Late adult–old age (age 45 years and older)	Integrity versus despair Ability to adapt to changes in lifestyle, functional level, and family structure	Later maturity Adjusting to decreasing physical strength and health Adjusting to retirement and reduced income Adjusting to death of a spouse Establishing an affiliation with one's age group Adopting and adapting social roles in a flexible way Satisfactory physical living space

- The microsystem consists of the immediate settings, activities, and personal relationships of the individual. Examples are family, classroom, workplace, and recreation group.
- The mesosystem is made up of the relationships between the different settings in which the person spends time. Examples are relationships between families and schools, between workplaces and schools, and between families and spiritual organizations (church parish, mosque, temple), and spiritual organizations and schools.
- The exosystem is a set of specific social structures that do not directly contain the individual but exert direct and indirect influence on individual development. Examples are the health care system, the education system, the justice system, and religious institutions.
- The macrosystem consists of all of the elements contained in the individual's microsystem, mesosystem, and exosystem, as well as the general underlying philosophy, cultural orientation, and values by which the person lives (Bronfenbrenner, 2009). Examples are overarching dimensions such as political orientation, economic model, and cultural values.

Mechanisms of the Bioecological Theory. Lev Semenovich Vygotsky (1896–1934) introduced a concept called the zone of proximal development, which is the key developmental mechanism of ecological theories. This zone is the space between the individual's potential and his or her actual developmental status (Green & Piel, 2016). For instance, a toddler may have a 10-word vocabulary but potentially could have a repertoire of hundreds of words. Activity that links those two states promotes development. For instance, parents who use joint referencing (looking at things that their toddlers are looking at and naming them) promote toddler vocabulary development within the zone of proximal development.

Bronfenbrenner's modern conception of developmental processes expands upon Vygotsky's idea of the zone of proximal development. In language acquisition, developmental support processes occur in all levels of the system. At the macrosystem level, a process supporting language development in young children would be the adoption of a national child care policy to support working parents. Such a policy would inform regulations concerning issues such as education level of child care workers, ratio of children to workers in child care centres, and space requirements per child.

Nursing Implications of the Bioecological Theory. An appropriate goal of nursing practice is to influence wellness by promoting health in all layers of the bioecological system. The ecological model applies to nursing practice beyond the individual level of health promotion to higher levels of the social context. Therefore, Bronfenbrenner's theory fits well with the current emphasis on primary health care (Box 21-4).

DIALECTICISM

In the dialectic tradition, all developmental theories are considered mutually interactive (Sameroff, 2010). Developmental theorists are increasingly proposing that change or development can occur within the framework of multiple theories. A key element of the dialectic tradition is the ability to incorporate multiple contexts. An example of a dialectic approach from the natural and biomedical sciences is the theory of gene expression or epigenetics. Epigenetics links genetics, the environment, and their influences on human development and disease. In the behavioural and social science disciplines, examples of dialectical thinking include the growing awareness of the effect of the economic environment on human development at the population level. Resilience theory is an approach in which the interaction between two processes, previously studied separately, is examined.

Keating and Hertzman's Population Health Theory

Human development has historically been considered an individual characteristic. According to Daniel P. Keating (1949–) and Clyde Hertzman's (1953–2013) (1999) population health approach, human development is a population phenomenon. These Canadian developmental theorists referred to the strong association between the health of a population, developmental outcomes, and the social and economic forces affecting the larger society. They based their developmental theory on epidemiological evidence that improved literacy (one marker of human development) is related to improvements in family economic status, in school community economic status, and in national economic status (Hertzman, 2011). Hertzman theorized that socioeconomic status created gradients in developmental health, a process he called "biological embedding" (Hertzman & Boyce, 2010).

Keating and Hertzman (1999) proposed that health, behaviour, and cognitive functions are largely set in early life and are then influenced further by succeeding events in the socioeconomic environment. Developmental health is defined as the physical and mental health, well-being, coping, and competence of human populations.

BOX 21-4 FOCUS ON PRIMARY HEALTH CARE

Bronfenbrenner's Ecological Theory and Primary Health Care

Three principles of primary health care are to (1) foster public participation, (2) educate the patient in order to promote health and prevent illness, and (3) foster intersectoral collaboration. Bronfenbrenner's ecological model of human development fits well with these principles. At each environmental layer, nurses can initiate actions to promote health:

- *Microsystem,* which includes the individual and his or her immediate setting (e.g., family, school, workplace, neighbourhood). As a nurse, you can help the individual develop personal skills, healthy lifestyles and activities, and supportive environments. For example, you can help teach family members caring for an elderly parent how to balance family care and self-care to keep themselves healthy.
- *Mesosystem,* which consists of relations among the individual's various immediate settings. To strengthen the mesosystem, you can work toward strengthening community action. You can link the family to community supports such as adult respite services and older persons' activities groups.
- *Exosystem,* which comprises relations among structures, sectors, services, and policies. The exosystem is strengthened when nurses promote healthy public policy. You are practising at this level when you help develop links between typically separate services such as the health care system and the social service system. For example, you can volunteer to be on planning committees and other decision-making bodies.
- *Macrosystem,* which consists of societal values. To promote optimum health at the macrosystem level, the nurse can be an advocate for social change. For example, if you believe that more value should be placed on older persons in society, you may advocate for higher standards and staff-to-resident ratios in long-term care facilities. Such advocacy might include writing letters to the editor, joining community or national advocacy groups, and lobbying politicians.

Developmental health is primarily a function of the overall quality of the social environment, including the national socioeconomic environment, civil society, and social network. Keating and Hertzman's population approach to human development is outlined in Figure 21-3.

Mechanisms of the Population Health Theory. Keating and Hertzman (1999) proposed three interrelated regulatory systems as the mechanisms for human population development: emotional regulation, attention regulation, and social regulation. Each regulatory system develops in interaction between the individual's biological processes and his or her multiple socioeconomic environments. *Emotional regulation,* which involves the modulation of emotional reactions, plays an important role in competent social functioning. *Attention regulation,* which involves regulation of arousal and reactivity of the brain, contributes to the ability to pursue goals and respond to challenges to those goals. *Social regulation* involves regulation of social interactions, including aspects such as mutual affection and warmth, particularly in nurturing relationships. Together, these three regulatory systems are thought to influence later competence as individuals interact reciprocally with their socioeconomic environments. Recent extensions of the work show that early developmental adversity actually affects gene expression or an individual's epigenetic profile and is linked to later heath and developmental outcomes (Essex, Boyce, Hertzman, et al., 2013; Suderman, Borghol, Pappas, et al., 2014).

Community Nursing Care Implications of the Population Health Theory. Community nurses have typically focused on the health and well-being of patients in a community context (see Chapter 4 for further information on caring for patients in the community). To promote well-being of individuals over their lifespan, community nurses need to understand how socioeconomic context affects health and implement practices that take into account socioeconomic impacts (Stanhope & Lancaster, 2015). The ecological levels of health promotion activities are directly applicable to the population health approach for community nurses. A population health approach helps identify these socioeconomic factors and provides direction for designing community nursing interventions that address them. Community health nurses can advocate for better environments for children affected by low socioeconomic status and work with their families to help address the risks to their children's development that can affect them for a lifetime.

Resilience Theory

Resilience is defined as the maintenance of positive adjustment under challenging life conditions (Cicchetti & Curtis, 2007). This approach arose in the field of child psychiatry when clinicians observed that some children and adolescents were able to thrive in severely adverse conditions (e.g., poverty, maternal depression, and paternal criminality), whereas others faltered (Luthar, 2003).

Mechanisms of Resilience. Resilience theory focuses on the interaction between protective processes and vulnerability processes. Vulnerability processes (physical illness, psychological stresses, social risk) and protective processes (self-efficacy, good parenting and problem solving, social support acquisition and maintenance) are examined together to understand and explain human growth and development. Individual factors found to promote resilience include self-efficacy, positive attitude, literacy, social competence, and a history of success. Family-level processes that protect from adversity include coherent response to crisis, social supports, stability, flexibility, effective parenting, and responsibilities outside the home (Rutter, 2005). Community-level processes that promote resilience include control over policy, collaborative and cooperative organization, widespread citizen participation in community, and volunteerism.

Resilience and family adaptation theory has been used to design interventions to support children and families at risk, focusing on protective processes within the context of key risk situations, usually defined by factors such as poverty, chronic illness, and civil conflict. This emphasis is a progression from the previous emphasis on only pathological processes, but the challenge is to design research that enables scholars to study both protective processes and vulnerability processes as they occur together.

Nursing Implications of Resilience. The focus of nursing practice is directly on the individual, family, and community factors that promote health. Nursing practice is usually used in situations that are stressful and challenging for individuals and families, such as illness and loss. Resilience theorists acknowledge the complexity of these moments and ask what nurses can use from these challenging situations that help the family succeed (Box 21-5). For example, a young single woman dealing with the birth of her first child will benefit from nursing interventions that focus both on protective processes (linking to support group, learning parenting skills) and on vulnerability processes (ensuring adequate health care, arranging for financial support).

DEVELOPMENTAL THEORIES AND NURSING

The diverse set of theories included in this chapter suggest that human behaviour is truly complex. No single theory successfully describes

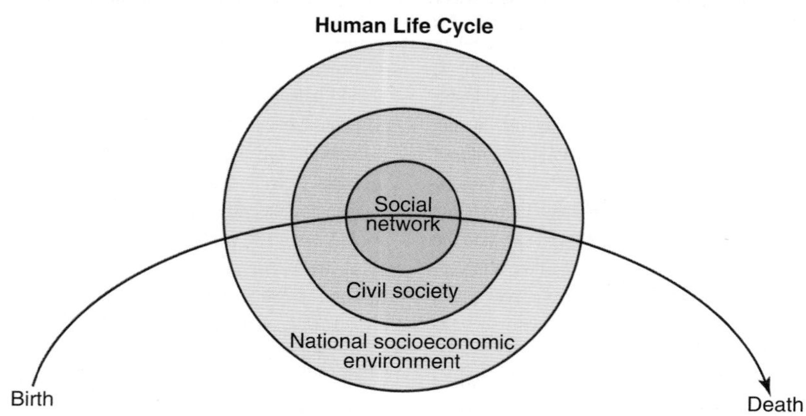

FIGURE 21-3 Framework for human development and the social determinants of health. Redrawn from Keating, D. P., & Hertzman, C. (Eds.). (1999). *Developmental health and the wealth of nations: Social, biological and educational dynamics* (p. 30). New York: Guilford Press.

BOX 21-5 RESEARCH HIGHLIGHT

Supporting Parents: Can Intervention Improve Mother–Child Relationships?

Research Focus

Healthy child development has been identified as one of the key determinants of health and resiliency in adulthood. Attachment security promotes healthy child development. In a systematic review by Letourneau, Tryphonopoulos, Giesbrecht, et al. (2015), researchers examined interventions aimed at improving the parent–child attachment security among children from a variety of groups, including those affected by maternal depression, financial stress, or marital problems.

Research Abstract

Early secure maternal–child attachment relationships lay the foundation for children's healthy social and mental development. Interventions targeting maternal sensitivity during the first year of infant life may be the key to promoting secure attachment. Letourneau et al. (2015) conducted a narrative systematic review and meta-analysis to examine the effectiveness of interventions aimed at promoting maternal sensitivity on maternal–child attachment security. Studies included mothers and their infants followed up to 36 months postpartum. Ten trials, involving 1 628 mother–infant pairs, were included. Examination of the trials showed that intervention designed to promote maternal sensitivity worked to improve maternal–child attachment security. The authors concluded that interventions aimed at improving maternal sensitivity alone or in combination with maternal reflection, implemented in the first year of infants' lives, are effective in promoting secure maternal–child attachments. Intervention aimed at highest-risk families produced the most beneficial effects.

Evidence-Informed Practice

- Helping parents become more sensitive and responsive to their infants to improve the quality of parent–child relationships is an important support mechanism for families at risk.
- Parent training and support have the potential to positively alter the style of interaction between parents and children.

Letourneau, N., Tryphonopoulos, P., Giesbrecht, G., Dennis, C. L., Bhogal, S., & Watson, B. (2015) Narrative and meta-analytic review of interventions aiming to improve maternal-child attachment security. *Infant Mental Health Journal, 36*(4), 366–387.

human growth and development in all its complexity. Theorists demonstrate their own values and beliefs in their focus and the subjects chosen for their work, and they work within cultural and historical perspectives. The theories described in this chapter are meant to provide the basis for meaningful thought and observation of an individual's pattern of growth and development and the role of environments in it. This observation and reflection provide you with a framework within which you can predict human responses to health and illness and recognize deviations from the norm.

Patterns of growth and development help determine future patterns of adjustment to life (Edelman et al., 2013). A clear understanding of these patterns and of the contexts within which they occur can assist you in planning questions for health screening and health history and in health teaching for patients of all ages. Nurses need to consider an individual's development within the context of his or her families, social relationships, communities, and the larger society.

Developmental theories help you as a nurse use critical thinking skills when you consider how and why people respond as they do. Your assessment of a patient requires a thorough analysis and interpretation of data to form accurate conclusions about a patient's developmental needs. To accurately identify patients' needs, you need the ability to consider developmental theory in data analysis. Typical developmental behaviours are compared with those projected by the developmental theory.

KEY CONCEPTS

- Nurses provide care for individuals and families throughout their lives. Developmental theories provide a basis for nurses to assess, interpret, and understand the responses seen in their patients.
- Development continues throughout life.
- Individuals have unique patterns of growth and development within broad limits.
- Development is not just a series of distinct linear tasks; it is also a process that varies across and within individuals.
- Three major categories of factors influence human growth and development: (1) genetic or natural forces within the person, (2) the environment in which the person lives, and (3) the interaction that takes place between these two.
- Theories within the organic tradition explore how individuals develop when mostly biological components are believed to stimulate developmental progress.
- Theories in the psychoanalytic and psychosocial tradition describe development of the human personality with regard to conflict resolution between the internal biological forces and the external societal and cultural forces.
- According to the mechanistic approach, human development and behaviour are responses to environmental forces rather than driven by internal causes such as maturation.
- Within the contextual tradition, the individual and the environment are viewed as mutually influential, acting on one another in dynamic interaction.
- In the dialectical tradition, the complete complexity of development is acknowledged. Theorists who work in this tradition strive to combine divergent ways of viewing human development.

CRITICAL THINKING EXERCISES

1. A 50-year-old woman is anxious because her children, 20 and 23 years of age, are no longer living at home. Her husband is still working full-time but planning to retire in 2 years. She is concerned that she is not needed, and she is bored with her life. Identify the developmental task of Erikson's theory that best fits this woman's situation. How will you assist this patient in changing her lifestyle while understanding her developmental tasks?
2. A community nurse conducting a routine assessment of an 18-month-old is concerned about the child being underweight for his age. Upon further discussion, the father reveals that he is not working at present and the family is having financial troubles. Using your knowledge of Bronfenbrenner's bioecological theory, what approach and subsequent strategies would be helpful for these parents?
3. Two 11-year-old girls are spending the day together at the mall. They exit one store, and one of the girls shows her friend a small purse that she stole from the store. Her friend is upset and wonders how she should respond. Use moral development theory to discuss this issue.

4. A woman visits her nurse practitioner at her local health clinic. The woman is struggling with depression and seeking to increase her medication dosage. She also reveals that she is struggling to cope with her 8-year-old son's problem behaviours, such as refusing to do homework and having tantrums when he fails to get his way. Using the dynamic maturational model of attachment, discuss how her mental health state could be influencing her child's behaviour.

REVIEW QUESTIONS

1. Children generally double their birth weight by 5 months of age. This is an example of
   1. Development
   2. Heredity
   3. State of health
   4. Physical growth
2. _________ development is the ability of an individual to distinguish right from wrong and to develop ethical values on which to base his or her actions.
   1. Moral
   2. Cognitive
   3. Psychosocial
   4. Psychoanalytic
3. Theories in the _________ tradition hold that development is a result of biology and adaptation.
   1. Organicism
   2. Psychoanalytic and psychosocial
   3. Contexualism
   4. Dialecticism
4. Which of the following factors is considered an environmental factor that affects human development?
   1. Family
   2. Heredity
   3. State of health
   4. Genetics
5. The developmental theorist who believed his or her research described a sequential process that resolved conflict between the internal life (personality) of adults and their outer world (culture) was
   1. Erikson
   2. Crittenden
   3. Freud
   4. Havighurst
6. The zone of proximal development is
   1. The space between the individual's potential and his or her actual developmental status
   2. Where sensitive caregivers should operate to promote development of their young children
   3. A concept described by Vygotsky
   4. All of the above
7. According to Piaget's theory of cognitive development, during what stage does the individual's moral thinking move to abstract and theoretical subjects, such as achieving world peace, finding justice, and seeking meaning in life?
   1. Formal operations
   2. Concrete operations
   3. Sensorimotor
   4. Preoperational
8. The nurse who is working with a school committee to develop playground safety guidelines is focusing on which level of the bioecological model?
   1. Mesosystem
   2. Microsystem
   3. Exosystem
   4. Macrosystem
9. Which of the following nursing interventions is representative of a population health approach?
   1. Parent teaching
   2. Developing a clinical practice guideline
   3. Participating in a community coalition to improve community housing
   4. Assisting an individual in obtaining funding support for home care
10. A resilient individual is able to experience positive development despite challenging life circumstances. For a young single mother with two young children, access to high-quality day care represents the following:
    1. A vulnerability process
    2. A critical period
    3. Attachment
    4. A protective process

Answers: 1. 4; **2.** 1; **3.** 1; **4.** 1; **5.** 4; **6.** 4; **7.** 1; **8.** 2; **9.** 3; **10.** 4

Rationales for the Review Questions appear at the end of the book.

RECOMMENDED WEBSITES

Canadian Institute of Child Health: http://www.cich.ca
The Canadian Institute of Child Health (CICH) is dedicated to improving the health of children and youth in Canada. Activities include research and policy recommendations and community development and resource building. The CICH focuses on four key areas of activity: supporting healthy pregnancy and childbirth, fostering healthy child development, ensuring that the environment is safe for children, and monitoring the state of children's health.

Centre for Health Promotion (CHP): http://www.phac-aspc.gc.ca/chhd-sdsh/index-eng.php
The CHP uses a life stages approach and is responsible for implementing policies and programs that enhance the conditions conducive to healthy development. The CHP addresses the determinants of health and facilitates successful movement through the life stages. The CHP acts through programs addressing healthy child development, families, aging and lifestyles, public information, and education (Canadian Health Network), as well as programs on issues related to rural health and support of the voluntary sector.

Centre of Excellence for Early Childhood Development: http://www.excellence-jeunesenfants.ca/home.asp?lang=EN
The mandate of the Centre of Excellence for Early Childhood Development (CEECD) is to foster the dissemination of scientific knowledge about the social and emotional development of young children and about the policies and services that influence this development. The CEECD also formulates recommendations for the services needed to ensure optimum early childhood development. This page of the CEECD website lists a variety of issues and behaviours common to children younger than 5 years, with links to articles on the subjects written by leading researchers in the field.

Infant Mental Health Promotion: http://www.imhpromotion.ca
Infant Mental Health Promotion (IMHP) is a coalition of professional representatives from service agencies that are dedicated to promoting optimal outcomes for infants and preschoolers, in collaboration with families and other caregivers. Programs and advocacy initiatives are rooted in sound knowledge of the origins of healthy development in children, based on attachment theory, theories of social-emotional development, and emerging neuroscience. They provide graduate certificates in infant and early child mental health and publish a quarterly newsletter, among other initiatives.

Nursing Child Assessment Satellite Training (NCAST): http://www.ncast.org/

Based in the University of Washington, this organization aims to give professionals, parents, and other caregivers the knowledge and skills to provide nurturing environments for young children. NCAST disseminates and develops research-informed products and training programs for practitioners and researchers in many disciplines and settings, which can be used with typically developing children, with those at risk for developmental delays, and with those in whom special health care needs have been identified.

REFERENCES

Ainsworth, M. D. S. (1979). Infant–mother attachment. *American Psychologist, 34*(10), 932–937. doi:10.1037/0003-066X.34.10.932.

Berk, L. (2008). *Exploring lifespan development.* Boston, MA: Allyn & Bacon.

Berk, L. (2013). *Child development* (9th ed.). Boston, MA: Pearson.

Bornstein, M., & Lamb, M. (2015). *Developmental psychology: An advanced textbook* (7th ed.). Hillsdale, NJ: Lawrence Erlbaum.

Bronfenbrenner, U. (2009). *The ecology of human development.* Boston, MA: Harvard University Press.

Bukatko, D. (2012). *Child development: A thematic approach* (6th ed.). Boston, MA: Houghton Mifflin.

Canadian Association of Schools of Nursing/Association Canadienne des Écoles de Sciences Infirmières (CASN/ACESI) (2015). *National Nursing Education Framework: Final Report.* Ottawa: Author.

Chess, S., & Thomas, A. (1995). *Temperament in clinical practice.* New York: Guilford Press.

Cicchetti, D., & Curtis, W. J. (2007). A multilevel approach to resilience [Special issue]. *Development and Psychopathology, 19*(3), 627–955. doi:10.1017/S0954579407000314.

Cicchetti, D., & Rogosch, F. (2012). Gene by environment interaction and resilience: Effects of child maltreatment and serotonin, corticotropin releasing hormone, dopamine, and oxytocin genes. *Development and Psychopathology, 24*(2), 411–427. doi:10.1017/S095457912000077.

Crandell, T., Crandell, C., & Vander Zanden, J. (2012). *Human development* (10th ed.). Whitby, ON: McGraw-Hill.

Crittenden, P. (2008). *Raising parents: Attachment, parenting and child safety.* Portland, OR: Willan Publishing.

Crittenden, P. M., & Claussen, A. H. (Eds.), (2003). *The organization of attachment relationships: Maturation, culture, and context.* Philadelphia, PA: Cambridge University Press.

Crittenden, P. M., & DiLalla, D. L. (1988). Compulsive compliance: The development of an inhibitory coping strategy in infancy. *Journal of Abnormal Child Psychology, 16*, 585–599. doi:10.1007/BF00914268.

Crittenden, P. M., & Kulbotten, G. R. (2007). Familial contributions to ADHD: An attachment perspective. *Tidsskrift for Norsk Psykologforening [Norwegian Journal of Psychology], 44*(10), 1220–1229.

Crittenden, P., & Landini, A. (2011). *Assessing adult attachment.* New York: W. W. Norton.

Douglas, V. (2013). *Introduction to Aboriginal health in Canada: Bridging health and healing.* New York: Springer.

Edelman, C., Kudzma, E., & Mandle, C. (2013). *Health promotion throughout the lifespan* (8th ed.). St. Louis, MO: Elsevier.

Erikson, E. (1993). *Childhood and society.* New York: W. W. Norton.

Erikson, E. (1997). *The lifecycle completed.* New York: W. W. Norton.

Essex, M. J., Boyce, T. W., Hertzman, C., et al. (2013). Epigenetic vestiges of early developmental adversity: Childhood stress exposure and DNA methylation in adolescence. *Child Development, 84*(1), 58–75. doi:10.1111/j.1467-8624.2011.01641.x.

Feeley, N., Zelkowitz, P., Westreich, R., et al. (2011). The evidence base for the cues program for mothers of very low birth weight infants: An innovative approach to reduce anxiety and support sensitive interaction. *Journal of Perinatal Education, 20*(3), 142–153. doi:10.1891/1058-1243.20.3.142.

Feldman, R. (2017). *Life span development: A topical approach* (3rd ed.). New York: Pearson.

Gesell, A. (1948). *Studies in child development.* New York: Harper.

Gesell, A., Ilg, F., & Bullis, A. (1949). *Vision: Its development in infant and child.* New York: Hoeber.

Gilligan, C. (1993). *In a different voice: Psychological theory and women's development.* Cambridge, MA: Harvard University Press.

Green, M. G., & Piel, J. A. (2016). *Theories of human development: A comparative approach* (2nd ed.). New York, NY: Routledge.

Greenwood, M., de Leeuw, S., Lindsay, N., et al. (2015). *Determinants of Indigenous peoples' health in Canada.* Toronto, ON: Canadian Scholars' Press.

Havighurst, R. (1972). *Developmental tasks and education* (3rd ed.). London: Longman Group.

Hertzman, C. (2011). Bringing a population health perspective to early biodevelopment: An emerging approach. In *Nature and nurture in early child development* (pp. 217–244). New York: Cambridge University Press.

Hertzman, C., & Boyce, T. (2010). How experience gets under the skin to create gradients in developmental health. *Annual Review of Public Health, 31*, 329–347. doi:10.1146/annurev.publhealth.012809.103538.

Hockenberry, M., & Wilson, D. (2015). *Wong's nursing care of infants and children* (10th ed.). St. Louis: Elsevier.

Keating, D., & Hertzman, C. (1999). *Developmental health and the wealth of nations: Social, biological, and educational dynamics.* New York: Guilford Press.

Klaczynski, P. (1990). Cultural-developmental tasks and adolescent development: Theoretical and methodological considerations. *Adolescence, 25*(100), 811–823.

Kliegman, R., Stanton, B., Geme, J., et al. (2016). *Nelson textbook of pediatrics* (20th ed.). Philadelphia, PA: Elsevier.

Kohlberg, L. (1981). *The philosophy of moral development: Moral stages and the idea of justice.* San Francisco: Harper & Row.

Laplante, D. P., Brunet, A., & King, S. (2016). The effects of maternal stress and illness during pregnancy on infant temperament: Project Ice Storm. *Pediatric Research, 79*(1–1), 107–113.

Letourneau, N., Tryphonopoulos, P., Giesbrecht, G., et al. (2015). Narrative and meta-analytic review of interventions aiming to improve maternal-child attachment security. *Infant Mental Health Journal, 36*(4), 366–387. doi:10.1002/imhj.21525.

Luthar, S. (2003). *Resilience and vulnerability: Adaptation in the context of childhood adversities.* New York: Cambridge University Press.

McCain, M., Mustard, F., & Shanker, S. (2007). *Early years study 2: Putting science into action.* Toronto: Council for Early Child Development.

National Scientific Council on the Developing Child (2012). *The science of neglect: The persistent absence of responsive care disrupts the developing brain: Working paper 12.* Boston, MA: Center on the Developing Child, Harvard University.

Nursing Child Assessment Satellite Training (NCAST) (1999). *Keys to caregiving.* Seattle, WA: NCAST Programs.

O'Connor, T. G., Bergman, K., Sarkar, P., et al. (2013). Prenatal cortisol exposure predicts infant cortisol response to acute stress. *Developmental Psychobiology, 55*(2), 145–155. doi:10.1002/dev.21007.

Patanella, D. (2011). Piaget's theory of moral development. In *Encyclopedia of child behavior and development* (pp. 1109–1111). New York: Springer. doi:10.1007/978-0-387-79061-9_2167.

Piaget, J. (2000). Piaget's theory of cognitive development. In K. Lee (Ed.), *Childhood cognitive development: The essential readings* (pp. 33–47). New York: Wiley-Blackwell.

Puig, J., Englund, M. M., Simpson, J. A., et al. (2013). Predicting adult physical illness from infant attachment: A prospective longitudinal study. *Health Psychology, 32*(4), 409. doi:10.1037/a0028889.

Rutter, M. (2005). The promotion of resilience in the face of adversity. In A. Clarke-Stewart & J. Dunn (Eds.), *Families count: Effects on child and adolescent development* (pp. 26–52). New York: Cambridge University Press.

Sameroff, A. (2010). A unified theory of development: A dialectic integration of nature and nurture. *Child Development, 81*(1), 6–22.

Seiffge-Krenke, I., & Gelhaar, T. (2008). Does successful attainment of developmental tasks lead to happiness and success in later development tasks? A test of Havighurst's (1948) theses. *Journal of Adolescence, 31*(1), 33–52.

Shonkoff, J. P., Garner, A. S., Siegel, B. S., et al. (2012). The lifelong effects of early childhood adversity and toxic stress. *Pediatrics, 129*(1), e232–e246. doi:10.1542/peds.2011-2663.

Slote, M. (2016). *Human development and human life.* Miami, FL: Springer.

Sroufe, A. (2005). Attachment and development: A prospective, longitudinal study from birth to adulthood. *Attachment & Human Development, 7*(4), 349–367.

Stanhope, M., & Lancaster, J. (2015). *Public health nursing: Population-centered health care in the community.* St. Louis, MO: Elsevier Health Sciences.

Suderman, M., Borghol, N., Pappas, J. J., et al. (2014). Childhood abuse is associated with methylation of multiple loci in adult DNA. *BMC Medical Genomics, 7*(1), 13. doi:10.1186/1755-8794-7-13.

Veríssimo, M., Santos, A. J., Fernandes, C., et al. (2014). Associations between attachment security and social competence in preschool children. *Merrill-Palmer Quarterly, 60*(1), 80–99.

Weizmann, F., & Harris, B. (2012). Arnold Gesell: The maturationist. In *Portraits of pioneers in developmental psychology* (Vol. 7). Hove, UK: Psychology Press.

22

Conception Through Adolescence

Canadian content written by Cynthia Murray, BN, MN, PhD
Original chapter by Jerrilee LaMar, PhD, RN, CNE

OBJECTIVES

Mastery of content in this chapter will enable you to:

- Define the key terms listed.
- Discuss physiological and psychosocial health concerns during the transition of the child from intrauterine to extrauterine life.
- Describe characteristics of physical growth of the fetus and of the child from birth to adolescence.
- Describe cognitive and psychosocial development from birth to adolescence.
- Describe the interactions that occur between parent and child.
- Explain the role of play in the development of the child.
- Identify factors that contribute to self-esteem in youth.
- Describe the influence of the school environment on the development of the child.
- Plan culturally appropriate health promotion activities for children of all backgrounds.
- Discuss ways in which you can help parents meet their children's developmental needs.

KEY TERMS

Adolescence, p. 387
Animism, p. 377
Apgar score, p. 362
Artificialism, p. 377
Blastocyst, p. 361
Bonding, p. 363
Classification, p. 383
Concrete operations, p. 382
Differentiation, p. 362
Embryo, p. 361
Estrogen, p. 387
Fertilization, p. 361
Fetus, p. 362
Fontanels, p. 364
Formal operations, p. 389
Hyperbilirubinemia, p. 366
Immanent justice, p. 377
Implantation, p. 361
Inborn errors of metabolism, p. 366
Infancy, p. 366
Lanugo, p. 362
Menarche, p. 387
Moulding, p. 364
Morula, p. 361
Nagele's rule, p. 361
Neonatal period, p. 361
Object permanence, p. 372
Organogenesis, p. 362
Placenta, p. 361
Prematurity, p. 365
Preoperational thought, p. 372
Preschool period, p. 376
Preterm labour, p. 363
Puberty, p. 381
Quickening, p. 362
School-age, p. 379
Sensorimotor period, p. 366
Sexually transmitted infections (STIs), p. 392
Teratogens, p. 363
Testosterone, p. 387
Toddlerhood, p. 371
Vernix caseosa, p. 362
Zygote, p. 361

MEDIA RESOURCES

http://evolve.elsevier.com/Canada/Potter/fundamentals/

- Audio Chapter Summaries
- Examination Review Questions
- Concept Map Creator
- Case Study with Questions
- Audio Glossary
- Content Updates
- Video Clips

It is imperative for nurses to have a foundational knowledge of human development and functioning (Canadian Association for Schools of Nursing [CASN], 2015). Human growth and development are continuous, intricate, complex processes that are divided into stages organized by age groups. This arbitrary, chronological division is used because it coincides with the timing and sequence of maturational changes that allow children to progress through a series of developmental stages and associated tasks (Box 22-1). This chapter focuses on the various physical, psychosocial, and cognitive changes. It also focuses on health risks and concerns during the various stages of growth and development (see Chapter 21 for further information about developmental theories).

BOX 22-1 Developmental Age Periods

Prenatal Period: Conception to Birth
Germinal: Conception to approximately 2 weeks
Embryonic: 2 to 8 weeks
Fetal: 8 to 40 weeks (birth)

Because of rapid growth rate and total dependency, this is one of the most mutable and vulnerable periods in the developmental process. The relationship between maternal health and certain manifestations of normalities and abnormalities in the newborn emphasizes the importance of adequate prenatal care to the health and well-being of the infant.

Infancy Period: Birth to Approximately 12 to 18 Months
Neonatal: Birth to 28 days
Infancy: 1 to approximately 12 to 18 months

The infancy period is one of rapid motor, cognitive, and social development. Through bonding with the parent or other caregiver, the infant establishes a basic trust in the world and the foundation for future interpersonal relationships. The critical first month of life, termed the **neonatal period**, although part of infancy, is often differentiated from the remainder of infancy because it is characterized by major physical adjustments to extrauterine existence and by the psychosocial adjustment of the parents to their new roles.

Early Childhood: 1 to 6 Years
Toddler: 1 to 3 years
Preschooler: 3 to 6 years

This period, which extends from the time children begin walking until school entry, is characterized by intense activity and discovery. It is a time of marked physical and psychosocial development. Motor development advances steadily. Children at this age acquire language and wider social relationships, learn role standards, gain self-control and skill mastery, develop increasing awareness of dependence and independence, and begin to develop a self-concept.

Middle Childhood: 6 to 12 Years

Frequently referred to as the *school age*, this period of development is one in which children expand relationships outside the family group and activities revolve around peer relationships. Physical, cognitive, and psychosocial development advances steadily, with emphasis on developing skill competencies. Social cooperation and early moral development take on more importance, with relevance for later life stages. This is a critical period in the development of a self-concept.

Adolescence: 12 to Approximately 19 Years

The period of rapid maturation and change known as adolescence is considered to be a transitional period that begins at the onset of puberty and extends to the point of entry into the adult world—in Canada, usually high school graduation. Biological and psychological maturation are accompanied by physical changes and emotional turmoil, and the self-concept is redefined. In the late adolescent period, children begin to internalize all previously learned values and to focus on an individual, rather than a group, identity.

Adapted from Hockenberry, M. J., & Wilson, D. (2015). *Wong's nursing care of infants and children* (10th ed.). St. Louis, MO: Mosby.

SELECTING A DEVELOPMENTAL FRAMEWORK FOR NURSING

Providing developmentally appropriate nursing care is easier when the care plan is based on a theoretical framework (see Chapter 21 for further information about theoretical frameworks). An organized, systematic approach ensures that children's needs are assessed and met by the plan. In a developmental approach, organized care is directed at an individual child's current level of functioning to motivate self-direction and health promotion; for example, the nurse might instruct parents to encourage toddlers to feed themselves in order to advance their developing independence and promote their sense of autonomy. Understanding an adolescent's need to be independent should prompt the nurse to negotiate with the adolescent to establish a contract about the care plan and its implementation. Also, parents may choose to have midwives, who provide developmentally appropriate individualized care, in their child-bearing experiences. All care must be planned so that it is culturally safe (see Chapter 9 for further information about providing culturally safe care), ethical and legal (see Chapters 7 and 8 for further information on providing ethical and legal care), and informed by the best evidence available (see Chapter 6 for further information on evidence-informed research).

CONCEPTION

From the moment of conception, human growth proceeds at a predictable and rapid rate. During the prenatal period, the embryo grows from a single cell to a complex, physiological being. All major organ systems develop in utero, and most function before birth.

Intrauterine Life

Intrauterine life that reaches full term usually lasts approximately 9 calendar months, or 40 weeks. The length of pregnancy is computed according to **Nagele's rule**, in which you count back 3 months from the first day of the pregnant woman's last menstrual period and then add 7 days. **Fertilization** occurs when a sperm penetrates the ovum and the material from both cell nuclei unites. The newly formed organism, known as a **zygote**, has its full genetic complement (1 pair of sex chromosomes and 22 pairs of autosomal chromosomes). The ovum and the sperm each contribute one chromosome to each pair. Through this mechanism, genetically determined characteristics (such as eye colour) are transmitted from parent to child and genetic conditions (such as Down syndrome) can result.

The zygote moves through the fallopian tube to the uterus within 3 to 4 days. During this time, the zygote continues to divide. Within 3 days, a solid ball of cells, the **morula**, has formed. The morula continues to develop and forms a central cavity, or **blastocyst**. Even at this early stage of development, cells begin to differentiate in structure and function. Cells at one end of the blastocyst develop into the **embryo**, and those at the opposite end form the **placenta**. Between days 6 and 10, some of the cells secrete enzymes that allow the blastocyst to burrow into the endometrium and become completely covered; this process is known as **implantation**. Chorionic villi—fingerlike projections that emerge from the outer sac surrounding the embryo—obtain oxygen and nutrition from the maternal blood supply and dispose of carbon dioxide and waste products.

The placenta produces essential hormones that maintain the pregnancy. It also provides nutrients to the developing fetus and removes wastes. Because the placenta is porous, noxious materials such as viruses and drugs can pass from mother to child. The effect of noxious agents on the fetus depends on the developmental stage in which exposure takes place; the embryonic stage (2 to 8 weeks after conception) is critical because the organ systems and the main external features are developing. The period of gestation is divided equally into three periods called *trimesters*.

First Trimester. During the first trimester, the first 3 calendar months, fetal cells continue to differentiate and develop into essential organ systems. As cellular change (**differentiation**) and rapid organ growth (**organogenesis**) occur, each organ is vulnerable to conditions in the environment. Interference with growth can cause the congenital absence of an organ system or extensive structural or functional alterations. Because several organ systems develop at the same time, disruption of one system often occurs with disruption of others. Toward the end of the first trimester, it is possible to detect fetal heart tones by fetoscopy or ultrasonography.

Second Trimester. During the second trimester, from the end of the third month to the end of the sixth month, the height of the mother's uterus above the symphysis pubis is an indicator of fetal growth and approximate gestational age. Between 16 and 20 weeks, the mother begins to feel fetal movement. This feeling of life is referred to as **quickening**.

By the end of the sixth month, most of the fetal organ systems are complete and can function. The **fetus** is therefore considered viable, or capable of life outside the uterus, if given intensive environmental support. Fingers and toes are differentiated, rudimentary kidneys function, and the genitalia are defined. The fetus is covered with **vernix caseosa**, a cheeselike substance coating the skin. **Lanugo**, or fine hair, covers most of the body. These substances protect the thin, fragile skin and decrease in amount as the pregnancy nears its completion; thus, infants born before 38 weeks' gestation have more of these protective coverings than do full-term infants.

Third Trimester. During the last 3 months of gestation, the fetus grows to approximately 50 cm in length. Subcutaneous fat is stored, and weight increases to between 3.2 and 3.4 kg. The skin thickens, lanugo begins to disappear, and the fetal body becomes rounder and fuller.

A tremendous spurt in brain growth begins during this trimester and lasts well into the first few years of life. The central nervous system has established its total number of neurons and connections between neurons, and myelination of nerve fibres progresses at a rapid rate.

At the end of the third trimester, the normal fetus is physically able to make the transition from intrauterine to extrauterine life. The circulatory system, which bypasses the right side of the heart (which, in turn, supplies the lungs with oxygen), can change its circulation to include the lungs. The lungs are capable of maintaining the inflated state for gas exchange. The primitive temperature maintenance systems, reflexes, and sensory organs are ready for use.

Health Promotion

As a nurse, you can address many topics with a pregnant patient to protect her health and that of the fetus. Such topics may vary, depending on the stage of pregnancy. Box 22-2 lists some of the topics to discuss with pregnant women and their partners. You can make a significant difference in supporting young families. After an assessment of the couple's strengths and weaknesses, you can direct parents to available services to enhance their coping skills (Halford, Petch, & Creedy, 2015).

TRANSITION FROM INTRAUTERINE TO EXTRAUTERINE LIFE

The transition from intrauterine to extrauterine life requires rapid changes in the newborn. As the nurse, you need to assess the newborn's ability to make these changes, and you should begin to plan before the birth for appropriate nursing interventions (Murray & McKinney, 2014). Circulatory, pulmonary, and thermal changes all contribute to the infant's adaptation to neonatal life. Gestational age and development, exposure to depressant drugs before or during labour, and the newborn's own behavioural style also influence the adjustment to the external environment. Therefore, initial assessment encompasses a variety of physical and psychosocial elements. You can also provide early opportunities for the parents and infant to develop close emotional bonds.

Physical Changes

The most extreme physiological change occurs when the newborn leaves the in utero circulation and assumes independent respiratory functioning. Nursing care is directed at maintaining an open airway, stabilizing and maintaining body temperature, and protecting the newborn from infection. The most widely used assessment tool is the **Apgar score**, in which heart rate, respiratory effort, muscle tone, reflex irritability, and colour are rated in order to determine overall status. The Apgar assessment is generally conducted at 1 and 5 minutes after birth and may be repeated until the newborn's condition stabilizes. Table 22-1 outlines the scoring criteria of physiological functioning. A total score of 0 to 3 signifies severe distress, a score of 4 to 6 represents moderate difficulty, and a score of 7 to 10 indicates little difficulty in adjusting to extrauterine life. Nurses can use the Apgar score to determine areas requiring further assessment and careful observation. In addition, nurses need to monitor and record the newborn's early elimination patterns (i.e., voiding and passage of meconium), as well as body temperature and other vital signs.

Psychosocial Changes

After conducting a physical evaluation and applying identification bracelets, it is important to promote the parents' and newborn's need for close physical contact. Early parent–child interaction encourages parent–child attachment or bonding. Physical factors (e.g., fatigue, hunger, and health) and emotional factors (e.g., needs for affection and for touch) are assessed.

Merely placing the family together does not promote closeness. The parents and newborn must be willing and able to respond to each other. Most healthy newborns are awake and alert for the first half-hour after birth. This is a good time for parent–child interaction to begin. Close body contact, often including skin-to-skin contact and breastfeeding, is a satisfying way for most families to start. If immediate contact is not possible, it should be incorporated into the care plan as

TABLE 22-1 Apgar Scoring

Sign	Score 0	Score 1	Score 2
Heart rate	Absent	Slow, <100 bpm	>100 bpm
Respiratory effort	Absent	Irregular, slow, weak cry	Strong cry
Muscle tone	Limp	Some flexion of extremities	Strong flexion of extremities
Reflex irritability	No response	Grimace	Cry, sneeze
Colour	Blue, pale	Body pink, extremities blue	Completely pink

bpm, Beats per minute.
Adapted from Hockenberry, M. J., & Wilson, D. (2015). *Wong's nursing care of infants and children* (10th ed., p. 247). St. Louis, MO: Mosby.

BOX 22-2 FOCUS ON PRIMARY HEALTH CARE

Health Promotion Topics for the Pregnant Patient

First-Trimester Health Concerns

Nutrition

Mothers with good nutritional practices have fewer complications of pregnancy and childbirth and bear healthier babies than do mothers with poor nutritional intake (Murray & McKinney, 2014). Inadequate prenatal nutrition has been associated with lower birth weight (Oats & Abraham, 2017), and infants with low birth weight have an increased risk for learning disorders, temperament problems, neurological and motor impairment, and developmental delays. Folic acid (vitamin B_9) intake must be adequate before and during pregnancy; the recommended daily dose is 0.4 mg. Mothers should eat foods rich in folic acid, such as green leafy vegetables, liver, lentils, and asparagus. Folic acid intake is believed to be responsible for decreasing the incidence of neural tube defects (Health Canada, 2011a). See Chapter 42 for a fuller description of the nutritional needs of the pregnant woman.

Teratogens

Agents capable of producing functional or structural damage to the developing fetus are called **teratogens**. Nurses need to educate the mother about avoiding exposure to teratogenic agents. One such teratogen is the rubella virus, which can cause stillbirth or congenital anomalies, primarily when exposure occurs in the first trimester. Many drugs are teratogenic during the first trimester. The nurse should assess the mother's past and current use of home remedies, medications (prescription and over-the-counter), and illegal drugs. The benefits of any drug needed to maintain the mother's health must be weighed against potential harm to the fetus.

Cigarette smoke and alcohol are also teratogens. Smoking during pregnancy has been shown to reduce birth weight and increase the incidence of premature birth, fetal death, and neonatal death (Murray & McKinney, 2014). It is also considered a risk factor for impaired growth and development among young children (Santrock, 2011). Alcohol consumed during pregnancy is known to cause fetal alcohol syndrome, fetal alcohol effects, and alcohol-related birth defects. Pregnant women must be educated about the risks of cigarette smoke and alcohol on the fetus.

Second-Trimester Health Concerns

Preterm Labour

Preterm labour is labour that begins before the thirty-seventh week of pregnancy. With technological advances, it is possible for 500 g babies of 24 to 26 weeks' gestation to survive; however, the risk of morbidity and disability is significant. Causes of preterm labour are poorly understood and may be the result of maternal or fetal problems. Maternal risk factors include physiological stresses such as renal and cardiovascular disease, diabetes mellitus, and uterine and cervical abnormalities. Urinary tract infections greatly increase the risk of preterm labour. Because of dramatic changes occurring in the maternal renal system, it is possible for a mother to have an asymptomatic urinary tract infection. Voiding habits should be discussed with the mother during this time. Mothers living in poverty, smokers, and mothers receiving poor prenatal care are at higher risk for preterm labour (Kliegman, Stanton, St. Geme, et al., 2016). The presence of multiple fetuses and fetal infections are two of the potential fetal factors for preterm labour. Interventions to prevent preterm labour include medications, intravenous fluids, and bed rest.

Third-Trimester Health Concerns

Choices of Birth Setting

In Canada, childbirth was gradually moved into hospital settings, starting in the early 1920s, and by 1950, approximately 76% of births occurred in hospitals (Mitchinson, 2002) because emergency backup was available in case of birth complications. Many hospitals have taken a family-centred approach to childbirth.

In some areas of the country, birthing centres are available for mothers who prefer a more homelike setting. Women delivering in this setting are required to attend childbirth classes, and the pregnancy must be considered low risk. Physicians and midwives with hospital privileges may attend births in these facilities. Mothers must understand that they may be transferred to a hospital if the conditions warrant.

A growing number of mothers choose to deliver at home when professional midwifery services are available. Control over the birth process and the desire for a more natural birth are common reasons why some mothers choose home births. Another reason is so that the entire family or other people close to the family can be part of the birth. Nurses can support the mother by offering information and resources to help her choose the birth setting.

early as possible, which may mean bringing the newborn to an ill parent or bringing the parents to an ill or premature child.

Bonding occurs when parents and newborn elicit reciprocal and complementary behaviour. Parental bonding behaviours include attentiveness and physical contact. Newborn bonding behaviour involves maintenance of physical contact with the parent. Preterm newborns, ill newborns, and ill mothers may have difficulty forming this bond if separation is prolonged; they need to be carefully assessed for any problems with attachment. The bonding process is further complicated if parents are unable to care for the infant. Nurses should give the parents support throughout the early bonding process, particularly if the newborn or mother is ill or if the newborn is separated from the parents.

The removal of nasopharyngeal and oropharyngeal secretions with suction or a bulb syringe ensures airway patency. Newborns are susceptible to heat loss and cold stress (Kliegman, Stanton, St. Geme, et al., 2016). Because hypothermia increases oxygen needs, the newborn's body temperature must be stabilized and maintained. The newborn may be placed directly on the mother's abdomen and covered in warm blankets; dried and wrapped in warm blankets, with the head well covered; or placed unclothed in an infant warmer with a temperature probe in place. For newborns unable to sustain adequate body temperature, isolettes and incubators, which supply radiant heat, are preferred.

Prevention of infection is a major concern in the care of the newborn, whose immune system is immature. Good hand hygiene technique is the most important factor in protecting the newborn and the nurse from infection. Once the blood and amniotic fluid have been removed from the infant's skin, the nurse does not need to wear cover gowns while providing care for the healthy newborn (Murray & McKinney, 2014). Other precautions include wearing gloves when touching mucous membranes or skin that is not intact (e.g., as a result of surgery or injury) and when drawing blood (e.g., heel stick).

The most commonly used prophylactic treatment against ophthalmic conjunctivitis is erythromycin (0.5%) because it prevents infections with *Neisseria gonorrhoeae* and other organisms, which can be transmitted during passage through an infected vaginal canal. This treatment should be applied during the newborn's initial assessment.

Vitamin K is administered in a single intramuscular injection shortly after birth. Vitamin K is important for the synthesis of prothrombin, necessary for clotting. Normally, the intestinal flora synthesizes vitamin K, and by about the third day, the infant should have enough intestinal flora to start to synthesize its vitamin K.

The stump of the moist umbilical cord is an excellent medium for bacterial growth. The cord should be cleansed with soap and water and dried at each diaper change. Until the stump dries and falls off, the diaper should be folded below the umbilicus to prevent accumulation of moisture.

NEWBORN

The neonatal period is the first month of life. During this stage, the newborn's physical functioning is mostly reflexive, and stabilization of the major organ systems is the body's primary task. Behaviour greatly influences interaction between the newborn and the environment and caregivers. For example, the average 2-week-old newborn may smile and is able to regard the mother's face. The effect of these reflexive behaviours is generally a surge of feelings of love that prompt the mother to cuddle the baby.

Nurses can apply their knowledge of this stage of growth and development to promote neonatal and parental health. If the nurse understands, for example, that the newborn's cry is usually a response to an unmet need (such as hunger), the nurse can assist parents in identifying ways to meet those needs, such as counselling the parents to feed their baby on demand rather than on a rigid schedule.

Physical Changes

A comprehensive nursing assessment is usually performed as soon as the newborn's physiological functioning is stable, generally within a few hours after birth. The infant's height, weight, head circumference, temperature, pulse, and respirations should be measured, and general appearance, body functions, sensory capabilities, reflexes, and responsiveness observed.

The average newborn weighs 3 400 g, is 50 cm in length, and has a head circumference of 35 cm. Up to 10% of birth weight is lost in the first few days after birth, primarily through fluid losses by respiration, urination, defecation, and low fluid intake. Birth weight is usually regained by the second week after birth, and a gradual pattern of increase in weight, height, and head circumference is evident. During the first month, weekly increases average 226 to 455 g in weight, 0.6 to 2.5 cm in length, and 2 cm in head circumference.

The newborn's heart rate ranges from 120 to 160 beats per minute. The average blood pressure is 85/54 mm Hg. The newborn's respiratory movements are primarily abdominal and vary in rate and rhythm, with an average rate of 30 to 60 breaths per minute. The axillary temperature ranges from 36°C to 37.5°C and generally stabilizes within 24 hours after birth.

Normal physical characteristics include the continued presence of lanugo on the skin of the back; cyanosis of the hands and feet for the first 24 hours; and a soft, protuberant abdomen. Skin colour varies according to racial and genetic heritage and gradually changes during infancy. **Moulding**, or overlapping of the soft skull bones, allows the fetal head to adjust to various diameters of the maternal pelvis and is a common occurrence with vaginal births. The bones readjust within a few days, producing a rounded appearance. The sutures and **fontanels** are usually palpable at birth. The diamond shape of the anterior fontanel and the triangular shape of the posterior fontanel between the unfused bones of the skull are shown in Figure 22-1.

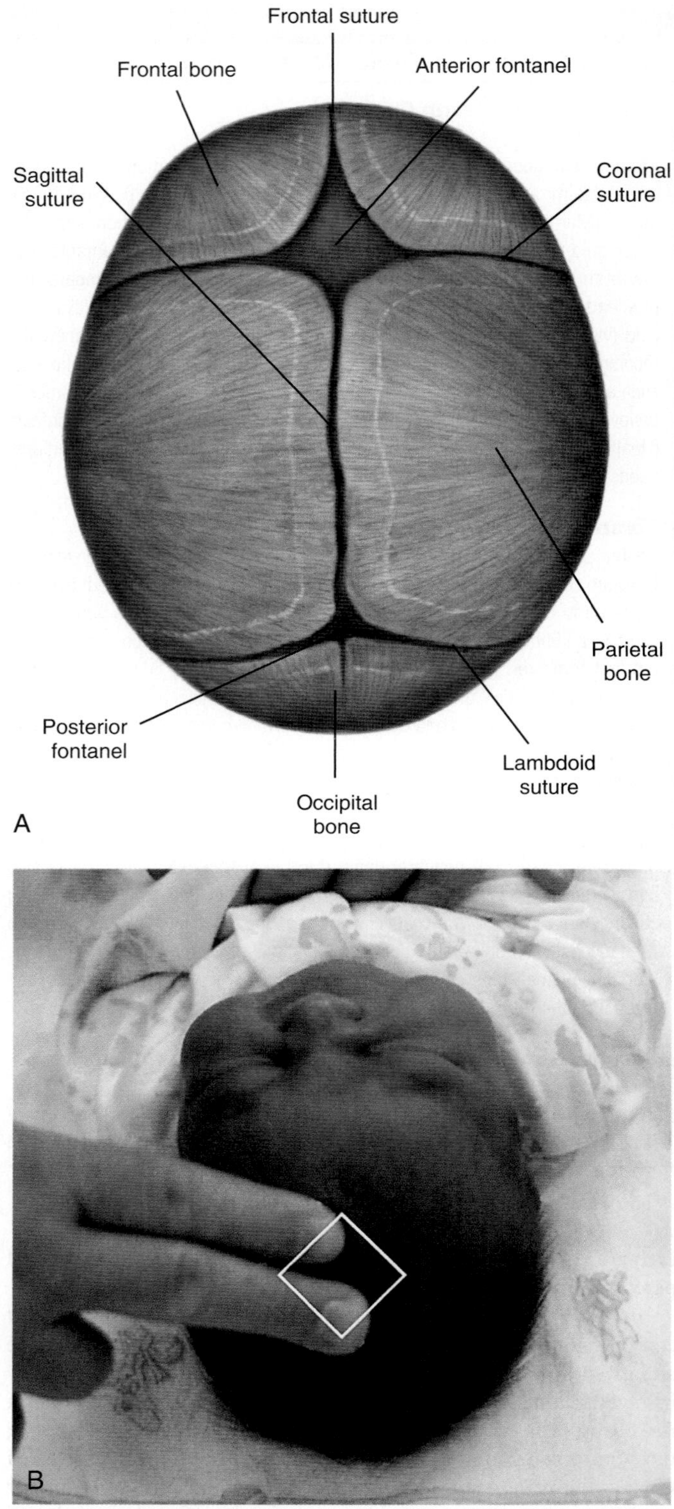

FIGURE 22-1 Fontanels and suture lines. (Adapted from Hockenberry, M. J., & Wilson, D. [2015]. *Wong's nursing care of infants and children* [10th ed., p. 261, Fig. 7-7]. St. Louis, MO: Mosby.)

To assess neurological function, the newborn's level of activity, alertness, irritability, responsiveness to stimuli, and reflexes should be observed. Normal reflexes include sucking, rooting, grasping, yawning, coughing, sneezing, hiccupping, blinking in response to bright lights, and startling (pulling arms and legs inward) in response to sudden,

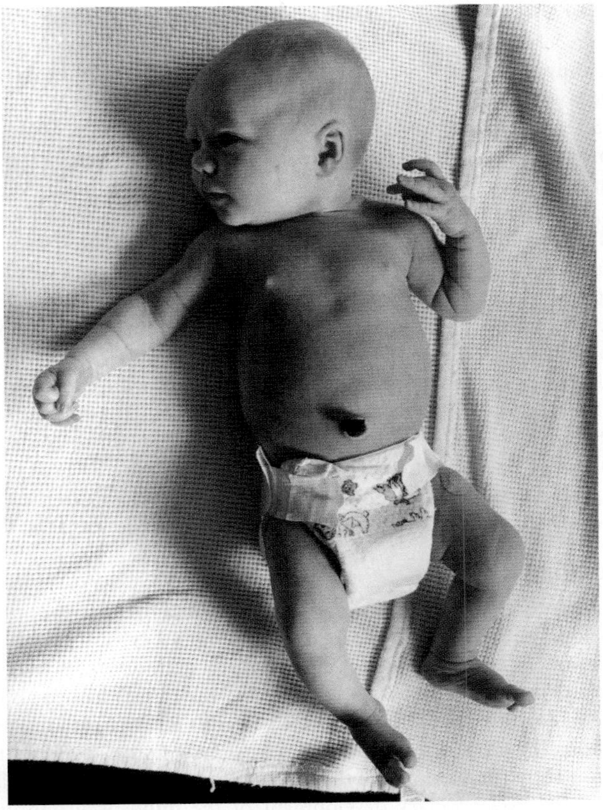

FIGURE 22-2 Tonic neck reflex. Newborns assume this position while supine. (From Hockenberry, M. J., & Wilson, D. [2015]. *Wong's nursing care of infants and children* [10th ed.]. St. Louis, MO: Mosby. Courtesy Paul Vincent Kuntz, Texas Children's Hospital.)

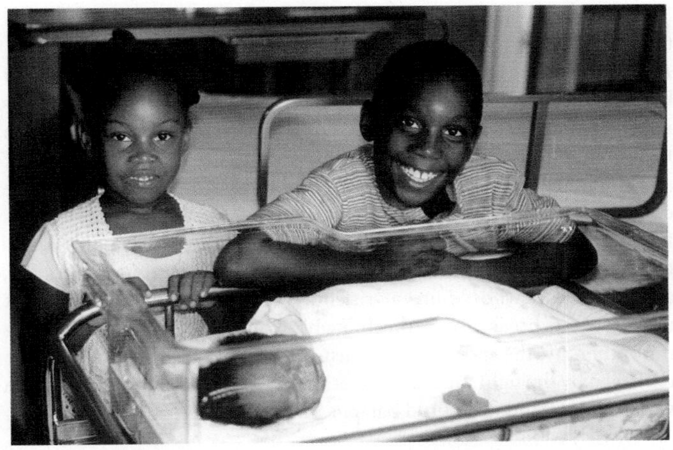

FIGURE 22-3 Older siblings with newborn. Siblings should be encouraged to visit with the newborn as soon as possible. (Courtesy Elaine Polan, RNC, BSN, MS.)

loud noises. An absence of any of these or other reflexes indicates prematurity, possible trauma, or central nervous system complications. Because the newborn depends largely on reflexes for survival and response to its environment, it is necessary to assess them. Figure 22-2 shows the tonic neck reflex: When newborns are lying supine, they reflexively turn the head to one side, extend the arm and leg on that side, and flex the opposite arm and leg.

Normal newborn behaviours include periods of sucking, crying, sleeping, and wakefulness. Movements are generally sporadic, but they are symmetrical and involve all four extremities. The relatively flexed fetal position of intrauterine life continues as the newborn attempts to maintain an enclosed, secure feeling. Newborns respond to sensory stimuli, particularly the primary caregiver's face, voice, and touch.

Except for the first hour after birth, when they are in a quietly alert state, newborns sleep almost continuously for the first 2 to 3 days to recover from the exhausting birth process. Thereafter, sleep periods vary from 20 minutes to 6 hours with little day–night differentiation.

Cognitive Changes

Early cognitive development begins with innate behaviour, reflexes, and sensory functions. Newborns initiate reflex activities and learn behaviours and desires. For example, newborns reflexively turn to the nipple (rooting) and learn that crying results in parents' response of feeding, diapering, and cuddling.

Sensory functions contribute to cognitive development in the newborn. At birth, children can fixate on moving objects about 20 to 25 cm from their faces (Hockenberry & Wilson, 2015). A preference for the human face is apparent. Auditory and vestibular (i.e., equilibrium) systems function from birth. These sensory capabilities allow newborns to elicit stimuli rather than simply receive them. Parents should be taught the importance of providing sensory stimulation, such as talking to their newborns and holding them to see their faces. This allows infants to seek or take in stimuli, thereby enhancing learning and promoting cognitive development.

Psychosocial Changes

During the first month of life, parents and newborns normally develop a strong bond that grows into a deep attachment. Interactions during routine care enhance or detract from the attachment process. The processes of feeding, changing, bathing, and comforting an infant promote interaction and provide a foundation for deep attachments. Early on, older siblings should have the opportunity to be involved with the newborn. Family involvement helps support growth and development and promotes nurturing (Figure 22-3).

If parents or newborns experience health complications after birth, bonding may be compromised. Infants' behavioural cues may be weak or absent, and caregiving may be less mutually satisfying. Tired, ill parents have difficulty interpreting and responding to their infants' cues. Children who have congenital anomalies are often too weak to be responsive to parental cues and require special supportive nursing care. For example, infants born with heart defects may tire easily during feedings. They may rest frequently after several bursts of sucking. They may awaken frequently, crying because they are hungry again. Mothers may think that they are inadequate as mothers or that the infants are being fussy. Both infants and mothers may feel frustrated. In this case, bonding is not enhanced and may even be reduced unless nursing intervention breaks the sequence of events.

For newborns, crying is a means of communication and provides cues to parents (Santrock, 2011). Although it can be a sign of distress, such as from pain, crying is an adaptive response to extrauterine life. Babies may cry because their diapers are wet, they are hungry, they want to be held, or they need a change in position or activity. Their crying may frustrate the parents if no cause is apparent. With help, parents can learn to recognize infants' cues and cry patterns and take appropriate action when necessary (Douglas, Miller, Bucetti, et al., 2015).

Health Risks

Hyperbilirubinemia is a condition in which an excessive amount of bilirubin accumulates in the blood, and it is characterized by a yellowish colouring of the skin, or jaundice. The accumulation occurs when the infant's immature liver is unable to balance the destruction of red blood cells with the use or excretion of by-products. The balance can be further upset by prematurity, inadequate intake during breastfeeding, excess production of bilirubin, certain disease states, or a disturbance in the liver. Bilirubin at high levels is highly toxic to neurons, and affected newborns are at risk for brain injury. Phototherapy is used to help break down the bilirubin for easier excretion. During phototherapy, the infant's eyes must be shielded because they can be damaged by the light. Because excretion of the extra bilirubin can cause watery stools, adequate fluid balance in the infant must be maintained.

Health Concerns

Screening. Screening tests and other laboratory tests should be coordinated as needed. Blood tests can determine inborn errors of metabolism. This term applies to genetic disorders caused by the absence or deficiency of a substance, usually an enzyme, essential to cellular metabolism that results in abnormal protein, carbohydrate, or fat metabolism. Although inborn errors of metabolism are rare, they account for a significant proportion of health problems in children. Neonatal screening can detect phenylketonuria (PKU), hypothyroidism, and galactosemia and thus allow appropriate treatment that can prevent permanent intellectual disability and other health problems. Routine screening of newborns for PKU is recommended (Kliegman et al., 2016). Other screening (e.g., for cystic fibrosis or hemophilia) may be necessary, depending on the family history.

Circumcision. Circumcision is "the surgical removal of some of the foreskin (prepuce) of the penis" (Kliegman et al., 2016, p. 890). It is controversial in this country and is not recommended as a routine procedure by the Canadian Paediatric Society (2015). The controversy surrounds the risks and benefits, especially with regard to pain control. Risks have been identified as hemorrhage, infection, adhesions, and meatal stenosis. Benefits include prevention of penile cancer, prevention of urinary tract infections, and preservation of male body image to be consistent with that of peers when circumcision is part of the culture (Hockenberry & Wilson, 2015). Parents must give informed consent before the procedure. Care of the circumcised site depends on the type of method used for the procedure. Circumcised newborns should be checked frequently for evidence of swelling, oozing, excessive bleeding, and the ability to void.

INFANT

Infancy, the period from 1 month to 1 year of age, is characterized by dramatic physical growth and change. Psychosocial development advances, and interactions between infants and the environment are greater and more meaningful. Infants who giggle and roll over in response to tickling are interacting more with their social environments than when they merely smile in response to a hug.

Physical Changes

Steady and proportional growth of the infant is more important than absolute growth values. The infant's growth can be compared with charts of normal age- and gender-related growth measurements. Using growth charts, nurses can also evaluate an infant's growth patterns by recording weight, length, and head circumference at selected intervals. Measurements recorded over time are the best way to monitor growth and identify problems. An infant with a growth problem may have measurements generally below the expected norms at all intervals or may experience an acute, brief interference with growth. An infant with a feeding problem or a genetic condition such as cystic fibrosis may have a weight below the expected norm.

Size increases rapidly during the first year; birth weight doubles in approximately 5 months and triples by 12 months. On average, weight gain is 680 g during the first 5 months and 340 g for months 7 to 12. Height increases an average of 2.5 cm during each of the first 6 months and 3.8 cm for the next 6 months. This 50% increase in birth height occurs primarily in the trunk, with the chest diameter approximating that of the head by the first birthday (Hockenberry & Wilson, 2015). The fontanels become smaller; the posterior fontanel closes at about 2 months.

Physiological functioning stabilizes, and by the end of the first year, the heart rate is 90 to 140 beats per minute, the blood pressure averages 95/65 mm Hg, and the respiratory rate is 30 to 35 breaths per minute. Patterns of body function also stabilize, as evidenced by predictable sleep, elimination, and feeding routines. Motor development proceeds steadily in a cephalocaudal direction (from the head toward the feet).

Cognitive Changes

The infant learns by experiencing and manipulating the environment. Developing motor skills and increasing mobility expand an infant's environment and, with developing visual and auditory skills, enhance cognitive development. For these reasons, Piaget (1952) named his first stage of cognitive development, which extends until around the third birthday, the sensorimotor period (see Chapter 21 for further information about developmental theories). Before the acquisition of language, the extraordinary development of the mind occurs through children's developing senses and motor abilities. Improved visual acuity and eye–hand coordination allow grasping and exploration of objects. In addition, rudimentary colour vision begins by age 2 months and improves throughout the first year, making the environment more interesting to see and explore. Infants' hearing also improves, allowing localization and discrimination of sounds.

Infants need opportunities to develop and use their senses. It is important to evaluate the appropriateness and adequacy of these opportunities. For example, ill or hospitalized infants may lack the energy to interact with their environments, and thus their cognitive development may be slowed. Infants need to be stimulated according to their temperament, energy, and age. Stimulation strategies can be used that maximize development of infants while conserving their energy and orientation. An example of this approach is talking to an infant and encouraging him or her to suck on a pacifier while administering a tube feeding.

Language. Speech is an important aspect of cognition that develops during the first year. Infants proceed from crying, cooing, and laughing to imitating sounds, comprehending the meaning of simple commands, and repeating words with knowledge of their meaning. By age 1 year, children recognize their own names and have two- or three-word vocabularies, usually including "Da-Da," "Ma-Ma," and "no." Nurses can promote language development by encouraging parents to name objects on which their infants' attention is focused.

Psychosocial Changes

Separation. During their first year, infants begin to differentiate themselves from other people, understanding that they are separate beings capable of acting on their own. Initially, infants are unaware of the boundaries of self, but through repeated experiences with the environment, they learn where the self ends and the external world begins. As infants determine their physical boundaries, they begin to respond to others.

At 2 or 3 months of age, infants begin to smile responsively rather than reflexively. Similarly, they can recognize differences in people when their sensory and cognitive capabilities improve. By 8 months, most infants can differentiate a stranger from a familiar person and respond differently to the two. Close attachment to the primary caregivers, most often parents, is usually established by this age. Infants seek out these people for support and comfort during times of stress. The ability to distinguish self from others allows children to interact and socialize within their environments. By age 9 months, for example, children play simple social games, such as patty-cake and peekaboo. More complex interactive games, such as hide-and-seek, involving objects, are possible by the age of 1 year. Erikson (1963) described the psychosocial developmental crisis for the infant as trust versus mistrust. If the infant's physical and emotional needs are met, then the infant begins to develop a sense of security (see Chapter 21 for further information about developmental theories).

Nurses should assess the availability and appropriateness of experiences contributing to psychosocial development. Hospitalized infants may have difficulty establishing physical boundaries because of repeated bodily intrusions and painful sensations. Limiting these negative experiences and providing pleasurable sensations are interventions that support early psychosocial development. Extended separations from parents complicate the bonding process and increase the number of caregivers with whom the infant must interact. Ideally, the parents should provide the majority of care during hospitalization. When parents are not present, an attempt should be made to limit the number of caregivers who have contact with the infant and to follow the parents' directions for care. These interventions will foster the infant's continuing development of trust.

Play. Play is a meaningful set of activities through which individuals interact with their environment and relate to others. Play provides opportunities for the infant to develop many motor skills. Much of infant play is exploratory, inasmuch as infants use their senses to observe and examine their own bodies and objects of interest in their surroundings. For example, placing their toes in their mouths provides infants with pleasure and information about their own body and helps form their early self-concept. Play becomes manipulative as children learn control of the hands. Adults can facilitate infant learning by planning activities that promote the development of milestones and by providing toys that are safe for infants to explore with the mouth and manipulate with the hands, such as rattles, blocks, stacking rings, and washable stuffed animals. Infants most frequently engage in solitary (one-sided) play, but they do enjoy watching others, particularly siblings. Infants need to be played with and stimulated through interactions with others.

Health Risks

Sudden Infant Death Syndrome. Sudden infant death syndrome (SIDS) is the sudden and unexpected death of an apparently healthy infant. SIDS is rare before 1 month of age, but its incidence peaks among infants between 2 and 4 months of age, and it can occur in infants up to a year old. Other terms for SIDS include sudden unexplained infant death (SUID) and sudden unexpected death in infancy (SUDI). SIDS is the main cause of death for babies between 1 and 12 months of age (Canadian Foundation for the Study of Infant Deaths: Baby's Breath Canada, 2015). The cause of SIDS is not understood, but the Public Health Agency of Canada (PHAC) (2014a) recommends the following precautions:

- Infants should sleep on their backs on a firm, flat surface alone (i.e., sharing any sleeping surface with another person is hazardous to the infant).
- A smoke-free environment should be provided before and after birth.
- A baby's crib must be free of such clutter as toys, bumper pads, pillows, blankets, and other loose bedding.
- The crib should be placed next to the adult's bed for the first 6 months.
- The infant should be dressed lightly to avoid overheating.
- Mothers should breastfeed if possible.

In research studies, the following maternal and antenatal risk factors were associated with a higher risk of SIDS: smoking, alcohol and illicit drug use, inadequate prenatal care, nutritional deficiency, low socioeconomic status, younger age, lower education, single marital status, shorter interpregnancy interval, intrauterine hypoxia, fetal growth restriction, and elevated second-trimester serum α-fetoprotein (Kliegman et al., 2016; Task Force on Sudden Infant Death Syndrome [SIDS], 2016). Infant risk factors included age (peak 2–4 months), male gender, race and ethnicity (Black, Indigenous, and other minorities), growth failure, no breastfeeding, no pacifier use, prematurity, prone and side sleep position, recent febrile illness, inadequate immunizations, smoking exposure, soft sleeping surface and/or bedding, bed sharing, thermal stress, overheating, colder season, and no central heating (Kliegman et al., 2016; Task Force on SIDS, 2016).

Accidental Injury. Injury is a major cause of death in children 6 to 12 months old. An understanding of the major developmental accomplishments during this period helps nurses plan for injury prevention. Box 22-3 lists the main types of injuries occurring in this age group and possible prevention strategies.

Child Maltreatment. As a nurse, you need to be aware that child maltreatment can occur during any stage of a child's life, beginning in infancy. *Child maltreatment* refers to violence, emotional or sexual mistreatment, or neglect of a child or adolescent. More children suffer from neglect than from any other type of maltreatment. Many suffer from more than one type of child maltreatment. In Canada, there are 14 confirmed cases of child abuse and neglect for every 1 000 children (Canadian Child Welfare Research Portal, 2011). Protection of children from maltreatment comes under the jurisdiction of a province or territory. If you suspect any type of maltreatment of children, you are legally required to report it. Document the location and a detailed description of all injuries, and include diagrams and photographs of the injuries using a measurement tool (Hockenberry & Wilson, 2015). Box 22-4 includes possible signs and symptoms of child maltreatment. These indications apply to children from infancy through adolescence.

A combination of signs and symptoms or a pattern of injury should arouse suspicion. It is important for you to be aware of certain birthmarks (e.g., Mongolian spots, which are flat, dark birthmarks that may look like bruises) and cultural practices (e.g., coining, in which the skin is rubbed or scratched with a coin to improve circulation or restore balance) that may mimic signs of maltreatment.

Health Concerns

Nutrition. The quality and quantity of nutrition influence the infant's growth and development. Nurses need to help parents select a nutritionally adequate diet for their infant. Nutrition is affected by many variables (e.g., culture, food preferences, slow eating, or food allergies), and no diet is effective for all children or for one age group.

Feeding Alternatives. Supplying essential nutrients to the infant is an important goal for parents. Nurses can support the parents' choice of feeding methods and facilitate a successful feeding process (Box 22-5). Canadian researchers have demonstrated the need for nurses to initiate and facilitate a discussion with parents regarding breastfeeding and their experiences of breastfeeding (Benoit, Goldberg, &

BOX 22-3 Injury Prevention During Infancy

Age: Birth to 4 Months

Major Developmental Accomplishments

Involuntary reflexes, such as the crawling reflex, may propel the infant forward or backward, and the startle reflex may cause the body to jerk.
The infant may roll over.
Eye–hand coordination improves, and the voluntary grasp reflex increases.

Injury Prevention

Aspiration

Aspiration is not as great a danger in this age group as in others, but caregivers should begin to practise safeguarding early (see "Age: 4 to 7 Months" section).
Hold the infant for bottle feeding; do not prop the bottle.
Know emergency procedures for choking.
Use pacifiers with one-piece construction and loop handle.

Suffocation and Drowning

Keep all plastic bags stored out of the infant's reach; discard large plastic garment bags after tying them in a knot.
Do not cover the infant's mattress with plastic.
Use a firm mattress; use no pillows or loose bedding.
Make sure crib design follows federal regulations and the mattress fits snugly; crib slats should be no farther than 6 cm apart. Do not use a drop-side crib.
Position the crib away from other furniture and away from radiators.
Do not tie a pacifier on a string around the infant's neck.
Remove bibs at bedtime.
Never leave the infant alone in a bath.
If the infant is younger than 12 months, do not leave him or her alone on an adult- or youth-sized mattress or on "beanbag"-type pillows.

Falls

Use a crib with fixed, raised rails.
Never leave the infant on a raised, unguarded surface.
When in doubt as to where to place the child, use the floor.
Restrain the child in an infant seat, and never leave him or her unattended while the seat is resting on a raised surface.
Avoid using a high chair until the child can sit well with support.

Poisoning

Poisoning is not as great a danger in this age group as in others, but caregivers should begin to practise safeguards early (see "Age: 4 to 7 Months" section).

Burns

Install smoke detectors in the home.
Avoid warming formula in a microwave oven; always check temperature of liquid before feeding.
Check bath water temperature.
Do not pour hot liquids when the infant is close by (e.g., sitting on lap).
Do not smoke cigarettes around the child.
Do not leave infant in the sun for more than a few minutes; keep exposed areas covered.
Wash flame-retardant clothes according to label directions.
Use cool-mist (rather than hot-mist) vaporizers.
Do not leave the child in a parked car.
Check the surface heat of the car restraint before placing the child in it.

Motor Vehicles

Transport the infant in a federally approved, rear-facing infant seat, in the back seat* (Figure 22-4).
Do not place infant on seat of car or in lap.
Never place an infant seat in the front passenger seat with an air bag.*
Do not place the child in a carriage or stroller behind a parked car.
Do not leave infant in a vehicle on a warm day.

Bodily Damage

Keep sharp, jagged objects out of child's reach.
Keep diaper pins closed and away from the infant.
Never shake a baby (which can cause shaken baby syndrome); advise caregivers to seek help if they feel irritated or overwhelmed by a baby's crying.

Age: 4 to 7 Months

Major Developmental Accomplishments

The infant rolls over.
The infant sits momentarily.
The infant grasps and manipulates small objects.
The infant picks up a dropped object.
The infant has well-developed eye–hand coordination.
The infant can focus on and locate very small objects.
The infant's tendency to put objects in his or her mouth is very prominent.
The infant can push up on hands and knees.
The infant crawls backward.

Injury Prevention

Aspiration

Keep buttons, beads, syringe caps, and other small objects out of the infant's reach.
Keep the floor free of any small objects.
Do not feed the infant hard candy, nuts, food with pits or seeds, or whole or circular pieces of hot dog.
Exercise caution when giving the infant teething biscuits, because large chunks may be broken off and aspirated.
Do not feed the infant while he or she is lying down.
Inspect toys for removable parts.

Suffocation

Keep all latex balloons out of the child's reach.
Remove all crib toys that are strung across the crib or playpen when the child begins to push up on hands or knees or is 5 months old.
Use only cribs with well-secured crib sides; do not use a drop-side cribs.

Falls

Restrain the child in a high chair.
Do not use baby walkers (baby walkers are no longer sold in or imported to Canada because of the high rate of injuries that they cause).

Poisoning

Make sure that paint for furniture or toys does not contain lead.
Hang plants, or place them on high surfaces rather than on the floor.
Store coinlike batteries and any toxic substances, such as cleaning fluid, paints, and pesticides, out of the reach of babies, on a high shelf or in a locked cabinet.
Discard used containers of poisonous substances.
Do not store toxic substances in food containers.
Store medication in a locked cabinet and keep cosmetic and personal products out of the child's reach.
Know the telephone number of the local poison control centre and add it to contacts list on mobile phone (usually listed in the beginning of telephone directories).

BOX 22-3 Injury Prevention During Infancy—cont'd

Burns

Keep faucets out of reach.
Place hot objects (candles, incense) on high surfaces.
Limit the child's exposure to sun; apply sunscreen.

Motor Vehicles

See "Age: Birth to 4 Months" section.

Bodily Damage

Give the child toys that are smooth and rounded, preferably made of natural wood or plastic.
Avoid long, pointed objects as toys.
Avoid toys that are excessively loud.
Keep sharp objects out of the infant's reach.
See also the "Age: Birth to 4 Months" section.

Age: 8 to 12 Months

Major Developmental Accomplishments

The child crawls and creeps.
The child stands, holding on to furniture.
The child stands alone.
The child cruises around furniture.
The child walks.
The child climbs.
The child pulls on objects.
The child throws objects.
The child is able to pick up small objects and has pincer grasp.
The child explores objects by putting them in his or her mouth.
The child dislikes being restrained.
The child explores away from parents.
The child's understanding of simple commands and phrases increases.

Injury Prevention

Aspiration

Keep lint and small objects off the floor, off furniture, and out of reach of children.
Take care in feeding solid table food to give very small pieces.
Do not use beanbag toys or allow the child to play with dried beans.
See also the "Age: 4 to 7 Months" section.

Suffocation and Drowning

Keep doors of appliances (ovens, dishwashers, refrigerators, coolers, and front-loading clothes washers and dryers) closed at all times.
If storing an unused appliance, such as a refrigerator, remove the door.
Supervise contact with inflated balloons; immediately discard popped balloons, and keep uninflated balloons out of children's reach.
Fence in swimming pools.
Always supervise the child when near any source of water, such as baths, cleaning buckets, drainage areas, and toilets.
Keep bathroom doors closed.
Eliminate unnecessary pools of water.
When swimming, keep child within arm's reach at all times.
Keep one hand on the child at all times when he or she is in the tub.

Falls

Gate the stairways at the top and bottom if the child has access to either end.
Dress the child in safe shoes (soles that do not "catch" on the floor, tied shoelaces) and clothing (pant legs that do not touch the floor).
Ensure that furniture is sturdy enough for the child to hold while pulling himself or herself to a standing position and cruising.

Poisoning

Never call medications "candy."
Avoid use of over-the-counter cough and cold preparations for infants.
Do not administer medications unless they are prescribed by a practitioner.
Put away medications and poisons immediately after use; put child-protector caps on properly.
Keep phone number for poison control centre readily available.

Burns

Place guards in front of or around any heating appliance, fireplace, or furnace.
Keep electrical wires hidden or out of the child's reach.
Place plastic guards over electrical outlets; place furniture in front of outlets.
Keep hanging tablecloths out of reach (the child may pull down hot liquids or heavy or sharp objects).

*Further information is available from Transport Canada (2017) and Health Canada (2012).
Adapted from Hockenberry, M. J., & Wilson, D. (2015). *Wong's nursing care of infants and children* (10th ed., pp. 443–444). St. Louis, MO: Mosby.

Campbell-Yeo, 2016). Since promotion of breastfeeding can contribute to maternal guilt, nurses need to develop a respectful, collaborative partnership with mothers when promoting breastfeeding, to minimize feelings of guilt (Benoit et al., 2016). Breastfeeding is considered the most complete nutritional source until the infant is about 6 months of age. Breast milk contains protein, fats, and carbohydrates, as well as immunoglobulins that bolster the infant's ability to resist infection. Breastfeeding has been associated with enhanced cognitive development and mother–infant bonding and a decreased frequency of respiratory tract illnesses, SIDS, type 1 and 2 diabetes, childhood leukemia, obesity, gastroenteritis, necrotizing enterocolitis, otitis media, atopic dermatitis, food allergies, and childhood internalizing behaviour problems (Hockenberry & Wilson, 2015; Kliegman et al., 2016; Liu, Leung, & Yang, 2013; PHAC, 2014b).

If breastfeeding is not possible or it is not desired by the parent, an acceptable alternative is commercially prepared formula that is fortified with iron. Formulas contain standard ingredients and are fortified with vitamins and minerals. Cow's milk and imitation milks are not recommended in the first year, because infants are not able to properly digest the contained fat. Cow's milk also contains more sodium and protein and less iron and essential nutrients than does formula (Hockenberry & Wilson, 2015). Because cow's milk has low levels of iron and high levels of calcium and phosphorus, absorption of iron may be decreased, causing anemia.

The average 1-month-old infant takes in approximately 540 to 630 mL of breast milk or formula per day. This amount increases slightly during the first 6 months and decreases when solid foods are introduced. The amount of formula per feeding and the number of feedings vary among infants.

Developmentally, infants are not ready for solid food until 6 months of age. Before 6 months, the infant's gastrointestinal tract cannot handle the complex nutrients in solid food, and the extrusion reflex causes food to be pushed out of the mouth. Also, early introduction to solid foods may cause food allergies.

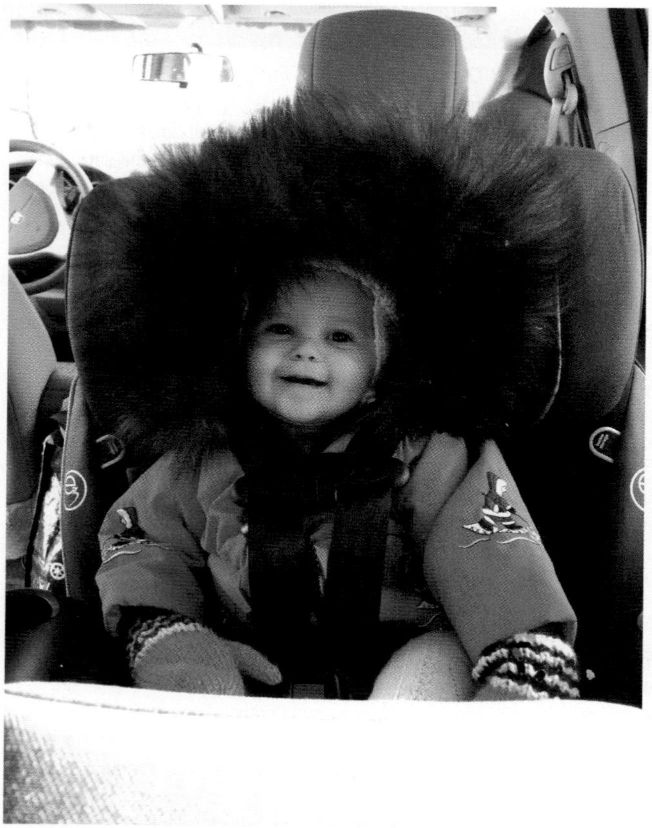

FIGURE 22-4 Federally approved infant car restraint. Note that the seat is rear facing in the back seat. (Courtesy Cynthia Murray, BN, MN, PhD.)

Cereals and well-cooked and puréed fruits, vegetables, and meats eaten during the second 6 months of life provide iron and additional sources of vitamins. These nutrients become especially important when infants stop consuming breast milk or formula and begin drinking whole cow's milk after the first birthday. Because the amount and frequency of feedings vary among infants, it is important to discuss differing feeding patterns with parents.

Honey has been used to sweeten water and coat pacifiers. However, honey should not be given to infants younger than 1 year because of the potential for infant botulism poisoning (Kliegman et al., 2016).

Supplementation. The need for dietary vitamin and mineral supplements depends on the infant's diet. Full-term infants are born with some iron stores. The breastfed infant absorbs adequate iron from breast milk during the first 4 to 6 months of life. After age 6 months, iron-fortified cereal is generally considered an adequate supplemental source. Because iron in formula is less readily absorbed than that in breast milk, formula-fed infants should receive iron-fortified formula throughout the first year. All Canadian infants who are breastfed need to receive a daily 400 IU vitamin D supplement to prevent rickets (PHAC, 2014b).

Adequate concentrations of fluoride to protect against dental caries are not available in human milk, so fluoridated water or supplemental fluoride is generally recommended. The presence of fluoride in formula depends on the type of formula and the source of water used in preparing the concentrated forms. Fluoride supplementation may be necessary.

Overfeeding and Infant Obesity. The association between overfeeding, infant obesity, and later adult obesity is controversial. However, early feeding experiences can influence later eating habits. Nurses should therefore emphasize balanced nutrition and good dietary habits, developed through feeding experiences that are mutually satisfying for parents and infant. Eating habits are frequently affected by the family's sociocultural background. Because some cultures consider an overweight baby to be a sign of good mothering, any suggestion to limit intake or slow weight gain may be seen as a threat. It is important for nurses to acquire an understanding of cultural influences in order to develop effective nursing interventions. For example, breastfeeding is associated with a reduced risk of childhood obesity, but some cultural beliefs may promote formula feeding. A traditional belief in the Somali culture is that breast milk spoils in the breast after several hours (Steinman, Doescher, Keppel, et al., 2009). Nurses working with pregnant or new mothers with a Somali cultural background need to educate these women and the Somali community about breastfeeding to counteract the cultural myth.

Dentition. The average age at which the first tooth erupts is 7 months, but considerable variation exists among infants because of their genetic endowment. Occasionally, an infant is born with a tooth, whereas others remain toothless at 1 year. The order of tooth eruption is fairly predictable: the lower central incisors are first to appear, closely followed by the upper central incisors. Most 1-year-olds have six teeth.

Teething may result in considerable discomfort for some infants and little or none for others. The inflammation of the gums before the tooth emerges may result in a low-grade fever and irritability. Some infants exhibit increased drooling, biting, or finger sucking. Biting on a frozen teething ring or ice cube wrapped in a washcloth may be soothing. Over-the-counter teething medications to rub on the inflamed gums and appropriate doses of acetaminophen are helpful when the infant is irritable and has difficulty eating or sleeping.

Most dentists recommend that parents cleanse their infant's teeth after each feeding. The parent can place a clean, wet washcloth or piece of gauze over a finger and use it to wipe the infant's teeth. Because of the risk of developing dental caries, prolonged breast- or bottle-feeding is discouraged, especially just before the infant goes to sleep because the infant is likely to leave milk in the mouth and around the teeth. The infant should never go to bed with a bottle of juice or milk (Kliegman et al., 2016).

Immunizations. The widespread use of immunizations has resulted in the dramatic decline of infectious diseases since the 1950s and is therefore an important factor in health promotion during childhood. Although most immunizations can be given to people of any age, the PHAC (2016a) recommended that the administration of the primary series begin soon after birth and be completed during early childhood. The Canadian national immunization guidelines for infants and children are presented in Table 22-2. However, publicly funded immunization schedules vary from province to province or territory. Therefore, nurses must know the specific immunization schedule for their jurisdiction. The PHAC (2015) maintains an online tool where parents can create a personal immunization schedule for their child based on age and provincial or territorial residence. Parents must receive instructions regarding the potential adverse effects of immunizations. Minor adverse effects may occur, but serious reactions are rare. High fever and extreme irritability should be reported to the health care provider.

As a result of complacency and fear regarding the adverse effects of certain vaccines, especially diphtheria and tetanus toxoids and pertussis vaccine (DTP), not all children receive appropriate immunizations (Hoekstra & Margolis, 2016). An important role for you as a nurse is to discuss the importance of vaccination for infants and children, provide up-to-date information to parents, and encourage

BOX 22-4 Clinical Manifestations of Potential Child Maltreatment

Physical Neglect

Suggestive Physical Findings

Failure to thrive (infants), signs of malnutrition (e.g., unhealthy looking skin and hair, sunken eyes or cheeks), evidence of poor health care (e.g., delayed immunization)
Poor personal hygiene, especially of teeth; unclean or inappropriate dress
Frequent injuries resulting from lack of supervision

Suggestive Behaviours

Dull and inactive (infants)
Self-stimulatory behaviours, such as finger sucking or rocking
Begging or stealing food, vandalism, or shoplifting
Absenteeism from school
Substance abuse in older children

Emotional Maltreatment and Neglect

Suggestive Physical Findings

Failure to thrive
Feeding disorders, such as rumination
Enuresis (bed wetting after toilet training has been established)
Sleep disorders

Suggestive Behaviours

Self-stimulatory behaviours such as biting, rocking, sucking
Stranger anxiety and lack of social smile (infants)
Withdrawal and unusual fearfulness
Antisocial behaviour, such as destructiveness, stealing, cruelty
Extremes of behaviour, such as overcompliance, passivity, aggressiveness, or being demanding
Lags in emotional and intellectual development, especially language
Suicide attempts

Physical Maltreatment

Suggestive Physical Findings

Bruises and welts on face, lips, mouth, back, buttocks, thighs, or areas of torso
Regular patterns on skin that are descriptive of certain objects, such as belt buckle; hand; wire hanger; chain; wooden spoon; squeeze or pinch marks; round cigar or cigarette burns; burns in the shape of an iron, radiator, or electric stove burner
Burns, injuries, fractures, lacerations, or bruises in various stages of healing on soles of feet, palms of hands, back, or buttocks
Presence of symmetrical burns in the absence of "splash" marks
Unusual symptoms, such as abdominal swelling, pain, and vomiting from punching
Marks such as those resembling human bites, or pulling out of hair
Unexplained repeated poisoning or unexplained sudden illness

Suggestive Behaviours

Wariness of physical contact with adults
Apparent fear of parents or of going home
Lying very still while surveying environment, lack of reaction to frightening events
Inappropriate reaction to injury, such as failure to cry from pain
Apprehensiveness when hearing other children cry
Indiscriminate friendliness and displays of affection, superficial relationships
Acting-out behaviour, attention-seeking behaviours
Withdrawn behaviour

Sexual Maltreatment

Suggestive Physical Findings

Bruises, bleeding, lacerations, or irritation of external genitalia, anus, mouth, or throat
Torn, stained, or bloody underclothing
Pain on urination or pain, swelling, and itching of genital area; penile discharge; unusual odour in the genital area
Sexually transmitted infection, nonspecific vaginitis, venereal warts, or presence of sperm
Difficulty in walking or sitting
Recurrent urinary tract infections
Pregnancy in a young adolescent

Suggestive Behaviours

Sudden emergence of sexually related problems, including excessive or public masturbation, age-inappropriate sexual play, promiscuity, or overtly seductive behaviour
Withdrawn behaviour, excessive daydreaming, preoccupation with fantasies, especially in play
Poor relationships with peers
Sudden changes, such as anxiety, loss or gain of weight, clinging behaviour
In incestuous relationships, a child's excessive anger at one parent for not protecting the child from the other parent
Regressive behaviour, such as bed-wetting or thumb-sucking
Sudden onset of phobias or fears, particularly fears of the dark, men, strangers, or particular settings or situations (e.g., undue fear of leaving the house, of staying at the day care centre, or of staying at the babysitter's house)
Running away from home
Substance abuse, particularly of alcohol or mood-elevating drugs
Profound and rapid personality changes, especially extreme depression, hostility, and aggression (often accompanied by social withdrawal)
Rapidly declining school performance
Suicidal attempts or ideation about suicide

Adapted from Hockenberry, M. J., & Wilson, D. (2015). *Wong's nursing care of infants and children* (10th ed., p. 562). St. Louis, MO: Mosby.

them to make an informed decision for their children. General contraindications to vaccination include moderate illness; allergic response to a previous dose of a particular vaccine; and, with live vaccines only, pregnancy, immunosuppression, and taking high doses of corticosteroids.

Sleep. Sleep patterns vary among infants, many having their days and nights "mixed up" until 3 to 4 months of age. By that age, most infants sleep between 9 and 11 hours a night. Total daily sleep averages 15 hours. Most infants take one or two naps a day by the end of the first year. Sleep disturbances with a physiological basis are rare, with the possible exception of colic. Common sleep disturbances among infants are described in Table 22-3.

TODDLER

Toddlerhood ranges from 12 to 36 months. Toddlers have increasing independence, physical mobility, and cognitive abilities. Toddlers become aware of their abilities to control their environments and are pleased with successful efforts. This success leads them to continue attempting to control their environments. Unsuccessful attempts at

BOX 22-5 RESEARCH HIGHLIGHT

Breastfeeding

Research Focus

Fathers are a key source of breastfeeding support. Nurses can play an important role in promoting breastfeeding by including fathers in breastfeeding education and interventions.

Research Abstract

Rempel and Rempel (2011) explored the role of involved fathers in breastfeeding families. The qualitative study was performed with a small sample of fathers ($n = 21$) in two regions of Ontario. The researchers found that the fathers viewed breastfeeding as a team endeavour. The fathering role consisted of supporting breastfeeding by becoming breastfeeding savvy, using their knowledge of breastfeeding to encourage and assist mothers in breastfeeding, valuing the breastfeeding mothers, and sharing housework and child care. The researchers concluded that nurses and other health care providers need to assist fathers in recognizing their unique contributions to the breastfeeding team.

Evidence-Informed Practice

- Assess the breastfeeding support of new mothers.
- Include the mother's partner in supporting and offering praise to the breastfeeding mother.
- Include fathers in breastfeeding education and interventions.
- Promote the unique role of the father on the breastfeeding team.

Rempel, L. A., & Rempel, J. K. (2011). The breastfeeding team: The role of involved fathers in the breastfeeding family. *Journal of Human Lactation, 27,* 115–121. doi:10.1177/0890334410390045.

control may result in the toddler refusing to do something, saying no frequently, or engaging in temper tantrums.

Physical Changes

The rapid development of motor skills allows toddlers to participate in self-care activities, such as feeding, dressing, and toileting. Initially, toddlers walk with a broad stance and gait, protuberant abdomen, and arms out to the sides for balance. Soon they begin to navigate stairs, using a rail or the wall to maintain balance. Locomotion skills eventually include running, jumping, standing on one foot for several seconds, and kicking a ball. Most toddlers can ride tricycles, climb ladders, and run well by their third birthday.

Fine motor capabilities move from scribbling spontaneously to drawing circles and crosses accurately. By age 3 years, children draw simple stick people and can usually stack a tower of small blocks. Increased locomotion skills, the ability to undress, and development of sphincter control allow toilet training if a toddler has developed the necessary language and cognitive abilities. Parents often consult nurses for an assessment of readiness for toilet training. A child's recognition of the urge to urinate and defecate is a crucial component in the child's mental readiness. At this stage, children usually show a willingness to please parents and take pride in their accomplishments (Santrock, 2011). Nurses must remind parents that patience, consistency, and a nonjudgemental attitude, in addition to child readiness, are essential for successful toilet training.

The cardiopulmonary system becomes stable in the toddler years. The heart and respiratory rates slow to an average of 110 beats and 25 breaths per minute, respectively, and the blood pressure varies slightly from infancy. The average blood pressure in toddlers is 90/50 mm Hg.

The anterior fontanel closes between 12 and 18 months of age, ending the period of the most rapid growth of the skull and brain. However, head circumference should be measured routinely until a toddler is 3 years of age.

The rate of increase in a toddler's weight and length slows. By age 2.5 years, children's weights are four times the birth weight. Height during the toddler years increases by approximately 7.5 cm a year, mainly as a result of increases in leg length. The average height of 2-year-olds is 85 cm. Slowed growth rates are accompanied by decreased caloric need, and smaller food intake leads some parents to worry about the adequacy of dietary intake. Parents need encouragement to offer appropriate servings of food, as recommended from *Eating Well With Canada's Food Guide* (Health Canada, 2011b), and to avoid force-feeding or allowing children to fill up on foods that have high levels of fat and sugar. Nurses can reassure parents that a child's nutrition is adequate by demonstrating the child's satisfactory status on a growth chart.

Cognitive Changes

Toddlers' completion of the development of object permanence, their ability to remember events, and their beginning ability to put thoughts into words at about 2 years of age signal their transition to Piaget's (1952) preoperational thought stage of cognitive development (see Chapter 21 for further information about development). Toddlers recognize that they are separate beings from their mothers, but they are unable to assume another person's point of view. They use symbols to represent objects, places, and people. This function is demonstrated when children imitate the behaviour of another person that they viewed earlier (e.g., pretend to shave like daddy), pretend one object is another (e.g., pretend that a doll is a baby), and use language to stand for absent objects (e.g., request a bottle).

Language. An 18-month-old child uses approximately 50 words (Santrock, 2011). A 24-month-old child has a vocabulary of up to 200 words and is generally able to speak in two-word sentences. "Who's that?" and "What's that?" typify questions asked during this period. First-person expressions such as "Me do it" and "That's mine" demonstrate 2-year-old children's use of pronouns and desire for independence and control. Despite the expanded vocabulary of older toddlers, the word they use most often is *no* until well into the third year. Offering choices to toddlers helps reduce their sense of frustration and builds their sense of independence (Santrock, 2011).

Because children's moral development is closely associated with their cognitive abilities, the moral development of toddlers is only beginning and is also egocentric. Toddlers do not understand concepts of right and wrong. However, they understand that some behaviours bring pleasant results and others elicit unpleasant results. Therefore, until toddlers achieve a higher level of cognitive function, they behave simply to avoid the unpleasant and seek out the pleasant (Hockenberry & Wilson, 2015).

Psychosocial Changes

According to Erikson (1963), a sense of autonomy emerges during the toddler years (see Chapter 21 for the developmental stages). Children strive for independence by using their developing muscles to do everything for themselves and control their bodily functions. Their strong wills are frequently exhibited in negative behaviour when caregivers attempt to direct their actions; for example, temper tantrums may result when toddlers are frustrated by parental restrictions. Parents need to provide toddlers with graded independence, allowing them to do things that do not result in harm to themselves or others. This strategy prevents them from doubting their abilities or feeling a sense of shame for what they have done. Firm consistent limits, patience, and support allow toddlers to develop socially acceptable behaviour and cope with the frustration of learning self-control (Santrock, 2011).

TABLE 22-2 Canadian Routine Childhood Immunization Schedule, Infants and Children (Birth to 17 Years of Age)

Vaccine*	Birth	2 mos	4 mos	6 mos	12 mos	15 mos	18 mos	23 mos	2 yrs	4 yrs	5 yrs	6 yrs	9 yrs	12 yrs	14 yrs	15 yrs	16 yrs	17 yrs
DTaP-IPV-Hib or DTaP-HB-IPV-Hib		A or B first dose	A or B second dose	A or B third dose	A or B fourth dose Generally at 18 months of age													
DTaP-IPV or Tdap-IPV										C								
Tdap															D			
Rot		E 2 or 3 doses Complete series before 8 months																
Pneu-C-13		F			F													
Men-C-C		G According to P/T schedule			G Generally at 12 months													
Men-C-C or Men-C-ACYW														H				
MMR and Var					I + J		I + J											
								OR										
MMRV					K		K Generally at 4-6 years											
HB	L 3 doses																	
								OR										
HB													M 2 or 3 doses					
HPV													N 2 or 3 doses					
								OR										
HPV																O 3 doses		
Inf				P 1 or 2 doses Recommended annually										P 1 dose Recommended annually				

A **Diphtheria toxoid–tetanus toxoid–acellular pertussis–inactivated polio–*Haemophilus influenzae* type b** (DTaP-IPV-Hib). For infants and children beginning primary immunization at 7 months of age and older, the number of doses of Hib vaccine required varies by age.

B **Diphtheria toxoid–tetanus toxoid–acellular pertussis–hepatitis B–inactivated polio–*Haemophilus influenzae* type b** (DTaP-HB-IPV-Hib). Alternative schedules may be used: DTaP-HB-IPV-Hib at 2, 4, and 12–23 months of age with DTaP-IPV-Hib vaccine at 6 months of age; or DTaP-HB-IPV-Hib at 2, 4, and 6 months of age with DTaP-IPV-Hib vaccine at 12–23 months of age.

Continued

TABLE 22-2 Canadian Routine Childhood Immunization Schedule, Infants and Children (Birth to 17 Years of Age)—cont'd

Vaccine*	Birth 2 mos 4 mos 6 mos 12 mos 15 mos 18 mos 23 mos 2 yrs 4 yrs 5 yrs 6 yrs 9 yrs 12 yrs 14 yrs 15 yrs 16 yrs 17 yrs
C	**Diphtheria toxoid–tetanus toxoid–acellular pertussis–inactivated polio** (DTaP-IPV) or **tetanus toxoid–reduced diphtheria toxoid–reduced acellular pertussis–inactivated polio** (Tdap-IPV).
D	**Tetanus toxoid–reduced diphtheria toxoid–reduced acellular pertussis** (Tdap). 10 years after last dose of DTaP- or Tdap-containing vaccine.
E	**Rotavirus** (Rot). Rotavirus pentavalent vaccine: 3 doses, 4 to 10 weeks apart; Rotavirus monovalent vaccine: 2 doses, at least 4 weeks apart. Give the first dose starting at 6 weeks and before 15 weeks of age. Administer all doses before 8 months of age.
F	**Pneumococcal conjugate 13-valent** (Pneu-C-13). Healthy infants beginning primary immunization at 2–6 months of age: 3- or 4-dose schedule. For a 3-dose schedule: 2, 4 months of age, followed by a booster dose at 12 months of age. For a 4-dose schedule: minimum of 8 weeks interval between doses beginning at 2 months of age, followed by a booster dose at 12–15 months of age. Healthy infants beginning primary immunization at 7–11 months of age: 2 doses, at least 8 weeks apart, followed by a booster dose at 12–15 months of age, at least 8 weeks after the second dose. Children who have received age-appropriate pneumococcal vaccination with a pneumococcal conjugate vaccine but not Pneu-C-13 vaccine: 12–35 months of age: 1 dose; 36–59 months of age and of Indigenous origin or attend group child care: 1 dose; other healthy children 36–59 months of age: consider 1 dose.
G	**Meningococcal conjugate monovalent** (Men-C-C). Children 12–48 months of age: 1 dose routinely provided at 12 months of age, regardless of any doses given during the first year of life. Immunization may be considered for unimmunized children 5–11 years of age.
H	**Meningococcal conjugate monovalent** (Men-C-C) **or meningococcal conjugate quadrivalent** (Men-C-ACYW). Early adolescence (around 12 years of age): 1 dose, even if meningococcal conjugate vaccine received at a younger age. Vaccine chosen depends on local epidemiology and programmatic considerations.
I	**Measles–mumps–rubella** (MMR). First dose at 12–15 months of age; second dose at 18 months of age or anytime thereafter, but should be given no later than around school entry.
J	**Varicella (chickenpox)** (Var). First dose at 12–15 months of age; second dose at 18 months of age or anytime thereafter, but should be given no later than around school entry.
K	**Measles–mumps–rubella–varicella** (MMRV). First dose at 12–15 months of age; second dose at 18 months of age or anytime thereafter, but should be given no later than around school entry.
L	**Hepatitis B** (HB). Months 0, 1, and 6 (first dose = month 0) with at least 4 weeks between the first and second dose, at least 2 months between the second and third dose, and at least 4 months between the first and third dose. Alternatively, can be administered as DTaP-HB-IPV-Hib vaccine, with first dose at 2 months of age.
M	**Hepatitis B** (HB). 9–17 years of age: months 0, 1, and 6 (first dose = month 0) with at least 4 weeks between the first and second dose, at least 2 months between the second and third dose, and at least 4 months between the first and third dose. 11–15 years of age: 2 doses; schedule depends on the product used.
N	**Human papillomavirus** (HPV). Girls, 9–14 years of age: HPV bivalent (HPV2) or HPV quadrivalent (HPV4) vaccine: months 0 and 6–12 (first dose = month 0). Alternatively, a 3-dose schedule may be used for HPV2 vaccine: months 0, 1, and 6 (first dose = month 0); for HPV4 vaccine: months 0, 2, and 6 (first dose = month 0); and HPV nonavalent (HPV9) vaccine: months 0, 2, and 6 (first dose = month 0). Boys, 9–14 years of age: HPV4 vaccine: months 0 and 6–12 (first dose = month 0). For a 2-dose schedule, the minimum interval between doses is 6 months. Alternatively, a 3-dose schedule may be used for HPV4 vaccine: months 0, 2, and 6 (first dose = month 0); and HPV9 vaccine: months 0, 2, and 6 (first dose = month 0).
O	**Human papillomavirus** (HPV). Girls, 15–17 years of age: HPV2 vaccine: months 0, 1, and 6 (first dose = month 0); HPV4 vaccine: months 0, 2, and 6 (first dose = month 0); or HPV9 vaccine: months 0, 2, and 6 (first dose = month 0). Boys, 15–17 years of age: HPV4 vaccine: months 0, 2, and 6 (first dose = month 0); or HPV9 vaccine: months 0, 2, and 6 (first dose = month 0). In individuals who received the first dose of HPV2 or HPV4 vaccine between 9 and 14 years of age, a 2-dose schedule can be used with the second dose administered at least 6 months after the first dose.
P	**Influenza** (Inf). Recommended annually for anyone 6 months of age and older without contraindications. Children 6 months to less than 9 years of age, receiving influenza vaccine for the first time: 2 doses, at least 4 weeks apart. Children 6 months to 8 years of age, previously immunized with influenza vaccine, and children 9 years of age and older: 1 dose.

*For abbreviations and brand names of vaccines refer to *Contents of Immunizing Agents Available for Use in Canada* in Part 1 of *Immunization Guide* (see https://www.canada.ca/en/public-health/services/publications/healthy-living/canadian-immunization-guide-part-1-key-immunization-information/page-15-contents-immunizing-agents-available-use-canada.html).

P/T, Provincial and territorial.

From Public Health Agency of Canada. (2016). *Canadian immunization guide.* Retrieved from http://healthycanadians.gc.ca/publications/healthy-living-vie-saine/1-canadian-immunization-guide-canadien-immunisation/index-eng.php?page=13#p1c12a2. *Canadian Immunization Guide.* Public Health Agency of Canada, 2016. Adapted and reproduced with permission from the Minister of Health, 2017.

TABLE 22-3 Selected Sleep Disturbances During Infancy and Early Childhood

Disorder and Description	Management
Nighttime Feeding	
Colic, irritability Prolonged need for bottle or breastfeeding at night Going to sleep at the breast or with a bottle Irregular sleep patterns Problems with returning to sleep after feeding; other comfort measures (e.g., rocking or holding) are usually ineffective	Soothe, rock for brief periods, offer pacifier. Gradually increase daytime feeding intervals to 4 hours or more. Offer last feeding as late as possible at night. Gradually increase amount of fluid during day. Offer no bottles in bed. Put child to bed when awake. When child is crying, check at progressively longer intervals each night; reassure child but do not hold, rock, take to parent's bed, or give bottle or pacifier.
Developmental Night Crying	
Child aged 6–12 months with undisturbed nighttime sleep now awakes abruptly; awakening may be accompanied by nightmares	Be assured that this phase is temporary. Enter room immediately to check on child, but keep reassurances brief. Avoid feeding, rocking, taking to parent's bed, or any other routine that may initiate trained nighttime crying.
Trained Night Crying (Inappropriate Sleep Associations)	
Child typically falls asleep in a place other than own bed (e.g., rocking chair or parent's bed) and is brought to own bed while asleep; on awakening, cries until usual routine is instituted (e.g., rocking)	Put child in own bed when child is awake. If possible, arrange sleeping area separate from other family members. Check crying child at progressively longer intervals each night; reassure child but do not resume usual routine.
Refusal to Go to Sleep	
Child resists bedtime and comes out of room repeatedly Nighttime sleep may be continuous, but frequent awakenings and refusal to return to sleep may occur and become a problem if parent allows child to deviate from usual sleep pattern	Evaluate whether bedtime is too early (child may resist sleep if not tired). Adopt consistent bedtime routine. If child persists in leaving bedroom, close door for progressively longer periods. Reinforce positive behaviour.
Nighttime Fears	
Child resists going to bed or wakes during the night because of fears	Evaluate whether bedtime is too early (child may fantasize when he or she has nothing to do but think in a dark room). Calmly reassure the frightened child; keeping a night light on may be helpful.
Child seeks parent's physical presence and falls asleep easily with parent nearby	Use reward system with child to provide motivation to deal with fears. Avoid patterns that can lead to additional problems (e.g., sleeping with child or taking child to parent's room).
Overwhelming fears	If child's fear is overwhelming, consider desensitization (e.g., progressively spending longer periods of time alone); obtain professional help for protracted fears. Distinguish between nightmares and sleep terrors (confused partial arousals).

Socially, toddlers remain strongly attached to their parents and fear separation from them. In their parents' presence, toddlers feel safe, and their curiosity is evident in their exploration of the environment. Children continue to engage in solitary play during toddlerhood, but also begin to participate in parallel play, which is playing beside rather than with another child. Toddlers who are just learning what belongs to them are often possessive of their toys. They learn the joy of sharing when they offer parents or caregivers toys to hold and the parents or caregivers express pleasure.

Health Risks

Their newly developed locomotion abilities and insatiable curiosity put toddlers at risk for injury. Toddlers need close supervision at all times, particularly when in environments that have not been child-proofed (Figure 22-5). Creating a safe, childproof environment in the home is essential for preventing accidental injuries.

Poisonings occur frequently in children nearing 2 years of age because they are interested in placing any object or substance in their mouths to learn about it. Parents must remove or lock up all possible poisons, including plants, cleaning materials, and medications. Lead poisoning can pose a health hazard for younger children (Hockenberry & Wilson, 2015). Health care providers need to educate families living in older homes about the risks, screening, and treatment of lead poisoning.

Because of toddlers' lack of awareness regarding the danger of water and their newly developed walking skills, drowning is a major cause of accidental death in this age group.

Toddlers can easily become separated from a parent because they often wander away. It is important to closely supervise toddlers, especially in an open public space. Setting limits is extremely important for toddlers' safety.

In automobiles, toddlers must remain in car seats. Under Canadian law, infants up to 9 kg must ride in rear-facing car seats, but it is safer

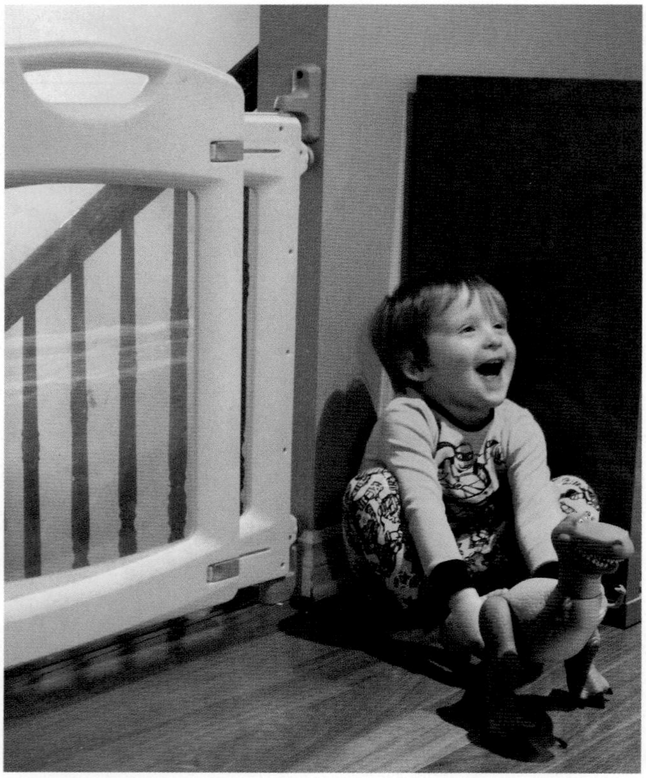

FIGURE 22-5 Creating a safe environment for toddlers. Safety precautions (such as child safety gates) should be provided for toddlers. (Courtesy Cynthia Murray, BN, MN, PhD.)

for children to remain in this position until they grow out of these seats (Transport Canada, 2017). The American Academy of Pediatrics (2011) recommends rear-facing car seats for all children under the age of 2. Children often learn to release the car restraints, and parents must be firm in their resolve not to drive unless the children are securely restrained. Toddlers depend completely on their parents for physical safety. Health care providers must educate parents on proper use of child passenger restraints.

Table 22-4 identifies developmental abilities acquired during this age period and injury prevention strategies.

Health Concerns

Nutrition. Most toddlers stop drinking breast milk or formula and begin drinking cow's milk. Nutritional requirements are increasingly met by solid foods. Because the consumption of more than 1 L of milk per day usually decreases children's appetite for these essential solid foods and results in inadequate iron intake, nurses should advise parents to limit milk intake to between 500 and 750 mL (two to three servings) per day. Children should not drink low-fat or skim milk until 2 years of age because they need the fat in whole milk for physical and intellectual growth. Healthy toddlers require a balanced daily intake of bread and grains, vegetables, fruit, dairy products, and proteins (see Chapter 42 for further information about nutrition). Because parents frequently overestimate the size of a normal serving for their child, nurses should discuss normal serving sizes with parents.

Special dietary considerations are required for children who are ill, are undergoing surgery, or have conditions involving ingestion, absorption, or use of nutrients. Alterations in the type of foods and caloric requirements may be necessary. Strict vegetarian diets for children also require careful planning to ensure adequate, balanced protein intake. Regardless of children's health status, several basic principles of nutrition apply. Mealtime has psychosocial and physical significance. If the parents struggle to control toddlers' dietary intake, problematic behaviour and conflicts may result. Toddlers often develop "food jags," or the desire to eat one food repeatedly. Rather than becoming disturbed by this behaviour, parents should be encouraged to offer a variety of nutritious foods at meals and to provide only nutritious snacks between meals. Serving finger foods to toddlers allows them to eat by themselves and to satisfy their need for independence and control. Small, reasonable servings enable toddlers to eat all of their meals.

PRESCHOOLER

The preschool period encompasses the years between 3 and 5 years of age. Children refine the mastery of their bodies and often are eager to begin school. Many people consider these the most intriguing years of parenting because children exhibit positive emotions and can more effectively share their thoughts, interact, and communicate. Physical development occurs at a slower pace than does cognitive and psychosocial development.

Physical Changes

Physical development continues in the preschool years. Heart and respiratory rates range from 60 to 100 beats and 23 to 25 breaths per minute, respectively. Blood pressure rises slightly to an average of 92/56 mm Hg. Children gain about 2.27 kg per year; the average weight is 14.5 kg at 3 years, 16.8 kg at 4 years, and about 18.6 kg at 5 years. Preschoolers grow 6 to 7.5 cm per year, double their birth length at about 4 years of age, and stand an average of 1 m tall by their fifth birthday. The elongation of the legs results in a more slender appearance. Little difference exists between the sexes, although boys are slightly larger with more muscle and less fatty tissue.

Large and fine muscle coordination improves. Preschoolers run well, walk up and down steps with ease, and learn to hop. By age 5 years, they can usually skip on alternate feet, can jump rope, and begin to skate and swim. Improvements in fine motor skills allow intricate manipulations. Children learn to copy crosses and squares. Triangles and diamonds are usually mastered between ages 5 and 6 years. Scribbling and drawing help children develop fine muscle skills and eye–hand coordination needed for the printing of letters and numbers.

Children need opportunities to learn and practise new physical skills. Early intervention programs are helpful in developing these skills, especially among disadvantaged children. Nursing care of healthy and ill children includes assessment of the availability of these opportunities. Although children with acute illnesses benefit from rest and exclusion from usual daily activities, children who have chronic conditions or have been hospitalized for long periods need ongoing exposure to developmental opportunities. With the parents, the nurse can weave these opportunities into the children's daily experiences depending on their abilities, needs, and energy level.

Cognitive Changes

Preschoolers continue to master the preoperational stage of cognition. The first phase of this period, known as *preconceptual thought* (2 to 4 years), is characterized by perception-bound thinking, in that children judge people, objects, and events by their outward appearance or what seems to be true (Piaget, 1952). For example, a child may think that a 240 mL glass full of fluid contains more than a 300 mL glass that also contains 240 mL of fluid because the smaller glass appears fuller. Even if they watch the fluid from the smaller glass being poured into the larger glass and the smaller glass refilled, they still assert that the full, smaller glass contains more.

Children's thinking is hindered by their limited attention and attending skills. **Artificialism**, the misconception that everything in the world has been created by humanity, may result in children's asking questions such as "Who built the mountains?" Another misconception of preschool thinking, **animism**, the attribution of animal life to inanimate objects, often results in statements such as "Trees cry when their branches are broken." A third misconception is a type of reasoning called **immanent justice**, the notion that if a built-in code of law and order is broken, punishment will occur immediately (Santrock, 2011). For example, a child might think that he became sick because he lied to his mother.

At about the age of 4 years, the intuitive phase of preoperational thought develops. Children's ability to think more complexly is demonstrated by their ability to classify objects according to size or colour and by questions such as "Why do they call it the 31st day of the month instead of the 30 last?" Egocentricity persists, but during these 3 years, it begins to be replaced with social interaction; for example, a 5-year-old child offers a bandage to a child with a cut finger. Children become

TABLE 22-4 Injury Prevention for Toddlers and Preschoolers

Developmental Abilities Related to Risk of Injury	Injury Prevention
	Motor Vehicles
• Walks, runs, and climbs • Is able to open doors and gates • Can ride tricycle • Can throw ball and other objects	• Continue to use federally approved car restraint. Until the age of 2, children should ride in rear-facing car seats. Then, toddlers weighing up to 18 kg should be placed in a forward-facing child seat that is anchored to the vehicle frame with a tether strap. A child weighing 18 to 36 kg should be seated in a booster seat. • Supervise child while he or she is playing outside, to prevent child from entering street. • Do not allow child to play on curb or behind a parked car. • Do not permit child to play in pile of leaves, snow, or anywhere that he or she is not visible. • Supervise tricycle riding. • Supervise child playing outside. • Teach children to obey pedestrian safety rules. • Supervise child when near traffic.
	Drowning
• Has great curiosity • Is helpless in water, unaware of its danger at any depth	• Supervise closely when child is near any source of water, including buckets. • Keep bathroom doors and lid on toilet closed. • Have fence around swimming pool, and lock gate. • Teach the child swimming and water safety (and continue to protect him or her from injury).
	Burns
• Is able to reach heights by climbing, stretching, standing on toes, and using objects as a ladder • Pulls objects • Explores any holes or openings • Can open drawers and closets • Is unaware of potential sources of heat or fire • Plays with mechanical objects	• Turn pot handles toward back of stove. • Place electric appliances, such as coffeemaker or frying pan, toward back of counter. • Place guard rails in front of radiators, fireplaces, and heating appliances. • Store matches and cigarette lighters in locked or inaccessible area; discard carefully. • Place burning candles, incense, hot foods, ashes, embers, and cigarettes out of reach. • Do not let tablecloth hang within child's reach. • Do not let electric cord from iron or other appliance hang within child's reach. • Cover electrical outlets with protective devices. • Keep electrical wires hidden or out of reach. • Do not allow child to play with electrical appliance, wires, or lighters. • Stress danger of open flames; teach child what "hot" means. • Always check bath water temperature; adjust hot-water heater temperature to 49°C or lower; do not allow child to play with faucets. • Apply a sunscreen with SPF 15 or higher when child is exposed to sunlight.
	Poisoning
• Explores by putting objects in mouth • Can open drawers, closets, and most containers • Climbs • Cannot understand warning labels	• Place all potentially toxic agents (including plants) in a locked cabinet or out of reach. • Put away medications and poisonous substances immediately after use; position (and tighten) child-resistant caps properly. • Refer to medications as "drugs," not as "candy." • Do not store large amounts of toxic agents. • Promptly discard empty poison containers; never reuse such containers to store a food item or other poison. • Teach child not to play in trash containers. • Never remove labels from containers of toxic substances. • Know number and location of nearest poison control centre (usually listed at beginning of telephone directories); add phone number to contacts on mobile phone.

Continued

TABLE 22-4 Injury Prevention for Toddlers and Preschoolers—cont'd

Developmental Abilities Related to Risk of Injury	Injury Prevention
	Falls
• Is able to open doors and some windows • Goes up and down stairs • Has unrefined depth perception	• Keep screen in window, nail securely, and install guard rail. • Place gates at top and bottom of stairs. • Keep doors locked or use child-resistant doorknob covers at entry to stairs, high porch, or other elevated area, such as laundry chute. • Remove unsecured or scatter rugs. • Apply nonskid mat in bathtub or shower. • Use a crib with fixed, raised rails. Keep mattress at lowest level. • Place carpeting under crib and in bathroom. • Keep large toys and bumper pads out of crib or playpen (child can use these as "stairs" to climb out). • Move child to youth bed when he or she is able to climb out of crib. • Dress child in safe clothing (soles that do not "catch" on floor, tied shoelaces, pant legs that do not hang on floor). • Never leave child unattended in shopping cart or stroller. • Supervise child at playgrounds; select play areas with soft ground cover and safe equipment.
	Choking and Suffocation
• Puts things in mouth • May swallow hard or nonedible pieces of food	• Do not give child large, round chunks of meat, such as whole hot dogs (instead, slice into thin pieces). • Do not give child fruit with pits, fish with bones, dried beans, hard candy, chewing gum, nuts, popcorn, grapes, or marshmallows. • Choose large, sturdy toys without sharp edges or small removable parts. • Discard unused refrigerators, unused ovens, and other unused appliances; if storing old appliance, remove doors. • Keep automatic garage door opener in inaccessible place. • Select safe toy boxes or chests without heavy, hinged lids. • Keep window blind strings out of child's reach. • Remove drawstrings from clothing.
	Bodily Damage
• Is still clumsy in many activities • Is easily distracted from tasks • Is unaware of potential danger from strangers or other people	• Avoid giving child sharp or pointed objects—such as knives, scissors, or toothpicks—especially when child is walking or running. • Do not allow lollipops or similar objects in the child's mouth when he or she is walking or running. • Teach safety precautions (e.g., to hold fork or scissors with pointed end away from face). • Store all dangerous tools, garden equipment, and firearms in locked cabinet. • Be alert to danger of animals, including household pets. • Use safety glass and decals on large glass areas, such as sliding glass doors. • Teach personal safety. • Teach child his or her name, address, and phone number, and teach child to ask for help from appropriate people (cashier, security guard, police officer) if lost; have identification on child (sewn in clothes, inside shoe). • Avoid dressing child in personalized clothing in public places. • Teach child to never go anywhere with a stranger. • Teach child to tell parents if anyone makes child feel uncomfortable in any way. • Always listen to child's concerns regarding others' behaviour. • Teach child to say no when confronted with uncomfortable situations.

Adapted from Hockenberry, M. J., & Wilson, D. (2015). *Wong's nursing care of infants and children* (10th ed., pp. 512–518). St. Louis, MO: Mosby.

aware of cause-and-effect relationships, as illustrated by the statement "The sun sets because people want to go to bed." Early causal thinking is also evident in preschoolers' transductive thoughts (reasoning occurs from one particular to another). If two events are related in time or space, children link them in a causal manner. A hospitalized child, for example, may reason, "I cried last night, and that's why the nurse gave me the shot." As children near the age of 5 years, they begin to use or can be taught to use rules to understand causation. They then begin to reason from the general to the particular. This development forms the basis for more formal logical thought. The hospitalized child now reasons, "I get a shot twice a day, and that's why I got one last night."

Preschoolers' knowledge of the world remains closely linked to concrete (perceived by the senses) experiences. Even their rich fantasy life is grounded in the perception of reality. The mixing of the two aspects can lead to many childhood fears, and adults may misinterpret children's stories as lying when children are actually presenting reality from their perspective.

The greatest fear of this age group appears to be that of bodily harm, and it can be seen in children's fear of the dark, thunderstorms, and medical personnel. This fear often makes children unwilling to allow nursing interventions such as measurement of vital signs. Preschoolers may cooperate if they are allowed to help the nurse measure the blood pressure of a doll or teddy bear or if they are allowed to handle the equipment the nurse will use.

Preschoolers' moral development expands to include a beginning understanding of behaviours considered socially right or wrong. Children continue to be motivated, however, by the wish to avoid punishment and the desire to obtain a reward. The primary difference between this stage of moral development and that of toddlers is that preschoolers are better able to identify behaviours that elicit rewards or punishment and begin to label these behaviours as right or wrong.

Language. Preschoolers' vocabularies continue to increase rapidly, and by the age of 6 years, children know more than 2 100 words and can construct sentences containing 5 to 6 words (Hockenberry & Wilson, 2015). Language is more social, and questions expand to "Why?" and "How come?" Phonetically similar words such as "die" and "dye" or "wood" and "would" might cause confusion in preschool children. Nurses should avoid such words when preparing children for procedures, and assess their comprehension of explanations.

Psychosocial Changes

The world of preschoolers expands beyond the family into the neighbourhood, where children meet other children and adults. Their curiosity and developing initiative lead to the active exploration of the environment, the development of new skills, and the making of new friends. Preschoolers have much energy, which enables them to plan and attempt many activities that may be beyond their capabilities, such as pouring milk into their cereal bowls. Guilt arises within children when they overstep the limits of their abilities and feel they have not behaved correctly. Children who in anger have wished their sibling were dead experience guilt if that sibling becomes ill. Children need to be taught that "wishing" for something to happen does not make it occur. Parents should allow preschoolers to perform tasks on their own, but must set firm limits and provide guidance.

During times of stress or illness, preschoolers may revert to bed-wetting or thumb-sucking and want the parents to feed, dress, and hold them. These dependent behaviours are often confusing and embarrassing to parents, who can benefit from a nurse's reassurance that they are the children's normal coping behaviours. Nurses should provide experiences that these children can master. Such successes help children return to their prior level of independent functioning. As language skills develop, children should be encouraged to talk about their feelings. Play is also an excellent way for preschoolers to vent frustration or anger and is a socially acceptable way to deal with stress.

Play. Children become more social after their third birthday as they shift from parallel to associative play. Children playing together engage in similar, if not identical, activity; however, no division of labour or rigid organization or rules exist. Most 3-year-old children are able to play with one other child in a cooperative manner in which they make something or play designated roles, such as mother and baby. By the age of 4 years, children play in groups of two or three, and by 5 years, the group has a temporary leader for each activity.

In many play activities, preschoolers display awareness of social context. Sex role identification is strengthening and children most often assume roles of people of their own sex. Children frequently mimic or repeat social experiences. This tendency is especially significant in hospitalized children. Through play, children may express questions, fears, anger, and misunderstanding about their illnesses and care. It is important to be alert to such clues and ensure that children can play within energy limits. Play can provide a healthy outlet for frustration, especially when children have been subjected to painful or restrictive experiences against their will.

Imaginary play depends on children's memory of things they have seen or heard. This sociodramatic play involving other children occupies about a third of 5-year-old children's playtime. Pretending allows children to learn to understand others' points of view, develop skills in solving social problems, and become more creative. Some children have imaginary playmates, which are a sign of creativity and healthy development.

Health Risks

As fine and gross motor skills develop, children become more coordinated with better balance; nevertheless, falls and other accidents remain a leading cause of injury. Guidelines for injury prevention in toddlers also apply to preschoolers (see Table 22-4). Nurses should alert parents of children in this age group to the risks of poisoning and pedestrian–motor vehicle accidents. The leading cause of death in Canadian children is unintentional injury. All of these injuries are preventable. Children should be taught about safety in the home, and this teaching should be reinforced early in elementary school.

Health Concerns

Nutrition. Nutrition requirements for preschoolers vary little from those for toddlers. The average daily intake is 1 800 calories. Parents may nonetheless worry about the amount of food their child is consuming. In most situations, however, the quality of the food is more important than quantity. Preschoolers consume about half of the average adult portions. Finicky eating habits are characteristic of 4-year-olds; in contrast, 5-year-olds are more interested in trying new foods. Parents should provide healthy food on a regular daily schedule of three meals and two snacks, while allowing the child to decide the amount to eat (Kliegman et al., 2016).

Sleep. Preschoolers average 12 hours of sleep a night and take infrequent naps. Sleep disturbances are common during these years. Disturbances may range from trouble getting to sleep to nightmares to prolonging bedtime with extensive rituals. Many preschoolers have had an overabundance of activity and stimulation during the day. Having children follow a set routine before bedtime helps them prepare for sleep.

Vision. Preschoolers should routinely be screened for vision problems. One of the common problems in the preschool period is amblyopia (blindness from disuse of an eye if a child has untreated strabismus). Early detection and treatment can improve vision for most children (Hockenberry & Wilson, 2015).

SCHOOL-AGE CHILDREN AND ADOLESCENTS

School-age children and adolescents lead demanding, challenging lives. The changes that occur between 6 and 19 years of age are diverse and span all areas of growth and development. Physical, psychosocial, cognitive, and moral skills are developed, expanded, refined, and synchronized. The environment in which the individual develops skills also expands and diversifies. Instead of only family and close friends, the environment now may include the school, community, and religious institution. Because of expectations for development, increasing skill and knowledge base, and environmental expansion, the individual experiences new difficulties and dilemmas. With age-specific assessment, nurses should review the appropriate developmental expectations for each age group. For example, before assessing risk-taking behaviours, recognize that adolescents normally strive to achieve a sense of identity while developing a moral code compatible with society.

Nurses can direct school-age children and adolescents toward normal developmental behaviours, assisting them in improving their abilities and using them to cope. Table 22-5 provides an overview of developmental behaviours typical of school-age children and

TABLE 22-5 Developmental Behaviours of School-Age Children and Adolescents

School-Age Children	Adolescents
Relationships With Parents	
Children gradually learn that parents are less than perfect; children can become disillusioned with parents and wish that friends' parents were their own. They still rely on parents for unconditional love, security, guidance, and nurturing.	Adolescents desire increasing independence and autonomy and yet continue needing some dependence and limit setting by parents; this conflict places strain on the parent–child relationship. Effective communication and democratic parenting are the best tools for meeting this challenge.
Relationships With Siblings	
Siblings seem to be at odds with one another at home, and yet they tend to be each other's best defenders away from home. Younger children often idolize older siblings, and this frequently leads to competition. Older children may envy attention that younger siblings require and can be quite bossy and somewhat abusive.	Younger siblings rarely understand their adolescent siblings' need for privacy. Adolescents often enjoy interacting with and guiding younger brothers and sisters when timing is convenient for them and they can remain in control.
Relationships With Peers	
During primary grades (6–7 years), children of both sexes play together, depending on who is available and interested. Around age 8, social groupings of same-sex peers form. These groups allow children to declare their independence from parental rules and establish their own rules of membership and behaviour. Preadolescent (ages 10–12 years) friendships are characterized by having a best friend of the same sex. These relationships may be transient, but they are intense and allow discussion of all areas of life. Childhood "crushes" are common.	Peer group is of critical influence on adolescents, who increasingly need recognition and acceptance. Companionship offered by peer groups provides a secure environment for individuals to try out new ideas and share similar feelings and attitudes. Adolescents often form cliques with peers with similar interests from the same socioeconomic group. Cliques, which are highly exclusive, help their members develop their identities.
Self-Concept	
Children's feelings of competence regarding mastery of tasks are key elements in forming self-esteem. Children need to receive positive feedback regarding their efforts. It is important for children to develop skills in at least one area, such as reading, music, or swimming.	Formal and informal peer groups are a primary force in shaping self-concept of group members. Popularity and recognition within the peer group enhance self-esteem and reinforce self-concept. Total immersion in the peer group may make it appear that adolescents have no original thoughts and are incapable of making decisions. Adolescents who withdraw from peers into isolation struggle with developing identity.
Fears	
Fears related to body safety decline. Fears of supernatural beings, such as ghosts and witches, persist and decline slowly. New fears related to school and family occur. Children fear ridicule from teachers and friends and disapproval and rejection of parents. They also become frightened about death and events that they hear on the news, such as war and destruction of the environment.	Fears in this age group centre on peer group acceptance, body changes, loss of self-control, and emerging sexual urges. Adolescents constantly examine their bodies for changes and signs of imperfection. Any defect, real or imagined, is a cause of endless worry.
Coping Patterns	
To deal with stress, school-age children use problem solving and defence mechanisms, such as denial and aggression. Several categories of coping behaviours of hospitalized school-aged children are inactivity (total silence, lack of activity, and apathy), orientation or precoping (looking and listening, walking around and exploring, and asking questions), cooperation (compliance with care), resistance (attempt to get away from the situation by turning away or making physical or verbal attacks), and controlling (assuming responsibility for self-care and suggesting how things could be done).	Coping behaviours expand with experiences adolescents have gained from life and from developing cognitive maturity. By age 15, most adolescents use a full range of defence mechanisms, including rationalization and intellectualization. Adolescents' problem-solving abilities have matured, and they can reason through philosophical discussions and complex situations that require abstract thinking and proposition of hypotheses. Some adolescents use avoidance coping strategies in which a problem is denied or repressed, and an attempt is made to reduce tension by engaging in substance abuse or avoiding people.
Morals	
Children learn rules from parents, but their understanding of rules or reasons for them is limited until about age 10 years. Before that, they are concerned with their own needs first and may cheat to win games. After 10 years of age, they advocate justice and believe that punishment should fit the crime (e.g., if children break something, they should pay to have it fixed).	According to Kohlberg (1964), as youths approach adolescence, they reach conventional level, where internalization of expectations of their family and society begins. Initially, youths exhibit considerable conformity to rules to win praise or approval from others and to avoid social disapproval or rejection; later, they seek to avoid criticism from people of authority in institutions.

TABLE 22-5 Developmental Behaviours of School-Age Children and Adolescents—cont'd

School-Age Children	Adolescents
Diversional Activities	
School-age children play cooperatively in group activities, such as sports and jumping rope. Play becomes competitive, and children often have difficulty learning to accept losing. Teasing, insults, dares, superstitions, and increased sensitivity are characteristics of this age.	Many teenagers develop special interests in certain sports and concentrate on developing maximal skills in them. Recreational activities are often determined by what is popular with peers and what can provide independence from parents (e.g., computers, cars).
Nutrition	
Children have definite likes and dislikes. Few nutritional deficiencies occur in this age group. Children have voracious appetites after school and need quality snacks, such as fruit and sandwiches, to avoid empty-calorie foods, such as chips and candy.	Total nutritional needs become greater during adolescence. Girls' caloric needs decrease and their need for protein increases slightly. Adolescents need to increase their consumption of iron-rich foods, and growth spurts increase calcium demand.

adolescents. Nurses must also increasingly involve children or adolescents in charting a developmental course. Not only can they describe their feelings about the changes, but they also can think through these changes. Problem solving becomes more purposeful and sophisticated and results in the achievement of the outcomes that they desire. This paced, active participation may initiate a style of involvement in lifelong self-care.

School-age children and adolescents must cope with many changes, and these can be a source of stress for children. For example, 6-year-old children beginning school are confronted with new authority figures, teachers, and rules and restrictions. They need to work and play cooperatively with a large group of children of various cultural backgrounds. School-age children must meet the challenge of developing cognitive skills that enhance their reasoning and allow them to learn to read, write, and manipulate numbers. Because of the stress of these changes, children may develop physical and psychosocial health problems (e.g., increased susceptibility to upper respiratory infections, inadequate peer relationships, or poor performance in school). It is important to design health promotion interventions that are based on an individual child's developmental stage.

SCHOOL-AGE CHILD

During these "middle years" of childhood, the foundation for adult roles in work, recreation, and social interaction is laid. In industrialized countries, this period begins when children start formal schooling at about the age of 6 years. **Puberty**, which occurs at about 12 years of age, signals the end of middle childhood. Great developmental strides are made during these years as children develop competencies in physical, cognitive, and psychosocial skills.

The school or educational experience expands children's world and is a transition from a life of relatively free play to a life of structured play, learning, and work. The school and home influence growth and development, necessitating adjustment by parents and children. Children must learn to cope with rules and expectations presented by the school and peers. Parents must learn to allow their children to make decisions, accept responsibility, and learn from life's experiences.

Physical Changes

The rate of growth during these early school years is slower than at any time since birth, but continues steadily. A particular child may not follow the pattern precisely. School-age children appear slimmer than preschoolers as a result of changes in fat distribution and thickness (Edelman, Kudzma, & Mandle, 2014). Growth accelerates at different times for different children. The average increase in height is 5 cm per year, and weight, which is more variable, increases by 2 to 3 kg per year. An average 6-year-old is 116 cm tall and weighs 21 kg; the average 12-year-old is 150 cm tall and weighs 40 kg. Many children double their weight during these middle childhood years (Hockenberry & Wilson, 2015).

School provides children with the opportunity to compare themselves with children of the same age. The physical examination is an excellent opportunity to discuss with a child and parents the influences of genetic endowment, nutrition, and exercise on height and weight. Annual measurement of height and weight may reveal alterations in growth that are symptoms of the onset of a variety of childhood diseases.

Boys are slightly taller and heavier than girls during these early school years. Approximately 2 years before puberty, children experience a rapid acceleration in skeletal growth. Girls, who generally reach puberty first, begin to surpass boys in height and weight, which causes embarrassment to both sexes. In North America, puberty occurs between the ages of 9 and 13 years in girls and 11 and 14 years in boys.

Cardiovascular functioning is refined and stabilized during the school years. The heart rate averages 75 to 100 beats per minute, the blood pressure normalizes to approximately 110/65 mm Hg, and the respiratory rate stabilizes to 20 to 30 breaths per minute. Lung growth is minimal, and respirations become slower, deeper, and more regular. However, by the end of this period, the heart is six times the size it was at birth and has generally reached its adult size.

School-age children become more graceful during the school years because their large-muscle coordination improves and their strength doubles. Most children practise the basic gross motor skills of running, jumping, balancing, throwing, and catching during play, which results in refinement of neuromuscular function and skills. Fine motor skills improve, and as control is gained over fingers and wrists, children become proficient in a wide range of activities, although much individual difference exists in the rate and degree of proficiency.

Most 6-year-olds can hold a pencil adeptly and print letters and words. By age 12 years, children can make detailed drawings and write sentences in script. Activities such as painting, drawing, playing computer games, and making models allow children to practise and improve newly refined skills. Parents should encourage children to pursue these activities. Table 22-6 describes specific gross motor and fine motor skills and their use in self-care activities.

The improved fine motor capabilities of school-age children allow them to become very independent in bathing, dressing, and taking care of other personal needs. They develop strong personal preferences in

TABLE 22-6 Average Motor Development in School-Age Children

Ages 6–7 Years	Ages 8–10 Years	Ages 11–12 Years
Fine Motor Skills		
• Uses knife to butter bread and learns to cut tender meat • Cuts, folds, and pastes paper • Prints with pencil • Draws person with 12–16 details • Copies triangle at age 6 years and diamond by age 7 years • Colours within lines of picture • Needs assistance to clean teeth thoroughly	• Uses knife and fork simultaneously • Learns to thread needle and tie knot • Uses hammer, saw, and screwdriver • Becomes proficient at cursive writing • Uses symbols in drawing (e.g., bird, star) • Builds simple models of cars and planes and does simple handicrafts • Can learn to floss teeth effectively and be independent in tooth care	• Learns to peel apples and potatoes • Sews simple garments on machine • Builds simple objects like birdhouse • Enjoys writing in decorative script • Begins to use creative and artistic talents • Builds complex models of cars and planes and does complex handicrafts • Learns to play musical instrument • Becomes proficient in caring for teeth with braces and other appliances
Gross Motor Skills		
• Remains in constant motion when awake • Moves more cautiously at age 7 years than at age 6 years • Hops and jumps into small squares • Learns to roller skate, skip rope, ride a bicycle, and swim	• Catches, throws, and hits a baseball • Engages in alternate rhythmic hopping • Engages in complex styles of skipping rope while reciting verbal jingles	• Can perform standing broad jump of 1.5 m • Can perform standing high jump of 1 m • Engages in sports involving simultaneous use of two or more complex motor skills, such as ice skating, skateboarding, or playing hockey
Self-Care		
• Takes bath without supervision • Often returns to finger feeding • Learns to brush and comb hair in acceptable manner without help • Puts on most clothes, but may need assistance with final adjustments	• Learns to clean bathroom after bath • Enjoys fixing own snacks and sack lunch • Learns to part hair and insert barrettes • Dresses self completely and can help younger siblings with clothes • Can make own bed	• Dusts, vacuums, and straightens own room • Learns to cook simply prepared foods • Washes, dries, and fixes own hair • Learns to sort, wash, dry, and press own clothing • Learns to care for fingernails and toenails

the way these needs are met. Illness and hospitalization threaten children's control in these areas; therefore, it is important to allow them to participate in care and maintain as much independence as possible. For example, children whose care mandates restriction of fluids cannot be allowed to decide the amount of fluids they will drink in 24 hours, but they can help decide the type of fluids and can help keep a record of intake.

Assessment of neurological development is often based on fine motor coordination. This assessment may include penmanship, stacking ability, and performance of sequential, rapid, alternating movements, such as touching the finger to the nose and then to the examiner's finger (smooth movement without tremors is the normal response). Fine motor coordination is crucial for academic success because children must be able to hold pencils and crayons, use scissors and rulers, and develop computer skills. The opportunity to practise these skills through schoolwork and play is essential for the acquisition of coordinated, complex behaviours.

Other physical changes take place during the school years. Steady skeletal growth in the trunk and extremities occurs, and small- and long-bone ossification is present, but not complete by age 12 years. Dental growth is prominent during the school years. The first permanent or secondary teeth begin to erupt at approximately 6 years of age. Development of the permanent teeth has, however, been occurring for some time before eruption. The root of a primary tooth is absorbed, leaving the crown, which causes the tooth to become loose and fall out, making room for the permanent tooth. Eruption of secondary teeth usually begins with the 6-year molars, and the others follow the same order as with the primary teeth. By 12 years, all primary teeth have been shed, and the majority of permanent teeth have erupted. Infrequent or inadequate dental care remains a persistent problem for many children.

As skeletal growth progresses, body appearance and posture change. Earlier posture, which was characterized by a stoop-shouldered, slight lordosis and prominent abdomen, changes to a more erect posture. It is essential that children, especially girls after the age of 12 years, be evaluated for scoliosis, the lateral curvature of the spine.

Eye shape alters because of skeletal growth. This improves visual acuity, and normal adult 20/20 vision is achievable. Screening for vision and hearing problems is easier, and results are more reliable because school-age children can more fully understand and cooperate with the test directions. The community health nurse typically assesses the dental, visual, and auditory status of school-age children and refers those with possible deviations to their family practitioner or pediatrician.

Cognitive Changes

Cognitive changes provide school-age children with the ability to think in a logical manner and to understand the relationship between things and ideas (Hockenberry & Wilson, 2015). The thoughts of school-age children are no longer dominated by their perceptions, and thus their ability to understand the world greatly expands. At about 7 years of age, children enter Piaget's (1952) third stage of cognitive development, known as **concrete operations**, in which they are able to use symbols to carry out operations (mental activities) in thought rather than in action. They begin to use logical thought processes with concrete materials (people, events, and objects they can touch and see).

Children in the concrete operational stage are considerably less egocentric than are younger children and develop the ability to concentrate on more than one aspect of a situation. School-age children now have the ability to recognize that the amount or quantity of a substance remains the same even when its shape or appearance changes. For instance, they can understand that two balls of clay of equal size retain the same amount of clay even when one is flattened and the other remains in ball shape.

The mental process of classification becomes more complex during the school years. Younger children can separate objects into groups according to shape or colour, whereas school-age children understand that the same element can exist in two classes at the same time. School-age children are becoming "thinkers" and are more capable of understanding another person's views and feelings (Santrock, 2011).

In middle childhood, youngsters can use their newly developed cognitive skills to solve problems. Some individuals are better than others at problem solving because of intelligence level, education, and experience, but all children can improve these skills. Children who are good problem solvers demonstrate the following characteristics: a positive attitude that the problem can be solved with persistence, a concern for accuracy, the ability to divide the problem into parts for study, and the ability to avoid guessing while searching for facts. Adults can help children improve their problem-solving strategies by helping them define the problem, plan a solution, and then evaluate their solution. Nurses can use these strategies to help hospitalized school-age children understand their illness and assume responsibility for their general health.

Language Development. Language growth is so rapid during middle childhood that these ages cannot be matched with language achievements. Children improve their use of language and expand their structural knowledge. They become more aware of the rules for linking words into phrases and sentences. They can also identify generalizations and exceptions to rules. They accept language as a means of representing the world in a subjective manner and realize that words have arbitrary, rather than absolute, meanings. They can use different words for the same object or concept, and they understand that a single word may have many meanings. Like younger children, school-age children watch parents and other adults to obtain clues about how to understand events (Santrock, 2011). Many school-age children use "bad language" to gain peer status and to shock adults. It often begins with bathroom language and progresses to sexual or genital words. Children begin to think about language, which enables them to appreciate jokes and riddles. Language acquisition is nurtured by social interactions with their parents and caretakers.

Psychosocial Changes

Erikson (1963) identified the developmental task for school-age children as industry versus inferiority (see Chapter 21 for further information about developmental theories). During this time, children strive to acquire competence and skills necessary for them to function as adults. School-age children who are positively recognized for success feel a sense of worth. Those faced with failure can feel a sense of unworthiness, which may result in withdrawal from school activities and peers.

Moral Development. The need for a moral code and social rules becomes more evident as school-age children's cognitive abilities and social experiences increase. For example, 12-year-old children are able to consider what society would be like without rules because of their ability to reason logically and their experiences with group play. They view rules as necessary principles of life, not just dictates from authorities. In the early school years, children strictly interpret and adhere to rules. As they grow older, their judgements become more flexible and they can evaluate rules for applicability to a given situation. School-age children consider motivations and behaviour when making judgements about the way their behaviours affect themselves and others. The abilities to be flexible when applying rules and to take the perspective of other people are essential in developing moral judgements. These abilities are present at times in earlier years, but are more consistently displayed in later school years.

Peer Relationships. Group and personal achievements are important to school-age children. Success is important in physical and cognitive activities. Play involves peers and the pursuit of group goals. Although solitary activities are not eliminated, they are overshadowed by group play. Learning to contribute, collaborate, and work cooperatively toward a common goal becomes a measure of success (Figure 22-6).

For the most part, school-age children prefer same-sex peers to opposite-sex peers. In general, girls and boys view the opposite sex negatively. Peer influence becomes diverse during this stage of development. Conformity is evidenced in mannerisms, clothing styles, and speech patterns, which are reinforced and influenced by contact with peers. During this period, clubs and peer groups become prominent. Group identity increases as school-age children approach adolescence. Also, during the "tween" years (i.e., ages 8 to 12), children are increasingly exposed to social media. To help tweens and teens safely navigate the online social world, the American Academy of Pediatrics (2013) recommends the following to parents:

- Learn about social media first-hand and monitor your child online.
- Require that you and your child "friend" each other.
- Speak to your child daily about his or her online habits.
- Place the home computer in a public room (e.g., family room).
- Emphasize that everything sent over the Internet and cellphone can be shared with the whole world.
- Discourage children from gossiping, spreading rumours, or bullying.
- Set time limits for cellphone and Internet use.
- Be vigilant about warning signs of trouble, such as dropping grades, and skipping activities and homework for social media.
- Speak to your child about "sexting" in a manner that is appropriate to your child's age.

Bullying is a significant problem in Canada. Approximately 15% of girls and 18% of boys report being bullied at least twice in the last few

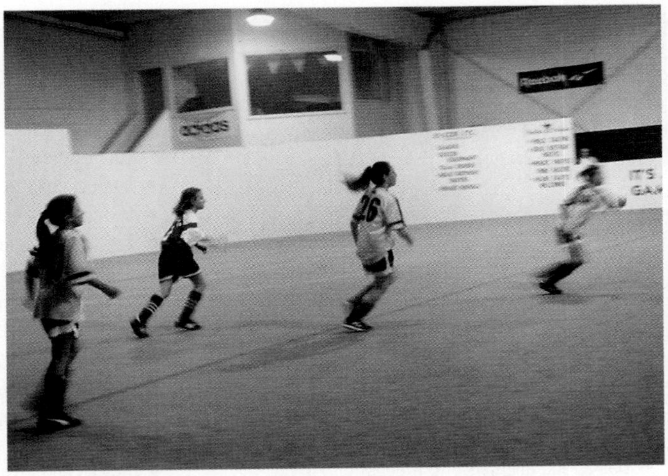

FIGURE 22-6 Peer relationships. School-age children gain a sense of achievement by working and playing with peers. (Courtesy Elaine Polan, RNC, BSN, MS.)

months (PREVNet, 2017). Bullied children have higher rates of academic, physical, and mental problems, including depression, anxiety, and suicide (PREVNet, 2017). According to Kub and Feldman (2015), there are four types of bullying: physical (e.g., hitting and pushing); verbal (e.g., insults and taunts); relational (e.g., spreading rumours and social exclusion); and cyber (e.g., sending mean or threatening text messages). Nurses can work with other professionals to create healthy public policy, build supportive and safe environments, strengthen community actions, develop personal skills, and reorient health services to help prevent and combat all forms of bullying (Kub & Feldman, 2015).

Sexual Identity. Sigmund Freud described middle childhood as the latency period because he believed that children of this age had little interest in their sexuality. Today, many researchers believe that school-age children have a great deal of curiosity about their sexuality. Some may experiment, but this play is usually temporary. Children's curiosity about adult magazines or meanings of sexually explicit words is also an example of their sexual interest. This is the time for children to have exposure to sex education, including information on sexual maturation, reproduction, and relationships (Edelman et al., 2014).

Health Risks

Accidents and injuries are major health problems affecting school-age children. Motor vehicle accidents and accidents related to recreational activities or equipment are the leading causes of death or injury from the age of 1 year to adulthood (Edelman et al., 2014). Nurses have an essential role in injury prevention initiatives. Also, nurses must respond competently and ethically to rapidly changing conditions (CASN, 2015) when accidents and injuries occur. Unintentional injuries account for nearly half of all childhood deaths, many of which can be prevented through use of precautionary measures (Table 22-7).

Although falls account for a major portion of pediatric hospital admissions, they account for less than 5% of pediatric deaths resulting from injury. Even though an accident may not result in death, it still can be a major cause of disability in children.

TABLE 22-7 Injury Prevention for School-Age Children

Developmental Abilities Related to Risk of Injury	Injury Prevention
	Motor Vehicles
• Is increasingly involved in activities away from home • Is excited by speed and motion • Can be reasoned with • Does not always perceive injury risk • Is easily distracted by environment	• Educate child regarding proper use of seat belts while a passenger in a vehicle. • Maintain discipline while a passenger in a vehicle (e.g., keep arms inside, do not lean against doors, do not interfere with driver). • Remind parents and children that no one should ride in the bed of a pickup truck. • Emphasize safe pedestrian behaviour. • Insist that child wear safety apparel (e.g., helmet) when applicable, such as when riding a bicycle or using a skateboard, all-terrain vehicle, or snowmobile.
	Drowning
• Is apt to overdo activities • May work hard to perfect a skill • Is cautious but not fearful	• Teach child to swim. • Teach basic rules of water safety. • Select safe and supervised places to swim. • Check sufficient water depth for diving. • Insist that child swim with a companion. • Use an approved flotation device in water or boat. • Learn cardiopulmonary resuscitation (CPR).
	Burns
• Demonstrates increasing independence • Is adventurous • Enjoys trying new things	• Make sure working smoke detectors are in homes. Set water heaters to 48.9°C to avoid scald burns. • Instruct child in behaviour in areas involving contact with potential burn hazards (e.g., gasoline, matches, bonfires or barbecues, lighter fluid, firecrackers, cigarette lighters, cooking utensils, chemistry sets). • Instruct child to avoid climbing or flying kites around high-tension wires. • Instruct child in proper behaviour in the event of fire (e.g., fire drills at home and school). • Teach child safe cooking (use low heat; avoid any frying; be careful of steam burns, scalds, or exploding foods, especially from microwaving). • Teach children about the danger of fire, and instruct them that if their clothing is on fire, they should "stop," "drop," and "roll."
	Substance Abuse and Poisoning
• May be easily influenced by peers • Adheres to group rules • Has strong allegiance to friends	• Educate child regarding hazards of taking nonprescription drugs and chemicals, including tobacco and alcohol. • Teach child to say no if he or she is offered illegal or dangerous drugs or alcohol. • Keep potentially dangerous products in properly labelled receptacles, preferably locked and out of child's reach.

TABLE 22-7 Injury Prevention for School-Age Children—cont'd

Developmental Abilities Related to Risk of Injury	Injury Prevention
	Bodily Damage
• Demonstrates increased physical skills • Needs strenuous physical activity • Is interested in acquiring new skills and perfecting attained skills • Is daring and adventurous, especially with peers • Frequently plays in hazardous places • Confidence often exceeds physical capacity • Desires group loyalty and has strong need for friends' approval • Attempts hazardous feats • Accompanies friends to potentially hazardous facilities • Delights in physical activity • Is likely to overdo activity • Has growth in height that exceeds muscular growth and coordination	• Help provide facilities for supervised activities. • Encourage playing in safe places. • Keep firearms safely locked up. • Teach proper care of, use of, and respect for devices with potential danger (e.g., power tools). • Teach children not to tease or surprise dogs, invade their territory, take dogs' toys, or interfere with dogs' feeding. • Stress use of eye, ear, or mouth protection when using potentially hazardous objects or devices or when engaged in potentially hazardous sports. • Do not permit use of trampolines except as part of supervised training. • Teach safety regarding use of corrective devices (glasses); if child wears contact lenses, monitor duration of wear to prevent corneal damage. • Stress careful selection, use, and maintenance of sports and recreation equipment such as skateboards and in-line skates. • Emphasize proper conditioning, safe practices, and use of safety equipment for sports or recreational activities. • Caution against engaging in hazardous sports, such as those involving trampolines. • Use safety glass and decals on large glassed areas, such as sliding glass doors. • Use window guards to prevent falls. • Teach name, address, and phone number and emphasize that child should ask for help from appropriate people (e.g., cashier, security guard, police) if lost; have identification on child (e.g., sewn in clothes, inside shoe). • Teach safety and stranger awareness. • Avoid personalized clothing in public places. • Caution child to never go anywhere with a stranger. • Have child tell parents if anyone makes child feel uncomfortable in any way. • Always listen to child's concerns regarding others' behaviour. • Teach child to say no when confronted with uncomfortable situations. • Help child avoid carrying more than 10–15% of body weight in a backpack, and teach child to always put backpack on in a way to evenly distribute weight; a lightweight backpack with wide shoulder straps, a waist strap, a padded back, and multiple compartments should be used.

Adapted from Hockenberry, M. J., & Wilson, D. (2015). *Wong's nursing care of infants and children* (10th ed., p. 601). St. Louis, MO: Mosby; and Kids Health. (2016). *Backpack safety*. Retrieved from http://kidshealth.org/parent/positive/learning/backpack.html.

More children die from automobile accidents than from all major preventable childhood diseases. The rates of injury and death have decreased since the institution of automobile child-restraint laws.

School-age children are also significantly affected by respiratory illnesses, especially asthma, cancer, and heart disease (Hockenberry & Wilson, 2015). In this age group, these problems have a relatively low mortality rate but a high morbidity rate in comparison with accidents. Cancers are the second leading cause of death in children 5 to 14 years of age (Hockenberry & Wilson, 2015). Leukemia is the most frequent type, and brain tumours and lymphoma are second and third, respectively.

Infections account for the majority of all childhood illnesses; respiratory infections are the most prevalent. The common cold remains the chief illness of childhood. Children living in poverty are more prone to disease and disability. Intellectual disabilities, learning disorders, sensory impairments, emotional difficulties, behavioural problems, and malnutrition are far more prevalent among children living in poverty (Campaign 2000, 2015).

Poverty and the prevalence of illness are highly correlated, probably because access to health promotion and preventive health care activities are minimal for children living in poverty. Poor nutrition and limited access to early intervention programs continue to be major health concerns for impoverished families. Education, social and health care reform, and environmental change are necessary to positively influence the health of children.

Children's developing cognitive and psychomotor skills make it possible for them to become more involved in health promotion and the management of chronic illness.

Health Concerns

During the school years, identity and self-concept become stronger and more individualized. School-age children are aware of their bodies and are sensitive about being exposed. In providing nursing care, it is important to ensure privacy and to offer explanations of common procedures. This approach helps foster children's self-esteem and lessens their fear of pain and intrusion (Hockenberry & Wilson, 2015).

Health Education. The school years are crucial for the acquisition of behaviours and health practices for a healthy adult life. Because cognition is advancing during the period, effective health education must be developmentally appropriate. Promotion of good health practices is a nursing responsibility. A comprehensive school health approach includes programs, activities, and services that take place in

BOX 22-6 Critical Functions of Comprehensive School Health

A comprehensive approach to promoting health in schools includes the following:

- Promote healthy habits and illness prevention measures, with attention to multicultural, linguistic, physical, cognitive, and emotional factors.
- Intervene to assist children and youth who are in need or at risk.
- Help support children who are already experiencing poor health.
- Foster parental education on health issues.
- Identify learning disabilities early, and begin appropriate interventions to foster learning and self-esteem.
- Facilitate growth and self-actualization.
- Emphasize positive health attitudes.
- Foster positive life skills that enhance successful coping.
- Encourage physical activity.
- Encourage involvement of individuals, families, and communities as active partners in the health care of school-age children.

Adapted from Canadian Association for School Health. (2007). *Canadian consensus statement (Revised 2007): Comprehensive school health.* Retrieved from http://www.cpha.ca/uploads/schoolhealth/2007_1.pdf.

schools and their surrounding communities in order to enable children and youth to improve their health and develop to their fullest potential (Canadian Association for School Health, 2007; Box 22-6).

School-age children should receive age-appropriate sexual health education that begins before the onset of sexual activity (Kliegman et al., 2016). Other topic areas for elementary health education curricula include the promotion of adequate nutrition, oral hygiene, and regular health supervision. School-age children should also be educated about prevention of tobacco, drug, and alcohol use (Edelman et al., 2014).

Nurses can instruct parents in health promotion that is appropriate for school-age children. Parents need to recognize the importance of annual checkups for immunizations, screenings, and dental care. When school-age children reach 10 years of age, it is recommended that their parents talk with the children about upcoming pubertal changes (Hockenberry & Wilson, 2015). Topics should include introductory information regarding menstruation, sexual intercourse, and reproduction. Nurses can provide age-appropriate written materials to aid parents in their efforts. The settings in which health promotion activities can occur are varied: the classroom, a school-based clinic, a community-based clinic, or community settings such as a public library or community centre.

Table 22-8 presents a list of possible health promotion interventions for school-age children.

Safety. Because accidents are the leading cause of death and injury in school-age children, safety is a priority health teaching consideration. Nurses can contribute to the general health of children by educating them about safety measures to prevent accidents. At this age, children should be encouraged to take responsibility for their own safety.

Nutrition. Nurses can contribute to the promotion of children's healthy lifestyle habits, including nutrition. School-age children should participate in educational programs that enable them to plan, select, and prepare healthy meals and snacks. These foods should be consistent with the recommendations in *Canada's Food Guide* (Health Canada, 2011b), which include limiting intake of fats and increasing intake of complex carbohydrates, fruits, and vegetables. Box 22-7 outlines several learning activities appropriate for this age group. In addition, it is important to encourage daily physical activity for all children.

Growth may slow down during the school years in comparison with infancy and adolescence. Obesity is the most common nutritional problem during childhood. Obesity is believed to begin in utero and during infancy and childhood (Edelman et al., 2014; Heindel, 2011). Obesity increases the risk for hypertension, diabetes, coronary heart disease, and psychosocial problems; some children with obesity have low self-esteem, poor body image, and reduced quality of life and interpersonal relationships (Sgrenci & Faith, 2011). Obesity may occur because children often rush into the home after school or play and eat

TABLE 22-8 Health Promotion for School-Age Children

School-Age Health Concerns	Health Promotion Interventions
Nutrition	Provide nutrition education that promotes healthy lifestyle—for example, limiting fat intake to 30% of calories, limiting saturated fat to 10% of calories, avoiding overeating.
Oral hygiene	• Provide examples of low-cariogenic snacks. • Review mechanics of dental hygiene: brushing, flossing. • Stress importance of biannual dental checkups.
Infections	• Provide immunization information and follow-up. • Teach infection prevention practices (hand hygiene, care of minor skin injuries). • Teach concepts of viral and bacterial illness. • Promote hand hygiene and regular bathing.
Tobacco, alcohol, and drug use	• Provide programs in preventing tobacco use. • Provide information regarding the hazards of alcohol and drug use.
Human sexuality	• Provide information about sexual maturation and reproduction in age-appropriate manner. • Encourage parents to view their children's sexual curiosity as part of the developmental process. • Discuss with parents the learning needs of their children regarding sexuality. Provide age-appropriate sexual health education.

BOX 22-7 Interventions to Promote Education About Nutrition

- Include healthy eating as part of the education programs at school.
- Make healthy foods available in school vending machines and at school sporting or other events.
- Encourage nutritious and nonfood items for school fundraising projects.
- Use positive messages to reinforce healthy eating and physical activity.
- Have teachers and school personnel model healthy eating habits.
- Limit access to unhealthy foods and beverages.
- Provide positive reinforcement for healthy food choices.
- Create a pleasant environment for eating.
- Promote safe food handling practices.
- Involve parents and the community in promoting healthy eating in schools.

Adapted from Knowledge Network. (n.d.). *Making it happen: Healthy eating at school.* Burnaby, BC: Author. Retrieved from http://healthyeatingatschool.ca/.

the most easily obtainable and appealing foods. Unfortunately, these foods are often high in calories and low in nutrition. Providing nutritious snacks is often the best way for a parent to ensure good nutritional intake. Caregivers should provide ready access to fresh fruit, raw vegetables, cheese, popcorn, and high-protein snacks such as skim-milk pudding and hot chocolate. When planning successful eating interventions, nurses need to consider cultural, economic, and social issues (Edelman et al., 2014).

Help families and children prevent obesity through proper nutrition and exercise. Many families often eat in fast-food restaurants in which the food is high in fat, calories, and salt. Nurses should encourage healthy food choices in these situations. Selections should include meats that are not breaded and are broiled, shakes that are made with low-fat yogurt or skim milk, and fruits and vegetables that are fresh or prepared in a low-calorie manner.

ADOLESCENCE

Adolescence is the period of development between childhood and adulthood, usually between 12 and 19 years of age. The term *adolescent* usually refers to psychological maturation of the individual, whereas *puberty* refers to the point at which reproduction becomes possible. The hormonal changes of puberty result in changes in the appearance of the young person: the primary sexual characteristic changes (maturation of the reproductive organs) and the secondary sexual characteristic changes (such as the development of pubic hair and female breasts). Mental development during puberty results in the ability to hypothesize and deal with abstractions. In addition, adolescents become much more social, and their behavioural patterns become much less predictable. Adjustments and adaptations are needed to cope with these simultaneous changes and the attempt to establish a mature sense of identity. Many people refer to adolescence as a stormy and stressful period filled with inner turmoil, but it is recognized that most teenagers successfully meet the challenges of this period. These challenges may cause adolescents to be moody and difficult. Within adolescence, three subphases exist: early adolescence, including puberty (ages 11 to 14 years), middle adolescence (ages 15 to 17 years), and late adolescence (ages 18 to 20 years). Opportunities, challenges, changes, skills, pressures, and physical, cognitive, and psychosocial development vary widely among the subphases (Table 22-9).

As a nurse, understanding of development provides a unique perspective for helping teenagers and parents anticipate and cope with the stresses of adolescence. Primary health care activities, particularly education, can promote healthy development. These activities occur in a variety of settings and can be directed at adolescents, parents, or both. For example, a nurse can conduct seminars in a high school to provide practical suggestions for solving problems of concern to a large group of students, such as treating acne or making responsible decisions about drugs or alcohol use. Similarly, a group education program for parents about how to cope with teenagers would promote parental understanding of adolescent development. These programs can be held in the school, clinic, private office, or community centre. To learn more about specific topics or problems, it is important to identify teenagers' needs and desires. Involvement produces more active, interested learners.

Physical Changes

Physical changes occur rapidly in adolescence. Sexual maturation occurs with the development of primary and secondary sexual characteristics. Four main focuses of the physical changes are as follows:

- Increased growth rate of skeleton, muscle, and viscera
- Sex-specific changes, such as changes in shoulder and hip width
- Alteration in distribution of muscle and fat
- Development of the reproductive system and secondary sex characteristics

The timing of physical changes associated with puberty varies widely between the sexes and within the same sex. Girls tend to begin their physical changes earlier than boys. Variations are more pronounced in boys (Kliegman et al., 2016). The sequence of pubertal growth changes is the same in most individuals (Table 22-10).

Changes are created by hormonal fluctuations within the body when the hypothalamus begins to produce gonadotropin-releasing hormones. This change sends the pituitary gland a signal to secrete gonadotropic hormones. Gonadotropic hormones stimulate ovarian cells to produce estrogen and testicular cells to produce testosterone. These hormones contribute to the development of secondary sex characteristics, such as hair growth and voice changes, and play an essential role in reproduction. The changing concentrations of these hormones are also linked to acne and body odour. Understanding these hormonal changes enables nurses to reassure adolescents and educate them about body care needs.

Boys who mature early have been shown by some researchers to be more poised, relaxed, good-natured, skilled in athletic activities, and likely to be school leaders than boys who mature late. In contrast, girls who mature early have been found to be less sociable and more shy and introverted, perhaps as a result of feeling conspicuous (Edelman et al., 2014). Such girls are more conscious of body development, such as breast development, and thus stand out from many of their peers.

Being like their peers is extremely important for adolescents. Nurses need to stress that normal sexual changes are quite variable. As with increases in height and weight, the pattern of sexual changes is more significant than their time of onset. Large deviations from normal patterns necessitate investigation.

Any deviation in the timing of the physical changes can be extremely difficult for adolescents to accept. It is important to provide emotional support for those undergoing early or delayed puberty. Even adolescents whose physical changes are occurring at the normal times may seek reassurance about their normality.

Height and weight usually increase during the prepubertal growth spurt. The growth spurt for girls generally begins between 8 and 14 years of age. Height increases 5 to 20 cm, and weight increases by 7 to 25 kg. The growth spurt in boys usually occurs between 10 and 16 years of age. Height increases approximately 10 to 30 cm, and weight increases by 7 to 30 kg. In both sexes, the final 20 to 25% of adult height and 50% of adult weight are attained during this time (Hockenberry & Wilson, 2015).

Girls attain 90 to 95% of their adult height by menarche (the onset of menstruation) and reach their full height by 16 to 17 years of age, whereas boys continue to grow taller until 18 to 20 years of age. Fat is redistributed into adult proportions as height and weight increase, and gradually the adolescent torso takes on an adult appearance. Despite individual and sex differences, growth follows a similar pattern for both sexes. Growth in the length of the extremities occurs earliest, making the hands and feet appear very large and the legs very long; the individual often appears awkward and clumsy. At the same time, the lower jaw and nose become longer and the forehead higher and wider as the baby face of childhood disappears. Next, the thighs widen; then the shoulders broaden, and growth of the trunk proceeds. The female hips widen and the male shoulders broaden throughout adolescence.

Personal growth curves can help a nurse in assessing physical development. The individual's sustained progression along the curve, however, is more important than a comparison of measurements with

TABLE 22-9 Growth and Development During Adolescence

Early Adolescence (11–14 Years)	Middle Adolescence (15–17 Years)	Late Adolescence (18–20 Years)
Growth		
Rapidly accelerating growth reaches peak velocity. Secondary sex characteristics appear.	Growth decelerates in girls. Stature reaches 95% of adult height. Secondary sex characteristics are well advanced.	The body is physically mature. Structural and reproductive growth are almost complete.
Cognition		
The person explores newfound ability for limited abstract thought. Clumsy groping for new values and energies occurs. One's "normality" is compared with that of peers of same sex.	Capacity for abstract thinking develops. Intellectual powers, often in idealistic terms, are increased. Concerns with philosophic, political, and social problems arise.	Abstract thought is established. The person can perceive and act on long-range options. The person is able to view problems comprehensively. Intellectual and functional identity are established.
Identity		
The person is preoccupied with rapid body changes. The person tries out various roles. Attractiveness is measured by acceptance or rejection by peers. Conformity to group norms is typical. Self-esteem declines.	Body image is modified. The person is very self-centred; narcissism is increased. A tendency toward inner experience and self-discovery develops. Fantasy life is rich. The person becomes idealistic. The person is able to perceive future implications of current behaviour and decisions, with variable application.	Body image and gender role definition are nearly secured. Sexual identity is mature. Identity is consolidated. Self-esteem increases. The person is comfortable with physical growth. Social roles are defined and articulated.
Relationships With Parents		
Independence–dependence boundaries are defined. The person has a strong desire to remain dependent on parents while trying to detach from them. No major conflicts over parental control occur.	Major conflicts over independence and control occur. This is the low point in the parent–child relationship. The person makes the greatest push for emancipation and disengagement. Emotional detachment from parents is final and irreversible; mourning occurs.	Emotional and physical separation from parents is completed. Independence is achieved from family with less conflict. Emancipation is nearly secured.
Relationships With Peers		
The person seeks peer affiliations to counter instability generated by rapid change. The person experiences an upsurge of close, idealized friendships with members of the same sex. Struggle for mastery takes place within the peer group.	The person has a strong need for identity to affirm self-image. Behavioural standards are set by peer group. Acceptance by peers is extremely important; rejection is feared. The person explores the ability to attract a sexual partner.	The peer group recedes in importance in favour of individual friendship. Male–female and same-sex relationships are tested against the possibility of permanent alliance. Relationships are characterized by giving and sharing.
Sexuality		
Self-exploration and evaluation occur. Dating is limited; the person usually socializes with a group. Intimacy is limited.	Multiple plural relationships are characteristic. The person decisively turns toward heterosexuality, bisexuality, or same-sex sexuality. "Self-appeal" is explored. Feeling of "being in love" is common. Relationships are tentatively established.	The person forms stable relationships and attachment to another person. The capacity for mutuality and reciprocity grows. Dating is common. The person may publicly identify herself or himself as gay, lesbian, bisexual, or transgender. Intimacy involves commitment rather than exploration and romanticism.
Psychological Health		
Wide mood swings occur. Intense daydreaming is characteristic. Anger is outwardly expressed with moodiness, temper outbursts, verbal insults, and name-calling.	A tendency toward inner experiences is exhibited; the person becomes more introspective. The person tends to withdraw when upset or when feelings are hurt. Emotions vacillate in time and range. Feelings of inadequacy are common; asking for help is difficult.	The person experiences more constancy of emotion. Anger is more apt to be concealed.

Adapted from Hockenberry, M. J., & Wilson, D. (2015). *Wong's nursing care of infants and children* (10th ed., p. 652). St. Louis, MO: Mosby.

TABLE 22-10 Average Sequences of Physiological Changes in Adolescence

	AGE RANGE (YEARS)	
Characteristics	**Girls**	**Boys**
Beginning of skeletal growth spurt	8–14.5 (peak: 12)	10.5–16 (peak: 14)
Beginning of breast development	8–13	—
Enlargement of testes and scrotal sac	—	10–13.5
Appearance of straight, pigmented pubic hair, which gradually becomes curly	8–14	10–15
Early voice changes (cracks)	—	11–14.5
Enlargement of penis and prostate gland	—	11–14.5
Menarche	10–18 (average: 12.25)	—
Spermatogenesis (ejaculation of sperm)	—	11–17 (average: 13.5)
Ovulation and completion of breast development	14–18 (average: 15.52)	—
Appearance of downy facial hair	—	12–17
Appearance of axillary (underarm) hair and increased output of oil and sweat-producing glands, which may lead to acne	10–16	12–17
Widening and deepening of female pelvis, with deposition of subcutaneous fat that gives rounded appearance to body	10–18	—
Increase in shoulder width	—	11–21
Deepening of male voice, with appearance of coarse and pigmented facial hair and appearance of chest and axillary hair as well as other body hair becoming more prominent, such as that on forearms and legs	—	16–21

the norm. To evaluate changes, the nurse should chart growth measurements during routine health assessments.

Adolescents are sensitive about physical changes that make them different from peers. For this reason, they are generally interested in the normal pattern of growth and in their personal growth curves. Therefore, nurses should share this information to reassure adolescents that their own patterns are normal.

Cognitive Changes

According to Piaget (1952), the changes that occur within the mind and the widening social environment of adolescents result in the highest level of intellectual development, known as **formal operations** (see Chapter 21 for further information on development). However, without an appropriate educational environment, some people may not attain this stage. Those who are guided toward developing rational thinking may reach this stage early.

Adolescents develop the ability to determine possibilities, rank possibilities, solve problems, and make decisions through logical operations. The teenager can deal effectively with hypothetical problems. When confronted with a problem, the teenager is able to consider an infinite variety of causes and solutions. Adolescents can move beyond the physical or concrete properties of a situation and use reasoning powers to understand the abstract. School-age children think about what is, whereas adolescents can imagine what might be. These newly developed abilities allow the individual to have more insight and skill in playing video games, computer games, and board games that require abstract thinking and deductive reasoning about many possible strategies. A teenager can solve problems by simultaneously manipulating several abstract concepts.

Development of the ability to reason abstractly is important in the pursuit of an identity. For example, newly acquired cognitive skills enable the teenager to define appropriate, effective, and comfortable sex role behaviours and consider their impact on peers, family, and society. The ability to think logically about these behaviours and their outcomes helps adolescents to develop personal thoughts and means of expressing sexual identity. In addition, because their level of cognitive functioning is higher, adolescents are receptive to more detailed and diverse information about sexuality and sexual behaviours. For example, sex education can include an explanation of physiological sexual changes and birth control measures.

By middle adolescence, an introspective quality emerges. At this time, adolescents believe that they are unique. They also may believe, because of their new physical skills, that they are invulnerable, and so they engage in risk-taking behaviours; many state that they "can drive fast and not get into an accident." Other typical adolescent behaviours include self-consciousness and the desire for privacy.

The complex development of thought during this period leads adolescents to question society and its values. Although adolescents have the capability to think as logically as adults, they do not yet have experiences from which to gain perspective. It is common for teenagers to consider their parents too narrow-minded or too materialistic. This perception can result in conflicts between teenagers and parents. Cognitive abilities and performance vary greatly among adolescents. In fact, an adolescent may perform at different levels in different situations on the basis of past experiences, formal education, and motivation in the use of logic and effective deductive reasoning.

Language Skills. Language development is fairly complete by adolescence, although vocabulary continues to expand. The primary focus becomes practising communication skills that can be used effectively in various situations. Adolescents need to communicate thoughts, feelings, and facts to others. The skills used in communication situations are varied. Adolescents must select the person with whom to communicate, decide on the message, and choose the way to transmit the message. For example, the way teenagers tell parents about failing grades is not the same as the way that they tell friends. Adolescents develop different skills and styles of communication and learn how and when to use them most effectively. These diverse communication skills are used and refined throughout life (Santrock, 2011). Good communication skills are crucial for overcoming peer pressure and unhealthy behaviours. The following are some hints for communicating with adolescents:

- Do not avoid discussing sensitive issues. Asking questions about sex, drugs, and school demonstrates your interest in their well-being and may open the channels for further discussion.
- Ask open-ended questions.
- Try to discern the meaning behind their words or actions.
- Be alert to clues to their emotional state.
- Involve other individuals and resources when necessary.

Psychosocial Changes

The search for personal identity is the major characteristic of adolescent psychosocial development. Teenagers must establish close peer relationships or risk remaining socially isolated. Erikson (1963) viewed identity (or role) confusion as the prime danger of this stage and suggested that the cliquishness and intolerance of differences seen in adolescent behaviour are defences against identity confusion (Erikson, 1968). Adolescents work at becoming emotionally independent from their parents, while retaining family ties. In addition, they need to develop their own ethical systems that are based on personal values. Choices about vocation, future education, and lifestyle must be made. The various components of identity evolve from these stages and compose a total adult personal identity that is unique to the individual. Indecisiveness and the inability to make an occupational choice are behaviours indicating the lack of resolution to certain developmental tasks.

Gender Identity. Achievement of gender identity is enhanced by the physical changes of puberty. According to Freud, these physiological changes of puberty stimulate the libido, the energy source that fuels the sex drive (see Chapter 21 for further information on development). This change is evidenced by teenagers' interest in romantic relationships and by their practice of masturbation. The physical evidence of maturity encourages the development of masculine and feminine behaviours. If these physical changes involve deviations, the person has more difficulty developing a comfortable sexual identity. Adolescents depend on these physical clues because they want assurance of maleness or femaleness and because they do not wish to be different from peers. Some adolescents are genderqueer, meaning they reject the traditional binary construct of gender, including gender labels, and may identify as neither girl/woman nor boy/man (Miller, 2016). Transgender adolescents have gender identities that are different from their biological sex and they may transition to their affirmed gender (Miller, 2016).

Other influences on gender identity are cultural attitudes and expectations of sex role behaviour and available role models. The masculine and feminine behaviours that teenagers see affect the way that they express sexuality.

Group Identity. Adolescents seek a group identity because they need esteem and acceptance (Figure 22-7). Similarity in dress, speech, or both is common in teenage groups. Popularity is a major concern for teenagers. Peer groups provide adolescents with a sense of belonging, approval, and the opportunity to learn acceptable behaviour. Popularity with both opposite-sex and same-sex peers is important. The strong need for group identity seems to conflict at times with the search for personal identity. It is as though adolescents require close bonds with peers so that they can later achieve a sense of individuality.

Family Identity. The movement toward stronger peer relationships contrasts with adolescents' movements away from parents. Although financial independence for adolescents is not the norm in Canadian society, many adolescents work part-time, using their income to bolster independence. When adolescents cannot have a part-time job because of studies, school-related activities, and other factors, parents can provide allowances for clothing and incidentals, which encourage adolescents to develop decision-making and budgeting skills.

Some adolescents and families have more difficulty during these years than others. Adolescents need to make choices, act independently, and experience the consequences of actions. This testing, however, is best done against the background of firm family support. The family needs to allow independence while providing a haven in which adolescents can contemplate actions. Families unable to provide this support complicate movement toward identity formation. Health care support of a family and an adolescent may be essential to their success.

Nurses can assist families in considering ways that are appropriate for them to foster the independence of their adolescent while maintaining family structure. Many of these discussions involve curfews, jobs, and participation in family chores. Emancipation from the immediate family is most successful when accomplished gradually and when it results in a balance between independence and family ties.

Vocational Identity. Selecting an occupation or a vocational direction in life is a goal for adolescents. Because of society's changing needs, adolescents must be future oriented when making these choices. However, adolescents do not know which jobs will be available and rewarding 10 or 20 years in the future, and selecting a career is thus a complicated task. Nurses need to be supportive to the family during this process and help adolescents select courses of action that promote self-satisfaction, identity, and continued opportunity for growth.

Moral Identity. The development of moral judgement depends heavily on cognitive and communication skills and peer interaction.

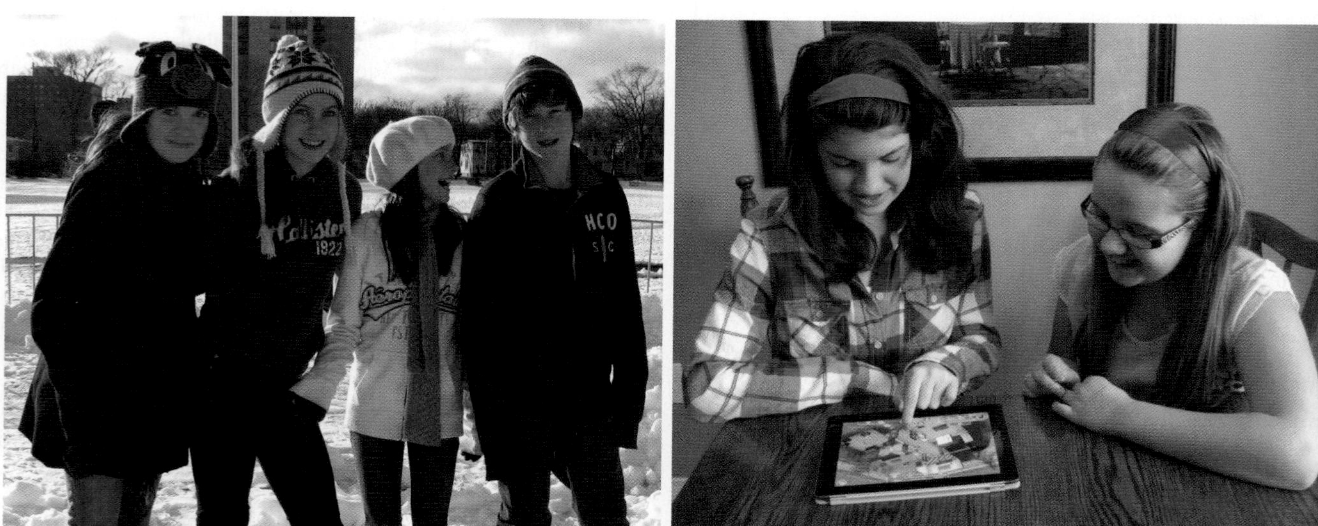

FIGURE 22-7 Social interactions strengthen a teenager's group identity. (Courtesy Cynthia Murray, BN, MN, PhD.)

Although moral development begins in early childhood, it is consolidated in adolescence because of the presence of certain skills. Adolescents learn that rules are cooperative agreements that can be modified to fit the situation, rather than absolute. Adolescents learn to use their own judgement rather than to use the rules to avoid punishment as in earlier years. Kohlberg (1964) explained moral development in terms of stages (see Chapter 21 for further information on development). At the highest level, morality is derived from individual principles of conscience. Adolescents judge themselves by internalized ideals; such judgement often leads to conflict between personal and group values. Group values become less significant in later adolescence.

Not all adolescents attain the same level of moral development; however, they generally advance through the stages of moral development, and the sequence of the stages is similar for all individuals, even though the time at achievement varies. Kohlberg's (1964) moral development theory focuses on justice based on reciprocity and equal respect. Adolescent girls have been found to be more likely to give caring responses to moral problems, whereas adolescent boys have been found to give more justice-oriented responses (Gilligan, 1982).

Health Identity. Healthy adolescents evaluate their own health according to feelings of well-being, ability to function normally, and absence of symptoms (Hockenberry & Wilson, 2015).

Interventions to improve health perception might, therefore, concentrate on the adolescent period. The rapid changes during this period make primary health care programs especially crucial. Adolescents try new roles, begin to stabilize their identity, and acquire values and behaviours from which their adult lifestyle will evolve.

Health Risks

Injuries. Injuries, including self-inflicted injuries and injuries caused by motor vehicle accidents and poisoning, are the leading causes of death in Canadian adolescents (PHAC, 2013). Feelings of being indestructible can lead to risk-taking behaviour. Many injuries are preceded by the use of alcohol (Hockenberry & Wilson, 2015). Nurses can play an important role in planning, implementing, and evaluating injury prevention strategies (CASN, 2014). For example, in partnership with community members and other stakeholders, a nurse might identify alcohol-related motor vehicle accidents among adolescents as a community health need and assist in the development, delivery, and evaluation of preventive programs and healthy public policies aimed at addressing the need.

Suicide. Suicide is increasing as a cause of death in adolescents between 15 and 19 years of age. Depression and social isolation commonly precede a suicide attempt, but suicidal thoughts probably result from a combination of several factors (Box 22-8).

A nurse must be able to identify the factors associated with adolescent suicide risk and precipitating events. In addition, the nurse should be alert to the following warning signs, which often occur for at least a month before suicide is attempted:

- Deterioration in school performance
- Social withdrawal
- Loss of initiative
- Loneliness, sadness, and crying
- Appetite and sleep disturbances
- Verbalization of suicidal thought

Immediate referrals to mental health providers are needed when assessment findings suggest that adolescents may be considering suicide. Guidance can help them focus on the positive aspects of life and strengthen coping abilities.

Substance Abuse. Adolescents may believe that mood-altering substances create a sense of well-being or improve level of performance. All adolescents are at risk for experimental or recreational substance use, but those with dysfunctional families are more at risk for chronic use and physical dependency. Some adolescents believe that substance use makes them more mature. They further believe they will look and feel better with drug usage. Alcohol is the substance most commonly used, followed by cannabis. Rates of opioid abuse and overdose are increasing in Canada, with the fastest rate of growth in hospitalizations for opioid poisoning occurring in adolescents and youth

BOX 22-8 Factors Associated With Suicide

History

Previous suicide attempt
Suicide attempt by family member or friend
History of child maltreatment
Past psychiatric hospitalization
Death of a parent when child was young

Individual Factors

Hopelessness
Marked, persistent depression
Alcohol or drug abuse
Impulsiveness
Difficulty tolerating frustration
Feelings of self-hatred, excessive guilt, or humiliation
Thinking disorder (wishes to join a deceased person, hears voices saying to kill self)
Physical, behavioural, developmental, or body image problems (delayed puberty, chronic illness, disability, attention deficit–hyperactivity disorder, learning disorders)
Gender identity or sexual orientation concerns; being gay, lesbian, bisexual, or transgender in an unsupportive environment
Seeing self as totally helpless: a victim of fate
Needing to do things perfectly

Family Factors

Difficult home situation: long, bitter parent–child conflict
Hostile parents
Overt rejection by one or both parents
Divorce or separation of parents
Recent or impending move
Family breakup or loss of parent
Stress of unrealistically high parental expectations
Parental indifference with very low expectations

Social and Environmental Factors

Firearms in the home
Incarceration
Lack of effective social support system
Isolation
Suicide of someone known
Few social, vocational, educational opportunities

Adapted from Hockenberry, M. J., & Wilson, D. (2015). *Wong's nursing care of infants and children* (10th ed., p. 751). St. Louis, MO: Mosby.

aged 15 to 24 (Canadian Institute for Health Information, 2017). Other substances frequently abused by teenagers include steroids, which are used to enhance athletic performances. It is believed that the use of these products may increase the likelihood of using other illicit drugs (Canadian Centre on Substance Abuse, 2014). Tobacco use, although decreasing, continues to be a problem among adolescents.

Eating Disorders. Weight extremes resulting from excessive or inadequate caloric intake are common during the adolescent years. The number of eating disorders is on the rise in adolescents, particularly among girls. If an adolescent's growth deviates radically from the usual pattern, further assessment is necessary to identify the cause. Items to include in the assessment are past and present diet history, food records, eating habits, attitudes, health beliefs, and socioeconomic and psychosocial factors (Hockenberry & Wilson, 2015). Knowledge of growth progression may be a way to discourage radical weight reduction activities. Allowing an adolescent to see when and how the weight curve changed can be a first step in identifying the problem and implementing dietary changes.

Although anorexia nervosa and bulimia are classified as separate eating disorders, manifestations of the two overlap (Enright, 2014). Anorexia nervosa is considered a clinical syndrome with both physical and psychosocial components. The majority of patients are adolescents and young women. Attending a highly competitive high school and being from a professional, upper-middle-class family increase the risk for this disorder. People with anorexia nervosa have an intense fear of gaining weight and refuse to maintain body weight at the normal minimum for their age and height.

Bulimia nervosa is most identified with binge eating and behaviours to prevent weight gain, including self-induced vomiting, misuse of laxatives and other medications, fasting, and excessive exercise (Hockenberry & Wilson, 2015). Because adolescents rarely volunteer information about behaviours to prevent weight gain, it is important to take a thorough dietary history. Society's expectations for thinness may have a strong influence on the development of these disorders. While eating disorders tend to be more common among girls, boys may also suffer from these disorders. Causes of eating disorders are the same for girls and boys.

Obesity and Physical Inactivity. Overweight and obesity, together with a decrease in physical activity, are becoming serious public health problems in Canada. Over the last 30 years, obesity rates have nearly tripled among Canadian children and adolescents (Government of Canada, 2016). A contributing factor is a lack of physical activity; children and adolescents spend more time watching television and using computers, especially playing computer games. Parents and other people working with adolescents must encourage greater physical activity among this age group, must monitor computer use, and must promote healthy nutrition.

Sexual Experimentation. Sexual experimentation is common among adolescents. Peer pressure, physiological and emotional changes, and societal expectations contribute to early heterosexual and same-sex relations. Two prominent consequences of adolescent sexual activity are sexually transmitted infections and pregnancy (Hockenberry & Wilson, 2015).

Sexually Transmitted Infections. The incidence of sexually transmitted infections (STIs) reported among adolescents (PHAC, 2016b) is increasing. Therefore, sexually active adolescents must be screened for STIs, even when they have no symptoms, because STIs can be asymptomatic. The annual physical examination of a sexually active adolescent should include a thorough sexual and genitourinary history and a careful examination of the genitalia so that genital warts, herpes, and other STIs are not missed. Recommended tests for women include Papanicolaou (Pap) smears, cervical cultures for gonorrhea and *Chlamydia* species, and syphilis tests; for men, urethral cultures for gonorrhea and *Chlamydia* species and syphilis tests are recommended. If men have participated in same-sex activities, rectal and pharyngeal cultures also need to be taken to check for gonorrhea. Because the human papillomavirus (HPV) is a common STI, all Canadian provinces and territories have HPV vaccine programs, whereby adolescent girls are given a vaccine that is effective against some HPV viruses associated with cervical cancer (PHAC, 2012). Health care providers can be proactive by using the patient interview process to identify risk factors in adolescents. Once risk factors are identified, corresponding strategies for prevention should be carried out.

The human immunodeficiency virus (HIV), which causes acquired immune deficiency syndrome (AIDS), is transmitted through unprotected sexual intercourse, the use of shared needles for injecting drugs, and infected blood products (see Chapter 27 for further information about HIV). Therefore, the risk-taking behaviours of sexual activity and drug use make adolescents vulnerable to the threat of AIDS and other STIs. Adolescents who have placed themselves at risk for AIDS should be tested for HIV infection. All adolescents need thorough and up-to-date knowledge about HIV and AIDS.

Pregnancy. Adolescent pregnancy occurs across socioeconomic classes, in public and private schools, among all ethnic and religious backgrounds, and in all parts of the country. Adolescent pregnancy with early prenatal supervision is considered less physically harmful to both mother and child than earlier believed. Pregnant teenagers need special education about nutrition, as well as health supervision and psychological support.

Health Concerns

Adolescents need to form healthy habits of daily living. Nurses should emphasize the importance of exercise, sleep, nutrition, and stress reduction and identify ways to convey these needs to each adolescent. To do this, the nurse must assess the individual's positive and negative habits and attitudes about health. Extensive and long-term follow-up is required if individualized interventions are to succeed. Nurses must be aware of the prevalence of health problems and make assessments accordingly.

Health Education. Community and school-based health programs for adolescents focus on health promotion and illness prevention. Nurses can become involved in these programs by providing screening and teaching for adolescents (Table 22-11). Developing and implementing programs to respond to adolescents' needs is another important strategy that nurses can be involved in. Helping adolescents make decisions about their health care strengthens their autonomy and promotes healthy behaviours. In any such programs, however, it is important to remember that adolescents must first feel comfortable and respected as individuals to reveal intimate information about their risk-taking behaviours, thus discussions with adolescents must be private and confidential.

A nurse can play an important role in preventing injuries and accidental deaths by taking part in such activities as injury prevention programs; organizations that promote responsible behaviour, including Mothers Against Drunk Driving (MADD) and Drug Abuse Resistance Education (DARE); and encouraging students to participate in organizations such as Students Against Drunk Driving (SADD). By stimulating adolescents to discuss alternatives to driving when under the influence of drugs or alcohol, you can prepare them to consider alternatives when such an occasion arises. It is also important to identify adolescents at risk for substance abuse, provide education to prevent accidents related to substance abuse, and provide counselling to patients in rehabilitation programs.

TABLE 22-11 Health Promotion for Adolescents

Adolescent Health Concerns	Health Promotion Intervention
Unintentional injuries	Advise the adolescent to take a driver's education course and to wear seat belts. Inform the adolescent of risk associated with drinking and driving and with use of drugs. Promote helmet use by adolescents who use bicycles, motorcycles, all-terrain vehicles, and snowmobiles. Ensure the adolescent receives proper orientation in the use of all sports equipment. Encourage the adolescent to swim with a "buddy."
Firearm use and violence	Teach conflict resolution skills.
Tobacco, alcohol, and drug use	Screen for tobacco (including smokeless), alcohol, and drug use, and inform the adolescent of risks of use.
Suicide	Offer suicide prevention information. Teach methods of dealing with a suicidal peer. Promote suicide alternatives.
Sexually transmitted infections	Provide the adolescent with information regarding disease, mode of transmission, and related symptoms. Encourage safer sexual practices, including abstinence from sexual activity or the use of condoms. Provide accurate information about the consequences of sexual activity.

The nurse can also play a strategic role in an antismoking movement, such as participating in a smoking prevention program initiated in a school. Communities may also involve nurses in creating and carrying out tobacco control policies at the local level (Douglas, Manion, Hall-Harper, et al., 2015).

Regardless of health setting, nurses need to provide sex education and counselling and can play a key role in counselling teenagers on ways to avoid pregnancies. Nurses can also assist adolescents in making decisions about pregnancies that do occur (e.g., becoming a parent, adoption, or abortion). Some schools have instituted day care programs so that adolescent mothers can continue their schooling after their babies are born. Whatever choice an adolescent makes, it is important that she receive appropriate health care, including counselling.

Extensive educational efforts to prevent the spread of AIDS and other STIs in this age group are a nursing responsibility. Formal or informal education, in a one-on-one or group setting, may be provided in the school or community. Speakers and organizations can be used to help in the educational process.

Adolescents in Rural Communities. Approximately 20% of Canadians live in rural areas and small towns; however, this percentage varies by province and territory. Although adolescents living in these areas have many of the same health needs as their urban counterparts, they also have some unique risks. For example, those living on farms are at increased risk for accidents because of exposure to heavy equipment, huge vehicles, and large animals (Government of Alberta, 2016). Other concerns for adolescents living in rural areas and small towns are limited availability of recreational facilities and limited access to specialized services.

Nurses can play an important role in improving the health of adolescents who live in rural areas by acting to decrease barriers to care, providing health promotion education, developing coping strategies for these adolescents, and assessing their health beliefs.

Minority Adolescents. By the next century, it is expected that minorities (non-White persons) as a group will become the majority. Minority adolescents have been identified as experiencing a greater percentage of health problems and barriers to health care.

Issues of concern that have been identified for minority adolescents living in a high-risk environment include learning or emotional difficulties, death related to violence (e.g., "honour killing" of a female relative on the perceived grounds that she has dishonoured the family [Amnesty International, 2014]), unintentional injuries, and increased rates of adolescent pregnancy and STIs, including AIDS. Poverty has a major negative effect on the lives of minority adolescents. Access to culturally appropriate health services is commonly limited. Nurses can make a significant contribution to improving access to appropriate health care for adolescents. Health promotion initiatives must be based on topics of concern for these adolescents.

As a nurse working in the community, it is important that they adopt culturally sensitive interventions to meet the needs of minority adolescents and their families (Hockenberry & Wilson, 2015). Culturally sensitive care encompasses knowledge and respect for different cultural world views, as well as self-awareness of your own biases, beliefs, and values (Edelman et al., 2014). You must be able to communicate in another language by speaking it or using an interpreter's services. Educational materials need to be written in the appropriate language. Information regarding health beliefs and healing practices must be assessed. With knowledge about various cultures and the means to care for minority adolescents, the nurse can act as an advocate to ensure accessibility of appropriate services.

Indigenous Adolescents. Health status and factors affecting it are generally worse for Canadian Indigenous adolescents (i.e., First Nations, Inuit, and Métis) than for any other adolescent populations (Canadian Human Rights Commission, 2013). In Canada, suicide rates are five to seven times higher among First Nations youth and 11 times higher among Inuit youth than among non-Indigenous youth (Health Canada, 2016). Indigenous adolescents are more likely to have crowded living conditions and to live in communities in which rates of alcohol abuse and substance abuse are high. Likewise, the incidence of unemployment and reported sexual and physical abuse is higher in Indigenous than in non-Indigenous communities (Canadian Human Rights Commission, 2013). Some problems, such as overcrowded living conditions and high rates of unemployment, persist for Indigenous people living in urban areas of Canada.

When working with Indigenous adolescents, nurses need to be aware of the unique factors that may affect these young people's health. First, nurses need to be aware that health beliefs and practices, as well as health problems, vary among Indigenous populations and communities. Nurses must be sensitive to culturally appropriate interventions. Many Indigenous communities take responsibility for their own health and well-being, develop their own health services, and include traditional methods of healing to improve well-being.

Lesbian, Gay, Bisexual, Transgender, Queer or Questioning, and 2 Spirit (LGBTQ2). Although research on LGBTQ2 youth is limited, special consideration must be given to the developmental and health challenges that may result from nonheterosexual orientations and societal attitudes toward those orientations (Hockenberry & Wilson, 2015). It may be difficult for adolescents to discuss some of these challenges because of the stigma associated with being LGBTQ2.

As a consequence, LGBTQ2 could be at greater risk for emotional distress, depression, and suicide, as well as for alcohol or other drug abuse. LGBTQ2 youth may need assistance with disclosing their sexual orientation and, before they disclose this information, a plan for dealing with negative and sometimes violent reactions from others who are nonaccepting of them. It is important to respond to these individuals in a sensitive and nonjudgemental way.

KEY CONCEPTS

- A developmental perspective helps the nurse understand commonalities and variations in each stage and the impact they have on the patient's health.
- During the intrauterine period, while embryo and fetus grow and develop, genetic factors and environmental factors (teratogens) may cause impairments in any body system.
- Physiological, cognitive, and psychosocial development continue from conception through adolescence, and nurses must be familiar with normal parameters to determine potential problems and promote normal development.
- Physical growth during the school years is slow and steady until the skeletal growth spurt just before puberty.
- The major psychosocial developmental task of school-age children is the development of a sense of competence.
- Cognitively, young school-age children develop the ability to think in a logical manner.
- The prepubertal growth spurt usually occurs 2 years earlier in girls than in boys.
- Adolescents move forward to the last stage of cognitive development, formal operations, in which they begin to think in an abstract manner, reflect on thought processes, and plan for the future.
- Adolescence begins with puberty, when the primary sexual characteristic changes (maturation of the reproductive organs) and the secondary sexual characteristic changes (such as the development of pubic hair and female breasts) begin.
- Adolescents are able to solve complex mental problems by using deductive reasoning.
- Adolescents' rapid change in physical appearance heightens self-consciousness and concerns regarding body image.
- Accidents are the major cause of death in all age groups up to adulthood.
- Motor vehicle accidents are the major cause of accidental death in adolescence.
- Adolescents begin the long process of emancipation from their parents and need parental support to accomplish this in a timely manner.

CRITICAL THINKING EXERCISES

1. Ms. Yeigh, who is in her first trimester of pregnancy, is attending the antepartum clinic for the first visit. What are the main health promotion topics you need to explore with her at this stage in her pregnancy?
2. The parents of 2-year-old Mark are concerned because his language does not seem to be at the same level as that of their neighbour's 2-year-old daughter. How would you reassure these parents and help them with language development?
3. Eight-year-old Lisa sometimes says to her parents that she feels "like a failure." According to Erickson's task for this stage of development, what measures can her parents and teacher use to help negate these feelings and help her meet this stage of development?
4. Twelve-year-old Maya is brought to the pediatric clinic for a physical examination. She is concerned about her lack of physical development in comparison with her peers. Discuss ways to educate Maya about puberty and the variations that occur.
5. Fifteen-year-old Ricardo wants very much to belong and to be accepted by his peers. He expresses concern when his peers begin to plan a party with alcohol and drugs. What should be discussed to help support his feelings and need to belong?

REVIEW QUESTIONS

1. A nurse monitors the growth and development of a child who had low birth weight. The nurse is cognizant that infants with low birth weight have an increased risk for which conditions? *(Select all that apply.)*
   1. Type 1 diabetes
   2. Developmental delays
   3. Temperament problems
   4. Neurological and motor impairment
2. A nurse weighs a 3-day-old, breastfed infant. The nurse notes that 5% of the infant's birth weight has been lost. What action should the nurse take?
   1. Inform the mother that the infant's weight is normal
   2. Notify the doctor about the infant's weight loss
   3. Instruct the mother to breastfeed the infant more frequently
   4. Instruct the mother to supplement breastfeeding with formula
3. A nurse administers the first dose of hepatitis B vaccine to a newborn baby. The nurse informs the parents that the second dose is administered at ____ month(s) of age and the third dose is administered at ____ month(s) of age.
   1. 6 months; 12 months
   2. 1 month; 6 months
   3. 3 months; 6 months
   4. 1 month; 3 months
4. A toddler pretends to shave after watching his father shave. This is an example of Piaget's
   1. Sensorimotor stage
   2. Intuitive phase of preoperational thought stage
   3. Autonomy stage
   4. Preoperational thought stage
5. A client asks the nurse about typical play behaviours among preschoolers. The nurse provides which information to the client? *(Select all that apply.)*
   1. Most 3-year-old children play cooperatively with another child.
   2. Most 5-year-old children only play alone.
   3. Preschoolers usually play side-by-side.
   4. Older preschoolers play in groups of two or three.
6. A nurse is assessing the suicide risk for a bullied child. Which findings are warning signs for suicide? *(Select all that apply.)*
   1. Loneliness, sadness, and crying
   2. Stable school performance
   3. Social withdrawal
   4. An increase in appetite
   5. A decrease in appetite
   6. Verbalization of suicidal thought
7. The school nurse observes bite marks and round burns on an 8-year-old child's arms. Upon questioning, the child tells the nurse, "Oh, that's nothing. I fell off my bike." Which action should the nurse take first?
   1. Speak to the child's teacher about the observed injuries
   2. Meet with the school principal about the observed injuries

3. Discuss the injuries with the child's parents
4. Report the incident to the authorities

8. A 10-year-old client attends an influenza vaccination clinic with a temperature of 37.5°C. For the last 24 hours, the client has had a minor, nonproductive cough. Which action should the nurse take?
   1. Hold the vaccine
   2. Check the client's temperature again in 15 minutes
   3. Administer the vaccine in one dose
   4. Administer the vaccine in two doses
9. A 12-year-old girl tells the school nurse that she is concerned because, unlike her friends, she has not started menstruating, although she has had some breast development. Which is the most likely reason for the client's concern?
   1. The client has a gynecological condition that is impeding menstruation.
   2. The client is in prepuberty.
   3. The client has an eating disorder that is impeding menstruation.
   4. The client is undergoing puberty at a normal rate.
10. The nurse gives a presentation to a group of parents on health risks for Canadian adolescents. Which parental statement indicates the need for more teaching about the health risks? *(Select all that apply.)*
    1. "The leading cause of death in adolescence is substance abuse."
    2. "The leading cause of death in adolescence is injuries."
    3. "Eating disorders are only a concern for parents with daughters."
    4. "The number of adolescents smoking cigarettes is increasing."

Answers: 1. 2, 3, 4; **2.** 1; **3.** 2; **4.** 4; **5.** 1, 4; **6.** 1, 3, 4, 5, 6; **7.** 4; **8.** 3; **9.** 4; **10.** 1, 3, 4

Rationales for the Review Questions appear at the end of the book.

RECOMMENDED WEBSITES

Campaign 2000: http://www.campaign2000.ca.
Campaign 2000 is a nonpartisan, cross-Canada coalition of more than 120 national, provincial, and community organizations committed to working together to end child and family poverty in Canada.

Canadian Institute of Child Health: http://www.cich.ca/.
The Canadian Institute of Child Health (CICH) is a national charitable organization dedicated to promoting the health of children and youth in Canada. The CICH works with government and industry to address children's safety and health care issues and to develop appropriate policies. This website offers evidence-informed resources of interest to health care providers, teachers, and parents.

Canadian Paediatric Society: Position Statements and Practice Points: http://www.cps.ca/en/documents.
This website includes the Canadian Paediatric Society's position statements on a variety of child health issues. It has updates as they are developed.

Immunize Canada: https://immunize.ca/.
Immunize Canada (formerly the Canadian Coalition for Immunization Awareness and Promotion) is a partnership of national nongovernmental, professional, health, consumer, government, and private-sector organizations focused on promoting the understanding and use of vaccines recommended by the National Advisory Committee on Immunization. This website provides evidence-informed resources on immunization for parents and health care providers.

REFERENCES

American Academy of Pediatrics. (2011). Policy statement: Child passenger safety. *Pediatrics, 127*, 788–793. doi:10.1542/peds.2011-0213.

American Academy of Pediatrics. (2013). *Talking to kids and teens about social media and sexting*. Retrieved from https://www.aap.org/en-us/about-the-aap/aap-press-room/news-features-and-safety-tips/Pages/Talking-to-Kids-and-Teens-About-Social-Media-and-Sexting.aspx.

Amnesty International. (2014). *Shocking: Surge of honor killings in Pakistan*. Retrieved from http://www.amnesty.ca/blog/shocking-surge-of-honor-killings-in-pakistan.

Benoit, B., Goldberg, L., & Campbell-Yeo, M. (2016). Infant feeding and maternal guilt: The application of a feminist phenomenological framework to guide clinician practices in breast feeding promotion. *Midwifery, 34*, 58–65. doi:10.1016/j.midw.2015.10.011.

Campaign 2000. (2015). *Let's do this: Let's end child poverty for good. 2015 Report card on child and family poverty in Canada*. Retrieved from http://www.cwp-csp.ca/resources/sites/default/files/resources/NationalReportCardEn2015.pdf.

Canadian Association for School Health. (2007). *Canadian consensus statement (Revised 2007): Comprehensive school health*. Retrieved from http://opha.on.ca/OPHA/media/Resources/Resource%20Documents/CSH_Consensus_Statement2007.pdf?ext=.pdf.

Canadian Association for Schools of Nursing (CASN). (2014). *Entry-to-practice public health nursing competencies for undergraduate nursing education*. Retrieved from http://casn.ca/wp-content/uploads/2014/12/FINALpublichealthcompeENforweb.pdf.

Canadian Association for Schools of Nursing (CASN). (2015). *National nursing education framework: Final report*. Retrieved from http://www.casn.ca/wp-content/uploads/2014/12/Framwork-FINAL-SB-Nov-30-20151.pdf.

Canadian Centre on Substance Abuse (2014). *The Canadian standards for youth substance abuse prevention*. Ottawa: Author.

Canadian Child Welfare Research Portal. (2011). *Frequently asked questions*. Retrieved from http://cwrp.ca/faqs.

Canadian Foundation for the Study of Infant Deaths: Baby's Breath Canada. (2015). *Parents and caregivers*. Retrieved from http://www.babysbreathcanada.ca/parentsandcaregivers.html.

Canadian Human Rights Commission (2013). *Report on equality rights of Aboriginal people* (Cat. No. HR4-22/2013E-PDF). Ottawa: Author. Retrieved from http://www.chrc-ccdp.gc.ca/sites/default/files/equality_aboriginal_report_2.pdf.

Canadian Institute for Health Information. (2017). *13 Canadians hospitalized each day for opioid poisoning*. Retrieved from https://www.cihi.ca/en/13-canadians-hospitalized-each-day-for-opioid-poisoning.

Canadian Paediatric Society. (2015). *Circumcision of baby boys: Information for parents*. Retrieved from http://www.caringforkids.cps.ca/handouts/circumcision.

Douglas, M. R., Manion, C. A., Hall-Harper, V. D., et al. (2015). Case studies from community coalitions: Advancing local tobacco control policy in a preemptive state. *American Journal of Preventive Medicine, 48*(Suppl. 1), 29–35. doi:10.1016/j.amepre.2014.09.020.

Douglas, P., Miller, Y., Bucetti, A., et al. (2015). Preliminary evaluation of a primary care intervention for cry-fuss behaviours in the first 3-4 months of life ('The Possums Approach'): Effects on cry-fuss behaviours and maternal mood. *Australian Journal of Primary Health, 21*(1), 38–45. doi:10.1071/PY13011.

Edelman, C. L., Kudzma, E. C., & Mandle, C. L. (2014). *Health promotion throughout the life span* (8th ed.). St. Louis, MO: Mosby Elsevier.

Enright, C. R. (2014). Feeding, eating, and elimination disorders. In M. J. Halter (Ed.), *Varcarolis' foundations of psychiatric mental health nursing: A clinical approach* (pp. 343–363). St. Louis, MO: Saunders/Elsevier.

Erikson, E. H. (1963). *Childhood and society* (2nd ed.). New York: W. W. Norton.

Erikson, E. H. (1968). *Identity: Youth and crises*. New York: W. W. Norton.

Gilligan, C. (1982). *In a different voice: Psychological theory and women's development*. Cambridge, MA: Harvard University Press.

Government of Alberta. (2016). *Farm safety for children*. Retrieved from https://myhealth.alberta.ca/Alberta/pages/keeping-your-child-safe-on-a-farm.aspx.

Government of Canada. (2016). *Childhood obesity*. Retrieved from http://healthycanadians.gc.ca/healthy-living-vie-saine/obesity-obesite/risks-risques-eng.php.

Halford, W. K., Petch, J., & Creedy, D. (2015). *Clinical guide to helping new parents: The Couple CARE for Parents Program*. New York: Springer.

Health Canada (2011a). *Canada's food guide: Pregnancy and breastfeeding*. Ottawa: Author. Retrieved from http://www.hc-sc.gc.ca/fn-an/food-guide-aliment/choose-choix/advice-conseil/women-femmes-eng.php.

Health Canada (2011b). *Eating well with Canada's food guide* (Catalogue No. H164-38/1-2011E). Ottawa: Author. Retrieved from https://www.canada.ca/en/health-canada/services/food-nutrition/reports-publications/eating-well-canada-food-guide-resource-educators-communicators-2007.html.

Health Canada (2012). *Is your child safe?* (Cat. No. H128-1/06-461-1E). Ottawa: Author. Retrieved from http://www.hc-sc.gc.ca/cps-spc/pubs/cons/child-enfant/safe-securite-eng.php.

Health Canada. (2016). *Suicide prevention*. Retrieved from http://www.hc-sc.gc.ca/fniah-spnia/promotion/suicide/index-eng.php.

Heindel, J. J. (2011). The obesogen hypothesis of obesity: Overview and human evidence. In R. H. Lustig (Ed.), *Obesity before birth: Maternal and prenatal influences on the offspring* (pp. 355–365). New York: Springer. doi:10.1007/978-1-4419-7034-3_17.

Hockenberry, M. J., & Wilson, D. (2015). *Wong's nursing care of infants and children* (10th ed.). St. Louis, MO: Mosby Elsevier.

Hoekstra, S., & Margolis, L. (2016). The importance of the nursing role in parental vaccine decision making. *Clinical Pediatrics, 55*(5), 401–403. doi:10.1177/0009922815627348.

Kids Health. (2016). *Backpack safety*. Retrieved from http://kidshealth.org/en/parents/backpack.html#.

Kliegman, R. M., Stanton, B. F., St. Geme, J. W., et al. (2016). *Nelson textbook of pediatrics* (20th ed.). St. Louis: Mosby Elsevier.

Kohlberg, L. (1964). Development of moral character and moral ideology. In M. L. Hoffman & L. N. W. Hoffman (Eds.), *Review of child development research* (Vol. 1). New York: Russell Sage Foundation.

Kub, J., & Feldman, M. A. (2015). Bullying prevention: A call for collaborative efforts between school nurses and school psychologists. *Psychology in the Schools, 52*(7), 658–671. doi:10.1002/pits.21853.

Liu, J., Leung, P., & Yang, A. (2013). Breastfeeding and active bonding protects against children's internalizing behavior problems. *Nutrients, 6*(1), 76–89. doi:10.3390/nu6010076.

Miller, S. J. (2016). Glossary of terms: Defining a common queer language. In S. J. Miller (Ed.), *Teaching, affirming, and recognizing trans and gender creative youth: A queer literacy framework* (pp. 299–309). New York: Palgrave Macmillan.

Mitchinson, W. (2002). *Giving birth in Canada 1900–1950*. Toronto: University of Toronto Press.

Murray, S. S., & McKinney, E. S. (2014). *Foundations of maternal-newborn and women's health nursing* (6th ed.). St. Louis, MO: Saunders Elsevier.

Oats, J., & Abraham, S. (2017). *Llewellyn-Jones fundamentals of obstetrics and gynaecology* (10th ed.). Toronto: Elsevier.

Piaget, J. (1952). *The origins of intelligence in children*. New York: International Universities Press.

PREVNet. (2017). *Bullying facts and solutions*. Retrieved from http://www.prevnet.ca/bullying/facts-and-solutions.

Public Health Agency of Canada. (2012). *Update on human papillomavirus (HPV) vaccines*. Retrieved from http://www.phac-aspc.gc.ca/publicat/ccdr-rmtc/12vol38/acs-dcc-1/index-eng.php.

Public Health Agency of Canada. (2013). *Leading causes of death, Canada, 2008*. Retrieved from http://www.phac-aspc.gc.ca/publicat/lcd-pcd97/pdf/lcd-pcd-t1-eng.pdf.

Public Health Agency of Canada (2014a). *Safe sleep for your baby brochure*. Ottawa: Author. Retrieved from http://www.phac-aspc.gc.ca/hp-ps/dca-dea/stages-etapes/childhood-enfance_0-2/sids/ssb_brochure-eng.php.

Public Health Agency of Canada. (2014b). *Breastfeeding and infant nutrition*. Retrieved from http://www.phac-aspc.gc.ca/hp-ps/dca-dea/stages-etapes/childhood-enfance_0-2/nutrition/index-eng.php.

Public Health Agency of Canada. (2015). *Immunization schedule tool*. Retrieved from http://healthycanadians.gc.ca/apps/schedule-calendrier/index-eng.php.

Public Health Agency of Canada. (2016a). *Canadian immunization guide*. Retrieved from http://healthycanadians.gc.ca/healthy-living-vie-saine/immunization-immunisation/canadian-immunization-guide-canadien-immunisation/index-eng.php.

Public Health Agency of Canada (2016b). *Canadian guidelines on sexually transmitted infections*. Ottawa: Author.

Public Health Agency of Canada. (2016c). *Canadian immunization guide chapter on influenza and statement on seasonal influenza vaccine for 2016-2017*. Retrieved from http://www.phac-aspc.gc.ca/naci-ccni/flu-2016-grippe-eng.php.

Rempel, L. A., & Rempel, J. K. (2011). The breastfeeding team: The role of involved fathers in the breastfeeding family. *Journal of Human Lactation, 27*(2), 115–121. doi:10.1177/0890334410390045.

Santrock, J. W. (2011). *Child development* (13th ed.). New York: McGraw-Hill.

Sgrenci, A. E., & Faith, M. S. (2011). Psychosocial aspects of childhood obesity. *Epidemiology of Obesity in Children and Adolescents, 2*, 419–429. doi:10.1007/978-1-4419-6039-9_23.

Steinman, L., Doescher, M., Keppel, G. A., et al. (2009). Understanding infant feeding beliefs, practices and preferred nutrition education and health provider approaches: An exploratory study with Somali mothers in the USA. *Maternal & Child Nutrition, 6*(1), 67–88. doi:10.1111/j.1740-8709.2009.00185.x.

Task Force on Sudden Infant Death Syndrome. (2016). SIDS and other sleep-related infant deaths: Evidence base for 2016 updated recommendations for a safe infant sleeping environment. *Pediatrics, 138*(5), e1. doi:10.1542/peds.2016-1124. Retrieved from http://pediatrics.aappublications.org/content/138/5/e20162940.

Transport Canada. (2017). *Buying a child car seat or booster seat*. Retrieved from https://www.canada.ca/en/services/transport/road/child-car-seat-safety/buying-child-car-seat-booster-seat.html.

23

Young to Middle Adulthood

Canadian content written by J. Craig Phillips, RN, ARNP, PhD, LLM, ACRN, FAAN
Original chapter by Patsy L. Ruchala, RN, DNSc

OBJECTIVES

Mastery of content in this chapter will enable you to:

- Define the key terms listed.
- Discuss major life events and developmental tasks of young and middle-aged adults.
- Discuss the significance of family in the life of the adult.
- Describe normal physiological changes in young and middle adulthood, including pregnancy.
- Discuss cognitive and psychosocial changes that occur during the adult years.
- Describe health concerns of young and middle-aged adults.
- Apply clinical decision making to administering care to young and middle-aged adults.

KEY TERMS

MEDIA RESOURCES

http://evolve.elsevier.com/Canada/Potter/fundamentals/

- Audio Chapter Summaries
- Examination Review Questions
- Concept Map Creator
- Case Study with Questions
- Audio Glossary
- Content Updates
- Video Clips

Young to middle adulthood is a period of challenges, rewards, and crises. Challenges may include the demands of working and raising families; rewards may include career, family, and personal successes; and crises may include job loss and caring for children or adolescents in crisis or for aging parents.

Adult developmental changes are unique to each individual. These changes are based on earlier characteristics and subsequent behaviours to adapt to these characteristics and new experiences. Young adulthood is the period between the late teens and the mid- to late 30s (Edelman, Kudzma, & Mandle, 2014). In 2016, young adults between 20 and 34 years of age constituted approximately 20.7% of the Canadian population (Statistics Canada, 2016a). During young adulthood, individuals move away from their families of origin, establish career goals, and decide whether to marry and begin families or to remain single.

Middle age is the period between the mid- to late 30s and the mid-60s. During this period, people become aware of changes in reproductive and physical abilities and may reassess life goals. In 2013, the median age of the Canadian population living in census metropolitan areas, where 70% of the population live, was 39 years of age, and it was 44.3 years of age in rural and remote communities outside census metropolitan areas (Statistics Canada, 2015a). This age group is growing because the baby-boom generation is maturing and in recent decades fertility rates have declined and life expectancy has increased (Statistics Canada, 2015a).

Developmental theories provide nurses with a basis for understanding the life events and developmental tasks of young and middle-aged adults. Developmental theorists Erikson (1963, 1982), Havighurst (1972), and Gilligan (1993) have described the phases of adulthood and related developmental tasks (see Chapter 21), and the Canadian Association of Schools of Nursing's (CASN, 2015) *National Nursing Education Framework* provides a competency framework to guide nurses in acquiring relevant knowledge and skills. This chapter provides foundational knowledge of human development and functioning over the lifespan, drawing from secondary education, natural and life sciences, and behavioural and social sciences. This foundational knowledge will help you develop "the ability to recognize and respond safely, competently and ethically to rapidly changing client-conditions and context" (CASN, 2015).

You may be a young or middle-aged adult yourself, coping with the demands of your own developmental period. As a nurse, you must be careful to recognize and respect the needs of your patients even if you are not experiencing the same challenges and events. You can help young and middle-aged adult patients achieve their potential by offering support and providing information and appropriate referrals.

YOUNG ADULTHOOD

Physical Changes

Most young adults have completed physical growth by 20 years of age. Young adults are usually quite active, experience fewer severe illnesses than do older age groups, tend to ignore physical symptoms of illness, and often postpone seeking health care. Physical characteristics of young adults begin to change as middle age approaches.

Patients in this developmental stage may benefit from a personal lifestyle assessment to identify habits that increase the risk for cardiac, malignant, pulmonary, renal, or other chronic diseases. A personal lifestyle assessment of the young adult includes assessment of general life satisfaction; hobbies and interests; habits (e.g., diet, sleep, exercise, sexual practices, caffeine use, alcohol, illicit drugs); home conditions (e.g., housing, finances); and occupational environment (e.g., type of work, exposure to hazardous substances, physical or mental strain).

Cognitive Changes

Cognitive changes are variations in reasoning and thinking. Critical thinking habits increase steadily through the young and middle adult years. Formal and informal education, life experiences, and work opportunities increase the individual's conceptual and problem-solving skills. Young adults with flexible decision-making processes cope most effectively by continually evolving and adjusting to changes in their home, workplace, and personal lives.

Choosing an occupation is a major task of young adults and involves knowing their skills, talents, and personality characteristics. The lack of resources or support systems to pursue higher education or develop work skills may limit occupational choices for many young adults.

By addressing health literacy issues (Box 23-1) and understanding how adults learn, nurses can develop relevant patient teaching plans (see Chapter 20 for further information about patient education). Adults enter learning situations with a background of unique life experiences, including illness. Therefore, nurses should always view each adult as an individual. When determining what amount of information the individual needs in order to make decisions about the prescribed course of therapy, nurses should consider factors that may affect the individual's adherence to the regimen, including educational level, socioeconomic factors, social context factors (Phillips, 2011), motivation, and desire to learn.

Psychosocial Changes

The emotional health of young adults is related to their ability to address and resolve personal and social tasks. Young adults often want to prolong adolescence and yet assume adult commitments. Between the ages of 23 and 28 years, people usually refine self-perception and capacity for intimacy. From ages 29 to 34 years, people usually focus on achieving personal and occupational goals and improving socioeconomic status. For many young adults, a dual-income family is needed in order to achieve and maintain middle-class status. Career and personal counselling can help individuals identify career choices and set realistic goals.

Ethnicity and gender issues influence an adult's life and can pose challenges for nursing care as each person holds culture-bound definitions of health and illness. An understanding of ethnicity, race, and gender differences enables nurses to provide individualized care (see Chapter 9 for further information about culture and context).

BOX 23-1 Health Literacy

Health literacy is an important health determinant for many health outcomes. Health literacy requires the patient to be able to access information, process that information to understand it, and act on that information to make good health decisions. People who are health literate are able to find the information they need; read, interpret, and understand the message conveyed; weigh their treatment options; navigate the available health services to determine which ones are appropriate; and understand instructions that health care providers give them.

Strategies that you as a nurse can use to increase health literacy include the teach-back technique. In this process you provide an initial teaching or explanation, followed by a summary of key information in manageable chunks, then check the patient's understanding and clarify any questions or concerns the patient has. When you seek to enhance your patients' health literacy, encourage questions by using body language that invites questions (e.g., position yourself at the patient's level), solicit questions (e.g., "Let me know when you have questions"), help the patient form questions, take time for questions, and check that teaching is complete (e.g., "Have all your questions been answered?").

Comprehending medical information is challenging. Assessing patients' health literacy and taking steps to help them understand the information presented to them and make informed decisions can improve health outcomes. Helping patients to become informed consumers will become a rewarding part of your nursing practice.

Adapted from McCall, J., & Wilson, C. (2015). Promoting health literacy in an HIV-infected population: Creating staff awareness. *Journal of the Association of Nurses in AIDS Care, 26*(4), 498–502. doi:10.1016/j.jana.2014.11.003.

Traditional gender roles of men and women have changed, resulting in alterations in traditional familial structures. Since the 1970s, women have been entering the workforce and pursuing careers outside the home in high numbers. In 2014, about 77% of Canadian women aged 25 to 54 years of age were employed (Statistics Canada, 2015b). Women contribute significantly to their families' incomes. As a result, many women deal with the stresses of being wife, mother, and employee. Likewise, men are assuming more parental and household responsibilities (Austin & Boyd, 2014). Some men choose to put careers on hold to be stay-at-home fathers.

Challenges may arise for young adults who do not conform to traditional gender roles. Gay, lesbian, bisexual, intersex, transgender, Two Spirit, queer, and questioning persons (LGBTQ2) may face challenges in navigating the health care system and social context to lead happy and healthy lives (Phillips & Saewyc, 2010). For transgender persons, this may be particularly challenging owing to "erasure"—the social process through which transsexuality is managed in cultures and institutions as being ultimately impossible (Bauer, Hammond, Travers, et al., 2009). Erasure describes how sexual minority identities are systematically "erased" from heteronormative society by allowing only gender binary (male/female) on health records and other documents (Bauer et al., 2009). For other sexual minorities, the common use of the epidemiological categories of men who have sex with men (MSM) and women who have sex with women (WSW) serves to "erase" the existence of gay and lesbian communities (Boellstorff, 2011; Prestage, 2011; Young & Meyer, 2005). Governmental apologies, such as the one delivered by Prime Minister Justine Trudeau on November 28, 2017 (Harris, 2017), acknowledge the structural challenges faced by LGBTQ2 persons and offer hope to members of those groups. This apology requires nurses to be vigilant in promoting equity in health care delivery to address the health disparities experienced by LGBTQ2 persons living in Canada (Harris, 2017).

Two Spirit is a term used to describe Indigenous people who assume cross- or multiple gender roles, attributes, dress, and attitudes for personal, spiritual, cultural, ceremonial, or social reasons. These roles are defined by each Indigenous cultural group and can be fluid over a person's lifetime. Some Indigenous people use terms such as *gay, lesbian, bisexual, transgender (GLBT), transsexual,* and *intersexed* (in combination with or exclusive to Two Spirit) to define who they are (Hunt, 2016).

Career. Young men and women hope to have fulfilling careers. They may formulate short- and long-term career goals. Successful employment ensures economic security and promotes friendships, social activities, support, and self-respect.

In many two-career partnerships, the benefits experienced (e.g., improved finances) may outweigh potential stressors (e.g., child care demands; household needs; increased physical, mental, or emotional demands). To reduce stress in a two-career family, neither partner should assume all household responsibilities. For some families, a solution is to hire a housekeeper. Others may set up an equal division of household and child care duties.

Sexuality. Young adults usually have the emotional maturity necessary to establish intimacy and develop fulfilling sexual relationships. Young adults who have failed to achieve the developmental tasks of adolescence may develop superficial relationships (Austin & Boyd, 2014).

For most young adults, the emotional aspect of sexual activity is as important as its type or frequency. Understanding the differences between sexual desire (i.e., responses to physical and mental stimuli during or in anticipation of sexual activity), sexual behaviour (i.e., how humans experience and express their sexuality), and sexual identity (i.e., how a person identifies their sexuality) will facilitate your work as a nurse with young adult patients. Recognizing the distinct differences between each of these categories and how they are influenced by internal and external factors will facilitate open dialogue and collaborative approaches to patient teaching about sexual health. This open dialogue has the capacity to reduce potential sexual health risks, including human immunodeficiency virus (HIV) and other sexually transmitted infections (Phillips & Saewyc, 2010). Adults should be encouraged to explore various aspects of their sexuality and be aware that their sexual needs and concerns evolve (see Chapter 27).

Singlehood. Social pressure to get married is not as great as it once was. During the 2011 to 2016 census period, families and living arrangements among Canadians continued to diversify. Married families accounted for more than half of all families. Common-law couples and lone-parent families continued to increase (Statistics Canada, 2016b). The 2011 census cycle was the first full cycle in which all areas of Canada recognized same-sex marriage, and the number of same-sex marriages increased by 42% between 2006 and 2011 (Statistics Canada, 2012). The number of same-sex marriages across Canada increased by an additional 16% between 2011 and 2016 (Statistics Canada, 2017a). Young adults who choose to remain single and maintain independence may consider siblings and parents as their family. However, close friends and associates may also be viewed as the individual's "family." Some single persons choose to become parents, either biologically or through adoption.

The single population is increasing partly because women have greater career opportunities than before and partly because single individuals often choose to live together and share housing costs rather than marry. In addition, many adults become single again after a marriage ends.

Marriage. Every married couple's relationship is unique, regardless of the gender makeup of the couple. Although no rules guarantee a successful marriage, some guidelines are useful for building a happy marriage. Before marriage, the couple ideally should (1) ensure that their emotions are based on love rather than physical attraction, (2) explore their motivations for marriage, (3) develop clear communication, (4) accept that behaviour and habits are unlikely to change after marriage, and (5) determine their compatibility in important beliefs and values.

When establishing a household and family, the married couple must work as a team. Individuals require maturity and self-esteem to accomplish the following major tasks of marriage: establishing an intimate relationship; deciding on and working toward mutual goals; establishing guidelines for decision-making issues; setting standards for social interactions; and choosing morals, values, and ideologies acceptable to both. Accomplishing these tasks provides the foundation for a stable relationship.

Marriage also requires the couple to learn patterns of sexual expression, establish roles, and practise effective conflict resolution and decision-making skills. Each partner may experience a sense of loss of individuality in the transition from being single to being married.

Child-Bearing Cycle. Conception, pregnancy, birth, and the puerperium (postpartum period) are phases of the child-bearing cycle. The changes during these phases are complex. Childbirth education classes can prepare the pregnant woman, her partner, and other supportive people to participate in the birthing process. Pregnant women and their families may benefit from a lay doula (support person).

Breastfeeding offers many advantages to both the new mother and baby (see Chapter 42). However, for the inexperienced mother, breastfeeding may cause anxiety and frustration. Women who have had no contact with newborns and other mothers who breastfeed may require assistance to breastfeed successfully. Nurses must be alert for signs that the mother needs information and assistance. By observing the mother while she breastfeeds, the nurse may catch problems such as improper positioning or ineffective sucking by the infant (Registered Nurses' Association of Ontario [RNAO], 2003). Regarding breastfeeding by transmasculine persons, MacDonald, Noel-Weiss, West, et al. (2016) highlight the need for nurses to be knowledgeable about lactation and chest care for these individuals and to be sensitive to their gender identity experiences.

The personal and social changes occurring in the lives of a couple after the birth of a baby cannot be underestimated. Nursing assessment of the couple's response to the birthing experience and parent–child attachment are discussed later in this chapter.

Parenthood. Contraception allows couples to decide when and whether to start a family. One factor influencing this decision is the reason for wanting a child. Social pressures may encourage a couple to have a child or may influence them to limit the number of children they have. Economic considerations frequently enter into the decision because raising children is expensive. Because couples are getting married later and are postponing pregnancies, general health status and age are also factors in whether a couple decides to have children.

Parenting roles must be defined and practised. Nurturing and socialization needs of children and adolescents can put pressure on the couple's relationship. In addition, parents' images of the "perfect parent" may conflict with reality. For example, mothers may be blamed for parental failures when an adolescent misuses substances. A qualitative literature synthesis highlighted mothers' experiences parenting an adolescent who misused substances and the complex social and familial factors that intersect with adolescent substance abuse (Katouziyan, Vandyk, & Phillips, in press).

Alternative Family Structures and Parenting. Norms and values about family life in Canada are evolving continuously, as demonstrated by judicial rulings on same-sex marriage since 2000. Greater numbers of infants are being born to cohabiting (common-law) couples (see Chapter 19). Families may take the form of a single parent and children, same-sex couples with or without children, or a combined family from previous relationships. Parents from alternative family structures may perceive a lack of support and bias from the health care system (McManus, Hunter, & Renn, 2006). Same-sex parents and their children may need support for adoption of children and the parenting role.

Hallmarks of Emotional Health

Most young adults have the physical and emotional resources and support systems to meet their many challenges, tasks, and responsibilities. During psychosocial assessment of young adults, nurses can assess for 10 hallmarks of emotional health that indicate successful maturation in this developmental stage (Box 23-2). If one or more of these hallmarks are not attained, further assessment and action may be required.

Social Support in Health and Illness

A current trend in health care is the use of a peer navigator (doula) to facilitate well-being (Figure 23-1). This trend is evident in states of health when a family uses the services of a doula to help a pregnant woman and her family to navigate the challenges of pregnancy. In chronic disease states such as cancer, mental illness, and HIV disease, peer navigators can help patients to navigate the complexities of the health care system and therapeutic regimens (Box 23-3).

BOX 23-2 10 Hallmarks of Emotional Health

- A sense of meaning and direction in life
- Successful negotiation through transitions
- Absence of feelings of being cheated or disappointed by life
- Attainment of several long-term goals
- Satisfaction with personal growth and development
- When married, feelings of love for partner; when single, satisfaction with social interactions
- Satisfaction with friendships
- Generally cheerful attitude
- Acceptance of constructive criticism
- No unrealistic fears

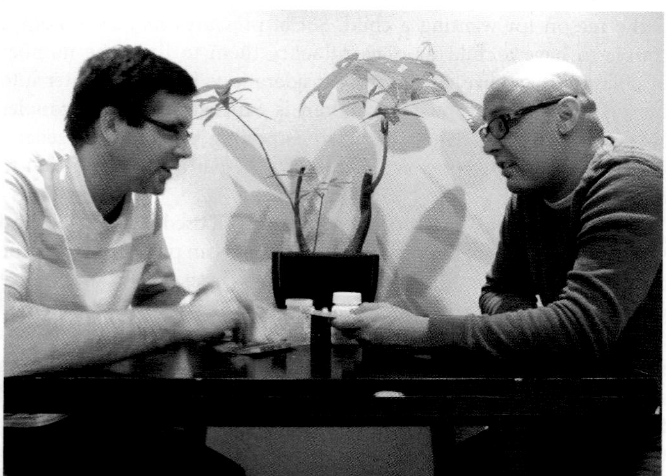

FIGURE 23-1 A peer navigator and patient discuss medication adherence strategies.

Health Risks

Health risk factors for a young adult originate in lifestyle patterns, family history, and the environment and occupation.

Lifestyle. Lifestyle habits such as poor food choices, smoking, stress, high-risk sexual behaviour, substance abuse, and inactivity increase the risk of illness. For example, prolonged stress can cause ulcers, emotional disorders, and infections (see Chapter 29 for further information about stress and adaptation). Smoking and second-hand smoke can cause lung cancer and pulmonary, cardiac, and vascular diseases. Computer-mediated communication (e.g., Internet dating, "sexting") can lead to high-risk sexual encounters and adverse health outcomes (Phillips & Saewyc, 2010). Your role as a nurse in health promotion is to identify lifestyle risk factors and provide education and support to reduce unhealthy behaviours.

Family History. A family history of a disease may put a young adult at risk for developing that disease in the middle or older adult years. For example, a family history of certain cancers or cardiovascular, renal, endocrine, or neoplastic disease increases the family member's risk of developing the disease.

Accidental Death and Injury. Accidents are the leading causes of injury and death in young adults (Lewis, Dirksen, Heitkemper, et al., 2014). Death and injury can result from motor vehicle or other

BOX 23-3 RESEARCH HIGHLIGHT

Engaging Vulnerable Persons to Address Health Challenges

Research Focus

Including patients as active participants in the development of interventions to address health challenges is essential to patient-centred care. For example, Phillips, Rowsell, Boomer, et al. (2016) collaborated with gay men living with HIV who smoke to develop elements for an online tailored smoking cessation intervention.

Research Abstract

The purpose of Phillips et al.'s study was to explore the perspectives of gay men living with HIV who smoke or have recently quit smoking, to inform the design and development of a web-based smoking reduction and cessation intervention. Participatory design techniques and qualitative methods were used to guide the creation of personas (composite representations of a person who would use the intervention). Findings indicated that an overarching theme of navigating life and seven other themes contributed to smoking reduction and cessation efforts for these men. The men described how triple stigma, anxiety about life, and apathy about life intersected with the complexities of managing their identity and HIV disease. The men described perceived benefits from smoking and that they had become immune to public health messages about smoking. This study highlights cultural differences between these men and mainstream society that should be considered in order to improve smoking reduction and cessation efforts with these men.

Evidence-Informed Practice

- Personas offer a mechanism for interpreting the experiences and traditions of vulnerable populations.
- Including patients in the development of interventions to address their health conditions may lead to greater intervention success.
- Smoking reduction and cessation interventions with gay men living with HIV must address their social realities and include tools to navigate life, disease, and social identity.

Phillips, J. C., Rowsell, D. J., Boomer, J., Kwon, J.-Y., & Currie, L. M. (2016). Personas to guide understanding traditions of gay men living with HIV who smoke. *Qualitative Health Research, 26*(1), 41–54.

accidents, physical assaults, and suicide attempts. In 2014, 29% of driver fatalities were among drivers between 20 and 34 years of age (Transport Canada, 2016).

Physical assault and violence may also cause injury or death. Canada's crime rate has steadily declined since 1991 (Statistics Canada, 2017b). However, firearm-related violent crime remains a significant public health and social issue. Nearly 80% of firearm-related deaths are the result of suicide, accident, or legal intervention; the remainder are attributed to criminal offenses (Statistics Canada, 2015c). Factors that may predispose to violence include poverty, breakdown of family relations, child abuse and neglect, and access to firearms. To detect personal and environmental risk factors for violence, it is important that nurses perform a thorough psychosocial assessment, including such factors as behavioural patterns, history of physical abuse and substance abuse, education, work history, and social support systems.

Substance Abuse. Substance abuse directly or indirectly contributes to mortality and morbidity in young adults. Regular heavy drinking (five or more drinks on one occasion) is most common among Canadians aged 20 to 34, and more men in this age group drink than do women in the same age range. Regular heavy drinking appears to be decreasing among both sexes, although more slowly in women compared to men in this age group (Statistics Canada, 2016c). Intoxication is often a factor in motor vehicle accidents.

Dependence on stimulants ("uppers") can result in overdose death by putting stress on the cardiovascular and nervous systems. Use of depressants ("downers") can lead to accidental or intentional overdose and death. Nurses can provide counselling and support for patients seeking treatment for substance abuse. Rates of opioid use are on the rise in the population and have reached epidemic proportions across North America.

Substance abuse cannot always be diagnosed, particularly in its early stages. Nonjudgemental questions about the use of legal drugs (prescribed drugs, over-the-counter drugs, tobacco, and alcohol), so-called soft drugs (marijuana), and illegal drugs (cocaine or heroin) should be a routine part of any physical assessment. Important information may be obtained by making specific inquiries about past medical problems, changes in food intake or sleep patterns, or problems of emotional lability. Reports of arrests because of driving while intoxicated, because of domestic or child abuse, or because of disorderly conduct should alert the nurse to the possibility of drug misuse or abuse.

Unplanned Pregnancies. Unplanned pregnancies, although more common among adolescents, also occur in young and middle adult Canadian women. Unplanned pregnancies are a source of stress that can result in adverse health outcomes for the mother, infant, and family. Many young adults have educational and career goals that take precedence over family development. Interference with these goals can affect future relationships and later parent–child relationships. When assessing the woman with an unplanned pregnancy, determination of the situational factors that affect pregnancy outcome is important. These include exploring issues such as family support systems; potential parenting disorders; depression; coping mechanisms; and possible financial, career, or housing problems.

Sexually Transmitted Infections. Sexually transmitted infections (STIs) are a major health problem in young adults (Public Health Agency of Canada [PHAC], 2013; Society of Obstetricians and Gynaecologists of Canada [SOGC], 2016). STIs include syphilis, chlamydia, gonorrhea, genital herpes, human papilloma virus (HPV) infection, and HIV disease (see Chapter 27 for further information about STIs). Zika virus is an emerging STI that has been detected in semen, and the duration of viral shedding is currently unknown. Men who have returned from a Zika virus risk area should be counselled about appropriate condom usage. Pregnant women and their male partners who must travel to risk areas are encouraged to practise abstinence or use condoms during sex. Couples who are planning a pregnancy need additional counselling if they are travelling to a risk area (Zika Working Group on behalf of the Committee to Advise on Tropical Medicine and Travel, 2016). STIs have immediate physical effects such as discharge and discomfort. STIs also can lead to chronic disorders (from genital herpes), infertility (from gonorrhea), or death. Many people have an STI without experiencing symptoms. Young adults need information about transmission, prevention, symptoms, and management of STIs.

Many young adults have misconceptions regarding transmission and treatment of STIs. Partners should be encouraged to know one another's sexual history and sexual practices. Nurses should be alert for STIs when patients come to clinics with complaints of urological or gynecological problems (see Chapter 32). Young adults should be assessed for their knowledge and use of safer sex practices and genital self-examinations.

Environmental or Occupational Factors. A common environmental or occupational risk factor is exposure to work-related hazards or agents. Diseases observed in workplaces include silicosis from inhalation of talcum and silicon dust, emphysema from inhalation of smoke, and hearing loss from noise exposure. Cancers resulting from occupational exposures may involve the lungs, liver, brain, blood, or skin. Environmental exposures with leisure activities include outdoor exposure to mosquitoes (which may transmit West Nile virus) and ticks (which may transmit Lyme disease). Questions regarding environmental and occupational exposures should be a routine part of nursing assessment.

Health Concerns

Infertility. Infertility refers to a lack of conception after a reasonable period of sexual intercourse without contraception (Assisted Human Reproduction Canada, 2012). Infertility affects as many as one in eight couples. For many couples, the use of infertility clinics can facilitate pregnancy, and the use of reproductive technologies is increasing in Canada (Bushnik, Cook, Yuzpe, et al., 2012). There are many causes of infertility that can affect couples, including female factors, such as ovulatory dysfunction or a pelvic factor, and male factors, such as sperm and semen abnormalities (Babycenter, 2017). Couples who delay conception until their mid-30s may experience fertility problems. For some infertile couples, a nurse may be the first resource contacted. Nursing assessment of infertile couples should include comprehensive histories of both partners to determine factors that may affect fertility, as well as pertinent physical findings (Lowdermilk, Perry, Cashion, et al., 2016).

Exercise. Exercise patterns can affect health status. Adults between 18 and 64 years of age should engage in moderate- to vigorous-intensity activity, in bouts of 10 minutes or more, for at least 150 minutes per week (Canadian Society for Exercise Physiology, 2011). Exercise improves cardiopulmonary function by decreasing blood pressure and heart rate. In addition, exercise decreases fatigue, insomnia, tension, and irritability. When assessing a patient's health status, nurses should conduct a thorough musculoskeletal assessment, including evaluations of joint mobility and muscle tone, and a psychosocial assessment for improved tolerance of stress to determine the effects of exercise.

Routine Health Screening. Routine screening examinations enable early detection of an illness and thus lower the risk of illnesses becoming severe. Patients should be encouraged to perform monthly skin, breast, or male genital self-examination (see Chapter 32). In Canada, cancer is the leading cause of death; more than half of all cases are prostate, breast, lung, or colorectal cancers. While

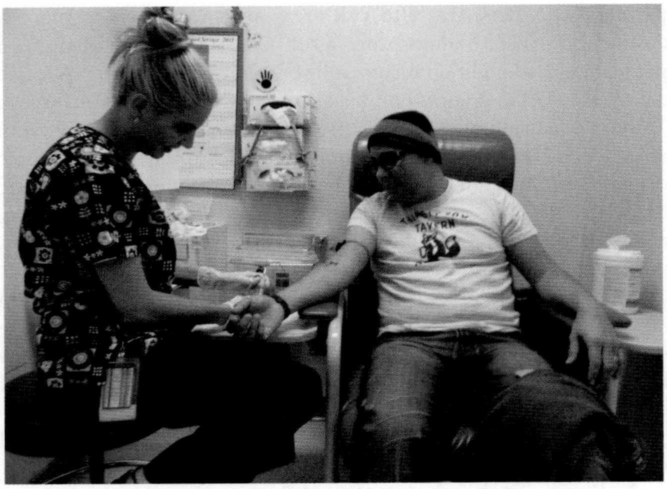

FIGURE 23-2 Routine health screening for persons living with chronic conditions.

the highest incidence of cancer is among persons over the age of 50, cancer contributes to illness and death in young and middle-aged adults (Canadian Cancer Society's Steering Committee, 2017). Breast and male genital cancers continue to be considerable issues in Canada. Therefore, your role as a nurse is extremely important in educating patients about breast self-examination and the current breast screening recommendations, and you must provide male patients with information about testicular self-examination and prostate cancer screening. In adolescence and early adulthood, prolonged exposure to ultraviolet rays from the sun or in tanning salons can increase the risk for development of skin cancer. Patients should be encouraged to undergo routine assessment of the skin for changes in colour or presence of lesions and changes in their appearance. Persons living with chronic conditions such as cancer, diabetes mellitus, or HIV may require specific condition-related screenings on a routine basis (Figure 23-2).

Job Stress. Job stress can occur every day or periodically. Most young adults are able to handle day-to-day crises. Situational job stress may occur when a new boss enters the workplace, a deadline is approaching, or the worker is given new responsibilities. Corporate restructuring may lead to layoffs and increased responsibilities for remaining employees and is a major source of stress. Job stress also occurs when a person becomes dissatisfied with a job. Because individuals perceive jobs differently, the types of job stressors vary from person to person. Your assessment of the young adult should include a description of the adult's work, including conditions and hours, duration of employment, changes in sleep or eating habits, and evidence of increased irritability or nervousness.

Family Stress. Family stressors can occur at any time in family life. Family life is a dynamic process that includes times when everyone in the family works together and times when everyone appears to pull apart. Situational stressors occur during events such as births, deaths, illnesses, marriages, and job losses. Because of changing relationships and structures in the emerging young adult family, stress levels are frequently high and may be related to a number of variables that can lead to family dysfunction. Stress and the possible resulting family dysfunction may account for high divorce rates during the first 3 to 5 years of marriage for young adult couples. When a patient seeks health care and exhibits stress-related symptoms, the nurse should ask whether the person has recently experienced a life-changing event.

Each family has certain predictable roles or jobs for members. These roles enable the family to function and be an effective part of society. One necessary role is the family leader. In most families, one parent is the leader or both parents act as co-leaders. In lone-parent families, the parent or, on occasion, a member of the extended family is the family leader. When this role changes as a result of illness, a situational crisis may occur. Nurses should assess environmental and familial factors, including support systems and coping mechanisms commonly used by family members.

Pregnancy. Although the physiological changes of pregnancy and childbirth occur only in women, cognitive and psychosocial changes and health concerns affect the entire child-bearing family. The entire family, therefore, needs education about pregnancy, labour, delivery, breastfeeding, and integration of the newborn into the family structure.

Women and men who are anticipating pregnancy benefit from good health practices before conception, including eating a balanced diet, exercising, attending regular dental checkups, and avoiding alcohol, drugs, and smoking. Women trying to become pregnant should not follow weight-reduction diets.

Prenatal Care. **Prenatal care** includes routine assessment of the pregnant woman by a nurse, family physician, obstetrician, nurse practitioner, or midwife. Health promotion interventions are important during the prenatal period and can improve the well-being of the woman and fetus (Box 23-4). Prenatal care includes a thorough physical assessment of the pregnant woman during regularly scheduled intervals; provision of information regarding STIs, vaginal infections, and urinary infections that could adversely affect the fetus; and counselling about exercise patterns, diet, and child care. Regular prenatal care can address health concerns that arise during the pregnancy.

BOX 23-4 CASE STUDY

Support During Pregnancy

Melinda was a 24-year-old woman pregnant with her first child. Her pregnancy was healthy and the fetus appeared to be growing well. Beginning in her sixth month of pregnancy, she enrolled in childbirth education classes, taught by a community health nurse. The nurse noticed that Melinda's boyfriend, Troy, accompanied her to the first class. During the second class, the nurse observed that Melinda was by herself and appeared a bit withdrawn. Concerned about whether Melinda would have adequate support during labour and birth, the nurse asked Melinda whether Troy was going to be coming back. Melinda replied that Troy had gone up north to work and would be gone for at least 3 months. She said she missed him already and was worried that he might miss the birth, because the camp where he worked was very remote. Because only a few flights a week were available, Melinda was not sure he would be able to leave when she went into labour. The nurse asked Melinda about other family members who might be able to support her. Melinda said she was estranged from her mother, but her 19-year-old sister might be able to be with her for the birth if she could take time off work. The nurse suggested that Melinda consider arranging to have a doula present during labour to offer physical, emotional, and informational support. The doula would meet with Melinda sometime before her due date to talk with her about what would be most helpful to her during labour and would be at her side through the birth. The nurse provided several names of doulas and encouraged Melinda to consider this as an additional support person in case her boyfriend or sister could not make it in time. During the next class, Melinda said that she had contacted a doula and made arrangements to meet with her. She stated that she was relieved to know that she would have labour support if Troy could not attend the birth. She was very appreciative of the nurse's help. Several months later, Melinda phoned the nurse to say that Troy caught a flight in time and that both he and the doula had really helped her during the birth and they were thrilled to have given birth to a healthy baby boy.

TABLE 23-1 Major Physiological Changes During Pregnancy

Signs and Symptoms	Causes
First Trimester	
Amenorrhea	Fertilization and implantation of egg Increases in hormone levels
"Morning sickness" (nausea, sometimes vomiting)	Increased serum hormone levels
Breast changes: enlargement, tenderness, darkened and enlarged nipples	Increased estrogen levels
Urinary frequency	Pressure of uterus on bladder
Fatigue	Increased nutritional demands Decreased nutritional intake resulting from morning sickness
Second Trimester	
Integumentary changes: pigment changes in nipple and breast, hyperpigmentation of abdominal line (linea nigra), mottling of cheeks or forehead (chloasma, or "mask of pregnancy"), localized or generalized pruritis	Increased levels of melanocyte-stimulating hormone
Hypertrophy of gums, causing gingival swelling and bleeding	Proliferation of interdental papillary blood vessels, caused by increased estrogen levels
Increasing height of uterine fundus	Growth of fetus
Sensation of movement or of abdominal gas (quickening)	Fetal movement
Third Trimester	
Braxton-Hicks contractions	Expansion and preparation of uterus for labour
Increased colostrum	Hormonal influence; preparation of breasts for lactation
Increased urinary frequency	Pressure on bladder from enlarged fetus
Shortness of breath	Pressure on diaphragm from enlarged uterus
Supine hypertension	Uterine pressure on inferior vena cava
Heartburn	Slower gastric emptying and esophageal reflux

Data from Lowdermilk, D. L., Perry, S. E., Cashion, M. C., & Alden, K. R. (2016). *Maternity and women's health care* (11th ed.). St. Louis, MO: Mosby.

TABLE 23-2 Major Psychosocial Changes During Pregnancy

Type of Change	Implications for Nursing Intervention
Body image	Morning sickness and fatigue may contribute to poor body image. Increase in breast size may make the woman feel more feminine and sexually appealing but may also be uncomfortable. The woman begins to "show" during the second trimester. The woman may experience a general feeling of well-being; she can feel the baby move and hear the baby's heartbeat.
Role changes	Both partners think about impending role changes and can have feelings of uncertainty about them. Both partners may have feelings of ambivalence about becoming parents and concern about their ability to be parents.
Sexuality	Partners need reassurance that sexual activity will not harm the fetus. Desire for sexual activity may be influenced by body image. Partners may desire cuddling and holding rather than sexual intercourse.
Coping mechanisms	Partners need reassurance that childbirth and child-rearing are natural and positive experiences but can also be stressful. Partners should be provided guidance in preparation for childbirth and encouraged to participate in childbirth classes.
Stresses during puerperium	Partners may return home from the hospital fatigued and unfamiliar with infant care. Partners may experience physical discomfort or feelings of anxiety. The woman may have to return to work soon after delivery, with subsequent feelings of guilt, anxiety, or, possibly, a sense of freedom or relief.
Postpartum blues and depression	Postpartum blues symptoms include transient emotional or mood disturbances such as weepiness, insomnia, anxiety, and poor concentration about 3 to 6 days after birth. Postpartum depression symptoms include extreme anxiety, sense of failure, feelings of guilt, sleep disturbances, appetite disorders, excessive concerns about the baby, and suicide ideation. Interventions include medication, therapy, counselling, and support.

Physiological Changes. The physiological changes and needs of the pregnant woman vary with each trimester (Table 23-1). Temporary changes in visual and hearing acuity, taste, and smell also occur. Nurses must be familiar with these physiological changes, their causes, and helpful interventions. All women experience some physiological changes in the first trimester, but some changes affect only certain women. During the second trimester, growth of the uterus and fetus results in some of the physical signs of pregnancy, and the woman will see her growing abdomen and feel fetal movements. During the third trimester, irregular, short contractions (**Braxton-Hicks contractions**), fatigue, and urinary frequency may occur. Close to the onset of labour, the woman may experience a burst of energy during which she prepares for the baby's arrival, a period called **nesting**.

The **puerperium** is a period of approximately 6 weeks after delivery. During this time, the woman's body reverts to its prepregnant physical status. Nurses should assess the woman's knowledge of and ability to care for both herself and her newborn. Assistance with infant feeding and care and assessment of parenting skills and mother–infant interactions are important. During this period, nurses should assess for postpartum depression, which may include maladaptive coping strategies and ineffective bonding interactions between mother and newborn.

Psychosocial Changes. Like the physiological changes of pregnancy, psychosocial changes may occur at various times during pregnancy and in the puerperium. Table 23-2 summarizes the major categories of psychosocial changes and implications for nursing intervention.

Acute Care. The young-adult years are generally a time of good physical and emotional health. Potential health hazards may be related to lifestyle. Acute care for young adults is frequently related to accidents, substance abuse, exposure to environmental and occupational hazards, stress-related illnesses, respiratory infections, gastroenteritis, influenza, urinary tract infections, and minor surgery.

An acute, minor illness can cause a disruption in the life activities of the young adult and increase stress in an already hectic lifestyle. Dependency and limitations posed by treatment regimens can also increase frustration for the young adult. To give young adults control of their health care choices, it is important for nurses to keep them informed about their health status and involve them in health care decisions. Acute phases of chronic illnesses may pose challenges for young adults.

Restorative and Continuing Care. Chronic conditions in young adulthood, although not common, do occur. Chronic illnesses such as hypertension, coronary artery disease, and diabetes may have their onset in young adulthood without being known to the young adult until later in life. Causes of chronic illness and disability in a young adult can include accidents, multiple sclerosis, rheumatoid arthritis, HIV, and cancer. Chronic illness and disability can affect the accomplishment of important developmental tasks in young adulthood. They can reduce a young adult's independence and require the person to change personal, family, and career goals. A young adult with chronic illness or disability may experience developmental problems related to sense of identity. The person needs support in the establishment of independence, reorganization of intimate relationships and family structure, and launching of a chosen career (Lewis et al., 2014).

MIDDLE ADULTHOOD

The middle adult years begin around the mid- to late-30s and lasts through the mid-60s. Personal and career achievements have often already been experienced. Many middle-aged adults enjoy assisting their children and other young people to become productive and responsible adults. Middle-aged adults may also begin to help aging parents. Using leisure time in satisfying and creative ways is a challenge that, if met satisfactorily, enables middle-aged adults to prepare for retirement. Socioeconomic instability brought on by corporate restructuring and economic realities, however, may leave many middle-aged adults either jobless or forced to accept lower-paying jobs.

Men and women must adjust to inevitable biological changes. Middle-aged adults need to adapt self-concept and body image to physiological realities and changes in physical appearance. Exercising, eating well, getting enough sleep, and practising good hygiene promote good health and a positive attitude toward physiological changes.

Physical Changes

Major physiological changes occur between the ages of 40 and 65 years. Table 23-3 summarizes normal developmental changes that are important to consider when conducting a physical examination. The most visible changes are greying of the hair, wrinkling of the skin, and thickening of the waist. Decreases in hearing and visual acuity are often noted during this period. These physiological changes may affect the person's self-concept and body image. For women, the most significant

TABLE 23-3 Physical Assessment Findings in the Middle-Aged Adult

Body System	Expected Findings
Integument	Intact condition Appropriate distribution of pigmentation Slow, progressive decrease in skin turgor Greying and loss of hair (baldness patterns in men are established by age 55; hair loss after this time might have other causes)
Head and neck	Symmetry of scalp, skull, and face
Eyes	Normal accessory organs of vision Visual acuity (according to Snellen chart) that is less than 20/50 Normal pupillary reaction to light and accommodation Normal visual fields and extraocular movements Normal retinal structures
Ears	Normal auditory structures and acuity
Nose, sinuses, and throat	Patent nares and intact sinuses, mouth, and pharynx Location of trachea at midline Nonpalpable lateral thyroid lobes
Thorax and lungs	Increased anteroposterior diameter Respiratory rate: 12–20 breaths per minute and regular Ratio of respiratory rate to heart rate: 1 : 4 Normal tactile fremitus, resonance, and breath sounds
Heart and vascular system	Normal heart sounds Systole: first heart sound loudest at apex Diastole: first heart sound loudest at base Point of maximal impulse: at fifth intercostal space in midclavicular line and 2 cm or less in diameter Temperature: 36.1°C–37.6°C Pulse: 60–100 bpm (in conditioned athlete, 50 bpm) Blood pressure: 130 mm Hg systolic, 85 mm Hg diastolic All pulses palpable
Breasts	Decreased size resulting from decreased muscle mass Normal nipples
Abdomen	No tenderness or organomegaly Decreased strength of abdominal muscles
Female reproductive system	Change in menstrual cycle and in duration and quality of menstrual flow to cessation of menses "Hot flashes"
Male reproductive system	Normal penis and scrotum Prostatic enlargement in some individuals
Musculoskeletal system	Decreased muscle mass Decreased range of joint motion
Neurological system	Appropriate affect, appearance, and behaviour Lucidity and appropriate level of cognitive ability Intact cranial nerves Adequate motor responses Responsive sensory system

bpm, Beats per minute.

physiological change during middle age is menopause. Men may also notice several sexual changes as androgen levels decrease, such as less firm erections and less frequent ejaculation (see Chapter 27). However, many middle-aged men are still capable of producing fertile sperm and fathering a child.

Perimenopause and Menopause. Menstruation and ovulation occur in a cyclical rhythm in women from adolescence into middle adulthood. Perimenopause is the period during which ovarian function declines, which results in a diminishing number of ova and irregular menstrual cycles. During this perimenopause time, however, women can still become pregnant. Menopause is the permanent cessation of menstruation. It occurs primarily because the ovaries stop producing the hormones estrogen and progesterone. Menopause typically occurs between the ages of 45 and 60 years. The presence and experience of menopausal symptoms, such as hot flashes and insomnia, varies among women from being asymptomatic to being severe enough to interfere with activities of daily living (Lowdermilk et al., 2016).

Cognitive Changes

Changes in the cognitive function of middle-aged adults are rare except with illness or trauma. The middle-aged adult can learn new skills and information. Some middle-aged adults enter educational or vocational programs to prepare themselves for entering the job market or changing jobs.

Psychosocial Changes

The psychosocial changes in middle-aged adults may involve expected events, such as children moving away from home, or unexpected events, such as a marital separation or the death of a loved one. Many middle-aged adults may find themselves in the so-called sandwich generation, simultaneously having the responsibilities of raising their own children and caring for aging parents. These changes may result in stress that can affect middle-aged adults' overall health. During middle age, the person examines life goals and relationships. Often a "midlife crisis" results, in which the person feels turmoil or anxiety about the course of his or her life and desires change. As a result, the person may change relationships, lifestyle, or occupation.

In assessing for psychosocial changes, nurses should assess the major life changes occurring in the middle-aged adult and the impact that the changes have on that person's state of health. The assessment should also include individual psychosocial factors such as coping mechanisms and sources of social support.

In the middle adult years, as children depart from the household, the family enters the postparental family stage. Time and financial demands on the parents decrease, and the couple faces the task of redefining their relationship. If grandchildren are born, grandparenting styles must be chosen. Many middle-aged adults begin to adopt a healthier lifestyle. Health promotion needs for the middle-aged adult include adequate rest, leisure activities, regular exercise, good nutrition, reduction or cessation in the use of tobacco or alcohol, and regular screening examinations. A middle-aged adult's social environment is also important, including relationship concerns; communication and relationships with children, grandchildren, and aging parents; and caregiver concerns with their own aging or disabled parents.

According to Erikson's (1968, 1982) developmental theory, the primary developmental task of the middle adult years is to achieve generativity (see Chapter 21). *Generativity* is the willingness to care for and guide others. Middle-aged adults can achieve generativity with their own children or other younger people. If middle-aged adults fail to achieve generativity, stagnation occurs, manifested by excessive concern with themselves or destructive behaviour toward their children and the community. For some Indigenous young adults, the medicine wheel teachings are also important to understanding their life stages (see Chapter 10 for information about the Medicine Wheel).

Career Transition. Career changes may occur by choice or as a result of changes in the workplace or society. Middle-aged adults change occupations for a variety of reasons, including limited upward mobility, decreasing availability of jobs, and to seek a more challenging occupation. In some cases, technological advances or other changes force middle-aged adults to seek new jobs. Some middle-aged adults choose not to retire and continue to work as long as they are able to work. Such changes, particularly when unanticipated, may result in stress that can affect health, family relationships, self-concept, and other dimensions. Assessing levels of coping and adaptation to work-related stress and changes is an essential part of the nurse's role.

Sexuality. After the departure of their last child from the home, many couples rejuvenate their relationships and find increased marital and sexual satisfaction during middle age. Onset of menopause can affect the sexual health of the middle-aged woman. A woman may desire increased sexual activity because pregnancy is no longer possible. Menopausal women may also experience vaginal dryness and dyspareunia or pain during sexual intercourse (see Chapter 27). During middle age, a man may notice changes in the strength of his erection and a decrease in his ability to experience repeated orgasm. This may result in the use of erectile function–enhancing agents (e.g., sildenafil citrate, tadalafil). Other factors influencing sexuality during this period include work stress, diminished health of one or both partners, and the use of prescription medications with adverse effects that may influence sexual desire or functioning (e.g., antihypertensive agents). Both partners may experience stresses related to sexual changes or a conflict between their sexual needs and self-perceptions and social attitudes or expectations. Assessing sexual functioning contributes to identification of potential risks for STIs and adverse health outcomes that can result from erectile function–enhancing agents.

Family Types. Psychosocial factors involving the family may include the stresses of singlehood, marital changes, family transition as children leave home, and the care of aging parents.

Singlehood. Many adults older than 35 years have never been married. Many of them have chosen to delay marriage and parenthood. Some single middle-aged adults, however, have chosen to become parents, either biologically or through adoption. Many single middle-aged adults may have no relatives but share a family type of relationship with close friends or work associates. Consequently, some single middle-aged adults may feel isolated during traditional "family" holidays. In times of illness, single adults may have to rely on relatives or friends. The nursing assessment of single middle-aged adults should include a thorough assessment of psychosocial factors, including the individual's definition of family and available support systems.

Marital Changes. Marital changes that may occur during middle age include death of a spouse, separation, divorce, and the choice of remarrying or remaining single. If a single, middle-aged adult decides to marry, the stressors of marriage are similar to those for the young adult. A widowed, separated, or divorced patient goes through a period of grief and loss in which it is necessary to adapt to the change in marital status. Normal grieving progresses through a series of phases, and the resolution of grief may take a year or more. Nurses should assess middle-aged adults' coping with the grief and loss associated with life's changes (see Chapter 25).

Family Transitions. Departure of the last child from the home may be a stressor. Many parents welcome freedom from child-rearing responsibilities, whereas others feel lonely or without direction because of this change (known as "empty-nest syndrome"). Eventually parents must reassess their marriage, resolve conflicts, and plan for the future.

On occasion, this readjustment phase may lead to marital conflicts, separation, and divorce.

Care of Aging Parents. Increasing lifespans have led to greater numbers of older persons in the population. Therefore, more middle-aged adults must address the personal and social issues confronting their aging parents, including becoming caregivers for their older parents.

Traditional social expectations between generations in families have changed because of housing, employment, health, and economic realities. Conflicts may arise between middle-aged adults and their older parents, who may strive to remain independent. Negotiations and compromises help in defining and resolving problems. As a nurse, you may encounter middle-aged and older persons in the community, in long-term care facilities, and in hospitals. You can help identify the health needs of both groups and can assist the multigenerational family in determining the health and community resources available to them as they make decisions and plans. You should also assess family relationships to determine family members' perceptions of responsibility and loyalty in relation to caring for older family members. It is also important to assess environmental resources (e.g., number of rooms in the house, stair rails, or handrails in bathrooms) needed for adults to care for their older parents.

Health Concerns

Physiological concerns for middle-aged adults include stress, level of wellness, obesity, and the formation of positive health habits. When adults seek health care, nurses' focus on the goal of wellness can guide patients to evaluate health behaviours, lifestyle, and environment. Patients' health can be undermined by alterable factors such as stress, obesity, tobacco use, excessive alcohol consumption, poor nutrition, and unsafe sexual practices. Drug use, abuse, and misuse may also occur. Attention to these risk factors can increase the quality of life and add years to it.

Stress and Stress Reduction. Middle-aged adults' perceptions of health and health behaviours are often important factors in maintaining health. Individuals are prone to stress-related illnesses such as heart attacks, hypertension, migraine headaches, ulcers, colitis, autoimmune disease, backache, arthritis, and cancer. Stress levels may also increase as the middle-aged adult tries to balance responsibilities related to employment, family life, care of children, and care of aging parents.

Throughout life, people are exposed to many stressors (see Chapter 29). After these stressors are identified, the nurse and patient can work together to intervene and modify the stress response. Stress can be reduced in three ways. First, the frequency of stress-producing situations can be minimized. Together, the nurse and patient should identify approaches to prevent stressful situations, such as habituation, change avoidance, time blocking, time management, and environmental modification. Second, stress resistance can be increased by psychophysiological preparation, such as increasing self-esteem, improving assertiveness, redirecting goal alternatives, and reorienting cognitive appraisal. Third, the physiological response to stress can be avoided. Nurses can teach patients relaxation techniques, imagery, and biofeedback to recondition their response to stress. Chapter 35 explains these general interventions in greater detail.

Levels of Wellness. Nurses need to be able to assess the health status of the middle-aged patient. Such assessment offers direction for planning nursing care and is useful in evaluating the effectiveness of nursing interventions. Table 23-3 shows the expected physical assessment findings of the middle-aged adult. Nurses should use standard assessment techniques as guides for physical assessment (see Chapter 32).

Obesity. *Obesity,* defined as having a body mass index of 30 or more, is a health concern for many middle-aged adults. Obesity peaks in middle age. Among Canadian adults, 25.4% are obese and an additional 36% are overweight (Standing Senate Committee on Social Affairs, Science & Technology, 2016). Health consequences of obesity include such conditions as high blood pressure, high blood cholesterol levels, type 2 (non-insulin-dependent) diabetes mellitus, coronary heart disease, osteoarthritis, and obstructive sleep apnea. Continued focus on the goal of wellness can assist patients in evaluating health behaviours and lifestyle that contribute to obesity during the middle adult years. Counselling related to physical activity and nutrition is an important component of the plan of care for overweight and obese patients.

Forming Positive Health Habits. A *habit* is a person's usual practice or manner of behaviour. This behaviour pattern is reinforced by frequent repetition until it becomes the individual's customary way of behaving. Some habits support health, such as exercise, eating a balanced diet, participating in routine screening and diagnostic tests (e.g., laboratory work for cholesterol, mammography), reducing stress, and daily brushing and flossing of teeth. Other habits involve behaviours harmful to health, such as smoking, consuming excessive alcohol, using illegal drugs, or eating foods with little or no nutritional value.

During assessment, nurses frequently obtain data about patients' positive and negative health behaviours. In the planning, implementation, and evaluation phases, nurses can help patients maintain habits that protect health and offer healthier alternatives to poor habits.

Health teaching and health counselling are often directed at improving health habits (Box 23-5). The more fully you understand the dynamics of behaviour and habits, the more likely your interventions will help the patient to achieve or reinforce health-promoting behaviours.

As a nurse, you can coach patients about forming positive health habits and improve their health literacy. By providing information about how the body functions and how habits are formed and changed, you raise patients' understanding of the impact of behaviour on health. You cannot change patients' habits; patients have control of and are

BOX 23-5 PATIENT TEACHING
Encouraging Positive Health Habits

Objective

- Patient will increase exercise patterns to include three 2-km walks per week to assist in weight loss and to improve cardiopulmonary functions.

Teaching Strategies

- Review with patient the daily work schedule and identify potential times for exercise.
- Inform patient about the effect of exercise on weight control and improved cardiac function.
- Demonstrate how to calculate target heart rate and assess pulse correctly.
- Provide warm-up and cool-down exercises, and demonstrate how to do them.
- Instruct patient about the importance of support shoes for walking exercises.

Evaluation

- Have patient keep log of exercise periods.
- Have patient demonstrate pulse measurement.
- Have patient demonstrate warm-up and cool-down exercises.
- Inspect patient's feet for blisters or sores.

BOX 23-6 Barriers to Health Literacy

External Barriers	Internal Barriers
Lack of facilities	Lack of knowledge
Lack of materials	Lack of motivation
Lack of social supports	Insufficient skills to effect change in health habits
	Undefined short- and long-term goals

responsible for their own behaviours. But you can explain psychological principles of changing habits and offer information about health risks. Ultimately, however, the patient decides which behaviours will become habits of daily living. Barriers to change exist (Box 23-6), and unless these barriers are minimized or eliminated, it is futile to encourage the patient to take actions that are going to be blocked.

As with adolescents and young adults, nurses need to continue educating middle-aged adults about STIs, substance abuse, and accident prevention.

Anxiety. *Anxiety* is a common response to change, conflict, and perceived control of the environment (Austin & Boyd, 2014). Adults often experience anxiety in response to the physiological and psychosocial changes of middle age. Such anxiety can motivate the adult to rethink life goals and can stimulate productivity. For some adults, however, this anxiety precipitates psychosomatic illness and preoccupation with death. Such middle-aged adults view life as being half or more over and think in terms of the time left to live.

Clearly, a life-threatening illness, marital transition, or job stressor increases the anxiety of the patient and family. Nurses may need to use crisis intervention or stress management techniques to help the patient adapt to the changes of the middle adult years (see Chapter 29).

Depression. *Depression* is a mood disorder that manifests itself in many ways. Although its onset occurs most frequently between the ages of 25 and 44 years, it is common among adults in the middle years and may have many causes (Austin & Boyd, 2014). The risk factors for depression include being female; disappointments or losses at work, at school, or in family relationships; departure of the last child from the home; and family history. The incidence of depression in women is twice that in men.

People experiencing mild depression describe feeling sad, "blue," downcast, "down in the dumps," and tearful. Other symptoms include changes in the amount (not sleeping [insomnia], sleeping too much [hypersomnia]) or quality of sleep (multiple awakenings), irritability, feelings of social disinterest, and decreased alertness. Physical changes such as weight loss or weight gain, headaches, or feelings of fatigue regardless of the amount of rest may also be depressive symptoms. Depression that occurs during the middle years is commonly characterized by moderate to high anxiety and physical complaints. Mood changes and depression are common phenomena during menopause. Depression may be worsened by the abuse of alcohol or other substances. Nursing assessment of a depressed middle-aged adult includes focused data collection regarding individual and family history of depression, mood changes, cognitive changes, behavioural and social changes, and physical changes. Assessment data should be collected from both the patient and his or her family. Family data may be particularly important, depending on the level of depression being experienced by the middle-aged adult.

Primary Health Care Programs. Primary health care programs for young and middle-aged adults are designed to prevent illness, promote health, and detect disease in the early stages. Nurses can make valuable contributions to the community's health by taking an active part in the planning of screening programs, teaching programs, and support groups for young and middle-aged adults.

BOX 23-7 CULTURAL ASPECTS OF CARE

Cultural safety is a concept that has been proposed as an approach to address health inequities. Cultural safety was originally developed by Indigenous nurse-scholars and educators as a way to provide more respectful care to Indigenous peoples. Cultural safety extends beyond cultural sensitivity and cultural competence to address the power imbalances, institutional discrimination, and inequitable positioning of certain groups (Pauly, McCall, Browne, et al., 2015).

Implications for Practice

- Recognize that some patients may choose to delay or avoid accessing health care because of perceived or actual adverse health encounters experienced by themselves or their friends, family, or community members.
- Be aware of cultural influences that may affect the experience of patients from vulnerable populations who seek assistance from health care providers.
- Educational materials that combine Western remedies with traditional approaches may be more easily accepted and utilized.
- It is important for nurses to critically reflect on how health issues are framed in health care and how that influences people's ability to access culturally safe health care.

Pauly, B., McCall, J., Browne A. J., Parker, J., & Mollison, A. (2015). Toward cultural safety: Nurse and patient perceptions of illicit substance use in a hospitalized setting. *Advances in Nursing Science, 38*(2), 121–135.

Family planning, birthing, and parenting skills are program topics in which adults might be interested. Health screening for diabetes, hypertension, eye disease, and cancer is a good opportunity for nurses to perform assessment and provide health teaching and health counselling.

Health education programs can promote changes in behaviour and lifestyle. As a health teacher, the nurse can offer information that enables the patient to make decisions about health practices and increase health literacy (see Box 23-1), or the ability to access, comprehend, evaluate, and communicate health information as a way to promote, maintain, and improve health in a variety of settings across the life course (PHAC, 2014). Educational programs must be culturally appropriate (Box 23-7) (Refer to Chapter 9 for information about cultural humility). Encouraging young to middle-aged adults to adopt more positive health practices during young and middle adulthood may lead to fewer or less complicated health problems during older adulthood. During health counselling, the patient and nurse should design a plan of action that addresses the patient's health and well-being. Through objective problem solving, the nurse can help the patient grow and change.

Acute Care. Acute illnesses and conditions experienced in middle adulthood may be similar to those in young adulthood. Injuries and acute illnesses in middle adulthood, however, may require a longer recovery period because of the slowing of recuperative processes. In addition, acute illnesses and injuries experienced in middle adulthood are more likely to become chronic conditions.

The incidence of HIV disease occurs across all age groups and is a consideration for middle-aged adults as well. Although typically thought of as occurring in earlier age groups, middle-aged adults should be assessed for risk factors and given information to help prevent HIV transmission.

Restorative and Continuing Care. Chronic illnesses such as diabetes mellitus, hypertension, rheumatoid arthritis, chronic obstructive pulmonary disease, or multiple sclerosis may affect the roles and responsibilities assumed by the middle-aged adult. Strained family relationships, modifications in family activities, increased health care tasks, increased financial stress, the need for housing adaptation, social isolation, medical concerns, and grieving may all result from chronic illness. The degree of disability and the patient's perception of both the illness and the disability determine the extent to which lifestyle changes will occur. A few examples of the problems experienced by patients who develop debilitating chronic illness during adulthood include role reversal, changes in sexual behaviour, and altered self-image. Nursing assessment of the chronically ill middle-aged adult includes assessment of his or her emotional, physical, social, and spiritual health status and the knowledge base of both the patient and family. This assessment should include the medical course of the illness and the prognosis for the patient. In addition, it is important to determine the coping mechanisms of the patient and family, their adherence to treatment and rehabilitation regimens, and the need for community and social services, along with appropriate referrals.

KEY CONCEPTS

- Adult development involves orderly and sequential changes that adults experience over time.
- Young adults are generally in a stable period of physical development, except for pregnancy-related changes.
- Cognitive development continues throughout the young and middle adult years.
- Increased health literacy among young and middle-aged adults can promote positive health outcomes for people in these stages of life.
- Emotional health of young adults is correlated with their ability to address and resolve personal and social problems.
- Young adults must choose a career and decide whether to remain single or marry and begin a family.
- Pregnant women need to understand physiological changes occurring during each trimester.
- Psychosocial changes and health concerns during pregnancy and the puerperium period affect the mother and the rest of the family.
- Health promotion interventions are important during the prenatal period and can improve the well-being of the woman and fetus.
- Midlife transition begins when a person becomes aware that physiological and psychosocial changes signify passage to another stage in life.
- Two significant physiological changes of the middle years are menopause in women and changes in sexual response in men.
- Cognitive changes are rare in middle age except in cases of illness or physical trauma.
- Psychosocial changes for middle-aged adults may be related to career transition, sexuality, marital changes, family transition, and care of aging parents.
- Health goals of middle-aged adults commonly involve preventing stress-related illnesses, participating in health assessments, and adopting positive health habits.

CRITICAL THINKING EXERCISES

1. Daoud is a 24-year-old gay man who smokes two packs of cigarettes per day. He began smoking when he was 14 years old. Daoud complains to you at the clinic, "I just can't seem to kick the habit, no matter how hard I try." What information do you need to know to assist Daoud in quitting smoking?
2. Ray-Jean, 48 years old, divorced, and the mother of 13- and 16-year-old sons, has recently had to assume the responsibility of caring for her 78-year-old father after he suffered a stroke. Describe your role in assisting Ray-Jean to care for her father.

REVIEW QUESTIONS

1. The nurse is assessing a 48-year-old patient with a history of coronary heart disease, osteoarthritis, and obstructive sleep apnea. The nurse suspects the patient is obese, based on which of the following assessment findings? *(Select all that apply.)*
   1. Fasting blood glucose level of 9 mmol/L
   2. Fasting blood glucose level of 5 mmol/L
   3. Body mass index (BMI) of 33 kg/m^2
   4. BMI of 28 kg/m^2
   5. Blood pressure of 125/85 mmHg
   6. Blood pressure of 145/90 mmHg
2. The nurse knows that young adults usually have good health and directs health care education in this population toward activities related to:
   1. Health promotion
   2. Primary prevention
   3. Secondary prevention
   4. Tertiary prevention
3. When planning the prescribed course of therapy, the nurse considers which of the following factors that may affect the individual's adherence with the regimen? *(Select all that apply.)*
   1. Gender
   2. Lifestyle
   3. Sexuality
   4. Education level
   5. Health literacy
   6. Motivation and desire to learn
4. The nurse caring for a patient in the second trimester of pregnancy instructs the patient to expect which common physiological change?
   1. Morning sickness
   2. Amenorrhea
   3. Increased colostrum
   4. Quickening
5. The nurse knows that firearm injuries are a major health concern in Canada. When caring for patients with firearm injuries, the nurse is aware that in Canada:
   1. Approximately 80% of firearm-related injuries are the result of criminal activity.
   2. Approximately 20% of firearm-related injuries are the result of criminal activity.
   3. Approximately 50% of suicides are carried out with firearms.
   4. Approximately 20% of suicides are carried out with firearms.
6. The nurse is developing a smoking reduction and cessation intervention with HIV-positive gay men. Which action demonstrates the use of cultural safety?
   1. The nurse invites several HIV-positive gay men to participate in intervention development to overcome stigma and power imbalances these men experience in the health care system.
   2. The nurse collaborates with the Medical Health Officer of the local health district to develop the intervention.
   3. The nurse engages with families of HIV-positive gay men to develop the smoking reduction and cessation intervention.
   4. The nurse acknowledges that HIV-positive gay men have unique cultural traditions and works to implement a standardized smoking reduction and cessation intervention.
7. A patient's father and paternal grandfather had myocardial infarctions (heart attacks) in their 50s. Therefore, the patient is at risk for a future myocardial infarction. The patient faces what type of health risk?

1. Lifestyle
2. Poor personal hygiene
3. Family history
4. Hereditary disease

8. A nurse is evaluating the effectiveness of health teaching about human lactation to the parents of a newborn. Which statement demonstrates that the family has increased health literacy?
   1. Parents teach back how to care for their breastfeeding newborn and describe where to find information about care and when they should contact a health care provider with concerns.
   2. Parents listen to the nurse describe how to care for their breastfeeding newborn and thank the nurse for sharing this knowledge with them.
   3. Parents teach back how to care for their breastfeeding newborn and are actively engaged in learning about the care of their newborn.
   4. Parents listen to the nurse and describe how to care for their breastfeeding newborn and report that they do not understand what the nurse has taught them.
9. A nurse is teaching a transmasculine patient about infant feeding options. Which statement demonstrates that the nurse is providing culturally safe care?
   1. I am here to teach you about lactation and infant feeding practices, including chestfeeding. How do you prefer I address you?
   2. Hi Jonah, I am here to teach you about lactation and breastfeeding your newborn.
   3. I refuse to provide care to transmasculine persons because it is against my philosophical and religious beliefs.
   4. I am here to teach you about lactation and infant feeding practices. I encourage you to formula feed your newborn.
10. To help recondition the patient's response to stress, the nurse can use: *(Select all that apply)*:
    1. Biofeedback
    2. Imagery
    3. Medication
    4. Time management strategies
    5. Relaxation techniques
    6. Assertiveness training

Answers: 1. 1, 3, 6; **2.** 1; **3.** 1, 2, 4, 5, 6; **4.** 4; **5.** 2; **6.** 1; **7.** 3; **8.** 1; **9.** 1; **10.** 1, 2, 5

Rationales for the Review Questions appear at the end of the book.

RECOMMENDED WEBSITES

Breastfeeding Committee for Canada: http://www.breastfeedingcanada.ca.
The Breastfeeding Committee for Canada was established in 1991 as a Health Canada initiative. This site addresses breastfeeding issues experienced among Canadians.

Canadian AIDS Treatment Information Exchange (CATIE): http://www.catie.ca/.
This site provides information about the treatment, management, and prevention of HIV and hepatitis C.

Canadian Cancer Society: http://www.cancer.ca.
This site provides information on specific cancers, clinical trials, support services, and ways to get involved.

Canadian Women's Health Network: http://www.cwhn.ca.
The goal of the Canadian Women's Health Network is to share information, resources, and strategies to improve women's health.

Institute of Aboriginal Peoples' Health: http://www.cihr-irsc.gc.ca/e/8668.html.
The Institute of Aboriginal Peoples' Health fosters the advancement of a national health research agenda to improve and promote the health of First Nations, Inuit, and Métis peoples in Canada, through research, knowledge translation, and capacity building.

La Leche League Canada: http://www.lllc.ca.
La Leche League Canada encourages, promotes, and provides mother-to-mother breastfeeding support and educational opportunities, thus contributing to the health of children, families, and society.

Movember Foundation: https://ca.movember.com/.
The Movember Foundation is the leading global organization for improving men's health.

Public Health Agency of Canada: http://www.phac-aspc.gc.ca/index-eng.php.
This site has links to topics concerning health issues of Canadians, including information on chronic diseases, infectious diseases, and healthy living.

REFERENCES

Assisted Human Reproduction Canada. (2012). *Your guide to infertility and assisted human reproduction (AHR).* Retrieved from http://publications.gc.ca/collections/collection_2012/sc-hc/H179-4-2012-eng.pdf.

Austin, W., & Boyd, M. A. (2014). *Psychiatric and mental health nursing for Canadian practice* (3rd ed.). Philadelphia, PA: Lippincott Williams & Wilkins.

Babycenter (2017). *Major Causes of Infertility* (chart). Retrieved from https://www.babycenter.ca/a6020/major-causes-of-infertility-chart.

Bauer, G. R., Hammond, R., Travers, R., et al. (2009). "I don't think this is theoretical; this is our lives": How erasure impacts health care for transgender people. *Journal of the Association of Nurses in AIDS Care, 20*(5), 348–361. doi:10.1016/j.jana.2009.07.004.

Boellstorff, T. (2011). But do not identify as gay: A proleptic genealogy of the MSM category. *Cultural Anthropology, 26*(2), 287–312. doi:10.1111/j.1548-1360.2011.01100.x.

Bushnik, T., Cook, J. L., Yuzpe, A. A., et al. (2012). Estimating the prevalence of infertility in Canada. *Human Reproduction, 27*(3), 738–746. doi:10.1093/humrep/der465.

Canadian Association of Schools of Nursing/Association Canadienne des Écoles de Sciences Infirmières (CASN/ACESI). (2015). *National nursing education framework: Final report.* Retrieved from http://www.casn.ca/wp-content/uploads/2014/12/Framwork-FINAL-SB-Nov-30-20151.pdf.

Canadian Cancer Society's Steering Committee (2017). *Canadian cancer statistics 2016.* Toronto: Author. Retrieved from http://www.cancer.ca/en/cancer-information/cancer-101/canadian-cancer-statistics-publication/?region=on.

Canadian Society for Exercise Physiology. (2011). *Canadian physical activity guidelines for adults 18-64 years.* Retrieved from http://www.csep.ca/CMFiles/Guidelines/CSEP_PAGuidelines_adults_en.pdf.

Edelman, C. L., Kudzma, E. C., & Mandle, C. L. (2014). *Health promotion throughout the lifespan* (8th ed.). St. Louis, MO: Mosby.

Erikson, E. (1963). *Childhood and society* (2nd ed.). New York: W. W. Norton.

Erikson, E. (1968). *Identity: Youth and crisis.* New York: W. W. Norton.

Erikson, E. (1982). *The life cycle completed: A review.* New York: W. W. Norton.

Gilligan, C. (1993). *In a different voice.* Cambridge, MA: Harvard University Press.

Harris, K. (2017). *'Our collective shame': Trudeau delivers historic apology to LGBT Canadians.* CBC. Retrieved from http://www.cbc.ca/news/politics/homosexual-offences-exunge-records-1.4422546.

Havighurst, R. (1972). Successful aging. In R. H. Williams, C. Tibbits, & W. Donahue (Eds.), *Process of aging* (Vol. 1). New York: Atherton.

Hunt, S. (2016). *An introduction to the health of two-spirit people: Historical, contemporary and emergent issues.* Prince George, BC: National Collaborating Centre for Aboriginal Health. Retrieved from https://www.ccnsa-nccah.ca/454/An_Introduction_to_the_Health_of_Two-Spirit_People.nccah.

Katouziyan, M., Vandyk, A., & Phillips, J. C. (in press). Mothering an adolescent who misuses substances: A qualitative evidence synthesis. In W. E. Peterson, L. L. Armstrong, & M. Foulkes (Eds.), *Mothers, addiction, and recovery: Finding meaning through the journey.* Demeter Press: Bradford, ON. [forthcoming 2018].

Lewis, S. L., Dirksen, S. R., Heitkemper, M. M., et al. (2014). *Medical surgical nursing in Canada: Assessment and management of clinical problems* (3rd ed.). Toronto: Elsevier Canada.

Lowdermilk, D. L., Perry, S. E., Cashion, M. C., et al. (2016). *Maternity and women's health care* (11th ed.). St. Louis, MO: Mosby.

MacDonald, T., Noel-Weiss, J., West, D., et al. (2016). Transmasculine individuals' experiences with lactation, chestfeeding, and gender identity: A qualitative study. *BMC Pregnancy and Childbirth, 16*, 106. doi:10.1186/s12884-016-0907-y. Retrieved from https://bmcpregnancychildbirth.biomedcentral.com/articles/10.1186/s12884-016-0907-y.

McManus, A., Hunter, L. P., & Renn, H. (2006). Lesbian experiences and needs during childbirth: Guidelines for health care providers. *Journal of Obstetric, Gynecologic, and Neonatal Nursing, 35*, 13–23.

Phillips, J. C. (2011). Antiretroviral therapy adherence: Testing a social context model among Black men who use illicit drugs. *Journal of the Association of Nurses in AIDS Care, 22*(2), 100–127. doi:10.1016/j.jana.2010.07.008.

Phillips, J. C., & Saewyc, E. M. (2010). HIV disease and gay, lesbian, bisexual, and transgender persons. In J. D. Durham & F. R. Lashley (Eds.), *The person with HIV/AIDS: Nursing perspectives* (4th ed., pp. 365–404). New York: Springer.

Prestage, G. (2011). *The term 'MSM' demeans us all.* New South Wales, Australia: The Kirby Institute, University of New South Wales. Retrieved from http://cbrc.net/sites/cbrc.net/files/MSM%20demeans%20us%20all.pdf.

Public Health Agency of Canada (PHAC) (2013). *Sexually transmitted infections—A continued public health concern.* Ottawa: Author. Retrieved from http://www.phac-aspc.gc.ca/cphorsphc-respcacsp/2013/sti-its-eng.php.

Public Health Agency of Canada (PHAC) (2014). *Health literacy.* Ottawa: Author. Retrieved from http://www.phac-aspc.gc.ca/cd-mc/hl-ls/index-eng.php#tabs-2.

Registered Nurses' Association of Ontario (RNAO) (2003). *Breastfeeding best practice guidelines for nurses.* Toronto: Author.

Society of Obstetricians and Gynaecologists of Canada (SOGC). (2016). *Sex & U.* Retrieved from http://www.sexandu.ca/.

Standing Senate Committee on Social Affairs, Science & Technology. (2016). *Obesity in Canada: A whole-of-society approach for a healthier Canada.* Retrieved from http://www.parl.gc.ca/content/sen/committee/421/SOCI/Reports/2016-02-25_Revised_report_Obesity_in_Canada_e.pdf.

Statistics Canada. (2012). *2011 census of population: Families, households, marital status, structural type of dwelling, collectives.* Retrieved from http://www.statcan.gc.ca/daily-quotidien/120919/dq120919a-eng.htm.

Statistics Canada. (2015a). *Annual demographic estimates: Canada, provinces and territories, 2015. Section 2: Population by age and sex.* Retrieved from http://www.statcan.gc.ca/pub/91-215-x/2015000/part-partie2-eng.htm.

Statistics Canada. (2015b). *Labour force characteristics by age and sex—Seasonally adjusted (Table 1). Labour force survey: Year-end review, 2014.* Retrieved from http://www.statcan.gc.ca/daily-quotidien/150128/t150128a001-eng.htm.

Statistics Canada (2015c). *Firearms and violent crime in Canada, 2012.* Ottawa: Author. Retrieved from http://www.statcan.gc.ca/pub/85-002-x/2014001/article/11925-eng.htm#a3.

Statistics Canada (2016a). *Population by sex and age group.* Ottawa: Author. Retrieved from http://www.statcan.gc.ca/tables-tableaux/sum-som/l01/cst01/demo10a-eng.htm.

Statistics Canada (2016b). *Population by marital status and sex.* Ottawa: Author. Retrieved from http://www.statcan.gc.ca/tables-tableaux/sum-som/l01/cst01/famil01-eng.htm.

Statistics Canada. (2016c). *Heavy drinking by age group and sex.* Retrieved from http://www.statcan.gc.ca/tables-tableaux/sum-som/l01/cst01/health79a-eng.htm.

Statistics Canada. (2017a). *Marital status and opposite- and same-sex status by sex for persons aged 15 and over living in private households for both sexes, total, presence and age of children, 2016 counts, Canada, provinces and territories, 2016 Census – 100% Data.* Retrieved from http://www12.statcan.gc.ca/census-recensement/2016/dp-pd/hlt-fst/fam/Table.cfm?Lang=E&T=11&Geo=00&SP=1&view=1&sex=1&presence=1.

Statistics Canada (2017b). *Canada's crime rate: Two decades of decline.* Ottawa: Author. Retrieved from http://www.statcan.gc.ca/pub/11-630-x/11-630-x2015001-eng.htm.

Transport Canada (2016). *Canadian motor vehicle traffic collision statistics, 2014.* Ottawa: Author. Retrieved from https://www.tc.gc.ca/media/documents/roadsafety/cmvtcs2014_eng.pdf.

Young, R. M., & Meyer, I. H. (2005). The trouble with "MSM" and "WSW": Erasure of the sexual-minority person in public health discourse. *American Journal of Public Health, 95*(7), 1144–1149. doi:10.2105/AJPH.2004.046714.

Zika Working Group on behalf of the Committee to Advise on Tropical Medicine and Travel. (2016). Canadian recommendations on the prevention and treatment of Zika virus: Update. *Canadian Communicable Diseases Report, 42*(5), 101–111. Retrieved from http://www.phac-aspc.gc.ca/publicat/ccdr-rmtc/16vol42/dr-rm42-5/ar-01-eng.php#a8.

24

Older Persons

Canadian content written by Sherry Dahlke, PhD, RN, GCN(C), Wendy Duggleby, RN, PhD
Original chapter by Gayle L. Kruse, RN, ACHPN, GCNS-BC

OBJECTIVES

Mastery of content in this chapter will enable you to:

- Define the key terms listed.
- Discuss demographic trends related to older persons in Canada.
- Identify common myths and stereotypes about older persons.
- List the types of community-based and institutional health care services available to older persons.
- Describe the concepts of aging well and quality of life.
- Discuss common developmental tasks of older persons.
- Describe common physiological changes associated with aging.
- Differentiate among delirium, dementia, and depression.
- Discuss issues related to psychosocial changes connected with aging.
- Describe selected health concerns of older persons.
- Identify nursing interventions related to the physiological, cognitive, and psychosocial changes of aging.

KEY TERMS

Age-friendly community, p. 421
Ageism, p. 413
Aging well, p. 413
Alzheimer's disease, p. 418
Cognitive stimulation, p. 427
Delirium, p. 418
Dementia, p. 418
Depression, p. 419
Elder abuse, p. 420
Functional status, p. 416
Long-term care, p. 414
Palliative care, p. 428
Personal care home, p. 414
Polypharmacy, p. 426
Reminiscence, p. 427
Restorative care, p. 428

MEDIA RESOURCES

http://evolve.elsevier.com/Canada/Potter/fundamentals/

- Audio Chapter Summaries
- Examination Review Questions
- Concept Map Creator
- Case Study with Questions
- Audio Glossary
- Content Updates
- Video Clips

The identification of 65 years of age as the start of older adulthood dates back to social reform in Germany in the nineteenth century. The age of 65 years continues to be used as the lower boundary to define older adulthood in demographics and social policy, although many older persons consider themselves to be "middle-aged" well into their 70s (Special Senate Committee on Aging, 2009). In Canada, the Special Senate Committee on Aging (2009) suggests that the term *older person* is the most appropriate term for persons over the age of 65 years. Sometimes the older age group is broken into groups of youngest old, old, and oldest old, with oldest old comprising people over 85. However, chronological age may have little relation to the reality of aging for an older person. Each person ages in his or her own way according to his or her own schedules and life histories. Even though generalizations are made in this chapter about the aging process and its effect on individuals, every older person is unique and must be treated by nurses as a unique individual.

The number of older persons in Canada is growing, both absolutely and as a proportion of the total population. On July 1, 2015, for the first time, there were more Canadians aged 65 and older than children 0–14 years of age (Statistics Canada, 2015a). Geographic variations in the aging population exist across Canada; the proportion of older persons is lowest in Nunavut (3.3%). Regarding the provinces, the lowest proportion of older people is in Alberta (11.6%) and highest in New Brunswick (19%) (Statistics Canada, 2015a). The number of older persons is expected to increase to 20.1% of the population by 2036 (Statistics Canada, 2015a). Part of that increase is a result of the extension of the average lifespan. In 2012, the average life expectancy at birth for Canadians was 81.1 years—78.8 years for men and 83.3 years for women (Statistics Canada, 2015b). Two other factors contribute to the projected increase in the number of older persons: the aging of the baby-boom generation and advances in health care practices to manage chronic diseases. The baby boomers are the large cohort of people born between 1946 and 1964. In 2011, the oldest baby boomers reached the age of 65 years and represented the fastest growing age group in Canada. By 2031, all baby boomers will have reached the age of 65 and will comprise of 23% of older persons in Canada. As baby boomers age, social and health care programs will need to expand to meet their needs, as well as the needs of the second fastest growing group of persons, those aged 100 years and older (Statistics Canada, 2015b). The numbers of centenarians have increased 25.7% since 2006, with a census count of 5 826 people in 2011.

The diversity of the population older than 65 years is also projected to increase, as future cohorts of older persons will be born outside of Canada (Statistics Canada, 2016a). Approximately 36% of Canadian older people over the age of 60 were born outside Canada. Most immigrated when young. In caring for older persons from these groups, nurses must account for diversity in cultures, values, and languages. Examples of culturally safe nursing approaches to older persons are respect for preferences in food, music, and religion; attentive listening; use of physical assessment norms appropriate for diverse groups; and asking about personal health practices, family customs, lifestyle preferences, and spiritual resources (Hirst, Lane, & Miller, 2015). Chapter 9 provides further information on culturally safe care. Before the 1950s, when the specialties of gerontology and geriatrics emerged, there was little differentiation between general principles of nursing care and nursing care of older people (Dahlke, 2011). The Canadian Gerontological Nurses Association (CGNA) demonstrated strong support for nursing care of older people through their establishment of Gerontological Nursing Competencies and Standards of Practice (CGNA, 2010).

VARIABILITY AMONG OLDER PERSONS

The nursing care of older persons poses special challenges because of the great variation in their physiological, cognitive, and psychosocial health. Levels of functional ability also vary widely among older persons. The majority of older persons are active and involved members of their communities. A smaller number have lost the ability to care for themselves, are confused or withdrawn, are unable to make decisions concerning their needs, or have a combination of these factors. Most older persons (93%) live in private homes, with only 7% residing in institutions such as nursing homes (Statistics Canada, 2015b). Age influences living arrangements: the proportion of older persons living with a spouse decreases with age, the proportion living alone increases with age, and the proportion living in an institution increases with age, with women being more likely than men to live in a communal setting (Milan, Wong, & Vezina, 2014).

Aging does not inevitably lead to disability and dependence. Most older people remain functionally independent despite the increasing prevalence of chronic disease. Nursing assessment, a complex and challenging process, can provide valuable clues to the effect a disease or illness is having on a patient's functional status. Chronic conditions add to the complexity of assessment and care of the older person. Approximately 91% of older persons report one or more chronic conditions; arthritis, hypertension, heart disease, vision impairment, and diabetes mellitus are the most common conditions in noninstitutionalized older persons (Canadian Institutes for Health Information [CIHI], 2011). These chronic conditions impose limitations on activities: slightly more than 22% of persons 65 to 74 years of age and nearly 50% of those 85 years or older report some limitations in activities.

The physical, cognitive, and psychosocial aspects of aging are closely related. For the older person, a reduced ability to respond to stress, the experience of multiple losses, and the physical changes associated with normal aging may combine to increase the risk for illness and functional deterioration. Although the interaction of these physical and psychosocial factors can be serious, nurses should not assume that all older persons have signs, symptoms, or behaviours representing disease and decline or that these are the only items to be assessed. An older person's strengths and abilities must also be identified during the assessment.

MYTHS AND STEREOTYPES

Despite ongoing research in the field of gerontology, false beliefs and myths about older persons persist. These stereotypes include beliefs about the physical and psychosocial characteristics and the lifestyles of older persons. Sometimes negative perceptions about older people are perpetuated through jokes, with up to half of jokes about getting old portraying a negative attitude toward aging and old people (Novak, Campbell, & Northcott, 2014). These negative perceptions about older people, in combination with the projected increases in numbers of older people, has led to concerns about older people using too many of our limited health care resources; however, increased costs in health care are often associated with the cost of health care technology rather than the age of the health care consumer (World Health Organization, 2015). However, negative stereotypes may adversely affect access to and the quality of the care provided to older patients (World Health Organization, 2015). Nurses, although personally susceptible to the myths and stereotypes held by society, have the responsibility to dispel the myths and replace the stereotypes with accurate information.

Older persons are sometimes stereotyped as ill and disabled. However, although many experience chronic conditions or have at least one disability that limits performance of activities of daily living (ADLs), only 23% of older persons describe their health as poor or fair (CIHI, 2011). Despite increased incidence of chronic diseases with age, 80% of older people are able to live independently, and three-quarters of older Canadians rate their mental health in positive terms (Chappell & Hollander, 2013). Other common misconceptions are that older persons are generally not interested in sex and that any interest in sexual activities is abnormal and should be discouraged. However, many older persons report continued enjoyment of sexual relationships. Another common misconception is that older persons are unable to use computers. More than half of older persons (aged 65 years and older) use the Internet (Figure 24-1), and 77% have a cell phone (Smith, 2014).

Some people believe that older persons are forgetful, confused, rigid, bored, unfriendly, and unable to understand and learn new information. However, centenarians, the oldest of the old, are described as having an optimistic outlook on life, good memories, broad social contacts and interests, and tolerance for others (Touhy, Jett, Boscart, et al., 2012). Although the process of learning may be affected by age-related changes in vision or hearing or by reduced energy and endurance, older persons are lifelong learners. When communicating with older persons nurses should use teaching techniques that

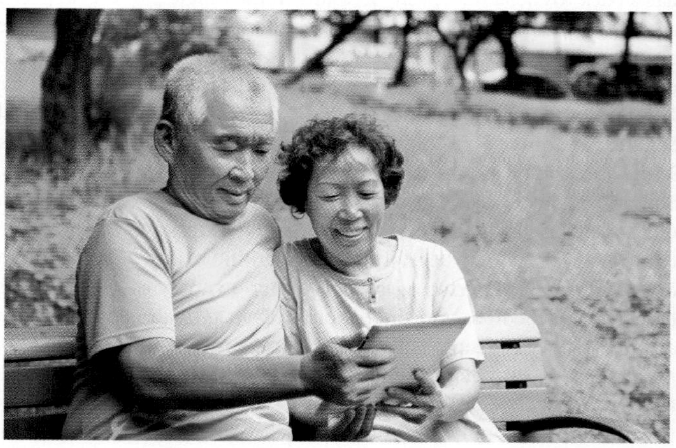

FIGURE 24-1 Most Canadian older persons use the Internet. (© tomwang/Can Stock Photo Inc.)

BOX 24-1 FOCUS ON OLDER PERSONS

Strategies for Communicating Effectively With Older Persons

- Try to find a quiet room with minimal outside noises for communication.
- Sit facing the patient so that he or she can watch your lip movements and facial expressions.
- If needed, make sure that glasses and hearing aids are being worn.
- Speak slowly and clearly (do not speak loudly).
- Keep your tone of voice low; older persons can hear low-frequency sounds better than high-frequency sounds.
- Periodically summarize what has been said to clarify that you have understood what the older person was saying, and repeat key points.
- Ask the older person to explain what he or she understood and invite questions to clarify information. There may also be cultural aspects related to communication. (Please refer to Chapter 17 for more information.)
- Emphasize and integrate emotional and personal values in the acquisition of skills and ideas.

Adapted from Hirst, S. P., Lane, A. M., & Miller, C. A. (2015). *Miller's nursing for wellness in older adults* (Canadian ed.). Philadelphia: Wolters Kluwer/ Lippincott Williams & Wilkins.

compensate for sensory changes, provide additional time for remembering and responding, and present concrete rather than abstract material to facilitate learning by older persons. Other effective teaching techniques draw from older persons' past experiences and correspond to their identified interests rather than to the content areas believed important by the health care provider. Box 24-1 presents communication strategies that you can use to address the learning needs of older persons.

In a society that values attractiveness, energy, and youth, these myths and stereotypes lead to the undervaluing of older persons. Some people believe that older persons are unattractive and become worthless to society after they leave the workforce. Others consider the knowledge and experience of older persons to be too old-fashioned to have any current value. These notions underlie the concept of **ageism**, which is discrimination against people because of increasing age, just as racism and sexism are discrimination based on skin colour and gender, respectively. Ageism has the potential to undermine the self-confidence of older persons, limit their access to care, and distort caregivers' understanding of the uniqueness of each older person (Hirst et al., 2015). By contrast, a society that values the contribution and wisdom of older people helps them to maintain decision making and function to their greatest ability.

NURSES' ATTITUDES TOWARD OLDER PERSONS

It is important for you as a nurse to assess your attitudes toward older persons, your own aging, and the aging of your family and friends. Your attitudes toward older persons result partly from your personal experiences with older persons, your education and employment experiences, attitudes of co-workers and employers, and your own age. Cultivation of positive attitudes toward older persons and specialized knowledge about aging and the health care needs of older persons are priorities for nurses.

Positive attitudes regarding older persons are based in part on a realistic portrayal of the characteristics and health care needs of older persons. In the past, negative attitudes about aging contributed to the persistence of stereotypes of older persons as dependent and less attractive than younger persons. Health care providers, under the influence of these attitudes, often lacked respect for older persons and ignored the opportunity to actively involve them in care decisions and activities. At times, hospitals and long-term care facilities have treated older persons as objects to be acted upon rather than as independent, dignified persons (Rozanova, Miller, & Welte, 2016). The time has come for all nurses to recognize and address ageism by questioning prevailing negative attitudes and stereotypes about older persons and advocating for them in all care settings.

BOX 24-2 Developmental Tasks for Older Persons

- Adjusting to decreasing health and physical strength
- Adjusting to retirement and reduced or fixed income
- Adjusting to the death of a spouse
- Accepting one's self as an aging person
- Maintaining satisfactory living arrangements
- Redefining relationships with adult children
- Finding ways to maintain quality of life

Adapted from Erikson, E. H., Erikson, J. M., & Kivnick, H. Q. (1986). *Vital involvement in old age: The experience of old age in our time.* New York: W. W. Norton.

Developmental Tasks for Older Persons

Although no two individuals age in the same way, either biologically or psychosocially, frameworks outlining developmentally appropriate tasks for older persons have been developed. Seven developmental tasks of older persons are listed in Box 24-2.

These developmental tasks are common to many older persons and are associated with varying degrees of change and loss. The more common losses involve health, significant others, a sense of being useful, socialization, income, and independent living. The ways that older persons adjust to the changes of aging are highly individualized. For some, adaptation and adjustment are relatively easy. For others, coping with the changes caused by aging may require the assistance of family, friends, and health care providers. As a nurse, you must be sensitive to the effect of such losses on older persons and their families and be prepared to offer support.

Older persons must also adjust to the physical changes that accompany aging. The extent and timing of these changes vary from individual to individual, but as body systems age, changes occur in appearance and functioning. These changes are not associated with a disease but are normal changes. The presence of disease may alter the timing of the changes or their impact on daily life. Structural and functional changes associated with aging are described in "Physiological Changes" later in the chapter.

AGING WELL AND QUALITY OF LIFE

More recently, theories of successful aging and developmental tasks have been integrated into the concept of aging well or active aging (Woods, Rillamas-Sun, Cochrane, et al., 2016). Older persons are considered to be "**aging well**" when they are achieving self-integration of all aspects of growing older. Faced with the changes that come with aging, older persons must find ways to maintain their quality of life. Existential issues and relationships are important aspects of quality of life for older persons (Register & Herman, 2010). However, the definition of quality of life varies from person to person. As a nurse you must listen to what an older person considers to be most important, rather than making assumptions about that individual's priorities. Together, you and the older person may set objectives for maintaining quality of life, whether quality of life is defined as maintenance of social relationships, continuing to live alone, or continuing activities such as driving or gardening or dancing.

COMMUNITY-BASED AND INSTITUTIONAL HEALTH CARE SERVICES

You may encounter older persons in a wide variety of community-based and institutional health care settings. Outside the acute care hospital setting, you and other nurses may care for older persons in private homes and apartments, adult day care centres, home care, assisted-living facilities (also known as *supportive housing*), long-term care facilities, and hospices. A **personal care home** is a private business that provides accommodation, meals, and supervision or assistance with personal care in a family-like atmosphere. In some provinces, personal care homes are offered as a type of assisted-living facility. Assisted-living facilities are designed for residents who need only minimal to moderate care. Residents live independently in their own apartments and are provided with support services such as homemaking or personal care. Some assisted-living facilities are small group homes where residents share common eating and living areas. Nursing services are not usually included in assisted-living facilities. **Long-term care** facilities provide accommodations, 24-hour nursing care, and support services for people who cannot care for themselves at home but do not need hospital care. Palliative care facilities such as hospices focus on providing care for persons who are dying. They can be publicly or privately funded.

Canadian older persons, because of their changing health status, will need different types of care options during their life. These include health care and social services (Box 24-3). Nurses can assist older persons and their families by providing information and answering questions as they make choices among care options. During the decision-making period, the actual move from a private home to an assisted-living or long-term care facility, and the time after the move, the nurse's role is to support the older person and the family. Nurses can provide information about the selection of a good assisted-living or long-term care facility. The best way to evaluate the quality of a facility is to visit it and inspect it personally (Hirst et al., 2015).

BOX 24-3 FOCUS ON OLDER PERSONS

Community Resources for Older Persons

- *Information and referral:* Local programs within communities offer an "info line" that provides information about agencies and services. Health Link is also a Canadian resource.
- *Senior centres:* Community-based centres provide services such as meals, limited transportation, and social and educational programming.
- *Home-delivered meals:* Programs that deliver hot meals to older person are run by community centres, churches, and hospitals.
- *Companions and friendly visitors:* Programs that offer socially focused home visitation and accompaniment for appointments are run by seniors centres, churches, and not-for-profit organizations.
- *Telephone reassurance:* Service providers make scheduled telephone calls to older people to provide support and reminders.
- *Personal emergency response systems:* An emergency response system that involves wearing a "call button" in a necklace or bracelet will initiate a phone call to designated support people when assistance is needed.
- *Energy assistance programs:* Provincial and territorial programs offer financial assistance to older people with limited income for paying utility bills.

ASSESSING THE NEEDS OF OLDER PERSONS

Gerontological nursing offers creative approaches for maximizing the potential of older persons. The standards of practice of the Canadian Gerontological Nursing Association (2010) were developed to define the uniqueness and scope of gerontological nursing practice, which includes functions such as assessment. With comprehensive assessment information regarding an older person's strengths, resources, and limitations, the nurse and the older person can identify needs and problems and select interventions that maintain their physical abilities and create an environment for psychosocial and spiritual well-being. To conduct a thorough assessment, nurses need to actively engage older persons and provide them with enough time to share important information about their health. Nurses should assess for changes in physiology, cognition, and psychosocial behaviour (please refer to Chapter 13 on nursing assessment and diagnosis for more information).

Nursing assessment must take into account five key points to ensure an age-specific approach: (1) the interrelation between physical and psychosocial aspects of aging, (2) the effects of disease and disability on functional status, (3) the decreased efficiency of homeostatic mechanisms, (4) the lack of standards for health and illness norms, and (5) altered manifestations of and responses to specific disease (Hirst et al., 2015). Obtaining a comprehensive assessment of an older person often takes more time than does an assessment of a younger person because of the longer life and medical history and the potential complexity of that history. By planning to spend extra time with the assessment, the nurse and an older person are less likely to feel rushed. During the physical examination, the nurse may find it necessary to allow rest periods or to conduct the assessment in several sessions because of the reduced energy and limited endurance experienced by some frail older persons.

Sensory changes may also affect data gathering. The choice of communication techniques is influenced by any visual or hearing impairment experienced by the older person. If older persons are unable to understand the nurse's visual or auditory cues, assessment data may be inaccurate or misleading. For example, if an older person has difficulty hearing the nurse's questions, his or her responses may be inappropriate, and the nurse may wrongly believe that he or she is confused.

Memory deficits, if present, will affect the accuracy and completeness of the data collected. Information contributed by a family member or other caregiver, such as a history of allergies and documentation of immunizations, may be necessary to supplement the older person's recollection of past medical events and information. Nurses must use tact when involving another adult in the assessment interview with an older person. The additional adult supplements the answers of the older person with his or her consent, but the older person remains the focus of the interview.

Interpreters or cultural brokers must be present when an older person does not speak the nurse's language. The spoken word must be interpreted within the context of the older person's culture. To ensure culturally safe means of communication during assessment, it is important to (1) identify how the older person wishes to be addressed (use culturally appropriate titles); (2) assess the health-related beliefs and practices of the older person; and (3) know the beliefs and practices of the older person's culture group with regard to spatial requirements, eye contact, and touch, and use them to establish rapport. (See Chapter 9 for more information on providing culturally safe care.)

In older patients, signs and symptoms of diseases and laboratory values may be different from those in younger persons; the classic signs and symptoms of diseases may be absent, blunted, or atypical in older persons (Hirst et al., 2015). These differences may result from age-related changes in organ systems and homeostatic mechanisms, from progressive loss of physiological and functional reserves, or from coexisting acute or chronic conditions. As a result, for example, an older person with a urinary tract infection may present with confusion, loss of appetite, weakness, dizziness, or fatigue instead of fever, dysuria, frequency, or urgency; an older person with pneumonia may have tachycardia, tachypnea, and confusion without the more common symptoms of fever and productive cough; and instead of substernal chest pain and diaphoresis, an older person with a myocardial infarction may experience epigastric discomfort, restlessness, hypotension, confusion, or referred or no pain. Variations from the usual norms for laboratory values may result from age-related changes in cardiac, pulmonary, renal, and metabolic function (Peters, 2010). Examples of laboratory values that may be increased by these changes include, but are not limited to, levels of alkaline phosphatase, serum cholesterol, triglycerides, serum glucose (postprandial), and serum uric acid. Examples of laboratory values that may be decreased by the aging process include, but are not limited to, levels of serum calcium and serum creatine kinase, as well as creatinine clearance.

It is important to recognize the early indicators of acute illness in older persons: change in mental status, falls, dehydration, decrease in appetite, loss of function, dizziness, and incontinence (Fedarko, 2011; Peters, 2010). Two key principles of providing age-appropriate nursing care are timely detection of these cardinal signs of illness and a focus on finding underlying causes so that treatment can begin (Box 24-4). Attention is often not paid to underlying causes because of mistaken assumptions about normal aging (Fedarko, 2011). Many health challenges can coexist, which adds to the difficulty in isolating the causes of symptoms. Mental status commonly changes as a result of disease and psychological issues, but more often in relation to drug toxicity or adverse drug events. A fall is a complex event, and careful investigation is necessary to find out whether it has environmental causes or is the symptom of a new-onset illness; such illnesses include cardiac, respiratory, musculoskeletal, neurological, urological, and sensory disorders. Dehydration is common in older persons because the thirst response is reduced, which results in less water intake, and because less free water is available as a consequence of decreased muscle mass. Vomiting and diarrhea can accompany the onset of an acute illness, and older persons are then at risk for further dehydration. Decrease in appetite is a common symptom with the onset of pneumonia, heart failure, and urinary tract infection. Loss of functional ability occurs either in a subtle manner over time or suddenly, depending on the underlying cause. Thyroid disease, infection, cardiac or pulmonary conditions, metabolic disturbances, and anemia are common causes of functional decline, so nurses need to identify them early and notify care providers so that proper treatment can be initiated. Dizziness is a common sign of various acute illnesses, including anemia, arrhythmia, infection, myocardial infarction, stroke, and brain tumour. New-onset urinary incontinence in an older person is often associated with a urinary tract infection, but it can also be a symptom of an electrolyte abnormality or adverse drug event.

BOX 24-4 Examples of Atypical Presentation of Illness

- Delirium (acute confusion) with an acute illness is considered a medical emergency.
- Depression without sadness
- Infectious disease without fever or tachycardia
- Myocardial infarction without chest pain
- Nondyspneic pulmonary edema
- Abdominal pain is absent or vague.
- Confusion is not inevitable. Look for neurological events, new medication, or the presence of risk factors for delirium.
- Many hospitalized older persons suffer from chronic dehydration accelerated by acute illness.
- Not all older persons have fevers with infection. Symptoms may include increased respiratory rate, falls, incontinence, or confusion.

Adapted from Peters, M. L. (2010). The older adult in the emergency department: Aging and atypical illness presentation. *Journal of Emergency Nursing, 36*(1), 29–34.

Physiological Changes

Perception of well-being can define quality of life. Understanding a patient's perceptions about health status is essential for the accurate assessment and development of clinically relevant interventions. Older persons' concepts of health generally depend on personal perceptions of functional ability. Therefore, older persons engaged in ADLs usually consider themselves healthy, whereas those whose activities are limited by physical, emotional, or social impairments may perceive themselves as ill.

Many observed physiological changes in older persons are called "normal." Finding such changes during an assessment is not unexpected. These physiological changes are not always pathological processes, but they may make older persons more vulnerable to some common clinical conditions and diseases. Some older persons experience all of these physiological changes, and others experience only a few. The body changes continuously with age, and specific effects on particular older persons depend on health, lifestyle, stressors, and environmental conditions. As a nurse, you should know about these commonly experienced changes in order to provide appropriate care for older persons and to assist with adaptation to the changes. Common physiological changes are summarized in Table 24-1.

General Survey. The general survey occurs during the initial encounter with an older person and includes a quick, but careful, head-to-toe scan of the client, which the nurse should document in a concise description. An initial inspection of an older person might reveal whether eye contact and facial expression are appropriate to the situation, as well as common aging changes such as facial wrinkles, grey hair, loss of body mass in the extremities, and an increase of body mass in the trunk.

Functional Changes

Declines in physical, psychological, cognitive, and social function that can occur with aging are usually linked to illness or disease and its degree of chronicity. However, the complex relationship among all of these areas ultimately influences an older person's functional abilities and overall well-being. It is difficult for older persons to accept the changes that occur in all the areas of their lives, which in turn have a profound effect on function. Some older people deny the changes and continue to expect the same performance from themselves regardless of age. Conversely, some overemphasize these changes and prematurely limit their activities and involvement in life. Also, the fear of becoming dependent is overwhelming for an older person who is experiencing functional decline as a result of aging.

Nurses need to educate older persons to promote understanding of age-related changes, appropriate lifestyle adjustments, and effective coping. Factors that promote the highest level of function in all the areas include a healthy, well-balanced diet; paced and appropriate activity; regularly scheduled visits with a health care provider; regular participation in meaningful activities; use of stress management techniques; and avoidance of alcohol, tobacco, and illicit drugs.

TABLE 24-1 Common Physiological Changes With Aging

System	Common Changes
Integumentary	Loss of skin elasticity with fat loss in extremities; pigmentation changes; glandular atrophy (oil, moisture, sweat glands); thinning hair, with hair turning grey-white (facial hair: decreased in men, increased in women); slower nail growth; atrophy of epidermal arterioles
Respiratory	Decreased cough reflex; decreased cilia; increased anterior–posterior chest diameter; increased chest wall rigidity; fewer alveoli, increased airway resistance; increased risk of respiratory infections
Cardiovascular	Thickening of blood vessel walls, narrowing of vessel lumen, loss of vessel elasticity, lower cardiac output, decreased number of heart muscle fibres, decreased elasticity and calcification of heart valves, decreased baroreceptor sensitivity, decreased efficiency of venous valves, increased pulmonary vascular tension, increased systolic blood pressure, decreased peripheral circulation
Gastrointestinal	Periodontal disease; decrease in saliva, gastric secretions, and pancreatic enzymes; smooth-muscle changes with decreased peristalsis and small intestinal motility; gastric atrophy; decreased production of intrinsic factor; increased stomach pH; loss of smooth muscle in the stomach; hemorrhoids; rectal prolapse; impaired rectal sensation
Musculoskeletal	Decreased muscle mass and strength, decalcification of bones, degenerative joint changes, dehydration of intervertebral disks, fat tissue increases, with loss of muscular-skeletal integrity postural kyphosis may occur
Neurological	Degeneration of nerve cells, decrease in neurotransmitters, decrease in rate of conduction of impulses
Sensory	
Eyes	Decrease in accommodation to near/far vision (presbyopia), difficulty adjusting to changes from light to dark, yellowing of the lens, altered colour perception, increased sensitivity to glare, smaller pupils
Ears	Loss of acuity for high-frequency tones (presbycusis), thickening of tympanic membrane, sclerosis of inner ear, buildup of earwax (cerumen)
Taste	Often diminished; often fewer taste buds
Smell	Often diminished
Touch	Decreased skin receptors
Proprioception	Decreased awareness of body positioning in space
Genitourinary	Fewer nephrons, 50% decrease in renal blood flow by age 80, decreased bladder capacity Male—enlargement of prostate Female—reduced sphincter tone
Reproductive	Male—sperm count diminished, smaller testes, erections less firm and slow to develop Female—decreased estrogen production, degeneration of ovaries, atrophy of vagina, uterus, and breasts
Endocrine	General—alterations in hormone production with decreased ability to respond to stress Thyroid—diminished secretions Cortisol, glucocorticoids—increased anti-inflammatory hormone Pancreas—increased fibrosis, decreased secretion of enzymes and hormones, decreased sensitivity to insulin
Immune system	Thymus decreases in size and volume T-cell function decreases Core temperature elevation is lowered

Modified from Jett K. (2014). Physiological changes. In T. Touhy & K. Jett (Eds.), *Ebersole and Hess' gerontological nursing and healthy aging* (4th ed.). St. Louis: Mosby.

Functional status in older persons ordinarily refers to the capacity and safe performance of ADLs and is a sensitive indicator of health or illness in older persons. ADLs are essential to independent living; therefore, nurses must carefully assess whether an older person has changed the way in which he or she completes these tasks. In fact, a sudden change in function, as evidenced by a decline or change in an older person's ability to perform any one or combination of ADLs, is often a sign of the onset of an acute illness, pain, or worsening of a chronic problem (Boltz, Resnick, & Galik, 2012). Pneumonia, urinary tract infection, dehydration, electrolyte disturbances, and delirium are examples of acute illnesses that may manifest as a change in function. Worsening of chronic conditions such as diabetes, cardiovascular disease, and chronic lung disease can also manifest as a change in function.

Various health care providers in a range of different settings are able to perform a functional assessment. Several standardized functional assessment tools are widely available; an online collection of tools is available at http://www.consultgeri.org. Some examples include Fulmer's SPICES overall assessment tool to promote optimal function in the older person (Hirst et al., 2015); assessment of urinary incontinence, which includes appropriate interventions (Dowling-Castronovo & Bradway, 2012); and mental status assessment to screen for cognitive impairment (Berstein, Laciritz, Barlow, et al., 2011). The SPICES tool directs the nurse to assess for sleep disorders, problems eating or feeding, incontinence, confusion, evidence of falls, and skin breakdown. When a decline in function is identified, nursing interventions should be focused on maintaining, restoring, and maximizing the older person's functional status so that he or she can maintain independence while preserving dignity.

Cognitive Changes

A common misconception about aging is that cognitive impairments are widespread among older persons. Forgetfulness is not an expected consequence of aging. Older persons often fear that they are, or soon will be, cognitively impaired. Younger persons often assume that older persons are confused and no longer able to handle their affairs. Structural and physiological changes within the brain—such as reduction in the number of cells, deposition of lipofuscin and amyloid in cells, and change in neurotransmitter levels—are normal with aging and are observed in older persons whether they do or do not have cognitive impairment. Symptoms of cognitive impairment such as disorientation, loss of language skills, loss of the ability to calculate, and poor judgement are not normal aging changes. When nurses identify these changes during the assessment, they must further investigate the underlying causes.

The three common conditions affecting cognition are delirium, dementia, and depression (Table 24-2). You may find that distinguishing among these three conditions is challenging, but it is essential for selecting appropriate nursing interventions. The Registered Nurses' Association of Ontario (RNAO, 2016) has published revised Best Practice Guidelines to screen for delirium, dementia, and depression in older persons. Appropriate nursing interventions specifically address the cause of the cognitive impairment.

TABLE 24-2 Comparison of Clinical Features of Delirium, Dementia, and Depression

	Delirium	Dementia	Depression
Definition	Delirium is a medical emergency. It is characterized by acute and fluctuating onset of confusion, disturbances in attention, disorganized thinking, and/or decline in consciousness. It can coexist with dementia. Older people with dementia have a higher risk of delirium.	Dementia is a gradual and progressive decline in mental processing ability that affects short-term memory, language, judgement, reasoning, and abstract thinking. It eventually affects long-term memory and the ability to perform familiar tasks. Some types of dementia are associated with changes in mood and behaviour.	*Depression* is a term used to describe when a cluster of depressive symptoms is present on most days, most of the time, for at least 2 weeks, and when the intensity of the symptoms is out of the ordinary for that person. It is a biologically based illness that affects a person's thoughts, feelings, behaviour, and even their physical health.
Onset and course	Sudden onset—it lasts hours to days. Often it is reversible with treatment of the underlying cause. Often it fluctuates over a 24-hour period and can be worse at night.	Gradual deterioration occurs over months to years. It has slow, chronic progression and is irreversible.	Recent unexplained changes in mood persist for at least 2 weeks. Usually it is reversible with treatment. Often it is worse in the morning.
Thinking	Fluctuations in alertness, cognition, perceptions, and thinking occur. The person may have misperceptions and delusions.	Cognitive decline with problems in memory occur plus one or more of the following: apraxia, agnosia, and/or executive functioning. The person may have paranoia and delusions of theft, and some types of dementia include hallucinations.	Reduced memory, concentration, and thinking occur, along with low self-esteem. The person may have delusions of poverty, feel guilt, and complain of somatic symptoms.
Mood	Fluctuations in emotions occur, with outbursts, anger, crying, and/or feeling fearful. Sleep may be disturbed, but there is no set pattern.	The person is depressed, especially in early stages. Apathy occurs. Sleep may be disturbed, with a pattern in the disturbance.	The person has depressed mood with decreased interest or experiences of pleasure. Changes in appetite occur, with possible suicidal ideation and/or feelings of hopelessness. Sleep is disturbed, with early morning waking.
Psychomotor activities	Hyperactive: agitation, restlessness, hallucinations Hypoactive: unarousable, very sleepy Mixed: combinations of hyper- and hypoactive manifestations	Wandering with exit seeking Agitation The person is withdrawn (which may be related to an existing depression).	Hyperactive: agitated Hypoactive: withdrawn, decreased motivation and interest
Screening tools	Confusion Assessment Method (CAM) If the person has features 1 and 2 plus either 3 or 4 he or she is positive for delirium. 1. Presence of acute onset and fluctuating course and 2. Inattention and either 3. Disorganized thinking or 4. Altered level of consciousness	Geriatric Depression Scale (GDS) Interpretation of the 15 GDS screen: Less than or equal to 4 = no depression 5–7 = borderline depression greater than 7 = probable depression	Folstein's Mini Mental Status Exam measures cognitive functioning. 25–30 = normal 20–24 = mild 10–20 = moderate less than 10 = severe cognitive impairment
Next steps	Notify the physician—delirium is considered a medical emergency. Determine and treat the underlying cause of the delirium (e.g., urinary tract infection, reaction to medication).	Management of behaviours should focus on nonpharmaceutical interventions.	Refer patient to a physician if there is suicidal risk. Refer to geriatric outreach teams.

Adapted from Registered Nurses' Association of Ontario (RNAO). (2016). *Delirium, dementia, and depression in older adults: Assessment and care* (2nd ed.). Toronto: Author. Retrieved from http://rnao.ca/sites/rnao-ca/files/bpg/RNAO_Delirium_Dementia_Depression_Older_Adults_Assessment_and_Care.pdf.

Delirium. Delirium, or acute confusional state, is a potentially reversible cognitive impairment that often has a physiological cause. Physiological causes of delirium include, but are not limited to, too many medications, dehydration, malnutrition, infection, pain, and stress (Bueckert, 2016). Delirium in older persons sometimes accompanies systemic infections and may be the presenting symptom for pneumonia or urinary tract infection. Delirium may also have environmental causes (e.g., sensory deprivation, unfamiliarity with surroundings) or psychosocial causes (e.g., emotional distress, pain). Although delirium may occur in any setting, an older person in the acute care setting is especially at risk because of predisposing factors (physiological, psychosocial, and environmental) in combination with the medical condition that led to the hospital admission. Older people who have dementia are at an increased risk of experiencing delirium.

The onset of delirium is typically sudden, and symptoms and severity fluctuate rapidly. Since delirium can fluctuate throughout the 24-hour period, it is important that nurses conduct frequent assessments. The presence of delirium necessitates prompt assessment and intervention. The cognitive impairment secondary to delirium is usually reversed once the cause of delirium is identified and treatment is started, unless permanent brain injury has occurred. The three main types of delirium are hypoactive, hyperactive, and mixed delirium; there is also a subsyndromal delirium in which the person presents with only some of the features of delirium. Scholars have also described a persistent delirium, which lasts longer than days and is associated with poor outcomes, such as increases in cognitive impairment and decreased functional ability (RNAO, 2016). Treatment of delirium is focused on determining causative factors; however, prevention of delirium is also important. To prevent delirium and maintain a patient's functioning, nurses must address the causative factors, which may be multidimensional.

The RNAO (2016) recommends that nurses establish and maintain person-centered and family-centered relationships with older patients in any setting. If the older person is experiencing cognitive changes, the family can be a resource in explaining whether or not this is a new onset of confusion and, thus, delirium and if a new medication was started. The family can also provide other nuances of the client's health history that can aid in determining the cause of the delirium.

Dementia. Dementia is an umbrella term for a variety of diseases that cause irreversible changes in the brain. The Alzheimer Society of Canada (2017) classifies five major types of dementia: Alzheimer's disease, diffuse Lewy body disease, frontotemporal dementia, Creutzfeldt-Jacob dementia, and vascular dementia. The symptoms of dementia include loss of memory, judgement, and reasoning and changes in mood, behaviour, and communication abilities. Deterioration of cognitive function leads to a decline in the ability to perform basic and instrumental ADLs. Unlike delirium, dementia is characterized by progressive, irreversible cerebral dysfunction. Because of the close resemblance of delirium to dementia, the presence of delirium must be ruled out whenever dementia is suspected. The most common form of dementia is Alzheimer's disease. In Canada, by sex, approximately 37.1% (females) and 28.7% (males) older than 85 years have dementia, in comparison with 2.8% (females) and 1.9% (males) in the age group 65 to 74 years (Alzheimer Society of Canada, 2017).

The cause of Alzheimer's disease is not known, and although several theories are being studied, none is definitive. Cholinesterase-inhibiting medications—memantine (Ebixa), donepezil (Aricept), rivastigmine (Exelon), and galantamine (Reminyl)—are currently prescribed to slow progression of symptoms. These medications prevent breakdown of the neurotransmitter acetylcholine by the enzyme cholinesterase (Anand & Singh, 2013). It is hypothesized that by increasing the amount of acetylcholine available to transmit impulses among neurons, cognition in some older persons with Alzheimer's disease will improve.

The characteristic progressive symptoms of Alzheimer's disease are loss of memory (amnesia), loss of the ability to recognize objects and people (agnosia), loss of the ability to perform familiar tasks (apraxia), and loss of language skills (aphasia). As Alzheimer's disease progresses, the affected person becomes more dependent on caregivers for assistance with ADLs. Safety issues must be addressed as the disease progresses and the ability to judge risks diminishes.

Like Alzheimer's disease, diffuse Lewy body disease is progressive. The features of diffuse Lewy body disease include dementia, fluctuating cognition, visual or auditory hallucinations (or both), and the motor features of Parkinsonism.

Frontotemporal dementia has an insidious onset and progresses slowly. Early symptoms include poor hygiene, lack of social tact, hyperorality, and sexual disinhibition. Incontinence is also an early symptom in frontotemporal dementia, whereas it is a late symptom in Alzheimer's disease. Repetitive behaviours (wandering, clapping, singing, picking up objects) are frequently observed. Safety and behaviour management are major concerns for caregivers.

A sudden onset of memory loss, behavioural changes, or difficulties with speech and movement occur with Creutzfeldt-Jakob disease (CJD). CJD is a rare, rapid, and fatal form of dementia caused by infectious agents called *prions.* Two types of CJD exist. *Classical CJD* (also called *sporadic CJD*) occurs at random. *Variant CJD* (vCJD) is a disease linked to eating beef products from cattle with bovine spongiform encephalopathy, also called "mad cow disease."

The cause of vascular dementia is interruption of blood supply to areas of the brain by thromboembolism, hemorrhage, or ischemia (RNAO, 2016). Symptoms of vascular dementia vary according to the areas of the brain affected. Progression of vascular dementia may be either stepwise, with repeated episodes of damage to the brain over time, or steadily progressive. Management of vascular dementia parallels the recommendations for cerebrovascular disease (i.e., reduction of risk factors by treatment of hypertension, hyperlipidemia, carotid disease, arrhythmias, diabetes mellitus, and polycythemia vera). Because the use of nicotine has been linked with vascular disease, older persons with vascular dementia should stop or reduce their use of tobacco products. If an older person has a cardiac arrhythmia such as atrial fibrillation, anticoagulant therapy may be indicated to reduce the risk of thromboembolism.

In the nursing management of older persons with any form of dementia, nurses must consider the needs of the patient and the needs of the family. Those needs change because the progressive nature of dementia leads to increased cognitive deterioration. In addition to the patient's physical needs, his or her safety needs and psychosocial needs must be considered. The patient's family requires information and support. Nursing care objectives are promotion of the use of remaining functional abilities and behavioural interventions to decrease the incidence of responsive behaviours.

The Alzheimer Society of Canada (2017) has compiled suggestions for care of persons with dementia. The most challenging behaviours are those that include verbal and physical aggression. When caring for patients with dementia, nurses should be calm and reassuring, look for an immediate cause, try distracting the patient, and, if safety is an issue, leave the situation and get assistance. Restraints cause physical harm and are not an efficacious alternative. Minimal restraint (policy of least restraint) for the shortest period of time should be used only as the last resort when safety is an issue. Unfortunately, older persons are "three times more likely to be restrained during an acute hospital admission than younger patients, even though this practice is associated with adverse effects" (Said & Kautz, 2013, p. 59). Before resorting

BOX 24-5 Readiness for Hospitalization of Older Persons With Dementia

The Alzheimer Society of Canada website (www.alzheimer.ca) offers a toolkit for families who have an older family member with dementia. This toolkit is the result of a research project funded by the Canadian Institutes of Health Research and the Alzheimer Society of Canada. It contains several downloadable documents that are designed for families to complete and keep with a "ready to go bag" in case of an emergency hospitalization. The documents provide information about the older person, a list of medications, his or her wishes regarding care (especially end-of-life care), and level of function needed to return home. The bag also contains necessities such as pajamas, warm blanket, and toiletries. This toolkit is designed to provide the information that care providers will need to know about the older person to provide optimal care and thus promotes improved care and helps the family navigate the hospital environment (http://www.alzheimer.ca/en/Living-with-dementia/Caring-for-someone/Hospital-visits).

The toolkit was developed on the basis of the study by Parke, Hunter, Strain, et al. (2013).

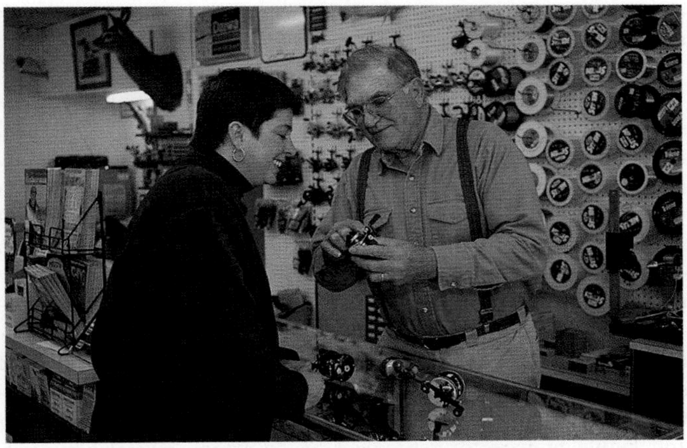

FIGURE 24-2 This older person works part-time at a sporting goods store.

to restraints, nurses should try nonpharmacological methods to meet the older person's needs. These include walking the person (if they are able), providing a distracting activity, asking family to sit and visit with the older person, or using a one-to-one nurse. Box 24-5 highlights resources that have been developed to facilitate improved care of older people with cognitive challenges should they end up in the hospital.

Depression. Late-life depression may be experienced by 15 to 20% of older persons who live in the community (RNAO, 2016). Depression reduces happiness and well-being, contributes to physical and social limitations, complicates the treatment of concomitant medical conditions, and increases the risk of suicide. The manifestation of depression in older persons differs from that in younger persons. Older persons are more likely to talk about being "blue" or "down in the dumps" and may express feelings of diminished life satisfaction (Hirst et al., 2015). Best Practice Guidelines for mental health treatment have been developed by the Canadian Coalition for Seniors' Mental Health (2016).

Delirium and depression, both reversible disorders, are often mistaken for irreversible dementia in older persons because cerebral dysfunction and cognitive impairment occur with these conditions, as well as with dementia. Careful and thorough assessment of older persons with cognitive impairment is essential to distinguish among delirium, dementia, and depression. People with dementia and depression have a higher risk of developing delirium (RNAO, 2016). As a beginning nurse, you may choose to consult with a clinical nurse specialist in gerontology. Accurate assessment is necessary to select appropriate nursing interventions.

Psychosocial Changes

The psychosocial changes that occur with aging involve changes in roles and relationships. Roles and relationships within the family change as parents become grandparents, as adult children become caregivers for aging parents, or as spouses become widows or widowers. Group membership roles and relationships change as older persons retire from work, move from a familiar neighbourhood, or stop attending social activities because of declining health status.

In an assessment, nurses should assess both the nature of the psychosocial changes facing an older person and the adaptation to those changes. It is important to ask the older person how he or she feels about himself or herself, in relation to self and others and as an aging person. Areas to be addressed during the assessment include the family, intimate relationships, past and current occupation, finances, housing, social networks, activities, and spirituality. Specific topics related to these areas include retirement, housing and environment, social isolation, abuse, sexuality, and death.

Retirement. The great majority of Canadian older people are retired; 13.4% of them are employed outside the home (Statistics Canada, 2016a). Some older people return to work after retirement for financial reasons, others prefer to work part-time hours; still other older people return to work for social reasons (McDonald & Donahue, 2011) (Figure 24-2).

Retirement is often mistakenly associated with passivity and seclusion. In actuality, it is a stage of life characterized by transitions and role changes. The psychosocial stresses of retirement may be related to role changes within the marital relationship or within the family and to loss of role. Older persons retired from employment outside the home may be challenged to cope with the loss of that work role. Older persons who worked at home and the spouses of those who worked outside the home also face role changes as they retire. Problems may also arise in relation to social isolation and finances. Retirement, which may be mandatory or voluntary, occurs at a variety of ages. Regardless of the age at retirement, it is one of the major turning points in life.

Planning for retirement is an important, advisable task for middle-aged individuals. People who plan in advance for retirement generally have a smoother transition into that stage of life. Financial planning for retirement, although important, is only one aspect of retirement planning. Planning begins with consideration of the "style" of retirement desired and includes an inventory of interests, current skills, and general health. Meaningful retirement planning is critical because retirement can last for 30 years or more.

Retirement has an impact on other individuals besides the retired adult. Spouses, adult children, and grandchildren are all affected. When the spouse is still working, the retired adult faces time alone. For example, the working spouse may have new ideas about the amount of participation in housework expected of the retired adult. Friction may develop when the plans of the retired adult conflict with the work responsibilities of the working spouse. The working spouse's expectations of the retired adult must be clarified. For couples, adjustment to retirement is affected by the quality of communication with each other, their process of decision making about issues such as money or activities, their adherence to either traditional or shared role orientations, and their level of affection and intimacy (Hirst et al., 2015). Adult children may expect the retired adult to become an automatic babysitter for grandchildren.

Loss of the work role has a major impact on some retired people. When so much of life has revolved around work and personal relationships at work, loss of the work role may be devastating. Personal identity may be rooted in the work role, and with retirement, a new identity must be constructed. The structure imposed on daily life by a work schedule is also lost, as are the social exchanges and interpersonal support that occur in the workplace. In the adjustment to retirement, older persons are challenged to develop a personally meaningful schedule and a supportive social network.

The most powerful factors that influence the retired person's satisfaction with life are health status, the option to continue working, and sufficient income (Hirst et al., 2015). Positive expectations also contribute to satisfaction in retirement. Nurses can help an older person and family prepare for retirement by discussing several key areas, including relationships with spouse and children, meaningful activities to replace the work role, adjusting or rebuilding social networks, issues related to the promotion and maintenance of income and health, and long-range planning, including wills and advance directives.

Social Isolation. Social isolation and loneliness are significant issues for older persons regardless of gender and geographic location (Dury, 2014). *Social isolation* is defined as the lack of a sense of belonging, social engagement, and quality relationships, whereas *loneliness* is a feeling of dissatisfaction with the level of social contact. Isolation exists in two forms: it may be a choice to not interact with others, or it may be a response to conditions that inhibit the ability or the opportunity to interact with others (Hirst et al., 2015). For example, geographic dispersion of families leads to decreased opportunities for interaction among family members. Regardless of whether isolation is a choice for older persons, they are vulnerable to its consequences.

Living alone and having multiple chronic illnesses are factors contributing to social isolation and loneliness (Dury, 2014). Some older persons may isolate themselves because of cognitive issues or concerns about incontinence or decreased mobility (Hirst et al., 2015). Nurses can assist lonely older persons to rebuild social networks and reverse patterns of isolation (Hirst et al., 2015). Many communities have outreach programs designed to make contact with isolated older persons. Outreach programs, such as Meals on Wheels, may help meet nutritional needs; daily telephone calls by volunteers may help meet socialization needs; and outings may help meet needs for activities. Social service agencies in most communities welcome older persons as volunteers and provide them with the opportunity to serve and to be served. Other organizations within communities such as religious institutions, colleges, and libraries offer a variety of programs for older persons that increase the opportunity to meet people with similar activities, interests, and needs.

Abuse. Elder abuse is the mistreatment of an older person by other people who are in a position of trust or power or who are responsible for the adult's care. Neglect is commonly associated with abuse. For example, elder abuse includes not performing an action (inaction) that a caretaker has a duty to perform, such as not providing medications to an older person who needs them (Canadian Network for the Prevention of Elder Abuse, 2017). Types of abuse are as follows:

- Physical abuse: use of physical force that may result in bodily injury, physical pain, or impairment
- Sexual abuse: nonconsensual sexual contact of any kind, which includes sexual contact with any person incapable of giving consent
- Psychological or emotional abuse: infliction of anguish, emotional pain, or distress through verbal or nonverbal acts
- Material abuse (financial abuse): illegal or improper exploitation of an older person's funds, property, or assets
- Neglect: the intentional or unintentional harmful behaviour on the part of an informal or formal caregiver in whom the older person has placed his or her trust
- Self-neglect: behaviour by an older person that threatens their health and safety, such as not eating

In most provinces in Canada, elder abuse must be reported. As a nurse, you play an important role in assessment, recognition, and reporting of elder abuse (Box 24-6), as well as its prevention, through education and resources for families.

Nurses often must put together clues to determine if elder abuse has occurred. By its nature, it is a hidden problem, and assessment begins with a suspicion that abuse may be occurring (see Case Study in Box 24-6 for an example).

Sexuality. Sexuality is increasingly recognized as an important factor in the lives of older persons. All older persons, whether healthy or frail, need to express sexual feelings. Sexuality involves love, warmth, sharing, and touching, not just the act of intercourse. Sexuality is linked with identity and validates the belief that people can give of themselves to others and have the gift appreciated.

Maintaining sexual health requires integration of somatic, emotional, intellectual, and social aspects of the sexual being. To help an older person achieve or maintain sexual health, nurses need to understand the physical changes in sexual response (see Chapter 27). They should provide privacy for any discussion of sexuality and should maintain a nonjudgemental attitude. Open-ended questions inviting the patient to explain sexual activities or concerns may elicit more information than do closed-ended questions about specific activities or symptoms. Older persons may appreciate information about the typical age-related changes in sexuality. Information about the prevention of sexually transmitted infections should be included when appropriate. The libido does not decrease in older persons, although frequency of sexual activity may decline. An older woman who does not understand physical changes affecting sexual activity may be concerned that her sex life is nearly over. The older man may feel the same when he discovers a change in the firmness of his erection, a decreased need for ejaculation with each orgasm, or a longer recovery period between episodes of intercourse.

In addition to the physical changes that affect sexual functioning, many older persons use prescription medications that depress libido, such as antihypertensives, antidepressants, sedatives, and hypnotics. Some drugs increase libido in older persons. For example, phenothiazines increase sexual desire in women, and levodopa has a similar effect in men.

While considering an older person's need for sexual expression, nurses must not ignore the important need to touch and be touched.

BOX 24-6 CASE STUDY

Elder Abuse

Mr. R. had been living alone in his home since his wife of 60 years had died. When the home care nurse first visited Mr. R., she noticed he was withdrawn and seemed fearful when she asked if his daughter had visited. The home care nurse also noted that his clothes were dirty and in need of repair. She was able to persuade him to allow her to take a blood pressure reading and noticed many bruises on his arms. He would not allow her to do a further assessment.

Thinking Points:

1. What types of abuse might this case represent?
2. What are some factors that contribute to this possible abuse situation?
3. What should the nurse do next?

Touch is an overt expression with many meanings and is an important part of sexuality in some cultures. Before using touch, nurses should respect the fact that it may not be appropriate for some older persons because of culturally associated meanings.

Experience in caring for older persons, in combination with the ability to establish therapeutic connection, will enable you to learn how to explore patients' sexual concerns. Knowing an older person's sexual needs can help you incorporate this information into the nursing care plan. In addition, improving communication and creating open and supportive environments of care will promote successful, healthy sexual expression.

The sexual preferences of older persons are as diverse as those of younger persons. Not all older persons are heterosexual. Although little is known about aging as a lesbian, gay, bisexual, or transsexual (LGBT) person, some scholars suggest that the LGBT community has increased health concerns, often due to social and economic issues (Emlet, 2016). To be effective caregivers for older LGBT persons, nurses need to be aware of their own beliefs about sexuality and the potential impact of those beliefs on their ability to provide care.

You may find that you are called on to advise older persons and help other health care providers understand the sexual needs of older persons. You may feel uncomfortable counselling older persons about sexual health and need not feel obligated to do so. But you should be prepared to refer older persons to appropriate professional counsellors.

Housing and Environment. Most Canadians want to stay in their communities as long as possible (Special Senate Committee on Aging, 2009). However, housing choices are strongly determined by an older person's ability to live independently. Changes in social roles, family responsibilities, health status, retirement, and income influence this ability. For example, physical impairments may necessitate relocation to a smaller, single-level home. Because of health problems, an older person may need to live with relatives or friends or move to an assisted-living or long-term care facility. A change in living arrangements may require an extended period of adjustment during which assistance and support from health care providers, friends, and family members are needed.

Some older persons choose to live with family members. Others prefer their own homes or apartments near their families. Leisure or retirement communities provide older people with living and social opportunities in a one-generation setting. Federally subsidized housing, where available, offers apartments with communal, social, and, in some cases, food service arrangements. There are Canadians, however, who because of poverty are unable to find adequate housing (Special Senate Committee on Aging, 2009). The Special Senate Committee on Aging (2009) has recommended that elimination of poverty for older persons be a goal of the Canadian government. When assisting older persons with housing needs, nurses should assess activity level, financial status, availability of access to public transportation and community activities, environmental hazards, and support systems. Housing choices should also account for anticipated future needs of older persons. For instance, a housing unit with only one floor and without exterior steps may be a prudent choice for an older person with severe arthritis who has already had some lower extremity joint replacement surgeries and anticipates the need for future surgeries.

Housing and environment have a major impact on the health of older persons. **Age-friendly community** is a concept that is spreading across Canada; it focuses on transportation, lighting, sidewalks, community centres, and supports that promote older people's ability to live independently (Keating, Eales, & Philips, 2013). The environment can support or hinder physical and social functioning, can enhance or drain energy, and can complement or tax existing physical changes such as vision and hearing. For example, older persons can most easily see the colours red, orange, and yellow; in contrast, they have difficulty distinguishing between green and blue and among pastel shades. To help older persons in health care settings find their rooms, pictures or other decorations near their doors can be used as landmarks. To improve perception of the boundaries of halls and rooms, door frames and baseboards should be painted in a colour that contrasts with the colour of the wall. Glare from highly polished floors, metallic fixtures, and windows is poorly tolerated.

Furniture should be comfortable and designed for the musculoskeletal changes of older persons. Older persons should examine furniture carefully for size, comfort, and function before purchasing it. Furniture should be easy to get into and out of and should provide back support. Dining room chairs should be tested for comfort during meals and height in relation to the table. Older persons may prefer transferring out of a wheelchair to another chair for meals because some styles of wheelchairs prevent sitting close enough to the table to eat comfortably. Raising the table to clear the wheelchair arms may bring the table closer to the adult but make it too high for comfortable use. To make getting out of bed easier and safer, the height of the bed should allow the adult's feet to be flat on the floor when the adult is sitting on the side of the bed.

The goal of nursing assessment of the environment is the promotion of independence and functional ability. Assessment of safety, a major component of an older person's environment, includes determining risks within the environment and the adult's ability to recognize and respond to the risks (see Chapter 37). Risks include factors leading to injury within the home (such as water heaters set at excessively hot temperatures or throw rugs that could cause a fall) and factors outside the home (such as deteriorating sidewalks and steps or a high incidence of street crime).

Death. Part of the life history of an older person is the experience of the death of family members and friends (see Chapter 25). As persons age, friends gradually die. The majority of older persons are faced with the death of a spouse. Some older persons must also cope with the death of children and grandchildren. All experience the deaths of friends. These deaths represent both losses and reminders of personal mortality. Nurses should not, however, assume that older persons are comfortable with the idea of death. Coming to terms with death is often difficult. As a nurse, you will play a key role in assisting older persons through the grieving process.

Older people have a wide variety of attitudes and beliefs about death. To support a patient at the end of life, you can use the Dignity in Care Toolkit (Manitoba Palliative Care Research Unit, 2016). This toolkit includes an assessment tool to assess a person's sense of dignity, as well as strategies to improve their dignity at the end of life. Another model of care that is available is a Living with Hope program (Duggleby, Cooper, Nekolaichuk, et al., 2016), which can be used to foster a patient's hope and improve quality of life. Such strategies to improve end-of-life care can be easily incorporated into everyday nursing practice. Nurses are often the one person to whom the older person and family members or friends turn for assistance in coping with death and loss. It is critical that you understand the grieving process, have excellent communication skills, understand the legal issues, are familiar with community resources, and are aware of your own feelings, limitations, and strengths as they relate to the care of older persons confronting death.

ADDRESSING THE HEALTH CONCERNS OF OLDER PERSONS

The two most common causes of death in Canadian older persons are cancer and heart disease. Other frequently reported causes of death are respiratory diseases, stroke, accidents or falls, diabetes, kidney disease, and liver disease (Statistics Canada, 2016a). For all these causes of death, preventive measures exist that could potentially reduce the frequency of these conditions and delay disability, death, or both. Box 24-7 is an example of a unique partnership to provide health care to older people.

Nursing interventions for older persons are directed toward improving or maintaining their health needs and concerns. Although various interventions cross all three levels of care—health promotion, acute care, and restorative care—approaches to each level are unique. When planning interventions, it is important to incorporate a patient's routines or rituals when possible because patients feel more secure when routines are continued. In general, the interventions are aimed at promoting independence and supporting self-care abilities. Box 24-8 outlines guidelines for prevention and health promotion interventions for older persons.

BOX 24-7 Collaborative Community Care for Seniors

The aim of Collaborative Community Care (C^3) for Seniors is to provide primary health care services for up to 5 500 older persons in the city of Edmonton, based on the best evidence for interprofessional primary health care teams. Clinical leadership is provided by nurse practitioners and a population health management approach is being used to focus on meeting the needs of older persons in Edmonton. This model was developed through a unique partnership between an academic nursing faculty (University of Alberta Nursing) and a large seniors' social service agency (Sage Seniors Association). This unique partnership provides an exceptional opportunity to incorporate teaching, research, and practice in an innovative, community-based model, as well as involve older people as research partners and participants. Engagement of older people, volunteers, and other important stakeholders, such as the board of directors and community partners, is viewed as critical to the success of the C^3 for Seniors project. This innovative project is set to begin January 2018. The physical renovations for the clinic have been completed.

Adapted from the presentation to Faculty of Nursing Caucus at the University of Alberta, Dr. Tammy O'Rourke, 2016.

Health Promotion and Maintenance: Physiological Health Concerns

Older persons, like persons of any age, vary in their desire to participate in health promotion activities; therefore, nurses should use an individualized approach, taking into account the person's beliefs about the importance of staying healthy and fit and remaining independent. Researchers have not fully identified the factors that lead to good health in advanced age, but four factors seem to be important: genetics, chance, good health habits, and preventive measures. As a nurse, you cannot alter an older person's genetic heritage or the chance occurrence of disease or injury, but you can promote health habits by establishing health maintenance programs, and you can recommend preventive measures. Health maintenance programs have been found to have a positive impact on the physical, mental, and social health of older persons. Community centres, houses of worship, schools, shopping malls, libraries, and hospital lobbies can be used as settings to conduct screening tests and present information on health topics. Using creative approaches, nurses can include health promotion activities for older persons in all health care settings.

Approximately 80% of older persons living at home have at least one chronic health condition. The most common conditions are arthritis, high blood pressure, back problems, chronic heart problems, cataracts, and diabetes (CIHI, 2011). The effect of chronic conditions on the lives of older persons varies widely, but, in general, chronic conditions diminish well-being and threaten independence of older persons. This is particularly the case when an older person has more than one chronic condition. Box 24-9 describes the impact on older persons of multiple chronic conditions.

Nursing interventions are often directed at the management of these conditions, but interventions can also focus on prevention. Nurses can recommend the following general preventive measures:

- Regular exercise
- Weight reduction if the older person is overweight
- Management of hypertension
- Smoking cessation
- Immunization for influenza, pneumococcal pneumonia, and tetanus

BOX 24-8 Guidelines for Prevention and Health Promotion Interventions for Older Persons

Screening for Healthy Older Persons

- Blood pressure checks at least annually
- Serum cholesterol every 5 years
- Fecal occult blood and rectal examination every 2 years after the age of 50 to screen for cancer
- Sigmoidoscopy every 5 years, ages 50–75
- Visual acuity and glaucoma screening every year
- Monthly breast self-examination for both men and women and annual breast examination by primary care practitioner
- Women should have a Pap smear and pelvic examination annually until three consecutive negative examinations, then every 3 years until age 69; after age 70 they may stop after three consecutive negative examinations. Women should also have a mammogram every 2–3 years.
- Men should have a digital rectal examination annually.

Screening for Older Persons With Risk Factors

- Blood glucose level
- Thyroid function
- Bone density
- Heart function
- Screening for dementia, depression, and substance use
- Fall assessment
- Medication review for drug interactions
- Functional assessment
- Men should have prostate-specific antigen blood test.

Health Promotional Counselling (for All Older Persons, Unless Contraindicated)

- Exercise 30 minutes a day
- Healthy food and nutritious intake that includes vitamins and minerals
- Dental care every 6 months
- Protective measures such as sunscreen and seatbelts

Adapted from Guidelines for prevention and health promotion interventions for older adults. In Hirst, S. P., Lane, A. M., & Miller, C. A. (2015). *Miller's nursing for wellness in older adults* (Canadian ed.). Philadelphia: Wolters Kluwer/Lippincott Williams & Wilkins.

BOX 24-9 EVIDENCE-INFORMED PRACTICE

Older Persons and Chronic Illness

Evidence Summary

Older people who have multiple chronic conditions (MCC) (three or more chronic conditions) have reported poor health status and high use of health care services. The purpose of this study (Ploeg, Matthew-Maich, Fraser, et al., 2017) was to explore the experience of managing MCC in the community from the perspectives of older persons with MCC, family caregivers, and health care providers. Using Thorne's interpretive description approach, 130 semi-structured interviews were conducted in two Canadian provinces with 41 community-living older persons, 47 family caregivers, and 42 health care providers. Participants described the experience of managing MCC as (a) overwhelming, draining, and complicated; (b) organizing pills and appointments; (c) being split into pieces; (d) doing what the doctor says; (e) relying on family and friends; and (f) having difficulty getting outside help. Participants expressed feeling an emotional impact of MCC, and there was a heavy reliance on family caregivers to provide support in the home.

Application for Nursing Practice

- Nurses should assess how older persons are dealing with MCC.
- Nurses need to use strategies that support the older person, as well as the family.
- Assessment and strategies need to have a holistic approach, as all aspects of the older person's life are affected by MCC.
- Improved communication between older persons with MCC and their health care providers is needed.
- The lack of services for older persons with MCC suggests a need to explore new care processes and innovative approaches.

Ploeg, J., Matthew-Maich, N., Fraser, K., Dufour, S., McAiney, C., Kaasalainen, S., Markle-Reid, M., Upshur, R., Cleghorn, L., & Emili, A. (2017). Managing multiple chronic conditions in the community: A Canadian qualitative study of the experiences of older adults, family caregivers and healthcare providers. *BMC Geriatrics, 17*(1), 40. doi:10.1186/s12877-017-0431-6

Approximately 12 200 hospitalizations and 3 500 deaths each year in Canada are attributed to influenza (Schanzer, Sevenhuysen, Winchester, et al., 2013). Annual immunization against influenza is strongly recommended for all older persons, especially residents of long-term care facilities and persons of any age with chronic cardiovascular, pulmonary, and metabolic disorders. Vaccination against pneumococcal pneumonia is recommended for all persons older than 65 years. Influenza vaccine is needed every year, whereas pneumococcal pneumonia vaccine is given only once (although some authorities recommend a booster vaccination 10 years after the initial vaccination). For tetanus immunization, booster injections every 10 years are recommended for persons who have received the primary series for tetanus immunization. However, not all older persons are up to date with their booster injections, and some have never received the primary series of injections. During assessment, nurses should ask older persons about the current status of all three types of immunizations, provide information about the immunizations, and make arrangements for the older person to receive the immunizations as needed. Older persons should also be referred for screening for the early detection of cancer and depression.

Most older persons are interested in their health and are capable of taking charge of their lives. They want to remain independent and to prevent disability. Initial screenings establish baseline data that can be used to determine wellness, identify health needs, and design health maintenance programs. After initial screening sessions, nurses can share information on nutrition, exercise, medications, and safety precautions with older persons. They may also provide information about specific conditions, such as hypertension or arthritis, or about self-care procedures, such as foot and skin care. By providing information about health promotion and self-care, nurses can significantly improve the health and well-being of older persons.

Cancer. Malignant neoplasms are the most common cause of death among older persons (Statistics Canada, 2017). Nurses may participate in programs to educate older persons about early detection, treatment, and risk factors. Examples include smoking cessation programs, teaching breast self-examination (see Chapter 4), and encouraging all older persons to have annual screening for fecal occult blood. It is also important to educate older persons about the signs of cancer and to encourage prompt reporting of nonhealing skin lesions, unexpected bleeding, change in bowel habits, and unexplained weight loss. Detection is complicated when cancer symptoms are mistakenly identified by patients and health care providers as part of the normal aging process, thus it is important to carefully distinguish between normal aging and pathological conditions.

Heart Disease. Heart disease is the second leading cause of death in older persons. Common cardiovascular disorders are hypertension and coronary artery disease. Hypertension is diagnosed when repeated diastolic blood pressure measurements are 90 mm Hg or greater and systolic measurements are 140 mm Hg or greater. Although over 22% of Canadians have elevated diastolic or systolic pressures or both (Statistics Canada, 2015a), the fact that hypertension is common does not mean it is normal or harmless. Research on treatment threshold in people older than 80 is limited; it is nonetheless suggested that blood pressure be 150/90 or less (Hirst et al., 2015). In coronary artery disease, partial or complete blockage of one or more coronary arteries leads to myocardial ischemia and myocardial infarction. Risk factors for both hypertension and coronary artery disease include smoking, obesity, lack of exercise, and stress. Additional risk factors for coronary artery disease include hypertension, hyperlipidemia, and diabetes mellitus. Nursing interventions for hypertension and coronary artery disease address weight reduction, exercise, dietary changes to limit salt and fat, stress management, and smoking cessation. Patient education includes information about medications, blood pressure monitoring, nutrition, stress reduction techniques, and the symptoms that indicate the need for emergency care.

Smoking. Cigarette smoking has been recognized as the major preventable cause of death and disease in Canada (Health Canada, 2011). Smoking cessation is a health promotion strategy as much for older persons as for younger persons. Older smokers can benefit from smoking cessation. In addition to reducing risk, smoking cessation may help stabilize existing conditions, such as chronic obstructive pulmonary disease. Smoking cessation may even contribute to the extension of life or of independent functioning. Use of the stages-of-change model has had success in smoking cessation (Hirst et al., 2015). The first stage in this model is pre-contemplation—when the person has not yet made a change but might be willing to read some information about his or her condition and how to improve it. The second stage is contemplation—the person is beginning to think about making some positive changes. In the third stage, preparation, the person is making an active plan about improving his or her health. Next the person puts the plan into action—the action stage. Finally, in the maintenance stage, the person is developing strategies to maintain healthy behaviours.

Alcohol Abuse. The numbers of older people engaged in heavy drinking has increased by 100 000 from 2013 to 2014 (Statistics Canada, 2016b). *Heavy drinking* is defined as five or more drinks for men and four or more drinks for women on one occasion at least once a month. Studies of alcohol abuse in older persons have revealed two patterns: a lifelong pattern of frequent heavy drinking and a late-onset pattern in which heavy drinking begins late in life. Frequently cited causes of excessive alcohol use are depression, loneliness, and lack of social support.

Abuse of alcohol may be underidentified in older people (Satre, 2015). Substance use, one of which is alcohol, is often associated with a chronic health challenge. Some older people initially use alcohol as a means to address pain. Signs of alcohol abuse are subtle, and the assessment may be complicated by coexisting dementia or depression. Alcohol abuse should be suspected when the older person has a history of repeated falls and accidents, exhibits a change in behaviour or personality, is socially isolated, has recurring episodes of memory loss and confusion, has a history of skipping meals or medications, and has difficulty managing household tasks and finances. When abuse of alcohol is suspected, treatment includes age-specific approaches in which the health care provider acknowledges the stresses experienced by the older person and encourages involvement in activities that match the person's interests and boost feelings of self-worth. The identification and treatment of coexisting depression is also important.

Nutrition. Lifelong eating habits and situational factors influence how older persons meet their needs for good nutrition. Such habits are based in tradition, ethnicity, and religion and influence choices of what foods are eaten and how those foods are prepared. Situational factors affecting nutrition include availability of access to food stores, finances, the physical and cognitive capability for food preparation, and a place to store food and prepare meals. Undernutrition can be a significant deterrent to healthy aging (Furman, 2006).

Nutritional needs of older persons are affected by levels of activity and by clinical conditions. Level of activity has implications for the total amount of calories: more sedentary older persons usually need fewer calories than more active older persons. However, caloric requirements are not determined solely by activity. Additional calories may be required in clinical situations such as recovery from surgery, whereas calories may be restricted when the patient is diabetic or overweight. Beyond caloric requirements, therapeutic diets may restrict fat, sodium, or simple sugars or may increase fibre or foods with high levels of calcium, iron, vitamin A, or vitamin C.

Good nutrition for older persons includes appropriate caloric intake and limited intake of fat, salt, refined sugars, and alcohol. Although the nutritional guidelines displayed in *Canada's Food Guide* (Health Canada, 2007) are the basic recommendations for nutrition in older persons (see Chapter 42), some older persons do not follow these guidelines. Protein intake may be lower than recommended if patients have reduced financial resources or limited access to grocery stores. Difficulty chewing meat may also limit protein intake. Fat intake may be higher than recommended because fast-food restaurant meals may be substituted for meals prepared at home or because methods of cooking may feature fried foods and sauces made with butter and cream. Extra salt and sugar may be used in cooking or at the table to compensate for a diminished sense of taste. Vitamin intake may be reduced if the adult has difficulty shopping for fresh fruits and vegetables. As a nurse, you should assess the nutritional status of older persons in all settings and identify interventions to improve their nutritional status (Furman, 2006).

Older persons with dementia have special nutritional needs. As memory and functional skills decline, they lose the ability to remember when to eat, how to prepare food, and, eventually, how to feed themselves. At the same time, caloric needs may increase because of the energy expended in pacing and wandering activities. Nurses and other caregivers of older persons with dementia should routinely monitor weight and food intake, serve food that is easy to eat, provide assistance with eating, and offer food supplements as needed to maintain weight (Keller, Carrier, Duizer, et al., 2014). Mealtime interventions for older persons with dementia provide opportunities for socialization and practice with functional skills.

Oral Health. Oral health is very important for older persons, as dental problems are common in older persons and include conditions involving natural teeth and dentures. Dental caries, gingivitis, broken or missing teeth, and ill-fitting or missing dentures may affect nutritional adequacy, cause pain, and lead to infection. Nurses can help prevent dental and gum disease through education about routine dental care (see Chapter 38). Nurses can also help older persons find dental services that offer reduced rates and that are accessible to patients with impaired mobility.

Exercise. Older persons should be encouraged to maintain physical exercise and activity. The primary benefits of exercise include maintaining and strengthening functional ability and promoting a sense of enhanced well-being. Mobility is important to older persons for maintaining their physical and psychological health (Webber, Porter, & Menec, 2010). An exercise such as walking builds endurance, increases muscle tone, improves joint flexibility, strengthens bones, reduces stress, and contributes to weight loss. Other benefits of an exercise program include improvement of cardiovascular function, improved plasma lipoprotein profiles, increased metabolic rate, increased gastrointestinal transit time, and improved quality of sleep.

An exercise program should meet physical needs while allowing for physical impairments, and nurses should encourage the older person to persevere with the program. Willingness to participate in and persevere with an exercise program is influenced by general beliefs about exercise, specific benefits from exercise, past experiences with exercise, personal goals, personality, and any unpleasant sensations associated with exercise. Walking is the preferred exercise of many older persons (Figure 24-3).

Walking and other low-impact exercises such as riding an exercise (stationary) bicycle or exercises in a swimming pool protect the musculoskeletal system and joints. Other exercises can be incorporated into an older person's ADLs. For example, the adult can perform arm and leg circles while watching television. However, before beginning an exercise program, the older person should have a physical examination. Exercise programs for sedentary older persons who have not been exercising regularly should begin conservatively and progress slowly. Safety considerations include wearing appropriate shoes and clothing, drinking water before and after exercising, avoiding outdoor exercise when the weather is very warm or very cold, and exercising with one or more partners. The older person should be instructed to stop exercising and seek help if he or she experiences tightness or pain in the chest, shortness of breath, dizziness or lightheadedness, or palpitations during exercise. Box 24-10 describes a program to encourage older persons to walk.

Arthritis. Arthritis is common in older persons, especially women. The degree to which the mobility of older persons is impaired depends on the extent of disease and which joints are affected. Changes in joint range of motion and stability, combined with the amount of pain experienced, affect quality of life. Arthritis has no cure, but pharmacological agents can decrease pain and swelling and therefore increase joint motion. Nursing interventions are aimed at promoting comfort,

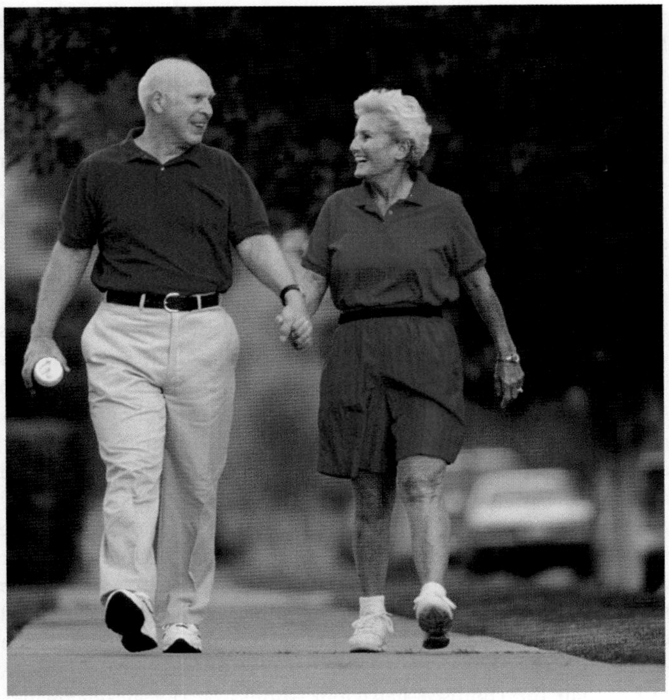

FIGURE 24-3 This couple enjoys walking together.

BOX 24-10 RESEARCH HIGHLIGHT

Walking in the Neighbourhood as a Means of Social Inclusion of Older Persons With Early-Onset Dementia

An ethnographic study by Phinney, Kelson, Baumbusch, et al. (2016) reports the social benefits and inclusion of people with dementia through their participation in Paul's Club, in Vancouver, B.C. Paul's Club is an independent social recreational club for people with young-onset dementia. Participants are able to leave their diagnosis at the door and engage in activities with other participants and volunteers. The group begins with coffee and casual conversation, reading newspapers and talking about current events, and a group activity such as yoga or dance, followed by lunch. After lunch, the group walks through the neighbourhood and ends their walk at a local ice cream shop. Walking the neighbourhood provides the opportunity to interact with shopkeepers, dogs they meet along the way, and with one another. The researchers explain that through their neighbourhood walks the group is constructing social citizenship by keeping the focus off dementia, creating a place of belonging, and claiming a place in community. The group's commitment to walking the neighbourhood aids members in participating in activities they consider "normal" and maintaining connection with community.

Phinney, A., Kelson, E., Baumbusch, J., O'Connor, D., & Purves, B. (2016). Walking in the neighbourhood: Performing social citizenship in dementia. *Dementia, 15*(3), 381–394.

functional ability, and safety. Education on self-care techniques, joint protection, and exercises for flexibility and strength is also important.

Falls. Falls are the leading cause of injuries among Canadians 65 years and over, with up to 30% of community-dwelling Canadian older persons experiencing a fall (Public Health Agency of Canada [PHAC], 2015). Falls are a safety concern and one of the most common causes of functional dependence in older persons. They may lead to fear of additional falls, withdrawal from usual activities, and loss of independence (see Chapter 36). Hospitalization and placement in a long-term care facility may be required. Falls account for 77% of unintentional injuries that result in hospitalization for older persons in Canada (Johnson, Kelly, & Rasaali, 2015). Falls are more frequent and have more serious consequences among persons older than 85 years.

Falls are caused by a combination of individual and environmental factors (Hirst et al., 2015). Individual factors include impaired vision; cardiovascular conditions, such as postural hypotension or syncope; conditions affecting mobility, such as arthritis, muscle weakness, and foot problems; conditions affecting balance; alterations in bladder function, such as frequency or incontinence; cognitive impairment; and adverse medication reactions. Medications can also have an impact on fall risk. Medications such as benzodiazepines and other hypnotics can impair an older person's central nervous system and affect gait. Environmental factors include, but are not limited to, poor lighting, slippery or wet floors, stairs or sidewalks in poor repair, shoes in poor repair or with slippery soles, and household items that could be tripped over, such as throw rugs, foot stools, and electric extension cords.

Multifactor falls-prevention programs such as "Keeping the elderly on their feet" have been found to significantly reduce falls in community-dwelling older people (Macpherson-Packard, Macfie, & Bate, 2015). This program is a 6-week education and exercise program that incorporates fall prevention, self-care, and cardiovascular and balance exercises. Nurses can encourage older persons to perform exercises aimed at increasing leg strength and balance, which also reduce the risk of falls. Simple interventions in the home, such as rearranging furniture to provide a clear pathway to the bathroom and providing a night light in the bathroom, can reduce falls related to nighttime trips to the toilet. Removing throw rugs and other items on the floor helps reduce slipping and tripping. Nurses can also instruct older persons in the safe use of assistive devices such as canes, walkers, and wheelchairs. Older persons taking medications that may have adverse effects such as postural hypotension, dizziness, or sedation can be instructed to be aware of these potential effects and to take precautions, such as changing position slowly or holding onto sturdy furniture if they are unsteady. Other health conditions such as ear infections can also contribute to falls. Box 24-11 describes a physical intervention to prevent falls among older people living in long-term care settings.

Sensory Impairments. Most older persons have changes in vision, hearing, taste, and smell as a result of normal aging. Chapter 47 describes in detail the nursing interventions used to maintain and improve sensory function.

Pain. National statistics reveal that pain increases with age, with Canadian women 65 and older reporting the highest rates of pain (Reitsma, Tranmer, Buchanan, et al., 2011). Causes of pain in older persons include acute and chronic conditions (e.g., trauma, infection, neuropathies). Consequences of persistent pain include depression, sleep difficulties, changes in gait and mobility, and decreased socialization. Older persons are most at risk of having their pain inadequately assessed and treated. Many factors influence the management of pain, including cultural influences on the meaning and expression of pain in older persons, fears related to the use of analgesic medications, and the problem of pain assessment with cognitively impaired older persons.

In caring for older persons, nurses must advocate for appropriate and effective pain management and for the use of standardized pain tools in assessing pain (see Chapter 31). The goal of nursing management of pain in older persons is to maximize function and improve quality of life.

BOX 24-11 EVIDENCE-INFORMED PRACTICE

Effect of the Sit-to-Stand Activity on Mobility, Function, and Quality of Life of Older Persons Residing in Long-Term Care Settings

Evidence Summary

After an admission to a nursing home the mobility of older residents declines because of sedentary behaviour and limited mobility. In this study by Slaughter, Wagg, Jones, and colleagues (2015), care staff received education about the importance of promoting function and independence in older people, as well as instructions on how to safely conduct the sit-to-stand activity. The time to complete the sit-to-stand activity was 30 seconds to 5 minutes. Older people's mobility, function, and quality of life were measured before the intervention and then at 3 and 6 months. Older people receiving the sit-to-stand activity over 6 months had less decline in their mobility and functional outcomes than did the control group. Moreover, the quality of life for the sit-to-stand group improved.

Application to Nursing Practice

- Nurses should assess older persons in nursing homes for functional decline.
- Promoting functional ability in older persons in nursing homes also increases their feelings of well-being.
- Nurses can use the sit-to-stand intervention when providing care to older persons.

Slaughter, S., Wagg, A. S., Jones, C. A., Schopflocher, D., Ickert, C., Bampton, E., Jantz, A., Milke, D., Schalm, C., Lycar, C., & Estabrooks, C. A. (2015). Mobility of vulnerable elders study: Effect of the sit-to-stand activity on mobility, function, and quality of life. *Journal of Post-Acute and Long-Term Care Medicine, 16*(2), 138–142.

Medication Use. Because older people tend to have more than one chronic health problem, they may receive multiple prescriptions or they may combine prescription drugs with over-the-counter products or with natural remedies. The combinations can cancel the benefits of any or all medications and produce adverse reactions, such as memory loss, sleepiness, agitation, and confusion. These effects have been associated with falls and other injuries (PHAC, 2015). The medications most commonly used are cardiovascular drugs, antihypertensives, analgesics, sedatives, tranquilizers, laxatives, and antacids. Polypharmacy (the concurrent use of many medications) increases the risk for adverse reactions. Although polypharmacy may reflect inappropriate prescribing, the concurrent use of multiple medications may be necessary if the older person has multiple acute and chronic conditions. However, a periodic and thorough review of all medications being used is important in helping older persons use the fewest necessary medications. The nurse's role with an older person is to ensure that the medications achieve the greatest therapeutic benefit with the least amount of harm. A good resource is the *Safe Living Guide for Seniors* (PHAC, 2015).

Older persons are at risk for adverse reactions because of age-related changes in the absorption, distribution, metabolism, and excretion of drugs (see Chapter 34). Medications may interact with one another; one drug may augment or negate the effect of another. Medications may also cause confusion; affect balance and mobility; cause dizziness, nausea, and vomiting; or lead to constipation, urinary frequency, or incontinence. Because of these effects, some older persons are unwilling to take medications, and others do not adhere to the prescribed dosing schedule.

Managing medications is a very important component of maintaining and promoting good health in old age. For some older persons taking large numbers of medications, safely managing medications can be a complex activity that can easily become overwhelming. Nurses can provide valuable assistance to these older persons as they carry out this important self-care activity.

As a nurse, you need to work collaboratively with an older person to ensure safe and appropriate use of prescribed and over-the-counter medications. The older person should be taught the names of all drugs being taken, when and how to take them, and the desirable and undesirable effects of the drugs. You should also teach how to avoid adverse effects and interactions of drugs and how to establish and follow an appropriate self-administration pattern. To reduce the risk for an adverse medication reaction, you should review the medications at each visit; examine for potential interactions with food or other drugs; simplify and individualize the drug regimen; take every opportunity to inform the older person and his or her family about all aspects of medication use; and encourage them to question the physician, advanced practice nurse, pharmacist, or all three about all prescribed and over-the-counter drugs.

When drugs are used in the management of confusion, special care is necessary. The sedatives and tranquilizers sometimes prescribed for acutely confused older persons may themselves cause or exacerbate confusion. These drugs should be carefully administered; age-related changes in body systems can affect the pharmacokinetic activity. When confusion has a physiological cause (such as an infection), the cause, rather than the confused behaviour, should be specifically treated. When confusion varies by time of day or is related to environmental factors, creative, nonpharmacological measures can be used, such as changing the environment to include things that are familiar to the older person, providing adequate light, encouraging use of assistive devices (glasses, hearing aids), or even encouraging the older person to make telephone calls to friends or family members to hear reassuring voices (Hirst et al., 2015).

Health Promotion and Maintenance: Psychosocial Health Concerns

Interventions supporting psychosocial health of older persons resemble those for other age groups. However, some interventions are more crucial for older persons experiencing social isolation, cognitive impairment, or stresses related to retirement, relocation, or approaching death. These interventions include therapeutic communication, touch, cognitive stimulation, reminiscence, and measures to improve body image.

Therapeutic Communication. With therapeutic communication, you perceive and respect the older person's uniqueness and meet his or her expectations. Older persons expect you to be attentive, caring, and knowledgeable. Being attentive means providing care in a timely manner and meeting the older person's expressed or unexpressed needs. As a caring nurse, you convey concern, kindness, and compassion. To show that you are knowledgeable, you need to demonstrate procedural competence and be adept at recognizing needs and relaying information. Older persons also expect others to respect their individuality. When you meet expectations and communicate effectively, they will accept you as someone who has a genuine concern for their welfare. However, you cannot simply enter an older person's environment and immediately establish a therapeutic relationship; you must first be knowledgeable and skilled in communication techniques (see Chapter 17).

Touch. Throughout life, touch tells people about their environment and the people around them. Gentle touch conveys affection and friendliness. A firm hand clasp may convey security. Touch is a therapeutic tool that nurses can use to help comfort older persons. Hume, Wright, Crocker, and colleagues (2010) found that agitation levels of older persons with dementia were significantly lower when they received a touch intervention. Touch can provide sensory stimulation, induce relaxation, provide physical and emotional comfort, orient the adult to reality, convey warmth, and communicate interest. It is a powerful physical expression of a relationship.

Older persons may be deprived of touching when separated from family or friends. An older person who is isolated, dependent, or ill; fears death; or lacks self-esteem has a greater need for touch. You may recognize touch deprivation by behaviours as simple as an older person reaching for your hand or standing close to you. When you use touch, you must be aware of cultural variations and individual preferences (see Chapter 9). Touch should convey respect and sensitivity; it should not be used in a condescending way, such as patting an older person on the head.

Cognitive Stimulation. Cognitive stimulation, in which persons engage in cognitive activities such as games, appears to show promise in improving cognitive function in persons with moderate to severe dementia (Forbes, Thiessen, Blake, et al., 2013). It is considered more effective and less confrontational than reality orientation techniques, although it does include some aspects of reality orientation. After conducting a systematic review of research, Woods and colleagues (2016) reported evidence from multiple trials that cognitive stimulation programs benefit cognition in people with mild to moderate dementia. These programs typically involved small groups of older people (five to seven) and their family in which family members were taught how to stimulate cognition using current information; topics of general interest; historical events; attention, memory, and visuospatial exercises; and clocks and calendars. Some older persons may benefit more from cognitive stimulation than others; however, this pattern still remains unknown. Until more information is available, nurses should be sensitive to individuals' responses. As a nurse, you should always be respectful, patient, and calm, and in communicating, you should answer questions simply, honestly, and with sensitivity.

Reminiscence. Reminiscence is recalling the past. Many older persons find enjoyment in sharing past experiences. In reminiscence as therapy, the recollection of the past is used to find meaning and understanding of the present and to resolve current conflicts. Remembering positive resolutions to problems reminds older persons of previous coping strategies used successfully. Reminiscing is also a way to express personal identity. Reflection on past achievements supports self-esteem. For some older persons, the process of remembering past events uncovers new meanings for those events and fosters hope (Duggleby et al., 2016). Researchers have developed software to aid older people to get in touch with their past (Sparks, 2015). The software enables older people to talk to other people and plays music and movies from decades past.

During the assessment process, nurses may use reminiscence to assess self-esteem, cognitive function, emotional stability, unresolved conflicts, coping ability, and expectations for the future. Reminiscence also occurs during direct care activities. Taking time to ask the older person questions about his or her experiences and listening attentively conveys to an older person an attitude of respect and concern.

Although reminiscence is often useful in a one-on-one situation with older persons, reminiscence can also be useful in group therapy for cognitively impaired or depressed older persons. A community nurse, for instance, can organize the group and select strategies to start a conversation (e.g., ask the group to discuss families or childhood memories). The group's size, structure, process, goals, and activities are then adapted to meet its members' needs.

Body-Image Interventions. The way that older persons present themselves influences body image and, potentially, feelings of isolation. Some physical characteristics of aging, such as distinguished-looking grey hair, may be socially desirable. Other features, such as a lined face that displays character or wrinkled hands that convey a lifetime of hard work, may also be impressive. Consequences of illness and aging that threaten the older person's body image include invasive diagnostic procedures, pain, surgery, loss of sensation in a body part, skin changes, loss of scalp hair, and incontinence. Body image is also affected by the use of devices such as dentures, hearing aids, artificial limbs, in-dwelling catheters, ostomy devices, and enteral feeding tubes.

The importance to the older person of presenting a socially acceptable image must be considered. When older persons have acute or chronic illnesses, the related physical dependence can make it difficult for them to maintain a healthy body image. Nurses can influence the older person's appearance by assisting with grooming and hygiene, such as combing hair, cleaning dentures, shaving, or changing clothing. Nurses should also be sensitive to odours in the environment. Odours may be created by urine and some illnesses. By controlling odours, nurses may encourage visitors to stay longer or visit more often.

OLDER PERSONS AND THE ACUTE CARE SETTING

Older persons in the acute care setting need special attention to help them adjust to the acute care environment and to meet their basic needs for comfort, safety, nutrition, hydration, and skin integrity. The acute care setting poses increased risk for adverse events such as delirium, dehydration, malnutrition, nosocomial infections, urinary incontinence, and falls.

The risk for delirium is increased when hospitalized older persons experience immobilization, infection, dehydration, pain, and hypoxia. Multiple medications and multiple medical diagnoses are also risk factors (Fedarko, 2011). Nonmedical causes include placement in unfamiliar surroundings, separation from supportive family members, and stress. Impaired vision or hearing contributes to confusion and interferes with nurses' attempts to reorient the patient. When prevention of delirium fails, the basis of nursing management is identification and treatment of the cause of delirium. Supportive interventions include encouraging family visits, providing memory cues (e.g., clocks, calendars, name tags), and compensating for sensory deficits. Reality orientation techniques may be useful.

Older persons are at greater risk for dehydration and malnutrition during hospitalization because of standard procedures such as limiting food and fluids in preparation for diagnostic tests. The risk for dehydration and malnutrition is also increased when older persons are unable to reach beverages or to feed themselves while in bed or connected to medical equipment. Interventions include getting the patient out of bed, providing beverages and snacks frequently, and including favourite foods and beverages in the diet plan.

The risk for health care–associated infections in older persons is increased by age-related reductions in immune system response. Of all health care agency–acquired infections, 65% occur in hospitalized patients older than 60 years; urinary catheter-related bacteriuria in older persons is the most common infection (Touhy et al., 2012). Other health care–associated infections include surgical site infection, pneumonia, and blood stream infections. Prevention begins with hand hygiene and measures to minimize the risk of infection from procedures (see Chapter 33). Prevention also includes measures to increase the older person's resistance to infection.

Older persons in acute care settings are also at risk for acquiring urinary incontinence (transient incontinence). Causes of transient urinary incontinence include delirium, untreated urinary tract infection, excessive urine production, medications, restricted mobility, and constipation or impaction. Interventions for transient urinary incontinence should be geared to correcting contributing factors. The interventions may include an individualized plan to provide voiding opportunities and modification of the environment to improve access to the toilet. In-dwelling urinary catheters should be avoided if possible. Skin breakdown should be prevented.

The risk for skin breakdown and the development of pressure injury is increased by changes in aging skin and situations that arise in the acute care setting, such as immobility, incontinence, and malnutrition. To prevent skin breakdown in older persons, nurses must avoid pressure on the skin, reduce shear forces and friction, provide skin care and moisture management, and provide nutritional support (see Chapter 42).

Older persons in the acute care setting are at risk for falling and sustaining injuries. Many of the falls occur as they get out of bed without assistance. Sedating medications may increase unsteadiness. Medications causing orthostatic hypotension may also increase the risk for falls because the blood pressure drops when the patient arises from a bed or chair. Diuretics increase the risk for falling because the adult must get out of bed often to void. Attempts to get out of bed when physically restrained may lead to injury if the patient becomes entangled in the restraint. Equipment such as wires from monitors, intravenous tubing, urinary catheters, and other medical devices become obstacles to safe ambulation. Impaired vision may prevent the patient from seeing tripping hazards such as garbage cans. Confused older persons, who may try to get out of bed although weak, unsteady, or drowsy, may benefit from the presence of family members and friends. Interventions to reduce the risk for falling include assistance with ambulation, strengthening exercises, medication monitoring, assistance with toileting, and removal of tripping hazards (see Chapter 37). Falls may be reduced by minimizing fall risk factors; through staff, patient, and family education; and through individualized fall-reduction interventions. The goal is to minimize the risk of falling without compromising mobility and functional independence.

Since the 1980s, many hospitals in Canada have established hospital acute care for elderly (ACE) units to provide specialized care for older people who have complex health care needs and to prevent functional decline (Hirst et al., 2015). Key elements of ACE units are patient-centred care, interprofessional team management, medical review, discharge planning, and assessments and interventions for common geriatric syndromes such as falls, incontinence, confusion, and skin integrity. The ACE principles can be applied to older patients regardless of which unit they are on, to promote best care practices.

OLDER PERSONS AND RESTORATIVE CARE

Restorative care consists of two types of ongoing care: (1) continuing the convalescence from acute illness or surgery that began in the acute care setting and (2) addressing chronic conditions that affect day-to-day functioning. Both types of care take place in private homes and long-term care settings.

Interventions during convalescence from acute illness or surgery are directed toward regaining or improving the prior level of independence in ADLs. Interventions that began in the acute care setting should be continued and later modified as convalescence progresses. To achieve this continuation, the acute care setting's discharge information should describe the ongoing interventions (e.g., exercise routines, wound care routines, medication schedules, vital sign monitoring, and blood glucose monitoring). To ensure that all the patient's needs are addressed, a team approach to discharge planning is important. Interventions should also address the restoration of interpersonal relationships and activities either at their previous level or at the level desired by the patient.

When restorative care addresses chronic conditions, the goals of care include stabilizing the chronic condition, promoting health, and promoting independence in ADLs. Interventions to stabilize the chronic condition may focus on regulation or prevention. An example of a regulatory intervention is the monitoring of blood glucose levels in diabetes. An example of promoting health is a smoking cessation program for older persons with chronic obstructive pulmonary disease.

Health promotion interventions for older persons, as addressed in this chapter, should occur in all health care settings. For example, nurse-directed programs in long-term care settings improve ambulation, reverse urinary incontinence, and reduce confusion.

Interventions to promote independence in ADLs address physical ability, cognitive ability, and safety. The physical ability to perform ADLs requires strength, flexibility, and balance. Impairments of vision, hearing, and touch must be accommodated. The cognitive ability to perform ADLs requires the ability to recognize, judge, and remember. Cognitive impairments, such as Alzheimer's disease, may interfere with the safe performance of ADLs, although the affected patient is still physically capable of the activities. Interventions to promote independence in ADLs adapt these requirements to the needs and lifestyle of the older person. Safety is always an important consideration. An older person should be able to perform the ADLs with the least amount of risk.

Beyond the basic ADLs, the older person's ability to perform instrumental ADLs must be assessed and appropriate interventions implemented. Instrumental ADLs are tasks such as using a telephone, preparing meals, shopping, doing laundry, cleaning the home, and driving an automobile. To remain independent at home or in assisted-living residences, older persons must be able to perform instrumental ADLs, be able to purchase services by outside workers, or have a supportive network of family and friends who assist with these tasks.

Restorative care measures focus on activities to prevent, improve, reduce, or eliminate problems. Priorities of care are established, patient goals and expected outcomes are determined, and appropriate interventions are selected. These are done with the patient's participation so that interventions are understood and conflicts in approaches or priorities can be avoided. An older person's lifetime experiences, values, and sociocultural background are the bases for planning individual care. When deterioration of the patient's cognitive status prevents participation in care decisions, family or significant others must be consulted. Family and friends are rich sources of data because they knew the patient before the impairment. Frequently they can provide explanations for the older person's behaviours and suggest methods of management. Thoughtful assessment and planning involve consideration of the influence of normal aging changes, facilitating an optimal level of comfort and coping, and promoting independence in self-care activities.

OLDER PERSONS AND PALLIATIVE CARE

As the proportion of older persons in Canada increases the number of deaths will double by 2056 (Statistics Canada, 2015a). Only 10% will die suddenly, leaving 90% of this cohort requiring some form of assistance during their final years. The World Health Organization (2017) describes the purpose of palliative care as improving overall quality of life for persons with life-limiting illness and their families. It includes good symptom management and interprofessional collaboration, with a focus on fostering patient and family hopes, and achieving their goals and expectations for illness management over time (Hennessy, Lown, Landzaat, et al., 2013). Often, this is viewed as happening in the last months, weeks, or days of life under the care of palliative care specialists. However, with the rising numbers of older persons worldwide, the Canadian Hospice and Palliative Care Association (2015) recommends that an integrated palliative approach be used to meet a person's and family's full range of needs at all stages of frailty or chronic illness, not just at the end of life. A palliative approach to care incorporates the ideals of palliative care for all patients and their families with chronic conditions, early on in the chronic disease trajectory as well as at the end of life, and is part of generalist health care practice in all settings (Sawatzky, Stajduhar, Porterfield, et al., 2014). As a nurse, you will be using the principles of the palliative approach for all of your patients who have chronic conditions.

KEY CONCEPTS

- The number of older persons, especially the number of older persons older than 85 years, is increasing.
- Because the nurse's attitudes toward older persons influence the quality of care, those attitudes should be based on accurate information about older persons, rather than on myths and stereotypes.
- Biological and psychosocial theories of aging offer possible explanations for the changes seen in aging, but every older person is a unique individual who ages in a unique way.
- The physical changes that accompany aging are considered normal, not pathological, although they may predispose older persons to disease.
- Cognitive impairment is not normal in older persons, and it necessitates assessment and intervention.
- Cognitive impairment includes acute, potentially reversible disorders (delirium) and chronic, irreversible, progressive disorders (dementia).
- Issues and events involving psychosocial changes related to aging include retirement, social isolation, change in housing, death of friends and family, sense of own mortality, and sexuality.
- Nursing interventions for psychosocial concerns include therapeutic communication, touch, cognitive stimulation, reminiscence, and interventions to improve body image.
- The leading causes of death in the older population are cancer, heart disease, stroke, lung disease, accidents and falls, diabetes, kidney disease, and liver disease.
- Health promotion recommendations for older persons include good nutrition, regular exercise, smoking cessation, measures to reduce the risk for falls, and measures to reduce adverse medication reactions.
- Acute care settings increase older persons' risk for delirium, dehydration, malnutrition, health care–associated infections, urinary incontinence, and falls.
- Restorative nursing interventions, whether accomplished in the older person's home or in long-term care institutions, stabilize chronic conditions, promote health, and promote independence in basic and instrumental ADLs.

CRITICAL THINKING EXERCISES

1. Mr. Brown, 73 years old, has come to the clinic for a routine check of his blood pressure. It is normal (130/80 mm Hg). He says that he wants to do everything he can to stay healthy. What advice can you give on health promotion and disease prevention?
2. Mrs. Shephard's daughter has come with her to the clinic. She is concerned about her mother's memory. She tells you that her mother's memory has been excellent but has suddenly become poor. Two days ago, Mrs. Shephard phoned her daughter six times in 2 hours, asking where her husband (the late Mr. Shephard) was, and, when told of his death 4 years ago, Mrs. Shephard denied this fact. When her daughter arrived at her house to check on her, she found that Mrs. Shephard had emptied the contents of all the closets onto the floor and accused her daughter of theft. Her daughter brought Mrs. Shephard to her own home that night because of concern about Mrs. Shephard's safety. From the daughter's report, you suspect delirium (acute confusional state). What questions should you ask, and what areas should you assess to identify the possible causes of Mrs. Shephard's confusion?
3. A nursing colleague tells you that she does not know very much about assessing older persons, and she asks for some pointers on how to perform a thorough assessment. What advice can you give her about the process of geriatric assessment?

REVIEW QUESTIONS

1. What two factors contribute to the projected increase in the number of older persons?
   1. Financial success and improved environment
   2. Fewer medical problems associated with aging
   3. Improved medication plan and increase in federal health care funding
   4. The aging of the "baby-boom" generation and the growth of the population segment older than 85 years
2. The three common conditions affecting cognition in older persons are:
   1. Stroke, heart attack, and cancer of the brain
   2. Cancer, Alzheimer's disease, and stroke
   3. Delirium, depression, and dementia
   4. Blindness, hearing loss, and stroke
3. Sexuality is recognized as a factor in the lives of older persons; thus:
   1. Any expression of sexuality should be discouraged.
   2. All older persons, whether healthy or frail, need to express sexual feelings.
   3. An older person's need for sexual expression decreases.
   4. The need to touch and be touched is decreased.
4. The libido does not decrease in older persons; however:
   1. Frequency of sexual activity may decline
   2. Physical changes do not usually affect sexual functioning
   3. The need to touch and be touched is decreased
   4. The sexual preferences of older persons are not as diverse
5. Visual acuity declines with age. Presbyopia is a progressive decline in:
   1. Distinguishing between blues and greens and among pastel shades
   2. The ability to see in darkness
   3. The ability to focus on near objects
   4. Adaptation to abrupt changes from darkness to light
6. A common age-related change in auditory acuity is called:
   1. Presbycusis
   2. Presbyopia
   3. Calcification
   4. Hypertrophy
7. Taste buds atrophy and lose sensitivity. Older persons are less able to discern:
   1. Salty, sweet, sour, and bitter tastes
   2. Hot and cold temperatures
   3. Moistness and dryness
   4. Spicy and bland tastes

8. Changes in the musculoskeletal system lead to changes in the configuration of the thorax. This is known as:
   1. Hypertrophy
   2. Calcification
   3. Presbycusis
   4. Kyphosis
9. Frontotemporal dementia has an insidious onset and progresses slowly. Early symptoms include:
   1. Poor hygiene, lack of social tact, and sexual disinhibition
   2. More involvement in surroundings and social situations
   3. Fluctuating cognition and visual or auditory hallucinations (or both)
   4. Motor features of Parkinsonism
10. A palliative approach to care includes:
    1. Persons with nonchronic conditions
    2. Older persons with noncancer and cancer diagnosis
    3. Specialist care
    4. Self-management of chronic illness

Answers: 1. 4; 2. 3; 3. 2; 4. 1; 5. 3; 6. 1; 7. 1; 8. 4; 9. 1; 10. 2

Rationales for the Review Questions appear at the end of the book.

RECOMMENDED WEBSITES

Alzheimer Society of Canada: http://www.alzheimer.ca
The Alzheimer Society of Canada provides current information about Alzheimer's disease, related dementias, caregiving, support, research, treatment, and programs and services.

Canadian Coalition for Seniors' Mental Health: http://ccsmh.ca
This website provides information on national guidelines, tools, and resources about older persons' mental health issues.

Canadian Gerontological Nursing Association: http://www.cgna.net
This website provides information about gerontological nursing practice in Canada, including current standards of practice.

Canadian Network of the Prevention of Elder Abuse: http://www.cnpea.ca
This website provides information about elder abuse in Canada and Best Practice Guidelines for the prevention of elder abuse.

Hartford Institute for Geriatric Nursing ConsultGeriRN.org: https://consultgeri.org/
This website provides continually updated evidence-informed protocols and assessment tools for nurses to use with older persons.

Public Health Agency of Canada, Division of Aging and Seniors: http://www.phac-aspc.gc.ca/seniors-aines/
This federal website provides links to new services, publications, and news releases on issues relevant to aging.

REFERENCES

Alzheimer Society of Canada. (2017). *What is dementia?* Retrieved from http://www.alzheimer.ca/en/About-dementia/What-is-dementia.

Anand, P., & Singh, B. (2013). A review on cholinesterase inhibitors for Alzheimer's disease. *Archives of Pharmacal Research, 36*(4), 375–399. doi:10.1007/s12272-013-0036-3.

Berstein, I. H., Laciritz, L., Barlow, C. F., et al. (2011). Psychometric evaluation of the Montreal Cognitive Assessment (MoCa) in three diverse samples. *Clinical Neuropsychologist, 25*(1), 119–126. doi:10.1080/13854046.2010.533196.

Boltz, M., Resnick, B., & Galik, E. (2012). Interventions to prevent functional decline in the acute care setting. In M. Boltz, E. Capezuti, T. Fulmer, et al. (Eds.), *Evidence-based geriatric nursing protocols for best practice* (4th ed., pp. 104–121). New York: Springer.

Bueckert, V. (2016). Demystifying delirium. *Alberta RN, 72*(2), 18–19.

Canadian Coalition for Seniors' Mental Health. (2016). *CCSMH strategic priorities: Promoting best practices in assessment and treatment.* Retrieved from http://ccsmh.ca/about/best-practices/.

Canadian Gerontological Nursing Association (CGNA). (2010). *Gerontological nursing competencies and standards of practice 2010.* Retrieved from http://www.cgna.net/Standards_of_Practice.html.

Canadian Hospice and Palliative Care Association. (2015). *The way forward national framework: A roadmap for an integrated palliative approach to care.* Retrieved from http://www.hpcintegration.ca/resources/the-national-framework.aspx.

Canadian Institutes for Health Information (CIHI). (2011). *Seniors and the health care system: What is the impact of multiple chronic conditions?* Retrieved from https://secure.cihi.ca/free_products/air-chronic_disease_aib_en.pdf.

Canadian Network for the Prevention of Elder Abuse. (2017). *What is elder abuse?* Retrieved from http://www.cnpea.ca/en/what-is-elder-abuse.

Chappell, N. L., Hollander, M. J., Mills, D. (2013). *Aging in Canada: Issues in Canada.* Ontario: Oxford University Press.

Dahlke, S. (2011). Examining nursing practice with older adults through a historical lens. *Journal of Gerontological Nursing, 27*(5), 41–48. doi:10.3928/00989134-20110106-06.

Dowling-Castronovo, A., & Bradway, C. (2012). Urinary incontinence. In M. Boltz, E. Capezuti, T. Fulmer, et al. (Eds.), *Evidence-based geriatric nursing protocols for best practice* (4th ed., pp. 393–397). New York: Springer.

Duggleby, W., Cooper, D., Nekolaichuk, C., et al. (2016). The psychosocial experiences of older palliative patients while participating in a Living with Hope program. *Journal of Palliative and Supportive Care, 14*(6), 672–679. doi:10.1017/S1478951516000183.

Dury, R. (2014). Social isolation and loneliness in the elderly: An exploration of some of the issues. *British Journal of Community Nursing, 19*(3), 125–128. doi:10.12968/bjcn.2014.19.3.125.

Emlet, C. A. (2016). Social, economic, and health disparities among LGBT older adults. *Journal of the American Society on Aging, 40*(2), 16–22.

Fedarko, N. S. (2011). The biology of aging and frailty. *Clinics in Geriatric Medicine, 27*(1), 27–37. doi:10.1016/j.cger.2010.08.006.

Forbes, D., Thiessen, E. J., Blake, C. M., et al. (2013). Exercise programs for people with dementia (Review). *Cochrane Database System Reviews,* (12), CD006489, doi:10.1002/14651858.CD006489.pub3.

Furman, E. F. (2006). Undernutrition in older adults across the continuum of care: Nutritional assessment, barriers, and interventions. *Journal of Gerontological Nursing, 32*(1), 22–27. doi:10.3928/0098-9134-20060101-11.

Health Canada (2007). *Eating well with Canada's food guide* (Catalogue No. H164-38/1-2007E). Ottawa: Author.

Health Canada. (2011). *Smoking and mortality.* Retrieved from http://www.hc-sc.gc.ca/hc-ps/tobac-tabac/legislation/label-etiquette/mortal-eng.php.

Hennessy, J. E., Lown, B. A., Landzaat, L., et al. (2013). Practical issues in palliative and quality-of-life care. *Journal of Oncology Practice, 9*(2), 78–80. doi:10.1200/JOP.2013.0000896.

Hirst, S. P., Lane, A. M., & Miller, C. A. (2015). *Miller's nursing for wellness in older adults* (Canadian ed.). Philadelphia: Wolters Kluwer/Lippincott Williams & Wilkins.

Hume, C., Wright, J., Crocker, T., et al. (2010). Non-pharmacological approaches for dementia that informal carers might try or access: A systematic review. *International Journal of Geriatric Psychiatry, 25*(7), 756–763. doi:10.1002/gps.2429.

Johnson, S., Kelly, S., & Rasaali, D. (2015). Differences in fall injury hospitalization and related survival rates among older adults across age, sex and areas of residence in Canada. *Injury Epidemiology, 2*(1), 24. doi:10.1186/s40621-015-0056-1. Retrieved from http://injepijournal.springeropen.com/articles/10.1186/s40621-015-0056-1.

Keating, N., Eales, J., & Philips, J. E. (2013). Age-friendly rural communities: Conceptualizing 'best-fit'. *Canadian Journal on Aging, 32*(4), 319–332. doi:10.1017/So714980813000408.

Keller, H., Carrier, N., Duizer, L., et al. (2014). Making the most of mealtimes (M3): Grounding mealtime interventions with a conceptual model. *Journal of American Medical Directors Association, 15*(3), 158–161. doi:10.1016/j.jamda.2013.12.001.

Macpherson-Packard, S., Macfie, B., & Bate, L. (2015). Keeping the elderly on their feet. *Nursing New Zealand, 21*(10), 16–17.

Manitoba Palliative Care Research Unit. (2016). *Dignity in care toolkit.* Retrieved from http://www.dignityincare.ca/en/toolkit.html#Dignity_Therapy_For_Dying_Patients.

McDonald, L., & Donahue, P. (2011). Retirement lost? *Canadian Journal on Aging, 30*(3), 401–422. doi:10.1017/S0713980811000298.

Milan, A., Wong, I., & Vezina, M. (2014). *Insights on Canadian society: Emerging trends in living arrangements and conjugal unions for current and future seniors* (Catalogue no. 75-006-X). Ottawa: Statistics Canada.

Novak, M., Campbell, L., & Northcott, H. C. (Eds.), (2014). *Aging and society: Canadian perspectives.* Toronto: Nelson.

Parke, B., Hunter, K. F., Strain, L. A., et al. (2013). Facilitators and barriers to safe emergency department transitions for community dwelling older people with dementia and their caregivers: A social ecological study. *International Journal of Nursing Studies, 50*(9), 1206–1218. doi:10.1016/j.ijnurstu.2012.11.005.

Peters, M. L. (2010). The older adult in the emergency department: Aging and atypical illness presentation. *Journal of Emergency Nursing, 36*(1), 29–34. doi:10.1016/j.jen.2009.06.014.

Phinney, A., Kelson, E., Baumbusch, J., et al. (2016). Walking in the neighbourhood: Performing social citizenship in dementia. *Dementia (Basel, Switzerland), 15*(3), 381–394. doi:10.1177/1471301216638180.
Ploeg, J., Matthew-Maich, N., Fraser, K., et al. (2017). Managing multiple chronic conditions in the community: A Canadian qualitative study of the experiences of older adults, family caregivers and healthcare providers. *BMC Geriatrics, 17*(1), 40. doi:10.1186/s12877-017-0431-6.
Public Health Agency of Canada (2015). *The safe living guide: A guide to safe living for seniors*. Ottawa: Author.
Register, M. E., & Herman, J. (2010). Quality of life revisited. The concept of connectedness in older adults. *Advances in Nursing Science, 33*(1), 53–63. doi:10.1097/ANS.0b013e3181c9e1aa.
Registered Nurses' Association of Ontario (RNAO) (2016). *Delirium, dementia, and depression in older adults: Assessment and care* (2nd ed.). Toronto: Author. Retrieved from http://rnao.ca/sites/rnao-ca/files/bpg/RNAO_Delirium_Dementia_Depression_Older_Adults_Assessment_and_Care.pdf.
Reitsma, M. L., Tranmer, J. E., Buchanan, D. M., et al. (2011). The prevalence of chronic pain and pain-related interference in the Canadian population from 1994-2008. *Chronic Diseases and Injuries in Canada, 31*(4), 157–164.
Rozanova, J., Miller, E. A., & Welte, T. (2016). Depictions of nursing home residents in US newspapers; sucessful ageing vs frailty. *Ageing & Society, 36*(1), 17–41. doi:10.107/SO1446586X14000907.
Said, A. A., & Kautz, D. D. (2013). Reducing restraint use for older adults in acute care. *Nursing, 2013*, 59–61. doi:10.1097/01.NURSE.0000437484.759992.ca.
Satre, D. D. (2015). Alcohol and drug use problems among older adults. *Clinical Psychology Science and Practice, 22*(3), 238–254. doi:10.1111/cpsp.12104.
Sawatzky, R., Stajduhar, K. I., Porterfield, P., et al. (2014). Demystifying a palliative approach. *Journal of Palliative Care, 30*(3), 248.
Schanzer, D., Sevenhuysen, C., Winchester, B., et al. (2013). Estimating influenza deaths in Canada, 1992-2009. *PLoS ONE*, doi:10.101371/journal.pone.0080481.
Slaughter, S., Wagg, A. S., Jones, C. A., et al. (2015). Mobility of vulnerable elders study: Effect of the sit-to-stand activity on mobility, function, and quality of life. *Journal of Post-Acute and Long-term Care Medicine, 16*(2), 138–143. doi:10.1016/j.jamda.2014.07.020.
Smith, A. (2014). *Older adults and technology use*. Pew Research Center. Retrieved from http://www.pewinternet.org/2014/04/03/older-adults-and-technology-use/.
Sparks, J. (2015). Technology helps patients get in touch with the past. *Nursing Older People, 27*(5), 7. doi:10.7748/nop.27.5.7.s7.
Special Senate Committee on Aging (2009). *Canada's aging population: Seizing the opportunity*. Ottawa: Parliament of Canada. Retrieved from https://sencanada.ca/content/sen/Committee/402/agei/rep/AgingFinalReport-e.pdf.
Statistics Canada. (2015a). *Canadian population estimates: Age and sex, July 1, 2015*. Retrieved from http://www.statcan.gc.ca/daily-quotidien/150929/dq150929b-eng.htm.
Statistics Canada. (2015b). *The Canadian population in 2011: Age and sex*. Retrieved from http://www12.statcan.ca/census-recensement/2011/as-sa/98-311-x/98-311-x2011001-eng.cfm.
Statistics Canada (2016a). *The contribution of immigration to the size and ethnocultural diversity of future cohorts of seniors*. Ottawa: Author. Retrieved from http://www.statcan.gc.ca/daily-quotidien/160309/dq160309a-eng.htm.
Statistics Canada (2016b). *Heavy drinking by age group and sex*; Retrieved from: http://www.statcan.gc.ca/tables-tableaux/sum-som/l01/cst01/health79a-eng.htm.
Statistics Canada (2017). *Fact Health Sheets; The 10 leading causes of death*. http://www.statcan.gc.ca/pub/82-625-x/2017001/article/14776-eng.htm.
Touhy, T., Jett, K., Boscart, V., et al. (2012). *Ebersole and Hess' gerontological nursing and healthy aging* (1st Cdn. ed.). Toronto: Elsevier Canada.
Webber, S., Porter, M., & Menec, V. (2010). Mobility in older adults: A comprehensive framework. *The Gerontologist, 50*(4), 443–450. doi:10.1093/geront/gnq013.
Woods, N., Rillamas-Sun, E., Cochrane, B., et al. (2016). Aging well: observations from the Women's Health Initiative Study. *Journals of Gerontology. Series A, Biological Sciences and Medical Sciences, 71*(Suppl. 1), S3–S12. doi:10.1093/Gerona/glv054.
World Health Organization (2015). *World report on ageing and health*. Geneva: Author.
World Health Organization. (2017). *Cancer: WHO definition of palliative care*. Retrieved from http://www.who.int/cancer/palliative/definition/en/.

25

The Experience of Loss, Death, and Grief

Canadian content written by Jim Hunter, RN, MSN
Original chapter by Emily L. McClung, MSN, RN, PhD(c)

OBJECTIVES

Mastery of content in this chapter will enable you to:

- Define the key terms listed.
- Identify your role in assisting patients who have experienced loss, death, and grief.
- Describe and compare the phases of grieving from Kübler-Ross (1969), Bowlby (1980), and Worden (1991).
- List and discuss the five categories of loss.
- Describe the types of grief.
- Describe the characteristics of a person experiencing grief.
- Discuss variables that influence a person's response to grief.
- Develop a nursing care plan for a patient or family experiencing loss and grief.
- Explain reasons for the need for improved end-of-life care for patients.
- Discuss principles of palliative care.
- Describe how to involve family members in palliative care.
- Describe the procedure for care of the body after death.
- Discuss your own experience of loss when caring for dying patients.

KEY TERMS

MEDIA RESOURCES

http://evolve.elsevier.com/Canada/Potter/fundamentals/

- Audio Chapter Summaries
- Examination Review Questions
- Concept Map Creator
- Case Study with Questions
- Audio Glossary
- Content Updates
- Video Clips

Loss and grief are experiences that affect not only patients and their families but also the nurses who care for them. In Canada and other Western societies, palliative and end-of-life care continues to develop its role in health care and gain acceptance, despite barriers that include a focus on the more dominant medical model, where the focus is on cure (Virdun, Luckett, Davidson, et al., 2015). Thus Canadians often deny the possibility of death, as well as the need to express grief and to feel the pain associated with a loss, both of which are beneficial to healing. Grief affects survivors physically, psychologically, socially, and spiritually because of very real concrete and perceived losses. Death of a patient, for example, may leave family, friends, and caregivers feeling powerless. Most nurses enter the profession with the intent of helping patients recover from illness, adjust to illness-related changes in lifestyle, and move toward restoration of health. It is often frightening to learn that knowledge, skill, and technology do not always result in recovery.

The nurse's role in facilitating the grief process includes assisting survivors to feel the loss, express the loss, and complete the stages of the grief process. To be effective, nurses must have a thorough understanding of a patient's loss, its significance and meaning to the patient and family, and how it affects the patient's and family's ability to carry on. Providing care for patients in crisis from loss or during the end of life requires knowledge, caring, and compassion to help bring comfort to patients and families, even when hope for a cure is gone. Helping patients to a peaceful, dignified death is an important aspect of nursing care. Although working with dying patients can be challenging, many nurses also find it to be a rewarding and often life-changing experience (Lopera, 2015).

SCIENTIFIC KNOWLEDGE BASE

Loss

Throughout their lives, people form attachments and suffer losses. They develop independence from their parents, start and leave school, change friends, begin careers, and form relationships. The growing-up process is natural and positive, and yet as people's lives unfold, they suffer necessary losses. **Necessary losses** are an integral part of each person's life. People expect their losses to be recovered and replaced by something different or better, but other losses cause an unbearable change in their sense of safety and security (Granek, 2012). Losses such as the death of a loved one, losses that come with a divorce, or loss of independence are significant and can have long-term effects on physical and psychological health. Loss comes in many forms, depending on the values and priorities learned within a person's sphere of influence, made up of family, friends, society, and culture. A person experiences loss in the absence of an object, person, body part or function, emotion, or idea that was formerly present (Table 25-1). Losses may be actual or perceived. An **actual loss** is any loss of a person or object that can no longer be felt, heard, known, or experienced by the individual. Examples are the loss of a body part, a child, a relationship, or a role at work. Lost objects that have been valued by a patient could be any possession that is worn out, misplaced, stolen, or ruined. For example, a child may grieve over the loss of a favourite toy. A **perceived loss** is any loss that is defined uniquely by the grieving patient. It may be less obvious to others. An example is the loss of confidence or prestige. Perceived losses are easily overlooked or misunderstood, and yet the process of grief follows the same sequence and progression as that for actual losses. Individual interpretation makes a difference in how the perceived loss is uniquely valued and the response that a person will have during grieving.

TABLE 25-1 Types of Loss

Definition	Implications of Loss
Loss of external objects (e.g., loss, misplacement, deterioration, theft, destruction by natural causes)	Extent of grieving depends on object's value, sentiment attached to it, and its usefulness.
Loss of known environment (e.g., moving from a neighbourhood, hospitalization, leaving or losing a job, moving out of Critical Care Unit)	Loss occurs through maturational or situational events and through injury or illness. Loneliness or newness of an unfamiliar setting threatens self-esteem and makes grieving difficult.
Loss of a significant other (e.g., through being promoted, moving, or running away; loss of a family member, friend, trusted nurse, acquaintance, or animal companion)	Significant other typically fulfills another person's need for psychological safety, love and belonging, and self-esteem.
Loss of an aspect of self (e.g., body part, psychological function, or physiological function)	Illness, injury, and developmental changes result in loss of an aspect of the self that causes grief and permanent changes in body image and self-concept.
Loss of life (e.g., death of family members, friend, or acquaintance; own death)	Loss of life creates grief for the survivors. The person facing death often fears pain, loss of control, and dependency on others.

Losses may also be maturational, situational, or both. A **maturational loss** is any change in the developmental process that is normally expected during a lifetime. One example would be a parent's feeling of loss as a child goes to school for the first time. Events associated with maturational loss are part of normal life transitions, but the feelings of loss persist as grieving helps a person cope with the change. **Situational loss** is any sudden, unpredictable external event. Often this type of loss includes multiple losses rather than a single loss; for example, an automobile accident may leave a driver paralyzed, unable to return to work, and grieving over the death of a passenger in the accident.

The type of loss and the perception of the loss influence the depth and duration of grief that a person experiences. Each individual responds to loss differently. It is incorrect to assume that the loss of an object does not generate the same level of grieving as the loss of a loved one. The value an individual places on the lost object (e.g., a family heirloom) determines the emotional response to the loss. As a nurse, you must assess the special meaning that a loss has for a patient and validate its effect on the patient's health and well-being.

Hospitalization, chronic illness, and disability are special circumstances that are associated with multiple losses. When patients enter a hospital, they lose their privacy, control over their daily routines, and any illusions that they may have about their personal indestructibility. In addition, modesty and control over bodily functions may be compromised. A chronic illness or disability often engenders concern over financial security. Furthermore, long-term illness may necessitate a job change, threaten independence, and force alterations in lifestyle. Even a brief illness or hospitalization necessitates temporary shifts in family role functioning. Chronic or debilitating illness may pose a major threat to the stability of relationships.

Death is the ultimate loss. Although death is part of the continuum of life and a universal and inevitable part of being human, it is also a mystical event that generates anxiety and fear. Death ends relationships and separates people. Even with a strong spiritual grounding, facing death is often difficult for the dying person, as well as for the person's family, friends, and caregivers. A person's terminal illness reminds close friends and associates of their own mortality. A person with an advanced, progressive, ultimately fatal illness, such as chronic renal failure, end-stage heart failure, amyotrophic lateral sclerosis, or metastatic cancer, faces many—often progressive—levels of suffering. It is difficult to be sick, and many people dislike seeking help from others; however, nearly all want companionship and want to strengthen relationships with significant others when death is imminent (Lopera, 2015).

When faced with death, feelings of guilt, anger, and fear can arise. It may cause family members and caregivers to withdraw at a time when the dying person needs a trusted, unhurried companion, acting with gentle advocacy and humility. Patients faced with death are increasingly choosing to die at home (National Consensus Project [NCP], 2013); thus family members are becoming more involved in the care of their loved one. The way a person approaches dying is influenced by personal fundamental beliefs and values, past experiences with death, culture, spirituality, and the quality of the human emotional support available.

Grief

Grief is the emotional response to a loss or death. Each individual responds to loss differently, grieving at an individual pace and pattern (Somers, McLennan, & MacCourt, 2016). Differences are based on individual experience, previously established coping strategies, cultural expectations, and spiritual beliefs (see Chapters 9 and 28) and involve the process of mourning and the process of adapting to a loss (Somers et al., 2016). It involves working through the grief until an individual accepts and adapts to his or her expectations to find meaning in the loss, and to go on in life without that which was lost (Rice, 2015).

Bereavement includes grief and mourning; it is the state of having lost a significant other to death (Waldrop, 2007). Survivors go through a bereavement period that is not linear. It does not proceed in sequential stages that can be precisely predicted, which may imply passivity on the part of the bereaved person. Rather, a survivor will move back and forth through a series of stages, tasks, or both many times, possibly over a period of several years, before the process is completed. Although no one really "gets over" a loss, the individual can heal and adapt to the loss. A useful analogy is to think of a new ring on a finger. Initially, the wearer is always aware that it is there, but over time, it will be less noticeable and yet still present. Several theorists have formulated stages of the grieving process as a series of tasks for survivors to work through their bereavement and adapt to life with a loss.

Selected Theories of Grief

Kübler-Ross's Stages of Grief. The framework for Kübler-Ross's (1969) theory is behaviour oriented and has five stages (Table 25-2). During **denial**, an individual acts as though nothing has happened and may refuse to believe or understand that a loss has occurred. In the **anger** stage, the individual resists the loss and may strike out at everyone and everything. During **bargaining**, the individual postpones awareness of the reality of the loss and may try to deal in a subtle or overt way as though the loss can be prevented. A person finally realizes the full impact and significance of the loss during the stage of **depression**, when the individual may feel overwhelmingly lonely and withdraw from interpersonal interaction. Finally, during the **acceptance** stage, the individual accepts the loss and begins to look to the future. Although these stages are valuable for novice nurses to understand the grief process, stage or phase theories may be seen as having limitations in some situations, because in reality, the stages and phases of grief may occur nonsequentially or may overlap (Miller, 2015).

Bowlby's Phases of Mourning. Bowlby's (1980) attachment theory is the foundation for his theory on mourning. *Attachment* is described as an instinctive behaviour that leads to the development of affectionate bonds between children and their primary caregiver. These bonds are present and active throughout the life cycle. Later, the bonds are generalized to other people with whom individuals form close relationships. Attachment behaviour ensures human survival because it keeps people in close contact with other people who can offer protection and support.

Bowlby (1980) described four phases of mourning (see Table 25-2). As in the case of the other grief theories, a person can move back and forth between any two of the phases while responding to the loss. The **numbing** phase may last from a few hours to a week or more and may be interrupted by periods of extremely intense emotion. It is the briefest phase of mourning. The grieving person may describe this phase as feeling "stunned" or "unreal." Numbing may serve to protect the body from the onslaught or consequence of the loss. The second phase of **yearning and searching** arouses emotional outbursts of tearful sobbing and acute distress in most people. Corless (2010) describes how it is necessary for the bereaved person to experience the pain of grief in order to finish the work of grief, through finding meaning in the loss. Therefore, anything that continually allows the person to avoid or suppress the pain can be expected to prolong the course of mourning. Common physical symptoms are tightness in the chest and throat, a shortness of breath, feelings of weakness and lethargy, insomnia, and loss of appetite. A person may also experience an intense yearning for the object or individual who is lost. This phase may last for months or years. During the phase of **disorganization and despair**, an individual may constantly examine how and why the loss occurred. It is common for the person to express anger at anyone who might be responsible. This examination gradually gives way to an acceptance that the loss is permanent. During the final phase of **reorganization**, which may require as much as a year or more, the person begins to accept unaccustomed roles, acquire new skills, and build new relationships. People experiencing this phase must be encouraged to find meaning and hope in their loss, without lessening its importance (Corless, 2010).

Worden's Four Tasks of Mourning. Worden's (1991) four tasks of mourning imply that people who mourn can be actively involved in helping themselves and can be assisted by outside intervention. Although the time spent working through the tasks varies greatly among individuals, typically it is a minimum of a full year.

- *Task 1: To accept the reality of the loss.* Even when a death has been expected, some period of disbelief and surprise that the event has really happened always occurs. This task involves the processes required to accept that the person or object is gone and will not return.
- *Task 2: To work through the pain of grief.* Even though people respond to loss differently, it is impossible to experience a loss and work through grief without emotional pain. Individuals who deny or shut off the pain prolong their grief.
- *Task 3: To adjust to the environment in which the deceased is missing.* According to Worden (1991), a person does not realize the full impact of a loss for at least 3 months. At this point, many friends and associates make less frequent contact, and the person is left to ponder the full impact of loneliness. People completing this task must take on roles formerly filled by the deceased, including some tasks that they never fully appreciated.
- *Task 4: To emotionally relocate the deceased and move on with life.* The goal of this task is not to forget the deceased or give up the relationship with the deceased but to have the deceased take a new, less prominent place in a person's emotional life. This is often the most difficult task to complete because people fear that if they make other attachments, they will forget their loved one or be disloyal. A person completes this stage after realizing it is possible to love other people without loving the deceased less.

Types of Grief. Knowledge of types of grief, which are based on characteristics or signs and symptoms of grief, enables you as a nurse to implement appropriate bereavement therapies.

Normal Grief. Normal or uncomplicated grief consists of the normal feelings, behaviours, and reactions to a loss, including resentment, sorrow, anger, crying, loneliness, and temporary withdrawal from activities. Often the "healthy" grief response to a loss can prove positive, helping an individual to mature and develop as a person as

TABLE 25-2 The Grief Process

Kübler-Ross's (1969) Five Stages of Grief	Bowlby's (1980) Four Phases of Mourning	Worden's (1991) Four Tasks of Mourning
Denial	Numbing	Accepting the reality of loss
Anger	Yearning and searching	Working through the pain of grief
Bargaining	Disorganization and despair	Adjusting to the environment without the deceased
Depression	Reorganization	Emotionally relocating the deceased and moving on with life
Acceptance		

he or she comes to terms with the changes that have occurred in his or her life and works to rearrange and reorganize internal models (Rice, 2015). This results in the development of adaptive coping strategies on which the person can rely in the future.

Anticipatory Grief. The process of disengaging, or "letting go," that occurs before an actual loss or death has occurred is called anticipatory grief (Shore, Gelber, Koch, et al., 2016). For example, once a person or family receives a terminal diagnosis, they begin the process of saying goodbye and completing life affairs. The process becomes more stressful when the patient is unable to make decisions as a result of the progression of illness. Unless guided by a patient's explicit decisions regarding end-of-life care, the family, in consultation with health care providers, assumes the responsibility of deciding whether to continue life-sustaining measures (Morris, King, Turner, et al., 2015). The family must weigh factors such as the patient's known values and choices, the medical facts, opinions and probabilities, the burden of treatment, the expected future quality of life for the patient, and the limitations of their own emotional resources.

When dying takes a long time, the patient's loved ones may exhibit few symptoms of grief once the death occurs. This seeming absence of grief symptoms may result because the family has engaged in the grief process over time. By the time the moment of death arrives, much of the shock, denial, and tearfulness has already been experienced.

Anticipatory grieving entails some risks. Family members may withdraw emotionally from the patient too soon, leaving the patient with no emotional support as death approaches. Complications may also arise if a person who was thought to be near death survives. Family members may then have difficulty reconnecting and may even be resentful that the person has lived past life expectancy.

Complicated Grief. When a person has difficulty progressing through the normal (generally accepted) phases or stages of grieving, bereavement becomes complicated and prolonged. In these cases, bereavement appears to "go wrong" and loss has not been adequately dealt with. This can impair function and threaten a person's relationships with others (Shear, 2015). Complicated grief includes these four types:

- *Chronic grief:* Active acute mourning characterized by normal grief reactions that do not subside and continue over very long periods and that becomes complicated mourning (Worden, 2009). Affected people verbalize an inability to "get past" the grief. This may also be known as unresolved grief, or complicated grief. Coping strategies implemented during complicated grief tend to be maladaptive (Worden, 2009).
- *Delayed grief:* Characterized by normal grief reactions that are suppressed or postponed and by the survivor's conscious or unconscious avoidance of the pain of the loss (Worden, 2009). Active grieving is held back, only to resurface later, usually in response to a trivial loss or upset. For example, a wife may appear to grieve for only a few weeks after the death of her spouse, but then she may become distraught and sad when a minor event triggers emotion. The extreme sadness is a delayed response to the death of her husband. Multiple losses can cause the grieving to be delayed (Worden, 2009).
- *Exaggerated grief:* Grief that overwhelms people to the point that they cannot function. This may be reflected in the form of severe phobias or self-destructive behaviour such as alcoholism, substance abuse, or suicide.
- *Masked grief:* Lack of awareness by survivors that behaviours that interfere with normal functioning are a result of their loss. For example, a person who is grieving may exhibit physical or psychiatric symptoms; some people have been known to exhibit delinquent behaviours (Worden, 2009).

Disenfranchised Grief. People experience grief when a loss is experienced and cannot always be openly acknowledged, socially sanctioned, or publicly shared due to stigmatization (Worden, 2009). Examples are the loss of a partner from an accidental fentanyl overdose, the loss of a child in utero or at birth, or the loss of a family member through suicide.

Application of Grief Theory to Other Types of Loss. Although grief theories apply mainly to the way that individuals cope with the death of a loved one, they also apply to other losses. The theories are relevant to the way people respond to a loss of body function, as in the case of organ transplantation or heart attack, and to disability, such as amputation of a limb or paralysis. Grief theory applies to individuals who progress through stages of mourning for lost independence, body integrity, and a change in body image. These individuals experience genuine emotional pain as they progress through the stages of grieving.

NURSING KNOWLEDGE BASE

Nursing knowledge has traditionally focused on the acute care setting, in which losses are more physical in nature. As you enter home and community settings, the definitions of loss are more comprehensive and in many ways different. You must develop interventions for each unique patient situation.

Factors Influencing Loss and Grief

The way that an individual perceives a loss and responds to it during bereavement is influenced by many factors.

Human Development. People of differing ages and stages of development display different and unique symptoms of grief. For example, toddlers are unable to understand loss or death, but they feel great anxiety over the loss of objects and separation from parents. School-aged children experience grief over the loss of a body part or function. They often associate misdeeds with causing death. Middle-aged adults usually begin to re-examine life and are sensitive to their own physical changes. Older persons often experience anticipatory grief because of aging and the possible loss of self-care abilities. Aging is frequently associated with losses such as physical changes, loss of employment, loss of social respect, loss of relationships, and threats to a sense of fulfillment and contributions made in life. Older persons are often resilient in responding to grief, despite its being a highly stressful process (Box 25-1); however, they are also more likely to experience dysfunctional grieving (Worden, 2009).

Psychosocial Perspectives of Loss and Grief. Loss and death are life experiences that each person faces. Death is an overwhelming experience that affects everyone involved in the loss situation or in the death of the individual. Culture can have a significant influence on people's views of death and how the dying person should be cared for. In each culture is a set of beliefs and values that are the result of positive and negative experiences, cultural influences, and spiritual beliefs (McLellan, 2015). As a nurse you are part of that same psychosocial environment and share many of the biases or perspectives gained during sociological development. Norms for psychosocial patterns of loss and grief are reflected in caregivers as well as in patients. You need to be aware of your own personal perspectives that may influence your approach and attitudes in caring for dying patients and their families (Wilson, Avalos, & Dowling, 2016).

An individual's expression of grief evolves as the person matures. Personal experiences shape the coping mechanisms that the individual uses to deal with stressors. As psychologists explain, the coping mechanisms that were effective in the past are repeated as a first response to the pain of a loss. When older coping strategies are unsuccessful, new coping mechanisms are attempted (see Chapter 29). When faced with a loss, a patient learns what is needed for his or her own coping through repetition that is based on the successes and failures of different coping mechanisms. Sometimes the number or depths of losses become overwhelming, and familiar coping styles are not successful. For example, in the case of disenfranchised grief, society has different expectations than the person who experiences the loss, and routine coping strategies become ineffective, unavailable, or maladaptive. Professional assistance is often required to help the patient and family understand and deal realistically with losses.

Socioeconomic Status. Socioeconomic status influences a person's ability to obtain options and use support mechanisms when coping with loss. In general, people feel greater burden from a loss when financial, educational, or occupational resources are lacking. For example, a patient with limited finances may not be able to replace a home lost in a fire or may not be able to purchase necessary medications to manage a newly diagnosed disease. These patients require referral to community social service and support agencies that can provide needed resources.

Personal Relationships. When loss involves a loved one, the quality and meaning of the relationship are critical in understanding a survivor's grief experience. It has been said that to lose parents is to lose the past, to lose a spouse is to lose the present, and to lose a child is to lose the future. When a relationship between two individuals has been very close, the one left behind can have great difficulty coping. Support from family and friends is based, in part, on the person's relationships with members of a social network and the manner and circumstances of the loss. People who do not receive support and compassion from others may have difficulty grieving.

Nature of the Loss. The ability to manage grief depends on the meaning of the loss and the situation surrounding the loss. A bereaved person's ability to accept help from others influences whether he or she will be able to cope. The visibility of a loss influences the support a person receives. For example, the loss of one's home from a fire prompts support from the community, whereas a private loss of an important possession may prompt less support from others. Some losses are not highly visible, such as reproductive loss (e.g., miscarriage, stillbirth, abortion, giving up a child for adoption, infertility).

The suddenness of a loss can delay resolution from grief. For example, a sudden and unexpected death is generally more difficult for a family to accept than death after a long-term chronic illness.

Culture and Ethnicity. A person's cultural background strongly influences attitudes toward life-sustaining treatments during terminal illness (McLellan, 2015). Cultural background and family practices also influence people's interpretation of a loss and expression of grief (Box 25-2). Culture affects how patients and their support systems or families respond to loss (see Chapter 9). For example, in the Western

BOX 25-1 FOCUS ON OLDER PERSONS
Bereavement

- Bereavement adjustments are multidimensional in that nearly every aspect of a person's life can be affected by a loss. Examples are decreased social support from friends and family, and potential changes in housing.
- The overall effect of bereavement on the physical and mental health of many older spouses is not as devastating as expected. Some losses at this stage are seen as more appropriate than for younger adults.
- Older bereaved spouses commonly experience both positive and negative feelings simultaneously; however, they are at increased risk for depression.
- Loneliness and problems associated with completing the tasks of daily living are two of the most common and difficult adjustments for older bereaved spouses. Older persons are more likely to have already lost siblings or other family members, which may affect available social support and social support networks.
- Older bereaved persons adjust to the deaths of spouses in diverse ways.

Data from Worden, J. W. (2009). *Grief counseling and grief therapy: A handbook for the mental health practitioner* (4th edition). New York: Springer.

BOX 25-2 CULTURAL ASPECTS OF CARE
End-of-Life Care

At the end of life, rituals, mourning practices, and specific expressions of grief are necessary for participants of all cultures in order to have a sense of acceptance and inner peace. Whether appropriate care at the end of life achieves a "good death" or an "acceptable death" for patients is controversial. Do patients achieve a sense of comfort and peace during the death experience? Most hospital policies and procedures support an "acceptable death"—nontheatrical, disciplined, and with minimal exchange of emotions—for the patient who is dying. This means providing basic standard levels of care and support, which may or may not take into account a patient's cultural beliefs and practices. A "good death" or "acceptable death" is also known as a "meaningful death" and can be defined as a dying process "with a focus on impeccable pain management, psychosocial and spiritual care, and an interdisciplinary team approach" (Stajduhar & Taylor, 2014). In contrast, Inbadas (2016) describes a desirable death in some family or cultural situations as one that allows social adjustments and personal preparations for the transition that will occur. A good death may be perceived by families as withholding painful truths from the family member. By withholding specific illness or treatment information, the family may feel they are trying to protect their relative from suffering (Gillick, 2009). In these situations, the value of autonomy may be in conflict with culture and tradition (Ayyub, 2015). The disengagement that occurs between the person who is dying and loved ones takes many forms because of cultural differences:

- Some Asian Americans, Latinos, and Orthodox Jews believe that telling a person that he or she has a terminal diagnosis will precipitate death.
- Asking patients if they would like more information on their condition or if they prefer the nurse or the physician to speak to the substitute decision maker may be a compromise between cultural values and patient autonomy.
- Families who try to conceal painful truths or otherwise seem at odds with core nursing values such as autonomy see themselves as trying to protect their family member from suffering.
- All cultures will hold individual and varying preferences regarding treatment, involvement of family, sharing of information, and care of the dying and deceased.

Implications for Practice
- Your nursing concept of social support must be broadened to include greater variation in the timing, form, and mode of support provided to grieving patients and families.
- Cultural beliefs influence who makes up a patient's support network and what support is acceptable to both give and receive during death.
- It is not important for you as a nurse to be an expert in all cultures, but it is a necessity to identify what is culturally important or significant for the individuals and families you are working with.

Data from Gillick, M. (2009). Decision making near life's end: A prescription for change. *Journal of Palliative Medicine, 12*(2), 121–125.

hemisphere, the grieving process is usually personal and private; individuals show restrained emotion. However, the ceremonies surrounding a person's death offer time for grief resolution and reminiscing. In Eastern hemisphere nations, such as the Philippines or China, respect for the dead is shown by wailing and physically demonstrating grief for a specified period. Despite these trends, members of the same ethnocultural background may respond to loss and death differently. Nurses must acquire an understanding and appreciation of each patient's cultural values as they apply to the experience of loss, death, and grieving.

Canada is a multicultural society, and as a nurse, you can anticipate many cultural contexts and responses to loss, death, and bereavement. You must be able to support and guide patients and families through the end-of-life process in a culturally informed and acceptable manner. Culturally sensitive practices are needed to guide the development of effective nursing interventions. When individuals lose control over aspects of their life because of illness, you need to provide respectful and appropriate culturally safe care to these patients. Such care is best achieved through asking specific questions of the patient or the family (Topp, 2015).

Spiritual Beliefs. Individuals' spirituality significantly influences their ability to cope with loss. Some of the spiritual resources on which patients may depend during a loss include faith in a higher power or influence, their community of fellowship with friends, their sources of hope and meaning in life, and their use of religious rituals and practices. Loss can sometimes cause internal conflicts about spiritual values and the meaning of life. Patients who have a strong interconnectedness with a higher power or others are often very resilient and able to face death with relatively minimal discomfort (see Chapter 28). Alternatively, patients faced with a life-threatening or terminal illness may begin to question their faith and wonder why this would be allowed to happen to them.

Coping With Grief and Loss

In order to support patients and families during loss, nurses must understand how people normally cope with grief and loss. Nursing interventions involve reinforcing the patient's successful coping mechanisms and introducing new coping approaches. Chapter 29 summarizes the nursing care principles for assisting patients in coping with stressful situations.

Hope. Hope is the anticipation of a continued good or of an improvement in, or lessening of, something unpleasant. It is a multidimensional concept that is energizing and provides comfort while a person endures life threats and personal challenges (Broadhurst & Harrington, 2016). Hope enhances coping skills by building on a patient's control. A person often reveals hope through an expression of expectations for life, the present, and the future. Many patients with terminal illness focus hope on milestones or something other than a prognosis (Ayyub, 2015). Spiritual distress is often based on the person's definition of hope or lack of hope. People may view hope as encouragement to work toward recovery. Other people may view hope more negatively by not being able to envision any future favourable outcomes.

Hope has purpose and direction and, in a palliative patient, can contribute to enhancing control, maintaining dignity, and sustaining relationships (Broadhurst & Harrington, 2016). The existence and maintenance of hope depend on a person's having strong relationships and a sense of emotional connectedness to others. Nurses and other health care providers may offer that personal connectedness essential to hope. Hope is often the basis from which patients find meaning in their illness. Hopefulness enables people to see life as enduring or having sustained meaning or purpose (Broadhurst & Harrington, 2016). Nurses have reported that they believe they make the greatest difference in patients' lives by helping them keep hope alive; by increasing a patient's awareness of what is possible, nurses can also maintain a renewed sense of purpose through hope (Griffiths, Ewing, Wilson, et al., 2015). Chapter 28 discusses the conceptual components of hope and related nursing care implications.

CRITICAL THINKING

Successful critical thinking involved in caring for patients who have experienced losses requires a synthesis of knowledge, previous experience with loss and grief, and information gathered from patients and families. To provide appropriate and responsive nursing care, nurses must apply both critical thinking qualities and intellectual and professional standards.

During assessment, nurses must analyze all sources of information in order to select appropriate nursing diagnoses (Figure 25-1). To understand the process of grief and its effect on the patient and family, the nurse integrates knowledge from nursing and other disciplines and from previous experiences in caring for patients suffering loss. Knowledge of the stages of grief, for example, enables you to better empathize with a patient and family and to understand the patient's behaviours. Through identification of the stages of grief, you are able

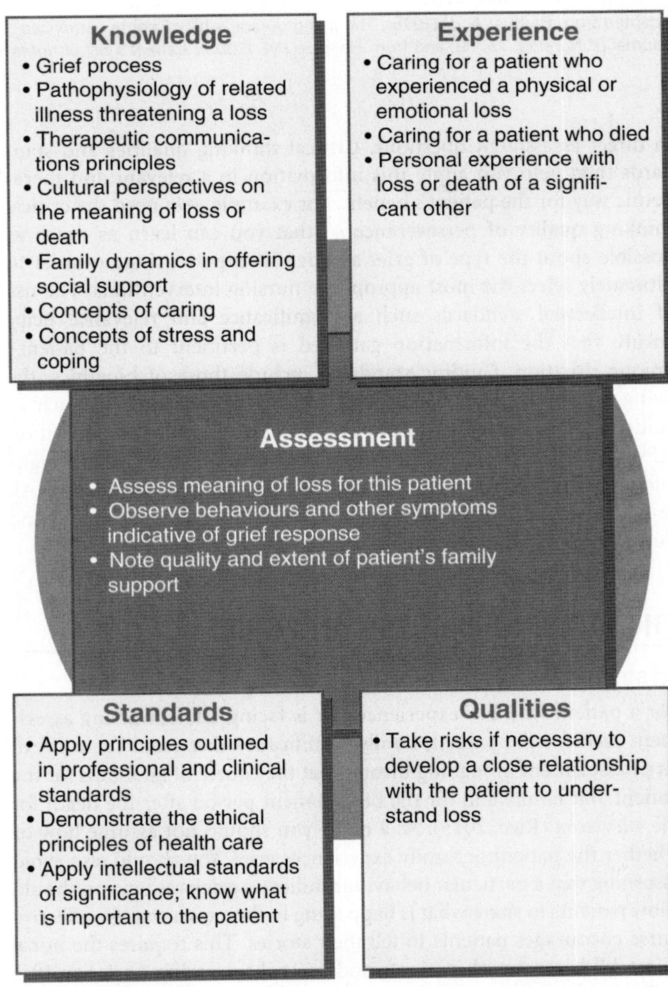

FIGURE 25-1 Critical thinking model for loss, death, and grieving assessment.

BOX 25-3 A Dying Person's Bill of Rights

I have the right to be in control.
I have the right to be treated as a living human being until I die.
I have the right to have a sense of purpose.
I have the right to be cared for by those who can maintain a sense of hopefulness.
I have the right to express my feelings and emotions about my approaching death in my own way.
I have the right to have a respected spirituality.
I have the right to participate in decisions about my care.
I have the right to expect continuing medical and nursing attention even though "cure" goals must be changed to "comfort" goals.
I have the right not to die alone.
I have the right to be comfortable.
I have the right to have my questions answered honestly.
I have the right not to be deceived.
I have the right to have help from and for my family in accepting my death.
I have the right to die in peace and dignity.
I have the right to laugh and to be angry and sad.
I have the right to retain my individuality and not be judged for my decisions that may be contrary to beliefs of others.
I have the right to be cared for by caring, sensitive, knowledgeable people who will try to understand my needs and will be able to gain some satisfaction in helping me face my death.

Adapted from Barbus, A. J. (1975). The dying person's bill of rights. *American Journal of Nursing, 75,* 99; and from Hospice RN. (2003). *Patient's bill of rights.*

to direct assessment questions. Critical thinking qualities and standards then help you apply this information in a relevant and therapeutic way for the patient's benefit. For example, you need the critical thinking quality of perseverance so that you can learn as much as possible about the type of grief a patient is experiencing, in order to ultimately select the most appropriate nursing interventions. The use of intellectual standards such as significance and relevance helps ensure that the information gathered is pertinent to the patient's unique situation. Guiding standards include those of bioethics, the dying person's bill of rights (Box 25-3), clinical standards such as guidelines for managing cancer pain, the Canadian Nurses Association (CNA, 2017) *Code of Ethics for Registered Nurses,* and provincial regulatory bodies' professional standards and practice standards. All provide evidence-informed guidelines for a thorough assessment and humane, compassionate nursing care.

THE NURSING PROCESS AND GRIEF

Assessment

For a patient who has experienced or is facing a loss, nursing assessment includes the patient, family, significant others, and the context. Grief assessment is ongoing throughout the course of an illness for the patient and family and for the bereavement period after the death for the survivors (Rice, 2015). As a nurse you should not assume how or whether the patient or family experiences grief. You should also avoid assuming that a particular behaviour indicates grief; rather, you should allow patients to share what is happening in their own way. An effective nurse encourages patients to tell their stories. This requires the nurse to establish trust with patients and to evoke a caring presence. It is helpful to have patients and families find a time and place to express their grief and describe their experiences (Figure 25-2). During an

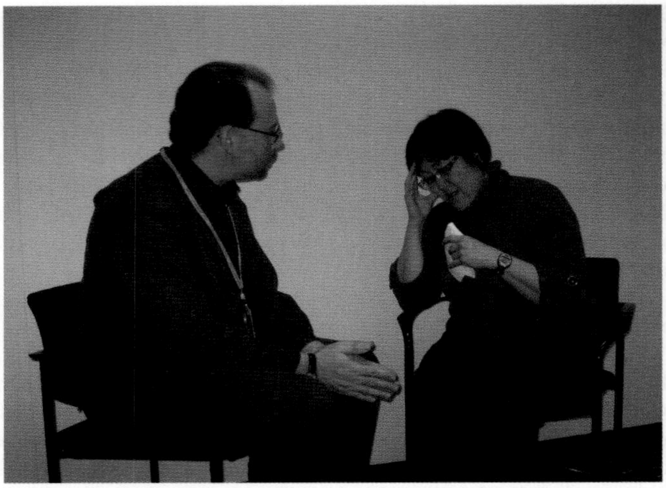

FIGURE 25-2 Nursing assistance in patient grief. A nurse finds a private place to listen to a patient expressing her grief.

assessment, patients and families should be interviewed separately unless a patient requests having family members present. A thorough and comprehensive approach to the assessment of grief will result in a well-designed plan of care that will facilitate patients' and families' abilities to work through grief.

Assessment begins by interviewing the patient and then the family, using honest and open communication. Listening carefully and observing the patient's responses and behaviours are important. Assume a neutral perspective and remain alert for nonverbal cues such as affect, facial expressions, voice tones, and topics that are avoided. While gathering data, summarize and validate any impressions formed with the patient and family so that appropriate nursing diagnoses can be made. Information from other health care workers, such as physicians, social workers, and providers of pastoral care, will contribute to the database.

Type and Stage of Grief. It is important to assess how a patient *is reacting* rather than how the patient *should be reacting.* The sequencing of stages or behaviours of grief may occur in order, they may be skipped, or they may recur. A single behaviour can be representative of any number of types of grief. Therefore, the identification of the type and stage of grief should be used only to guide the assessment and not to judge the outcomes of the grieving process. By understanding a theorist's phase of grief, nurses can accurately assess a situation. For example, if a patient is complaining of loneliness and difficulty falling asleep, consider all factors surrounding the loss. When did the loss occur? What type of loss occurred? The patient may be experiencing a normal grief reaction, or, if the loss occurred 2 years ago, the patient may be experiencing chronic grief.

Ask patients to describe their loss and how it has affected them: "Tell me how your diagnosis of heart disease makes you feel." You can anticipate characteristics or responses during a phase of grieving, but you should allow patients to describe their feelings as thoroughly as possible: "How has this change in your life affected you today?" "Tell me more." Then probe and validate feelings expressed in the patient's emotions: "You seem angry; tell me more …," "You seem sad; tell me …," "What are your feelings about … ?" Avoid premature assumptions about the phase of grief that a patient might be experiencing, so that you do not terminate the assessment too early.

Grief Reactions. Nurses use psychological and physical assessment skills to compile a complete database about the patient, family,

BOX 25-4 Symptoms of Normal Grief

Feelings
Sadness
Anger
Guilt or self-reproach
Anxiety
Loneliness
Fatigue
Helplessness
Shock or numbness (lack of feeling)
Yearning
Feeling of emancipation or relief

Cognitions (Thought Patterns)
Disbelief
Confusion
Preoccupation about the deceased
Sense of the presence of the deceased
Auditory hallucinations
Perceptual disturbances
Hopelessness ("I'll never be okay again")

Physical Sensations
Hollowness in the stomach
Tightness in the chest
Tightness in the throat
Oversensitivity to noise
Depersonalization ("Nothing seems real")
Shortness of breath
Muscle weakness
Lack of energy
Dry mouth
Headache
Abdominal pain

Behaviours
Sleep pattern changes
Appetite disturbances
Absent-minded behaviour
Dreams about the deceased
Sighing
Emotional lability
Carrying objects that belonged to the deceased

or both. Although no two people grieve exactly the same way, most people who grieve have at least some outward signs and symptoms (Box 25-4). Clinical reasoning is needed to analyze the data and cues collected and to determine the appropriate related cause. For example, a patient who is experiencing dysfunctional grieving may have a changing affect, lowered activity level, somatic complaints such as headache or upset stomach, and alterations in sleep patterns, memory, and concentration. You might associate these symptoms with any number of problems such as anxiety, gastrointestinal disturbances, or even impaired memory. However, the focus is to assess the patient's symptoms in context. What are the meaning and significance of the loss, and how are they affecting the patient in physical and psychological ways? With what does the patient associate the symptoms? In what way are the symptoms related to one another when they occur? What symptoms are observed when the patient openly expresses grief? Over what time period have the symptoms been present: before the loss or during the loss? Careful analysis refines your ability to make judgements about the patient's condition.

A loss takes place in a social context. When the primary provider in a family has a terminal illness, the family begins to reorganize itself as soon as the patient is no longer able to fulfill the same number and types of roles. When a person is disabled, the patient and family undergo similar reorganization, realigning roles and responsibilities to meet demands. During this time, patients and families can experience a variety of physical and psychological symptoms. Nurses need to assess the entire family's response to loss, recognizing that family members may be dealing with aspects of grief different from those of the patient. Good interviewing and physical assessment skills guide you as caregiver and as an advocate of the patient in planning appropriate nursing care. It is important to assess for any changes in family relationships or interactions during a patient's illness. Terminal illness may bring distant family members together, which can result in additional stressors on families. An awareness of this potential allows you to identify strategies for adaptive family coping if they are required.

Factors That Affect Grief. Because a number of factors influence loss and the grief response, it helps to discuss the meaning of loss to the patient and family. This discussion usually elicits information that allows you as their nurse to explore a number of topics in detail, such as personal characteristics of the person experiencing loss, the nature of family relationships, support systems, and cultural and spiritual beliefs (Table 25-3). You must then apply assessment skills from appropriate specialty areas (e.g., family or spiritual assessment; see Chapters 19 and 28, respectively) to acquire a thorough understanding of the patient's loss.

End-of-Life Decisions. Serious illness or loss can add a stressful and difficult element to decision making. Time to make decisions or consider all options may be limited, or the patient may be unable to fully participate in the decision-making process (Griffiths et al., 2015). In order to preserve patient autonomy, many people are using advance directives. Advance directives may include living wills or the designation of a **health care proxy**. The CNA (2015), along with other national health organizations, developed a Joint Position Statement, *The Palliative Approach to Care and the Role of the Nurse,* which includes a statement on advance care planning. In this document, the CNA states, "Nurses should encourage all people to reflect on, communicate and document their values (i.e., personal, cultural, religious and those that constitute a legacy for enduring and sustaining life), in addition to health and personal care wishes that include end-of-life care" (p. 5). An advance directive documents a person's preferences regarding life-sustaining treatment and communicates these preferences if the person becomes incapable of doing so for himself or herself (CNA, 2015). This upholds the nursing professional value of autonomy. There are some disadvantages to advance directives. A living will or instructional directive limits treatment (CNA, 2015); however, instructions in a living will may not adequately cover the uniqueness of each potential situation. A **substitute decision-maker** is designated in advance by the patient, knows the patient's wishes regarding treatment and life-sustaining procedures, and, ideally, would live locally (CNA, 2015). As a nurse, you must be aware of the legal status of advance directives in your province or territory as living wills or other advance directives may not be recognized legally in all provinces. You also need to know the laws regarding a person's competence to consent to treatment, as

TABLE 25-3 Assessment of Factors That Influence Grieving

Factor	Areas, Suggestions, and Questions to Explore
Nature of relationships	Functions of the family, community, and society *Examples:* "How long have you known your friend?" "What role has your mother played in your family?" "What is your relationship? Will it change?" "How will family relationships change as a result of the loss?"
Social support system	Availability of family, friends, health care providers *Examples:* Who is present? Absent? Supportive? Nonsupportive? What do family and friends do that is most meaningful? Are family and friends available when needed? Are health care providers accepting and exploring ways to preserve the patient's dignity and lifestyle?
Nature of loss	Actual versus perceived; death issues; impact on roles *Examples:* "Tell me what the loss means to you." "What factors help you to grieve?" "What factors interfere with grieving?" "What past experiences or outcomes have you had with loss?"
Cultural and spiritual beliefs	Values, cultural norms, spirituality, customs, attitudes *Examples:* "What is your belief about death? About the meaning of life?" "What customs do you value at the time of death?" "How is this loss viewed by other people of your culture or religious group?" "Do medical treatments interfere with religious practices?" "Who has the right to say yes or no to life-sustaining measures?"
Loss of personal life goals	Actual or perceived individual losses affecting future decisions and options *Examples:* "What is your goal in life for … ?" "How has this goal changed as a result of your diagnosis?" "How will your role change your personal goals?" "What planning have you and your family made for your own life?"
Family's grief	Relationships, involvement with the dying process *Examples:* Observe patient and family's level of grief, patterns of behaviour, rank of leadership or power. What has helped family members deal with problems in the past? What was not helpful? What are the family's strengths and weaknesses?
Survivor risk factors	High risk, such as sudden death, violent death, loss of a child *Examples:* "Describe your feelings at this time." "Let's talk about why you think you could have prevented this. Are you feeling guilty because … ?" "What are unresolved issues or perceptions toward others?"
Hope	Goals, worth, adaptation to future changes *Examples:* "Tell me what you think about your treatment plan." "What do you expect will happen to you?" "How does this illness affect your goals in life?' "What are you hoping for after your surgery?"

well as legislation regarding the selection and responsibilities of substitute decision makers or a health care proxy (see Chapter 8).

When a person has a terminal illness, family members must face end-of-life decisions that have ethical, legal, and practical implications. Families may experience higher levels of stress, discomfort, or even guilt when deciding whether to initiate or withdraw life-sustaining treatments. Some treatments may offer symptom relief but simultaneously prolong life, which creates conflict or dilemmas for families and caregivers. Although some patients may have advance directives, it is important for family members to know in advance a patient's wishes in regard to life-sustaining measures. At times, family members may disagree with each other about treatment plans, or the values of the family may be in conflict with those of the health care provider. Situations such as these often result in ethical dilemmas for families, nurses, or other care providers. Decision making related to ethical situations should consider the primary nursing values from the CNA (2017) *Code of Ethics for Registered Nurses*. Ethicists and ethical decision-making models may be used if agreement on treatment is not possible.

The *Code of Ethics for Registered Nurses* (CNA, 2017) identifies three values that are pertinent to nurses assisting individuals in end-of-life decision making:

1. *Promoting health and well-being:* Nurses must ensure that an individual's wishes as stated in an advance directive are respected and that continuing care and support are provided.
2. *Promoting and respecting informed decision making:* Nurses must respect and promote the autonomy of individuals, help patients express their needs and values, and help patients obtain appropriate care.
3. *Preserving dignity:* Nurses must advocate on the patient's behalf and examine biological, psychological, social, cultural, and spiritual factors that affect end-of-life treatment decisions.

Responsibility statements associated with each value in the code give more direction to nurses in upholding the values. For example, the value "health and well-being" includes this responsibility statement:

When a person receiving care is terminally ill or dying, nurses foster comfort, alleviate suffering, advocate for adequate relief of discomfort and pain, and assist people in meeting their goals of culturally and spiritually appropriate care. This includes providing a palliative approach to care for the people they interact with across the lifespan and the continuum of care, support for the family during and following the death, and care of the person's body after death (CNA, 2017, p. 13).

The National Consensus Project (NCP, 2013) has articulated a set of major domains and clinical practice guidelines regarding end-of-life care. Nurses must assess the patient's and family's wishes for end-of-life care, including the preferred place for death, the use and extent of life-sustaining measures, cultural-specific expectations, and expectations regarding pain control and symptom management (Box 25-5). Does the patient want to try all available treatments? Does the family or patient insist on the use of a feeding tube for continued nutritional support after the patient stops eating? When life support requires use of a mechanical ventilator, is this something the patient wants? Does the family feel comfortable in administering analgesics? Nurses must give the patient and family time to discuss their preferences. Often it is necessary to return to a conversation on a subsequent day or visit. If you feel uncomfortable in assessing a patient's wishes, it is important to find a health care provider who is experienced with discussing end-of-life issues and can assist in communicating a patient's preferences to the health care team. For example, physicians may be helpful when discussing issues related to probability or futility, or a social worker may be able to help with decision making with regard to family roles, responsibilities, and relationships.

Some patients may request medical assistance in dying (MAID). This is also known as physician-assisted death. The *Criminal Code* was amended in 2016 by the Supreme Court of Canada to allow some people to make decisions about when they want their life to end. Patients must meet certain very specific criteria, including experiencing enduring suffering as a result of an illness, disease, or disability that is grievous and irremediable (Léonard, 2016). The role of nurses (except for nurse practitioners) is limited to aiding in the provision of MAID, but nurses may not actually administer a substance that induces death (College of Registered Nurses of British Columbia [CRNBC], 2016). Provincial governments, health authorities, and professional associations are still in the process of determining exact roles and processes required for individuals' participation with MAID. Each nurse should check with his or her own provincial regulatory body about limits and conditions regarding their own involvement with MAID.

End-of-life care is one of the more significant topics you will discuss with patients (Box 25-6). Good interdisciplinary teamwork is essential to provide quality end-of-life care. Thus, you must communicate what is known about patient preferences and decisions in change-of-shift reports, health team conferences, written care plans, documentation in the patient's record, and ongoing consultation with physicians and other health team members.

Nurses' Experience With Grief. When caring for grieving patients, you must assess your own emotional well-being. Self-reflection, which is a part of critical thinking, is a valuable tool in assessing whether a person's sadness is related to the patient, to unresolved personal experiences from the past, or to a combination

BOX 25-5 RESEARCH HIGHLIGHT

Family Perception of End-of-Life Care

Research Focus

Family members are often involved in providing care during a dying person's last month of life, regardless of the setting (home, hospice, or hospital). Their perspectives of how the person's last days of life are spent provide valuable insight into the quality of end-of-life care.

Research Abstract

Morris, King, Turner, et al. (2015) conducted a narrative literature review of the perceptions of family caregivers providing end-of-life care in the home. The researchers obtained information from 28 empirical studies and literature reviews were included. Data about the emotional burden and experiences of families regarding end-of-life decision making, the illness experience, and the dying process were collected. Findings suggested that there need to be increased financial and societal incentives to ensure that family caregivers are supported adequately. Although the family plays a central role in a person's dying at home, there remain questions regarding how these family caregivers can best be supported as well as gaps in this support. Some families may not regard home deaths as possible; they identified some practical and moral concerns about home death, such as having limited family members to provide care, the quality of the care being delivered, and the practicality of dying at home for someone with poor housing conditions.

Evidence-Informed Practice

- It is important to learn directly from patients and families their understanding of the illness.
- Families of dying patients may have great difficulty making decisions about moral and practical issues related to the patient dying at home.
- Nurses should recognize that family members carry a significant emotional, financial, and societal burden, particularly with respect to caregiving, and will need nursing support.
- Nurses should provide guidance and support to help families understand the dying process. Families need to know in advance what they may expect to see throughout the dying process.

Morris, S., King, C., Turner, M., & Payne, S. (2015). Family carers providing support to a person dying in the home setting: A narrative literature review. *Palliative Medicine, 29*(6), 487–495. doi:10.1177/0269216314565706

BOX 25-6 CASE STUDY

Nursing Roles With Loss, Grief, and End-of-Life Issues: John's Story

Nurses from many areas and disciplines are involved in the experiences of loss, death, and grief. John is an 81-year-old with recurrent small-cell lung cancer and is considered eligible for palliative care. Several years ago, he received a diagnosis of limited-stage small-cell lung cancer. A course of chemotherapy and radiotherapy resulted in a remission of several years' duration. Subsequent follow-up revealed that the cancer had returned, and John's condition was considered terminal. Throughout John's experience with his illness, he has interacted with many nurses with varying roles and responsibilities. Although these nurses all had different roles, functions, and work areas, they were all involved and sharing with John and his family's sense of loss, grief, celebrations, and eventual preparation for death.

Initially, John interacted with the clinic nurse at his family physician's office. Although not involved directly in his care, this nurse was able to provide support, reassurance, and encouragement each time John visited the office. While John was receiving his treatments at the cancer centre, he relied on the chemotherapy clinic nurses to check on how he was feeling, and he counted on them to be caring but not gloomy, to keep his spirits up, and to encourage him to keep "fighting" while it was beneficial. One nurse in particular had frequent contact with John, and he looked forward to seeing her. She was a clinical trials research nurse, and John had enrolled in a medication trial. This advanced practice nurse was, to John, like his own private nurse, someone who wanted to see him regularly, took a genuine interest in him, and provided tremendous support to him and his family.

Home care nurses also played an important role in John's experience. The initial home assessment, enrollment in a community palliative care program, and discussion of "do not resuscitate" protocols were managed in a caring and compassionate manner.

John's health is now relatively stable and appears to have reached a plateau in the disease course. Each time the home care nurse visits and performs her assessment and documentation, John sees this as a "social" visit but finds the support to be very important. Being a reserved person, John finds it easier to discuss some of his issues with a professional. John has not decided yet whether he wishes to die at home or in a hospital; however, caring and compassionate palliative care nurses will at that point become key components of John's and his family's experience.

John's story is not unique. Most nurses are involved in the experience of loss, death, and grief, regardless of the area of practice. Having a sound understanding of these concepts will enable you to provide supportive, understanding, and compassionate care to your patients, anywhere along the continuum of life, loss, grief, and, eventually, death.

BOX 25-7 NURSING DIAGNOSTIC PROCESS

Assessment Activities	Defining Characteristics	Nursing Diagnosis
Ask patient to discuss future goals and plans.	Patient sighs and says, "I have no future."	*Hopelessness related to failing physical condition*
Observe patient's nonverbal behaviour.	Patient becomes passive with little affect and turns away from speaker.	*Ineffective individual coping related to low mood, and inability to manage loss*
Offer patient choices and observe responses.	Patient shrugs and says, "What does it matter?"	*Powerlessness related to perceived poor outcomes*
Assess activity level.	Patient refuses to eat. Patient sleeps all the time, keeping blinds closed and lights out. Patient refuses to participate in care.	*Self-care deficit related to inability to perform activities of daily living* *Social isolation related to inability to cope with loss*

of both. It is normal to have personal feelings and emotions about certain illnesses and death. However, it is inappropriate to emphasize your personal family situations and values over those of the patient. Talking with friends and professional colleagues may help you resolve conflicts about caring for dying patients. Some nurses choose to work in a specialty area in which deaths are usual. Close bonds between nurses and patients often develop in these situations. Part of being a professional involves knowing yourself and when to move away from a situation. Nurses who choose to work in palliative care settings obtain support from their peers, as well as from interdisciplinary team debriefings. Nurses may not always identify maladaptive coping behaviours themselves, and the entire team has a responsibility to recognize and support ineffective coping in their colleagues (Ek, Lars, Prahl, et al., 2014).

Patient Expectations. Nurses must assess the patient's and family's expectations for nursing care. Patient perceptions and expectations can influence how the nurse prioritizes nursing diagnoses. For example, if patients perceive their pain and discomfort as severe, they will be less attentive to attempts to discuss the significance and meaning of their loss. Before the nurse can begin meaningful discussion or counselling, the patient must be comfortable. On occasion, patients are hesitant to accept, and families reluctant to administer, narcotic analgesics because of fears of addiction.

Significant medication teaching may be required in these situations. Once the patient is assessed as comfortable and the patient considers the pain level acceptable or under control, the nurse should assess the patient's expectations within the context of the loss by asking questions such as "How can we help you cope with your loss?" "What do you feel is necessary from us for you to be able to manage the grief you feel?" "What is most important that we do for you while you are under our care?"

It is important to give family members the chance to explain how they perceive the nurse's role, explain what they think are the goals of the health care team, and ask any questions they may have. This helps nurses clarify any misunderstandings that might exist. For example, the family may have unrealistic expectations regarding the treatment available to the patient and the anticipated effects, or different family members may have conflicting opinions.

◆ Nursing Diagnosis

From data collected during the assessment, the nurse can identify a nursing diagnosis that accurately reflects the needs of the patient or family experiencing the loss. Critical thinking skills are the tools used to apply concepts of assessment, clustering of cues, and drawing a conclusion of the actual or perceived needs of the patient. The nurse clusters defining characteristics and identifies the nursing diagnosis applicable to the patient's situation (Box 25-7). Clustering of patient or family behaviours, actual or potential losses, the patient's attempts at coping, and data involving the nature and meaning of the loss will lead to individualized nursing diagnoses, such as the following:

- *Anticipatory grieving*
- *Anxiety*
- *Caregiver role strain*
- *Compromised family coping*
- *Dysfunctional grieving*
- *Fear*
- *Hopelessness*
- *Ineffective coping*
- *Ineffective denial*
- *Powerlessness*
- *Readiness for enhanced spiritual well-being*
- *Social isolation*
- *Spiritual distress*

The presence of one or two defining characteristics is usually insufficient for an accurate diagnosis. As a nurse you must carefully review the data to consider whether competing diagnoses exist. For example, if a dying person cries, displays anger, and reports nightmares, this could signal several possible nursing diagnoses, as these characteristics are common to more than one diagnosis. Possibilities include *pain, ineffective coping,* and *spiritual distress.* It is important to examine all available data and inquire about and observe for the presence of other behaviours and symptoms until you can identify an accurate diagnosis.

Part of the diagnostic process is to identify the appropriate related factor for each diagnosis. For example, *dysfunctional grieving related to the loss of the ability to walk from paralysis* necessitates different interventions than does *dysfunctional grieving related to the loss of a job.*

In order to promote a holistic approach to care, wellness-oriented diagnoses need to be included, such as *readiness for enhanced spiritual well-being.* These diagnoses allow for recognizing and drawing from patient strengths. In addition, the nursing diagnostic process is continual because the patient situation will change.

When identifying nursing diagnoses for the dying patient, other problems are identified separately according to specific standards of care. Other nursing diagnoses can include *disturbed body image, impaired physical mobility,* or *ineffective role performance.* More physical nursing diagnoses are identified when the patient begins to experience physical changes accompanying the progression of illness, including *impaired urinary elimination and/or bowel incontinence, acute pain, nausea, disturbed sensory perception,* and *ineffective breathing pattern.* The comfort of dying patients, including specialized pain control and acceptance of the dying process by the family, is a realistic expectation. With terminal illness, physical assessment of the dying process is ongoing so that nurses can adapt or validate the actual nursing diagnoses with the patient's changing condition.

◆ Planning

Grieving is the natural response to loss and thus has therapeutic value. The focus in planning nursing care is to support the patient physically, emotionally, developmentally, and spiritually in the expression of grief. Figure 25-3 illustrates the interrelatedness of critical thinking factors during the planning phase of the nursing process. Through critical thinking, nurses ensure a well-designed plan in which they support a patient's personhood, self-esteem, and autonomy by including the patient in making decisions about the plan of care. When caring for the dying patient, it is important to devise a plan that helps a patient die with dignity and offers family members the assurance that their loved one is cared for compassionately (Box 25-8). The care planning process is highly individual to the patient and family, and when possible, both must be included as active participants in a nurse's planning, goal setting, and development of realistic interventions and timelines.

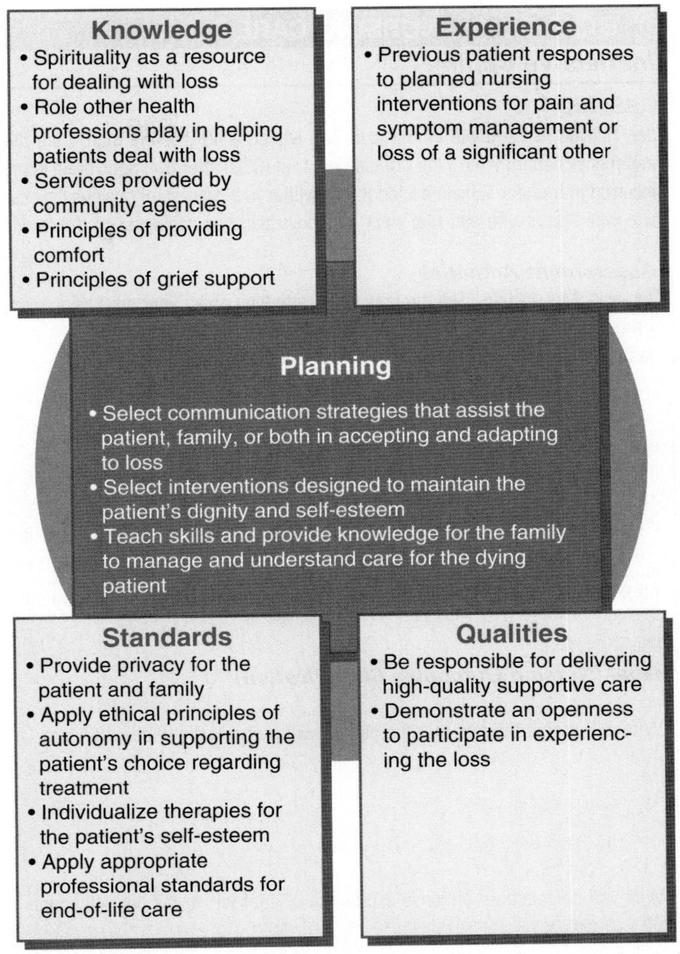

FIGURE 25-3 Critical thinking model for loss, death, and grief planning.

Goals and Outcomes. Realistic goals and expected outcomes are established on the basis of a patient's nursing diagnoses. Patient resources such as physical energy and activity tolerance, supportive family members, spiritual faith, and methods for coping are integrated into the plan of care. For example, if a patient with a life-threatening illness has the diagnosis *powerlessness related to planned cancer therapy,* a goal of "Patient will be able to discuss expected course of disease" is realistic if the patient is able to remain attentive and participate in educational discussions without becoming fatigued. In contrast, the expected outcome "Patient will participate in series of short planned teaching discussions about disease" accounts for the patient's need for teaching sessions to be short to avoid exhaustion.

Goals of care for a patient dealing with loss might be long or short term, depending on the nature of the loss, the patient's phase of grieving, and the nature of the illness. Many terminally ill patients experience plateaus (periods of relatively stable health) interspersed with periods of exacerbation of symptoms. Because a patient may move back and forth between phases of grief, nurses may need to revise goals and outcomes to ensure that they remain relevant. Help from the patient's partner in deciding which goals are relevant is important. General nursing care goals for patients with a loss include

BOX 25-8 NURSING CARE PLAN

Ineffective Coping

ASSESSMENT

Jan Runyon is the nurse who admits Mr. Miller, a 48-year-old man, from the emergency department to the Critical Care Unit (CCU) after traumatic brain injury incurred in a motor vehicle accident. Mr. Miller is a successful business executive who has a wife and two sons. The physician has explained to the family that Mr. Miller's prognosis is poor. Tests are underway to determine the extent of brain injury. Mrs. Miller and the children are in the CCU waiting area, waiting on word about Mr. Miller.

Assessment Activities	*Findings and Defining Characteristics*
Jan asks Mrs. Miller, "Tell me how you are feeling about your discussion with the physician."	"I know they are doing everything they can. He is going to be okay, I just know he is. He has never been sick a day in his life."
Jan observes Mrs. Miller's interaction with her children.	Mrs. Miller has difficulty problem solving. The family has posed several questions to her as to what she plans to say to Mr. Miller's employees. Mrs. Miller is unable to decide what to say at this time.
Jan overhears Mrs. Miller on the phone in the waiting area.	Mrs. Miller states over the phone, "Don't worry, he's having some tests right now. I know Bill; he'll be back in the office before you know it. Tell the staff everything will be okay."
Jan accompanies the transplant coordinator, who asks Mrs. Miller if the family has ever discussed organ donation.	Mrs. Miller responds, "Bill will be fine. That's not important right now!"

NURSING DIAGNOSIS: Ineffective coping related to husband's traumatic brain injury and poor prognosis

PLANNING

*Goal (Nursing Outcomes Classification)**	*Expected Outcomes*
	Grief Resolution
Wife will accept the fact that the patient will probably die within 48 hours.	Wife will verbalize to caregiver within the next 6 hours that her husband's death is actually imminent. Wife will inform children within 24 hours of their father's likely death. Wife will make a decision about organ donation within the next 12 hours. Wife will discuss immediate lifestyle changes that will occur as a result of her husband's death over the next 48 hours.
Wife will demonstrate effective expression of grief within the next 48 hours.	Wife will discuss with her children their concerns about what they need to do as a family to prepare for their father's impending death within the next 48 hours. Wife will discuss effects that loss has on her personally with caregiver within the next 48 hours.

*Outcomes classification label from Moorhead, S., Johnson, M., & Maas, M. L. (2013). *Nursing outcomes classification (NOC)* (5th ed.). St. Louis, MO: Mosby.

INTERVENTIONS

Interventions (Nursing Interventions Classification)[†]	*Rationale*
Presence	
Display interest in wife's situation and accept her behaviours of denial.	Recognizing denial (based on Kübler-Ross's [1969] theory) gives the staff direction for planning unique interventions based on grief theory (Griffiths et al., 2015).
Establish trust and a positive regard by creating an atmosphere of sharing. Offer privacy and security.	Privacy offers a place of security to exhibit personal needs and to work through feelings. Anxiety about losing dignity when expressing grief will hinder an honest expression of feelings (Ayyub, 2015).
Grief Work Facilitation	Grief work may be effective, particularly for those with complicated grief disorders. A variety of online and in-person approaches are available (Rice, 2015).
Offer wife encouragement to explore and verbalize feelings of grief.	Encouragement refocuses on current needs and assists in initiating grief process.
Identify personal coping strategies used in the past; assess their effectiveness and promote them when appropriate.	Previously successful coping strategies are the first to be used when a person is under stress (Rice, 2015). Discouraging maladaptive behaviours helps minimize dysfunctional grieving.
Determine wife's acceptance of available community resources and initiate as appropriate: significant other (business partner), children, clergy, or other health care providers.	Professionals can use their expertise to direct the grieving process (Simonsen & Cooper, 2015). Trust in relationships already formed will speed the therapeutic communication process.

[†]Intervention classification labels from Bulechek, G. M., Butcher, H. K., Dochterman, J. M., & Wagner, C. (2013). *Nursing interventions classification (NIC)* (6th ed.). St. Louis, MO: Mosby.

BOX 25-8 NURSING CARE PLAN

Ineffective Coping—cont'd

EVALUATION

Nursing Actions	***Patient Response and Finding***	***Achievement of Outcome***
Say to patient's wife, "This has been a difficult time. Your husband's injury has been so sudden."	Wife responds, "I still cannot believe it. The doctors do not believe he will live through the night."	Wife begins to acknowledge patient's impending death.
Ask, "Tell me how you are feeling now."	Wife explains, "I am worried about my kids. Both boys are close to their dad. I feel this unbelievable sadness."	Wife is able to express normal grieving behaviours.
Observe wife's behaviour when with children. Wife discusses decisions that must be made.	Wife discusses decisions that must be made because of impending death of her husband. She allows the children to express their sadness.	Wife is able to express grief with family; maintains role as supportive mother.

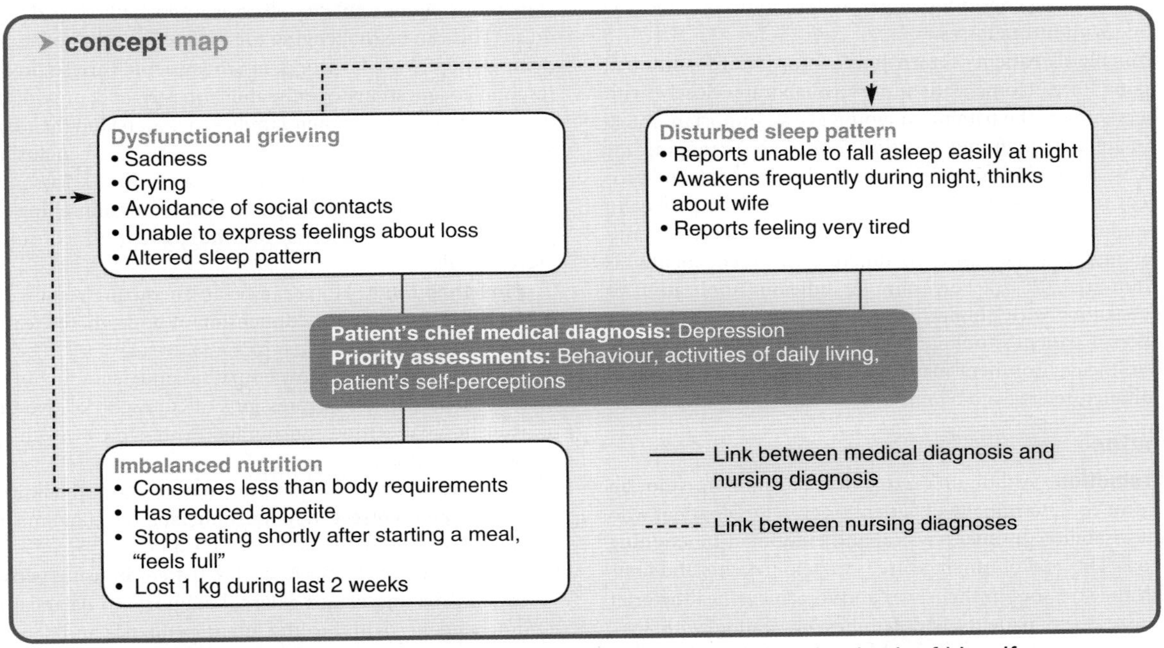

FIGURE 25-4 Concept map for a patient with depression after the death of his wife.

accommodating grief, accepting the reality of a loss, and renewing regular relationships. When a patient has a terminal illness, controlling pain and symptoms, maintaining autonomy, and achieving spiritual comfort are important goals. For the goal "achieving a sense of dignity for a parent diagnosed with cancer," expected outcomes might include the following:

- Patient will be able to continue parental responsibilities in care of toddler.
- Patient will express hopefulness that cancer treatment will control symptoms.
- Patient will engage in playing chess with friends on a weekly basis.

Setting Priorities. When a patient has multiple nursing diagnoses, the problems cannot be addressed simultaneously. At any given time, two or three problems dominate the nurse's attention. Figure 25-4 is a concept map developed for a patient with a medical diagnosis of depression after the death of his wife 6 months previously. As a result of the patient's medical condition, associated health problems include the nursing diagnoses *dysfunctional grieving, disturbed sleep pattern,* and *imbalanced nutrition: less than body requirements.* The nurse must determine which of the three diagnoses necessitates greater attention. The continuing grief experienced by the patient might be the focus. Until the patient is able to accept his loss and begin resolving his grief, he may be unable to attend to interventions that will improve his nutritional intake and sleep status.

Patients' conditions always change. In the ongoing assessment of a patient's condition, nurses can quickly discover a new problem. You must always consider which of the patient's most urgent physical or psychological needs require immediate intervention. The patient's expectations and preferences also need to be taken into account when determining the priorities of care. If a terminally ill patient's priorities include controlling pain and maintaining self-esteem, pain control is the priority when analgesics become ineffective and the patient experiences acute distress. If the patient is progressing as desired, you may refocus priorities to address unmet needs. For example, the patient suffering depression caused by his wife's death also has problems of imbalanced nutrition and disturbed sleep pattern. If the patient reports improved appetite and has shown weight stabilization since the last clinic visit, you can focus more attention on the sleep pattern disturbance. If a terminally ill patient places more emphasis on spiritual support than on other priorities, such as learning about planned treatments, you must attend to the patient's priorities. Meeting patient priorities may allow you to then address other needs more effectively with less effort.

Continuity of Care. Interdisciplinary teams work to help identify and meet the needs of people who experience losses. Dietitians, clergy, physicians, social workers, physiotherapists, psychologists, chaplains, and other specialty health care providers can assist a patient and family in their grief. A coordinated team approach to managing a patient's needs results in a well-managed care plan. When a patient of yours dies, the loss that you and your colleagues experience can be shared within the interprofessional group. Support is needed to promote healing for all who worked with the dying patient and the family. Conflicts and differences can be discussed openly and solutions found in a healthy manner with the patient as the primary focus. For example, ethical conflicts may have arisen related to proposed or performed medical treatments or interventions. Through working together, the sharing of experiences, feelings, alternatives, and solutions becomes the basis for dealing with future losses.

Many terminally ill patients return home and require continued intensive nursing care. Home care nurses collaborate closely with family members to meet the patient's ongoing needs. Important interventions to include in planning a return home are arranging for main-floor access, arranging appropriate medical equipment, and providing sufficient family respite. When it is realistic for the patient to remain independent, therapeutic strategies should bolster the patient's sense of autonomy and the ability to function as independently as possible (Virdun et al., 2015). For example, judicious application of orthotic devices, along with physiotherapy and occupational therapy, can often bolster a patient's functional capacity. In the home, safety issues related to the environment may exist, and patients often benefit from nurse-initiated referrals to community occupational therapists.

◆ Implementation

Health Promotion. Although a return to full function is not an expected outcome for a terminally ill patient or even for a patient who has significant disability, optimal physical and emotional functioning is a realistic goal. The goal of nursing care is to help patients and families cope with the stressors in their lives and to achieve healthy grief resolution. Nurses help patients and families in dealing with loss, making decisions about the patient's health care, and adjusting to any disappointment, frustration, and anxiety created by their loss.

Therapeutic Communication. Nursing care of the grieving patient and family begins with establishing a caring presence and determining the significance of their loss. This is difficult if the patient is unwilling or unable to express feelings or is experiencing numbing or denial. Therapeutic communication strategies can be used that enable patients to discuss their loss and find ways to work through it. A nurse's presence, attentive listening, and use of open-ended questions enable patients to freely share their thoughts and concerns. Closed-ended questions often reflect only what the person asking the question presumes is the problem. For example, in response to the question "Does knowing you have cancer make you fearful?" a patient will probably not reveal as much as to "Tell me how your diagnosis of cancer is making you feel." You should acknowledge the patient's grief and show support by demonstrating caring behaviours throughout the discussion (see Chapter 18). You will gain the patient's trust by showing a desire to enter into a caring, therapeutic relationship with the patient. Listening attentively to the patient can be very therapeutic for the patient, and you may discover details that help you plan effective care.

If a patient chooses not to share feelings or concerns, you should convey a willingness to be available when needed. If you are reassuring and respectful of the patient's need for dignity and privacy, a therapeutic relationship will probably develop. Sometimes patients need to begin resolving their grief before they can discuss their loss.

Some patients will not discuss feelings about their loss, or sometimes a patient does not want to discuss loss, symptoms, or impending death. In this case, you must observe for expressions of anger, denial, depression, or guilt. You must also know your own feelings before encouraging patients to express their anger. Individuals may express anger toward family, staff, or physicians. Patients can also become demanding and accusing. Nurses must remain supportive by letting patients and family members know that feelings such as anger are normal. For example, you might say, "You are obviously upset. I just want you to know I am here to talk with you if you want." You must avoid barriers to communication such as denying the patient's grief, providing false reassurance, or avoiding discussion of sensitive issues (see Chapter 17).

No topic that a dying patient wishes to discuss should be avoided. When the patient wants to talk, it is important for you to find time to do so. This can be challenging for a nurse with limited experience with dying patients or who works in a busy acute care setting. You should respond to questions openly and honestly and provide information that helps patients and their families to understand their condition, the trajectory or future course of their disease, the benefits and burdens of treatment, and values and goals (Topp, 2015). In some cases, you may recognize the need for pastoral care or counselling services, and you can initiate a referral for the patient to consult with such professionals.

Promoting Hope. Hope can be an energizing resource for patients experiencing loss. For each dimension of hope, there are nursing strategies that promote hope.

- *Affective dimension:* Show empathic understanding of the patient's strengths. Reinforce expressions of courage, positive thinking, and realistic goal setting. Encourage expression of both positive and negative feelings.
- *Cognitive dimension:* Offer information about the illness and treatments, and correct any misunderstanding or misinformation. Clarify or modify the patient's perceptions.
- *Behavioural dimension:* Assist the patient in using personal resources and making use of external supports to balance the need for independence with healthy interdependence and dependence.
- *Affiliative dimension:* Encourage patients to foster supportive relationships with others.
- *Temporal dimension:* Focus on short-term goals as life expectancy diminishes.
- *Contextual dimension:* Encourage development of achievable goals. Allow time to reminisce about achievements or positive moments.

Facilitating Mourning. Nursing care strategies can be used to help patients move through uncomplicated grief (Worden, 2009). The following guidelines are helpful for people who are mourning a death, facing death, or grieving over an actual loss:

- *Help the patient accept that loss is real.* Discuss how the loss or illness occurred or was discovered, when, under what circumstances, who told the patient about it, and other similar topics to help make the event real and to place it in perspective.
- *Support efforts to live without the deceased person or in the presence of disability.* A problem-solving approach is often helpful. Have patients or the family make a list of their problems, help them prioritize the problems, and then lead them step by step through a discussion of how they might tackle each one. Encourage them to rely on other family members, community resources, or other people who can help.
- *Encourage establishment of new relationships.* Many people fear that establishing new relationships would be disloyal. They need

reassurance that new relationships do not mean that they are replacing the person who has died. Encourage the patient to become involved in nonthreatening social relationships (e.g., religious gatherings, volunteer activities).

- *Allow time to grieve.* It is common to have "anniversary reactions" around the time of the loss in subsequent years. Some people worry that they are mentally or emotionally unstable when sadness or other signs of grief recur after a period of relative calm. Encourage the patient to reminisce.
- *Interpret "normal" behaviour.* Being distractible, having difficulty sleeping or eating, thinking one has heard the deceased's voice, or dreaming about the deceased are common after loss. These symptoms do not mean an individual has an emotional problem or is becoming ill in some way. Reinforce the fact that these occurrences are normal and will resolve over time.
- *Provide continuing support.* Patients and their families may need to talk and may look to you for support for many months or years after a loss. If you have occasion to see the patient or family after an extended time, it is appropriate to ask about how they are coping or adjusting. This gives them the opportunity to talk if they need to.
- *Be alert for signs of ineffective coping.* Be aware of coping mechanisms that may be maladaptive, such as increased alcohol or substance use, which can include excessive use of over-the-counter pain medications or sleep aids.

Acute Care.

Palliative Care. For people who face life-threatening illnesses, medical and technological advances are available to reverse the course of the disease or prolong life. For patients with serious life-limiting illness, it becomes important for health care providers to find ways to help patients approach the end of life. The aim of palliative care is to relieve suffering and improve the quality of living and dying (Stajduhar & Tayler, 2014). Not all patients and families who would benefit from palliative care services will receive them. Some patients and families will "leave no stone unturned" and therefore will not accept that the patient is dying. In situations where patients become suddenly ill or symptoms do not appear until late-stage terminal illness, the patient and family have not had time to grieve the loss and subsequently accept the impending death. In other cases, palliative care resources may be limited, may not be available in a timely manner, or may not be available at all.

Palliative care is for any age, any diagnosis, and at any time, not just during the last few months of life. Stajduhar and Tayler (2014) explain that when preservation of dignity becomes the goal of palliation, care options encompass the physical, psychological, social, spiritual, and existential aspects of the patient's illness. Palliative care thus allows patients to make more informed choices, better alleviate symptoms, and have more opportunity to manage unfinished business. Ferris, Balfour, Bowen, and colleagues (2013) designed the *Model to Guide Hospice Palliative Care,* which provides a comprehensive approach for palliative caregiving with nationally accepted principles and norms of practice.

According to the World Health Organization (2017), when health care providers supply palliative care, they do the following:

- Provide relief from pain and other distressing symptoms
- Affirm life and regard dying as a normal process
- Neither hasten nor postpone death
- Integrate psychological and spiritual aspects of patient care
- Offer a support system to help patients live as actively as possible until death
- Offer a support system to help families cope during the patient's illness and their own bereavement
- Enhance the quality of life

Stajduhar and Tayler (2014) add that palliative care also helps promote "early interventions aimed at having conversations with patients and their family members about their goals of care, comfort measures, and needs and wishes" (p. 144) and promote "applying the principles of palliative care earlier in the illness trajectory" (p. 144).

Palliative care is a philosophy of total care. A palliative care approach ensures that a patient experiences a "meaningful death," free of avoidable pain and suffering, in accordance with the patient's and family's wishes, and is the difference between technically competent symptom management and a holistic approach to end-of-life care (Stajduhar & Tayler, 2014). Palliative care is highly dependent on an interdisciplinary team–based approach, in which each team member has individual expertise and makes an individual commitment to common goals. The team includes physicians, nurses, social workers, pastoral care providers, physiotherapists, occupational therapists, and pharmacists. Massage therapists, music therapists, or art therapists—who provide alternative therapies—might also be a part of the team (see Chapter 35). Volunteers may be part of the team and can provide additional psychosocial support and simple comfort measures.

The Canadian Hospice Palliative Care Association Nursing Standards Committee (2014) has developed nursing standards of practice for hospice palliative care. The aim of these nursing norms is to ensure that knowledgeable and skilled caregivers are available and are supported. Goals of the guidelines include revealing any gaps in the care of a patient and giving guidance to management of the health care resources consistent with the palliative care philosophy.

Palliative care is compassionate care and supportive of dying people and their families. Nurses play a key role in providing care to the dying because of the intimate nature of the nurse's work and the fact that they are present with the patient and families, often for 8 or 12 hours at a time, depending on the context. Thus, one of the most important skills that you as a nurse in palliative care can provide is establishing a caring relationship with both patient and family. It also becomes very important for you to provide appropriate symptom-control measures for maintaining the patient's dignity and self-esteem, to prevent feelings of abandonment or isolation, and to provide a comfortable and peaceful environment at the time of death.

Symptom control. Comfort for a dying patient requires management of symptoms of disease and therapies. For many patients, symptom distress is characteristic of the dying experience (Lopera, 2015). *Symptom distress* is the experience of discomfort or anguish related to the progression of a disease. Patients experience anguish from not knowing or being unaware of aspects of their health status or treatment. Worry and fear are common among patients and may heighten their perception of discomfort. Nurses need to assess the character of a patient's symptoms carefully in order to select appropriate therapies. Chapter 31 details the assessment of pain. By providing information about treatment options or the anticipated course of an illness, nurses help preserve the dignity of patients and families (Griffiths et al., 2015). Complementary therapies are sometimes used for symptom management—for example, therapeutic touch, massage, aromatherapy, music therapy, biofeedback, homeopathy, acupuncture, and relaxation therapy. On occasion, patients may inquire about culture-specific complementary therapies. Many hospice programs offer complementary therapies, the most popular being massage, music therapy, energy healing, guided imagery, and aromatherapy. Chapter 35 discusses complementary therapies in more depth.

One symptom common among terminally ill patients is dyspnea (air hunger). The sense of suffocation can cause anxiety or panic in the patient and significant stress in the caregiver. As the patient's anxiety increases when he or she is unable to breathe adequately, the dyspnea worsens. Family who are in attendance and observing these changes may likely become more anxious as well. Topp (2015) has worked with family members of terminally ill patients and found that collaborative decision making, including the patient's views, helps the patient maintain a sense of control and decrease the emotional burden on the family related to decision making. For example, a patient may choose to switch oxygen devices, even though they deliver the same concentration of oxygen. However, if the patient believes that a different device makes a difference, the switch might be enough to relieve the dyspnea at least briefly. A patient who is breathing by mouth may receive more benefit from a mask than from a nasal cannula; however, a mask can also increase anxiety, which results in worsening dyspnea. When options in respiratory therapy exist, it helps to give the patient a choice.

Management of air hunger also involves the judicious administration of morphine and antianxiolytics for relief of respiratory distress. Table 25-4 summarizes nursing care measures for additional symptoms of terminal disease. Because therapies and clinical practice standards are constantly evolving, nurses must stay current in this area.

Maintaining dignity and self-esteem. The notion of dignity varies from patient to patient and between one circumstance and the next, and it is an overarching value or goal inherent in palliative care. Personal dignity may revolve around a person's positive sense of self-regard, is individualistic, and is closely linked with the patient's personal goals and social contexts (Virdun et al., 2015). Dignity may also revolve around the extent to which patients feel valued and how they are treated by caregivers.

Nurses can promote a patient's self-esteem and dignity by conveying respect for the patient as a whole person who has feelings, accomplishments, and passions independent of the illness experience (Ayyub, 2015). Giving importance to autonomy, acceptance, resilience, and maintaining hope acknowledges individual personhood; it also strengthens the empathic, therapeutic communication between the patient, the patient's family, and the nurse. Providing time for patients to share their life experiences, particularly about what has been meaningful, enables you as their nurse to know patients better. Knowing patients then facilitates choice of therapies that promote patient decision making and autonomy.

For many patients, receiving spiritual comfort helps preserve dignity and self-esteem. Facilitating connections to a spiritual practice or community and supporting the expression of culturally held beliefs are both very important. Patients may also benefit by being assured that some aspect of their lives may transcend death. In other words, the patient gains comfort from knowing that something of his or her life will continue after death. Participating in a life project such as making an audio or video recording for the family, writing letters, or keeping a journal can offer patients the comfort of knowing that something of their essence will survive (Virdun et al., 2015). Chapter 28 further discusses some of the spiritual practices and religious rituals that can support people in need of spiritual comfort.

Basic to promoting self-esteem and dignity is attending to the patient's appearance and surroundings. Cleanliness, absence of body odours, attractive clothing, and personal grooming all contribute to a sense of worth. When helping a patient tend to bodily functions, the nurse should always show respect, even when the patient becomes dependent. It is important to keep the patient's immediate surroundings pleasant by opening curtains and letting light change from the bright of day to the dark of night. The quick removal of liquid stool or vomitus will help avoid unpleasant odours.

Disabilities experienced by the patient may threaten dignity, especially when caregivers take control of the patient's life. Patients should be allowed to participate in nursing care decisions (e.g., how and when to administer personal hygiene, diet preferences, and timing of nursing therapies). The nurse should keep the patient and family well informed about planned therapies, their purpose, and anticipated effects. It is also important to provide the patient with privacy during nursing care procedures and when the patient and family need time together.

Preventing abandonment and isolation. Many terminally ill patients are fearful of dying alone. Therefore, it is important for you as their nurse to answer the call light quickly and to explain when staff will be giving care and performing assessments throughout the day and night. You should establish presence and use appropriate touch when performing care measures. You must be available to answer questions, even if data are not needed, no further decisions are left to make, or no further curative interventions are available (Virdun et al., 2015). Patients may feel a sense of involvement when sharing a room and interacting with staff. Patients can share conversation and companionship with roommates and visitors. The choice of private or shared room should be discussed with the patient and family whenever possible.

Family is always considered as the unit of care in palliative care. If family members have difficulty accepting the patient's impending death, they may avoid visitation, exhibit denial, or express unrealistic expectations. When family members do visit, it is important to talk with them and keep them informed of the patient's progress. It may be useful to give family members helpful hints about what to discuss with patients. For example, you can help improve a family member's communication skills by role-modelling attentive listening and offering reassurance. You should encourage the family to discuss activities other family members are involved in, reminisce about enjoyable times, and inquire about the patient's concerns. It is important to advocate for the patient to ensure that the patient does not become exhausted by visits. A useful strategy is to establish a schedule for family to be in attendance or to suggest family or friends visit two at a time. It is also helpful to find simple and appropriate care activities for the family to perform, such as feeding the patient, washing the patient's face, combing hair, and filling out the patient's menu. Older persons often become particularly lonely at night and may feel more secure if a family member stays at the bedside during the night. Visitors should be allowed to remain with dying patients at any time if the patient wants them. Also, nurses must know how to contact family members at any time if the patient requests a visit or if the patient's condition worsens.

Providing a comfortable and peaceful environment. At all times the patient should be kept comfortable through frequent and regular repositioning, keeping bed linens dry, and controlling extraneous environmental noise. Pictures, cherished objects, cards or letters from family members and friends, and plants and flowers create an environment that is more familiar and comforting. The nurse can offer the patient frequent back, lower leg, and foot massage, or guided imagery exercises, and allow the patient time to listen to preferred types of music. A comfortable, pleasant environment helps patients relax, which promotes the ability to sleep and minimizes severity of symptoms.

Fear of dying and death. People are afraid of dying and death for many different reasons: the process of dying, with its associated pain and loss of dignity; not knowing what will happen after death; and dying before fulfilling dreams and goals. The intensity of the fear varies with each person and his or her circumstances, including age, culture, sex, personal experiences, family situation, social supports, and religious beliefs. Lamprell-Josephs (2016) points out that nurses need to

TABLE 25-4 Promoting Comfort in Terminally Ill Patients

Symptoms	Characteristics or Causes	Nursing Interventions
Discomfort	Any source of physical irritation may worsen pain.	Provide thorough skin care—including daily baths, lubrication of skin, and dry, clean bed linens—to reduce irritants. Assess for appropriateness of special mattresses.
	As the patient approaches death, the mouth remains open, tongue becomes dry and edematous, and lips become dry and cracked.	Provide oral care at least every 2 to 4 hours. Use foam or premoistened swabs for frequent mouth care. Apply a light film of water-soluble lubricant to lips and tongue (see Chapter 38).
	Blinking reflexes diminish near death, which causes drying of the cornea.	Remove crusts from eyelid margins. Administer artificial tears to reduce corneal drying.
Fatigue	Metabolic demands of a cancerous tumour cause weakness and fatigue.	Help patient identify values or desired tasks; then help patient conserve energy for only those tasks. Promote frequent rest periods in a quiet environment.
	Exhaustion phase of the general adaptation syndrome causes energy depletion.	Time and pace nursing care activities (ensure periods of rest between blocks of care). Encourage use of energy-saving devices such as mobility aids.
Nausea	Nausea may occur as an adverse effect of medications and as a result of severe pain, as a symptom of certain illnesses, or as a result of palliative chemotherapy or radiation therapy.	Administer antiemetics: provide oral care at least every 2 to 4 hours; offer clear-liquid diet and ice chips; avoid liquids that increase stomach acidity, such as coffee, milk, and citric acid juices. Encourage high-calorie nutritional supplements (e.g., Ensure, Boost).
Constipation	Narcotic medications and immobility slow peristalsis.	Provide preventive care, which is most effective: increase fluid intake; include bran, whole-grain products, and fresh vegetables in diet; encourage exercise (see Chapter 42).
	Lack of bulk in diet or reduced fluid intake may occur with appetite changes.	Administer prophylactic stool softeners on a regular basis.
	Constipation can add to discomfort.	Administer laxatives as necessary.
Diarrhea	Diarrhea results from disease process (e.g., colon cancer), from complications of treatment or medications, or from fecal impaction caused by constipation.	Assess for fecal impaction (if sudden liquid stool occurs) and treat if required. Provide thorough perineal care if required. Administer antidiarrheals as needed. Confer with physician to change medication if possible. Provide low-residue diet.
Urinary incontinence	Incontinence results from progressive disease (e.g., involvement of spinal cord, reduced level of consciousness).	Protect skin from irritation or breakdown. Implement use of barrier creams to help protect skin integrity. Use disposable incontinence briefs if appropriate. Use in-dwelling urinary catheter or condom catheters if appropriate (see Chapter 43).
Inadequate nutrition	Nausea and vomiting can decrease appetite.	Serve smaller portions and bland foods, which may be more palatable. Encourage intake of nutritional supplements.
	Depression from grieving may cause anorexia.	Allow home-cooked meals, which may be preferred by the patient and gives the family a chance to participate in care.
Dehydration	As disease progresses, patient is less willing or able to maintain oral fluid intake.	Remove factors causing decreased intake; give antiemetics, and apply topical analgesics to oral lesions. Reduce discomfort from dehydration; provide mouth care at least every 4 hours; offer ice chips or moist cloth to lips.
Ineffective breathing patterns (e.g., dyspnea, shortness of breath)	Disease progression that involves lung tissue (e.g., progression of cancer, pneumonia, pulmonary edema) may affect breathing.	Treat or control underlying cause. For example, in some cases of pulmonary edema, a diuretic may be appropriate and may temporarily relieve symptoms. Provide reassurance and comfort measures to the patient. Place patient in a semi-Fowler's position, which will help.
	Anemia reduces oxygen-carrying capacity.	Maximize patient's oxygenation (e.g., place the patient in a semi-Fowler's position or upright; provide supplemental oxygen; maintain a patent airway; reduce anxiety or fever).
	Anxiety increases oxygen demand.	Administer medications such as bronchodilators, inhaled steroids, or narcotics and antianxiolytics to suppress cough, ease breathing, and alleviate apprehension.
	Fever increases oxygen demand.	Administer antipyretics as needed. Promote comfort through measures such as removing some clothing and bedding.
Confusion, disorientation, and restlessness	These manifestations may be caused by hypoxia, metabolic changes, brain metastases, or medication adverse effects.	Ensure a safe environment. Monitor patient frequently. Reorient the patient as needed. Administer medications as prescribed and as needed.

BOX 25-9 PATIENT TEACHING

Preparing the Dying Patient's Family

Objectives

- Improve the family's ability to provide appropriate physical care for the dying patient in the home.
- Improve the family's ability to provide appropriate psychological support to the dying patient.

Teaching Strategies

- Describe and demonstrate feeding techniques and selection of foods to facilitate the patient's ease of chewing and swallowing.
- Demonstrate bathing, mouth care, and other hygiene measures, and allow the family to perform return demonstration.
- Show the family a video on simple transfer techniques to prevent injury to themselves and the patient; help the family practise these techniques.
- Instruct the family on the need to take rest periods.
- Teach the family to recognize signs and symptoms to expect as the patient's condition worsens, and provide information on whom to call in an emergency.
- Discuss ways to support the dying patient, and listen to needs and fears.
- Solicit questions from the family, and provide information as needed.

Evaluation

- Ask the family members to demonstrate physical care techniques (e.g., turning, feeding, mouth care).
- Ask the family members to describe how they vary approaches to care when the patient has symptoms such as pain or fatigue.
- Ask the family to discuss how they feel about their ability to support the patient.

help patients realistically appraise these fears. Nurses also need to listen and understand as patients express their emotions.

Support for the Grieving Family. The family may be the primary caregivers when the patient chooses to die at home. Family members need support, and they benefit from being taught ways to care for their loved one (Box 25-9). Caring for a family member can be emotionally stressful and physically exhausting for the family caregiver. Not all families can manage care on their own. In the home setting, nurses provide the opportunity for the family to be temporarily relieved of duties so that they can rest. Such respite care is a resource available through hospice programs, in which respite workers can come into the home, or a patient can go to a facility for a respite stay.

Families also need to be informed of home care, hospice, and community service options so they can choose among the resources available. The Saint Elizabeth Health Care Foundation in Canada has sponsored a free-of-charge publication, *Family Hospice Care: Pre-Planning and Care Guide,* that is a practical and informative resource to help families meet the needs of terminally ill loved ones (van Bommel, 2006). Each province and health region has varying resources; therefore, nurses are required to know what is available to them in the individual family's jurisdiction. In some cases, families may need assistance and support in making the decision about placement in a health care facility.

Nurses must keep the family informed so that they can anticipate the type of symptoms the patient will probably experience and the implications for care. Family members should be encouraged to express their grief openly with the patient and to give the patient the opportunity to discuss any remaining concerns or requests. The family also needs personal time to share their concerns with nursing staff and to ask questions about treatment options, the course of the patient's disease, and the meaning of the patient's behaviours. It is wise for nurses to communicate news of the patient's impending death when the family is together, if possible, as family members can provide support for one another. The nurse should convey the news in a private area and be willing to remain with the family as needed. In some situations in which families are large or cannot all be together, it may be beneficial to have a designated family spokesperson or representative through whom information can be relayed.

It is also important to educate the family regarding the signs of impending death. Tissue perfusion becomes impaired, which results in cool and clammy skin. Alterations in heart rate or rhythms, hypotension, and pooling of blood in dependent areas may occur. The extremities often have a mottled appearance. Breathing patterns may be impaired. Patients may exhibit shortness of breath or increased secretions. Later signs include increasingly longer and more frequent periods of apnea, alternating with hyperpnea; this pattern is known as *Cheyne-Stokes respirations.* Patients may exhibit alterations in level of consciousness and changes in behaviour; for example, disorientation and restlessness may occur. Urine output decreases, and incontinence may occur. In addition, periods of sleep increase, and eventually some patients may become unconscious as death nears.

In the hospital setting, nurses assist in planning a visitation schedule for family members to keep the patient and family from excessive fatigue. Young children should visit dying parents. During the final moments of a patient's life, the nurse can help the family to stay in communication with the patient through their frequent visits, caring silence, attentive listening, touch, and telling the patient of their love. After the patient's death, the family should be encouraged to remain with the deceased for as long as they feel they need to. Nurses are required to provide support and assist the family with decision making, such as notification of a funeral home or mortician, transportation of additional family members, and collection of the patient's belongings.

Hospice Care. Hospice care is an alternative care delivery model for terminally ill patients. It is one phase of palliative care. **Hospice** is not necessarily a facility but a concept for family-centred care designed to assist the patient in being comfortable and maintaining a satisfactory lifestyle until death. Hospice services are available in the home, hospital, stand-alone facilities, and long-term care settings. Availability and accessibility vary across Canada. Hospice care programs include the following components:

- Patient and family as the unit of care
- Coordinated home care with access to beds in available inpatient and long-term care facilities
- Control of symptoms (physical, sociological, psychological, and spiritual)
- Physician-directed services
- Provision of an interdisciplinary care team of physicians, nurses, spiritual advisors, social worker, and counsellors
- Availability of medical and nursing services at all times
- Bereavement follow-up after a patient's death
- Use of trained volunteers for frequent visitation and respite support

Canada's first hospice was established in Toronto in 1979. Casey House in Toronto and the John Gordon home in London, Ontario, provide hospice care for people dying from AIDS. Canuck Place, in

Vancouver, was the first freestanding children's hospice in North America and provides a continuum of care that comprises three components: respite, palliative, and bereavement.

The nurse's role in hospice care is to meet the primary wishes of the dying patient and to be amenable to individual desires of each patient. Nurses support a patient's choice in maintaining comfort and dignity. Whether the patient ultimately dies at home or in a health care facility, the patient's wishes are followed as much as possible. When options are complicated by family needs, hospice professionals will try to work with the patient's wishes.

A hospice program emphasizes palliative care in which the patient and family are active participants. Patient care goals are mutually set, and all participants need to fully understand the options and desires of the patient. The hospice team attempts to meet the patient's desires and to encourage the family to stay within those guidelines. One or more bereavement visits are often made by the staff of the hospice team to the family even after the death of the patient, to help the family move through the grieving process successfully.

It is important that the hospice team know the patient's preference regarding where his or her death should take place. Many patients prefer to die at home in a familiar setting, whereas others, not wishing to burden their families, choose to die in a hospital or long-term care facility. Some families are ill-prepared or unable to care for a patient at home (Griffiths et al., 2015), and some patients suffer physical ailments that prevent them from being cared for at home. The health and welfare issues involved in hospice care are viewed from a broader perspective than just the patient's desires. The concern for family needs is also taken into consideration by the hospice team.

A patient receiving hospice care may be hospitalized because of a change in condition or exacerbation of symptoms, and the health care team coordinates care between the home and inpatient setting. An effort is always made to keep patients at home for as long as possible (or as long as they desire). The family provides basic supportive care. However, if the family cannot meet all of the patient's needs, a nurse is available to coordinate and administer symptom management therapies. The goal of the interdisciplinary team is 24-hour accessibility as needed. As a patient's death becomes imminent, members of the hospice team are available to give support to the patient and family.

Care After Death. When a patient dies in a hospital setting, nurses provide **postmortem care**. Nurses are responsible for coordination of all aspects of care surrounding a patient's death. Box 25-10 summarizes the nurse's and physician's responsibilities for care of the body after

BOX 25-10 PROCEDURAL GUIDELINE

Care of the Body After Death

Delegation Considerations

Care of the body after death can be delegated to unregulated care providers except in cases of organ or tissue donation. Check agency policy for which staff member is authorized to remove any invasive tubes or catheters.

Equipment

Bath towels, washcloths, wash basin, scissors, shroud kit with name tags, bed linen, room deodorizer, documentation forms

Procedure

1. Physicians must complete the death certificate: cause of death, time when death was pronounced, therapy used, and actions taken. In some provinces, such as British Columbia, nurses may pronounce the death but may not complete the death certificate. (This may not be the policy in all agencies. Follow your agency's policy.)
2. Physicians may request an autopsy, especially for deaths under unusual circumstances.
3. Trained staff members offer survivors the option of donating the organs or tissue of the deceased; personal, religious, and cultural needs should be included during this process.
4. Nurses work with sensitivity to preserve the patient's and family's dignity.
   a. Check orders for any specimens or special orders needed by the physician.
   b. Make arrangements for staff, spiritual advisor, or others to stay with the family while the body is being prepared for viewing; find out whether survivors have special requests for viewing (e.g., shaving, a special gown, Bible in hand, rosary at the bedside).
   c. Before shaving of male patient: Determine whether the family wishes the patient to remain unshaven if it was his custom to wear a beard. Determine whether patient's religion or culture has a preference regarding facial hair.
   d. Remove all equipment, tubes, supplies, and dirty linens according to agency protocol. Exceptions to this process include organ donation (leave support systems in place), and sudden or unexpected deaths that necessitate coroner involvement or investigation (leave tubings and lines in situ, but cut them near the body and clamp them).
   e. Cleanse the body thoroughly, apply clean sheets, and remove all trash from the room.
   f. Brush and comb the patient's hair. Apply any personal hairpiece.
   g. Position according to protocol: The eyes should be closed by gently holding the patient's eyelids closed for a few minutes; dentures should be in the patient's mouth to maintain facial alignment.
   h. Cover the body with a clean sheet up to the chin with arms outside covers if possible.
   i. Lower the lighting, and spray a deodorizer if possible to remove unpleasant odours.
   j. Give the family the option to view or not to view the dead body; clarify that either option is acceptable.
   k. If family members choose to view the dead body, go with them.
   l. Encourage the family to say goodbye through both touch and talk.
   m. Do not rush the goodbye process. Once the family is more comfortable, ask if they would like to be left alone. Remind them that they can call you if they need to.
   n. Clarify which personal belongings should stay with the body and who will take personal items; documentation requires both a descriptor of the objects (i.e., rings, jewellery, electronics) and the name of each person who received them, with the time and date.
   o. Do not discard items found after the family is gone; call the family and tell them what was found and ask who might pick it up. Descriptions of the articles help the patient's family make decisions accordingly.
   p. Apply name tags according to protocol, such as on the wrist, on the right big toe, or outside a shroud.
   q. Complete documentation in the nursing notes. Documents vary, depending on the agency (see Box 25-11).
   r. Remain sensitive to other hospitalized patients or visitors when transporting the body, such as covering the body with a clean sheet, temporarily and gently closing doors to patients' rooms, and watching to avoid visitors when moving the body to another part of the hospital or to the exit for the funeral home.
   s. Follow all protocol and policies to meet all legal requirements in caring for the body.

death. Nurses need to be familiar with institutional policies and procedures that are established for postmortem care. Many of these practices also depend on the individual's unique experiences and preferences. In all cases, it is important to care for the patient's body with dignity and sensitivity and in a manner consistent with the patient's religious or cultural beliefs. After death, the body undergoes many physical changes. For that reason, care must be provided as soon as possible to prevent tissue damage or disfigurement of body parts.

Patients' and families' cultural beliefs are very important in postmortem care (see Chapter 9). Maintaining the integrity of rituals and mourning practices helps families accept the patient's death and achieve inner peace. The ethical decisions that surround a patient's death are based on the values of a culture. Health care providers must determine the makeup of a family network and which members should be involved in decisions such as organ donation and end-of-life care.

Hospitals are required to formulate policies and procedures that are based on current provincial and territorial laws to validate death, identify potential organ or tissue donors, and provide postmortem care. For transplantation of organs, the patient must be maintained in a Critical Care Unit on ventilatory and circulatory support until vital organs are harvested. The family must clearly understand that the patient is "brain dead" and that the equipment (i.e., ventilator and vasopressor medications) is not keeping the patient alive but keeping the physical body in a state so that the organs will not be damaged before being harvested.

Support of the family is crucial at the time of the patient's death. If family members are not present at that time, the assigned nurse (or another staff member who knows the family) makes contact with the family. If you are the assigned nurse, you inform the family of the death and respond to any immediate questions from the family. It is important that you find out from the family whether they will come to the facility to view the deceased and to collect any personal belongings. Make a note of which family members will come and when. In some situations, family members may be too distraught to safely drive themselves and need to be encouraged to have someone else drive or to take alternative transportation. After a death, it is acceptable to lower the head of the bead, to straighten the body, and attempt to gently close the eyes and mouth. Once the family has arrived to view the deceased, it is beneficial, before they view the body, for the nurse to explain to the family what they may expect to see. Typically, a deceased person has a peaceful expression (as facial muscles have relaxed); however, the body feels cool to touch and appears greyish-white. Within several hours, the body begins to stiffen as rigor mortis sets in. The body may have areas of pooled blood that appear bruised. The eyes and mouth may be partially open, but mucous membranes will appear dry. This appearance may be difficult for some family members to observe.

Nurses can be very helpful in supporting families through the organ and tissue request process. It is important to provide a private area in which to discuss all issues with the family. The staff member designated to make a request, such as a formal transplant coordinator, a social worker, chaplain, or nurse, must offer the family clarification of what defines brain death because support systems must remain in place even after the patient is pronounced "dead" for vital organ retrieval (i.e., heart, lungs, kidneys, and liver). Nurses reinforce explanations throughout the organ retrieval process. The family must know who legally can give final consent, the options for organ or tissue donation, any associated costs, and how donation will affect burial or cremation. Nonvital tissues such as corneas, skin, long bones, and middle ear bones can be harvested when the patient is proclaimed dead, without artificially maintaining vital functions. If the patient did not make specific documented requests before death, the family must agree on organ and tissue donation. Nurses should review the organ retrieval laws in the family's province or territory, as well as the institution's policy and procedure regarding the formal consent process.

Another topic that can create tension or anxiety is autopsy. The physician usually asks for permission for an autopsy, but nurses are often the professionals who answer questions and support the family's choices. It is very difficult to approach a grieving family with such a request; ideally, the topics of autopsy and donation are discussed before the patient's death. The value of an autopsy is that it may improve knowledge in the field of medicine or bring answers or clarification for the family. To help the living, the autopsy can lead to new therapies or new understanding of diseases. The more reasons nurses can think of to support organ donation, tissue donation, or autopsy, the more the family will be helped to realize the good that can be accomplished by either donation or research autopsy.

The family becomes the primary patient when the actual death has occurred, and the shift of concern moves from the deceased patient to the living family. At this time, it is important to appropriately use the resources that are available. For example, pastoral care staff can be a helpful resource to assist the family even before the actual death, if no bereavement team is available. However, it is important to know whether the family chooses to have spiritual counsellors present. Some families prefer to grieve alone, whereas others may desire the support of other people. Social workers and counsellors can also offer assistance. If the family's expectations for support are unknown, any professional who assists the family can ask the simple questions and make suggestions for assistance.

Documentation of all the events surrounding a patient's death is important for avoiding misunderstandings and clarifying final events in a patient's life. Each facility's policies and procedures support legal guidelines that must be followed and accurately documented. Box 25-11 lists the content to be documented about end-of-life care. Documentation validates the success of meeting goals identified for the patient or provides a justification for failure to meet any goals. Complete and accurate documentation offers a summary of activities that can become the focus for risk management or legal investigations.

A physician or coroner must sign some of the medical forms, but the registered nurse must record most of the forms. Gathering of information for the forms may be delegated to unregulated care providers, but a nurse must chart the data in the nurse's notes. A licensed professional should witness the signing of forms.

BOX 25-11 Documentation of End-of-Life Care

The following items must be documented at the end of a patient's life:

- Time of death and actions taken to prevent death, or cardiac arrest record, if applicable
- The name of the person who pronounced the patient's death
- Any special preparation and type of donation, including time, staff, and company
- The name of the family member or friend who was called and who came to the hospital: donor organization, morgue, funeral home, chaplain, and individual family members making any decisions
- Personal articles left on the body and taped to skin, or tubes left in
- Personal items given to the family: specific names and descriptors of items
- Time of discharge and destination of the body
- Location of name tags on the body
- Special requests made by the family
- Any other statements that might be needed to clarify the situation

In cases of legal matters, the family expects a clear, concise description of what occurred in the care of the patient at the time of death. Opinions must be avoided, and facts are stated in a nonjudgemental, objective manner. Provincial and territorial guidelines direct the type of information that is to be charted and when it is to be charted. Patients have the right to access their health records. Copies of parts of the chart can be given to family members upon written request and the approval of the physician and hospital (see your employer's guidelines). Nurses must understand and uphold the legal guidelines of documentation at all times (see Chapter 15).

The Grieving Nurse. When nurses have cared for a patient for a period of time, it is possible to have deep personal feelings of loss and sadness when the patient dies. It is common for nurses to want to hold the hand of the patient who is dying. By being present at the time of the patient's death, nurses are able to "let go."

You, as a nurse, can attempt in many ways to cope with the loss of a dying patient. Attending the viewing at the mortuary or funeral is one way to say goodbye. Writing a letter of sympathy to the family can prove helpful. Some agencies routinely send out sympathy cards from the interdisciplinary team, in which you can write an individual note. It is natural for you to go through the grieving process. When you work in an area in which multiple losses occur, it is easy for bereavement overload to develop unless you have ways to process grief. You might feel frustration, anger, guilt, sadness, or anxiety. Often nurses seek out other nurses or health care providers to discuss their own grief (Figure 25-5). It is important for you to develop your own support systems that allow time away from the care setting and provide opportunities to share personal feelings.

Stress management techniques (see Chapter 29) can help restore a nurse's energy and continued enjoyment in caring for patients. Your self-care is crucial for your survival and recovery from loss, not only for your sake but also for the sake of future patients. Interdisciplinary team debriefings regarding complex or ethical issues are valuable in helping nurses cope with loss. Nurse managers and administrators have a responsibility to ensure that the working environment is supportive (Phillips, 2016).

◆ Evaluation

Patient Care. Nurses care for patients and families at every phase of the grief process. This requires nurses to remain aware of signs and symptoms of grief, even when patients are not specifically seeking care directly related to a loss. These signs and symptoms help in evaluation of whether a patient is able to deal with a loss and progress through the grief process. Critical thinking ensures that the evaluation process is thorough and relevant to the patient's situation (Figure 25-6).

In order for you to determine the effectiveness of nursing interventions, you must refer to the goals and expected outcomes established in the plan of care. By comparing actual patient behaviours with expected outcomes, you evaluate the patient's health status and whether the plan needs to be revised. For example, if the goal is to have the patient communicate a sense of hope with family members, you evaluate the verbal and nonverbal communication process for cues related to hope. The patient's responses indicate whether new therapies are needed or whether existing therapies should be revised. You would continue to evaluate the progress of the patient, the effectiveness of interventions, and the interactions between the family and patient. It

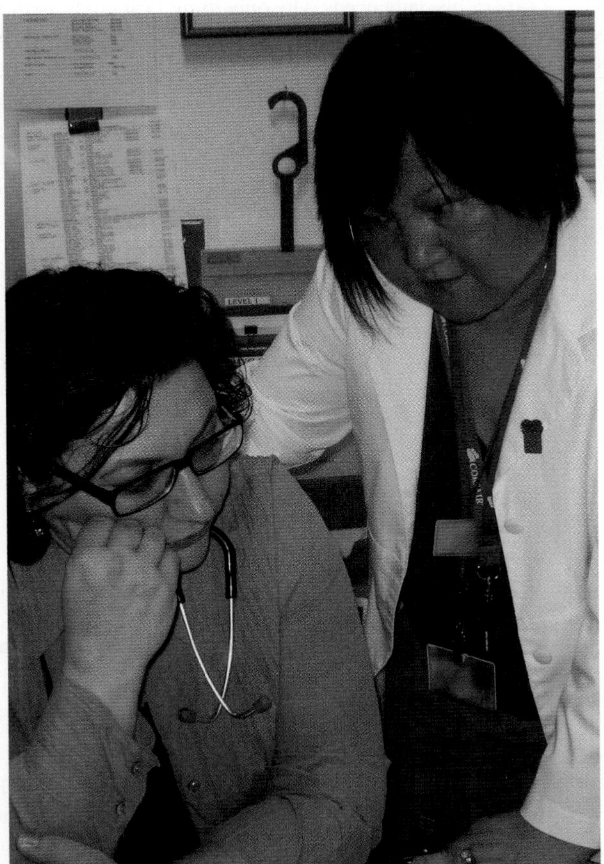

FIGURE 25-5 Nurses benefit from support of colleagues during their time of loss.

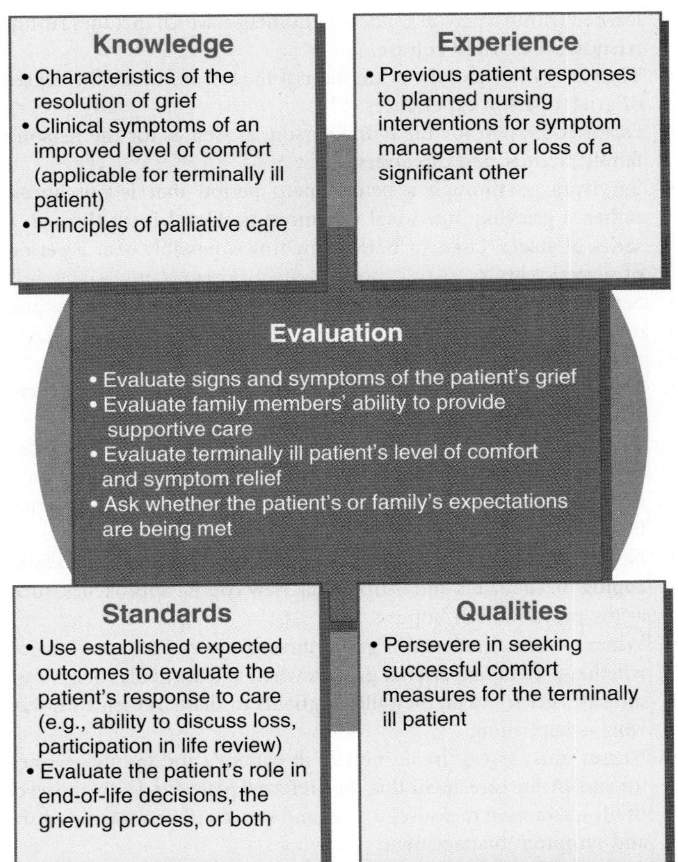

FIGURE 25-6 Critical thinking model for loss, death, and grieving evaluation.

is important for the patient and family to share experiences and be active participants in the evaluation process.

Patient Expectations. Patients expect individualized care, including relief of symptoms, preservation of dignity, and support of the family to maximize quality of life. The success of the evaluation depends partially on the bond that the nurse forms with the patient. If the patient does not trust you as the nurse, he or she is not likely to share personal expectations or desires with you. It thus becomes important for you to take the time to talk with the patient and learn whether expectations are being met. The following are examples of questions that will validate whether patient expectations have been achieved:

- "Am I helping you in the way you have hoped?"
- "Would you like me to assist you in a different way?"
- "Do you have a specific request that I have not yet met?"
- "What is most important for us to do for you at this time?"
- "Are we dealing with your problems in a timely manner?"

Through communication and evaluation, you can continue to determine whether outcome criteria were met to support the goals of care. It is often easy to evaluate the patient's needs, but evaluating the family's needs is more complex. Once rapport is established, you must be vigilant to avoid problems that threaten that rapport.

KEY CONCEPTS

- When caring for patients who have experienced a loss, nurses facilitate the grieving process by assisting survivors in feeling the loss, expressing the loss, and moving through the tasks of the grieving.
- Loss comes in many forms, depending on the values and priorities learned within a person's sphere of influence, which includes family, friends, society, and culture.
- The type of loss and the perception of the loss influence the degree of grief a person experiences.
- Death is difficult for the dying person, as well as for the person's family, friends, and caregivers.
- Survivors go through a bereavement period that is not linear; rather, a grieving individual will move back and forth through a series of stages, tasks, or both many times, possibly over a period of several years.
- Several theorists have formulated stages of the grieving process and a series of tasks for survivors to successfully complete their bereavement and adapt to life with a loss.
- Nurses' knowledge of the types of grief enables them to implement appropriate bereavement therapies.
- The way an individual perceives and responds to a loss is influenced by development, psychosocial perspectives, socioeconomic status, personal relationships, the nature of the loss, culture, and spiritual beliefs.
- Nursing interventions involve reinforcing patients' successful coping mechanisms and introducing new coping approaches, such as the promotion of hope.
- When assessing patients in grief, nurses must not assume how or whether patients experience grief or whether a particular behaviour indicates grief; rather, they allow patients to share in their own way what is happening.
- Nurses must assess the terminally ill patient's and family's wishes for end-of-life care, including the preferred place for death, the level of life-sustaining measures to use, and expectations regarding pain and symptom management.
- A plan of care is developed by integrating patients' resources such as physical energy and activity tolerance, supportive family members, spiritual faith, and methods for coping.
- Nurses need to establish a caring presence and use therapeutic communication strategies that enable patients to discuss their loss and find ways to manage it.
- Palliative care enables patients to make more informed choices, better alleviate symptoms, and have more opportunity to manage unfinished business.
- Nurses can promote a patient's self-esteem and dignity by conveying respect for the patient as a whole person.
- Hospice is not a facility but a concept for family-centred care designed to assist the patient in being comfortable and maintaining a satisfactory lifestyle until death.

CRITICAL THINKING EXERCISES

1. Mr. Singh visits the community health clinic and tells you, "I don't know what's wrong with me. I lost my wife 6 months ago and I still get angry that God let her die. I still miss her so much. I have been going out with friends, but I just don't enjoy it that much. Sometimes I wake up at night and I think my wife is still here. What is wrong with me? I thought I would be feeling better by now." How could you respond to Mr. Singh?
2. You are assigned to care for Mrs. Nester. She has bone cancer and has experienced ongoing deep pain in her back and hips, with some discomfort also in her lower extremities. Discuss the management of pain for Mrs. Nester.
3. A nursing colleague is discussing her patient with you. She says, "My patient is a 48-year-old man with a degenerative neurological disease. The disease is progressive. He is having trouble walking and taking care of his daily needs. The only thing I can do is assist him with bathing, feeding, and walking. He really is not a candidate yet for palliative care." What would be your response to your colleague?

REVIEW QUESTIONS

1. A child is grieving over the loss of a pet. This is an example of:
   1. An actual loss
   2. A perceived loss
   3. A situational loss
   4. A maturational loss
2. A middle-aged man comes to a community clinic for his annual flu shot. In the discussion, you learn that he still works at a local law firm. However, he has recently lost two important cases, and his boss has been pressuring him "to turn it around." The patient may be experiencing:
   1. An actual loss
   2. A perceived loss
   3. A situational loss
   4. A maturational loss
3. The community health nurse's job is to provide grief counselling for the residents of a community in which a major flood has occurred. The loss associated with flooding is best described as:
   1. An actual loss
   2. A perceived loss
   3. A situational loss
   4. A maturational loss
4. A patient has received a diagnosis of terminal brain cancer. When you visit him during rounds, he asks you whether the cancer could have been caused by something he ate or by exposure to some chemical toxin. The patient is probably experiencing:
   1. Bowlby's phase of numbing
   2. Kübler-Ross's stage of acceptance

3. Worden's tasks of emotionally relocating
4. Bowlby's phase of disorganization and despair

5. According to Kübler-Ross's stages of dying, a patient may feel overwhelmingly lonely and withdraw from interpersonal interaction during this phase:
   1. Denial
   2. Anger
   3. Bargaining
   4. Depression
6. Since the death of his wife, the patient has assumed full responsibility for the care of his children. He has noticed over the past few weeks that friends are calling less often. He is most likely in which of the following phases of mourning?
   1. Anticipatory grieving
   2. Worden's task 3 of mourning
   3. Kübler-Ross's phase of bargaining
   4. Bowlby's phase of disorganization and despair
7. Which of the following is one of the most common and difficult issues faced by older bereaved spouses?
   1. Adjusting to physical problems
   2. Overcoming mental health problems
   3. Completing the tasks of daily living
   4. Managing finances
8. "Patient will express hopefulness that cancer treatment will control symptoms" is an example of:
   1. A goal
   2. An intervention
   3. A plan
   4. An expected outcome
9. A 16-year-old patient has been admitted to the Critical Care Unit after suffering a closed-head injury. The patient is soon declared brain dead. The physician and nurse are preparing to approach the family to consider donation of the patient's heart and lungs. When working with families in this situation, it is important to explain that:
   1. The ventilator is being used to prevent brain death.
   2. The ventilator maintains organ perfusion until time for harvesting.
   3. Tissues such as corneas can be harvested only if the patient remains ventilated.
   4. Organ donation can occur only if the patient has made a request to donate organs in the past.
10. Which of the following types of care allows patients to make more informed choices, achieve better alleviation of symptoms, and have more opportunity to manage unfinished business?
   1. Acute care
   2. Mourning care
   3. Palliative care
   4. Terminal care

Answers: 1. 1; **2.** 2; **3.** 3; **4.** 4; **5.** 4; **6.** 2; **7.** 3; **8.** 4; **9.** 2; **10.** 3

Rationales for the Review Questions appear at the end of the book.

RECOMMENDED WEBSITES

Bereaved Families of Ontario: http://www.bereavedfamilies.net.
This website provides support programs and resources for people of all ages who have lost a family member.

Canadian Hospice Palliative Care Association (CHPCA): http://www.chpca.net/index.
The Canadian Hospice Palliative Care Association is a national organization that promotes excellence in care for people approaching death. One of its goals is to advocate for improved hospice palliative care policy, resource allocation, and supports for caregivers.

Edmonton Zone Palliative Care Program: http://www.palliative.org.
The objective of this program is to provide information to health care providers that will help them to reflect on their practice with persons who are terminally ill. This website offers palliative care tips, nursing notes, a caregiver guide, and links to publications and other resources.

Government of Canada, End of Life Care: http://www.hc-sc.gc.ca/hcs-sss/palliat/index-eng.php.
This federal government website includes information on the involvement of the federal government in palliative care and contains links to publications and other related resources.

Victoria Hospice: http://www.victoriahospice.org/.
This website has many useful resources and tools for families, patients, volunteers, and professionals. Literature may be downloaded and ordered from this site.

REFERENCES

Ayyub, R. (2015). An ethical challenge for health care professionals to answer the patient question: Am I dying? *I-managers Journal on Nursing*, *5*(1), 34–37.

Bowlby, J. (1980). *Attachment and loss: Vol. 3. Loss, sadness, and depression*. New York: Basic Books.

Broadhurst, K., & Harrington, A. (2016). A mixed method thematic review: The importance of hope to the dying patient. *Journal of Advanced Nursing*, *72*(1), 18–32. doi:10.1111/jan.12765.

Canadian Hospice Palliative Care Association Nursing Standards Committee (2014). *Hospice palliative care nursing standards of practice*. Ottawa: Canadian Hospice Palliative Care Association.

Canadian Nurses Association (CNA) (2015). *The palliative approach to care and the role of the nurse* [Position statement]. Ottawa: Author. Retrieved from https://www.cna-aiic.ca/~/media/cna/page-content/pdf-en/the-palliative-approach-to-care-and-the-role-of-the-nurse_e.pdf.

Canadian Nurses Association (2017). *Code of ethics for registered nurses*. Ottawa: Author.

College of Registered Nurses of British Columbia (CRNBC). (2016). *Medical assistance in dying*. Retrieved from https://www.crnbc.ca/Standards/resourcescasestudies/beinganurse/MAID/Pages/Default.aspx.

Corless, J. B. (2010). Bereavement. In B. R. Ferrel & N. Coyle (Eds.), *Textbook of palliative nursing* (3rd ed., pp. 597–611). New York: Oxford University Press.

Ek, K., Lars, W., Prahl, C., et al. (2014). Death and caring for dying patients: Exploring first-year nursing students' descriptive experiences. *International Journal of Palliative Nursing*, *20*(10), 509–515. doi:10.12968/ijpn.2014.20.10.509.

Ferris, F. D., Balfour, H. M., Bowen, K., et al. (2013). A model to guide patient and family care: Based on nationally accepted principles and norms of practice. *Journal of Pain and Symptom Management*, *24*, 106–123. doi:10.1016/S0885-3924(02)00468-2.

Gillick, M. R. (2009). Decision making near life's end: a prescription for change. *Journal of Palliative Medicine*, *12*(2), 121–125. doi:10.1089/jpm.2008.0240.

Granek, L. (2012). Disciplinary wounds: Has grief become the identified patient for a field gone awry? *Journal of Loss and Trauma*, *18*(3), 275–288. doi:10.1080/15325024.2012.688708.

Griffiths, J., Ewing, G., Wilson, C., et al. (2015). Breaking bad news about transitions to dying: A qualitative exploration of the role of the district nurse. *Palliative Medicine*, *29*(2), 138–146. doi:10.1177/0269216314551813.

Inbadas, H. (2016). History, culture and traditions, The silent spaces in the study of spirituality at the end of life. *Journal of Advanced Nursing*, *72*(1), 18–32. doi:10.3390/rel7050053.

Kübler-Ross, E. (1969). *On death and dying*. New York: Macmillan.

Lamprell-Josephs, S. (2016). Do spiritual beliefs influence coping mechanisms for dealing with death and dying? *European Journal of Palliative Care*, *22*(5), 248–251.

Léonard, C. (2016). Medical assistance in dying: What can nurses expect after. *Canadian Nurse*, *112*(4), 25–27. June 6.

Lopera, M. A. (2015). Nursing care of patients during the dying process: A painful professional and human function. *Investigación y Educación en Enfermería*, *33*(2), 297–304. doi:10.17533/udea.iee.v33n2a12.

McLellan, J. (2015). Religious responses to bereavement, grief, and loss among refugees. *Journal of Loss and Trauma*, *20*, 131–138. doi:10.1080/15325024.2013.833807.

Miller, E. (2015). The grieving process; A necessary step toward healing. *Association of Rehabilitation Nursing*, *40*(4), 207–208. doi:10.1002/rnj.220.

Morris, S., King, C., Turner, M., et al. (2015). Family carers providing support to a person dying in the home setting: A narrative literature review. *Palliative Medicine*, *29*(6), 487–495. doi:10.1177/0269216314565706.

National Consensus Project. (2013). *Clinical practice guidelines for quality palliative care* (3rd ed.). Retrieved from https://www.hpna.org/multimedia/NCP_Clinical_Practice_Guidelines_3rd_Edition.pdf.

Phillips, J. (2016). Exemplary nursing leadership is central to improving care of the dying. *Journal of Nursing Management, 24*(1), 1–3. doi:10.1111/jonm.12353.

Rice, A. (2015). Common therapeutic factors in bereavement groups. *Death Studies, 39*, 165–172. doi:10.1080/07481187.2014.946627.

Shear, M. (2015). Complicated grief. *New England Journal of Medicine, 372*, 153–160. doi:10.1056/NEJMcp1315618.

Shore, J., Gelber, M., Koch, L., et al. (2016). Anticipatory grief: An evidence-based approach. *Journal of Hospice and Palliative Nursing, 18*(1), 15–19. doi:10.1097/NJH.0000000000000208.

Simonsen, G., & Cooper, M. (2015). Helpful aspects of bereavement counselling: An interpretive phenomenological analysis. *Counselling and Psychotherapy Research, 15*(2), 119–127. doi:10.1002/capr.12000.

Somers, S., McLennan, M., & MacCourt, P. (2016). Education on grief, loss and dementia for family caregivers. *Canadian Nurse, 112*(7), 26–27.

Stajduhar, K., & Tayler, C. (2014). Taking an "upstream" approach in the care of dying cancer patients: The case for a palliative approach. *Canadian Oncology Nursing Journal, 24*(3), 144–148.

Topp, M. (2015). Comforting the dying. *Kai Tiaki Nursing New Zealand, 21*(4), 28.

van Bommel, H. (2006). *Family hospice care: Pre-planning and care guide.* Scarborough, ON: Resources Supporting Family and Community Legacies.

Virdun, C., Luckett, T., Davidson, P., et al. (2015). Dying in the hospital setting: A systematic review of quantitative studies identifying the elements of end-of-life care that patients and their families rank as most important. *Palliative Medicine, 29*(9), 774–796. doi:10.1177/0269216315583032.

Waldrop, D. (2007). Caregiver grief in terminal illness and bereavement: A mixed methods study. *Health and Social Work, 32*, 197–206.

Wilson, O., Avalos, G., & Dowling, M. (2016). Knowledge of palliative care and attitudes toward nursing the dying patient. *British Journal of Nursing, 25*(11), 600–605. doi:10.12968/bjon.2016.25.11.600.

Worden, J. W. (1991). *Grief counseling and grief therapy: A handbook for the mental health practitioner* (2nd ed.). New York: Springer.

Worden, J. W. (2009). *Grief counseling and grief therapy: A handbook for the mental health practitioner* (4th ed.). New York: Springer.

World Health Organization. (2017). *WHO definition of palliative care.* Retrieved from http://www.who.int/cancer/palliative/definition/en/.

26

Self-Concept

Canadian content written by Judee E. Onyskiw, RN, BScN, MN, PhD
Original chapter by Victoria N. Folse, APN, PMHCNS-BC, LCPC, PhD

OBJECTIVES

Mastery of content in this chapter will enable you to:

- Define the key terms listed.
- Discuss factors that influence the following components of self-concept: identity, body image, and role performance.
- Identify stressors that affect self-concept and self-esteem.
- Describe the components of self-concept as related to psychosocial and cognitive developmental stages.
- Explore ways in which a nurse's self-concept and nursing actions can affect a client's self-concept and self-esteem.
- Incorporate research findings to promote evidence-informed practice for identity confusion, disturbed body image, low self-esteem, and role conflict.
- Examine cultural considerations that affect self-concept.
- Apply the nursing process to promote a client's self-concept.

KEY TERMS

Body image, p. 460
Identity, p. 459
Identity confusion, p. 463
Role ambiguity, p. 463
Role conflict, p. 463
Role overload, p. 463
Role performance, p. 460
Role strain, p. 463
Self-concept, p. 457
Self-esteem, p. 461
Sick role, p. 463

MEDIA RESOURCES

http://evolve.elsevier.com/Canada/Potter/fundamentals/

- Audio Chapter Summaries
- Examination Review Questions
- Concept Map Creator
- Case Study with Questions
- Audio Glossary
- Content Updates
- Video Clips

Self-concept is the mental image that one has of oneself. It is subjective and a complex mixture of conscious and unconscious thoughts, attitudes, and perceptions that a person has about his or her own identity. *Self-concept and self-esteem* are two independent but related terms that are often used interchangeably, but in fact, there is a difference in the meanings of these terms. *Self-concept* is often considered the cognitive aspect of self, whereas *self-esteem* refers to the affective or emotional aspect of self. Self-esteem refers to the extent to which we like, accept, approve of, or value ourselves. In other words, self-concept asks the question "Who am I?" whereas self-esteem really focuses on "Am I worthy?" Nurses facilitate communication and ensure that the nursing care plan is individualized to meet each client's needs when these terms are used appropriately.

Self-concept comprises several domains: social, emotional, physical, and academic. Self-concept affects how people adapt to health challenges, difficult situations, and relationships. Individuals with a positive self-concept and self-esteem are better able to cope with illness and stressful life circumstances and events. They are also more likely to choose healthy behaviours and participate in activities to promote their health and prevent illness.

Nurses care for clients with a variety of health problems that can threaten their self-concept and self-esteem. The loss of a bodily function, a decline in activity tolerance, and difficulty managing a chronic illness are all situations that can potentially affect a client's self-concept. Nurses need to assess clients to determine if they have a healthy self-concept and to develop nursing strategies to meet a client's needs. Nurses play a vital role in helping clients adjust to alterations in self-concept and in supporting components of self-concept that enable clients to cope with difficulties.

SCIENTIFIC KNOWLEDGE BASE

The development of self-concept and self-esteem is a lifelong process, beginning in early childhood and continuing across the lifespan. In general, self-concept and self-esteem levels are high in childhood, decrease in adolescence, rise gradually throughout adulthood, peak at about 50 to 60 years, and then decline in old age (Orth & Robins, 2014; Trzesniewski, Donnellan, & Robins, 2013). The development of a child's self-concept is influenced by interactions with parents and other family members, as well as relationships with others such as teachers and friends. Other factors that influence the development of self-concept are the child's gender, developmental stage, socioeconomic status, culture, and environment (Figure 26-1). Young children start out with reasonably high levels of self-concept (Orth & Robins, 2014;

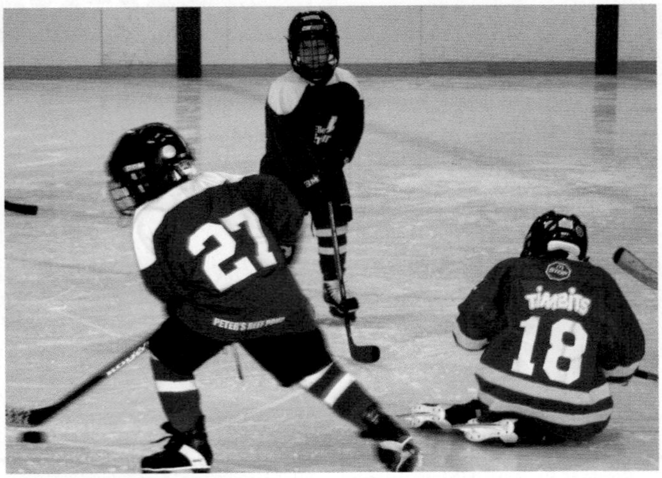

FIGURE 26-1 Participating in group activities can foster children's self-esteem. (From https://morguefile.com/search/morguefile/3/hockey/pop.)

Zeigler-Hill & Myers, 2012). In childhood, children tend to rate themselves higher on measures of self-concept than they rate other children, which is perhaps a reflection of their egocentric view of the world. The biological, social, and cognitive changes of late childhood take a toll on children's positive view of themselves. Self-concept begins to decline by preadolescence and gender differences appear. Adolescence is a particularly critical time, when many factors affect self-concept. The adolescent experience appears to adversely affect girls more than boys (Trzesniewski et al., 2013). For girls, adolescence brings overt physical changes, such as the development of breasts, a gain in body fat, and the onset of menarche with its associated symptoms. As a result, adolescent girls may be more sensitive to their appearance and how others view them. For boys, there are no sudden physical changes to indicate puberty. Maturational changes are generally regarded as more positive.

Self-esteem generally increases from adolescence to middle adulthood. A large number of studies using different samples and measures provide evidence that both men and women show age-related increases in self-concept and self-esteem from late adolescence to middle adulthood, with men reporting higher levels of self-esteem than women (for reviews, see Orth & Robins, 2014; Trzesniewski et al., 2013). Job satisfaction and job performance are linked to self-esteem. When individuals lose a job, they lose their position-related identity, and their self-perceptions may be altered or diminished. They may not be motivated to be active socially or may even become depressed. Underemployment also can affect role identity and self-esteem (McKee-Ryan, 2011). A developmental goal of adulthood is to establish a sense of self that is stable and transcends relationships and situations.

In older persons, self-concept declines and the gender gap narrows and may even disappear (Orth & Robins, 2014; Zeigler-Hill & Myers, 2012). The sense of self may be negatively affected by declines in health, cognitive abilities, and socioeconomic status associated with aging. When older persons develop a health problem or lose a partner, for example, they may experience negative changes in independence or social interaction. These changes may alter their perceptions of themselves.

Ethnic and cultural differences in self-concept and self-esteem have also been demonstrated. Findings from cross-cultural research show similarities with previous research from Westernized samples that show age and gender differences in self-concept and self-esteem (Orth & Robins, 2014). Across all nations, males consistently reported higher levels of self-esteem than did females, and both men's and women's self-esteem increased from late adolescence to middle adulthood. Despite these broad cross-cultural similarities, the cultures differed significantly in the magnitude of the age and gender differences. These differences were associated with cultural differences in socioeconomic, sociodemographic, gender-equality, and cultural value indicators (Bleidorn, Arslan, Denissen, et al., 2016). Nurses must be sensitive to factors that affect self-concept and self-esteem in the diverse cultures that make up the fabric of Canadian society, in order to ensure a patient-centred approach to nursing care.

Individuals' perceptions of themselves and of their health are closely related. Clients' beliefs about their personal health can enhance their self-concept. Statements such as "I can get through anything" or "I've never been sick a day in my life" indicate that a person's thoughts about personal health are positive. Self-concept is also affected by illness, hospitalization, and surgery. Chronic illness may affect the ability to provide financial support, thereby affecting an individual's self-esteem and perceived roles within the family. Negative perceptions regarding health status may be reflected in such statements as "It's not worth it anymore" or "I'm just a burden to my family." Chronic illness can affect identity and body image. This is reflected in statements such as "I'll never get any better" or "I can't stand to look at my body this way."

What individuals think and how they feel about themselves affect the way they care for themselves physically and emotionally and the way they care for others. How a person behaves is generally consistent with both self-concept and self-esteem. Individuals who have poor self-concept and poor self-esteem often do not feel in control of situations and may not feel worthy of care, which can influence decisions regarding health care. Knowledge of variables that affect both self-concept and self-esteem are crucial for providing effective treatment.

NURSING KNOWLEDGE BASE

Knowledge developed from medical and social sciences, humanities, and psychology, as well as knowledge from nursing research and clinical practice, is used to provide clients with evidence-informed practice. This broad knowledge base allows nurses to have a holistic view of clients, which promotes quality client care that best meets the self-concept needs of each client.

Development of Self-Concept

Self-concept develops throughout the lifespan and involves many factors. Erik Erikson's psychosocial theory of development (1963) helps us understand key tasks that individuals face at various stages of development. Each stage builds on the tasks of the previous stage, and successful mastery of each stage leads to a positive sense of self (Box 26-1).

Most individuals master each stage; however, individuals can regress during times of major stress or illness. Nurses learn to recognize an individual's failure to achieve an age-appropriate developmental stage or an individual's regression to an earlier stage in a period of crisis. This understanding enables nurses to individualize care and determine appropriate nursing interventions. Self-concept is always changing and is based on the following:

- Sense of competency and mastery of prior and new experiences
- Perceived reactions of other people to one's body
- Ongoing perceptions and interpretations of other people's thoughts and feelings
- Personal and professional relationships

BOX 26-1 Self-Concept: Erikson's Developmental Tasks

Trust Versus Mistrust (Birth to Age 1 Year)
Develops trust from consistency in caregiving and nurturing interactions of parents and others
Distinguishes self from environment

Autonomy Versus Shame and Doubt (Ages 1 to 3 Years)
Begins to communicate likes and dislikes
Is increasingly autonomous in thoughts and actions
Appreciates body appearance and function
Develops self through modelling, imitation, and socialization

Initiative Versus Guilt (Ages 3 to 6 Years)
Takes initiative
Identifies with a gender
Gains enhanced self-awareness
Increases language skills, including identification of feelings
Is sensitive to family feedback

Industry Versus Inferiority (Ages 6 to 12 Years)
Incorporates feedback from peers and teachers
Increases self-esteem with new skill mastery (e.g., reading, math, sports, music)
Experiences strengthening of sexual identity
Is aware of strengths and limitations

Identity Versus Role Confusion (Ages 12 to 20 Years)
Accepts body changes and maturation
Examines attitudes, values, and beliefs; establishes goals for the future
Feels positive about expanded sense of self
Interacts with people whom he or she finds sexually attractive or intellectually stimulating

Intimacy Versus Isolation (Ages Mid-20s to Mid-40s)
Has intimate relationships with family and significant others
Has stable, positive feelings about self
Experiences successful role transitions and increased responsibilities

Generativity Versus Self-Absorption (Ages Mid-40s to Mid-60s)
Accepts changes in appearance and physical endurance
Reassesses life goals
Shows contentment with aging

Ego Integrity Versus Despair (Ages Late 60s and Older)
Feels positive about own life and its meaning
Is interested in providing a legacy for the next generation

- Collective beliefs and images one holds about oneself
- Academic and employment-related identity
- Racial and ethnic identity
- Gender and sexual identity
- Personality structure
- Perceptions of events that have an impact on the self
- Personal appearance and physical attractiveness
- Current feelings about the physical, emotional, and social self
- Self-expectations

Components and Interrelated Terms of Self-Concept

A positive self-concept provides a sense of meaning, wholeness, and clarity. A healthy self-concept has a high degree of stability, generates positive feelings toward the self, and helps individuals adapt positively to stressors. There are many components of self-concept. Social scientists refer to a bundle of interrelated concepts when speaking of self-concept. Those particularly relevant to nurses are identity, body image, and role performance.

Identity. Identity involves the internal sense of individuality, wholeness, and consistency of a person over time and in various circumstances. Our identity distinguishes us from others. Identity is influenced by age, gender, sexuality, social class, ethnicity, and culture. Establishing an individual identity is an important developmental task from childhood to adolescence to young adulthood. Identity develops over time and ends in the "uniqueness" of each individual. A child learns culturally and socially accepted values, behaviours, and roles through observing other people and modelling their behaviour. Identity is often gained from self-observation and from what individuals are told about themselves (Stuart, 2013). A child first identifies with parental figures and later with teachers, peers, and role models. To form an identity, a child must be able to integrate learned behaviours and expectations into a coherent, consistent, and unique whole (Erikson, 1963).

Achieving one's identity is necessary for developing intimate relationships, because individuals express identity in relationships with others (Stuart, 2013). Sexuality is part of one's identity. Gender identity is a person's internal psychological sense of being male or female and includes a person's sexual orientation. It is one of the most central aspects of self-concept (Rathus, Nevid, Fichner-Rathus, et al., 2016). This image and its meaning depend on culturally determined values of gender-appropriate behaviour that are affected by socialization (see Chapter 22). Gender identity is a complex concept that is based partly on a person's anatomy (i.e., sexual organs), and partly on the psychology of the individual, which is influenced by culture and tradition.

Traditionally, children have been raised to have a female or male gender identity in accordance with their assigned genital anatomy. This rigidity in how society classifies gender is referred to as *gender binary*, a classification system that assumes either a male or female gender identity and ignores the fact that there are variations in gender identification (Rathus et al., 2016). While most people identify with the sexual anatomy they were born with, other individuals do not identify with their sexual anatomy and struggle to find an expression of their gender identity that is comfortable for them. *Transgender* is the term used to describe individuals whose gender identity, expression, or behaviour differs from those typically associated with their assigned sex at birth (Rathus et al., 2016).

Religious faith also may foster identity formation through participation in traditions and rituals (Blazek & Besta, 2012). Associating with others in a religious community provides strong identity experiences that influence an individual's sense of self.

Racial-ethnic or cultural identity is a sense of commitment or belonging to an identified racial or ethnic group, as well as participation and pride in its cultural traditions. Racial or cultural identity develops from identification and socialization within an established group, as well as through the experience of integrating the response of individuals outside the cultural or racial group into a person's sense of self. Differences in ethnic identity (e.g., Polish Canadian, Lebanese Canadian) exist through participation in traditions, customs, and rituals. The evolution of cultural identity may be challenging for some individuals. For example, the children of Chinese immigrants who are

BOX 26-2 CULTURAL ASPECTS OF CARE

Racial and Cultural Background

Racial and cultural identity are important components of a person's self-concept. Early in growth and development, an individual develops racial and cultural identity within the family context. As the individual grows, the cultural aspects of their self-concept may be reinforced through family, social, cultural, or religious experiences. An individual's self-concept may be strengthened or challenged through political, social, or cultural influences experienced in school or work environments. Positive or negative cultural role modelling and past experiences also influence self-concept.

Implications for Practice

- To improve a client's self-concept, develop an open, nonrestrictive attitude when assessing for and encouraging cultural or religious practices.
- Ask clients what they think is important to help them feel better or gain a stronger sense of self.
- Encourage cultural identity by individualizing self-care practices, dietary choices, and clothing to meet each client's self-concept needs.
- Facilitate culturally sensitive health promotion activities identified through evidence-informed practice that address at-risk behaviors (such as smoking, substance abuse, premature sexual experiences).

Neblett, E., Terzian, M., & Harriott, V. (2010). From racial discrimination to substance abuse: The buffering effects of racial socialization. *Child Development Perspectives, 4,* 131–137; Trzesniewski, K., Donnellan, B., & Robins, R. W. (2013). Development of self-esteem. In V. Zeigler-Hill (Ed.), *Self-esteem* (pp. 60–79). New York: Psychology Press; Usborne, E., & Taylor, D. M. (2010). The role of cultural identity clarity for self-concept clarity, self-esteem, and subjective well-being. *Personality and Social Psychology Bulletin, 36*(7), 883–897.

born in Canada may experience two different environments on a daily basis—a traditional Chinese home and a largely White school environment. Indigenous peoples recognize the pivotal role of personal and cultural identity and the losses suffered due to governmental practices that forced assimilation with the dominant Canadian culture, such as removing children from their parents and communities to attend residential schools. Indigenous peoples have engaged in strategies to reclaim their culture by revitalizing their language, history, customs, and the traditional practices that support their identity (Usborne & Taylor, 2010, p. 895). See Chapter 10 for further discussion of Indigenous identity. A strong racial-cultural identity generally buffers against the effects of prejudice and discrimination (Neblett, Terzian, & Harriott, 2010) and is positively related to self-concept, self-esteem, and psychological health and well-being and engaging in positive health practices (Usborne & Taylor, 2010). Cultural differences in self-concept exist and may also demonstrate some age- and gender-specific trends (Box 26-2).

Body Image. Body image involves attitudes related to the body, including physical appearance, structure, or function. Feelings about body image include those related to femininity and masculinity, youthfulness, sexuality, health, and vitality. These mental images are not always consistent with a person's actual physical structure or appearance. Some body image distortions have psychological origins, such as those that occur in an eating disorder (e.g., anorexia nervosa). Other alterations occur as a result of situational events, such as an amputation of a limb as a result of trauma or a scar due to surgery.

The majority of men and women experience some degree of body dissatisfaction, which can affect body image and overall self-concept. Disturbances in body image can be exaggerated when a change in health status occurs. The way other people view a person's body and the feedback offered are also influential. For example, a controlling, violent husband might tell his wife that she is ugly and that no one else would want her. Over time, with repeated humiliation and degradation, she may incorporate this devalued image into her self-concept.

Body image is affected by cognitive growth and physical development. Normal developmental transitions such as puberty or menopause can affect body image. Body image is influenced by hormonal changes during adolescence. The development of secondary sex characteristics and changes in body fat distribution affect an adolescent's self-concept. In the older adult, changes associated with aging, such as decreasing visual acuity and hearing, can affect body image.

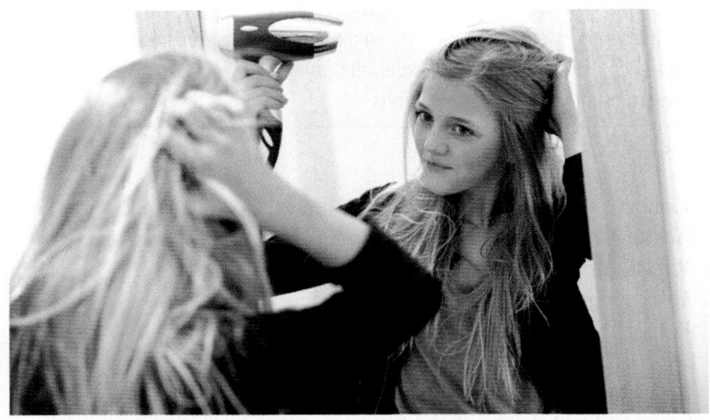

FIGURE 26-2 An individual's appearance influences self-concept. (From iStock.com/stocknroll.)

Cultural and societal attitudes and values also influence body image. Culture and society dictate accepted norms for body image that can influence a person's attitudes (Figure 26-2).

Values such as ideal body weight and shape, as well as attitudes toward body markings, piercing, and tattoos, are culturally based. In North American culture, people have been socialized to fear the aging process. Youth, beauty, and vitality are emphasized in actors who appear in television programs, movies, and advertisements. The media play an important role in creating and perpetuating unrealistic standards of thinness, youth, and physical attractiveness that are difficult or impossible for individuals to attain. Exposure to societal messages that reflect the sociocultural norm has been shown to have a negative impact on both females and males (Spurr, Berry, & Walker, 2013).

Body image depends only partly on reality. When physical changes occur, individuals may or may not incorporate these changes into their body image. For example, people who have experienced significant weight loss may not perceive themselves as thin and thus may have a distorted body image. Body image issues are often associated with impaired self-concept and self-esteem.

Role Performance. Role performance is the way in which individuals perceive their ability to carry out significant roles. Common roles include parent, child, spouse, employee, and student. Some roles are temporary (e.g., student or client role) while others are permanent (e.g., child or parent). An individual's perception of competency in a role may or may not match other people's evaluation. Roles that individuals follow in given situations involve socialization to expectations or standards of behaviour. Individuals learn behaviours that are approved by society through the following processes:

- *Reinforcement-extinction:* Certain behaviours become common or are avoided, depending on whether they are approved and reinforced or are discouraged and punished.
- *Inhibition:* An individual learns to refrain from certain behaviours, even when tempted to engage in them.
- *Substitution:* An individual replaces one behaviour with another, which provides the same personal gratification.
- *Imitation:* An individual acquires skills or behaviours by observing and then imitating the skills and behaviours of other members of the family or other social or cultural groups.
- *Identification:* An individual internalizes the beliefs, behaviours, and values of role models into a personal, unique expression of self.

Ideal societal role behaviours are often hard to achieve in real life. Individuals have multiple roles and personal needs that often conflict. For example, an individual may be a mother of small children, a daughter of elderly parents, a student, and an employee. Each role involves meeting certain expectations. To function effectively in multiple roles, a person must know the expected behaviour and values, desire to conform to them, and be able to meet the role requirements. Successful adults learn to distinguish between ideal role expectations and realistic possibilities. Fulfillment of these expectations leads to an enhanced sense of self. Difficulty or failure in meeting role expectations leads to deficits in the sense of self and often contributes to decreased self-esteem or altered self-concept.

Self-Esteem. **Self-esteem** is an individual's overall sense of self-worth or the emotional appraisal of self-concept. It represents the overall judgement of personal worth or value. Self-esteem is positive when a person feels capable, worthwhile, and competent (Rosenberg, 1965). Self-esteem is shaped by the individual's appraisals of how he or she is perceived by significant others.

According to Erikson (1963), young children begin to develop a sense of usefulness or industry by learning to act on their own initiative. Children's self-esteem is related to their personal evaluation of their effectiveness at school, within the family, and in social settings. The evaluation of other significant people such as parents, teachers, and peers has a profound influence on children's self-esteem.

Global self-esteem levels tend to be highest in childhood, possibly because children's sense of self is inflated by a variety of positive sources (Orth & Robins, 2014). Self-esteem tends to decline in adolescence. This may be partially understood in the context of maturational changes associated with puberty and increased expectations associated with the transition from primary to secondary school. This decline may also be associated with a shift to more realistic information about the self. Some gender differences exist in the adolescent years, with boys reporting greater self-esteem than girls (Bleidorn et al., 2016; Orth & Robins, 2014).

Several factors have been shown to be positively associated with self-esteem in adolescents: for example, family cohesion, greater number of siblings, parental support, and social and emotional support from other adult role models (Orth & Robins, 2014). Supportive and caring relationships will help foster self-esteem in adolescents. Other factors related to greater self-esteem include family income above the poverty level, safe and nurturing environments, and religious community. Participating in physical activity that is developmentally appropriate and enjoyable can lead to positive self-esteem in adolescents (Beasley & Garn, 2013; Guèvremont, Findlay, & Kohen, 2014).

Self-esteem levels rise gradually during adulthood and decline sharply in old age (Orth & Robins, 2014). In general, this pattern holds true across gender, socioeconomic status, and ethnicity. Erikson's (1963) emphasis on the generativity stage (see Chapter 21) may explain the increase in self-esteem and self-concept in adulthood. The individual is focused on being increasingly productive and creative at work, while at the same time promoting and guiding the next generation. Other than childhood, the mid-60s represents the highest level of self-esteem across the lifespan. At around 70 years of age, self-esteem declines sharply, which, according to Erikson's theory of psychosocial development (1963), reflects a diminished need for self-promotion and a shift in self-concept to a more modest and balanced view of the self.

Safety Alert Adolescence marks a time when youth begin to experiment with risky behaviours, such as engaging in substance abuse, premature sexual activity, and unprotected sex. These risks threaten adolescents' health and have implications for health care interventions. A decline in self-esteem during adolescence is often associated with an increased need for attention, which may be demonstrated by engaging in risky behaviours. In addition, the influence of peers is strong during adolescence. Research has shown, however, that adolescents with a stronger sense of identity are not as susceptible to the influence of peers, and are not as likely to engage in risky behaviours as are adolescents with a weaker sense of identity (Dumas, Ellis, & Wolfe, 2012).

To better understand self-esteem, consider the relationship between a person's self-concept and the ideal self. The *ideal self* is a representation of the attributes the person would like to have—an image of the person ideally. The ideal self acts as a motivator that gives the individual an incentive for future behaviour—providing an image of what he or she wants to be or not be. The ideal self is also used as a standard to evaluate the actual self. The ideal self originates in the preschool years and develops throughout life. Early in life, parents set ideals for their children to have certain attributes, such as honesty, intelligence, and success. Through socialization practices, children often internalize their parents' ideals. The ideal self is also influenced by other factors, such as school, peer relations, and the media. Self-evaluation is an ongoing mental process. In general, a person whose self-concept comes close to matching the ideal self has high self-esteem, whereas a person whose self-concept varies widely from the ideal self tends to have low self-esteem.

A positive sense of self-esteem is an important variable in determining how an individual functions in the world. A person's ability to contribute to society in a meaningful way often affects self-concept and self-esteem. Once established, basic feelings about the self tend to be constant, although they may fluctuate somewhat. A situational crisis may temporarily affect one's self-esteem. Individuals who are sick and unable to be involved in society may feel worthless. Accepting a client as an individual with worth and dignity can help maintain and improve the client's self-esteem.

Stressors Affecting Self-Concept

A self-concept stressor is any real or perceived change that threatens identity, body image, or role performance (Figure 26-3). A stressor challenges a person's adaptive capacities. The most important factor in determining an individual's response is the individual's perception of the stressor. The ability to re-establish balance is related to numerous factors, including the number, intensity, and duration of the stressors, and health status (see Chapter 29). The normal process of maturation and development itself is a stressor. Changes that occur in physical, spiritual, emotional, sexual, familial, and sociocultural health can affect

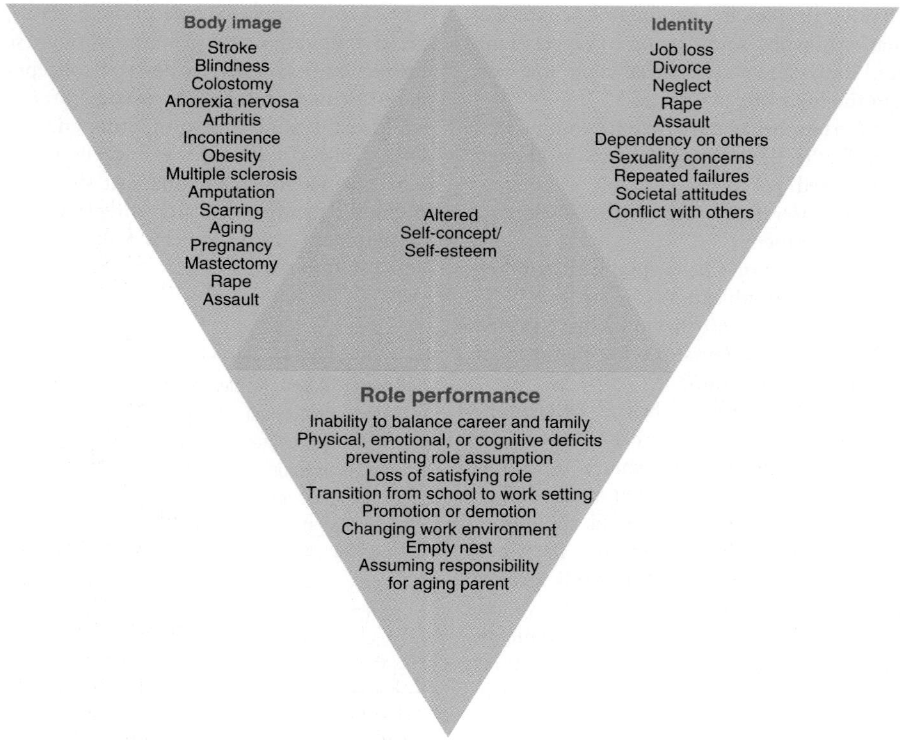

FIGURE 26-3 Common stressors that influence self-concept.

self-concept. Being able to adapt to stressors is likely to lead to a positive sense of self, whereas failure to adapt may lead to a negative sense of self.

Any change in health can be a stressor that potentially affects self-concept. A physical change can alter body image, thereby affecting identity and self-esteem. Chronic illnesses often alter role performance, which may affect identity and self-esteem. An essential process in adjusting to loss is the development of a new self-concept. The following case study illustrates the interrelationships among the various components of self-concept.

Amil, a 48-year-old man, has a sudden, unexpected stroke. He had not even been aware that he was hypertensive. Amil awakens in the hospital to find that he cannot move his right hand. He cannot care for himself and is unable to turn himself for days. With the nurses' and physiotherapists' constant encouragement, he is finally able to pull himself out of bed and into a chair. He wonders about his future. Amil's body image has dramatically changed. While he used to think of himself as physically strong, he now feels weak and helpless. He worries about his family. His older child is away at college, and his younger child is still in high school. Although his wife works, they need both incomes to meet their monthly expenses and to educate their children. If his condition does not improve, Amil's role as the primary financial provider for his family will drastically change.

Amil's self-esteem diminishes as his recovery and rehabilitation progress slowly. His self-concept has changed from someone who was self-sufficient to someone who must rely on others. Although he returns home and is in rehabilitation, Amil is not able to perform tasks for his family and must wait until his wife and child get home to help him with activities that require strength. Amil's physician tells him that he is fortunate to be alive, but his adaptation capabilities are stretched to the maximum. His identity is not clear to him anymore. He has no clear role within the family, his body image has been radically altered, and his self-esteem is low.

Amil continues with physiotherapy. Even simple tasks require significant time and energy. Slowly, he begins to gain some strength. After months of rehabilitation and support from an interprofessional team of health care providers, he is able to return to work, with some modifications to ensure his safety. He has some diminished mental agility and muscle weakening, but he is able to perform most aspects of his job. His self-esteem and body image improve. Although he still feels weaker, his physical capabilities closely resemble those he had before the stroke.

Guiding Questions

- *Try to put yourself in the patient's place. How would you cope with these changes? What if this happened to a relative who was the same age as your patient? How would these changes affect him or her? Ask questions to help you gain an understanding of the experience from your patient's perspective and point of view. How does he describe his experience?*
- *Give the patient the opportunity to express his feelings. How has this sudden alteration in his health affected his life, his image of himself, and his ability to lead the lifestyle he was used to before his stoke?*
- *Ask the patient about other health challenges or major obstacles in his life that he has had in the past. Can he identify strengths and capabilities that he has used previously to help him in his present situation?*

Crisis occurs when a person cannot overcome obstacles with his or her usual methods of problem solving and adaptation. Any crisis potentially threatens self-concept and self-esteem. Some crises, such as the one described in the preceding case study, directly affect all components of self-concept. The stressors created by a crisis—identity confusion, disturbed body image, low self-esteem, role conflict, role strain, role ambiguity, and role overload—may result in illness. During self-concept crises, supportive and educative resources can help a person learn new ways of coping and responding to the stressful event or situation in order to maintain or enhance self-concept.

Identity Stressors. Developmental markers such as puberty, menopause, retirement, and decreasing physical abilities may affect identity. Identity, like body image, is closely related to appearance and abilities. An individual's identity is affected by stressors throughout life, but it is particularly vulnerable during adolescence, a time characterized by physical, emotional, and mental changes of increasing maturity, which can result in insecurity and anxiety. It is also a time when adolescents are developing psychosocial competence, including coping strategies (see Chapter 29). A positive self-concept in adolescence enhances psychological and physical health in young adulthood.

Adults generally have a more stable identity and thus a more firmly developed self-concept than do younger people. Cultural and social stressors, rather than personal stressors, may have more effect on an adult's identity. For example, an adult may have to balance career and family or make choices regarding religious or cultural traditions. Retirement may mean the loss of an important means of achievement and continued success. People at retirement may begin to re-evaluate their identities and accomplishments. Loss of a significant other can lead the surviving individual to re-examine aspects of his or her identity.

Identity confusion results when people do not maintain a clear, consistent, and continuous consciousness of personal identity. It may occur at any stage of life if a person is unable to adapt to identity stressors. Under extreme stress, an individual may experience disturbed personal identity, a state in which the differences between the self and others cannot be determined. One example of identity confusion is when an adolescent realizes that some of his or her feelings and behaviours are focused on an individual of the same sex. A period of anxiety and confusion begins regarding sexuality and gender expectations. The person must adjust and accept this new identity of the self.

Body Image Stressors. Changes in appearance, structure, or function of a body part requires an adjustment in body image. An individual's perception of the change and the relative importance placed on body image affects the significance of the loss of function or change in appearance. For example, if a woman's body image incorporates reproductive functions as the ideal, a hysterectomy to treat uterine cancer may be a significant alteration and may result in a perceived loss of femininity or wholeness. Changes in body appearance, such as an amputation, facial disfigurement, or scars from burns or surgery, are physically obvious stressors affecting body image. Mastectomy and colostomy are surgical procedures that alter body appearance and function; although these changes are usually undetected by other people, they nonetheless have a significant effect on the individual. Even elective changes such as breast augmentation or reduction can affect body image. Chronic illnesses such as heart and renal disease affect body image because the body no longer functions at an optimal level. Anticipated body changes resulting from developmental processes can also affect body image. In addition, the effects of pregnancy, significant weight gain or loss, pharmacological management of illness, or radiation therapy change body image. Negative body image can lead to adverse health outcomes.

Many people associate success with a specific body part or function. For example, athletes may consider their bodies and physical activities to be the focus of personal success. Adaptation and rehabilitation may be affected if they can never again participate in athletics as they know it because of an accident or injury. To a surgeon, an amputation of a finger would significantly alter his or her ability to perform surgery. This change may affect the person's perception of his or her self-worth. Body image changes necessitate the revision of long-accepted self-perceptions, as well as alterations in lifestyle. To regain a positive self-concept and self-esteem, each person must adapt to his or her body image stressors.

Society's response to an individual's physical changes may be affected by the conditions surrounding the alteration. For example, an individual may be treated as a hero and praised for self-sacrifice when paralysis is the result of military duty, whereas an individual who was paralyzed as a result of driving intoxicated may elicit a very different response from others.

Role Performance Stressors. Throughout life, a person undergoes numerous role changes. Normal changes associated with growth and maturation result in developmental transitions. Situational transitions occur when parents, spouses, children, or friends die or when people move, marry, divorce, or change jobs. A health–illness transition is changing from a state of health or well-being to one of illness. A shift along the continuum from illness to wellness is as stressful as a shift from wellness to illness. Any of these transitions may lead to role conflict, role ambiguity, role strain, or role overload.

Role conflict results when a person simultaneously assumes two or more roles that are inconsistent, contradictory, or mutually exclusive. For example, when a middle-age woman with teenage children assumes responsibility for caring for her older parents, conflicts may arise in relation to being both the adult child and the parents' caregiver. Role conflicts can occur when trying to balance time and energy between her children and parents. The perceived importance of each conflicting role influences the degree of conflict experienced. The **sick role** involves the expectations of other people and society about how a person should behave when sick. Role conflict may occur when general societal expectations ("Take care of yourself and you will get better") conflict with the expectations of co-workers ("The job needs to get done"). The conflict of taking care of oneself while getting everything done can be a major challenge.

Role ambiguity involves unclear role expectations. When expectations are unclear, people may be unsure about what to do or how to behave. Such situations are often stressful and confusing. Role ambiguity is common in adolescence. Parents, peers, and the media pressure adolescents to assume adultlike roles, but many adolescents may still lack the resources to move beyond the role of dependent children. Role ambiguity can occur in employment situations. Employees may become unsure about job expectations in complex, rapidly changing, or highly specialized organizations.

Role strain is the stress or frustration experienced by an individual when behaviours, expectations, or obligations associated with a single social role are incompatible. Individuals who feel inadequate or unsuited for a new social role may experience role strain. For example, individuals who marry someone with children often feel unprepared to suddenly assume the parental role.

Role overload involves having more roles or responsibilities within a role than are manageable. It is frequently reflected in unsuccessful attempts to meet the demands of work and family while still having some personal time. During periods of illness or change, the people involved, either as the person who is ill or as a significant other, often find themselves in role overload.

Self-Esteem Stressors. Individuals with high self-esteem are generally more resilient and are better able to cope with demands and stressors than are those with low self-esteem. High self-esteem is associated with more optimal mental and physical health, greater control over circumstances, and greater adaptation and productivity in adulthood (Trzesniewski et al., 2013). Low self-worth can contribute to feeling unfulfilled and isolated from others and can result in depression and unremitting uneasiness or anxiety. Illness, surgery, or accidents that change life patterns can also influence feelings of self-worth. Chronic illnesses such as diabetes, arthritis, and cardiac dysfunction necessitate changes in accepted and long-assumed behavioural patterns. The more the chronic illness interferes with the ability to engage in activities contributing to feelings of worth or success, the more it affects self-esteem.

Self-esteem stressors vary with developmental stages. Perceived inability to meet parental expectations, harsh criticism, inconsistent discipline, and unresolved sibling rivalry may reduce children's sense of self-worth. Ineffective parenting also is associated with low self-esteem in children. Low self-esteem takes a toll on children. Children with low self-esteem and self-worth are more likely to experience internalizing disorders such as depression and anxiety. They are also more likely to bully other children and are more likely to be bullied (Coloroso, 2010) (Box 26-3). Low self-esteem in adolescence is one of the strongest predictors of depression (Hymel & Swearer, 2015). A developmental milestone such as pregnancy also introduces unique self-concept stressors and has significant implications for health. Low self-esteem is one of the strongest predictors of postpartum depression (Beck, 2008). In older adults, self-concept stressors include health problems, reduced functional ability, and stressful life events and circumstances (Box 26-4).

The Family's Effect on the Development of Self-Concept

The family plays a key role in creating and maintaining each family member's self-concept. Children develop a basic sense of who they are from their caregivers. Bowlby's (1982) attachment theory suggests that the quality of the attachment that children develop with their caregivers influences the development of a set of expectations about the self, their interpretations of the actions of other people, and ideas about how to respond to them. Attachment theory suggests that children who experience sensitive and supportive caring will develop expectations that they are worthy of other people's love and that other people are supportive. The quality of parenting interactions also influences children's development. Parents who respond in a firm, consistent, and warm manner promote positive self-esteem in their children (Coloroso, 2010). Parents who are harsh, behave inconsistently, or have low self-esteem themselves may foster negative self-concepts in their children. Even well-meaning parents can cultivate negative self-concepts in children. To assist clients in developing a positive self-concept, it is important to assess the family's style of relating (see Chapter 19).

BOX 26-3 RESEARCH HIGHLIGHT

Bullying and Self-Concept

Research Focus

Bullying is defined as physical, psychological, or verbal intimidation or attack, or a combination of these meant to cause distress, harm, or both to an intended victim. School-aged children report being bullied in the classroom, schoolyard, or playground, and more recently on social media and the Internet (i.e., cyberbullying). Bullying is a serious problem both for the victims and for the children who bully others.

Bullying has always been a concern among parents, educators, and health care providers because of the serious impact on children's health and well-being. Public concern increased dramatically after the tragic death of Reena Virk, a 14-year-old who was bullied by her peers and then murdered. Two Canadian teens who committed suicide (Amanda Todd and Rehtaeh Parsons) have also increased public awareness in recent years about the link between bullying and suicide in teens. Participation in bullying also increases the risk of suicidal ideas in youth.

Hymel and Swearer (2015) conducted a review of research to better understand the complexity of bullying among youth and to provide some directions for future research and intervention efforts. They found that while prevalence rates vary greatly across studies, 10 to 33% of students report victimization by peers, and 5 to 13% report bullying others. This rate increases to 61% for those who identify as a sexual minority (i.e., lesbian, gay, bisexual, or transgender) (Blais, Gervais, & Hébert, 2014). Both boys and girls engage in bullying; however, there are some gender differences. The most consistent finding was boys' greater involvement in physical bullying and girls' greater use of relational, verbal aggression and cyberbullying. Children can simultaneously be victims of bullies and bullies of other children, such as their younger siblings (Hymel & Swearer, 2015).

Victimization has been linked with a host of negative mental health outcomes such as depression and anxiety and suicidal ideation, as well as having a negative influence on academic functioning, social relationships, and self-perception (Hymel & Swearer, 2015). There are negative long-term adjustment difficulties in adulthood for individuals who were victimized in their youth (McDougall & Vaillancourt, 2015).

The reasons why children bully other children are complex and multifaceted (Hymel & Swearer, 2015). One explanation for why children bully other children focuses on self-concept. Studies have shown that children with a positive self-concept are less likely to bully other children, engage in delinquent behaviour, or be instigators of peer conflict (Coloroso, 2010). In addition, children with a positive self-concept are less likely to be bullied. The quality of the family environment, particularly a lack of responsive parenting, negatively influences children's self-concept. Lower self-concept is associated with an increase in bullying behaviour.

Evidence-Informed Practice

- Building children's self-concept is an important strategy to prevent bullying behaviour in children and to prevent being victimized by a bully.
- Parents must be helped to understand how children are affected by parenting behaviour in particular and the family environment.
- It is important to involve the entire family system in the intervention process when children are identified as victims or bullies.
- Youth are reluctant to report bullying. Positive relationships between parents and their children may enhance the likelihood that children will report bullying.
- Referral to other health care providers may be necessary to assist vulnerable children and families.

Note: The articles by Hymel and Swearer (2015) and McDougall and Vaillancourt (2015) are two of six in the 2015 special issue (May-June) of *American Psychologist* on "School Bullying and Victimization."

Blais, M., Gervais, J., & Hébert, M. (2014). Internalized homophobia as a partial mediator between homophobic bullying and self-esteem among youths of sexual minorities in Quebec (Canada). *Ciênc. Saúde Coletiva, 19*(3), 727–735. doi:10.1590/1413-81232014193.16082013; Hymel, S., & Swearer, S. M., (2015). Four decades of research on school bullying: An introduction. *American Psychologist*, 70(4), 293–299. doi.org10.1037a0038928; McDougall, P., & Vaillancourt, T. (2015). Long-term adult outcomes of peer victimization in childhood and adolescence: Pathways to adjustment and maladjustment. *American Psychologist*, 70(4), 300–310. doi:org10.1037a0039174.

BOX 26-4 FOCUS ON OLDER PERSONS

Promoting a Positive Self-Concept

Promoting a positive self-concept in all older persons is essential, but it is especially important for those experiencing disability, frailty, or reduced functional capacity.

- Examples of activities to help older persons feel a sense of self-worth while providing a legacy for younger family members include conducting a life review or participating in a reminiscence group, recording an oral history, or making a photo scrapbook of meaningful life events (Eliopoulos, 2013).
- Potential threats to an older person's self-esteem may arise from the institutional environments where they receive care. These threats can include dependence, devaluation, depersonalization, functional impairments, and lack of control over one's environment. Nursing interventions directed toward reducing or eliminating these threats can improve an older person's quality of life.
- Self-concept may be negatively affected in older adulthood by a number of life changes, including health problems, reduced functional ability, declining income or socioeconomic status, spousal loss or bereavement, loss of social support, and decline in achievement experiences after retirement (Stuart, 2013).
- Health care providers should be alert to an older person's preoccupation with physical complaints; they should conduct a comprehensive assessment and encourage clients to verbalize needs, feelings, and emotions such as fear, insecurity, and loneliness (Stuart, 2013).
- By actively listening and accepting the person's feelings; being respectful; praising health-seeking behaviours; and recognizing, acknowledging, and praising accomplishments, health care providers convey respect for the older person's worth.

BOX 26-5 RESEARCH HIGHLIGHT

Professional Identity and Nursing

Evidence Summary

A person's professional identity is a component of his or her overall identity. It is a sense of self that is derived and perceived from the role we take on in the career, occupation, or work that we choose to do. A positive and healthy professional identity is critically important for nurses to function skillfully and competently, and it ultimately benefits the patients and families in nurses' care. Although a professional identity is separate from self-concept, it is inextricably linked to self-concept. Nurses feeling positively about themselves can support patient care in a positive health care environment and enhance job satisfaction and retention rates in nursing. Johnson, Cowin, Wilson, and colleagues (2012) explored the factors that influence professional identity in nurses.

Key Findings

- Nurses' professional identities start prior to entering their formal nursing education as potential students have some preconceived values and beliefs about the profession.
- Nurses' professional identities develop throughout the years of educational preparation and continue to develop in their nursing careers.
- The education period is a critical time for nursing students because during this time, students gain the knowledge and skills to gain entry into the profession and to self-identify with the profession.
- The different educational contexts all play a vital role in constructing a professional identity. While nurse educators are a key influence, clinical preceptors in clinical learning environments have significant influence in helping students develop a professional identity.
- Professional identity is a key issue in the transition from being a student to becoming a practising nurse. Students need to feel comfortable and confident as they assume their new positions after graduation.
- Professional identity is not static but continually evolving. Nurses undergo constant reshaping of professional identity throughout their careers, with frequent advances occurring in nursing, health, and medical knowledge as well as changes in technology, roles, and client expectations.
- Gaining advanced education in nursing through certifications, specialization, and graduate education further enhances professional identity (Miskelly & Duncan, 2014).

Johnson, M., Cowin, L. S., Wilson, I. & Young., H. (2012). Professional identity and nursing: Contemporary theoretical developments and future research challenges. *International Nursing Review, 59*, 562–569; Miskelly, P., & Duncan, L. (2014). "I'm actually the grown-up now": Leadership, maturity and professional identity development. *Journal of Nursing Management, 22*, 38–48. doi:10.1111/jonm.12030.

The Nurse's Effect on the Client's Self-Concept

As a nurse, your acceptance of a client with an altered self-concept helps promote positive change. When a client's physical appearance has changed, likely both the client and the family will observe your verbal and nonverbal responses and reactions. You need to be aware of your own feelings, ideas, values, expectations, and judgements. Self-awareness is critical in initially understanding and accepting others. Nurses who are secure in their own identities more readily accept and thus reinforce clients' identities (Box 26-5). It is important to assess and clarify the following self-concept issues:

- Thoughts and feelings about lifestyle, health, and illness
- Awareness of how nonverbal communication may affect clients and families
- Personal values and expectations and how they affect clients
- Ability to convey a nonjudgemental attitude toward clients
- Preconceived attitudes toward cultural differences in self-concept and self-esteem

Some clients with a change in body appearance or function are very sensitive to health care providers' verbal and nonverbal responses. A positive and matter-of-fact approach to care can provide a model for the client and family to follow. You can have a positive effect by conveying genuine interest and acceptance. By recognizing and including self-concept issues in planning and delivering care, you can positively influence client outcomes. By building a trusting nurse–client relationship and appropriately involving the client and family in decision making, you can enhance self-concept. An individualized approach may highlight a client's unique needs, including incorporating alternative health care practices or methods of spiritual expression.

You also can significantly influence a client's body image. For example, for a woman who has undergone a mastectomy, you can positively affect her body image by showing acceptance of the mastectomy scar. Clients closely watch other people's reactions to their wounds and scars. A facial expression of shock or disgust can contribute to the client developing a negative body image. It is important to monitor your responses. Statements such as "Your wound is healing nicely" or "The tissue looks healthy" will be affirming to the client. Nonverbal behaviours help to convey caring for a client and can affect self-esteem (Figure 26-4). For example, the self-concept of an incontinent client can be threatened by the perception that the caregivers find the situation unpleasant. A good practice is to anticipate personal reactions, acknowledge them, and focus on the client instead of on the unpleasant task or situation. Imagining yourself in the client's position will help you find strategies and measures to ease your client's embarrassment, frustration, and anger.

Preventive measures, early identification, and appropriate treatment can minimize the intensity of self-esteem stressors and the potential effects on the client and family. Learn to design specific self-concept interventions to fit a client's profile of risk factors. Assess the client's perception of a problem and work collaboratively with the client and with other members of the health care team to resolve issues related to self-concept (Box 26-6).

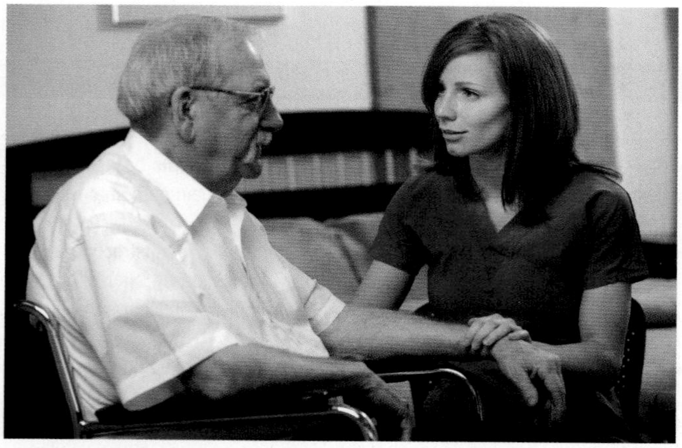

FIGURE 26-4 Nurses can use touch and eye contact to enhance a client's self-esteem.

CRITICAL THINKING

Self-concept profoundly influences a person's response to illness. A critical thinking approach to nursing care is essential. This approach requires synthesis of knowledge, experience, information gathered from clients and families, critical thinking abilities, and knowing and adhering to professional standards. Solid clinical judgement requires anticipating the required information, collecting and analyzing the data, and making appropriate decisions regarding client care.

In the case of self-concept, it is essential to integrate knowledge from nursing and other disciplines, including self-concept theory and communication principles, and to consider cultural and developmental factors. Previous experience in caring for clients with alterations in self-concept can assist you in individualizing your care for each client. The nursing process continues until the client's self-concept is improved, restored, or maintained.

SELF-CONCEPT AND THE NURSING PROCESS

Assessment

In assessing self-concept, nurses must focus on the various components of self-concept: identity, body image, role performance, and self-esteem. Assessment should include observing behaviours suggestive of an altered self-concept (Box 26-7), actual and potential self-concept stressors (see the earlier case study), and coping patterns. Nurses need to be sensitive to the effect that cultural influences have on the client's behaviours and needs. Some behaviours suggestive of an altered self-concept for someone in one culture may be normal for

BOX 26-6 RESEARCH HIGHLIGHT

Adolescence and Body Image

Research Focus

Sociocultural norms in North American society strongly suggest to individuals that their value is determined by their appearance. The media typically play an important role in depicting individuals as thin, youthful, and beautiful. Adolescents for whom this standard is unrealistic feel self-conscious and dissatisfied with their bodies. The extent to which they internalize society's standards for thinness is associated with body dissatisfaction and represents a risk factor for eating disorders.

Research Abstract

Spurr, Berry, and Walker (2013) conducted two studies using a qualitative approach to explore adolescent views of psychological wellness and healthy bodies. They held nine focus groups with a total of 46 adolescents from two high schools in one mid-Western Canadian province. There were 28 females and 18 males aged 16 to 19 years of age who participated in the two studies. Data were analyzed using thematic analysis. The most common themes emerging from the focus group discussions in both studies included the negative impact of media on adolescent body image and pressure to conform to Western views of physical appearance. Their findings illustrate the need for nurses to understand the influence of the media on both male and female adolescents' views of their body image and to incorporate protocols for assessment, education, and counselling of adolescents on the healthy usage of media into their pediatric and mental health clinical practice.

Evidence-Informed Practice

- Promoting empowerment, building self-esteem, and developing positive self-concept are important health promotion strategies.
- Body weight concerns and coping strategies are important issues for nurses to address with adolescents.
- Nurses should increase clients' awareness of the role of the media and popular culture in promoting unrealistic and unhealthy standards.
- Nurses need to understand the influence of the media on adolescents' views of their body image and incorporate into their pediatric clinical practice protocols for assessment, education, and counselling of adolescents on the healthy usage of media.
- Nurses have a critical role to play in developing and implementing healthy public policies that encourage adolescents to have healthy views of body image.

Spurr, S., Berry, L., & Walker, K. (2013). Exploring adolescent views of body image: The influence of media. *Issues in Comprehensive Nursing, 36*(1-2), 17–36.

BOX 26-7 Behaviours Suggestive of Altered Self-Concept

- Avoidance of eye contact
- Slumped posture
- Unkempt appearance
- Being overly apologetic
- Hesitant speech
- Being overly critical or angry
- Frequent or inappropriate crying
- Negative self-evaluation
- Being excessively dependent
- Hesitancy in expressing views or opinions
- Lack of interest in what is happening
- Passive attitude
- Difficulty in making decisions

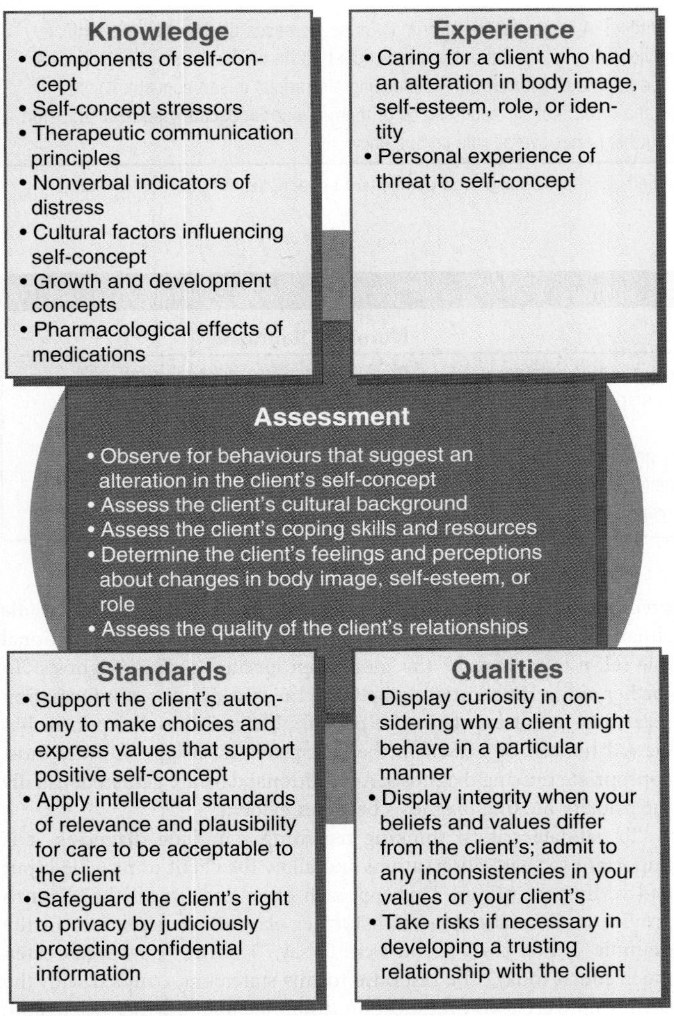

FIGURE 26-5 Critical thinking model to assess self-concept.

individuals in other cultures. For example, in many Indigenous and Asian cultures, eye contact is a sign of disrespect. In order to gather comprehensive assessment, information from multiple sources must be synthesized critically (Figure 26-5).

At appropriate times, you will need to ask specific questions to assess your client's self-concept, paying close attention to their responses (Table 26-1). It is critically important to closely observe nonverbal behaviour. Note the manner in which clients talk about significant people in their lives. This can provide clues to both stressful and supportive relationships, as well as to key roles that the client assumes. Using knowledge of developmental stages to determine what areas are likely to be important to the client, inquire about these aspects of the person's life. For example, ask an older client about his or her life and what has been important to him or her. At this stage of development, individuals are examining their lives and considering the effects they have had in the world. The individual's conversation will probably provide data relating to role performance, identity, self-esteem, stressors, and coping patterns.

Coping Behaviours. Nursing assessment should also include consideration of previous coping behaviours; the nature, number, and intensity of the stressors; and the client's internal and external resources. Knowledge of how a client has handled past stressors can enable insight into the client's style of coping. People do not address all issues in the same way, but they often use a familiar coping pattern for newly encountered stressors. As previous coping patterns are identified, it is useful to determine whether these patterns have contributed to healthy functioning or created more problems. For example, abused women sometimes use alcohol or drugs to cope with the abuse, but the use of these harmful substances only creates additional stressors (see Chapter 29).

Exploring resources and strengths, such as the availability of significant others or prior use of community resources, can be important when developing a realistic and effective plan. It is also critical to understand how a client views a situation. For example, older women may be more accustomed to changes in their health status because of the aging process in general, and experiencing heart disease may be one more aspect of growing older. On the other hand, a cardiac event occurring in middle age may be less expected and more problematic for women because of family and career responsibilities and may thus elicit greater anxiety.

Significant Others. Significant others can help identify changes in a client's behaviour that may suggest alterations in self-concept. These individuals may have insights into the client's way of dealing with stressors or knowledge about what is important to the client's self-concept. The way a significant other talks about the client and the significant other's nonverbal behaviours may provide information about what kind of support is available for the client.

Clients' Expectations. The client's expectations are another important factor to consider when assessing self-concept. Asking a client what he or she thinks you can do to help is important. Collaborating with clients is essential so that interventions are acceptable to them. Asking a client how he or she thinks the interventions will make a difference elicits useful information regarding the client's expectations and provides an opportunity to discuss the client's goals. For example, while working with a client who is experiencing anxiety related to an upcoming diagnostic test, you might ask about the relaxation exercise that he or she has been practising. The client's response provides valuable information about his or her beliefs and attitudes regarding the efficacy of the intervention, as well as the potential need to modify the nursing approach.

❖ NURSING DIAGNOSIS

Carefully consider the assessment data to identify a client's actual or potential problem areas. Rely on knowledge and experience, apply appropriate professional standards, and look for clusters of defining characteristics that indicate a nursing diagnosis. Although multiple nursing diagnostic labels exist for altered self-concept, the following

TABLE 26-1 Nursing Assessment of Client's Self-Concept

Assessment Questions*	Responses Reflecting Difficulties With Self-Concept
Identity	
"How would you describe yourself?"	Derogatory answers (e.g., "I don't know; not too much is worth mentioning") should raise concern.
Body Image	
"What aspects of your appearance do you like?" "Would you like to change any aspects of your appearance? If yes, describe the changes you would make."	Most people can identify something positive about their appearance (e.g., "I have nice eyes"). If a person cannot identify any positive characteristic, this may suggest a negative body image and poor self-esteem. Most people have something that they would like to change (e.g., "My nose is too big" or "My hips are too large"), but a long list of problem areas may suggest difficulties with self-concept.
Self-Esteem	
"Tell me about the things you do that make you feel good about yourself." "How do you feel about yourself?"	Statements about not having any strengths or being able to do anything well should raise concern. Statements that are very negative about the client should raise concern (e.g., "I am hopeless" or "I have never felt good about myself").
Role Performance	
"Tell me about your primary roles (e.g., partner, parent, friend, sister, employee, volunteer). How effective are you at carrying out each of these roles?"	Listen for the different roles identified. A large number of primary roles increases the risk for role conflict and role overload. As with previous questions, if the client indicates that he or she does not believe that these roles are adequately covered, the client may be experiencing alterations in self-concept. Most people carry out several roles and often feel as though some of them are not adequately addressed; listen for the client's perception about his or her overall role competency.

*In addition to the client's verbal response, note any nonverbal behaviours. A negative self-concept is suggested by hesitant speech, lack of interest in what is happening, and slumped posture.

BOX 26-8 NURSING DIAGNOSTIC PROCESS

Assessment Activities	Defining Characteristics	Nursing Diagnosis
Observe client's behaviour during conversation.	Client demonstrates restlessness, inability to maintain eye contact, facial tension, increased perspiration, and self-preoccupation.	Anxiety related to accidental injury, pain, uncertainty of outcome of upcoming surgery
Empathically communicate, "Tell me how you are coping" or "How are you feeling about tomorrow's procedure?"	Client replies, "I'm scared. They may amputate my leg tomorrow. I don't know how I'll manage. I was awake all night. I just kept thinking about everything."	

list (Herdman & Kamitsuru, 2014) provides examples of self-concept–related nursing diagnoses:

- *Disturbed body image*
- *Caregiver role strain*
- *Disturbed personal identity*
- *Ineffective role performance*
- *Chronic low self-esteem*
- *Situational low self-esteem*
- *Risk for situational low self-esteem*
- *Readiness for enhanced self-concept*

Making nursing diagnoses about self-concept is complex. Often, isolated data could be the defining characteristics for more than one nursing diagnosis (Box 26-8). For example, a client might express feelings of uncertainty and inadequacy. These are defining characteristics for both anxiety and situational low self-esteem. If the client is demonstrating defining characteristics for more than one nursing diagnosis, then gather specific data to validate and differentiate the underlying problem. To further assess the possibility of anxiety as the nursing diagnosis, you might consider whether the client has any of the following defining characteristics: Is the person experiencing increased muscle tension, shakiness, a sense of being "rattled," or restlessness? These symptoms may suggest anxiety rather than low self-esteem. On the other hand, if the person expresses a predominantly negative self-appraisal, including inability to handle situations or events and difficulty making decisions, then situational low self-esteem may be the more appropriate nursing diagnosis. To further aid in differentiating between the two diagnoses, information regarding recent events in the person's life and how the person has viewed himself or herself in the past provides insight into the most appropriate nursing diagnosis. As additional data are gathered, usually the priority nursing diagnosis becomes evident.

To validate critical thinking regarding a nursing diagnosis, it is important to share observations and allow the client to provide input and verify perceptions. This approach often encourages the client to provide additional data, which further clarifies the situation. In the example in Box 26-8, if you were to say, "I notice you haven't eaten much lunch today," the response to this statement, coupled with the client's nonverbal communication, could facilitate further discussion. An alternative approach may be to state, "I notice you jumped when I came up behind you. Are you feeling uneasy today?" This statement allows the client to verify whether he or she is in fact anxious and to discuss any concerns.

◆ Planning

Planning involves synthesizing knowledge, experience, critical thinking qualities, and standards (Figure 26-6). Critical thinking ensures that

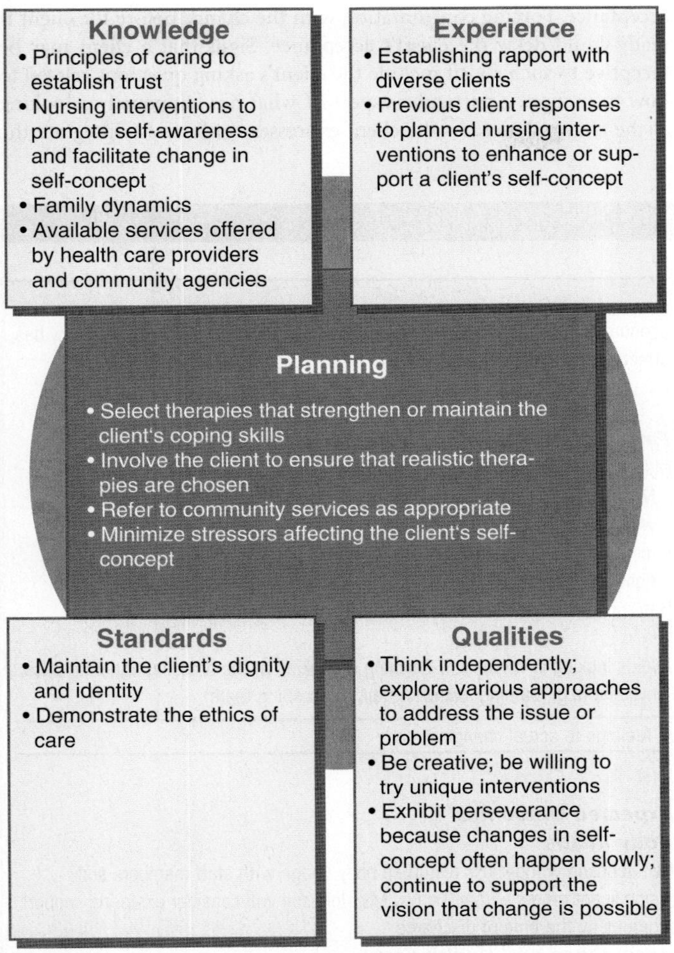

FIGURE 26-6 Critical thinking model for self-concept planning.

the nursing care plan integrates all that you know about the individual, as well as key critical thinking elements (Box 26-9). Professional standards are especially important to consider when you develop a plan of care. These standards often establish ethical or evidence-informed practice guidelines for selecting effective nursing interventions.

Another method used to help plan nursing care is a concept map. The concept map illustrated in Figure 26-7 shows the relationship between a medical diagnosis, postoperative reconstruction of severe facial scars, and the four nursing diagnoses. The concept map also links the nursing diagnoses and shows how they are interrelated. In this example, disturbed body image is related to situational low self-esteem. As the client's facial scars improve, she should begin to feel better about her appearance.

Goals and Outcomes. In collaboration with the client, you should develop an individualized plan of care for each nursing diagnosis. Goals should be established that are individualized, are realistic, and have measurable outcomes. It is important to consult with the client about whether the goals are perceived as realistic. By consulting with the client and with significant others, mental health clinicians, and community resources, you can design a more comprehensive and workable plan. Once a goal has been formulated, consider how the data that illustrated the problem would change if the problem were diminished. These changes should be reflected in the outcome criteria. For example, a client receives a diagnosis of *situational low self-esteem related to a recent job layoff.* You and the client establish a goal: "Client's self-esteem and self-concept should begin to improve in 2 weeks." Examples of expected outcomes directed toward that goal include the following:

- The client will discuss a minimum of three areas of his or her life in which he or she is functioning well.
- The client will be able to voice the recognition that losing the job is not reflective of his or her worth as a person.
- The client attends a support group for out-of-work individuals.

Setting Priorities. The care plan lists the goals, expected outcomes, and interventions for a client with an alteration in self-concept. Interventions focus on helping the client adapt to the stressors that led to the disturbance in self-concept and on supporting successful coping. A client may perceive a situation as overwhelming and may feel hopeless about returning to the previous level of functioning. The client may need time to adapt to physical changes.

Establishing priorities may include therapeutic communication to address self-concept issues to ensure that the client's ability to address physical needs is maximized. It is important to look for strengths in both the client and the family and to provide resources and education to assist the client in changing limitations into strengths. Client teaching creates an understanding of the normality of certain situations (e.g., the nature of a chronic disease, change in a relationship, or the effect of a loss). Often, once this is understood, the sense of hopelessness and helplessness decreases.

Continuity of Care. The perceptions of significant others must be incorporated into the plan of care. Clients who have experienced deficits in self-concept before the current episode of treatment may have established a system of support that includes mental health clinicians, clergy, and other community resources. Before involving the family, consider the client's desires for the family's involvement and cultural norms regarding who most frequently makes decisions in the family.

◆ Implementation

As with all the steps of the nursing process, a therapeutic nurse–client relationship is central to the implementation phase. Once the goals and outcome criteria have been developed, consider nursing interventions to promote a healthy self-concept and help the client move toward achieving the goals. To develop effective nursing interventions, consider the nursing diagnosis and broad interventions that address the diagnosis. These broad, standard interventions should be tailored to the individual client. Regardless of the health care setting, it is important to work with clients and their families or significant others to promote a healthy self-concept. For example, nursing interventions may include strategies to help clients regain or restore the elements that contribute to a strong and secure sense of self. The approaches that you choose will vary according to the level of care required.

Health Promotion. Work with clients to help them develop healthy lifestyle behaviours that contribute to a positive self-concept (Box 26-10).

Acute Care. In the acute care setting, some clients experience potential threats to their self-concept because of the nature of the treatment and diagnostic procedures. Threats to a person's self-concept can result in anxiety or fear. Numerous stressors, including unknown diagnoses, the need to make changes in lifestyle, and change in functioning, may be present and need to be addressed. In the acute care setting, more than one stressor is often present, which increases the overall stress level for the client and family.

Nurses in the acute care setting also encounter clients who are faced with the need to adapt to an altered body image as a result of surgery, accidents, or other physical change. Sometimes, threats to self-concept and the need to adapt result in aggressive behaviour. Often a visit by someone who has experienced similar changes and adapted to them (e.g., someone who has undergone a laryngectomy or a mastectomy) may be helpful. The timing of such a visit is important. Because addressing these needs may be difficult while the client is in an acute care setting, appropriate follow-up and referrals, including home care, are essential. It is important to remain sensitive to the client's level of acceptance. Forcing confrontation with the change before the client is ready could delay the client's acceptance. Signs that a client may be receptive to such a visit include the client's asking questions related to how to manage a particular aspect of what has happened or looking at the changed area. As the client expresses readiness to integrate the

BOX 26-9 NURSING CARE PLAN

Disturbed Body Image

ASSESSMENT

You have been assigned to care for Ms. Johnson, a 45-year-old married woman who underwent a unilateral radical mastectomy because of malignancy. Ms. Johnson's physical assessment has been completed, and she has received adequate medication for pain. You sit down to discuss how the mastectomy has affected Ms. Johnson's self-concept.

Assessment Activities	Findings and Defining Characteristics
Assess identity concerns (e.g., sexual role, femininity).	Ms. Johnson looks away, shakes her head, and states, "I don't feel feminine. My husband says it won't affect how he feels about me, but I'm sure it will."
Ask Ms. Johnson how the mastectomy is affecting her sense of self.	Intermittent eye contact, frequent crying when alone, pulling hospital gown tightly across chest
Observe Ms. Johnson's mood and interactions with others, including family members.	Has superficial conversations with staff and family members
Determine Ms. Johnson's participation in self-care activities.	Avoids looking in mirror and touching or looking at the dressing; ignoring basic hygiene (e.g., bathing, combing hair, or brushing teeth)

NURSING DIAGNOSIS: Disturbed body image related to negative thoughts and feelings to actual change in body

PLANNING

Goal (Nursing Outcomes Classification)*	Expected Outcomes
Ms. Johnson will identify and express feelings verbally and nonverbally.	***Body Image*** Ms. Johnson will discuss disturbed body image with staff members and significant others within 3 days. Ms. Johnson will consider exploring support groups by the time of discharge.
Ms. Johnson will participate in self-care related to mastectomy.	***Acceptance and Health Status*** Ms. Johnson will look at tissue surrounding surgical site within 2 days. Ms. Johnson will begin to attend to basic hygiene needs within 2 days.
Ms. Johnson will identify and use resources outside the hospital.	***Social Involvement*** Ms. Johnson will verbalize commitment to participating in community resources (e.g., mastectomy support group) by the time of discharge. By postoperative visit, Ms. Johnson will determine whether she wishes to attend support group.

*Outcome classification labels from Moorhead, S., Johnson, M., Maas, M., & Swanson, E. (Eds.). (2012). *Nursing outcomes classification (NOC)* (5th ed.). St. Louis, MO: Mosby.

INTERVENTIONS

Interventions (Nursing Interventions Classification)†	Rationale
Initially assign the same staff members to work with Ms. Johnson.	Continuity in care will facilitate the establishment of a therapeutic relationship; familiarity and trust will enhance communication.
Approach Ms. Johnson and initiate conversation; use silence and active listening to promote communication.	Ms. Johnson's ability to initially find the words for what she is experiencing may be limited.
Remain aware of your own feelings regarding Ms. Johnson's bodily changes and physical appearance.	Inadvertently communicating your own discomfort or negativity will interfere with Ms. Johnson's ability to openly communicate her feelings.
Have Ms. Johnson spend time alone and with supportive family members for crying, recording in her journal, reflection, or prayer.	This use of time encourages expression of thoughts and feelings, including depression, grief, resentment, and fear of rejection. Family involvement is an essential element of comprehensive care.
Facilitate evaluation of overall self-concept.	The effect on body image may influence other aspects of self-concept and self-esteem, including perception of identity and role performance.
Involve Ms. Johnson's husband in discussion of uncomfortable issues, such as sexual concerns.	Sexuality is a basic need and concern for both men and women, and yet it can be one of the most difficult discussions for clients to initiate.
Assist Ms. Johnson in identifying and using appropriate support systems outside the hospital, including home health care.	Support can assist the client in feeling normal again and in integrating a new body image into her self-concept.

†Intervention classification labels from Bulechek, G. M., Butcher, H. K., Dochterman, J. M., & Wagner, C. (Eds.). (2013). *Nursing interventions classification (NIC)* (6th ed.). St Louis, MO: Mosby.

BOX 26-9 NURSING CARE PLAN

Disturbed Body Image—cont'd

EVALUATION

Nursing Actions	***Client Response and Finding***	***Achievement of Outcome***
Ask Ms. Johnson how effective she feels in her ability to identify and express feelings verbally and nonverbally.	Ms. Johnson responds, "It's hard for me to talk about myself, but I have really made an effort to talk about what the loss of my breast means to me."	Ms. Johnson reports improvement in communication skills and success with discussing disturbed body image with primary nurse and husband.
Observe Ms. Johnson's participation in self-care related to mastectomy.	Ms. Johnson assumes responsibility for basic hygiene immediately after establishing the goal and has used a mirror to examine her mastectomy scar.	Ms. Johnson has increased her independence and has begun to integrate body image change into her self-concept.
Assist Ms. Johnson in identifying resources outside the hospital; secure a commitment to use resources.	Ms. Johnson verbalizes commitment to participating in community resources (e.g., mastectomy support group).	Outcome has not been completely achieved; Ms. Johnson has expressed hesitancy in attending a support group but is receptive to home care. Home care nurse will ensure that goal is re-evaluated and addressed as appropriate.

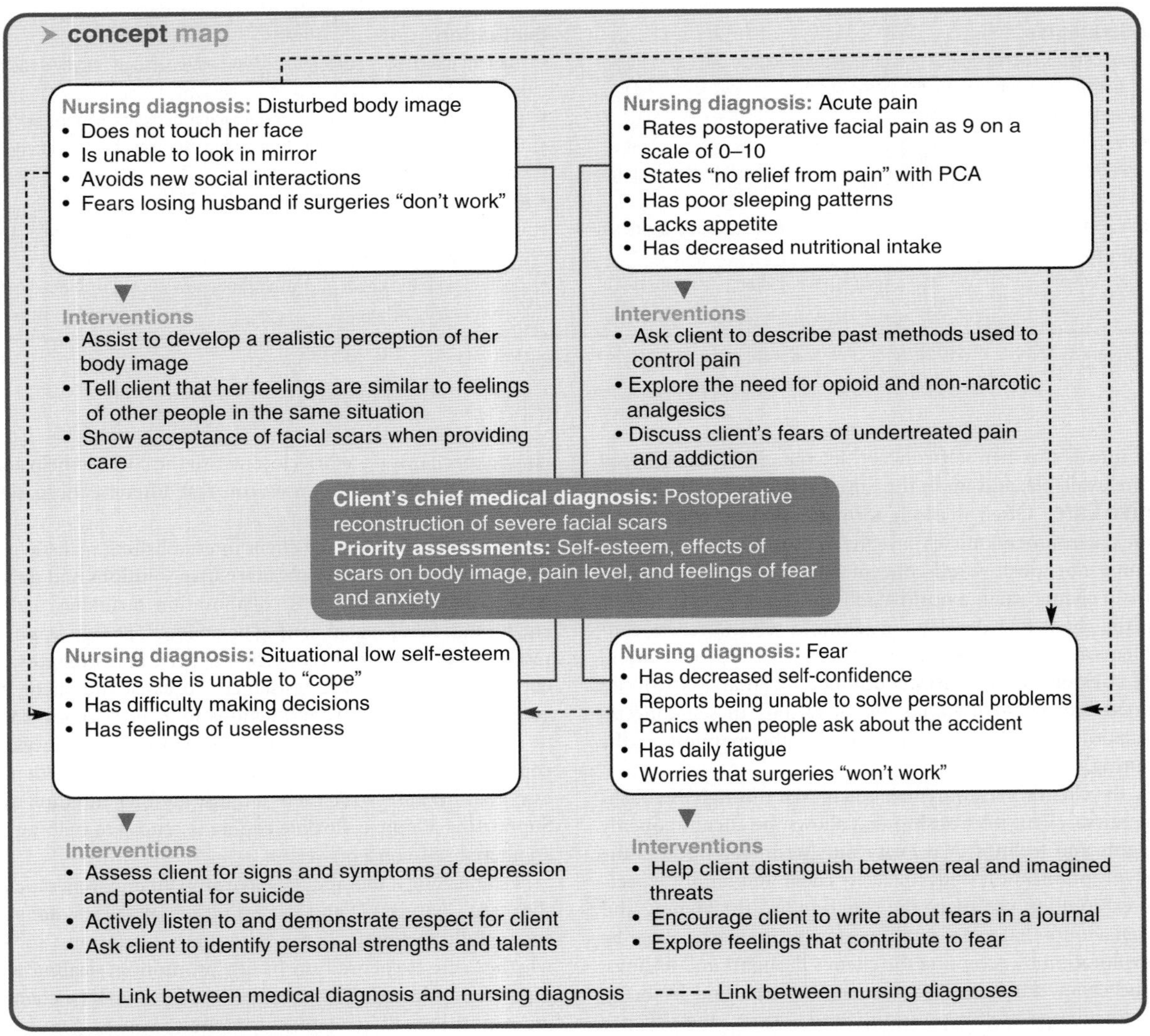

FIGURE 26-7 Concept map for client after surgical reconstruction of severe facial scars. *PCA,* Patient (client)-controlled analgesia.

BOX 26-10 FOCUS ON PRIMARY HEALTH CARE
Promoting Client's Self-Concept

The focus of primary health care is to promote health and prevent illness by stressing client education and self-care. Measures that contribute to a healthy self-concept and therefore promote health and well-being include those that support adaptation to stress, such as proper nutrition and regular exercise within the client's capabilities; those that facilitate adequate sleep and rest; and those that reduce stress.

Nurses are in a unique position to identify lifestyle practices that put a client's self-concept at risk or are suggestive of an altered self-concept. For example, a young adult visits a clinic with complaints of being unable to sleep and experiencing anxiety attacks. In gathering the health history, you may learn of lifestyle practices such as excessive use of alcohol or nonprescription drugs, too little rest, or a large number of life changes occurring simultaneously. These data, when taken together, may suggest actual or potential self-concept disturbances. In this situation, you determine how the client views the various lifestyle elements so that you can facilitate the client's insight into behaviours. If necessary, you provide needed health teaching or make appropriate referrals to other community services. Clients who are experiencing threats to or alterations in self-concept often benefit from mental health and community resources to promote increased awareness. Knowledge of available community resources enables you to make appropriate referrals.

BOX 26-11 PATIENT TEACHING
Alterations in Self-Concept

Objective
- Risks for situational low self-esteem will be reduced in the home care setting.

Teaching Strategies
- Reinforce the client's expression of thoughts and feelings; clarify meaning of verbal and nonverbal communication.
- Encourage opportunities for self-care.
- Elicit the client's perceptions of strengths and weaknesses.
- Convey verbally and behaviourally that the client is responsible for his or her own behaviour.
- Identify relevant stressors with the client, and ask for the client's appraisal of these stressors.
- Explore the client's adaptive and maladaptive coping responses to problems.
- Collaboratively identify alternative solutions; encourage the client to use alternatives not previously tried.
- Continue to reinforce the client's strengths and successes.

Evaluation
- Confirm the client's perception of and actual use of improved communication skills.
- Observe the client's level of participation in decisions that affect care.
- Confirm with the client and family that the increase in activities and tasks has been a positive experience.
- Observe the client's establishment of a simple routine.
- Observe the client take necessary action to change maladaptive coping responses and maintain adaptive responses.
- Confirm with the client and family how new coping resources can be applied to continued change.

Modified from Stuart, G. W. M. T. (2013). *Principles and practice of psychiatric nursing* (10th ed.). St. Louis, MO: Mosby.

body change into his or her self-concept, let the client know about groups that are available, and make the initial contact.

Restorative Care. Often, in a long-term nurse–client relationship in a home care environment, nurses have the opportunity to work with clients to attain a more positive self-concept (Box 26-11). Interventions designed to help clients attain a positive self-concept are based on the premise that the client first develops insight and self-awareness concerning problems and stressors and then acts to solve the problems and cope with the stressors. This approach, outlined by Stuart (2013), can be incorporated into client teaching for alterations in self-concept, including situational low self-esteem, which might manifest in the home care setting.

Increasing the client's self-awareness is achieved through establishing a trusting nurse–client relationship that allows the client to openly explore thoughts and feelings. A priority nursing intervention is the expert use of communication skills to clarify client and family expectations. Open exploration can make the situation less threatening and encourages behaviours that expand self-awareness. You encourage the client's self-exploration by accepting the client's thoughts and feelings, by helping the client clarify interactions with others, and by being empathetic. Encourage self-expression, and stress the client's self-responsibility. To promote the client's self-evaluation, help the client to define problems clearly, and identify positive and negative coping mechanisms. Work closely with the client to help analyze adaptive and maladaptive responses, contrast different alternative responses, and discuss outcomes.

Collaborating with the client in establishing realistic goals involves helping the client to identify alternative solutions and develop realistic goals based on them. This collaboration facilitates real change and encourages further goal-setting behaviours. Design opportunities that result in success, reinforce the client's skills and strengths, and help the client to obtain needed assistance. To assist the client in becoming committed to decisions and actions to achieve goals, teach the client to stop using ineffective coping mechanisms and develop successful coping strategies. Supporting attempts that are health promoting is essential, because with each success, another attempt can be made. Supporting adaptive, flexible coping is crucial to helping a client with an altered self-concept.

Establishing a therapeutic environment and a therapeutic relationship (see Chapter 17) and increasing self-awareness are also critical in successfully helping clients who have alterations in self-concept, whether care is focused on health promotion, dealing with an acute process, or addressing restorative care. To support a client in developing a positive self-concept, nurses must convey genuine caring (see Chapter 18) and establish a partnership with the client to address underlying problems.

Evaluation

Client Care. Critical thinking is needed to evaluate success in meeting each client's goal and the established expected outcomes (Figure 26-8). Frequent evaluation of client progress is recommended so that changes can be instituted if necessary. Use knowledge of behaviours and characteristics of a healthy self-concept when you review the client's behaviours. This method determines whether outcomes have been met.

Expected outcomes for a client with a self-concept disturbance may include nonverbal behaviours indicating a positive self-concept, statements of self-acceptance, and acceptance of change in appearance or function. Nonverbal behaviours can be key indicators of clients' self-concept. For example, a client who has had difficulty making eye contact may demonstrate a more positive self-concept by making more frequent eye contact. Social interaction, adequate self-care, acceptance of the use of prosthetic devices, and statements indicating understanding of teaching all indicate progress. A positive attitude toward rehabilitation and increased movement toward independence facilitate a return to preexisting roles at work or at home. Patterns of interacting can also reflect changes in self-concept. For example, a client who has been hesitant to express his or her views may more readily offer opinions and ideas as self-esteem increases. The goals of care may be unrealistic or inappropriate as the client's condition changes. The plan may need to be revised, to reflect on successful experiences with other clients. Client adaptation to major changes may take a year or longer, but such length is not suggestive of problems with adaptation. Look for signs that the client has reduced some stressors and that some behaviours have become more adaptive. Changes in self-concept take time. For some clients, the sense of hopelessness and helplessness may persist. Referral to other mental health specialists may be necessary.

Client Expectations. If you have a good rapport with the client, the client may be able to share how things are going from his or her perspective. You may be able to facilitate this sharing by initiating a review of what has happened over time. This offers the opportunity to share perceptions and encourages clients to consider and voice how they have conceptualized any changes.

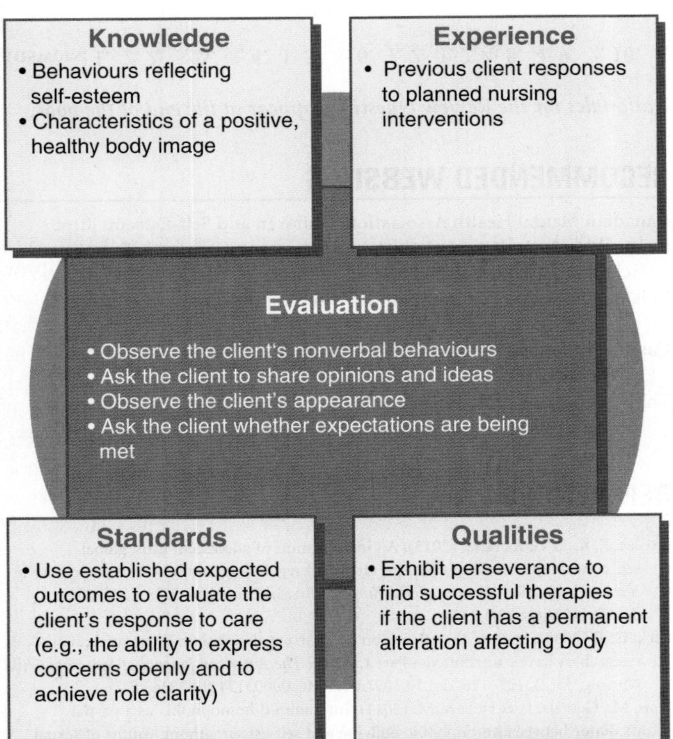

FIGURE 26-8 Critical thinking model for self-concept evaluation.

KEY CONCEPTS

- Self-concept is an integrated set of conscious and unconscious attitudes and perceptions about the self.
- Components of self-concept are identity, body image, and role performance.
- Each developmental stage involves factors that are important to developing a healthy, positive self-concept.
- Identity is particularly vulnerable during adolescence.
- Body image is the mental picture of a person's own body and is not necessarily consistent with a person's actual body structure or appearance.
- Body image stressors include changes in physical appearance, structure, or functioning that are caused by normal developmental changes or illness.
- Self-esteem is the emotional appraisal of self-concept and reflects the overall sense of being capable, worthwhile, and competent.
- Self-esteem stressors include developmental and relationship changes, illness (particularly chronic illness involving changes in what were normal activities), surgery, accidents, and the responses of other individuals to changes resulting from these events.
- Role stressors, including role conflict, role ambiguity, and role strain, may originate in unclear or conflicting role expectations and may be aggravated by illness.
- The nurse's self-concept and nursing actions can have an effect on a client's self-concept.
- Planning and implementing nursing interventions for self-concept disturbance involve increasing the client's self-awareness, encouraging self-exploration, aiding in self-evaluation, helping formulate goals for adaptation, and assisting the client in achieving those goals.

CRITICAL THINKING EXERCISES

1. You are assigned to care for a 23-year-old Chinese Canadian client who sustained multiple fractures to his face and femur 4 days ago in a motor vehicle accident. He had surgery the evening of admission to repair his femur but was admitted to wait for surgery to his face. The client lives with his girlfriend and their 7-month-old daughter and works as a janitor in the local university. He left China with his mother when he was a young child and has grown up in Canada. You have been with him for most of the morning. He was given an analgesic for his pain. His pain rating decreased from 6 to 3 on a scale of 0 to 10, but the morphine left him drowsy. During the morning, he shared with you some of his concerns about when he will be able to return to work. You are in the room when the surgeon tells him about his upcoming surgery. A temporary tracheotomy is planned because of the extensive surgery needed in the nasal and throat area. After the surgeon leaves, the client tells you that he does not want the tracheotomy. He indicates that he is unclear about what it actually entails, even though the surgeon explained it in fairly simple terms. He states, "I just want to get back to normal." How would you address this comment and his lack of understanding regarding the tracheotomy?
2. A 16-year-old girl is preparing for discharge from the hospital after giving birth a day earlier. She is unmarried, is uninvolved with the

baby's father, and has minimal support from her family to help her care for her newborn. Before admission, she arranged to give the baby up for adoption. She reaffirms this as a good decision because she will be able to return to school and still graduate with her peers. The client confides in you that her biggest concerns right now are how she feels about herself and how she looks. Taking into account the developmental needs of this adolescent, how will you collaborate with her to establish priority interventions to address her self-concept difficulties?

3. As a part of your community health experience, you are assigned to visit a 75-year-old woman who has gone to live with her daughter after being hospitalized for agitation and aggression secondary to Alzheimer's disease. When you go to their home, you find the 55-year-old daughter tearful. She says, "I just don't know if I can do this. She is so confused. She calls me two or three times a night but often doesn't recognize me when I come to her. I've been missing a lot of work. Even when I'm there, I'm not as productive because I'm so tired." What additional assessment data would be important to gather? What provisional nursing diagnosis could be made for the daughter?

REVIEW QUESTIONS

1. When a nurse is caring for a patient after a mastectomy, interventions to promote physiological stability and pain control are necessary. What other nursing interventions would the nurse need to develop?
   1. Interventions to improve the client's mobility
   2. Interventions to improve the client's self-concept
   3. Interventions to improve the client's activity tolerance
   4. Interventions to improve the client's ability to perform self-care activities
2. Adolescents are at risk for body image disturbance. Which of the following is an accurate statement about body image?
   1. Body image is not influenced by the opinions of others.
   2. Body image refers to the external features of a person.
   3. Body image includes actual and perceived perceptions of one's body.
   4. Physical changes during adolescence are quickly incorporated into the person's body image.
3. What age group is particularly vulnerable to stressors that can affect an individual's identity because it is a time of great change?
   1. Infants
   2. Children
   3. Adolescents
   4. Adults
4. What is the possible outcome when a person does not maintain a clear, consistent, and continuous consciousness of personal identity?
   1. Identity confusion
   2. Low self-esteem
   3. Low self-concept
   4. Body image difficulties
5. What is the nurse assessing for when she or he asks the client, "How do you feel about yourself?"
   1. Identity
   2. Body image
   3. Self-esteem
   4. Role performance
6. Which of the following would help increase a client's self-awareness?
   1. Establishing a trusting nurse–client relationship that allows the client to explore his or her thoughts and feelings
   2. Accepting the client's thoughts and feelings
   3. Helping the client to define his or her problems clearly
   4. Having the client identify his or her positive and negative coping mechanisms
7. Which of the following findings from your nursing assessment suggest a negative self-concept? *(Select all that apply.)*
   1. The client avoids eye contact.
   2. The client has a stooped or slumped posture.
   3. The client shows independence in self-care.
   4. The client has an untidy or unkempt appearance.
   5. The client requests a visit from the hospital chaplain.
8. The nurse is caring for a patient after back surgery. He states, "I'm a construction worker. I won't be able to work and provide for my family." Which component of self-concept does this statement address?
   1. Identity
   2. Body image
   3. Self-esteem
   4. Role performance
9. The nurse is assessing a 16-year-old who has been diagnosed with a sexually transmitted infection. The nurse realizes that risk-taking behaviours (e.g., unprotected sex) may be associated with:
   1. Peer pressure
   2. Poor self-esteem
   3. Social expectation
   4. Lack of information
10. Which of the following questions would be appropriate to assess the client's satisfaction and dissatisfaction associated with role responsibilities and relationships? *(Select all that apply).*
    1. How do you feel about yourself?
    2. What are your responsibilities in your family?
    3. Are you comfortable discussing your surgery?
    4. What are your relationships like with your relatives?
    5. What changes in your body are you expecting after surgery?

Answers: 1. 2; **2.** 3; **3.** 3; **4.** 1; **5.** 3; **6.** 1; **7.** 1, 2, 4; **8.** 4; **9.** 2; **10.** 2, 4

Rationales for the Review Questions appear at the end of the book.

RECOMMENDED WEBSITES

Canadian Mental Health Association: Children and Self-Esteem: http://cmha.calgary.ab.ca/mental-health/understanding-mental-illness/children-and-youth/children-self-esteem/.

This web page offers advice about how to promote positive self-esteem in children.

Canadian Women's Health Network: Body Image and the Media: http://www.cwhn.ca/node/40776.

This site contains a discussion of the impact of the media on body image, and it provides advice to help young women have a healthy body image.

REFERENCES

Beasley, E. K., & Garn, A. C. (2013). An investigation of adolescent girls' global self-concept, physical self-concept, identified regulation, and leisure-time activity in physical education. *Journal of Teaching in Physical Education, 32*(3), 237–252. doi:10.1123/jtpe.32.3.237.

Beck, C. T. (2008). State of the science on postpartum depression: What nurse researchers have contributed—Part 1. *MCN. The American Journal of Maternal Child Nursing, 33*(2), 121–126. doi:10.1097/01.NMC.0000313421.97236.cf.

Blais, M., Gervais, J., & Hébert, M. (2014). Internalized homophobia as a partial mediator between homophobic bullying and self-esteem among youths of sexual minorities in Quebec (Canada). *Ciênc. Saúde Coletiva, 19*(3), 727–735. doi:10.1590/1413-81232014193.16082013.

Blazek, M., & Besta, T. (2012). Self-concept clarity and religious orientations: Prediction of purpose in life and self-esteem. *Journal of Religion and Health, 51*(3), 947–960. doi:10.1007/s10943-010-9407-y.

Bleidorn, W., Arslan, R. C., Denissen, J. A., et al. (2016). Age and gender differences in self-esteem—A cross-cultural window. *Journal of Personality and Social Psychology, 111*(3), 396–410. doi:10.1037/pspp0000078.

Bowlby, J. (1982). *Attachment and loss: Vol. 1. Attachments* (2nd ed.). New York: Basic Books.

Coloroso, B. (2010). *The bully, the bullied, and the bystander: From preschool to high school—How parents and teachers can help break the cycle.* Toronto: HarperCollins.

Dumas, T. M., Ellis, W. E., & Wolfe, D. A. (2012). Identity development as a buffer of adolescent risk behaviors in the context of peer group pressure and control. *Journal of Adolescence, 35*(4), 917–927. doi:10.1016/j.adolescence.2011.12.012.

Eliopoulos, C. (2013). *Gerontologic nursing* (8th ed.). Philadelphia, PA: Lippincott.

Erikson, E. (1963). *Childhood and society* (2nd ed.). New York: W. W. Norton.

Guèvremont, A., Findlay, L., & Kohen, D. (2014). Organized extracurricular activities: Are in-school and out-of-school activities associated with different outcomes for Canadian youth? *Journal of School Health, 84*(5), 317–325. doi:10.1111/josh.12154.

Herdman, T. H., & Kamitsuru, S. (Eds.), (2014). *NANDA International: NANDA International nursing diagnoses: Definitions and classifications, 2015–2017*. Oxford, UK.: Wiley-Blackwell.

Hymel, S., & Swearer, S. M. (2015). Four decades of research on bullying: An introduction. *American Psychologist, 70*(4), 293–299. doi:10.1037/a0038928.

Johnson, M., Cowin, L. S., Wilson, I., et al. (2012). Professional identity and nursing: Contemporary theoretical developments and future research challenges. *International Nursing Review, 59*(4), 562–569. doi:10.1111/j.1466-7657.2012.01013.x.

McDougall, P., & Vaillancourt, T. (2015). Long-term adult outcomes of peer victimization in childhood and adolescence: Pathways to adjustment and maladjustment. *American Psychologist, 70*(4), 300–310. doi:10.1037/a0039174.

McKee-Ryan, F. M. (2011). "I have a job, but…": A review of underemployment. *Journal of Management, 37*(4), 962–996. doi:10.1177/0149206311398134.

Miskelly, P., & Duncan, L. (2014). "I'm actually the grown-up now": Leadership, maturity and professional identity development. *Journal of Nursing Management, 22*(1), 38–48. doi:10.1111/jonm.12030.

Neblett, E., Terzian, M., & Harriott, V. (2010). From racial discrimination to substance abuse: The buffering effects of racial socialization. *Child Development Perspectives, 4*(2), 131–137. doi:10.1111/j.1750-8606.2010.00131.x.

Orth, U., & Robins, R. W. (2014). The development of self-esteem. *Current Directions in Psychological Science, 23*(5), 381–387. doi:10.1177/0963721414547414.

Rathus, S. A., Nevid, J. S., Fichner-Rathus, L., et al. (2016). *Human sexuality in a world of diversity* (5th ed.). Toronto: Pearson Canada.

Rosenberg, M. (1965). *Society and the adolescent self-image.* Princeton, NJ: Princeton University Press.

Spurr, S., Berry, L., & Walker, K. (2013). Exploring adolescent views of body image: The influence of media. *Issues in Comprehensive Pediatric Nursing, 36*(1–2), 17–36. doi:10.3109/01460862.2013.776145.

Stuart, G. W. (2013). *Principles and practice of psychiatric nursing* (10th ed.). St. Louis, MO: Mosby.

Trzesniewski, K., Donnellan, B., & Robins, R. W. (2013). Development of self-esteem. In V. Zeigler-Hill (Ed.), *Self-esteem* (pp. 60–79). New York: Psychology Press.

Usborne, E., & Taylor, D. M. (2010). The role of cultural identity clarity for self-concept clarity, self-esteem, and subjective well-being. *Personality and Social Psychology Bulletin, 36*(7), 883–897. doi:10.1177/0146167210372215.

Zeigler-Hill, V., & Myers, E. M. (2012). A review of gender differences in self-esteem. In S. P. McGeown (Ed.), *Psychology of gender differences* (pp. 131–143). Hauppauge, NY: Nova.

27

Sexuality

Canadian content written by Jason Woytas, RN, MN, BSN
Original chapter by Kathy Lever, MSN, WHNP-BC

OBJECTIVES

Mastery of content in this chapter will enable you to:

- Define the key terms listed.
- Discuss the nurse's role in maintaining or enhancing a patient's sexual health.
- Discuss the complexities of sexual identity, gender identity, and sexual orientation.
- Describe key concepts of sexual development across the lifespan.
- Describe the sexual response cycle.
- Identify high-risk and safer sex behaviours.
- Identify common sexually transmitted infections (STIs).
- Identify major types of sexual dysfunction and potential causes.
- Assess a patient's sexuality.
- Define appropriate nursing diagnoses for patients with alterations in sexuality.
- Identify and describe nursing interventions to promote sexual health.
- Evaluate a patient's sexual health.
- Identify potential referral resources for patients' sexual concerns outside the nurse's level of expertise.
- Use critical thinking skills to assist patients in meeting their sexual needs.

KEY TERMS

Bisexuality, p. 477
Consent, p. 484
Contraception, p. 481
Dyspareunia, p. 478
Gender identity, p. 477
Heterosexuality, p. 477
Homophobia, p. 477
Homosexuality, p. 477
Infertility, p. 483
LGBTQ2S, p. 477
Queer, p. 477
Safer sex, p. 479
Same-sex relationship, p. 477
Sexual assault, p. 484
Sexual dysfunction, p. 484
Sexual health, p. 476
Sexual identity, p. 477
Sexual orientation, p. 477
Sexual response cycle, p. 478
Sexuality, p. 476
Sexually transmitted infections (STIs), p. 477
Transsexuality, p. 477
Two-spirited, p. 477
Vasocongestion, p. 478

MEDIA RESOURCES

http://evolve.elsevier.com/Canada/Potter/fundamentals/

- Audio Chapter Summaries
- Examination Review Questions
- Concept Map Creator
- Case Study with Questions
- Audio Glossary
- Content Updates
- Video Clips

Sexuality and its expression are vital elements to the wholeness we feel as human beings. **Sexuality** is seen as "a central aspect of being human throughout life and encompasses sex, gender, identities and roles, sexual orientation, eroticism, pleasure, intimacy, and reproduction" (Wagner, Bondil, Dabees, et al., 2005). People's view of themselves and others as sexual beings is influenced by their cultural, ethnic, and religious beliefs and practices. Sexuality also concerns people's sexual relationships with others and how they are perceived by others (van der Riet, 1998). Sexual functioning is seen as what people *do* as sexual beings; it is thought to consist of the four phases of the sexual response cycle as conceived by Masters and Johnson (1966; Barton, Wilwerding, Carpenter, et al., 2004). Sexual functioning, according to this definition, is the same as sexual behaviour; sexual dysfunction is thought to occur when behaviour does not follow some predetermined path and is seen as wrong or abnormal or necessitating intervention.

The World Health Organization (WHO) defines **sexual health** as "a state of physical, emotional, mental and social well-being related to sexuality; it is not merely the absence of disease, dysfunction or infirmity. Sexual health requires a positive and respectful approach to sexuality and sexual relationships, as well as to the possibility of having pleasurable and safe sexual experiences, free of coercion, discrimination and violence. For sexual health to be attained and maintained, the sexual rights of all persons must be respected, protected and fulfilled" (WHO, 2016, paragraph 4).

Nurses have a role in the promotion of positive, healthful sexuality for youth, adolescents, young and middle-aged adults, and older persons. Nurses can also educate patients to help prevent adverse outcomes such as unwanted pregnancy, sexually transmitted infections (STIs), sexual dysfunction, or abusive behaviour related to sexual activity (Health Canada, 2006; Pessango, 2013).

Religious teachings, culturally prescribed gender roles, beliefs about sexual orientation, and social and environmental climates influence both the patient's and the health care provider's value systems. As a nurse, you need to explore your own beliefs and prejudices and strive to develop a nonjudgemental and caring approach that integrates sexual health care into everyday practice.

SCIENTIFIC KNOWLEDGE BASE

To assist patients in meeting their sexual needs, nurses must have a sound scientific knowledge base about sexual and gender identity, sexual orientation, sexual development, the sexual response cycle, high-risk and safer sex behaviours, STIs, contraception, and abortion.

Sexual and Gender Identity

Sexual identity is the objective labelling of a person as male or female. In most cases this is based on the appearance of their genitalia. In some cases, individuals may not fully fit with society's notions of masculinity or femininity, but still relate to their assigned gender (Meyer-Bahlburg, 2013). However, people do not always fit neatly within these systems of sexual identification. Variations in genitalia, gonads, chromosomes, or hormones occur in an estimated 17 of 1 000 births in Canada (Johnson, 2007). For example, some people are born with ambiguous genitalia, which makes determining the sex of the infant difficult. Several genetic conditions can disrupt development of the fetus in such a way that the baby is neither fully male nor fully female (Meyer-Bahlburg, 2013). A child with an androgen disorder may have male-appearing genitalia and might genetically be a girl; another child might have male hormones and the external appearance of a girl.

Gender identity is the degree to which a person identifies as male, female, or some combination thereof. It begins in early childhood as the child becomes aware of the differences of the sexes and perceives that he or she is male or female. Gender identity is usually consistent with physical sex at birth; however, this is not always the case. For example, in transsexuality, the physical body is incongruous with the gender identity. A transsexual person may have a female body but feel like a man or may have a male body but feel like a woman (Merryfeather & Bruce, 2014). More broadly, the trans community encompasses a diverse group of people who express or identify with gender differently than what is normally expected by society and includes people who identify as transsexual, transitioned, trans, queer, or Two-spirited (University of Toronto, Centre for Addiction and Mental Health, 2017).

Gender surgery is an option for some members of the trans community. Generally speaking, *sex reassignment surgery* (Egale Canada Human Rights Trust, 2015) and *gender-affirming surgeries* (Transgender Health Information Program, 2017) refer to a variety of procedures that help alter the body of someone who is experiencing gender dysphoria. The types of surgeries that are performed and covered in each province vary, though some provinces cover some costs for some of these out-of-province surgeries.

Sexual Orientation

Sexual orientation describes the predominant gender preference of a person's sexual attraction over time. Heterosexuality is sexual preference for members of the opposite sex; homosexuality is sexual preference for members of the same sex; however, this type of relationship is more commonly referred to as a same-sex relationship. As *homosexuality* is considered to be an outdated and broad term, it is generally preferred to use more specific terms, like *lesbian* (a female attracted to another female) or *gay man* (a man who is attracted to another gay man) (Community Foundation of Canada, 2017). Bisexuality is an equal or almost equal preference for both sexes. In a recent Statistics Canada (2016) survey, 1.7% of Canadians aged 18 to 59 identified themselves as gay or lesbian, and about 1.3% of respondents identified themselves as bisexual. The survey found that people who identified as homosexual or bisexual accessed health services at a similar rate as heterosexuals, with the exception of having also consulted a psychologist. The same survey found that 33.4% of people identifying as homosexual or bisexual reported most of their days as being stressful, as compared to 26.7% of heterosexuals, and were more likely than heterosexuals to feel they needed health care in the previous 12 months but did not receive it. As a nurse, you must not assume that you know your patients' gender identity or sexual orientation. Anyone could be lesbian, gay, bisexual, transsexual, or heterosexual. If you learn a patient's sexual orientation, you should not assume that you may tell anyone else or include it in the medical record without the patient's knowledge. Some people might want to keep their sexual orientation confidential.

LGBTQ2S is a term that is frequently used to refer to people who identify as lesbian, gay, bisexual, transgender or transsexual, queer, or Two-spirited. Often, it refers to a number of different communities and groups of people who hold diverse and fluid sexual orientations and identities. The term is used to help bring awareness to the needs and experiences of people who identify with the LGBTQ2S community (University of Toronto, Centre for Addiction and Mental Health, 2017). Queer, while seen as offensive and derogatory in many situations, is starting to be reclaimed by some members of this community as a synonym for lesbian, gay man, bisexual, or trans. The term Two-spirited is attributed to Albert Macleod, who described it as having roots in many First Nations traditions, to describe an individual who has a masculine and feminine spirit and who may have same-sex attraction and a wide variety of gender variance.

Earlier thinking about sexual orientation led many to believe that heterosexuality was normal and mentally healthy and that all other orientations were abnormal or signs of a psychological disorder. Today, this theory is summarily rejected; scientists agree that homosexuality, transsexuality, and bisexuality are not disorders and are not associated with mental illness or abnormal psychological functioning. Nevertheless, homophobia—the prejudicial treatment of or negative attitudes about lesbian, gay, bisexual, or transsexual people and those who are perceived to have these gender or sexual identities—still exists. However, support for LGBTQ2 individuals has increased in recent years, with a number of Pride associations doing advocacy and awareness campaigns regarding issues faced by LGBTQ2 communities. Pride associations located in many cities across Canada, including Toronto, Edmonton and Vancouver, have hosted large parades in support of this community for many years.

The Community Foundations of Canada (2017) has put forth some guidelines around the use of terminology when talking about sexual orientation. They suggest that terms like *homosexual* are outdated and that broad terms like *gay* or *homosexual* are too broad, that more specific terms like *lesbian, gay man, bisexual woman* be used. To help foster inclusivity, they suggest using gender-neutral terms to help reduce bias. For example, instead of using *husband* or *wife*, use *spouse* or *partner*, or use the term *their* instead of *him* or *her*. Organizations like the Canadian Centre for Diversity and Inclusion (CCDI) have worked to build more inclusive environments and equity for members of the LGBTQ2s community. Issues around pay equity, spousal benefits, and job promotion have been areas where members of this community have faced discrimination in the past.

Sexual Development

As a person grows and develops, so does his or her sexuality. Each stage of development brings changes in sexual functioning and in the role of sexuality in relationships.

Infancy and Childhood. Beginning at early ages, young children start to explore their sexuality through various means (Balter, van Rhijn, & Davies, 2016). They are socialized into cultural, societal, and familial norms through interactions with parents, caregivers, and peers. Sexual development can be influenced by the ease with which parents and caregivers are able to communicate with children in terms of their sexuality. This can include the naming of genital parts, learning about appropriate behaviours for boys and girls, exploring their bodies while in the washroom, and learning about personal spatial limits and gender through play (such as learning about the body parts of the opposite gender).

Puberty and Adolescence. This is a developmental period in which social and emotional changes are also significant. Peer group attachments are strong; sexual attraction to other people is common (Figure 27-1). Often, peer groups can encourage or reinforce adolescents' decisions about whether or not to engage in sexual activity. Decisions about sexual activity can also be influenced as the adolescent moves from thinking concretely (where only the here and now is important) to thinking abstractly (often considering the future). Promoting safe, healthy group interactions with adolescents of both genders as adolescents develop (such as watching movies or listening to music) can help promote healthy relationships (Wisnieski & Matzo, 2013). Many adolescents who engage in sexual activity are influenced by the amount of sexual activity they perceive their peers to partake in, as well as perceiving their activities to be low risk in nature. Adolescents involved in risky sexual behaviour are often influenced by the use of drugs and alcohol, and sensation seeking. The tendency toward risky sexual behaviour increases when adolescents are in a relationship.

Public health care providers have been alarmed by the trend toward greater sexual activity at increasingly younger ages, particularly because

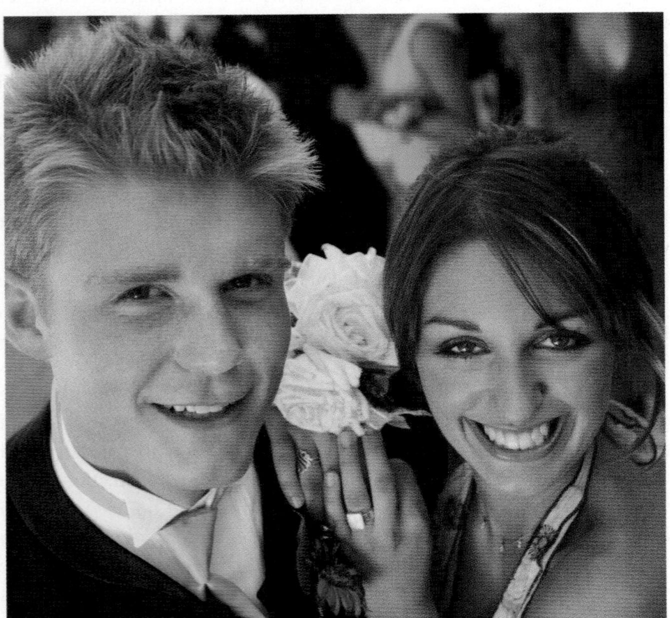

FIGURE 27-1 Adolescents with peers. Adolescents function within a powerful network of peers as they explore their sexual and gender identity. (Credit © sirtravelalot/Shutterstock.)

of the adverse consequences. According to Rotermann (2012), two-thirds of 15- to 24-year-olds have been sexually active at least once, with a third of these having had sex before the age of 17. In 2010, a third of sexually active 15- to 24-year-olds reported having more than one partner in the previous year. While condom use has increased, it was typically with people being active with just one partner. According to Bushnik (2016), the rates of chlamydia and gonorrhea have risen in Canada over the past 20 years.

Support for adolescents who have questions or concerns around their sexuality should be well rounded. Interventions should match the adolescent's cognitive development, address the effects of peer pressure and common misconceptions regarding sexuality, and emphasize the importance of family, friends, and extended family in building healthy relationships (Wisnieski & Matzo, 2013). Providing sex education is often controversial in school settings—while sex education is present and supported in some school settings, it is opposed by educators and parents in other schools because of the belief that it encourages adolescents to engage in early and risky sexual behaviour.

Adulthood. Adults have matured physically but continue to explore and define emotional maturation in relationships. Intimacy and sexuality are issues for all adults of all sexual orientations, whether they are in a sexual relationship, choose to abstain from sex, are single, are widowed, or are divorced—whatever circumstances arise. People can be sexually healthy in numerous ways.

Through middle adulthood, physical changes can affect sexual functioning. Decreasing levels of estrogen in perimenopausal women (during the years leading up to menopause) and menopausal women (after menstruation has ceased) may result in diminished vaginal lubrication and decreased vaginal elasticity. Both of these changes may lead to **dyspareunia**, which is painful intercourse. Declining levels of testosterone result in decreased desire for sexual activity. Suggestions such as using vaginal lubrication and creating time for caressing and tenderness can help patients adjust to normal changes related to aging.

As men age, they are likely to experience an increase in the post-ejaculatory refractory period, delayed ejaculation, and erectile dysfunction. Advising patients of these normal changes related to aging can ease concerns regarding functioning. Aging adults may also need to adjust to the effects of chronic illness, medications, aches, pains, and other health concerns that affect sexuality.

Older Personhood. As people age, some shift their priority from genital sex to other ways of expressing sexual desire. Activities that promote affection, romance, intimacy, and companionship may be enough to satisfy the sexual needs of some older persons (Figure 27-2). However, not all older persons experience a decline in interest in sex. Often nurses and older persons are hesitant to speak about sexuality due to embarrassment and cultural restraint (Buttaro, Koeniger-Donohue, & Hawkins, 2014). However, many issues can and should be addressed with sexually active older persons, including body image, erectile dysfunction, and STIs. Studies have shown that a number of misconceptions exist in regard to sexuality with older persons (Abeykoon & Lucyk, 2015). Often, health care providers avoid discussing with them issues around sex unless the issue is obvious. As well, many clinical trials around STIs don't include people from this age group. However, with medications like Viagra, Cialis, Levitra, and various progesterone and estrogen products, people are remaining sexually active for longer periods of time, and rates of STIs have increased in this population.

Sexual Response Cycle. Masters and Johnson (1966) developed a four-stage model explaining the human **sexual response cycle**. The model suggested that major similarities exist between men and women. The four stages of the model are excitement, plateau, orgasm, and resolution, and they represent episodes of **vasocongestion** (swelling of tissues) and muscle contractions.

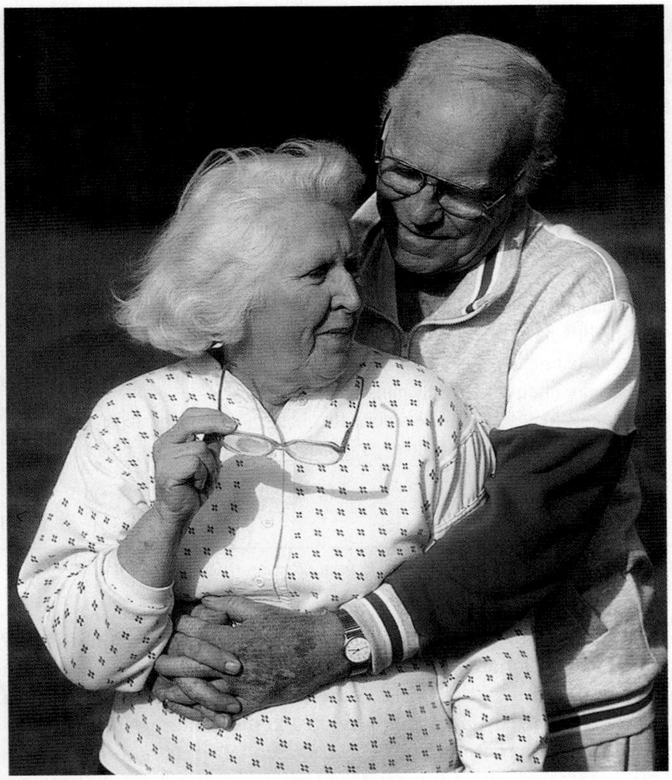

FIGURE 27-2 Intimacy and affection are important to older persons. (From Sorrentino, S. A. [2004]. *Mosby's Canadian textbook for the support worker* [p. 166]. Toronto: Elsevier.)

In the *excitement* stage, the heart rate and blood pressure increase, and blood flows into the sexual organs. In women, the breasts enlarge in size, and a reddish flush may be seen over the upper torso. The nipples become more erect. Increased blood flow to the genitalia results in enlargement of the clitoris; engorgement of the labia majora, which flatten and spread outward; and swelling of the labia minora. The upper two-thirds of the vagina enlarge, and the vaginal walls thicken. The vaginal walls also secrete a fluid that allows for penile penetration. In men, the penis becomes erect as blood flows into the spongy tissues. The skin of the scrotum thickens, and the testicles swell; the scrotum elevates, and the testicles move in toward the body.

The *plateau* phase is a state of advanced arousal. Blood pressure and heart rate continue to increase, and breathing may become rapid. In women, the lower third of the vagina (at the entry to the vagina) swells. The upper vagina continues to expand, and the uterus moves into an upright position. The labia minora become more engorged with blood and become a darker colour. The clitoris shortens and withdraws below the clitoral hood. The breasts continue to increase in size. In men, the testicles continue to enlarge. The head or glans of the penis changes to a deeper colour.

Orgasm is the phase of significant muscular contractions. During this phase, respiration and heart rates peak, and subjective feelings of intense pleasure radiate through the body. Most of the major muscles in the body contract and may go into spasm. In women, the pelvic muscles contract between 3 and 15 times. The muscles of the anal sphincter and the uterus itself contract. Orgasm in the male occurs in two stages; in the first phase, seminal fluid is forced into the bulb of the penis by contractions of the vas deferens, the two seminal vesicles, the ejaculatory ducts, and the prostate gland. The bladder neck closes off to prevent urine from mixing with the semen. The second stage of orgasm for the man occurs when the muscles around the urethra contract and fluid is propelled along the urethra and out of the urethral meatus. These contractions are accompanied by subjective feelings of intense pleasure.

In the *resolution* phase, vasocongestion diminishes, and the rest of the body returns to its normal state: muscle tension is reduced within minutes, and heart rate, blood pressure, and respiration rate return to normal. During this phase in women, blood flow to the pelvic organs is reduced. The breasts return to their normal size, and flushing of the skin disappears. In men, the penis loses its rigidity, and the testicles and scrotum shrink in size. In men, this phase is followed by a refractory period during which orgasm and ejaculation are physiologically impossible. In young men, the refractory period may last a few minutes, but as men age, this period lasts longer, and older men may not be able to have another orgasm or ejaculation for many hours or even days. Women do not experience a refractory period; they may have multiple orgasms with continued stimulation.

Kaplan (1979) introduced the idea of desire in her description of the human sexual response cycle. Her model comprises three parts: desire, excitement, and orgasm. In Kaplan's model, emotion and cognition, which lead to the subjective feeling of desire, are an important part of sexual response. Excitement and orgasm in this model are as described in Masters and Johnson's (1966) model. Kaplan did not include resolution in her model; she suggested that the cycle has three independent phases. Also, according to this model, it is possible to experience excitement without having experienced desire first.

More recently, Basson (2005) described an alternative model of the female sexual response cycle. It relies heavily on psychoemotional processes, as opposed to the more physiological basis of Masters and Johnson's (1966) and Kaplan's (1979) models. In her model, desire (or *libido*) is thought to occur at a variety of points in the sexual response cycle. The female sexual response cycle is conceptualized as a circular rather than linear process as described in the two previous models. Basson suggests that women rely on different reasons to be receptive to or instigators of sexual activity; rewards such as emotional intimacy, feelings of well-being, and lack of negative feelings resulting from avoiding sex are all factors that may cause a woman to feel desire. With varied motivations for sexual activity, women respond to sexual stimuli from a partner. When the woman receives these stimuli, they are processed psychologically and physically; this may then lead to subjective feelings of arousal and a responsive feeling of desire. Sexual satisfaction is thought to further increase motivation and willingness to be receptive at a future time. Basson reasoned that satisfaction does not necessarily mean orgasm; she suggests that for many women, feelings of closeness and intimacy and the partner's satisfaction may be enough to cause satisfaction for the woman.

Sexual Behaviour

Sexual behaviour typically comprises the broad array of sexual activities people participate in, such as masturbation, hugging, kissing, manual stimulation of a partner, vaginal or anal penetration, oral-genital stimulation, oral-anal stimulation, sexual excitement while looking at erotica, and telephone or "cyber" sex (Society of Obstetricians and Gynaecologists of Canada [SOGC], 2017). It is difficult to define "normal" and "abnormal" because wide variation exists between cultures and at different times in society. An inclusive attitude is that whatever people find pleasurable is "normal" as long as it occurs between consenting adults who engage in sexual behaviour by choice, in a safe environment where rules and boundaries are negotiated and respected (Box 27-1).

High-Risk Sexual Behaviour. Because body fluids can be transferred between partners, unprotected sex can result in pregnancy or the transmission of STIs. Safer sex refers to sexual activities that present minimal or reduced risk for disease transmission or unintended

BOX 27-1 RESEARCH HIGHLIGHT

A Quantitative Study of "Friends With Benefits" Relationships

This study examined the experiences of undergraduate university students who have either been or currently are in a "friends with benefits" relationship.

Research Focus

The focus of this study was to examine the relationship between the reasons for and expectations of this type of relationship, and the eventual outcome of the relationship.

Research Abstract

Gusarova, Fraser, and Alderson (2012) provided 146 male and 135 female undergraduate students with questionnaires that asked about their "friends with benefits relationships" (FWBR). Although most respondents had positive (38%) or neutral (37%) experiences, 40% would not enter this relationship again. Relationships that had emotional complications (22%) strongly predicted negative outcomes. Women were found to be more likely to hope that this type of relationship would result in dating.

Evidence-Informed Practice

- FWBR (two friends who engage in sexual activity without formally dating) has been increasingly studied in recent years but there is still a lot to be studied.
- FWBR relationships are generally seen as being more stable and less risky than people who "hook-up" for sexual intercourse with someone they don't know well, as hook-ups are more likely to involve a risk of pressure into unwanted sexual activities.
- As FWBR relationships are generally not exclusive, and communication about expectations of the relationship often doesn't occur, the emotional and social needs are often not strongly met.
- Being aware and open to communicate about these relationships can be an important aspect of the nurse–patient relationship and can provide some valuable assessment data.

Gusarova, I., Fraser, V., & Alderson, K. G. (2012). A quantitative study of "friends with benefits" relationships. *Canadian Journal of Human Sexuality, 21*(1), 41–59.

pregnancy. *Unsafe sex* refers to activities through which risk for infection, unintended pregnancy, or injury is increased. Unsafe sex includes anal-penile or vaginal-penile intercourse without a condom (Van Ouytsel, Walrave, Ponnet, et al., 2015). Without the use of barriers such as condoms or latex dental dams, penile-anal intercourse is probably the riskiest activity, followed by penile-vaginal intercourse, oral-anal sex, and oral-genital sex.

The dynamics of sexual risk taking are not fully understood, but numerous studies have revealed that drug and alcohol use, peer pressure, and sensation seeking are highly correlated with unsafe sex, especially among adolescents (Gusarova, Fraser, & Alderson, 2012; Wisnieki & Matzo, 2013).

Sexually Transmitted Infections

A number of STIs are of concern to public health officials and health care providers. In Canada, health officials report increases in all of the infections that, by law, must be reported, including chlamydia, gonorrhea, and syphilis (Government of Canada, 2017). There is some variance between provinces in terms of which STIs are reported and how they are reported. Nurses need to be aware of the mandatory reporting requirements in their province.

A major problem in dealing with STIs is finding and treating the people who have them. Because symptoms may be absent or go unnoticed, some people may not even know that they are infected. Sexual behaviour may include the whole body rather than just the genitalia; therefore, many parts of the body are potential sites for an STI. The mouth, tongue, and throat are commonly used for sexual pleasure. The vagina, perineum, anus, and rectum are also frequently included in sexual activity. Furthermore, any contact with another person's body fluids near an open lesion on the skin, anus, or genitalia can result in transmission of an STI.

Sometimes people do not seek treatment because they are embarrassed to discuss sexual symptoms or concerns. They may also hesitate to talk about their sexual behaviour if they believe that it is not "normal." This hesitation to seek help often hinders the detection of an STI.

Human Papillomavirus. Human papillomavirus (HPV) is the most common STI in the world according to the Society of Obstetrics and Gynaecologists of Canada (2017). It is strongly linked with cervical cancer, and it may be manifested as external genital warts that occur on the penis, scrotum, perineum, vulva, and perianal area; they usually appear as small, hard, painless bumps. These warts can also occur in the vagina, on the cervix, inside the urethra, and inside the anus. If untreated, they may grow and develop a fleshy, cauliflowerlike appearance. Because they are caused by a virus, genital warts cannot be cured. They are treated with a topical drug (applied to the skin), by freezing, or, if they recur, with injections of medication. If the warts are very large, they can be removed surgically. A preventive vaccine for HPV has been approved which offers protection against seven HPV types. The recommendation is that girls and women between the ages of 9 and 45 be offered this vaccine; it is important that the vaccine be given before the initiation of sexual activity. Women who are sexually active may receive the vaccine but, because they may have already been exposed to some strains of HPV, are less likely to benefit from it. The HPV vaccine has also been shown to be effective in men aged 9 to 26 years.

HPV is the leading cause of oropharyngeal cancers. HPV subtype 18 is most often associated with oral cancer, and the virus is readily spread through mucosal contact. White, non-smoking males between 35 and 55 are most at risk, outnumbering females 4 to 1 (Oral Cancer Foundation, 2017).

Chlamydia. Chlamydia is one of the most common of all bacterial STIs (SOGC, 2017). Chlamydial infection may cause an abnormal genital discharge and burning with urination; however, it is often asymptomatic. It is treated by an antibiotic.

Chlamydia produces many serious complications in women. If undetected and thus untreated, it can progress to pelvic inflammatory disease (PID) in women, a very painful and sometimes debilitating disease that is linked to infertility. An untreated chlamydial infection may cause scarring of the uterine tubes, which increases the risk for ectopic pregnancy and infertility. Research findings suggest that chlamydial infection can also cause another form of STI called *lymphogranuloma venerum*, also known as LGV, or venereal disease. It may also lead to miscarriage, preterm birth, and an infant's low birth weight for women who are pregnant (SOGC, 2017).

Syphilis. Syphilis, a bacterial infection, can be transmitted through oral, vaginal–penile, or anal sex with an infected person. A pregnant woman with syphilis can pass it on to her baby, which can lead to birth defects or death in the baby. Syphilis also can be transmitted through injection drug use or through broken skin or sores, although transmission by these routes is not common. Syphilis can be diagnosed with a simple blood test and is easily treated with antibiotics. If it is not treated, syphilis can affect the brain, blood vessels, heart, and bones. It can also cause death. Males older than 30 years account for the majority of syphilis cases in Canada (SOGC, 2017), and local outbreaks are reported periodically across the country.

Gonorrhea. Gonorrhea is easily transmitted during vaginal-penile intercourse, anal-penile intercourse, and oral sex (SOGC, 2017). Infection rates are on the rise in Canada; it is currently the second most common STI, and is often found as a co-infection with chlamydia. It can affect the penis, cervix, rectum or anus, throat, and eyes. Pain during sex or during urination, or unusual discharge, may be indications of a gonorrheal infection. Gonorrhea must be treated with antibiotics. If left untreated, it may cause serious health problems, including infertility. It can also cause blood, joint, and eye infections in a baby born to an infected woman.

Genital Herpes. Genital herpes, caused by the herpes simplex virus, is the most common manifestation of genital ulceration and is transmitted by people who have no visible or symptomatic lesions in up to 70% of cases (SOGC, 2017). Genital herpes can cause extensive ulceration (painful blisters or open sores) with severe pain. The infection can be passed on from mother to baby during birth and can cause lesions and possibly life-threatening infections of the central nervous system for the baby. Without treatment, episodes can last for 3 or more weeks, and many people with herpes have recurrent episodes. At present, the viral infection is incurable; antiviral drugs can only control the symptoms and suppress transmission.

Human Immunodeficiency Virus Infection. Human immunodeficiency virus (HIV) is the virus that causes acquired immune deficiency syndrome (AIDS). Essentially, HIV destroys the body's ability to defend against infection. Many people do not have symptoms when they first are infected with HIV, although some may have a flulike illness within 1 to 2 weeks after exposure. More persistent or severe symptoms may not appear for 10 years or more after infection. During the asymptomatic period, however, the virus is actively multiplying, infecting, and killing cells of the immune system. As the immune system weakens, various complications occur (SOGC, 2017).

AIDS represents the most advanced stage of HIV infection. The syndrome can result in many infections that do not usually affect healthy people. In people with AIDS, these infections are often severe and sometimes fatal. People with AIDS are particularly prone to developing cancers, especially those caused by viruses (such as Kaposi's sarcoma or cervical cancer) and those of the immune system (such as lymphomas).

In an infected person, HIV is present in the majority of body fluids. For transmission to occur, therefore, some exchange of body fluid, particularly blood, must occur. Primary routes of transmission include contaminated intravenous needles, unprotected sexual activity (anal intercourse, vaginal intercourse, and oral-genital sex), and transfusion of blood and blood products. HIV can also be spread from infected mothers to their babies during pregnancy, at birth, or during breastfeeding. HIV has not been proved to be transmitted through sweat, tears, saliva, or urine.

Rates of HIV continue to rise in Canada, affecting approximately 75 500 people by 2014 estimates. Approximately 20% of people who have HIV are unaware they are affected (SOGC, 2017). For people who are knowingly going to have sex with an HIV-positive partner or otherwise be exposed to contaminated bodily fluids, pre-exposure prophylaxis may be available in some circumstances. Post-exposure prophylaxis is also available (i.e., for needlestick injuries) but must be started within 72 hours to be most effective. While there is no cure for HIV, antiretroviral medication is frequently used to slow the progression of the disease.

Prevention of Sexually Transmitted Infections. People most likely to be infected with an STI are those who have unprotected sex. Exposure to multiple partners or to a sexual partner who has many partners increases the risk of acquiring an STI. Injection drug users are also a high-risk group because they share blood by sharing needles. Primary prevention of STIs starts with changing the sexual behaviour that heightens the risk for infection. Health promotion must be targeted toward high-risk groups and must emphasize education and counselling regarding safer sexual behaviour. STIs often occur together, and screening is usually performed for all STIs at the same time.

Safer Sex. *Safer sex* refers to the sexual practices and behaviour that reduce the risk of contracting and transmitting STIs, especially HIV. When a partner is infected or when the infection status of a partner is not known, it is crucial to practise safer sex. For vaginal-penile and penile-anal intercourse, partners should use condoms. Safer sex practices are also necessary for oral sex; if one of the partners is a woman, a thin piece of rubber, a latex dental dam, a female condom, or an unlubricated male condom cut open to form a flat piece of latex should be placed between the other partner's mouth and the woman's vulva before any oral contact is made. Male partners should cover their penis with an unlubricated condom before any oral contact is made (SOGC, 2017).

Using Condoms. Condoms were originally sold to promote birth control. However, when used correctly, they also provide protection against STIs. A condom acts as a barrier to keep blood, semen, and vaginal fluids from passing from one person to another. In Canada, condoms are free at many public health clinics and readily available from drugstores and supermarkets. Condoms can be made from latex, polyurethane, or natural membranes such as sheepskin or lambskin. Latex and polyurethane condoms reduce the risk of most STIs (including HIV) and help protect against pregnancy. Natural membrane condoms do not protect against STIs because some bacteria and viruses can pass through small pores in the material (Healthwise Staff, 2016).

A female condom is a strong, soft, clear sheath made of polyurethane with two rings at either end. It is placed inside the vagina before sex and protects against pregnancy and STIs (including HIV). When placed correctly, one end covers the cervix and the other end covers part of the external genitalia (Healthwise Staff, 2016) although the U.S. Centers for Disease Control and Prevention (CDC) (2015) state that the efficacy of using female condoms during anal intercourse is unknown.

Contraception

Contraception is a crucial facet of sexual health to avoid unwanted pregnancies. Some forms of contraception require a health care provider's intervention: hormonal contraceptives (e.g., birth control pills or patch, injectable contraceptives), intrauterine devices (IUDs), the diaphragm, the vaginal contraceptive ring, and the cervical cap. Surgical procedures that provide permanent contraception are also available to men (vasectomy) and women (tubal ligation). Other forms of contraception do not require a prescription or intervention from a health care provider: condoms, contraceptive sponges, vaginal spermicides, and fertility awareness methods (i.e., timing of intercourse in relation to the menstrual cycle). Table 27-1 summarizes some of the contraceptive choices available.

Effective contraception involves factors relating to the sexually active couple, the method of contraception, the couple's understanding of the contraceptive method, the consistency of contraceptive use, and the compliance with the requirements of the chosen method. Personal characteristics that have been identified as positively influencing

TABLE 27-1 Available Contraceptives

Type	Effectiveness	Description
Male condom	82–98%	A thin, skin-tight sheath placed on an erect penis to stop sperm from entering a partner's body. Water-based lubricants can make them more comfortable, increase sensation, and reduce the risk of breakage.
Female condom	79–95%	A lubricated pouch that is placed in the vagina before penile insertion; it stops sperm from entering the woman's body. It may break or slip, and some women may have difficulty placing it correctly.
Birth control pills	91–99%	Pills taken every day that contain a low dose of hormones (estrogen and progestin or progestin alone). The ovaries are prevented from releasing an egg for fertilization, eggs are prevented from implanting, and the mucus around the cervix is thickened, which makes entry of the sperm more difficult. They are available only by prescription.
Cervical cap	Previous childbirth: 68–74% No previous vaginal childbirth: 84–91%	A small, flexible cup that is inserted into the vagina before penile insertion. It covers the cervix and prevents sperm from entering the uterus. The caps are available in different sizes; proper fitting by a trained health care provider is required.
Intrauterine device (IUD) (both hormonal and copper IUD)	99.2–99.9%	A small piece of plastic or copper that is inserted into the uterus by a physician. Sperm is prevented from fertilizing an egg, or, if an egg is fertilized, the egg is prevented from implanting in the uterus. Some IUDs also release hormones to prevent pregnancy. IUDs can stay in place for 1–8 years.
Birth control patch	91–99%	A thin, 2 cm × 2 cm patch that can be worn on the lower abdomen, buttock, upper arm, or upper torso. The patch is applied once a week for 3 consecutive weeks; the fourth week is patch free. The mechanism of action is the same as that of oral contraceptives.
Injectable contraceptive	94–99%	Progestin is injected into a woman's arm or buttocks once every 12 weeks. The hormone prevents the ovaries from releasing eggs. A physician or nurse administers the injections.
Vaginal contraceptive ring	91–99%	A soft, flexible, transparent ring that is self-inserted into the vagina and delivers hormones over 3 weeks, after which time the ring is removed for 1 week. A new ring is then inserted.
Contraceptive sponge	Woman who has had children: 68–80% Woman who has not had children: 84–91%	A soft sponge that is filled with spermicide and placed in the vagina before vaginal–penile intercourse. It is effective for 24 hours after placement. The sponge must be kept in place for 6 hours after intercourse.
Vaginal spermicides	72–82%	Gels, films, and suppositories, which contain a spermicidal agent, that are inserted into the vagina before vaginal–penile intercourse. The agent kills sperm and acts as a physical barrier to prevent any surviving sperm cells from entering the cervix. This approach may be used by women who are at low risk for STIs and whose partners are at low risk.
Fertility awareness method	76–95%	A woman can monitor her fertility patterns and know, on the basis of daily observations of body temperature and cervical mucus, when she is most likely and least likely to conceive. She must abstain from vaginal–penile intercourse when she is most likely to conceive. This method can also be used to achieve pregnancy.
Tubal ligation	99%	A surgical procedure in which a woman's uterine tubes are tied into a loop and then cut. This procedure is performed with the woman under general anaesthesia, and its effects should be considered permanent.
Vasectomy	99%	A minor surgical procedure for men in which the vas deferens that carry the sperm are cut, "tied," cauterized, or otherwise interrupted. The semen no longer contains sperm after the tubes are cut, and conception cannot occur. The procedure can be performed in a physician's office with a local anaesthetic. The results of this procedure should be considered permanent.

Adapted from HealthWise Staff. (2016). Retrieved from https://myhealth.alberta.ca/Pages/default.aspx.

contraceptive use include motivation to avoid unplanned pregnancy, ability to plan, comfort with sexuality, and previous contraceptive use (Running & Berndt, 2003). Cultural and religious background may permit certain practices and prohibit others. For example, the teachings of the Roman Catholic Church prohibit the use of contraception except for the fertility awareness method.

Emergency Contraception. There are two types of emergency contraception currently available in Canada. Commonly referred to as Plan B or the morning-after pill, medication is available in two forms: LNG-EC pills are available without a prescription from a pharmacy and are most effective within 24 hours of unprotected intercourse but can be taken up to 5 days after. A body mass index (BMI) of greater than 25 may decrease their effectiveness (SOGC, 2017). UPA-EC pills remain more effective for a longer period of time (5 days) and appear to be equally effective for those who have a higher BMI. However, the most effective method is the use of a copper intrauterine device, which is inserted by a doctor within 7 days of unprotected intercourse. This method also provides ongoing secure birth control.

As of 2005, Canadian pharmacists may dispense emergency contraception pills (ECPs) (LNG-EC pills) without a physician's prescription; however, pharmacists have the right to refuse to do so if it conflicts with their personal beliefs. ECPs are available for free or at minimum cost at many university health services, sexual health clinics, birth control clinics, Planned Parenthood clinics, and women's health clinics. Adolescent girls do not require parental consent to obtain ECPs, and no medical examination is required.

Abortion

Since 1988, Canada has been one of the few countries without any legal restrictions on abortion. Canada has no requirements for waiting periods, parental or spousal consent, gestational limits, or restrictions on types of elective abortion. Abortion is also a safe procedure, especially if performed within the first trimester of pregnancy. Some provinces fully fund all elective abortions; others fund only those performed in hospitals. However, access to abortion services is often a problem for women living outside major cities. Abortion rates declined between 2007 and 2014, with 58.5% of abortions occurring in abortion clinics and 41.5% occurring in hospitals (Abortion Rights Coalition of Canada, 2017). In Prince Edward Island, no hospitals provide abortions.

Abortion continues to be a hotly debated issue. Women and their partners faced with an unwanted pregnancy may consider an elective abortion. As a nurse, you can provide an environment in which the issue of abortion can be discussed openly and various options with an unwanted pregnancy can be explored. You should discuss religious, social, and personal issues in a nonjudgemental manner with patients. Reasons for choosing an elective abortion vary and may include terminating an unwanted pregnancy or aborting a fetus known to have abnormalities. When abortion is chosen as a way of dealing with an unwanted pregnancy, the woman, and often her partner, may experience a sense of loss, grief, or guilt or a combination of these. Guilt may surface immediately, or it may be more covert and manifest as sexual dysfunction.

Health care providers must reflect on their own personal values related to abortion. The health care provider is entitled to personal views and should not be forced to participate in counselling or procedures contrary to beliefs and values. Nurses should choose specialties or places of employment in which their personal values are not compromised and the health care that a patient needs is not jeopardized.

NURSING KNOWLEDGE BASE

In planning to help patients address sexual needs, nurses should use critical thinking skills and basic nursing knowledge. Nurses may draw from the following areas of nursing knowledge: sociocultural dimensions of sexuality; how to discuss sexual issues; alterations in sexual health (infertility, sexual abuse, sexual dysfunction); and conditions that create sexual health concerns (pregnancy, surgery, illness, disability).

Sociocultural Dimensions of Sexuality

Sexuality is influenced by cultural rules and norms that determine which behaviour is acceptable within the culture. Society plays a powerful role in shaping sexual values and attitudes and in supporting specific expression of sexuality in its members. Each cultural and social group has its own set of rules and norms that guide the behaviour of its members. These rules become an integral part of an individual's thinking and underlie sexual behaviour; they include, for example, how people find partners, their choices of partners, how they relate to one another, how often they have sex, and what they do when they have sex.

It is widely suggested that nurses include information about sexual health and the implications for sexuality when they care for patients. Nurses should also routinely ask patients whether they have any sexual concerns related to their condition or treatments (Albaugh & Kellog-Spadt, 2003). However, this question is frequently omitted, and a valuable opportunity to be proactive and holistic in the care provided is thus missed (Haboubi & Lincoln, 2003). Some nurses may feel that asking about sexuality is an invasion of patients' privacy (Bartlik, Rosenfeld, & Beaton, 2005), or they may think that gender is a barrier (Burd, Nevadunsky, & Bachmann, 2006). Nurses appear to be more likely to wait for the patient to initiate the discussion than to assess this routinely (Guthrie, 1999). Nurses may think that the patient does not expect them to ask questions about this (Magnan, Reynolds, & Galvin, 2005), or they may believe that it is the physician's responsibility (Herson, Hart, Gordon, et al., 1999). As a result, sexual problems may not be recognized and thus may be ignored. Some nurses may presume that because of the seriousness of the patient's disease or because of the patient's stage of life, sexuality is not an important issue (Huang, 1999); this presumption can have consequences, such as lack of education for the patient.

Discussing Sexual Issues

Sexuality is a significant part of each person's being; however, sexual assessment and interventions are not always included in health care. The area of sexuality can be emotionally charged for nurses as well as for patients. Discomfort with talking about sexual issues, lack of information, and differences between a patient's values and the nurse's values may prevent the nurse from discussing issues of sexuality with patients. The most valuable tool that nurses can develop for providing care in areas of sexuality is effective, nonjudgemental communication. If you as a nurse have difficulty discussing topics related to sexuality, you should understand why, and you should develop a plan for addressing your discomfort.

Discussing matters of a sexual nature can also be embarrassing for patients. Often, patients do not mention sexual health issues; they may worry about looking stupid, using incorrect words, or being offensive, or they may simply have no way of describing their concerns. It is crucial that nurses be comfortable in asking questions about sexuality and in responding to issues that arise from such questioning. By using a perceptive and educated approach to talking about sexuality, nurses can offer the support that many patients require.

Effective communication about sexuality requires caring, sensitivity, tact, compassion, the use of appropriate language, and nondiscriminatory attitudes. When talking with patients about sexuality, it is important not to have preconceived notions about their sexual identity or activity. Lesbians, gay men, and bisexual people may not receive adequate health care if health care providers assume heterosexual sexual orientation and fail to obtain complete sexual histories. Older persons' sexual health may also be overlooked if health care providers stereotype these patients as asexual.

Alterations in Sexual Health

Infertility. Infertility is the inability of a couple to conceive after 1 year of unprotected intercourse and affects one in six couples. Generally, infertility is caused by either hormonal or structural causes, including fallopian tube damage and sperm dysfunction. Primary care nurses often provide support and education around obesity management, smoking cessation, and alcohol and drug use, all of which can affect fertility. In some cases, surgery, assisted conception, or both may help (Massey, 2015).

Choices for the infertile couple include medical assistance with fertilization, adoption, or exploring the possibility of remaining childless. Nurses can give emotional support and refer couples to infertility support groups that can provide couples with further emotional and educational help.

Sexual Abuse. Sexual abuse is a widespread health problem. Abuse crosses all gender, socioeconomic, age, and ethnic groups. Most often, this abuse is perpetrated by a former intimate partner or by a family member. Sexual abuse has far-ranging effects on physical and psychological functioning (Sabella, 2016). Increasingly, sexual abuse is occurring through the Internet: sexual predators recruit victims on social networking sites and then arrange to meet the victims, after which the abuse begins.

Evidence of sexual abuse in children may be uncovered during history taking or physical examination (see Chapter 32). Symptoms that should raise suspicion of sexual abuse include a child showing an early, exaggerated awareness of sex or exhibiting seductive behaviour toward adults; swelling or bruising of the external genitalia, anus, breasts, or buttocks; lacerations of or a foreign substance in the vagina or anus; and an STI in a child younger than 15 years. In Canada, nurses are required by law to report suspected child abuse to child protection authorities. Signs and symptoms of sexual abuse are listed in Box 27-2.

When sexual abuse is recognized, support needs to be mobilized for the victim and the family. All family members may require therapy in situations of incest, to promote healthy interactions and relationships. Rape victims may need to come to terms with the crisis before feeling comfortable with intimate expressions of affection. The victim's partner may need support in understanding this process and ways to assist the victim. Children who have been sexually abused need to understand that they are not at fault for the incident. The parents must understand that their response is critical to how the child reacts and adapts. As a nurse, you may come in contact with patients confronting these stressors. You are in an ideal position to assess occurrences of sexual violence and to educate individuals about community services. You should be aware of resources for referral and support in the community.

Consent is described as the voluntary agreement to engage in sexual activity and can be demonstrated verbally and/or by a person's conduct without undue pressure; the person must be capable of consent. A person needs to be 16 years old to consent to sexual activity as an adult. A person who is under 16 years of age cannot consent to sexual activities with someone 5 or more years older than him or her, and if under 14 years of age, the person is unable to consent to sexual activity with someone who is 2 or more years older.

Sexual assault is seen as an assault on the sexual nature or the sexual identity of an individual (Edmonton Police Service, 2014). While it is often seen as unwanted physical touching, sexual assault may also involve language, gestures, or actions that violate the sexual integrity of the individual. According to the Department of Justice Canada (2017), it is estimated that only 5% of sexual assaults are reported and that 87% of self-reported sexual assault victims are women, of which less than half (43%) of cases going to trial result in a guilty verdict.

Sexting is a newer trend in which people send sexually suggestive or explicit content to each other via computerized devices (i.e., cellphones, computers, electronic tablets) through such means as text messaging, social media, or other communication applications (Champion & Pedersen, 2015). While many who participate in sexting view it as being satisfying (i.e., providing immediate gratification) and safer than sex (no chance of developing an STI or getting pregnant), there are some risks associated with it. Those who use sexting to recruit sexual partners tend to take part in riskier sexual activities, have higher rates of substance use, and are at risk of having nude photos of themselves being shared with individuals the pictures were not intended for. The threat of pictures being shared publically can potentially be dangerous and has led many schools to add online safety to the curriculum. The popularity and anonymity of many online social groups make it easy to potentially hurt, silence, and oppress individuals and cause them distress when someone threatens to share their sexually explicit pictures with family or friends or on the Internet (Schneider, O'Donnell, Stueve, et al., 2012; Slane, 2013).

BOX 27-2 Signs and Symptoms That May Indicate Current or Previous Sexual Abuse

- Irritation or injury (such as cuts and bruises or scarring) of the thighs, perineum, or breasts
- Trauma to mouth and throat, including petechiae of the oral cavity
- Oral sexually transmitted infections
- Intense fear of bathing or perineal care
- Vaginal discharge, genital odour, and painful urination
- Difficulty walking or sitting
- Avoidance of casual touching
- Sleep pattern disturbances
- Nightmares
- Depression
- Anxiety
- Decreased self-esteem
- Difficulties with intimate relationships
- Substance abuse
- Frequent visits to health care providers
- Headaches
- Gastrointestinal problems
- Eating disorders
- Abdominal pain
- Vaginal pain
- Dysmenorrhea

Adapted from Bohn, D., & Holz, K. (1996). Sequelae of abuse: Health effects of childhood sexual abuse, domestic battering, and rape. *Journal of Nurse-Midwifery, 41*(6), 442.

Sexual Dysfunction. **Sexual dysfunction** is a common, complex problem that arises because of biological, psychological, and interpersonal factors (Table 27-2). Sexual problems and dysfunction are often associated with health problems such as heart disease, diabetes, cancer, and mental illness. It is not known how many people experience sexual dysfunction, and it is most probably a minority who seek help. Researchers estimate that between 10 and 52% of men and 25 and 63% of women have sexual problems, although the prevalence of sexual dysfunctions that meet the diagnostic criteria of the fifth edition of the *Diagnostic and Statistical Manual of Mental Disorders* (American Psychiatric Association, 2013) is lower (Heiman, 2002). For most people, sexual dysfunction is perplexing and emotionally disturbing, and it adversely affects their primary relationship.

Sexual dysfunction can usually be treated with either medical interventions (mostly pharmacological) or psychological interventions (e.g., cognitive and behavioural methods). The aim is typically to achieve changes in physical (genital response, orgasms) or subjective (greater desire, ease of orgasm) responses (Heiman, 2002).

Sexual Dysfunction in Women. Loss of sexual desire is the most common reason that women seek help for sexual dysfunction (Butcher, 1999a). Despite considerable research, sexual desire is poorly understood. Medical conditions (including depression), stress, and fatigue affect sexual desire. Painful intercourse is another common sexual dysfunction in women. Recurring sexual pain can produce a cycle in which trepidation because of previous pain leads to avoidance of the sexual activity that produced it, which leads to lack of arousal, failure to achieve orgasm, and loss of sexual desire (Butcher, 1999b). This cycle can evolve to avoidance of sexual activity altogether.

Sexual Dysfunction in Men. One of the most common types of sexual dysfunction for men is erectile dysfunction. It is estimated that

TABLE 27-2 Types of Sexual Dysfunction

Category	Type*	Definition
Sexual desire disorders	Hypoactive sexual desire disorder	Persistent or recurrent deficiency or absence of sexual fantasies and desire for sexual activity
	Sexual aversion disorder	Persistent or recurrent extreme aversion to, and avoidance of, all or almost all genital sexual contact with a sexual partner
Sexual arousal disorders	Female sexual arousal disorder	Failure in a woman to attain or maintain the lubrication-swelling response or to experience a subjective sense of sexual excitement and pleasure during sexual activity
Male erectile dysfunction		Persistent or recurrent inability to attain an adequate erection or to maintain an adequate erection until completion of the sexual activity
Orgasmic disorders	Female orgasmic disorder (anorgasmia)	The recurrent and persistent inhibition of the female orgasm, as manifested by the absence or delay of orgasm after a period of sexual excitement the clinician judges adequate in intensity and duration to produce such a response
	Male orgasmic disorder (retarded ejaculation)	Persistent or recurrent delay in, or absence of, orgasm after a normal sexual excitement phase during sexual activity that the clinician, taking into account the man's age, judges to be adequate in focus, intensity, and duration
	Male orgasmic disorder (premature ejaculation)	Persistent or recurrent ejaculation with minimal sexual stimulation before, upon, or shortly after penetration and before the man wishes it
Sexual pain disorders	Dyspareunia	Recurrent or persistent genital pain in either a man or a woman before, during, or after sexual intercourse that is not associated with vaginismus or with lack of lubrication
	Vaginismus	An involuntary constriction of the outer third of the vagina that prevents penile insertion and intercourse
Sexual dysfunction resulting from drug use or diseases		Sexual dysfunction judged to be caused by the direct physiological effects of a general medical condition or use of a substance

*According to American Psychiatric Association. (2013). *Diagnostic and statistical manual of mental disorders* (5th ed.). Washington, DC: Author.

about 27% of sexually active Canadian men experience erectile dysfunction, which is the repeated inability to achieve or maintain an erection (Auld & Brock, 2002). Erectile dysfunction can be caused by any health problem, including heart disease, hypertension (or its treatment), diseases of the prostate, diabetes mellitus, multiple sclerosis, and depression. Erectile dysfunction itself might be a warning sign of undiagnosed cardiovascular disease.

Patients With Particular Sexual Health Concerns

Pregnant and Postpartum Women. Female sexual interest tends to fluctuate during pregnancy; it increases during the second trimester and often decreases during the first and third trimesters. The decrease in libido during the first trimester may be caused by nausea, fatigue, and breast tenderness. During the second trimester, blood flow to the pelvic area is increased to supply the placenta, and sexual enjoyment and libido accordingly increase. During the third trimester, increased abdominal size may make finding a comfortable position difficult.

The most prevalent sexual problem during pregnancy is fear of harming the fetus. However, pregnancy and birth complications are not associated with sexual intercourse (von Sydow, 1999). If women have a history of miscarriages or premature labour, they may be advised to avoid sexual intercourse during the later months of pregnancy. Other restrictions such as no orgasms or no sexual arousal may be necessary to protect high-risk pregnancies (Mayo Foundation for Medical Education and Research, 2015).

Patients Recovering From Surgery. Surgeries that result in disfigurement, especially of the face, breasts, genitalia, and reproductive organs, frequently have harmful effects on a patient's self-image and sexuality (de Marquiegui & Huish, 1999). The effects of surgery, whether temporary or permanent, are often not fully anticipated and may not be fully manifested until after discharge from the hospital. Patients' partners might also have adjustments to make and may find it difficult to resume sexual activity. Coping with anxiety, fear, or depression about the surgery is essential. Nurses need to support patients to discuss their concerns, especially sexual anxieties, because problems can become deep-rooted, complicated, and more difficult to resolve over time (de Marquiegui & Huish, 1999). Patients who have had ileostomies, colostomies, or urostomies are particularly concerned about possible loss of control, unpleasant smells or sounds, seepage or broken bags, and their partners' responses (see Chapter 44). Perioperative counselling and support are essential for these patients.

Patients With Illness or Disabilities. Illness and disability often affect sexual health. During periods of illness, individuals may experience major physical changes, the effects of drugs or treatments, the emotional stress of a prognosis, concern about future functioning, and separation from significant others. Situational stressors could include a heart attack (myocardial infarction); cancer diagnosis and treatment; or chronic disease such as diabetes, multiple sclerosis, or Parkinson's disease. Nurses should not assume, because of a patient's age or severity of prognosis, that sexual functioning is not a concern. In some instances, patients may wrongly believe that their condition prohibits sexual activity, or they may need some guidance to promote satisfactory sexual functioning (Nusbaum, Hamilton, & Lenahan, 2003).

Many myths are prevalent about people with a disability, including the idea that they are asexual or somehow different. Long-term disability can have profound effects on a person's sense of sexuality and sexual function. Congenital or birth impairments commonly affect sexual development; for example, for people with disabilities who require assistance in activities of daily living, the resulting lack of privacy and independence may mean that they miss out on typical sexual experiences (Glass & Soni, 1999). Acquired disabilities may have different implications: impairments sustained in youth may bring about low social and sexual confidence, and people who sustain disabilities as adults may be far more aware of what they have lost. It is important that health care providers validate a disabled person's sexuality. Nurses can do this by sensitively initiating conversations about sexual function and safer sex practices.

CRITICAL THINKING

Successful critical thinking requires synthesis of knowledge, experience, information gathered from patients, critical thinking qualities, and intellectual and professional standards. Clinical judgement requires nurses to anticipate the information necessary, analyze the data, and make appropriate decisions regarding patient care. Figure 27-3 depicts numerous critical thinking elements, as well as patient assessment data, that contribute to appropriate nursing diagnoses regarding sexuality.

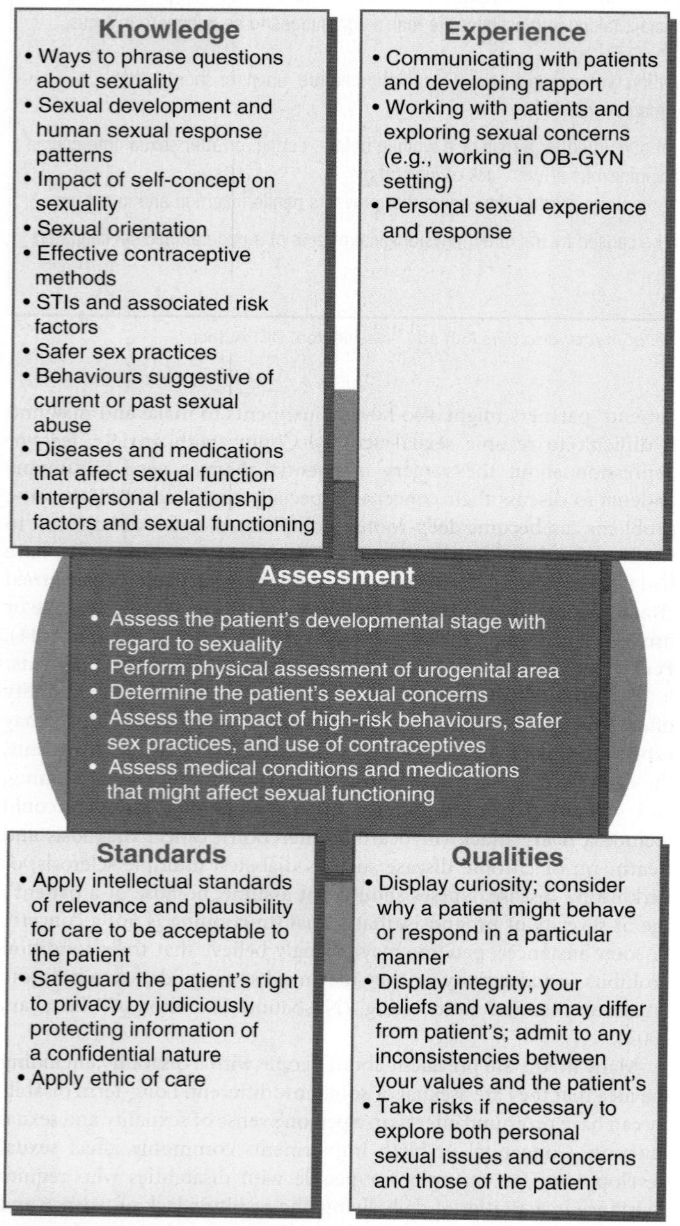

FIGURE 27-3 Critical thinking model for sexuality assessment. *OB-GYN,* Obstetrical-gynecological; *STIs,* sexually transmitted infections.

In the case of sexuality, nurses need to integrate knowledge from nursing and other disciplines. Nurses must have a good understanding, for example, of the human sexual response cycle, safer sex practices, and the taxonomy of sexual problems, as well as solutions to these, to anticipate how to assess a patient and then how to interpret findings. Previous experience in caring for patients whose sexuality becomes threatened can help nurses approach the next patient in a more reflective and helpful way. Patients may have customs and values different from those of the nurse. Professional standards require that nurses respect each patient as an individual.

SEXUALITY AND THE NURSING PROCESS

A person's sexuality has physical, psychological, social, and cultural elements. Nurses must assess all relevant elements to determine a patient's sexual well-being. Nurses should build a sound knowledge base and be willing to explore personal issues regarding sexuality. The nursing role in addressing sexual concerns can range from ongoing assessment to providing information to counselling to referral.

Assessment

Factors Affecting Sexuality. In gathering a sexual history, nurses should consider physical, functional, relationship, lifestyle, and self-esteem factors that may influence sexual functioning.

Sexual Health History. When taking a health history, it is good to include a few questions related to sexual functioning to determine whether the patient has any sexual concerns. Nurses can incorporate these questions in the review of systems and address them in a routine, matter-of-fact manner. Any mention a patient makes of sexual activity offers a good opportunity to open a discussion about this topic. The nurse should use language that is appropriate to the age and educational level of the patient and be mindful of cultural issues, as the patient may be hesitant to talk to a nurse who is of the opposite gender or is much older or younger than the patient. Asking open-ended questions will help encourage patients to ask questions and use words they are comfortable with. Nurses need to let patients know that they are about to ask a few questions to obtain a sexual health history and that these questions are asked of all patients, as this can help break the ice and assure patients that the questions are routine (Pessango, 2013).

When taking a health history, it is beneficial to think of the five Ps:

- Partners
- Practices
- Protection from STIs
- Past history of STIs
- Prevention of pregnancy

Conducting a sexual assessment of children and adolescents provides special challenges for health care providers, including issues of language, of promoting normal development while not minimizing problems, and of screening for sexual concerns while not unduly alarming children. In addition, the sexual counselling of minors raises ethical and legal issues regarding the patient's rights to health care and education on the one hand, and the parents' or guardian's right to supervise information on the other. When introducing sexual questions, it helps to use an open, positive, interested disposition. The nurse should inform parents that he or she is going to be discussing this in private with their child or teenager and that this is a normal part of the nursing assessment.

When caring for older persons, nurses may adjust their assessment approach. When gathering a sexual history, it is important to keep in mind that the older person may have difficulty discussing intimate details with health care providers because of cultural and social norms for their age group. Nurses have a responsibility to help maintain healthy sexuality of older persons by offering the opportunity to discuss any concerns or to seek information. Often, asking questions on the topic of sexuality in a comfortable, relaxed manner facilitates older persons' discussion of their sexual needs.

Because of the prevalence of domestic violence and sexual abuse, questions relating to abusive relationships can be important. Questions that address domestic violence or abuse should be addressed to the patient in private. A question such as "Are you in a relationship in which someone is hurting you?" may encourage a patient to reveal current or previous abuse. An additional question such as "Has anyone ever forced you to have sex when you did not wish to participate?" may more specifically encourage the patient to discuss concerns. Recognizing both subjective and objective signs and symptoms of abuse can aid in recognition of this too-common problem (see Box 27-2). If a person identifies sex abuse as a current or past problem, appropriate referrals need to be made with the patient's permission.

While documenting the sexual history of a patient, it is also helpful to explore the patient's use of contraceptives and safer sex practices as appropriate. Adolescents may respond to a comment that reassures them that having questions related to sexuality is normal. A lead-in could be "Many teenagers have questions about whether their bodies are developing at the right rate. Do you have any questions about sex or your body?"

Some individuals are too embarrassed or do not know how to ask questions about sexuality. If a patient makes a sexual joke or expresses concern about relations with his or her partner, he or she may have questions. Observing for and listening to concerns about sexuality takes practice. With experience, you will develop skill in clarifying and paraphrasing to help patients express their sexual concerns. By including sexuality in the health history, you are acknowledging that sexuality is an important part of health and creating an opportunity for the patient to discuss sexual concerns.

Physical Assessment. The physical examination is important in evaluating the cause of sexual concerns or problems; however, this is beyond the scope of the generalist nurse and more appropriate for the advanced practice nurse or physician. Talking about sexuality at the time of the genital examination is not appropriate and can be misconstrued by the patient and may make him or her feel uncomfortable. Discussions about sexuality are best held when the patient is fully clothed and sitting comfortably in a private room.

Patient Expectations. As in the case of any patient assessment, it is important to understand the patient's expectations regarding his or her care. Questions such as "What would you like to have happen in regard to [expressed concern]?" and "What initial steps might you take?" can help the person identify desired outcomes. It is important for the nurse to set aside personal views and not assume what a patient's expectations might be.

◆ Nursing Diagnosis

After completing an assessment and applying critical thought to the diagnostic process (Box 27-3), the nurse selects diagnoses applicable to the patient's needs. Possible nursing diagnoses related to sexual functioning (NANDA International, 2009) are as follows:

- *Anxiety*
- *Ineffective coping*
- *Interrupted family processes*
- *Deficient knowledge (about contraception or STIs or both)*
- *Sexual dysfunction*
- *Ineffective sexuality patterns*
- *Social isolation*
- *Risk for other-directed violence*
- *Risk for self-directed violence*

Clues that may signal risk or an actual nursing diagnosis related to sexuality include a history of surgery involving the reproductive organs, changes in appearance, past or current physical or sexual abuse, chronic illness, and developmental milestones such as puberty or menopause. Before making nursing diagnoses related to sexual dysfunction, the nurse must first assess anatomical, physiological, sociocultural, and situational issues thoroughly.

When making a nursing diagnosis in regard to sexuality, the nurse must clarify with the patient that the defining characteristics do in fact exist and that the patient perceives a problem with regard to sexuality. Determining the etiological or contributing factors is important in order to focus effective planning and to select appropriate nursing interventions. For example, the nursing interventions appropriate for the nursing diagnosis *chronic low self-esteem* would be different from those appropriate for other etiological factors. For *self-esteem disturbance related to chronic, recurring herpes infection,* the appropriate interventions include counselling and education on how to maintain safer sexual practices. In contrast, *self-esteem disturbance related to sexual abuse* would necessitate counselling and referral to community resources (e.g., crisis services or a sexual abuse support group).

BOX 27-3 NURSING DIAGNOSTIC PROCESS

Assessment Activities	Defining Characteristics	Nursing Diagnosis
Observe readiness to discuss sexual concerns through verbalization (e.g., "When can I return to life as normal?" or "There goes my love life") or behaviour (e.g., exhibitionism).	Patient verbalizes concern that sexual activity may cause another myocardial infarction or death.	Ineffective sexuality patterns related to fear of recurrent myocardial infarction or death during intercourse.
Ask patient and spouse about previous level and method of sexual expression (e.g., frequency, initiator).		
Observe for affectionate behaviour (e.g., touching, hand holding, kissing).	Patient's spouse exhibits reluctance to touch patient.	
In privacy, ask spouse about perceptions of patient's recovery and return to full functioning.	Spouse verbalizes concern that patient will need continuous care, attention, and protection.	
Observe for anxiety (e.g., hand wringing).	Patient maintains eye contact, shifts position frequently.	

◆ Planning

Goals and Outcomes. During planning, nurses again synthesize information from multiple resources (Figure 27-4). Critical thinking skills are used to integrate professional standards and knowledge about the patient's sexuality into the care plan. It is especially important to maintain a patient's dignity and identity when developing the care plan. For example, nurses can convey respect for a gay patient by including the help of his or her partner in the plan to the degree that the partner can assist the patient in maintaining his or her identity and dignity.

Nurses develop an individualized care plan for each nursing diagnosis (Box 27-4). Together, the nurse and the patient set realistic goals for care. Expected outcomes must be individualized and realistic. For example, for a patient with a nursing diagnosis of *sexual dysfunction related to dyspareunia,* the nurse and the patient would develop a goal to be free from pain or discomfort during sexual intercourse. Expected outcomes for this goal may be as follows:

- The patient will report decreased anxiety and greater satisfaction with sexual activity.
- The patient will consistently use a water-soluble lubricant with sexual intercourse.
- The patient will avoid the use of feminine hygiene products that destroy the natural flora and secretions of the vaginal walls.

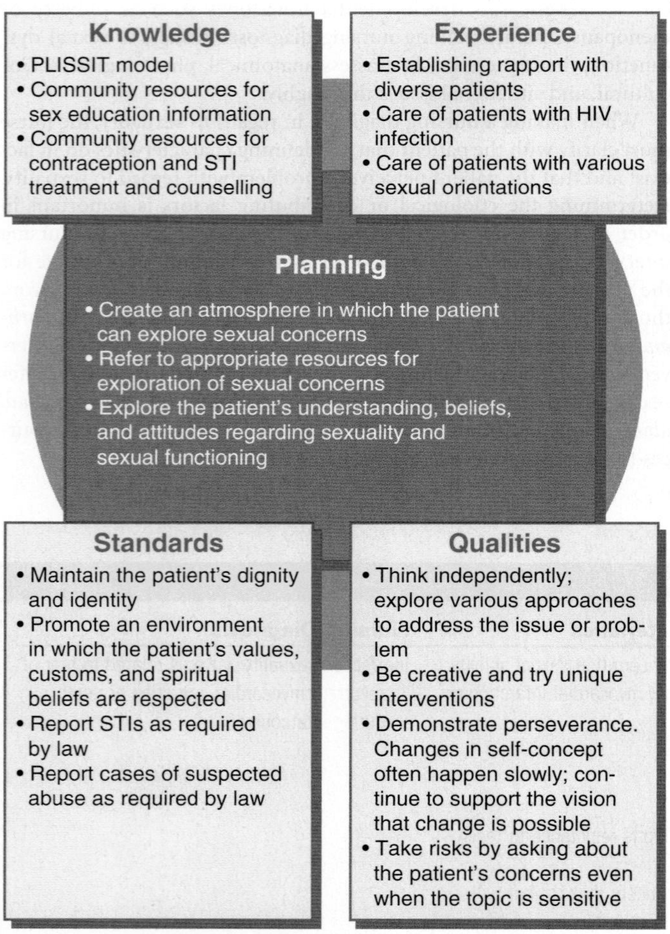

FIGURE 27-4 Critical thinking model for sexuality planning. *HIV,* Human immunodeficiency virus; *PLISSIT,* permission giving, limited information, specific suggestions, and intensive therapy; *STI,* sexually transmitted infection.

A concept map is useful for organizing patient care (Figure 27-5). A concept map shows the relationship of a medical diagnosis (e.g., decreased libido and depression) with the four nursing diagnoses identified from the patient assessment data. The map also shows links and relationship with the nursing diagnosis. For example, ineffective coping affects and contributes to social isolation; as long as the patient has ineffective coping, social isolation continues or perhaps worsens.

Setting Priorities. A framework useful in guiding planning is the "PLISSIT" model, developed by Annon (1976). In this model, levels of intervention are progressively more involved. *P* stands for "permission giving." During assessment, the nurse can bring up the topic of sexuality and give the individual permission to talk about sexual concerns. *LI* stands for "limited information," which is basic information regarding sexuality and sexual functioning. An example is discussing nocturnal emissions with a prepubescent boy to minimize fear that might develop if the boy did not know this was a normal part of development. *SS* stands for "specific suggestions"—in this case, specific suggestions regarding a sexual concern or issue. For example, a postmenopausal woman might be concerned about her lack of vaginal lubrication, and the nurse might suggest use of a water-based lubricant during sexual intercourse. If the nurse is not equipped to address a particular concern, he or she should refer the patient to another qualified health care provider. *IT* stands for "intensive therapy." At this level of intervention, the nurse's role is to refer the patient to a qualified practitioner, such as a social worker or sexuality counsellor, for individualized therapy. The level of intervention that nurses plan depends in part on their own experience and knowledge. When a patient requires specific suggestions or intensive therapy, the nurse may recommend referral to a specialist.

Continuity of Care. Planning in the area of sexuality may include referrals to community resources (Box 27-5). Sexual conflicts in marriage or trauma related to sexual abuse or incest may necessitate intensive treatment with a mental health care provider or certified sex therapist. For women in abusive relationships, most communities have battered women's shelters that provide counselling and serve as a safe haven while they plan for their future.

◆ Implementation

Health Promotion. Because of their education, clinical expertise, and wellness orientation, nurses are among the professionals best situated to develop and implement sexual health initiatives. Nurses can promote sexual health by identifying patients at increased risk, providing appropriate information, helping individuals gain insight into their problems, and exploring methods to deal with problems effectively. A health promotion perspective ought to guide nurses in designing a number of programs: informal educational opportunities, continuing education, peer learning activities for adolescents, community and political initiatives, and health care provider education (Beitz, 1998). Topics for education vary, depending on the nursing diagnosis (Box 27-6).

Acute Care. In general, nursing interventions that address alterations in sexuality are aimed at raising awareness, assisting in clarification of issues or concerns, providing information, or performing a combination of these. Nurses who have pursued specialized education in sexual functioning and counselling may provide more intensive sex therapy. Nurses should recognize when an individual's needs exceed their the nurses' expertise, in which case they should provide an appropriate referral.

In the initial intervention, the nurse often explores current sexual practices of the patient. The patient should be encouraged to investigate and acknowledge social and ethical values and consider the role of sexuality in his or her self-concept. When significant discrepancy

BOX 27-4 NURSING CARE PLAN

Sexual Dysfunction

ASSESSMENT

Mr. Clements is a 46-year-old patient who was last seen in the office 2 months ago, when he was found to have mild hypertension and was given a prescription for propranolol (Inderal). His blood pressure today is 122/82 mm Hg.

Jack, a nursing student, talks with Mr. Clements after reading his records, which include the recent diagnosis of mild hypertension, the order for propranolol, and the current blood pressure reading of 122/82 mm Hg. The record also indicates that Mr. Clements is married and living with his wife.

Jack tells Mr. Clements of the improvement in his blood pressure since his last visit. He inquires whether Mr. Clements is taking his medication regularly.

Mr. Clements reports that he has been taking his medication regularly. He relates that it scared him when his blood pressure was up because both his parents had died of strokes. Jack then inquires whether Mr. Clements has noted any adverse effects from the medicine. Mr. Clements says that he has not, except that he may be a little more tired than he used to be. Jack then states, "Some people find that certain blood pressure medications affect their sexual performance. Have you noticed any changes in sexual functioning since you began your medication?" Mr. Clements replies that he has had some problems achieving an erection since starting the medication.

Assessment Activities	*Findings and Defining Characteristics*
Ascertain when Mr. Clements began noticing his inability to have an erection.	He responds that it was at about the same time he started taking propranolol.
Ask Mr. Clements about his sexual relationship with his wife before taking propranolol.	He states they used to have intercourse one to three times per week.
Ask Mr. Clements whether he has noticed any changes in his desire for sex.	He states that he has the same level of interest as before.
Ask Mr. Clements whether he has made any changes to his lifestyle since the first of the year.	He denies any changes.

NURSING DIAGNOSIS: Erectile dysfunction related to adverse effects of antihypertensive medication

PLANNING

*Goal (Nursing Outcomes Classification)**	*Expected Outcomes*
	Sexual Functioning
Patient will be able to achieve satisfactory erections.	Patient will talk to his physician about this problem, and a change of medication may be warranted.

*Outcome classification label from Moorhead, S., Johnson, M., Maas, M. L., & Swanson, E. (Eds.). (2008). *Nursing outcomes classification (NOC)* (4th ed.). St. Louis, MO: Mosby.

INTERVENTIONS

Interventions (Nursing Interventions Classification)†	*Rationale*
Sexual Counselling	
Establish trust and respect with patient. Offer privacy during conversations.	Conveys sense of caring, increasing likelihood of patient's ability to express concerns fully (Ross, Channon-Little, & Rosser, 2000)
Discuss possible effects of antihypertensive on sexual functioning, and encourage patient to discuss sexual concerns with physician.	Helps patient understand possible cause for sexual difficulties and gives patient important options to review with physician (Klein, 2015)
Encourage patient to discuss concerns with his wife. Role-play so that patient can practise ways to approach concerns.	Many of the sexual problems in relationships involve poor communication (Klein, 2015)
Anxiety Reduction	Anxiety and embarrassment can be difficult, and can interfere with adult-to-adult relationships (Klein, 2015)
Assure patient that other blood pressure medications are available to maintain blood pressure control that do not negatively affect sexual function.	Knowing that options exist and that blood pressure can continue to be safely managed gives patient sense of control (Running & Berndt, 2003)

†Intervention classification labels from Bulechek, G. M., Butcher, H. K., & Dochterman, J. M. (2008). *Nursing interventions classification (NIC)* (5th ed.). St. Louis, MO: Mosby.

EVALUATION

Nursing Actions	*Patient Response and Finding*	*Achievement of Outcome*
At his next visit, ask Mr. Clements whether his problems have been resolved.	He responds that since he has been on new medication, he has had no trouble having an erection.	Mr. Clements reports sexual function with the new medication.

exists between values and past or current practices, the patient may need referral for more intensive counselling.

Major developmental milestones (e.g., puberty or menopause) should prompt education about potential effects on sexuality. Situational crises such as a life change with pregnancy, illness, extreme financial stress, placement of a spouse in a long-term care facility, or loss and grief affect sexuality. Effects may last for days, months, or years and can generate performance anxieties that lead to continued sexual dysfunction. If an individual is prepared for possible changes in sexual functioning, performance anxieties may be minimized.

When concerns are assessed and identified, they can be addressed in the context of the patient's value system. In response to identified concerns, the nurse may initiate discussion in pertinent areas. It may be appropriate to discuss sexual practices such as oral-genital sex or mutual masturbation as methods of expressing intimate affection when vaginal-penile intercourse is contraindicated. Often, if a

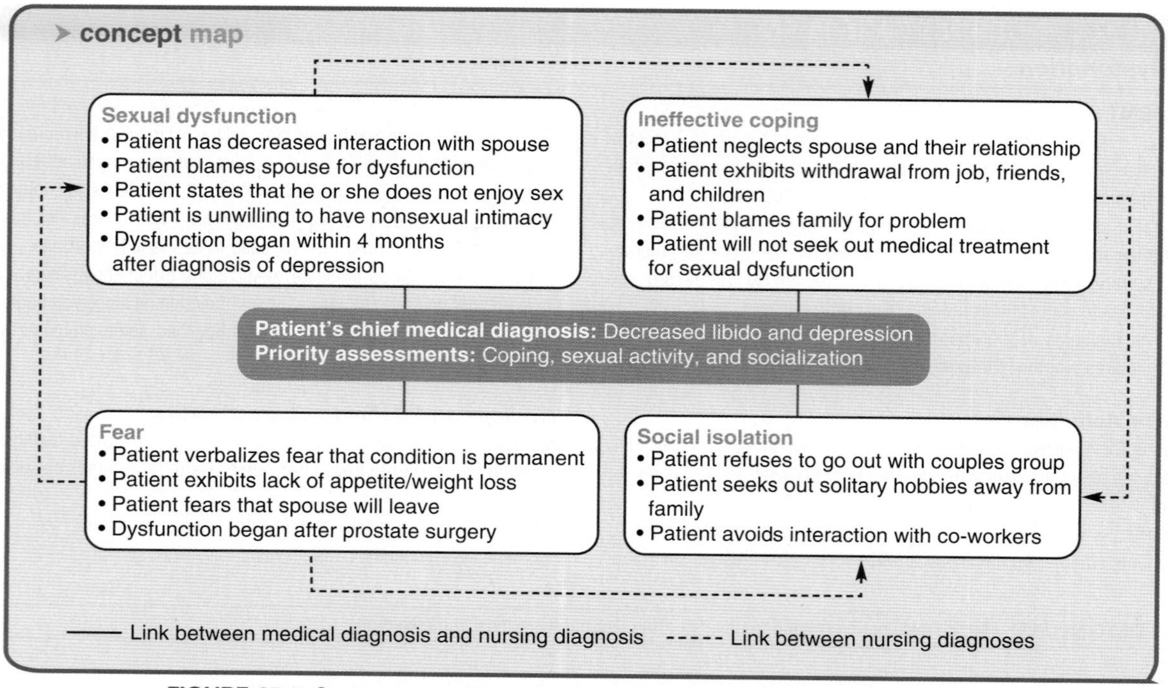

FIGURE 27-5 Concept map for patient with decreased libido and depression.

BOX 27-5 Community Resources Relating to Sexuality

Planned Parenthood
Sex therapists
Clinical psychologists
Social workers
Health department (often for both family planning and treatment of STIs)

Groups that provide education and services for those with particular conditions include the following:

- Diabetes Canada
- Heart and Stroke Foundation of Canada
- Muscular Dystrophy Canada
- Sexual abuse support groups
- Women's shelters (for those who have been physically abused, sexually abused, or both)
- Hotlines for help (which have lists of community support resources)

partner's abilities (physical and/or mental) change, dealing with sexuality needs to be addressed with both partners. Dealing with issues of fatigue, a change in sensory perceptions, pain, and limited motion may require a change in positioning, touch, and so on. Often, counselling is needed to deal with these kinds of changes (Klein, 2015).

Restorative Care. In the patient's home, the nurse can help create an environment that is comfortable for sexual activity. This may involve recommending ways to arrange the bedroom to accommodate an individual's limitations. For example, a patient in a wheelchair may prefer to move the chair close to the side of the bed at an angle that allows for more ease in touching and caressing. Suggestions regarding how to accommodate barriers such as Foley catheters or drainage tubes can contribute to enhanced sexual activity.

In the long-term care setting, many facilities support spouses sharing rooms, but have a harder time dealing with residents who develop relationships once they have already moved into the facility (Bell, 2013). Staff generally identify three types of sexual expression in these settings: love and caring, romance, and eroticism. While the first two are generally supported by staff, eroticism generally isn't, which usually results in staff separating the two residents, often at the insistence of their families. This is even more prevalent when facing LGBTQ relationships, or when at least one of the residents has a cognitive impairment. Often policies are not present to guide staff in how to react in such situations. It is important to explore possibilities for dealing with such issues, including the possibility of having a semi-private room that provides for both visual and auditory privacy, should the need arise.

◆ Evaluation

Patient Care. To determine whether patient goals and outcome criteria have been met, nurses review patients' responses to interventions (Figure 27-6). Using critical thinking, nurses apply what they know about sexuality and the patient's unique situation.

In follow-up discussions with the patient or spouse, the nurse determines whether goals and outcomes have been achieved. Patients can be asked to relate risk factors, verbalize concerns, share stories of their experiences, and clarify their level of satisfaction. Nurses can also observe behavioural cues, such as eye contact, posture, and extraneous hand movements, that indicate comfort or are suggestive of continued anxiety or concern as topics are addressed. As outcomes are evaluated, the nurse, the patient, and the spouse may need to modify expectations or establish time frames in which to achieve the target goals. All involved may need to be reminded of the individual nature of sexual expression and the multiple factors that affect perceptions and responses. Sexual wellness is not an absolute. An individual must define what is acceptable and satisfying. The partner's level of sexual satisfaction must also be considered. Sexual performance is seldom the exclusive focus of sexual satisfaction. Open communication and positive self-esteem are essential factors in effectively resolving concerns.

BOX 27-6 FOCUS ON PRIMARY HEALTH CARE

Sexual Health Education Topics

- Guidelines for normal development: For example, you might talk to a toddler's mother about preparing the toddler for a new baby, to a school-aged child about the appearance of pubic hair, or to a 60-year-old man about erectile difficulties. Details of physiological changes should be described as a part of general health care. Providing patient education gives permission for a patient to raise questions or concerns regarding personal functioning.
- Contraception, when talking with a patient of child-bearing age: The discussion should include such topics as the desire for children, usual sexual practices, acceptable methods of contraception, frequency of sexual activity, comfort with genital touching, comfort with sharing contraceptive responsibility with the partner, and comfort with interruption of sexual acts. You might ask, "Are you using contraceptives with your partner now?" and then follow up, on the basis of the patient's answer. For a patient who does not have a regular contraceptive method, does not have a reliable contraceptive method, or is not satisfied with the current method, the various methods of contraception should be reviewed to provide necessary information for an informed choice. The best method is the one that the patient will use consistently.
- Safer sex practices, when talking with a sexually active adolescent, with a patient who has more than one sex partner, or with a patient whose partner has multiple sexual partners: You should provide information regarding STI symptoms and transmission, use of condoms, and risky sexual activities (e.g., trauma from penile–anal sex). A topic to consider in discussing sexual relating is the emotional risks within a relationship. Role-play can be a useful educational tool for helping a person learn to say no or negotiate with a partner to use a condom.
- The need for regular physical examinations: Regular health examinations are important for maintaining sexual health. The annual health examination also provides an easy opportunity to discuss contraception and safer sex practices. Regular clinical breast examinations, mammography, and Papanicolaou (Pap) smears are important for women, as are testicular self-examinations for men.

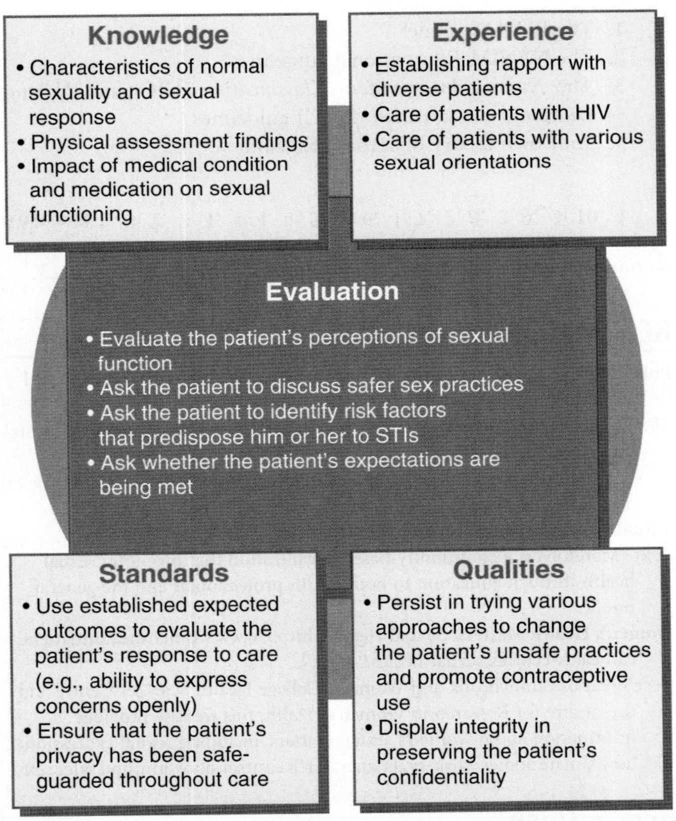

FIGURE 27-6 Critical thinking model for sexuality evaluation. *HIV,* Human immunodeficiency virus; *STI,* sexually transmitted infection.

Patient Expectations. In evaluating the outcomes of interventions related to sexuality, the nurse must consult with the patient. Resolution of sexual concerns must meet the patient's perceptions of improvement. A patient must define what is acceptable and satisfying. In considering the status of sexual health, the patient's partner's perceptions of sexual satisfaction are also significant.

KEY CONCEPTS

- Sexuality is related to all dimensions of health; therefore, as a part of nursing care, sexual concerns or problems should be addressed.
- Sexuality is a part of each individual's identity and includes sexual identity, gender identity, and sexual orientation.
- Attitudes toward sexuality vary widely and are influenced by religious beliefs, society's values, the family, and other factors.
- Nurses' attitudes toward sexuality also vary and may differ from those of patients; nurses should be sensitive to patients' sexual preferences and needs.
- Sexual development is a process beginning in infancy and involves some level of sexual behaviour or growth in all developmental stages.
- The physiological sexual response changes with aging, but aging does not lead to diminished sexuality.
- Sexual health involves physical and psychosocial aspects and contributes to an individual's sense of self-worth and positive interpersonal relationships.
- Sexual dysfunction can have an easily identified cause or varied and complex causes.
- Interventions for sexual dysfunctions depend on the condition and the patient; interventions may include giving information, teaching specific exercises, improving communication between partners, and referral to a knowledgeable professional.
- Choice and use of contraceptive methods are affected by desire for children, usual sexual practices, acceptable methods of contraception, frequency of sexual activity, comfort with genital touching, comfort with sharing contraceptive responsibility with the partner, and comfort with interruption of sexual acts.
- A brief review of sexuality should be included in every nursing assessment of a patient's level of wellness.
- Most nursing interventions to enhance a patient's sexual health involve providing information and education.

CRITICAL THINKING EXERCISES

1. Your current clinical experience is in a community health care setting. You are conducting the initial interview with a 48-year-old

man who started taking antihypertensive medications 2 weeks ago. You take his blood pressure and find it to be 136/74 mm Hg. You ask him how he has been doing since his last visit. He looks down at the floor and says, "Oh, okay, I guess. Seems like I'm just getting old now." What kind of follow-up would be indicated on the basis of this information?

2. You are assigned to care for a 15-year-old girl who was admitted after a motor vehicle accident. Yesterday she underwent internal fixation of a fractured ankle. In gathering her nursing history, you explore sexuality and learn that she has just recently become sexually active with her boyfriend of 3 months. When you ask about safer sex and the use of birth control, she tells you that she knows she does not have to worry about STIs with him because he is just not one of those kinds of boys. In regard to birth control, she says that her boyfriend has reassured her that because he is pulling out before ejaculation, she does not risk becoming pregnant. How would you proceed?
3. You are working on a rehabilitation unit and caring for a 67-year-old man who had a stroke 3 weeks ago. He shares a room with another man who is recovering from a stroke. Your patient has been progressing in his self-care skills and is now able to get around with a cane, feed himself, and perform most of his bathing. His wife is in fairly good health, and the plan is for him to return home within the next 1 to 2 weeks. As you work with him one morning, he says to you, "You know, one of the things that is hardest about being here is not being able to sleep in the same bed as Greta. I miss her so much. Even though she visits every day, it is just not the same." How would you explore his comment, and what planning would you consider?

REVIEW QUESTIONS

1. Gender identity is the individual's:
   1. Sexual behaviour
   2. Sexual orientation
   3. Sense of being male, female, or some combination thereof
   4. Sense of preferring one sex over the other
2. Sexual health refers to:
   1. Having no STIs
   2. Awareness of and positive attitudes toward sexual functioning
   3. Using contraception consistently
   4. Sexual activity with multiple partners
3. Inability or difficulty in sexual functioning caused by numerous factors is called:
   1. Sexual behaviour
   2. Sexual response
   3. Sexual orientation
   4. Sexual dysfunction
4. A major problem in dealing with STIs is that:
   1. Symptoms are often absent or go unnoticed
   2. Most STIs cannot be treated with antibiotics
   3. Little is known about how they are transmitted
   4. Little can be done to help
5. The most common bacterial STI is:
   1. Syphilis
   2. Genital chlamydia
   3. Gonorrhea
   4. HIV infection and AIDS
6. Of the following methods of contraception, which *two* require a health care provider's intervention?
   1. Diaphragm and intrauterine device (IUD)
   2. Condoms and hormones
   3. Cervical caps and condoms
   4. Sterilization and vaginal spermicidals
7. Which of the following is the most effective contraception method for women?
   1. Female condom
   2. Birth control pill
   3. Contraceptive sponge
   4. Vaginal spermicide
8. The most valuable tool that you can use when providing sexual health care is:
   1. Knowledge of right and wrong sexual behaviours
   2. Effective, nonjudgemental communication
   3. Nursing diagnoses
   4. Firm personal convictions about what constitutes normal sexual behaviour
9. When you are gathering a sexual history from an older person, you must keep in mind that:
   1. Older persons do not usually participate in sexual activity
   2. Older men always lose fertility
   3. Older persons may have difficulty discussing intimate matters
   4. Both older men and women are sexually dysfunctional
10. A useful framework for the nurse to guide planning and set priorities about sexual activity for a patient is
    1. The PLISSIT model
    2. The NANDA International guidelines
    3. The *Nursing Interventions Classification* (NIC) and *Nursing Outcomes Classification* (NOC) guidelines
    4. Your own theory of sexual behaviour

Answers: 1. 3; 2. 2; 3. 4; 4. 1; 5. 2; 6. 1; 7. 2; 8. 2; 9. 3; 10. 1

Rationales for the Review Questions appear at the end of the book.

RECOMMENDED WEBSITES

Public Health Agency of Canada: Sexual Health and Sexually Transmitted Infections: http://www.phac-aspc.gc.ca/index-eng.php.

The Public Health Agency of Canada works with provinces, nongovernmental organizations, and health care providers to improve and maintain the sexual health and well-being of Canadians. This website offers links to sexual health and STI information, publications, and resources.

Sexual Education Resource Centre MB: http://www.serc.mb.ca/.

SERC Manitoba is a community-based organization that promotes sexual health through education to both health professionals and the general public.

Women's Health Matters: Sexual Health: http://www.womenshealthmatters.ca/health-centres/sexual-health/.

Developed by Sunnybrook and Women's College Health Sciences Centre and the Centre for Research in Women's Health, this website provides information about women's sexual matters, including sexual expression, how female bodies work, pregnancy, birth control, abortion, and safer sex.

REFERENCES

Abeykoon, H., & Lucyk, K. (2015). Sex and seniors: A perspective. *CPHA Health Digest, Winter 2015/2016*. Retrieved from https://www.cpha.ca/sex-and-seniors-perspective.

Abortion Rights Coalition of Canada. (2017). *Statistics—abortions in Canada*. Retrieved from http://www.arcc-cdac.ca/backrounders/statistics-abortion-in-canada.pdf.

Albaugh, J., & Kellog-Spadt, S. (2003). Sexuality and sexual health: The nurse's role and initial approach to patients. *Urologic Nursing, 23*(3), 227–228.

American Psychiatric Association. (2013). *Diagnostic and statistical manual of mental disorders* (5th ed.). (DSM-5). Washington, DC: Author.

Annon, J. S. (1976). The PLISSIT model: A proposed conceptual scheme for the behavioral treatment of sexual problems. *Journal of Sex Education and Therapy, 2*(1), 1–15.

Auld, R. B., & Brock, G. (2002). Sexuality and erectile dysfunction: Results of a national survey. *Journal of Sexual & Reproductive Medicine, 2*, 50–54.

Balter, A. S., van Rhijn, T. M., & Davies, A. W. J. (2016). The development of sexuality in childhood in early learning settings: An exploration of early childhood educators' perceptions. *Canadian Journal of Human Sexuality, 25*(1), 30–40. doi:10.3138/cjhs.251-A3.

Bartlik, B., Rosenfeld, S., & Beaton, C. (2005). Assessment of sexual functioning: Sexual history taking for health care practitioners. *Epilepsy & Behavior, 7*(Suppl. 2), S15–S21. doi:10.1016/j.yebeh.2005.08.027.

Barton, D., Wilwerding, M., Carpenter, L., et al. (2004). Libido as part of sexuality in female cancer survivors. *Oncology Nursing Forum, 31*(3), 599–609. doi:10.1188/04.ONF.599-609.

Basson, R. (2005). Women's sexual dysfunction: Revised and expanded definitions. *Canadian Medical Association Journal, 172*(10), 1327–1333. doi:10.1503/cmaj.1020174.

Beitz, J. M. (1998). Sexual health promotion in adolescents and young adults: Primary prevention strategies. *Holistic Nursing Practice, 12*(2), 27–37. doi:10.1097/00004650-199801000-00006.

Bell, J. (2013). Book review: Gayle Appel Doll: Sexuality & long-term care: Understanding and supporting the needs of older adults. *Social Work in Health Care, 52*(1), 99–102. doi:10.1080/00981389.2012.728913.

Burd, I., Nevadunsky, N., & Bachmann, G. (2006). Impact of physician gender on sexual history taking in a multispecialty practice. *Journal of Sexual Medicine, 3*(2), 194–200. doi:10.1111/j.1743-6109.2005.00168.x.

Bushnik, T. (2016). *Women in Canada: A gender based statistical report* (Catalogue No. 89-503-X). Ottawa: Statistics Canada.

Butcher, J. (1999a). ABC of sexual health: Female sexual problems. I: Loss of desire—What about the fun? *British Medical Journal, 318*(7175), 41–43.

Butcher, J. (1999b). ABC of sexual health: Female sexual problems. II: Sexual pain and sexual fears. *British Medical Journal, 318*(7175), 110–112.

Buttaro, T. M., Koeniger-Donohue, R., & Hawkins, J. (2014). Sexuality and quality of life in aging: Implications for practice. *Journal for Nurse Practitioners, 10*(7), doi:10.1016/j.nurpra.2014.04.008.

Centers for Disease Control and Prevention [CDC]. (2015). *2015 Sexually transmitted diseases treatment guidelines.* Retrieved from https://www.cdc.gov/std/tg2015/clinical.htm.

Champion, A. R., & Pedersen, C. L. (2015). Investigating differences between sexters and non-sexters on attitudes, subjective norms, and risky sexual behaviours. *Canadian Journal of Human Sexuality, 24*(3), 205–214. doi:10.3138/cjhs.243-A5.

Community Foundations of Canada. (2017). *Diversity at work: Inclusive language guidelines.* Retrieved from http://hrcouncil.ca/hr-toolkit/diversity-language-guidelines.cfm.

de Marquiegui, A., & Huish, M. (1999). ABC of sexual health: A woman's sexual life after an operation. *British Medical Journal, 318*(7177), 178–181.

Department of Justice Canada. (2017). *Improving the reporting, charging and prosecution of sexual assaults against adults.* Ottawa: Author. Retrieved from https://www.canada.ca/en/department-justice/news/2017/03/improving_the_reportingchargingandprosecutionofsexualassaultsaga.html.

Edmonton Police Service. (2014). *What is sexual assault?* Edmonton: Author. Retrieved from http://www.edmontonpolice.ca/CommunityPolicing/PersonalPropertyCrimes/SexualAssault/WhatisSexualAssault.aspx.

Egale Canada Human Rights Trust. (2015). *Sex reassignment surgery (SRS) backgrounder.* Retrieved from http://egale.ca/sex-reassignment-surgery-srs-backgrounder/.

Glass, C., & Soni, B. (1999). ABC of sexual health: Sexual problems of disabled patients. *British Medical Journal, 318*(7182), 518–521.

Government of Canada. (2017). *List of nationally notifiable diseases.* Retrieved from http://diseases.canada.ca/notifiable/diseases-list.

Gusarova, I., Fraser, V., & Alderson, K. G. (2012). A quantitative study of "friends with benefits" relationships. *Canadian Journal of Human Sexuality, 21*(1), 41–59.

Guthrie, C. (1999). Nurses' perceptions of sexuality relating to patient care. *Journal of Clinical Nursing, 8*(3), 313–321. doi:10.1046/j.1365-2702.1999.00253.x.

Haboubi, N. H., & Lincoln, N. (2003). Views of health professionals on discussing sexual issues with patients. *Disability and Rehabilitation, 25*(6), 291–296.

Health Canada. (2006). *Sexually transmitted infections (STIs).* Ottawa: Author. Retrieved from https://www.canada.ca/en/health-canada/services/health-concerns/diseases-conditions/sexually-transmitted-infections.html.

Healthwise Staff. (2016). *Effectiveness rate of birth control methods.* Retrieved from https://myhealth.alberta.ca/health/pages/conditions.aspx?Hwid=tw9416.

Heiman, J. R. (2002). Sexual dysfunction: Overview of prevalence, etiological factors, and treatments. *Journal of Sex Research, 39*(1), 73–78. doi:10.1080/00224490209552124.

Herson, L., Hart, K. A., Gordon, M. J., et al. (1999). Identifying and overcoming barriers to providing sexuality information in the clinical setting. *Rehabilitation Nursing, 24*(4), 148–151.

Huang, C. (1999). Discussing sex with disabled patients. *Western Journal of Medicine, 171*(2), 76–77.

Johnson, O. S. (2007). *The sexual spectrum: Exploring human diversity* (updated edition). Vancouver: Raincoast Books.

Kaplan, H. S. (1979). *Disorders of sexual desire.* New York: Simon & Schuster.

Klein, M. J. (2015). *Sexuality and disability.* WebMD. Retrieved from http://emedicine.medscape.com/article/319119-overview#showall.

Magnan, M. A., Reynolds, K. E., & Galvin, E. A. (2005). Barriers to addressing patient sexuality in nursing practice. *Medsurg Nursing, 14*(5), 282–289.

Massey, M. T. (2015). Managing infertility in primary care. *Practice Nurse, 45*(3), 32–37.

Masters, W. H., & Johnson, V. E. (1966). *Human sexual response.* Boston: Little, Brown.

Mayo Foundation for Medical Education and Research. (2015). *Sex during pregnancy: What's OK, what's not.* Retrieved from http://www.mayoclinic.org/healthy-lifestyle/pregnancy-week-by-week/in-depth/sex-during-pregnancy/art-20045318.

Merryfeather, L., & Bruce, A. (2014). The invisibility of gender diversity: Understanding transgender and transsexuality in nursing literature. *Nursing Forum, 49*(2).

Meyer-Bahlburg, H. (2013). Sex steroids and variants of gender identity. *Endocrinology and Metabolism Clinics, 42*(3), 435–452. doi:10.1016/j.ecl.2013.05.011.

NANDA International. (2009). *NANDA International nursing diagnoses: Definitions and classification, 2009–2011.* Chichester, UK: John Wiley & Sons.

Nusbaum, M. R., Hamilton, C., & Lenahan, P. (2003). Chronic illness and sexual functioning. *American Family Physician, 67*(2), 347–354.

Oral Cancer Foundation. (2017). *HPV/ Oral cancer facts.* Retrieved from http://oralcancerfoundation.org/understanding/hpv/hpv-oral-cancer-facts/.

Pessango, R. A. (2013). Don't be embarrassed: Taking a sexual health history. *Nursing, 43*(9), 60–64. doi:10.1097/01.NURSE.0000431139.82532.b3.

Ross, M. W., Channon-Little, L. D., & Rosser, B. R. (2000). *Sexual health concerns: Interviewing and history taking for health practitioners* (2nd ed.). Philadelphia, PA: F. A. Davis.

Rotermann, M. (2012). *Sexual health and condom use of 15- to 24-year-olds in 2003 and 2009/2010* (Catalogue No. 82-003-XPE), *Health Reports, 23*(1). Ottawa: Statistics Canada. Retrieved from http://www.statcan.gc.ca/pub/82-003-x/2012001/article/11632-eng.pdf.

Running, A., & Berndt, A. (2003). *Management guidelines for nurse practitioners working in family practice.* Philadelphia, PA: F. A. Davis.

Sabella, D. (2016). Revisiting child sexual abuse and survivor issues. *American Journal of Nursing, 116*(3), 48–54. doi:10.1097/01.NAJ.0000481280.22557.45.

Schneider, S. K., O'Donnell, L., Stueve, A., et al. (2012). Cyberbullying, school bullying, and psychological distress: A regional census of high school students. *American Journal of Public Health, 102*(1), 171–177. doi:10.2105/AJPH.2011.300308.

Slane, J. (2013). Sexting and the law in Canada. *Canadian Journal of Human Sexuality, 22*(3), 117–122. doi:10.3138/cjhs.22.3.C01.

Society of Obstetricians and Gynaecologists of Canada [SOGC]. (2017). *Sexual activity.* Retrieved from http://www.sexandu.ca/sexual-activity/.

Statistics Canada. (2016). *Same-sex couples and sexual orientation … By the numbers.* Ottawa: Author. Retrieved from http://www.statcan.gc.ca/eng/dai/smr08/2015/smr08_203_2015.

Transgender Health Information Program. (2017). *Gender-affirming surgeries.* Retrieved from http://transhealth.phsa.ca/medical-options/surgeries.

University of Toronto, Centre for Addiction and Mental Health. (2017). *Re:searching for LGBTQ health.* Retrieved from http://lgbtqhealth.ca/.

van der Riet, P. (1998). The sexual embodiment of the cancer patient. *Nursing Inquiry, 5*(4), 248–257. doi:10.1046/j.1440-1800.1998.00244.x.

Van Ouytsel, J., Walrave, M., Ponnet, K., et al. (2015). The association between adolescent sexting, psychosocial difficulties and risk behaviors: Integrative review. *The Journal of School Nursing, 31*(1), 54–69. doi:10.1177/1059840514541964.

von Sydow, K. (1999). Sexuality during pregnancy and after childbirth: A metacontent analysis of 59 studies. *Journal of Psychosomatic Research, 47*(1), 27–49.

Wagner, G., Bondil, P., Dabees, K., et al. (2005). Ethical aspects of sexual medicine. *Journal of Sexual Medicine, 2*(2), 163–168. doi:10.1111/j.1743-6109.2005.20225.x.

Wisnieski, D. M., & Matzo, M. (2013). Promoting healthy sexual behavior in adolescents. *American Journal of Nursing, 113*(6), 67–70. doi:10.1097/01.NAJ.0000431279.98524.f8.

World Health Organization. (2016). *Sexual and reproductive health: Defining sexual health.* Geneva, Switzerland: Author. Retrieved from http://www.who.int/reproductivehealth/topics/sexual_health/sh_definitions/en/.

28

Spirituality in Health and Health Care

Written by Barbara Pesut, RN, PhD, Jeanette Vinek, RN, RScP, BScN, MHScN

OBJECTIVES

Mastery of content in this chapter will enable you to:

- Define the key terms listed.
- Describe the historical influences of spirituality and religion on nursing.
- Discuss research findings that suggest a relationship between spiritual practices and patients' health status.
- Discuss the relationship between spirituality and nursing theory.
- Compare and contrast the concepts of religion and spirituality.
- Describe how spirituality may facilitate coping during times of illness or suffering over the life journey.
- Describe the relational attributes that facilitate spiritual nursing care.
- Discuss the process and qualities of spiritual nursing care.
- Discuss an ethical approach to spiritual nursing care.
- Discuss the role of the nurse in providing spiritual nursing care.
- Describe a process for understanding patients' spirituality.
- Discuss appropriate ways to facilitate patients' spiritual practices.
- Describe when it is necessary to involve a spiritual leader or pastoral care.
- Reflect on how to determine if your spiritual care has been therapeutic.

KEY TERMS

MEDIA RESOURCES

http://evolve.elsevier.com/Canada/Potter/fundamentals/

- Audio Chapter Summaries
- Examination Review Questions
- Concept Map Creator
- Case Study with Questions
- Audio Glossary
- Content Updates
- Video Clips

The word *spirituality* is derived from the Latin word *spiritus*, which refers to breath or wind. The spirit gives life to, or animates, a person. Spirituality has been defined as "a way of being in the world in which a person feels a sense of connectedness to self, others, and/or a higher power or nature; a sense of meaning in life; and transcendence beyond self, everyday living, and suffering" (Weathers, McCarthy, & Coffey, 2015, p. 93). Spirituality can help individuals achieve the balance needed to maintain health and well-being and to cope with illness. Caring for a patient's spiritual needs means caring for the whole person, accepting his or her beliefs and experiences, and helping with issues concerning meaning and hope.

HISTORICAL PERSPECTIVES

Nursing has a rich spiritual heritage. Within this heritage, spirituality was most recognizable within religion. Organized nursing originated from religious orders in which nuns were primarily responsible for providing nursing care. In Canada, the earliest nurses belonged to Roman Catholic orders devoted to care of the sick—most notably, the Sisters of Charity of Montreal (Grey Nuns), an order founded by Marie Marguerite d'Youville in 1737 (Paul, 2000). The Sisters of Charity were responsible for bringing a Judeo-Christian model of nursing care to the most remote areas of western and northern Canada. Florence Nightingale's ideas of modern nursing were first taught in London in 1860. Her model of Western nursing, rooted in Christianity, was spread around the world during the colonial era (Paul, 2000). Canadian missionary nurses were among those who brought Florence Nightingale's ideas of modern nursing methods to China, India, Japan, and Korea in the first half of the twentieth century (Grypma, 2008).

Religion was at the core of early nursing philosophies and practice until the nineteenth century (McSherry, 2001). But during the late nineteenth and early twentieth centuries, confidence in religion was replaced by confidence in medical science. Religious aspects of care became less visible. However, many nurses became dissatisfied with a medical approach to care that neglected spirituality, in part because a purely scientific approach could not answer the existential questions raised by patients (McSherry, 2001). Nurses began to find ways to articulate and incorporate spirituality into practice and research. Between 1980 and 2000, renewed interest in spirituality was reflected by an increase in nursing literature on spirituality, as well as a growing interest in parish nursing as a way for faith communities in Canada to reclaim their healing mission (Miller, 2004; Olson, Simington, & Clark, 1998).

Canadian nursing scholarship has made important contributions to this renewed interest by emphasizing the relationship between spirituality, religion, health, and culture. This is important because of Canada's cultural diversity. For example, in their study of spirituality and health in Punjabi Sikh living in British Columbia, Labun and Emblen (2007) explored how the interplay of spirituality, religion, and health informs culturally competent care. More recently, Reimer-Kirkham and colleagues have used a social justice lens to explore how religious and spiritual diversity is negotiated in Canadian health care (e.g., Reimer-Kirkham, 2014; Reimer-Kirkham & Cochrane, 2016). Just as Canadian nurses must understand cultural influences in health and illness, they must also recognize the need for sensitive, safe, and ethical nursing care in which patients' spiritual needs and resources are recognized and supported.

Spirituality and Health: Empirical Evidence

The Canadian Nurses Association (CNA) recognizes spirituality as an essential dimension of overall health (CNA, 2010). Spiritual needs may increase as health declines (Bruce, Shields, & Molzahn, 2011). There is increasing evidence that spirituality plays a role in personal capacities, illness-coping strategies, and positive health behaviours. For example, research involving 263 patients with cancer found that those who reported healthy inner spirituality, spiritual coping, and spiritual well-being were less likely to experience depression and intrapersonal and interpersonal conflicts (Vespa, Jacobsen, Spazzafumo, et al., 2011). A meta-analysis of data from studies of youth with chronic physical and mental health conditions indicated that positive spiritual coping was an important strategy for overall well-being (Reynolds, Mrug, Schwebel, et al., 2016). Similarly, an exploration of the beliefs of 228 hospitalized patients in Australia found that 80% of respondents felt that religious and spiritual beliefs aided in the healing process by providing psychological support, an improved sense of well-being, and support in maintaining a healthy lifestyle (Hilbers, Haynes, & Kivikko, 2010, p. 5). A recent review of the evidence of the impact of religious and spiritual interventions in mental health care indicated such interventions may help to reduce clinical symptoms (Goncalves, Lucchetti, Menezes, et al., 2015). Studies such as these suggest that spirituality is an important consideration in personal health and health care more generally.

SPIRITUALITY AND NURSING THEORY

Nursing theory is a logical structuring of ideas that help us to think about what we believe nursing to be and how nurses do their work. One of the first nursing theorists was Florence Nightingale. Her theoretical thinking was informed by her beliefs about God and natural law (Calabria & Macrae, 1994). Theoretical thinking in nursing developed during the late 1950s and early 1960s. During these two decades, nurses produced over 20 new nursing models (Thorne, 2003), some of which included spirituality as an aspect of nursing practice (Martsolf & Mickley, 1998). Even though spirituality was not explicitly addressed in many of these models, spirituality and religion still informed nursing theory in important ways. This is because nursing theory attempts to answer basic questions about the nature of persons, about health, and about the environment (Meleis, 1997). Thinking about the environment that surrounds nursing practice naturally led to nurses speculating about the nature of the world we live in, including its spiritual dimensions. For example, Rosemary Parse's (2014) humanbecoming theory specifies beliefs about the world in relation to meaning, rhythmicity, and transcendence. Jean Watson's (2011) caring science theory offers beliefs about the unity and connectedness of all the world and the role that caring plays in that connectedness. Meehan's (2003, 2012a, 2012b) careful nursing theory outlines 10 key concepts including disinterested love, contagious calmness, trustworthy collaboration, and power derived from service. These theories, and others similar to them, draw on a broad range of spiritual, religious, and philosophical beliefs to describe the nature of persons, health, and the environment. However, it is important to remember that these theories adopt particular beliefs about the world that may or may not resonate with the beliefs that nurses or patients hold, and so may have varying applicability to practice.

In contrast, mid-range theories are meant to be more "immediately useful, concrete, and meaningful to practitioners" (Risjord, 2010, p. 141). An example of a mid-range theory is that of dignity therapy. Dignity is a critical part of human spirituality. Chochinov's dignity model provides an empirical framework by which nurses can elicit and address important aspects of patient spirituality (Sinclair & Chochinov, 2012a). This model includes a dignity inventory by which nurses can better understand patient distress and an intervention designed to enhance meaning and purpose. Further, this model provides pragmatic theoretical guidance for how nurses and other practitioners can preserve dignity through specific attitudes, behaviours, compassion, and dialogue (Sinclair & Chochinov, 2012b) (Box 28-1). Other mid-range theories include Dobratz's (2016) mid-range theory of adaptive spirituality and White's (2016) mid-range theory of spirituality and spiritual self-care.

Conceptualizing Spirituality and Religion

Conceptualizing is an important part of nursing theory. Conceptual work consists of creating definitions that become tools for nurses that bridge between the broader world of ideas and the unique nurse–patient interaction (Thorne, 2005). Over the past two decades, nurses have created many definitions of **spirituality** for nursing practice. Several integrative reviews of spirituality in health care literature have identified the following common themes: meaning, purpose, connectedness,

BOX 28-1 CASE STUDY

Application of Mid-Range Theory of Dignity

Meghan is a home care nurse working with Tom, who is receiving palliative care. As Tom nears death, he often expresses despair over the meaninglessness of his life. Meghan knows that dignity therapy is an evidence-based intervention that has the potential to support Tom's spiritual health. She works with a hospice volunteer, who in turn spends time with Tom doing dignity therapy. The volunteer uses a dignity interview through which Tom is encouraged to share his memories and wisdom. The hospice volunteer records the interviews, transcribes them, and then produces a legacy document that summarizes the interviews. Meghan and the volunteer meet together with Tom and his family to share this living legacy. It is a healing and tearful time. After this intervention, Meghan notices that Tom rarely talks about meaninglessness and seems more at peace.

Thinking Points

- Dignity therapy is just one example of a mid-range theory. Explore White's (2016) mid-range theory and think about how it might apply to your practice.
- How might a nurse's ideas about the environment and the nature of persons influence how he or she chooses a mid-range theory to apply in practice?

relationship, transcendence, healing, and intuitive sense (Ramezani, Ahmadi, Mahommadi, et al., 2014; Weathers et al., 2015). However, trying to define spirituality has been challenging. If we try to include all of the diverse ideas about what spirituality is, the concept becomes too vague to be useful for nursing practice or knowledge development (Paley, 2008). You only have to think about the themes just identified to realize that they cover the entire human experience. This has been a problem for the development of practice-based knowledge about spirituality.

Many people use the terms *religion* and *spirituality* interchangeably. Although closely associated, these terms are not synonymous. **Religion** is an organized system of beliefs concerning the cause, nature, and purpose of the universe, especially belief in or the worship of a God or gods (Andrews & Boyle, 2007). A person might describe himself or herself as spiritual but not religious, as both spiritual and religious, or as neither spiritual nor religious. Few would characterize themselves as religious but not spiritual, as spirituality is an inherent part of religion. Although nursing defines spirituality and religion differently, these differences may be less clear in practice. Individuals who describe themselves as spiritual but not religious may draw on religious ideas and practices as they grow in their spiritual journey. As a result, nurses need to know how to give skillful spiritual and religious care (Pesut, 2016).

Another common term individuals use to express their spirituality is that of **faith**. Faith is often used in two ways: as a cultural or institutional religion, such as Judaism, Buddhism, Islam, or Christianity; and as a relationship with a divinity, a higher power, an authority, or a spirit. Faith may also involve a sense of **transcendence**: an awareness of something that a person cannot see or know in ordinary physical ways (Perry, 2004) or an experience of fullness that goes beyond daily life (Taylor, 2007). This experience does not necessarily need to be understood in relation to God—it may be in relation to the universe, nature, or humanity.

A patient-centred approach to spirituality respects this diversity. Part of respecting diversity is recognizing that some individuals might be offended by the claim often made in nursing literature that all individuals are spiritual (Pesut, Fowler, Reimer-Kirkham, et al., 2009). Some individuals either do not believe in the existence of God (**atheist**) or believe that any ultimate reality is unknown (**agnostic**) and so may resist the idea that all persons have a spiritual nature because of spirituality's long association with religion. Thorne (2005) has encouraged nurses to remember that the purpose of conceptualizing is to support nursing's service to society. Part of that service is remembering that the definitions we create, and the claims we make, must serve a diverse society.

SPIRITUALITY AND THE LIFE JOURNEY

Children's ideas of a higher power or supreme being are often based on what is presented to them in their homes or spiritual community. Their spirituality develops as they learn about themselves in relationship with others. Adolescents may reconsider their childhood concept of a spiritual power and, in the search for an identity, may question values and practices. Many adults experience spiritual growth by entering into lifelong relationships. An ability to care meaningfully for others and the self is evidence of a healthy spirituality. Older persons often turn to important relationships and the giving of themselves to others as spiritual tasks. As people mature, they often turn inward to enduring values and to a concept of a supreme being or a higher meaning that has been sustaining and meaningful. A healthy spirituality in older persons is one that gives peace to and acceptance of the self.

Becoming a nurse is also part of the life journey in which spirituality may play an important role. Many students enter nursing because they desire to make a meaningful contribution to life by helping to alleviate the suffering of others. However, nursing is a challenging profession. Immersion in the suffering of others and challenging work environments can influence how students feel about the profession, which in turn can influence their meaning and purpose in life. Nursing students need strategies to develop their own spiritual resources to ensure that they stay well in the context of practice (Box 28-2).

Developing and Maintaining Spirituality

Understanding one's own spirituality is a lifelong process. It shifts and changes with life experience. Maintaining and increasing our understanding of spirituality is a contemplative and reflective process. Learning to recognize what gives one's life meaning and purpose and cultivating opportunities to experience this feeling of purpose are ways to develop one's spirituality. Consider for a moment the things that bring the greatest meaning to your life, the times when you feel peace, you feel joy, you feel purpose. What were you doing right before you experienced these feelings? Did you pause for a moment and take a breath? Did you recognize the beauty of the garden outside your window? Did you feel gratitude for the meal before you? Did you recognize the humanity in a face before you? These are all spiritual experiences and can be nurtured and grown once they are brought to awareness. Through this awareness, one can choose to consciously connect and be fully present in the moment. Being fully present in the moment, or "presence," facilitates spiritual care (Swinton & Pattison, 2010).

Reflective journalling; paying attention to our thoughts, emotions, and sensations; noticing when we feel most connected to those around us; and reflecting on what was occurring for us in that moment can

BOX 28-2 RESEARCH HIGHLIGHT

The Role of Spirituality in Coping With the Demands of Hospital Culture Among Fourth-Year Nursing Students

Cilliers and Terblanche (2014) explored the role of spirituality in helping nursing students at one faith-based university cope with hospital culture. They analyzed written essays of 14 nursing students about their experiences with the demands of working in a hospital setting. Students described an idealized approach to nursing and hospital care that was replaced by a sense of disappointment and confusion as they dealt with the realities of practice. As a result, they needed to face realities of nursing they had not anticipated, and this affected their spirituality. They described feeling exhausted, sad, and out of balance. Further, it was difficult to talk to friends and family about what they were experiencing. Under these circumstances, students found comfort in a greater power. Nurturing their own spiritual life was an important way to develop hope and courage amidst potential despair.

Evidence-Informed Practice

- Nursing students need to be prepared for some reality shock as they enter the real world of nursing practice.
- It is useful to develop supportive networks within which nursing students can share their experiences.
- Nursing students should explore ways to develop their own spiritual resources as they prepare for practice.

Cilliers, F., & Terblanche, L. (2014). The role of spirituality in coping with the demands of the hospital culture amongst fourth-year nursing students. *International Review of Psychiatry, 26*(3), 279–288. doi:10.3109/09540261.2014.890922

help us understand our spirituality. In addition, it is useful to take time for contemplation on life's big questions—spend time in meditation, join a spiritual community, ask questions. Look for new ways to experience the feeling of transcendence, spend time in nature, and then practise what works for you. If you feel a sense of peace from meditation, then meditate. If a walk in nature creates a sense of connection, then walk in nature. If quiet contemplation or prayer provides a feeling of transcendence, then pray. Each person will have a unique experience of spirituality, and learning to recognize when you are most connected to all things around you and seeking out these opportunities will expand and deepen your understanding of spirituality and enhance your ability to understand the spiritual needs of your patients. It is important to nurture this awareness, as nurses who have a spiritual base or identity are more likely to facilitate spiritual practices and provide spiritual care in practice (Cockell & McSherry, 2012).

Mindfulness. Mindfulness can be an important strategy for developing spiritual practice, both for yourself and for others. Mindfulness is "awareness, cultivated by paying attention in a sustained and particular way: on purpose, in the present moment, and non-judgmentally" (Kabat-Zinn, 2013, p. 1). There are seven attitudinal factors at the foundation of mindfulness practice (Kabat-Zinn, 2013):

- An attitude of nonjudgement
- An attitude of patience (both with yourself and the process), allowing things to unfold at their own pace
- An attitude of open curiosity, approaching each moment as if encountering everything for the first time
- An attitude of trust in ourselves
- An attitude of nonstriving, relinquishing the tendency to strive toward a goal in exchange for a willingness to pay attention to whatever arises in each moment
- An attitude of acceptance—an acceptance of the present moment as it is, accepting what we notice without trying to make it different
- An attitude of letting-go or nonattachment; we let things be as they are in the present moment, without grasping or pushing away

Adopting these attitudes of mindfulness helps create an environment that is safe for patients to express their spirituality.

Research examining the effectiveness of mindfulness programs with university students demonstrated that it is beneficial for stress reduction and improves quality of life. Students who learned mindfulness had an increased nonjudgemental and nonreactive stance toward feelings, thoughts, and emotions; thus mindfulness can be an effective intervention to support mental health (Canby, Cameron, Calhoun, et al., 2015; de Bruin, Meppelink, & Bögels, 2015). As the acuity and complexity in health care increase and demands on nurses grow, reducing nurses' stress in practice has become ever more important. Research with health care providers who have received mindfulness training has found that levels of burnout and stress were reduced, mental well-being improved, and patient satisfaction increased (Goodman & Schorling, 2012; Horner, Piercy, Eure, et al., 2014; Smith, 2014). Mindfulness is one way to develop one's own spiritual awareness while facilitating the spiritual practices of others.

Spirituality and Illness

Few individuals experience life's journey without facing an unexpected or chronic illness or injury resulting in suffering and loss. Such events can lead to both spiritual challenges and transformation. Spiritual dimensions of the illness experience may include reconsidering beliefs about life; maintaining spiritual or religious practices; connecting with God and significant others; and finding balance, courage, and growth (Van Leeuwen, Tiesinga, Jochemasen, et al., 2007).

In the face of suffering, individuals may feel alone or even abandoned by a higher power. They may question their spiritual values and beliefs, raising questions about their way of life and purpose for living. Anger is not uncommon, and patients may express anger toward God, their families, themselves, or health care providers. People also look for ways to remain faithful to their beliefs during their suffering. They may pray, attend religious services, or reflect on the positive aspects of their lives. A review of the experiences of persons living with multiple chronic conditions indicated that spiritual strategies were used to maintain emotional health. Further, a sense of life purpose was motivation for engaging in self-management strategies (Coventry, Small, Panagioti, et al., 2015).

Terminal illness marks the end of the life journey and brings unique struggles. As the physical body is in the process of dying, individuals are confronted with questions about the meaning of their life and what comes after life. Fears of physical pain, isolation, and losing control are common, both for oneself and for one's family. Spiritual beliefs and practices often provide a source of comfort and strength, and individuals may experience the end of life as a time of positive spiritual transformation. For example, a review that included studies representing 178 patients at the end of life indicated that relationships with self, others, nature, music, and God or a higher power were important during this time. Common spiritual needs were to finish business, to maintain involvement and control, and to keep a positive outlook (Edwards, Pang, Shiu, et al., 2010).

The spiritual framework of coping illustrated in Figure 28-1 provides an overview of how spirituality relates to coping and health. An illness or injury would constitute a stressor. The experience of that illness or injury is shaped both by personal factors and how one appraises the event. For example, an individual might attribute the cause of an illness to a punishment by God for a sin they committed and this would magnify the stressor. The effect of the stressor is also determined by personality factors, such as problem-solving styles or hope, and religious influences, such as doctrinal beliefs and religious orientation. Perceptions of God, and in particular whether God is more likely to be punishing or loving in the face of suffering, greatly influence appraisals of illness. How one appraises the stressor contributes to the effect of that stressor. Individuals can then enact spiritual coping behaviours, both corporate and private, and work to establish spiritual connections. These coping strategies may in turn contribute to enhanced meaning-making and well-being.

What do patients expect from nurses in the area of spiritual care (Box 28-3)? Although nurses are not typically seen as primary spiritual care providers, patients do appreciate having nurses know about their spirituality and showing concern in this regard. This is most often the case if spirituality is important to the patient, in the context of life-threatening illness, and if there is a relationship between the patient and nurse (Johnston Taylor, 2007). In a study of Chinese individuals with terminal illness, participants suggested that although they did not expect nurses to provide spiritual care, a compassionate environment that promoted hope and acceptance supported their spirituality (Mok, Wong, & Wong, 2010). The review involving end-of-life patients cited earlier indicated that a patient-centred approach to spiritual care involved having nurses who were kind, compassionate, comforting, and gentle; who affirmed patients as persons; and who sought to allow patients to set the agenda and make choices in accordance with their values and wishes (Edwards et al., 2010).

CRITICAL THINKING

At the core of nursing, and indeed at the core of all human service professions, is a commitment to caring for each person as a unique and inherently valuable individual. In the case of spirituality, this

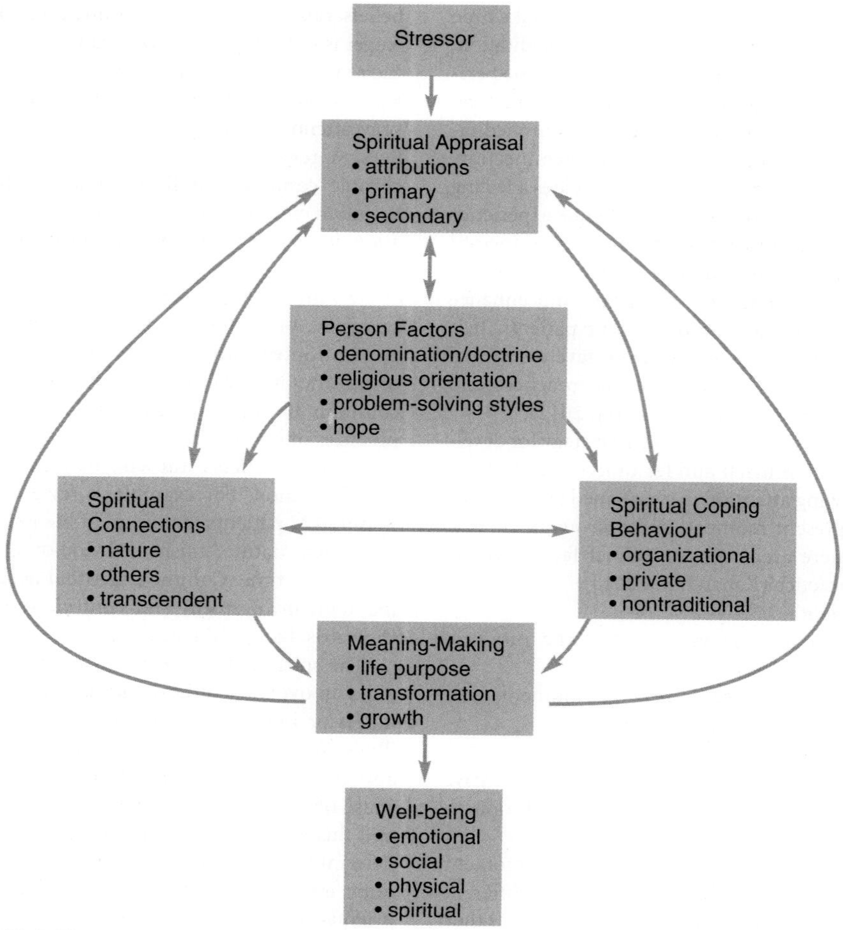

FIGURE 28-1 The spiritual framework of coping (an adaptation and application of the transactional model). (From Gall, T. L., Charbonneau, C., Clarke, N. H., Grant, K., Joseph, A., & Shouldice, L. [2005]. Understanding the nature and role of spirituality in relation to coping and health: A conceptual framework. *Canadian Psychology, 46*[2], 88–104. Copyright © 2005, Canadian Psychological Association. Permission granted for use of material.)

BOX 28-3 RESEARCH HIGHLIGHT

Spiritual Support for Persons With End-Stage Heart Failure and Their Carers

Ross and Austin (2015) explored the spiritual needs and preferences of persons living with end-stage heart failure and those of their carers. The authors conducted 47 interviews with participants at 3-month intervals for up to 1 year. They learned that these individuals experienced spiritual needs related to love and belonging, hope and coping, meaning and purpose, faith and belief, and existential issues. Over the course of the illness, individuals transitioned from fighting the disease to focusing on quality of life. Participants desired spiritual support in the form of having someone to talk to who would support them and foster hope. A home visiting service, preferably led by a nurse or other member of the heart failure team, was recommended by patients.

Evidence-Informed Practice

- Nurses need to be alert to spiritual needs in this population and take the time to listen to concerns.
- Spiritual needs will change over time.
- Fostering hope is an important spiritual care strategy.
- A single individual who can provide support for spiritual issues at home would help to meet the needs of this population.

Ross, L., & Austin, J. (2015). Spiritual needs and spiritual support preferences of people with end-stage heart failure and their carers: implications for nurse managers. *Journal of Nursing Management, 23,* 87–95.

commitment begins with a respect for each person's beliefs. Differences exist in the ways people experience the world and find meaning in that experience. Critical thinking in the context of spiritual care entails two important processes. First, it means gaining an understanding of the patient. This includes the person's spiritual and religious values, beliefs, and experiences and how those are influenced by his or her current circumstances. Naturally, the depth of this assessment must be sensitive to the circumstances (e.g., patients coming in for day surgery as opposed to palliative care) and the depth of the nurse–patient relationship. Second, a critical thinking approach to spiritual care entails ensuring that the care provided is both ethical and based on the best available evidence.

Understanding Patients' Spirituality

You will note that we have chosen not to use the language of assessing spirituality. Spiritual care is different from the physical aspects of care. Spirituality contains an element of mystery that cannot be assessed and treated in the same way that you might treat a physical problem, such as a pressure injury. Diagnosing and intervening in a patient's spirituality could be considered disrespectful and intrusive. Instead, nurses should think about *understanding* rather than assessing patients' spirituality (Box 28-4). It could be thought of as a series of conversations whereby nurses seek to understand what is important and meaningful to individuals. The depth of that conversation will rest largely on the circumstances the patient is facing and the extent of relational development.

BOX 28-4 RESEARCH HIGHLIGHT

Discerning the Healing Path

Giske and Cone (2015) examined 22 nurses' experiences with spiritual care with the aim of gaining insight into how nurses understand and practise spiritual care. They characterized this process of care as discerning the healing path, which consisted of three stages. In stage one, nurses looked for signs and cues that spirituality might be important to the patient. In stage two, nurses uncovered patients' deeper concerns by finding time to spend with patients and gently probing for such concerns while respecting patients' privacy. In stage three, they facilitated the healing process through several strategies, including attentive engagement. Throughout these stages, it was important for nurses to build a relationship of trust with the patient and to go outside their comfort zone.

Evidence-Informed Practice

- Nurses need to look for cues that spirituality is important to patients.
- In practising spiritual care it is important to build relationships of trust.
- Nurses need to recognize that they may feel out of their comfort zone when discerning the patient's healing path.
- Creating time and a climate of privacy for conversation fosters patients' expression of deeper concerns.
- The nurse's attentive engagement aids in a patient's healing process.

Giske, T., & Cone, P.H. (2015). Discerning the healing path—How nurses assist patient spirituality in diverse health care settings. *Journal of Clinical Nursing, 24*, 2926–2935. doi:10.1111/jocn.12907

But even more important, the nurse should discover those values and beliefs that are important to take into account in health care. Does the patient have beliefs that will influence important health care decisions? Are there religious rituals or restrictions that should inform care? Without knowing these details, the nurse risks harming the patient. For example, a nurse who removes sacramental garb or provides food that is prohibited may actually be contributing to the breaking of religious law and thus be seen to be harming that individual's spirit.

In these conversations, the nurse is not the expert but rather a co-learner in the mysteries of life. This kind of work generally consists of quiet conversations, effective listening, and communication through presence and touch. Sinclair and Chochinov (2012c) have proposed the pneumonic SACR-D to provide guidance for how health care providers should communicate about spiritual and existential issues. The framework consists of self-awareness, assessing the patient, compassionate presence, referring to additional spiritual support, and dialogue.

In many cases, nurses would say that they are the learners in such conversations. Patients teach them about life as they share their stories of transition and suffering. Above all, the process of learning about a patient's spirituality should be grounded in an understanding of compassion. Sinclair, Raffin Bouchal, Chochinov, et al. (2014) define **compassion** as "a virtuous response that seeks to address the suffering and needs of a person through relational understanding and action" (p. 195). To practise compassion, a nurse requires virtue, relational skills, and a commitment to responding with action to the spiritual concerns that arise (Sinclair, McClement, Raffin Bouchal, et al., 2016).

However, even though understanding is a relational and evolving process, it is still important that the nurse have some form of systematic approach to ensure that critical information is obtained. When patients enter the health care system, it is essential to obtain information about their religious and spiritual beliefs and practices. This has been referred to as a spiritual screening and seeks to discern whether spirituality and religion are important to the individual and, if so, what beliefs or practices are most important to take into account in the context of care.

Numerous tools are available to enable nurses to gain a deeper understanding of patients' spirituality. A helpful tool for clinical practice is the FICA Spiritual History Tool, developed by Puchalski and Romer (2000) (see Box 28-5 for a systematic process of understanding a patient's spirituality). Remember that how this tool is used will depend on the circumstances. The key is to be sensitive to what patients

BOX 28-5 PROCEDURAL GUIDELINE

Understanding a Patient's Spirituality: FICA

F—Faith and Belief

"Do you consider yourself spiritual or religious?" or "Is spirituality something important to you?" or "Do you have spiritual beliefs that help you cope with stress and difficult times?" (Contextualize to reason for visit if it is not the routine history.) If the patient responds "No," the health care provider might ask, "What gives your life meaning?" Sometimes patients respond with answers such as family, career, or nature. (The question of meaning should also be asked even if people answer "Yes" to spirituality.)

I—Importance

"What importance does your spirituality have in your life? Has your spirituality influenced how you take care of yourself and your health? Does your spirituality influence you in your health care decision making (e.g., advance directives, treatment, etc.)?"

C—Community

"Are you part of a spiritual community?" Communities such as churches, temples, and mosques or a group of like-minded friends, family, or yoga can serve as strong support systems for some patients. This can be explored further: "Is this of support to you? How? Is there a group of people you really love or who are important to you?"

A—Address in Care

"How would you like me, your health care provider, to address these issues in your health care?" (With the newer models including diagnosis of spiritual distress, *A* also refers to the assessment and plan of patient spiritual distress or issues within a treatment or care plan.)

The George Washington Institute for Spirituality and Health. *FICA Spirituality History Tool.* Retrieved from https://smhs.gwu.edu/gwish/clinical/fica/spiritual-history-tool

want to tell you and to be a good listener. If you are a compassionate and open listener, you will be more likely to gain meaningful information.

Further, it is important to think about how and when the information will be gathered and recorded. Numerous nurses are involved in one patient's care and having all of these nurses inquire using this tool is not appropriate. For each nursing context, it is important to ask the following questions and to create policies and procedures that address these questions.

- Who should be collecting this data?
- How extensive should the assessment be in light of the clinical context?
- At what point in the care trajectory should this information be obtained?
- Which responses should be documented so that the information is available to all health care providers and which responses should be held in confidence?

Pondering and answering these questions in the health care context is part of expert nursing thinking and critical judgement.

This more in-depth understanding of a patient's spirituality has certain goals that should guide these conversations (Puchalski, Ferrell, Virani, et al., 2009):

- Invite patients to share their spiritual beliefs and values.
- Learn about those beliefs and values.
- Open an opportunity for compassionate care.
- Empower patients to draw on their resources for healing and acceptance.
- Identify practices and beliefs that are important for the plan of care.
- Identify those patients who would benefit from a referral to a spiritual care provider.

ETHICAL SPIRITUAL CARE

The *Code of Ethics for Registered Nurses* (Canadian Nurses Association, 2017) requires nurses to treat all patients with dignity and respect. In providing nursing care, you must not discriminate on the basis of spiritual beliefs, age, ethnicity, marital status, gender, race, sexual orientation, health status, or disability. However, for many, discrimination is not a conscious process but rather an unchallenged set of biases that cause us to react to others in less than caring ways. Therefore, an important part of ethical spiritual care is constantly working with your own potential biases as a nurse. This is more commonly known as reflective practice. In the process of delivering care, the nurse remains open to internal dialogues and feelings that have the potential to violate patients' dignity or respect. Once the nurse identifies those internal feelings, he or she can do the hard work of trying to understand the origins of those feelings so that engagement with patients can grow ethically. This is particularly important in the context of religion and spirituality, as society tends to polarize over religious beliefs. If you are a "believer," do you judge harshly the "unbeliever"? If you are agnostic or atheist, do you dismiss the believer? Box 28-6 provides some questions that are useful for you to reflect on.

In a study led by Canadian scholar Reimer-Kirkham, one of the key strategies of successful spiritual care was identifying points of commonality across diversity. Health care providers spoke of finding a human connection that transcended differing belief systems (Pesut & Reimer-Kirkham, 2010). This approach means identifying the common values that make people human and respecting the commitments and values that make humans unique. Love, trust, hope, forgiveness, meaning, and community are needs of all people.

Beyond a foundational approach of respect, there are two important ethical issues when nurses engage in spiritual care. The first is understanding and respecting appropriate nurse–patient boundaries. The second is ensuring that you are competent to engage in spiritual care and knowing when you are beyond your competency, so that you can refer to a spiritual care provider or social worker. Spiritual care requires an interdisciplinary approach. Nursing is a relational process and so it is not always easy to discern where the professional boundaries lie. This is particularly relevant in spiritual care. When we establish a relationship with patients and we discern that they want to share the more intimate aspects of their spiritual lives with us, it is not always easy to know what is appropriate to do. Here is where questions arise, such as the following:

- Is it appropriate to share my own beliefs with patients, particularly if they are different from theirs?
- Is there a role for proselytizing in nursing, or what do I do if patients try to proselytize me?
- Should I participate in religious practices like prayer if patients request it of me?
- How do I respond to what I perceive to be unhelpful spiritual beliefs (e.g., when individuals feel that they are being punished by God or resist health care treatment because they believe they will be divinely healed)?

The answers to these questions are complex, and the responses will vary according to the context. This is why expert nursing judgement is so important. The *Code of Ethics for Registered Nurses* (Canadian Nurses Association, 2017) provides some important guidelines:

- Nurses provide care directed first and foremost toward the health and well-being of persons receiving care, recognizing and using the values and principles of primary health care (p. 16).
- Nurses are sensitive to the inherent power differentials between care providers and persons receiving care. They do not misuse that power to influence decision-making (p. 17).
- Nurses provide education to support the informed decision-making of capable persons. They respect the decisions a person makes, including choice of lifestyles or treatment that are not conducive to good health, and continue to provide care in a non-judgmental manner (p. 17).

BOX 28-6 Nursing Care Reflective Exercises

Take a few moments to reflect on the following questions:

- Do you believe that there is a God or ultimate authority in the universe? If so, how does that belief influence your behaviour and, ultimately, your nursing care?
- How do you feel about religion? Should religious beliefs be accounted for in the context of nursing care?
- Why does suffering happen in the world? How should individuals respond to suffering?
- What behaviours, practices, or lifestyles do you consider immoral or wrong? What patients might you look after who would exhibit those behaviours and how might your beliefs influence your ability to give care?
- Do you come from a religious background and does that background encourage you to share your beliefs and possibly to convert others to those beliefs? How might that influence your practice? Should patients be allowed to try to convert you to their beliefs?
- What happens to you after you die?

Although these may seem like questions unrelated to nursing practice, understanding more about what you believe will help you to deal more authentically with the beliefs of others. It will also help you to think through issues that will ultimately arise in the context of your practice. It is also important to know that nursing practice itself might challenge you to rethink and reframe your beliefs. That is an important part of growing as a person.

- In health-care decision-making, in treatment and in care, nurses work with persons receiving care to take into account their values, customs and spiritual beliefs, as well as their social and economic circumstances without judgment or bias (p. 18).
- If nursing care is requested that is in conflict with the nurse's moral beliefs and values but in keeping with professional practice, the nurse provides safe, compassionate, competent, and ethical care until alternative care arrangements are in place to meet the person's needs or desires (p. 23).

As you study these guidelines, you can see that there are some important principles to adopt in relation to boundaries and spiritual care. First, it is always the patient's best interest that should be foremost. In the case of sharing your own values and beliefs, the first question should be whose interests does this serve, yours or the patient's. Second, patients have a right to make decisions about their health care on the basis of spiritual and religious beliefs that we as nurses may not agree with. Our role is to inform them of the best evidence in relation to their decision. They have the right to choose. Third, as a nurse, you, too, have the right to abstain from health care situations that violate your religious or spiritual beliefs, provided you ensure that alternative arrangements can be made. The following quotation, taken from a consensus report on spiritual care in palliative care, is an excellent statement on boundaries in the context of nurse–patient relationships:

> *The health care professional–patient relationship is often a one-way relationship that lacks equality and reciprocity. Boundaries allow for compassionate presence in the healing encounter. Health care professionals are more vulnerable to crossing these boundaries when they are overworked, stressed, or have experienced chronic losses or grief. Thus, it is critical that institutions and individual professionals make opportunities for appropriate self-care and reflection to avoid these risks.*
>
> ***(Puchalski et al., 2009, p. 901)***

The situations described above are just a few illustrations of how important it is to ensure that, as a nurse, you are competent to engage in spiritual care. Competencies for spiritual care include establishing therapeutic relationships, understanding the meanings of diverse spiritualities and their implications for care, and knowing when to refer to spiritual care providers (see Safety Alert). Although many nursing studies have suggested nurses feel ill-prepared to provide spiritual care, these studies often suggest that spiritual care is a discrete domain of care rather than an aspect of care that is embedded within the caring relationship in nursing. Thus, nurses are already well prepared to engage in the types of authentic and trusting relationships that provide a good context for spiritual care.

However, what nurses are often less confident about is providing care across diverse religious and spiritual traditions. This is a valid concern in light of the risk for harm if nurses fail to take into account these beliefs. For example, taking off the sacred garb of a baptized Sikh has important religious implications. Although doing so is often unavoidable in health care, it requires sensitivity to the implications and assistance, if necessary, with reconnecting them with their religious community for restoration of their baptized state. This is just one of many examples of religious implications for care. Unfortunately, many of these situations have been downplayed in nursing because of the desire to recognize spirituality apart from religion and to not stereotype individuals within religious traditions. These are certainly valid concerns. However, it is possible both to recognize the validity of spirituality and religion and to understand the possible implications of religious traditions without stereotyping.

Safety Alert One of the most important competencies for nurses is knowing when to refer to a spiritual care provider (the term *spiritual care provider* refers here to both health care chaplains and spiritual leaders from the community who provide spiritual oversight to a group). Although nurses can provide a caring context for patients' spirituality, this should not in any way be misconstrued to suggest that nurses have expertise in spiritual care (unless they have additional education in this field). Part of excellent care is understanding when patients require expert assistance, either from a spiritual leader from their tradition or from a social worker if they do not adhere to a religious tradition (Pesut et al., 2009).

Fowler (2002), a nurse, theologian, and health care chaplain, has suggested that spiritual care has layers, somewhat like an onion. At the outermost layers are public and semipublic information that most individuals willingly share. However, as the layers get peeled away, you encounter more intimate layers when individuals struggle with troubling feelings, guilt, and concerns and encounter challenges that should be dealt with only by a trusted religious leader. Nurses are competent to deal with the more public layers and should be concerned about things such as the influence of their own tradition on health, healing, decision making, and beliefs about illness, suffering, and end of life. However, for a nurse to go beyond those layers to the deeper spiritual struggles is risky both for the nurse and for the patient. Fowler likens it to a nonswimmer jumping in to save a drowning person. Nurses are not educated to address health-related spiritual beliefs. If those beliefs are unhealthy (e.g., when individuals feel that God is punishing them), the nurse may not have the expertise to provide a reframing of those beliefs toward a healthy outcome. Therefore, it is critical that nurses know who their referral persons are and be quick to refer to them if they sense that the spiritual struggles are beyond their expertise.

Fowler, M. (2002). *Spiritual care in nursing.* Course lectures in graduate course, Azusa Pacific University, Azusa, CA; Pesut, B., Fowler, M., Reimer-Kirkham, S., Johnston Taylor, E., & Sawatzky, R. (2009). Particularizing spirituality in points of tension: Enriching the discourse. *Nursing Inquiry, 16*(4), 1–10.

Table 28-1 provides *possible* care considerations for some of the most common religious traditions. Naturally, it is important to remember that this is just a starting point. This allows nurses to enter the caregiving situation with some background knowledge, but is it essential to clarify with each individual the practices he or she adheres to within his or her tradition. There is great variability even among common religions, and individuals will pick and choose the practices they adhere to within that religion. You need not be afraid to ask. Many religious individuals will gladly talk about their faith and practices if you are open. Take the time to be present and to be curious. Think of yourself as an explorer among the mystery of sacred stories and commitments that characterizes persons' lives (Pesut, 2016).

PROVIDING SPIRITUAL CARE

Spiritual care is often overlooked in the provision of care (Epstein-Peterson, Sullivan, Enzinger, et al., 2015). Some barriers to nurses offering spiritual care are time constraints, lack of privacy, inadequate training, and role confusion (Balboni, Sullivan, Enzinger, et al., 2014; Hood, Olson, & Allen, 2007). A recent review of studies exploring spirituality in nursing education indicated that spiritual awareness is an important quality for student nurses to have, and that education can enhance feelings of preparedness for spiritual care (Lewinson, McSherry, & Kevern, 2015).

Spiritual nursing care, at its foundation, is an expression of self (Sawatzky & Pesut, 2005). To engage in spiritual care, nurses must first

TABLE 28-1 Religious Beliefs About Health

Religious or Cultural Background	Possible Health Care Beliefs and Practices	Nursing Implications
Hinduism	Modern medical science is accepted. Illness is caused by past sins. Holy days are celebrated with fasting, prayer, and feasting.	Privacy is needed for prayer and meditation. Modesty in clothing is important, and hospital gowns may be considered indecent; same-sex caregivers are preferred. Important sacraments are associated with birth, naming, puberty, and death. Religious symbols should not be removed.
Sikhism	Modern medical science is accepted. Baptized and nonbaptized Sikhs have different religious requirements.	Prayers are said twice a day; privacy is preferred. Modesty in clothing is important, and hospital gowns may be considered indecent; same-sex caregivers are preferred. Religious symbols include uncut hair, comb, steel bracelet, symbolic dagger, undershorts, and turban; these should not be removed. Cleanliness during eating and prayers is important.
Buddhism	Modern medical science is accepted. Understanding, rather than belief, is emphasized. Dharma, the law of nature, teaches that life is impermanent and all people have to age and die. Death is usually accepted as the last stage of life, and withdrawal of life support may be permitted. Buddhists may believe in rebirth after death.	Treatment may be refused on holy days. Prayers may occur five times daily. Privacy is needed for meditation. The patient may want a Buddhist monk in attendance for spiritual support.
Islam	Muslims must be able to practise the Five Pillars of Islam. Muslims may have a fatalistic view of health. Faith healing is used. Withdrawal of life support may be permitted. Autopsies are generally forbidden.	Prayers are said five times per day, facing toward Mecca. Privacy is important. Fasting may occur on holy days. Modesty in clothing is important, and hospital gowns are considered indecent; same-sex caregivers are required.
Judaism	Jews believe in the sanctity of life. God and medicine must have a balance. Observance of the Sabbath is important.	Prayers are said three times per day; men may wear prayer shawl and skull cap. Treatment may be refused on the Sabbath.
Christianity	Modern medical science is accepted. Many Christians follow complementary alternative medicine (see Chapter 35). Prayer and faith healing are used; some Christians use laying on of hands.	Times of prayer vary between individuals; privacy is preferred. Sacraments of Holy Communion and the Anointing of the Sick may be practised. Religious symbols may include cross and prayer beads.
Hutterian	Modern science is accepted. About 80% of Hutterians seek alternative therapies. All things are shared communally. Hutterians live on colonies to help avoid earthly distractions that impede spiritual practice and devotion. Praying for good health is not appropriate; rather, prayers may be for wisdom to live a healthy life or bear suffering without complaint. Created order is God over man, man above woman, elder adult above younger adult, and parent over child.	Education about health is appreciated. Straightforward discussions are preferred. Health providers are respected. Families expect to be involved in health care discussions. Decision-making processes about what health concerns are important for the colony are made by the leaders. Individual decisions regarding medical treatment may be made in consultation with other members of the colony.
Ojibway (Anishinabe)	Central value is that everything belongs to everyone in extended family. Health is a spiritual experience. Disease and illness may be caused by soul loss or spiritual intrusion.	Families generally want to be involved in health care decisions and may wish to stay with the ill individual. They desire to get to know the nurse before sharing problems. They may use Western medicine blended with traditional healing practices.

be comfortable with hearing about patients' spirituality. **Spiritual care** is an altruistic, interpersonal, intuitive, and integrative process by which the nurse seeks to understand and reflect the patient's spiritual values, beliefs, and experiences (Figure 28-2; Sawatzky & Pesut, 2005): altruistic in that it requires that the nurse put the patient's need first; relational in that patients feel their spirituality is supported through an interpersonal relationship of care; intuitive in that the mysterious nature of spirituality cannot always be understood through rational thought; and integrative in that spirituality should not be considered separate from the other aspects of care. The relief of suffering through

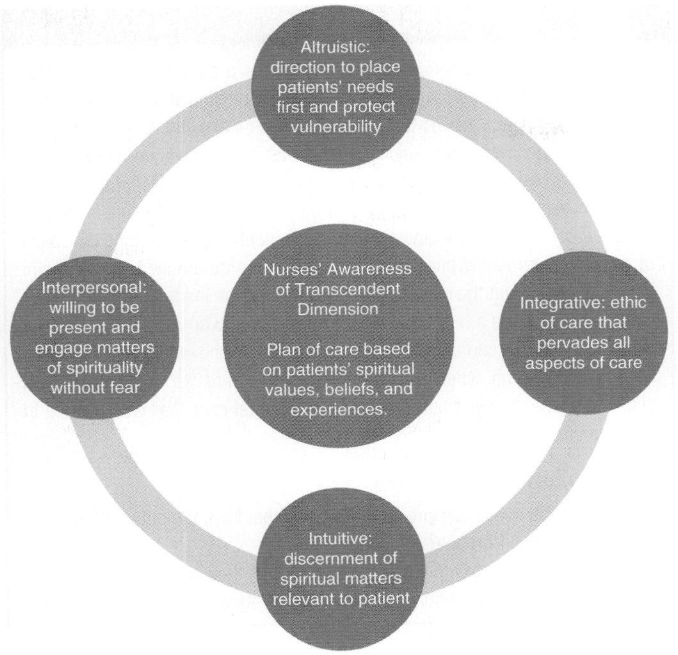

FIGURE 28-2 Attributes of spiritual care in nursing practice. (Adapted from Sawatzky, R., & Pesut, B. [2005]. Attributes of spiritual care in nursing practice. *Journal of Holistic Nursing, 23,* 19–33. Copyright © 2005. Reprinted by permission of SAGE Publications.)

BOX 28-7 The Five Cs of Relational Practice in Spiritual Care

Doane and Varcoe (2015) suggest that every nurse needs a relational inquiry tool kit. Part of this toolkit are nurses' obligations and capacities. They have framed these obligations and capacities in terms of five Cs: compassion, curiosity, commitment, competence, and corresponding. Here are some questions to ask yourself about these five Cs as you think about your own obligations to spiritual care:

Compassion: Am I willing to share in the suffering of others and to work to alleviate that suffering? Do I have compassion for myself as I do that work?

Curiosity: Am I curious about the spirituality and religiousness of others? Do I take the time to ask about it and explore what is meaningful to them? Am I okay with hearing "truths" that are different than mine?

Commitment: Have I thought about what my most cherished values are? Do I consistently make choices that align with those values? Are my values open to new interpretations as I gain more wisdom in life?

Competence: Am I competent to provide spiritual and religious care? Do I invest time and energy in developing that competence? Do I know when I need to refer to another member of the interdisciplinary team?

Corresponding: Do I provide spiritual care in a way that is patient-centred? In other words, do I work to understand and base my practice on what is meaningful to them?

Doane, G., & Varcoe, C. (2015). *How to nurse: relational inquiry with individuals and families in changing health and health care contexts.* Baltimore, MD: Lippincott Williams & Wilkins.

excellent pain management contributes to spiritual well-being because persons are holistic.

Nurses often have questions about how to "do" spiritual care. Sinclair and colleagues explored how expert clinicians provide spiritual care at the end of life. They conducted interviews and participant observation at five Canadian sites. They discovered that spiritual care is more about the qualities that health care providers bring to the clinical setting than it is about specific skills or knowledge. They identified five core themes that typified these qualities: listening intuitively, seeing soulfully, speech through taming the tongue, touch that embodied spiritual care, and presence that was characterized by vulnerability and reciprocity. Findings from this study suggest that the essence of spiritual care is knowing how to be in a way that supports spiritual well-being in patients (Sinclair et al., 2014). This way of being is typical of all high-quality relational practice.

Relational practice is a process of respectful, compassionate, and authentic inquiry into the experience of another (Doane & Varcoe, 2015). Many of the relational capacities taught throughout nursing curricula offer support to nurses as they provide nursing care that includes the patient's spirituality (see Box 28-7 for the five Cs of relational practice). The relational skills that undergird all of nursing practice are the same skills that create the foundation of spiritual care. Recognizing this may help offset feelings of inadequacy that arise when nurses think about providing spiritual care (Pesut, 2008). According to Sawatzky and Pesut (2005), "Spiritual expressions such as love, hope and compassion constitute the most basic and universal approach to spiritual care and can be integrated into all aspects of nursing care" (p. 23).

Facilitating Spiritual Practices

Physical health is affected by beliefs, expectations, and thoughts. Although the mechanisms are not yet fully understood, body, mind, and spirit are interconnected; when one facet of a person faces a challenge or receives support, the others are affected. This idea is commonly referred to as **holism**. Recent research on wound healing and stress found that both psychological and physiological stress delay wound healing and increase the potential for wound infection (Gouin & Keicolt-Glaser, 2011). Research such as this suggests that spiritual and religious practices may do more than just provide a comforting effect. Prayer, meditation, contemplation, sacraments, rituals, and other practices that support spiritual and religious expression may indeed reduce stress and support health and healing. Thoughts and beliefs mediate chemical responses in the body that support or inhibit health and healing (Lidstone & Stoessl, 2007). Try the exercise in Box 28-8 to get a sense of the mind–body connection.

BOX 28-8 Mind–Body Connection: Try It for Yourself

Settle back and gently close your eyes. Imagine a plump, juicy, yellow lemon. Holding the image of the luscious lemon in your mind, imagine picking up the lemon and smelling it. Imagine cutting the lemon in half, with the juices squirting out. In your mind's eye, bring half of the cut lemon to your lips and squeeze the juice into your mouth.

What happened? Did you salivate? Some people even experience a puckering of their mouths.

This is an example of the mind–body connection that demonstrates the effect of a thought on the body. Spiritual practices, which support feelings of transcendence, connection, well-being, and calm, support healing.

Rituals that bring meaning to life are spiritual practices. Many spiritual practices are integrated throughout a person's daily activities and do not necessarily take place in a church or formal setting. What is considered spiritual practice varies greatly from person to person, even for people of the same spiritual or religious tradition. These may be as varied as practices or sacraments associated with a person's religion, such as prayer, daily readings, or communion, and informal

BOX 28-9 Examples of Spiritual Practices

Meditation	Active listening, guidance
Contemplation	Journalling
Prayer	Service
Gratitude	Exercise
Presence	Listening to music
Mantra	Worship
Yoga	Affirmations
Tai chi	Solitude
Qi gong	Study
Reflection	Fasting
Ritual participation	Simplicity
Sacred readings	Confession
Incense use	

The spiritual practice of prayer is a part of most faith traditions. The processes and practices of the prayer may vary, but the common thread is communion with a higher power. This communion occurs through reciting memorized prayer, chanting, singing, dancing, meditation, supplication, stream-of-consciousness, or silence. Sharma, Reimer-Kirkham, and Cochrane (2013) drew on research to explore the ways that prayer is enacted in health care contexts. They suggest that prayer can be used to support or challenge dominant religious and health care views. How prayer is enacted or ignored can reveal where power differences are. Prayer can also provide an important way to bridge religious differences. This is important for nurses to think about, as patients commonly ask nurses to pray with or for them.

Sharma, S., Reimer-Kirkham, S., & Cochrane, M. (2013). Prayer as transgressions: stories from healthcare. In. G. Giordan, & L. Woodhead (Eds.), *Prayer in Religion and Spirituality* (pp. 189–204). Boston, MA: Brill Press.

BOX 28-10 CASE STUDY

The meaning held in a simple act of respect for a patient's important religious symbol was taught to me by two first-year nursing students. On a busy morning in residential care, Maria,* an elderly female resident, was distracted and anxious because the religious medals that she always wore next to her heart were missing. The two students found out from the staff that the medals had been missing for several days, and they were advised to simply get the patient dressed and to the dining room. The students, understanding the sense of peace these medals brought to Maria, became determined to find them. They did indeed find the medals. As they returned the medals to their special place next to Maria's heart, her affect turned from worry to joy. Maria was transformed by the caring actions of the students. In the weeks that followed, Maria's face lit up when these students came into her room. With this simple act, the students had provided the spiritual care that was needed in the moment.

Thinking Points

- What simple things can you do for patients that have the potential to make a meaningful difference?
- When was the last time someone went out of their way to help you with something that was important to you? What effect did that have on you?

*Pseudonym.

practices, such as enjoying a sense of connectedness with others or enjoying the beauty of nature (Box 28-9 provides examples of spiritual practices). Demystifying spiritual practice and recognizing those places in everyday life where spiritual practices are present, but not identified as such, creates awareness of them.

Food and nutrition are important aspects of patient care and often are an important component of some religious observances. Food and the rituals surrounding the preparation and serving of food can be important to a person's spirituality. Nurses can consult with a dietitian to integrate the patient's dietary preferences into daily care. In the event that an agency cannot prepare food in the preferred way, the family may be asked to bring meals that accommodate dietary restrictions. Personal care of the patient should be planned to allow time for spiritual readings, visits by spiritual advisors, or attendance at religious services.

Some churches and synagogues offer audio recordings of their services for those members who cannot attend in person. Family members can plan a prayer session or an organized reading of spiritual material on a regular basis. Arrangements may need to be made with spiritual care staff for the patient and family to receive the sacraments. Clergy will routinely offer to make home visits for people unable to attend religious services. Recorded meditations, classical or spiritual music, and televised spiritual services are other options. Nurses should be respectful of icons, medals, prayer rugs, or crosses that patients bring to a health setting and ensure that they are not accidentally lost, damaged, or misplaced (Box 28-10).

REFLECTING ON NURSES' SPIRITUAL CARE

Personal growth along the journey of spirituality is a lifelong pursuit and one that is not easily evaluated by others. Particularly during times of illness and suffering, patients need to clarify values, reshape philosophies, strengthen relationships, and live experiences that help to shape their purpose in life. It is not normally within the nursing role to "evaluate" whether patients achieve connectedness, meaning, peace, hope, or other indicators of spirituality. Meaning-making during suffering is often a mysterious, highly personal experience. As nurses, we can always be present for patients in their suffering and we can do everything within our power to alleviate distress. We should aggressively treat pain and other symptoms. We should provide a hospitable climate for those who are most important in patients' lives. We should put great effort into ensuring that patients can continue with their religious and spiritual practices. We should know the values and beliefs that are important to take into account as part of the overall picture of care. These are all spiritual "interventions." But we need to be cautious about entering into the areas of mystery, particularly if we are sensing our own need to explain or control patients' suffering.

In this aspect of nursing care, it is appropriate to reflect on your own contributions to a healing relationship. Were patients' spiritual practices respected? Was the relationship characterized by caring and support? Does the patient express trust and confidence in you? Is the patient able to discuss important issues or topics? Is the patient comfortable expressing spiritual needs to you? That sense of rapport that develops within a nurse–patient relationship is often the best indicator that you have helped to provide a safe context within which patients can live their spiritual journey.

KEY CONCEPTS

- Spirituality is highly personal and unique to each individual.
- Nurses must be aware of their own spirituality in order to recognize the spirituality of others.
- Canadian nursing practice has a rich spiritual heritage that has influenced contemporary practice.
- Spirituality may have beneficial health outcomes.
- Nursing theories can guide nurses in providing spiritual care.

- Faith is a relationship with God or a higher power or authority that enables action and gives purpose and meaning to an individual's life.
- Religion is a system of organized beliefs and worship that a person practises to express spirituality outwardly.
- Spirituality is a lifelong journey that may reflect the age and life experiences of the patient, as well as his or her current context.
- When patients experience acute or chronic illness or a terminal disease, spiritual resources either help a person recover or spiritual concerns develop.
- Spiritual practices are varied and may include private worship, prayer, meditation, sacraments, singing, use of rosary or prayer beads, and reading religious texts.
- Critical thinking in spiritual care includes an understanding of the unique perspective of the patient.
- A spiritual assessment is most successful when nurses attempt to understand rather than assess patients' spirituality, allowing the development of the relationship.
- Spiritual assessment tools should be flexible, and the depth of the assessment must be sensitive to the circumstances.
- The personal nature of spirituality requires open communication and the establishment of trust between nurse and patient.
- Ethical care includes respecting appropriate nurse–patient boundaries and knowing when patients should be referred to a spiritual care provider or social worker.
- Certain religions may have dietary restrictions or beliefs and practices of health care that may have implications for nursing practice.
- Spiritual care is an expression of self; how nurses learn to be with patients and the qualities that nurses bring are important to nursing care.
- Spiritual practices may be an effective coping resource for physical and psychological symptoms.
- Spiritual care cannot be evaluated like other aspects of nursing practice. Rather, nurses should focus on being present for patients while seeking to alleviate suffering.

CRITICAL THINKING EXERCISES

1. Mr. Gadacz is a 40-year-old businessman with more than 100 employees. A 12-hour workday is not unusual for him. He is married, has four teenage children, and is solely responsible for providing financially for the family. Last evening, he was admitted to the cardiac care unit with severe chest pain resulting from a myocardial infarction (heart attack). He is now stabilized but frequently asks about his diagnostic tests and what he needs to do to be able to go home. He tells his nurse, "My doctor tells me I will need surgery once I am more stable. I hope he can do that soon. I just can't believe this is happening. I worry about what will happen to my business while I am gone and to my family if I can't keep my business going." He asks you, "Could I die from this?" You notice that Mr. Gadacz has devotional literature at his bedside. How might you go about conducting a spiritual health assessment for Mr. Gadacz?
2. Tejal is a new graduate nurse caring for Ms. Rosenbaum for the first time. Ms. Rosenbaum is 27 years old and has recently received a diagnosis of uterine cancer. She is scheduled for an abdominal hysterectomy. Tejal notices from the patient chart that Ms. Rosenbaum has identified herself as Jewish. What factors might be important to consider in relation to Ms. Rosenbaum's spirituality or religion for the plan of care? How might Tejal determine which factors are relevant for Ms. Rosenbaum?
3. Critical thinking is an ongoing process. When you learn that you are assigned to care for Fangzhou Lin, you note that the Kardex information includes his religion (Buddhist) and his place of birth (Hong Kong). A colleague tells you he can speak some English. The patient is 80 years old and reportedly has a hearing deficit. What knowledge might you wish to reflect on critically before beginning a spiritual assessment of this patient?

REVIEW QUESTIONS

1. Which of the following answers *best* demonstrates caring for a patient's spiritual needs?
   1. Having the same beliefs as the patient
   2. Praying for the patient
   3. Accepting the patient's beliefs and experiences
   4. Calling for a religious leader if the nurse determines a need
2. Which of the following answers *best* describes a patient who does not believe in the existence of God?
   1. Agnostic
   2. Atheist
   3. Anarchist
   4. Agenie
3. Which statements are *true* when considering the spiritual practices of the patient? *(Select all that apply.)*
   1. They have no place in the health care setting.
   2. They provide structure and support for the patient.
   3. They can be a barrier to providing nursing care.
   4. There are many different types.
   5. They are dependent on religious beliefs.
4. Which of the following statements *best* describes establishing presence with a patient?
   1. Offering a closeness—physically, psychologically, and spiritually
   2. Offering touch
   3. The nurse sharing his or her own spiritual beliefs
   4. Performing procedures
5. Which of the following are important to consider when providing care to a patient from the Hindu tradition? *(Select all that apply.)*
   1. Modern medical practice is not accepted.
   2. Followers may be adhering to fast days.
   3. Same-sex caregivers are preferred.
   4. Removing religious symbols is permitted.
   5. Prayer is public and shared.
6. Which of the following *best* describes spirituality?
   1. A structured search for God
   2. A different word to describe religion
   3. An appropriate term to describe atheists
   4. Commonly identified as meaning, purpose, and connectedness
7. Based on research findings, which of the following interventions by the nurse are appreciated by the patient? *(Select all that apply.)*
   1. Intimate interventions like meditation and journalling
   2. Support of the patient's spiritual practices
   3. Sharing of the nurse's personal beliefs and practices
   4. An attitude of open curiosity regarding the patient's spiritual beliefs and spiritual concerns
   5. Sharing of the nurse's religious beliefs
8. Which of the following may be *most* beneficial to a patient who is experiencing a terminal illness or has suffered a recent disability because of a disease or injury?
   1. Grief work
   2. Diet therapy
   3. Acupuncture
   4. Values clarification

9. Which of the following *best* describes spiritual assessment?
   1. It is structured and follows a specific process.
   2. It can only be done by a spiritual care provider.
   3. It should be flexible, and the depth of the assessment is dependent on the circumstances.
   4. It is the first component of the nursing assessment.
10. Which of the following *best* describe relational practice? *(Select all that apply.)*
    1. Creates the environment for spiritual care
    2. Allows the nurse to create clear boundaries
    3. Is unlikely if the patient and nurse hold different spiritual beliefs
    4. Is not a component of spiritual care
    5. Is respectful, compassionate, and authentic inquiry into the experience of another

Answers: 1. 3; **2.** 2; **3.** 2, 4; **4.** 1; **5.** 2, 3; **6.** 4; **7.** 2, 3, 4; **8.** 4; **9.** 3; **10.** 1, 5

Rationales for the Review Questions appear at the end of the book.

RECOMMENDED WEBSITES

Canadian Association for Parish Nursing Ministry: http://www.capnm.ca.
The Canadian Association for Parish Nursing Ministry is committed to the development of parish nursing as a health and ministry resource within Canada.

Center for Spirituality and Healing: https://www.csh.umn.edu.
Established in 1995 at the University of Minnesota in the United States, the Center for Spirituality and Healing provides education about integrative medicine, combining biomedical, complementary, cross-cultural, and spiritual care.

Center for Spirituality, Theology and Health: https://spiritualityandhealth.duke.edu/.
The purpose of this centre, which is part of Duke University in the United States, is to conduct research on the effects of spirituality on physical and mental health.

Dignity in Care: http://www.dignityincare.ca/en/.
The website provides a wealth of resources on dignity therapy.

Global Network for Spirituality and Health: http://smhs.gwu.edu/gwish/global-network.
This network provides a way for members to work together internationally toward high-quality comprehensive and compassionate spiritual care.

Institute for the Bio-Cultural Study of Religion: http://www.ibcsr.org/index.php/irr-basicinfo/ibcsr-research-review.
This organization produces a regular annotated bibliography of the recent research in the field.

Living with Hope: http://www.nurs.ualberta.ca/livingwithhope/.
This website is an excellent resource for supporting patients to live with hope.

Nurses Christian Fellowship: http://www.ncf-jcn.org.
Nurses Christian Fellowship, a US institution, is a Christian organization with the goal of integrating Christianity into nursing care. This website contains information about the scope and trend of research related to spiritual care. The Canadian chapter of Nurses Christian Fellowship can be found at http://www.ncfcanada.ca/.

Spirituality in Health-Care Network: http://www.spiritualityinhealthcare.net/links.html.
This site provides links to a number of other resources.

REFERENCES

Andrews, M. M., & Boyle, J. S. (2007). *Transcultural concepts in nursing care* (5th ed.). Philadelphia, PA: Lippincott.

Balboni, M. J., Sullivan, A., Enzinger, A. C., et al. (2014). Nurse and physician barriers to spiritual care provision at the end of life. *Journal of Pain and Symptom Management, 48*(3), 400–410. doi:10.1016/j.painsymman.2013.09.020.

Bruce, A., Shields, L., & Molzahn, A. (2011). Language and the (im)possibilities of articulating spirituality. *Journal of Holistic Nursing, 29*(1), 44–52. doi:10.1177/0898010110381116.

Calabria, M. D., & Macrae, J. A. (Eds.), (1994). *Suggestions for thought by Florence Nightingale*. Philadelphia, PA: University of Pennsylvania Press.

Canadian Nurses Association (CNA) (2010). *Position statement: Spirituality, health and nursing practice*. Ottawa: Author. Retrieved from https://www.cna-aiic.ca/~/media/cna/page-content/pdf-en/ps111_spirituality_2010_e.pdf?la=en.

Canadian Nurses Association (CNA) (2017). *Code of ethics for registered nurses*. Ottawa: Author. Retrieved from https://cna-aiic.ca/en/on-the-issues/best-nursing/nursing-ethics.

Canby, N. K., Cameron, I. M., Calhoun, A. T., et al. (2015). A brief mindfulness intervention for health college students and its effects on psychological distress, self-control, meta-mood and subjective vitality. *Mindfulness, 6*(5), 1071–1081. doi:10.1007/s12671-014-0356-5.

Cilliers, F., & Terblanche, L. (2014). The role of spirituality in coping with the demands of the hospital culture amongst fourth-year nursing students. *International Review of Psychiatry, 26*(3), 279–288. doi:10.3109/09540261.2014.890922.

Cockell, N., & McSherry, W. (2012). Spiritual care in nursing: An overview of published international research. *Journal of Nursing Management, 20*(8), 958–969. doi:10.1111/j.1365-2834.2012.01450x.

Coventry, P. A., Small, N., Panagioti, M., et al. (2015). Living with complexity; marshalling resources: A systematic review and qualitative meta-synthesis of lived experience of mental and physical multimorbidity. *BMC Family Practice, 16*(171), 1–12. doi:10.1186/s12875-015-0345-3.

de Bruin, E. I., Meppelink, R., & Bögels, S. M. (2015). Mindfulness in higher education: Awareness and attention in university students increase during and after participation in a mindfulness curriculum course. *Mindfulness, 6*, 1137–1142. doi:10.1007/s12671-014-0364-5.

Doane, G., & Varcoe, C. (2015). *How to nurse: Relational inquiry with individuals and families in changing health and health care contexts*. Baltimore, MD: Lippincott Williams & Wilkins.

Dobratz, M. C. (2016). Building a middle-range theory of adaptive spirituality. *Nursing Science Quarterly, 29*(2), 146–153. doi:10.1177/0894318416630090.

Edwards, A., Pang, N., Shiu, V., et al. (2010). The understanding of spirituality and the potential role of spiritual care in end-of-life and palliative care: A meta-study of qualitative research. *Palliative Medicine, 24*(8), 753–770. doi:10.1177/0269216310375860.

Epstein-Peterson, Z. D., Sullivan, A. J., Enzinger, A. C., et al. (2015). Examining forms of spiritual care provided in the advanced cancer setting. *The American Journal of Hospice & Palliative Care, 32*(7), 750–757. doi:10.1177/1049909114540318.

Fowler, M. (2002). *Spiritual care in nursing*. Course lectures in graduate course, Azusa Pacific University, Azusa, CA.

Giske, T., & Cone, P. H. (2015). Discerning the healing path—how nurses assist patient spirituality in diverse health care settings. *Journal of Clinical Nursing, 24*(19–20), 2926–2935. doi:10.1111/jocn.12907.

Goncalves, J. P. B., Lucchetti, G., Menezes, P. R., et al. (2015). Religious and spiritual interventions in mental health care: A systematic review and meta-analysis of randomized controlled trials. *Psychological Medicine, 45*, 2937–2949. doi:10.1017/S0033291715001166.

Goodman, M. J., & Schorling, J. B. (2012). A mindfulness course decreases burnout and improves well-being among healthcare providers. *International Journal of Psychiatry in Medicine, 43*(2), 119–128.

Gouin, J., & Keicolt-Glaser, J. (2011). The impact of psychological stress on wound healing: Methods and mechanisms. *Immunology and Allergy Clinics of North America, 31*(1), 81–93. doi:10.1016/j.iac.2010.09.010.

Grypma, S. (2008). *Healing Henan: Canadian nurses at the North China Mission, 1888–1947*. Vancouver: University of British Columbia Press.

Hilbers, J., Haynes, A. S., & Kivikko, J. G. (2010). Spirituality and health: An exploratory study of hospital patients' perspectives. *Australian Health Review, 34*(1), 3–10.

Hood, L. E., Olson, J. K., & Allen, M. (2007). Learning to care for spiritual needs: Connecting spiritually. *Qualitative Health Research, 17*(9), 1198–1206. doi:10.1177/1049732307306921.

Horner, J. K., Piercy, B. S., Eure, L., et al. (2014). A pilot study to evaluate mindfulness as a strategy to improve inpatient nurse and patient experiences. *Applied Nursing Research, 27*(3), 198–201.

Johnston Taylor, E. (2007). Client perspectives about nurse requisites for spiritual caregiving. *Applied Nursing Research, 20*(1), 44–46. doi:10.1016/j.apnr.2006.06.005.

Kabat-Zinn, J. (2013). *Full catastrophe living: Using the wisdom of your body and mind to face stress, pain, and illness*. New York: Bantam Books.

Labun, E., & Emblen, J. (2007). Spirituality and health in Punjabi Sikh. *Journal of Holistic Nursing, 25*(3), 141–148. doi:10.1177/0898010106293592.

Lewinson, L. P., McSherry, W., & Kevern, P. (2015). Spirituality in pre-registration nurse education and practice: A review of the literature. *Nurse Education Today, 35*, 806–814. doi:10.1016/j.nedt.2015.01.011.

Lidstone, S. C., & Stoessl, A. J. (2007). Understanding the placebo effect: Contributions from neuroimaging. *Molecular Imaging and Biology*, *9*(4), 176–185. doi:10.1007/s11307-007-0086-3.

Martsolf, D. S., & Mickley, J. R. (1998). The concept of spirituality in nursing theories: Differing worldviews and extent of focus. *Journal of Advanced Nursing*, *27*(2), 294–303.

McSherry, W. (2001). Spiritual crisis? Call a nurse. In H. Orchard (Ed.), *Spirituality in health care contexts* (pp. 107–117). London: Jessica Kingsley Publishers.

Meehan, T. C. (2003). Careful nursing: A model for contemporary nursing practice. *Journal of Advanced Nursing*, *44*(1), 99–107.

Meehan, T. C. (2012a). The careful nursing philosophy and professional practice model (2012). *Journal of Clinical Nursing*, *21*(19–20), 2905–2916.

Meehan, T. C. (2012b). Spirituality and spiritual care from a careful nursing perspective. *Journal of Nursing Management*, *20*(8), 990–1001. doi:10.1111/j.1365-2834.2012.01462.x.

Meleis, A. I. (1997). *Theoretical thinking and practical wisdom: Challenges for the future* (3rd ed.). Philadelphia, PA: Lippincott.

Miller, L. W. (2004). *Faith and health: A framework for Christian nurses*. Victoria, BC: Trafford Publishing.

Mok, E., Wong, F., & Wong, D. (2010). The meaning of spirituality and spiritual care among the Hong Kong Chinese terminally ill. *Journal of Advanced Nursing*, *66*(2), 360–370. doi:10.1111/j.1365-2648.2009.05193.x.

Olson, J., Simington, J. A., & Clark, M. B. (1998). Educating parish nurses. *The Canadian Nurse*, *94*(8), 40–44.

Paley, J. (2008). Spirituality in nursing: A reductionist approach. *Nursing Philosophy*, *9*(1), 3–18. doi:10.1111/j.1466-769X.2007.00330.x.

Parse, R. R. (2014). *The humanbecoming paradigm: A transformational worldview*. Pittsburgh, PA: Discovery International Publications.

Paul, P. (2000). The history of the relationship between nursing and faith traditions. In M. B. Clark & J. K. Olson (Eds.), *Nursing within a faith community: Promoting health in times of transition* (pp. 147–159). Thousand Oaks, CA: Sage Publication.

Perry, D. J. (2004). Self-transcendence: Lonergan's key to integration of nursing theory, research, and practice. *Nursing Philosophy*, *5*(1), 67–74. doi:10.1111/j.1466-769X.2004.00166.x.

Pesut, B. (2008). Spirituality and spiritual care in nursing fundamentals textbooks. *The Journal of Nursing Education*, *47*(4), 167–173.

Pesut, B. (2016). There be dragons: Effects of unexplored religion on nurses' competence in spiritual care. *Nursing Inquiry*, *23*(3), 191–199. doi:10.1111/nin.12135.

Pesut, B., Fowler, M., Reimer-Kirkham, S., et al. (2009). Particularizing spirituality in points of tension: Enriching the discourse. *Nursing Inquiry*, *16*(4), 1–10. doi:10.1111/j.1440-1800.2009.00462.x.

Pesut, B., & Reimer-Kirkham, S. (2010). Situated clinical encounters in the negotiation of religious and spiritual plurality: A critical ethnography. *International Journal of Nursing Studies*, *47*(7), 815–825. doi:10.1016/j.ijnurstu.2009.11.014.

Puchalski, C. M., Ferrell, B., Virani, R., et al. (2009). Improving the quality of spiritual care as a dimension of palliative care: The report of the consensus conference. *Journal of Palliative Medicine*, *12*(10), 885–904. doi:10.1089/jpm.2009.0142.

Puchalski, C., & Romer, A. L. (2000). Taking spiritual history allows clinicians to understand patients more fully. *Journal of Palliative Medicine*, *3*(1), 129–137. doi:10.1089/jpm.2000.3.129.

Ramezani, M., Ahmadi, F., Mohammadi, E., et al. (2014). Spiritual care in nursing: A concept analysis. *International Nursing Review*, *61*(2), 211–219. doi:10.1111/inr.12099.

Reimer-Kirkham, S. (2014). Nursing research on religion and spirituality through a social justice lens. *ANS. Advances in Nursing Science*, *37*(3), 249–257. doi:10.1097/ANS.0000000000000036.

Reimer-Kirkham, S., & Cochrane, M. (2016). Resistant, reluctant or responsible? The negotiation of religious and cultural plurality in Canadian healthcare. In S. Sharma & D. Llewellyn (Eds.), *Religion, equality, and inequalities* (pp. 65–76). Surrey, UK: Ashgate.

Reynolds, N., Mrug, S., Schwebel, D., et al. (2016). Spiritual coping, psychosocial adjustment, and physical health in youth with chronic illness: A meta-analytic review. *Health Psychology Review*, *10*(2), 226–243. doi:10.1080/17437199.2016.1159142.

Risjord, M. (2010). *Nursing knowledge: Science, practice and philosophy*. Oxford, UK: Wiley-Blackwell.

Ross, L., & Austin, J. (2015). Spiritual needs and spiritual support preferences of people with end-stage heart failure and their carers: Implications for nurse managers. *Journal of Nursing Management*, *23*(1), 87–95. doi:10.1111/jonm.12087.

Sawatzky, R., & Pesut, B. (2005). Attributes of spiritual care in nursing practice. *Journal of Holistic Nursing*, *23*(1), 19–33. doi:10.1177/0898010104272010.

Sharma, S., Reimer-Kirkham, S., & Cochrane, M. (2013). Prayer as transgressions: Stories from healthcare. In G. Giordan & L. Woodhead (Eds.), *Prayer in religion and spirituality* (pp. 189–204). Boston, MA: Brill Press.

Sinclair, S., & Chochinov, H. M. (2012a). Dignity: A novel path into the spiritual landscape of the human heart. In M. Cobb, C. M. Puchalski, & B. Rumbold (Eds.), *Oxford textbook of spirituality in healthcare* (pp. 145–150). Oxford, UK: Oxford University Press.

Sinclair, S., & Chochinov, H. M. (2012b). Dignity conserving care: Research evidence. In M. Cobb, C. M. Puchalski, & B. Rumbold (Eds.), *Oxford textbook of spirituality in healthcare* (pp. 285–292). Oxford, UK: Oxford University Press.

Sinclair, S., & Chochinov, H. M. (2012c). Communicating with patients about existential and spiritual issues: SACR-D work. *Progress in Palliative Care*, *20*(2), 72–78. doi:10.1179/1743291X12Y.0000000015.

Sinclair, S., McClement, S., Raffin-Bouchal, S., et al. (2016). Compassion in health care: An empirical model. *Journal of Pain and Symptom Management*, *51*(2), 193–203.

Sinclair, S., Raffin Bouchal, S., Chochinov, H., et al. (2014). Spiritual care: How to do it. *BMJ Supportive and Palliative Care*, *2*(4), 319–327. doi:10.1136/bmjspcare-2011-000191.

Smith, S. A. (2014). Mindfulness-based stress reduction: An intervention to enhance the effectiveness of nurses' coping with work-related stress. *International Journal of Nursing Knowledge*, *25*(2), 119–130.

Swinton, J., & Pattison, S. (2010). Moving beyond clarity: Towards a thin, vague, and useful understanding of spirituality in nursing care. *Nursing Philosophy*, *11*(4), 226–237. doi:10.1111/j.1466-769X.2010.00450.x.

Taylor, C. (2007). *A secular age*. Cambridge, MA: Harvard University Press.

Thorne, S. (2003). Theoretical issues in nursing. In J. Ross-Kerr & M. J. Wood (Eds.), *Canadian nursing: Issues and perspectives* (pp. 116–134). Toronto: Mosby.

Thorne, S. (2005). Conceptualizing in nursing: What's the point? Guest Editorial. *Journal of Advanced Nursing*, *51*, 107.

Van Leeuwen, R., Tiesinga, L. J., Jochemasen, H., et al. (2007). Aspects of spirituality concerning illness. *Scandinavian Journal of Caring Sciences*, *21*(4), 482–489. doi:10.1111/j.1471-6712.2007.00502.x.

Vespa, A., Jacobsen, P. B., Spazzafumo, L., et al. (2011). Evaluation of intrapsychic factors, coping styles, and spirituality of patients affected by tumors. *Psycho-Oncology*, *20*(1), 5–11. doi:10.1002/pon.1719.

Watson, J. (2011). *Human caring science. A theory of nursing* (2nd ed.). Boston: Jones and Bartlett.

Weathers, E., McCarthy, G., & Coffey, A. (2015). Concept analysis of spirituality: An evolutionary approach. *Nursing Forum*, *51*(2), 79–96. doi:10.1111/nuf.12128.

White, M. L. (2016). Spirituality self-care practices as a mediator between quality of life and depression. *Religions*, *7*(54), 1–10. doi:10.3390/rel7050054.

29

Stress and Adaptation

Canadian content written by Tanya Park, RN, PhD
Original chapter by Matthew R. Sorenson, PhD, APN, ANP-C

OBJECTIVES

Mastery of content in this chapter will enable you to:

- Define the key terms listed.
- Describe how stress is conceptualized.
- Define the key biological systems involved in stress responses.
- Describe how overwhelming stress or chronic stress can affect health.
- Differentiate acute stress disorder and post-traumatic stress disorder.
- Discuss the integration of stress theory with nursing theories.
- Formulate nursing diagnoses from assessment data.
- Describe stress management techniques beneficial for coping with stress.
- Discuss the process of crisis intervention.
- Develop a care plan for patients experiencing stress.
- Discuss how stress in the workplace can affect health care providers.

KEY TERMS

Acute stress disorder, p. 512
Adaptation, p. 508
Alarm reaction, p. 509
Appraisal, p. 509
Burnout, p. 521
Coping, p. 509
Crisis, p. 509
Crisis intervention, p. 521
Developmental crises, p. 509
Distress, p. 511
Endorphins, p. 511
Eustress, p. 511
Exhaustion stage, p. 509
Fight-or-flight response, p. 509
Flashbacks, p. 512
General adaptation syndrome, p. 509
Homeostasis, p. 509
Post-traumatic growth, p. 512
Post-traumatic stress disorder (PTSD), p. 512
Primary appraisal, p. 509
Resistance stage, p. 509
Secondary appraisal, p. 509
Situational crises, p. 509
Stress, p. 508
Stressor, p. 508
Trauma, p. 512

MEDIA RESOURCES

http://evolve.elsevier.com/Canada/Potter/fundamentals/

- Audio Chapter Summaries
- Examination Review Questions
- Concept Map Creator
- Case Study with Questions
- Audio Glossary
- Content Updates
- Video Clips

Stress: Everyone has experienced it, but the term **stress** is difficult to define and is often loosely used. It has been used to describe a stimulus, a process, a response, and a state, which leads to confusion and ambiguity (Le Moal, 2007). In this chapter, the term **stressor** is used to describe an event that activates stress response systems—that is, it acts as a stimulus. This activation of multiple biological systems and psychological schemas has a collective goal of maintaining a state of dynamic equilibrium. Stressors can arise in the external environment and range from motivational prompts, such as taking a school examination, to devastating personal events, such as a life-threatening illness, a motor vehicle crash, a sexual assault, or a natural disaster (e.g., an earthquake or a tornado). Internal stressors, such as hunger or infection, can also activate stress response systems. Behavioural responses to stressors presumably reflect the activation of numerous biological systems. Behavioural responses can change over time, inasmuch as previous stressful experiences and individual contextual factors can produce **adaptation** in stress response systems. Among animals, biological systems help alert the animal to some type of threat in the environment and prepare it to mount a defence. These systems also turn off when the threat is past. For humans, in addition to acute threats to body integrity, psychological well-being and sense of self-worth can be threatened. Physical and psychological health can be severely affected by serious or chronic stressors, and these effects can be long-standing and pervasive. It is important for health care providers to understand conceptual frameworks that have been developed to explain the relationship between stress (overwhelming or chronic) and health.

CONCEPTUALIZATIONS OF STRESS

Physiological Conceptualizations

Walter Cannon was one of the pioneers of the early twentieth century who laid the groundwork for regulatory physiology and concepts of adaptation. He demonstrated that the sympathetic–adrenal–medullary (SAM) system acted to maintain homeostasis of the internal environment. He first coined the term **fight-or-flight response**, in 1915, to describe an animal's response to threats through the activation of the SAM system (Figure 29-1; Le Moal, 2007). Hans Selye, another pioneer, focused on maladaptation and the pathology of stress. He demonstrated the existence of a biological stress syndrome, which he called the **general adaptation syndrome** (Selye, 1974; Figure 29-2). This three-stage syndrome occurs in response to serious stressors. The first stage is the **alarm reaction**, analogous to Cannon's fight-or-flight response to stress. In this stage, complex physiological changes help the organism mobilize energy and react to the stressor. The second stage of the general adaptation syndrome is the **resistance stage**. During resistance, the organism maintains arousal while the body works to defend against and adapt to the stressor and maintain homeostasis. Should the stressors continue for an extended period, organisms use up their finite ability to adapt, and they enter a third stage of the adaptation syndrome, called the **exhaustion stage**. This is a pathological state in which organisms start showing diverse health consequences, which may eventually result in death. Selye was also the first to emphasize the role of the pituitary–adrenal axis in the pathological processes of stress.

At this point, two systems for stress were proposed: (1) the SAM system for behavioural fight-or-flight responses to stress and immediate adaptation and (2) the pituitary–adrenal axis for maintaining homeostasis. The concept of the pituitary–adrenal axis was expanded to the hypothalamic–pituitary–adrenal (HPA) axis; this axis is thought to mediate a bidirectional brain–body communication during physiological and psychological stress and is activated to promote homeostasis and to adapt to threatening or stressful situations (Engelmann & Ludwig, 2004). Bruce McEwen (2007), elaborating on the concept of **homeostasis** (the return of systems to a stable set point), used the term *allostasis* to describe how serious stressors can change physiological set points through adaptation. In this way, organisms are readied to respond and adapt to future stressors, but maintaining this state of readiness has an energy cost. This cost is termed *allostatic load*, which refers to the physiological burden of repeated stressors and enduring a heightened stress response system. When this load becomes too great, stress responses change from adaptation to health problems and stress-related disorders.

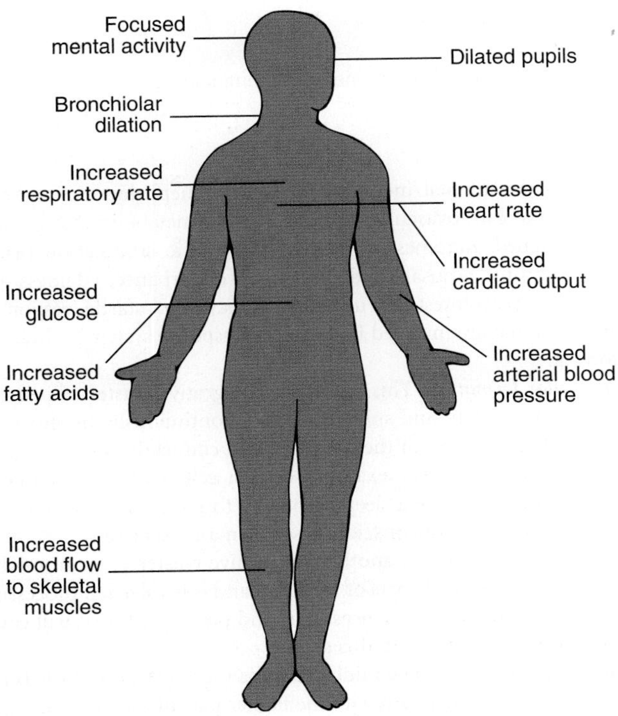

FIGURE 29-1 Fight-or-flight response.

Psychological Conceptualizations

In addition to physiological models of stress and stress responses, cognitive approaches to stress were also studied. The general adaptation syndrome and fight-or-flight responses to stress did not explicitly take into account perceptions and appraisals of stress in humans. Researchers began to look at the relationship between the person and the environment. The roles of perception and appraisal in stress responses are integral in the framework of stress proposed by Richard Lazarus. Lazarus (1999) maintained that a person is under stress only if the person evaluates the event or circumstance as personally significant. **Appraisal** of an event or circumstance is an ongoing perceptual process (Aguilera, 1998). Evaluating an event for its personal meaning is called **primary appraisal**. If as a result of primary appraisal the person identifies the event or circumstance as a harm, loss, threat, or challenge, the person experiences stress. If stress is present, **secondary appraisal** focuses on possible coping strategies. **Coping** is the active process of managing taxing circumstances, expending effort to solve personal and interpersonal problems, and seeking to master, minimize, reduce, or tolerate stress or conflict. Balancing factors contribute to restoring equilibrium.

If previous ways of coping are not effective, a **crisis** may occur, in which the person faces a turning point in life and the person must change. Caplan (1981) distinguished two types of crises: those associated with changing developmental levels, or **developmental crises**, and **situational crises**. Examples of developmental crises could be related to mastering developmental tasks as an individual (independence in adolescence) or as a family (children leaving home, caregiving to elderly parents). Examples of situational crises could include natural disasters like floods or famine, the end of an intimate relationship, or loss of work transportation through a motor vehicle crash. The frame of reference for a crisis is the viewpoint of the person experiencing the crisis. According to Aguilera's (1998) crisis theory, the vital questions for a person in crisis are "What does this mean to you?" and "How is it going to affect your life?" A basic assumption of crisis theory is that a person can either advance or regress as a result of a crisis, depending on how the crisis is managed. Feedback cues lead to ongoing reappraisals of original perceptions. Therefore, coping behaviours constantly change as new information is perceived.

Later work in the important role of appraisal and perception focused on the contribution of age and gender to responses to stressful events. Coping strategies, meaning attached to events, and responses to stressors change with age (Nosek, Kennedy, Beyene, et al., 2010). Gender differences may be conceptualized as an interaction between biologically based sex differences and an individual's social context (Desbonnet, Garrett, Daly, et al., 2008; Kimerling, Clum, & Wolfe, 2000). Women and men may perceive a stressor differently, may attach different meanings to that stressor, and thus may have different responses and reactions (Davis, Matthews, & Twamley, 1999; Liu & Alloy, 2010). For example, Taylor (2006) has theorized that women

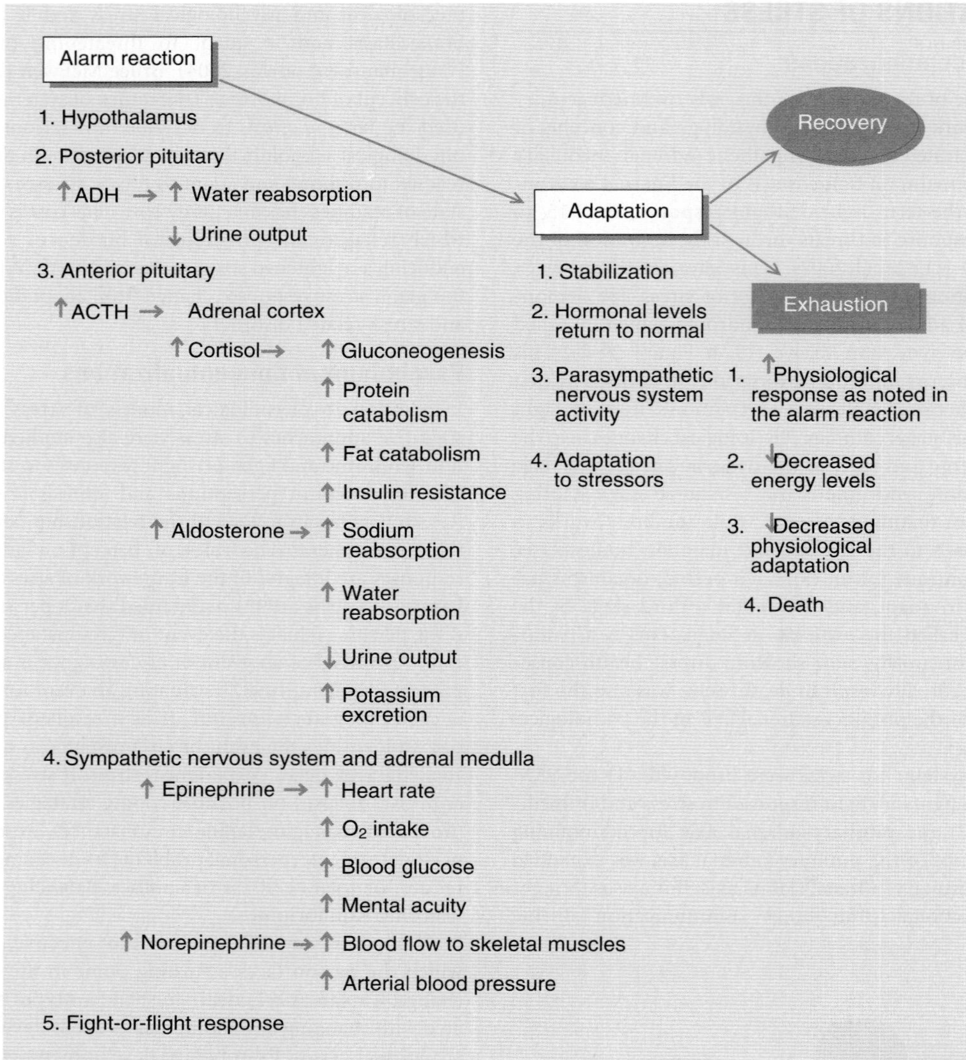

FIGURE 29-2 General adaptation syndrome. *ACTH,* Adrenocorticotropic hormone; *ADH,* antidiuretic hormone.

more often show nurturing and support-seeking behaviours in response to stress, rather than fight–flight behaviours.

In summary, individual differences in response to stressors can be affected by previous vulnerabilities and experiences, coexisting health problems, age, gender, allostatic load, and coping resources. Psychological and biological conceptualizations are not mutually exclusive. Indeed, the integration of the various frameworks helps explain the complexity of the relationship between stress and health.

STRESS RESPONSE SYSTEMS

Sympathetic–Adrenal–Medullary System

Activation of the SAM system results in increased heart rate, diversion of blood from the intestines to the brain and skeletal muscles, increased blood pressure, bronchodilation and increased respiratory rate, and increases in blood glucose levels (Chrousos, Loriaux, & Gold, 1988; Selye, 1991). All these changes are meant to prepare for fight-or-flight responses. A stressor activates specific cells in the brain stem that release norepinephrine into the bloodstream. Norepinephrine stimulates the adrenal medulla to release epinephrine. Epinephrine produces the cardiovascular, respiratory, and metabolic changes and the heightened awareness or alertness. Chronic stimulation brings about a chronic arousal state, with sleep disturbance, edginess and irritability, gastrointestinal upset, and increased startle responses. Brain areas that are involved in this stress response system include the following:

- *Reticular formation:* This is a small, integrative cluster of neurons in the brain stem and spinal cord that continuously monitors the physiological status of the body through connections with sensory and motor tracts. For example, certain cells within the reticular formation can cause a sleeping person to regain consciousness or increase the level of consciousness when a need arises.
- *Limbic system:* This is another integrative cluster of neurons that interconnect several parts of the brain and is involved in processing strong emotional experiences. Fear and perceived threat will cause increased activity within this system.
- *Midbrain and pons:* The midbrain joins the lower part of the brain stem and the spinal cord with the higher part of the brain and acts as a reflex centre for certain auditory, visual, and postural stimuli.

The pons mainly relays impulses to and from the medulla oblongata to other parts of the brain and the peripheral nervous system, and it also controls the rate and depth of breathing.

- *Medulla oblongata:* This brain region controls vital functions necessary for survival, including heart rate, blood pressure, and respiration. Impulses travelling to and from the medulla oblongata can increase or decrease these vital functions. For example, heart rate is regulated by sympathetic or parasympathetic nervous system impulses travelling from the medulla oblongata to the heart. The rate increases in response to pulses from sympathetic fibres and decreases with impulses from parasympathetic fibres.

Hypothalamic–Pituitary–Adrenal Axis

Activation of the HPA axis results in the release of a cascade of hormones (Dunn, 1989). A stressor activates the hypothalamus to release a corticotrophin-releasing hormone (CRH). This hormone activates receptors in the anterior pituitary, which signals the release of adrenocorticotropic hormone (ACTH) into the bloodstream. ACTH interacts with its receptors in the adrenal cortex to release glucocorticoids. In humans, the major glucocorticoid is cortisol. Cortisol has effects similar to those of epinephrine, contributing to the increase in heart rate and blood pressure, causing shunting of blood to skeletal muscles, and increasing the availability of glucose in the bloodstream. This stress response system is tightly controlled by negative feedback, whereby rising cortisol levels activate receptors in the hypothalamus and the pituitary gland, shutting off further release of CRH and ACTH (Brunello, Davidson, Deahl, et al., 2001). Other brain chemicals, such as β-endorphin (Kageyama, Tamasawa, & Suda, 2011), arginine vasopressin (Yayou, Nakamura, & Ito, 2009), and oxytocin (Olff, Langeland, Witteveen, et al., 2010), are also involved in the regulation of the HPA axis.

This part of the endocrine system interacts with other parts that regulate sex hormone levels, thyroid hormones, electrolyte and fluid balance, and insulin release. Therefore, overwhelming or chronic stressors can have diverse and complex impacts on health. The following brain areas are involved in this stress response system:

- *Hypothalamus:* This region of the brain is involved with many basic physiological processes, including appetite, sexual drive, sleeping, motor activity, and mood states (all of which are affected by stress). The hypothalamus is highly interconnected with many other areas of the brain. Dysregulation of the hypothalamus is thought to be involved in depression.
- *Pituitary gland:* This small gland, attached to the hypothalamus, produces and releases hormones that control vital functions. It is divided into the anterior and posterior portions. The anterior pituitary releases stress-, thyroid-, growth-, and reproduction-related hormones, whereas the posterior pituitary releases hormones related to electrolyte and water balance, as well as oxytocin. Both the pituitary gland and the hypothalamus can produce endorphins. **Endorphins** are hormones that produce a sense of well-being and reduce pain (Lazarus, 1999).
- *Adrenal glands:* One of these glands rests atop each kidney, and they are fundamental to stress responses. Each is composed of two very different regions. The outer region, or cortex, is where glucocorticoids such as cortisol are produced and released, and the inner region, or medulla, is where epinephrine is produced and released.

STRESS AND THE IMMUNE SYSTEM

Physiological responses to stress also include immunological responses, although the mechanisms through which stress affects the immune system are not fully understood (Aldwin, 2000; Box 29-1). The immune system differentiates between self and non-self material, so that, under normal conditions, one's own cells are not treated as threats in the way that bacteria, viruses, parasites, or toxins are treated. An antigen on the surface of bacteria cells identifies them as invaders. After being exposed to a particular antigen, the immune system remembers how to respond to that antigen and is prepared to respond with antibodies when the same antigen appears at a later time. Autoimmune illnesses such as multiple sclerosis, fibromyalgia, or insulin resistance can occur when the immune system misinterprets the body's own cells as foreign. Glucocorticoids are powerful anti-inflammatory agents and play a role in the cascade of homeostatic immune responses that are activated by infection or inflammation and clinical depression. Dysregulation or chronic activation of the SAM system and the HPA axis may increase the risk of stress-related mental illnesses, as well as cardiovascular disease, insulin resistance (which in turn can increase risk for type 2 diabetes), metabolic syndromes, and autoimmune illnesses.

BOX 29-1 Factors Influencing the Response to Stressors

Aspects of a Stressor That Influence the Stress Response

Intensity
Scope
Duration
Number and nature of other stressors
Past exposure to serious stressors
Predictability

Characteristics of the Individual That Influence the Stress Response

Age
Gender
Perception of personal control or inescapability
Availability of social supports
Feelings of competence
Cognitive appraisal

THE RELATIONSHIP BETWEEN TYPE OF STRESSOR AND HEALTH

Selye (1974) identified two types of stress: **distress**, or damaging stress, and **eustress**, or stress that protects health. Eustress is motivating energy, such as happiness, hopefulness, and purposeful movement (Halter, Pollard, Ray, et al., 2014). Eustress is a positive, healthy adaptation to stressors in daily life. In reference to this concept, Selye (1974) wrote the book *Stress Without Distress.* However, Aldwin (2000) wrote that the idea of healthy stress is controversial because it is difficult to tell whether a person has benefited from stress or is coping by denying the stress in some way.

Distressing events can be categorized in many ways, including work stressors, family stressors, chronic stressors, acute stressors, daily hassles, trauma, and crisis: "Work and family stress interact, family being the background for work stress, and work the background for family stress" (Lazarus, 1999). Women who have preschool children, for example, may experience full-time work as stressful when their child cannot go to day care because the child is ill and their spouse's job involves extended periods away from home. It is difficult to categorize some events, like the horrific devastation and loss of life experienced as a result of the March 2011 earthquake in Japan, and to predict what long-term health implications there will be for, in this case, the Japanese population. Chronic stress can arise also from stressful roles, such as being a caregiver for a spouse with Alzheimer's disease, or persistent physical or psychological conflict. Another example of chronic stress is living with a long-term illness. Conversely, acute stress is provoked by time-limited events that are threatening for a relatively brief period. In the context of chronic or acute stress, daily hassles, such as commuting to work, maintaining a home, social and personal interactions, and managing money, can become more difficult to manage. Trauma can refer to any physical damage to the body or, in psychological terms, can refer to feelings of fear, threat, and persistent reliving after witnessing or experiencing an emotionally painful, distressful, or shocking event or series of events. Severe stressors such as natural disasters or interpersonal events such as family violence or child maltreatment are often considered traumatic events; however, as in other types of stressors, perception plays a major role in the individual's response to such events. Indeed, for some people, serious stressors can lead to positive change or personal growth, leading in turn to greater self-knowledge, improved coping skills, stronger social ties, and positive changes in values and perspectives (Wendt, Tuckey, & Prosser, 2011). There is an emerging body of knowledge regarding positive change, called post-traumatic growth, defined as "positive psychological change experienced as a result of the struggle with highly challenging life circumstances" (Tedeschi & Calhoun, 2004).

Stress-Related Disorders

Prolonged exposure to a serious stressor or an acute stressor that overwhelms the ability to cope can lead to stress-related disorders (Box 29-2). However, even if an individual's stress-related symptoms do not meet full criteria for a stress disorder, it is important to recognize that those symptoms may have a significant impact on the individual's functioning and relationships with others. If interventions are not implemented, these symptoms can decrease quality of life and increase the risk of developing the full disorder. Early emerging stress-related symptoms include poor sleep, tension and jitteriness, and inability to concentrate, to a degree that day-to-day activities are affected.

Although stress-related psychiatric disturbances are usually considered to be acute stress disorder and post-traumatic stress disorder (PTSD), these are only two potential health outcomes. It is important to recognize the diversity of health effects from serious stressors. Indeed, clinical depression, chronic pain syndromes, somatization disorder, and irritable bowel syndrome have all been linked to chronic stress (Blackburn-Munro & Blackburn-Munro, 2001; Matthews, Gump, & Owens, 2001). Health providers need to perform thorough, multifaceted assessments to identify the full range of health effects.

Acute Stress Disorder. Acute stress disorder is caused by exposure to one or more traumatic events and lasts at least 3 days to 1 month after experiencing, witnessing, or being confronted with a traumatic event; the reaction is one of intense fear, helplessness, or horror (American Psychiatric Association, 2013). Other criteria of acute stress disorder are the presence of the following symptoms: (1) The patient displays acute dissociative symptoms; (2) the patient has at least one recurring symptom (intense memories, flashbacks [recurring, intensely vivid mental images of a past traumatic experience], or distressing dreams); (3) the patient displays marked avoidance of stimuli that arouse memories of the trauma; (4) the patient shows marked hyperarousal; and (5) the patient experiences arousal symptoms such as sleep disturbance, irritable behaviour, and angry outbursts. These symptoms must have a significant effect on the individual's occupational, social, or personal functioning to meet full criteria for acute stress disorder. Examples of traumatic events that lead to acute stress disorder are motor vehicle crashes, natural disasters, violent personal assault, emergency service work experiences, and military combat. Nurses are also not immune to acute stress disorder. Treatment usually focuses on symptoms, to aid in sleeping and to relieve the jitteriness and irritability. If the trauma-related symptoms persist longer than 1 month, the individual will likely meet the criteria for post-traumatic stress disorder.

Post-Traumatic Stress Disorder (PTSD). Symptoms of post-traumatic stress disorder (PTSD) are more persistent, having endured for at least 1 month (American Psychiatric Association, 2013). The symptom clusters are similar to those of acute stress disorder, with less emphasis on dissociative symptoms (Breslau & Kessler, 2001). The diagnosis of PTSD was formulated from research with men returning from the Vietnam War and was first thought to be quite rare. Ongoing community-based studies showed it to be more prevalent, with lifetime prevalence rates of 9.2% in Canada (Van Ameringen, Mancini, Patterson, et al., 2008). Treatment guidelines for PTSD have been published and include multimodal interventions with drug therapy and targeted psychotherapy (Forbes, Creamer, Bisson, et al., 2010).

BOX 29-2 RESEARCH HIGHLIGHT

Understanding Risks for Developing Psychological Distress

Research Focus

When caring for patients with a chronic illness, nurses must focus on the whole patient, and this includes the effects of living with a chronic illness, such as stress and stress-related disorders. It is important to note that stressful events attributed to historical events like colonialism continue to be prevalent for Indigenous women. The project reported by Benoit, Cotnam, Raboud, et al. (2016) highlights this important issue.

Research Abstract

Benoit and colleagues reported on phase 1 of a large study in their 2016 article. This article presents the findings from measurements of stress, depression, and post-traumatic stress disorder (PTSD) levels among urban Indigenous women living with and without human immunodeficiency virus (HIV) in Ontario, Canada. Participants of the study included 30 Indigenous women living with HIV and 60 without HIV, aged 18 years or older. The authors concluded that, with or without HIV, Indigenous women reported elevated levels of stress and physical and mental health concerns. Interventions to mitigate these findings need to include interprofessional collaboration and diversity of health care support.

Evidence-Informed Practice

- Regardless of HIV status, Indigenous women are at higher risk for stress, depression, and post-traumatic stress disorder.
- Nurses must include holistic health care practices if they are going to mitigate the risk for stress and stress-related disorders in this vulnerable population.
- Health care providers must recognize the ongoing impact of historical events on the health of Indigenous women.

Benoit, A. C., Cotnam, J., Raboud, J., Greene, S., Beaver, K., Zoccole, A., ...Loutfy, M. (2016). Experiences of chronic stress and mental health concerns among urban Indigenous women. *Archives of Women's Mental Health, 19*(5), 809–823.

NURSING KNOWLEDGE BASE

Nurses have proposed theories related to stress and coping. Because stress plays a role in vulnerability to disease, symptoms of stress often necessitate nursing intervention.

Nursing Theory and the Role of Stress

Neuman's (1995) systems model is based on the concepts of stress and reaction to stress. Nurses are responsible for developing interventions to prevent or reduce stressors on the patient or to make them more bearable for the patient (Neuman, 1995). Because Neuman's model is a systems model, it is applied to understand not only patients' individual responses to stressors but also families' and communities' responses. All systems experience multiple stressors, each of which has a differing potential to disturb the person's, family's, or community's dynamic balance. Every person has developed a set of responses to stress that constitute the "normal line of defence" (Neuman, 1995). This line of defence helps maintain health and wellness. However, when "physiological, psychological, sociocultural, developmental, or spiritual influences" are unable to buffer stress, the normal line of defence is broken, and disease can result. Neuman's systems model coincides with Selye's (1974) general adaptation syndrome and McEwen's (2007) concept of allostatic load.

Neuman's (1995) systems model stresses the importance of accuracy in assessment and interventions that promote optimal wellness through the use of primary, secondary, and tertiary prevention strategies. According to Neuman's theory, the goal of primary prevention is to promote patient wellness by stress prevention and reduction of risk factors. Secondary prevention occurs after symptoms appear. The nurse helps the patient determine the meaning of the illness and stress and finds resources available to handle them. Tertiary prevention begins when the patient is becoming more stable and recovering. At the tertiary level of prevention, the nurse supports rehabilitation processes involved in healing, moving the patient back to wellness, and the primary level of disease prevention.

In their health promotion model, Pender, Murdaugh, and Parsons (2002) proposed that health promotion is directed toward increasing the level of well-being of an individual or group. Conversely, primary, secondary, and tertiary types of prevention (health protection) focus on avoiding negative events. Pender and colleagues considered stress reduction strategies important to reducing threats to well-being, helping people fulfill their potential, and shaping and maintaining health behaviours. To change behaviour, the patient must initiate the change and behave differently in interactions. On the basis of core assumptions regarding the capability and desire of people to be healthy, Pender and colleagues suggested strategies for prevention and health promotion related to stress management.

Situational, Maturational, and Sociocultural Factors

Multiple factors affect the types of potential stressors and coping mechanisms. Age is one; for example, adolescence, adulthood, and old age bring different stressors (Andersen & Teicher, 2008). Appraisal of stressors, amount and type of social support, and coping strategies are other factors that affect appraisal of stressors, as are previous life experiences (Aguilera, 1998).

Situational Factors. Situational stress can arise from a person's current circumstances, such as moving, changing jobs (stressful job changes include promotions, transfers, downsizing, restructuring, and changes in supervisors and/or responsibilities), and adjusting to a chronic illness or condition. Common diseases and conditions that can be exacerbated by stress are obesity, hypertension, diabetes, depression, asthma, and coronary artery disease. Being a family caregiver may also cause situational stress, although the source of stress may be not necessarily the caregiving but other factors in the caregiver's life, such as work, finances, or lack of respite (Merluzzi, Philip, Vachon, et al., 2011). Spouses and other family members also experience stress when a loved one is ill (Box 29-3).

BOX 29-3 RESEARCH HIGHLIGHT

Spousal Support for Psychological Distress

Research Focus

People with chronic illnesses who require care are most often cared for by family members. In Canada, there are more than 8 million caregivers who are providing care to a family member or friend with a chronic illness (Penning & Wu, 2016). The impact of caregiving on the caregiver's health is often overlooked by health care providers. While caregiving can be a rewarding experience, the stress of caring for a family member may increase the carer's risk for mental health issues and disorders, such as anxiety, depression, and acute stress disorder.

Research Abstract

The purpose of Penning and Wu's study was to compare the stress and mental health implications of caregiving. The authors looked at the experiences of middle-aged and older male and female caregivers when caring for a spouse, children, siblings, other family members, friends, and others. The study design used a multivariate regression analysis on a subsample of caregivers aged 45 and older from the 2007 Canadian General Social Survey data. The 2007 Canadian General Social Survey, Cycle 21 (GSS-21), conducted by Statistics Canada, is an annual national survey that gathers individual- and household-level data to monitor changes in social conditions and the well-being of Canadians (Statistics Canada, 2009). The results of the multivariate regression analysis revealed that being a caregiver was stressful and detrimental to a person's mental health. Caring for a spouse or child was more stressful and detrimental to the mental health of women carers than was caring for parents. Interestingly, there were similar results for men; however, unlike for women in the study, men's overall mental health was not adversely affected. Similarly, for men, caring for a spouse and for children was more stressful than caring for others but did not adversely affect overall mental health. Another interesting finding was that over 40% of caregivers reported experiencing activity limitations, and over 50% reported having at least one chronic illness, with women reporting higher rates of chronic illness. The researchers concluded that despite limitations in the study, their findings are notable in arguing for the differential implications of caregiving for the mental health of spouses, parents, children, and other caregivers.

Evidence-Informed Practice

- The findings suggest that spousal caregiving and child caregiving tend to be more rather than less stressful and detrimental to middle-aged and older caregivers' mental health than is caregiving to most others,
- Gender differences need to be considered regarding the effects of caregiving on the carer, as the findings show that women's mental health is more detrimentally affected than men's mental health when caring for a spouse or child.
- Nurses need to consider the cost to the caregivers' health when working with people with chronic illness. Support for carers needs to be prioritized when working with people with chronic illness.

Penning, M. J., & Wu, Z. (2016). Caregiver stress and mental health: Impact of caregiving relationship and gender. *The Gerontologist, 58*(6), 1102–1113.

Maturational Factors. Stressors vary with life stage and are not necessarily related to negative events. Important individual and family developmental milestones can be anticipated with excitement but can nonetheless be stressful. Preadolescents may experience stress related to self-esteem issues, changes in family structure as a result of divorce or death of a parent, or hospitalizations. As adolescents search for their identity with peer groups and separate from their families, they may view these developmental tasks as stressors. In addition, they must make decisions about using mind-altering substances, peer pressure, sexuality, jobs, school, and career choices; the decision-making process may also be viewed as stressful. Stress for adults can arise from major changes in individual and family life circumstances (Aguilera, 1998). These changes include the many milestones of beginning a family and a career, losing parents, helping children leave home, and accepting physical aging. In old age, stressors include the loss of autonomy and mastery, as a result of general frailty or health problems that limit mobility, stamina, and strength, and the loss of a spouse, close friends, and family that provided social support over the years (Box 29-4).

Sociocultural Factors. Low socioeconomic status is not necessarily associated with more stress than better financial status is. Nurses must not make assumptions about the sources of stress for an individual or family. However, some circumstances create higher risk of experiencing serious stressors or trauma. For example, living under conditions of continuing violence, living in disintegrated neighbourhoods, and homelessness can be damaging, especially for young people (Pender et al., 2002).

A person's cultural background also greatly influences the perception of and reaction to stress (Aldwin, 2000). Cultural context must be integrated into any assessment. Differences are observed from culturally distinct groups within the general population, such as Indigenous cultures, as well as from immigrant populations. It is important to recognize that Indigenous culture is not singular. Indeed, potential stressors vary by geographic region (e.g., whether patients live in urban centres, rural areas, or remote parts of Canada); by historical events, such as residential schooling; and by the financial status of a specific Indigenous group. Although stressors related to immigration have been well described, ongoing stressors also may influence the health of families for generations, or intergenerational stress. Initial stressors can include career and financial issues related to underemployment, loss of extended family supports, language barriers, and unfamiliarity regarding accessing health services (Mollica, Sarajlic, Chernoff, et al., 2001; Shen & Takeuchi, 2001). Later stressors can be related to raising children in a dual context (between cultural norms of the country of origin and the current environment) (Beiser, Hamilton, Rummens, et al., 2010). An example of intergenerational stress and how this may influence mental health is discussed in Box 29-5.

CRITICAL THINKING

When caring for a patient who is experiencing stress, the nurse needs to integrate knowledge from nursing and other disciplines, previous experiences, and information gathered from the patient to understand

BOX 29-4 FOCUS ON OLDER PERSONS

Stress

- Older persons are incorrectly presumed to be more vulnerable to the psychosocial effect of stressors (Kasl, 1992). However, the diurnal pattern of hypothalamic–pituitary–adrenal (HPA) axis activity does change with age, with higher evening levels of cortisol (Magri, Cravello, Barili, et al., 2006). As a result, sleep patterns may be altered, memory may be impaired (Lupien, Fiocco, Wan, et al., 2005), and immune system functioning may be blunted (Graham, Christian, & Kiecolt-Glaser, 2006). These changes can lead to increasing physical and mental frailty (Butcher & Lord, 2004).
- A study of stress and coping in patients aged 75 to 91 years revealed that such patients, in comparison with patients of other ages, were less likely to view their lives as having problems, and they expended less effort in coping (Aldwin, Sutton, Chiara, et al., 1996). This view may arise from multiple factors, including life experiences and perspectives of older persons that make most problems seem insignificant, having acquired appropriate stress management techniques and increased acceptance of daily hassles.
- The timing of stress-inducing events can significantly influence older persons' ability to cope. Many older people experience several stressful events (e.g., loss of a spouse and new medical diagnosis) within a brief time frame, which may result in reduced coping ability.
- Older people with strong spiritual beliefs effectively use religious coping in response to medical illness and disasters (Foster, 1997).
- Major depressive disorder and anxiety disorders are the most prevalent mental health disorders in later life (Chapman & Perry, 2008; Skultety & Rodriguez, 2008).

BOX 29-5 CULTURAL ASPECTS OF CARE

Intergenerational Trauma and Indigenous Women: Implications for Mental Health

Understanding the consequences of intergenerational trauma is important for nurses who work with diverse cultural groups. *Intergenerational trauma* is described as trauma that occurs as a result of historical occurrences, such as colonization, and that has an impact on health for many generations after the original events took place (Sotero, 2006, cited in Roy, 2014). Maladaptive patterns of usually destructive behaviour (e.g., addictions, suicide, violence) were created in response to the original trauma and are absorbed into the culture and transmitted as learned behaviour from generation to generation (Sotero, 2006, cited in Roy, 2014). Coping strategies are influenced by culture. Cultures vary in their emotion-focused and problem-focused coping strategies. For example, according to some cultures, emotions should be controlled; according to others, they should be expressed.

Implications for Practice

- Realize that intergenerational stress can affect health and stress-related illness for many generations.
- Use introspection to examine your own experiences and perceptions of stress and coping.
- Assess the influence of culture on a patient's appraisal of stress.
- Determine the available resources within a patient's culture that may facilitate coping.

Roy, A. (2014). Intergenerational trauma and Aboriginal women: Implications for mental health during pregnancy. *First Peoples Child and Family Review, 9*(1), 8–21.

the particular stressor, its meaning for the patient and family, and current and past events that influence their responses to this stressor. Nurses must know the neurophysiological changes that occur in response to overwhelming or chronic stress. Nurses must also be able to determine the patient's perception of the situation and help the patient identify and use coping strategies that have helped in the past. If the patient's usual coping skills are unsuccessful or support systems are inadequate, the nurse must implement crisis intervention counselling (see "Crisis Intervention").

As a nurse, you should be confident in the belief that you can help the patient manage the current situation effectively. Patients who are overwhelmed and perceive events as being beyond their capacity to cope rely on you as their guide to action. Through a nurse's expert advice and counsel, many patients gain confidence in their own ability to manage the consequences of the recent event. Standards of practice can help nurses make an accurate assessment of the level of a patient's stress, previously successful coping mechanisms, and available support systems before intervening.

❖ NURSING PROCESS

◆ Assessment

When assessing a patient's stress level and coping resources, the nurse must ask the patient to share personal and sensitive information. Therefore, the nurse must first establish a trusting nurse–patient relationship. By asking open-ended questions, listening carefully, observing the patient's nonverbal behaviour, and observing the patient's environment, the nurse can learn about the patient's stress. Nurses use critical thinking skills to synthesize and analyze information (Figure 29-3). Often patients have difficulty expressing what is troubling them until they have the opportunity to talk with someone who has time to listen.

Subjective Findings. When assessing a patient's level of stress and coping resources, it is important to arrange a nonthreatening physical environment, without a desk as a barrier, for the interaction (Halter et al., 2014). The nurse assumes the same height as the patient, arranging the interview environment so that eye contact can be comfortably maintained or avoided. Placing chairs at a 90-degree angle or side by side can help reduce the intensity of the interaction (Halter et al., 2014). The interview is used to determine the patient's view of the stress, past successful coping resources, any possible maladaptive coping, and adherence to prescribed medical recommendations, such as medication or diet (Monat & Lazarus, 1991; Table 29-1). If the patient is using denial as a coping mechanism, the nurse must be alert to whether the patient is overlooking necessary information. Other patients may state that they feel overwhelmed and unable to cope, but with help, they can reduce their multiple interacting stressors to manageable pieces. As in all patient interactions, nurses must respect the confidentiality and sensitivity of the information shared.

Safety Alert Medical conditions such as sleep apnea and thyroid dysfunction that are common in older people can initially cause symptoms that mimic stress-related symptoms. For this reason, a thorough physical assessment of an older person who appears stressed or anxious is necessary to rule out potentially serious medical disorders. In addition, in older people, signs of stress and crisis must be differentiated from emerging dementia and also from acute confusion, a condition that can be life-threatening.

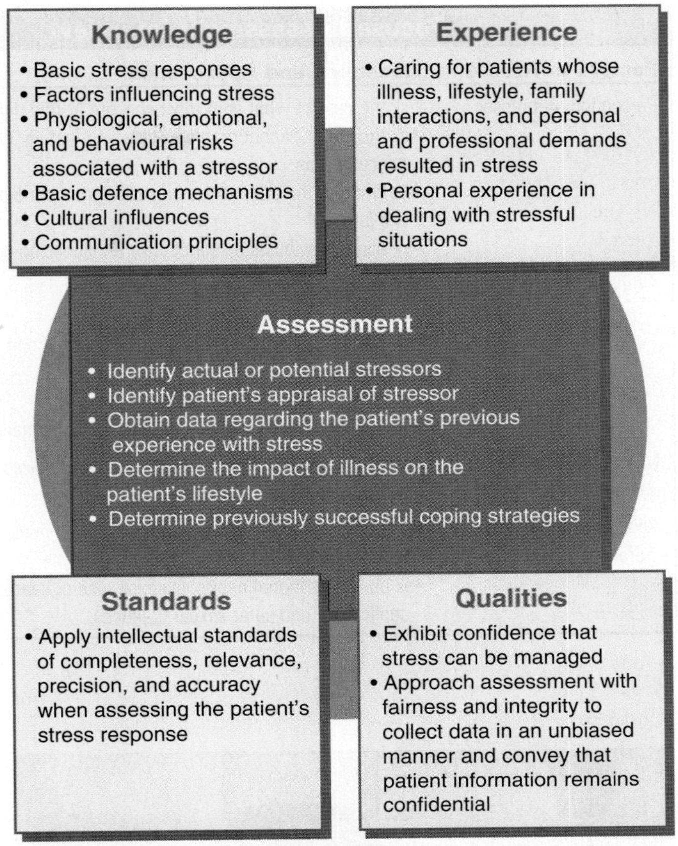

FIGURE 29-3 Critical thinking model for stress and coping assessment.

Objective Findings. Nurses obtain further findings about stress and coping by observing the patient's appearance and nonverbal behaviour during the interview, including grooming and hygiene, handshake and gait, body language, speech quality, eye contact, and attitude. However, it is important to consider that someone who is experiencing stress may not be behaving as "usual" when meeting a health care provider for the first time, so care should be exercised in making judgements at this time. During the assessment, depending on the patient's anxiety level, the nurse takes basic vital signs to assess for physiological signs of stress, such as elevated blood pressure, heart rate, or respiratory rate (Figure 29-4).

Patient Expectations. It is crucial that nurses understand the meaning the patient attaches to the precipitating event and how stress responses are affecting the patient's life. Nurses must allow the patient time to express priorities for coping. For example, if a woman has just been told that a breast mass was identified on a routine mammogram, the nurse must discern what the patient wants and needs most from the nurse. Some patients identify an immediate need for information about biopsy or mastectomy; others need guidance and support on how to share the news with family members. In some cases, when nothing can be done to change or improve the situation, just being with the patient can be helpful. Once the nurse understands patient expectations, it is important to support the patient in meeting his or her identified needs.

◆ Nursing Diagnosis

Nurses cluster data that indicate a potential or actual stressor and the patient's response. Keeping in mind previous knowledge and

TABLE 29-1 Focused Assessment Interview

Factors to Assess	Questions and Approaches	Physical Assessment Strategies
Perception of stressor	Ask the patient what is of most concern at this time. Ask the patient about problems sleeping, eating, working, and concentrating. Ask whether the patient has had accidents in the home, in the car, or on the job. Ask about previous stressors that are influencing current appraisals.	Observe nonverbal behaviour and expressions of feelings that indicate anxiety, fear, anger, irritability, or tension.
Available coping resources	Ask the patient about current friendships and contacts with family members. Ask what the patient has done in the past to cope with similar problems or stress. Ask how the patient spends leisure time. Ask the patient to describe any specific stress management techniques.	Observe whether the patient is alone or with others. Observe grooming and hygiene. Observe the patient's communication skills. Determine whether the patient is able to ask for help. Observe developmental level and sociocultural circumstances.
Maladaptive coping used	Assess current and past patterns of use of tobacco, prescription or over-the-counter drugs, and caffeine.	Observe for effects of heavy use of tobacco, alcohol, illegal drugs, and caffeine.
Adherence to healthy practices	Ask whether the patient visits a physician or nurse practitioner regularly for checkups. Ask about nutritional habits, exercise, use of seat belts, helmets (if applicable), and safer sexual practices.	Monitor pulse, blood pressure, weight. Observe nonverbal behaviour.

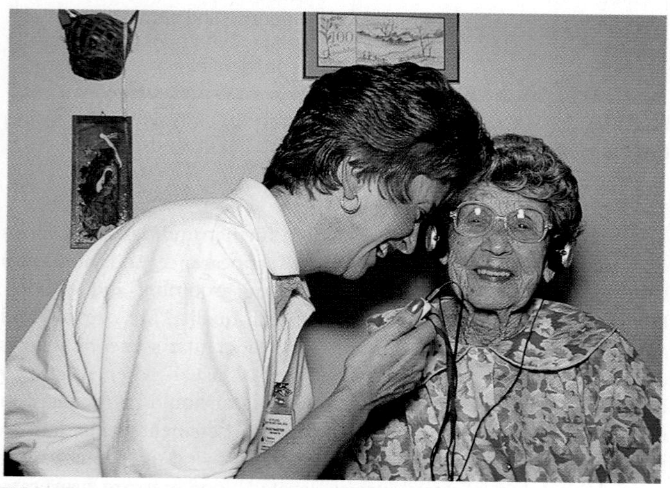

FIGURE 29-4 Sharing a joke or laughing with patients can reduce stress and support a therapeutic relationship.

BOX 29-6 NURSING DIAGNOSTIC PROCESS

Assessment Activities	Defining Characteristics	Nursing Diagnosis
Ask patient about change in sleeping patterns.	Sleep disturbance; difficulty falling asleep at night or staying asleep Nightmares or disturbing dreams Sighing	*Anxiety*
Ask patient to complete a sleep diary for 2 weeks.	Excessive sleeping	
Observe patient's behaviour and response to questions during assessment.	Fatigue Inability to concentrate Inaccurate response to questions Inappropriate laughing or crying	
Observe patient's appearance.	Poor grooming Self-harm	
Ask patient about changes in eating patterns.	Weight gain or loss Lack of interest in food	

experiences with patients under stress, nurses then make individualized nursing diagnoses (Box 29-6).

Nursing diagnoses for people experiencing stress generally focus on coping. Major defining characteristics of *ineffective coping* include verbalization of both an inability to cope and an inability to ask for help. Defining characteristics are identified by asking patients what currently concerns them most and allowing them sufficient time to answer. The nurse observes for nonverbal signs of anxiety, fear, anger, irritability, and tension. Other defining characteristics include the presence of life stressors, an inability to meet role expectations and basic needs, alteration in societal participation, self-destructive behaviour, change in usual communication patterns, high rate of accidents, excessive food intake, drinking, smoking, and sleep disturbances. Stress can result in multiple nursing diagnoses, such as the following:

- *Anxiety*
- *Caregiver role strain*
- *Chronic pain*
- *Post-traumatic stress disorder*
- *Powerlessness*

Crises differ from stressors in the degree of severity, although stressors and crises have many similarities. A patient who perceives a situation as stressful, who is unable to cope in ways that have worked before, and who has insufficient support is experiencing a crisis. A crisis can be devastating and requires the nurse to help mobilize all resources available (Aguilera, 1998).

◆ Planning

Goals and Outcomes. Desirable outcomes for people experiencing stress are (1) effective coping, (2) coping by their family, (3) emotional health of the caregiver, and (4) psychosocial adjustment to life changes (Moorhead, Johnson, & Maas, 2008). Nurses may select interventions for stress and improved coping such as coping enhancement or crisis intervention, which are in the *Nursing Interventions Classification (NIC)* (Bulechek et al., 2013. In addition, nurses select individualized interventions after considering the nursing diagnosis, the resources available to the patient, and the goals identified by the patient and nurse (Figure 29-5).

Nursing interventions may be designed within the framework of primary, secondary, and tertiary prevention. At the primary level of prevention, individuals and populations who may be at risk for stress are identified (Stuart & Wright, 1995). At the secondary level, nursing actions are directed at symptoms, such as decreasing the frequency or intensity of specific symptoms. At the tertiary level, nursing interventions assist the patient in readapting and might include relaxation training and time management training (Box 29-7). Another method of planning care involves using a concept map (Figure 29-6). The nurse creates the map after identifying relevant nursing diagnoses from the assessment database. In this example, the nursing diagnoses are linked to the patient's medical diagnosis of PTSD. The concept map shows the relationships with the nursing diagnoses: PTSD, *ineffective coping, anxiety, and risk for other-directed violence.* In this approach, nurses use critical thinking skills to organize patient data and plan for patient-centred care.

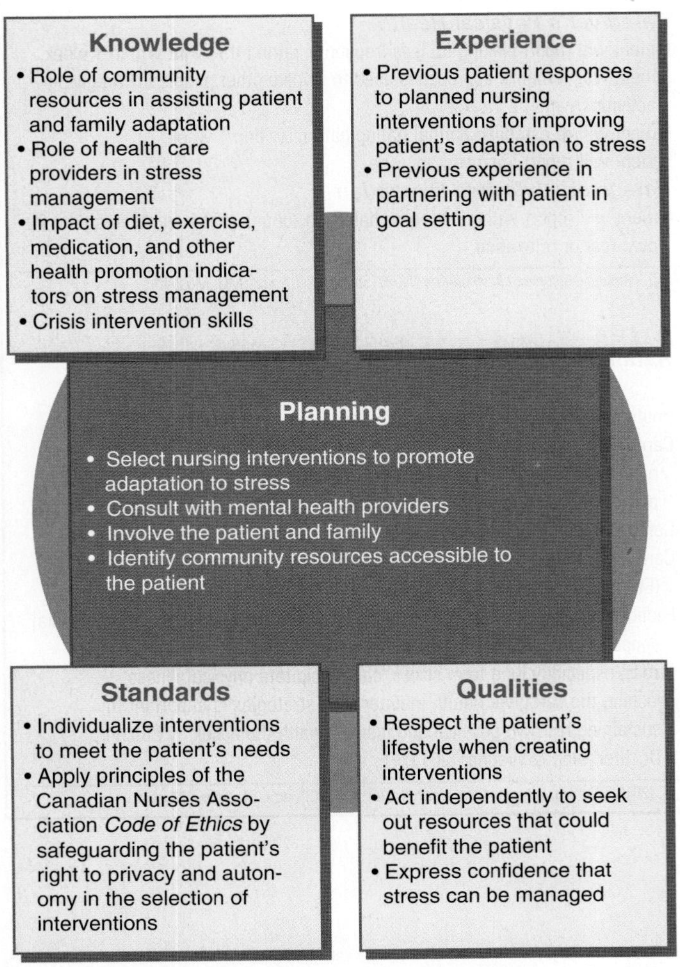

FIGURE 29-5 Critical thinking model for stress and coping planning.

Just as the nursing assessment of stress and coping depends on patient perception of the problem and coping resources, interventions focus on a partnership of the nurse with the patient and support system, usually the family. In the case of a family or community stressor and impaired family or community coping, the view of the situation and resources is broader.

Setting Priorities. When nurses prioritize needs for a person experiencing stress or a crisis, the first question to be answered is "What is happening in your life that you needed to come today?" or "What happened in your life that is *different*?" This question requires the patient to focus. The nurse should then assess the patient's perception of the event, situational supports, and what the patient usually does when faced with a problem (Aguilera, 1998). As in all areas of nursing, safety of the patient and family is the first priority.

> **Safety Alert** Direct questions help to determine whether a person is suicidal or homicidal. The nurse might ask, "Have you thought that life is not worth living? Are those thoughts with you most of the day?" "Have you thought your problems would be solved if that other person were not around anymore?" If the patient answers "yes" to any of these questions, the nurse should calmly determine whether the patient has a plan and determine how lethal the means are. If suicide or homicide is not an issue, the nurse should consider other threats to the safety of people who are under the patient's care and provide for their temporary care or supervision if necessary. When immediate assessment is completed and safety is ensured, the problem-solving process should begin (Aguilera, 1998).

Continuity of Care. Sometimes the scope of nursing practice is insufficient to meet all of the patient's needs. For patients experiencing stress from medical conditions or psychiatric disorders, nurses must consult with advanced practice mental health nurses, psychiatrists, psychologists, psychiatric social workers, or other mental health experts. An interprofessional approach to care is often most effective in addressing the holistic needs of the patient and should be included in the planning of care. The nurse's role is to recognize the need for collaboration and consultation, inform the patient about potential resources, and make arrangements for interventions, such as consultations, group sessions, or therapy as needed.

◆ Implementation

Health Promotion. Three primary modes of intervention for stress are to decrease stress-producing situations, increase resistance to stress, and learn skills that reduce physiological and psychological responses to stress (Pender et al., 2002). Nurses are in a position to educate patients and families about the importance of health promotion (Boxes 29-8 and 29-9). Several strategies help increase resistance to stress and reduce response to stress.

Regular Exercise. A regular exercise program improves muscle tone and posture, controls weight, reduces tension, and promotes relaxation. In addition, exercise improves mood and immune

BOX 29-7 NURSING CARE PLAN

Caregiver Role Strain

ASSESSMENT

When the professional nurse first goes to Carl's house, she finds the home to be in slight disarray. The lawn is overgrown, dirty dishes are in the sink, and an empty can of soup is sitting on the kitchen counter. Carl is standing in the living room, folding clothes from a laundry basket, and Evelyn, Carl's wife, is sitting in a chair watching TV. Evelyn recently received a diagnosis of Alzheimer's disease.

Assessment Activities	*Findings and Defining Characteristics*
Ask Carl about his recent stressors and coping strategies.	He continues to fold clothes during the visit, stating, "There's so much to do that I don't even know where to begin." Carl describes being awakened three to four times per night to find Evelyn wandering in the house. He states that he has no outside activities and his children live in other provinces. He does have several close friends who live nearby, but he does not know of community resources.
Observe Carl's grooming and hygiene.	Carl is unshaven and appears dishevelled.
Ask Carl about his sleep and nutrition patterns.	Carl states that he has lost 9 kg in the past 6 months and that his appetite has been poor.
Assess Carl's mood and affect by asking how he is feeling.	Carl states, "I feel very tired. Everything feels overwhelming."
Assess Carl's suicide potential.	Carl denies being suicidal.
Assess health status and health care status.	Carl has not seen a nurse practitioner or physician for his own health in over a year.

NURSING DIAGNOSIS: Caregiver role strain related to recent diagnosis of wife's Alzheimer's disease

PLANNING

*Goal (Nursing Outcomes Classification)**	*Expected Outcomes*
	Caregiver's Physical Health
Patient will appear rested in 1 month.	Patient will report waking up less frequently during the night within 1 week. Patient will verbalize approaches used to involve other people in caregiving activities within 2 weeks.
Patient will maintain a stable weight over next 4 weeks.	Patient will re-establish normal eating pattern within 1 week. Patient will report improved appetite.
	Caregiver's Lifestyle Disruption
Patient will state that he has resumed one outside activity within 1 month.	Patient will report within 1 week a balanced routine that incorporates time for own rest or relaxation.

*Outcome classification labels from Moorhead, S., Johnson, M., Maas, M. L., & Swanson, E. (Eds.). (2012). *Nursing outcomes classification (NOC)* (5th ed.). St. Louis, MO: Mosby.

INTERVENTIONS

Interventions (Nursing Interventions Classification)†	*Rationale*
Caregiver Support	
Assist patient in establishing a consistent care routine.	Routines can help tasks be simplified and more time efficient.
Discuss ways that patient agrees will simplify care routine, such as hiring a teenage neighbour to mow the lawn, buying frozen meals, having groceries delivered, and having a cleaning service twice a month.	Caregivers experience stress outside of their caregiving roles. Frequently, providing ways to assist the caregiver with home maintenance, meal planning, and shopping assists caregivers with stress management.
Identify sources of respite care by encouraging patient to identify available friends who can assist with caregiving.	Caregiving cannot normally be successful if it involves only one caregiver. Caregiver may be hesitant to ask for help because of past family conflict (Etters, Goodall, & Harrison, 2008).
Explore community resources such as home care, adult day care, and Meals on Wheels with patient.	Feelings of burden have been found to be lower among caregivers with social supports (Solomon & Draine, 1995).
Teach patient stress-management techniques.	Stress, especially long-term stress, can precipitate physical illness.
Set up monthly health checks for patient that include vital sign and weight measurements.	Teaching the caregiver health maintenance strategies is important for sustaining his own physical and mental health (Bulechek, & Butcher, Dochtermann & Wagner (2013).

†Intervention classification labels from Bulechek, G. M. & Butcher, H.K., Dochterman, J. M., & Wagner, C. (2013). *Nursing interventions classification (NIC)* (6th ed.). St. Louis,: Mosby.

BOX 29-7 NURSING CARE PLAN

Caregiver Role Strain—cont'd

EVALUATION

Nursing Actions	***Patient Response and Finding***	***Achievement of Outcome***
Observe for signs of fatigue.	Carl states he feels more rested and less depressed.	Carl is able to sleep for 6 hours during night and takes a 30-minute nap in the afternoon.
Review new care routines. Ask patient what other modifications may need to be made.	Carl buys frozen meals to use when he is busy with other caregiving responsibilities.	Carl has reduced his personal expectation that he must cook every meal himself.
Ask patient about how community and additional family support is helping to relieve stress.	Meals on Wheels delivers lunch 5 days per week. A neighbour mows the lawn for Carl.	Carl is mobilizing community resources.
Ask patient to compare past and current energy levels.	Carl reports having more energy and smiles spontaneously.	Carl has improved balance between Evelyn's and his own routines.
Weigh patient regularly.	Carl reports gaining 2 kg in 1 month.	Carl has resumed a normal eating pattern.
Ask patient about recent food intake.	Carl reports having eaten lunch with Evelyn on the day of the visit.	Carl has been able to sustain reasonable food intake recently.

BOX 29-8 FOCUS ON PRIMARY HEALTH CARE

Preventing Stress

Nurses address their patient's stress or potential stress in many different primary health care settings. In a community setting, the nurse might work with a group of teenage mothers on how to care for their newborns and themselves. The goal is to improve the health and safety of the babies and mothers and to prevent stress, health breakdown, and crises in their lives. In a home setting, the nurse might help the family of a patient who has cancer to recognize and deal with symptoms of stress in their lives. At a community clinic, the nurse might assess the stress in the life of a patient with sleep problems and plan interventions with the patient to help improve their sleep. Nurse practitioners who work in primary health care settings can provide a range of services related to family health and ongoing management of chronic health problems.

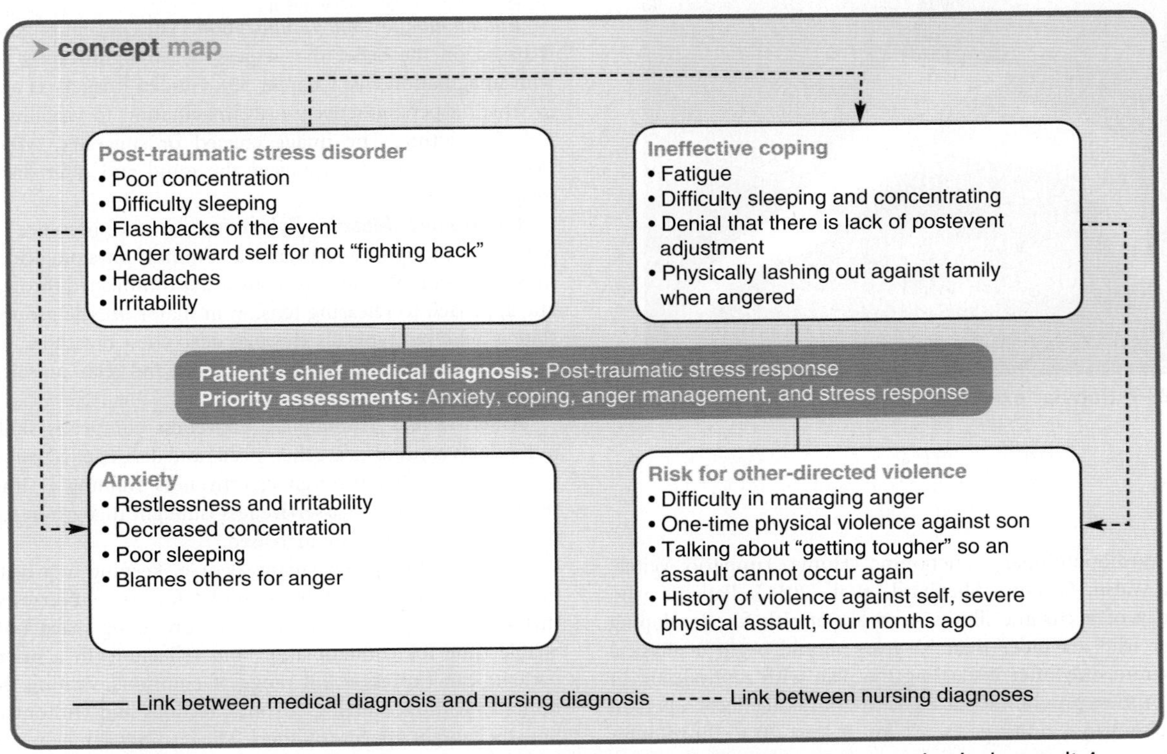

FIGURE 29-6 Concept map for patient with PTSD after experiencing a severe physical assault 4 months ago.

BOX 29-9 PATIENT TEACHING

Stress Management Strategies

Objective

- Improved coping with daily hassles in the workplace (such as a depending on others for transportation to work, chronically late co-worker, multiple competing work demands, intense work demands at specific times)

Teaching Strategies

- Teach the patient how to break down hassles into specific aspects in order to begin coping with them.
- Advise the patient to avoid impulsive changes in lifestyle when stressed.
- Assist the patient with time management skills and setting priorities.
- Assist the patient in examining lifestyle issues that may serve as stress relievers, such as walking.
- Assist the patient in examining dietary sources of increased tension, such as excessive caffeine intake (e.g., coffee, tea, chocolate).
- Assist the patient in building a network of social support.
- Teach the patient relaxation techniques, such as rhythmic breathing.

Evaluation

- Observe the patient for signs of active coping strategies.
- Ask the patient to keep a record of hours of sleep.
- Ask the patient to list activities that are soothing or enjoyable.

Data from Pender, N. J., Murdaugh, C., & Parsons, M. A. (2002). *Health promotion in nursing practice* (4th ed.). Upper Saddle River, NJ: Haworth Press.

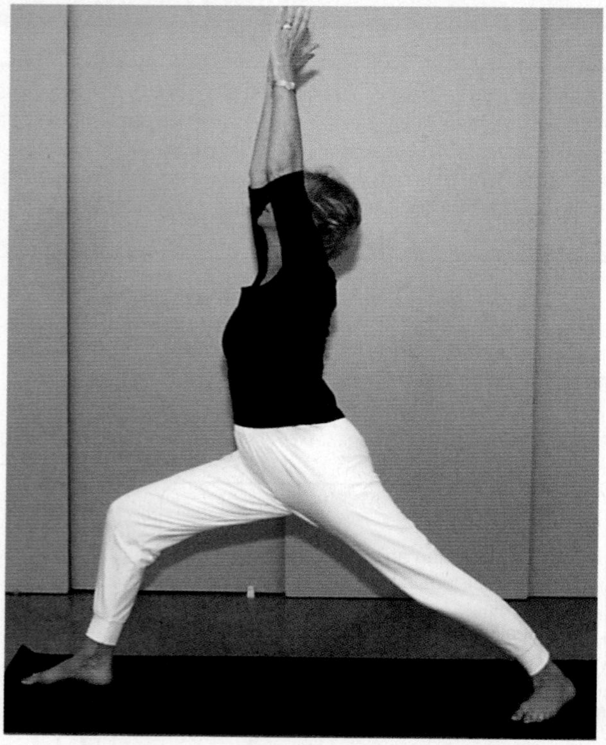

FIGURE 29-7 Regular exercise assists in coping with stress.

system and cardiopulmonary functioning (Hume, Timperio, Veitch, et al., 2011; Walsh, Gleeson, Shephard, et al., 2011). Patients who have a history of a chronic illness, who are at risk for developing an illness, or who are older than 35 years should begin a physical exercise program only after discussing the plan with a physician. In general, for a fitness program to have positive physical effects, a person should exercise 3 to 4 times per week for at least 20 to 30 minutes (Figure 29-7).

Support Systems. A support system of family, friends, and colleagues who listen, offer advice, and provide emotional support may be of benefit to patients experiencing stress. Many support groups are available to individuals, such as those sponsored by the Heart and Stroke Foundation of Canada, the Canadian Cancer Society, local hospitals and churches, and mental health organizations.

Time Management. Time management techniques include developing lists of tasks to be performed in order of priority: for example, tasks that require immediate attention, those that are important but can be delayed, and those that are routine and can be accomplished when time becomes available. In many cases, setting priorities helps individuals identify tasks that are not necessary or perhaps can even be delegated to someone else.

Guided Imagery and Visualization. The concept of guided imagery is based on the belief that a person can significantly reduce stress with imagination (see Chapter 35). Guided imagery is a relaxed state in which a person actively uses imagination to visualize a soothing, peaceful setting. The image created or suggested typically evokes many sensory words to engage the mind and offer distraction and relaxation.

Progressive Muscle Relaxation. In the presence of anxiety-provoking thoughts and events, a common physiological symptom is muscle tension. Physiological tension is diminished through a systematic approach to releasing tension in major muscle groups. A relaxed state is achieved typically through deep chest breathing, and then the patient is directed to alternately tighten and relax muscles in specific groupings (see Chapter 35).

Assertiveness Training. Assertiveness comprises skills that help individuals communicate their needs and desires effectively. The ability to resolve conflict through assertiveness training is important for reducing stress. When assertiveness is taught in a group setting, benefits of the experience are increased.

Journal Writing. For many people, keeping a private, personal journal provides a therapeutic outlet for stress. Nurses can suggest this activity to patients and assist by providing space and privacy to enable time for contemplation and reflection. In a private journal, patients can express a full range of emotions, venting their feelings honestly without hurting anyone's feelings and without concern for how they might appear to others. The writings can help individuals by increasing their awareness of situations through self-reflection. Journal

BOX 29-10 CASE STUDY

Missing What Is Important

I was so keen! I wanted to be such a good nurse. Thus, in the second year of my nursing program, I began my first day on an assessment unit within our provincial psychiatric hospital with eager anticipation of testing my newly learned communication techniques, mixed with some curiosity and admitted anxiety about how I would react to patients. As it turned out, what I was stressed about was so far off the mark! I was so concerned about how I would react to patients that I did not consider how patients would react to me. We were to complete verbatim reports regarding our interactions with our patients. However, my assigned patient was a middle-aged man with paranoid schizophrenia who apparently was suspicious of new people. It was suggested that I "hang around" the unit for a few days, so that my patient could get used to seeing me before I actually approached him. But what about those verbatim reports? How could I initiate the first conversation? Maybe discreet observations could fill in for the time being. I was caught up in my role as an unobtrusive staff member. On the second day, the patient abruptly approached me and in an angry tone stated, "You have been following me and watching me for 2 days!" So much for my discretion. In focusing only on my perceptions and needs, I had thought little about how perception, like communication, can be different for the participants. My spontaneous response was, "You're right, I have. I just didn't know how to approach you." His anger dissolved into a laugh at my awkwardness. That clear, honest response was the start of a very rewarding nurse–patient relationship that spanned the entire 2-month rotation. He taught me so much about mental health nursing: how perceptions about potential stressors affected our interactions, how spontaneity could be powerful in interactions, and how my self-perceptions needed to be checked against the perceptions of my patients, regardless of diagnosis. I subsequently enjoyed mental health as a career choice, which spanned more than 30 years. I worked with many different clinical populations over the years, but I still remember my stress and distress over my first patient and how it made me blind to what was really going on.

entries can also be shared with health care providers to help plan interventions.

Stress Management in the Workplace. Rapid changes in health care technology, diversity in the workforce, organizational restructuring, and changing work systems can place stress on nurses (Bauman, O'Brien-Pallas, Armstrong-Sassen, et al., 2001; Manning, Curtis, & McMillen, 1999). Additional causes of job stress include particular job assignments (Box 29-10), challenging schedules, such as two different work shifts within a short period of time, working predominantly night shifts, fear of failure, and inadequate support services (Manning et al., 1999). **Burnout** occurs as a result of chronic stress. Burnout is "a syndrome of emotional exhaustion, depersonalization of others, and perceptions of reduced personal accomplishment, resulting from intense involvement with people in a caregiving environment" (Cuneo, Cooper, Drew, et al., 2011; Gibbons, 2010). This can be reflected in high rates of sick leave, irritability with co-workers, increased risk of errors at work, and increased home stress. Nurses are not immune to maladaptive coping, such as use of alcohol, in response to chronic stress or burnout.

Primary prevention is essential to addressing risk for burnout and is important for all health providers. Personal stress management strategies need to be a part of professional practice; they can include working on crafts, scheduled social outings with friends, participation in a team sport or an individual recreational or physical activity, limiting amount of overtime worked, taking an art class, or reading for pleasure. If nurses recognize feelings of burnout, they can engage in some of the same strategies that help patients: increase their own self-reflections regarding potential sources of stress, use daily journal writing to increase recognition of contextual factors, seek a colleague or mentor to help with their reflections, create an inventory of available personal and support resources, and devise a plan for addressing the various stressors in a manageable and positive manner. An important step is identifying the limits and scope of responsibilities at work (Cuneo et al., 2011; Gibbons, 2010). It is essential that nurses recognize the areas over which they have control and can change and those for which they do not have responsibility.

Acute Care

Crisis Intervention. When stress overwhelms a person's usual coping mechanisms and all available resources must be mobilized, the situation becomes a crisis. A crisis creates a turning point in a person's life because it changes the direction of a person's life in some way. According to Aguilera (1998), the precipitating event usually occurs 1 to 2 weeks before the individual seeks help, but it may have occurred within the past 24 hours. In general, a crisis is resolved in some way within approximately 6 weeks. The aim of crisis intervention is to return the person to a pre-crisis level of functioning and to promote growth (Figure 29-8). The use of unfamiliar strategies can result either in a heightened awareness of previously unrecognized strengths and resources or in deterioration in functioning. Thus, a crisis is often referred to as a situation of both danger and opportunity. Some people or families emerge from a crisis state functioning more effectively, whereas others are weakened, and still others are rendered completely dysfunctional. Although there are a variety of crisis intervention models (Jackson-Cherry & Erford, 2010), Figure 29-8 presents an example of a crisis intervention model that is widely and currently used.

Crisis intervention is a specific type of brief psychotherapy with prescribed steps (Jackson-Cherry & Erford, 2010). Crisis intervention is more directive than traditional psychotherapy or counselling and can be used by any member of the health care team who has been trained in its techniques. The basic approach is problem solving, and the focus is on only the problem presented by the crisis.

When using a crisis intervention approach, the nurse helps the patient make the mental connection between the stressful event and the patient's reaction to it. This is crucial because the patient may be unable to envision the whole situation clearly. The nurse can help the patient become aware of current feelings, such as anger, grief, or guilt, in order to reduce tension. The nurse can also assist the patient in exploring coping mechanisms, perhaps identifying ways of coping that the patient had not thought of. Finally, the nurse may help increase the patient's social contacts if the patient has been internally focused and isolated.

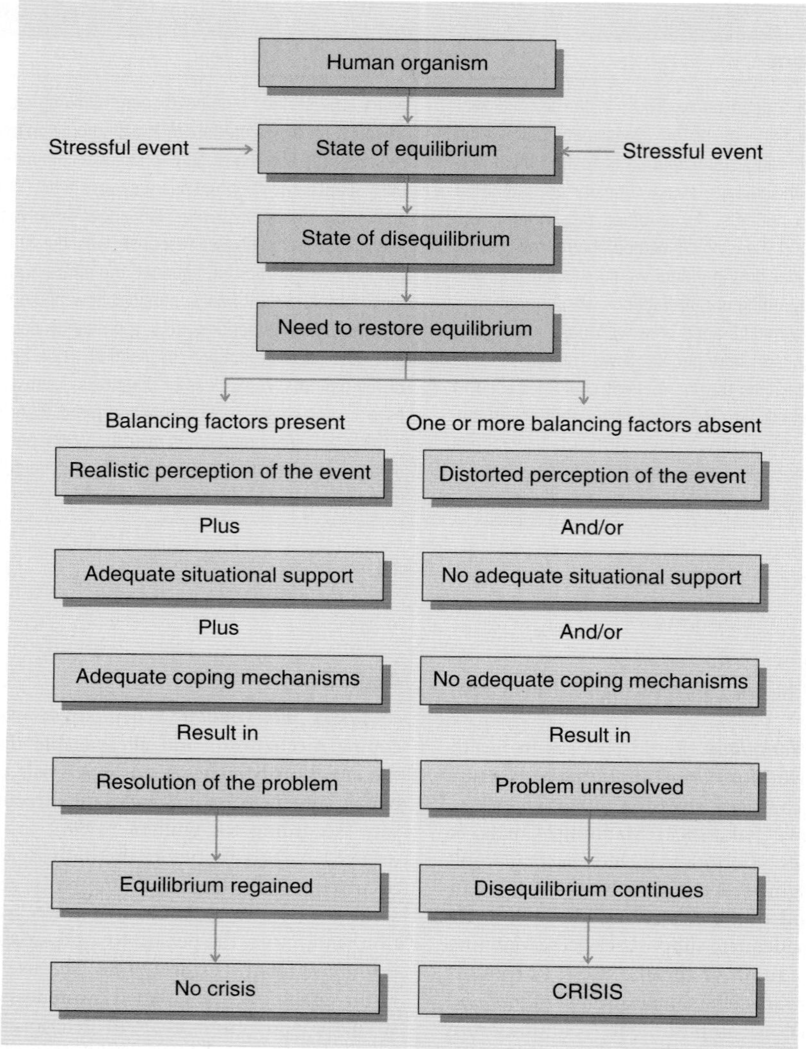

FIGURE 29-8 Crisis intervention model. (Redrawn from Aguilera, D. C. [1998]. *Crisis intervention: Theory and methodology* [8th ed.]. St. Louis, MO: Mosby.)

Restorative and Continuing Care. A person under stress recovers when the stress is removed or coping strategies are successful; however, a person who has experienced a crisis has changed, and the effects may last for years or for the rest of the person's life (Walsh et al., 2011). The final stage of adapting to a crisis is acknowledgement of the long-term implications of the crisis.

◆ Evaluation

Patient Care. By evaluating the goals and expected outcomes of care, the nurse knows whether the nursing interventions were effective and whether the patient is coping with the identified stress. The nurse needs to review the measurable goals and assess whether the patient has met the criteria for success as stated in the outcomes. If the nursing interventions have not been effective in helping the patient achieve targeted goals, the nurse must re-evaluate the strategies implemented and revise the care plan in light of the patient's current health status (Figure 29-9).

To evaluate whether goals and outcomes of care have been achieved, nurses observe patient behaviours and interactions between the patient and family, if appropriate. If the nurse's contact with a patient ends before goals have been achieved, the patient should be referred to appropriate resources so that progress is not delayed or interrupted.

Patient Expectations. It is crucial to maintain ongoing communication with patients in regard to the care plan. Patients under severe stress or trauma often feel powerless and vulnerable. Nurses can help reduce these feelings by actively involving patients and families in assessment, prioritizing, goal setting, and evaluation. Being involved enables patients to direct their energy positively and encourages them to take responsibility for their health. It also facilitates open communication, which makes it easier for the patient to report on interventions that are successful and helps nurses better understand why some interventions fail to meet the patient's goals.

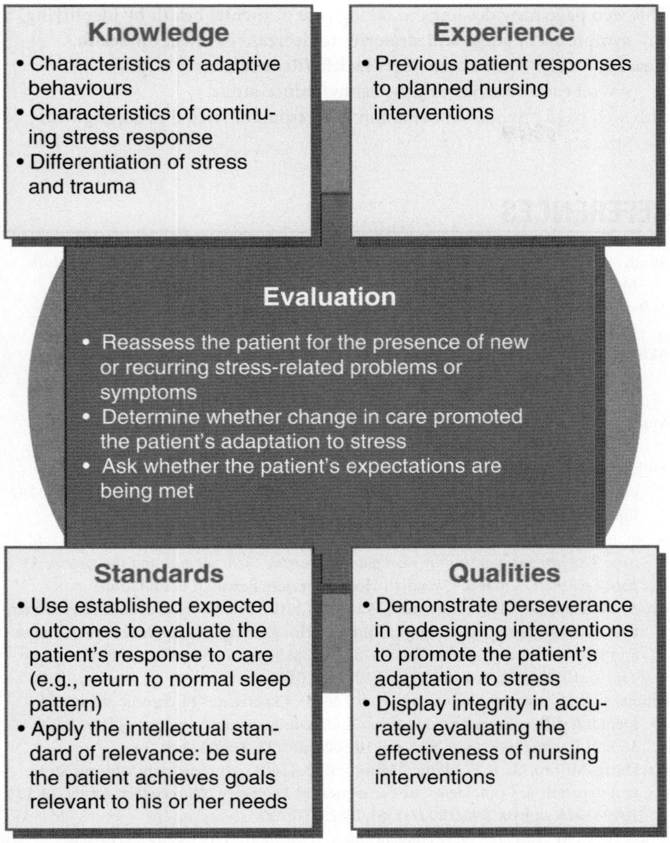

FIGURE 29-9 Critical thinking model for stress and coping evaluation.

KEY CONCEPTS

- Physiological and psychological frameworks have been developed to describe how stress affects biological systems and psychological well-being.
- Overwhelming or chronic stress can increase the risks of (1) serious and long-standing physical and mental health problems; (2) choosing coping strategies that are unhealthy, such as isolating oneself, not getting enough rest or a proper diet, or using tobacco, alcohol, or caffeine; (3) ignoring warning signs of illness; and (4) neglecting to take prescribed medicines or treatments.
- A person is under psychological stress only if the person evaluates the event or circumstance as personally significant. Such an evaluation of an event for its personal meaning is called *primary appraisal.*
- Several types of stressors are work stressors, family stressors, chronic stressors, acute stressors, daily hassles, traumatic events, and crisis.
- Rapid changes in health care technology, diversity in the workforce, organizational redesign, and changing work systems can place nurses at risk for stress-related symptoms and burnout.
- Potential stressors and coping mechanisms vary across the lifespan: from childhood through adolescence, adulthood, and old age.
- Coping is a means of managing psychological stress and reflects a dynamic process in response to the current situation, past experiences, and available resources.
- Three primary modes for stress intervention are to decrease stress-producing situations, increase resistance to stress, and learn skills that reduce physiological response to stress.
- If stress is so severe that the patient is unable to cope in any ways that have worked before, the patient is experiencing a crisis.
- A crisis is a turning point in life and can be developmental or situational.
- In general, a crisis is resolved in some way within approximately 6 weeks. Crisis intervention aims to return the person to a pre-crisis level of functioning and to promote growth.

CRITICAL THINKING EXERCISES

1. You are caring for a 30-year-old woman who has recently had surgery as a first step in her treatment for metastatic breast cancer. She is the lone parent and sole provider for three young children (all younger than 7 years). What additional information do you need to know about the patient to develop a discharge plan? Consider and discuss the various stressors that must be considered when you write an appropriate discharge plan.
2. A patient comes to the primary health care clinic complaining of dizziness, which is not related to any physical findings on examination. During the health history, the patient reports that her life is very stressful and she is barely coping. She finalized her divorce 3 months ago, is working 32 hours per week, and is attending college. Her ex-husband recently lost his job and can no longer pay child support. She tearfully confesses that she thinks she might be pregnant but does not want her ex-husband to know. Develop nursing diagnoses related to this situation.
3. An older man is admitted to the hospital with a fractured hip. Before his injury, he lived with his wife, who has advancing Alzheimer's disease. While he is hospitalized, she is staying with a niece who lives 50 km away, but this cannot be a permanent situation because her niece is also in frail health. The patient has no children who can help when he returns home. He is concerned about who will care for his wife after he is discharged. What approach would be the best to take in establishing goals for treatment?

REVIEW QUESTIONS

1. The vital functions necessary for survival, which include heart rate, blood pressure, and respiration, are controlled by the:
   1. Medulla oblongata
   2. Reticular formation
   3. Pituitary gland
   4. Limbic system
2. While assessing a person for effects of the general adaptation syndrome, the nurse should be aware that:
   1. Heart rate increases in the adaptation state.
   2. Blood volume increases in the exhaustion stage.
   3. Vital signs return to normal in the exhaustion stage.
   4. Blood glucose level increases during the alarm reaction stage.
3. When performing an assessment of a young woman who was in an automobile accident 6 months before, the nurse learns that the woman has vivid images of the crash whenever she hears a loud, sudden noise. The nurse recognizes that these reactions are flashbacks, which are symptoms of:
   1. Social phobia
   2. Acute anxiety
   3. Post-traumatic stress disorder
   4. Borderline personality disorder

4. A man is adjusting to a chronic illness; the chronic illness can be considered:
    1. A sociocultural stressor
    2. A maturational stressor
    3. A situational stressor
    4. An environmental stressor
5. A child who has been in a house fire comes to the emergency department with her parents. The child and parents are upset and tearful. During your first assessment for stress, what should you say?
    1. "Tell me who I can call to help you."
    2. "Tell me what upsets you most about this experience."
    3. "I will contact someone who can help get you temporary housing."
    4. "I will sit with you until other family members can come help you get settled."
6. You are evaluating the coping strategies of a patient experiencing stress from receiving a new diagnosis of multiple sclerosis and psychomotor impairment. You realize that the patient is coping successfully when the patient makes which of the following statements?
    1. "I am going to learn to drive a car so I can be more independent."
    2. "My sister says she feels better when she goes shopping, so I will go shopping."
    3. "I have always felt better when I go for a long walk. I will do that when I get home."
    4. "I am going to attend a support group to learn more about multiple sclerosis and what I will be able to do."
7. The nurse knows that the patient is recovering from the stress of an emergency surgery when the patient makes which of the following statements?
    1. "I am going to change jobs."
    2. "I am learning progressive relaxation training."
    3. "I plan to have plastic surgery while I am here in the hospital."
    4. "I am planning to sell my house and move within the next 6 weeks."
8. A staff nurse is talking with her nursing supervisor about the stress she feels from having transferred to a new inpatient unit. The supervising nurse recognizes that:
    1. Nurses who feel stress usually pass the stress along to their patients.
    2. A nurse who feels stress is ineffective as a nurse and should not be working.
    3. Nurses who talk about feeling stress are unprofessional and should calm down.
    4. Nurses frequently experience stress with the rapid changes in health care technology and organizational restructuring.
9. In general, a person's crisis is resolved in some way within approximately:
    1. 6 weeks
    2. 1 month
    3. 6 months
    4. 2 weeks

Answers: 1. 1; **2.** 4; **3.** 3; **4.** 3; **5.** 2; **6.** 4; **7.** 2; **8.** 4; **9.** 1

Rationales for the Review Questions appear at the end of the book.

RECOMMENDED WEBSITES

Health Canada: Mental Health—Coping With Stress: http://www.hc-sc.gc.ca/hl-vs/iyh-vsv/life-vie/stress-eng.php.

This web page provides links to taking care of mental health by identifying symptoms of stress and strategies to decrease its effect on health.

Heart & Stroke Foundation: Get Healthy/Reduce Stress: https://www.heartandstroke.ca/get-healthy/reduce-stress.

This web page provides information and resources related to coping with stress.

REFERENCES

Aguilera, D. C. (1998). *Crisis intervention: Theory and methodology* (8th ed.). St. Louis, MO: Mosby.

Aldwin, C. M. (2000). *Stress, coping, and development: An integrative perspective.* New York: Guilford Press.

Aldwin, C. M., Sutton, K. J., Chiara, G., et al. (1996). Age differences in stress, coping, and appraisal: Findings from the Normative Aging Study. *Journals of Gerontology, Series B, Psychological Sciences and Social Sciences, 51*(4), P179–P188.

American Psychiatric Association (2013). *Diagnostic and statistical manual of mental disorders* (5th ed.). Washington, DC: Author.

Andersen, S. L., & Teicher, M. H. (2008). Stress, sensitive periods and maturational events in adolescent depression. *Trends in Neuroscience, 31*(4), 183–191. doi:10.1192/bjp.177.2.144.

Bauman, A., O'Brien-Pallas, L., Armstrong-Sassen, M., et al. (2001). *Commitment and care: The benefits of a healthy workplace for nurses, their patients and the system. A policy synthesis.* Ottawa: Canadian Health Services Research Foundation.

Beiser, M., Hamilton, H., Rummens, J. A., et al. (2010). Predictors of emotional problems and physical aggression among children of Hong Kong Chinese, Mainland Chinese and Filipino immigrants to Canada. *Social Psychiatry and Psychiatric Epidemiology, 45*(10), 1011–1021. doi:10.1007/s00127-009-0140-3.

Benoit, A. C., Cotnam, J., Raboud, J., et al. (2016). Experiences of chronic stress and mental health concerns among urban Indigenous women. *Archives of Women's Mental Health, 19*(5), 809–823. doi:10.1007/s00737-016-0622-8.

Blackburn-Munro, G., & Blackburn-Munro, R. E. (2001). Chronic pain, chronic stress and depression: Coincidence or consequence? *Journal of Neuroendocrinology, 13*(12), 1009–1023. doi:10.1046/j.0007-1331.2001.00727.x.

Bulechek, G. M., Butcher, H. K., Dochterman, J. M., et al. (Eds.), (2013). *Nursing interventions classification (NIC)* (6th ed.). St. Louis, MO: Mosby.

Breslau, N., & Kessler, R. C. (2001). The stressor criterion in *DSM-IV* posttraumatic stress disorder: An empirical investigation. *Biological Psychiatry, 50*(9), 699–704. doi:10.1016/S0006-3223(01)01167-2.

Brunello, N., Davidson, J. R., Deahl, M., et al. (2001). Posttraumatic stress disorder: Diagnosis and epidemiology, comorbidity and social consequences, biology and treatment. *Neuropsychobiology, 43*(3), 150–162. doi:10.1159/000054884.

Butcher, S. K., & Lord, J. M. (2004). Stress responses and innate immunity: Aging as a contributing factor. *Aging Cell, 3*(4), 151–160. doi:10.1111/j.1474-9728.2004.00103.x.

Caplan, G. (1981). Mastery of stress: Psychosocial aspects. *American Journal of Psychiatry, 138*(4), 413–420. doi:10.1176/ajp.138.4.413.

Chapman, D. P., & Perry, G. S. (2008). Depression as a major component of public health for older adults. *Prevalent Chronic Diseases, 5*(1), A22.

Chrousos, G. P., Loriaux, L., & Gold, P. W. (1988). The concept of stress and its historical development. In G. P. Chrousos, L. Loriaux, & P. W. Gold (Eds.), *Mechanisms of physical and emotional stress* (pp. 3–10). New York: Plenum Press.

Cuneo, C. L., Cooper, C., Drew, C. S., et al. (2011). The effect of Reiki on work-related stress of a registered nurse. *Journal of Holistic Nursing, 29*(1), 33–43. doi:10.1177/0898010110377294.

Davis, M. C., Matthews, K. A., & Twamley, E. W. (1999). Is life more difficult on Mars or Venus? A meta-analytic review of sex differences in major and minor life events. *Annals of Behavioral Medicine, 21*(1), 83–97. doi:10.1007/BF02895038.

Desbonnet, L., Garrett, L., Daly, E., et al. (2008). Sexually dimorphic effects of maternal separation stress on corticotrophin releasing factor and vasopressin systems in the adult rat brain. *International Journal of Developmental Neuroscience, 26*(3–4), 259–268. doi:10.1016/j.ijdevneu.2008.02.004.

Dunn, A. J. (1989). CRF as mediator of stress responses. Neurochemical and behavioral aspects. In L. Bueno, S. Collins, & J.-L. Junien (Eds.), *Stress and digestive motility* (pp. 13–22). London: John Libbey.

Engelmann, M., & Ludwig, M. (2004). The activity of the hypothalamo-neurohypophysial system in response to acute stressor exposure: Neuroendocrine and electrophysiological observations. *Stress (Amsterdam, Netherlands), 7*(2), 91–96. doi:10.1080/10253890410001677240.

Etters, L., Goodall, D., & Harrison, B. E. (2008). Caregiver burden among dementia patient caregivers: A review of the literature. *Journal of the Academy of Nurse Practitioners, 20*(8), 423–428. doi:10.1111/j.1745-7599.2008.00342.x.

Forbes, D., Creamer, M., Bisson, J. I., et al. (2010). A guide to guidelines for the treatment of PTSD and related conditions. *Journal of Traumatic Stress, 23*(5), 537–552. doi:10.1002/jts.20565.

Foster, J. (1997). Successful coping, adaptation and resilience in the elderly: An interpretation of epidemiological data. *Psychiatric Quarterly*, *68*(3), 189–219. doi: 10.1023/A:1025432106406.

Gibbons, C. (2010). Stress, coping and burn-out in nursing students. *International Journal of Nursing Studies*, *47*(10), 1299–1309. doi:10.1016/j.ijnurstu.2010.02.015.

Graham, J. E., Christian, L. M., & Kiecolt-Glaser, J. K. (2006). Stress, age, and immune function: Towards a lifespan approach. *Journal of Behavioral Medicine*, *29*(4), 389–400. doi:10.1007/s10865-006-9057-4.

Halter, M. J., Pollard, C. L., Ray, S. L., et al. (Eds.), (2014). *Varcarolis's Canadian Psychiatric Mental Health Nursing: A clinical approach*. Toronto: Elsevier.

Hume, C., Timperio, A., Veitch, J., et al. (2011). Physical activity, sedentary behaviour, and depressive symptoms among adolescents. *Journal of Physical Activity and Health*, *8*(2), 152–156.

Jackson-Cherry, L. R., & Erford, B. T. (2010). *Crisis intervention and prevention*. Englewood Cliffs, NJ: Pearson Education, Inc.

Kageyama, K., Tamasawa, N., & Suda, T. (2011). Signal transduction in the hypothalamic corticotrophin-releasing factor system and its clinical implications. *Stress (Amsterdam, Netherlands)*, *14*(4), 357–367. doi:10.3109/10253890.2010.536279.

Kasl, S. V. (1992). Stress and health among the elderly: An overview of issues. In M. Wykle, E. Kahava, & J. Kowal (Eds.), *Stress and health among the elderly* (pp. 5–35). New York: Springer.

Kimerling, R., Clum, G. A., & Wolfe, J. (2000). Relationships among trauma exposure, chronic posttraumatic stress disorder symptoms, and self-reported health in women: Replication and extension. *Journal of Trauma Stress*, *13*(1), 115–128. doi: 10.1023/A:1007729116133.

Lazarus, R. (1999). *Stress and emotion: A new synthesis*. New York: Springer.

Le Moal, M. (2007). Historical approach and evolution of the stress concept: A personal account. *Psychoneuroendocrinology*, *32*(Suppl. 1), S3–S9. doi:10.1016/j.psyneuen.2007.03.019.

Liu, R. T., & Alloy, L. B. (2010). Stress generation in depression: A systematic review of the empirical literature and recommendations for future study. *Clinical Psychology Reviews*, *30*(5), 582–593.

Lupien, S. J., Fiocco, A., Wan, N., et al. (2005). Stress hormones and human memory function across the lifespan. *Psychoneuroendocrinology*, *30*(3), 225–242. doi:10.1016/j.psyneuen.2004.08.003.

Magri, F., Cravello, L., Barili, L., et al. (2006). Stress and dementia: The role of the hypothalamic–pituitary–adrenal axis. *Aging Clinical and Experimental Research*, *18*(2), 167–170.

Manning, G., Curtis, K., & McMillen, S. (1999). *Stress: Living and working in a changing world*. Duluth, MN: Whole Person Associates.

Matthews, K. A., Gump, B. B., & Owens, J. F. (2001). Chronic stress influences cardiovascular and neuroendocrine responses during acute stress and recovery, especially in men. *Health Psychology*, *20*(6), 403–410. doi:10.1037/0278-6133.20.6.403.

McEwen, B. (2007). Physiology and neurobiology of stress and adaptation: Central role of the brain. *Physiology Reviews*, *87*(3), 873–904. doi:10.1152/physrev.00041.2006.

Merluzzi, T. V., Philip, E. J., Vachon, D. O., et al. (2011). Assessment of self-efficacy for caregiving: The critical role of self-care in caregiver stress and burden. *Palliative Support Care*, *9*(1), 15–24. doi:10.1017/S1478951510000507.

Mollica, R. F., Sarajlic, N., Chernoff, M., et al. (2001). Longitudinal study of psychiatric symptoms, disability, mortality, and emigration among Bosnian refugees. *JAMA: Journal of the American Medical Association*, *286*(5), 546–554. doi:10.1001/jama.286.5.546.

Monat, A., & Lazarus, R. (1991). *Stress and coping: An anthology*. New York: Columbia University Press.

Moorhead, S., Johnson, M., & Maas, M. (Eds.), (2008). *Nursing outcomes classification (NOC)* (4th ed.). St. Louis, MO: Mosby.

Neuman, B. (1995). *The Neuman systems model* (3rd ed.). Stamford, CT: Appleton & Lange.

Nosek, M., Kennedy, H. P., Beyene, Y., et al. (2010). The effects of perceived stress and attitudes toward menopause and aging on symptoms of menopause. *Journal of Midwifery and Women's Health*, *55*(4), 328–334. doi:10.1016/j.jmwh.2009.09.005.

Olff, M., Langeland, W., Witteveen, A., et al. (2010). A psychobiological rationale for oxytocin in the treatment of posttraumatic stress disorder. *CNS Spectrums*, *15*(8), 522–530.

Pender, N. J., Murdaugh, C., & Parsons, M. A. (2002). *Health promotion in nursing practice* (4th ed.). Upper Saddle River, NJ: Haworth Press.

Penning, M. J., & Wu, Z. (2016). Caregiver stress and mental health: Impact of caregiving relationship and gender. *The Gerontologist*, *58*(6), 1102–1113. doi:10.1093/geront/gnv038.

Roy, A. (2014). Intergenerational trauma and Aboriginal Women: Implications for mental health during pregnancy. *First Peoples Child and Family Review*, *9*(1), 8–21.

Selye, H. (1974). *Stress without distress*. New York: J. B. Lippincott.

Selye, H. (1991). History and present status of the stress concept. In A. Monat & R. Lazarus (Eds.), *Stress and coping: An anthology* (pp. 21–35). New York: Columbia University Press.

Shen, B. J., & Takeuchi, D. T. (2001). A structural model of acculturation and mental health status among Chinese Americans. *American Journal of Community Psychology*, *29*(3), 387–418. doi:10.1023/A:1010338413293.

Skultety, K. M., & Rodriguez, R. L. (2008). Treating geriatric depression in primary care. *Current Psychiatry Reports*, *10*(1), 44–50. doi:10.1007/s11920-008-0009-2.

Solomon, P., & Draine, J. (1995). Adaptive coping among family members of persons with serious mental illness. *Psychiatric Services*, *46*(11), 1156–1160. doi:10.1176/ps.46.11.1156.

Sotero, M. (2006). A conceptual model of historical trauma: implications for public health practice and research. *Journal of Health Disparities Research and Practice*, *1*(1), 93–108.

Statistics Canada (2009). *General Social Survey, 2007: Cycle 21—Family, Social Support, and Retirement Main Survey Questionnaire*. Ottawa: Author.

Stuart, G., & Wright, L. (1995). Applying the Neuman systems model to psychiatric nursing practice. In B. Neuman (Ed.), *The Neuman systems model* (3rd ed.). Norwalk, CT: Appleton & Lange.

Taylor, S. E. (2006). Tend and befriend: Biobehavioral bases of affiliation under stress. *Current Directions in Psychological Science*, *15*(6), 273–277.

Tedeschi, R. G., & Calhoun, L. G. (2004). Post-traumatic growth: Conceptual foundations and empirical evidence. *Psychological Inquiry*, *15*(1), 1–18. doi:10.1207/s15327965pli1501_01.

Van Ameringen, M., Mancini, C., Patterson, B., et al. (2008). Post-traumatic stress disorder in Canada. *CNS Neuroscience & Therapeutics*, *14*(3), 171–181. doi:10.1111/j.1755-5949.2008.00049.

Walsh, N. P., Gleeson, M., Shephard, R. J., et al. (2011). Position statement. Part one: Immune function and exercise. *Exercise Immunology Review*, *17*, 6–63.

Wendt, S., Tuckey, M. R., & Prosser, B. (2011). Thriving, not just surviving, in emotionally demanding fields of practice. *Health and Social Care in the Community*, *19*(3), 317–325. doi:10.1111/j.1365-2524.2010.00983.x.

Yayou, K., Nakamura, M., & Ito, S. (2009). Effects of AVP V1a and CRH receptor antagonist on psychological stress responses to frustrating condition in sheep. *Journal of Veterinary Medical Science*, *71*(4), 431–439. doi:10.1292/jvms.71.431.

30

Vital Signs

Written by Tracy Stephen, RN, MN

OBJECTIVES

Mastery of content in this chapter will enable you to:

- Define the key terms listed.
- Explain the principles and mechanisms of thermoregulation.
- Describe nursing measures that promote heat loss and heat conservation.
- Discuss physiological changes associated with fever.
- Accurately assess temperature via multiple routes: tympanic, oral, temporal, rectal, and axillary.
- Accurately assess pulse, respirations, oxygen saturation, and blood pressure.
- Explain the physiology of normal regulation of blood pressure, pulse, oxygen saturation, and respirations.
- Describe factors that cause variations in body temperature, pulse, oxygen saturation, respirations, and blood pressure.
- Describe ethnic variations in blood pressure.
- Identify ranges of acceptable vital sign values for an infant, a child, and an adult.
- Explain variations in technique used to assess an infant's, a child's, and an adult's vital signs.
- Describe the benefits and precautions involving self-measurement of blood pressure.
- Identify when vital signs should be measured.
- Accurately record and report vital sign measurements.
- Appropriately delegate vital sign measurement to unregulated care providers.

KEY TERMS

Afebrile, p. 530
Antipyretics, p. 541
Auscultatory gap, p. 566
Basal metabolic rate (BMR), p. 528
Blood pressure, p. 557
Bradycardia, p. 547
Cardiac output, p. 542
Celsius, p. 532
Conduction, p. 529
Convection, p. 529
Core temperature, p. 528
Diaphoresis, p. 529
Diastolic (blood pressure), p. 557
Diffusion, p. 549
Dysrhythmia, p. 548
Eupnea, p. 549
Evaporation, p. 529
Febrile, p. 530
Fever, p. 530
Fever of unknown origin, p. 531
Frostbite, p. 531
Heat exhaustion, p. 531
Heatstroke, p. 531
Hematocrit, p. 557
Hypertension, p. 557
Hyperthermia, p. 531
Hypotension, p. 559
Hypothalamus, p. 528
Hypothermia, p. 531
Hypoxemia, p. 549
Malignant hyperthermia, p. 531
Masked hypertension, p. 559
Nonshivering thermogenesis, p. 529
Orthostatic hypotension, p. 560
Perfusion, p. 549
Postural hypotension, p. 560
Pulse deficit, p. 548
Pulse oximeter, p. 553
Pulse pressure, p. 557
Pyrexia, p. 530
Pyrogens, p. 530
Radial pulse, p. 542
Radiation, p. 529
Shivering, p. 528
Sphygmomanometer, p. 560
Stroke volume, p. 542
Systolic (blood pressure), p. 557
Tachycardia, p. 547
Thermoregulation, p. 528
Tidal volume, p. 549
Ventilation, p. 549
Vital signs (VS), p. 527
White coat hypertension, p. 559

ⓔ MEDIA RESOURCES

http://evolve.elsevier.com/Canada/Potter/fundamentals/

- Audio Chapter Summaries
- Examination Review Questions
- Concept Map Creator
- Case Study with Questions
- Audio Glossary
- Content Updates
- Video Clips

The most frequent measurements obtained by health care providers are those of temperature, pulse, blood pressure, respiratory rate, and oxygen saturation. These measurements indicate the effectiveness of circulatory, respiratory, neural, and endocrine body functions. Because of their importance, they are referred to as **vital signs (VS)**. Many factors such as pain, environmental temperature, physical state, activities, or illness can cause vital signs to change, sometimes to values outside an acceptable range. Recently, pain has been referred to as the "fifth vital sign," demonstrating the importance of its assessment not only as a factor that influences the standard vital signs but as an indicator of the necessity to ensure the inclusion of its assessment as part of baseline data (see Chapter 31 for further information about pain assessment).

Vital signs provide important data to determine the usual state of health (baseline data). A change in vital signs indicates a change in physiological function, which may signal the need for medical or nursing intervention. Measuring vital signs is a quick and efficient way of monitoring a patient's condition, identifying problems, or evaluating responses to interventions. With knowledge of the physiological variables influencing vital signs and recognition of the relationship of vital signs changes to other physical assessment findings, precise determinations of health are made. Inspection, palpation, and auscultation are used to determine vital signs. These simple skills should not be taken for granted. Careful measurement techniques ensure accurate and consistent findings. Vital signs and other physiological measurements are the basis for clinical problem solving.

GUIDELINES FOR MEASURING VITAL SIGNS

Vital signs are an important part of all assessments. Data are obtained during a complete physical assessment (see Chapter 32 for further information about conducting a physical assessment) and as needed to assess a patient's condition. Vital sign measurements during a routine physical examination provide a baseline for future assessments. The patient's needs and condition determine when, where, how, and by whom vital signs are measured. The nurse must measure vital signs correctly or delegate their measurement appropriately. Values must be understood, and knowledge of the person's developmental stage and functioning over the lifespan is vital to correct interpretation (Canadian Association of Schools of Nursing [CASN], 2015). Then findings must be communicated appropriately and interventions begun as needed. Often the prioritization of interventions can be determined in part by vital signs, using the acronym ABC, which stands for airway, breathing, and circulation. Box 30-1 lists acceptable adult values.

Use the following guidelines to incorporate vital sign measurement into your nursing practice:

- Unregulated care providers may measure selected vital signs (i.e., in stable patients), and then the nurse responsible for the patient may interpret and act on these measurements.
- Use equipment that is functional and appropriate for the size and age of the patient to ensure accurate findings (e.g., an oral thermometer is not appropriate for use in an infant).
- Select equipment on the basis of the patient's condition and characteristics (e.g., an adult-size blood pressure cuff should not be used for a child).
- Minimize environmental factors that may affect vital signs (e.g., assessing the patient's temperature in a warm, humid room may yield a value that is not a true indicator of the patient's condition).
- Use an organized, step-by-step approach to ensure accuracy.
- Approach the patient in a calm, caring manner while demonstrating proficiency in handling supplies needed for vital sign measurement. The manner of approach can alter vital signs.
- Follow guidelines cited in Box 30-2 to decide frequency of vital sign assessment. Increase the frequency of vital sign assessment if the patient's condition warrants it (i.e., frequency of vital signs ordered by the prescribing health care provider is the *minimum* number of times that they should be checked).
- Use vital sign measurements to determine indications for prescribed medication administration (e.g., certain cardiac medications are given only if pulse or blood pressure values are in a certain range; antipyretics are administered only when temperature is elevated outside the acceptable range for the patient).
- Analyze the results of vital sign measurement by considering the patient's usual values, medical history, therapies, and prescribed medications. A patient's usual values may differ from the acceptable range for that age or physical state. Some illnesses or treatments cause predictable changes in vital signs. Some medications affect

BOX 30-1 Vital Signs: Acceptable Readings for Adults

Temperature Range: 36°C to 38°C*

Average oral/tympanic/temporal: 37°C
Average rectal: 37.5°C
Average axillary: 36.5°C

Pulse

60–100 beats per minute

Respirations

10–20 breaths per minute

Blood Pressure

Systolic: 120–139 mm Hg
Diastolic: 80–89 mm Hg
Pulse pressure: 30–50 mm Hg

*Hooper, V., Chard, R., Clifford, T., et al. (2009). ASPAN's evidence-based clinical practice guideline for the promotion of perioperative normothermia. *Journal of Perianesthesia Nursing, 24*(5), 271–287.

BOX 30-2 When to Measure Vital Signs

Upon admission to a health care facility
During a home care visit
According to the prescribing health care provider's order or the health facility's standards of practice
Before, during, and after a surgical procedure or an invasive diagnostic procedure
Before, during, and after the administration of blood products
Before, during, and after administration of medications that affect cardiovascular, respiratory, and temperature-control function
When patient's general physical condition changes (e.g., loss of consciousness or increased pain)
Before and after nursing interventions that affect a vital sign (e.g., before a patient previously on bed rest ambulates or before a patient performs range-of-motion exercises)
When a patient reports nonspecific symptoms of physical distress (e.g., feeling "funny" or "different")
Before a patient is sent home on a day or weekend pass and when the person returns to the floor

one or more vital signs. The nurse is often in the best position to assess all clinical findings about a patient and must be knowledgeable of related physical signs or symptoms and the patient's ongoing health status.

- Baseline measurements allow the identification of changes in vital signs. When vital signs appear abnormal, it is useful to have another nurse repeat the measurement. Verify, document, and communicate significant changes in vital signs to the prescribing health care provider or nurse in charge.
- Involve the patient and/or caregiver in vital sign assessment and the significance of findings through implementation of teaching plans as necessary.

BODY TEMPERATURE

Physiology

Body temperature is the difference between the amount of heat produced by body processes and the amount lost to the external environment. Despite extremes in environmental conditions and physical activity, temperature-control mechanisms keep the body's core temperature (temperature of structures deep within the body) relatively constant (Figure 30-1), whereas body surface temperature fluctuates, depending on blood flow to the skin and the amount of heat lost to the external environment. Because of these surface temperature fluctuations, acceptable body temperature ranges from 36°C to 38°C, a narrow range in which the body's tissues and cells function best.

The measurement of body temperature is aimed at obtaining an average temperature of core body tissues. Sites reflecting core temperatures are more reliable indicators of body temperature than are sites reflecting surface temperatures (Box 30-3). The temperature value

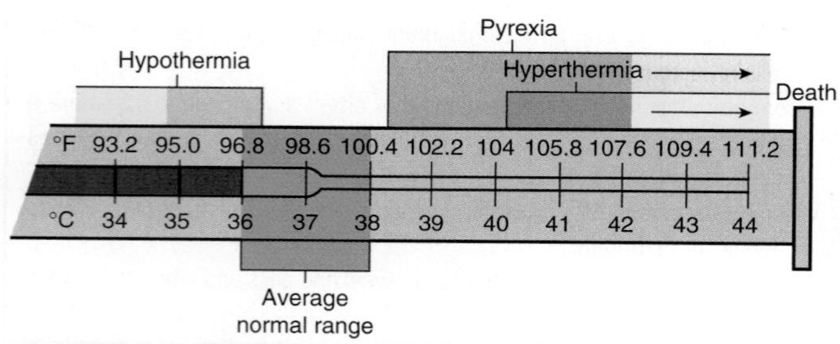

FIGURE 30-1 Ranges of normal temperature values and physiological consequences of abnormal body temperature.

BOX 30-3 Sites of Measurement of Core and Surface Temperature

Core Temperature
Rectum
Tympanic membrane
Temporal artery
Esophagus
Pulmonary artery
Urinary bladder

Surface Temperature
Skin
Mouth
Axillae

obtained may also differ between one measurement site and another. In clinical practice, nurses learn the temperature range of individual patients, recognizing that no single temperature reading is normal for all people.

Regulation. The balance between heat lost and heat produced, or thermoregulation, is precisely regulated by physiological and behavioural mechanisms. For body temperature to stay constant and within an acceptable range, the relationship between heat production and heat loss must be closely maintained. This relationship is regulated by neurological and cardiovascular mechanisms. To regulate patients' temperatures, knowledge of temperature-control mechanisms is applied.

Neural and Vascular Control. The hypothalamus, located between the cerebral hemispheres, controls body temperature the same way that a thermostat works in a building. A comfortable temperature is the *set point* at which a heating system operates. In the building, a decrease in environmental temperature activates the furnace, whereas a rise in temperature shuts the system down. The hypothalamus is like the building's furnace; it senses minor changes in body temperature. The anterior hypothalamus controls heat loss, and the posterior hypothalamus controls heat production.

When nerve cells in the anterior hypothalamus become heated above the set point, impulses are sent to reduce body temperature. Mechanisms of heat loss include sweating, vasodilation (widening) of blood vessels, and inhibition of heat production. Blood is redistributed to surface vessels to promote heat loss. If the posterior hypothalamus senses that the body's temperature is lower than the set point, heat conservation mechanisms are instituted: vasoconstriction (narrowing) of blood vessels reduces blood flow to the skin and extremities. Compensatory heat is produced through voluntary muscle contraction and muscle shivering. When vasoconstriction is ineffective in preventing additional heat loss, shivering begins. Disease or trauma to the hypothalamus or to the spinal cord, which carries hypothalamic messages, can cause serious alterations in temperature control.

Heat Production. Thermoregulation depends on the normal function of heat production processes. Heat is produced in the body as a by-product of metabolism, the chemical reaction in all body cells. Food is the primary fuel source for metabolism. Activities requiring additional chemical reactions increase metabolic rate. As metabolism increases, additional heat is produced. When metabolism decreases, less heat is produced. Heat production occurs during rest, voluntary movements, involuntary shivering, and nonshivering thermogenesis.

Basal metabolism accounts for the heat produced by the body at absolute rest. The average basal metabolic rate (BMR) depends on the body surface area. Thyroid hormones also affect the BMR. By promoting the breakdown of body glucose and fat, thyroid hormones increase the rate of chemical reactions in almost all cells of the body. When large amounts of thyroid hormones are secreted, the BMR can increase 100% above normal. Absence of thyroid hormones can reduce the BMR by half, causing a decrease in heat production. The male sex hormone testosterone increases BMR. Men have a higher BMR than do women. Voluntary movements such as muscular activity during exercise require additional energy. Metabolic rates can increase up to 2 000 times normal during exercise. Heat production can increase up to 50 times normal.

Shivering is an involuntary body response to temperature differences in the body. The skeletal muscle movement during shivering requires significant energy. In vulnerable patients, shivering can seriously deplete energy sources, which results in further physiological deterioration. Shivering can increase heat production four to five times greater than normal. The heat produced assists in equalizing body temperature, and shivering ceases. Newborns and older persons are less able to generate heat by shivering or preserve heat by vasoconstriction, putting them at an increased risk for hypothermia (Cheshire, 2016, p. 97).

Nonshivering thermogenesis occurs primarily in newborns and is the main source of heat generation due to their inability to shiver. Sympathetic nerve endings secrete norepinephrine in response to chilling, which stimulates fat metabolism in the richly vascularized brown adipose tissue to produce internal heat that is conducted to surface tissues through the blood (Hockenberry & Wilson, 2015, p. 341).

Heat Loss. Heat loss and heat production occur simultaneously. The skin's structure and exposure to the environment result in constant, normal heat loss through radiation, conduction, convection, and evaporation.

Radiation is the transfer of heat from the surface of one object to the surface of another without direct contact between the two. Up to 85% of the human body's surface area radiates heat to the environment. Peripheral vasodilation increases blood flow from internal organs to the skin to increase radiant heat loss. Peripheral vasoconstriction minimizes radiant heat loss. Radiation increases as the temperature difference between the objects increases. If the environment is warmer than the skin, the body absorbs heat through radiation.

Heat loss is increased through radiation by removing clothing or blankets. The patient's position enhances radiation heat loss (e.g., standing exposes a greater radiating surface area, and lying in a fetal position minimizes heat radiation). Covering the body with dark, closely woven clothing also reduces the amount of heat lost from radiation.

Conduction is the transfer of heat from one object to another through direct contact. Heat is conducted through contact with solids, liquids, and gases. When warm skin touches a cooler object, heat is lost. Conduction normally accounts for a small amount of heat loss. Interventions such as applying a cool cloth increase conductive heat loss. Applying several layers of clothing reduces conductive loss. The body gains heat by conduction when contact is made with materials warmer than skin temperature (e.g., application of an aquathermia pad).

Convection is the transfer of heat away from the body by air movement. A fan promotes heat loss through convection. Convective heat loss increases when moistened skin comes into contact with slightly moving air.

Evaporation is the transfer of heat energy when a liquid is changed to a gas. The body continuously loses heat by evaporation. About 600 to 900 mL per day evaporates from the skin and lungs, resulting in water and heat loss. By regulating perspiration (sweating), the body promotes additional evaporative heat loss. Millions of sweat glands located in the dermis of the skin secrete sweat through tiny ducts on the skin's surface. When body temperature rises, the anterior hypothalamus signals the sweat glands to release sweat. Sweat evaporates from the skin surface, which results in heat loss. During exercise and emotional or mental stress, sweating is one way to lose excessive heat produced by the increased metabolic rate.

Diaphoresis is visible perspiration, which occurs primarily on the forehead and upper thorax, although it can be seen elsewhere on the body. Excessive evaporation can cause skin scaling and itching, as well as drying of the nares and pharynx. Lowered body temperature inhibits sweat gland secretion. People who have a congenital absence of sweat glands or a serious skin disease that impairs sweating are unable to tolerate warm temperatures because they cannot cool themselves adequately.

Skin in Temperature Regulation. The skin regulates temperature through insulation of the body, vasoconstriction (which affects the amount of blood flow and heat loss to the skin), and temperature sensation. The skin, subcutaneous tissue, and fat keep heat inside the body. When blood flow between skin layers is reduced, the skin alone is an excellent insulator. People with more body fat have more natural insulation than do slim and muscular people.

In the human body, the internal organs produce heat. During exercise or increased sympathetic stimulation, the amount of heat produced is greater than the usual core temperature. Blood flows from the internal organs, carrying heat to the body surface. The skin is well supplied with blood vessels, especially the areas of the hands, feet, and ears. Blood flow through these vascular areas of skin may vary from minimal flow to as much as 30% of the blood ejected from the heart. Heat transfers from the blood through vessel walls to the skin's surface and is lost to the environment through the heat-loss mechanisms. The body's core temperature remains within safe limits.

The degree of vasoconstriction determines the amount of blood flow and heat loss to the skin. If the core temperature is too high, the hypothalamus inhibits vasoconstriction. As a result, blood vessels dilate, and more blood reaches the skin's surface. On a hot, humid day, the blood vessels in the hands are dilated and easily visible. In contrast, if the core temperature becomes too low, the hypothalamus initiates vasoconstriction and blood flow to the skin lessens, thus conserving body heat.

Behavioural Control. Healthy individuals voluntarily act to maintain a comfortable body temperature when exposed to temperature extremes. A person's ability to control body temperature depends on (1) the degree of temperature extreme, (2) the person's ability to sense feeling comfortable or uncomfortable, (3) thought processes or emotions, and (4) the person's mobility or ability to remove or add clothes. Body temperature control is difficult if any of these abilities is absent. Infants can sense uncomfortably warm conditions but cannot change their environment. Older persons and people with spinal cord injuries may need assistance in detecting cold environments and minimizing heat loss. Illness, altered levels of consciousness, or impaired thought processes result in an inability to recognize the need to change behaviour for temperature control. In extreme temperatures, health-promoting behaviours, such as removing or adding clothing, have a limited effect on controlling temperature. It is important for the nurse to assess for factors that place patients at high risk for ineffective thermoregulation.

Factors Affecting Body Temperature

Many factors affect body temperature. Changes in body temperature within an acceptable range occur when the relationship between heat production and heat loss is altered by physiological or behavioural variables. Nurses need to be aware of these factors when assessing temperature variations and evaluating deviations from normal.

Age. At birth, the newborn leaves a warm, relatively constant environment and enters one in which temperatures fluctuate widely. Temperature-control mechanisms are immature. An infant's temperature may respond dramatically to changes in the environment, requiring extra care to protect the newborn. Body coverings must be adequate, and exposure to temperature extremes must be avoided. A newborn loses up to 30% of body heat through the head and thus needs to wear a cap to prevent heat loss. When protected from environmental extremes, the newborn's core and peripheral body temperature can be normally maintained between 36.5°C and 37.6°C.

Temperature regulation is unstable until children reach puberty. The normal temperature range gradually drops as individuals approach older adulthood. Older persons have a lower and narrower range of body temperatures than do younger adults. An oral temperature of 35°C is not unusual for older persons in cold weather. However, the average body temperature of older persons is approximately 36°C.

Older persons are particularly sensitive to temperature extremes because of deterioration in control mechanisms, particularly poor vasomotor control (control of vasoconstriction and vasodilation), reduced amounts of subcutaneous tissue, reduced sweat gland activity, and reduced metabolism.

Exercise. Muscle activity requires increases in blood supply and in carbohydrate and fat breakdown. This increased metabolism causes an increase in heat production. Any form of exercise can increase heat production and thus body temperature. Prolonged strenuous exercise, such as long-distance running, can temporarily raise body temperatures up to 41°C.

Hormone Level. Women generally experience greater fluctuations in body temperature than men. Hormonal variations in progesterone during the menstrual cycle cause body temperature fluctuations. When progesterone levels are low, the body temperature is a few tenths of a degree below the baseline level. This lower temperature persists until ovulation occurs. During ovulation, greater amounts of progesterone enter the circulatory system and raise the body temperature to previous baseline levels or higher. These temperature variations can be used to predict a woman's most fertile time to achieve pregnancy.

Body temperature changes also occur during menopause (cessation of menstruation). Menopausal women may experience times of intense body heat and sweating, lasting anywhere from 30 seconds to 5 minutes. Skin temperature may increase intermittently by up to 4°C, which is known as a *hot flash.* These increases in temperature result from the instability of the vasomotor controls for vasodilation and vasoconstriction.

Circadian Rhythm. Body temperature normally changes 0.5°C to 1°C during a 24-hour period. In persons who are awake during the day and sleep during the night, the temperature is usually lowest between 0100 and 0400 hours (Figure 30-2). During the day, body temperature rises steadily, until a maximum temperature value is reached at about 1800 hours, and then declines back down to early morning levels. It takes 1 to 3 weeks for temperature patterns to reverse in people who work at night and sleep during the day. In general, the circadian temperature rhythm does not change with age.

Stress. Physical and emotional stress increases body temperature through hormonal and neural stimulation. These physiological changes increase metabolism, which increases heat production. The patient who is anxious about entering a hospital or undergoing a procedure may register a higher normal temperature.

Environment. Environment influences body temperature. If body temperature is measured in a very warm room, a patient may be unable to regulate body temperature by heat-loss mechanisms, resulting in the elevation of body temperature. If the patient has just been outside in the cold without warm clothing, body temperature may be low because of extensive radiant and conductive heat loss. Infants, older persons, and those with spinal cord injuries are most likely to be affected by environmental temperatures, because their temperature-regulating mechanisms are less efficient. Body temperature often adjusts to the room temperature in people with spinal cord injuries; this is called *poikilothermia*. The degree of poikilothermism depends on the level of injury, with high cervical injuries having a greater loss of ability to regulate temperature (Lewis, Ruff-Dirkson, Heitkemper, et al., 2014, p. 1776).

Temperature Alterations. Body temperatures outside the usual range affect the hypothalamic set point. Such changes can be related to excess heat production, excessive heat loss, minimal heat production, minimal heat loss, or any combination of these alterations. The nature of the change affects the type of clinical problems experienced.

Fever. **Pyrexia**, or **fever**, occurs because heat-loss mechanisms are unable to keep pace with excess heat production; as a result, body temperature rises to an abnormal level. A fever is usually not harmful if it stays below 39°C, and a single temperature reading may not indicate a fever. In addition to physical signs and symptoms of infection, determination of fever is based on several temperature readings at different times of the day that are compared with the usual value for that person at those times.

A true fever results from an alteration in the hypothalamic set point. **Pyrogens** such as bacteria and viruses cause a rise in body temperature. Pyrogens act as antigens, triggering immune system responses. The hypothalamus reacts to raise the set point, and the body responds by producing and conserving heat. Several hours may pass before the body temperature reaches the new set point. During this period, the person experiences chills, shivers, and feels cold, even though the body temperature is rising (Figure 30-3). The chill phase resolves when the new set point, a higher temperature, is achieved. During the next phase, the plateau, the chills subside, and the person feels warm and dry. If the new set point is "overshot" or the pyrogens are removed (e.g., destruction of bacteria by antibiotics), the third phase of a febrile episode occurs. The hypothalamus set point drops, initiating heat loss responses. The skin becomes warm and flushed because of vasodilation. Diaphoresis assists in evaporative heat loss. When the fever "breaks," the person becomes **afebrile.**

Fever is an important defence mechanism. Temperature elevations up to 38°C enhance the body's immune system. During a **febrile** episode, white blood cell production is stimulated. Increased temperature reduces the concentration of iron in the blood plasma, suppressing the growth of bacteria. Fever also fights viral infections by

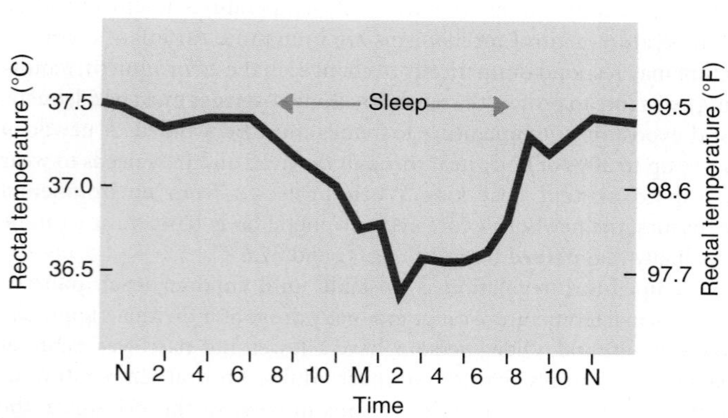

FIGURE 30-2 Temperature cycle for 24 hours.

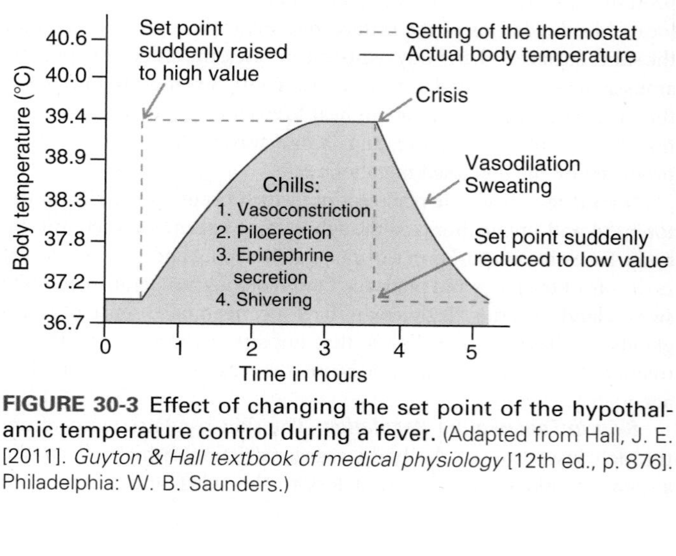

FIGURE 30-3 Effect of changing the set point of the hypothalamic temperature control during a fever. (Adapted from Hall, J. E. [2011]. *Guyton & Hall textbook of medical physiology* [12th ed., p. 876]. Philadelphia: W. B. Saunders.)

stimulating production of interferon, the body's natural virus-fighting substance.

By analyzing a fever pattern, health care providers can make diagnoses. Fever patterns differ, depending on the causative pyrogen. The increase or decrease in pyrogen activity results in fever spikes and declines at different times of the day. The duration and degree of fever depend on the strength of the pyrogen and the ability of the individual to respond. The term fever of unknown origin refers to a fever that does not have a determined cause.

During a fever, cellular metabolism increases and oxygen consumption rises. Heart and respiratory rates increase to meet the increased metabolic needs of the body for nutrients. The increased metabolism entails the use of energy that produces additional heat. If the patient has a cardiac or respiratory problem, the stress of a fever can be great. A prolonged fever can weaken a person by exhausting energy stores. Increased metabolism requires additional oxygen. If the demand for additional oxygen cannot be met, cellular hypoxia (inadequate oxygenation) occurs. Myocardial hypoxia produces angina (chest pain); cerebral hypoxia produces confusion. Interventions during a fever may include oxygen therapy. Water loss through increased respiration and diaphoresis can be excessive, placing a patient at risk for fluid volume deficit. Dehydration is a serious problem for older persons and for children with low body weight. Maintaining optimum fluid volume status is an important nursing intervention (see Chapter 40 for further information about fluid and electrolytes).

Hyperthermia. Hyperthermia is body temperature that is elevated as a result of the body's inability to promote heat loss or reduce heat production. Whereas fever is an upward shift in the set point, hyperthermia results from an overload of the body's thermoregulatory mechanisms. Any disease or trauma to the hypothalamus can impair heat-loss mechanisms. Malignant hyperthermia is an inherited genetic condition that manifests when susceptible individuals are exposed to certain anaesthetics. Once exposed, the individual will rapidly develop hyperthermia along with hemodynamic instability, rigidity, and signs of rhabdomylosis (Heytens, Forget, Scholtès, et al., 2015, p. 508).

Heatstroke. Prolonged exposure to the sun or high environmental temperatures can overwhelm the body's heat-loss mechanisms. Heat also depresses hypothalamic function. These conditions cause heatstroke, a dangerous heat emergency with a high mortality rate. Patients at risk include the very young, older persons, and those who have cardiovascular disease, hypothyroidism, diabetes, spinal cord injury, or alcoholism. Also at risk are patients who take medications that decrease the body's ability to lose heat (e.g., phenothiazines, anticholinergics, diuretics, amphetamines, and β-adrenergic receptor antagonists) and those who exercise or engage in strenuous physical labour (e.g., athletes, construction workers, and farmers).

Signs and symptoms of heatstroke include confusion, delirium, excess thirst, nausea, muscle cramps, visual disturbances, giddiness, and incontinence. The most important sign is hot, dry skin. Patients with heatstroke do not sweat because of severe electrolyte loss and hypothalamic malfunction. Vital signs reveal a body temperature sometimes as high as 45°C, with an increase in heart rate and lowering of blood pressure. If the condition progresses, unconsciousness can occur. Permanent neurological damage may result unless cooling measures are rapidly started.

Heat Exhaustion. Heat exhaustion occurs when profuse diaphoresis results in excessive water and electrolyte loss. The patient exhibits signs and symptoms of fluid volume deficit (see Chapter 40 for further information about fluid and electrolytes). Treatment includes transporting the patient to a cooler environment and restoring fluid and electrolyte balance.

TABLE 30-1 Classification of Hypothermia

Description	Temperature (°C)
Mild	34–36
Moderate	30–34
Severe	<30

Hypothermia. Heat loss during prolonged exposure to cold overwhelms the body's ability to produce heat, causing hypothermia. Hypothermia is classified by core temperature measurements (Table 30-1). It can be unintentionally induced (e.g., by falling through the ice of a frozen lake) or intentionally induced (e.g., during specific surgical procedures) to reduce metabolic demand and the body's need for oxygen. Accidental hypothermia usually develops gradually and may go unnoticed for several hours. When body temperature drops to 35°C, uncontrolled shivering, loss of memory, depression, and poor judgement occur. As the body temperature falls below 34.4°C, heart rate, respiratory rate, and blood pressure fall and the skin becomes cyanotic. If hypothermia progresses, cardiac dysrhythmias, loss of consciousness, and unresponsiveness to painful stimuli occur. In cases of severe hypothermia, clinical signs similar to death (e.g., lack of response to stimuli and extremely slow respirations and pulse) are demonstrated. The assessment of core temperature is critical when hypothermia is suspected. A special thermometer that displays low readings may be required because most standard devices do not register below 35°C.

Frostbite occurs when the body is exposed to subnormal temperatures. Ice crystals forming inside cells can result in permanent circulatory and tissue damage. Areas on the body particularly susceptible to frostbite are the earlobes, tip of the nose, fingers, and toes. The injured area becomes white, waxy, and firm to the touch and loss of sensation occurs in the affected area. Intervention includes gradual warming measures, analgesia, and protection of the injured tissue.

NURSING PROCESS AND THERMOREGULATION

Knowledge of the physiology of body temperature regulation is essential for assessing and evaluating the patient's response to temperature alterations and for intervening safely. Independent measures can be implemented to increase or minimize heat loss, promote heat conservation, and increase comfort. These measures complement the effects of medically ordered therapies. Many measures can be taught to family members, parents of children, and other caregivers.

Assessment

Sites. Core and surface body temperature may be measured at several sites. The core temperatures of the pulmonary artery, esophagus, and urinary bladder are measured in intensive care settings. These measurements require the use of invasive devices placed in body cavities or organs that continuously display readings on an electronic monitor.

Intermittent temperature measurements are obtained invasively from the sites of the mouth, rectum, and tympanic membrane or noninvasively from the axilla and temporal artery sites. Chemically prepared thermometer patches can also be applied to the skin. In order to measure oral, rectal, axillary, and skin temperature, blood circulation at the measurement site must be effective so that the heat of the blood is conducted to the thermometer probe. Tympanic temperature relies on the radiation of body heat to an infrared sensor. Temporal artery thermometers measure the naturally emitted infrared heat from the temporal arterial supply (Allegaert, Casteels, van Gorp, et al., 2014). Because they share the same arterial blood supply as the hypothalamus, tympanic and temporal artery temperature measurements can be considered core temperatures (Purssell, While, & Coomber, 2009).

Correct measuring technique must be used at each site (Skill 30-1) to ensure accurate readings. The temperature obtained varies according to the site used but should remain between 36.0°C and 38.0°C. Rectal temperatures are usually 0.5°C higher than oral temperatures, and axillary temperatures are usually 0.5°C lower than oral temperatures. Each measurement site has advantages and disadvantages (Box 30-4). The rectal site was traditionally chosen because of the close replication of core body temperature but is now less routinely measured given the availability of less invasive and accurate alternative measurement devices such as the temporal thermometer. The safest and most effective site should be chosen for each patient. When possible, the same site should be used when measurements must be repeated.

Thermometers. Two types of thermometers are commonly available for measuring body temperature: electronic and disposable. A third type, the mercury-in-glass thermometer, was once the standard device for the clinical setting. Most municipalities have now prohibited the sale or use of mercury-containing medical devices because of potential toxins associated with mercury spills, in addition to the potential hazards associated with glass breakage during temperature measurement.

Temperature is recorded according to the Celsius scale. Electronic thermometers allow conversion to alternative scales by activating a switch.

Electronic Thermometer. The electronic thermometer consists of a rechargeable battery-powered display unit, a thin wire cord, and a temperature-processing probe covered by a disposable plastic cover

SKILL 30-1 MEASURING BODY TEMPERATURE

Delegation Considerations

The task of measuring temperature can be delegated to unregulated care providers (UCPs). The nurse is responsible for assessing the impact of changes in body temperature; therefore, when the task of measuring temperature is delegated, it is important to *inform the unregulated care provider* about the following:

- The appropriate route and device to measure temperature
- Patient-specific factors that can falsely raise or lower temperature
- Appropriate precautions when positioning the patient
- Frequency of temperature measurement for the patient
- Usual values for patient
- Abnormalities that should be reported to the health care provider

Equipment

- Appropriate thermometer
- Soft tissue or wipe
- Alcohol swabs
- Lubricant (for rectal measurements only)
- Pen and either vital sign flow sheet or documentation form
- Disposable gloves
- Plastic thermometer sleeve or disposable probe cover

PROCEDURE

STEPS	RATIONALE
1. Assess for signs and symptoms of temperature alterations and for factors that influence body temperature.	• Physical signs and symptoms may indicate abnormal temperature. You can accurately assess the nature of variations.
2. Determine previous activity that would interfere with accuracy of temperature measurement. Wait before measuring oral temperature in the following situations: 2 minutes after patient has smoked, 5 minutes after patient has chewed gum, and 20 minutes after patient has ingested hot or cold liquids or foods.	• The oral temperature can be affected by the temperature of the smoke, liquids, or food.
3. Determine appropriate temperature site and device for patient.	• This choice is based on advantages and disadvantages of each site (see Box 30-4) (Mains, Coxall, & Lloyd, 2008). Use a disposable, single-use thermometer for a patient who has isolation precautions.
4. Explain to patient the route by which temperature will be measured and the importance of maintaining proper position until the reading is complete.	• Patients are often curious about measurements and should be cautioned against prematurely removing the thermometer to read results.
5. Perform hand hygiene.	• Hand hygiene reduces transmission of microorganisms between the patient and the nurse.
6. Obtain temperature reading. **A.** Oral temperature measurement with electronic thermometer **(1)** Put on disposable gloves (optional).	• Use of oral probe cover, removed without physical contact, minimizes the need to wear gloves.
(2) Remove thermometer pack from charging unit. Attach oral probe (blue tip) to thermometer unit. Grasp top of probe stem, being careful not to press the ejection button.	• Charging provides battery power. Removal of hand-held unit from base prepares it to measure temperature. Pressing ejection button releases plastic probe cover from tip.

STEPS	RATIONALE
(3) Slide disposable plastic probe cover over thermometer probe until cover locks in place (see Step 6A[3] illustration).	• Soft plastic cover will not break in patient's mouth and it prevents transmission of microorganisms between patients.
(4) Have patient sit or lie in bed. Ask patient to open mouth; gently place thermometer probe under patient's tongue in posterior sublingual pocket lateral to centre of lower jaw (see Step 6A[4] illustration).	• Heat from superficial blood vessels in sublingual pocket produces temperature reading. Temperatures in right and left posterior sublingual pockets are significantly higher than in area under front of tongue.

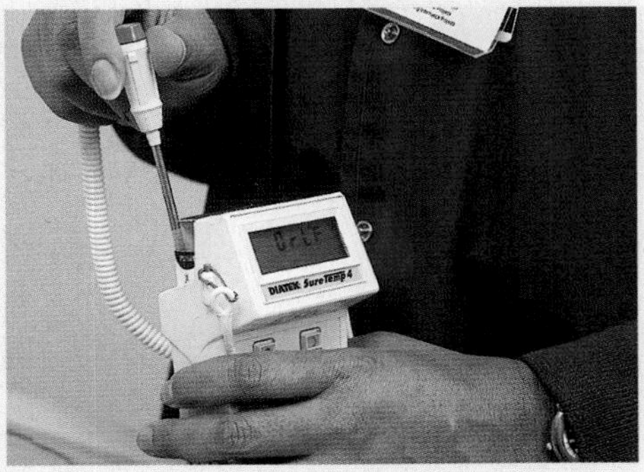

STEP 6A(3) Inserting thermometer stem into plastic probe cover.

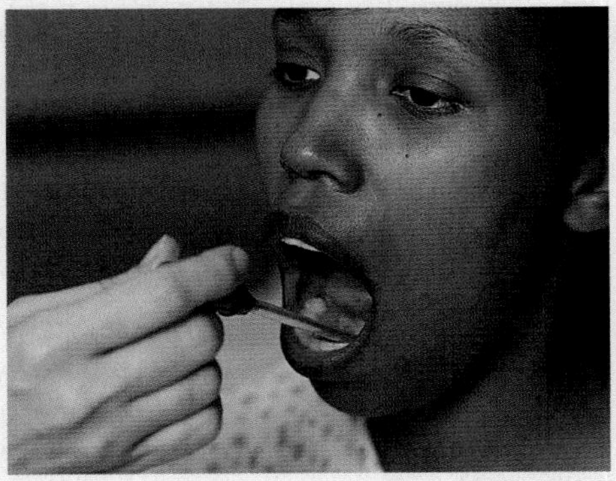

STEP 6A(4) Probe under tongue in posterior sublingual pocket.

STEPS	RATIONALE
(5) Ask patient to hold thermometer probe with lips closed.	• Holding the probe this way helps maintain proper position of thermometer during recording.
(6) Leave thermometer probe in place until audible signal occurs and patient's temperature appears on digital display; remove thermometer probe from under patient's tongue.	• Probe must stay in place until signal occurs, to ensure accurate reading.
(7) Push ejection button on thermometer stem to discard plastic probe cover into appropriate receptacle.	• Discarding probe cover reduces transmission of microorganisms between patients.
(8) Return thermometer stem to storage well of recording unit.	• Proper storage protects probe from damage. Returning probe automatically causes digital reading to disappear.
(9) If gloves were worn, remove and dispose in appropriate receptacle. Perform hand hygiene.	• Glove disposal and hand hygiene reduce transmission of microorganisms between patients.
(10) Return thermometer to charger.	• Charging provides battery power.
B. Rectal temperature measurement with electronic thermometer	
(1) Prepare patient for procedure.	
(a) Draw curtain around patient's bed or close room door, or do both.	
(b) Assist patient in a side-lying or Sims' position with upper leg flexed.	• Provides appropriate access for insertion of rectal probe.
(c) Move aside bed linen to expose only anal area. Keep patient's upper body and lower extremities covered with sheet or blanket.	• These actions maintain patient's privacy, minimize embarrassment, and promote comfort. Anal area is exposed for correct thermometer placement.
(d) Remind patient to remain in position until procedure is complete.	
(2) Put on disposable gloves.	• Gloves help maintain standard precautions during exposure to items soiled with body fluids (e.g., feces).
(3) Remove thermometer pack from charging unit. Attach rectal probe (red tip) to thermometer unit. Grasp top of probe stem, being careful not to press the ejection button.	• Charging provides battery power. Removal of hand-held unit from base prepares it to measure temperature. Pressing the ejection button releases plastic probe cover from tip.
(4) Slide disposable plastic probe cover over thermometer probe until cover locks in place.	• Probe cover prevents transmission of microorganisms between patients.
(5) Squeeze liberal portion of lubricant on tissue. Dip thermometer's blunt end into lubricant, covering 2.5–3.5 cm for adult patient or 1.2–2.5 cm for infant or child.	• Lubrication minimizes trauma to rectal mucosa during thermometer insertion. Tissue avoids contamination of remaining lubricant in container.
(6) With nondominant hand, separate patient's buttocks to expose anus. Ask patient to breathe slowly and relax.	• Separating buttocks fully exposes anus for thermometer insertion. Relaxing anal sphincter facilitates thermometer insertion.
(7) Gently insert thermometer into patient's anus in direction of umbilicus, 3.5 cm for adult patient. Do not force thermometer.	• Insertion in this direction ensures adequate exposure against blood vessels in rectal wall.
(8) If resistance is felt during insertion, withdraw thermometer.	• This action prevents trauma to mucosa.

CRITICAL DECISION POINT: *If thermometer cannot be adequately inserted into rectum, remove thermometer and consider alternative method for obtaining temperature.*

Continued

SKILL 30-1 MEASURING BODY TEMPERATURE—cont'd

STEPS	RATIONALE
(9) Once positioned, thermometer probe should be left in place (see Step 6B[9] illustration) until audible signal occurs and patient's temperature appears on digital display; remove thermometer probe from anus.	• Probe must stay in place until signal occurs, to ensure accurate reading.

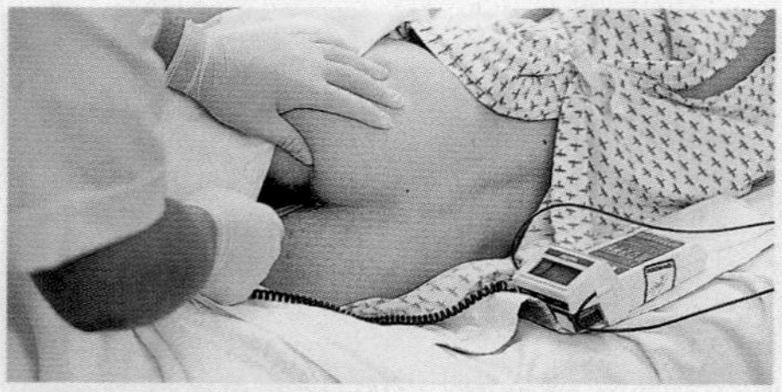

STEP 6B(9) Probe positioned in anus.

STEPS	RATIONALE
(10) Push ejection button on thermometer stem to discard plastic probe cover into appropriate receptacle. Wipe probe adequately with alcohol swab, paying particular attention to ridges where probe cover is connected to probe.	• Discarding probe cover reduces transmission of microorganisms between patients.
(11) Return thermometer stem to storage well of recording unit.	• Proper storage protects probe from damage. Returning probe automatically causes digital reading to disappear.
(12) Wipe patient's anal area with soft tissue to remove lubricant or feces, and discard tissue. Assist patient to assume a comfortable position and be sufficiently covered with linens.	• These actions provide for comfort and hygiene.
(13) Remove and dispose of gloves in appropriate receptacle. Perform hand hygiene.	• Glove disposal and hand hygiene reduce transmission of microorganisms between the patient and the nurse.
(14) Return thermometer unit to charger. Verify that charger and probes are wiped with alcohol daily (in isolation areas, they are wiped whenever they are removed from the room).	• Charging provides battery power. Wiping with alcohol reduces transmission of microorganisms between the patient and the nurse.
C. Axillary temperature measurement with electronic thermometer	
(1) Prepare patient for procedure.	
(a) Draw curtain around patient's bed or close room door, or do both.	• These actions maintain patient's privacy, minimize embarrassment, and promote comfort.
(b) Assist patient to a supine or sitting position.	• These positions enable easy access to axilla.
(c) Move clothing or gown away from patient's shoulder and arm.	• This action exposes axilla for correct thermometer probe placement.
(2) Remove thermometer pack from charging unit. Ensure oral probe (blue tip) is attached to thermometer unit. Grasp top of probe stem, being careful not to press the ejection button.	• Charging provides battery power. Removal of hand-held unit from base prepares it to measure temperature. Pressing ejection button releases plastic cover from probe.
(3) Slide disposable plastic probe cover over thermometer probe until cover locks in place.	• Soft plastic cover prevents transmission of microorganisms between patients.
(4) Raise patient's arm away from torso; inspect for skin lesions and excessive perspiration. Insert probe into centre of patient's axilla, lower patient's arm over probe (see Step 6C[4] illustration).	• Maintains proper position of probe against blood vessels in axilla.

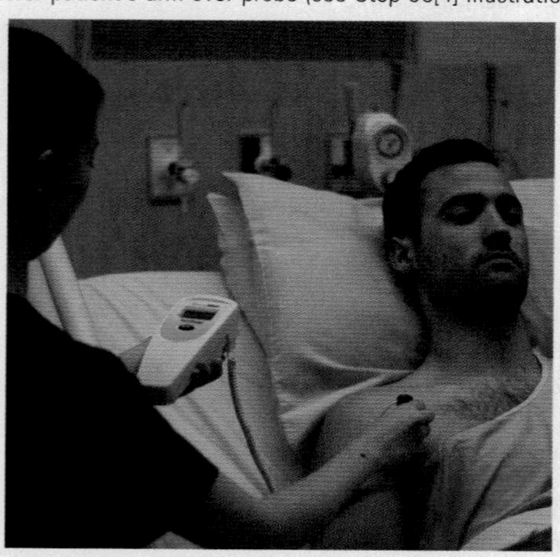

STEP 6C(4) Proper placement of thermometer tip in patient's axilla. (Courtesy Barbara J. Astle, RN, PhD.)

STEPS	RATIONALE
CRITICAL DECISION POINT: *Do not use axilla if skin lesions are present because local temperature may be altered and area may be painful to touch. Wipe off excessive perspiration.*	
(5) Hold probe in place until audible signal occurs and temperature appears on digital display.	• Probe must stay in place until signal occurs, to ensure accurate reading.
(6) Remove probe from patient's axilla.	
(7) Push ejection button on thermometer stem to discard plastic probe cover into appropriate receptacle.	• Discarding probe cover reduces transmission of microorganisms between the patient and the nurse.
(8) Return thermometer stem to storage well of recording unit.	• Proper storage protects probe from damage. Returning probe automatically causes digital reading to disappear.
(9) Assist patient to assume a comfortable position, and move linen or gown back over patient's shoulder.	• These actions restore comfort and promote privacy.
(10) Perform hand hygiene.	• Hand hygiene reduces transmission of microorganisms between the patient and the nurse.
(11) Return thermometer to charger.	• Charging provides battery power.
D. Tympanic membrane temperature measurement with electronic thermometer	
(1) Assist patient in assuming comfortable position with head turned to side, away from nurse. Right-handed caregivers should obtain temperature from patient's right ear. Left-handed caregivers should obtain temperature from patient's left ear.	• This positioning ensures comfort and exposes auditory canal for accurate temperature measurement. The less acute the angle of approach, the better the probe seal.
(2) Check for the presence of obvious cerumen in the patient's ear canal.	• To ensure clear optical pathway, lens cover of speculum must not be impeded by cerumen. Switch to other ear or select alternative measurement site if necessary.
(3) Remove thermometer hand-held unit from charging base, being careful not to press the ejection button.	• Charging provides battery power. Removal of hand-held unit from base prepares it to measure temperature. Pressing ejection button releases plastic probe cover from tip.
(4) Slide clean disposable speculum cover over otoscope-like lens tip until it locks into place; be careful not to touch lens cover.	• Lens cover must be clear of dust, fingerprints, and cerumen to ensure clear optical pathway.
(5) Insert speculum into patient's ear canal in accordance with manufacturer's instructions for tympanic probe positioning:	• Correct positioning of the probe with regard to ear canal ensures accurate readings. Operator errors cause false readings.
(a) Pull patient's pinna backward, up, and out. For children younger than 3 years, pull pinna down and back.	• The speculum does not get a panoramic view of the ear canal unless it is straightened because the canal is curved (Hockenberry & Wilson, 2015, p. 131).
(b) Fit otoscope probe snugly into canal and do not move (see Step 6D[5](b) illustration).	• Gentle pressure seals ear canal from ambient temperature, which can alter readings as much as 2.8°C.

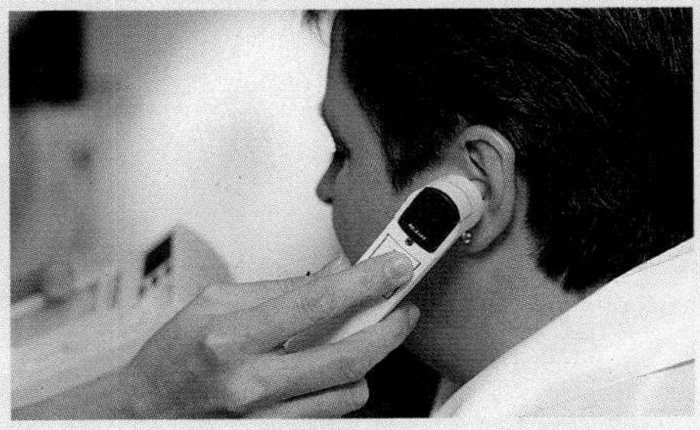

STEP 6D(5)(b) Tympanic thermometer with probe cover inserted into auditory canal.

STEPS	RATIONALE
(c) Point speculum tip toward patient's nose.	
(6) When probe is in place, press scan button on hand-held unit. Leave thermometer probe in place until audible signal occurs and patient's temperature appears on digital display.	• When scan button is pressed, probe detects infrared energy. Otoscope tip must stay in place until signal occurs, to ensure accurate reading.
(7) Carefully remove speculum from auditory canal.	• Careful removal prevents rubbing of sensitive outer ear lining.
(8) Push ejection button on hand-held unit to discard plastic probe cover into appropriate receptacle.	• Discarding probe cover reduces transmission of microorganisms between the patient and the nurse and automatically causes digital reading to disappear.
(9) If a second reading is necessary, replace probe lens cover and wait 2 to 3 minutes before inserting probe tip.	• Lens cover must be free of cerumen to maintain optical path. Time allows auditory canal to regain usual temperature.
(10) Return hand-held unit to charging base.	• Proper storage protects probe from damage.
(11) Assist patient to assume a comfortable position.	• This action restores comfort and sense of well-being.
(12) Perform hand hygiene.	• Hand hygiene reduces transmission of microorganisms between the patient and the nurse.

Continued

SKILL 30-1 MEASURING BODY TEMPERATURE—cont'd

STEPS	RATIONALE
7. Discuss findings with patient as needed.	• Such discussion promotes patient's participation in care and understanding of health status.
8. If patient's temperature is being assessed for the first time and is within normal range, document temperature as baseline.	• Baseline is used to compare future temperature measurements.
9. Compare current temperature reading with patient's previous baseline and with acceptable temperature range for patient's age group.	• Normal body temperature fluctuates within narrow range; comparison helps reveal presence of abnormality. Improper placement or movement of thermometer causes inaccuracies. Second measurement confirms initial findings of abnormal body temperature.

UNEXPECTED OUTCOMES	RELATED INTERVENTIONS
Temperature 1°C above usual range	• Assess possible sites (e.g., central line catheter, wounds) for localized infection and for related data suggestive of a systemic infection. • Implement appropriate nursing measures (see Box 30-9).
Persistent fever	• Notify appropriate health care provider and administer antipyretic and antibiotics as prescribed.
Temperature 1°C below usual range	• Remove any drafts, wet clothing, or damp linens. • Apply extra blankets, and, unless contraindicated, offer warm liquids.

RECORDING AND REPORTING

- Record temperature on vital sign flow sheet. Document temperature after administration of specific therapies in nurses' narrative notes.
- Report abnormal findings to nurse in charge or to prescribing health care provider.

HOME CARE CONSIDERATIONS

- Assess temperature and ventilation of patient's environment to determine existence of any environmental condition that may influence outcome of patient's temperature.
- In the home, patients may continue to use mercury-in-glass thermometers (see Box 30-6). Educate patient and caregiver about mercury hazards and encourage replacement with an electronic thermometer.

(Figure 30-4). Separate unbreakable probes are available for oral and rectal use. The oral probe can also be used for axillary temperature measurement. Electronic thermometers provide two modes of operation: a 4-second predictive temperature and a 3-minute standard temperature. When the first mode is used, a reading appears on the display unit within 20 to 50 seconds of insertion. A signal is sounded when the peak temperature reading has been measured.

Another form of electronic thermometer is used exclusively for tympanic temperature. An otoscope-like speculum with an infrared sensor tip detects heat radiated from the tympanic membrane. Within 2 to 5 seconds after the speculum is placed in the auditory canal, a reading appears on the display unit. A signal is sounded when the peak temperature reading has been measured.

Newer to the market is an electronic thermometer that measures the temperature of the superficial temporal artery. A hand-held scanner with an infrared sensor tip detects the temperature of cutaneous blood flow: the sensor is swept across the forehead and just behind the ear (Figure 30-5). Once scanning is complete, a reading appears on the display. Temporal artery temperature is a reliable and noninvasive measure of core temperature and has become an institutional standard in many health care settings (Box 30-5).

The greatest advantages of electronic thermometers are that they can be used immediately and read easily within seconds. The plastic sheath is unbreakable, making these devices ideal for use in children. Their expense is a major disadvantage. Maintaining cleanliness of the

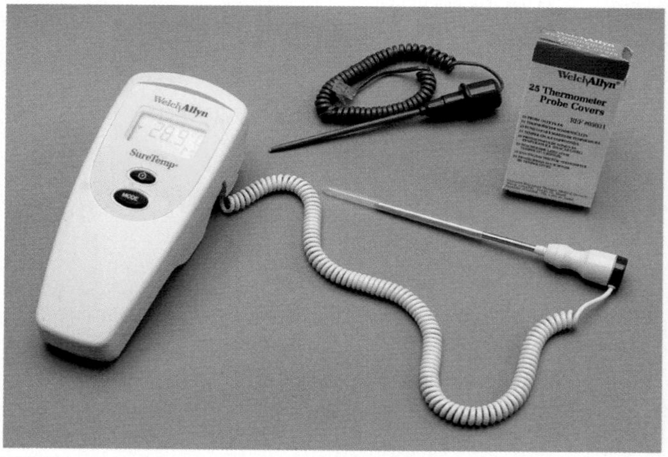

FIGURE 30-4 Electronic thermometer. The blue probe is for oral or axillary use. The red probe is for rectal use.

probes is important. If a rectal probe is not properly cleaned between patients, contamination of the rectal probe by gastrointestinal disease organisms can be a vector of disease transmission. The thermometer must be wiped frequently with alcohol, and the thermometer probe must be wiped with an alcohol swab after each use. Particular attention

BOX 30-4 Advantages and Disadvantages of Select Temperature Measurement Sites

Tympanic Membrane

Advantages

Site is easily accessible; minimal patient repositioning is required. Temperature reading can be obtained without disturbing or waking patient.
Device provides core reading, as the eardrum is close to the hypothalamus.
Measurement is very rapid (2 to 5 seconds).
Measurement is unaffected by oral intake of food or fluids or by smoking.
Device can be used for tachypneic patients without affecting breathing.
Device can be used in newborns to reduce handling of infants and subsequent heat loss.

Disadvantages

Measurement is more variable with this device than with other core temperature devices.
Hearing aids must be removed before measurement.
Site cannot be used in patients following surgery of the ear or tympanic membrane.
Readings are altered by cerumen impaction and otitis media.
Disposable probe cover comes in only one size.
Device does not accurately measure core temperature changes during and after exercise. Accuracy of results is influenced by the size of the probe (most are 8 mm). This may be a problem in young children, due to the small diameter of their ear canal (Hockenberry & Wilson, 2015, p. 119).
Inaccuracies can result from incorrect positioning of unit (Maxton, Justin, & Gillies, 2004).
Obtaining continuous measurement is not possible.
Temperature readings are affected by ambient temperature devices such as incubators, radiant warmers, and fans.

Rectum

Advantages

Site is argued to be more reliable when oral temperature cannot be obtained.

Disadvantages

Measurement at this site lags behind those at sites of core temperature during rapid temperature changes (Maxton et al., 2004).
Site should not be used in patients with diarrhea, rectal surgery, a rectal disorder, or bleeding tendencies.
Site should not be used for routine measurement of vital signs in newborns.
Given the invasiveness of this approach and the positioning that is required, this may be a source of patient discomfort, embarrassment, and anxiety.
Impacted stool alters readings (Maxton et al., 2004).
Measurement at this site carries risk of exposure to body fluids.
Lubrication is required.

Mouth

Advantages

Site is accessible, and no position change is required.
Measurement is comfortable for patients.
Measurement provides accurate reading of surface temperature.
Measurement reflects rapid change in core temperature.

Disadvantages

Readings are affected by ingestion of fluids or foods, smoking, and oxygen delivery.
Site is not suitable for patients who have had oral surgery, have suffered trauma, have a history of epilepsy, or have shaking chills.
Site should not be used for infants and small children or in confused, unconscious, or uncooperative patients.
Measurement at this site carries risk of exposure to body fluids.

Axilla

Advantages

Site is safe and noninvasive.
Appropriate for use in newborns and in uncooperative or unconscious patients.

Disadvantages

Measurement time is long.
Measurement at this site necessitates continuous positioning by nurse.
Measurement time lags behind those at sites of core temperature during rapid temperature changes.
Requires exposure of thorax, which can result in temperature loss, especially in newborns.
Readings are affected by exposure to environment during device placement (Maxton et al., 2004).
Not recommended for detecting fever in infants and young children.

Skin

Advantages

Continuous reading can be obtained.
Site is safe and noninvasive.
Requires minimal disturbance to patient.
Appropriate site for newborn measurement.

Disadvantages

Measurement time lags behind those at other sites during temperature changes, especially during hyperthermia.
Adhesion of the thermometer can be impaired by diaphoresis or sweat.
Measurement at this site can be affected by environmental temperature.
Cannot be used for patients who have allergy to adhesive.

Temporal Artery

Advantages

Provides a considerable reduction in required nursing time to measure (Isler, Aydin, Tutar, et al. 2014).
Measurement reflects rapid change in core temperature.
Site is easy to access without changing the patient's position.
Measurement is comfortable and eliminates need to remove clothing.
Measurement is useful in premature infants, newborns, and children.

Disadvantages

Measurement is not effective through head covering (e.g., dressing) or hair.
Results are affected by diaphoresis or sweating.
Continuous measurement is not possible.
Fails to detect fever at the two critical temperature points of 38°C or greater, and 39°C in children younger than 36 months (Hoffman, Etwaru, Dreisinger, et al., 2013).

must be paid to the probe hub, which has ridges, where the probe cover is secured to the probe.

Chemical Strip Thermometers. Single-use or reusable chemical strip (or dot) thermometers are thin strips of plastic containing a temperature sensor at one end. The sensor consists of chemically impregnated dots that change colour at different temperatures in increments of 0.1°C between 35.5°C and 40.4°C (Figure 30-6). Most of these devices are intended for single use, but the dots on reusable strips return to their original colour in seconds. The devices are used for measuring oral or axillary temperatures, particularly in children, and may be used rectally in a special sheath. The thermometer is removed after 60 seconds and read after another wait of 10 seconds to ensure that the temperature reading has stabilized. Research has shown that disposable single-use thermometers tend to overestimate or underestimate true temperature readings. The device is recommended only for screening purposes. When an abnormal temperature is suspected, the temperature should be confirmed with an electronic thermometer. The chemical strip thermometers are useful in caring for patients with isolation precautions (see Chapter 33 for further information about infection control), to avoid the need to take electronic instruments into these patients' rooms.

Another type of disposable thermometer is a temperature-sensitive patch or tape. Applied to the forehead or abdomen, the patch changes colour at different temperatures. These thermometers are also useful for screening patients, especially infants, for altered temperature. If an abnormal temperature is suspected, the temperature must be confirmed with an electronic temperature device. Disposable thermometers are not appropriate for monitoring temperature therapies.

Glass Thermometers. The traditional glass thermometer is a glass tube sealed at one end and with a mercury—or more recently, due to safety factors, an alcohol-filled—bulb at the other end of the device. Exposure of the bulb to heat causes the internal fluid to expand and rise in the enclosed tube. The length of the thermometer is marked with centigrade (Celsius) calibrations from which the temperature reading is obtained. The thermometer must be positioned properly at the oral, rectal, or axillary site and must be maintained for the appropriate length of time to obtain an accurate reading (Box 30-6). There are many disadvantages to the use of this type of device. In addition to the time delay (approximately 3 minutes with the device held in place), the mercury-in-glass device is easily breakable and, when broken, releases the contents, which may include hazardous mercury. With the potent toxicities associated with mercury spills, in addition to injuries from the use of glass thermometers, most health care agencies no longer supply these devices. The World Health Organization

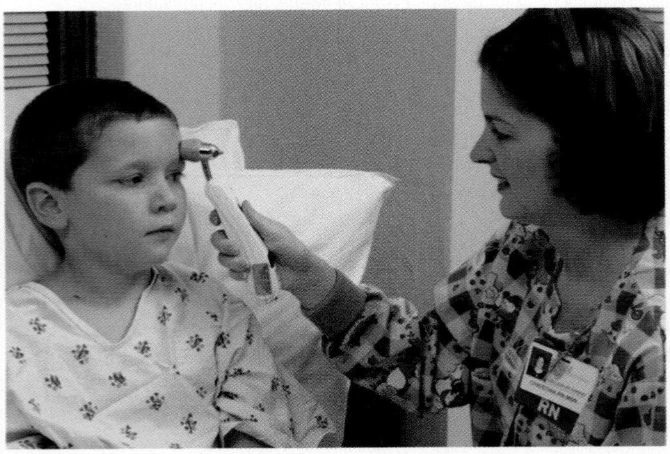

FIGURE 30-5 Temporal artery thermometer scanning the child's forehead.

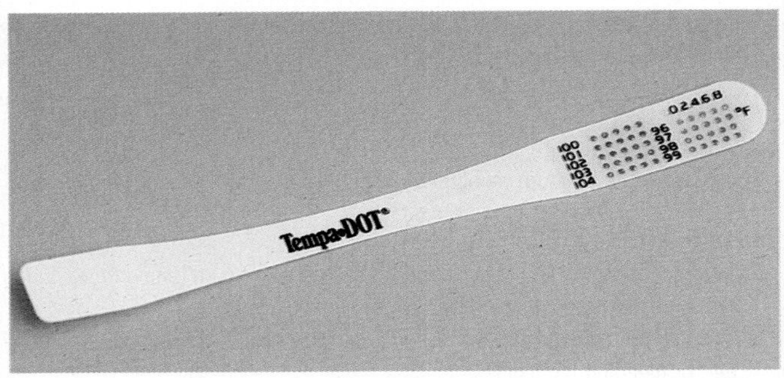

FIGURE 30-6 Disposable, single-use thermometer strip.

BOX 30-5 PROCEDURAL GUIDELINE

Measurement of Temporal Artery Temperature

Delegation Considerations

The measurement of temporal artery temperature can be delegated to unregulated care providers. The nurse is responsible for assessing the impact of changes on body temperature; therefore, when measurement of temporal artery temperature is delegated, it is important to *inform the unregulated care provider* about the following:

- Frequency of temperature measurement
- Factors that falsely raise or lower temperature readings
- Reporting abnormalities to the nurse for further assessment

Equipment

Temporal artery thermometer, alcohol wipes or probe cover (optional).

Procedure

1. Perform hand hygiene.
2. Ensure that the patient's forehead is dry; wipe it with a towel if it is moist.
3. Place the probe flush on the patient's forehead to avoid measuring ambient temperature.
4. Press the red scan button with your thumb. Scanning for the highest temperature will be continuous until you release the scan button.
5. Slowly slide the thermometer straight across the patient's forehead while keeping the probe flush on the patient's skin.
6. Keeping scan button pressed, lift the probe from the patient's forehead, and touch the probe to the patient's neck just behind the earlobe (the area where perfume is typically applied).
7. While the probe is scanning, a clicking sound occurs; this sound stops when peak temperature is scanned.
8. Release the scan button; read and record the temperature. Reading remains on the screen for 15 seconds after the button is released.
9. Clean the probe with an alcohol wipe, or, if a probe cover was used, remove and dispose of the probe cover.

BOX 30-6 PROCEDURAL GUIDELINE

Use of a Glass Thermometer

Delegation Considerations

Patient, family, or unregulated care provider will safely perform temperature measurement.

Equipment

Glass thermometer (rectal or oral), plastic sleeve, lubricating jelly (rectal only), disposable gloves

Procedure

1. Perform hand hygiene. Apply disposable gloves to avoid contact with body fluids (e.g., saliva, stool).
2. Hold the nonbulbed end of the glass thermometer (if colour-coded, tip will be blue or red) with your fingertips to reduce contamination of the bulb.
3. Read the internal fluid level while gently rotating the thermometer at eye level. If the fluid is above the desired level, grasp the tip of the thermometer securely, stand away from solid objects, and sharply flick your wrist downward. Brisk shaking lowers the fluid level in the glass tube. Continue shaking the thermometer until the reading is below 35.6°C. The thermometer reading must be lower than the patient's actual temperature before the thermometer is used.
4. Insert the thermometer into a plastic sleeve cover, if available, to protect it from body secretions (e.g., saliva, stool). For rectal use, apply lubricant to cover 2.5 cm to 3.5 cm of the rectal thermometer.
5. Place the thermometer according to the technique appropriate for the oral, rectal, or axillary site (see Skill 30-1).
6. Leave the thermometer in place 3 minutes for oral or rectal temperature, 5 minutes for axillary temperature, or according to agency policy.
7. Remove the thermometer. Carefully discard the plastic sleeve. Wipe off secretions with a clean tissue, moving toward the bulb, or follow institutional cleaning policies. If the device has been used without a plastic sleeve, ensure that the thermometer is cleansed with warm, soapy water or rubbing alcohol after use. Store the thermometer in its storage container. Remove your gloves, and perform hand hygiene.
8. Read the thermometer at eye level. Record the findings. Store the thermometer in its storage container. Remove your gloves, and perform hand hygiene.

(2017a) recommends phasing out the use of mercury-containing thermometers and all other nonessential mercury-containing products, implementing safe use and disposal of these products.

Patients may have mercury-in-glass thermometers in their homes. It is important to teach patients and their families what to do in the event of breakage of a mercury-in-glass thermometer and encourage replacement with an electronic thermometer. Guidelines on how to clean up and dispose of small mercury spills can be found on the Environment Canada website: https://www.ec.gc.ca/mercure-mercury/default.asp?lang=En&n=D2B2AD47-1.

Despite the gradual phasing out of mercury-in-glass thermometers they are still in use, especially in developing countries (Oncel, Tekgunduz, Ozdemir, et al., 2013, p. 193). Therefore, it is important to understand the correct procedure on how to use them in practice.

◆ Nursing Diagnosis

Nurses identify assessment findings and cluster defining characteristics to form a nursing diagnosis. Nursing diagnoses for patients with body temperature alterations include the following:

- *Risk for imbalanced body temperature*
- *Hyperthermia*
- *Hypothermia*
- *Ineffective thermoregulation*

For example, an increase in body temperature, flushed skin, skin warm to touch, and tachycardia are indicative of the diagnosis *hyperthermia.* The nursing diagnosis is stated as either an at-risk or an actual temperature alteration. If the patient has risk factors for temperature alterations, the nurse should minimize or eliminate them.

Once the diagnosis is established, the nurse accurately determines the related factor or cause (Box 30-7). The related factor directs the selection of appropriate nursing interventions. In the example of hyperthermia, a related factor of vigorous activity will result in interventions much different from those for a related factor of decreased ability to perspire.

◆ Planning

During planning, nurses integrate knowledge gathered from assessment and patient history to develop and modify a person-centred plan of care (CASN, 2015) (Box 30-8). It is important to match a patient's needs with interventions that are supported and recommended in the clinical research literature.

Goals and Outcomes. The care plan for a patient with alteration in temperature must include realistic and individualized goals along with relevant outcomes. The nurse needs to collaborate closely with the patient in setting goals and outcomes and choosing nursing interventions. Expected outcomes are established to gauge progress toward returning the body temperature to an acceptable range. Goals may be short term, such as regaining normal range of body temperature in 24 hours, or long term, such as helping the patient modify the environment, (e.g., obtaining appropriate clothing to wear in cold weather). Outcomes must be related to what is learned about the patient.

Setting Priorities

The severity of temperature alteration and its effects, together with the patient's general health status, influence care priorities. Safety is a top priority. In many cases, other medical problems complicate the care plan. For instance, alterations in body temperature affect the body's requirements for fluids. Patients with cardiac disease may have difficulty tolerating required fluid replacement therapy.

Continuity of Care. Patients at high risk for alterations in body temperature require an individualized care plan directed at maintaining normothermia (normal body temperature) and reducing risk factors. For example, the outcome of care may be that the patient can explain actions to take during a heat wave. The nurse should teach the patient and caregiver the importance of thermoregulation and actions to take during very hot weather. Education is particularly important for parents who need to know how to take action at home when an infant or child develops temperature alteration.

◆ Implementation

Health Promotion. Health promotion for patients at risk for altered body temperature is directed toward promoting balance between heat production and heat loss. Patient activity, temperature of the environment, and clothing are all considered. In the prevention of hyperthermia, nurses teach patients to avoid strenuous exercise in hot, humid weather; to drink fluids such as water or clear fruit

BOX 30-7 NURSING DIAGNOSTIC PROCESS

Assessment Activities	Defining Characteristics	Nursing Diagnosis
Measure vital signs, including temperature, pulse, respirations, and pulse oximetry (SpO_2).	Increased body temperature above usual range Tachycardia Tachypnea Hypoxemia	*Ineffective thermoregulation related to aging and inability to adapt to environmental temperature*
Palpate skin.	Warm, dry skin	
Observe patient's appearance and behaviour while talking and resting.	Restlessness Confusion Flushed appearance	
Review medical history.	Location (e.g., found in unventilated apartment during heat wave) and other patient characteristics (e.g., 85 years old with history of dementia)	

BOX 30-8 NURSING CARE PLAN

Hyperthermia

ASSESSMENT

Mr. Coburn is a 45-year-old teacher who arrives at the outpatient clinic complaining of malaise. His medical history includes a past urinary tract infection. Several of his students have had colds lately. He has been feeling unwell for the past 3 days.

Assessment Activities	***Findings and Defining Characteristics***
Palpate skin.	Skin *warm* and *dry* to touch
Observe patient's behaviour when talking and resting.	Breathing appears laboured; face is *flushed*
Measure vital signs.	Blood pressure: right arm, 116/62 mm Hg; left arm, 114/64 mm Hg Right radial pulse: 128 *beats per minute,* regular and bounding Respiratory rate regular at 26 *breaths per minute* SpO_2: 98% on room air Oral temperature: 39.2°C
Review medical history.	Smokes one pack of cigarettes per day and recently began expectorating *yellow-green sputum* *Tired* for past 3 days and dizzy upon rising in the morning

NURSING DIAGNOSIS: Hyperthermia related to infectious process

PLANNING

Goal (Nursing Outcomes Classification)* ***Thermoregulation***	***Expected Outcomes***
Patient will regain normal range of body temperature within next 24 hours.	Body temperature will decline at least 1°C within next 8 hours.
Patient will attain sense of comfort and rest within next 48 hours.	Patient will verbalize increased satisfaction with rest and sleep pattern. Patient will report increase in energy level within next 3 days.

*Outcome classification label from Moorhead, S., Johnson, M., Maas, M. L., & Swanson, E. (2012). *Nursing outcomes classification (NOC)* (5th ed.). St. Louis, MO: Mosby.

INTERVENTIONS

Interventions (Nursing Interventions Classification)†	***Rationale***
Fever Treatment	
Instruct patient to reduce external coverings and keep clothing and bed linen dry.	Heat loss is promoted through conduction and convection.
Instruct patient to monitor temperature at home frequently and take acetaminophen every 4 hours as ordered for temperature higher than 38°C.	Antipyretics reduce set point.
Instruct patient to limit physical activity and increase frequency of rest periods over next 2 days.	Activity and stress increase metabolic rate, contributing to heat production.

†Intervention classification label from Bulechek, G. M., Butcher, H. K., Dochterman, J. M., & Wagner, C. (Eds.). (2013). *Nursing interventions classification (NIC)* (6th ed.). St. Louis, MO: Mosby.

EVALUATION

Nursing Actions	***Patient Response and Finding***	***Achievement of Outcome***
Obtain body temperature measurement.	Body temperature: 37.8°C	Body temperature is within normal limits.
Ask Mr. Coburn whether his energy level has changed since the last visit.	He responds, "I am sleeping much better and have returned to work with a lot more energy."	Rest and sleep pattern have improved, and energy level has increased.

juices before, during, and after exercise; to wear light, loose-fitting, light-coloured clothes; to avoid exercising in areas with poor ventilation; to wear a protective covering over the head when outdoors; and, when entering hot climates, to expose themselves to the heat gradually.

Prevention is key for patients at risk for hypothermia and involves educating not only the patients but family members and friends. Patients most at risk are the extremes of age—very young, very old—and people debilitated by trauma, spinal cord injury, stroke, diabetes, drug or alcohol intoxication, sepsis, and Raynaud's disease. Mentally ill and disabled patients may acquire hypothermia because they are unaware of the dangers of cold conditions. People without adequate home heating, shelter, diet, or clothing are also at risk. Fatigue, skin colour (dark-skinned patients are more susceptible), malnutrition, hypoxemia, and body piercing can contribute to the risk of frostbite.

Acute Care

Fever. When body temperature is elevated, it is important to initiate interventions to treat fever. The objective of therapy is to increase heat loss, reduce heat production, and prevent complications.

The procedures used to intervene and treat the temperature depend on the cause; any adverse effects; and the strength, intensity, and duration of the elevation. The nurse plays a key role in assessing and implementing temperature-reducing strategies (Box 30-9). The prescribing health care provider may try to determine the cause of the elevated temperature by isolating the causative pyrogen. Necessary culture specimens for laboratory analysis, such as urine, blood, sputum, and tissue from wound sites (see Chapter 33 for further information about infection control), may need to be obtained. After the cultures have been sent, the prescribing health care provider orders administration of antibiotic medications, to destroy pyrogenic bacteria and eliminate the cause of the elevated temperature.

In children, most fevers are caused by viruses, last only briefly, and have limited effects. Children still have immature temperature-control mechanisms so temperatures can rise rapidly. Dehydration and febrile seizures can occur while temperatures are rising in children between 6 months and 6 years of age. Febrile seizures are unusual in children older than 6 years. The actual temperature, often exceeding 38.8°C, seems to be more important than the rapidity of the temperature increase. Children are at particular risk for fluid volume deficit because they can quickly lose large amounts of fluids in proportion to their body weight. It is important to maintain accurate intake and output records and encourage fluid consumption.

A fever may also indicate a hypersensitivity response to a medication. Drug fevers can be accompanied by other symptoms of allergy, such as rash or pruritus. Treatment involves withdrawing the particular medication.

Antipyretics are medications that reduce fever. Nonsteroidals such as acetaminophen, salicylates, indomethacin, and ketorolac reduce fever by increasing heat loss. Corticosteroids reduce heat production by interfering with the immune system and can mask signs of infection. Corticosteroids are not used to treat a fever. However, be aware of their effect on suppressing the patient's ability to develop a fever in response to a pyrogen.

Nonpharmacological therapy for fever involves methods that increase heat loss by evaporation, conduction, convection, or radiation. Blankets cooled by circulating water delivered by motorized units increase conductive heat loss. The manufacturer's instructions for applying these hypothermia blankets must be followed because of risk for skin breakdown and "freeze burns." Placing a bath blanket between the patient and the hypothermia blanket and wrapping distal extremities (fingers, toes, and genitalia) are recommended to reduce the risk of injury to the skin and tissue from hypothermia therapy. Traditional methods such as tepid sponge baths, bathing with alcohol water solutions, applying ice packs to axillae and groin areas, and cooling fans should be used cautiously because they lead to shivering. These methods have no demonstrated advantage over antipyretic medications. Nursing measures to enhance body cooling must attempt to avoid stimulating shivering. Shivering is counterproductive and increases energy expenditure up to 400%. Wrapping the patient's extremities has been recommended to reduce the incidence and intensity of shivering.

Heatstroke. Heatstroke is an emergency. Treatment for heatstroke includes moving the patient to a cooler environment; reducing clothing covering body; placing cool, wet towels over skin; and using oscillating fans to increase convective heat loss. Emergency medical treatment may include intravenous fluids and irrigation of the stomach and lower bowel with cool solutions, in addition to cooling blankets.

Hypothermia. The priority of treatment for hypothermia is to prevent a further decrease in body temperature. Removing wet clothes and replacing with dry clothes and wrapping the patient in blankets are key interventions. In health care settings, forced-air warming blankets can actively rewarm hypothermic patients. Away from a health care setting, the patient should be laid under blankets next to a warm person. A conscious patient should drink hot liquids (e.g., soup) and avoid alcohol and caffeine. It is important to keep the patient's head

BOX 30-9 Nursing Measures for Patients With a Fever

Assessment

- Obtain core temperature during each phase of a febrile episode.
- Assess for contributing factors such as dehydration, infection, and environmental temperature.
- Identify physiological response to temperature.
- Measure all vital signs.
- Observe skin colour.
- Assess skin temperature.
- Observe for shivering and diaphoresis.
- Assess the patient's comfort and well-being.
- Determine phase of fever: chill, plateau, or fever break.

Interventions (Unless Contraindicated)

- Obtain blood cultures when ordered: Blood specimens are obtained to coincide with temperature spikes when the antigen-producing organism is most pervasive.
- Minimize heat production: Reduce frequency of activities that increase oxygen demand, such as excessive turning in bed; allow rest periods; limit physical activity.
- Maximize heat loss: Reduce external covering on patient's body to promote heat loss through radiation and conduction without inducing shivering; keep clothing and bed linen dry to increase heat loss through conduction and convection.
- Meet requirements for increased metabolic rate: Provide oxygen as ordered to improve oxygen delivery to body cells; provide measures to stimulate appetite; offer well-balanced meals; provide fluids (3 L per day for patient with normal cardiac and renal function) to replace fluids lost through insensible water loss and sweating.
- Promote patient comfort: Encourage the patient to practise oral hygiene for dry oral mucous membranes; control environmental temperature without inducing shivering (between 21°C and 27°C).
- Identify febrile episode phases: Examine previous temperature measurements to identify trends.
- Initiate health teaching as indicated.

covered, place the patient near a fire or in a warm room, or place heating pads next to areas of the patient's body (head and neck) that lose heat most rapidly.

Restorative and Continuing Care. A patient who has been febrile should be educated about the importance of taking and continuing antibiotics as directed until the course of treatment is completed. Children and older persons are at risk for fluid volume deficit because they can quickly lose large amounts of fluids in proportion to their body weight. Intake of preferred fluids should be encouraged.

◆ Evaluation

All nursing interventions are evaluated by comparing the patient's actual response with the expected outcomes of the care plan. This evaluation reveals whether goals of care have been met or whether the plan must be revised. After any intervention, the nurse should measure the patient's temperature to evaluate for change. Other evaluative measures such as palpation of the skin and assessment of pulse and respirations can be used. If therapies are effective, body temperature will return to an acceptable range, other vital sign measurements will stabilize, and the patient will report a sense of comfort.

PULSE

The pulse is the bounding of arterial blood flow that is palpable at various points on the body. Blood flows through the body in a continuous circuit. The pulse is an important indicator of the status of the circulatory system.

Physiology and Regulation

Electrical impulses originating from the sinoatrial node travel through heart muscle to stimulate cardiac contraction. Approximately 60 to 70 mL of blood enters the aorta with each ventricular contraction (stroke volume). With each stroke volume ejection (blood pushed out of the heart), the walls of the aorta distend, creating a pulse wave that travels rapidly toward the distal ends of the arteries. When a pulse wave reaches a peripheral artery, it can be felt by palpating the artery lightly against underlying bone or muscle. The number of pulsing sensations occurring in 1 minute is the *pulse rate.*

The volume of blood pumped by the heart during 1 minute is the cardiac output: the product of heart rate and ventricular stroke volume. In an adult, the heart pumps about 5 000 mL of blood per minute (e.g., if heart rate is 70 beats per minute and stroke volume is 70 mL, the cardiac output is 4 900 mL per minute). A change in heart rate or stroke volume does not always change the heart's output or the amount of blood in the arteries. Mechanical, neural, and chemical factors regulate the strength of heart contractions and its stroke volume. When these factors are unable to alter stroke volume, the heart rate changes to subsequently adjust blood pressure (BP). As heart rate increases, the heart has less time to fill. Without a change in stroke volume, blood pressure decreases. As the heart rate slows, filling time is increased, and blood pressure increases. The inability of blood pressure to respond to increases or decreases in heart rate may indicate a health deviation and must be reported to the prescribing health care provider. An abnormally slow, rapid, or irregular pulse alters cardiac output. It is important to be able to assess the ability of the patient's heart to meet the demands of the body tissues for nutrients by palpating a peripheral pulse or by using a stethoscope to listen to heart sounds (apical rate).

Assessment of Pulse

Any artery can be assessed for pulse rate, but the radial artery is commonly used because it is easily palpated. When a patient's condition suddenly worsens, the carotid artery is the recommended site for quickly finding a pulse. The heart will continue delivering blood through the carotid artery to the brain as long as possible. When cardiac output declines significantly, peripheral pulses weaken and are difficult to palpate. Nurses most commonly assess the radial and apical pulses in adult patients, but people who are learning to monitor their own heart rates use the radial or carotid pulse (e.g., athletes, patients taking medications for cardiac disease, and patients starting a prescribed exercise regimen). If the radial pulse at the wrist is abnormal or intermittent, or if it is inaccessible because of a dressing or cast, the apical pulse should be assessed. When a patient takes medication that affects the heart rate, the apical pulse provides a more accurate assessment of cardiac function. In infants or young children, it is best to assess the brachial or apical pulse because other peripheral pulses are deep and difficult to palpate accurately.

Assessment of other peripheral pulse sites, such as the popliteal or femoral, is unnecessary in routine measurement of vital signs. These alternative peripheral pulses are assessed during a complete physical examination, when surgery or treatment has impaired blood flow to a body part, or when a patient has clinical indications of impaired peripheral blood flow (see Chapter 32). Table 30-2 summarizes pulse sites and criteria for measurement. Skill 30-2 outlines pulse rate assessment. Table 30-3 lists acceptable pulse rate ranges.

Use of a Stethoscope. A stethoscope is used to assess the apical rate (Figure 30-7). The five major parts of the stethoscope are the earpieces, binaurals, tubing, bell chest piece, and diaphragm chest piece.

The plastic or rubber earpieces fit snugly and comfortably in the ears. The binaurals are angled and strong enough so that the earpieces stay firmly in the ears without causing discomfort. To ensure the best reception of sound, the earpieces follow the contour of the ear canal, pointing toward the face when the stethoscope is in place. Stethoscopes can have single or dual tubes. The tubing has thick walls and is flexible yet moderately rigid to eliminate transmission of environmental noise and to prevent the tubing from kinking. Tubing that is longer than 30 to 40 cm decreases the transmission of sound waves, making it more difficult to accurately auscultate sounds.

The chest piece consists of a bell and a diaphragm that are typically rotated from one to the other into position. The diaphragm or bell must be in proper position to hear sounds through the stethoscope. The position of the chest piece can be tested by tapping lightly on the diaphragm to determine which side is functioning. The diaphragm is the circular, flat portion of the chest piece and is covered by a thin plastic disk. It transmits high-pitched sounds created by the high-velocity movement of air and blood. Lung, heart, and bowel sounds are best auscultated by using the diaphragm. The diaphragm is positioned to make a tight seal against the patient's skin (Figure 30-8). Enough pressure should be exerted to leave a temporary red ring on the patient's skin when the diaphragm is removed.

The bell is the bowl-shaped chest piece usually surrounded by a rubber ring. The ring avoids chilling the patient with cold metal when the chest piece is placed on the skin. The bell transmits low-pitched sounds created by the low-velocity movement of blood. Heart and vascular sounds are auscultated through the bell. The nurse should apply the bell lightly, resting the chest piece on the patient's skin (Figure 30-9). Compressing the bell against the skin reduces low-pitched sound amplification and creates a "diaphragm of skin." Some stethoscopes have just one chest piece that combines the features of the bell and diaphragm. With the use of light pressure, the chest piece acts as a bell; with more pressure, it acts as a diaphragm.

The stethoscope is a delicate instrument and requires proper care for optimal function. The earpieces should be removed regularly and

TABLE 30-2 Pulse Sites

Site (Artery)	Location	Use and Assessment Criteria
Temporal	Over temporal bone of head, above and lateral to eye	Of significance in the diagnosis of temporal arteritis
Carotid	Along medial edge of sternocleidomastoid muscle in neck	During physiological shock or cardiac arrest, when other sites are not palpable
Apical	Fourth to fifth intercostal space at left midclavicular line	Auscultation is performed to obtain apical pulse
Brachial	Groove between biceps and triceps muscles at antecubital fossa	Provides status of circulation to lower arm; to auscultate blood pressure
Radial	Radial or thumb side of forearm at wrist	Common site to assess peripheral pulse and status of circulation to hand
Ulnar	Ulnar side of forearm at wrist	Assess status of circulation to hand; also to perform Allen's test (test for patency of radial artery)
Femoral	Below inguinal ligament, midway between symphysis pubis and anterior superior iliac spine	Appropriate location to assess pulse during physiological shock or cardiac arrest when other pulses are not palpable; to assess status of circulation to leg
Popliteal	Behind knee in popliteal fossa	Assess status of circulation to lower leg
Posterior tibial	Inner side of ankle, below medial malleolus	Assess status of circulation to foot
Dorsalis pedis	Along top of foot, between extension tendons of the great toe and next toe	Assess status of circulation to foot

SKILL 30-2 ASSESSING THE RADIAL AND APICAL PULSES

Delegation Considerations

The task of pulse measurement can be delegated to unregulated care providers (UCPs). The nurse is responsible for assessing changes in pulse; therefore, when the task of pulse measurement is delegated, it is important to *inform the unregulated care provider* about the following:

- Patient's history or risk for irregular pulse
- Frequency of pulse measurement in patient
- Patient's usual pulse values
- Abnormalities that should be reported to the health care provider

Equipment

- Stethoscope (for measurement of apical pulse only)
- Watch or clock with second hand or digital display
- Pen and either vital sign flow sheet or documentation record
- Alcohol swab

PROCEDURE

STEPS	RATIONALE
1. Determine need to assess radial or apical pulse.	• Use clinical judgement to determine need for assessment.
A. Note risk factors for alterations in apical pulse.	• Certain conditions heighten risk for pulse alterations (e.g., cardiac disease, cardiac dysrhythmias, sudden chest pain or acute pain from any site, invasive cardiovascular diagnostic tests, surgery, sudden infusion of large volume of intravenous fluid, hemorrhage, administration of medications that alter cardiac function).
B. Assess for signs and symptoms of altered stroke volume and cardiac output, such as dyspnea, fatigue, chest pain, orthopnea, syncope, palpitations (unpleasant awareness of heartbeat), jugular venous distension, edema of dependent body parts, and cyanosis or pallor of skin.	• Physical signs and symptoms may indicate alteration in cardiac function.
2. Assess for factors that normally influence pulse rate and rhythm: age, exercise, position changes, fluid balance, medications, temperature, sympathetic nervous system stimulation.	• These assessments enable you to accurately evaluate the presence and significance of pulse alterations. Acceptable range of pulse rate changes with age (see Table 30-3).
3. Determine previous baseline apical rate (if available) from patient's record. Otherwise, note baseline radial rate.	• By comparing rates you can assess for change in patient's condition and evaluate future apical pulse measurements.
4. Explain to patient that pulse or heart rate is to be assessed. If patient was active, wait 5–10 minutes before taking his or her pulse. Encourage patient to relax and not to speak.	• Activity and anxiety elevate heart rate. The patient's voice interferes with your ability to hear sound when you measure apical pulse. Measuring pulse rates at rest allows for objective comparison of values.

Continued

SKILL 30-2 ASSESSING THE RADIAL AND APICAL PULSES—cont'd

STEPS	RATIONALE
5. Perform hand hygiene.	• Hand hygiene reduces transmission of microorganisms between the patient and the nurse.
6. If necessary, draw curtain around patient's bed or close room door, or do both.	• These actions maintain patient's privacy, minimize embarrassment, and promote comfort.
7. Obtain pulse measurement.	
A. Radial pulse	
(1) Assist patient to assume a supine or sitting position.	• These positions enable easy access to pulse sites.
(2) If patient is supine, place patient's forearm straight alongside body, across lower chest, or across upper abdomen with wrist extended straight (see Step 7A[2] illustration). If patient is sitting, bend patient's elbow 90 degrees and support lower arm on chair or on your arm. Slightly flex patient's wrist with palm down (see Step 7A[3] illustration).	• Relaxed position of lower arm and slight flexion of wrist promotes exposure of artery to palpation without restriction.
(3) Place tips of your first two or middle three fingers over groove along radial or thumb side of patient's inner wrist (see Step 7A[3] illustration).	• Fingertips are the most sensitive parts of the hand to palpate arterial pulsation. The thumb has pulsations that may interfere with accuracy.

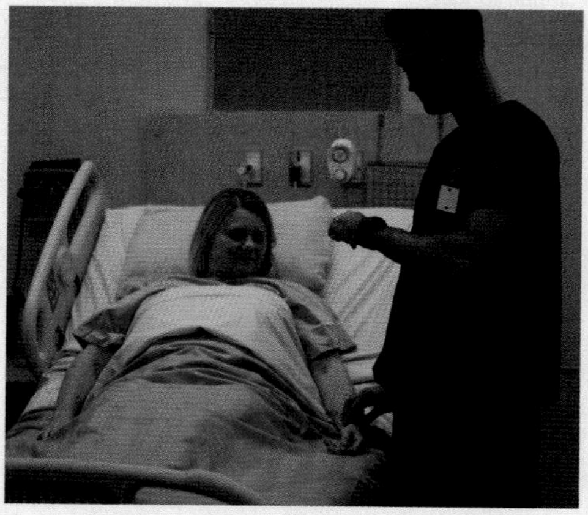

STEP 7A(2) Pulse check with patient's forearm at side with wrist extended. (Courtesy Barbara J. Astle, RN, PhD.)

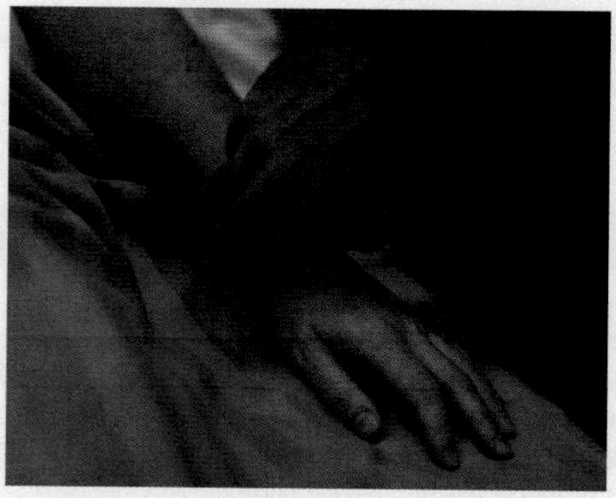

STEP 7A(3) Hand placement for pulse checking radial pulse. (Courtesy Barbara J. Astle, RN, PhD.)

STEPS	RATIONALE
(4) Lightly compress your fingertips against patient's radius, obliterate pulse initially, and then relax pressure so that pulse becomes easily palpable.	• Pulse is more accurately assessed with moderate pressure. Too much pressure occludes pulse and impairs blood flow.
(5) Determine strength of pulse. Note whether thrust of vessel against your fingertips is bounding (+4), strong (+3), weak (+2), thready (+1), or absent (0).	• Strength reflects volume of blood ejected against arterial wall with each heart contraction. Accurate description of strength improves communication among health care providers, although keep in mind this is subjective data.
(6) After you can feel a regular pulse, look at watch and begin to count pulse rate when second hand reaches a number on watch dial; start counting pulse with "one," then "two," and so on.	• You can determine pulse rate accurately only after you can palpate the pulse. Count of "one" is the first beat palpated after you begin timing.
(7) If pulse is regular, count rate for 30 seconds and multiply total by 2.	• A 30-second count is accurate for rapid, slow, or regular pulse rates.
(8) If pulse is irregular, count rate for 1 minute (60 seconds). Assess frequency and pattern of irregularity. Compare bilateral radial pulses.	• Inefficient contraction of heart fails to transmit pulse wave, interfering with cardiac output, resulting in irregular pulse. Longer measurement time ensures accurate count.

CRITICAL DECISION POINT: *If pulse is irregular, assess apical or radial pulse to detect a pulse deficit. Count apical pulse rate while a colleague counts radial pulse rate. Begin apical pulse count out loud to simultaneously assess pulses. If pulse count differs by more than two, a pulse deficit exists; this can indicate altered cardiac output.*

STEPS	RATIONALE
B. Apical pulse	
(1) Perform hand hygiene; clean earpieces and diaphragm of stethoscope with alcohol swab.	• These actions reduce transmission of microorganisms between patients and when stethoscopes are shared.
(2) Draw curtain around patient's bed or close room door, or do both.	• These actions maintain patient's privacy, minimize embarrassment, and promote comfort.
(3) Assist patient to supine or sitting position. Move aside bed linen and gown to expose sternum and left side of chest.	• Expose portion of patient's chest wall to select auscultatory site.

STEPS	RATIONALE
(4) Locate anatomical landmarks to identify the *point of maximal impulse* (PMI), also called the *apical impulse* (see Steps 7B[4](a) to 7B[4](d); illustrations). Heart is located behind and to left of sternum with base at top and apex at bottom. Find angle of Louis just below suprasternal notch between sternal body and manubrium; it can be palpated as a bony prominence (see Step 7B[4](a) illustration). Slip fingers down each side of angle to find second intercostal space (ICS; see Step 7B[4](b) illustration). Carefully move fingers down left side of sternum to fifth ICS (see Step 7B[4](c) illustration) and laterally to the left midclavicular line (MCL; see Step 7B[4](d) illustration). A light tap felt in an area within 1 to 2 cm of the PMI is reflected from the apex of the heart.	• Use of anatomical landmarks allows correct placement of stethoscope over apex of heart, enhancing ability to hear heart sounds clearly. In a patient with large breasts, ask the patient to move the breast aside so that you can access the PMI site. If you are unable to palpate the PMI, reposition patient on left side. In the presence of severe cardiac disease, the PMI may be located to the left of the MCL or at the sixth ICS.
(5) Place diaphragm of stethoscope in palm of your hand for 5 to 10 seconds.	• By warming metal or plastic diaphragm, you avoid startling patient and promote patient's comfort.
(6) Place diaphragm of stethoscope over PMI at the fifth ICS, at left MCL, and auscultate for normal S_1 and S_2 heart sounds (heard as "lub-dub" see Step 7B[6] illustrations).	• Allow stethoscope tubing to extend straight without kinks that would distort sound transmission. Normally, S_1 and S_2 heart sounds are high-pitched and best heard with the diaphragm.

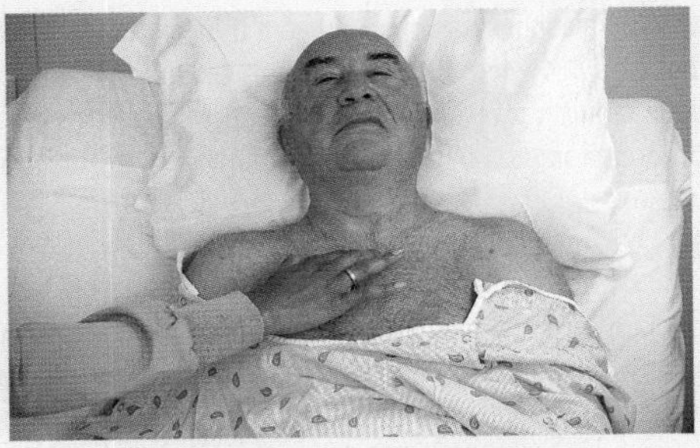

STEP 7B(4)(a) Locating the angle of Louis.

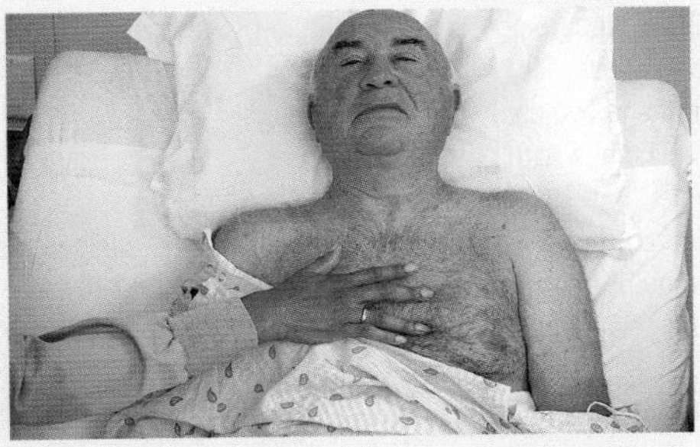

STEP 7B(4)(c) Locating the fifth intercostal space.

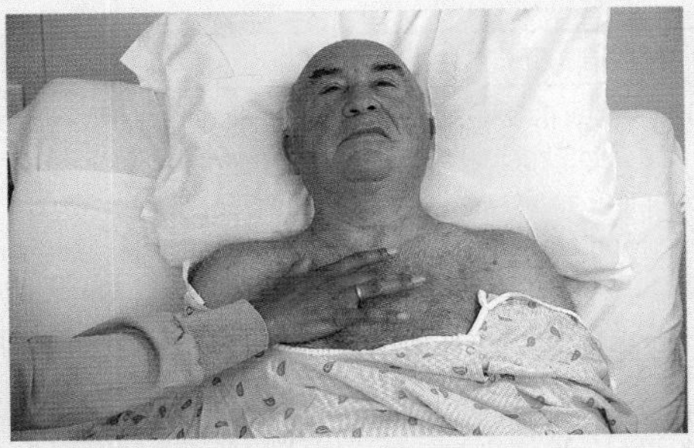

STEP 7B(4)(b) Locating the second intercostal space.

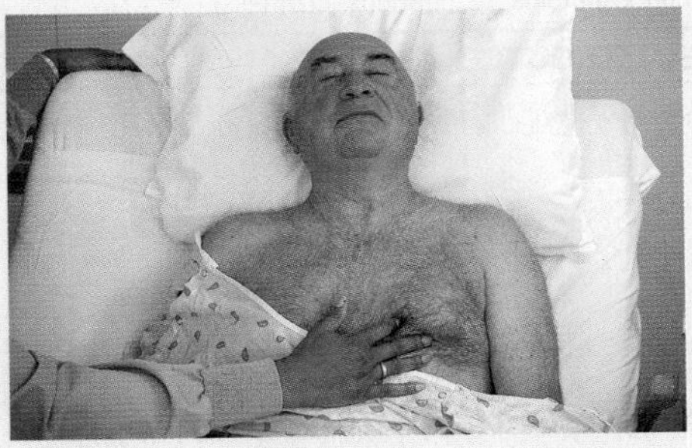

STEP 7B(4)(d) Identifying the midclavicular line.

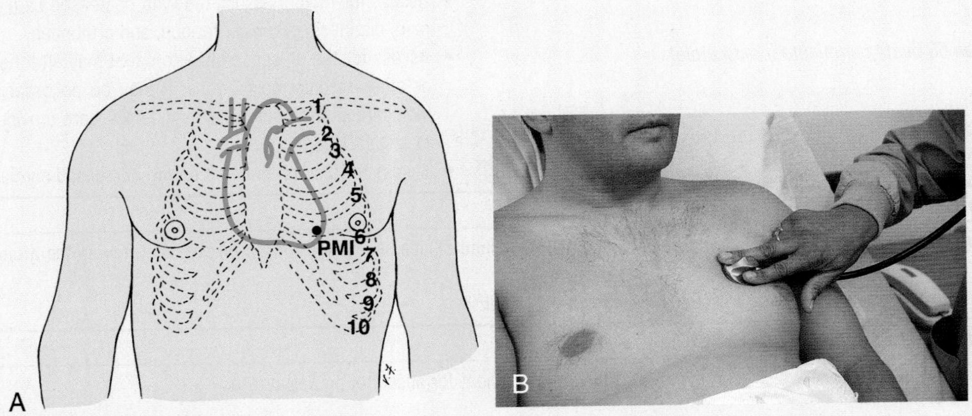

STEP 7B(6) A, Location of point of maximal impulse (PMI) in adult. **B,** Stethoscope placement over PMI.

Continued

SKILL 30-2 ASSESSING THE RADIAL AND APICAL PULSES—cont'd

STEPS	RATIONALE
(7) When S_1 and S_2 are heard with regularity, look at watch and begin to count rate: when second hand reaches a number on watch dial, start counting with "one," then "two," and so on.	• You can accurately determine apical rate only after you can auscultate sounds clearly. Count of "one" is first sound auscultated after timing begins.
(8) If apical rate is regular, count for 30 seconds and multiply by 2.	• Regular apical rate can be assessed within 30 seconds.

CRITICAL DECISION POINT: *If heart rate is irregular or if patient is receiving cardiac medication, count for 1 minute (60 seconds). An irregular rate is more accurately assessed when measured over a longer interval.*

STEPS	RATIONALE
(9) If heart rate is irregular, or patient is receiving certain cardiovascular medications, for example digoxin, count for a full 1 minute (60 seconds) and describe pattern of irregularity (S_1 and S_2 occurring early or later after previous sequence of sounds; e.g., every third or every fourth beat is skipped). Digoxin is held if the apical rate is less than 60.	• Regular occurrence of dysrhythmia within 1 minute may indicate inefficient contraction of heart and alteration in cardiac output.
(10) Replace patient's gown and bed linen; assist patient to return to comfortable position.	• These actions restore patient's comfort and promote sense of well-being.
(11) Clean earpieces and diaphragm of stethoscope with alcohol swab as necessary.	• Cleaning with an alcohol swab helps prevent transmission of microorganisms between patients and when the stethoscope is shared.
8. Perform hand hygiene.	• Hand hygiene reduces transmission of microorganisms between patients.
9. Discuss findings with patient as needed.	• Such discussion promotes patient's participation in care and understanding of health status.
10. Compare current readings with previous baseline measurement or acceptable range of heart rate for patient's age (see Table 30-3).	• Evaluate for change in condition and alterations.
11. Compare peripheral pulse rate with apical rate, and note any discrepancy.	• Differences between measurements indicate pulse deficit and possibly cardiovascular compromise. Abnormalities may necessitate therapy.
12. Compare radial pulse equality between arms, and note any discrepancy.	• Differences between radial arteries indicate compromised peripheral vascular system.
13. Correlate pulse rate with data obtained from blood pressure and related signs and symptoms (palpitations, dizziness).	• Pulse rate and blood pressure are interrelated.

UNEXPECTED OUTCOMES	RELATED INTERVENTIONS
Radial pulse is weak or thready	• Assess both radial pulses and compare findings. Local obstruction to one extremity (e.g., clot, edema) may decrease peripheral blood flow. • Perform complete assessment of all pulses (see Chapter 32). • Observe for symptoms associated with decreased tissue perfusion, such as pallor and cool skin temperature of tissue distal to the weak pulse. • Measure apical and radial pulse simultaneously to determine presence of pulse deficit.
Apical pulse is greater than 100 beats per minute (tachycardia)	• Assess for presence of fever, anxiety, pain, recent exercise, hypotension, decreased oxygenation, or dehydration, all of which can elevate pulse. • Measure all vital signs. • Assess for factors associated with decreased cardiac output, such as chest pain, dizziness, cyanosis, fatigue, and orthopnea.
Apical pulse is less than 60 beats per minute (bradycardia)	• Assess for the presence of factors that may alter heart rate, such as digoxin or other cardiac medications. It may be necessary to withhold prescribed medications until the prescribing health care provider can evaluate the need to adjust dosage. • Assess for factors associated with decreased cardiac output.

RECORDING AND REPORTING

- Record pulse rate with assessment site in nurses' notes or vital signs flow sheet. Document pulse rate in nurses' narrative notes after administration of specific therapies.
- *Report abnormal findings* to nurse in charge or prescribing health care provider.

HOME CARE CONSIDERATIONS

- Assess home environment to determine which room will afford quiet environment for auscultating apical rate.

TABLE 30-3 Normal Resting Pulse Rates Across Age Groups

Age/Condition	Average (Beats Per Minute)	Normal Limits
Newborn	120	70–190
1 yr	120	80–160
2 yr	110	80–120
4 yr	100	80–120
6 yr	100	75–115
8 yr	90	70–110
10 yr	90	70–110
12 yr		
Female	90	70–110
Male	85	65–105
14 yr		
Female	85	65–105
Male	80	60–100
16 yr		
Female	80	60–100
Male	75	55–95
18 yr		
Female	75	55–95
Male	70	50–90
Well-conditioned athlete	May be 50–60	50–100
Adult	74–76	60–100
Older person	74–76	60–100

Jarvis, C., Browne, A. J., MacDonald-Jenkins, J., & Luctkar-Flude, M. (2014). *Physical examination & health assessment* (2nd Canadian ed., p. 158, Table 10-1). Toronto: Elsevier.

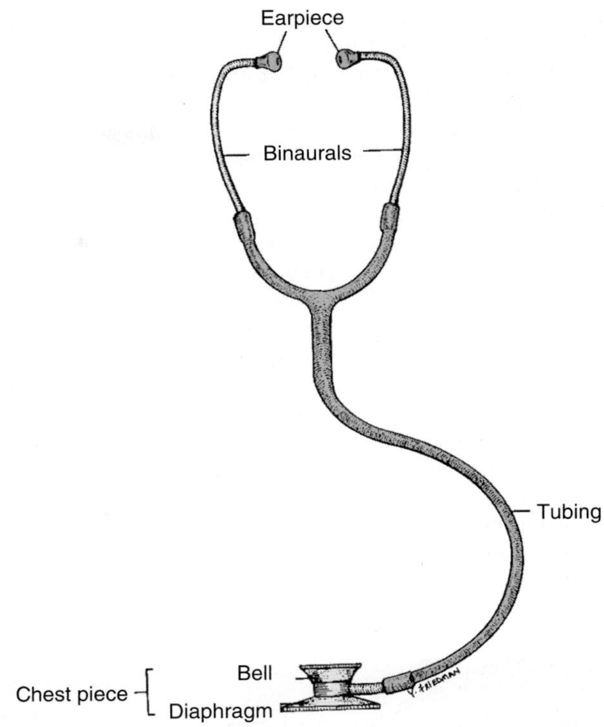

FIGURE 30-7 Parts of a stethoscope.

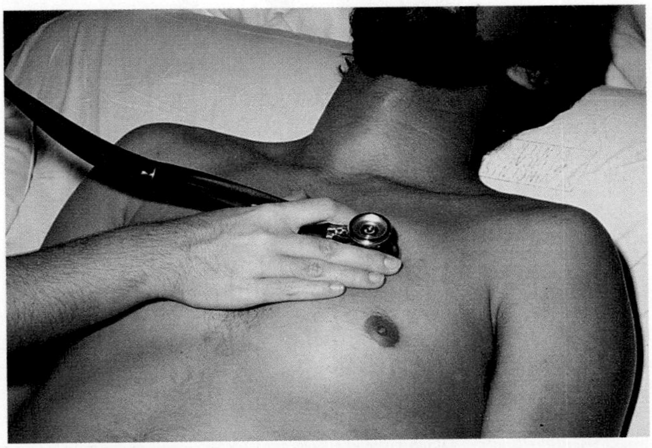

FIGURE 30-8 Positioning the diaphragm of the stethoscope firmly and securely when high-pitched heart sounds are auscultated.

cleaned according to the manufacturer's instructions (to remove cerumen). The bell and diaphragm need to be cleaned (to remove dust, lint, and body oils) routinely with alcohol to help prevent transmission of microorganisms. The tubing can be cleaned with mild soap and water. Nurses are encouraged to have their own stethoscope. If several nurses use the same stethoscope, the earpieces should be cleansed with an antiseptic prior to each use.

Character of the Pulse

Assessment of the radial pulse includes measurement of the rate, rhythm, strength, and bilateral equality. When auscultating an apical pulse, the nurse assesses rate and rhythm only.

Rate. Before measuring a pulse, the patient's baseline rate should be reviewed for comparison (see Table 30-3). Some practitioners make baseline measurements of the pulse rate with the patient sitting, standing, and lying. Changes in posture cause changes in pulse rate because of alterations in blood volume and sympathetic nervous system activity. The heart rate temporarily increases when a person changes from a lying to a sitting or standing position.

It is important to always consider the variety of factors influencing the pulse rate (Table 30-4). A single factor or a combination of factors can cause significant changes. If the nurse detects an abnormal rate while palpating a peripheral pulse, the next step is to assess the apical rate. This requires auscultation of heart sounds, which provides a more accurate assessment of cardiac contraction (see Chapter 32).

The nurse should identify the first and second heart sounds (S_1 and S_2). At normal slow rates, S_1 is low-pitched and dull, sounding like a "lub." S_2 is higher pitched and shorter, creating the sound "dub." Each set of "lub-dub" is counted as one heartbeat. Using the diaphragm or bell of the stethoscope, the nurse counts the number of "lub-dubs" occurring in 1 minute.

Peripheral and apical pulse rate assessment may reveal variations in heart rate. Two common abnormalities in pulse rate are tachycardia and bradycardia. **Tachycardia** is an abnormally fast heart rate, more than 100 beats per minute in adults. **Bradycardia** is a slow heart rate, less than 60 beats per minute in adults.

An inefficient contraction of the heart that fails to transmit a pulse wave to the peripheral pulse site creates a pulse deficit. Two people are required to detect a pulse deficit; one to assess either the radial or apical rate, and the second to simultaneously assess the other rate. Then the two rates are compared. The difference between the apical and radial pulse rates is the pulse deficit. For example, if the apical rate is 92 beats per minute and the radial rate is 78 beats per minute, the pulse deficit is 14 beats per minute. Pulse deficits are frequently associated with abnormal rhythms.

Rhythm. Normally, a regular interval occurs between each pulse or heartbeat. An interval interrupted by an early or late beat or a missed beat indicates an abnormal rhythm, or dysrhythmia. Dysrhythmia threatens the heart's ability to provide adequate cardiac output, particularly if it occurs repetitively. Dysrhythmia is identified by palpating an interruption in successive pulse waves or auscultating an interruption between heart sounds. If dysrhythmia is present, the nurse should assess the regularity of its occurrence and auscultate the apical rate (see Chapter 32 for further information about conducting a health assessment). Dysrhythmias are described as "regularly irregular" or "irregularly irregular."

To document a dysrhythmia, a prescribing health care provider may order electrocardiography, Holter monitoring, or telemetry. In electrocardiography, the electrical activity of the heart is recorded for a 12-second interval. The Holter monitor records 24 hours of electrical activity in a small recorder that the patient wears. In cardiac telemetry, the heart's electrical activity is monitored continuously, and the data are transmitted to a stationary monitor. Telemetry enables observation of heart rhythm during all the patient's daily activities and thus allows for immediate treatment if the rhythm becomes erratic or unstable.

Strength. The strength of a pulse reflects both the volume of blood ejected against the arterial wall with each heart contraction and the condition of the arterial vascular system leading to the pulse site. Normally, the pulse strength remains the same with each heartbeat. Pulse strength may be graded or described as bounding, strong, weak, thready, or absent. It is included during assessment of the vascular system (see Chapter 32 for further information about conducting a health assessment).

Equality. Pulses on both sides of the body should be assessed to compare their characteristics. A pulse in one extremity may be unequal to the pulse in the other extremity in strength, or it may be absent in many disease states (e.g., thrombus [clot] formation). All symmetrical pulses can be assessed simultaneously except for the carotid pulses, which should never be measured simultaneously because excessive pressure may occlude blood supply to the brain or trigger carotid reflexes that may result in altered cardiac output.

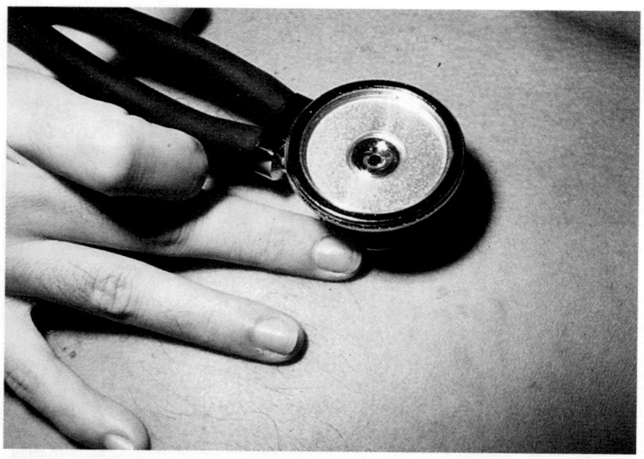

FIGURE 30-9 Positioning the bell of the stethoscope lightly on the skin to hear low-pitched heart sounds.

❖ NURSING PROCESS AND PULSE DETERMINATION

Pulse assessment helps to determine the general state of cardiovascular health and the body's response to other system imbalances. Tachycardia, bradycardia, and dysrhythmia are defining characteristics of many nursing diagnoses, including the following:

- *Activity intolerance*
- *Anxiety*
- *Decreased cardiac output*
- *Deficient/excess fluid volume*
- *Impaired gas exchange*
- *Hyperthermia*
- *Hypothermia*
- *Acute pain*
- *Ineffective tissue perfusion*

The nursing care plan includes interventions specific for the nursing diagnosis identified and its related factors. For example, the defining characteristics of an abnormal heart rate, exertional dyspnea, and a

TABLE 30-4 Factors Influencing Pulse Rates

Factor	Increases Pulse Rate	Decreases Pulse Rate
Exercise	Short-term exercise	Long-term exercise, which conditions the heart and results in a lower resting pulse and a quicker return to resting level after exercise
Temperature	Fever and heat	Hypothermia
Emotions	Anxiety increases sympathetic stimulation, affecting heart rate	Relaxation
Pain	Acute pain, which increases sympathetic stimulation and thereby increases heart rate; the effect of chronic pain on heart rate varies	Unrelieved severe pain, which increases parasympathetic stimulation and thereby affects heart rate
Medications	Positive chronotropic medications such as epinephrine	Negative chronotropic medications such as digitalis, β-adrenergic blockers, and calcium channel blockers
Hemorrhage	Loss of blood increases sympathetic stimulation	
Postural changes	Standing or sitting	Lying down
Pulmonary conditions	Diseases causing poor oxygenation, such as asthma and chronic obstructive pulmonary disease (COPD)	

patient's verbal report of fatigue lead to a diagnosis of *activity intolerance.* When the related factor is "inactivity after a prolonged illness," interventions focus on increasing the patient's daily exercises. Patient outcomes are evaluated by assessing the pulse rate, rhythm, strength, and equality after each intervention.

RESPIRATION

Human survival depends on the ability of oxygen (O_2) to reach body cells and of carbon dioxide (CO_2) to be removed from the cells. Respiration is the mechanism that the body uses to exchange gases between the atmosphere and the blood and between the blood and the cells. Respiration involves **ventilation** (the movement of gases in and out of the lungs), **diffusion** (the movement of oxygen and carbon dioxide between the alveoli and the red blood cells), and **perfusion** (the distribution of red blood cells to and from the pulmonary capillaries). To analyze respiratory efficiency, assessment data must be integrated from all three processes. Ventilation is assessed by determining respiratory rate, respiratory depth, and respiratory rhythm. Diffusion and perfusion are assessed by determining oxygen saturation.

Physiological Control

Breathing is generally a passive process; a person thinks little about it. The respiratory centre in the brain stem regulates the involuntary control of respirations. Adults normally breathe in a smooth, uninterrupted pattern, 12 to 20 times a minute.

Ventilation is regulated by levels of carbon dioxide, oxygen, and hydrogen ion concentration (pH) in the arterial blood. The most important factor is the level of CO_2 in the arterial blood. An elevation in the CO_2 level causes the respiratory control system in the brain to increase the rate and depth of breathing. The increased ventilatory effort removes excess CO_2 (which is the state of hypercarbia) by increasing exhalation. However, patients with chronic lung disease have ongoing hypercarbia. For them, chemoreceptors in the carotid artery and aorta become sensitive to **hypoxemia**, or low levels of arterial O_2. If arterial O_2 levels fall, these receptors signal the brain to increase the rate and depth of ventilation. Hypoxemia helps control ventilation in patients with chronic lung disease. Because low levels of arterial O_2 provide the stimulus that allows the patient to breathe, administration of high oxygen levels can be dangerous for these patients.

Mechanics of Breathing

Although breathing is normally passive, muscular work is involved in moving the lungs and chest wall. Inspiration is an active process. During inspiration, the respiratory centre sends impulses along the phrenic nerve, causing the diaphragm to contract. Abdominal organs move downward and forward, increasing the length of the chest cavity to move air into the lungs. The diaphragm moves approximately 1 cm, and the ribs retract upward from the body's midline approximately 1.2 to 2.5 cm. During a normal, relaxed breath, a person inhales 500 mL of air. This amount is referred to as the **tidal volume**. During expiration, the diaphragm relaxes and the abdominal organs return to their original positions. The lung and chest wall return to a relaxed position (Figure 30-10). In contrast to inhalation, expiration is a passive process. The normal rate and depth of ventilation, **eupnea**, is interrupted by sighing. The sigh, a prolonged deeper breath, is a protective physiological mechanism for expanding small airways and alveoli not ventilated during a normal breath.

The accurate assessment of respiration depends on the recognition of normal thoracic and abdominal movements. During quiet breathing, the chest wall gently rises and falls. Contraction of the accessory muscles of breathing (i.e., the intercostal muscles between the ribs and the muscles in the neck and shoulders) is not visible. During normal quiet breathing, diaphragmatic movement causes the abdominal cavity to rise and fall slowly.

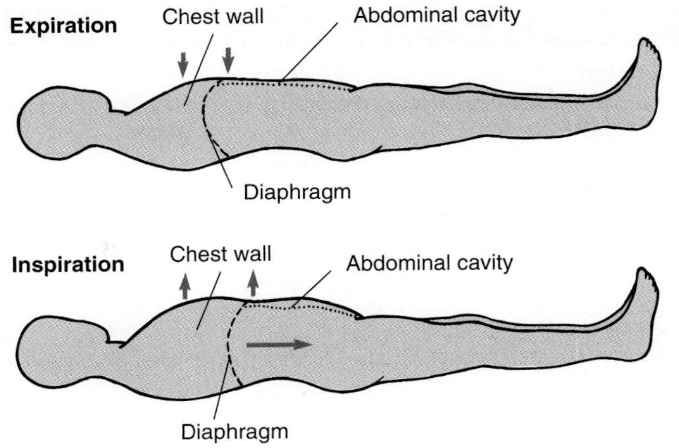

FIGURE 30-10 Illustration of diaphragmatic and chest wall movement during inspiration and expiration.

Assessment of Ventilation

Special equipment is not needed to measure respirations, but measurement must not be haphazard. Accurate measurement requires observation and palpation of chest wall movement.

A sudden change in the character of respirations is important. Because respiration is tied to the function of numerous body systems, all variables need to be considered when changes occur (Box 30-10). For example, abdominal trauma may injure the phrenic nerve, which is responsible for diaphragmatic contraction. The extent of the injury and the implications for the respiratory system are important to understand.

In a nursing assessment, you should try to not let the patient know that you are assessing his or her respiration. A patient aware of your intentions may consciously alter the rate and depth of breathing. The best time to measure respiration is immediately after measuring the pulse while your hand remains on the patient's wrist as it rests over the chest or abdomen. When assessing, keep in mind the patient's usual ventilatory rate and pattern, the influence any disease or illness has on respiratory function, the relationship between respiratory and cardiovascular function, and the influence of therapies on respiration. The objective measurements in assessing respiratory status include the rate and depth of breathing and the rhythm of ventilatory movements (Skill 30-3).

Respiratory Rate. The nurse should observe both inspiration and expiration when counting ventilation or respiration rate. The respiratory rate varies with age (Table 30-5) and usually decreases with age.

An apnea monitor is a respiratory monitoring device that aids in respiratory assessment. Leads that sense movement are attached to the patient's chest wall. Absence of chest wall movement triggers the apnea alarm. Apnea monitoring is used frequently with infants in hospitals and at home to observe for prolonged apneic events.

Ventilatory Depth. Depth of respiration is assessed by observing the degree of excursion or movement in the patient's chest wall. Ventilatory movements can be described as "deep," "normal," or "shallow." A deep respiration involves full expansion of the lungs with full exhalation. Respirations are shallow when only a small quantity of air passes through the lungs and ventilatory movement is difficult to

BOX 30-10 Factors Influencing Character of Respiration

Exercise

Exercise increases respiratory rate and depth to meet body's need for additional O_2 and to rid body of CO_2.

Acute Pain

Pain alters rate and rhythm of respiration; breathing becomes shallow.

Patient inhibits or splints chest wall movement when pain is in area of chest or abdomen.

Anxiety

Anxiety increases respiratory rate and depth as a result of sympathetic stimulation.

Smoking

Chronic smoking changes pulmonary airways, resulting in increased rate of respirations at rest when the person is not smoking.

Body Position

A straight, erect posture promotes full chest expansion.

A stooped or slumped position impairs ventilatory movement.

Lying flat prevents full chest expansion.

Medications

Opioids, general anaesthetics, and sedative hypnotics depress respiratory rate and depth.

Amphetamines and cocaine may increase respiratory rate and depth.

Bronchodilators slow respiratory rate by causing airway dilation.

Neurological Injury

Injury to the brain stem impairs the respiratory centre and inhibits respiratory rate and rhythm.

Hemoglobin Function

In the state of anemia, decreased hemoglobin levels reduce O_2-carrying capacity of the blood, which results in increases in respiratory rate.

Increased altitude lowers the amount of saturated hemoglobin, which increases respiratory rate and depth.

Abnormalities in blood cell function (e.g., sickle cell disease) reduce ability of red blood cells to carry oxygen, which results in increases in respiratory rate and depth.

SKILL 30-3 ASSESSING RESPIRATIONS

Delegation Considerations

The task of measuring respiration can be delegated to unregulated care providers (UCPs). The nurse is responsible for assessing for change in respiration rate, rhythm, and depth; therefore, when the task of measuring respiration is delegated, it is important to *inform the unregulated care provider* about the following:

- The patient's history or risk for abnormal respiratory status
- The frequency of respiration measurement for a specific patient
- Abnormalities that should be reported to the health care provider

Equipment

- Watch with second hand or digital display
- Pen and either vital sign flow sheet or record form

PROCEDURE

STEPS	RATIONALE
1. Determine need to assess patient's respiration.	• Use clinical judgement to determine need for assessment.
A. Note presence of risk factors for respiratory alterations.	• Conditions that heighten risk for alterations in ventilation—detected by changes in respiratory rate, depth, and rhythm—include fever, pain, anxiety, diseases of chest muscles, constrictive chest or abdominal dressings, gastric distension, chronic pulmonary diseases, traumatic chest injury, presence of a chest tube, respiratory infection, pulmonary edema and emboli, anemia, and head injury with damage to brain stem.
B. Assess for signs and symptoms of respiratory alterations, such as bluish (cyanotic) appearance of nail beds, lips, mucous membranes, and skin; restlessness, irritability, confusion, and reduced level of consciousness; pain during inspiration; laboured or difficult breathing; adventitious breath sounds (see Chapter 32 for further information about conducting a health assessment), inability to breathe spontaneously; thick, frothy, blood-tinged, or copious sputum produced on coughing.	• Physical signs and symptoms indicate alterations in respiratory status related to ventilation.
2. Assess pertinent laboratory values.	
A. Arterial blood gases (normal values may vary slightly between institutions): *pH:* 7.35–7.45 mm Hg *$PaCO_2$:* 35–45 mm Hg *PaO_2:* 80–100 mm Hg *SaO_2:* 95%–100%	• Arterial blood gases measure arterial blood pH, partial pressure of O_2 (PaO_2) and CO_2 ($PaCO_2$), and arterial O_2 saturation (SaO_2), which reflects patient's oxygenation status.

STEPS	RATIONALE
B. Pulse oximetry (SpO_2): Normal levels are 95–100%; 85–89% may be acceptable for certain chronic disease conditions; less than 85% is abnormal (see Skill 30-4).	• Although 95% is considered normal, 90% can be considered acceptable in patients with disorders such as sleep apnea. SpO_2 less than 85% is often accompanied by changes in respiratory rate, depth, and rhythm.
C. Specific tests of the complete blood cell count (CBC): (normal values for adults may vary between institutions and references consulted): *Hemoglobin:* 135–180 g/L in male patients; 120–160 g/L in female patients *Hematocrit:* 0.43–0.49 in male patients; 0.38–0.44 in female patients *Red blood cell count:* $4.7–5.74 \times 10^{12}$/L in male patients; $4.2–4.87 \times 10^{12}$/L in female patients	• Hemoglobin, hematocrit, and red blood cell count (three of several CBC tests) measure the concentration of hemoglobin volume of red blood cells, and red blood cell count, all of which reflect patient's capacity to carry O_2.
3. Determine previous baseline respiratory rate (if available) from patient's record.	• This enables the ability to assess for changes in patient's condition and provides comparison with future respiratory measurements.
4. Perform hand hygiene.	• Hand hygiene reduces transmission of microorganisms between the patient and the nurse.
5. Draw curtain around patient's bed or close room door, or do both.	• Drawing the curtain and closing the room door maintains patient's privacy, minimizes embarrassment, and promotes comfort.

CRITICAL DECISION POINT: *Patients with difficulty breathing (dyspnea), such as those with heart failure, with abdominal ascites, or in late stages of pregnancy, should be assessed in the position of greatest comfort. Repositioning may increase the work of breathing, which increases respiratory rate.*

STEPS	RATIONALE
6. Ensure patient is in comfortable position, preferably sitting or lying with the head of the bed elevated 45 to 60 degrees. Move bed linen or gown to be sure patient's chest is visible.	• Sitting erect promotes full ventilatory movement. A clear view of the chest wall and abdominal movements is needed for assessment.
7. Place patient's arm in relaxed position across his or her abdomen or lower chest, or place your hand directly over patient's upper abdomen (see Step 7 illustration).	• A similar position used during pulse assessment allows you to assess respiratory rate inconspicuously. The patient's hand or your hand rises and falls during respiratory cycle.

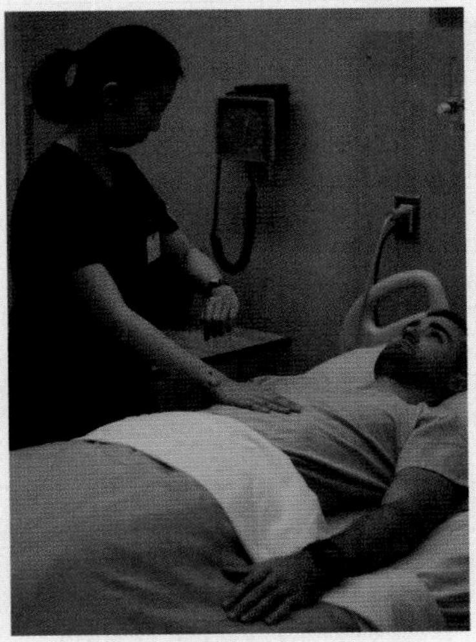

STEP 7 Nurse's hand over patient's abdomen to check respiration. (Courtesy Ouni Liao.)

STEPS	RATIONALE
8. Observe complete respiratory cycle (one inspiration and one expiration).	• You can determine rate accurately only after you have viewed the patient's respiratory cycle.
9. After observing cycle, look at watch's second hand. When second hand reaches a number on watch dial, begin counting respiratory cycles, starting with "one" for the first full cycle, then "two," and so on.	• Timing begins with count of one. Respirations occur more slowly than pulse.
10. If rhythm is regular, count number of respiratory cycles in 30 seconds and multiply by 2. If rhythm is irregular, slower than 12 per minute, or faster than 20 per minute, count for 1 full minute.	• Respiratory rate is equivalent to number of respiratory cycles per minute. Suspected irregularities necessitate assessment for at least 1 minute.

Continued

SKILL 30-3 ASSESSING RESPIRATIONS—cont'd

STEPS	RATIONALE
11. Note depth of respirations, which you subjectively assess by observing degree of chest wall movement while counting respiratory rate. You can also objectively assess respiratory depth by palpating patient's chest wall excursion or auscultating the posterior thorax after respiratory rate has been counted (see Chapter 32). Depth is described as "shallow," "normal," or "deep."	• Character of ventilatory movement may reveal specific disease state restricting volume of air from moving into and out of the lungs.
12. Note rhythm of ventilatory cycle. Normal breathing is regular and uninterrupted. Sighing should not be confused with abnormal rhythm.	• Character of ventilations can reveal specific types of alterations. Without being aware of it, people periodically take single deep breaths or sigh to expand small airways prone to collapse.

CRITICAL DECISION POINT: *Any irregular respiratory pattern or period of apnea (the cessation of respiration for several seconds) in an adult is a symptom of underlying disease and must be reported to the prescribing health care provider or nurse in charge. Further assessment may be required (see Chapter 32), and immediate intervention may be needed. An irregular respiratory rate and short apneic spells are normal only in newborns.*

STEPS	RATIONALE
13. Move back bed linen and patient's gown.	• This action restores patient's comfort and promotes sense of well-being.
14. Perform hand hygiene.	• Hand hygiene reduces transmission of microorganisms between patients.
15. Discuss findings with patient as needed.	• Such discussion promotes patient's participation in care and understanding of health status.
16. If patient's respiration is assessed for the first time, document rate, rhythm, and depth as baseline values.	• These data are used for comparing data from future respiratory assessments.
17. Compare respiration data with patient's previous baseline values and with normal values for rate, rhythm, and depth.	• These data allow you to assess for changes in patient's condition and for presence of respiratory alterations.

UNEXPECTED OUTCOMES	RELATED INTERVENTIONS
Patient's respiratory rate is less than 12 (bradypnea) or more than 20 (tachypnea) breaths per minute, depth is increased or decreased, rhythm is irregular, or patient feels "short of breath"	• Observe for related factors, including obstructed airway, abnormal breath sounds, productive cough, restlessness, irritability, anxiety, and confusion. • Position patient in a supported sitting position (semi-Fowler's or high Fowler's), unless contraindicated. • Provide oxygen as ordered. • When possible, remove respiratory irritants from the environment, such as second-hand smoke and perfumes.

RECORDING AND REPORTING

- Record respiratory rate and character in nurses' notes or vital sign flow sheet. Indicate type and amount of oxygen therapy if it was used by the patient during assessment. Document respiratory rate in nurses' narrative notes after administration of specific therapies.
- Report abnormal findings to nurse in charge or to prescribing health care provider.

HOME CARE CONSIDERATIONS

- Assess for environmental factors in the home that may influence patient's respiration, such as second-hand smoke, poor ventilation, or gas fumes.

see. Objective techniques are used if chest excursion is unusually shallow (see Chapter 32). Table 30-6 summarizes breathing pattern alterations.

Ventilatory Rhythm. Breathing pattern can be determined by observing the chest or the abdomen. Diaphragmatic breathing results from the contraction and relaxation of the diaphragm and is best observed by watching abdominal movements. Healthy men and children usually demonstrate diaphragmatic breathing. Women tend to use thoracic muscles to breathe; therefore, movements are best observed in the upper chest. Laboured respirations involve use of the accessory muscles of respiration visible in the neck. When a foreign body interferes with the movement of air in and out of the lungs, the intercostal spaces in the rib cage retract during inspiration, indicating increased respiratory effort. A longer expiration phase is evident when the outward flow of air is obstructed (e.g., as in asthma). In infants, additional indicators of respiratory distress are nasal flaring, grunting, and wheezing, making it important to look, listen, and feel when assessing breathing patterns in this population.

With normal breathing, a regular interval occurs after each respiratory cycle. Infants tend to breathe less regularly. The young child may breathe slowly for a few seconds and then suddenly breathe more rapidly. In assessment, the nurse should estimate the time interval after each respiratory cycle. Respiration is regular or irregular in rhythm.

Assessment of Diffusion and Perfusion

To evaluate the respiratory processes of diffusion and perfusion, the oxygen saturation of the blood is measured. Blood flow through the pulmonary capillaries contains red blood cells for oxygen attachment. After oxygen diffuses from the alveoli into the pulmonary blood, most of the oxygen attaches to hemoglobin molecules in red blood cells. The red blood cells then carry the oxygenated hemoglobin molecules through the left side of the heart and out to the peripheral capillaries, where the oxygen detaches, depending on the needs of the tissues.

The percentage of hemoglobin that is bound with oxygen in the arteries is the percentage of saturation of hemoglobin (SaO_2). This value is usually between 95 and 100%. SaO_2 is affected by factors that interfere with ventilation, perfusion, or diffusion (see Chapter 39). The saturation of venous blood (SvO_2) is lower because the tissues have removed some of the oxygen from the hemoglobin molecules. A normal value for SvO_2 is 70%. SvO_2 is affected by factors that interfere with or increase the tissue's need for oxygen.

Measurement of Arterial Oxygen Saturation. A pulse oximeter permits the indirect measurement of oxygen saturation (Skill 30-4). This device contains a probe with a light-emitting diode (LED) and photo detector connected by cable to an oximeter (Figures 30-11 and 30-12). The LED emits light wavelengths that are absorbed differently by oxygenated and deoxygenated hemoglobin molecules. The photo detector detects the amount of oxygen bound to hemoglobin molecules; the oximeter calculates the pulse saturation (SpO_2).

The photo detector is in the oximeter probe. The appropriate probe should be selected to reduce measurement error. Digit probes are spring-loaded and conform to various sizes. Earlobe probes have greater accuracy at lower saturations and are least affected by

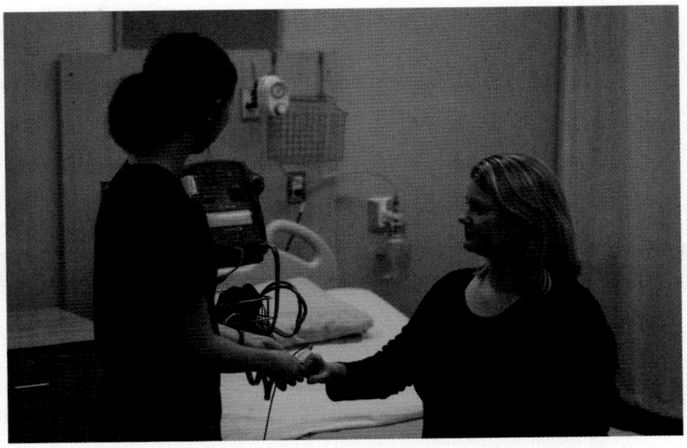

FIGURE 30-11 **Portable pulse oximeter.** (Courtesy Barbara J. Astle, RN, PhD.)

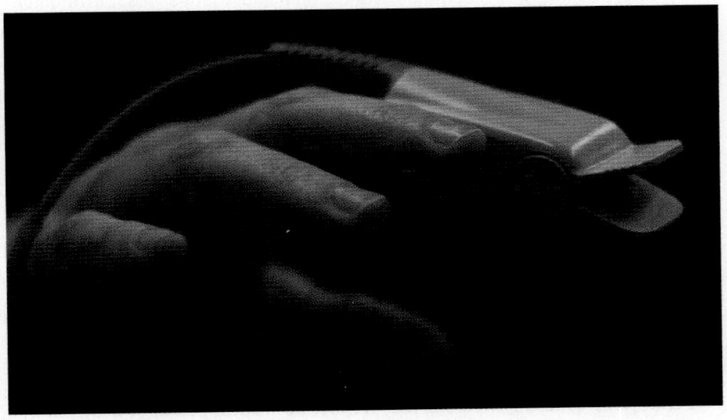

FIGURE 30-12 **Spring tension oximeter probe.** (Courtesy Barbara J. Astle, RN, PhD.)

TABLE 30-5 Acceptable Ranges of Respiratory Rates by Age

Age	Rate (Breaths per Minute)
Newborn	30–60
Infant (6 months)	30–50
Toddler (2 years)	25–32
Child and preadolescent (3–12 years)	20–30
Adolescent (13–18 years)	16–19
Adult (older than 18 years)	10–20

TABLE 30-6 Alterations in Breathing Pattern

Alteration	Description
Bradypnea	Rate of breathing is regular but abnormally slow (<12 breaths per minute).
Tachypnea	Rate of breathing is regular but abnormally rapid (>20 breaths per minute).
Hyperpnea	Respirations are laboured, increased in depth, and increased in rate (>20 breaths per minute). This occurs normally during exercise.
Apnea	Respirations cease for several seconds and then resume. Persistent cessation results in respiratory arrest.
Hyperventilation	Rate and depth of respirations increase. Hypocarbia may occur.
Hypoventilation	Respiratory rate is abnormally low, and depth of ventilation may be depressed. Hypercarbia may occur.
Cheyne-Stokes respiration	Respiratory rate and depth are irregular, characterized by alternating periods of apnea and hyperventilation. Respiratory cycle begins with slow, shallow breaths that gradually increase to abnormal rate and depth. The pattern reverses, breathing slows and becomes shallow, climaxing in apnea before respiration resumes.
Kussmaul's respiration	Respirations are abnormally deep, regular, and increased in rate.
Biot's respiration	Respirations are abnormally shallow for two to three breaths, followed by irregular periods of apnea.

SKILL 30-4 MEASURING OXYGEN SATURATION (PULSE OXIMETRY)

Delegation Considerations

The task of measuring oxygen saturation can be delegated to unregulated care providers (UCPs). The nurse is responsible for assessing the effect of changes in oxygen saturation; therefore, when the task of measuring oxygen saturation is delegated, it is important to *inform the unregulated care provider* about the following:

- The importance of notifying the nurse immediately of any reading lower than SpO_2 of 90%
- How to select appropriate sensor site and probe for measurement of oxygen saturation
- The frequency of oxygen saturation measurements for the patient
- Factors that can falsely lower SpO_2 (see Box 30-11)

Equipment

- Oximeter
- Oximeter probe appropriate for patient and recommended by manufacturer
- Acetone or nail polish remover, if needed
- Pen and either vital sign flow sheet or documentation form

PROCEDURE

STEPS	RATIONALE
1. Determine need to measure patient's oxygen saturation.	• Clinical judgement is used to determine need for assessment.
A. Note risk factors, including acute or chronic compromised respiratory function; recovery from general anaesthesia or monitored sedation; traumatic injury to chest; ventilator dependence; activity intolerance; and changes in supplemental oxygen therapy.	• Certain conditions heighten risk for decreased oxygen saturation.
B. Assess for signs and symptoms such as altered respiratory rate, depth, or rhythm; adventitious breath sounds (see Chapter 32 for further information about conducting a health assessment); cyanotic appearance of nail beds, lips, mucous membranes, and skin; restlessness, irritability, or confusion; reduced level of consciousness; and laboured or difficult breathing.	• Physical signs and symptoms may be indicative of abnormal oxygen saturation.
2. Assess for factors that normally influence measurement of SpO_2 (see Box 30-11), such as oxygen therapy, hemoglobin level, temperature, and medications (e.g., bronchodilators).	• This assessment enables you to accurately assess oxygen saturation variations. Peripheral vasoconstriction related to hypothermia can interfere with SpO_2 determination.
3. Review patient's medical record for pulse oximetry order, or consult agency policy or procedure manual for standard of care for measurement.	• Medical order may be needed to assess oxygen saturation.
4. Determine site most appropriate for sensor probe placement (e.g., digit, earlobe) by assessing capillary refill (see Chapter 32 for further information about conducting a health assessment) and skin condition. If capillary refill is less than 3 seconds, choose another site.	• Sensor requires pulsating vascular bed to identify hemoglobin molecules that absorb emitted light. Changes in SpO_2 are reflected in the circulation of the finger capillary bed within 30 seconds and the capillary bed of earlobe within 5–10 seconds.
A. Site needs to have adequate circulation and be free of moisture.	• Moisture prevents the sensor from detecting SpO_2 levels.
B. If peripheral digit is selected, it must be free of polish or artificial nail.	• Artificial nails and nail polish interferes with accuracy of readings. Opaque coatings decrease light transmission; nail polish containing blue pigment can absorb light emissions and falsely alter saturation measurement.
C. If tremors are present, use earlobe as site.	• Motion artifact is the most common cause of a false reading.
D. If patient is obese, clip-on probe may not fit; obtain a single-use tape-on probe.	
5. Determine previous baseline SpO_2 (if available) from patient's record.	• Baseline information provides basis for comparison and assists in assessment of current status and evaluation of interventions.
6. Explain purpose of procedure to patient and how oxygen saturation will be measured.	• Explaining procedures promotes patient's cooperation and increases compliance.
7. Perform hand hygiene.	• Hand hygiene reduces transmission of microorganisms between the patient and the nurse.
8. Position patient comfortably. If finger is chosen as monitoring site, support patient's lower arm.	• This positioning enables probe positioning and decreases motion artifact that interferes with SpO_2 determination.
9. Use acetone to remove any fingernail polish from digit to be assessed.	• Nail polish can interfere with accuracy of readings. Opaque coatings decrease light transmission; polish containing blue pigment can absorb light emissions and falsely alter oximetry measurements.
10. Instruct patient to breathe normally.	• Normal breathing prevents large fluctuations in respiratory rate and depth and prevents possible errors in SpO_2 reading.

STEPS	RATIONALE
11. Attach sensor probe to monitoring site. Inform patient that clip-on probe feels like a clothespin on the finger but will not hurt.	• To avoid startling patient, prepare patient to feel pressure of sensor probe's spring tension on a peripheral digit or earlobe.

CRITICAL DECISION POINT: ***Do not attach probe to finger, ear, or bridge of nose if area is edematous or skin integrity is compromised. Do not attach probe to hypothermic fingers. Select ear or bridge of nose if adult patient has history of peripheral vascular disease. Do not use sensors on earlobe and bridge of nose in infants and toddlers because of skin fragility. Do not use disposable adhesive probes if patient has latex allergy. Do not place probe on same extremity as electronic blood pressure cuff because blood flow to finger is temporarily interrupted when cuff inflates; this results in inaccurate readings that trigger alarms.***

STEPS	RATIONALE
12. Once sensor is in place, turn on oximeter. Observe pulse waveform and intensity display, and listen for audible beep. Correlate oximeter pulse rate with patient's radial pulse. Oximeter pulse rate and patient's radial pulse should be the same. If differences are present, re-evaluate oximeter probe placement, and reassess pulse rates.	• Pulse waveform and intensity display enables detection of valid pulse to SpO_2 value. Double-checking pulse rate ensures oximeter accuracy.
13. Leave probe in place until oximeter readout reaches constant value and pulse display reaches full strength during each cardiac cycle. Inform patient that oximeter alarm will sound if probe falls off or if patient moves probe. Read SpO_2 on digital display.	• Reading takes 10 to 30 seconds, depending on site selected.
14. If SpO_2 monitoring is to be continuous, verify SpO_2 alarm limits and alarm volume, which are preset by the manufacturer at a minimum of 85% and a maximum of 100%. Determine limits for SpO_2 and pulse rate alarms on the basis of each patient's condition. Verify that alarms are functional. Assess skin integrity under sensor probe every 2 hours. Relocate sensor probe at least every 4 hours and more frequently if skin integrity is altered or tissue perfusion compromised.	• Alarms must be set at appropriate limits and volumes to avoid frightening patients and visitors. • Spring tension of sensor probe or sensitivity to disposable sensor probe adhesive can cause skin irritation and lead to disruption of skin integrity.
15. Assist patient to return to comfortable position.	• This action restores patient's comfort and promotes sense of well-being.
16. Perform hand hygiene.	• Hand hygiene reduces transmission of microorganisms between the patient and the nurse.
17. Discuss findings with patient as needed.	• Such discussion promotes patient's participation in care and understanding of health status.
18. If SpO_2 measurements are intermittent or spot-checked, remove probe and turn oximeter power off between measurements. Store probe in appropriate location.	• Batteries will be depleted if oximeter is left on. Sensor probes are expensive and vulnerable to damage.
19. Compare SpO_2 readings with patient's baseline and acceptable values.	• Comparison reveals presence of abnormality.
20. Correlate SpO_2 with SaO_2 obtained from arterial blood gas measurements (see Chapter 40) if available.	• Reliability of noninvasive assessments is documented.
21. Correlate SpO_2 reading with data obtained from assessment of respiratory rate, depth, and rhythm (see Skill 30-3).	• Measurements of ventilation, perfusion, and diffusion are interrelated.

UNEXPECTED OUTCOMES	RELATED INTERVENTIONS
SpO_2 is less than 90%	• Verify that oximeter probe is intact and that outside light transmission does not influence measurement. • Observe for signs associated with decreased oxygenation (e.g., anxiety, restlessness, tachycardia, cyanosis) (see Box 30-12). • Verify that supplemental oxygen delivery system is delivered as ordered and is functioning properly. • Minimize factors that alter SpO_2 (e.g., lung secretions, increased activity, hyperthermia). • Position patient to promote optimal ventilation (e.g., high Fowler's position for obese patient). • Recheck SpO_2 after interventions, and notify physician if still below 90%.
Pulse rate indicated on oximeter is lower than patient's radial or apical pulse	• Reposition sensor probe to alternative site with increased blood flow. • Assess patient for signs of altered cardiac output (e.g., decreased blood pressure, cool skin, confusion).

Continued

SKILL 30-4 MEASURING OXYGEN SATURATION (PULSE OXIMETRY)—cont'd

STEPS	RATIONALE

RECORDING AND REPORTING

- Record SpO_2 value on nurses' notes or vital sign flow sheet, indicating type and amount of oxygen therapy used by patient during assessment. Record any signs and symptoms of oxygen desaturation in nurses' narrative notes. Report abnormal findings to nurse in charge or prescribing health care provider.
- Document SpO_2 in nurses' narrative notes after administration of specific therapies.
- Record in nurses' notes patient's use of continuous or intermittent pulse oximetry.

HOME CARE CONSIDERATIONS

- Pulse oximetry is used in home care to noninvasively monitor oxygen therapy or changes in oxygen therapy.
- Instruct caregivers to examine oximeter site before applying sensor.
- Instruct caregivers on procedure to implement when oxygen saturation is not within acceptable values.

peripheral vasoconstriction. Disposable sensor pads can be applied to a variety of sites, even the bridge of an adult's nose or the sole of an infant's foot. Factors that affect light transmission or peripheral arterial pulsations also affect the ability of the photo detector to measure SpO_2 (Box 30-11). Control of these factors allows accurate interpretation of abnormal SpO_2 measurements.

NURSING PROCESS AND RESPIRATORY VITAL SIGNS

Measurements of respiratory rate, pattern, and depth, along with SpO_2, enable the assessment of ventilation, diffusion, and perfusion. Other assessments also involve respiratory status (see Chapter 32). Each measurement provides clues in determining the nature of a patient's problem. Respiratory assessment data are defining characteristics of many nursing diagnoses, including the following:

- *Activity intolerance*
- *Ineffective airway clearance*
- *Anxiety*
- *Ineffective breathing pattern*
- *Impaired gas exchange*
- *Acute pain*
- *Ineffective tissue perfusion*
- *Dysfunctional ventilatory weaning response*

The nursing care plan includes interventions specific for the nursing diagnosis identified and the related factors (Box 30-12). For example, the defining characteristics of tachypnea, changes in depth of respirations, use of accessory muscles, cyanosis, and a decline in SpO_2 lead to

BOX 30-11 Factors Affecting Determination of Pulse Oxygen Saturation (SpO_2)

Interference With Light Transmission

Outside light sources interfere with oximeter's ability to process reflected light.

Carbon monoxide (caused by smoke inhalation or poisoning) artificially elevates SpO_2 by absorbing light in a way similar to oxygen.

Patient motion interferes with oximeter's ability to process reflected light.

Jaundice interferes with oximeter's ability to process reflected light.

Intravascular dyes (e.g., methylene blue) absorb light in a way similar to deoxyhemoglobin and artificially lower saturation.

Nail polish, artificial nails, and metal studs in nails interfere with light absorption and the ability of the oximeter to process reflected light.

Dark skin pigment sometimes results in signal loss or overestimation of saturation.

Reduction of Arterial Pulsations

Peripheral vascular disease (atherosclerosis) reduces pulse volume.

Hypothermia at assessment site decreases peripheral blood flow.

Pharmacological vasoconstrictors (epinephrine, dopamine) decrease peripheral pulse volume.

Low cardiac output and hypotension decrease blood flow to peripheral arteries.

Peripheral edema obscures arterial pulsation.

Tight probe records venous pulsations in the finger that compete with arterial pulsations.

BOX 30-12 CASE STUDY

Oxygen Therapy and Palliative Care

During my nursing assessment of a palliative patient who had requested comfort care only, I noted that her oxygen saturation level was below 90%; therefore, as I had been taught, I immediately initiated oxygen therapy with nasal prongs at 2 L. Her SpO_2 came up to normal levels immediately, so I left the oxygen on and proceeded with my other patient assessments. Her physician came in to see her later that day and he immediately questioned why she was hooked up to oxygen. I explained about her low saturation levels, certain that he would agree with my intervention. Instead, he asked me, "Did she appear uncomfortable before you put the oxygen on? Was she struggling to breathe?" I had to reply, "No, she was very peaceful and resting." Then he said that if she was not uncomfortable, oxygen therapy was unnecessary, as she is on "comfort measures only." Honestly, that thought had never occurred to me, as I had been trained that if oxygen levels are low, you put oxygen on. This challenged me in my future practice to not look only at the saturation levels but also to assess the patient: Is the patient in distress? Struggling to breathe? Showing other signs of discomfort? It also challenged me to truly pursue greater knowledge about, and advocate for, comfort care with palliative patients.

a diagnosis of *impaired gas exchange.* Related factors may include lung surgery, history of chronic obstructive lung disease, and history of heavy smoking. Patient outcomes are evaluated by assessing the respiratory rate, ventilatory depth, rhythm, and SpO_2 after each intervention.

BLOOD PRESSURE

Blood pressure is the force exerted on the walls of an artery by the pulsing blood under pressure from the heart. Blood flows throughout the circulatory system because of pressure changes. It moves from an area of high pressure to an area of low pressure. Systemic or arterial blood pressure (the blood pressure in the system of arteries in the body) is a good indicator of cardiovascular health. The heart's contraction forces blood under high pressure into the aorta. The peak of maximum pressure when ejection occurs is the systolic blood pressure. When the ventricles relax, the blood remaining in the arteries exerts diastolic blood pressure, which is the minimal pressure exerted against the arterial walls at any time.

The standard unit for measuring blood pressure is millimetres of mercury (mm Hg). The measurement indicates the height to which the blood pressure can raise a column of mercury. It is recorded as the systolic reading over the diastolic reading (e.g., 120/80). The difference between systolic and diastolic pressure is the pulse pressure. For a blood pressure of 120/80, the pulse pressure is 40. This parameter has been recently considered a potential indicator of cardiovascular disease, given its relationship to compliance or stiffening of the arteries.

Physiology of Arterial Blood Pressure

Blood pressure reflects the interrelationships of cardiac output, peripheral vascular resistance, blood volume, blood viscosity, and artery elasticity. Knowledge of these hemodynamic variables helps in the assessment of blood pressure alterations.

Cardiac Output. Blood pressure depends on cardiac output. When volume increases in an enclosed space, such as a blood vessel, the pressure in that space rises. As cardiac output increases, more blood is pumped against arterial walls, causing the blood pressure to rise. Cardiac output increases as a result of an increase in heart rate, greater heart muscle contractility, or an increase in blood volume. Changes in heart rate can occur faster than changes in heart muscle contractility or blood volume. A rapid or significant increase in heart rate decreases the heart's ability to fill, resulting in blood pressure decreasing.

Peripheral Resistance. Blood pressure depends on peripheral vascular resistance. Blood circulates through a network of arteries, arterioles, capillaries, venules, and veins. Arteries and arterioles are surrounded by smooth muscle that contracts or relaxes to change the size of the lumen. Normally, arteries and arterioles remain partially constricted to maintain a constant flow of blood. The size of arteries and arterioles changes to adjust blood flow to the needs of local tissues. For example, when a major organ requires more blood, the peripheral arteries constrict, decreasing their supply of blood. More blood then becomes available to the major organ because of the resistance change in the periphery. Peripheral vascular resistance is the resistance to blood flow determined by the tone of the vascular musculature and diameter of blood vessels. The smaller the lumen of a vessel, the greater the resistance to blood flow. As resistance rises, arterial blood pressure rises. As vessels dilate and resistance falls, blood pressure subsequently decreases.

Blood Volume. The volume of blood circulating within the vascular system affects blood pressure. Most adults have a circulating blood volume of approximately 5 000 mL. Normally, this blood volume remains constant. However, if volume increases, more pressure is exerted against arterial walls. For example, the rapid, uncontrolled infusion of intravenous fluids would typically increase blood pressure. When circulating blood volume decreases, as with hemorrhage or dehydration, blood pressure would subsequently decrease.

Viscosity. The thickness or viscosity of blood affects the ease with which blood flows through the small vessels. The hematocrit, or percentage of red blood cells in the blood, determines blood viscosity. When the hematocrit rises and blood flow slows, the heart must contract more forcefully to move the viscous blood through the circulatory system. This results in arterial blood pressure increasing.

Elasticity. Normally, the walls of an artery are elastic and easily distensible. As pressure within the arteries increases, the diameter of the vessel walls increases to accommodate the rising pressure change. Arterial distensibility prevents wide fluctuations in blood pressure. However, in certain diseases, such as arteriosclerosis, vessel walls lose their elasticity and are replaced by fibrous tissue that cannot stretch as well. With reduced elasticity, resistance to blood flow is greater. As a result, when the left ventricle ejects its stroke volume, the vessels no longer yield to pressure. Instead, a given volume of blood is forced through the rigid arterial walls, and systemic pressure rises. Systolic pressure is more significantly elevated than diastolic pressure as a result of reduced arterial elasticity.

Most importantly, each hemodynamic factor significantly affects the others. For example, as arterial elasticity declines, peripheral vascular resistance increases. The complex control of the cardiovascular system normally prevents any single factor from permanently changing the blood pressure. For example, if the blood volume falls, the body compensates with increased vascular resistance.

Factors Influencing Blood Pressure

Blood pressure is not constant; it is continually influenced by many factors. One measurement cannot adequately reflect a patient's blood pressure. Blood pressure changes from heartbeat to heartbeat. Blood pressure trends, not individual measurements, guide nursing interventions. By understanding these factors, you can more accurately interpret blood pressure readings.

Age. Normal blood pressure levels vary throughout life. Blood pressure increases during childhood. The level of a child's or adolescent's blood pressure is assessed with regard to body size and age. An infant's systolic blood pressure ranges from 65 to 115 systolic, and the diastolic pressure ranges from 42 to 80. The normal systolic blood pressure for a 7-year-old is 87 to 117, and the normal diastolic pressure is 48 to 64. Larger children (heavier and/or taller) have higher blood pressures than do smaller children of the same age. During adolescence, blood pressure continues to vary according to body size.

An adult's blood pressure tends to increase with advancing age. Canadian guidelines indicate that blood pressure should be assessed at all appropriate health care visits. In most people, including those with nondiabetic chronic kidney disease, blood pressure should be treated to lower than 140/90 mm Hg. In those people with diabetes, blood pressure should be treated to below 130/80 mm Hg (Table 30-7). Those with high normal blood pressure should be followed up annually to assess for risk of early-onset hypertension (Leung, Daskalopoulou, Dasgupta, et al., 2017). Older persons may have a rise in systolic pressure that is related to decreased vessel elasticity; however, blood pressure higher than 140/90 is defined as hypertension and increases an older person's risk for hypertension-related illness.

Stress. Anxiety, fear, pain, and other emotional stress result in stimulation of the sympathetic nervous system, which increases heart rate, cardiac output, and peripheral vascular resistance. These alterations, in turn, increase blood pressure. Anxiety can raise blood pressure by as much as 30 mm Hg.

Ethnicity. The incidence of hypertension is higher among ethnic groups such as South Asian, First Nations, Métis, Inuit, and in people of African descent. Genetic and environmental factors are believed to be contributing factors (Heart & Stroke Foundation, 2017).

Gender. Males and females do not have clinically significant differences in blood pressure levels. After puberty, boys tend to have higher blood pressure readings. After menopause, women tend to have higher levels of blood pressure than do men of similar ages.

Daily Variation. A daily peak and trough, the diurnal rhythm, occurs in blood pressure. Blood pressure rises into late afternoon and early evening then declines into early morning when it is at its lowest (Jarvis, Browne, MacDonald-Jenkins, et al., 2014, p. 160).

Medications. During blood pressure assessment, it is important to determine if the patient is on any type of medications, as some can directly or indirectly affect blood pressure. Antihypertensive or other cardiac medications may lower blood pressure (Table 30-8). Opioid analgesics can lower blood pressure. Vasoconstrictors and an excess of intravenous fluids can increase blood pressure. It is therefore critical to always assess blood pressure before administering any of these medications.

Activity, Weight, and Smoking. Blood pressure can be reduced for several hours after a period of exercise. Older persons often experience a 5- to 10-mm Hg fall in blood pressure about 1 hour after eating. Increases in oxygen demanded by the body during activity leads to increases in blood pressure. Obesity is a factor in hypertension. Smoking results in vasoconstriction. Blood pressure rises when a person is smoking, and it returns to baseline 15 minutes after smoking ceases.

TABLE 30-7 Blood Pressure Treatment Targets

Setting	Location or Condition	TARGET SBP mm Hg	TARGET DBP mm Hg
Home	Home blood pressure and daytime ABPM	<135/85	<85
Office	High risk*	≤120	N/A
	Diabetes	<130	<80
	All others (including chronic kidney disease)	<140	<90

**High risk:* Having at least one of the following factors: ((a) clinical or subclinical cardiovascular disease, (b) chronic kidney disease (nondiabetic nephropathy, proteinuria <1 g/d, estimated glomerular filtration rate 20–59 mL/min/1.73 m^2), (c) estimated 10-year global Framingham risk >15%, or (d) age ≥75 years.
ABPM, Ambulatory blood pressure monitoring; *DBP,* diastolic blood pressure; *SBP,* systolic blood pressure.
To keep up to date with the latest evidence and resources for the prevention and control of hypertension, go to http://www.htnupdate.ca.
Hypertension Canada. (2017). *What's new? Hypertension Canada 2017 Hypertension Canada guidelines for the management of hypertension* (slide 11). Retrieved from https://www.hypertension.ca/images/CHEP_2017/HTN_Whats_New_2017_EN.pdf.

Hypertension

The most common alteration in blood pressure is hypertension. Hypertension is often asymptomatic. Hypertension is associated with thickening and loss of elasticity in the arterial walls. Peripheral vascular resistance increases within thick, inelastic vessels. The heart must continually pump against greater resistance. As a result, blood flow to vital organs such as the heart, brain, and kidney decreases.

According to Hypertension Canada (Leung et al., 2017), one elevated blood pressure measurement does not usually qualify as a diagnosis of hypertension unless the office blood pressure measurement (OBPM) or automated office blood pressure (AOBP) measurements' means are systolic blood pressure ≥180 mm Hg and/or diastolic blood pressure ≥110 mm Hg (Figure 30-13). However, if an elevated manual reading (e.g., ≥140/90 mm Hg) is obtained during the first blood pressure measurement, two subsequent readings should be taken. If using non-AOBP measurement, the first reading should be discarded and the additional readings are then averaged. If an AOPB measurement is taken, the blood pressure calculated and displayed by the device is used. If the AOPB and subsequent manual blood pressure results remain elevated, further medical follow-up, such as home blood pressure monitoring and ambulatory blood pressure monitoring, are required to confirm the diagnosis of hypertension (Leung et al., 2017) (see Figure 30-13). Nurses need to incorporate these blood pressure measurement recommendations into practice, in order to correctly interpret blood pressure and minimize error. Box 30-13 describes a nursing example.

TABLE 30-8 Antihypertensive Medications

Medication Type	Names	Action
Diuretics	Furosemide (Lasix), spironolactone (Aldactone), metolazone, polythiazide, triamterene (Dyazide)	Reduce kidneys' reabsorption of sodium and water, thus lowering circulating fluid volume
β-Adrenergic blockers	Atenolol (Tenormin), nadolol (Corgard), propranolol (Inderal), metoprolol (Lopressor)	Combine with β-adrenergic receptors in the heart, arteries, and arterioles to block response to sympathetic nerve impulses; this results in reduced heart rate and thus cardiac output
Vasodilators	Hydralazine hydrochloride (Apresoline), minoxidil (Loniten)	Act on arteriolar smooth muscle to cause relaxation and reduce peripheral vascular resistance
Calcium channel blockers	Diltiazem (Cardizem, Dilacor XR), verapamil hydrochloride (Calan SR), nifedipine (Procardia)	Reduce peripheral vascular resistance by systemic vasodilation
Angiotensin-converting enzyme (ACE) inhibitors	Ramipril (Altace), captopril (Capoten), enalapril (Vasotec), lisinopril (Prinivil, Zestril), benazepril (Lotensin)	Block the conversion of angiotensin I to angiotensin II, which prevents vasoconstriction; also reduces aldosterone production and fluid retention, thereby lowering circulating fluid volume
Angiotensin II receptor blockers	Losartan (Cozaar), olmesartan (Benicar)	Block the binding of angiotensin II, which prevents vasoconstriction

Home measurement of blood pressure is an important facet in the diagnosis of white coat hypertension and masked hypertension. In **white coat hypertension**, blood pressure is elevated during a visit to a health care provider. Affected patients are more likely to develop true hypertension over time. In **masked hypertension**, the blood pressure reading is normal while the patient is with a health care provider but becomes elevated at home (Hypertension Canada, 2015). People with a family history of hypertension are at significant risk for developing hypertension and cardiovascular disease. Cardiovascular disease is a noncommunicable disease (NCD) that accounts for most NCD deaths—17.5 million people annually (World Health Organization, 2017b) (Box 30-14). Modifiable risk factors linked to hypertension include obesity, cigarette smoking, heavy alcohol consumption, high sodium (salt) intake, sedentary lifestyle, and continued exposure to stress. Hypertension is a major factor underlying deaths from strokes and is a factor contributing to myocardial infarctions (heart attacks). When hypertension is diagnosed, the patient and family need to be educated about hypertension and its treatment, correct blood pressure measurement technique and normal values, and the importance of adhering to a treatment plan (Hypertension Canada, 2015).

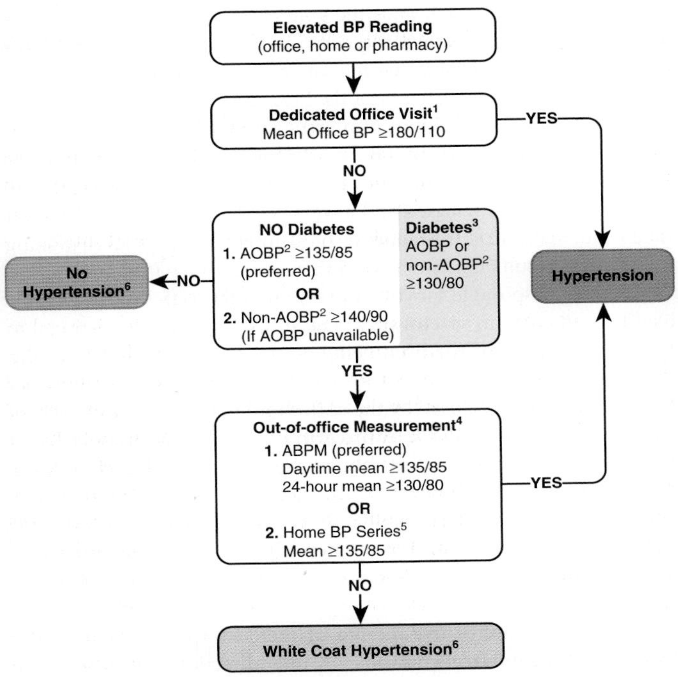

FIGURE 30-13 Criteria for the diagnosis of hypertension and recommendations for follow-up: overview. Measurement using electronic (oscillometric) upper arm devices is preferred over auscultation. *ABPM,* Ambulatory blood pressure measurement; *AOBP,* automated office blood pressure; *BP,* blood pressure; *HBPM,* home blood pressure measurement; *OBPM,* office blood pressure measurement. (Reprinted from Leung, A. A., Daskalopoulou, S. S., Dasgupta, K., McBrien, K., Butalia, S., Zarnke, K. B., ... & Rabi, D. M. [2017]. Hypertension Canada's 2017 guidelines for diagnosis, risk assessment, prevention, and treatment of hypertension in adults. *Canadian Journal of Cardiology 33*[5], p. 557-579.)

Hypotension

Hypotension is considered present when the systolic blood pressure decreases to 90 mm Hg or lower. Some adults may have a low blood pressure normally; however, for the majority of people, low blood pressure is an abnormal finding associated with illness.

BOX 30-14 Cardiovascular Disease (CVD)—A Noncommunicable Disease: Key Facts

- CVDs are the number one cause of death globally: More people die annually from CVDs than from any other cause.
- An estimated 17.5 million people died from CVDs in 2012, representing 31% of all global deaths. Of these deaths, an estimated 7.4 million were due to coronary heart disease and 6.7 million were due to stroke.
- Over three-quarters of CVD deaths take place in low- and middle-income countries.
- Out of the 16 million deaths under the age of 70 due to noncommunicable diseases, 82% occur in low- and middle-income countries, and 37% are caused by CVDs.
- Most CVDs can be prevented by addressing behavioural risk factors, such as tobacco use, unhealthy diet and obesity, physical inactivity, and harmful use of alcohol, using population-wide strategies.
- People with CVD or who are at high cardiovascular risk (due to the presence of one or more risk factors such as hypertension, diabetes, hyperlipidemia, or already established disease) need early detection and management, through counselling and medicines, as appropriate.

World Health Organization. (2017). *Cardiovascular diseases (CVDs) fact sheet.* Retrieved from http://www.who.int/mediacentre/factsheets/fs317/en/.

BOX 30-13 CASE STUDY

White Coat Hypertension

Between the ages of 45 and 49, my neighbour, M. J., had a blood pressure reading of approximately 140/85 during her annual checkups. After each visit, I informed her that she may have white coat hypertension and recommended that she monitor her blood pressure at home because individuals who have white coat hypertension are at risk of developing true hypertension. I advised her to reduce her sodium dietary intake and to exercise regularly; she did not drink alcohol. I monitored her blood pressure at home; results were all below 135/85. At her annual checkup after her 50th birthday, her blood pressure was 140/86; at a follow-up visit 2 months later, it was 142/88. During that time, her blood pressure at home ranged between 136 and 140 (systolic) and 82 and 86 (diastolic). She went to the hypertension clinic to have a 24-hour blood pressure monitor applied. I informed her that this test would provide the physician with information to make treatment decisions. Because of high readings during the test, Dyazide (triamterene), 25 mg daily, was prescribed. I continued to monitor her blood pressure at home, but because her results remained in the hypertensive range, enalapril (Vasotec) 2.5 mg was added to her blood pressure drug regimen at her next visit 4 months later. Since then, all of her blood pressure readings, both at home and in the physician's office, have been below 126 (systolic) and 82 (diastolic). Four years later, M. J.'s blood pressure continues to be controlled.

Hypotension occurs because of the dilation of the arteries in the vascular bed, the loss of a substantial amount of blood volume (e.g., hemorrhage), or the failure of the heart muscle to pump adequately (e.g., myocardial infarction). Hypotension associated with pallor, skin mottling, clamminess, confusion, increased heart rate, or decreased urine output is life-threatening and should be reported to a prescribing health care provider immediately.

Orthostatic hypotension, also referred to as **postural hypotension,** occurs when a normotensive person (a person with normal blood pressure) develops symptoms of low blood pressure when rising to an upright position. When a healthy individual changes from lying down to a sitting or standing position, the peripheral blood vessels in the legs constrict. Vasoconstriction in the lower extremities during standing prevents the pooling of blood in the legs caused by gravity. Thus, no symptoms are normally felt when standing. In contrast, when patients have a decreased blood volume, their blood vessels are already constricted. When a volume-depleted patient stands, blood pressure drops significantly, and heart rate increases to compensate for the drop in cardiac output. Patients who are dehydrated, are anemic, or have experienced prolonged bed rest or recent blood loss are at risk for orthostatic hypotension.

To assess for orthostatic hypotension, during vital sign measurements, blood pressure and pulse are obtained with the patient supine, sitting, and standing. The readings are obtained 1 to 3 minutes after the patient changes position. In most cases, orthostatic hypotension is detected within a minute of standing up. If it occurs, assist the patient to a lying position and notify the prescribing health care provider or nurse in charge. While obtaining orthostatic measurements, it is important to observe for other symptoms of hypotension, such as fainting, weakness, or light-headedness. When recording orthostatic blood pressure measurements, the nurse records the patient's position, in addition to the blood pressure measurement—for example, "140/80 supine, 132/72 sitting, 108/60 standing." Because the skill of orthostatic measurements requires advanced reasoning and ongoing nursing judgement, the nurse *should not delegate this procedure* to unregulated care providers.

Measurement of Blood Pressure

Arterial blood pressure may be measured either directly (invasively) or indirectly (noninvasively). The direct method requires the insertion of a thin catheter into an artery. Tubing connects the catheter to electronic monitoring equipment. The monitor displays a constant arterial pressure waveform and reading. Because of the risk of sudden blood loss from an artery, invasive blood pressure monitoring is used only in intensive care settings. For noninvasive blood pressure measurement, the 2015 Canadian Hypertension Education Program (CHEP) now recommends that validated oscillometric devices be used, because they minimize errors caused by the use of auscultation, such as provider hearing deficits, rounding the reading to a 0 or 5, and rapid deflation. Other concerns are that mercury sphygmomanometers are being phased out and aneroid sphygmomanometers are less likely to remain calibrated (Hypertension Canada, 2015). Despite these concerns, the auscultatory method is still often being utilized. According to a survey of Canadian family physicians, 52% of them still use aneroid or mercury devices with auscultation to manually measure blood pressure, instead of following the current Canadian guidelines (Kaczorowski, Myers, Gelfer, et al. 2017). It is important that electronic measurement of blood pressure be encouraged; however, until manual blood pressure is no longer being used, it is important for nurses to know proper technique (Skill 30-5).

Blood Pressure Equipment. Before assessing blood pressure, make sure that you know how to use a sphygmomanometer and stethoscope. A **sphygmomanometer** includes a pressure manometer, an occlusive cloth or vinyl cuff that encloses an inflatable rubber bladder, and a pressure bulb with a release valve that inflates the bladder. Manometers are of two types: aneroid (Figure 30-14) and mercury. Aneroid manometers have the advantages of being safe, lightweight, portable, and compact. The aneroid manometer contains a glass-enclosed circular gauge with a needle that registers millimetre calibrations. Before using the aneroid model, ensure that the needle is pointing to zero and that the manometer is correctly calibrated. Aneroid sphygmomanometers require regular calibration, otherwise their use can lead to inaccurate results (Hypertension Canada, 2015).

Mercury manometers, once the gold standard, are less commonly used because they contain mercury, a hazardous substance. Most municipalities have prohibited the sale or use of mercury-containing devices because of potential hazards. Pressure created by the inflation of the cuff moves the column of mercury upward against the force of gravity. Millimetre calibrations mark the height of the mercury column. To ensure accurate readings, the mercury column should fall freely as pressure is released and always remain at zero when the cuff is deflated. Measure at the meniscus of the mercury at eye level; looking up or down results in distorted readings.

Cloth or disposable vinyl compression cuffs contain an inflatable bladder and come in several sizes. The size selected is proportional to the circumference of the limb being assessed (Figure 30-15). Ideally, the width of the cuff should be 40% of the circumference of the upper arm. The bladder, enclosed by the cuff, should encircle at least 80% of the arm of an adult and the entire arm of a child. The lower edge of the cuff should be positioned above the patient's antecubital fossa, allowing room for placement of the stethoscope bell or diaphragm. Many adults require a large-sized cuff. Using the forearm when a large cuff is not available is not recommended. Blood pressure measurements are not accurate unless the correct size cuff is applied appropriately (Table 30-9).

The release valve of the aneroid or mercury sphygmomanometer should be clean and freely movable in either direction. The valve, when closed, holds the pressure constant. A sticky valve makes pressure cuff deflation hard to regulate. The pressure bulb should be free of leaks.

Auscultation. The best environment for blood pressure measurement by auscultation is a quiet room at a comfortable temperature. Although the patient may lie or stand, sitting is the preferred position. In most patients, blood pressure readings obtained in the supine, sitting, and standing positions are similar.

Patient position should be consistent during routine blood pressure measurements to enable meaningful comparison of values. Before measuring blood pressure, attempt to control factors responsible for artificially high readings, such as pain, anxiety, or exertion. It is important to minimize the patient's perceptions that the physical or interpersonal environment is stressful in order to reduce any effect on blood pressure measurement.

During the initial assessment, measure and record the blood pressure in both arms. Normally, pressures in the arms differ by 5 to 10 mm Hg. In subsequent assessments, the blood pressure in the arm with the higher pressure is measured. Pressure differences greater than 10 mm Hg indicate vascular problems and should be reported to the prescribing health care provider or nurse in charge.

The patient should be asked to state his or her usual blood pressure. If the patient does not know, inform the patient of his or her blood pressure reading after measuring and recording the blood pressure. It is important to educate the patient about optimal values of blood pressure, the risk factors for developing hypertension, and the dangers of hypertension.

SKILL 30-5 MEASURING BLOOD PRESSURE

Delegation Considerations

In most provinces and territories, the task of measuring blood pressure can be delegated to unregulated care providers (UCPs). The nurse is responsible for assessing changes in blood pressure; therefore, when the task of measuring blood pressure is delegated, it is important to *inform the unregulated care provider* about the following:

- Selection of appropriate limb for blood pressure measurement—typically the arm, but can also be measured on leg
- Selection of appropriate-size blood pressure cuff for designated extremity
- Frequency of blood pressure measurement for patient
- Patient's usual values
- Abnormalities that should be reported to the health care provider

Equipment

- Aneroid sphygmomanometer
- Cloth or disposable vinyl pressure cuff of appropriate size for patient's extremity
- Stethoscope
- Alcohol swab
- Pen and either vital sign flow sheet or documentation form

PROCEDURE

STEPS	RATIONALE
1. Determine need to assess patient's blood pressure.	• Use clinical judgement to determine need for assessment.
A. Note risk factors for alteration in blood pressure, including cardiovascular disease, renal disease, diabetes, circulatory shock, acute or chronic pain, rapid intravenous infusion of fluids or blood products, increased intracranial pressure, postoperative conditions, and toxemia of pregnancy.	• Certain conditions heighten risk for blood pressure alteration.
B. Observe for signs and symptoms of blood pressure alterations. **(1)** High blood pressure (hypertension): headache (usually occipital), flushing of face, nosebleed, and fatigue (older persons): often asymptomatic until pressure is very high **(2)** Low blood pressure (hypotension): dizziness, mental confusion; restlessness; pale, dusky, or cyanotic skin and mucous membranes; and cool, mottled skin over extremities	• Physical signs and symptoms may indicate alterations in blood pressure.
2. Determine best site for blood pressure assessment. Avoid applying cuff to extremity where intravenous fluids are infusing; where an arteriovenous shunt or fistula is present; on the side where breast or axillary surgery has been performed; and when extremity has been traumatized, is diseased, or requires a cast or bulky bandage (Box 30-15). Use lower extremities when the brachial arteries are inaccessible.	• Inappropriate site selection results in poor amplification of sounds, causing inaccurate readings. Application of pressure from inflated cuff bladder temporarily impairs blood flow and can exacerbate existing impairment of circulation in extremity.
3. Determine previous baseline blood pressure (if available) from patient's record.	• Baseline measurement enables the assessment of change in patient's condition and provides comparison with future blood pressure measurements.
4. Identify factors likely to interfere with accuracy of blood pressure measurement (e.g., acute anxiety, stress, pain). Encourage patient to avoid caffeine and tobacco for 60 minutes before blood pressure is assessed, and avoid exercise 30 minutes before (Hypertension Canada, 2015).	• Exercise and smoking cause false elevations in blood pressure. Smoking increases blood pressure immediately, with the effect lasting up to 15 minutes. Caffeine (e.g., in coffee) increases blood pressure for up to 3 hours.
5. Explain to patient that blood pressure is to be assessed, and have patient rest at least 5 minutes before blood pressure is measured in sitting or lying position; wait 1 minute if patient is standing. Ask patient not to speak when blood pressure is being measured.	• These preparations allow patients to relax and help avoid falsely elevated readings. Blood pressure readings taken at different times can be objectively compared with readings taken with patient at rest. Talking to a patient when the blood pressure is being assessed affects the accuracy of the readings (Hypertension Canada, 2015).

BOX 30-15 CASE STUDY

Blood Pressure Measurement in Patients With Mastectomies

I was assessing vital signs during my morning rotation as a student nurse and was just about to measure a female patient's vital signs when I noted a sign above her bed that said "no blood pressure on arms, please." This puzzled me and made me nervous as to what I should do. I had never been faced with this situation before, and so far, I had only been taught how to take blood pressure on the arm. Thankfully, I found an experienced registered nurse (RN) and, despite the fact that I felt like it was a silly question, asked how I was supposed to measure this patient's blood pressure and why it could not be done on her arms. I then took her blood pressure on her thigh as the RN instructed. Prior to this, the thought had actually occurred to me that it probably wouldn't hurt the patient to take her blood pressure on her arm, but I discovered later that this is not true, and that the pressure of the cuff on her arm could actually lead to lymphedema. When lymph nodes are removed from the axilla, as often happens with mastectomies, they can no longer return fluid to central circulation. Instead, the fluid can accumulate in the arm, thereby putting pressure on the veins and venous return. This can cause numbness, pain, impaired motor function, and many other complications (Lewis et al., 2014, p. 1503).

Continued

SKILL 30-5 MEASURING BLOOD PRESSURE—cont'd

STEPS	RATIONALE
6. Select appropriate cuff size.	• Improper cuff size results in inaccurate readings. If cuff is too small or comes loose when inflated, this may result in falsely high readings. A cuff that is too large may produce falsely low readings.
7. Ensure proper functioning of cuff components: release valve should be clean and freely movable in either direction; inflation bulb and tubing should be intact and free of leaks.	• Improper functionality results in difficulty with regulation of cuff inflation and deflation.
8. Perform hand hygiene.	• Hand hygiene reduces transmission of microorganisms between the patient and the nurse.
9. Have patient assume sitting or lying position. Be sure room is warm, quiet, and relaxing.	• These actions maintain patient's comfort during measurement. The patient's perceptions that the physical or interpersonal environment is stressful affect the blood pressure measurement.
10. With patient sitting or lying, position patient's forearm at heart-level position with patient's thigh flat (provide support as needed). To measure at patient's arm, turn palm up (see Step 10 illustration); to measure at patient's thigh, position with knee slightly flexed. If patient is sitting, the legs should not be crossed and feet should be touching the floor.	• If extremity is unsupported, patient may perform isometric exercise that increases diastolic blood pressure. Leg crossing falsely elevates blood pressure (Peters, Binder, & Campbell, 1999).
11. Expose patient's extremity arm, or the leg in certain medical situations, by fully removing constricting clothing.	• Exposure ensures proper cuff application.
12. Palpate patient's brachial artery (arm; see Step 12A illustration) or popliteal artery (leg). With cuff fully deflated, apply bladder of cuff above artery by centring cuff over artery. If no centre arrows appear on the cuff, estimate the centre of the bladder and place this centre over artery. Position cuff 2.5 cm above site of pulsation (antecubital or popliteal space). Wrap cuff evenly and snugly around extremity (see Step 12B illustrations). Do not place blood pressure cuff over clothing.	• Inflating bladder directly over artery ensures that proper pressure is applied during inflation. Loose-fitting cuff causes false high readings.

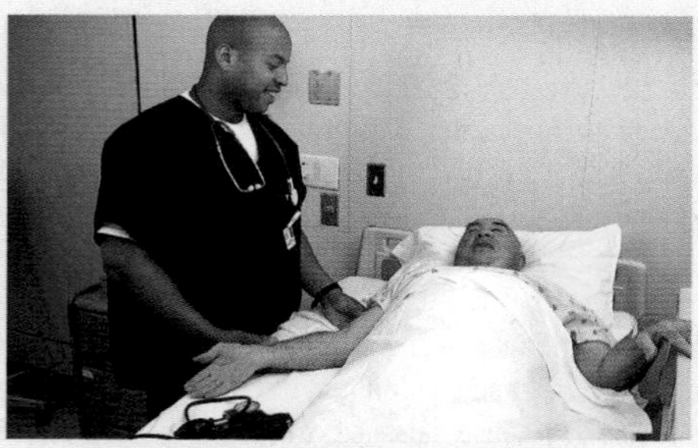

STEP 10 Patient's forearm supported in bed.

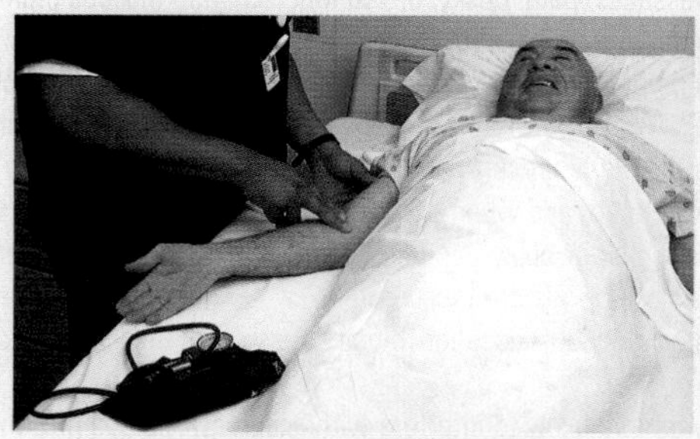

STEP 12A Palpating patient's brachial or popliteal artery.

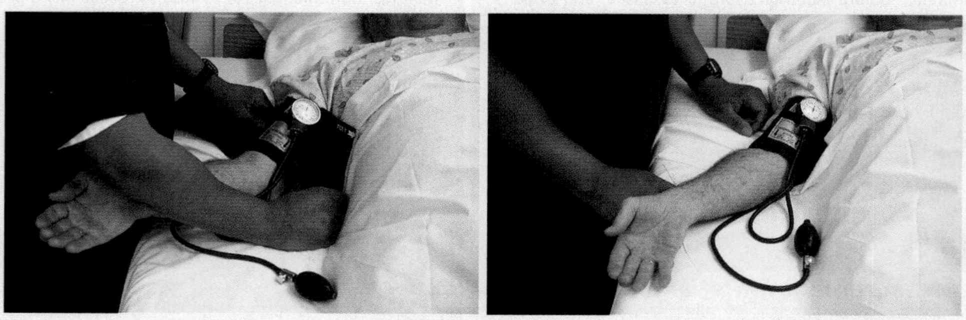

STEP 12B **Left,** Bladder of cuff centred above artery. **Right,** Blood pressure cuff wrapped around upper arm.

STEPS	RATIONALE
13. Position aneroid manometer gauge no further than 1 metre away.	• Gauge indicates correct readings.
14. Measure blood pressure.	
A. Two-step method	• Provides estimate of systolic pressure, which assists in level of cuff inflation particularly when baseline blood pressure is unknown.
(1) Relocate patient's brachial or popliteal pulse. Palpate the artery distal to the cuff with fingertips of nondominant hand while inflating cuff rapidly to pressure 30 mm Hg above the point at which the pulse disappears. Slowly deflate cuff, and note reading when the pulse reappears. Deflate cuff fully and wait 1 minute.	• Relocating prevents false low readings. Maximal inflation point for accurate reading can be determined by palpation. If you are unable to palpate artery because of weakened pulse, an ultrasonic stethoscope can be used (see Chapter 32). Completely deflating cuff prevents venous congestion and false high readings.

STEPS	RATIONALE
(2) Place stethoscope earpieces in your ears, and be sure sounds are clear, not muffled.	• Each earpiece should follow angle of ear canal to facilitate hearing.
(3) Relocate patient's brachial or popliteal pulse and place bell or diaphragm chest piece of stethoscope over it. Do not allow chest piece to touch cuff or clothing (see Step 14A[3] illustration).	• Proper stethoscope placement ensures optimal sound reception. An improperly positioned stethoscope causes muffled sounds that often result in false low systolic readings and false high diastolic readings.
(4) Close valve of pressure bulb clockwise until it is tight.	• Tightening of valve prevents air leak during inflation.
(5) Rapidly inflate cuff to 30 mm Hg above previously palpated systolic pressure (patient's estimated systolic pressure; see Step 14A[5] illustration).	• Rapid inflation ensures accurate measurement of systolic pressure.

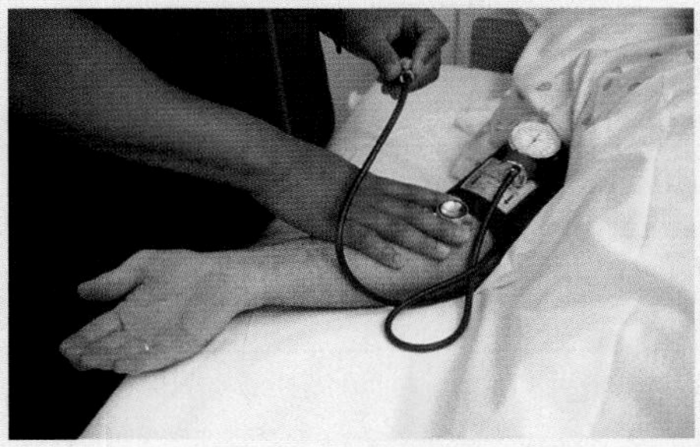

STEP 14A(3) Stethoscope over brachial artery to measure blood pressure.

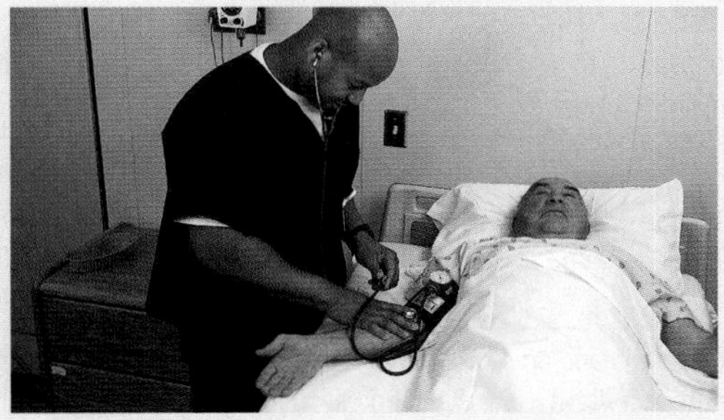

STEP 14A(5) Inflating blood pressure cuff.

STEPS	RATIONALE
(6) Slowly release pressure bulb valve, and allow needle of manometer gauge to fall at rate of 2–3 mm Hg/second. Make sure no extraneous sounds are audible.	• Too rapid or slow a decline in pressure can cause inaccurate readings. Noise interferes with precise determination of Korotkoff phases.
(7) Note point on manometer when first clear sound is heard. The sound will slowly increase in intensity.	• First Korotkoff sound indicates systolic pressure.
(8) Continue to deflate cuff, noting point at which sound becomes muffled or dampened.	• Fourth Korotkoff sound is distinctly muffled and is indication of diastolic pressure in children.
(9) Continue to deflate cuff gradually, noting point at which sound disappears in adults. Listen for 10–20 mm Hg after the last sound, and then allow remaining air to escape quickly.	• Beginning of the fifth Korotkoff sound is indication of diastolic pressure in adults. Cuff is deflated as soon as possible because continuous cuff inflation causes arterial occlusion, resulting in numbness and tingling sensation in patient's arm.
B. One-step method	• Used for frequent measurements and when there is previous awareness of systolic inflation level.
(1) Place stethoscope earpieces in your ears, and be sure sounds are clear, not muffled.	• Each earpiece should follow angle of ear canal to facilitate hearing.
(2) Relocate patient's brachial or popliteal artery, and place bell or diaphragm chest piece of stethoscope over it. Do not allow chest piece to touch cuff or clothing.	• Proper stethoscope placement ensures optimal sound reception. Improper positioning of stethoscope causes muffled sounds that often result in false low systolic readings and false high diastolic readings.
(3) Close valve of pressure bulb clockwise until tight. Quickly inflate cuff to 30 mm Hg above palpated systolic pressure.	• Tightening of valve prevents air leak during inflation. Inflation above systolic level ensures accurate measurement of systolic pressure.
(4) Slowly release pressure bulb valve, and allow needle of manometer gauge to fall at rate of 2–3 mm Hg/second.	• Too rapid or slow a decline in pressure can cause inaccurate readings.
(5) Note point on manometer when first clear sound is heard (first Korotkoff sound). The sound will slowly increase in intensity.	• First Korotkoff sound indicates systolic pressure.
(6) Continue to deflate cuff, noting point at which sound becomes muffled or dampened (fourth Korotkoff sound).	• Fourth Korotkoff sound is distinctly muffled and indicates diastolic pressure in children.
(7) Continue to deflate cuff gradually, noting point at which the sound disappears (fifth Korotkoff sound) in adults. Listen for 10–20 mm Hg after the last sound, and then allow remaining air to escape quickly.	• Beginning of the fifth Korotkoff sound is indication of diastolic pressure in adults. Cuff is deflated as soon as possible because continuous cuff inflation causes arterial occlusion, resulting in numbness and tingling sensation in patient's arm.
15. Hypertension Canada recommends that for auscultation, at least three measurements should be taken in the same arm with the patient in the same position. The first reading should be discarded, and the latter two averaged (Leung et al., 2017).	• Multiple readings increase accuracy of blood pressure measurement.
16. Remove cuff from extremity unless measurement must be repeated. If patient's blood pressure is being assessed for the first time, repeat blood pressure assessment on other extremity.	• By comparing blood pressure in both extremities, circulation problems can be detected. (Difference of 5–10 mm Hg between extremities is normal.)

Continued

SKILL 30-5 MEASURING BLOOD PRESSURE—cont'd

STEPS	RATIONALE
17. Assist patient to return to comfortable position, and cover patient's upper arm if it was previously clothed.	• These actions restore patient's comfort and promote sense of well-being.
18. Wipe the blood pressure cuff with disinfectant or, if disposable, keep in patient's room until no longer needed; then dispose of the cuff according to agency policy.	• Cleaning or disposing of the blood pressure cuff helps reduce the transmission of microorganisms between patients.
19. Discuss findings with patient as needed.	• Such discussion promotes patient's participation in care and understanding of health status.
20. Perform hand hygiene.	• Hand hygiene reduces transmission of microorganisms between the patient and the nurse.
21. Compare reading with previous baseline value, acceptable value of blood pressure for patient's age, or both.	• Evaluate for change in condition and alterations.

CRITICAL DECISION POINT: *In some situations (e.g., critically ill patients or those with peripheral vascular disease), it is often necessary to compare blood pressure readings in both arms, both legs, or all four extremities. If using upper extremities, use the arm with the higher pressure for subsequent assessments, unless this is contraindicated.*

STEPS	RATIONALE
22. Correlate blood pressure with data obtained from pulse assessment and other related cardiovascular signs and symptoms.	• Blood pressure and heart rate are interrelated.

UNEXPECTED OUTCOMES	RELATED INTERVENTIONS
Blood pressure reading cannot be obtained	• Determine whether any immediate crisis is present by measuring pulse and respiratory rate. • Assess for signs of decreased cardiac output (e.g., weak or thready pulse, confusion, pallor, or cyanosis). If any sign is present, notify nurse in charge or prescribing health care provider immediately. • Use alternative sites or procedures to obtain blood pressure. Auscultate blood pressure in lower extremity; use a Doppler ultrasonic instrument or a palpation method to obtain systolic measurement. • Repeat blood pressure measurement with sphygmomanometer. Electronic blood pressure devices are less accurate in conditions of low blood flow.
Blood pressure is not sufficient for adequate perfusion and oxygenation of tissues	• Compare blood pressure value with baseline value. A systolic reading of 90 mm Hg is an acceptable value for some patients. • Position patient in supine position to enhance circulation, and restrict activity if this is the cause of blood pressure to decrease. • Assess for signs of decreased cardiac output (e.g., weak or thready pulse, confusion, pallor, or cyanosis). If any sign present, notify nurse in charge or prescribing health care provider immediately. • Increase rate of intravenous infusion, or administer vasoconstrictor medications if ordered.
Blood pressure is elevated above acceptable range	• Repeat measurement in patient's other arm, and compare findings. Verify correct size and placement of cuff. • Ask colleague to repeat measurement in 2 minutes. • Observe for related symptoms (e.g., headache, confusion), although symptoms are sometimes not apparent until blood pressure is extremely elevated. • Report elevated blood pressure to nurse in charge or prescribing health care provider immediately. • Administer antihypertensive medications as ordered.

RECORDING AND REPORTING

- Inform patient of value and need for periodic reassessment of blood pressure.
- Record blood pressure in nurses' notes or vital sign flow sheet. Document blood pressure in nurses' narrative notes after administration of specific therapies.
- Report abnormal findings to nurse in charge or prescribing health care provider.

HOME CARE CONSIDERATIONS

- Assess home noise level to determine which room will provide the quietest environment for assessing blood pressure.
- Consider using electronic blood pressure cuff in the home if patient has hearing difficulties, adequate financial resources, and adequate dexterity.

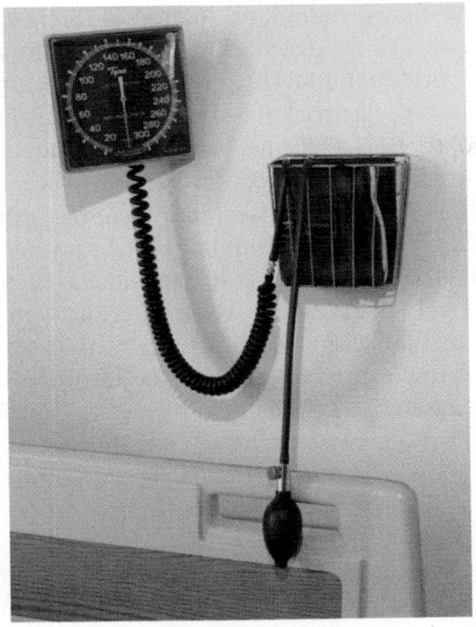

FIGURE 30-14 Wall-mounted aneroid sphygmomanometer.

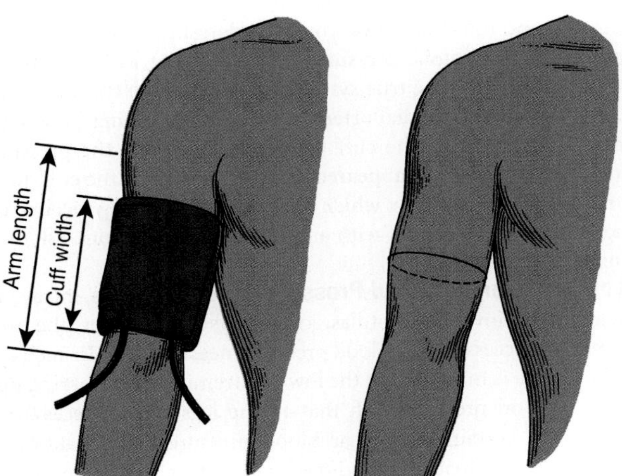

FIGURE 30-15 Guidelines for proper blood pressure cuff size. Bladder length should cover 80 to 100% of arm circumference, and bladder width should be close to 40% of arm circumference (Hypertension Canada, 2015).

Indirect measurement of arterial blood pressure works on a basic principle of pressure: blood flows freely through an artery until an inflated cuff applies pressure to tissues and causes the artery to collapse. After the cuff pressure is released, the point at which blood flow returns and sound appears through auscultation is the systolic pressure.

In 1905, Nikolai Korotkoff, a Russian surgeon, first described the sounds heard over an artery distal to the blood pressure cuff. The first Korotkoff sound is a clear rhythmical tapping that corresponds to the pulse rate and gradually increases in intensity. Onset of the sound corresponds to the systolic pressure. A blowing or swishing sound occurs as the cuff continues to deflate; this is the second Korotkoff sound. As the artery distends, blood flow becomes turbulent. The third Korotkoff sound is a crisper and more intense tapping. The fourth Korotkoff sound is muffled and low-pitched as the cuff is further deflated. At this point, the cuff pressure has fallen below the pressure within the vessel walls; this sound is the diastolic pressure in infants

TABLE 30-9 Common Mistakes in Blood Pressure Assessment

Error	Effect
Bladder or cuff too wide	False low reading
Bladder or cuff too narrow or too short	False high reading
Cuff wrapped too loosely or unevenly	False high reading
Deflating cuff too slowly	False high diastolic reading
Deflating cuff too quickly	False low systolic reading and false high diastolic reading
Arm below heart level	False high reading
Arm above heart level	False low reading
Arm not supported	False high reading
Stethoscope fits poorly or impairment of the examiner's hearing, causing sounds to be muffled	False low systolic reading and false high diastolic reading
Stethoscope applied too firmly against antecubital fossa	False low diastolic reading
Cuff inflating too slowly	False high diastolic reading
Repeating assessments too quickly	False high systolic reading
Inadequate inflation level	False low systolic reading
Multiple examiners using different Korotkoff sounds for diastolic readings	False high systolic reading and low diastolic reading

and children. The fifth Korotkoff "sound" is actually the disappearance of sound. In adolescents and adults, the fifth sound corresponds to the diastolic pressure (Figure 30-16). In some patients, the sounds are clear and distinct. In other patients, only the beginning and ending sounds are clear. When recording numbers for blood pressure measurement, note the point on the manometer when the first sound is heard (systolic reading), and the point on the manometer when the fifth sound is heard (diastolic reading). Some institutions recommend recording the point when the fourth sound is heard as well, especially for patients with hypertension. The numbers are presented by slashed lines (e.g., "120/80" or "120/100/80"). The arm used to measure the blood pressure (e.g., "right arm [RA] 130/70") and the patient's position (e.g., "sitting") should be noted.

Blood pressure findings prompt many medical decisions and nursing interventions concerning a patient's health care. Obtaining an accurate blood pressure measurement is essential. Error can arise from several sources (see Table 30-9). When unsure of a reading, it is good to ask a colleague to reassess the blood pressure.

Assessment in Children. All children 3 years of age through adolescence should have blood pressure checked at least yearly. Blood pressure in children changes with growth and development. Nurses can help parents understand the importance of this routine screening in children who may be at risk for hypertension.

The measurement of blood pressure in infants and children is difficult for several reasons:

- Different arm sizes necessitate careful selection of appropriate cuff size. Do not choose a cuff on the basis of the name of the cuff; for example, an "infant" cuff may be too small for some infants.

- Readings are difficult to obtain in restless or anxious infants and children. Allow a delay of at least 15 minutes to recover from recent activities and apprehension.
- Preparing the child for the blood pressure cuff's unusual sensation can increase cooperation. Most children understand the analogy of a "tight hug on your arm."
- Placing the stethoscope too firmly on the antecubital fossa causes errors in auscultation.
- Korotkoff sounds are difficult to hear in children because of low frequency and amplitude. A pediatric stethoscope bell can be helpful. The fourth Korotkoff sound, which is typically quite muffled, represents the diastolic pressure in infants and children.

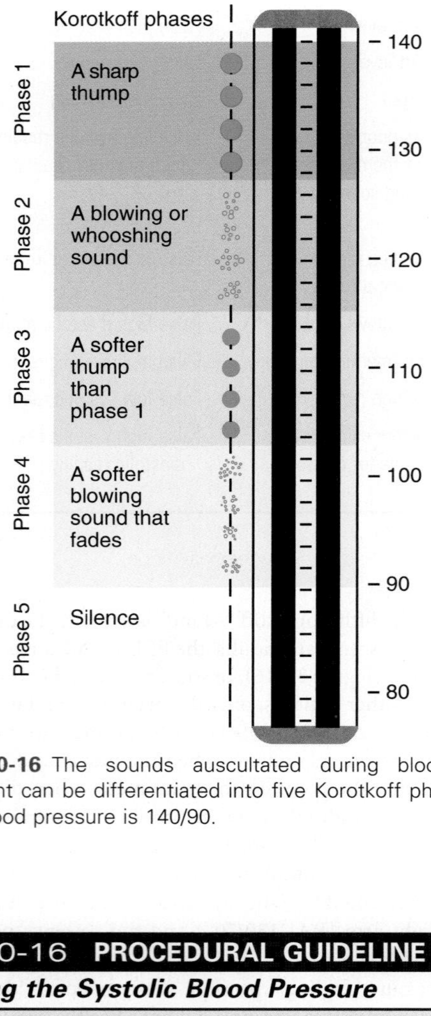

FIGURE 30-16 The sounds auscultated during blood pressure measurement can be differentiated into five Korotkoff phases. In this example, blood pressure is 140/90.

Ultrasonic Stethoscope. If you are unable to auscultate sounds because of a weakened arterial pulse, an ultrasonic stethoscope can be used (see Chapter 32 for further information about conducting a health assessment). This stethoscope enables you to hear low-frequency systolic sounds. It is commonly used for measuring the blood pressure of infants, children, and adults with low blood pressure.

Palpation. The indirect palpation technique is useful for patients whose arterial pulsations are too weak to create Korotkoff sounds. Severe blood loss and decreased heart contractility are examples of conditions that result in blood pressure too low to auscultate accurately. In these cases, the systolic blood pressure can be assessed by palpation; the diastolic pressure, however, is difficult to assess by palpation (Box 30-16). When using the palpation technique, record the systolic value and how it was measured (e.g., "RA 90/—, palpated, supine").

The palpation technique can be used with auscultation. In some hypertensive patients, the sounds usually heard over the brachial artery when the cuff pressure is high disappear as pressure is reduced, and then they reappear at a lower level. This temporary disappearance of sound is the **auscultatory gap**. It typically occurs between the first and second Korotkoff sounds. The gap in sound may cover a range of 40 mm Hg and thus may cause you to underestimate systolic pressure or overestimate diastolic pressure. It is important to inflate the cuff high enough to hear the true systolic pressure before the auscultatory gap. Palpation of the radial artery helps in determining how high to inflate the cuff. Inflate the cuff to 30 mm Hg above the pressure at which the radial pulse disappeared and rapidly deflate the cuff. Record the range of pressures in which the auscultatory gap occurs (e.g., "blood pressure RA 180/94 with an auscultatory gap from 180 to 160, sitting").

Lower Extremity Blood Pressure. Dressings, casts, intravenous catheters, arteriovenous fistulas, or shunts can render the upper extremities inaccessible for blood pressure measurement. In such cases, blood pressure is measured in the lower extremities. Comparing upper extremity blood pressure with that in the legs is also necessary for patients with certain cardiac or blood pressure abnormalities. The popliteal artery, palpable behind the knee in the popliteal space, is the site for auscultation. The cuff must be wide and long enough to allow for the larger girth of the thigh. Placing the patient in a prone position is best. If such a position is impossible, ask the patient to flex the knee

BOX 30-16 PROCEDURAL GUIDELINE

Palpating the Systolic Blood Pressure

Delegation Considerations

The skill of palpation of blood pressure *may not be delegated* to unregulated care providers.

Equipment

Sphygmomanometer

Procedure

1. Perform hand hygiene.
2. Apply the blood pressure cuff to the patient's extremity selected for measurement.
3. Continually palpate the pulse of the patient's brachial, radial, or popliteal artery with fingertips of one of your hands.
4. Rapidly inflate the blood pressure cuff 30 mm Hg above the point at which the patient's pulse cannot be palpated.
5. Slowly release the valve and deflate the cuff at a rate of 2 to 3 mm Hg per second.
6. Note the manometer reading when the pulse is again palpable; this is the systolic blood pressure.
7. Deflate the cuff rapidly and completely. Remove the cuff from the patient's extremity unless repeat measurement is needed.
8. Perform hand hygiene. Record pressure as "[systolic]/—" and palpated (e.g., "blood pressure 108/—, palpated").

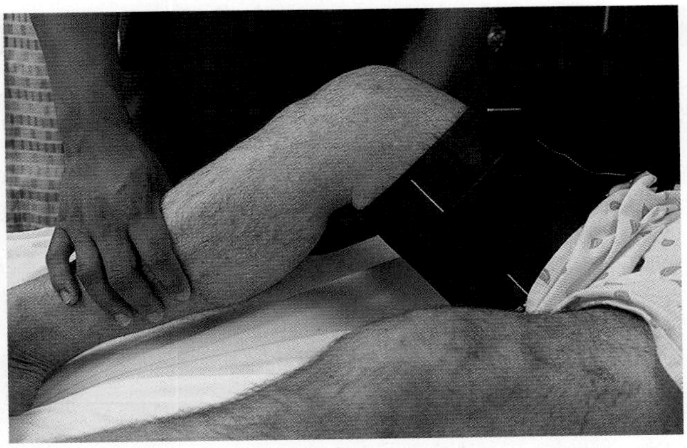

FIGURE 30-17 A lower extremity blood pressure cuff is positioned above the popliteal artery at midthigh with the knee flexed. (Courtesy St. Mary's Health Center. St. Louis, MO.)

slightly for easier access to the artery. Position the cuff 2.5 cm above the patient's popliteal artery with the bladder over the posterior aspect of the midthigh (Figure 30-17). The procedure is identical to that for brachial artery auscultation. Systolic pressure in the legs is usually 10 to 40 mm Hg higher than in the brachial artery, but the diastolic pressure should be the same.

Automatic Blood Pressure Devices. Many styles of electronic devices are available to determine an automatic blood pressure assessment rather than a manual one (Figure 30-18). For example, some devices rely on an electronic sensor to detect the vibrations caused by the rush of blood through an artery. When the cuff deflates, the sensor determines the initial burst of vibrations and translates the information into a systolic pressure reading. When the vibrations are lowest, just before they stop, the diastolic pressure is determined.

Hypertension Canada (2015) recommends the use of automated blood pressure measurement over manual measurement, and AOBP measurement is the preferred method as it provides a more standardized assessment of blood pressure. The AOBP method has multiple preprogrammed measurements, each administered 1 minute apart over 4–7 minutes while the patient is alone in a quiet room. Alarm limits can be programmed to alert the nurse if the blood pressure measurement is outside desired parameters. The use of AOPB measurement reduces the risk of white coat hypertension and lowers the prevalence of masked hypertension (Box 30-17).

Automatic devices are easy to use and efficient, and knowledge about how to use a stethoscope is not required. The automated device enables assessment of blood pressure during interpersonal interactions (Figure 30-19). AOBP measurement limits interaction because the patient is alone while the measurements are being taken. The AOBP method can thus decrease the risk of nursing error related to blood pressure measurement, as talking to a patient when blood pressure is being assessed interferes with the accuracy of the reading (Hypertension Canada, 2015).

Self-Measurement of Blood Pressure. More people measure their own blood pressure because of improved technology in home-monitoring devices and a greater interest in health promotion. Portable home devices include aneroid sphygmomanometers and the now recommended electronic digital readout devices that do not require use of a stethoscope. The electronic devices inflate and deflate cuffs with the push of a button, and their use minimizes or eliminates many auscultation-induced errors (Hypertension Canada, 2015).

Stationary automatic blood pressure devices can be found in public places such as grocery stores, drug stores, fitness clubs, airports, and

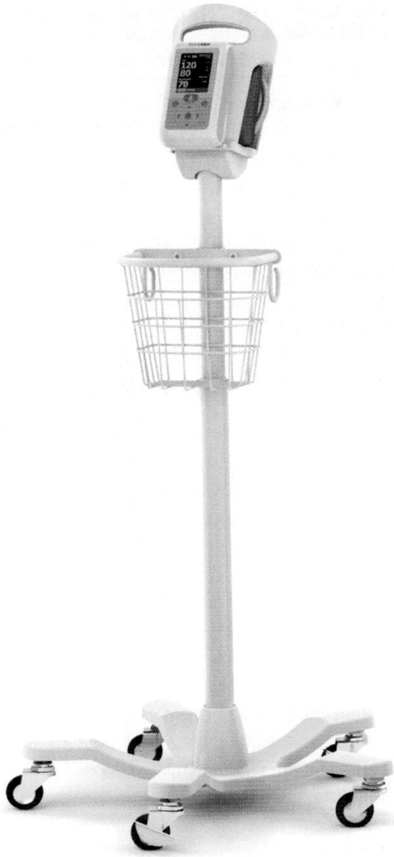

FIGURE 30-18 Automatic blood pressure monitor. (Photo courtesy Welch Allyn, http://www.welchallyn.com.)

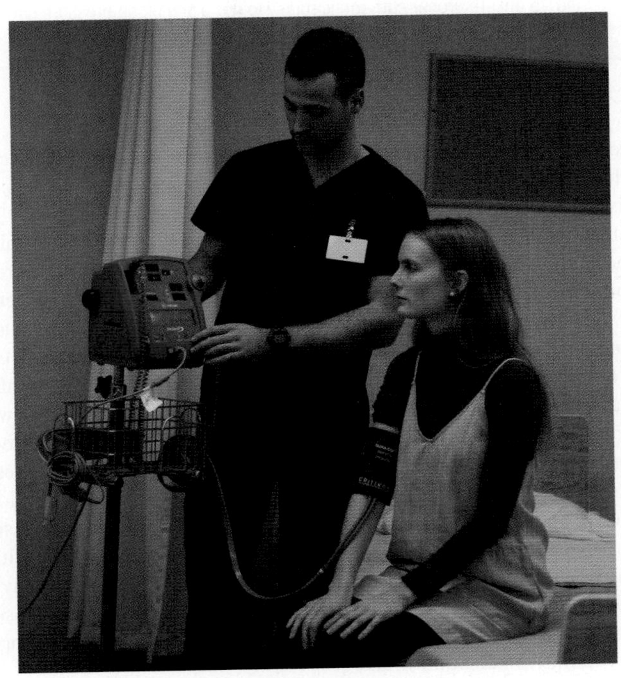

FIGURE 30-19 Taking an electronic blood pressure measurement. (Courtesy Barbara J. Astle, RN, PhD.)

BOX 30-17 PROCEDURAL GUIDELINE

Electronic Blood Pressure Measurement

Delegation Considerations

The task of obtaining an electronic blood pressure measurement can be delegated to an unregulated care provider unless the patient is considered unstable or needs close monitoring. The nurse is responsible for assessing the impact of changes in blood pressure; therefore, when the task of obtaining an electronic blood pressure measurement is delegated, it is important to *ensure that the unregulated care provider* performs the following tasks:

- Selects appropriate limb for measurement
- Selects appropriate-size cuff for designated limb
- Selects blood pressure cuff recommended by manufacturer
- Obtains blood pressure measurement for patient with ordered frequency
- Reports abnormalities

Equipment

Electronic blood pressure machine and blood pressure cuff of appropriate size as recommended by manufacturer

Procedure

1. Determine appropriateness of using electronic blood pressure measurement. This device is not suitable for use in patients with irregular heart rates, peripheral vascular disease, seizures, tremors, or shivering.
2. Determine best site for cuff placement (see Skill 30-5, Step 2).
3. Select appropriate cuff size for patient's extremity and appropriate cuff for machine. The electronic blood pressure cuff and machine are matched by the manufacturer and are not interchangeable.
4. Assist patient to comfortable position, either lying or sitting. Plug in device, and place near patient, ensuring that the connector hose between the cuff and machine will reach the patient.
5. Prepare blood pressure cuff by manually squeezing all air out of the cuff and connecting cuff to connector hose.
6. Turn on machine to enable device to perform a self-test on internal computer systems.
7. Expose patient's extremity for measurement by removing restrictive clothing, to ensure proper cuff application. Do not place blood pressure cuff over clothing.
8. Wrap flattened cuff snugly around patient's extremity, verifying that only one finger fits between cuff and patient's skin. Make sure the "artery" arrow marked on the outside of the cuff is correctly placed.
9. Verify that connector hose between cuff and machine is not kinked. Kinking prevents proper inflation and deflation of cuff.
10. In accordance with manufacturer's directions, set frequency control to automatic or manual, and then press "start" button. The first blood pressure measurement will pump the cuff to a pressure of about 180 mm Hg. After this pressure is reached, the machine begins a deflation sequence that helps measure the blood pressure. The first reading is the peak pressure inflation for additional measurements.
11. When deflation is complete, digital display provides most recent values and flashes time (in minutes) that has elapsed since measurement occurred (see Figure 30-19).
12. Set frequency of blood pressure measurements and upper and lower alarm limits for systolic, diastolic, and mean blood pressure readings. Intervals between blood pressure measurements can be set from 1 to 90 minutes. Determine measurement frequency and alarm limits on the basis of patient's acceptable range of blood pressure, your nursing judgement, and health care provider's order.
13. Obtain additional readings at any time by pressing the start button. (Sometimes you need these readings for unstable patients.) Pressing the "cancel" button immediately deflates the cuff.
14. If blood pressure determinations must be frequent, leave the cuff in place. Remove cuff at least every 2 hours to assess underlying skin integrity, and, if possible, alternate blood pressure sites. Patients with abnormal bleeding tendencies are at risk for microvascular rupture from repeated inflations. When electronic blood pressure machine is no longer needed, clean or dispose of cuff according to facility policy to reduce transmission of microorganisms between patients.
15. Record blood pressure and site assessed on vital sign flow sheet or in nurses' notes. Record associated signs of blood pressure alterations in nurses' progress notes. Report abnormal findings to nurse in charge or health care provider.

worksites. Users rest their arm within the machine's inflatable cuff, which contains a pressure sensor. The cuff fits over clothing. A visual display tells users their blood pressure within 60 to 90 seconds. The reliability of the stationary machines is limited. Blood pressure values (both systolic and diastolic) may vary by 5 to 10 mm Hg or more in comparison with values measured by a manual sphygmomanometer.

Self-measurement of blood pressure has several benefits. Elevated blood pressure may be detected in people previously unaware of a problem. People with high normal blood pressure can provide information about the pattern of blood pressure values. Patients with hypertension can benefit from actively participating in their treatment through self-monitoring, which may subsequently enhance adherence to treatment. Self-monitoring also helps to confirm elevated blood pressure readings related to white coat hypertension (Hypertension Canada, 2015). The disadvantages of self-measurement include improper use of the device and inaccurate readings. A patient may be needlessly alarmed by one elevated reading. Patients with hypertension may become overly conscious of their blood pressure and inappropriately adjust medication intake.

Patients can learn to use self-measurement devices if they have the information needed to perform the procedure correctly and know when to seek medical attention. Patients should be advised that because of possible inaccuracies in the blood pressure devices, they must not adjust their medication regimens without consulting the health care provider. It is important to teach patients the meaning and implications of readings and ensure understanding of proper measurement techniques.

❖ NURSING PROCESS AND BLOOD PRESSURE DETERMINATION

In assessing blood pressure and pulse, the patient's general state of cardiovascular health and responses to other system imbalances can be evaluated. Hypotension, hypertension, orthostatic hypotension, and narrow (small difference) or wide (large difference) pulse pressures are defining characteristics of certain nursing diagnoses, including the following:

- *Activity intolerance*
- *Anxiety*
- *Decreased cardiac output*
- *Deficient/excess fluid volume*
- *Risk for injury*

- *Acute pain*
- *Ineffective tissue perfusion*

The nursing care plan includes interventions specific for the nursing diagnosis identified and the related factors. For example, the defining characteristics of hypotension, dizziness, pulse deficit, and dysrhythmia lead to a diagnosis of *decreased cardiac output.* Related factors may include poor oral intake, excessive heat exposure, and a history of valvular heart disease. The related factor guides the choice of nursing interventions. The nurse evaluates patient outcomes by assessing the blood pressure after each intervention.

HEALTH PROMOTION AND VITAL SIGNS

The emphasis on health promotion and health maintenance, as well as early discharge from hospital settings, has resulted in an increased need for patients and their families to monitor vital signs in the home. CASN (2015) also underlines the importance of health teaching in its statement that says that baccalaureate nursing graduates should have "the ability to counsel and educate clients to promote health, symptom and disease management"(p.13). Therefore, teaching regarding all vital sign measurements in order to promote and maintain health should be incorporated within the patient's plan of care (Box 30-18).

Recording Vital Signs

Measurements of vital signs can be recorded on graphic flow sheets (and/or in progress notes) or, in some institutions, using electronic medical records (EMR) (Figure 30-20). Improved patient safety and decreased medication errors in practice have been noted with the use of information systems such as the EMR (Gardner & Jones, 2012). It is important to identify institutional procedures for documenting and to remember that timely documentation is critical. In one study, nurses who memorized the vital signs because they did not have the time to document in the patient's electronic or paper record or interim paper notes created additional errors, compromised the data, and potentially jeopardized the safety of the patient (Yeung, Lapinsky, Granton, et al., 2012). In addition to the actual vital sign values, it is important to record in the progress notes any accompanying or precipitating symptoms, such as chest pain and dizziness with abnormal blood pressure, shortness of breath with abnormal respiration, cyanosis with hypoxemia, or flushing and diaphoresis with elevated temperature. Document any interventions initiated as a result of abnormal vital sign measurements, such as administration of oxygen therapy or an antihypertensive medication.

For patients for whom critical paths or care maps are used, vital sign values may be listed as outcomes (see Chapter 13 for further information about nursing assessments). If a vital sign value is higher or lower than the anticipated outcomes, a variance note should be written to explain the nature of the variance and the nurse's course of action. For example, a care map for a patient who has undergone a thoracotomy may list a postoperative outcome of "afebrile." If the patient has a fever, the nurse's variance note addresses possible sources of fever (e.g., retained pulmonary secretions) and nursing interventions (e.g., increased suctioning, postural drainage, or hydration).

BOX 30-18 FOCUS ON PRIMARY HEALTH CARE

Health Promotion and Vital Signs

Temperature

- Identify patient's ability to initiate preventive health care and recognize alteration in body temperature. Educate patient and caregiver about ways to prevent body temperature alterations.
- Teach patient risk factors for hypothermia and frostbite: fatigue; malnutrition; hypoxemia; cold, wet clothing; and alcohol intoxication.
- Teach patient risk factors for heat stroke: strenuous exercise in hot, humid weather; sudden exposure to hot climates; insufficient fluid intake before, during, and after exercise.
- Teach patient importance of taking and continuing to take antibiotics as directed until course of treatment is completed (e.g., to decrease chance of resurgence of infection or the development of antibiotic-resistant organisms).

Pulse Rate

- Patients taking certain cardiac medications need to learn to assess their own pulse rates to detect adverse effects.
- Patients undergoing cardiac rehabilitation need to learn to assess their own pulse rates to determine their response to exercise.

Blood Pressure

- Patients with family history of hypertension are at significant risk for hypertension. Teach risk factors for hypertension: obesity, cigarette smoking, heavy alcohol consumption, high blood cholesterol and triglyceride levels, and continued exposure to stress.
- Patients with hypertension need to learn about their blood pressure values, long-term follow-up care and therapy, the lack of obvious symptoms indicative of high blood pressure, the ability of therapy to control but not cure hypertension, and benefits of consistently following the treatment plan.
- Teach patient importance of appropriate-sized blood pressure cuff and recommend electronic measurement for home use.
- Instruct patient or primary caregiver to measure blood pressure at same time each day and after patient has had a brief rest. Patients should measure blood pressure while sitting or lying down, and they should use the same position and arm each time they measure pressure.
- Recommend electronic measurement of blood pressure, but if auscultation is all that is available, instruct patient or primary caregiver that if it is difficult to hear the pressure, the cuff may be too loose, not big enough, or too narrow; the stethoscope is not over arterial pulse; the cuff was deflated too quickly or too slowly; or the cuff was not pumped high enough for systolic readings.

Respirations

- Patients who demonstrate decreased ventilation benefit from learning deep breathing and coughing exercises (see Chapter 48 for further information about care of surgical patients).
- Instruct patient or caregiver to contact home care nurse or prescribing health care provider if unusual fluctuations in respiratory rate occur.
- Teach patient signs and symptoms of hypoxemia: headache, somnolence, confusion, dusky colour of skin and mucous membranes, shortness of breath, and dyspnea.
- Teach patient effect of high-risk behaviours on respiratory function—cigarette smoking, environmental pollutants, etc.

When considering how to teach patients and their families about vital sign measurements and their importance and significance, the patient's age is an important factor. Because of the increase in the population of older persons, caregivers must be more aware of changes that are unique to older persons. Box 30-19 identifies some of these variations.

BOX 30-19 FOCUS ON OLDER PERSONS

Vital Signs

Temperature

- Normal body temperature ranges from 36°C to 36.8°C orally and 36.6°C to 37.2°C rectally. Temperatures considered to be within normal range sometimes reflect a fever in an older person.
- Older persons are very sensitive to slight changes in environmental temperature because their thermoregulatory systems are not as efficient (Touhy, Jett, Boscart, et al., 2012, p. 201).
- Sweat gland reactivity decreases in older persons; as a result, sweating may not occur until temperatures are very high, leading to hyperthermia and heatstroke.
- Loss of subcutaneous fat reduces the insulating capacity of the skin; older men are at especially high risk for hypothermia.
- For older persons, be especially attentive to subtle temperature changes and other manifestations of fever, such as tachypnea, anorexia, falls, delirium, and decline in overall function.

Pulse Rate

- If it is difficult to palpate the pulse of an older person or an obese patient, a Doppler device provides a more accurate reading.
- In older persons, it takes longer for the pulse rate to rise to meet sudden increased demands that result from stress, illness, or excitement. Once elevated, the pulse rate of an older person takes longer to return to normal resting rate (Touhy et al., 2012, pp. 77–78).
- Heart sounds are sometimes muffled or difficult to hear in older persons because of an increase in air space in the lungs.

Blood Pressure

- In older persons with decreased upper arm mass, blood pressure cuff size must be selected especially carefully.
- Accurate assessment of blood pressure in older persons may be more difficult than in younger persons, for several reasons. A couple of these are as follows: blood pressure has a tendency to fluctuate in response to postural changes; older persons commonly have pseudohypertension. Pseudohypertension is caused by the inability of the external cuff to compress the arteries in people with arteriosclerosis, resulting in elevated systolic readings despite normal diastolic readings and no evidence of end-organ damage (Miller, 2015).
- Older adults commonly have pseudohypertension, which is the phenomenon of elevated systolic blood pressure readings that result from the inability of the external cuff to compress the arteries in older people with arteriosclerosis. This phenomenon explains the findings of extremely elevated systolic blood pressure readings in people without any evidence of end-organ damage and with normal diastolic blood pressure readings. (Miller, 2015, p. 415).
- Instruct older persons to change position slowly and wait after each change before beginning activity, to avoid orthostatic hypotension and prevent injuries.

Respirations

- Aging causes ossification of costal cartilage and causes the ribs to slant downward, which results in more rigidity of the rib cage, which in turn reduces chest wall expansion. Kyphosis and scoliosis that can occur in older persons restrict chest expansion and decrease tidal volume.
- Older persons depend more on accessory abdominal muscles during respiration than on weaker thoracic muscles.
- The respiratory system matures by the time a person reaches the age of 20 and then begins to decline. Despite this decline, older persons are able to perform customary life activities with little or no effort under usual conditions. Sudden events that increase demand for oxygen (e.g., stress, exercise, illness) may cause a respiratory deficit to become evident in the older person (Touhy et al., 2012, p. 78).
- Identifying an acceptable site for the pulse oximeter probe may be difficult in older persons because of the likelihood of peripheral vascular disease, decreased cardiac output, cold-induced vasoconstriction, and anemia.

KEY CONCEPTS

- Vital sign measurement includes the physiological measurement of temperature, pulse, blood pressure, respiration, and oxygen saturation.
- Vital signs are measured as part of either a complete physical examination or a review of a patient's condition.
- Changes in vital signs are evaluated with other physical assessment findings; clinical judgement is used to determine frequency of measurement.
- Knowledge of the factors influencing vital signs assists in determining and evaluating abnormal values.
- Vital signs provide a basis for evaluating response to nursing and medical interventions.
- Vital signs should be measured when the patient is inactive and the environment is controlled for comfort.
- Patients should be assisted in maintaining body temperature by interventions that promote heat loss, production, or conservation.
- A fever is one of the body's normal defence mechanisms.
- Measurement of temperature with the temporal artery is the least invasive, most accurate method of obtaining core temperature.
- Respiratory assessment includes determining the effectiveness of ventilation, perfusion, and diffusion.
- Assessment of respiration involves observing ventilatory movements through the respiratory cycle.
- Variables affecting ventilation, perfusion, and diffusion influence oxygen saturation.
- Pulse rate and rhythm, measured at the radial or apical pulses, are documented to assess cardiac function. Hypertension is diagnosed immediately if the mean of electronic measurement is systolic blood pressure ≥180 mm Hg and/or diastolic blood pressure ≥110 mm Hg; however, if the electronic measurement mean is lower than these but is still considered high, additional out-of-office measurements are required for diagnosis (Leung et al., 2017).
- Hypertension Canada (Leung et al., 2017) encourages the use of validated electronic digital oscillometric devices over auscultation for blood pressure measurement.
- Improperly selecting and applying the blood pressure cuff results in measurement errors.
- Changes in one vital sign often influence characteristics of the other vital signs.

CRITICAL THINKING EXERCISES

1. A patient is visiting the health clinic for a routine physical examination by the nurse practitioner. The unregulated care provider

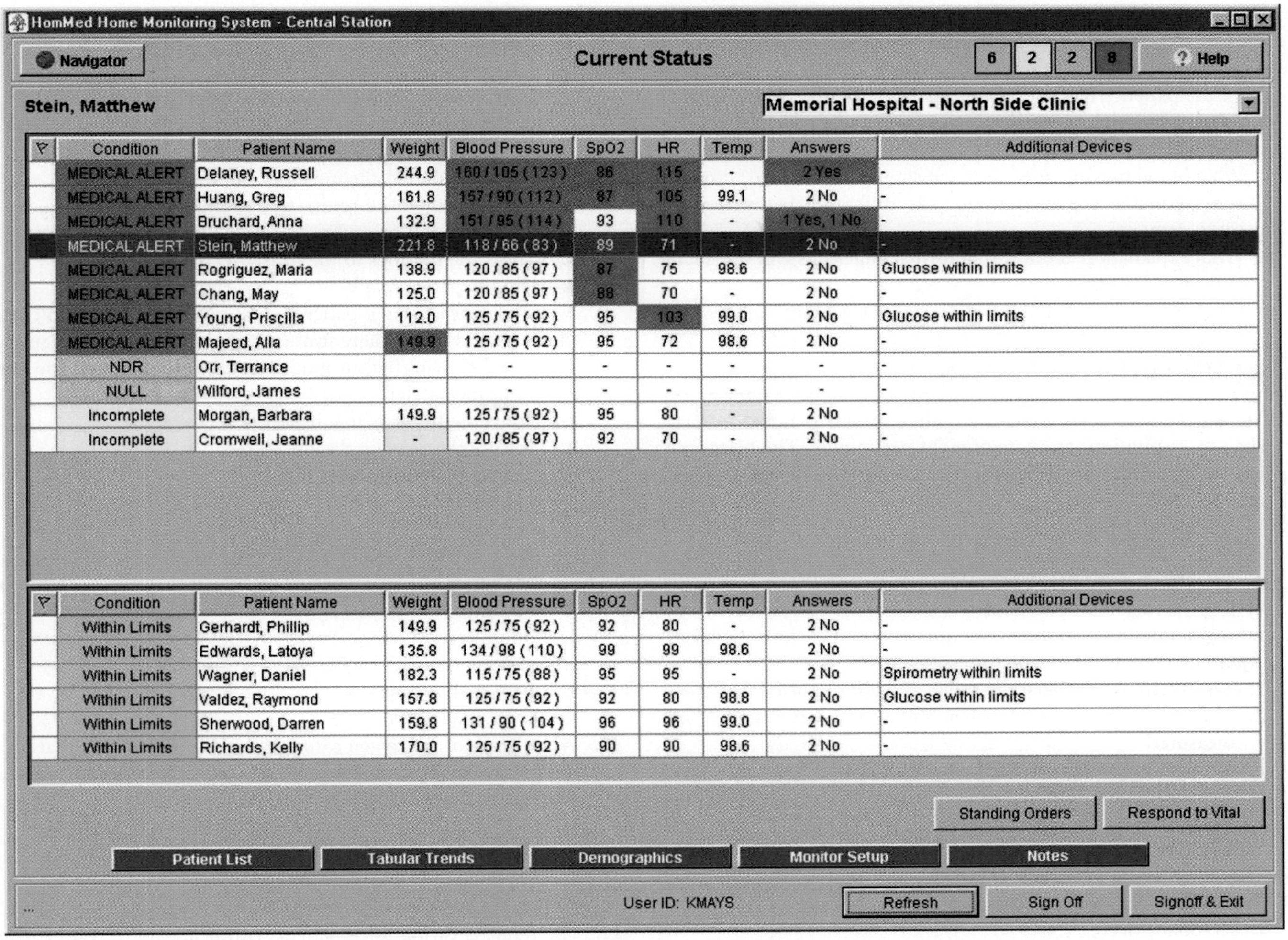

Condition	Patient Name	Weight	Blood Pressure	SpO2	HR	Temp	Answers	Additional Devices
MEDICAL ALERT	Delaney, Russell	244.9	160 / 105 (123)	86	115	-	2 Yes	-
MEDICAL ALERT	Huang, Greg	161.8	157 / 90 (112)	87	105	99.1	2 No	-
MEDICAL ALERT	Bruchard, Anna	132.9	151 / 95 (114)	93	110	-	1 Yes, 1 No	-
MEDICAL ALERT	Stein, Matthew	221.8	118 / 66 (83)	89	71	-	2 No	-
MEDICAL ALERT	Rogriguez, Maria	138.9	120 / 85 (97)	87	75	98.6	2 No	Glucose within limits
MEDICAL ALERT	Chang, May	125.0	120 / 85 (97)	88	70	-	2 No	-
MEDICAL ALERT	Young, Priscilla	112.0	125 / 75 (92)	95	103	99.0	2 No	Glucose within limits
MEDICAL ALERT	Majeed, Alla	149.9	125 / 75 (92)	95	72	98.6	2 No	-
NDR	Orr, Terrance	-	-	-	-	-	-	-
NULL	Wilford, James	-	-	-	-	-	-	-
Incomplete	Morgan, Barbara	149.9	125 / 75 (92)	95	80	-	2 No	-
Incomplete	Cromwell, Jeanne	-	120 / 85 (97)	92	70	-	2 No	-

Condition	Patient Name	Weight	Blood Pressure	SpO2	HR	Temp	Answers	Additional Devices
Within Limits	Gerhardt, Phillip	149.9	125 / 75 (92)	92	80	-	2 No	-
Within Limits	Edwards, Latoya	135.8	134 / 98 (110)	99	99	98.6	2 No	-
Within Limits	Wagner, Daniel	182.3	115 / 75 (88)	95	95	-	2 No	Spirometry within limits
Within Limits	Valdez, Raymond	157.8	125 / 75 (92)	92	80	98.8	2 No	Glucose within limits
Within Limits	Sherwood, Darren	159.8	131 / 90 (104)	96	96	99.0	2 No	-
Within Limits	Richards, Kelly	170.0	125 / 75 (92)	90	90	98.6	2 No	-

FIGURE 30-20 Image of an electronic medical record of vital signs. (From http://www.aaronnursing.com/Telehealth.asp.)

obtains the following vital sign measurements: tympanic temperature, 36.9°C; right radial pulse rate, 96 beats per minute and irregular; blood pressure, sitting, right arm, 162/82 mm Hg, and left arm, 150/70 mm Hg; SpO_2, 95% on room air; respiratory rate, 22 breaths per minute.

a. As the admitting nurse, what questions would you ask this patient to evaluate his risk for hypertension?
b. On the basis of these vital sign measurements, what actions should you take?

2. A mother brings her child into the Care Centre and notes that the child has been fussy, has not had much of an appetite, and is "not his active self." The child is crying and struggling to get out of the mother's lap during the interview. You note that the child is small for his age but his physical development appears normal.
   a. Describe the sequence you would use for obtaining vital signs.
   b. When you select the appropriate equipment for measuring the vital signs, what, if any, special considerations are needed?
   c. The unregulated care provider reports she has obtained a temperature reading of 37.7°C. What additional information do you request from the unregulated care provider?
3. A patient is admitted to the medical unit for chronic dyspnea and discomfort in her left chest with deep breathing and coughing. She has been smoking for 35 years and has a 20-year history of emphysema. Over the past 4 months, she has lost 4.5 kg and currently weighs 50 kg.
   a. When delegating the measurement of vital signs to an unregulated care provider, what information and directions should you provide?
   b. The blood pressure and heart rate are within acceptable ranges. The temperature is 37.5°C, obtained with an oral electronic thermometer; the respiratory rate is 32 breaths per minute and shallow; and the SpO_2 is 89%. On the basis of these results, list your actions in priority order.
4. A resident in a subacute extended-care facility is being treated for pneumonia with antibiotics. The resident has been on bed rest for the past 2 days. He has a history of hypertension, treated with diuretics, but is otherwise healthy. He has been afebrile for the past 24 hours and is eager to walk to the activity room. Their activity orders are "up ad lib."
   a. Should an unregulated care provider be delegated to assist with ambulation?
   b. What places this patient at risk for a fall?
   c. What precautions need to be taken to prevent a fall?
5. A woman arrives at the prenatal clinic for her first visit. She is 8 months pregnant. The unregulated care provider assesses her vital signs, height, and weight. The patient weighs 104 kg and is 160 cm

tall; blood pressure in her right arm is 210/92 mm Hg; her heart rate is 104 beats per minute; her respiratory rate is 24 breaths per minute; her tympanic temperature is 37.1°C. You are concerned about the patient's blood pressure. In repeating the measurement, you obtain 148/86 mm Hg in the right arm and 144/84 mm Hg in the left arm.

a. What blood pressure measurement should be recorded? Provide some possible explanations for the difference between your measurements.
b. What explanation about the abnormal vital signs will you share with the patient?
c. What will be included in your discharge teaching?

REVIEW QUESTIONS

1. During a nursing assessment, an adult patient is noted to have shallow respirations at a rate of eight per minute. The heart rate is 46 beats per minute. The patient's vital signs would be described as:
   1. Bradycardia and apnea
   2. Tachycardia and apnea
   3. Bradycardia and bradypnea
   4. Tachycardia and bradypnea
2. During a nursing assessment the nurse notes that the patient has a pulse deficit. A pulse deficit is:
   1. The difference between the radial and apical pulse rates
   2. The digital pressure felt when radial and ulnar pulses are measured
   3. The amount of pressure felt when radial and ulnar pulses are measured
   4. The difference between the systolic and diastolic blood pressure readings
3. The nurse recognizes that as individuals approach older adulthood, body temperature tends to:
   1. Gradually decrease
   2. Gradually increase
   3. Fluctuate
   4. Remain the same
4. The nurse is to administer the scheduled metoprolol to an adult patient. The vital signs reveal the pulse rate at 70 beats per minute, blood pressure at 140/96, and respirations at 12 per minute. Which nursing action should the nurse take?
   1. Hold the metoprolol and notify the physician.
   2. Retake the blood pressure in 15 minutes
   3. Administer the metoprolol as scheduled.
   4. Assist the patient to change positions and recheck blood pressure in the opposite arm.
5. While the nurse assesses a patient's vital signs, the patient states that she feels short of breath, and the nurse notes that she has a respiratory rate of 24 breaths per minute. Which action should the nurse take first?
   1. Notify the physician with the results immediately.
   2. Provide supplemental oxygen at a rate of 2 L per nasal prongs.
   3. Position the patient in a supported semi-Fowler's or high Fowler's position, then retake the respiratory rate.
   4. Note that the respiratory rate is within the normal range.
6. When the nurse teaches the patient about the management of hypertension, which of the following topics should be included in the teaching? *(Select all that apply.)*
   1. Diet modification
   2. Self-measurement of blood pressure and acceptable range of results
   3. Self-adjustment of antihypertensive medications
   4. Stress management
7. An older person recently on bed rest is assisted out of bed. The nurse measures his blood pressure as the patient changes position, and the results are as follows: 140/80 supine, 132/72 sitting, 108/60 standing. The patient also mentions that he feels light-headed. Which action should the nurse take first?
   1. Assist the patient to return to a supine position.
   2. Obtain a blood pressure measurement in the other arm.
   3. Report the findings to the nurse in charge.
   4. Help the patient walk.
8. A nurse is measuring a patient's vital signs. The nurse notes that the radial pulse is initially strong, diminishes in intensity, and has an interruption in rhythm about every four to six beats. The nurse should immediately:
   1. Report the findings to a health care provider.
   2. Measure the apical pulse for 60 seconds.
   3. Connect the patient to a cardiac monitor.
   4. Measure apical and radial pulse rates simultaneously for 60 seconds.
9. After assessing the patient's pulse, the nurse recognizes that poor oxygenation of the blood ordinarily affects the pulse rate, causing it to become:
   1. Bounding
   2. Irregular
   3. Faster than normal
   4. Slower than normal
10. When measuring oxygen saturation, the nurse recalls that all of the following can influence the reading, resulting in inaccurate results, except for:
    1. Rapid heart rate, reduced circulation to extremities
    2. Nail polish, tremors
    3. Decreased respiratory depth and effort
    4. Bright light near measuring site
11. The nurse is caring for a patient with heart failure who is complaining of chest pain. The nursing assessment reveals that the patient is newly confused with tachypnea, tachycardia, decreased blood pressure, and a fever. The nurse would question which physician's order?
    1. IV normal saline at 100 mL/hour
    2. Oxygen per nasal prongs at 2 L/m
    3. Metoprolol 50 mg PO STAT
    4. Electrocardiogram (ECG) STAT

Answers: 1. 3; 2. 1; 3. 1; 4. 3; 5. 3; 6. 1, 2, 4; 7. 1; 8. 2; 9. 2; 10. 3; 11. 3.

Rationales for the Review Questions appear at the end of the book.

RECOMMENDED WEBSITES

British Columbia Ministry of Health Services, Guidelines and Protocols Advisory Committee (GPAC): Hypertension—Detection, Diagnosis and Treatment of Hypertension: https://www2.gov.bc.ca/gov/content/health/practitioner-professional-resources/bc-guidelines

Part of the British Columbia Ministry of Health Services, the Guidelines and Protocols Advisory Committee developed several documents to recommend proper blood pressure management, including the recommended technique for measuring blood pressure. Other topics are home blood pressure monitoring, dietary approaches, and a patient guide.

Canadian Heart & Stroke Foundation: http://www.heartandstroke.ca/

This website provides information about stroke and heart disease.

Centre for Chronic Disease Prevention and Control: Cardiovascular Disease: https://www.canada.ca/en/public-health/services/chronic-diseases/cardiovascular-disease.html

This web page, part of the website of the Public Health Agency of Canada, provides links to a variety of Canadian resources on cardiovascular health, including the Canadian Association of Cardiovascular Prevention and Rehabilitation and the Canadian Stroke Strategy, Heart and Stroke Foundation of Canada and the Canadian Stroke Network.

Hypertension Canada: http://guidelines.hypertension.ca/

This website offers information on hypertension to health providers and the public. The mission of Hypertension Canada is to advance health through the prevention and control of high blood pressure and its complications. CHEP is a volunteer, nonprofit hypertension education program that provides annually updated, relevant, evidence-informed hypertension guidance. All sites provide educational tools.

REFERENCES

Allegaert, K., Casteels, K., van Gorp, I., et al. (2014). Tympanic, infrared skin, and temporal artery scan thermometers compared with rectal measurement in children: A real-life assessment. *Current Therapeutic Research, 76*, 34–38. doi:10.1016/j.curtheres.2013.11.005.

Canadian Association of Schools of Nursing (CASN/ACESI). (2015). *National nursing education framework: Final report.* Retrieved from http://www.casn.ca/wp-content/uploads/2014/12/Framwork-FINAL-SB-Nov-30-20151.pdf.

Cheshire, W. P. (2016). Thermoregulatory disorders and illness related to heat and cold stress. *Autonomic Neuroscience: Basic and Clinical, 196*, 96–104. doi:10.1016/j.autneu.2016.01.001.

Gardner, C., & Jones, S. (2012). Utilization of academic electronic medical records in undergraduate nursing education. *Online Journal of Nursing Informatics (OJNI), 16*(2). Retrieved from http://ojni.org/issues/?p=1702.

Heart and Stroke Foundation. (2017). *Heart/risk & prevention.* Retrieved from http://www.heartandstroke.ca/heart/risk-and-prevention.

Heytens, L., Forget, P., Scholtès, J. L., et al. (2015). The changing face of malignant hyperthermia: Less fulminant, more insidious. *Anaesthesia and Intensive Care, 43*(4), 506–511.

Hockenberry, M. J., & Wilson, D. (2015). *Wong's nursing care of infants and children* (10th ed.). St. Louis, MO: Mosby.

Hoffman, R. J., Etwaru, K., Dreisinger, N., et al. (2013). Comparison of temporal artery thermometry and rectal thermometry in febrile pediatric emergency department patients. *Pediatric Emergency Care, 29*(3), 301–304. doi:10.1097/PEC.0b013e3182850421.

Hypertension Canada. (2015). *Hypertension Canada guidelines.* Retrieved from http://guidelines.hypertension.ca.

Isler, A., Aydin, R., Tutar Güven, S., et al. (2014). Comparison of temporal artery to mercury and digital temperature measurement in pediatrics. *International Emergency Nursing, 22*(3), 165–186. doi:10.1016/j.ienj.2013.09.003.

Jarvis, C., Browne, A. J., MacDonald-Jenkins, J., et al. (2014). *Physical examination and health assessment* (2nd Cdn ed.). Toronto: Elsevier Canada.

Kaczorowski, J., Myers, M. G., Gelfer, M., et al. (2017). How do family physicians measure blood pressure in routine clinical practice? National survey of Canadian family physicians. *Canadian Family Physician, 63*(3), e193–e199. Retrieved from http://www.cfp.ca/content/63/3/e193#ref-16.

Leung, A. A., Daskalopoulou, S. S., Dasgupta, K., et al. (2017). Hypertension Canada's 2017 guidelines for diagnosis, risk assessment, prevention, and treatment of hypertension in adults. *Canadian Journal of Cardiology, 33*(5), 557–576. doi:10.1016/j.cjca2017.03.005.

Lewis, S. L., Ruff-Dirksen, S., Heitkemper, M., et al. (2014). *Medical-surgical nursing in Canada: Assessment and management of clinical problems* (3rd Cdn. ed.). Toronto: Elsevier Canada.

Mains, J. A., Coxall, K., & Lloyd, H. (2008). Measuring temperature. *Nursing Standard, 22*(39), 44–47.

Maxton, F. J., Justin, L., & Gillies, D. (2004). Estimating core temperature in infants and children after cardiac surgery: A comparison of six methods. *Journal of Advanced Nursing, 45*(2), 214–222. doi:10.1046/j.1365-2648.2003.02883.x.

Miller, C. A. (2015). *Nursing for wellness in older adults* (7th ed.). Philadelphia: Wolters Kluwer.

Oncel, M. Y., Tekgunduz, K. S., Ozdemir, R., et al. (2013). A comparison of different methods of temperature measurement by mothers and physicians in healthy newborns. *Indian Journal of Pediatrics, 80*(3), 190–194. doi:10.1007/s12098-012-0790-0.

Peters, G. L., Binder, S. K., & Campbell, N. R. (1999). The effect of crossing legs on blood pressure: A randomized single-blind cross-over study. *Blood Pressure Monitoring, 4*(2), 97–101.

Purssell, E., While, A., & Coomber, B. (2009). Tympanic thermometry—Normal temperature and reliability. *Paediatric Nursing, 21*(6), 40–43.

Touhy, T. A., Jett, K., Boscart, V., et al. (2012). *Ebersole and Hess' gerontological nursing & healthy aging* (1st Cdn ed.). Toronto: Elsevier.

World Health Organization (WHO). (2017a). *Mercury and health fact sheet.* Retrieved from http://www.who.int/mediacentre/factsheets/fs361/en.

World Health Organization (WHO). (2017b). *Cardiovascular diseases (CVDs) fact sheet.* Retrieved from http://www.who.int/mediacentre/factsheets/fs317/en/.

Yeung, M. S., Lapinsky, S. E., Granton, J. T., et al. (2012). Examining nursing vital signs documentation workflow: Barriers and opportunities in general internal medicine units. *Journal of Clinical Nursing, 21*(7–8), 975–982. doi:10.1111/j.1365-2702.2011.03937.x.

31

Pain Assessment and Management

Canadian content written by Monakshi Sawhney, RN(EC), PhD, Brenda L. Martelli, RN(EC), MEd
Original chapter by Maureen F. Cooney, DNP, FNP-BC

OBJECTIVES

Mastery of content in this chapter will enable you to:

- Define the key terms listed.
- Discuss common misconceptions about pain.
- Describe the physiology of pain.
- Identify components of the pain experience.
- Explain how the physiology of pain relates to selecting interventions for pain relief.
- Describe the components of pain assessment.
- Perform an assessment of a patient experiencing pain.
- Explain how cultural factors influence the pain experience.
- Describe the appropriate nursing diagnoses, outcomes, and interventions for a patient with pain.
- Describe guidelines for selecting and individualizing pain interventions.
- Explain the various pharmacological approaches to treating pain.
- Describe applications for the use of nonpharmacological pain interventions.
- Discuss nursing implications for administering analgesics.
- Identify barriers to effective pain management.
- Evaluate a patient's response to pain interventions.

KEY TERMS

Acupuncture, p. 595
Acute pain, p. 579
Addiction, p. 603
Adjuvants, p. 598
Anaesthetics, p. 582
Analgesics, p. 582
Biofeedback, p. 594
Breakthrough pain, p. 579
Chordotomy, p. 601
Chronic pain, p. 579
Cutaneous stimulation, p. 595
Dorsal rhizotomy, p. 601
Drug tolerance, p. 603
Epidural analgesia, p. 600
Epidural space, p. 600
Guided imagery, p. 594
Local anaesthesia, p. 600
Modulation, p. 577
Nociception, p. 576
Opioids, p. 597
Pain, p. 575
Pain threshold, p. 578
Pain tolerance, p. 580
Patient-controlled analgesia (PCA), p. 598
Perception, p. 577
Physical dependence, p. 603
Placebos, p. 604
Pseudoaddiction, p. 579
Regional anaesthesia, p. 600
Reiki, p. 595
Relaxation, p. 594
Therapeutic touch, p. 595
Transcutaneous electrical nerve stimulation (TENS), p. 596
Transduction, p. 576
Transmission, p. 576

MEDIA RESOURCES

http://evolve.elsevier.com/Canada/Potter/fundamentals/

- Audio Chapter Summaries
- Examination Review Questions
- Concept Map Creator
- Case Study with Questions
- Audio Glossary
- Content Updates
- Video Clips

Pain is a common reason why people seek health care. Despite being a commonly occurring symptom, even experienced by premature infants, pain is not well understood and is inconsistently and inadequately addressed (Stevens, Abbott, Yamada, et al., 2011). Pain is defined as "an unpleasant, subjective sensory *and* emotional experience associated with actual or potential tissue damage, or described in terms of such damage" (International Association for the Study of Pain Subcommittee on Taxonomy [IASP], 1994). This definition recognizes the physical and psychological nature of the pain experience. Pain is a highly personal experience, which can be accurately described only by the individual experiencing it (Pasero & McCaffery, 2011). This concept has endured for more than 40 years, when McCaffery first defined pain as "whatever the experiencing person says it is, existing whenever he says it does" (McCaffery, Herr, & Pasero, 2011, p. 21). In recent years, definitions of pain have evolved to include the notion that a person's inability to verbally communicate does not preclude the possibility that pain is present or negate the responsibility of health care providers to treat it (Herr, Coyne, Key, et al., 2006).

Almost all acute and cancer pain can be relieved, and most patients with chronic non-cancer pain can be helped (Canadian Pain Society [CPS], 2010). Yet, in Canada, acute pain in hospitalized infants (Johnston, Barrington, Taddio, et al., 2011), children (Stinson, Yamada, Dickson, et al., 2008), and adults (Roth, Kling, Gockel, et al., 2005) and chronic pain in children (Palmero, 2009), adults (Schopflocher, Taenzer, & Jovey, 2011), and older persons (Ramage-Morin, 2008) continue to be undermanaged. Nurses are ethically responsible to promote the health and well-being of individuals, families, and communities in their care; this includes assessing and managing pain through the use of appropriate, evidence-informed measures (Canadian Nurses Association, 2017). Responsive, evidence-informed pain management can reduce pain and improve quality of life, and it promotes earlier mobilization and return to work, resulting in fewer hospital and clinic visits, shortened hospital stays, and reduced health care costs.

SCIENTIFIC KNOWLEDGE BASE

Pain is part of the human experience. In the past, pain was viewed simply as a symptom of an illness or condition. Now, pain is understood to be complex, and chronic pain is considered to be a disease in its own right (Brookoff, 2000).

Nature of Pain

Pain is more than a physical sensation caused by a specific stimulus. An individual's perception of pain includes *affective* (emotional), cognitive, behavioural, and sensory components that are shaped by past experience, culture, and situational factors (Mehta & Chan, 2008). The nature of the stimulus for pain can be physical, psychological, or a combination of both.

Physiology of Pain

Pain is a multifaceted experience that involves both the peripheral and central nervous systems. Pain can be classified by its inferred pathophysiology: nociceptive (physiological) pain or neuropathic pain. *Nociceptive pain* is the experience of pain that occurs in response to tissue injury. It involves the neural processing of noxious stimuli that occurs when nociceptors (pain-sensing nerves) are activated by tissue damage or inflammation (Latremoliere & Woolf, 2009). *Neuropathic pain* involves the abnormal processing of stimuli due to a lesion or disease in the peripheral or central nervous system (Fornasari, 2012; IASP, 2012; Rodriguez, 2015).

Nociception has four specific processes: transduction, transmission, perception, and modulation (Rodriguez, 2015). Patients in pain cannot discriminate among these four processes. However, understanding them will help you as a nurse to recognize factors that can cause pain, symptoms that accompany pain, and the rationale and actions of a selected treatment plan.

The first process involved in nociception is **transduction**. When tissue cells are damaged by either thermal stimuli (e.g., burn), mechanical stimuli (e.g., cut), or chemical stimuli (e.g., chemotherapy), the damaged cells release pain-sensitizing and inflammatory substances including prostaglandins, bradykinin, histamine, prostaglandins, serotonin, and substance P (Box 31-1). These substances activate nociceptors, resulting in transduction, or the generation of electrical activity in peripheral terminals (an action potential) (Fornasari, 2012; Rodriguez, 2015).

In the second process, **transmission**, these pain-sensitizing and inflammatory substances surround the pain nerve fibres in the extracellular fluid, creating the spread of the pain message via the afferent peripheral nerve fibres to the dorsal horn of the spinal cord. Within the dorsal horn of the spinal cord, a synaptic transmission from the *afferent* (sensory) peripheral nerve to the spinothalamic tract nerves occurs through a complex neurophysiological and neurochemical mechanism, resulting in the relay of the signal to various higher brain centres (Fornasari, 2012; Rodriguez, 2015; Figure 31-1).

Two types of afferent peripheral nerve fibres conduct painful stimuli: the fast, myelinated A-delta fibres, and the very small, slow, unmyelinated C fibres. The A fibres send sharp, localized, and distinct sensations that focus the source of the pain and detect its intensity. The C fibres relay impulses that are poorly localized, burning, and persistent (Fornasari, 2012). For example, after stepping on a nail, a person initially feels a sharp, localized pain, which is a result of A-fibre transmission. Within a few seconds, the pain becomes more diffuse

BOX 31-1 Neurophysiology of Pain: Neuroregulators

Neurotransmitters (Excitatory)

Substance P

Found in the pain neurons of the dorsal horn (excitatory peptide)
Needed to transmit pain impulses from the periphery to the higher brain centre
Causes vasodilation and edema

Serotonin

Released from the brain stem and dorsal horn to inhibit pain transmission

Prostaglandins

Generated from the breakdown of phospholipids in cell membranes
Believed to increase sensitivity to pain

Neuromodulators (Inhibitory)

Endorphins and Dynorphins

Function as the body's natural supply of morphine-like substances
Activated by stress and pain
Located within the brain, spinal cord, and gastrointestinal tract
Cause analgesia when they attach to opiate receptors in the brain
Present in higher levels in people who have less pain than others with a similar injury

Bradykinin

Released from plasma that leaks from surrounding blood vessels at the site of tissue injury
Binds to receptors on peripheral nerves, increasing pain stimuli
Binds to cells that cause the chain reaction–producing prostaglandins

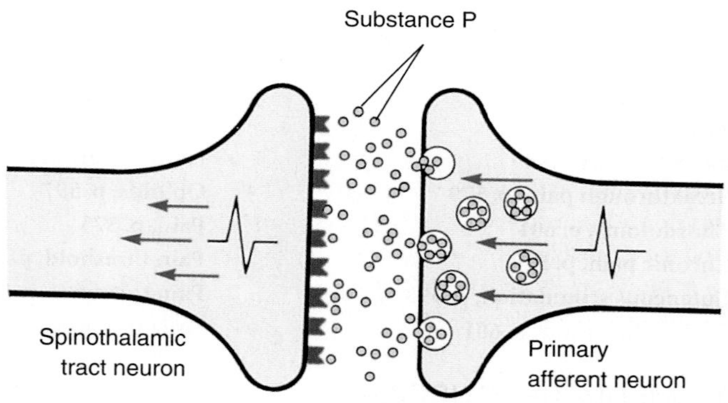

FIGURE 31-1 Substance P and other neurotransmitters are released from primary afferent fibres that terminate in the dorsal horn of the spinal cord. (Paice, J. A. [1991]. Unraveling the mystery of pain. *Oncology Nursing Forum, 18*[5], 843.)

and widespread, until the whole foot aches, as a result of C-fibre innervation.

Pain stimuli continue to travel through nerve fibres in the spinothalamic tracts that cross to the opposite side of the spinal cord. Pain impulses then travel up the spinal cord. Figure 31-2 shows the normal pain reception pathway. After the pain impulse ascends the spinal cord, information is quickly transmitted by the thalamus to higher centres in the brain. These centres include the reticular formation, limbic system, somatosensory cortex, and association cortex. It only takes microseconds for the pain signal to be transmitted from the site of injury to the brain.

Perception, the third nociceptive process, is the conscious awareness of pain. Once a pain stimulus reaches the cerebral cortex, the brain interprets the intensity, quality, and character of the pain, and information from past experiences. As well, psychological, social, spiritual, and cultural associations are used to process the perception of the pain (Arnstein, 2010). The somatosensory cortex identifies the location and intensity of the pain, and the association cortex determines how we feel about the pain. There are cells within the limbic system that are believed to control emotion, particularly anxiety. Thus, the limbic system may play an active role in processing the emotional reaction to pain and the memory of the pain experience (Shyu & Vogt, 2009). However, the human ability to experience and remember pain does not depend on *cognitive ability* (explicit memory). The experience of pain is remembered by even the youngest of infants, including those born prematurely (Grunau & Tu, 2007).

As a person becomes aware of pain, a complex reaction unfolds. Psychological and cognitive factors interact with neurophysiological factors in the perception of pain. Perception gives awareness and meaning to pain so that a person can then react. The reaction to pain is the physiological and behavioural responses that occur after pain is perceived.

Modulation of pain is the final nociceptive phase and refers to the increase or decrease in pain signal intensity that can occur before, during, and after pain is perceived (Arnstein, 2010, p. 42). For example, once the brain perceives the pain, inhibitory neurotransmitters are released (see Box 31-1); these include endogenous opioids (endorphins and enkephalins), serotonin, norepinephrine, and gamma aminobutyric acid, which work to hinder the transmission of pain and help produce an analgesic effect (Arnstein, 2010).

A protective reflex response may also occur with pain reception (Figure 31-3). A-delta fibres send sensory impulses to the spinal cord,

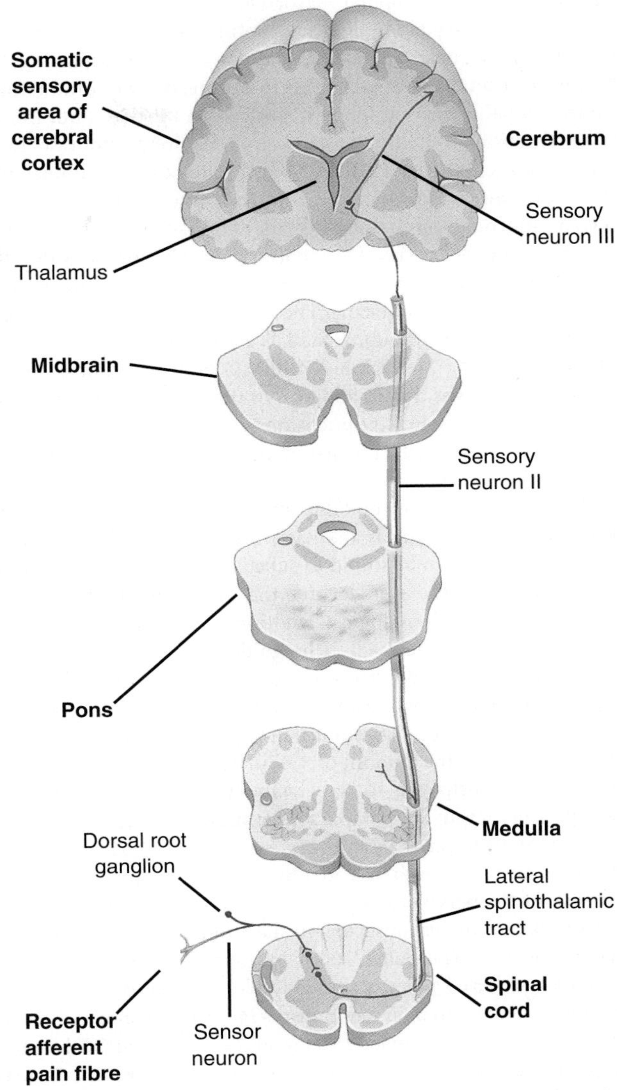

FIGURE 31-2 Spinothalamic pathway that conducts pain stimuli to the brain.

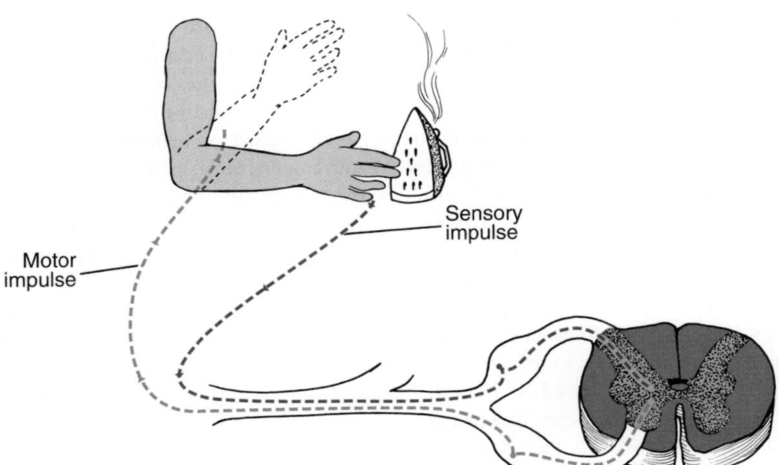

FIGURE 31-3 Protective reflex to pain stimulus.

where they synapse with spinal motor neurons. The motor impulses travel via a reflex arc along *efferent* (motor) nerve fibres back to a peripheral muscle near the site of stimulation, thus bypassing the brain. Contraction of the muscle leads to a protective withdrawal from the source of pain. For example, when a person touches a hot iron, a burning sensation is felt, but the hand also reflexively withdraws from the iron's surface. When superficial fibres in the skin are stimulated, a person moves away from the pain source. If internal tissues such as muscle or mucous membranes become stimulated, tightening and guarding of muscles occur. This reflex is usually absent below the injury in patients with spinal cord injuries. However, patients with spinal cord injuries can still experience pain above the level of injury (Widerström-Noga, Finnerup, & Siddall, 2009).

Theory of Pain. Melzack and Wall's (1965) gate-control theory was the first to suggest that in addition to the physical sensation, pain has emotional and cognitive dimensions and that pain impulses can be regulated or even blocked by gating mechanisms located along the central nervous system. The theory suggests that pain impulses pass through when a gate is open and that impulses are blocked when a gate is closed. Closing the gate is the basis for pain-relief interventions. Gating mechanisms can be found in substantia gelatinosa cells within the dorsal horn of the spinal cord, thalamus, and limbic system. Understanding what physiological, emotional, and cognitive processes can influence these gates will help guide your approach to pain management. For example, stress, exercise, and other factors increase the release of endorphins, raising an individual's **pain threshold**, or the minimal intensity of a stimulus that is perceived as painful (IASP, 2012). Knowing that the amount of modulating substances varies with each person will help you to understand why pain intensity varies among patients, even for comparable stimuli, and why individuals exhibit different responses to pain.

More recently, research has identified neuronal modifiability or "plasticity" of the nervous system. This refers to the nervous system's ability to change in response to repeated intense stimuli (Julius & Basbaum, 2001; Woolf & Salter, 2000). In response to repeated noxious stimuli, or unrelieved pain, neurons develop a memory of the pain. This leads to changes to pain mechanisms in the peripheral and central nervous system, called *peripheral* and *central sensitization*. With central sensitization, dorsal horn spinal cord neurons may become increasingly sensitive and responsive to all stimuli, leading to chronic pain (Basbaum & Julius, 2006; Kehlet, Jensen, & Woolf, 2006). This means that unrelieved acute pain can lead to chronic pain.

Physiological Responses. As pain impulses ascend the spinal cord toward the brain stem and thalamus, the autonomic nervous system (ANS) becomes stimulated, as part of the stress response (see Chapter 29). Stimulation of the sympathetic branch of the ANS results in physiological responses (Table 31-1) (Hamunen, Kontinen, Hakala, et al., 2012). If the pain is continuous, severe, or deep, typically involving the visceral organs (e.g., with a myocardial infarction or colic from gallbladder or renal stones), the parasympathetic nervous system goes into action. Sustained physiological responses to pain could cause serious harm to an individual, such as altered immune response (Rittner, Brack, & Stein, 2008). However, most people reach a level of adaptation in which physical signs return to normal. Therefore, patients in pain will *not* always have changes in their vital signs. Although nurses need to consider a person's physiological responses to pain, they should avoid using them as sole measures to infer pain.

Behavioural Responses. Once pain is perceived, if it is not managed effectively, a cycle of events begins that can significantly diminish the meaning and quality of a person's life. Pain, especially intense acute pain or chronic pain, is physically and emotionally exhausting and can interfere, short or long term, with the ability to function and engage with others. Anxiety is a common initial response to pain, while depression, irritability, and chronic fatigue often accompany persistent pain (Turk, Fillingim, Ohrbach, et al., 2016). These responses to pain help explain why pain management can be so challenging.

TABLE 31-1 Physiological Reactions to Pain

Response	Cause or Effect
Sympathetic Stimulation*	
Dilation of bronchial tubes and increased respiratory rate	Provides increased oxygen intake
Increased heart rate	Provides increased oxygen transport
Peripheral vasoconstriction (pallor, elevation in blood pressure)	Elevates blood pressure with shift of blood supply from periphery and viscera to skeletal muscles and brain
Increased blood glucose level	Provides additional energy
Diaphoresis	Controls body temperature during stress
Increased muscle tension	Prepares muscles for action
Dilation of pupils	Affords better vision
Decreased gastrointestinal motility (nausea, vomiting)	Frees energy for more immediate activity
Parasympathetic Stimulation†	
Pallor	Causes blood supply to shift away from periphery
Muscle tension	Results from fatigue
Decreased heart rate and blood pressure	Results from vagal stimulation
Rapid, irregular breathing	Causes body defences to fail under prolonged stress of pain
Weakness or exhaustion	Results from expenditure of physical energy

*Superficial pain and pain of low to moderate intensity.
†Severe or deep pain.

Unrelieved pain affects physical, psychological, social, and spiritual well-being (Turk et al., 2016). Patient factors may contribute to unrelieved pain. For example, some patients will endure severe pain without asking for assistance, and some patients may not report pain if they believe their pain may inconvenience others or signals a loss of self-control. To ensure optimal health outcomes and minimize the impact on activities of daily living, it is important to discuss the benefits of using effective pain-management strategies.

Nonverbal or behavioural indicators of pain may include body movements, facial expressions, and vocalizations. Bracing, splinting or protecting the painful part, rocking, body stiffening, jaw clenching, grimacing, frowning, crying, moaning, or screaming may indicate pain is present. Affective responses can include social withdrawal, changes in eating or sleep patterns, stoicism, fear, anxiety, anger, or feelings of hopelessness (Hadjistavropoulos, Herr, Prkachin, et al., 2014). Valid and reliable tools exist to assist in the assessment of pain in people who are unable to self-report their pain. Lack of pain expression does not necessarily mean that a person has no pain. For example, premature and full-term infants sometimes do not cry, and they may exhibit few motor movements, especially after excessive and repeated exposure to pain (Stevens, McGrath, Gibbins, et al., 2007). Similarly, opioids can blunt the behavioural expression of pain by sedating the patient. Yet, the patient who is sedated or sleeping can still be in pain (Pasero & Portenoy, 2011).

Types of Pain

Pain may be categorized by its duration, such as acute and chronic pain, or by its pathology, such as cancer pain and noncancer pain (e.g., pain associated with arthritis, diabetic neuropathy, low back pain, and headache) or by the process of action (nociceptive or neuropathic).

Acute Pain. Acute pain usually has an identifiable cause, either somatic, visceral, or nociceptive (Arnstein, 2010), and is of short duration (usually less than 6 months). Acute pain has a predictable ending (healing) and an identifiable cause, and eventually it resolves with or without treatment after a damaged area heals. Evidence, however, suggests that unrelieved acute pain may have development- and age-related consequences. For instance, significant and repeated exposure to acute pain during epochs of rapid early infant brain development may alter an infant's pain response (Taddio & Katz, 2005). Untreated or poorly treated intraoperative and postoperative pain and stress can also increase infant mortality and morbidity (Fitzgerald & Walker, 2009). Unrelieved moderate to severe postoperative pain can lead to the development of chronic pain (Althaus, Arranz Becker, & Neugebauer, 2013; Kehlet et al., 2006).

No matter what the age, unrelieved acute pain can have a negative impact on recovery from illness or surgery, resulting in prolonged hospitalization, increased risk of complications from immobility (see Chapter 45), and delayed rehabilitation. When pain is not relieved, physical or psychological recovery can be delayed because the patient's prime focus may be on achieving pain relief. Although it may not be possible to completely eliminate the pain, working with the patient and members of the interprofessional health care team to reduce pain to an acceptable level is realistic. The nurse's primary goals should be to prevent pain whenever possible and to effectively manage pain so that patients can participate in their own recovery.

Chronic Pain. Chronic pain is defined as pain that persists past the normal time of healing (IASP, 2012). It is distinctly different than acute pain. Chronic pain can be intermittent (occurs in a pattern) or persistent (lasting more than 12 hours daily) (Canadian Pain Coalition, 2011), experienced at any point in life, including early childhood (Stinson, Finley, Dick, et al., 2016), and lead to great personal suffering. Chronic pain may be nonmalignant or related to cancer. Chronic noncancer pain is usually not life-threatening. However, patients with chronic noncancer pain are often frustrated because they cannot predict how they will feel from day to day, and the pain they experience may be unrelenting. The pain may result from an injured area that healed long ago but continues to be nonresponsive to treatment. Chronic noncancer pain may be experienced along with other symptoms such as sleep disturbances, depression, anxiety, and anger (Turk et al., 2016). This type of pain may be a major cause of psychological and physical disability, leading to problems such as job loss, the inability to perform simple daily activities, sexual dysfunction, and social isolation from family and friends.

Despite the fact that Canadians are among the largest opioid users per capita in the world, undertreated chronic noncancer pain is a challenge faced by patients and health care providers alike (Busse, Guyatt, Carrasco, et al., 2017). Now, more than ever, health care providers may be reluctant to treat chronic noncancer pain with opioids. Patients with chronic noncancer pain who exhibit behaviours seen in addictive disease, such as increasing demands for larger doses of opioids, are mistakenly diagnosed with addiction (i.e., pseudoaddiction) (Pasero, Quinn, Portenoy, et al., 2011). They may actually be seeking pain relief as a result of undertreated pain. To help break the cycle of poor pain management, nurses should inform patients about concerns raised when they seek help from multiple health care providers and refer the patient to a pain team or chronic pain clinic, if available. The current Canadian guideline for chronic noncancer pain addresses the challenges with assessment and management of chronic noncancer pain, and it provides recommendations and tools for safe and responsible selection, prescription, titration, and monitoring of opioids (Busse et al., 2017).

The coping strategies used by individuals with chronic pain, as well as their personal beliefs, may determine how they will function with and adjust to pain. Esteve, Ramírez-Maestre, and López-Martínez (2007) found that individuals who believed they could control their pain, avoided viewing their condition as a tragedy, and believed that they were not severely disabled appeared to function better than those who did not. When managing pain, a comprehensive approach that includes both nonpharmacological and pharmacological strategies should be utilized. The use of evidence-informed adaptive coping strategies is encouraged, such as cognitive-behavioural therapy, relaxation techniques, positive thinking, visual imagery, and distraction (Registered Nurses' Association of Ontario [RNAO], 2013).

Cancer Pain. Pain in a patient with cancer may be acute, chronic, or both. The pain may also be nociceptive, neuropathic, or both. Cancer pain may be caused by tumour progression and its related pathological process, invasive procedures, toxicities of treatment, infection, and physical limitations. It can be sensed at the actual site of the tumour or distant to the site. When pain is sensed at a site that is distant to the area of tissue damage it is called *referred pain.* For example, a patient who has pancreatic cancer may sense the pain from a pancreatic tumour in the lower back. Referred pain can occur in patients experiencing cancer pain or noncancer pain.

Any new report of pain by a patient with existing pain needs to be investigated. Although the need for treatment of cancer pain has become increasingly evident, the issue of undertreatment continues (Caraceni, Martini, Zecca, et al., 2004). Many individuals with cancer pain live at home in their community, and pain is managed by themselves, by their families or both. Research findings suggest that accessing community resources when pain is not well managed may be difficult for these families and that the stress of caring for a loved one with cancer pain can affect the health of family caregivers (Harrison, Young, Price, et al., 2009). The importance of establishing an organized, systematic, and comprehensive approach to pain assessment and treatment, as well as communicating with and supporting patients' families, cannot be overemphasized; nurses have the potential to play pivotal roles in these endeavours.

Pain by Inferred Pathology Process. Identifying the cause of pain is one of the first steps in successfully managing pain. Nociceptive pain is pain caused by tissue damage and is subdivided into *somatic* (musculoskeletal) and *visceral* (internal organ) pain. Neuropathic pain arises from abnormal or damaged pain nerves (Table 31-2). Each of these pathological processes has distinct pain characteristics (IASP, 2012) that are discussed later under "Assessment" in the "Nursing Process and Pain" section.

Breakthrough Pain. Some patients experience occasional, transitory exacerbations of their baseline pain, called breakthrough pain, because the pain "breaks through" the regular pain medication or treatment that adequately controls the baseline pain. Research has shown that breakthrough pain is not routinely recognized, evaluated, or treated (Portenoy, Bennett, Rauck, et al., 2006). When breakthrough pain is brief and precipitated by an activity-related action, such as movement, sneezing, or coughing, it is referred to as *incident pain* (Pasero, Quinn et al., 2011, p. 310). *Idiopathic pain*, another subtype of breakthrough pain, is not associated with an identifiable cause and has a longer duration than that of incident pain (p. 310) (Box 31-2).

TABLE 31-2 Classification of Pain by Inferred Pathology: Two Major Types of Pain

I. **Nociceptive pain:** Normal processing of stimuli that damages normal tissues or has the potential to do so if prolonged; usually responsive to nonopioids, opioids, or both.	II. **Neuropathic pain:** Abnormal processing of sensory input by the peripheral or central nervous system; treatment usually includes adjuvant analgesics.
A. **Somatic pain:** Arises from bone, joint, muscle, skin, or connective tissue. It is usually aching or throbbing in quality and is well localized.	A. **Centrally generated pain** 1. Deafferentation pain. Injury to either the peripheral or central nervous system. Examples: Phantom pain may reflect injury to the peripheral nervous system; burning pain below the level of a spinal cord lesion reflects injury to the central nervous system.
	2. Sympathetically maintained pain. Associated with dysregulation of the autonomic nervous system. Examples: May include some of the pain associated with complex regional pain syndrome (type I, type II).
B. **Visceral pain:** Arises from visceral organs, such as the gastrointestinal tract and pancreas. This may be subdivided: 1. Tumour involvement of the organ capsule, which causes aching and fairly well-localized pain. 2. Obstruction of hollow viscus, which causes intermittent cramping and poorly localized pain.	B. **Peripherally generated pain** 1. Painful polyneuropathies. Pain is felt along the distribution of many peripheral nerves. Examples: Diabetic neuropathy, alcohol-nutritional neuropathy, and those associated with Guillain-Barré syndrome. 2. Painful mononeuropathies. Usually associated with a known peripheral nerve injury, and pain is felt at least partly along the distribution of the damaged nerve. Examples: Nerve root compression, nerve entrapment, trigeminal neuralgia.

Pasero, C., & McCaffery, M. (2011). *Pain assessment and pharmacological management* (p. 2). St. Louis, MO: Mosby/Elsevier. Copyright © 2011, Pasero C., McCaffery, M. May be duplicated for use in clinical practice. Data from Max, M. B., & Portenoy, R. K. (2003). Methodological challenges for clinical trials of cancer pain treatments. In C. R. Chapman & K. M. Foley (Eds.), *Current and emerging issues in cancer pain: Research and practice.* New York: Raven Press; Portenoy, R. K. (1996). Neuropathic pain. In R. K. Portenoy & R. M. Kanner (Eds.), *Pain management: Theory and practice.* Philadelphia, PA: F. A. Davis.

BOX 31-2 Subtypes of Breakthrough Pain

1. Incident pain: Cause of pain is generally identifiable but occurrence may be unpredictable.
   a. Predictable incident pain: Something identifiable, such as movement, predictably causes the pain.
   b. Unpredictable incident pain: Occurrence of pain is unpredictable and may be caused by events such as bladder spasm. This pain occurs spontaneously.
2. Idiopathic pain: Cause is not readily identifiable.
3. End-of-dose pain: An increase in baseline pain that occurs prior to a scheduled dose of around-the-clock analgesic. Onset is usually gradual, and duration may be longer than that of incident or idiopathic pain.

Pasero, C., & McCaffery, M. (2011). *Pain assessment and pharmacological management* (p. 101). St. Louis., MO: Mosby/Elsevier. Data from Bennett, D., Burton, A. W., Fishman, S., Fortner, B., McCarberg, B., Miaskowski, C., et al. (2005). Consensus panel recommendations for the assessment and management of breakthrough pain: Part 1: Assessment. *Pharmacology & Therapeutics, 30*(5), 296–301.

NURSING KNOWLEDGE BASE

In *Notes on Nursing: What It Is and What It Is Not* (1859/1969), Florence Nightingale stated that "pain ... perpetuates and intensifies itself." Thus, nurses have a long history of dealing with the effects of pain on patients. In this section, factors that influence pain are explored.

Knowledge, Attitudes, and Beliefs

Pain assessment and management may be influenced by the nurses' or members of the interprofessional team's personal beliefs, attitudes, or pain-related myths (McCaffery et al., 2011, p. 39). There are many factors that influence clinicians' belief in patients' reports of pain. It is important to acknowledge that the knowledge, attitudes, and preferences of health care providers, including your own, will influence pain care decision making. A patient's tolerance to pain and response to pain may influence your perception of the patient's degree of discomfort (McCaffery, Pasero, & Ferrell, 2007). Patients deemed to have a low **pain tolerance**, which is the greatest level of pain an individual is prepared to endure in a given situation (IASP, 2012), may be perceived as complainers. To avoid making judgements about another's pain, it is important to acknowledge your own beliefs about pain. Consider the immediate context in which a patient is experiencing pain, as well as his or her past pain experiences. Base your pain assessment and pain care decision making on a variety of sources and observations, such as the patient's self-report, information from family and significant others, the patient's behaviour and physiology, and internal and external environmental factors.

Numerous studies on how clinicians judge the pain of others have indicated that, when compared with patients' self-reports, health care providers tend to underestimate or, on occasion, overestimate the patient's pain (Prkachin, Solomon, & Ross, 2007; Ung, Yenna, Hu, et al., 2016). For example, it has been demonstrated that nurses tend to overestimate pain when patients report no pain and underestimate pain when patients report mild to intense pain (Heikkinnen, Salanterä, Kettu, et al., 2005) or when they are told that patients might be faking pain to obtain opioids (Kappesser, Williams, & Prkachin, 2006). Differences in pain ratings may also result from the type of tool used for pain assessment (Chambers, Hardial, Craig, et al., 2005). Nurses are often unaware of the process of inferring pain in others, yet nurses' judgements guide their actions. For example, a nurse's personal opinion about the patient's report of pain may affect the titration of opioid doses (McCaffery et al., 2011).

Making assumptions about patients in pain may seriously limit a nurse's ability to offer pain relief. Too often, nurses allow misconceptions about pain (Box 31-3) to affect their willingness to intervene. Some even avoid acknowledging a patient's pain because of their own fear and denial. Nurses have their personal beliefs; however, they must accept the patient's report of pain and act according to professional guidelines, standards, position statements, policies and procedures, and evidence-informed research findings. To help differentiate between personal beliefs and the patient's experience, nurses need to view the experience of pain from the patient's perspective by becoming an active, knowledgeable observer of the patient in pain. In your own nursing practice, this will assist you in being more objective, and it will allow you to provide a more holistic and effective approach to your pain care decision making and actions. These expressions of professionalism will be meaningful to the individual and improve his or her pain outcomes.

Factors Influencing Pain

Pain is complex and involves physiological, social, spiritual, psychological, and cultural influences. Each individual's pain experience is different. Nurses need to consider all factors that affect the patient in pain.

Physiological Factors

Age. Age is an important variable that influences pain, particularly in infants, children, and older people. Developmental differences among these age groups influence how children and older people perceive and react to pain. Young children have difficulty understanding the procedures that nurses perform that may cause pain. Cognitively, toddlers and preschoolers are often unable to recall explanations about pain, or they associate pain with experiences that can occur in various situations. They may also have difficulty expressing their pain or may use verbal descriptors that differ from those used by older individuals (Stanford, Chambers, Craig, 2005). When assessing pain in a child, consider adapting your approaches (including what to ask and the behaviours to observe). Help prepare the child for a painful procedure. Ask the child and parents about the terms most often used by the child to describe the pain experience and pain treatment, and then use those terms when communicating about pain with the child. For instance, children have developed words for pain by the age of 18 months and may describe pain as an "ache" or "hurt." As cognitive development matures, so does the ability for a toddler to report the degree of pain, such as it hurts a lot or a little. School-age children and adolescents are capable of seriation, hence can better rate their pain intensity using validated pain tools (Franck, Greenberg, & Stevens, 2000).

Older persons may be more sensitive to severe pain as a result of structural, biochemical, and functional changes (Hadjistavropoulos et al., 2014). Older patients may experience cognitive impairment, confusion, or memory loss, either from pathology or medication, which can be compounded by sight and hearing impairment. Mobility, activities of daily living (ADLs), social activities outside the home, and activity tolerance may all be reduced in older persons. Therefore, pain in an older person requires careful, comprehensive assessment, diagnosis, and management (American Geriatric Society, 2009) (Box 31-4).

The ability of older patients to interpret pain can be complicated by the presence of multiple diseases with vague symptoms that affect similar parts of the body. Nurses need to undertake a detailed assessment when a patient has more than one source of pain (Herr, 2002a, 2002b). The manifestations of different diseases can cause atypical presentations of painful conditions. Different diseases can also cause similar symptoms. For example, chest pain does not always indicate a heart attack; it may be a symptom of arthritis of the spine or of an abdominal disorder. Not all older people experience cognitive impairment. However, when older persons are confused, they may not be able to recall and explain details of pain experiences. Misconceptions about pain management in the very young and in older persons may seriously hamper effective pain management for these populations (Tables 31-3 and 31-4).

Sleep. Sleep disturbances, including insomnia and sleep interruption, can heighten pain perception, increase pain intensity, and decrease coping abilities. Sleep disturbance and fatigue is a common problem

BOX 31-3 Common Biases and Misconceptions About Pain

The following statements are false:

People who misuse drugs and alcohol overreact to discomfort.

Patients with minor illnesses have less pain than those with severe physical alterations.

The amount of tissue damage in an injury can accurately indicate pain intensity.

Health care providers are the best authorities on the nature of a patient's pain.

Psychogenic pain is not real.

Chronic pain is psychological.

Patients should expect to have pain during a hospital stay.

Patients who cannot speak do not feel pain.

Infants are incapable of experiencing pain.

BOX 31-4 FOCUS ON OLDER PERSONS

Factors Influencing Pain

With aging, muscle mass decreases, body fat increases, and the percentage of body water decreases. This results in the potential for an increased concentration of water-soluble drugs, such as morphine. Also, the volume of distribution for fat-soluble drugs, such as fentanyl, increases (Pergolizzi, Böger, Budd, et al., 2008).

- Older persons frequently eat poorly, resulting in them having low serum albumin levels. Many drugs are highly protein bound. In the presence of low serum albumin, more of the active form of a drug remains unbound, which increases the risk for adverse effects, toxic effects, or both (American Geriatric Society, 2009).
- Decline of hepatic and renal function is a natural occurrence with aging. This results in reduced metabolism and excretion of drugs. Hence, older people often experience a greater peak effect and longer duration of analgesics (Pergolizzi et al., 2008).
- Age-related changes in the skin, such as thinning and loss of elasticity, could affect the absorption rate of topical analgesics. However, transdermal analgesics have been proven beneficial for older patients and are particularly suitable for those with impaired gastrointestinal function (Pergolizzi et al., 2008).
- Patient-controlled analgesia (PCA) and regional analgesia are not contraindicated in older persons, but frequent assessment for pain and the adverse effects of analgesics and of cognition are necessary to ensure the efficacy and safety of PCA (Chou, Gordon, de Leon-Casasola, et al., 2016).
- The loss of the efficiency of homeostatic mechanisms puts older persons at risk for falls or delirium after the administration of sedative drugs or regional anaesthesia (American Geriatric Society, 2009).

TABLE 31-3 Pain in Infants

Misconception	Correction
Infants cannot feel pain or are less sensitive to pain because of an immature nervous system.	Infants can feel pain. Their immature inhibitory capacities can enhance the pain experience (Rodkey & Pillai Riddell, 2013). Complete myelination is not required in order for infants to feel pain (Twycross, 2009).
Infants are incapable of expressing pain.	Behavioural cues, such as facial expression and motor movements, along with responses such as crying and physiological cues such as vagal tone can be indicators of pain and have led to the development of validated pain assessment tools for infants. Infants can react to pain via afferent/efferent pathways but cannot cognitively modulate the pain (Stevens, Pillai Riddell, Oberlander, et al., 2007).
Infants must learn about pain from previous painful experiences.	Emotional processing and cognitive abilities are maturational in nature and can influence the expression of pain and the ability to cope with pain. However, pain is present with the first insult; it need not be learned from an earlier painful experience (Grunau & Tu, 2007).
Pain cannot be accurately assessed in infants.	Behavioural responses, primarily facial expressions, can be reliably and validly assessed. Specific facial expressions are acknowledged as the most specific indicator of pain in response to acute noxious stimuli (Stevens, Pillai Riddell, et al., 2007). Numerous behavioural validated pain-assessment tools have been developed to use with infants (Stevens, Pillai Riddell, et al., 2007).
Because infants cannot demonstrate cognitive awareness, they are insensible and lack memory for pain.	Early and repeated exposure to noxious stimuli can affect the infant's future responses to painful events (Grunau & Tu, 2007).
Analgesics and anaesthetics cannot be safely given to infants and neonates because of their immature capacity to metabolize and eliminate drugs, as well as their sensitivity to opioid-induced respiratory depression.	Infants older than 1 month of age metabolize drugs in the same manner as older infants and children. Careful selection of the drug, dosage, administration route, and time; frequent monitoring for desired and undesired effects; and drug titration and weaning can minimize the adverse effects of opioids and nonopioids for pain management in neonates (Taddio, 2007).

Twycross, A. (2009). Why managing pain in children matters. In A. Twycross, S. J. Dowden, & E. Bruce (Eds.), *Managing pain in children: A clinical guide* (p. 5). Oxford, UK: Wiley-Blackwell; Rodkey, E. N., & Pillai Riddell, R. (2013). The infancy of infant pain research: The experimental origins of infant pain denial. *Journal of Pain, 14*(4), 338–350.

for patients with long-term illnesses or as a result of treatment. If fatigue occurs along with sleeplessness, the perception of pain may be even greater (Schuh-Hofer, Wodarski, Pfau, et al., 2013).

Heredity. Increasingly, research has provided evidence that genetic information can influence our ability to metabolize pain medicine, our pain threshold, pain tolerance, and susceptibility to develop chronic pain (James, 2013).

Neurological Function. A patient's neurological function can influence the pain experience. Any factor that interrupts or influences normal pain reception or perception affects the patient's awareness of and response to pain. For example, patients who have a spinal cord injury, peripheral neuropathy (as in the case of diabetes mellitus), or a neurological disease (e.g., multiple sclerosis) experience altered pain sensation. Certain pharmacological medications influence pain perception and response. Analgesics (medications that relieve pain), sedatives, and anaesthetics (medications that cause temporary loss of sensation) depress functions of the central nervous system. Because patients at risk for pain insensitivity could suffer injury, they require preventive nursing care that includes neurological assessment (see Chapter 32).

Social Factors

Attention. The degree to which a patient focuses on pain can influence pain perception. Increased attention has been associated with increased pain, whereas distraction has been associated with a diminished pain response (Uman, Chambers, McGrath, et al., 2008). This is a concept that nurses use when applying nonpharmacological pain-relief interventions such as relaxation and massage. By focusing a patient's attention and concentration on other stimuli, his or her awareness of pain temporarily declines.

Previous Experience. Prior painful experiences may shape how a patient responds to subsequent painful events. If a person has had frequent episodes of pain, or severe pain, without relief, pain-related anxiety or fear may occur. In contrast, if a person has had repeated experiences with the same type of pain but the pain has been successfully relieved, it becomes easier to interpret the pain sensation and the patient is better prepared to take actions to relieve the pain.

When patients have no prior exposure to a particular pain-inducing event, they may be unprepared to manage their pain, and this may impair their coping abilities. For example, incisional pain is common after abdominal surgery. When a patient knows to expect pain, he or she may view the incisional pain as a serious complication of surgery. As a result, the person may tense up and breathe shallowly and become anxious. It is important to inform patients of the type of pain that might be experienced as a result of surgery or other procedures or illnesses and of methods to reduce it.

Family and Social Support. People in pain often depend on family or friends for support, assistance, or protection. A loved one can help minimize loneliness and fear. An absence of support can make the pain experience more stressful. The presence of parents is especially important for children with pain. Nurses should explain to parents that children typically want their parents with them during a pain event, but warn them that a parent's own anxiety and responses may influence how the child experiences and responds to pain (Chambers, Craig, & Bennett, 2002). Parents should be provided with information about the procedure, and the nurse should involve them by explaining how they can use pain-related distraction strategies with their child during the painful procedure. For example, skin-to-skin contact or kangaroo care is a useful strategy to use with preterm infants experiencing procedural pain. The parent or caregiver and the infant are chest to chest

TABLE 31-4 Pain in Older Persons

Misconception	Correction
Pain is a natural outcome of growing old.	Older persons are at greater risk than younger adults for many painful conditions; however, in the absence of disease, pain is not a normal part of aging.
Pain perception, or sensitivity, decreases with age.	Some studies suggest that greater age brings a higher threshold for painful electrical, thermal, and mechanical stimuli to the skin, while others have reported that older patients have alterations in the sensorineural apparatus, thus diminishing the perception of pain (Delgado-Guay & Bruera, 2008).
If the older patient does not report pain, he or she does not have pain.	Older patients commonly underreport pain. Reasons include expecting to have pain with increasing age; not wanting to alarm loved ones; being fearful of losing independence; not wanting to distract, anger, or bother caregivers; and believing that caregivers know that the older patient has pain and are doing all that can be done to relieve it. The absence of a report of pain does not mean the absence of pain.
If an older patient appears to be occupied, asleep, or otherwise distracted from pain, he or she does not have pain.	Older patients often believe it is unacceptable to show pain and have learned to use a variety of ways to cope with it instead (e.g., many patients use distraction successfully for short periods of time). Sleeping may be a coping strategy or may indicate exhaustion, not pain relief. Assumptions about the presence or absence of pain cannot be made solely on the basis of a patient's behaviour.
The potential adverse effects of opioids make them too dangerous to use to relieve pain in older persons.	Opioids may be used safely in older persons. Although the opioid-naïve older person may be more sensitive to opioids, this does not justify withholding their use in pain management for this population. Potentially dangerous opioid-induced adverse effects can be prevented with slow titration; regular, frequent monitoring and assessment of the patient's response; and adjustment of dose and interval between doses when adverse effects are detected. If necessary, clinically significant respiratory depression can be reversed by an opioid antagonist drug.
Patients with Alzheimer's disease and other cognitive impairments do not feel pain, and their reports of pain are most likely invalid.	No evidence exists that cognitively impaired older persons experience less pain or that their reports of pain are less valid than those of individuals with intact cognitive function. It is probable that patients with dementia or other deficits of cognition suffer significant unrelieved pain and discomfort. Assessment of pain in these patients is challenging, but possible. The best approach is to accept the patient's report of pain and treat the pain as it would be treated in an individual with intact cognitive function.

Adapted from McCaffery, M., & Pasero, C. (1999). *Pain: Clinical manual* (2nd ed.). St. Louis, MO: Mosby; Data from American Geriatrics Society. (2009). Pharmacological management of persistent pain in older persons. *Journal of American Geriatrics Society, 57*, 1331–1346. doi:10.1111/j.1532-5415.2009.02376.x; Delgado-Guay, M. O., & Bruera, E. (2008). Management of pain in the older person with cancer, Part 1: Pathophysiology, pharmacokinetics, and assessment. *Oncology, 22*(1), 56–61. Retrieved from http://www.cancernetwork.com/oncology-journal/management-pain-older-person-cancer-part-1-pathophysiology-pharmacokinetics-and-assessment; Hanks-Bell, M. N., Halvey, K., & Paice, J. A. (2004). Pain assessment and management in aging. *Online Journal of Issues in Nursing, 9*(3). Retrieved from http://www.nursingworld.org/MainMenuCategories/ANAMarketplace/ANAPeriodicals/OJIN/TableofContents/Volume92004/No3Sept04/ArticlePreviousTopic/PainAssessmentandManagementinAging.aspx.

with skin-to-skin contact. This is a powerful nonpharmacological strategy for preterm infants, who typically undergo 10–16 painful invasive procedures daily (Cong, Cusson, Walsh, et al., 2012). Also, breastfeeding should be encouraged as a means of pain reduction for procedural pain in infants, as evidenced by a recent Cochrane review (Harrison, Reszel, Bueno, et al., 2016).

Psychological Factors

Anxiety. The relationship between pain and anxiety is complicated. Anxiety is associated with many types of pain; however, the cause-and-effect relationship has not been established (McCaffery et al., 2011). Pain often causes anxiety, but it is not clear that anxiety increases the intensity of pain. However, pain-related anxiety can result in the avoidance of activities that a patient fears may cause pain. When anxiety goes unnoticed, it may be difficult to manage pain effectively. The management of anxiety through the use of nonpharmacological and pharmacological approaches is appropriate. However, anxiolytic medications should not be used as a substitute for analgesia.

Meaning of Pain. The meaning of pain affects the experience of pain and how one adapts to it. A person will perceive pain differently if it suggests a threat, loss, punishment, or challenge. For example, a woman in labour may perceive pain differently than a woman with a history of cancer who experiences new pain and fears recurrence.

Spiritual Factors. Religion and spirituality help individuals become part of a community or feel connected with nature or the universe. In some traditions, pain is viewed as retribution from God, or an opportunity to demonstrate the strength of character that will be rewarded after death. Prayer, hope, and seeking spiritual support, such as attendance at church, have been linked to less suffering associated with pain (Closs, Edwards, Swift, et al., 2013; Wachholtz, Pearce, & Koenig, 2007). But severe or prolonged pain can permeate the very essence of the person, eroding what is important, often challenging established beliefs and values, which may result in poorer pain outcomes (Rippentrop, Altmaier, Chen, et al., 2005). Similarly, for those who view humans as irreducible energy fields in continual interaction with universal sources of energy, pain may be intensified or lessened as a result of changes in energy patterns.

Spiritual assessment tools such as FICA (*F*aith, belief, meaning; *I*mportance and *I*nfluence; *C*ommunity; and Address/*A*ction in care) are available (Maxwell, Brouch, & Jungquist, 2005). It is good to explore potential religious and spiritual coping strategies with patients, such as meaning-making, distraction, spiritual supports, and relaxation techniques. For example, for patients whose faith or spirituality is based in a religious tradition, suggest a visit from a clergyperson. Or, support the choice of meditation, therapeutic touch, Reiki, or acupuncture as restorative modalities designed to improve energy-flow patterns. Providing interventions designed to holistically heal is essential for the best possible pain management.

Cultural Factors. Culture shapes individuals' responses, behaviours, and attitudes about pain and how they react to and cope with

BOX 31-5 CULTURAL ASPECTS OF CARE

Assessing Pain

Culture affects behavioural responses to pain and treatment preferences. For example, the Chinese culture includes Confucianism, which maintains that pain is an essential element of life and is a trial or a sacrifice (Chen, Miaskowski, Dodd, et al., 2008). Thus, a patient with this belief would rather endure pain and not report it to a clinician, although the person may report it to a family member. Although it is important that, as a nurse, you become culturally competent in order to understand the characteristics of a culture, this knowledge does not tell you what to expect of a particular patient (McCaffery et al., 2011). Therefore, we encourage you to be sensitive to the differences among all individuals by seeking information from each patient and family about their specific beliefs. Remember to be mindful of the fact that the more difference there is between you and your patient, the more difficult it is for you to assess and treat the patient.

Implications for Practice

- Emotional and cognitive responses to pain (overt, stoic) vary between and within cultures.
- Words used to express pain vary among cultures (hurt, ache, discomfort).
- Personal and social meanings of pain and past pain experiences affect pain perception.
- The meaning of pain may influence the perception of pain intensity.
- Health care providers' beliefs and expectations regarding pain expression influence the use of pain management strategies.
- Therapeutic goals of pain management are influenced by cultural beliefs.
- Be aware of perceived causal factors of pain (fate, lifestyle, punishment, witchcraft).
- Believe patients' reports about their perceived pain; do not act on your own beliefs about a patient's pain.
- Seek information about the cultural backgrounds of your patients through discussion with your patients and families and research of the best published evidence.

Data from Al-Atiyyat, N. M. H. (2009). Cultural diversity and cancer pain. *Journal of Hospice and Palliative Nursing, 11*(3), 154–164. doi:10.1097/NJH.0b013e3181a1aca3; Davidhizar, R., & Giger J. N. (2004). A review of the literature on care of patients in pain who are culturally diverse. *International Nursing Review, 51*(1), 47–55. doi:10.1111/j.1466-7657.2003.00208.x; Lai, D. W. L., & Surood, S. (2009). Chinese health beliefs of older Chinese in Canada. *Journal of Aging and Health, 21*(1), 38–62. doi:10.1177/0898264308328636; Lasch, K. (2000). Culture, pain, and culturally sensitive pain care. *Pain Management Nursing, 1*(3 Suppl. 1), S16–22; Pasero, C., & McCaffery, M. (Eds.). (2011). *Pain assessment and pharmacological management.* St. Louis, MO: Elsevier/Mosby.

pain. People learn what is expected and accepted by their culture. Based on your own cultural beliefs, as a nurse you may also expect that others will or should respond to pain in a particular manner. However, by understanding that pain has different meanings for different cultures, you can design culturally sensitive care.

Some cultures are demonstrative about pain; others are introverted. Your knowledge of the level of a patient's assimilation into Canadian society may be helpful. For example, if several generations of an Asian patient's family have lived in Canada, the influence of the Asian culture may be limited. In contrast, a recent immigrant from another culture may have different beliefs from those of the larger Canadian population. Explore the impact of cultural differences on the patient's pain experience, and adjust the plan of care (Box 31-5). Work with the patient and family to facilitate communication about the assessment and management of pain. Find a culturally appropriate assessment tool, and communicate the use of that tool to other health care providers.

CRITICAL THINKING

Critical thinking requires synthesizing knowledge, experience, patient information, critical thinking attitudes, and professional standards. Clinical judgements require that nurses anticipate the information needed, analyze the data, and make decisions about patient care. A patient's condition or situation is always changing; thus, it is essential during pain assessments for nurses to consider all critical elements that will enable them to make a nursing diagnosis.

Knowledge about pain physiology and factors that influence pain will help you as a nurse to manage patients' pain effectively. With experience, you will become more skilled at assessing pain and choosing effective therapies. Successful pain management does not necessarily mean pain elimination, but rather the attainment of mutually agreed-upon pain-relief goals that allow patients to manage their pain and maintain function and quality of life.

NURSING PROCESS AND PAIN

The nursing process provides nurses with a systematic approach to understanding and treating a patient's pain. An important aspect of effective pain management is establishing a trusting relationship with the patient and family. Pain management extends beyond pain relief; it encompasses the patient's quality of life and ability to work and play productively, and to function normally within the family and society (Arnstein, 2010).

Your application of the nursing process can be optimized by framing it around readily available clinical pain guidelines, which are based on best evidence and are continuously updated (see the Recommended Websites at the end of this chapter).

Assessment

Pain assessment is the basis of all pain management. The patient's pain should be consistently monitored along with other assessments such as vital signs, especially if the pain is not well controlled. Establishing a nursing diagnosis, deciding on appropriate interventions, and evaluating the patient's response to the interventions are contingent on a timely and accurate pain assessment (Figure 31-4). Effective and unbiased pain assessment is best achieved by using a validated pain assessment tool appropriate to the patient (McCaffery et al., 2011; RNAO, 2013).

Factors to consider when choosing an assessment tool include the age and developmental stage of the patient, patient condition, type of pain, culture, cognitive ability, preference, and ease of use for both the patient and the nurse (Arnstein, 2010; Wells et al., 2008). Specific tools are available that are appropriate for patients across the lifespan, from preterm neonates to cognitively impaired older persons. Pain assessment should include obtaining a pain intensity, determining pain location, pain descriptors, and the effects of pain on function and mood. The type of assessment will depend on the needs of the patient.

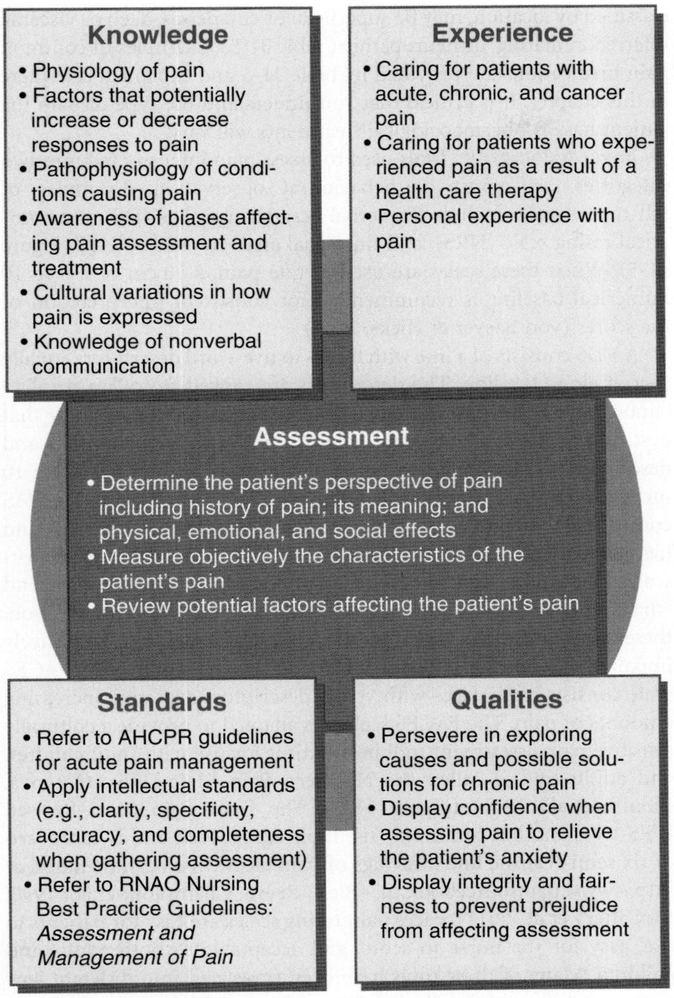

FIGURE 31-4 **Critical thinking model for pain and comfort assessment.** *AHCPR,* Agency for Health Care Policy and Research; *RNAO,* Registered Nurses' Association of Ontario.

Establishing a pain management goal with the patient enables nurses to interpret the pain assessment data collected. Pain management goals should be "SMART"— *S*pecific, *M*easurable, *A*chievable, *R*ealistic, and have a *T*ime frame associated with them. When a SMART pain management goal is established, the nurse can help support the patient in achieving this goal. For patients with chronic or complex pain conditions, thorough assessment of pain should include affective, cognitive, and behavioural dimensions of the pain experience as well as a pain history (Turk, Wilson, Cahana, 2011). The nurse's assessment of chronic noncancer complex pain should focus on the relationship between pain, function, quality of life, and treatment side effects, because complete pain relief may not be possible. In the home setting, family members may assist with pain assessment. The OPQRSTUV approach to pain can be used to remember the essential components of effective pain care for all patients (Box 31-6).

Failure of clinicians to assess a patient's pain, accept the findings, and treat the report of pain is a common cause of unrelieved pain and suffering (McCaffery et al., 2011). Nurses need to use the right tools and methods to avoid errors, and choose the best pain interventions. It is important to become aware of possible errors in pain assessment (Box 31-7).

BOX 31-6 Obtaining a Pain History: OPQRSTUV Mnemonic

O = Onset/Origin: When/where did it start?

P = Palliation/Provocation: What makes the pain better/worse?

Q = Quality: What does the pain feel like (i.e., sharp, dull, continuous, intermittent)

R = Region/Radiation: Where is your pain and does it radiate?

S = Severity: Score pain using a validated pain tool, such as 4/10 on 0–10 scale. Obtain pain assessment at rest and with activity.

T = Timing: When did pain begin or end and how long did it last?

U = Understanding: What do you believe is causing this symptom? How is this symptom affecting you, your family, or both?

V = Value: Are there any other views or feelings about this symptom that are important to you or your family? (This may include cultural and religious values.)

From Fraser Health. (2017). *Symptom assessment acronym.* Surrey, BC: Author. Retrieved from http://www.fraserhealth.ca/media/SymptomAssessmentRevised_Sept09.pdf.

BOX 31-7 Sources of Error When Assessing Pain

- Bias, which causes nurses to consistently overestimate or underestimate their patients' pain
- Unclear assessment questions, which lead to unreliable assessment data (see OPQRSTUV mnemonic in Box 31-6 to optimize pain history taking and assessment)
- Use of pain assessment tools that have no established reliability or validity
- Expecting self-reports of pain from individuals who cannot rate their pain using a pain scale or who cannot provide a complete verbal account of their pain
- Not considering the pain context and the trajectory or change in an individual's expression of pain over time

Expression of Pain. A patient's self-report of pain is considered the gold standard and, as such, is the single most reliable indicator of the existence and intensity of pain (CPS, 2005; Jovey, Ennis, Gardner-Nix, et al., 2003). Many patients fail to report or discuss pain; at the same time, many nurses believe that patients will report pain. If patients sense that the nurse doubts their pain, they will share little or minimize their report of pain. It is important to establish a caring, therapeutic, trusting relationship that allows open communication about pain.

Patients unable to communicate their pain because of their age, medical condition, language requirements, or cognitive disability require special consideration throughout the pain assessment and treatment process. A self-report or behavioural observation pain assessment tool should be selected that is appropriate for age, language, and condition of the patient. The nurse should assess and document pain and comfort behaviours before and after pain management interventions to gauge the effectiveness of treatments.

Cognitively impaired patients might require simple assessment approaches involving close observation of behaviour changes, especially with movement. Feldt (2000) designed the Checklist of Nonverbal Pain Indicators (CNPI), which focuses on behaviours for use with cognitively impaired older persons. The Pain Assessment in Advanced Dementia (PAINAD) provides a clinically relevant and easy-to-use pain assessment tool for individuals with advanced dementia (Warden, Hurley, & Volicer, 2003) The r-FLACC tool is validated for cognitively impaired children, as they cannot report or quantify the severity of their pain (Voepel-Lewis, Milviya, Tait, et al., 2008).

Characteristics of Pain. Assessment of common pain characteristics will help you as a nurse to understand the type and pattern of pain and aid in choosing interventions. When you assess pain and when you ask the patient for his or her self-report of pain, it is important to remember that using instruments to quantify the intensity and characteristics of pain depends on having a good fit between the needs of the patient and the attributes of the assessment tool. Developmental level, cognitive ability, language, and culture are a few factors to consider when assessing pain characteristics.

Onset, Duration, and Sequence of Pain. Ask questions to determine the onset, duration, and sequence of pain. When did the pain begin? How long has it lasted? Does it occur at the same time each day? How often does it recur? Is there frequent breakthrough pain or prolonged pain recovery? Understanding the pattern and cycles of pain will enable you to intervene before the pain occurs or worsens (refer to the OPQRSTUV mnemonic presented earlier in this chapter; see Box 31-6).

Provocation/Pain Pattern. Various factors affect the pain pattern. It is important to assess for factors that precipitate or aggravate pain. Ask the patient to describe activities that cause or increase pain—for example, specific actions such as turning or bending. The low back pain and radiation down the leg associated with a ruptured intravertebral disc are usually aggravated by bending or lifting. Similarly, swallowing and talking typically aggravate the pain of pharyngitis. Asking the patient if the pain is worse at certain times of day, or if it is intermittent, constant, or a combination of both, will help you to plan effective interventions.

Palliation/Relief Measures. Ask the patient what pain-relief measures he or she uses and which measures are found to be most effective. Patients with chronic, complex pain often have a number of pharmacological and nonpharmacological measures that help relieve pain. Physical and cognitive modalities such as heat or cold, exercise, gentle stretching, massage, acupuncture, imagery, relaxation, distraction, or music are components of a tool kit of pain-relief measures (Henwood & Ellis, 2004). Patients will often know what works best for them, and they appreciate that you are willing to listen and to try their techniques. You should also identify practitioners whose services the patient has used for pain management (e.g., orthopedist, acupuncturist, chiropractor, massage therapist, or naturopath).

Quality. Another subjective characteristic of pain is its quality; the descriptors that patients use will vary according to their habits, culture, age, and preference. For example, some patients may use "hurt" and "ache" for mild pain but reserve the word "pain" for severe discomfort. The patient may describe the pain as crushing, throbbing, sharp, or dull. Certain pain descriptors are typically associated with certain conditions or injuries. For example, patients will often describe pain associated with a myocardial infarction as crushing or viselike, and the pain of a surgical incision as dull, aching, and throbbing. Neuropathic pain is typically described as burning, shooting, or electric shocks (Williams, 2006). The words that patients use to describe their pain will help to determine the type of pain they are experiencing and, in turn, will dictate the best treatment.

Radiation/Location. To assess location, ask the patient to point to painful areas using his or her own body as a guide or provide a body outline to record pain. When describing and recording pain location, use anatomical landmarks and descriptive terminology. The statement "The pain is localized in the upper right abdominal quadrant" is more specific than "The patient states that the pain is in the abdomen." Pain, classified by location, may be superficial or cutaneous, deep or visceral, referred, radiating, or neuropathic (Table 31-5). Examples of common pain medications are provided in Table 31-5 and explained elsewhere in this chapter. It is critical that you understand the type of pain the patient has, as pharmacological treatments will vary.

Severity/Intensity. Tools used to assess pain intensity fall into two categories, self-report or behavioural observation. Examples of self-report scales include the verbal descriptor scale (VDS), the numerical rating scale (NRS), and the visual analogue scale (VAS) (Figure 31-5). When these scales are used to rate pain, a 10 cm or a 0 to 10 numerical baseline is recommended for consistent interpretation of the scores (von Baeyer & Hicks, 2000).

A VDS consists of a line with three- to five-word descriptors equally spaced along the line. The descriptors are ranked from "no pain" to "unbearable pain." The patient is asked to choose the descriptor that best reflects his or her current pain. An NRS has both numbers and descriptors to guide pain assessment. The scale anchors of 0 and 10 include verbal descriptors such as "no pain" and "most pain." The VAS consists of a straight line, representing a continuum of intensity, and has verbal descriptors at each end. Faces scales are validated self-report scales that can be used by children as young as 3 or 4 years of age and who do not understand numbers (Stanford et al., 2006). In addition, these scales are often well understood and acceptable to cognitively impaired older persons (Taylor & Herr, 2003). The Wong-Baker FACES scale consists of six faces with verbal descriptors depicting increasing amounts of pain. The FACES scale was adapted to provide a culturally sensitive pain assessment tool in Inuktitut for use with Inuit children and adults and is called the Northern Pain Scale (Ellis, Ootoova, Blouin, et al., 2011) (Figure 31-6). The Faces Pain Scale–Revised (FPS-R) is another commonly used self-report scale and is composed of six semi-realistic line drawings of pain faces which can be found at http://www.painsourcebook.ca. (Bieri, Reeve, Champion, et al., 1990; McCaffery et al., 2011). Faces pain rating scales are easy for patients to use, easy for the nurse to score, and acceptable to both adults and children. Many of these tools have been translated into different languages and may be duplicated for use in your clinical practice (see Chapter 3 in Pasero & McCaffery, 2011).

If the patient cannot provide a pain intensity rating, choose a behavioural observation tool. These tools prompt you to observe your patient

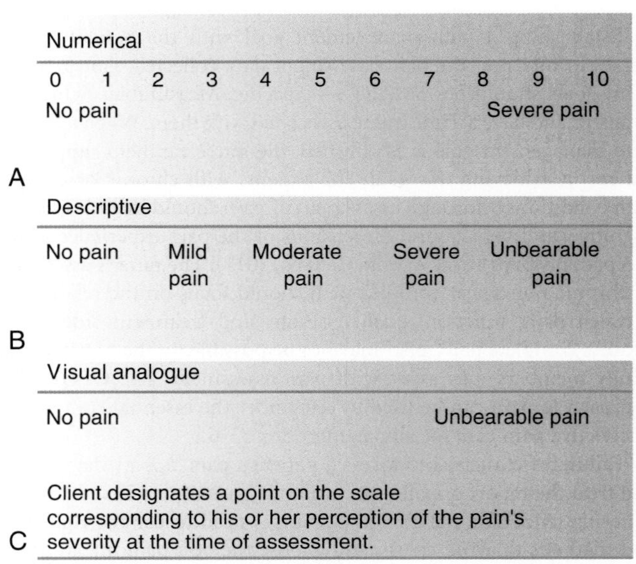

FIGURE 31-5 Sample pain scales. **A,** Numerical rating scale. **B,** Verbal descriptive scale. **C,** Visual analogue scale.

TABLE 31-5 Classification of Pain by Location

Location	Characteristics	Examples of Causes	Examples of Common Medications
Superficial or Cutaneous			
Pain resulting from stimulation of skin	Pain is localized and of short duration. It is usually a sharp sensation.	Needle-stick; small cut or laceration	Topical analgesics and anaesthetics (e.g., Ametop or EMLA for infants >37 weeks gestational age or Pain Ease topical spray for children >3 years of age given prior to painful procedures such as venipunctures or intravenous initiation (CHEO, 2016c) Lidoderm patch for cutaneous neuropathic pain in adults
Deep or Visceral			
Pain resulting from stimulation of internal organs	Pain is diffuse and may radiate in several directions. Duration varies, but it usually lasts longer than superficial pain. Pain may be sharp, dull, or unique to organ involved.	Crushing sensation (e.g., angina pectoris); burning sensation (e.g., gastric ulcer)	Opioids such as morphine, hydromorphone
Referred			
Common phenomenon in visceral pain because many organs themselves have no pain receptors; entrance of sensory neurons from affected organ into same spinal cord segment as neurons from areas where pain is felt; perception of pain is in unaffected areas	Pain is felt in a part of the body separate from the source of pain and may assume any characteristic.	Myocardial infarction (MI), which may cause referred pain to jaw, left arm, and left shoulder; kidney stones, which may refer pain to groin	Opioids for acute MI.
Radiating			
Sensation of pain extending from initial site of injury to another body part	Pain feels as though it travels down or along the body part. It may be intermittent or constant.	Low back pain from ruptured intravertebral disc, accompanied by pain radiating down leg from sciatic nerve irritation	Temporary treatment with one-time epidural injection of a steroid; injections of anaesthetics (e.g., xylocaine or bupivacaine)
Neuropathic*			
Arises from abnormal or damaged pain nerves as a result of prior injury or disease; certain nerves may continue to send pain messages to the brain even though no ongoing tissue damage is present (see Table 31-2)	Pain is usually described as burning, shooting, numbing, or electric-like.	Consequence of disease or prior injury to either the peripheral or central nervous system Complex regional pain syndrome, type I, type II, stroke, spinal cord injury, multiple sclerosis; diabetic neuropathy, alcohol-nutritional neuropathy, and those associated with Guillain-Barré syndrome; nerve root compression, nerve entrapment, trigeminal neuralgia; post-thoracotomy, herniorrhaphy, mastectomy; herpes zoster	Opioids, tricyclic antidepressants (e.g., nortriptyline/amitriptyline), anticonvulsants (e.g., gabapentin/pregabalin), and topical lidocaine

*Based on Charlton, E. J. (Ed.). (2005). *Neuropathic pain. Core curriculum for professional education in pain* (pp. 1–8). Seattle, WA: IASP Press.

and score typical pain behaviours that sum to a pain intensity score. The Neonatal Infant Pain Scale (NIPS) (Lawrence, Alcock, McGrath, et al., 1993) and the Premature Infant Pain Profile (Stevens, Johnston, Petryshen, et al., 1996) specifically focus on the pain behaviours of premature and term babies. With the FLACC Postoperative Pain Tool, five categories of behaviour are scored: facial expression (F), leg movement (L), activity (A), cry (C), and consolability (C) (Manworren & Hynan, 2003; Merkel, Voepel-Lewis, Shayevitz, et al., 1997).

A pain scale should be easy for the patient to use and easy for the nurse to score and record in the patient's chart. The nurse should use the same scale for the same patient consistently. A pain scale should be used before and after an intervention to gauge the effectiveness of the

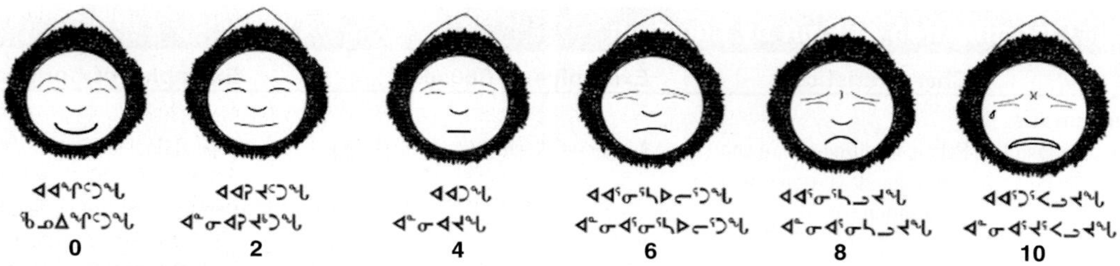

FIGURE 31-6 Northern pain scale. Brief word instructions: Point to each face using words to describe the pain intensity. Ask the child to choose the face that describes his or her own pain and record the appropriate number. (From Ellis, J. A., Ootoova, A., Blouin, R., Rowley, B., Taylor, M., DeCourtney, C., Joyce, M., Greenley, W., & Gaboury, I. [2011]. Establishing the psychometric properties and preferences for the Northern Pain Scale. *International Journal of Circumpolar Health, 70*[3], 274–285. Ellis/Ootoova is an adapted version of the Wong/Baker FACES Pain Rating Scale from Hockenberry, M. J., & Wilson, D. [2006]. *Wong's nursing care of infants and children* [8th ed., p. 1876]. St. Louis, MO: Elsevier Mosby.)

BOX 31-8 CASE STUDY
Pediatric Pain Management

Your patient assignment includes a 6-kg ex-premature infant who is now 47 weeks corrected age. He has undergone a laparotomy for a bowel anastomosis. How would you optimally manage his pain?

The anaesthesiologist and pain service has opted for nurse-controlled analgesia with a basal infusion of morphine 20 mcg/kg/hr with the ability to offer breakthrough doses of 0.04 mg/kg/dose every 20 minutes as needed. Nonsteroidal anti-inflammatory drugs are contraindicated with this patient, as are other adjuncts, including Tylenol rectally, as foundational analgesia.

Check your learning:

1. What validated pain scale would you use to assess pain in this infant?
2. What nonpharmacological strategies could you offer for procedural pain during blood work for this infant?
3. Why is nurse-controlled analgesia (NCA) a good modality for this patient?

Responses:

1. The NIPS or FLACC scale could be used to measure pain.
2. Kangaroo care, breastfeeding, and sucrose are nonpharmacological approaches that can be used to address procedural pain.
3. NCA allows for a basal infusion with stable opioid levels and can be used to provide breakthrough doses and pre-emptive doses before performance of painful procedures such as turning and positioning.

Howard, R. F., Lloyd-Thomas, A., Thomas, M., Williams, D. G., Saul, R., Bruce, E., & Peters, J. (2010). Nurse controlled analgesia (NCA) following major surgery in 10,000 patients in a children's hospital. *Pediatric Anesthesia, 20,* 126–134. doi:10.1111/j.1460-9592.2009.03242.x.

intervention. A rating of 5 or more on a 0-to-10 scale requires immediate attention. However, a pain intensity score is only one component of best practice pain care. Box 31-8 describes one nurse's effective solutions in caring for a young patient who has undergone a laparotomy for a bowel anastomosis.

Contributing Symptoms. Symptoms such as depression, anxiety, fatigue, nausea, anorexia, sleep disruption, spiritual distress, or guilt may increase suffering and aggravate pain. It is important to assess for pain-associated symptoms and evaluate their effects on the patient's pain perception and pain tolerance. Monitoring and treating these symptoms contributes to effective pain management and improved quality of life. A referral to psychology or psychiatry may be warranted for workup of depression and anxiety as well as physiotherapy referral to optimize function and address any deconditioning.

Effects of Pain. Pain is a physiological, psychological, and psychosocial stressor that negatively affects all aspects of a patient's life. Unrelieved acute pain prolongs hospital stays, delays healing, and may lead to chronic pain. Poorly controlled procedural pain from needle-sticks may lead to "needle phobia" that sets the stage for treatment refusal or delay. Chronic and complex pain can severely challenge a patient's ability to function in all domains of his or her life (Henwood, Ellis, Logan, et al., 2010).

Behavioural effects and nonverbal indicators. When a patient has pain, the nurse needs to assess verbalization, vocal response, facial and body movements, and social interaction. For patients who cannot provide a verbal report of pain (e.g., infants, unconscious patients, disoriented, confused, aphasic patients, and patients who speak a foreign language), it is important to assess behaviours that are indicative of pain. Grimacing, moaning, crying, inability to settle and rest, poor appetite, and negative emotions such as anger, fear, and anxiety are cues that the patient may be experiencing pain. Also, the patient may exhibit behaviours when in pain that may not be an intuitive pain behaviour; hence, it is important to consult with the parents or caregivers to ascertain typical pain behaviours for that patient (e.g., a cognitively impaired child may rub his or her ear continuously when in pain) (Box 31-9). For patients who are unable to speak either French or English, an interpreter should be used to translate the child's pain assessment and to enable health care providers to outline the treatment plan.

Some nonverbal expressions characterize sources of pain. A person with chest pain often grabs or holds the chest. A person with severe abdominal pain often assumes a fetal position. The nonverbal expression of pain may support or contradict other information about pain. If a woman reports that her labour pains are occurring

BOX 31-9 Behavioural/Nonverbal Indicators of Pain

Vocalizations
- Moaning
- Crying
- Gasping
- Grunting

Facial Expressions
- Grimacing
- Clenched teeth
- Wrinkled forehead
- Tightly closed or widely opened eyes
- Lip biting

Body Movement
- Restlessness
- Immobilization
- Muscle tension
- Increased hand and finger movements
- Pacing activities
- Rhythmic or rubbing motions
- Protective movement of body parts

Social Interaction
- Avoidance of conversation
- Focused only on activities for pain relief
- Avoidance of social contacts
- Reduced attention span
- Withdrawn
- Despondent—failure to interact purposefully and meaningfully with immediate environment

more frequently and begins to massage her abdomen more frequently, her report is confirmed. If a patient complains of severe abdominal pain but grasps the chest, a more detailed assessment may be necessary, including an assessment for referred pain. For some patients, vocalizations are culturally acceptable ways to communicate and do not necessarily indicate a higher severity of pain or reduced pain tolerance.

Premature and full-term infants in pain often display characteristic facial actions. The Neonatal Facial Coding System (NFCS) (Grunau & Craig, 1987) is a coding tool for assessing pain-related changes in facial actions, such as brow lowering, eyes squeezing shut, chin quivering, mouth stretching vertically or horizontally, and lip pursing. Some infants, especially extremely preterm infants, may not cry or move in response to a painful stimulus (Stevens, McGrath, et al., 2007). This lack of pain response may also occur in older children and adults. Pain may result in the patient attending to the discomfort and fighting it or to giving in to the discomfort and withdrawing socially.

Influence on activities of daily living. Patients who have daily pain may not be able to carry out routine activities. Inactivity leads to physical deconditioning. The primary goal of pain management should be to improve the patient's function. Pain can also affect sleep, and impaired sleep can increase pain. It is important to ask patients if pain interferes with their ability to sleep, if it awakens them, or if it keeps them awake (see Chapter 40). Nonpharmacological or pharmacological pain-management interventions may be needed to aid sleep.

Depending on the location of the pain, the patient may have difficulty performing activities of daily living, including basic hygiene, dressing, and grooming activities. For example, patients with severe arthritis may experience pain when grasping eating utensils or lowering themselves to a toilet seat. The nurse should assess the patient's need for assistance with self-care activities and collaborate with members of the health care team (e.g., occupational therapist) to augment their functioning. The need for family members or friends to assist the patient with basic hygiene should also be considered.

Pain can affect sexual activity. Fear of worsening pain, arousal, confidence, performance, difficulty finding a comfortable position, and relationship problems are frequently reported pain-related problems (Josefsson & Gard, 2010; Kwan & Roberts, 2005). Prolonged use of opioids for chronic pain or cancer pain may affect sexual function and libido, as can the use of some adjuvant analgesics such as antidepressants (Pasero, Polomano, Portenoy, et al., 2011). It is important not to neglect sexual issues when discussing pain. The nurses needs to explore with the patient pain-related sexual issues and determine his or her preference for information and/or individual or group discussion to address these concerns. It is important to convey a willingness to have a discussion regarding pain and sexual health regardless of the patient's sexual orientation.

Pain also affects the ability of a patient to work or, for children and adolescents, to perform school work. The more physical activity required in a job, the greater the risk of discomfort when the pain is associated with musculoskeletal and certain visceral alterations. Pain may increase if the job is stressful. The nurse should inquire about the patient's work and assess whether pain affects his or her ability to function in the job. The daily chores of homemakers should be assessed in the same manner. Nurses should also assess whether it is necessary for patients to stop activity occasionally because of pain, and then help patients select ways of minimizing or controlling the pain so that they are able to remain productive.

It is also important to include an assessment of the effect of pain on social activities. The pain may be so debilitating that the patient becomes too exhausted to socialize. The nurse should identify the patient's normal social activities, the extent to which they have been disrupted, and the patient's desire to participate. Grief over lost goals or unfilled desires may augment pain. For an adolescent with pain, the nurse can explore options such as having a peer over to watch a movie, rather than participating in a group activity such as a volleyball game that may exacerbate the adolescent's pain.

Patient Expectations. Patients who seek health care assistance with pain as a major symptom may have experienced the pain for many hours or days. Hospitalized patients may expect and even accept some pain. Asking patients to describe an acceptable pain level is a first step in encouraging them to take control of their pain. Assessing previous pain experiences and effective home interventions provides a treatment care foundation on which the nurse can build. Patients expect that nurses will believe their reports of pain and be prompt in meeting their comfort needs.

◆ Nursing Diagnosis

Nurses should not diagnose pain simply because they assume that a patient will have discomfort. The nurse will make an accurate diagnosis only after having performed a complete assessment. The development of an accurate nursing diagnosis of pain results from thorough data collection and analysis (Box 31-10). Careful assessment, which should include examination of the patient's history for recent procedures or preexisting painful conditions, will reveal the presence of or potential for pain.

The nursing diagnosis focuses on the nature of the pain so that the nurse can identify the best interventions for relieving pain and minimizing its effect on function. Accurate identification of related factors

BOX 31-10 NURSING DIAGNOSTIC PROCESS

Utilize OPQRSTUV Mnemonic

Assessment Activities	Defining Characteristics	Nursing Diagnosis
Have patient describe pain intensity.	Pain is constant; 5 out of 10	*Potential chronic pain related to chronic physical disability*
Assess onset and location of pain.	Present for 7 months in lower lumbar area	
Observe patient behaviours.	Grimaces and grunts with movement, rubs flanks frequently; reduced movement with sitting and standing	
Assess effect of pain on activities of daily living (ADLs).	Appetite poor; gets little sleep; difficulty bathing and dressing	
Review medical history and history of pain management treatments.	Previous trauma Previous analgesic trials including opioids and nonopioids and note their effectiveness. Determine previous non-pharmacological treatment trials including physiotherapy, acupuncture, massage therapy or chiropractic services and note their effectiveness.	

ensures that appropriate nursing interventions will be chosen. For example, *acute pain related to physical trauma versus acute pain related to natural low-risk childbirth processes* require very different nursing interventions, such as "monitoring of vital signs for possible shock" versus "controlled breathing techniques." Examples of other diagnoses that may be applicable to patients at risk for pain are the following:

- *Anxiety*
- *Ineffective coping*
- *Fatigue*
- *Fear*
- *Hopelessness*
- *Impaired physical mobility*
- *Imbalanced nutrition: less than body requirements*
- *Acute pain*
- *Chronic pain*
- *Powerlessness*
- *Ineffective role performance*
- *Self-care deficit*
- *Chronic low self-esteem*
- *Situational low self-esteem*
- *Risk for situational low self-esteem*
- *Sexual dysfunction*
- *Disturbed sleep pattern*
- *Impaired social interaction*
- *Spiritual distress*

◆ Planning

The care plan integrates key patient information, critical thinking elements (Figure 31-7), and professional standards, which provide the best evidence for selecting nursing interventions (Box 31-11). Professional standards of care regarding pain management are available as agency policies or through professional organizations such as the RNAO or the Canadian Pain Society and its affiliated special interest groups. See the "Recommended Websites" section at the end of this chapter.

A concept map helps with care planning. Patients in pain frequently have interrelated problems. As one problem worsens, others also change. The concept map shows how nursing diagnoses link to one another and to medical diagnoses. For example, when planning care for the patient with arthritis, the nurse notes the relationships between *acute pain, impaired physical mobility, self-care,* and *fatigue* (Figure 31-8). Understanding these relationships helps the nurse to develop a holistic and patient-centred care plan.

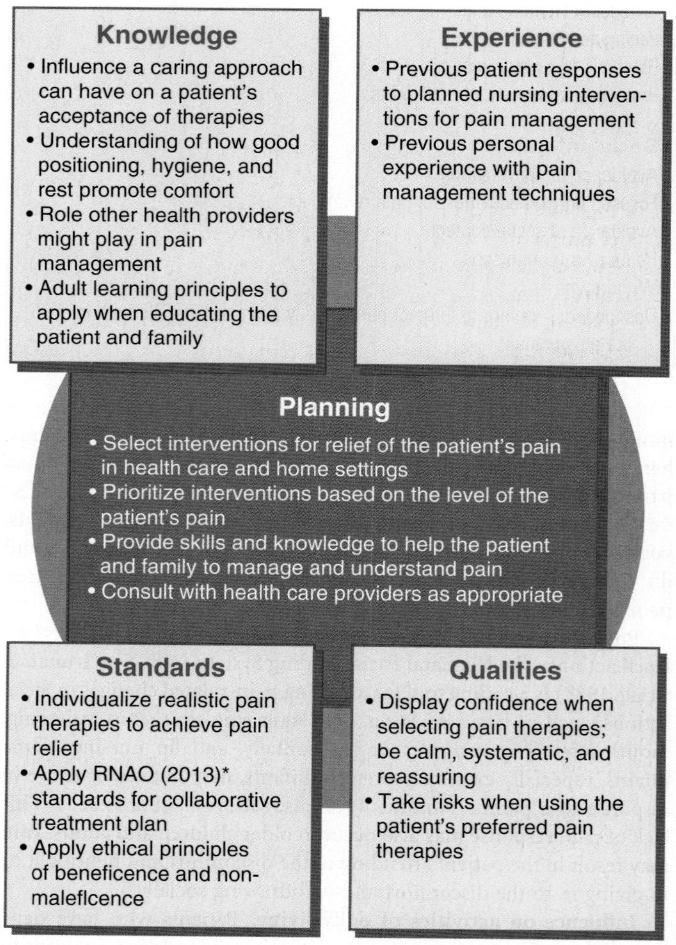

FIGURE 31-7 Critical thinking model for comfort planning. *Registered Nurses' Association of Ontario (RNAO) (2013). *Assessment and management of pain* (3rd ed.). Toronto, ON: Author. Retrieved from http://rnao.ca/sites/rnao-ca/files/AssessAndManagementOfPain_15_WEB-_FINAL_DEC_2.pdf

Goals and Outcomes. Pain management goals permit the patient to function to the best possible extent. The nurse should determine with the patient what the pain has prevented the patient from doing and decide on a realistic and acceptable level of pain that will allow a return of function. Success is determined through attainment of goals and positive outcomes. For example, if the goal is "the patient will achieve a satisfactory level of pain relief within 24 hours," the following are possible outcomes:

- Reporting that pain is a 3 or less on a scale of 0 to 10, or does not interfere with ADLs
- Identifying factors that intensify pain, and modifying behaviour accordingly
- Using pain-relief measures safely, both pharmacotherapies and nonpharmacological supports

Setting Priorities. When setting priorities in pain management, the nurse needs to consider the type of pain the patient is experiencing and the effects pain has on various body functions. The nurse should discuss with the patient the selected interventions appropriate for the nature and effects of the pain. For example, if a patient has had acute pain but an analgesic has brought relief, attention is focused on how the pain is influencing activity, appetite, and sleep. In contrast, when a patient's pain continues to be severe, immediate pain relief is the obvious priority. Nursing priorities will change as the patient's pain experience changes. Plans should take into account expected occurrences of pain.

Collaborative Pain Care. A comprehensive plan includes a variety of resources and all members of the interprofessional team to work together for pain control. This includes staff nurses, advanced practice nurses and nurse practitioners, pharmacists, physiotherapists, occupational therapists, psychologists, social workers, and pastoral and spiritual care. For children, child life specialists can also assist with pain management. For chronic cancer pain, an oncology advanced practice nurse knows the pharmacological and nonpharmacological interventions that work best. Pharmacists are knowledgeable about the effects, interactions, and adverse effects of multiple drug regimes often required to treat pain. Physiotherapists can plan exercises that strengthen muscle groups and lessen pain in affected areas. Occupational therapists can devise splints to support painful body parts. Child life specialists can plan social and play activities that reflect the developmental needs of the child. Psychologists can assist with augmenting coping behaviours for chronic pain or for patients with chronic pain and an acute exacerbation. The family should also be involved in the care plan because they may need to administer care in the home after discharge. The home care instructions should be both verbal and written. If the pain management plan is not successful, the nurse should discuss the need for a change in treatment plan with the most responsible physician, consult a pain service, or both. Nurse practitioners working on pain management teams can be instrumental in providing holistic care by adjusting modalities or managing unbearable side effects during the trajectory of the patient's hospitalization (Kaasalainen, DiCenso, Donald, et al., 2007).

◆ Implementation

The nature of the pain and how much it affects well-being determines the choice of interventions. Pain therapy requires an individualized approach, perhaps more so than any other patient problem. The nurse, the patient, and the family must be partners in using pain-control measures. Nurses administer and monitor pain treatments ordered by a physician, but should consider using other complementary comfort measures. Patient remedies are often successful, especially when the patient has already had experience with pain. Generally, the least invasive and safest therapy should be tried first.

Health Promotion. The Ottawa Charter for Health Promotion (https://www.who.int/healthpromotion/conferences/previous/ottawa/en/) defines health promotion as the process of enabling individuals to gain control over and to improve their health and well-being (World Health Organization [WHO], 2008). Chronic pain and suffering diminish quality of life; thus, relieving pain and promoting self-control become important. Once pain is controlled to an acceptable level, patients and their families need to be provided with education and information about pain so that they can participate in the pain care decision-making process. This will help reduce anxiety and increases a patient's sense of control. For example, patients who are in the hospital for the first time may know that they require tests but do not understand them. As a result, they may become anxious and fearful. Fear increases the perception of painful stimuli. Health promotion

BOX 31-11 NURSING CARE PLAN

Acute Pain

ASSESSMENT

Ms. Mays was diagnosed with a cancerous tumour in her left lung 8 months ago. After treatment, she was taking oral analgesics on an as-needed (prn) basis. She can no longer tolerate taking medications orally and is now hospitalized with uncontrollable chest pain and possible pneumonia. Her husband is with her. A patient-controlled analgesia (PCA) of morphine 0.5 mg on-demand dose with a 10-minute lockout is begun.

Assessment Activities	*Findings and Defining Characteristics*
Onset: Ask her when the pain began. Review her past medical and nursing history.	Her pain started 6 months ago but has gotten worse over the last 2 weeks. Her past history of illness describes her cancer diagnosis and the treatments she has received over the past 8 months.
Palliative/Provoking factors: Ask Ms. Mays what she did at home to control her pain. Ask her what makes the pain worse.	Her pain escalated from a 3 to a 10, so she doubled her medication and went to bed. This did not help. Lying flat and coughing make the pain worse.
Quality: Ask Ms. Mays what the pain feels like.	She describes her pain as constant and dull. It becomes sharp when she coughs.
Radiating: Ask Ms. Mays where the pain is located and if it travels anywhere.	She states the pain is in her left-side thoracic area. She states it radiates to her upper back when she coughs.
Severity: Ask Ms. Mays what her pain intensity is now, both at rest and with movement. Observe Ms. Mays's nonverbal behaviours.	On a scale of 0 to 10, currently she reports a 9 at rest, and >10/10 with movement. She is restless and unfocused during the history-taking.

Continued

BOX 31-11 NURSING CARE PLAN

Acute Pain—cont'd

Assessment Activities	Findings and Defining Characteristics
Timing: Ask Ms. Mays if there is a time of day when the pain is worse, or if the pain increases when she is doing a particular task.	She states the pain is worse at night when she is lying down.
Understanding: Ask Ms. Mays what she believes is causing the pain.	She believes she has a recurrent tumour in her left lung that is causing the pain.
Value: Ask Ms. Mays what her pain has prevented her from doing. Ask her if she has any personal beliefs that may affect how pain is managed.	She responds that she is unable to complete her own hygiene activities or sleep well. She explains that she has been taught to not complain about pain and to be stoic.
Ask Ms. Mays about her pain intensity goal (out of 10).	She says that a pain intensity of 5 out of 10 would help her function better now. A goal of 3 would be preferred.

NURSING DIAGNOSIS: Acute pain related to a biological injuring agent (tumour).

PLANNING

Goals (Nursing Outcomes Classification)*	Expected Outcomes
Pain Control	
Patient will obtain an acceptable level of comfort as soon as possible.	Patient will report pain at stated goal or below prior to discharge.
Husband will assist in restoring Ms. Mays to a more comfortable state.	Husband will provide selected comfort measures to Ms. Mays before bedtime.
Pain: Disruptive Effects	
Patient will actively participate in ADLs.	Ms. Mays will report sleeping for 5 to 6 hours without interruption from pain. Perhaps a sleep aid can be initiated while in the hospital if disrupted sleep persists. She will complete her own hygiene with minimal assistance. She will walk the hallway with her husband every 4 hours for 15 minutes.
Medication Response	
Ms. Mays will be assessed for adverse effects of opioids. If she experiences opioid adverse effects they will be managed.	Ms. Mays will be assessed for nausea, pruritus, constipation, and sedation. Her bowel pattern will be maintained and she will have a normal bowel movement every other day or similar to her baseline routine. Consideration will be given for starting a bowel agent before discharge for the period of time she is taking opioids. Any adverse effects will be managed with the appropriate treatment options.

*Outcome classification labels from Moorhead, S., Johnson, M., Maas, M. L., & Swanson, E. (Eds.). (2012). *Nursing outcomes classification (NOC)* (5th ed.). St. Louis, MO: Mosby/Elsevier.

INTERVENTIONS

Interventions (Nursing Interventions Classification)†	Rationale
Pain Management	
Begin PCA at prescribed dose. Explain to patient and spouse how to use the PCA. Emphasize the importance of only the patient pushing the button, not the husband; she knows best when she is having pain and she can pre-emptively activate the button prior to mobilization.	Patient is experiencing an acute episode of her cancer pain. Discouraging the husband from pushing the button will minimize potential oversedating effects of the opioid because the patient must be awake to perceive the pain and push the button (Wuhrman, Cooney, Dunwoody, et al., 2007).
Monitor intravenous (IV) PCA opioid use. Explain to patient and spouse the action of the medication, potential adverse effects, and the importance of reporting if the pain is not relieved.	Pain is easier to prevent than to treat. Provide patient and spouse with written instructions regarding the use of the PCA pump. Instruct the husband to inform staff of unrelieved pain or unmanageable adverse effects (Pasero, Quinn, et al., 2011).
Administer nonopioid analgesics as prescribed.	Nonopioid analgesics can effectively assist in the management of pain and also result in a decrease in opioid dose required to manage pain.
Have patient select nonpharmacological interventions that have relieved pain in the past (e.g., distraction, music, simple relaxation therapy, or massage).	Personal control allows a patient to shape immediate circumstances through his or her own actions. Nonpharmacological interventions augment pharmacological strategies but should not be used in place of analgesics (Pasero & McCaffery, 2011).

†Intervention classification labels from Bulechek, G. M., Butcher, H. K., Dochterman, J. M., & Wagner, C (Eds.). (2013). *Nursing interventions classification (NIC)* (6th ed.). St Louis, MO: Mosby/Elsevier.

EVALUATION

Nursing Actions	Patient Response and Finding	Achievement of Outcome
Ask Ms. Mays if she attained her pain-relief goal most of the time.	She responds, "My pain usually runs around a 3, which is my goal, except when I start walking."	Ms. Mays reports an acceptable level of comfort, which is a change from the level that indicated unacceptable pain. Instruct her to push her button pre-emptively about 5 minutes before ambulating.

BOX 31-11 NURSING CARE PLAN

Acute Pain—cont'd

Nursing Actions	Patient Response and Finding	Achievement of Outcome
Observe Ms. Mays's ability to perform ADLs, walk, and sleep.	She is dressed for breakfast and is walking the hallway every 4 hours with her husband. The night nurse's notes indicate Ms. Mays slept through the night.	Ability to perform ADLs and sleep has improved. Continue to monitor.
Ask Mr. Mays if he was able to give his wife a back massage.	He reported that she did not want a back rub but preferred to have her feet rubbed, which he was happy to do. "She said it made her feel more relaxed."	Nonpharmacological intervention was successful, but the nursing care plan was updated.
Ask Ms. Mays the time and consistency of her last bowel movement.	She has not had a bowel movement in 3 days.	Assess her abdomen for bowel sounds and distension. Inquire about passing flatus. As constipation is the most common opioid adverse effect, consult with her physician about starting a stool softener and mild peristaltic stimulant. It is recommended to start these agents as soon as possible (Pasero, Quinn, et al., 2011).

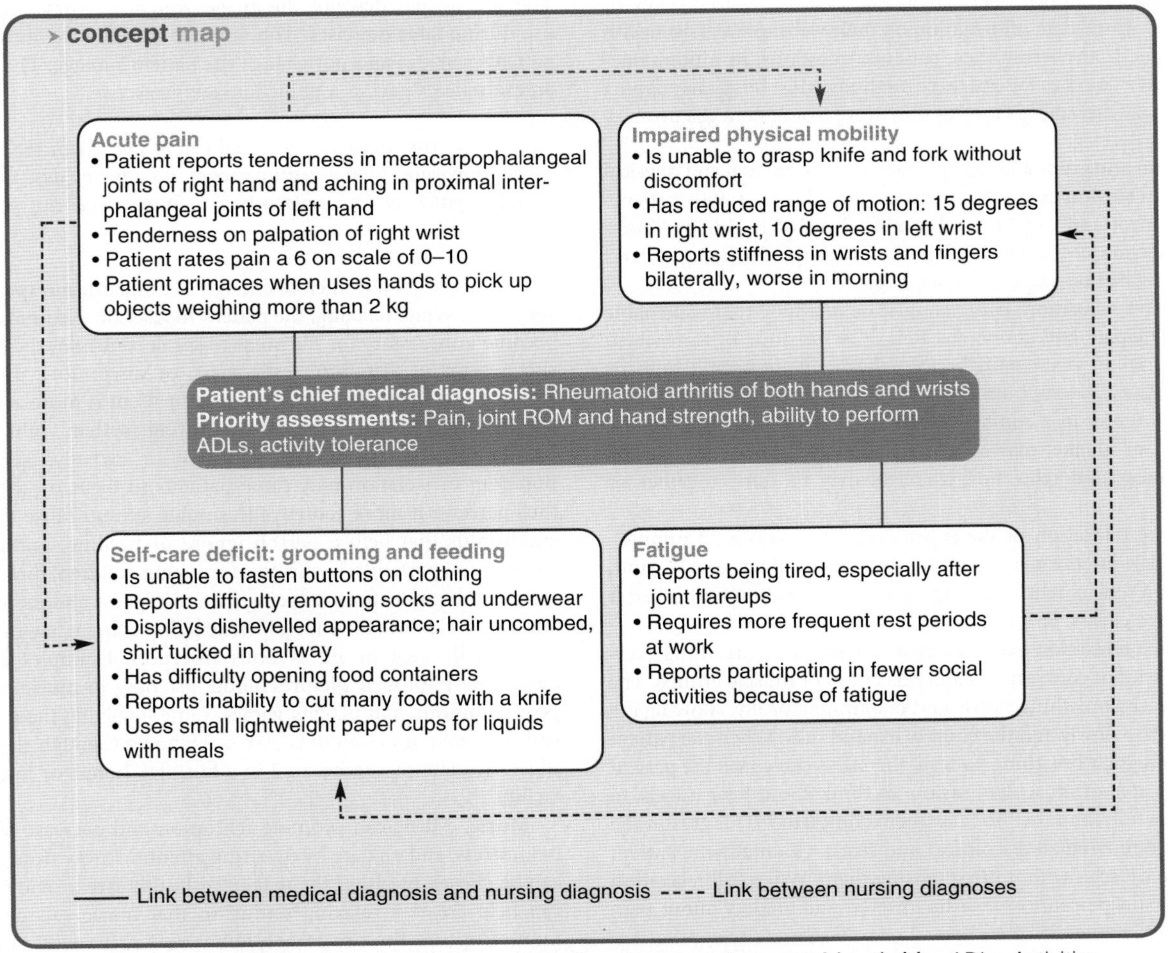

FIGURE 31-8 Concept map for patient with pain related to rheumatoid arthritis. *ADLs,* Activities of daily living; *ROM,* range of motion.

goes beyond teaching, however. Nurses can use the Ottawa Charter for Health Promotion document (Canadian Public Health Association, Health and Welfare Canada, & WHO, 1986)—a seminal and still useful document for today's public health practice (Hancock, 2007)—as a framework to develop their skills in creating a supportive environment, using the strategies of enabling, mediating, and advocating for better pain-management services.

Nonpharmacological Pain-Relief Interventions. Several nonpharmacological interventions do not need a physician's order but are initiated by nurses. These approaches are used in addition to, not in place of, pharmacological measures (Gruener & Lande, 2006). Nonpharmacological interventions include cognitive-behavioural and physical approaches.

The goals of cognitive-behavioural interventions, such as relaxation and guided imagery, are to change pain perceptions, alter pain behaviour, and provide a greater sense of control. Physical agents aim to provide comfort, correct physical dysfunction, alter physiological responses, and reduce fears associated with pain-related immobility. Complementary and alternative medicine (CAM) therapies, such as herbal supplements, energy therapies, and manipulation or body-based therapies, are also available. The National Center for Complementary and Integrative Health (NCCIH) and the Canadian Health Network, a health promotion service operated by the Public Health Agency of Canada, offer up-to-date information on their websites to assist health care providers in answering their patients' questions, in a nonjudgemental manner, about the use of these methods. Most hospitals support complementary therapies as long as they serve to augment the primary therapy.

Relaxation and guided imagery. Relaxation is mental and physical freedom from tension or stress. Relaxation techniques provide patients with self-control and can be used at any phase of health or illness. Relaxation techniques include meditation, yoga, guided imagery, and progressive relaxation exercises (see Chapter 35).

For effective relaxation, patients must be in a state that will enable them to participate and cooperate. Relaxation is difficult to teach to patients who are in severe pain, because they may not be able to focus and concentrate. The environment should be quiet and free of stimuli. The patient may sit in a comfortable chair or lie in bed (Box 31-12). A light sheet or blanket may help the patient feel more comfortable. Guided imagery and relaxation exercises may be done together or separately.

Progressive relaxation of the entire body takes about 15 minutes. The patient pays attention to the body, noting areas of tension. Warmth and relaxation replace tension in these areas. Some patients relax better with their eyes closed. Soft background music can help.

Progressive relaxation exercises involve controlled breathing exercises and a series of contractions and relaxation of muscle groups. The patient begins by breathing slowly and diaphragmatically, allowing the abdomen to rise slowly and the chest to expand fully. When the patient establishes a regular breathing pattern, the nurse can coach the patient to locate any area of muscular tension, to think about how it feels, to tense muscles fully, and then to relax them completely. This creates the sensation of removing all discomfort and stress. Gradually the patient can relax the muscles without first tensing them. When full relaxation is achieved, pain perception may be lowered and anxiety about pain may decrease. Chapter 35 offers several relaxation exercise approaches.

If a patient becomes agitated or uncomfortable, it is best to stop the exercise. If the patient has difficulty relaxing any part of the body, it is best to slow the progression of the exercise and concentrate on the tensed body part. The patient must know that the exercise can be stopped at any time. With practice, the patient can soon perform relaxation exercises independently.

BOX 31-12 Body Positions for Relaxation

Sitting

Sit with entire back resting against back of chair.
Place feet flat on the floor.
Keep legs separated.
Hang arms at the side or rest on chair arms.
Keep head aligned with spine.

Lying

Keep legs separated with toes pointed slightly outward.
Rest arms at sides without touching sides of body.
Keep head aligned with spine.
Use thin, small pillow under head.

In guided imagery, the patient creates an image in his or her mind, concentrates on that image, and gradually becomes less aware of pain. The nurse coaches the patient in forming the image and concentrating on the sensory experience. Initially, the patient is asked to think of a pleasant scene or experience that promotes the use of all of the senses. The patient may describe the image, which the nurse may record for use during later exercises. The nurse should use the information the patient provides and not change the patient's image. The following is an example of part of a guided imagery exercise:

> *Imagine you are lying on a cool bed of grass with the sounds of rushing water from a nearby stream. It's a balmy day. You turn to see a patch of blue wildflowers in bloom and can smell their fragrance.*

The nurse should sit close enough to be heard, and speak in a calm, soft voice. While relaxing, the patient focuses on the image, and it will become unnecessary for the nurse to speak continuously. If the patient shows signs of agitation, restlessness, or discomfort, the exercise is stopped and then tried again when the patient is more at ease.

Distraction. The reticular activating system inhibits painful stimuli if a person receives sufficient or excessive sensory input. Boredom or isolation may cause patients to focus on their pain and thus perceive it more acutely. Pleasurable stimuli cause the release of endorphins that help a person ignore or become unaware of pain. Distraction, particularly effective for young children, directs attention to something else, thus reducing pain awareness and increasing tolerance. It works best for short, intense pain lasting a few minutes, such as a needle-stick or intravenous insertion. Examples are praying, describing photos or pictures aloud, listening to music, using therapeutic humour, and playing games, some involving the use of virtual reality technology (Dahlquist, Weiss, Dillinger Clendaniel, et al., 2009). Most distractions can be used in a hospital, home, or long-term care facility.

Music. Music can promote relaxation and decrease physiological pain, stress, and anxiety by diverting attention away from pain. Music can be chosen by either the patient or health care provider. The nurse can help create a relaxing setting so that music can be listened to uninterrupted. The use of earphones may assist with concentration and block out ambient noise. Although some benefits can be achieved with music therapy, the evidence is weak to moderate regarding the effects of music therapy on reducing acute pain (Wells, McCaffery, & Pasero, 2008).

Biofeedback. Biofeedback is a behavioural therapy that involves giving individuals information about physiological responses (e.g., blood pressure or tension) and ways to exercise voluntary control over those responses (Rakel & Faass, 2006). It is used to produce deep relaxation and may be effective for managing regional pain syndrome (Bruehl & Chung, 2006) and migraine headaches (Damen, Bruijn, Koes, et al., 2006). In the treatment of headaches, electrodes are attached externally over each temple. The electrodes measure skin tension in microvolts. A polygraph machine visibly records the tension level for the patient to see. The patient learns to achieve optimal relaxation by lowering the actual level of tension experienced, using feedback from the polygraph. The therapy takes several weeks to learn. Chapter 35 describes the benefits and limitations of biofeedback. A referral to a psychologist will be warranted to initiate biofeedback within the hospital.

Acupuncture. Acupuncture, traditionally embedded in naturalistic theories and in Chinese medicine dating back 2 500 years, may help reduce chronic and acute pain (Chou & Huffman, 2007) and, if properly performed, is a safe procedure. Acupuncture involves the insertion of acupuncture needles into specific "acupuncture points" (acupoints) on the patient's body followed by the twisting of the needle up and down by hand. Evidence from numerous systematic reviews indicates that acupuncture is potentially effective for emesis developing after surgery or chemotherapy in adults, for nausea associated with pregnancy, and for relieving dental pain. During the last decades, our understanding of how acupuncture analgesia works has undergone considerable development. Acupuncture activates endogenous opioid mechanisms and may stimulate gene expression of neuropeptides (Zhao, 2008). The training and provision of acupuncture care in Canada is rapidly expanding. Chapter 35 describes the benefits and limitations of acupuncture.

Cutaneous stimulation. Cutaneous stimulation, also referred to as touch healing (TH) therapies, is the stimulation of the skin to relieve pain. A massage, warm bath, ice bag, and transcutaneous electrical nerve stimulation (TENS) are simple ways to reduce pain perception. How cutaneous stimulation works is unclear. It has been suggested that TH therapies involve mechanisms of neural plasticity in somatosensory maps, thus resulting in sensory reorganization (Kerr, Wasserman, & Moore, 2007).

An advantage to cutaneous stimulation is that the measures can be used in the home, giving patients and families some control over pain symptoms and treatment. The proper use of cutaneous stimulation can reduce pain perception and help reduce muscle tension that might otherwise increase pain. The practitioner first helps the patient get into a comfortable position and explains the purpose of the therapy. Cutaneous stimulation should not be used directly on sensitive skin areas (e.g., burns, bruises, skin rashes, inflammation, underlying bone fractures).

Massage is a safe and effective way to reduce anxiety and minimize tension (Figure 31-9). Massage involves the manipulation of the soft tissues by either mechanical or physical means. Recent literature suggests that hand and foot massage can be an option for reducing pain, along with back or body massage. The recommended duration of massage is 5 to 20 minutes (Wells et al., 2008). Massages communicate caring and are easy for family members or health care providers to learn and adopt (Box 31-13).

Tactile stimulation such as rubbing or stroking using moderate intensity can be used just prior to and during the vaccination of children over 4 years of age. This works within the framework of the gate control theory whereby touch competes with pain in routing the message to the brain, thereby reducing pain (Taddio, Appelton, Bortolussi, et al., 2010).

Therapeutic touch (TT) and Reiki are classified as biofield, training-specific therapies, the medical use of subtle energy fields in and around the body for positive health effects. TT and Reiki involve the practitioner's use of hands to help strengthen the body's ability to heal. TT was developed in the 1970s by a nurse, Dr. Dolores Krieger (1979), and Reiki is an ancient practice believed to have originated thousands of years ago (Vitale, 2007). In recent years, nursing has been instrumental in exploring the benefits of energy work. Although there is still a lack of empirically based investigations to support these practices, nurses and others have reported clinical observations that the use of TT and Reiki has relaxation effects and stress management benefits, lessens pain, and promotes inner healing (Aghabati, Mohammadi, & Esmaiel, 2010; Lee, Pittler, & Ernst, 2008; Vitale, 2007). Energy work has been endorsed as a valid modality for nursing intervention by a number of nursing groups across Canada, such as the Canadian Holistic Nurses Association and the Registered Nurses' Association of Ontario's Complementary Therapies Nurses' Interest Group. Please see Chapter 35 for additional information.

Cold and heat applications have been shown to relieve pain and promote healing. The choice of heat or cold varies with patients' condition and preference. Use of either method may require a physician's order (Wells et al., 2008). Moist heat can help relieve pain from a tension headache, and cold applications can reduce acute pain from inflamed joints. To avoid injury, it is important to check the temperature and avoid direct application of cold or heat to the skin. Patients at most risk for injury include those with spinal cord or other neurological injury, older people, and confused patients.

Application of cold packs may be effective for pain relief in certain conditions. Cold is particularly effective for dental pain and has been used to relieve pain associated with coughing and breathing in post-cardiac surgery (Chaillier Ellis, Stolarick, et al., 2010). Cold applications are also useful before needle-stick procedures. Cold may be placed either near or distal to the pain site. The cold should be applied for 20 minutes to achieve maximum effect. Placement of a cold pack near the actual site of pain tends to provide the most relief.

Heat application is another option for relieving pain. Heating pads or hot water bottles may be used, as can commercial pillows that are warmed in the microwave and contour to the body. These methods are ideal at home; disposable heat and warmth solutions are used in the hospital to help prevent spread of infection.

Although heat and cold applications are methods to consider when promoting comfort, few studies have been published addressing their impact on pain or functional qualities (Wells et al., 2008). Refer to

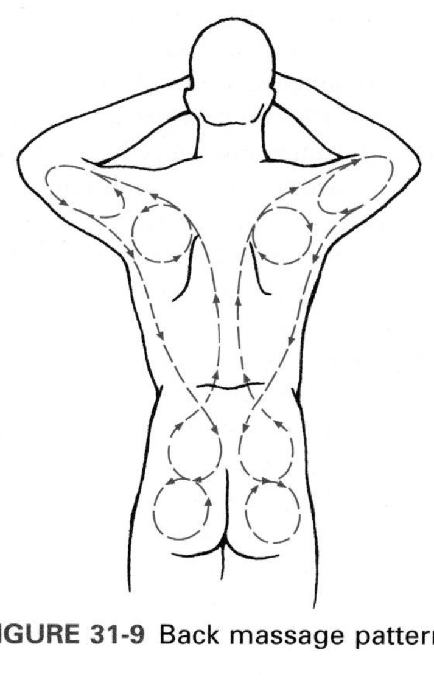

FIGURE 31-9 Back massage pattern.

BOX 31-13 PROCEDURAL GUIDELINE

Massage

Delegation Considerations

The nurse is responsible for assessing contraindications and patient response to massage. Administering a massage may be delegated to an unregulated care provider (UCP), provided that the patient is stable. Before delegation, you must do the following:

- Instruct the UCP about which body parts to massage.
- Instruct the UCP about the importance of not massaging reddened skin areas.
- Clarify the early signs of impaired skin integrity for select patients, and instruct the UCP to report changes in the patient's skin.

Equipment

- Moisturizing lotion
- Bath towel or blanket

Procedure

1. Assist patient to assume a comfortable position.
2. Dim room lights, turn on soft music, or both, according to patient preference.
3. Perform hand hygiene. Warm lotion in hands or place container in warm water.
4. Adjust or remove patient's bed clothing.
5. Place small amount of lotion in your hands.
6. Massage each body part for at least 10 minutes.
   A. *Back:* Begin a sacral area massage with a circular motion (see Figure 31-9), moving upward from buttocks to shoulders. Use a firm, smooth stroke over the scapula. Continue in one smooth stroke to upper arms and laterally along sides of back, down to iliac crests. Use long, gliding strokes along muscles of spine. Knead any muscles that feel tense or tight. Knead skin by gently grasping tissue between thumb and fingers. Knead upward along one side of the spine from buttocks to shoulders, around nape of neck. Knead or stroke downward toward sacrum. Repeat along other side of back.
   B. *Neck:* Support neck at the hairline with one hand and massage upward with a gliding stroke. Knead muscles on one side. Switch hands to support neck, and knead other side. Stretch the neck slightly, with one hand at the top and the other at the bottom.
   C. *Arms:* Use a gliding stroke to massage upward from patient's wrist or forearm. With thumb and forefinger of both hands, knead muscles from forearm to shoulder. Continue kneading bicep, deltoid, and triceps muscles. Finish with gliding strokes from wrists to shoulder.
   D. *Hands:* Slowly open patient's palm, and glide fingers over the palmar surface. Use thumbs to apply friction to palm and move thumbs in a circular motion. Stretch the palm outward. Massage each finger, using a cork-screw-like motion from the base of the finger to the tip. Gently knead each muscle in patient's fingers. Glide hands smoothly from fingertips to wrists. Repeat for other hand.
   E. *Feet:* Gently massage top and bottom of each foot. Using gliding motion, massage from heel to toe. Gently massage the dorsal surface of the foot and each toe. Repeat for other foot.
7. Wipe excess lotion off patient's back, neck, or extremity. If necessary, assist patient to dress and resume a comfortable position.
8. Ask patient about level of comfort. Note any areas of muscle pain or tension.

Perry and Potter's (2017) textbook *Nursing Skills and Techniques* (9th ed.) for further guidance on the application of warm and cold therapy and the necessary safety precautions for use.

Another form of cutaneous stimulation, sometimes called *counter-stimulation*, is **transcutaneous electrical nerve stimulation (TENS)**. TENS involves stimulation of the skin with a mild electrical current passed through external electrodes (Melzack & Wall, 2003). This therapy requires a physician's order. The TENS unit consists of a battery-powered transmitter, lead wires, and electrodes. The electrodes are placed directly over or near the pain site. Hair or skin preparations should be removed before attaching the electrodes. When a patient feels pain, the transmitter is turned on and a buzzing or tingling sensation is created. The patient may adjust the intensity and quality of skin stimulation. The tingling sensation can be applied until pain relief occurs. TENS may be effective for postsurgical pain control and reduction of pain caused by postoperative procedures. Physiotherapy should be consulted for TENS assessment and application.

Herbal supplements. Herbal supplements have not been sufficiently studied to be recommended for pain relief; however, many patients self-medicate using supplements such as echinacea, ginseng, ginkgo biloba, and garlic supplements (Wirth, Hudgins, & Paice, 2005). Some herbal products may interact with prescribed analgesics; in particular, ginkgo biloba may decrease the ability of blood to clot after surgery. The patient should be asked to report all substances taken to relieve pain and this should be part of the medication reconciliation while the patient is in the hospital (Yoon & Schaffer, 2006) (see Chapter 35).

Reducing pain perception. One simple way to promote comfort is to remove or prevent painful stimuli (Box 31-14). As a nurse you can take steps to reduce patients' pain by paying attention to the way you perform procedures. This is especially important for patients who are immobilized or have difficulty in expressing themselves. Consider a patient's condition and the aspects of the procedure that are uncomfortable. Use techniques to avoid pain-producing situations. For example, in a patient with severe arthritic knee pain, know that extreme flexion of the knee can cause pain. Before walking the patient to the bathroom, make sure that an elevated toilet seat is available. The patient can then be seated and can rise with minimal discomfort.

BOX 31-14 Controlling Painful Stimuli in the Patient's Environment

Tighten and smooth wrinkled bed linen.
Loosen constricting bandages (unless specifically applied as a pressure dressing).
Change wet dressings and linens.
Position patient in correct anatomical alignment.
Check temperature of hot or cold applications, including bath water.
Lift patient in bed—do not pull.
Position patient correctly on bedpan.
Avoid exposing skin or mucous membranes to irritants (e.g., urine, stool, wound drainage).
Prevent urinary retention by keeping Foley catheters patent and free flowing.
Prevent constipation with stool softeners, fluids, diet, and exercise.
Reduce lighting and ambient sound.

Acute Pain Management. Some patients have acute pain from invasive procedures (e.g., surgery or endoscopy), trauma, or cancer. The key to successful pain relief is ongoing evaluation of interventions. In caring for the patient the nurse needs to ask the following questions:

Is relief obtained? Do the medications cause any unacceptable adverse effects? It is the responsibility of the health care team to collaborate in order to find the combination of therapy that works best for the patient.

Pharmacological Pain-Relief Interventions. The ideal analgesic has yet to be developed, but many opioid and nonopioid pain-relieving medications are available. Most require a physician's order.

> **Safety Alert** As a nurse, your critical thinking and judgement in the selection and administration of analgesics helps to ensure safe and effective pain relief.
> - Be cognizant of the pain diagnosis, the patient's physical characteristics (e.g., age), and severity of the illness; know that some analgesics will be contraindicated.
> - Employ the 10 rights (person, drug, dose, route, time, documentation, reason, evaluation, patient education, and right to refuse) of medication administration.
> - When dispensing opioids, be sure to check the dose and drug type, as the names of some common medications sound alike. Some institutions employ an independent double-check policy for high-alert medications, including opioids.
> - Administer all analgesics using standardized guidelines.
> - Evaluate analgesic effectiveness, and report and document any adverse effects.

Analgesics. Analgesics are a common and effective method of pain relief. Although analgesics can effectively relieve pain, nurses and physicians still tend to undertreat patients' pain.

Three types of analgesics exist: (1) nonsteroidal anti-inflammatory drugs (NSAIDs) and nonopioids, (2) **opioids**, and (3) co-analgesics, a variety of medications that enhance analgesics or have analgesic properties.

Acetaminophen (Tylenol) has no anti-inflammatory effects and works peripherally and centrally, but its action is unknown. Its major adverse effect is hepatotoxicity. It is in a variety of over-the-counter (OTC) cold, flu, and allergy remedies. The maximum 24-hour dose for an adult is 4 g (the same dose limitation as Aspirin) and is weight-dependent for infants and children. Acetaminophen does not affect platelet function and has minimal impact on the gastrointestinal tract (Arnstein, 2010). For postoperative or severe pain, it is often combined with opioids (e.g., Hydromorphone, morphine, Percocet, Vicodin, Lortab, and Ultracet) because it reduces the dose of opioid needed to achieve successful pain control. An overdose of acetaminophen can be fatal and is treated with acetylcysteine (Mucomyst).

Nonselective NSAIDs, such as Aspirin and ibuprofen, provide relief for mild to moderate acute pain resulting from trauma or an inflammatory process (Arnstein, 2010). NSAIDs are believed to act by inhibiting the synthesis of prostaglandins (Pasero, Portenoy, & McCaffery, 2011) and thus the cellular responses to inflammation. Most NSAIDs act on peripheral nerve receptors to reduce transmission of pain stimuli. Unlike opioids, NSAIDs do not depress the central nervous system, nor do they interfere with bowel or bladder function (Pasero, Portenoy, & McCaffery, 2011).

Salicylates or Aspirin are typically avoided in pediatrics, especially during the antecedent illness, as they can contribute to the development of Reye's syndrome, caused by failure of the mitochondria, which can cause agitation, delirium, and confusion (McGovern, Glasgow, & Stewart, 2001).

Chronic NSAID use in older patients is associated with more frequent adverse effects (e.g., gastrointestinal bleeding and renal insufficiency) and should be avoided (Arnstein, 2010). Taking NSAIDs with food reduces the likelihood of gastrointestinal upset (Arnstein, 2010).

Nonselective NSAIDs have been found to be safe when taken for short periods of time. Celecoxib is the only selective cyclooxygenase-2 (COX-2) inhibitor currently available in Canada; however, it should not be used in patients with a sulfa allergy. Some patients with asthma or an allergy to Aspirin are also allergic to NSAIDs (CPS, 2005). Some NSAIDs are available OTC; patients should be advised to discuss using OTC NSAIDs for managing pain with their primary health provider (D'Arcy, 2006).

Codeine is a weak opioid used for moderate to severe pain. Although codeine has been widely prescribed for pain relief, recent advances in our understanding of the pharmacogenetics of codeine have forced a more rigorous investigation of its properties and adverse effects, particularly in the pediatric age group. Codeine is a prodrug. A *prodrug* is a drug that must undergo chemical and enzymatic conversion to morphine to have an analgesic effect. Codeine's pharmacokinetics are variable and, in some patients, unpredictable.

Genetic variations exist that affect how the isoenzyme CYP2D6 converts codeine to morphine. Some patients may be ultrafast metabolizers, rapidly converting codeine to morphine. This places them at risk for oversedation and respiratory depression that could result in death. One case report details the death of a breastfed infant who died after receiving breast milk from a mother who had been prescribed codeine postpartum (Madadi, Koren, Cairns, et al., 2006). Two other young children died when they received codeine following a routine tonsillectomy procedure (MacDonald & MacLeod, 2010). Guidelines for infants, young children, and breastfeeding mothers should be modified until further research can be undertaken to better understand codeine and alternative pharmacological drugs used (MacDonald & MacLeod, 2010). As a result of several pediatric deaths secondary to codeine ingestion, most pediatric hospitals have removed it from their formulary. Health Canada has issued a recommendation that codeine-containing cough medications should not be administered to children under 13 years of age because of rare yet fatal adverse effects (Health Canada, 2013).

Opioid or opioid-like analgesics are generally prescribed for moderate to severe pain. These analgesics act by binding with opiate receptors to modify the perception of pain. An uncommon but potentially fatal adverse effect of opioids is oversedation and respiratory depression (Pasero, Quinn, et al., 2011). Respiratory depression caused by opioids can be prevented by using careful titration of opioids, close monitoring of sedation scores, and conducting a thorough respiratory assessment that includes the depth, quality, and regularity of the respirations (Pasero, Quinn, et al., 2011). In some pediatric hospitals, protocols exist for monitoring requirements (nurse in room or constant observation) for children under 1 year of age with basal infusions or epidural infusions.

If a patient experiences respiratory depression, an opioid antagonist such as naloxone can be administered. The dose must be titrated carefully and given as per physician order. Administering naloxone too quickly or administering too much can reverse the analgesic effect and produce severe pain that may be difficult to control. In addition, rapid administration can increase the sympathetic response and the patient may experience tachycardia, dysrythmias, hypertension, pulmonary edema, and even cardiac arrest (Pasero, Quinn, et al., 2011). Nurses need to carefully assess and reassess patients every 15 minutes for 2 hours after drug administration because of the risk of renarcotization and the return of respiratory depression. Naloxone is also used in smaller doses (1–2 mcg/kg IV) for the treatment of pruritus (Brislin & Rose, 2005). In pediatrics, some preprinted order sets have infusion options for naloxone infusions in the range of 0.25–2 mcg/kg/dose, and this low dose will not reverse the opioid (Children's Hospital of Eastern Ontario [CHEO], 2016a).

Common adverse effects of opioids include nausea, vomiting, constipation, sedation, pruritus, and confusion. Less common effects include urinary retention, dry mouth, sweating, orthostatic hypotension, and seizures (Pasero, Quinn, et al., 2011). Most adverse effects are dose related; hence, a reduction in the opioid dose may treat the adverse effect or allow it to be more tolerable (Pasero, Quinn, et al., 2011). If intolerable adverse effects persist, sometimes an opioid rotation will reduce the adverse effects such that intractable nausea with morphine patient-controlled analgesia (PCA) may be minimized or eliminated with a rotation to hydromorphone or Dilaudid PCA.

Around-the-clock (ATC) dosing should be considered when pain exists for 12 out of 24 hours (Pasero, Quinn, et al., 2011). The benefits of ATC dosing include prevention in delay of timely medication administration and avoidance of the peaks and valleys of pain and analgesic blood levels associate with as-needed (prn) regimens.

As-needed dosing can be used to treat breakthrough pain; however, this method requires the patient's participation, as he or she needs to request analgesia. Undertreatment of pain can occur if prn dosing is used for continuous pain. As-needed dosing is most useful when initiating opioid therapy to treat moderate to severe escalating pain or when pain is diminishing (Pasero, Quinn, et al., 2011).

The proper use of analgesics requires careful assessment and critical thinking in the application of pharmacological principles and logic. A patient's response to an analgesic is highly individualized. An NSAID can be as effective as or more effective than an opioid for some patients if the pain is caused by inflammation. An orally administered analgesic usually has a longer onset and duration of action than an injectable form. In addition, controlled- or extended-release opioid formulations (MS Contin, H Contin, OxyContin, Kadian, Avinza, and methadone) are available for administration every 8 to 12 hours ATC with short-acting breakthrough dosing ordered. Physicians should not order these long-acting formulations on a prn basis. Typically, the long-acting opioids are calculated on the basis of the previous 24-hour requirements and are adjusted according to the amount of breakthrough doses required. Special licenses are required to prescribe methadone and physicans wishing to prescribe methadone must apply for a special exemption through Health Canada (Government of Canada https://www.canada.ca/en/health-canada/services/health-concerns/controlled-substances-precursor-chemicals/exemptions/methadone-program.html).

It is essential that nurses know the comparative potencies of analgesics in both oral and injectable forms. In addition, it is important to know the route of administration most effective for a patient so that controlled, sustained pain relief can be achieved. If nurses on different shifts choose alternative routes for the same doses, the patient will not receive the same level of analgesia, and pain control will be poor. *Equianalgesic charts* are charts that convert one opioid to another (e.g., morphine to hydromorphone) or parenteral forms of opioids to oral forms (or vice versa). They are available online or by contacting pharmacy team members. To see an example of an equianalgesic chart and pocket tool developed by the Canadian Pharmacists Association go to RxTx (https://www-e-therapeutics-ca.) and look for the Opioids general monograph (2017). For example, morphine 1 mg given orally is equivalent to morphine 2 to 3 mg given intravenously (IV). An equianalgesic chart provides this type of information.

Before administering opioids, it is important to consider the patient's situation, including current treatments, diseases and conditions, and kidney and liver function. Opioid doses often need adjusting according to patient circumstances. Patients requiring special consideration include opioid-naïve patients, breastfeeding mothers, patients on dialysis, persons with neurological or respiratory conditions, and patients with recent abdominal surgery. Pharmacists are instrumental in assisting with specific dosing requirements in special circumstances, such as renal impairment.

Adjuvants, or co-analgesics, are drugs that were originally developed to treat conditions other than pain but have been shown to have analgesic properties. Adjuvants, used for acute or chronic pain, can be employed as additional therapies or as a primary therapy for some specific painful conditions. Classes of drugs considered as adjuvant therapy include the following: anticonvulsants, such as gabapentin for neuropathic pain; antidepressants such as amitriptyline for neuropathic pain; corticosteroids; alpha$_2$-adrenergic agonists, such as clonidine; cannabinoids; and topical analgesics (Pasero, Polomano, et al., 2011).

Patient-controlled analgesia. Patients benefit from having control over their own pain therapy. When patients depend on nurses for prn analgesia, an erratic cycle of alternating pain and analgesia often occurs. The patient feels pain and asks for medication, but the nurse must first assess the patient and then prepare the medication. Within an hour, analgesia finally occurs, but adequate pain relief may last only 30 to 60 minutes. The patient's discomfort then gradually escalates, and the cycle is repeated.

A drug delivery system called **patient-controlled analgesia (PCA)** is a safe method for pain management that allows patients to self-administer opioid doses (e.g., morphine, hydromorphone, fentanyl) on demand with minimal risk of overdose. PCA allows patients to control when they request analgesia and avoids the delay in waiting for pain relief. The goal is to maintain a constant plasma level of analgesic so that the problems of prn dosing are avoided. Systemic PCA typically pertains to IV administration, but PCA devices are also used to deliver pain medication via subcutaneous, epidural, intrathecal, and transdermal routes (Pasero, Quinn, et al., 2011). PCAs are portable computerized infusion pumps containing a chamber for a syringe, cartridge (Figure 31-10), or bag that delivers a small, preset dose of medication. To receive a bolus dose, the patient activates a button attached to the PCA pump. To minimize overdoses, the system is designed with a preset "lockout" interval, typically 6–8 minutes, based on the pharmacotherapies of the drug. The system is designed to deliver a specified number of doses every hour as required and demanded by the patient. PCA can be used on demand only or with a basal or continuous infusion (Pasero, Quinn, et al., 2011). PCA dosing is based strictly on weight, and dosing for any pediatric patient over 50 kg is based on adult dosing. Pediatric patients typically need to be older than 6 years of age so that they have the comprehension to use PCA. For patients under 6 years of age or those with cognitive impairment, a nurse-controlled analgesia (NCA) modality can be administered using the same principles of weight-based dosing as for PCA, with the option of a basal infusion. The advantage of NCA includes pre-emptive analgesia by the nurse, by activating the pump before the patient undergoes a painful procedure such as turning, positioning, or suctioning.

> **Safety Alert** Remember to perform an independent double-check with a nurse colleague to ensure that the medication and the pump settings (e.g., basal rate, bolus dose, loading dose, and lockout interval and total hourly dose) are the same as those ordered by the physician and are congruent with the appropriate documentation sources and medication administration record.

PCA is beneficial in many ways. The patient gains control over his or her pain, and pain relief does not depend on nurse availability.

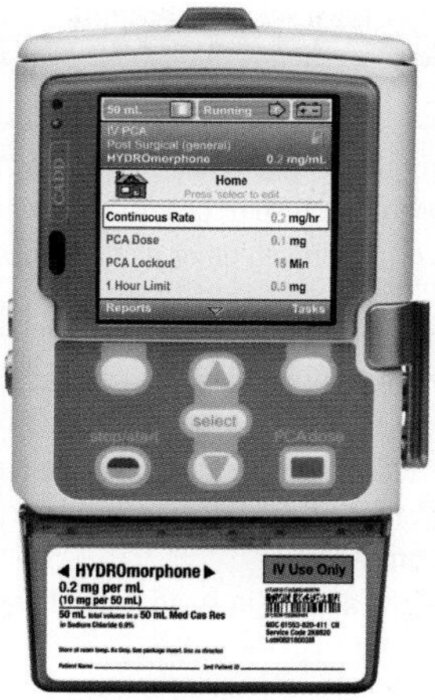

FIGURE 31-10 Ambulatory patient-controlled analgesia (PCA) pump. (Smith Medical: CADD Solis Ambulatory PCA Pump: https://www.smiths-medical.com/brands/cadd.)

Patients can also access medication when they need it. This can decrease patient anxiety and lead to decreased medication use. Small doses of medications are delivered at short intervals, stabilizing serum drug concentrations for sustained pain relief.

Patients who do not favour PCA are those who feel they do not understand how to use the technology. Nurses view PCA as inappropriate when it is ordered for patients with short-term memory loss or states of confusion (King & Walsh, 2007). Patient suitability, preparation, and teaching are, therefore, critical to the safe and effective use of PCA devices (Box 31-15). It is important to teach patients how to use the technology and determine if they are physically able to locate and press the button to deliver the dose. Family members need to be reminded they must not press the button for patients, as this is deemed unauthorized administration of a dose by another person, referred to as *PCA by proxy*. Nurses need to check to ensure that their institution has established a policy that safeguards against PCA by proxy (Pasero, Quinn, et al., 2011).

The IV line and PCA device need to be checked regularly to ensure proper functioning. Errors in pump programming can occur that put the patient at risk for an overdose, resulting in oversedation and respiratory depression. In addition, opioid-naïve patients should be monitored carefully for both of these adverse effects at the initiation of PCA therapy (Pasero, Quinn, et al., 2011).

The first mechanical device for oral medications, Medication on Demand (MOD), recently became available. This device allows patients access to their own oral prn medications, including opioids and other analgesics, antiemetics, and anxiolytics, at the bedside. Research has shown that this system is satisfying to patients, and there have been no reports of medication loss or inappropriate use (Rosati, Gallagher, Shook, et al., 2007).

Local analgesic infusion pump. Postoperatively, such as following cardiac (White, Rawal, Latham, et al., 2003) and orthopedic surgeries (Liu, Richman, Thirlby, et al., 2006), an infusion of a local anaesthetic into the operative site may be effective for pain management and help to avoid systemic adverse effects of oral or intravenous analgesics. A catheter from the wound, placed during surgery, is connected to a pump containing a local anaesthetic, such as Marcaine. The infusion is usually left in place for 48 hours and may be set to either demand or continuous modes. Oral analgesics may still be needed by the patient, but the total dose is often reduced. Either single-shot nerve blocks or continuous nerve blocks can be used in pediatrics. Some pediatric patients who qualify can be discharged home on an ambulatory nerve block pump that is discontinued by the patient or family within 48 hours of discharge. Patient satisfaction scores are high, and pain is well controlled with nerve blocks. The block can reduce opioid requirements and reduce length of stay. Children's Hospital of Eastern Ontario has an outpatient program and has developed a teaching video that provides an overview of the pump, troubleshooting, and removal instructions (refer to http://www.cheo.on.ca/en/Video-Outpatient-Catheter-Therapy).

Topical analgesics and anaesthetics. Topical analgesics such as ELA-Max/LMX and EMLA (eutectic mixture of local anaesthetics) are available for both children and adults (Eidelman, Weiss, Lua, et al., 2005). EMLA is applied to the skin, via a disc or as thick cream, 30 to 60 minutes before minor procedures (e.g., IV start) or anaesthetic infiltration of soft tissue. EMLA should not be placed around the eyes, on the tympanic membrane, or over large skin surfaces. The Lidoderm patch is a topical analgesic effective for cutaneous neuropathic pain in adults. Three patches, cut to size, are placed on and around the pain site using a 12-hour-on, 12-hour-off schedule to avoid lidocaine toxicity. Other topical analgesics include ketoprofen patches and capsaicin lotion (Pasero, Polomano, et al., 2011).

Sucrose. Oral sucrose is an effective strategy to reduce pain while procedures are carried out in infants (Harrison, Yamada, Adams-Weber, et al., 2015) (Box 31-16). Sweet taste is thought to trigger a release of endogenous opioids. Small volumes of sucrose are required, given in small doses throughout the duration of the painful procedure.

BOX 31-15 Preparation for Patient-Controlled Analgesia

Objectives

- Patient will be able to explain the purpose of patient-controlled analgesia (PCA) in managing pain.
- Patient will use the PCA device correctly.
- Patient will achieve pain control.

Teaching Strategies

Some institutions employ both written and verbal instructions with PCA and offer instructions in advance for using PCA with elective surgery so that the patient is not learning this modality in the post–anaesthetic care unit for the first time. The Children's Hospital of Eastern Ontario (CHEO) created an instructional video (CHEO, 2016b) in both English and French for the use of PCA; it is posted on their website for patients to view preoperatively before the surgery and postoperatively as required to reinforce concepts. The video script was vetted via the youth forum for feedback and suggestions prior to final production. Refer to http://www.cheo.on.ca/en/acute-pain-service.

- Teach the use of PCA before it is needed so that the patient can understand how to use it after awakening from anaesthesia or sedation. Reinforce as needed.
- Instruct patient on the purpose of PCA, emphasizing that the patient controls medication delivery.
- Explain that the lockout interval prevents the risk of overdose.
- Tell family members or friends that they should not operate the PCA device for the patient.
- Ask the patient to demonstrate use of the PCA delivery button.

Evaluation

- Ask patient to tell you the purpose of the PCA device.
- Observe the patient administering a dose.
- Evaluate the severity of the patient's pain, both at rest and with movement, with PCA and determine if the patient's preset pain goal has been achieved.
- Evaluate and treat any adverse effects.

BOX 31-16 RESEARCH HIGHLIGHT

Sucrose for Reducing Pain in Infants

Research Focus

Infants undergo painful procedures during their first year of life. Even healthy infants require blood sampling for newborn screening and receive injections for scheduled childhood immunization. Effective management of pain during these procedures is vital for the well-being of the developing infant. Canadian researchers have contributed substantially to the development of effective pain-management strategies for infants and have demonstrated analgesic effects of sweet-tasting solutions in diverse infant populations (Harrison, Yamada, Adams-Weber, et al., 2015). Using evidence in your practice will help you provide the best care possible to patients of all ages.

Research Abstract

The purpose of the systematic review by Stevens and colleagues (Stevens, Yamada, Ohlsson, et al., 2016) was to review all published studies of analgesic effects of sweet solutions in infants aged 1 to 12 months to determine if sweet solutions reduced pain during scheduled childhood immunization. Fourteen studies were included in the review. Results were that small volumes of sucrose and glucose, when given to infants to suck before their injections, reduced crying during and after the procedure. The authors recommended that health care providers advocate for use of sucrose or glucose in their clinical practice when administering injections or performing other painful procedures on infants.

Evidence-Informed Practice

- Effective management of pain during painful procedures is important to the well-being of infants.
- Small volumes of sucrose or glucose significantly reduce pain during administration of medical procedures in infants up to 1 year of age, provided up to 2 minutes before the procedure.
- Sweet solutions need to be given in small doses before and throughout the procedure.
- Other pain-management strategies can be used in addition to sweet solutions, such as offering the infant a pacifier if this is a normal part of the infant's care.
- Support mothers to help their infants during immunization. For example, support mothers to breastfeed during immunization and/or to provide kangaroo care.

Stevens, B., Yamada, J., Ohlsson, A., Haliburton, S. & Shorkey. A. (2016). Sucrose for analgesia in newborn infants undergoing painful procedures. *Cochrane Database of Systematic Reviews, 7*, CD001069. doi:10.1002/14651858.CD001069.pub5.

Non-nutritive sucking, as with use of a pacifier, may further assist with pain management. The efficacy of sucrose has been well demonstrated in infants undergoing painful procedures; however, further studies are required to determine efficacy in young children (Stevens, Yamada, Ohlsson, et al., 2016).

Local and regional anaesthetics and analgesics. Local anaesthesia is the infiltration of a local anaesthetic medication to induce loss of sensation to a localized body part. Physicians use local anaesthesia during brief surgical procedures, such as the removal of a skin lesion or suturing a wound. The local anaesthetic is topically applied on skin and mucous membranes, or injected subcutaneously or intradermally to anaesthetize a body part. The drugs produce temporary loss of sensation by inhibiting nerve conduction. Local anaesthetics can also block motor and autonomic functions, depending on the amount used and the location and depth of an injection. Smaller sensory nerve fibres are more sensitive to local anaesthetics than are large motor fibres. As a result, the patient loses sensation before losing motor function and, conversely, motor activity returns before sensation.

Local anaesthetics can cause adverse effects, depending on their absorption into the circulation. Itching or burning of the skin or a localized rash is common after topical applications. Application to vascular mucous membranes increases the chance of systemic effects, such as a change in heart rate.

Regional anaesthesia is the injection of a local anaesthetic to block a group of sensory nerve fibres. Tissues are anaesthetized layer by layer as the surgeon or anaesthesiologist introduces the agent into deeper structures of the body. Some types of regional anaesthesia are epidural anaesthesia, nerve blocks, and spinal anaesthesia.

Whereas epidural anaesthesia induces temporary loss of sensation, epidural analgesia permits control or reduction of severe pain without the more serious sedative effects of parenteral or oral narcotics. Epidural analgesia is commonly used for the treatment of acute post-operative pain, labour and delivery pain, and chronic pain, especially when associated with cancer (Sawhney, 2012). Epidural catheters can be placed via the caudal, lumbar, or thoracic region (Brislin & Rose, 2005). However, intraspinal opioids can produce the same adverse effects of nausea, mental clouding, and sedation because they are absorbed via the cerebrospinal fluid into the circulation of the epidural vascular plexus. Epidural analgesia can be short or long term, depending on the patient's condition and life expectancy. Short-term therapy is used for pain after intrathoracic, abdominal, and orthopedic surgery. Long-term therapy is particularly useful for intractable cancer pain (Raffaeli, Andruccioli, Righetti, et al., 2006).

Epidural analgesia is administered into the epidural space, which lies between the dura mater and the vertebrae (Figure 31-11). The physician inserts a needle into the level of the vertebral interspace nearest to the dermatomal area requiring analgesia (Sawhney, 2012). When the needle reaches the space, preservative-free local anaesthetic and opioids may be injected and a small catheter may be passed into the space. Once a catheter is advanced into the epidural space and the needle is removed, the remainder of the catheter is secured with a dressing and taped along the back of the patient (Figure 31-12). If the catheter is only temporary, it is connected to tubing positioned along the spine and over the patient's shoulder. The end of the catheter can then be placed on the patient's chest for the nurse's access. Patients may also be given control of the demand dose, which is known as patient-controlled epidural analgesia (PCEA). When PCEA is used, the basal rate is intended to meet the patient's analgesic requirements and the PCEA bolus doses are intended to control periods of breakthrough pain (Pasero, Quinn, et al., 2011). Infants may benefit from a single caudal block whereby a one-time dose of local anaesthetic is administered to manage surgical pain, specifically with procedures below the level of the umbilicus (Verghese & Hannallah, 2005).

Nursing implications. Nurses can provide emotional support to patients receiving local or regional anaesthesia by explaining the procedure to them and warning them that they will temporarily lose sensory function. Patients commonly fear paralysis because epidural and spinal injections come close to the spinal cord. To reassure a patient, the nurse should explain that numbness, tingling, and coldness are common.

After administration of a local anaesthetic, the patient should be protected from injury until full sensory and motor function return. Patients are at risk for injuring the anaesthetized body part without knowing it. For example, after an injection into a joint, the nurse needs to warn the patient to avoid using the joint until function returns. For patients with topical anaesthesia, heat or cold should not be applied to numb areas. After spinal anaesthesia, the patient should be instructed to stay in bed until sensory and motor function return. The nurse needs to assist the patient during the first attempt at getting out of the bed and ensure that the patient is wearing proper footwear to prevent falls and to optimize stability.

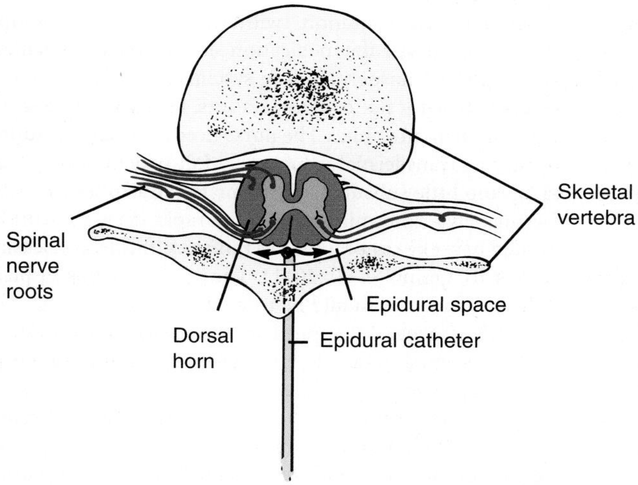

FIGURE 31-11 Anatomical drawing of epidural space.

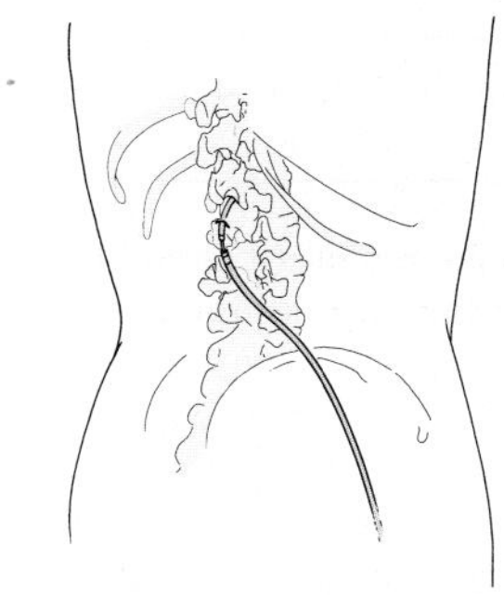

FIGURE 31-12 Epidural catheter taped in place.

When managing epidural infusions, the nurse connects the catheter to an infusion pump, a port, or a reservoir or caps it off for bolus injections. To reduce the risk of accidental epidural injection of drugs intended for IV use, the catheter should be clearly labelled as an "epidural catheter." The nurse should always administer continuous infusions through electronic infusion devices for proper control. Because of the catheter location, surgical asepsis is used to prevent a serious and potentially fatal infection. The nurse must notify the physician immediately of any signs or symptoms of infection or pain at the insertion site. Thorough hygiene is necessary during nursing procedures to keep the catheter system clean and dry. Nursing implications for managing epidural analgesia are summarized in Table 31-6.

Supplemental doses of opioids or sedatives (hypnotics) are avoided because they have additive effects that can be detrimental to the central nervous system. Monitoring of medication adverse effects differs, depending on whether infusions are intermittent or continuous. If opioids are to be administered, mu-agonist opioids, such as morphine, fentanyl, and hydromorphone, are the most common choices (Pasero, Quinn, et al., 2011). Adverse reactions can be related to the opioid or the local anaesthetic agent. Nurses should refer to their specific institutional protocols for monitoring standards.

Patients should be instructed about the action of the medication, advantages and disadvantages of the epidural route of medication, and potential adverse effects. They should be instructed to notify a health provider if they develop any adverse effects. If the patient requires long-term epidural use, the nurse should inform him or her that a permanent catheter may be tunnelled through the skin and exit at the patient's side. Nurses need to teach patients who are on long-term therapy how to safely administer infusions in the home with minimal ongoing intervention by the nurse. For these patients, home care will likely be required.

Invasive Interventions for Pain Relief. When pain is severe, invasive interventions may give relief when more conservative treatment is neither tolerated nor effective. These interventions include intrathecal implantable pumps or injections, spinal cord stimulators, deep brain stimulation, neuroablative procedures (e.g., **chordotomy**, **dorsal rhizotomy**, thalamotomy), trigger point injections, radiofrequency ablation, cryoablation,

TABLE 31-6 Nursing Care for Patients With Epidural Infusions

Goal	Actions
Prevent catheter displacement	Secure catheter (if not connected to implanted reservoir) carefully on skin.
Maintain catheter function	Check external dressing around catheter site for dampness or discharge. (Leak of cerebrospinal fluid may develop.) Use transparent dressing to secure catheter and to aid inspection. Inspect catheter for breaks. Note the epidural catheter marking at the skin so any dislodgments or migration can be easily recognized.
Prevent infection	Use strict aseptic technique when caring for catheter (see Chapter 33). Do not routinely change dressing over site. Change infusion tubing every 24 hours, or as per institutional policy.
Monitor for respiratory depression	Monitor vital signs, especially respirations, per institutional policy. Pulse oximetry and apnea monitoring may be used, as per institutional policy. Within pediatrics, infants under 1 year of age are often placed in a constant observation (nurse-monitored) room for closer observation and monitoring.
Prevent and treat complications	Assess for potential adverse effects, such as pruritus, nausea, and vomiting. Administer appropriate treatments to manage adverse effects as ordered and required.
Maintain urinary and bowel function	Monitor intake and output. Assess for bladder and bowel distension. Protect lumbar epidural catheters from soilage with infants who are diapered or patients who are incontinent to avoid contamination of the catheter. Assess for discomfort, frequency, and urgency. Some institutions will place a Foley catheter with lumbar epidurals, which remains until the epidural is discontinued.

intradiscal electrothermal (IDET) annuloplasty, vertebroplasty, intraspinal medications (e.g., opioids, steroids, local anaesthetics, alpha agonists), and others (Vanni & Rehm, 2010). It is not acceptable to tell a patient with severe unrelieved pain that "there is nothing more we can do for you." Patients with pain unresponsive to medications need consultation with a pain expert or an interprofessional pain team.

Procedure Pain Management. The Thunder Project II (Puntillo, 2003) identified several procedures in critical care patients that cause pain:

- *Turning*
- *Wound drain removal*
- *Tracheal suctioning*
- *Femoral catheter removal*
- *Placement of central line*
- *Changing of wound dressings*

Premedicating patients before painful procedures may assist them in cooperating during the procedure and may help to reduce the experience of pain. This is also true for patients who present in the emergency department with abdominal pain. The American Pain Society (2003) recommends medicating patients in pain before conducting an extensive physical examination or diagnostic procedures.

Cancer Pain Management. Cancer pain may be chronic or acute or a combination of the two. A number of key organizations across Canada, such as Cancer Care Ontario's Cancer-Related Pain Management Guideline Panel (Green, Zwaal, Beals, et al., 2010), the Canadian Pain Society (2005), and Cancer Care Nova Scotia (2005), have released evidence-informed clinical practice guidelines for the management of cancer pain. These guidelines are designed to treat cancer pain in a more comprehensive and aggressive manner and to provide patients and families with options for pain relief. The choice of treatment may change as the patient's condition and the characteristics of pain change. Effective pain management is best achieved when pharmacological and nonpharmacological pain interventions are used together and is part of an interprofessional collaborative team approach.

Various medications and routes of administration provide relief for patients with cancer pain. Long-acting or controlled-release medications have been successful in managing all types of chronic pain. These controlled-released medications (e.g., MS Contin, H Contin, Roxanol SR, OxyContin) relieve pain for 8 to 12 hours. A 72-hour fentanyl patch is also available. Management of most chronic pain can be achieved with oral or patch medications.

Administering analgesics to treat chronic noncancer and cancer pain requires principles different from those used to treat acute pain. The WHO (1996) recommends a three-step approach to managing cancer pain (Figure 31-13). Therapy begins with using NSAIDs, adjuvants, or both and progresses to strong opioids if pain persists. However, when a patient with cancer first experiences pain, it is recommended to begin with a higher dosage than will be needed for continued pain relief. The physician can then slowly decrease the dosage to the amount needed, ensuring immediate pain relief. Adverse effects of analgesia, such as nausea, pruritus and constipation, can be aggressively treated so that analgesia can be continued. Patients may become tolerant to the adverse effects of nausea, but not to the constipating effects of analgesics. Stimulant laxatives should be routinely administered both to prevent and to treat constipation.

Patients with persistent pain requiring prolonged opioid administration sometimes develop an opioid tolerance. As a result, higher doses of opioids are required to attain pain relief. The higher opioid dose is not lethal because patients also develop a tolerance to the medication. For patients with chronic pain, it is necessary to give required analgesics on a regular, ATC basis, even when the pain subsides. Prescribing analgesics on a prn basis for chronic pain is likely to be ineffective and result in more suffering. Regular administration maintains therapeutic drug blood levels for ongoing pain control. Helping patients to understand this will help prevent breakthrough pain and loss of pain control.

The transdermal route is useful when patients are unable to take drugs orally. Patients find these systems easy to use, and they allow for continuous opioid administration without needles or pumps. Self-adhesive patches release the medication slowly over time, achieving effective analgesia. Transdermal drug systems administer fentanyl at predetermined doses for up to 48 to 72 hours. Fentanyl is about 100 times more potent than morphine. The nurse needs to exercise caution when administering transdermal patches to adult patients who weigh less than 45 kg (too little subcutaneous tissue for absorption) or who are hyperthermic. Hyperthermia causes more rapid drug absorption. The patch should never be cut or folded as this alters the drug-releasing mechanism (Pasero, Quinn, et al., 2011). The patch remains in place for 48 to 72 hours, and sites should be rotated with each change. The transdermal patch is generally applied to the back, flank, chest, or upper arm and is deemed to be safe for long-term therapy. Care providers should wear plastic gloves while manipulating the patches so as to avoid inadvertent absorption of the fentanyl. Medication disposal procedures should be followed within institutions and proper disposal in the home environment to avoid the potential for misuse by other parties and to minimize environmental contamination (Pasero, Quinn, et al., 2011).

> **Safety Alert** Fentanyl should be used only in patients who are opioid tolerant and is not used for acute pain.

A transmucosal fentanyl "unit" (it resembles a lozenge on a handle) has been developed to treat breakthrough pain—a transient flare of

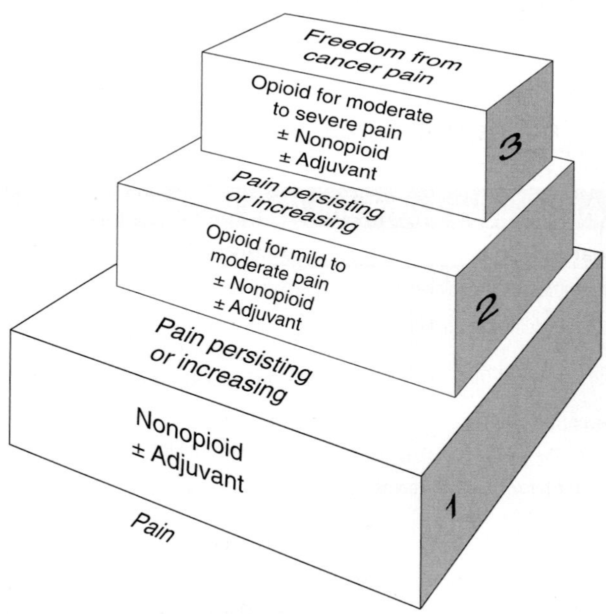

FIGURE 31-13 World Health Organization's pain relief ladder. This is a three-step approach to using drugs in cancer pain management. +/–, with or without medications. (From World Health Organization. [1996]. *Cancer pain relief with a guide to opioid availability*. Geneva, Switzerland: Author. Retrieved from http://apps.who.int/iris/bitstream/10665/37896/1/9241544821.pdf. Figure also available at http://www.who.int/cancer/palliative/painladder/en/.)

moderate to severe pain superimposed on continuous or persistent pain—in opioid-tolerant patients. The unit is placed in the mouth and swabbed over the buccal mucosa and lower gums. The unit must remain intact to dissolve in the mouth, allowing 15 minutes for absorption. No more than two units per breakthrough pain episode should be used. If the patient's pain is not relieved after two units, the nurse should notify the physician.

Analgesics may be given rectally when patients have nausea and vomiting or are fasting before or after surgery (Pasero, Quinn, et al., 2011). This route is contraindicated if patients have diarrhea or if cancerous lesions involve the anus or rectum. Morphine, hydromorphone, and oxymorphone are available as suppositories.

Another way to treat severe cancer pain in the home or acute care setting is with continuous infusions or a basal rate on a PCA device. This provides improved, uniform pain control with fewer peaks and valleys in plasma concentration, more effective drug action, and lower drug dosages overall. Candidates for continuous infusions include patients with severe pain for whom oral and injectable medications provide minimal relief, patients with severe nausea and vomiting, and patients unable to swallow oral medications. The intramuscular route should not be used for controlling cancer pain because the injection itself is painful and absorption of the drug is inconsistent and erratic.

When a patient is first given continuous-drip morphine, it is essential that the IV access be patent and that the IV site be without complications (see Chapter 40). A central-line catheter such as a Groshong or Hickman catheter, an implanted venous access port, or a peripherally inserted central catheter (PICC) is usually best suited for long-term IV infusion. When IV access is poor, the subcutaneous route with a concentrated dose is possible.

Barriers to Effective Pain Management. Barriers to effective pain management are complex and can involve the patient, health care provider, and health care system (Box 31-17). A deep-seated and often inappropriate concern shared by health care providers and patients is the fear of addiction when long-term opioid use is prescribed to manage pain. Differences exist between **physical dependence**, **addiction**, and **drug tolerance** (Box 31-18). Experiencing a physical dependency does not imply addiction, and drug tolerance in and of itself does not constitute addiction. Nurses and other health care providers need to avoid labelling patients as "drug seeking" because this term is poorly defined and may negatively affect their care. If the nurse is concerned that a patient is abusing opioids, the nurse has a responsibility to assess addictive issues and engage in a frank discussion with the patient. The nurse should also notify the primary health care provider, explaining the reasons for unease. The nurse and the health care team could consider using an opioid contract, a written agreement between a sole prescribing physician and the patient that outlines key points regarding opioid therapy or daily dispensing with a maximum number of pills allotted per day (Busse et al., 2017). Mehta and Langford (2006) have published recommendations for the management of acute pain in patients who are dependent on opioids but not necessarily addicted.

Individuals with an active addictive disorder or a history of substance abuse are at increased risk of poorly managed pain because of clinicians' attitudes, inadequate knowledge about addiction, and fears of exacerbating addiction by administering opioids. Poorly managed pain in these populations results in increased length of hospital stays and more frequent readmissions and outpatient and emergency department visits (Grant, Cordis, & Doberman, 2007). Estimates of addiction in patients are difficult to determine. Nicholoson and Passik (2007) have suggested that the rate of addiction to opioids and alcohol is approximately the same as it is in the general population, ranging from 6 to 10%. In the acute care setting, the prevalence is higher

BOX 31-17 Barriers to Effective Pain Management

Barriers for Patients

- Previous experience with poorly controlled pain
- Fear of addiction
- Worry about adverse effects
- Fear of tolerance (drug will not continue to work when needed)
- Concern that patient takes too many pills already
- Fear of injections
- Concern about not being a "good" patient
- Not wanting to worry family and friends
- More tests may be needed
- Belief that one needs to suffer to be cured
- Belief that pain is punishment for past indiscretions
- Inadequate education
- Reluctance to discuss pain
- Belief that pain is inevitable
- Belief that pain is part of aging
- Fear of disease progression
- Belief that health care team members are already doing all that they can
- Fear that patient will forget to take analgesics
- Fear of distracting physicians from treating illness
- Belief that physicians have more important or ill patients to see
- Belief that suffering in silence is noble and expected

Barriers for Health Care Providers

- Concern that patient did not receive adequate pain assessment
- Concern about addiction
- Opiophobia (fear of opioids)
- Fear of legal repercussions
- No visible cause of pain exists
- Belief that patients must learn to live with pain
- Reluctance to deal with adverse effects of analgesics
- Not believing patient's report of pain
- Fear of giving a dose that will kill the patient
- Time constraints
- Belief that opioids may "mask" symptoms
- Belief that pain is part of aging or disease progression
- Overestimation of risks of respiratory depression
- Not viewed as ethical obligation to properly treat pain

Barriers for the Health Care System

- Concern with creating "addicts"
- Ability to fill prescriptions
- Nurse practitioners and physician assistants unable to prescribe opioids
- Extensive documentation requirements
- Poor pain policies and procedures regarding pain management
- Lack of resources and education
- Inadequate access to pain clinics; long waiting lists for chronic pain clinics, for both pediatric and adult patients
- Poor understanding of economic impact of unrelieved pain

BOX 31-18 Definitions Related to the Use of Opioids for Pain Treatment

Physical Dependence

A state of adaptation that is manifested by a class-specific drug withdrawal syndrome that can be produced by abrupt cessation, rapid dose reduction, decreasing blood level of the drug, or administration of an antagonist. It is not the same as addiction.

Drug Tolerance

A state of adaptation in which exposure to a drug induces changes that result in a diminution of one or more of the drug's effects over time. It is not the same as addiction.

Addiction

A neurobiological disease that has genetic, psychosocial, and environmental factors influencing its development and manifestations. It is characterized by behaviours that include one or more of the following: impaired control over drug use, compulsive use, continued use despite harm, and craving.

Pseudoaddiction

Patient drug-seeking behaviours that may occur when pain is undertreated.

Approved by the Boards of Directors of the American Academy of Pain Medicine, The American Pain Society, and the American Society of Addiction Medicine. February 2001.
See also Centre for Addiction and Mental Health. Health Information: Addiction. Retrieved on from: http://www.camh.ca/en/hospital/health_information/a_z_mental_health_and_addiction_information/drug-use-addiction/Pages/addiction.aspx and
Pereira, J., & Bruera, E., (Eds.) (2001). Appendix F: Opioid analgesics—Pharmacokinetics. In *Alberta hospice palliative care resource manual* (2nd ed., p. 80) [Electronic version]. Calgary: Alberta Cancer Board. Retrieved from http://www.palliative.org/NewPC/_pdfs/education/ACB%20Hospice%20Palliative%20Manual.pdf.

because many medical illnesses such as cancer are complications of addictive disease (McCaffery et al., 2011).

Any treatment thought not to have a specific effect is considered a placebo (Sullivan, Terman, Peck, et al., 2005). **Placebos** may be defined as "any medication or procedure, including surgery, that produces an effect in a patient because of its implicit or explicit intent, not because of its specific physical or chemical properties" (McCaffery et al., 2011, p. 42). Placebos may be appropriately used as controls in randomized controlled drug trials. However, the use of placebos, without patient consent, to treat pain is considered unethical (McCaffery et al., 2011) and sets up an adversarial relationship between the care providers and the patient and his or her family. If a placebo is prescribed, the nurse should question the prescription and ask, "Why?" Many health care agencies have policies that limit placebo use only to research.

Restorative and Continuing Care

Pain Clinics, Palliative Care, and Hospices. In recent years, health care providers have recognized pain as a significant health problem and, as a result, a number of programs and pain clinics have been developed. A comprehensive pain centre can treat patients on an inpatient or outpatient basis, conduct research into new treatments, and train professionals. Clinicians from various health disciplines, such as pharmacists, nurses, physicians, physiotherapists, psychologists, pastoral care workers, nutritionists, and social workers, work with patients to discover effective pain-relief measures from a holistic perspective. Many hospitals have palliative care teams to assist patients and families in managing their chronic or end-of-life pain and symptoms from diseases. Learning to live life fully with an incurable condition is one goal of palliative care (see Chapter 25). Patients and their family members need ongoing assistance in managing the patient's pain at home. Some palliative care programs have a pain and symptom management team that may be consulted for complex pain and symptom problems.

In Canada, palliative and end-of-life care are burgeoning practice and research fields. The Canadian Institutes of Health Research (CIHR) support research and program development in these clinical areas. A hospice provides specialized end-of-life care in the patient's home or at a facility (see Chapter 25), helping patients with life-limiting illnesses to continue to live at home in comfort and privacy, with effective pain control as one of the priorities (Mehta, Cohen, Ezer, et al., 2010). Under the guidance of hospice nurses, families learn to monitor patients' symptoms and become the patients' primary caregivers. A hospice patient may become hospitalized in the event of a brief, acute care crisis or family problem. The Canadian Virtual Hospice is an online resource for patients, families, and health care providers.

◆ Evaluation

Patient Care. Evaluating pain is one of many nursing responsibilities that require critical thinking (Figure 31-14). The patient's behavioural responses to pain-relief interventions are not always obvious. Evaluating the effectiveness of a pain intervention requires that the nurse be an intent observer and know what responses to anticipate on the basis of the type of pain, the type of intervention, the timing of the intervention, the physiological nature of the injury or disease, the pharmacotherapies used, and the patient's previous responses. The nurse's input should be extracted from the three Ps or domains of pain management: physiotherapies, psychological therapies and support, and pharmacotherapies.

If a patient continues to have discomfort after an intervention, the nurse can try a different approach. For example, if an analgesic provides only partial relief, relaxation or guided-imagery exercises might be added. The nurse should consult with the physician about increasing the dosage, decreasing the interval between doses, or trying different analgesics. The nurse should also evaluate tolerance to therapy and the overall relief obtained. If an intervention aggravates discomfort, it should be stopped immediately and an alternative sought. Time and patience are necessary to maximize the effectiveness of pain management. Nurses need to evaluate the entire pain experience to determine the most effective interventions and times for medication administration.

Patient Perceptions. The patient, if able, is the best resource for evaluating the effectiveness of pain-relief measures. Nurses must continually assess whether the character of the patient's pain changes. The family can be a valuable resource, particularly if the patient has cancer or is noncommunicative and may not be able to express discomfort during the latter stages of terminal illness. Treating pain is successful when the patient's expectations of pain relief are met. Recall, however, that some patients may experience pain needlessly because they accept suffering and because they lack knowledge of available pain-relief interventions.

Pain assessment and responses to intervention should be accurately documented so that they can be communicated to the health care team. Communication occurs from nurse to nurse, shift to shift, and nurse to other health care providers. The nurse caring for the patient is responsible for reporting and documenting what has been effective for managing pain. Various bedside tools, such as validated pain tools and a pain management flow sheet, help centralize information about pain management. Patients expect the nurse to be sensitive to their pain and

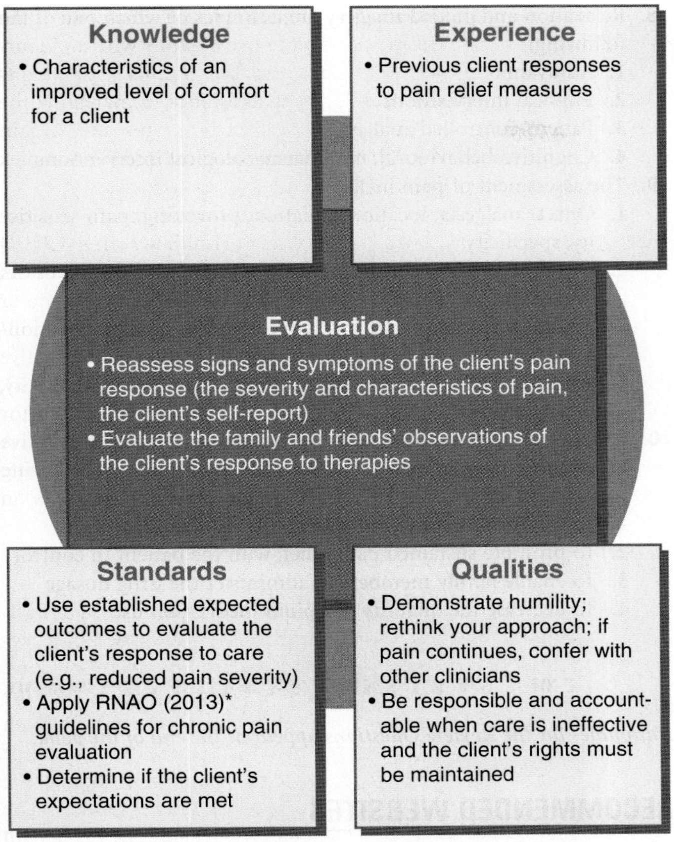

FIGURE 31-14 Critical thinking model for pain relief evaluation.
*Registered Nurses' Association of Ontario (RNAO) (2013). *Assessment and management of pain* (3rd ed.). Toronto, ON: Author. Retrieved from http://rnao.ca/sites/rnao-ca/files/AssessAndManagementOfPain_15_WEB-_FINAL_DEC_2.pdf

to be diligent in managing that pain. Because pain relief is a team effort, it is vital to communicate effectively with all members, including the patients' family and significant others, seek a collaborative approach, and determine optimal treatment goals (Box 31-19).

KEY CONCEPTS

- Pain is a purely subjective physical and psychosocial experience.
- A nurse's misconceptions about pain may result in doubt about the degree of the patient's suffering and in unwillingness to provide relief.
- Knowledge of the nociceptive pain processes of the pain experience—transmission, transduction, perception, and modulation—provides the nurse with guidelines for determining pain-relief measures.
- An interaction of psychological and cognitive factors affects pain perception.
- A person's cultural background influences the meaning of pain and how it is expressed.
- It is common for older patients not to report pain.
- Patients who have chronic pain are unlikely to show behavioural changes.
- An in-depth pain history should not be collected when the patient is experiencing severe discomfort.
- Pain can cause physical signs and symptoms similar to the signs and symptoms of other diseases.

BOX 31-19 Establishing a Collaborative Team Approach to Pain Management

1. Establish common goals for pain relief and optimal functioning.
2. Use common language regarding pain assessment and management.
3. Use validated pain-rating scales.
4. Secure a common knowledge base and encourage the use of clinical practice guidelines.
5. Optimize regular team communication opportunities for direct communication and problem solving.
6. Assess patient and caregiver expectations regarding pain control.

Data from Arnstein, P. (2010). *Clinical coach for effective pain management.* Philadelphia, PA: F. A. Davis; Pasero, C., & McCaffery, M. (2011). *Pain assessment and pharmacological management.* St. Louis, MO: Mosby/Elsevier.

- The nurse individualizes pain interventions by collaborating closely with the patient, using assessment findings, and trying a variety of multimodal interventions.
- Eliminating sources of painful stimuli is a basic nursing measure for promoting comfort.
- A regular schedule should be used for analgesic administration, as this is more effective than an as-needed schedule in controlling pain.
- A patient-controlled analgesic device gives patients pain control, with low risk of overdose.
- While caring for a patient who receives local anaesthesia, the nurse should protect the affected limb from injury.
- When administering epidural analgesia, the nurse needs to take steps to prevent infection and monitor closely for respiratory depression.
- The nurse's primary goal in pain management is to anticipate and prevent pain, rather than to treat it.
- In evaluating the effectiveness of a pain intervention, the nurse needs to consider the changing character of pain, the patient's response to the intervention, and the patient's perceptions of a therapy's effectiveness.
- Nurses must report any unexpected change in analgesia usage, or in the site, severity, or character of the pain.

CRITICAL THINKING EXERCISES

1. Do you have a friend or family member who lives with cancer and is willing to talk about it? If so, ask the individual to tell you about different painful experiences he or she may have had and what he or she would recommend to help nurses provide better care during these painful events.
2. Madeleine Tremblay is a 40-year-old woman newly diagnosed with fibromyalgia. She is married and has a daughter and son who are 2 and 5 years old, respectively. Her husband travels frequently and is often home only on weekends. Mrs. Tremblay tells the nurse: "The pain is so bad at night that I only get 3 or 4 hours of sleep. I have no opportunity to rest during the day because I'm busy caring for my children. I am so tired that I don't know how I am going to cope with this pain long term." Identify two follow-up care plan components that would be important when considering Mrs. Tremblay's concerns regarding the management of her pain.
3. Alexis, aged 3 years, is admitted to the pediatric unit for a third-degree burn to her right lower extremity. How would you proceed in assessing this child's pain?
4. Mrs. Gorsky, an 83-year-old woman with metastatic breast cancer to the bone, has been receiving intravenous morphine for a week

for severe back and leg pain. Her frequently increased infusion of morphine is not reducing her pain to an acceptable level, and she is becoming increasingly sedated. What other pharmacological interventions might be considered?

REVIEW QUESTIONS

1. As one of the strategies used to help relieve Ms. Bouclair's pain during a dressing change, the nurse encourages her to concentrate on a favourite vacation setting. What is this nonpharmacological pain intervention known as?
   1. Recall
   2. Distraction
   3. Imagery
   4. Relaxation exercises
2. A patient complains of pain in a site that is different from where the pain originates. How does the nurse document this pain?
   1. Transient pain
   2. Superficial pain
   3. Phantom pain
   4. Referred pain
3. Jacobie is a cooperative 5-year-old Inuit boy who had abdominal surgery 24 hours ago. Which of the following validated pain assessment tools would be most appropriate for the nurse to use to assess this child's pain?
   1. FLACC
   2. Numerical Rating Scale
   3. The Northern Pain Scale
   4. Wong-Baker FACES Scale
4. Which one of the following responses would the nurse expect to be corroborative data with respect to the patient experiencing moderate pain?
   1. Restlessness
   2. Decreased heart rate
   3. Increased blood pressure
   4. Protection of the painful area
5. Mr. Kumar, an 82-year-old man with Alzheimer's disease, is restless and moaning. His daughter states that he did not sleep well most of the night. Which one of the following actions is the most appropriate initial nursing response?
   1. Obtain a psychiatric evaluation.
   2. Administer pain medication as ordered.
   3. Recommend giving the patient sleeping medication.
   4. Assess and document physical and behavioural data.
6. Mrs. Young requests medication for her abdominal incision pain, which she rates as 5 (scale of 0 to 10, with 10 being the worst pain). One hour after administration of her pain medication, she is able to walk in the hall for 10 minutes and rates her pain as a 2/10. Which one of the following interpretations about the dosage of pain medications is the most appropriate?
   1. Adequate
   2. Excessive
   3. Insufficient
   4. Unnecessary
7. Which one of the following nursing actions is the most appropriate when a patient is anticipating a painful procedure?
   1. Discuss analgesic options with the physician.
   2. Inform the patient that the discomfort will be minimal.
   3. Teach about the procedure and its associated discomfort.
   4. Provide education about the procedure but avoid the associated discomfort.
8. Relaxation and guided imagery are examples of which one of the following?
   1. Adjuvants
   2. Physical interventions
   3. Patient-controlled analgesia
   4. Cognitive-behavioural, nonpharmacological interventions
9. The assessment of pain includes:
   1. Onset, analgesia, location/radiation, provoking, pain sensitivity, specificity
   2. Onset, analgesia, complementary therapies, passive motion, understanding, value
   3. Onset, provoking and palliative factors, quality, location/radiation, severity, timing, understanding, and value
   4. Onset, pain tolerance, location/radiation, pain sensitivity, timing, value
10. Patient-controlled analgesia (PCA) is often used for postoperative and cancer pain management for which one of the following reasons?
    1. To improve nursing control over opioid administration
    2. To promote sustained pain relief, with the patient in control
    3. To enable family members to administer the drug dosage
    4. To decrease the quantity of opioid medication use

Answers: 1. 3; **2.** 4; **3.** 3; **4.** 3; **5.** 4; **6.** 3; **7.** 3; **8.** 4; **9.** 3; **10.** 2

Rationales for the Review Questions appear at the end of the book.

RECOMMENDED WEBSITES

Canadian Cancer Society: http://www.cancer.ca.
This site is an educational resource to help cancer patients and their caregivers. It has the most up-to-date knowledge and tools available related to cancer prevention, diagnosis, treatments, and supports and services. It also features a number of pain management publications, which include information on traditional and complementary therapies.

Canadian Hospice Palliative Care Association: http://chpca.net/index.
This site is intended as an educational resource for professional and informal caregivers and interest groups. It includes an extensive listing of online resources for those interested in palliative and end-of-life care, including cancer, clinical, and research sites.

Canadian Pain Coalition: http://prc.canadianpaincoalition.ca/en/index.html.
The Canadian Pain Coalition is a partnership of pain consumer groups, health professionals who care for people in pain, and scientists studying better ways of treating pain.

Canadian Pain Society: http://www.canadianpainsociety.ca.
The Canadian Pain Society is an association whose members include physicians, nurses, and other clinicians involved with the management of pain. Its aim is to foster and encourage research on pain, to promote education and training in the field of pain, and to improve the management of patients with acute and chronic pain.

Canadian Virtual Hospice: http://www.virtualhospice.ca/en_US/Main+Site+Navigation/Home.aspx.
This site is a resource for patients, families, caregivers, and health care providers who would like more information on palliative care or end-of-life care.

Health Canada: http://www.hc-sc.gc.ca/index-eng.php.
Health Canada provides an extensive listing of clinical guidelines for nurses in primary care. It provides the public, clinicians, and researchers with information on pain and other public health concerns. If you search this site you will find a document outlining questions, issues, and research surrounding neuropathic pain. (http://www.collectionscanada.gc.ca/obj/thesescanada/vol2/OKQ/TC-OKQ-1762.pdf)

International Association for the Study of Pain (IASP): http://www.iasp-pain.org/.

The IASP is the leading professional forum for science, practice, and education in the field of pain. IASP brings together scientists, clinicians, health care providers, and policymakers to stimulate and support the study of pain and to use that knowledge for improved pain relief worldwide.

Mayday Pain Project: http://www.painandhealth.org/.

The Mayday Pain Project's goal is to improve pain assessment and care of patients nationally and internationally, particularly for those living in rural, isolated areas. The site presents well-researched resources in a professional manner for educational purposes only.

Pain Treatment Topics: https://www.painbc.ca/pain-treatment-topics.

This site is a noncommercial resource for health care providers and their patients, providing open access to clinical news, information, research, and education for a better understanding of evidence-informed pain-management practices.

Registered Nurses' Association of Ontario: Assessment and Management of Pain: http://www.rnao.org/Page.asp?PageID=924&ContentID=720.

The Registered Nurses' Association of Ontario's website is specific to nursing and is available in English and French. It features a number of Best Practice Guidelines, including those for the assessment and management of pain.

University of Toronto Centre for the Study of Pain: http://sites.utoronto.ca/pain/.

The University of Toronto Centre for the Study of Pain is a partnership involving the faculties of dentistry, medicine, nursing, and pharmacy. The mission of the centre is to lead, both nationally and internationally, in pain research, education, knowledge translation, networking, and sustainability.

REFERENCES

Aghabati, N., Mohammadi, E., & Esmaiel, Z. P. (2010). The effect of therapeutic touch on pain and fatigue of cancer patients undergoing chemotherapy. *Evidence-based complementary and alternative medicine: eCAM*, *7*(3), 375–381. doi:10.1093/ecam/nen006.

Althaus, A., Arranz Becker, O., & Neugebauer, E. (2013). Distinguishing between pain intensity and pain resolution: Using acute post-surgical pain trajectories to predict chronic post-surgical pain. *European Journal of Pain*, *18*(4), 1532–2149. doi:10.1002/j.1532-2149.2013.00385.x.

American Geriatric Society. (2009). Pharmacological management of persistent pain in older adults. *Journal of the American Geriatric Society*, *57*(8), 1331–1346. doi: 10.1111/j.1532-5415.2009.02376.x.

American Pain Society. (2003). *Principles of analgesic use in the treatment of acute and cancer pain* (4th ed.). Glenview, IL: Author.

Arnstein, P. (2010). *Clinical coach for effective pain management*. Philadelphia, PA: F. A. Davis.

Basbaum, A. I., & Julius, D. (2006). Toward better pain control. *Scientific American*, *294*, 60–67.

Bieri, D., Reeve, R., Champion, G., et al. (1990). The FACES Pain Scale for the self-assessment of the severity of pain experienced by children: Development, initial validation, and preliminary investigation for ratio scale properties. *Pain*, *41*(2), 139–150.

Brislin, R. P., & Rose, J. B. (2005). Pediatric acute pain management. *Anesthesiology Clinics of North America*, *23*(4), 789–814. doi:10.1016/j.atc.2005.07.002.

Brookoff, D. (2000). Chronic pain: 1. A new disease? *Hospital Practice*, *35*(7), 45. doi:10.3810/hp.2000.07.205.

Bruehl, S., & Chung, O. Y. (2006). Psychological and behavioral aspects of complex regional pain syndrome management. *The Clinical Journal of Pain*, *22*(5), 430–437. doi:10.1097/01.ajp.0000194282.82002.79.

Busse, J., Guyatt, G. H., Carrasco, A., et al. (2017). *The 2017 Canadian guideline for opioids for chronic non-cancer pain*. Hamilton, ON. Retrieved from http://nationalpaincentre.mcmaster.ca/documents/Opioid%20GL%20for%20CMAJ_01may2017.pdf.

Canadian Nurses Association (CNA). (2017). *Code of ethics for registered nurses*. Ottawa: Author.

Canadian Pain Coalition. (2011). *Conquering pain for Canadians (booklet)*. Retrieved from http://www.canadianpaincoalition.ca/index.php/en/help-centre/conquering-pain.

Canadian Pain Society (CPS). (2005). *Accreditation pain standard: Making it happen!* Whitby, ON: Authors. Retrieved from https://c.ymcdn.com/sites/canadianpainsociety.site-ym.com/resource/resmgr/Docs/accreditation_manual.pdf.

Canadian Pain Society (CPS). (2010). *Position Statement*. Retrieved from http://www.canadianpaincoalition.ca/index.php/en/about-us/the-charter.

Canadian Pharmacists Association. (2017). *Opioids General Monograph. RxTx*. Retrieved from https://www-e-therapeutics-ca.

Canadian Public Health Association, Health and Welfare Canada, and the World Health Organization. (1986). *Ottawa Charter for Health Promotion*. Retrieved from http://www.who.int/healthpromotion/conferences/previous/ottawa/en/.

Cancer Care Nova Scotia. (2005). *Best practice guidelines for the management of cancer-related pain in adults: Cancer Care Nova Scotia (CCNS)*. Halifax: Author. Retrieved from http://www.cancercare.ns.ca/media/documents/CancerPainApprovedDec05.pdf.

Caraceni, A., Martini, C., Zecca, E., et al. (2004). Breakthrough pain characteristics and syndromes in patients with cancer pain. An international survey. *Palliative Medicine*, *18*(3), 177–183. doi:10.1191/0269216304pm890oa.

Chaillier, M., Ellis, J., Stolarick, A. J., et al. (2010). Cold therapy for the management of pain associated with deep breathing and coughing–post–cardiac surgery. *Canadian Journal of Cardiovascular Nursing*, *20*(2), 18–24.

Chambers, C. T., Craig, K. D., & Bennett, S. M. (2002). The impact of maternal behavior on children's pain experiences: An experimental analysis. *Journal of Pediatric Psychology*, *27*(3), 293–301. doi:10.1093/jpepsy/27.3.293.

Chambers, C. T., Hardial, J., Craig, K. D., et al. (2005). Faces Scales for the measurement of postoperative pain intensity in children following minor surgery. *The Clinical Journal of Pain*, *21*(3), 277–285.

Chen, L., Miaskowski, C., Dodd, M., et al. (2008). Concepts within the Chinese culture that influence the cancer pain experience. *Cancer Nursing*, *31*(2), 103–108. doi:10.1097/01.NCC.0000305702.07035.4d.

Children's Hospital of Eastern Ontario (CHEO). (2016a). *Medical directives for application of topical anesthetics prior to painful procedures #2051*. Ottawa: Author.

Children's Hospital of Eastern Ontario (CHEO). (2016b). *PCA teaching video*. Ottawa. Retrieved from http://www.cheo.on.ca/en/acute-pain-service.

Children's Hospital of Eastern Ontario (CHEO). (2016c). *Pre-printed order for epidural analgesia #2014*. Ottawa: Author.

Chou, R., Gordon, D., de Leon-Casasola, O., et al. (2016). Guidelines on the management of post-operative pain. *Journal of Pain*, *17*(2), 131–157. doi:10.1016/j.jpain.2015.12.008.

Chou, R., & Huffman, L. H. (2007). Nonpharmacologic therapies for acute and chronic low back pain: A review of the evidence for an American Pain Society/American College of Physicians Clinical Practice Guideline. *Annals of Internal Medicine*, *147*(7), 492–504.

Closs, S. J., Edwards, J., Swift, C., et al. (2013). Religious identity and the experience and expression of chronic pain: A review. *Journal of Religion, Disability & Health*, *17*(2), 91–124. doi:10.1080/15228967.2013.778515.

Cong, X., Cusson, R. M., Walsh, S., et al. (2012). Effects of skin to skin contact on autonomic pain responses in preterm infants. *Journal of Pain*, *13*(7), 636–645. doi:10.1016/j.jpain.2012.02.008.

Dahlquist, L. M., Weiss, K. E., Dillinger Clendaniel, L., et al. (2009). Effects of videogame distraction using a virtual reality type head-mounted display helmet on cold pressor pain in children. *Journal of Pediatric Psychology*, *34*(5), 574–584. doi:10.1093/jpepsy/jsn023.

Damen, L., Bruijn, J., Koes, B. W., et al. (2006). Prophylactic treatment of migraine in children. Part 1. A systematic review of non-pharmacological trials. *Cephalalgia: An International Journal of Headache*, *26*(4), 373–383. doi:10.1111/j.1468-2982.2005.01046.x.

D'Arcy, Y. (2006). Hot topics in pain management: Using NSAIDs safely. *Nursing*, *35*(2), 22.

Delgado-Guay, M. O., & Bruera, E. (2008). Management of pain in the older person with cancer, Part 1: Pathophysiology, pharmacokinetics, and assessment. *Oncology*, *22*(1), 56–61. Retrieved from www.globalaging.org/health/us/2008/cancerolder.pdf.

Eidelman, A., Weiss, J. M., Lua, J., et al. (2005). Topical anaesthetics for dermal instrumentation: A systematic review of randomized, controlled trials. *Annals of Emergency Medicine*, *46*(4), 343–351. doi:10.1016/j.annemergmed.2005.01.028.

Ellis, J. A., Ootoova, A., Blouin, R., et al. (2011). Establishing the psychometric properties and preferences for the Northern Pain Scale. *International Journal of Circumpolar Health*, *70*(3), 274–285.

Esteve, R., Ramírez-Maestre, C., & López-Martínez, A. E. (2007). Adjustment to chronic pain: The role of pain acceptance, coping strategies, and pain-related cognitions. *Annals of Behavioral Medicine*, *33*(2), 179–188. doi:10.1007/BF02879899.

Feldt, K. S. (2000). The checklist of nonverbal pain indicators (CNPI). *Pain Management Nursing*, *1*(1), 13–21. doi:10.1053/jpmn.2000.5831.

Fitzgerald, M., & Walker, S. M. W. (2009). Infant pain management: A developmental neurobiological approach. *Nature Reviews. Neurology*, *5*, 35–50. doi:10.1038/ncpneuro0984.

Fornasari, D. (2012). Pain mechanisms in patients with chronic pain. *Clinical Drug Investigations*, *32*(Suppl. 1), 45–52. doi:10.2165/11630070-000000000-00000.

Franck, L. S., Greenberg, C. S., & Stevens, B. (2000). Pain assessment in infants and children. *Pediatric Clinics of North America, 47*(3), 487–512.

Grant, M. S., Cordis, G. A., & Doberman, D. J. (2007). Acute pain management in hospitalized patients with current opioid abuse. *Topics in Advanced Practice Nursing eJournal, 7*(1).

Green, E., Zwaal, C., Beals, C., et al. (2010). Cancer-related pain management: A report of evidence-based recommendations to guide practice. *The Clinical Journal of Pain, 26*(6), 449–462. doi:10.1097/AJP.0b013e3181dacd62.

Gruener, D., & Lande, S. (2006). *Pain control in the primary care setting*. Glenview, IL: American Pain Society.

Grunau, R. E., & Tu, M. T. (2007). Long-term consequences of pain in human neonates. In K. J. S. Anand, B. J. Stevens, & P. J. McGrath (Eds.), *Pain in neonates and infants* (3rd ed., pp. 45–55). St. Louis, MO: Elsevier.

Grunau, R. V., & Craig, K. (1987). Pain expression in neonates: Facial action and cry. *Pain, 28*, 395–410.

Government of Canada. *Methadone Program*. (Accessed on 13 November 2017) From: https://www.canada.ca/en/health-canada/services/health-concerns/controlled-substances-precursor-chemicals/exemptions/methadone-program.html.

Hadjistavropoulos, T., Herr, K., Prkachin, K. M., et al. (2014). Pain assessment in elderly adults with dementia. *The Lancet. Neurology, 13*(12), 1216–1227. doi:10.1016/S1474-4422(14)70103-6.

Hamunen, K., Kontinen, V., Hakala, E., et al. (2012). Effect of pain on autonomic nervous system indices derived from photoplethysmography in healthy volunteers. *British Journal of Anaesthesia, 108*(5), 838–844. doi:10.1093/bja/aes001.

Hancock, T. (2007). Creating environments for health—20 years on. *International Journal of Health Promotion and Education, 14*(Suppl. 2), 7–8.

Harrison, D., Reszel, J., Bueno, M., et al. (2016). Breastfeeding for procedural pain in infants beyond the neonatal period (review). *The Cochrane Database of Systematic Reviews*, (10), Art. No.: CD011248, doi:10.1002/14651858.CD011248.pub2.

Harrison, D., Yamada, J., Adams-Weber, T., et al. (2015). Sweet tasting solutions for reduction of needle-related procedural pain in children aged one to 16 years. *The Cochrane Database of Systematic Reviews*, (5), CD008408, doi:10.1002/14651858.CD008408.pub3.

Harrison, J. D., Young, J. M., Price, M. A., et al. (2009). What are the unmet supportive care needs of people with cancer? A systematic review. *Supportive Care in Cancer, 17*(8), 1117–1128. doi:10.1007/s00520-009-0615-5.

Health Canada (2013). *Codeine recommendations*. Ottawa: Author. Retrieved from http://healthycanadians.gc.ca/recall-alert-rappel-avis/hc-sc/2013/33915a-eng.php.

Heikkinnen, K., Salanterä, S., Kettu, M., et al. (2005). Prostatectomy patients' postoperative pain assessment in the recovery room. *Journal of Advanced Nursing, 52*(6), 592–600. doi:10.1111/j.1365-2648.2005.03631.x.

Henwood, P., & Ellis, J. A. (2004). Chronic neuropathic pain in spinal cord injury: The patient's perspective. *Pain Research & Management, 9*(1), 39–45.

Henwood, P., Ellis, J. A., Logan, J., et al. (2010). Acceptance of chronic neuropathic pain in spinal cord injured persons: A qualitative approach. *Pain Management Nursing, 13*(4), 215–222. doi.org/10.1016/j.pmn.2010.05.005.

Herr, K. (2002a). Chronic pain: Challenges and assessment strategies. *Journal of Gerontological Nursing, 28*(1), 20–27.

Herr, K. (2002b). Chronic pain in the older patient: Management strategies. *Journal of Gerontological Nursing, 28*, 28–34.

Herr, K., Coyne, P. J., Key, T., et al. (2006). Pain assessment in the nonverbal patient: Position statement with clinical practice recommendations. *Pain Management Nursing, 7*(2), 44–52. doi:10.1016/j.pmn.2006.02.003.

International Association for the Study of Pain, Task Force on Taxonomy. (1994). *IASP taxonomy*. Retrieved from https://www.iasp-pain.org/Taxonomy.

International Association for the Study of Pain, Task Force on Taxonomy. (2012). *IASP taxonomy*. Retrieved from https://www.iasp-pain.org/Taxonomy.

James, S. (2013). Human pain and genetics: some basics. *British Journal of Pain, 7*(4), 171–178. doi:10.1177/2049463713506408.

Johnston, C., Barrington, K., Taddio, A., et al. (2011). Pain in Canadian NICUs: Have we improved over the past 12 years? *The Clinical Journal of Pain, 27*(3), 225–232. doi:10.1097/AJP.0b013e3181fe14cf.

Josefsson, K. A., & Gard, G. (2010). Women's experience of sexual health when living with rheumatoid arthritis—an exploratory qualitative study. *BMC Musculoskeletal Disorders, 11*, 240. doi:10.1186/1471-2474-11-240. Retrieved from http://www.biomedcentral.com/1471-2474/11/240.

Jovey, R. D., Ennis, J., Gardner-Nix, J., et al. (2003). Use of opioid analgesics for the treatment of chronic noncancer pain: A consensus statement and guidelines from the Canadian Pain Society. *Pain Research & Management, 8*(Suppl.A), 3A–14A.

Julius, D., & Basbaum, A. I. (2001). Molecular mechanisms of nociception. *Nature, 413*(6852), 203–209. doi:10.1038/35093019.

Kaasalainen, S., DiCenso, A., Donald, F. C., et al. (2007). Optimizing the role of the nurse practitioner to improve pain management in long-term care. *Canadian Journal of Nursing Research, 39*(2), 14–31.

Kappesser, J., Williams, A. C., & Prkachin, K. M. (2006). Testing two accounts of pain underestimation. *Pain, 124*(1), 109–116. doi:10.1016/j.pain.2006.04.003.

Kehlet, H., Jensen, T. S., & Woolf, C. (2006). Persistent post-surgical pain: Risk factors and prevention. *Lancet, 367*, 1618–1625.

Kerr, C. E., Wasserman, R. H., & Moore, C. I. (2007). Cortical dynamics as a therapeutic mechanism for touch healing. *Journal of Alternative and Complementary Medicine, 13*(1), 59–66. doi:10.1089/acm.2006.5245.

King, S., & Walsh, K. (2007). I think PCA is great, but ...—Surgical nurses' perceptions of patient-controlled analgesia. *International Journal of Nursing Practice, 13*, 276–283. doi:10.1111/j.1440-172X.2007.00638.x.

Krieger, D. (1979). *The therapeutic touch: How to use your hands to help or heal*. Englewood Cliffs, NJ: Prentice-Hall.

Kwan, K. S. H., & Roberts, L. J. (2005). Sexual dysfunction and chronic pain: The role of psychological variables and impact on quality of life. *European Journal of Pain, 9*(6), 643–652. doi:10.1016/j.ejpain.2004.12.008.

Latremoliere, A., & Woolf, C. (2009). Central sensitization: A generator of pain hypersensitivity by central neural plasticity. *Journal of Pain, 10*(9), 895–926.

Lawrence, J., Alcock, D., McGrath, P., et al. (1993). The development of a tool to assess neonatal pain. *Neonatal Network, 12*(6), 59–66.

Lee, M. S., Pittler, M. H., & Ernst, E. (2008). Effects of Reiki in clinical practice: A systematic review of randomised clinical trials. *International Journal of Clinical Practice, 62*(6), 947–954. doi:10.1111/j.1742-1241.2008.01729.x.

Liu, S. P., Richman, J. M., Thirlby, R. C., et al. (2006). Efficacy of continuous wound catheters delivering local anesthetic for postoperative analgesia: A quantitative and qualitative systematic review of randomized controlled trials. *Journal of the American College of Surgeons, 203*(6), 914–932. doi:10.1016/j.jamcollsurg.2006.08.007.

MacDonald, N., & MacLeod, S. M. (2010). Has the time come to phase out codeine? *Canadian Medical Association Journal, 182*(17), 1825. doi:10.1503/cmaj.101411.

Madadi, P., Koren, G., Cairns, J., et al. (2006). Maternal codeine is not safe for all breast-fed infants. *Canadian Pharmacists Journal, 139*(6), 56–50.

Manworren, R., & Hynan, L. (2003). Clinical validation of FLACC: Preverbal patient pain scale. *Pediatric Nursing, 29*(2), 140–146.

Maxwell, T., Brouch, M., & Jungquist, C. (2005). *Palliative and end-of-life pain management: Self-directed learning module*. Pensacola, FL: American Society for Pain Management Nursing.

McCaffery, M., Herr, K., & Pasero, C. (2011). Misconceptions that hamper assessment and treatment of patients who report pain. In C. Pasero & M. McCaffery (Eds.), *Pain assessment and pharmacological management* (pp. 20–48). St. Louis, MO: Mosby/Elsevier.

McCaffery, M., Pasero, C., & Ferrell, B. R. (2007). Nurses' decisions about opioid dose. *American Journal of Nursing, 107*(12), 35–39. doi:10.1097/01.NAJ.0000301016.18877.19.

McGovern, M. C., Glasgow, J. F. T., & Stewart, M. C. (2001). Reye's syndrome and Aspirin: Lest we forget. *British Medical Journal, 15*, 91–92.

Mehta, A., & Chan, L. S. (2008). Understanding of the concept of "total pain": A prerequisite for pain control. *Journal of Hospice and Palliative Nursing, 10*(1), 26–32.

Mehta, A., Cohen, S. R., Ezer, H., et al. (2010). Striving to respond to palliative care patients' pain at home: A puzzle for family caregivers. *Oncology Nursing Forum, 38*(1), E37–E45. doi:10.1188/11.ONF.E37-E45.

Mehta, V., & Langford, R. (2006). Acute pain management for opioid dependent patients. *Anaesthesia, 61*, 269. doi:10.1111/j.1365-2044.2005.04503.x.

Melzack, R., & Wall, P. D. (1965). Pain mechanisms: A new theory. *Science, 150*, 971–979.

Melzack, R., & Wall, P. D. (2003). *Handbook of pain management*. London: Churchill Livingstone.

Merkel, S. I., Voepel-Lewis, T., Shayevitz, J. R., et al. (1997). The FLACC: A behavioral scale for scoring postoperative pain in young children. *Pediatric Nursing, 23*(3), 293–297.

Nicholoson, B., & Passik, S. D. (2007). Management of chronic noncancer pain in the primary care setting. *Southern Medical Journal, 100*(10), 1028–1036.

Nightingale, F. (1969). *Notes on nursing: What it is and what it is not*. New York: Dover. (Original work published 1859).

Palmero, T. M. (2009). Assessment of chronic pain in children: Current status and emerging topics. *Pain Research & Management, 14*(1), 21–26.

Pasero, C., & McCaffery, M. (2011). *Pain assessment and pharmacological management*. St. Louis, MO: Mosby.

Pasero, C., Polomano, R. C., Portenoy, R. K., et al. (2011). Adjuvant analgesics. In C. Pasero & M. McCaffery (Eds.), *Pain assessment and pharmacological management* (pp. 623–652). St. Louis, MO: Mosby/Elsevier.

Pasero, C., & Portenoy, R. K. (2011). Neurophysiology of pain and analgesia and the pathophysiology of neuropathic pain. In C. Pasero & M. McCaffery (Eds.), *Pain assessment and pharmacological management* (pp. 1–12). St. Louis, MO: Mosby/Elsevier.

Pasero, C., Portenoy, R. K., & McCaffery, M. (2011). Nonopioid analgesics. In C. Pasero & M. McCaffery (Eds.), *Pain assessment and pharmacological management* (pp. 177–276). St. Louis, MO: Mosby/Elsevier.

Pasero, C., Quinn, T. E., Portenoy, R. K., et al. (2011). Opioid analgesics. In C. Pasero & M. McCaffery (Eds.), *Pain assessment and pharmacological management* (pp. 277–282). St. Louis, MO: Mosby/Elsevier.

Pergolizzi, J., Böger, R. H., Budd, K., et al. (2008). Opioids and the management of chronic severe pain in the elderly: Consensus statement of an international expert panel with focus on the six clinically most often used World Health Organization Step III opioids (buprenorphine, fentanyl, hydromorphone, methadone, morphine, oxycodone). *Pain Practice*, *8*(4), 287–313. doi:10.1111/j.1533-2500.2008.00204.x.

Perry, A. G., & Potter, P. A. (2017). *Clinical nursing skills and techniques* (9th ed.). St. Louis, MO: Mosby/Elsevier.

Portenoy, R. K., Bennett, D. S., Rauck, R., et al. (2006). Prevalence and characteristics of breakthrough pain in opioid-treated patients with chronic noncancer pain. *Journal of Pain*, *7*(8), 583–591. doi:10.1016/j.jpain.2006.02.003.

Prkachin, K. M., Solomon, P. E., & Ross, J. (2007). Underestimation of pain by health-care providers: Towards a model of the process of inferring pain in others. *Canadian Journal of Nursing Research*, *39*(2), 88–106.

Puntillo, K. (2003). Pain assessment and management in the critically ill: Wizardry or science? *American Journal of Critical Care*, *12*(4), 310–316.

Raffaeli, W., Andruccioli, J., Righetti, D., et al. (2006). Intraspinal therapy for the treatment of chronic pain: A review of the literature between 1990 and 2005 and suggested protocol for its rational and safe use. *Neuromodulation: Technology at the Neural Interface*, *9*(4), 290–308. doi:10.1111/j.1525-1403.2006.00071.x.

Rakel, D. P., & Faass, N. (2006). *Complementary medicine in clinical practice*. Sudbury, MA: Jones & Bartlett.

Ramage-Morin, P. (2008). Chronic pain in Canadian seniors. *Health Reports*, *19*(1), 37.

Registered Nurses' Association of Ontario. (2013). *Assessment and management of pain* (3rd ed.). Toronto, ON: Author. Retrieved from http://rnao.ca/sites/rnao-ca/files/AssessAndManagementOfPain_15_WEB-_FINAL_DEC_2.pdf.

Rippentrop, E. A., Altmaier, E. M., Chen, J. J., et al. (2005). The relationship between religion/spirituality and physical health, mental health, and pain in a chronic pain population. *Pain*, *116*(3), 311–321. doi:10.1016/j.pain.2005.05.008.

Rittner, H. L., Brack, A., & Stein, C. (2008). Pain and the immune system. *British Journal of Anesthesia*, *101*(1), 40–44. doi:10.1093/bja/aen078.

Rodkey, E. N., & Pillai Riddell, R. (2013). The infancy of infant pain research: The experimental origins of infant pain denial. *Journal of Pain*, *14*(4), 338–350.

Rodriguez, L. (2015). Pathophysiology of pain: Implications for perioperative nursing. *AORN Journal*, *101*(3), 338–344.

Rosati, J., Gallagher, M., Shook, B., et al. (2007). Evaluation of an oral patient-controlled analgesia device for pain management in oncology inpatients. *Journal of Supportive Oncology*, *5*(9), 443–448.

Roth, W., Kling, J., Gockel, I., et al. (2005). Dissatisfaction with post-operative pain management—A prospective analysis of 1071 patients. *Acute Pain*, *7*(2), 75–83. doi:10.1016/j.acpain.2005.05.001.

Sawhney, M. (2012). Epidural analgesia: What nurses need to know. *Nursing*, *42*(8), 36–41.

Schopflocher, D., Taenzer, P., & Jovey, R. (2011). The prevalence of chronic pain in Canada. *Pain Research and Management*, *16*(6), 445–450.

Schuh-Hofer, S., Wodarski, R., Pfau, D. P., et al. (2013). One night of total sleep deprivation promotes a state of generalized hyperalgesia: A surrogate pain model to study the relationship of insomnia and pain. *Pain*, *154*, 1613–1621.

Shyu, B., & Vogt, B. A. (2009). Short-term synaptic plasticity in the nociceptive thalamic-anterior cingulate pathway. *Molecular Pain*, *5*, 51–71. doi:10.1186/1744-8069-5-51.

Stanford, A. E., Chambers, C. T., & Craig, K. D. (2005). A normative analysis of the development of pain-related vocabulary in children. *Pain*, *114*, 278–284. doi:10.1016/j.pain.2004.12.029.

Stanford, A. E., Chambers, C. T., & Craig, K. D. (2006). The role of developmental factors in predicting young children's use of a self-report scale for pain. *Pain*, *120*(1), 16–23. doi:10.1016/j.pain.2005.10.004.

Stevens, B., Abbott, L., Yamada, J., et al. (2011). Epidemiology and management of painful procedures in hospitalized children across Canada. *Canadian Medical Association Journal*, *183*(7), E403–E410. doi:10.1503/cmaj.101341.

Stevens, B., Johnston, C., Petryshen, P., et al. (1996). Premature infant pain profile: Development and initial validation. *The Clinical Journal of Pain*, *12*(1), 13–22.

Stevens, B., McGrath, P., Gibbins, S., et al. (2007). Determining behavioral and physiological responses to pain in infants at risk for neurological impairment. *Pain*, *127*(1–2), 94–102. doi:10.1016/j.pain.2006.08.012.

Stevens, B., Pillai Riddell, R. R., Oberlander, T., et al. (2007). Assessment of pain in neonates and infants. In K. J. S. Anand, B. J. Stevens, & P. J. McGrath (Eds.), *Pain in neonates and infants* (3rd ed., pp. 67–90). St. Louis, MO: Elsevier.

Stevens, B., Yamada, J., Ohlsson, A., et al. (2016). Sucrose for analgesia in newborn infants undergoing painful procedures. *The Cochrane Database of Systematic Reviews*, (7), Art. CD001069, doi:10.1002/14651858.CD001069.pub5.

Stinson, J., Finley, A., Dick, B., et al. (2016). *Kids get chronic pain too: Assessment and management of paediatric chronic pain*. Retrieved from https://ken.caphc.org/xwiki/bin/view/Other/Assessment+and+Management+of+Paediatric+Chronic+Pain.

Stinson, J., Yamada, J., Dickson, A., et al. (2008). Review of systematic reviews on acute procedural pain in children in the hospital setting. *Pain Research & Management*, *13*(1), 51–57.

Sullivan, M., Terman, G. W., Peck, B., et al. (2005). APS position statement on the use of placebos in pain management. *Journal of Pain*, *6*(4), 215–217. doi:10.1016/j.jpain.2005.01.347.

Taddio, A. (2007). Evidence for systemic morphine and fentanyl analgesia. In K. J. S. Anand, B. J. Stevens, & P. J. McGrath (Eds.), *Pain in neonates and infants* (3rd ed., pp. 141–154). St. Louis, MO: Elsevier.

Taddio, A., Appelton, M., Bortolussi, R., et al. (2010). Reducing the pain of childhood vaccinations: An evidence-based clinical practice guideline. *Canadian Medical Association Journal*, *182*(18), 1–13. doi:10.1503/cmaj.101720.

Taddio, A., & Katz, J. (2005). The effects of early pain experience in neonates on pain responses in infancy and childhood. *Pediatric Drug*, *7*(4), 245–257.

Taylor, L. J., & Herr, K. (2003). Pain intensity assessment: A comparison of selected pain intensity scales for use in cognitively impaired African American older adults. *Pain Management Nursing*, *4*(2), 87–95. doi:10.1016/S1524-9042(02)54210-7.

Turk, D., Fillingim, R. B., Ohrbach, R., et al. (2016). Assessment of psychosocial and functional impact of chronic pain. *Journal of Pain*, *17*(9), Suppl 2, T21–T49. doi:10.1016/j.jpain.2016.02.006.

Turk, D. C., Wilson, H. D., & Cahana, A. (2011). Treatment of chronic non-cancer pain. *The Lancet*, *377*(9784), 2226–2235.

Twycross, A. (2009). Why managing pain in children matters. In A. Twycross, S. J. Dowden, & E. Bruce (Eds.), *Managing pain in children: A clinical guide*. Oxford, UK: Wiley-Blackwell.

Uman, L. S., Chambers, C. T., McGrath, P. J., et al. (2008). A systematic review of randomized controlled trials examining psychological interventions for needle-related procedural pain and distress in children and adolescents: An abbreviated Cochrane review. *Journal of Pediatric Psychology*, *33*(8), 842–854. doi:10.1093/jpepsy/jsn031.

Ung, A., Yenna, S., Hu, W., et al. (2016). Assessing knowledge, perceptions and attitudes to pain management among medical and nursing students: A review of the literature. *British Journal of Pain*, *10*(1), 8–21. doi:10.1177/2049463715583142.

Vanni, L., & Rehm, M. N. (2010). Cancer pain management. In B. St. Marie (Ed.), *Core curriculum for pain management nursing* (2nd ed., pp. 461–479). Dubuque, IA: Kendall Hunt Professional.

Verghese, S. T., & Hannallah, R. S. (2005). Postoperative pain management in children. *Anesthesiology Clinics of North America*, *23*(1), 163–184. doi:10.1016/j.atc.2004.11.008.

Vitale, A. (2007). An integrative review of Reiki touch therapy research. *Holistic Nursing Practice*, *21*(4), 167–179. doi:10.1097/01.HNP.0000280927.83506.f6.

Voepel-Lewis, T., Milviya, S., Tait, A. R., et al. (2008). A comparison of the clinical utility of pain assessment tools for children with cognitive impairment. *Pediatric Anesthesiology*, *106*(1), 72–76.

von Baeyer, C., & Hicks, C. (2000). Support for a common metric for pediatric pain intensity scales. *Pain Research and Management*, *4*(2), 157–160.

Wachholtz, A. B., Pearce, M. J., & Koenig, H. (2007). Exploring the relationship between spirituality, coping, and pain. *Journal of Behavioral Medicine*, *30*(4), 311–318. doi:10.1007/s10865-007-9114-7.

Warden, V., Hurley, A. C., & Volicer, L. (2003). Development and psychometric evaluation of the Pain Assessment in Advanced Dementia (PAINAD) Scale. *Journal of the American Medical Directors*, *Jan/Feb*, 9–15.

Wells, N., McCaffery, M., & Pasero, C. (2008). Improving the quality of care through pain assessment and management. In R. Hughes (Ed.), *Patient safety and quality: An evidence-based handbook for nurses* (pp. 474–502). AHRQ Publication No. 08-0043. Rockville, MD: Agency for Healthcare Research & Quality. Retrieved from https://archive.ahrq.gov/professionals/clinicians-providers/resources/nursing/resources/nurseshdbk/nurseshdbk.pdf.

White, P. F., Rawal, S., Latham, P., et al. (2003). Use of a continuous local anesthetic infusion for pain management after median sternotomy. *Anesthesiology*, *99*(4), 918–923.

Widerström-Noga, E. G., Finnerup, N. B., & Siddall, P. J. (2009). Biopsychosocial perspective on a mechanisms-based approach to assessment and treatment of pain following spinal cord injury. *Journal of Rehabilitation Research & Development*, *46*(1), 1–12. doi:10.1682/JRRD.2008.03.0038.

Williams, H. (2006). Assessing, diagnosing and managing neuropathic pain. *Nursing Times*, *102*(16), 22–24.

Wirth, J. H., Hudgins, J. C., & Paice, J. A. (2005). Use of herbal therapies to relieve pain: A review of efficacy and adverse effects. *Pain Management Nursing*, *6*, 145–167. doi:10.1016/j.pmn.2005.08.003.

Woolf, C. J., & Salter, M. J. (2000). Neuronal plasticity: Increasing the gain in pain. *Science*, *9*, 1765–1768.

World Health Organization (1996). *Cancer pain relief with a guide to opioid availability*. Geneva: Author. Retrieved from http://apps.who.int/iris/bitstream/10665/37896/1/9241544821.pdf, http://www.who.int/cancer/palliative/painladder/en/.

World Health Organization (2008). *Cancer control: Knowledge to action. WHO guide for effective programmes (diagnosis and treatment)*. Geneva, Switzerland: Author. Retrieved from http://www.who.int/cancer/modules/FINAL_Module_4.pdf.

Wuhrman, E., Cooney, M. F., Dunwoody, C. J., et al. (2007). Authorized and unauthorized ("PCA by proxy") dosing of analgesic infusion pumps: Position statement with clinical practice recommendations. *Pain Management Nursing, 8*(1), 4–11.

Yoon, S., & Schaffer, S. (2006). Herbal, prescribed, and over-the-counter drug use in older women: Prevalence of drug interactions. *Geriatric Nursing, 27*, 118. doi:10.1016/j.gerinurse.2006.02.014.

Zhao, Z. (2008). Neural mechanism underlying acupuncture analgesia. *Progress in Neurobiology, 85*(4), 355–375. doi:10.1016/j.pneurobio.2008.05.004.

32

Health Assessment and Physical Examination

Canadian content written by Mary Ellen Andrews, RN(NP), PhD, Janet Luimes RN(NP), MScN
Original chapter by Patricia A. Stockert, RN, BSN, MS, PhD

OBJECTIVES

Mastery of content in this chapter will enable you to:

- Discuss the purposes of physical assessment.
- Discuss cultural diversity, cultural competency, and cultural safety as these relate to the provision of culturally competent health and physical assessment and improved patient health outcomes.
- Identify data to collect from the nursing history before a physical examination.
- Describe environmental preparations necessary prior to a physical examination.
- List techniques used to prepare a patient physically and psychologically before and during an examination.
- Demonstrate the techniques used with each physical assessment skill.
- Describe physical measurements made in assessing each body system.
- Discuss normal physical findings in young, middle-aged, and older persons.
- Identify preventive screenings and the appropriate age(s) for each screening to occur.
- Identify self-screening examinations commonly performed by patients.
- Discuss ways to incorporate health promotion and health teaching into the examination.
- Identify how nurses use physical assessment skills during routine nursing care.

KEY TERMS

Acromegaly, p. 631
Adventitious sounds, p. 646
Alopecia, p. 627
Aneurysm, p. 663
Aphasia, p. 675
Apical impulse, p. 648
Arcus senilis, p. 633
Atherosclerosis, p. 652
Atrophy, p. 645
Basal cell carcinoma, p. 625
Benign (fibrocystic) breast disease, p. 660
Borborygmi, p. 662
Bronchophony, p. 646
Bruit, p. 652
Capillary refill, p. 630
Caries, p. 638
Cerumen, p. 636
Chancre, p. 665
Cherry angiomas, p. 625
Cholecystitis, p. 663
Cirrhosis, p. 630
Clubbing, p. 656
Conjunctivitis, p. 633
Cyanosis, p. 623
Dermatitis, p. 625
Distension, p. 613
Dysrhythmia, p. 650
Ectropion, p. 632
Eczema, p. 625
Edema, p. 625
Entropion, p. 632
Erythema, p. 624
Excoriation, p. 637
Exophthalmos, p. 631
Exostosis, p. 639
Hemorrhoids, p. 668
Hepatitis B, p. 662
Hernia, p. 661
Hirsutism, p. 627
Hydrocephalus, p. 631
Hypertonicity, p. 672
Hypotonicity, p. 672
Indurated, p. 625
Integument, p. 622
Jaundice, p. 624
Kyphosis, p. 670
Leukoplakia, p. 639
Lordosis, p. 670
Melanoma, p. 622
Metastasize, p. 659
Murmurs, p. 650
Nystagmus, p. 634
Occlusion, p. 652
Ophthalmoscope, p. 633
Orthopnea, p. 644
Osteoporosis, p. 670
Otoscope, p. 636
Ototoxicity, p. 636
Palpation, p. 613
Pancreatitis, p. 663
Papanicolaou (Pap) smear, p. 665
Paralytic ileus, p. 662
Peristalsis, p. 662
Peritonitis, p. 662
PERRLA, p. 633
Petechiae, p. 625
Phlebitis, p. 656
Pigmentation, p. 624
Point of maximal impulse (PMI), p. 648
Polyps, p. 637
Ptosis, p. 632
Pulse deficit, p. 650
Scoliosis, p. 670
Senile keratosis, p. 625
Squamous cell carcinoma, p. 625
Stenosis, p. 652
Strabismus, p. 631
Striae, p. 661
Syncope, p. 652
Tactile fremitus, p. 645
Thrill, p. 651
Turgor, p. 625
Varicosities, p. 639
Ventricular gallop, p. 650
Vocal fremitus, p. 645
Whispered pectoriloquy, p. 646

MEDIA RESOURCES

http://evolve.elsevier.com/Canada/Potter/fundamentals/

- Audio Chapter Summaries
- Examination Review Questions
- Concept Map Creator
- Case Study with Questions
- Audio Glossary
- Content Updates
- Video Clips

A holistic assessment of a patient's health status involves the collection of a broad range of data that includes information about the emotional, intellectual, physical, psychosocial, and spiritual (see Chapter 13) and cultural dimensions (see Chapter 9). The process for collecting data about a patient includes a thorough health history and the physical examination. The physical exam, although primarily focused on physiological function, may also include assessment of cognition, mood, and functional status.

Nurses are often the first person with whom patients are in contact when they are provided with health care services. It is, therefore, extremely important that nurses be able to detect changes in a patient's condition. Whether the nurse is conducting health assessments in a primary care clinic, in acute care agencies, or in a patient's home, nurses continuously seek information about patients' health status. For this reason, the ability to critically think and interpret the meaning of a patient's behaviour and physiological status is a skill that is important in professional nursing practice.

The skills of physical assessment and examination provide powerful tools to detect subtle, as well as obvious, changes in a patient's health. Physical assessment enables the nurse to assess patterns reflecting health problems and to evaluate the patient's progress following therapy. Health screenings may focus on a specific physical problem or assess cognition, mood, and functional status. For example, nurses perform blood pressure screenings to detect the risk for high blood pressure. If screening determines that a patient has a risk for a hypertension, the nurse refers the patient for a more complete physical examination.

A complete health assessment involves a nursing history (see Chapter 13), behavioural and physical examination, and a cultural assessment (see Chapter 9). The focus of this chapter is an introduction to the skills necessary to perform a physical examination. For more information on physical examination and health assessment, nursing students and health care providers should access comprehensive textbooks such as Jarvis, Browne, MacDonald-Jenkins, et al.'s (2014) *Physical Examination and Health Assessment* (2nd Canadian ed.) or Ball, Dains, Flynn, et al.'s (2015a) *Seidel's Guide to Physical Examination* (8th ed.).

A complete physical examination is a head-to-toe review of each body system that offers objective information about the patient. This enables the nurse to make clinical judgements and develop the plan for nursing care. The patient's condition and response affect the extent of the examination. The accuracy of the physical assessment will influence the choice of therapies a patient receives and the evaluation of the response to those therapies. Continuity in health care improves when the nurse makes an ongoing, objective, and comprehensive assessment.

SOCIAL AND CULTURAL CONSIDERATIONS

Culturally competent health and physical assessment requires the nurse to be culturally aware and sensitive (see Chapter 9). The nurse demonstrates cultural competence, in part, by respecting patient preference when completing an examination. It is important to remember that social or cultural background may influence a patient's behaviour and beliefs about health. Integrating cultural assessment with health and physical assessment for every patient provides the nurse with the background data needed to facilitate a culturally competent physical examination. Assessment data about the use of complementary or folk therapies, dietary preferences, family relationships (including extended family), and past experiences with health care offer important clues to help the nurse better understand how to perform physical assessment in ways that are respectful of these preferences and help build relational practice. Ethnohistorical, biocultural, and socioeconomic assessment data may provide important information about potential health risks.

Cultural assessment data inform a culturally safe physical assessment, by providing information that helps the nurse think critically about the political, social, and economic contexts of patients' lives and how inequities in power and access to resources for health influence the health of individuals (see Chapter 9; Browne & Varcoe, 2014). Applying a cultural safety lens will help the nurse avoid stereotyping patients on the basis of gender or ethnicity. Nurses need to learn to recognize common biocultural variations of normal as well as disorders that may be more common in certain populations in the community. For example, infants of Indigenous, Asian, or African descent may exhibit Mongolian spots, which is a normal variation of hyperpigmentation seen in newborns (Jarvis & MacDonald-Jenkins, 2014a). Canadians of Indigenous, African, or South Asian ancestry may be more likely to exhibit the signs and symptoms of high blood pressure or diabetes (Jarvis & MacDonald-Jenkins, 2014b). Providing culturally competent care leads to greater patient satisfaction and improved clinical outcomes (Galanti, 2014).

Purposes of Physical Examination

Examinations are designed to address the patient's needs. In an acutely ill patient, the nurse assesses only the involved body system(s). When a patient who has asthma is having an acute episode with difficulty breathing, the nurse initially focuses on assessing the pulmonary and cardiac systems. Then a more comprehensive examination about the patient's total health status is completed when the patient is physiologically more stable. Commonly, a complete physical examination is performed for routine screening to promote wellness behaviours and preventive health care measures, such as the annual medical exam. Additionally, a complete medical exam is often required to determine eligibility for extended health insurance, military service, or a specialized driver's license; as a pre-employment medical exam for a new job; with initiating care by a new practitioner; for a presurgical assessment; and for the admission process to a hospital or long-term care facility.

A complete physical examination provides valuable information for all members of the patient's interprofessional health care team. Thorough examination and documentation contribute to the following essential elements for comprehensive evidence-informed care:

- Gather baseline data about the patient's health history and present status
- Supplement, confirm, or refute data obtained in the history
- Confirm and identify nursing diagnoses

- Make clinical judgements about a patient's changing health status and management
- Evaluate the outcomes of care

To assist in learning about the physical assessment of body systems, it is helpful to review anatomy and physiology. There are many anatomy and physiology textbooks available that will assist you in the identification of the structures and functions of the human body and interconnectedness of the physiological systems. For example, to conduct an assessment of cranial nerves, it is important to develop an understanding of the function of each nerve and the motor and sensory pathways innervated by these nerves.

Gathering a Health History

The main objective of interacting with patients is to find out what their concerns are and to help them find solutions. As a nurse you must pay close attention to a patient's concerns. Direct the interview and examination so that you can create a clear picture of the patient's condition. The collection of health history and physical examination data requires patience and a dedication to thoroughness and detail. Conducting a successful interview and physical examination is based on several principles, relational practice being foremost (see Chapters 9, 13, and 17). The interview allows for the formation of a partnership with the patient. Orient the interview to the patient, not to a disease. For example, a patient is not a "diabetic"; rather he or she is "a person who has diabetes." Make sure you know your own idiosyncrasies (e.g., wanting to be liked, fear of catching a disease) so you are able to prevent these feelings from affecting the therapeutic relationship you will develop with the patient.

Developing Nursing Diagnoses and a Care Plan

After gathering information about the patient's health from the health history, a subsequent physical assessment can reveal information that refutes, confirms, or supplements the history. As a nurse you need to think critically about the information the patient provides, apply knowledge from previous clinical care, and methodically conduct the examination to create a clear picture of the patient's health status. For example, if a patient complains of back pain, ask the patient several questions to clarify the nature of the pain. During the examination, look carefully for the source of the pain (e.g., discomfort when changing position or a bruise across the patient's back) to rule out a variety of potential conditions (e.g., back strain, contusions, trauma, scoliosis). It is important to remember that one assessment finding (e.g., back pain) does not conclusively reveal the nature of an abnormality. A complete assessment is necessary to form a definitive nursing or medical diagnosis. Grouping significant findings into clusters of data assists in revealing actual or "risk for" nursing diagnoses (see Chapter 13). In addition, each abnormal finding suggests the need to gather additional information.

Information gathered during the initial history and physical assessment provides a baseline for the patient's functional abilities. This baseline is a record of findings identified when the patient was first assessed that can be used as a comparison for future assessment findings. Thus, the comprehensiveness and attention to detail in the documentation enable the nurse and others to determine changes in a patient's condition during subsequent assessments.

The accuracy of the database allows for the development of an individualized nursing diagnosis. Physical assessment findings determine the etiology of the diagnosis so that the selection of interventions is appropriate for the care plan. It is important to view physical assessment as an ongoing process; thus the care plan changes with changes in the patient's condition. Ongoing monitoring of the patient's progress and responses to therapies and treatments necessitate a review of the nursing diagnoses and plan of care as health conditions resolve or deteriorate, and when new health problems arise.

Managing Patient Problems

When caring for patients, the nurse assesses and performs a variety of interventions. Yet the nurse's success in giving care depends on the ability to recognize a change in status and to modify interventions so that patients gain the most desirable outcomes. Physical assessment skills enable nurses to judge the status of patients' health and direct the management of care. For example, the nurse inspects the skin during a routine bath and finds it excessively dry. The nurse does not use soap, and applies body lotion to the skin. The nurse revises the written care plan so that other nurses know the type of skin care to provide and instructs the patient about skin care. Performing the mechanics of physical assessment is relatively simple. The more difficult challenge lies in using findings to make decisions.

Evaluating Nursing Care

Nurses demonstrate accountability for their nursing care through evaluating the results of nursing interventions. Physical assessment skills enhance the evaluation of nursing measures through monitoring physiological and behavioral outcomes of care. Nurses use physical assessment skills to assess a condition (e.g., palpation of the patient's pulse) and evaluate a patient's response to care (e.g., an evaluation of a patient's tolerance to an exercise plan). Accurate, detailed, objective documentation of measurements through physical assessment assists in determining whether the expected outcomes of care are met.

SKILLS OF PHYSICAL ASSESSMENT

A comprehensive physical examination involves the use of five skills: inspection, palpation, percussion, auscultation, and olfaction.

Inspection

Inspection is the use of vision and hearing to distinguish normal from abnormal findings. It is important to know what to consider normal for patients of different age groups. Nurses need experience to recognize normal variations among patients. Inspection is a simple technique that can provide valuable clues about a patient's health status. The quality of an inspection depends on the nurse's willingness to spend time doing a thorough job. To inspect body parts accurately, follow these principles:

- Make sure adequate lighting is available.
- Position and expose body parts so all surfaces can be viewed.
- Inspect each area for size, shape, colour, symmetry, position, drainage, and abnormalities.
- When possible, compare each area inspected with the same area on the opposite side of the body.
- Use additional light (e.g., a penlight) to inspect body cavities.
- Do not hurry inspection. Pay attention to detail.

After inspection of a body part, findings sometimes indicate the need for further examination. Palpation should be used with or after visual inspection.

Palpation

Palpation involves the use of the hands to touch body parts to make sensitive assessments. Palpation is used to examine all accessible parts of the body. For example, the skin is palpated for temperature, moisture, texture, turgor, tenderness, and thickness. The abdomen is palpated for tenderness, **distension** (swelling), or masses. Different parts of the hand are used to detect characteristics such as texture, temperature, and perception of movement (Table 32-1).

TABLE 32-1 Examples of Characteristics Measured by Palpation

Area Examined	Criteria Measured	Portion of Hand to Use
Skin	Temperature	Dorsum of hand/fingers
	Moisture	Palmar surface
	Texture	Palmar surface/pads of fingertips
	Turgor and elasticity	Grasping with fingertips
	Tenderness	Palmar surface/pads of fingertips
	Thickness	Palmar surface/pads of fingertips
Organs (e.g., liver and intestine)	Size	Entire palmar surface of hand or palmar surface of fingers
	Shape	Palmar surface/pads of fingertips
	Tenderness	Entire palmar surface of hand or palmar surface of fingers
	Absence of masses	Palmar surface/pads of fingertips
Glands (e.g., thyroid and lymph)	Swelling	Pads of fingers
	Symmetry and mobility	Palmar surface/pads of fingertips
Blood vessels (e.g., carotid or femoral artery)	Pulse amplitude	Palmar surface/pads of fingertips
	Elasticity	
	Rate	
	Rhythm	
Thorax	Excursion	Palmar surface
	Tenderness	Finger pads/palmar surface of fingers
	Fremitus	Palmar or ulnar surface of entire hand

Palpation is conducted as follows: Before palpation, help the patient relax and be comfortable because muscle tension during palpation impairs effective assessment. To promote relaxation, have the patient take slow, deep breaths and place the arms along the side of the body. *Palpate tender areas last.* Be sure to ask the patient to point out the more sensitive areas. Watch the patient's facial expressions and body movements and note any nonverbal signs of discomfort.

Palpation requires warm hands, short fingernails, and a gentle approach. Perform palpation slowly, gently, and deliberately. Light, intermittent pressure is best when palpating; heavy, prolonged pressure causes a loss of sensitivity in the hand. To avoid injuring a patient, do not attempt deep palpation without clinical supervision. Caution is the rule. Use the most sensitive parts of the hand, the palmar surface of the fingers and finger pads, to determine position, texture, size, consistency, masses, fluid, and crepitus. Measure temperature using the dorsal surface or back of the hand. The ulnar surface of the hand and finger is more sensitive to vibration. Measure position, consistency, and turgor by lightly grasping the body part with the fingertips.

Do not palpate without considering the patient's condition. For example, if the patient has a fractured rib, use extra care to locate the painful area. Do not palpate a vital artery with pressure that obstructs blood flow. Also consider the body area being palpated, as well as the reason for using palpation.

Percussion

Percussion involves tapping the body with the fingertips to produce a vibration that travels through body tissues. The character of the sound determines the location, size, and density of underlying structures to verify abnormalities assessed by palpation and auscultation. This vibration is transmitted through body tissues, and the character of the sound heard depends on the density of the underlying tissue. By knowing the way various densities influence sound, the nurse locates organs or masses, maps their boundaries, and determines their size. An abnormal sound suggests a mass or substance such as air or fluid within an organ or body cavity. The skill of percussion requires dexterity and is usually used by advanced practitioners.

Auscultation

Auscultation involves listening to sounds the body makes to detect variations from normal. Some sounds can be heard without assistance, but most will require a stethoscope.

First, learn the normal sounds created by the cardiovascular, respiratory, and gastrointestinal (GI) systems, such as the passage of blood through an artery. Recognize abnormal sounds after learning normal variations. To become more proficient in auscultation one needs to know the types of sounds each body structure makes and the location in which the sounds are heard best. Also, it is good to learn which areas do not normally emit sounds.

To auscultate correctly, the nurse needs to hear well, have a good stethoscope, and know how to use it properly. For those with a hearing disorder, a stethoscope with greater sound amplification should be used. The stethoscope is always placed directly on the skin, because clothing obscures sound. Chapter 30 describes the parts of the stethoscope and general use. The bell is best for low-pitched sounds, such as vascular and certain heart sounds, and the diaphragm is best for high-pitched sounds, such as bowel and lung sounds.

Be familiar with the stethoscope before attempting to use it. Practise using the stethoscope. Extraneous sounds created by movement of the tubing or chest piece interfere with auscultation of body organ sounds. By deliberately producing these sounds, learn to recognize and disregard them during the actual examination.

Learn to recognize the following characteristics of sounds:

- Frequency, or the number of sound wave cycles generated per second by a vibrating object. The higher the frequency, the higher the pitch of a sound, and vice versa.
- Loudness, or the amplitude of a sound wave. Auscultated sounds are loud or soft.
- Quality, or sounds of similar frequency and loudness from different sources. Terms such as *blowing* or *gurgling* describe the quality of sound.
- Duration, or the length of time that sound vibrations last. The duration of sound is short, medium, or long. Layers of soft tissue dampen the duration of sounds from deep internal organs.

Auscultation requires concentration and practice. Always consider the part of the body auscultated and the cause of the sound. For example, closure of the mitral valve causes the first heart sound. Learn where to hear the sounds best. Typically, the first heart sound is heard best when auscultated at the left fifth intercostal space along the midclavicular line. It is also important to learn the characteristics of normal sounds. The first heart sound has the quality of a loud "lub," whereas the second sound is a "dub." After understanding the cause and character of normal auscultated sounds, it becomes easier to recognize abnormal sounds and their origins.

Olfaction

While assessing a patient, it is good to become familiar with the nature and source of body odours (Table 32-2). Olfaction helps in detecting abnormalities that cannot be recognized by any other means. For example, if a patient's cast has a sweet, heavy, thick odour, this indicates an underlying infection. Findings from olfaction and other assessment skills should prompt the nurses to investigate the origin of the odour as it may indicate abnormalities.

PREPARATION FOR EXAMINATION

Proper preparation of the environment, equipment, and patient ensures a smooth physical examination with few interruptions. A disorganized approach when preparing for a physical examination will cause errors and incomplete findings.

Infection Control

During an examination, some patients will present with open skin lesions or weeping wounds. Use standard precautions throughout the examination (see Chapter 33) as appropriate. It is necessary to wear gloves during palpation and percussion of patients presenting with open skin lesions or weeping wounds to reduce contact with microorganisms. If a patient has excessive drainage or risk of spray from a wound, wear a gown and other personal protective equipment as needed. Always use hand hygiene before initiating and after completing a physical assessment.

Environment

A physical examination requires privacy. A well-equipped examination room is preferable, but often the examination occurs in the patient's hospital or tertiary care room. In the home, nurses will often perform an examination in the patient's bedroom. Any examination room needs to be well equipped for all necessary procedures. Adequate lighting is necessary for proper illumination of body parts. Ideally, an examination room is soundproof so that patients feel comfortable discussing their conditions. The nurse needs to eliminate sources of noise, take precautions to prevent interruptions from others, and make sure the room is warm enough to maintain comfort.

Sometimes it is difficult to perform a complete examination when patients are in beds or on stretchers. Special examination tables make patients easily accessible and help them assume special positions. Patients need to be carefully assisted so that they do not fall while getting on and off the examination table. Do not leave a confused, combative, or uncooperative patient unsupervised on an examination table.

Examination tables are often hard and uncomfortable. When the patient lies supine, raise the head of the table about 30 degrees. Also give the patient a small pillow to use. When examining a patient in bed, raise the bed to reach the patient's body parts more easily. Remember to use proper body mechanics to ensure your physical safety and the safety of the patient while performing an exam (see Chapter 45).

Equipment

Before equipment preparation and the examination, perform thorough hand hygiene. Set up equipment so it is readily available and arranged in order for easy use. Keep equipment as warm as appropriate. Rub the diaphragm of the stethoscope briskly between the hands before applying it to the skin. If assisting with a vaginal exam, run warm water over the vaginal speculum just before using. The ophthalmoscope and otoscope require good batteries and light bulbs. Check all equipment to ensure that it functions properly. Box 32-1 lists typical assessment equipment used to perform a complete physical examination.

TABLE 32-2 Assessment of Characteristic Odours

Odour	Site or Source	Potential Causes
Alcohol	Oral cavity	Ingestion of alcohol, diabetes
Ammonia	Urine	Urinary tract infection, renal failure
Body odour	Skin, particularly in areas where body parts rub together (e.g., underarms and under breasts)	Poor hygiene, excess perspiration (hyperhidrosis), foul-smelling perspiration (bromhidrosis)
	Wound site	Wound abscess
	Vomitus	Abdominal irritation, contaminated food
Feces	Vomitus/oral cavity (fecal odour)	Bowel obstruction
	Rectal area	Fecal incontinence
Foul-smelling stools in infant	Stool	Malabsorption syndrome
Halitosis	Oral cavity	Poor dental and oral hygiene, gum disease
Sweet, fruity ketones	Oral cavity	Diabetic acidosis
Stale urine	Skin	Uremic acidosis
Sweet, heavy, thick odour	Draining wound	*Pseudomonas* (bacterial) infection
Musty odour	Casted body part	Infection inside cast
Fetid, sweet odour	Tracheostomy or mucous secretions	Infection of bronchial tree (*Pseudomonas* bacteria)

Physical Preparation of the Patient

The patient's physical comfort is vital for an accurate examination. Before starting, ask if the patient needs to use the restroom. An empty bladder and bowel facilitate examination of the abdomen, genitalia, and rectum. Collection of urine or fecal specimens occurs at this time if needed. Be sure to explain the proper method for collecting specimens, and label each specimen properly according to the policies of the receiving laboratory.

Physical preparation involves being sure the patient is dressed and draped properly. The patient in the hospital will likely be wearing only a simple gown. An outpatient will have to undress and wear a light cover gown. If the examination is limited to certain body systems, it is not always necessary for the patient to undress completely. The patient should be given privacy and plenty of time during undressing. Walking into the room as the patient undresses causes embarrassment. Drapes and gowns are made of linen or disposable paper. After patients have undressed and put on a gown, they sit or lie down on the examination table with the drape over the lap or lower trunk. Make sure the patient stays warm by eliminating drafts, controlling room temperature, and providing warm blankets. Routinely ask if the patient is comfortable.

BOX 32-1 Equipment and Supplies for Physical Assessment

- Cervical brush, broom, or spatula devices (if needed)
- Cotton applicators
- Disposable pad/paper towels
- Drapes
- Eye chart (e.g., Snellen chart)
- Flashlight and spotlight
- Forms (e.g., physical, laboratory)
- Gloves (sterile and clean)
- Gown for patient
- Ophthalmoscope
- Otoscope
- Papanicolaou (Pap) slides (labelled with patient information) and cytological fixative (if needed), or liquid cytology
- Percussion (reflex) hammer
- Pulse oximeter
- Ruler
- Scale with height measurement rod
- Specimen containers (e.g., tissue or urine samples)
- Sphygmomanometer and cuff
- Sterile swabs (e.g., for culture or viral collection)
- Stethoscope
- Tape measure
- Thermometer
- Tissues
- Tongue depressors
- Tuning fork
- Vaginal speculum (if needed)
- Water-soluble lubricant
- Wristwatch with second hand or digital display

Positioning. During the examination, ask the patient to assume proper positions so that body parts are accessible and the patient stays comfortable. Table 32-3 lists the preferred positions for each part of the examination and contains figures illustrating these positions. Patients' abilities to assume positions will depend on their physical strength, mobility, ease of breathing, age, and degree of wellness. Explain the positions, and assist patients in assuming them. Adjust the drapes so that the area examined is accessible, making sure not to unnecessarily expose a body part. A patient may assume more than one position. To decrease the number of times the patient changes positions, organize the examination so that all techniques requiring a sitting position are performed first, then perform those that require a supine position next, and so forth. It is important to use extra care when positioning older patients, because they are more prone to having disabilities and postural limitation.

Psychological Preparation of the Patient

Many patients find an examination stressful or tiring, or they experience anxiety about possible findings. A thorough explanation of the purpose and steps of each assessment lets patients know what to expect and what to do so that they can cooperate. Explanations should be kept simple and in understandable terms. As the examiner, you can help patients to feel free to ask questions and mention any discomfort. As each body system is examined, give a more detailed explanation. Convey an open, professional approach while remaining relaxed. A still, formal demeanour will inhibit the patient's ability to communicate, but a style that is too casual will fail to assure the patient (see Chapter 17, Communication).

When the patient and nurse are of opposite gender, it helps to have a third person of the patient's gender in the room. The presence of a third person assures the patient that the examiner will behave ethically. This person is also a witness to the examiner's conduct and the patient's.

During the examination, watch the patient's emotional responses. Observe whether the patient's facial expression shows fear or concern and if body movements show anxiety. Remain calm, and explain each step clearly. It is sometimes necessary to stop the examination and ask how the patient feels. Do not force the patient to continue. Postponing the examination is advantageous because the findings may be more accurate when the patient can cooperate and relax. If the patient's fears result from misconceptions, clarify the purpose of the examination and how you will perform it.

Assessment of Age Groups

It is necessary to use different interview styles and approaches to physical examination for patients of different age groups. When assessing children, the nurse must be sensitive and anticipate the child's reaction to the examination as a strange and unfamiliar experience. Routine pediatric examinations focus on health promotion and illness prevention, particularly for the care of well children who have no serious health problems (Perry, Hockenberry, Lowdermilk, et al., 2017). This examination focuses on growth and development, sensory screening, dental examination, and behavioural assessment. Children who are chronically ill or disabled, foster children, or adopted children sometimes require additional examination visits. When examining children, the following tips assist in data collection:

- Gather all or part of the histories on infants and children from parents or guardians.
- Perform the examination in a nonthreatening area; provide time for play to become acquainted.
- Because parents sometimes think the examiner is testing them, offer support during the examination and do not pass judgement.
- Call children by their first name, and address the parents as "Mr.," Mrs.," or "Ms." rather than by their first names.
- Use open-ended questions to allow parents to share more information and describe more of the children's problems. This also enables observation of parent–child interactions. Interview older children, who often provide details about their health history and severity of symptoms.
- Treat adolescents as adults and individuals because they tend to respond best when treated as such.
- Remember that adolescents have the right to confidentiality. After talking with parents about historical information, make an opportunity to speak alone with adolescents.

Pediatric (Box 32-2) and geriatric (Box 32-3) assessment tools are used to document and evaluate changes in health status. The Rourke assists in the examination of normal growth and development in children. In the geriatric population, a functional assessment, evaluation of activities of daily living, might determine the need for assistance in the home.

ORGANIZATION OF THE EXAMINATION

The complete physical examination is made up of assessments for each body system. Patients with specific symptoms or returning for follow-up care typically require a focused examination of specific body systems. For example, a patient who comes to a clinic with symptoms of a severe chest cold requires a focused assessment of the ears, nose,

TABLE 32-3 Positions for Examination

Position	Areas Assessed	Rationale	Limitations
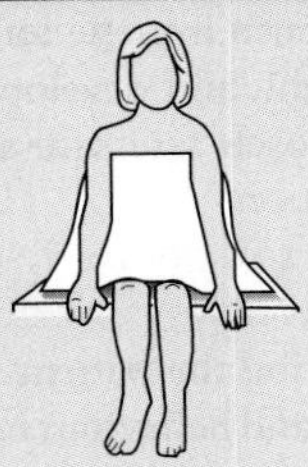 Sitting	Head and neck, back, anterior and posterior thorax and lungs, breasts, axillae, heart, vital signs, and upper extremities	Sitting upright provides full expansion of lungs and provides better visualization of symmetry of upper body parts.	A physically weakened patient is sometimes unable to sit. Use supine position with head of bed elevated instead.
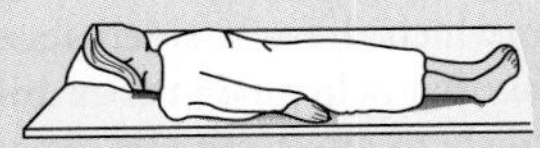 Supine	Head and neck, anterior thorax and lungs, breasts, axillae, heart, abdomen, extremities, pulses	This is the most normally relaxed position. It provides easy access to pulse sites.	If patient becomes short of breath easily, raise the head of bed.
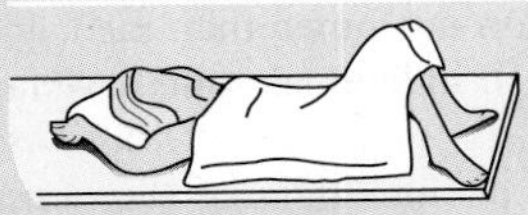 Dorsal recumbent	Head and neck, anterior thorax and lungs, breasts, axillae, heart, abdomen	Position is for abdominal assessment because it promotes relaxation of abdominal muscles.	Patients with painful disorders are more comfortable with knees flexed.
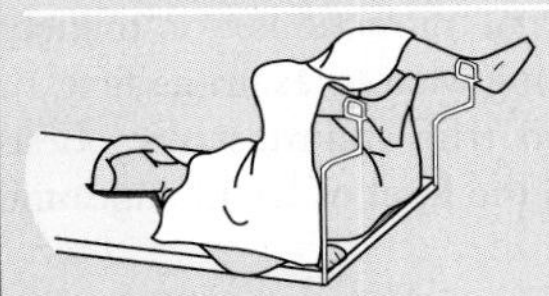 Lithotomy*	Female genitalia and genital tract	This position provides maximal exposure of genitalia and facilitates insertion of vaginal speculum.	Lithotomy position is embarrassing and uncomfortable, so examiner should minimize time that patient spends in it. Patient should be kept well draped.
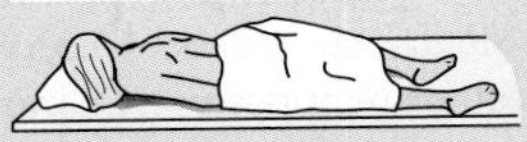 Sims'	Rectum and vagina	Flexion of hip and knee improves exposure of rectal area.	Joint deformities hinder patient's ability to bend hip and knee.
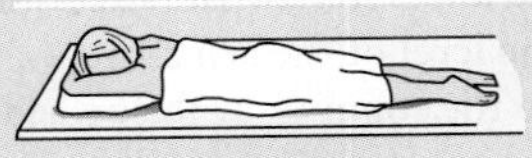 Prone	Musculoskeletal system	This position is only for assessing extension of hip joint, skin, buttocks.	Patients with respiratory difficulties do not tolerate this position well.
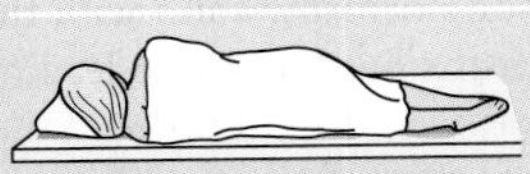 Left lateral recumbent	Heart	This position aids in detecting murmurs.	Patients with respiratory difficulties do not tolerate this position well.
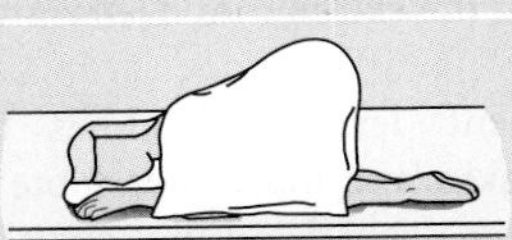 Knee–chest*	Rectum	This position provides maximal exposure of rectal area.	This position is embarrassing and uncomfortable.

*Some patients with arthritis or other joint deformities are unable to assume this position.

throat, respiratory and cardiovascular systems, but will not routinely require a neurological assessment. When a patient is admitted to the hospital, a complete examination is performed. A patient who is receiving a routine health promotion examination undergoes specific preventive screenings, depending on the patient's age or health risk (Table 32-4). Nurses need to use judgement to ensure that an examination involves assessment of relevant body systems and that the correct observations are documented.

The performance of a complete health assessment follows the format of the nursing history interview review of body systems. The nurse should obtain information from the history to focus attention on specific parts of the examination. Findings from the history generally reveal a pattern of related signs and symptoms. The physical examination supplements information from the history to confirm or refute the data.

Nurses need to be systematic and well organized about the examination so that they do not miss important assessment findings. A head-to-toe approach includes all body systems and helps to anticipate each step. In an adult, the examination begins by assessing the head and neck structures, including hair and skin, and progressing methodically down the body to incorporate all body systems. The following tips help keep an examination well organized:

- Compare both sides of the body for symmetry. A degree of asymmetry is normal (e.g., the biceps muscles in the dominant arm are

BOX 32-2 Developmental Assessment of Infants and Children

A good Canadian resource for the assessment of children is the Rourke Baby Record (Rourke, Leduc, & Rourke, 2014). This tool provides information about growth and developmental milestones for children from birth to 5 years of age. The tool combines helpful information on nutrition, child safety, and the childhood immunization schedule. A Rourke Baby Record can be downloaded free from the website http://www.rourkebabyrecord.ca/index.html. Information about the tool development and associated evidence is also accessible from this website. Additionally, infant and child growth charts for Canada can be accessed from the Canadian Paediatric Society website, with additional information for the use of these tools: http://www.cps.ca/tools-outils/who-growth-charts.

BOX 32-3 Geriatric Assessment Tools

A number of assessment tools are used with older persons to assess functional independence. Functional independence is the ability to perform basic personal care and activities and support independent living. Most often, functional assessment tools are used to assess older persons; however, younger individuals with spinal cord injuries or head injuries can be assessed using these tools as well.

Many screening tools are available that help nurses to assess an older person's independence in the home, or their level of functioning on return home from the hospital. Nurses who work with older persons should increase their knowledge about functional assessment tools. A good online resource for functional assessment tools can be found at Hartford Institute for Geriatric Nursing ConsultGeri https://consultgeri.org/try-this/general-assessment/issue-4. The Katz Index (Katz, Ford, Moskowitz, et al., 1963), although published a number of years ago, provides a simple screening evaluation of activities of daily living. Access to this tool is free from many sources online.

sometimes more developed than the same muscles in the nondominant arm).

- If a patient is seriously ill, first assess the systems of the body more at risk for being abnormal. For example, a patient with chest pain first undergoes a cardiovascular assessment.
- If a patient becomes fatigued, offer rest periods between assessments.
- Perform painful procedures near the end of the examination.
- Record assessments in specific terms on a physical assessment form or in the nurses' notes.
- Use common and accepted medical abbreviations to keep notes brief and concise.
- Record quick notes during the examination to avoid keeping the patient waiting. Complete any observations at the end of the examination.
- A physical assessment form allows the nurse to record information in the same sequence as it was gathered.

A guide for the performance of a complete physical assessment can be found in Jarvis and Luctkar-Flude's (2014a) chapter in Jarvis and colleagues' (2014) text. A good source of information on recording the history and physical exam can be found in a chapter by Ball, Dains, Flynn, et al. (2015b).

GENERAL SURVEY

Assessment begins when first meeting the patient. Determine the patient's reason for seeking health care. Initial data from the general survey begins with a review of the patient's primary health problems. Make mental notes of the patient's behaviour and appearance. Begin the examination with a general survey. The survey provides information about characteristics of an illness, a patient's hygiene and body image, emotional state, recent changes in weight, and developmental status. If there are abnormalities or problems, closely assess the affected body system later during the physical examination.

General Appearance and Behaviour

Assess appearance and behaviour while preparing the patient for the examination. The review of general appearance and behaviour includes the following:

- *Age and gender:* A person's gender and age affect the type of examination performed and the manner in which the assessments are made. Physical characteristics offer clues that help guide the examination. Certain conditions are more likely to affect individuals of a specific gender or who have certain physical characteristics; for example, breast cancer is more common in women than men, and the incidence of skin cancer is higher in individuals who have fair complexions.
- *Signs of distress:* There are sometimes obvious signs or symptoms indicating pain (grimacing, splinting painful area) or difficulty in breathing (shortness of breath, sternal retractions) or anxiety. These signs establish priorities regarding what to examine first.
- *Body type:* Observe if a patient appears trim and muscular, obese, or excessively thin. Body type reflects the level of health, age, and lifestyle.
- *Posture:* Normal standing posture is an upright stance with parallel alignment of the hips and shoulders. Normal sitting posture involves some degree of rounding of the shoulders. Observe whether the patient has a slumped, erect, or bent posture. Posture often reflects mood or pain. Many older people assume a stooped, forward-bent posture, with the hips and knees somewhat flexed and the arms bent at the elbows, raising the level of the arms.
- *Gait:* Observe the patient walking into the room or at the bedside (if the patient is ambulatory). Note whether movements are coordinated or uncoordinated. A person normally walks with the arms swinging freely at the sides, with the head and face leading the body.
- *Body movements:* Observe whether movements are purposeful, and note if there are any tremors involving the extremities. Determine if any body parts are immobile.
- *Hygiene and grooming:* Note the patient's level of cleanliness by observing the appearance of the hair, skin, and fingernails. Note if the patient's clothes are clean. Grooming depends on the activities being performed just before the examination, as well as the patient's occupation. Also note the amount and type of cosmetics used.
- *Dress:* Culture, lifestyle, socioeconomic level, and personal preference affect the type of clothes worn. Note if the type of clothing worn is appropriate for the temperature and weather conditions. Depressed or mentally ill individuals are often unable to choose proper clothing. An older person tends to wear extra clothing because of the sensitivity to cold.
- *Body odour:* An unpleasant body odour often results from physical exercise, poor hygiene, or certain disease states.
- *Affect and mood:* Affect is a person's feelings as they appear to others. Patients express mood or emotional state verbally and nonverbally. Note if verbal expressions match nonverbal behaviour. Observe if mood is appropriate for the situation. Observe facial expressions while asking questions.
- *Speech:* Normal speech is understandable and moderately paced. It shows an association with the person's thoughts. Note if the patient

TABLE 32-4 Recommended Preventive Screenings

Screening Measure	Ages 19–49	Ages 50–64	Ages 65+
Breast cancer	Screening may be considered in high-risk individuals (e.g., first-degree relative with *BRCA* gene)	Mammogram every 2–3 years	Mammogram every 2–3 years
Colon/rectal cancer	Screening may be considered in individuals at high risk (e.g., first-degree relative with colon/rectal cancer prior to age 50)	Fecal immunochemical test (FIT) or fecal occult blood test (FOBT) every 2 years or flexible sigmoidoscopy every 10 years	FIT or FOBT every 2 years or flexible sigmoidoscopy every 10 years until 75 years
Diabetes	Fasting blood glucose and/or HbA1c every 3 years in all individuals age 40 and older Fasting blood glucose and/or HbA1c every 3 years in people at higher risk for diabetes (i.e., CANRISK calculator) Screen individuals at high risk more often HbA1c screening not recommended during pregnancy or in children, adolescents, or those with suspected type I diabetes	Fasting blood glucose and/or HcA1c every 3 years Screen individuals at high risk more often	Fasting plasma glucose and/or HbA1c every 3 years Screen individuals at high risk more often
Vision	Every 2–5 years	Every 2–3 years	Every year
Lipid disorders	Ages 19–39: Screen based on risk assessment with lipid profile (blood test) Ages 40–49: Screen men and menopausal woman with lipid profile	Screen men and women with lipid profile	Screen based on risk assessment with lipid profile
Blood pressure	Measure blood pressure at each appropriate visit to primary care provider	Measure blood pressure at each appropriate visit to primary care provider	Measure blood pressure at each appropriate visit to primary care provider
Obesity/body mass index (BMI)	Height, weight, BMI and waist circumference every year	Height, weight, BMI and waist circumference every year	Height, weight, BMI and waist circumference every year
Oral cavity/ pharyngeal disorders	Dental exam every 6 months	Dental exam every 6 months	Dental exam every 6 months
Prostate cancer	Consider for individuals age 40 and older who are at high risk and with at least 10-year life expectancy, after discussing strengths and limits of available screening with patient. Recommended screening is annual prostate-specific antigen level (PSA) AND digital rectal exam (DRE)	Consider for individuals with at least 10-year life expectancy, after discussing strengths and limits of available screening with patient. Recommended screening is annual PSA and DRE	Consider for individuals with at least 10-year life expectancy, after discussing strengths and limits of available screening with patient. Recommended screening is annual PSA and DRE
Skin cancer	Routine self-exam and annual health care provider exam for those at high risk	Routine self-exam and annual health care provider exam for those at high risk	Routine self-exam and annual health care provider exam for those at high risk
Testicular cancer	Males age 15 and older: Regular testicular self-examination (TSE)	Regular TSE	Regular TSE
Cervical cancer	Sexually active women age 25 and older: Papanicolaou (Pap) test every 3 years if results are normal	Papanicolaou (Pap) test every 3 years if results are normal	Papanicolaou (Pap) test every 3 years if results are normal; stop at age 69 if three normal results in last 10 years
Osteoporosis		Screen those with history of previous fragility fracture or Osteoporosis Risk Assessment Instrument score ≥9 for bone mineral density with dual energy X-ray absorptiometry (DEXA)	Screen women and men age 65 and older not more than once every two years for bone mineral density with DEXA
Sexually transmitted infections	Gonorrhea, chlamydia, venereal disease research laboratory (VDRL) test, human immunodeficiency virus (HIV), and hepatitis B virus (HBV) if high risk or history of previous sexually transmitted infection (STI)	Gonorrhea, chlamydia, VDRL, HIV, and HBV if high risk or history of previous STI	Gonorrhea, chlamydia, VDRL, HIV, and HBV if high risk or history of previous STI
Domestic abuse/ intimate partner violence	Screen all women of child-bearing age for intimate partner violence and offer referral to intervention services for women who screen positive		

Based on Canadian Task Force on Preventive Health Care. (2016); Hypertension Canada (2015); Canadian Diabetes Association Clinical Practice Guidelines Expert Committee (2013); Shimizu, Bouchard, & Mavriplis (2016).

speaks rapidly or slowly. Emotions or neurological impairment sometimes cause an abnormal pace. Observe whether the patient speaks in a normal tone with clear inflection of words.

- *Patient abuse:* Abuse of children, women, and older persons is a growing health problem. Obvious physical injury or neglect are signs of possible abuse (e.g., evidence of malnutrition or presence of bruising on the extremities or trunk). Assess for the patient's fear of the spouse or partner, caregiver, parent, or adult child. Note if the partner or caregiver has a history of violence, alcoholism, or drug abuse. Is the person unemployed, ill, or frustrated in caring for the patient? Most provinces mandate a report to a social service agency if a health care provider suspects abuse or neglect (Box 32-4). During an assessment, if you suspect abuse, interview the patient in private. It is difficult to detect abuse, because victims often will not complain or report that they are in an abusive situation (Varcoe, 2014). Patients are more likely to reveal any problems when the suspected abuser is absent from the room.

Safety Alert The risk for further abuse is high once the victim has reported the abuse or tries to leave the abusive situation. Provide counselling options for these individuals.

- *Substance abuse:* Substance abuse affects all socioeconomic groups. A single visit to a clinic does not always reveal the problem. Several visits often reveal behaviours that nurses can confirm with a well-focused history and physical examination. The patient should be approached in a caring and nonjudgemental way, because issues of substance abuse involve both emotional and lifestyle issues. Box 32-5 lists characteristics of patients that may raise suspicion of substance abuse. When substance abuse is suspected, ask the patient the following CAGE questions (CAGE is an acronym for the following):
    - Have you ever felt the need to **C**ut down on your drinking or drug use?
    - Have people **A**nnoyed you by criticizing your drinking or drug use?
    - Have you ever felt bad or **G**uilty about your drinking or drug use?
    - Have you ever used or had a drink first thing in the morning as an **E**ye-opener to steady your nerves or feel normal?

BOX 32-4 Clinical Indicators of Abuse

Physical Findings	Behavioural Findings
Child Sexual Abuse	
Vaginal or penile discharge Blood on underclothing Pain, itching, or unusual odour in genital area Genital injuries Difficulty sitting or walking Pain while urinating; recurrent urinary tract infections Foreign bodies in rectum, urethra, or vagina Sexually transmitted infections Pregnancy in young adolescent	Problem in sleeping or eating Fear of certain people or places Play activities recreate the abuse situation Regressed behaviour Sexual acting out Knowledge of explicit sexual matters Preoccupation with others' or own genitals Profound and rapid personality changes Rapidly declining school performance Poor relationship with peers
Domestic Abuse	
Injuries and trauma are inconsistent with reported cause Multiple injuries involving head, face, neck, breasts, abdomen, and genitalia (black eyes, orbital fractures, broken nose, fractured skull, lip lacerations, broken teeth, strangulation marks) X-ray films show old and new fractures in different stages of healing Abrasions, lacerations, bruises/welts Burns Human bites	Attempted suicide Eating or sleeping disorders Anxiety Panic attacks Pattern of substance abuse (follows physical abuse) Low self-esteem Depression Sense of helplessness Guilt Increased forgetfulness Stress-related complaints (headache, anxiety)
Older Person Abuse	
Injuries and trauma are inconsistent with reported cause (cigarette burn, scratch, bruise, or bite) Hematomas Bruises at various stages of resolution Bruises, chafing, excoriation on wrist or legs (restraints) Burns Fractures inconsistent with cause described Dried blood	Dependent on caregiver Physically or cognitively impaired, or both Combative Wandering Verbally aggressive Minimal social support Prolonged interval between injury and medical treatment

Data from Perry, S. E., Hockenberry, M. J., Lowdermilk, D. L., Wilson, D., Sama, C., & Keenan-Lindsay, L. (Eds.). (2017). *Maternal Child Nursing Care in Canada* (2nd ed.). St. Louis, MO: Mosby; Varcoe, C. (2014). Interpersonal violence assessment. In C. Jarvis, A. J. Browne, J. MacDonald-Jenkins, & M. Luctkar-Flude (Eds.), *Physical examination and health assessment* (2nd Cdn. ed., pp. 120–137). Toronto: Elsevier Canada.

Vital Signs

Assessment of vital signs (see Chapter 30) is the first part of the physical examination.

Height and Weight

Height and weight reflect a person's general level of health. Weight is a routine measure during health screenings and clinical visits. Both measures are routine when patients are admitted to a health care setting. Health care providers measure an infant or child's height and weight to assess growth and development. In older persons, height and weight are usually coupled with a nutritional assessment to determine possible causes or contributions to the treatment of chronic diseases, or help to identify the older person who has difficulty with eating and other functional activities. It is important to look for overall trends in height and weight, as changes can be indicative of health problems.

Assessments screen for significant changes in weight. A patient's weight will normally vary daily because of fluid loss or retention. A downward trend in a frail older person indicates serious reduction in nutritional reserves. The nursing history helps to focus on possible causes for a change in weight (Table 32-5). When measuring a patient's height and weight, first ask the patient his or her current height and weight. Also assess for weight gains or losses. A weight gain of 2.3 kg (5 lb) in a day indicates fluid retention problems. If the patient has lost more than 5% of body weight in a month or 10% in 6 months, the loss is considered significant.

Body mass index (BMI) tables are used to help determine the normal expected weight range for a patient at a given height (Figure 32-1). With the BMI, waist circumference of adults is used to measure the health risk associated with obesity. A patient's waist is measured midway between the costal margin and the iliac crest. Measurement should be taken to the nearest 0.5 cm at the end of expiration. The tape measure should fit snugly but should not compress soft tissue. Locating the intersection of the patient's height and weight on the BMI table will indicate the patient's BMI. The risk for health problems based on this value can be assessed using the BMI categories. Patients at high risk should be encouraged to seek the care of a health care practitioner for weight loss, dietary changes, and exercise programs.

Patients should always be weighed at the same time of day, on the same scale, and in the same clothes to allow an objective comparison of subsequent weights. Accuracy of weight measurement is important because health care providers will base medical and nursing decisions (e.g., drug dosage determinations, lifting, and positioning) on changes. Patients capable of bearing their own weight use a standing scale. A standard platform scale is calibrated by moving the large and small weights to zero. When measuring a patient's weight, make the balance beam level and steady by adjusting the calibrating knob. The patient stands on the scale platform and remains still. Move the largest weight to the 22.5 kg increment under the patient's weight. Then adjust the smaller weight to balance the scale at the nearest 0.1 kg. Electronic scales automatically display the weight within seconds. Electronic scales are automatically calibrated each time they are used.

Stretcher and chair scales are available for patients unable to bear weight. After the patient is transferred to the scale, a hydraulic device lifts the patient above the bed and measures the weight on a balance beam or digital display. Use caution when transferring patients to and from the scales.

Infants should always be weighed in baskets or on platform scales. To weigh the infant, remove the infant's clothing, and weigh the infant in dry, disposable diapers. Adjust the measurement later for the weight of the diaper, ensuring an accurate reading. Keep the room warm to prevent chills. A light cloth or paper placed on the scale's surface prevents cross-infection from urine or feces. When placing infants in baskets or on platforms, hold a hand lightly above to prevent accidental falls. An infant's weight is measured in grams.

To measure the height of weight-bearing patients, have them remove their shoes. A measuring stick or tape is attached vertically to the weight scales or wall. Have the patient stand erect. The platform scale has a metal rod attached to the back of the scale; this swings out and over the crown of the head. When a scale is unavailable, you can also place a measuring stick or flat book on the head. With the rod or stick placed level horizontally at a 90-degree angle to the measuring stick, measure the patient's height in centimetres.

Remove the shoes of a non–weight-bearing patient, and position the patient (such as an infant) supine on a firm surface. Portable

BOX 32-5 Red Flags for Suspicion of Substance Abuse

- Patients who frequently miss appointments
- Patients who frequently request written excuses for absence from work
- Patients who have chief complaints of insomnia, "bad nerves," or pain that does not fit a particular pattern
- Patients who often report lost prescriptions (e.g., tranquilizers or pain medications) or ask for frequent refills
- Patients who make frequent emergency department visits
- Patients who have a history of changing health care providers or who bring in medication bottles prescribed by several different providers
- Patients with a history of gastrointestinal bleeds, peptic ulcers, pancreatitis, cellulitis, or frequent pulmonary infections
- Patients with frequent sexually transmitted infections (STIs), complicated pregnancies, multiple abortions, or sexual dysfunction
- Patients who complain of chest pains or palpitations or who have a history of admissions to rule out myocardial infarctions
- Patients who give histories of activities that place them at risk for human immunodeficiency virus (HIV) infection (multiple partners, multiple rapes)
- Patients with a family history of addiction; history of childhood sexual, physical, or emotional abuse; or social and financial or marital problems
- If two or more of the CAGE questions are positive, strongly suspect substance abuse and consider how to motivate the patient to seek treatment.

Data from American Psychiatric Association. (2013). *Diagnostic and statistical manual of mental disorders* (5th ed.). Washington, DC: Author; Reis, R. K., Fiellin, D. A., Miller, S. C., & Saitz, R. (Eds.). (2014). *The ASAM principles of addiction medicine* (5th ed.). Philadelphia, PA: Lippincott Williams & Wilkins.

TABLE 32-5 Nursing History for Weight Assessment

Assessment Category	Rationale
Ask about total weight lost or gained; compare with usual weight; note time period for loss (e.g., gradual, sudden, desired, or undesired).	Determines severity of problem and reveals if weight change is related to disease process, change in eating pattern, or pregnancy.
If weight loss is desired, ask about eating habits, diet plan followed, food preparation, calorie intake, appetite, exercise pattern, support group participation, weight goal.	Aids in determining appropriateness of diet plan followed.
If weight loss is undesired, ask about anorexia, vomiting, diarrhea, thirst, frequent urination, and change in lifestyle, activity, and stress levels.	Focuses on problems that cause weight loss (e.g., gastrointestinal problems).
Assess if patient has noted changes in social aspects of eating: more meals in restaurants, rushing to eat meals, stress at work, or skipping meals.	Lifestyle changes sometimes contribute to weight changes.
Assess if patient takes chemotherapy, diuretics, insulin, fluoxetine, prescription and nonprescription appetite suppressants, laxatives, oral hypoglycemics, and herbal supplements (weight loss); steroids, oral contraceptives, antidepressants, insulin (weight gain).	Weight gain or loss is an adverse effect of these medications.
Assess for preoccupation with body weight or body shape, such as with fasting, never feeling thin enough, unusually strict caloric intake or restrictions, laxative abuse, induced vomiting, amenorrhea, excessive exercise, excessive alcohol intake.	Indicates an eating disorder.

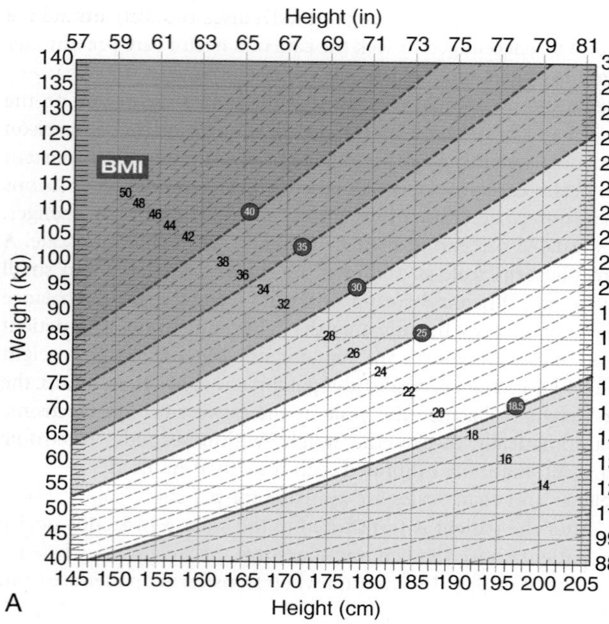

A

Waist circumference	BMI category: Normal 18.5–24.9 kg/m²	Overweight 25–29.9 kg/m²	Obese class I 30–34.9 kg/m²
Men: < 102 cm Women: < 88 cm	Least risk	Increased risk	High risk
Men: ≥ 102 cm Women: ≥ 88 cm	Increased risk	High risk	Very high risk

B

FIGURE 32-1 Height and weight measures: Weights for people over 18 years (excluding pregnant or lactating women).

- Weight and height are required to measure a person's body mass index (BMI), which is calculated by dividing weight (kg) by height squared (m^2).
- Weight is measured with the patient wearing light clothing and no footwear and is recorded to the nearest 0.2 kg.
- Height is measured with the person wearing no shoes, standing in an erect position, looking straight ahead with feet together and heels against a wall or measuring board. A horizontal bar or other similar device should be lowered so that it rests flat on top of the person's head. Height is recorded to the nearest 0.5 cm.
- For a quick determination of BMI, use a straight-edge to help locate the point on the chart below where height and weight intersect. Read the number on the dashed line closest to this point. For example, a person who weighs 69 kg and is 173 cm tall has a BMI of about 23.

NOTE: The BMI cannot be used to distinguish between increased body weight due to adiposity or fluid retention (e.g., peripheral edema), although this distinction should be apparent clinically. The BMI may have limitations in people who are very muscular or very lean, in those who are very tall or very short, in people with long limb lengths relative to trunk size (e.g., those with Marfan syndrome), and in people with short limb lengths relative to trunk size (e.g., those with achondroplasia). (**A,** Health Canada [2016]. *Canadian guidelines for body weight classification in adults* [Catalogue no. H49-179/2003E; p. 37]. Ottawa: Health Canada. Retrieved from http://www.hc-sc.gc.ca/fn-an/nutrition/weights-poids/guide-ld-adult/cg_quick_ref-ldc_rapide_ref-eng.php. **B,** Douketis, J. D., Paradis, G., Keller, H., & Martineau, C. [2005]. Canadian guidelines for body weight classification in adults: Application in clinical practice to screen for overweight and obesity and assess disease risk. *Canadian Medical Association Journal, 172*[8], 995–998.)

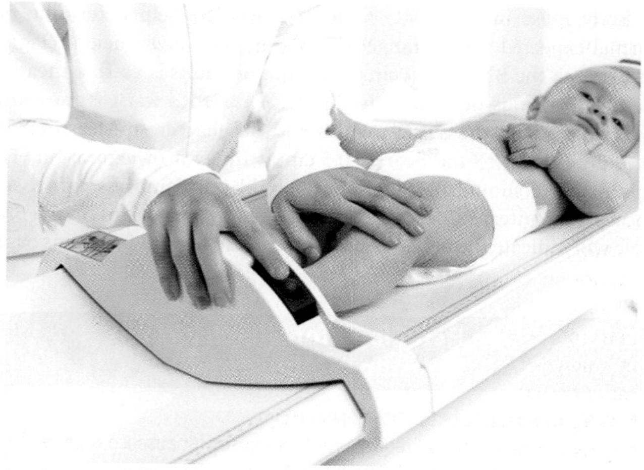

FIGURE 32-2 Measurement of infant length. (From Ball, J. W., Dains, J. E., Flynn, J. A., Solomon, B. S., & Stewart, R. W. [2015]. *Seidel's guide to physical examination* [8th ed., p. 84]. St. Louis, MO: Mosby. Courtesy seca GmbH, Hamburg, Germany.)

devices are available that provide a reliable means to measure height. Place the infant on the device, having the parent hold the infant's head against the headboard. With the infant's legs straight at the knees, place the footboard against the bottom of the infant's feet (Figure 32-2). Record the infant's length to the nearest 0.5 cm.

THE INTEGUMENTARY SYSTEM: SKIN, HAIR, AND NAILS

The **integument** consists of the skin, hair, scalp, and nails. Developing a routine approach to physical assessment helps to ensure the completeness of your exam. The approach to patient assessment might begin with the inspection of all skin surfaces. Alternatively, as your assessment skills develop, you may choose to assess the skin gradually while examining other body systems (e.g., inspecting the skin of the torso while assessing the respiratory, cardiovascular, and abdominal systems). Use the skills of inspection, palpation, and olfaction to assess the integument's function and integrity.

Skin

Assessment of the skin reveals changes in oxygenation, circulation, nutrition, local tissue damage, and hydration. In a hospital setting, the majority of patients are older persons, debilitated patients, or young and seriously ill patients. There are significant risks for skin lesions resulting from trauma to the skin during administration of care, from exposure to pressure during immobilization, or from reaction to various medications used in treatment. Patients at high risk are persons who are neurologically impaired or chronically ill, and orthopedic patients. Others at risk are patients with diminished mental status, poor tissue oxygenation, low cardiac output, or inadequate nutrition. In nursing homes and extended-care facilities, patients are often at risk for many of the same problems, depending on their level of mobility and the presence of chronic illness. It is important to routinely assess the skin for development of primary or initial lesions. Without proper care, primary lesions can deteriorate to become secondary lesions that require more extensive nursing care. The development of a pressure ulcer for example, will lengthen a hospital stay unless the nurse prevents or discovers it early and treats it properly (see Chapter 46).

In 2016, it was estimated that approximately 6 800 new cases of **melanoma**, an aggressive form of skin cancer, were diagnosed and that

12 000 Canadians would die from melanoma (Canadian Cancer Society [CCS] Steering Committee, 2017). Cutaneous malignancies are the most common neoplasms seen in patients. It is thus important to incorporate a thorough skin assessment on all patients and to educate them about self-examination (Box 32-6).

The condition of the patient's skin reveals the need for nursing intervention. Use assessment findings to determine the type of hygiene measures required to maintain integrity of the integument (see Chapter 38). Adequate nutrition and hydration become goals of therapy if an alteration in the integument's status is identified (see Chapter 42).

To accurately observe a patient's skin, adequate lighting is required. The recommended choice is natural or halogen lighting. For detecting skin changes in the dark-skinned patient, sunlight is the best choice (Marks & Miller, 2014). Room temperature also affects skin assessment. A room that is too warm causes superficial vasodilation, resulting in an increased redness of the skin. A cool environment causes the sensitive patient to develop cyanosis (bluish discoloration) around the lips and nail beds.

Use disposable gloves for palpation if open, moist, or draining lesions are present. Although each part of the body is inspected during an examination, it is helpful to make a brief but careful overall visual sweep of the entire body. This provides a good assessment of the distribution and extent of any lesions, as well as the overall symmetry of skin colour. Because you need to inspect all skin surfaces, the patient will assume several positions. Table 32-6 outlines the nursing history for skin assessment. If you notice abnormalities during an examination, palpate the involved areas. Skin odours are usually apparent in the folds of the skin, such as the axillae or under the female patient's breasts.

Colour. Skin colour varies from body part to body part and from person to person. Despite individual variations, skin colour is usually uniform over the body. Table 32-7 lists common variations. Normal

BOX 32-6 PATIENT TEACHING

Skin Assessment

Objectives

- Patient will perform a monthly self-examination of the skin.
- Patient will identify factors that increase the risk of skin cancer.
- Patient will follow hygiene practices aimed at maintaining skin integrity.

Teaching Strategies

- Instruct patient to conduct a complete monthly self-examination of all skin surfaces, noting moles, blemishes, and birthmarks. Cancerous melanomas start as small, molelike growths that increase in size, change colour, become ulcerated, and bleed (see Box 32-8).
- Tell patient to report any change in skin lesions, lesion that bleeds or fails to heal, or a sore that does not heal to a health care provider. Especially instruct older persons, who tend to have delayed wound healing.
- To treat excessively dry skin, patient should avoid hot water, harsh soaps, and drying agents such as rubbing alcohol. Tell patient to use a superfatted (Dove) soap, and pat rather than rub the skin after bathing.
- Instruct patient to apply moisturizers (mineral oil) to the skin regularly to reduce itching and drying, and wear cotton clothing (Marks & Miller, 2014).

Evaluation

- Observe patient performing a skin assessment.
- Have the patient describe signs of skin cancer and measures to take to prevent skin cancer.
- Ask the patient to describe methods for keeping the skin lubricated and supple.

TABLE 32-6 Nursing History for Skin Assessment

Assessment Category	Rationale
Ask patient about history of changes in the skin: dryness, pruritus, sores, rashes, lumps, colour, texture, odour, lesion that does not heal.	Patient is the best source to recognize change. Usually skin cancer is first noticed as a localized change in skin colour.
Consider if the patient has the following history: fair, freckled, ruddy complexion; light-coloured hair or eyes; tendency to burn easily.	Characteristics are risk factors for skin cancer.
Determine whether patient works or spends excessive time outside. If so, ask whether patient wears sunscreen, other protective clothing, or both.	Exposed areas such as face and arms will be more pigmented than rest of body. The Canadian Task Force on Preventive Health Care (2016) recommends use of sunscreen and protective clothing.
Determine whether patient has noted lesions, rashes, or bruises.	Most skin changes do not develop suddenly. Change in character of lesion possibly indicates cancer. Bruising indicates trauma or bleeding disorder.
Question patient about frequency of bathing and type of soap used.	Excessive bathing and use of harsh soaps cause dry skin.
Ask if patient has had recent trauma to skin.	Some injuries cause bruising and changes in skin texture.
Determine whether patient has history of allergies.	Skin rashes commonly occur from allergies.
Ask if patient uses topical medications or home remedies on skin.	Incorrect use of topical agents causes inflammation or irritation.
Ask if patient goes to tanning parlours, uses sun lamps, or takes tanning pills.	Overexposure of skin to these irritants may cause skin cancer.
Ask if patient has family history of serious skin disorders such as skin cancer or psoriasis.	Family history may reveal information about patient's condition.
Determine if patient works with creosote, coal, tar, petroleum products, arsenic compounds, or radium.	Exposure to these agents creates risk for skin cancer.

TABLE 32-7 Skin Colour Variations

Colour	Condition	Causes	Assessment Locations
Bluish (cyanosis)	Increased amount of deoxygenated hemoglobin (associated with hypoxia)	Heart or lung disease, cold environment	Nail beds, lips, mouth, skin (severe cases)
Pallor (decrease in colour)	Reduced amount of oxyhemoglobin Reduced visibility of oxyhemoglobin resulting from decreased blood flow	Anemia Shock	Face, conjunctivae, nail beds, palms of hands Skin, nail beds, conjunctivae, lips
Loss of pigmentation	Vitiligo	Congenital or autoimmune condition causing lack of pigment	Patchy areas on skin over face, hands, arms
Yellow-orange (jaundice)	Increased deposit of bilirubin in tissues	Liver disease, destruction of red blood cells	Sclera, mucous membranes, skin
Red (erythema)	Increased visibility of oxyhemoglobin caused by dilation or increased blood flow	Fever, direct trauma, blushing, alcohol intake	Face, area of trauma, sacrum, shoulders, other common sites for pressure ulcers
Tan-brown	Increased amount of melanin	Suntan, pregnancy	Areas exposed to sun: face, arms, areolae, nipples

skin **pigmentation** ranges in tone from ivory or light pink to ruddy pink in light skin and from light to deep brown or olive in dark skin. In older persons, pigmentation increases unevenly, causing discoloured skin. While inspecting the skin, be aware that cosmetics or tanning agents sometimes mask colour.

The assessment of colour first involves areas of the skin not exposed to the sun, such as the palms of the hands. Note if the skin is unusually pale or dark. Areas exposed to the sun, such as the face and arms, will be darker. It is more difficult to note changes such as pallor or cyanosis in patients with dark skin tones. Usually colour hues are seen best in the palms, soles of the feet, lips, tongue, and nail beds. Areas of increased colour (hyperpigmentation) and decreased colour (hypopigmentation) are common. Skin creases and folds are darker than the rest of the body in the dark-skinned patient.

Inspect sites where you are able to identify abnormalities more easily. For example, you can see pallor more easily in the face, buccal (mouth) mucosa, conjunctiva, and nail beds. Observe for cyanosis in the lips, nail beds, palpebral conjunctivae, and palms. In recognizing pallor in the dark-skinned patient, observe that normal brown skin appears to be yellow-brown and normal black skin appears to be ashen grey. Also assess the lips, nail beds, and mucous membranes for generalized pallor; if pallor is present, the mucous membranes will be ashen grey. Assessment of cyanosis in the dark-skinned patient requires observation of areas where pigmentation occurs the least (conjunctiva, sclera, buccal mucosa, tongue, lips, nail beds, and palms and soles). In addition, verify these findings with clinical manifestations (Marks & Miller, 2014).

The best site to inspect for **jaundice** (yellow-orange discoloration) is the patient's sclera. Normal reactive hyperemia, or redness, can be seen most often in regions exposed to pressure, such as the sacrum, heels, and greater trochanter. Inspect for any patches or areas of skin colour variation. Localized skin changes, such as pallor or **erythema** (red discoloration), indicate circulatory changes. For example, an area of erythema is due to localized vasodilation resulting from a sunburn, inflammation, or fever. It is difficult to observe erythema in the dark-skinned patient, so palpate the area for heat and warmth to note the presence of skin inflammation (Jarvis et al., 2014). An area of an extremity that appears unusually pale results from arterial occlusion or edema. Be sure to ask if the patient has noticed any changes in skin colouring.

There is also a pattern of physical assessment findings of the skin that is indicative of substance abuse in some patients who are chemically dependent or are intravenous (IV) drug abusers (Table 32-8). It is sometimes difficult to recognize signs and symptoms after one examination. A patient who takes repeated IV injections has edematous, reddened, and warm areas along the arms and legs. This pattern suggests recent injections. Evidence of old injection sites appears as hyperpigmented and shiny or scarred areas.

TABLE 32-8 Physical Findings of the Skin Indicative of Substance Abuse

Body System	Commonly Associated Drug
Diaphoresis	Sedative hypnotic (including alcohol)
Spider angiomas	Alcohol, stimulants
Burns (especially fingers)	Alcohol
Needle marks	Opioids
Contusion, abrasions, cuts, scars	Alcohol, other sedative hypnotics
"Homemade" tattoos	Cocaine, intravenous (IV) opioids (prevents detection of injection sites)
Increased vascularity of face	Alcohol
Red, dry skin	Phencyclidine (PCP)

Data from Reis, R. K., Fiellin, D. A., Miller, S. C., & Saitz, R. (Eds.). (2014). *Principles of addiction medicine* (5th ed.). Philadelphia, PA: Lippincott Williams & Wilkins.

Moisture. The hydration of skin and mucous membranes helps to reveal body fluid imbalances, changes in the skin's environment, and regulation of body temperature. Moisture refers to wetness and oiliness. The skin is normally smooth and dry. Skin folds such as the axillae are normally moist. Minimal perspiration or oiliness is often present (Jarvis et al., 2014). Increased perspiration is sometimes associated with activity, warm environments, obesity, anxiety, or excitement. Use ungloved fingertips to palpate skin surfaces and observe for dullness, dryness, crusting, and flaking. Flaking is the appearance of flakes resembling dandruff when the skin surface is lightly rubbed. Scaling involves fishlike scales that are easily rubbed off the skin's surface. Both flaking and scaling indicate abnormally dry skin. Excessively dry skin is common in older persons and individuals who use excessive amounts of soap during bathing. Other factors causing dry skin include lack of humidity, exposure to sun, smoking, stress, excessive perspiration, and dehydration. Excessive dryness worsens existing skin conditions such as eczema and dermatitis.

Temperature. The temperature of the skin depends on the amount of blood circulating through the dermis. Increased or decreased skin temperature indicates an increase or decrease in blood flow. An increase in skin temperature often accompanies localized erythema or redness of the skin. A reduction in skin temperature reflects a decrease in blood flow. It is important to remember that if an examination room is cold, this will affect the patient's skin temperature and colour.

Accurately assess temperature by palpating the skin with the dorsum, or back of the hand. Compare symmetrical body parts. Normally the skin temperature is warm. Sometimes skin temperature is the same throughout the body, and other times it varies in one area. Always assess skin temperature for patients at risk of having impaired circulation, such as after a cast application or vascular surgery. A stage I pressure ulcer can be identified early by noting warmth and erythema on an area of the skin (see Chapter 46).

Texture. The character of the skin's surface and the feel of deeper portions are its texture. Determine whether the patient's skin is smooth or rough, thin or thick, tight or supple, and indurated (hardened) or soft by stroking it lightly with the fingertips. The texture of the skin is normally smooth, soft, even, and flexible in children and adults. However, the texture is usually not uniform throughout. The palms of the hand and soles of the feet tend to be thicker. With advancing age, the skin becomes wrinkled and leathery because of a decrease in collagen, subcutaneous fat, and sweat glands.

Localized changes result from trauma, surgical wounds, or lesions. When finding irregularities in texture such as scars or induration, ask the patient if a recent injury to the skin has occurred. Deeper palpation sometimes reveals irregularities such as tenderness or localized areas of induration commonly caused by repeated injections.

Turgor. Turgor is the skin's elasticity. Edema or dehydration diminishes turgor. Normally the skin loses its elasticity with age. To assess the skin turgor, grasp a fold of skin on the back of the forearm or sternal area with the fingertips and release. Normally the skin lifts easily and snaps back immediately to its resting position. The back of the hand is not the best place to test for turgor, because the skin is normally loose and thin (Ball et al., 2015a). The skin stays pinched when turgor is poor. Note the ease with which the skin moves and the speed at which it returns to place. Failure of the skin to reassume its normal contour or shape indicates dehydration. The patient with poor skin turgor does not have a resilience to the normal wear and tear on the skin. A decrease in turgor predisposes the patient to skin breakdown.

Vascularity. The circulation of the skin affects colour in localized areas and the appearance of superficial blood vessels. With aging, capillaries become fragile. Localized pressure areas, found after a patient has remained in one position, appear reddened, pink, or pale (see Chapter 46). Petechiae are pinpoint-sized, red or purple spots on the skin caused by small hemorrhages in the skin layers. Petechiae do not blanch but may indicate serious blood-clotting disorders, drug reactions, or liver disease.

Edema. Areas of the skin become swollen or edematous from a buildup of fluid in the tissues. Direct trauma and impairment of venous return are two common causes of edema. Inspect edematous areas for location, colour, and shape. The formation of edema separates the skin's surface from the pigmented and vascular layers, masking skin colour. Edematous skin also appears stretched and shiny. Palpate edematous areas to determine mobility, consistency, and tenderness. When pressure from the examiner's fingers leaves an indentation in the edematous area, it is called *pitting edema*. To assess the degree of pitting edema, press the edematous area firmly with the thumb for several seconds and release. The depth of pitting, recorded in millimetres, determines the degree of edema (Ball et al., 2015a). For example, 1+ edema equals a 2-mm depth, 2+ edema equals a 4-mm depth, 3+ equals 6 mm, and 4+ equals 8 mm (see Figure 32-40).

Lesions. The skin is normally free of lesions, except for common freckles or age-related changes such as skin tags, senile keratosis (thickening of skin), cherry angiomas (ruby-red papules), and atrophic warts. Lesions are primary (occurring as initial spontaneous manifestations of a pathological process), such as an insect bite, or secondary (resulting from later formation or trauma to a primary lesion), such as a pressure ulcer. When a lesion is detected, inspect it for colour, location, texture, size, shape, type, grouping (clustered or linear), and distribution (localized or generalized). Observe any exudate for colour, odour, amount, and consistency. Measure the size of the lesion by using a small, clear, flexible ruler divided in centimetres. Comparing a lesion with a household measure, such as a coin or eraser, is not reliable (Ball et al., 2015a). Measure lesions in height, width, and depth.

Palpation determines the lesion's mobility, contour (flat, raised, or depressed), and consistency (soft or indurated). Certain types of lesions present a characteristic pattern. For example, a tumour is usually an elevated, solid lesion larger than 1 cm. Primary lesions, such as macules and nodules, come from some stimulus to the skin (Box 32-7). Secondary lesions, such as ulcers, occur as alterations in primary lesions. Upon identifying a lesion, closely inspect it in good lighting. Palpate gently, covering the entire area of the lesion. If the lesion is moist or draining fluid, wear gloves during palpation.

Note if the patient complains of tenderness during palpation. Cancerous lesions frequently undergo changes in colour and size (Box 32-8). Basal cell carcinoma is most common in sun-exposed areas and frequently occurs in a background of sun-damaged skin; it almost never spreads to other parts of the body. Squamous cell carcinoma is more serious than basal cell and develops on the outer layers of sun-exposed skin; these cells may travel to lymph nodes and throughout the body. Report abnormal lesions to the health care provider for further examination.

Every nurse should be able to perform a complete examination of the skin and recognize abnormalities. Box 32-9 presents patient education that nurses should communicate while performing an examination of the integumentary system and in discussions about health screening.

> **Safety Alert** Individuals exposed to the sun through sunbathing or artificial means increase their risk for development of skin cancer. Provide appropriate teaching to inform patients of ways to decrease their risk (see Boxes 32-6 and 32-9).

Hair and Scalp

The following types of hair cover the body: terminal hair (long, coarse, thick hair easily visible on the scalp, axillae, pubic areas, and in the beard in men) and vellus hair (small, soft, tiny hairs covering the whole body except for the palms and soles). Inspecting the condition and distribution of hair and the integrity of the scalp requires good lighting.

Inspection. During inspection, explain that it is necessary to separate parts of the hair to detect abnormalities. If lesions or lice are probable, wear clean gloves to avoid infection. Table 32-9 describes the nursing history for assessment of the hair and scalp.

BOX 32-7 Types of Primary Skin Lesions

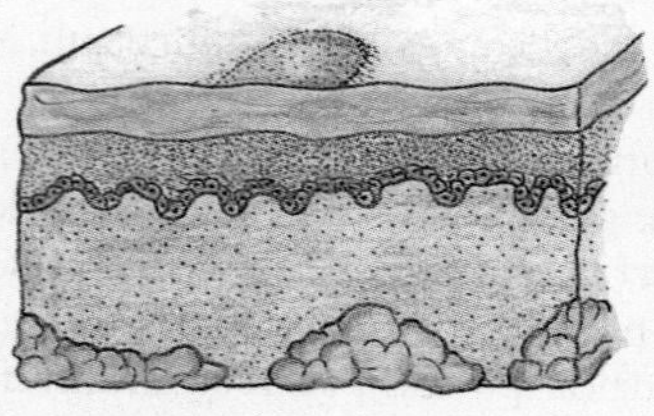

Macule: Flat, nonpalpable change in skin colour, smaller than 1 cm (e.g., freckle, petech)

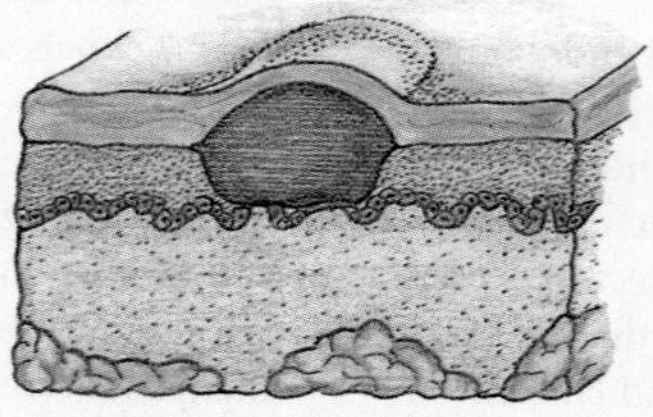

Papule: Palpable, circumscribed, solid elevation in skin, smaller than 1 cm (e.g., elevated nevus)

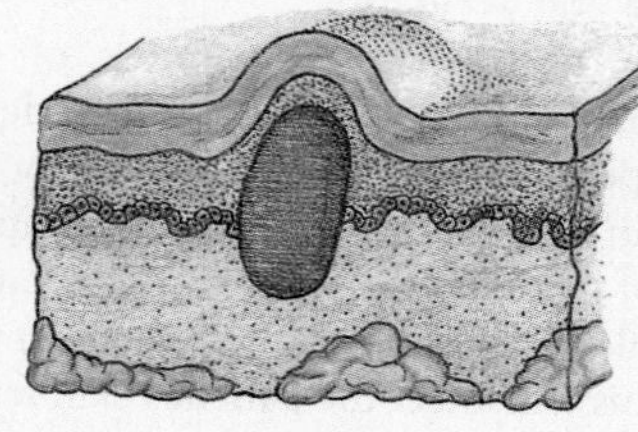

Nodule: Elevated solid mass, deeper and firmer than papule, 1–2 cm (e.g., wart)

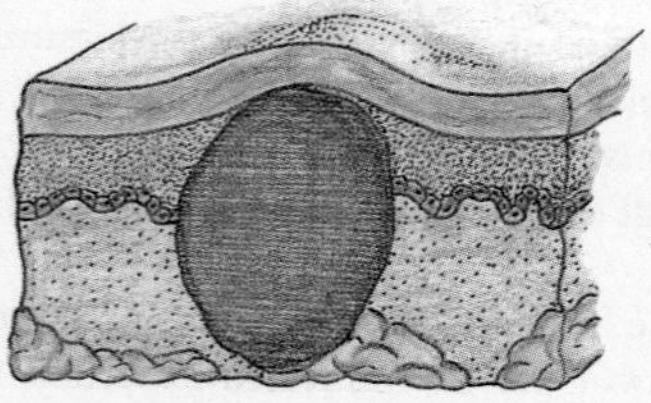

Tumour: Solid mass that extends deep through subcutaneous tissue, larger than 1–2 cm (e.g., epithelioma)

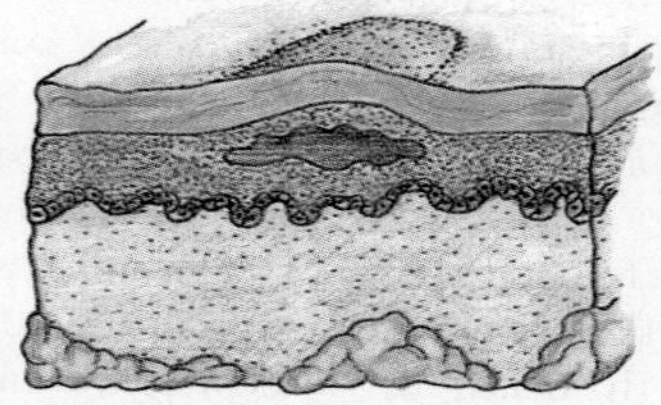

Wheal: Irregularly shaped, elevated area or superficial localized edema; varies in size (e.g., hive, mosquito bite)

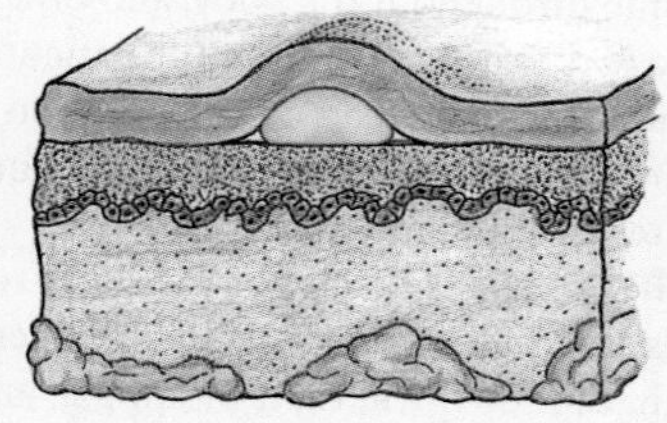

Vesicle: Circumscribed elevation of skin filled with serous fluid, smaller than 1 cm (e.g., herpes simplex, chicken pox)

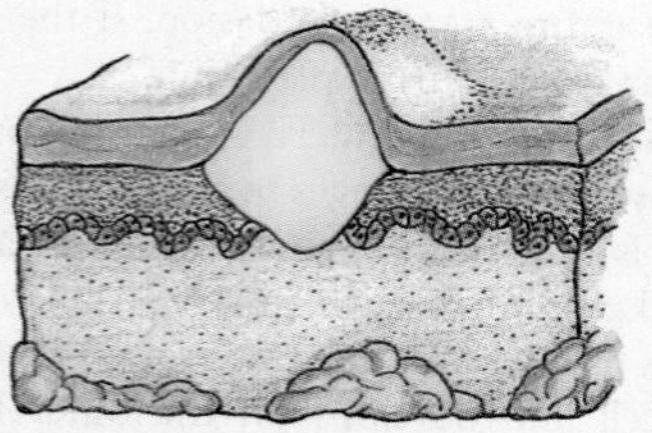

Pustule: Circumscribed elevation of skin similar to vesicle but filled with pus; varies in size (e.g., acne, staphylococcal infection)

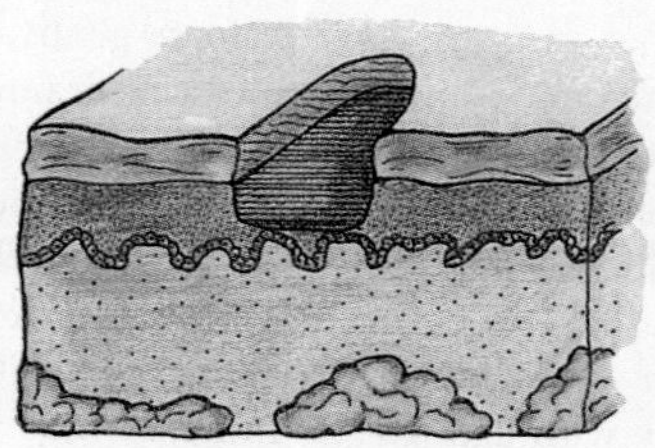

Ulcer: Deep loss of skin surface that extends to dermis and frequently bleeds and scars; varies in size (e.g., venous stasis ulcer)

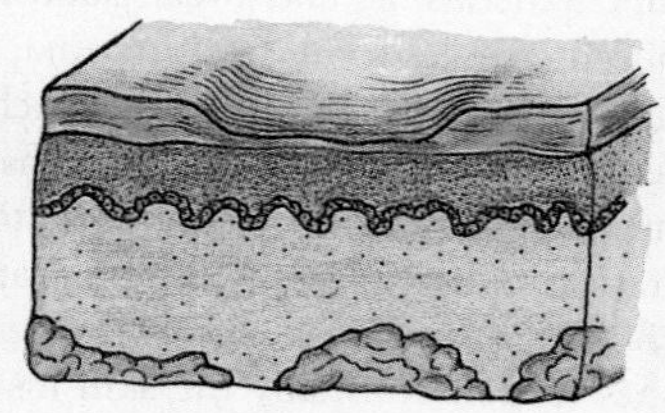

Atrophy: Thinning of skin with loss of normal skin furrow, with skin appearing shiny and translucent; varies in size (e.g., arterial insufficiency)

TABLE 32-9 Nursing History for Hair and Scalp Assessment

Assessment Category	Rationale
Ask patient if he or she is wearing a wig or hairpiece, and ask him or her to remove it.	Wigs or hairpieces interfere with inspection of hair and scalp. (Patient sometimes requests to omit this part of examination.)
Determine if patient has noted change in growth or loss of hair; change in texture or colour.	Change often occurs slowly over time.
Identify type of hair care products used for grooming.	Excessive use of chemical agents and burning of hair cause drying and brittleness.
Determine if patient has recently had chemotherapy (drugs that cause hair loss) or taken a vasodilator (minoxidil) for hair growth.	Chemotherapeutic agents kill cells that rapidly multiply, such as tumour cells and normal hair cells. Minoxidil causes excessive hair growth.
Has patient noted changes in diet or appetite?	Nutrition influences condition of hair.

First inspect the colour, distribution, quantity, thickness, texture, and lubrication of body hair. Scalp hair is coarse or fine; curly or straight; and should be shiny, smooth, and pliant. While separating sections of scalp hair, observe characteristics of colour and coarseness. Colour varies from very light blond to black to grey and sometimes shows alterations from rinses or dyes. In older persons, the hair becomes dull grey, white, or yellow. The hair also thins over the scalp, axillae, and pubic areas. Older men often lose facial hair, whereas some older women develop hair on the chin and upper lip.

Be aware of the normal distribution of hair growth in a man and a woman. At puberty, a change in the amount and distribution of hair

BOX 32-8 Skin Malignancies

Basal Cell Carcinoma

0.5- to 1.0-cm crusted lesion that is flat or raised and has a rolled, somewhat scaly border.

Frequently there are underlying, widely dilated blood vessels that appear within the lesion.

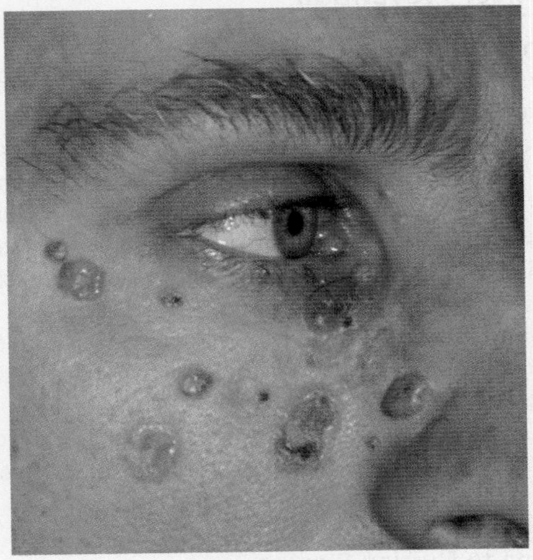

Basal cell carcinoma

Squamous Cell Carcinoma

Occurs more often on mucosal surfaces and nonexposed areas of skin, compared with basal cell.

0.5- to 1.5-cm scaly lesion is sometimes ulcerated or crusted. Appears frequently and grows more rapidly than basal cell.

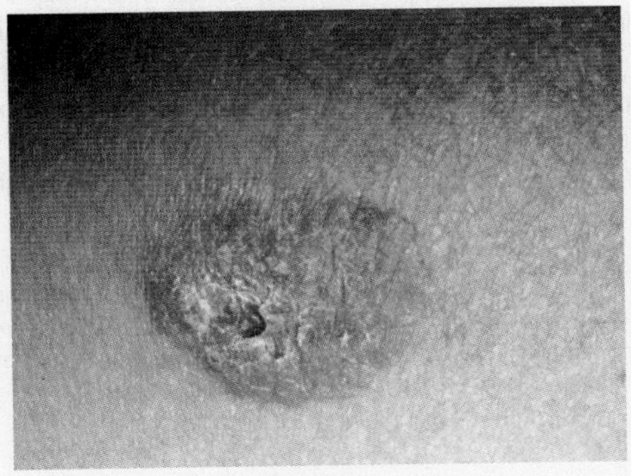

Basal squamous cell carcinoma

Melanoma

0.5- to 1.0-cm brown, flat lesion that appears on sun-exposed or nonexposed skin. Variegated pigmentation, irregular borders, and indistinct margins.

Ulceration, recent growth, or recent changes in long-standing mole are ominous signs.

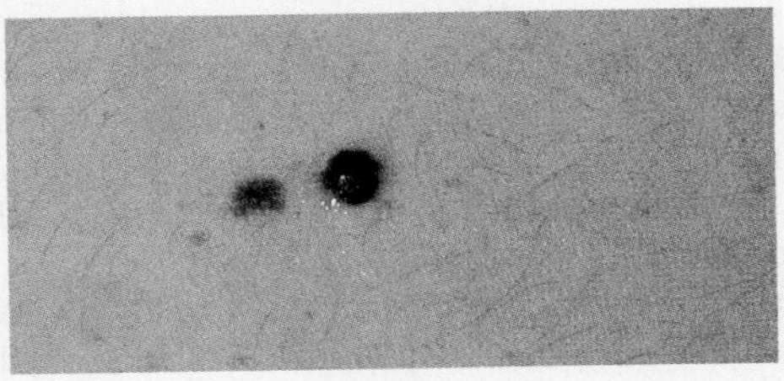

Melanoma

Illustrations from Marks, J., & Miller, J. (Eds.) (2014). *Lookingbill and Mark's principles of dermatology* (5th ed.). Philadelphia, PA: Elsevier; *Basal cell:* p. 65, Fig. 5-14A; *Squamous cell:* p. 63, Fig. 5-12. *Melanoma:* From Paller, A. S., & Mancini, A. J. (2011). *Hurwitz clinical pediatric dermatology* (4th ed., p. 192, Fig. 9.18). Edinburgh: Elsevier/Saunders.

growth occurs. Some patients with hormone disorders experience an unusual distribution and growth. A woman with **hirsutism** has hair growth on the upper lip, chin, and cheeks, with vellus hair becoming coarser over the body. For some, a change in hair growth negatively affects body image and emotional well-being.

Some changes occur in the thickness, texture, and lubrication of scalp hair. Disturbances such as a febrile illness or scalp disease sometimes result in hair loss. Conditions such as thyroid disease alter the condition of the hair, making it fine and brittle. Hair loss (**alopecia**) or thinning of the hair is usually related to genetic tendencies and endocrine disorders such as diabetes, thyroiditis, and even menopause. Poor nutrition causes stringy, dull, dry, and thin hair. The oil of sebaceous glands lubricates the hair. Excessively oily hair is associated with androgen hormone stimulation. Dry, brittle hair occurs with aging and with excessive use of chemical agents.

The amount of hair covering the extremities is sometimes reduced as a result of aging. Arterial insufficiency is most common over the lower extremities and results in hair loss.

Inspect the scalp for lesions. The scalp is normally smooth and inelastic, with even colouration. By carefully separating strands of hair, thoroughly examine the scalp for lesions. Note the characteristics of any scalp lesion. If you find lumps or bruises, ask if the patient has experienced recent head trauma. Moles on the scalp are common. Warn the patient that combing or brushing sometimes causes a mole

BOX 32-9 EVIDENCE-INFORMED PRACTICE GUIDELINE

Skin Cancer Prevention

Research Summary

What is cancer? More specifically, what is skin cancer? Cancer, by definition, is an "uncontrolled growth and spread of abnormal cells" (CCS Steering Committee, 2017). Therefore, skin cancer is characterized by abnormal skin cells, which can spread and invade other tissues. More importantly, what can we do about skin cancer? As nurses, it becomes our responsibility to assess for and educate patients about all types of skin cancers, especially for the most serious form, called melanoma. There are several risk factors for melanoma—major factors are positive family history of melanoma, a prior melanoma, and multiple or unusual moles. Other factors include fair complexion or skin that is sensitive to the sun, excessive exposure to the sun (especially before age 18), and the use of tanning beds or booths.

Research has indicated that when detected early and treated properly, skin cancer is highly curable (CCS Steering Committee, 2017). Therefore, early assessment and intervention are of utmost importance.

Application to Nursing Practice

Nurses have a responsibility to screen for cancer. Promoting and teaching self-screening of skin, hair, and nails to all patients and their family members is one way in which nurses can help prevent skin cancer.

- Instruct patients to conduct a complete monthly self-examination of the skin and scalp, noting moles, blemishes, and birthmarks.
  - Perform the examination after a bath or shower, including a head-to-toe check.
  - Use a well-lit room and mirrors to examine all skin surfaces. If necessary, ask a family member or significant other to aid in the investigation.
  - Remember the warning signs of skin cancer by using the ABCD mnemonic: *A* is for asymmetry—look for uneven shape; *B* is for border irregularity—look for edges that are blurred, notched, or ragged; *C* is for colour—pigmentation is not uniform; blue, black, brown variegated and areas of pink, white, grey, blue, or red are abnormal; and *D* is for diameter—greater than the size of a typical pencil eraser.
- Instruct patients to contact their health care provider if a skin lesion or mole starts to bleed or ooze or feels different (swollen, hard, lumpy, itchy, or tender to the touch). Stress this point to older persons, who tend to have delayed wound healing.
- Inform patients of ways to prevent skin cancer by avoiding overexposure to the sun:
  - Wear wide-brimmed hats and long sleeves.
  - Apply broad-spectrum sunscreens with SPF of 15 or greater to protect against ultraviolet B (UVB) and ultraviolet A (UVA) rays, approximately 15 minutes before going into the sun and after swimming or perspiring.
  - Avoid tanning under the direct sun at midday (10 a.m. to 4 p.m.).
  - Do not use indoor sunlamps, tanning parlours, or tanning pills.
- Inform patients who are on medications that make the skin more sensitive to the sun (e.g., oral contraceptives, antibiotics, anti-inflammatories, antihypertensives, immunosuppressives) to take extra precautions when spending time in the sun.
- Instruct patients to protect their children from the sun. Severe sunburns in childhood greatly increase melanoma risk later in life.

These interventions will provide the patient with self-screening measures to detect, prevent, and seek early treatment for skin cancer.

Data from Canadian Cancer Society. (2017). *Melanoma.* Retrieved from http://www.cancer.ca/en/cancer-information/cancer-type/skin-melanoma/melanoma/?region=on

to bleed. Dandruff or psoriasis frequently causes scaliness or dryness of the scalp.

Careful inspection of hair follicles on the scalp and pubic areas can possibly reveal lice or other parasites. The three types of lice are *Pediculus humanus capitis* (head lice), *Pediculus humanus corporis* (body lice), and *Pediculus pubis* (crab lice). Head and crab lice attach their eggs to hair. The tiny eggs look like oval particles of dandruff. The lice themselves are difficult to see. Head and body lice are very small with greyish white bodies. Crab lice have red legs. Observe for bites or pustular eruptions in the hair follicles and in areas where skin surfaces meet, such as behind the ears and in the groin. The discovery of lice requires immediate treatment (Box 32-10).

Nails

The condition of the nails reflects general health, state of nutrition, a person's occupation, and level of self-care. Nail biting can reveal a person's psychological state. Before assessing the nails, gather a brief history (Table 32-10). The most visible portion of the nails is the nail plate, the transparent layer of epithelial cells covering the nail bed (Figure 32-3). The vascularity of the nail bed creates the nail's underlying colour. The semilunar, whitish area at the base of the nail bed is called the *lunula,* from which the nail plate develops.

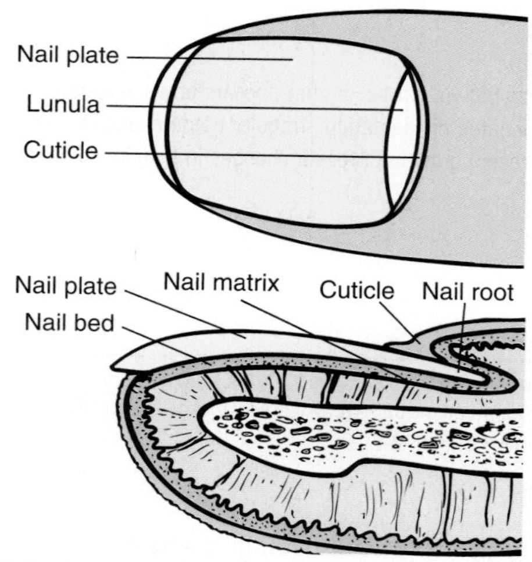

FIGURE 32-3 Components of the nail unit. (From Lewis, S. L., Bucher, L., Heitkemper, M. M., et al. [2014]. *Medical-surgical nursing* [9th ed.]. St. Louis: Mosby.)

Inspection and Palpation. Inspect the nail bed for colour, cleanliness, and length; the thickness and shape of the nail, the texture of the nail; the angle between the nail and the nail bed; and the condition of the lateral and proximal nail folds around the nail. Also palpate the nail base. Inspecting the nails can give the examiner a quick sense about the patient's hygiene practices. The nails are normally transparent, smooth, well rounded, and convex, with a nail bed angle of about 160 degrees. The surrounding cuticles are smooth, intact, and without inflammation. If the nails are ragged, dirty, and poorly kept, this is a good indication that either the patient practices infrequent nail care or is physically unable to perform care. However, consider the patient's profession, because some individuals have dirty nails as part of their

BOX 32-10 PATIENT TEACHING

Hair and Scalp Assessment

Objective

- Patient and/or family will perform proper hygiene practices for care of the hair and scalp.

Teaching Strategies

- Teach patient and family about basic hygiene practices for care of the hair and scalp (see Chapter 38).
- Inform patient and family about signs and symptoms of lice and how to check for infestations. Dispel myths regarding lice, emphasizing that they are a common occurrence in school-aged children and are not associated with poor hygiene.
- Discuss treatment options for lice. Currently in Canada, there are three different types of pharmacotherapy available for lice: topical insecticides (pyrethrins, permethrins), noninsecticidal agents (isopropyl myristate/ST-cyclomethicone, silicone oil dimethicone [NYDA], benzyl alcohol lotion), and oral medications (trimethoprim-sulfamethoxazole). Both topical insecticides and noninsecticidal agents can be purchased over the counter at drug stores and are the preferred treatment options. There is little evidence to support the efficacy of oral medications for head lice treatment, and they require a written prescription.
  - Pyrethrins and permethrins are approved for children 2 months of age and older with confirmed head lice.
  - Silicone oil demethicone is approved for use in children 2 years of age and older.
  - Myristate/ST-cyclomethicone is approved for use in children 4 years of age and older.
  - Benzyl alcohol lotion is approved for use in children 6 months of age and older and is more expensive than other agents.
  - Because of its neurotoxic effects, lindane is no longer recommended for treatment of lice.
  - Household products such as petroleum jelly, oil, and mayonnaise are NOT recommended for treating lice as their efficacy of killing lice is low.
- Upon selection of a pharmacological treatment option, instruct patient and family to follow the directions on the product box, as treatment methods vary by product type. A second treatment 7–10 days after initial treatment is recommended for all cases where a live infestation is found (i.e., live lice).
- Inform patient and family that pediculicides can cause scalp itching, rash, and mild burning sensation. This does not indicate reinfestation; reinfestation must be diagnosed by presence of live lice or eggs.
- There is little evidence to support the added benefit of wet combing after application of lice products. However, some patients may choose to do wet combing as a precautionary measure, to remove detectable nits and eggs.
- Inform patient and family that lice and nits do not live long away from the skin. Therefore, thorough environmental cleaning and disinfecting after a household infestation may not be necessary. However, items that have been in close contact with the head or body hair of an infested individual should be decontaminated to prevent reinfestation and transmission. Such items can be decontaminated by:
  - Washing items in hot water (≥66°C) and drying them in a hot dryer for 15 minutes.
  - Dry-cleaning, or sealing nonwashable items in a plastic bag for 14 days.
  - Soaking combs, brushes, and hair accessories in lice-killing products for 1 hour or in boiling water for 10 minutes.
- Instruct patient and family about ways to reduce transmission of lice:
  - Do not share personal-care items with others (e.g., brushes, hats, hair bands).
  - Use thorough hand hygiene practices.
  - If lice were sexually transmitted, patient needs to notify his or her partner.
  - Avoid close physical contact with infested individuals, especially head-to-head or skin-to-skin contact.
  - Generally, there is no medical rationale to exclude individuals with lice from school, day care, or work. Rather, the Canadian Paediatric Society recommends a full course of treatment and avoiding close head-to-head activities.

Evaluation

- Have patient or parents describe methods used to care for the hair and scalp.
- Have patient or parents explain the steps to take to reduce lice transmission in the home.
- Have patient or parents explain the steps to treat lice infestations in the home.

Data from Centers for Disease Control and Prevention (CDC). (2013). *Parasites—Lice.* Retrieved from https://www.cdc.gov/parasites/lice/index.html; Cummings, C., Finlay, J. C., MacDonald, N. E., & the Canadian Paediatric Society Community Paediatrics Committee. (2016). *Head lice infestations: A clinical update.* Retrieved from https://www.cps.ca/en/documents/position/head-lice.

TABLE 32-10 Nursing History for Nail Assessment

Assessment Category	Rationale
Ask if patient has experienced recent trauma or changes in nails (splitting, breaking, discoloration, thickening).	Trauma changes shape and growth of nail. Systemic conditions cause changes in colour, growth, and shape.
Has the patient had other symptoms of pain, swelling, presence of systemic disease with fever, or psychological or physical stress?	Alterations sometimes occur slowly over time.
Question patient's nail care practices. Determine if patient has acrylic nails or silk wraps.	Helps to determine if change in nails is due to local or systemic problem. Acrylic nails and silk wraps are areas for fungal growth. Chemical agents cause drying of nails. Improper care damages nails and cuticles.
Determine if patient has risks for nail or foot problems (e.g., diabetes, peripheral vascular disease, obesity).	Vascular changes associated with diabetes and peripheral vascular disease reduce blood flow to peripheral tissues; foot lesions and thickened nails are common. Some older persons have trouble performing foot and nail care because of poor vision, incoordination, or inability to bend over. Obese patients have difficulty bending over.

employment (e.g., mechanics, coal miners, and farmers) despite excellent nail care. Jagged, bitten, or broken nail edges or cuticles predispose a patient to localized infection. Report any abnormalities such as erythema or swelling.

> **Safety Alert** Patients with impaired circulation are at greater risk for localized infection. It is important to observe the condition of hand and foot nails and nail beds to identify risks for and early signs of infection.

In light-skinned individuals, nail beds are pink with translucent white tips. In dark-skinned patients, nail beds are darkly pigmented with a blue or reddish hue. A brown or black pigmentation is normal with longitudinal streaks. Trauma, cirrhosis, diabetes mellitus, and hypertension cause splinter hemorrhages. Vitamin, protein, and electrolyte changes cause various lines or bands to form on the nail beds.

Nails normally grow at a constant rate, but direct injury or generalized disease impairs growth. With aging, the nails of the fingers and toes become harder and thicker. Longitudinal striations develop, and the rate of nail growth slows. Nails become more brittle, dull, and opaque and turn yellow in older persons because of insufficient calcium. Also with age, the cuticle becomes less thick and wide.

Inspection of the angle between the nail and nail bed normally reveals an angle of 160 degrees (Box 32-11). A larger angle and softening of the nail bed indicate chronic oxygenation problems. Palpate the nail base to determine firmness and the condition of circulation. The nail base is normally firm.

To palpate, gently grasp the patient's finger and observe the colour of the nail bed. Next, apply gentle, firm, quick pressure with the thumb to the nail bed and release and observe capillary refill. As you apply pressure, the nail bed will appear white or blanched; however, the pink colour should return immediately on release of pressure. Capillary refill is measured in seconds; less than 2 seconds is brisk, while greater than 4 seconds is sluggish. Failure of the pinkness to return promptly indicates circulatory insufficiency. An ongoing bluish or purplish cast to the nail bed occurs with cyanosis. A white cast or pallor results from anemia.

Calluses and corns are commonly found on the toes or fingers. A callus is flat and painless, resulting from a thickening of the epidermis. Friction and pressure from shoes cause corns, usually over bony prominences. During the examination, the patient should be instructed in proper nail care (Box 32-12).

BOX 32-11 Abnormalities of the Nail Bed

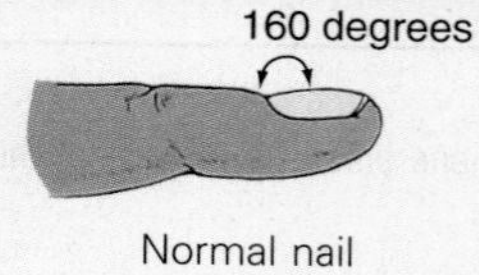

Normal nail: Approximately 160-degree angle between nail plate and nail

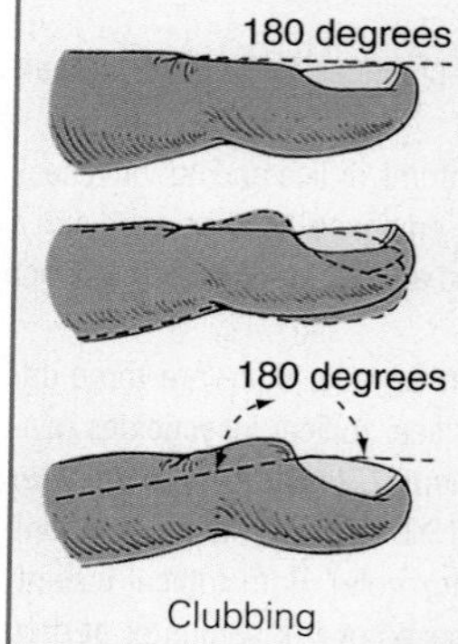

Clubbing: Change in angle between nail and nail base (eventually larger than 180 degrees); nail bed softening, with nail flattening; often, enlargement of fingertips
Causes: Chronic lack of oxygen: heart or pulmonary disease

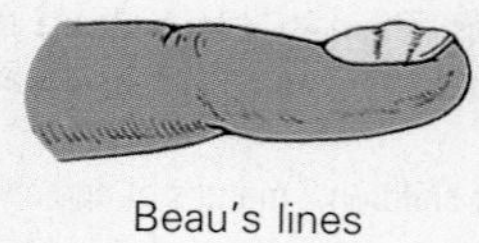

Beau's lines: Transverse depressions in nails indicating temporary disturbance of nail growth (nail grows out over several months)
Causes: Systemic illness such as severe infection; nail injury

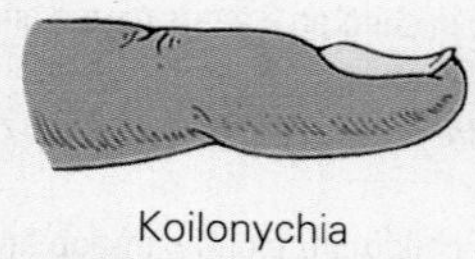

Koilonychia (spoon nail): Concave curves
Causes: Iron deficiency anemia, syphilis, use of strong detergents

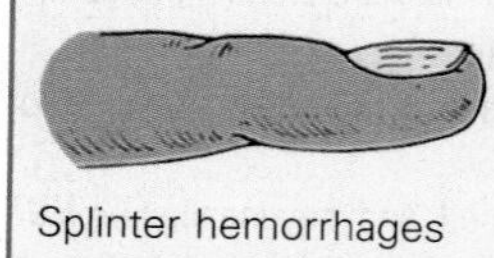

Splinter hemorrhages: Red or brown linear streaks in nail bed
Causes: Minor trauma, subacute bacterial endocarditis, trichinosis

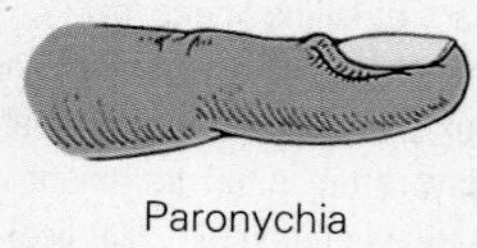

Paronychia: Inflammation of skin at base of nail
Causes: Local infection, trauma

BOX 32-12 PATIENT TEACHING

Nail Assessment

Objective

- Patient properly cares for fingernails, feet, and toenails.

Teaching Strategies

- Instruct patient to cut nails only after soaking them about 10 minutes in warm water. (Exception: Diabetic patients are warned against soaking nails because this dries the hands and feet out; dry skin leads to infection.)
- Caution patient against over-the-counter preparations to treat corns, calluses, or ingrown toenails.
- Tell the patient to cut nails straight across and even with the tops of the fingers or toes. If patient has diabetes, tell patient to file rather than cut the nails (see Chapter 38).
- Instruct patient to shape nails with a file or emery board.
- *If patient is diabetic:*
  - Wash feet daily in warm water, and carefully dry them, especially between the toes. Inspect feet each day in good lighting, looking for dry places and cracks in the skin. Soften dry feet by applying a cream or lotion such as Nivea, Eucerin, or Alpha Keri.
  - Do not put lotion between the toes; moisture between the toes allows microorganisms to grow, leading to infections.
  - Caution patient against using sharp objects to poke or dig under the toenail or around the cuticle.
  - Have patient see a podiatrist for treatment of ingrown toenails and nails that are thick or tend to split.

Evaluation

- Inspect nails during subsequent patient interactions.
- Have patient explain steps to take to avoid injury.

TABLE 32-11 Nursing History for Head Assessment

Assessment Category	Rationale
Determine if patient has experienced recent head trauma. If so, assess state of consciousness after injury (immediately on return and 5 minutes later), duration of unconsciousness, and predisposing factors (e.g., seizure, poor vision, blackout).	Trauma is a major cause of lumps, bumps, cuts, bruises, or deformities of scalp or skull. Loss of consciousness after head injury indicates possible brain injury.
Ask if patient has history of headache; note onset, duration, character, pattern, and associated symptoms.	Character of headache helps in determining causative factors, such as sinus infection, migraine, or neurological disorders.
Determine length of time patient has experienced neurological symptoms.	Duration of signs or symptoms indicates severity of problem.
Review patient's occupational history for use of safety helmets.	Nature of some occupations creates a risk for head injury.
Ask if patient participates in contact sports.	These activities require use of safety helmets.

HEAD AND NECK

An examination of the head and neck includes assessment of the head, eyes, ears, nose, mouth, pharynx, and neck (lymph nodes, carotid arteries, thyroid gland, and trachea). This assessment is commonly referred to in clinical documentation under EENT (eyes, ears, nose, and throat) and includes all of the associated physical structures (e.g., peripheral arteries and carotid arteries). Assessment of the head and neck requires inspection, palpation, and auscultation, with inspection and palpation often done simultaneously.

Head

Inspection and Palpation. The nursing history involves screening for intracranial injury and local or congenital deformities (Table 32-11). This starts with inspecting the patient's head, noting the position, size, shape, and contour. The head is normally held upright and midline to the trunk. The patient holding the head tilted to one side is perhaps an indication of unilateral hearing or visual loss. A horizontal jerking or bobbing indicates a tremor.

Note the patient's facial features, looking at the eyelids, eyebrows, nasolabial folds, and mouth for shape and symmetry. It is normal for slight asymmetry to exist. If there is facial asymmetry, note if all features on one side of the face are affected or if only a portion of the face is involved. Various neurological disorders (e.g., facial nerve paralysis) affect different nerves that innervate muscles of the face.

Examine the size, shape, and contour of the skull. The skull is generally round with prominences in the frontal area anteriorly and the occipital area posteriorly. Trauma typically causes local skull deformities. In infants, a large head results from congenital anomaly or the buildup of cerebrospinal fluid in the ventricles (hydrocephalus). Some adults have enlarged jaws and facial bones resulting from acromegaly, a disorder caused by excessive secretion of growth hormone. Palpate the skull for nodules or masses. Gently rotate the fingertips down the midline of the scalp and then along the sides of the head to identify abnormalities. Then palpate the temporomandibular joint (TMJ) space bilaterally. Place the fingertips just anterior to the tragus of each ear. The fingertips should slip into the joint space as the patient's mouth opens, to gently palpate the joint spaces. Normally, the movements should be smooth, although it is not unusual to hear or feel a clicking or snapping in the TMJ (Ball et al., 2015a, p. 516).

Eyes

Examination of the eyes includes inspection of external and internal eye structures and extraocular movement and the assessment of visual acuity and visual fields. Figure 32-4 shows a cross-section of the eye. Through assessment, visual alterations are detected and the level of assistance that patients require when ambulating or performing self-care activities is determined. Some patients with visual problems also need special aids for reading educational materials or instructions (e.g., medication labels). Table 32-12 outlines the nursing history for an eye examination. Box 32-13 describes common types of visual problems.

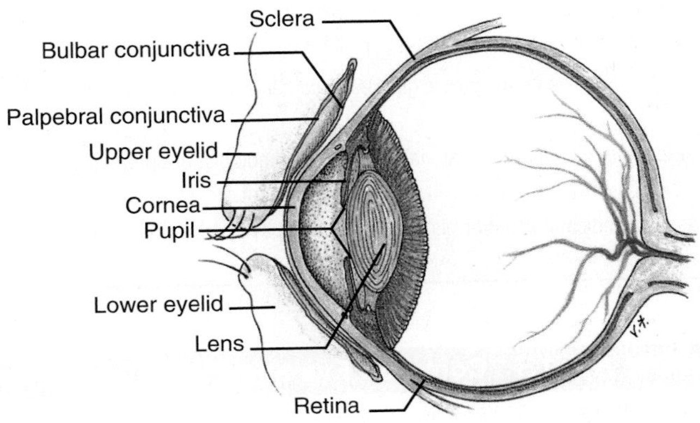

FIGURE 32-4 Cross-section of the eye.

External Eye Structures. To inspect external eye structures, stand directly in front of the patient at eye level and ask the patient to look at your face.

Position and Alignment. Assess the position of the eyes in relation to one another. Normally, they are parallel to each other. Bulging eyes (exophthalmos) usually indicate hyperthyroidism. The crossing of eyes (strabismus) results from neuromuscular injury or inherited abnormalities. Tumours or inflammation of the orbit often cause abnormal eye protrusion.

For the remainder of the eye examination, have the patient remove glasses or contact lenses.

Eyebrows. Inspect the eyebrows for size, extension, texture of hair, alignment, and movement. Normally, the eyebrows are symmetrical. Coarseness of hair and failure to extend beyond the temporal canthus possibly reveals hypothyroidism. If the brows are thinned, this is possibly a result of waxing or plucking. Aging causes loss of the lateral third of the eyebrows. Have the patient raise and lower the eyebrows. The brows normally raise and lower symmetrically. An inability to move the eyebrows indicates a facial nerve paralysis (cranial nerve VII).

Eyelids. Inspect the eyelids for position, colour, condition of the surface, condition and direction of the eyelashes, and the patient's ability to open, close, and blink. When the eyes are open in a normal

TABLE 32-12 Nursing History for Eye Assessment

Assessment Category	Rationale
Determine if patient has history of eye disease, (e.g., glaucoma, retinopathy, cataracts), eye trauma, diabetes, hypertension, or eye surgery.	Some diseases or trauma cause risk for partial or complete visual loss. Patient may have had surgery for a visual disorder.
Determine problems that prompted patient to seek health care. Ask patient about eye pain, photophobia (sensitivity to light), burning or itching, excess tearing or crusting, diplopia (double vision) or blurred vision, awareness of a "film" or "curtain" over field of vision, floaters (small, black spots that seem to float across field of vision), flashing lights, or halos around lights.	Common symptoms of eye disease indicate need for health care provider.
Determine whether there is family history of eye disorders or diseases.	Certain eye problems such as glaucoma or retinitis pigmentosa are inherited.
Review patient's occupational history and recreational hobbies; are safety glasses worn?	Performance of close, intricate work causes eye fatigue. Working with computers causes eye strain. Certain occupational tasks (e.g., working with chemicals) and recreational activities (e.g., fencing, motorcycle riding) place people at risk for eye injury unless patients take precautions.
Ask patient if he or she wears glasses or contacts and if so, how often.	Patients need to wear glasses or contacts during certain portions of examination for accurate assessment.
Determine when patient last visited an ophthalmologist or optometrist.	Date of last eye examination indicates level of preventive care patient takes.
Assess medications patient is taking, including eye drops or ointment.	Determines need to assess patient's knowledge of medications. Certain medications cause visual symptoms.

BOX 32-13 Common Eye and Visual Problems

Hyperopia
Hyperopia is farsightedness, a refractive error in which rays of light enter the eye and focus behind the retina. Individuals are able to clearly see distant objects but not close objects.

Myopia
Myopia is nearsightedness, a refractive error in which rays of light enter the eye and focus in front of the retina. Individuals are able to clearly see close objects but not distant objects.

Presbyopia
Presbyopia is impaired near vision in middle-aged and older persons, caused by loss of elasticity of the lens and associated with the aging process.

Retinopathy
Retinopathy is a noninflammatory eye disorder resulting from changes in retinal blood vessels. It is a leading cause of blindness.

Strabismus
Strabismus is a congenital condition in which both eyes do not focus on an object simultaneously; these eyes appear crossed. Impairment of the extraocular muscles or their nerve supply causes strabismus.

Amblyopia
Amblyopia is a congenital condition, commonly referred to as a "lazy eye," which occurs when the nerve pathway in one eye does not develop in early childhood. This weakness to one eye can result in blurred vision, distortion of depth perception, or progressive vision loss to the affected eye. Early screening and referral of children for amblyopia and strabismus is important to correct and preserve vision.

Cataracts
A cataract is an increased opacity of the lens, which blocks light rays from entering the eye. Cataracts sometimes develop slowly and progressively after age 35 or suddenly after trauma. Cataracts are one of the most common eye disorders. Most older persons (age 65 years and older) have some evidence of visual impairment from cataracts. Protection of the eyes from the sun's rays and trauma through the use of sunglasses and protective eyewear when there is an occupational or recreational risk for eye injury is an important factor in the prevention of cataracts.

Glaucoma
Glaucoma is intraocular structural damage resulting from elevated intraocular pressure. Obstruction of the outflow of aqueous humor causes this. Without treatment, the disorder will lead to blindness.

Macular Degeneration
Macular degeneration is blurred central vision often occurring suddenly, caused by a progressive degeneration of the centre of the retina. It is the most common visual impairment of individuals over age 50 and the most common cause of blindness in older persons. There is no cure.

position, the lids do not cover the pupil and the sclera cannot be seen above the iris. The lids are also close to the eyeball. An abnormal drooping of the lid over the pupil is called **ptosis** (pronounced "toe-sis"), caused by edema or impairment of the third cranial nerve. In the older person, ptosis results from a loss of elasticity that accompanies aging. Observe for defects in the position of the lid margins. An older person frequently has lid margins that turn out (**ectropion**) or in (**entropion**). An entropion sometimes leads to the lashes of the lid irritating the conjunctiva and cornea, increasing the risk of infection. The eyelashes are normally distributed evenly and curved outward away from the eye. An erythematous or yellow lump (hordeolum or sty) on the follicle of an eyelash indicates an acute suppurative inflammation.

To inspect the surface of the upper lids, ask the patient to close his or her eyes. Then raise both eyebrows gently with the thumb and index finger to stretch the skin. The lids are normally smooth and the same colour as the skin. Redness indicates inflammation or infection. Lid edema is sometimes due to allergies or to heart or kidney failure. Edema of the eyelids prevents them from closing. Inspect lesions for typical characteristics and discomfort or drainage. Wear clean gloves if drainage is present.

The lids normally close symmetrically. Failure of the lids to close exposes the cornea to drying. This condition is common in unconscious patients or in those with facial nerve paralysis. Ask the patient to open the eyes for inspection of the lower lids. Assess the same characteristics noted for the upper lids. Normally a patient blinks involuntarily and bilaterally up to 20 times a minute. The blink reflex lubricates the cornea. Report absent or infrequent, rapid, or monocular (one-eyed) blinking.

Lacrimal Apparatus. The lacrimal gland (Figure 32-5), located in the upper outer wall of the anterior part of the orbit, is responsible for tear production. Tears flow from the gland across the eye's surface to the lacrimal duct, which is in the nasal corner or inner canthus of the eye. The lacrimal gland is sometimes the site of tumours or infections. Inspect this area for edema and redness. Palpate the gland gently to detect tenderness. Normally the gland cannot be felt.

The nasolacrimal duct sometimes becomes obstructed, blocking the flow of tears. Observe for evidence of edema in the inner canthus. Gentle palpation of the duct at the lower eyelid just inside the lower orbital rim causes a regurgitation of tears.

Conjunctivae and Sclerae. The bulbar conjunctiva covers the exposed surface of the eyeball up to the outer edge of the cornea. Observe the sclera under the bulbar conjunctiva; it normally has the colour of white porcelain in White patients and light yellow in dark-skinned patients. Sclerae become pigmented and appear either yellow or green if liver disease is present.

Take care when inspecting the conjunctivae. For adequate exposure of the bulbar conjunctiva, retract the eyelids without placing pressure directly on the eyeball. Gently retract both lids, with the thumb and index finger pressed against the lower and upper bony orbits. Ask the patient to look up, down, and from side to side. Many patients begin to blink, making the examination difficult. Inspect for colour, texture, and the presence of edema or lesions. Normally the conjunctivae are free of erythema. The presence of redness indicates an allergic or infectious conjunctivitis. Bright red blood in a localized area surrounded by normal-appearing conjunctiva usually indicates subconjunctival hemorrhage. Conjunctivitis is a highly contagious infection. It is easy to spread the crusty drainage that collects on eyelid margins from one eye to the other. Wear clean gloves during the examination. Performing proper hand hygiene is necessary before and after the examination.

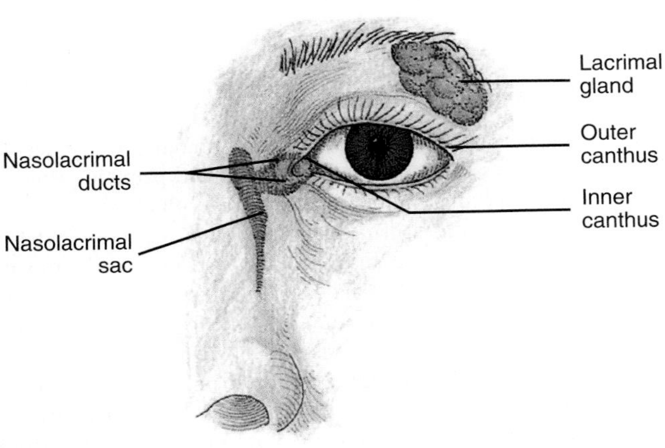

FIGURE 32-5 The lacrimal apparatus secretes and drains tears, which moisten and lubricate eye structures.

Corneas. The cornea is the transparent, colourless portion of the eye covering the pupil and iris. While the patient looks straight ahead, inspect the cornea for clarity and texture while shining a penlight obliquely across the cornea's entire surface. The cornea is normally shiny, transparent, and smooth. In an older person, the cornea loses its lustre. Any irregularity in the surface indicates an abrasion or tear that requires further examination by a health care provider. Both conditions are very painful. Note the colour and details of the underlying iris. The iris becomes faded in an older person. A thin white ring along the margin of the iris, called an arcus senilis, is common with aging but is abnormal in anyone under age 40. To test for the corneal blink reflex, see the cranial nerve test section of this chapter.

Pupils and Irises. Observe the pupils for size, shape, equality, accommodation, and reaction to light. The pupils are normally black, round, regular, and equal in size (3 to 7 mm in diameter) (Figure 32-6). The iris should be clearly visible.

Cloudy pupils indicate cataracts. Dilated pupils result from glaucoma, trauma, neurological disorders, eye medications (e.g., atropine), or withdrawal from opioids. Inflammation of the iris or use of drugs (e.g., pilocarpine, morphine, or cocaine) causes constricted pupils. Pinpoint pupils are a common sign of opioid intoxication. Shining a beam of light through the pupil and onto the retina stimulates the third cranial nerve and causes the muscles of the iris to constrict. Any abnormality along the nerve pathways from the retina to the iris alters the ability of the pupils to react to light. Changes in intracranial pressure, lesions along the nerve pathways, locally applied ophthalmic medications, and direct trauma to the eye alter pupillary reaction.

Test pupillary reflexes (to light and accommodation) in a dimly lit room. While the patient looks straight ahead, bring a penlight from the side of the patient's face, directing the light onto the pupil. If the patient looks at the light, there will be a false reaction to accommodation. A directly illuminated pupil constricts, and the opposite pupil constricts consensually. Observe the quickness and equality of the reflex. Repeat the examination for the opposite eye.

To test for accommodation, ask the patient to gaze at a distant object (the far wall) and then at a test object (finger or pencil) held approximately 10 cm from the bridge of the patient's nose. The pupils normally converge and accommodate by constricting when looking at close objects. The pupillary responses should be equal. Testing for accommodation is important only if the patient has a defect in the pupillary response to light (Jarvis et al., 2014, p. 299). If assessment of pupillary reaction is normal in all tests, record the abbreviation PERRLA (pupils equal, round, reactive to light, and accommodation).

Internal Eye Structures. The examination of the internal eye structures through the use of an ophthalmoscope is beyond the scope of new graduate nurses' practice. Advanced nurse practitioners use the ophthalmoscope to inspect the fundus, which includes the retina,

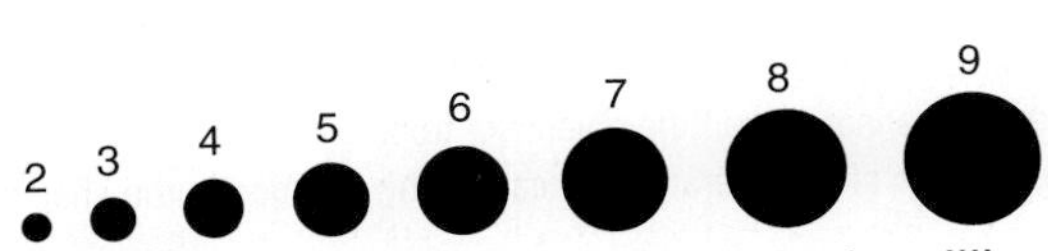

FIGURE 32-6 Chart depicting pupillary size in millimetres.

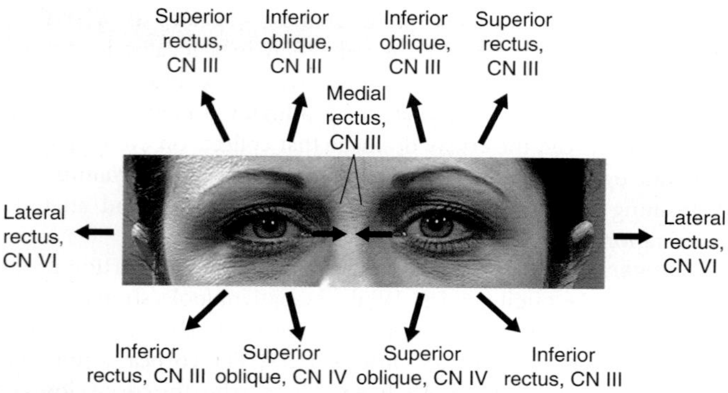

FIGURE 32-7 Six directions of gaze. Direct the patient to follow finger movement through each gaze. *CN*, cranial nerve. (From Ball et al. [2015]. *Seidel's guide to physical examination* [8th ed., p. 215]. St. Louis, MO: Mosby.)

choroid, optic nerve disc, macula, fovea centralis, and retinal vessels. Patients in greatest need of an examination are those with diabetes, hypertension, and intracranial disorders.

Extraocular Movements. Six small muscles guide the movement of each eye. Both eyes move parallel to each other in each of the six directions of gaze (Figure 32-7). To assess extraocular movements, have the patient sit or stand 60 cm away, facing you. Hold a finger at a comfortable distance (15 to 30 cm) from the patient's eyes. Have the patient maintain his or her head in a fixed position facing forward and follow the movement of the finger with the eyes only. Have the patient look to the right, to the left, and diagonally up and down to the left and right. The finger moves smoothly and slowly within the normal field of vision.

As the patient gazes in each direction, observe for parallel eye movement, the position of the upper eyelid in relation to the iris, and the presence of abnormal movements. As the eyes move through each direction of gaze, the upper eyelid covers the iris only slightly. **Nystagmus**, an involuntary, rhythmical oscillation of the eyes, is assessed by periodically stopping movement of the finger. To initiate nystagmus in patients with normal eye movements, have them gaze to the far left or right. Disturbances in eye movement reflect local injury to eye muscles and supporting structures or a disorder of the cranial nerves innervating the muscles.

Visual Fields. As a person looks straight ahead, he or she is normally able to see all objects in the periphery. To assess visual fields, have the patient stand or sit 60 cm away, facing you at eye level. The patient gently closes or covers one eye (e.g., the left) and looks at your eye directly opposite. Close the opposite eye (in this case, the right) so that the field of vision is superimposed on that of the patient. Move a finger equidistant from you and the patient outside the field of vision, then slowly bring it back into the visual field. Ask the patient to tell when he or she is able to see the finger. If you see the finger before the patient does, a portion of the patient's visual field is reduced. To test temporal field vision, the object should be slightly behind the patient. (Note: The nurse can see the finger.) Repeat the procedure for each field of vision for the other eye.

> **Safety Alert** Some patients with visual field problems are at risk for injury because they cannot see all the objects in front of them. Older persons commonly have loss of peripheral vision caused by changes in the shape of the lens.

Visual Acuity. The assessment of visual acuity, the ability to see small details, involves testing central vision. The easiest way to assess near vision is to ask patients to read printed material under adequate lighting. If patients wear glasses or contact lenses, they should wear them during assessment. It is important to determine the language the patient speaks and reading ability. Asking patients to read aloud will help determine literacy. If the patient has difficulty reading, move to the next step.

Assessment of distance vision requires using a Snellen chart (paper chart or projection screen). The chart should be well lit. Vision without corrective lenses is tested first. Have the patient sit or stand 6.1 m (20 feet) away from the chart and try to read all the letters beginning at any line with both eyes open. Then have the patient read the line with each eye separately (the patient covers the opposite eye with an index card or eye cover). The patient should avoid applying pressure to the eye. Note the smallest line in which the patient is able to read all the letters correctly, and record the visual acuity for that line. Repeat the test with the patient wearing corrective lenses. Complete the test rapidly enough so that the patient does not memorize the chart (Jarvis et al., 2014).

If a patient is unable to read, use an *E* chart or one with pictures of familiar objects. Instead of reading letters, patients tell which direction each *E* is pointing or the name of the object. The visual acuity score for each eye and for both eyes is then recorded.

The Snellen chart has standardized numbers at the end of each line of the chart. The numerator is the number 20, or the distance the patient stands from the chart. The denominator is the distance from which the normal eye is able to read the chart. Normal vision is 20/20. The larger the denominator, the poorer the patient's visual acuity. For example, a value of 20/40 means that the patient, standing 6.1 m (20 feet) away, can read a line that a person with normal vision can read from 40 feet away. Visual acuity is recorded as O.D. (right eye) and O.S. (left eye) as well as *sc* (without correction) or *cc* (with correction), depending on whether the patient wears glasses or contact lenses.

If patients cannot read even the largest letters or figures of a Snellen chart, test their ability to count upraised fingers or to distinguish light. Hold a hand 30 cm from the patient's face, and have the patient count the upraised fingers. To check light perception, shine a penlight into the eye and then turn the light off. If the patient notes when the light is turned on or off, light perception is intact.

Near vision is assessed by asking the patient to read a hand-held card containing a vision screening chart. Instruct the patient to hold the card a comfortable distance (5 to 6 cm) from the eyes and read the smallest line possible. This portion of the examination is a good time to discuss the need for routine eye examinations (Box 32-14).

Ears

The three parts of the ear are the external, middle, and inner ear (Figure 32-8). Assessment involves inspecting and palpating external ear structures, inspecting middle ear structures with an otoscope, and testing the inner ear by measuring the patient's hearing acuity. External ear structures consist of the auricle, outer ear canal, and tympanic membrane (eardrum). The ear canal is normally curved and approximately 2.5 cm long in an adult. It is lined with skin containing fine hairs, nerve endings, and glands secreting cerumen. The middle ear is an air-filled cavity containing the three bony ossicles (malleus, incus, and stapes). The eustachian tube connects the middle ear to the nasopharynx. Pressure between the outer atmosphere and the middle ear is stabilized through the eustachian tube. The inner ear contains the cochlea, vestibule, and semicircular canals.

BOX 32-14 PATIENT TEACHING

Eye Assessment

Objectives

- Patient follows recommendations for regular eye examinations.
- Patient recognizes warning signs and symptoms of eye disease.
- Patient takes appropriate safety precautions for visual deficits.

Teaching Strategies

- Inform adult patients that people between ages 19 and 49 need to have a complete eye examination every 2–5 years (or more often if family history reveals risk factors, such as diabetes or hypertension, for eye disorders).
- Inform adult patients that people between ages 50 and 64 need to have an eye examination every 2–3 years, and people over 65 years of age need to have an eye exam annually, to screen for conditions that may develop without symptoms (e.g., glaucoma).
- Inform patient that people with diabetes should have an eye exam every 1–2 years because of increased risk of retinopathy.
- Describe the typical symptoms of eye disease (see Box 32-13).
- Instruct older persons to take the following precautions because of normal visual changes:
  - Avoid or use caution while driving at night.
  - Increase lighting in the home to reduce risk of falls.
  - Paint the first and last steps of a staircase and the edge of each step in between a bright colour to aid depth perception.

Evaluation

- Ask patient or family member to report on patient's most recent visit to an ophthalmologist.
- Have patient describe when to have an eye examination.
- Ask patient to describe common symptoms of eye disease.
- Observe the home environment of a patient with visual deficits.

Canadian Diabetes Association Clinical Practice Guideline Expert Committee (2013); Canadian Ophthalmological Society (2016); Shimizu, Bouchard, & Mavriplis, (2016).

BOX 32-15 PATIENT TEACHING

Ear Assessment

Objectives

- Patient uses proper technique for cleaning the ears.
- Patient follows preventive guidelines for screening of hearing loss.
- Patient with hearing loss communicates effectively.

Teaching Strategies

- Instruct patient in the proper way to clean the outer ear (see Chapter 38), avoiding use of cotton-tipped applicators and sharp objects such as hairpins, which cause impaction of cerumen deep in the ear canal or cause trauma.
- Tell patient to avoid inserting pointed objects into the ear canal.
- Encourage patients over age 65 to have regular hearing checks. Explain that a reduction in hearing is a normal part of aging (see Chapter 47).
- Instruct family members of patients with hearing loss to avoid shouting and instead speak in low tones, and to be sure the patient is able to see the speaker's face.

Evaluation

- Ask patient to explain the proper technique for cleaning the ears.
- In a follow-up visit, question patient about frequency of hearing checks.
- Observe patient with hearing loss interacting with family members.

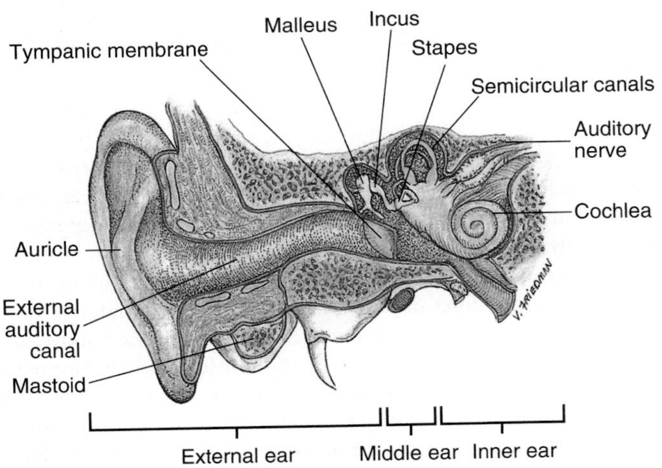

FIGURE 32-8 Structures of the external, middle, and inner ear.

Assessment of the ears helps in determining the integrity of ear structures and the condition of hearing (Box 32-15). Nursing history data (Table 32-13) aid in identifying risks for hearing disorders.

Understanding the mechanisms for sound transmission helps in identifying the nature of hearing disorders. Sound travels through the ear by air and bone conduction; the following explains the steps of hearing:

1. Sound waves in the air enter the external ear, passing through the outer ear canal.
2. The sound waves reach the tympanic membrane, causing it to vibrate.
3. Vibrations are transmitted through the middle ear by the bony ossicular chain to the oval window at the opening of the inner ear.
4. The cochlea receives the sound vibration.
5. Nerve impulses from the cochlea travel to the auditory (eighth cranial) nerve and to the cerebral cortex.

Disorders of the ear result from several types of problems, including mechanical dysfunction (blockage by earwax or foreign body), trauma (foreign bodies or noise exposure), neurological disorders (auditory nerve damage), acute illnesses (viral infection), and toxic effects of medications.

Auricles. With the patient sitting comfortably, inspect the auricle's size, shape, symmetry, landmarks, position, and colour. The auricles are normally of equal size and level with each other. The upper point of attachment is in a straight line with the lateral canthus, or corner of the eye. The position of the auricle is almost vertical. Ears that are low-set or at an unusual angle are a sign of chromosome abnormality (e.g., Down syndrome) or may indicate the possibility of fetal alcohol affects or syndrome. Ear colour is usually the same as that

TABLE 32-13 Nursing History for Ear Assessment

Assessment Category	Rationale
Ask if patient has experienced ear pain, itching, discharge, vertigo, tinnitus (ringing in ears), or change in hearing.	These signs and symptoms indicate infection or hearing loss.
Assess risks for hearing problem. *Infants/children:* Hypoxia at birth, meningitis, birth weight less than 1500 g, family history of hearing loss, congenital anomalies of skull or face, nonbacterial intrauterine infections (rubella, herpes), maternal drug use, excessively high bilirubin, head trauma *Adults:* Exposure to industrial or recreational noise, genetic disease (Meniere disease), neurodegenerative disorder	Risk factors predispose patient to permanent hearing loss. It is difficult to assess an infant's hearing status with examination only.
Determine patient's exposure to loud noises at work and availability of protective devices.	Prolonged noise exposure causes temporary or permanent hearing loss.
Note behaviours indicative of hearing loss, such as failure to respond when spoken to, requests to repeat comments, leaning forward to hear, and child's inattentiveness or use of monotonous voice tone.	Individuals with hearing loss cope with sensory deficit through a variety of behavioural cues.
Assess if patient takes large doses of aspirin or other ototoxic drugs (e.g., aminoglycosides, furosemide, streptomycin).	Medications have adverse effects of hearing loss.
Determine whether patient uses hearing aid.	Determining this informs nurse to assess ability to care for device and informs nurse to adjust voice tone to communicate.
If patient had recent hearing problem, note onset, contributing factors, affected ear, and effect on activities of daily living.	Helps determine nature and severity of hearing problem.
Determine whether patient has repeated history of cerumen buildup in ear.	Cerumen impaction is a common cause for conduction deafness.

of the face, without moles, cysts, deformities, or nodules. Redness is a sign of inflammation or fever. Extreme pallor indicates frostbite. Deformities of the ear can be a sign that there may be other organ abnormalities that occurred during fetal development (e.g., kidney).

Palpate the auricles for texture, tenderness, and skin lesions. Auricles are normally smooth and without lesions. If the patient complains of pain, gently pull the auricle, press on the tragus, and palpate behind the ear over the mastoid process. If palpating the external ear increases the pain, an external ear infection is likely. If palpation of the auricle and tragus does not influence the pain, the patient possibly has a middle ear infection. Tenderness in the mastoid area indicates mastoiditis.

Inspect the opening of the ear canal for size and presence of discharge. If discharge is present, wear clean gloves during the examination. A swollen or occluded meatus is not normal. **Cerumen**, a yellow, waxy substance, is common. Yellow or green, foul-smelling discharge indicates infection or a foreign body.

Ear Canals and Eardrums. Deeper structures of the external and middle ear are assessed with the use of an **otoscope**. The examination of the internal ear structures through the use of an otoscope is beyond the scope of new graduate nurses' practice. Advanced nurse practitioners use the otoscope to inspect the ear canal, tympanic membrane, and bony landmarks. Patients in greatest need of an examination are those with a possible foreign body in the ear canal, pain, swelling, or injury near the ear or patients with disorders related to balance. A detailed presentation of an otoscope examination of the inner ear can be found in the textbook by Jarvis and colleagues (2014, pp. 351–353).

Hearing Acuity. A patient with a hearing loss often fails to respond to conversation. The three types of hearing loss are conduction, sensorineural, and mixed. A conduction loss interrupts sound waves as they travel from the outer ear to the cochlea of the inner ear because the sound waves are not transmitted through the outer and middle ear structures. Examples of causes of a conduction loss are swelling of the auditory canal or tears in the tympanic membrane. A sensorineural loss involves the inner ear, auditory nerve, or hearing centre of the brain. Sound is conducted through the outer and middle ear structures, but the continued transmission of sound becomes interrupted at some point beyond the bony ossicles. A mixed loss involves a combination of conduction and sensorineural loss.

> **Safety Alert** Patients working or living around loud noises are at risk for hearing loss. In addition, adolescents are at risk for premature hearing loss from continued exposure to loud music in their car or home or at concert events. The use of iPods, MP3 players, and smartphones also increases the risk for hearing loss in all patients.

Older persons experience an inability to hear high-frequency sounds and consonants (e.g., *S, Z, T,* and *G*). Deterioration of the cochlea and thickening of the tympanic membrane cause older persons to gradually lose hearing acuity. They are especially at risk for hearing loss due to **ototoxicity** (injury to auditory nerve) resulting from high-maintenance doses of antibiotics (e.g., aminoglycosides).

To conduct a hearing assessment, have the patient remove any hearing aid, if worn. Note the patient's response to questions. Normally, the patient responds without excessive requests to have the questions repeated. If hearing loss is suspected, check the patient's response to the whispered voice. Test one ear at a time while the patient occludes the other ear with a finger. Ask the patient to gently move the finger up and down during the test. While standing 30 to 60 cm from the testing ear, cover the mouth so that the patient is unable to read lips. After exhaling fully, whisper softly toward the unoccluded ear, reciting random numbers with equally accented syllables, such as *nine-four-ten.* If necessary, gradually increase voice intensity until the patient correctly repeats the numbers. Then test the other ear for comparison. Ball and colleagues (2015a) reported that patients normally hear numbers clearly when whispered, responding correctly at least 50% of the time. If a hearing loss is present, patients are referred for an audiometric assessment. While there are tests that can be performed using a tuning fork (Weber and Rinne tests), these are a gross screening tool and not as reliable as audiometry.

Nose and Sinuses

The integrity of the nose and sinuses is assessed through inspection and palpation. The patient sits during the examination. Use of a penlight enables gross examination of each naris. A more detailed examination requires use of a nasal speculum to inspect the deeper nasal turbinates. Table 32-14 lists components of the nursing history. Box 32-16 describes teaching guidelines during nose and sinus assessment.

Nose. When inspecting the external nose, observe for shape, size, skin, colour, and the presence of deformity or inflammation. The nose is normally smooth and symmetrical with the same colour as the face. Recent trauma sometimes causes edema and discoloration. If swelling or deformities exist, gently palpate the ridge and soft tissue of the nose by placing one finger on each side of the nasal arch and gently moving the fingers from the nasal bridge to the tip. Note any tenderness, masses, or underlying deviations. Nasal structures are usually firm and stable.

Air normally passes freely through the nose when a person breathes. To assess patency of the nares, place a finger on the side of the patient's nose and occlude one naris. Ask the patient to breathe with the mouth closed. Repeat the procedure for the other naris.

While illuminating the anterior nares, inspect the mucosa for colour, lesions, discharge, swelling, and evidence of bleeding. If discharge is present, apply gloves. Normal mucosa is pink and moist without lesions. Pale mucosa with clear discharge indicates allergy. A mucoid discharge indicates rhinitis. A sinus infection results in yellowish or greenish discharge. Habitual use of intranasal cocaine and opioids causes puffiness and increased vascularity of the nasal mucosa. For the patient with a nasogastric tube, routinely check for local skin breakdown (**excoriation**) of the naris, characterized by redness and skin sloughing.

To view the septum and turbinates, have the patient tip the head back slightly to provide a clear view. Illuminate the septum and observe for alignment, perforation, or bleeding. Normally the septum is close to the midline, and thicker anteriorly than posteriorly. The turbinates are covered with mucous membranes that warm and moisten inspired air. Normal mucosa is pink and moist, without lesions. A deviated septum obstructs breathing and interferes with passage of a nasogastric tube. Perforation of the septum often occurs after repeated use of intranasal cocaine. Note any **polyps** (tumour-like growths) or purulent drainage.

Sinuses. Examination of the sinuses involves palpation. In cases of allergies or infection, the interior of the sinuses becomes inflamed and swollen. The most effective way to assess for tenderness is by externally palpating the frontal and maxillary facial areas (Figure 32-9). Palpate the frontal sinus by exerting pressure with the thumb up and under the patient's eyebrow. Gentle, upward pressure elicits tenderness

TABLE 32-14 Nursing History for Nose and Sinus Assessment

Assessment Category	Rationale
Ask if patient has had trauma to nose.	Trauma causes septal deviation and asymmetry of external nose.
Ask if patient has history of allergies, nasal discharge, epistaxis (nosebleeds), or postnasal drip.	History is useful in determining source or nature of nasal and sinus drainage.
If there is history of nasal discharge, assess colour, amount, odour, duration, and associated symptoms (e.g., sneezing, nasal congestion, obstruction, or mouth breathing).	Aids in ruling out presence of infection, allergy, or drug use.
Assess for history of nosebleed, including site, frequency, amount of bleeding, treatment, and difficulty stopping bleeding.	Characteristics sometimes reveal trauma, medication use, or excessive dryness as causative factors.
Ask if patient uses nasal spray or drops, including amount, frequency, and duration of use.	Overuse of over-the-counter nasal preparations causes physical change in mucosa.
Ask if patient snores at night or has difficulty breathing.	Difficulty with breathing or snoring indicates septal deviation or obstruction.

BOX 32-16 PATIENT TEACHING

Nose and Sinus Assessment

Objectives

- Patient will safely use over-the-counter nasal sprays.
- Parents will take proper measures to stop a child's nosebleed.
- Older persons will take safety precautions with loss of olfaction.

Teaching Strategies

- Caution patient against overuse of over-the-counter nasal sprays, which leads to "rebound" effect, causing excess nasal congestion.
- Instruct parents in care of a child with nosebleeds: have child sit up and lean forward to avoid aspiration of blood, apply pressure to the anterior nose with the thumb and forefinger as the child breathes through the mouth, and apply ice or a cold cloth to the bridge of the nose if pressure fails to stop bleeding.
- Instruct all patients to install smoke detectors on each floor of their home.
- Instruct older persons to always check dated labels on food to ensure against spoilage.

Evaluation

- Have patient explain proper use of over-the-counter nasal sprays.
- Have parents demonstrate and describe technique for stopping a nosebleed.
- Inspect patient's home during visit, and look for smoke detectors. Ask to check some food items in the refrigerator.

easily if sinus irritation is present. Do not apply pressure to the eyes. If tenderness of sinuses is present, the sinuses may be transilluminated.

Mouth and Pharynx

The mouth and pharynx are assessed to detect signs of overall health, determine oral hygiene needs, and develop therapies for patients with dehydration, restricted intake, oral trauma, or oral airway obstruction. To assess the oral cavity, use a penlight and tongue depressor or a single gauze square. Wear clean gloves during the examination. Have the patient sit or lie down during the examination. The oral cavity can also be assessed while administering oral hygiene (see Chapter 38). Table 32-15 describes the nursing history for assessment of the mouth and pharynx.

Lips. Have patients wearing lipstick remove it before the examination. Inspect the lips for colour, texture, hydration, contour, and lesions. With the patient's mouth closed, view the lips from end to end.

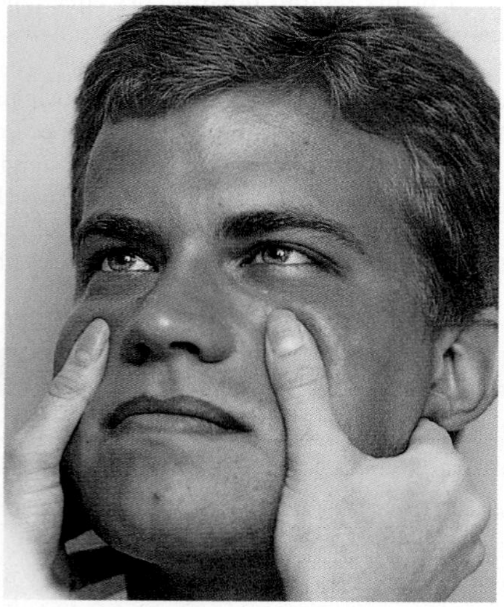

FIGURE 32-9 Palpation of maxillary sinuses.

Normally they are pink, moist, symmetrical, and smooth. Lip colour in dark-skinned patients varies from pink to plum. Anemia causes pallor of the lips, with cyanosis caused by respiratory or cardiovascular problems. Cherry-coloured lips indicate carbon monoxide poisoning. Any lesions such as nodules or ulcerations are related to infection, irritation, or skin cancer.

Buccal Mucosa, Gums, and Teeth. Ask the patient to clench the teeth and smile so that teeth occlusion can be observed. The upper molars normally rest directly on the lower molars, and the upper incisors slightly override the lower incisors. A symmetrical smile reveals normal facial nerve function.

Inspect the teeth to determine the quality of dental hygiene (Box 32-17). Note the position and alignment of the teeth. To examine the posterior surface of the teeth, have the patient open the mouth with the lips relaxed. Use a tongue depressor to retract the lips and cheeks, especially when viewing the molars. Note the colour of teeth and presence of dental caries (cavities), tartar, and extraction sites. Normal, healthy teeth are smooth, white, and shiny. A chalky white discoloration of the enamel is an early indication of caries formation. Brown or black discolorations indicate the formation of caries. A stained yellow colour is from tobacco use, whereas coffee, tea, and colas cause a brown stain. In the older person, loose or missing teeth are common because bone resorption increases. An older person's teeth often feel rough when tooth enamel calcifies. Yellow or darkened teeth are also common in the older person because of the general wear and tear that exposes the darker, underlying dentin.

To view the mucosa and gums, ask the patient to first remove any dental appliance. View the inner oral mucosa by having the patient open and relax the mouth slightly and then gently retract the patient's lower lip away from the teeth (Figure 32-10). Repeat this process for the upper lip. Inspect the mucosa for colour, hydration, texture, and lesions such as ulcers, abrasions, or cysts. Normally the mucosa is a glistening pink, smooth, and moist. Some common small, yellow-white raised lesions on the buccal mucosa and lips are Fordyce spots, or ectopic sebaceous glands (Ball et al., 2015a). If lesions are present, palpate them gently with a gloved hand for tenderness, size, and consistency.

TABLE 32-15 Nursing History for Mouth and Pharyngeal Assessment

Assessment Category	Rationale
Determine if patient wears dentures or retainers and if they are comfortable.	Patient needs to remove dentures for nurse to visualize and palpate gums. Ill-fitting dentures chronically irritate mucosa and gums.
Determine if patient has had recent change in appetite or weight.	Symptoms result from painful mouth conditions or poor hygiene.
Determine if patient uses tobacco products:	
Smoking of cigarette, cigar, or pipe	Smoking of these products increases risk for lung, oral cavity, larynx, and esophageal cancers (Canadian Cancer Society Steering Committee [CCS], 2017).
Smokeless tobacco: use of chewing tobacco and snuff	Smokeless tobacco causes various cancers and noncancerous oral disorders. Long-term snuff users have increased risk for cancer of the gums and cheeks (CCS, 2017c).
Review history for alcohol consumption.	Excessive alcohol consumption appears to put a person at greater risk for oral cavity and pharynx cancer. Effects of alcohol are independent of tobacco use.
Assess dental hygiene practices, including use of fluoride toothpaste, frequency of brushing and flossing, and frequency of dental visits.	Assessment reveals patient's need for education, financial support, or both. Periodontal disease has a higher prevalence in older persons who have a history of high plaque buildup, use tobacco, and visit the dentist infrequently.
Ask if patient has pain from chewing or eating. If so, ask if mouth lesions are present, including duration and associated symptoms.	Pain is often associated with a broken tooth, tooth grinding, or temporomandibular joint problems. Extra care is needed during oral hygiene administration.

BOX 32-17 PATIENT TEACHING

Mouth and Pharyngeal Assessment

Objectives

- Patient will practise proper oral hygiene measures and dental care.
- Patient will describe warning signs of oral cancer.
- Older patient will maintain normal solid food intake.

Teaching Strategies

- Discuss proper techniques for oral hygiene, including brushing and flossing (see Chapter 38).
- Explain the early warning signs of oral cavity and pharynx cancer: a sore that bleeds easily and does not heal, a lump or thickening, and a red or white patch on the mucosa that persists. Difficulty chewing, swallowing, or moving the tongue or jaw are late symptoms (Canadian Cancer Society, 2017c).
- Encourage regular dental examination every 6 months for children, adults, and older persons.
- Identify older persons who have difficulty chewing and changes in the teeth. Teach patients to eat soft foods and cut food into small pieces.

Evaluation

- Ask patient to demonstrate brushing.
- Have patient identify when to have regular dental checkups.
- Have patient identify the warning signs of oral cavity and pharynx cancer.
- Ask older patient to keep a diet record for 3 days.

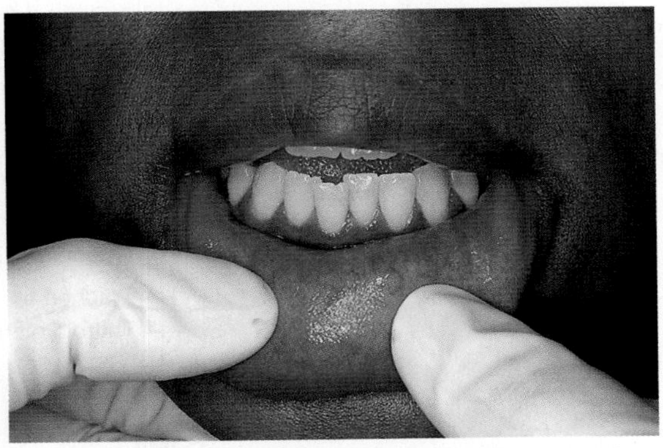

FIGURE 32-10 Inspection of inner oral mucosa of the lower lip.

To inspect the buccal mucosa, ask the patient to open the mouth, and then gently retract the cheeks with a tongue depressor or gloved finger covered with gauze (Figure 32-11). View the surface of the mucosa from right to left and top to bottom. A penlight illuminates the most posterior portion of the mucosa. Normal mucosa is glistening, pink, soft, moist, and smooth. Varying shades of hyperpigmentation are normal in 10% of light-skinned patients after age 50 and up to 90% of dark-skinned patients by the same age. For patients with normal pigmentation, the buccal mucosa is a good site to inspect for jaundice and pallor. In older persons, the mucosa is normally dry because of reduced salivation. Thick white patches (**leukoplakia**) are often a precancerous lesion seen in heavy smokers and alcoholics. Palpate for any buccal lesions by placing the index finger within the buccal cavity and the thumb on the outer surface of the cheek.

Safety Alert Patients who smoke cigarettes, cigars, or pipes and those who use smokeless tobacco have an increased risk of oral, laryngeal, and esophageal cancer. These individuals may have leukoplakia or other lesions anywhere in their oral cavity (e.g., lips, gums, tongue) at an early age.

Inspect the gums (gingivae) for colour, edema, retraction, bleeding, and lesions while retracting the cheeks. Healthy gums are pink, smooth, and moist and tightly fit around each tooth. Dark-skinned patients often have patchy pigmentation. In older persons, the gums are usually pale. Using clean gloves, palpate the gums to assess for lesions, thickening, or masses. Normally there is no tenderness. Spongy gums that bleed easily indicate periodontal disease and vitamin C deficiency. If the patient has loose or mobile teeth, swollen gums, or pockets containing debris at the tooth margins, suspect periodontal disease or gingivitis.

Tongue and Floor of Mouth. Carefully inspect the tongue on all sides, as well as the floor of the mouth. Have the patient relax the mouth and stick the tongue out halfway. Note any deviation, tremor, or limitation in movement. This tests hypoglossal nerve function. If the patient protrudes the tongue too far, this will elicit the gag reflex. When the tongue protrudes, it lies midline. To test for tongue mobility, ask the patient to raise the tongue up and move it from side to side. The tongue should move freely.

Using a penlight for illumination, examine the tongue for colour, size, position, texture, and coatings or lesions. A normal tongue is medium or dull red in colour, moist, slightly rough on the top surface, and smooth along the lateral margins. The undersurface of the tongue and the floor of the mouth are highly vascular (Figure 32-12). Take extra care to inspect this area, a common site for oral cancer lesions. The patient lifts the tongue by placing its tip on the palate behind the upper incisors. Inspect for colour, swelling, and lesions such as nodules or cysts. The ventral surface of the tongue is pink and smooth, with large veins between the frenulum folds. To palpate the tongue, explain the procedure and ask the patient to protrude the tongue. Grasp the tip with a gauze square and gently pull it to one side. With a gloved hand, palpate the full length of the tongue and the base for any areas of hardening or ulceration. **Varicosities** (swollen, tortuous veins) are common in the older person and rarely cause problems.

Palate. Have the patient extend the head backward, holding the mouth open to inspect the hard and soft palates. The hard palate, or roof of the mouth, is located anteriorly. The whitish hard palate is dome shaped. The soft palate extends posteriorly toward the pharynx. It is normally light pink and smooth. Observe the palates for colour, shape, texture, and extra bony prominences or defects (Figure 32-13). A bony growth, or **exostosis**, between the two palates is common.

Pharynx. Perform an examination of pharyngeal structures to rule out infection, inflammation, or lesions. Have the patient tip the head back slightly, open the mouth wide, and say "Ah" while you place the tip of a tongue depressor on the middle third of the tongue. Take care not to press the lower lip against the teeth. By placing the tongue depressor too far anteriorly, the posterior part of the tongue mounds up, obstructing the view. Placing the tongue depressor on the posterior tongue elicits the gag reflex.

With a penlight, first inspect the uvula and soft palate (Figure 32-14). Both structures, which are innervated by the tenth cranial

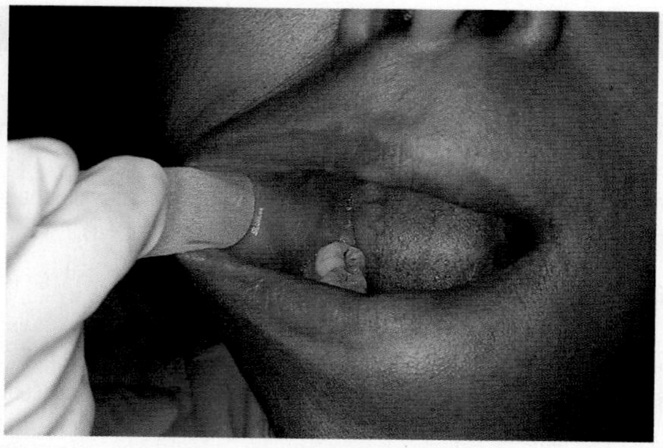

FIGURE 32-11 Retraction of the buccal mucosa allows for clear visualization.

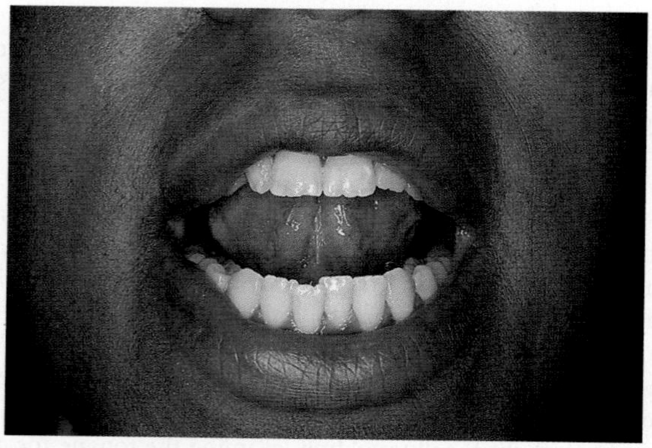

FIGURE 32-12 The undersurface of the tongue is highly vascular.

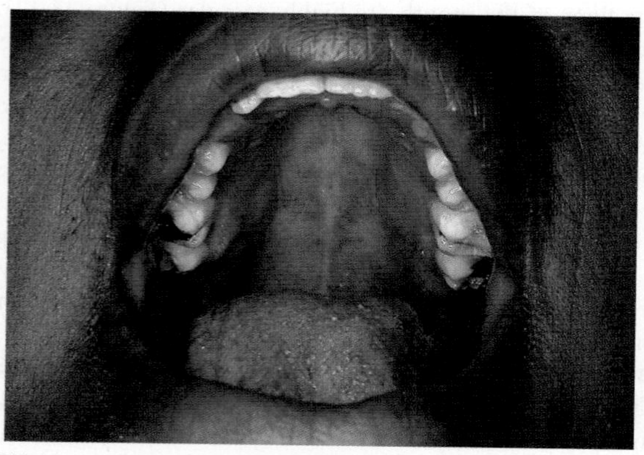

FIGURE 32-13 The hard palate is located anteriorly in the roof of the mouth.

(vagus) nerve, should rise centrally as the patient says "Ah." Examine the anterior and posterior pillars, soft palate, and uvula. View the tonsils in the cavities between the anterior and posterior pillars and note the presence or absence of tissue. The posterior pharynx is behind the pillars. Normally, pharyngeal tissues are pink and smooth and well hydrated. Small irregular spots of lymphatic tissue and small blood vessels are normal. Note edema, petechiae (small hemorrhages), lesions, or exudate. Patients with chronic sinus problems frequently exhibit a clear exudate that drains along the wall of the posterior pharynx. Yellow or green exudate indicates infection. A patient with a

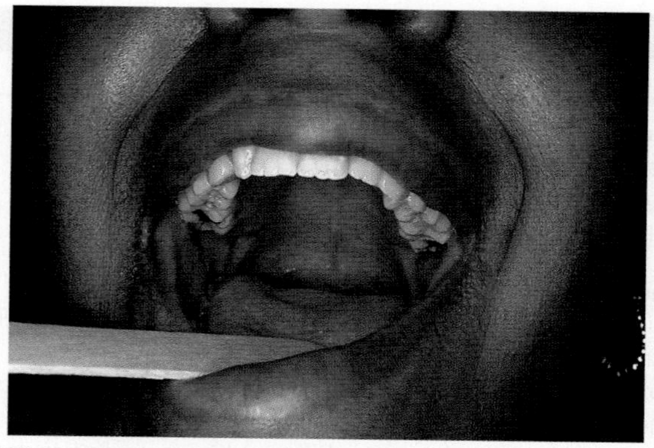

FIGURE 32-14 Use of a penlight and tongue depressor enables visualization of the uvula and posterior soft palate.

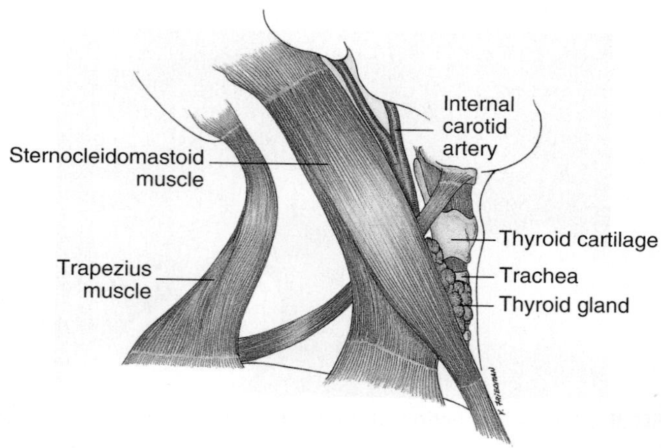

FIGURE 32-15 Anatomical position of the major neck structures. Note the triangles formed by the sternocleidomastoid muscle, lower jaw, and anterior neck anteriorly and by the sternocleidomastoid muscle, trapezius muscle, and lower neck posteriorly.

typical sore throat has a red and edematous uvula and tonsillar pillars with possible presence of yellow exudate.

Neck

Assessment of the neck includes assessment of the neck muscles, lymph nodes of the head and neck, carotid arteries, jugular veins, thyroid gland, and trachea (Figure 32-15). The examination of the jugular veins and carotid arteries is included under the vascular system assessment. Inspection and palpation of the neck are performed to determine the integrity of the neck structures and to examine the lymphatic system. The lymphatic system is examined region by region during the assessment of body systems (head and neck, breast, genitalia, and extremities). An abnormality of superficial lymph nodes sometimes reveals the presence of an infection or malignancy. Examination of the thyroid gland and trachea also aids in ruling out malignancies. This examination is carried out with the patient sitting. The sternocleidomastoid and trapezius muscles outline the areas of the neck, dividing each side of the neck into two triangles. The anterior triangle contains the trachea, thyroid gland, carotid artery, and anterior cervical lymph nodes. The posterior triangle contains the posterior lymph nodes. Table 32-16 reviews the nursing history for the head and neck examination.

TABLE 32-16 Nursing History for Neck Assessment

Assessment Category	Rationale
Assess for history of recent cold or infection or enlarged lymph nodes, exposure to radiation or toxic chemicals.	Colds or infections (e.g., mononucleosis) cause temporary or permanent lymph node enlargement. Lymph nodes are also enlarged in various diseases such as cancer.
If there is an enlarged lymph node, consider reviewing history of intravenous drug use, hemophilia, sexual contact with people infected with human immunodeficiency virus (HIV), history of blood transfusion, multiple and indiscriminate sexual contacts, or male with homosexual or bisexual activities.	These are risk factors for HIV infection.
Ask if patient has had history of neck pain with restriction in movement.	Indicates muscle strain, head injury, local nerve injury, or enlarged or swollen lymph node.
Ask if patient has had change in temperature preference (more or less clothing); swelling in neck; change in texture of hair, skin, or nails; or change in emotional stability.	Symptoms indicative of thyroid disease.
Ask if patient has history of hypothyroidism or hyperthyroidism or takes thyroid medication or has a family history of thyroid disease.	Disease or medications influence tissue growth of gland.
Review medical history of pneumothorax (collapsed lung) or bronchial tumour.	Conditions place patient at risk for tracheal displacement or lateral deviation.

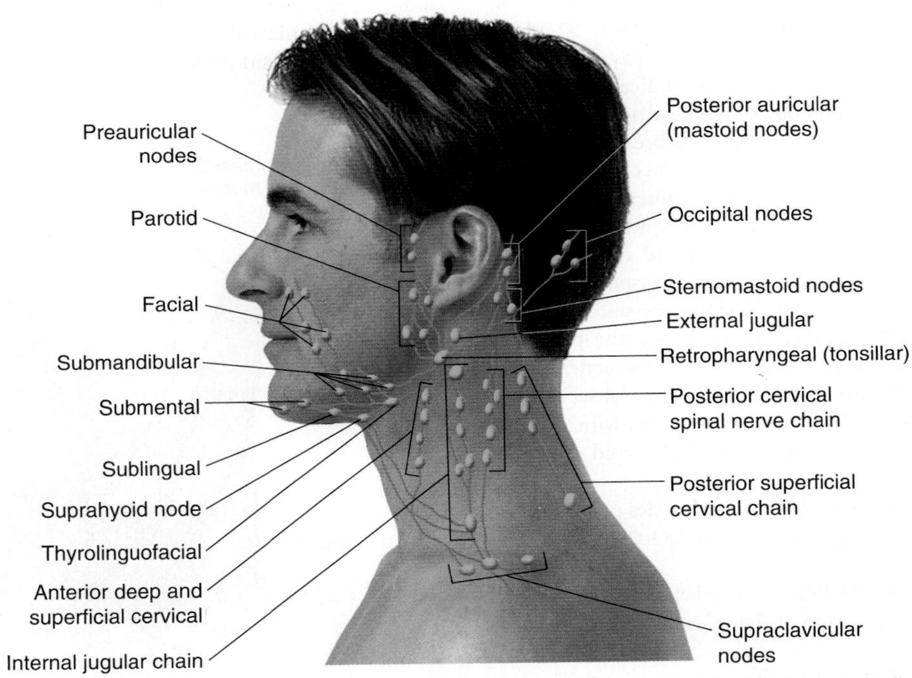

FIGURE 32-16 Palpable lymph nodes in the head and neck. (From Ball et al. [2015]. *Seidel's guide to physical examination* [8th ed., p. 169]. St. Louis, MO: Mosby.)

Neck Muscles. The neck is inspected first in the usual anatomical position, with slight hyperextension. Observe for symmetry of the neck muscles. Ask the patient to flex the neck with the chin to the chest, hyperextend the neck backward, and move the head laterally to each side and then sideways with the ear moving toward the shoulder. This tests the sternocleidomastoid and trapezius muscles. The neck normally moves without discomfort. Tests that assess muscle strength and function can be performed during assessment of the head and neck, although the description of these tests is included in the assessment of the musculoskeletal system.

Lymph Nodes. An extensive system of lymph nodes collects lymph from the head, ears, nose, cheeks, and lips (Figure 32-16). The immune system protects the body from foreign antigens, removes damaged cells from the circulation, and provides a partial barrier to growth of malignant cells within the body. Assessing the lymph nodes requires competence when caring for patients with suspected immunoincompetence, which is often linked to allergies, human immunodeficiency virus (HIV) infection, autoimmune disease (e.g., lupus erythematosus), lymphomas or serious infection.

With the patient's chin raised and head tilted slightly, first inspect the area where lymph nodes are distributed and compare both sides. This position stretches the skin slightly over any possible enlarged nodes. Inspect visible nodes for edema, erythema, or red streaks. Nodes are not normally visible.

Use a methodical approach to palpate the lymph nodes to avoid overlooking any single node or chain. The patient relaxes with the neck flexed slightly forward. Inspect and palpate both sides of the neck for comparison. During palpation, either face or stand to the side of the patient for easy access to all nodes. Using the pads of the middle three fingers of each hand, gently palpate in a rotary motion over the nodes. Check each node methodically in the following sequence: occipital, postauricular nodes, preauricular, retropharyngeal, submandibular, and submental. Try to detect enlargement and note the location, size, shape, surface characteristics, consistency, mobility, tenderness, and warmth of the nodes. If the skin is mobile, move the skin over the area of the nodes. It is important to press underlying tissue in each area and not simply move the fingers over the skin. However, if excessive pressure is applied, it is easy to miss small nodes and destroy palpable nodes.

To palpate supraclavicular nodes, ask the patient to bend the head forward and relax the shoulders. Palpate these nodes by hooking the index and third finger over the clavicle, lateral to the sternocleidomastoid muscle. Palpate the deep cervical nodes only with the fingers hooked around the sternocleidomastoid muscle.

Normally lymph nodes are not easily palpable. However, small, mobile, nontender nodes are common. Lymph nodes that are large, fixed, inflamed, or tender indicate a problem such as local infection, systemic disease, or neoplasm (Jarvis et al., 2014) (Box 32-18). If enlarged nodes are found, explore the adjacent areas and regions drained by the nodes. Tenderness almost always indicates inflammation. A problem involving a lymph node of the head and neck means an abnormality in the mouth, throat, abdomen, breasts, thorax, or arms. These are the areas drained by the head and neck nodes.

Thyroid Gland. The thyroid gland lies in the anterior lower neck, in front of and to both sides of the trachea. The gland is fixed to the trachea with the isthmus overlying the trachea and connecting the two irregular, cone-shaped lobes (Figure 32-17). Inspect the lower neck overlying the thyroid gland for obvious masses, symmetry, and any subtle fullness at the base of the neck. Ask the patient to hyperextend the neck, which helps tighten the skin for better visualization. Offer the patient a glass of water, and, while observing the neck, have the patient swallow. This manoeuvre helps with visualizing an abnormally enlarged thyroid. Normally, the thyroid cannot be visualized.

For information about palpating for enlarged nodes or masses, see the textbook by Jarvis and colleagues (2014, pp. 282–283) or that by Ball and colleagues (2015, pp. 193–195).

Carotid Artery and Jugular Vein. This portion of the examination is described under examination of the vascular system (see later section).

Trachea. The trachea is a part of the upper respiratory system that the examiner directly palpates. It is normally located in the midline above the suprasternal notch. Masses in the neck or mediastinum and pulmonary abnormalities cause displacement laterally. Have the patient sit or lie down during palpation. Determine the position of the trachea by palpating at the suprasternal notch, slipping the thumb and index fingers to each side. Note if the finger and thumb shift laterally. Do not apply forceful pressure because this elicits coughing.

THORAX AND LUNGS

Accurate physical assessment of the thorax and lungs requires review of the ventilatory and respiratory functions of the lungs. If disease is affecting the lungs, this will affect other body systems as well. For example, reduced oxygenation causes changes in mental alertness because of the brain's sensitivity to lowered oxygen levels. Data from all body systems are used to determine the nature of pulmonary alterations.

Before assessing the thorax and lungs, be familiar with the landmarks of the chest (Figure 32-18). These landmarks help in identifying findings and using assessment skills correctly. The patient's nipples, angle of Louis, suprasternal notch, costal angle, clavicles, and vertebrae are key landmarks that provide a series of imaginary lines for sign identification. Keep a mental image of the location of the lobes of the lung and the position of each rib (Figure 32-19). The proper orientation to anatomical structures ensures a thorough assessment of the anterior, lateral, and posterior thorax.

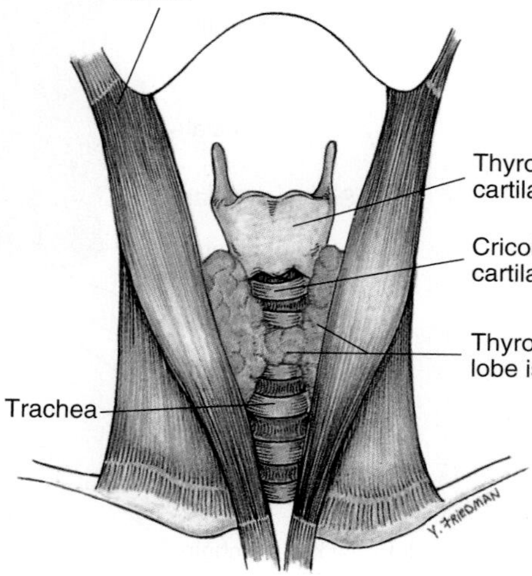

FIGURE 32-17 Anatomical position of the thyroid gland.

BOX 32-18 PATIENT TEACHING

Neck Assessment

Objective

- Patient takes proper preventive action if he or she notices a mass in the neck.

Teaching Strategies

- Stress importance of regular adherence to medication schedule to patients with thyroid disease.
- Instruct patient about the lymph nodes and how infection commonly causes node tenderness.
- Instruct patient to call a health care provider when he or she notices an enlarged lump or mass in the neck.
- Teach patient risk factors for human immunodeficiency virus (HIV) infection and other sexually transmitted infections.

Evaluation

- Have patient explain when to notify a health care provider about a neck mass.

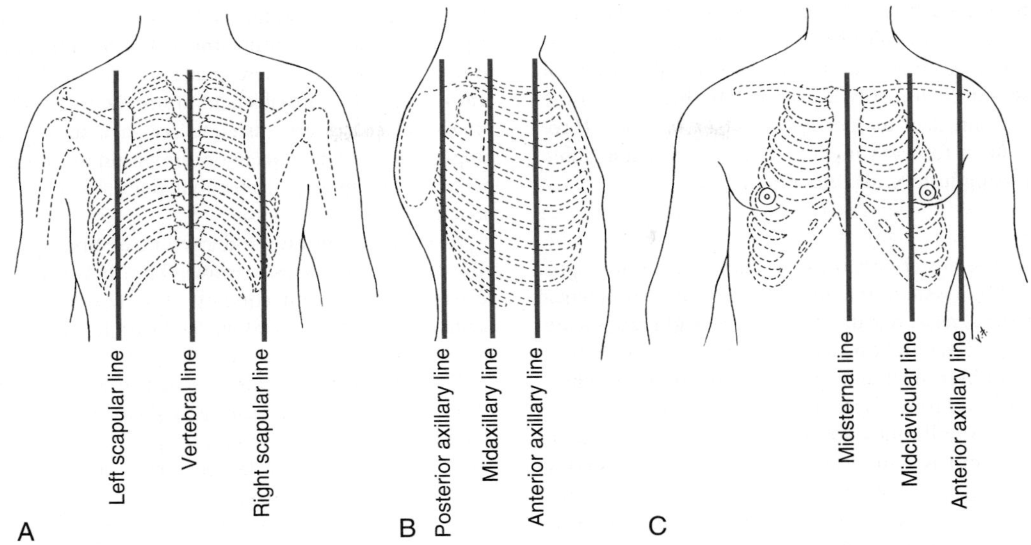

FIGURE 32-18 Anatomical chest wall landmarks. **A,** Posterior chest landmarks. **B,** Lateral chest landmarks. **C,** Anterior chest landmarks.

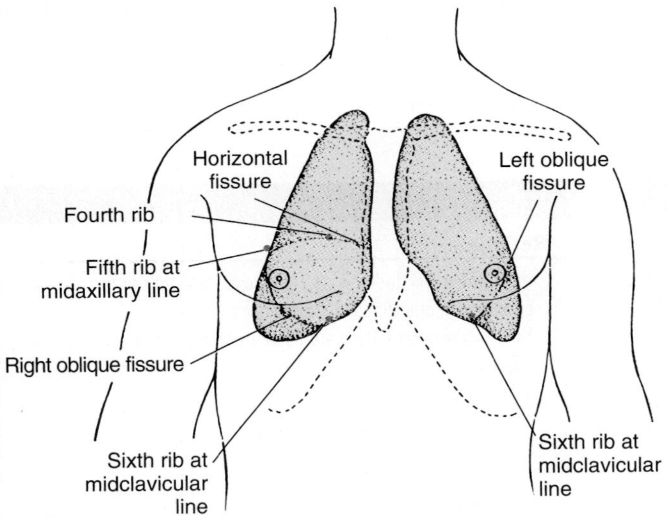

FIGURE 32-19 Anterior position of lung lobes in relation to anatomical landmarks.

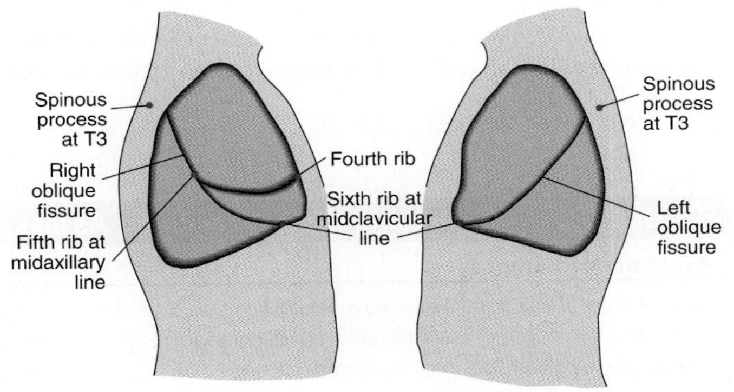

FIGURE 32-20 Lateral position of lung lobes in relation to anatomical landmarks.

Locating the position of each rib is critical to visualizing the lobe of the lung being assessed. To begin, locate the angle of Louis at the manubriosternal junction. The angle is a visible and palpable angulation of the sternum and is the point at which the second rib articulates with the sternum. Count the ribs and intercostal spaces (between the ribs) from this point. The number of each intercostal space corresponds with that of the rib just above it. The spinous process of the third thoracic vertebra and the fourth, fifth, and sixth ribs helps to locate the lung's lobes laterally. The lower lobes project laterally and anteriorly (Figure 32-20). Posteriorly, the tip or inferior margin of the scapula lies approximately at the level of the seventh rib (Figure 32-21). After identifying the seventh rib, count upward to locate the third thoracic vertebra, and align it with the inner borders of the scapula to locate the posterior lobes.

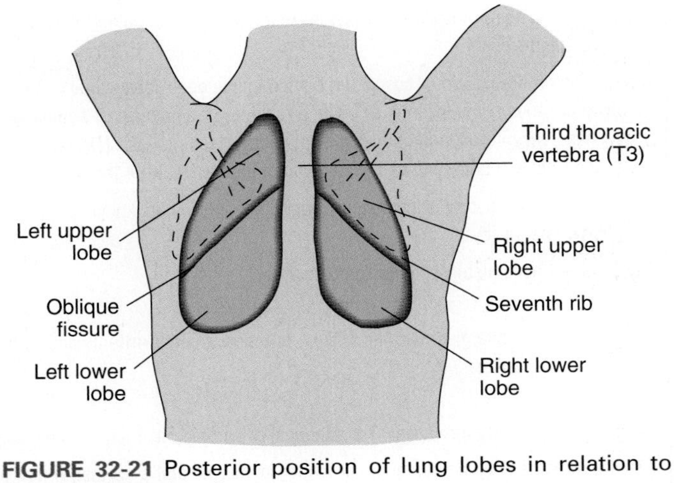

FIGURE 32-21 Posterior position of lung lobes in relation to anatomical landmarks.

The examination requires the patient to be undressed to the waist, with good lighting. Assess patients at risk for pulmonary problems, such as the patient confined to bed rest or the patient with chest pain who cannot fully expand the lungs. The examination begins with the patient sitting for assessment of the posterior and lateral chest. Have the patient sit or lie down for assessment of the anterior chest. Table 32-17 reviews the nursing history for lung examination.

Posterior Thorax

Begin examination of the posterior thorax by observing for any signs or symptoms in other body systems that indicate pulmonary problems. Reduced mental alertness, nasal flaring, somnolence, and cyanosis are examples of signs assessed that indicate oxygenation problems. Inspect the posterior thorax by observing the shape and symmetry of the chest from the patient's back and front. Note the anteroposterior diameter. Body shape or posture significantly impairs ventilatory movement. Normally the chest contour is symmetrical, with the anteroposterior diameter one-third to one-half of the transverse, or side-to-side, diameter. A barrel-shaped chest (anteroposterior diameter equals transverse diameter) characterizes aging and chronic lung disease. Infants have an almost round shape. Congenital and postural alterations cause abnormal contours. Some patients lean over a table or splint the side of the chest because of a breathing problem. Splinting or holding the chest wall because of pain causes a patient to bend toward the side affected. Such a posture impairs ventilatory movement.

Standing at a midline position behind the patient, look for deformities, position of the spine, slope of the ribs, retraction of the intercostal spaces during inspiration, and bulging of the intercostal spaces during expiration. The scapulae are normally symmetrical and closely attached to the thoracic wall. The normal spine is straight without lateral deviation. Posteriorly, the ribs tend to slope across and down. The ribs and intercostal spaces are easier to see in a thin person. Normally, no bulging or active movement occurs within the intercostal spaces during breathing. Bulging indicates that the patient is using great effort to breathe.

Also assess the rate and rhythm of breathing (see Chapter 30). Observe the thorax as a whole. The thorax normally expands and relaxes regularly with equality of movement bilaterally. In healthy adults, the normal respiratory rates vary from 12 to 20 respirations per minute.

The posterior thorax is palpated to assess further characteristics. Palpate the thoracic muscles and skeleton for lumps, masses, pulsations, and unusual movement. If the patient notes pain or tenderness, avoid deep palpation. Fractured rib fragments could be displaced against vital organs. Normally the chest wall is not tender. If there is a suspicious mass or swollen area, lightly palpate it for size, shape, and the typical qualities of a lesion.

To measure chest excursion or depth of breathing, stand behind the patient and place the thumbs along the spinal processes at the tenth rib, with the palms lightly contacting the posterolateral surfaces (Ball et al., 2015a). Place thumbs 5 cm apart, pointing toward the spine and fingers pointing laterally (Figure 32-22, *A*). Press the hands toward the spine so that a small skin fold appears between the thumbs. Do not slide the hands over the skin. Instruct the patient to take a deep breath

TABLE 32-17 Nursing History for Lung Assessment

Assessment Category	Rationale
Assess history of tobacco or marijuana use, including type of tobacco, duration and amount (pack-years = number of years smoked × number of packs per day), age started, and efforts to quit and length of time since smoking stopped.	Smoking is a risk factor for lung cancer, heart disease, cerebrovascular disease, emphysema, or chronic bronchitis. Smoking accounts for a significant percentage of all cancer deaths.
Ask if patient has had a *persistent cough* (productive or nonproductive), *sputum streaked with blood, voice change, chest pain,* shortness of breath, orthopnea, dyspnea during exertion or at rest, poor activity tolerance, or *recurrent attacks of pneumonia or bronchitis.*	Symptoms of cardiopulmonary alterations help localize objective physical findings. (Warning signals for lung cancer are in italic type.)
Determine if patient works or lives in an environment containing pollutants (e.g., asbestos, arsenic, coal dust) or requiring exposure to radiation. Does patient have exposure to second-hand smoke?	These risk factors increase chance for various lung diseases.
Review history for known or suspected human immunodeficiency virus (HIV) infection, substance abuse, low income, or being a resident or employee of a nursing home or shelter, homeless, recent prison inmate, family member of tuberculosis (TB) patient, or immigrant to Canada from a country where TB is prevalent (Public Health Agency of Canada, 2016a).	These are risk factors for HIV.
Ask if patient has history of persistent cough, hemoptysis, unexplained weight loss, fatigue, night sweats, or fever.	These are risk factors for both TB and HIV infection.
Does patient have history of chronic hoarseness?	Hoarseness indicates laryngeal disorder or abuse of cocaine or opioids (sniffing).
Assess history of allergies to pollens, dust, or other airborne irritants and to foods, drugs, or chemical substances.	Symptoms such as choking feeling, bronchospasm with respiratory stridor, wheezes on auscultation, and dyspnea are often caused by allergic response.
Review family history for cancer, TB, allergies, or chronic obstructive pulmonary disease.	Conditions place patient at risk for lung disease.
Ask if patient has had a pneumonia or influenza vaccine and a TB test; if not, educate patient on need to do so.	The very young, the very old, and those with chronic respiratory problems or with immunosuppressive diseases are at increased risk for respiratory disease.

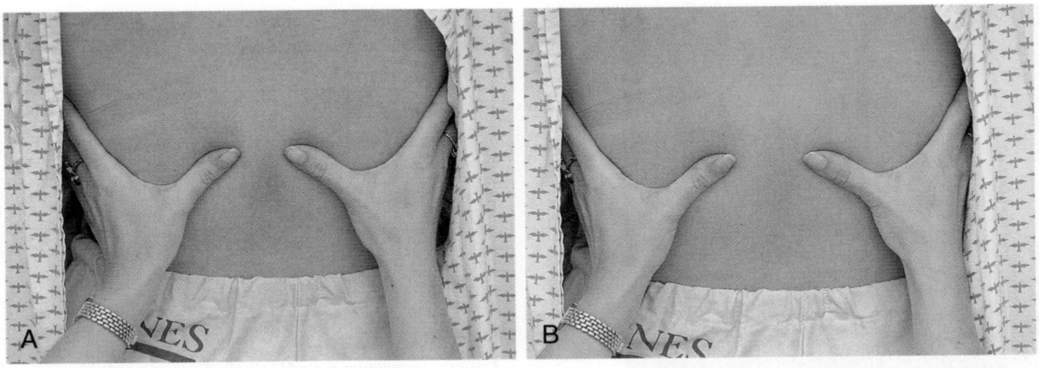

FIGURE 32-22 **A,** Hand position for palpation of posterior thorax excursion. **B,** As patient inhales, movement of chest excursion separates the thumbs.

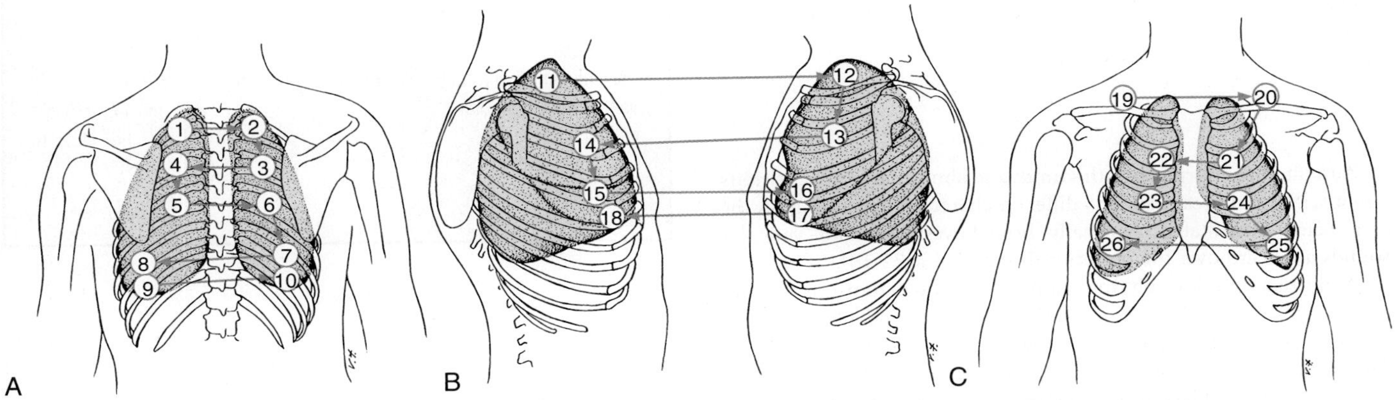

FIGURE 32-23 **A-C,** A systematic pattern (posterior-lateral-anterior) is followed when palpating and auscultating the thorax. (From Ball et al. [2015]. *Seidel's guide to physical examination* [8th ed., p. 275]. St. Louis, MO: Mosby.)

after exhaling. Note movement of the thumbs (Figure 32-22, *B*). Chest excursion is symmetrical, separating the thumbs 3 to 5 cm. Reduced chest excursions may be caused by pain, postural deformity, or fatigue. In the older person, chest movement normally declines because of costal cartilage calcification and respiratory muscle atrophy (reduction in size).

During speech, the sound created by the vocal cords is transmitted through the lung to the chest wall. The sound waves create vibrations that are palpated externally. These vibrations are called vocal fremitus or tactile fremitus. Accumulation of mucus, collapse of lung tissue, or presence of lung lesions blocks the vibrations from reaching the chest wall.

To palpate for tactile fremitus, place the palmar surfaces of the fingers or the ulnar part of the hand over symmetrical intercostal spaces, beginning at the lung apex (Figure 32-23, *A*), using a firm, light touch. Ask the patient to say "ninety-nine" or "one-one-one." Palpate both sides simultaneously and symmetrically (from top to bottom) for comparison, or use one hand, quickly alternating between the two sides (Ball et al., 2015a). Normally, a faint vibration is present as the patient speaks. If fremitus is faint, ask the patient to speak in a louder or lower tone of voice. Normally, fremitus is symmetrical. Vibrations are strongest at the top, near the level of the tracheal bifurcation. In a crying infant, assess strong vibrations through the chest wall.

Auscultation is used to assess the movement of air through the tracheobronchial tree and detect mucus or obstructed airways. Normally, air flows through the airways in an unobstructed pattern. In recognizing the sounds created by normal airflow, the examiner can detect sounds caused by airway obstruction.

Place the diaphragm of the stethoscope firmly on the skin, over the posterior chest wall between the ribs (Figure 32-24). The patient folds the arms in front of the chest and keeps the head bent forward while taking slow, deep breaths with the mouth slightly open. Listen to an entire inspiration and expiration at each position of the stethoscope. If sounds are faint, as in the obese patient, ask the patient to breathe harder and faster temporarily. Breath sounds are much louder in children because of their thin chest walls. In children, the bell, or a pediatric stethoscope, works best because of a child's small chest. Use a systematic pattern comparing lung sounds in one region on one side of the body with sounds in the same region on the opposite side. It is impossible to remember the quality of all sounds noted on one side of the body and then compare them with sounds on the other side (see Figure 32-22, *A*).

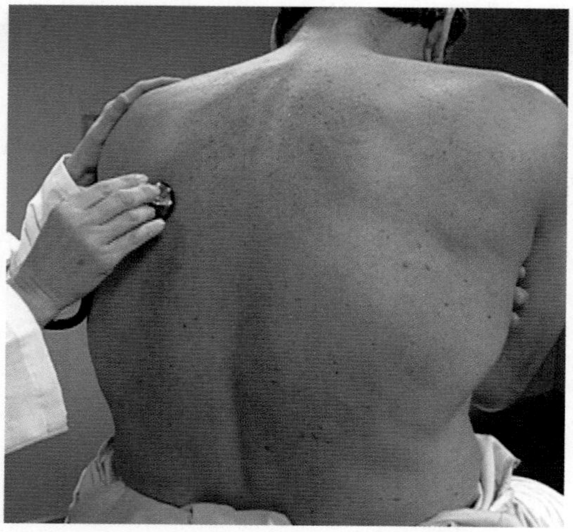

FIGURE 32-24 Use the diaphragm of the stethoscope to auscultate breath sounds. (From Ball et al. [2015a]. *Seidel's guide to physical examination* [8th ed., p. 276]. St. Louis, MO: Mosby.)

TABLE 32-18 Normal Breath Sounds

Description	Location	Origin
Vesicular		
Vesicular sounds are soft, breezy, and low-pitched. Inspiratory phase is three times longer than expiratory phase.	Best heard over lung's periphery (except over scapula)	Created by air moving through smaller airways
Bronchovesicular		
Bronchovesicular sounds are blowing sounds that are medium-pitched and of medium intensity. Inspiratory phase is equal to expiratory phase.	Best heard posteriorly between scapulae and anteriorly over bronchioles lateral to sternum at first and second intercostal spaces	Created by air moving through large airways
Bronchial		
Bronchial sounds are loud and high-pitched with hollow quality. Expiration lasts longer than inspiration (3 : 2 ratio).	Heard only over trachea	Created by air moving through trachea close to chest wall

Auscultate for normal breath sounds and abnormal or **adventitious sounds.** Normal breath sounds differ in character, depending on the area being auscultated. Normally bronchovesicular and vesicular sounds are heard over the posterior thorax (Table 32-18).

Abnormal sounds result from air passing through moisture, mucus, or narrowed airways. They also result from alveoli suddenly reinflating or from an inflammation between the pleural linings of the lung. Adventitious sounds often occur superimposed over normal sounds. The four types of adventitious sounds are crackles, rhonchi, wheezes, and pleural friction rub. A specific entity causes each sound, and each has typical auditory features (Table 32-19). During auscultation, note the location and characteristics of the sounds, and listen for the absence of breath sounds (found in patients with collapsed or surgically removed lobes).

If there are abnormalities in tactile fremitus or auscultation, perform the vocal resonance tests (spoken and whispered voice sounds). Place the stethoscope over the same locations used to assess breath sounds, and have the patient say "ninety-nine" in a normal voice tone. Normally, the sound is muffled. If fluid is compressing the lung, the vibrations from the patient's voice are transmitted to the chest wall and the sound becomes clear (**bronchophony**). Then ask the patient to whisper "ninety-nine." The whispered voice is usually faint and indistinct. Certain lung abnormalities cause the whispered voice to become clear and distinct (**whispered pectoriloquy**). Bronchophony and whispered pectoriloquy can be indicative of lung disorders such as pneumonia, asthma, chronic obstructive pulmonary disease (COPD), and lung tumours and suggest the need for diagnostic assessment (Box 32-19).

Lateral Thorax

Assessment of the posterior thorax is extended to the lateral sides of the chest. The patient sits during examination of the lateral chest. Have the patient raise the arms, to improve access to lateral thoracic structures. Use inspection, palpation, and auscultation skills to examine the lateral thorax (see Figure 32-23, *B*). Do not assess excursion laterally. Normally, the breath sounds heard are vesicular.

Anterior Thorax

The anterior thorax is inspected for the same features as the posterior thorax. The patient sits or lies down with the head elevated. Observe the accessory muscles of breathing: sternocleidomastoid, trapezius, and abdominal muscles. The accessory muscles move little with normal passive breathing. When an adult patient requires effort to breathe as a result of strenuous exercise or disease (e.g., COPD), the accessory muscles and abdominal muscles contract. Some patients produce a grunting sound. In children, an increased effort to breathe can cause an increased use of accessory muscles of the neck and chest, resulting in nasal flaring, tracheal tug (indrawing of the suprasternal area), and chest wall retractions. Children sometimes produce an audible wheeze or barking sounds.

Observe the width of the costal angle; it is usually larger than 90 degrees between the two costal margins. Observe the breathing pattern. Normal breathing is quiet and barely audible near the open mouth. Most often, respiratory rate and rhythm are assessed anteriorly (see Chapter 30). The male patient's respirations are usually diaphragmatic, whereas a female's are more costal. Accurate assessment occurs as a patient breathes passively.

Palpate the anterior thoracic muscles and skeleton for lumps, masses, tenderness, or unusual movement. The sternum and xiphoid are relatively inflexible. Place the thumbs parallel along the costal margin approximately 6 cm apart with the palms touching the anterolateral chest. Push the thumbs toward the midline to create a skin fold. As the patient inhales deeply, the thumbs normally separate approximately 3 to 5 cm, with each side expanding equally.

Assess tactile fremitus over the anterior chest wall. Anterior findings differ from posterior findings because of the heart and female breast

TABLE 32-19 Adventitious Breath Sounds

Sound	Site Auscultated	Cause	Character
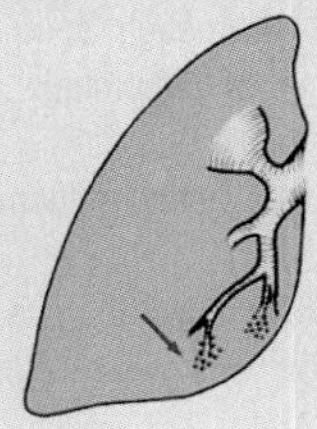 Crackles	Are most common in dependent lobes: right and left lung bases	Random, sudden reinflation of groups of alveoli; disruptive passage of air through small airways	Fine crackles are high-pitched fine, short, interrupted crackling sounds heard during end of inspiration, usually not cleared with coughing. Medium crackles are lower, more moist sounds heard during middle of inspiration; not cleared with coughing. Coarse crackles are loud, bubbly sounds heard during inspiration; not cleared with coughing.
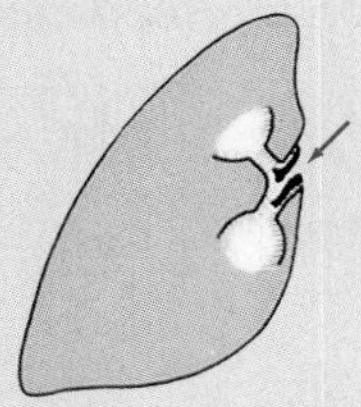 Rhonchi (sonorous wheeze)	Are primarily heard over trachea and bronchi; if loud enough, can be heard over most lung fields	Muscular spasm, fluid, or mucus in larger airways, new growth or external pressure causing turbulence	Loud, low-pitched, rumbling coarse sounds heard most often during inspiration or expiration; sometimes cleared by coughing.
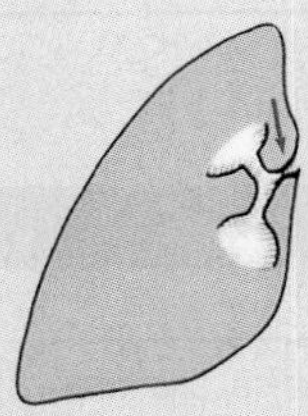 Wheezes (sibilant wheeze)	Heard over all lung fields	High-velocity airflow through severely narrowed or obstructed airway	High-pitched, continuous musical sounds like a squeak heard continuously during inspiration or expiration; usually louder on expiration.
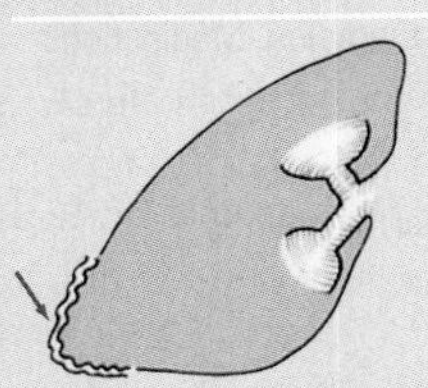 Pleural friction rub	Heard over anterior lateral lung field (if patient is sitting upright)	Inflamed pleura, parietal pleura rubbing against visceral pleura	Has dry, rubbing, or grating quality heard during inspiration or expiration; does not clear with coughing; heard loudest over lower lateral anterior surface.

Data from Ball, J. W., Dains, J. E., Flynn, J. A., Solomon, B. S., & Stewart, R. W. (2015). *Seidel's guide to physical examination* (8th ed. p. 278). St. Louis, MO: Mosby.

tissue. Fremitus is felt next to the sternum at the second intercostal space, at the level of the bronchial bifurcation. It decreases over the heart, lower thorax, and breast tissue.

Auscultation of the anterior thorax follows a systematic pattern (see Figure 32-23, *C*). Have the patient sit, if possible, to maximize chest expansion. Give special attention to the lower lobes, where mucous secretions commonly gather. Listen for bronchovesicular and vesicular sounds above and below the clavicles and along the lung periphery. Auscultate also for bronchial sounds, which are loud, high-pitched, and hollow sounding, with expiration lasting longer than inspiration (3 : 2 ratio). Normally this sound is heard over the trachea.

Use a systematic pattern when comparing the right and left sides (see Figure 32-23). Compare lung sounds in one region on one side of the body with sounds in the same region on the opposite of the body.

HEART

Findings from the assessment of heart function are compared with findings from the vascular assessment (see later section). Alterations in either system sometimes manifest as changes in the other. Some patients with signs or symptoms of cardiac problems have a life-threatening condition requiring immediate attention. In this case, it is vital to act quickly and conduct only the portions of the examination that are absolutely necessary. When a patient is more stable, a more thorough assessment can be conducted. The nursing history (Table 32-20) provides data to help interpret physical findings.

Cardiac function is assessed through the anterior thorax. In the adult, the heart is located in the centre of the chest (precordium), behind and to the left of the sternum, with a small section of the right atrium extending to the right of the sternum. The base of the heart is

BOX 32-19 PATIENT TEACHING

Lung Assessment

Objectives

- Patient describes warning signs of lung disease.
- Children receive routine childhood immunizations.
- Older persons receive influenza and pneumonia vaccines annually.
- Patients will verbalize an understanding of air pollutants in the home and the importance of a smoke-free environment at home and in the community.
- Patient with chronic obstructive pulmonary disease (COPD) clears airways more effectively and reports less shortness of breath.

Teaching Strategies

- Explain risk factors for chronic lung disease and lung cancer, including cigarette smoking, history of smoking for over 20 years, exposure to environmental pollution, and radiation exposure from occupational, medical, and environmental sources. Exposure to radon and asbestos also increases risk, especially for cigarette smokers. Other risk factors include certain metals (arsenic, cadmium, chromium), some organic chemicals, and tuberculosis. Exposure to second-hand cigarette smoke increases risk for nonsmokers.
- Share brochures on lung cancer from the Canadian Cancer Society with patient and family.
- Discuss warning signs of lung cancer, such as a persistent cough, sputum streaked with blood, chest pains, and recurrent attacks of pneumonia or bronchitis.
- Counsel parents of young children on benefits from receiving annual influenza and routine childhood vaccinations.
- Counsel older persons on benefits from receiving annual influenza and pneumonia vaccinations because of a greater susceptibility to respiratory infection.
- Instruct patient with COPD in coughing and pursed-lip breathing exercises.
- Refer individuals at risk for tuberculosis who visit clinics or health care centres for skin testing.

Evaluation

- Have patient describe risk factors for lung disease and cancer.
- Ask patient to identify any known risks for cancer.
- Ask patient to name warning signs for cancer.
- In a follow-up visit, review patient's immunization record.
- Observe patient performing breathing exercises and coughing.

TABLE 32-20 Nursing History for Heart Assessment

Assessment Category	Rationale
Determine history of smoking, alcohol intake, caffeine intake, use of prescriptive and recreational drugs, exercise habits, and dietary patterns and intake (including fat and sodium intake).	Smoking, alcohol ingestion, cocaine use, lack of regular exercise, and intake of foods high in carbohydrates, fats, and cholesterol are risk factors for cardiovascular disease. Caffeine can cause heart dysrhythmias.
Determine if patient is taking medications for cardiovascular function (e.g., antidysrhythmics, antihypertensives) and if patient knows their purpose, dosage, and adverse effects.	Knowledge enables nurse to assess adherence to drug therapies. Medications sometimes affect vital sign values.
Assess for chest pain or discomfort, palpitations, excess fatigue, cough, dyspnea, leg pain or cramps, edema of feet, cyanosis, fainting, and orthopnea. Ask if symptoms occur at rest or during exercise.	These are key symptoms of heart disease. Cardiovascular function is sometimes adequate during rest but not during exercise.
If patient reports chest pain, determine if it is cardiac in nature. Angina pain is usually a deep pressure or ache that is substernal and diffuse, radiating to one or both arms, neck, or jaw.	Determines nature of pain and need to initiate care immediately.
Determine whether patient has a stressful lifestyle. What physical demands or emotional stress exists?	Repeated exposure to stress increases risk for heart disease.
Assess family history for heart disease, diabetes, high cholesterol levels, hypertension, stroke, or rheumatic heart disease.	Factors increase risk for heart disease.
Ask patient about history of heart trouble (e.g., heart failure, congenital heart disease, coronary artery disease, dysrhythmias, murmurs).	Knowledge reveals patient's level of understanding of condition. Preexisting condition influences examination techniques used, as well as findings to expect.
Determine whether patient has preexisting diabetes, lung disease, obesity, or hypertension.	These disorders alter heart function.

the upper portion, and the apex is the bottom tip. The surface of the right ventricle composes most of the heart's anterior surface. A section of the left ventricle shapes the left anterior side of the apex. The apex actually touches the anterior chest wall at approximately the fourth to fifth intercostal space just medial to the left midclavicular line. This is where the **apical impulse** can be palpated, also referred to as the **point of maximal impulse (PMI)**.

An infant's heart is positioned more horizontally. The apex of the heart is at the third or fourth intercostal space, just to the left of the midclavicular line. By the age of 7 years, a child's PMI is in the same location as the adult's. In tall, slender individuals, the heart hangs more vertically and is positioned more centrally. With increased stockiness and shortness, the heart tends to lie more to the left and horizontally (Jarvis et al., 2014).

To assess heart function, a clear understanding of the cardiac cycle and associated physiological events is of utmost importance. The heart normally pumps blood through its four chambers in a methodical, even sequence. Events on the left side occur just before those on the right. As blood flows through each chamber, the valves open and close, the pressures within the chambers rise and fall, and the chambers contract. Each event creates a physiological sign. Both sides of the heart function in a coordinated fashion.

There are two phases to the cardiac cycle: systole and diastole. During systole, the ventricles contract and eject blood from the left ventricle into the aorta and from the right ventricle into the pulmonary artery. During diastole, the ventricles relax and the atria contract to move blood into the ventricles and fill the coronary arteries.

Heart sounds occur in relation to physiological events in the cardiac cycle. As systole begins, ventricular pressure rises and closes the mitral and tricuspid valves. Valve closure causes the first heart sound (S_1), often described as "lub." The ventricles then contract, and blood flows through the aorta and pulmonary circulation. After the ventricles empty, ventricular pressure falls below that in the aorta and pulmonary artery. This allows the aortic and pulmonic valves to close, causing the second heart sound (S_2), described as "dub." As ventricular pressure continues to fall, it drops below that of the atria. The mitral and tricuspid valves reopen to allow ventricular filling. Rapid ventricular filling creates a third heart sound (S_3), heard more often in children and young adults. An S_3 is also an abnormality in adults over 30 years of age. A fourth heart sound (S_4) occurs when the atria contract to enhance ventricular filling. An S_4 is heard in healthy older persons, children, and athletes, but it is not normal in adults. Because S_4 also indicates an abnormal condition, it needs to be reported to a health care provider.

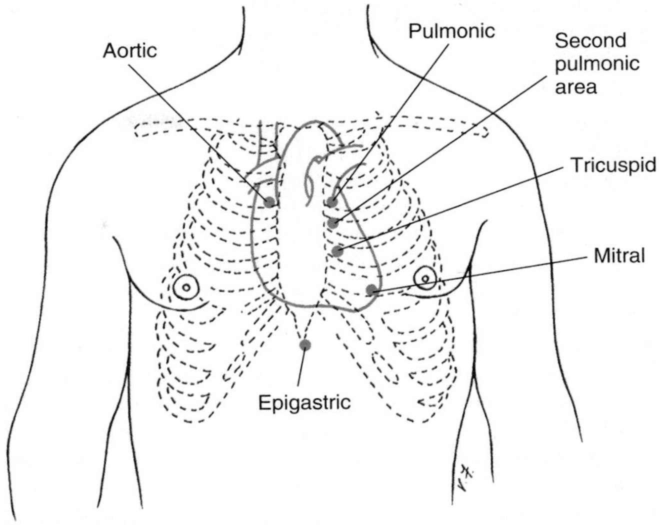

FIGURE 32-25 Anatomical sites for assessment of cardiac function.

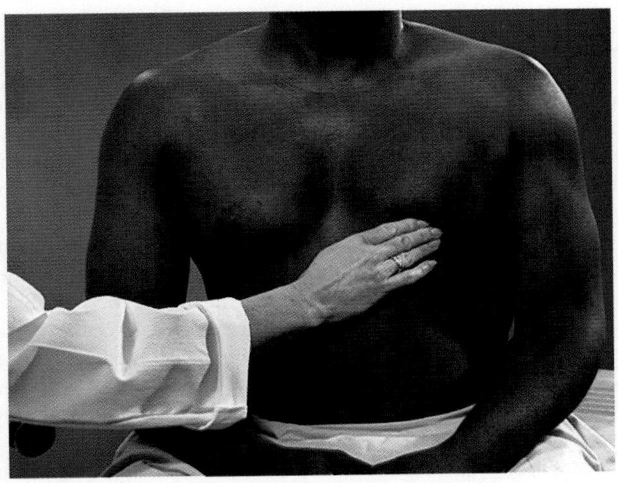

FIGURE 32-26 Palpation of apical pulse. (From Ball et al. [2015]. *Seidel's guide to physical examination* [8th ed., p. 305]. St. Louis, MO: Mosby.)

Inspection and Palpation

Before the examination, ensure that the patient is relaxed and comfortable. Explain the procedure to relieve the patient's anxiety. An anxious or uncomfortable patient will have mild tachycardia, which will lead to inaccurate findings.

Use the skills of inspection and palpation simultaneously. The examination begins with the patient in the supine position or with the upper body elevated 45 degrees because patients with heart disease frequently suffer shortness of breath while lying flat. Stand at the patient's right side. Do not let the patient talk, especially when auscultating heart sounds. Good lighting in the room is essential.

During inspection and palpation, look for visible pulsations and exaggerated lifts, and palpate for the apical impulse and any source of vibrations (thrills). Follow an orderly sequence, beginning with assessment of the base of the heart and moving toward the apex. First inspect the angle of Louis, which lies between the sternal body and manubrium, and feel the ridge in the sternum approximately 5 cm below the sternal notch. Slip the fingers along the angle on each side of the sternum to feel adjacent ribs. The intercostal spaces are just below each rib. The second intercostal space allows identification of each of the six anatomical landmarks (Figure 32-25). The second intercostal space on the right is the aortic area, and the left second intercostal space is the pulmonic area. Deeper palpation is needed to feel the spaces in obese or heavily muscled patients. After locating the pulmonic area, move the fingers down the patient's left sternal border to the third intercostal space, called the *second pulmonic area.* The tricuspid area is located at the fourth or fifth intercostal space along the sternum. To find the apical or mitral area, locate the fifth intercostal space just to the left of the sternum and move the fingers laterally, to the left midclavicular line. Locate the apical area with the palm of the hand or the fingertips. Normally, the apical pulse is felt as a light tap in an area 1 to 2 cm in diameter at the apex (Figure 32-26). Another landmark is the epigastric area at the tip of the sternum. Typically, this is used to palpate for aortic abnormalities.

Locate the six anatomical landmarks of the heart, and inspect and palpate each area. Look for the appearance of pulsations, viewing each area over the chest at an angle to the side. Normally, pulsations will not be seen, except perhaps at the PMI in thin patients or at the epigastric area as a result of abdominal aorta pulsation. Use the proximal halves of the four fingers together, and then alternate this with the ball of the hand to palpate for pulsations. Touch the areas gently to allow movements to lift the hand. Normally, no pulsations or vibrations are felt in the second, third, or fourth intercostal spaces. Loud murmurs cause a vibration. Time palpated pulsations or vibrations and their occurrence in relation to systole or diastole by auscultating heart sounds simultaneously.

The apical impulse or PMI should be felt easily. If it is hard to find, have the patient roll onto the left side, moving the heart closer to the chest wall. Estimate the size of the heart by noting the diameter of the PMI and its position relative to the midclavicular line. In cases of serious heart disease, the cardiac muscle enlarges, with the PMI found to the left of the midclavicular line. The PMI is sometimes difficult to find in the older person because the chest deepens in its anteroposterior diameters. It is also difficult to find in muscular or overweight patients. An infant's PMI is usually found near the third or fourth intercostal space. It is easy to palpate because of the child's thin chest wall.

Auscultation

Auscultation of the heart enables detection of normal heart sounds, extra heart sounds, and murmurs. Concentrate on detecting low-intensity sounds created by valve closures. To begin auscultation, eliminate all sources of room noise and explain the procedure to the patient to reduce his or her anxiety. Follow a systematic pattern beginning at the aortic area and inching the stethoscope across each of the anatomical sites (Figure 32-27). Listen for the complete cycle ("lub-dub") of heart sounds clearly at each location. Then repeat the sequence using the bell of the stethoscope. Sometimes the patient will assume three different positions during the examination (see Figure 32-27): sitting up and leaning forward (good for all areas and to hear high-pitched murmurs), supine (good for all areas), and left lateral recumbent (good for all areas; best position for hearing low-pitched sounds in diastole).

Learn to identify the first (S_1) and second (S_2) heart sounds. At normal rates, S_1 occurs after the long diastolic pause and preceding the short systolic pause. S_1 is high-pitched, dull in quality, and heard best at the apex. If it is difficult to hear S_1, time it in relation to the carotid pulsation. S_2 follows the short systolic pause and precedes the long diastolic pause; it is best heard at the aortic area.

Auscultate for rate and rhythm after hearing both sounds clearly. Each combination of S_1 and S_2 or "lub-dub" counts as one heartbeat. Count the rate for 1 minute, and listen for the interval between S_1 and S_2, and then the time between S_2 and the next S_1. A regular rhythm involves regular intervals of time between each sequence of beats. There is a distinct silent pause between S_1 and S_2. Failure of the heart to beat at regular successive intervals is a **dysrhythmia**. Some dysrhythmias are life-threatening.

When assessing an irregular heart rhythm, compare apical and radial pulse rates simultaneously to determine if a pulse deficit exists. Auscultate the apical pulse first, and then immediately palpate the radial pulse (one-examiner technique). Assess the apical and radial rates at the same time when two examiners are present. When a patient has a **pulse deficit**, the radial pulse is slower than the apical pulse because ineffective contractions fail to send pulse waves to the periphery. Report a difference in pulse rates to the health care provider immediately.

Assess for extra heart sounds at each auscultatory site. Use the bell of the stethoscope, and listen for low-pitched extra heart sounds such as S_3 and S_4 gallops, clicks, and rubs. Auscultate over all anatomical areas. S_3, or a **ventricular gallop**, occurs just after S_2 at the end of ventricular diastole. This is due to a premature rush of blood into a ventricle that is stiff or dilated as a result of heart failure and hypertension. The combination of S_1, S_2, and S_3 sounds like "Ken-tuck′-y."

S_4, or an atrial gallop, occurs just before S_1 or ventricular systole. The sound of an S_4 is similar to that of "Tenn′-es-see." Physiologically, it is due to an atrial contraction pushing against a ventricle that is not accepting blood because of heart failure or other alterations. Extra heart sounds are heard more easily with the patient lying on the left side and the stethoscope at the apical site.

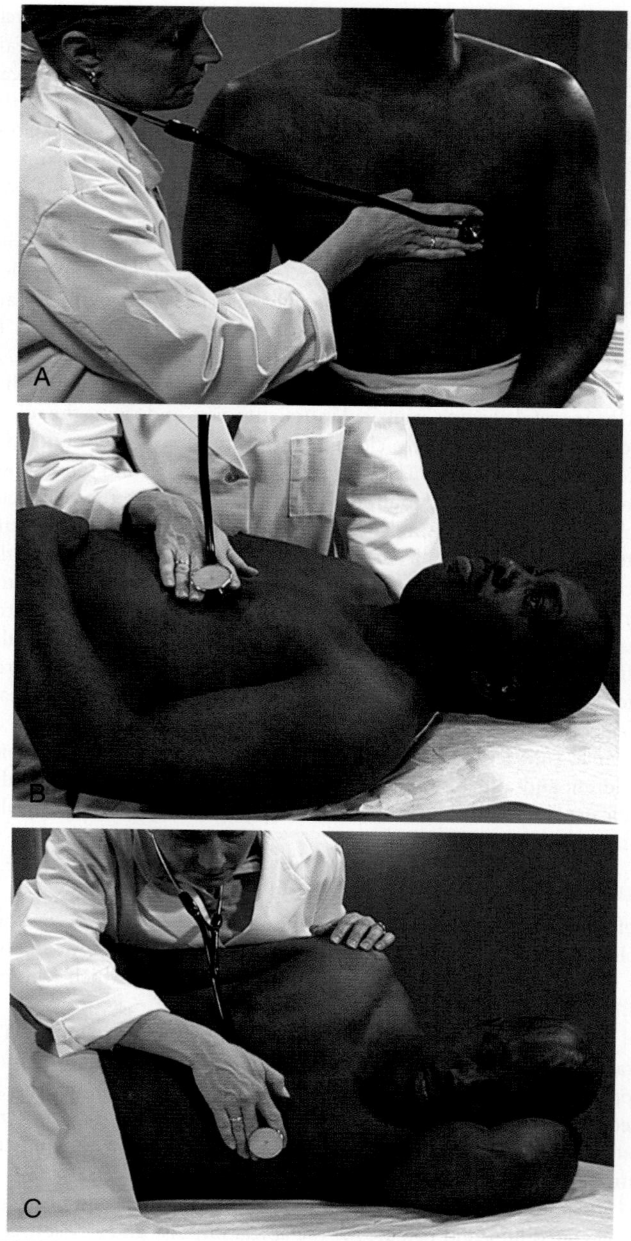

FIGURE 32-27 Sequence of patient positions for heart auscultation. **A,** Sitting. **B,** Supine. **C,** Left lateral recumbent. (From Ball et al. [2015]. *Seidel's guide to physical examination* [8th ed., p. 308]. St. Louis, MO: Mosby.)

The final portion of the examination includes assessment for heart murmurs. **Murmurs** are sustained swishing or blowing sounds heard at the beginning, middle, or end of the systolic or diastolic phase. They are due to increased blood flow through a normal valve, forward flow through a stenotic valve or into a dilated vessel or heart chamber, or backward flow through a valve that fails to close. A murmur is asymptomatic or a sign of heart disease (Box 32-20). Murmurs are common in children. The following factors should be kept in mind when auscultating to detect murmurs:

- When a murmur is detected, auscultate the mitral, tricuspid, aortic, and pulmonic valve areas for placement in the cardiac cycle

BOX 32-20 PATIENT TEACHING

Heart Assessment

Objectives

- Patient describes risk factors for cardiovascular disease (CVD) and takes appropriate steps to eliminate risks from lifestyle.
- Patient with risk for CVD will seek support from appropriate caregivers.

Teaching Strategies

- Explain risk factors for CVD, including diabetes, arterial hypertension, chronic kidney disease, obesity, abdominal aortic aneurysm, clinical evidence of atherosclerosis, current smoking, inflammatory bowel disease, human immunodeficiency virus (HIV), hypertensive disorder of pregnancy, erectile dysfunction, chronic obstructive pulmonary disease, high dietary intake of saturated fat or cholesterol, lack of regular aerobic exercise, stressful lifestyle, and family history of premature CVD or dyslipidemia (Anderson, Grégoire, Pearson, et al., 2016).
- Refer patient (if appropriate) to resources available for controlling or reducing risks (e.g., nutritional counselling, exercise class, stress reduction programs).
- Explain that lifestyle interventions play an important role in preventing and reducing risk of CVD. For example, research shows that achieving and maintaining a healthy body weight, healthy diet (e.g., Mediterranean diet, DASH diet), regular physical activity, smoking cessation, moderate alcohol consumption, and sufficient sleep duration are associated with CVD prevention and risk reduction (Anderson et al., 2016).
- Encourage patients with risk factors for CVD and individuals 40 years of age and older to have lipid testing as part of risk assessment for CVD (Allan, Linblad, Comeau, et al., 2015; Anderson et al., 2016).
- Explain the components of lipid testing and results to patient. Common components of lipid testing include low-density lipoprotein (LDL) cholesterol, high-density lipoprotein (HDL) cholesterol, and triglycerides.
  - LDL cholesterol is often referred to as "bad cholesterol" as too much of it can lead to atherosclerotic plaques and CVD. In individuals with moderate to high risk for CVD, target LDL levels are ≤2.0 mmol/L.
  - HDL cholesterol is known as "good" cholesterol because it carries cholesterol from other parts of the body to the liver where it can be broken down and eliminated. Target HDL levels are generally ≥1.2 mmol/L.
  - Triglycerides are a type of fat the body uses. High levels of triglycerides and LDL can increase risk for CVD. Generally, target triglyceride levels are ≤1.7 mmol/L.
  - Cardiovascular risk can be assessed using the Framingham Risk Score (calculator accessible at https://www.cvdriskchecksecure.com/framinghamriskscore.aspx).
- Advise patient to avoid cigarette smoke because nicotine causes vasoconstriction.
- Advise patient to quit smoking because this lowers the risk for CVD.

Evaluation

- Ask patient to identify risk factors for CVD.
- Have patient develop and implement lifestyle interventions to reduce risk of CVD.
- Monitor patient's cholesterol level during follow-up appointments at the clinic or with a health care provider.

(timing), the place it is heard best (location), radiation, loudness, pitch, and quality.

- If a murmur occurs between S_1 and S_2, it is a systolic murmur. If it occurs between S_2 and the next S_1, it is a diastolic murmur.
- The location of a murmur is not necessarily directly over the valves. With experience, you will learn where each type of murmur is best heard. For example, mitral murmurs are heard best at the apex of the heart.
- To assess for radiation, listen over areas beside where it is heard best. Murmurs are also heard over the neck or back.
- Intensity or loudness is related to the rate of blood flow through the heart or the amount of blood regurgitated. In serious murmurs, feel for a thrust or intermittent palpable sensation at the auscultation site. A **thrill** is a continuous palpable sensation like the purring of a cat. Intensity is recorded in the following grades (Ball et al., 2015a, p. 313):

  Grade 1: Barely audible in a quiet room
  Grade 2: Clearly audible but quiet
  Grade 3: Moderately loud
  Grade 4: Loud, with associated thrill
  Grade 5: Very loud, thrill easily palpable
  Grade 6: Louder, may be heard without stethoscope, thrill palpable and visible
- A murmur is low, medium, or high in pitch, depending on the velocity of blood flow through the valves. A low-pitched murmur is heard best with the bell of the stethoscope. If it is heard best with the diaphragm, the murmur is high pitched.

The quality of a murmur refers to its characteristic pattern and sound. A crescendo murmur starts softly and builds in loudness. A decrescendo murmur starts loudly and then becomes less intense.

VASCULAR SYSTEM

Examination of the vascular system includes measuring the blood pressure (see Chapter 30) and assessing the integrity of the peripheral vascular system. Table 32-21 reviews the nursing history data collected before the examination. The skills of inspection, palpation, and auscultation are used to assess the vascular system, and portions of the vascular examination are performed during other body systems assessments. For example, the carotid pulse is checked after palpating the cervical lymph nodes. Signs and symptoms of arterial and venous insufficiency are noted when assessing the skin.

Blood Pressure

Blood pressure readings can vary by as much as 5–10 mm Hg between the arms (Jarvis et al., 2014, p. 162). The higher reading should be recorded. Systolic readings that differ by 10–15 mm Hg or more suggest atherosclerosis or arterial obstruction.

Carotid Arteries

When the left ventricle pumps blood into the aorta, the arterial system transmits pressure waves. The carotid arteries reflect heart function better than peripheral arteries because their pressure correlates with that of the aorta. The carotid artery supplies oxygenated blood to the head and neck (Figure 32-28). The overlying sternocleidomastoid muscle protects the carotid artery.

To examine the carotid arteries, have the patient sit or lie supine with the head of the bed elevated 30 degrees. Examine one carotid artery at a time. If both arteries are simultaneously occluded during palpation, the patient will lose consciousness as a result of inadequate circulation to the brain. The carotid arteries should not be palpated

TABLE 32-21 Nursing History for Vascular Assessment

Assessment Category	Rationale
Determine if patient experiences leg cramps, numbness or tingling in extremities, sensation of cold hands or feet, pain in legs, or swelling or cyanosis of feet, ankles, or hand.	These signs and symptoms indicate vascular disease.
If patient experiences leg pain or cramping in lower extremities, ask if walking or standing for long periods, or during sleep, aggravates or relieves it.	Relationship of symptoms to exercise will clarify whether problem is vascular or musculoskeletal. Pain caused by vascular condition tends to increase with activity. Musculoskeletal pain is not usually relieved when exercise ends.
Ask patients if they wear tight-fitting leg wear or hosiery and sit or lie in bed with legs crossed.	Tight hosiery around lower extremities and crossing legs can impair venous return.
Reconsider previous heart risk factors (e.g., smoking, exercise, nutritional problems).	These predispose patient to vascular disease.
Assess medical history for heart disease, hypertension, phlebitis, diabetes, or varicose veins.	Circulatory and vascular disorders influence findings gathered during examination.

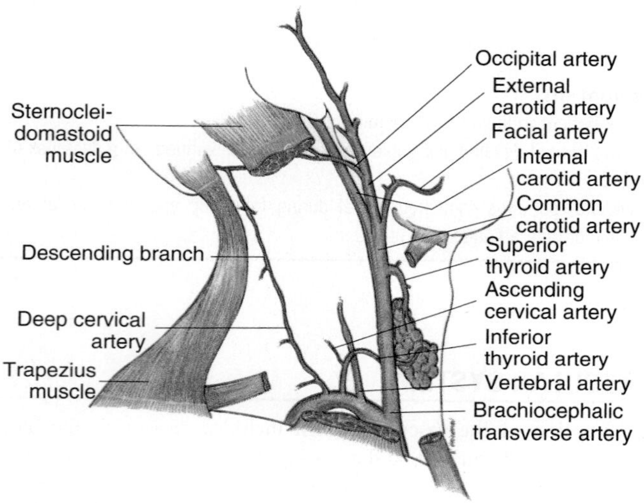

FIGURE 32-28 Anatomical position of the carotid artery.

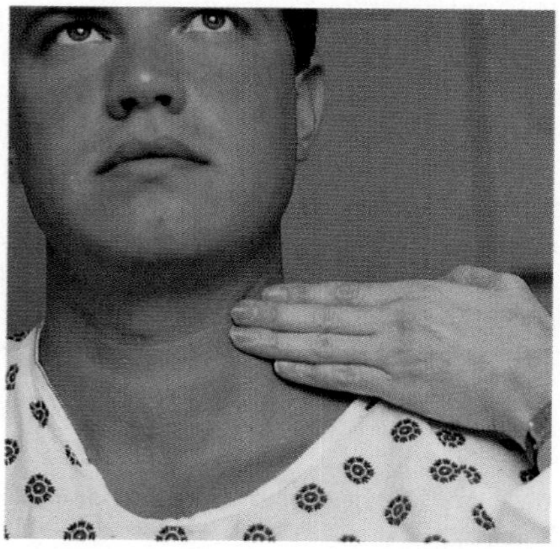

FIGURE 32-29 Palpation of internal carotid artery along the margin of the sternocleidomastoid muscle.

or massaged vigorously because the carotid sinus is located at the bifurcation of the common carotid arteries in the upper third of the neck. This sinus sends impulses along the vagus nerve. Its stimulation causes a reflex drop in heart rate and blood pressure, which causes syncope or circulatory arrest. This is a particular problem for older persons.

Begin inspection of the neck for obvious pulsation of the artery. Have the patient turn the head slightly away from the artery being examined. Sometimes the wave of the pulse is visible. The carotid is the only site for assessing the quality of a pulse wave. An absent pulse wave indicates arterial occlusion (blockage) or stenosis (narrowing).

To palpate the pulse, ask the patient to look straight ahead or turn the head slightly toward the side being examined. Turning relaxes the sternocleidomastoid muscle. Slide the tips of the index and middle fingers around the medial edge of the sternocleidomastoid muscle. Gently palpate to avoid occlusion of circulation (Figure 32-29).

The normal carotid pulse is localized rather than diffuse. As a strong pulse, the carotid has a thrusting quality. As the patient breathes, no change occurs. Rotation of the neck or a shift from a sitting to a supine position does not change the carotid artery's quality. Both carotid arteries are normally equal in pulse rate, rhythm, and strength and are equally elastic. Diminished or unequal carotid pulsations indicate atherosclerosis or other forms of arterial disease.

The carotid is the most commonly auscultated pulse. Auscultation is especially important for middle-aged or older patients suspected of having cerebrovascular disease. When the lumen of a blood vessel is narrowed, this disturbs blood flow. As blood passes through the narrowed section, this creates turbulence, causing a blowing or swishing sound. The blowing sound is called a bruit (pronounced "brew-ee").

Place the bell of the stethoscope over the carotid artery at the lateral end of the clavicle and the posterior margin of the sternocleidomastoid muscle. Have the patient turn the head slightly away from the side being examined (Figure 32-30). Ask the patient to hold the breath for a moment so that breath sounds do not obscure a bruit. Normally, no sounds are heard during carotid auscultation. Palpate the artery lightly for a thrill (palpable bruit) if a bruit is audible.

Jugular Veins

The most accessible veins for examination are the internal and external jugular veins in the neck. Both veins drain bilaterally from the head and neck into the superior vena cava. The external jugular vein lies superficially and is just above the clavicle. The internal jugular vein lies deeper, along the carotid artery.

It is best to examine the right internal jugular vein because it follows a more direct anatomical path to the right atrium of the heart. The column of blood inside the internal jugular vein serves as a manometer, reflecting pressure in the right atrium. The higher the column, the greater the venous pressure. Raised venous pressure reflects right-sided heart failure.

Normally, when a patient lies in the supine position, the external jugular vein distends and becomes easily visible. In contrast, the jugular veins normally flatten when the patient is in a sitting or standing position. Some patients with heart disease, however, have distended jugular veins when sitting.

To measure venous pressure, inspect the jugular veins. Blood volume, the capacity of the right atrium to receive blood and send it to the right ventricle, and the ability of the right ventricle to contract and force blood into the pulmonary artery all influence venous pressure. Any factor resulting in greater blood volume within the venous system results in elevated venous pressure. Assess venous pressure by using the following steps:

1. Ask the patient to lie supine with the head elevated 30 to 45 degrees (semi-Fowler's position).
2. Expose the neck and upper thorax. Use a pillow to align the head. Avoid neck hyperextension or flexion, to ensure that the vein is not stretched or kinked (Figure 32-31).
3. Usually pulsations are not evident with the patient sitting up. As the patient slowly leans back into a supine position, the level of venous pulsations begins to rise above the level of the manubrium as much as 1 or 2 cm as the patient reaches a 45-degree angle. Measure venous pressure by measuring the vertical distance between the angle of Louis and the highest level of the visible point of the internal jugular vein pulsation.
4. Use two rulers. Line up the bottom edge of a regular ruler with the top of the area of pulsation in the jugular vein. Then take a centimetre ruler and align it perpendicular to the first ruler at the level of the sternal angle. Measure in centimetres the distance between the second ruler and the sternal angle (Figure 32-32).
5. Repeat the same measurement on the other side. Bilateral pressures higher than 2.5 cm are considered elevated and are a sign of right-sided heart failure. One-sided pressure elevation is due to obstruction.

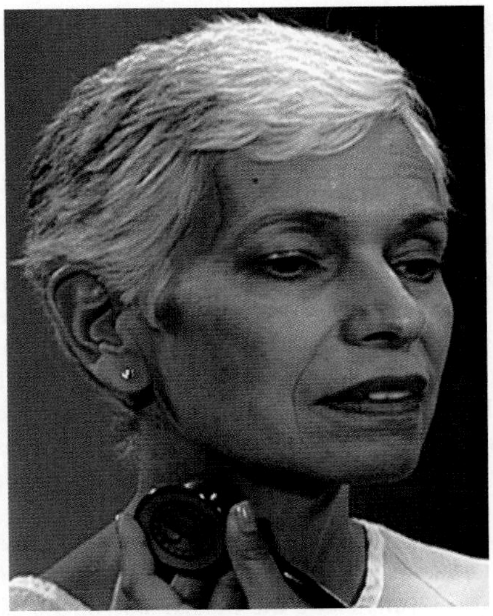

FIGURE 32-30 Auscultation for carotid artery bruit. (From Ball et al. [2015]. *Seidel's guide to physical examination* [8th ed., p. 342]. St. Louis, MO: Mosby.)

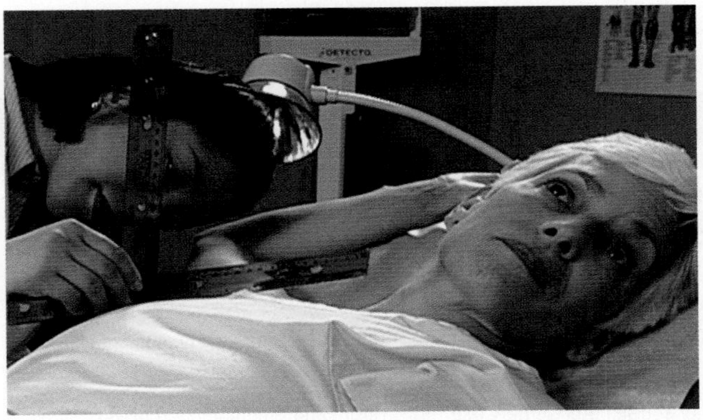

FIGURE 32-32 Measuring jugular venous pressure. (From Ball et al. [2015]. *Seidel's guide to physical examination* [8th ed., p. 343]. St. Louis, MO: Mosby.)

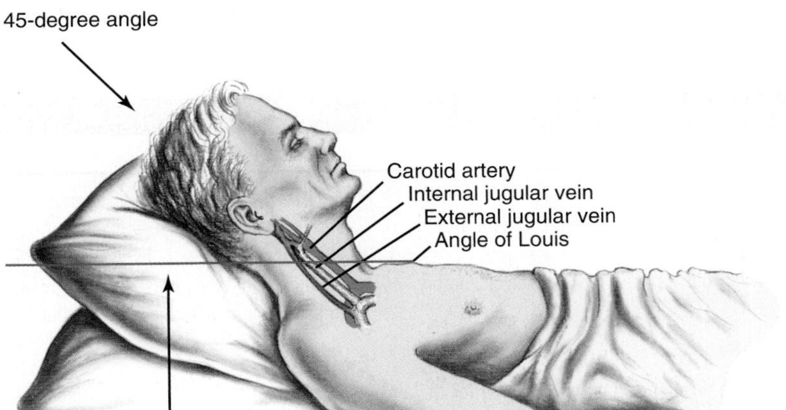

FIGURE 32-31 Position of patient to assess jugular vein distension. (From Ball et al. [2015]. *Seidel's guide to physical examination* (8th ed., p. 337). St. Louis, MO: Mosby.)

Peripheral Arteries and Veins

To examine the peripheral vascular system, first assess the adequacy of blood flow to the extremities by measuring arterial pulses and inspecting the condition of the skin and nails. Next assess the integrity of the venous system. Assess the arterial pulses in the extremities to determine sufficiency of the entire arterial circulation.

Factors such as coagulation disorders, local trauma or surgery, constricting casts or bandages, and systemic diseases impair circulation to the extremities (Table 32-22). Discuss risk factors and ways to monitor for circulatory problems with the patient (Box 32-21).

Peripheral Arteries. Each peripheral artery is examined using the distal pads of the second and third fingers. The thumb helps anchor the brachial and femoral artery. Apply firm pressure but avoid occluding a pulse. When a pulse is difficult to find, it helps to vary pressure and feel all around the pulse site. Be sure not to palpate your own pulse.

Routine vital signs usually include assessment of the rate and rhythm of the radial artery because it is easily accessible. Count the pulse for either 30 seconds or a full minute, depending on the character of the pulse. Always count an irregular pulse for 60 seconds. With palpation, normally the pulse wave is felt at regular intervals. When an interval is interrupted by an early, late, or missed beat, the pulse rhythm is irregular. In emergencies, health care providers usually assess the carotid artery because it is accessible and most useful in evaluating heart activity. To check local circulatory status of tissues, palpate the peripheral arteries long enough to note that a pulse is present.

Assess each peripheral artery for elasticity of the vessel wall, strength, and equality. The arterial wall is normally elastic, making it easily palpable. After depressing the artery, it will spring back to shape when the pressure is released. An abnormal artery is hard, inelastic, or calcified.

The strength of a pulse is a measurement of the force at which blood is ejected against the arterial wall. Some examiners use a scale rating from 0 to 4+ for the strength of a pulse (Ball et al., 2015a, p. 340):

0 Absent, not palpable
1+ Pulse diminished, barely palpable
2+ Expected/normal
3+ Full pulse, increased
4+ Bounding pulse

All peripheral pulses need to be measured for equality and symmetry. Compare the left radial pulse with that of the right, and so on. Lack of symmetry indicates impaired circulation, such as a localized obstruction or an abnormally positioned artery.

In the upper extremities, the brachial artery channels blood to the radial and ulnar arteries of the forearm and hand. If circulation in this artery becomes blocked, the hands will not receive adequate blood flow. If circulation in the radial or ulnar arteries becomes impaired, the hand will still receive adequate perfusion. An interconnection between the radial and ulnar arteries guards against arterial occlusion.

To locate pulses in the arm, have the patient sit or lie down. Find the radial pulse along the radial side of the forearm at the wrist. Thin individuals have a groove lateral to the flexor tendon of the wrist. Feel the radial pulse with light palpation in the groove (Figure 32-33). The ulnar pulse is on the opposite side of the wrist and feels less prominent (Figure 32-34). Palpate the ulnar pulse only when evaluating arterial insufficiency to the hand.

To palpate the brachial pulse, find the groove between the biceps and triceps muscle above the elbow at the antecubital fossa (Figure 32-35). The artery runs along the medial side of the extended arm. Palpate the artery with the fingertips of the first three fingers in the muscle groove.

The femoral artery is the primary artery in the leg, delivering blood to the popliteal, posterior tibial, and dorsalis pedis arteries. An interconnection between the posterior tibial and dorsalis pedis arteries guards against local arterial occlusion.

TABLE 32-22 Indicators for Assessing Local Blood Flow

Indicator	Rationale
Systemic diseases (e.g., arteriosclerosis, atherosclerosis, diabetes)	Diseases result in changes in integrity of walls of arteries and smaller blood vessels.
Coagulation disorders (e.g., thrombosis, embolus)	Blood clot causes mechanical obstruction to blood flow.
Local trauma or surgery (e.g., contusion, fracture, vascular surgery)	Direct manipulation of vessels or localized edema impairs blood flow.
Application of constricting devices (e.g., casts, dressings, elastic bandages, restraints)	Constriction causes tourniquet effect, impairing blood flow to areas below site of constriction.

BOX 32-21 PATIENT TEACHING

Vascular Assessment

Objectives

- Patient will know normal blood pressure range for age and compare it with own blood pressure readings to identify normalcy of blood pressure.
- Patient with vascular insufficiency will avoid activities that worsen circulatory status.

Teaching Strategies

- Tell patient the blood pressure reading. Explain the normal reading for the patient's age. Discuss implications of abnormalities.
- Instruct patient with risk or evidence of vascular insufficiency in the lower extremities to avoid tight clothing over the lower body or legs, to avoid sitting or standing for long periods, to walk regularly, and to elevate feet when sitting.
- Advise patient to avoid cigarette smoking because nicotine causes vasoconstriction.
- Identify patients with hypertension; they sometimes benefit from regular monitoring of blood pressure (daily, weekly, or monthly). Teach patients how to use home-monitoring kits (see Chapter 30).

Evaluation

- Ask patient to identify if blood pressure reading is within normal limits for age.
- Have patient with vascular insufficiency describe precautions to take to avoid further circulatory deficiency.
- Have patient demonstrate self-monitoring of blood pressure.

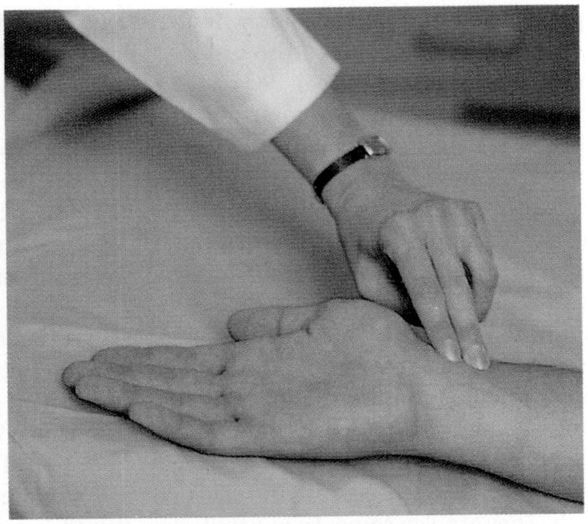

FIGURE 32-33 Palpation of radial pulse.

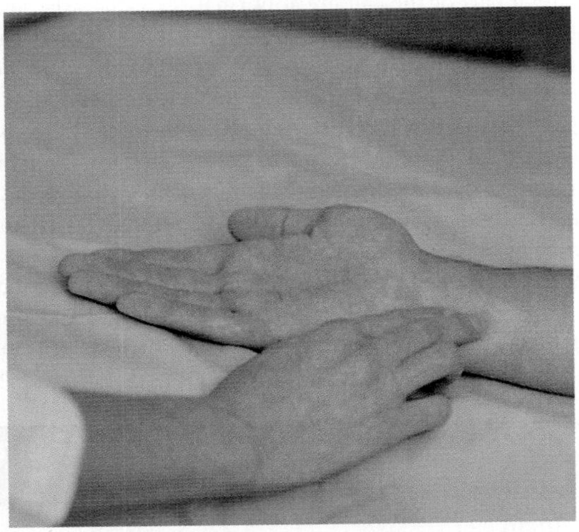

FIGURE 32-34 Palpation of ulnar pulse.

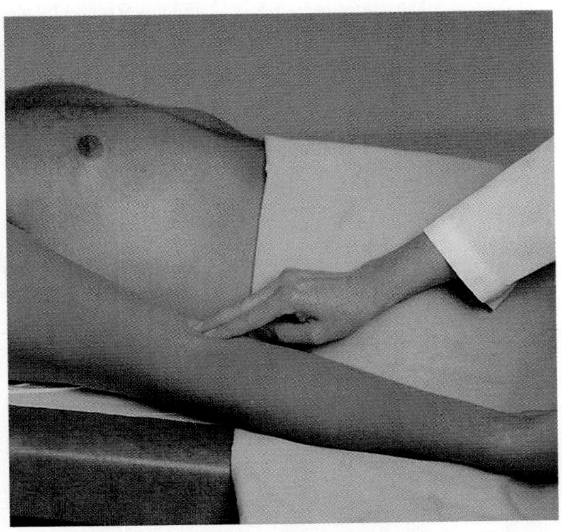

FIGURE 32-35 Palpation of brachial pulse.

Find the femoral pulse with the patient lying down with the inguinal area exposed (Figure 32-36). The femoral artery runs below the inguinal ligament, midway between the symphysis pubis and the anterosuperior iliac spine. Sometimes deep palpation is required to feel the pulse. Bimanual palpation is effective in obese patients. Place the fingertips of both hands on opposite sides of the pulse site. A pulsatile sensation is felt when the arterial pulsation pushes the fingertips apart.

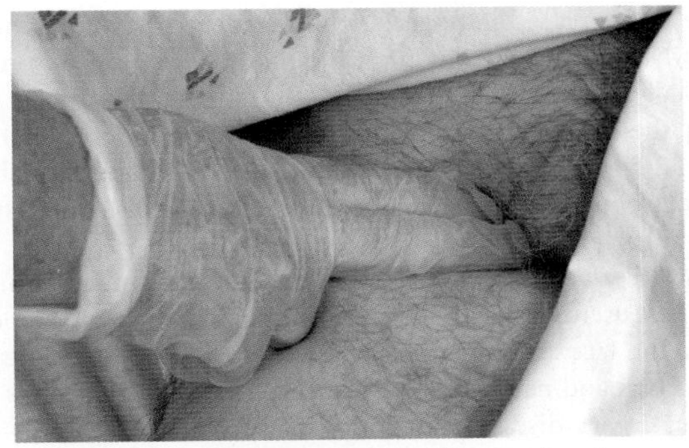

FIGURE 32-36 Palpation of femoral pulse.

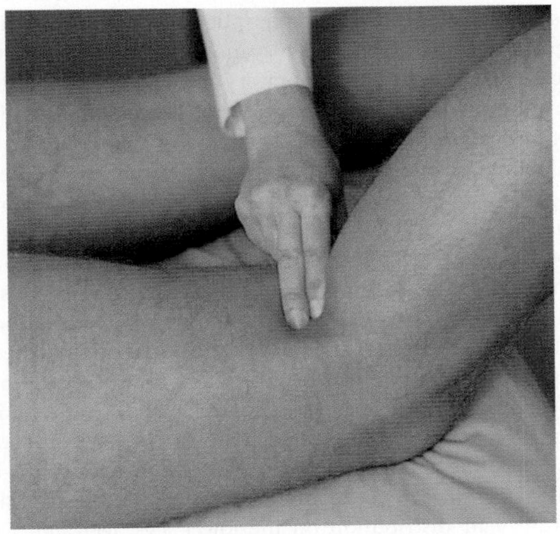

FIGURE 32-37 Palpation of popliteal pulse.

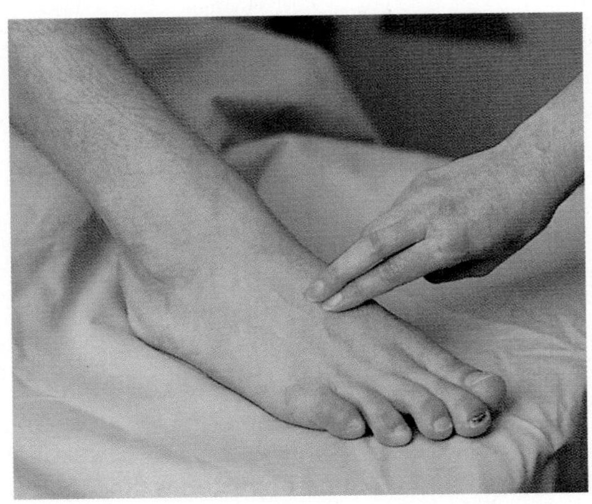

FIGURE 32-38 Palpation of dorsalis pedis pulse.

The popliteal pulse runs behind the knee. Have the patient slightly flex the knee, with the foot resting on the examination table, or assume a prone position with the knee slightly flexed (Figure 32-37). Instruct the patient to keep leg muscles relaxed. Palpate with the fingers of both hands deeply into the popliteal fossa, just lateral to the midline. The popliteal pulse is difficult to locate.

With the patient's foot relaxed, locate the dorsalis pedis pulse. The artery runs along the top of the foot in line with the groove between the extensor tendons of the great toe and first toe (Figure 32-38). To find the pulse, place the fingertips between the first and second toes and slowly move up the dorsum of the foot. This pulse is sometimes congenitally absent.

Find the posterior tibial pulse on the inner side of each ankle (Figure 32-39). Place the fingers behind and below the medial malleolus (ankle bone). With the patient's foot relaxed and slightly extended, palpate the artery.

Tissue Perfusion. The condition of the skin, mucosa, and nail beds offers useful data about the status of circulatory blood flow. Examine the face and upper extremities, looking at the colour of the skin, mucosa, and nail beds. The presence of cyanosis requires special attention. Heart disease sometimes causes central cyanosis, which indicates poor arterial oxygenation. Some characteristics of this are a bluish discoloration of the lips, mouth, and conjunctivae. Blue lips, earlobes, and nail beds are signs of peripheral cyanosis, which indicates peripheral vasoconstriction. When cyanosis is present, consult with a health care provider to have laboratory testing of oxygen saturation to determine the severity of the problem. Examination of the nails involves inspection for **clubbing**, a bulging of the tissues at the nail base. Clubbing is due to insufficient oxygenation at the periphery resulting from conditions such as chronic emphysema and congenital heart disease.

Inspect the lower extremities for changes in colour, temperature, and condition of the skin indicating either arterial or venous alterations (Table 32-23). This is a good time to ask the patient about any history of pain in the legs. If an arterial occlusion is present, the patient has signs resulting from an absence of blood flow. Pain will be distal to the occlusion. The *Ps*—pain, pallor, pulselessness, paresthesias, and paralysis—characterize an occlusion. Venous congestion causes tissue changes indicating an inadequate circulatory flow back to the heart.

During examination of the lower extremities, also inspect skin and nail texture; hair distribution on the lower legs, feet, and toes; the venous pattern; and scars, pigmentation, or ulcers. Palpate the legs and feet for colour and temperature. Also assess capillary refill. Measure capillary refill by blanching the nail bed with a substantial pressure for several seconds. Release the pressure, and observe the time elapsed before the nail regains its full colour. An acceptable capillary refill time is less than 2 seconds (Jarvis et al., 2014, p. 239).

The absence of hair growth over the legs indicates circulatory insufficiency. Chronic recurring ulcers of the feet or lower legs are a serious sign of circulatory insufficiency and require a health care provider's intervention.

Peripheral Veins. The status of the peripheral veins is assessed by asking the patient to assume sitting and standing positions. Assessment includes inspection and palpation for varicosities, peripheral edema, and phlebitis. Varicosities are superficial veins that become dilated, especially when the legs are in a dependent position. They are common in older persons because the veins normally fibrose, dilate, and stretch. They are also common in people who stand for prolonged periods. Varicosities in the anterior or medial part of the thigh and the posterolateral part of the calf are abnormal.

Dependent edema around the area of the feet and ankles is a sign of venous insufficiency or right-sided heart failure. Dependent edema is common in older persons and individuals who spend a lot of time standing (e.g., waitresses, security guards, and nurses). To assess for pitting edema, use the index finger to press firmly for several seconds and then release over the medial malleolus or the shins. A depression left in the skin indicates edema. Grading 1+ through 4+ characterizes the severity of the edema (Figure 32-40).

Phlebitis is an inflammation of a vein that occurs commonly after trauma to the vessel wall, infection, immobilization, and prolonged insertion of IV catheters (see Chapter 39). Phlebitis promotes clot

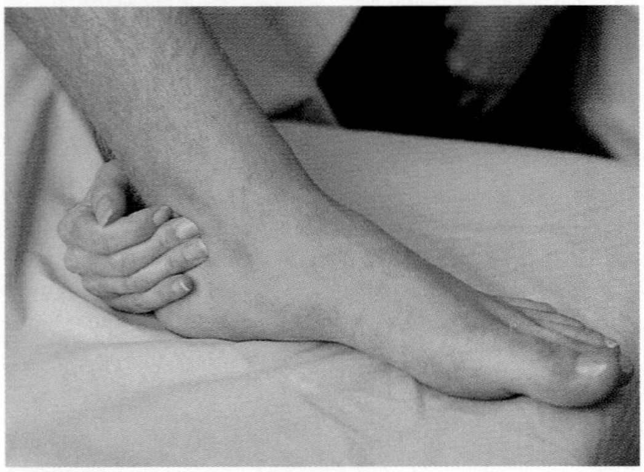

FIGURE 32-39 Palpation of posterior tibial pulse.

TABLE 32-23 Signs of Venous and Arterial Insufficiency

Assessment Criterion	Venous	Arterial
Colour	Normal or cyanotic	Pale; worsened by elevation of extremity; dusky red when extremity is lowered
Temperature	Normal	Cool (blood flow blocked to extremity)
Pulse	Normal	Decreased or absent
Edema	Often marked	Absent or mild
Skin changes	Brown pigmentation around ankles	Thin, shiny skin; decreased hair growth; thickened nails

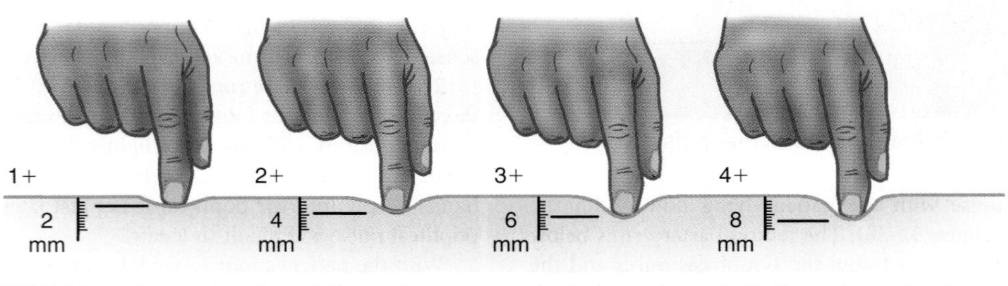

FIGURE 32-40 Assessing for pitting edema. (From Ball et al. [2015]. *Seidel's guide to physical examination* [8th ed., p. 344]. St. Louis, MO: Mosby.)

formation, a potentially dangerous situation because a clot within a deep vein of the leg can become dislodged and travel through the heart, causing a pulmonary embolus. To assess for phlebitis, inspect the calves for localized redness, tenderness, and swelling over vein sites. Gentle palpation of calf muscles reveals warmth, tenderness, and firmness of the muscle. Unilateral edema of the affected leg is one of the most reliable findings of phlebitis (Day, 2003). Determine if dorsiflexion of the foot (Homan sign) causes pain in the calf. However, Homan sign is not always a reliable indicator of phlebitis and is present in other conditions (Day, 2003). Performing the Homan sign test is contraindicated in patients with deep vein thrombosis. If a clot is present, it may become dislodged from its original site during this test, resulting in a pulmonary embolism.

Lymphatic System

Lymphatic drainage of the lower extremities is assessed during examination of the vascular system or during the female or male genital examination. Superficial and deep nodes drain the legs, but only two groups of superficial nodes are palpable. With the patient supine, palpate the area of the superficial inguinal nodes in the groin area (Figure 32-41). Then move the fingertips toward the inner thigh, feeling for any inferior nodes. Use a firm but gentle pressure when palpating over each lymphatic chain. Multiple nodes are not normally palpable, although a few soft, nontender nodes are not unusual. Enlarged, hardened, tender nodes reveal potential sites of infection or metastatic disease.

BREASTS

It is important to examine the breasts of female and male patients. Males have a small amount of glandular tissue, a potential site for the growth of cancer cells, in the breast. In contrast, the majority of the female breast is glandular tissue.

Female Breasts

Researchers predicted that new cases of invasive breast cancer would affect 26315 women and 206 men in Canada in 2017 (CCS Steering Committee, 2017). The disease is second to lung cancer as the leading cause of death in women. Early detection is the key to cure.

Recently published clinical practice guidelines have moved away from routine recommendation of annual clinical breast examinations (CBEs) by health care providers, as research has not proven CBEs to be an effective screening tool. However, CBE may still help detect abnormalities in breast tissue. Women are also encouraged to be aware of what is normal in their own breasts, through use of breast self-examination (BSE), so they can detect an abnormality (Shimizu, Bouchard, & Mavriplis, 2016). For a detailed overview of teaching BSE please see the textbook by Jarvis and colleagues (2014, pp. 421–422).

The patient's history (Table 32-24) should note normal developmental changes, as well as signs of breast disease. Because of its glandular structure, the breast undergoes changes during a woman's life. Knowing these changes (Box 32-22) is important to a complete an accurate assessment. Both men and women should be encouraged to observe their breasts for changes.

Inspection. Have the patient remove the top gown or drape to allow simultaneous visualization of both breasts. Have the patient stand or sit with her arms hanging loosely at her sides. If possible, place a mirror in front of the patient during inspection so she can see what to look for when performing a BSE. To recognize abnormalities, the patient needs to be familiar with the normal appearance of her breasts. Describe observations or findings in relation to imaginary lines that divide the breast into four quadrants and a tail. The lines cross at the centre of the nipple. Each tail extends outward from the upper outer quadrant (Figure 32-42).

Inspect the breasts for size and symmetry. Normally, the breasts extend from the third to the sixth ribs, with the nipple at the level of the fourth intercostal space. It is common for one breast to be smaller. However, inflammation or a mass causes a difference in size. As the woman becomes older, the ligaments supporting the breast tissue weaken, causing the breasts to sag and the nipples to lower.

Observe the contour or shape of the breasts, and note masses, flattening, retraction, or dimpling. Breasts vary in shape and can be convex, pendulous, or conical. Retraction or dimpling results from invasion of underlying ligaments by tumours. The ligaments fibrose and pull the overlying skin inward toward the tumour. Edema also changes the contour of the breasts. To bring out retraction or changes in the shape of breasts, ask the patient to assume three positions: raise arms above the head, press hands against the hips, and extend arms

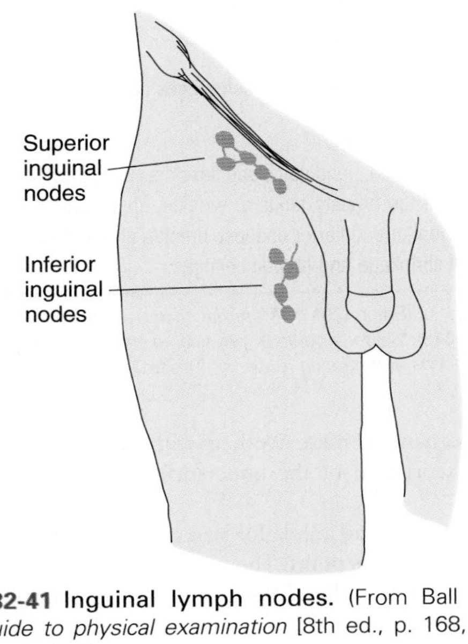

FIGURE 32-41 Inguinal lymph nodes. (From Ball et al. [2015]. *Seidel's guide to physical examination* [8th ed., p. 168, Fig. 9-3]. St. Louis, MO: Mosby.)

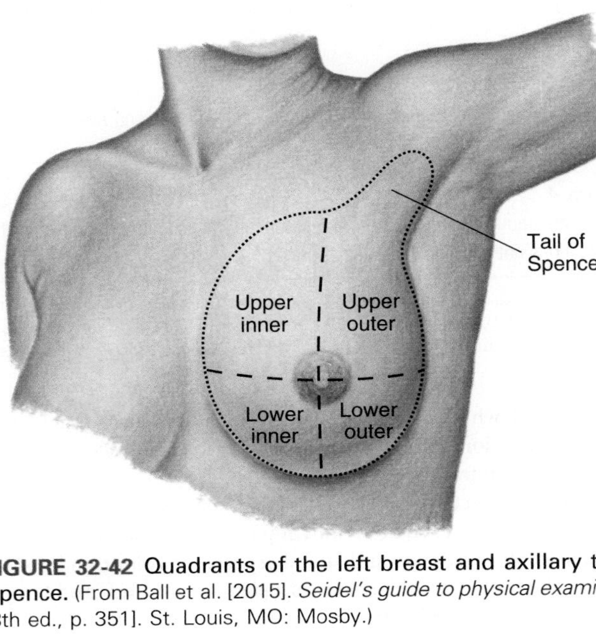

FIGURE 32-42 Quadrants of the left breast and axillary tail of Spence. (From Ball et al. [2015]. *Seidel's guide to physical examination* [8th ed., p. 351]. St. Louis, MO: Mosby.)

TABLE 32-24 Nursing History for Breast Assessment

Assessment Category	Rationale
Determine if woman is over age 50; has a personal or family history of breast cancer or other cancer; has a personal or family history of *BRCA* gene mutations; has dense breasts; is of Ashkenazi Jewish ancestry; has been exposed to ionizing radiation (i.e., cancer treatment); has been on hormone replacement therapy; has atypical hyperplasia; drinks more than one alcoholic beverage per day; is overweight or obese; is high socioeconomic status; has early-onset menarche (before age 13) or late-age menopause (after age 52); never had children or gave birth to first child after age 30; or has used oral contraceptives.	These are risk factors for breast cancer (Canadian Cancer Society, 2017b).
Ask if patient (both sexes) has noticed lump, thickening, pain, or tenderness of breast; discharge, distortion, retraction, or scaling of the nipple; or change in size of breast.	Potential signs and symptoms of breast cancer help nurse to focus on specific areas of breast during assessment.
Determine patient's use of medications (oral contraceptives, digitalis, diuretics, steroids, or estrogen). Determine patient's caffeine intake.	Some medications cause nipple discharge. Hormones and caffeine cause fibrocystic changes in breast.
Determine patient's level of activity, alcohol intake, and weight.	Breast cancer incidence rates correlate with being overweight or obese (postmenopausal), physical inactivity, use of oral contraceptives, and consumption of one or more alcoholic beverages per day (Canadian Cancer Society, 2017b).
Ask if patient performs breast self-examination (BSE). If so, determine time of month she performs examination in relation to menstrual cycle. Have patient describe or demonstrate method used.	Nurse's role is to educate patient about breast cancer and techniques for BSE.
If patient reports a breast mass, ask about length of time since patient first noticed the lump. Does lump come and go, or is it always present? Have there been changes in the lump (e.g., size, relationship to menses), and are there associated symptoms?	Information helps in determining nature of mass (e.g., breast cancer or fibrocystic disease).

BOX 32-22 Normal Changes in the Breast During a Woman's Lifespan

Puberty (8 to 20 Years)

Tanner staging (1–5) is a method of assessment for sexual maturity of adolescents (Jarvis et al., 2014; Tanner, 1962). Breasts mature in five stages. One breast may grow more rapidly than the other. The ages at which changes occur and rate of developmental progression vary.

Stage 1 (Preadolescent)

This stage involves elevation of the nipple only.

Stage 2

The breast and nipple elevate as a small mound, and the areolar diameters enlarge.

Stage 3

There is further enlargement and elevation of the breast and areola, with no separation of contour.

Stage 4

The areola and nipple project into the secondary mound above the level of the breast (does not occur in all girls).

Stage 5 (Mature Breast)

Only the nipple projects, and the areola recedes (varies in some women).

Young Adulthood (20 to 30 Years)

Breasts reach full (nonpregnant) size. Shape is generally symmetrical. Breasts are sometimes unequal in size.

Pregnancy

Breast size gradually enlarges to two to three times the previous size. Nipples enlarge and become erect. Areolae darken, and diameters increase. Superficial veins become prominent. The nipples expel a yellowish fluid (colostrum).

Menopause

Breasts shrink. Tissue becomes softer, sometimes flabby.

Older Women

Breasts become elongated, pendulous, and flaccid as a result of glandular tissue atrophy. The skin of the breasts tends to wrinkle, appearing loose and flabby. Nipples become smaller and flatter and lose erectile ability. Nipples sometimes invert because of shrinkage and fibrotic changes.

Data from Perry, S. E., Hockenberry, M. J., Lowdermilk, D. L., Wilson, D., Sama, C., & Keenan-Lindsay, L. (Eds.). (2017). *Maternal child nursing care in Canada* (2nd ed.). St. Louis, MO: Mosby.; Ball, J. W., Dains, J. E., Flynn, J. A., Solomon, B. S., & Stewart, R. W. (2015). *Seidel's guide to physical examination* (8th ed.). St. Louis, MO: Mosby; and Touhy, T. A. &, Jett, K. F. (2016). *Ebersole & Hess' towards healthy aging: Human needs and nursing response* (9th ed.). Philadelphia, PA: Elsevier.

straight ahead while sitting and leaning forward. Each manoeuvre causes a contraction of the pectoral muscles, which will accentuate the presence of any retraction.

Carefully inspect the skin for colour; venous pattern; and the presence of lesions, edema, or inflammation. Lift each breast when necessary to observe lower and lateral aspects for colour and texture changes. The breasts are the colour of neighbouring skin, and venous patterns are the same bilaterally. Venous patterns are easily visible in thin or pregnant women. Women with large breasts often have redness and excoriation of the undersurfaces caused by rubbing of skin surfaces.

Inspect the nipple and areola for size, colour, shape, discharge, and the direction the nipples point. The normal areolae are round or oval and nearly equal bilaterally. Colour ranges from pink to brown. In light-skinned women, the areola turns brown during pregnancy and remains dark. In dark-skinned women, the areola is brown before pregnancy (Ball et al., 2015a, p. 356). Normally, the nipples point in symmetrical directions, are everted, and have no drainage. If the nipples are inverted, ask if this has been a lifetime history. A recent inversion or inward turning of the nipple indicates an underlying growth. Rashes or ulcerations are not normal on the breast or nipples. Note any bleeding or discharge from the nipple. Clear yellow discharge 2 days after childbirth is common. While inspecting the breasts, explain the characteristics you see. Teach the patient the significance of abnormal signs or symptoms.

Palpation. Palpation is used to assess the condition of underlying breast tissue and lymph nodes. Breast tissue consists of glandular tissue, fibrous supportive ligaments, and fat. Glandular tissue is organized into lobes that end in ducts that open onto the nipple's surface. The largest portion of glandular tissue is in the upper outer quadrant and tail of each breast. Suspensory ligaments connect to skin and fascia underlying the breast to support the breast and maintain its upright position. Fatty tissue is located superficially and to the sides of the breast.

A large portion of lymph from the breasts drains into axillary lymph nodes. If cancerous lesions **metastasize** (spread), the nodes commonly become involved. Study the location of supraclavicular, infraclavicular, and axillary nodes (Figure 32-43). The axillary nodes drain lymph from the chest wall, breasts, arms, and hands. A tumour of one breast sometimes involves nodes on the opposite side, as well as those on the same side.

To palpate the lymph nodes, have the patient sit with her arms at her sides and muscles relaxed. While facing the patient and standing on the side being examined, support the patient's arm in a flexed position and abduct the arm from the chest wall. Place the free hand against the patient's chest wall and high in the axillary hollow. With the fingertips, press gently down over the surface of the ribs and muscles. Palpate the axillary nodes with the fingertips gently rolling soft tissue. Palpate four areas of the axilla: at the edge of the pectoralis major muscle along the anterior axillary line, the chest wall in the midaxillary area, the upper part of the humerus, and the anterior edge of the latissimus dorsi muscle along the posterior axillary line.

Normally lymph nodes are not palpable. Carefully assess each area, and note their number, consistency, mobility, and size. The presence of one or two small, soft, nontender palpable nodes is normal. A palpable node feels like a small mass that is hard, tender, and immobile. Also palpate along the upper and lower clavicular ridges. Reverse the procedure for the patient's other side.

It is sometimes difficult for patients to learn to palpate for lymph nodes. Lying down with the arm abducted makes the area more accessible. Instruct the patient to use her left hand for the right axillary and clavicular areas. Take the patient's fingertips and move them in the proper fashion. Then have the patient use her right hand to palpate for nodes on the left side.

With the patient lying supine and one arm behind the head (alternating with each breast), palpate the patient's breast tissue. The supine position allows the breast tissue to flatten evenly against the chest wall. The patient raises her hand and places it behind the neck to further stretch and position breast tissue evenly. Place a small pillow or towel under the patient's shoulder blade to further position breast tissue.

The consistency of normal breast tissue varies widely. The breasts of a young patient are firm and elastic. In an older patient, the tissue sometimes feels stringy and nodular. The patient's familiarity with the texture of her own breasts is very important. Patients gain this familiarity through BSE (Box 32-23).

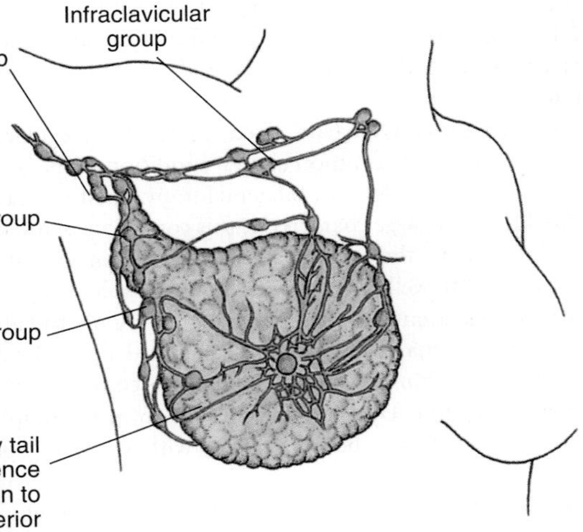

FIGURE 32-43 Anatomical position of axillary and clavicular lymph nodes.

BOX 32-23 PATIENT TEACHING

Female Breast Assessment

Objectives

- Patient will perform breast self-examination (BSE).
- Patient will have screening mammography performed at recommended intervals, beginning at age 50.
- Patient will identify signs and symptoms of breast cancer.
- Patient will identify signs and symptoms of benign (fibrocystic) breast disease.
- Patient will follow a low-fat diet.

Teaching Strategies

Instruct patient on how to perform BSE

- Have patient perform return demonstration of BSE, and offer the opportunity to ask questions.
- Explain recommended frequency of mammography and assessment by a health care provider.
- Discuss signs and symptoms of breast cancer.
- Discuss signs and symptoms of benign (fibrocystic) breast disease.
- Inform a woman who is obese or who has a family history of breast cancer that she is at higher risk for the disease (Canadian Cancer Society, 2017b). Encourage dietary changes, including limiting meat consumption to well-trimmed, lean beef, pork, or lamb; removing skin from cooked chicken before eating it; selecting tuna and salmon packed in water and not oil; and using low-fat dairy products.

Evaluation

- Have patient demonstrate BSE.
- During follow-up visit, determine whether patient has had mammography performed.
- Ask patient to explain frequency of mammography.
- Have patient describe signs and symptoms of breast cancer compared with those of benign (fibrocystic) breast disease.

If the patient complains of a mass, examine the opposite breast to ensure an objective comparison of normal and abnormal tissue. Use the pads of the first three fingers to compress breast tissue gently against the chest wall, noting tissue consistency. Perform palpation systematically in one of three ways: (1) clockwise or counterclockwise, forming small circles with the fingers along each quadrant and the tail; (2) using a vertical technique with the fingers moving up and down each quadrant; or (3) palpating from the centre of the breast in a radial fashion, returning to the areola to begin each spoke. Whatever approach used, be sure to cover the entire breast and tail, directing attention to any areas of tenderness.

When palpating large, pendulous breasts, use a bimanual technique. Support the inferior portion of the breast in one hand while using the other hand to palpate breast tissue against the supporting hand.

During palpation, note the consistency of breast tissue. It normally feels dense, firm, and elastic. With menopause, breast tissue shrinks and becomes softer. The lobular feel of glandular tissue is normal. The lower edge of each breast sometimes feels firm and hard. This is the normal inframammary ridge and not a tumour. It helps to move the patient's hand so that she can feel normal tissue variations. Palpate abnormal masses to determine location in relation to quadrants, diameter in centimetres, shape (e.g., round or discoid), consistency (soft, firm, or hard), tenderness, mobility, and discreteness (clear or unclear boundaries).

Cancerous lesions are hard, fixed, nontender, irregular in shape, and usually unilateral. A common benign condition of the breast is **benign (fibrocystic) breast disease**. Bilateral lumpy, painful breasts and sometimes nipple discharge characterize this condition. Symptoms are more apparent during the menstrual period. When palpated, the cysts (lumps) are soft, well differentiated, and movable. Deep cysts feel hard.

Pay special attention when palpating the nipple and areola to assess for nodules, edema, ulceration or discharge. Palpate the entire surface gently. Use the thumb and index finger to compress the nipple, and note any discharge. During the examination of the nipple and areola, the nipple sometimes becomes erect with wrinkling of the areola. These changes are normal.

After completing the examination, have the patient demonstrate self-palpation. Observe the patient's technique, and emphasize the importance of a consistent and systematic approach. Urge the patient to see her health care provider if she discovers an abnormal mass during self-examination. She also needs to know all of the signs and symptoms of breast cancer.

Male Breasts

Examination of the male breast is relatively easy. Inspect the nipple and areola for nodules, edema, and ulceration. An enlarged male breast results from obesity or glandular enlargement. Breast enlargement in young males results from steroid use. Fatty tissue feels soft, whereas glandular tissue is firm. Use the same techniques to palpate for masses as those used in examination of the female breast.

> **Safety Alert** Men, especially men who have a first-degree relative (e.g., mother, sister) with breast cancer, are at risk for breast cancer and need to palpate their breasts at regular intervals. In discussion with their health care provider, these men may also be scheduled for routine mammograms.

ABDOMEN

The abdominal examination is complex because of the number of organs located within and near the abdominal cavity. A thorough nursing history (Table 32-25) helps with interpretation of physical signs. The examination includes an assessment of structures of the lower GI tract in addition to the liver, stomach, uterus, ovaries, kidneys, and bladder. Abdominal pain is one of the most common symptoms that patients report when seeking medical care. An accurate assessment requires matching patient history data with a careful assessment of the location of physical symptoms.

The organs are assessed anteriorly and posteriorly. A system of landmarks helps map out the abdominal region. The xiphoid process (tip of the sternum) is the upper boundary of the anterior abdominal region. The symphysis pubis marks the lower boundary. Divide the abdomen into four imaginary quadrants (Figure 32-44, *A*), and refer to assessment findings and record them in relation to each quadrant. Posteriorly, the lower ribs and heavy back muscles protect the kidneys, which are located from the T12 to L3 vertebrae (Figure 32-44, *B*). The costovertebral angle formed by the last rib and vertebral column is a landmark used during kidney and liver palpation.

During the abdominal examination, the patient needs to relax. A tightening of abdominal muscles hinders palpation. Ask the patient to void before beginning. Be sure the room is warm, and drape the upper chest and legs. The patient lies supine or in a dorsal recumbent position with the arms at the sides and knees slightly bent. Place small pillows beneath the knees. If the patient places the arms under the head, the abdominal muscles tighten. Proceed calmly and slowly, being sure that there is adequate lighting. Expose the abdomen from just above the xiphoid process down to the symphysis pubis. Warm hands and stethoscope further promote relaxation. Ask the patient to report pain and point out tender areas. Assess tender areas last.

The order of an abdominal examination differs slightly from previous assessments. Begin with inspection and follow with auscultation. By using auscultation before palpation there is less chance of altering

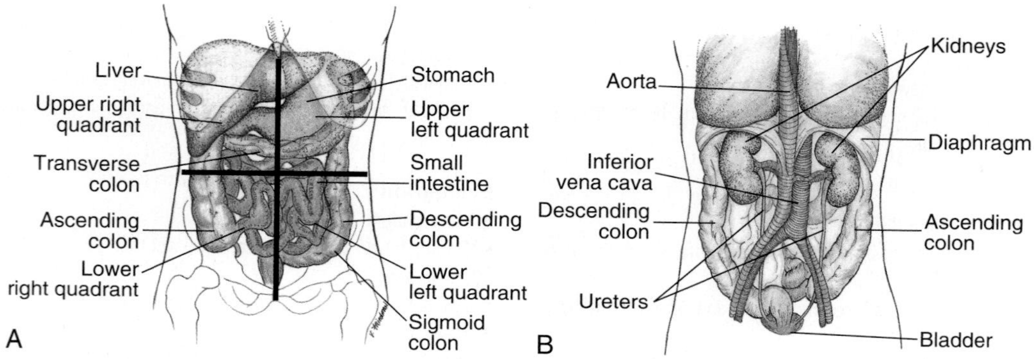

FIGURE 32-44 **A,** Anterior view of abdomen divided by quadrants. **B,** Posterior view of abdominal section.

TABLE 32-25 Nursing History for Abdominal Assessment

Assessment Category	Rationale
If patient has abdominal or low back pain, assess character of pain in detail (location, onset, frequency, precipitating factors, aggravating factors, type of pain, severity, course).	Pattern of characteristics of pain helps determine its source.
Carefully observe patient's movement and position, including lying still with knees drawn up, moving restlessly to find comfortable position, and lying on one side or sitting with knees drawn to chest.	Positions assumed by patient reveal nature and source of pain, including peritonitis, renal stone, and pancreatitis.
Assess normal bowel habits and stool character; ask if patient uses laxatives.	Data compared with physical findings help in identifying cause and nature of elimination problems.
Determine if patient has had abdominal surgery, trauma, or diagnostic tests of gastrointestinal (GI) tract.	Surgical or traumatic alterations of abdominal organs cause changes in expected findings (e.g., position of underlying organs). Diagnostic tests change character of stool.
Assess if patient has had recent weight changes or intolerance to diet (e.g., nausea, vomiting, cramping, especially in last 24 hours).	Data possibly indicate alterations in upper GI tract (stomach or gallbladder) or lower colon.
Assess for difficulty in swallowing, belching, flatulence (gas), bloody emesis (hematemesis), black or tarry stools (melena), heartburn, diarrhea, or constipation.	These characteristic signs and symptoms indicate gastrointestinal alterations.
Ask if patient takes anti-inflammatory medication (e.g., aspirin, ibuprofen, steroids) or antibiotics.	Pharmacological drugs cause GI upset or bleeding.
Ask patient to locate tender areas before examination begins.	Assess painful areas last to minimize discomfort and anxiety.
Inquire about family history of cancer, kidney disease, alcoholism, hypertension, or heart disease.	Data possibly reveal risk for alterations identifiable during examination.
Determine if female patient is pregnant; note last menstrual period.	Pregnancy causes changes in abdominal shape and contour.
Assess patient's usual intake of alcohol.	Chronic alcohol ingestion causes gastrointestinal and liver problems.
Review patient's history for the following: health care occupation, hemodialysis, intravenous drug user, household or sexual contact with hepatitis B virus (HBV) carrier, more than one sex partner in previous 6 months, international traveller in area of high HBV infection rate.	These are risk factors for HBV exposure.

the frequency and character of bowel sounds. Be sure to have a tape measure and marking pen available during the examination.

Inspection

Make it a habit to observe the patient during routine care activities. Note the patient's posture and look for evidence of abdominal splinting: lying with the knees drawn up or moving restlessly in bed. A patient free from abdominal pain will not guard or splint the abdomen. To inspect the abdomen for abnormal movement or shadows, stand on the patient's right side and inspect from above the abdomen. To assess abdominal contour, sit down to look across the abdomen. Direct the examination light over the abdomen.

Skin. Inspect the skin over the abdomen for colour, scars, venous patterns, lesions, and striae (stretch marks). The skin is subject to the same colour variations as the rest of the body. Venous patterns are normally faint, except in thin patients. Striae result from stretching of tissue by obesity or pregnancy. Artificial openings indicate drainage sites resulting from surgery (see Chapter 48) or an ostomy (see Chapters 43 and 44). Scars reveal evidence of past trauma or surgery that has created permanent changes in underlying organ anatomy. Bruising indicates accidental injury, physical abuse, or a type of bleeding disorder. Ask the patient about self-administered injections (e.g., low-molecular-weight heparin or insulin). Unexpected findings include generalized colour changes such as jaundice or cyanosis. A glistening, taut (tight) appearance indicates ascites.

Umbilicus. Note the position; shape; colour; and signs of inflammation, discharge, or protruding masses. A normal umbilicus is flat or concave with the colour the same as that of the surrounding skin. Underlying masses cause displacement of the umbilicus. An everted (pouched-out) umbilicus usually indicates distension. A hernia (protrusion of abdominal organs through the muscle wall) causes upward protrusion of the umbilicus. Normally the umbilical area does not emit discharge.

Contour and Symmetry. Inspect for contour, symmetry, and surface motion of the abdomen, noting any masses, bulging, or distension. A flat abdomen forms a horizontal plane from the xiphoid process to the symphysis pubis. A round abdomen protrudes in a convex sphere from the horizontal plane. A concave abdomen appears to sink into the muscular wall. Each of these findings is normal if the abdomen's shape is symmetrical. In the older person, there is often an overall increased distribution of adipose tissue. The presence of masses on only one side, or asymmetry, possibly indicates an underlying pathological condition.

Intestinal gas, a tumour, or fluid in the abdominal cavity causes distension. When distension is generalized, the entire abdomen protrudes. The skin often appears taut, as if it were stretched over the abdomen. When gas causes distension, the flanks do not bulge. However, if fluid is the source of the problem, the flanks bulge. Ask the patient to roll onto one side. A protuberance forms on the dependent side if fluid is the cause of the distension. Ask the patient if the abdomen feels unusually tight. Be careful not to confuse distension with obesity. In obesity, the abdomen is large, rolls of adipose tissue are often present along the flanks, and the patient does not complain of tightness in the abdomen. If abdominal distension is expected, measure the abdomen by placing a tape measure around the abdomen at the level of the umbilicus. Consecutive measurements will show any increase or decrease in distension. Use a marking pen to indicate the location of tape measure.

Enlarged Organs or Masses. Observe the contour of the abdomen while asking the patient to take a deep breath and hold it. Normally, the contour remains smooth and symmetrical. This manoeuvre forces the diaphragm downward and reduces the size of the abdominal cavity. Any enlarged organs in the upper abdominal cavity (e.g., liver or spleen) will descend below the rib cage to cause a bulge. Perform a closer examination with palpation.

To evaluate the abdominal musculature, have the patient raise his or her head off the examination table. This position causes superficial abdominal wall masses, hernias, and muscle separations to become more apparent.

Movement or Pulsations. Inspect for movement. Normally, men breathe abdominally and women breathe more costally. A patient with severe pain has diminished respiratory movement and tightens the abdominal muscles to guard against the pain. Closely inspect for peristaltic movement and aortic pulsation by looking across the abdomen from the side. These movements are visible in thin patients; otherwise, no movement is present.

Auscultation

During the abdominal assessment, auscultation is performed before palpation because manipulation of the abdomen alters the frequency and intensity of bowel sounds. The patient should be asked not to talk so that the examiner can hear bowel sounds. Patients with GI tubes connected to suction need them temporarily turned off before beginning the examination.

Bowel Motility. Peristalsis, or the movement of contents through the intestines, is a normal function of the small and large intestine. Bowel sounds are the audible passage of air and fluid that peristalsis creates. To perform auscultation, place the warmed diaphragm of the stethoscope lightly over each of the four quadrants. Normally, air and fluid move through the intestines, creating soft gurgling or clicking sounds that occur irregularly 5 to 30 times per minute (Jarvis & Luctkar-Flude, 2014b, p. 560). Sounds usually last from half a second to several seconds. It takes 5 minutes of continuous listening before determining that bowel sounds are absent. Auscultate all four quadrants to be sure not to miss any sounds. The best time to auscultate is between meals. Sounds are generally described as normal, audible, absent, hyperactive, or hypoactive. Absent sounds indicate a lack of peristalsis, possibly due to late-stage bowel obstruction, paralytic ileus, or peritonitis. Normally, absent or hypoactive bowel sounds occur postoperatively following general anaesthesia. Hyperactive sounds are loud, "growling" sounds called borborygmi, which indicate increased gastrointestinal motility. Inflammation of the bowel, anxiety, diarrhea, bleeding, excessive ingestion of laxatives, and reaction of the intestines to certain foods cause increased motility (Box 32-24).

Vascular Sounds. Bruits indicate narrowing of the major blood vessels and disruption of blood flow. The presence of bruits in the abdominal area will possibly reveal aneurysms or stenotic vessels. Use the bell of the stethoscope to auscultate in the epigastric region and each of the four quadrants. Normally there are no vascular sounds over the aorta (midline through the abdomen) or femoral arteries (lower quadrants). Renal artery bruits are heard by placing the stethoscope over each upper quadrant anteriorly or over the costovertebral angle posteriorly. If a bruit is detected, report it immediately to a health care provider.

Kidney Tenderness. With the patient sitting or standing erect, use direct or indirect percussion to assess for kidney inflammation. With the ulnar surface of the partially closed fist, percuss posteriorly the costovertebral angle at the scapular line. If the kidneys are inflamed, the patient feels tenderness during percussion.

Palpation

Palpation is used primarily to detect areas of abdominal tenderness, distension, or masses. As their skill base increases, nurses learn to palpate for specific organs. Both light and deep palpation are used.

Light palpation is performed over each abdominal quadrant. Initially, areas previously identified as problem spots should be avoided. Lay the palm of the hand with fingers extended and approximated lightly on the abdomen. Explain the manoeuvre to the patient, and then with the palmar surface of the fingers depress approximately 1 cm in a gentle dipping motion (Jarvis & Luctkar-Flude, 2014b, p. 564) (Figure 32-45). Avoid quick jabs, and use smooth, coordinated movements. For ticklish patients, first place the patient's hand on the abdomen with your hand on the patient's; continue this until the patient tolerates palpation.

BOX 32-24 PATIENT TEACHING

Abdominal Assessment

Objectives

- Patient will maintain normal bowel elimination.
- Patient will achieve pain relief.
- Patients at high risk for hepatitis B virus (HBV) will receive immunization.
- Patient will identify signs and symptoms of colon cancer.

Teaching Strategies

- Explain factors that promote normal bowel elimination, such as diet, regular exercise, limited use of over-the-counter drugs causing constipation, establishment of regular elimination schedule, and a good fluid intake (see Chapter 44). Stress importance for older persons.
- Caution patients about dangers of excessive use of laxatives or enemas.
- Instruct patient to have acute abdominal pain evaluated by a health care provider.
- If patient has persistent pain, explain measures used for pain relief (e.g., relaxation exercises, positioning) (see Chapter 31).
- If patient is a health care worker or has contact with blood or fluids of infected persons, encourage patient to receive the series of three HBV vaccine doses.
- Instruct patient about warning signs of colon cancer, including rectal bleeding, cramping pain in lower abdomen, black or tarry stools, blood in stool, and a change in bowel habits (constipation or diarrhea).

Evaluation

- Reassess patient's bowel elimination pattern and stool character after therapies begin.
- Observe patient using pain-relief measures and reassess character of pain.
- During follow-up clinic or office visit, check patient's compliance with HBV vaccine schedule.
- Ask patient to state signs and symptoms of colon cancer.

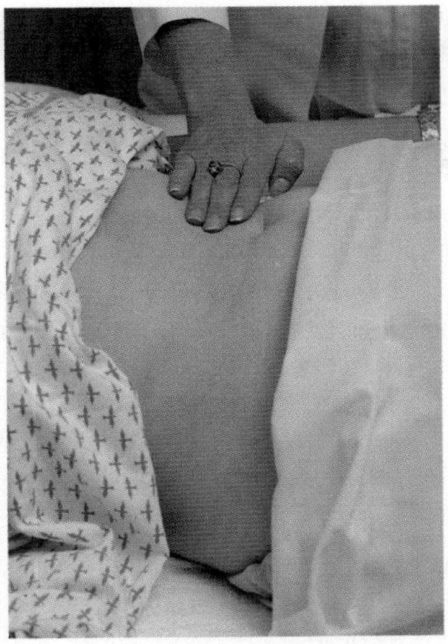

FIGURE 32-45 Light palpation of abdomen.

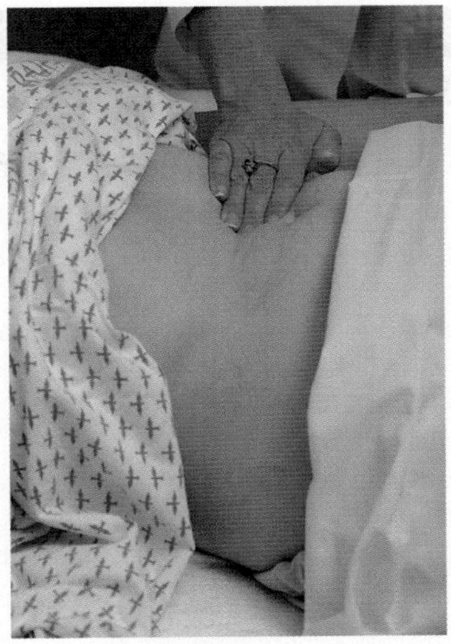

FIGURE 32-46 Deep palpation of abdomen.

Use a systematic palpation approach for each quadrant and assess for muscular resistance, distension, tenderness, and superficial organs or masses. Observe the patient's face for signs of discomfort. The abdomen is normally smooth with consistent softness and nontender without masses. The older person often lacks abdominal tone. Guarding or muscle tenseness sometimes occurs while palpating a sensitive area. If tightening remains after the patient relaxes, peritonitis, acute cholecystitis, or appendicitis is sometimes the cause. It is easy to detect a distended bladder with light palpation. Normally the bladder lies below the umbilicus and above the symphysis pubis. Routinely check for a distended bladder if a patient has been unable to void (e.g., because of anaesthesia or sedation) or has been incontinent, or if an in-dwelling urinary catheter is not draining well.

With practice and experience, nurses perform deep palpation to delineate abdominal organs and to detect less obvious masses. For deep palpation nurses must have short fingernails. It is important for the patient to be relaxed while the hands depress approximately 5 to 8 cm into the abdomen (Jarvis & Luctkar-Flude, 2014b, pp. 565–566) (Figure 32-46). Deep palpation should never be done over a surgical incision or over extremely tender organs. It is also unwise to use deep palpation on abnormal masses. Deep pressure causes tenderness in the healthy patient over the cecum, sigmoid colon, aorta, and the midline near the xiphoid process.

Each quadrant is surveyed systematically. Palpate masses for size, location, shape, consistency, tenderness, pulsation, and mobility. Test for rebound tenderness by pressing a hand slowly and deeply into the involved area and then letting go quickly. The test is positive if the patient feels pain with the release of the hand. Rebound tenderness occurs in patients with peritoneal irritation such as occurs in appendicitis; pancreatitis; or any peritoneal injury causing bile, blood, or enzymes to enter the peritoneal cavity.

Aortic Pulsation. To assess aortic pulsation, palpate with the thumb and forefinger of one hand deeply into the upper abdomen, just left of the midline. Normally a pulsation is transmitted forward. If there is enlargement of the aorta from an aneurysm (localized dilation of a vessel wall), the pulsation expands laterally. A pulsating abdominal mass should not be palpated. In obese patients it is often necessary to palpate with both hands, one on each side of the aorta.

> **Safety Alert** When enlargement from an aneurysm is present, only someone with advanced education and experience should perform palpation of this area.

FEMALE GENITALIA AND REPRODUCTIVE TRACT

Examination of the female genitalia can be embarrassing to the patient, so the nurse needs to use a calm, relaxed approach. The gynecological examination is also one of the most difficult experiences for adolescents. Cultural background further adds to apprehension. In some cultures, a strong social value may exist where women do not expose their bodies to men or even to other women. In other cultures, the examination of genitalia may be considered offensive. Cultural expression of these values, and the level of emotional or physical comfort with the procedure, needs to be explored prior to any genital exam. The lithotomy position assumed during the examination is an added source of embarrassment. It is often the nurse's role to provide a thorough explanation for the examination and the procedures that will be used. The nurse can also assess the patient's level of anxiety regarding a genital exam while obtaining the nursing history (Table 32-26). Patient acceptance and comfort can be augmented through correct positioning and draping. Adolescents sometimes choose to have parents present in the examination room.

Sometimes a patient requires a complete examination of the female reproductive organs: assessment of the external genitalia and a vaginal examination. The nurse will examine external genitalia while performing routine hygiene measures or preparing to insert a urinary catheter. An internal examination, to assess for signs of cancer or other disorders, is part of each woman's preventive health care because ovarian cancer causes more deaths than any other cancer of the female reproductive system (CCS Steering Committee, 2017). Adolescents and young adults are examined because of the growing incidence of sexually transmitted infections (STIs).

Preparation of the Patient

As a beginning nurse, your responsibility will be assisting the patient's health care provider with the examination (Jarvis & Luctkar-Flude, 2014bc, pp. 753–766). For a complete examination, the following

TABLE 32-26 Nursing History for Female Genitalia and Reproductive Tract Assessment

Assessment Category	Rationale
Determine if patient has had previous illness, including sexually transmitted infections (STIs), or surgery involving reproductive organs.	Illness or surgery influences appearance and position of organs being examined.
Determine if patient has received a human papillomavirus (HPV) vaccine.	HPV vaccine is recommended for females (ages 9–26) to prevent cervical cancer (Public Health Agency of Canada, 2016b). HPV increases patient's risk for development of cervical cancer.
Review menstrual history, including age at menarche, frequency and duration of menstrual cycle, character of flow (e.g., amount, presence of clots), presence of dysmenorrhea (painful menstruation), pelvic pain, dates of last two menstrual periods, and premenstrual symptoms.	This information is useful to determine level of reproductive health, including normalcy of menstrual cycle.
Ask patient to describe obstetrical history, including each pregnancy and history of abortions or miscarriages.	Observed physical findings will vary, depending on woman's history of pregnancy.
Ask patient to describe current and past contraceptive practices and problems encountered. Determine whether patient uses safer sex practices. Discuss risk of STIs and HIV infection.	Use of certain types of contraceptives influences reproductive health (e.g., sensitivity reaction to spermicidal jelly). Sexual history reveals risk for and understanding of STIs.
Assess if patient has signs and symptoms of vaginal discharge, painful or swollen perianal tissues, or genital lesions.	These signs and symptoms may indicate an STI or other pathological condition.
Determine if patient has symptoms or history of genitourinary problems, including burning during urination, frequency, urgency, nocturia, hematuria, incontinence, or stress incontinence (see Chapter 43).	Urinary problems are associated with gynecological disorders, including STIs.
Ask if patient has had signs of bleeding outside of normal menstrual period or after menopause or has had unusual vaginal discharge.	These are warning signs for cervical and endometrial cancer or vaginal infection.
Determine if patient has history of HPV (condyloma acuminatum, herpes simplex, or cervical dysplasia); has multiple sex partners; smokes cigarettes; has had multiple pregnancies; or was young at first intercourse.	These are risk factors for cervical cancer. Vaccines are available for HPV for females 9–26 years of age.
Determine if patient is older than 40, is obese, and has history of ovarian dysfunction, breast or endometrial cancer, irradiation of pelvic organs, or endometriosis; has family history of ovarian, breast, or colon cancer; has history of infertility or nulliparity; or uses estrogen (alone) or as part of hormone replacement therapy.	These are risk factors for ovarian cancer.
Determine if patient is postmenopausal, obese, or infertile; had early menarche; had late menopause; has history of hypertension, diabetes, gallbladder disease, or polycystic ovary disease; has family history of endometrial, breast, or colon cancer; or has a history of estrogen-related exposure (estrogen replacement therapy, tamoxifen use).	These are risk factors for endometrial cancer.

special equipment is needed: examination table with stirrups, vaginal speculum of correct size, adjustable light source, sink, clean disposable gloves, sterile cotton swabs, glass slides, plastic or wooden spatula, cervical brush or broom device, cytological fixative, and culture plates or media.

The equipment needs to be ready before the examination begins. Ask the patient to empty her bladder so that the uterus and ovaries are readily palpable. Often it is necessary to collect a urine specimen. Assist the patient to the lithotomy position, in bed or on an examination table, for the external genitalia assessment. Help the patient place her feet into stirrups for a speculum examination. Have the woman stabilize each foot in a stirrup and then have her slide the buttocks down to the edge of the examining table. Place a hand at the edge of the table and instruct the patient to move until touching the hand. The patient's arms should be at her sides or folded across the chest to prevent tightening of abdominal muscles.

Some women who suffer from pain or deformity of the joints are unable to assume a lithotomy position. In this situation, the patient need abduct only one leg, or another person can assist in separating the patient's thighs. The side-lying position can also be used, with the patient lying on the left side with the right thigh and knee drawn up to her chest.

Give the patient a square drape or sheet: She holds one corner over her sternum, the adjacent corners fall over each knee, and the fourth corner covers the perineum. After the examination begins, lift the drape over the perineum. A male examiner always needs to have a female attendant present during the examination. A female examiner may prefer to work alone but should have a female attendant present if the patient is particularly anxious or emotionally unstable.

External Genitalia

The perineal area needs to be well illuminated to be examined. The examiner must wear clean gloves on both hands to help prevent contact with infectious organisms. The perineum is extremely sensitive and tender; this area should not be touched suddenly without warning the patient. It is best to touch the neighbouring thigh first before advancing to the perineum.

As the examiner, while the patient is sitting at the end of the examination table or bed, inspect the quantity and distribution of hair growth. Preadolescents have no pubic hair. During adolescence, hair grows along the labia, becoming darker, coarser, and curlier. In an adult, hair grows in a triangle over the female pubis and along the medial surfaces of the thighs. Hair should be free of nits and lice. The underlying skin should be free of inflammation, irritation, or lesions.

An increasingly common practice among younger women is the removal of genital hair by means of waxing or shaving. The genital region in these patients should be assessed for abrasion, ingrown hair, irritation from clothing, and signs of infection. Patients who remove the hair in their genital region should be instructed to use increased hygiene practices (Centers for Disease Control and Prevention, 2013).

Inspect surface characteristics of the labia majora. The skin of the perineum is smooth, clean, and slightly darker than other skin. The mucous membranes appear dark pink and moist. The labia majora are gaping or closed and appear dry or moist. They are usually symmetrical. After childbirth, the labia majora separate, causing the labia minora to become more prominent. When a woman reaches menopause, the labia majora become thinned. With advancing age, they become atrophied (reduced in size). The labia majora are normally without inflammation, edema, lesions, or lacerations.

To inspect the remaining external structures, use the nondominant hand and gently place the thumb and index finger inside the labia minora and retract the tissues outwardly (Figure 32-47). Be sure to have a firm hold to avoid repeated retraction against the sensitive tissues. Use the other hand to palpate the labia minora between the thumb and second finger. On inspection, the labia minora are normally thinner than the labia majora, and one side is sometimes larger. The tissue feels soft on palpation and without tenderness. The size of the clitoris is variable, but it normally does not exceed 2 cm in length and 0.5 cm in width. Look for atrophy, inflammation, or adhesions. If inflamed, the clitoris will be a bright cherry red. In young women, it is a common site for syphilitic lesions, or **chancres**, which appear as small open ulcers that drain serous material. Some older women have malignant changes that result in dry, scaly, nodular lesions.

Inspect the urethral orifice carefully for colour and position. It is normally intact without inflammation. The urethral meatus is anterior to the vaginal orifice and is pink. It appears as a small slit or pinhole opening just above the vaginal canal. Note any discharge, polyps, or fistulas.

Inspect the vaginal orifice (introitus) for inflammation, edema, discoloration, discharge, and lesions. Normally the introitus is a thin, vertical slit or a large orifice. The tissue is moist. While inspecting the vaginal orifice, note the condition of the hymen, which is just inside the introitus. In a virgin, the hymen restricts the opening of the vagina. Only remnants of the hymen remain after sexual intercourse.

Inspect the anus, looking for lesions and hemorrhoids. After completion of the external examination, dispose of examination gloves and offer the patient perineal hygiene.

Patients who are at risk for contracting a sexually transmitted infection (STI) need to learn to perform a genital self-examination (GSE) (Box 32-25). The purpose of the examination is to detect any signs or

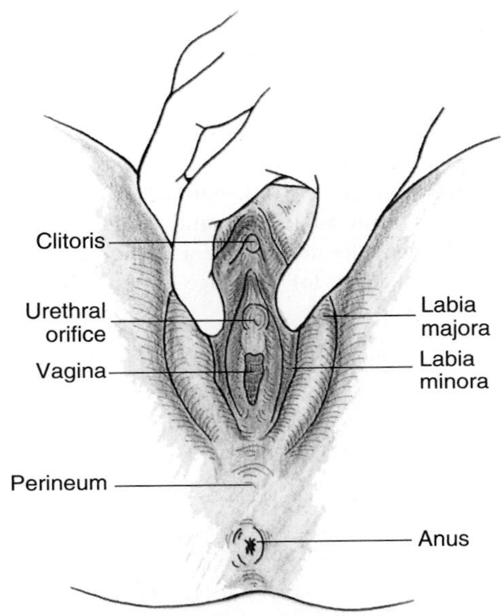

FIGURE 32-47 Female external genitalia.

BOX 32-25 PATIENT TEACHING

Female Genitalia and Reproductive Tract Assessment

Objectives

- Patient will pursue routine gynecological examinations based on her level of risk for cervical cancer and other gynecological pathology.
- Patient with a sexually transmitted infection (STI) will follow safer sex practices.
- Patient will use measures to prevent acquisition and transmission of STIs.

Teaching Strategies

- Teach patient about purpose and recommended frequency of **Papanicolaou (Pap) smears** and gynecological examinations. Explain that the Pap smear is relatively painless and needed with a pelvic examination for women who are over the age of 25 and sexually active. Pap smear screening is recommended every 3 years when results are normal, and more often when results are abnormal (Canadian Task Force on Preventive Health Care, 2016).
- Counsel patient with an STI about diagnosis and treatment.
- Instruct patient in genital self-examination (GSE): Using a mirror, position self in order to examine the area covered by the pubic hair. Spread the hair apart, looking for bumps, sores, or blisters. Also, look for any warts, which appear as small, bumpy spots and that enlarge to fleshy, cauliflower-like lesions. Next, spread the outer vaginal lips apart and look at the clitoris for bumps, blisters, sores, or warts. Also look at both sides of the inner vaginal lips. Inspect the area around the urinary and vaginal opening for bumps, blisters, sores, or warts.
- Explain warning signs of STIs: pain or burning on urination, pain during sex, pain in pelvic area, bleeding between menstruation, itchy rash around vagina, and abnormal vaginal discharge.
- Teach measures to prevent STIs: male partner's use of condoms, restricting number of sexual partners, avoiding sex with individuals who have several other partners, and perineal hygiene measures.
- Tell patients with an STI to inform sexual partners of the need for an examination and treatment.
- Reinforce the importance of performing perineal hygiene (as appropriate).

Evaluation

- Ask patient to explain when she should routinely have a gynecological examination and Pap test.
- Have patient describe ways to prevent transmission of STIs.
- For patient with an STI, determine during follow-up visit if patient has followed safe sexual practices (use nonthreatening inquiry).

symptoms of an STI. Many people do not know they have an STI (e.g., chlamydia), and some STIs (e.g., syphilis) remain undetected for years.

Speculum Examination of Internal Genitalia

An examination of the internal genitalia requires skill and practice. Advanced practice nurses and primary care providers will perform this examination. Beginning students will more than likely only observe the procedure or assist the examiner by helping the patient with positioning, handing off specimen supplies, and supporting the patient. A detailed presentation of the internal genital exam can be found in the textbook by Jarvis and colleagues (2014, pp. 757–765). The examination involves use of a plastic or metal speculum, consisting of two blades and an adjustment device. The examiner inserts the speculum into the vagina to assess the internal genitalia for cancerous lesions and other abnormalities. During the examination, the examiner will collect a specimen for a Papanicolaou (Pap) test for cervical cancer.

MALE GENITALIA

An examination of the male genitalia is done to assess the integrity of the external genitalia (Figure 32-48), inguinal ring, and canal. Because the incidence of STIs in adolescents and young adults is high, an assessment of the genitalia needs to be a routine part of any health maintenance examination for this age group (Box 32-26). The examination begins by having the patient void. The examination room should be warm. The patient lies supine with the chest, abdomen, and lower legs draped or stands during the examination. The examiner must wear clean gloves.

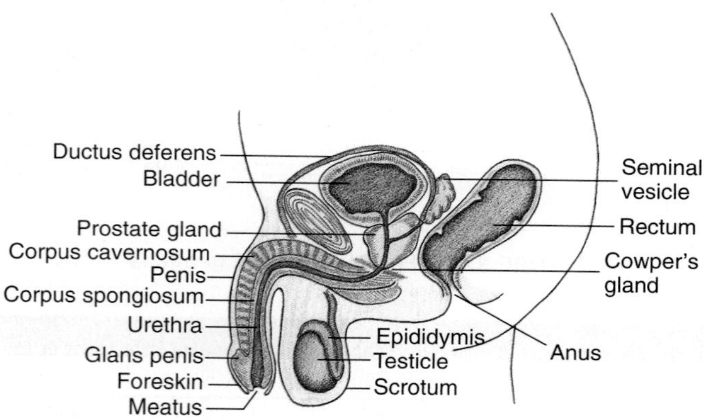

FIGURE 32-48 External and internal male sex organs.

Using a calm, gentle approach can lessen the patient's anxiety. The position and exposure of the body during the examination is embarrassing for some patients. To minimize the patient's anxiety, it often helps to offer explanations of the steps of examination so the patient can anticipate all actions. The genitalia should be manipulated gently to avoid causing erection or discomfort. A thorough history (Table 32-27) is obtained before the examination to ensure that the assessment is complete.

Sexual Maturity

First, note the sexual maturity of the patient by observing the size and shape of the penis and testes; the size, colour, and texture of the scrotal skin; and the character and distribution of pubic hair. Use Tanner stages to assess and document sexual maturation (Jarvis & Luctkar-Flude, 2014d, p. 719). In stage 1, the penis and scrotum show no change in size and there is no evidence of pubic hair. In stage 2, the testes first increase in size during preadolescence. At this time there is little to no pubic hair. At stage 3, the scrotal hair becomes coarse and dark and the penis begins to enlarge. Further growth and coverage of the pubic area occur in stage 4 and the glans penis matures and scrotum darkens. By the end of stage 5, the testes and penis enlarge to adult size and shape and scrotal skin darkens and becomes wrinkled. The penis has no hair, and the scrotum has very little hair (Figure 32-49). Also inspect the skin covering the genitalia for lice, rashes, excoriations, or lesions. Normally the skin is clear, without lesions.

Penis

To inspect penile surfaces thoroughly, manipulate the genitalia or have the patient assist. Inspect the shaft, corona, prepuce (foreskin), glans, and urethral meatus. The dorsal vein is apparent on inspection. In uncircumcised males, retract the foreskin to reveal the glans and urethral meatus. The foreskin usually retracts easily. A small amount of white, thick smegma sometimes collects under this foreskin. Obtain a culture if abnormal discharge is present. The urethral meatus is slitlike and is positioned on the ventral surface just millimetres from the tip of the glans. In some congenital conditions, the meatus is displaced along the penile shaft. The area between the foreskin and glans is a common site for venereal lesions. Gently compress the glans between thumb and index finger; this opens the urethral meatus for inspection

BOX 32-26 PATIENT TEACHING

Male Genitalia Assessment

Objectives

- Patient will describe methods to prevent transmission of sexually transmitted infections (STIs).
- Patient will perform genital self-examination.
- Patient with an STI will follow safer sex practices.

Teaching Strategies

- Counsel patient with an STI about diagnosis and treatment.
- Explain warning signs of STIs: pain on urination and during sex, abnormal penile discharge (different from usual), swollen lymph nodes, or rash or ulcer on skin or genitalia.
- Teach measures to prevent STIs: use of condoms, avoiding sex with an infected partner, restricting number of sexual partners, avoiding sex with individuals who have multiple partners, and using regular perineal hygiene.
- Tell patients with an STI to inform their sexual partners of the need to have an examination and treatment.
- Instruct patient to seek treatment as soon as possible if partner becomes infected with an STI.
- Instruct patient in how to perform genital self-examination (see Box 32-27).

Evaluation

- Ask patient to describe methods for preventing and treating STI.
- During a follow-up visit, determine whether patient with an STI has used safer sex practices.

TABLE 32-27 Nursing History for Male Genitalia Assessment

Assessment Category	Rationale
Review normal urinary elimination pattern, including frequency of voiding; history of nocturia; character and volume of urine; daily fluid intake; symptoms of burning, urgency, and frequency; difficulty starting stream; and hematuria (see Chapter 43).	Urinary problems are directly associated with genitourinary problems because of anatomical structure of men's reproductive and urinary systems.
Assess patient's sexual history and use of safer sex habits (multiple partners, infection in partners, failure to use condom).	Sexual history reveals risk for and understanding of sexually transmitted infections (STIs) and human immunodeficiency virus (HIV).
Determine if patient has had previous surgery or illness involving urinary or reproductive organs, including STI.	Alterations resulting from disease or surgery are sometimes responsible for symptoms or changes in organ structure or function.
Ask if patient has noted penile pain or swelling, genital lesions, or urethral discharge.	These signs and symptoms may indicate STI.
Determine if patient has noticed heaviness or painless enlargement of testis or irregular lumps.	These signs and symptoms are early warning signs for testicular cancer.
If patient reports an enlargement in inguinal area, assess if it is intermittent or constant, associated with straining or lifting, and painful, and whether pain is affected by coughing, lifting, or straining at stool.	Signs and symptoms reflect potential inguinal hernia.
Ask if patient has difficulty achieving erection or ejaculation; also review whether patient is taking diuretics, sedatives, antihypertensives, or tranquilizers.	These medications influence sexual performance.

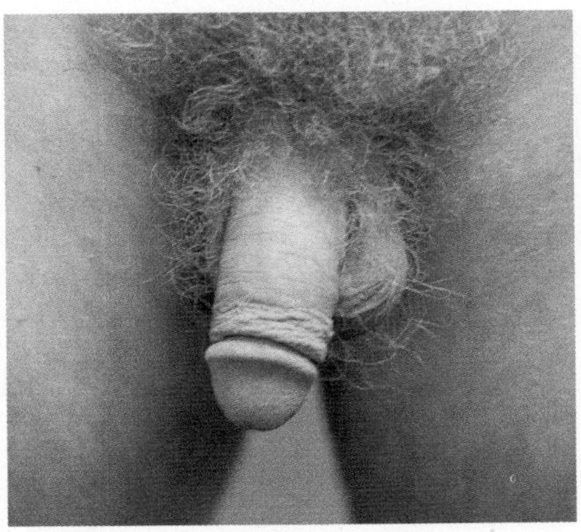

FIGURE 32-49 Normal male genitalia (circumcised). (From Ball et al. [2015]. *Seidel's guide to physical examination* [8th ed., p. 471, Fig. 19-5A]. St. Louis, MO: Mosby.)

of lesions, edema, and inflammation. Normally the opening is glistening and pink, without discharge. Palpate any lesion gently to note tenderness, size, consistency, and shape. When inspection and palpation of the glans is complete, pull the foreskin down to its original position.

Continue by inspecting the entire shaft of the penis, including the undersurface, looking for lesions, scars, or edema. Palpate the shaft between the thumb and first two fingers to detect localized areas of hardness or tenderness. A patient who has lain in bed for a prolonged time sometimes develops dependent edema in the penis shaft.

It is important for any male patient to learn to perform a GSE to detect signs or symptoms of STIs. Many people who have an STI do not know it. Self-examination is a routine part of self-care (Box 32-27).

Scrotum

The examiner should be particularly cautious while inspecting and palpating the scrotum because the structures lying within the scrotal sac are very sensitive. The scrotum is divided internally into two halves. Each half contains a testicle, epididymis, and the vas deferens, which travels upward into the inguinal ring. Normally, the left testicle is lower than the right. Inspect the scrotum's size, shape, and symmetry while observing for lesions or edema. Gently lift the scrotum to view the posterior surface. The scrotal skin is usually loose, and the surface is coarse. The scrotal skin is more deeply pigmented than body skin. Tightening, loss or wrinkling indicates edema. The size of the scrotum normally changes with temperature variations because the dartos muscle contracts in cold and relaxes in warm temperatures. Lumps in the scrotal skin are commonly sebaceous cysts.

The testes are normally sensitive but not tender. The underlying testicles are normally ovoid and approximately 2 to 4 cm in size. Gently palpate the testicles and epididymis between the thumb and first two fingers. The testes feel smooth, rubbery, and free of nodules. The epididymis is resilient. Note the size, shape, and consistency of the organs. The most common symptoms of testicular cancer are a painless enlargement of one testis and the appearance of a palpable, small, hard lump, about the size of a pea, on the front or side of the testicle. In the older male, the testicles decrease in size and are less firm during palpation. Continue to palpate the vas deferens separately as it forms the spermatic cord toward the inguinal ring, noting nodules or swelling. It normally feels smooth and discrete.

Testicular cancer is a solid tumour common in young men ages 15 to 29 years (Canadian Cancer Society, 2017a). Early detection is critical. Testicular self-examination (TSE) should be explained to the patient while he is being examined. Further details on teaching TSE can be found in the textbook by Jarvis and colleagues (2014, pp. 729–730).

Inguinal Ring and Canal

The external inguinal ring provides the opening for the spermatic cord to pass into the inguinal canal. The canal forms a passage through the abdominal wall, a potential site for hernia formation. A hernia is a protrusion of a portion of intestine through the inguinal wall or canal. Sometimes an intestinal loop enters the scrotum. Often hernias are asymptomatic. However, complications of hernias can be serious, including severe pain and bowel obstruction. Physical examination of

BOX 32-27 Male Genital Self-Examination

All men aged 15 years and older need to perform this examination on a regular basis using the following steps.

Genital Examination

Perform the examination after a warm bath or shower, when the scrotal skin is less thick.

Stand naked in front of a mirror, and hold the penis in your hand and examine the head. Pull back the foreskin if uncircumcised to expose the glans.

Inspect and palpate the entire head of the penis in a clockwise motion, looking carefully for any bumps, sores, or blisters (bumps and blisters may be light coloured or red, resemble pimples) (see illustration). Look also for any genital warts.

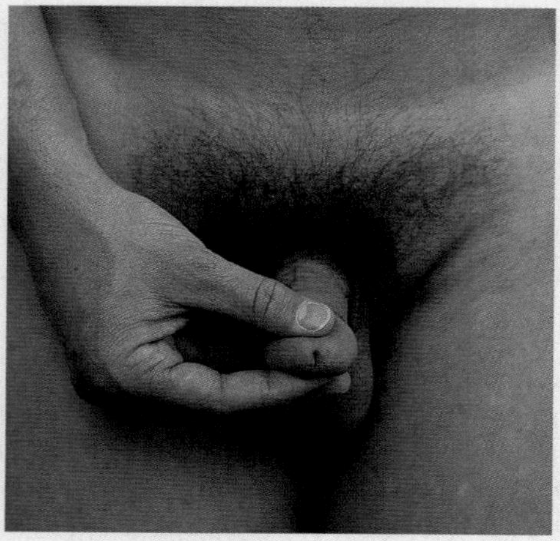

Male genital examination.

Look at the opening (urethral meatus) at the end of the penis for discharge.

Look along the entire shaft of the penis for the same signs.

Be sure to separate pubic hair at the base of the penis and carefully examine the skin underneath.

Testicular Self-Examination

Look for swelling or lumps in the skin of the scrotum while looking in the mirror.

Use both hands, placing the index and middle fingers under the testicles and the thumb on top (see illustration).

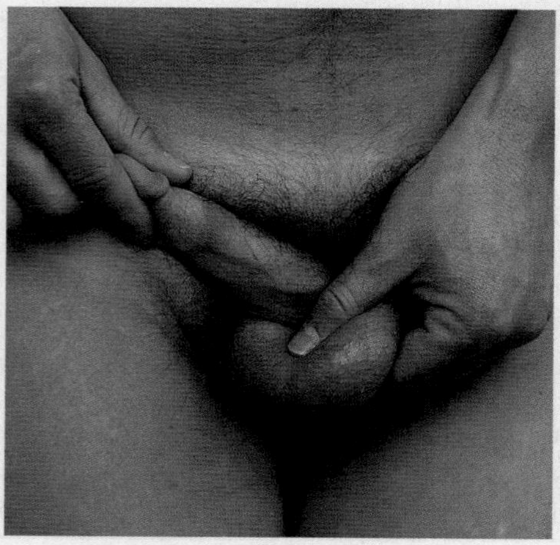

Testicular self-examination.

Gently roll the testicle, feeling for lumps, swelling, soreness, or a change in consistency (hardening).

Find the epididymis (a cordlike structure on the top and back of the testicle; it is not a lump).

Feel for small, pea-sized lumps on the front and side of the testicle. The lumps are usually painless and are abnormal.

Call your health care provider if you are uncertain whether you have detected any abnormal findings.

Photos from Ball, J. W., Dains, J. E., Flynn, J. A., Solomon, B. S., & Stewart, R. W. (2015). *Seidel's guide to physical examination* (8th ed., pp. 472–474). St. Louis, MO: Mosby.

inguinal hernias is an advanced practice nursing skill. A detailed overview of this examination can be found in the textbook by Jarvis and colleagues (2014, pp. 727–728).

RECTUM AND ANUS

The rectal examination is usually performed after the genital examination. It is not commonly performed during the examination in young children or adolescents. A rectal examination may detect colorectal cancer in its early stages. In men, the rectal examination is also used to detect prostatic tumours. A thorough history (Table 32-28) is collected to determine the patient's risk for bowel or rectal disease or prostatic disease.

An examination of the rectum and anus requires much skill and practice; advanced nurse practitioners and primary care providers will perform this examination. Beginning students will more than likely only observe the procedure or assist the examiner by helping the patient with positioning, handing off specimen supplies, and comforting the patient. A detailed presentation of the anus, rectum, and prostate exams can be found in the textbook by Jarvis and colleagues (2014, pp. 583–598).

The rectal examination is uncomfortable, so explaining all steps to the patient can help the patient relax. A calm, slow-paced, gentle approach should be used during the examination. Female patients remain in the dorsal recumbent position following genitalia examination or they assume a side-lying (Sims') position. The best way to examine men is to have the patient stand and bend over forward with hips flexed and upper body resting across the examination table. A nonambulatory patient is examined in Sims' position. The examiner must use disposable gloves.

Inspection

Using the nondominant hand, the examiner gently retracts the buttocks to view the perianal and sacrococcygeal areas. Perianal skin is smooth and more pigmented and coarser than skin over the buttocks. Anal tissue is inspected for skin characteristics, lesions, external **hemorrhoids** (dilated veins that appear as reddened protrusions), ulcers, fissures and fistulas, inflammation, rashes, or excoriation. Anal tissues are moist and hairless, and the voluntary external muscle sphincter holds the anus closed. Next, the examiner asks the patient to bear down as though having a bowel movement. Any internal hemorrhoids or fissures will appear at this time. Clock reference (e.g., 3 o'clock, 8

TABLE 32-28 Nursing History for Rectal and Anal Assessment

Assessment Category	Rationale
Determine whether patient has experienced bleeding from rectum, black or tarry stools (melena), rectal pain, or change in bowel habits (constipation or diarrhea).	These are warning signs of colorectal cancer* or other gastrointestinal alterations.
Determine whether patient has personal or strong family history of colorectal cancer, polyps, or chronic inflammatory bowel disease. Ask if patient is over age 40.	These are risk factors for colorectal cancer.*
Assess dietary habits, including high fat intake, diet high in processed or red meats, or deficient fibre content (inadequate fruits and vegetables).	Bowel cancer is often linked to dietary intake of fat or insufficient fibre intake.*
Determine if patient is obese, is physically inactive, smokes, or consumes alcohol.	These are risk factors for colorectal cancer.
Determine whether patient has undergone screening for colorectal cancer (digital examination, fecal immunochemical test [FIT], fecal occult blood test [FOBT], flexible sigmoidoscopy, and colonoscopy).	Undergoing this screening reflects understanding of and adherence to preventive health care measures.
Assess medication history for use of laxatives or cathartic medications.	Repeated use causes diarrhea and eventual loss of intestinal muscle tone.
Assess for use of codeine or iron preparations.	Codeine causes constipation. Iron turns the color of feces black and tarry.
Ask male patient if he has experienced weak or interrupted urine flow, inability to urinate, difficulty in starting or stopping urine flow, polyuria, nocturia, hematuria, or dysuria. Does patient have continuing pain in lower back, pelvis, or upper thighs?	These are warning signs of prostatic cancer.* Symptoms also suggest infection or prostate enlargement.

*Data from Canadian Cancer Society. (2017). *Colorectal cancer.* Retrieved from http://www.cancer.ca/en/cancer-information/cancer-type/colorectal/colorectal-cancer/?region=on

BOX 32-28 PATIENT TEACHING

Rectal and Anal Assessment

Objectives

- Patient will have a regular digital examination performed appropriate to age and symptom presentation.
- Patient will be able to identify symptoms of colorectal and prostatic cancer.
- Patient will follow a nutritiously sound diet.

Teaching Strategies

- Discuss the Canadian Task Force on Preventive Health Care (2016) recommendations for early detection of colorectal cancer and preventive health screening methods.
- Individuals at increased risk should discuss options with their health care provider.
- Discuss warning signs of colorectal cancer (see Table 32-28).
- Discuss dietary planning and healthy lifestyle choices to maintain or improve colon health.
- Warn patient against problems caused by overuse of laxatives, cathartic medications, codeine, or enemas.
- Discuss with male patients the Canadian Urological Association (Izawa, Klotz, Siemens, et al., 2011) guidelines for early detection of prostatic cancer. These guidelines recommend discussing the risks and benefits of screening for prostate cancer with all men 50 years and older with a presumed life expectancy of 10 years or greater. If, after weighing the risks and benefits, a patient wishes to continue with screening, digital rectal examination (DRE) and prostate-specific antigen (PSA) level tests are recommended every 1–5 years (Izawa et al., 2011).
- Inform male patients that men with a first-degree relative diagnosed with prostate cancer need to begin testing earlier.
- Discuss the warning signs of prostatic cancer.

Evaluation

- During follow-up visits, determine whether patient has had a rectal examination performed.
- Have patient explain warning signs of colorectal and prostatic cancer.
- Ask patient to describe appropriate lifestyle and food choices for a healthy colon.

o'clock) is used to describe location of findings. Normally there is no protrusion of tissue.

Digital Palpation

The anal canal and sphincters are examined with digital palpation, and in male patients, the prostate gland is palpated to rule out enlargement (Box 32-28). A detailed presentation of the anus, rectum, and prostate exams can be found in the textbook by Jarvis and colleagues (2014, pp. 583–598).

MUSCULOSKELETAL SYSTEM

The musculoskeletal assessment can be conducted as a separate examination or integrated into other portions of the total physical examination. Assessment can be performed during other nursing care measures such as bathing or positioning. The assessment of musculoskeletal function focuses on determining range of joint motion, muscle strength and tone, and joint and muscle condition. The assessment of musculoskeletal integrity is especially important when the patient reports pain or loss of function in a joint or muscle. Frequently, muscular disorders are the result of neurological disease. For this reason, health care providers often conduct a neurological assessment simultaneously.

While examining the patient's musculoskeletal function, it helps to visualize the anatomy of bone and muscle placement and joint structure (see Chapter 45). Joints vary in their degree of mobility. The spinal vertebrae are examples of slightly movable joints in comparison to the hinge joint movement of the knee or elbow.

For a complete examination, the muscles and joints should be exposed so they are able to move without restriction from clothing and so that they are easy to visualize. The patient assumes a sitting, supine, prone, or standing position while certain muscle groups are assessed. Table 32-29 lists the information gathered in the nursing history.

General Inspection

To begin assessment, observe the patient's gait when he or she enters the examination room. When a patient is unaware of the nature of the observation, gait is more natural. Later, a more formal test has the patient walk in a straight line away and then return to point of origin. Note how the patient walks, sits, and rises from a sitting position. Normally, patients walk with the arms swinging freely at the sides and the head leading the body. Older persons often walk with smaller steps and a wider base of support. Any foot dragging, limping, or shuffling and the position of the trunk in relation to the legs should be noted.

Observe the patient from the side in a standing position. The normal standing posture is upright with parallel alignment of the hips and shoulders. There is an even contour of the shoulders, level scapulae and iliac crests, alignment of the head over the gluteal folds, and symmetry of extremities. Looking sideways at the patient, note the normal cervical, thoracic, and lumbar curves. Holding the head erect is normal. As the patient sits, some degree of rounding of the shoulders is normal. Older persons tend to assume a stooped, forward-bent posture with the hips and knees somewhat flexed and arms bent at the elbows, raising the level of the arms.

Common postural abnormalities include lordosis, kyphosis, and scoliosis. **Kyphosis**, or hunchback, is an exaggeration of the posterior curvature of the thoracic spine. This postural abnormality is common in the older person. **Lordosis**, or swayback, is an increased lumbar curvature. A lateral spinal curvature is called **scoliosis**. Loss of height is frequently the first clinical sign of osteoporosis, in which height loss occurs in the trunk as a result of vertebral fracture and collapse. **Osteoporosis** is a metabolic bone disease that causes a decrease in quality and quantity of bone. One in three women and one in five men will experience an osteoporotic fracture in their lifetime (Osteoporosis Canada, 2016). Osteoporosis affects not only adults; it strikes any age group, including children. Although a small amount of height loss is to be expected with aging, if the amount of loss is great, osteoporosis is likely (Box 32-29). As men and women age, they are more likely to have osteoporotic fractures of the forearm or wrists, hips, and vertebrae (Osteoporosis Canada, 2016).

During general inspection, the examiner looks at the extremities for overall size, gross deformity, bony enlargement, alignment, and symmetry. Normally, there is bilateral symmetry in length, circumference, alignment, and position and in the number of skin folds (Ball et al., 2015a, p. 510). A general review pinpoints areas requiring specialized assessment.

TABLE 32-29 Nursing History for Musculoskeletal Assessment

Assessment Category	Rationale
Determine if patient is involved in competitive sports (particularly involving collision and contact), fails to warm up adequately, is in poor physical condition, or has had a rapid growth spurt (adolescents).	These are risk factors for sports injury.
Review patient history for use of alcohol and caffeine; cigarette smoking; constant dieting; calcium intake less than 500 mg daily; thin and light body frame; nulliparous status; menopause before age 45; estrogen deficiency; postmenopause status; family history of osteoporosis; advanced age; history of fractures or falls; sedentary lifestyle; chronic diseases (Cushing's hyperthyroidism and hypothyroidism, malabsorption or malnutrition disorders, neoplasm); long-term use of corticosteroids, methotrexate, phenytoin, aluminum-containing antacids; lack of weight-bearing exercise; lack of exposure to sunlight or inadequate vitamin D intake.	These are risk factors for osteoporosis.
Ask patient to describe history of problems in bone, muscle, or joint function (e.g., recent fall, trauma, lifting of heavy objects, history of bone or joint disease with sudden or gradual onset, location of alteration).	History assists in assessing nature of musculoskeletal problem.
Assess nature and extent of pain, including location, duration, severity, predisposing and aggravating factors, relieving factors, and type.	Pain frequently accompanies alterations in bone, joints, or muscle. This has implications for not only comfort but also ability to perform activities of daily living.
Assess patient's normal activity pattern, including type of exercise routinely performed.	Provides baseline in assessment. Sedentary lifestyle and lack of appropriate exercise increase bone loss and risk of fractures.
Determine how alteration influences ability to perform activities of daily living (e.g., bathing, feeding, dressing, toileting, ambulating) and social functions (e.g., household chores, work, recreation, sexual activities).	The extent to which patient is able to perform self-care will determine the level of nursing care. Type and degree of restriction in continuing social activities influence topics for patient education and ability of nurse to identify alternative ways to maintain function.
Assess height loss of women over age 50 by subtracting current height from recall of maximum adult height.	Measurement is useful screening tool to predict osteoporosis.

BOX 32-29 PATIENT TEACHING

Musculoskeletal Assessment

Objectives

- Patient will follow measures to prevent or minimize osteoporosis.
- Patient will assume proper body posture.
- Patient will be able to perform self-care measures.

Teaching Strategies

- Instruct patient in correct postural alignment. Consult with physical therapist to provide patient with exercises for improving posture.
- Recommend to women and men age 50 and older that they should undergo routine screening for osteoporosis (Papaioannou, Morin, Cheung, et al., 2010).
- To reduce bone demineralization, instruct older persons in a proper exercise program (e.g., weight-bearing, muscle-strengthening, and balance-training exercise) to be followed three or more times a week.
- Encourage intake of calcium to meet the recommended daily allowance. Increased vitamin D will aid calcium absorption.
  - Recommendation for daily calcium intake: age 4 to 8 years (800 mg), 9 to 18 years (1300 mg), 19 to 50 years (1000 mg), and 50+ years (1200 mg) (Osteoporosis Canada, 2016). If supplementing to achieve recommended calcium intake, instruct patient to take no more than 600 mg of calcium at one time.
  - Recommended vitamin D supplementation is 400 to 1 000 IU for low-risk adults and 800 to 2 000 IU for individuals considered at high risk (Osteoporosis Canada, 2016).
- Explain to patients with low back pain that they will benefit from modification of worker risk factors (e.g., lifting heavy weights, use of protective equipment), regular aerobic exercise, exercises that strengthen the back and increase trunk flexibility, and learning how to lift properly.
- Instruct older persons and those with osteoporosis in proper body mechanics and range-of-motion and moderate weight-bearing exercises (e.g., swimming and walking), to minimize trauma and subsequent fracture of bones.
- Instruct patient in use of assistive devices (e.g., zippers on clothing instead of buttons; elevation of chairs to minimize bending of knees and hips) when patient is unable to perform activities of daily living.
- Instruct older patients to pace activities to compensate for loss in muscle strength and to avoid falls.

Evaluation

- Observe patient's posture.
- Ask patient to describe therapies for preventing osteoporosis.
- Observe patient perform range-of-motion exercises.
- Have patient keep log of regular weight-training exercises.
- Ask patient or family members to describe patient's use of self-care aids.

Palpation

During a complete examination, the examiner applies gentle palpation to all bones, joints, and surrounding muscles. In a focused assessment, the involved area and adjacent muscle groups or joints are examined. Any heat, tenderness, edema, or resistance to pressure is noted. The patient should not feel any discomfort upon palpation. Muscles should be firm.

Range of Joint Motion

The examination includes comparison of both active and passive range of motion (ROM); the patient puts each major joint through active and passive full ROM (see Chapter 45). Beginning students need to learn the correct terminology for the movements that the joints are capable of making (Table 32-30) and know how to instruct the patient in how to move through each ROM. ROM should be demonstrated to the patient when possible. To assess ROM passively, ask the patient to relax and then passively move the extremities through their ROM. Compare the same body parts for bilateral equality and symmetry in movement. Figure 32-50 shows an example of ROM positions for the hand and wrist. A joint must not be forced into a painful position. Examiners must know the normal range of each joint and the extent to which they can move the patient's joints. ROM is equal between contralateral joints. Ideally, the patient's normal range should be assessed to determine a baseline for assessing later change.

Joints are typically free from stiffness, instability, swelling, or inflammation. There should be no discomfort when applying pressure to bones and joints. In older patients, joints often become swollen and stiff with reduced ROM resulting from cartilage erosion and fibrosis of synovial membranes (see Chapter 45). If a joint appears swollen and inflamed, it should be palpated for warmth.

TABLE 32-30 Terminology for Normal Range-of-Motion Positions

Term	Range of Motion	Examples of Joints
Flexion	Movement decreasing angle between two adjoining bones; bending of limb	Elbow, fingers, knee
Extension	Movement increasing angle between two adjoining bones	Elbow, knee, fingers
Hyperextension	Movement of body part beyond its normal resting extended position	Head
Pronation	Movement of body part so that front or ventral surface faces downward	Hand, forearm
Supination	Movement of body part so that the front or ventral surface faces upward	Hand, forearm
Abduction	Movement of extremity away from midline of body	Leg, arm, fingers
Adduction	Movement of extremity toward midline of body	Leg, arm, fingers
Internal rotation	Rotation of joint inward	Knee, hip
External rotation	Rotation of joint outward	Knee, hip
Eversion	Turning of body part away from midline	Foot
Inversion	Turning of body part toward midline	Foot
Dorsiflexion	Flexion of toes and foot upward	Foot
Plantar flexion	Bending of toes and foot downward	Foot

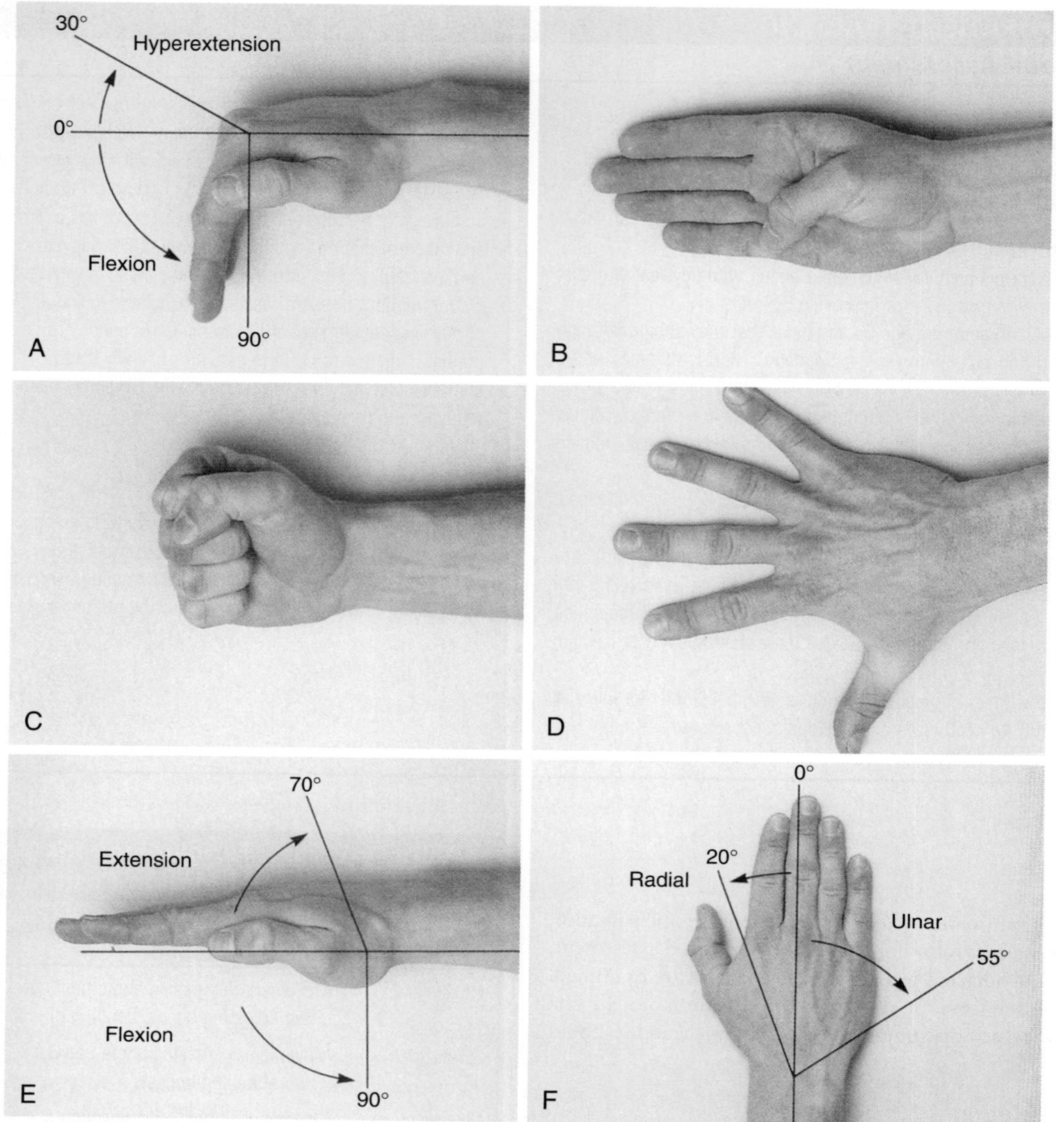

FIGURE 32-50 Range of motion of the hand and wrist. A, Metacarpophalangeal flexion and hyperextension. **B,** Finger flexion: thumb to each fingertip and to the base of the little finger. **C,** Finger flexion, fist formation. **D,** Finger abduction. **E,** Wrist flexion and hyperextension. **F,** Wrist radial and ulnar movement. (From Ball et al. [2015]. *Seidel's guide to physical examination* [8th ed., p. 515]. St. Louis, MO: Mosby.)

Muscle Tone and Strength

Muscle strength and tone are assessed during ROM measurement. These findings are integrated with those from the neurological assessment. Muscle tone is noted through the slight muscular resistance felt as the examiner moves the relaxed extremity passively through its ROM.

To assess muscle tone, ask the patient to allow an extremity to relax or hang limp. This is often difficult, particularly if the patient feels pain in the extremity. Support the extremity, and grasp each limb, moving it through the normal ROM. Normal tone causes a mild, even resistance to movement through the entire range.

If a muscle has increased tone, or hypertonicity, the examiner will meet considerable resistance with any sudden passive movement of a joint. Continued movement eventually causes the muscle to relax. A muscle that has little tone (hypotonicity) feels flabby. The involved extremity hangs loosely in a position determined by gravity.

For assessment of muscle strength, the patient assumes a stable position. The patient performs manoeuvres demonstrating strength of major muscle groups (Table 32-31). Symmetrical muscle pairs are compared for strength on the basis of a grading scale of 0 to 5 (Table 32-32). The arm on the dominant side is normally stronger than the arm on the nondominant side. In older persons, a loss of muscle mass causes bilateral weakness, but muscle strength remains greater in the dominant arm or leg.

Each muscle group needs to be examined. To start, ask the patient to first flex the muscle being examined and then to resist when you apply an opposing force against that flexion. It is important to not allow the patient to move the joint. Gradually increase pressure to a muscle group (e.g., elbow extension). Have the patient resist the pressure applied by attempting to move against resistance (e.g., elbow flexion). The patient resists until instructed to stop. Vary the amount of pressure applied, then observe the joint move. If you identify a

TABLE 32-31 Manoeuvres to Assess Muscle Strength

Muscle Group	Manoeuvre
Neck (sternocleidomastoid)	Place hand firmly against patient's upper jaw. Ask patient to turn head laterally against resistance.
Shoulder (trapezius)	Place hand over midline of patient's shoulder, exerting firm pressure. Have patient raise shoulders against resistance.
Elbow	
Biceps	Pull down on forearm as patient attempts to flex arm.
Triceps	As you flex patient's arm, apply pressure against forearm. Ask patient to straighten arm.
Hip	
Quadriceps	When patient is sitting, apply downward pressure to thigh. Ask patient to raise leg up from table.
Gastrocnemius	Patient sits, while examiner holds shin of flexed leg. Ask patient to straighten leg against resistance.

TABLE 32-32 Assessing Muscle Strength

Muscle Function Level	Grade
No evidence of movement	0
Trace of movement	1
Full range of motion, but not against gravity*	2
Full range of motion against gravity, but not against resistance	3
Full range of motion against gravity and some resistance, but weak	4
Full range of motion against gravity, full resistance	5

*Passive movement.

From Ball, J. W., Dains, J. E., Flynn, J. A., Solomon, B. S., & Stewart, R. W. (2015). *Seidel's guide to physical examination* (8th ed., Table 21-1). St. Louis, MO: Mosby.

weakness, compare the size of the muscle with its opposite counterpart by measuring the circumference of the muscle body with a tape measure. A muscle that has atrophied feels soft and boggy when palpated.

NEUROLOGICAL SYSTEM

The neurological system is responsible for many functions, including initiation and coordination of movement, reception and perception of sensory stimuli, organization of thought processes, control of speech, and storage of memory. A close integration exists between the neurological system and all other body systems. For example, urine production relies in part on the adequacy of blood flow to the kidneys, and the size of arterioles supplying the kidneys is under neural control.

An assessment of neurological function alone is quite time consuming. For efficiency, neurological measurements should be integrated with other parts of the physical examination. For example, cranial nerve function is tested during the survey of the head and neck. Mental and emotional status is observed during the initial interview.

Many variables need to be considered when deciding the extent of the examination. A patient's level of consciousness influences the ability to follow directions. General physical status influences tolerance to assessment. The patient's chief complaint also helps determine the need for a thorough neurological assessment. If the patient complains of headache or a recent loss of function in an extremity, the patient will need a complete neurological review. Table 32-33 reviews the data collected in the nursing history. For a complete examination, the following special equipment is needed:

- Reading material
- Vials containing aromatic substances (e.g., vanilla extract and coffee)
- Opposite tip of cotton swab or tongue blade broken in half
- Snellen eye chart
- Penlight
- Vials containing sugar or salt
- Tongue blade
- Two test tubes, one filled with hot water and the other with cold water
- Cotton balls or cotton-tipped applicators
- Tuning fork
- Reflex hammer

Mental and Emotional Status

Nurses learn a great deal about a patient's mental capacities and emotional state by simply interacting with the patient. They ask questions during an examination to gather data and observe the appropriateness of emotions and thoughts. There are special screening tools designed to assess a patient's mental status. A widely used tool in the screening for cognitive impairment is the Montreal Cognitive Assessment, which is focused on the assessment of mild cognitive impairment (Julayanont, Phillips, Chertkow, et al., 2013); available at http://www.mocatest.org/). The Mini-Mental State Examination (MMSE) is another screening instrument that measures orientation and cognitive function (Mitchell, 2013). The MMSE is available online from numerous sources. The maximum score on the MMSE is 30; patients with scores of 21 or less generally have cognitive impairment requiring further evaluation.

To ensure an objective assessment, nurses need to consider the patient's cultural and educational background, values, beliefs, and previous experiences. Such factors influence responses to questions. An alteration in mental or emotional status reflects a disturbance in cerebral functioning. The cerebral cortex controls and integrates intellectual and emotional functioning. Primary brain disorders, medication, and metabolic changes are examples of factors that change cerebral function.

Delirium is an acute mental disorder characterized by confusion, disorientation, and restlessness. The acute condition is often misdiagnosed as a form of dementia, a more progressive, organic mental disorder such as in Alzheimer's disease. Thus, many health care providers miss the underlying cause of the condition. Delirium is often overlooked in older persons because of a failure to adequately assess mental status. Fortunately, the condition often reverses when it is correctly assessed and the underlying cause is treated (central nervous system, metabolic, and cardiopulmonary disorders; systemic illnesses; and sensory deprivation or overload) (Stuart, 2013). Delirium may occur with older persons but also may occur in children having surgery (20%) and hospitalized children (8%) (Stuart, 2013). It is important to obtain a good history of the patient's behaviour before delirium develops so as to recognize the condition early. Family members are usually a good resource. Box 32-30 summarizes clinical criteria for delirium.

TABLE 32-33 Nursing History for Neurological Assessment

Assessment Category	Rationale
Determine if patient uses analgesics, alcohol, sedatives, hypnotics, antipsychotics, antidepressants, nervous system stimulants, or recreational drugs.	These medications alter level of consciousness or cause behavioural changes. Abuse sometimes causes tremors, ataxia, and changes in peripheral nerve function.
Determine if patient has recent history of seizures or convulsions: clarify sequence of events (aura, fall to ground, motor activity, loss of consciousness); character of any symptoms; and relationship of seizure to time of day, fatigue, or emotional stress.	Seizure activity often originates from central nervous system alteration. Characteristics of seizure aid in determining its origin.
Screen patient for symptoms of headache, tremors, dizziness, vertigo, numbness or tingling of body part, visual changes, weakness, pain, or changes in speech. Presence of any symptom requires more detailed review (onset, severity, precipitating factors, or sequence of events).	These symptoms frequently originate from alterations in central nervous system or peripheral nervous system function. Identification of specific patterns aids in diagnosis of pathological condition.
Discuss with patient's family any recent changes in patient's behaviour (e.g., increased irritability, mood swings, memory loss, change in energy level).	Behavioural changes sometimes result from intracranial pathological states.
Assess patient for history of change in vision, hearing, smell, taste, or touch.	Major sensory nerves originate from the brain stem. These symptoms help in localizing nature of problem.
If an older person displays sudden acute confusion (delirium), review history for drug toxicity (anticholinergics, diuretics, digoxin, cimetidine, sedatives, antihypertensives, antiarrhythmics), serious infections, metabolic disturbances, heart failure, and severe anemia.	This is one of the most common mental disorders in older people. The condition is always potentially reversible (see Box 32-30).
Review past history for head or spinal cord injury, meningitis, congenital anomalies, neurological disease, or psychiatric counselling.	Factors cause neurological symptoms or behavioural changes to develop, focusing assessment on possible cause.

BOX 32-30 Clinical Criteria for Delirium

- *Definition:* An acute disturbance of attention (i.e., reduced ability to direct, focus, sustain and shift attention) and awareness (i.e., reduced orientation to the environment) that is accompanied by a change in cognition. It is not due to a preexisting or evolving dementia, substance withdrawal or intoxication, exposure to a toxin, or multiple etiologies. Delirium develops over a short period of time, usually hours to days, and tends to fluctuate during the course of the day. It is usually a direct physiological consequence of a general medical condition. It is most common in older persons, but occurs occasionally in younger patients.
- There is reduced clarity of awareness of the environment.
- Ability to focus, sustain, or shift attention is impaired (questions must be repeated).
- Irrelevant stimuli easily distract the person.
- There is an accompanying change in cognition (memory impairment, disorientation, or language disturbance).
- Dementia commonly affects recent memory.
- Disorientation usually occurs, with patient disoriented to time, place, or person.
- Language disturbance involves impaired ability to name objects or ability to write; speech is sometimes rambling.
- Perceptual disturbances include misinterpretations, delusions, or visual and auditory hallucinations. Neurological signs include tremor, unsteady gait, asterixis, or myoclonus.

Modified from American Psychiatric Association. (2013). *Diagnostic and statistical manual of mental disorders* (5th ed.). Washington, DC: Author; Stuart, G. (2013). *Principles and practice of psychiatric nursing* (10th ed.). St. Louis, MO: Mosby.

TABLE 32-34 Glasgow Coma Scale

Action	Response	Score
Eyes open	Spontaneously	4
	To speech	3
	To pain	2
	None	1
Best verbal response	Oriented	5
	Confused	4
	Inappropriate words	3
	Incomprehensible sounds	2
	None	1
Best motor response	Obeys commands	6
	Localized pain	5
	Flexion withdrawal	4
	Abnormal flexion	3
	Abnormal extension	2
	Flaccid	1
	TOTAL SCORE	15

Level of Consciousness. A person's level of consciousness exists along a continuum from full awakening, alertness, and cooperation to unresponsiveness to any form of external stimuli. To assess level of consciousness, the nurse talks with the patient, asking questions about events involving the patient or concerns about any health problems. A fully conscious patient responds to questions quickly and expresses ideas logically. With a lowering of the patient's consciousness, the Glasgow Coma Scale (GCS) is used for an objective measurement of consciousness on a numerical scale (Table 32-34). The patient needs to be as alert as possible before testing. One should use caution when using the scale if a patient has sensory losses (e.g., vision, hearing). The GCS allows evaluation of a patient's neurological status over time. The higher the score, the better the patient's neurological function. Short, simple questions are asked, such as "What is your name?" "Where are you?" and "What day is this?" The patient is also asked to follow simple commands, such as "Move your toes."

If a patient is not conscious enough to follow commands, the nurse can try to elicit the pain response. To do this, apply firm pressure with the thumb over the root of the patient's fingernail. The normal response to the painful stimuli is withdrawal of the body part from the stimulus. A patient with serious neurological impairment exhibits abnormal posturing in response to pain. A flaccid response indicates the absence of muscle tone in the extremities and severe injury to brain tissue.

Behaviour and Appearance. Behaviour, moods, hygiene, grooming, and choice of dress reveal pertinent information about mental status. Nurses need to remain perceptive of a patient's mannerisms and actions during the entire physical assessment. Nonverbal and verbal behaviours are noted. Does the patient respond appropriately to directions? Does the patient's mood vary with no apparent cause? Does the patient show concern about appearance? Is the patient's hair clean and neatly groomed, and are the nails trim and clean? The patient should behave in a manner expressing concern and interest in the examination. The patient should make eye contact with the nurse and express appropriate feelings that correspond to the situation. Normally, the patient will show some degree of personal hygiene.

Choice and fit of clothing reflect socioeconomic background or personal taste rather than deficiency in self-concept or self-care. It is important to avoid being judgemental and to focus assessment on the appropriateness of clothing for the weather. Older persons sometimes neglect their appearance because of a lack of energy, finances, mobility, or reduced vision.

Language. Normal cerebral function allows a person to understand spoken or written words and to express the self through written words or gestures. Thus, to assess cerebral function, the patient's voice inflection, tone, and manner of speech are assessed. Normally, the patient's voice has inflections, is clear and strong, and increases in volume appropriately. Speech is fluent. When communication is clearly ineffective (e.g., omission or addition of letters and words, misuse of words, or hesitations), the nurse should assess for **aphasia**, as injury to the cerebral cortex results in aphasia.

The two types of aphasia are sensory (or receptive) and motor (or expressive). With receptive aphasia, a person cannot understand written or verbal speech. With expressive aphasia, a person understands written and verbal speech but cannot write or speak appropriately when attempting to communicate. A patient sometimes suffers a combination of receptive and expressive aphasia. Language capabilities should be assessed when it is clear that ineffective communication with the patient exists. Some simple assessment techniques are the following:

- Point to a familiar object, and ask the patient to name it.
- Ask the patient to respond to simple verbal and written commands, such as "Stand up" or "Sit down."
- Ask the patient to read simple sentences out loud.

Normally, a patient names objects correctly, follows commands, and reads sentences correctly.

Intellectual Function

Intellectual function includes memory (recent, immediate, and past), knowledge, abstract thinking, association, and judgement. Testing each aspect of function involves a specific technique. However, because cultural and educational background influences the ability to respond to test questions, questions related to concepts or ideas with which the patient is unfamiliar should not be asked.

Memory. To assess memory, immediate recall and recent and remote memory are assessed. Patients demonstrate immediate recall by repeating a series of numbers (e.g., *7, 4, 1*) in the order they are presented or in reverse order. Patients normally recall a series of five to eight digits forward and four to six digits backward.

Assessment begins with the nurse first asking the patient permission to test his or her memory. Then the nurse states clearly and slowly the name of three unrelated objects. After mentioning all three, the patient is asked to repeat each. The nurse continues until the patient is successful. Then, later in the assessment, the patient is asked to repeat the three words again. The patient should be able to identify the three words. Another test for recent memory involves asking the patient to recall events occurring during the same day (e.g., what was eaten for breakfast). Information can be validated with a family member.

To assess past memory, the patient is asked to recall the maiden name of the patient's mother, a birthday, or a special date in history. It is best to ask open-ended questions rather than simple yes/no questions. A patient usually has immediate recall of such information. With an older person, hearing loss should not be interpreted as confusion. Good communication techniques are essential throughout the examination to ensure that the patient clearly understands all directions and testing.

Knowledge. Knowledge is assessed by asking how much the patient knows about his or her illness or the reason for seeking health care. By assessing a patient's knowledge, the nurse can determine a patient's ability to learn or understand. If there is an opportunity to teach, the patient's mental status can be tested by asking for feedback during a follow-up visit.

Abstract Thinking. Interpreting abstract ideas or concepts reflects the capacity for abstract thinking. An individual requires a higher level of intellectual function to explain phrases that are common to them such as "A stitch in time saves nine" or "Don't count your chickens before they're hatched." Note whether the patient's explanations are relevant and concrete. The patient with altered mental status will probably interpret the phrase literally or merely rephrase the words.

Association. Another higher level of intellectual functioning involves finding similarities or associations between concepts: a dog is to a beagle as a cat is to a Siamese. The nurse names related concepts and asks the patient to identify their associations. Questions are appropriate to the patient's level of intelligence. Using simple concepts is sufficient.

Judgement. Judgement requires a comparison and evaluation of facts and ideas to understand their relationships and to form appropriate conclusions. A patient's ability to make logical decisions may be measured using questions such as "Why did you seek health care?" or "What would you do if you became ill at home?" Normally a patient makes logical decisions.

Cranial Nerve Function

A physical examination can involve the assessment of all 12 cranial nerves or a single nerve or related group of nerves. A dysfunction in one nerve reflects an alteration at some point along the distribution of the cranial nerve. Measurements used to assess the integrity of organs within the head and neck also assess cranial nerve function. A complete assessment involves testing the 12 cranial nerves in order of their numbers. To remember the order of the nerves, use this simple phrase: "On old Olympus' towering tops, a Finn and German viewed some hops." The first letter of each word in the phrase is the same as the first letter of the names of the cranial nerves listed in order (Table 32-35).

TABLE 32-35 Cranial Nerve Function and Assessment

Number	Name	Type	Function	Method
I	Olfactory	Sensory	Sense of smell	Ask patient to identify different nonirritating aromas such as coffee and vanilla.
II	Optic	Sensory	Visual acuity	Use Snellen chart, or ask patient to read printed material while wearing glasses.
III	Oculomotor	Motor	Extraocular eye movement	Assess directions of gaze.
IV	Trochlear	Motor	Pupil constriction and dilation	Measure pupillary reaction to light reflex and accommodation.
			Upward and downward movement of eyeball	Assess directions of gaze.
V	Trigeminal	Sensory and motor	Sensory nerve to skin of face	Lightly touch cornea with wisp of cotton. Assess corneal reflex. Measure sensation of light pain and touch across skin of face.
			Motor nerve to muscles of jaw	Palpate temples as patient clenches teeth.
VI	Abducens	Motor	Lateral movement of eyeballs	Assess directions of gaze.
VII	Facial	Sensory and motor	Facial expression	As patient smiles, frowns, puffs out cheeks, and raises and lowers eyebrows, look for asymmetry.
			Taste	Have patient identify salty or sweet taste on front of tongue.
VIII	Auditory	Sensory	Hearing	Assess ability to hear spoken word.
IX	Glossopharyngeal	Sensory and motor	Taste	Ask patient to identify sour or sweet taste on back of tongue.
			Ability to swallow	Use tongue blade to elicit gag reflex.
X	Vagus	Sensory and motor	Sensation of pharynx	Ask patient to say "ah." Observe movement of palate and pharynx.
			Movement of vocal cords	Assess speech for hoarseness.
XI	Spinal accessory	Motor	Movement of head and shoulders	Ask patient to shrug shoulders and turn head against passive resistance.
XII	Hypoglossal	Motor	Position of tongue	Ask patient to stick out tongue to midline and move it from side to side.

Sensory Function

The sensory pathways of the central nervous system conduct sensations of pain, temperature, position, vibration, and crude and finely localized touch. Different nerve pathways relay the sensations. Most patients require only a quick screening of sensory function unless there are symptoms of reduced sensation, motor impairment, or paralysis.

> **Safety Alert** The risk of skin breakdown is greater in a patient with impaired sensation. When assessing decreased sensation, complete a skin and tissue assessment of the area affected by the sensory loss. In addition, teach the patient to avoid pressure, thermal, and chemical trauma to the area.

Normally a patient has sensory responses to all stimuli that are tested. A patient feels sensations equally on both sides of the body in all areas. To assess the major sensory nerves the nurse must know the sensory dermatome zones (Figure 32-51). Some areas of the skin are innervated by specific dorsal root cutaneous nerves. For example, if assessment reveals reduced sensation when checking for light touch along an area of the skin (e.g., the lower neck), this determines, in general, where a neurological lesion exists (e.g., fourth cervical spinal cord segment).

All sensory testing is done with the patient's eyes closed so that the patient is unable to see when or where a stimulus strikes the skin (Table 32-36). Then stimuli are applied in a random, unpredictable order to maintain the patient's attention and prevent detection of a predictable pattern. The nurse asks the patient to describe when, what, and where he or she feels each stimulus. Symmetrical areas of the body are compared while applying stimuli to the patient's arms, trunk, and legs.

Motor Function

An assessment of motor function includes measurements made during the musculoskeletal examination. In addition, cerebellar function is assessed. The cerebellum coordinates muscular activity, maintains balance and equilibrium, and controls posture.

Coordination. To avoid confusion, it is good to demonstrate each manoeuvre and then have the patient repeat it, observing for smoothness and balance in the patient's movements (Box 32-31). In older persons, normally slow reaction time causes movements to be less rhythmical.

To assess fine motor function, have the patient extend the arms out to the sides and touch each forefinger alternately to the nose (first with eyes open, then with eyes closed). Normally the patient alternately touches the nose smoothly. Performing rapid, rhythmical, alternating movements demonstrates coordination in the upper extremities. While sitting, the patient begins by patting the knees with both hands. Then the patient alternately turns up the palm and back of the hands while continuously patting the knees. Normally patients perform the manoeuvre smoothly and regularly with increasing speed.

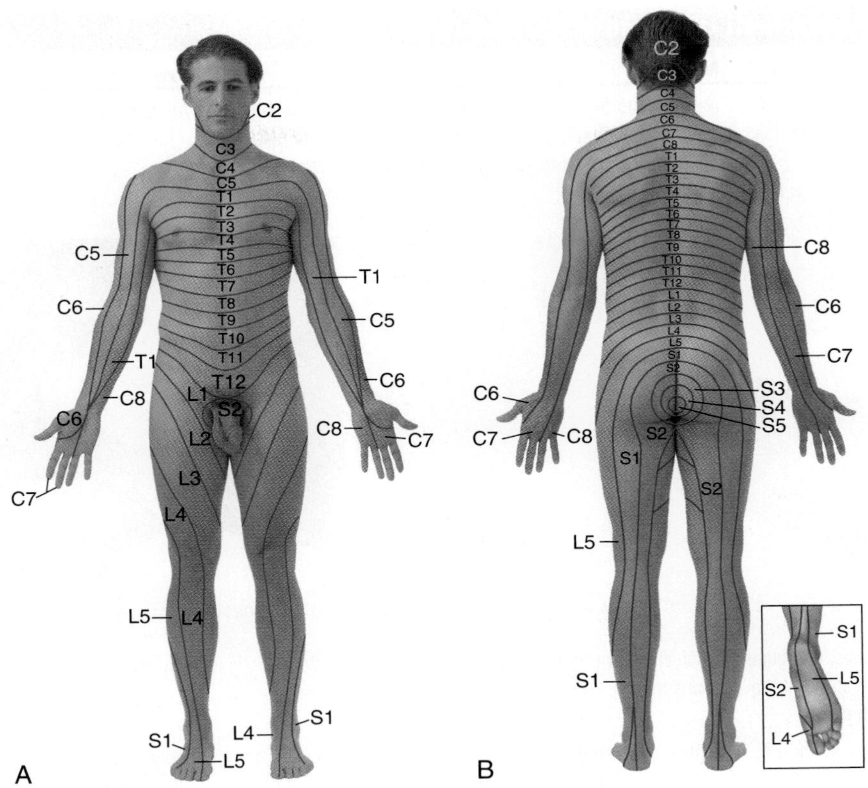

FIGURE 32-51 Dermatomes of the body, the body surface areas innervated by particular spinal nerves. C1 usually has no cutaneous distribution. **A,** Anterior view. **B,** Posterior view. It appears that there is a distinct separation of surface area controlled by each dermatome, but there is almost always overlap between spinal nerves. (From Ball et al. [2015]. *Seidel's guide to physical examination* [8th ed., p. 549]. St. Louis, MO: Mosby.)

An additional manoeuvre for upper extremity coordination involves touching each finger with the thumb of the same hand in rapid sequence. The patient moves from the index finger to the little finger and back, with one hand tested at a time. The patient's dominant hand is slightly less awkward when performing this movement. Movement is smooth and in succession.

To test lower extremity coordination the patient lies supine, legs extended. Place a hand at the ball of the patient's foot. The patient taps the hand with the foot as quickly as possible. Test each foot for speed and smoothness. The feet do not move as rapidly or evenly as the hands.

Balance. Use one or two of the following tests to assess balance and gross motor function:

- Have the patient perform a Romberg test by standing with feet together, arms at the sides, both with eyes open and eyes closed. Protect the patient's safety by standing at the side, observe for swaying. Expect slight swaying of the body in the Romberg test. A loss of balance (positive Romberg) causes a patient to fall to the side. Normally the patient does not break the stance.
- Have the patient close the eyes, with arms held straight at the sides, and stand on one foot and then the other. Normally patients are able to maintain balance for 5 seconds with slight swaying.
- Ask the patient to walk a straight line by placing the heel of one foot directly in front of the toes of the other foot.

> **Safety Alert** When examining an older person's gait, be aware of the risk for falls. Some older people need assistance with this portion of the examination.

Reflexes

Eliciting reflex reactions provides data about the integrity of sensory and motor pathways of the reflex arc and specific spinal cord segments. Assessment of reflexes does not determine higher neural centre functioning. Figure 32-52 traces the pathway of the reflex arc. Each muscle contains a small sensory unit called a *muscle spindle*, which controls muscle tone and detects changes in the length of muscle fibres. Tapping a tendon with a reflex hammer stretches the muscle and tendon, lengthening the spindle. The spindle sends nerve impulses along afferent nerve pathways to the dorsal horn of the spinal cord segment. Within milliseconds, the impulses reach the spinal cord and synapse to travel to the efferent motor neuron in the spinal cord. A motor nerve sends the impulses back to the muscle, causing the reflex response.

The two categories of normal reflexes are deep tendon reflexes, elicited by mildly stretching a muscle and tapping a tendon, and cutaneous reflexes, elicited by stimulating the skin superficially. Table 32-37 summarizes common deep tendon and cutaneous reflexes. Reflexes are graded as follows (Jarvis et al., 2014, p. 681):

0 No response
1+ Sluggish or diminished
2+ Active or expected response
3+ More brisk than expected, slightly hyperactive
4+ Brisk and hyperactive with intermittent or transient clonus

When assessing reflexes, have the patient relax as much as possible to avoid voluntary movement or tensing of muscles. Position the limbs to slightly stretch the muscle being tested. Hold the reflex hammer loosely between the thumb and fingers so that it is able to swing freely, and tap the tendon briskly (Figure 32-53). Compare the responses on

TABLE 32-36 Assessment of Sensory Nerve Function

Function	Equipment	Method	Precautions
Pain	Broken tongue blade or wooden end of cotton applicator	Ask patients to voice when they feel dull or sharp sensation. Alternately, apply sharp and blunt ends of tongue blade to skin's surface. Note areas of numbness or increased sensitivity.	Areas where skin is thick, such as heel or sole of foot, are less sensitive to pain.

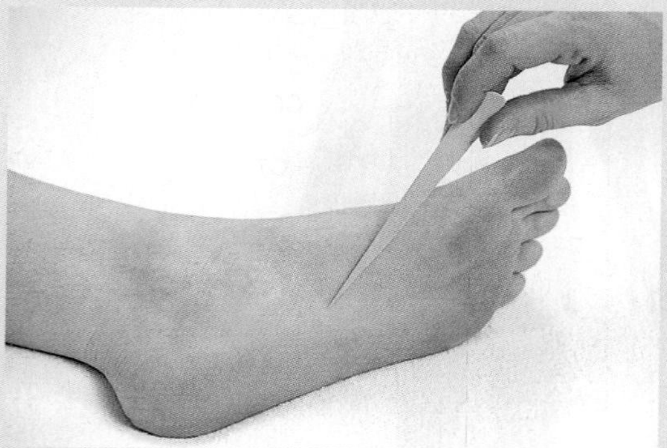

Assessing sensory nerve function in foot.

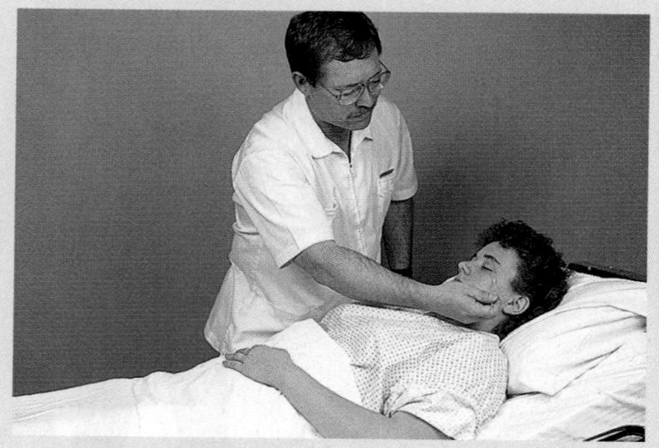

Assessing sensory nerve function in face.

Function	Equipment	Method	Precautions
Temperature	Two test tubes, one filled with hot water and the other with cold	Touch skin with tube. Ask patient to identify hot or cold sensation.	Omit test if pain sensation is normal.
Light touch	Cotton ball or cotton-tip applicator	Apply light wisp of cotton to different points along skin's surface. Ask patient to voice when feeling a sensation.	Apply at areas where skin is thin or more sensitive (e.g., face, neck, inner aspect of arms, top of feet and hands).
Vibration	Tuning fork	Apply stem of vibrating fork to distal interphalangeal joint of fingers and interphalangeal joint of great toe, elbow, and wrist. Have patient voice when and where vibration is felt.	Be sure patient feels vibration and not merely pressure.
Position		Grasp finger or toe, holding it by its sides with thumb and index finger. Alternate moving finger or toe up and down. Ask patient to state when finger is up or down. Repeat with toes.	Avoid rubbing adjacent appendages as you move finger or toe. Do not move joint laterally; return to neutral position before moving again.
Two-point discrimination	Two broken tongue blades	Lightly apply one or both tongue blade tips simultaneously to the skin's surface. Ask patient whether one or two pricks are felt. Find the distance at which patient can no longer distinguish two points.	Apply blade tips to same anatomical site (e.g., fingertips, palm of hand, or upper arms). Minimum distance at which patient discriminates two points varies (2 to 8 mm on fingertips).

BOX 32-31 PATIENT TEACHING

Neurological Assessment

Objectives

- Patient's family will understand relationship of patient's behavioural and mental changes to physical status.
- Patient with sensory or motor impairment will select safety measures for self-care.
- Older person will routinely inspect skin for injuries.

Teaching Strategies

- Explain to family or friends the implications of any behavioural or mental impairment shown by patient.
- If patient has sensory or motor impairments, explain measures to ensure safety (e.g., use of ambulation aids or safety bars in bathrooms or stairways).
- Teach an older person to plan enough time to complete tasks because reaction time is slow.
- Teach an older person to observe skin surfaces for areas of trauma, because perception of pain is reduced.

Evaluation

- Ask family to discuss patient behaviours that result from neurological impairments.
- Have patient explain safety measures used to avoid injury from sensory and motor limitations.
- Have older patient explain reason for inspecting skin surface routinely.

corresponding sides. Normally, older persons present with diminished reflexes. Stick figures are sometimes used to record reflexes.

AFTER THE EXAMINATION

Findings from the physical assessment are recorded during the examination or at the end. Special forms are available to record data. It is good to review all findings before assisting the patient with dressing, in case any information needs to be rechecked or additional data gathered. Physical assessment findings should be integrated into the plan of care.

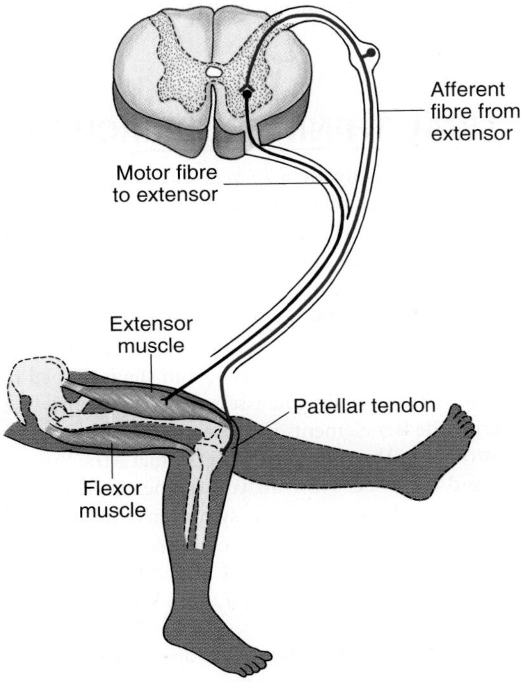

FIGURE 32-52 Pathway of the reflex arc.

After completing the assessment, give the patient time to dress. The hospitalized patient sometimes needs help with hygiene and returning to bed. When the patient is comfortable, it helps to share a summary of the assessment findings. If the findings have indicated serious abnormalities, such as a mass or highly irregular heart rate, consult the patient's health care provider before revealing any findings. It is the health care provider's responsibility to make definitive medical diagnoses. Explain the type of abnormality found and the need for the health care provider to conduct an additional examination.

When cleaning the examination area, use infection-control practices in removing materials or instruments soiled with potentially infectious wastes. If the patient's bedside was the examination site, clear away soiled items from the bedside table, and make sure that the bed linen is dry and clean. The patient will appreciate a clean gown and the opportunity to wash the face and hands. Afterward, be sure to perform hand hygiene.

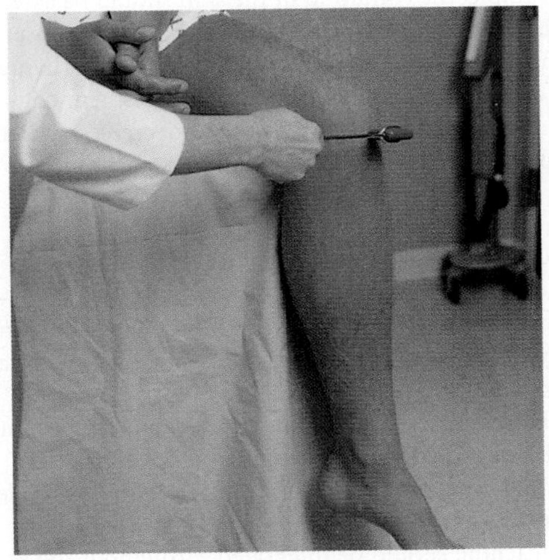

FIGURE 32-53 Position for eliciting the patellar tendon reflex. The lower leg normally extends.

TABLE 32-37 Assessment of Common Reflexes

Type	Procedure	Normal Reflex
Deep Tendon Reflexes		
Biceps	Flex patient's arm up to 45 degrees at elbow with palms down. Place your thumb in antecubital fossa at base of biceps tendon and your fingers over biceps muscle. Strike triceps tendon with reflex hammer.	Flexion of arm at elbow
Triceps	Flex patient's arm at elbow, holding arm across chest, or hold upper arm horizontally and allow lower arm to go limp. Strike triceps tendon just above elbow.	Extension at elbow
Patellar	Have patient sit with legs hanging freely over side of table or chair, or have patient lie supine and support knee in a flexed 90-degree position. Briskly tap patellar tendon just below patella.	Extension of lower leg
Achilles	Have patient assume same position as for patellar reflex. Slightly dorsiflex patient's ankle by grasping toes in palm of your hand. Strike Achilles tendon just above heel at ankle malleolus.	Plantar flexion of foot
Cutaneous Reflexes		
Plantar	Have patient lie supine with legs straight and feet relaxed. Take handle end of reflex hammer and stroke lateral aspect of sole from heel to ball of foot, curving across ball of foot toward big toe.	Plantar flexion of all toes
Gluteal	Have patient assume side-lying position. Spread buttocks apart and lightly stimulate perineal area with cotton applicator.	Contraction of anal sphincter
Abdominal	Have patient stand or lie supine. Stroke abdominal skin with base of cotton applicator over lateral borders of rectus abdominis muscle toward midline. Repeat test in each abdominal quadrant.	Contraction of rectus abdominis muscle with pulling of umbilicus toward stimulated side

Be sure to record a complete assessment. If you delayed entering any items into the assessment form, record them at this time to avoid forgetting any important information. If you made entries periodically during the examination, review them for accuracy and thoroughness. Communicate significant findings to appropriate medical and nursing personnel, either verbally or in the patient's written care plan.

The patient often needs a number of ancillary examinations, such as X-ray examinations, laboratory tests, or ultrasonography, after a physical examination. The tests provide additional screening information to rule out the presence of abnormalities and help in the diagnosis of specific abnormalities found during the examination. Explain the purpose of these tests and the sensations that the patient will experience.

INTEGRATION OF PHYSICAL ASSESSMENT WITH NURSING CARE

It is important to learn to integrate an examination into routine patient care. For example, the condition of the skin should be assessed during a bed bath, or a patient's gait, ROM, and balance observed as the patient ambulates. Assisting with activities of daily living offers an additional opportunity to obtain cognitive assessment data. This practice makes more efficient use of time and decreases anxiety involved in formal physical assessment examinations.

KEY CONCEPTS

- Baseline assessment findings reflect the patient's functional abilities and serve as the basis for comparison with subsequent assessment findings.
- Physical assessment of a child or infant requires application of the principles of growth and development.
- The normal process of aging affects physical findings collected from an older person.
- Patient teaching should be integrated throughout the examination to help patients learn about health promotion and disease prevention.
- Inspection requires good lighting, full exposure of the body part, and a careful comparison of the part with its counterpart on the opposite side of the body.
- Palpation involves the use of parts of the hand to detect different types of physical characteristics.
- Auscultation is used to assess the character of sounds created in various body organs.
- A physical examination is performed only after proper preparation of the environment and equipment and after preparing the patient physically and psychologically.
- Throughout the examination the patient should be kept warm and comfortable and should be informed of each step of the process.
- A competent examiner is systematic while combining assessment of different body systems simultaneously.
- Information from the history helps focus the assessment on body systems likely to be affected.
- When assessing a seriously ill patient, the nurse concentrates on the body systems most likely to be affected.
- Creating a mental image of internal organs in relation to external anatomical landmarks enhances accuracy in assessing the thorax, heart, and abdomen.
- When assessing heart sounds, it helps to imagine events occurring during the cardiac cycle.
- The carotid arteries should never be palpated simultaneously.
- When examining a woman's breasts, the nurse should explain the techniques for breast self-examination.
- The abdominal assessment differs from other portions of the examination in that auscultation follows inspection.
- During assessment of the genitalia, the technique for genital self-examination should be explained.
- An assessment of musculoskeletal function is conducted when observing the patient ambulate or participate in other active movements.
- Mental and emotional status is assessed by interacting with the patient throughout the examination.
- At the end of the examination, the nurse provides for the patient's comfort and then documents a detailed summary of physical assessment findings.

CRITICAL THINKING EXERCISES

You are caring for Mrs. Brown, a 75-year-old woman of First Nations ancestry who underwent repair of a right fractured femur attributed to osteoporosis. Mrs. Brown was transferred to your hospital from the health centre in her small rural home community. This is her first postoperative day on your clinical unit. The night nurse reported that the patient had an "uneventful" night. She has an intravenous line (IV) for fluids and medication, a right hip dressing, a Jackson-Pratt drain, and a Foley (urethral) catheter to gravity and she is on bed rest.

1. What body systems would you assess for this patient?
   a. Describe the key elements in these assessments.
2. Upon entrance to the room, you observe that Mrs. Brown appears agitated and confused. How do you further evaluate her mental status? What condition may these symptoms indicate?
3. After you reorient Mrs. Brown, she allows you to continue with your assessment. On auscultation of her posterior lung field bases, you hear a crackling noise on inspiration. What is this sound, and what does it indicate?
4. You next assess her cardiac status. Her apical heart rate is 72 beats per minute, rhythm regular. You interpret this finding as
   a. Abnormal
   b. Bradycardia
   c. Normal
   d. Tachycardia
5. You are performing neurovascular checks of the lower extremities. Describe how you would evaluate for capillary refill.
6. How will you demonstrate cultural competency in your care and assessment of Mrs. Brown?

REVIEW QUESTIONS

1. What nursing assessment is done as part of the general survey?
   1. Appearance and behaviour
   2. Measurement of vital signs
   3. Observing specific body systems
   4. Conducting a detailed health history
2. The parents of a 7-year-old patient report that the child has a fever. What is the most appropriate way for the nurse to assess the skin temperature of the child?
   1. Palpate the child's forehead with the base of the hands
   2. Palpate the child's head and neck with the fingertips of the hands
   3. Palpate the child's skin with the dorsal surface of the hands
   4. Obtain a rectal temperature on the child

3. The nurse is teaching the patient to inspect all skin surfaces for abnormal skin pigmentation and lesions. Which of the following abnormalities should the patient be instructed to report to a health care provider? *(Select all that apply.)*
   1. An asymmetrical, flat lesion that is 10 mm × 6 mm diameter
   2. A symmetrical, flat lesion that is uniform in colour
   3. A flat, brown coloured lesion with irregular borders
   4. A symmetrical, raised lesion that is 8 mm × 8 mm in diameter
   5. A raised lesion with irregular borders that is 3 mm × 4 mm in diameter
   6. A symmetrical, purple coloured lesion with regular borders
4. When auscultating an adult patient's lungs, the nurse hears a loud, low-pitched, rumbling coarse sound during inspiration and expiration. What do these sounds indicate?
   1. Crackles, caused by increased fluid in the airways
   2. Normal breath sounds
   3. Rhonchi, caused by secretions in the bronchial airways
   4. Wheezes, a normal variation in adults with chronic obstructive pulmonary disease
5. When auscultating heart sounds, what does the S_2 sound correlate with?
   1. Closure of the aortic and mitral valves
   2. Closure of the mitral and tricuspid valves
   3. Opening of the aortic and pulmonic valves
   4. Opening of the tricuspid and pulmonic valves
6. A patient has a suspected fracture of the left scaphoid bone. Which pulse is a priority for the nurse to assess?
   1. The dorsalis pedis
   2. The radial
   3. The posterior tibialis
   4. The apical
7. The nurse assesses a patient with abdominal pain. Place in correct order the assessment techniques employed during this examination.
   1. Palpation
   2. Inspection
   3. Percussion
   4. Auscultation
8. The nurse is teaching a patient how to perform a testicular self-examination. What is the correct information to provide the patient?
   1. "The testes are normally round, movable, and have a lumpy consistency."
   2. "Contact your health care provider if you feel a painless pea-sized nodule."
   3. "The best time to do a testicular self-examination is before you bathe or shower."
   4. "Perform a testicular self-examination weekly to detect signs of testicular cancer."
9. When the nurse is assessing range of motion of a patient's knee, what movements are assessed? *(Select all that apply.)*
   1. Flexion
   2. Extension
   3. Abduction
   4. Adduction
   5. Internal rotation
   6. External rotation
10. The nurse asks the patient to interpret the saying "Don't count your chickens before they're hatched." What does the patient's response reveal?
    1. Judgement
    2. Knowledge
    3. Association
    4. Abstract reasoning
11. The nurse is assessing the patient's visual direction of gaze. What cranial nerve(s) does this assessment evaluate? *(Select all that apply.)*
    1. II—Optic
    2. III—Oculomotor
    3. IV—Trochlear
    4. VI—Abducens
    5. VII—Facial
    6. XI—Spinal accessory
12. The nurse recognizes which of the following as common biocultural variations of normal physical exam findings? *(Select all that apply.)*
    1. Darker skin creases on the body of a patient with a dark complexion
    2. Dry, flaky cerumen in the ear canal of a child of First Nations descent
    3. Elevated blood pressure in an individual of African ancestry
    4. Dark brown areolae in a fair-complexioned woman aged 45 years

Answers: 1. 1; **2.** 3; **3.** 1, 3, 4, 5; **4.** 3; **5.** 3; **6.** 2; **7.** 2, 3, 4, 1; **8.** 2; **9.** 1, 2; **10.** 4; **11.** 2, 3, 4; **12.** 1, 3, 4

Rationales for the Review Questions appear at the end of the book.

RECOMMENDED WEBSITES

Canadian Cancer Society (CCS): http://www.cancer.ca/.

This website is a source of general information about all types of cancers, including Canadian statistics on the prevalence, mortality, and survival rates for specific cancers. Please note that screening guidelines for cancer vary slightly from region to region. Students are encouraged to consult with the guidelines of their local region and to be aware of national guidelines for cancer screening and prevention.

Canadian Diabetes Association (CDA): http://www.diabetes.ca/.

The Canadian Diabetes Association website contains a wealth of resources on diabetes and evidenced-informed guidelines for patient care. The site contains information about risk factors and associated disease processes and conditions.

Canadian Task Force on Preventive Health Care (CTFPHC): http://www.canadiantaskforce.ca/.

This site provides information on health prevention and evidence-informed recommendations.

Choosing Wisely Canada: https://www.choosingwiselycanada.org/.

This site provides information for patients and health care providers on unnecessary tests and treatments, with the intent of increasing awareness of effective, high-quality, patient-centred care.

Montreal Cognitive Assessment: http://www.mocatest.org/.

This site provides access to the Montreal Cognitive Assessment (MoCA) and research on cognitive impairment.

NurseONE.ca: http://www.nurseone.ca/.

This website is a good resource for information about nursing practice in Canada. NurseONE also provides a broad range of resource materials for nurses looking to expand their practice knowledge. Information on nursing student access to NurseONE can be found at the following link: http://cnsa.ca/what-is-nurseone-and-how-do-i-register/.

Osteoporosis Canada: https://www.osteoporosis.ca/.

The Osteoporosis Canada website provides information and support to individuals who have osteoporosis. The site contains links to information on calcium and vitamin D, as well as health promotion and prevention recommendations.

Public Health Agency of Canada (PHAC): http://www.phac-aspc.gc.ca/index-eng.php.

The Public Health Agency of Canada is a repository of a wealth of information on infectious and chronic diseases, immunization, food and travel safety, and emergency preparedness. The site also provides daily updates on current concerns (e.g., flu virus tracking) and other health promotion and disease prevention issues.

Rourke Baby Record: http://www.rourkebabyrecord.ca/.

The Rourke Baby Record website provides information about children's first 5 years of life. Literature and research that contributed to the development of this tool are linked to the website. This tool and the website offer information about pediatric assessment.

REFERENCES

Allan, G. M., Linblad, A. J., Comeau, A., et al. (2015). Simplified lipid guidelines. Prevention and management of cardiovascular disease in primary care. *Canadian Family Physician, 61*(10), 857–867. Retrieved from http://www.cfp.ca/content/61/10/857.full.pdf+html.

Anderson, T. J., Grégoire, J., Pearson, G. J., et al. (2016). 2016 Canadian Cardiovascular Society Guidelines for the management of dyslipidemia for the prevention of cardiovascular disease in the adult. *Canadian Journal of Cardiology, 32*(11), 1263–1283. doi:10.1016/j.cjca.2016.07.510.

Ball, J. W., Dains, J. E., Flynn, J. A., et al. (2015a). *Seidel's guide to physical examination* (8th ed.). St. Louis, MO: Mosby.

Ball, J. W., Dains, J. E., Flynn, J. A., et al. (2015b). Recording information. In *Seidel's guide to physical examination* (8th ed., pp. 616–631). St. Louis, MO: Mosby.

Browne, A. J., & Varcoe, C. (2014). Cultural and social considerations in health assessment. In C. Jarvis, A. J. Browne, J. MacDonald-Jenkins, et al. (Eds.), *Physical examination and health assessment* (2nd Canadian ed., pp. 27–44). Toronto: Elsevier Canada.

Canadian Cancer Society (CCS). (2017a). *Testicular cancer*. http://www.cancer.ca/en/cancer-information/cancer-type/testicular/risks/?region=sk.

Canadian Cancer Society (CCS). (2017b). *Breast cancer. Risk factors for breast cancer*. Retrieved from http://www.cancer.ca/en/cancer-information/cancer-type/breast/risks/?region=on.

Canadian Cancer Society (CCS). (2017c). *Oral cancer*. Retrieved from http://www.cancer.ca/en/cancer-information/cancer-type/oral/oral-cancer/?region=on.

Canadian Cancer Society (CCS) Steering Committee (2017). *Canadian cancer statistics 2017*. Toronto, ON: Canadian Cancer Society. Retrieved from http://www.cancer.ca/en/cancer-information/cancer-101/canadian-cancer-statistics-publication/?region=on.

Canadian Task Force on Preventive Health Care. (2016). *Published guidelines*. Retrieved from http://canadiantaskforce.ca/.

Centers for Disease Control and Prevention (CDC). (2013). *Lice*. Retrieved from https://www.cdc.gov/parasites/lice/index.html.

Day, M. W. (2003). Recognizing and managing deep vein thrombosis. *Nursing, 33*(5), 36–42.

Galanti, G. (2014). *Caring for patients from different cultures* (5th ed.). Philadelphia, PA: University of Pennsylvania Press.

Izawa, J. I., Klotz, L. K., Siemens, D. R., et al. (2011). Prostate cancer screening: Canadian guidelines 2011. *Canadian Urological Association Journal, 5*(4), 235–240. doi:10.5489/cuaj.11134.

Jarvis, C., Browne, A., MacDonald-Jenkins, J., et al. (Eds.), (2014). *Physical examination and health assessment* (2nd Canadian ed.). Toronto: Elsevier Canada.

Jarvis, C., & Luctkar-Flude, M. (2014a). The complete health assessment: Putting it all together. In C. Jarvis, A. J. Browne, J. MacDonald-Jenkins, et al. (Eds.), *Physical examination and health assessment* (2nd Canadian ed., pp. 782–803). Toronto: Elsevier Canada.

Jarvis, C., & Luctkar-Flude, M. (2014b). The abdomen. In C. Jarvis, A. J. Browne, J. MacDonald-Jenkins, et al. (Eds.), *Physical examination and health assessment* (2nd Canadian ed., pp. 546–582). Toronto: Elsevier Canada.

Jarvis, C., & Luctkar-Flude, M. (2014c). Female genitourinary system. In C. Jarvis, A. J. Browne, J. MacDonald-Jenkins, et al. (Eds.), *Physical examination and health assessment* (2nd Canadian ed., pp. 744–781). Toronto: Elsevier Canada.

Jarvis, C., & Luctkar-Flude, M. (2014d). Male genitourinary system. In C. Jarvis, A. J. Browne, J. MacDonald-Jenkins, et al. (Eds.), *Physical examination and health assessment* (2nd Canadian ed., pp. 715–743). Toronto: Elsevier Canada.

Jarvis, C., & MacDonald-Jenkins, J. (2014a). Skin, hair and nails. In C. Jarvis, A. J. Browne, J. MacDonald-Jenkins, et al. (Eds.), *Physical examination and health assessment* (2nd Canadian ed., pp. 219–268). Toronto: Elsevier Canada.

Jarvis, C., & MacDonald-Jenkins, J. (2014b). Heart and neck vessels. In C. Jarvis, A. J. Browne, J. MacDonald-Jenkins, et al. (Eds.), *Physical examination and health assessment* (2nd Canadian ed., pp. 475–518). Toronto: Elsevier Canada.

Julayanont, P., Phillips, N., Chertkow, H., et al. (2013). Montreal Cognitive Assessment (MoCA): Concept and clinical review. In A. J. Lamer (Ed.), *Cognitive screening instruments* (Chapter 6, pp. 111–151). London: Springer-Verlag. doi:10.1007/978-1-4471-2452-8_6.

Katz, S., Ford, A. B., Moskowitz, R. W., et al. (1963). Studies of illness in the aged: The index of ADL: A standardized measure of biological and psychosocial function. *Journal of the American Medical Association, 185*(12), 914–919. doi:10.1001/jama.1963.03060120024016.

Marks, J., & Miller, J. (Eds.), (2014). *Lookingbill and Mark's principles of dermatology* (5th ed.). Philadelphia, PA: Saunders Elsevier.

Mitchell, A. J. (2013). The Mini-Mental State examination (MMSE): An update on its diagnostic validity for cognitive disorders. In A. J. Lamer (Ed.), *Cognitive screening instruments* (Chapter 2, pp. 15–46). London: Springer-Verlag. doi:10.1007/978-1-4471-2452-8_2.

Osteoporosis Canada. (2016). *Gary's workout: Part I—Lower body exercises*. Retrieved from https://www.osteoporosis.ca/garys-workout-part-1-lower-body-exercises/.

Papaioannou, A., Morin, S., Cheung, A. M., et al. (2010). 2010 Clinical practice guidelines for the diagnosis and management of osteoporosis in Canada: Summary. *Canadian Medical Association Journal, 182*(17), 1864–1873. doi:10.1503/cmaj.100771.

Perry, S. E., Hockenberry, M. J., Lowdermilk, D. L., et al. (Eds.), (2017). *Maternal child nursing care in Canada* (2nd ed.). St. Louis, MO: Mosby.

Public Health Agency of Canada (2016a). Human immunodeficiency virus infections. In *Canadian guidelines on sexually transmitted infections. Section 5—Management and treatment of specific infections—Human immunodeficiency virus infections*. Ottawa: Author. Retrieved from http://www.phac-aspc.gc.ca/std-mts/sti-its/cgsti-ldcits/section-5-8-eng.php.

Public Health Agency of Canada (2016b). *Canadian immunization guide* (7th ed.). Ottawa: Author. Retrieved from https://www.canada.ca/en/public-health/services/canadian-immunization-guide.html.

Rourke, L. L., Leduc, D. G., & Rourke, J. T. B. (2014). Rourke baby record 2014: Collaboration in action. *Canadian Family Physician, 47*, 333–334.

Shimizu, T., Bouchard, M., & Mavriplis, C. (2016). Update on age-appropriate preventive measures and screening for Canadian primary care providers. *Canadian Family Physician, 62*, 131–138. Retrieved from http://www.cfp.ca/content/62/2/131.full.pdf+html.

Stuart, G. (2013). *Principles and practice of psychiatric nursing* (10th ed.). St. Louis, MO: Mosby.

Tanner, J. M. (1962). *Growth at adolescence* (2nd ed.). Oxford, UK: Blackwell Scientific.

Varcoe, C. (2014). Interpersonal violence assessment. In C. Jarvis, A. J. Browne, J. MacDonald-Jenkins, et al. (Eds.), *Physical examination and health assessment* (2nd Canadian ed., pp. 120–137). Toronto: Elsevier Canada.

33

Infection Control

Canadian content written by Colleen M. Astle, RN, BScN, MN, CNeph(C), Deborah Hobbs, RN, BScN, CIC
Original chapter by Lorri A. Graham, RN

OBJECTIVES

Mastery of content in this chapter will enable you to:

- Define the key terms listed.
- Explain the relationship between the chain of infection and the transmission of infection.
- Identify the body's normal defences against infection.
- Discuss the events in the inflammatory response.
- Describe the signs and symptoms of a localized and a systemic infection.
- Identify patients most at risk for infection.
- Explain conditions that promote the transmission of health care–associated infection.
- Explain the difference between medical and surgical asepsis.
- Give an example of preventing infection for each element of the infection chain.
- Perform proper procedures for hand hygiene.
- Explain the rationale and components of routine practices.
- Explain the rationale and practices for additional (isolation) precautions.
- Explain how infection-control measures in the home may differ from those in the hospital.
- Properly don a surgical mask, sterile gown, and sterile gloves.

KEY TERMS

Aerobic, p. 685
Anaerobic, p. 685
Asepsis, p. 697
Broad-spectrum antibiotics, p. 688
Carriers, p. 684
Colonizing, p. 684
Communicable, p. 684
Disinfection, p. 698
Edema, p. 689
Endogenous infection, p. 689
Epidemiology, p. 711
Exogenous infection, p. 689
Exudates, p. 689
Hand hygiene, p. 700
Handwashing, p. 700
Health care–associated infection (HAI), p. 689
Immune response, p. 687
Immunocompromised, p. 684
Inflammatory response, p. 688
Invasive, p. 684
Isolation precautions, p. 705
Leukocytosis, p. 689
Localized, p. 687
Medical asepsis, p. 697
Microorganisms, p. 684
Necrotic, p. 688
Normal flora, p. 687
Nosocomial infection, p. 689
Pathogenicity, p. 687
Pathogens, p. 684
Phagocytosis, p. 689
Purulent, p. 689
Routine practices, p. 705
Sanguineous, p. 689
Serosanguineous, p. 689
Serous, p. 689
Sterile field, p. 714
Sterilization, p. 698
Superinfection, p. 688
Surgical asepsis, p. 712
Susceptibility, p. 687
Systemic, p. 687
Virulence, p. 684

MEDIA RESOURCES

http://evolve.elsevier.com/Canada/Potter/fundamentals/

- Audio Chapter Summaries
- Examination Review Questions
- Concept Map Creator
- Case Study with Questions
- Audio Glossary
- Content Updates
- Video Clips

Good health depends in part on a safe environment. Practices or techniques that control or prevent transmission of infection help to create an environment that protects patients and health care workers from disease. Patients in all health care settings are at risk for acquiring infections because they often have lower resistance to infectious microorganisms and increased exposure to numbers and types of disease-causing microorganisms, and they sometimes undergo invasive procedures wherein a body cavity or organ is entered by either puncture or incision. Microorganisms can only be seen with the aid of a microscope and are typically a single cell. They include bacteria, protozoans, certain types of algae, and fungi. In acute care or ambulatory care facilities, patients can be exposed to pathogens, some of which may be resistant to most antibiotics. By practising infection prevention and control techniques, nurses can avoid spreading microorganisms to patients.

In all settings, patients and their families must be able to recognize sources of infections and be able to institute protective measures. Patient teaching should include information concerning infections, modes of transmission, and methods of prevention.

Health care workers can protect themselves from contact with infectious materials or exposure to communicable diseases by having knowledge of the infectious process and appropriate barrier protections. The spread of diseases such as hepatitis B and C, acquired immune deficiency syndrome (AIDS), sudden acute respiratory syndrome (SARS), tuberculosis, and, more recently, Ebola, have resulted in a greater emphasis on infection control techniques. Infection control has two purposes: (1) protecting patients from acquiring infections and (2) protecting health care workers from becoming infected. Many of the techniques used to protect patients also provide effective protection for nurses. Nurses must remain constantly vigilant to prevent the spread of infection while providing care.

SCIENTIFIC KNOWLEDGE BASE

Microorganisms live and grow on inanimate objects and in air, water, food, soil, plants, and animals. They also live and grow in and on people. Most microorganisms are nonpathogens, meaning that they do not cause a person to be ill; however, some are pathogens, meaning that they are capable of causing disease. An infection is a disease state resulting from the entry and multiplication of a pathogen in the tissues of a host, causing the body to manifest clinical signs and symptoms. If the infection can be transmitted from one person to another, it is a communicable (infectious, contagious) disease. Resident skin microorganisms are usually nonpathogenic. However, they can cause serious infection when surgery or other invasive procedures allow them to enter deep tissues, or when a patient is severely immunocompromised (has an impaired immune system).

Chain of Infection

The presence of a pathogen does not mean that an infection will begin. The development of an infection occurs in a cycle that depends on the presence of all the following elements:

- An infectious agent (pathogen)
- A reservoir (source for pathogen growth)
- A portal of exit from the reservoir
- A mode of transmission
- A portal of entry to a host
- A susceptible host

An infection develops if this chain remains intact (Figure 33-1). Nurses need to follow infection prevention and control practices to break the chain so that infections do not develop.

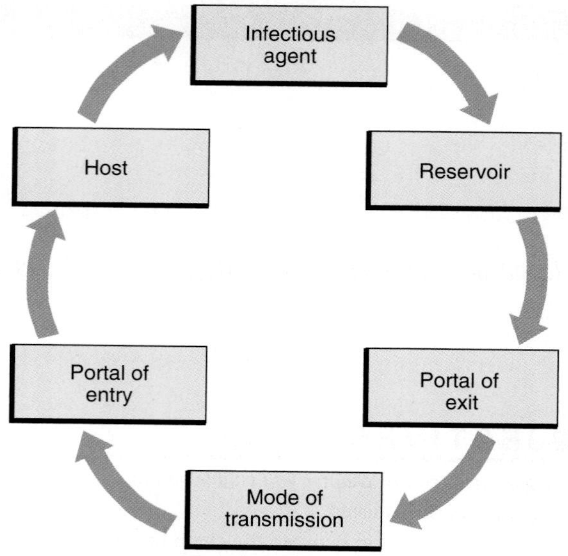

FIGURE 33-1 Chain of infection.

Infectious Agents. Microorganisms include bacteria, viruses, fungi, and protozoa (Table 33-1). Microorganisms on the skin are called *resident* or *transient flora.* Resident organisms are considered permanent residents of the skin, where they survive and multiply without causing harm. They are not easily removed by handwashing with plain soaps unless considerable friction is used. Resident microorganisms in deep skin layers are usually killed only by performing hand hygiene with products containing antimicrobial ingredients.

Transient microorganisms attach to the skin when a person has contact with another person or object. For example, when you touch a bedpan or a contaminated dressing, transient bacteria adhere to your skin. The organisms attach loosely to the skin in dirt and grease and under fingernails. These organisms may be readily transmitted unless removed by proper handwashing or hand hygiene (Centers for Disease Control and Prevention [CDC], 2012).

The potential for microorganisms to cause disease depends on the following factors:

- A sufficient number of organisms
- Virulence, or the ability to produce disease
- The ability to enter and survive in the host
- The susceptibility of the host

Reservoir. A *reservoir* is a place where a pathogen can survive but may or may not multiply. For example, hepatitis A virus survives in shellfish but does not multiply; *Pseudomonas* organisms can survive and multiply in nebulizer reservoirs used in the care of patients with respiratory problems. The most common reservoir is the human body. A variety of microorganisms live on the skin and within body cavities, fluids, and discharges. When a pathogen is present on or in the body but does not cause harm, the pathogen is colonizing the site. Carriers are animals or persons who show no symptoms of illness but who have pathogens on or in their bodies that can be transferred to others. For example, a person can be a carrier of hepatitis B virus without having any signs or symptoms of infection. Animals, food, water, insects, and even inanimate objects can also be reservoirs for infectious organisms. For example, the bacterium *Legionella pneumophila,* which causes Legionnaires' disease, lives in contaminated water and water systems. To thrive, pathogens require a reservoir that provides food, oxygen (or no oxygen, depending on the pathogen), water, an appropriate temperature and pH, and minimal light.

TABLE 33-1 Common Pathogens and Resulting Major Infections

Organism	Major Reservoir(s)	Major Infections
Bacteria		
Clostridium difficile	Colon	Colitis, diarrhea
Escherichia coli	Colon	Gastroenteritis, urinary tract infection
Staphylococcus aureus	Skin, hair, anterior nares	Wound infection, pneumonia, food poisoning, cellulitis, bacteremia, meningitis, osteomyelitis, septic arthritis
Streptococcus (β-hemolytic group A) organisms	Oropharynx, skin, perianal area	"Strep throat," rheumatic fever, scarlet fever, impetigo, wound infection, glomerulonephritis (Wong & Yuen, 2012)
Streptococcus (β-hemolytic group B) organisms	Adult genitalia	Urinary tract infection, wound infection, postpartum sepsis, neonatal sepsis
Mycobacterium tuberculosis	Droplet nuclei from lungs	Tuberculosis
Neisseria gonorrhoeae	Genitourinary tract, rectum, mouth	Gonorrhea, pelvic inflammatory disease, infectious arthritis, conjunctivitis
Rickettsia rickettsii	Wood tick	Rocky Mountain spotted fever
Staphylococcus epidermidis	Skin	Wound infection, bacteremia
Viruses		
Hepatitis A virus	Feces	Hepatitis A
Hepatitis B virus	Blood and body fluids	Hepatitis B
Hepatitis C virus	Blood	Hepatitis C
Herpes simplex virus (type 1)	Lesions of mouth or skin, saliva, genitalia	Cold sores, aseptic meningitis, genital herpes, herpetic whitlow
Human immunodeficiency virus	Blood, semen, vaginal secretions, breast milk (has also been isolated in saliva, tears, and urine, but these have not proved to be sources of transmission)	Acquired immune deficiency syndrome
Fungi		
Aspergillus organisms	Soil, dust, construction dust, decaying or organic matter	Sinusitis or skin, lung, wound, or central nervous system infection (Baumgardner, 2012)
Candida albicans	Mouth, skin, colon, genital tract	Candidiasis, pneumonia, sepsis
Protozoan		
Plasmodium falciparum	Blood	Malaria

Food. Microorganisms require nourishment. Some—such as *Clostridium perfringens,* the microbe that causes gas gangrene—thrive on organic matter. Others, such as *Escherichia coli,* consume undigested food in the bowel. Carbon dioxide and inorganic materials such as soil provide nourishment for other organisms.

Oxygen. Aerobic bacteria require oxygen to survive and to multiply sufficiently to cause disease. Aerobic organisms cause more infections than do anaerobic organisms (i.e., organisms that can survive only in the absence of oxygen). Examples of aerobic organisms are *Staphylococcus aureus* and strains of *Streptococcus* organisms.

The gastrointestinal tract is colonized by large numbers of anaerobic bacteria that can cause infections if the bowel is damaged. Infections deep within the pleural cavity, in a joint, or in a deep sinus tract are typically caused by anaerobes. Bacteria that cause tetanus, gas gangrene, and botulism are anaerobes.

Water. Most organisms require water or moisture for survival. For example, microorganisms thrive in the moist drainage from a surgical wound. However, some bacteria assume a form called a *spore.* Spores remain viable even when deprived of water and are resistant to drying. Spore-forming bacteria, such as those that cause anthrax, botulism, and tetanus, can live without water.

Temperature. Microorganisms can live only in certain temperature ranges. The ideal temperature for most pathogens in humans is 35°C to 37°C; however, some can survive temperature extremes that would be fatal to humans (Rossvoll, Ronning, Granum, et al., 2014). Cold temperatures tend to prevent the growth and reproduction of bacteria.

pH. The acidity of an environment determines the viability of microorganisms. Most microorganisms prefer an environment within a pH range of 5 to 8. Bacteria in particular thrive in urine with an alkaline pH. Most organisms cannot survive the acidic environment of the stomach. In patients receiving acid-reducing medications (e.g., antacids and histamine 2 blockers), these can cause an overgrowth of gastrointestinal organisms, which can contribute to nosocomial pneumonia (Ramsay, Pratt, Ryan, et al., 2013).

Minimal Light. Microorganisms thrive in dark environments, such as those under dressings and within body cavities. Ultraviolet light may be effective in killing certain forms of bacteria (e.g., *Mycobacterium tuberculosis*).

Portal of Exit. After microorganisms find a site in which to grow and multiply, they must find a portal of exit if they are to enter another host and cause disease. *A portal of exit* is the path by which the pathogen leaves the reservoir (CDC, 2012). Exits in the human body include body openings (mouth, nose, rectal, vaginal, and urethral openings; and artificial openings such as those resulting from ostomies), breaks in the skin (a scrape, cut, or other wound), and breaks in the mucous membranes (the skin in the mouth, eyes, nose, vagina, and rectum). Pathogens are carried through portals of exit by blood, body fluids, excretions, and secretions (e.g., urine, stool, vomitus, saliva, mucus, pus, vaginal discharge, semen, wound drainage, bile, and sputum). For example, pathogens that infect the respiratory tract, such as *M. tuberculosis,* can be released from the body through the mouth and nose when an infected person sneezes, coughs, talks, or even breathes. In patients with artificial airways such as tracheostomy or endotracheal tubes (see Chapter 39), organisms easily exit the respiratory tract through these devices. Similarly, when a patient has a urinary tract infection, microorganisms exit during urination or through urinary diversions such as ileal conduits, urostomies, and suprapubic drains (see Chapter 43).

Modes of Transmission. Microorganisms can be transmitted from the reservoir to the host in many ways. Certain infectious diseases tend to be transmitted more commonly by specific modes (Table 33-2). However, a microorganism may be transmitted by more than one mode. For example, human chicken pox virus may be spread by the airborne route or through direct contact.

Indirect contact is a major mode of transmission in health care facilities. The health care worker's hands can easily pick up microbes from one person, place, or thing and then transmit them to other people, places, or things. However, almost any object within the environment (e.g., a stethoscope or thermometer) can be a mode of indirect transmission of pathogens. Some organisms, such as *Clostridium difficile,* which can produce spores, can live in hospital environments for months. *C. difficile* can be spread by direct or indirect contact. All health care workers providing direct care (e.g., nurses, physiotherapists, and physicians) or performing diagnostic and support services (e.g., laboratory technicians, respiratory therapists, and dietary workers) must follow practices to minimize the spread of infection. Each group follows procedures for handling equipment and supplies used by a patient. For example, respiratory therapists perform hand hygiene before working with each patient and dispose of contaminated therapy equipment in a prescribed manner. Certain medical devices and diagnostic procedures provide avenues for the spread of pathogens. Invasive procedures such as cystoscopy (the use of an endoscope to visualize the bladder) facilitate the diagnosis of

TABLE 33-2 Modes of Transmission

Mode of Transmission	Examples of Organisms
Contact Transmission The transfer of microbes by physical touch; may be by direct contact, indirect contact, or droplet	
Direct Contact Physical skin-to-skin contact between an infected or colonized individual and a susceptible host (e.g., via touching patient)	*Clostridium difficile, Staphylococcus,* herpes simplex virus, methicillin-resistant *Staphylococcus aureus* (MRSA), vancomycin-resistant enterococci (VRE), carbapenemase-producing organisms (CPO)
Indirect Contact Contact between a susceptible host and a contaminated intermediate object (e.g., via touching soiled linen, equipment, or dressings; transferring pathogens to a patient via hands that are not washed between handling patients)	*Clostridium difficile, Staphylococcus,* respiratory syncytial virus (RSV), *Pseudomonas,* MRSA, VRE, CPO
Droplet Transmission Large particles (droplets) from the respiratory system of an infected source propelled up to 2 m through the air and deposited onto a susceptible host (e.g., droplets produced via coughing, sneezing, or talking)	Influenza virus, rubella virus, RSV, *Neisseria meningitis*
Airborne Transmission Small airborne particles (droplet nuclei) containing microbes remain suspended in the air for long periods of time (e.g., droplets and aerosolized airborne particles produced via coughing and sneezing); air currents transmit these particles long distances (>2 m); susceptible host inhales them	*Mycobacterium tuberculosis* (causes tuberculosis), varicella-zoster virus (causes chicken pox), measles virus
Vehicle Transmission A single contaminated source (e.g., water, drugs, intravenous fluid, food, equipment) transmits infection to multiple hosts, possibly resulting in an outbreak	*Pseudomonas* (via water, drugs), *Escherichia coli* (via food, water), *Enterobacter cloacae* (via intravenous fluid), *Salmonella* (via food)
Vectorborne Transmission Insects (fleas, mites, ticks, mosquitoes) or pests (e.g., mice) transmit microbes to humans	*Vibrio cholerae, Plasmodium falciparum* (causes malaria), West Nile virus, Lyme disease

Data from Public Health Ontario & Provincial Infectious Diseases Advisory Committee. (2015). *Infection prevention and control for clinical office practice.* Toronto: Queen's Printer for Ontario. Retrieved from https://www.publichealthontario.ca/en/eRepository/IPAC_Clinical_Office_Practice_2013.pdf.

problems but also increase the risk of infection transmission. Because so many factors can promote the spread of infection to a patient, all health care workers must be conscientious about using infection control practices, such as performing proper hand hygiene and ensuring that equipment has been adequately cleaned, disinfected or sterilized.

Portal of Entry. Organisms can enter the body through the same routes they use to exit (i.e., body openings and breaks in the skin or mucous membranes). For example, organisms enter the body when a needle pierces the skin. As long as the device is in place, more organisms are able to enter the body. In patients with a urinary catheter, any obstruction to the flow of urine allows organisms to travel up the urethra. Factors that reduce the body's defences enhance the chances of pathogens entering the body.

Susceptible Host. Whether a person acquires an infection is related to his or her susceptibility to an infectious agent—susceptibility depends on the individual's degree of resistance to a pathogen. Although everyone is constantly in contact with large numbers of microorganisms, an infection does not develop until an individual becomes susceptible to the strength and numbers of microorganisms capable of producing infection. The more virulent an organism is, the greater the likelihood that a person will be susceptible to it. Organisms with resistance to antibiotics are becoming more common in acute care settings—this is believed to be associated with the frequent and sometimes inappropriate use of antibiotics. A person's resistance to an infectious agent may be enhanced by receiving an appropriate vaccine or actually contracting the disease.

Infectious Process

By understanding the chain of infection, you can intervene to prevent infections from developing. If a patient is at risk for acquiring an infection, you should observe for signs and symptoms of infection and take appropriate actions to prevent its spread. Infections follow a progressive course (Box 33-1). The severity of a patient's illness depends on the extent of the infection, the ability of the microorganism to cause disease (pathogenicity of the microorganisms), and the susceptibility of the host (patient).

If infection is localized, or restricted to a limited area (e.g., a wound infection), proper care controls the spread and minimizes the illness. The patient may experience localized symptoms such as pain and tenderness at the wound site. An infection that affects the entire body instead of just a single organ or part is systemic and can be fatal.

The course of an infection influences the level of nursing care provided. Nurses are responsible for properly administering antibiotics and monitoring the response to drug therapy (see Chapter 34). Supportive therapy includes providing adequate nutrition and rest to bolster the patient's defences against the infectious process. The complexity of care depends on body systems affected by the infection.

Regardless of whether an infection is localized or systemic, nurses play a critical role in minimizing its spread. For example, an organism causing a simple wound infection can spread to involve an intravenous needle–insertion site if the nurse uses an improper technique when changing a dressing at this site. Nurses who have breaks in their own skin can also acquire infections from patients if their techniques for controlling infection transmission are inadequate.

BOX 33-1 Course of Infection by Stage

Incubation Period

- Interval between the entrance of the pathogen into the body and the appearance of first symptoms (e.g., in chicken pox, 2 to 3 weeks; in the common cold, 1 to 2 days; in influenza, 1 to 3 days; in mumps, 15 to 18 days).

Prodromal Stage

- Interval from the onset of nonspecific signs and symptoms (malaise, low-grade fever, and fatigue) to more specific symptoms (during this time, microorganisms grow and multiply and the patient may be more capable of spreading disease to others).

Illness Stage

- Interval when the patient manifests signs and symptoms specific to type of infection (e.g., the common cold is manifested by a sore throat, sinus congestion, and rhinitis; mumps is manifested by an earache, a high fever, and parotid and salivary gland swelling).

Convalescence

- Interval when the acute symptoms of infection disappear and the body tries to replenish its resources and return to a state of homeostasis; the length of recovery depends on the severity of the infection and the patient's general state of health (may take several days to months).

Defences Against Infection

The body has several mechanisms that protect it against infection. Normal body flora that reside inside and outside the body protect a person from several pathogens. Each organ system has defence mechanisms that fight infectious microorganisms. The immune response is a protective reaction that neutralizes pathogens and repairs body cells. The immune system is composed of cells and molecules that help the body resist disease; certain responses of the immune system are nonspecific and protect against microorganisms regardless of prior exposure (e.g., normal flora, body system defences, and inflammation), whereas others are specific defences against particular pathogens. If any of the body's defences fail, an infection can quickly progress to a serious health problem.

Normal Flora. The body normally contains microorganisms that reside on the surface and in deep layers of skin, in the saliva and oral mucosa, and in the gastrointestinal and genitourinary tracts. A person normally excretes trillions of microbes daily through the intestines. The skin also has a large population of resident flora—these normal flora do not typically cause disease when residing in their usual area of the body but, instead, participate in maintaining health.

Normal flora of the large intestine exist in great numbers without causing injury. Normal flora may assist in fighting infection and inflammation and maintaining homeostasis. Gut microorganisms change dietary fibre into fatty acids, which are reabsorbed by the large bowel and synthesize vitamins B and K, bile acids, and sterols; this synthesis has a benefit to both the host and the flora. Bile has antibacterial properties as well as fatty acids that stabilize the normal flora populations and prevent invasion of pathogens (Brestoff & Artis, 2015). When the normal flora are disrupted, disease-causing organisms can proliferate. The skin's normal flora exert a protective action by inhibiting the multiplication of organisms landing on the skin. The mouth and pharynx are also protected by flora that impair the growth of invading microbes. The mass of normal flora maintains a sensitive balance with other microorganisms to prevent infection. Any factor that disrupts this balance places a person at increased risk for acquiring an infectious disease. For example, according to studies, when a patient acquires microorganisms within the hospital, the person's resident flora change, which may lead to an infection (Graham, 2015).

TABLE 33-3 Normal Defence Mechanisms Against Infection

Defence Mechanisms	Action	Factors That May Alter Defence
Skin		
Intact multilayered surface (body's first line of defence against infection)	Provides barrier to microorganisms and antibacterial activity	Cuts, abrasions, wounds, areas of maceration (softening of the skin due to moisture), burns, or penetration by invasive devices
Shedding of outer layer of skin cells	Removes organisms that adhere to skin's outer layers	Failure to bathe regularly
Sebum	Contains fatty acid that kills some bacteria	Excessive bathing
Mouth		
Intact multilayered mucosa	Provides mechanical barrier to microorganisms	Lacerations, trauma, extracted teeth
Saliva	Washes away particles containing microorganisms, contains microbial inhibitors (e.g., lysozyme)	Poor oral hygiene, dehydration
Eye		
Tearing and blinking	Blinking prevents entry of particles containing pathogens, and tearing helps to wash particles away	Injury
Respiratory Tract		
Cilia lining upper airway, coated with mucus	Trap inhaled microbes and sweep them outward in mucus to be expectorated or swallowed	Smoking, high concentration of oxygen and carbon dioxide, decreased humidity, cold air
Macrophages	Engulf and destroy microorganisms that reach the lung's alveoli	Smoking
Urinary Tract		
Flushing action of urine flow	Washes away microorganisms on lining of bladder and urethra	Obstruction to normal flow by urinary catheter placement, obstruction from growth or tumour, delayed micturition
Intact multilayered epithelium	Provides barrier to microorganisms	Introduction of urinary catheter, continual movement of catheter in urethra
Gastrointestinal Tract		
Acidity of gastric secretions	Acids destroy some microorganisms	Administration of antacids to neutralize acids
Increased peristalsis in small intestine	Prevents retention of bacterial contents	Delayed motility resulting from impaction of fecal contents in large bowel or mechanical obstruction by masses
Vagina		
At puberty, normal flora causing vaginal secretions to achieve low pH	Inhibit growth of many microorganisms	Use of antibiotics or oral contraceptives, which disrupt normal flora

In addition, the use of **broad-spectrum antibiotics** for the treatment of infection can lead to a **superinfection**, which develops when broad-spectrum antibiotics eliminate a wide range of microorganisms, not just those causing infection. Normal bacterial flora are eliminated, reducing the body's defences and thus allowing disease-producing microorganisms to multiply (Lee, Cho, Jeong, et al., 2013).

Body System Defences. A number of the body's organ systems have unique defences against infection (Table 33-3). The skin, respiratory tract, and gastrointestinal tract are easily accessible to microorganisms: pathogenic organisms easily adhere to the skin's surface, are inhaled into the lungs, or are ingested with food. Each organ system has defence mechanisms physiologically suited to its structure and function. For example, the lungs cannot completely control the entrance of microorganisms; however, the airways are lined with hair-like projections (cilia) that rhythmically beat to move a blanket of mucus and adherent or trapped organisms up to the pharynx to be removed. Conditions that impair an organ's specialized defences increase the person's susceptibility to infection.

Inflammation. Inflammation is the body's cellular response to injury or infection. Inflammation is a protective vascular reaction that delivers fluid, blood products, and nutrients to interstitial tissues in an area of injury. The process neutralizes and eliminates pathogens or **necrotic** (dead) tissues and establishes a means of repairing body cells and tissues. Signs of localized inflammation are swelling, redness, heat, pain or tenderness, and loss of function in the affected body part. When infection becomes systemic, other signs and symptoms develop, including fever, leukocytosis, malaise, anorexia, nausea, vomiting, and lymph node enlargement.

The **inflammatory response** may be triggered by physical agents, chemical agents, or microorganisms. Mechanical trauma, temperature extremes, and radiation are examples of physical agents. Chemical agents include external and internal irritants, such as harsh poisons and gastric acid.

After tissues are injured, the inflammatory response, a series of well-coordinated events, occurs:

- Vascular and cellular responses
- The formation of inflammatory exudates (fluid and cells that are discharged from cells or blood vessels, e.g., pus or serum)
- Tissue repair

Vascular and Cellular Responses. Acute inflammation is an immediate response to cellular injury. Arterioles supplying the infected or injured area dilate, allowing more blood into the local circulation. The increase in local blood flow causes the characteristic redness of inflammation. The symptom of localized warmth results from a greater volume of blood at the inflammatory site. Local vasodilation enables blood and white blood cells (WBCs) to travel to the injured tissues.

Injury causes tissue necrosis, and, as a result, the body releases histamine, bradykinin, prostaglandin, and serotonin. These chemical mediators increase the permeability of small blood vessels, allowing fluid, protein, and cells to enter interstitial spaces. Accumulated fluid appears as localized swelling (edema).

Another symptom of inflammation is pain—the swelling of inflamed tissues increases the pressure on nerve endings, causing pain. Chemical substances such as histamine stimulate nerve endings. As a result of physiological changes occurring with inflammation, the involved body part usually undergoes a temporary loss of function. For example, a localized infection of the hand causes the fingers to become swollen, painful, and discoloured. Joints may become stiff as a result of the swelling, but the function of the fingers returns when inflammation subsides.

The cellular response of inflammation involves WBCs arriving at the site. These cells pass through the blood vessels and into the tissues. Through the process of phagocytosis, specialized WBCs, called *neutrophils* and *monocytes,* ingest and destroy microorganisms and other small particles. As inflammation becomes systemic, other signs and symptoms develop. Leukocytosis, or an increase in the number of circulating WBCs, is the body's response to WBCs leaving blood vessels. A serum WBC count is normally 5 000/mm^3 to 10 000/mm^3 but may rise to 15 000/mm^3 or even higher during inflammation. Fever is caused by the phagocytic release of pyrogens from bacterial cells that cause a rise in the hypothalamic set point (see Chapter 30).

Inflammatory Exudates. The accumulation of fluid, dead tissue cells, and WBCs forms an exudate at the site of inflammation (see Chapter 46). The exudate may be serous (clear, watery plasma), sanguineous (bloody drainage), serosanguineous (thin, watery drainage that is blood tinged), or purulent (thick drainage that contains pus). Eventually, the exudate is cleared away through lymphatic drainage. Platelets and plasma proteins such as fibrinogen form a meshlike matrix at the site of inflammation to prevent the spread of infection.

Tissue Repair. When tissues are injured, healing involves the inflammation, proliferation, and remodelling stages (see Chapter 46). Damaged cells are eventually replaced with healthy new ones, which undergo a gradual maturation until they take on the same structural characteristics and appearance as the previous cells. However, unless a wound is minor, the healed wound does not usually have the tensile strength of the tissue it replaces and scarring may occur.

Health Care–Associated Infections

Patients in health care settings have an increased risk of acquiring infections. A health care–associated infection (HAI), also known as nosocomial infection or *iatrogenic infection,* is an infection acquired after admission to a health care facility that was not present or incubating at the time of admission. Patients in hospitals are at risk for infections because they may have a high acuity of illness and frequently undergo aggressive treatments, many of which compromise immunity (Public Health Agency of Canada [PHAC], 2013a). Transmission of antibiotic-resistant organisms also can occur in health care facilities because a large population of susceptible people who frequently receive antibiotics are in close proximity to each other.

Clostridium difficile infection (CDI) is one of the most common and costly HAIs. *C. difficile* is a Gram-positive, spore-forming, anaerobic bacillus that produces two toxins, A and B, which cause diarrhea and colitis in patients whose bacterial flora have been disrupted by prior antibiotic use. Pseudomembranous colitis (PMC) is a more severe form of CDI, in which patients have a colitis characterized by the presence of pseudomembranes on the colon surface seen during endoscopy. Infection control measures to prevent transmission of *C. difficile* to patients include placing the patient on contact isolation, good hand hygiene (preferably with soap and water for patients who have diarrhea), gloves and gowns, as well as thorough environmental cleaning. Another important preventative measure is good antibiotic stewardship.

HAIs can result from a diagnostic or therapeutic procedure, such as a urinary tract infection that develops after catheter insertion. The incidence of nosocomial infections can be reduced if nurses use critical thinking when practising aseptic techniques. Nurses should always consider the patient's risks for infection and anticipate how the approach to care may increase or decrease the chances of infection transmission (Box 33-2).

HAIs may be exogenous or endogenous. An exogenous infection arises from microorganisms external to the individual that do not exist as normal flora; examples are *Salmonella* organisms and *Clostridium tetani.* An endogenous infection can occur when some of the patient's flora become altered and overgrowth results. Examples are infections caused by enterococci, yeasts, and streptococci. When sufficient numbers of microorganisms normally found in one body cavity or lining are transferred to another body site, an endogenous infection develops. For example, the transmission of enterococci, normally found in fecal material, from the hands to the skin is a common cause of wound infections. The number of microorganisms needed to cause an infection depends on the virulence of the organism, the host's susceptibility, and the site affected.

A patient's risk of infection is influenced by the number of health care workers having direct contact with the patient, the type and number of invasive procedures, the therapy received, and the length of hospitalization. Major sites for HAI are surgical and traumatic wounds, urinary and respiratory tracts, and the bloodstream (Box 33-3).

Older persons have an increased susceptibility to HAIs because they are more likely to have a chronic disease and because of the effects of the aging process itself (Box 33-4). Extended stays in health care institutions, increased disability, and prolonged recovery times are all potential outcomes of HAIs. HAIs decrease the patient's quality of life and increase costs to the health care system. Therefore, their prevention is an important part of managed care.

❖ NURSING PROCESS IN INFECTION CONTROL

◆ Assessment

When considering infection prevention, the nurse must assess a patient's defence mechanisms, susceptibility, and knowledge of infections. A review of disease history with the patient and family may reveal an exposure to a communicable disease. A thorough review of the patient's clinical condition may allow the nurse to detect signs and symptoms of an infection or a risk for infection. Information about the patient's defences against infection can be determined by an analysis of laboratory findings. By knowing the factors that increase susceptibility or risk for infection, nurses are better able to plan preventive therapy that includes aseptic techniques. Recognizing early signs and symptoms of infection allows nurses to alert others on the health care team to the potential need for therapy and to initiate supportive nursing measures.

Status of Defence Mechanisms

Nurses can determine the status of a patient's normal defence mechanisms against infection through a review of the physical assessment findings and the patient's medical condition. For example, any break in the skin or mucosa is a potential site for infection. Similarly, a chronic smoker is at greater risk for acquiring a respiratory tract

BOX 33-2 NURSING CARE PLAN

Perils of Central Venous Catheters

ASSESSMENT

Susan Serious is a 48-year-old woman in end-stage renal failure secondary to focal segmental glomerulosclerosis, diagnosed 2 months previously. She is dialysis dependent, which required the insertion of a central venous catheter. Susan was admitted to the nephrology service on Friday evening from the emergency department with complaints of chills, nausea, vomiting, headache, and fatigue. She stated that she had felt well until the end of her dialysis treatment that day.

Susan related that she is allergic to co-trimoxazole (Bactrim). Her medication list is composed of amlodipine (Norvasc), ramipril (Altace), furosemide (Lasix), prednisone, calcium carbonate, multivitamins (Replavite), ferrous gluconate, and darbepoetin alpha (Aranesp).

Assessment Activities	*Findings and Defining Characteristics*
Review signs and symptoms of localized and systemic infections.	Signs of localized infection include swelling, redness, heat, pain, or tenderness and loss of function in the affected body part. Signs and symptoms of systemic infection include fever, leukocytosis, malaise, anorexia, nausea, vomiting, and lymph node enlargement.
Research susceptibility to infection in patients with end-stage renal failure.	The literature shows that infections are a significant cause of morbidity and mortality in patients with end-stage renal failure, in part due to the clinical setting where treatment is received, the type of dialysis access, and the use of immunosuppressive medications (Collier & Davenport, 2014). Susan has been taking prednisone 30 mg daily.
Review effects of medications.	Prednisone suppresses the body's response to infection.

NURSING DIAGNOSIS: Risk for infection related to disease, immunosuppressive medications, and the use of a central venous catheter.

PLANNING

Goals	*Expected Outcomes*
Susan will be treated for infection and will remain free of future infections.	Follow-up results of chest radiographs, complete blood count with differential, and blood cultures with attending nephrologist to diagnose and treat existing infection. Initiate intravenous (IV) antibiotics, as ordered, to treat existing infection. Arrange to have the tunnelled central venous catheter removed for 48 hours while receiving antibiotics as ordered, to eliminate the source of infection. After 48 hours, the catheter may be reinserted using sterile technique. Susan will recover from existing infection and will not develop signs or symptoms of new infections.
Susan will become knowledgeable of infection risks.	Susan will self-monitor for signs and symptoms of infection, report these to health care providers, and observe for good aseptic technique during catheter care by the health care providers. Review the use and dosage of prednisone with Susan to increase her understanding of immunosuppressive medications.

INTERVENTIONS

Prevention and Early Detection	*Rationale*
Monitor Susan's temperature and vital signs, and inspect the central venous catheter exit site for evidence of infection.	Interventions are designed to prevent and ensure early detection of infection.
Practise hand hygiene before and after catheter care. Teach Susan to perform hand hygiene.	Handwashing reduces bacterial counts on hands (PHAC, 2012b).
Teach Susan about her catheter: aseptic technique, infection rates, care, and indications of infection.	Increased knowledge will aid in the early detection of infection.
Teach Susan about her medications, indications, adverse effects, and dosages.	Increased knowledge will increase adherence to the medication regimen and reporting of any related issues.

BOX 33-2 NURSING CARE PLAN

Perils of Central Venous Catheters—cont'd

EVALUATION

Nursing Actions	Patient Response and Finding	Achievement of Outcome
Compare Susan's temperature, vital signs, and physical findings with baseline data.	Susan remains afebrile, free of signs and symptoms of infection.	Susan has no active infection at this time.
Ask Susan to review knowledge of catheter-related infections.	Susan is able to identify signs and symptoms of catheter-related infections.	Susan has demonstrated a good knowledge base of catheter-related infections.
Ask Susan to explain the importance of hand hygiene related to catheter care.	Susan is able to relate that hand hygiene helps to reduce microorganisms that may contribute to infections.	Susan understands the principles and rationale of hand hygiene.
Ask Susan to discuss central venous catheters and the use of aseptic technique during care of the catheters.	Susan is able to describe aseptic technique during catheter care.	Susan has demonstrated knowledge of catheter care.
Ask Susan to review the medications she is currently using.	Susan is able to list and explain the use of her current medications.	Susan has demonstrated an understanding of her medications regarding their use, effects, and potential concerns.

BOX 33-3 Sites for and Causes of Health Care–Associated Infections

Surgical and Traumatic Wounds

Improper skin preparation (shaving) before surgery
Failure to cleanse skin surface properly
Failure to use aseptic technique during dressing changes
The use of contaminated antiseptic solutions
Improper hand hygiene

Urinary Tract

Inappropriate and unsterile catheterization techniques
Inadequate monitoring of in-dwelling urinary catheters
Obstruction or blockages in tubing
An improper specimen-collection technique
Urine in the catheter or drainage tube being allowed to re-enter bladder (reflux)
Improper hand hygiene

Respiratory Tract

Contaminated respiratory therapy equipment
Failure to use aseptic technique while suctioning airway
Improper disposal of secretions
Improper hand hygiene

Bloodstream

Contamination of intravenous fluids by tubing or needle changes
The insertion of drug additives to intravenous fluid
The addition of a connecting tube or stopcocks to an intravenous system
Improper care of a needle-insertion site
Improper insertion technique
Contaminated needles or catheters
Failure to change the intravenous access site when inflammation first appears
Improper technique during the administration of multiple blood products
Improper care of peritoneal or hemodialysis catheters
Improper hand hygiene

BOX 33-4 FOCUS ON OLDER PERSONS

Immune Function

- An age-related decline in immune system function, termed *immune senescence,* increases the body's susceptibility to infection and lessens the strength of the overall immune response (Reuben, 2016).
- Age-related changes alter the response to infection resulting in atypical signs and symptoms.
- Chronic disease, prevalent among older persons, allows infectious agents to readily invade; hospitalization and institutionalization as a result of chronic disease also increase older persons' exposure to pathogens (Boraschi et al., 2013; Reuben, 2016).
- Risks associated with the development of infections in older patients include poor nutrition, unintentional weight loss, and low serum albumin levels (Amarya, Singh, & Sabharwall, 2015; Reuben, 2016).
- Age-related changes in immunity contribute to the increased risk for acquiring pneumonia and influenza in older adulthood, both of which have significant age-related increases in mortality rates (Boraschi et al., 2013; Reuben, 2016).
- Older persons present with an altered response to infection with atypical signs and symptoms such as confusion.

Data from Reuben, D. B. (2016). Geriatric assessment. In Goldman, L., & Schafer, A. I. (Eds.), *Cecil essentials of medicine* (25th ed., pp. 102–106). Philadelphia, PA: Saunders.

BOX 33-5 Risk Factors for Infection

Inadequate Primary Defences

Broken skin or mucosa
Traumatized tissue
Decreased ciliary action
Obstructed urine outflow
Altered peristalsis
A change in the pH of secretions
Decreased mobility

Inadequate Secondary Defences

A reduced hemoglobin level
The suppression of white blood cells (WBCs) (drug or disease related)
A suppressed inflammatory response (drug or disease related)
A low WBC count (leukopenia)

infection after general surgery because the cilia of the lung are less likely to propel retained mucus from the lung's airways. Any reduction in the body's primary or secondary defences against infection places a patient at risk (Box 33-5).

Patient Susceptibility

Many factors influence susceptibility to infection. Nurses need to gather information about each factor through the patient's and family's history.

Age. Throughout the lifespan, susceptibility to infection changes. An infant has immature defences against infection. Born with only the antibodies provided by the mother, the infant's immune system is incapable of producing the necessary immunoglobulins and WBCs to adequately fight some infections. However, breastfed infants have greater immunity than do bottle-fed infants because they receive the mother's antibodies through the breast milk. As the child grows, the immune system matures; however, the child is still susceptible to organisms that cause the common cold, intestinal infections, and, if the child is not vaccinated, infectious diseases such as mumps and measles.

The young or middle-aged adult has refined defences against infection. Normal flora, body system defences, inflammation, and the immune response provide protection against invading microorganisms. Viruses are the most common cause of infectious illness in young and middle-aged adults.

Defences against infection change with aging (Boraschi, Aquado, Dutel, et al., 2013). The immune response, particularly cell-mediated immunity, declines. Older persons also undergo alterations in the structure and function of the skin, urinary tract, and lungs. For example, the skin loses its turgor and the epithelium thins; as a result, the skin is more easily abraded or torn. This increases the potential for invasion by pathogens (Table 33-4).

Nutritional Status. When protein intake is inadequate as a result of poor diet or debilitating disease, the rate of protein breakdown exceeds that of tissue synthesis (see Chapter 42). A reduction in the intake of protein and other nutrients such as carbohydrates and fats reduces the body's defences against infection and impairs wound healing (see Chapter 42). Patients with illnesses or problems that increase protein requirements are at further risk. These problems include traumatic injury, extensive burns, and conditions causing fever. Patients who have had surgery also require increased protein.

Nurses need to assess patients' dietary intake and ability to tolerate solid foods. Patients who have difficulty with swallowing, who experience alterations in digestion, or who are too confused or weak to feed themselves are at risk for inadequate dietary intake. A dietitian may be called in to assess the nutritional adequacy of a patient's diet. When preparing a patient for discharge, the nurse should evaluate the patient's and family's understanding of nutritional needs.

Stress. The general adaptation syndrome is the body's response to emotional or physical stress (see Chapter 29). During the alarm stage, the basal metabolic rate increases as the body uses energy stores. Adrenocorticotropic hormone acts to increase serum glucose levels and decrease unnecessary anti-inflammatory responses through the release of cortisone. If stress continues or becomes intense, elevated cortisone levels result in a decreased resistance to infection. Continued stress leads to exhaustion, wherein energy stores are depleted and the body has no resistance to invading organisms. The same conditions that increase nutritional requirements, such as surgery or trauma, also increase physiological stress. Chronic diseases also increase risk for infections. Examples of chronic diseases and how they increase risk for infection are presented in Box 33-6.

Disease Process. Patients with diseases of the immune system are at particular risk for infection. Leukemia, AIDS, lymphoma, and aplastic anemia are conditions that compromise a host by weakening defences against infectious organisms. Patients with leukemia, for

BOX 33-6 Chronic Diseases

Chronic diseases are diseases of slow progression and long duration. They primarily occur in people over 65 years of age and affect quality of life and mobility.

Chronic diseases include the following:

- Coronary artery disease (CAD)
- Stroke (accounts for more than 30% of all deaths each year)
- Cancer (claims more than 500 000 lives each year)
- Chronic obstructive pulmonary disease (COPD)
- Diabetes mellitus (DM) II (leading cause of kidney failure, amputations, and blindness)
- Arthritis (most common cause of disability)
- Neurodegenerative disease
- Renal failure (accounted for 62% of all deaths worldwide in 2011)

Risk factors for infection:

1. Compromised host defenses (cancer, arthritis, respiratory diseases, renal failure, hematological and hepatic disorders, diabetes, AIDs, alcoholism, immunosuppression)
2. Compromised circulation (obesity, peripheral vascular disease, lymphedema)
3. Compromised host defenses (radiation, medication and organ transplant, burns)
4. Treatment (surgery, invasive lines, dialysis, intubation, total parenteral nutrition)
5. Personal and environmental factors related to compromised host defense (history of infection, immobility, stress, increased hospital stay, smoking)
6. Factors specific to site invasion (skin folds, trauma, bites, thermal injuries)

Four health-damaging but modifiable behaviours that contribute to chronic illness and are responsible for much of this illness, disability, and premature deaths include tobacco use, insufficient physical activity, poor nutrition, and excessive alcohol use.

Data from Larsen, P. D. (2016). *Chronic illness, impact and intervention* (9th Ed.). Burlington, MA: Jones & Bartlett Learning; Centers for Disease Control and Prevention (CDC). (2017). *Chronic disease prevention and health promotion.* Retrieved from www.cdc.gov/chronicdisease; Carpenito, L. J. (2013). Risk for infection. In *Handbook of nursing diagnosis* (14th ed., pp. 338–350). Philadelphia, PA: Blackwell Publishing.

TABLE 33-4 Assessing the Risk of Infection in Older Persons

Component	Possible Changes With Age	Possible Outcomes
Skin	Thinner dermal and epidermal layers, decreased collagen strength, decreased skin elasticity, decreased sweating	Pressure injuries
Peripheral nerves	Reduced sensitivity, particularly in patients with a history of alcohol abuse, vitamin B_{12} deficiency, and diabetes mellitus	Pressure injuries, patients unaware of trauma to skin, leading to infection
Circulation	Heart failure, calcified mitral and aortic valves	Pneumonia, bacterial endocarditis
Peripheral circulation	Loss of elasticity of veins (prone to distension), less effective venous valves, blood pooling in lower extremities	Venous stasis ulcers
Mouth	Dehydration, reduction in saliva production, functional inability to maintain oral hygiene	Parotid gland infection, periodontal disease, localized abscess, bacteremia (i.e., bacteria in the blood)
Gastrointestinal tract	Loss of ability to secrete stomach acid in 30% of persons older than 70 years	*Salmonella* diarrhea
Pulmonary system	Increased colonization of oropharynx, impaired mucociliary clearance, decreased macrophage function, decreased cough reflex	Viral and bacterial pneumonia
Genitourinary tract	Prostatic hypertrophy or hyperplasia, urethral strictures, age-related hormonal changes in vaginal wall, pelvic floor relaxation, ureterocele or cystocele, degeneration of nerves leading to neurogenic bladder, use of tricyclic antidepressants results in urinary retention, dehydration	Asymptomatic bacteriuria (i.e., bacteria in the urine), cystitis, pyelonephritis
Nutrition	Malnutrition, vitamin deficiency (vitamin A, vitamin C, pyridoxine, and riboflavin), protein and caloric deficiencies	Impaired immune response to infection
Drug therapy	Corticosteroid and cytotoxic drugs	Impaired immune response to infection in patients already at risk for decline in immune system function
Long-term care residency	Age-related changes are multifactorial and include changes in all systems of the body that contribute to the risk of infection. The increasing use of invasive devices, antimicrobials, and multiple medications contribute to infections in this population. The elderly population and the health care setting may provide a setting that promotes the development and spread of infections. Preventive measures should be instituted, such as increased hand hygiene, reduced use of in-dwelling catheters, increased efforts to reduce aspiration, increased administration of vaccines, and prudent use of antibiotics	Frequent serious infection, increased risk of pneumonia and urinary tract infections. Increased risk of acquiring a multidrug-resistant organism

Evans, N., & Ness, S. (2014). *Older adult care. Online continuing education course.* Wild Iris Continuing Medical Education, Inc. Retrieved from www.nursingceu.com/courses/472/index_nceu.html; Grota, P. (2014). *APIC text of infection control and epidemiology* (4th ed., pp 401–407). Washington DC: Association for Professionals in Infection Control and Epidemiology (APIC).

example, are unable to produce normal WBCs to effectively ward off infection (see Box 33-6).

Patients with chronic diseases such as coronary artery disease (CAD), diabetes mellitus, arthritis, and multiple sclerosis are also more susceptible to infection because of general debilitation and nutritional impairment. Cancer and end-stage renal failure (which alters the immune response), peripheral vascular disease (which reduces blood flow to injured tissues), and diseases that impair body system defences, such as emphysema and bronchitis (COPD) (which impair ciliary action and thicken mucus), increase susceptibility to infection (see Box 33-6). Patients with burns have a very high susceptibility to infection because of the damage to skin surfaces. The greater the depth and extent of the burns, the higher the risk for infection.

Medical Therapy. Some drugs and medical therapies compromise immunity to infection. Nurses need to assess their patients' history to determine whether they take medications at home that increase infection susceptibility. A review of therapies received within the health care setting may further reveal risks. Adrenal corticosteroids, prescribed for several conditions, are anti-inflammatory drugs that cause protein breakdown and impair the inflammatory response against bacteria and other pathogens. Cytotoxic or antineoplastic drugs attack cancer cells but cause adverse effects such as depression of bone marrow activity and normal cell toxicity. When bone marrow activity is depressed, the body is unable to produce lymphocytes and sufficient WBCs. When normal cells become altered by antineoplastic agents, cellular defences against infection fail. Cyclosporine and other immunosuppressant drugs, which decrease the body's immune response, are commonly taken by organ transplant recipients. The immunosuppressants prevent organ and tissue rejection, but they also increase the recipients' susceptibility to infection.

Patients with cancer who are receiving radiotherapy are at risk for infection. The massive doses of radiation that destroy cancerous cells can also depress bone marrow activity and destroy normal cells.

Clinical Appearance

The signs and symptoms of infection may be local or systemic. Localized infections are most common in areas of skin or mucous membrane breakdown, such as surgical and traumatic wounds, pressure injuries, and mouth lesions. Infections also develop locally in cavities beneath the skin; an example is an abscess.

To assess an area for localized infection, the nurse should first inspect the area for redness and swelling caused by inflammation. Because drainage from open lesions or wounds may occur, nurses must wear disposable gloves. Infected drainage may be yellow, green, or brown, depending on the pathogen. Ask the patient about pain or tenderness around the site. The patient may complain of tightness and pain caused by edema. If the infected area is large enough, movement of a body part may be restricted. Gentle palpation of an infected area usually results in some degree of tenderness.

Systemic infections cause more generalized symptoms than do local infections. Systemic infections usually result in fever, fatigue, and malaise. Lymph nodes that drain the area of infection often become enlarged, swollen, and tender during palpation. For example, an abscess in the peritoneal cavity may cause the enlargement of the lymph nodes in the groin. An infection of the upper respiratory tract may cause cervical lymph node enlargement. If an infection is serious and widespread, all major lymph nodes may enlarge. Systemic infections commonly cause a loss of appetite, nausea, and vomiting.

Systemic infections may develop after treatment for a localized infection has failed. Nurses should be alert for changes in a patient's level of activity and responsiveness. As systemic infections develop, the patient may become lethargic and complain of a loss of energy. An elevation in body temperature may lead to episodes of increased heart and respiratory rates and low blood pressure. The involvement of major body systems may produce specific signs. For example, a pulmonary infection may result in a productive cough with purulent sputum. A urinary tract infection may result in cloudy, foul-smelling urine.

In older persons, infection may not present with typical signs and symptoms. Fever, pain, and swelling are often absent in older people because they tend to have lower body temperatures, decreased pain sensation, and less immune response to infection. As a result, in older persons, infection is often advanced before it is identified. Atypical symptoms such as a change in behaviour (e.g., new or increased confusion, incontinence, or agitation) may be the only symptoms of an infectious illness (Reuben, 2016). For example, as many as 20% of older persons with pneumonia do not have the typical signs and symptoms of fever, shaking, chills, and "rusty" productive sputum. The only symptoms present may be an increased heart rate with no apparent reason, confusion, or generalized fatigue.

Laboratory Data

A review of laboratory test results may confirm infection (Table 33-5). However, laboratory values alone are not sufficient to detect infection; other clinical signs must be assessed. Factors other than infection may alter test values. For example, trauma and physical stress can cause an elevation in the number of neutrophils. A culture may show the growth of an organism in the absence of overt signs of infection.

Patients With Infection

A patient with infection may have a variety of health problems. Nurses need to assess ways that the infection affects the patient's and family's needs—these may be physical, psychological, social, or economic. For example, a patient with a chronic disease such as AIDS may experience serious psychological problems as a result of self-imposed isolation or rejection by family and friends. Using a case-management approach, the nurse can determine the patient's and family's ability to adjust to the disease and the resources available to help them manage health care challenges (Trehearne, Fishman, & Lin, 2014).

◆ Nursing Diagnosis

During assessment, nurses gather objective findings, such as an open incision or a reduced caloric intake, and subjective data, such as a

TABLE 33-5 Laboratory Tests to Screen for Infection

Laboratory Value	Normal (Adult) Values	Indication of Infection
White blood cell (WBC) count	5–10 × 10⁹/L	Increased in acute infection, neoplasm, allergy neoplasm, or immunosuppression, decreased in certain viral or overwhelming infections
Erythrocyte sedimentation rate (ESR) Westergren method	Up to 15 mm/hour for men and 20 mm/hour for women	Elevated in presence of inflammatory process, acute and chronic infection, tissue necrosis or infarction
Iron level	8–25 mcmol/L	Decreased in chronic infection
C-reactive protein	<10 mg/L	An acute-phase reactant protein that is elevated in the presence of an acute inflammatory process
Cultures of urine and blood	Normally sterile, without microorganism growth	Presence of infectious microorganism growth
Cultures and Gram stain of wound, sputum, and throat	No WBCs on Gram stain, possible normal flora	Presence of infectious microorganism growth and WBCs on Gram stain
WBC	**Differential Count (Percentage of Each Type of WBC)**	**Indication of Infection**
Neutrophils	55–70%	Increased in acute suppurative infection, decreased in overwhelming bacterial infection (older persons)
Lymphocytes	20–40%	Increased in chronic bacterial and viral infection, decreased in sepsis
Monocytes	2–8%	Increased in protozoal, rickettsial, and tuberculosis infections
Eosinophils	1–4%	Increased in parasitic infection
Basophils	0.5–1%	Normal during infection

Data from Pagana, K. D., Pagana, T. J., & Pike-MacDonald, S. A. (2013). *Mosby's Canadian manual of diagnostics and laboratory tests* (1st Canadian ed.) Toronto: Mosby/Elsevier.

patient's complaint of tenderness over a surgical wound site (Box 33-7). The nurse then interprets the data carefully, looking for clusters of defining characteristics or risk factors that create a pattern suggesting a specific nursing diagnosis. The following are examples of nursing diagnoses that may apply:

- *Disturbed body image*
- *Risk for infection*
- *Risk for injury*
- *Imbalanced nutrition—less than body requirements*
- *Impaired oral mucous membrane*
- *Risk for impaired skin integrity*
- *Social isolation*
- *Impaired tissue integrity*

It may be necessary for the nurse to validate data (e.g., by inspecting the integrity of a wound more carefully). Likewise, additional data such as laboratory findings may be helpful. The proper selection of appropriate nursing diagnoses depends on the correct analysis and organization of data.

The diagnosis must have the correct etiological factor for a nurse to establish an appropriate and well-thought-out plan. For example, minimizing the risk for infection related to broken skin requires good hygiene measures and wound care; minimizing the risk for infection related to malnutrition requires good nutritional support and fluid balance.

Nurses may diagnose a risk for infection or make diagnoses that result from the effects of infection on the patient's health status. Nurses' success in planning appropriate nursing interventions depends on the accuracy of the diagnosis and their ability to meet the patient's needs.

BOX 33-7 NURSING DIAGNOSTIC PROCESS

Assessment Activities	Defining Characteristics	Nursing Diagnosis
Check results of laboratory tests.	WBC count 3.9×10^9/L	*Risk for infection related to neutropenia*
Review current medications.	Patient receiving azathioprine (Imuran), an immunosuppressant	
Identify potential sites of infection.	Intravenous catheter in right forearm in place for 3 days Foley catheter draining amber-coloured urine	

◆ Planning

Goals and Outcomes. The patient's care plan is based on each nursing diagnosis and related factors (Box 33-8). The nurse develops a plan that sets attainable outcomes so that interventions are purposeful and directed. For example, if you are caring for a patient with the nursing diagnosis *risk for infection related to broken skin,* you must implement skin and wound care measures to promote healing. The expected outcomes "reduction in wound size by 1 cm" and "absence of drainage" represent targets for measuring the patient's improvement. Once outcomes are met, the goal of "skin intact and without drainage" can be reached. Interventions are selected in collaboration with the patient, the family, and others on the health care team. Nurses direct the care in the acute care setting; care may also involve other professionals in assisting with instructions on post-discharge procedures. Common goals of care relating to infection include the following:

- Preventing exposure to infectious organisms
- Controlling or reducing the extent of the infection
- Maintaining resistance to infection
- Educating the patient and family about infection control techniques

Setting Priorities. In collaboration with the patient, the nurse establishes priorities for the goals of care. For example, for a patient who has an open wound and cancer and cannot tolerate solid foods, the priority of administering therapies that promote wound healing exceeds the goal of educating the patient to assume self-care therapies at home. When the patient's condition improves, the priorities will change, and patient education will become an essential intervention.

Continuity of Care. The development of a care plan includes infection prevention practices. Nurses may initiate appropriate referrals, such as to a dietitian, infection control professional, or home care nurse, to collaborate in a patient's care. When care is being administered in the home, the nurse should ensure that the environment supports good infection control practices. For example, if a patient does not have running water, the nurse needs to bring a waterless antimicrobial solution during visits to ensure adequate hand hygiene. Educating patients and families is also an important aspect of prevention.

◆ Implementation

By recognizing and assessing a patient's risk factors and implementing appropriate measures, nurses can reduce the risk of infection.

BOX 33-8 NURSING CARE PLAN

Risk for Infection

ASSESSMENT

Mrs. Spicer was admitted to the medical nursing unit 3 days ago with a diagnosis of lymphoma. She received her first dose of multiagent chemotherapy yesterday.

Jess Ralston is the student nurse caring for Mrs. Spicer. He begins his shift by conducting a focused assessment.

Assessment Activities	*Findings and Defining Characteristics*
Review patient's chart for laboratory data reflecting immune function.	Data show a reduction in number of white blood cells (WBCs) (leukopenia).
Ask patient to describe appetite and review food intake for past 24 hours. Weigh patient. Measure height.	Mrs. Spicer reports she has not had interest in eating for a couple of weeks. She has lost approximately 2.5 kg. Her current weight is 57 kg, and her height is 170 cm. Her food intake yesterday consisted of a small cup of applesauce, a half bowl of soup, some crackers, and two glasses of juice. Mrs. Spicer states, "I get full easily and lose interest in food."
Palpate patient's cervical and clavicular lymph nodes.	Lymph nodes are enlarged and painless.
Review effects of chemotherapy in drug reference.	Multiagent chemotherapy causes drug-induced pancytopenia.

Continued

BOX 33-8 NURSING CARE PLAN

Risk for Infection—cont'd

NURSING DIAGNOSIS: Risk for infection related to immunosuppression and reduced food intake.

PLANNING

*Goals (Nursing Outcomes Classification)**	*Expected Outcomes*
	Risk Detection
Patient will remain free of infection.	Patient will remain afebrile. Patient will develop no signs or symptoms of local infection (e.g., will remain free of cough, cloudy or foul-smelling urine, and purulent drainage from open wound or normal body opening).
	Knowledge: Infection Control
Patient will become knowledgeable of infection risks.	Patient will identify routines to follow in the home that reduce the transmission of microorganisms. Patient will identify signs and symptoms indicating infection to report to her health care provider.

*Outcome classification labels from Moorhead, S., Johnson, M., Maas, M. L, & Swanson, E. (Eds.). (2013). *Nursing outcomes classification (NOC)* (5th ed.). St. Louis, MO: Mosby.

INTERVENTIONS

Interventions (Nursing Intervention Classification)†	*Rationale*
Prevention and Early Detection	
Monitor patient's body temperature routinely, inspect oral cavity for lesions, inspect urethral and vaginal orifices for drainage or discharge, inspect intravenous access site for drainage, and observe patient for evidence of cough.	Interventions are designed to prevent and ensure early detection of infection in a patient at risk (Carpenito, 2013).
Practice hand hygiene routinely before caring for a patient, between patients, and before any invasive procedures.	Rigorous hand hygiene reduces bacterial counts on the hands (PHAC, 2012b).
Teach patient how to perform hand hygiene correctly.	Patient can easily come in contact with infectious agents that can cause infection.
Consult with dietitian about providing a high-calorie, high-protein, low-bacteria diet. Minimize intake of salads, undercooked meat, pepper, paprika, and raw fruits and vegetables. Offer small, frequent meals.	Maintaining calorie and protein intake will prevent weight loss. Foods high in bacteria should be avoided because they increase the risk for gastrointestinal infection (Carpenito, 2013).
Infection Control	
Instruct patient to report the following to the physician: temperature >38°C, persistent cough with or without sputum, pus or foul-smelling drainage from the body site, the presence of an abscess, urine that is cloudy or foul smelling, or burning on urination.	Signs and symptoms are indicative of local or systemic infection.
Teach patient to follow these activities at home: • Avoid crowds and large gatherings of persons. • Bathe daily. • Do not share personal hygiene items with family members (e.g., toothbrush, washcloth, and deodorant stick). • Take your temperature twice daily. • Do not drink water that has been standing for >15 minutes. • Do not reuse cups or glasses without washing.	These measures are designed to prevent infection in patients with impaired immune function (Carpenito, 2013).

†Nursing Intervention classification labels from Bulechek, G. M., Butcher, H. K., Dochterman, J. M., & Wagner, C. M. (Eds.). (2013). *Nursing interventions classification (NIC)* (6th ed.). St. Louis, MO: Mosby.

EVALUATION

Nursing Actions	*Patient Response and Finding*	*Achievement of Outcome*
Compare patient's body temperature and other physical findings with baseline data.	Mrs. Spicer remains afebrile and denies having cough or burning on urination. No signs of drainage or discharge from body site are evident.	Mrs. Spicer has no active infection at this time.
Ask patient to describe signs and symptoms to report to health care provider.	Mrs. Spicer is able to identify the temperature range to report. She is able to describe cough. She is unable to identify signs of urinary infection or local discharge.	Mrs. Spicer has a partial understanding of signs and symptoms to report. She will need additional instruction and an information sheet.
Ask patient to explain the measures to take at home to reduce exposure to infectious agents.	Mrs. Spicer is able to discuss the need to avoid sharing personal hygiene articles. She has asked for a list of other precautions and requested that her husband be included in discussion.	Mrs. Spicer has a partial understanding of restrictions. I will obtain printed guidelines and include her husband in discussion this evening.

Health Promotion. Nurses may prevent an infection from developing or spreading by minimizing the numbers and kinds of organisms transmitted to potential infection sites. Eliminating reservoirs of infection, controlling portals of exit and entry, and avoiding actions that transmit microorganisms prevent pathogens from finding a new site in which to grow. The proper use of sterile supplies, barrier protection, and proper hand hygiene are examples of methods that nurses use to control the spread of microorganisms. A further preventive measure is to strengthen a potential host's defences against infection. Nutritional support, rest, maintenance of physiological protective mechanisms, and receipt of recommended immunizations (Box 33-9) protect a patient from invasion by pathogens.

Being vigilant about infection control helps nurses to apply good medical–surgical aseptic practices at the right time and in the right clinical situation. When a patient develops an infection, the nurse needs to continue preventive care so that health care personnel and other patients are not exposed to the infection. Isolation precautions may be necessary for patients with communicable diseases; the environment is controlled by barriers against the transmission of infection (see "Isolation Guidelines" section).

Acute Care Measures. Treatment of an infectious process includes eliminating the infectious organisms and supporting the patient's defences. To identify the causative organism, nurses may collect specimens of body fluids or drainage from infected body sites for cultures. When the disease process or causative organism has been identified, the physician prescribes the treatment that is most effective for the situation. Nurses properly administer antibiotics and other treatments, watch for adverse reactions, and assess the progress of the infection.

Systemic infections necessitate measures to prevent complications of fever (see Chapter 30). Maintaining the patient's intake of fluids prevents dehydration resulting from diaphoresis. Because of the patient's increased metabolic rate, adequate nutritional intake must be ensured. Rest preserves energy for the healing process.

Localized infections often necessitate measures to remove debris to promote healing. Nurses need to apply the principles of wound care to remove any infected drainage from the wound site and support the integrity of healing wounds. Special dressings can be applied to facilitate the removal of infectious drainage and promote healing of wound margins. Drainage tubes may be inserted to remove infected drainage from body cavities. Nurses must use medical and surgical aseptic techniques to manage wounds and ensure correct handling of all drainage or body fluids (see Chapter 46).

During the course of infection, nurses can support the patient's body defence mechanisms. For example, if a patient has infectious diarrhea, the nurse must maintain skin integrity to prevent breakdown and the entrance of microorganisms. Other routine hygiene measures such as bathing and oral care protect the skin and mucous membranes from invasion and overgrowth of microorganisms.

Asepsis

Nurses' efforts to minimize the onset and spread of infection are based on the principles of aseptic technique. **Asepsis** is the process for keeping away disease-producing microorganisms. *Aseptic technique* refers to practices designed to render an area and objects as free from microorganisms as possible. The two types of aseptic technique are medical asepsis and surgical asepsis.

Medical asepsis, or clean technique, includes procedures used to reduce and prevent the spread of microorganisms. Hand hygiene, using clean gloves (i.e., disposable gloves) to prevent direct contact with blood or body fluids, and cleaning the environment routinely are examples of medical asepsis. The principles of medical asepsis are commonly followed in the home, as in washing hands before preparing food.

After an object becomes unsterile or unclean, it is considered *contaminated.* In medical asepsis, an area or object is considered contaminated if it contains or is suspected of containing microorganisms. For example, a used bedpan, the floor, and a used dressing are contaminated.

Nurses need to follow certain principles and procedures, including routine practices, to prevent infection and control its spread (see "Isolation Guidelines" section). During daily routine care, nurses use basic medical aseptic techniques to break the infection chain. Because infections are readily transmitted between patients and caregivers, it may become necessary for the nurse to follow isolation precautions as appropriate (see "Isolation Guidelines" section).

Nurses are responsible for providing the patient with a safe environment. The effectiveness of infection control practices depends on the nurse and his or her colleagues' conscientiousness and consistency in using effective aseptic technique. It is easy to forget key procedural steps or, in a hurry, to take shortcuts that break aseptic procedures. However, a nurse's failure to be meticulous places the patient at risk for an infection that can seriously impair recovery or lead to death.

Control or Elimination of Infectious Agents. Proper cleaning, disinfection, and sterilization of contaminated objects significantly reduce and often eliminate microorganisms. In health care centres,

BOX 33-9 FOCUS ON PRIMARY HEALTH CARE

Immunizations

Immunizations are an essential component of disease prevention. Nurses should encourage proper immunization of infants, children, individuals at risk, and older persons. In Canada, most provinces provide free-of-charge immunization to infants against measles, mumps, rubella, diphtheria, tetanus, acellular pertussis, and poliomyelitis. Parents may be required to pay to have their infant or child vaccinated against *Haemophilus influenzae* type b (Hib), human papillomavirus (HPV), varicella, and hepatitis B. The HPV vaccine is available in Canada for both male and female patients 9 to 26 years of age. For maximum benefit, it should be given before the patient becomes sexually active.

Older persons and those who have underlying medical conditions are at risk for influenza and pneumonia and are therefore offered influenza vaccines each year and pneumococcal vaccines as per the recommended schedule, which varies according to the recipient's age. Nurses should remind patients of the importance of having a tetanus–diphtheria booster vaccination every 10 years. Health care workers who care for persons at high risk for complications from influenza should be immunized for influenza yearly as well.

In most provinces and territories, public health nurses or community nurses hold free immunization clinics for patients at risk during an outbreak of a potentially deadly infection such as bacterial meningitis.

Public Health Agency of Canada. (2016). *Canadian immunization guide* (8th ed.). Ottawa: Public Health Agency of Canada. Retrieved from https://www.canada.ca/en/public-health/services/canadian-immunization-guide.html

a sterile processing department disinfects and sterilizes reusable supplies. However, nurses also may be required to perform these functions. Many principles of cleaning and disinfection also apply to the home.

Cleaning. *Cleaning* is the physical removal of foreign material (e.g., dust, soil, and organic material such as blood, secretions, excretions, and microorganisms) from objects and surfaces (Provincial Infectious Diseases Advisory Committee [PIDAC], 2013). In general, cleaning involves the use of water and mechanical action with detergents or enzymatic products. When an object comes in contact with infectious or potentially infectious material, the object is contaminated. Reusable objects must be cleaned thoroughly before reuse and then either disinfected or sterilized according to the manufacturer's recommendations.

When cleaning equipment that is soiled by organic material such as blood, fecal matter, mucus, or pus, nurses should take appropriate measures to protect themselves against contamination. These may include wearing a mask and protective eyewear (or a face shield) and waterproof gloves. These barriers provide protection from infectious organisms. A brush and detergent or soap are needed for cleaning.

The following steps ensure that an object is clean:

1. Rinse a contaminated object or article with cold running water to remove organic material. Hot water causes the protein in organic material to coagulate and stick to objects, making removal difficult.
2. After rinsing, wash the object with soap and warm water. Soap or detergent reduces the surface tension of water and emulsifies the dirt or remaining material. Rinse the object thoroughly to remove the emulsified dirt.
3. Use a brush to remove dirt or material in grooves or seams. Friction dislodges the contaminated material for easy removal. Open any hinged items for cleaning.
4. Rinse the object in warm water.
5. Dry the object and prepare it for disinfection or sterilization if indicated by the intended use of the item.
6. The brush, gloves, and sink in which the equipment is cleaned should be considered contaminated and should be cleaned and dried.

Disinfection and Sterilization. **Disinfection** is the elimination of all pathogens except bacterial spores (Alberta Health, 2012; PIDAC, 2013). Disinfectants are used on inanimate objects; antiseptics are used on living tissue. Disinfection usually involves chemicals, heat, or ultraviolet light. An item must be thoroughly cleaned before it is disinfected. Examples of disinfectants are alcohols, chlorines, glutaraldehydes, phenols, and quaternary ammonium compounds. These chemicals can be caustic and toxic to tissues. Some disinfectants are indicated for use only on noncritical items; nurses should read the label and follow the manufacturer's recommendations for use.

Sterilization is the destruction of all microorganisms, including spores. Steam under pressure, ethylene oxide gas, hydrogen peroxide plasma, and chemicals are the most common sterilizing agents. Items must be cleaned thoroughly before they can be sterilized.

Whether an item is to be simply cleaned, or cleaned and disinfected or sterilized, depends on the intended use of the item. Devices are classified in three categories (Box 33-10). Nurses should be familiar with their agency's policy and procedures for cleaning, handling, and delivering care items for eventual disinfection and sterilization. Workers especially trained in disinfection and sterilization should perform most of the procedures. Efficacy of the disinfecting or sterilizing method is influenced by the following factors:

- *Concentration of solution and duration of contact.* A weakened concentration or shortened exposure time may lessen effectiveness.
- *Type and number of pathogens.* Certain organisms are killed more easily than others by disruption. Higher numbers of pathogens on an object necessitate longer disinfecting time.
- *Surface areas to treat.* All dirty surfaces and areas must be fully exposed to disinfecting and sterilizing agents.
- *Temperature of the environment.* Disinfectants tend to work best at room temperature.
- *Presence of soap.* Soap may cause certain disinfectants to be ineffective. Thorough rinsing of an object is necessary before disinfecting.
- *Presence of organic materials.* Disinfectants can become inactivated unless blood, saliva, pus, or body excretions are already washed off.

Table 33-6 lists processes for disinfection and sterilization and their characteristics. Selection of the method for disinfecting or sterilizing an item depends on the intended use and nature of the item (e.g., some delicate instruments cannot tolerate steam and must be sterilized with gas or plasma).

Control or Elimination of Reservoirs. To control or eliminate reservoir sites for infection, nurses need to eliminate or control sources of body fluids, drainage, or solutions that might harbour microorganisms. Nurses must also carefully discard articles that become contaminated with infectious material (Box 33-11). All health care institutions must have guidelines for the disposal of infectious waste according to provincial or territorial laws.

Control of Portals of Exit. Nurses need to follow several measures to minimize or prevent infectious organisms from exiting the

BOX 33-10 Categories for Sterilization, Disinfection, and Cleaning

Critical Items

Critical items are instruments and devices that enter sterile tissue or the vascular system. They present a high risk of infection if the items are contaminated with microorganisms, including bacterial spores. Critical items must be thoroughly cleaned and sterilized. Examples of these items follow:

- Surgical instruments
- Intravascular catheters
- Urinary catheters
- Needles

Semicritical Items

Semicritical items are devices that come in contact with mucous membranes or nonintact skin but do not penetrate them. These items also present a risk of infection and must be free of all microorganisms (except bacterial spores). Semicritical items must be thoroughly cleaned and disinfected.

The following are examples of these items:

- Electronic thermometers
- Respiratory therapy equipment
- Endotracheal tubes
- Gastrointestinal endoscopes
- Vaginal and nasal specula

Noncritical Items

Noncritical items are items that either touch only intact skin but not mucous membranes or do not directly touch the patient. Noncritical items must be cleaned or cleaned and disinfected. Examples of these items follow:

- Bedpans, urinals, and commodes
- Blood pressure cuffs
- Linens
- Stethoscopes
- Some eating utensils

TABLE 33-6 Examples of Disinfection and Sterilization Processes

Characteristics	Examples of Use
Moist Heat Steam is moist heat under pressure. When exposed to high pressure, water vapour can attain a temperature above the boiling point to kill pathogens and spores.	An autoclave is used to sterilize surgical instruments and dressings.
Chemicals A number of chemical disinfectants are used in health care, including alcohols, chlorines, formaldehyde, glutaraldehydes, hydrogen peroxide, iodophors, phenolics, and quaternary ammonium compounds. Each product performs in a unique manner and is used for a specific purpose.	Chemicals are used for the disinfection of instruments and equipment such as thermometers and endoscopes. Use the appropriate facility-approved disinfectant in a safe manner (e.g., with gloves, proper ventilation) for the approved purpose.
Ethylene Oxide Gas Ethylene oxide gas destroys spores and microorganisms by altering cells' metabolic processes. Fumes are released within an autoclave-like chamber. This gas is toxic to humans, and aeration time varies with products.	This gas sterilizes some rubber and plastic items.
Boiling Water Boiling is the least expensive method of sterilization for use in the home. Bacterial spores and some viruses resist boiling. It is not used in hospitals.	The items (e.g., glass baby bottles) should be boiled for at least 15 minutes.

BOX 33-11 Infection Control to Reduce Reservoir Sites

Bathing
Use soap and water to remove drainage, dried secretions, or excess perspiration.

Dressing Changes
Change dressings that become wet or soiled (see Chapter 46).

Contaminated Articles
Place tissues, soiled dressings, and soiled linen in moisture-resistant bags for proper disposal.

Contaminated Needles
Engage the safety features of all sharp devices and dispose of them in a puncture-proof container. Place syringes, uncapped hypodermic needles, and intravenous needles in puncture-proof containers, which should be located in patient rooms or treatment areas so that exposed, contaminated equipment need not be carried a distance (see Chapter 34). *Do not recap needles* or attempt to break them.

Bedside Unit
Keep table surfaces clean and dry.

Bottled Solutions
Do not leave bottled solutions open for prolonged periods. Keep solutions tightly capped. Date bottles when opened and discard according to your facility's policy.

Surgical Wounds
Keep drainage tubes and collection bags patent to prevent the accumulation of serous fluid under the skin surface.

Drainage Bottles and Bags
Empty and dispose of drainage suction bottles according to your health agency's policy. Empty all drainage systems on each shift unless otherwise ordered by a physician. Never raise a drainage system (e.g., urinary drainage bag) above the level of the site being drained unless the drainage system is clamped off.

body. To control organisms exiting via the respiratory tract, the nurse should wear a mask as needed, avoid talking directly into patients' faces, and never talk, sneeze, or cough directly over surgical wounds or sterile dressing fields. The nurse should cover the mouth or nose when sneezing or coughing. Nurses are also responsible for teaching patients to protect others when they sneeze or cough and for providing patients with disposable wipes or tissues to control the spread of microorganisms.

Nurses who have an upper respiratory tract infection should consider not working; they may be required to remain at home. Nurses who continue to work with patients should wear a mask when working closely with a patient and pay special attention to hand hygiene. Nurses should not be caring for patients who are highly susceptible to infection (e.g., an immunosuppressed patient or a neonate).

Another way of controlling the exit of microorganisms is through the careful handling of blood, body fluids, secretions, or excretions (e.g., urine, feces, vomitus, and exudate). Contaminated fluids can easily splash while being discarded or cleaned up. Nurses should always wear disposable gloves when handling blood, body fluids, secretions, or excretions. Masks, gowns, and protective eyewear should be worn if splashing or contact with any fluids is possible. Disposable soiled items should be appropriately disposed of in impervious plastic bags. Laboratory specimens from all patients are handled as if they were infectious.

Control of Transmission. Effective control of infection requires nurses to remain aware of the modes of transmission and ways to control them. In the hospital, home, or long-term care facility, a patient should have a personal set of care items. The sharing of bedpans, urinals, bath basins, and eating utensils can easily lead to transmission of infection. Thermometers, even when individually used, warrant special care. Because the patient's own mucus can become a source of microorganism growth, the electronic thermometer is used with a disposable sheath over the probe; the sheath is discarded after each use. Single-use chemical strip thermometers present less risk of infection than do other thermometers. Use of electronic thermometers for rectal temperatures has been associated with nosocomial diarrhea (CDC, 2015). The organism *C. difficile* is able to survive on inanimate surfaces such as a thermometer probe for weeks to months. In institutions where nosocomial diarrhea occurs, electronic thermometers are not recommended for rectal temperatures.

To prevent transmission of microorganisms through indirect contact, soiled items and equipment must not touch the nurse's clothing. A common error is to carry dirty linen in the arms against the uniform. Fluid-resistant linen bags should be used, or soiled linen should be carried with hands held out from the body. Laundry hampers should be replaced before they are overflowing.

Hand Hygiene. Hand hygiene is the most important and most basic technique in preventing the transmission of infections. Hand hygiene includes using an instant alcohol hand antiseptic before and after providing patient care, handwashing with soap and water when hands are visibly soiled, and performing a surgical scrub when necessary. The components of good handwashing include using an adequate amount of soap, rubbing the hands together to lather the soap and create friction, and rinsing under a stream of water (CDC, 2015). The purpose is to remove soil and transient organisms from the hands and to reduce total microbial counts over time.

Contaminated hands are a prime cause of cross-infection. For example, imagine you are caring for a patient who has excessive pulmonary secretions, and you assist the patient in expectorating mucus and disposing of the tissues in a bedside container. The patient's roommate asks you to open containers of food on the meal tray. You then leave the patient's room to pour a dose of medication that is to be taken in 5 minutes. If you fail to perform hand hygiene before opening the containers of food or pouring the medication, organisms from the first patient's mucus can easily be transmitted to the roommate's food and to the medication container. Decreased nosocomial infection rates have been reported with improved hand hygiene compliance (Hammer, 2013).

The decision regarding when and what type of hand hygiene should occur depends on the following: the intensity of contact with patients or contaminated objects, the degree or amount of contamination that could occur with that contact, the susceptibility of the patient or the health care worker to infection, and the procedure or activity to be performed (PIDAC, 2013). For example, after prolonged and direct contact with a patient's wound drainage, the nurse must perform thorough hand hygiene.

It takes 40–60 seconds to clean hands by washing with soap and water (PIDAC, 2013). If the hands are visibly soiled, more time may be needed. Routine handwashing may be performed with plain soap. Plain soap with water can physically remove a certain level of microbes, but antiseptic agents are necessary to kill or inhibit microorganisms and reduce the level still further (PIDAC, 2013). Skill 33-1 lists the steps for hand hygiene.

The use of alcohol-based waterless antiseptics is recommended (by PIDAC, 2013) to improve hand hygiene practices, protect health care workers' hands, and reduce the transmission of pathogens to patients and personnel in health care settings. Alcohols have excellent germicidal activity and are more effective than either plain soap or antimicrobial soap and water. Emollients are added to alcohol-based antiseptics to prevent drying of the skin. Researchers have found that these antiseptics may be more effective than water because they are used quickly and are available at the bedside (CDC, 2015).

The CDC (2017a) recommends that hands be washed with plain soap when hands are visibly soiled. If the hands are not visibly soiled, an alcohol-based waterless antiseptic agent can be used for routine decontamination of hands in all other clinical situations:

- Before direct contact with each patient (e.g., taking a pulse or blood pressure, lifting a patient)
- After direct contact with each patient
- Before donning sterile gloves
- After removing gloves (i.e., after removing sterile gloves or clean, nonsterile gloves)
- After contact with body fluids or excretions, mucous membranes, nonintact skin, or wound dressings, as long as hands are not visibly soiled (if visibly soiled, wash with soap and water)
- When moving from a contaminated body site to a clean body site during patient care
- After contact with inanimate objects (including medical equipment) in the immediate vicinity of the patient

Alternatively, if alcohol-based hand rub is not available, health care workers may wash hands in all clinical situations (CDC, 2017a). Also, health care workers are advised to wash their hands with soap and water if patient exposure to *C. difficile* is suspected or proven. The physical action of washing and rinsing hands under such circumstances is recommended because alcohol-based hand rub has poor activity against spores (Association for Professionals in Infection Control and Epidemiology [APIC], 2013; World Health Organization [WHO], 2009).

Nurses need to instruct patients and visitors about the proper technique and times for hand hygiene. Nurses should ensure that patients and visitors understand the importance of cleaning under their nails and that artificial nails should not be worn because they harbour increased numbers of pathogens. Teaching proper hand hygiene is particularly important if health care is to continue at home. Patients should wash their hands before eating or handling food; after handling contaminated equipment, linen, or organic material; and after elimination. Visitors are encouraged to wash their hands before eating or handling food, after coming in contact with infected patients, and after handling contaminated equipment or organic material.

Control of Portals of Entry. Many measures that control the exit of microorganisms likewise control their entrance. Maintaining the integrity of skin and mucous membranes reduces the chances of microorganisms reaching a host. The patient's skin should be kept well lubricated by using lotion as appropriate. Immobilized and debilitated patients are particularly susceptible to skin breakdown. Patients should not be positioned on tubes or objects that might cause breaks in the skin. Dry, wrinkle-free linen also reduces the chances of skin breakdown. Frequent turning and positioning are needed in order to prevent a patient's skin from becoming reddened. Frequent oral hygiene prevents the drying of mucous membranes. A water-soluble ointment keeps the patient's lips well lubricated.

After elimination, a woman should clean the rectum and perineum by wiping from the urinary meatus toward the rectum. Cleansing in a direction from the least to the most contaminated area helps reduce genitourinary infections. Meticulous and frequent perineal care is especially important in women who wear incontinence pads.

Patients, health care workers, and even housekeepers are at risk for acquiring infections from accidental needle sticks. After administering an injection or inserting an intravenous catheter, the nurse should engage any safety device and carefully dispose of needles in a puncture-resistant box (see Chapter 34). A stray needle lying in the bed linen or carelessly thrown into a wastebasket is a prime source of

SKILL 33-1 HAND HYGIENE

Delegation Considerations

- Monitor an unregulated care provider (UCP) to ensure that he or she is using the proper method of hand hygiene.
- Instruct the UCP to report any skin irritation from soaps or antimicrobials.

Equipment

- Easy-to-reach sink with warm running water
- Antimicrobial or regular soap
- Alcohol-based waterless antiseptic
- Paper towels or air dryer
- Clean plastic nail stick

PROCEDURE

STEPS	RATIONALE
1. Inspect surface of hands for breaks or cuts in skin or cuticles. Report and cover lesions before providing patient care.	• Open cuts or wounds can harbour high concentrations of microorganisms. Agency policy may prevent you from caring for high-risk patients. If dermatitis occurs, additional interventions may be needed.
2. Inspect hands for visible soiling.	• Lengthier handwashing is needed if soiling is heavy.
3. Inspect nails for length and presence of artificial acrylics or chipped nail polish.	• Nails should be short and filed because most microbes on hands come from beneath the fingernails. Nails should be free of artificial applications and chipped or old nail polish (CDC, 2017a).
4. Assess patient's risk for, or extent of, infection (e.g., white blood cell count, extent of open wounds, known medical diagnosis).	• Use of alcohol-based waterless antiseptic is encouraged if you will be working with patients who are immunosuppressed (CDC, 2017b).
5. Push wristwatch and long uniform sleeves above wrists. Avoid wearing rings. If worn, remove for the duration of the procedure.	• Provide complete access to fingers, hands, and wrists. Wearing of rings increases number of microorganisms on hands (CDC, 2017a).
6. If hands are visibly dirty or contaminated with protein-containing material, use water and plain soap or antimicrobial soap for handwashing:	
A. Stand in front of sink, keeping hands and uniform away from sink surface. (If hands touch sink during handwashing, repeat procedure.)	• Inside of sink is a contaminated area. Reaching over the sink increases the risk of touching the edge, which is contaminated.
B. Turn on water. Turn faucet on or push knee pedals laterally or press pedals with foot to regulate flow and temperature (see Step 6B illustration).	

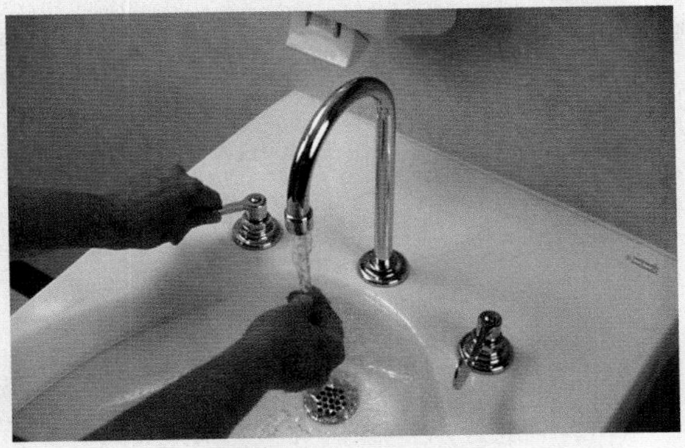

STEP 6B Turn on water.

STEPS	RATIONALE
C. Avoid splashing water against uniform.	• Microorganisms travel and grow in moisture.
D. Regulate flow of water so that temperature is warm.	• Warm water removes less of the protective oils than does hot water.
E. Wet hands and wrists thoroughly under running water. Keep hands and forearms lower than elbows during washing.	• Hands are the most contaminated parts to be washed. Water flows from least to most contaminated area, rinsing microorganisms into the sink.
F. Apply a small amount of soap, lathering thoroughly (see Step 6F illustration). Soap granules and leaflet preparations may be used.	• Antimicrobial soaps used exclusively can be drying to hands and can cause skin irritations. The decision of whether to use an antimicrobial soap or alcohol-based hand antiseptic should depend on the procedure to be performed and the patient's immune status.

Continued

SKILL 33-1 HAND HYGIENE—cont'd

STEPS	RATIONALE
G. Wash hands using plenty of lather and friction for at least 10 to 15 seconds. Interlace fingers and rub palms and back of hands with circular motion at least five times each. Keep fingertips down to facilitate removal of microorganisms. Rub knuckles of one hand into the palm of the other; repeat with other hand (see Step 6G illustration).	• Soap cleanses by emulsifying fat and oil and lowering the surface tension of water. Friction and rubbing mechanically loosen and remove dirt and transient bacteria. Interlacing fingers and thumbs and rubbing knuckles ensure that all surfaces are cleansed.

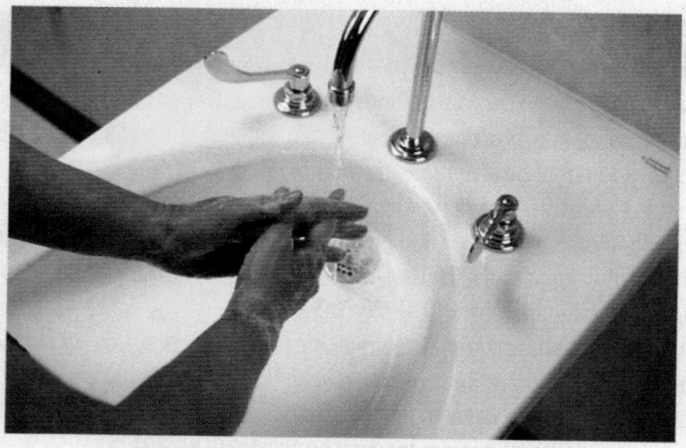

STEP 6F Lather hands thoroughly.

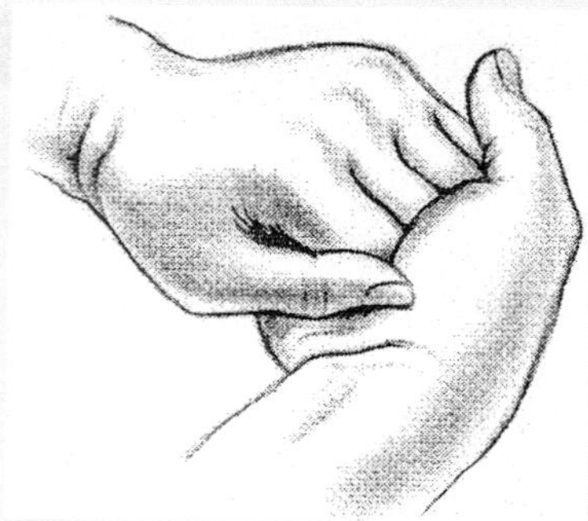

STEP 6G Rub the knuckles of one hand into the palm of the other. (Redrawn from World Health Organization. [2009]. World Alliance for Patient Safety, *WHO Guidelines on hand hygiene in health care. First global patient safety challenge: Clean care is safer care* [Handwashing technique with soap and water, p. 60, Step 15]. Retrieved from whqlibdoc.who.int/publications/2009/9789241597906_eng.pdf.)

STEPS	RATIONALE
H. Rub thumb on one hand with the palm of the other hand; repeat with other hand (see Step 6H illustration).	• Thumbs are frequently missed areas.
I. Work the fingertips on one hand into the palm of the other. Massage soap into nail spaces; repeat with other hand (see Step 6I illustration).	• Fingertips are frequently missed areas.

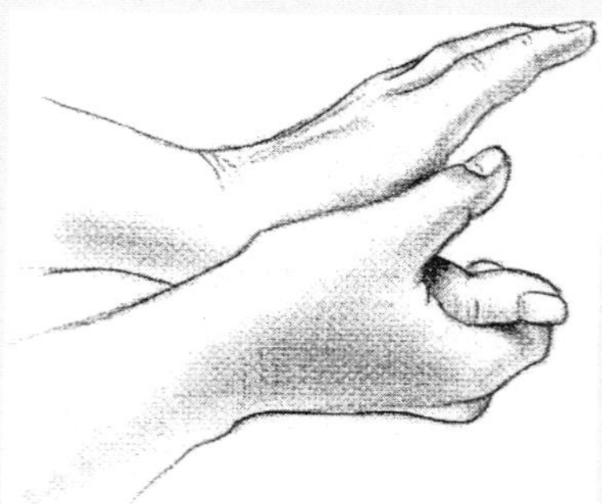

STEP 6H Rub the thumb into the palm of the other hand. (Redrawn from World Health Organization. [2009]. World Alliance for Patient Safety, *WHO Guidelines on hand hygiene in health care. First global patient safety challenge: Clean care is safer care* [Handwashing technique with soap and water, p. 60, Step 16]. Retrieved from whqlibdoc.who.int/publications/2009/9789241597906_eng.pdf.)

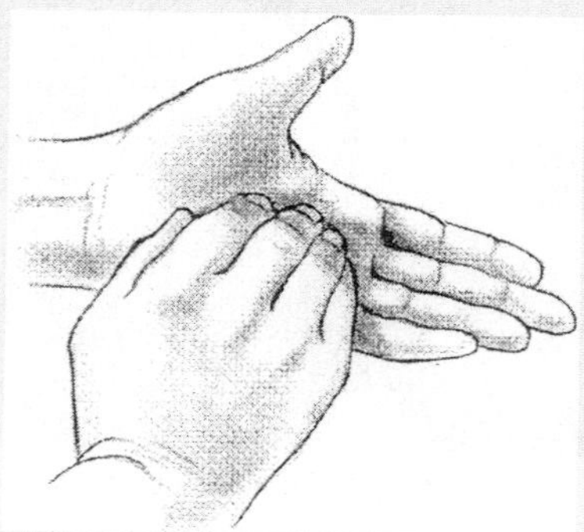

STEP 6I Work the fingertips into the palm of the other hand. (Redrawn from World Health Organization. [2009]. World Alliance for Patient Safety, *WHO Guidelines on hand hygiene in health care. First global patient safety challenge: Clean care is safer care* [Handwashing technique with soap and water, p. 59, Step 2]. Retrieved from whqlibdoc.who.int/publications/2009/9789241597906_eng.pdf.)

STEPS	RATIONALE
J. Areas under fingernails are often soiled. Clean them with orangewood stick or fingernails of other hand and additional soap.	• Areas under nails can be highly contaminated, which increases the risk of infection.

CRITICAL DECISION POINT: *Do not tear or cut skin under or around nail.*

STEPS	RATIONALE
K. Rinse hands and wrists thoroughly, keeping hands down and elbows up (see Step 6K illustration).	• Rinsing mechanically washes away dirt and microorganisms.
L. Optional: Repeat steps A through J and extend period of washing if hands are heavily soiled.	
M. Dry hands thoroughly from fingers to wrists and forearms with paper towel, single-use cloth, or warm-air dryer.	• Drying from cleanest (fingertips) to least clean (forearms) area avoids contamination. Drying hands prevents chapping and roughened skin.
N. If paper towel is used, discard it in proper receptacle.	• Prevents transfer of microorganisms.
O. Turn off water with foot or knee pedals. To turn off hand faucet, use clean, dry paper towel; avoid touching handles with hands (see Step 6O illustration).	• Faucets are contaminated. Using paper towels to touch faucet prevents contamination of hands.

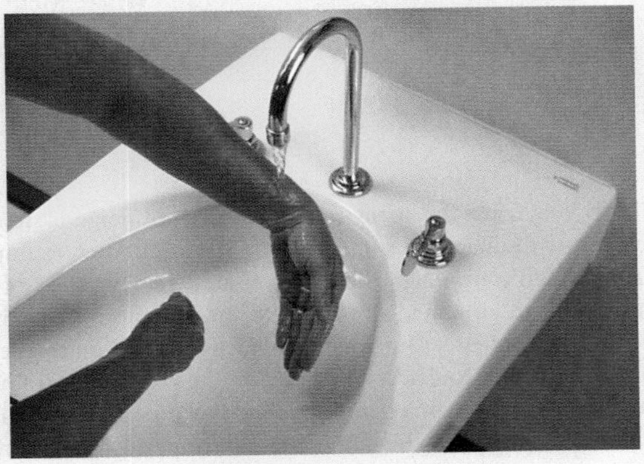

STEP 6K Rinse hands.

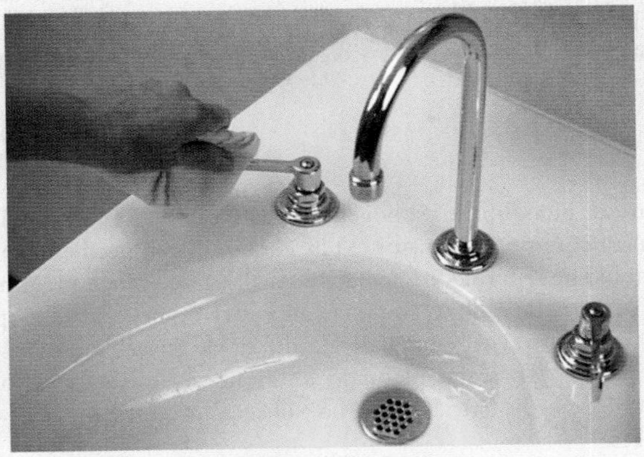

STEP 6O Turn off faucet.

STEPS	RATIONALE
P. If hands are dry or chapped, a small amount of lotion or barrier cream can be applied.	• Use agency-provided container of lotion because many lotions may interfere with antimicrobial action or disintegrate gloves.
Q. Inspect surfaces of hands for obvious signs of soil or other contaminants.	• Determine whether handwashing is adequate.
R. Inspect hands for dermatitis or cracked skin.	• The presence of these conditions indicates complications from excessive handwashing.
7. If hands are not visibly soiled, use an alcohol-based waterless antiseptic for routine decontamination of hands in all clinical situations.	
A. Apply an ample amount of product to palm of one hand (see Step 7A illustration).	• Enough product is needed to thoroughly cover the hands.
B. Rub hands together, covering all surfaces of hands and fingers with antiseptic (see Step 7B illustration).	• Complete coverage of the hands and fingers by using friction ensures antimicrobial effect.

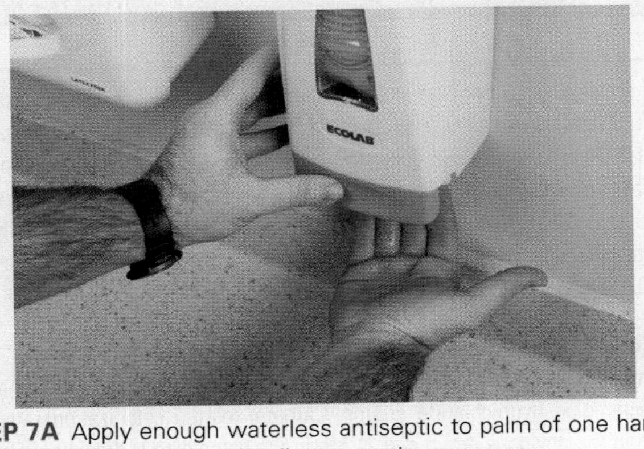

STEP 7A Apply enough waterless antiseptic to palm of one hand to cover all hand surfaces—usually two to three pumps.

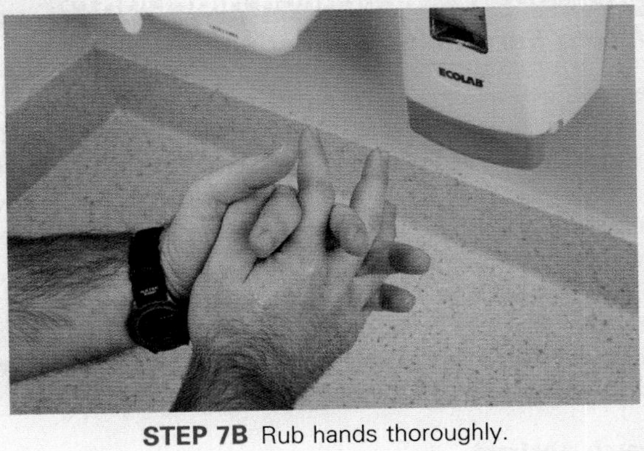

STEP 7B Rub hands thoroughly.

STEPS	RATIONALE
C. Rub hands together for several seconds until alcohol is dry. Allow hands to dry before applying gloves.	• Drying ensures full antiseptic effect (Public Health Agency of Canada, 2012b).
D. If hands are dry or chapped, a small amount of lotion or barrier cream can be applied.	• Use the agency-provided container of lotion because many lotions may interfere with antimicrobial action or disintegrate gloves.

Continued

SKILL 33-1 HAND HYGIENE—cont'd

STEPS	RATIONALE

RECORDING AND REPORTING

- It is not necessary to record or report this procedure.
- Report any dermatitis to employee health or infection control per agency policy.

HOME CARE CONSIDERATIONS

- Evaluate the handwashing facilities in the home to determine the possibility of contamination, the proximity of the facilities to the patient, and available supplies in the area.
- Evaluate the availability of warm running water and soap when conducting home visits, and anticipate the need for alternative handwashing products such as alcohol-based hand rubs and antiseptic wipes.
- Instruct the patient and primary caregiver in the proper techniques and situations for handwashing.

exposure to bloodborne pathogens. Hepatitis B and C are the infections most commonly transmitted by contaminated needles. A needle stick should be reported immediately. Health care agencies require the victim of a needle stick to complete an injury report and seek appropriate treatment. The Canadian Needle Stick Surveillance Network (PHAC, 2013b) has the mandate to monitor health care workers exposed to needle sticks and the subsequent outcomes of these exposures.

Another cause of microorganism entrance into a host is improper handling and management of urinary catheters and drainage sets (see Chapter 43). The point of connection between a catheter and drainage tube should remain closed and intact. As long as such systems are closed, their contents are considered sterile. Outflow spigots on drainage bags should also remain closed to prevent the entrance of bacteria. Movement of the catheter at the urethra should be minimized by stabilizing the catheter with tape to reduce chances of microorganisms ascending the urethra into the bladder. Urine-measuring containers should not be shared between patients.

Nurses may care for patients with closed drainage systems that collect wound drainage, bile, or other body fluids. In each example, the site from which a drainage tube exits should remain clear of excess moisture and accumulated drainage. All tubing should remain connected throughout use. Drainage receptacles should be opened only when it is necessary to discard or measure the volume of drainage.

At times, nurses will obtain specimens from drainage tubes or intravenous tubing ports. First, the nurse must perform hand hygiene; then tubes and ports are disinfected by wiping the surface outward with alcohol, iodine, or a chlorhexidine alcohol solution before entering the system (Box 33-12). Temporarily placing squares of sterile gauze around the ends of an open drainage tube, such as a urinary catheter, adds further protection against bacteria. However, keeping drainage tubes closed and secure is the best practice.

A final method for reducing the entrance of microorganisms is the technique for cleansing wounds (see Chapter 46). A surgical wound is considered to be sterile. To prevent the entrance of microorganisms into the wound, clean outward from a wound site. When applying an

BOX 33-12 RESEARCH HIGHLIGHT

Reducing Surgical Site Infections

Research Focus

Advances in medical technology have led to the creation of intravascular devices for the purpose of fluid and drug administration, hemodynamic monitoring, hemodialysis, and other functions that have improved the ability to deliver care. These catheters, though necessary, put the patients at risk for complications such as local skin infections, catheter-related bloodstream infections, septic thrombophlebitis, endocarditis, and metastatic infection. These conditions increase morbidity, mortality, length of stay, and cost of care. The intent of the double-blinded study discussed here was to compare the effects of three antiseptics in preventing catheter-related infections.

Research Abstract

Bilir, Yelken, and Erkan (2013) randomly assigned 57 Critical Care Unit (CCU) and anaesthetic patients who had undergone 109 intravascular catheter insertions (57 arterial catheters and 52 central venous catheters) to receive 10% povidone iodine (19), 4% chlorhexidine gluconate (19), or octenidine hydrochloride (19) as the skin antiseptic. The aim of the study was to compare the effects of the three antiseptics on bacterial colonization and local infection on the insertion site. The skin was cleansed with the antiseptic at the time of catheter insertion and daily thereafter for the duration of the study: Group I, 7.2 days; Group II, 7.8 days; and Group III, 7.5 days. The skin was observed for inflammation, infection, and allergic reactions to the antiseptics. There was a statistically significant difference between groups in catheter-related sepsis and colonization ($p < 0.001$).

Evidence-Informed Practice

Documented catheter-related sepsis was 10.5% in the povidone iodine group and octenidine hydrochloride groups. Catheter-related colonization rate was 26.3% in the povidone group and 21.5% in the octenidine hydrochloride group. In the chlorhexidine group, there was no catheter-related sepsis or colonization. The use of 4% chlorhexidine demonstrated a reduced incidence of catheter-related infection in the adult population who had catheter insertion in the CCU and anaesthetic setting.

Bilir, A., Yelken, B., & Erkan, A. (2013). Chlorhexidine, octenidine or povidone iodine for catheter related infections: A randomized controlled trial. *Journal of Research in Medical Science, 18*(6), 510–512.

antiseptic or cleaning with soap and water, wipe around the wound edge first and then clean outward away from the wound. Clean gauze should be used for each revolution around the wound's circumference.

Protection of the Susceptible Host. Patients' resistance to infection improves as nurses protect patients' normal body defences against infection. Nurses can intervene to maintain the body's normal reparative processes (Box 33-13). Nurses must also protect themselves and others by following their agency's isolation guidelines.

Isolation Guidelines. The risk of transmitting an HAI or infectious disease among patients is high. When a patient has a suspected or known infection, health care workers are alerted and follow infection control practices. However, sometimes health care workers are not aware that patients have infections. The majority of organisms causing nosocomial infections are found in the colonized body substances of patients regardless of whether a culture has confirmed infection and a diagnosis has been made (Siegel, Rhinehart, Jackson, et al., 2007). Body substances such as feces, saliva, mucus, and wound drainage always contain potentially infectious organisms.

The CDC issued isolation guidelines in 1996 that contain a two-tiered approach (Garner, 1996). These guidelines were updated and expanded on in 2007 and have been adopted by most health care agencies. Some health care agencies have adopted Health Canada's isolation guidelines (1999), which contain a similar two-tiered approach. The Health Canada guidelines were written to accommodate acute, long-term, home, and ambulatory care settings, whereas the CDC guidelines were written specifically for acute care settings. Nevertheless, the CDC guidelines and Health Canada's guidelines are essentially interchangeable.

The first tier of the isolation guidelines contains practices designed to care for all patients in any setting, regardless of their diagnosis or presumed infectiousness (Table 33-7). In Health Canada's guidelines, it is called *routine practices*. Routine practices apply when a health care worker is or potentially may be exposed to (1) blood; (2) all body fluids, secretions, and excretions except sweat; (3) nonintact skin; or (4) mucous membranes. Routine practices include the appropriate use of gowns, gloves, masks, eyewear, and other protective devices or clothing. Barrier protection is indicated for use with all patients because every patient has the potential to transmit infection via blood and body fluids and the risk for infection transmission can be unknown. Routine practices also include rules on appropriate handwashing, cleaning of equipment, and disposal of contaminated linen and sharps.

The second tier of the isolation guidelines is additional precautions. These precautions are designed to contain pathogens in one area, usually the patient's room; therefore, they are often called isolation precautions. Only patients infected or colonized with certain highly transmissible or epidemiologically significant pathogens are placed under isolation precautions. These precautions are followed in addition to routine practices. Isolation precautions are categorized in three ways: airborne, droplet, and contact precautions (see Table 33-7). The precautions used depend on how the pathogen is spread. For example, a patient diagnosed with (or suspected of having) active tuberculosis would require the use of airborne precautions, using a special mask and ventilated room, in conjunction with routine practices.

Regardless of the category of isolation precaution (Box 33-14), nurses must observe the following basic principles:

- Observe thorough hand hygiene before entering and leaving the room of a patient in isolation.
- Dispose of contaminated supplies and equipment in a manner that prevents the spread of microorganisms to other persons as indicated by the mode of transmission of the organism.
- Apply knowledge of a disease process and the mode of infection transmission when using protective barriers.
- Ensure that all persons who might be exposed during transport of a patient outside the isolation room are protected.

Psychological implications of isolation precautions. A patient required to be in isolation in a private room may become lonely because normal social relationships are disrupted. This situation can be psychologically harmful, especially for children (Box 33-15).

Patients' body image may be altered as a result of the infectious process. Patients may feel unclean, rejected, lonely, or guilty. Infection prevention and control practices further intensify these feelings of difference or undesirability. Isolation in a private room limits sensory contact. Unless nurses act to minimize feelings of psychological and physical isolation, patients' emotional state can interfere with their recovery.

Before isolation measures are instituted, a patient and family must understand the nature of the disease or condition, purposes of isolation, and steps for carrying out specific precautions. If they are able to participate in maintaining infection prevention, the chances of reducing the spread of infection are increased. The patient and family should be taught to perform hand hygiene and use barrier protection if appropriate. Each procedure should be demonstrated, and the patient and family should be given an opportunity to practise it. It is also important to explain how infectious organisms can be transmitted so that the patient understands the difference between contaminated and clean objects.

Nurses should take measures to improve the patient's sensory stimulation during isolation. The room environment should be clean and pleasant. Drapes or shades should be opened, and excess supplies and equipment removed. Nurses must listen to the patient's concerns or interests. If the nurse hurries through care or shows a lack of interest, the patient will feel rejected and even more isolated. Mealtime is a particularly good opportunity for conversation. Providing comfort measures such as repositioning, a back massage, or a tepid sponge bath increases physical stimulation. If appropriate for the patient's condition, the nurse should encourage the patient to walk and to sit up in a

BOX 33-13 Infection Control: Protecting the Susceptible Host

Protecting Normal Defence Mechanisms

Regular bathing removes transient microorganisms from the skin's surface. Lubrication helps keep the skin hydrated and intact.

Regular oral hygiene removes proteins in the saliva that attract microorganisms. Flossing removes tartar and plaque that can cause infection.

Maintenance of adequate fluid intake promotes normal urine formation and a resultant outflow of urine to flush the bladder and urethral lining of microorganisms.

For physically dependent or immobilized patients, nurses should encourage routine coughing and deep breathing to keep patients' lower airways clear of mucus.

Nurses should encourage proper immunization of children and adult patients (see Box 33-9).

Maintaining Healing Processes

Nurses need to encourage the intake of adequate fluids and a well-balanced diet containing essential proteins, vitamins, carbohydrates, and fats. Nurses should also use measures to increase the patient's appetite.

A patient's comfort and sleep need to be promoted as both are vital to replenishing energy stores on a daily basis.

Nurses can assist a patient in learning techniques to reduce stress.

TABLE 33-7 Health Canada Routine Practices and Additional Precautions

Routine Practices

Routine practices and precautions are for the care of all patients; they incorporate previous precautions against bloodborne pathogens (Universal Precautions) and body substance isolation.

Hand hygiene must be performed before and after direct patient contact; before and after contact with the patient's environment; after contact with blood, body fluids, secretions, and excretions and after contact with equipment or articles contaminated by them; before gloves are put on and immediately after gloves are removed. (Refer to the agency's policy for use of alcohol-based waterless antiseptics.)

Gloves are worn when touching blood, body fluids, secretions, excretions, nonintact skin, mucous membranes, or contaminated items. Gloves should be removed and hand hygiene performed between care of patients. Gloves should also be changed and hand hygiene performed between procedures on the same patient and after contact with material that may be highly contaminated.

Masks, eye protection, or face shields are worn if patient care activities or procedures may generate splashes or sprays of blood or body fluid.

Gowns should be used to protect uncovered skin and prevent soiling of clothing during procedures and patient care activities likely to generate a splash or spray of blood or body fluid.

Reusable patient care equipment is properly cleaned and reprocessed before use in the care of another patient. Single-use items are discarded.

All soiled linen from health care facilities should be handled the same way for all patients. If the bag soaks through, an additional bag should be used.

Used sharp instruments and needles are discarded in a puncture-resistant container, which is located in the area where the item is used.

Generally, a single room is unnecessary for routine patient care. Patients who visibly soil the environment or for whom appropriate hygiene cannot be maintained should be placed in a single room with dedicated toileting facilities.

ADDITIONAL (ISOLATION) PRECAUTIONS (TIER TWO)

Category	Description and Disease	Barrier Protection
Airborne precautions	For known or suspected infections caused by microbes transmitted by airborne droplets; examples: measles, chicken pox (varicella), disseminated zoster, tuberculosis	Private room (room door kept closed), negative-pressure airflow of at least six exchanges per hour, respiratory protection device (e.g., N95 respirator) must be worn when the patient has tuberculosis or when the patient has varicella, disseminated zoster, or measles and the worker is not immune
Droplet precautions	For known or suspected infections caused by microbes transmitted by droplets produced by coughing, sneezing, or talking; examples: diphtheria (pharyngeal), rubella, influenza, pertussis, mumps, meningococcal pneumonia, sepsis	Private room or cohort patients (room door closed unless bed is more than 2 m from the door), mask is worn when within 2 m of the patient
Contact precautions	For known or suspected infections caused by direct or indirect contact; examples: colonization or infection with multidrug-resistant organisms; *C. difficile*; major wound infections; gastrointestinal, respiratory, or skin infections	Private room or cohort patients (door can be open); gloves and gown upon entry into isolation room; limiting patient movement outside isolation room to necessary medical treatments or procedures; cleaning and disinfecting or discarding items before removal from isolation room

Adapted from Canadian Committee on Antibiotic Resistance. (2007). *Infection prevention and control best practices for long term care, home and community care including health care offices and ambulatory clinics.* Retrieved from http://www.designit.ca/ccar/english/pdfs/IPC-BestPractices-June2007.pdf.

BOX 33-14 PROCEDURAL GUIDELINE

Caring for a Patient on Isolation Precautions

Delegation Considerations

Care of a patient in isolation can be delegated to an unregulated care provider (UCP) when necessary procedures are within the UCP's competence.

Equipment

- Barrier protection determined by type of isolation
- Supplies necessary for procedures performed in room

Procedure

1. Assess isolation indications (e.g., current laboratory test results or the patient's history of exposure).
2. Review agency policies and precautions necessary for the specific isolation category, and consider care measures to be performed while in the patient's room.
3. Review nurses' notes or confer with colleagues regarding the patient's emotional state and adjustment to isolation.
4. Perform hand hygiene and prepare all equipment to be taken into the patient's room.
5. Prepare for entrance into isolation room:
   A. Perform hand hygiene.
   B. Apply gown (when needed), making sure it covers you from neck to knees. Pull sleeves down to wrist. Tie securely at neck and waist (see Step 5B illustration).

BOX 33-14 PROCEDURAL GUIDELINE

Caring for a Patient on Isolation Precautions—cont'd

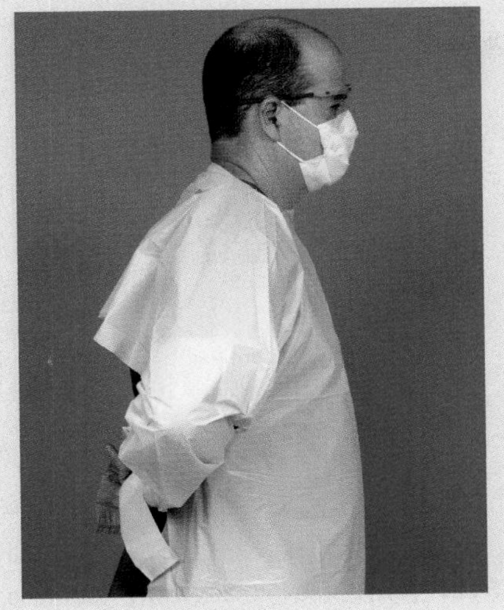

STEP 5B Tie gown at waist.

C. Apply either surgical mask or respirator around mouth and nose when needed. (Type will depend on type of isolation and facility policy.)

D. Apply eyewear or goggles snugly and adjust to fit around face and eyes (when needed).

E. Apply disposable nonsterile gloves for isolation. (Note: Unpowdered, latex-free gloves should be worn if the patient or the health care worker has a latex allergy.) If gloves are worn with a gown, bring the glove cuffs over edge of the gown sleeves.

6. Enter the patient's room. Arrange supplies and equipment. (If equipment will be removed from room for reuse, place it on a clean paper towel.)
7. Explain purpose of isolation and necessary precautions to the patient and family. Offer an opportunity to ask questions. Assess for evidence of emotional problems that may be caused by being in isolation.
8. Assess vital signs:
   A. If patient is infected or colonized with a resistant organism (e.g., methicillin-resistant *Staphylococcus aureus* [MRSA]), the equipment remains in room. Proceed to assess vital signs. Avoid contact of stethoscope or blood pressure cuff with infectious material.
   B. If stethoscope is to be reused, the entire stethoscope must be thoroughly cleaned after leaving the room. You may use a few alcohol swabs to clean and disinfect the stethoscope. (Ideally, equipment is dedicated for the use of the patient with an antibiotic-resistant organism and remains in the room.) Clean diaphragm or bell with alcohol. Set aside on clean surface.
   C. Individual or disposable thermometers should be used.
9. Administer medications:
   A. Give oral medication in wrapper or cup.
   B. Dispose of wrapper or cup in plastic-lined receptacle.
   C. Administer injection.
   D. Discard syringe and uncapped needle or sheathed needle into special container.
   E. If gloves are not worn and hands contact contaminated article or body fluids, wash hands immediately.
10. Administer hygiene measures, encouraging the patient to discuss questions or concerns about isolation. Informal teaching can be used at this time:
    A. Prevent the gown from becoming wet.
    B. Remove linen from the bed; avoid contact with the gown. Place linen in an impervious bag.
    C. Change gloves and wash your hands if they become excessively soiled and further care is necessary.
11. Collect specimens:
    A. Place specimen containers on a clean paper towel in the patient's bathroom.
    B. Follow procedure for collecting specimen of body fluids.
    C. Transfer specimen to the container without soiling the outside of the container. Place the container in a plastic bag, and place a label on the outside of the bag or as per agency policy.

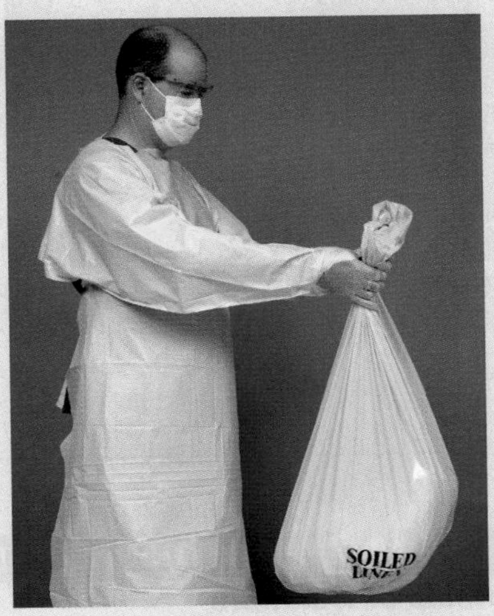

STEP 12B Tie linen bag securely.

12. Dispose of linen and garbage bags as they become full:
    A. Use sturdy, moisture-resistant single bags to contain soiled articles.
    B. Tie bags securely at the top in a knot (see Step 12B illustration).
13. Resupply room as needed.
14. When leaving isolation room, remove personal protective equipment, except for N95 respirator, inside doorway or in anteroom. Remove N95 respirator after leaving the patient's room and closing the door.
    A. Remove gloves. Remove one glove by grasping the cuff and pulling the glove inside out over the hand. Discard the glove. With the ungloved hand, tuck a finger inside the cuff of the remaining glove and pull it off, inside out.
    B. Perform hand hygiene.
    C. Untie waist and neck strings of the gown. Allow the gown to fall from your shoulders. Remove hands from sleeves without touching the outside of the gown (see Step 14C illustration). Hold the gown inside at shoulder seams and fold inside out; discard in laundry bag.

Continued

BOX 33-14 PROCEDURAL GUIDELINE

Caring for a Patient on Isolation Precautions—cont'd

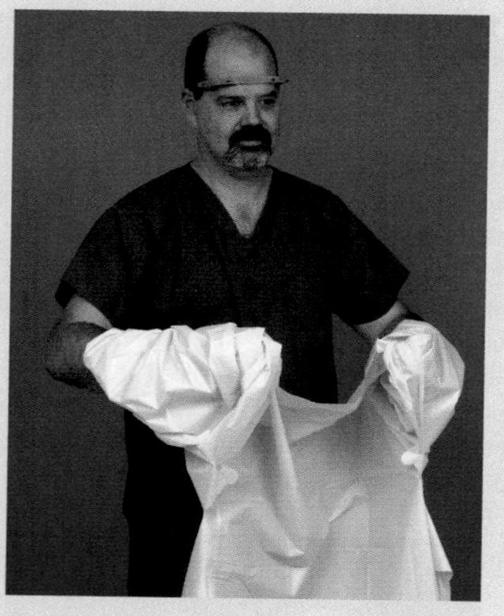

STEP 14C Remove hands from sleeves without touching outside of the gown.

D. Perform hand hygiene.
E. Untie first bottom mask string and then top strings; pull the mask away from your face, and drop the mask into a waste receptacle (see Step 14E illustration). (Do not touch outer surface of mask.)

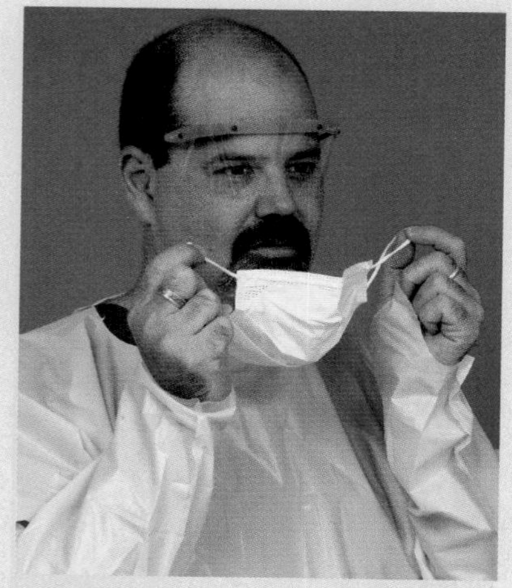

STEP 14E Remove mask away from face.

F. Remove eyewear or goggles.
G. Perform handwashing and hand hygiene.
H. Explain to the patient when you plan to return to the room. Ask whether the patient requires any personal-care items, books, or magazines.
I. Leave the room and close the door, if necessary. (Door should be closed if airborne precautions are being used.)
J. All contaminated supplies and equipment should be disposed of in a manner that prevents the spread of microorganisms to other individuals (see your agency's policy).

BOX 33-15 RESEARCH HIGHLIGHT

Adverse Effects of Isolation

Research Focus

Antonio and Jensen (2014) reviewed the impact of isolation due to antibiotic-resistant organisms on hospitalized elderly patients and on nursing care.

Research Abstract

Twenty-eight research articles were retrieved from Medline, Cumulative Index to Nursing and Allied Health Literature (CINAHL), Ovid EBMR Reviews, and Scopus databases looking at the impact of isolation on persons older than 65 years of age. Adverse psychological consequences of isolation included depression, anxiety, anger, hostility, loneliness, neglect, and low self-esteem. Adverse physiological effects included falls, malnutrition, the development of pressure injuries, and fluid and electrolyte imbalances. Secondarily, inattention from health care staff was noted, including taking longer to answer the call bell, lack of explanations, and less time being spent with the patients, resulting in increased incontinence. Decreased physiotherapy and occupational and recreational therapies were also noted.

Evidence-Informed Practice

- Nurses must be extra vigilant to ensure the standard of care is similar for all patients, including those on isolation precautions.
- Nurses should ensure that both physical and psychological factors are addressed when planning and carrying out care for isolated patients.
- Nurses must be sure to record observations and complete nursing notes for all patients, including those in isolation.

Antonio, N., & Jensen, L. (2014). Improving clinical practice in the management of elderly patients hospitalized with antimicrobial resistant organisms. *Journal of Nursing Education and Practice, 4*(8), 107–114.

chair. Recreational activities such as board games or cards may be an option to keep the patient mentally stimulated.

Nurses must explain to the family the patient's risk for depression or loneliness. Visiting family members should be taught the principles of isolation and encouraged to avoid expressions or actions that convey revulsion, fear, or disgust. Ways to provide meaningful stimulation should also be discussed.

Protective Environment. Private rooms used for isolation may have negative-pressure airflow to prevent infectious particles from flowing out of the room. Special rooms with positive-pressure airflow are used for highly susceptible patients, such as organ transplant recipients. On the door or wall outside the room, the nurse needs to post a card listing the precautions for the isolation category according to the agency's policy. The card is a handy reference for health care workers and visitors, and it alerts anyone who might enter the room that special precautions must be followed.

The isolation room should contain hand hygiene, bathing, and toilet facilities. Soap and water and alcohol-based hand rub must be made available. Personnel and visitors perform hand hygiene before approaching the patient's bedside and again before leaving the room.

If toilet facilities are unavailable, special procedures for handling portable commodes, bedpans, or urinals must be followed. Personal protective equipment should be stored in an anteroom between the room and hallway or in a convenient location close to the point of use.

All patient care rooms, including those used for isolation, contain an impervious bag for soiled or contaminated linen as well as a waste receptacle with plastic liners. Impervious receptacles stop the transmission of microorganisms by preventing seepage and soiling of the outside surface. A disposable rigid container should be available in the room for discarding of used needles, syringes, and sharp objects.

Nurses should remain aware of infection prevention and control techniques while working with patients in protected environments. Depending on the microorganism and the mode of transmission, the nurse must evaluate what articles or equipment may be taken into an isolation room. For example, the Public Health Agency of Canada (2012a) recommends the dedicated use of articles such as stethoscopes, sphygmomanometers, and rectal thermometers in the isolation room of a patient infected or colonized with methicillin-resistant *Staphylococcus aureus* (MRSA). These devices should not be used on other patients unless the devices are first adequately cleaned and disinfected. If the nurse brings an article into the room, exposes the article to infected material, and then touches or removes the article, the nurse increases the risk of transmitting infection to other patients or personnel.

Personal protective equipment. Personal protective equipment (gowns, masks, protective eyewear, and gloves) should be readily available. The primary reason for gowning is to prevent the contamination of clothes during contact with the patient. Gowns and cover-ups protect health care workers and visitors from coming in contact with infected material, blood, or body fluid. Gowns may also be required for contact precautions, depending on the expected amount of exposure to infectious material. Gowns used for barrier protection are made of a fluid-resistant material and should be changed immediately if damaged or heavily contaminated.

Isolation gowns usually open at the back and have ties or snaps at the neck and waist to keep the gown closed and secure. They should be long enough to cover all outer garments. Long sleeves with tight-fitting cuffs provide added protection. No special technique is required for applying clean gowns as long as they are fastened securely. However, nurses must be careful when removing a gown to minimize the contamination of their hands and uniform. Isolation gowns are disposable or reusable, depending on the agency's policy.

Full face protection (with eyes, nose, and mouth covered) should be worn when splashing or spraying of blood or body fluid into the face is possible. Masks and eye protection should also be worn when working with a patient placed on droplet precautions; they protect the wearer from inhaling microorganisms from a patient's respiratory tract and prevent the transmission of pathogens from the wearer's respiratory tract to the patient. Surgical masks protect a wearer from inhaling large-particle aerosols that travel short distances (2 m). Eye protection protects a wearer from receiving large-particle droplets to the eye. Prescription eye glasses are not considered suitable eye protection. At times, a patient who is susceptible to infection wears a mask to prevent inhalation of pathogens. Patients on droplet or airborne precautions who are transported outside their rooms should wear masks to protect other patients and personnel. According to the CDC (2017b), masks may prevent the transmission of infection through direct contact with mucous membranes. In addition, masks discourage the wearer from touching the eyes, nose, or mouth.

A properly applied mask fits snugly over the mouth and nose so that pathogens and body fluids cannot enter or escape through the sides (Box 33-16). If a person wears glasses, the top edge of the mask fits below the glasses so that the glasses do not cloud over as the person exhales. Talking should be kept to a minimum while wearing a mask to reduce respiratory airflow—a mask that has become moist may not provide a barrier to microorganisms and should be discarded. A mask should never be reused. Patients and family members should be warned that a mask can cause a sensation of smothering. If family members

BOX 33-16 PROCEDURAL GUIDELINE

Donning a Surgical-Type Mask

Procedure

1. Find top edge of the mask (usually has a thin metal strip). The pliable metal fits snugly against bridge of nose.
2. Hold the mask by the top two strings or loops. Tie the two top ties at the top of back of the head (see Step 2 illustration), with ties above ears (alternative: slip loops over each ear).

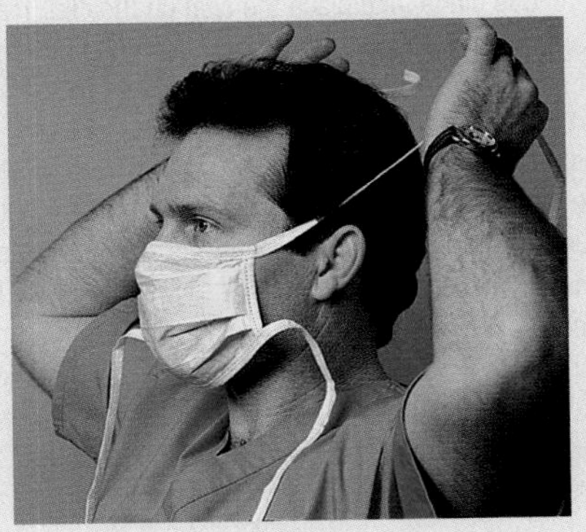

STEP 2 Tie two top ties at top of back of head.

3. Tie the two lower ties snugly around the neck, with mask well under chin (see Step 3 illustration).

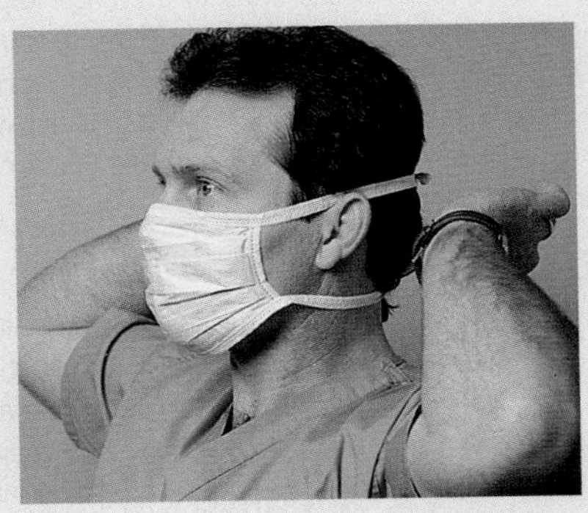

STEP 3 Tie two lower ties snugly around the neck.

4. Gently pinch upper metal band around bridge of nose.

Note: Mask should be changed if it becomes wet, moist, or contaminated.

become uncomfortable wearing a mask, they should leave the room and discard the mask.

Specially fitted respiratory protective devices or N95 masks are required when nurses care for a patient with known or suspected tuberculosis or when the patient has varicella, disseminated zoster, or measles and the worker is not immune. The mask must have a higher filtration rating than the regular surgical mask and be fitted snugly to the wearer's face to prevent leakage around the sides. Nurses should be aware of their agency's policy regarding the type of respiratory protective device required.

Gloves help to prevent the transmission of pathogens by direct and indirect contact. Clean, nonsterile gloves (also called disposable gloves) should be worn when contact with blood, body fluid, secretions, excretions, or contaminated items is possible. Clean gloves should be donned just before touching mucous membranes and nonintact skin. Gloves should be changed between tasks and procedures on the same patient after contact with material that may contain a high concentration of microorganisms. Gloves should be removed promptly after use, before touching noncontaminated items and environmental surfaces, and before going to another patient. Hand hygiene should be performed immediately after removing the gloves to avoid the transfer of microorganisms to other patients and environments. Facilities provide nonlatex gloves for health care staff who are allergic or sensitive to latex. When full protective apparel is needed, the nurse must first perform hand hygiene, apply a mask and eyewear or goggles (as needed), apply a gown, and then put on gloves. Disposable gloves are easily applied and are designed to fit either hand. The glove cuffs should be pulled up over the wrists or over the cuffs of the gown. The gloves' thin rubber can be easily torn; if a break or tear is detected in a glove while providing care, the nurse should change gloves if care is not completed. If no additional contact with the patient is planned, reapplying gloves is unnecessary.

Family members visiting patients who are in isolation that necessitates the use of gloves must know when and how to apply gloves properly. Nurses need to demonstrate the application of gloves to family members and explain the reason for glove use, placing emphasis on the importance of hand hygiene after the removal of gloves.

When participating in a procedure that may create droplets or splashing or spraying of blood or other body fluids, nurses must wear protective eyewear and a mask or a face shield (PHAC, 2012a). Examples of such procedures are the irrigation of a large abdominal wound or the insertion of an arterial catheter in which the nurse assists a physician. Eyewear may be available in the form of plastic glasses or goggles. They should fit snugly around the face so that fluids cannot enter between the face and the glasses.

Specimen collection. Often, many laboratory studies are required when a patient is suspected of having an infectious disease. Body fluids and secretions suspected of containing infectious organisms are collected for culture and sensitivity tests. The specimen is placed in a medium that promotes the growth of organisms. A laboratory technologist then identifies the microorganisms growing in the culture. Additional test results indicate antibiotics to which the organisms are resistant or sensitive, and sensitivity reports determine the antibiotics to be used in treatment.

Nurses need to obtain all culture specimens using disposable gloves and sterile equipment. Collecting fresh material from the site of the infection, such as wound drainage, ensures that the specimen is not contaminated by neighbouring microbes. All specimen containers should be sealed tightly to prevent spillage and contamination of the outside of the container. Box 33-17 describes the techniques for collecting specimens from a patient with a suspected infection.

Bagging waste or linen. Nurses should use special bagging procedures when removing contaminated items from a patient's environment. Bagging contaminated items and ensuring that the outside of the bag is not contaminated prevents accidental exposure of personnel and contamination of the surrounding environment.

The Public Health Agency of Canada (2012a) recommends using a single bag for discarding items if the bag is impervious and sturdy and if the article can be placed in the bag without contaminating the outside of the bag. Soiled linen should be placed in an impervious laundry bag in the patient's room. Double bagging is recommended *only* if it is impossible to prevent the contamination of the bag's outer surface. Studies have shown that double bagging is otherwise not necessary to control infection (Maki, Alvarado, & Hassemer, 1986).

BOX 33-17 Specimen Collection Techniques*

Wound Specimen

Clean the site with sterile water or saline before wound specimen collection. Wear gloves and use a cotton-tipped swab or a syringe to collect as much drainage as possible. Set a clean test tube or culture tube on a clean paper towel close by. After swabbing the centre of the wound site, grasp the collection tube by holding it with a paper towel. Carefully insert the swab without touching the outside of the tube. After securing the tube's top, transfer the tube into a bag for transport and then perform hand hygiene.

Blood Specimen

Wearing gloves, use a syringe and culture media bottles to collect up to 10 mL of blood per culture bottle (check your agency's policy about exact amounts required). After prepping the patient, perform a venipuncture at two different sites to decrease the likelihood of both specimens being contaminated with skin flora. Place the blood culture bottles on the bedside table or another surface; swab off the bottle tops with alcohol. Inject the appropriate amount of blood into each bottle. Transfer the specimen into a clean, labelled bag for transport and remove gloves. Perform hand hygiene.

Stool Specimen

Wearing gloves, use a clean cup with sealing top (it does not need to be sterile) and a tongue blade to collect a small amount of stool, approximately the size of a walnut: place the cup on a clean paper towel in the patient's bathroom; using the tongue blade, collect the needed amount of feces from the patient's bedpan; transfer the feces to the cup without touching the cup's outside surface. Dispose of the tongue blade, and place the seal on the cup. Transfer the specimen into a clean bag for transport. Remove gloves and perform hand hygiene.

Urine Specimen

Wearing gloves, use a syringe and sterile cup or tube to collect 1 to 5 mL of urine. Place the cup or tube on a clean towel in the patient's bathroom. If the patient has a urinary catheter, use the syringe to collect the specimen. If the patient is not catheterized, have the patient follow the procedure to obtain a clean voided specimen (see Chapter 43). Transfer the urine into a sterile container by injecting urine from the syringe or by pouring it from the collection cup. Secure the top of the container and transfer the specimen into a clean, labelled bag for transport. Remove gloves and perform hand hygiene.

*Agency policies may differ on the type of containers and amount of specimen material required.
Data from Pagana, K. D., Pagana, T. J., & Pike-MacDonald, S. A (2013). *Mosby's Canadian manual of diagnostic and laboratory tests* (1st Canadian ed.). Toronto: Mosby/Elsevier.

The use of one standard-sized linen bag that is not overfilled, is tied securely, and is intact is adequate to prevent infection transmission. The same rule applies to garbage bags.

Transporting patients. Before transferring patients to wheelchairs or stretchers, the nurse should have the patients perform hand hygiene and give the patients clean gowns and robes. Patients infected with organisms transmitted by the airborne route should leave their rooms only for essential purposes, such as diagnostic procedures or surgery. These patients must also wear masks. Personnel transporting these patients may also need to wear barrier protection depending on the amount of contact they will be having with the patient.

At times, a patient being transported may drain body fluids onto a stretcher or wheelchair. When this occurs, the nurse must be sure to have the equipment cleaned and, if necessary, disinfected after the patient returns to the room. An extra layer of sheets may be used to cover the stretcher or seat of the wheelchair.

Personnel in diagnostic or procedural areas or the operating room should be notified that the patient is on isolation precautions. Record the type of isolation on the patient's chart. Explain to the patient ways that he or she can help prevent the transmission of infection during transport. A patient on airborne or droplet isolation is provided with a mask and given tissues and a bag to allow for the proper disposal of secretions.

Role of the Infection Control Professional. Many hospitals employ professionals who are specially trained in infection prevention and control; most of these professionals are nurses. These individuals are responsible for advising hospital personnel regarding infection prevention and control and for monitoring infections within the hospital. Infection Prevention and Control Canada (IPAC–Canada) is a voluntary multidisciplinary association of infection-control professionals. Its mission is to promote excellence in the practice of infection prevention and control (IPAC–Canada, 2017). The duties of an infection-control professional include the following:

- Provide staff with education on infection prevention and control.
- Develop and review infection prevention and control policies and procedures.
- Recommend appropriate isolation procedures.
- Screen patient records for community-acquired infections that may be reportable to the public health department.
- Consult with employee health departments concerning recommendations to prevent and control the spread of infection among personnel, such as tuberculosis testing.
- Gather statistics regarding the epidemiology (cause and effect) of HAIs.
- Notify the public health department of incidents of communicable diseases within the facility.
- Confer with all hospital departments to investigate unusual events or clusters of infection.
- Recommend education for patients and families.
- Identify infection-control problems related to equipment.
- Monitor antibiotic-resistant organisms in the institution.
- Monitor construction sites in hospitals to ensure that appropriate dust containment measures are used.

An infection-control professional can be a valuable resource for nurses in controlling HAIs.

Infection Prevention and Control for Hospital Personnel. Health care workers are continually at risk of exposure to infectious microorganisms. Each agency has protocols in place to advise staff and to monitor infection protocols. Hospitals offer regularly scheduled staff education programs. Each province and territory has rules and procedures to ensure that health care workers are not unnecessarily exposed to pathogens.

Patient Education. Often patients must learn to use infection control practices at home (Box 33-18). Preventive technique will become almost second nature to you as a nurse if practised daily, but your patients will be less aware of factors that promote the spread of

BOX 33-18 PATIENT TEACHING

Infection Control

Objective

- Patient will perform self-care using proper infection control techniques.

Teaching Strategies

- Instruct patient to clean equipment using soap and water and disinfect it with an appropriate disinfectant.
- Demonstrate proper hand hygiene, explaining that it should be done before and after all treatments and when infected body fluids are contacted.
- Inform patient of the signs and symptoms of wound infection.
- For patients who receive tube feedings at home, explain the importance of following instructions regarding how long formula can be prepared ahead of time and left unrefrigerated. Tell patient that contaminated enteral feedings can cause infections. Teach patient to care for the feeding bag and tubing as per the organizations protocol.
- Instruct patient to place contaminated dressings and other disposable items containing infectious body fluids in impervious plastic bags and to place needles in a puncture-proof and leak-proof container, such as an empty bleach bottle with the opening taped shut or a coffee can with the lid taped closed. Glass containers should not be used. Ensure that the patient knows to contact the local municipality or public health department before disposing of contaminated items (Provincial Infection Control Network of British Columbia [PICNet], 2014).
- Instruct patient (or family) to separate noticeably soiled linen from other laundry, wash it in water that is as hot as the fabric will tolerate, add 250 mL of bleach to detergent, and set the dryer temperature as high as the fabric will allow.

Evaluation

- Ask patient or family member to describe techniques used to reduce the transmission of infection.
- Ask patient to demonstrate select techniques.
- Ask patient to explain the risks for infection based on the condition.

After patients are at home, nurses need to educate them about infection and techniques to prevent or control its spread, and nurses need to determine their compliance with infection control practices. Family members caring for patients must be involved in the teaching plan—patients and family members should be taught a common-sense approach to controlling and preventing infection. Topics to address in a teaching session include the following:

- The patient's susceptibility to infection
- The chain of infection, with specific reference to the means of transmission
- Hygienic practices that minimize organism growth and spread; emphasize hand hygiene
- Preventive health care (e.g., proper diet, immunizations, and exercise)
- The proper methods for handling and storage of food
- An awareness of family members who are at risk for acquiring infection

infection and ways to prevent its transmission. The home environment does not always lend itself to infection prevention—often you must help patients adapt according to the resources available to maintain hygienic techniques. However, patients in a home care setting generally have a lower risk of infection than do patients in a hospital because they have less exposure to resistant organisms and undergo fewer invasive procedures.

Surgical Asepsis. Surgical asepsis, or sterile technique, requires precautions different from those of medical asepsis. Surgical asepsis includes procedures used to eliminate all microorganisms, including spores, from an object or area. In surgical asepsis, an area or object is considered contaminated if touched by any object that is not sterile. When nurses are working with a sterile field or with sterile equipment, they must understand that the slightest break in technique results in contamination. Surgical asepsis should be used in the following situations:

- During procedures that require the intentional perforation of the patient's skin (e.g., the insertion of intravenous catheters or administration of injections)
- When the skin's integrity is broken as a result of trauma, surgical incision, or burns
- During procedures that involve the insertion of catheters or surgical instruments into sterile body cavities

Although surgical asepsis is commonly practised in the operating room, labour and delivery area, and major diagnostic areas, nurses may also use surgical aseptic techniques at the patient's bedside; for example, when inserting intravenous or urinary catheters, suctioning the tracheobronchial airway, or reapplying sterile dressings. In an operating room, nurses must follow a series of steps to maintain sterile technique, including applying a mask, protective eyewear, and a cap; performing a surgical hand scrub; and applying a sterile gown and gloves. In contrast, when performing a dressing change at a patient's bedside, nurses may only perform hand hygiene and apply sterile gloves (see "Principles of Surgical Asepsis" section). When using the principles of surgical asepsis, nurses need to remember that they are trying to prevent infections. For more information on infection control, see Box 33-19.

Patient Preparation. Because surgical asepsis necessitates exact techniques, the nurse must have the patient's cooperation. Therefore, the nurse must prepare the patient before any procedure. Some patients may fear moving or touching objects during a sterile procedure, but others may try to assist. Nurses need to explain how a procedure is to be performed and what the patient can do to avoid contaminating sterile items, including the following:

- Avoid sudden movements of body parts covered by sterile drapes.
- Refrain from touching sterile supplies, drapes, or the nurse's gloves and gown.
- Avoid coughing, sneezing, or talking over a sterile area.

Certain sterile procedures may take an extended period of time. The nurse should assess the patient's needs and anticipate factors that may disrupt a procedure. If a patient is in pain, the nurse should try to administer analgesics no more than half an hour before a sterile procedure begins. The patient should be given the opportunity to void. Often patients must assume uncomfortable positions during sterile procedures; the nurse can help the patient to assume the most comfortable position possible. Finally, the patient's condition may result in actions or events that contaminate a sterile field. For example, a patient with a respiratory infection transmits organisms by coughing or breathing; the nurse needs to anticipate such a problem and offer the patient a mask.

Principles of Surgical Asepsis. When beginning a surgically aseptic procedure, nurses must follow certain principles to ensure the maintenance of asepsis. Failure to follow these principles places patients at risk for infection. The following principles are important:

1. *A sterile object remains sterile only when touched by another sterile object.* This principle guides nurses in the placement of sterile objects and how to handle them.
   A. Sterile objects that touch sterile objects remain sterile; for example, sterile gloves are worn or sterile forceps are used to handle objects on a sterile field.
   B. Sterile objects that touch clean objects become contaminated; for example, if the tip of a syringe or other sterile object touches the surface of a clean disposable glove, the object is contaminated.
   C. Sterile objects that touch contaminated objects become contaminated; for example, when you touch a sterile object with an ungloved hand, the object is contaminated.
   D. Sterile objects that touch questionable objects are considered contaminated; for example, when a tear or break in the covering or packaging of a sterile object is found, the object is discarded regardless of whether the object itself appears untouched.
2. *Only sterile objects may be placed on a sterile field.* All items are properly sterilized before use. Sterile objects are kept in clean, dry storage areas. The package or container holding a sterile object must be intact and dry—a package that is torn, punctured, wet, or open is considered to be contaminated.

BOX 33-19 Surgical Asepsis: Infection Control

Objective

- The goal of surgical asepsis or aseptic technique is to prevent microorganisms from becoming introduced to a susceptible site. It should also prevent transmission of microorganisms to other patients or to staff.

Principles

- Ensure that all required supplies are gathered and that there is a clear and dry field to carry out the procedure.
- Movement within or around a sterile field should be done in a manner that does not contaminate the sterile field.
- Sterile fields should be prepared as close to the time of use as possible; the potential for environmental contamination from dust and particles in the ambient environment that settle on surfaces increases over time.
- Conversation in a sterile field should be kept to a minimum to reduce contamination by means of respiratory droplets.
- Perform hand hygiene prior to setting up a sterile field.
- Ensure that the sterile barrier covering the supplies is intact, with no punctures or evidence of moisture damage.
- If there is any question of the item's sterility, the item must be considered unsterile.
- Open sterile packs carefully to prevent contamination of the contents of the pack.
- All items in a sterile field must be sterile.
- Once a sterile package is opened, a 2.5-cm border around the edges is considered unsterile.
- Pour solutions into receptacles on the sterile field slowly to avoid splashing. Splashing can cause strike-through or splash-back from nonsterile surfaces to the sterile field.
- An object is considered to be no longer sterile if it is below a person's waist or if it is out of the range of vision.
- Wear sterile gloves for the procedure to prevent the introduction of microorganisms to the site and to protect the wearer from coming into contact with body fluids.

3. *A sterile object or field out of the range of vision or an object held below a person's waist is contaminated.* You must never turn your back on a sterile tray or leave it unattended. Contamination can occur accidentally by a dangling piece of clothing, falling hair, or an unknowing patient touching a sterile object. Any object held below waist level is considered contaminated because it cannot be viewed at all times. Sterile objects should be kept in front of you with your hands as close together as possible.
4. *A sterile object or field becomes contaminated by prolonged exposure to air.* Nurses need to avoid activities that may create air currents, such as excessive movements or rearranging linen after a sterile object or field becomes exposed. When sterile packages are being opened, it is important to minimize the number of persons walking into the area. Microorganisms travel by droplets through the air; therefore, no one should talk, laugh, sneeze, or cough over a sterile field or when gathering and using sterile equipment. Microorganisms travelling through the air can fall on sterile items or fields if the nurse reaches over the work area. When opening sterile packages, hold the item or piece of equipment as close as possible to the sterile field without touching the sterile surface. Keeping the movement or rearranging of sterile items to a minimum also reduces contamination by air transmission.
5. *When a sterile surface comes in contact with a wet, contaminated surface, the sterile object or field becomes contaminated by capillary action.* If moisture seeps through a sterile package's protective covering, microorganisms travel to the sterile object. When stored sterile packages become wet, the objects must be discarded immediately or the equipment sent for resterilization. When working with a sterile field or tray, the nurse may have to pour sterile solutions. Any spill can be a source of contamination unless the object or field rests on a sterile surface that cannot be penetrated by moisture. Urinary catheterization trays contain sterile supplies that rest in a sterile, plastic container. In this example, sterile solutions spilled within the container will not contaminate the catheter or other objects. In contrast, if the nurse places a piece of sterile gauze in its wrapper on a patient's bedside table and the table surface is wet, the gauze is considered contaminated.
6. *Fluid flows in the direction of gravity.* A sterile object becomes contaminated if gravity causes a contaminated liquid to flow over the object's surface. To avoid contamination during a surgical hand scrub, the nurse holds his or her hands above the elbows. This allows water to flow downward without contaminating the hands and fingers. This is also the reason for drying from the fingers to elbows with hands held up, after the scrub.
7. *The edges of a sterile field or container are considered to be contaminated.* Frequently, sterile objects are placed on a sterile towel or drape (Figure 33-2). Because the edge of the drape touches an unsterile surface, such as a table or bed linen, a 2.5-cm border around the drape is considered contaminated. Objects placed on the sterile field must be inside this border. The edges of sterile containers become exposed to air after they are open and are thus contaminated. After a sterile needle is removed from its protective cap or after forceps are removed from a container, the objects must not touch the container's edge. The lip of an opened bottle of solution also becomes contaminated after it is exposed to air. When pouring a sterile liquid, first pour a small amount of solution to wash away microorganisms on the bottle lip. This small amount of solution is then discarded; pour a second time on the same side to fill a container with the desired amount of solution.

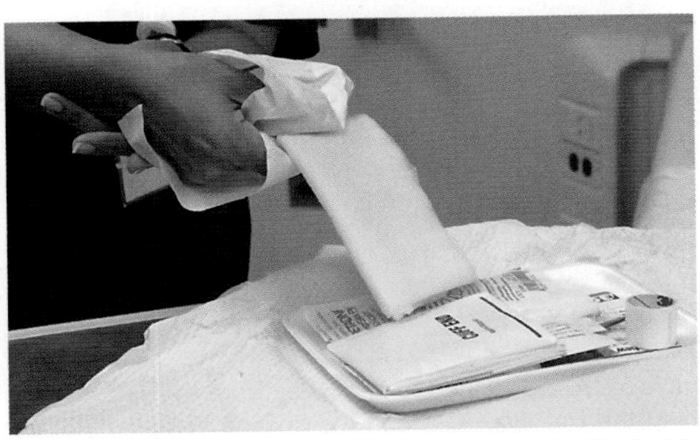

FIGURE 33-2 Placing sterile item on a sterile field.

Performing Sterile Procedures. All necessary equipment should be assembled before a procedure to avoid having to leave a sterile area to obtain equipment. A few extra supplies should be available in case objects accidentally become contaminated. Before the sterile procedure, each step should be explained so that the patient can cooperate fully. If an object becomes contaminated during the procedure, it should be discarded immediately.

Donning and removing caps, masks, and eyewear. For sterile procedures on a general nursing division, nurses may wear a surgical mask and eyewear without a cap. Eyewear is worn as a part of standard precautions or routine practices if fluid or blood could splash into the nurse's eyes. For sterile surgical procedures, the nurse must first apply a clean cap that covers all the hair and then put on the surgical mask and eyewear. The mask must fit snugly around the face and nose to prevent contamination by droplet nuclei. After a mask is worn for several hours, the area over the mouth and nose often becomes moist. Because moisture promotes the spread of microorganisms, the mask should be changed if it becomes moist.

Protective glasses or goggles should fit snugly around the forehead and face to fully protect the eyes. Eyewear needs to be worn only for procedures that create the risk of body fluids splashing into the eyes.

Before removing a mask, eyewear, and cap, remove the gloves to prevent contamination of the hair, neck, and facial area. After untying the mask, hold it by the ties and discard it with the cap. Masks should not be worn hanging from the neck after removal from the face. Eyewear is removed and cleaned later for reuse. After removing all protective wear, perform hand hygiene.

Opening sterile packages. Sterile items such as syringes, gauze dressings, and catheters are packaged in paper or plastic containers that are impervious to microorganisms as long as they are dry and intact. Some institutions wrap reusable supplies in a double thickness of paper, linen, or muslin. These packages are permeable to steam and thus allow for steam autoclaving. Sterile items are kept in clean, enclosed storage cabinets and are separated from nonsterile equipment.

Sterile supplies carry chemical tapes indicating that a sterilization process has taken place. The tapes change colour during the sterilization process; if the tapes do not change colour, the item is not sterile. A sterile item should never be used if the integrity of the packaging is compromised. Health care facilities may apply the date processed and a lot number to the item after processing ("event-related expiration"), or they may apply an expiration date ("date-related expiration") to the item. With either system, it is important for nurses to check the integrity of the packaging before using an item.

Before opening a sterile item, perform thorough hand hygiene. Inspect the supplies for package integrity and sterility and assemble the supplies in the work area, such as the bedside table or treatment room, before opening the packages. A cleaned bedside table or countertop provides a large, clean working area for opening items. The work area should be above waist level. Sterile supplies should not be opened in a confined space where a dirty object might fall on or strike them.

Opening a sterile item on a flat surface. Sterile packaged items must be opened without contaminating the contents. Commercially packaged items are usually designed so that the user has to tear away or separate only the paper or plastic cover. The item is held in one hand while the wrapper is pulled away with the other (Figure 33-3). Take care to keep the inner contents sterile before use. When opening items processed by the facility and packed in paper or linen, observe the following steps:

1. Place the item flat in the centre of the work surface.
2. Remove the sterilization tape or seal.
3. Grasp the outer surface of the tip of the outermost flap.
4. Open the outer flap away from the body, keeping the arm outstretched and away from the sterile field (Figure 33-4, *A*).
5. Grasp the outside surface of the first side flap.
6. Open the side flap, allowing it to lie flat on the table surface. Keep your arm to the side and not over the sterile surface (see Figure 33-4, *B*). Do not allow the flaps to spring back over the sterile contents.
7. Grasp the outside surface of the second side flap and allow it to lie flat on the table surface (see Figure 33-4, *C*).
8. Grasp the outside surface of the last and innermost flap.
9. Stand away from the sterile package and pull the flap back, allowing it to fall flat on the surface (see Figure 33-4, *D*).
10. Use the inner surface of the package (except for the 2.5-cm border around the edges) as a sterile field to add additional sterile items. The 2.5-cm border can be grasped to manoeuvre the field on the table surface.

If the sterile supplies are not for immediate use, you can close the sterile package. In this case, touch only the wrapper's outside surface. To close a package, the order of unwrapping is reversed, and you should not touch the inside contents or reach over the field.

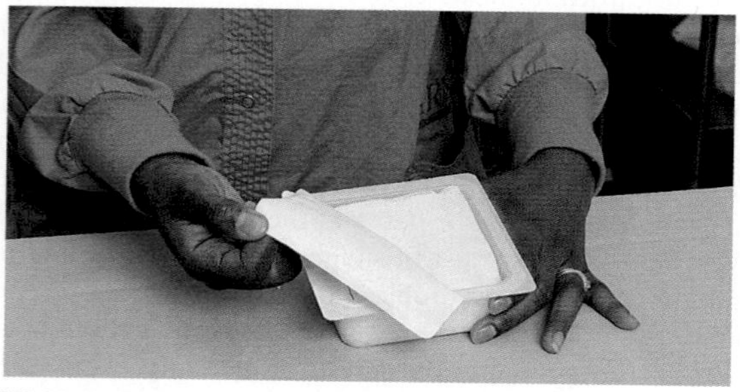

FIGURE 33-3 Opening a sterile package on a cleaned work area above waist level.

Opening a sterile item while holding it. To open a small, sterile item, hold the package in your nondominant hand. Using the dominant hand, carefully open the side and top flaps away from the enclosed sterile item in the order previously mentioned. Open the item in a hand so that the item can be handed to a person wearing sterile gloves or transferred to a sterile field.

Preparing a sterile field. When performing sterile procedures, nurses need a sterile work area that provides room for the handling and placing of sterile items. A **sterile field** is an area free of microorganisms and prepared to receive sterile items. The field may be prepared by using the inner surface of a sterile wrapper as the work surface or by using a sterile drape or dressing tray. Skill 33-2 describes preparation of a sterile field. After the surface for the field is created, add sterile items by carefully placing them directly on the field or by transferring them with a sterile forceps. A sterile object that comes in contact with the 2.5-cm border must be discarded.

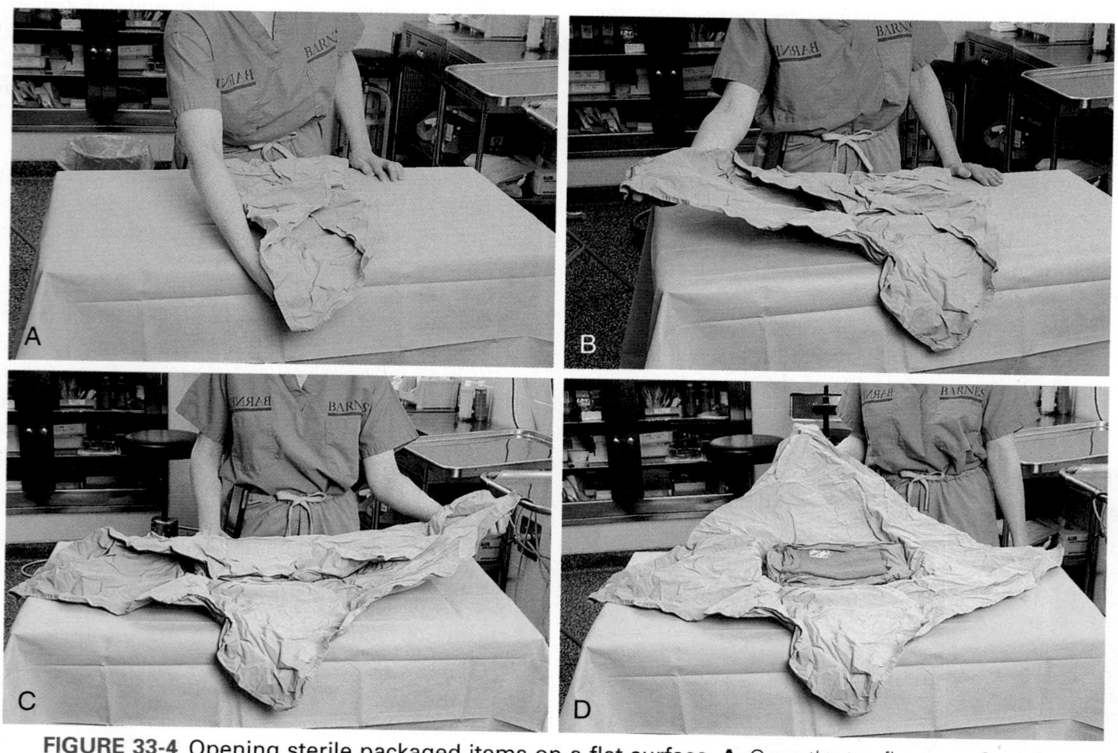

FIGURE 33-4 Opening sterile packaged items on a flat surface. **A**, Open the top flap away from the body. **B**, Keep your arm away from the sterile field while opening the side flap. **C**, Open the second side flap. **D**, Open the back flap.

SKILL 33-2 PREPARATION OF A STERILE FIELD

Delegation Considerations

Delegation of the preparation of a sterile field is inappropriate unless you are delegating to an unregulated care provider (UCP) who has received specialized training. Operating room technicians are usually trained for this skill.

Equipment

- Sterile drape
- Assorted sterile supplies

PROCEDURE

STEPS	RATIONALE
1. Prepare sterile field just before planned procedure. Supplies are to be used immediately.	• Prevents exposure of sterile field and supplies to air and contamination.
2. Select clean work surface above waist level.	• A once-sterile object held below the waist is considered contaminated.
3. Assemble necessary equipment.	• Preparation of equipment in advance prevents a break in the technique.
4. Check dates or labels on supplies for sterility of equipment.	• Equipment stored beyond expiration date is considered unsterile.
5. Perform hand hygiene. Option: Procedure may be performed with gloves on.	• Reduces microbial counts on skin.
6. Place pack containing sterile drape on work surface and open as described in Figure 33-4.	• Ensures sterility of packaged drape.
7. With fingertips of one hand, pick up folded top edge of sterile drape.	• The 2.5-cm border around drape is unsterile and may be touched with fingers or clean gloves.
8. Gently lift drape up from its outer cover and let it unfold by itself without touching any object. Discard outer cover with your other hand.	• If sterile object touches any nonsterile object, it becomes contaminated.
9. With your other hand, grasp adjacent corner of drape and hold it straight up and away from your body (see Step 9 illustration).	• Drape can now be properly placed while using two hands. Drape must be held away from unsterile surfaces.
10. Holding drape, first position and lay bottom half over intended work surface (see Step 10 illustration).	• Prevents reaching over sterile field.

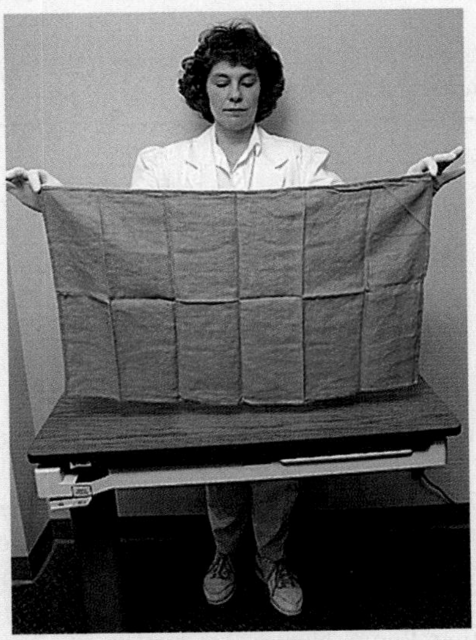

STEP 9 Hold drape straight up and away from body.

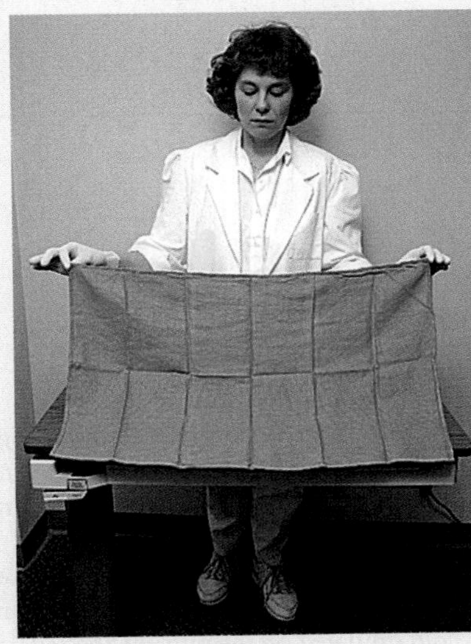

STEP 10 Lay bottom half of drape over work surface.

STEPS	RATIONALE
11. Allow top half of drape to be placed over work surface last (see Step 11 illustration).	• Creates flat sterile work surface.
12. Grasp 2.5-cm border around edge to position as needed.	• Assists in differentiating and organizing the sterile surface.
Adding Sterile Item	
13. Open sterile item (according to package directions) while holding outside wrapper in nondominant hand.	• Frees dominant hand for unwrapping outer wrapper.
14. Carefully peel wrapper onto nondominant hand. Do not shake item onto sterile field.	• Item remains sterile.

Continued

SKILL 33-2 PREPARATION OF A STERILE FIELD—cont'd

STEPS	RATIONALE
15. Being sure wrapper does not fall down on sterile field, place item onto field at angle. Do not hold arm over sterile field (see Step 15 illustration).	• Prevents reaching over field and contaminating its surface.

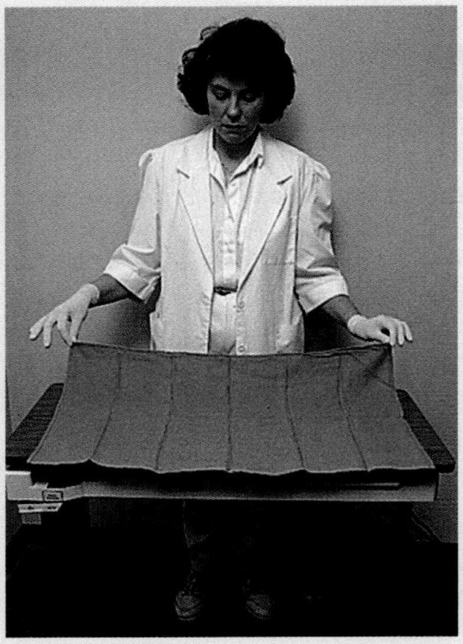

STEP 11 Place top half of drape over work surface.

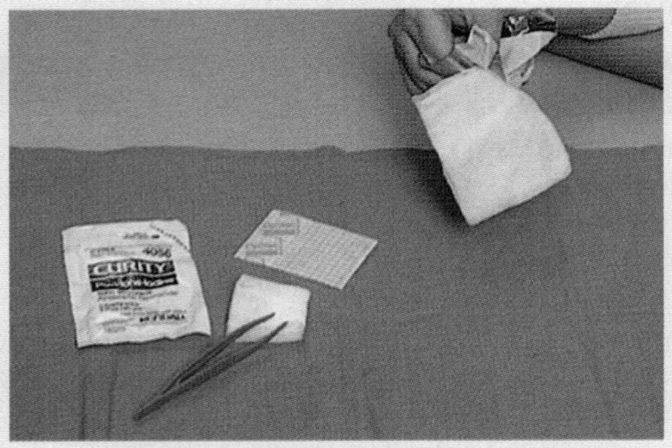

STEP 15 Adding item to sterile field.

STEPS	RATIONALE
16. Dispose of outer wrapper.	• Prevents accidental contamination of sterile field.
17. Perform procedure using sterile technique.	• Prevents transmission of infection to patient.

RECORDING AND REPORTING

• It is not necessary to record or report this procedure.

You may choose to wear sterile gloves while preparing items on the field. If this is done, you can touch the entire drape, but sterile items must be handed over by an assistant. Your gloves cannot touch the wrappers of sterile items.

Pouring sterile solutions. Often nurses must pour sterile solutions into sterile containers. A bottle containing a sterile solution is sterile on the inside and contaminated on the outside; the outside neck of the bottle is also contaminated, but the inside of the bottle cap is considered sterile. After the cap or lid is removed, it is held in the hand or placed sterile side (inside) up on a clean surface. This means that the inside of the lid can be seen as it rests on the table surface. A bottle cap or lid should never rest on a sterile surface, even though the inside of the cap is sterile. The outer edge of the cap is unsterile and would contaminate the sterile surface. Likewise, placing a sterile cap down on an unsterile surface increases the chances of the inside of the cap becoming contaminated.

It is important to check the label of the bottle to ensure it is the correct solution. Then hold the bottle with its label in the palm of the hand to prevent the possibility of the solution wetting and fading the label. The edge of the bottle is kept away from the edge or inside of the receiving container. Pour the solution slowly to avoid splashing the underlying drape or field. The bottle should never be held so high above the container that even slow pouring will cause splashing. The bottle should be held outside the edge of the sterile field.

Surgical hand scrub. Patients undergoing operative procedures are at an increased risk for infection. When working in operating rooms, nurses must decontaminate their hands to decrease and suppress the growth of skin microorganisms, in case the glove tears (Operating Room Nurses Association of Canada [ORNAC], 2014).

During surgical hand antisepsis before an operation, scrub from the fingertips to the elbows with an antiseptic soap. The optimum duration of the surgical hand scrub is unclear, although research indicates that it may be dependent on the type of antimicrobial product. Either an antimicrobial surgical scrub agent intended for surgical hand antisepsis or an alcohol-based antiseptic surgical hand rub that has persistent and cumulative activity is acceptable to use as a surgical scrub. For a traditional scrub, a 3- to 5-minute scrub should be performed to allow adequate contact time with the product, using the manufacturer's written instructions (Association of periOperative Registered Nurses [AORN], 2014a). Nurses should follow their agency's policy for length of scrub time. A study by Edmonds, Zapka, Kasper, and colleagues (2013) suggested that neither a brush nor a sponge is necessary to reduce bacterial counts on the hands, especially when an alcohol-based product is used.

For maximum elimination of bacteria, all jewellery should be removed, including wristwatches, and the nails should be kept clean and short (AORN, 2014b). Artificial nails, or any fingernail enhancements should not be worn because they may harbour a greater number of bacteria. Similarly, nail polish should be avoided because it conceals soil under the nails and because chipped nail polish may increase the bacterial load (AORN, 2014b). Nurses who have active skin infections, open lesions or cuts, or respiratory infections should be excluded from the surgical team. Skill 33-3 describes the steps for surgical hand hygiene.

Applying sterile gloves. Sterile gloves are an additional barrier to bacterial transfer. Nurses who work on general nursing divisions use *open gloving* before procedures such as dressing changes and urinary catheter insertions. *Closed gloving,* which is performed after applying sterile gowns, is practised in operating rooms and special treatment areas. The proper glove size should be selected; the glove should not stretch so tightly that it can easily tear, yet it should be tight enough that objects can be picked up easily.

Donning a sterile gown. Nurses must wear a sterile gown when assisting at the sterile field in an operating room, delivery room, or special treatment areas so that sterile objects can be comfortably handled with less risk of contamination. The circulating nurse usually does not wear a sterile gown. The sterile gown acts as a barrier to decrease the shedding of microorganisms from skin surfaces into the air, thus preventing wound contamination. Nurses may also wear a sterile gown if they are caring for a patient with a large open wound or assisting a physician during a major invasive procedure (e.g., inserting an arterial catheter).

After the nurse has applied a mask and surgical cap and performed the surgical hand scrub, the nurse dons a sterile gown. The gown is picked up from a sterile pack, or the nurse can ask an assistant to hand the gown to him or her. Only a certain portion of the gown—the area

SKILL 33-3 SURGICAL HAND SCRUB: PREPARING FOR GOWNING

Delegation Considerations

The role of the scrub nurse can be delegated to a surgical technologist or licensed practical nurse. Unregulated care providers (UCPs) can help the registered nurse in the circulating nurse role by opening sterile supplies, setting up sterile fields, and running errands under the direction of the registered nurse.

Equipment

- Deep sink with foot or knee controls for dispensing water and soap (faucets should be high enough for hands and forearms to fit comfortably)
- Antimicrobial surgical scrub agent or alcohol-based waterless antiseptic, according to agency policy (product should be nonirritating, broad spectrum, fast acting, and effective in reducing skin microorganisms and have a residual effect) (Association of periOperative Registered Nurses [AORN], 2014b)
- Surgical scrub sponge (if using traditional surgical hand scrub) and a disposable nail cleaner
- Paper mask and cap or hood
- Sterile towel
- Proper scrub attire
- Protective eyewear (goggles or face shield)

PROCEDURE

STEPS	RATIONALE
1. Consult your agency's policy regarding required length of scrub time and antiseptic to use for hand antisepsis.	• Guidelines vary regarding ideal time needed and antiseptic to use for surgical scrub.
2. Be sure fingernails are short, clean, and healthy. Artificial nails should be removed. Natural nails should be less than 0.5 cm long.	• Long nails and chipped or old polish increase number of bacteria residing on nails. Long fingernails can puncture gloves, causing contamination. Artificial nails are known to harbour Gram-negative microorganisms and fungus (AORN, 2014a).

CRITICAL DECISION POINT: *Remove nail polish if chipped or worn longer than 4 days because it may harbour microorganisms (AORN, 2014a).*

STEPS	RATIONALE
3. Inspect hands for presence of abrasions, cuts, or open lesions.	• These conditions increase the likelihood of microorganisms residing on skin surfaces.
4. Apply surgical shoe covers, cap or hood, face mask, and protective eyewear.	• Mask prevents escape into air of microorganisms that can contaminate hands. Other protective wear prevents exposure to blood and body fluid splashes during the procedure.
5. Surgical hand hygiene:	
A. Turn on water-activating sensor or use knee or foot controls.	
B. Wet hands and arms under running water and lather with detergent to 5 cm above elbows. (Hands need to be above elbows at all times.)	• Water runs by gravity from fingertips to elbows flowing from least to most contaminated areas. Hands become cleanest part of upper extremity. Washing a wide area reduces risk of contaminating overlying gown that you later apply.
C. Rinse hands and arms thoroughly under running water. **Remember to keep hands raised above elbows.**	• Rinsing removes transient bacteria from fingers, hands, and forearms.

Continued

SKILL 33-3 SURGICAL HAND SCRUB: PREPARING FOR GOWNING—cont'd

STEPS	RATIONALE
D. Under running water, clean under nails of both hands with nail pick. Discard after use (see Step 5D illustration).	• Removes dirt and organic material that harbour large numbers of microorganisms.
E. Wet clean sponge and apply antimicrobial detergent. Scrub nails of one hand with 15 strokes. Holding sponge perpendicular, scrub palm, each side of thumb and fingers, and posterior side of hand with 10 strokes each. The arm is mentally divided into thirds, and each third is scrubbed 10 times (see Step 5E illustrations). The duration of scrub is determined by the manufacturer's recommendations for the scrub agent used, which is usually 2 to 6 minutes (AORN, 2014a). Rinse sponge and repeat sequence for other arm. A two-sponge method may be substituted. Check your agency's policy.	• Friction loosens resident bacteria that adhere to skin surfaces. Technique ensures coverage of all surfaces. Scrubbing is performed from cleanest area (hands) to marginal area (upper arms).

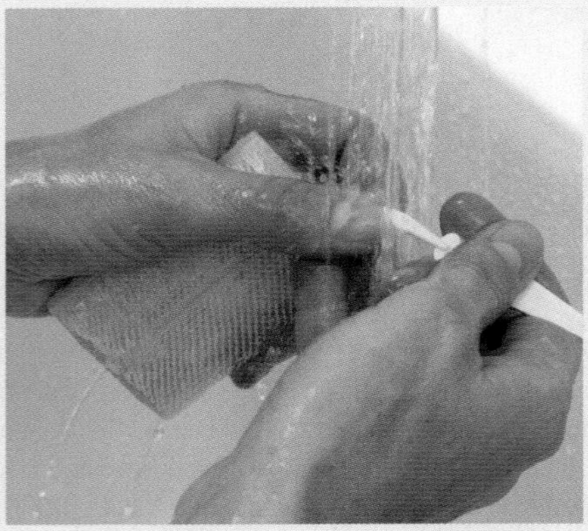

STEP 5D Clean under fingernails.

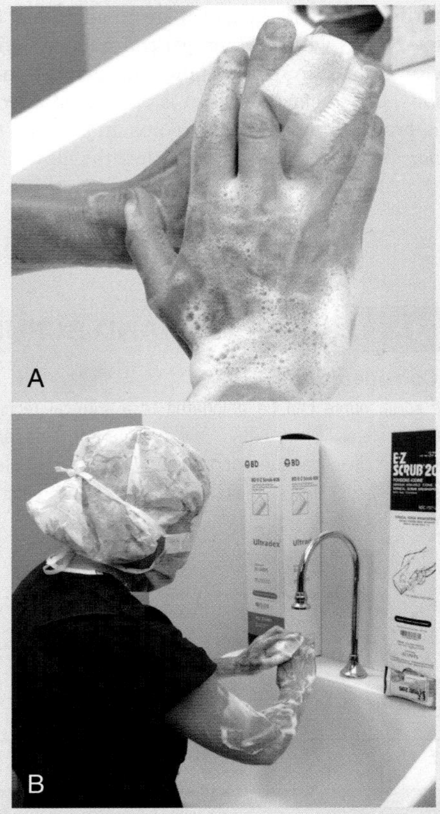

STEP 5E A, Scrub side of fingers. **B,** Scrub forearms.

STEPS	RATIONALE
F. Discard sponge and rinse hands and arms thoroughly (see Step 5F illustration). Turn off water with foot or knee control and back into room entrance with hands elevated in front of and away from the body.	• After touching skin, the sponge is considered contaminated. Rinsing removes resident bacteria. Using foot or knee tap control and backing into room prevent accidental contamination.

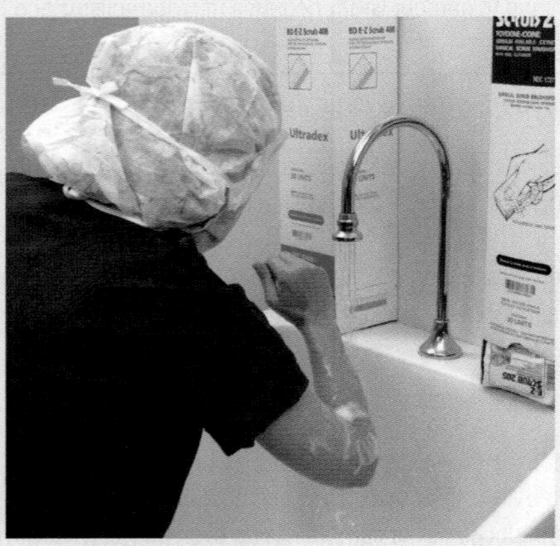

STEP 5F Rinse arms.

STEPS	RATIONALE
G. Walk up to sterile tray and lean forward slightly to pick up a sterile towel (see Step 5G [A] illustration). Dry one hand thoroughly, moving from fingers to elbow. Dry in a rotating motion. Dry from cleanest to least clean area (see Step 5G [B] illustration).	• Drying prevents chapping and facilitates donning of gloves. Leaning forward prevents accidental contact of arms with scrub attire.

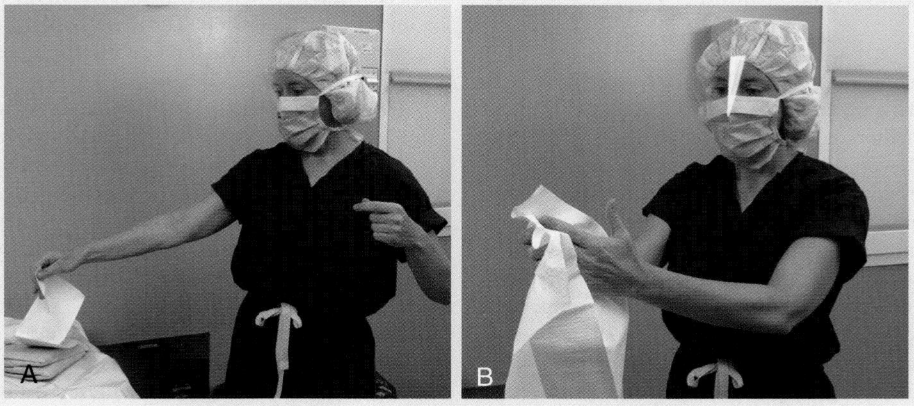

STEP 5G A, Grasping sterile towel. **B,** Drying sequence.

H. Repeat drying method for other hand by carefully reversing towel or using a new sterile towel.	• Prevents accidental contamination.
I. Discard towel.	• Prevents accidental contamination.
J. Proceed with sterile gowning (see Skill 33-4).	
6. Alternative method of surgical hand hygiene using alcohol-based antiseptic:	
A. Wash hands with soap and water for at least 15 seconds to remove soil.	• Removes dirt and organic material that harbour large numbers of microorganisms.
B. Under running water, clean under nails of both hands with disposable nail cleaner. Discard after use and dry hands with paper towel.	
C. Apply enough alcohol-based waterless antiseptic to one palm to cover both hands thoroughly (see Step 6C illustration). Spread the antiseptic over all surfaces of the hands and fingernails. Follow product instructions for length of time to rub over hand surfaces. Allow to air-dry.	• Ensures coverage of all surfaces. Air-drying ensures complete antisepsis is achieved.

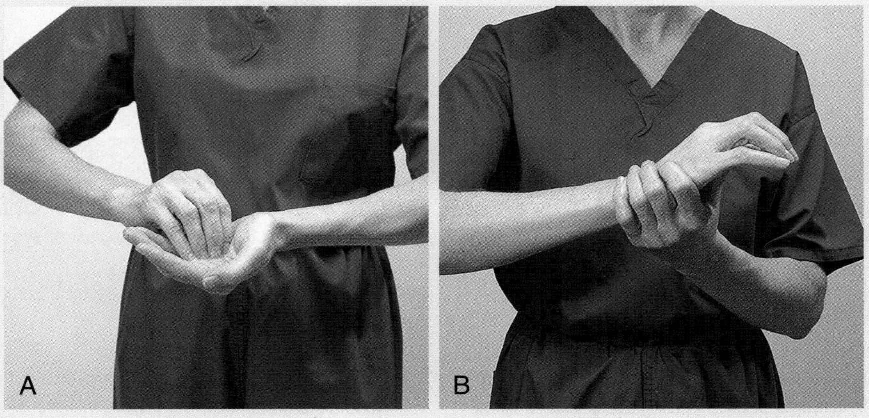

STEP 6C Application of antimicrobial agent for brushless hand scrub. This nurse is using 3M Avagard. Photo courtesy of 3M Health Care.

D. Repeat the process and allow hands to air-dry before applying sterile gloves.

RECORDING AND REPORTING

- It is not necessary to record or report this procedure.
- Report any dermatitis to employee health or infection control per your agency's policy.

from the anterior waist to, but not including, the collar and the anterior surface of the sleeves—is considered sterile. The back of the gown, the area under the arms, the collar, the area below the waist, and the underside of the sleeves are not sterile because the nurse cannot keep these areas in constant view and ensure their sterility. Skill 33-4 reviews the steps for applying a sterile gown and closed gloving, and Skill 33-5 reviews the method of open gloving.

◆ Evaluation

Nurses' success when practising infection control techniques is measured by determining whether the goals for reducing or preventing infection are achieved. By comparing the patient's response, such as the absence of fever or development of wound drainage, with expected outcomes, nurses determine the success of nursing interventions. Similarly, nurses determine whether interventions should be revised or eliminated. Correctly assessing wounds for healing and conducting a physical assessment of body systems (see Chapter 32) are important skills in evaluation. Nurses need to closely monitor patients, especially those at risk, for signs and symptoms of infection. For example, a patient who has undergone a surgical procedure is at risk for infection at the surgical site, as well as at sites of invasive procedures such as a venipuncture or central line insertion. In addition, the patient is at risk for a respiratory tract infection as a result of decreased mobility and for a urinary tract infection if an in-dwelling catheter is present. Nurses must closely monitor all invasive and surgical sites for swelling, erythema, and purulent drainage. Breath sounds are monitored for changes, and sputum character is checked for purulence. Laboratory test results are reviewed for leukocytes in the urine, which may indicate a urinary tract infection. The absence of signs or symptoms of infection is the expected outcome of infection prevention and monitoring activities.

The patient at risk for infection must understand the measures needed to reduce or prevent microorganism growth and spread. Providing patients or family members with the opportunity to discuss infection control measures and to demonstrate procedures will increase their ability to adhere to therapy. Nurses may determine that patients require new information or that previously instructed information needs reinforcement.

The nurse needs to document the patient's response to therapies for infection control. A clear description of any signs and symptoms of systemic or local infection is necessary to give all nurses a baseline for comparative evaluation. The efficacy of any intervention in reducing infection must be reported.

SKILL 33-4 APPLYING A STERILE GOWN AND PERFORMING CLOSED GLOVING

Delegation Considerations

The role of the scrub nurse can be delegated to a surgical technician.

Equipment

- Surgical cap
- Surgical mask
- Eye protection
- Foot covers
- Sterile gown (prepared by circulating nurse)

PROCEDURE

STEPS	RATIONALE
1. Before entering operating room or treatment area, apply cap, face mask, and eyewear. Foot covers are also required in operating room.	• Prevent hair and air droplet nuclei from contaminating sterile work areas. Eyewear protects mucous membranes of eye. Foot covers are paper or cloth and fit over work shoes.
2. Perform thorough surgical hand hygiene (see Skill 33-3).	• Removes transient and resident bacteria from fingers, hands, and forearms.
3. Ask circulating nurse to assist by opening sterile pack containing sterile gown (folded inside out).	• Gown's outer surface remains sterile.
4. Have circulating nurse prepare glove package by peeling outer wrapper open while keeping inner contents sterile. Inner glove package is then placed on sterile field created by sterile outer wrapper.	• This action keeps gloves sterile and allows the nurse who has scrubbed to handle sterile items.
5. Reach down to sterile gown package; lift folded gown directly upward and step back away from table.	• This action provides a wide margin of safety, avoiding contamination of gown.
6. Holding folded gown, locate neckband. With both hands, grasp inside front of gown just below neckband.	• Clean hands may touch inside of gown without contaminating outer surface.
7. Allow gown to unfold, keeping inside of gown toward body. Do not touch outside of gown with bare hands or allow it to touch the floor.	• Outside of gown will remain sterile surface.
8. With hands at shoulder level, slip both arms into armholes simultaneously (see Step 8 illustration). Ask circulating nurse to bring gown over shoulders by reaching inside to arm seams and pulling gown on, leaving sleeves covering hands.	• Careful application prevents contamination. Gown covers hands to prepare for closed gloving.

STEPS	RATIONALE
9. Have circulating nurse securely tie back of gown at neck and waist (see Step 9 illustration). (If gown is a wraparound style, sterile flap to cover gown is not touched until you have gloved.)	• Gown must completely enclose underlying garments.

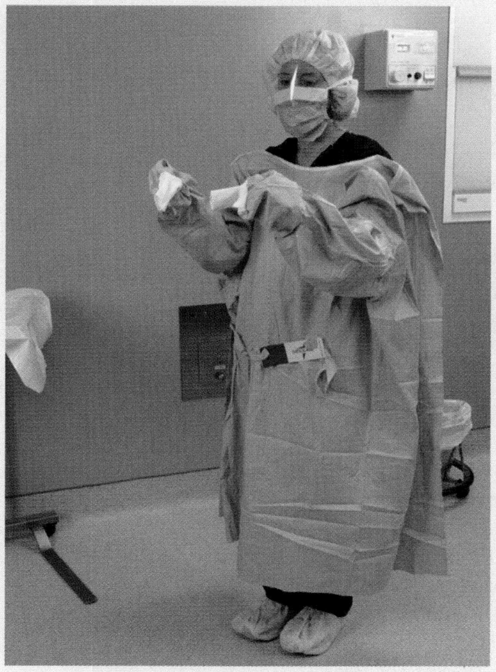

STEP 8 Place arms in sleeves.

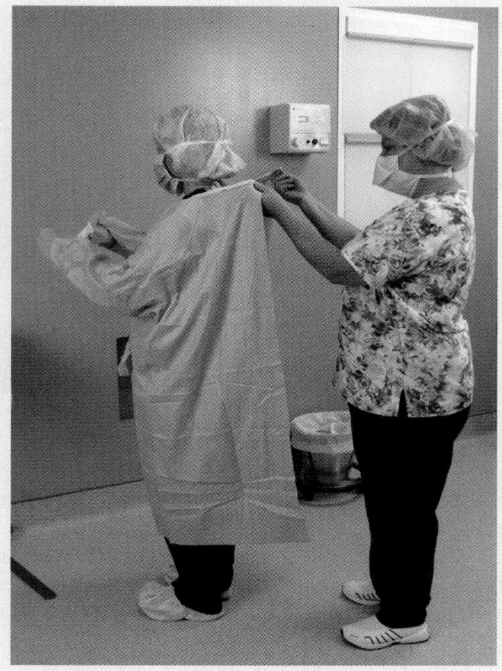

STEP 9 Circulating nurse ties scrub gown.

STEPS	RATIONALE
10. Closed gloving:	
A. With hands covered by gown sleeves, open inner sterile glove package (see Step 10A illustration).	• Hands remain clean. Sterile gown cuff will touch sterile glove surface.
B. With dominant hand inside gown cuff, pick up glove for nondominant hand by grasping folded cuff.	• Sterile gown touches sterile glove.
C. Extend nondominant forearm with palm up and place palm of glove against palm of nondominant hand. Glove fingers will point toward elbow.	• Position glove for application over cuffed hand, keeping glove sterile.
D. Grasp back of glove cuff with covered dominant hand and turn glove cuff over end of nondominant hand and gown cuff (see Step 10D illustration).	• Seal that is created by glove cuff over gown prevents exit of microorganisms over operative sterile field.

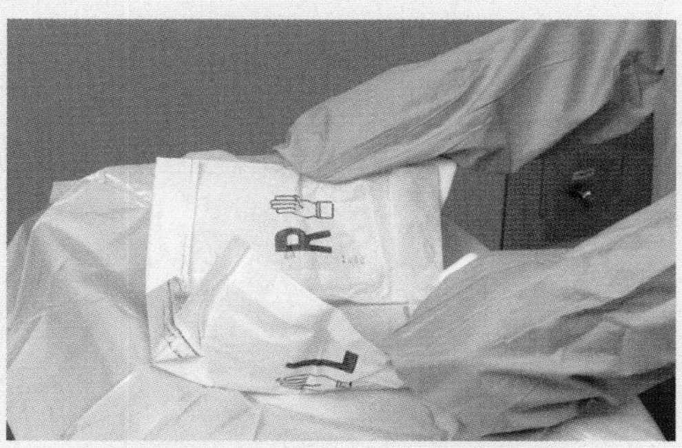

STEP 10A Open glove package.

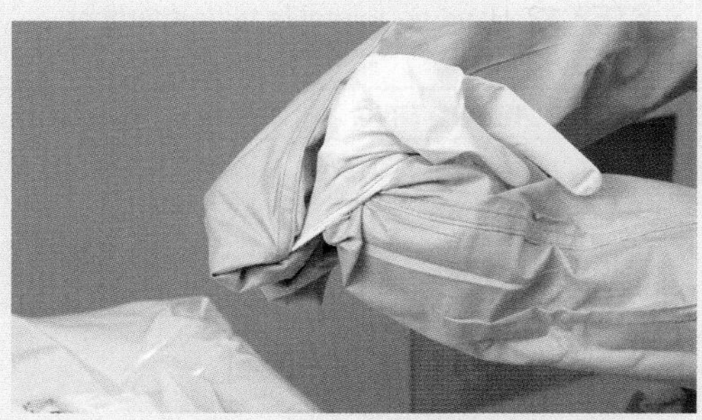

STEP 10D Apply glove to nondominant hand, keeping dominant hand inside cuff.

E. Grasp top of glove and underlying gown sleeve with covered dominant hand. Carefully extend fingers into glove, being sure glove's cuff covers gown's cuff.

Continued

SKILL 33-4 APPLYING A STERILE GOWN AND PERFORMING CLOSED GLOVING—cont'd

STEPS	RATIONALE
F. Glove dominant hand in same manner, reversing hands (see Step 10F illustration). Use gloved nondominant hand to pull on glove. Keep hand inside sleeve (see Step 10F illustration).	• Sterile object touches sterile object and therefore stays sterile. Touching the sterile sleeve with the sterile gloved hand allows the gloved hands to remain sterile.

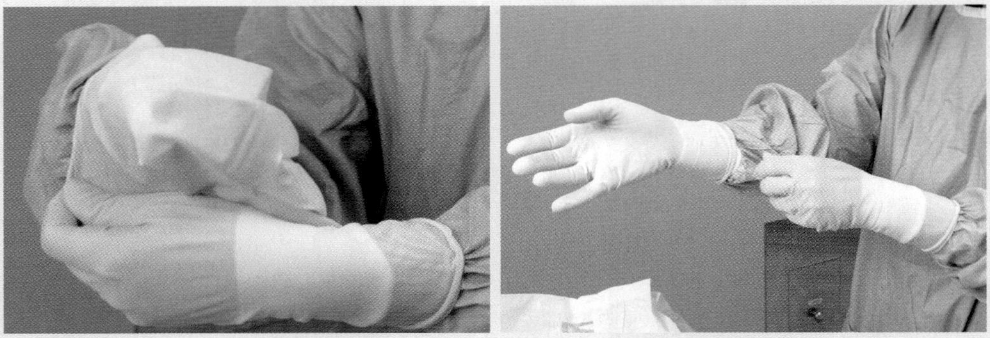

STEP 10F Apply second glove.

STEPS	RATIONALE
G. Be sure fingers are fully extended into both gloves.	• Ensure that you have full dexterity while using gloved hand.
11. For wraparound sterile gowns, take gloved hand and release fastener or ties in front of gown.	• Front of gown is sterile.
12. Hand tie to sterile team member, who stands still (see Step 12 illustration). Allowing margin of safety, turn around to the left, covering back with extended gown flap. Take back tie from team member and secure tie to gown.	• Contact with team member could contaminate gown and gloves. Garments worn under the gown must be enclosed.

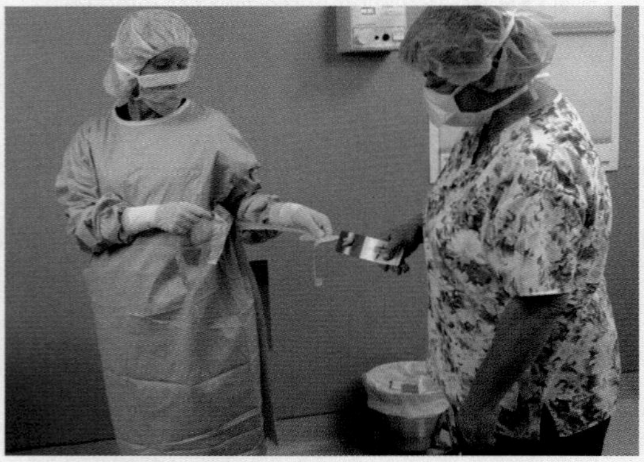

STEP 12 Hand tie to sterile team member.

RECORDING AND REPORTING

- It is not necessary to record or report this procedure.

SKILL 33-5 OPEN GLOVING

Delegation Considerations

Delegation of open gloving depends on whether an unregulated care provider (UCP) has received special training and is competent to perform the sterile procedure.

Equipment

- Sterile gloves (proper size)

PROCEDURE

STEPS	RATIONALE
1. Perform thorough hand hygiene.	• Removes bacteria from skin surfaces and reduces risk of transmitting infection.
2. Remove outer glove package wrapper by carefully separating and peeling apart sides.	• Prevents inner glove package from accidentally opening and touching contaminated objects.
3. Grasp inner package and lay it on clean, dry, flat surface just above waist level. Open package, keeping gloves on wrapper's inside surface (see Step 3 illustration).	• Sterile object held below the waist is contaminated. Inner surface of glove package is sterile.

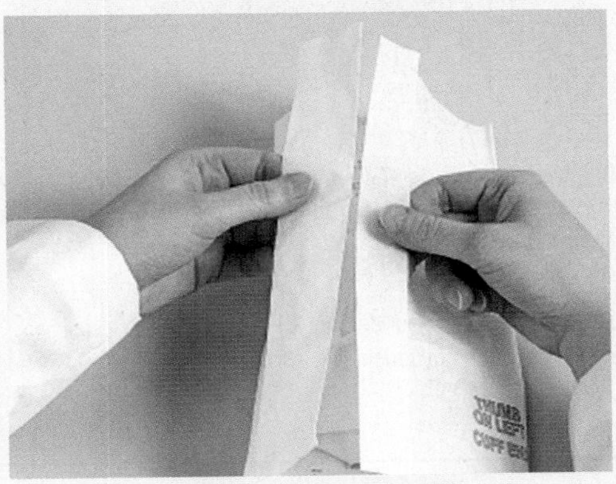

STEP 3 Open package.

STEPS	RATIONALE
4. If gloves are not pre-powdered, take packet of powder and apply lightly to hands over sink or wastebasket.	• Powder allows gloves to slip on easily. (Some staff members do not use powder for fear of promoting growth of microorganisms.)
5. Each glove has cuff approximately 5 cm wide. Glove dominant hand first.	• Proper identification of gloves prevents contamination by improper fit. Gloving of dominant hand first improves dexterity.
6. With thumb and first two fingers of nondominant hand, grasp edge of cuff of glove for dominant hand. Touch only glove's inside surface.	• Inner edge of cuff will lie against skin and is thus not sterile.
7. Carefully pull glove over dominant hand, being sure cuff does not roll up wrist. Be sure thumb and fingers are in proper spaces (see Step 7 illustration).	• If glove's outer surface touches hand or wrist, then it is contaminated.
8. With gloved dominant hand, slip fingers underneath second glove's cuff (see Step 8 illustration).	• Cuff protects gloved fingers. Sterile surface touching sterile surface prevents glove contamination.

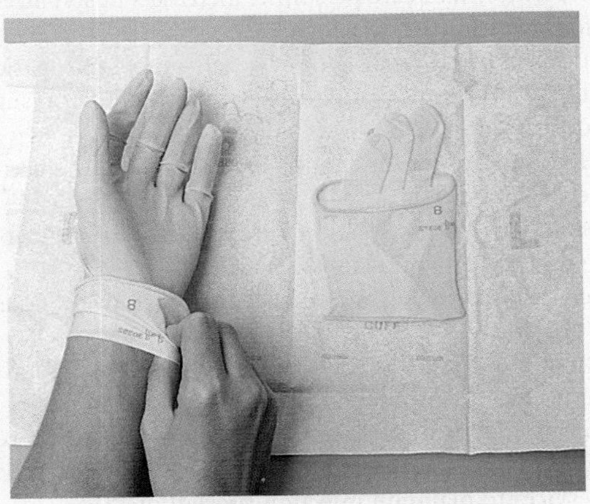

STEP 7 Pull glove over dominant hand.

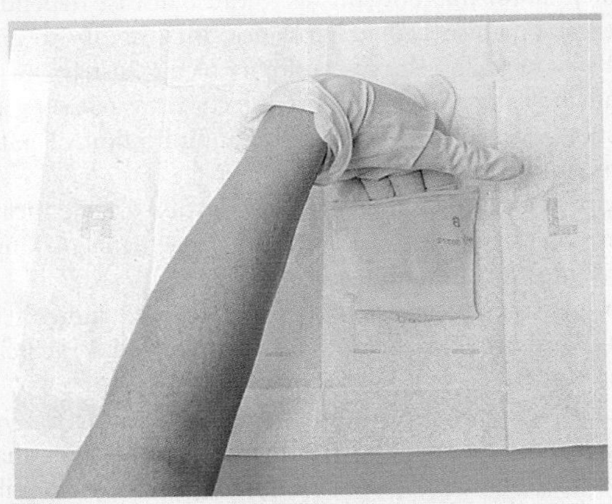

STEP 8 Slip fingers underneath second glove's cuff.

Continued

SKILL 33-5 OPEN GLOVING—cont'd

STEPS	RATIONALE
9. Carefully pull second glove over nondominant hand. Do not allow fingers and thumb of gloved dominant hand to touch any part of exposed nondominant hand. Keep thumb of dominant hand abducted back (see Step 9 illustration).	• Contact of gloved hand with exposed hand results in contamination.
10. After second glove is on, interlock hands. The cuffs usually fall down after application. Be sure to touch only sterile sides (see Step 10 illustration).	• Ensure smooth fit over fingers.

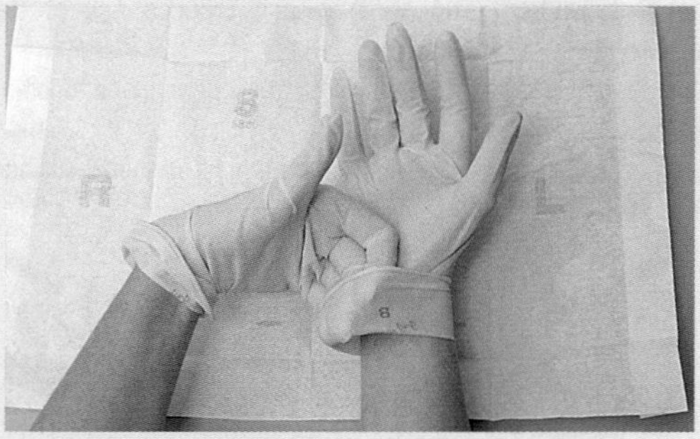

STEP 9 Pull second glove over nondominant hand.

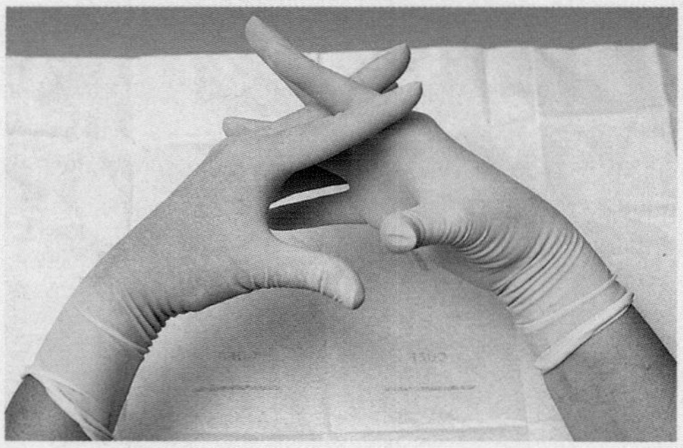

STEP 10 Interlock hands. Gloved hands must be kept above waist level within the visual field at all times or clasped together above elbow level.

Glove Disposal

STEPS	RATIONALE
11. Grasp outside of one cuff with other gloved hand; avoid touching wrist.	• Minimize contamination of underlying skin.
12. Pull glove off, turning it inside out. Discard in receptacle.	• Outside of glove does not touch skin surface.
13. Take fingers of bare hand and tuck inside remaining glove cuff. Peel glove off, inside out. Discard in receptacle. Perform hand hygiene.	

RECORDING AND REPORTING

- It is not necessary to record or report this procedure.

KEY CONCEPTS

- Hand hygiene is the most important technique to use in preventing and controlling the transmission of infection.
- The potential for microorganisms to cause disease depends on the number of organisms, their virulence, their ability to enter and survive in a host, and the susceptibility of the host.
- Normal body flora help to resist infection by releasing antibacterial substances and inhibiting the multiplication of pathogenic microorganisms.
- The signs of local inflammation and infection are identical.
- An infection can develop as long as the six elements making up the chain of infection are uninterrupted.
- Microorganisms are transmitted by direct and indirect contact, droplets, airborne particles, and contaminated vehicles and vectors.
- Advancing age, poor nutrition, stress, diseases of the immune system, chronic disease, and treatments or conditions that compromise the immune response increase a person's susceptibility to infection.
- The major sites for HAI are the urinary and respiratory tracts, the bloodstream, and surgical or traumatic wounds.
- The CDC now recommends the use of alcohol-based waterless antiseptics as an alternative to handwashing to more effectively reduce the transmission of microorganisms.
- Invasive procedures, medical therapies, long hospitalization, and contact with health care personnel increase a hospitalized patient's risk for acquiring an HAI.
- Isolation practices may prevent personnel and patients from acquiring infections and may prevent the transmission of microorganisms.
- Standard precautions or routine practices entail the use of generic barrier techniques in the care of all patients.
- Transmission-based (isolation) precautions are used for patients with specific, highly transmissible infections.
- Proper cleansing involves the mechanical removal of soil from an object or area.
- A patient in isolation is subject to sensory deprivation because of the restricted environment.
- An infection-control professional monitors the incidence of infection within an institution and provides educational and consultative services to maintain infection prevention.
- Surgical asepsis necessitates more stringent techniques than does medical asepsis and is directed at eliminating all microorganisms.

- Surgical aseptic practices are followed if the skin is broken or if the nurse performs an invasive procedure in a body cavity that is normally free of microorganisms.

CRITICAL THINKING EXERCISES

1. Mrs. Jaycock had an in-dwelling urethral catheter for 1 week. The catheter has now been out for 24 hours. She complains of frequency of and pain on urination. Mrs. Jaycock suggests that the catheter be reinserted so that she does not need to get up frequently. What can frequency of or pain on urination indicate? Should the catheter be reinserted? Why or why not? Describe at least one appropriate assessment measure and independent nursing action for Mrs. Jaycock.
2. You are caring for Mr. Huang, who has a large, open, draining abdominal wound. You notice another health care worker changing Mr. Huang's dressing without wearing gloves or using sterile supplies or sterile technique. When you question the health care worker regarding this practice, the person says, "Don't worry, the wound is already infected, and the antibiotics and draining will take care of any contaminants." How would you respond to this comment? What would your next steps be in following up on this incident?
3. Mrs. Niles is 83 years of age and lives alone. She has difficulty walking and relies on a church volunteer group to deliver lunches during the week. Her fixed income limits her ability to buy food. Last week, Mrs. Niles's 79-year-old sister died. The two sisters had been very close. Explain the factors that might increase Mrs. Niles's risk for infection.
4. Mr. Vargas is admitted to your facility with a history of recent weight loss, a cough that has persisted for 2 months, and hemoptysis. His chest X-ray film shows a cavity in one lung, and his physician suspects tuberculosis. What type of isolation precautions would you use for Mr. Vargas? What protection would you use when providing care? What education would you provide for the patient and his family?

REVIEW QUESTIONS

1. If an infection can be transmitted from one person to another, it is a:
   1. Communicable disease
   2. Portal of entry to a host
   3. Portal of exit from a reservoir
   4. Susceptible host
2. The mode of transmission for methicillin-resistant *Staphylococcus aureus* (MRSA) is:
   1. Direct and indirect contact
   2. Droplet transmission
   3. Airborne transmission
   4. Vectorborne transmission
3. The interval when a patient manifests signs and symptoms specific to a type of infection is the:
   1. Incubation period
   2. Convalescence stage
   3. Prodromal stage
   4. Illness stage
4. The most important and basic way to break the chain of infection is by:
   1. Wearing gloves
   2. Practising hand hygiene
   3. Placing patients in isolation
   4. Providing private rooms for patients
5. The minimum handwashing time with soap and water necessary to remove most transient microorganisms is:
   1. 1.5 seconds
   2. 15 seconds
   3. 40–60 seconds
   4. 3 minutes
6. A patient is on isolation precautions for pulmonary tuberculosis. The nurse notes that the patient seems to be angry but knows this is a normal response to isolation. The nurse's best intervention is to:
   1. Provide a dark, quiet room to calm the patient
   2. Explain the isolation procedures and provide meaningful stimulation
   3. Reduce the level of precautions to keep the patient from becoming angry
   4. Limit family and other caregiver visits to reduce the risk of spreading the infection
7. A gown should be worn when:
   1. The patient's hygiene is poor
   2. The patient has AIDS or hepatitis
   3. The nurse is assisting with medication administration
   4. Blood or body fluids may get on the nurse's clothing from a task the nurse plans to perform
8. You have dressed a patient's wound and now plan to administer a medication (which is currently in the room) to the patient. It is important to:
   1. Remove your gloves and perform hand hygiene before leaving the room
   2. Remove your gloves and perform hand hygiene before administering the medication
   3. Leave your gloves on to administer the medication
   4. Leave the medication on the bedside table to avoid having to remove your gloves before leaving the patient's room
9. A patient on your unit develops diarrhea, which is confirmed to be caused by *C. difficile*. What type of isolation should this patient be placed on?
   1. Airborne isolation
   2. Contact precautions
   3. Standard precautions or routine practices
   4. Droplet precautions
10. When performing surgical hand hygiene, the nurse's hands must be kept:
    1. Above the elbows
    2. Below the elbows
    3. At a 45-degree angle
    4. In a comfortable position

Answers: 1. 1; **2.** 1; **3.** 4; **4.** 2; **5.** 3; **6.** 2; **7.** 4; **8.** 2; **9.** 2; **10.** 1

Rationales for the Review Questions appear at the end of the book.

RECOMMENDED WEBSITES

Infection Prevention and Control Canada: https://ipac-canada.org/.
Infection Prevention and Control Canada (IPAC–Canada) is a national, multidisciplinary, voluntary association of infection-control professionals committed to improving infection prevention and control.

Public Health Agency of Canada: http://www.phac-aspc.gc.ca.
This federal government site provides links to documents related to infection control practices, including the *Canada Communicable Disease Report.*

REFERENCES

Alberta Health. (2012). *Standards for cleaning, disinfection, and sterilization of reusable medical devices for health care facilities and settings*. Edmonton: Author. Retrieved from https://open.alberta.ca/dataset/b9dd9349-6d5b-48aa-b83b-d206210a9f97/resource/7ef701ba-1e58-4a5d-b2a4-4f3d5e5de1fa/download/IPC-Medical-Device-Cleaning-2012.pdf.

Amarya, S., Singh, K., & Sabharwall, M. (2015). Changes during aging and their association with malnutrition. *Journal of Clinical Gerontology and Geriatrics*, *6*(3), 78–84. doi:10.1016/j.jcgg.2015.05.003.

Antonio, N., & Jensen, L. (2014). Improving clinical practice in the management of elderly patients hospitalized with antimicrobial resistant organisms. *Journal of Nursing Education and Practice*, *4*(8), 107–114.

Association of periOperative Registered Nurses (AORN). (2014a). Hand antisepsis, surgical. In *Standards, recommended practices, and guidelines*. Denver, CO: Author.

Association of periOperative Registered Nurses (AORN). (2014b). *Perioperative standards and recommended practices*. Denver, CO: Author.

Association for Professionals in Infection Control and Epidemiology (APIC). (2013). Guide to preventing *Clostridium difficile* infections. *(APIC implementation guide)*. Washington, DC: Author. Retrieved from http://apic.org/Resource_/EliminationGuideForm/59397fc6-3f90-43d1-9325-e8be75d86888/File/2013CDiffFinal.pdf.

Baumgardner, D. J. (2012). Soil-related bacterial and fungal infections. *Journal of the American Board of Family Medicine*, *25*(5), 734–744. doi:10.3122/jabfm.2012.05.110226.

Bilir, A., Yelken, B., & Erkan, A. (2013). Chlorhexidine, octenidine or povidine iodine for catheter-related infections: A randomized controlled trial. *Journal of Research in Medical Science*, *18*(6), 510–512.

Boraschi, D., Aquado, M. T., Dutel, C., et al. (2013). The gracefully aging immune system. *Science Translational Medicine*, *5*(185), 185ps8. doi:10.1126/scitranslmed.3005624.

Brestoff, J. R., & Artis, D. (2015). Commensal bacteria at the interface of host metabolism and the immune system. *Nature Immunology*, *14*(7), 676–684. doi:10.1038/ni.2640.

Carpenito, L. J. (2013). Risk for infection. In *Handbook of Nursing Diagnosis* (14 ed., pp. 338–350). Philadelphia, PA: Blackwell Publishing.

Centers for Disease Control and Prevention (CDC). (2012). An introduction to applied epidemiology and biostatistics. Section 10: Chain of infection. In *Principles of epidemiology in public health practice* (3rd ed.). Atlanta: Author. Retrieved from https://www.cdc.gov/ophss/csels/dsepd/ss1978/ss1978.pdf.

Centers for Disease Control and Prevention (CDC). (2015). *Clostridium difficile infection information for patients*. Atlanta: CDC. Retrieved from https://www.cdc.gov/hai/organisms/cdiff/cdiff-patient.html.

Centers for Disease Control and Prevention (CDC). (2017a). *Handwashing: Clean hands save lives*. Atlanta: CDC. Retrieved from https://www.cdc.gov/handwashing/index.html.

Centers for Disease Control and Prevention (CDC). (2017b). *Chronic diseases: Prevention and health promotion*. Retrieved from https://www.cdc.gov/chronicdisease/index.htm.

Collier, S., & Davenport, A. (2014). Reducing the risk of infection in end-stage kidney failure patients treated by dialysis. *Nephrology, Dialysis, Transplantation*, *29*(12), 2158–2161.

Edmonds, S. L., Zapka, C., Kasper, D., et al. (2013). Effectiveness of hand hygiene for removal of *Clostridium difficile* spores from hands. *Infection Control and Hospital Epidemiology*, *34*(3), 302–305. doi:10.1086/669521.

Garner, J. S. (1996). Guideline for isolation precautions in hospitals. The Hospital Infection Control Practices Advisory Committee. *Infection Control and Hospital Epidemiology*, *17*(1), 54–80.

Graham, L. (2015). Infection prevention and control. In P. A. Potter, A. G. Perry, P. Stockert, et al. (Eds.), *Essentials in Nursing Practice* (8th ed., p. 243). St. Louis, MO: Elsevier Mosby.

Hammer, S. (2013). *Handwashing: Reducing nosocomial infections*. Ithaca, NY: Cayuga Medical Center. Retrieved from http://iwsp.human.cornell.edu/files/2013/09/Hand-Washing-Reducing-Nosocomial-Infections-2j1mlfb.pdf.

Health Canada. (1999). Infection control guidelines: Routine practices and additional precautions for preventing the transmission of infection in health care. *Canada Communicable Disease Report*, *25*(Suppl. 4), 83–111.

Infection Prevention and Control (IPAC) Canada. (2017). *Home page*. Retrieved from https://ipac-canada.org/.

Lee, C. R., Cho, I. H., Jeong, B. C., et al. (2013). Strategies to minimize antibiotic resistance. *International Journal of Environmental Research and Public Health*, *10*(9), 4274–4305. doi:10.3390/ijerph10094274.

Maki, D. G., Alvarado, C., & Hassemer, C. (1986). Double-bagging items from isolation rooms is unnecessary as an infection control measure: A comparative study of surface contamination with single- and double-bagging. *Infection Control*, *7*, 535–537.

Operating Room Nurses Association of Canada (ORNAC). (2014). *Recommended standards, guidelines and position statements for perioperative registered nursing practice* (11th ed.). Ottawa: Author.

Provincial Infection Control Network of British Columbia (PICNet). (2014). *Infection prevention and control guidelines for providing health care to clients in the community*. Vancouver: Author. Retrieved from https://www.picnet.ca/wp-content/uploads/PICNet_Home_and_Community_Care_Guidelines_2014_.pdf.

Provincial Infectious Diseases Advisory Committee (PIDAC). (2013). *Best practices for cleaning, disinfection and sterilization of medical equipment devices in all health care settings* (3rd ed.). Vancouver: Author. Retrieved from https://www.publichealthontario.ca/en/eRepository/PIDAC_Cleaning_Disinfection_and_Sterilization_2013.pdf.

Public Health Agency of Canada (PHAC). (2012a). *Routine practices and additional precautions for preventing the transmission of infection in health care settings*. Retrieved from http://publications.gc.ca/collections/collection_2013/aspc-phac/HP40-83-2013-eng.pdf.

Public Health Agency of Canada (PHAC). (2012b). *Hand hygiene practices in health care settings*. Ottawa: Author. Retrieved from http://publications.gc.ca/collections/collection_2012/aspc-phac/HP40-74-2012-eng.pdf.

Public Health Agency of Canada (PHAC). (2013a). *The Chief Public Health Officer's report on the state of public health in Canada, 2013: Infectious disease—the never-ending threat*. Ottawa: Author. Retrieved from www.phac-aspc.gc.ca/cphorsphc-respcacsp/2013/infections-eng.php.

Public Health Agency of Canada (PHAC). (2013b). *Canadian Needle Stick Surveillance Network: Analysis of occupational exposures to blood, body fluids and bloodborne pathogens (1 January 2008 to 30 June 2012). Final program report*. Retrieved from http://publications.gc.ca/collections/collection_2014/aspc-phac/HP40-88-2013-eng.pdf.

Public Health Agency of Canada (PHAC). (2016). *Canadian immunization guide*. Ottawa: Author. Retrieved from https://www.canada.ca/en/public-health/services/canadian-immunization-guide.html.

Ramsay, E. N., Pratt, N. L., Ryan, P., et al. (2013). Proton pump inhibitors and the risk of pneumonia: A comparison of cohort and self-controlled case series designs. *BMC Medical Research Methodology*, *13*, 82. doi:10.1186/1471-2288-13-82.

Reuben, D. B. (2016). Geriatric assessment. In L. Goldman & A. I. Schafer (Eds.), *Cecil essentials of medicine* (25th ed., pp. 102–106). Philadelphia, PA: Saunders.

Rossvoll, E., Ronning, H. T., Granum, P. E., et al. (2014). Toxin production and growth of pathogens subjected to temperature fluctuations simulating consumer handling of cold cuts. *International Journal of Food Microbiology*, *185*, 82–92. doi:10.1016/j.ijfoodmicro.2014.05.020.

Siegel, J. D., Rhinehart, E., Jackson, M., et al. (2007). *Guidelines for isolation precautions: Preventing transmission of infectious agents in health care settings*. Retrieved from https://www.cdc.gov/infectioncontrol/pdf/guidelines/isolation-guidelines.pdf.

Trehearne, B., Fishman, P., & Lin, E. H. B. (2014). Role of the nurse in chronic illness management. *Nurse Economics*, *32*(4), 178–184.

Wong, S. S., & Yuen, K. Y. (2012). Streptococcus pyrogens and re-emergence of scarlet fever as a public health problem. *Emerging Microbes and Infections*, *1*, e2. doi:10.1038/emi.2012.9.

World Health Organization (WHO). (2009). *WHO guidelines on hand hygiene in health care: First global patient safety challenge: Clean care is safer care*. Geneva, Switzerland: Author. Retrieved from http://apps.who.int/iris/bitstream/10665/44102/1/9789241597906_eng.pdf.

34

Medication Administration

Canadian content written by Sharon Kaasalainen, RN, PhD

Original chapter by Amy M. Hall, RN, BSN, MS, PhD, CNE, Wendy R. Ostendorf, RN, MS, EdD, CNE

OBJECTIVES

Mastery of content in this chapter will enable you to:

- Define the key terms listed.
- Examine the nurse's role and responsibilities regarding medication administration.
- Describe the physiological mechanisms of medication action, including absorption, distribution, metabolism, and excretion of medications.
- Differentiate among different types of medication actions.
- Discuss developmental factors that influence pharmacokinetics.
- Discuss factors that influence medication actions.
- Discuss methods of educating a patient about prescribed medications.
- Compare and contrast the roles of the physician, the pharmacist, and the nurse in medication administration.
- Implement nursing actions to prevent medication errors.
- Describe factors to consider when choosing routes of medication administration.
- Calculate a prescribed medication dose.
- Discuss factors to use when assessing a patient's needs for and response to medication therapy.
- Explain the rights of medication administration.
- Prepare and administer subcutaneous, intramuscular, and intradermal injections; intravenous medications; hypodermoclysis infusions; oral and topical skin preparations; eye, ear, and nose drops; vaginal instillations; rectal suppositories; and inhalants.
- Describe the importance of safe medication techniques.
- Describe the importance of establishing and adhering to agency policies and procedures when administering medications.
- Identify and describe how principles of primary health care are applied to medication administration in nursing practice.

KEY TERMS

Absorption, p. 731
Adverse effects, p. 732
Anaphylactic reactions, p. 732
Biotransformation, p. 731
Buccal, p. 734
Concentration, p. 733
Controlled substances, p. 730
Culture of safety, p. 743
Detoxify, p. 731
Hypodermoclysis, p. 810
Idiosyncratic reaction, p. 732
Infusions, p. 733
Inhalation, p. 736
Injection, p. 734
Instillation, p. 762
Intra-articular, p. 736
Intracardiac, p. 736
Intradermal (ID), p. 734
Intramuscular (IM), p. 734
Intraocular, p. 736
Intravenous (IV), p. 734
Irrigations, p. 737
Medication allergy, p. 732
Medication error, p. 743
Medication interaction, p. 733
Medication reconciliation, p. 744
Metered-dose inhalers (MDIs), p. 768
Metric system, p. 736
Narcotics, p. 730
Ophthalmic, p. 764
Parenteral administration, p. 734
Peak concentration, p. 733
Pharmacokinetics, p. 731
Polypharmacy, p. 754
Prescription, p. 739
Serum half-life, p. 733
Side effects, p. 732
Solution, p. 737
Subcutaneous, p. 734
Sublingual, p. 734
Synergistic effect, p. 733
Therapeutic effect, p. 732
Toxic effects, p. 732
Transdermal disc, p. 736
Verbal order, p. 739
Z-track method, p. 794

MEDIA RESOURCES

http://evolve.elsevier.com/Canada/Potter/fundamentals/

- Audio Chapter Summaries
- Examination Review Questions
- Concept Map Creator
- Case Study with Questions
- Audio Glossary
- Content Updates
- Video Clips

Patients who have acute or chronic diseases or conditions use a variety of strategies to restore or maintain their health. A medication is a substance used in the prevention, diagnosis, relief, treatment, or cure of health alterations. Medications are a primary treatment that patients associate with restoration of health. No matter where patients receive their health care—in hospitals, at clinics, or at home—nurses play an essential role in preparing and administering medications, teaching patients about medications, and evaluating patients' responses to medications. In the primary health care setting, patients often self-administer their medications. As a nurse, you are responsible for evaluating the effects of the medications on the patient's health status, teaching patients about their medications and their adverse drug events, promoting patient adherence to the medication regimen, and evaluating the patient's technique for all routes of medication delivery. Additionally, you must assess the relationship between a patient's medication regime and socioenvironmental influences, including accessibility to resources (e.g., financial and geographical). Consistent with principles of primary health care, nurses can implement interventions to address barriers to effective medication management.

In both acute and restorative health care settings, nurses spend a great deal of time administering medications to patients and ensuring that patients are adequately prepared to self-administer medications when they are discharged. If patients cannot administer their own medications when they are at home, family members or support persons can take responsibility for this task. As a nurse, you assess the effect of the medications in restoring or maintaining health and continue to educate the patient, the patient's family, and home care personnel about the medication's purpose, regimen, and adverse reactions.

SCIENTIFIC KNOWLEDGE BASE

Medications are administered to patients to prevent, diagnose, or treat disease and health conditions. Because medication administration and evaluation are essential to nursing practice, you need to understand the actions and effects of the medications your patients take. To safely and accurately administer medications, you must have an understanding of pharmacology, pharmacokinetics (the study of how medications enter, affect, and exit the body), human growth and development, human anatomy, pathophysiology, psychology, nutrition, and mathematics. You need to apply your cumulative nursing knowledge when administering medications. The nursing process provides the framework for you to organize your thoughts and actions, and it is the foundation for medication administration.

Pharmacological Concepts

Drug Names. A medication may have as many as three different names. A medication's chemical name provides an exact description of the medication's composition and molecular structure. Chemical names are rarely used in clinical practice. For example, the chemical name N-acetyl-para-aminophenol is commonly known as Tylenol. The generic, or nonproprietary, name is given by the manufacturer that first develops the medication. Acetaminophen is the generic name for Tylenol. The generic name becomes the official name under which the medication is listed in official publications, such as the *Compendium of Pharmaceuticals and Specialties (CPS),* the *Canadian Formulary (CF),* or the *United States Pharmacopeia (USP).* In addition to the drug name, all drug products approved for distribution in Canada have an eight-digit number, which is assigned by the Health Protection Branch of the federal government. This Drug Identification Number (DIN) is used by various groups and agencies to track drug information across Canada.

The trade name, brand name, or proprietary name is the name under which a manufacturer markets a medication. The trade name is followed by the symbol ™, which indicates that the manufacturer has trademarked the medication's name (e.g., Tempra™, Motrin™). Manufacturers choose trade names that are easy to pronounce, spell, and remember so that laypersons will remember the medication names. A medication may be produced by many different companies, and similarities in their trade names can be confusing. Because similarities in drug names are a common cause of medical errors, the Joint Commission (2017) in the United States publishes on its website a list of drugs whose names look like or sound like other drug names as well as recommendations for nurses, prescribers, other health care providers, and health care organizations to prevent drug errors related to look-alike and sound-alike names of medications. Medications are available under a variety of different nomenclatures, or names, and as a nurse you must be careful to obtain the exact name and spelling for the particular medications you administer. For a listing of prescription drugs, both their trade and generic names, commonly used in Canada see http://www.medbroadcast.com/drug.

Classification. Medication classification indicates the effect of the medication on a body system, the symptoms that the medication relieves, or the medication's desired effect. For example, patients who have type 2 diabetes often take medications to control their blood glucose level. *Sulfonylureas* are one classification of medications often used by these patients. At least seven different medications are included in the sulfonylurea classification (McKenry, Tessier, & Hogan, 2005). A prescriber chooses a particular medication on the basis of the patient's characteristics; the medication's cost, efficacy, and dosing frequency; and the prescriber's experience with the medication. Some medications belong to more than one class. For example, aspirin is an analgesic, an antipyretic, and an anti-inflammatory medication. Classification of medications is important in discerning their respective effects and nursing considerations (Box 34-1).

Medication Forms. Medications are available in a variety of forms, or preparations (Figure 34-1). The form of the medication

BOX 34-1 Clinical Tip

Adverse effects, nursing considerations, and patient teaching are commonly shared by medications in the same class. Students and new practitioners are often overwhelmed by the number of medications they need to know. Using classification of medications simplifies the process of identifying adverse effects of medications, nursing considerations, and patient teaching. Patient safety is also increased.

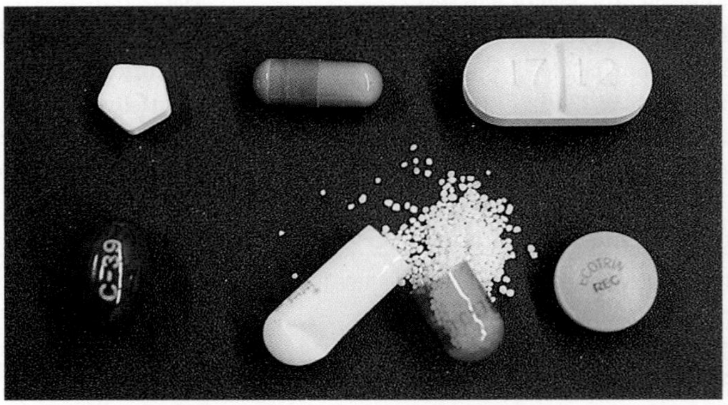

FIGURE 34-1 Forms of oral medications. **Top row:** Uniquely shaped tablet, capsule, scored tablet. **Bottom row:** Gelatin-coated liquid, extended-release capsule, enteric-coated tablet.

TABLE 34-1 Forms of Medication

Form	Description
Medication Forms Commonly Prepared for Administration by Oral Route	
Solid Forms	
Caplet	Shaped like a capsule and coated for ease of swallowing
Capsule	Medication encased in a gelatin shell
Tablet	Powdered medication compressed into a hard disc or cylinder; in addition to primary medication, contains binders (adhesives that allow the powder to stick together), disintegrators (to promote tablet dissolution), lubricants (for ease of manufacturing), and fillers (to make a convenient size for swallowing)
Enteric-coated tablet	Coated tablet that does not dissolve in stomach; coatings dissolve in intestine, where medication is absorbed
Pill	Contains one or more medications; shaped into globules, ovoids, or oblongs; rarely used because most pills have been replaced by tablets
Liquid Forms	
Elixir	Clear fluid containing medication and either water or alcohol, or both; often sweetened
Extract	Syrup or dried form of pharmacologically active medication, usually made by evaporating the solution
Aqueous solution	Medication dissolved in water
Aqueous suspension	Finely divided drug particles dispersed in a liquid medium; when the suspension is left standing, particles settle to the bottom of the container
Syrup	Medication dissolved in a concentrated sugar solution
Tincture	Medicinal alcoholic extract from a plant or vegetable
Other Oral Forms and Terms Associated With Oral Preparations	
Troche (lozenge)	Flat, round tablet that dissolves in the mouth to release medication; not intended for ingestion.
Aerosol	Aqueous medication sprayed and absorbed in the mouth and upper airway; not intended for ingestion
Sustained release	Tablet or capsule that contains small particles of a medication coated with material that requires time to dissolve
Medication Forms Commonly Prepared for Administration by Topical Route	
Ointment (salve or cream)	Semisolid, externally applied preparation, usually containing one or more medications
Liniment	Preparation that usually contains medication and alcohol, oil, or soapy emollient; applied to the skin
Lotion	Liquid suspension that usually protects, cools, or cleanses skin and can contain medication
Paste	Thick ointment; absorbed through the skin more slowly than ointment; often used for skin protection
Transdermal disc or patch	A disc or patch from which medication is absorbed through the skin slowly over a long period of time (e.g., 24 hours, 1 week)
Medication Forms Commonly Prepared for Administration by Parenteral Route	
Solution	Sterile preparation that contains water with one or more dissolved medicinal compounds
Powder	Sterile particles of medication that are dissolved in a sterile liquid (e.g., water or normal saline) before administration
Medication Forms Commonly Prepared for Instillation Into Body Cavities	
Solution	Medication dissolved in water or other liquid
Intraocular disc	Small, flexible oval (similar to a contact lens) consisting of two soft, outer layers and a middle layer containing medication; slowly releases medication when moistened by ocular fluid
Suppository	Solid medicine dosage mixed with gelatin and shaped into a pellet for insertion into a body cavity (rectum or vagina); melts at body temperature to release medication

determines its route of administration. The composition of a medication is designed to enhance its absorption and metabolism. Many medications are made in several forms, such as tablets, capsules, elixirs, and suppositories. When administering a medication, the nurse must be certain to use the proper form (Table 34-1).

Medication Legislation and Standards

Canadian Drug Legislation. Regulation of drug standards began in Canada in 1884, when the *Adulteration Act* set the conditions under which a drug could be adulterated. The *Food and Drugs Act* of 1920 replaced this Act and, with amendments in 1950, gave the federal government control of the manufacture and sale of all drugs (except narcotics), all food, all cosmetics, and certain medical devices.

The federal government first attempted to control narcotic substances in 1908 through the *Opium Act.* Cocaine and morphine came under the jurisdiction of this Act in 1911. In 1961, the *Narcotic Control Act,* which controls the manufacture, distribution, and sale of narcotic drugs, was enacted. This Act was repealed in 1996 and replaced by the

Controlled Drugs and Substances Act. The federal government has also passed legislation that regulates the manufacture and sale of herbs and other natural health products. This legislation addresses the content of these products as well as the products' packaging, labelling, distribution, and storage.

Drug Standards. Official publications, such as the *British Pharmacopoeia (BP)* and the *Canadian Formulary*, set standards for drug strength, quality, purity, packaging, safety, labelling, and dosage form. Physicians, nurses, and pharmacists depend on these standards to ensure that patients receive pure drugs in safe and effective dosages.

Accepted standards must be met in the following areas:

- *Purity*: Manufacturers must meet purity standards for the type and concentration of substances allowed in drug products.
- *Potency*: The concentration of the active drug in the preparation affects its strength, or potency.
- *Bioavailability*: The ability of a drug to be released from its dosage form and to be dissolved, absorbed, and transported by the body to the drug's site of action.
- *Efficacy*: Detailed laboratory studies help determine a drug's effectiveness.
- *Safety*: All drugs need to be continually evaluated to determine their adverse reactions.

Control. Administration of the *Food and Drugs Act* and the *Controlled Drugs and Substances Act* is carried out by the Health Protection Branch (HPB) of the federal government. Before a new drug can be marketed in Canada, an application for approval must be made to the HPB. After intensive testing to ensure the drug's effectiveness and safety in humans, the HPB reviews the application. The HPB issues a DIN and Notification of Compliance, which allow the drug to be sold in Canada. Stringent controls are applied to this new drug until sufficient information has been accumulated to ensure its safety and efficacy. Only then is the drug released for general use. Monitoring of the drug is ongoing to report adverse effects, safety concerns, or changes in the indications for a particular drug's use.

Provincial, Territorial, and Local Regulation of Medication. The provincial and territorial governments do not directly regulate the manufacture or sale of drugs. However, because the provincial and territorial governments have most of the legislative responsibility for health care, provincial and territorial legislation indirectly affects the use and sale of drugs within provincial and territorial boundaries. In addition, each province and territory has legislation regarding medical, dental, pharmacy, and nursing practice that dictates each health care provider's role in the ordering, dispensing, and administration of drugs. In particular, some provincial and territorial pharmacy legislation includes schedules that indicate the drugs that can be sold without prescription, over the counter, and by prescription only. The National Association of Pharmacy Regulatory Authorities facilitates the activities of the regulatory authorities of all provinces and Yukon and promotes the harmonization of the practice of drug sales across the country.

Health care institutions establish policies that conform to federal and provincial regulations. The size of an institution, the types of services it provides, and the types of professional personnel it employs influence an institution's policies for drug control, distribution, and administration. Because an institution is primarily concerned with preventing health problems resulting from drug use, institutional policies are often more restrictive than government controls. For example, a common institutional policy is the automatic discontinuation of antibiotic therapy after a predetermined number of days. Although a prescriber may reorder an antibiotic, this policy helps to control unnecessarily prolonged drug therapy, which may lead to drug sensitivity or toxic reactions.

Medication Regulation and Nursing Practice. In Canada, nurses must be familiar with both the federal and provincial or territorial regulations affecting drug administration in their practice areas. If a nurse moves from one province or territory to another, he or she may discover significant differences in the laws governing drug administration. For example, laws vary concerning the prescription and administration of drugs. In the past, only physicians could prescribe medications. Today, most provinces have amended their nursing practice acts to include the prescription of medications by nurses in advanced practice. In most cases, this privilege is limited to nurse practitioners, clinical nurse specialists, and nurse midwives.

Provincial nursing organizations have developed regulations that guide nursing practice with regard to medication administration—for example, the College of Nurses of Ontario *Practice Standard on Medication* (2017), the College and Association of Registered Nurses of Alberta *Medication Administration Guidelines for Registered Nurses* (2015), and the Saskatchewan Registered Nurses' Association *Medication Management for Registered Nurses: A Patient-Centered Decision-Making Framework* (2015). Such guidelines are intended to promote safe medication administration practices for nurses.

Nurses are responsible for following legal provisions when administering **controlled substances** (drugs that affect the mind or behaviour), which can be dispensed only with a prescription. Violations of the *Narcotic Control Act* are punishable by fines, imprisonment, and loss of nursing licence or nursing registration. Hospitals and other health care institutions have policies for the proper storage and distribution of controlled substances, including narcotics (Box 34-2). **Narcotics** are natural opioid drugs or semi-synthetic or synthetic substitutes for these drugs.

Pharmacokinetics as the Basis of Medication Actions

For medications to be therapeutic, they must be taken into a patient's body, where they are absorbed and distributed to cells, tissues,

BOX 34-2 Guidelines for Safe Narcotic Administration and Control

- Store all narcotics in a locked, secure cabinet or container. (Cabinets with computer-controlled locking devices are preferred.)
- Count narcotics frequently. Count and record inventories on a continuous basis, especially when narcotic drawers are opened and when nursing shifts change.
- Report discrepancies in narcotic counts immediately.
- Use a special inventory record each time a narcotic is dispensed. Records are often kept electronically and provide an accurate ongoing count of narcotics used, narcotics remaining, and information about narcotics that are wasted.
- After dispensing a narcotic, use the record to document the patient's name, the date and time of medication administration, the name of the medication, the dose, and your signature.
- If you dispense only part of a premeasured dose of a controlled substance, a second nurse must witness disposal of the unused portion. If paper records are kept, both you and the nurse who witnesses the wastage are required to sign the form. Computerized systems record the nurses' names electronically. Do not place wasted portions in the sharps containers.
- Medications are not to be disposed of into a sink, toilet, or garbage can. Instead, wasted medications are returned to the pharmacy or disposed of in a pharmacy-designated container. Wasted controlled liquid medications are never left in their vials; they are drawn up using a needleless syringe and disposed of as a liquid.

or a specific organ, and they must alter physiological functions. Pharmacokinetics is the study of how medications enter the body, reach their site of action, metabolize, and exit the body. Nurses must use their knowledge of pharmacokinetics when timing medication administration, selecting the route of administration, considering the patient's risk for alterations in medication action, and evaluating the patient's response.

Absorption. Absorption refers to the passage of medication molecules into the blood from the medication's site of administration. Medication absorption is affected by the route of administration, the ability of the medication to dissolve, blood flow to the site of administration, the patient's body surface area, and lipid solubility (maximum concentration of a chemical that will dissolve in fatty substances) of medication.

Route of Administration. Each route of medication administration has a different rate of absorption. When medications are applied to the skin, absorption is slow due to the physical makeup of the skin. Medications placed on the mucous membranes and respiratory airways are quickly absorbed because these tissues are highly vascular. Because orally administered medications must pass through the gastrointestinal (GI) tract to be absorbed, the overall rate of absorption is usually slow. Intravenous (IV) injection produces the most rapid absorption because this route provides immediate access to systemic circulation.

Ability of the Medication to Dissolve. The ability of an oral medication to dissolve depends on its form or preparation. Solutions and suspensions in a liquid state are absorbed more readily than tablets or capsules. Acidic medications pass through the gastric mucosa rapidly. Medications that have a base pH are not absorbed before reaching the small intestine.

Blood Flow to the Site of Administration. When the site of administration contains a rich blood supply, the body absorbs medications more rapidly. As blood comes in contact with the site of administration, the medication is absorbed. Therefore, areas that have more blood supply will experience enhanced absorption, facilitating the passage of the medication into the bloodstream.

Body Surface Area. When a medication is in contact with a large surface area, the medication will be absorbed at a faster rate. This characteristic explains why most medications are absorbed in the small intestine, not in the stomach.

Lipid Solubility of a Medication. Because the cell membrane has a lipid layer, highly lipid-soluble medications easily cross the cell membrane and are absorbed quickly. The absorption of medication is also affected by the presence of food in the stomach. Some oral medications are absorbed more easily when administered between meals or on an empty stomach because food can change the structure of a medication and impair its absorption. When you administer medications, you should be aware of potential medication–medication interactions listed in the *CPS*, in drug manuals, and on drug packaging. If medications that interact are ordered at the same time, notify the prescriber immediately to revise medication administration times.

Safe medication administration requires knowledge of factors that may alter or impair the absorption of the prescribed medications. This information is based on an understanding of the medication's pharmacokinetics, the patient's history, the physical examination of the patient, and knowledge gained through daily interactions with patients. Use this knowledge to ensure that you administer all prescribed medications at the correct time. Consult and collaborate with the patient's prescribers to ensure the patient achieves the therapeutic effect of all medications. Before administering any medication, check pharmacology books or drug references and package inserts, or consult with pharmacists to identify medication–medication interactions or medication–nutrient interactions. Furthermore, because the safe delivery of many medications (e.g., blood pressure–lowering agents, blood glucose–lowering medications, and anti-arrhythmics) is dependent on nursing assessments, ensure that physical assessment data are collected and interpreted before administering medications.

Distribution. After a medication is absorbed by the body, it is distributed to tissues and organs and to its specific site of action. The rate and extent of distribution depend on the physical and chemical properties of the medications and the physiology of the person taking the medication.

Circulation. After a medication enters the bloodstream, it is carried throughout the body's tissues and organs. The speed at which it reaches the site depends on the vascular content of the tissues and organs. Conditions that limit blood flow or blood perfusion inhibit the distribution of a medication. For example, patients who have experienced heart failure have impaired circulation, which also impairs medication delivery to the intended site of action. Therefore, the efficacy of medications in heart failure patients can be delayed or altered.

Membrane Permeability. For a medication to be distributed to an organ, it must pass through all the organ's tissues and biological membranes. Some membranes serve as barriers to the passage of medications. For example, the blood–brain barrier allows only fat-soluble medications to pass into the brain and cerebral spinal fluid. Therefore, central nervous system (CNS) infections require treatment with antibiotics that selectively cross the blood–brain barrier. This change in the permeability of the blood–brain barrier can lead to confusion and other adverse effects in some older patients. The placental membrane also has a nonselective barrier to medications. Fat-soluble and non–fat-soluble agents can cross the placenta and result in fetal deformities, respiratory depression, and, when combined with narcotic use, withdrawal symptoms.

Protein Binding. Most medications bind to proteins to some extent. The degree to which medications bind to serum proteins, such as albumin, affects the medication's distribution. Medications bound to albumin cannot exert pharmacological activity. The unbound, or free, medication is the active form of the medication. Older persons have a decrease in albumin in their bloodstream, which is probably the result of a change in their liver function. The same is true for patients who have liver disease or malnutrition, who, along with older persons, have the potential for more medication being unbound and thus may be at risk for an increase in medication activity or toxicity, or both.

Metabolism. After a medication reaches its site of action, it metabolizes into a less active or inactive form that is more easily excreted. Biotransformation occurs when enzymes detoxify, degrade (break down), and remove the biologically active chemicals. Most biotransformation occurs within the liver, although the lungs, kidneys, blood, and intestines also metabolize medications. The liver is especially important because its specialized structure oxidizes and transforms many toxic substances. The liver degrades many harmful chemicals before they are distributed to the tissues. If a decrease in liver function occurs, a medication is usually eliminated more slowly and results in an accumulation of the medication. If the organs that metabolize medications are altered, patients are at risk for medication toxicity. For example, a small sedative dose of a barbiturate may cause a patient with liver disease to lapse into a hepatic coma.

Excretion. After medications are metabolized, they exit the body through the kidneys, liver, bowel, lungs, or exocrine glands. The chemical makeup of a medication determines the organ of excretion. Gaseous and volatile compounds, such as nitrous oxide and alcohol, exit through the lungs. Deep breathing and coughing (see Chapter 48) help the postoperative patient to eliminate anaesthetic gases more rapidly. The exocrine glands excrete lipid-soluble medications. When medications exit through the sweat glands, the skin often becomes irritated. Nurses can assist the patient in good hygiene practices (see Chapter 38) to promote cleanliness and skin integrity. If a medication is excreted through the mammary glands, a nursing infant is at risk of ingesting the chemicals. Nurses need to check on the safety of any medication used by breastfeeding women.

The GI tract is another route for medication excretion. Many medications enter the hepatic circulation where they are broken down by the liver and excreted into the bile. After chemicals enter the intestines through the biliary tract, they may be reabsorbed by the intestines. Factors that increase peristalsis (e.g., laxatives and enemas) accelerate medication excretion through the feces, whereas factors that slow peristalsis (e.g., inactivity and improper diet) may prolong a medication's effects.

The kidneys are the main organs for medication excretion. Some medications escape extensive metabolism and exit unchanged in the urine. Other medications must undergo biotransformation in the liver before being excreted by the kidneys. If renal function declines, a patient is at risk for medication toxicity. If the kidneys cannot adequately excrete a medication, the dose may need to be reduced. Maintenance of an adequate fluid intake (50 mL/kg/day) promotes proper elimination of medications for the average adult.

Types of Medication Action

Medications vary considerably in the way they act and in their types of action. Factors other than characteristics of the medication also influence medication actions. A patient does not always respond in the same way to each successive dose of a medication. Sometimes, the same medication causes very different responses in different patients. Therefore, nurses need to understand all the effects that medications can have on patients.

Therapeutic Effects. The **therapeutic effect** is the expected or predictable physiological response that a medication causes. Each medication has a desired therapeutic effect, which is the reason it is prescribed. For example, nitroglycerine reduces the body's cardiac workload and increases myocardial oxygen supply. A single medication may have more than one therapeutic effect. For example, aspirin reduces platelet aggregation (clumping) and is an analgesic, an antipyretic, and an anti-inflammatory drug. With knowledge of the desired therapeutic effect for each medication, nurses are better able to provide patient education to accurately evaluate the medication's desired effect.

Side Effects. **Side effects** are the unintended, secondary effects that a medication predictably will cause. Side effects may be harmless or injurious. For example, opioids sometimes cause pruritus, with the absence of a rash or other allergic symptoms. If the side effects are serious enough to negate a medication's intended beneficial effects, the prescriber may decide to discontinue the medication. Patients often stop taking medications because of side effects.

Adverse Effects. **Adverse effects** are severe, negative responses to medication. For example, a patient may become comatose after ingesting a drug. When adverse responses to medications occur, the prescriber immediately discontinues the medication. Some adverse effects are unexpected effects that were not discovered during drug testing. When this situation occurs, health care providers should report the adverse effect to the Health Protection Branch of the federal government (http://www.hc-sc.gc.ca/dhp-mps/medeff/report-declaration/index-eng.php#a2). This reporting system is voluntary.

Toxic Effects. **Toxic effects** develop after prolonged intake of a medication or after a medication accumulates in the blood because of impaired metabolism or impaired excretion. Excess amounts of a medication within the body may have lethal effects, depending on the medication's action. For example, toxic levels of morphine, which is an opioid, may cause severe respiratory depression and death. Antidotes are available to treat specific types of medication toxicity. For example, Narcan is used to reverse the effects of opioid toxicity.

Idiosyncratic Reactions. Medications sometimes cause unpredictable effects, such as an **idiosyncratic reaction**, which occurs when a patient overreacts or underreacts to a medication or has a reaction different from the normal reaction. For example, a child receiving an antihistamine (Benadryl) may become extremely agitated or excited instead of becoming drowsy. It is not always possible to predict whether a patient will have an idiosyncratic response to a medication.

Allergic Reactions. Allergic reactions are unpredictable responses to a medication. Some patients become immunologically sensitized to the initial dose of a medication. After repeated administration of the medication, the patient develops an allergic response to the medication, its chemical preservatives, or a metabolite. The medication or chemical acts as an antigen, triggering the release of the body's antibodies. A patient's **medication allergy** symptoms may vary, depending on the individual and the medication (Table 34-2). Among the different classes of medications, antibiotics cause a high incidence of allergic reactions.

Anaphylactic reactions are severe reactions that are life-threatening and are characterized by sudden constriction of bronchial muscles, edema of the pharynx and larynx, severe wheezing, shortness of breath, and circulatory collapse. Immediate use of antihistamines, epinephrine, or bronchodilators is required to treat anaphylactic reactions. Emergency resuscitation measures are sometimes required. A patient with a known history of an allergy to a medication needs to avoid exposure to that medication and must wear a bracelet or medal engraved with emergency medical information, including medication allergies (e.g., a MedicAlert bracelet, Figure 34-2). These bracelets and medals alert health care workers to the patient's medical information, including allergies, if the patient is unable to communicate this information when receiving medical care. Additionally, some patients with allergies leading to anaphylactic reactions carry their own epinephrine pens.

TABLE 34-2 Mild Allergic Reactions

Symptom	Description
Urticaria	Raised, irregularly shaped skin eruptions with varying sizes and shapes; eruptions have reddened margins and pale centre
Rash	Small, raised vesicles that are usually reddened; often distributed over entire body
Pruritus	Itching of skin; accompanies most rashes
Rhinitis	Inflammation of mucous membranes lining nose; causes swelling and clear, watery discharge

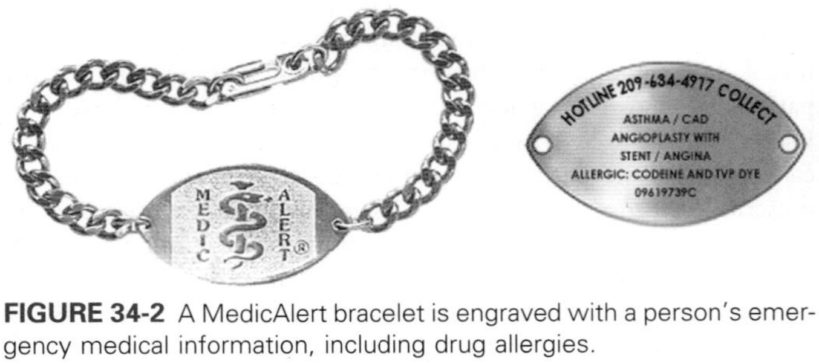

FIGURE 34-2 A MedicAlert bracelet is engraved with a person's emergency medical information, including drug allergies.

Medication Interactions

When one medication modifies the action of another medication, a medication interaction occurs. Medication interactions are common in patients who take several medications. Some medications increase or diminish the action of other medications or may alter the way another medication is absorbed, metabolized, or eliminated from the body. When two medications have a synergistic effect, the combined effect of the two medications is greater than the effect of the medications when given separately. For example, alcohol acts as a depressant on the central nervous system and has a synergistic effect on antihistamines, antidepressants, barbiturates, and narcotic analgesics.

Sometimes a medication interaction is desired. Prescribers combine medications to create an interaction that will have a beneficial effect on the patient's condition. For example, a patient with high blood pressure may be prescribed several medications, such as diuretics and vasodilators, which act together to control blood pressure when one medication alone is not effective.

Medication Dose Responses

After administration, a medication undergoes absorption, distribution, metabolism, and excretion. Except when administered intravenously, medications take time to enter the bloodstream. The quantity and distribution of a medication in different body compartments change constantly. When a medication is prescribed, the goal is to achieve a constant blood level of the medication within a safe therapeutic range. Repeated doses are required to achieve a constant therapeutic concentration of a medication because a portion of a drug is always being excreted. The highest serum concentration (peak concentration) of a medication usually occurs just before the body absorbs the last of the medication (McKenry et al., 2005). After peaking, the serum medication concentration falls progressively. After IV infusions, the peak concentration occurs quickly, but the serum level also begins to fall immediately (Figure 34-3). The point at which the lowest amount of drug is detected in the serum is called the *trough concentration*. Some medications doses (e.g., vancomycin) are based on peak and trough serum levels. The trough level is generally drawn 30 minutes before the drug is administered, and the peak level is drawn whenever the drug is expected to reach its peak concentration. The time a drug takes to reach its peak concentration varies depending on the medication's pharmacokinetics.

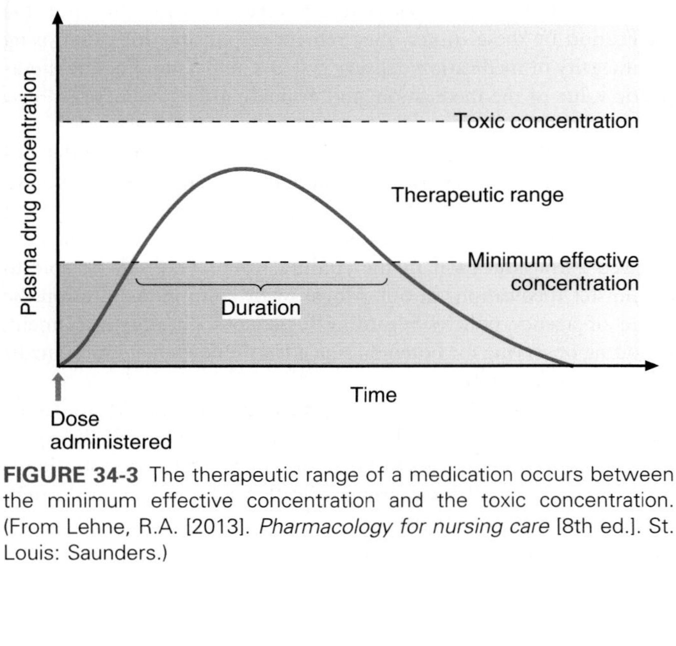

FIGURE 34-3 The therapeutic range of a medication occurs between the minimum effective concentration and the toxic concentration. (From Lehne, R.A. [2013]. *Pharmacology for nursing care* [8th ed.]. St. Louis: Saunders.)

All medications have a serum half-life, which is the time it takes for the excretion processes to lower the serum medication concentration by half. To maintain a therapeutic plateau, the patient needs to receive regular fixed doses. For example, current evidence indicates that pain medications are most effective when they are given "around the clock" to maintain an almost constant level of pain medication rather than being given when the patient intermittently complains of pain. After an initial medication dose, the patient receives each successive dose when the previous dose reaches its half-life.

Together with the patient, nurses need to follow regular dosage schedules and adhere to prescribed doses and dosage intervals (Table 34-3). Some agencies set schedules for medication administration. However, nurses are able to alter this schedule on the basis of knowledge about a medication. For example, at some agencies, medications prescribed to be taken once a day are given at 9:00 a.m. However, if a medication works best when given before bedtime, the medication should be administered before the patient goes to sleep.

When teaching patients about dosage schedules, use language that is familiar to the patient. For example, when teaching a patient about medication dosing twice a day, instruct the patient to take a medication in the morning and again in the evening. Use knowledge about the time intervals of medications to anticipate a medication's effect and to educate the patient about when to expect a response. Table 34-4 lists common terms associated with medication actions.

Routes of Administration

The route prescribed for administering a medication depends on the medication's properties, the medication's desired effect,

TABLE 34-3 Common Dosage Administration Schedules

Dosage Schedule	Abbreviation or Notation*
Before meals	AC, ac
As desired	ad lib
Twice a day	BID, bid
Hour	h, hr
At bedtime	hs
After meals	PC, pc
Whenever there is a need	prn
Every morning, every a.m.	qam
Every day, daily	*(formerly OD, but short form no longer to be used)**
Every hour	qh
Every 2 hours	q2h
Every 4 hours	q4h
Every 6 hours	q6h
Every 8 hours	q8h
Four times a day	QID, qid
Every other day	*(formerly QOD, but short form no longer to be used)**
Give immediately	STAT
Three times a day	TID, tid

*For some terms, it is safer to write out the term than to abbreviate it (see Table 34-7). Follow your agency's policy regarding the use of abbreviations.

TABLE 34-4 Terms Associated With Medication Actions

Term	Meaning
Onset	The time it takes for a medication to produce a response after it has been administered.
Peak	The time it takes for a medication to reach its highest effective concentration.
Trough	Minimum blood serum concentration of medication, typically reached just before the next scheduled dose.
Duration	The time during which a medication is present in sufficient concentration to produce a response.
Plateau	Blood serum concentration of a medication has been reached and is maintained after repeated fixed doses.

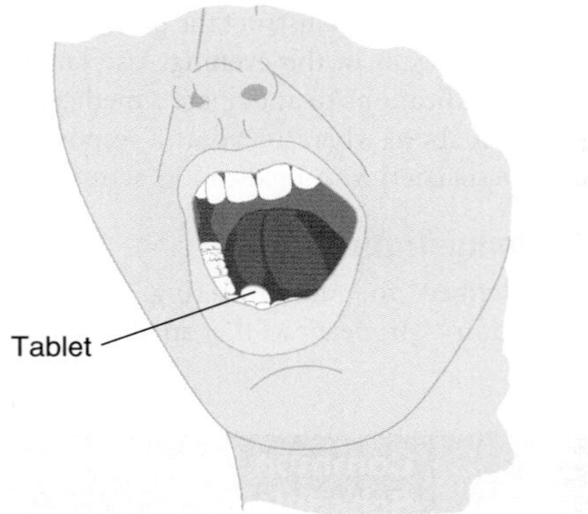

FIGURE 34-4 Sublingual administration of a tablet.

and the patient's physical and mental condition (Table 34-5). It is good to collaborate with the prescriber to determine the best route for a patient's medication, as in the following hypothetical situation:

Mr. Huels's temperature is 39.2°C. He complains of nausea and is unable to tolerate oral fluids. The nurse checks Mr. Huels's orders, which read, "Acetaminophen 650 mg orally for temperature above 38.5°C." Based on the nurse's assessment of Mr. Huels's nausea, the nurse determines that he will not be able to tolerate acetaminophen orally. The nurse consults the prescriber and receives an order for acetaminophen per rectum. By using a rectal suppository, the nurse is able to administer the acetaminophen without increasing the patient's symptoms of nausea.

Oral Routes. The oral route is the easiest and the most commonly used route of administering medication. Medications are given by mouth and swallowed with fluid. Oral medications have a slower onset of action and a more prolonged effect than parenteral medications. In general, patients prefer taking medication orally.

Sublingual Administration. Some medications are designed to be readily absorbed after being placed under the tongue to dissolve (Figure 34-4). A medication given by the sublingual route should not be swallowed because the medication will not have the desired effect.

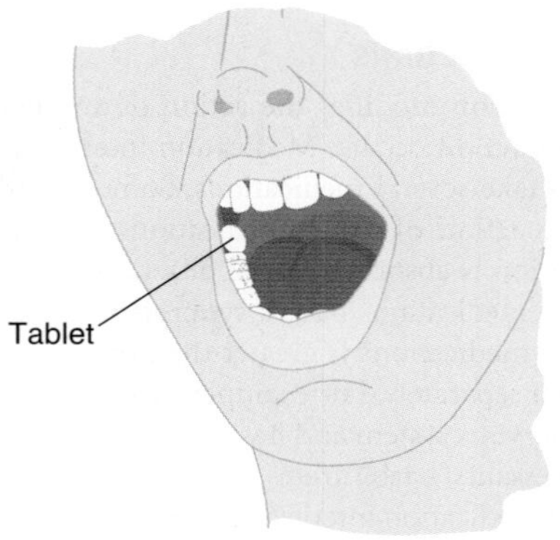

FIGURE 34-5 Buccal administration of a tablet.

Nitroglycerine is commonly given sublingually. After giving a sublingual medication, the nurse should avoid giving the patient liquids; the patient is instructed not to drink anything until the medication is completely dissolved.

Buccal Administration. Administration of a medication by the buccal route involves placing solid medication in the mouth and against the mucous membranes of the cheek until the medication dissolves (Figure 34-5). To avoid mucosal irritation, teach patients to alternate cheeks with each subsequent dose. Advise patients not to chew or swallow the medication or to take any liquids with it. A buccal medication acts locally on the mucosa or systemically when it is dissolved in a person's saliva.

Parenteral Routes. Parenteral administration involves injecting a medication into body tissues. The following are the four major sites of injection (which is the insertion of liquid into the body with a syringe):

Intradermal (ID): Injection into the dermis just under the epidermis
Subcutaneous (subcu): Injection into tissues just below the dermis
Intramuscular (IM): Injection into a muscle
Intravenous (IV): Injection into a vein

Some medications are administered into body cavities other than these four sites. These other routes of medication administration include epidural, intrathecal, intraosseous, intraperitoneal, intrapleural, and intra-arterial routes. Depending on agency policy, additional education or certification may be required for nurses to administer medications through some routes. Whether nurses actually administer the medication by these routes, they remain responsible for monitoring the integrity of medication delivery systems, understanding the therapeutic value of the medication, and evaluating the patient's response to the therapy.

Epidural Route. Epidural medications are administered in the epidural space via a catheter, which is put in place by an anaesthesiologist. This route is often used for the administration of analgesia both intraoperatively and postoperatively (see Chapter 31). If you have received extra education in the epidural route, you will be able to administer medications in bolus form or by continuous infusion. Be aware of agency policies regarding a patient's physical assessment, including observing for potential side effects following epidural medication administration.

Intrathecal Route. Intrathecal medications are administered through a catheter that has been placed into the subarachnoid space or into one of the ventricles of the brain. Intrathecal administration is often associated with long-term medication administration through surgically implanted catheters.

TABLE 34-5 Factors Indicating Choice of Administration Routes

Advantages	Disadvantages or Contraindications
Oral, Buccal, and Sublingual Routes	
Convenient and comfortable for patient	Avoid when patient has alterations in gastrointestinal function (e.g., nausea, vomiting), reduced motility (after general anaesthesia or bowel inflammation), or surgical resection of a portion of the gastrointestinal tract.
Economical	Gastric secretions destroy some medications. Oral administration is contraindicated in patients who are unable to swallow (e.g., patients with neuromuscular disorders, esophageal strictures, mouth lesions).
Easy to administer	Oral medications may irritate the lining of the gastrointestinal tract, discolour teeth, or leave an unpleasant taste.
Medications may produce local or systemic effects.	An unconscious or confused patient may be unable or unwilling to swallow or hold medication under the tongue.
Rarely cause anxiety for patient	Oral medications cannot be given when the patient has gastric suction. Oral medications are contraindicated in patients before some medical tests and surgeries.
Subcutaneous, Intramuscular (IM), Intravenous (IV), and Intradermal (ID) Routes	
An alternative means of administration when oral medications are contraindicated	Risk of introducing infection. Some medications are expensive. Some patients experience pain from repeated needle sticks. Subcutaneous, IM, and ID routes are avoided in patients who have bleeding tendencies.
More rapid absorption than with topical or oral routes	Risk of tissue damage with subcutaneous injections.
IV infusion provides medication delivery when patient is critically ill or when long-term therapy is required. IV infusion is useful to maintain therapeutic levels of a medication over time (e.g., IV antibiotics, patient-controlled analgesia). If peripheral perfusion is poor, IV route is preferred over injections.	IM and IV routes have higher absorption rates, which places the patient at higher risk for reactions. Anxiety is caused in many patients, especially children.
Dermal Route	
Topical Medications	
Primarily provide local effects	Patients with skin abrasions are at risk for rapid medication absorption and systemic effects.
Painless	Medications slowly absorb through the skin.
Limited side effects	
Transdermal Medications	
Prolonged systemic effects with limited adverse effects	Leaves oily or pasty substance on skin and may soil clothing.
Mucous Membranes*	
Therapeutic effects are provided by local application to the affected sites	Mucous membranes are highly sensitive to some medication concentrations.
Aqueous solutions are readily absorbed and capable of causing systemic effects	Insertion of rectal and vaginal medication often causes embarrassment.
An alternative means of administration when oral medications are contraindicated	Patients with ruptured eardrums cannot receive irrigations. Rectal suppositories are contraindicated if patient has had rectal surgery or if active rectal bleeding is present.
Inhalation Routes	
Provides rapid relief for local respiratory problems	Some local inhalants can cause serious health effects.
Used for introduction of general anaesthetic gases	

*Includes mouth (buccal, sublingual), eyes, ears, nose, vagina, rectum, and ostomy.

Intraosseous Route. This method of medication administration involves the infusion of medication directly into the bone marrow. Intraosseous routes are most commonly used in infants and toddlers because their intravascular space is difficult to access. This method is most often used when an emergency arises and IV access is impossible. The physician inserts an intraosseous infusion needle into the bone, usually the tibia, for the administration of medication by the nurse.

Intraperitoneal Route. Medications are administered into the peritoneal cavity, where they are absorbed into the circulation system. Intraperitoneal routes are used to administer chemotherapeutic agents, insulin, and antibiotics.

Intrapleural Route. An injection or a chest tube is used to administer intrapleural medications directly into the pleural space. Chemotherapeutic agents are the most common medications administered by this method.

Intra-Arterial Route. Intra-arterial medications are administered directly into the arteries and are commonly used to deliver tissue plasminogen activators in patients who have arterial clots. Often, intra-arterial medications are delivered through in-dwelling catheters. Nurses are responsible for monitoring the integrity of infusions systems and evaluating patients for adverse responses to these medications, including systemic and gastrointestinal bleeding. Nurses must be familiar with agency protocols, policies, and procedures for patient assessment.

Other methods of medication administration that are usually limited to administration by a physician are intracardiac routes, in which medication is injected directly into cardiac tissue, and intra-articular routes, in which medication is injected into a joint.

Topical Administration. Medications applied to the skin and to mucous membranes usually result in local effects. Gloves should be worn to prevent absorbing medication through the applier's skin and for hygienic reasons. Topical medications are administered by painting or spreading the medication over the skin, applying moist dressings, soaking body parts in a solution, or giving medicated baths. Systemic effects often occur if a patient's skin is thin or broken down, if the medication concentration is high, or if the medication's contact with the skin is prolonged.

A transdermal disc or patch (i.e., an adhesive-backed patch that releases nitroglycerine, scopolamine, or estrogens) has systemic effects. The disc secures the medicated ointment to the skin. These topical applications may be applied for as few as 12 hours or as long as 7 days.

Medications can be applied to mucous membranes in a variety of ways: (1) by directly applying a liquid or ointment (e.g., using eye drops, gargling, swabbing the throat); (2) by inserting a medication into a body cavity (e.g., placing a suppository in the rectum or vagina or inserting medicated packing into the vagina); (3) by instilling fluid into a body cavity (e.g., use of ear drops, nose drops, or bladder and rectal instillation, and fluid is retained); (4) by irrigating a body cavity (e.g., flushing with medicated fluid the eye, ear, vagina, bladder, or rectum, and fluid is not retained); and (5) by spraying (e.g., instillation into the nose or throat).

Inhalation Route. The deeper passages of the respiratory tract provide a large surface area for medication absorption. Medications can be administered through the nasal passages, the oral passage, or endotracheal or tracheostomy tubes. Endotracheal tubes are inserted into the patient's mouth and extend to the trachea (Figure 34-6), whereas tracheostomy tubes directly enter the trachea through an incision in the patient's neck. Medications that are administered by the inhalation route are readily absorbed and work rapidly because of the rich vascular alveolar–capillary network present in the pulmonary tissue. Inhaled medications may have either local or systemic effects.

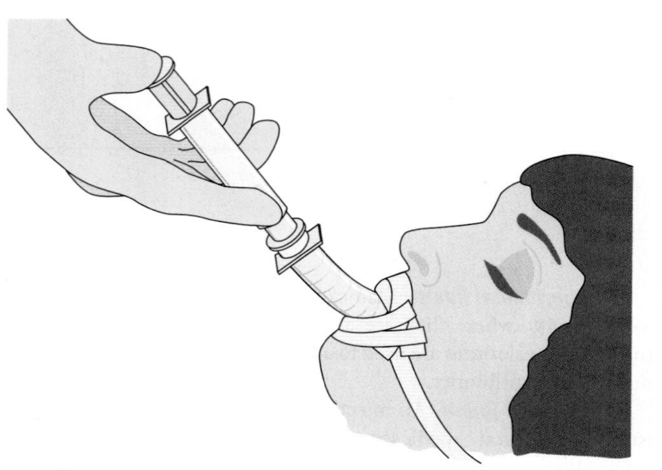

FIGURE 34-6 Medication being instilled through an endotracheal tube.

Intraocular Route. In intraocular medication delivery, a medication in a form similar to a contact lens is inserted directly into the patient's eye. The eye medication disc has two soft outer layers that enclose the medication. The disc can remain in the patient's eye for up to 1 week. Pilocarpine, a medication used to treat glaucoma, is the most common medication delivered through the intraocular route.

Systems of Medication Measurement

The proper administration of a medication depends on the nurse's ability to compute medication doses accurately and to measure medications correctly. Mistakes can lead to a fatal error. Nurses are responsible for checking the accuracy of the dose before giving a medication. The metric, apothecary, and household systems of measurement are used in medication therapy. Most nations, including Canada, use the metric system as their standard of measurement. Household measurements are used by health care providers when they write prescriptions to be self-administered by patients.

Metric System. Because it is a decimal system, the metric system (Système Internationale d'Unités [SI]) is the most logically organized system of measurement. Metric units can easily be converted and computed through simple arithmetic, such as multiplication and division. Each basic unit of measurement is organized into units of 10. Secondary units are formed by multiplying or dividing by 10. In multiplication, the decimal point moves to the right; in division, the decimal moves to the left. For example:

$$10\text{ mg} \times 10 = 100\text{ mg}$$

$$10\text{ mg}/10 = 1\text{ mg}$$

When designating a metric dosage, *do not write a zero* alone after a decimal point (e.g., write 5 mg, not 5.0 mg) and always include a zero before the decimal point (e.g., 0.1 mg) to comply with current guidelines (Institute for Safe Medication Practices, 2015; Joint Commission, 2017). The basic units of measurement in the metric system are the metre (length), the litre (volume), and the gram (weight). For medication calculations, use only the measurements for volume and weight. In the metric system, the basic units are designated by the use of lowercase or uppercase letters:

Gram = g or Gm

Litre = L or l

Lower-case letters are used for abbreviations for other units:

Milligram = mg

Millilitre = mL

A system of Latin prefixes designates a subdivision of the basic units: *deci-* (1/10 or 0.1), *centi-* (1/100 or 0.01), and *milli-* (1/1 000 or 0.001). Greek prefixes designate multiples of the basic units: *deka-* (10), *hecto-* (100), and *kilo-* (1 000). When medication doses are written in metric units, prescribers and nurses use either divisions or multiples of a unit. Convert any fractions to the decimal form.

500 mg or 0.5 g, not 1/2 g

10 mL or 0.01 L, not 1/100 L

Solutions. Solutions of various concentrations are used for injections, irrigations, and infusions. A solution is a given mass of solid substance dissolved in a known volume of fluid or a given volume of liquid dissolved in a known volume of another fluid. When a solid is dissolved in a fluid, the concentration is expressed in units of mass per units of volume (e.g., g/mL, g/L, mg/mL). A concentration of a solution may also be expressed as a percentage. A 10% solution, for example, is 10 g of solid dissolved in 100 mL of solution. A proportion also expresses concentrations. A 1/1 000 solution represents a solution containing 1 g of solid in 1 000 mL of liquid or 1 mL of liquid mixed with 1 000 mL of another liquid.

Household Measurements. Household measures include drops, teaspoons, tablespoons, cups, pints, and quarts (or litres) for volume, and ounces and pounds (or grams and kilograms) for weight. Although ounces and pounds are considered household measures, they are also used in the apothecary system. The advantage of household measurements is their convenience and familiarity. When the accuracy of a medication dose is not critical, household measures can be safely used. For example, many over-the-counter (OTC) medications can safely be measured by this method. To calculate medications accurately, nurses need to be familiar with the common equivalents of metric and household units (Table 34-6). The disadvantage of household measures is their inaccuracy. Household utensils, such as teaspoons and cups, often vary in size. The scales used to measure pints or quarts are often not well calibrated.

NURSING KNOWLEDGE BASE

The Institute of Medicine (IOM) (2003) published the book *To Err Is Human: Building a Safer Health System,* in 1999. According to this report, in any given year, an estimated 98 000 people die from medical errors that occur in hospitals; more people die from medical errors than from motor vehicle accidents, breast cancer, and workplace injuries; and medication-related errors for hospitalized patients cost approximately $2 billion annually.

Nurses play an important role in patient safety, especially in the area of medication administration. To safely administer medications, ensure that you know how to calculate medication doses accurately, strictly adhere to agency policy and procedure, and report any medication errors that occur. Be aware of the different roles that members of the health care team play in prescribing and administering medications. Remember to apply your previous learning to medication administration. The nursing process provides the framework for organizing your thoughts and actions, and it is the foundation for medication administration (Box 34-3).

Clinical Calculations

To administer medications safely, nurses need an understanding of basic arithmetic to calculate medication doses, mix solutions, and perform a variety of other activities. This skill is important because medications are not always dispensed in the unit of measure in which they are ordered (Box 34-4). This discrepancy occurs because medication companies package and bottle certain standard dosages. For example, the prescriber may order 20 mg of a medication that is

TABLE 34-6 Equivalents of Measurement

Metric Measurement	Household Measurement
1 mL	15 drops (gtt)
4–5 mL	1 teaspoon (tsp)
15 mL	1 tablespoon (tbsp)
30 mL	2 tablespoons (tbsp)
250 mL	1 cup (c)
480 mL (approximately 500 mL)	1 pint (pt)
960 mL (approximately 1 L)	1 quart (qt)
3840 mL (approximately 4 L)	1 gallon (gal)

BOX 34-3 EVIDENCE-INFORMED PRACTICE

Reducing Distractions During Medication Administration

Evidence Summary

Many medication errors occur when nurses become distracted or lose focus during medication administration (Raban & Westbrook, 2014). Errors also occur when nurses fail to follow standard nursing protocols and procedures related to medication administration. Nurses experience multiple interruptions and distractions in today's health care environment. Systems need to be put in place to help nurses avoid these distractions and subsequent medication errors. In a synthesis of systematic reviews, Lapkin, Levett-Jones, Chenoweth, and colleagues (2016) reported a number of approaches that helped reduce interruptions during medication administration, including having quiet zones for medication preparation, standardized checklists, and reminders such as "Do Not Interrupt" signs or vests worn by nurses during medication rounds. Other strategies that appeared to reduce interruptions included (a) diversion strategies, which involved other staff attending to phone calls and non-emergency requests; (b) storing medications closer to the patients (e.g., cupboards or drawers in patient's rooms); and (c) the use of a designated nurse for medication administration (Lapkin et al., 2016). Using these strategies, nurses were better able to follow the medication administration procedure, and they perceived fewer distractions during medication administration.

Application to Nursing Practice

- Consistently following nursing protocols for medication administration decreases medication errors.
- Nurses who experience fewer distractions during medication administration experience fewer medication errors.
- Placing "Do Not Disturb" signs in medication preparation areas helps reduce distractions and errors.
- Nurses need to investigate strategies that will decrease distractions, enhance their ability to follow nursing protocols, and improve their focus during medication administration.

Raban, M., & Westbrook, J. (2014). Are interventions to reduce interruptions and errors during medication administration effective? A systematic review. *BMJ Quality and Safety, 23*(5), 414–421; Lapkin, S., Levett-Jones, T., Chenoweth, L., & Johnson M. (2016). The effectiveness of interventions designed to reduce medication administration errors: A synthesis of findings from systematic reviews. *Journal of Nursing Management, 24*(7), 845–858.

BOX 34-4 Common Reasons for Measurement Conversions

- Needing to convert fluid ounces to millilitres for measurement of intake and output
- Needing to convert body weight from pounds to kilograms and vice versa
- Needing to convert volume equivalents to calculate intravenous flow rates and to prepare wound irrigation solutions, enemas, or bladder irrigations

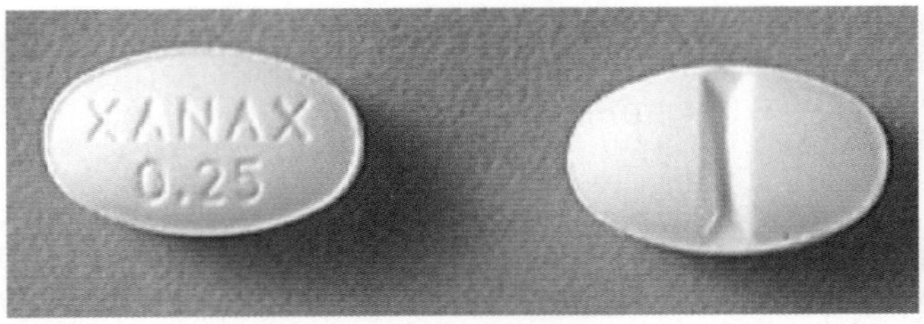

FIGURE 34-7 Scored medication tablet. (Courtesy Sharon Kaasalainen, RN, PhD.)

available only in 40-mg vials. Nurses frequently need to convert available units of volume and weight to the prescribed doses. Therefore, be aware of approximate equivalents in all major measurement systems.

Conversions Within One System. To convert units of measurement in the metric system, divide or multiply. To change milligrams to grams, divide by 1 000, moving the decimal three places to the left.

$$1000 \text{ mg} = 1 \text{ g}$$

$$350 \text{ mg} = 0.35 \text{ g}$$

To convert litres to millilitres, multiply by 1 000 or move the decimal three places to the right.

$$1 \text{ L} = 1000 \text{ mL}$$

$$0.25 \text{ L} = 250 \text{ mL}$$

To convert units of measurement within the apothecary system or the household system, consult an equivalence table. For example, when converting fluid ounces to quarts, recall that 32 ounces is the equivalent of 1 quart. To convert 8 ounces to a quart measurement, divide 8 by 32 to get the equivalent, which is 0.25 quart.

Dose Calculations. Many formulas can be used to calculate medication doses. Apply the following basic formula when preparing solid or liquid doses of a medication:

$$\text{Dose ordered/Dose on hand} \times \text{Amount on hand} = \text{Amount to administer}$$

The dose ordered is the amount of medication prescribed. The dose on hand is the dose of medication supplied by the pharmacy (e.g., milligrams, units) and is expressed on the medication label as the contents of a tablet or capsule or as the amount of medication dissolved per unit volume of liquid. The amount on hand is the basic unit or quantity of the medication that contains the dose on hand. For solid medications, the amount on hand may be one capsule; the amount of liquid on hand may be a millilitre or litre, depending on the container. For example, a liquid medication comes in the strength of 125 mg per 5 mL. Thus, 125 mg is the dose on hand, whereas 5 mL is the amount on hand. The amount to administer is the actual amount of medication the nurse will administer. Always express the amount to administer in the same unit as the amount on hand.

The following example illustrates how to apply the formula. The prescriber orders the patient to receive morphine 2 mg IV. Thus, the dose ordered is 2 mg. The medication is available in a vial containing 10 mg per millilitre, and the amount on hand is 1 mL. The formula is applied as follows:

$$2 \text{ mg}/10 \text{ mg} \times 1 \text{ mL} = \text{Amount in millilitres to administer}$$

To simplify the 2/10 fraction to decimal form, divide numerator and denominator by 2:

$$1/5 \times 1 \text{ mL} = 1/5 \text{ mL or } 0.2 \text{ mL to administer}$$

Syringes are calibrated only in decimals. After converting the fraction 1/5 to 0.2 mL, prepare the correct dose.

The following is an example of how the formula applies when calculating solid dose forms. The prescriber orders 0.125 mg orally (PO) of digoxin. The medication is available in tablets containing 0.25 mg of digoxin.

$$0.125 \text{ mg}/0.250 \text{ mg} \times 1 \text{ tablet} = \text{Number of tablets to administer}$$

The fraction 0.125/0.250 equals 1/2 or 0.5. Therefore,

$$0.5 \times 1 \text{ tablet} = 0.5 \text{ or } \tfrac{1}{2} \text{ tablet to be administered}$$

Many tablets are manufactured with scores, or indentations, across the centre of the tablet (Figure 34-7). If half a tablet is required, then pharmacy should split the tablet using a splitting device, label the package, and send the proper dose of medication to the unit since nurses splitting tablets in half on the unit, even if they are prescored, leads to medication errors (Niemann, Bertsche, Meyrath, et al., 2015).

Often, liquid medications are manufactured in volumes greater than 1 mL. In applying the formula, be careful to use the correct concentration to avoid a medication error. For example, a medication order is for "erythromycin suspension 250 mg PO." The pharmacy delivers 100 mL bottles with the label stating "5 mL contains 125 mg of erythromycin." Thus, to obtain the correct dose of medication, the appropriate concentration is 125 mg in 5 mL.

$$250 \text{ mg}/125 \text{ mg} \times 5 \text{ mL} = \text{Volume to administer}$$

The fraction 250/125 equals 2. Therefore,

$$2 \times 5 \text{ mL} = 10 \text{ mL to administer}$$

Some agencies require a nurse to double-check calculations with another nurse before administering the medication, especially when the risk of administering the wrong medication dose is high (e.g., heparin or insulin). As a nurse, always double-check your calculations or confer with another nurse or health care provider if an answer to your calculation seems unreasonable.

Pediatric Doses. Nurses must use caution when calculating children's medication doses. Children metabolize medications at different rates than adults. For example, premature and newborn infants are especially vulnerable to adverse effects of medications because their livers and kidneys have not matured to full functioning levels. After the newborn period, the liver metabolizes some drugs more quickly, which may require that the child receive either larger doses or more frequent doses (Hockenberry & Wilson, 2014). Medication dosages for children are also affected by difficulty in evaluating whether the medication has the desired effect and the hydration status of the child. In most cases, the prescriber will calculate the dose for a child before ordering the medication. However, nurses are responsible for the safe dose range for any medication administered to a child. Be aware of the formulas used to calculate pediatric doses and recheck all doses before administration. Drug package inserts or medication references often list the normal ranges for pediatric doses. Various formulas are used to determine the appropriate medication dosages for children. These formulas are often calculated on the basis of the child's age, weight, body surface area, and the medication amount. The most accurate method of calculating pediatric doses is based on a child's body surface area (Hockenberry & Wilson, 2014). Mosteller's formula or the standard nomogram (e.g., the West nomogram) is used to estimate a child's body surface area (Figure 34-8).

The following formula is used to calculate a pediatric dose. The formula is a ratio of the child's body surface area compared with the body surface area of an average adult, which is 1.7 square metres, or 1.7 m^2.

$$\text{Child's dose} = \text{Surface area of child}/1.7\ m^2 \times \text{Normal adult dose}$$

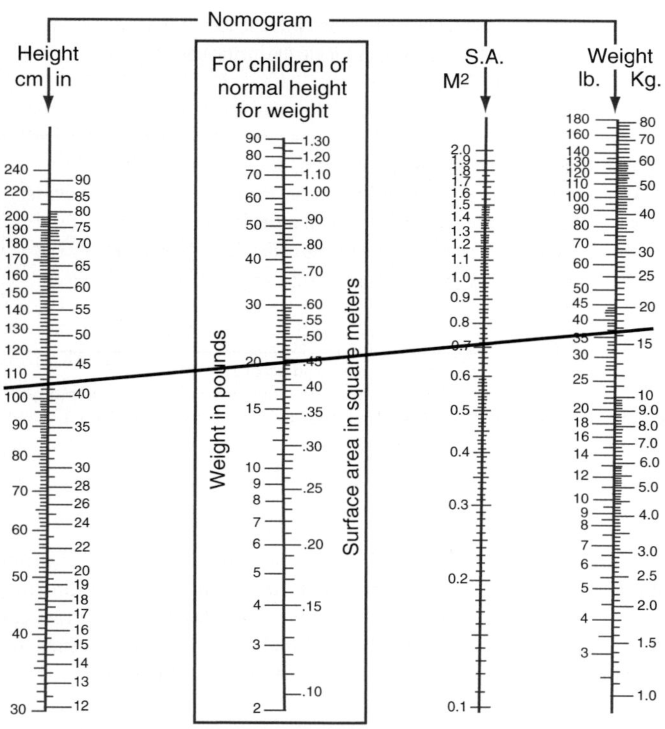

Alternative (Mosteller's formula):

$$\text{Surface area } (m^2) = \sqrt{\frac{\text{Height (cm)} \times \text{Weight (kg)}}{3600}}$$

FIGURE 34-8 West nomogram used to estimate the body surface area of children. A straight line is drawn between a child's height and weight. The point where the line crosses the surface area *(S.A.)* column is the child's estimated body surface area. (From Behrman, R. E., Kliegman, R., & Jenson, H. B. [2004]. *Nelson textbook of pediatrics* [17th ed.]. Philadelphia, PA: Saunders.)

For example, a prescriber orders ampicillin for a child weighing 12 kg. The normal adult dose for ampicillin is 250 mg. According to the West nomogram (see Figure 34-8), a child weighing 12 kg has a surface area of 0.54 m^2. Using this information, calculate the appropriate child's dose:

$$\text{Child's dose} = 0.54\ m^2/1.7\ m^2 \times 250\ mg$$

The m^2 units are cancelled out.

$$\text{Child's dose} = 0.54/1.7 \times 250\ mg$$

$$0.54/1.7 = 0.3$$

$$\text{Child's dose} = 0.3 \times 250\ mg = 75\ mg$$

An alternative method to determine medication doses for children involves basing the amount of medication to administer (usually in milligrams) on the weight of the child (usually in kilograms). For example, a prescriber orders 5 mg/kg to be given to a child weighing 14 kg. Using this information, calculate the appropriate dosage based on the following calculation:

$$\text{Child's dose} = 5\ mg/kg \times 14\ kg = 70\ mg \text{ to be delivered}$$

Collectively, the prescriber and the pharmacist help to ensure the right medication is delivered to the right patient. Most often the prescriber is a physician, but he or she can also be a nurse practitioner or pharmacist depending on individual provincial legislation in this area. For example, Bill 179, the *Regulated Health Professions Statute Law Amendment Act,* gives Ontario nurse practitioners and pharmacists open prescribing privileges. Other provinces, like Alberta, also allow pharmacists to prescribe medications.

As a nurse, when you administer medications, you are accountable for knowing which medications are prescribed, their therapeutic and nontherapeutic effects, and any nursing implications associated with the medications. You are responsible for performing a physical assessment of the patient (e.g., monitoring and interpreting blood pressure before administering an antihypertensive medication) and, on the basis of data from the physical assessment, for determining whether a medication is safe to administer. You should also know why the patient needs the medication and be able to determine whether the patient needs supervision when taking the medication or education about the medication and its effects. Always monitor the effect of the drug after it is administered and report any reactions to the prescriber.

Prescriber's Role

The physician, nurse practitioner, or, in some provinces, the pharmacist prescribes the patient's medication by writing a medication order (**prescription**) on a form in the patient's medical record, in an order book, or on a legal prescription pad; by transmitting the information on a paper form through a facsimile (fax) machine (rarely done today); or by sending the information through a computer terminal. For each medication ordered, prescribers must document the patient's diagnosis, condition, or indication for use. A prescriber may also order a medication by talking directly to the nurse or by telephone. A medication or medical treatment ordered in this way is called a **verbal order** (most common in settings where physicians tend to be offsite most of the time; e.g., in long-term care, and in rural and remote settings). When the nurse receives a verbal order, he or she must read it back and receive confirmation from the prescriber to ensure accuracy (Box 34-5). The nurse immediately enters

BOX 34-5 Recommendations Designed to Reduce Medication Errors Associated With Verbal Medication Orders and Prescriptions

National Coordinating Council for Medication Error Reporting and Prevention Recommendations to Reduce Medication Errors Associated With Verbal Medication Orders and Prescriptions

Adopted February 20, 2001
Revised February 24, 2006
Revised May 1, 2015

Preamble

Confusion over the similarity of drug names accounts for approximately 25% of all reports to the *USP* Medication Errors Reporting (MER) Program. To reduce confusion pertaining to verbal orders and to further support the council's mission to minimize medication errors, the following recommendations have been developed.

In these recommendations, verbal orders are prescriptions or medication orders that are communicated as oral, spoken communications between senders and receivers face to face, by telephone, or by other auditory device.

Recommendations

1. Verbal communication of prescription or medication orders should be limited to urgent situations where immediate written or electronic communication is not feasible.
2. Health care organizations* should establish policies and procedures that
   - Describe limitations or prohibitions on use of verbal orders
   - Provide a mechanism to ensure validity/authenticity of the prescriber
   - List the elements required for inclusion in a complete verbal order
   - Describe situations in which verbal orders may be used
   - List and define the individuals who may send and receive verbal orders
   - Provide guidelines for clear and effective communication of verbal orders
3. Leaders of health care organizations should promote a culture in which it is acceptable, and strongly encouraged, for staff to question prescribers when there are any questions or disagreements about verbal orders. Questions about verbal orders should be resolved before the preparation, or dispensing, or administration of the medication.
4. Verbal orders for antineoplastic agents should *not* be permitted under any circumstances. These medications are not administered in emergency or urgent situations, and they have a narrow margin of safety.
5. Elements that should be included in a verbal order include
   - Name of patient
   - Age and weight of patient, when appropriate
   - Drug name
   - Dosage form (e.g., tablets, capsules, inhalants)
   - Exact strength or concentration
   - Dose, frequency, and route
   - Quantity and duration
   - Purpose or indication (unless disclosure is considered inappropriate by the prescriber)
   - Specific instructions for use
   - Name of the prescriber and, when appropriate, the telephone number
   - Name of individual transmitting the order, if different from the prescriber
6. The content of verbal orders should be clearly communicated:
   - The name of the drug should be confirmed by any of the following:
     - Spelling
     - Providing both the brand and generic names of the medication
     - Providing the indication for use
   - To avoid confusion with spoken numbers, a dose such as 50 mg should be dictated as "fifty milligrams ... five zero milligrams" to distinguish from "fifteen milligrams ... one five milligrams."
   - To avoid confusion with drug name modifiers, such as prefixes and suffixes, additional spelling-assistance methods should be used (i.e., S as in Sam).
   - Instructions for use should be provided without abbreviations. For example, do not record "1 tab TID"; communicate the instruction as "Give one tablet three times daily."
   - Whenever possible, the receiver of the order should *write* down the complete order to enter it into a computer, then *read* it back, and receive confirmation from the individual who gave the order or test result.
7. All verbal orders should be committed immediately to writing and the written record should be signed by the individual receiving the order.
8. Verbal orders should be documented in the patient's medical record, reviewed, and countersigned by the prescriber as soon as possible.

*Health care organizations include community pharmacies, physicians' offices, hospitals, nursing homes, home care agencies, and so on.

From *Recommendations to reduce medication errors associated with verbal medication orders and prescriptions.* (2015). Retrieved from http://www.nccmerp.org/recommendations-reduce-medication-errors-associated-verbal-medication-orders-and-prescriptions.

the order into the patient's medical record and records the time and the name of the prescriber who gave the order (Joint Commission, 2017). Lastly, the nurse signs the record. Most institutions require a prescriber's signature within 24 hours after the order is made. Institutional policies vary regarding the personnel who are authorized to receive verbal or telephone orders. Nursing students cannot receive these types of medication orders. Nursing students give newly ordered medications only after the order has been written and verified by a registered nurse.

Common abbreviations are used when writing orders. Abbreviations indicate dosage frequencies or times, routes of administration, and special information for administering the medication (see Table 34-3). Caution must be exercised when using abbreviations because some shortened forms can lead to confusion and the potential for medication errors (Table 34-7). It is important for nurses to know their agency's policies on abbreviations. Nurses must not use error-prone abbreviations when documenting medication orders or other information about medications (Institute for Safe Medication Practices, 2015; Joint Commission, 2017; National Coordinating Council for Medication Error Reporting and Prevention [NCCMERP], 2015).

Types of Orders

Five types of medication orders are common in acute care settings: routine, "prn," single (one-time), "STAT," and "now" orders. Medication orders are based on the frequency and the urgency of medication administration. Some conditions change the status of a patient's medication orders. For example, in some agencies, the patient's preoperative medications are automatically discontinued after surgery, and the health care provider needs to write new medication orders (see Chapter 48). The prescriber should review the medications and write new

TABLE 34-7 Abbreviations, Symbols, and Dose Designations With Potential for Errors in Medication Administration

Intended Abbreviation	Meaning	Misinterpretation	Correction
U or u	Unit	Can be mistaken for the number 0 or 4, causing a 10-fold overdose or greater (e.g., "4U" can be misread as "40," or "4u" can be misread as "44"); can be mistaken for "cc," causing the dose to be administered in volume instead of in units (e.g., "4u" can be misread as "4 cc")	Write out "unit"
IU	International unit	Can be mistaken for "IV" (intravenous) or "10" (ten)	Write out "international unit"
Q.D., q.d., QD, or qd	Every day	Can be mistaken for "q.i.d.," especially if the period after the letter "q" or the tail of the letter "q" is misunderstood as the letter "I"	Write out "daily"
Q.O.D., q.o.d., QOD, or qod	Every other day	Can be mistaken for "q.d." (daily) or "q.i.d." (four times daily) if the letter "o" is poorly written	Write out "every other day"
MS, MSO_4	Morphine sulphate	Can be mistaken for magnesium sulphate	Write out the complete drug name
$MgSO_4$	Magnesium sulphate	Can be mistaken for morphine sulphate	Write out the complete drug name
µg	Microgram	Can be mistaken for "mg" (milligram)	Write the abbreviation "mcgram"
hs	At bedtime, hours of sleep (hora somna)	Can be mistaken for "half-strength"	Write out "bedtime" or "half-strength"
T.I.W. or tiw	3 times a week	Can be mistaken for 3 times a day or twice in a week	Write out "three times weekly"
S.C., S.Q., SC, and SQ	Subcutaneous	SC can be mistaken for S.L. (sublingual); SQ can be mistaken for the words "5 every": the letter "q" in "sub q" can be mistaken for the word "every" (e.g., a heparin dose ordered "sub q 2 hours before surgery" can be misunderstood as being required every 2 hours before surgery)	Write the abbreviation "subcut" or the term "subcutaneously"
D/C	Discharge or discontinue	When "discharge" is intended, can be mistaken for premature "discontinuation of medications," especially when followed by a list of discharge medications	Write out "discharge" and "discontinue"
cc	Cubic centimetres	Can be mistaken for the letter "u" (units)	Use the abbreviation "mL"

Adapted from The Joint Commission for Accreditation of Health Care. (2015). *2015 National patient safety goals: FAQs.* Retrieved from https://www.ismp.org/Tools/errorproneabbreviations.pdf.

orders when a patient is transferred to another health care agency, relocated to a different service within a hospital, or discharged.

Routine Medication Orders. A routine order is carried out until the prescriber cancels it by writing a new order or until a prescribed number of days have elapsed. A routine order may indicate a final date or the total number of treatments or doses. Many institutions have policies for automatically discontinuing routine orders. The following are examples of routine orders: "tetracycline 500 mg PO q6h" and "Decadron 10 mg daily × 5 days."

As-Needed (prn) Orders

According to a *prn* order, a medication is to be given only when a patient requires it. Nurses need to use their skills in objective and subjective assessment and discretion when determining whether the patient needs the medication. Often, the prescriber sets minimum intervals for the time of administration, which requires the medication not be given more often than a prescribed period of time. An example is "morphine sulphate 5 mg subcutaneously q3–4 h prn for incisional pain." This order indicates that the patient needs to wait at least 3 hours between doses. When administering medications, document the assessment made and the time of medication administration. Make frequent evaluation of the effectiveness of the medication and record your findings in the appropriate record.

Single (One-Time) Orders. A prescriber will often order a medication to be given only once at a specified time. This order is common for preoperative medications or medications given before diagnostic examinations: for example, "Versed 25 mg IM on call to OR" and "Valium 10 mg PO at 0900."

STAT Orders. A STAT order signifies that a single dose of a medication is to be given immediately and only once. STAT orders are often written for emergencies when the patient's condition changes suddenly: for example, "Give Apresoline 10 mg IV STAT."

Now Orders. A "now" order is more specific than a one-time order; it is used only once, when a patient needs medication quickly but not immediately, as in a STAT order. When a nurse receives a "now" order, he or she has up to 90 minutes to administer the medication. An example of a "now" order is "Give Vancomycin 1 g IV piggyback now."

Prescriptions. The prescriber writes prescriptions for patients who are to be administered medications outside of the hospital setting. The prescription includes more detailed information than a regular order because the patient must understand how to take the medication and when to refill the prescription if a refill is necessary. The parts of a prescription are illustrated in Figure 34-9. Nurses need to assess the patient's accessibility to pharmacies and other health care resources to determine whether the patient needs additional support in the community.

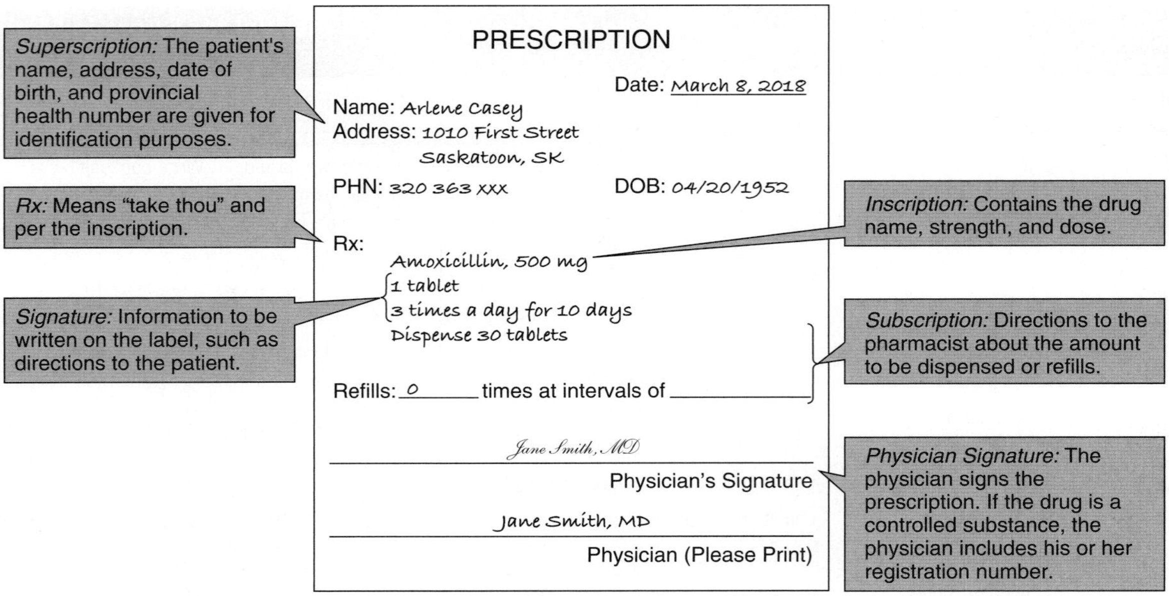

FIGURE 34-9 Sample medication prescription.

Pharmacist's Role

The pharmacist prepares and distributes prescribed medications. Pharmacists work with nurses, physicians, and other health care providers to evaluate the efficacy of patients' medication. The pharmacist is responsible for filling prescriptions accurately and for ensuring the prescriptions are valid. The pharmacist in a health care agency rarely needs to mix compounds or solutions, except in the case of IV solutions. Most medication companies deliver medications in a form that is ready for use. The pharmacist's main task is dispensing the correct medication in the proper dosage and amount and labelling the medication accurately. The pharmacist also provides information about medication side effects, toxicity, interactions, and incompatibilities.

Distribution Systems

Systems for storing and distributing medications vary. Pharmacists provide the medications, but nurses distribute the medications to patients. Institutions that provide nursing care reserve a special area for stocking and dispensing medications. Examples of medication storage areas are special medication rooms, portable locked carts, medication cabinets with computer-controlled locking devices, and individual storage units next to patients' rooms. Nurses need to ensure that all medications are in locked containers in a room (e.g., a medication room) or are under constant surveillance.

Stock Supply System. In a stock system, medications are available in quantity, in large, multidose containers. The stock system is time-consuming and costly because a nurse must dispense each medication separately for each patient. This type of medication delivery has been associated with a high rate of medication errors and is not commonly used today.

Unit-Dose System. The unit-dose system uses portable carts containing a drawer with a 24-hour supply of medications for each patient. Each drawer is labelled with the name of a patient. The unit dose is the ordered dose of medication the patient receives at one time. Each tablet or capsule is wrapped in a foil or paper container. At a designated time each day, the pharmacist or a pharmacy technician refills the drawers in the cart with a fresh supply. The cart also contains limited amounts of "prn" and stock medications. Controlled substances are not kept in the individual patient drawers; they are kept in a larger locked drawer. The unit-dose system is designed to reduce the number of medication errors and to save the steps required when dispensing medications.

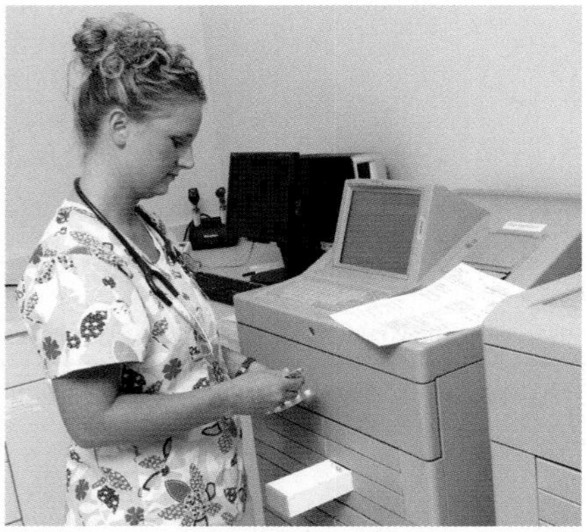

FIGURE 34-10 Nurse using automated medication dispensing system.

Automated Dispensing Systems. Automated medication dispensing systems (AMDS) are used successfully throughout Canada (Figure 34-10). These systems use computerized controls to dispense narcotics and unit-dose medication. Each nurse accesses the system by entering a security code. All procedures connected to an AMDS are controlled electronically via a patient's profile. The patient's name and drug profile must be accessed before the AMDS will dispense a medication. The nurse enters the patient's identification number into the computer and selects the desired medication, the correct dose, and the route from a display on the computer screen. The system opens the drawer containing the medication and records the transaction. Nurses may also scan bar codes to identify the patient, medication (name, dose, route), and the nurse administering the medication. This information is then automatically recorded in a computerized database.

BOX 34-6 CASE STUDY

Medication Error

June, who is a nurse working in a long-term care facility, has been asked by the director of care to work a few additional hours after her shift to administer medications to residents during dinner, since the evening nurse has called in sick and a replacement cannot be found. June is tired, having worked a full day shift, but agrees to keep working as she feels obligated to help and knows that the residents need their medications. During her dinner medication rounds, she is called away to assess another resident who has just fallen. When she returns, she is rushed and quickly finishes her medication rounds. Afterward, she realizes that she may have given a medication to the wrong patient. June feels that she needs to report this as she is worried about the consequences for both patients, but also worries that she will be disciplined by her director of care.

Thinking Points:

1. If you were in this situation, what would you do?
2. Who would you communicate this possible error to?
3. What actions would you take immediately?
4. What assessments would you make?
5. What actions could June have taken to avoid this possible medication error?

Computers on wheels (COWs) are used in many hospital units and offer a more cost-effective and efficient way to track patient admissions and records, including information about medications. COWs are carts or desks on wheels that have a laptop mounted on top. Nurses, who are the main users of COWs, can travel from room to room in the hospital to see patients at the bedside and have access to diagnostic information (e.g., vital signs, laboratory results) and treatment supplies. Nurses scan a patient's bracelet to ensure the patient's identity and then afterward scan a bar code for each prescribed medication. This gives nurses the ability to track and verify medications and decrease the chance of medication errors.

Nurse's Role

Administering medications to patients requires knowledge and skills that are unique to nurses. As a nurse you must first determine that the medication ordered is the correct medication. Do not assume that all medications in the patient's drawer or pill box are to be given to the patient. Collect and interpret physical assessment data to determine whether a patient should receive a medication at a given time, administer medications correctly, and monitor the effects of prescribed medications. Assess the patient's ability to self-administer medications. An integral part of your role is educating the patient and the patient's family about proper medication administration and monitoring. Do not delegate any part of the medication administration process to unregulated care providers, and use the nursing process to integrate medication therapy into nursing care.

Medication Errors

A **medication error** is any event that could cause or lead to a patient either receiving inappropriate medication therapy or failing to receive appropriate medication therapy. Most errors made by nurses are medication errors. A medication error can cause or lead to inappropriate medication use or patient harm. A medication error can occur when nurses neglect routine procedures, such as checking dose calculations; administer unfamiliar medications; neglect to administer an ordered medication; fail to comply with the rights of medication administration (see the section "Standards" for a sample list of common rights); and fail to perform necessary assessments before medication administration (e.g., monitoring the patient's blood glucose levels or blood pressure). Additional system issues that can lead to medication errors include distraction, illegible orders, transcription errors, and inappropriate use of abbreviations (Parry, Barriball, & While, 2015). Hospital medication delivery systems should be designed so that a system of checks and balances helps reduce medication errors. The most common types of medication administration errors made by students include (a) omission (i.e., a patient does not receive a prescribed medication), (b) a patient is given the improper dose or quantity, (c) the patient is given the medication at the wrong time, (d) the patient is given an extra dose, or (e) the medication is given to the wrong patient (Wolf, Hicks, & Serembus, 2006).

Medication errors are difficult for nurses to manage (Box 34-6). Many nurses experience psychological trauma and feel worried, guilty, or terrified that the medication error might create serious negative effects for a patient, leading to a loss of confidence in their clinical practice abilities (Mayo & Duncan, 2004). Sometimes nurses blame others for their mistake, which contributes to a "passing the blame" approach, rather than dealing with it constructively and collaboratively with their unit staff.

To demonstrate accountability and acting responsibly in professional practice, nurses need to acknowledge their errors when they occur. Because nurses play an essential role in the preparation and administration of medications, they need to be vigilant in preventing medication errors (Box 34-7) and advocate for work environments that are conducive to safe medication administration (Box 34-8).

Medication errors can also result from the design of health care products or from procedures and systems, such as product labelling and distribution. When an error occurs, the patient's safety and well-being is top priority. The nurse should assess the patient's condition and notify the physician or prescriber of the medication error as soon as possible. The nurse may need to take measures to counteract the error. After the patient's condition has stabilized, the incident should be reported to the appropriate person in the institution (e.g., a manager or supervisor).

When a medication error occurs, the nurse is responsible for preparing a written occurrence or incident report, which usually needs to be filed within 24 hours of the error. The report includes the patient identification information; the location and time of the incident; an accurate, factual description of the error that occurred and measures taken to address the error; and the nurse's signature. The occurrence report is not a permanent part of the patient's medical record and is not referred to in the record (see Chapters 8 and 17), which legally protects the health care provider and the institution. Institutions use occurrence reports to track incident patterns and to address quality improvement and risk-management issues. Many institutions have procedures in place for disclosing incidents to patients or their family members.

All medication errors, including errors that do not cause obvious or immediate harm and near misses, must be reported. It is important for you as a nurse to feel comfortable in reporting an error and not fear repercussions from managerial staff. Even when a patient suffers no harm from a medication error, the institution can still learn why the mistake occurred and what steps can be taken to avoid similar errors in the future. Creating a **culture of safety** through strategies such as "good catch" or "near miss" reporting is becoming a popular

BOX 34-7 Steps to Take to Prevent Medication Errors

- Follow the rights of medication administration.
- Be sure to read labels at least three times (comparing medication administration record with label) before, during, and after administering the medication.
- Use at least two patient identifiers whenever administering a medication.
- Do not allow any other activity to interrupt administration of medication to a patient.
- Double-check all calculations, and verify with another nurse.
- Do not interpret illegible handwriting; clarify with the prescriber.
- Question unusually large or small doses.
- Document all medications as soon as they are given.
- When you have made an error, reflect on what went wrong and ask how you could have prevented the error.
- Evaluate the context or situation in which a medication error occurred. This helps to determine whether you have the necessary resources for safe medication administration.
- When repeated medication errors occur within a work area, identify and analyze the factors that may have caused the errors and take corrective actions.
- Attend in-service programs that focus on the medications commonly administered.

Adapted from National Coordinating Council for Medication Error Reporting and Prevention. (2014). *Recommendations for health care professionals to reduce medication errors associated with the label, labeling and packaging of pharmaceutical (drug) products and related devices.* Retrieved from http://www.nccmerp.org/recommendations-health-care-professionals-reduce-medication-errors-associated-labeling. Reprinted with permission of the National Coordinating Council for Medication Error Reporting and Prevention.

BOX 34-8 Informatics and Medication Safety

Many medication errors occur when the nurse incorrectly administers medications at the patient's bedside. The following innovations and advances in technology help to reduce the number of medication errors in nursing practice:

- Networked computers allow all the patient's health care providers to see a current list of ordered and discontinued medications.
- Internet and intranet access allow nurses and other health care providers to access current information about medications (e.g., indications, desired effects, adverse effects) and specific agency policies that address medication administration (e.g., how fast to administer an intravenous [IV] push medication, how to administer medications through a nasogastric tube).
- In some agencies, prescribers enter medication orders directly into a networked computer system or a personal hand-held computer.
- Automated medication dispensing systems and electronic medication administration records help with medication reconciliation, administration, and documentation (Manno, 2006; Paoletti, Suess, Lesco, et al., 2007).
- Bar-coding technology requires nurses to scan the medication, the patient's identification bracelet, and the nurse's identification badge before administering the medication. This process helps to ensure compliance with the rights of medication administration (Mills, Neily, Mims, et al., 2006; Paoletti et al., 2007; Skibinski, White, Lin, et al., 2007).

Application to Nursing Practice

- Actively participate in the selection and evaluation of advanced technologies and the creation of nursing policies and protocols used for medication administration.
- Always follow agency policies when administering medications.
- Implement agency policies for when the technology cannot be used (e.g., during computer down time or power outages).
- Follow the manufacturer's guidelines for care of electronic equipment and report problems with technology immediately.

method for addressing medication safety. Table 34-8 outlines error-prone conditions that lead to student nurse–related errors and specific strategies for avoiding these errors.

Medication errors often occur when a patient is transferred to a different unit within a hospital or to another health care agency. Therefore, reconciling the list of a patient's medications during the transfer process is an important part of ensuring safe patient care (Joint Commission, 2017). Nurses play an essential role in medication reconciliation (Box 34-9).

When admitting a patient to any health care setting, the nurse should compare the medications the patient took in the previous setting (e.g., at home or in another nursing unit) with the patient's current medication orders (Ptasinski, 2007). When a patient is discharged, the nurse reviews the patient's current medications with the health care providers in the new setting. This action, **medication reconciliation**, may be time-consuming, but it is an essential step in ensuring medication safety. When reconciling medications, the nurse needs to consult with the patient, the patient's caregivers and family members, the physician or advanced practice nurse, and the pharmacist (World Health Organization [WHO], 2014).

BOX 34-9 Process for Medication Reconciliation

1. Verify: Obtain a current list of the patient's medications.
2. Clarify: Ensure the accuracy of the medications, dosages, and frequencies; clarify the content of the list with as many people as necessary (e.g., the patient, caregivers, health care providers, pharmacists).
3. Reconcile: Compare new medication orders against the current list; investigate any discrepancies by contacting the patient's health care provider.
4. Transmit: Communicate the updated and verified list to caregivers and the patient as appropriate.

Adapted from Ptasinski, C. (2007). Develop a medication reconciliation process. *Nurse Manager, 38,* 18.

CRITICAL THINKING

Knowledge

To understand why a particular medication has been prescribed for a patient and how the medication will alter the patient's physiology and have a therapeutic effect, nurses use knowledge they have acquired from many disciplines. For example, from physiology, they learn that potassium is a major intracellular ion. When patients do not have enough potassium in their body (hypokalemia), they experience signs and symptoms such as muscle fatigue or weakness. In some cases, severe hypokalemia is fatal because of the dysrhythmias that may occur as a result. To restore the patient's potassium level to normal, medications may be prescribed, which will also relieve the patient's signs and symptoms of hypokalemia.

Nurses administer a wide variety of medications, and new medications are constantly being approved for dispensation. As a result, nurses

TABLE 34-8 Error-Prone Conditions Leading to Student Nurse–Related Errors

Condition	Description	Strategies to Prevent Error
Preparing drugs for multiple patients	Preparing medications for multiple patients increases the risk of administering medications to the wrong patient.	Organize the medication process by preparing medications for one patient at a time. When preparing medications for multiple patients, apply patient labels to medication cups, removable needle caps of syringes, and IV bags. Use two unique identifiers to verify the correct patient before administering medications.
Nonstandard times	Medications scheduled for administration during nonstandard or less commonly used times are prone to dose omissions.	Student nurses develop a proactive plan with staff nurses to clarify the responsibility for administration of each ordered medication and how new medication orders received during the shift will be handled. Instructors and staff nurses should monitor the patient's MARs and review potential omissions with the student nurses.
Documentation	When both staff nurses and student nurses are assigned to the same patients, neglecting to document or review previously administered medications can lead to dose omissions or extra doses.	Both student nurses and staff nurses should use the same MAR. The patient's MAR should be taken to the patient's bedside and the drug administration should be documented immediately after the patient has been administered the medications. Review all sources of documented drug administration, especially for patients who are transferred from a different unit. Student nurses need to be involved in all verbal reports about the patients they are caring for.
MARs unavailable or not referenced	Neglecting to take the MAR to the patient's bedside when administering medications can lead to errors.	Always use MARs when preparing and administering medications; worksheets should not be used. Prepare medications in accordance only with the original MAR, and take the MAR to the patient's bedside for verification before administering medications. Always use two unique identifiers to verify the correct patient before administering medications.
Partial drug administration	Depending on the year of study, student nurses may not be involved in administering all of the prescribed medications to patients, such as IV medications.	For each unit that hosts student nurses, nursing instructors should provide a daily report that indicates the types of medications that the student nurses will and will not be administering. At the beginning of a shift, the student nurse confirms with the staff nurse responsible for patient assignment the types of medications the student nurse will and will not be administering. Student nurse reports medications that are not given when due.
Held or discontinued medications	Drugs that have been placed on hold or have been discontinued may be mistakenly administered when student nurses are unfamiliar with an agency's processes for holding and discontinuing medications.	Agencies should annually review their procedures for holding medications and make necessary revisions to ensure that the process is clear and reliable. Student nurses consult with nursing instructors and staff nurses regarding processes for holding or discontinuing medications.
Monitoring issues	Errors occur when nurses are unaware of medications that require vital signs monitoring or lab values assessment before medication administration.	Student nurses ensure that they know how to access the most recent lab values. Student nurses ensure that they know which medications require vital signs monitoring (e.g., antihypertensive medications) and lab values assessment (e.g., warfarin) before being administered.
Nonspecific doses dispensed	Excessive doses have been administered when student nurses expect the drug is provided in a patient-specific dose, but the pharmacy has dispensed the drug in a larger dose or quantity.	The pharmacy should dispense medications in ready-to-use, patient-specific doses whenever possible; otherwise, provide further instructions on the MAR and the dose itself. On MARs, the patient-specific dose should be listed first, as in the following example: "Lopressor 25 mg," followed by "25 mg = 1/2 of a 50-mg tab."
Oral liquids in parenteral syringes	Preparation of oral or enteral solutions in parenteral syringes can lead to nursing students incorrectly administering these products by the IV route.	Pharmacists should dispense all oral liquid products in oral syringes. Medication areas should be stocked with oral syringes. Use only oral syringes to prepare oral medications.

MAR, Medical administration record.

Adapted from Institute for Safe Medication Practices. (2007). *Error-prone conditions that lead to student nurse–related errors.* Retrieved from https://www.ismp.org/newsletters/acutecare/articles/20071018.asp.

may not always have knowledge about the medications they are asked to administer. Responsible nurses admit what they do not know and acquire the knowledge needed to safely administer unfamiliar medications by consulting a medication book, electronic computer manuals, the prescriber, or a pharmacist.

Experience

Nursing students often have limited experience with medication administration as it applies to professional practice. Clinical experiences provide nursing students with the opportunity to apply the nursing process to medication administration. As you gain experiences in medication administration, your psychomotor skills (the steps you take to complete the task) become more refined; however, psychomotor skills represent only a small part of medication administration. The patient's attitudes, knowledge, physical and mental status, and responses can make medication administration a complex experience.

Cognitive and Behavioural Attributes

Every step of safe medication administration requires a disciplined attitude and a comprehensive, systematic approach. To be consistent with professional, ethical, and legal nursing standards, you must always accept full responsibility for all your actions related to medication administration. When administering a medication to a patient, ensure that your nursing actions do not harm the patient in any way. Do not assume that the medication ordered for the patient is the correct medication or the correct dose. You can be held accountable for administering an ordered medication that is knowingly inappropriate for the patient. Thus, for all medications that you administer, you need to be familiar with the therapeutic effect, usual dosage, laboratory references, and adverse effects. Before administering medications, you must conduct a comprehensive physical assessment of the patient and critically analyze the assessment data. You are also responsible for ensuring that patients who will self-administer medications have been properly informed about all aspects of self-administration.

Institutional policy may limit nurses' ability to administer medications in certain units in acute care settings. Nurses may be limited by certain medication routes or by certain dosages. In most institutions, nursing procedure manuals list the institution's policies that define the classes of medications that nurses may and may not administer. The types and doses of medications that nurses may deliver can also vary from unit to unit within the same facility. For example, Dilantin, a powerful medication that is prescribed to treat seizures, may be administered by mouth or by IV push. In large doses, Dilantin can affect the rhythm of the heart. Therefore, when a nursing unit does not have the ability to monitor the patient's heart rate and rhythm, some institutions limit the amount of Dilantin that can be given to a patient. To ensure safe medication administration, nurses must adhere to evidence-informed practice guidelines and agency policy and procedure. Not all prescribers are aware of the limitations of all health care institutions and may prescribe medications that cannot be given in a particular health care setting. Nurses must recognize this possibility and ensure that the prescriber is informed of any limitations.

Standards

Standards are actions that ensure safe nursing practice. In Canada, the activity of medication administration by registered nurses is governed by the Canadian Nurses Association's (2017) *Code of Ethics* and professional practice standards set by provincial and territorial nursing associations. Nurses are legally and ethically responsible to acquire the knowledge needed to administer medications and to uphold the patient's rights, dignity, and uniqueness in the process. To ensure safe nursing practice, each time a nurse administers a medication, he or she must be aware of the rights of medication administration. All medication errors can be linked, in some way, to an inconsistency in adhering to the following rights of medication administration:

1. The right medication
2. The right dose
3. The right patient
4. The right route
5. The right time and frequency
6. The right documentation
7. The right reason
8. The right to refuse
9. The right patient education
10. The right evaluation

Right Medication. A medication order is required for every medication administered to a patient. When medications are first ordered, compare the medication administration record or computer order with the prescriber's written order. Always verify new medication information when new orders are written or when patients transfer from one nursing unit or health care facility to another (Joint Commission, 2017). When preparing medications, compare the label of the medication container with the medication form. Check the label against the medication form three times: (1) before removing the container from the drawer or shelf, (2) when the amount of medication ordered is removed from the container, and (3) before returning the container to storage. Never prepare medications from unmarked containers or from containers with illegible labels (Joint Commission, 2017). When you are using unit-dose prepackaged medications, check the label against the medication administration record when taking medications out of the medication dispensing system. After you determine that the information on the patient's medication administration record is accurate, the record is used to prepare and administer the medications. Verify all medications against the medication administration record at the patient's bedside before opening the medication packages and delivering the medications to the patient.

Administer only the medications that you prepare. If an error occurs, the nurse who administers the medication is responsible. If a patient questions the medication, do not ignore the patient's concerns. An alert patient will know whether a medication is different from one previously received. In most cases, the patient's medication order has been changed; however, the patient's questions might reveal an error. If an error does occur, withhold the medication and recheck it against the prescriber's orders.

Patients who self-administer medications should keep the medications in their original labelled containers, separate from other medications, to avoid confusion. Many hospitals request that all medication in the hospital setting be administered by nurses, rather than allowing patients to self-administer; this process ensures that patients do not receive double doses of medication. If a patient refuses a medication, the nurse should discard it; it should not be returned to the original container. Unit-dose packaged medications can be saved if they are unopened. However, because of infection control, some agencies require medication to be discarded if it has been taken into a patient's room. If a patient refuses narcotics, follow the proper hospital procedure of having another nurse witness the wastage of the medication.

Right Dose. The unit-dose system is designed to minimize errors. The chance of error increases when a medication must be prepared from a larger volume or strength than needed or when the prescriber, in ordering a medication, uses a system of measurement different from what the pharmacist supplies. When performing a medication calculation or conversion, ensure that another nurse verifies the calculated dose.

After confirming the calculated dose, prepare the medication by using standard measurement devices. Use graduated cups, syringes, and scaled droppers to measure medications accurately. At home, patients should use measuring spoons and cups, not household spoons and cups, which vary in volume.

Only tablets that are scored by the manufacturer should be broken. When a scored tablet needs to be broken, ensure the break is even. A tablet can be cut in half by using a knife or a pill-cutting device. Discard tablets that do not break evenly. Some agencies allow nurses to save the unadministered portion of the scored medication tablet for subsequent doses if the remaining tablet is repackaged and labelled. Nurse should verify with agency policy before administering a tablet that has been opened, cut, and repackaged. In the home care setting, pill splitting is particularly problematic. The Institute for Safe Medication Practices (2006) has developed suggestions to help with this process. It is important to determine whether the patient has both the motor dexterity and visual acuity needed to split tablets. If possible, prescribers need to avoid ordering medications that require splitting.

Often a nurse prepares a tablet by crushing it so that it can be mixed in food. The crushing device should always be cleaned completely before the tablet is crushed. Remnants of previously crushed medications may increase a medication's concentration or result in the patient receiving a portion of an unprescribed medication. Crushed medications should be mixed with very small amounts of food or liquid but should not be mixed with the patient's favourite foods or liquids because a medication may alter the taste of the food or liquid and thereby decrease the patient's desire for them. This is particularly important when administering crushed medications to pediatric patients.

Safety Alert Not all medications can be crushed. Some medications, such as timed-release or extended-release capsules, are coated with special material to prevent the medication from being absorbed too quickly. Before crushing a medication, refer to a medication manual or another medication reference to ensure that the medication can be safely crushed.

Right Patient. Medication errors often occur because one patient receives a medication intended for another patient. An important step in administering medications safely is to ensure medications are given to the right patient. Remembering every patient's name and face is difficult. To identify a patient correctly, check the medication administration record against the patient's identification bracelet and ask the patient to state his or her name, to ensure that the patient's identification bracelet has the correct information (Figure 34-11).

If an identification bracelet is missing or the text is smudged or illegible, acquire a new bracelet for the patient. When asking the patient's name, one should not merely speak the name and assume that the patient's response indicates that he or she is the right person. Instead, ask the patient to state his or her full name. To avoid making the patient feel uneasy, simply explain that the question is routine for giving a medication.

Right Route. If a prescriber's order does not designate a route of administration, or if the specified route is not the recommended route, always consult with the prescriber.

When administering injections, take precautions to ensure that the medications are given correctly. Prepare injections only from preparations designed for parenteral use. The injection of a liquid designed for oral use can produce local complications, such as a sterile abscess, or fatal systemic effects. Medication companies label parenteral medications "for injectable use only."

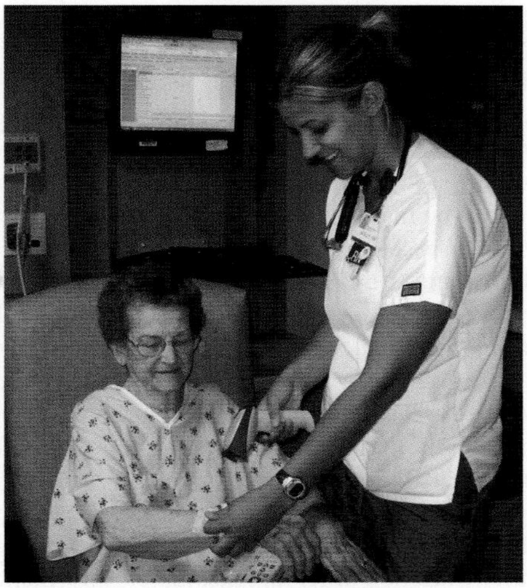

FIGURE 34-11 Nurse using a bar code scanner to identify patient during medication administration.

Right Time and Frequency. Nurses must know why a medication is ordered for certain times of the day and whether the time schedule can be altered. For example, two medications are ordered: one q8h (every 8 hours) and the other three times a day. Both medications are scheduled three times within a 24-hour period. The prescriber intends the q8h medication to be given around the clock to maintain therapeutic blood levels of the medication. In contrast, the nurse needs to give the three-times-a-day medication during the waking hours. Each institution has a recommended time schedule for medications ordered at frequent intervals. Nurses may alter these recommended times if necessary or appropriate.

The prescriber often gives specific instructions for the timing of administration of a medication. For example, when a preoperative medication is to be given "on call," the nurse needs to administer the medication when the operating room notifies the nursing unit that the patient can be transferred for surgery. A medication ordered pc (after meals) is to be given within half an hour after a meal, when the patient has a full stomach. A STAT medication is to be given immediately.

Priority is given to medications that must act at certain times. For example, insulin should be administered at a precise interval before a meal. Antibiotics should be administered on time around the clock to maintain therapeutic blood levels. All routinely ordered medications should be given within 60 minutes of the times for which they are ordered (i.e., 30 minutes before or after the prescribed time).

Some medications require nurses to use their clinical judgement to determine the proper time for administration. A "prn" sleeping medication should be administered when the patient is prepared for bed or at another time appropriate for maximum benefit. When administering "prn" analgesics, use your judgement. For example, you may need to obtain a STAT order from the prescriber if the patient requires a medication before the "prn" interval has elapsed. Always document your calls to the patient's prescriber that were made to obtain a change in the medication order.

Before a patient is discharged from the hospital setting, the nurse evaluates the patient's need for home care, especially if the patient was admitted to the hospital as the result of a problem with medication self-administration. Patients often leave the hospital with a basic knowledge of their medications but are unable to retrieve and implement this knowledge after they return home. Before discharge, the nurse evaluates whether medications are adequate or are prescribed at therapeutic levels for the patient. At home, a patient may need to take several medications throughout the day. Nurses can help patients to plan their schedules on the basis of preferred medication intervals, the medications' pharmacokinetics, and the patients' own daily schedule. For patients who have difficulty remembering when to take medications, a chart can be made that lists the times when each medication is to be taken or a special container prepared to hold each timed dose.

Right Documentation. Nurses and other health care providers use accurate documentation to communicate with each other. Correct documentation is essential to ensure safe medication administration. Because medication errors may result from inaccurate documentation, it is vital to ensure that the documentation is appropriate before giving the medications. Appropriate documentation includes the patient's name; the name of the ordered medication written out in full (no medication name abbreviations); the time the medication was administered; and the medication's dose, route, and frequency. Common problems with medication orders are incomplete information, inaccurate dose form or strength, illegible orders or signatures, incorrect placement of decimals leading to the wrong dosage, and nonstandard terminology (Hughes & Ortiz, 2005). If any pieces of information are missing, contact the prescriber to verify the order. The prescribing health care provider is responsible for providing accurate, complete, and understandable medication orders.

After administering a medication, complete the medication administration record according to agency policy to verify that the medication was administered as ordered. Nurses are also responsible for documenting any preassessment data regarding the administration of certain medications (e.g., antihypertensive medications, blood glucose–lowering agents, and medications for pain management). Inaccurate documentation of medications, such as failing to document an administered medication or documenting an incorrect dose, can lead to errors in subsequent decisions about the patient's care. For example, errors in documentation about insulin often result in negative patient outcomes. Consider the following situation: a patient receives insulin at breakfast, but the nurse who gave the insulin neglected to document it. The nurse goes home, and a new nurse is assigned to care for the patient. The new nurse notices that the previous nurse did not document the insulin and assumes that the ordered insulin was not given. Therefore, the new nurse gives the patient another dose of insulin. Two hours later, the patient experiences a low blood glucose level that causes the patient to experience seizures. Timely and accurate documentation would have prevented this situation.

Right Reason. Nurses are professionally responsible for obtaining the rationale for prescribed medications. If you are unaware of a new medication, you have the professional responsibility to research the medication by using the following sources: the *Compendium of Pharmaceuticals and Specialties (CPS)*, drug manuals, or electronic drug information databases. When retrieving information about a medication, be attentive to nursing implications, including routes of administration, preadministration physical assessments, expected onset of action, contraindications, and follow-up nursing assessments and evaluation for both adverse effects and desired responses. Nurses are professionally obligated to contact the prescriber for verification in any of the following situations: a prescriber orders a drug that the nurse identifies as contraindicated on the basis of either the patient's medical history or the patient's current condition, the ordered dose exceeds the recommended limits, or the ordered route is contraindicated for the patient. Being vigilant in critically assessing a patient's medication regimes is essential to maintaining patient safety.

Right to Refuse. With the emerging focus on patient-centred care and the recognition that patients are not passive recipients of care, more attention has been given to ensuring that the rights of patients are also upheld during the medication administration process (MacDonald, 2010). Thus, it is important to remember that a patient has the right to refuse a medication. Patients need to be informed that they have this right, but at the same time, they also need to be fully informed about the potential consequences of their refusal. If a patient refuses medication therapy, the nurse should not become defensive, and instead recognize that every person of consenting age has the autonomous right to refuse a medication (Box 34-10).

Right Patient Education. In order for patients to be fully informed about their medication and the consequences of refusing to take it, it is imperative that they receive the right education about their medications and their overall treatment plan. For some patients, education may be required for family members as well, particularly if they are involved in helping patients manage their medications at home. Education should include providing information about the drug being given, such as the reason for taking it, its action, and possible adverse effects that the patient might experience while taking it. This information is important for patients and their family members to know to ensure patient safety (Bastable, 2013). Patients and their family members need to be involved in the decision-making process about managing and administering medications and, to achieve this, they need the right information.

Right Evaluation. Patients also need to have the right evaluation at the appropriate times. Before a medication is given, the nurse needs to check to make sure that the medication order is correct and that the medication is available and accessible to the patient. Nurses need to follow up with the pharmacy or prescriber if they have any concerns or questions about the medication.

Nurses also need to make sure that any special assessments that are required have been completed, such as taking a pulse or blood pressure or checking important laboratory results that are necessary for a particular medication. If a nurse is working in the community, it is essential to ensure that patients and/or their family members have the necessary equipment and resources that facilitate safe and effective administration of medications. This assessment should include a thorough functional and cognitive assessment since many older people are faced with several conditions, such as cognitive impairments and

BOX 34-10 CASE STUDY

The Right to Refuse Medication

You have been caring for Joe, who has paranoid schizophrenia, for over 2 years now as a community mental health outreach nurse. During one of your visits with him, he tells you that he has stopped taking his antipsychotic medications because he feels he is doing much better now. You worry that this will set Joe back and wonder what you should do, although you understand that Joe has the right to refuse medications.

Thinking Points:

1. What should be your immediate response to Joe?
2. What clinical assessments are needed?
3. Who should you communicate this issue to?
4. How will this change your visits with Joe in the future?

physical limitations, which may affect their ability to manage their medications properly.

Once a medication has been given, careful monitoring of the effectiveness of the medication, its adverse effects, and signs of adverse reactions and/or drug interactions is necessary. If the medication has not achieved its desired effect, additional follow-up is needed. Within a collaborative model of care, nurses should be working closely with pharmacists and physicians if further follow-up or assessments are necessary (MacDonald, 2010).

Risk Management: Agency Policy and Procedure. Most institutions have nursing policy and procedure manuals to guide nursing practice. These manuals are updated annually on the basis of current evidence-informed practice literature. Policy and procedure manuals contain vital information for medication administration, including the types of medications nurses are permitted to administer, the preparation of medications, the administration of medications, and guidelines for evaluating patients' response to medications. For example, some agencies require nurses to complete specialized training to qualify them to safely administer IV chemotherapeutic agents. Furthermore, the administration of certain medications (e.g., IV inotropic medications for regulating a patient's blood pressure) are prohibited on general medicine and surgery units and permitted only in critical care areas where the patient is continuously monitored for responses to medication therapy.

Maintaining Patients' Rights. Because of the potential risks related to medication administration, patients have the right to the following:

- To be informed of the medication's name, purpose, action, and potential undesired effects
- To refuse a medication regardless of the consequences
- To have qualified nurses or physicians assess their medication history, including allergies and use of herbal therapies (Box 34-11)
- To be properly advised of the experimental nature of medication therapy and to give written consent for its use
- To receive labelled medications safely without discomfort in accordance with the rights of medication administration
- To receive appropriate supportive therapy in relation to medication therapy
- To not receive unnecessary medications
- To be informed whether medications are part of a research study

Nurses need to be aware of these rights and handle all inquiries by patients and their families courteously and professionally.

BOX 34-11 Nursing Assessment Questions

- What prescription and nonprescription medications do you take, when do you take them, and how do you take them? Do you have a list of medications from your pharmacy or your health care provider?
- What are your medications for?
- What adverse effects have you experienced?
- Have you ever stopped taking your medications? If so, why did you stop taking them?
- How do you help yourself to remember to take your medications?
- Do you have any allergies to medications or foods? If so, describe what happens when you take the medication or eat the food.
- Describe your normal eating patterns. What foods do you eat, and at what times do you normally eat?
- How do your religious or cultural beliefs influence your beliefs about your medications?
- How do you pay for your medications? Do you have additional insurance through your employer or pension plan to help cover the costs of your medication? Do you live close to a pharmacy? How do you access prescription medications in your community?
- What questions do you have about your medications?

NURSING PROCESS AND MEDICATION ADMINISTRATION

Assessment

To determine the need for and potential response to medication therapy, nurses assess many factors. To ensure safe medication administration, nurses must perform thorough physical assessments of all patients before administering medications.

History. Before administering medications, the nurse needs to obtain or review the patient's medical history. A patient's medical history provides indications or contraindications for medication therapy. A patient who has disease or illness is at risk for adverse medication effects. For example, if a patient has a gastric ulcer, compounds containing aspirin will increase the likelihood of bleeding. If a patient has a long-term health condition, such as diabetes or arthritis, the patient requires medications to treat these conditions. A patient's surgical history may also indicate the use of medications. For example, after a thyroidectomy, a patient may require hormone replacement.

History of Allergies. If the patient has a history of contact allergies or allergies to medication or food, the nurse needs to inform the other members of the health care team. Food allergies should be carefully documented because many medications include ingredients also found in food sources. For example, a patient who is allergic to shellfish may also be sensitive to any product containing iodine, such as Betadine or dyes used in radiological testing. To ensure patient safety, when patients are admitted to a hospital, they are issued an identification band that lists the medications they are allergic to. All allergies must be noted on the nurse's admission notes, the medication records, and the physician's documentation of the patient's history.

Medication Data. Nurses must assess information about each medication that the patient takes, including length of time the medication has been taken, the current dosage, and whether the patient has experienced any adverse effects. They must review the medication data, including the action, purpose, normal dosages, routes, adverse effects, and nursing implications for administration and monitoring. Common questions to ask include the following: Is the smallest possible dose ordered? (A question pertinent for medications ordered for older persons.) Can a certain medication interact with other medications the patient is taking? Are special instructions required for administering the medication? Often, several resources must be consulted to gather the information needed. Some valuable resources are pharmacology textbooks, nursing journals, the *Compendium of Pharmaceuticals and Specialties* (*CPS*), online medication manuals, medication package inserts, nursing journals, and the pharmacist. As a nurse you are responsible for knowing as much as possible about each medication you administer. Many nursing students prepare or purchase cards containing medication data to use as a quick resource.

Diet History. A diet history reveals the patient's normal eating patterns and food preferences. Nurses can then plan the dosage schedule more effectively and advise patients to avoid foods that may interact with their medications. It is important to be aware of patients' cultural preferences for food, and if these foods interact with medications, provide the patients and their families with comprehensive, respectful explanations.

Patient's Perceptual or Coordination Problems. For a patient with limited perceptual, fine motor, or coordination skills, self-administration of medication may be difficult. For example, a patient with arthritis who takes insulin to manage blood glucose levels may have difficulty manipulating a syringe. Nurses must always assess the patient's ability to prepare doses and take medications correctly. If the patient is unable to self-administer medications, the nurse must determine whether a family member or friend will be available to assist the patient, or collaborate with the interdisciplinary team to refer the patient to a home care service that can assist in medication administration.

Patient's Current Condition. The physical or mental status of a patient may affect whether a medication is given or how it is administered. The nurse must carefully assess a patient before giving any medication. For example, the patient's blood pressure should be checked before giving an antihypertensive medication. A patient who is nauseated may be unable to swallow a tablet. Assessment findings also serve as a baseline in evaluating the effects of medication therapy.

Patient's Attitude Toward Medication Use. The patient's attitude about medications may reveal the patient's level of medication dependence or drug avoidance. Patients may not express their feelings about taking a particular medication, particularly if they have become dependent on it. It is good to observe the patient's behaviour for evidence of medication dependence or avoidance. Nurses also need to be aware that the patient's cultural beliefs about Western medicine could interfere with medication adherence (Box 34-12 and see Chapter 9).

Patient's Knowledge and Understanding of Medication Therapy. The patient's knowledge and understanding of medication therapy influence the willingness or ability to follow a medication regimen. Adherence is unlikely unless a patient understands the medication's purpose, the importance of regular dosage schedules and proper administration methods, and the medication's possible adverse effects. When assessing a patient's knowledge of a medication, ask, "What is it for? How is it taken? When is it taken? What adverse effects have you experienced? Have you ever stopped taking doses? Is there anything else you do not understand about the medication but would like to know?" When the patient has a history of poor adherence, review resources available for the purchase of medications.

Patient's Learning Needs. Nurses must determine the need for instruction by assessing the patient's level of knowledge about a medication and the resources available to help the patient to take medications regularly. The nurse may need to explain the action and purpose of the medication, the expected adverse effects, the correct administration techniques, and steps the patient can take to remember the medication regimen. If a patient has a newly prescribed medication, the instruction will need to be more involved.

◆ Nursing Diagnosis

Assessment of the patient provides data about the patient's condition, the ability to self-administer medications, medication management (e.g., diabetic management), and medication use patterns, which can be used to determine actual or potential problems with medication therapy. Certain data are defining characteristics; when clustered together, they reveal nursing diagnoses. For example, nonadherence related to a medication regimen may be indicated when a patient admits that he or she is not taking prescribed medications correctly, or when evidence shows that a medication has not reversed symptoms as expected. The following nursing diagnoses may be observed during the administration of medications:

- *Anxiety*
- *Ineffective health maintenance*
- *Health-seeking behaviours*
- *Deficient knowledge of medications*
- *Nonadherence to prescribed medications*
- *Disturbed visual sensory perception*
- *Impaired swallowing*
- *Effective therapeutic regimen management*
- *Ineffective therapeutic regimen management*

After the patient's diagnosis has been selected, the nurse needs to identify the related factors, which guide the selection of nursing interventions. For example, the related factors of inadequate resources and lack of knowledge require different interventions. If the patient's nonadherence is related to inadequate finances, the nurse needs to collaborate with the patient's family members, social workers, or community agencies to ensure that the patient receives the necessary medications. If the related factor is lack of knowledge, referrals are initiated to ensure that home care nurses follow up with the patient and that they implement an extensive teaching plan.

◆ Planning

Nurses organize care activities to ensure the safe administration of medications. Hurrying to give patients medications can lead to errors.

BOX 34-12 CULTURAL ASPECTS OF CARE

Influences on Medication

Administration

Health beliefs vary by culture and often influence how patients manage and respond to drug therapy. Differences in values, beliefs, and attitudes affect a patient's adherence to drug therapy. For example, cultures attach different symbolic meanings to medications and drug therapy.

Herbal remedies and alternative therapies are common in some cultures and ethnic groups and can interfere with prescribed medications. In addition, differences between the health beliefs of health care providers and their patients can affect a patient's adherence to medical therapy.

Demographic changes in both age and race can affect the nursing practice in medication administration. In addition to the psychosocial aspect of medication therapy, pharmacological research has shown that some ethnic and racial groups experience differences in drug response, metabolism, and adverse effects.

Implications for Practice

- Assess a patient's cultural beliefs, attitudes, and values when administering medications and teach patients about their medications.
- Resolve conflicts between medications and cultural beliefs to achieve optimal patient outcomes.
- Ask whether the patient practises any alternative therapies or takes any herbal preparations.
- If a patient is not responding to drug therapy as expected, consider whether cultural influences affect the drug response, the rate at which it is metabolized, and adverse effects. Bear in mind that a change in the patient's medication is sometimes necessary.
- Always exercise awareness of your personal beliefs and distinguish between your values and the patients'.

Data from Blazquez, A., Mas, S., Plana, M. T., Lafuente, A., & Lázaro, L. (2012). Fluoxetine pharmacogenetics in child and adult populations. *European Child & Adolescent Psychiatry, 21*(11), 599–610; Li, W., Kuo, C. T., Hwang, S. L., & Hsu, H. T. (2012). Factors related to medication non-adherence for patients with hypertension in Taiwan. *Journal of Clinical Nursing, 21*(13/14), 1816–1824; Polinski, J. M., Kesselheim, A. S., Frolkis, J. P., Wescott, P., Allen-Coleman, C., & Fischer, M. A. (2014). A matter of trust: Patient barriers to primary medication adherence. *Health Education and Research, 29*(5), 755–763.

When preparing and administering medications, it is important to minimize distractions and interruptions (Pape, Guerra, Muzquiz, et al., 2005).

Goals and Outcomes. Setting goals and related outcomes will help you to use your time wisely during medication administration. For example, establish the following goal and related outcomes for a patient with newly diagnosed type 2 diabetes:

Goal: The patient will safely administer all ordered medications before discharge.

Outcomes:

- The patient will express an understanding of the desired effects and the adverse effects of medications.
- The patient will state the signs, symptoms, and treatment of hypoglycemia.
- The patient will be able to monitor and interpret blood glucose levels to determine medication management or treatment for hypoglycemia.
- The patient will establish a daily routine that will coordinate timing of medication with mealtimes.

Setting Priorities. Nurses need to prioritize care when administering medications. They use information gathered from their assessment of the patient to determine whether the administration of medications is appropriate and, if it is, which medication should be given first. For example, if a patient is in pain, pain medication needs to be provided as soon as possible. If the patient is experiencing an elevated blood pressure, antihypertensive medications should be administered before other medications. Nurses must establish priorities when providing patient education about medications; the most important information about the medications should be provided first. For example, because hypoglycemia is a serious adverse effect of insulin, the patient must be able to identify and treat hypoglycemia before learning how to administer an insulin injection.

Collaborative Care. Nurses collaborate with a variety of health care providers when administering medications. It is also important when giving instruction to collaborate with the patient's family or friends, who can reinforce the importance of medication regimens in the patient's home setting. Interdisciplinary collaboration with the prescriber, the pharmacist, and the home care case manager helps to ensure that the patient receives medications safely. Patients need to be able to read both medication labels and printed teaching sheets. Nurses collaborate with community resources (e.g., the home care nurse, social workers) if patients have difficulty in understanding medication management, adhering to medication routines because of functional ability, or accessing resources because of physical or financial restrictions.

When patients are hospitalized, their medication and discharge instructions should not be postponed until the day of discharge. For the patient to understand medications and self-administration guidelines, the nurse must allow sufficient time for questions and discussion. Early planning is critical. Whether a patient attempts self-administration or a nurse assumes responsibility for administering medications, the following goals and expected outcomes must be met: (a) the patient and the patient's family understand the medication therapy; (b) the patient gains the therapeutic effect of the prescribed medications without discomfort or complications; (c) the patient experiences no complications related to the route of administration; and (d) the patient can safely self-administer the prescribed medications.

◆ Implementation

Health Promotion. When working with patients to promote and maintain their health, nurses need to identify factors that may improve or diminish their well-being. Beliefs about health, personal motivations, socioeconomic factors, and habits (e.g., smoking) can influence the patient's compliance with the medication regimen.

Teaching the patient and the patient's family about the benefit of a medication and the knowledge needed to take it correctly is an essential component of primary health care and can promote adherence to the medication regimen (Box 34-13). Integrating the patient's health beliefs and cultural practices into the treatment plan can assist in establishing a schedule or routine with the patient. The nurse may make referrals to community resources if the patient cannot afford to purchase the necessary medications, or if the patient cannot arrange transportation to obtain the necessary medications. Nurses should teach all patients the basic guidelines for medication safety. These

BOX 34-13 FOCUS ON PRIMARY HEALTH CARE

Improving Drug Adherence

When a patient is discharged from hospital or sent home from a visit to a clinic, the ongoing treatment may include regularly taking medications at home. In cases of chronic illness, the success of the treatment may depend on the patient's adherence to drug therapy. Nurses can play an important role in assisting patients to adhere to their medication regimen.

The following suggestions may improve patient adherence:

- Ensure that the patient and the patient's family understand the reason for the medication, proper administration of the medication, and the possible consequences of nonadherence.
- Ensure that the patient and the patient's family and friends are able to recognize symptoms of medication adverse effects or toxicity, such as physiological changes and alterations in behaviour. Because the patient's family members and friends are often the first people to recognize such effects in the patient, they are an important resource for ensuring patient adherence.
- Teach proper self-administration of medications to patients for all routes. For example, demonstrate how to accurately measure a liquid medication. Show the patient how to prepare and administer an injection correctly by using aseptic technique. Assess the patient's ability to self-administer injections. If a patient cannot independently self-administer injections, family members or friends can be taught to administer the injections. Alternatively, collaborate with community and home care services to administer injections when patients are discharged to their home. Provide specially designed equipment as necessary, such as syringes with enlarged calibrated scales for easier reading or Braille-labelled medication vials.
- Help the patient to address any economic issues that might affect adherence.
- Explore with the patient any factors that will influence his or her ability to adhere to treatment; for some patients, keeping a daily medication log may be helpful.
- Provide a written schedule that includes the name of the medication, the dose, and a description or picture of the medication.
- Encourage patients to take their medication in conjunction with an activity they do every day, such as brushing their teeth or having breakfast.
- Help patients to organize their pills into a box with daily dividers. If adherence is a major concern, home care nurses or family members can check the box and refill it on a weekly basis.
- Work with the patient's pharmacist to ensure the pharmacy calls to remind the patient when a refill is required.

BOX 34-14 PATIENT TEACHING

Safe Insulin Administration

Objective

- The patient will correctly administer subcutaneous insulin.

Teaching Strategies

- Teach the patient how to determine that insulin is not out of date.
- Instruct the patient to keep insulin in its original labelled container.
- Instruct the patient to keep insulin refrigerated if necessary.
- Assess the patient's visual acuity to ensure that he or she is able to prepare the appropriate amount of insulin.
- Demonstrate how to rotate the location of insulin injection sites.
- Help the patient to determine the amount of insulin required, based on the results of home capillary glucose monitoring, as ordered by the patient's health care provider.
- Observe the patient's ability to correctly assess the results of capillary blood glucose monitoring.
- Demonstrate to the patient how to prepare a single insulin preparation.
- Demonstrate to the patient how to administer a subcutaneous insulin injection.
- Show the patient how to keep a daily log book to record insulin injections, including results of home capillary glucose monitoring, type and amount of insulin given, expiration date on insulin vial, time of insulin injection, and injection site used.

Evaluation

- Ask the patient to describe the signs and symptoms of hypoglycemia and the associated interventions.
- Ask the patient to describe the procedure used at home for determining the correct dose of insulin needed and the injection site.
- Observe the patient preparing an insulin dose on the basis of the results of capillary glucose monitoring.
- Observe the patient selecting the injection site and self-administering the insulin injection.
- Review the information recorded in the patient's log book for completeness.

guidelines ensure the proper use and storage of medications in the home (Box 34-14).

Acute Care. Patients are often hospitalized to receive expert nursing observation and documentation of their responses to medications. When receiving a medication order, several nursing interventions are essential for safe and effective medication administration.

Receiving Medication Orders. A medication order is required for any medication to be administered by a nurse. Before any other interventions, the nurse must ensure that the medication order contains all the elements in Box 34-15. If the medication order is not complete, the nurse must inform the prescriber and ensure completeness before carrying out the medication order.

Correct Transcription and Communication of Orders. Nurses or a designated unit secretary sometimes write the prescriber's complete order on the appropriate medication form, the medication administration record. The transcribed order includes the patient's name, identification number, room, bed number, allergies, and the medication name, dose, frequency, and route of administration. Each time a medication dose is prepared, the nurse refers to the medication form. When the unit-dose system is used, only one transcription is necessary, which limits the opportunity for errors. When transcribing orders, the nurse must ensure that names, doses, and symbols are legible, and rewrite any smudged or illegible transcriptions.

Some institutions have prescribed order entry. The prescriber enters an order directly into the computer, which avoids the need for the transcription of orders. Computer interfaces transfer the order to the medication administration record, the pharmacy record, and the automated dispensing system. The computer printout may be used as the medication administration record (Figure 34-12).

As a nurse you must always check all transcribed orders against the original order for accuracy and thoroughness. If an order is incorrect or inappropriate, consult the prescriber. If you give the wrong medication or an incorrect dose, you are legally responsible for the error. Other health care providers involved in the error are also legally responsible.

Accurate Dose Calculation and Measurement. When measuring liquid medications, use a standard measuring container to reduce the chance of error. Calculate each dose when preparing the medication, pay close attention to the process of calculation, and avoid interruption from other nursing activities (Pape et al., 2005).

BOX 34-15 Components of Medication Orders

A complete medication order includes all the following information:

- Patient's full name: The patient's full name distinguishes the patient from other persons with the same last name. In an acute care setting, patients may also be assigned a special identification number (e.g., a medical record number) to help differentiate patients with the same names. This number may be included on the order form.
- Date and time the order is written: The day, month, year, and time must be listed. Designating the time that an order is written helps to clarify when certain orders are to stop automatically. If an incident occurs involving a medication error, documentation is easier when this information is available.
- Medication name: The prescriber will order a medication by its generic or trade name. Correct spelling is essential to prevent confusion with medications with similar spelling.
- Dose: The amount or strength of the medication is included.
- Route of administration: The prescriber uses accepted abbreviations to indicate the medication routes. Accuracy is important because some medications can be administered by more than one route.
- Time and frequency of administration: Nurses need to know when to initiate medication therapy. Orders for multiple doses establish a routine schedule for medication administration.
- Signature of prescriber: The prescriber's signature makes the order a legal request.

Consult with other nurses when calculating a new or unusual dose.

Correct Administration. To help ensure safe administration, use aseptic techniques and proper procedures when handling and giving medications. Verify the patient's identity by using at least two patient identifiers (Joint Commission, 2017) and perform the necessary assessments (e.g., assessing heart rate before giving antidysrhythmic medications). Carefully monitor the patient's response to medication,

Saint Francis Medical Center

MEDICATION ADMINISTRATION RECORD

Room: 3700-03

Patient: PDM, Pharmacy
Birth: 11/30/79 Admit: 01/01/XX
MRN: 2000403 Acct: 900015
Doctor: Jim Smith

Age: 39 y Ht: 5 ft 2 in Wt: 125.2 lbs
Metric: Ht: 1 m 57 cm Wt: 56.79 kg

Date: 01/18/XX – 01/19/XX

ADEs/Nondrug allergies: Latex – Zosyn – Amoxicillin – Insulins – Darvocet – Lugols soln. – Antihi +

Medication	0800	0900	1000	1100	1200	1300	1400	1500	1600	1700	1800	1900	2000	2100	2200	2300	2400	0100	0200	0300	0400	0500	0600	0700
P00014 Bacitracin ointment AKA: Bacitracin ointment Dose: Apply STRGH: 30 gm/tube TID Topical: Right lower leg For external use only Testing			RL 10																					
P00029 Insulin/human regular AKA: Humulin R Dose: 15 units STRGH: 1 ml = 100 units AC Sub-Q	RL 0730																							
P00030 Fexofenadine 60 mg/pseudo 120 mg AKA: Allegra–D Sr Tab Dose: 1 tab STRGH: 60/120/tab BID Oral Auto Sub: 1 Allegra–D Tab bid For Claritin–D 12 hr and 24 hr Per P&T Comm			RL 10																					
P00036 Aspirin AKA: Aspirin 325 mg Tab Dose: 2 tab 650 mg STRGH: 325 mg/tab Q3–4h Oral Testing						RL 1315			RL 1615															
P00039 Haloperidol tablet AKA: Haldol 0.5 mg tab Dose: 1 mg STRGH: 1 mg/tab QHS Oral																								
P00035 Zolpidem AKA: Ambien 5 mg tab Dose: 5 mg STRGH: 5 mg/tab QHS PRN Oral MR × 1 Testing																								

Circle = Dose not given
Initials = Dose given
Deltoid = R.D., L.D.
Vastus Lateralis = R.V.L., L.V.L.
Lower Abdominal = R.L.A., L.L.A.
Anterior Gluteal = R.A.G., L.A.G.
Posterior Gluteal = R.P.G., L.P.G.

Page: 01 (continued)

Initials and signature Rita Lassater RL	**Initials and signature**	**Initials and signature**
Initials and signature	**Initials and signature**	**Initials and signature**
Initials and signature	**Initials and signature**	**Initials and signature**

FIGURE 34-12 Example of a medication administration record. *AC,* Active control; *ADEs*, adverse drug events; *AKA*, also known as; *BID*, twice a day; *MR,* medication record; *PRN,* as needed; *Q3–4h*, every 3 to 4 hours; *QHS*, before bed; *STRGH,* strength; *TID*, three times a day.

especially when administering the first dose of a new medication. Document the patient's response on the appropriate record forms.

Recording Medication Administration. After administering a medication, record it immediately on the appropriate record form (see Figure 34-12). Never chart a medication before administering it. Recording the medication immediately after its administration prevents errors.

The recording of a medication includes writing the name of the medication, the dose, the route, and the exact time of administration. Record assessment parameters (e.g., blood glucose level, blood pressure, pain score) and the site of any injections, in accordance with agency policy.

If a patient refuses a medication or undergoes tests or procedures that result in a missed dose, the reason the medication was not given must be recorded in both the medication administration record and nurse's notes.

Restorative Care. Medication administration activities vary among the numerous types of restorative care settings. Patients with functional limitations may require the nurse to fully administer all medications. In the home setting, patients usually administer their own medications. Regardless of the type of medication activity, nurses are responsible for instructing patients and their families in medication action, administration, and adverse effects. Additionally, the nurse needs to monitor the patient's adherence to medication and determine the effectiveness of medications that have been prescribed.

Special Considerations for Administering Medications to Specific Age Groups. A patient's developmental level affects the way that nurses administer medications. Nurses' knowledge of a patient's developmental needs helps them to anticipate responses to medication therapy.

Infants and Children. Children vary in age, weight, body surface area, and their ability to absorb, metabolize, and excrete medications. Children's medication doses are lower than doses for adults; therefore, special caution is needed when preparing medications for children. Medications are usually not prepared and packaged in standardized dose ranges for children. Preparing an ordered dose from an available amount of medication requires careful calculation.

All children require special psychological preparation before receiving medications. The child's parents are valuable resources for learning the best way to administer medications to their child. Sometimes the child will experience less trauma if a parent administers the medication and the nurse supervises.

Supportive care is needed if a child is expected to cooperate. When administering medication to a child, explain the procedure to the child, using short words and simple language appropriate to the child's level of comprehension. Long explanations may increase the child's anxiety, especially for painful procedures such as an injection. Nurses need to administer medications to children even when they refuse to cooperate or resist consistently despite explanation and encouragement. If the child is uncooperative, administer the medication to the child quickly and carefully (Hockenberry & Wilson, 2014). If you are able to involve the child, you may have greater success giving a medication. For example, when you say, "It's time to take your tablet now. Do you want it with water or juice?" you are allowing the child to make a choice. Do not give the child the option of not taking a medication. After a medication is given, praise the child; you may even offer a simple reward such as a star or a token. Tips for administering medications to children are listed in Box 34-16.

Older Persons. Older persons also require special consideration during medication administration (Box 34-17). In addition to physiological changes of aging (Figure 34-13), behavioural and economic factors influence an older person's use of medications.

BOX 34-16 Tips for Administering Medications to Children

Oral Medications

- Use liquid forms when available. They are safer for children to swallow and they help to avoid aspiration.
- Use droppers to administer liquids to infants.
- If older children have difficulty swallowing pills, suggest that they put the pill in their mouth and then sip liquid through a straw. The suction action pulls the liquid up the straw and makes it easier to swallow the pill.
- Offer juice, a soft drink, or a frozen juice bar after a medication is swallowed.
- To reduce nausea, pour carbonated beverages over finely crushed ice.
- When medications are mixed with palatable flavourings, such as syrup or applesauce, use only a small amount. Avoid mixing a medication with foods or liquids that the child enjoys, because the child may in turn refuse them.
- A plastic, disposable syringe is the most accurate device for preparing liquid doses, especially doses of less than 10 mL (cups, spoons, and droppers are inaccurate.)
- When administering liquid medications, use a spoon, a plastic cup, or an oral syringe (without needle).

Injections

- Use caution when selecting intramuscular injection sites for infants and small children. The deltoid muscle, which can be used for adults and older children, is underdeveloped and should not be used in infants and small children.
- Children can be unpredictable and uncooperative. Ensure that someone (preferably another nurse) is available to restrain a child if physical control is needed. The parent should act as a comforter, not a restrainer.
- Always awaken a sleeping child before giving him or her an injection.
- Distracting the child with conversation, a ringing bell, or a toy may reduce the child's perception of pain.
- Give the injection quickly and do not argue with the child.
- If time allows, use a eutectic mixture of local anaesthetics (EMLA) cream.

Polypharmacy. Polypharmacy occurs when the patient takes two or more medications to treat the same illness, when the patient takes two or more medications from the same chemical class, when the patient uses two or more medications with the same or similar actions to treat several disorders simultaneously, or when a patient mixes nutritional supplements or herbal products with medications (Brager & Soland, 2005; Touhy, Jett, Boscart, et al., 2012). Older persons also often experience polypharmacy when they self-medicate to seek relief from a variety of symptoms (e.g., pain, constipation, insomnia, and indigestion) by using OTC preparations, traditional folk medicines, or herbal remedies. OTC medications contain many different ingredients; when used inappropriately, they can cause adverse effects and adverse reactions, or they may be contraindicated by the patient's condition.

Because many older people suffer chronic health problems, polypharmacy is common. The patient who experiences polypharmacy is at increased risk of adverse reactions and medication interactions with other medications and food.

Polypharmacy can be divided into two types: rational polypharmacy and irrational polypharmacy. Rational polypharmacy occurs when patients need to take several medications to treat their health conditions, which is often the case for older persons. For example, many older people take multiple medications to lower their blood pressure. Irrational polypharmacy occurs when the patient takes more

BOX 34-17 FOCUS ON OLDER PERSONS

Medication Administration

- Simplify the drug therapy plan whenever possible (McKenry et al., 2005).
- Keep instructions clear and simple and provide written material in large print (Touhy et al., 2012).
- Assess the patient's functional status to determine whether the patient requires assistance in taking medications (McKenry et al., 2005).
- Have the patient drink a little fluid before taking oral medications, to ease swallowing. Encourage the patient to drink at least 150 to 180 mL of fluid after taking medications (Touhy et al., 2012).
- Older persons may have a greater sensitivity to drugs, especially drugs that act on the central nervous system. Therefore, nurses need to carefully monitor patients' responses to medications and anticipate dosage adjustments as needed (Meiner, 2014).
- If the patient has difficulty swallowing a capsule or tablet:
  - Ask the physician to substitute a liquid medication, if possible (Touhy et al., 2012).
  - Ask the patient to sit up straight and to tuck in the chin to decrease risk of aspiration (McKenry et al., 2005).
- Teach alternatives to medications, such as proper diet in place of vitamins and exercise in place of laxatives (Touhy et al., 2012).
- On a frequent basis, review the patient's medication history, including over-the-counter medications (Meiner, 2014).

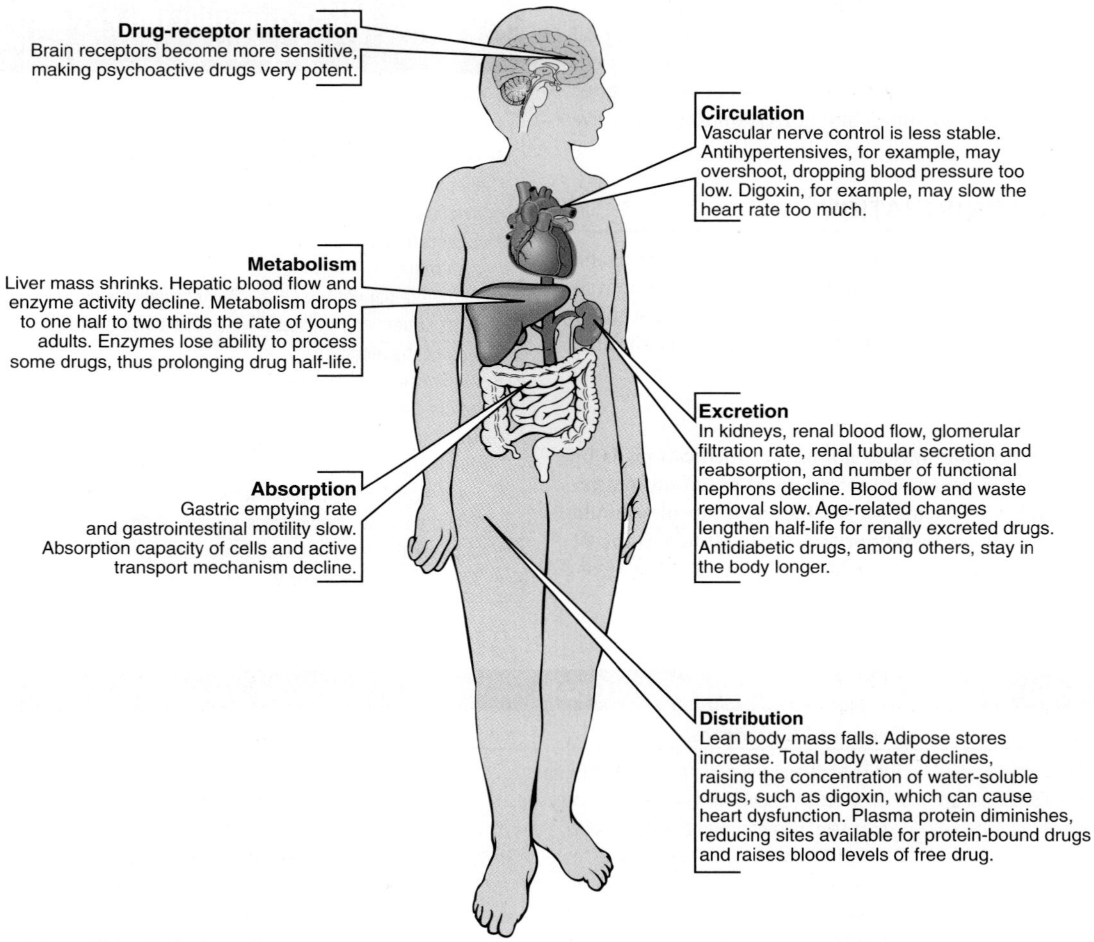

FIGURE 34-13 The aging body and drug use. (From Lewis, S. M., Dirksen, S. R., Heitkemper, M. M., Bucher, L. L., & Camera, I. M. [Eds.]. [2011]. *Medical-surgical nursing: Assessment and management of clinical problems* [8th ed., p. 76; Fig. 5-10]. St. Louis, MO: Mosby.)

medications than needed. Irrational polypharmacy results from several causes. For example, some older people need to see more than one health care provider to treat their different health conditions. When health care providers fail to take an accurate medication history or do not communicate with each other, the result can be patients taking many different medications, which increases their risk of polypharmacy (Brager & Soland, 2005).

Nonadherence. *Nonadherence* is defined as a deliberate misuse of medication, such as not taking a prescribed medication or altering the dose of a medication. In general, nonadherence occurs either because of drug ineffectiveness, uncomfortable adverse effects, or the prohibitive cost of the medicine.

◆ Evaluation

Nurses monitor patient responses to medications on an ongoing basis. For each medication, nurses require knowledge of the desired effect, the therapeutic action, and the common adverse effects. A change in a patient's condition can be physiologically related to health status, medications, or both. Nurses must be alert for reactions in a patient who takes several medications. To achieve the goal of safe and effective medication administration, a careful evaluation of both the patient's response to therapy and the patient's ability to assume responsibility for self-care is required.

To evaluate the effectiveness of nursing interventions in meeting established goals of care, nurses use evaluative measures to identify whether patient outcomes were met. Various evaluation measures are applied in the context of medication administration, including direct observation of the patient's behaviour or response, rating scales and checklists, and oral questioning. Physiological measurement is the most common method of evaluation. Examples of physiological measures are blood pressure, heart rate, and visual acuity. Patient statements can also be used as evaluative measures. Table 34-9 gives examples of goals, expected outcomes, and corresponding evaluative measures.

MEDICATION ADMINISTRATION

Medication administration is an essential part of nursing practice and requires a sound knowledge base in anatomy, physiology, pathophysiology, pharmacology, psychology, and research. The following sections illustrate the steps involved in administering medications through various routes.

Oral Administration

The easiest and most desirable way to administer medications is by mouth (Skill 34-1). Patients usually are able to ingest or self-administer oral medications with few problems. Most tablets and capsules should be administered and swallowed with approximately 60 to 100 mL of fluid (as allowed). Some situations contraindicate administering medications by mouth.

The primary contraindications to giving oral medications include the presence of GI alterations, the inability of the patient to swallow food or fluids, and the use of gastric suction. An important precaution to take when administering any oral preparation is to protect patients from aspiration. Aspiration occurs when food, fluid, or medication intended for GI administration is inadvertently administered into the respiratory tract. The nurse must protect the patient from aspiration by assessing the patient's ability to manage oral medications. Box 34-18 describes techniques used to protect the patient from aspirating. Properly positioning the patient is also essential in preventing aspiration. The patient is in a seated position when receiving oral medications, if such a position is not contraindicated by the patient's condition. Having the patient slightly flex the head in a chin-down position usually reduces aspiration (Metheny, 2006). It is good to use a multidisciplinary approach (e.g., consult with a speech therapist, a dietitian,

BOX 34-18 Protecting the Patient From Aspiration

- Determine the patient's ability to swallow.
- Assess the patient's cough.
- Determine the presence of a gag reflex.
- Prepare oral medications in the form that is easiest for the patient to swallow.
- Ensure that the patient is in a side-lying or upright position, to prevent aspiration.
- Allow the patient to self-administer medications, if possible.
- If the patient has unilateral weakness, place the medication in the stronger side of the mouth.
- Administer pills one at a time, ensuring that each pill is properly swallowed before the next one is introduced.
- Thicken regular liquids or offer fruit nectars if the patient cannot tolerate thin liquids.
- Have the patient hold and drink from a cup, if possible.
- When possible, medications should be timed to coincide with mealtimes or when the patient is well rested and awake.
- Administer medications through another route if risk of aspiration is severe.

TABLE 34-9 Example Evaluation for Patient Goals

Goals	Expected Outcomes	Expected Outcomes
The patient and the patient's family understand the patient's medication therapy.	The patient and the patient's family describe information about the medication, its dosage, schedule, purpose, and adverse effects.	Written measurement: Ask the patient to write out the medication schedule for a 24-hour period.
		Oral questioning: Ask the patient to describe the purpose, dosage, and adverse effects of each prescribed medication.
	The patient and the patient's family identify situations that require medical intervention.	Oral questioning: Ask the patient's family to describe what to do if the patient has adverse effects from a medication.
	The patient and the patient's family demonstrate the appropriate administration technique.	Direct observation: Ask the patient to demonstrate the filling of an insulin syringe and self-injection.
The patient safely self-administers medications.	The patient follows a prescribed treatment regimen.	Anecdotal notes: Have the patient's family keep a log of the patient's adherence to therapy for 1 week.
	The patient performs administration techniques correctly.	Direct observation: Observe while the patient instills eye drops.
	The patient identifies available resources for obtaining the necessary medication.	Oral questioning: Ask the patient's family to identify how to contact the local pharmacy or community clinic to obtain the patient's medications.

SKILL 34-1 ADMINISTERING ORAL MEDICATIONS

Delegation Considerations

The administration of oral medications cannot be delegated to unregulated care providers (UCPs). Instruct UCPs to report the occurrence of medication adverse effects immediately.

Equipment

- Medication cart or tray
- Disposable medication cups
- Patient identification labels
- Glass of water, juice, or preferred liquid
- Drinking straw
- Pill-crushing device (optional)
- Medication administration record or computer printout

PROCEDURE

STEPS	RATIONALE
1. Check the accuracy and completeness of each medication administration record (MAR) or computer printout against the prescriber's original medication order. Check the patient's name and the medication name, dosage, route, and time for administration. Copy or rewrite any portion of the MAR that is difficult to read.	• The order sheet is the most reliable source and only legal record of medications the patient is to receive. Adherence to the order ensures the patient receives the correct medications. Illegible MARs are a source of medication errors.
2. Assess the patient for any contraindications to receiving oral medication: Is the patient experiencing nausea or vomiting? Has the patient received a diagnosis of bowel inflammation or reduced peristalsis? Has the patient undergone recent gastrointestinal (GI) surgery? Does the patient have gastric suction? Is the patient restricted to nothing by mouth (NPO)? Check the patient's reflexes for swallowing, coughing, and gagging.	• Alterations in GI function interfere with a medication's ability to be distributed, absorbed, and excreted. Patients with GI suction might not receive benefit from medications because they are suctioned from the GI tract before they can be absorbed. Patients with impaired swallowing are at risk for aspiration (Metheny, 2006).
3. Assess the patient's medical history, history of allergies, medication history, and diet history. List the patient's food and drug allergies on each page of the MAR and prominently display the allergies on the patient's medical record. This information may also be added to an identification bracelet.	• The information reflects the patient's need for medications and the potential responses to medications. Communication of the patient's potential food and drug interactions and allergies is essential for safe, effective care.
4. Gather information from the patient's physical examination and laboratory data that may influence medication administration (e.g., vital signs, blood glucose levels, electrolyte levels, laboratory findings related to blood clotting times and to renal and liver function).	• Physical examination or laboratory data may contraindicate medication administration. Poor liver and kidney functions affect the metabolism and excretion of medications (McKenry et al., 2005).

CRITICAL DECISION POINT: *If the patient has any contraindications for receiving oral medications, or if you are in doubt of the patient's ability to swallow oral medications, temporarily withhold medication and inform the prescriber.*

STEPS	RATIONALE
5. Assess the patient's knowledge regarding health and medication use.	• This assessment helps to determine the patient's need for medication education and whether the patient adheres to medication therapy at home. The assessment may reveal difficulties with medication use problems, such as medication intolerance, nonadherence, abuse, addiction, or dependence.
6. Assess the patient's preferences for fluids. Maintain fluid restriction when applicable.	• Offering fluids during medication administration increases the patient's fluid intake. Fluids ease swallowing and facilitate absorption from the GI tract. Fluid restrictions must be maintained when applicable.
7. Prepare medications:	
A. Perform hand hygiene.	• Proper hygiene reduces the transfer of microorganisms.
B. If a medication cart is used, move it to a location outside the patient's room.	• Organization of equipment saves time and reduces the chance for error.
C. Unlock the medicine drawer or cart or log on to the automated medication dispensing system.	• Medications are safeguarded when locked in a cabinet or cart. Storage in a locked area prevents preparation error.
D. Prepare medication for one patient at a time. If you are using paper copies of the MAR, keep all pages for one patient together. If you are using the patient's medication administration on the computer, view only one computer screen at a time.	• Preventing distractions limits preparation errors (Pape et al., 2005).

Continued

SKILL 34-1 ADMINISTERING ORAL MEDICATIONS—cont'd

STEPS	RATIONALE
E. Select the correct medication from a stock supply or a unit-dose drawer. Compare the label on the medication with the MAR (see Step 7E illustration) or the computer screen. Check the expiration date on all medication labels.	• Comparing the labels on the medication with the transcribed orders reduces the chance for error. *This is the first accuracy check.*
F. Calculate the medication dose as necessary. Double-check all calculations, and verify your calculations with another nurse.	• Double-checking reduces the risk of error.
G. If you are preparing a controlled substance, check the patient's MAR or computer record to determine the last time the medication was administered. Check the record for the previous medication count and compare the current count with the supply available.	• Checking the medication count reduces the risk of double-dosing if the patient is receiving controlled substances on a prn (as needed) schedule. • Controlled substance laws require nurses to carefully monitor and count any dispensed narcotics.
H. To prepare tablets or capsules from a floor stock bottle, pour the required number into the bottle cap and transfer the medication to a medication cup. Do not touch the medication with your fingers. Return extra tablets or capsules to the bottle. Break scored medications. If necessary, use a clean pillating device. Identify scored tablets by looking for a line that divides the tablet in half.	• A clean technique is required of medication administration. Cleaning the pillating (or pill-cutting) device ensures that prior medications are cleaned out of the device and cannot contaminate this tablet. To ensure that you give the accurate dose to patient, split only those tablets that are scored.
I. To prepare unit-dose tablets or capsules, place the packaged tablet or capsule directly into a medicine cup. Do not remove the wrapper (see Step 7I illustration.)	• Wrappers maintain the cleanliness of medications and allow the nurse to identify the medication name and dose at the patient's bedside.

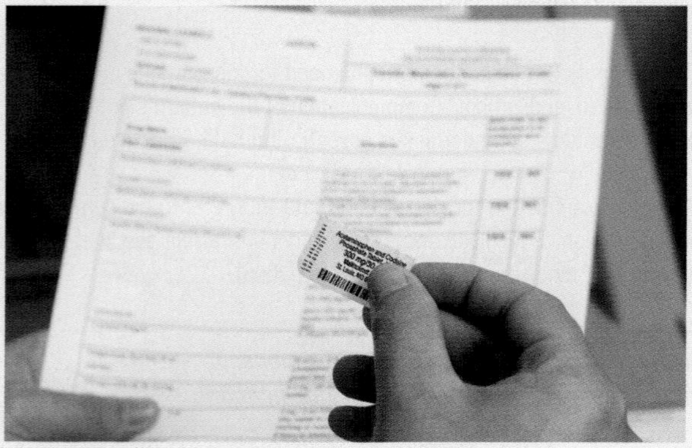

STEP 7E The nurse verifies each medication with the MAR.

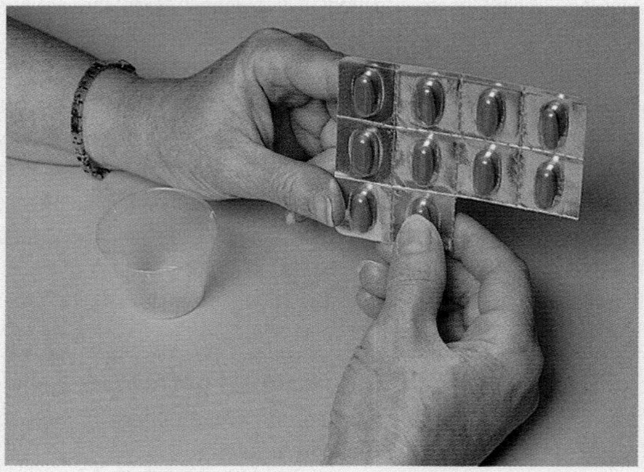

STEP 7I Place tablet into medicine cup without removing wrapper.

CRITICAL DECISION POINT: *If you are preparing narcotics, check the narcotic record for the previous drug count and compare it against the supply available. You are responsible for being aware of and upholding laws regarding the use of controlled substances.*

STEPS	RATIONALE
J. Place all tablets or capsules to be given to patient in one medicine cup, with the patient's identification label attached, except for those medications that require preadministration assessments (e.g., pulse rate or blood pressure); keep medications in their wrappers. After medication administration, remove the patient's identification label and discard the label in the appropriate confidential waste disposal receptacle.	• Labelling the patient's medication cup reduces the risk of administering medications to the incorrect patient. • Keeping medications that require preadministration assessments separate from other medications makes it easier for the nurse to withhold medications as necessary. • Disposing of the patient's label in confidential waste receptacles is necessary to protect patient confidentiality.

CRITICAL DECISION POINT: *Not all medications can be crushed (e.g., capsules and enteric-coated drugs). When in doubt whether a medication can be crushed, consult your pharmacist. When pills are crushed, the patient is more likely to experience choking or aspiration of particles of medication or soft food. Please see the ISMP document at http://www.ismp.org/tools/donotcrush.pdf for information about crushing pills if the pharmacy is not available or is closed.*

STEPS	RATIONALE
K. If the patient has difficulty swallowing, and liquid medications are not an option, use a pill-crushing device, such as a mortar and pestle, to grind the pills (see Step 7K illustration). Before using a mortar and pestle, clean them. If a pill-crushing device is not available, place the tablet inside a medication cup, place another medication cup on top of it, and press on the top cup with a blunt instrument until the pill is crushed. Mix the ground tablet in small amount of soft food (custard or applesauce).	• Large tablets can be difficult to swallow. A ground tablet mixed with palatable soft food is usually easier to swallow. Cleaning pill-crushing devices ensures that contamination of medications does not occur.

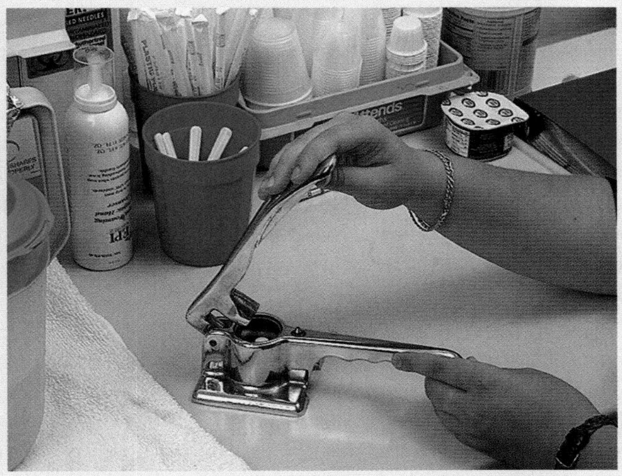

STEP 7K Pill-crushing device used to crush pills when necessary.

STEPS	RATIONALE
L. To prepare liquids:	
(1) Gently shake the container. If the medication is in a unit-dose container with the correct amount to administer, no further preparation is needed. If the medication is in a multidose bottle, remove the bottle cap from the container and place the cap so that the inside of the cap is not exposed.	• Shaking the container ensures the medication is mixed before administration. Correct placement of the cap of the bottle avoids contamination.
(2) Hold a multidose bottle with the label against the palm of your hand while pouring.	• Hold the bottle so that any spilled liquid will not soil or fade the label.
(3) Hold the medication cup at eye level and fill to the desired level on the scale (see Step 7L[3] illustration). The scale should be even with the fluid level at its surface or the base of the meniscus, not at its edges. Draw up volumes of less than 10 mL in a syringe without a needle (see Step 7L[3] illustration).	• Filling medication properly ensures accuracy of measurement. The use of a syringe enables greater accuracy for small doses of medication.

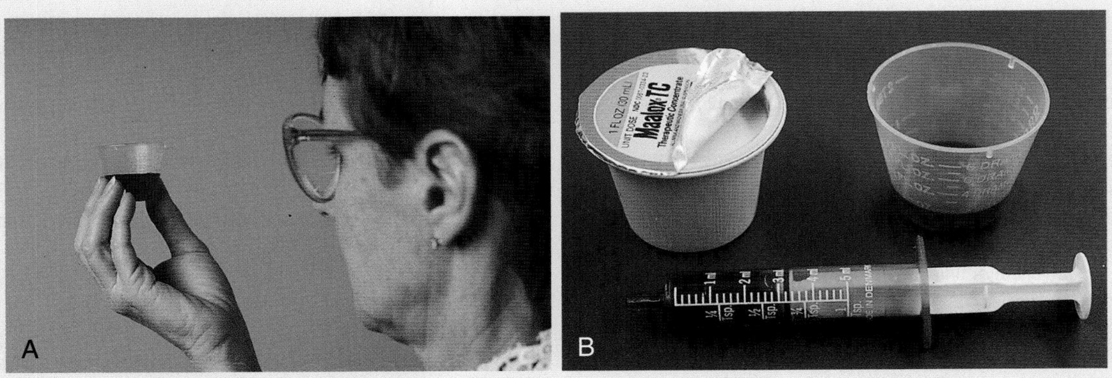

STEP 7L(3) **A,** Pour the desired volume of liquid so that the base of the meniscus is level with the line on the scale. **B,** Use a needleless syringe to draw up volumes of less than 10 mL.

STEPS	RATIONALE
(4) Discard any excess liquid into the appropriate receptacle. Wipe the lip and neck of the multidose bottle with a paper towel.	• Prevents contamination of the bottle's contents and prevents the bottle cap from sticking to the counter. • Avoids unnecessary manipulation of the dose.

Continued

SKILL 34-1 ADMINISTERING ORAL MEDICATIONS—cont'd

STEPS	RATIONALE
M. Compare the MAR, computer printout, or computer screen with the prepared medication and container.	• Reading labels a second time reduces the chance for error. *This is the second accuracy check.*
N. Return stock containers or unused unit-dose medications to the storage shelf or drawer and read the labels again.	• The *third accuracy check* of medication labels in multiple-dose containers further reduces administration errors.
O. Do not leave medications unattended.	• Nurses are responsible for the safekeeping of drugs.
8. Administering medications:	
A. Take medications to the patient at the correct time.	• Medications are administered within 30 minutes before or after the prescribed time to ensure the intended therapeutic effect. Give STAT medications immediately or single-order medications at the time they are ordered.
B. Identify the patient by using at least two patient identifiers. Compare the patient's name and one other identifier (e.g., the hospital identification number) on the MAR, computer printout, or computer screen with information on the patient's identification bracelet. Ask the patient to state his or her name, if possible, for a third identifier.	• These steps comply with the Joint Commission's (2017) requirements and improve medication safety. In most acute care settings, the patient's name and identification number on an armband and the MAR is used to identify patients. Identification bracelets are made at the time of the patient's admission and are the most reliable source of identification. The patient's room number is not an acceptable identifier.

CRITICAL DECISION POINT: *Replace patient identification bracelets that are missing, illegible, or faded.*

STEPS	RATIONALE
C. Compare labels of the medications with the MAR at the patient's bedside.	• Perform a final check of medication labels against the MAR at the patient's bedside to reduce medication administration errors.
D. Explain to the patient the purpose of each medication and its action. Encourage the patient to ask any questions about the drugs.	• The patient has the right to be informed; questions often indicate the need for teaching and reveal nonadherence to therapy or potential medication errors. A patient's understanding of the purpose of each medication improves adherence to medication therapy.
E. Assist the patient to a sitting position (or side-lying position if sitting is contraindicated).	• A sitting position prevents aspiration during swallowing (Metheny, 2006).
F. Administer medications:	
(1) *For tablets:* The patient may wish to hold solid medications in the hand or in a cup before placing them in the mouth.	• The patient can become familiar with medications by seeing each drug.
(2) Offer water or juice to help the patient swallow the medications. Give cold carbonated water if it is available and not contraindicated.	• Offering a choice of fluids promotes the patient's comfort and can improve fluid intake. Carbonated water helps passage of the tablet through the esophagus.
(3) *For sublingual-administered medications:* Have the patient place the medication under the tongue and allow it to dissolve completely (see Figure 34-4). Caution the patient against swallowing the tablet.	• Medication is absorbed through the blood vessels of the undersurface of the tongue. If medication is swallowed, it is destroyed by gastric juices or detoxified by the liver so rapidly that therapeutic blood levels are not attained.
(4) *For buccal medications:* Have the patient place the medication in the mouth against the mucous membranes of the cheek until it dissolves (see Figure 34-5). Avoid administering liquids until the buccal medication has dissolved.	• Buccal medications act locally on mucosa or systemically as they are swallowed in saliva.
(5) *For powdered medications:* Mix with liquids at bedside and give to the patient to drink.	• When prepared in advance, powdered medications may thicken and even harden, which makes swallowing difficult.
(6) Caution the patient against chewing or swallowing lozenges.	• Medication acts through slow absorption through oral mucosa, not gastric mucosa.
(7) Give effervescent powders and tablets immediately after they have dissolved.	• Effervescence improves the unpleasant taste of the medication and often relieves GI problems.
G. If the patient is unable to hold medications in the hand or in a cup, place the medication cup to the patient's lips and gently introduce each drug into the mouth, one at a time. Do not rush.	• Administering a single tablet or capsule eases swallowing and decreases the risk of aspiration.
H. If a tablet or capsule falls to the floor, discard it and repeat the preparation.	• Medication is contaminated when it touches the floor.
I. Stay at the bedside until the patient has completely swallowed each medication. If you are uncertain whether the medication was swallowed, ask the patient to open the mouth.	• The nurse is responsible for ensuring that the patient receives the ordered dose. If left unattended, the patient may not take the dose or may save medications, which could cause a risk to health.
J. For highly acidic medications (e.g., aspirin), offer the patient a nonfat snack (e.g., crackers) if it is not contraindicated by the patient's condition.	• A nonfat snack reduces the possible gastric irritation from highly acidic medication.
K. Assist the patient in returning to a comfortable position.	• The patient's comfort is maintained.
L. Replenish the stock, such as cups and straws. If a medication cart was used, return the cart to the medication room. Clean the work area.	• A clean and organized work space helps other staff to complete their duties efficiently.

STEPS	RATIONALE
9. Evaluate the patient's response to medications at times that correlate with the medication's onset, peak, and duration.	• The nurse can evaluate the medication's therapeutic benefit and detect the onset of adverse effects or allergic reactions.
10. Ask the patient or the patient's family member to identify the medication name and explain the purpose, action, dosage schedule, and potential adverse effects of the drug.	• The nurse can determine the level of knowledge gained by the patient and the patient's family.

UNEXPECTED OUTCOMES	RELATED INTERVENTIONS
Adverse effects (e.g., toxic effects, allergic reactions)	• Symptoms such as urticaria, rash, pruritus, rhinitis, and wheezing may indicate an allergic reaction. • Withhold further doses, and add allergy information to the patient's health record • Always notify the prescriber and the pharmacy when the patient exhibits adverse effects.
Patient refuses medication	• Explore reasons why the patient does not want the medication. • If misunderstandings of the medication therapy are apparent, address the misconceptions by educating the patient. • Do not force the patient to take the medication; patients have the right to refuse treatment. • If the patient continues to refuse medication despite attempts to educate the patient, record on patient's chart why the drug was withheld and notify the prescriber.

RECORDING AND REPORTING

- Record the administration of oral medications on the computerized or paper copy of the MAR immediately after administering the medications. If you are using a paper copy of the MAR, include your initials or signature.
- Record the reason any drug was withheld and follow the agency's policy for proper recording.
- Record and report your evaluation of the medication's effect to the prescriber if required (e.g., report urine output following administration of a diuretic if ordered by the prescriber).

HOME CARE CONSIDERATIONS

- To ensure safe medication administration at home, instruct patients on all aspects of medication administration, including dosage, desired effect, when to take the medications, proper storage of the medications, anticipated adverse effects, and whether to take medication with or without food.
- Evaluate the patient's ability to safely self-administer medications. If the patient needs assistance in self-administration, introduce nursing interventions, such as a chart or pillbox. If interventions fail and the patient still is unable to safely administer medications, notify the prescriber.

and an occupational therapist) with patients who have difficulty swallowing (Morris, 2006).

For patients with nasogastric feeding tubes, liquid medications are preferred, but some tablets can be crushed and some capsules can be opened to mix in a solution for administration (Box 34-19).

Topical Medication Applications

Topical medications are medications that are applied locally, most often to intact skin but also to mucous membranes. They are prepared in many forms, including lotions, pastes, and ointments (see Table 34-1).

Skin Applications. Because many locally applied medications, such as lotions, pastes, and ointments, cause both systemic and local effects, these medications are applied with the use of gloves and applicators. Use sterile techniques if the patient has an open wound. Skin encrustation and dead tissues harbour microorganisms and block contact of the medications from the tissues to be treated. Before applying medications, clean the area to be treated thoroughly by washing the skin gently with soap and water, soaking an involved site, or locally debriding tissue (see Chapter 46).

Apply each type of topical medication according to the directions to ensure proper penetration and absorption. When applying ointments or pastes, spread the medication evenly over the involved surface and cover the area well without applying an overly thick layer. Prescribers may order a gauze dressing to be applied over the medication to prevent soiling of clothes and wiping away of the medication. Lightly spread lotions and creams onto the skin's surface; rubbing often causes irritation. Apply a liniment by rubbing it gently but firmly into the skin. After that, dust a powder lightly to cover the affected area with a thin layer. During any application, assess the skin thoroughly. When recording the administration, note the area where the medication was applied, the name of the medication, and the condition of the skin.

Some topical medications are applied in the form of a transdermal patch that remains in place for an extended period of time (e.g., 12 hours or 7 days). Many patches are clear, which makes them difficult to see. Nurses and patients may inadvertently leave old transdermal patches in place, which results in the patient receiving an overdose of the medication. Therefore, it is important to carefully assess the patient's skin and ensure that the existing patch is removed before applying a new patch. The following guidelines are used to ensure safe administration of transdermal or topical medications (Institute for Safe Medication Practices, 2007):

1. Document on the medication administration record or computer record the area where the medication was applied.
2. When applying a transdermal patch, ask the patient whether he or she has an existing patch.

BOX 34-19 PROCEDURAL GUIDELINE

Giving Medications Through a Nasogastric Tube, Intestinal Tube, Gastrostomy Tube, or Small-Bore Feeding Tube

Delegation Considerations:

The administration of medications through a nasogastric tube, intestinal tube, gastrostomy tube, or small-bore feeding tube cannot be delegated. Instruct unregulated care providers to report the occurrence of adverse effects immediately.

Equipment:

- 60-mL syringe (catheter tip for large-bore tubes, Luer-Lok tip for small-bore tubes)
- Gastric pH test strips (scale of 0.0 to 11.0 or 14.0 preferred)
- Graduated container
- Water
- Medication to be administered
- Pill crusher, if medication is in tablet form
- Medication administration record
- Clean gloves

Procedure:

1. Check the accuracy and completeness of each medication administration record against the prescriber's written medication order: check the patient's name, the drug name and dosage, and the route and time of administration.
2. Investigate and, if possible, use alternative routes of medication administration (e.g., intravenous, transdermal, rectal).
3. Avoid complicated medication regimens that frequently interrupt enteral feedings.
4. Prepare medication (see Skill 34-1, Steps 7A–G and M–O). Check the label of the medication with the medication administration record three times.
5. Avoid giving elixirs or medications that have a pH of less than 4.
6. Never add medications directly to a feeding tube. Before administering a medication, determine if it needs to be given on an empty stomach or if it is compatible with the enteral feeding. The amount of time the enteral feeding needs to be held before administration varies with the medication. Verify with agency policy or with a pharmacist the amount of time that you hold a feeding.
7. Verify tube placement before administering medications (see Chapter 42).
8. Administer medications in a liquid form (suspension, elixir, or solution) when possible to prevent tube obstruction.
9. Before crushing tablets, ensure that they are crushable. Buccal, sublingual, enteric-coated, or sustained-release medications cannot be crushed. Read medication labels carefully before crushing a tablet or opening a capsule.
10. Take medications to the patient at the correct time, and perform hand hygiene.
11. Identify the patient by using at least two patient identifiers. Compare the patient's name and one other identifier (e.g., the hospital identification number) on the identification bracelet with the medication administration record. Ask the patient to state his or her name, if possible, for a third identifier.
12. Compare the labels on the medications against the medication administration record one more time at the patient's bedside.
13. Explain the procedure and the medications to the patient.
14. Dissolve crushed tablets, gelatin capsules, and powders in 15 to 30 mL of warm water. Dissolve each medication separately.
15. Do not give whole or undissolved medications through the feeding tube.
16. Put on clean, disposable gloves.
17. Verify the placement of any tube that enters the mouth or nose by using pH testing (see Chapter 42).
18. Assess gastric residual (see Chapter 42).
19. Draw up medication in syringe. Do not mix medications together.
20. Connect the syringe with medication to a nasogastric tube, G-tube, J-tube, or small-bore feeding tube. Do not use the pigtail vent for irrigation or instillation of fluid.
21. Administer medication either by pushing the medication through the tube by depressing the plunger of the syringe or by allowing the medication to flow into the body freely by using gravity. Administer each medication separately.
22. Flush the tube with 15 to 30 mL of warm water between each medication. Unless contraindicated, the total amount of liquid volume administered to the patient is approximately 60 mL.
23. After giving all the medications, flush the tube once more with 30 to 60 mL of warm water.
24. Remove gloves and perform hand hygiene.
25. Document administration of medications on the medication administration record.
26. Continually evaluate the patient's response to medication therapy. If the desired effect is not achieved, a different medication or a different route of administration may be indicated because of problems with the drug bioavailability when given by the enteral route.

Adapted from Jordan, S., Griffiths, H., & Griffin, R. (2003). Administration of medicines. II. Pharmacology. *Nursing Standard, 18*(3), 45–55.

3. Do not assume that a patch has fallen off or has already been removed. Assess the skin thoroughly before administering the medication.
4. When taking a medication history or reconciling medications, specifically ask the patient whether he or she takes any medications in the form of patches, topical creams, or any route other than the oral route.
5. If the dressing or patch is difficult to see (e.g., it is clear), apply a noticeable label to the patch.
6. Document removal of the patch or medication on the medication administration record or computer record.

Nasal Instillation. Patients with nasal sinus alterations may receive medications by spray, drops, or tampons (Box 34-20). The most commonly administered form of nasal instillation (administration of a liquid) is a decongestant spray or drops, which are used to relieve symptoms of sinus congestion and colds. Caution patients to avoid abuse of medications because overuse can lead to a rebound effect in which the nasal congestion worsens. When excess decongestant solution is swallowed, serious systemic effects can develop, especially in children. Saline drops are safer as a decongestant for children than nasal preparations that contain sympathomimetics (e.g., Afrin or Neo-Synephrine).

Self-administering sprays is easier because the patient can control the spray and inhale as it enters the nasal passages. For patients who use nasal sprays repeatedly, check the nares for irritation. Position patients to permit the medication to reach the affected sinus.

Eye Instillation. Common eye medications used by patients are eye drops and ointments, including OTC preparations, such as

BOX 34-20 PROCEDURAL GUIDELINE

Administering Nasal Instillations

Delegation Considerations:
The administration of nasal drops and ointments cannot be delegated. Instruct unregulated care providers to report the occurrence of medication adverse effects immediately.

Equipment:

- Prepared medication with a clean dropper or spray container
- Facial tissue
- Small pillow (optional)
- Washcloth (optional)
- Clean, disposable gloves (if patient has extensive nasal drainage)
- Medication administration record
- Penlight (to inspect nares; if ointment is to be applied to a specific lesion inside the nares)

Procedure:

1. Check the accuracy and completeness of each medication administration record (MAR) or computer printout against the prescriber's original medication order. Check the patient's name and the medication name, dosage, route, and time for administration. Copy or rewrite any portion of the MAR that is difficult to read.
2. If nasal drops are to be administered, refer to the medical record to determine which sinus is affected, so that you can position the patient appropriately for drug instillation.
3. Assess the patient's medical history (e.g., cardiovascular disease, hyperthyroidism). Medical conditions can contraindicate the use of decongestants that stimulate the central nervous system. Adverse effects may occur, such as transient hypertension, tachycardia, palpitations, and headache.
4. List the patient's food and drug allergies on each page of the MAR and prominently display the allergies on the patient's medical record as per agency policy. Determine whether the patient has any allergies to medications delivered via nasal instillation.
5. Review the physician's order, including the patient's name and the medication name, dosage, route, time of administration, and indication.
6. Take the medication to the patient at the correct time, and perform hand hygiene. Using a penlight, inspect the condition of the nose and sinuses. Palpate sinuses for tenderness.
7. Assess the patient's knowledge regarding the use of nasal instillations and the technique for instillation, and determine whether the patient is willing to learn self-administration.
8. Prepare the medication (see Skill 34-1, Steps 7A–G, M–O). Ensure that you compare the label of the medication against the MAR at least two times while preparing the medications.
9. Identify the patient by using at least two identifiers. Compare the patient's name and one other identifier (e.g., the hospital identification number) on the MAR, computer printout, or computer screen with information on the patient's identification bracelet. Ask the patient to state his or her name, if possible, for a third identifier.
10. Compare the MAR with the medication labels at the patient's bedside.
11. Explain the procedure to the patient regarding the positioning and the sensations to expect, such as a burning or stinging of the mucosa, or a choking sensation as the medication trickles into the throat.
12. Arrange the supplies and medications at the bedside. Put on gloves if the patient has nasal drainage.
13. Gently roll or shake the medication container.
14. Instruct the patient to clear or blow the nose gently unless contraindicated (e.g., risk of increased intracranial pressure or nosebleeds). Clearing the nose helps to remove mucus and secretions that can block medication distribution.
15. Administer nasal drops:
    A. Assist the patient to a supine position and position the head properly to facilitate access to the nasal passages.
        (1) To access the posterior pharynx, tilt the patient's head backward.
        (2) To access the ethmoid and sphenoid sinuses, tilt the head back over the edge of the bed or place a small pillow under the patient's shoulder and tilt the head back (see Step 15A[2] illustration).
        (3) To access the frontal and maxillary sinuses, tilt the head back over the edge of the bed or pillow with the head turned toward the side to be treated (see Step 15A[3] illustration). This position will allow the medication to drain into the affected sinus.
    B. Support the patient's head with your nondominant hand to prevent the straining of neck muscles.
    C. Instruct the patient to breathe through the mouth, which reduces the chance of aspirating nasal drops into the trachea and lungs.

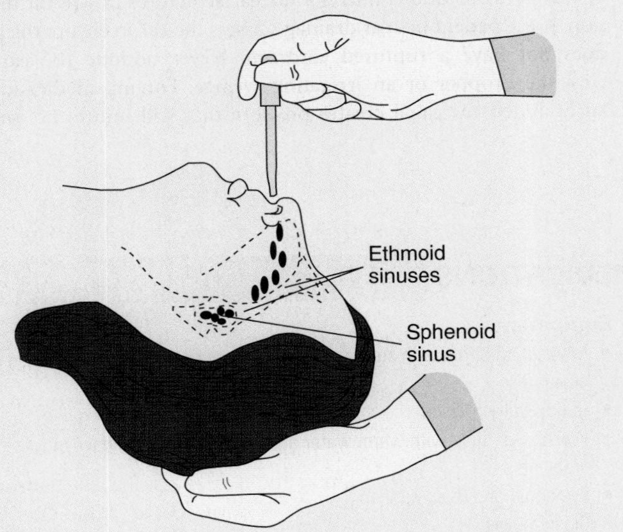

STEP 15A(2) Position for instilling nose drops into the ethmoid and sphenoid sinuses.

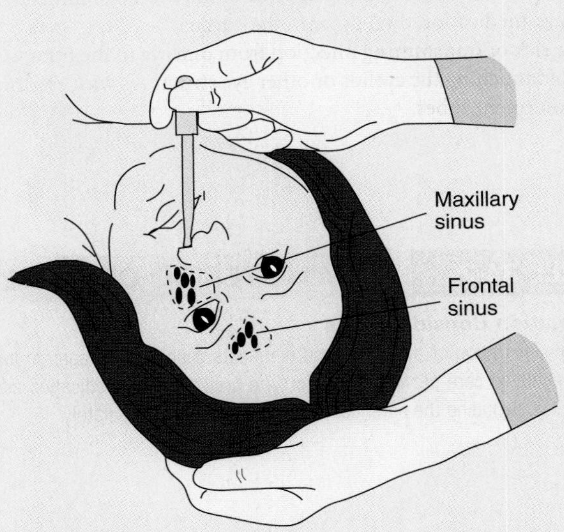

STEP 15A(3) Position for instilling nose drops into the frontal and maxillary sinuses.

Continued

BOX 34-20 PROCEDURAL GUIDELINE
Administering Nasal Instillations—cont'd

- **D.** Hold the dropper 1 cm above the nares to avoid contamination of the dropper. Instill the prescribed number of drops toward midline of the ethmoid bone to facilitate distribution of medication over the nasal mucosa.
- **E.** Have the patient remain in a supine position for 5 minutes to prevent premature loss of medication through the nares.
- **F.** Offer a facial tissue to blot a runny nose, but caution the patient against blowing the nose for several minutes.

16. Assist the patient to a comfortable position after the medication is absorbed.
17. Administering nasal spray:
- **A.** Assist the patient to a comfortable high Fowler's position or a sitting position.
- **B.** Administer the nasal spray with the patient's head upright. Tipping the opening of the nasal spray container downward will cause the medication to be administered in a stream, not a spray, and will deliver more medication than the prescribed order.
- **C.** Offer a facial tissue to blot a runny nose, but caution the patient against blowing the nose for several minutes.

18. Dispose of soiled supplies in the proper container, and perform hand hygiene.
19. Document administration of medication on the MAR or in the computer.
20. Observe the patient for the onset of adverse effects 15 to 30 minutes after administration. Drugs absorbed through mucosa can cause a systemic reaction.
21. Ask whether the patient is able to breathe through the nose after decongestant administration to determine the drug's effectiveness. Sometimes the patient will need to occlude one nostril at a time and breathe deeply.
22. Evaluate the patient's response to the medications at times that correlate with the medication's onset, peak, and duration. Evaluate the patient for both desired effects and adverse effects. Re-inspect the condition of the nasal passages between the instillations.
23. Ask the patient to review the risks of overuse of decongestants and methods for administration.
24. Have the patient demonstrate self-medication.

artificial tears and vasoconstrictors (e.g., Visine and Murine). Many patients receive prescribed ophthalmic medications for eye conditions, such as glaucoma, and after cataract extraction. In older persons, the ease with which eye medications can be self-administered can be affected by gerontological changes, including poor vision, hand tremors, and difficulty grasping or manipulating containers. Instruct patients and their family members about the proper techniques for administering eye medications (Skill 34-2). Determine the ability of the patient and the patient's family members to administer the eye medication by demonstrating the procedure. Showing patients each step of the procedure for instilling eye drops can improve their compliance. Follow these principles when administering eye medications:

- The cornea of the eye is richly supplied with pain fibres and thus is very sensitive to anything applied to it. Avoid instilling any form of eye medication directly onto the cornea.
- The risk of transmitting infection from one eye to the other is high. Avoid touching the eyelids or other eye structures with eyedroppers or ointment tubes.
- Use eye medication only for the patient's affected eye.
- Never allow a patient to use another patient's eye medications.

Intraocular Administration. Some medications are administered intraocularly (see Skill 34-2). Intraocular medications resemble a contact lens. Place the medication into the conjunctival sac, where it remains in place for up to 1 week. Medications such as pilocarpine are administered this way. Patients need to be taught about monitoring for adverse reactions to the disc. Patients also need to be taught how to insert and remove the disc.

Ear Instillation. Internal ear structures are very sensitive to temperature extremes. Failure to instill ear drops or irrigating fluid at room temperature may cause vertigo (severe dizziness) or nausea. Although the structures of the outer ear are not sterile, sterile drops and solutions are used in case the eardrum is ruptured. The entrance of nonsterile solutions into middle ear structures can result in infection. If the patient has ear drainage, assess the ear to ensure the patient does not have a ruptured eardrum. Never occlude the ear canal with the dropper or an irrigating syringe. Forcing medication into an occluded ear canal creates pressure that will injure the eardrum.

SKILL 34-2 ADMINISTERING OPHTHALMIC MEDICATIONS

Delegation Considerations

The administration of eye drops and ointments cannot be delegated. Instruct unregulated care providers to report the occurrence of medication adverse effects, including the potential for visual difficulty, immediately.

Equipment

- Medication bottle with sterile eyedropper, ointment tube, or medicated intraocular disc
- Cotton ball or tissue
- Washbasin filled with warm water and washcloth if eyes have crust or need drainage
- Eye patch and tape (optional)
- Clean gloves
- Medication administration record (MAR) or computer printout

PROCEDURE

STEPS	RATIONALE
1. Check the accuracy and completeness of each MAR or computer printout against the prescriber's medication order. Check the patient's name, the medication name and dosage (e.g., number of drops, if a liquid), the eye to be treated (e.g., right, left, or both eyes), and the route and time of administration. Copy or rewrite any portion of the MAR that is difficult to read.	
2. Assess the condition of the patient's external eye structures. (This may also be assessed just before drug instillation.)	• This assessment provides a baseline to help determine whether the medication causes a local response. The assessment also indicates the need to clean the eye before medication application.
3. Determine whether the patient has any known allergies to eye medications. Also ask whether the patient has an allergy to latex.	
4. Determine whether the patient has any symptoms of visual alterations.	• Certain eye medications act to either decrease or increase these symptoms. Determining the patient's visual alteration status ensures that the nurse is able to recognize a change in the patient's condition after the medication is administered.
5. Assess the patient's level of consciousness and ability to follow directions.	• A patient who becomes restless or combative during the procedure is at a greater risk of accidental eye injury.
6. Assess the patient's knowledge regarding medication therapy and the desire to self-administer medication.	
7. Assess the patient's ability to manipulate and hold an eye dropper.	
8. Prepare medication (see Skill 34-1, Steps 7A–G and M–O): Ensure that you check the label of the medication against the MAR at least two times while preparing the medication.	
9. Take the medication to the patient at the correct time, and perform hand hygiene.	
10. Identify the patient by using at least two patient identifiers. Compare the patient's name and one other identifier (e.g., the hospital identification number) on the MAR, computer printout, or computer screen with information on patient's identification bracelet. Ask the patient to state his or her name, if possible, for a third identifier.	
11. Compare labels of medications with the MAR or computer printout at the patient's bedside.	
12. Arrange the medication supplies at the bedside and put on clean gloves. If eye drops are stored in the refrigerator, allow them to reach room temperature before instilling them.	• The use of gloves reduces the transmission of microorganisms and follows standards to prevent accidental exposure to body fluids. Warming the eye drops reduces irritation to the eye.
13. Gently roll the container.	• Rolling the container ensures that the medication is mixed before administration. Shaking the bottle causes bubbles, which makes medication administration difficult.
14. Explain the procedure to the patient, including the positioning and sensations to expect, such as burning or stinging.	
15. Ask the patient to lie supine or to sit back in a chair with the head slightly hyperextended.	• This position provides easy access to the eye for medication instillation and minimizes drainage of medication through the tear duct.
16. If crusts or drainage are present along the eyelid margins or the inner canthus, gently wash them away. Soak any crusts that are dried and difficult to remove by applying a damp washcloth or cotton ball over the eye for a few minutes. Always wipe from the inner canthus to the outer canthus.	• Crusts or drainage harbours microorganisms. Soaking enables easy removal of the crusts and prevents pressure from being applied directly over the eye. Cleansing from the inner canthus to the outer canthus helps prevent entrance of microorganisms into the lacrimal duct.
17. Hold a cotton ball or clean tissue in your nondominant hand.	• Cotton or tissue absorbs the medication that escapes the eye.
18. With the tissue or cotton resting below the lower lid, gently press downward with your thumb or forefinger against the bony orbit.	• This technique exposes the lower conjunctival sac. Retraction against the bony orbit prevents pressure and trauma to the eyeball and prevents your fingers from touching the eye.
19. Ask the patient to look at the ceiling, and explain the steps to the patient.	• When the patient looks toward the ceiling, this action retracts the sensitive cornea up and away from the conjunctival sac and reduces stimulation of the blink reflex.
A. Instill the eye drops: **(1)** With your dominant hand resting on the patient's forehead, hold the filled medication eyedropper or the ophthalmic solution approximately 1–2 cm above the conjunctival sac (see Step 19A[1] illustration).	• This technique helps to prevent accidental contact of the eyedropper with eye structures, thus reducing risk of both injury to the eye and transfer of infection to dropper. Ophthalmic medications are sterile.
(2) Instill the prescribed number of medication drops into the conjunctival sac.	• The conjunctival sac normally holds one or two drops, which provides even distribution of medication across the eye.

Continued

SKILL 34-2 ADMINISTERING OPHTHALMIC MEDICATIONS—cont'd

STEPS	RATIONALE
(3) If the patient blinks or closes the eye, or if the drops land on the outer lid margins, repeat the procedure.	• The patient obtains the therapeutic effect of the drug only when the eye drops enter the conjunctival sac.
(4) After instilling the drops, ask the patient to close the eye gently.	• Closing the eye helps to distribute the medication. Squinting or squeezing of eyelids forces medication from the conjunctival sac (Safe Medication [n.d.]).
(5) When administering medications that cause systemic effects, apply gentle pressure with your finger and a clean tissue on the patient's nasolacrimal duct for 30–60 seconds.	• This action prevents the overflow of medication into the nasal cavity.
B. Instill eye ointment:	
(1) Ask the patient to look at the ceiling.	• This action retracts the sensitive cornea up and away from the conjunctival sac and reduces stimulation of the blink reflex.
(2) Holding the ointment applicator above the lower lid margin, apply a thin stream of ointment evenly along the inner edge of the lower eyelid on the conjunctiva (see Step 19B[2] illustration) from the inner canthus to outer canthus.	• This technique distributes the medication evenly across the eye and lid margin.

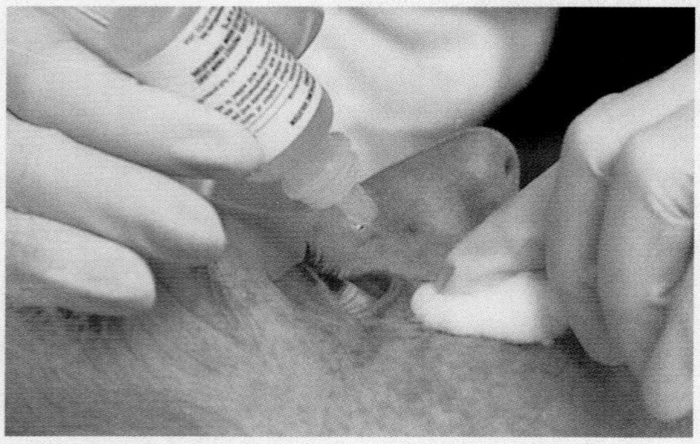

STEP 19A(1) Hold the eyedropper above the conjunctival sac.

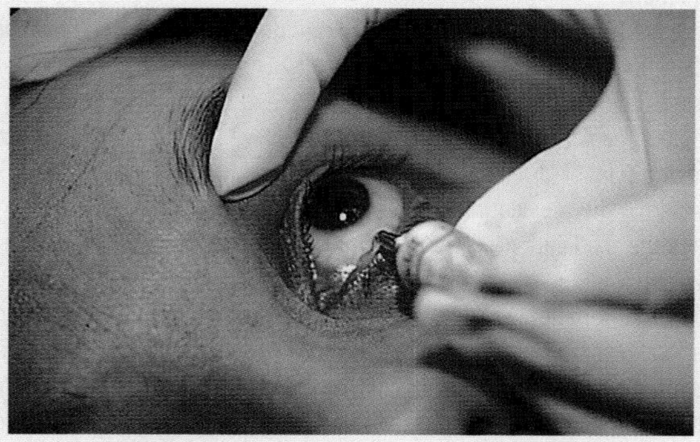

STEP 19B(2) Apply ointment along the lower eyelid.

STEPS	RATIONALE
(3) Have the patient close the eye and use a cotton ball to rub the lid lightly in a circular motion, if rubbing is not contraindicated.	• This action further distributes the medication without traumatizing the eye.
C. Intraocular disc	
(1) Application:	
(a) Open the package containing the disc. Gently press your fingertip against the disk so that it adheres to your finger. Position the convex side of the disc on your fingertip (see Step 19C[1][a] illustration).	• These actions enable the nurse to inspect the disc for damage or deformity.
(b) With your other hand, gently pull the patient's lower eyelid away from the eye. Ask the patient to look up.	• This action prepares the conjunctival sac for receiving the medicated disc.
(c) Place the disc in the conjunctival sac, so that it floats on the sclera between the iris and the lower eyelid (see Step 19C[1][c] illustration).	• This placement ensures delivery of the medication.

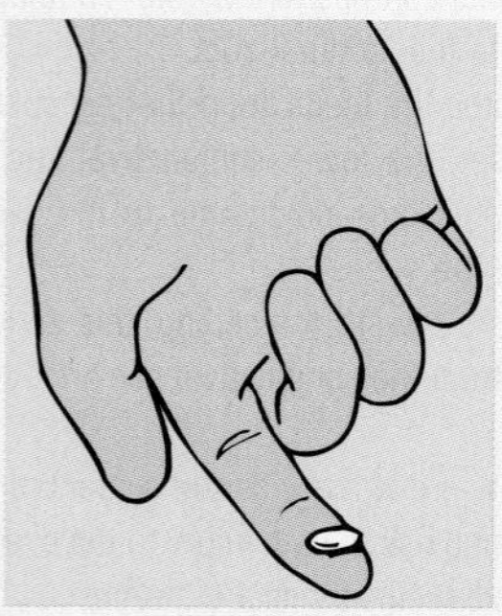

STEP 19C(1)(a) Gently position the convex side of the disc against your fingertips.

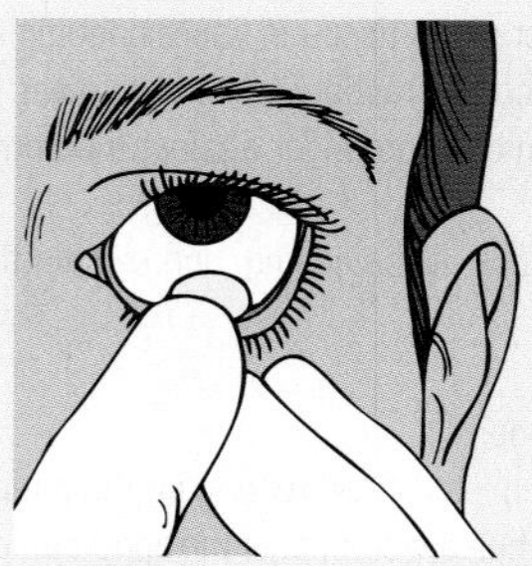

STEP 19C(1)(c) Place the disc in the conjunctival sac between the iris and the lower eyelid.

STEPS	RATIONALE
(d) Pull the patient's lower eyelid out and over the disc (see Step 19C[1][d] illustration).	• This action ensures accurate medication delivery.

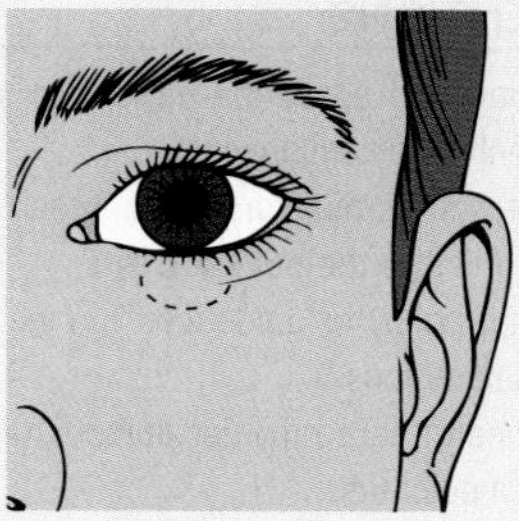

STEP 19C(1)(d) Gently pull the lower eyelid over the disc.

CRITICAL DECISION POINT: *You should not be able to see the disc at this time. If you can see the disc, repeat step 19C(1)(d).*

(2) Removal:

(a) Perform hand hygiene and put on gloves.

(b) Explain the procedure to the patient.

(c) Gently pull on the patient's lower eyelid to expose the intraocular disc.

(d) Using your forefinger and thumb of the opposite hand, pinch the disc and lift it out of the patient's eye (see Step 19C[2][d] illustration).

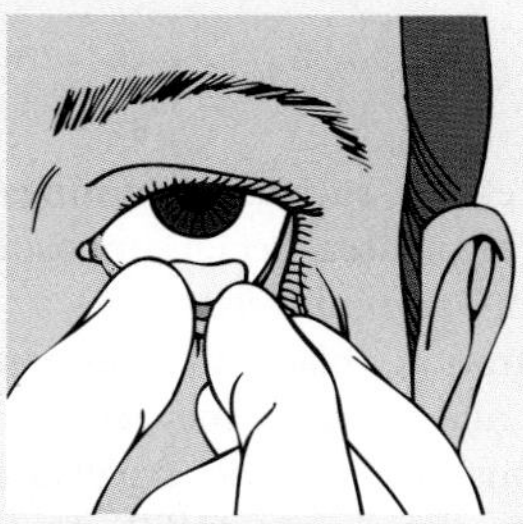

STEP 19C(2)(d) Carefully pinch the disc to remove it from the patient's eye.

STEPS	RATIONALE
20. If excess medication is on the eyelid, gently wipe it from the inner canthus to outer canthus.	• Wiping away of excess medication promotes the patient's comfort and prevents trauma to eye (Safe Medication [n.d.]).
21. If the patient wears an eye patch, apply a clean patch by placing it over the affected eye so that the entire eye is covered. Tape securely without applying pressure to eye.	• A clean eye patch reduces the chance of infection.

CRITICAL DECISION POINT: *If the patient receives more than one eye medication to the same eye at the same time, wait at least 5 minutes before administering the next medication to avoid interaction between medications (Safe Medication [n.d.]).*

STEPS	RATIONALE
22. If the patient receives eye medication to both eyes at the same time, use a different tissue or cotton ball for each eye.	• The use of separate tissues or cotton balls prevents cross-contamination between eyes.
23. Remove gloves, dispose of soiled supplies in proper receptacle, and perform hand hygiene.	
24. Note the patient's response to instillation; ask whether the patient felt any discomfort.	• The patient's response determines whether the procedure was performed correctly and safely and whether the patient is experiencing adverse effects of the medication.
25. Observe the patient's response to the medication by assessing any visual changes and noting any adverse effects.	
26. Ask the patient to discuss the medication's purpose, action, adverse effects, and the technique of administration.	
27. Have the patient demonstrate self-administration of the next dose.	

Continued

SKILL 34-2 ADMINISTERING OPHTHALMIC MEDICATIONS—cont'd

STEPS	RATIONALE

UNEXPECTED OUTCOMES	RELATED INTERVENTIONS
Inability of patient to instill drops without supervision	• Reinforce your teaching and allow the patient to self-administer drops as often as possible to enhance confidence. • If the patient cannot self-administer drops, teach others, such as family members, to instill drops into the patient's eye.
Signs of reaction to medication, such as allergic reaction (e.g., tearing, reddened sclera) or systemic response (e.g., bradycardia)	• Follow the institutional policy or guidelines for the reporting of adverse or allergic reaction to medications. • Notify the patient's health care provider immediately, and withhold further administration of the medication. • Add information about the allergy to the patient's medical record, according to agency policy.

RECORDING AND REPORTING

- Document on the MAR or the computer record the medication, concentration, number of drops, time of administration, and the eye (left, right, or both) that received medication.
- Record the appearance of the eye in the nurses' notes.

HOME CARE CONSIDERATIONS

- Patients with chronic health care problems should consult with their health care provider before they use over-the-counter eye medication.
- When they use eye drops at home, patients should not share medications with other family members because the risk of infection transmission is high.

Box 34-21 provides guidelines for administering ear drops and ear irrigations and describes the differences in straightening the ear canal for children and adults.

The external ear structures of children differ from those of adults. When instilling drops or irrigating solutions, first straighten the ear canal. In infants and young children, straighten the cartilaginous canal by grasping the auricle of the ear and pulling it gently down and backward. In adults, the ear canal is longer and composed of underlying bone. The adult ear canal is straightened by pulling the auricle upward and outward. Failure to straighten the canal properly may prevent medicinal solutions from reaching the deeper external ear structures.

Vaginal Instillation. Vaginal medications are available as suppositories, foam, jellies, and creams. Suppositories are individually packaged in foil wrappers and are sometimes stored in a refrigerator to prevent the solid, oval-shaped suppositories from melting. After a suppository is inserted into the vaginal cavity, body temperature causes it to melt and be distributed and absorbed. Foam, jellies, and creams are administered with an applicator inserter (Box 34-22). A suppository is given with a gloved hand in accordance with standard precautions and routine practices (see Chapter 33). Patients often prefer administering their own vaginal medications, which requires privacy. After instillation of the medication, a patient may wish to wear a perineal pad to collect the drainage. Because vaginal medications are often given to treat infection, the discharge may be foul smelling. Follow aseptic techniques and offer the patient frequent opportunities to maintain her perineal hygiene (see Chapter 38).

Rectal Instillation. Rectal suppositories are thinner and more bullet-shaped than vaginal suppositories. The rounded end prevents anal trauma during insertion. Rectal suppositories contain medications that exert local effects, such as promoting defecation, or systemic effects, such as reducing nausea. Rectal suppositories are usually stored in the refrigerator until administered.

During administration, place the suppository past the internal anal sphincter and against the rectal mucosa (Box 34-23). Otherwise, the suppository may be expelled before it can dissolve and be absorbed into the mucosa. With practice, you will learn to recognize the sensation of the sphincter relaxing around the finger. Do not force the suppository into a mass of fecal material. If necessary, clear the rectum with a small cleansing enema before inserting a suppository.

Administering Medications by Inhalation

Medications administered by hand-held inhalers are dispersed through an aerosol spray, mist, or powder that penetrates the lung airways. The alveolocapillary network absorbs medications rapidly. Metered-dose inhalers (MDIs), dry powder inhalers (DPIs), and slow-stream inhaler devices usually produce local effects, such as bronchodilatation; however, some medications can lead to serious systemic side effects.

Patients who receive medications by inhalation frequently have chronic respiratory disease, such as chronic asthma, emphysema, or bronchitis. Medications given by inhalation provide these patients with control of their airway obstruction. Inhaled medications are often described as "rescue" or "maintenance" medications. Rescue medications are short-acting medications that are taken for immediate relief of acute respiratory distress. Maintenance inhalers are used on a daily scheduled basis to prevent acute respiratory distress. The effects of maintenance inhalers start within hours of administration and last for a longer period of time than rescue inhalers. Because these patients depend on these medications for disease control, they must learn

BOX 34-21 PROCEDURAL GUIDELINE

Administering Ear Medications

Delegation Considerations:
The administration of ear medications cannot be delegated. Instruct unregulated care providers about the potential adverse effects of ear medications and the need to report their occurrence immediately.

Equipment:
- Medication administration record (MAR)
- Clean gloves if patient has drainage from the ear
- Medication bottle with dropper, cotton-tipped applicator, and cotton ball (optional) if ear drops are being administered
- Irrigating syringe, kidney-shaped basin, and towel if ear is to be irrigated

Procedure:
1. Check the accuracy and completeness of each MAR or computer printout against the prescriber's original medication order. Check the patient's name and the medication name, dosage, route, and time for administration. Copy or rewrite any portion of the MAR that is difficult to read.
2. Prepare the medication. Ensure that you compare the label of the medication against the MAR at least two times during the medication preparation.
3. Take the medication to the patient at the correct time, and perform hand hygiene. Put on gloves if drainage is present.
4. Identify the patient by using at least two patient identifiers. Compare the patient's name and one other identifier (e.g., the hospital identification number) on the MAR, computer printout, or computer screen with information on the patient's identification bracelet. Ask the patient to state his or her name, if possible, for a third identifier.
5. Compare the label on the medication with the MAR one more time at the patient's bedside.
6. Explain the procedure to the patient regarding positioning and the sensations to expect, such as hearing bubbling or feeling water in the ear as medication trickles into the ear.
7. Teach the patient about the medication.
8. Administer the ear drops:
   - A. Have the patient assume a side-lying position (if this position is not contraindicated by patient's condition) with the ear to be treated facing up. Alternatively, the patient may sit in a chair or at the bedside.
   - B. Perform hand hygiene. Put on gloves if drainage is present.
   - C. Straighten the ear canal by pulling the auricle down and back (for children under 3 years of age) or upward and outward (for adults).
   - D. Hold the dropper 1 cm above the ear canal and instill the prescribed drops (see Step 8D illustration).

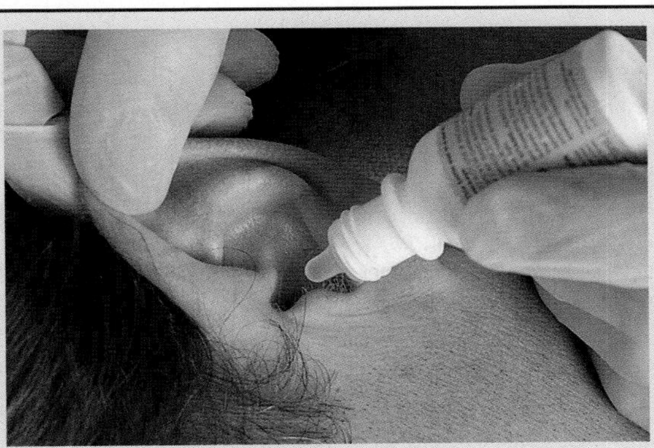

STEP 8D Placing ear drop in ear.

   - E. Ask the patient to remain in a side-lying position for 2 to 3 minutes. Apply gentle massage or pressure to the tragus of the ear with your finger unless contraindicated due to pain.
   - F. If a cotton ball is needed, place the cotton ball into the outermost part of the ear canal. Do not press cotton deep into the canal. Remove cotton after 15 minutes.
9. Administer ear irrigations:
   - A. Assess the tympanic membrane or review the medical record for a history of eardrum perforation, which would contraindicate ear irrigation.
   - B. Assist the patient in assuming a sitting or lying position with the head tilted or turned toward the affected ear. Place a towel under the patient's head and shoulder and have the patient hold a kidney-shaped basin under the affected ear.
   - C. Perform hand hygiene. Put on gloves if drainage is present.
   - D. Fill the irrigating syringe with approximately 50 mL of the solution.
   - E. Gently grasp the auricle and straighten the ear canal by pulling it down and back (for children under 3 years of age) or upward and outward (for children 4 years of age and older and adults).
   - F. Slowly instill the irrigating solution by holding the tip of the syringe 1 cm above the opening of the ear canal. Allow the fluid to drain out during instillation. Continue until the canal is clean or until all solution is used.
10. Clean the work area and put the medication supplies away.
11. Remove gloves and perform hand hygiene.
12. Document medication administration on the MAR or computer record.
13. Evaluate the patient's response to the medication.

BOX 34-22 PROCEDURAL GUIDELINE

Administering Vaginal Medications

Delegation Considerations:
The administration of medications by the vaginal route cannot be delegated. Instruct unregulated care providers to report new or increased vaginal discharge or bleeding and occurrence of potential adverse effects of the medications immediately.

Equipment:
- Vaginal cream, foam, jelly, or suppository, or irrigating solution with applicator (if required)
- Clean, disposable gloves
- Towels, or a washcloth, or both
- Paper towels
- Perineal pad
- Drape or sheet
- Water-soluble lubricating jelly
- Medication administration record (MAR) or computer printout

Procedure:
1. Check the accuracy and completeness of each MAR or computer printout against the prescriber's original medication order. Check the patient's name and the medication name, form (cream, foam, jelly, or suppository), route, dosage, time of administration, and drug indication.

Continued

BOX 34-22 PROCEDURAL GUIDELINE

Administering Vaginal Medications—cont'd

2. Review the patient's history of allergies, including allergies to latex. Prepare the medication (see Skill 34-1, Steps 7A–G and M–O). Compare the label of the medication with the MAR two times while preparing the medication.
3. Take the medication to the patient at the correct time, and perform hand hygiene.
4. Identify the patient by using at least two patient identifiers. Compare the patient's name and one other identifier (e.g., the hospital identification number) on the MAR, computer printout, or computer screen with information on the patient's identification bracelet. Ask the patient to state her name, if possible, for a third identifier.
5. Allow the patient to empty or attempt to empty her bladder before administration of vaginal medication. To facilitate adequate absorption, the patient needs to lie quietly for at least 10 minutes.
6. Compare the label on the medication with the MAR one more time at the patient's bedside.
7. Teach the patient about the medication. Explain to the patient the procedure for positioning and the sensations she can expect, such as feelings of moisture or wetness in the vaginal area. Assess the patient's ability to manipulate the applicator or suppository and to position herself to insert the medication. Explain the procedure to the patient. Especially if the patient plans to self-administer the medication, it is important to be specific in your explanation.
8. Close the room curtain or door and arrange the supplies at the bedside.
9. Assist the patient to lie in a dorsal recumbent position. This position provides full exposure and easy access to the vaginal canal and allows the suppository to dissolve without escaping through an orifice.
10. Put on clean, disposable gloves.
11. Keep the abdomen and lower extremities draped.
12. Ensure that the lighting is adequate to visualize the vaginal opening. Inspect the condition of external genitalia and the vaginal canal, noting the appearance of any discharge. Clean the area with a towel or washcloth if necessary.
13. Insert the vaginal suppository:
    - A. Remove the suppository from its foil wrapper. Apply a liberal amount of sterile water-based lubricating jelly to the smooth or rounded end of the suppository. Lubricate the gloved index finger of your dominant hand.
    - B. With your nondominant gloved hand, expose the vaginal orifice by gently retracting the labial folds.
    - C. With your dominant gloved hand, gently insert the rounded end of the suppository along the posterior wall of the vaginal canal for the entire length of your finger (7.5 to 10 cm) to ensure equal distribution of the medication along the walls of the vaginal cavity (see Step 13C illustration).
    - D. Withdraw your finger and wipe any remaining lubricant from around the orifice and labia.
14. Administer the cream or foam:
    - A. Fill the cream or foam applicator, as described on the package directions.
    - B. With your nondominant gloved hand, expose the vaginal orifice by gently retracting the labial folds.
    - C. With your dominant gloved hand, insert the applicator approximately 5 to 7.5 cm. Push the applicator plunger to deposit the medication into the vagina to allow equal distribution of medication (see Step 14C illustration).
    - D. Withdraw the applicator and place it on a paper towel. Wipe residual cream from the labia or vaginal orifice.
15. Dispose of supplies, remove gloves, and perform hand hygiene.
16. Instruct the patient to remain on her back for at least 10 minutes.
17. Document the medication administration on the MAR or computer record.
18. If the applicator was used, wear gloves to wash it with soap and warm water, rinse, and store for future use.
19. Offer the patient a perineal pad when she resumes ambulation, to prevent vaginal discharge from spreading to clothing.
20. Inspect the appearance of discharge from the vaginal canal and the condition of external genitalia between applications to evaluate the medication's effectiveness.

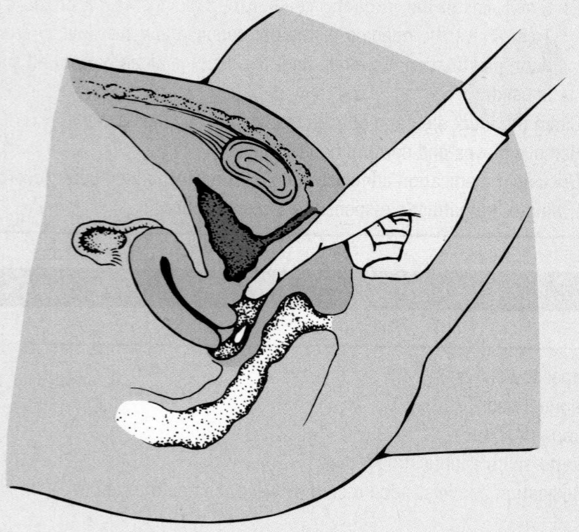

STEP 13C Insertion of a suppository into the vaginal canal.

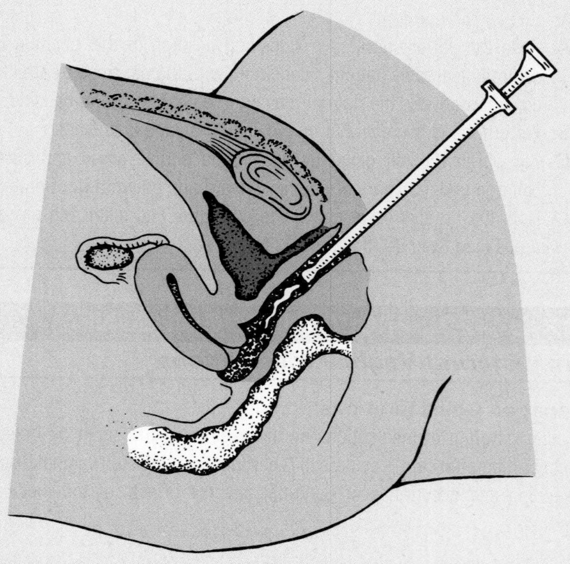

STEP 14C Instillation of medication in the vaginal canal.

BOX 34-23 PROCEDURAL GUIDELINE

Administering Rectal Suppositories

Delegation Considerations:

The administration of medications by the rectal route cannot be delegated. Instruct unregulated care providers to expect and report fecal discharge or a bowel movement and to report the occurrence of potential adverse effects or medications immediately.

Equipment:

- Rectal suppository
- Water-soluble lubricating jelly
- Clean gloves (two pair)
- Drape or sheet
- Tissue
- Medication administration record (MAR) or computer printout

Procedure:

1. Check the accuracy and completeness of each MAR or computer printout against the prescriber's original medication order. Check the patient's name and the medication name, route, dosage, and time of administration. Copy or rewrite any portion of the MAR that is difficult to read.
2. Review the medical record for information on rectal surgery, bleeding, and for a history of allergies.
3. Prepare medication (see Skill 34-1, Steps 7A–G and M–O). Ensure that you compare the label of the medication with the MAR two times during medication preparation.
4. Take the medication to the patient at the correct time, and perform hand hygiene.
5. Identify the patient by using at least two patient identifiers. Compare the patient's name and one other identifier (e.g., the hospital identification number) on the MAR, computer printout, or computer screen with information on the patient's identification bracelet. Ask the patient to state his or her name, if possible, for a third identifier.
6. Compare the label of the medication with the MAR or computer printout one more time at the patient's bedside.
7. Teach the patient about the medication. Explain the procedure to the patient regarding the positioning and the sensations to expect, such as feelings of needing to defecate. Ensure that the patient understands the procedure and that he or she can self-administer the medication.
8. Close the room curtain or door and arrange supplies at the bedside.
9. Put on clean gloves.
10. Assist the patient in assuming Sims' position to expose the anus and facilitate relaxation of the external anal sphincter. Keep the patient draped with only the anal area exposed.
11. Ensure the lighting is adequate to visualize the anus. Check for evidence of active rectal bleeding. Examine the condition of the anus externally and palpate the rectal walls to assess for presence of feces, which may interfere with the suppository placement (see Chapter 32). Dispose of gloves in proper receptacle if they are soiled.
12. Put on a new pair of disposable gloves (if previous gloves were discarded).
13. Remove the suppository from its wrapper and lubricate the rounded end (see Step 13 illustration) with a sterile water-soluble lubricating jelly to reduce the friction when the suppository enters the rectal canal. Lubricate the index finger of your dominant hand with a water-soluble lubricant.

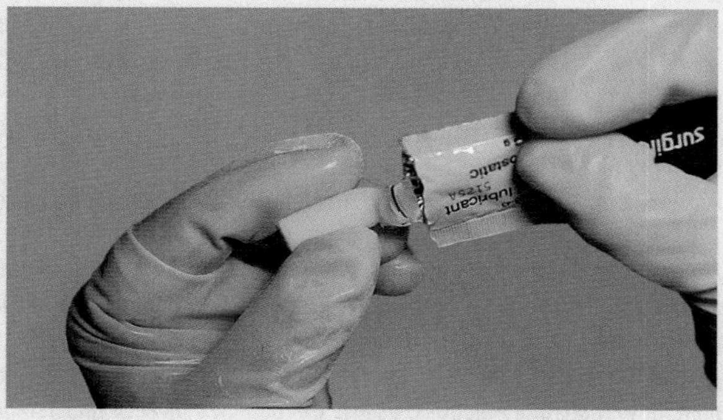

STEP 13 Remove the suppository from its wrapper.

14. Ask the patient to take slow, deep breaths through the mouth and relax the anal sphincter.
15. Retract the buttocks with your nondominant hand. Insert the suppository gently through the anus, past the internal sphincter and against the rectal wall, 10 cm in adults, 5 cm in children and infants. Apply gentle pressure to hold the buttocks together momentarily, if necessary, to keep medication in place and to facilitate medication distribution and absorption.
16. Withdraw your finger and wipe the anal area with tissue.
17. Remove gloves and dispose of medication supplies in the appropriate receptacle and perform hand hygiene.
18. Ask the patient to remain flat or on the side for 5 minutes, to prevent expulsion of the suppository.
19. If the suppository contains a laxative or fecal softener, place a call light within the patient's reach.
20. Document medication administration on the MAR or computer record.
21. Evaluate the effectiveness of the medication by observing the patient for a response to the suppository (e.g., bowel movement, relief of nausea) at times that correlate with the medication's onset, peak, and duration.

about the inhalers and how to administer them safely (Skill 34-3). If a patient uses more than one type of inhaler, the bronchodilator is given first.

An MDI delivers a measured dose of medication with each push of the canister. Chemical propellants (e.g., hydrofluorocarbons) push the medication out of the MDI. MDIs are either squeeze-and-breathe inhalers or inhalers activated by the patient's breath. The squeeze-and-breathe MDI requires the application of approximately 2 to 5 kg of pressure to the top of the canister to administer the medication. To use this type of MDI, the patient must have hand strength, which often diminishes as a result of aging or the effects of chronic respiratory disease. Lack of sufficient hand strength can restrict the patient's ability to self-administer medication via MDIs. Breath-activated MDIs release the medication when the patient inhales. Release of the medication is dependent on the strength of the patient's breath on inspiration (Capriotti, 2005). The MDI can be used with a spacer to allow the particles of medication to slow down and break into smaller pieces, which improves the drug's absorption in the patient's airway. Spacers are equipped with a face mask when they are used by infants and children younger than 4 years of age. Spacers are especially helpful for patients who have difficulty coordinating the steps involved in self-administering inhaled medications. When patients do not use

SKILL 34-3 USING METERED-DOSE OR DRY POWDER INHALERS

Delegation Considerations

The administration of a metered-dose inhaler (MDI) or dry powder inhaler (DPI) and the supervision of patients who self-administer these medications cannot be delegated to unregulated care providers (UCPs). Instruct UCPs to report changes in the patient's respiratory status, increased coughing, or the occurrence of potential adverse effects immediately.

Equipment

- MDI or DPI
- Spacer (optional with MDI)
- Facial tissues (optional)
- Washbasin or sink with warm water
- Paper towel
- Medication administration record (MAR) or computer printout

PROCEDURE

STEPS	RATIONALE
1. Check the accuracy and completeness of each MAR or computer printout against the prescriber's original medication order. Check the patient's name and the medication name, route, dosage, and time of administration. Copy or rewrite any portion of the MAR that is difficult to read.	
2. Assess the patient's respiratory pattern, auscultate the patient's breath sounds.	• Assessment of the patient's respiratory pattern establishes the baseline of airway status for comparison during and after treatment.
3. Assess the patient's ability to hold, manipulate, and depress the canister. Assess the patient's strength of inhalation.	• Any impairment in the ability to grasp, to breathe, or to coordinate movements interferes with the patient's ability to use the MDI or DPI correctly.
4. Assess the patient's readiness to learn—for example, whether the patient asks questions about the medication, disease, or complications; requests education in use of inhaler; is mentally alert; participates in self-care.	• The patient's readiness to learn affects the ability to understand explanations and actively participate in the learning process (Bastable, 2013).
5. Assess the patient's ability to learn: the patient should not be fatigued, in pain, or in respiratory distress; assess the patient's level of understanding of technical terms.	• The patient's mental or physical limitations affect the ability to learn and the methods the nurse can use for instruction (Bastable, 2013).
6. Assess the patient's knowledge and understanding of the disease and the purpose and action of the prescribed medications.	• Knowledge of disease is essential for the patient to understand the proper use of the inhaler.
7. Determine the medication schedule and the number of inhalations prescribed for each dose.	• The medication schedule influences the explanations the nurse provides for use of inhaler.
8. Prepare the medication (see Skill 34-1, Steps 7A–G and M–O). Ensure that you compare the label of the medication with the MAR two times during medication preparation.	
9. Identify the patient by using at least two patient identifiers. Compare the patient's name and one other identifier (e.g., the hospital identification number) on the MAR, computer printout, or computer screen with information on the patient's identification bracelet. Ask the patient to state his or her name, if possible, for a third identifier.	
10. Compare the label on medications with the MAR one more time at the patient's bedside.	
11. Instruct the patient in a comfortable environment, for example, by sitting in a chair in the hospital room or sitting at a kitchen table in the patient's home.	• The patient will be more likely to remain receptive to education if he or she is in a comfortable environment (Bastable, 2013).
12. Provide adequate time for the teaching session.	
13. Perform hand hygiene and arrange the equipment needed.	
14. Allow the patient an opportunity to manipulate the inhaler, the canister, and the spacer device. Explain and demonstrate how the canister fits into the inhaler.	• Manipulating the various items facilitates the patient's familiarity with the equipment.

CRITICAL DECISION POINT: *If the patient is using an MDI with or without a spacer and the inhaler is new or has not been used for several days, push a "test spray" into the air (MayoClinic.com, 2007). A test spray is not needed for a DPI.*

STEPS	RATIONALE
15. Explain to the patient what a metered dose is and warn the patient about overuse of the inhaler, including medication adverse effects.	• The patient must not arbitrarily administer excessive inhalations because of the risk of serious adverse effects. If medication is given in recommended doses, adverse effects are uncommon.
16. Explain the steps for administering squeeze-and-breathe inhaled dose of medication of MDI (demonstrate steps when possible):	• Use of simple, step-by-step explanations allows the patient to ask questions at any point during the procedure.
A. Insert the MDI canister into the holder.	
B. Remove the mouthpiece cover from the inhaler.	
C. Shake the inhaler vigorously five or six times.	• Shaking the inhaler ensures that fine particles are aerosolized.

STEPS	RATIONALE
D. Have the patient take a deep breath and exhale.	• A deep breath followed by an exhalation empties the lungs and prepares the patient's airway to receive the medication.
E. Instruct the patient to position the inhaler in one of two ways. **(1)** Close the mouth around the MDI with the opening toward the back of the throat (see Step 16E[1] illustration). **(2)** Position the device 2–4 cm in front of the mouth (see Step 16E[2] illustration).	• This position directs the aerosol spray toward the airway. Positioning the mouthpiece in front of the mouth is considered the best way to deliver the medication.

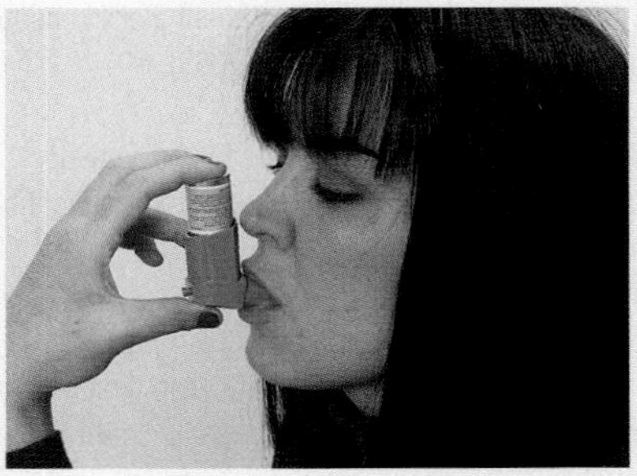

STEP 16E(1) The patient opens lips and places inhaler in mouth with opening toward back of throat.

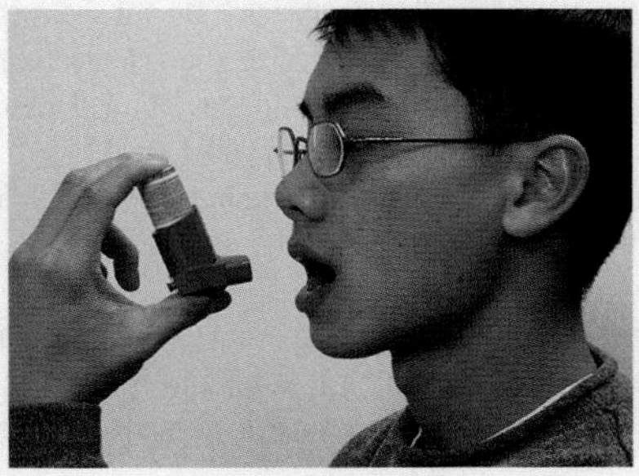

STEP 16E(2) The patient positions the mouthpiece 2 to 4 cm away from the mouth. This placement is considered the best way to deliver the medication.

STEPS	RATIONALE
F. With the inhaler properly positioned, have patient hold the inhaler with thumb at the mouthpiece and the index finger and middle finger at the top. This arrangement is called a three-point or lateral hand position.	• MDIs work best when patients use a three-point or lateral hand position to activate the canister.
G. Instruct the patient to tilt the head back slightly and inhale slowly and deeply through the mouth for 3–5 seconds while depressing the canister fully.	• Medication is distributed to airways during inhalation. Inhalation through the mouth rather than the nose draws medication more effectively into airways.
H. Instruct the patient to hold the breath for approximately 10 seconds.	• Holding the breath allows tiny drops of aerosol spray to reach the deeper branches of the airways.
I. Instruct the patient to remove the MDI from the mouth and to exhale through pursed lips.	• Using pursed lips keeps the small airways open during exhalation.
17. Explain the steps to administer MDI by using a spacer, such as an AeroChamber (demonstrate when possible):	
A. Remove the mouthpiece cover from the MDI and the mouthpiece of the spacer. Inspect the spacer for foreign objects. If the spacer has a valve, ensure the valve is intact.	
B. Insert the MDI into the end of the spacer.	• The spacer traps medication released from the MDI; the patient then inhales the drug from the device. These devices break up and slow down the medication particles, enhancing the amount of medication received by the patient (Vella & Grech, 2005).
C. Shake the inhaler vigorously five or six times.	• Shaking the inhaler ensures the fine particles are aerosolized.
D. Have the patient exhale completely before closing the mouth around the mouthpiece of the spacer. Avoid covering small exhalation slots with the lips (see Step 17D illustration).	

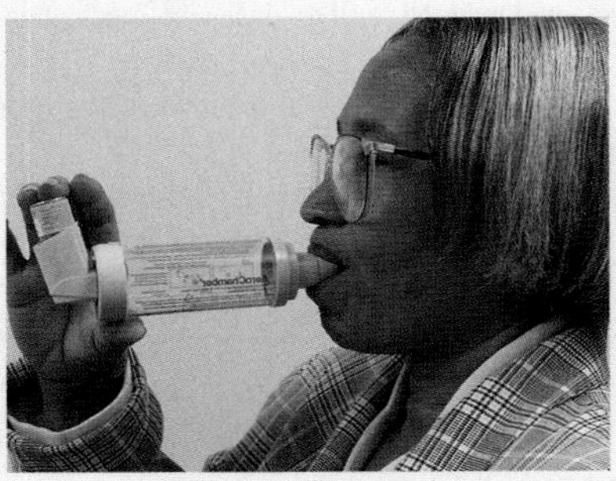

STEP 17D Have the patient place the mouthpiece in the mouth and close the lips, being careful to keep the exhalation slots exposed.

STEPS	RATIONALE
E. Have the patient depress the medication canister, spraying one puff into the spacer.	• The spacer emits a spray that allows finer particles to be inhaled. • Large droplets are retained in the spacer.

Continued

SKILL 34-3 USING METERED-DOSE OR DRY POWDER INHALERS—cont'd

STEPS	RATIONALE
F. Instruct the patient to inhale deeply and slowly through the mouth for 3–5 seconds.	• Deep inhalations maximize the amount of medication that enters the lungs.
G. Instruct the patient to hold the breath for 10 seconds.	• Holding the breath ensures full medication distribution.
H. Instruct the patient to remove the MDI and spacer before exhaling.	• Removing the MDI and spacer allows the patient to exhale normally.
18. Explain the steps to administer DPI or breath-activated MDI (demonstrate when possible):	
A. Remove the cover from the mouthpiece. Do not shake the inhaler.	
B. Prepare the medication as directed by the manufacturer (e.g., hold the inhaler upright and turn the wheel to the right and then to the left until a click is heard, load the medication pellet, etc.).	• Preparing the medication properly primes the inhaler to ensure the medication will be delivered to the patient (Capriotti, 2005).
C. Instruct the patient to exhale away from the inhaler before inhalation.	• Exhaling before using the inhaler prevents loss of powder.
D. Position the mouthpiece between the patient's lips.	• Properly positioning the mouthpiece prevents the medication from escaping through the mouth.
E. Instruct the patient to inhale deeply and forcefully through the mouth.	• Deep inhalations create aerosol.
F. Instruct the patient to hold the breath for 5–10 seconds.	• Holding the breath ensures full medication distribution.
19. Instruct the patient to wait at least 20–30 seconds between inhalations of medications.	• Medications must be inhaled sequentially. The first inhalation opens the airways and reduces inflammation. The second or third inhalation penetrates the deeper airways.

CRITICAL DECISION POINT: *If two medications are to be administered, give the bronchodilator first.*

STEPS	RATIONALE
20. Instruct the patient in cleaning the inhaler:	
A. Once a day, the inhaler and its cap should be rinsed in warm running water. The inhaler must be completely dry before use.	• Accumulation of spray around the mouthpiece can interfere with proper distribution during use.
B. Twice a week, the L-shaped plastic mouthpiece should be washed with mild dishwashing soap and warm water. Rinse and dry well before placing the canister back inside the mouthpiece (Canadian Lung Association, n.d.).	• Regular cleaning removes residual medication. Do not place inhalers holding cromolyn, nedocromil, or HFA (hydrofluoroalkane) in water.
21. Ask whether the patient has any questions.	• The patient has an opportunity to clarify misconceptions or misunderstandings.
22. Have the patient explain and demonstrate the steps in the use of an inhaler.	• A return demonstration provides feedback for measuring the patient's learning.
23. Ask the patient to explain the medication schedule, adverse effects, and when to call health care providers.	• Reviewing the medication requirements improves the likelihood of adherence to the therapy.
24. Ask the patient to calculate how many days the inhaler will last.	• This calculation helps the patient to determine when to reorder a prescription.
25. After the medication has been taken, assess the patient's respiratory status, including the ease of respirations, auscultation of lungs, and the use of pulse oximetry to assess the patient's oxygenation status.	• Assessment of the respiratory status determines the status of the patient's breathing pattern and adequacy of ventilation.

UNEXPECTED OUTCOMES	RELATED INTERVENTIONS
Need for a bronchodilator more frequently than every 4 hours	• Respiratory problems are indicated. The type of medication and delivery methods need to be reassessed. Notify the health care provider if respiratory status does not improve.
Cardiac dysrhythmias, especially in patient receiving β–adrenergics	• If the patient experiences symptoms with dysrhythmias (e.g., lightheadedness, syncope), withhold all further doses of medication and notify the prescriber.
Inability of patient to self-administer medication properly	• Explore alternative delivery routes or alternative methods of medication administration.
Paroxysms of coughing	• Aerosolized particles irritate the posterior pharynx. Notify the prescriber; reassess the type of medication or the delivery method.

RECORDING AND REPORTING

- Document the skills that you taught the patient and the patient's ability to perform these skills.
- Document on the MAR or computer record the medication, time of administration, and number of puffs.
- Report any undesirable effects from the medication.

HOME CARE CONSIDERATIONS

- Remind patients to carry their prescribed inhalers to use immediately in case of an acute asthma attack.

their inhalers and spacers correctly, they do not receive the full effect of the medication. Therefore, patient education is essential.

DPIs hold dry, powdered medication and create an aerosol when the patient inhales through a reservoir that contains a dose of the medication. DPIs require less manual dexterity than MDIs, and because the device is activated by the patient's breath, the patient does not need to coordinate puffs with inhalation, as required when an MDI is used. DPIs do not require use of a spacer; however, the medication inside the DPI may clump if the DPI is used in a humid climate, and some patients cannot inspire at the speed needed to administer the entire dose of the medication.

One important aspect of patient teaching is to help the patient determine when the MDI or DPI is empty and needs to be replaced. Floating the MDI to determine the amount of medication remaining is no longer recommended because extra propellant may cause buoyancy even if no medication remains in the inhaler. Furthermore, MDIs with hydrofluoroalkanes (HFA) should never be immersed (Capriotti, 2005). Some DPIs have mechanisms that indicate the number of doses remaining; however, these mechanisms are not always accurate. To calculate how long the medication in an MDI or DPI will last, divide the capacity of the canister by the number of doses the patient takes per day. For example, a patient is to take albuterol, a β-adrenergic agonist bronchodilator. The ordered dose is two puffs four times a day. The canister has a total of 200 puffs. Complete the following calculations to determine how long the MDI will last:

$$2 \text{ puffs} \times 4 \text{ times a day} = 8 \text{ puffs per day}$$

$$200 \text{ puffs} \div 8 \text{ puffs per day} = 25 \text{ days}$$

The canister in this example will last 25 days. To ensure the patient does not run out of medication, teach the patient to refill the medication prescription at least 7 to 10 days before it is expected to run out (MayoClinic.com, 2016).

Administering Medications by Irrigations

Some medications irrigate or wash out a body cavity and are delivered through a stream of solution. Irrigations most commonly use sterile water, saline, or antiseptic solutions to irrigate the eye, ear, throat, vagina, or urinary tract. Use aseptic technique if the patient has a break in the skin or mucosa. When the cavity to be irrigated is not sterile, as in the case of the ear canal (see Box 34-21) or vagina, use a clean technique. In health care settings, sterile solutions are usually used. Irrigations are used to clean an area, instill a medication, or apply heat or cold to injured tissue.

Administering Parenteral Medications

Parenteral administration of medications is the administration of medications by injection. Parenteral administration is an invasive procedure that must be performed with aseptic techniques (Box 34-24). After a needle pierces the skin, the patient is at risk of infection. Each type of injection requires the application of specific skills to ensure the medication reaches the proper location. The effects of a parenterally administered medication develop rapidly, depending on the rate of medication absorption. The nurse must always closely observe the patient's response.

Equipment. A variety of syringes and needles are available, each designed to deliver a precise volume of medication to a specific type of tissue. Use nursing judgement when determining the syringe or needle that will be most effective.

Syringes. Syringes consist of a close-fitting plunger and a cylindrical barrel with a tip designed to fit the hub of a hypodermic needle.

BOX 34-24 Preventing Infection During an Injection

- To prevent contamination of the solution, draw the medication from the ampule quickly. Do not allow it to stand open.
- To prevent needle contamination, avoid letting the needle touch a contaminated surface (e.g., the outer edges of the ampoule or vial, the outer surface of the needle cap, your hands, a countertop, a table surface).
- To prevent syringe contamination, avoid touching the length of the plunger or the inner part of the barrel. Keep the tip of the syringe covered with a cap or needle.
- To prepare the skin, wash skin soiled with dirt, drainage, or feces with soap and water and then dry. Use friction and a circular motion to clean the skin with an antiseptic swab. Swab from centre of site and move outward in a 5-cm radius.

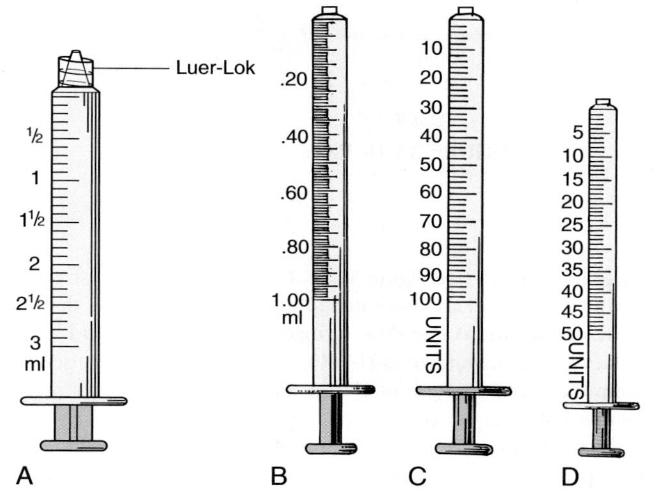

FIGURE 34-14 Types of syringes. **A,** Luer-Lok syringe marked in 0.1 (tenths). **B,** Tuberculin syringe marked in 0.01 (hundredths) for doses of less than 1 mL. **C,** Insulin syringe marked in units (100). **D,** Insulin syringe marked in units (50).

Syringes, in general, are classified as being Luer-Lok or non–Luer-Lok. This nomenclature is based on the design of the syringe's tip. Luer-Lok syringes (Figure 34-14, *A*) require special needles, which are twisted onto the tip and lock in place. This design prevents the inadvertent removal of the needle. Non–Luer-Lok syringes (Figure 34-14, *B–D*) require needles that slip onto the tip. In clinical settings, all syringes now have safety devices to prevent needle-stick injuries.

Fill the syringe by aspiration, by pulling the plunger outward while the needle tip remains immersed in the prepared solution. You may handle the outside of the syringe barrel and the handle of the plunger. To maintain sterility, avoid letting any unsterile object touch the tip or the inside of the barrel, the hub, the shaft of the plunger, or the needle (Figure 34-15).

Syringes come in numerous sizes, from 0.5 mL to 60 mL. A 1- to 3-mL syringe is usually adequate for a subcutaneous or IM injection. The use of a syringe larger than 5 mL is unusual for an injection. The larger volume creates discomfort. Instead, larger syringes are used to administer certain IV medications, to add medications to IV solutions, and to irrigate wounds or drainage tubes. Syringes may be prepackaged with a needle attached; however, the needle size may be changed depending on the route of administration and the size of the patient.

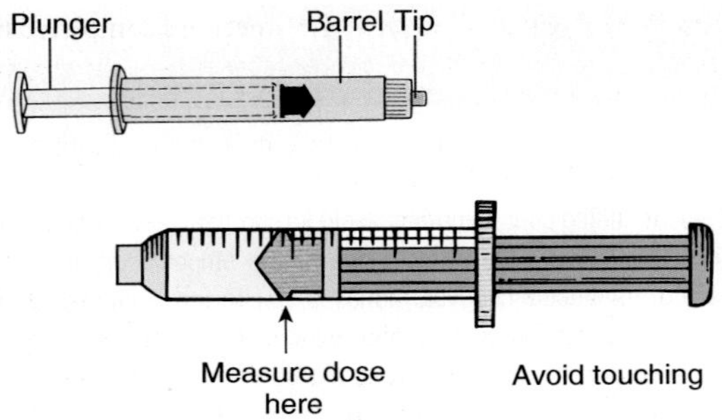

FIGURE 34-15 Parts of a syringe.

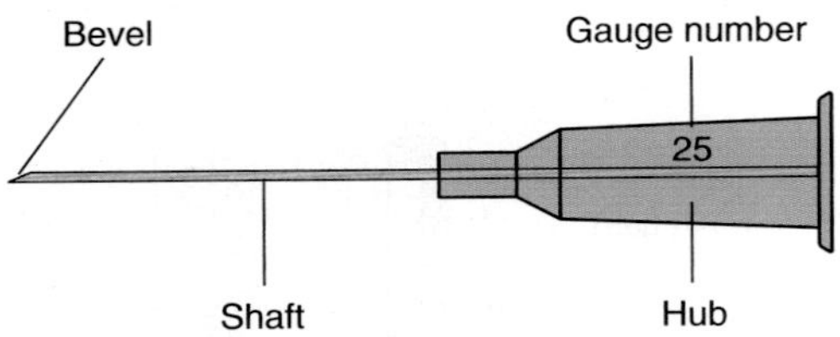

FIGURE 34-16 Parts of the needle.

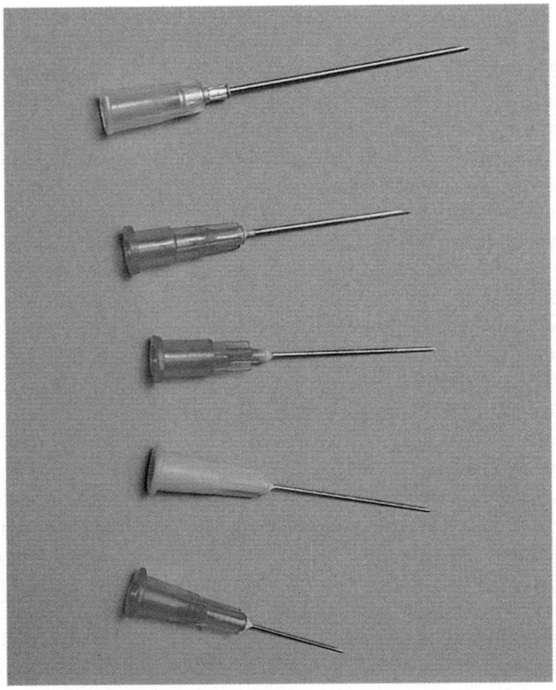

FIGURE 34-17 Needles. **Top to bottom:** 19 gauge, 3.8 cm length; 20 gauge, 2.5 cm length; 21 gauge, 2.5 cm length; 23 gauge, 2.5 cm length; and 25 gauge, 1.6 cm length.

Insulin syringes (see Figure 34-14, *C-D*) are available in sizes from 0.3 mL to 1 mL and are calibrated in units. Insulin syringes that hold 0.3 mL are known as low-dose syringes (30 units per 0.3 mL). Most insulin syringes are known as U-100s and are designed to be used with insulin that has a strength of U-100. Each millilitre of U-100 insulin contains 100 units of insulin.

The tuberculin syringe (see Figure 34-14, *B*) has a long, thin barrel with a preattached thin needle. The syringe is calibrated in sixteenths of a minim and in hundredths of a millilitre and has a capacity of 1 mL. Use a tuberculin syringe to prepare small amounts of medications (e.g., intradermal or subcutaneous injections). A tuberculin syringe is also useful when preparing small, precise doses for infants or young children.

Needles. Needles are packaged in individual sheaths to allow flexibility in choosing the right needle for a patient. Some needles are preattached to standard-sized syringes. Most needles are made of stainless steel and are disposable.

The needle has three parts: the hub, which fits onto the tip of a syringe; the shaft, which connects to the hub; and the bevel, or slanted tip (Figure 34-16). The tip of a needle, or the bevel, is always slanted. The bevel creates a narrow slit when it is injected into tissue.

When the needle is removed, the slit quickly closes to prevent leakage of medication, blood, or serum. Long bevelled tips are sharper and narrower to minimize discomfort to the patient when entering tissue used for subcutaneous or IM injections.

Needles vary in length from 0.6 to 7.6 cm (Figure 34-17). Although metric measurement is preferred in Canada, most needles used here come from the United States and likely will not appear in metric sizes. Choose the needle length according to the patient's size and weight and the type of tissue into which the medication is to be injected. In general, a child or slender adult requires a shorter needle. Use longer needles (2.5 to 3.8 cm) for IM injections and use a shorter needle (1 to 1.6 cm) for subcutaneous injections.

Needle diameter is measured by gauge. As the gauge becomes smaller, the needle diameter becomes larger (see Figure 34-17). Gauge selection depends on the viscosity of fluid to be injected or infused. An IM injection usually requires an 18- to 27-gauge needle (most commonly used is a 21- to 23-gauge needle), depending on the viscosity of the medication. Subcutaneous injections require small-diameter needles, such as a 25-gauge needle. A 26-gauge needle is used for an intradermal injection. The standard length of a needle for IM injections is 3.8 cm (1.5 inches); however, this needs to be adjusted based on the size of the patient and the location to be injected.

Disposable Injection Units. Disposable, single-dose, prefilled syringes are available for some medications. It is important to check the medication and concentration because all prefilled syringes look very similar. When using these syringes, the nurse does not have to prepare medication doses, except perhaps to expel portions of unneeded medications.

The Tubex and Carpuject injection systems include reusable plastic mechanisms that hold prefilled, disposable, sterile cartridge-needle units (Figure 34-18). To prepare these systems, slip the cartridge into the syringe, secure it (by following the package directions), and check for air bubbles in the syringe. Advance the plunger to expel excess medication as you would with a regular syringe. A new type of injection system involves screwing a plungerlike device into the end of a prefilled vial that contains a needle. After the medication is given, safely dispose of the entire unit in a puncture-proof and leakproof receptacle. The design of these injection systems reduces the risk of needle-stick injuries.

Preparing an Injection From an Ampule. Ampules contain single doses of medication in a liquid. Ampules are available in several sizes, from 1 mL to 10 mL or more (Figure 34-19, *A*). An ampule is made of glass with a constricted neck that must be snapped off to access the medication. A coloured ring around the neck indicates where the ampule is scored to be broken easily. Aspiration of the

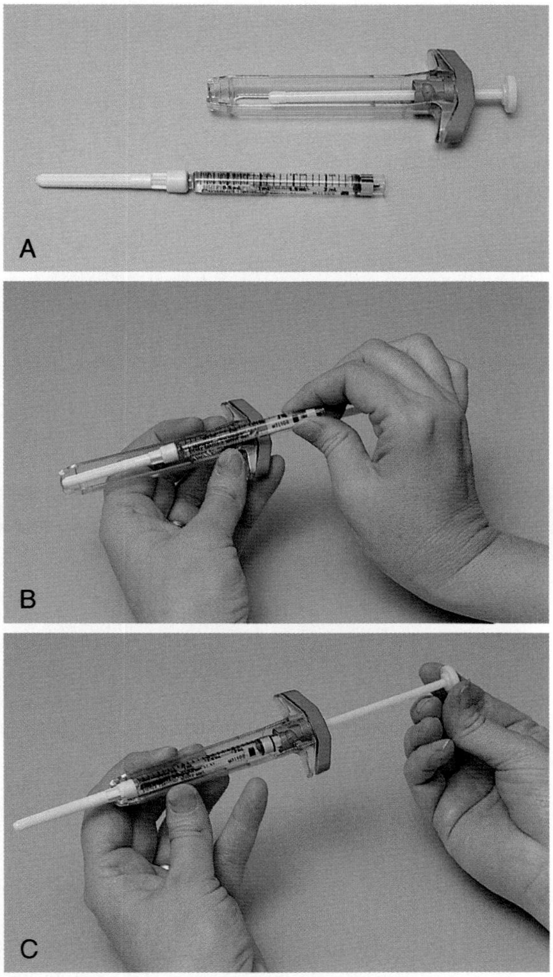

FIGURE 34-18 Disposable injection unit. **A,** Carpuject syringe and prefilled sterile cartridge with needle. **B,** Assembling the Carpuject system. **C,** Cartridge locks at needle end; plunger screws into opposite end.

medication into a syringe (Skill 34-4) is sometimes completed by using a filter needle to prevent small glass fragments from entering the syringe (Stein, 2006). Change the filter needle to an appropriate-sized needle for the actual injection.

Preparing an Injection From a Vial. A vial is a single-dose or multidose container with a rubber seal at the top (see Figure 34-19, *B*). A metal cap protects the seal until it is ready to be used. Vials contain liquid or dry forms of medications. Medications that are unstable in solution are packaged dry. The vial label specifies the solvent or diluents to be used to dissolve the medication and the amount of diluents needed to prepare a desired medication concentration. Normal saline and sterile distilled water are solutions commonly used to dissolve medications.

Unlike the ampule, the vial is a closed system, and air must be injected into the vial to permit easy withdrawal of the solution. Failure to inject air creates a vacuum within the vial that makes withdrawal difficult (see Skill 34-4). To avoid drawing up parts of the rubber stopper or other particles into the syringe, use a filter needle when preparing medications from vials (Nicoll & Hesby, 2002).

To prepare a powdered medication, draw up the amount of diluents or solvent recommended on the vial's label. Inject the diluent into the vial in the same manner used for injecting air into the vial. Most powdered medications dissolve easily, but you may need to withdraw the needle to mix the contents thoroughly. If this step is needed, remove the needle and gently roll the vial between your hands to dissolve the powdered medication, then reinsert the needle to draw up the dissolved medication. After mixing multidose vials, make a label that records the date and time of the mixing and indicates the concentration of medication per millilitre. Multidose vials may require refrigeration after the contents are reconstituted.

Mixing Medications. If two medications are compatible, they can be mixed in one injection if the total dose is within accepted limits. When two or more medications are mixed, the patient will not have to receive more than one injection at a time. Most nursing units keep charts that list common compatible medications. If you have any uncertainty about medication compatibilities, consult a pharmacist.

Mixing Medications From Two Vials. Apply the following principles when mixing medications from two vials:

1. Do not contaminate one medication with another.
2. Ensure the final dose is accurate.
3. Maintain an aseptic technique.

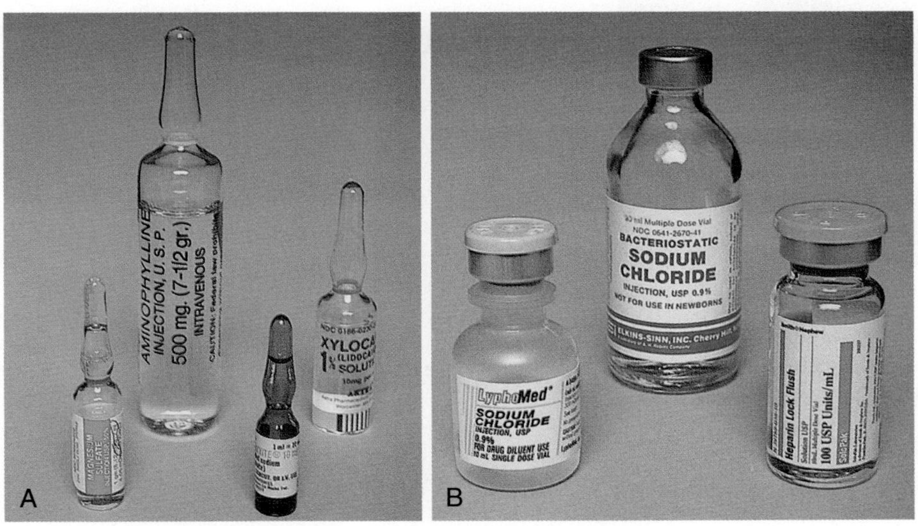

FIGURE 34-19 **A,** Medication in ampules. **B,** Medication in vials.

SKILL 34-4 PREPARING INJECTIONS

Delegation Considerations

The preparation of injections cannot be delegated to unregulated care providers.

Equipment

- Medication administration record (MAR) or computer printout
- Medication in an ampule
- Syringe, needle, and filter needle
- Small gauze pad or unopened alcohol swab
- Medication in a vial
- Syringe
- Needles:
  - Blunt-tip vial access cannula (if a needleless system used)
  - Filter needle (if indicated)
  - Needle for drawing up medication (if needed) and needle for injection
- Small gauze pad or alcohol swab
- Diluent (e.g., normal saline or sterile water) (if indicated)

PROCEDURE

STEPS	RATIONALE
1. Check the accuracy and completeness of each MAR or computer printout against the prescriber's original medication order. Check the patient's name and the medication name, route, dosage, and time of administration. Copy or rewrite any portion of the MAR that is difficult to read.	
2. Review the pertinent information related to the medication, including its action, purpose, adverse effects, and nursing implications.	
3. Assess the patient's body build, muscle size, and weight.	• The patient's body type determines the type and size of the syringe and the needles for injection.
4. Perform hand hygiene and assemble the medication supplies.	
5. Check the date of expiration on the medication vial or ampule.	• Medication potency may increase or decrease when medications are expired.
6. Prepare medication (see Skill 34-1, Steps 7A–G and M–O): Ensure that you compare the label of the medication with the MAR at least two times while preparing the medication.	
A. Ampule preparation	
(1) Tap the top of the ampule lightly and quickly with your finger until the fluid moves from the neck of the ampule (see Step 6A[1] illustration).	• Tapping the ampule dislodges any fluid that collects above the neck of the ampule. All solution moves into the lower chamber of the ampule.

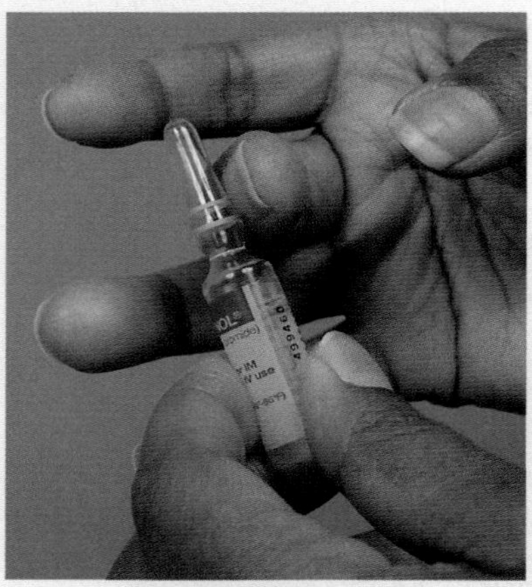

STEP 6A(1) Tapping the ampule moves the fluid down the neck of the ampule.

STEPS	RATIONALE
(2) Place a small gauze pad or an unopened alcohol swab around the neck of the ampule (see Step 6A[2] illustration).	• Placing a pad around the neck of the ampule protects the user's fingers from injury when the glass tip is broken off.

STEPS	RATIONALE
(3) Snap the neck of the ampule quickly and firmly away from the hands (see Step 6A[3] illustration).	• Snapping the neck quickly and firmly protects the user's fingers and face from the shattering glass.

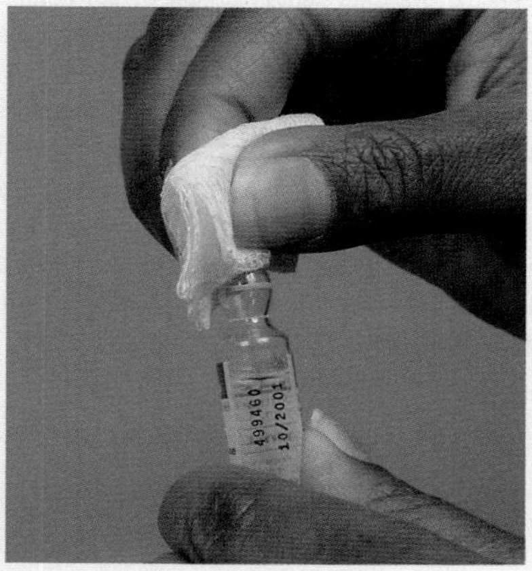

STEP 6A(2) Gauze pad placed around the neck of the ampule.

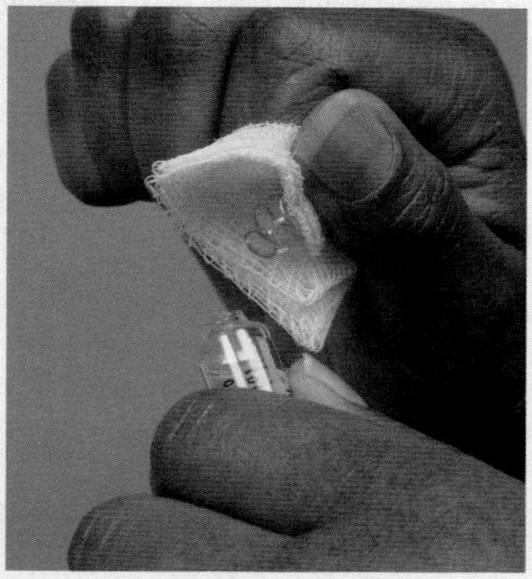

STEP 6A(3) Snapping the neck of the ampule away from the hands.

STEPS	RATIONALE
(4) Draw up the medication quickly, using a filter needle long enough to reach the bottom of the ampule.	• The injection system is vulnerable to airborne contaminants. The needle must be long enough to access the medication for preparation. Filter needles are used to sift out any fragments of glass (Stein, 2006).
(5) Hold the ampule upside down, or set it on a flat surface. Insert the filter needle into the centre of the ampule opening. Do not allow the needle tip or shaft to touch the rim of the ampule.	• The broken rim of the ampule is considered contaminated. When the ampule is inverted, the solution dribbles out if the needle tip or shaft touches the rim of the ampule.
(6) Aspirate the medication into the syringe by gently pulling back on the plunger (see Step 6A[6] illustrations).	• Withdrawal of the plunger creates negative pressure within the syringe barrel, which pulls the fluid into the syringe.

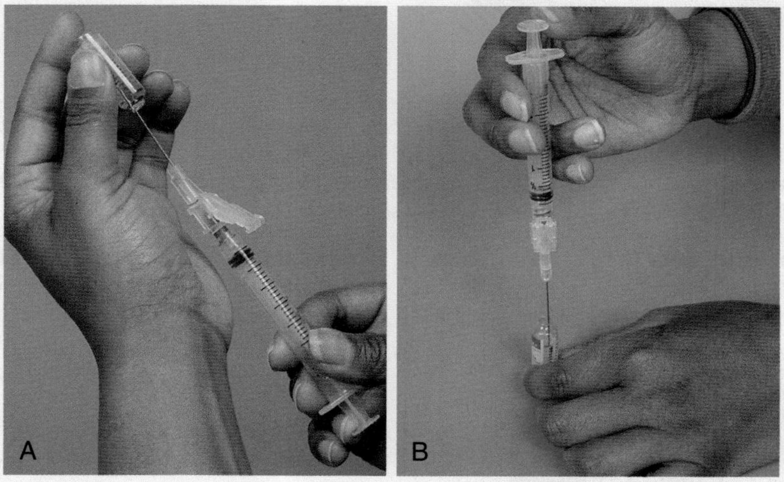

STEP 6A(6) A, Medication aspirated with the ampule inverted. **B,** Medication aspirated with the ampule on a flat surface.

STEPS	RATIONALE
(7) Keep the needle tip under the surface of the liquid. Tip the ampule to bring all fluid within reach of the needle.	• Keeping the needle tip under the surface of the liquid prevents the aspiration of air bubbles.
(8) If air bubbles are aspirated, do not expel the air into the ampule.	• Expelling air into the ampule may force fluid out of the ampule, which could lead to loss of the medication.
(9) To expel excess air bubbles, remove the needle from the ampule. Hold the syringe with the needle pointing up. Tap the side of the syringe to cause the bubbles to rise toward the needle. Draw back slightly on the plunger, then push the plunger upward to eject the air. Do not eject any fluid.	• Withdrawing the plunger too far will remove it from the barrel. Holding the syringe vertically allows fluid to settle in the bottom of the barrel. Pulling back on the plunger allows the fluid within the needle to enter the barrel so that fluid is not expelled. Air at the top of the barrel and within the needle is then expelled.
(10) If the syringe contains excess fluid, dispose of it in the appropriate receptacle. Hold the syringe vertically with the needle tip up and slanted slightly toward the receptacle. Recheck the fluid level in the syringe by holding it vertically. Do not dispose of excess liquids into a sink, toilet, or garbage can.	• The position of the needle allows the medication to be safely expelled without flowing down the needle shaft. Rechecking the fluid level ensures the proper dose.

Continued

SKILL 34-4 PREPARING INJECTIONS—cont'd

STEPS	RATIONALE
(11) Cover the needle with its safety sheath or cap. Replace the filter needle with a needle or a needleless access device for injection.	• Covering the needle prevents contamination of the needle and minimizes needle-stick injuries. Filter needles cannot be used for injection.
B. Vial containing a solution	
(1) Remove the cap covering the top of the unused vial to expose the sterile rubber seal. If a multidose vial has been previously used, the cap has already been removed. Firmly and briskly wipe the surface of the rubber seal with an alcohol swab and allow it to dry.	• The vial comes packaged with a seal that cannot be replaced after the cap has been removed. Not all drug manufacturers guarantee that caps of unused vials are sterile. Therefore, seals must be swabbed with alcohol before preparing the medication. Allowing the alcohol to dry prevents the needle from being coated with alcohol, which could mix with the medication.
(2) Pick up the syringe and remove the needle cap or the cap covering the needleless vial access device (see Step 6B[2] illustration). Pull back on the plunger to draw an amount of air into the syringe equivalent to the volume of medication to be aspirated from the vial.	• Inject air into the vial to prevent the buildup of negative pressure in the vial when aspirating medication.

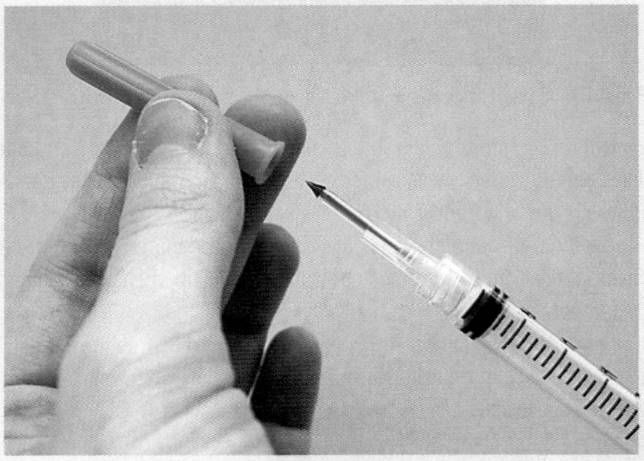

STEP 6B(2) Syringe with needleless adapter.

CRITICAL DECISION POINT: *Some medications require that a filter needle be used when preparing medications from a vial. The same policy is required by some institutions. Check the agency policy to determine whether the use of a filter needle is indicated (Nicoll & Hesby, 2002). If using a filter needle to aspirate the medication, use an appropriately sized needle to administer the medication.*

STEPS	RATIONALE
(3) With the vial on a flat surface, insert the tip of the needle. Ensure the bevelled tip enters first, through the centre of the rubber seal (see Step 6B[3] illustration). Apply pressure to the tip of the needle during insertion.	• The centre of the seal is thinner and easier to penetrate than the sides of the seal. Injecting the bevelled tip of the needle first and using firm pressure prevents coring of the rubber seal, which could enter the vial or needle.

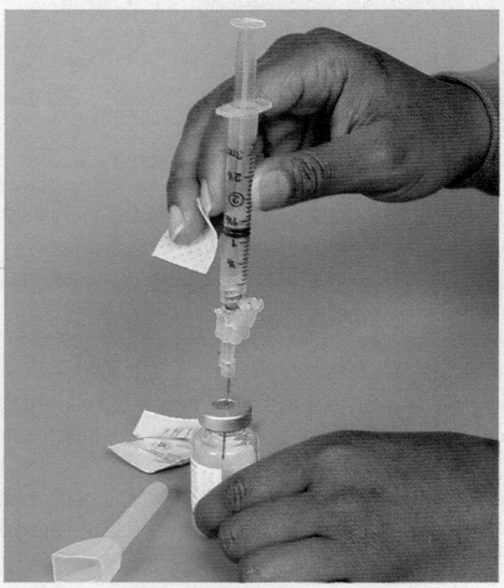

STEP 6B(3) Insert the tip of the needle through the centre of the vial diaphragm (with the vial flat on the table).

STEPS	RATIONALE
(4) Inject air into the vial's airspace, holding on to the plunger. Hold the plunger with firm pressure; the plunger may be forced backward by air pressure within the vial.	• Injecting air before aspirating the fluid creates a vacuum that is needed to allow the medication to flow into the syringe. Injecting air into the vial's airspace prevents the formation of bubbles, which can lead to an inaccurate dose.
(5) Invert the vial while keeping a firm hold on the syringe and plunger (see Step 6B[5] illustration). Hold the vial between your thumb and the middle fingers of your nondominant hand. Grasp the end of the syringe barrel and plunger with the thumb and forefinger of your dominant hand to counteract pressure in the vial.	• Inverting the vial allows the fluid to settle in the lower half of the container. Correct positioning of your hands prevents forceful movement of the plunger and permits easy manipulation of the syringe.

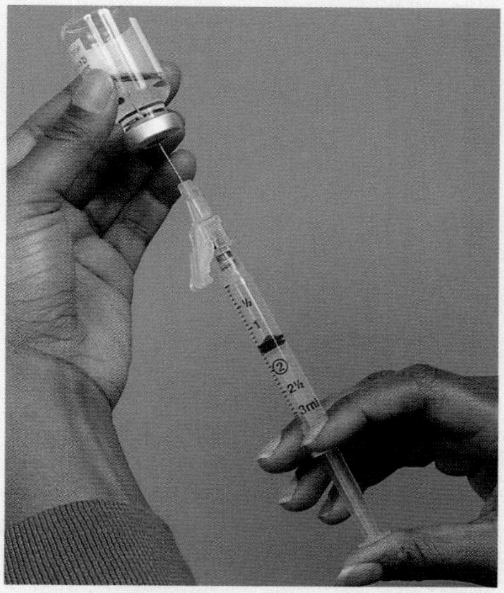

STEP 6B(5) Withdraw fluid with the vial inverted.

STEPS	RATIONALE
(6) Keep the tip of the needle below the fluid level.	• Keeping the needle tip under the surface of the liquid prevents the aspiration of air.
(7) Allow air pressure from the vial to fill the syringe gradually with medication. If necessary, pull back slightly on the plunger to obtain the correct amount of solution.	• Positive pressure within the vial forces the fluid into the syringe (unless the vial has been used several times).
(8) When the desired volume of solution is obtained, position the needle into the vial's airspace; tap the side of the syringe barrel carefully to dislodge any air bubbles. Eject any air remaining at the top of the syringe into the vial.	• Forcefully striking the barrel while the needle is inserted in the vial may bend the needle. The accumulation of air displaces the medication and can lead to dose errors.
(9) Remove the needle from the vial by pulling back on the barrel of the syringe.	• Accidentally pulling the plunger instead of the barrel can cause the plunger to separate from the barrel, which can result in the loss of medication.

Continued

SKILL 34-4 PREPARING INJECTIONS—cont'd

STEPS	RATIONALE
(10) Hold the syringe at eye level, at a 90-degree angle, to ensure the correct volume has been obtained and no air bubbles are present. Remove any remaining air by tapping the barrel to dislodge the air bubbles (see Step 6B[10] illustration). Draw back slightly on the plunger; then push the plunger upward to eject the air. Do not eject the fluid. Recheck the volume of the medication.	• Holding the syringe vertically allows fluid to settle in the bottom of the barrel. Pulling back on the plunger allows the fluid within the needle to enter the barrel so that fluid is not expelled. Air at the top of the barrel and within the needle is then expelled.

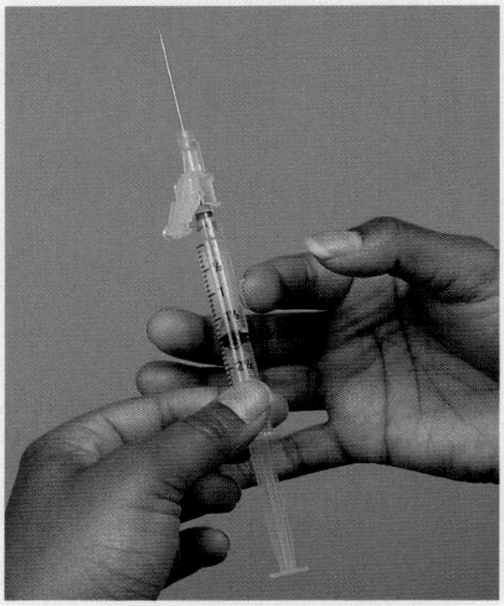

STEP 6B(10) Hold the syringe upright and tap the barrel to dislodge air bubbles.

STEPS	RATIONALE
(11) If medication is to be injected into a patient's tissue, change the needle to one of the appropriate gauge and length according to the route of medication and the patient's size and weight.	• Inserting a needle through a rubber stopper may dull the bevelled tip. New needles are sharper. Because no fluid remains along the shaft, the needle will not track medication through the tissues.
(12) For a multidose vial, make a label that includes the date of mixing, the concentration of the medication per millilitre, and your initials.	• Labelling ensures that future doses will be prepared correctly. Some medications must be discarded after a certain number of days have elapsed since the mixing of the vial.
C. Vial containing a powder (reconstituting medications)	
(1) Remove the cap covering the vial of powdered medication and the cap covering the vial of proper diluent. Firmly wipe both seals with the alcohol swab and allow to dry.	• Not all drug manufacturers guarantee that caps of unused vials are sterile. Therefore, seals must be swabbed with alcohol before preparing the medication. Allowing the alcohol to dry prevents the needle from being coated with alcohol, which could mix with the medication.
(2) Draw up diluent into the syringe following the Steps 6B(2) through 6B(10).	• Drawing up the diluent prepares the diluent for injection into a vial containing powdered medication.
(3) Insert the tip of the needle through the centre of the rubber seal on the vial of powdered medication. Inject the diluent into the vial. Remove the needle.	• The diluent begins to dissolve and reconstitute medication.
(4) Mix the medication thoroughly. Roll the vial in your palms. Do not shake.	• Rolling ensures proper dispersal of medication throughout the solution. Shaking produces bubbles.
(5) Reconstituted medication in the vial is ready to be drawn into a new syringe. Read the label carefully to determine the dose after reconstitution.	• After the diluent has been added, the concentration of medication (mg/mL) determines the dose to be given.
(6) Prepare medication in syringe following Steps 6B(2) through 6B(12).	

CRITICAL DECISION POINT: *Some institutions may require prepared parenteral medications to be verified for accuracy by another nurse. Check the agency policy before administering medication.*

STEPS	RATIONALE
7. Dispose of all soiled supplies. Place broken ampule vials, used vials, and used needles in a puncture-proof and leak-proof container. Clean the medication work area and perform hand hygiene.	• Proper disposal of glass and needle prevents accidental injury to staff and controls the transmission of infection.

UNEXPECTED OUTCOMES	RELATED INTERVENTIONS
Air bubbles remaining in syringe	• Expel air from the syringe and add medication to the syringe until the correct dose is prepared.
Incorrect dose prepared	• Discard the prepared dose and prepare the corrected new dose.

To mix medications from two vials, use only one syringe with a needle or use a syringe with a needleless access device attached (Figure 34-20). Aspirate a volume of air equivalent to the first medication's dose (vial A). Inject the air into vial A, ensuring the needle does not touch the solution. Withdraw the needle and aspirate a volume of air equivalent to the second medication's dose (vial B). Inject the air into vial B. Immediately withdraw the medication from vial B into the syringe, then insert the needle back into vial A, being careful not to push the plunger and expel the medication in the syringe into the vial. Withdraw the desired amount of medication from vial A into the syringe. After withdrawing the necessary amount, withdraw the needle from the syringe. Insert into the syringe a new needle or a needleless access device suitable for injection.

Mixing Medications From One Vial and One Ampule. When mixing medication from a vial and an ampule, prepare medication from the vial first and then use the same syringe and filter needle to withdraw medication from the ampule. Prepare the medication combination in this order because you do not need to add air to withdraw medication from an ampule.

Insulin Preparation. Insulin is the hormone used to treat diabetes in some patients. Although inhaled insulin has recently been approved for use, insulin is most commonly administered by injection. Because insulin is a protein, if it were taken orally, it would break down and be destroyed in the gastrointestinal tract. Most patients who have diabetes that requires them to take insulin learn to self-administer the injections. In Canada, health care providers usually prescribe insulin in concentrations of 100 units per millilitre of solution, which is called U-100 insulin. Make sure to use the correct syringe when preparing insulin. For example, use a 100-unit insulin syringe to prepare U-100 insulin.

Prefilled insulin pens are becoming more commonly used in hospitals to minimize errors in dosing and type of insulin administered (Table 34-10). Insulin pens are easy to use but they take more time to inject the insulin compared to a syringe. The insulin pen type must match the insulin brand ordered.

Insulin is classified by its rate of action: rapid-acting, short-acting, intermediate-acting, or long-acting. Each type has a different onset, peak, and duration of action (Table 34-11). Only regular (short-acting) insulin can be administered intravenously. Orders for insulin injections attempt to imitate the normal pattern of a patient's insulin release from the pancreas. Some insulins come in a stable premixed solution (e.g., "30/70 insulin" comprises 30% regular or short-acting insulin to 70% NPH [neutral protamine Hagedorn] or intermediate-acting insulin). Patients receiving premixed insulins do not need to mix insulins.

A patient with diabetes may require more than one type of insulin. For example, by receiving both a short-acting insulin and an intermediate-acting insulin, a patient receives a more sustained control of blood glucose levels over 24 hours.

Insulin is ordered either by a specific dose at select times or by a sliding scale. A sliding scale dictates a certain dose on the basis of the

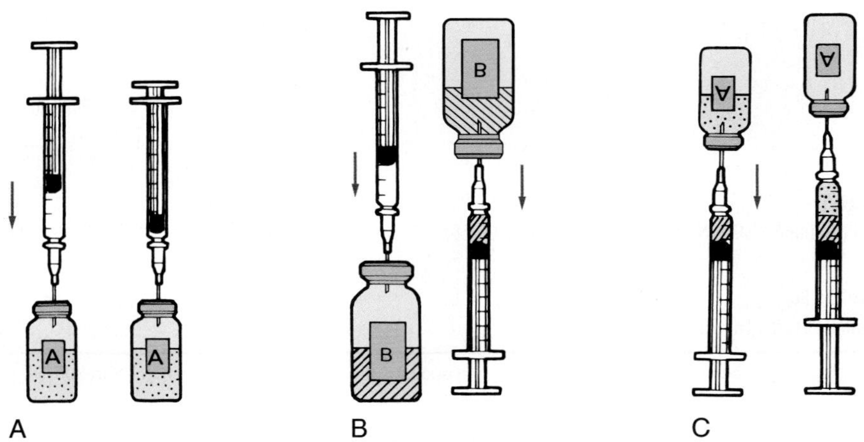

FIGURE 34-20 **Mixing medications from two vials. A,** Injecting air into vial A. **B,** Injecting air into vial B and withdrawing the dose. **C,** Withdrawing medication from vial A; the two medications are now mixed.

TABLE 34-10 Preparing a Preloaded Pen Device

Loading	Please refer to the pen manufacturer's instruction sheets.
Appropriate mixing	NPH and premixed insulins. Roll 10 times – tip 10 times and visually check that insulin has a consistent milky appearance.
Priming shot	A priming shot is required when changing a cartridge or using a new needle. Typically, it is recommended to use two units to prime the pen; however, please refer to the pen instruction sheets from the manufacturer.
Dialing up dose	Dial-up units of insulin required.
Delivery of insulin	Inject insulin at a 90-degree angle in desired injection site when using a shorter needle (4, 5, or 6 mm). A 45-degree angle may be needed if the person is thin or if a longer needle (>8 mm) is being used. A proper skin lift should also be used in thin individuals or when using longer needles. Hold the injection for 10 seconds to ensure full delivery of dose.

From the Canadian Diabetes Association. (2016). *Clinical practice guidelines: Insulin pen start checklist help sheet* (p. 2). Retrieved from http://guidelines.diabetes.ca/BloodGlucoseLowering/InsulinChecklist.

patient's blood glucose level (Box 34-25). Usually, rapid-acting or short-acting insulins are used for sliding scales. Before drawing up the insulin doses, gently roll all cloudy insulin preparations between the palms of the hands (or rotate the vial for at least 1 minute) to resuspend the insulin. Do not shake insulin vials; shaking causes the formation of bubbles, which take up space in the syringe and thereby alter the dose. If more than one type of insulin is required to manage the patient's diabetes, two different types of insulin can be mixed in one syringe *if they are compatible* (Box 34-26), by following the steps demonstrated in Figure 34-20. When two types of insulin are mixed, the single injection minimizes the patient's discomfort that is associated with multiple injections. In hospitals, when taking capillary blood samples for blood glucose monitoring, always swab the patient's anticipated sample site (e.g., the fingertip) with an alcohol swab before taking the sample. Use of an aseptic technique prevents the introduction of microorganisms and protects patients from infection while in the hospital. Although diabetic patients are commonly educated not to use alcohol swabs in the home care setting, their use is essential to

BOX 34-25 Example of a Sliding Scale Insulin Order

Give regular insulin subcutaneously:
- 2 units for glucose 11.1–13.3 mmol/L
- 4 units for glucose 13.4–13.8 mmol/L
- 6 units for glucose 13.9–16.7 mmol/L

For glucose greater than 16.8 mmol/L, call physician.

TABLE 34-11 A Comparison of Insulin Preparations

Type of Insulin	Onset	Peak	Duration
Rapid-Acting and Short-Acting (Clear)			
Insulin glulisine (Apidra)	10–15 minutes	1–2 hours	3–5 hours
Insulin lispro (Humalog)	10–15 minutes	1–2 hours	3.5–4.75 hours
Insulin aspart (NovoRapid)	10–15 minutes	1–1.5 hours	3–5 hours
Regular insulin (short-acting insulin)* (Humulin-R, Novolin ge Toronto)	30 minutes	2–3 hours	6.5 hours
Intermediate-Acting (Cloudy)			
Isophane insulin suspension (Novolin ge NPH insulin, Humulin N)	1–3 hours	5–8 hours	Up to 18 hours
Long-Acting (Clear)			
Insulin glargine (Lantus)†	90 minutes	Plateau	24 hours
Insulin detemir (Levemir)†	90 minutes	"Peakless"	16–24 hours
Premixed Insulins (Cloudy)‡			
Premixed regular insulin—NPH (Humulin 30/70, Novolin ge 30/70, 40/60, 50/50)	30–60 minutes	2–12 hours	18–24 hours
Premixed insulin analogues • Biphasic insulin aspart (NovoMix 30) • Insulin lispro/lispro protamine (Humalog Mix25 and Mix50)	30–60 minutes	2–12 hours	18–24 hours

*Regular insulin is the only insulin for intravenous use; when administered intravenously, the onset of action is within 10 to 30 minutes and the peak effect is within 20 to 30 minutes.
†Cannot be mixed with other insulins.
‡A single vial or cartridge contains a fixed ratio of insulin (% of rapid-acting or short-acting insulin to % of intermediate-acting insulin).
Based on Canadian Diabetes Association. (2013). *Clinical practice guidelines for the prevention and management of diabetes in Canada.* Retrieved from http://guidelines.diabetes.ca/fullguidelines.

BOX 34-26 PROCEDURAL GUIDELINE

Mixing Two Kinds of Insulin in One Syringe

Delegation Considerations:
The mixing of two kinds of insulin in one syringe cannot be delegated.

Equipment:
- Insulin vials
- Insulin syringe
- Alcohol swabs
- Medication administration report (MAR) or computer printout

Procedure:
1. Check the accuracy and completeness of each MAR or computer printout against the prescriber's original medication order. Check the patient's name and the medication name, dosage, route, and time for administration. Copy or rewrite any portion of the MAR that is difficult to read.
2. Carefully verify the insulin labels; compare the medication labels against the MAR before preparing the dose to ensure that the correct type of insulin is prepared.
3. Perform hand hygiene.
4. If the insulin is cloudy, roll the bottle of insulin between your hands to resuspend the insulin preparation.
5. Wipe the tops of both insulin vials with the alcohol swabs.
6. Verify the insulin dosage against the MAR a second time.
7. If mixing rapid- or short-acting insulin with intermediate- or long-acting insulin, take the insulin syringe and aspirate a volume of air equivalent to the dose of insulin to be withdrawn from the intermediate- or long-acting insulin first. If two intermediate- or long-acting insulins are mixed, either vial can be prepared first.
8. Insert the needle and inject air into the vial of the intermediate- or long-acting insulin. Do not let the tip of the needle touch the insulin.
9. Remove the syringe from the vial of the intermediate- or long-acting insulin without aspirating the insulin.
10. With the same syringe, inject a volume of air that is equivalent to the dose of insulin to be withdrawn into the vial of the rapid- or short-acting insulin. Withdraw the correct dose into the syringe.
11. Remove the syringe from the rapid- or short-acting insulin vial after carefully removing air bubbles in the syringe to ensure the correct dose.
12. After verifying the insulin dosage with the MAR a third time, show the insulin preparation in the syringe to another nurse to verify that the correct dose of insulin was prepared. Determine which point on the syringe scale represents the total of the combined units of insulin by adding the number of units of both insulins together (e.g., 3 units regular insulin + 10 units NPH insulin = 13 units total insulin).
13. Place the needle of the syringe back into the vial of the intermediate- or long-acting insulin. Be careful not to push the plunger, which would inject the insulin in the syringe into the vial.
14. Invert the vial, and carefully withdraw the desired amount of insulin into the syringe.
15. Withdraw the needle and check the fluid level in the syringe. Keep the needle of the prepared syringe sheathed or capped until you are ready to administer the medication. Show the syringe to another nurse to verify the correct dose was prepared.
16. Dispose of soiled medication supplies in the proper receptacle and perform hand hygiene.
17. Because rapid- or short-acting insulin binds with intermediate- or long-acting insulin, which reduces the action of the faster-acting insulin, administer the mixture within 5 minutes of preparing it.

Adapted from the Canadian Diabetes Association. (n.d.). *Blood Sugar & Insulin.* Retrieved from https://www.diabetes.ca/diabetes-and-you/healthy-living-resources/blood-sugar-insulin.

maintain asepsis and infection control standards in hospital settings. Always consult with agency protocol for special care required when treating diabetic patients.

Administering Injections

Each injection route differs depending on the type of tissues the medication enters. The characteristics of the tissues influence the rate of medication absorption and thus the onset of medication action. Before injecting a medication, the nurse must know the volume of the medication to administer, the medication's characteristics and viscosity, and the location of anatomical structures underlying the injection sites (Skill 34-5).

If injections are not administered correctly, negative patient outcomes can result. Failure to select an injection site in relation to anatomical landmarks can result in nerve or bone damage during needle insertion. An inability to maintain stability of the needle and syringe unit can result in pain for the patient and possible tissue damage. If the nurse fails to aspirate the syringe before injecting an IM medication, the medication may accidentally be injected directly into an artery or vein. Injecting too large a volume of medication for the site selected causes the patient extreme pain and may result in local tissue damage.

Many patients, particularly children, fear injections. Patients with serious or chronic illness often are given several injections daily. Nurses may be able to minimize the patient's discomfort in the following ways:

- Using a sharp-bevelled needle in the smallest suitable length and gauge
- Positioning the patient as comfortably as possible, to reduce muscular tension
- Selecting the proper injection site, by using anatomical landmarks
- Diverting the patient's attention from the injection by asking open-ended questions
- Inserting the needle quickly and smoothly to minimize tissue pulling
- Holding the syringe steady while the needle remains in the tissues
- Injecting the medication slowly and steadily

Subcutaneous Injections. Subcutaneous injections involve administering medications into the loose connective tissue under the dermis (see Skill 34-5). Because subcutaneous tissue is not as richly supplied with blood as the muscles, medication given by subcutaneous injection is absorbed more slowly than medication given by IM injections; however, medications injected subcutaneously are absorbed completely if the patient's circulatory status is normal. Because subcutaneous tissue contains pain receptors, the patient may experience some discomfort.

SKILL 34-5 ADMINISTERING INJECTIONS

Delegation Considerations

The administration of injections cannot be delegated to an unregulated care provider (UCP). Instruct UCPs to report the occurrence of potential medication adverse effects or any changes in the patient's vital signs or level of consciousness (e.g., sedation) immediately.

Equipment

- Proper size syringe and needle:
  - *Subcutaneous:* Syringe (1–3 mL) and needle (25–27 gauge, 1–1.6 cm)
  - *Subcutaneous U-100 insulin*: Insulin syringe (0.3, 0.5, or 1 mL) with pre-attached needle (28–31 gauge)
  - *IM:* Syringe 2–3 mL for adult, 0.5–1 mL for infants and small children
- Needle, with length corresponding to the site of injection and the age of the patient according to the following guidelines (Nicoll & Hesby, 2002):
  - *Any site (children):* 1.6–3.2 cm (depending on the size of the child)
  - *Vastus lateralis (adults):* 2.5–3.8 cm
  - *Deltoid (adults):* 2.5–3.8 cm
  - *Ventrogluteal (adults):* 3.8 cm
- Small gauze pad, or alcohol swab, or both
- Vial or ampule of medication or skin test solution
- Clean gloves
- Medication administration record (MAR) or computer printout

PROCEDURE

STEPS	RATIONALE
For All Injections	
1. Check the accuracy and completeness of each MAR or computer printout against the prescriber's original medication order. Check the patient's name and the medication name, route, dosage, and time of administration. Copy or rewrite any portion of the MAR that is difficult to read.	• The order sheet is the most reliable source and only legal record of printout against the prescriber's original medication order. Check the MAR and the original medication order to ensure that the patient receives the correct medications. Illegible MARs are a source of medication errors.
2. Assess the patient's medical history, medication history, and history of allergies. Determine whether the patient is allergic to any substances and the normal allergic reaction they have experienced.	• Certain substances have similar compositions; never administer a substance to which a patient has a known allergy.
3. Check the date of expiration for the medication.	• Drug potency may increase or decrease when medications are expired.
4. Observe the patient's verbal and nonverbal responses to receiving the injection.	• Injections can be painful. Some patients have anxiety, which can increase their experience of pain.
5. Assess the patient for contraindications.	
A. *For subcutaneous injections:* Assess the patient for factors such as circulatory shock and reduced local tissue perfusion. Assess the adequacy of the patient's adipose tissue.	• Reduced tissue perfusion interferes with medication absorption and distribution. Physiological changes of aging and the patient's health may affect the amount of the patient's subcutaneous tissue. The amount of subcutaneous tissue influences the methods chosen for administering injections.
B. *For intramuscular injections:* Assess the patient for muscle atrophy, reduced blood flow, and circulatory shock.	• Atrophied muscles absorb medication poorly. Factors that interfere with blood flow to muscles will impair the medication's absorption.

CRITICAL DECISION POINT: *Because of documented adverse effects to intramuscular injections, other routes of medication administration are safer. Verify that an intramuscular injection is necessary and explore alternative medication routes if possible (Nicoll & Hesby, 2002; World Health Organization [WHO], 2016).*

STEPS	RATIONALE
6. Aseptically prepare the correct medication dose from an ampule or vial (see Skill 34-4). Ensure that all air is expelled from the syringe. Check the label of medication against the MAR three times while preparing the medication. Create a removable label that shows the patient's name, the name of the drug, and the dosage. Apply the label to the removable needle cap.	• Aseptic preparation ensures that the medication is sterile. Preparation techniques differ for ampules and vials. Checking the label against the MAR ensures that the right medication is prepared for the right patient.
7. Take the medication to the patient at the right time, and perform hand hygiene.	• Taking the medication according to schedule ensures the patient receives the effect of the medication at the right time. Hand hygiene reduces the transfer of microorganisms.
8. Close the room curtain or door.	• Closing the curtain or door provides privacy and avoids distractions.

STEPS	RATIONALE
9. Identify the patient using at least two patient identifiers. Compare the patient's name and one other identifier (e.g., the hospital identification number) on the MAR, computer printout, or computer screen against information on the patient's identification bracelet. Ask the patient to state his or her name, if possible, for a third identifier.	• This process complies with the Joint Commission's (2017) requirements and improves medication safety. In most acute care settings, the name and identification number on the patient's armband and the MAR are used to identify patients. Identification bracelets are made at the time of the patient's admission and are the most reliable source of information. The patient's room number is *not* an acceptable identifier.
10. Compare the label on the medication with the MAR one more time at the patient's bedside.	• The final check of medication labels against the MAR at the patient's bedside reduces medication administration errors.
11. Describe the steps of procedure and inform the patient that the injection will cause a slight burning or stinging sensation.	• Describing the process to the patient helps to minimize the patient's anxiety.
12. Perform hand hygiene; put on disposable gloves.	• Hand hygiene and the wearing of gloves reduces the transfer of microorganisms.
13. Keep a sheet or gown draped over the patient's body parts that do not need to be exposed.	• Use of a sheet or gown respects the dignity of the patient while only the area to be injected is exposed.
14. Select an appropriate injection site. Inspect the skin surface over the injection site for bruises, inflammation, and edema.	• Injection sites should be free of abnormalities that may interfere with medication absorption. Injection sites that are used repeatedly can become hardened from lipohypertrophy (increased growth in fatty tissue). Do not inject an area that is bruised or shows signs associated with infection.
A. *Subcutaneous injection:* Palpate the injection site for masses or tenderness. Avoid these areas. For patients who require daily insulin, rotate the injection site daily. Ensure the needle is the correct size by grasping a skin fold at the injection site with your thumb and forefinger. Measure across the skin fold. The needle should be one-half the distance across the fold to give it at a 90-degree angle.	• Subcutaneous injections can be inadvertently given in the muscle, especially when the injection site is in the abdomen or thigh (Annersten & Willman, 2005). Use of the appropriate size of needle ensures that medication will be injected in the subcutaneous tissue (Hunter, 2008; King, 2003).
B. *Intramuscular injection:* Note the integrity and size of the muscle and palpate for tenderness or hardness. Avoid these areas. If injections are given frequently, rotate the injection sites. Use the ventrogluteal site if possible.	• Unless contraindications exist for this site, the ventrogluteal site is the preferred injection site for adults and children, but for infants the vastus lateralis site should be used. (Cook & Murtagh, 2006; Hockenberry & Wilson, 2014; Nicoll & Hesby, 2002; Small, 2004).
C. *Intradermal injection:* Note any lesions or discolorations of the patient's forearm. Select an injection site three to four fingerwidths below the antecubital space and a handwidth above the wrist. If the forearm cannot be used, inspect the patient's upper back. If necessary, sites for subcutaneous injections may be used.	• An intradermal site should be free from lesions or discolorations so that results of a skin test can be seen and interpreted correctly.
15. Assist the patient to a comfortable position:	
A. *Subcutaneous injection:* Have the patient relax the arm, leg, or abdomen, depending on the site chosen for injection.	• Relaxation of the injection site minimizes the patient's discomfort.
B. *Intramuscular injection:* Position the patient depending on the site chosen (e.g., have the patient sit, lie flat, lie on one side, or lie prone).	• The position of the patient can reduce strain on the patient's muscle and minimize the discomfort of the injection.
C. *Intradermal injection:* Have the patient extend the elbow and support the elbow and forearm on a flat surface.	• The position of the patient stabilizes the injection site for easy accessibility.
D. Speak with the patient about a subject of interest. Ask open-ended questions.	• Distraction reduces anxiety.

CRITICAL DECISION POINT: *Ensure that the patient's position is not contraindicated by a medical condition.*

16. Relocate the injection site using anatomical landmarks.	• Injection into the correct anatomical site prevents injury to nerves, bones, and blood vessels.

Continued

SKILL 34-5 ADMINISTERING INJECTIONS—cont'd

STEPS	RATIONALE
17. Clean the injection site with an antiseptic swab. Touch the swab to the centre of the site and rotate outward in a circular direction for about 5 cm (see Step 17 illustration).	• The mechanical action of the swab removes secretions containing microorganisms.
18. Hold the swab or gauze between the third and fourth fingers of your non-dominant hand.	• The gauze or swab is readily accessible when the needle is withdrawn.
19. Remove the needle cap or sheath from the needle by pulling it straight off.	• Preventing the needle from touching the sides of the cap avoids the risk of contamination.
20. Hold the syringe between the thumb and forefinger of your dominant hand. **A.** *Subcutaneous injection:* Hold the syringe as if you were holding a dart, palm down; or hold the syringe across the tops of your fingertips (see Step 20A illustration).	• Quick, smooth injection requires proper manipulation of the syringe parts.

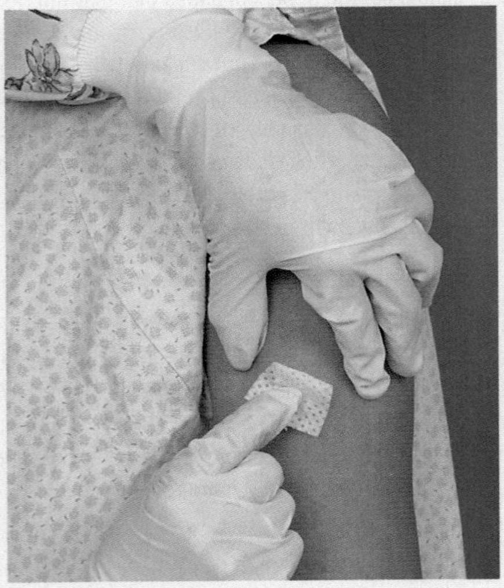

STEP 17 Clean the injection site by using a circular motion.

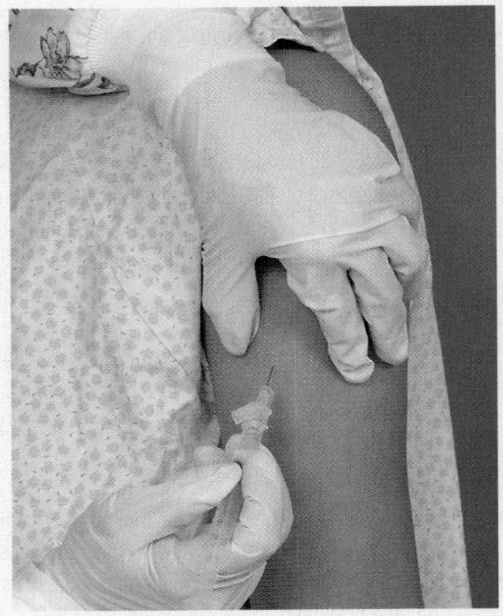

STEP 20A Hold the syringe as if grasping a dart.

STEPS	RATIONALE
B. *Intramuscular injection:* Hold the syringe as if you were holding a dart, palm down.	
C. *Intradermal injection:* Hold the bevel of the needle pointing up.	• With the bevel pointing up, the medication is less likely to be deposited into tissues below dermis.
21. Administer the injection: **A.** Subcutaneous injection **(1)** For an average-sized patient, spread the skin tightly across the injection site or pinch the skin with your nondominant hand.	• The needle penetrates tight skin easier than loose skin. Pinching the skin elevates the subcutaneous tissue and may desensitize the area.
(2) Inject the needle quickly and firmly at a 45- to 90-degree angle. Hold the skin fold until the needle has been withdrawn from the skin (Frid, Hirsch, Gaspar, et al., 2010).	• Quick, firm insertion minimizes the patient's discomfort. (Injecting medication into compressed tissue irritates the nerve fibres.) Injecting at the correct angle prevents accidental injection into the muscle. Injecting into a raised skin fold is thought to result in a more diffuse depot of insulin, in contrast to a compact bolus injected without a pinch up (King, 2003).
(3) For an obese patient, pinch the skin at the injection site and insert the needle at a 90-degree angle below the tissue fold.	• It is important to ensure that the injection is given in the subcutaneous adipose tissue rather than intradermally (just under the epidermis) or into the muscle (Hunter, 2008).

CRITICAL DECISION POINT: *Piercing a blood vessel during a subcutaneous injection is very rare, so aspiration is not necessary when administering subcutaneous injections.*

STEPS	RATIONALE

(4) Inject the medication slowly (see Step 21A[4] illustration).

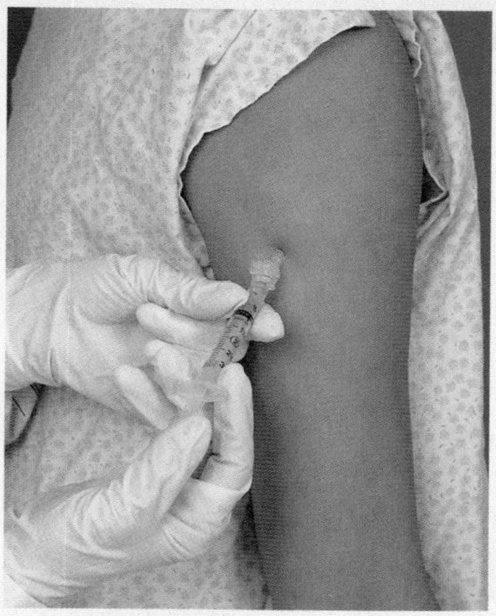

STEP 21A(4) Inject the medication slowly.

B. Intramuscular injection

(1) Position your nondominant hand at the proper anatomical landmarks and pull the skin down approximately 2.5–3.5 cm or laterally with the ulnar side of your hand to administer the injection in a Z-track. Hold this position until the medication is injected. Use your dominant hand to insert the needle quickly at a 90-degree angle into the muscle.

- The Z-track creates a zigzag path through the tissues to seal the needle track and avoid tracking of the medication. The Z-track should be used for all intramuscular injections (smaller needles may be needed for smaller muscles) (Hopkins & Arias, 2013; Nicoll & Hesby, 2002; Ogston-Tuck, 2014; WHO, 2016).

(2) If the patient's muscle mass is small, grasp a body of muscle between your thumb and fingers.

- Grasping the muscle ensures that the medication reaches the muscle mass (Hockenberry & Wilson, 2014).

(3) After the needle pierces the skin, grasp the lower end of the syringe barrel with your nondominant hand to stabilize the syringe. Continue to hold the skin tightly with your nondominant hand. Move your dominant hand to the end of the plunger. Do not move the syringe.

- Smooth manipulation of the syringe reduces the patient's discomfort from needle movement. The skin must remain pulled until after the drug is injected to ensure Z-track administration.

CRITICAL DECISION POINT: *If blood appears in the syringe, remove the needle and dispose of the medication and syringe properly. Prepare another dose of medication for injection.*

(4) Wait 10 seconds, and then smoothly and steadily withdraw the needle and release the skin. Apply gentle pressure with dry gauze if desired.

- A wait of 10 seconds allows time for the medication to absorb into the muscle before removal of the syringe and prevents the medication from leaking back out through the track created by the needle (Nicoll & Hesby, 2002).

C. Intradermal injection

(1) With your nondominant hand, stretch the skin over the injection site with your forefinger or thumb.

- The needle pierces tight skin more easily than loose skin.

(2) With the needle almost against the patient's skin, insert it slowly with the bevel pointed up at a 5- to 15-degree angle until resistance is felt. Advance the needle through the epidermis to approximately 3 mm below the skin surface. The needle tip can be seen through skin.

- This technique ensures the needle tip is in the dermis.

(3) Inject the medication slowly. Normally, resistance is felt. If resistance is not felt, the needle is in too deep; remove and begin again. Your nondominant hand can stabilize the needle during the injection.

- Slow injection minimizes the discomfort at the injection site. The dermal layer is tight and does not expand easily when the solution is injected. Stabilizing the needle prevents unnecessary movements and decreases the patient's discomfort.

Continued

SKILL 34-5 ADMINISTERING INJECTIONS—cont'd

STEPS	RATIONALE
(4) While injecting medication, notice that a small bleb of approximately 6 mm in diameter (resembling a mosquito bite) appears on the skin's surface (see Step 21C[4] illustration). Instruct the patient that this bleb is a normal finding.	• The bleb indicates the medication is deposited in the dermis.

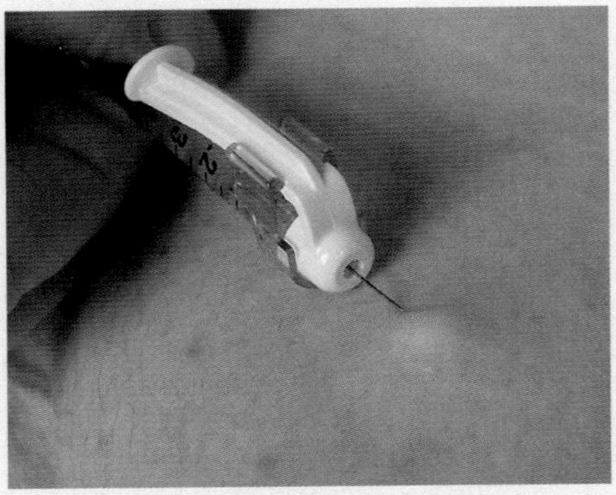

STEP 21C(4) The injection creates a small bleb.

STEPS	RATIONALE
22. Withdraw the needle while wiping an alcohol swab or gauze gently over the injection site.	• Support of tissue around the injection site minimizes the patient's discomfort during withdrawal of the needle. Dry gauze may minimize the patient's discomfort associated with the use of alcohol on nonintact skin.
23. Apply gentle pressure. Do not massage the injection site. Put on a bandage if needed.	• Massage may cause underlying tissue damage. Massage of the intradermal site may disperse the medication into underlying tissue layers and thereby alter the test results.
24. Assist the patient to a comfortable position.	• Helping the patient to a comfortable position gives the patient a sense of well-being.
25. Discard into a puncture- and leak-proof receptacle the uncapped needle or the needle enclosed in safety shield and attached to the syringe. Do *not* recap the needle.	• Proper needle disposal prevents injury to patients and health care personnel. Recapping the needle increases the risk of needle-stick injury (Health Canada, 2004).
26. Remove disposable gloves and perform hand hygiene.	• Proper hygiene reduces the transmission of microorganisms.
27. Stay with the patient for 3–5 minutes to observe for any allergic reactions.	• Severe anaphylactic reaction is characterized by dyspnea, wheezing, and circulatory collapse and is a life-threatening emergency.
28. Periodically return to the patient's room to ask whether the patient feels any acute pain, burning, numbness, or tingling at the injection site.	• Continued discomfort may indicate injury to underlying bones or nerves.
29. Inspect the injection site, noting any bruising or induration.	• Bruising or induration indicates a complication associated with the injection. Document your findings and notify the patient's health care provider. Provide a warm compress to the site.
30. Observe the patient's response to medication at times that correlate with the medication's onset, peak, and duration.	• Intramuscular medications are rapidly absorbed. Adverse effects of parenteral medications may develop rapidly. The nurse's observations are to evaluate the efficacy of the medication action.
31. Ask the patient to explain the purpose and effects of the medication.	• Questioning the patient will help to evaluate the patient's understanding of the information just taught.
32. For intradermal injections, use a skin pencil and draw a circle around the perimeter of the injection site. Read the site within an appropriate amount of time, which is determined by the type of medication or skin test administered.	• The pencil mark makes the injection site easy to find. Results of skin testing are read at various times, on the basis of the type of medication used or the type of skin test completed. Refer to the manufacturer's directions to determine when to read the test's results.

UNEXPECTED OUTCOMES	RELATED INTERVENTIONS
Raised, reddened, or hard zone (induration) around intradermal test site	• Notify the patient's health care provider. • Document the patient's sensitivity to the injected allergen or the positive test if tuberculin skin testing was completed. • Do not use this site for future injections.
Hypertrophy of skin, resulting from repeated subcutaneous injections	• Instruct patient not to use the injection site for 6 months.
Signs and symptoms of allergy or adverse effects	• Follow the institutional policy or guidelines for the appropriate response to adverse drug reactions. • Notify the patient's health care provider immediately. • Add allergy information to the patient's medical record.

STEPS	RATIONALE
Complaints of localized pain, numbness, tingling, or burning sensation at injection site, indicating possible injury to nerve or tissues	• Assess the injection site. • Document your findings. • Notify the patient's health care provider.

RECORDING AND REPORTING

- Chart the medication dose, route, site, time, and date of injection on the MAR immediately after giving medication, as per agency policy.
- Document if the scheduled medication is withheld and record the reason as per agency policy.
- Report any undesirable effects from the medication to the prescriber.
- Record the patient's response to medications in the nurses' notes and report to prescriber if required.

HOME CARE CONSIDERATIONS

- Assess the patient's readiness to learn before instructing him or her on how to administer self-injections. Some patients are hesitant to administer injections to themselves; relieve any anxiety before teaching this skill to a patient.
- Patients can often purchase or obtain sharps boxes for home use. If this purchase is not feasible, a hard plastic bottle that is nontransparent (e.g., a fabric softener bottle or a detergent bottle) may be used to safely store syringes after use. Disposal of needles used in the home varies among communities. Check with local authorities to verify how to appropriately dispose of needles.

The best subcutaneous injection sites are the outer posterior aspect of the upper arms, the abdomen from below the costal margins to the iliac crests, and the anterior aspects of the thighs (Figure 34-21). The site most frequently recommended for heparin injections is the abdomen (Figure 34-22). Other recommended sites are the scapular areas of the upper back and the upper ventral or dorsal gluteal areas. The injection site chosen should be free of skin lesions, bony prominences, and large underlying muscles or nerves.

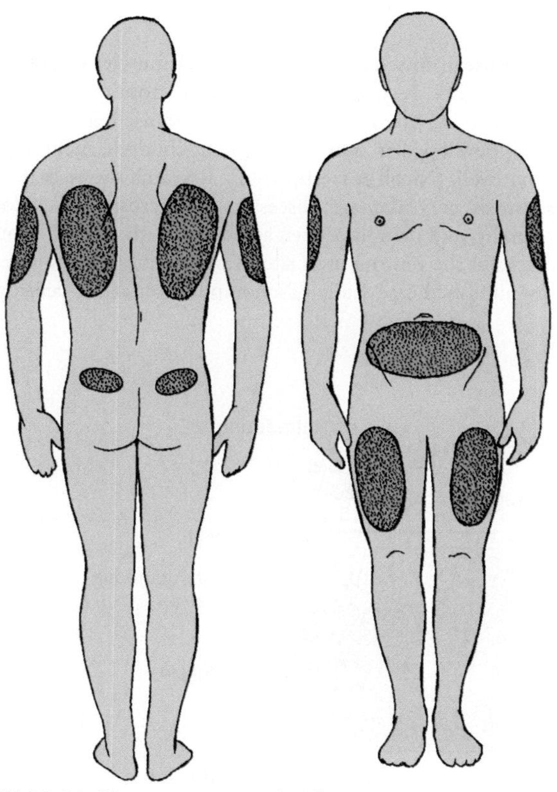

FIGURE 34-21 Sites recommended for subcutaneous injections.

The administration of low-molecular-weight heparin (LMWH) (e.g., enoxaparin) requires special considerations. The injection site is the right or left side of the abdomen at least 5 cm from the umbilicus. Administer LMWH in its prefilled syringe with the attached needle; do not expel the air bubble in the syringe before giving the medication. The needle should be introduced into a skin fold held between the thumb and forefinger; the skin fold should be held throughout the injection. To minimize bruising, do not rub the injection site after injection (Sanofi, 2016). New evidence suggests that a slower injection rate of 30 seconds should be used, to reduce bruising and pain (Akbari Sari, Janani, Mohammady, et al., 2014; Sanofi, 2016).

When giving U-100 insulin, use U-100 insulin syringes with preattached 26- to 31-gauge needles (Canadian Diabetes Association Clinical Practice Guidelines Expert Committee, 2013). Recommended sites for insulin injections include the upper arm and the anterior and lateral portions of the thigh, buttocks, and abdomen. Patients with diabetes who inject insulin should practise intrasite rotation (rotating injection sites within the same body part) to provide greater consistency in the absorption of insulin. For example, if the morning

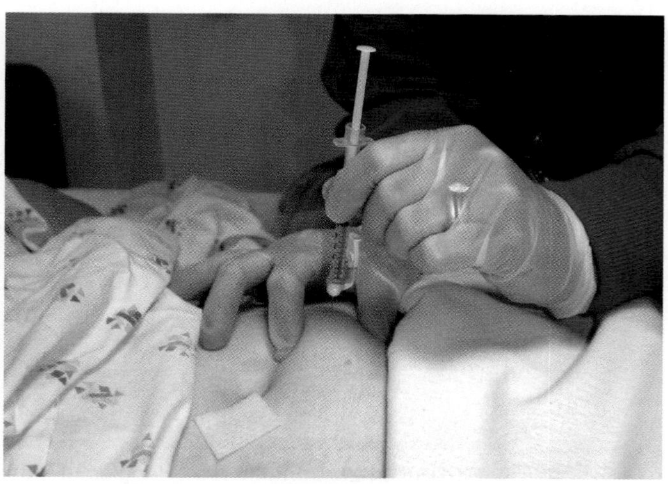

FIGURE 34-22 Giving subcutaneous heparin in the abdomen.

insulin is injected into the patient's arm, then a subsequent injection should also be given in the arm but at least 2.5 cm away from the previous site. No injection site should be used again for at least 1 month. The rate of insulin absorption varies depending on the site: the abdomen has the quickest absorption, followed by the arms, thighs, and buttocks (Canadian Diabetes Association, 2013; McCulloch, 2016). For subcutaneous injections of insulin, pinch the skin and insert the needle at a 90-degree angle; inject the insulin, then release the pinched skin, count 5 to 6 seconds and remove the needle.

Only small doses (0.5 to 1 mL) of water-soluble medications should be given subcutaneously because the tissue is sensitive to irritating solutions and large volumes of medications. Medications can collect within the tissues to cause sterile abscesses, which appear as hardened, painful lumps under the skin.

A patient's body weight indicates the depth of the subcutaneous layer. Therefore, choose the needle length and angle of insertion based on the patient's weight and an estimation of the amount of subcutaneous tissue (Annersten & Willman, 2005). In general, medications can be injected in the subcutaneous tissue of a normal-sized patient using a 25-gauge 1.6-cm needle inserted at a 45-degree angle (Figure 34-23) or a 1.3-cm needle inserted at a 90-degree angle. A child may require only a 1.3-cm needle. If the patient is obese, pinch the tissue and use a needle long enough to insert through the fatty tissue at the base of the skinfold. The preferred needle length is one-half the width of the skinfold; the angle of insertion may be between 45 and 90 degrees. Thin patients may have insufficient tissue for subcutaneous injections; the upper abdomen is the best injection site for these patients. To ensure a subcutaneous medication reaches the subcutaneous tissue, follow this rule: if you can grasp 5 cm of tissue, insert the needle at a 90-degree angle; if you can grasp 2.5 cm of tissue, insert the needle at a 45-degree angle (Rushing, 2004).

Intramuscular Injections. The intramuscular (IM) route provides faster medication absorption than the subcutaneous route because of a muscle's greater vascularity; however, IM injections are associated with many risks. Therefore, when administering a medication by the IM route, it is important to first verify that the injection is justified (Dayananda, Belaval, Raina, et al., 2014; WHO, 2016). In many cases, such as influenza and pneumonia vaccinations, no alternative routes exist to administer the medication.

A longer and heavier-gauge needle is used to pass through the subcutaneous tissue and penetrate the deep muscle tissue (see Skill 34-5). The patient's body weight and the amount of adipose tissue can influence the selection of a needle size. For example, an obese patient may require a needle 7.5 cm long, whereas a thin patient may require a 1.3- to 2.5-cm needle. It is not necessary to aspirate during the administration of an IM injection (Sisson, 2015).

The angle of insertion for an IM injection is 90 degrees (see Figure 34-23). Muscle is less sensitive to irritating and viscous medications. A normal, well-developed patient can tolerate 3 mL of medication into a larger muscle without severe muscle discomfort. A larger volume of medication is unlikely to be absorbed properly. Children, older people, and thin patients can tolerate only 2 mL of an IM injection. Do not give more than 1 mL to small children and older infants, and do not give more than 0.5 mL to smaller infants (Hockenberry & Wilson, 2014).

Assess the muscle integrity of the selected site before giving an injection. The muscle should be free of tenderness. Repeated injections in the same muscle can cause severe discomfort. Ensure that the patient is relaxed, then palpate the muscle to rule out any hardened lesions. Discomfort can be minimized during an injection by helping the patient to assume a position that will help reduce muscle strain. Other interventions, such as distraction and applying pressure to the IM site, may be used to decrease pain during an IM injection.

Sites. When selecting an IM site, consider the following: Is the area free of infection or necrosis? Do local areas show signs of bruising or abrasions? Where is the location of underlying bones, nerves, and major blood vessels? What volume of medication is to be administered? Each site has certain advantages and disadvantages. The characteristics of each IM site and the indications for use of each site are listed in Box 34-27.

> **Safety Alert** Researchers who have investigated complications associated with intramuscular injection sites indicate that the ventrogluteal site is the preferred site for most injections administered to adults and children, including infants of any age (Cook & Murtagh, 2006; Hockenberry & Wilson, 2014; Nicoll & Hesby, 2002).

Ventrogluteal muscle. The ventrogluteal muscle, which involves the gluteus medius, is situated deep and away from major nerves and blood vessels. It is a safe site for all patients because it is a large muscle that is well developed in adults and young children, including those who do not walk (Nicoll & Hesby, 2002). Research shows that injuries such as fibrosis, nerve damage, abscess, tissue necrosis, muscle contraction, gangrene, and pain have been associated with all of the common IM sites except the ventrogluteal site (Kara, Uzelli, & Karaman, 2015). The only published case study of a complication at the ventrogluteal

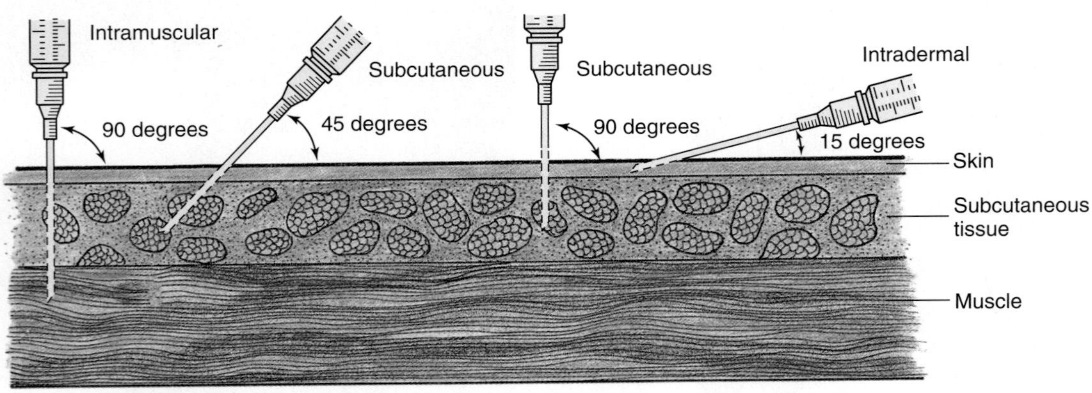

FIGURE 34-23 Comparison of angles of insertion for intramuscular (90 degrees), subcutaneous (45 and 90 degrees), and intradermal (15 degrees) injections.

BOX 34-27 Characteristics of Intramuscular Sites and Indications for Usage

Vastus Lateralis Muscle
- Lacks major nerves and blood vessels
- Facilitates rapid drug absorption
- Used frequently with infants (younger than 12 months old) receiving immunizations
- May also be used in older children and toddlers receiving immunizations

Ventrogluteal Muscle
- Offers a deep site, situated away from major nerves and blood vessels
- Offers less chance of contamination in incontinent patients and infants
- Identified easily by prominent bony landmarks
- Is preferred site for medications (e.g., antibiotics) that are larger in volume, more viscous, and irritating for adults, children, and infants

Deltoid Muscle
- Is easily accessible but the muscle is not well developed in most patients
- May be used for small amounts of medications
- Not used in infants or children with underdeveloped muscles
- Use of the muscle involves potential for injury to the brachial artery and to the radial and ulnar nerves
- May be used for immunizations of toddlers, older children, and adults
- Recommended site for hepatitis B vaccine and rabies injections

site when done correctly reported a local reaction to the medication, which is not a complication associated with the site itself (Nicoll & Hesby, 2002).

To locate the ventrogluteal muscle, place the heel of your hand over the greater trochanter of the patient's hip with the wrist perpendicular to the femur. Use your right hand for the left hip, and your left hand for the right hip. Point your thumb toward the patient's groin and point your fingers toward the patient's head; point your index finger to the anterior superior iliac spine, and extend your middle finger back along the iliac crest toward the buttocks. The index finger, the middle finger, and the iliac crest form a V-shaped triangle; the injection site is the centre of the triangle (Figure 34-24). The patient may lie on his or her side or back. Flexing of the knee and hip helps the patient to relax this muscle.

Vastus lateralis muscle. This thick and well-developed muscle is located on the anterior lateral aspect of the thigh and extends in an adult from a handbreadth above the knee to a handbreadth below the greater trochanter of the femur (Figure 34-25). Use the middle third of the muscle for injection. The width of the muscle usually extends from the midline of the thigh to the midline of the thigh's outer side. When administering injections to young children or cachectic patients, grasp the body of the muscle during injection to ensure the medication is deposited in the muscle tissue. To help relax the muscle, ask the patient to assume a sitting position or to lie flat with leg extended. The vastus lateralis site is often used when infants, toddlers, and children are administered biologicals (e.g., immune globulins, vaccines, or toxoids) (Nicoll & Hesby, 2002).

Dorsogluteal muscle. In the past, the dorsogluteal muscle has been a traditional site for IM injections. However, the exact location of the sciatic nerve varies from one person to another. If a needle hits the sciatic nerve, the patient may experience permanent or partial paralysis of the involved leg. Therefore, do *not* use the dorsogluteal site (Cook & Murtagh, 2006; Kara et al., 2015).

Deltoid muscle. Although the deltoid site is easily accessible, the muscle is not well developed in many patients. A potential for injury

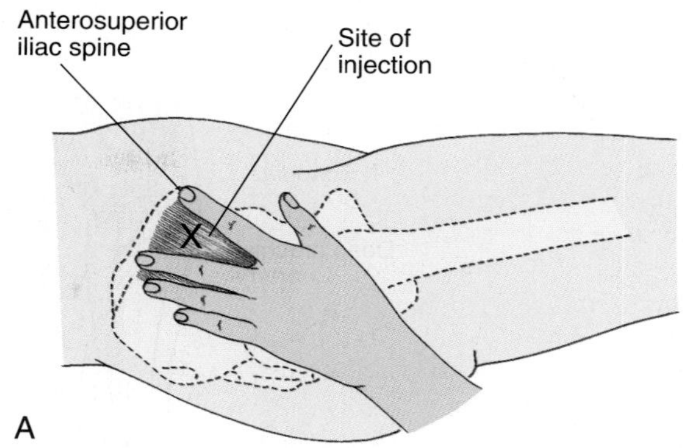

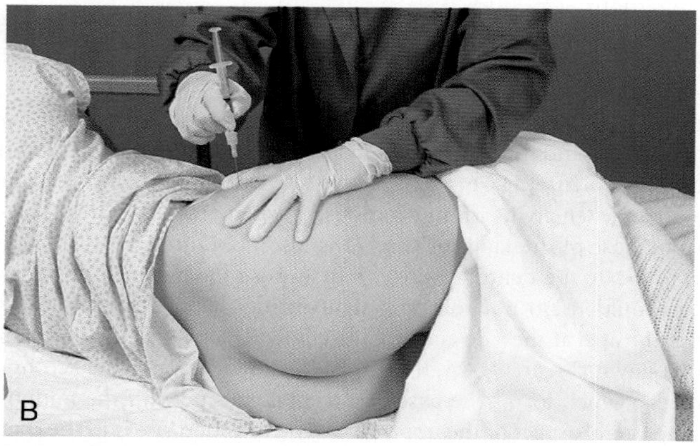

FIGURE 34-24 A, Landmarks for the ventrogluteal site. **B,** Giving intramuscular injection in the ventrogluteal muscle.

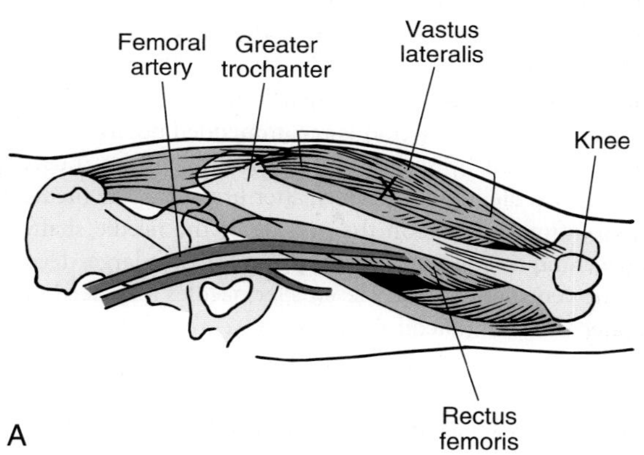

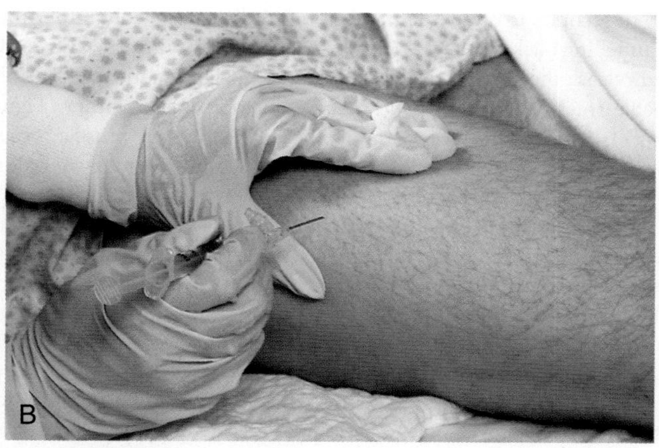

FIGURE 34-25 A, Landmarks for the vastus lateralis site. **B,** Giving intramuscular injection in the vastus lateralis muscle.

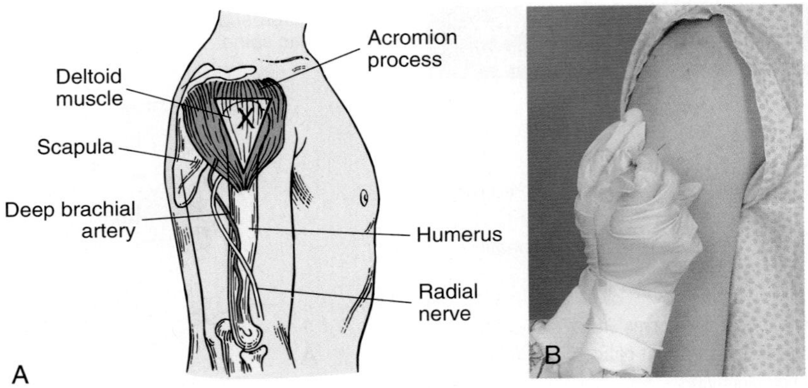

FIGURE 34-26 **A,** Landmarks for the deltoid site. **B,** Giving intramuscular injection in the deltoid muscle.

exists when using this site because the axillary, radial, brachial, and ulnar nerves and the brachial artery lie within the upper arm along the humerus (Figure 34-26, *A*). Use this site only for small medication volumes, when giving immunizations, or when other sites are inaccessible because of dressings or casts (Davidson & Rourke, 2013).

To locate the deltoid muscle, fully expose the patient's upper arm and shoulder. Do not roll up a tight-fitting sleeve. Have the patient relax the arm at the side and flex the elbow. The patient may sit, stand, or lie down (Figure 34-26, *B*). Palpate the lower edge of the acromion process, which forms the base of a triangle in line with the midpoint of the lateral aspect of the upper arm. The injection site is in the centre of the triangle, approximately 3 to 5 cm below the acromion process (Davidson & Rourke, 2013). The site can also be located by placing four fingers across the deltoid muscle, with your top finger along the acromion process. The injection site is then three fingerwidths below the acromion process.

Technique for Intramuscular Injections. When administering IM injections, the Z-track method is recommended because it minimizes local skin irritation by sealing the medication in the muscle tissue. Insert a new needle into the syringe after preparing the medication so that no solution remains on the outside of the needle shaft. For the Z-track technique, select an IM site, preferably in a large, deep muscle, such as the ventrogluteal muscle; smaller needles may need to be used for smaller muscles (Nicoll & Hesby, 2002). After preparing the site with an antiseptic swab, pull the overlying skin and subcutaneous tissues approximately 2.5 to 3.5 cm laterally to the side. Holding the skin taut with the nondominant hand, insert the needle deep into the muscle, and slowly inject the medication. The needle remains inserted for 10 seconds to allow the medication to disperse evenly rather than channelling back up the track of the needle. Then, withdraw the needle and release the skin. This technique leaves a zigzag path that seals the needle track where the tissue planes slide across each other (Figure 34-27). The medication cannot escape from the muscle tissue. Injections using this technique cause less discomfort and fewer lesions at the injection site (Nicoll & Hesby, 2002).

Intradermal Injections. Intradermal injections are commonly performed for skin testing (e.g., tuberculin screening and allergy tests). Because these medications are potent, they are injected into the dermis, where blood supply is reduced and medication absorption occurs slowly. If the medications enter the circulation too rapidly, a patient may have a severe anaphylactic reaction.

For accurate skin testing, the nurse must be able to see the injection site clearly to detect changes in colour and tissue integrity. Intradermal sites should be lightly pigmented, free of lesions, and relatively hairless. The inner forearm and upper back are ideal locations.

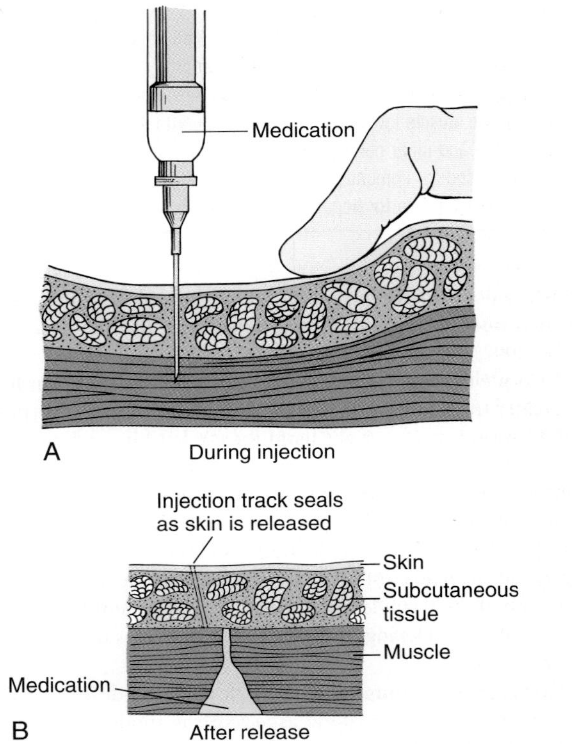

FIGURE 34-27 **A,** Pulling on the overlying skin during intramuscular injection moves tissue to prevent later tracking. **B,** The Z-track left after injection prevents the deposit of medication through sensitive tissue.

Use a tuberculin or small hypodermic syringe for skin testing. The angle of insertion for an intradermal injection is 5 to 15 degrees (see Figure 34-23), with the bevel of the needle pointed up. As the medication is injected, a small bleb resembling a mosquito bite should appear on the skin's surface (see Skill 34-5). If a bleb does not appear or if the site bleeds after withdrawal of the needle, the medication may have entered the subcutaneous tissues. In this case, the test results will not be valid.

Safety in Administering Medications by Injection

Needleless Devices. Needle-stick injuries occur frequently in all health care settings. Some hospitals report that one-third of nursing staff suffer needle-stick injuries each year (Canadian Centre for

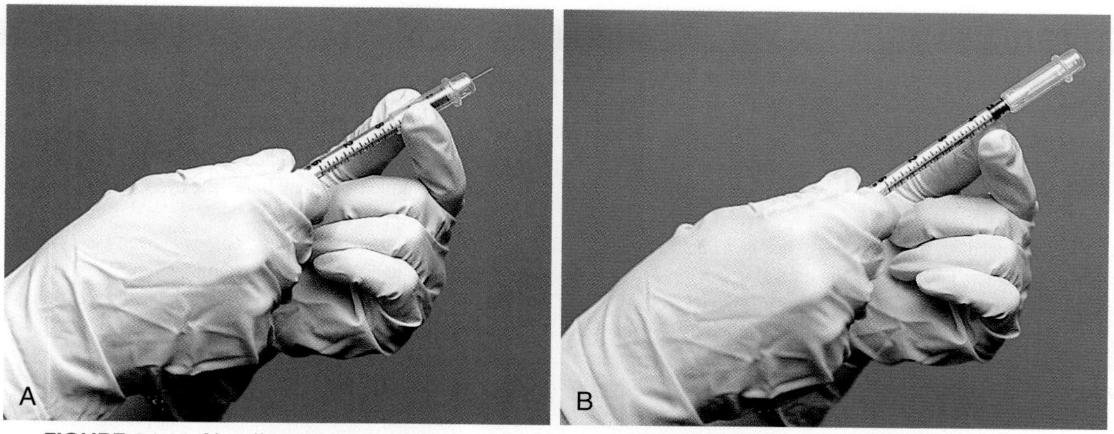

FIGURE 34-28 **Needle with plastic guard to prevent needle sticks. A,** Position of guard before injection. **B,** After injection, the guard locks in place, covering the needle.

Occupational Health and Safety [CCOHS], 2014). However, because many workers do not report their injuries, the incidence of needle-stick injuries is probably higher. Needle-stick injuries commonly occur when needles are recapped, IV lines and needles are mishandled, or needles are left at a patient's bedside. The risk of exposure of health care workers to bloodborne pathogens has led to the development of "needleless devices" or special needle safety devices.

Special syringes are designed with a sheath or guard that covers the needle after it is withdrawn from the skin (Figure 34-28). The needle is immediately covered to eliminate the possibility of a needle-stick injury. The syringe and sheath are disposed of together in a receptacle. Needleless devices should be used whenever possible to reduce the risk of injury from needle sticks and sharps (CCOHS, 2014; Health Canada, 2004; Occupational Safety and Health Administration [OSHA], n.d.).

Needles and other instruments that are considered "sharps" are always disposed of into clearly marked containers that are puncture-proof and leak-proof (Figure 34-29). A needle should never be forced into a needle disposable receptacle that is full. Nurses should never place used needles and syringes in a wastebasket, in their pocket, on a patient's meal tray, or at the patient's bedside. Box 34-28 summarizes recommendations for the prevention of needle-stick injuries.

Intravenous Administration. Medications are administered intravenously by the following methods:

1. As mixtures within large volumes of IV fluids
2. By injection of a bolus, or small volume, of medication through an existing IV infusion line or intermittent venous access (heparin or saline lock)
3. By "piggyback" infusion of a solution containing the prescribed medication and a small volume of IV fluid through an existing IV line

In all three methods, the patient has either an existing IV infusion line or an IV access site (sometime called a heparin or saline lock). In most institutions, policies and procedures list the persons who may give IV medications and the situations in which these medications may be given. These policies are based on the medication, capability, and availability of staff, and the type of monitoring equipment available.

Chapter 40 describes the technique for performing venipuncture and establishing continuous IV fluid infusions. Medication administration is only one reason for supplying IV fluids. IV fluid therapy is used primarily for fluid replacement in patients unable to take oral fluids and as a means of supplying the patient with electrolytes and nutrients.

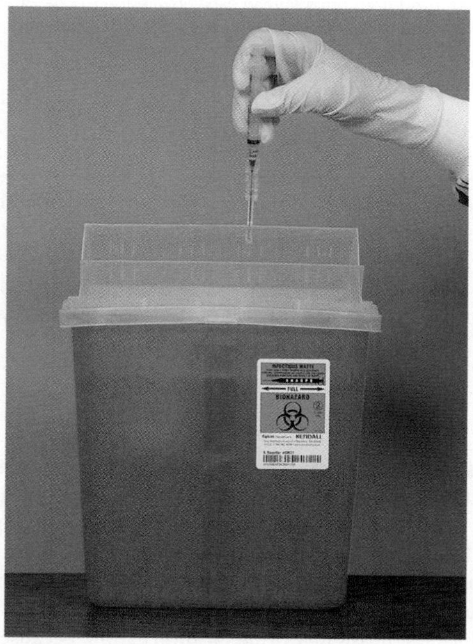

FIGURE 34-29 **Sharps disposal using only one hand.**

When using any method of IV medication administration, patients should be closely monitored for symptoms of adverse reactions. After a medication enters the bloodstream, it begins to act immediately, and its action cannot be stopped. Thus, nurses need to take special care to avoid errors in dose calculation and preparation. They must carefully follow the rights of safe medication administration, double-check their medication calculations with another nurse, and know the desired action and adverse effects of every medication administered. If the medication has an antidote, it must be available during administration. When administering potent medications, the patient's vital signs are assessed before, during, and after infusion.

Administering medications by the IV route has advantages. The IV route is used in emergencies when a fast-acting medication must be delivered quickly. The IV route is also preferred when constant therapeutic blood levels need to be established. Some medications are highly alkaline and irritating to the muscle and subcutaneous tissue. These medications cause less discomfort when given intravenously.

BOX 34-28 Recommendations for the Prevention of Needle-Stick Injuries

- Avoid using needles when effective needleless systems or sharps with engineered sharps injury protections (SESIP) safety devices are available.
- Never recap needles.
- Never move an exposed needle tip toward an unprotected hand.
- Plan safe handling and safe disposal of needles before beginning the procedure.
- Immediately dispose of needles, needleless systems, and SESIP into puncture-proof disposal containers located near the area of use.
- Maintain occupational health and safety standards that include the following:
  - Assessment and implementation of innovations in procedures and technological developments to reduce risks of exposure to contaminated sharps
  - Employee training to address the risks, hazards, and recommended precautions, and the importance of hepatitis B vaccination, where appropriate
  - Documentation of consideration and use of appropriate, commercially available, and effective safer devices
  - Selection of devices that do not jeopardize patient or employee safety and are determined to be medically advisable
  - Documentation of input from employees regarding methods to reduce exposure
  - Annual re-examination of occupational health and safety standards
- Maintain a needle-stick injury reporting protocol that protects the privacy of persons who have had sharps injuries and includes the following information:
  - Type and brand of device involved in the incident
  - Location of the incident (e.g., name of the department or work area)
  - Description of the incident
  - Protection of privacy for both the employee and patient involved in the needle-stick injury

Data from Occupational Safety and Health Administration (OSHA). (2012). Bloodborne pathogens standard; Corrections and technical amendment, *Federal Register, 77, 19933*. Retrieved from https://www.osha.gov/FedReg_osha_pdf/FED20120403.pdf; World Health Organization (WHO). (2012). *Injection safety*. Retrieved from http://www.wpro.who.int/mediacentre/factsheets/fs_20120204/en/.

Safety Alert Because IV medications are immediately available to the bloodstream after they are administered, verify the prescribed rate of administration with a drug reference manual or a pharmacist before giving any IV medication. This step ensures that the medication is administered safely over the appropriate amount of time. Patients can experience severe adverse reactions if IV medications are administered too quickly.

Large-Volume Infusions. Of the three methods of administering IV medications, mixing medications in large volumes of fluids is the safest and easiest. Medications are diluted in large volumes (500 mL or 1000 mL) of compatible IV fluids, such as normal saline or lactated Ringer's solution (Skill 34-6). In most institutions, the pharmacist adds medications to the primary container of IV solution to ensure asepsis and to reduce the possibility of medication errors. Because the medication is not in a concentrated form, the risk of adverse effects or fatal reactions is minimal when infused over the prescribed time frame. Vitamins and potassium chloride are two types of medications commonly added to IV fluids. However, continuous infusion presents risks: if the IV fluid is infused too rapidly, the patient may suffer circulatory fluid overload.

Intravenous Bolus. An IV bolus, or "push," involves the introduction of a concentrated dose of a medication directly into the patient's systemic circulation (Skill 34-7). A bolus has the advantage of requiring only a small amount of fluid to deliver the medication; therefore, the bolus is useful when the patient is on restricted fluids. However, an IV bolus, or "push," is the most dangerous method for administering medications because the nurse has no time to correct an error. Also, a bolus may cause direct irritation to the lining of the blood vessels. Before administering a bolus, confirm the placement of the IV line by obtaining a blood return through the IV catheter or needle. The inability to obtain a blood return suggests that the needle or catheter is in the patient's tissues or is resting against the vein wall. Never give a medication intravenously if the insertion site appears puffy or edematous or if the IV fluid cannot flow at the proper rate. Accidental injection of a medication into the tissues around a vein can cause pain, sloughing of tissues, and abscesses, depending on the medication's composition.

The rate of administration of an IV bolus medication is determined by the amount of medication that can be given per minute. For example, if a patient is to receive 4 mL of a medication over 2 minutes, give 2 mL of the IV bolus medication every minute. Research each medication to determine the recommended concentration and rate of administration. When delivering a medication IV push, consider the purpose for which a medication is prescribed and any potential adverse effects related to the rate or route of administration.

Volume-Controlled Infusions. IV medications can also be administered through small amounts (50 to 100 mL) of compatible IV fluids. The fluid is within a secondary fluid container separate from the primary fluid bag. The container connects directly to the primary IV line or to separate tubing that inserts into the primary line. Three types of containers are volume-control administration sets (e.g., Volutrol or Pediatrol): piggyback sets, tandem sets, and mini-infusors. The use of volume-controlled infusions has several advantages:

- The risk of rapid-dose infusion by IV push is reduced. Medications are diluted and infused over longer time intervals (e.g., 30 to 60 minutes).
- Medications that are stable for only a limited time in solution (e.g., antibiotics) can be administered.
- IV fluid intake can be controlled.

Volume-Control Administration. Volume-control administration (e.g., Volutrol, Buretrol, Pediatrol) sets are small (50 to 150 mL) containers that attach just below the primary infusion bag or bottle. The set is attached and filled in a manner similar to the procedure used with a regular IV infusion; however, the priming or filling of the set is different and depends on the type of filter (floating valve or membrane). A Buretrol or Volutrol is used to deliver IV fluids in a safe manner to children in many agencies even when infusion pumps are used. Follow package directions for priming sets (see Chapter 40).

Piggyback. A piggyback is a small (25 to 250 mL) IV bag or bottle that connects to short tubing lines that, in turn, connect to the upper

SKILL 34-6 ADDING MEDICATIONS TO INTRAVENOUS FLUID CONTAINERS

Delegation Considerations

Adding medications to IV fluid containers cannot be delegated to unregulated care providers (UCPs). (In some institutions, the pharmacist may add medications to the primary containers of IV solutions to promote safe medication administration and ensure asepsis.)

Equipment

- Vial or ampule of prescribed medication
- Syringe of appropriate size (5–20 mL)
- Sterile needle (2.5–3.8 cm, 19–21 gauge) with special filters (if required)
- Diluent as indicated (e.g., sterile water, normal saline)
- Sterile IV fluid container (bag or bottle, 25–1000 mL in volume)
- Alcohol or antiseptic swab
- Label to attach to IV bag or bottle
- Medication administration record (MAR) or computer printout

PROCEDURE

STEPS	RATIONALE
1. Check the accuracy and completeness of each MAR or computer printout against the prescriber's original medication order. Check the patient's name and the medication name, route, dosage, and time of administration. Copy or rewrite any portion of the MAR that is difficult to read.	
2. Assess the patient's medical history.	
3. Collect information necessary to administer the drug safely, including the medication's action, purpose, adverse effects, normal dose, time of peak onset, and nursing implications.	
4. When more than one medication is to be added to the IV solution, assess for compatibility of the medications.	• Medications often are incompatible when mixed together. Chemical reactions that occur result in clouding or crystallization of IV fluids. Check the hospital policy for a list of approved medication compatibilities.
5. Assess the patient's systemic fluid balance, as evidenced by skin hydration and turgor, body weight, pulse, blood pressure, and ratio of fluid intake to urinary output.	• Continuous IV infusions can lead to fluids that infuse too rapidly, thereby causing circulatory overload, especially in children and older persons (Touhy et al., 2012; Hockenberry & Wilson, 2014).
6. Assess the patient's history of medication allergies.	• The IV administration of medications causes rapid effects. Allergic response can be immediate.
7. Perform hand hygiene.	
8. Assess the IV insertion site for signs of infiltration or phlebitis (see Chapter 40).	• An intact, properly functioning site ensures medication is given safely.
9. Assess the patient's understanding of the purpose of the medication therapy.	
10. Prepare the prescribed medication (see Skill 34-4); use aseptic techniques. Ensure that you compare the label of the medication with the MAR two times while preparing the medication.	• Proper technique ensures the medication is sterile; preparation techniques differ for ampules and vials.
11. Perform hand hygiene.	
12. Compare the labels of the medication and the IV fluid bag with the MAR or computer printout.	• Checking the labels ensures that the correct medication is injected into the correct IV fluid.
13. Add the medication to a new container (usually in the medication room or at medication cart):	
A. *Solution in a bag:* Locate the medication injection port on the plastic IV solution bag. The port has a small rubber stopper at the end. Do not select the port for the IV tubing insertion or the air vent.	• The medication injection port is self-sealing to prevent introduction of microorganisms after repeated use. • Accidental injection of medication through the main tubing port or the air vent can alter the pressure within the bottle and cause fluid leaks through the air vent. The cap seals the bottle to maintain its sterility.
B. *Solution in a bottle:* Locate the injection site on the IV solution bottle, which is often covered by a metal or plastic cap.	
C. Wipe the port or injection site with alcohol or an antiseptic swab (see Step 13C illustration).	• Cleaning the port of injection site reduces the risk of introducing bacteria into the port.

Continued

SKILL 34-6 ADDING MEDICATIONS TO INTRAVENOUS FLUID CONTAINERS—cont'd

STEPS / **RATIONALE**

D. Remove the needle cap or sheath from the syringe and insert the needle of the syringe or the needleless device through the centre of injection port or site; inject the medication (see Step 13D illustration).

- Injection of the needle into the sides of the port may cause a leak and lead to fluid contamination.

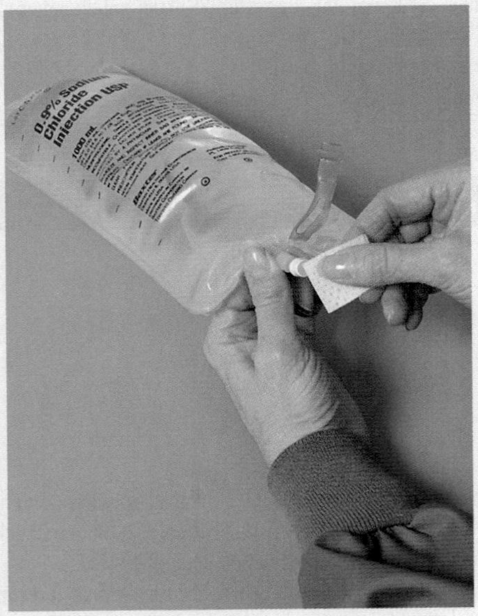

STEP 13C Clean the injection port with an antiseptic swab.

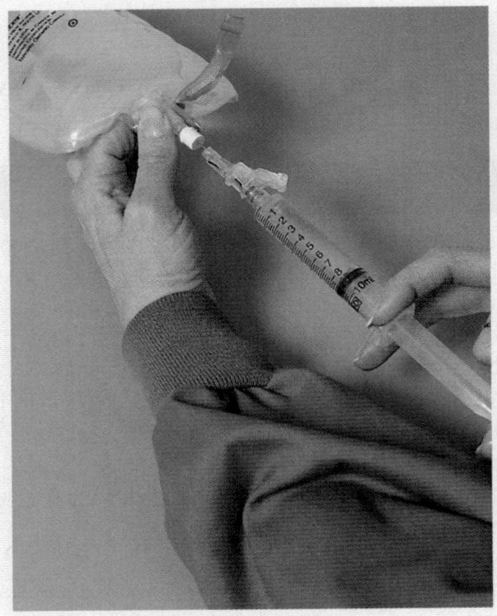

STEP 13D Inject the medication through the port.

E. Withdraw the syringe from the bag or bottle.

- When the syringe is withdrawn, the injection port self-seals to prevent the introduction of microorganisms.

F. Mix the medication and the IV solution by holding the bag or bottle and turning it gently end to end.

- Gently turning the bag or bottle allows even distribution of the medication.

G. Complete the medication label by printing the name and dose of the medication, the date and time of administration, and your initials. Apply the label to the bottle or bag, being careful not to cover any essential information preprinted on the bottle or bag. Spike the bag or bottle with the IV tubing.

- The label informs other health care providers of the contents of the bag or bottle.
- Concealing important information on the IV bag can lead to medication errors.

14. Take the assembled items to the patient's bedside at the right time.

15. Identify the patient using at least two patient identifiers. Compare the patient's name and one other identifier (e.g., the hospital identification number) on the MAR, computer printout, or computer screen against information on the patient's identification bracelet. Ask the patient to state his or her name, if possible, for a third identifier.

16. Prepare the patient by explaining that the medication is to be given through the existing IV line or a new line that will be started. Explain that no discomfort should be felt during the medication infusion. Encourage the patient to report symptoms of discomfort.

- Most IV medications do not cause discomfort when diluted; however, potassium chloride is irritating. Pain at the insertion site may be an early indication of infiltration.

17. Connect the infusion tubing or spike container to the existing tubing. Regulate the infusion at the ordered rate.

- Properly regulated infusion prevents rapid infusion of fluid.

CRITICAL DECISION POINT: *Some medications (e.g., potassium chloride) can cause serious adverse reactions, including fatal cardiac dysrhythmias. These medications should be infused on an IV pump. Check the institutional guidelines or policies indicating which IV medications require administration on an IV pump.*

18. Add the medication to the existing container.

CRITICAL DECISION POINT: *Because you cannot know exactly how much IV fluid remains in an existing hanging IV container, you are unable to determine the exact concentration of the medication in the IV solution. Therefore, it is recommended that medications be added to new IV fluid containers whenever possible.*

STEPS	RATIONALE
A. Prepare a vented IV bottle or plastic bag:	
(1) Check the volume of the solution remaining in the bottle or bag.	• Proper minimal volume (see drug insert) is needed to dilute the medication adequately.
(2) Close off the IV infusion clamp.	• Closing the clamp prevents medication from directly entering the patient's circulation system when it is injected into the bag or bottle.
(3) Wipe the medication port with an alcohol or antiseptic swab.	• Cleaning the port mechanically removes microorganisms that could enter container during needle insertion.
(4) Remove the needle cap or sheath from the syringe; insert the syringe needle or needleless device through the injection port and inject the medication.	• The injection port is self-sealing and prevents fluid leaks.
(5) Withdraw the syringe from the bag or bottle.	
(6) Lower the bag or bottle from the IV pole and gently mix the medication and the IV solution by holding the bag or bottle and turning it gently end to end. Rehang the bag or bottle.	• Gently turning the bag or bottle ensures the medication is evenly distributed.
B. Complete the medication label and apply it to the unprinted side of the IV solution bag or bottle. Do not cover the imprinted label of the solution.	• The label informs other health care providers of the contents of the bag or bottle. Concealing important information on the IV bag can lead to medication errors.
C. Regulate the infusion to the desired rate. Use an IV pump if indicated.	• Proper regulated infusion prevents rapid infusion of fluid.
19. Properly dispose of equipment and supplies. Do not recap the needle or syringe. Discard the specially sheathed needles as a unit with the needle covered.	• Proper disposal of the needle prevents injury to both the nurse and the patient. Capping of needles increases risk of needle-stick injuries.
20. Perform hand hygiene.	
21. Observe the patient for signs or symptoms of medication reaction.	• IV medications can cause rapid effects.
22. Observe the patient for signs and symptoms of fluid volume excess.	• Rapid uncontrolled infusion can cause circulatory overload.
23. Periodically return to the patient's room to assess the IV insertion site and the rate of infusion.	• Over time, the IV site may become infiltrated or the needle may become malpositioned. The flow rate may change according to patient's body position or the volume of solution left in the container.
24. Observe the patient for signs or symptoms of IV infiltration.	• Infiltrated medications can injure tissue.
25. Ensure that a label is applied to the IV tubing; the label must state the date and time that the IV tubing was opened and must be attached to the IV infusion system. Consult with agency policy regarding frequency of changing the IV tubing.	• Most agencies have policies indicating that IV tubing should be changed every 72 hours. The frequency of changing IV tubing may increase on the basis of the solution being administered (e.g., antibiotics, or total parental nutrition [TPN]) or the type of in-dwelling IV catheter (e.g., central line). Changing the IV tubing helps to prevent nosocomial infections.
26. Assess the IV tubing frequently for integrity and occlusions.	• Disruptions in the integrity of the IV tubing can lead to the patient not receiving the required IV therapy or medication and may lead to infection.
27. Ask the patient to explain the purpose and effects of the medication therapy.	

UNEXPECTED OUTCOMES	RELATED INTERVENTIONS
Adverse or allergic reaction to medication	• Follow institutional policy or guidelines for your appropriate response to and reporting of adverse drug reactions. • Notify the patient's health care provider immediately. • Add the allergy information to the patient's medical record.
Signs of fluid volume overload (e.g., abnormal breath sounds, shortness of breath, intake greater than output)	• Assess the patient for compromised circulatory regulation (vital signs, input:output, focused respiratory and cardiac assessments). • Stop the IV infusion. • Notify the patient's health care provider immediately.
Swelling, warmth, redness, and tenderness at intravenous site, indicating phlebitis (see Chapter 40)	• Stop IV infusion and discontinue IV. • Treat the IV site as indicated by institutional policy. • If continuation of IV therapy is indicated, insert a new IV.
Coolness, pallor, and swelling at intravenous site, indicating infiltration (see Chapter 40)	• Some IV medications are extremely harmful to the subcutaneous tissue. • Provide IV extravasation care as indicated by institutional policy, or use a medication reference manual or consult a pharmacist to determine the appropriate follow-up care.

RECORDING AND REPORTING

- Record the solution and medication added to parenteral fluid on the appropriate form.
- Report any adverse effects to the patient's health care provider, and document adverse effects according to institutional policy.

SKILL 34-7 ADMINISTERING MEDICATIONS BY INTRAVENOUS BOLUS

Delegation Considerations

The administration of medications by IV bolus cannot be delegated to unregulated care providers (UCPs). Instruct UCPs to report immediately any unexpected drug reactions, discomfort at the infusion site, and changes in any required vital signs.

Equipment

- A watch with a second hand
- Medication administration record (MAR) or computer printout
- Clean gloves
- Antiseptic swab
- IV push (existing line):
  - Medication in a vial or ampule
  - Syringe for medication preparation
  - Needleless device or sterile needle (21–25 gauge)
- IV lock:
  - Syringe and needleless device (21–25 gauge) for medication preparation
  - Vial of the appropriate flush solution (saline is most common, but heparin may also be used; if heparin is used, the most common concentration is 10 to 100 units; check agency policy)

PROCEDURE

STEPS	RATIONALE
1. Check the accuracy and completeness of each MAR or computer printout against the prescriber's original medication order. Check the patient's name and the medication name, route, dosage, and time of administration. Copy or rewrite any portion of the MAR that is difficult to read.	

CRITICAL DECISION POINT: *Some IV medications can be pushed safely only when the patient is being continuously monitored for dysrhythmias, blood pressure changes, or other adverse effects. Therefore, some medications can be pushed only in specific areas within a health care agency. Confirm the institutional guidelines regarding requirements for special monitoring and verify that these requirements are available before giving medication.*

STEPS	RATIONALE
2. Collect the information necessary to administer the medication safely, including action, purpose, adverse effects, normal dose, time of peak onset, the pace at which to give the medication, and nursing implications, such as the need to dilute the medication or to administer it through a filter.	
3. If pushing the medication into an IV line, determine the compatibility of the medication both with the IV fluids and any additives in the IV solution.	• IV medications are not always compatible with IV solutions and additives.
4. Perform hand hygiene. Assess the IV or saline (heparin) lock insertion site for signs of infiltration or phlebitis (see Chapter 40).	• Confirming the placement of the IV catheter and the integrity of the surrounding tissue ensures the medication is administered safely.
5. Check the patient's medical history and allergies.	• The IV bolus delivers medication rapidly. Allergic reactions can be fatal.
6. Check the date of expiration for the medication vial or ampule.	• Drug potency sometimes increases or decreases when medications are expired.
7. Assess the patient's understanding of the purpose of medication therapy.	
8. Prepare the ordered medication from the vial or ampule using aseptic technique (see Skill 34-4). Check the label of the medication carefully with the MAR two times. Apply a removable label indicating the patient's name and the medication name and dosage to the removable needle cap.	

CRITICAL DECISION POINT: *Some IV medications require dilution before administration. Verify the dilution requirements with the agency policy. If a small amount of medication is given (e.g., less than 1 mL), dilute the medication in 5 to 10 mL of normal saline or sterile water so that the medication does not collect in the "dead spaces" (e.g., the Y-site injection port or IV cap) of the IV delivery system.*

STEPS	RATIONALE
9. Take the medication to the patient at the correct time.	
10. Identify the patient using at least two patient identifiers. Compare the patient's name and one other identifier (e.g., the hospital identification number) on the MAR, computer printout, or computer screen against information on the patient's identification bracelet. Ask the patient to state his or her name, if possible, for a third identifier.	
11. Compare the label of the medication with the MAR at the patient's bedside.	• The *third check* of the medication label against the MAR at bedside reduces medication administration errors.

STEPS	RATIONALE
12. Explain the procedure to the patient. Encourage the patient to report symptoms of discomfort at the IV site.	• Asking the patient to report symptoms of discomfort helps in early identification of infiltration.
13. Perform hand hygiene. Apply gloves.	• Hand hygiene reduces the transmission of infection. During IV bolus administration, the risk of blood exposure is low. However, you may need to manipulate the IV dressing or expose the site while you complete other activities. Gloves reduce your exposure.
14. Administer the medication by IV push (through the existing IV line):	
A. Select the injection port of the IV tubing closest to patient. Whenever possible, the injection port should accept a needleless syringe. Use the IV filter if required by a medication reference manual or agency policy.	• The WHO (2016), Public Health Agency of Canada (2014), and US Occupational Safety and Health Administration (OSHA) (2012), strongly recommend that all IV injection sites be needleless to prevent needle-stick injuries.
B. Wipe the injection port with an antiseptic swab. Allow to dry.	• Wiping with an antiseptic swab helps prevent the introduction of microorganisms during needle insertion.
C. Connect the syringe to the IV line. Insert the needleless tip or a small-gauge needle of a syringe containing the prepared drug through the centre of the injection port (see Step 14C illustration).	• This procedure prevents damage to the port's diaphragm and subsequent leakage.
D. Occlude the IV line by pinching the tubing just above the injection port (see Step 14D illustration).	• This step is the *final check* that the medication is being delivered into the bloodstream.

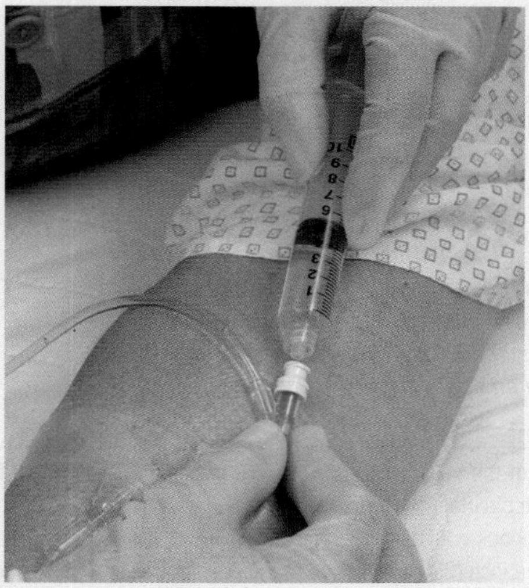

STEP 14C Connecting the syringe to the IV line with a blunt needleless cannula tip.

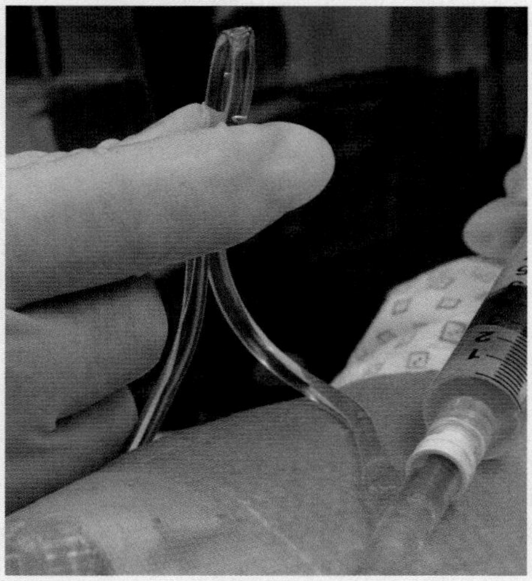

STEP 14D Intravenous line pinched above the injection port for medication infusion.

CRITICAL DECISION POINT: *In some cases, especially with a smaller-gauge IV needle or a needleless device, the blood return may not be aspirated, even if the IV is patent (open and unblocked). If the IV site does not show signs of infiltration, and the IV fluid is infusing without difficulty, proceed with the IV push.*

Continued

SKILL 34-7 ADMINISTERING MEDICATIONS BY INTRAVENOUS BOLUS—cont'd

STEPS	RATIONALE
E. Release the tubing and inject the medication within the amount of time recommended by institutional policy, the pharmacist, or a medication reference manual. Use your watch to time the administration (see Step 14E illustration). The IV line may be pinched while pushing medication and released when not pushing medication (see Step 14E illustration). Allow the IV fluids to infuse when the medication is not being pushed.	• Following the proper procedure ensures safe medication infusion. Rapid injection of IV medication can prove fatal. Allowing the IV fluids to infuse while not pushing the IV drug enables medications to be delivered to the patient at a prescribed rate.

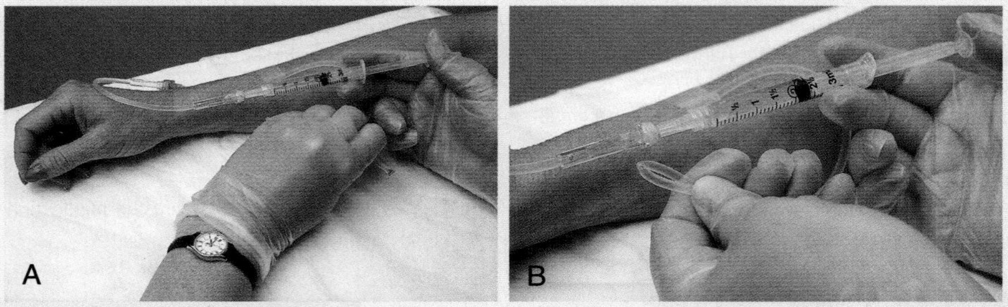

STEP 14E A, Timing the IV push medication. **B,** The IV line is pinched off for medication infusion (optional).

CRITICAL DECISION POINT: *If the IV medication is incompatible with IV fluids, stop the IV fluids, clamp the IV line, flush with 10 mL of normal saline or sterile water, give the IV bolus over the appropriate amount of time, flush with another 10 mL of normal saline or sterile water at the same rate as the medication was administered, and then restart the IV fluids at the prescribed rate. If the IV that is currently hanging is a medication, disconnect the IV, and administer the IV push as outlined in Step 14. This step avoids giving the patient a sudden bolus of the medication in the existing IV line and avoids creating potential risks associated with IV incompatibilities. Some IV medications and fluids cannot be stopped. Verify the institutional policy regarding the temporary stopping of IV fluids or continuous IV medications. If unable to stop the IV infusion, start a new IV site and administer the medication using the IV lock method.*

STEPS	RATIONALE
F. After injecting the medication, release the tubing, withdraw the syringe, and recheck the fluid infusion rate.	• Injection of the bolus may alter the rate of fluid infusion. Rapid fluid infusion can cause circulatory overload.
15. Administer medications by IV push (IV lock or a needleless system): **A.** Prepare the flush solutions according to agency policy. Ensure that a syringe with the correct barrel width is used. Consult with agency policy regarding syringes for delivering IV bolus medications.	• Small syringes with narrow bores (e.g., 1 mL or 3 mL) create greater pressure per square inch (PSI) when used to inject solutions into an IV line. A high PSI can damage the lumen of certain types of in-dwelling IV catheters (central lines and peripherally inserted central catheter [PICC] lines). Ensure that you consult with agency policy to ensure safe maintenance of these lines.
(1) Saline flush method (preferred method):	• Normal saline has been found to be effective in keeping IV locks patent and is compatible with a wide range of medications.
(a) Prepare two syringes with 2–3 mL of normal saline (0.9%) in a syringe.	
(2) Heparin flush method (traditional method):	
(a) Prepare one syringe with the ordered amount of heparin flush solution.	
(b) Prepare two syringes with 2–3 mL of normal saline.	
B. Administer medication: **(1)** Wipe the lock's injection port with an antiseptic swab.	• Wiping the injection port prevents introduction of microorganisms during the needle insertion.

STEPS	RATIONALE
(2) Insert a syringe containing normal saline into the injection port of the IV lock (see Step 15B[2] illustration).	

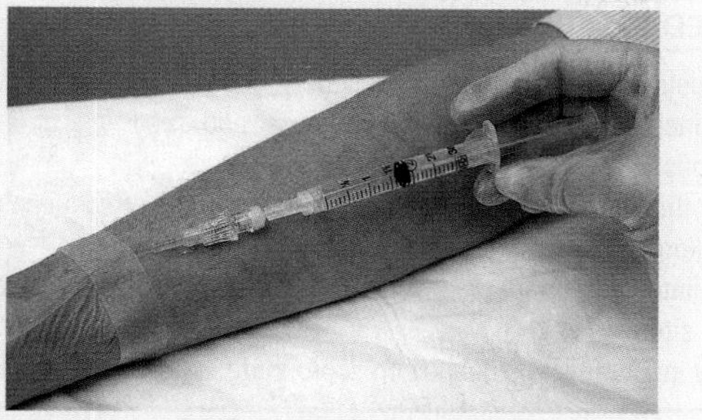

STEP 15B(2) Syringe inserted into the injection port.

STEPS	RATIONALE
(3) Pull back gently on the syringe plunger and look for blood return.	• This step determines whether the IV needle or catheter is positioned in the vein.

CRITICAL DECISION POINT: *Sometimes a saline (or heparin) lock will not yield a blood return even though the lock is patent. If the IV site does not show signs of infiltration, proceed with the IV push.*

STEPS	RATIONALE
(4) Flush the IV lock with normal saline by pushing slowly on the plunger.	• Flushing the IV lock clears it of blood.

CRITICAL DECISION POINT: *Observe closely the area of skin above the IV catheter. As the IV lock is flushed, note any puffiness or swelling, which could indicate infiltration into the vein, and thereby require removal of the catheter.*

STEPS	RATIONALE
(5) Remove the saline-filled syringe.	
(6) Clean the lock's injection port with an antiseptic swab.	• Cleaning the injection port prevents transmission of infection.
(7) Insert the syringe containing the prepared medication into the injection port of the IV lock.	
(8) Inject the medication within the amount of time recommended by institutional policy, the pharmacist, or a medication reference manual. Use a watch to time the administration.	• Rapid injection of the IV medication can result in death. Following the guidelines for IV push rates promotes patient safety (Karch & Karch, 2003).
(9) After administering the bolus, withdraw the syringe.	
(10) Clean the lock's injection port with an antiseptic swab.	• Cleaning the injection port helps prevent transmission of microorganisms.
(11) Attach the syringe with normal saline and inject the normal saline flush at the same rate that the medication was delivered.	• Irrigation with saline prevents occlusion of the IV access device and ensures that all medication is delivered. Flushing the IV site at the same rate as the medication ensures that any medication remaining within the IV needle is delivered at the correct rate.
(12) *Heparin flush option:* Insert the needle of the syringe containing the heparin through the diaphragm.	• Inserting the needle through the diaphragm maintains the patency of the IV catheter and tubing by inhibiting clot formation. Use the SASH method: **S**aline, **A**dministration of medication, **S**aline, **H**eparin.
16. Dispose of uncapped needles and syringes in puncture-proof and leak-proof container.	• Proper disposal reduces the risk of accidental needle sticks.
17. Remove and dispose of gloves. Perform hand hygiene.	• Proper hygiene reduces the transmission of microorganisms.
18. Observe the patient closely for adverse reactions while the medication is administered and for several minutes thereafter.	• IV medications act rapidly.
19. Observe the IV site during injection for sudden swelling.	• Swelling indicates infiltration into tissues surrounding the vein.
20. Observe the patient's status after administering the medication to evaluate the effectiveness of medication.	• IV bolus medications often cause rapid changes in the patient's physiological status. Some medications require careful monitoring and assessment and possible laboratory testing (e.g., vasopressors require the monitoring of blood pressure and heart rate; Dilantin requires laboratory studies to determine whether it is at a therapeutic level).
21. Consult with agency policy with regard to the frequency of saline flushes.	• To maintain patency of IV catheters (peripheral or central), IV devices require routine flushing. Short-term peripheral angiocatheters are flushed every 12 hours with a normal saline solution. Consult with agency policy with regard to protocols for flushing central lines.
22. Ask the patient to explain the medication's purposes and adverse effects.	

Continued

SKILL 34-7 ADMINISTERING MEDICATIONS BY INTRAVENOUS BOLUS—cont'd

STEPS	RATIONALE

UNEXPECTED OUTCOMES	RELATED INTERVENTIONS
Adverse reaction to medication	• Stop delivering medication immediately and follow institutional policy or guidelines for the appropriate response and reporting of adverse drug reactions. • Notify the patient's health care provider of adverse effects immediately. • Add allergy information to the patient's medical record.
Symptoms of infiltration or phlebitis at intravenous site	• Immediately discontinue administration of the injection and discontinue use of the site. • Follow institutional guidelines on appropriate extravasation care.

RECORDING AND REPORTING

- Record the medication, dose, time, and route on the appropriate form (MAR) or in computer record.
- Report any adverse reactions immediately to the health care provider because the reactions could be life-threatening. The patient's response may indicate the need for additional medical therapy.
- Record the patient's response to medication in the nurses' notes.

Y-port of a primary infusion line or to an intermittent venous access (Figure 34-30). The piggyback tubing is a microdrip or macrodrip system (see Chapter 40). The set is called a *piggyback* because the small bag or bottle is set higher than the primary infusion bag or bottle. In the piggyback setup, the main line does not infuse when the piggybacked medication is infusing. The port of the primary IV line contains a back-check valve that automatically stops flow of the primary infusion when the piggyback infusion flows. After the piggyback solution infuses and the solution within the tubing falls below the level of the primary infusion drip chamber, the back-check valve opens and the primary infusion again flows.

Tandem. A tandem setup is a small (25- to 100-mL) IV bag or bottle connected to a short tubing line that connects to the lower Y-port of a primary infusion line or to an intermittent venous access. The tandem set is placed at the same height as the primary infusion bag or bottle. In the tandem setup, the tandem and the main line infuse simultaneously. The tandem setup must be monitored closely. If it is not immediately clamped when the medication is infused, the IV solution from the primary line will back up into the tandem line.

Mini-Infusion Pump. The mini-infusion pump is battery operated and allows medications to be given in very small amounts (5 to 60 mL) within controlled infusion times using standard syringes (Skill 34-8).

Intermittent Venous Access. An intermittent venous access (commonly called a heparin lock or saline lock) is an IV catheter with a small chamber covered by a rubber diaphragm or a specially designed cap (Figure 34-31). Special rubber-seal injection caps accept the needleless safety devices and can be inserted into most IV catheters (see Chapter 40). Advantages to intermittent venous access include the following:

- Reduced risk of the patient developing fluid volume excess
- Increased mobility, safety, and comfort for the patient

Before administering an IV bolus or piggyback medication, assess the patency and placement of the IV site. After the medication has been administered through an intermittent venous access, the access must be flushed with a solution to keep it patent. In general, normal saline is an effective flush solution for peripheral catheters. Some institutions require the use of heparin. Verify and follow the institution's policies regarding the care and maintenance of the IV site.

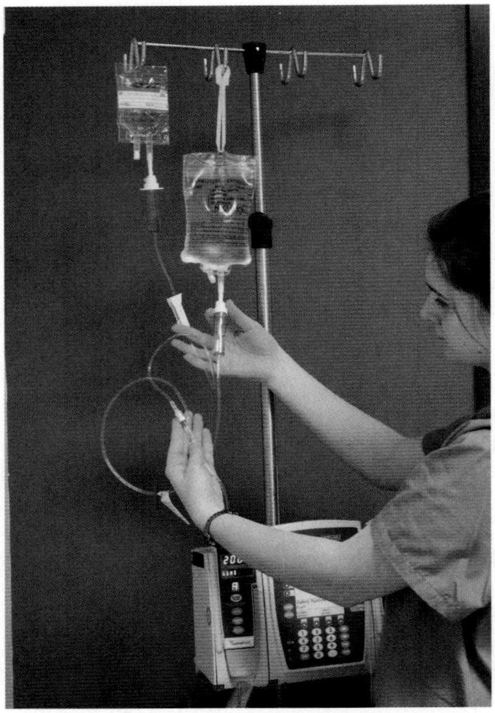

FIGURE 34-30 Piggyback setup. (Courtesy Sharon Kaasalainen, RN, PhD.)

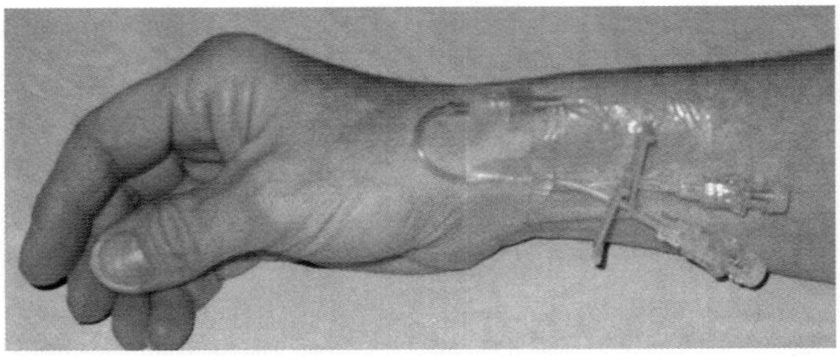

FIGURE 34-31 Intermittent lock covered with a rubber diaphragm.

SKILL 34-8 ADMINISTERING INTRAVENOUS MEDICATIONS BY PIGGYBACK, INTERMITTENT INTRAVENOUS INFUSION SETS, AND MINI-INFUSION PUMPS

Delegation Considerations

The administration of medications by IV fluid by piggyback, intermittent IV infusion sets, and mini-infusion pumps cannot be delegated to unregulated care providers (UCPs). Instruct UCPs to report any unexpected drug reactions or discomfort at the infusion site as soon as possible.

Equipment

- Antiseptic swab
- IV pole
- Medication administration record (MAR) or computer printout
- Medication labels
- Piggyback, tandem, or mini-infusion pump:
- Medication prepared in 5- to 150-mL labelled infusion bag or syringe
- Short microdrip or macrodrip tubing set for piggyback (may have needleless system attachment)
- Needleless device or stopcocks if available
- Needles (21 or 23 gauge, only if stopcocks or other needleless methods are not available)
- Mini-infusion pump
- Adhesive tape (optional)
- Volume-control administration set
- Volutrol, Buretrol, or Pediatrol
- Infusion tubing (may have needleless system attachment)
- Syringe (1–20 mL)
- Vial or ampule of ordered medication

PROCEDURE

STEPS	RATIONALE
1. Check the accuracy and completeness of each MAR or computer printout against the prescriber's original medication order. Check the patient's name and the medication name, route, dosage, and time of administration. Copy or rewrite any portion of the MAR that is difficult to read.	• The order sheet is the most reliable source and only legal record of medications patients are to receive. Checking the accuracy of the medication order ensures that the patient receives the correct medications. Illegible MARs are a source of medication errors.
2. Determine the patient's medical history.	
3. Collect the information necessary to administer the medication safely, including the action, purpose, adverse effects, normal dose, time of peak onset, and nursing implications.	• Information about the medication indicates the type of appropriate IV solution to use and helps to ensure safe and accurate medication administration.
4. Assess the compatibility of the drug with the existing IV solution.	• Drugs that are incompatible with IV solutions may result in clouding or crystallization of the solution in IV tubing, which may harm the patient.

CRITICAL DECISION POINT: *Never administer IV medications through tubing that is infusing blood, blood products, or parenteral nutrition solutions.*

STEPS	RATIONALE
5. Assess the patency of the patient's existing IV infusion line by noting the infusion rate of the main IV line.	• The IV line must be patent and fluids must infuse easily for medication to reach the venous circulation effectively.

CRITICAL DECISION POINT: *If the patient's IV site is saline locked, clean the port with alcohol and assess the patency of the IV line by flushing it with 2–3 mL of sterile normal saline. Attach the appropriate IV tubing to the saline lock and administer the medication via piggyback, tandem, mini-infusion, or volume-control administration set. When the infusion is completed, disconnect the tubing, clean the port with alcohol, and flush the IV line with 2–3 mL sterile normal saline. Maintain sterility of the IV tubing between intermittent infusions.*

STEPS	RATIONALE
6. Perform hand hygiene. Assess the IV insertion site for signs of infiltration or phlebitis: redness, pallor, swelling, tenderness on palpation.	• Confirmation of placement of IV needle or catheter and integrity of surrounding tissues ensures medication is administered safely.
7. Assess the patient's history of medication allergies.	• The effects of medications can develop rapidly after IV infusion. Nurses should be aware of patients who are at risk for an allergic reaction.
8. Assess the patient's understanding of purpose of medication therapy.	
9. Prepare the medication. Ensure that you compare the label of the medication with the MAR two times while preparing the medication.	• Ensure that correct medication is given to patient. First and second checks for accuracy ensure that the correct medication is administered.
10. Assemble the supplies at the bedside. Prepare the patient by explaining that the medication will be given through the IV equipment.	
11. Perform hand hygiene.	

Continued

SKILL 34-8 ADMINISTERING INTRAVENOUS MEDICATIONS BY PIGGYBACK, INTERMITTENT INTRAVENOUS INFUSION SETS, AND MINI-INFUSION PUMPS—cont'd

STEPS	RATIONALE
12. Identify the patient using at least two patient identifiers. Compare the patient's name and one other identifier (e.g., the hospital identification number) on the MAR, computer printout, or computer screen against information on the patient's identification bracelet. Ask the patient to state his or her name, if possible, for a third identifier.	• This process complies with the Joint Commission's (2017) requirements and improves medication safety. In acute care settings, the patient's name and identification number on an armband and the MAR are usually used to identify patients. Identification bracelets are made at the time of the patient's admission and are the most reliable source of information. The patient's room number is *not* an acceptable identifier.
13. Compare medication label with MAR at patient's bedside.	• *This is the third accuracy check.*
14. Explain to the patient the purpose of the medication and its adverse effects. Encourage the patient to report symptoms of discomfort at the IV site.	• Communication with the patient keeps the patient informed of planned therapies. Patients who can verbalize pain at the IV site can help detect IV infiltrations early, reducing the possibility of damage to the surrounding tissues.
15. Administer the infusion:	
A. Piggyback or tandem infusion	• The infusion tubing should be filled with solution and free of air bubbles to prevent an air embolus.
(1) Connect the infusion tubing to the medication bag (see Chapter 40). Allow the solution to fill the tubing by opening the regulator flow clamp. Once the tubing is full, close the clamp and cap the end of the tubing.	
(2) Hang the piggyback medication bag above the level of the primary fluid bag. (A hook may be used to lower the main bag.) Hang the tandem infusion at the same level as the primary fluid bag.	• The height of the fluid bag affects the rate of medication flow to the patient.
(3) Connect the tubing of the piggyback or tandem infusion to the appropriate connector on the primary infusion line:	
(a) *Stopcock:* Wipe the stopcock port with an alcohol swab and connect the tubing. Turn the stopcock to the open position.	
(b) *Needleless system:* Wipe the needleless port, and insert the tip of the piggyback or tandem infusion tubing (see Step 15A[3][b] illustrations).	• The WHO (2016), Health Canada (2004), and US OSHA (2012) strongly recommend that all IV injection sites be needleless to prevent needlestick injuries. The needleless system establishes the route for IV medication to enter the main IV line.

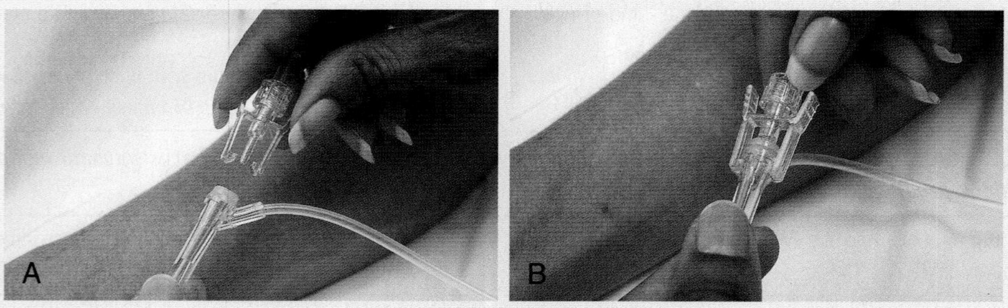

STEP 15A(3)(b) A, Needleless lever lock cannula system. **B,** The blunt-ended cannula inserts into the port and locks.

STEPS	RATIONALE
(c) *Tubing port:* Connect the sterile needle to the end of the piggyback or tandem infusion tubing, remove the cap, clean the injection port on the main IV line, and insert the needle or needleless access device through the centre of the port. Secure by taping the connection.	• Use this step *only* if the needleless system is not available. The tubing port helps prevent the introduction of microorganisms during needle insertion.
(4) Regulate the flow rate of the medication solution by adjusting the regulator clamp. (Infusion times vary. Refer to a medication reference manual or institutional policy for the safe flow rate.)	• The proper flow rate provides a slow, intermittent infusion of medication and maintains therapeutic blood levels.

STEPS	RATIONALE
(5) After medication has infused, check the flow regulator on the primary infusion. The primary infusion should automatically begin to flow after the piggyback or tandem solution is empty.	• The back-check valve on the piggyback stops the flow of the primary infusion until the second medication infuses. The tandem and primary infusions flow together until the tandem set empties. Monitoring the flow rate ensures the proper administration of IV fluids.
(6) Regulate the main infusion line to the desired rate, if necessary.	• The infusion of the piggyback may interfere with the main line infusion rate.
(7) Leave the IV piggyback bag and tubing in place for future medication administration or discard in appropriate containers.	• The establishment of a secondary line produces a route for microorganisms to enter the main line. Repeated changes in the tubing increase the risk of infection transmission (check agency policy).
B. Volume-control administration set (e.g., Volutrol)	
(1) Assemble the supplies in the medication room.	• Use of the medication room controls the risk of contaminating the IV solution.
(2) Prepare medication from a vial or ampule (see Skill 34-4).	• Following proper procedure ensures the medication is sterile.
(3) Fill the Volutrol with the desired amount of fluid (50–100 mL) by opening the clamp between the Volutrol and the main IV bag (see Step 15B[3] illustration).	• Use of a small volume of fluid dilutes the IV medication and reduces the risk of too-rapid infusion.

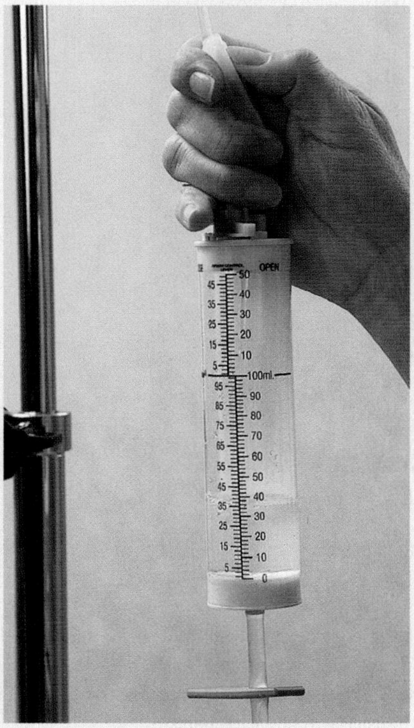

STEP 15B(3) Filling the volume-control administration device.

STEPS	RATIONALE
(4) Close the clamp and ensure the clamp on the air vent of the Volutrol chamber is open.	• This prevents additional leakage of fluid into the Volutrol. The air vent allows fluid in the Volutrol to exit at a regulated rate.
(5) Clean the injection port on the top of the Volutrol with an antiseptic swab.	• Cleaning the injection port prevents the introduction of microorganisms during needle insertion.

Continued

SKILL 34-8 ADMINISTERING INTRAVENOUS MEDICATIONS BY PIGGYBACK, INTERMITTENT INTRAVENOUS INFUSION SETS, AND MINI-INFUSION PUMPS—cont'd

STEPS	RATIONALE
(6) Remove the needle cap or sheath and insert the syringe needle through the port, then inject the medication (see Step 15B[6] illustrations). Gently rotate the Volutrol between your hands.	• Rotating mixes the medication with the solution in the Volutrol to ensure equal distribution.

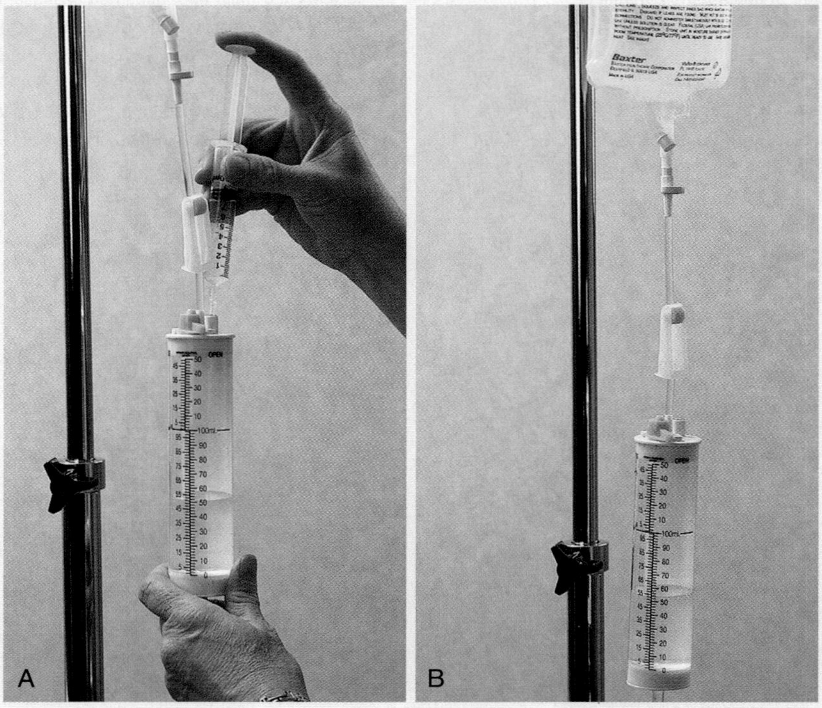

STEP 15B(6) **A,** Medication injected into the device. **B,** The prepared device.

STEPS	RATIONALE
(7) Regulate the IV infusion rate to allow the medication to infuse in the time recommended by institutional policy, a pharmacist, or a medication reference manual.	• For optimal therapeutic effect, the medication should infuse in the prescribed time interval.
(8) Label the Volutrol with the name of the medication, the dosage, the total volume (including the diluent), and the time of administration.	• Proper labelling alerts nurses to medication being infused and prevents other medications from being added to the Volutrol.
(9) Dispose of the uncapped needle or the needle enclosed in safety shield and syringe in a proper container. Perform hand hygiene.	• Proper disposal prevents accidental needle-stick injuries. Hand hygiene reduces the transmission of microorganisms.
C. Mini-infusion administration	
(1) Connect the prefilled syringe to the mini-infusion tubing.	• The special tubing is designed to fit the syringe to deliver the medication to the main IV line.
(2) Carefully apply pressure to the syringe plunger, allowing the tubing to fill with medication.	• Applying pressure ensures that the tubing is free of air bubbles to prevent an air embolus.

STEPS	RATIONALE
(3) Place the syringe into a mini-infusor pump (follow product directions). Ensure the syringe is secure (see Step 15C[3] illustration).	

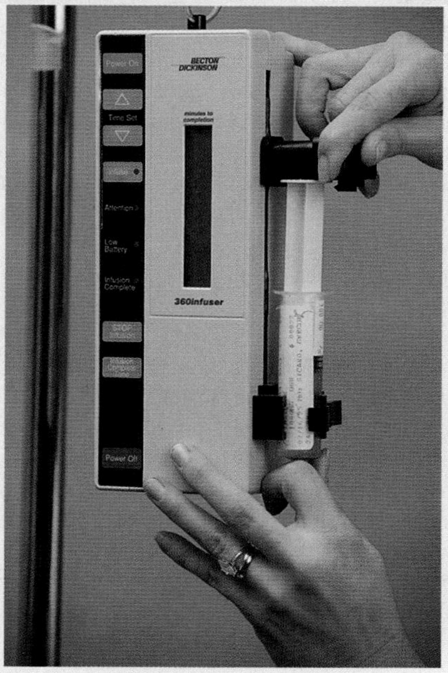

STEP 15C(3) Securing the syringe into a mini-infusor.

STEPS	RATIONALE
(4) Connect the mini-infusion tubing to the main IV line.	
(a) *Stopcock:* Wipe the stopcock port with an alcohol swab and connect the tubing. Turn the stopcock to the open position.	• Use of the stopcock reduces the risk of needle-stick injuries.
(b) *Needleless system:* Wipe the needleless port and insert the tip of the mini-infusor tubing.	
(c) *Tubing port:* Connect the sterile needle to the mini-infusion tubing, remove the cap, clean the injection port on the main IV line, and insert the needle through the centre of the port. Consider placing tape where the IV tubing enters the port to secure the connection.	• Cleaning reduces the transmission of microorganisms.
(5) Explain the purpose of the medication and the adverse effects to the patient and explain that the medication is to be given through the existing IV line. Ask the patient to report any symptoms of discomfort at the IV site.	• Proper communication informs the patient of planned therapies.
(6) Hang the infusion pump with the syringe on the IV pole alongside the main IV bag. Set the pump to deliver medication within the time recommended by institutional policy, the pharmacist, or a medication reference manual. Press the button on the pump to begin infusion. Optional: Set the alarm.	• The pump automatically delivers medication at a safe, constant rate, on the basis of the volume in the syringe. (An alarm is used if the medication is delivered into a heparin or saline lock.)
(7) After medication has infused, check the flow regulator on the primary infusion. The infusion should automatically begin to flow once the pump stops. Regulate the main infusion line to the desired rate as needed. (Note: If the stopcock is used, turn off the mini-infusion line.)	• Proper flow maintains the patency of primary IV line.
16. Observe the patient for signs of adverse reactions.	• IV medications act rapidly.
17. During infusion, periodically check the infusion rate and the condition of the IV site.	• The IV must remain patent for proper medication administration. If infiltration develops, discontinue the infusion.
18. Ask the patient to explain the purpose and side effects of the medication.	• Asking the patient about the medication evaluates the patient's understanding of the instructions.

Continued

SKILL 34-8 ADMINISTERING INTRAVENOUS MEDICATIONS BY PIGGYBACK, INTERMITTENT INTRAVENOUS INFUSION SETS, AND MINI-INFUSION PUMPS—cont'd

UNEXPECTED OUTCOMES	RELATED INTERVENTIONS
Adverse drug reaction	• Stop medication infusion immediately. • Follow institutional policy or guidelines for the appropriate response, assessments, and reporting of adverse drug reactions. • Notify the patient's health care provider of adverse effects immediately. • Document the allergy in the patient's medical record.
Medication does not infuse over desired period	• Determine the reason for the lack of infusion (e.g., improper calculation of flow rate, wrong positioning of the IV needle at the insertion site, or infiltration). • Take corrective action as indicated.
Swelling, warmth, reddening, and tenderness at intravenous site, indicating phlebitis (see Chapter 40)	• Stop IV infusion. • Discontinue IV. • Treat the IV site as indicated by the institutional policy. • Select a new IV site if continuation of therapy is indicated.
Coolness, pallor, and swelling at intravenous site (see Chapter 40)	• Signs of infiltration are indicated. • Some IV medications are extremely harmful to subcutaneous tissue. • Provide IV extravasation care as indicated by institutional policy; or use a medication reference manual or consult a pharmacist to determine the appropriate follow-up care.

RECORDING AND REPORTING

- Record the medication, dose, route, and time administered on the MAR or computer printout.
- Record the intake and output from the volume of fluid in the medication bag or Volutrol.
- Report any adverse reactions to the nurse in charge or the physician.

HOME CARE CONSIDERATIONS

- Teach the patient and caregiver to dispose of needles and contaminated equipment in puncture-proof containers (e.g., a coffee can).
- Instruct the patient's family about community resources for obtaining supplies.
- Collaborate with the interdisciplinary team to facilitate access to supplies for patients who have both physical and geographical barriers.

Administration of IV Therapy in the Home. Sometimes patients are discharged from an acute care setting and continue to receive IV therapy in the home setting. Medications such as antibiotics, chemotherapy, total parenteral nutrition, pain medications, and blood transfusions may be given in the home. Most patients who have home IV therapy will have a central venous catheter inserted before their discharge (see Chapter 40). In addition, patients who need to receive IV therapy in the home have home care nurses who assist in the management of the IV therapy.

However, patients and their families need to be carefully assessed for their ability to manage this therapy at home. Instruction on IV care management must be provided while the patient is still in the hospital. Patients and their families need to be taught how to recognize problems and what to do when these problems occur. It is important for the patient's family to recognize signs of infection and complications and to know that when these signs occur, the home care nurse or physician must be notified. In addition, patients and their families need information regarding the maintenance of IV administration equipment, including the infusion pump.

Subcutaneous Butterfly Catheters. Subcutaneous butterfly catheters provide a route for both subcutaneous medication administration and hypodermoclysis (Box 34-29). As a route for medication administration, subcutaneous butterfly catheters reduce the frequency of breaking the skin barrier to inject a medication. This route is used for patients requiring longer-term therapy with medication that is administered via subcutaneous injection. **Hypodermoclysis** is the administration of fluids through a butterfly catheter and is commonly used for patients with limited IV access, palliative care patients, and patients at risk for or with mild dehydration.

A fine-gauge needle (e.g., 24-gauge) is inserted into the patient's subcutaneous tissue. The preferred site for subcutaneous butterfly catheters is the subcutaneous tissue of the abdomen. Other appropriate sites include the subcutaneous tissue of the upper arms, upper back (scapular area), anterior thighs, and the anterior upper chest (avoiding the breast and axilla). A subcutaneous butterfly catheter must not be inserted into tissues that have recently been irradiated or where a rash, bruising, or scar tissue is present. After inserting a subcutaneous butterfly catheter, only one type of medication can be injected (e.g., morphine).

Contraindications to using the hypodermoclysis route for IV fluid administration include cardiac failure, prerenal or renal failure, low platelet or coagulation disorders, and existing fluid overload or marked edema (see Chapter 40). If a patient is severely dehydrated, the IV route is preferred for fluid administration.

BOX 34-29 PROCEDURAL GUIDELINE

Subcutaneous Butterfly Catheters and Hypodermoclysis

Delegation Considerations:

The insertion of subcutaneous butterfly catheters cannot be delegated. Instruct unregulated care providers to report the occurrence of adverse effects of medications immediately.

Equipment:

- Butterfly catheter with 24-gauge, 19-mm needle (the smallest and shortest gauge should be used)
- Interline injection site
- Antiseptic swab
- Occlusive dressing (Tegaderm or Opsite)
- Tape
- Clean gloves

Subcutaneous Medication Administration

- Ordered medication
- Syringe and needleless access device

Hypodermoclysis

- Ordered intravenous (IV) fluid
- IV administration set

Procedure:

1. Check the accuracy and completeness of each medication administration record (MAR) or computer printout against the prescriber's original medication order. Check the patient's name and the medication name, route, dosage, and time of administration. Copy or rewrite any portion of the MAR that is difficult to read.
2. Assess the patient's medical history, medication history, and history of allergies; know the substances the patient is allergic to and the allergic reaction.
3. Check the date of expiration for the medication.
4. Assess the adequacy of adipose tissue and any contraindications, such as rash, bruising, or scar tissue.
5. Remove the butterfly catheter from the package (see Step 5 illustration). Replace the existing cap with an interlink injection site.
6. *Subcutaneous medication administration:* Aseptically prepare the correct medication dose from an ampule or vial (see Skill 34-4). Ensure all air is expelled. Check the label of the medication with the MAR two times while preparing the medication. Replace the needle with a needleless injection device, clean the interlink injection port with an aseptic swab, and prime the subcutaneous catheter tubing.
   Hypodermoclysis: Attach the IV line to the interlink injection site on the subcutaneous butterfly catheter device and prime the unit.

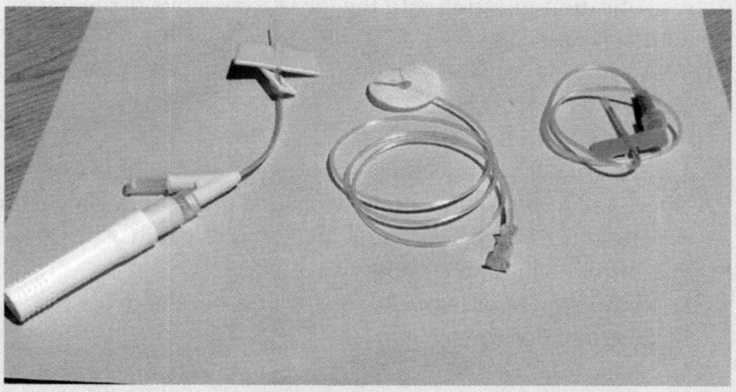

STEP 5 Subcutaneous butterfly catheters. (Courtesy Lynne Thibeault, Confederation College, Thunder Bay, ON.)

7. Take the medication to the patient at the right time, and perform hand hygiene.
8. Close the room curtain or door to provide privacy.
9. Identify the patient, using at least two identifiers. Compare the patient's name and one other identifier (e.g., the hospital identification number) on the MAR, computer printout, or computer screen against information on the patient's identification bracelet. Ask the patient to state his or her name, if possible, as a third identifier.
10. Compare the label of the medication with the MAR one more time at the patient's bedside.
11. Explain to the patient the steps of the procedure and the sensations to expect, including a slight burning or stinging when the catheter is inserted. Inform the patient that the catheter will remain and will be used for medication administration of a particular medication.
12. Keep a sheet or gown draped over the body parts not requiring exposure.
13. Apply clean gloves.
14. Select an appropriate injection site. Inspect the skin surface over the sites for bruises, inflammation, or edema.
15. Palpate the sites for masses or tenderness. Avoid these areas.
16. Assist the patient into a comfortable position; have the patient relax the abdomen, thigh, or upper arm, depending on selected site.
17. Locate the site using appropriate anatomical landmarks.
18. Clean the site with an antiseptic swab. Apply the swab at the centre of the site and rotate outward in a circular direction for about 5 cm.
19. Remove the sheath from the catheter needle by pulling it straight off.
20. Hold the subcutaneous butterfly wings between the thumb and forefinger of your dominant hand with the palm down.
21. Ensure that the bevel of the needle is pointed upward.
22. Using the thumb and index finger of your nondominant hand, gently pinch the patient's skin around the selected injection site to create a roll of skin 1.25 to 2.5 cm in diameter.
23. Insert the full length of the needle through the skin at a 30-degree angle.
24. Assess for blood return into the catheter tubing. If blood return occurs, withdraw the needle and repeat the procedure at a new site.
25. Release the catheter wings and stabilize them on the skin surface with your thumb and index finger.
26. Apply an occlusive dressing (e.g., Tegaderm, Opsite) over the insertion site and some of the tubing. Reinforce the dressing with tape.
27. Apply a label to the occlusive dressing that shows the date and time of administration and your initials.
28. *Subcutaneous medication administration:* Wipe the interlink injection port with an antiseptic swab and administer the medication.
    Hypodermoclysis: Adjust the flow rate of IV fluids according to the physician's order.
29. Dispose of the syringe with the needleless injection device into a sharps container.
30. Remove gloves and discard. Perform hand hygiene.
31. Document the procedure, including the site, type, and gauge of subcutaneous butterfly catheter; the date and time of insertion; the patient's response to the insertion; and your initials.

KEY CONCEPTS

- Learning the medication classifications improves a nurse's understanding of nursing implications for administering medications with similar characteristics.
- Federal medication legislation regulates the production, distribution, prescription, and administration of medications.
- All controlled substances are handled according to strict procedures that account for each medication.
- The nurse applies his or her understanding of the physiology of medication action when physically assessing a patient before medication, timing the administration, selecting routes, initiating actions to promote medication efficacy, and observing responses to medications.
- The older person's body undergoes structural and functional changes that alter medication actions and influence the way in which medication therapy is provided.
- Children's medication doses are computed on the basis of body surface area and weight.
- Medications given parenterally are absorbed more quickly than medications administered by other routes.
- Each medication order should include the patient's name; the order date; the medication name, dosage, route, time of administration, and indication; and the prescriber's signature.
- A medication history reveals allergies, medications that the patient is taking, and the patient's compliance with therapy.
- The nursing process should be used when administering medication.
- The rights of medication administration ensure accurate preparation and administration of medication doses.
- The rights of medication administration are the right medication, right dose, right patient, right route, right time and frequency, right documentation, and right reason, right evaluation (or assessment), right patient education, and right to refuse.
- The nurse should administer only the medications that he or she prepares; prepared medications must never be left unattended.
- The nurse needs to avoid distractions and follow the same routines when preparing medications to reduce the chance of medication errors.
- Needles should never be recapped.
- To prevent medication errors, the nurse must document immediately all medications he or she administers.
- The nurse must use clinical judgement to determine the best time to administer "prn" (when needed) medications.
- Medication errors must be reported immediately.
- When preparing medications, the nurse checks the medication container label against the medication administration record three times.
- The Z-track method for intramuscular injections protects the subcutaneous tissues from irritating parenteral fluids.
- Failure to select injection sites by anatomical landmarks may lead to tissue, bone, or nerve damage.

CRITICAL THINKING EXERCISES

1. Mrs. Nguyen, a 69-year-old woman, has recently experienced a stroke and has right-sided weakness. The neurological clinical nurse specialist wrote orders to start oral medications today. What steps do you take to ensure that this patient can safely receive her oral medications? What do you do if the patient is unable to swallow?
2. Marissa is a 25-year-old woman who recently delivered a healthy infant. She is to receive WinRho 300 mcg IM today. What size needle and which injection site and technique do you use to administer this medication?
3. Jack, a 70-year-old retired farmer, has been experiencing new respiratory difficulties. His physician has ordered him to start using an albuterol inhaler with a spacer. What steps do you take to ensure that he can self-administer his metered-dose inhaler?
4. You receive an order to give furosemide (Lasix) 40 mg IV push. You have never given this medication on this unit. What steps do you take before administering the Lasix?

REVIEW QUESTIONS

1. Which of the following rights is the most recent right to be added to the list of rights of medication administration?
   1. Right to refuse
   2. Right route
   3. Right medication
   4. Right patient
2. The nurse is having difficulty reading a physician's order for a medication. She knows the physician is very busy and does not like to be called. What does the nurse do?
   1. Call a pharmacist to interpret the order.
   2. Call the physician to have the order clarified.
   3. Consult the unit manager to help interpret the order.
   4. Ask the unit secretary to interpret the physician's handwriting.
3. A patient has a gastrointestinal alteration. Which method of medication administration should *not* be used?
   1. Oral
   2. Topical
   3. Inhalation
   4. Injection
4. Most medication errors occur when the nurse:
   1. Fails to follow routine procedures
   2. Is responsible for administering numerous medications
   3. Is caring for too many patients
   4. Is administering unfamiliar medications
5. A patient is to receive cephalexin (Keflex) 500 mg PO. The pharmacy has sent 250 mg tablets. How many tablets should the nurse give?
   1. 0.5 tablet
   2. 1 tablet
   3. 1.5 tablets
   4. 2 tablets
6. A medication injection into the loose connective tissue under the dermis is known as what kind of injection?
   1. An intramuscular injection
   2. An intravenous injection
   3. A subcutaneous injection
   4. An intradermal injection
7. Nurses are responsible for following legal provisions when administering controlled substances or narcotics. What may be the result of a nurse's failure to comply?
   1. Fines, imprisonment, and loss of nurse licensure
   2. Loss of employment
   3. Medication errors
   4. Poor health outcomes resulting from narcotic use
8. Pharmacokinetics is the study of how medications:
   1. Are derived from plants
   2. Enter the body, reach their site of action, are metabolized, and exit the body
   3. Are used for certain disease processes
   4. Are manufactured and distributed to pharmaceutical companies

9. Which of the following is an official publication that sets standards for medication strength, quality, purity, packaging, safety, labelling, and dose form?
   1. *Physicians Reference Guide*
   2. *Nurse's Drug Guide*
   3. *Narcotic Control Act*
   4. *The Canadian Formulary (CF)*
10. Who is responsible for the administration of the *Food and Drugs Act* and the *Controlled Drugs and Substances Act*?
    1. Health Protection Branch (HPB)
    2. Nurse or physician dispensing and prescribing medications
    3. *Canadian Formulary*
    4. Health care institutions

Answers: 1. 1; **2.** 2; **3.** 1; **4.** 1; **5.** 4; **6.** 3; **7.** 1; **8.** 2; **9.** 4; **10.** 1

Rationales for the Review Questions appear at the end of the book.

RECOMMENDED WEBSITES

Canadian Pharmacists Association: http://www.pharmacists.ca
The Canadian Pharmacists Association (CPhA) is a national organization of pharmacists. CPhA's website provides links to drug information, patient information, and resources.

Institute for Safe Medication Practices (ISMP) Canada: https://www.ismp-canada.org/index.htm
This website has information about medication error prevention and reporting as well as information about products and educational programs about medication safety.

Health Canada: Drug Product Database: http://www.hc-sc.gc.ca/dhp-mps/prodpharma/databasdon/index-eng.php/
This website provides access to government reports, resources, and programs about the safety and effectiveness of pharmaceutical drugs and other therapeutic products.

Health Canada: Therapeutic Products Directorate: http://www.hc-sc.gc.ca/ahc-asc/branch-dirgen/hpfb-dgpsa/tpd-dpt/index-eng.php
Health Canada's Therapeutic Products Directorate is the Canadian federal authority that regulates pharmaceutical drugs and medical devices for human use. This website provides access to information on reporting adverse reaction information.

University of Saskatchewan: medSask: http://medsask.usask.ca/
medSask, operating from the University of Saskatchewan, aims to give health care providers and laypersons access to objective and concise information on drugs and drug therapy.

REFERENCES

Akbari Sari, A., Janani, L., Mohammady, M., et al. (2014). Slow versus fast subcutaneous heparin injections for preventing bruising and site-pain intensity. *The Cochrane Database of Systematic Reviews*, (7), CD008077, doi:10.1002/14651858.CD008007.pub3.

Annersten, M., & Willman, A. (2005). Performing subcutaneous injections: A literature review. *Worldviews on Evidence-based Nursing*, *2*(3), 122–130. doi:10.1111/j.1741-6787.2005.00030.x.

Bastable, S. (2013). *Nurse as educator: Principles of teaching and learning for nursing practice* (4th ed.). Sudbury, MA: Jones & Bartlett.

Brager, R., & Soland, E. (2005). The spectrum of polypharmacy. *Nurse Practitioner*, *30*(6), 44–50. doi:10.1097/00006205-200506000-00008.

Canadian Centre for Occupational Health and Safety (CCOHS). (2014). *Needlestick injuries*. Retrieved from http://www.ccohs.ca/oshanswers/diseases/needlestick_injuries.html.

Canadian Diabetes Association Clinical Practice Guidelines Expert Committee. (2013). Canadian Diabetes Association 2013 clinical practice guidelines for the prevention and management of diabetes in Canada. *Canadian Journal of Diabetes*, *37*(Suppl. 1), S1–S212.

Canadian Lung Association. (n.d.). *How to use your inhaler*. Retrieved from https://www.lung.ca/lung-health/get-help/how-use-your-inhaler.

Canadian Nurses Association (CNA). (2017). *Code of ethics for registered nurses*. Ottawa: Author.

Capriotti, T. (2005). Changes in inhaler devices for asthma and COPD. *Medsurg News*, *14*(3), 185–194.

College and Association of Registered Nurses of Alberta. (2015). *Medication guidelines*. Retrieved from http://www.nurses.ab.ca/content/dam/carna/pdfs/DocumentList/Guidelines/MedicationGuidelines_Mar2015.pdf.

College of Nurses of Ontario. (2017). *Practice standard: Medication*. Retrieved from http://www.cno.org/globalassets/docs/prac/41007_medication.pdf.

Cook, I. F., & Murtagh, J. (2006). Ventrogluteal area: A suitable site for intramuscular vaccination of infants and toddlers. *Vaccine*, *24*(13), 2403–2408. doi:10.1016/j.vaccine.2005.11.065.

Davidson, K., & Rourke, L. (2013). Teaching best-evidence: deltoid intramuscular injection technique. *Journal of Nursing Education and Practice*, *3*(7), 122.

Dayananda, L., Belaval, V. V., Raina, A., et al. (2014). Intended intramuscular gluteal injections: are they truly intramuscular? *Journal of Postgraduate Medicine*, *60*(2), 175–178. doi:10.4103/0022-3858.132334.

Frid, A., Hirsch, L., Gaspar, R., et al. (2010). New injection recommendations for patients with diabetes. *Diabetes & Metabolism*, *36*(Suppl. 2), S3–S18. doi:10.1016/S1262-3636(10)70002-1.

Health Canada. (2004). *Trends in workplace injuries, illnesses, and policies in healthcare across Canada*. Ottawa: Author. Retrieved from http://www.hc-sc.gc.ca/hcs-sss/pubs/hhrhs/2004-hwi-ipsmt/index-eng.php.

Hockenberry, M. J., & Wilson, D. (2014). *Wong's nursing care of infants and children* (10th ed.). St. Louis, MO: Mosby.

Hopkins, U., & Arias, C. (2013). Large-volume IM injections: a review of best practices. *OncologyNurseAdvisor.com*, 32–37. Retrieved from http://www.oncologynurseadvisor.com/chemotherapy/large-volume-im-injections-a-review-of-best-practices/article/281208/. January/February 2013.

Hughes, R. G., & Ortiz, E. (2005). Medication errors: Why they happen, and how they can be prevented. *American Journal of Nursing*, *105*(3), 14–24.

Hunter, J. (2008). Subcutaneous injection technique. *Nursing Standard*, *21*(22), 41–44.

Institute for Safe Medication Practices. (2006). Tablet splitting: Do it only if you "half" to, and then do it safely. *ISMP Medication Safety Alert!* Retrieved from https://www.ismp.org/newsletters/acutecare/articles/20060518.asp.

Institute for Safe Medication Practices. (2007). Patches: What you can't see can harm patients. *Nurse Advise-ERR*, *5*(4), 1.

Institute for Safe Medication Practices. (2015). *ISMP list of error-prone abbreviations, symbols, and dosage designations*. Retrieved from http://www.ismp.org/Tools/errorproneabbreviations.pdf.

Institute of Medicine. (2003). *Report brief. To err is human: Building a safer health system*. Retrieved from http://www.nationalacademies.org/hmd/~/media/Files/Report%20Files/1999/To-Err-is-Human/To%20Err%20is%20Human%201999%20%20report%20brief.pdf.

Joint Commission. (2017). *2018 national patient safety goals*. Retrieved from https://www.jointcommission.org/standards_information/npsgs.aspx.

Kara, D., Uzelli, D., & Karaman, D. (2015). Using ventrogluteal site in intramuscular injections is a priority or an alternative? *International Journal of Caring Sciences*, *8*(2), 507–513.

Karch, A. M., & Karch, F. E. (2003). Not so fast! IV push drugs can be dangerous when given too rapidly. *American Journal of Nursing*, *103*(8), 71.

King, L. (2003). Subcutaneous insulin injection technique. *Nursing Standard*, *17*(34), 45–52.

Lapkin, S., Levett-Jones, T., Chenoweth, L., et al. (2016). The effectiveness of interventions designed to reduce medication administration errors: a synthesis of findings from systematic reviews. *Journal of Nursing Management*, *24*(7), 845–858. doi:10.1111/jonm.12390.

MacDonald, M. (2010). Patient safety: Examining the adequacy of the 5 rights of medication administration. *Clinical Nurse Specialist*, *24*(4), 196–203. doi:10.1097/NUR.0b013e3181e3605f.

Manno, M. S. (2006). Preventing adverse drug events. *Nursing*, *36*(3), 56–61.

Mayo, A., & Duncan, D. (2004). Nurse perceptions of medication errors: what we need to know for patient safety. *Journal of Nursing Care Quality*, *19*(3), 209–217.

MayoClinic.com. (2016). *Asthma*. Retrieved from http://www.mayoclinic.com/health/asthma/DS00021.

McCulloch, D. (2016). General principles of insulin therapy in diabetes mellitus. *UpToDate, 2015*. Retrieved from http://www.uptodate.com/contents/general-principles-of-insulin-therapy-in-diabetes-mellitus.

McKenry, L. M., Tessier, E., & Hogan, M. A. (2005). *Mosby's pharmacology in nursing* (22nd ed.). St. Louis, MO: Mosby.

Meiner, S. (2014). *Gerontologic nursing* (5th ed.). St. Louis, MO: Mosby.

Metheny, N. A. (2006). Preventing aspiration in older adults with dysphagia. *Medsurg Nursing*, *15*(2), 110–111.

Mills, P. D., Neily, J., Mims, E., et al. (2006). Improving the bar-coded administration system at the Department of Veteran Affairs. *American Journal of Health Systems and Pharmacy*, *63*(15), 1442–1447.

Morris, H. (2006). Managing dysphagia in older people. *Primary Health Care, 16*(6), 34–36.
National Coordinating Council for Medication Error Reporting and Prevention. (2015). *Council recommendations to reduce medication errors associated with verbal medication orders and prescriptions*. Retrieved from http://www.nccmerp.org/recommendations-reduce-medication-errors-associated-verbal-medication-orders-and-prescriptions.
Nicoll, L. H., & Hesby, A. (2002). Intramuscular injection: An integrative research review and guideline for evidence-based practice. *Applied Nursing Research, 15*(3), 149–162.
Niemann, D., Bertsche, A., Meyrath, D., et al. (2015). A prospective three-step intervention study to prevent medication errors in drug handling in paediatric care. *Journal of Clinical Nursing, 24*(1–2), 101–114. doi:10.1111/jocn.12592.
Occupational Safety and Health Administration (OSHA). (n.d.). *Bloodborne pathogens and needlestick prevention*. Retrieved from https://www.osha.gov/SLTC/bloodbornepathogens/.
Ogston-Tuck, S. (2014). Intramuscular injection technique: an evidence-based approach. *Nursing Standard, 29*(4), 52–59. doi:10.7748/ns.29.4.52.e9183.
Paoletti, R. D., Suess, T. M., Lesco, M. G., et al. (2007). Using bar-code technology and medication observation methodology for safer medication administration. *American Journal of Health Systems Pharmacy, 64*(5), 536–543. doi:10.2146/ajhp060140.
Pape, T. M., Guerra, D. M., Muzquiz, M., et al. (2005). Innovative approaches to reducing nurses' distractions during medication administration. *Journal of Continuing Nursing Education, 36*(3), 108–116.
Parry, A., Barriball, K., & While, A. (2015). Factors contributing to registered nurse medication administration error: a narrative review. *International Journal of Nursing Studies, 52*(1), 403–420. doi:10.1016/j.ijnurstu.2014.07.003.
Ptasinski, C. (2007). Develop a medication reconciliation process. *Nurse Manager, 38*(3), 18.
Public Health Agency of Canada. (2014). *Routine practices and additional precautions for preventing the transmission of infection in health care [Electronic version]* (pp. 1–195). Ottawa: Public Health Agency of Canada. Retrieved from http://www.phac-aspc.gc.ca/nois-sinp/guide/summary-sommaire/tihs-tims-eng.php.
Raban, M., & Westbrook, J. (2014). Are interventions to reduce interruptions and errors during medication administration effective? A systematic review. *BMJ Quality and Safety, 23*(5), 414–421. doi:10.1136/bmjqs-2013-002118.
Rushing, J. (2004). Clinical do's and don'ts. How to administer a subcutaneous injection. *Nursing, 34*(6), 32.
Safe Medication (n.d.). *How to use eye drops properly*. Retrieved from http://www.safemedication.com/safemed/MedicationTipsTools/HowtoAdminister/HowtoUseEyeDropsProperly.aspx.
Sanofi. (2016). *Lovenox subcutaneous injection*. Retrieved from http://www.lovenox.com/hcp_default.aspx.
Saskatchewan Registered Nurses' Association. (2015). *Medication management for RNs: A patient-centred decision-making framework*. Retrieved from http://www.srna.org/images/stories/Nursing_Practice/Resources/Medication_Management_for_RNs_FINAL_2015_09_03_Rev_2015_09_30_Web.pdf.
Sisson, H. (2015). Aspirating during the intramuscular injection procedure: a systematic literature review. *Journal of Clinical Nursing, 24*(17–18), 2368–2375. doi:10.1111/jocn.12824.
Skibinski, K. A., White, B. A., Lin, L., et al. (2007). Effects of technological interventions on the safety of a medication-use system. *American Journal of Health Systems Pharmacy, 64*(1), 90–96. doi:10.2146/ajhp060060.
Small, S. P. (2004). Preventing sciatic nerve injury from intramuscular injections: Literature review. *Journal of Advanced Nursing, 47*(3), 287–296. doi:10.1111/j.1365-2648.03092.x.
Stein, H. G. (2006). Glass ampules and filter needles: An example of implementing the sixth "R" in medication administration. *Medsurg Nursing, 15*(5), 290–294.
Touhy, T., Jett, K., Boscart, V., et al. (2012). *Ebersole and Hess' gerontological nursing and healthy aging* (Canadian ed.). Toronto: Elsevier Canada.
Vella, C., & Grech, V. (2005). Assessment of use of spacer devices for inhaled drug delivery to asthmatic children. *Pediatric Allergy and Immunology, 16*(3), 258–261. doi:10.1111/j.1399-3038.2005.00253.x.
Wolf, Z. R., Hicks, R., & Serembus, J. F. (2006). Characteristics of medication errors made by students during the administration phase: A descriptive study. *Journal of Professional Nursing, 22*(1), 39–51. doi:10.1016/j.profnurs.2005.12.008.
World Health Organization (WHO). (2016). *WHO guideline on the use of safety-engineered syringes for intramuscular, intradermal and subcutaneous injections in health care settings*. Retrieved from http://apps.who.int/iris/bitstream/10665/250144/1/9789241549820-eng.pdf?
World Health Organization (WHO). (2014). *The high 5s project standard operation protocol: Assuring medication accuracy at transitions in care: Medication reconciliation*. Retrieved from http://www.who.int/patientsafety/implementation/solutions/high5s/h5s-sop.pdf.

35

Complementary and Alternative Approaches in Health Care

Written by Deborah Gibson, RN, MSN

OBJECTIVES

Mastery of content in this chapter will enable you to:

- Define the key terms listed.
- Identify the differences between complementary and alternative approaches in health care.
- Describe the various treatments associated with complementary and alternative medicine.
- Explain the scope of naturopathic and chiropractic medicine.
- Understand how complementary and alternative approaches assist in health promotion and disease prevention.
- Recognize botanical treatments as an approach to complementary and alternative medicine.
- Understand the nurse's role in interprofessional collaboration in relation to complementary and alternative medicine.

KEY TERMS

Acupoints, p. 823
Acupuncture, p. 823
Allopathic medicine, p. 815
Alternative approaches, p. 816
Biofeedback, p. 822
Botanicals, p. 824
Chiropractic medicine, p. 822
Complementary and alternative medicine (CAM), p. 815
Complementary approaches, p. 816
Complementary health care, p. 815
Energy flow, p. 823
Holistic health, p. 815
Imagery, p. 821
Integrative medicine, p. 816
Meditation, p. 821
Meridians, p. 823
Mindfulness, p. 818
Natural health products, p. 825
Naturopathic medicine, p. 823
Nutrition, p. 824
Prayer, p. 818
Qi, p. 823
Relaxation, p. 821
Stress response, p. 821
Therapeutic touch, p. 822
Traditional Chinese medicine (TCM), p. 822
Yin and yang, p. 822
Yoga, p. 818

MEDIA RESOURCES

http://evolve.elsevier.com/Canada/Potter/fundamentals/

- Audio Chapter Summaries
- Examination Review Questions
- Concept Map Creator
- Case Study with Questions
- Audio Glossary
- Content Updates
- Video Clips

Interest in wellness and integrative medicine has been gaining momentum in Canada, with an increasing number of Canadians turning to complementary health care options including **complementary and alternative medicine (CAM)** approaches for the treatment of chronic pain, health concerns, and health promotion (Dewar, Gregg, White, et al., 2009; Hollenberg, Tsasis & Kelley, 2011; Keshet, Ben-Ayre, & Schiff, 2012; Public Health Agency of Canada [PHAC], 2008; Singer & Adams, 2011, 2014). The philosophy of **holistic health** is not new. "Health is derived from the old English word *Hal* which means whole, soundness or spiritual wellness" (Micozzi, 2015; Rakel & Weil, 2012, p. 6). Holistic health takes into account all aspects of a person's psychological, physical, spiritual, and social needs. Aristotle first proposed that the body and mind could not be separated and that a healer must observe and reflect upon the total person. Ancient civilizations dating from 5000 B.C., including the Egyptians and Chinese, were employing and recording the effects of various herbal and energy healing traditions on the body. Despite the Dark Ages (1493–1541), characterized by a loss of interest in science and an increase in magic to explain the world environment, interest in the human condition continued to grow. The roots of twentieth-century conventional medicine (**allopathic medicine**) can be traced to René Descartes (1595–1650), a deeply religious mathematician and philosopher who believed that the mind and body must be separated to protect the "spirit" from scientific inquiry. Consequently, the development of medicine focused exclusively on physical function and reduction of the larger whole into examination of the smaller parts (Rakel & Weil, 2012). This is still evident, as seen by the various fields of specialization that occur within modern medical practices. Florence Nightingale (1820–1910), the founder of modern nursing, practised a holistic approach to health. She incorporated various healing modalities along with cleanliness, sanitation, fresh air, light, and compassionate and spiritual care while providing nursing care to soldiers during the Crimean War.

At the middle of the twentieth century, broad cultural shifts and paradigm changes occurred in Canada. Social activism grew, and attitudes toward traditional health care delivery systems changed. These social movements coincided with demographic changes, increased cultural diversity, and global mobility. Ultimately, these forces led consumer interest toward a person-centred, empowered approach to health. People desired a different kind of health care: one that embraced healing, acknowledgement of the spiritual dimensions of health and illness, and openness toward alternative medical systems. A variety of heath care systems highlight the importance of imbalance as opposed to disease, with the goal of restoring balance (Cassidy, 2015). Today, the public has enormous access to information and to organizations that promote personal, holistic, complementary, and integrative health through the Internet (e.g., http://www.chna.ca; http://www.cand.ca/; http://www.chiropractic.ca).

COMPLEMENTARY, ALTERNATIVE, AND INTEGRATIVE APPROACHES IN HEALTH CARE

CAM approaches complement conventional medicine and include numerous care approaches based on paradigms of health and healing. CAM approaches are primarily focused on the underlying causes of illness and imbalance in the body instead of on disease symptoms (Micozzi, 2015). While CAM approaches of Indigenous healing, traditional Chinese medicine, chiropractic, naturopathic medicine, massage, and relaxation therapy offer a wide range of complexity in their approach to health, these approaches share and emphasize the medical model of wellness (Micozzi, 2015). Common characteristics of CAM approaches are listed in Box 35-1.

The terms *complementary* and *alternative* are often used interchangeably and as an "adjunct to" as opposed to a "replacement for conventional medical care" (Micozzi, 2015, p. 13). **Complementary approaches** align with or contribute to and enhance conventional medical treatments, whereas **alternative approaches** may be used instead of a conventional medical treatment (Micozzi, 2015). Many complementary approaches, such as naturopathic and chiropractic medicine, require diagnostic and therapeutic treatments specific to their discipline, whereas other complementary approaches, such as imagery, do not require diagnostic examination. It is important for nurses to be knowledgeable about the safety and efficacy of the various CAM approaches in order to advise and support patients in their decision making. According to Thomson, Jones, Browne, and colleagues (2014), age, education, perceived control over health, and spirituality are important predictors of exploring CAM before conventional medicine.

CAM approaches have become a growing consumer movement, with favourable patient-reported outcomes (Micozzi, 2015). CAM is often used interchangeably with integrative medicine; however these terms are not synonymous. **Integrative medicine** or health care is a combination of best practices from conventional, complementary, and alternative approaches (National Center for Complementary and Integrative Health [NCCIH], 2016; Rakel & Weil, 2012) in which health and healing can be facilitated with safety and effectiveness (Koopsen & Young, 2009; Young & Koopsen, 2009). One major premise of this concept is the belief that all health care providers must provide the best treatment for their patients while respecting their health care choices. In this way, integrative medicine focuses on healing, rather than disease, and allows for interdisciplinary care.

Complementary and alternative approaches are often organized into six categories that researchers find useful (Box 35-2). Some categories and examples of complementary and alternative approaches

BOX 35-1 Characteristics of CAM Approaches

- Complementary and alternative medicine (CAM) approaches:
  - Work in conjunction with the body's own self-healing mechanisms
  - Are "holistic" (i.e., they view the whole person as unique with his or her own inner resources)
  - Focus on disease prevention and well-being
- Nutrition and natural products are fundamental to maintain tissue and cell growth.
- Each person's body heals itself. The focus is on the healed body instead of the healer.
- Knowledge is shared between the patient and the practitioner. Both are active participants in the interaction.

From Micozzi, M. S. (2015). Translation from conventional medicine. In M. S. Micozzi, *Fundamentals of complementary and alternative medicine* (5th ed., pp. 13–21). St. Louis, MO: Saunders; Health Canada. (2003, November). Complementary and alternative health care: The other mainstream? *Health Policy Research Bulletin, 7*. Ottawa: Author. Retrieved from http://www.hc-sc.gc.ca/sr-sr/alt_formats/hpb-dgps/pdf/pubs/hpr-rps/bull/2003-7-complement/2003-7-complement-eng.pdf.

BOX 35-2 Categories and Examples of Complementary and Alternative Approaches

Natural Products

Approaches use substances found in nature.

Examples: herbal medicine (botanicals), vitamins, minerals, dietary supplements, probiotics

Mind–Body Approaches

Interventions use a variety of techniques to enhance the mind's ability to affect body functions and symptoms.

Examples: imagery, meditation, yoga, music therapy, prayer, journalling, biofeedback, humour, tai chi, art therapy, acupuncture

Manipulative and Body-Based Approaches

Approaches are based on manipulation or movement of one or more parts of the body.

Examples: chiropractic medicine, massage

Energy Approaches

Approaches focus on the use of energy fields, such as magnetic and biofields, that are believed to surround and permeate the body.

Examples: healing touch, therapeutic touch, Reiki, external qi gong, magnets

Systems of Care

Whole systems of care are built on theory and practice and often evolved apart from and earlier than Western medicine. Each has its own approaches and practices.

Examples: traditional Chinese medicine, Ayurvedic medicine, naturopathy, homeopathy

Traditional Healers

Healers use methods from Indigenous theories, beliefs, and experiences. An example is the Indigenous healer or shaman.

From Lindquist, R., Snyder, M., & Tracy, M. (Eds.). (2014). *Complementary & alternative approaches in nursing* (7th ed., p. 5). New York: Springer.

are presented in Table 35-1. This list is not exhaustive and does not address issues of safety and efficacy.

Public Interest in Complementary and Alternative Medicine Approaches

Integrative medicine programs provide health care consumers with access to both allopathic and complementary practitioners. In some institutions, nurses may practise massage, reiki, and therapeutic touch. An increasing popularity and demand for alternative health care services and providers has been growing nationally and globally (Tovey, Chatwin, Masey, et al., 2003). A study released by the Fraser Institute indicated that 54% of respondents had used at least one form of complementary or alternative approach and that 74% of Canadians had used CAM at some point during their lifetime (Esmail, 2007, p. 4; Micozzi, 2015). Commonly used approaches include chiropractic and naturopathic medicine, massage, prayer, acupuncture, relaxation techniques, and botanical approaches. Furthermore, individuals with asthma, diabetes, and migraines visited a CAM provider at a

TABLE 35-1 Complementary and Alternative Approaches

Types	Mechanism or Philosophy of Action
Whole Medical Systems	
Complementary health care	A health care system augmented with approaches directed towards the underlying causes and preventative measures as opposed to only the symptoms of disease.
Complementary approaches	Health care approaches used in addition to conventional medical treatment that contribute to and/or enhance overall well-being.
Ayurveda	A traditional Hindu system of medicine that dates to ancient India. Ayurveda practitioners use a combination of remedies, such as herbs, purgatives, and oils to treat disease.
Latin American practices	The curanderismo medical system includes a humoral model (used by Hippocrates to explain disease) for classifying food, activity, drugs, illnesses, and a series of folk illnesses.
Traditional Indigenous medicine	A healing practice promotes harmony within a community and in the physical and spiritual worlds through sweating and purging, herbal remedies, and shamanic healing.
Naturopathic medicine	Naturopathic medicine views disease as a process instead of an entity, recognizing the body's inherent healing abilities. Approaches include botanical medicine, nutrition, hydrotherapy, naturopathic manipulation, traditional Chinese medicine, and acupuncture.
Traditional Chinese medicine	Traditional and systematic techniques promote health and treat disease through acupuncture, herbal remedies, massage, acupressure, qigong (balancing energy flow through movement), and moxibustion (the use of heat from burning herbs).
Biologically Based Approaches (Natural Health Products)	
Botanicals/Plants	Botanicals are used singly or in mixtures, offering a therapeutic benefit. They provide a source of nutrients, essential oils, and energy and have biomedical guidelines for nutrition and disease prevention.
Homeopathic medicines	A system of medicinal treatments based on the theory that certain diseases can be cured with small doses of substances that, in a healthy person, would produce symptoms similar to the symptoms of disease. The prescribed remedies are made from naturally occurring plant, animal, or mineral substances.
Vitamins and minerals (megavitamin therapy)	Megavitamin therapy involves the increased intake of nutrients, such as vitamins B, C, D, and beta carotene. The treatment focus is on a variety of health concerns, including cancer, schizophrenia, and coronary artery disease.
Traditional medicines (Ayurvedic remedies) (traditional Chinese herbal remedies)	Ayurvedic remedies use a combinations of herbs, purgatives, and rubbing oils to treat disease. Herbs and medicinal plants, considered the backbone of medicine, have been studied extensively.
Probiotics	These live microorganisms are orally administered to confer a protective benefit on the immune system of the small intestine.
Amino acids, essential fatty acids (EFAs), and antioxidant supplements	These products, packaged as tablets or capsules, reduce the body's inflammatory response and limit oxidative stress within the body.
Nutrition as Medicine	
Gerson therapy	Disease is believed to be caused by the accumulation of toxic substances that disrupt the body's immune system. This therapy advocates a low-salt, high-potassium organic diet of fruit juices, raw vegetables, and nutritional supplements and is primarily used in the treatment of cancer.
Macrobiotic diet	A predominantly vegan diet (white meat fish, occasional fruits, seeds, and nuts) believed to have anticancer properties. The diet consists of 40–60% whole cereal grain, 20–30% vegetables, and 5–10% beans.
Mediterranean diet	This diet, characteristic of people living in the Mediterranean region, is high in whole grains, nuts, fruits, vegetables, and omega-3 essential fatty acids, producing a protective benefit for cardiac health and various inflammatory diseases.

Continued

TABLE 35-1 Complementary and Alternative Approaches—cont'd

Types	Mechanism or Philosophy of Action
Manipulative and Body-Based Approaches	
Acupressure	A therapeutic technique, digital pressure is applied in a specified way on designated body points to relieve pain, produce analgesia, or regulate bodily function.
Chiropractic medicine	This practice emphasizes that the body has an inherent recuperative ability to restore and maintain health and well-being through the evaluation and conservative treatment of neuromuscular disorders. Care includes therapeutic adjustments of the spinal column and counselling patients on lifestyle choices of diet, nutrition, exercise, and stress management (Bergmann & Peterson, 2011).
Tai chi	This technique incorporates breath, movement, and meditation to cleanse, strengthen, and circulate vital energy and blood. Tai chi helps to stimulate the immune system and maintain balance.
Massage therapy	The manipulation of soft tissue through stroking, rubbing, or kneading increases the body's circulation and improves muscle tone and relaxation.
Simple touch	Touching the patient in appropriate, gentle ways is used to stimulate a connection, display acceptance, and give appreciation.
Mind–Body Interventions	
Aromatherapy	Essential plant oils are used to promote relaxation or stimulation, thereby enhancing overall well-being.
Art therapy	Art is used to reconcile emotional conflicts and foster self-awareness and creativity.
Biofeedback	Instruments are used to provide a person with visual or auditory information about autonomic physiological body functions, such as muscle tension, skin temperature, and brain wave activity. Biofeedback highlights the relationships between thoughts, feelings, and physiological responses.
Breath work	A variety of breathing patterns are used to relax, invigorate, or open the emotional channels. The emphasis of breath in Ayurvana uses *prana* (the essence of breath), whereas in yoga, breath control is referred to as *pranayama* (Mayor, 2015).
Dance therapy	Dance is used as an intervention for social, emotional, cognitive, or physical difficulties.
Hypnotherapy	The induction of trance states and the use of therapeutic suggestion are used to treat paralysis, headaches, addictions, pain, and phobias.
Imagery	This therapeutic technique is used to treat pathological conditions by concentrating on an image or series of images.
Labyrinth meditation	Labyrinths are ancient spiritual symbols found in religious traditions. Walking the labyrinth is regarded as a spiritual act of meditation, reflection, and prayer and as a pilgrimage.
Meditation	Meditation is a self-directed practice that relaxes the body and calms the mind by focusing on rhythmic breathing.
Mindfulness	Drawing from Buddhist psychology, **mindfulness** helps to build awareness of the present moment with an attitude of openness. "Mindfulness is a way of being in the present moment, on purpose, non-judgementally" (Kabat-Zinn, 2003, cited in Rakel & Fortney, 2012, p. 20)
Music therapy	Music therapy supports the physical, psychological, cognitive, and social needs of individuals with disabilities and illness. Music therapy is used to manage pain and to improve physical movement, communication, emotional expression, and memory.
Prayer	**Prayer** is a method of communication (verbal, silent, within a group or solitary) for one's desires and needs and is often identified as an important source of help in managing physical and spiritual pain (Clarke, 2012). A variety of techniques are used in many cultures to incorporate caring, compassion, love, and empathy.
Psychotherapy	Mental and emotional disorders are treated by the use of psychological techniques.
Yoga	**Yoga** involves exercise, poses, regulated breathing (pranayama breathing, associated with yoga practices), and meditation to attain physical and mental well-being through inner awareness and focus on the present moment and breathwork. The goal of yoga is to challenge oneself without becoming overwhelmed (Harvard Medical School, 2015). The practice focuses on the body's musculature, posture, breathing, and consciousness.
Energy Medicine	
Qigong	Qigong is derived from the ancient Chinese practice of breathing, movement, and meditation and involves the assuming of basic postures. This practice promotes strength, balance, and optimal body functioning and is used to treat stress-related conditions, fatigue, and musculoskeletal stiffness.
Reiki therapy	Reiki is derived from ancient Buddhist practices in which a practitioner places a hand on or above the body and transfers "universal life energy" to the patient. The energy from this therapy provides strength, harmony, and balance to treat health issues.
Therapeutic touch	Practitioners direct balanced energies toward the energies of a patient by laying the hands on or close to a patient's body.

significantly higher rate than did individuals within the general population (Metcalfe, Williams, McChesney, et al., 2010).

The Canadian Interdisciplinary Network for CAM Research was created in 2004 to foster CAM research and disseminate information. Objectives include providing information that reflects a Canadian perspective on the safety and efficacy of various CAM approaches.

Although CAM approaches are less expensive and more cost-effective for the health care system, patients (or their private insurance plans) must pay for these services. Despite this, more than 50% of the population from Europe, North America, and other industrialized regions and 70% of Canadians have sought assistance from alternative or complementary medicine at least once (Mpinga, Kandolo, Verloo, et al., 2013, p. 45; PHAC, 2008).

Complementary and Alternative Medicine Approaches and Holistic Nursing

The goals of CAM and holistic nursing care are similar. The practice of holistic nursing regards the patient's mind, body, and spirit, whereas complementary approaches regard the whole person—physical, emotional, mental, and spiritual—with the goal of creating balance for the person (Snyder, Niska, & Lindquist, 2014). Nurses use holistic interventions such as relaxation therapy, imagery, music therapy, simple touch (which is especially helpful with older patients; Box 35-3), massage, and prayer (Box 35-4). Such interventions affect the whole person and are economical, noninvasive, nonpharmacological complements to traditional medical care. Holistic interventions can augment standard treatments, replace ineffective or debilitating interventions, and promote and maintain health (Dossey & Keegan, 2013). The Canadian Holistic Nurses Association (2008) developed standards of practice for holistic nursing and promotes holistic nursing practice, education, research, and administration. These standards are currently under revision. The Canadian Association of Schools of Nursing (CASN, 2015) released a national nursing education framework highlighting nursing competency domains that emphasize necessary degree-level outcomes related to complementary and alternative approaches in health care. Key competencies related to CAM are shown in Table 35-2.

Growing appreciation for the importance of healing the spirit and body has influenced the development of hospital programs, such as music, art, and recreation therapy. At the University of Alberta Hospital, the Artists on the Wards program connects local artists with individual patients at the bedside, assisting patients in developing their creativity and aiding in physical, spiritual, emotional, and mental healing. The hospital also houses the McMullen Art Gallery (Figure 35-1), which

BOX 35-3 FOCUS ON OLDER PERSONS

Touch

- Touch is a primary need and as necessary to humans as food, growth, and shelter. Healing touch refers to a broad range of techniques for the purposes of reducing pain, reducing anxiety, and promoting optimal health (Anderson & Taylor, 2011).
- Older persons need touch as much as or more than other age groups. Loneliness resulting from lack of touch can be acute among older persons, who often have fewer family members or friends to provide touch.
- Simple touch can be an enhanced form of communication when the other senses are reduced (Dossey & Keegan, 2013).
- Simple touch helps older persons feel more connected to their environment and accepted by those around them. The act of touching can enhance the older person's self-esteem and sense of worth.

BOX 35-4 Focus on Palliative Care

A complementary therapy pilot project (Berger, Tavares, & Berger, 2013) was developed to explore the potential benefits of massage, therapeutic touch (TT), aromatherapy, and Reiki for patients in an Ontario hospital's palliative care unit. The intentions of the study were to expand patients' and families' "experience of quality and satisfaction with end of life care" and to establish if complementary approaches could "enhance symptom management" (p. 1294). The data analysis indicated a "significant decrease in severity of pain, anxiety, low mood, restlessness, and discomfort ($p < 0.01$, 95% CI) and significant increase in inner stillness/peace ($p < 0.01$, 95% CI) and comfort." Conclusions from this study showed that an integrated approach to complementary therapy improves symptom management, increases comfort, and is a "valuable addition to interdisciplinary care" (p. 1294). Furthermore, TT programs in a geriatric palliative care unit highlighted TT as safe and beneficial in helping patients to relax (Senderovicha, Ip, Beralla, et al., 2016).

Further research studies on the use of complementary and alternative therapy in palliative care units are warranted.

TABLE 35-2 CASN Competency Domains for CAM Approaches in Health Care

Domain 1: Knowledge	Competency 1.2: Foundational knowledge of human development and functioning over the lifespan that builds on secondary education, from natural and life sciences and from behavioural and social sciences (anatomy, physiology, microbiology, biochemistry, pharmacology, nutrition, pathophysiology, genetics, psychology, sociology [p. 10])
Domain 3: Nursing Practice	Competency 3.1: Holistic and comprehensive assessment of diverse clients, to plan and provide competent, ethical, safe, and compassionate nursing care (p. 13) Competency 3.8: Engagement and leadership in the provision of comfort care including pain and symptom management (p. 13)
Domain 5: Professionalism	Competency 5.2: An understanding of the significance of fitness to practice as it relates to self-care and lifelong learning (p. 16)

CAM, Complementary and alternative medicine; *CASN,* Canadian Association for Schools of Nursing.

From Canadian Association for Schools of Nursing/Association Canadienne des Écoles de Sciences Infirmières [CASN/ACESI]. (2015). *National nursing education framework: Final report.* Retrieved from http://www.casn.ca/wp-content/uploads/2014/12/Framwork-FINAL-SB-Nov-30-20151.pdf

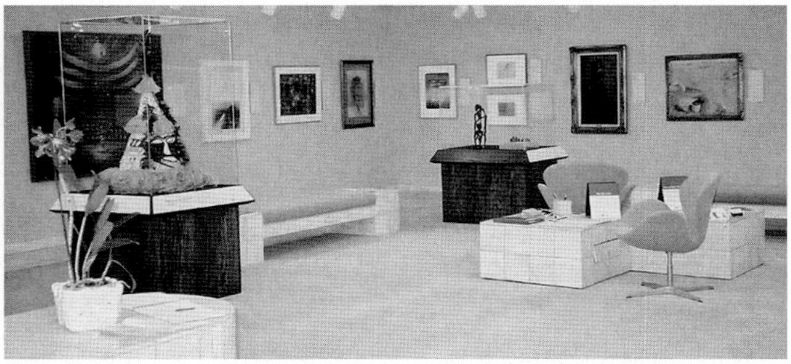

FIGURE 35-1 McMullen Art Gallery, University of Alberta Hospital, is accessible for patients, visitors, and staff. (Courtesy University of Alberta Hospital, Edmonton, Alberta.)

provides space for spiritual practice and access to chaplains as members of the health care team. The University of Alberta Hospital also offers patients and families both a chapel and a teepee (Figure 35-2). The teepee, built specifically for Indigenous patients and their families, is used for prayer, reflection, and healing ceremonies. A few hospitals have or are considering the construction of labyrinths on their grounds. Patients and visitors can use these labyrinths for walking, meditation, and prayer (see Table 35-1).

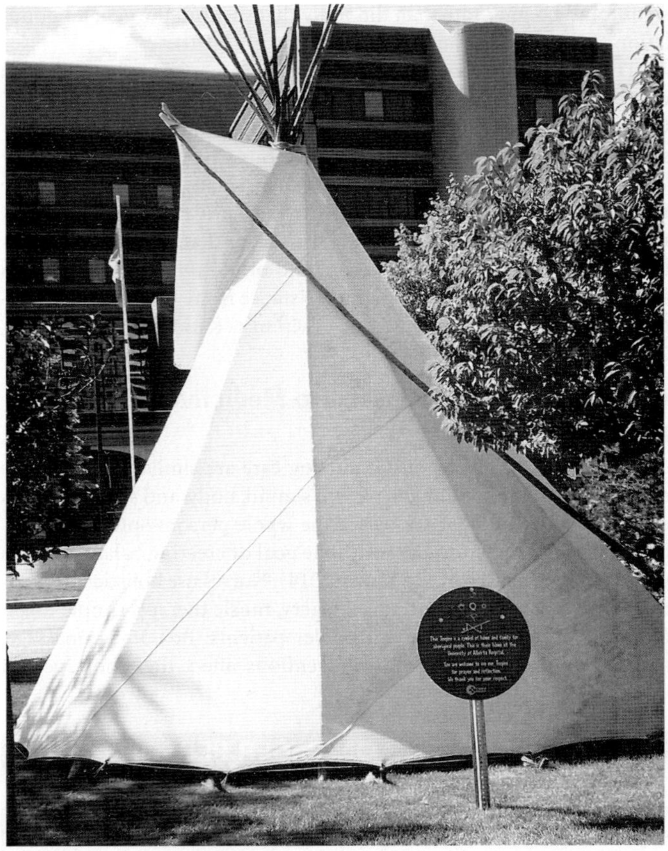

FIGURE 35-2 This teepee outside the University of Alberta Hospital provides space for prayer and healing. (Courtesy University of Alberta Hospital.)

NURSING-ACCESSIBLE APPROACHES

Nurses have practised a variety of approaches such as imagery, meditation, support groups, music therapy, journalling, massage, and therapeutic touch for patients with acute and chronic conditions (Snyder, et al., 2014). These techniques are easily learned and provided for patients within independent nursing practice (Dossey & Keegan, 2013). Good assessment, along with a patient's permission, are prerequisites for implementation. Some CAM approaches may alter physiological responses, thus physician-prescribed approaches (e.g., medication dosages) may need to be adjusted. CAM approaches should be chosen according to the patient's functional status, beliefs or religious perspectives, access to health care, and insurance coverage (Box 35-5).

These approaches are designed to teach patients how they can change their behaviour to alter their physical responses to stress and relieve associated symptoms such as muscle tension, gastrointestinal discomfort, pain, and sleep disturbances. A key principle of this approach is that the individual must be actively involved in the treatment plan. Patients achieve better responses if they practise the techniques or exercises daily and commit to implementing and maintaining the planned approach for realization of the desired outcome.

BOX 35-5 CASE STUDY

A Holistic Approach to Health

As the nurse at an integrative medicine clinic, you are responsible for completing initial assessments, counselling, and advising new patients about complementary and alternative approaches. You meet Mrs. Lorimer, a 48-year-old female, who is employed as a teacher. She indicates that she has anxiety and is currently taking anti-anxiety medication. Her primary reason for visiting the clinic is to learn about complementary approaches for treatment of her anxiety, as an alternative to additional pharmaceutical medication.

Key Points

Past history: Mrs. Lorimer indicates that her mother has a history of anxiety and depression.

Social history: Her relationships with her children and husband are strong. She attends church regularly and expresses a connection to her faith.

Medications: She currently takes a selective serotonin reuptake inhibitor (SSRI) medication for her anxiety (as prescribed by her general practitioner).

Attitude toward health: She cries during the interview and expresses feelings of loss and sadness about her perceived inability to control her anxiety. She expresses that her occupation and family activities are stressful and feels she has little time or energy at the end of the day.

Approaches

First, ask open-ended assessment questions to gain an understanding and broader perspective of Mrs. Lorimer's concerns, social determinants of health, and current health status. What is the patient's medical diagnosis? Is it correct? Could other medical problems be contributing to her anxiety? Have all the conventional medical approaches been thoroughly explored or considered? Has she discussed alternative treatment plans with her health care provider? It is important to explore the patient's attitude, frame of mind, coping strategies, support systems, and goals. Key strengths include her strong social support system and her faith. She will need to regularly communicate and connect with her family members to further understand triggers for the anxiety, and plan strategies for family activities and, ultimately, her health.

Take a collaborative approach with Mrs. Lorimer to explore practical steps that she and her family can take to assist in decreasing her stress and anxiety, including limiting activities, creating a schedule so that all family members assist with daily household activities, and taking time for self-care. These elements must be combined with realistic goals for reducing stress and anxiety, including a structured follow-up. Review dietary supplementation, eating habits, sleep patterns, self-care patterns, and asking for assistance when needed. Emphasize the importance of sharing this information with her primary health care provider to determine whether these patterns are beneficial or harmful to her health. Discuss potential relaxation strategies such as relaxation, music therapy, and breathwork.

In developing her plan of care, create a realistic program that combines the benefits of exercise and other mind–body approaches, including journal writing, guided imagery with visualization, and meditation (e.g., through a prayer group at her church). Additional supportive resources might include appropriate self-help books, and website resources (such as those on mindfulness) that provide additional reflection and insight into psychological, physical, and emotional lifestyle challenges associated with stress and anxiety.

Relaxation Therapy

People are exposed to stressful situations in everyday life that evoke a stress response (see Chapter 29 for further information about stress and adaptation). The biochemical functions of major organ systems are modulated by the mind. Thoughts and feelings influence the production of chemicals (i.e., neurotransmitters, neurohormones, and peptides) that circulate in the body and convey messages to various body systems. Physiologically, the stress response can cause increased heart, respiratory, and metabolism rates; tightened muscles; and a general sense of foreboding, fear, nervousness, irritability, and negative mood. Other physiological responses include elevated blood pressure, dilated pupils, stronger cardiac contractions, and increased levels of blood glucose, serum cholesterol, circulating free fatty acids, and triglycerides. Although these responses effectively prepare a person for short-term stress, long-term stress can cause structural damage and chronic illness, such as angina, tension headaches, cardiac arrhythmias, pain, and ulcers (Dossey & Keegan, 2013).

Relaxation is a state of overall decreased cognitive, physiological, and behavioural arousal. The process of relaxation reduces the neural impulses sent to the brain, thus decreasing the brain's activity. Relaxation is characterized by decreases in heart and respiratory rates, blood pressure, and oxygen consumption and increases in muscle relaxation and alpha-wave brain activity.

Clinical Applications of Relaxation Therapy. Relaxation techniques can lower heart rate and blood pressure, decrease muscle tension, improve perceived well-being, and reduce symptom distress in individuals experiencing a variety of situations from medical concerns to loss and grief. The type of relaxation intervention should be matched to the individual's functional status, the energy expenditure of the relaxation technique, and the motivation of the individual for frequent practice.

Relaxation therapy, either alone or in combination with deep breathing, imagery, biofeedback, yoga (Figure 35-3), or music, can bring about healthy physiological changes such as pain reduction, decreased anxiety, a decrease in blood pressure and heart rate, and alleviation of tension headaches (Huang, Moser, & Hwang, 2016; Micozzi & Jawer, 2015). In a prospective, randomized control study, Huang and colleagues (2016) examined the effect of biofeedback-assisted relaxation (BFAR) therapy in patients with heart failure. The results showed that BFAR was effective in improving physical symptoms.

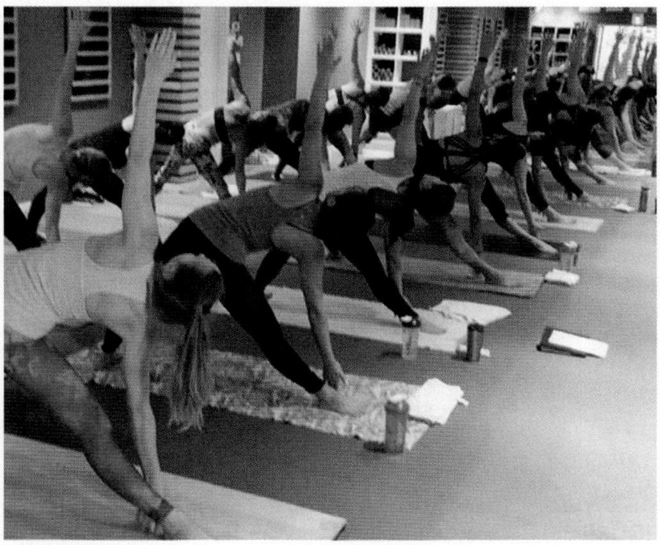

FIGURE 35-3 Yoga focuses on muscles, posture, breathing, and consciousness. (Courtesy Deborah Gibson, RN, MSN.)

Meditation and Breathing

Meditation is any activity that limits stimulus input by directing the attention to a single unchanging or repetitive stimulus (Rakel & Faass, 2012); it can enhance attention, cognitive ability, and mental health (Lim, Condon, & DeSteno, 2015). *Meditation* refers to a range of practices that relax the body and still the mind. The root word, *meditari*, means "to consider." In 1975, Dr. Herbert Benson's book *The Relaxation Response* drew the attention of Western health care practitioners to the physical and psychological benefits of relaxation. As Benson noted, the components of meditation are simple: a quiet space, a comfortable position, a receptive attitude, and a focus of attention. He described meditation as a process that anyone can use to calm down, to cope with stress, and, for those with spiritual inclinations, to feel at one with God or the universe. Most meditation techniques involve slow, relaxed, deep, usually abdominal, breathing. Meditation evokes a restful state, lowers oxygen consumption, reduces respiratory and heart rates, and decreases anxiety.

Clinical Applications of Meditation. A variety of conditions are indications for meditation therapy. Meditation improves breathing patterns in patients with asthma, assists in managing stress-related illnesses (Merkes, 2010), and is indicated for the following conditions: anxiety or tension, chronic bereavement, chronic fatigue syndrome, chronic pain, substance use, hypertension, low self-esteem, depression, and sleep disorders. Furthermore, meditation in conjunction with yoga has been found to lower diastolic and systolic blood pressure; thus this combination is an effective alternative to pharmacotherapy (Park & Han, 2017).

Imagery

Imagery or visualization techniques, which are frequently used with relaxation training, help a person create mental images, to stimulate physical changes, improve perceived well-being, and enhance self-awareness. Imagery can be either self-directed or guided by a practitioner (Dossey & Keegan, 2013). "Guided imagery works by eliciting the benefits of a relaxed state of mind through the use of suggestions and affirmations that enable one to integrate relaxation feelings into daily living" (Greene & Greene, 2012, p. 152). For example, the patient may be directed to begin slow, abdominal breathing while focusing on the rhythm of the breath. The patient is then guided to visualize ocean waves washing onto a shore with each inhalation, then receding with each exhalation. Next, the patient is encouraged to notice the smells, sounds, and temperatures that he or she is experiencing. As the session progresses, the patient may be instructed to visualize warmth entering the body during inspiration and tension leaving the body during expiration. Imagery scenarios can be individualized for each patient or left to the patient to develop.

Clinical Applications of Imagery. Imagery is used to control or relieve pain or stress, to achieve calmness and serenity, and to visualize cancer cells being destroyed by immune system cells. Imagery is also used in the treatment of chronic conditions, such as asthma, hypertension, functional urinary disorders, menstrual and premenstrual syndromes, and rheumatoid arthritis, and of gastrointestinal disorders, such as irritable bowel syndrome (Dossey & Keegan, 2013). A recent study measured the impact of cognitive-behavioural therapy with relaxation versus imagery on test anxiety in university settings. Results indicated that group treatments along with imagery provided an effective method of treating test anxiety (Reiss, Warnecke, Tolgou, et al., 2017).

COMPLEMENTARY AND ALTERNATIVE MEDICINE APPROACHES REQUIRING EDUCATION

CAM treatments may be administered by nurses, but only after the completion of a specific course of study. A nurse must have a certification, degree, or license beyond a registered nursing degree to administer most of these approaches, such as biofeedback, therapeutic touch, and massage therapy.

Biofeedback

Biofeedback techniques are frequently used in addition to relaxation interventions to assist individuals in learning how to control specific autonomic nervous system responses. Biofeedback is a therapeutic procedure that uses electronic or electromechanical instruments to measure, process, and provide rapid and accurate information about neuromuscular and autonomic nervous system activity. This feedback is provided in physical, physiological, auditory, and visual measurements through a pneumograph. Biofeedback practitioners help patients to develop awareness of and voluntary control over physiological responses and thereby change behaviour or activity to improve health (Peek, 2016; Schwartz, Collura, Kamiya, et al., 2016). For example, in audio feedback, patients may hear a sound if their pulse rate or blood pressure increases out of their therapeutic zone. This form is helpful as information is transmitted without the need for visual attention (Peek, 2016). It is considered to complement traditional relaxation programs because it can immediately demonstrate to patients their ability to control some physiological responses.

Clinical Applications of Biofeedback. Biofeedback has numerous applications, including treatment for migraine headaches, rehabilitation for victims of stroke, and treatment for hypertonicity and spasticity (Bolek, Rosenthal, & Sherman, 2016).

Therapeutic Touch and Healing Touch

Therapeutic touch (TT) is a training-specific therapy that was developed in the 1970s by a nurse, Dr. Dolores Krieger. Although the philosophical and religious assumptions of TT differ from those of other Eastern healing modalities, both practices involve trained practitioners who attempt to direct their own balanced energies in an intentional and motivated manner toward the patient (DeLany, 2015; Krieger, Peper, & Ancoli, 1979). TT consists of the practitioner's hands being placed either on or close to a person's body. The practitioner scans the patient's body and diagnoses areas of accumulated tensions. The practitioner then attempts to redirect these energies to bring the person's energy back into balance (DeLany, 2015; Krieger, 1975; Krieger et al., 1979).

Clinical Applications of Therapeutic Touch and Healing Touch. In a randomized, prospective control pilot study, Lu, Hart, Lutgendorf, and colleagues (2016) sought to to identify the efficacy of healing touch and relaxation therapy for adults with advanced cancer undergoing stem cell transplant. Results indicated that although the healing touch modality was better tolerated than relaxation therapy, both interventions improved mood and function in these patients. Further research is needed to determine the impact these modalities have on length of hospital stay and to discern which patients tolerate relaxation therapy (Lu et al., 2016).

Chiropractic Medicine

Chiropractic medicine was developed in the late 1890s and has become the third-largest independently practised health profession in the Western world (Bergmann & Peterson, 2011; Rakel & Faass, 2012). Practitioners of chiropractic medicine graduate from a 4-year program and must pass four national board examinations for licensure (Bergmann & Peterson, 2011). The broad chiropractic model of health care is committed to a holistic approach that focuses on the assessment and treatment of the spine, joints, nervous system, and musculoskeletal system. The basic principles of chiropractic therapy incorporate the idea that human beings have an innate healing potential; harnessing this potential is the goal of this healing profession.

The central tenet of chiropractic treatment is to correct the body's alignment and improve function through spinal manipulation (manual or manipulative approaches), postural and exercise education, ergonomic training, nutrition consultation, and ultrasound and laser approaches (Figure 35-4). This model theorizes that joint dysfunction or subluxation operates as an irritant that lowers the body's ability to resist disease (Bergmann & Peterson, 2011; Redwood, 2011). *Manipulation* is defined as a therapeutic movement of the spine or a quick but strong pressure on a joint between two vertebrae of the spine which rotates the joint beyond its normal range of motion. Additional components of chiropractic medicine in patient management and health promotion include dietary modification, nutritional supplementation, physiotherapies, and regular exercise to optimize overall health and proper body function (Bergmann & Peterson, 2011; Fontaine, 2015; Micozzi, 2015; Redwood, 2011).

Clinical Applications of Chiropractic Therapy. The basic goals of chiropractic therapy focus on restoring the body's structural and functional imbalances that may result in pain. One of the major structural distortions that chiropractors treat is vertebral subluxation, in which joint mobility is decreased due to slight changes in the position of the articulating bones. Subluxation exists when joint motion is restricted or malpositioned. Chiropractic interventions treat musculoskeletal abnormalities, headaches, dysmenorrhea, disorders of blood pressure, vertigo, tinnitus, and visual disorders (Bergmann & Peterson, 2011; Micozzi, 2015).

Traditional Chinese Medicine

Traditional Chinese medicine (TCM), from the mid-twentieth century, blends several healing modalities, including herbal remedies, acupuncture, diet, exercise, and meditation, with scientific theoretical principles (Micozzi, 2015). A major concept in Chinese medicine is yin and yang, which represent opposing, yet complementary, phenomena that exist in a state of dynamic equilibrium. Examples of yin and yang are night and day, hot and cold, and shade and sun. Yin represents shade, cold, and inhibition, whereas yang represents fire, light, and excitement. Yin also represents the inner part of the body, specifically

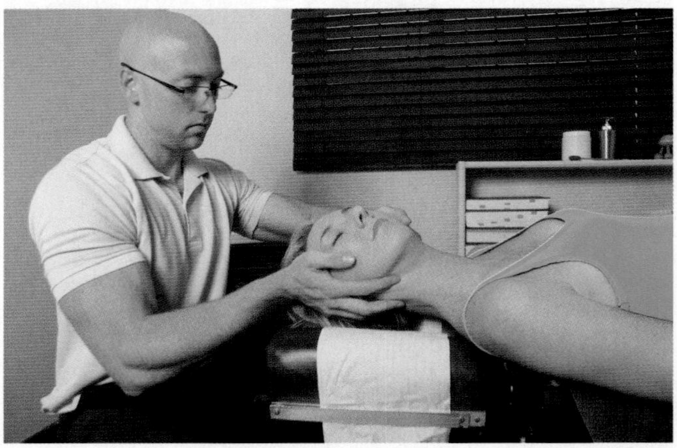

FIGURE 35-4 The central tenet of chiropractic treatment is the spinal manipulation directed at specific joints. (From Adobe Stock Photos.)

the viscera, liver, heart, spleen, lungs, and kidneys, whereas yang represents the outer part, specifically the bowels, stomach, and bladder. According to TCM, when an imbalance occurs in these paired opposites, disease can emerge (Fontaine, 2015; Micozzi, 2015).

Qi (pronounced *chee*) is translated as the body's vital energy that has the qualities of "flow and balance" (Micozzi, 2015, p. 18). Disease is classified into three major categories: external causes, internal causes, and neither internal nor external causes. Regardless of the cause, when yin and yang are out of balance, the movement of qi is altered. The body has several forms of qi that directly influence its physiological functions and help maintain homeostasis.

Another important component of Chinese medicine involves five elements: earth, metal, water, wood, and fire. Various health phenomena are organized according to these elements and interact with each other. In Chinese medicine, outward manifestations reflect the internal environment. Two primary areas assessed in Chinese medicine are the tongue and several pulses. The colour, shape, and coating of the tongue reflect the general condition of the internal organs. The pulses provide information about the condition and balance of qi, blood, yin and yang, and internal organs (Fontaine, 2015; Micozzi, 2015).

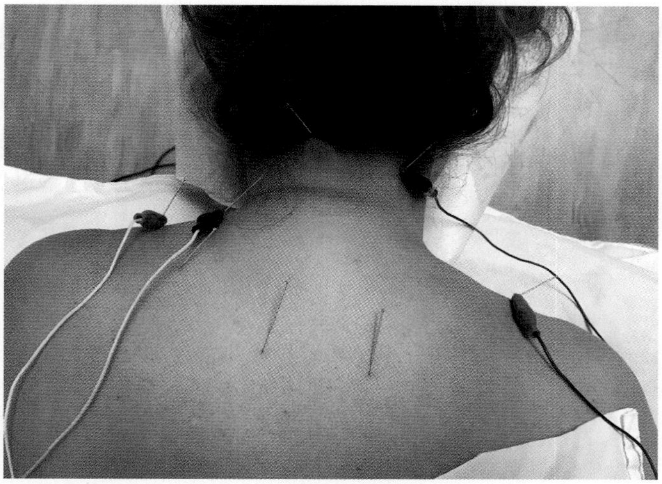

FIGURE 35-5 Acupuncture involves the insertion of special needles to regulate the flow of energy. Electric current connected to the needles enhances the flow and healing. (Courtesy Deborah Gibson, RN, MSN.)

Naturopathic Medicine

Naturopathic medicine is becoming a popular and "authentic" paradigm for "integrative primary health care" (Pizzorno, Snider, & Micozzi, 2015, p. 347), providing individualized management of care though evidence-informed practice (Wardle & Sarris, 2017). Naturopathic doctors graduate from a 4-year program and write national board examinations for licensure. They offer a new perspective of safe and effective methods of health restoration through a variety of health promotion and preventative and treatment approaches. These treatments integrate traditional and natural approaches with modern scientific knowledge and medicines, including botanical (plant) medicine, to stimulate healing and treat underlying causes of diseases (Canadian Association of Naturopathic Doctors [CAND], 2016). Acupuncture, nutritional counselling and supplementation, cupping, and hydrotherapy are also used.

Clinical Applications of Naturopathic Medicine. Breed and Berenznay (2017) studied the impact and quality of care for patients with anxiety and depression who were seen by naturopathic physicians in a community centre. Study results identified significant improvement in patients' symptoms of depression and anxiety ($p < 0.0001$) and future implications for the treatment of anxiety and depression within the context of an integrative community centre.

Acupuncture

According to Chinese medicine, channels of energy run in regular patterns throughout the body and over its surface. These channels, called meridians, are like rivers flowing through the body. An obstruction of these meridians functions like a dam, backing up the flow in one part of the body and restricting the flow in other parts, eventually leading to disease. Located along the channels are acupoints, or holes through which qi can be influenced by the insertion of needles, a process known as acupuncture.

Acupuncture is a method of stimulating certain points (acupoints) on the body by the insertion of special needles to modify the perception of pain, normalize physiological functions, or treat or prevent disease (Figure 35-5). Acupuncture is used to regulate the flow of qi (Micozzi, 2015). According to Chinese traditional medicine, acupuncture needles unblock obstructed energy flow and re-establish the flow of qi through the meridians, thereby stimulating the skin and underlying muscles, leading to afferent nerve excitement. The sensory information is then transported to the central nervous system, which ultimately affects visceral function (Uchida, Kagitani, & Sato-Suzuki, 2017). The effects of the acupuncture needles may be enhanced by applying heat or weak electrical currents to the needles.

Clinical Applications of Acupuncture. Acupuncture is the primary treatment used by practitioners of Chinese medicine and naturopathic doctors who have learned Chinese medicine theory. Other health care providers must receive additional training for certification in acupuncture.

Acupuncture is used to treat back and neck pain, myofascial pain, headaches, tennis elbow, osteoarthritis, and musculoskeletal sprains. Other problems that have been successfully treated are sinusitis, gastrointestinal disorders, menstrual symptoms, neurological disorders, chronic pulmonary diseases (including asthma), hypertension, smoking and other addictions, anxiety, and clinical depression (Ergil & Ergil, 2015).

Cupping

Cupping is a therapeutic approach originating in China that is used in Chinese medicine and by naturopathic doctors. Practitioners use a small glass cup that is placed on the body's acupuncture points and then applied to the skin using a vacuum or suction technique to stimulate qi and, ultimately, healing for chronic neck pain, upper or lower back pain, and improved range of motion (Ergil, 2015) (Figure 35-6). Patients with chronic neck pain were enrolled into a randomized control trial to "test the efficacy of cupping massage in patients with chronic neck pain" (Saha, Schumann, Cramer, et al., 2017, p. 26). Results indicated that cupping massage is effective in relieving pain, facilitating movement, improving mental health, and improving function and quality of life for patients with chronic nonspecific neck pain.

Massage Therapy

Practitioners of massage therapy, a recognized health care profession in Canada, offer assessment, treatment, and prevention for pain of soft tissue and joints. Therapists use manipulation and stimulation of pressure receptors in an effort to augment physical functioning and promote pain relief (Field, 2016; Kania-Richmond, Reece, Suter, et al., 2014) (Figure 35-7).

Clinical Applications of Massage Therapy. Patient-reported outcomes suggest that massage therapy offers therapeutic benefits for individuals experiencing medical conditions across the lifespan.

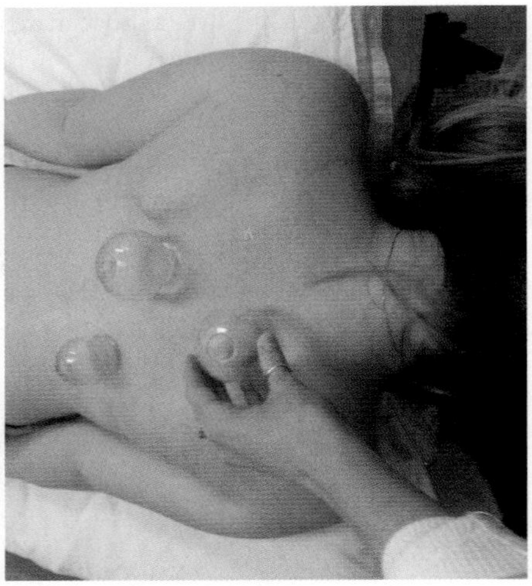

FIGURE 35-6 Cupping is a complementary approach used to stimulate qi and alleviate pain. (Courtesy Dr. Annie Gibson, ND.)

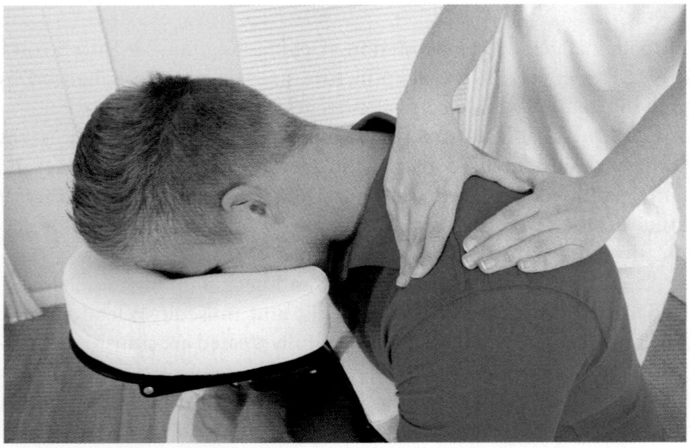

FIGURE 35-7 Massage therapy is used to relieve symptoms from health concerns. (From Adobe Stock Photos.)

Conditions treated include, but are not limited to, prenatal and postnatal depression; anxiety and clinical depression; stimulation with preterm and full-term infants; autism; skin conditions; arthritis; fibromyalgia; hypertension; autoimmune conditions, including asthma and multiple sclerosis; immune conditions, including human immunodeficiency virus (HIV) and breast cancer; and aging problems, including Parkinson's disease and dementia (Field, 2016).

HEALTH PROMOTION: NUTRITION IN DISEASE PREVENTION

A growing body of scientific research done over the past few decades and currently ongoing has explored the relationship between nutrition and its effect on disease. Substantial evidence from epidemiological studies indicates that the relationship between diet, nutrition, diabetes, cancer, and cardiovascular disease is directly linked to lifestyle and nutritional choices (Wolever, Reeds, Mansuri, et al., 2016; World Health Organization [WHO], 2017). A recent report stated that "diet is the most important risk factor for illness ... globally" (Horton, 2016, p. 1706). The necessity to address nutrition in disease prevention was underscored in a study by Ezzati, Obermeyer, Tzoulaki, and colleagues (2015) which tracked obesity trends in 200 countries from 1975 to 2014. Research findings predicted increased rates of obesity for one in five men and women by 2025. Furthermore, the Lancet (2016) found the diabetes prevalence in adults had increased since 1980. "Together with population growth and ageing, this rise has led to a near quadrupling of the number of adults with diabetes worldwide" (p. 1513). The prevalence of diseases such as type 2 diabetes, which previously was rarely seen in young children, is now increasing in this population.

In nutritional science aimed at prevention of disease, quality, not quantity, of nutritional intake is emphasized, and a shift toward a Mediterranean diet high in nuts, olive oil, fish, fruits, vegetables, yogurt, and whole grains is recommended. An increased intake of whole grains and dietary fibre is inversely associated with insulin resistance and type 2 diabetes (Li & Uppal, 2010) and may reduce incidence of coronary artery disease. It is important to note that a number of CAM professionals, such as naturopathic and chiropractic physicians, are required to take nutritional science courses as part of their program of study; nutritional science should also be integrated in medical school curriculum. In addition, further research is needed for developing protective nutritional strategies against cancer resulting from increasing exposure to environmental carcinogenic agents and for supporting the health of aging populations worldwide (Dinkova-Kostova, 2007; Thorogood, Simera, Dowler, et al., 2007).

A single fruit or vegetable contains many protective chemicals and nutrients that cannot be sourced from a supplement alone. These plant chemicals, commonly called *phytochemicals* or antioxidants, destroy free radicals, protect cells from damage, and offer defence against disease. The Canadian Cancer Society (2017) addresses key dietary sources of phytochemicals and advises choosing a variety of colourful foods each day. Examples include dark green and orange (carrots, spinach, oranges); red and blue or purple (beets, red peppers, blueberries); and white, brown, and tan (cauliflower, garlic, bananas).

Botanicals/Natural Health Products

An estimated 25 000 plant species are used as medicinal approaches globally. Botanical therapy, the oldest form of medicine, was widespread for thousands of years, but its popularity declined with the development of modern scientific medicine in the early eighteenth century. However, because approximately 80% of the world's population lives in developing countries, herbal medicine constitutes a prominent approach to health care worldwide. In countries that use predominantly allopathic medicine, an increased interest in herbal medicine has developed from consumer interest in natural foods and growing concern about the complications and limitations of scientific medicine. Statistics indicate that 71% of Canadians have used natural health products such as vitamins and minerals, herbal products, and homeopathic medicines (Health Canada, 2011, 2016).

Botanicals are extracted from plants, animals, and microorganisms, and the active ingredients are prepared in tinctures or extracts, elixirs, syrups, capsules, pills, tablets, lozenges, powders, ointments or creams, drops, and suppositories. As with other medications, some herbal substances contain powerful chemicals and can cause harm or adverse effects. As such, botanicals and herbs should be examined for interaction and compatibility with other prescribed or nonprescribed substances. Botanical products are, in general, classified as beneficial, harmful, or neutral, in which case they have no effects on the specific ailment. Health Canada (2008) establishes safety and quality for all foods and drugs sold in Canada through the *Canada Food and Drugs Act* and regulations.

The philosophy of botanical therapy differs from the philosophy of conventional drug therapy. The goal of botanical therapy is to restore balance within the individual by facilitating the self-healing ability.

Drug therapy, by contrast, is aimed at the treatment of a specific disease or symptoms.

Health Canada regulates all over-the-counter **natural health products** (NHPs) and botanicals for safety, effectiveness, and quality. NHPs include herbs, probiotics, essential fatty acids, vitamins, minerals, and homeopathics that are used to "diagnose, treat, prevent disease; restore or correct function, maintain or promote health" (Health Canada, 2011). These regulations include good manufacturing practices and guidelines for obtaining a product license. Botanicals/NHPs approved for sale under the new regulations have been assigned a Drug Identification Number (DIN; DIN-HM for homeopathic medicines) or natural product number (NPN). These numbers certify that the product has passed a review of its formulation, labelling, and instructions for use. Health Canada advises Canadians to use only health products that carry a DIN, DIN-HM, or NPN on the label.

Clinical Applications of Botanicals/Natural Health Products. Numerous NHPs have been determined to be safe and effective for a variety of conditions (Table 35-3). Milk thistle, for example, can effectively treat certain liver and gallbladder conditions; its antioxidant properties are believed to protect the liver and facilitate regeneration of liver cells. St. John's wort has been found to be effective as a tricyclic antidepressant agent and more effective than placebo (Linde, Berner, & Kriston, 2008).

Limitations of Botanicals/Natural Health Products. Although botanicals have been shown to provide beneficial effects for a variety of conditions, a number of concerns may exist. Concentrations of active ingredients can vary, and contamination may occur with prescription medication and other herbs or chemicals, including pesticides and heavy metals. Some herbs have been found to contain toxic products associated with cancer. Comfrey, for example, has been used for its wound-healing properties; however, some species of comfrey contain highly carcinogenic pyrrolizideine alkaloids and have produced liver cancer in small animals. Other unsafe botanicals (NHPs) are listed in Table 35-4.

Not all companies follow strict quality-control and manufacturing guidelines, which set standards for acceptable levels of pesticides, residual solvents, bacterial levels, and heavy metals. For this reason, botanicals/NHPs should only be purchased from reputable

TABLE 35-3 Botanicals/Natural Health Products Commonly Used and Considered Safe

Common Name	Effects	Indications*	Warnings†	Other
Black cohosh	Estrogen-like effects	Menopausal hot flashes Premenstrual syndrome	Significant estrogenic activity has not been found but not recommended if patient has a history of breast cancer	Is promising for the relief of moderate hot flashes related to menopause
Chamomile (German or Hungarian)	Topically: Anti-inflammatory Orally: Anti-inflammatory, antiestrogenic effects	Chemotherapy-induced mucositis Dyspepsia Colic Inflammatory conditions Insomnia Menstrual disorders	Contraindicated if allergies to the daisy family May potentiate the effect of anticoagulants and CNS depressants	Avoid confusion with Roman chamomile
Echinacea	Topically: Anaesthetic and anti-inflammatory, wound healing Orally: Stimulates the immune system	Upper respiratory infections Colds Urinary tract infections	Contraindicated in patients receiving cancer treatments and for people with autoimmune diseases, multiple sclerosis, tuberculosis, diabetes, asthma, leukemia, HIV/AIDS, lupus, or allergies to the daisy family Not to be used longer than 8 weeks	Chemical constituents differ among roots, leaves, and flowers
Evening primrose oil	Anti-inflammatory constituents omega-6 and gamma-linoleic acids	Mastalgia Atopic dermatitis Premenstrual syndrome (PMS) Menopausal hot flashes Rheumatoid arthritis	Contraindicated in patients with seizure disorders Large doses may cause loose stools and abdominal pain	Studies have shown positive effects on relieving mastalgia (cyclic breast pain)
Fish oil	Omega-3 essential fatty acids are believed to have anti-inflammatory properties	Rheumatoid arthritis Prevention of cardiovascular disease and cancer	Possible increase of INR with warfarin (Coumadin) Avoid doses greater than 3 gm/day to avoid inhibiting blood coagulation Quality of product should be monitored for cancer-causing pollutants, such as dioxin and PCBs	Effective in reducing triglyceride levels The Mediterranean diet, which is rich in fish, has been associated with lower rates of cancers. May improve overall cognitive functioning and behaviour in children with attention deficit–hyperactivity disorder (ADHD)

Continued

TABLE 35-3 Botanicals/Natural Health Products Commonly Used and Considered Safe—cont'd

Common Name	Effects	Indications*	Warnings[†]	Other
Garlic	Major constituent allicin reduces oxidative stress and stimulates the immune system Inhibits platelet aggregation	Hypertension Cold and flu prevention Athlete's foot (topically)	May prolong bleeding time Possible interactions with anticoagulants Topical application may cause skin irritation	Supplementation not recommended for use during pregnancy due to its effect on bleeding time
Ginger	Antiemetic Antibiotic	Motion/morning sickness Nausea and vomiting Vertigo	May enhance the effects of Coumadin, aspirin, and NSAIDs	Recent studies indicate no fetal harm when used for morning sickness
Ginkgo biloba	Contains flavonoids and organic acids that have anti-inflammatory/antioxidant effects Inhibits platelet-activating factor	Dementia Poor circulation Poor memory	Ingestion may increase the risk of serious bleeding, especially in patients taking anticoagulants or NSAIDs Can cause contact dermatitis High doses can cause seizures	Potential promise in enhancing cognitive functions in people with dementia and improving peripheral arterial disease
Glucosamine (Hydrochloride/ sulphate)	Naturally occurring amino sugar that stimulates the synthesis of proteins responsible for cartilage growth and maintenance	Joint pain Osteoarthritis	May increase the anticoagulant effects of Coumadin	Mounting evidence for pain reduction and disease-modifying effects in osteoarthritis
Milk thistle	Silymarin, the active constituent, is a potent inhibitor of tumour necrosis factor (TNF), which reduces toxicity to the liver and reduces inflammation	Chronic hepatitis Cirrhosis, gastrointestinal upset	Reports on significant decrease in fasting blood glucose in diabetics using conventional diabetic therapy	Do not confuse with blessed thistle. Mixed evidence on effectiveness in managing hepatitis or cirrhosis
Saw palmetto	Androgen receptor blocker Anti-inflammatory	Benign prostatic hyperplasia (BPH) Urinary problems	Increased risk of bleeding if on anticoagulants	Evidence suggests that it provides mild improvement for urinary problems
St. John's wort	Inhibits reuptake of serotonin, dopamine, and norepinephrine neurotransmitters Wound healing (topical)	Depression Sedative Menopausal symptoms	Not appropriate for severe depression May enhance the effects of SSRIs and other antidepressants Significant interactions with many medications (warfarin, antiretrovirals, cyclosporine, oral contraceptive therapy) Photosensitivity with chronic use	Studies support its use in treating mild to moderate depression
Valerian	Valepotriate constituents have sedative-hypnotic and smooth muscle effects	Muscle spasms Sleep disorders Restlessness	May cause headaches or gastrointestinal disturbances Patient must avoid using concurrently with other sedatives	Studies support its use in treating insomnia and improving sleep quality

CNS, Central nervous system; *INR,* international normalized ratio; *NSAIDs,* nonsteroidal anti-inflammatory drugs; *PCBs,* polychlorinated biphenyls; *SSRIs,* selective serotonin reuptake inhibitors.

*Unless otherwise noted, these natural health products have not shown sufficient evidence to rate their effectiveness for all stated indications.

[†]Data do not support the use of these herbs in infants or children or during pregnancy or lactation.

Adapted from Skidmore-Roth, L. (2010). *Skidmore-Roth Mosby's herbs and natural supplements* (4th ed.). St. Louis, MO: Mosby; The Pharmacist's Letter. (2010). *Natural medicines comprehensive database* (12th ed.). Stockton, CA: Therapeutic Research Faculty; and University of Maryland Medical Center. (2015). *Herbal medicine.* Retrieved from http://www.umm.edu/altmed/articles/herbal-medicine-000351.htm.

manufacturers (Box 35-6). In addition, labels on herbal products should include the scientific name of the botanical, the name and address of the manufacturer, the batch or lot number, the date of manufacture, the expiration date, and the DIN-HM or NPN identifying safety and effectiveness.

NURSING ROLE FOR INTERPROFESSIONAL COLLABORATION IN CAM

The integrative medicine approach is consistent with the nursing holistic approach. Indeed, many nurses already practise the use of simple

TABLE 35-4 Unsafe Botanicals/Natural Health Products

Common Name	Uses	Comments
Aconite (Aconitum, blue monkshood root)	Pain and inflammation (joint pain, gout, etc.)	Nausea, vomit Contains alkaloids toxic to the heart, lungs and central nervous system (CNS) Most common type of severe herbal poisoning in Hong Kong
Coltsfoot (British tobacco, coughwort)	Bronchitis Asthma Sore throat	Liver damage, contains large number of hepatotoxic pyrrolizidine alkaloids that are carcinogenic
Comfrey (blackwort, slippery root)	Relieves cough, heavy menstrual periods, stomach problems, chest pain, may be used to treat cancer	Liver damage, contains large number of toxic hepatotoxic pyrrolizidine alkaloids that can cause cancer
Country mallow (heartleaf, white mallow)	Asthma Colds and nasal congestion	Contains ephedrine similar to the stimulant ephedra, which can cause heart attack and seizure (unauthorized for sale as a natural health product by Health Canada)
Greater celandine (celandine, *Chelidonii herba*)	Dyspepsia Irritable bowel syndrome (IBS) Gastric cancer	Liver damage
Ephedra (ma huang, herbal Ecstasy)	Weight loss Athletic performance enhancer	Unsafe for people with hypertension, diabetes, or thyroid disease because of stimulant effects Many interactions with herbs and drugs Health Canada (2010) advisory against use of any product containing this substance
Kava	Anxiety and stress, improves insomnia	Hepatotoxicity and liver failure, may exacerbate Parkinson's and depression Issues related to contaminants in product Health Canada (2010) advisory against use
Lobelia (asthma weed, Indian tobacco)	Improves respiratory problems such as asthma, bronchitis, whooping cough	Nausea, vomiting, CNS overstimulation may cause tachycardia, hypotension, coma and possibly death
Yohimbe	Used to treat low libido or impotence	Hypertension, tachycardia, headache, seizures, liver and kidney problems, and cardiac conduction disorders

Adapted from Consumer Reports. (March 2017). *15 supplemental ingredients to always avoid.* Retrieved from https://www.consumerreports.org/vitamins-supplements/15-supplement-ingredients-to-always-avoid/; and The Pharmacist's Letter. (2010). *Natural medicines comprehensive database* (12th ed.). Stockton, CA: Therapeutic Research Faculty.

BOX 35-6 FOCUS ON PRIMARY HEALTH CARE

Patient Education: Purchasing Botanicals/NHPs

Individuals purchasing botanicals may be unaware of the lack of regulation regarding the manufacturing and sale of such products. It is difficult to make informed decisions when faced with hundreds of products. When patients choose to use botanicals/NHPs, they should purchase these products only from reputable manufacturers to ensure safety, appropriate use, and response.

Patients can be assisted in making informed choices about botanicals/NHPs by offering them the following guidelines:

- Avoid hype: Be wary of supplements that offer a "cure" or a "secret formula."
- All product labels should indicate the following:
  - The scientific name of the botanical, the quantity, concentration, expiration date, and manufacturer's name, the purpose, dosage form, route of administration, and warnings of possible adverse reactions, the names of other key ingredients and the natural product number (NPN) or Drug Identification Number (DIN-HM), indicating that the formulation has been reviewed by Health Canada.
- Ensure that the product is supported by published research. Avoid "multi-ingredient" formulations when possible; otherwise, determining potential reactions with other medicines will be difficult. Consumers often pay more for secondary products that may not be present in established therapeutic levels.
- Look for well-educated service staff who can answer consumers' questions.
- Be cautious about "mega" doses of anything: even excess ingestion of certain vitamins can be toxic.
- Be skeptical about cheap herbal remedies. Consumers must pay for the manufacturer's investments in ensuring quality and purity. Very inexpensive herbal products are often of inferior quality.

NHPs used for weight loss, body building, sleep problems, and diabetes have become a worldwide problem because of their use in addition to prescription and nonprescription drugs. Purchasing unauthorized NHPs through the Internet may increase patients' risks for unsafe products.

touch; this includes a variety of practice modalities designed to promote the health and well-being of the patient. The use of these modalities is based on the assumption that nurses practise within the scope of practice, as defined by the provincial nursing regulatory body, Canadian Nurses Association (CNA) (2015), and Canadian Holistic Nurses Association (2008). As health care participants, nurses who provide CAM approaches must possess the knowledge and skill necessary to provide safe and ethical care through continued education and certificate courses offered by universities, colleges, and professional associations or through study with expert practitioners. Nurses should understand provincial and territorial legislation regarding complementary approaches, practise within the scope of these laws, and be able to make appropriate recommendations about CAM approaches to allopathic primary care providers. Nursing resources on nursing scope of practice in relation to CAM have been developed and are available through a variety of professional associations, including the Canadian Holistic Nurses Association, provincial nursing regulatory bodies such as the College of Registered Nurses of British Columbia (2013), and CNA (2015). These resources assist in understanding professional responsibilities, ethics related to implementation and advisement of CAM, as well implications for nurses.

It is important for nurses to remain current on Best Practice Guidelines as well as current research in the field of CAM approaches in order to provide accurate information to patients and other health care providers. For example, the Canadian Interdisciplinary Network for Complementary and Alternative Medicine Research has been created to foster excellence in CAM research.

Nurses are in an opportune position to advise patients about the appropriate times to use conventional or CAM approaches. Since patients often trust nurses to provide sound advice on the use of different approaches, it is important that nurses maintain knowledge of both the potential benefits and risks associated with different CAM approaches. Furthermore, nurses are in a unique position to become familiar with patients' religious and cultural viewpoints and to determine CAM approaches that would be best suited to individuals' beliefs.

Patients should be reminded to inform their health care providers about the medications and approaches they receive. In particular, complete information about the use of botanicals and NHPs should be added to the medical record to prevent potential drug and herb interactions. See Chapter 18 for further information about interprofessional collaboration.

KEY CONCEPTS

- An increasing number of Canadians are using complementary and alternative health care and natural health products to treat illness and promote health.
- Complementary therapy is used in conjunction with allopathic medicine, whereas alternative therapy is generally used without the addition of conventional health care methods.
- Integrative medicine uses a multidisciplinary (both allopathic and complementary) treatment approach.
- Stress is an adaptive response that allows individuals to react to demanding situations.
- Chronic stress may be maladaptive, thereby leading to chronic muscle tension and changes in mood and immunity.
- Relaxation is a beneficial state characterized by improved mood, relaxed muscle tension, lowered blood pressure, and slower pulse and respiratory rates.
- To promote effectiveness and beneficial outcomes, complementary and alternative medicine approaches require collaboration and active participation with the patient.
- Complementary and alternative medicine (CAM) approaches should be chosen according to the patient's functional status, belief or religious perspectives, access to health care, and insurance coverage.
- Some CAM approaches may alter physiological responses, thereby requiring changes in routine medication doses.
- Imagery is usually visual but can also involve the auditory, gustatory, and olfactory senses.
- Many CAM approaches are thought to be effective on the basis of increasing scientific research and observed positive outcomes in a number of patients currently using CAM approaches. Many of the approaches are supported by research published in professional nursing and medical journals.
- Current research supports various nutritional practices as a form of health promotion and disease prevention.
- Not all natural health products are safe.

CRITICAL THINKING EXERCISES

Patient profile: Margaret is a 76-year-old Catholic woman who has received a diagnosis of a slow-growing renal tumour. Surgery is scheduled to take place in 2 weeks, and Margaret is afraid of both the procedure and the outcome. Is it cancer? Will the surgery result in a disability?

1. What specific nursing-accessible complementary and alternative medicine interventions can you offer Margaret to reduce her anxiety and prepare her for the surgery?
2. After surgery, Margaret becomes depressed. What complementary and alternative medicine approaches may be appropriate to assist Margaret with her depression?

REVIEW QUESTIONS

1. Despite the success of allopathic medicine (traditional Western medicine), many patients find complementary approaches provide relief for which of the following conditions?
   1. Heart disease and pancreatitis
   2. Ulcers and hepatitis
   3. Chronic back pain and arthritis
   4. Lupus and diabetes
2. Many complementary approaches, such as acupuncture, have diagnostic and therapeutic methods specific to their field. Which approach can be easily learned and used as part of independent nursing practice?
   1. Massage therapy
   2. Chinese medicine
   3. Shamanism
   4. Imagery
3. Which of the following statements best describes the experience of Canadians who have used a complementary and alternative medicine?
   1. Most have used complementary and alternative medicine therapy to prevent illness or maintain wellness.
   2. Few found these approaches helpful.
   3. Most had their complementary and alternative medicine covered through health care coverage.
   4. Most are from lower socioeconomic backgrounds.
4. Which of the following is representative of holistic nursing care?
   1. Mind, body, and spirit
   2. Disease, spirit, and family
   3. Desires and emotions
   4. Muscles, nerves, and spine disorders
5. After a nurse completes an assessment of a patient, whose permission is required before implementing complementary and alternative medicine therapy?
   1. The physician
   2. The patient
   3. The family
   4. No permission is required.
6. According to the principles of complementary and alternative medicine approaches, which of the following statements best describes the individual who receives treatment?

1. Actively involved in the treatment
2. A complete believer in what is being taught
3. Submissive to the practitioner
4. Less competent in his or her own care

7. Which of the following describes the most effective use of St. John's wort?
   1. Antioxidant
   2. Anti-inflammatory
   3. Mild antidepressant
   4. Vasodilator
8. Meditation may augment the effects of which of the following medications?
   1. Antihypertensive medications
   2. Insulin and vitamins
   3. Prednisone
   4. Cough syrups and aspirin
9. Acupuncture techniques are frequently used to:
   1. Bring the patient's body back into balance through the transfer of energy
   2. Stimulate and activate the body's self-healing abilities
   3. Treat diseases of the spine and joints.
   4. Create a state of relaxation through reduction of neural impulses sent to the brain
10. Therapeutic touch is a training-specific therapy that was developed by which profession?
    1. Medicine
    2. Physiotherapy
    3. Occupational therapy
    4. Nursing

Answers: 1. 3; **2.** 4; **3.** 1; **4.** 1; **5.** 2; **6.** 1; **7.** 3; **8.** 1; **9.** 2; **10.** 4

Rationales for the Review Questions appear at the end of the book.

RECOMMENDED WEBSITES

Canadian College of Naturopathic Medicine (CCNM): http://www.ccnm.edu

This website provides detailed information about the 4-year, full-time program offered by this professional college of naturopathic medicine. The site includes a resource centre with links to other websites.

Canadian Interdisciplinary Network for Complementary and Alternative Research (IN-CAM): http://www.incamresearch.ca/index.php?home&lng=en

This network facilitates research, knowledge, and education about CAM in Canada. Links to other associated networks and institutions are provided.

Canadian Nursing Association: https://www.cna-aiic.ca/

This website provides resources on professional practice and professional development.

Chinese Medicine and Acupuncture Association of Canada: http://www.cmaac.ca/

This organization aims to raise the profile and reputation of Chinese medicine and acupuncture. The site includes the organization's history and a Canada-wide members' index.

College of Chiropractors of British Columbia: http://www.chirobc.com/

This website provides information from the governing body that regulates chiropractors in British Columbia.

College of Chiropractors of Ontario: http://cco.on.ca/En

The College of Chiropractors of Ontario is the governing body that regulates chiropractors in Ontario.

College of Nurses of Ontario: Practice Guideline: Complementary Therapies: http://www.cno.org/Global/docs/prac/41021_CompTherapies.pdf

This document provides information on complementary approaches and their application to nursing practice in Ontario, including guidelines for practice.

ConsumerLab.com: http://www.consumerlab.com/

The quality and quantity of ingredients in various brands of NHPs are independently tested by this organization. General use is free, but a small yearly fee is required to access the entire database.

M. D. Anderson Cancer Center: Complementary, Alternative & Integrative Medicine: https://www.mdanderson.org/treatment-options/complementary-and-integrative-medicine.html

The information provided here about complementary medicine and how it can be integrated with allopathic medicine is useful to both health care providers and the public.

National Center for Complementary and Alternative Medicine: http://nccam.nih.gov/

This centre provides information on various natural health products, research, and ongoing clinical trials related to CAM. It also gives links to a variety of other resources and institutions related to complementary and alternative medicines.

Natural and Non-prescription Health Products: https://www.canada.ca/en/health-canada/services/drugs-health-products/natural-non-prescription.html

This directorate is Health Canada's regulating authority for NHPs for sale in Canada. The site includes information on the regulatory practices, definitions related to NHPs, and an index of various health-related issues.

Public Health Agency of Canada: https://www.canada.ca/en/public-health.html

The agency's focus is on efforts to prevent chronic diseases, injuries, and public health emergencies. The agency works closely with provinces and territories to keep Canadians healthy and reduce pressures on the health care system.

REFERENCES

Anderson, J. G., & Taylor, A. G. (2011). The effects of healing touch in clinical practice: A systematic review of randomized clinical trials. *Journal of Holistic Nursing, 29*(2), 221–228. doi:10.1177/0898010110393353.

Benson, H. (1975). *The relaxation response.* New York: Avon.

Berger, L., Tavares, M., & Berger, B. (2013). The Canadian experience of integrating complementary therapy in a hospital palliative care unit. *Journal of Palliative Medicine, 16*(10), 1294–1298. doi:10.1089/jpm.2013.0295.

Bergmann, T. F., & Peterson, D. H. (2011). *Chiropractic technique: Principles and procedures* (3rd ed.). St. Louis, MO: Elsevier Mosby.

Bolek, J. E., Rosenthal, R. L., & Sherman, R. A. (2016). Advanced topics in surface electromyography: Instrumentation and applications. In M. S. Schwartz & F. Andrasik (Eds.), *Biofeedback: A practitioner's guide* (4th ed., pp. 68–84). New York: Guilford Press.

Breed, C., & Berenznay, C. (2017). Treatment of depression and anxiety by naturopathic physicians: An observational study of naturopathic medicine within an integrated multidisciplinary community health center. *Journal of Alternative and Complementary Medicine (New York, N.Y.), 23*(5), 348–354. doi:10.1089/acm.2016.0232.

Canadian Association for Schools of Nursing/Association Canadienne des Écoles de Sciences Infirmières (CASN/ACESI). (2015). *National nursing education framework: Final report.* Retrieved from http://www.casn.ca/wp-content/uploads/2014/12/Framwork-FINAL-SB-Nov-30-20151.pdf.

Canadian Association of Naturopathic Doctors (CAND). (2016). *About naturopathic medicine: What can it do for you?* Retrieved from http://www.cand.ca/what-can-it-do-for-you/.

Canadian Cancer Society. (2017). *Make Healthy Choices: Eat Well.* Retrieved from http://www.cancer.ca/en/prevention-and-screening/reduce-cancer-risk/make-healthy-choices/eat-well/?region=bc.

Canadian Holistic Nurses Association. (2008). *Standards of practice.* Retrieved from http://chna.ca/standards-of-practice/.

Canadian Nurses Association. (2015). *Framework for the practice of registered nurses in Canada* (2nd ed.). Ottawa: Author. Retrieved from https://cna-aiic.ca/~/media/cna/page-content/pdf-en/framework-for-the-pracice-of-registered-nurses-in-canada.pdf?la=en.

Cassidy, C. M. (2015). Social and cultural factors in medicine. In M. S. Micozzi (Ed.), *Fundamentals of complementary and alternative medicine* (5th ed.). St. Louis, MO: Saunders/Elsevier.

Clarke, J. (2012). Christianity and nursing. In M. D. Fowler, S. Reimer-Kirkham, R. Sawatzky, et al. (Eds.), *Religion, religious ethics, and nursing*. New York: Springer.

College of Registered Nurses of British Columbia. (2013). *Complementary and alternative health care*. Vancouver, BC: Author. Retrieved from https://www.crnbc.ca/Standards/Lists/StandardResources/437CompandAlternativeHealthCare.pdf.

DeLany, J. (2015). Massage, bodywork and touch therapies. In M. S. Micozzi (Ed.), *Fundamentals of complementary and alternative medicine* (5th ed.). St. Louis, MO: Saunders/Elsevier.

Dewar, A., Gregg, K., White, M., et al. (2009). Navigating the health care system: Perceptions of patients with chronic pain. *Chronic Diseases in Canada, 29*(4). Retrieved from http://www.phac-aspc.gc.ca/publicat/hpcdp-pspmc/29-4/ar_03-eng.php.

Dinkova-Kostova, A. T. (2007). Chemoprotection against cancer: An idea whose time has come. *Alternative Therapies in Health and Medicine, 13*(2), S122–S127.

Dossey, B., & Keegan, L. (2013). *Holistic nursing: A handbook for practice* (6th ed.). Sudbury, MA: Jones & Bartlett.

Ergil, K. V. (2015). Traditional medicine of China and East Asia. In M. Micozzi (Ed.), *Fundamentals of complementary and alternative medicine* (5th ed., pp. 477–507). St. Louis, MO: Saunders/Elsevier.

Ergil, K. V., & Ergil, M. C. (2015). Classical acupuncture. In M. Micozzi (Ed.), *Fundamentals of complementary and alternative medicine* (5th ed., pp. 508–543). St. Louis, MO: Saunders/ Elsevier.

Esmail, N. (2007). Complementary and alternative medicine in Canada: Trends in use and public attitudes, 1997–2006. *Public Policy Sources, 87*. Vancouver, BC: The Fraser Institute. Retrieved from https://www.fraserinstitute.org/sites/default/files/ComplementaryAlternativeMedicine.pdf.

Ezzati, M., Obermeyer, Z., Tzoulaki, I., et al. (2015). Contributions of risk factors and medical care to cardiovascular mortality trends. *Nature Reviews. Cardiology, 12*, 508–530. doi:10.1038/nrcardio.2015.82.

Field, T. (2016). Massage therapy research review. *Complementary Therapies in Clinical Practice, 24*, 19–21. doi:10.1016/j.ctcp.2016.04.005.

Fontaine, K. (2015). *Complementary and alternative therapies for nursing practice* (4th ed.). Englewood Cliffs, NJ: Pearson.

Greene, C., & Green, B. (2012). Efficacy of guided imagery to reduce stress via the Internet: A pilot study. *Journal of Holistic Nursing, 26*(3), 150–165. doi:10.1097/HNP.0b013e31824ef55a.

Harvard Medical School. (2015). *Yoga—Benefits beyond the mat*. Retrieved from http://www.health.harvard.edu/staying-healthy/yoga-benefits-beyond-the-mat.

Health Canada. (2008). *Canada's Food and Drugs Act & Regulations*. Ottawa: Author. Retrieved from http://www.hc-sc.gc.ca/fn-an/legislation/acts-lois/act-loi_reg-eng.php.

Health Canada. (2010). *Unauthorized natural choice health products found on the Canadian market*. Ottawa: Author. Retrieved from http://www.marketwired.com/press-release/unauthorized-natural-choice-health-products-found-on-the-canadian-market-1109550.htm.

Health Canada. (2011). *Natural health product tracking survey 2010. Ipsos-Reid survey*. Ottawa: Author. Retrieved from http://www.int4life.ca/uploads/5/1/5/1/5151557/2010_report.pdf.

Health Canada. (2016). *About natural health products*. Ottawa: Author. Retrieved from http://www.hc-sc.gc.ca/dhp-mps/prodnatur/about-apropos/cons-eng.php.

Hollenberg, D., Tsasis, P., & Kelley, N. (2011). CAM in Canadian hospitals: The new frontier. *Journal of Complementary & Integrative Medicine, 8*(1), 1553–3840. doi:10.2202/1553-3840.1466.

Horton, R. (2016). Offline: Medicine and nutrition: "That's insane". *Lancet, 387*(10029), 1706. Retrieved from http://www.thelancet.com/journals/lancet/article/PIIS0140-6736(16)30300-2/fulltext.

Huang, T., Moser, D. K., & Hwang, S. (2016). The short-term and long-term effects of biofeedback-assisted relaxation therapy in patients with heart failure: A randomized control study. *Sage Open Nursing, 2*, 1–6. Retrieved from http://journals.sagepub.com/doi/pdf/10.1177/2377960816680825.

Kania-Richmond, A., Reece, B., Suter, E., et al. (2015). The professional role of massage therapists in patient care in Canadian urban hospitals—A mixed methods study. *BMC Complementary and Alternative Medicine, 15*(20). Retrieved from https://bmccomplementalternmed.biomedcentral.com/articles/10.1186/s12906-015-0536-4.

Keshet, Y., Ben-Ayre, E., & Schiff, E. (2012). Can holism be practiced in a biomedical setting? A qualitative study of the integration of complementary medicine to a surgical department. *Health (London, England: 1997), 16*(6), 585–601. doi:10.1177/1364593112438566.

Koopsen, C., & Young, C. (2009). *Integrative health: A holistic approach for health professionals*. Boston: Jones & Bartlett.

Krieger, D. (1975). Therapeutic touch: The imprimatur of nursing. *The American Journal of Nursing, 75*(5), 784–787.

Krieger, D., Peper, E., & Ancoli, S. (1979). Therapeutic touch: Searching for evidence of physiological change. *The American Journal of Nursing, 79*(4), 660–662.

Li, C., & Uppal, M. (2010). Canadian National Nutrition Committee clinical update on dietary fibre in diabetes: Food sources to physiological effects. *Canadian Journal of Diabetes, 34*(4), 355–356. doi:10.1016/S1499-2671(10)44010-1.

Lim, D., Condon, P., & DeSteno, D. (2015). Mindfulness and compassion: An examination of mechanism and scalability. *PLoS ONE, 10*(2), e0118221. doi:10.1371/journal.pone.0118221.

Linde, K., Berner, M. M., & Kriston, L. (2008). St. John's wort for major depression. *Cochrane Database of Systematic Reviews*, (4), CD000448.

Lu, D., Hart, L., Lutgendorf, S., et al. (2016). Effects of healing touch and relaxation therapy on adult patients undergoing hematopoietic stem cell transplant: A feasibility pilot study. *Cancer Nursing, 39*(3), E1–E11. doi:10.1097/NCC.0000000000000272.

Mayor, D. (2015). Vitalism. In M. S. Micozzi (Ed.), *Fundamentals of complementary and alternative medicine* (5th ed.). St. Louis, MO: Saunders/Elsevier.

Merkes, M. (2010). Mindfulness-based stress reduction for people with chronic diseases. *Australian Journal of Primary Health, 16*(3), 200–210. doi:10.1071/PY09063.

Metcalfe, A., Williams, J., McChesney, J., et al. (2010). Use of complementary and alternative medicine by those with a chronic disease and the general population: Results of a national population based survey. *BMC Complementary and Alternative Medicine, 10*, 58. doi:10.1186/1472-6882-10-58.

Micozzi, M. S. (2015). Translation from conventional medicine. In M. S. Micozzi (Ed.), *Fundamentals of complementary and alternative medicine* (5th ed., pp. 13–21). St. Louis, MO: Saunders/Elsevier.

Micozzi, M. S., & Jawer, M. A. (2015). Mind-body therapies, stress, and psychometrics. In M. S. Micozzi (Ed.), *Fundamentals of complementary and alternative medicine* (5th ed.). St. Louis, MO: Saunders/Elsevier.

Mpinga, E. K., Kandolo, T., Verloo, H., et al. (2013). Traditional/alternative medicines and the right to health: Key elements for a convention on global health. *Health and Human Rights, 15*(1), 44–57.

National Center for Complementary and Integrative Health (NCCIH). (2016). *Complementary, alternative or integrative health: What's in a name?* Washington, DC: National Institutes of Health. Retrieved from https://nccih.nih.gov/health/integrative-health#moreinfo.

NCD Risk Factor Collaboration (NCD-RisC). (2016). Worldwide trends in diabetes since 1980: A pooled analysis of 751 population-based studies with 4·4 million participants. *Lancet, 387*(10027), 1513–1530. doi: http://dx.doi.org/10.1016/S0140-6736(16)00618-8.

Park, S., & Han, K. (2017). Blood pressure response to meditation and yoga: A systematic review and meta-analysis. *Journal of Alternative and Complementary Medicine (New York, N.Y.), 23*(9), 685–695. doi:10.1089/acm.2016.0234.

Peek, C. J. (2016). The primer of biofeedback instrumentation. In M. S. Schwartz & F. Andrasik (Eds.), *Biofeedback: A practitioner's guide* (4th ed., pp. 35–67). New York: Guilford Press.

Pizzorno, J. E., Snider, P., & Micozzi, M. S. (2015). Nature cure, naturopathy and natural medicine. In M. S. Micozzi (Ed.), *Fundamentals of complementary and alternative medicine* (5th ed., pp. 347–365). St. Louis, MO: Saunders/Elsevier.

Public Health Agency of Canada (PHAC). (2008). *Complementary and alternative health*. Ottawa: Author. Retrieved from http://www.phac-aspc.gc.ca/chn-rcs/cah-acps-eng.php.

Rakel, D., & Faass, N. (2012). *Complementary medicine in clinical practice*. Sudbury, MA: Jones & Bartlett.

Rakel, D., & Fortney, L. (2012). The healing encounter. In D. Rakel (Ed.), *Integrative medicine* (3rd ed., pp. 20–25). Philadelphia: Sanders/Elsevier.

Rakel, D., & Weil, A. (2012). Chapter 1: Philosophy of integrative medicine. In D. Rakel (Ed.), *Integrative medicine* (3rd ed., pp. 3–13). Philadelphia, PA: Saunders/Elsevier.

Redwood, D. (2011). Chiropractic. In T. F. Bergmann & D. H. Peterson (Eds.), *Chiropractic technique: Principles and procedures* (3rd ed.). St. Louis, MO: Mosby/Elsevier.

Reiss, N., Warnecke, I., Tolgou, T., et al. (2017). Effects of cognitive behavioral therapy with relaxation vs. imagery rescripting on test anxiety: A randomized controlled trial. *Journal of Affective Disorders, 208*, 483–489. doi:10.1016/j.jad.2016.10.039.

Saha, F. J., Schumann, S., Cramer, H., et al. (2017). The effects of cupping massage in patients with chronic neck pain—A randomized controlled trial. *Complementary Medicine Research, 24*(1), 26–32. doi:10.1159/000454872.

Schwartz, M. S., Collura, T. F., Kamiya, J., et al. (2016). Theory and definitions of biofeedback and applied psychophysiology. In M. S. Schwartz & F. Andrasik (Eds.), *Biofeedback: A practitioner's guide* (4th ed., pp. 3–23). New York: Guilford Press.

Senderovicha, H., Ip, M., Beralla, M., et al. (2016). Therapeutic Touch in a geriatric palliative care unit—A retrospective review. *Complementary Therapies in Clinical Practice, 24*, 134–138. doi:10.106/j.ctcp.2016.06.002.

Singer, J., & Adams, J. (2011). The place of complementary approaches in an integrated model of refugee health care: Counsellors' and refugee clients' perspectives. *Journal of Refugee Studies, 24*(2), 351–375. doi:10.1186/1472-6882-14-167.

Singer, J., & Adams, J. (2014). Integrating complementary and alternative medicine into mainstream healthcare services: The perspectives of health service managers. *BMC Complementary and Alternative Medicine, 14*, 167. doi:10.1186/1472-6882-14-167.

Snyder, M., Niska, K., & Lindquist, R. (2014). Evolution and use of complementary and alternative therapies. In R. Lindquist, M. Snyder, & M. Tracy (Eds.), *Complementary & alternative approaches in nursing* (7th ed., pp. 3–16). New York: Springer.

Thomson, P., Jones, J., Browne, M., et al. (2014). Why people seek complementary and alternative medicine before conventional medical treatment: A population based study. *Complementary Therapies in Clinical Practice, 20*(4), 339–346. doi:10.1016/j.ctcp.2014.07.008.

Thorogood, M., Simera, I., Dowler, E., et al. (2007). A systematic review of population and community dietary interventions to prevent cancer. *Nutrition Research Reviews, 20*(1), 74–88.

Tovey, P., Chatwin, J., Mason, W., et al. (2003). *The Mediation of CAM in and by cancer user groups, charities and informal networks in the UK & Pakistan*. Retrieved from https://www.york.ac.uk/res/iht/projects/l218252053.htm.

Uchida, S., Kagitani, F., & Sato-Suzuki, I. (2017). Somatoautonomic reflexes in acupuncture therapy: A review. *Autonomic Neuroscience: Basic & Clinical, 203*, 1–8. doi:10.1016/j.autneu.2016.11.001.

Wardle, J., & Sarris, J. (2017). Introduction: Evidence-based clinical naturopathic practice. In J. Wardle & J. Sarris (Eds.), *Clinical naturopathy: In practice*. Chatswood, NSW. Australia: Elsevier.

Wolever, T., Reeds, J., Mansuri, S., et al. (2016). Dietary patterns and type 2 diabetes mellitus in a First Nations community. *Canadian Journal of Diabetes, 40*(4), 304–310. doi:10.1016/j.jcjd.2016.05.001.

World Health Organization (WHO). (2017). *Global health estimates: Deaths by cause, age, sex and country, 2000–2015*. Geneva: Author. Retrieved from http://www.who.int/healthinfo/global_burden_disease/estimates/en/index1.html.

Young, C., & Koopsen, C. (2009). *Spirituality, health, and healing: An integrative approach* (2nd ed.). Burlington, MA: Jones & Bartlett Learning.

36

Activity and Exercise

Canadian content written by Jill Vihos, RN, BScN, MN, PhD
Original chapter by Judith A. McCutchan, RN, ASN, BSN, MSN, PhD

OBJECTIVES

- Define the key terms listed.
- Describe the role of the musculoskeletal and nervous systems in the regulation of activity and exercise.
- Discuss physiological and pathological influences on body alignment and joint mobility.
- Describe how to maintain and use proper body mechanics.
- Describe the evidence that supports regular activity and exercise in patient care.
- Describe the benefits of implementing an exercise program for the purpose of health promotion.
- Describe the benefits of implementing exercise and activity during the acute, restorative, and continuing care of patients.
- Describe important factors to consider when planning an exercise program for patients across the lifespan and for those with specific chronic illnesses.
- Describe how to assess patients for activity intolerance.
- Describe how to assess patients for complications related to immobility.
- Formulate nursing diagnoses for patients who experience impaired mobility and activity intolerance.
- Develop a nursing care plan for a patient with impaired mobility and activity intolerance.
- Describe the interventions for maintaining activity tolerance and mobility during the acute, restorative, and continuing care of patients.
- Evaluate the nursing care plan for maintaining activity and exercise for patients across the lifespan and with specific chronic illnesses.
- Describe how to use proper body mechanics and ergonomics to prevent musculoskeletal injuries.
- Discuss the importance of no-lift policies for patients and health care providers.
- Describe equipment needed for safe patient handling and movement.
- Discuss the impact of national patient safety resources, initiatives, and regulations in relation to patient handling and movement.

KEY TERMS

Activities of daily living (ADLs), p. 836
Activity tolerance, p. 833
Antagonistic muscles, p. 836
Antigravity muscles, p. 836
Cartilage, p. 835
Cartilaginous joints, p. 834
Centre of gravity, p. 833
Ergonomics, p. 847
Exercise, p. 833
Fibrous joints, p. 834
Friction, p. 833
Gait, p. 854
Isometric contraction, p. 834
Isotonic contraction, p. 834
Joint, p. 834
Ligaments, p. 834
Mobility, p. 854
Muscle tone, p. 833
Pathological fractures, p. 834
Posture, p. 836
Proprioception, p. 836
Range of motion (ROM), p. 834
Synarthrotic joint, p. 834
Synchondrodial joint, p. 834
Syndesmodial joint, p. 834
Synergistic muscles, p. 836
Synovial joints, p. 834
Tendons, p. 834

MEDIA RESOURCES

http://evolve.elsevier.com/Canada/Potter/fundamentals/

- Audio Chapter Summaries
- Examination Review Questions
- Concept Map Creator
- Case Study with Questions
- Audio Glossary
- Content Updates
- Video Clips

Regular physical activity and exercise contribute to patients' physical and emotional well-being (Edelman, Kudzma, & Mandle, 2013; Esposito & Fitzpatrick, 2011). This is a principle that you, as a nurse, should apply in the care of patients in all settings. Functional decline (the loss of the ability to perform self-care or activities of daily living) may result not only from illness but also from deconditioning associated with inactivity, the negative effects of which can be seen over short periods of time. Deconditioning involves physiological changes following a period of inactivity, bed rest, or sedentary lifestyle. It is a particular risk for hospitalized patients who spend most of their time in bed, even when they are able to walk. As a result, nurses play an important role in helping to increase the overall activity of inpatients to minimize the risk of deconditioning.

A program of regular physical activity and exercise has the potential to enhance all dimensions of a patient's health (Box 36-1). This chapter provides you with knowledge of exercise and activity as it relates to health promotion, the acute phase of illness, and the restorative and continuing care of patients. Applying knowledge about exercise and activity will allow you to plan nursing strategies for individualized exercise and activity programs. Knowing the function of the musculoskeletal system in maintaining posture, balance, body mechanics, and movement, and implementing evidence-informed knowledge about safe patient handling, are essential in protecting the safety of both the patient and the nurse (see Chapter 45).

BOX 36-1 Effects of Exercise

Cardiovascular System
- Increased cardiac output
- Improved myocardial contraction, thereby strengthening cardiac muscle
- Decreased resting heart rate
- Improved venous return

Pulmonary System
- Increased respiratory rate and depth followed by a quicker return to resting state
- Improved alveolar ventilation
- Decreased work of breathing
- Improved diaphragmatic excursion

Metabolic System
- Increased basal metabolic rate
- Increased use of glucose and fatty acids
- Increased triglyceride breakdown
- Increased gastric motility
- Increased production of body heat

Musculoskeletal System
- Improved muscle tone
- Increased joint mobility
- Improved muscle tolerance to physical exercise
- Possible increase in muscle mass
- Reduced bone loss

Activity Tolerance
- Improved tolerance
- Decreased fatigue

Psychosocial Factors
- Improved tolerance to stress
- Reports of "feeling better"
- Reports of decrease in illness (e.g., colds, influenza)

Based on Huether, S. E., & McCance, K. L. (2012). *Understanding pathophysiology* (5th ed.). St. Louis, MO: Mosby; Hoeman, S. P. (2008). *Rehabilitation nursing: Process, application, and outcomes* (4th ed.). St. Louis, MO: Mosby.

SCIENTIFIC KNOWLEDGE BASE

It is important for nurses to understand the physiology and regulation of body mechanics, exercise, and activity, as it helps nurses to provide individualized patient care.

Overview of Exercise and Activity

The coordinated efforts of the musculoskeletal and nervous systems maintain balance, posture, and body alignment during lifting, bending, moving, and performing activities of daily living. Proper balance, posture, and body alignment reduce the risk of injury to the musculoskeletal system and facilitate body movements, allowing physical mobility without muscle strain and excessive use of muscle energy (see Chapter 45).

Body Alignment. *Body alignment* refers to the relationship of one body part to another body part along a horizontal or vertical line. Correct alignment involves positioning in such a way that no excessive strain is placed on a person's joints, tendons, ligaments, or muscles, thereby maintaining adequate muscle tone and contributing to balance (see Chapter 45). Muscle tone is the internal state of muscle tension within an individual muscle or muscle groups.

Body Balance. Body balance is achieved when a centre of gravity is balanced over a stable base of support and is enhanced using proper posture (Patton & Thibodeau, 2012). You can use balance to maintain proper body alignment and posture by taking two simple actions: (1) widening the base of support by separating your feet to a comfortable distance, and (2) bringing the centre of gravity closer to the base of support; do this by bending your knees and flexing your hips until you are squatting yet maintaining proper back alignment by keeping your trunk erect. For example, the nurse raises the height of a hospital bed when performing a procedure such as changing a dressing to prevent bending too far at the waist and shifting the base of support.

Friction. Friction is a force that occurs in a direction to oppose movement. It increases a patient's risk for skin and tissue damage and potential pressure injuries (see Chapter 46). Friction is reduced by following some basic principles:

- Avoid lifting or moving patients manually. Using a mechanical lift completely prevents friction.
- In situations when you must assist a patient to move manually, use a friction-reducing device such as a slider sheet, slide board, or transfer board to reduce friction.
- When possible, use some of the patient's strength and mobility to assist with transferring or moving the patient in bed. For instance, if patients can bend their knees as you assist them in moving up in bed, friction is decreased. Explain the procedure and tell the patient when to move (see Chapter 45).
- The greater the surface area of the object to be moved, the greater the friction. If a patient is unable to assist in moving up in bed, placing the patient's arms across the chest decreases surface area and reduces friction.

Exercise and Activity. Exercise is physical activity for the purpose of conditioning the body, improving health, and maintaining fitness, or it may be used as a therapeutic measure. When a person exercises, physiological changes occur in body systems (see Box 36-1). The exercise program chosen and developed for a patient depends on that individual's activity tolerance, or the kind and amount of exercise or activity that the individual is able to perform. Physiological, emotional, and developmental factors influence the patient's activity tolerance.

An active lifestyle is important for promoting and maintaining health and is also an essential treatment modality for chronic illnesses (Combs, Diehl, Chrzastowski, et al., 2013). Regular physical activity and exercise enhance functioning of all body systems, including cardiopulmonary functioning (endurance), musculoskeletal fitness (strength, flexibility, and bone integrity), weight control and maintenance (body image), and psychological well-being (Edelman et al., 2013).

The best program of physical activity includes a combination of exercises that produce different physiological and psychological benefits. Isotonic, isometric, and resistive isometric are three categories of exercise classified according to the type of muscle contraction involved. Isotonic exercises cause muscle contraction and changes in muscle length (isotonic contraction). Walking, swimming, dance aerobics, jogging, bicycling, and moving arms and legs with light resistance are examples of isotonic exercises. Isotonic exercises enhance circulatory and respiratory functioning, increase muscle mass, tone, and strength; and promote osteoblastic activity (activity by bone-forming cells) to combat osteoporosis.

Isometric exercises involve tightening or tensing muscles without moving body parts (isometric contraction) (see Chapter 45). Isometric exercises are especially helpful to people who are recovering from injuries or procedures that limit range of motion. An example is quadriceps set exercises—pressing the knee toward the bed and holding—an exercise commonly done after knee surgery. Isometric exercises are ideal for patients who are unable to tolerate the increased activity. A patient who is immobilized in bed can perform isometric exercises. Benefits of isometric exercises include minimized potential for muscle wasting by increasing muscle mass, tone, and strength, thus decreasing the potential for muscle wasting; increased circulation to the involved body part; and increased osteoblastic activity.

Resistive isometric exercises are those in which the individual contracts the muscle while pushing against a stationary object or resisting the movement of an object (Resnick, Boltz, Galick, et al., 2012). A gradual increase in the amount of resistance and in the length of time that the muscle contraction is held will increase muscle strength and endurance. Examples of restrictive isometric exercises include the plank (for abdominal strengthening) and the wall push-up (for chest, triceps, and shoulder strengthening). The patient who is in a sitting position may do hip lifting, in which the hands push against a surface such as the seat of a chair to raise the hips. Resistive isometric exercises help to promote muscle strength and provide sufficient stress against bone to promote osteoblastic activity.

Regulation of Movement

Coordinated body movement involves the integrated functioning of the skeletal, muscular, and nervous systems. Because these three systems cooperate so closely in mechanical support of the body, they are often considered a single functional unit.

Skeletal System. The skeletal system or bones perform five functions in the body: support, protection, movement, mineral storage, and hematopoiesis (blood cell formation). In a discussion of body mechanics, two of these functions—support and movement—are most important (Patton & Thibodeau, 2012). Bones provide the framework for support and contribute to shape, alignment, and positioning of body parts.

Bones are further characterized by firmness, rigidity, and elasticity. Firmness results from inorganic salts, such as calcium and phosphate, that are laid down in the bone matrix. Firmness is related to the bone's rigidity, which is necessary to keep long bones straight and enables bones to bear weight. In addition, bones have a degree of elasticity and flexibility that changes with age. For example, newborns have a large amount of cartilage and are highly flexible, but their bones are unable to support weight. Toddlers' bones are more pliable than those of older people and thus are better able to withstand falls. Older persons, especially women, are more susceptible to bone loss (resorption) and osteoporosis. Osteoporosis Canada (2017) estimates that there are approximately 2 million Canadians with osteoporosis. One in three women and one in five men will break a bone due to osteoporosis in their lifetime.

Bones protect vital organs (e.g., the skull around the brain; the ribs around the heart and lungs). They also aid in calcium regulation, store calcium, and release calcium into the body's circulation as needed. Patients with decreased calcium regulation and metabolism are at risk for developing osteoporosis and pathological fractures (fractures caused by weakened bone tissue) (Walker, 2008). Eighty percent of fractures in Canadians over 60 are related to osteoporosis (Osteoporosis Canada, 2017). In addition, the internal structure of bones contains bone marrow, which participates in red blood cell (RBC) production (hematopoiesis) and acts as a reservoir for blood. Patients with altered bone marrow function or diminished RBC production are usually weakened and fatigue easily, which decreases their mobility and places them at risk of falling.

Joints, ligaments, tendons, and cartilage permit strength and flexibility of the skeleton. Strength enables the skeletal system to support the body.

Joints. Joints or articulations are the connections between bones. Each joint is classified according to its structure and degree of mobility. Joints are classified as four types: synarthrotic, cartilaginous, fibrous, and synovial (Huether & McCance, 2012). A person's flexibility is demonstrated through range of motion (ROM), which is the range of normal movement for a joint.

In a synarthrotic joint, bones are jointed by bones. No movement is associated with this type of joint, and the bony tissue that forms between the bones provides strength and stability. The classic example of this type of joint is the sacrum, in which vertebrae are joined (Figure 36-1, *A*).

The cartilaginous joint, or synchondrodial joint, has little movement but is elastic and uses cartilage to unite body surfaces. Cartilaginous joints are found when bones are exposed to constant pressure, such as the costosternal joints between the sternum and ribs (Figure 36-1, *B*).

The fibrous joint, or syndesmodial joint, is a joint in which two bony surfaces are united by a ligament or membrane. The fibres of ligaments are flexible and stretch, permitting a limited amount of movement. For example, the paired bones of the lower leg (tibia and fibula) are fibrous joints (Huether & McCance, 2012) (Figure 36-1, *C*).

The synovial joint is a freely movable joint in which contiguous bony surfaces are covered by articular cartilage and connected by ligaments lined with a synovial membrane. Joining of the humeral radius and ulna by cartilage and ligaments forms a pivotal joint (Figure 36-1, *D*). Other types of synovial joints are the ball-and-socket joints (e.g., hip joint) and the hinge joints (e.g., interphalangeal joints of the fingers).

Ligaments, Tendons, and Cartilage. Ligaments are white, shiny, flexible bands of fibrous tissue that support the skeletal system. Ligaments bind joints together and connect bones and cartilage. Ligaments are elastic and aid joint flexibility and support (Figure 36-2). In addition, some ligaments have a protective function. For example, ligaments between the vertebral bodies and the ligamentum flavum prevent damage to the spinal cord during movement of the back.

Tendons are white, glistening, fibrous bands of tissue that connect muscle to bone. Tendons are strong, flexible, and inelastic, and they

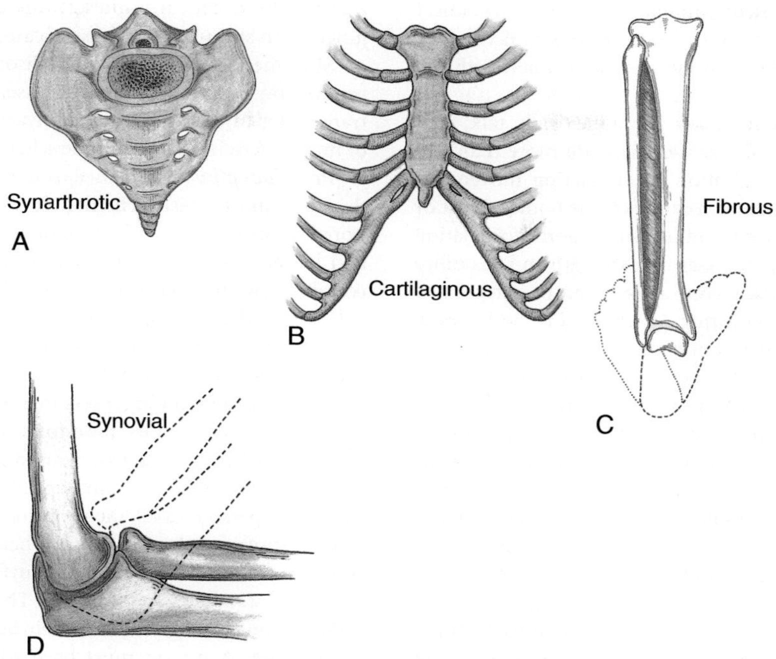

FIGURE 36-1 **Joint types. A,** Synarthrotic. **B,** Cartilaginous. **C,** Fibrous. **D,** Synovial.

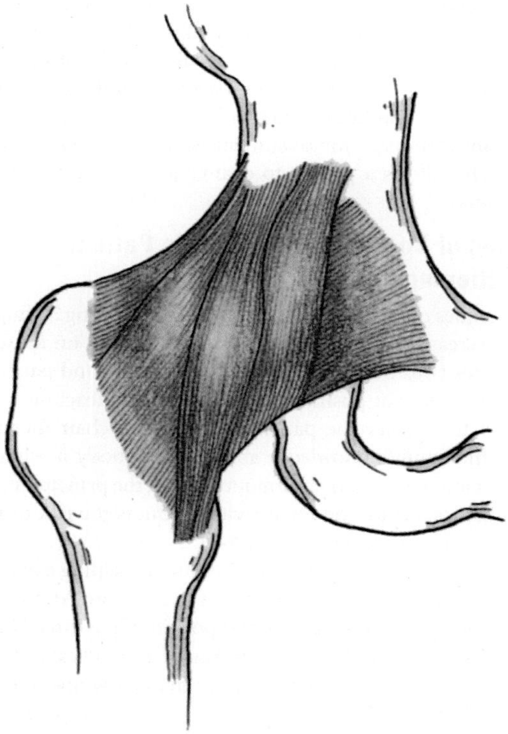

FIGURE 36-2 Ligaments of the hip joint.

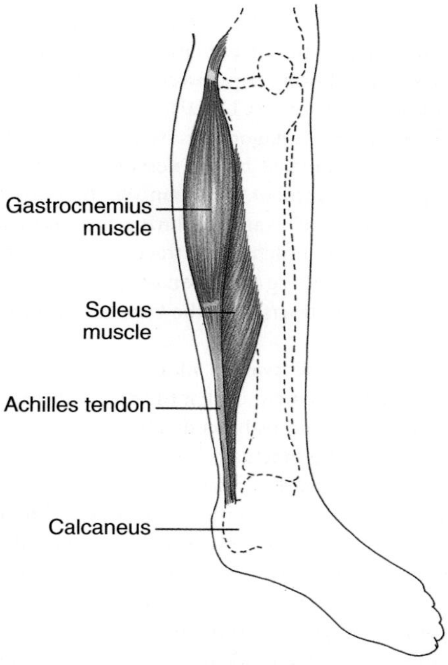

FIGURE 36-3 Tendons and muscles of the lower leg.

occur in various lengths and thicknesses. The Achilles tendon (tendo calcaneus) is the thickest and strongest tendon in the body. It begins near the middle of the posterior of the calf and attaches the gastrocnemius and soleus muscles in the calf to the calcaneal bone in the back of the foot (Figure 36-3).

Cartilage is nonvascular, supporting connective tissue with flexibility similar to that of firm plastic. The gristle-like nature of cartilage permits it to sustain weight and to serve as a shock absorber between articulating bones. It is located chiefly in the joints and thorax, trachea, larynx, nose, and ear. The fetus has a large amount of temporary cartilage, which is replaced by bone developed during infancy. Permanent cartilage is unossified (not hardened), except in advanced age and in diseases such as osteoarthritis. Strength and flexibility do not result entirely from joints, ligaments, tendons, and cartilage. Adequate skeletal muscle is also necessary.

Skeletal Muscle. Muscles are made of fibres that contract when stimulated by an electrochemical impulse that travels from the nerve to the muscle across the neuromuscular junction. The electrochemical impulse causes the filaments (predominantly protein molecules of myosin and actin) within the fibre to slide past each other, with the filaments changing length.

Contraction of skeletal muscles allows people to walk, talk, run, breathe, and participate in physical activity. There are more than 600 skeletal muscles in the body. In addition to facilitating movement, these muscles determine the form and contour of our bodies. Most of our muscles span at least one joint and attach to both articulating bones. Adequate skeletal muscle is necessary for strength and flexibility (Patton & Thibodeau, 2012). Muscle contractions can be categorized by functional purpose: moving, resisting, or stabilizing body parts. Muscle action necessary for active movement is referred to as dynamic or isotonic contraction. In contrast, static or isometric contraction causes an increase in muscle tension or muscle work but with no active movement of the muscle (e.g., instructing the patient in tightening and relaxing a muscle group, as in quadriceps set exercises or pelvic floor muscle exercises). Voluntary movement is a combination of isotonic and isometric contractions. For example, when you lift a patient up in bed, the patient's weight causes increased tension in the muscles of your arms until the tension (isometric) is equal to the weight to be lifted and the weight of your lower arms. When this equilibrium is reached, continued stimulation of the muscles results in muscle shortening (isotonic) and bending of the elbows (active movement), and the patient is lifted off the bed.

Isometric contraction and exercise increases energy expenditure. As a nurse, you must recognize the energy expenditure (increased respiratory rate and increased work on the heart) associated with isometric exercises, because these types of exercises may be contraindicated in certain illnesses or conditions (e.g., myocardial infarction or chronic obstructive pulmonary disease [COPD]).

Muscle Groups. The antagonistic, synergistic, and antigravity muscle groups are coordinated by the nervous system and maintain posture and initiate movement. **Antagonistic muscles** bring about movement at the joint. For example, during flexion of the arm, the active mover (the biceps brachii) contracts and its antagonist (the triceps brachii) relaxes. During extension of the arm, the active mover (the triceps brachii) contracts and the new antagonist (the biceps brachii) relaxes.

Synergistic muscles are two or more muscles that contract to accomplish the same movement. When the arm is flexed, the strength of the contraction of the biceps brachii is increased by contraction of the synergistic muscle, the brachialis.

Antigravity muscles work to stabilize joints. These muscles continuously oppose the effect of gravity on the body and permit a person to maintain an upright or sitting posture. In an adult, the antigravity muscles are the extensors of the leg—the gluteus maximus, the quadriceps femoris, and the soleus muscles—and the muscles of the back.

Skeletal muscles support posture and carry out voluntary movement. These muscles are attached to the skeleton by tendons, which provide strength and permit motion. The movement of the extremities is voluntary and requires coordination from the nervous system.

Nervous System. Movement and posture are regulated by the nervous system. The major voluntary motor area, located in the cerebral cortex, is the precentral gyrus, or motor strip. Motor fibres descend from the motor strip and cross at the level of the medulla. Motor fibres from the right motor strip initiate voluntary movement for the left side of the body, and the motor fibres from the left motor strip initiate voluntary movement for the right side of the body.

Transmission of the impulse from the nervous system to the musculoskeletal system is an electrochemical event and requires a neurotransmitter. *Neurotransmitters* are chemicals (e.g., acetylcholine) that transfer the electrical impulse from the nerve across the myoneural junction to stimulate the muscle, causing movement.

Movement can be impaired by disorders that alter neurotransmitter production, as in Parkinson's disease; alter transfer from the neurotransmitter to the muscle, as in myasthenia gravis; or alter activation of muscle activity, as in multiple sclerosis (Huether & McCance, 2012).

Proprioception. **Proprioception** is the awareness of the position of the body and its parts (Huether & McCance, 2012). Position is monitored by proprioceptors located on nerve endings in muscles, tendons, and joints. **Posture** is regulated by the nervous system and requires coordination of proprioception and balance. As a person carries out **activities of daily living (ADLs)**, proprioceptors monitor muscle activity and body position. For example, the proprioceptors on the soles of the feet contribute to correct posture during standing or walking. During standing, pressure is continuous on the bottom of the feet. The proprioceptors monitor the pressure, communicating this information through the nervous system to the antigravity muscles. The standing person remains upright until deciding to change position. As a person walks, the proprioceptors on the bottom of the feet monitor pressure changes. Thus, when the bottom of the moving foot comes in contact with the walking surface, the individual automatically moves the stationary foot forward. The proprioceptors allow people to walk without having to watch their feet.

Balance. A person must have adequate balance when standing, running, lifting, or performing ADLs. Balance is controlled by the nervous system, specifically by the cerebellum and the inner ear. The cerebellum coordinates all voluntary movement, particularly highly skilled movements, such as those required in skiing.

Within the inner ear are the semicircular canals, three fluid-filled structures that assist in maintaining balance. Fluid within the canals has inertia. When the head is suddenly rotated in one direction, the fluid remains stationary for a moment, whereas the canal turns with the head. This allows a person to change position suddenly without losing balance.

Principles of Body Mechanics, Safe Patient Transfer, and Positioning Techniques

Using principles of safe patient transfer and positioning during routine activities decreases work effort and places less strain on musculoskeletal structures (Box 36-2). Nurses teach colleagues and patients' families how to transfer or position patients properly. Teaching a patient's family how to transfer the patient from bed to chair increases and reinforces the family's knowledge about proper body mechanics, and safe transfer and positioning techniques. Using the principles of proper body mechanics during routine activities reduces the risk of injury to the nurse and the patient (see Box 36-2).

Whether moving a patient who is immobile, helping a patient from the bed to the chair, or teaching a patient to carry out ADLs efficiently, knowledge of safe patient transfer and positioning is vital. Nurses also incorporate knowledge of physiological and pathological influences on body alignment and mobility. Nurses are frequently involved in activities that include standing or sitting at desks and computers to document care, and preparing equipment and supplies. All of these activities require as much attention to proper body mechanics as to hands-on patient care.

Pathological Influences on Body Mechanics and Movement

Many pathological conditions affect body alignment, body movement, and the capacity for exercise and activity. These conditions include congenital abnormalities, degenerative diseases, and episodic illnesses affecting bones, joints, muscles, and the central nervous system.

BOX 36-2 Quality Improvement: Principles of Body Mechanics, Safe Patient Transfer, and Patient Positioning

- Mechanical lifts are essential when a patient is unable to assist.
- When transferring a patient, perform six check points:
  1. Three for the top: *Ears (1)* in line with *shoulders (2)*, shoulders in line with *hips (3)*.
  2. Three for the bottom: *Tighten stomach (1)* and *push your buttocks back (2)* while keeping your *body weight over the heels (3)*. Move your trunk forward, bending at the hips, not the waist.
  3. Elbows are tucked in to your sides.
  4. Use palms-up grip.
  5. Work in your comfort zone: Bend and tuck elbows into your sides, move hands from shoulders to hips.
  6. Weight transfer: Stand with a stable base of support, transfer weight side to side and front to back.
- When a patient is unable to assist, remember the following principles:
  - The wider the base of support, the greater the stability.
  - The lower the centre of gravity, the greater the stability.
  - Facing the direction of movement prevents abnormal twisting of the spine.
  - Dividing balanced activity between arms and legs reduces the risk of back injury.
  - Leverage, rolling, turning, or pivoting requires less work than lifting.
  - Use transfer sheets to reduce friction between the patient and the surface over which the patient is moved, to reduce the force required to reposition the patient.
  - Reducing the force of work reduces the risk of injury.
  - Maintaining good body mechanics reduces fatigue of the muscle groups.
  - Alternating periods of rest and activity helps reduce fatigue.
- When transferring a patient who is in the supine position with another health care provider, always work at the height of the taller person.

Adapted from Alberta Health Services. (2017). *Ergonomics training*. Retrieved from http://www.albertahealthservices.ca/careers/Page12772.aspx.

Chronic diseases affecting the internal organs can also affect an individual's capacity for activity and exercise.

Congenital Abnormalities. Congenital abnormalities affect musculoskeletal alignment, balance, and appearance. For example, osteogenesis imperfecta is an inherited disorder characterized by bones that are porous, short, bowed, and deformed; as a result, children with this disorder experience curvature of the spine and shortness of stature. Scoliosis is a structural curvature of the spine associated with vertebral rotation. Muscles, ligaments, and other soft tissues become shortened as a result. Balance and mobility are affected in proportion to the severity of abnormal spinal curvatures (Hockenberry & Wilson, 2014).

Disorders of Bones, Joints, and Muscles. Osteoporosis, a well-publicized disorder of aging, results in the reduction of bone density or mass. The cause is uncertain, and theories vary from hormonal imbalances to insufficient intake of nutrients (Huether & McCance, 2012).

Joint mobility is altered by inflammatory and noninflammatory joint diseases and articular disruption. Inflammatory joint disease (e.g., arthritis) is characterized by inflammation or destruction of the synovial membrane and articular cartilage and the systemic signs of inflammation. Noninflammatory diseases have none of these characteristics, and the synovial fluid is normal (Huether & McCance, 2012). Joint degeneration, which can occur with inflammatory and noninflammatory disease, is marked by changes in articular cartilage combined with overgrowth of bone at the articular ends. Degenerative changes commonly affect weight-bearing joints such as the hips and knees.

Articular disruption involves trauma to the articular capsules and ranges from mild, such as a tear resulting in a sprain, to severe, such as a separation leading to dislocation. Articular disruption also includes disorders such as developmental dysplasia of the hip (Hockenberry and Wilson, 2014).

Central Nervous System Damage and Disorders. Damage to any part of the central nervous system that regulates voluntary movement causes impaired body alignment and immobility (see Chapter 31). For example, a patient with a traumatic head injury experiences damage in the motor strip in the cerebrum. The amount of voluntary impairment is directly related to the amount of destruction of the motor strip. A patient with a complete spinal cord injury in the lumbar region has permanent damage below the level of the injury and retains control of trunk muscles, but not the lower extremity muscles.

It is important to understand which type of voluntary and involuntary movement is present after damage to the central nervous system. This information affects the type of interventions selected to maximize a patient's activity level.

Degenerative diseases of the central nervous system affect an individual's health and abilities over time. Degenerative diseases of the nervous system such as Parkinson's disease or multiple sclerosis can affect an individual's control of movement and balance.

Musculoskeletal Trauma. Musculoskeletal trauma often results in bruises, contusions, sprains, and fractures. A *fracture* is a disruption of bone tissue continuity. Fractures most commonly result from direct external trauma. They also occur because of some deformity of the bone (e.g., with pathological fractures of osteoporosis) (see Chapter 31). These often result in a period of reduced mobility followed by a period of rehabilitation and thus are described in more detail in Chapter 45.

Other Chronic Diseases. Many chronic diseases of the internal organs also affect an individual's ability to be active and exercise. Diseases of the heart such as coronary artery disease and heart failure can alter tissue perfusion and hence activity tolerance. Chronic diseases of the lungs such as asthma and COPD can impair gas exchange, thus also affecting activity tolerance. Diabetes, chronic renal impairment, and various cancers can all similarly affect one's ability to exercise.

NURSING KNOWLEDGE BASE

Application of knowledge about activity and exercise enables nurses to think critically about the holistic needs of patients. Nursing knowledge as it pertains to activity and exercise helps nurses to assess, identify, and intervene when patients have decreased activity tolerance or physical limitation that affects their mobility, ability to exercise, or both (see Chapter 45).

Deconditioning

In acute care settings, intervening to increase inpatients' activity and mobility levels as soon as possible to prevent deconditioning and other complications of immobilization is essential (Table 36-1). In a study involving 78 adults who were admitted to a respiratory unit for diagnostic or preoperative evaluation and who were able to walk and were not confined to bed rest, functional capacity decreased over a 5-day period in six assessment areas: upper limb muscle strength, respiratory muscle strength, lung function, chest wall expansion, submaximal exercise tolerance, and spinal and trunk mobility (Suesada et al. (2007).

Additional physical benefits of inpatient mobilization include less delirium, pain, urinary discomfort, urinary tract infection, fatigue,

TABLE 36-1 Risks Associated With Deconditioning

Body System	Adverse Effects	Potential Complications	Nursing Actions
Respiratory	Decreased lung expansion Hypoventilation Impaired gas exchange Pulmonary secretion pooling	Atelectasis Pneumonia Hypoxemia Pulmonary edema Pulmonary embolism	Frequent respiratory system assessment, including rate, rhythm, depth, quality, effort of respiration, SpO_2, and auscultation of anterior and posterior lung fields. Positioning in bed to facilitate maximum lung expansion Encourage deep breathing and coughing exercises Encourage incentive spirometry Chest physiotherapy Daily ambulation
Circulatory	Venous pooling and peripheral edema in extremities as a result of decreased systemic vascular resistance Decreased cardiac output	Thrombus formation Orthostatic hypotension	Frequent circulatory system assessment, including pulse, blood pressure, skin colour, assessment of extremities for colour, sensation, movement, temperature, edema and peripheral pulses, and auscultation of heart sounds. Application and ongoing assessment of compression stockings Passive range-of-motion exercises Assessment of blood pressure before ambulating, to prevent injury Daily ambulation
Integumentary	Decreased delivery of oxygen and nutrients to tissues Inflammation over bony prominences Shearing of skin during movement Tissue ischemia due to pressure between bony prominences and bed or chair	Skin breakdown Abrasions/excoriation Pressure injuries Infection	Frequent assessment of posterior skin surfaces to identify inflammation and skin breakdown Repositioning patients every 2–3 hours Assessment and management of skin to ensure integument is clean and dry Application of skin barriers to prevent skin breakdown
Musculoskeletal	Reduced muscle mass Decreased muscle strength Impaired joint mobility Decreased endurance	Fatigue Muscle atrophy Decreased stability and balance Joint contractures	Isotonic and isometric exercises Passive range-of-motion exercises Daily ambulation Application of splints to prevent joint contractures
Gastrointestinal	Decreased peristalsis Decreased fluid intake Decreased appetite	Abdominal distension Constipation Ileus Aspiration	Frequent abdominal assessment, including inspection, auscultation, and palpation Assessment of fluid intake and output Assessment of oral intake Assessment of daily bowel activity Daily ambulation High-protein diet

SpO_2, Peripheral capillary oxygen saturation.
Adapted from Crawford, A., & Harris, H. (2016). Caring for adults with impaired physical mobility. *Nursing, 46*(12), 36–41. doi:10.1097/01.NURSE.0000504674.19099.1d; Kalisch, B. J., Lee, S., & Dabney, B. W. (2013). Outcomes of inpatient mobilization: a literature review. *Journal of Clinical Nursing, 23*, 1486–1501. doi:10.1111/jocn.12315.

deep vein thrombosis, and pneumonia, and improved ability to void (Kalisch, Lee, & Dabney, 2013). Longer periods of hospitalization inevitably lead to more severe deconditioning, slower recovery, more functional decline, and longer length of hospital stay (Kalisch et al., 2013; Suesada, Martins, & Carvalho, 2007). These findings support the promotion of early mobility in hospitalized patients.

Safety Guidelines for Nursing Skills

Ensuring patient safety is an essential role of the professional nurse. To ensure patient safety, communicate clearly with members of the health care team, assess and incorporate the patient's priorities of care and preferences, and use the best evidence when making decisions about your patient's care. When performing the skills in this chapter, remember the following points to ensure safe patient handling and individualized patient-centred care.

- Mentally review the transfer steps before beginning the procedure; this ensures both your safety and that of the patient.
- Prior to transferring a patient, perform a functional assessment to determine the patient's mobility, strength, and the assistance that he or she is able to offer during transfer. Stand on the patient's weak side when assisting (Pierson & Fairchild, 2013).
- Determine the amount and type of assistance required for transfer, including the type of transfer equipment and the number of personnel to safely transfer and prevent harm to the patient and health care providers.
- Raise the side rail on the side of the bed opposite where you are standing to prevent the patient from falling out of bed on that side.
- Arrange equipment (e.g., intravenous lines, feeding tube, in-dwelling catheter) in such a way that it does not interfere with the positioning or transfer process.
- Evaluate the patient for correct body alignment and pressure risks after the transfer.
- Make sure that all personnel understand how the equipment functions before it is used.

- Educate patients about how equipment functions, to reduce their anxiety and enlist their cooperation.

Safe Patient Handling

Nurses are exposed to the hazards related to lifting and transferring patients in many settings, such as inpatient nursing units, long-term care facilities, and the operating room (Griffis, 2012). In most health care facilities, quality improvement programs and no-lift policies have been implemented. Manually lifting and transferring patients contributes to the high incidence of work-related musculoskeletal problems and back injuries in nurses and members of the health care team. Current evidence shows that many nurses frequently transfer to different positions and leave the profession because of work-related injuries (Griffis, 2012). Implementing evidence-informed interventions and programs can reduce the number of work-related injuries, which improves the health of the nurse and reduces indirect costs to the health care system.

Many provinces have implemented occupational health and safety legislation regarding lifting and moving loads. For instance, in Alberta the law requires that employers provide equipment and training and that employees use that equipment and training (*Occupational Health and Safety Act Alberta* [Government of Alberta, 2016]). Health boards are implementing comprehensive safe patient-handling programs in all parts of Canada. Comprehensive safe patient-handling programs include the following elements (VISN 8 Patient Safety Center, 2015):

- An ergonomics assessment protocol for health care environments
- Patient assessment criteria and algorithms for safe patient handling and movement
- Special equipment kept in convenient locations to help transfer patients
- Back-injury resource nurses
- An "after-action" review that allows the health care team to apply knowledge about moving patients safely in different settings
- A no-lift policy

It is the responsibility of the nurse not only to implement existing safe handling policies within the workplace but also to advocate for enhancements to safety (Skill 36-1). This includes identifying unsafe situations such as broken equipment or the improper techniques of others. It involves reviewing literature and government policy to remain current on best practices. Nurses need to assume an active role in their workplaces to ensure that a culture of safety exists and that appropriate patient-handling equipment is readily available for use (Hunter, Branson, & Davenport, 2010). The nurse must advocate for change within the workplace when safer options exist, for the benefit of all staff and patients.

SKILL 36-1 USING SAFE AND EFFECTIVE TRANSFER TECHNIQUES

Delegation Considerations

The skill of effective transfer techniques can be delegated to unregulated nursing personnel (UNP). Patients who are transferred for the first time after prolonged bed rest, extensive surgery, critical illness, or spinal cord trauma usually require supervision by the nurse. Instruct the UNP about:

- Seeking assistance when moving or transferring a patient (e.g., when the patient is overweight, medicated, or confused).
- Patient limitations (e.g., changes in blood pressure, mobility restrictions) that affect safe transfer techniques.

Equipment

- Transfer belt, sling, or lapboard (as needed)
- Nonskid shoes, transfer sheets, and pillows
- Wheelchair (Position chair at 45- to 60-degree angle to bed, lock brakes, remove footrests, and lock bed brakes.)
- Stretcher (Position next to bed, lock brakes on stretcher, lock brakes on bed.)
- Mechanical/hydraulic lift (Use frame, canvas strips or chains, and hammock or canvas strips.)
- Stand-assist lift device

ASSESSMENT

STEPS	RATIONALE
1. Identify patient using two identifiers (e.g., name and birthday or name and medical record number) according to agency policy. Explain procedure.	• Ensures correct patient. Complies with The Joint Commission standards and improves patient safety (Joint Commission, 2017).
2. Assess physiological capacity to transfer:	• Provides information relative to patient's abilities, physical status, ability to comprehend, and number of individuals needed to provide safe transferring.
A. Muscle strength (legs and upper arms)	• Immobile patients have decreased muscle strength, tone, and mass. Affects ability to bear weight or raise body.
B. Joint mobility (range of motion [ROM]) and contracture formation	• Immobility or inflammatory processes (e.g., arthritis) sometimes lead to contracture formation and impaired joint mobility.
C. Paralysis or paresis (spastic or flaccid)	• Patient with central nervous system damage often has bilateral paralysis (requiring transfer by swivel bar, sliding bar, or mechanical lift) or unilateral paralysis, which requires belt transfer to "best" side. Weakness (paresis) requires stabilization of knee while transferring. Flaccid arm needs to be supported with sling during transfer.
D. Bone continuity.	• Patients with trauma to one leg or hip may be non–weight bearing during transfer. Amputees may use slide board to transfer.
3. Assess for weakness, dizziness, or orthostatic (postural) hypotension or risk for orthostatic hypotension (e.g., previously on bed rest, first time arising from supine position following surgical procedure, history of dizziness when arising)	• Determines risk of fainting or falling during transfer. Immobilized patients have decreased ability for autonomic nervous system to equalize blood supply, resulting in drop of 20 mm Hg systolic or more in blood pressure when rising from sitting position (Fedorowski & Melander, 2013; Lewis et al., 2013).
4. Activity tolerance, noting for fatigue during activity	• Determines ability of patient to help with transfer.

Continued

SKILL 36-1 USING SAFE AND EFFECTIVE TRANSFER TECHNIQUES—cont'd

STEPS	RATIONALE
5. Assess proprioceptive function (awareness of posture and equilibrium), including ability to maintain balance while sitting in bed or on side of bed and tendency to sway toward one side.	• Determines stability of patient's balance for transfer and risk for falls.
6. Assess sensory status, including central and peripheral vision, adequacy of hearing, and presence of peripheral sensation loss.	• Determines influence of sensory loss on ability to make transfer. Visual field loss decreases patient's ability to see in direction of transfer. Peripheral sensation loss decreases proprioception. Patients with visual and hearing losses need transfer techniques adapted to deficits. Patients with a cerebrovascular accident (CVA) sometimes lose area of visual field, which profoundly affects vision and perception.

CRITICAL DECISION POINT: *Patients with hemiplegia also often "neglect" one side of the body (inattention to or unawareness of one side of body or environment), which distorts perception of the visual field. If patient experiences neglect of one side, instruct him or her to scan all visual fields when transferring.*

STEPS	RATIONALE
7. Assess level of comfort (e.g., joint discomfort, muscle spasm) and measure level of pain on a 0–10 scale. Offer prescribed analgesic 30 minutes before transfer.	• Pain reduces patient's motivation and ability to be mobile. Pain relief before transfer enhances patient participation (Christo, Li, Gibson, et al., 2011).
8. Assess vital signs.	• Vital sign changes such as increased pulse and respiration and drop in blood pressure indicate activity intolerance (see Chapter 30).
9. Assess patient's cognitive status, including ability to follow verbal instructions, short-term memory, and recognition of physical deficits and limitations to movement.	• Determines patient's ability to follow directions and learn transfer techniques.

CRITICAL DECISION POINT: *Patients with head trauma or cerebrovascular accident may have perceptual cognitive deficits that create safety risks. If the patient has difficulty comprehending, simplify instructions by providing one step at a time and maintain consistency.*

STEPS	RATIONALE
10. Assess patient's level of motivation such as eagerness versus unwillingness to be mobile and perception of value of exercise.	• Altered physiological and psychological conditions reduce a patient's desire to engage in activity.
11. Assess patient's specific risk for falling or being injured during transfer (e.g., neuromuscular deficits, visual loss, motor weakness, fear of falling, or bone loss).	• Causes risk for tripping, losing balance.
12. Assess previous mode of transfer (if applicable).	• Determines mode of transfer and assistance required to provide continuity.
13. Assess patient's specific risk of falling or being injured when transferred (e.g., neuromuscular deficits, motor weakness, calcium loss from bones, cognitive and visual dysfunction, altered balance).	• Certain conditions increase risk of falling or potential injury.
14. Assess special transfer equipment needed for home setting and previous mode of transfer (if applicable).	• Prior teaching of family and support people, assessing home for safety risks and functionality, and providing applicable aids greatly enhance transfer ability at home.

PLANNING

STEPS	RATIONALE
1. Gather appropriate equipment.	
2. Determine number of people needed to assist with transfer by referring to proper algorithm. Do not start procedure until all caregivers are available.	• Ensures safe patient transfer. Algorithms for safe patient handling and movement are provided at https://www.lmcins.com/media/cms/Safe_Patient_Handling__Movement_Alg_E3527ACCC721E.pdf
3. Perform hand hygiene. Verify that bed brakes are locked.	• Reduces transmission of microorganisms. Promotes patient and caregiver safety.
4. Explain procedure to patient.	• Increases patient participation.

IMPLEMENTATION

1. Transfer patient.

A. Assisting cooperative patient to sitting position in bed:

CRITICAL DECISION POINT: *Careful assessment of the patient's ability to assist in the following position technique is extremely important. Consider the use of a mechanical lift. Your role in helping the patient to a sitting position is to be a guide and to instruct. If the patient can bear weight and move to a sitting position independently, allow him or her to do so and offer assistance (VISN 8 Patient Safety Center, 2015).*

STEPS	RATIONALE
(1) Raise bed to waist level. Place patient in supine position.	• Enables nurse to assess patient's body alignment continually.
(2) Face head of bed at 45-degree angle and remove pillows.	• Proper positioning reduces twisting of nurse's body when moving patient. Pillows cause interference when patient is sitting up in bed.
(3) Place your feet in wide base of support, with one foot closer to bed in front of other foot.	• Improves balance and allows transfer of body weight as patient is moved to sitting position.
(4) Place arm nearer head of bed under patient's shoulders, supporting his or her head and cervical vertebrae.	• Maintains alignment of head and cervical vertebrae and allows for even lifting of patient's upper trunk.
(5) Place other hand on bed surface.	• Provides support and balance.
(6) Raise patient to sitting position by shifting weight from front to back leg.	• Improves balance, overcomes inertia, and transfers weight in the direction patient is being moved.
(7) Push against bed using arm that is placed on bed surface.	• Divides activity between arms and legs and protects back from strain. By bracing one hand against mattress and pushing against it as you lift patient, you transfer weight away from your back muscles through your arm onto mattress.
B. Assisting cooperative patient who can partially bear weight to sitting position on side of bed:	
(1) With bed flat and waist high, turn patient to a side-lying position with assistance of another caregiver if necessary. Patient needs to face nurse on side of bed that patient will be sitting on (see illustration, Step 1B[1]).	• Decreases amount of work needed by nurse and patient.
(2) Raise head of bed 30 degrees.	• Facilitates raising patient to sitting position and protects him or her from falling.
(3) Stand opposite patient's hips. Turn diagonally so you face patient and far corner of head of bed.	• Places the nurse's centre of gravity nearer patient. Reduces twisting of nurse's body because the nurse is facing direction of movement.
(4) Place feet apart with foot closest to bed in front of other foot (see illustration for Step 1B[4]).	• Increases balance and allows transfer of body weight as nurse moves patient to a sitting position.

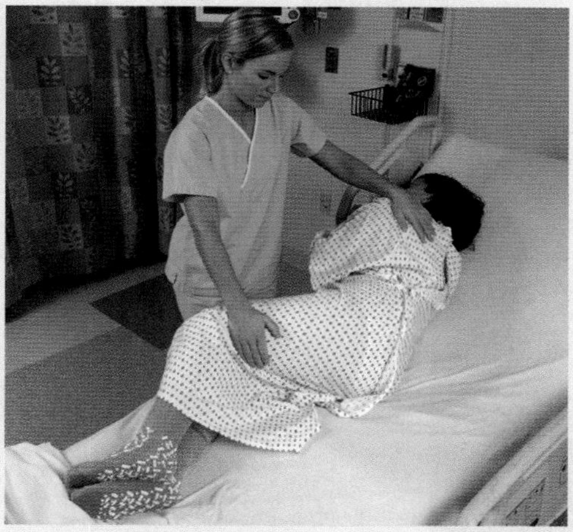

STEP 1B(1) Side-lying position.

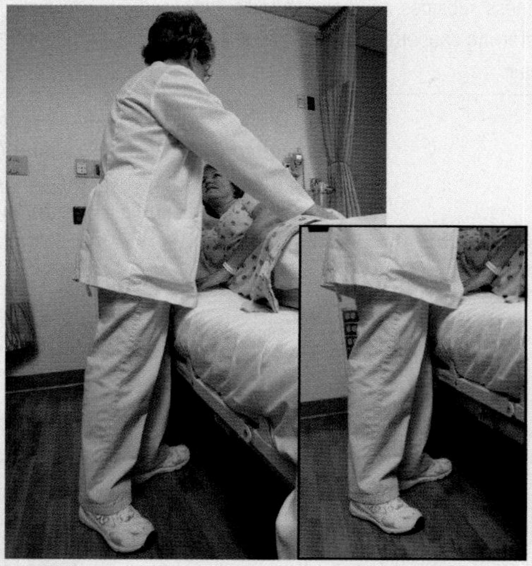

STEP 1B(4) Proper foot placement.

STEPS	RATIONALE
(5) Place arm nearer head of bed under patient's shoulders, supporting head and cervical vertebrae.	• Maintains alignment of head and cervical vertebrae and allows for even lifting of patient's trunk.

Continued

SKILL 36-1 USING SAFE AND EFFECTIVE TRANSFER TECHNIQUES—cont'd

STEPS	RATIONALE
(6) Place other arm over patient's thighs (see illustration for Step 1B[6]).	• Supports hip and prevents patient from falling backward during procedure.
(7) Move patient's lower legs and feet over side of bed. Pivot toward rear leg, allowing patient's upper legs to swing downward. At same time, shift weight to back leg and elevate patient (see illustration for Step 1B[7]).	• Decreases friction and resistance. Weight of patient's legs when off bed allows gravity to lower legs, and weight of legs helps to pull to sitting position.

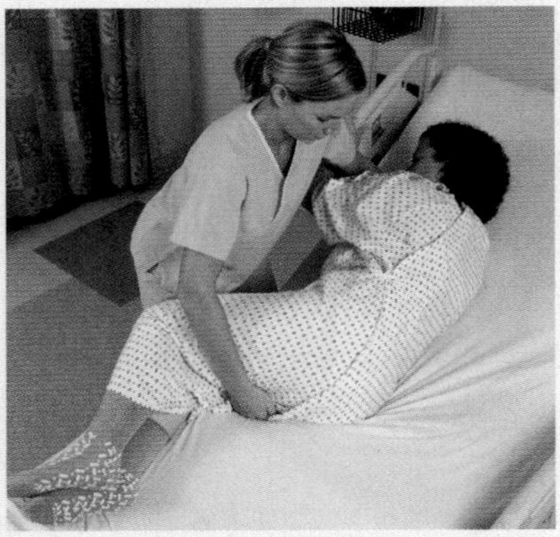

STEP 1B(6) Nurse places arm over patient's thighs.

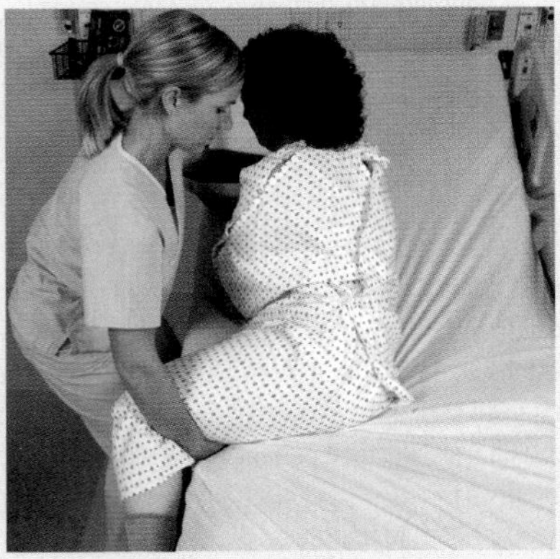

STEP 1B(7) Nurse shifts weight to rear leg and elevates patient.

STEPS	RATIONALE
(8) Allow patient to dangle on side of bed for a few minutes. Have patient alternately flex and extend feet and move lower legs. Ask if patient feels dizzy. Have patient relax and take a few deep breaths until dizziness subsides and balance is gained.	• Determines ability to tolerate standing. Dizziness that lasts more than 60 seconds may indicate orthostatic hypotension; return patient to bed (Myszenski, 2017). Recheck blood pressure.
C. Transferring cooperative patient who is partially weight bearing from bed to chair:	

CRITICAL DECISION POINT: *Allow patient to transfer independently if able to fully bear weight. Stand by as needed to promote safe transfer (VISN 8 Patient Safety Center, 2015). If patient has partial weight bearing with upper-body strength and caregiver must lift more than 115.9 kg (35 lbs) of patient weight, use a stand-assist lift device and follow manufacturer instructions (Step 1C).*

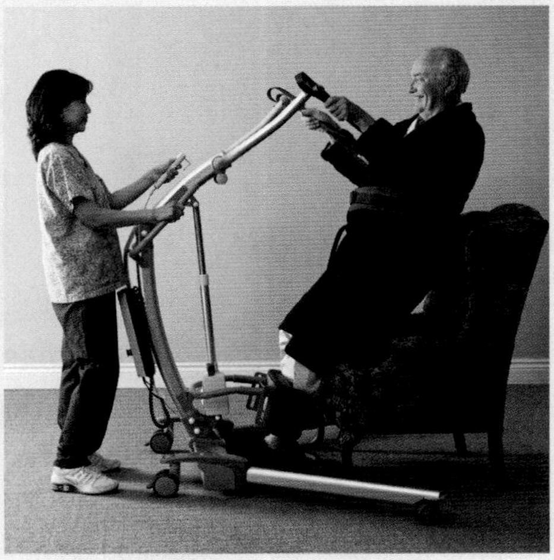

STEP 1C Stand-assist device.

STEPS	RATIONALE
(1) Help patient to sitting position on side of bed (see Step 1B). Have chair placed next to bed at 45-degree angle on patient's strong side. Allow patient to sit on side of bed (dangling) for a few minutes before transferring. Ask if patient feels dizzy. Do not leave unattended while patient is dangling.	• Positions chair within easy access for transfer. Placing chair on patient's stronger side allows patient to help with transferring. Dangling helps equilibrate blood pressure, reducing risk for dizziness or fainting when standing.

STEPS	RATIONALE
(2) Apply transfer belt or other transfer aids. Be sure it completely circles patient's waist. Place the belt low and be sure it is snug. You may need to adjust belt once patient stands.	• Transfer belt maintains stability of patient during transfer and reduces risk for falling (Pierson & Fairchild, 2013; VISN 8 Patient Safety Center, 2015). Patient's arm needs to be in sling if flaccid paralysis is present.
(3) Ensure that patient has stable nonskid shoes. Weight-bearing or strong leg is forward, with weak foot back.	• Nonskid soles decrease risk of slipping during transfer. Always have patient wear shoes during transfer; bare feet increase risk of falls. Patient stands on stronger, or weight-bearing, leg.
(4) Spread feet apart.	• Ensures balance with wide base of support.
(5) Flex hips and knees, aligning knees with patient's knees (see illustration for Step 1C[5]).	• Flexing knees and hips lowers centre of gravity to object to be raised; aligning knees with those of patient allows for stabilization of knees when patient stands.
(6) Grasp transfer belt from underneath along patient's sides.	• Provides movement of patient at centre of gravity. Never lift patients with upper-extremity paralysis or paresis by or under arms (VISN 8 Patient Safety Center, 2015).

CRITICAL DECISION POINT: *Use a transfer belt or walking belt with handles in place of the under-axilla technique. The under-axilla technique is physically stressful for nurses and uncomfortable for patients (Pierson & Fairchild, 2013).*

(7) Rock patient up to standing position on count of three while straightening hips and legs and keeping knees slightly flexed (see illustration for Step 1C[7]). Unless contraindicated, instruct patient to use hands to push up if applicable.	• Rocking motion gives patient's body momentum and requires less muscular effort to lift him or her.

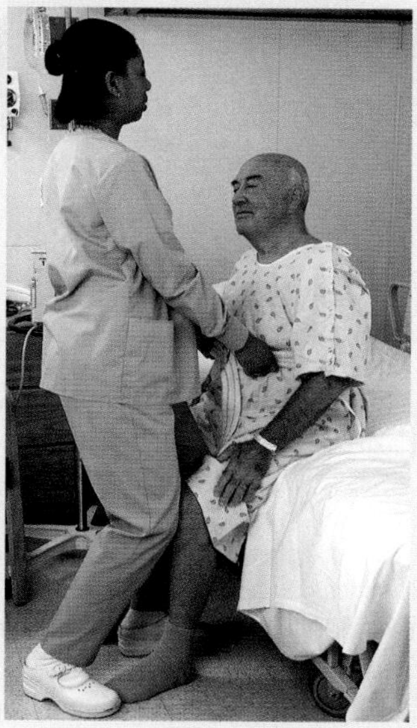

STEP 1C(5) Nurse flexes hips and knees, aligning knees with patient's knees.

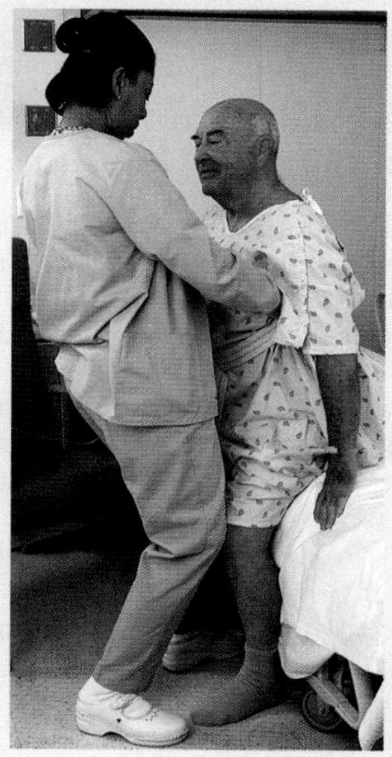

STEP 1C(7) Nurse rocks patient to standing position.

(8) Maintain stability of patient's weak or paralyzed leg with knee.	• Often patient maintains ability to stand on paralyzed or weak limb with support of knee to stabilize (Pierson & Fairchild, 2013).
(9) Pivot on foot farther from chair.	• Maintains support of patient while allowing adequate space for patient to move.
(10) Instruct patient to use armrests on chair for support and ease into chair (see illustration for Step 1C[10]).	• Increases patient stability.

Continued

SKILL 36-1 USING SAFE AND EFFECTIVE TRANSFER TECHNIQUES—cont'd

STEPS	RATIONALE
(11) Flex hips and knees while lowering patient into chair (see illustration for Step 1C[11]).	• Prevents injury to nurse from poor body mechanics.

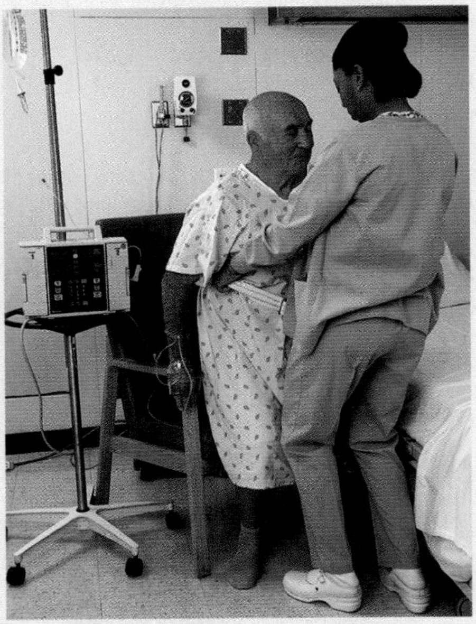

STEP 1C(10) Patient uses armrests for support.

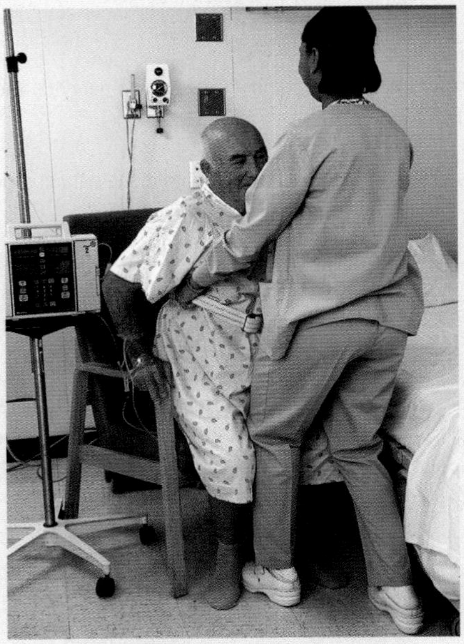

STEP 1C(11) Nurse eases patient into chair.

STEPS	RATIONALE
(12) Assess patient for proper alignment for sitting position. Provide support for paralyzed extremities. Lapboard or sling supports flaccid arm. Stabilize leg with bath blanket or pillow.	• Prevents injury to patient from poor body alignment.
(13) Praise patient's progress, effort, or performance.	• Continued support and encouragement provide incentive for patient perseverance.
D. Using mechanical lift and full-body sling to transfer uncooperative patient who can bear partial weight or patient who cannot bear weight and is either uncooperative or does not have upper-body strength to move from bed to chair:	• Mechanical lift devices prevent musculoskeletal injuries to health care workers (Pelczarski, 2012).
(1) Position lift properly at bedside (see equipment instructions).	• Ensures safe elevation of patient off bed. (Before using lift, be thoroughly familiar with its operation.)
(2) Position chair near bed and allow adequate space to manoeuvre lift.	• Prepares environment for safe use of lift and subsequent transfer.
(3) Raise bed to high position with mattress flat. Lower side rail.	• Maintains nurses' alignment during transfer.
(4) Keep side rail up on side opposite from you.	• Maintains patient safety.
(5) Roll patient away from you.	• Positions patient for use of lift sling.
(6) Place sling under patient. Place lower edge under patient's knees (wide piece) and upper edge under patient's shoulders (narrow piece).	• Allows positioning of patient on mechanical/hydraulic sling. Places sling under patient's centre of gravity and greatest part of body weight.
(7) Roll patient to opposite side and pull body sling through.	• Completes positioning of patient on mechanical/hydraulic sling.
(8) Roll patient supine onto canvas seat.	• Sling needs to extend from shoulders to knees (hammock) to support patient's body weight equally.
(9) Remove patient's glasses if appropriate.	• Swivel bar is close to patient's head and can break eyeglasses.
(10) If using a transportable hydraulic lift, place horseshoe-shaped base of lift under side of bed (on side with chair).	• Positions hydraulic lift efficiently and promotes smooth transfer.
(11) Lower upper horizontal bar to sling level following manufacturer directions. Some lifts require valve to be locked.	• Positions lift close to patient. Locking valve prevents injury to patient.
(12) Attach hooks on strap to holes in sling. Short straps hook to top holes of sling; longer straps hook to bottom of sling.	• Secures hydraulic lift to sling.
(13) Elevate head of bed.	• Positions patient in sitting position.
(14) Fold patient's arms over chest.	• Prevents injury to paralyzed arms.
(15) Use lift to raise patient off bed (see illustration for step 1D[15]).	• Moves patient off bed.
(16) Use steering handle to pull lift from bed and manoeuvre to chair.	• Moves patient from bed to chair.
(17) Move lift to chair.	• Positions lift in front of chair.

STEPS	RATIONALE
(18) Position patient and lower slowly into chair following manufacturer guidelines (see illustration for Step 1D[18]).	• Safely guides patient into back of chair as seat descends.

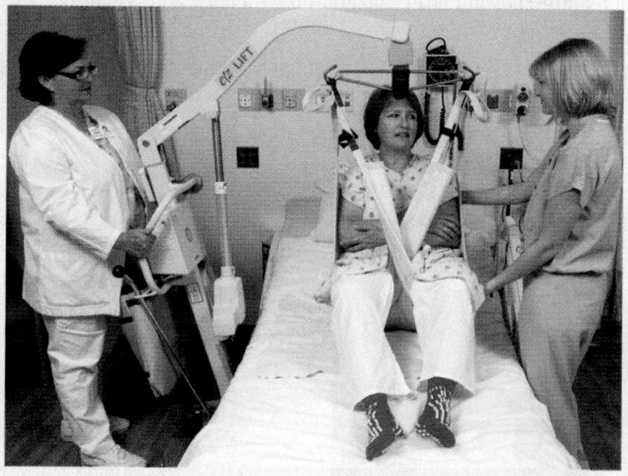

STEP 1D(15) Use mechanical lift to raise patient off bed.

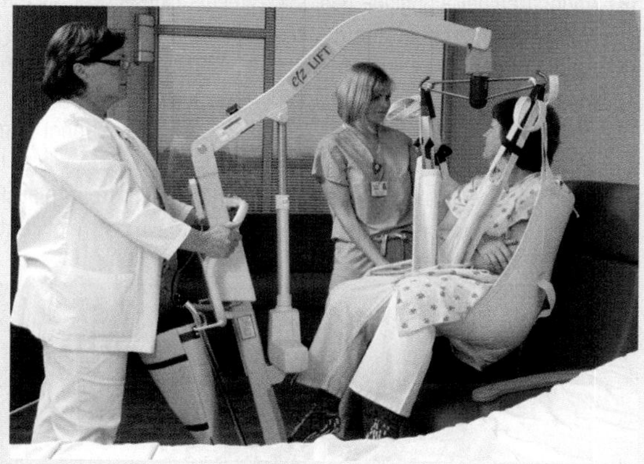

STEP 1D(18) Use mechanical lift to lower patient into chair.

STEPS	RATIONALE
(19) Remove straps and mechanical/hydraulic lift.	• Prevents damage to skin and underlying tissues from canvas or hooks.
(20) Check patient's sitting alignment and correct if necessary.	• Prevents injury from poor posture.
E. Transferring patient from bed to stretcher (bed at stretcher level):	
(1) Raise bed to height of stretcher.	• Bed and stretcher need to be at same level to allow patient to slide from bed to stretcher.
(2) Lower head of bed as much as patient can tolerate. Cross patient's arms on chest. Ensure that bed brakes are locked.	• Prevents injury to arms during transfer.
(3) Lower side rails. Two caregivers stand on side where stretcher will be; third caregiver stands on other side.	• Minimizes caregivers' stretching. Prevents patient from falling out of bed and promotes safety.
(4) Two caregivers help patient roll onto side toward them (use of drawsheet is optional) with smooth, continuous motion.	• Positions patient for placing friction-reducing lateral transfer device.
(5) Place slide board under drawsheet or follow manufacturer guidelines (see illustrations for Step 1E[5]). Gently roll patient back onto slide board.	• Patient needs to be placed on transfer device properly to allow safe transfer.

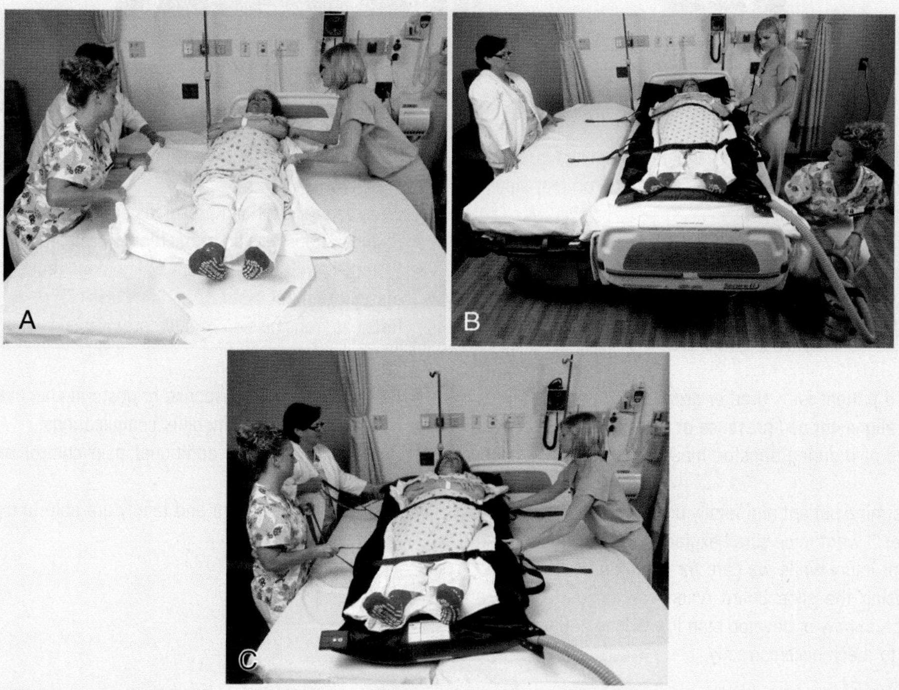

STEP 1E(5) **A,** Transfer of patient from bed to stretcher using slide board. **B,** Inflating air-assisted transfer device. **C,** Transfer of patient using air-assisted transfer device.

Continued

SKILL 36-1 USING SAFE AND EFFECTIVE TRANSFER TECHNIQUES—cont'd

STEPS	RATIONALE
(6) Align stretcher alongside bed. Lock wheels of stretcher once it is in place. Instruct patient not to move.	• Positions stretcher in correct position for transfer and prevents patient from falling out of bed.
(7) All three caregivers place feet widely apart with one foot slightly in front of the other and grasp friction-reducing device.	• Prepares for transfer. Wide base of support allows nurse to shift weight and minimizes back strain.
(8) On count of three, two caregivers pull drawsheet or patient from bed onto stretcher while third person holds slide board in place. Using the friction-reducing slide board, shift weight from front to back foot (see illustration for Step 1E[8]). Position patient in centre of stretcher.	• Transfers patient smoothly and efficiently to the stretcher.

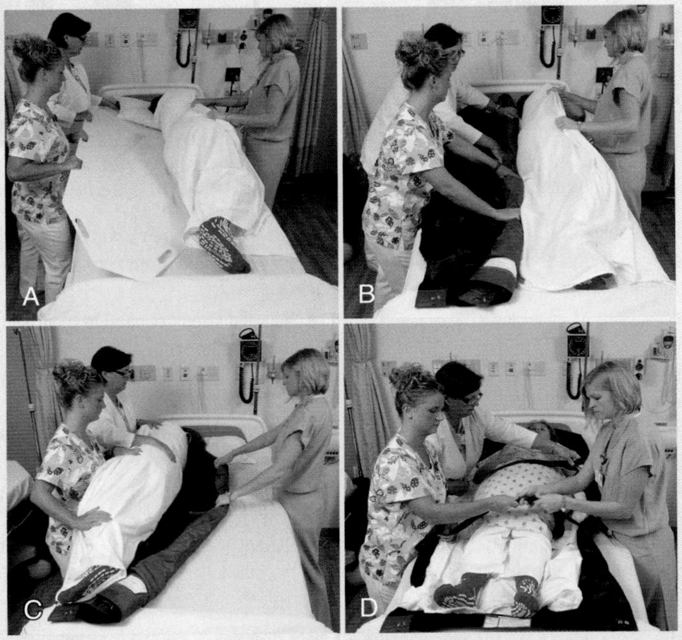

STEP 1E(8) **A,** Two caregivers position slide board under patient. **B,** Two caregivers place air-assisted device under patient. **C,** Patient rolls to opposite side while other caregiver unrolls air-assisted device. **D,** Secure safety straps.

STEPS	RATIONALE
(9) Put up side rail of stretcher on side where caregivers are, roll stretcher away from side of bed, and put side rail up on that side.	• Side rails prevent patient from falling off stretcher.
(10) Cover patient with sheet or blanket.	• Promotes comfort and preserves patient dignity.
(11) Perform hand hygiene.	• Reduces transmission of microorganisms.
(12) Following transfer, evaluate patient's body alignment.	• Prompt identification of poor alignment reduces risks to patient's skin and musculoskeletal systems.
2. Perform hand hygiene.	• Reduces transmission of microorganisms.

EVALUATION

1. Evaluate vital signs. Ask if patient feels tired or dizzy.	• Evaluates patient's response to postural changes and activity.
2. Observe for correct body alignment and presence of pressure points on skin.	• Minimizes risk for immobility complications.
3. Ask if patient experienced pain during transfer; measure current pain level.	• Determines need for additional pain control or alteration of technique of transferring.
4. Use **Teach Back** to determine patient and family understanding about safe transfer techniques. State, "I want to be sure I explained how using the slide board prevents the risk for injury while we care for you. Can you explain to me the importance of using the slide board when we transfer you to a stretcher?" Revise instruction now or develop plan for revised patient teaching if patient is not able to teach back correctly.	• Evaluates what patient and family are able to explain or demonstrate.

STEPS	RATIONALE

UNEXPECTED OUTCOMES	RELATED INTERVENTIONS
Patient sustains injury on transfer	• Evaluate incident that caused injury (e.g., assessment inadequate, change in patient status, improper use of equipment). • Complete occurrence report according to institution policy.
Patient's level of weakness does not permit active transfer	• Obtain help from additional nursing personnel. • Increase bed activity and exercise to heighten tolerance.
Patient transfers well on some occasions, poorly on others	• Assess patient for factors that affect ability to transfer (e.g., pain, fatigue, confusion) before transfer. • Allow for a rest period before transferring, medicate for pain if indicated, or reorient patient.

RECORDING AND REPORTING

- Record procedure, including pertinent observations: weakness, ability to follow directions, weight-bearing ability, balance, ability to pivot, number of personnel needed to assist, and amount of assistance (muscle strength) required in nurses' notes.
- Report any unusual occurrence to nurse in charge. Report transfer ability and assistance needed to next shift or other caregivers. Report progress or transfer difficulties to rehabilitation staff (physiotherapist or occupational therapist).
- Document your evaluation of patient learning.

HOME CARE CONSIDERATIONS

- Teach family how to use safe patient-handling equipment if necessary.
- Teach patient and family about the importance of safety while helping patients with mobility.

Transfer Techniques. Nurses often provide care for immobilized patients whose position must be changed, who must be moved up in bed, or who must be transferred from a bed to a chair or from a bed to a stretcher. Body mechanics alone do not protect nurses from injury to their musculoskeletal systems when they move or transfer patients. Although nurses use many transfer techniques, knowledge of ergonomics and safe patient handling is crucial in maintaining caregiver and patient safety. **Ergonomics** is an applied science concerned with designing and arranging workplace settings in such a way that people interact more effectively with the objects they encounter in that environment.

Nurses must assess every situation that involves patient handling and movement, to minimize risk of injury (Box 36-3). After completing the assessment, the nurse will use an algorithm (Figures 36-4 to 36-6) to guide decisions about safe patient handling (VISN 8 Patient Safety Center, 2015). Skill 36-1 describes the steps commonly used in

BOX 36-3 CASE STUDY

Activity and Exercise

I have been in nursing for over 40 years. For more than 30 years of that time, before moving into teaching, I worked as a hospital staff nurse providing direct care to patients. I worked mainly in areas where patients were unable to assist themselves very much, such as in the birthing and critical care units. As is the case with most nurses, the wear and tear of lifting, turning, and transferring patients took a toll on my body, primarily on my back, knees, and feet. But for as long as it was part of my role, I was able to do work.

Several years later, after I began teaching a nursing fundamentals course, my physical activity related to nursing consisted of demonstrating fundamental skills in the laboratory setting and of providing assistance to students with their practice. During my fifth year of teaching that course, I was taken by surprise at how difficult I found it to lift, position, or transfer my volunteer "patients," and at how extremely tired and sore I was at the end of each day. What was happening to me?

Upon reflection, I realized that two factors were involved. The first was normal change resulting from aging: the decrease in strength and endurance that occurs after age 40 among women. The second factor was the relatively sedentary lifestyle I had led since I had left bedside nursing. Mine was a classic case of functional decline from disuse, a major concern as aging occurs. As I thought further about it, I remembered that I had noticed groceries becoming heavier and stair climbing feeling more difficult. At the rate I was changing, I had little hope of maintaining my independence well into old age. In the shorter term, if I expected to keep teaching for a few more years, I would need to do something about my fitness level quickly!

My strategies? To use my gym membership (neglected for months and never attended routinely) four times per week from June through August and at least three times per week throughout the academic year, and to walk for no less than 30 minutes every day. No more avoiding stairs, either! I decided to walk up one floor and down two or three until that became easier and then increase stair climbing from there.

How will I know whether my plan has been effective? Although I don't expect to be as strong as I once was as a clinical nurse, I will be able to accomplish my teaching activities and my normal daily routines effortlessly, with minimal backaches and energy to spare.

Although it was a shock to recognize that aging had affected my personal and professional life, the ingrained nursing habits of reflection and of establishing goals helped me feel confident that I could manage these changes.

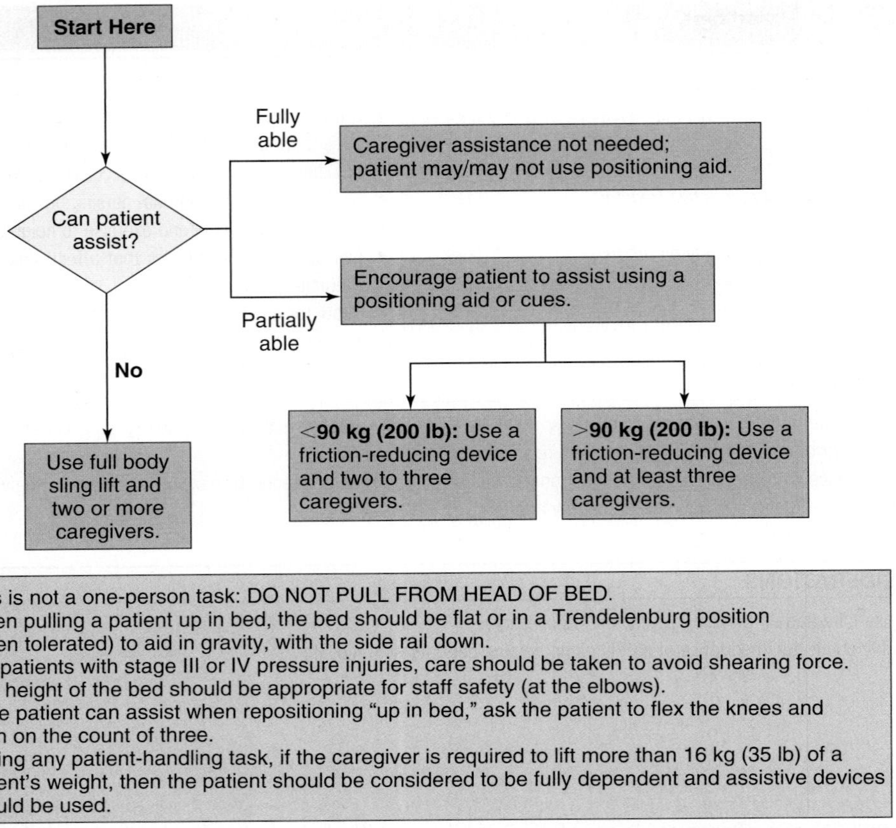

FIGURE 36-4 **Algorithm used to reposition patient in bed.** (Modified from VISN 8 Patient Safety Center [VISN 8]. [2015]. *Safe patient handling and movement algorithms.* Retrieved from https://www.lmcins.com/media/cms/Safe_Patient_Handling__Movement_Alg_E3527ACCC721E.pdf.)

transferring patients safely and effectively. When transferring a patient, it is helpful to encourage maximum patient involvement. The nurse should use a patient's strength when lifting, transferring, or moving, when possible. Involving the patient has the additional benefit of increasing participation in self-care and can promote a sense of accomplishment.

Factors Influencing Activity and Exercise

Factors influencing activity and exercise include developmental changes, behavioural aspects, environmental issues, cultural and ethnic influences, and family and social support. Nurses need to consider these areas of knowledge and incorporate them into the plan of care, whether the patient is seeking health promotion, acute care, or restorative and continuing care.

Developmental Changes. Throughout the lifespan, the body's appearance and functioning undergo change. The greatest change and impact on the maturational process are observed at both ends of the developmental spectrum.

Infants Through School-Aged Children. The newborn infant's spine is flexed and lacks the anteroposterior curves of the adult. The first spinal curve occurs when the infant extends the neck from the prone position. As growth and stability increase, the thoracic spine straightens and the lumbar spinal curve appears, which allows sitting and standing.

The toddler's posture is awkward because of the slight swayback and protruding abdomen. As the child walks, the legs and feet are usually far apart and the feet are slightly everted. Toward the end of toddlerhood, posture appears less awkward, curves in the cervical and lumbar vertebrae are accentuated, and foot eversion disappears.

By the third year, the body is slimmer, taller, and better balanced. Abdominal protrusion is decreased, the feet are not as far apart, and the arms and legs have increased in length. The child appears more coordinated. The musculoskeletal system continues to grow and develop through adolescence (see Chapter 22).

Adolescence. Adolescent growth is often sporadic and uneven. As a result, the adolescent may appear awkward and uncoordinated. Adolescent girls usually grow and develop earlier than boys do. In girls, hips widen and fat is deposited in the upper arms, thighs, and buttocks. The adolescent boy's changes in shape are usually a result of long-bone growth and increased muscle mass (see Chapter 22).

Young to Middle-Aged Adults. A healthy adult also has the necessary musculoskeletal development and coordination to carry out ADLs. Normal changes in posture and body alignment in adulthood occur mainly in pregnant women. These changes result from the body's adaptive response to weight gain and the growing fetus (see Chapter 23). When pregnant, the woman's centre of gravity shifts toward the anterior. As a result, the pregnant woman leans back and is slightly swaybacked. Pregnant women frequently experience back pain.

Older Persons. In older persons, a progressive loss of bone mass occurs as a result of decreased physical activity, hormonal changes, and increased osteoclastic activity (activity by cells responsible for bone tissue absorption). Bone loss leads to weaker bones. Vertebrae become softer and long shaft bones become less resistant to bending. Changes

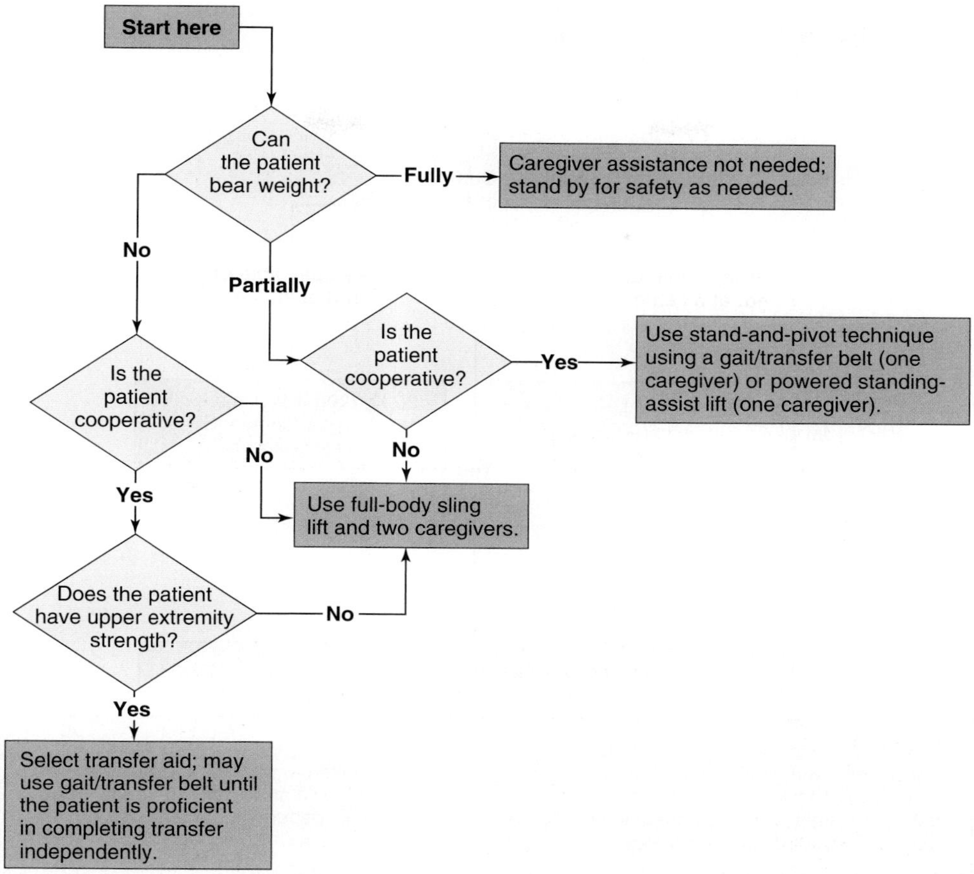

- For seated transfer aid, must have chair with arms that recess or are removable.
- For full-body sling lift, select a lift that is specifically designed to access a patient from the car (if the car is the starting or ending destination).
- If patient has partial weight-bearing capacity, transfer toward stronger side.
- Toileting slings are available for toileting.
- Mesh slings are available for bathing.
- During any patient-transferring task, if any caregiver is required to lift more than 16 kg (35 lb) of a patient's weight, then the patient should be considered to be fully dependent and assistive devices should be used for the transfer.

FIGURE 36-5 **Algorithm used to transfer patient to and from bed to chair, chair to toilet, chair to chair, or car to chair.** (Modified from VISN 8 Patient Safety Center [VISN 8]. [2015]. *Safe patient handling and movement algorithms.* Retrieved from https://www.lmcins.com/media/cms/Safe_Patient_Handling__Movement_Alg_E3527ACCC721E.pdf.)

in muscle tissue also occur as adults age, beginning as early as during the 20s for men and during the 40s for women. Muscle fibres shrink and have reduced tone and contractility. Strength and endurance change; fatigue occurs more readily, and overall energy may be reduced (Paterson & Warburton, 2010).

Older persons may walk more slowly and appear less coordinated. They also may take smaller steps, keeping their feet closer together, which decreases their base of support. Thus, body balance may become unstable, and they are at greater risk for falls and injuries (see Chapter 24). It is important to encourage or plan physical activities for older persons. Exercise programs are important for socialization, independence, and maintaining core body strength. Physical exercise can improve endurance, coordination, and muscle stability and reduce risk for falls and injuries.

Safety Alert Falls among older persons are a significant health concern in Canada. More than one-third of older persons experience falls. Falls are the leading cause of injury for older persons and can result in disability, chronic pain, loss of independence, reduced quality of life, and even death. In Canada, the direct health care costs for falls are an estimated $2 billion annually (Canadian Patient Safety Institute, 2016). Use of fall risk assessment tools (Figure 36-7) and fall prevention initiatives (Box 36-4) can help to identify persons at risk for falls and implement prevention strategies.

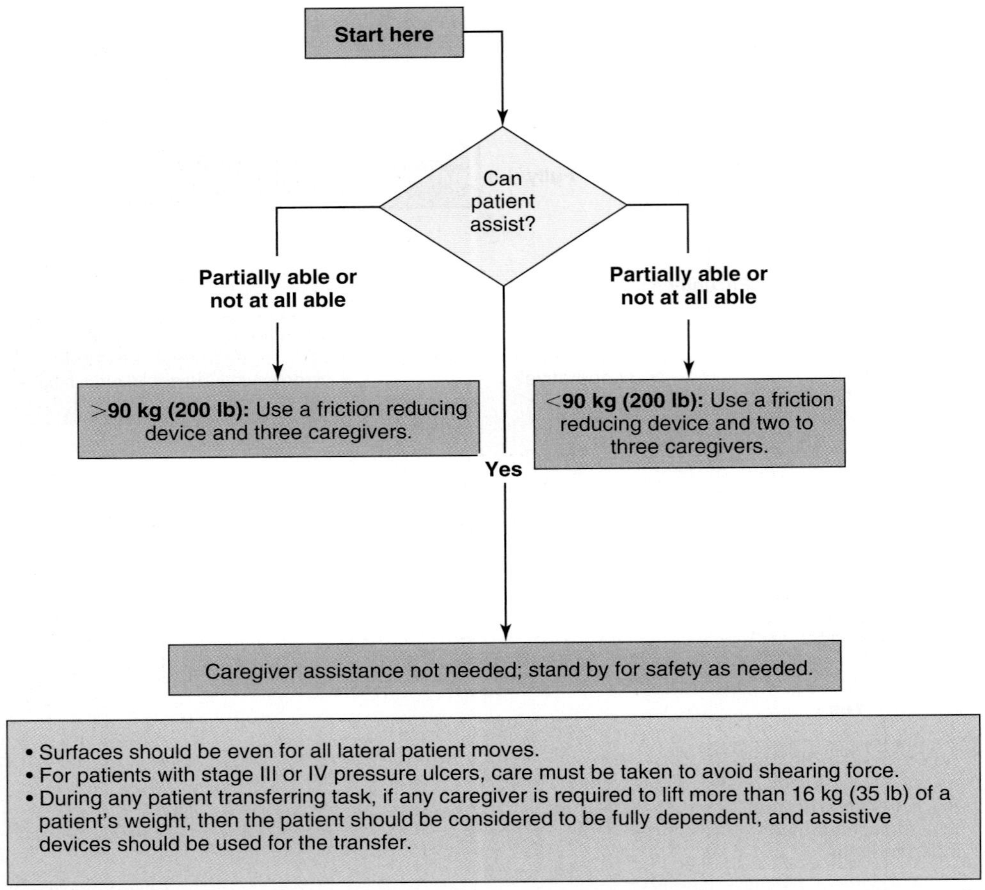

FIGURE 36-6 Algorithm used to complete lateral transfer to and from bed to stretcher, trolley. (Modified from VISN 8 Patient Safety Center [VISN 8]. [2015]. *Safe patient handling and movement algorithms.* Retrieved from https://www.lmcins.com/media/cms/Safe_Patient_Handling__Movement_Alg_E3527ACCC721E.pdf.)

BOX 36-4 Unit Standard Fall Prevention Protocol

Use for all patients at risk for falls:

- Use appropriate orientation strategies.
- Use clear communication.
- Assist patients with sensory aids (i.e., hearing aids, glasses).
- Do comfort rounds every 2–3 hours (toileting needs, hydration, position changes).
- Teach patient and family about fall risk and prevention strategies.
- Ensure that call bell, personal items, and walking aids are within easy reach.
- Assess patients' understanding of the call bell system and determine if patient is able to use call bell.
- Remind patients to call for help when transferring, ambulating, and toileting.
- Assess whether patient is using assistive devices correctly.
- Have patient wear nonslip footwear for all transfers and ambulation.
- Clear barriers (e.g., clutter in room) prior to ambulating.

Alberta Health Services. (2013). *Take action: Prevent a fall before it happens.* Retrieved from http://www.albertahealthservices.ca/assets/programs/ps-1051701-falls-prevention-guide.pdf

Behavioural Aspects. Physical activity benefits a person's overall health and is reported to reduce stress (Childs & de Wit, 2014). Patients are more likely to incorporate an exercise program into their daily lives if it is supported and assisted by family and friends, nurses, physicians, and other members of the health care team. Nurses should take into consideration the patient's knowledge of exercise and activity, barriers to a program of exercise and physical activity, and current exercise habits.

Patients are more open to developing an exercise program if they are at the stage of being ready to change their behaviour. Prochaska and DiClemente's (1986) transtheoretical model of behaviour change has been the most utilized model of understanding and facilitating behaviour change since it was developed in the 1980s. It identifies five stages individuals go through in implementing a lifestyle change: precontemplation, contemplation, preparation, action, and maintenance. Information on the benefits of regular exercise may be helpful to the patient in the contemplation stage. Patients' decisions to change behaviour and include a daily exercise routine in their lives may occur gradually with the provision of repeated information that is individualized to their needs and lifestyle (Box 36-5). Once the patient has reached the action stage, the nurse must develop, in collaboration with the patient, an exercise program that is customized to fit his or her needs. The nurse then must provide continued follow-up support and assistance until the exercise program becomes a daily routine.

Alberta Health Services **Schmid Fall Risk Assessment Tool – Acute Care**	HRN: Site: DOB: yyyy/mon/dd Last Name: First and Additional Names: PHN: Gender: Age in Years: Admitting Physician: Encounter #: Address: Street, City, Province, Postal Code Telephone Number: Date of Admission: yyyy/mon/dd Family Physician:
To be completed on all patients upon admission, post-fall, and/or when the patient's status changes. Score each area relating to patient's current status. Weights are in parenthesis. Total weight at bottom.	

Date of **Initial** Assessment: yyyy/mon/dd **Unit:** ____________

Select only **one indicator for each category.

Mobility	Score	Score
(0) Ambulates with no gait disturbance		
(1) Ambulates or transfers with assistive devices		
(1) Ambulates with unsteady gait and no assistance		
(0) Unable to ambulate or transfer		
Mentation	Score	Score
(0) Alert oriented × 3		
(1) Periodic confusion		
(1) Confusion at all times		
(0) Comatose/unresponsive		
Elimination	Score	Score
(0) Independent in elimination		
(1) Independent with frequency or diarrhea		
(1) Needs assistance with toileting		
(1) Incontinence		
Prior Fall History (within past 6 months)	Score	Score
(1) Yes – Before admission (Home or previous inpatient care)		
(2) Yes – During this admission		
(0) No		
(0) Unknown		
Current Medications	Score	Score
(1) A score of I is given if the patient is on I or more of the following medications: Anti-convulsants/sedatives or psychotropics/hypnotics *(consider all medication side effects and role in fall risk)*		
	Score	Score
Total Score:		
Completed By: (signature/designation)		
Date: (yyyy/mon/dd)		

Total Score:

Score of 3 or more: Patient is at risk for falls and fall prevention interventions should be implemented–**see reverse side**

FIGURE 36-7 Schmid Fall Risk Assessment Tool—Acute Care. (Nancy A. Schmid, MS, RN, NEA-BC.)

BOX 36-5 General Strategies for Initiating and Maintaining an Exercise Program

Five steps to beginning an exercise program:

Step 1: Assess Fitness Level
- Seek approval from a health care provider to begin. Are there any limitations to consider before determining the exercises in the fitness program?
- Record baseline fitness scores such as pulse rate before and after walking 1 km, how long it takes to walk 1 km, number of push-ups that can be done at a time, how far you are able to reach forward while seated on floor with legs outstretched in front, waist circumference, and body mass index.

Step 2: Design the Fitness Program
- Consider fitness goals. Make goals attainable.
- Develop a balanced routine of aerobic activity and strength training.
- Plan a logical progression of activities that goes at your own pace, record it on paper, and keep track.
- Build a program that includes different activities into a daily routine.
- Allow time for recovery.

Step 3: Assemble Equipment
- Choose athletic shoes designed for the chosen exercise.
- If choosing to exercise at home, try equipment at a fitness centre before purchasing.

Step 4: Get Started
- Start slowly and build up a routine gradually.
- Divide exercise time throughout the day if time or fatigue is a barrier. Ten minutes of exercise three times a day instead of a single 30-minute workout may be better for some patients' schedules and medical conditions.
- Take rest periods.

Step 5: Monitor Progress
- Retake fitness assessment at 6 weeks and then every 3 to 6 months.
- If losing motivation: set new goals, exercise with a friend, or incorporate new activities.

Adapted from Mayo Clinic. (2016). *Healthy living fitness program: 5 steps to getting started.* Retrieved from http://www.mayoclinic.com/healthy-living/fitness/in-depth/fitness/art-20048269?pg=1.

Environmental Issues

Work Sites. A common barrier for many patients is the lack of time needed to engage in a daily exercise program. Work sites have the potential to help their employees overcome the obstacle of time constraints by offering opportunities, reminders, and rewards for those committed to physical fitness (McGann, Jancey, & Tye, 2013). Signs could be used to encourage employees to use the stairs instead of elevators. Rewards such as free parking or discounted parking fees could be given to employees who walk from distant lots.

Schools. Children today are less active, resulting in an increase in childhood obesity (Bammann, Peplies, De Henauw, et al., 2014; Grossklaus & Marvicsin, 2014). Daily physical activity or physical education has been mandated in elementary schools across Canada. Children aged 5 to 11 years old should participate in at least 1 hour of moderate- to vigorous-intensity physical activity daily (Public Health Agency of Canada [PHAC], 2012a). Schools can provide a foundation for lifetime commitment to exercise and physical fitness by incorporating physical activity into a child's daily routine.

Community. The community's support of physical fitness can be instrumental in promoting the health of its members. Examples of community involvement to promote physical fitness are the provision of walking trails and track facilities in community parks and physical fitness classes offered by trained professionals. Success in implementing physical fitness programs depends on a collaborative effort between public health agencies, parks and recreational associations, provincial and local government agencies, health care agencies, and community members (Combs et al., 2013; Wallace, Lees, Minou, et al., 2014).

Cultural and Ethnic Influences. When developing a physical fitness program for culturally diverse populations, it is important to consider what motivates individuals to take up exercise and physical activity and what they see as appropriate, enjoyable, and beneficial. Variables that can influence participation, frequency, and duration when participating in exercise, such as religious fasting periods, need to be considered. It is also important to know epidemiological statistics for specific chronic disease entities that are associated with different cultural and ethnic origins (Box 36-6).

Family and Social Support

Social support can be used as a motivational tool to encourage and promote exercise and physical fitness. The patient can engage a friend or a significant other to participate in a "buddy system" whereby they walk together each day at a specified time. This companionship provides socialization and increases the enjoyment for some patients. It may lead to the development of a lifelong commitment to physical fitness. Parents can support their children in sports and physical activity by providing encouragement, praise, and transportation and by participating themselves (Rhodes & Pfaeffli, 2010).

CRITICAL THINKING

Providing competent care requires a synthesis of knowledge, experience, and information gathered from patients; critical thinking attitudes; and intellectual and professional standards. Patients' conditions are always changing. Clinical judgements require nurses to anticipate the information necessary, analyze the data, and make decisions regarding patient care.

To understand activity tolerance and physical fitness and their impact on a patient, nurses must integrate knowledge from nursing and other disciplines, previous experiences, and information gathered from patients. As nurses begin the process of problem solving for patient care, a variety of concepts must be considered together to provide the best outcome for the patient. The foundation for planning and decision making is knowledge of the musculoskeletal system and of health alterations that create problems for the patient in the area of activity, exercise, and body mechanics. In addition, nurses must stay current on and incorporate various guidelines, such as those supplied by the Canadian Diabetes Association (2013) and the *Canadian Physical Activity Guidelines* developed by the Canadian Society for Exercise Physiology (2011).

Nurses' experiences and ability to think creatively enhance their approach to each new patient situation. For patients with limited exercise capacity or activity tolerance, nurses need to develop the nursing care plan to include interventions that maintain the present level of function with the goal of increasing the level of function. It is important to remember that patients have the capacity for improvement in spite of the impairments. Encouragement, support, commitment, creativity, and perseverance are important attitudes in critical thinking for these patients.

Perseverance is necessary when caring for patients who depend on nurses for assistance with ambulation or exercise. In addition,

BOX 36-6 CULTURAL ASPECTS OF CARE

Physical Activity

Epidemiological studies of ethnic groups indicate that physical inactivity is one of the risk factors associated with noninsulin-dependent diabetes mellitus (NIDDM). Historically, activity was a fundamental part of everyday life for all Canadians, as a mechanism for transportation, acquiring food, and labour. Rapid advances in technology are contributing to an increasingly sedentary lifestyle. In Canada, NIDDM is between 3.6 and 5.3 times more prevalent within the Indigenous population. Introduction of new technology has influenced traditional activity patterns of Indigenous peoples. Physical activity has been identified as playing an important role in the prevention and treatment of NIDDM, yet the Indigenous population has a disproportionate number of poor, unemployed, and disadvantaged individuals who lack access to recreation and leisure activities.

Implications for Practice

- Because physical inactivity is a modifiable risk factor for the development of NIDDM, prevention and treatment programs need to focus heavily on exercise and be tailored to the activity tolerance of the individual patient.
- Motivational factors incorporated into the exercise program, such as providing a healthy snack or meal for participants and giving each patient a log to monitor weight loss and blood glucose levels, will enhance compliance.
- Promotion of physical activity should be supported by recognizing that a symbiotic relationship exists between cultural values and traditional leisure pursuits. Patients with a strong spiritual connection to the land may enjoy outdoor or wilderness recreation in the form of traditional games and activities, such as lacrosse and hunting.
- Ensure that members of Indigenous groups collaborate in the planning of educational program initiatives.
- Development of an exercise or prevention program, or both, should attempt to remove potential barriers, such as transportation and cost, to facilitate commitment to the program.

Adapted from Chui, K., & Austin, G. in Edelman, C. L., Kudzma, E. C., & Mandle, C. L. (2013). *Health promotion throughout the lifespan* (8th ed.). St. Louis, MO: Mosby; Government of Alberta. (2007). *Cultural diversity: Including everyone in physical activity.* Retrieved from http://www.healthyalberta.com/HealthyPlaces/642.htm; National Collaborating Centre for Aboriginal Health. (2013). *Physical activity fact sheet.* Retrieved from https://www.ccnsa-nccah.ca/495/Physical_Activity_Fact_Sheet.nccah?id=72.

responsibility for positioning often becomes repetitive, and nurses must recognize its importance (see Chapter 45). Perseverance is especially important in delegating these activities to other personnel and being sure they are completed. Making certain that the task is performed correctly is also an essential nursing function. Problems with activity and mobility are often prolonged; creativity is necessary when designing interventions for improving activity tolerance and mobility skills.

NURSING PROCESS

Assessment

Assessment of body alignment and posture is completed with the patient standing, sitting, or lying down. Assess normal physiological changes in growth and development; deviations related to poor posture, trauma, muscle damage, or nerve dysfunction; and any learning needs of patients. Provide patients with opportunities to observe their posture and obtain important information about other factors that contribute to poor alignment, such as inactivity, fatigue, malnutrition, and psychological problems. To gather relevant information, ask questions related to the patient's exercise and activity tolerance. During assessment (Figure 36-8), consider all the elements that contribute to making appropriate nursing diagnoses.

Put the patient at ease so that unnatural or rigid positions are not assumed. When assessing body alignment of a patient who is immobilized or unconscious, remove pillows and positioning supports from the bed if not contraindicated, and place the patient in the supine position.

Patient Expectations

To ensure patient-centred care, assess a patient's expectations, values, and beliefs concerning activity and exercise and determine individual perceptions of what is normal or acceptable when developing a care plan. Perceived self-efficacy influences a person's willingness to engage in exercise. The outcomes people anticipate depend on their

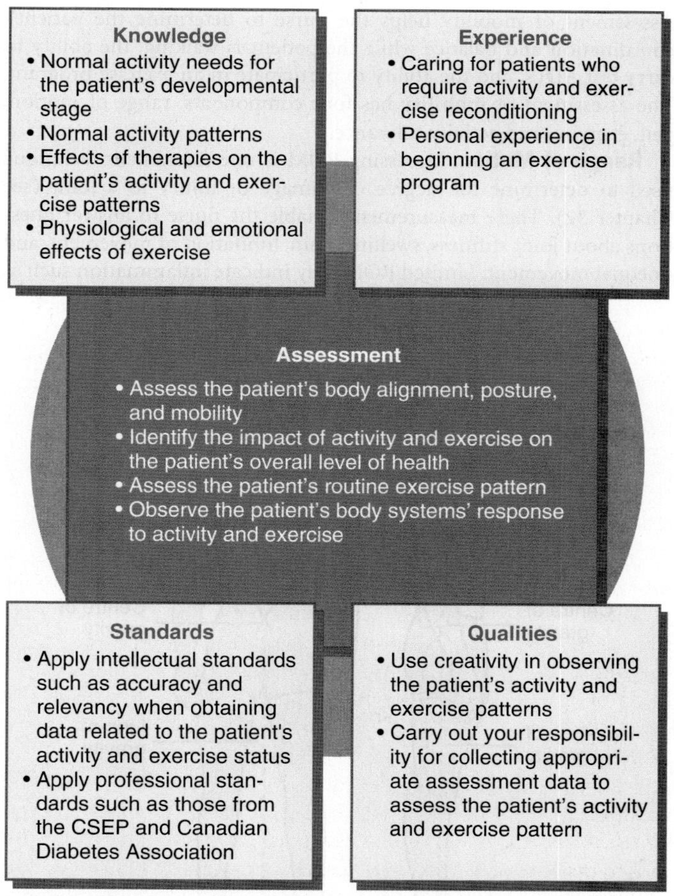

FIGURE 36-8 Critical thinking model for activity and exercise assessment. *CSEP,* Canadian Society for Exercise Physiology.

judgements of how well they will be able to perform in given situations (Bandura, 2006). Ask the patient to what extent he or she enjoys exercising and his or her belief in the ability to exercise. This is a factor positively associated with adult physical activity (PHAC, 2012b). For example, pain and fatigue are factors that influence physical activity. When patients experience pain or fatigue following exercise, they may be unable to commit to exercise programs.

Body Alignment

Standing. Assessment of the standing patient includes the following: the head is erect and midline; body parts are symmetrical; the spine is straight with normal curvatures (cervical concave, thoracic convex, lumbar concave); the abdomen is comfortably tucked; the knees are in a straight line between the hips and ankles and slightly flexed; the feet are flat on the floor and pointed directly forward and slightly apart to maintain a wide base of support; and the arms hang comfortably at the sides (Figure 36-9). The patient's centre of gravity is in the midline, and the line of gravity is from the middle of the forehead to a midpoint between the feet. Laterally, the line of gravity runs vertically from the middle of the skull to the posterior third of the foot (Wilson & Giddens, 2013). During assessment, the nurse needs to identify deviations from expected findings. Self-assessment of body alignment when standing is also important for the nurse, to optimize body mechanics for safe patient handling to prevent personal injury.

Mobility

Assessment of mobility helps the nurse to determine the patient's coordination and balance while the patient is walking, the ability to carry out ADLs, and the ability to participate in an exercise program. The assessment of mobility has four components: range of motion, gait, exercise, and activity tolerance.

Range of Motion. Assessing ROM is one assessment technique used to determine the degree of damage or injury to a joint (see Chapter 32). These measurements enable the nurse to answer questions about joint stiffness, swelling, pain, limitation of movement, and unequal movement. Limited ROM may indicate inflammation such as arthritis, fluid in the joint, altered nerve supply, or contractures. Increased mobility (beyond normal) of a joint may indicate connective tissue disorders, ligament tears, or possible joint fractures.

Gait. Gait is the manner or style of walking, and includes rhythm, cadence, and speed. Walking with a limp is a gait. Propulsive, scissors, spastic, steppage, and waddling are descriptive names for other common gaits. Assessing gait allows you as the nurse to draw conclusions about balance, posture, and the ability to walk without assistance. Note conformity; a regular, smooth rhythm; symmetry in the length of leg swing; smooth swaying related to the gait phase; and a smooth, symmetrical arm swing (Wilson & Giddens, 2013).

Exercise and Activity. Regular exercise conditions the body, improves health, maintains fitness, and provides therapy to correct a deformity or restore the overall body to a maximal state of health. Daily activity is a measure for a patient's functional status. Determine how much exercise and the types of exercise that the patient participates in regularly. Ask the patient to describe the types of activities he or she does in a typical day or week. For greater accuracy, have the patient keep a diary of exercise activities for a week and review it together.

Activity Tolerance. Activity tolerance is the response a person has to the type and amount of exercise or activity that he or she is able to perform. Before a patient starts ambulation or other planned activities, the nurse should obtain a patient's vital signs, observe skin colour, and ask about level of comfort and current energy level or sense of fatigue. Nurses need to assess activity tolerance when planning physical activity for health promotion and for patients with acute or chronic illness. This assessment provides baseline data about a patient's activity patterns and assists in determining which factors (physical, psychological, or motivational) are affecting activity tolerance. Box 36-7 lists factors that affect activity tolerance. Box 36-8 lists nursing assessment questions to ask.

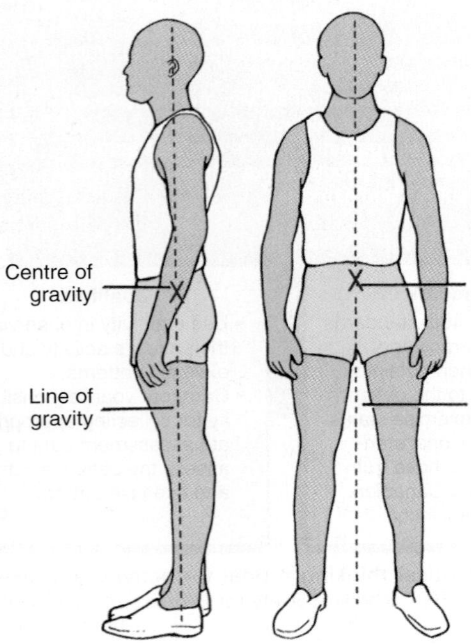

FIGURE 36-9 Correct body alignment when standing.

BOX 36-7 Factors Influencing Physical Activity Tolerance

Physiological Factors
Skeletal abnormalities
Muscular impairments
Endocrine or metabolic illnesses (e.g., diabetes mellitus or thyroid disease)
Hypoxemia
Decreased cardiac function
Decreased endurance
Impaired physical stability
Pain
Sleep pattern disturbance
Prior exercise patterns
Infectious processes and fever

Emotional Factors
Anxiety
Depression
Chemical addictions
Motivation

Developmental Factors
Age
Gender

Pregnancy
Physical growth and development of muscle and skeletal support

Modified from Lewis, S. L., et al. (2013). *Medical-surgical nursing assessment and management of clinical problems* (9th ed.). St. Louis, MO: Mosby.

BOX 36-8 Nursing Assessment Questions

Nature of the Problem
- Tell me about the types of problems you are having with physical activities and exercise.
- How much do you exercise each day?
- Describe your typical day. What types of activities do you do?
- What types of exercise do you prefer?
- How long do you exercise at any given time?

Signs and Symptoms
- Do you have any muscle or joint pain during or after exercise?
- Do you have shortness of breath during any activity?
- Do you ever feel chest discomfort or pain during exercise or physical activity?

Onset and Duration
- Which activities cause you to become short of breath?
- How long does it take to resume normal breathing after exercise or physical activity?

Severity
- How far do you walk before the pain in your legs begins?
- On a scale of 0 to 10 (with 10 being the worst discomfort), rate your leg pain.
- Describe your shortness of breath as minimal, moderate, or severe after physical activities or exercise, or both.

Barriers to Exercise and Activity
- Do you have any chronic illnesses that affect your ability to carry out daily activities such as grocery shopping, washing clothes, or daily walking?
- Do you have any physical limitations that prevent you from exercising on a daily basis?
- Do you have access to a community walking path or exercise equipment, or both?
- What prevents you from exercising 30 minutes each day?

Patient Values
- Tell me what you believe about the importance of regular exercise.
- How confident are you in being able to perform the exercises your health care provider has recommended?

Effect on Patient
- Has the lack of an exercise routine affected your weight?
- Do you feel more tired since you have not been able to exercise on a routine basis?
- Have you noticed any increase in shortness of breath when performing activities that require little exertion?

BOX 36-9 NURSING DIAGNOSTIC PROCESS

Impaired Physical Mobility

Assessment Activities	Defining Characteristics
Observe patient's gait.	Shuffled gait Uncoordinated gait Patient reports slower walking speed
Observe patient performing tasks such as eating, dressing, or recreational activities.	Uncoordinated movements Limited fine motor coordination
Measure range of joint motion.	Reduced joint motion in lower and/or upper extremities Stiffness in joints
Measure patient's strength.	Has difficulty rising to sitting position or exiting bed

◆ Nursing Diagnosis

Assessment of the patient's activity tolerance, physical fitness, body alignment, and joint mobility provides related clusters of data or defining characteristics that help the nurse identify a nursing diagnosis. Nurses must be accurate when identifying diagnoses. For example, a patient who reports being tired or weakened potentially could be diagnosed as having *activity intolerance or fatigue.* Defining characteristics are used to lead to the definitive diagnosis. For example, a finding of abnormal heart rate or dyspnea would lead the nurse to the diagnosis of activity intolerance, not to fatigue.

When activity and exercise are problems for a patient, nursing diagnoses often focus on the individual's ability to move. The diagnostic label should direct nursing interventions. This requires the correct selection of the related factors. For example, *activity intolerance related to excess weight gain* requires very different interventions than if the related factor is prolonged bed rest. Box 36-9 provides an example of how the diagnostic process leads to accurate diagnosis selection. The following are examples of nursing diagnoses related to activity and exercise:

- *Health-seeking behaviours*
- *Readiness for enhanced self-care*
- *Activity intolerance*
- *Ineffective coping*
- *Impaired gas exchange*
- *Risk for injury*
- *Impaired physical mobility*
- *Imbalanced nutrition: more than body requirements*
- *Acute or chronic pain*

◆ Planning

During planning, nurses need to synthesize information from multiple resources (Figure 36-10). The nurse's critical thinking ensures that the patient's care plan integrates all patient information. Best practice guidelines are especially important to consider when developing a care plan, as these documents establish scientifically based guidelines for selecting effective nursing interventions.

Concept maps assist in the planning of care. Figure 36-11 shows the relationship between a patient's medical diagnosis of heart failure and the identified nursing diagnosis.

Goals and Outcomes

Once the nurse has identified the nursing diagnoses, the nurse and the patient can set goals and expected outcomes to direct interventions. The plan includes consideration of preexisting health concerns and of any risks of injury to the patient. It is especially important to have knowledge of the patient's home environment when planning therapies to maintain or improve activity, body alignment, and mobility. For some patients with alterations in joint mobility, family members may be the providers of care. It is important to include the patient's family in the care plan. Family caregivers play critical roles in the home environment, motivating and coaching patients to stay active. The

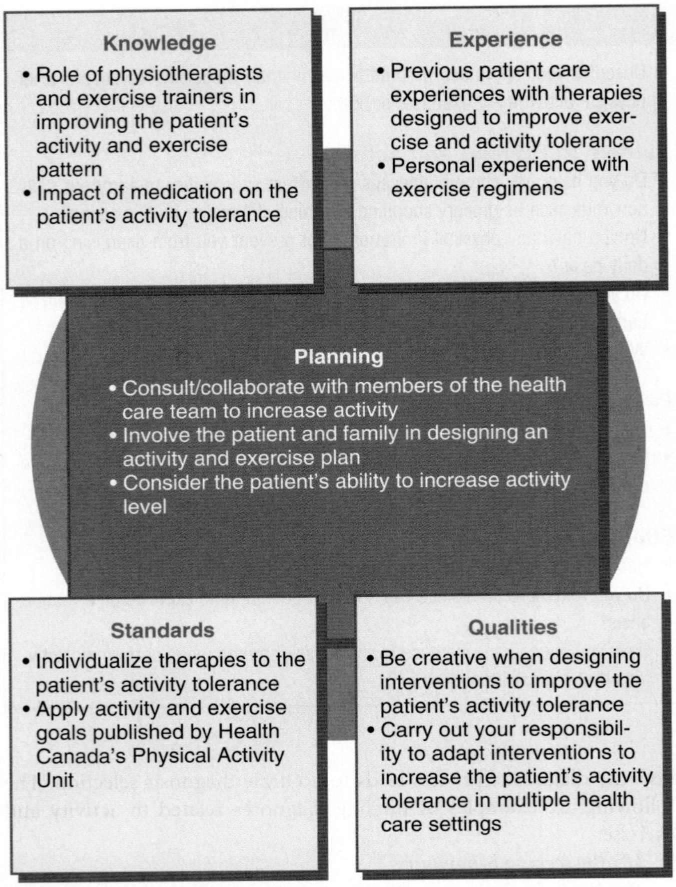

FIGURE 36-10 Critical thinking model for activity and exercise planning.

general goal related to exercise and activity is to improve or maintain the patient's motor function and independence. The following are examples of outcomes for patients with deficits in activity and exercise (Ackley & Ladwig, 2014):

- Participates in prescribed physical activity while maintaining appropriate heart rate, blood pressure, and breathing rate
- Verbalizes an understanding of the need to increase activity gradually according to tolerance and symptoms
- Expresses understanding of balancing rest and activity

Setting Priorities

Care planning is patient centred, taking into consideration the patient's most immediate needs. Nurses need to determine the immediacy of any problem by its effect on the patient's mental and physical health. For example, a patient may have chronic diseases such as diabetes and hypertension, which would be improved with an increase in exercise. However, if that same patient has recently experienced angina, immediate investigation and treatment of the angina is the priority.

Teamwork and Collaboration

Planning involves understanding a patient's need to maintain function and independence. To ensure comprehensive patient-centred care, nurses need to collaborate with the multidisciplinary team. Contributions from physicians, physiotherapists, kinesiologists, and occupational therapists are essential in planning care. The nurse must always individualize a care plan to meet the actual and potential needs of the patient (Box 36-10).

◆ Implementation

Health Promotion A sedentary lifestyle contributes to the development of health-related problems. As a nurse, you can promote health by encouraging patients to engage in a regular exercise program in any setting (Box 36-11). Discuss the recommendations for physical activity and fitness with the patient (Box 36-12). Design a program of exercise in collaboration with the patient, taking into account, age, developmental (see Box 36-12 and Box 36-13) and cultural factors. Collaborate with the patient's physician, physiotherapist, occupational therapist, and other members of the health care team to ensure patient-centred care.

Before starting an exercise program, teach patients to calculate their maximum heart rate by subtracting their current age in years from 220 and then determine their target heart rate by calculating 60 to 90% of this maximum rate, depending on their health care provider's recommendation. Patients should be taught to monitor their pulse during exercise and to exercise so that the heart rate is maintained within the target range.

Regardless of the exercise prescription implemented by the patient, warm-up and cool-down periods must be included in the program (Edelman et al., 2013). The warm-up period usually lasts 5 to 10 minutes and may include stretching, calisthenics, and subsequent aerobic activity performed at a lower intensity. The warm-up period prepares the body and decreases the potential for injury. The cool-down period follows the exercise routine and usually lasts 5 to 10 minutes. The cool-down period allows the body to readjust to baseline functioning gradually and provides an opportunity to combine movement such as stretching with relaxation-enhancing mind–body awareness (Edelman et al., 2013).

Many patients find it difficult to incorporate an exercise program into their daily routines because of time constraints. For these patients, it is beneficial to reinforce that exercise can be incorporated in small amounts—as little as 10 minutes at a time. Activities such as taking a short walk at lunch or walking to the corner store instead of driving can help increase total exercise. A more active lifestyle can involve taking the stairs instead of the elevator and parking farther from the entrance.

Other patients may benefit from a prescribed exercise and physical fitness program carefully designed to meet their needs and expectations. A comprehensive exercise prescription incorporates a combination of aerobic exercise, stretching and flexibility exercises, and resistance training. Aerobic exercise includes such activities as walking, running, bicycling, aerobic dance, jumping rope, and cross-country skiing. Recommended frequency of aerobic exercise is three to five times per week, or every other day. For a patient who prefers to exercise every day, cross-training is recommended. For example, the patient may run one day and do yoga on the next day.

Stretching and flexibility exercises include active ROM exercises that allow for stretching of all muscle groups and joints. This form of exercise is ideal for warm-up and cool-down periods. Benefits include increased flexibility, improved circulation and posture, and an opportunity for relaxation.

Resistance training increases muscle strength and endurance and is associated with improved performance of daily activities and avoidance of injuries and disability. Formal resistance training includes weight training, but the same benefits can be obtained by performing ADLs such as pushing a vacuum cleaner, raking leaves, shovelling snow, and kneading bread. Some patients may use weight training to bulk up their muscles. However, the purpose of weight training from a health perspective is to develop tone and strength and to stimulate and maintain healthy bones (O'Donovan, Blazevich, Boreham, et al., 2010).

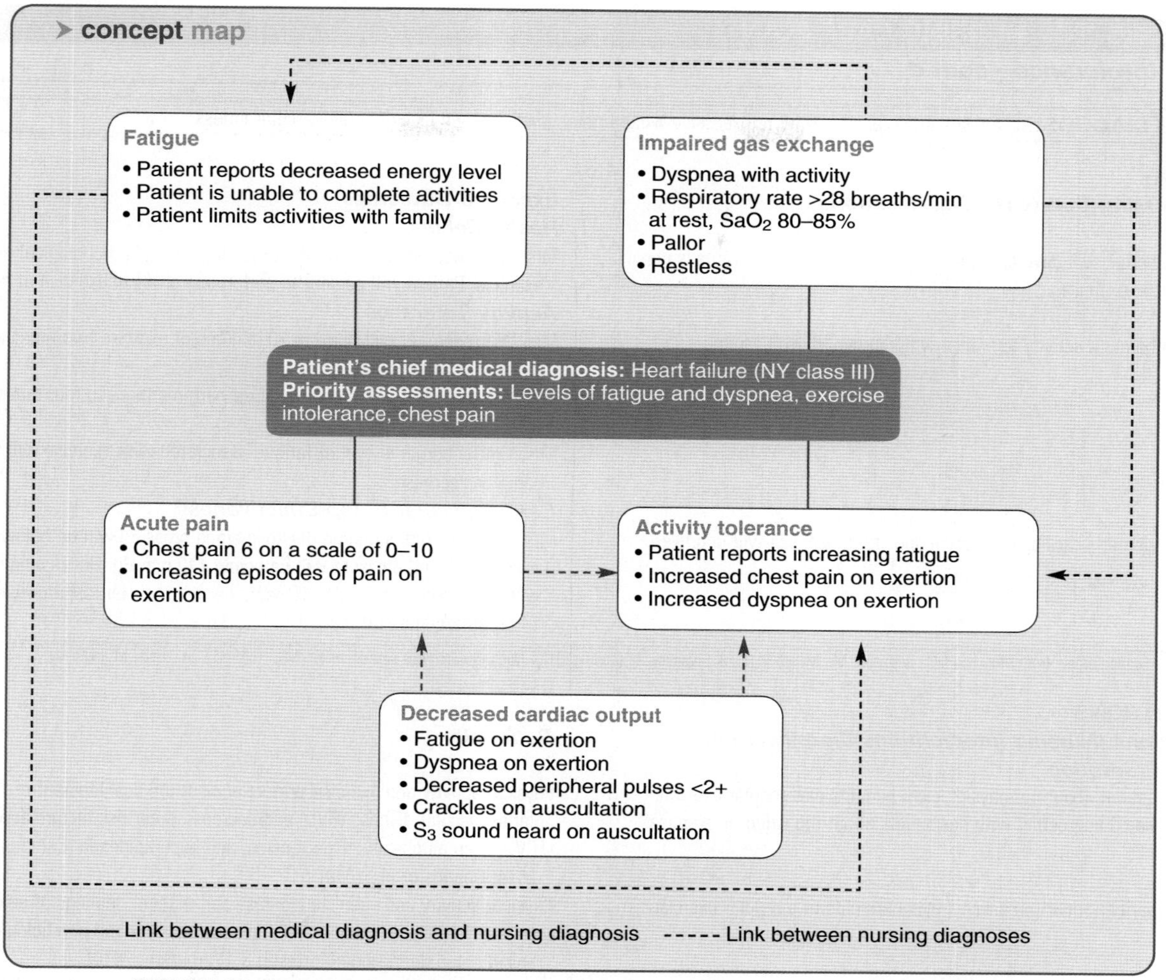

FIGURE 36-11 Concept map for a patient with heart failure and decreased activity.

BOX 36-10 NURSING CARE PLAN

Activity Intolerance

ASSESSMENT

Mrs. Mary Wertenberger is a 45-year-old homemaker. She has enrolled in a cardiovascular disease prevention (CDP) program prescribed by her physician and conducted by Eric Sieple, a registered nurse. Mrs. Wertenberger has several risk factors associated with cardiovascular disease. She expresses feelings of stress resulting from excessive demands on her time. Eric's assessment included a discussion of Mrs. Wertenberger's current health problems as well as a pertinent physical examination.

Assessment Activities	***Findings and Defining Characteristics****
Ask Mrs. Wertenberger what prompted her physician to recommend a CDP program.	She responds, "I *gained 23 kg* over the past year. I become *fatigued* easily and lack the energy to keep up with even simple household chores. I don't want to leave the house anymore."
Ask Mrs. Wertenberger about her exercise and eating habits.	She responds, "I want to exercise but with the demands of child care and caring for my aging parents, I just don't feel like it. I feel pulled in every direction, that increases my stress, and then I want to eat, eat, eat!"
Perform baseline assessment.	Height: 160 cm Weight: *102 kg* Blood pressure: *152/90 mm Hg (at rest)* Pulse: 96 beats per minute (at rest) Breathing rate: 20 breaths per minute (at rest) Blood pressure: *164/96 mm Hg (climbing 10 steps)* Pulse: *120 beats per minute (climbing 10 steps)* Breathing rate: *36 breaths per minute (climbing 10 steps)*

*Defining characteristics are shown in italics.

Continued

BOX 36-10 NURSING CARE PLAN

Activity Intolerance—cont'd

NURSING DIAGNOSIS: Activity intolerance related to excessive weight gain, inactivity, and lack of cardiovascular fitness

PLANNING

Goals (Nursing Outcomes Classification)[†]	*Expected Outcomes*
	Health Beliefs
Mrs. Wertenberger will develop a plan of exercise that incorporates isotonic and isometric exercises.	Mrs. Wertenberger will state the physiological and psychological effects of exercise. Patient will commit to performing physical exercise at home.
	Activity Tolerance
Mrs. Wertenberger's activity tolerance will improve above baseline.	Mrs. Wertenberger will perform 20 minutes of exercise two times a week over the next 2 weeks. Mrs. Wertenberger will record exercise patterns three to four times over the next 2 weeks. Mrs. Wertenberger's level of fatigue associated with exercise will remain the same or decrease.
	Cardiovascular Pump Effectiveness
Mrs. Wertenberger's cardiopulmonary response to exercise will improve.	Mrs. Wertenberger's resting diastolic blood pressure will be below 80 mm Hg. Her systolic blood pressure will be below 140 mm Hg. Her resting heart rate will range between 75 and 85 beats per minute. Her respiratory rate will be 14 breaths/minute (at rest).

[†]Outcome classification labels from Moorhead, S., Johnson, M., Maas, M. L., & Swanson, E. (Eds.). (2013). *Nursing outcomes classification (NOC)* (5th ed.). St. Louis, MO: Mosby.

INTERVENTIONS

Interventions (Nursing Interventions Classification)[‡]	*Rationale*
Exercise Promotion	
Instruct the patient about the physiological benefits of a regular exercise program. Match instruction with her beliefs about the value of exercise.	Physical activity and exercise protect against the development of cardiovascular disease (CVD) and decrease other risk factors associated with CVD, such as obesity, hypertension, and hyperlipidemia (Campos-Outcalt, 2014; Donges et al., 2010).
Instruct the patient about the psychological benefits of a regular exercise program.	Physical activity and exercise increase self-esteem, feelings of enjoyment, self-confidence, and mood and decrease physical and psychological stress, anxiety, and depression (Paterson & Warburton, 2010).
Develop a progressive plan of exercise with the patient, such as 3 to 5 km or 20 minutes of brisk walking and quadriceps, biceps, and gluteal muscle isometric exercises three to four times per week.	Cross-training (a combination of exercise activities) provides variety to combat boredom and increases potential for total body conditioning (Edelman et al., 2013).
Instruct the patient to use an exercise log and to record the day, time, duration, and responses (pulse, feelings, shortness of breath, daily weight).	Keeping a log may increase adherence to exercise prescription.
Schedule weekly meetings with Mrs. Wertenberger for follow-up and review of exercise log, progress, and barriers.	Patients are more likely to increase physical activity and remain adherent to an exercise program if they are counselled by a health care provider (Edelman et al., 2013).

[‡]Intervention classification labels from Bulechek, G. M., Butcher, H. K., & Dochterman, J. M. (Eds.). (2013). *Nursing interventions classification (NIC)* (6th ed.). St. Louis, MO: Mosby.

EVALUATION

Nursing Actions	*Patient Responses and Findings*	*Achievement of Outcomes*
Review Mrs. Wertenberger's exercise log at each visit.	She responds, "I make time to exercise because of this log. I hate missing a day and leaving a blank page; this represents failure. I want to succeed." Exercise log documents activity four times per week.	Mrs. Wertenberger reports enjoying exercise, as well as observing some personal benefits of exercise. The exercise log is facilitating adherence to the exercise prescription.
Record weight, blood pressure, and pulse.	Weight, 95 kg. Resting heart rate between 80 and 85 beats per minute. Blood pressure, 146/86 mm Hg.	Improved cardiovascular effects of exercise: • Heart rate is within normal range. • Blood pressure is lower but not at expected range. Monitor blood pressure as patient continues to lose weight.
Ask Mrs. Wertenberger if exercise is helping to lower fatigue level.	Mrs. Wertenberger responds, "At first, finding time to exercise was hard, but once I started feeling less tired and even less stressed, it was easy to integrate exercise into my daily activities."	Achieved improved activity tolerance with exercise.

Body Mechanics. The Canadian Centre for Occupational Health and Safety (2017) has published numerous guidelines related to ergonomic standards for preventing musculoskeletal injuries in the workplace. More than half of all back pain in health care settings is associated with manual lifting tasks (Workers Health and Safety Centre, 2013). Back injuries are often the direct result of improper lifting and bending. The most common back injury is strain on the muscle group around the lumbar vertebrae. Injury to this area affects the ability to bend forward, backward, and from side to side. The ability to rotate the hips and lower back is also decreased (Lin, Tsai, Chen, et al., 2012). Body mechanics alone are not sufficient to prevent musculoskeletal injuries when lifting or transferring patients (Waters, Nelson, Hughes, et al., 2009).

Before repositioning a patient, assess the weight to be moved and what assistance the patient can provide. Never attempt to lift a patient without assistance. When using mechanical lifts, a second person is always required to assist. Use mechanical lifts, friction-reduction devices, slide boards, and other handling aids available in the workplace (Alberta Health Services, 2017). Many health care agencies have a no-lift policy, in which manual lifting of the whole or a large part of the weight of the patient by a health care worker is prohibited, except in exceptional or life-threatening situations. Some agencies also have lift teams (Table 36-2).

BOX 36-11 Promoting Exercise

Nurses can do the following to help patients participate in exercise:

- Educate patients about the importance of exercise in preserving health.
- Encourage patients to pace activities and increase speed and intensity gradually to avoid pain.
- Administer prescribed anti-inflammatory medications 1 to 2 hours before starting an exercise program.
- Encourage patients to balance rest and activity and to get plenty of sleep.
- Teach patients how to use canes or walkers to assist with walking as needed.
- Encourage patients to choose smooth and even walking surfaces.
- Advise patients not to force joints past the point of resistance or pain.
- Instruct patients to check legs and feet daily for redness, swelling, blisters, or broken skin.
- Instruct patients to wear properly fitting shoes with nonslip soles.
- Encourage patients to walk with a companion or group so that exercise is socially rewarding.

Acute Care

Patients who are hospitalized should be encouraged to do stretching exercises, active ROM exercises, and low-intensity walking. Physiotherapists can also assist patients with isometric exercises. When patients cannot participate in active ROM, the nurse can maintain joint mobility and prevent contractures by implementing passive ROM into the plan of care. If needed, patients can be medicated for pain 30 minutes before exercise. An analgesic that makes the patient feel dizzy should not be used.

Musculoskeletal System. Nurses can help maintain the musculoskeletal system in patients in acute care by encouraging the use of stretching and isometric exercises. The nurse should review the patient's chart and collaborate with physiotherapy and the health care

BOX 36-12 Recommendations for Exercise

Children 5–11 and Youths 12–17 Years of Age

Preamble

- Should be physically active as part of play, games, sports, transportation, recreation, physical education, or planned exercise in the context of family, school, and community
- Activity can improve cholesterol levels, blood pressure, body composition, bone density, cardiorespiratory, musculoskeletal fitness, and aspects of mental health
- May be appropriate for children with a disability or medical condition

Guidelines

- At least 60 minutes of moderate- to vigorous-intensity physical activity daily
- Vigorous-intensity activities at least 3 days per week
- Activities that strengthen muscle and bone at least 3 days per week
- More daily physical activity provides greater health benefits

Adults 18–64 Years of Age

Preamble

- Can meet guidelines through planned exercise sessions, transportation, recreation, sports, or occupational demands, in the context of family, work, volunteer, and community activities
- Activity can reduce the risk of premature death, coronary heart disease, stroke, hypertension, colon cancer, breast cancer, type 2 diabetes, and osteoporosis and improve fitness, body composition, and indicators of mental health (Warburton, Charlesworth, Ivey, et al., 2010)
- Guidelines may be available for those who are pregnant or have a disability or medical condition

Guidelines

- At least 150 minutes of moderate- to vigorous-intensity aerobic physical activity per week, in bouts of 10 minutes or more
- Add muscle- and bone-strengthening activities using major muscle groups, at least 2 days per week

Adults 65 and Older

Preamble

- Should be physically active beyond the incidental physical activities accumulated in the course of daily living
- Following guidelines may reduce the risk of chronic disease and premature death, maintain functional independence and mobility, and improve fitness, body composition, bone health, cognitive function, and indicators of mental health
- May be appropriate for older persons with frailty, a disability, or medical condition

Guidelines

- Accumulate at least 150 minutes of moderate- to vigorous-intensity aerobic physical activity per week in bouts of 10 minutes or more
- Add muscle- and bone-strengthening activities using major muscle groups at least 2 days per week
- Those with poor mobility should perform physical activities to enhance balance and prevent falls

Adapted from Canadian Society for Exercise Physiology. (2011). *Canadian physical activity guide.* Retrieved from http://www.csep.ca/cmfiles/guidelines/canadianphysicalactivityguidelinesstatements_e_2012.pdf.

BOX 36-13 FOCUS ON OLDER PERSONS

Helping the Older Person Initiate and Maintain an Exercise Program

Nurses should base an older patient's exercise program on individual assessment data (underlying conditions, medications, present activity level). Before an older person starts an exercise program, the nurse needs to consult the physician for exercise restrictions. Modification of the exercise program is based on the individual's responses. The nurse can use the following guidelines to counsel the patient:

- It is never too late to begin an exercise program (Edelman et al., 2013; Elliot, 2011). Ensure that patients consult a health care provider before beginning an exercise program, particularly if the patient has heart or lung disease or other chronic illnesses.
- Use assessment data and consult with physiotherapy to determine when you need to adjust exercise programs for older persons.
- Recommend resistance-and-agility training programs. These forms of exercise reduce fear of falling and increase a sense of well-being in older persons (Kwun, Laufgraben, & Gopalakrishnan, 2012).
- Provide resources for planned exercise programs. Weight-bearing and resistance exercise slows bone loss and prevents fractures in older persons (Roush, 2011).
- Encourage older persons to avoid prolonged sitting and to get up and stretch. Frequent stretching decreases the risk of developing joint contractures.
- Encourage older persons to maintain proper body alignment when sitting, to minimize joint and muscle stress.
- Teach patients how to use stronger joints and larger muscle groups. Efficient distribution of the workload decreases joint stress and pain.
- Instruct patients to use correct body mechanics, wear appropriate clothing and footwear, and maintain sufficient hydration.
- Encourage older persons who are unable to participate in a formal exercise program to improve joint mobility and enhance circulation by simply stretching and exaggerating movements during the performance of routine activities of daily living.

Further instructions for older persons regarding exercise are as follows:

- Perform a gradual, extended exercise warm-up (e.g., 15 minutes) to maximize flexibility and decrease the chance of muscle injury.
- Begin at a low level (40 to 50% of predicted maximal heart rate; maximal heart rate is estimated as the number 220 minus patient's age) and to follow gentle exercise progression.
- Avoid sudden twisting movements, rapid movements, and rapid transitions from one movement to the next.
- Avoid exercises that tax vision and balance.
- Avoid sustained isometric contractions of >10 seconds.
- Avoid exercise during acute viral infections.
- Stop exercising if cardiac dysrhythmias, angina, or excessive breathlessness occurs.
- Perform cool-down exercises until the heart rate returns to resting level to decrease postural hypotension and cardiac dysrhythmias.

Adapted from Touhy, T., Jett, K., Boscart, V., & McCleary, L. (2012). *Ebersole & Hess' gerontological nursing and healthy aging* (1st Canadian ed.). Toronto: Elsevier Canada.

TABLE 36-2 Safe Client Handling for Health Care Workers

Action	Rationale
When planning to move a patient, arrange for adequate help.	Ensures that caregiver has adequate assistance to prevent injury to self and patient.
Use patient-handling equipment and devices, such as height-adjustable beds, ceiling-mounted lifts, friction-reducing slide sheets, and air-assisted devices (Hunter et al., 2010; Tullar, Brewer, Amick, et al., 2010).	These devices help to reduce the caregiver's muscular strain during patient handling.
Encourage patient to assist as much as possible.	This promotes patient's independence and strength and minimizes workload.
Take position close to patient (or object being lifted).	Keeps patient or object in same plane as lifter and close to caregiver's centre of gravity. Reduces horizontal reach and stresses on caregiver's back.
Tighten abdominal muscles and keep back, neck, pelvis, and feet aligned. Avoid twisting.	Reduces risk of injury to lumbar vertebrae and muscle groups. Twisting increases risk of injury (Lin et al., 2012).
Bend at knees; keep feet wide apart.	A broad base of support increases stability and maintains centre of gravity.
Use arms and legs (not back).	Leg muscles are stronger, larger muscles capable of greater work without injury.
Slide patient toward your body, using a pull sheet or slide board. When transferring a patient onto a stretcher or bed, a slide board is more appropriate.	Sliding requires less effort than lifting. A pull sheet minimizes shearing forces, which can damage patient's skin.
The person with the heaviest load coordinates efforts of the team involved by counting to three.	Simultaneous lifting minimizes the load for any one lifter.

provider to identify possible contraindications before initiating isometric exercises. A physiotherapist will design an isometric exercise program for the specific needs of a patient. The nurse's role is to follow that program and assist patients accordingly. For example, an exercise program includes isometric exercises of the biceps and triceps to prepare a patient for crutch walking. The patient should be instructed to stop the activity if pain, fatigue, or discomfort is experienced.

During isometrics, a patient tightens or contracts a muscle group for 10 seconds and then completely relaxes for several seconds (Resnick et al., 2012). Repetitions are increased gradually for each muscle group until the isometric exercise is repeated 8 to 10 times. Patients should be instructed to perform the exercises slowly and increase repetitions as their physical condition improves. A patient needs to do isometric exercise for quadriceps and gluteal muscle groups, which are used for walking, four times per day until a patient is ambulatory.

Joint Mobility. The easiest intervention to maintain or improve joint mobility for patients and one that can be coordinated with other activities is the use of ROM exercises (see Chapter 45). In active ROM exercises, patients are able to move their joints independently. With passive ROM exercises, the nurse moves each joint in patients who are unable to perform these exercises themselves. The use of ROM exercises provides data to systematically assess and improve the patient's mobility.

Joints that are not moved periodically are at risk for *contractures*, a permanent shortening of a muscle followed by the eventual shortening of associated ligaments and tendons. Over time the joint becomes fixed in one position, and the patient loses normal use of it. Passive ROM exercises are the exercises of choice for patients who do not have voluntary motor control.

Some older persons who experience a decline in physical activity and changes in joints often have limited mobility and joint flexibility. A variety of recommended approaches can be used to help older persons use proper body mechanics and prevent injury.

Unless contraindicated, the nursing care plan includes exercising each joint through as nearly a full ROM as possible. Passive ROM exercises should be initiated as soon as the patient loses the ability to move the extremity or joint. Chapter 45 details ROM exercises for each area and illustrates the motion of each joint.

Walking. Walking increases joint mobility and can be measured by length of time or distance walked. The nurse should measure distances walked in meters instead of charting "ambulated to nurses' station and back." Illness or trauma usually reduces activity tolerance, resulting in the need for help with walking or the use of assistive devices such as crutches, canes, or walkers. Patients who increase their walking distance before discharge improve their ability to independently perform basic ADLs, increase activity tolerance, and have a faster recovery after surgery.

Helping a Patient Walk

Helping a patient walk requires preparation. The patient's strength, coordination, baseline vital signs, and balance need to be assessed in order to determine the type of assistance needed. As the nurse helping a patient to walk, assess orientation and determine if there are any signs of distress. Postpone walking if you determine that the patient cannot walk safely. Evaluate the environment for safety before ambulation (e.g., removal of obstacles, a clean and dry floor, and the identification of rest points in case the patient's activity tolerance becomes less than expected or if the patient becomes dizzy). Have the patient wear supportive, nonskid shoes.

Help the patient to a position of sitting at the side of the bed and dangling the legs over the side of the bed for 1 to 2 minutes before standing. Some patients experience orthostatic hypotension (i.e., a drop in blood pressure that occurs with they change from a horizontal to vertical position) (Fedorowski & Melander, 2013; Lewis, Heitkemper, Dirksen, et al., 2013). Those at higher risk are patients who are immobilized, patients who are on prolonged bed rest, older persons, and patients with chronic diseases such as diabetes mellitus and cardiovascular disease. Signs and symptoms of orthostatic hypotension include dizziness, lightheadedness, nausea, tachycardia, pallor, and even fainting. Orthostatic hypotension usually stabilizes quickly, but if the patient develops dizziness lasting 60 seconds, the patient should be returned to bed (Myszenski, 2017; Perme & Chandrashekar, 2009).

Dangling a patient's legs before standing is an intermediate step that allows assessment of the patient before changing positions to maintain safety and prevent injury to the patient. In some instances the nurse will need to take the patient's blood pressure while the patient is sitting on the side of the bed.

Several methods are used to help a patient ambulate. Always provide support at the waist with a gait belt so that the patient's centre of gravity remains midline. A gait belt encircles the patient's waist snugly. The nurse holds the back of the belt behind the patient (Figure 36-12).

If the patient has a fainting (syncope) episode or begins to fall, assume a wide base of support with one foot in front of the other; this helps to support the patient's body weight (Figure 36-13, *A*). Extend one leg, let the patient slide against the leg and gently lower the patient to the floor, protecting the head (Figure 36-13, *B, C*). When the patient attempts to ambulate again, proceed more slowly, monitor for reports of dizziness, and take the patient's blood pressure before, during, and after ambulation.

Restorative and Continuing Care

Restorative and continuing care involves implementing activity and exercise strategies to assist the patient regaining mobility and activity capacity after acute care is no longer needed. Restorative and continuing care also includes activities and exercises that restore and promote optimal functioning in patients with specific chronic illnesses, such as coronary heart disease (CHD), hypertension, COPD, and diabetes mellitus (Table 36-3). Remaining active while living with chronic diseases improves outcomes, including prevention of complications, improved function, and enhanced quality of life. Given the degree of physical compromise individuals with one or more chronic diseases may experience, consultation with the patient's primary care provider, medical specialist, or both is prudent before implementation of an

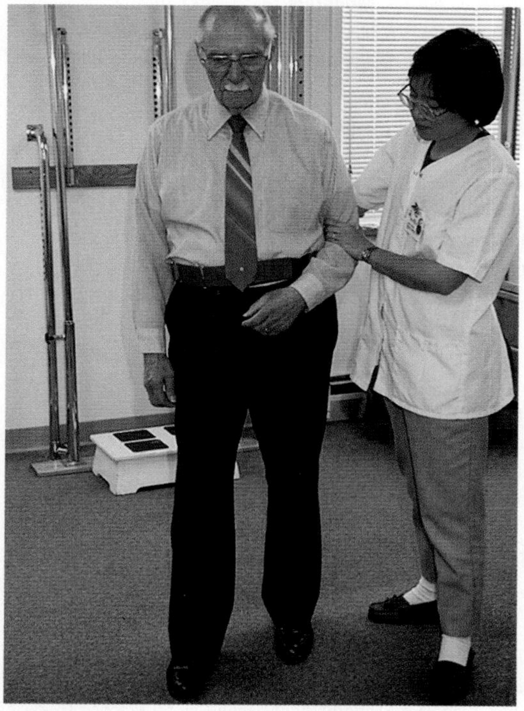

FIGURE 36-12 When helping a patient walk, the nurse uses a gait belt and walks slightly behind the patient's side. (From Sorrentino, S. A., Wilk, M. J., & Newmaster, R. (2009). *Mosby's Canadian textbook for the support worker* (2nd ed., p. 439, Fig. 24-22). Toronto: Elsevier.)

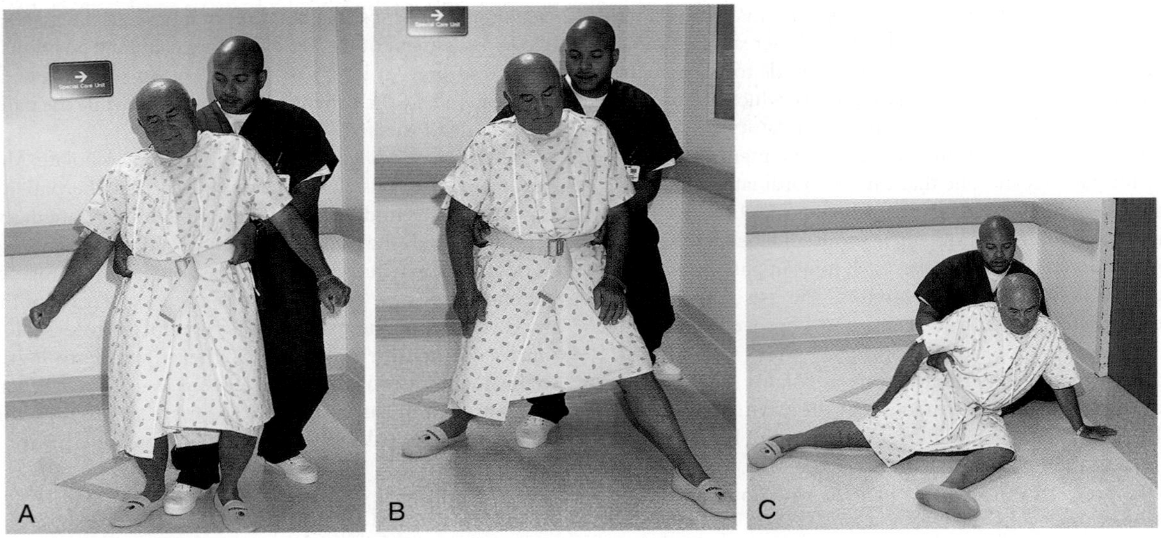

FIGURE 36-13 Safe patient handling: Fall **A,** Stand with feet apart to provide a broad base of support. **B,** Extend one leg and let patient slide against it to the floor. **C,** Bend knees to lower body as patient slides to the floor.

TABLE 36-3 Physical Activity and Exercise—Recommendations From the Clinical Practice Guidelines for the Prevention and Management of Diabetes in Canada

Definition and Recommended Frequency	Intensity	Examples
Aerobic Exercise		
Rhythmic, repeated and continuous movements of the same large muscle groups for at least 10 minutes at a time	**Moderate** 50–70% of person's maximum heart rate	Biking Brisk walking Continuous swimming Dancing Water aerobics
Recommended for a minimum of 150 minutes per week (moderate intensity)	**Vigorous** >70% of person's maximum heart rate	Brisk walking up an incline Jogging Aerobics Hockey Basketball Fast swimming Fast dancing
Resistance Exercise		
Activities that use muscular strength to move a weight or work against a resistance load	**3 times per week** Start with one set of 15–20 repetitions at moderate weight Progress to two sets of 10–15 repetitions Progress to three sets of 8 repetitions at heavier weight	Exercise with weight machines Weight lifting

Adapted from Canadian Diabetes Association Clinical Practice Guidelines Expert Committee. (2013). Canadian Diabetes Association 2013 clinical practice guidelines for the prevention and management of diabetes in Canada. *Canadian Journal of Diabetes, 37*(Suppl. 1), S1–S212. Retrieved from http://guidelines.diabetes.ca/app_themes/cdacpg/resources/cpg_2013_full_en.pdf.

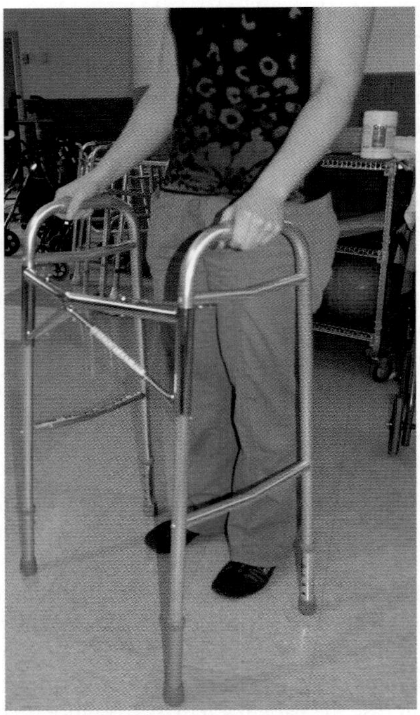

FIGURE 36-14 Patient using a standard walker.

exercise plan. Some patients' chronic disease process may be so advanced that they are unable to participate in even the most modest of exercise programs.

Assistive Devices for Walking

In collaboration with other members of the health care team, such as physiotherapists, nurses can promote activity and exercise by teaching the proper use of canes, walkers, or crutches, depending on the assistive device most appropriate for the patient's condition.

Walkers. A walker is a lightweight, movable device that stands waist high and consists of a metal frame with handgrips, four widely placed sturdy legs, and one open side (Figure 36-14). Because it has a wide base of support, the walker provides great stability and security during walking. A walker can be used by a patient who has problems with balance. Walkers with wheels are useful for patients who have difficulty lifting and advancing the walker as they walk because of limited balance or endurance (Figures 36-15 and 36-16). To determine if the walker is the correct size, instruct the patient to relax the arms at the side of the body and stand up straight. The top of the walker should line up with the crease on the inside of the patient's wrist. Elbows should be flexed about 15 to 30 degrees when standing inside the walker, with hands on the handgrips. To ambulate using a walker, the patient holds the handgrips on the upper bars, takes a step, moves the walker forward, and takes another step. Teach patients how to use walkers safely and how to avoid the risk of falling.

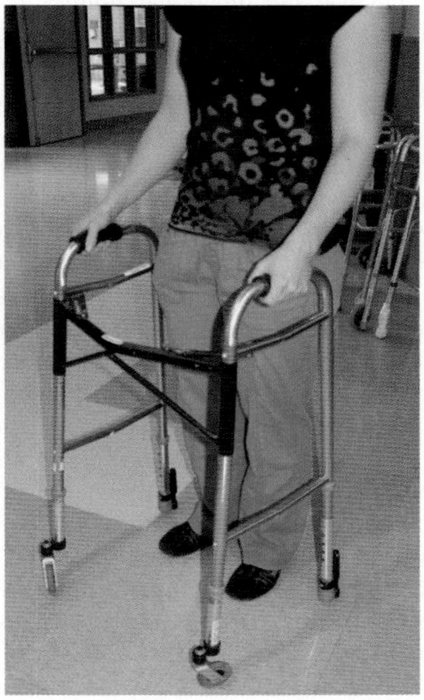

FIGURE 36-15 Patient using a two-wheeled walker.

Canes. Canes are lightweight, easily movable devices made of wood or metal. They provide less support than a walker and are less stable. To determine the correct cane length for a patient, measure the distance from the patient's greater trochanter to the floor (Pierson & Fairchild, 2013). Two common types of canes are the straight-legged cane and the quad cane. The straight-legged cane is more common and is used to support and balance a patient with decreased leg strength. The patient should keep the cane on the stronger side of the body. Teach the following three steps to promote maximum support when walking: First, instruct the patient to place the cane forward 15 to 25 cm, keeping body weight on both legs. Second, coach the patient to move the weaker leg forward to the cane so body weight is divided between the cane and the stronger leg. Third, have the patient advance the stronger leg past the cane so the cane supports the body weight and weaker leg. During walking the patient continually repeats these three steps. Assess the patient's knowledge to ensure that he or she knows that two points of support, such as both feet or one foot and the cane, are on the floor at all times.

The quad cane provides the most support and is used when there is partial or complete leg paralysis or some hemiplegia (Figure 36-17). The patient is taught the same three steps that are used with the straight-legged cane.

Crutches. Crutches are often needed to increase mobility. A crutch is a wooden or metal staff. The use of crutches is often temporary (e.g., after ligament damage to the knee). However, some patients with paralysis of the lower extremities need them permanently.

The two types of crutches are the double adjustable or forearm crutch and the axillary wooden or metal crutch (which is the most common type) (Figure 36-18). The metal band and handgrip are adjusted to fit the patient's height. The axillary crutch has a padded curved surface at the top, which fits under the axilla. A handgrip in the form of a crossbar is held at the level of the palms to support the body.

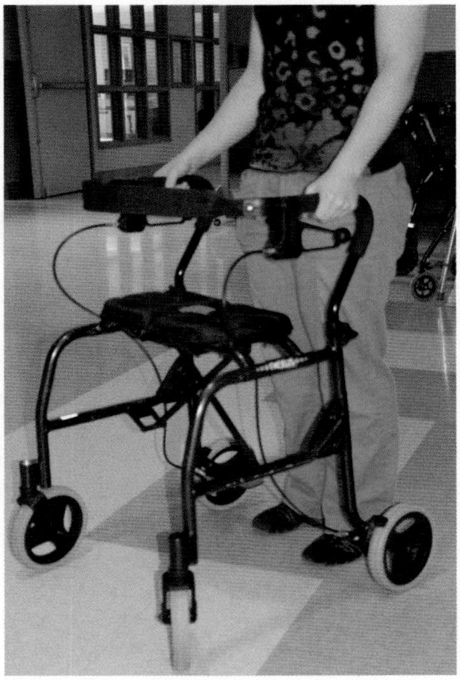

FIGURE 36-16 Patient using a rollator walker.

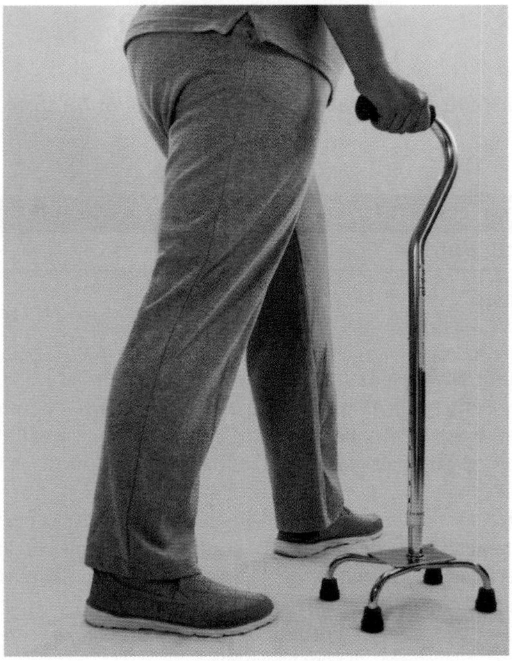

FIGURE 36-17 Patient using a quad cane.

It is important to measure crutches for the appropriate length and to teach patients how to use their crutches safely to achieve a stable gait, ascend and descend stairs, and rise from a sitting position. Begin crutch instruction with guidelines for safe use (Box 36-14).

Measuring for Crutches. Measurement for the axillary crutch includes the patient's height, the angle of elbow flexion, and the distance between the crutch pad and the axilla. When crutches are fitted, the length of the crutch needs to be two to three fingerwidths from the axilla and the tips positioned approximately 5 cm lateral and 10 to 15 cm anterior to the front of the patient's shoes (Figure 36-19).

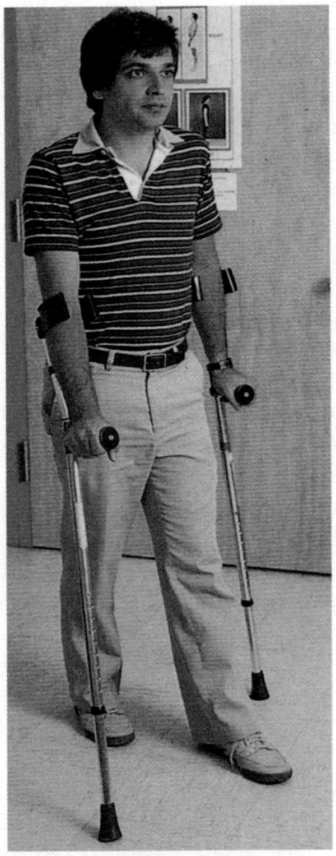

FIGURE 36-18 Double adjustable Lofstrand, or forearm, crutch.

When fitting a patient with crutches, position the handgrips so the axillae are not supporting the patient's body weight. Pressure on the axillae increases the risk to underlying nerves, which sometimes results in partial paralysis of the arm. Determine the correct position of the handgrips with the patient upright, supporting weight by the handgrips with the elbows slightly flexed at 20 to 25 degrees. Elbow flexion may be verified with the goniometer. When determining the height and placement of the handgrips, verify that the distance between the crutch pad and the patient's axilla is approximately 5 cm (two or three fingerwidths) (Figure 36-20).

Crutch Gait. Patients assume a gait by alternately bearing weight on one of both legs and on the crutches. Determine the gait by assessing the patient's physical and functional abilities and the disease or injury that resulted in the need for crutches. This section summarizes the basic crutch stance and the four standard gaits: four-point alternating gait, three-point alternating gait, two-point gait, and swing-through gait.

The basic crutch stance is the tripod position, formed when the crutches are placed 15 cm in front of and 15 cm to the side of each foot (Figure 36-21). This position improves the patient's balance by providing a wider base of support. The body alignment of the patient in the tripod position includes an erect head and neck, straight vertebrae, and extended hips and knees. The axillae should not bear any weight. The patient assumes the tripod position before crutch walking.

Four-point alternating, or four-point, gait gives stability to the patient but requires weight bearing on both legs. Each leg is moved alternately with each opposing crutch, so three points of support are on the floor at all times (Figure 36-22, *A*).

Three-point alternating, or three-point, gait requires the patient to bear all of the weight on one foot. In a three-point gait the patient bears weight on both crutches and then on the uninvolved leg, repeating the sequence (see Figure 36-22, *B*). The affected leg does not touch the

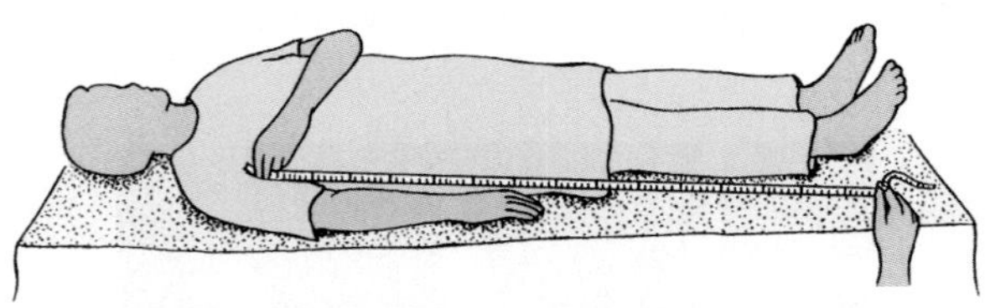

FIGURE 36-19 Measuring crutch length.

BOX 36-14 PATIENT TEACHING

Crutch Safety

Objective

- Patient will describe and demonstrate safe crutch walking.

Teaching Strategies

- Teach patient with axillary crutches about the dangers of pressure on the axillae, which occurs when leaning on the crutches to support body weight.
- Explain why the patient must use crutches that were measured for him or her.
- Show the patient how to routinely inspect crutch tips. Rubber tips should be securely attached to the crutches. When tips become worn out, they should be replaced. Rubber crutch tips increase surface friction and help prevent slipping.
- Explain that the crutch tips should remain dry. Water decreases surface friction and increases the risk of slipping.
- Explain that the patient should wear nonslip shoes and not wear an open gown or other long, flowing clothing to decrease the risk of falls.
- Show patient how to inspect the structure of the crutches.
- Cracks in a wooden crutch decrease its ability to support weight. Bends in aluminum crutches can alter body alignment.
- Provide patient with a list of medical supply companies in the community where repairs, new rubber tips, handgrips, and crutch pads can be obtained.
- Instruct patient to have spare crutches and spare tips readily available.

Evaluation

- Patient can describe principles of crutch safety.
- Patient correctly demonstrates proper use of crutches.

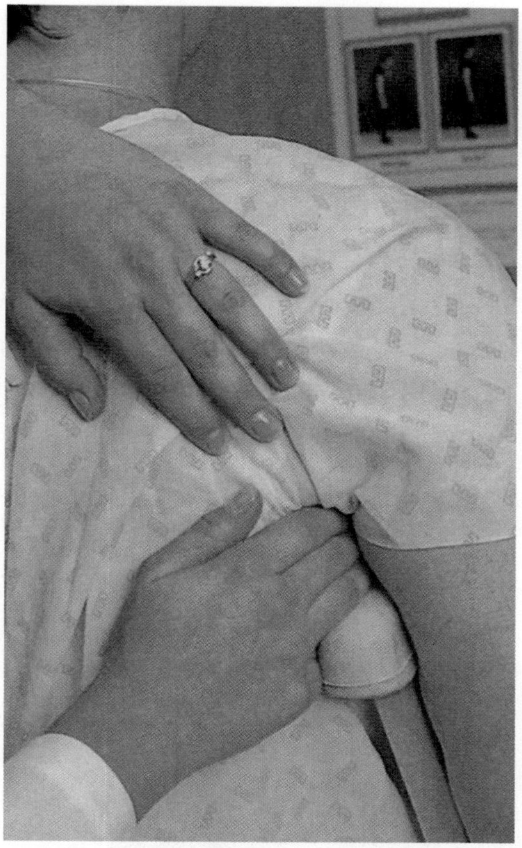

FIGURE 36-20 Verifying correct distance between crutch pads and axilla.

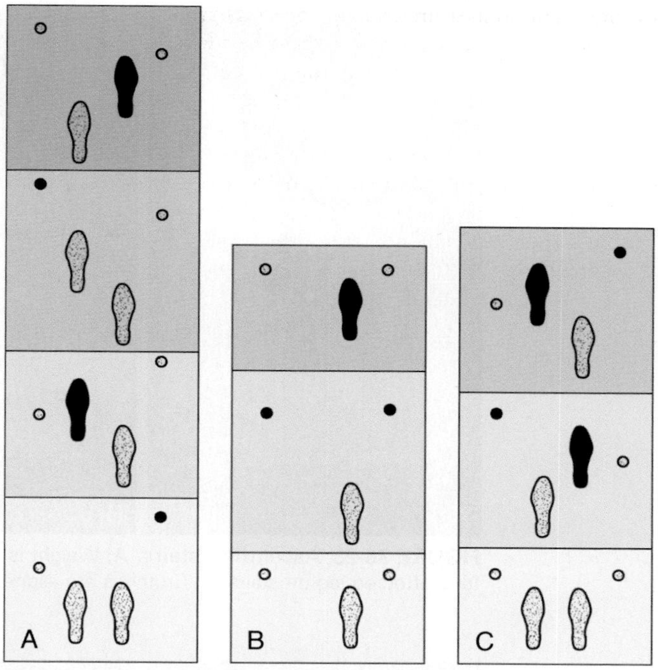

FIGURE 36-22 A, Four-point alternating gait. Solid feet and crutch tips show the order of foot and crutch tip movement in each of the four phases. *(Read from bottom to top.)* **B,** Three-point gait with weight borne on unaffected leg. Solid foot and crutch tips show weight bearing in each phase. *(Read from bottom to top.)* **C,** Two-point gait with weight borne partially on each foot and each crutch advancing with opposing leg. Solid areas indicate leg and crutch tips bearing weight. *(Read from bottom to top.)*

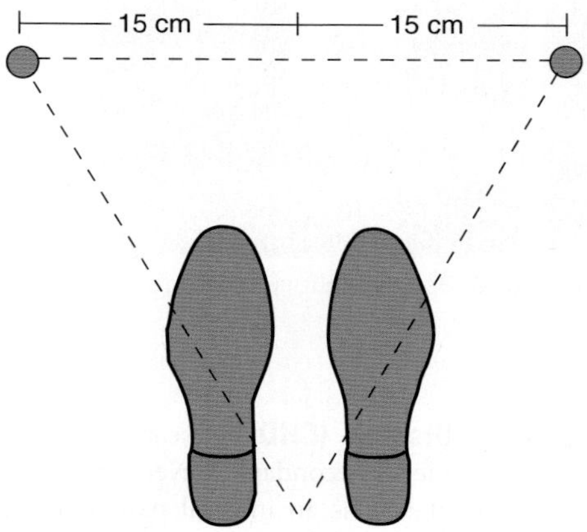

FIGURE 36-21 Tripod position, basic crutch stance.

ground during the early phase of the three-point gait. Gradually the patient progresses to touch-down and full weight bearing on the affected leg.

The two-point gait requires at least partial weight bearing on each foot (see Figure 36-22, *C*). The patient moves a crutch at the same time as the opposing leg, so the crutch movements are similar to arm motion during normal walking.

Individuals with paraplegia who wear weight-supporting braces on their legs frequently use the swing-through gait. With weight placed on the supported legs, the patient places the crutches one stride in front and then swings to or through them while supporting his or her weight.

Crutch Walking on Stairs. When ascending stairs on crutches, the patient usually uses a modified three-point gait (Figure 36-23). The patient stands at the bottom of the stairs and transfers body weight to the crutches. The person then advances the unaffected leg between the crutches and the stairs. The patient then shifts weight from the crutches to the unaffected leg. Finally, the person aligns both crutches on the stairs. The patient repeats this sequence until he or she reaches the top of the stairs.

A three-point sequence is also used to descend the stairs (Figure 36-24). The patient transfers body weight to the unaffected leg. The person then places the crutches on the stairs and begins to transfer body weight to the crutches, moving the affected leg forward. Finally, the patient moves the unaffected leg to the stairs with the crutches. The patient repeats the sequence until reaching the bottom of the stairs.

Because in most cases patients need to use crutches for some time, they need to be instructed to use them on the stairs before discharge. This teaching applies to all patients who are dependent on crutches, not just those who have stairs in their homes. Nurses will frequently collaborate with physiotherapists to provide instruction about crutch walking.

Sitting in a Chair With Crutches. As with crutch walking and crutch walking up and down stairs, the procedure for sitting in a chair involves phases and requires the patient to transfer weight

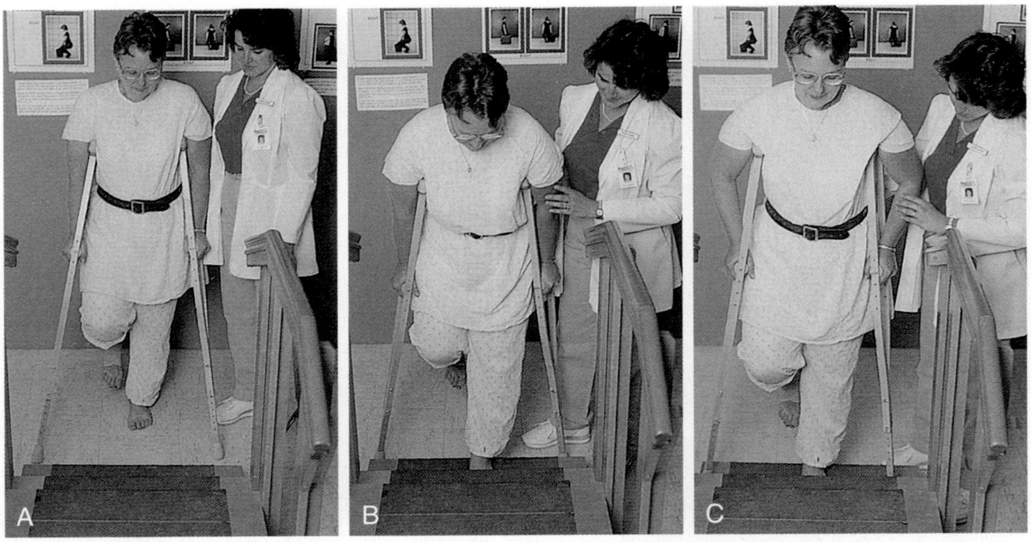

FIGURE 36-23 Ascending stairs. **A,** Weight is placed on crutch. **B,** Weight is transferred from crutches to unaffected leg on stairs. **C,** Crutches are aligned with unaffected leg on stairs.

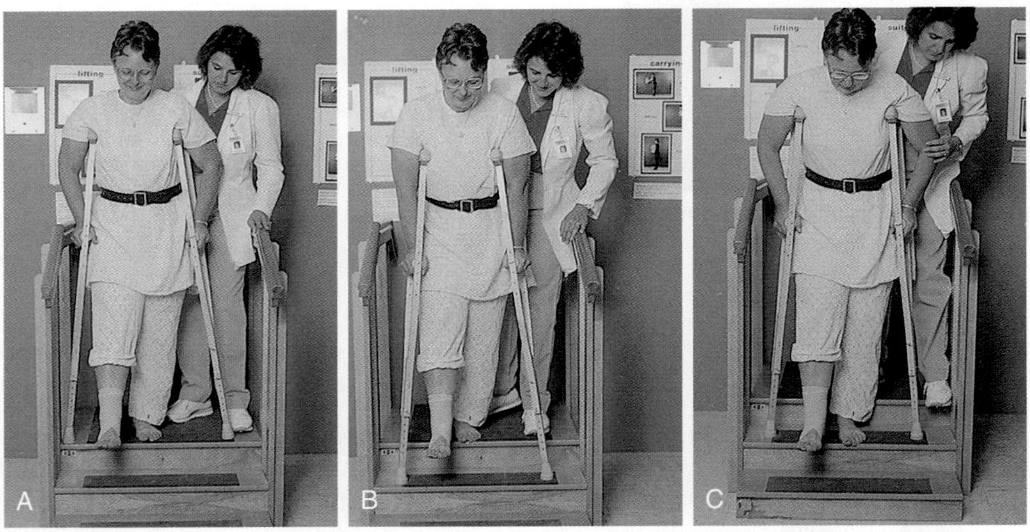

FIGURE 36-24 Descending stairs. **A,** Body weight is on unaffected leg. **B,** Body weight is transferred to crutches. **C,** Unaffected leg is aligned on stairs with crutches.

(Figure 36-25). First the patient positions himself or herself at the centre front of the chair with the posterior aspect of the legs touching the chair. Then the patient holds both crutches in the hand opposite the affected leg. If both legs are affected, as with a person with paraplegia who wears weight-supporting braces, the patient holds the crutches in the hand of his or her stronger side. With both crutches in one hand, the patient supports body weight on the unaffected leg and the crutches. While still holding the crutches, the patient grasps the arm of the chair with the remaining hand and lowers the body into it. To stand, the procedure is reversed, and the patient, when fully upright, assumes the tripod position before beginning to walk.

Restoration of Activity and Chronic Illness

Nurses design care plans to increase activity and exercise in patients with specific disease conditions and chronic illnesses such as CHD, hypertension, COPD, and diabetes mellitus.

Coronary Heart Disease (CHD). Research shows that activity and exercise play a role in secondary prevention or recurrence of CHD. Cardiac rehabilitation is an integral part of the comprehensive care of patients who have been diagnosed with CHD. Nurses are involved in many aspects of cardiac rehabilitation and assist patients in developing exercise programs that fit their needs and levels of functioning. Increased physical activity appears to benefit individuals with myocardial infarction, angina pectoris, or heart failure, as well as those who have had a coronary artery bypass graft (CABG) or percutaneous transluminal coronary angioplasty (PCTA). Patients with CHD benefit from exercise and activity and can experience reduced mortality and morbidity, improved quality of life, increased psychological well-being, improved left ventricular function, increased functional capacity, decreased blood lipids and apolipoproteins, and psychological well-being (Campos-Outcalt, 2014; Donges, Duffield, & Drinkwater, 2010).

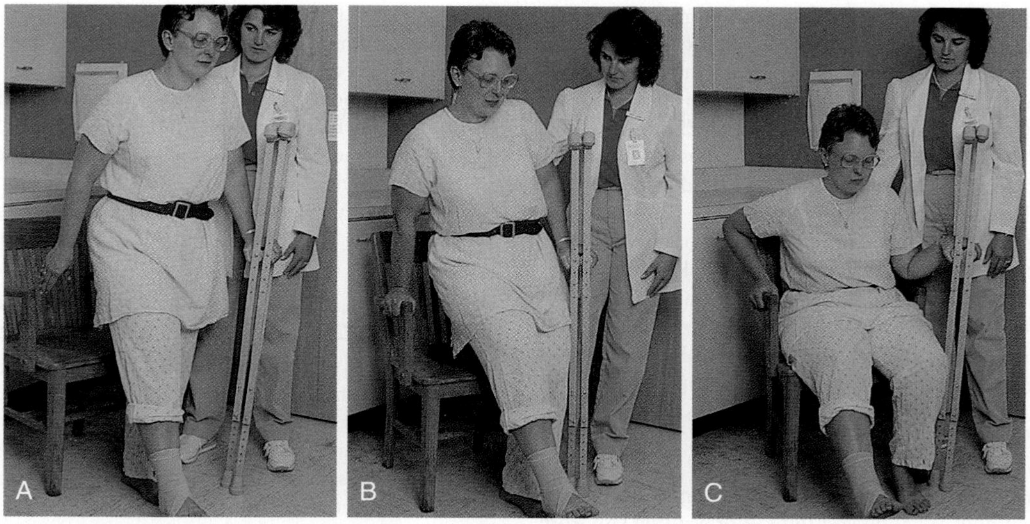

FIGURE 36-25 Sitting in a chair. A, Both crutches are held by one hand. Patient transfers weight to crutches and unaffected leg. **B,** Patient grasps arm of chair with free hand and begins to lower herself into chair. **C,** Patient completely lowers herself into chair.

Hypertension. Exercise has the effect of reducing systolic and diastolic blood pressure readings. Research shows that low- to moderate-intensity aerobic exercise (e.g., brisk walking, bicycling) is the most effective exercise for lowering blood pressure. In addition, a tai chi exercise program has demonstrated a significant reduction in systolic and diastolic blood pressure (Edelman et al., 2013; Lo, Yeh, Chang, et al., 2012).

Chronic Obstructive Pulmonary Disease (COPD). Pulmonary rehabilitation helps patients reach an optimal level of functioning. Some patients are fearful of participating in exercise because of the potential of worsening dyspnea (difficulty breathing). This aversion to physical activity sets up a progressive deconditioning in which minimal physical exertion results in dyspnea. Pulmonary rehabilitation provides a safe environment for monitoring patients' progress. In addition, they receive encouragement and support to increase activity and exercise (Berry, Rejeski, Miller, et al., 2010; Salhi, Troosters, Behaegel, et al., 2010).

Diabetes Mellitus. Along with diet, glucose monitoring, and medication, exercise is an important component in the care of patients with diabetes mellitus. It is recommended that persons with diabetes have at least 150 minutes per week of aerobic exercise, in addition to at least two sessions per week of resistance exercise (Canadian Diabetes Association (2013). Endurance and resistance exercise appear to be equally effective in improving the control of metabolism in patients with type 2 and type 1 diabetes. Individuals with type 1 diabetes are encouraged to exercise because exercise leads to improved glucose control, cardiovascular fitness, and psychological well-being. Exercise lowers blood sugar levels, and the effects of exercise on blood sugar levels often last for at least 24 hours. The patient with type 1 diabetes should be instructed about certain risks and precautions regarding exercise. Instruction includes the need for a pre-exercise comprehensive physical examination; patients also should be instructed to perform low- to moderate-intensity exercises, to carry a concentrated form of carbohydrates (e.g., sugar packets, hard candy), and to wear a medical alert bracelet.

Exercise must occur on a regular basis to have the desired continued benefits in the management of blood glucose levels, lipids, and overall quality of life (Hameed, Shereff, & Hussain, 2011).

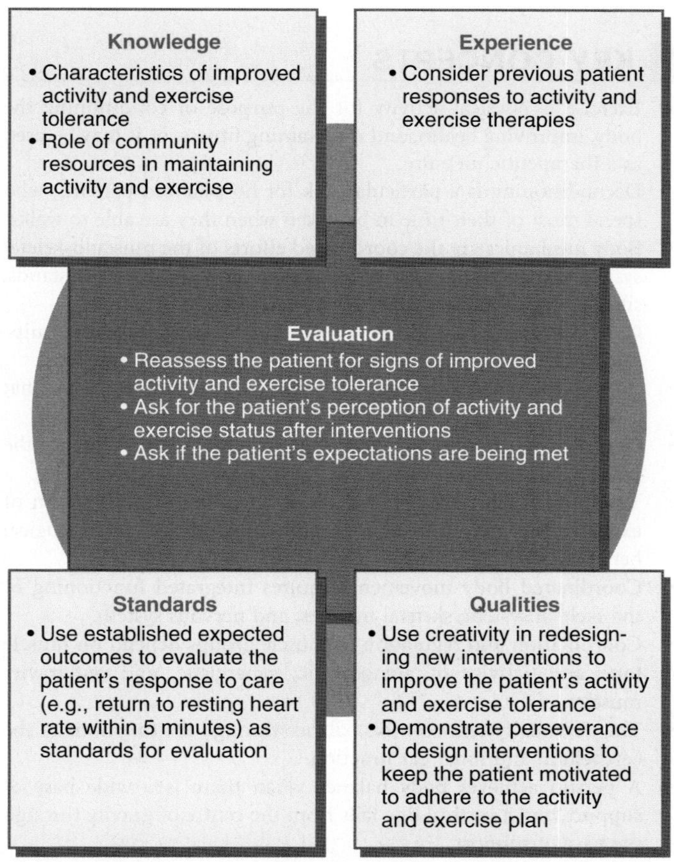

FIGURE 36-26 Critical thinking model for activity and exercise evaluation.

◆ Evaluation

Patient Expectations. For activity and exercise, nurses measure the effectiveness of nursing interventions by the success in meeting the patient's expected outcomes and goals of care. The patient is the only one who will experience the effectiveness and benefits of activity and exercise (Figure 36-26). Working closely with the patient will enable the nurse to identify goals and strategies that can be met realistically within the limits of the patient's priorities, capabilities, and health treatment (see Figure 36-26). The nurse should ask the patient questions such as, "How well did you tolerate walking, and is that what you expected?" and "You have been walking regularly for a month now, how has it made you feel?" Continuous evaluation helps to determine whether new or revised therapies are required, and whether new nursing diagnoses have developed.

Patient Outcomes. To evaluate the effectiveness of nursing interventions in enhancing activity and exercise, nurses make comparisons with baseline measures that include pulse, blood pressure, oxygen saturation, strength, fatigue, and psychological well-being. Actual outcomes are compared with expected outcomes to determine the patient's health status and progression. The following is an example of questions a nurse might ask when a patient does not meet his or her expected outcomes:

- The last time we met you planned to walk outside for 20 minutes 3 days a week. However, you report that you are only able to walk twice a week right now. What do you think is preventing you from meeting your goal?
- You state that you experience leg pain after walking short distances. Describe your pain. Which pain-relieving measures have you tried?

KEY CONCEPTS

- Exercise is physical activity for the purpose of conditioning the body, improving health, and maintaining fitness, or it may be used as a therapeutic measure.
- Deconditioning is a particular risk for hospitalized patients, who spend most of their time in bed even when they are able to walk.
- Body mechanics are the coordinated efforts of the musculoskeletal system and nervous system as the person moves, lifts, bends, stands, sits, lies down, and completes daily activities.
- Careful attention to body mechanics and use of appropriate equipment is critical in the prevention of musculoskeletal injuries.
- Activity tolerance is the kind and amount of exercise or work that a person is able to perform.
- Physiological, emotional, and developmental factors influence the patient's activity tolerance.
- The best program of physical activity includes a combination of exercises that produce different physiological and psychological benefits.
- Coordinated body movement requires integrated functioning of the skeletal system, skeletal muscles, and nervous system.
- Coordination and regulation of muscle groups depend on muscle tone and activity of antagonistic, synergistic, and antigravity muscles.
- The nervous system controls balance through the functions of the cerebellum and inner ear function.
- A person achieves body balance when there is a wide base of support, and a vertical line falls from the centre of gravity through the base of support.
- Developmental changes, behavioural aspects, environmental issues, cultural and ethnic influences, and family and social support affect the patient's perception of and motivation to engage in physical activity and exercise.
- Ability to engage in normal physical activity and exercise depends on intact and functioning nervous and musculoskeletal systems.
- The nursing process is used to provide care for patients who are experiencing or are at risk for activity intolerance and impaired physical mobility.
- After identifying nursing diagnoses, nurses plan and implement interventions to increase activity and exercise, in collaboration with the patient, when possible.
- Range-of-motion (ROM) exercises incorporated into daily activities can include one or all of the body's joints.
- The nurse needs to apply proper algorithms when transferring and lifting patients.
- Assistive devices to promote walking include canes, walkers, and crutches.

CRITICAL THINKING EXERCISES

Mrs. Smith has experienced some success in losing weight. She states, "I feel like I should have lost more weight by now." However, she expresses concern about how to incorporate exercise into her daily routine to maintain weight and assist with future weight loss.

1. Mrs. Smith states, "It is hard for me to determine exactly how much exercise I get doing my usual activities." She also expresses feelings of overwhelming stress and excessive demands on her time. Which interventions would you suggest to Mrs. Smith to help assess her current level of exercise?
2. Recognizing the challenges Mrs. Smith has voiced in balancing the excessive demands on her time and incorporating an exercise program, develop some strategies to help her initiate and maintain daily exercise.
3. Develop a feedback method for Mrs. Smith, emphasizing her success in exercising and maintaining a healthy weight.

REVIEW QUESTIONS

1. A nurse is instructing a patient who has decreased leg strength on the left side how to use a cane. Which action indicates proper cane use by the patient?
   1. The patient keeps the cane on the left side of the body.
   2. The patient slightly leans to one side while walking.
   3. The patient keeps two points of support on the floor at all times.
   4. After the patient places the cane forward, the patient then moves the right leg forward to the cane.
2. The body alignment of the patient in the tripod position includes the following: (*Select all that apply.*)
   1. An erect head and neck
   2. Straight vertebrae
   3. Extended hips and knees
   4. Axillae resting on the crutch pads
   5. Bent knees and hips
3. A patient is experiencing some problems with joint stability. The doctor has prescribed crutches for the patient to use while being allowed to bear weight on both legs. Which of the following gaits should the patient be taught to use?
   1. Four-point
   2. Three-point
   3. Two-point
   4. Swing-through
4. Which of the following *most* motivates a patient to participate in an exercise program?
   1. Providing a patient with a pamphlet on exercise
   2. Providing information to the patient when he or she is ready to change behaviour
   3. Explaining the importance of exercise at the time of diagnosis of chronic disease

4. Providing the patient with a booklet with examples of exercises
5. Providing the patient with a prescribed exercise program

5. Which of the following are principles of proper body mechanics when lifting or carrying objects? *(Select all that apply.)*
   1. Keep the knees in a locked position.
   2. Bend at the waist to maintain a centre of gravity.
   3. Maintain a wide base of support.
   4. Hold objects away from the body for improved leverage.
   5. Encourage the patient to help as much as possible.
6. The nurse recognizes that the older person's progressive loss of total bone mass and tendency to take smaller steps with feet kept closer together will most likely:
   1. Increase the patient's risk for falls and injuries.
   2. Result in less stress on the patient's joints.
   3. Decrease the amount of work required for patient movement.
   4. Allow for mobility, in spite of the aging effects on the patient's joints.
7. A nurse plans to provide education to the parents of school-age children, which includes the increased prevalence of ___________ as a result of children being less physically active outside of school.
   1. Diabetes
   2. Musculoskeletal injury
   3. Childhood obesity
   4. Depression
8. An unregulated care provider asks for help in transferring a patient who is 56.8 kg (125 lbs) from the bed to a wheelchair. The patient is unable to help. What is the nurse's best response?
   1. "As long as we use proper body mechanics, no one will get hurt."
   2. "The patient only weighs 56.8 kg. You don't need my assistance."
   3. "Call the lift team for additional assistance."
   4. "The two of us can lift the patient easily."
9. Which of the following statements made by an older person reflects the best understanding of the need to exercise regardless of age?
   1. "You are never too old to begin an exercise program."
   2. "My granddaughter and I walk together around the recreation centre track three times a week."
   3. "I purchased a subscription to a runner's magazine for my grandson for his birthday."
   4. "When I was a child, I exercised more than I see kids doing today."
10. Which is the correct gait when a patient is ascending stairs on crutches?
    1. A modified two-point gait. (The affected leg is advanced between the crutches to the stairs.)
    2. A modified three-point gait. (The unaffected leg is advanced between the crutches to the stairs.)
    3. A swing-through gait
    4. A modified four-point gait. (Both legs advance between the crutches to the stairs.)
11. Before transferring a patient from the bed to a stretcher, which assessment data does the nurse need to gather? *(Select all that apply.)*
    1. Patient's weight
    2. Patient's level of consciousness
    3. Patient's ability to assist
    4. Presence of medical equipment
    5. Nutritional intake
12. A patient with a right knee replacement is prescribed no weight bearing on the right leg. The nurse reinforces crutch walking knowing that which of the following crutch gaits is most appropriate for this patient?
    1. Two-point gait
    2. Three-point gait
    3. Four-point gait
    4. Swing-through gait
13. Which of the following indicates that additional assistance is needed to transfer the patient from the bed to the stretcher?
    1. The patient is 167 cm and weighs 48 kg.
    2. The patient speaks and understands English.
    3. The patient is returning to the unit from the recovery room after a procedure requiring conscious sedation.
    4. The patient received analgesia for pain 30 minutes ago.
14. The nurse encourages a patient with type 2 diabetes to engage in a regular exercise program primarily to improve the patient's:
    1. Gastric motility, thereby facilitating glucose digestion.
    2. Respiratory affect, thereby decreasing activity intolerance.
    3. Overall cardiac output, thereby resuming heart rate.
    4. Use of glucose and fatty acids, thereby decreasing blood glucose level.
15. Musculoskeletal disorders are the most prevalent and debilitating occupational hazards for nurses. To reduce the risk for these injuries, the Canadian Institute for Patient Safety advocates which of the following?
    1. Mandate that physiotherapists do all patient transfers
    2. Require adequate staffing levels in health care organizations
    3. Require the use of assistive equipment and devices
    4. Require an adequate number of staff to be involved in all patient transfers

Answers: **1.** 3; **2.** 1, 2, 3; **3.** 1; **4.** 2; **5.** 3, 5; **6.** 1; **7.** 3; **8.** 3; **9.** 2; **10.** 2; **11.** 1, 2, 3, 4; **12.** 2; **13.** 3; **14.** 4; **15.** 3

Rationales for Review Questions can be found at the end of the book.

RECOMMENDED WEBSITES

Active Living Alliance for Canadians with a Disability: https://ala.ca/.
This organization is an alliance of individuals, agencies, and national associations that together promote, support, and enable Canadians with disabilities, across all settings and environments, to lead active and healthy lives.

Canadian Centre for Activity and Aging: http://www.uwo.ca/ccaa/.
The centre is a research and community resource institution whose mandate is to investigate the interrelationship of physical activity and aging and to develop strategies, based on research, to promote the independence of older persons.

Canadian Fitness and Lifestyle Research Institute: http://www.cflri.ca/.
The institute addresses the well-being of Canadians through research on and communication of information about physically active lifestyles to the public and private sectors.

Canadian Society for Exercise Physiology (CSEP): www.csep.ca.
CSEP is the principal body for physical activity, health and fitness research, and personal training in Canada. It provides high-quality research, education, and training related to exercise physiology and science. It is the gold standard of health and fitness professionals and is dedicated to getting Canadians active safely by providing customized and specialized physical activity and fitness programs, as well as guidance and advice based on extensive training and evidence-informed research.

Fitness Vancouver: http://www.fitnessvancouver.ca/.
This website's Exercise Library contains an abundance of clearly described and well-illustrated exercises that any nurse could use to establish a fitness program.

Government of Canada: Health Promotion: http://www.phac-aspc.gc.ca/hp-ps/index-eng.php.

The Public Health Agency of Canada maintains this website, which contains many useful health promotion resources and guides that will aid health care providers and community leaders in encouraging Canadians to take a more active role in improving their health.

Health & Safety Ontario: http://www.healthandsafetyontario.ca/HSO/Home.aspx.

Health & Safety Ontario provides Ontario's public-service sector with information and strategies about how to achieve safer and healthier work environments for their workers. Regional and on-site prevention training, risk assessment, and safety consulting are used to identify and reduce workplace risks and hazards while preventing workplace injuries, illness, and disease.

Public Health Agency of Canada: https://www.canada.ca/en/public-health.html.

The role of this federal agency is to protect the health and safety of Canadians, focusing on preventing chronic diseases, preventing injuries, and responding to public health emergencies, such as outbreaks of infectious diseases.

REFERENCES

Ackley, B. J., & Ladwig, G. B. (2014). *Nursing diagnosis handbook: An evidence-based guide to planning care* (10th ed.). St. Louis, MO: Mosby.

Alberta Health Services. (2017). *Ergonomics training*. Retrieved from http://www.albertahealthservices.ca/careers/Page12772.aspx.

Bammann, K., Peplies, J., De Henauw, S., et al. (2014). Early life course risk factors for childhood obesity: The IDEFICS case-control study. *PLoS ONE, 9*(2), e86914. doi:10.1371/journal.pone.0086914.

Bandura, A. (2006). Guide for constructing self-efficacy scales. In F. Pajares & T. Urdan (Eds.), *Self-efficacy beliefs of adolescents*. Charlotte, NC: Information Age Publishing.

Berry, M. J., Rejeski, W. J., Miller, M. E., et al. (2010). A lifestyle activity intervention in patients with chronic obstructive pulmonary disease. *Respiratory Medicine, 104*(6), 829. doi:10.1016/j.rmed.2010.02.015.

Campos-Outcalt, D. (2014). The new cardiovascular disease prevention guidelines: What you need to know. *Journal of Family Practice, 63*(2), 89–93.

Canadian Centre for Occupational Health and Safety. (2017). *OSH answers fact sheets: Work-related musculoskeletal disorders (WMSDs)—Risk factors*. Retrieved from http://www.ccohs.ca/oshanswers/ergonomics/risk.html.

Canadian Diabetes Association Clinical Practice Guidelines Expert Committee. (2013). Canadian Diabetes Association 2013 clinical practice guidelines for the prevention and management of diabetes in Canada. *Canadian Journal of Diabetes, 37*(Suppl. 1), S1–S212. Retrieved from http://guidelines.diabetes.ca/app_themes/cdacpg/resources/cpg_2013_full_en.pdf.

Canadian Patient Safety Institute. (2016). *Falls*. Retrieved from http://www.patientsafetyinstitute.ca/en/Topic/Pages/Falls.aspx.

Canadian Society for Exercise Physiology. (2011). *Canadian physical activity guidelines*. Retrieved from http://www.csep.ca/cmfiles/guidelines/canadianphysicalactivityguidelinesstatements_e_2012.pdf .

Childs, E., & de Wit, H. (2014). Regular exercise is associated with emotional resilience to acute stress in healthy adults. *Frontiers in Physiology: Clinical and Translational Physiology, 5*, 1. doi:10.3389/fphys.2014.00161.

Christo, P. J., Li, S., Gibson, S. J., et al. (2011). Effective treatments for pain in the older patient. *Current Pain and Headache Reports, 15*(1), 22–34. doi:10.1007/s11916010-0164-0.

Combs, S. A., Diehl, M. D., Chrzastowski, C., et al. (2013). Community-based group exercise for persons with Parkinson disease: A randomized controlled trial. *Neurorehabilitation, 32*(1), 117–124. doi:10.3233/NRE-130828.

Donges, C. E., Duffield, R., & Drinkwater, E. J. (2010). Effects of resistance or aerobic exercise training on interleukin-6, C-reactive protein, and body composition. *Medicine & Science in Sports & Exercise, 42*(2), 304–313. doi:10.1249/MSS.0b013e3181b117ca.

Edelman, C. L., Kudzma, E. C., & Mandle, C. L. (2013). *Health promotion throughout the lifespan* (8th ed.). St. Louis, MO: Mosby.

Elliot, M. (2011). Taking control of osteoporosis to cut down on risk of fracture. *Nursing Older People, 23*(3), 30–35. doi:10.7748/nop2011.04.23.3.30.c8422.

Esposito, E., & Fitzpatrick, J. (2011). Registered nurses' beliefs of the benefits of exercise, their exercise behaviour, and their patient teaching regarding exercise. *International Journal of Nursing Practice, 17*(4), 351–356. doi:10.1111/j.1440-172X.2011.01951.x.

Fedorowski, A., & Melander, O. (2013). Syndrome of orthostatic intolerance: A hidden danger. *Journal of Internal Medicine, 273*(4), 322–335. doi:10.1111/joim.12021.

Government of Alberta. (2016). *Occupational Health and Safety Act*. Retrieved from www.qp.alberta.ca/documents/acts/o02.pdf.

Griffis, H. (2012). Adverse risk: A dynamic interaction model of patient moving and handling. *Journal of Nursing Management, 20*(6), 713–736. doi:10.1111/j.1365-2834.2011.01276.x.

Grossklaus, H., & Marvicsin, D. (2014). Parenting efficacy and its relationship to the prevention of childhood obesity. *Pediatric Nursing, 40*(2), 69–86.

Hameed, U. A., Shereff, M. Y., & Hussain, M. E. (2011). Structured exercise interventions for type 2 diabetes mellitus: Strength of current evidence. *Journal of Medicine and Allied Science, 1*(2), 61–68.

Hockenberry, M., & Wilson, D. (2014). *Wong's nursing care of infants and children* (10th ed.). St. Louis, MO: Mosby.

Huether, S. E., & McCance, K. L. (2012). *Understanding pathophysiology* (5th ed.). St. Louis, MO: Mosby.

Hunter, B., Branson, M., & Davenport, D. (2010). Saving costs, saving health care providers' backs, and creating a safe patient environment. *Nursing Economics, 28*(2), 130–134.

Joint Commission (TJC). (2017). *2018 National patient safety goals*. Oakbrook Terrace, IL: Author. Retrieved from http://www.jointcommission.org/standards_information/npsgs.aspx.

Kalisch, B. J., Lee, S., & Dabney, B. W. (2013). Outcomes of inpatient mobilization: A literature review. *Journal of Clinical Nursing, 23*, 1486–1510. doi:10.1111/jocn.12315.

Kwun, S., Laufgraben, M. J., & Gopalakrishnan, G. (2012). Prevention and treatment of postmenopausal osteoporosis. *Obstetrician and Gynaecologist, 14*(4), 251–256. doi:10.1111/j.1744-4667.2012.00135.x.

Lewis, S. L., Heitkemper, M. M., Dirksen, S. R., et al. (2013). *Medical-surgical nursing in Canada: Assessment and management of clinical problems* (2nd Cdn. ed.). Toronto: Elsevier Canada.

Lin, P. H., Tsai, Y. A., Chen, W. C., et al. (2012). Prevalence, characteristics, and work-related risk factors of low back pain among hospital nurses in Taiwan: A cross-sectional survey. *International Journal of Occupational Medical and Environmental Health, 25*(1), 41–50. doi:10.2478/s13382-012-0008-8.

Lo, H. M., Yeh, C. Y., Chang, S. C., et al. (2012). A tai chi exercise programme improved exercise behavior and reduced blood pressure in outpatients with hypertension. *International Journal of Nursing Practice, 18*(6), 545–551. doi:10.1111/ijn.12006.

McGann, S., Jancey, J., & Tye, M. (2013). Taking the stairs instead: The impact of workplace design standards on health promotion strategies. *Australasian Medical Journal, 6*(1), 23–28. doi:10.4066/AMJ.2013.1584.

Myszenski, A. (2017). *The role of lab values in clinical decision making and patient safety for the acutely ill patient*. Retrieved from https://www.physicaltherapy.com/articles/essential-role-lab-values-and-3637.

O'Donovan, G., Blazevich, A. J., Boreham, C., et al. (2010). The ABC of physical activity for health: A consensus statement from the British Association of Sport and Exercise Sciences. *Journal of Sports Science, 28*(6), 573–591. doi:10.1080/02640411003671212.

Osteoporosis Canada. (2017). *What is osteoporosis? About the disease*. Retrieved from https://osteoporosis.ca/about-the-disease.

Paterson, D., & Warburton, D. (2010). Physical activity and functional limitations in older adults: A systemic review related to Canada's physical activity guidelines. *International Journal of Behavioural Nutrition and Physical Activity, 7*, 1–12. doi:10.1186/1479-5868-7-38.

Patton, E. T., & Thibodeau, G. A. (2012). *Anatomy and physiology* (8th ed.). St. Louis, MO: Mosby.

Pelczarski, K. M. (2012). Back in action: Design considerations for safe patient handling. *Health Facilities Management, 25*(8), 21–25.

Perme, C., & Chandrashekar, R. (2009). Early mobility and walking program for patients in intensive care units: Creating a standard of care. *American Journal of Critical Care, 18*(3), 212–221. doi:10.4037/ajcc2009598.

Pierson, F., & Fairchild, S. (2013). *Principles and techniques of patient care* (5th ed.). St. Louis, MO: Saunders.

Prochaska, J. O., & DiClemente, C. C. (1986). Toward a comprehensive model of change. In W. Miller & N. Heather (Eds.), *Treating addictive behaviors: Process of change*. New York: Springer. doi:10.1007/978-1-4613-2191-0_1.

Public Health Agency of Canada. (2012a). *Physical activity tips for children (5–11 years)*. Retrieved from https://www.phac-aspc.gc.ca/hp-ps/hl-mvs/pa-ap/05paap-eng.php.

Public Health Agency of Canada. (2012b). *Physical activity tips for adults (18–64 years)*. Retrieved from https://www.phac-aspc.gc.ca/hp-ps/hl-mvs/pa-ap/07paap-eng.php.

Resnick, B., Boltz, M., Galick, E., et al. (2012). *Restorative care nursing for older adults: A guide for all care settings* (2nd ed.). New York: Springer.

Rhodes, R., & Pfaeffli, L. (2010). Mediators of physical activity behaviour change among adult non-clinical populations: A review update. *International Journal of Behavioural Nutrition and Physical Activity, 7*, 1–11. doi:10.1186/1479-5868-7-37.

Roush, K. (2011). Prevention and treatment of osteoporosis in postmenopausal women: A review. *American Journal of Nursing, 111*(8), 26–35. doi:10.1097/01.NAJ.0000403358.44058.f7.

Salhi, B., Troosters, T., Behaegel, M., et al. (2010). Effects of pulmonary rehabilitation in patients with restrictive lung diseases. *Chest, 137*(2), 273–279. doi:10.1378/chest.09-0241.

Suesada, M. M., Martins, M. A., & Carvalho, C. R. (2007). Effect of short-term hospitalization on functional capacity in patients not restricted to bed. *American Journal of Physical and Rehabilitation Medicine, 86*(6), 455–462.

Tullar, J. M., Brewer, S., Amick, B. C., et al. (2010). Occupational safety and health interventions to reduce musculoskeletal symptoms in the health care sector. *Journal of Occupational Rehabilitation, 20*(2), 199–219. doi:10.1007/s10926-010-9231-y.

VISN 8 Patient Safety Center. (2015). *Safe patient handling and movement algorithms.* Retrieved from https://www.lmcins.com/media/cms/Safe_Patient_Handling__Movement_Alg_E3527ACCC721E.pdf.

Walker, J. (2008). Osteoporosis: Pathogenesis, diagnosis, and management. *Nursing Standard, 22*(17), 48–56.

Wallace, R., Lees, C., Minou, M., et al. (2014). Effects of a 12-week community exercise programme on older people. *Nursing Older People, 26*(1), 20–26. doi:10.7748/nop2014.02.26.1.20.e508.

Warburton, D., Charlesworth, S., Ivey, A., et al. (2010). A systematic review of the evidence for Canada's physical activity guideline for adults. *International Journal of Behavioral Nutrition and Physical Activity, 7*, 1–220. doi:10.1186/1479-5868-7-39.

Waters, T., Nelson, A., Hughes, N., et al. (2009). *Safe patient handling training for schools of nursing.* Retrieved from https://www.cdc.gov/niosh/docs/2009-127/pdfs/2009-127.pdf.

Wilson, S. F., & Giddens, J. F. (2013). *Health assessment for nursing practice* (5th ed.). St. Louis, MO: Mosby.

Workers Health and Safety Centre. (2013). *Patient Handling.* Retrieved from https://www.whsc.on.ca/What-s-new/News-Archive/New-MOL-Document-Highlights-Employer-Obligations-R.

37

Quality and Patient Safety

Canadian content written by Chantal Backman RN, MHA, PhD
Original chapter by Michelle Aebersold, PhD, RN

OBJECTIVES

Mastery of content in this chapter will enable you to:

- Define the key terms listed.
- Discuss the domains of quality of care.
- Discuss the importance of "benchmarks" for public reporting of patient safety incidents.
- Discuss methods to prevent and reduce safety risks.
- Discuss strategies to maintain patient and staff safety.
- Describe the most common safety risks in health care.
- Recognize adverse events and know how to respond effectively to minimize harm to the patient.
- Understand the importance of reporting safety incidents.
- Disclose adverse events.
- Understand various approaches to improve quality and safety.
- Describe assessment activities designed to identify patients' physical, psychosocial, and cognitive statuses as they pertain to his or her safety.
- Identify relevant nursing diagnoses associated with risks to safety.
- Develop a nursing care plan for patients whose safety is threatened.
- Describe nursing interventions specific to patients' age for reducing safety risks.
- Describe methods to evaluate interventions designed to maintain or promote safety.
- Define the knowledge, skills, and attitudes necessary to promote safety in a health care setting.

KEY TERMS

MEDIA RESOURCES

http://evolve.elsevier.com/Canada/Potter/fundamentals/

- Audio Chapter Summaries
- Examination Review Questions
- Concept Map Creator
- Case Study with Questions
- Audio Glossary
- Content Updates
- Video Clips

Over the past several decades, quality and patient safety have become increasingly critical issues in health care. The Institute of Medicine's (IOM) report, *To Err Is Human: Building a Safer Health System* (IOM, 1999), was a pivotal publication that brought patient safety to the forefront of health care in the United States. In 2002, the Canadian National Steering Committee on Patient Safety published a report entitled *Building a Safer System*. That report outlined a national, integrated strategy for improving patient safety in the Canadian health care system.

Quality of care is defined as "the degree to which health care services for individuals and populations increase the likelihood of desired health outcomes and are consistent with current professional knowledge" (IOM, 1999). Quality of care incorporates the following six domains: (1) **accessibility**: right care, received at the right time, in the right setting, and by the right health care provider; (2) **effectiveness**: care received that achieves the expected benefit and is based on the best available scientific evidence; (3) **efficiency**: care received that is waste free, including the waste of supplies, equipment, time, ideas, and information; (4) **patient safety**: care received where harm is avoided; (5) **patient-centred care**: care received that is respectful and responsive to individual patient preferences, needs, cultural traditions, and values; and (6) **equitable**: care received regardless of gender, ethnicity, geographic location, and socioeconomic status (IOM, 1999).

Patient safety, one of the quality domains, is defined as "the pursuit of the reduction and mitigation of unsafe acts within the health care system, as well as the use of best practices shown to lead to optimal patient outcomes" (Canadian Patient Safety Dictionary, 2003). The occurrence of adverse events is remarkably prevalent in hospitals. Yearly, approximately 185 000 patients experience an adverse event in Canadian hospitals, 70 000 of which are potentially preventable (Baker Norton, Flintoft, et al., 2004). Between 9 000 and 23 000 people in Canada, and between 44 000 and 98 000 people in the United States, die annually as a result of preventable adverse events (Baker et al., 2004; IOM, 1999). The most common errors are related to medications, transfusions, surgeries, restraints, falls, burns, pressure injuries, and patient mix-ups (IOM, 1999).

A recent report released by the Canadian Institute for Health Information (CIHI) indicated that in 2014–15, "1 in 18 hospital stays in Canada involved at least one harmful event (138,000 out of 2.5 million hospital stays). Of those, 30,000 (or one in five) involved more than one form of harm. While most patients experience safe care, sometimes, harmful events happen that affect patients. Many of these events are preventable" (CIHI, 2016).

A **patient safety incident** (or **adverse event**) is "an event or circumstance that could have resulted, or did result, in unnecessary harm to a patient" (Canadian Patient Safety Institute, 2015). There are three types of patient safety incidents defined by the Canadian Patient Safety Institute:

- **Harmful incident**: an incident that resulted in patient harm (previously known as "preventable adverse event")
- **Near miss**: an incident that did not reach the patient (no harm resulted)
- **No-harm incident**: an incident that reached the patient, but no discernible harm resulted

As part of the health care team, nurses are professionally responsible for engaging in activities that support a patient-centred safety culture. The IOM defines patient-centred care as health care that establishes a partnership among practitioners, patients, and their families (when appropriate) to ensure that decisions respect patients' wants, needs, and preferences and that patients have the education and support they need to make decisions and participate in their own care (IOM, 1999). Considerable emphasis is placed on improving the education of nursing students so they become competent in promoting safe health care practices. The Canadian Patient Safety Institute's Safety Competencies Framework includes the following key concepts for nurses and other health care providers: (1) contribute to a culture of patient safety, (2) work in teams for patient safety, (3) communicate effectively for patient safety, (4) manage safety risks, (5) optimize human and environmental factors, and (6) recognize, respond to, and disclose adverse events (Frank & Brien, 2008).

Providing health care in a safe manner and in a safe community environment is essential for a patient's survival and well-being. By incorporating critical thinking skills when following the nursing process, nurses assume responsibility for assessing the patient and the environment for safety hazards as well as for planning and intervening appropriately to maintain a safe environment. By paying attention to patient safety, nurses are functioning not only as providers of safe care but also as an active participants in health promotion. Equally important is that nurses must ensure their own safety as they provide patient care.

In an effort to improve patient safety, many organizations focus on developing and monitoring key health care safety metrics as well as providing information to health care organizations and to the public. Health care organizations foster a patient-centred safety culture by:

- Continually focusing on performance-improvement programs;
- Acting on risk-management findings and safety reports;
- Providing current reliable technology;
- Integrating evidence-informed practice into procedures;
- Designing a safe work environment and atmosphere; and
- Providing continuing education and access to appropriate resources for staff (Box 37-1).

BOX 37-1 Resources Related to Safety and Safety Initiatives

- Canadian Patient Safety Institute: http://www.patientsafetyinstitute.ca
- Accreditation Canada: https://accreditation.ca
- Canadian Foundation for Healthcare Improvement: http://www.cfhi-fcass.ca/
- The Joint Commission: http://www.jointcommission.org/
- The Agency for Healthcare Research and Quality: http://www.ahrq.gov/
- The Institute for Healthcare Improvement: http://www.ihi.org/
- The U.S. Department of Veterans Affairs: VA National Center for Patient Safety: http://www.patientsafety.va.gov

SCIENTIFIC KNOWLEDGE BASE

Factors Influencing Safety

Health care takes place in a high-risk and complex environment. While specialization allows a wider range of patient treatments and services, it also provides greater opportunities for things to go wrong and adverse events to occur. Karsh, Holden, Alper, and colleagues (2006) have described some factors that may influence safety, including patient and provider factors, task factors, technology factors, and environmental factors.

Patient and Provider Factors. Patient and provider factors are characteristics of individuals such as health, age, weight, needs, mood, personality, knowledge and experience, intelligence, language, and cultural background. Some characteristics may vary depending on the situation (e.g., mood, fatigue, and stress).

Task Factors. Task factors are characteristics of the tasks health care providers must perform; this includes the tasks themselves as well as their characteristics (e.g., workflow, time pressure, and workload).

Technology Factors. These factors refer to the technologies (and their quantity and quality) available within an organization. Such factors include (1) the number of technologies, (2) the types of technologies, (3) their availability, and (4) their location. The design of the technologies includes their integration with other technologies, propensity to breakdown, responsiveness, and other design characteristics.

Environmental Factors. Environmental factors are the features of the work environment. These features include lighting, noise, physical space, and layout. A safe environment reduces the risk for illness and injury and helps to contain the cost of health care by preventing extended lengths of treatment or hospitalization, or both; improving or maintaining a patient's functional status; and increasing a patient's sense of well-being. A safe environment affords protection to the staff as well, allowing them to function at an optimal level.

Physical hazards in the environment place patients at risk for accidental injury and death. In Canada, unintentional injuries are the leading cause of death for individuals between the ages of 1 and 34 years (Public Health Agency of Canada, 2008) and are also a major cause of disability. Specific causes of injury and death include poisoning, suffocation, drowning, fires, burns, and machinery accidents. Among adults aged 65 and over, falls are the most common cause of unintentional injury (CIHI, 2013). Many physical hazards, especially those contributing to falls, can be minimized through adequate lighting, the reduction of obstacles, and the implementation of security measures.

Organizational Factors. Organizational factors are the structural, cultural, and policy-related characteristics of the institution (e.g., leadership characteristics, culture, policies, hierarchy, and span of control).

Karsh and colleagues (2006) explain that "none of these factors may be important to patient safety in and of itself; rather, it is typically the interaction between inputs that can influence patient safety. For example, lighting is not good or bad by itself, but lighting can be problematic for certain tasks or create glare on certain displays. Similarly, a technology such as computerized physician order entry may or may not influence patient safety; rather, it will have a positive or negative impact on safety depending on many factors such as (a) how well it is integrated into the physical environment and the workflow, (b) how much training is provided to end users, and (c) how end users perceive its ease of use and usefulness" (p. i60).

Systems Thinking and Quality Improvement

Systems in health care are highly complex and are "characterized by multiple actors, multiple choices, multiple hand-offs...no ownership, no natural team and no one with hospital-wide authority to make changes and insure quality" (Leape, 1997). In Reason's Swiss cheese model (Reason, 1997), each slice of cheese represents a barrier put in place to try to make the health care system safer (Figure 37-1). Each safeguard inherently contains a number of weaknesses, which are represented by the holes in the cheese. The holes in the slices of cheese are continuously moving around and often a subsequent barrier is able to stop a hazard from reaching the patient, but when the holes line up in certain combinations, hazards have the opportunity to sneak through the safeguards that have been put in place and find their way to the patient. The holes at the end of the system, which come into contact with the patient, are termed *active failures* and generally involve those directly involved in patient care (e.g., nurses, physicians).

The core principle of most "accident" frameworks is that multiple factors are involved in the accident, such as individual situational factors, workplace conditions, and/or latent organizational and management decisions. More complex processes and structures usually present greater potential for multiple factors and latent errors in the system. Health care providers who are directly in contact with patients most often identify the multiple failures that are cascading to cause the harm, but these individuals are fallible and, eventually, a patient may be harmed.

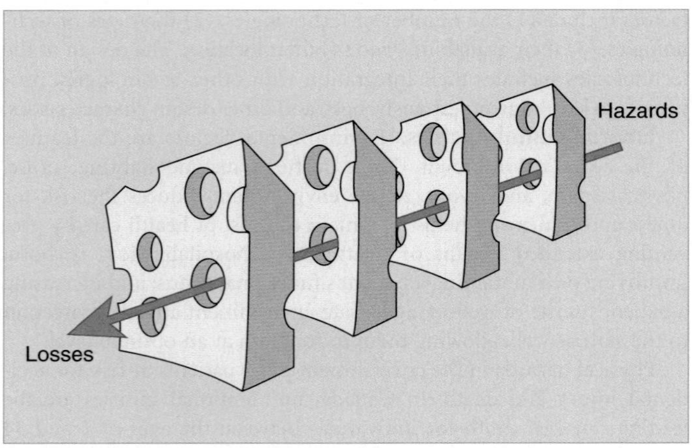

FIGURE 37-1 The Swiss cheese model of how defences, barriers, and safeguards may be penetrated by an accident trajectory. (From Reason, J. [2000]. Human error: models and management. *British Medical Journal, 320*[7237], 768–770.)

Reason (1997) states that only a systems approach (as opposed to an individual approach) will create a safer culture. His theory is strongly supported by evidence from other high-risk industries, which show the benefits of built-in defenses, safeguards, and barriers. Defensive systems can either be "engineered" (referring to automated defensive systems such as automatic shut-downs [e.g., alarms, forcing functions, physical barriers]) or involve people dependent on defensive systems that rely on the skills and knowledge of the individual, such as pilots, surgeons, and anaesthetists. Policies and procedures are also defensive layers. For Reason, the pivotal post-incident question is why safeguards fail, rather than who caused the incident.

Safety Analysis or Safety Improvement Techniques. In the effort to ensure patient safety, many methods and techniques are applied, such as root cause analysis, failure mode and effect analysis, and Lean Six Sigma methodologies, to reduce or prevent errors. All of these methods provide different ways of analyzing and improving system design. But if nurses and other health care providers do not have training in systems thinking, any of those methods can lead to the wrong results.

Root cause analysis (RCA) is a retrospective approach to find out what underlying features of a situation contributed to a patient safety incident. Adopting the idea that the immediate cause of an event is almost always the end result of multiple systems failures, RCA is used to seek to identify and understand all contributing causes in order to redesign the system to make it safer in the future.

Health care facilities often conduct a *failure mode and effect analysis (FMEA)* to identify problems with processes and products before they occur. FMEA is a prospective approach used to anticipate and prevent patient safety incidents through safe design. FMEA is an engineering approach—usually taken early in the development of a product—with the aim of imaginatively identifying potential failures and their effects. Knowledge from past failures may contribute to a designer's ability to foresee possible failures in their design. Designs are then adjusted to make failure less likely. FMEA is used to analyze every aspect of a system's design.

Human Factors. "Human factors" is a discipline dedicated to identifying and correcting incompatibility between people, their tools, and their environment. By identifying and correcting the elements leading to this incompatibility, an improvement in patient safety, efficiency, technology adoption, and user experience, as well as a reduction in the need for user training, can be achieved. To reiterate what James Reason, the eminent British psychologist and human factors expert, said, "we cannot change the human condition, but we can change the conditions under which humans work" (Reason, 1997).

Many organizations use human factor principles (e.g., forcing functions) to modify equipment (Cafazzo & St-Cyr, 2012). Forcing functions are built in the design of technologies to reduce or avoid errors and to ensure that the person will not miss key information or steps in a process. Furthermore, the goal of human factors engineering is to improve human performance. For example, by automating processes, fewer nurses are needed to collect the same information, the information is more complete and timely, the risk of data entry error is greatly reduced, and the need to retranscribe information from paper into a database has been eliminated (Backman, Vanderloo, d'Entremont, et al., 2015). Despite the importance of human factors engineering in health care, the adoption and evaluation of these approaches have been slow in progressing. Some exceptions to this slow uptake include leading organizations such as Healthcare Human

Factors group in Toronto, Ontario (http://humanfactors.ca/) and the Armstrong Institute for Patient Safety and Quality at Johns Hopkins Hospital in Baltimore, Maryland (https://www.hopkinsmedicine.org/armstrong_institute/index.html).

Interdisciplinary Teamwork, Communication and Feedback Skills. TeamSTEPPS is a program that has been developed to provide health providers with a range of strategies and techniques for improving teamwork (Agency for Healthcare Research and Quality, 2017b). Effective teamwork does just not happen; it requires understanding of factors such as the characteristics of a successful team, how teams function, and ways to maintain good teamwork. Identifying the team members at the start of each episode of care is key in knowing the strengths and weaknesses of all team members. TeamSTEPPS is being widely incorporated into health care training and simulations.

NURSING KNOWLEDGE BASE

A nurse must be aware of common safety precautions and of the special risks to safety that are found in health care settings. A nurse must also be familiar with a patient's developmental level, mobility, sensory and cognitive statuses, and lifestyle choices.

Risks in Health Care Settings

Patient safety incidents occur when something that was planned as part of medical care does not work out, or when an inappropriate care plan was used. These incidents occur in all health care settings. Nurses must be aware of regulatory and organizational safety initiatives and individual patient risk factors. The Agency for Healthcare Research and Quality (AHRQ) (2017a) lists 20 tips to help prevent medical errors. These tips can be viewed on the AHRQ website, http://www.ahrq.gov/patients-consumers/care-planning/errors/20tips/. The Joint Commission (TJC) and the Centers for Medicare and Medicaid Services (CMS) emphasize error prevention and patient safety. Their "Speak Up" campaign encourages patients to take a role in preventing health care errors by becoming active, involved, and informed participants on the health care team. For example, patients are encouraged to ask health care workers if they have washed their hands before providing care. The National Patient Safety Goals of The Joint Commission (2017) are specifically directed to reduce the risk of medical errors (Box 37-2). The goals highlight specific improvements in patient safety and ongoing problematic areas in health care. These evidence-informed recommendations require health care facilities to focus their attention on a series of specific actions.

When an actual or potential adverse event occurs, the nurse or health care provider who was involved completes an incident report. An incident report is a confidential document that completely describes any patient incident occurring on the premises of a health care organization. Reporting allows an organization to identify trends or patterns throughout the facility and areas to improve. Focusing on the root cause of an event instead of the individual involved promotes a "culture of safety" that helps in specifically identifying what contributed to an error. The probability of an accident occurring declines when health care providers adhere to evidence-informed principles of safety (Taylor-Adams, Brodie, & Vincent, 2008).

BOX 37-2 The Joint Commission 2017 National Patient Safety Goals

- Identify patients correctly
- Improve staff communication
- Use medicines safely
- Use alarms safely
- Prevent infection
- Prevent mistakes in surgery

From The Joint Commission. (2017). *Critical access hospital national patient safety goals.* Retrieved from https://www.jointcommission.org/assets/1/6/2017_NPSG_CAH_ER.pdf.

Staff Safety

Environmental Risk. Various forms of chemicals used in health care settings are a source of environmental risk for both the patient and the health care worker. Chemicals such as mercury and those found in some medications, anaesthetic gases, cleaning solutions, and disinfectants are potentially toxic if ingested or inhaled. The Workplace Hazardous Materials Information System (WHMIS) sets the standards for the control of hazardous substances in workplaces across Canada (Health Canada, 2015). A hazardous substance is any product or material that could cause physical or medical problems. WHMIS consists of three main elements: worker education programs, cautionary labelling of products, and the provision of Material Safety Data Sheets (MSDSs). Cautionary labels display the product's physical and health hazards and safety and first aid measures, and identify the types of hazard that the product presents (Figure 37-2). MSDSs provide detailed information about the substance, any health hazards imposed, precautions for safe handling and use, and steps to take if the substance is released or spilled. Nurses must understand WHMIS labelling requirements and be aware of the location of MSDSs where they work.

Infection Prevention and Control. Controlling the spread of infection through the consistent use of routine practices maintains the safety of patients, staff, and visitors (see Chapter 33). The importance of these measures was illustrated during the outbreak of severe acute respiratory syndrome (SARS) in Toronto in 2003. The illness began with one individual admitted to an emergency department and spread to several patients and staff before its infectious nature was recognized and precautions were instituted.

Violence. Violence may be directed toward nurses from patients or patients' family members. Factors that can contribute to abusive situations include insufficient staffing levels, violation of patients' personal space due to lack of privacy, and the provision of care that requires close physical contact (Canadian Nurses Association, 2015). Violence toward nurses can take the form of threats, intimidation, and physical behaviours, such as throwing objects. Nurses should seek assistance from co-workers to help them manage abusive situations (College of Nurses of Ontario, 2017a). Incidents of workplace violence should be reported, as this is essential to the development of effective strategies to reduce such occurrences.

Patient Safety. Specific risks to a patient's safety within the health care environment include falls, procedure-related accidents, and equipment-related accidents. The nurse assesses for these potential problem areas, considers the developmental level of the patient, and takes steps to prevent or minimize accidents.

Falls. Falls account for up to 90% of all reported incidents in hospitals. In addition to age, a history of previous falls, gait disturbance, balance and mobility problems, postural hypotension, sensory impairment, urinary and bladder dysfunction, use of medications, and certain medical diagnostic categories (e.g., cancer and cardiovascular, neurological, and cerebrovascular diseases) increase the risk of falling. One of the more common factors precipitating a fall is a patient's attempt to get out of bed to use the toilet.

Hip fractures are among the most serious fall-related injuries. Between April 2003 and March 2006, the rate of hip fracture in Canadian older persons during admission to hospital was close to 1 in 1 000 (CIHI, 2007). Older persons with a hip fracture may have a long

Symbol	Name	Description
	Flammable and combustible material	Product may catch fire when exposed to heat, sparks, or flame.
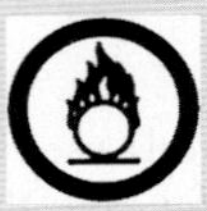	Oxidizing material	Product may cause a fire or explosion if exposed to combustible material.
	Compressed gas	Product is under high pressure. May explode or burst when heated, dropped, or damaged.
	Corrosive material	Product can cause burns to eyes, skin, or respiratory system.
	Dangerously reactive material	Product may react with light, heat, extreme temperatures, or vibration causing explosion, fire, or release of poisonous gases.
	Poisonous and infectious material: immediate and serious toxic effects	Product may be fatal or cause serious or permanent damage if exposed to even once.
	Poisonous and infectious material: other toxic effects	Product may cause cancer, birth defects, or other permanent damage if exposed to repeatedly.
	Poisonous and infectious material: biohazardous and infectious material	Product may cause disease, serious illness, or death.

FIGURE 37-2 Workplace Hazardous Materials Information System hazard symbols. (Adapted from the Canadian Centre for Occupational Health and Safety. [2012]. *WHMIS labelling requirements.* Retrieved from https://www.ccohs.ca/topics/legislation/WHMIS/.)

period of recovery and may not be able to return to their previous level of functioning, even losing their ability to live independently (SMARTRISK, 2009).

Falls that result in injuries can extend a patient's length of stay in the health care environment, placing the patient at a greater risk for other complications. Nurses can implement multifaceted interventions to reduce the risk of falls, including assessment and communication about patient risks, staff assignments in close proximity, signage, improved patient hand-offs, nurse toilet and comfort safety rounds, and involving the patient and family (Spoelstra, Given, & Given, 2012).

Procedure-Related Accidents. Procedure-related accidents are those that occur during therapy. They include medication and fluid administration errors, the improper application of external devices, and accidents related to the improper performance of procedures (e.g., incorrect urinary catheter insertion).

In a study of Canadian hospitals, Baker, Norton, Flintoft, and colleagues (2004) found that 7.5% of patients were affected by medical errors during their hospital stay. The most common errors were related to surgical procedures and drug or fluid administration. In 15.9% of these cases, the errors resulted in the death of a patient. Etchells, Juurlink, and Levinson (2008) stress that although medication errors cannot be avoided completely, systems can be designed to minimize the possibility and severity of errors. In order to reduce the likelihood of medication error, nurses must be aware and stay current on "look-alike" names; nurses can post signs to this effect in medication rooms; and hospitals can choose to buy medication with labels that have tall man lettering to reduce the risk of making errors (e.g., dimenhyDRINATE, and diphenhydramine [Institute for Safe Medication Practices, 2016]). Nurses and health care facilities must build safety into processes of care and take a systems approach when making efforts to reduce medical errors (Canadian Nurses Association & University of Toronto Faculty of Nursing, 2004).

Nurses are able to prevent many procedure-related accidents by adhering to organizational policy and procedures and standards of nursing practice (Box 37-3). For example, proper preparation and administration of medications, use of patient and medication bar coding, and "smart" intravenous (IV) pumps reduce medication errors (see Chapters 33 and 42). All nurses and other staff need to be aware that distractions and interruptions contribute to procedure-related accidents and need to be limited, especially during high-risk procedures such as medication administration. The potential for infection is reduced when surgical asepsis is used for sterile dressing changes or any invasive procedure such as insertion of a urinary catheter. Finally, correct use of safe patient handling techniques and equipment reduces the risk of injuries when moving and lifting patients (see Chapter 36).

BOX 37-3 Nine Life-Saving Patient Safety Solutions

- *Be aware of look-alike and sound-alike medication names.* Carefully review the medication orders of these drugs and use the 10 rights of medication safety.
- *Use patient identification.* Use two forms of patient identification, such as a hospital armband and medical record number.
- *Communicate during patient handover.* Communicate critical information, provide time for health care personnel to ask and resolve questions, and involve the patient and family during a handover process.
- *Perform correct procedure at correct body site.* Mark the operative site and take a "time out" to verify that it is the correct patient, operative site, and procedure before initiating the procedure.
- *Control concentrated electrolyte solutions.* Use the six rights of medication administration, and follow the organization's protocols for these solutions.
- *Ensure medication accuracy at transitions in care.* Perform medication reconciliation at each health care transition. More specifically, during admission, transfer, and discharge, nurses should compare all medications a patient is taking against the medical order and against the patient's "home medication list."
- *Avoid catheter and tubing misconnections.* Nurses should be meticulous in the verification of the catheter and tubing connections, they should verify that the correct size catheter is in use, and they should verify that the correct connection tubing is being used. Nurses should label tubing and connections when a patient has multiple catheters.
- *Do not reuse single-use injection devices.* Nurses should never reuse needles, injection devices, or intravenous catheters.
- *Improve hand hygiene to prevent health care–associated infections.* Nurses should perform hand hygiene before and after each patient encounter and after contact with contaminated objects (even when gloves are worn). Family and visitors should be encouraged to perform hand hygiene before and after visits.

Courtesy World Health Organization Collaborating Centre on Patient Safety Releases. (2007, May 2). *WHO launches nine patient safety solutions.* Retrieved from http://www.who.int/mediacentre/news/releases/2007/pr22/en/index.html.

Safety Alert Always follow agency policy when using lifting devices, and do not use them alone. Student nurses should always work with qualified personnel when using these devices.

Equipment-Related Accidents. Accidents that are equipment related result from the malfunction, disrepair, or misuse of equipment, or from an electrical hazard. To avoid rapid infusion of IV fluids, all general-use and patient-controlled analgesic pumps need to have free-flow protection devices.

To avoid accidents, nurses should not operate monitoring or therapy equipment without adequate instruction. If faulty equipment is found, the nurse should place a tag on it to prevent it from being used on another patient and should promptly report any malfunctions. In health care settings, the clinical engineering staff are responsible for making regular safety checks of equipment.

Risks at Developmental Stages

A patient's developmental stage presents specific threats to safety. Patients throughout all developmental stages may be subject to abuse. Child abuse, domestic violence, and abuse of older persons are serious threats to safety. These topics are discussed in Chapters 23, 24, and 32.

BOX 37-4 Changes Associated With Aging That Increase the Risk of Accidents

Musculoskeletal Changes
Muscle strength and function decrease, joints become less mobile, bones are more brittle due to osteoporosis, postural changes (e.g., kyphosis) are common, and range of motion is limited.

Nervous System Changes
All voluntary or automatic reflexes slow to some extent, the ability to respond to multiple stimuli decreases, and sensitivity to touch is decreased.

Sensory Changes
Peripheral vision and lens accommodation decrease, lenses may develop opacity (cataracts), the stimuli threshold for light touch and pain increases, the transmission of hot and cold impulses is delayed, and hearing is impaired as high-frequency tones become less perceptible.

Genitourinary Changes
Nocturia and occurrences of incontinence increase with age.

Adapted from Ebersole, P., Hess, P., Touhy, T. A., Jett, K., & Luggen, A. (2016). *Toward healthy aging: Human needs and nursing response* (9th ed.). St. Louis, MO: Mosby.

Infants and Children. Unintentional injuries are the leading cause of death in Canadian children between the ages of 1 and 14 years; each year 1 of every 230 children is hospitalized for treatment of unintentional injuries (Safe Kids Canada, 2007). The nature of the injuries sustained is related to normal growth and development. Small children are curious and trusting of their environment and do not perceive themselves to be in danger. The incidence of poisoning is highest in late infancy and toddlerhood because of children's increased level of oral activity and growing ability to explore the environment. Toddlers and preschoolers, who are attracted to water but do not perceive its dangers, are at a greater risk for drowning. Childhood injuries are also reflective of adults' perceptions of the causes of accidents and their ability to prevent them. For example, the incorrect use of vehicle restraints for children aged 5 to 14 places these children at greater risk of death from injuries sustained in motor vehicle accidents (the leading cause of death from injury in this age group) (Safe Kids Canada, 2007).

Adolescents. As children enter adolescence, they develop greater independence and begin to develop a sense of identity and their own values. Adolescents start to separate emotionally from their families, and peers generally have a stronger influence on them. The struggle for identity may cause a teenager to experience shyness, fear, and anxiety, with resulting dysfunction at home or school. In an attempt to relieve the tensions associated with physical and psychosocial changes, as well as peer pressures, adolescents may begin to act impulsively and engage in risk-taking behaviours such as smoking and substance use. In addition to the health risks posed by nicotine and other substances (e.g., alcohol, drugs, glue), the ingestion of such substances increases the incidence of accidents such as drowning and motor vehicle accidents.

Adults. Threats to an adult's safety are frequently related to lifestyle habits. For example, a patient who consumes excessive alcohol is at greater risk for motor vehicle accidents. A long-term smoker has a greater risk of cardiovascular and pulmonary diseases. Likewise, an adult experiencing a high level of stress is more likely to have an accident or illnesses such as headaches, gastrointestinal disorders, and infections.

Older Persons. The physiological changes that occur during the aging process increase a patient's risk for injury (Box 37-4). Changes in vision, hearing, mobility, reflexes, circulation, and the ability to make quick judgements predispose older persons to falls (see Chapter 24). When a patient is hospitalized, confusion, multiple medical problems, medications, immobility, urinary urgency, age-related sensory changes, postural instability, and an unfamiliar environment further contribute to the risk of falls (Meiner & Leuckenotte, 2015). Certain disease states common to older persons, such as arthritis and cerebrovascular accidents, also increase the chances of injury. In 2007–08, unintentional falls were the most common cause of injury in adults aged 65 years and older, with 70% of injuries in this age group caused by falls (CIHI, 2013). Patients most often fall while transferring from beds, chairs, and toilets; while getting into or out of a bathtub; by tripping over carpet edges or doorway thresholds; by slipping on wet surfaces; and while descending stairs. Icy walkways and obstacles in the yard are also common causes of outdoor falls in older persons.

Individual Risk Factors

Other risk factors posing threats to safety are lifestyle, impaired mobility, sensory or communication impairment, and a lack of safety awareness.

Impaired Mobility. Impaired mobility due to muscle weakness, paralysis, or poor coordination or balance is a major factor in patient falls. Immobilization predisposes a patient to additional physiological and emotional hazards, which can in turn further restrict mobility and independence.

Sensory or Communication Impairment. Patients with visual, hearing, tactile, or communication impairment, such as aphasia or a language barrier, are at greater risk for injury. Such patients may not be able to perceive a potential danger or express their need for assistance (see Chapter 47).

Lack of Safety Awareness. Some patients are unaware of safety precautions, such as keeping medicine or poisons away from children or observing the expiration date on food products. A complete nursing assessment, including a home inspection, can help nurses identify a patient's level of knowledge regarding home safety so that deficiencies can be corrected with an individualized nursing care plan.

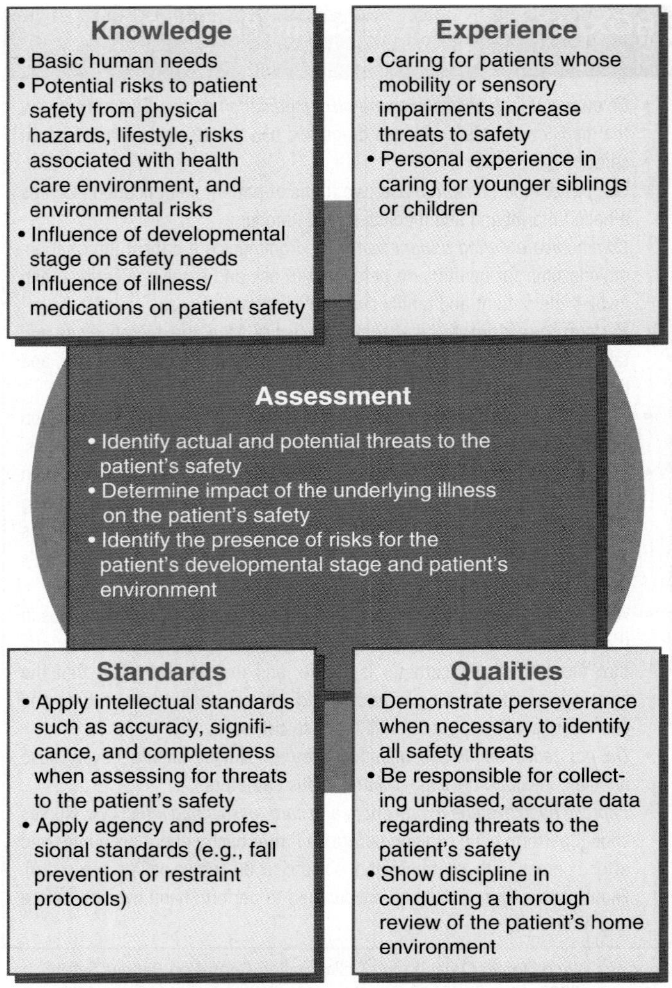

FIGURE 37-3 Critical thinking model for safety assessment.

CRITICAL THINKING

Successful critical thinking requires a synthesis of a nurse's knowledge and experience, as well as of information gathered from patients, combined with professional standards. Clinical judgements require nurses to anticipate necessary information, analyze the data, and make decisions regarding patient care. Critical thinking is an ongoing process. During an assessment (Figure 37-3), a nurse should consider all critical thinking elements and information about the specific patient to make appropriate nursing diagnoses.

In the case of safety, a nurse integrates knowledge from nursing and other scientific disciplines with previous experiences in caring for patients who were at risk for or had an injury. This is combined with critical thinking attitudes such as responsibility and discipline, and any standards of practice that are applicable. Agency guidelines and professional nursing associations provide standards for nursing activities such as medication administration, fall-prevention steps, and infection control to guide nurses in the provision of safe care. One such set of standards is the Registered Nurses' Association of Ontario (RNAO) (2005) *Prevention of Falls and Fall Injuries in the Older Adult.* For example, while assessing a patient's home environment, the nurse needs to consider typical locations within the home where dangers commonly exist. For a patient who has a visual impairment, the nurse applies previous experience in caring for patients with visual changes to anticipate how to thoroughly assess the patient's needs. Critical thinking directs the nurse to anticipate what needs to be assessed and how to make conclusions about available data.

❖ SAFETY AND THE NURSING PROCESS

A nurse is responsible for incorporating critical thinking skills when using the nursing process, assessing each patient and his or her environment for hazards that threaten safety, and planning and intervening appropriately to maintain a safe environment. The nursing process provides a clinical decision-making approach to develop and implement an individualized plan of safe patient care.

◆ Assessment

To conduct a thorough patient assessment, nurses must consider possible threats to a patient's safety, including the patient's immediate environment, as well as any individual risk factors.

Health History. By conducting a health history, the nurse gathers data about the patient's level of wellness to determine if any underlying conditions exist that pose threats to safety. For example, nurses should give special attention to assessing the patient's gait, muscle strength and coordination, balance, and vision. A review of the patient's developmental status must be considered as assessment information is analyzed. A nurse must also review whether the patient has been exposed to any environmental hazards or is taking medications or undergoing procedures that pose risks. For example, the use of diuretics increases the frequency of voiding and may result in the patient having to use toilet facilities more often. This may then increase the likelihood of a fall, as these often occur when patients get out of bed quickly because of urinary urgency.

Patient's Home Environment. When caring for a patient in the home, a home hazard assessment is necessary. The nurse should walk through the home with the patient and discuss how the patient normally conducts daily activities. Key areas to inspect are the bathroom, kitchen, and areas with stairs. For example, when assessing the adequacy of the lighting, the nurse should inspect areas where the patient moves and works, such as outside walkways, steps, interior halls, and doorways. Getting a sense of the patient's routine helps the nurse recognize less obvious hazards.

Health Care Environment. When a patient is being cared for within a health care facility, a nurse must determine if any hazards exist in the immediate care environment. Does the placement of equipment or furniture pose barriers to ambulation? Does the positioning of the patient's bed allow the patient to reach items on a bedside table? Does the patient need assistance with ambulation? Is the patient aware of activity restrictions? Has the patient been taught to use the call bell, and is it within reach? Collaboration with clinical engineering staff is essential to make sure that equipment has been assessed and is in proper functioning condition.

Risk for Falls. Assessment of the patient's fall risk factors is essential in determining specific needs and targeting interventions to prevent falls. A fall assessment tool (Table 37-1) can help determine potential risks before accidents and injuries result. The tool shown in Table 37-1 is the Hendrich II Fall Risk Model. This tool is intended for use in acute care settings and takes into account the patient's ability to move independently as well as other factors that can increase the risk for falls, such as certain types of medications (Hendrich, 2016). Nurses should familiarize themselves with the fall assessment tool used in their clinical area, as such tools vary among agencies. Patients should be assessed for their risk of falls on admission to the health care setting. An assessment should also be completed after a fall to determine why the fall occurred, as patients who have fallen are at much greater risk of falling again (Hendrich, 2016; RNAO, 2005). In many cases, family members can be significant resources in assessing a patient's fall risk. Families are often able to report on the patient's level of confusion and ability to ambulate.

Risk for Medical Errors. Nurses should always be alert to factors within the environment that create conditions in which medical errors are more likely to occur. Studies indicate that overwork and fatigue cause a significant decrease in alertness and concentration, leading to errors (Trinkoff, Geiger-Brown, Brady, et al., 2006). Nurses need to be aware of these factors and include checks and balances when working under stressful conditions. For example, checking the patient's

TABLE 37-1 Hendrich II Fall Risk Model™

Risk Factor	Risk Point	Score
Confusion/Disorientation/Impulsivity	4	
Symptomatic Depression	2	
Altered Elimination	1	
Dizziness/Vertigo	1	
Gender (Male)	1	
Any Administered Antiepileptics (Anticonvulsants): carbamazepine, divalproex sodium, ethotoin, ethosuximide, felbamate, fosphenytoin, gabapentin, lamotrigine, mephenytoin, methsuximide, phenobarbital, phenytoin, primidone, topiramate, trimethadione, valproic acid*	2	
Any Administered Benzodiazepines:† alprazolam, chloridiazepoxide, clonazepam, clorazepate dipotassium, diazepam, flurazepam, halazepam, lorazepam, midazolam, oxazepam, temazepam, triazolam	1	
Get-Up-and-Go Test: "Rising from a Chair" If unable to assess, monitor for change in activity level, assess other risk factors, document both on patient chart with date and time.		
Ability to rise in a single movement—No loss of balance with steps	0	
Pushes up, successful in one attempt	1	
Multiple attempts but successful	3	
Unable to rise without assistance during test If unable to assess, document this on the patient chart with the date and time	4	
(A score of 5 or greater = High Risk)	Total Score	

Ongoing medication review updates:

*Levetiracetam (Keppra) was not assessed during the original research conducted to create the Hendrich Fall Risk Model. As an antiepileptic, levetiracetam does have side effects of somnolence and dizziness, which contribute to its fall risk and should be scored (effective June 2010).

†The study did not include the effect of benzodiazepine-like drugs since they were not on the market at that time. However, due to their similarity in drug structure, mechanism of action, and drug effects, they should also be scored (effective June 2010).

identification bracelet before beginning any procedure or administering any medication can reduce the risk for error.

The National Steering Committee on Patient Safety (2002) made recommendations to improve the safety of Canada's health care system. At the core of these recommendations was the need to nurture a culture of safety within the system. The Canadian Patient Safety Institute (CPSI) was established in 2003 to provide leadership in the development of such a culture.

Patient Expectations. Patients generally expect to be safe in their home and in the health care setting. However, a patient's viewpoint of what is safe may differ from the nurse's viewpoint. For this reason, any assessment must include the patient's understanding of his or her perception of risk factors. This information will be important later if changes are needed in the patient's environment. Patients usually do not purposefully put themselves in jeopardy. When patients are uninformed or inexperienced, threats to their safety can occur. Patients must always be consulted on ways to reduce hazards in their environment.

◆ Nursing Diagnosis

After completing an assessment of a patient's safety status, nurses should review any clusters of data to identify patterns suggesting that safety is threatened. By identifying the defining characteristics and related factors from the data, nurses should be better able to make appropriate nursing diagnoses (Box 37-5).

The related factors become the basis for selecting nursing therapies. For example, *risk for injury related to impaired mobility* and *risk for injury related to barriers in the home environment* require different nursing interventions. The patient with altered mobility may require ambulatory aids and physiotherapy. When the related factor is barriers in the home, a nurse might recommend changes that will create a safer environment. At times, as in the example in Box 37-5, multiple related factors may apply. Examples of nursing diagnoses that may apply for patients whose safety is threatened are the following:

- *Impaired home maintenance—risk for injury*
- *Disturbed thought processes—risk for trauma*

BOX 37-5 NURSING DIAGNOSTIC PROCESS

Assessment Activities	Defining Characteristics	Nursing Diagnosis
Observe patient's mobility and body alignment.	Uncoordinated gait Poor posture	*Risk for injury related to impaired mobility, decreased vision, poorly lit home, and cluttered environment*
Ask patient about visual acuity.	Reports difficulty seeing at night Reports tripping over rugs and furniture	
Complete a home hazard appraisal.	Poorly lit home Rooms filled with small items Excessive amount of furniture for size of room Rugs not secure	

◆ Planning

During planning, the nurse critically synthesizes information from multiple sources (Figure 37-4). Critical thinking ensures that the patient's care plan integrates all that the nurse has learned about the patient, as well as the key critical thinking elements. For example, nurses should reflect on knowledge regarding the services that other disciplines (e.g., occupational therapy) can provide in helping the patient return home safely, as well as on any previous experience in which a patient benefited from safety interventions. These experiences can help nurses adapt approaches to suit new patients. Applying critical thinking qualities such as creativity helps the nurse and the patient collaborate in planning interventions that are relevant and helpful, particularly when changes are being made in the home environment.

Goals and Outcomes. Planning and goal setting need to be done in collaboration with the patient, family, and other members of the health care team (Box 37-6). The patient who is an active participant in reducing threats to safety will be more alert to potential hazards. Goals and outcomes must be measurable and realistic, with consideration to the resources available to the patient. The overall goal for a patient with a threat to safety is to remain free from injury. The

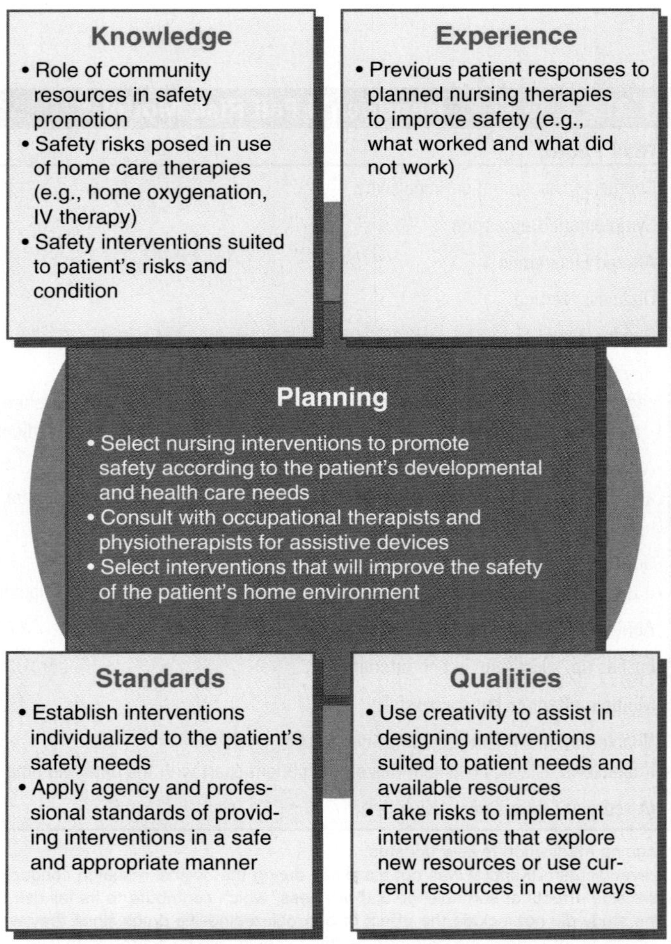

FIGURE 37-4 Critical thinking model for safety planning.

BOX 37-6 NURSING CARE PLAN

Risk for Injury

ASSESSMENT

The following is a scenario for developing a nursing care plan to mitigate against the risk of patient injuries. Mr. Key, a visiting nurse, is seeing Ms. Cohen, an 85-year-old woman, at her home. The patient has been recovering from a mild stroke affecting her left side. Ms. Cohen lives alone but receives regular assistance from her daughter and son, who both live within 16 km. Mr. Key's assessment includes a discussion of Ms. Cohen's health problem and how the stroke has affected her, as well as a pertinent physical examination.

Assessment Activities	***Findings and Defining Characteristics***
Ask Ms. Cohen how the stroke has affected her mobility.	She responds, "I bump into things, and I'm afraid I'm going to fall."
Conduct a home hazard assessment.	Cabinets in the kitchen are in disarray and full of breakable items that could fall out. Throw rugs are on floors; bathroom lighting is poor (40-watt bulb); bathtub lacks safety strips and grab bars; and home is cluttered with furniture and small objects.
Observe Ms. Cohen's gait and posture.	Ms. Cohen has kyphosis and has a hesitant, uncoordinated gait. She frequently holds walls for support.
Assess Ms. Cohen's muscle strength.	The left arm and leg are weaker than the right.
Assess visual acuity with corrective lenses.	Ms. Cohen has trouble reading and seeing familiar objects at a distance while wearing current glasses.

NURSING DIAGNOSIS: Risk for injury related to impaired mobility, decreased visual acuity, and physical environmental hazards

PLANNING

Goals (Nursing Outcomes Classification)*	***Expected Outcomes***
	Risk Control
Home will be free of hazards within 1 month.	Modifiable hazards in kitchen and hallway will be reduced in the home within 1 week. Revisions to bathroom will be completed in 1 month.
	Knowledge: Personal Safety
Patient and family will be knowledgeable of potential hazards for patient's age group within 1 week.	Patient and her daughter will identify risks and the steps to avoid them in the home at the conclusion of a teaching session next week.
	Fall Prevention Behaviour
Patient will express greater sense of feeling safe from falls in 1 month.	Patient will report improved vision with the aid of new eyeglasses within 1 week.
Patient will be free of injury within 2 weeks.	Patient will be able to safely ambulate throughout the home and perform personal care activities within 2 weeks.

*Outcome classification labels from Moorhead, S., Johnson, M., Maas, M. L., & Swanson, E. (Eds.). (2008). *Nursing outcomes classification (NIC)* (4th ed.). St. Louis, MO: Mosby.

INTERVENTIONS

Interventions (Nursing Interventions Classification)†	***Rationale***
Fall Prevention	
Review findings from home hazard assessment with patient and her daughter.	Fall risks for homebound older persons include visual disturbances, unsteady gait, and postural changes (Meiner & Lueckenotte, 2015). Evaluation of home hazards will highlight extrinsic factors that may lead to falls.
Establish a list of priorities to modify. Have patient's son assist in installing bathroom safety devices.	Modification of environment reduces fall risk (McCullagh, 2006).
Install lighting (75-W bulbs, nonglare) throughout the home. Have patient's son install blinds over kitchen windows.	With aging, the pupil loses the ability to adjust to light, causing sensitivity to glare. Glare can make it difficult to clearly see a walking path (Meiner & Lueckenotte, 2015).
Discuss with patient and daughter the normal changes of aging, effects of recent stroke, associated risks for injury, and how to reduce risks.	Education regarding management of hazards can reduce fear of falling (Ebersole, Hess, Touhy, et al., 2016).
Encourage daughter to schedule patient's vision testing for new prescription within 2–4 weeks.	Improved visual acuity reduces incidence of falls (Edelman & Mandle, 2013).
Refer patient to a physiotherapist to assess need for assistive devices for kyphosis, left-sided weakness, and gait.	Exercise often improves gait, balance, and flexibility. Modifying gait problems by increasing lower extremity strength reduces fall risk.

†Intervention classification labels from Bulechek, G. M., Butcher, H. K., & Dochterman, J. M. (Eds.). (2008). *Nursing interventions classification (NIC)* (5th ed.). St. Louis, MO: Mosby.

Continued

BOX 37-6 NURSING CARE PLAN

Risk for Injury—cont'd

EVALUATION

Nursing Actions	***Patient Response and Finding***	***Achievement of Outcome***
Ask patient and family to identify risks.	Ms. Cohen and her daughter are able to identify risks during a walk through the home and expressed a greater sense of safety as a result of changes made.	Ms. Cohen and her daughter are more knowledgeable of potential hazards.
Observe environment for elimination of hazards.	Throw rugs have been removed. Lighting has been increased to 75 watts, except in the bathroom and bedroom.	Environmental hazards have been partially reduced.
Reassess Ms. Cohen's visual acuity.	Ms. Cohen has new glasses and says she can read better and see distant objects more clearly.	Ms. Cohen's vision has improved, enabling her to ambulate more safely.
Observe Ms. Cohen's gait and posture.	Ms. Cohen's gait remains hesitant and uncoordinated; she reports that her daughter has not had time to take her to the physiotherapist.	The outcome of safe ambulation has not been totally achieved; continue to encourage Ms. Cohen and daughter to go to physiotherapy appointment.

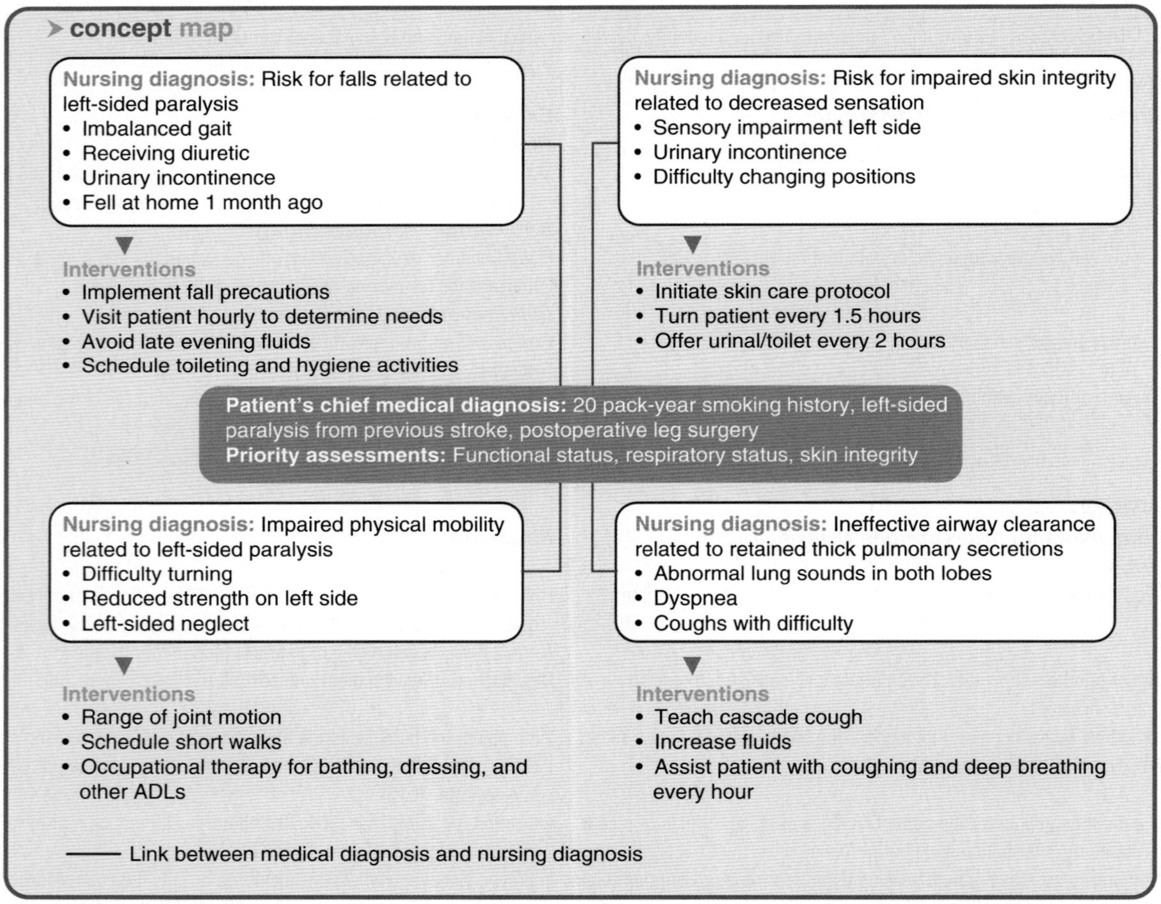

FIGURE 37-5 Concept map for a patient with a cerebrovascular accident 3 months previously with left-sided paralysis, 2 days after right femoral–popliteal bypass. *ADLs*, Activities of daily living.

following are examples of expected outcomes that focus on a patient's need for safety:

- Modifiable hazards will be reduced in the home environment by 100% within 1 month.
- The patient will not suffer a fall or injury.
- The patient will identify risks associated with visual impairment.

Setting Priorities. Nursing interventions are prioritized to provide safe and efficient care. For example, the patient described in the concept map (Figure 37-5) has several nursing diagnoses. The patient's mobility problem is an obvious priority because of its influence on skin integrity and the risk for falls. A nurse should plan individualized interventions based on the severity of risk factors and the

BOX 37-7 CULTURAL ASPECTS OF CARE

Cultural phenomena affecting health and safety include attitudes toward personal space, social organizations, communication, and environmental control. While conducting a home assessment for risks to safety, nurses must remember that they have entered the patient's territory and that the patient's attitude toward his or her residence and belongings must be appreciated. For example, some patients may be considered aloof and distant with regard to personal space. It may be very difficult for them to have an outsider in their home who suggests changes regarding their personal belongings to reduce physical hazards. It is particularly difficult to determine a patient's attitude toward his or her home environment when the patient's primary language and that of the health care provider differ.

Another culturally sensitive issue involves the patient's sense of environmental control. Nurses must be aware of health beliefs and practices that will affect the outcome of interventions. For example, a reliance on family and religious organizations, as opposed to community resources, may affect the patient's compliance with nursing interventions and referrals.

Nurses must learn to ask questions sensitively and to show respect for different cultural beliefs. Adapting to different cultural beliefs and practices requires flexibility. Respect for the belief systems of others and the effects of those beliefs on the patient's well-being are critically important to competent health care. The nurse must have the ability and knowledge to communicate about and to understand health behaviours influenced by culture.

Implications for Practice

- Resistance to change long-standing habits can interfere with a cultural group's acceptance of injury-prevention practices. Nurses should include family members who have a strong influence, such as a dominant man or older woman, when providing safety education.
- Nurses should evaluate the use of traditional ethnic remedies or foods that contain lead as these can increase a patient's risk for lead poisoning.
- Nurses should remember that living in rural areas and in manufactured housing places the patient at greater risk for fire-related injuries and death.
- Nurses should stress the importance of having fully functioning smoke detectors and a multipurpose fire extinguisher.
- Nurses should assess the patient's smoking and drinking habits. Residential fire deaths are often attributed to the use of cigarettes and alcohol.
- Patients who live in poverty and have low educational levels are at greater risk for injury and disease. Nurses should assist the patient and family in identifying community resources, such as the local health office or clinic.
- Nurses also need to be aware of family patterns and how the patient and family interact with each other. Family disruption and weak intergenerational ties can increase a patient's risk for injury from violent behaviour.

Adapted from Giger, J. N., & Davidhizar, R. (2002). The Giger and Davidhizar transcultural assessment model. *Journal of Transcultural Nursing 13,* 185.

patient's developmental stage, level of health, lifestyle, and culture (Box 37-7). Planning also involves understanding the patient's need to maintain independence within physical and cognitive capabilities. The nurse and the patient collaborate to establish ways of maintaining the patient's active involvement within the home and health care environment. Educating the patient and family is also an important intervention to reduce safety risks over the long term.

Continuity of Care. Patients need to learn how to identify and select resources within their community that enhance safety (e.g., block parent homes, local police departments, and neighbours willing to check on a patient's well-being). Collaboration with the patient and family and other disciplines such as social work, occupational therapy, and physiotherapy may become an important part of the plan of care. For example, a hospitalized patient may need to go to a rehabilitation facility to gain strength and endurance before being discharged home. Nurses need to ensure that the patient and family understand the need for these types of resources and are willing to make changes that will promote the patient's safety.

◆ Implementation

Nursing interventions are directed toward ensuring a patient's safety in all settings and include health promotion, developmental interventions, environmental interventions, and limiting specific risks to patient safety.

Health Promotion. To promote a patient's health, it is necessary for the individual to be in a safe environment and to practise a lifestyle that minimizes the risk of injury. Edelman and Mandle (2013) have described passive and active strategies aimed at health promotion. *Passive strategies* are implemented through public health and government legislative interventions (e.g., sanitation and clean water laws). *Active strategies* are those in which the individual is actively involved through changes in lifestyle (e.g., wearing a seat belt or installing outdoor lighting) and participation in wellness programs. The nurse can participate by supporting legislation and working in community-based settings. Because environmental and community values have the greatest influence on health promotion, community and home health nurses assess and recommend safety measures in the home, school, neighbourhood, and workplace.

Developmental Interventions. Accidents involving children are mostly preventable, thus parents need to be aware of specific dangers at each stage of growth and development. Accident prevention requires health education for parents and the removal of dangers whenever possible. Nurses are frequently in a position to educate parents about reducing the risks of injuries for young children (see Chapter 22). Nurses working in prenatal and postpartum settings can incorporate safety into the care plan of the child-bearing family. Community health nurses can assess the home and show parents how to promote safety in their homes (Table 37-2). The following discussion highlights some specific risks at different developmental stages.

Infants, Toddlers, and Preschoolers. Small children must be protected from accidental poisoning. Strategies for prevention of the accidental ingestion of poisonous materials are outlined in Table 37-2. In any instance of accidental poisoning, guidelines for intervening (Box 37-8) should be adhered to. The poison control centre phone number should be visible on the telephone in homes with young children and on a parent's smartphone, and the centre should be called immediately if poisoning is suspected.

School-Aged Children. School-aged children increasingly explore their environment (see Chapter 22). They may travel to and from school on foot or by school bus, and they may have friends outside their immediate neighbourhood. They may also become more active in extracurricular activities. Parents, teachers, and nurses must instruct children in safe practices to follow at school and play. Table 37-2 lists nursing interventions to help guide parents in providing for the safety of school-aged children. Using examples when discussing safe practices is an effective way to teach school-aged children.

TABLE 37-2 Interventions to Promote Safety for Children and Adolescents

Intervention	Rationale
Infants and Toddlers	
Ensure that infants sleep on their backs. Teach parents the mnemonic "back to sleep."	Sleeping on the back is associated with the lowest risk of sudden infant death syndrome (SIDS) (Canadian Paediatric Society, 2016).
Ensure that parents do not fill cribs with pillows, large stuffed toys, or comforters. Sheets should fit snugly.	Infants may become entwined in sheets and other bedding and suffocate (Canadian Paediatric Society, 2016).
Ensure that pacifiers are not attached to a string or ribbon and placed around a child's neck.	Strangulation may occur.
Ensure that all instructions for preparing and storing formula are being followed.	Proper formula preparation and storage prevents contamination. A formula may come in a concentrated form, or it may already be diluted and ready to use. Following directions ensures the proper concentration of the formula. Undiluted formula can cause fluid and electrolyte disturbances; overly diluted formula does not provide sufficient nutrients.
Ensure that only large, soft toys without small parts such as buttons are being used.	Small parts can become dislodged, and choking and aspiration are possible.
Teach parents that playpens with mesh sides should not be left with a side down; spaces between crib slats should be <6 cm apart.	A child's head may become wedged in the lowered mesh side or between crib slats, and asphyxiation may occur.
Teach parents to never leave crib sides down or leave babies unattended on change tables or in infant seats, swings, strollers, or high chairs.	Infants and toddlers can roll or move and fall from change tables or out of accessories such as infant seats or swings.
Teach parents to discontinue using accessories such as infant seats and swings when the child becomes too active or physically too big.	When physically active or too big, the child can fall out of or tip over these accessories and suffer an injury.
Teach parents to never leave a child alone in the bathroom, in the tub, or near any water source (e.g., a pool).	Accidental drowning may occur.
Teach parents strategies to baby-proof the home: • Install safety locks on floor-level cabinets • Use child-resistant caps • Place small or sharp objects, medications, and cleaning agents out of children's reach • Leave potentially poisonous materials in their original containers • Remove poisonous plants from the home Also ensure that parents are aware that poisoning can result from swallowing miniature button or disc batteries, commonly found in games, cameras, calculators, and watches.	Babies explore their world with their hands and mouth. Choking and poisoning may occur.
Teach parents to remove plastic bags from the cleaners or grocery store from the home.	Suffocation may occur if plastic covers the nose and mouth.
Ensure that electrical outlets are protected by covers.	Crawling babies may insert objects into outlets and experience an electrical shock.
Ensure that window guards are on all windows.	Guards prevent children from falling out of windows.
Ensure that keyless locks (e.g., deadbolts) have been installed on doors above a child's reach (even when they are standing on a chair).	Keyless locks prevent a toddler from leaving the house and wandering off. Death from exposure, car accidents, and drowning may occur if a toddler wanders away. Keyless locks allow for rapid exit in the case of fire.
Teach parents that children weighing <36 kg must always be in an age- and weight-appropriate car seat that has been installed according to the manufacturer's instructions. This includes car seats and booster seats. Children under 13 years should be in the back seat of the car. All passengers should wear their seat belts (Canadian Paediatric Society, 2017).	In case of a sudden stop or crash, an unrestrained child may suffer severe head injuries and death.
Encourage caregivers to learn cardiopulmonary resuscitation and the Heimlich manoeuvre.	Caregivers should be prepared to intervene in acute emergencies, such as choking.
Preschoolers	
Encourage parents to teach children to swim at an early age, but always provide supervision near water.	Swimming is a useful skill that may someday save a child's life. However, all children need constant supervision near water.
Encourage parents to teach children how to cross streets and walk in parking lots. Instruct them to never run out into the street after a ball or toy.	Pedestrian accidents involving young children are common.

TABLE 37-2 Interventions to Promote Safety for Children and Adolescents—cont'd

Intervention	Rationale
Encourage parents to teach children not to talk to, go with, or accept any item from a stranger. Children should also be taught not to go with a known adult unless they have their parent's permission (Child Find Canada, 2006).	This precaution reduces the risk of exploitation and abduction.
Encourage parents to teach children basic physical safety rules, such as the proper use of safety scissors, never running with an object in their mouth or hand, and never attempting to use the stove or oven unassisted.	The risk of injury is lower if children are taught basic safety procedures.
Encourage parents to teach children not to eat items found in the street or grass.	Poisoning may occur.
Teach parents to remove doors from unused refrigerators and freezers and to instruct children not to play or hide in a car trunk or unused appliances.	If a child cannot freely exit from an appliance or car trunks, asphyxiation may occur.
School-Aged Children	
Encourage parents to teach children the safe use of equipment for play and work.	Children need to learn the safe, appropriate use of implements to avoid injury.
Encourage parents to teach children proper bicycle safety, including the use of a helmet and rules of the road.	These safety precautions may reduce injuries from falling off a bike or being hit by a car.
Encourage parents to teach children proper techniques for specific sports, as well as the need to wear proper safety gear (e.g., eyewear or mouth guards).	The use of proper sports techniques, the correct equipment, and protective gear prevents injuries.
Encourage parents to teach children not to operate electrical equipment while unsupervised.	If an electrical mishap were to occur, no one would be available to help.
Teach parents that children should never have access to firearms or other weapons. All firearms should be kept in locked cabinets.	Children are often fascinated by firearms and weapons and may attempt to play with them.
Encourage parents to teach children safe use of the Internet.	Children are vulnerable to being exploited by predators over the Internet.
Adolescents	
Encourage enrollment in driver's education classes.	Many injuries in this age group are related to motor vehicle accidents.
Provide information about the effects of using alcohol, drugs, or other substances (e.g., glue, aerosols, or gasoline).	Adolescents are prone to risk-taking behaviours and are subject to peer pressure.
Provide sex education, including safer sex practices, birth control, and abstinence.	Many adolescents begin sexual relationships. Pregnancy and sexually transmitted infections may result.
Refer adolescents to community and school-sponsored activities.	Adolescents need to socialize with peers yet need some supervision.
Encourage mentoring relationships between adults and adolescents.	Adolescents are in need of role models after whom they can pattern their behaviour.
Teach adolescents the safe use of the Internet.	Safe use of the Internet avoids overuse and possible exposure to inappropriate websites.

Adapted from Hockenberry, M., & Wilson, D. (2014). *Wong's nursing care of infants and children* (8th ed.). St. Louis, MO: Mosby.

BOX 37-8 PROCEDURAL GUIDELINE

Interventions for Accidental Poisoning

Nurses should teach parents to call 911 or emergency services immediately if their child is unconscious, not breathing, or having convulsions or seizures due to poison contact or ingestion. If they think that their child has come in contact with poison and has mild or no symptoms, they should call their local poison control centre. Phone numbers for poison control centres across Canada can be accessed at http://www.aboutkidshealth.ca/En/HealthAZ/TestsAndTreatments/Resources/Pages/Poison-Information-Centres-in-Canada.aspx (AboutKidsHealth.ca, 2017).

Different types and methods of poisoning require different, immediate treatment:

- Swallowed poison—Remove the item from the child, and have the child spit out any remaining substance. Do not make the child vomit. Do not use syrup of ipecac.
- Skin poison—Remove the child's clothes and rinse the skin with lukewarm water for at least 15 minutes.
- Eye poison—Flush the child's eye by holding the eyelid open and pouring a steady stream of room-temperature water into the inner corner.
- Poisonous fumes—Take the child outside or into fresh air immediately. If the child has stopped breathing, start cardiopulmonary resuscitation (CPR) and do not stop until the child breathes on his or her own, or until someone can take over (American Academy of Pediatrics/Healthy Children.org, 2017).

Because school-aged children participate in more activities outside their home and neighbourhood environments, they are at greater risk of injury from strangers. Children should be warned repeatedly not to accept candy, food, gifts, or rides from strangers and not to go anywhere with a known adult unless they have their parent's permission. In addition, children need to know what to do if a stranger approaches. Frequently, neighbourhoods have a "block parent" program. The owner of a block parent home ensures that an adult is home during the times when children are walking to and from school. If a stranger approaches a child, the child can run to that home (identified by a sign), and the adult will protect the child and call the proper authorities. A nurse may work with school systems or neighbourhoods to initiate such a system to protect children.

Sports safety is stressed in school sports, and parents and health care providers can reinforce these safety tips by insisting that children wear protective gear while participating in sports such as skateboarding and snowboarding. For example, schools provide hard batting helmets for baseball games, and parents should also provide this equipment when children are playing baseball in their own backyards.

Bicycle- and scooter-related injuries are a major cause of death and disability among children. Bikes should be in good working order and the proper size for the child. Children under the age of 10 years should not be permitted to ride their bike on the road, as they have not yet developed the combined physical and cognitive skills to do this safely (Parachute Canada, 2017). They should also be cautioned not to engage in dangerous stunts or activities while bike riding. A properly fitted helmet should be worn, as it can decrease the risk of head injury by up to 85% (Parachute Canada, 2017). Because most fatalities from bicycle accidents are related to head injuries, most provinces have implemented laws requiring that children wear bicycle helmets while cycling (Figure 37-6).

Adolescents. Risks to the safety of adolescents involve many factors outside the home environment, particularly their almost constant involvement with their peers (see Chapter 22). Adults serve as role models for adolescents and, through providing examples, setting expectations, and providing education, can help adolescents minimize risks to their safety. For example, adolescents who are considering getting a body piercing or tattoo need information about the risks for complications with these procedures and strategies for minimizing these risks. This age group has a high incidence of suicide because of feelings of decreased self-worth and hopelessness. Nurses should be aware of the risks posed at this time and be prepared to teach adolescents and their parents measures to prevent accidents and injury (see Table 37-2).

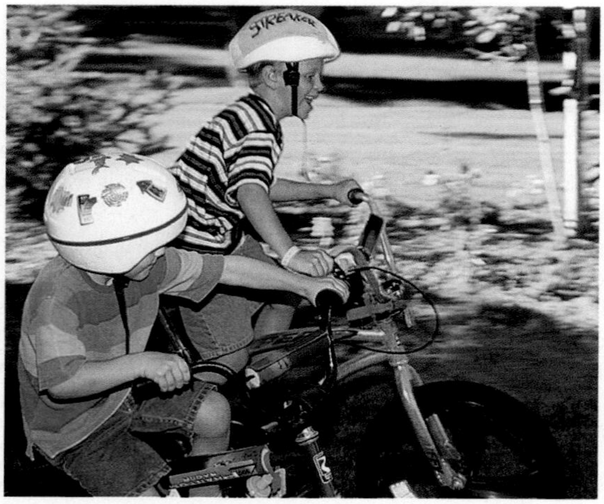

FIGURE 37-6 Proper bicycle safety equipment for school-aged children.

When adolescents learn to drive, their environment expands, and so does their risk for injury. The potential for motor vehicle accidents is higher among teen drivers than in any other age group. Teens are more likely to speed, run red lights, and drive while intoxicated. The young driver must be taught to comply with rules and regulations when using a car.

Safety Alert Nurses should reinforce to new drivers and their parents the need to consistently wear safety belts and to never ride in a car with a driver who may be intoxicated. Assist parents and their teen in developing a plan of action to be used if the teen finds himself or herself with a driver who has been drinking or has used other substances.

Because adolescence is a time when mature sexual physical characteristics develop, adolescents may begin to have physical relationships with others. They need prompt, accurate instruction to prevent pregnancy and the spread of sexually transmitted infections (see Chapter 27).

Adults. Risks to young and middle-aged adults frequently result from lifestyle factors such as postpartum depression, high stress levels, inadequate nutrition, excessive alcohol intake, and substance abuse (see Chapter 23). In our fast-paced society, there appears to be more expression of anger, which can quickly precipitate accidents (e.g., "road rage"). Adults need to have the opportunity to discuss the choices they have made in their life and the types of threats to safety that exist. Given information about threats to their well-being, adults may make the necessary modifications to their lifestyle practices. Useful resources are stress-management centres, employee-assistance programs, and health-promotion activities, which can be found in many communities and hospitals. In addition, neighbourhood centres, community clinics, and outpatient clinics are equipped to assist adults in modifying lifestyle habits that present risks to their health (e.g., smoking, overeating, lack of exercise, alcoholism).

Older Persons. Nursing interventions for older persons are designed to reduce the risk of falls and other accidents and to compensate for the physiological changes of aging (Box 37-9).

In older persons, diminished eyesight and impaired memory may result in an accidental overdose or missed doses of prescribed medications. The use of medication organizers that are filled once a week by the patient or family can help to prevent such errors. These organizers have the day and time on each box so that the patient knows when and what to take at any given time (Figure 37-7). They can be purchased at any drugstore at a very reasonable cost. Medication not in use or out of date should be taken to a pharmacy or municipal waste disposal depot for proper disposal (Government of Canada, 2014).

Burns and scalds are also more apt to occur with older individuals because they may become confused when turning the dials on a stove or other heating appliance. Nursing measures for preventing burns are designed to minimize the risk presented by impaired vision. Hot water faucets and dials can be colour coded to make it easier for the adult to know what has been turned on. Lowering the thermostat setting on the water heater reduces the risk of scalding.

Older persons are more likely to have motor vehicle accidents because of three specific physiological changes. First, changes in visual

BOX 37-9 FOCUS ON OLDER PERSONS

Physiological Changes of Aging

- Older persons experience alterations in vision and hearing. Encourage yearly vision and hearing examinations and frequent cleaning of glasses and hearing aids as a means of preventing falls and burns.
- Older persons may have slower reaction times. Nurses should teach patient safety tips for avoiding motor vehicle accidents. Driving may need to be restricted to daylight hours or suspended altogether.
- Range of motion, flexibility, and strength are decreased. Nurses should encourage supervised exercise classes for older persons and teach them to seek assistance with household tasks as needed. Nurses should assess whether safety features, such as grab bars in the bathroom, are needed.
- Reflexes are slowed, and the ability to respond to multiple stimuli is reduced. Nurses should provide adequate, meaningful stimuli but prevent sensory overload.
- Nocturia and incontinence are more frequent in older persons. Nurses should institute a regular toileting schedule for the patient. A recommended frequency is every 3 hours. Diuretics are generally given in the morning; however, nurses should speak with the patient about his or her response to the drug to determine the best timing. Assistance should be provided, along with adequate lighting, to patients who need to use the bathroom at night.
- The family plays a significant role in the care of older persons. Often, family members serve as informal caregivers for older persons. In Canada in 2006, 30% of women and 22% of men between the ages of 45 and 54 provided informal care to an older person (Vanier Institute of the Family, 2010). Encourage the family to allow the older person to remain as independent as possible and to provide help for only those things that are necessary.
- The high prevalence of chronic conditions in older persons results in the use of a high number of prescription and over-the-counter medications. Coupled with age-related changes in pharmacokinetics, this presents a greater risk of serious adverse effects. Medications typically prescribed for older persons include anticholinergics, diuretics, anxiolytic and hypnotic agents, antidepressants, antihypertensives, vasodilators, analgesics, and laxatives, all of which may themselves pose risks or interact with other medications to increase the risk for falls. Review the patient's drug profile to ensure that any of the above noted drugs are used cautiously, and assess the patient regularly for any adverse effects that may increase the risk for falls.

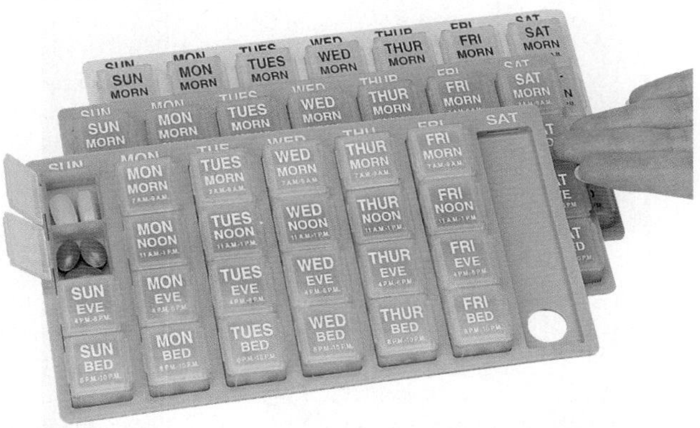

FIGURE 37-7 The One-Day-At-A-Time medicine organizer. (Courtesy Apothecary Products, Inc. Burnsville, MN.)

acuity, depth perception, and peripheral vision prevent these patients from quickly observing situations in which an accident is likely to occur. Second, decreased hearing acuity alters older persons' ability to hear emergency vehicle sirens or car and truck horns. Third, because of a decreased nervous system response, older persons may be unable to react as quickly as they once could to avoid an accident. A decline in these skills may account for the most common types of accidents, including right-of-way and turning accidents. Nurses should educate these patients regarding safe driving practices (e.g., driving shorter distances or only in daylight, using side- and rear-view mirrors carefully, and looking back toward their "blind spot" before changing lanes). If hearing is a problem, patients might try keeping a window rolled down while driving or reducing the volume of the radio or music.

Eventually, counselling may be necessary to help a patient make the decision as to when to stop driving. This is not an easy decision as it can have implications for the patient's self-concept and self-esteem. It also has practical implications—the individual who has been accustomed to driving to daily activities will have to find alternative transportation. As a result, the patient may resist giving up his or her driver's licence and vehicle. Nurses can support the decision to stop driving by offering anticipatory guidance when an illness with progressive impairment is diagnosed, working with family members to determine how to approach the issue with the patient, and providing information about objective assessment of driver ability (Dobbs, Pidborochynski & Linsdell, M. (2015) When a patient makes this decision, nurses should help them locate resources in the community that provide transportation.

Pedestrian accidents can be reduced by persuading individuals to wear reflectors on garments when walking at night; to stand on the sidewalk and not in the street when waiting to cross; to always cross at corners and not in the middle of the block (particularly on a major street); to cross with the traffic light and not against it; and to look left, right, and left again before entering the street or crosswalk.

Environmental Interventions. Nurses can implement specific interventions aimed at maintaining a safe environment. Particularly important are measures for preventing fires and dealing with them if they do occur. Other environmental interventions are those that address basic needs, physical hazards, and the transmission of pathogens. Many communities now maintain registries with their public security agencies so that the community is aware if there is a vulnerable individual living either alone or with a family. Should there be an extended power outage, leaving some individuals vulnerable, such as a person requiring supplemental oxygen who may have limited tank time (as usually they use electricity-driven units in the home), the city or community has services organized to check on these individuals and, if necessary, transport them to shelters or other appropriate locations.

Other Environmental Interventions. Nurses can contribute to a safer environment by helping patients meet basic needs related to oxygen, humidity, nutrition, and temperature. To ensure that oxygen availability is not threatened, nurses should recommend to patients living at home that they have annual inspections of the heating system, chimney, and appliances. Carbon monoxide detectors are available for home use at a reasonable cost but should not be considered a replacement for the proper use and maintenance of fuel-burning appliances. To achieve a comfortable level of humidity in the home, patients can attach a humidifier to the furnace or, in the case of patients who have

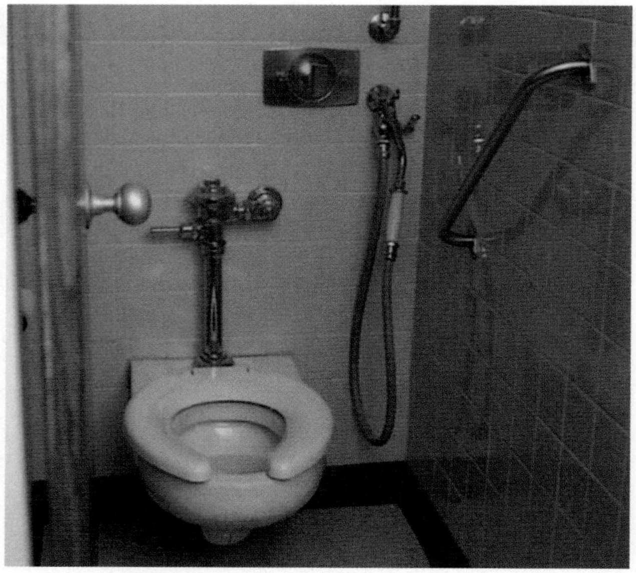

FIGURE 37-8 Safety bars beside a toilet and shower.

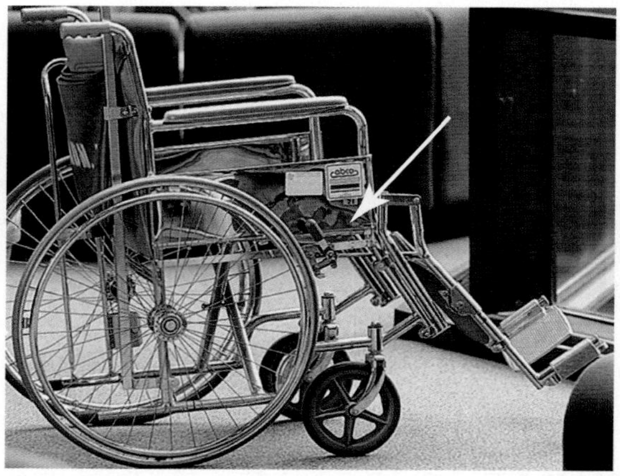

FIGURE 37-9 Safety wheel locks *(arrow)* on a wheelchair.

upper respiratory tract infections, use a room humidifier where they sleep. Nurses should teach basic techniques for food handling (e.g., handwashing and checking for spoilage) and preparation (e.g., keeping food refrigerated before serving) so that nutritional needs are met safely. It is also helpful for family members to write the date on packages of leftovers. Older persons who have difficulty preparing their own food may benefit from Meals on Wheels, an organization that provides fresh, nutritious meals in the home. Patient education for older persons and patients who enjoy outdoor activities should include ways to prevent and treat frostbite, hypothermia, heatstroke, and heat exhaustion (see Chapter 30).

Adequate lighting and security measures in and around the home, including the use of night-lights, exterior lighting, and good-quality locks on windows and doors, enable patients to reduce the risk of injury from crime. Local police departments and community organizations often have safety classes available to teach residents how to take precautions to minimize the chance of becoming involved in a crime. Some useful tips include always parking the car near a bright light or in a busy public area, carrying a whistle attached to the car keys, keeping car doors locked while driving, and always paying attention while driving to notice if anyone starts to follow the car. Patients should be encouraged to join block associations and work closely with law enforcement personnel to reduce crime in their neighbourhoods.

To prevent the transmission of pathogens, nurses should teach aseptic practices. Patients and family members need to learn thorough hand hygiene practices (handwashing or the use of hand sanitizer) and when to use it (e.g., before and after caring for a family member, before food preparation, before preparing a medication for a family member, and after contacting any body fluids). When patients require dressing changes or the use of syringes and needles, families should be shown how to properly dispose of contaminated items in the home as most communities have regulations regarding the disposal of biohazardous waste.

Limiting Specific Risks to Patient Safety

A number of specific safety measures are applicable to patients in the home or health care settings. Nurses should take actions to help patients avoid injuries related to falls, the use of restraints and side rails, electrical hazards, and radiation. Special precautions are necessary to prevent injury in patients susceptible to having seizures.

Falls. Easy modifications in the home and health care environment can reduce the risk of falls (Table 37-3). A heavy or debilitated patient in a bed or wheelchair or on a toilet should be properly supported and secured. Side rails may be necessary. Safety bars near toilets, locks on beds and wheelchairs, and call lights are additional safety features found in health care settings (Figures 37-8 and 37-9). Excess furniture and equipment should be removed. Weakened patients should wear rubber-soled shoes or slippers when walking or transferring. For patients who use assistive aids such as canes, crutches, or walkers, it is important to routinely check the condition of rubber tips and the integrity of the aid.

In the health care setting, injuries may occur when patients attempt to address self-care needs independently despite encouragement to call for assistance. One way to minimize the occurrence of such incidents is to check in on patients frequently during the day. A formal routine of nursing rounds, during which nurses visit patients every hour and provide necessary assistance, has been found to decrease the incidence of falls and increase patient satisfaction (Box 37-10).

Restraints. A **restraint** is a physical, chemical, or environmental means of controlling an individual's behaviour or actions (College of Nurses of Ontario, 2017b). The use of restraints is controversial as they have been associated with negative consequences, including injury and death. Nurses need to familiarize themselves with the legal aspects of restraint use. Nurses must also follow guidelines and standards provided by their provincial nursing governing body as well as policies and procedures set by their clinical practice setting. A least-restraint approach is recommended to ensure highest-quality care. This approach ensures that all alternative interventions are attempted before moving to the use of restraints, and that the form of restraint selected is the one that addresses a patient's needs in the least restrictive way (College of Nurses of Ontario, 2017b).

It is imperative that nurses try alternative measures (Box 37-11) as the application of a restraint should always be a measure of last resort. The use of restraints must be guided by a patient's needs and requires a thorough assessment by the nurse and other members of the multidisciplinary team involved in the patient's care. A restraint-use algorithm provides evidence-informed guidelines for determining whether a restraint is appropriate and what interventions might be used (Figure 37-10).

The use of any type of restraint involves a psychological adjustment for the patient and family. If restraints must be used, the nurse must assist family members and the patient by explaining the purpose of the restraints, the patient's expected care while restrained,

TABLE 37-3 Measures to Prevent Falls by Older Persons

Measure	Rationale
Stairs	
Install treads with a uniform depth of 22.5 cm and 22.5 cm risers (vertical face of steps).	If stairs are of uniform size, older persons do not need to continually adjust their vision.
Install uniform-textured or plain-coloured surfaces on each tread, and mark the edges of treads with a contrasting colour.	Uniform textures or colour helps to decrease vertigo. Marking the edges of treads provides obvious visual cues to end of stairs.
Ensure proper lighting of each tread. Block glare from the sun or a light bulb with translucent shades or a screen, or use lower-wattage or nonglare bulbs.	Older persons' vision is unable to adjust quickly to changes in lighting.
Ensure adequate headroom so that patients do not have to duck to negotiate stairs.	Sudden changes in head position may result in dizziness.
Remove protruding objects from staircase walls.	Decreased peripheral vision may prevent the patient from seeing an object.
Maintain outdoor walkways and stairs in good condition and free of holes, cracks, and splinters.	Decreased visual acuity can prevent the patient from seeing any structural defect.
Handrails	
Install a smooth but slip-resistant handrail at least 5 cm from wall.	A 5-cm distance allows the patient to grasp the handrail firmly for support.
Secure the handrail firmly so that the patient's weight is supported, especially at bottom and top of stairway.	Older persons have the greatest risk of falling at top and bottom of stairs because their centre of gravity is being shifted and balance is unstable.
Install grab rails in bathroom near the toilet and tub.	These measures enable the patient to have support while rising from a sitting to standing position.
Install an elevated toilet seat with armrests and nonslip strips.	
Floors	
Ensure that patients wear properly fitting shoes or slippers with a nonskid surface.	Such footwear reduces the chances of slipping.
Secure all carpeting, mats, and tiles; place nonskid backing under small rugs.	A sudden slip may cause dizziness and an inability to regain balance.
Place bath mats or nonskid, coloured strips on bathtub or shower stall floors and on the floor in front of the toilet.	Wet surfaces increase the risk of falling.
Secure electrical cords against the baseboards.	This measure prevents tripping.
Maintain proper illumination inside and outside where the patient moves and walks.	This measure reduces the risk of falling due to eye strain.
Health Care Facility Orientation	
Place disoriented patients in a room near the nurses' station.	Proximity provides for more frequent observation by nursing staff.
Supervise confused patients closely.	Confused patients often attempt to wander out of bed or the room.
Show the patient how to use the call light at the bedside and in the bathroom, and place it within easy reach.	The location and use of the call light are essential to patient safety.
Place bedside tables and overbed tables close to the patient.	This measure prevents the patient from searching or overreaching for items such as eyeglasses, dentures, a hearing aid, or the telephone.
Remove clutter from bedside tables, hallways, bathrooms, and grooming areas.	This measure eliminates potential hazards and promotes patient independence.
Leave one side rail up and one down on the side where the oriented and ambulatory patient gets out of bed.	The patient can use the side rail for support when getting in and out of bed and to position self once in bed.
Transport	
Lock beds and wheelchairs when transferring a patient from a bed to a wheelchair or back to bed.	The locks provide stability and support during transfer.
Place side rails in the up position and secure safety straps around the patient when transporting him or her by stretcher.	This measure prevents the patient from rolling off the stretcher.

Adapted from Chang, J. T., Morton, S. C., Rubenstein, L. Z., Mojica, W. A., Maglione, M., Suttorp, M. J., et al. (2004). Interventions for the prevention of falls in older adults: Systematic review with meta-analysis of randomized clinical trials. *British Medical Journal, 328*, 680.

BOX 37-10 RESEARCH HIGHLIGHT

Effects of Nursing Rounds

Research Focus

Hospitalized patients often require assistance with basic activities of daily living such as eating, toileting, and ambulating. Patients usually communicate their needs by use of a call light. Not meeting a patient's needs in a timely fashion decreases patient satisfaction and places him or her at greater risk for injury. The nurse plays a key role in the prevention of falls and injuries related to falls.

Research Abstract

Mitchell, Lavenberg, Trotta, and colleagues (2014) wanted to know the effectiveness of nursing rounds on reducing call light usage, increasing patient satisfaction, and reducing the frequency of patient falls. In their systematic literature review, they found 16 articles that met their inclusion criteria. The studies varied in how they measured their findings. However, the evidence demonstrated that, overall, nursing rounds improved patient satisfaction, reduced patient falls, and reduced call light usage. The common actions performed during nursing rounds included pain management, toileting, positioning, and placing items such as the call light, telephone, television remote, bed light switch, tissues, and water within reach and the garbage can next to bed. In addition, before leaving the room, the nurse asked, "Is there anything else I can do for you before I leave? I have time while I'm here in the room." The patient was also told that a staff member would be back in 1 (or 2) hours.

Evidence-Informed Practice

- Nursing rounds performed at set intervals positively affect patient satisfaction and safety and lead to fewer distractions for the staff.
- Nurses' ability to meet patients' needs affects patients' perception of the quality of nursing care.
- Nurses can anticipate patient needs by performing rounds, including specific nursing actions, at 1-hour intervals.

Mitchell, M. D., Lavenberg, J. G., Trotta, R., & Umscheid, C. A. (2014). Hourly rounding to improve nursing responsiveness: A systematic review. *Journal of Nursing Administration, 44*(9), 462–472. doi:10.1097/NNA.0000000000000101.

BOX 37-11 Alternatives to Restraints

- Orient patients and families with the care environment; explain all procedures and treatments.
- Provide companionship and supervision; use trained sitters or adjust staffing.
- Offer diversionary activities, such as listening to music or having something to hold; enlist support and input from the family.
- Assign confused or disoriented patients to rooms near the nurses' station; observe these patients frequently.
- Use calm, simple statements and physical cues as needed.
- Use de-escalation, time-outs, and other verbal intervention techniques when managing aggressive behaviours.
- Provide appropriate visual and auditory stimuli (e.g., family pictures, a clock, or a radio).
- Remove cues that promote leaving (e.g., sight of elevators, stairs, or street clothes).
- Promote relaxation techniques and normal sleep patterns.
- Institute exercise and ambulation schedules as allowed by patients' conditions; consult a physiotherapist for mobility and exercise programs.
- Attend to the patient's toileting, food, and fluid needs.
- Camouflage intravenous lines with clothing, a stockinette, or a Kling dressing.
- Evaluate all medications the patients are receiving, and ensure effective pain management.
- Reassess the physical status of patients, and review laboratory findings connected with their health.

Adapted from Joint Commission Resources. (2006). *Strategies for avoiding restraint related errors.* Retrieved from http://www.jcrinc.com; American Nurses Association. (2006). Geriatric nursing resources for care of older adults. *Physical restraints.* Retrieved from https://consultgeri.org/geriatric-topics/physical-restraints.

the precautions to be taken to avoid injury, and the temporary and protective aspects of restraints. Informed consent from family members may also be required before using restraints. The case study in Box 37-12 demonstrates family involvement in a decision about restraints.

A physical restraint immobilizes a patient or a patient's extremity (College of Nurses of Ontario, 2017b). The optimal goal with all patients is to avoid the use of physical restraints, and alternatives must always be considered. However, patients who are at risk for injury to self or others may need physical restraints temporarily. Physical restraints do not prevent falls and may actually increase the severity of an injury from a fall (RNAO, 2005).

Whenever patients are physically restrained, there is a natural tendency for them to try to remove the restraint, and this can lead to injury. Restrained patients can easily become entangled in a restraint device when attempting to get out of it. In some cases, death has resulted from strangulation or asphyxiation. As a result, long-term care facilities and many health care facilities have banned the use of the jacket (vest) restraint. The use of any physical restraint is also associated with serious complications, including pressure injuries, constipation, pneumonia, urinary and fecal incontinence, and urinary retention. Contractures, nerve damage, and circulatory impairment are also potential hazards. In addition, restrained patients can experience humiliation, fear, anger, and a loss of self-esteem.

Safety Alert Routine assessment of a patient in a physical restraint is critical to prevent injury. The restraint must be moved and the patient repositioned at regular intervals, according to the agency's policy. Restraints should be used only after other alternatives have been tried, and the least restrictive method of restraint should be used. The use of restraints must be part of the patient's medical treatment. Restraints are considered a short-term intervention, and once they have been applied, regular assessments are needed to determine whether they should be continued. All assessments and interventions must be clearly documented according to the agency's policy.

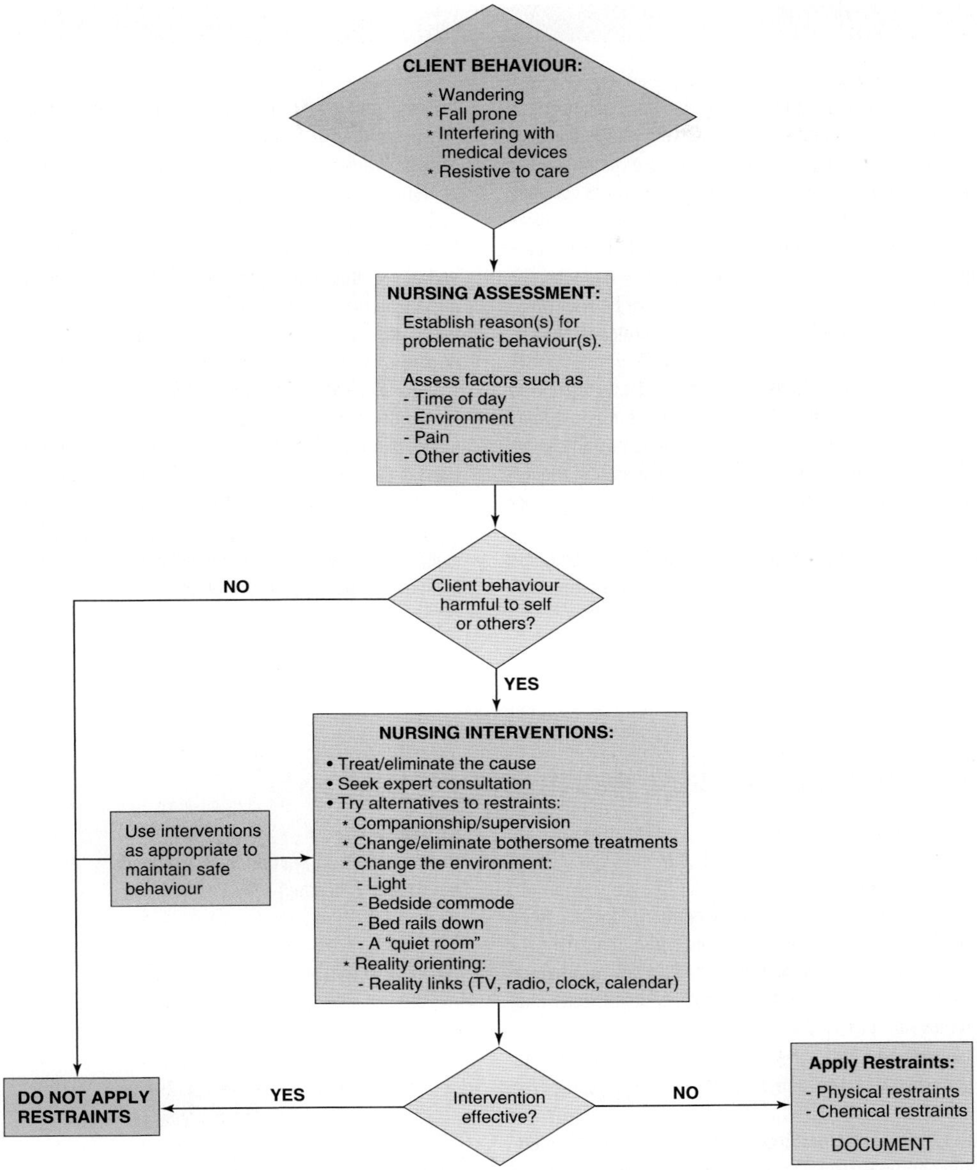

FIGURE 37-10 Algorithm for the use of restraints. (Developed from Ledford, L., & Mentals, J. [Written 1996; revised November 2005]. *"Restraints"—A research-based protocol.* Iowa City, IA: University of Iowa Gerontological Nursing Interventions Research Center. Copyright © The University of Iowa Gerontological Nursing Interventions Research Center, Research Translation and Dissemination Core.)

For legal purposes, nurses must know the agency's policy and procedures for the appropriate use and monitoring of physical restraints. The use of a restraint must be clinically justified and be a part of the patient's prescribed medical treatment and care plan. A physician's order may be required, depending on provincial or territorial legislation and agency policy—in some settings, nurses may order restraints. Requirements for ordering restraints may vary depending on the circumstances of a patient's situation and the type of restraint needed; nurses must comply with the agency's policies. Assessment of patients who are restrained must be ongoing. Proper documentation, including the behaviours that necessitated the application of restraints, the procedure used in restraining, the condition of the body part restrained (e.g., circulation to the patient's hand), and the evaluation of the patient response, is essential. Restraints should be removed periodically and the patient should be assessed to determine if the restraints continue to be needed.

Skill 37-1 includes guidelines for the proper use and application of restraints. Use of restraints must meet the following objectives:

- Reduce the risk of patient injury
- Prevent the interruption of therapy, such as traction, IV infusion, nasogastric tube feeding, or Foley catheterization
- Prevent the confused or combative patient from removing life-support equipment
- Reduce the risk of injury to others by the patient

In keeping with current trends toward health promotion, improved assessment techniques and modifications of the environment are offered as alternatives to physical restraints. An **Ambularm** is a device worn on the leg that signals when the leg is in a dependent position,

BOX 37-12 CASE STUDY

David's Mittens

Katherine has been caring for David, a 6-month-old boy who has been hospitalized for several weeks. David has a complex health problem and is currently experiencing severely dry, itchy skin associated with his illness. Katherine has noticed that anti-itch medications decrease David's discomfort but do not eliminate the itch entirely. As a result, he continues to scratch, and even with regularly trimmed nails, he has scratched himself hard enough to cause bleeding. David's mother plays with him to distract him from the itch, and when he tries to scratch, she gently holds his hands. However, she cannot be with David at all times in the hospital. Another concern is that David scratches his skin while sleeping.

Katherine discusses the situation with David's mother, and they decide to use mitten restraints to protect David's skin. They agree to use the restraints when David sleeps and when he is awake and alone. Katherine notes this decision in David's care plan, implements the required documentation according to her hospital's policy, and applies the restraints according to the proper procedure.

Katherine returns to work after 2 days off and finds that David's restraints have been applied improperly, leaving him at risk for injury. Recognizing that this may reflect a knowledge gap on the part of staff involved in David's care, she posts the instructions for the proper application of restraints at David's bedside, where they will be easily seen. Katherine also notes in David's care plan the need for proper use of restraints.

The need for the mitten restraints is reassessed daily, including feedback from David's mother. Volunteers visit him at the times he is most likely to be awake and alone, thus minimizing the need for restraints. Regular assessment and documentation are maintained according to the hospital's protocol. With continued treatment of David's illness, his skin condition improves, and within 5 days, the mitten restraints are discontinued.

Katherine and David's mother are pleased to see that David sustained no further scratch injuries once the restraints were implemented. David's mother states that although she does not like to see her baby restrained, she knows it is in his best interest. She appreciates the volunteers' efforts to spend time with David as well as everyone's diligence in applying the restraints properly. Katherine reflects on this situation and decides that the next time she implements the use of restraints, she will post instructions for their use at the bedside immediately upon implementation.

SKILL 37-1 APPLYING PHYSICAL RESTRAINTS

Delegation Considerations

The application of physical restraints may be delegated to trained unregulated care providers (UCPs). Review the following with the UCP:

- Ask the UCP to inform you of any skin redness or excoriation, constriction of circulation under the restraint, or change in the patient's breathing.
- Review the correct placement of the restraint with the UCP and ask him or her to request assistance if the patient has any mobility restrictions that might affect how to remove or reapply a restraint.
- Instruct the UCP when and how to change the patient's position and to provide range-of-motion exercises, skin care, toileting, and opportunities for socialization.

However, nurses are always responsible for the assessment of a patient's safety needs, selection of appropriate alternative interventions, evaluation of the effectiveness of restraint, and ongoing assessment to prevent complications of restraint use.

Equipment

- Proper restraint: mitten, belt, extremity
- Padding (if needed)

PROCEDURE

STEPS	RATIONALE
1. Assess whether the patient needs a restraint. Does the patient continually try to interrupt needed therapy? Is the patient at risk for injuring self or others?	• Restraints are used only when other measures have failed to prevent the interruption of therapy such as traction, intravenous (IV) infusions, or nasogastric tube feedings; to prevent a confused or combative patient from self-injury by falling out of bed or a wheelchair; to prevent a patient from removing a urinary catheter, surgical drain, or life-support equipment; and to reduce the risk of injury to others by the patient.
2. Assess the patient's behaviour, such as confusion, disorientation, agitation, restlessness, combativeness, or inability to follow directions. Consult with a gerontological nurse specialist if available.	• If patient's behaviour continues despite attempts to eliminate the cause of behaviour, use of physical restraint may be necessary.
3. Review agency's policies regarding restraints. Consider the purpose, type, location, and duration of restraint. Determine whether signed consent for the use of restraint is needed.	• The least restrictive type of restraint must be ordered. A physician's order may be necessary—check provincial or territorial legislation and agency policy. Because restraints limit the patient's ability to move freely, the nurse must make clinical judgements appropriate to the patient's condition and the agency policy.

STEPS	RATIONALE
4. Review manufacturer's instructions before entering the patient's room. Determine the most appropriate size restraint.	• Nurses should be familiar with all devices used for patient care and protection. Incorrect application of a restraining device may result in patient injury or death.
5. Perform hand hygiene and gather equipment.	• Reduces transmission of microorganisms; promotes organization.
6. Introduce yourself to the patient and family. Assess their feelings about restraint use. Explain that restraint is temporary and designed to protect the patient from injury.	• Helps minimize patient anxiety during the application of the device, and helps minimize family concern during the maintenance of restraint.
7. Inspect the area where the restraint is to be placed. Assess the condition of skin underlying where the restraint is to be applied.	• Restraints may compress and interfere with the functioning of devices or tubes. Inspection provides baseline assessment data regarding skin integrity.
8. Approach the patient in a calm, confident manner. Check the patient's identification using two identifiers. Explain what you plan to do.	• Reduces patient anxiety and promotes cooperation.
9. Adjust the bed to proper height, and lower the side rail on the side of patient contact.	• Allows nurse to use proper body mechanics and prevent injury.
10. Provide privacy. Make sure the patient is comfortable and in proper body alignment. Drape patient as needed.	• Privacy protects self-esteem. Proper body alignment promotes comfort and prevents contractures and neurovascular injury.
11. Pad the skin and bony prominences (if necessary) before applying restraints.	• Padding reduces friction and pressure on skin and underlying tissues.
12. Apply the appropriate-size restraint, making sure it is not over an IV line or other device (e.g., dialysis shunt) and that it does not cover the patient's identification or allergy bracelet.	• IV lines and other therapeutic devices may become occluded. The patient's ID and allergy information must always be visible and accessible.
A. Belt restraint: This device secures the patient to a bed or stretcher. Apply it over the patient's clothes or gown. Remove wrinkles from the front and back of the restraint while placing it around the patient's waist. Bring ties through slots in the belt. Avoid placing the belt across the chest or too tightly across the abdomen (see Step 12A illustration).	• Restrains centre of gravity and prevents the patient from rolling off the stretcher or sitting up while on stretcher or from falling out of bed. Tight application may interfere with ventilation.

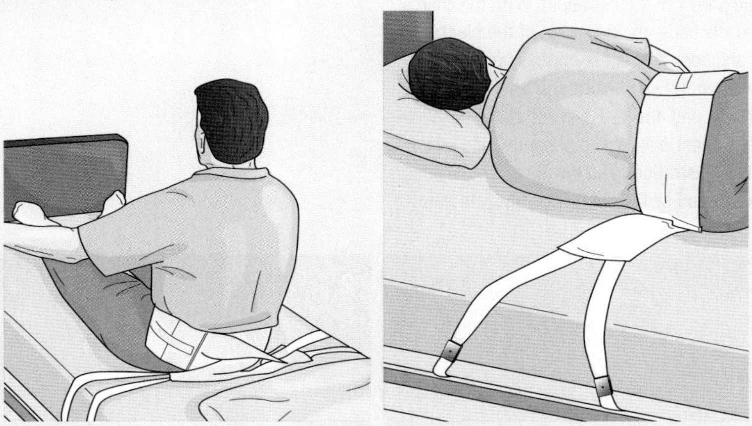

STEP 12A Belt restraint is tied to the bed frame and to an area that does not cause the restraint to tighten when the side rail is raised or lowered. (From Sorrentino, S. A. [2004]. *Mosby's textbook for nursing assistants* [7th ed., p. 193]. St. Louis, MO: Mosby.)

STEPS	RATIONALE
B. Extremity (ankle or wrist) restraint: This restraint is designed to immobilize one or all extremities. Commercially available limb restraints are composed of sheepskin or foam padding (see Step 12B illustration). The limb restraint is wrapped around the wrist or ankle with the soft part toward the skin and is secured snugly in place with Velcro straps.	• Maintains immobilization of the extremity to protect the patient from injury from a fall or accidental removal of a therapeutic device (e.g., IV tube or Foley catheter). Tight application may interfere with circulation.

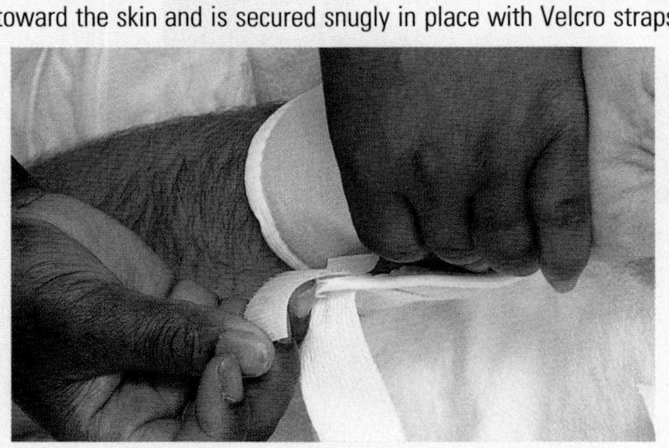

STEP 12B Extremity restraint being applied to the wrist.

Continued

SKILL 37-1 APPLYING PHYSICAL RESTRAINTS—cont'd

STEPS	RATIONALE
C. **Mitten restraint:** This thumbless mitten device is used to restrain the patient's hands (see Step 12C illustration). Place a hand in the mitten, being sure the mitten end is brought all the way over the wrist.	• Prevents patients from dislodging invasive equipment, removing dressings, or scratching, yet allows greater movement than a wrist restraint.
D. **Elbow restraint:** This piece of fabric with slots has tongue blades placed so that the elbow joint remains rigid (see Step 12D illustration).	• Commonly used with infants and children to prevent elbow flexion (e.g., when an IV line is in place).

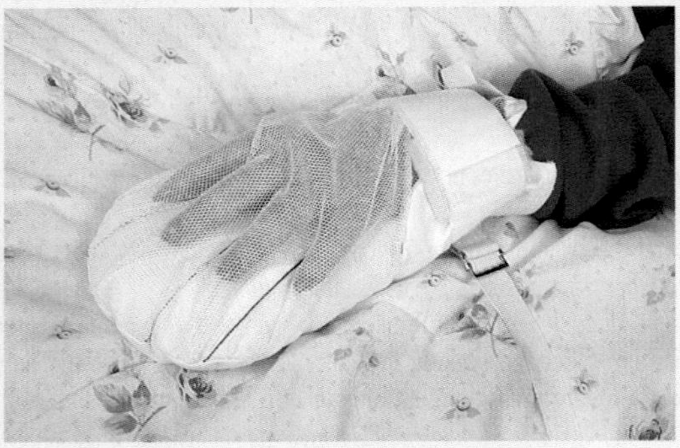

STEP 12C Mitten restraint.

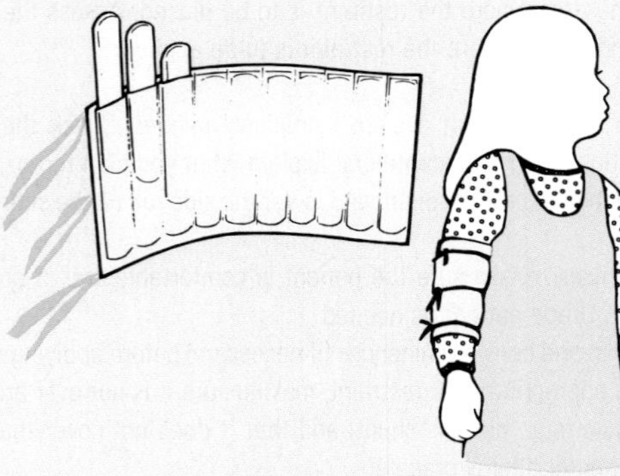

STEP 12D Elbow restraint.

STEPS	RATIONALE
E. **Mummy restraint:** The mummy restraint consists of a blanket or sheet. It is opened on the bed or crib with one corner folded toward the centre. The child is placed on the blanket with shoulders at the fold and feet toward the opposite corner (see Step 12E-1 illustration). With the child's right arm straight down against the body, the right side of the blanket is pulled firmly across the right shoulder and chest and secured beneath the left side of the body (see Step 12E-2 illustration). The left arm is placed straight against the body, and the left side of the blanket is brought across the shoulder and chest and locked beneath child's body on the right side (see Step 12E-3 illustration). The lower corner is folded and brought over the body and tucked or fastened securely with safety pins (see Step 12E-4 illustration).	• Maintains short-term restraint of small child or infant for an examination or treatment involving the head and neck. Effectively controls movement of torso and extremities.

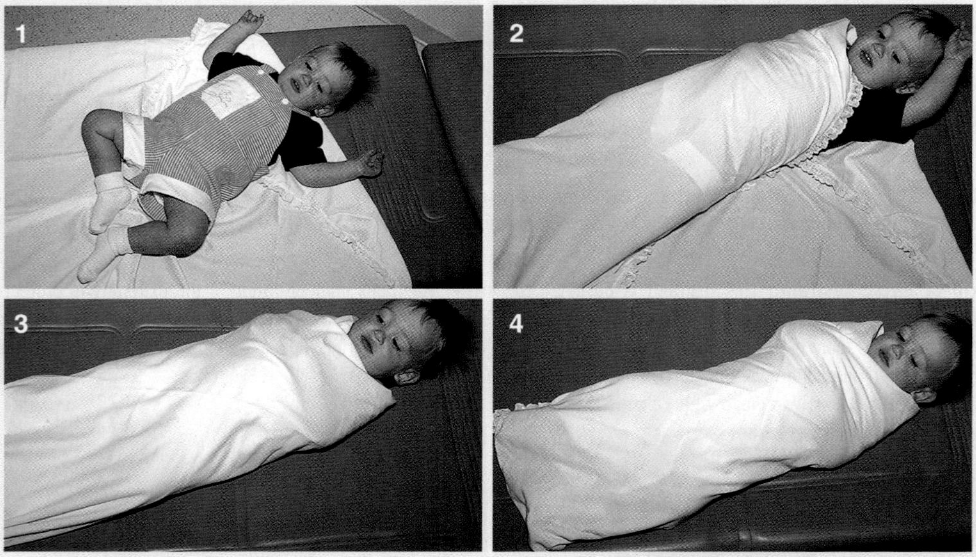

STEP 12E Mummy restraint.

STEPS	RATIONALE
13. Attach restraints to the bed frame, which moves when the head of the bed is raised or lowered (see Step 13 illustration).	• Patient may be injured if restraint is secured to side rail and it is lowered.

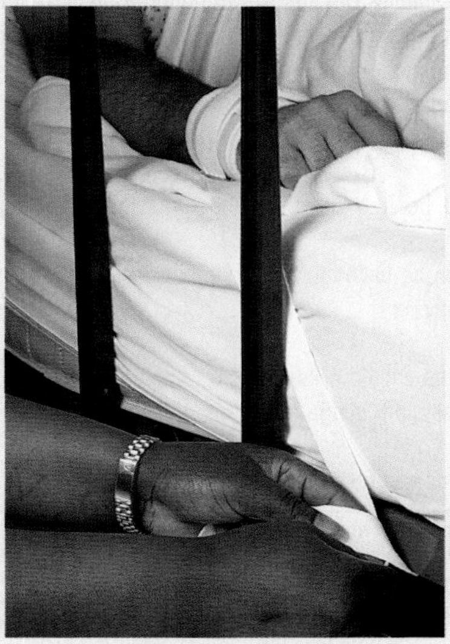

STEP 13 Tie restraint strap to the bed frame.

CRITICAL DECISION POINT: *Do not attach end of restraint to side rails.*

STEPS	RATIONALE
14. Secure restraints with a quick-release tie (see Step 14 illustration). Do not tie in a knot.	• Allows for quick release in an emergency.
15. Insert two fingers under the secured restraint (see Step 15 illustration).	• A tight restraint may cause constriction and impede circulation. Checking for constriction prevents neurovascular injury.

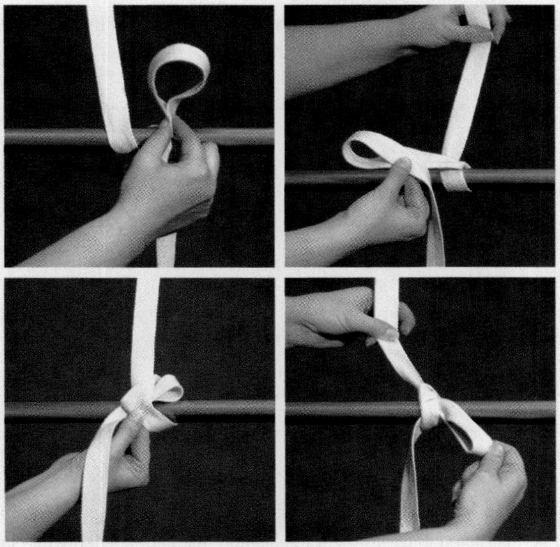

STEP 14 The Posey quick-release tie. (Courtesy J.T. Posey Co., Arcadia, CA.)

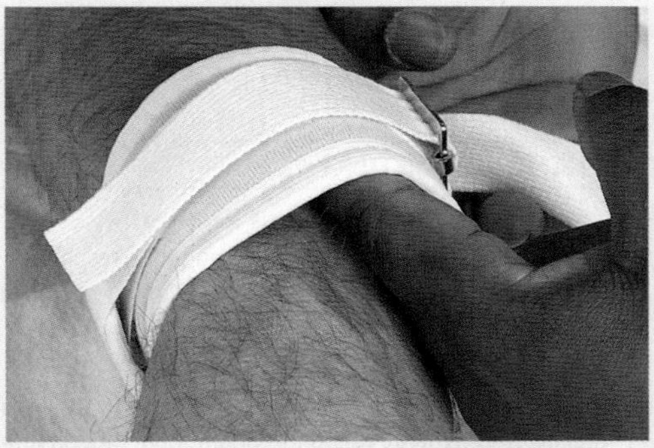

STEP 15 Place two fingers under the restraint to check tightness.

STEPS	RATIONALE
16. The proper placement of the restraint, skin integrity, pulses, temperature, colour, and sensation of the restrained body part should be assessed at least every hour or according to agency's policy.	• Frequent assessments prevent complications, such as suffocation, skin breakdown, and impaired circulation.
17. Restraints should be removed at regular intervals (see agency policy). If the patient is violent and noncompliant, remove one restraint at a time or have staff assist while removing the restraints. The patient should not be left unattended at this time.	• Provides opportunity to change patient's position and perform full range of motion, toileting, and exercise and to provide food or fluids.

Continued

SKILL 37-1 APPLYING PHYSICAL RESTRAINTS—cont'd

STEPS	RATIONALE
18. Secure a call light or intercom system within the patient's reach.	• Allows patient, family, or caregiver to obtain assistance quickly.
19. Leave the bed or chair with wheels locked. The bed should be in its lowest position.	• Locked wheels prevent the bed or chair from moving if the patient attempts to get out. If the patient falls when the bed is in lowest position, the chances of injury are reduced.
20. Perform hand hygiene.	• Reduces transmission of microorganisms.
21. Reassess the patient's status and needs.	
A. Inspect the patient for any injuries, including all hazards of immobility, while restraints are in use.	• Patient should be free of injury and not exhibit any signs of immobility complications.
B. Observe IV catheters, urinary catheters, and drainage tubes to ensure that they are positioned correctly and that therapy remains uninterrupted.	• Reinsertion can be uncomfortable and can increase the risk of infection or interrupt therapy.
C. Regularly reassess the patient's need for continued use of the restraint (for medical or surgical reason) with the intent of discontinuing the restraint at the earliest possible time (see agency-specific policy).	• Use of restraints should be seen as a temporary measure and discontinued as soon as possible (College of Nurses of Ontario, 2017b).
D. Provide appropriate sensory stimulation and reorient patient as needed.	• Use of restraints can further increase disorientation.

UNEXPECTED OUTCOMES	RELATED INTERVENTIONS
Patient has signs of impaired skin integrity	• Assess skin and provide appropriate therapy. • Notify the physician and reassess the need for continued use of the restraint. • Ensure the correct application of restraint. Pad the skin under the restraint, and remove restraint more often.
Patient has altered neurovascular status in an extremity (cyanosis, pallor, coldness of skin, or complaints of tingling, pain, or numbness)	• Remove the restraint immediately, stay with the patient, and notify the physician. • Protect the extremity from further injury (e.g., pressure from tubing or encumbrance, positioning).
Patient is increasingly confused, disoriented, or agitated	• Identify the reason for this change in behaviour, and attempt to eliminate the cause. • Attempt a restraint alternative.
Patient escapes from restraint device and suffers fall or injury	• Attend to the patient's immediate physical needs, and inform the physician. • Reassess the type of restraint used, the correct application, and if alternatives can be used.

RECORDING AND REPORTING

- Record behaviours that place patient at risk for injury.
- Describe restraint alternatives attempted and patient's response.
- Record patient's and family's understanding of and consent to restraint application.
- Record type and location of the restraint and time applied.
- Record time of assessments and releases.
- Document the patient's behaviour after the application of the restraint.
- Document specific assessments related to orientation, oxygenation, skin integrity, circulation, and positioning.
- Describe the patient's response when restraints were removed.

HOME CARE CONSIDERATIONS

- Plan care with family. If possible, use of an Ambularm may free patient from physical restraints.
- Instruct family members (or other caregivers) in the use of alternatives to restraints (see Box 37-11).
- A physical restraint may require a physician order. The restraint should not be sent home with family unless the device is needed to protect the patient from injury. If physical restraints are necessary, the family members (or other caregivers) must be instructed in their proper application, the care needed while in restraints, and the complications for which to look. Also inform caregivers whom to contact if any abnormal findings occur.
- A patient who needs to be restrained in bed should have a hospital bed and will require constant supervision in the home.

such as over the side rail or on the floor (Figure 37-11). The Bed-Check bed exit alarm system (Figure 37-12) uses a weight-sensitive sensor mat that can be placed on the patient's mattress or chair. This device sounds an audible alarm at the bedside when pressure is released off the sensor mat. Such devices are useful for patients who tend to climb out of bed unassisted but are in danger of falling. Other alarms can be placed on doors to alert staff or family members when a confused patient, prone to wandering, opens a door.

Another alternative form of restraint is the Posey Bed Enclosure (Figure 37-13), a soft-sided, self-contained enclosed bed. It allows for freedom of movement and thus reduces the side effects caused by physical restraints such as pressure injuries and loss of dignity. The Posey Bed Enclosure works well for patients who are restless and unpredictable, cognitively impaired, and at risk for injury if they were to fall or get out of bed, such as patients on anticoagulant therapy at risk for intracranial bleeding. The bed may also be a safer alternative to side rails.

A long-term care setting may be designed to include environmental restraints, such as locked nursing units. Residents with dementia may be at risk for injury if they wander away from their unit or building. A locked nursing unit can be designed to permit individuals the freedom to wander safely around their unit and can include exits to secure, enclosed outdoor spaces when weather permits. A locked unit is still a form of restraint and should be implemented only after alternatives to restraint have proven unsuccessful.

In some situations, chemical restraints may be indicated. Chemical restraint is defined as "any form of psychoactive medication used, not to treat illness, but to intentionally inhibit a particular behaviour or movement" (College of Nurses of Ontario, 2017b, p. 4). For example, it may be necessary to sedate a patient who is consistently pulling out a nasogastric tube. As with any other restraint, chemical restraints should be implemented only after nonrestraining measures (e.g., distraction, use of a sitter) have proven ineffective and with the informed consent of the patient or their substitute decision maker. Proper adherence to medication administration guidelines is vital to the safe use of chemical restraints, and the patient's response to and need for these medications must be assessed on a regular basis.

Side Rails. Side rails may help to increase a patient's mobility and stability when in bed or when moving from the bed to a chair. Side rails also help prevent the unconscious patient from falling out of bed or off a stretcher (Figure 37-14). However, raised side rails that

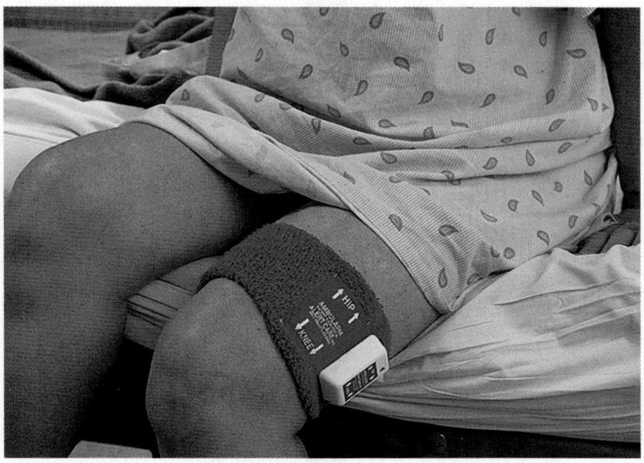

FIGURE 37-11 Patient wearing an Ambularm device.

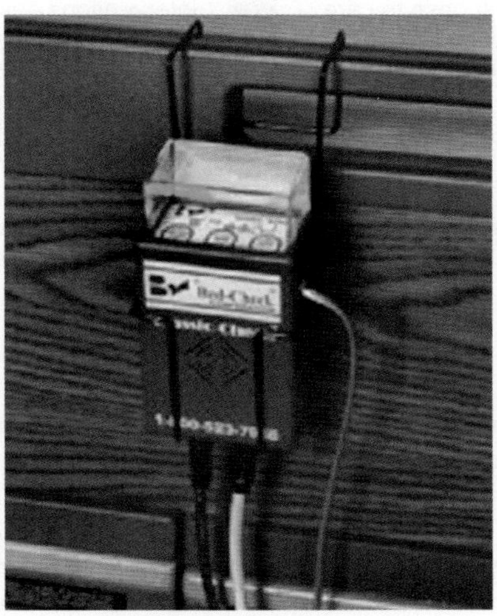

FIGURE 37-12 The Bed-Check bed exit alarm. (Courtesy Bed-Check Corp.)

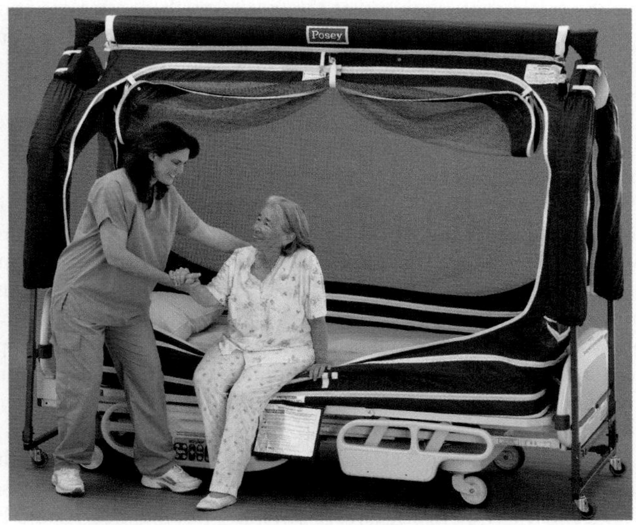

FIGURE 37-13 The Posey Bed enclosure. (Courtesy J. T. Posey Co., Arcadia, CA.)

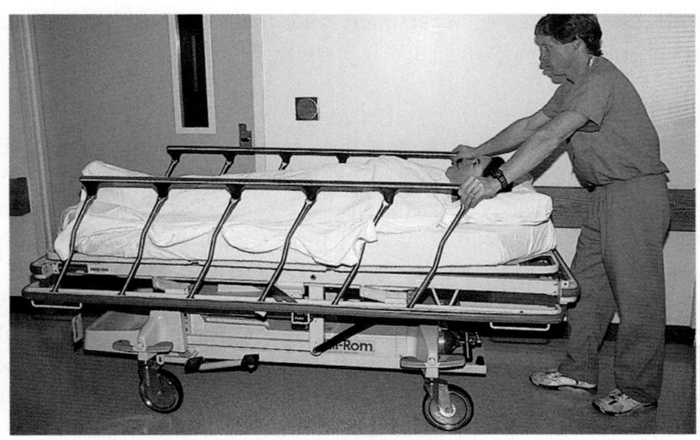

FIGURE 37-14 Side rails in the up position on a stretcher.

BOX 37-13 PATIENT TEACHING

Prevention of Electrical Hazards in the Home

Objective
- Patient will recognize electrical hazards in the home and eliminate them.

Teaching Strategies
- Discuss grounding appliances and other equipment.
- Provide examples of common hazards: frayed cords, damaged equipment, and overloaded outlets.
- Discuss guidelines to prevent electrical shocks:
  - Use extension cords only when necessary, and use electrical tape to secure the cord to the floor where it will not be stepped on.
  - Do not run wires under carpeting.
  - Teach the patient to grasp the plug, not the cord, when unplugging items.
  - Teach the patient to keep electrical items away from water.
  - Teach the patient not to operate equipment with which he or she is unfamiliar.
  - Teach the patient to disconnect items before cleaning them.

Evaluation
- Have patient list electrical hazards existing in the home.
- Review with the patient the steps he or she will take to eliminate these hazards.
- Reassess the home after the patient has had an opportunity to eliminate the hazards.

cannot be opened by the patient are considered a restraint (College of Nurses of Ontario, 2017b). The use of side rails for a disoriented patient may cause more confusion and further injury. A confused patient who is determined to get out of bed may attempt to climb over the side rail or climb out at the foot of the bed, often resulting in a fall or injury. Nursing interventions to reduce a patient's confusion should first focus on the cause of the confusion. Frequently, a patient's attempt to explore his or her environment or to self-toilet is mistaken as confusion. A thorough assessment is essential. Whenever side rails are used, the bed should be maintained in the lowest position possible.

Electrical Hazards. Electrical equipment must be maintained in good working order and should be grounded. The third (longer) prong in an electrical plug is the ground. Theoretically, the ground prong carries any stray electrical current back to the ground—hence, its name. The other two prongs carry the power to the piece of electrical equipment. Improperly grounded or malfunctioning electrical equipment increases the risks of electrical injury and fire. Educating both the patient and the family can reduce the risk for electrical hazards in the home environment (Box 37-13).

If a patient receives an electrical shock in a health care setting, the nurse must immediately determine whether the patient has a pulse. If the patient has no pulse, cardiopulmonary resuscitation should be initiated and emergency personnel should be notified. If the patient has a pulse and remains alert and oriented, the nurse needs to quickly obtain vital signs and assess the skin for signs of thermal injury. The patient's physician must be notified. If an electrical shock occurs in the home, the nurse follows the same procedure but has the patient go to the emergency department and then notifies the patient's physician.

◆ Evaluation

Patient Care. The components of critical thinking should be applied to the evaluation step of the nursing process (Figure 37-15). The actual care delivered by the health care team is evaluated on the basis of expected outcomes. If the patient's goals have been met, the nursing interventions can be considered effective and appropriate. If not, the nurse must determine whether new risks to the patient have developed or whether previous risks remain. The patient and family need to participate in this process to find permanent ways to reduce risks to safety. Nurses need to continually assess the patient's and family's need for additional support services, such as home care, physiotherapy, counselling, and further teaching.

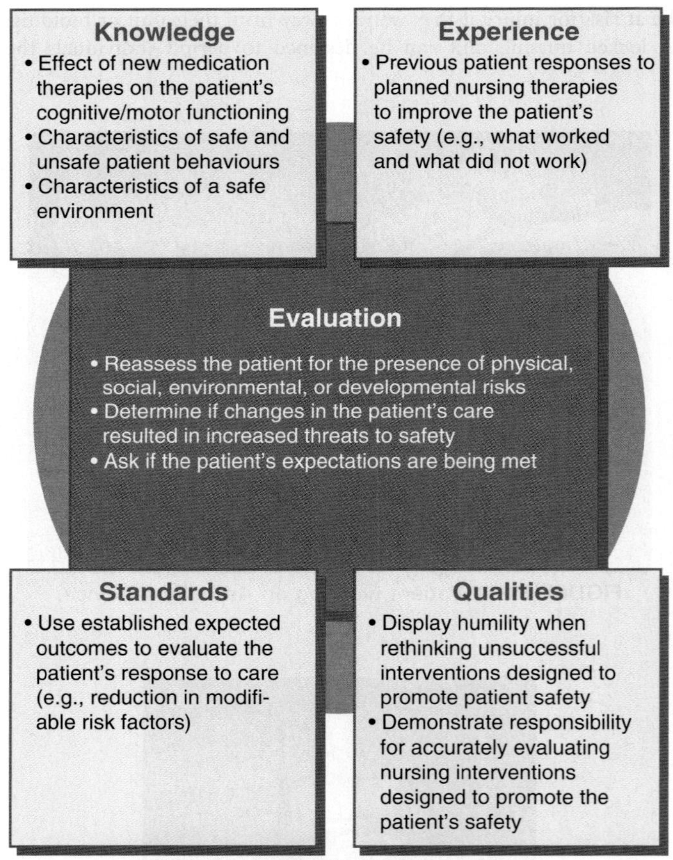

FIGURE 37-15 Critical thinking model for safety evaluation.

Patient Expectations

Nurses who have developed a good relationship with a patient whereby the patient feels safe and secure in the environment are more likely to have a patient with high levels of satisfaction regarding their care. Nurses must determine if patient expectations have been met. Is the patient satisfied with any changes made to the environment? Does the patient believe that his or her safety is ensured? If patient expectations have not been met, nurses must reassess not only the patient and the environment but also the patient's expressed desires.

KEY CONCEPTS

- A safe environment is essential to promoting, maintaining, and restoring health.
- Nurses must maintain their own safety in order to provide safe care to patients.
- In the community, a safe environment is one in which basic needs are achievable, physical hazards are reduced, the transmission of pathogens is reduced, pollution is controlled, and sanitation is maintained.
- In a health care agency, a safe environment is one that minimizes falls, patient-inherent accidents, procedure-related accidents, and equipment-related accidents.
- A factor that reduces atmospheric oxygen is the presence of high carbon monoxide levels, which may result from an improperly functioning furnace.
- Prolonged exposure to extreme environmental temperatures can cause patient injury or even death.
- The reduction of physical hazards in the environment includes providing adequate lighting, decreasing clutter, and securing the home.
- The transmission of pathogens is reduced through medical and surgical asepsis, immunization, adequate food sanitation, insect and rodent control, and the appropriate disposal of human waste.
- Children less than 5 years of age are at the greatest risk for home accidents that may result in severe injury and death.
- The school-aged child is at risk for injury at home, at school, and while travelling to and from school.
- Adolescents are at risk for injury from automobile accidents, suicide, and substance abuse.
- Threats to an adult's safety are frequently associated with lifestyle habits.
- Risks of injury for older patients are directly related to the physiological changes of the aging process; falls are the greatest cause of accidental injury in older persons.
- By incorporating critical thinking skills in the application of the nursing process, nurses assess the patient and the environment to determine risk factors for injury; cluster risk factors; formulate a nursing diagnosis; and plan specific interventions, including patient education.
- Nursing interventions for promoting safety are individualized for developmental stage, lifestyle, and environment.
- Nursing interventions are developed to modify the environment for protection from falls, fires, poisoning, and electrical hazards.
- The expected outcomes include a safe physical environment, a patient whose expectations have been met and who is knowledgeable about safety factors and precautions, and a patient free of injury.

CRITICAL THINKING EXERCISES

1. Mrs. Santiago, who is 88 years old and has been functioning independently at home, was recently admitted to the hospital. Through your admission assessment, you learn that she experiences urinary frequency and urgency and occasional dizziness. When you perform the "Get up and Go" test, you find that she can get up on her own successfully after multiple attempts. Use the Hendrich II Fall Risk Model (see Table 37-1) to determine Mrs. Santiago's risk for a fall, and design specific interventions to ensure her safety in the hospital.
2. Mrs. Patel, a 76-year-old long-term care resident with Alzheimer's disease, has been refusing food and fluids for the past month. The family has agreed to the placement of a nasogastric tube to improve her fluid and nutritional statuses. Shortly after the first tube feeding was started, Mrs. Patel became more restless, and she has been picking at the tube.
   a. What might be precipitating Mrs. Patel's behaviour of picking at the tube?
   b. What approaches can be used to eliminate interference with the treatment?
   c. If a restraint is necessary to avoid the disruption of therapy, what interventions are required to ensure the patient's safety while in restraints?
3. A family member of a patient reports that, just a few minutes ago, a lit cigarette dropped on the patient's mattress but that the small fire was put out. What actions are needed to ensure the safety of this patient?

REVIEW QUESTIONS

1. Accidental injuries are the leading cause of death for which age group?
   1. 1 to 12 months
   2. 1 to 34 years
   3. 45 to 64 years
   4. 65 years and over
2. Adolescents are at a greater risk for injury from:
   1. Poisoning, drowning, motor vehicle accidents
   2. Motor vehicle accidents, suicide, and substance abuse
   3. Home accidents, motor vehicle accidents, fire
   4. Falls, suicide, drowning
3. The physiological changes caused by aging increase the older patient's risk for:
   1. Falls
   2. Suicide
   3. Alcoholism
   4. Seizures
4. WHMIS is a system to control hazardous substances in the workplace and includes:
   1. Environmental interventions and cautionary labelling of products
   2. Worker education programs and the provision of MSDSs
   3. Patient education programs and worker education programs
   4. Risk assessment and the provision of MSDSs
5. Medication and fluid administration errors and the improper application of external devices are examples of:
   1. Patient-inherent accidents
   2. Procedure-related accidents
   3. Equipment-related accidents
   4. Environmental-related accidents
6. Which of the following statements about restraints is *not* true?
   1. Restraints are used only after other alternatives have been tried.
   2. The least restrictive method of restraint should be used.
   3. Restraints are considered a long-term intervention.
   4. If a restraint is used, it must be part of the patient's medical treatment.
7. When teaching parents about responding to poisoning in children, the nurse should instruct them to:
   1. Give oral fluids
   2. Induce vomiting
   3. Call the local poison control centre
   4. Drive the child to the emergency department

8. All of the following are acceptable alternatives to the use of restraints, *except:*
   1. Attending to needs for toileting, food, and liquid
   2. Offering diversionary activities, such as music or something to hold
   3. Camouflaging IV lines with clothing or a stockinette
   4. Ensuring that a family member is with the patient at all times

Answers: 1. 2; **2.** 2; **3.** 1; **4.** 2; **5.** 2; **6.** 3; **7.** 3; **8.** 4

Rationales for the Review Questions appear at the end of the book.

RECOMMENDED WEBSITES

Canadian Patient Safety Institute: http://www.patientsafetyinstitute.ca/en/Pages/default.aspx

Part of Health Canada, the Canadian Patient Safety Institute has been a leader in addressing patient safety issues in Canadian health care agencies. This website provides links to various topics relevant to promoting patient safety.

Canada Safety Council: http://canadasafetycouncil.org/

The Canada Safety Council is a national, nongovernmental, charitable organization dedicated to providing safety education. Its mission is to reduce preventable deaths and injuries in public and private places throughout Canada.

DriveABLE: http://driveable.com/

This website is a useful resource for nurses working with patients who need to make a decision to stop driving. DriveABLE is an Alberta-based company that provides objective and evidence-informed approaches to assessing driver ability, as well as resources for supporting individuals and families through this process.

Parachute: http://www.parachutecanada.org/

Parachute is a national nonprofit organization dedicated to preventing injuries and saving lives. Parachute's injury prevention program has become one of the leading injury-prevention groups in Canada.

Workplace Hazardous Materials Information System: http://www.hc-sc.gc.ca/ewh-semt/occup-travail/whmis-simdut/index-eng.php

This website is developed and maintained by Health Canada's WHMIS Division and includes policies and information related to WHMIS.

REFERENCES

AboutKidsHealth.ca. (2017). *Poison information centres in Canada.* Retrieved from http://www.aboutkidshealth.ca/En/HealthAZ/TestsAndTreatments/Resources/Pages/Poison-Information-Centres-in-Canada.aspx.

Agency for Healthcare Research and Quality. (2017a). *20 tips to help prevent medical errors: Patient fact sheet.* Retrieved from http://www.ahrq.gov/patients-consumers/care-planning/errors/20tips/.

Agency for Healthcare Research and Quality. (2017b). *About TeamSTEPPS®.* Rockville, MD: Author. Retrieved from http://www.ahrq.gov/teamstepps/about-teamstepps/index.html.

American Academy of Pediatrics/Healthy Children.org. (2017). *Poison prevention & treatment tips.* Retrieved from http://www.healthychildren.org/English/news/Pages/Tips-for-Poison-Prevention-and-Treatment.aspx.

Backman, C., Vanderloo, S., d'Entremont, B., et al. (2015). Implementation of an electronic data collection tool to monitor nursing-sensitive indicators in a large academic health sciences centre. *Canadian Journal of Nursing Leadership, 28*(3), 77–91.

Baker, G. R., Norton, P. G., Flintoft, V., et al. (2004). The Canadian Adverse Events Study: The incidence of adverse events among hospital patients in Canada. *Canadian Medical Association Journal, 170,* 1678–1686.

Cafazzo, J. A., & St-Cyr, O. (2012). From discovery to design: the evolution of human factors in healthcare. *Healthcare Quarterly, 15*(Special issue), 24–29.

Canadian Institute for Health Information (CIHI). (2007). *Patient safety in Canada: An update.* Retrieved from https://secure.cihi.ca/estore/productFamily.htm?pf=PFC1088&lang=en&media=0.

Canadian Institute for Health Information (CIHI). (2013). *National trauma registry report: Major injury in Canada.* Retrieved from https://secure.cihi.ca/estore/productSeries.htm?pc=PCC46.

Canadian Institute for Health Information (CIHI). (2016). *1 in 18 patients experiences harm in Canadian hospitals.* Retrieved from https://www.cihi.ca/en/health-system-performance/quality-of-care-and-outcomes/1-in-18-patients-experiences-harm-in-canadian-hospitals.

Canadian Nurses Association. (2015). *Workplace violence and bullying.* Ottawa: Author. Retrieved from http://cna-aiic.ca/~/media/cna/page-content/pdf-en/Workplace-Violence-and-Bullying_joint-position-statement.pdf.

Canadian Nurses Association & University of Toronto Faculty of Nursing. (2004). *Nurses and patient safety: A discussion paper.* Retrieved from https://www.cna-aiic.ca/~/media/cna/page-content/pdf-fr/patient_safety_discussion_paper_e.pdf?la=en.

Canadian Paediatric Society. (2016). *Safe sleep for babies.* Retrieved from https://www.caringforkids.cps.ca/handouts/safe_sleep_for_babies.

Canadian Paediatric Society. (2017). *Car seat safety.* Retrieved from http://www.caringforkids.cps.ca/handouts/car_seat_safety.

Canadian patient safety dictionary. (2003). Retrieved from http://www.royalcollege.ca/portal/page/portal/rc/common/documents/publications/patient_safety_dictionary_e.pdf.

Canadian Patient Safety Institute (CPSI). (2015). *Patient safety incident.* Retrieved from http://www.patientsafetyinstitute.ca/en/topic/pages/patient-safety-incident.aspx.

Child Find Canada. (2006). *Educating your children about strangers: The exploiter or abductor: Not a stranger.* Retrieved from http://www.childfind.ca/safety/parents2.php.

College of Nurses of Ontario. (2017a). *Conflict prevention and management.* Toronto: Author. Retrieved from http://www.cno.org/Global/docs/prac/47004_conflict_prev.pdf.

College of Nurses of Ontario. (2017b). *Practice standard: Restraints.* Toronto: Author. Retrieved from http://www.cno.org/Global/docs/prac/41043_Restraints.pdf.

Dobbs, B., Pidborochynski, T., & Lindsdell, M. (2015). *The senior driver myths & facts: information for health care professionals, patients, and families on assessment and referral issues.* 3rd ed. Retrieved from https://driveable.com/images/driveable/pdf's/Myths_and_Facts_Senior_Drivers_2015_pdf.

Ebersole, P., Hess, P., Touhy, T. A., et al. (2016). *Toward healthy aging: Human needs and nursing response* (9th ed.). St. Louis, MO: Mosby.

Edelman, C. L., & Mandle, C. L. (2013). *Health promotion throughout the lifespan* (8th ed.). St. Louis, MO: Mosby.

Etchells, E., Juurlink, D., & Levinson, W. (2008). Medication errors: The human factor. *Canadian Medical Association Journal, 178*(1), 63–64. doi:10.1503/cmaj.071658.

Frank, J. R., & Brien, S. (Eds.), (2008). *The safety competencies: Enhancing patient safety across the health professions.* Ottawa, ON: Canadian Patient Safety Institute.

Government of Canada. (2014). *Safe disposal of prescription drugs.* Retrieved from http://healthycanadians.gc.ca/drugs-products-medicaments-produits/buying-using-achat-utilisation/disposal-defaire-eng.php.

Health Canada. (2015). *Workplace Hazardous Materials Information System.* Retrieved from http://www.hc-sc.gc.ca/ewh-semt/occup-travail/whmis-simdut/about-a_propos_e.html.

Hendrich, A. (2016). Fall risk assessment for older adults: The Hendrich II Fall Risk Model. *Try this: Best practices in nursing care to older adults, Issue 8.* New York: The Hartford Institute for Geriatric Nursing, New York University. Retrieved from https://consultgeri.org/try-this/general-assessment/issue-8.pdf.

Institute for Safe Medication Practices. (2016). *FDA and ISMP lists of look-alike drug names with recommended tall man letters.* Retrieved from https://www.ismp.org/Tools/tallmanletters.pdf.

Institute of Medicine (IOM). (1999). *To err is human: Building a safer health system.* Retrieved from http://www.nationalacademies.org/hmd/Reports/1999/To-Err-is-Human-Building-A-Safer-Health-System.aspx.

Karsh, B. T., Holden, R. J., Alper, S. J., et al. (2006). A human factors engineering paradigm for patient safety: designing to support the performance of the healthcare professional. *Quality and Safety in Health Care, 15*(Suppl. 1), i59–i65. doi:10.1136/qshc.2005.015974.

Leape, L. L. (1997). A systems analysis approach to medical error. *Journal of Evaluation in Clinical Practice, 3*(3), 213–222.

McCullagh, M. C. (2006). Home modification: How to help patients make their homes safer and more accessible as their abilities change. *The American Journal of Nursing, 106*(10), 54.

Meiner, S., & Lueckenotte, A. (2015). *Gerontologic nursing* (5th ed.). St. Louis, MO: Mosby.

Mitchell, M. D., Lavenberg, J. G., Trotta, R., et al. (2014). Hourly rounding to improve nursing responsiveness: A systematic review. *The Journal of Nursing Administration, 44*(9), 462–472. doi:10.1097/NNA.0000000000000101.

National Steering Committee on Patient Safety. (2002). *Building a safer system: A national integrated strategy for improving patient safety in Canadian health care.* Retrieved from http://www.royalcollege.ca/portal/page/portal/rc/common/documents/advocacy/building_a_safer_system_e.pdf.

Parachute Canada. (2017). *Wheeled activities.* Retrieved from http://www.parachutecanada.org/injury-topics/topic/C108.

Public Health Agency of Canada. (2008). *Leading causes of death, Canada, 2008, males and females combined.* Ottawa: Author. Retrieved from http://www.phac-aspc.gc.ca/publicat/lcd-pcd97/pdf/lcd-pcd-t1-eng.pdf.

Reason, J. (1997). *Managing the risks of organizational accidents.* Aldershot, UK: Ashgate.
Registered Nurses' Association of Ontario (RNAO). (2005). *Prevention of falls and fall injuries in the older adult* (Revised). Toronto: Author. Retrieved from http://rnao.ca/sites/rnao-ca/files/Prevention_of_Falls_and_Fall_Injuries_in_the_Older_Adult.pdf.
Safe Kids Canada. (2007). *Child and youth unintentional injury: 10 years in review: 1994–2003.* Retrieved from http://www.parachutecanada.org/downloads/research/Child_and_Youth_Unintentional_Injury_-_1994-2003.pdf.
SMARTRISK. (2009). *The economic burden of injury in Canada.* Retrieved from www.parachutecanada.org/downloads/research/reports/EBI2009-Eng-Final.pdf.
Spoelstra, S. L., Given, B. A., & Given, C. W. (2012). Fall prevention in hospitals: an integrative review. *Clinical Nursing Research, 21*(1), 92–112.
Taylor-Adams, S., Brodie, A., & Vincent, C. (2008). Safety skills for clinicians: An essential component of patient safety. *Journal of Patient Safety, 4*(3), 141–147.
Trinkoff, A., Geiger-Brown, J., Brady, B., et al. (2006). How long and how much are nurses working? *The American Journal of Nursing, 106*(4), 60–71.
Vanier Institute of the Family. (2010). *Families count: Profiling Canada's families IV.* Ottawa: Author. Retrieved from http://vanierinstitute.ca/resources/families-count/.

38

Hygiene

Canadian content written by Jim Hunter, RN, MSN
Original chapter by Patricia A. O'Connor, RN, MSN, CNE

OBJECTIVES

Mastery of content in this chapter will enable you to:

- Define the key terms listed.
- Discuss common factors that influence personal hygiene practices.
- Discuss the role that the nursing process and critical thinking play in the provision of hygiene care.
- Conduct a comprehensive assessment of a patient's total hygiene needs.
- Understand the importance of foot care for the diabetic patient.
- Describe conditions that place the patient at risk for problems related to the hair, scalp, integument, feet, nails, eyes, ears, nose, mouth, and throat and discuss their related interventions.
- Describe how hygiene care for the older patient may differ from that for the younger patient.
- Discuss the different approaches used in maintaining a patient's comfort and safety during hygiene care.
- Successfully perform hygiene for care of the integument; perineum; feet, hands, and nails; mouth; and eyes, ears, and nose.

KEY TERMS

Acne, p. 911
Alopecia, p. 908
Buccal mucosa, p. 903
Cerumen, p. 910
Complete bed bath, p. 917
Cuticle, p. 903
Dermis, p. 904
Enucleation, p. 939
Epidermis, p. 903
Gingivitis, p. 904
Halitosis, p. 908
Lunula, p. 903
Maceration, p. 903
Mastication, p. 904
Neuropathy, p. 907
Partial bed bath, p. 918
Perineal care, p. 926
Periodontal disease, p. 904
Stomatitis, p. 908
Xerostomia, p. 913

MEDIA RESOURCES

http://evolve.elsevier.com/Canada/Potter/fundamentals/

- Audio Chapter Summaries
- Examination Review Questions
- Concept Map Creator
- Case Study with Questions
- Audio Glossary
- Content Updates
- Video Clips

Personal hygiene affects an individual's comfort, safety, and physical and psychological well-being. Individuals who are well are capable of meeting their own hygiene needs, but those who are ill or have disabilities may require various levels of assistance. Many personal, social, environmental, and cultural factors can influence hygiene practices. In agency or home settings, nurses must determine a patient's ability to perform self-care and provide hygiene care according to the patient's needs and preferences. In the home setting, nurses can assist in helping the patient and family to adapt hygiene techniques, equipment, and approaches.

Because hygiene care requires close contact with a patient, therapeutic communication skills should be used (see Chapter 17) to build and promote a caring therapeutic relationship and to assist nurses in providing patients with teaching or delivery of hygiene care. Other nursing activities can be integrated during hygiene care, including patient assessment and interventions, such as integumentary assessment, assessment of mood or affect, range-of-motion exercises, the application of dressings, and the inspection and care of intravenous (IV) sites. During hygiene care, nurses need to encourage and promote the patient's independence as much as possible, ensure privacy, convey respect, and maintain and support physical comfort and safety.

SCIENTIFIC KNOWLEDGE BASE

Proper hygiene care requires an understanding of the anatomy and physiology of the integument, oral cavity, eyes, ears, nose, hands, feet, and nails. The skin and mucosal cells exchange oxygen, nutrients, and fluids with underlying blood vessels. The cells require adequate nutrition, hydration, and circulation to resist injury and disease. Good hygiene techniques assist in promoting the normal structure and function of body tissues.

In addition, knowledge of pathophysiology is applied to provide skilled preventive hygiene care. As a nurse, you need to learn to recognize disease states that create changes in the integument, oral cavity, and sensory organs. For example, diabetes mellitus results in chronic vascular changes that impair healing of the skin and mucosa. In the early stages of untreated acquired immune deficiency syndrome (AIDS), fungal infections of the oral cavity are common. Stroke can result in paralysis of the trigeminal nerve, which eliminates the blink reflex, increasing the risk for corneal drying. In the presence of conditions such as these, hygiene practices are adapted to anticipate patient needs and minimize harmful effects. By integrating knowledge of anatomy, physiology, and pathophysiology during hygiene care, nurses can recognize abnormalities and initiate appropriate actions to prevent further injury.

The Skin

The skin is an active organ with the functions of protection, secretion, excretion, temperature regulation, and sensation (Table 38-1). The skin has three primary layers: epidermis, dermis, and subcutaneous (see Chapter 32). Bacteria commonly reside on the outer layer (the **epidermis**). These resident bacteria are normal flora (see Chapter 33); they do not cause disease but instead inhibit the multiplication of disease-causing microorganisms.

The skin can provide crucial information regarding a patient's health status and provide important information regarding the functioning of other systems and organs (see Chapter 32).

The Feet, Hands, and Nails

The feet, hands, and nails often require special attention to prevent infection. Any injury or deformity to the foot, including growths or injuries to the overlying skin and nails, can be painful and thus interfere with a patient's normal ability to walk and weight-bear.

The hand, in contrast to the foot, is constructed largely for manipulation rather than support. Dexterity exists in the hand because of the wide range of movement between the thumb and fingers. Any condition that interferes with the movement of the hand (e.g., superficial or deep pain or joint inflammation) can impair a patient's self-care abilities.

The nails are epithelial tissues that grow from the root of the nail bed, which is in the skin at the nail groove and hidden by the fold of skin called the **cuticle**. The visible part of the nail is the nail body. It has a crescent-shaped white area known as the **lunula**. Under the nail lies a layer of epithelium called the *nail bed* (Figure 38-1). In light-skinned individuals, a healthy nail is transparent, smooth, and convex, with a pink nail bed and translucent white tip. Some disease processes can cause changes in the shape, thickness, and curvature of the nail (see Chapter 32).

The Oral Cavity

The oral cavity extends from the lips to the anterior pillars of the tonsils. It is the structure for taste, mastication, and speech articulation. The **buccal mucosa** (oral mucosa) are normally light pink and moist.

TABLE 38-1 Function of the Skin and Implications for Care

Function and Description	Implications for Care
Protection	
The epidermis is relatively impermeable and protects the body from environmental stress (e.g. trauma, pathogens) and environmental factors (e.g. heat, cold).	Weakening of the epidermis occurs by scraping or stripping its surface (e.g., using dry razors, tape or dressing removal, or improper turning or positioning techniques resulting in shearing). Excessive dryness causes cracks and breaks in the skin and mucosa that allow bacteria to enter. Emollients soften the skin and prevent moisture loss, and hydration of the mucosa prevents dryness. Constant exposure of skin to moisture can cause **maceration** (softening), which interrupts dermal integrity and promotes ulcer formation and bacterial growth. Bed linen and clothing should be kept fresh and dry. Overuse of soaps, detergents, cosmetics, and deodorants can cause chemical irritation. Alkaline soaps neutralize the protective acid condition of skin. Cleaning the skin removes excess oil, sweat, dead skin cells, and dirt that can promote bacterial growth. Bath water should not be excessively hot or cold.
Sensation	
The skin contains sensory organs for touch, pain, temperature, and pressure.	Friction should be minimized to avoid the loss of the stratum corneum, which can result in the development of pressure injuries. Smoothing linen removes sources of mechanical irritation. To prevent accidental injury of the patient's skin, nurses should remove their own jewellery before giving care.
Temperature Regulation	
Body temperature is controlled by evaporation of perspiration, radiation, and conduction of heat from the body when blood vessels of the skin are vasodilated through lack of perspiration and vasoconstriction.	Factors that interfere with heat loss can alter temperature control. Wet bed linens or gowns interfere with convection, conduction, and evaporation. Excess blankets or bed coverings can interfere with heat loss through radiation and conduction and promote heat conservation.
Absorption and Secretion	
The skin allows limited excretion of some metabolic wastes and by-products such as minerals, sugars, and uric acid. Sebum lubricates and softens the skin and hair and decreases the amount of heat loss from the skin.	Perspiration and oil can harbour microorganisms. Bathing removes excess body secretions; however, excessive bathing can cause drying of the skin.

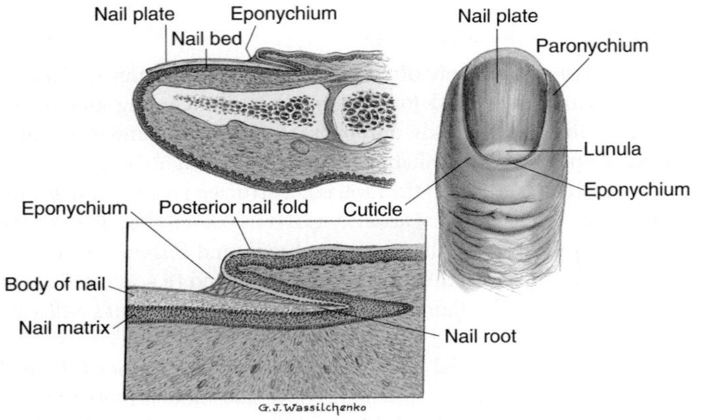

FIGURE 38-1 Anatomical structure of a normal nail. (From McFarland, G. K., Hirsch, J. E., Tucker, S. M., & Thompson, J. M. [Eds.]. [2002]. *Mosby's clinical nursing* [5th ed.]. St. Louis, MO: Mosby.)

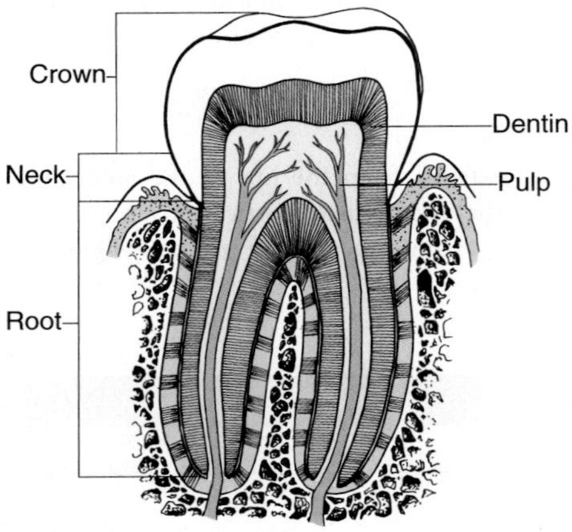

FIGURE 38-2 A normal tooth.

The floor of the mouth and the undersurface of the tongue are richly supplied with blood vessels, which allows for rapid absorption of sublingual medications (e.g., nitroglycerin). Any type of ulceration or trauma to the area can result in significant bleeding. The mouth also contains three pairs of salivary glands that start the digestive process by releasing enzymes, protect the mucosa from heat and chemical irritants, transmit taste information, and provide lubrication for the movement of food. Salivary secretion can be decreased by medications and disease processes.

There are 32 permanent teeth for chewing, or **mastication**. They are designed to cut, tear, and grind food so that it can be mixed with saliva and swallowed. A normal tooth consists of a crown, neck, and root (Figure 38-2). The periodontal membrane lies just below the gum margins, surrounds a tooth, and holds it firmly in place. Healthy teeth are free from cavities and are properly aligned.

Difficulty with chewing can develop when gum tissues become inflamed or infected or when teeth are lost or become loose. Regular oral hygiene is necessary to maintain the integrity of tooth surfaces and to prevent **gingivitis** (gum inflammation) and **periodontal disease**.

The Hair

Hair is produced by hair follicles located in the **dermis** (Figure 38-3). Hair growth, distribution, and pattern can indicate a person's general health status. Hormonal changes, emotional and physical stresses, aging, infection, and certain illnesses can affect hair colour and condition. The hair shaft itself is inert and cannot be directly affected by physiological factors. However, changes in its colour or condition are caused by hormonal or nutrient deficiencies of the hair follicle (see Figure 38-3).

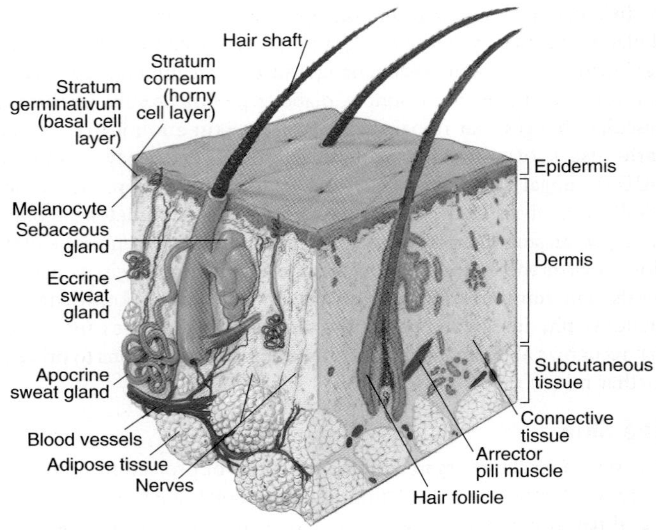

FIGURE 38-3 Hair follicles and relationship of follicles and their related structures to the epidermal and dermal layers of the skin. (From Lewis, S. M., Heitkemper, M. M., Dirksen, R. R., et al. [2014]. *Medical–surgical nursing in Canada: Assessment and management of clinical problems* [3rd Canadian ed., p. 541, Fig. 25-1]. Toronto: Elsevier/Mosby.)

The Eyes, Ears, and Nose

The eyes, ears, and nose require careful attention during the provision of hygiene. Chapter 32 describes the structure and function of these organs. Cleaning these sensitive sensory tissues should be done in a way that prevents injury and discomfort for the patient, such as being careful not to get soap in the patient's eyes. In addition, the time spent with a patient during hygiene provides an excellent opportunity to ask whether he or she has experienced any changes in vision, hearing, or sense of smell.

NURSING KNOWLEDGE BASE

Hygiene care is never routine; the care requires intimate contact with patients, and good communication skills are necessary to build and promote a therapeutic relationship. No two individuals perform hygiene in the same manner, and it is important to individualize care from knowledge about the patient's unique hygiene practices and preferences.

While providing hygiene care, nurses can learn about patients' health promotion practices and needs, emotional needs, and needs pertaining to health care education. A patient's personal preferences for hygiene can be influenced by several factors.

Social Practices

Social groups influence hygiene preferences and practices, including the type of hygiene products used and the nature and frequency of personal care. During childhood, hygiene is influenced by family customs, including, for example, the frequency of bathing, the time of day bathing is performed, and the type of oral hygiene practised. As children enter their adolescent years, personal hygiene may be influenced by peer group behaviour, and they may become more interested in their personal appearance. For example, girls may begin to wear makeup, and boys may begin shaving. During the adult years, involvement with friends and work groups shapes the expectations individuals have about their personal appearance. Older persons' hygiene practices may change because of living conditions, health status, and available resources.

Personal Preferences

Each patient has individual preferences about when to bathe, shave, and perform hair care. Patients select different products according to personal preferences and needs. These preferences should assist nurses in delivering individualized care for patients. In addition, nurses should assist patients in developing new hygiene practices when necessitated by an illness or condition.

Body Image

Patients' general appearance may reflect the importance that hygiene holds for them. Body image is a person's subjective concept of his or her physical appearance (see Chapter 26), and it can change frequently. When patients undergo surgery, illness, a change in physical or mental health status, or simply age, body image can alter dramatically. For this reason, effort should be made to promote patients' hygienic comfort and appearance.

Body image affects the way in which hygiene is maintained. If patients are neatly groomed, nurses should consider the details of grooming when planning care and consult with the patients before making decisions about how hygiene care is to be provided. Patients who appear unkempt or uninterested in hygiene may require an assessment of their hygiene practices, their mental status, or additional education about the importance of hygiene.

Socioeconomic Status

A person's economic resources can influence the type and extent of hygiene practices used. Nurses should be sensitive in considering whether a patient's economic status influences his or her ability to regularly maintain hygiene. When patients have the added problem of a lack of resources, it becomes difficult to participate and take a responsible role in health promotion activities such as basic hygiene.

When basic care items are not affordable, alternatives need to be considered. It is also important to assess whether the use of these products is an acceptable practice among patients' social or cultural group. For example, not all patients may choose to use deodorant or cosmetics.

Health Beliefs and Motivation

Knowledge about the importance of hygiene and its implications for well-being influences hygiene practices. However, knowledge alone is not enough. According to Cowdell and Steventon (2015), individual characteristics such as personal factors (psychological, sociocultural, and biological) directly influence an individual's health promotion activities.

It is important to know, for example, whether patients perceive that they are at risk for dental disease, that dental disease is serious, and that brushing and flossing are effective in reducing this risk. When patients recognize that a risk is present and that reasonable action can be taken to reduce the risk, they are more receptive to counselling and teaching efforts.

Cultural Variables

Patients' cultural beliefs and personal values can influence hygiene care (Box 38-1). Individuals from diverse cultural backgrounds follow different self-care practices (see Chapter 9). Feelings of disapproval must not be conveyed when nurses are caring for patients whose hygienic practices are different from their own. In some cultures, it is customary to bathe once a week; in North America, it is common to bathe or shower daily.

BOX 38-1 Cultural Influences on Hygiene

Patients need a culturally competent plan for hygiene care. For some, hygiene practices are influenced by culture and are a potential source of conflict or stress in a hospital environment. Hygiene is a very personal matter and bathing, perineal hygiene, and hair care practices can be sensitive issues. Using knowledge from theoretical models enables the health care provider to provide culturally sensitive care that respects and incorporates the patient's cultural background.

Implications for Practice

- Maintain privacy, especially for women from cultures that value female modesty.
- Be aware that in some cultures, touch has many different meanings: touching the shoulder of a Japanese man can cause feelings of humiliation; Asian women do not shake hands with other women or men; for some Indigenous people, touch can mean a prevention of harm.
- Be aware that to the patient of Asian descent, silence can be interpreted as a sign of respect.
- Provide gender-congruent caregivers as needed or requested. If a gender-congruent caregiver is not available, ask the family for assistance.
- Do not cut or shave a patient's hair or beard without prior discussion with the patient or family.
- Be aware that some cultures (e.g., Chinese, Filipino) discourage bathing for 7 to 10 days after childbirth.
- Bear in mind that some cultures (e.g., Chinese, Japanese, Korean, Hindu) consider the top parts of the body cleaner than the lower parts.
- Be aware that among Hindus and Muslims, the left hand is used for cleaning and the right hand is used for eating and praying.

Data from Galanti, G. A. (2015). *Caring for patients from different cultures* (5th ed.). Philadelphia, PA: University of Pennsylvania; Giger, J., & Davidhizar, R. E. (2013). *Transcultural nursing: Assessment and intervention* (6th ed.). St. Louis, MO: Mosby Elsevier.

Physical Condition

Patients with certain types of physical limitations, disabilities, or pain often lack the physical energy, dexterity, and range of motion to perform hygiene care. A patient in traction or a cast or who has an IV line or other device connected to the body needs assistance with hygiene. Patients under the effects of sedation do not have the mental clarity or coordination to perform self-care. Chronic illnesses, such as cardiac disease, cancer, neurological disorders, and certain psychiatric conditions, may exhaust or incapacitate a patient. A weakened grasp resulting from arthritis, stroke, or muscular disorders can prevent a patient from using a toothbrush, washcloth, or comb.

CRITICAL THINKING

Successful critical thinking requires the synthesis of knowledge, experience, information gathered from patients, critical thinking qualities, and intellectual and professional standards. Clinical judgements require nurses to anticipate the information necessary to analyze data and make decisions regarding patient care. Patients' conditions are always changing, requiring ongoing critical thinking. During assessment, nurses must consider all contributing factors needed to make a nursing diagnosis (Figure 38-4).

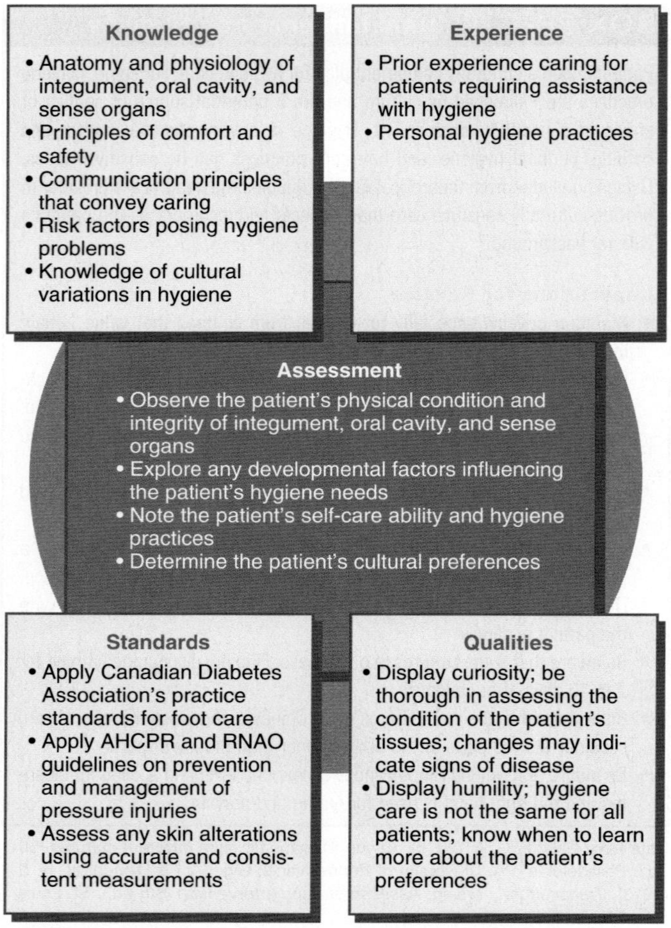

FIGURE 38-4 Critical thinking model for hygiene assessment. *AHCPR,* Agency for Health Care Policy and Research; *RNAO,* Registered Nurses' Association of Ontario.

Because hygiene care is so important for patients to feel comfortable, refreshed, and renewed, nurses should avoid making hygiene care a simple routine. Instead, nurses need to integrate knowledge from nursing and other disciplines, previous experiences, and information gathered from patients. In addition, attributes such as curiosity and humility are useful when designing a plan of care that will meet patients' hygiene needs. Agency and professional nursing standards and guidelines, such as those from the Registered Nurses' Association of Ontario (RNAO), are used when planning care to meet the patient's hygiene needs.

❖ NURSING PROCESS

◆ Assessment

Important considerations for assessment include the patient's ability to perform self-care, usual hygiene practices, and preferences with special attention to balance, coordination, strength, range of motion, and activity tolerance. Nursing assessment is an ongoing process. It involves all phases of the nursing process, including goal setting, planning, intervention, and evaluation. Not all body regions need to be assessed before administering hygiene; however, routine assessment of a patient's condition is undertaken whenever patient care is provided. For example, during oral care, the condition of the teeth and mucosa can be inspected. If the patient has had a repeated problem (e.g., dry skin or inflamed oral mucosa), it is important to conduct an assessment before care is administered because variations in technique may be necessary.

Physical Examination. While assisting a patient with personal hygiene, carefully assess the integument, oral cavity structures, and the eyes, ears, and nose (see Chapter 32). Using the skills of inspection and palpation, look for alterations in the integrity and function of tissues. Assessment can also be used to determine the type and extent of hygiene care required and the need for specialized equipment (e.g., grab bars, tub chair). Special attention should be given to the structures most influenced by hygiene measures. Is the skin intact, especially over bony prominences? Is the skin dry from too much bathing or from other factors? Are calluses present on the feet, which may benefit from soaking? Is a coating of the tongue present, which necessitates frequent oral care? Over time, the nurse's assessment provides the baseline for determining whether hygienic measures maintain or improve the patient's condition.

The Skin. While inspecting the skin, thoroughly examine its colour, texture, thickness, turgor, temperature, and hydration. The skin should be smooth, warm, and supple and have good turgor. Pay special attention to the presence and condition of any lesions (see Chapter 32), and assess for dryness indicated by flaking, redness, scaling, and cracking. Certain common skin problems affect how hygiene is administered (Table 38-2). Assess tattoos and body piercings for potential health risks such as skin irritation and infection, which are the most prevalent associated complications. Serious complications such as hepatitis B or C, HIV/AIDS, or even death can also result from body piercings and tattoos (Halloran, 2015). Be alert to the possibility of hidden or unexpected piercings. Careful attention should be paid in assessing less obvious or difficult-to-reach skin surfaces, such as under the female patient's breasts, under the male patient's scrotum, or around the female's perineal tissues. Observed skin problems should be documented and explained to the patient; teaching on proper skin care and specific hygiene techniques should also be discussed with the patient.

Certain conditions place patients at risk for impaired skin integrity (Box 38-2). Nurses must be particularly alert when assessing patients with reduced sensation, vascular insufficiency, or immobility. Both extremities should be assessed and patients assisted in turning so that skin surfaces can be fully viewed. The development of pressure injuries is a common complication that can extend hospital stays and threaten the well-being of long-term care patients. Tools such as the Braden Scale (Sardo, Simões, Alvarelhão, et al., 2015) are available to determine those patients who may be at risk for impaired skin integrity. When caring for patients with darkly pigmented skin, nurses should be aware of assessment techniques and skin characteristics unique to highly pigmented skin (Box 38-3).

The Feet and Nails. When assessing the feet, perform a thorough examination of all skin surfaces, including the areas between the toes and over the soles of the feet. The heels, soles, sides of the feet, and "knuckles" of the toes are prone to irritation from poorly fitting shoes. In addition, inspect the shape and size of the toes, as well as the shape of the foot. The toes are normally straight and flat. The feet should be in straight alignment with the ankle and tibia. Inspect the feet for lesions and note areas of dryness, inflammation, or cracking.

Assess the patient's gait. Painful foot disorders or decreased sensation can cause limping or an unnatural gait. Inquire whether the patient has foot discomfort and determine factors that aggravate the pain. Foot problems may result from bone or muscular alterations or wearing poor-fitting footwear, rather than skin disorders.

Patients with peripheral vascular disease, diabetes mellitus, and other diseases that affect peripheral circulation and sensation should

TABLE 38-2 Common Skin Problems

Characteristics	Implications	Interventions
Dry Skin		
Flaky, rough texture on exposed areas such as hands, arms, legs, or face	Skin may become infected if epidermal layer is allowed to crack.	Bathing should be less frequent and the skin rinsed of all soap residue, because if left on the skin, soap can cause irritation and skin breakdown. Increase and encourage fluid intake, if permitted. Use a nonallergenic moisturizing cream, to help form a protective barrier and assist with keeping fluid within the skin. Use creams to clean skin that is dry or if patient is allergic to soaps or detergents.
Acne		
Inflammatory, papulopustular skin eruption, usually involving bacterial breakdown of sebum; appears on face, neck, shoulders, and back	Infected material within pustule can spread if area is squeezed or picked. Permanent scarring can result.	Wash hair and skin thoroughly each day with soap to remove excess oil and prevent secondary infections. Use cosmetics sparingly, as oily cosmetics and creams accumulate in pores and tend to worsen the condition. Use prescribed topical or oral antibiotics.
Skin Rashes		
Skin eruption that may result from overexposure to sun or moisture or from an allergic reaction (may be flat or raised, localized or systemic, pruritic or nonpruritic)	If skin is continually scratched, inflammation and infection may occur.	Wash the area thoroughly and apply an antiseptic spray or lotion to prevent further itching and aid in the healing process. Apply warm or cold compresses to relieve inflammation, if indicated.
Contact Dermatitis		
Inflammation of skin characterized by abrupt onset with erythema, pruritus, pain, and appearance of scaly oozing lesions (seen on face, neck, hands, forearms, and genitalia)	Dermatitis is often difficult to eliminate because the person is usually in continual contact with the substance causing the skin reaction, and it may be hard to identify this substance.	Avoid causative agents (e.g., cleaners and soaps).
Psoriasis		
Noncontagious, chronic skin condition characterized by an abnormal growth of keratinocytes (a type of skin cell) and an inflammatory reaction that results in the formation of thick, silvery, scaly, inflamed patches of skin; commonly seen on the scalp, knees, elbows, and chest	The cause of psoriasis is unknown, and no cure exists. It is often difficult to diagnosis as it has similar symptoms to eczema and atopic dermatitis.	Treatment options are aimed at reducing the extent and severity of the condition and improving quality of life. The patient should avoid trigger agents such as smoking, stress, excessive alcohol, and skin injury (e.g., sunburn).
Abrasion		
Scraping or rubbing away of epidermis that may result in localized bleeding and later weeping of serous fluid	Infection occurs easily because of the loss of this protective skin layer.	Caregivers should trim their fingernails and not wear jewellery when providing patient care. Clean the area and dry thoroughly and gently. Observe for retained moisture in dressings or bandages—excess moisture can increase the risk of infection. Lift—do not pull—when transferring or repositioning a patient (see Chapter 45).

be assessed for the adequacy of circulation to the feet (see Chapter 32). Inspection and daily foot care can help prevent the development of a foot ulcer. Foot ulcerations are a predisposing factor for lower extremity amputations in individuals with diabetes mellitus (Pemayun, Naibaho, Novitasari, et al., 2015).

Palpation of the dorsalis pedis and posterior tibial pulses is used to determine whether adequate or reduced blood flow is reaching peripheral tissues. Edema and changes in skin colour, texture, and temperature can indicate whether patients require special hygiene care. Individuals with diabetes mellitus should also be assessed for **neuropathy**—degeneration of the peripheral nerves characterized by a loss of sensation, which can lead to injury. Patients' sensation to light touch, pain, and temperature should be assessed.

Inspect the condition of the fingernails and toenails, looking for lesions, dryness, inflammation, and cracking (Table 38-3). The nail is surrounded by a cuticle, which slowly grows over the nail

BOX 38-2 Risk Factors for Skin Impairment

Immobilization

When restricted from moving freely, patients' dependent body parts are exposed to pressure, reducing circulation to the affected body parts. Nurses should know which patients require assistance to turn and reposition.

Reduced Sensation

Patients with paralysis, circulatory insufficiency, or local nerve damage are unable to sense an injury to the skin. While bathing a patient, assess the status of sensory nerve function by checking for pain, tactile sensation, and temperature sensation.

Nutrition and Hydration Alterations

Patients with limited caloric and protein intake can develop thinner, less elastic skin, with a loss of subcutaneous tissue. This can result in impaired or delayed wound healing.

Secretions and Excretions on the Skin

Moisture on the skin's surface serves as a medium for bacterial growth and can cause irritation, soften epidermal cells, and lead to skin breakdown. The presence of perspiration, urine, fecal material, or wound drainage on the skin can also result in breakdown or infection, or both.

Vascular Insufficiency

Inadequate arterial supply to tissues and impaired venous return decrease the circulation to the extremities. Inadequate blood flow can cause ischemia and tissue breakdown. The risk of infection also exists because the delivery of nutrients, oxygen, and white blood cells to injured tissues is inadequate.

External Devices

An external device applied to or around the skin exerts pressure and friction on the skin. Assess all surfaces exposed to casts, cloth restraints, bandages and dressings, tubing, or orthopedic braces.

BOX 38-3 Skin Assessment and Implications for Practice

Identifying changes in skin colour is important in evaluating patients' risks for skin breakdown and pressure injuries (see Chapter 46). When a patient's natural skin contains more melanin, it is more difficult to determine hyperemia and cyanosis. Some hyperpigmentation areas are normal, such as slate grey nevus, which may be on the sacrum of African, Aboriginal, and Asian patients. These areas should not be confused with skin colour changes such as hyperemia or cyanosis.

Implications for Practice

For dark-skinned patients, assess baseline skin tone by asking the patient or family to point out an area of baseline skin colour for that person. Assess the oral mucosa, over the cheekbones, and conjunctivae in the dark-skinned patient, and the nail beds and lips in light-skinned patients.

Assess localized skin changes:

- Colour darker than surrounding skin colour; purplish, bluish (cyanosis), eggplant
- Taut skin
- Shiny skin
- Induration (hardening of the tissues)
- Use natural light sources when possible because fluorescent light can give the skin a bluish tone
- Examine body sites with the least amount of melanin for underlying skin colour identification

Assess for edema (nonpitting, pitting) (see Chapter 32).

Assess skin temperature, using the back of the hand; if the patient's condition permits, do not use gloves when doing this assessment:

- Initially may feel warmer than surrounding skin
- Subsequently may feel cooler than surrounding skin

Data from Estes, M. E., & Buck, M. (2008). *Health assessment and physical assessment* (1st Canadian. ed.). Toronto: Thomson Nelson; MacDonald-Jenkins, J. (2014). Skin, hair, and nails. In C. Jarvis, A. Browne, J. MacDonald-Jenkins, & M. Luctkar-Flude (Eds.), *Physical examination and health assessment* (2nd Canadian ed.). Toronto: Elsevier Canada; Stephen, T. C. (2015). Assessment of integumentary function. In R. A. Day, P. Paul., & B. Williams (Eds.), *Brunner & Suddarth's textbook of Canadian medical-surgical nursing* (3rd ed.). Philadelphia, PA: Lippincott Williams & Wilkins.

and must be regularly pushed back. The skin around the nail beds and cuticles should be smooth and without inflammation. Women should be asked whether they frequently polish their nails and use polish remover because chemicals in these products can cause excessive nail dryness and discoloration. Disease can change the shape and curvature of the nails. Inflammatory lesions and fungus of the nail bed can cause thickened, horny nails, which can separate from the nail bed.

The Oral Cavity. All areas of the oral cavity need to be inspected carefully for colour, hydration, texture, and lesions (see Chapter 32). Patients who do not follow regular oral hygiene practices may have receding gum tissue, gingivitis, a coated tongue, discoloured teeth (particularly along the gum margins), dental caries, missing teeth, and halitosis (bad breath). Localized pain and infection are common symptoms of periodontal disease and certain tooth disorders.

Some patients in acute care settings require a complete oral assessment. The identification of risks for infection and other conditions can suggest the type and frequency of oral care. Proper oral care has been shown to decrease the risk of aspiration and nosocomial infections in ventilated patients (Gupta, Gupta, Singh, et al., 2016). It is also well established that Gram-negative bacteria (e.g., *Pseudomonas aeruginosa*) found in dental plaque can result in pneumonia in hospitalized older persons. It is especially important to examine the oral cavity of patients receiving radiation or chemotherapy. Both treatments can reduce the amount of saliva, resulting in drying and stomatitis (inflammation of the oral mucosal tissues). The assessment serves as a basis for preventive care for patients as they undergo treatment.

The Hair. Before performing hair care, assess the condition of the hair and scalp. Healthy hair is clean, shiny, and untangled; the scalp is free of lesions. The hair of dark-skinned patients is usually thicker, drier, and curlier than that of lighter-skinned patients. Table 38-4 summarizes hair and scalp problems that may be identified during the assessment. In community and home care settings, it is particularly important to inspect the hair for pediculosis capitis (head lice) so that the appropriate treatment can be provided. If head lice are suspected, guard against self-infestations by handwashing and using gloves or tongue blades to inspect the patient's hair. A loss of hair (alopecia) can result from the effects of chemotherapy medications, hormonal changes, improper hair care practices, or may be idiopathic. Patients at risk for scalp problems are those who have experienced head trauma and those who practise poor hygiene.

The Eyes, Ears, and Nose. The condition and function of the eyes, ears, and nose need to be examined (see Chapter 32). Normally the eyes are free of infection and irritation. The sclerae are visible anteriorly as the white portion of the eye. The conjunctivae (the lining of the eyelids) are clear, pink, and without inflammation. The eyelid

TABLE 38-3 Common Foot and Nail Problems

Characteristics	Implications	Interventions
Callus		
A thickened portion of the epidermis consisting of a mass of horny, keratotic cells. It is usually flat, painless, and found on the undersurface of the foot or on the palm of the hand. It is caused by local friction or pressure.	The condition may cause discomfort when wearing tight shoes.	Advise the patient to wear gloves when using tools or objects that may create friction on palmar surfaces, and to wear soft-soled shoes with insoles. Soak callus in warm water and magnesium sulphate (Epsom salts) to soften the cell layers. Apply cream or lotion to reduce reformation. Encourage the patient to see a podiatrist (ensure that the patient is aware of the associated cost).
Keratosis (corn)		
Corns are caused by chronic friction and pressure from ill-fitting or loose shoes. They are seen mainly on or between toes or over a bony prominence. A corn is usually cone shaped, round, and raised. Soft corns are macerated.	The conical shape compresses the underlying dermis, making it thin and tender. The pain worsens when tight shoes are worn. Corns can become soft and macerated by perspiration. The patient may suffer an alteration in gait resulting from pain.	Surgical removal may be necessary, depending on the severity of pain and size of the corn. The patient should avoid the use of oval corn pads, which can increase pressure on toes and reduce circulation. Use warm water soaks to soften the corns before gentle rubbing with a callus file or pumice stone (consult with physician or podiatrist). Wider and softer shoes are suggested.
Plantar Wart		
A fungating lesion caused by the papillomavirus that appears on the sole of the foot.	Warts may be contagious, are painful, and can make walking difficult.	Treatment ordered may include applications of salicylic acid, electrodessication (burning with electrical spark), or freezing with solid carbon dioxide.
Athlete's Foot (Tinea Pedis)		
A fungal infection of the foot; scaliness and cracking of skin occurs between the toes and on the soles of feet. Small blisters containing fluid may appear. The problem can be caused by wearing constricting footwear.	Athlete's foot can spread to other body parts, especially the hands. It is contagious and frequently recurs.	Feet should be well ventilated. Drying feet well after bathing and applying powder helps to prevent infection. Wearing clean socks or stockings reduces the incidence. The physician or nurse practitioner may prescribe antifungal topical applications.
Ingrown Nail		
An ingrown toenail or fingernail grows inward into the soft tissue around nail. An ingrown nail often results from improper nail trimming.	Ingrown nails can cause localized pain when pressure is applied and can lead to infection.	Treatment is frequent hot soaks in an antiseptic solution and removal of the portion of nail that has grown into skin. Instruct the patient in proper nail-trimming techniques, and provide a referral to a podiatrist. (Ensure that the patient is aware of the associated cost.)
Ram's Horn Nail		
An unusually long, curved, thickened nail.	Attempts to cut ram's horn nails may result in damage to the nail bed with an increased risk of infection.	Refer the patient to a podiatrist. (Ensure that the patient is aware of the associated cost.)
Paronychia		
Inflammation of tissue surrounding the nail, after a hangnail or other injury. It occurs in individuals who frequently have their hands in water and is common in patients with diabetes.	Infection	Treatment can include hot compresses or soaks, or topical or oral antibiotics. Paronychia can be prevented by careful manicuring.
Foot Odour		
Results from excess perspiration, promoting microorganism growth.	The condition may cause discomfort because of excess perspiration and odour, and increases patients' risk for infection.	Frequent washing, using foot deodorants and powders, and wearing clean footwear prevents or reduces the problem.

TABLE 38-4 Problems of Head and Body Hair and Scalp

Characteristics	Implications	Interventions
Dandruff		
Scaling of the scalp is accompanied by itching. In severe cases, dandruff can be found on eyebrows.	Dandruff causes individuals embarrassment and if it enters the eyes, conjunctivitis may develop.	Shampoo regularly with a medicated shampoo. In severe cases, obtain a physician's advice.
Ticks		
Small, grey-brown parasites that burrow into the skin and suck the blood.	Ticks transmit several diseases to individuals. The most common are Rocky Mountain spotted fever, tularemia, and Lyme disease.	Do not pull ticks quickly from the skin because their sucking apparatus remains and may cause infection. Ticks can be removed slowly with tweezers.
Pediculosis Capitis (Head Lice)		
Head lice require a source of human blood to survive. Transmission is by direct contact (e.g., head to head). The parasite is found near the scalp, attached to hair strands. Eggs look like oval particles, similar to dandruff. Bites or pustules may be observed behind the ears and at the hairline. Itching at the hairline is the most common symptom.	Contacts of the patients (e.g., family members and classmates) should be examined and treated. Although no current evidence exists of transmission by shared articles, families may wish to wash bedding and combs in hot water. Dry-cleaning, or storing items in occlusive plastic bags for approximately 2 weeks is also effective (Cummings, Finlay, MacDonald, et al., 2016).	Check the entire scalp. Use a medicated shampoo to eliminate lice. Follow the product directions carefully; a repeat application is required 7–10 days later to ensure that surviving eggs are destroyed. Seek physician advice if treatment is ineffective; a new medication may be required for effective chemical eradication. Some products can cause neurotoxicity and should not be used with children under 6 years of age. Do not use products containing lindane. This product has been withdrawn for use in some countries. Use a fine-toothed comb to assist with the manual removal of nits (the empty eggshell) and lice.
Pediculosis Corporis (Body Lice)		
Body lice differ from head lice in that they tend to cling to clothing and may not be easily seen. They suck blood and lay eggs on clothing and furniture.	The patient itches constantly. Scratches seen on the skin may become infected. Hemorrhagic spots may appear on skin where lice are sucking blood.	Ask the patient to bathe or shower thoroughly. After the skin is dried, apply a recommended pediculicide lotion. After 8–12 hours, have the patient take another bath or shower. Bag infested clothing or linen until laundered in hot water. Vacuum rooms thoroughly and throw away the bag after completion.
Pediculosis Pubis (Crab Lice)		
Crab lice parasites are found in pubic hair. Crab lice are greyish white with red legs.	Lice may be spread via bed linen, clothing, or furniture, or via sexual contact.	Clean pubic hair to remove body lice. Treatment of sexual partners is recommended.
Hair Loss (Alopecia)		
Alopecia occurs in individuals of all races. Balding patches are seen at the periphery of the hairline. Hair becomes brittle and broken. The condition can be caused by genetics, the use of hair curlers or hair picks, tight braiding, and some medications.	Patches of uneven hair growth and loss alter the patient's appearance and affect self-image.	Advise the patient to stop any hair care practices that might be further damaging the hair.

margins are in close approximation with the eyeball, and the lashes are turned outward. The lid margins are without inflammation, drainage, or lesions. The eyebrows are symmetrical.

It is important to determine whether the patient wears contact lenses. This is especially significant for patients who enter hospitals or other agencies unresponsive or in a confused state. To determine whether a contact lens is present, stand to the side of the patient's eye and observe the cornea for the presence of a soft or rigid lens; if you do not see one, observe the sclera to detect whether a contact lens has shifted off the patient's cornea. An undetected lens can cause severe corneal injury if left in place too long.

Inspect the external ear structures (auricle, helix, and earlobe), and use an otoscope to inspect the external auditory canal and tympanic membrane. While performing hygiene measures, nurses are most concerned with noting the presence of accumulated **cerumen** or drainage in the ear canal, local inflammation, tenderness on palpation, or the patient's report of pain (see Chapter 32).

Inspect the nares for signs of inflammation, discharge, lesions, edema, and deformity (see Chapter 32). The nasal mucosa is normally pink and clear and has little or no discharge. A clear, watery discharge may be the result of allergies. If patients have any form of tubing exiting the nose (e.g., nasogastric tube), inspect the naris surfaces that come in contact with the tubing for tissue sloughing, localized tenderness, inflammation, and bleeding.

Developmental Changes. The normal process of aging influences the condition of body tissues and structures and, thus, the manner in which hygiene measures are performed. Chapter 47 addresses the changes in hearing, vision, and olfaction across the lifespan as a result of growth and development.

The Skin. Neonates' skin is relatively immature at birth. The epidermis and dermis are loosely bound together, and the skin is very thin. Friction against the skin layers can cause bruising, so neonates must be handled carefully during bathing. Any break in the skin can easily lead to infection.

Toddlers' skin layers are more tightly bound together. Thus, children have a greater resistance to infection and skin irritation. However, because of children's active play and the absence of established hygiene habits, greater attention is needed from parents and caregivers to provide thorough hygiene and to begin teaching good hygiene habits.

During adolescence, the growth and maturation of the integument increases. In girls, estrogen secretion causes the skin to become soft, smooth, and thicker, with increased vascularity. In boys, male hormones produce an increased thickness of the skin with some darkening in colour. Sebaceous glands become more active, predisposing adolescents to acne. Eccrine and apocrine sweat glands become fully functional during puberty. Adolescents usually begin to use deodorants, and more frequent bathing and shampooing become necessary to reduce body odours and eliminate oily hair. Sweating is usually more pronounced in boys.

The condition of adults' skin depends on hygiene practices and exposure to environmental irritants. Normally, the skin is elastic, well hydrated, firm, and smooth. When adults practise frequent bathing or are exposed to an environment with low humidity, the skin can become very dry and flaky.

With aging, the skin loses its resiliency and moisture, and sebaceous and sweat glands become less active. The epithelium thins, and elastic collagen fibres shrink, making the skin fragile and subject to bruising and breaking. These changes in the outer epidermis or stratum corneum (Dulan, Sheridan, & Laucher, 2016), warrant caution when turning and repositioning older persons. Typically, older persons' skin becomes drier and wrinkled. Because the skin may be excessively dry, older persons should avoid bathing daily and using very hot water or harsh soaps.

The Feet and Nails. When we stand, the feet provide support and absorb shock. With aging, they begin to show signs of wear and tear. This may occur earlier if individuals have failed to wear comfortable, supportive footwear. The cushioning layer of fat on the soles of the feet becomes thin.

Chronic foot problems are a common result of poor foot care, improperly fitting footwear, aging, and systemic disease. Older persons often have dry feet because of a decrease in sebaceous gland secretion, dehydration of epidermal cells, and poor condition of footwear. Callus formation and decreased sensation place the patient at a high risk for the development of foot ulcers (Bateman, 2014). Painful feet can be the result of congenital deformities, weak structure, injuries, and diseases such as diabetes, rheumatoid arthritis, or osteoarthritis. After 55 years of age, arthritis is a common cause of changes in the feet. Additional common foot problems are hammer toes, hallux valgus (bunions), corns, and ingrown toenails.

Fungal infections can occur under toenails, causing dark yellow streaks or total discoloration. The nails can also become opaque, scaly, and hypertrophied. If foot or nail problems stay unresolved, patients can easily become disabled. Nurses must apply knowledge of typical changes in the feet and nails when anticipating the type of hygiene that patients will require.

The Oral Cavity. Infants begin teething at approximately 6 to 8 months of age (Mitchell & Shoemaker, 2017). The first permanent (secondary) teeth erupt at about 6 years of age. From adolescence, when all of the permanent teeth are in place, through middle adulthood, the teeth and gums remain healthy if individuals avoid fermentable carbohydrates and sticky sweets. Regular dental care and hygiene practices such as brushing and flossing help to prevent caries and periodontal disease.

As individuals grow older, numerous factors can result in poor oral care. These include age-related changes of the mouth, chronic disease such as diabetes, physical disabilities involving hand grasp or strength affecting the ability to perform oral care, lack of attention to oral care, and prescribed medications that affect the buccal (oral) mucosa. Aging teeth become brittle, drier, and darker. Teeth can become uneven, jagged, and fractured. Gums lose vascularity and tissue elasticity, which can cause dentures to fit poorly. Many older persons are edentulous and wear complete or partial dentures. It is important to determine whether older patients wear dentures and the condition of underlying supportive gum tissue.

The Eyes, Ears, and Nose. Although the structure of the eyes does not have marked developmental changes, altered visual acuity can occur at several points during the aging process; for example, when children start school or when patients reach middle age, visual acuity may change. As patients age, they are also at risk for changes in visual clarity (e.g., caused by glaucoma or cataracts) and visual field losses (e.g., caused by macular degeneration or glaucoma).

Structures of the ears do not change as patients age; however, changes in hearing acuity or balance may occur with aging. In young children, changes in hearing acuity may result from a foreign object being placed in the ear—this may be a temporary change, resolved once the object is removed. Changes may also result from repeated ear infections or exposure to loud noise, such as when children listen to loud music on headphones.

Older persons may have changes in the structure and function of the small bones in the inner ear that affect hearing acuity. Aging may result in increased cerumen production, which can also impede hearing acuity. In addition, the movement of fluid through the semicircular canals may change with age, and patients may experience positional dizziness or balance problems.

Although changes in the sense of smell can occur at any time, they seem to be more common in older persons. These changes may also affect taste and patients' appetite.

New and acute changes in the structure and function of the eyes, ears, and nose must be fully assessed and evaluated. Timely evaluation of these changes may result in effective treatments or confirm that they are age related.

Use of Sensory Aids. When patients wear eyeglasses, contact lenses, artificial eyes, or hearing aids, nurses need to assess their knowledge and ask them to describe the methods that are used for routine care (Box 38-4). The information gathered is then compared with the proper care technique for these devices. Any differences between patient practice and standard practice may indicate a need for patient education.

Self-Care Ability. Patients with physical or cognitive impairments need assistance with all or some aspects of personal hygiene. Assessment of patients' physical and cognitive statuses determines specifically which aspects of hygiene care can be performed independently, which require some assistance, and which require total assistance.

The assessment must include the measurement of patients' muscle strength, flexibility and dexterity, balance, coordination, and activity

BOX 38-4 Assessing a Patient's Use of Sensory Aids

Eyeglasses

Ask about purpose for wearing glasses (e.g., reading, distance, or both)

Ask about methods used to clean glasses

Ask about presence of symptoms (e.g., blurred vision, photophobia, headaches, irritation)

Contact Lenses

Determine type of lens worn

Ask about frequency and duration of time lenses are worn (including sleep time)

Ask about presence of symptoms (e.g., burning, excess tearing, redness, irritation, swelling, or sensitivity to light)

Ask about techniques used by the patient to cleanse, store, insert, and remove lenses

Ask about use of eye drops or ointments

Determine whether patient has an emergency identification bracelet or card that alerts others to remove patient's lenses in case of emergency

Artificial Eye

Ask about method used to insert and remove eye

Ask about method for cleansing eye

Ask about presence of symptoms (e.g., drainage, inflammation, or pain involving the orbit)

Hearing Aid

Ask about type of aid worn

Ask about methods used to cleanse aid

Ask about patient's ability to change battery and adjust hearing aid volume

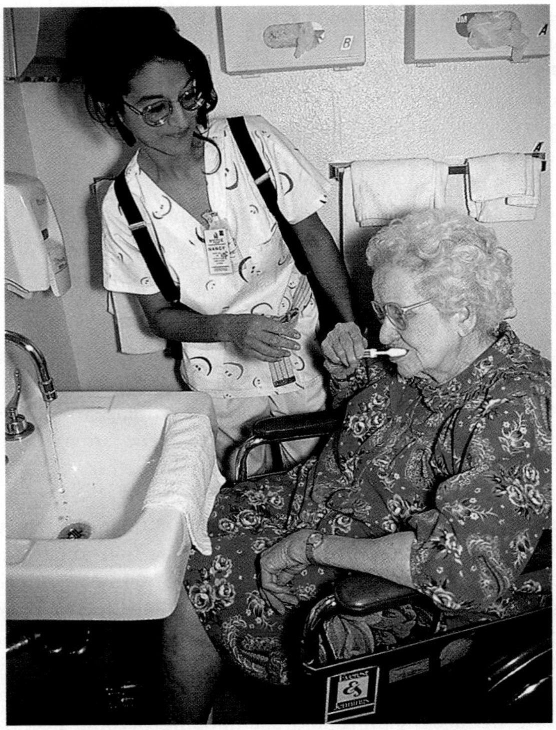

FIGURE 38-5 Observe the patient brushing teeth. Observation helps the nurse determine how much assistance the patient may need.

tolerance—these qualities are needed to perform activities such as bathing, brushing teeth, and bending over to inspect the feet. The degree of assistance needed by patients during hygiene care may also depend on vision, their ability to sit without support, their hand grasp strength, the range of motion in their extremities, or the presence of equipment such as an IV line, dressings, or traction. Painful conditions of the upper extremities pose special problems. Self-care ability is assessed by asking patients to perform activities such as brushing their teeth or combing their hair. The nurse needs to observe carefully as the patient carries out the activity and note whether the patient can perform the task thoroughly and correctly (Figure 38-5).

When a patient has self-care limitations, part of the assessment is to determine whether family or friends are available to assist. Assisting with hygiene measures can at times be unpleasant, so the assessment should include how the family members assist, how often this assistance is provided, and what their feelings are about being a caregiver. In addition, it is important to assess the home environment and its influence on the patient's hygiene practices. Does the home environment contain barriers that may affect the patient's self-care abilities? Water faucets that are too tight to easily adjust, bathtubs with high sides, and a bathroom too small to fit a wheelchair or walker in front of a sink are a few examples.

Hygiene Practices. An assessment of hygiene practices reveals a patient's grooming preferences. For example, a patient may choose to groom the hair in a certain style or to trim nails a certain way. When a patient has a physical disability, special precautions may be needed to perform grooming without injury. Asking the patient to assist or teach how to perform preferred grooming practices gives the patient a greater sense of independence and helps the nurse to avoid causing the patient discomfort or injury.

Cultural Factors. A patient's cultural background is an influential factor when determining hygiene needs. Culture plays a role not only in hygiene practices and preferences but also in sensitivity regarding personal space (see Chapter 9). For example, some patients may view tasks associated with closeness and touch as being offensive or impolite. Nurses need to ask patients what would make them feel most comfortable during a bath. Instead of a full bath, perhaps a patient would prefer only a partial bath, with a family member performing the bathing of private body areas. The patient may also defer part of the hygiene care. If, in the nurse's judgement, hygiene is critical to prevent developing or worsening problems, such as skin breakdown, the nurse must take the time to understand the patient's concerns and negotiate a mutually satisfactory solution to the problem.

Patients at Risk for Hygiene Problems. Some patients present risks that require more attentive and rigorous hygiene care (Table 38-5). These risks may result from adverse effects of medications, a lack of knowledge, an inability to perform hygiene, or a physical condition that potentially injures the skin or other structures. An immobilized patient who has a fever, for example, requires more frequent bathing to minimize perspiration on the skin, and more frequent turning and positioning to reduce the risk of skin breakdown.

Nurses need to anticipate whether a patient is predisposed to such risks and follow through with a complete assessment. For example, if a patient is receiving chemotherapy, the treatment has a risk of destroying the normal flora in the mouth, allowing for the overgrowth of

TABLE 38-5 Health Risks and Implications for Hygiene

Risks	Hygiene Implications
Oral Problems	
Inability to use upper extremities due to paralysis, weakness, or restriction (e.g., cast or dressing)	Patient lacks upper extremity strength or dexterity needed to brush teeth.
Dehydration, inability to take fluids or food by mouth	Dehydration causes excess drying and fragility of the mucosa, and increases the accumulation of secretions on the tongue and gums.
Presence of nasogastric or oxygen tubes; mouth breathers	These cause drying of the mucosa.
Chemotherapeutic drugs	Drugs kill rapidly multiplying cells, including normal cells lining the oral cavity. Ulcers and inflammation can develop.
Other medications (antihistamines)	These can cause a decrease in saliva production, which leads to thicker mucus and dryness of the oral mucosa (**xerostomia**).
Over-the-counter lozenges, cough drops, antacids, and chewable vitamins	Medications may contain large amounts of sugar. Repeated use increases sugar or acid content in mouth.
Radiation therapy to head and neck	Radiation therapy decreases the function of the salivary glands, which can contribute to stomatitis (Gupta & West, 2016).
Oral surgery, trauma to mouth, placement of an oral airway	These cause trauma to the oral cavity with swelling, ulcerations, inflammation, and bleeding.
Immunosuppression; altered blood clotting	These conditions predispose to inflammation and bleeding gums.
Diabetes mellitus	Patients with diabetes are prone to dryness of the mouth, gingivitis, periodontal disease, and tooth loss.
Skin Problems	
Immobilization	Dependent body parts are exposed to pressure from underlying surfaces. The inability to turn or change position increases the risk for pressure injuries.
Reduced sensation due to stroke, spinal cord injury, diabetes, local nerve damage	There is interruption in transmission of nerve impulses when excessive heat or cold, pressure, friction, or chemical irritants are applied to skin.
Limited protein or caloric intake and reduced hydration (e.g., caused by fever, burns, gastrointestinal alterations, poorly fitting dentures)	Limited caloric and protein intakes predispose to impaired tissue synthesis. The skin becomes thinner, less elastic, and smoother, with a loss of subcutaneous tissue. Poor wound healing may result. Reduced hydration impairs skin turgor.
Excessive secretions or excretions on the skin from perspiration, urine, watery fecal material, and wound drainage	Moisture is a medium for bacterial growth and can cause local skin irritation, softening of epidermal cells, and skin maceration.
Presence of external devices (e.g., casts, restraint, bandage, dressing)	A device can exert pressure or friction against the skin's surface.
Vascular insufficiency	Arterial blood supply to tissues is inadequate, or venous return is impaired, causing decreased circulation to the extremities. Tissue ischemia and breakdown may occur. The risk for infection is high.
Foot Problems	
Inability to bend over or see clearly	Patient is unable to fully visualize the entire surface of each foot, impairing his or her ability to adequately assess the condition of skin and nails.
Eye Care Problems	
Reduced dexterity and hand coordination	Physical limitations create an inability to safely insert or remove contact lenses.

opportunistic bacteria. Therefore, the oral examination should be more thorough and detailed, involving all surfaces of the tongue and mucosa. If a patient is diaphoretic, special attention should be given to body areas such as underneath the breasts and the perineal area, where moisture may collect and irritate skin surfaces. Nurses should anticipate problems created by these risks and provide appropriate preventive care. Their assessment should include a review of the patient's medical and surgical histories, medications, and specific risk factors.

Special Considerations in Hygiene Assessment. Depending on the type of hygiene the nurse is planning to provide, the nurse should conduct certain focused assessments. Before giving foot care, the nurse should assess the type of footwear worn by a patient. Children or young adults who frequently fail to wear socks may have excess perspiration that promotes fungal growth. Tight or poorly fitting shoes, socks, garters, or knee-high nylon stockings may cause skin irritation and interfere with circulation to the feet. Nurses should also assess whether patients wear clean footwear daily, because repeated use of soiled footwear can lead to infection. If patients have diabetes mellitus or another peripheral vascular disease, it is extremely important that they wear appropriate footwear. Extra-wide and extra-deep shoes accommodate bunions or hammer toes. Cushioned inner soles help redistribute pressure on the metatarsal head. Patients may need to be referred to a podiatrist and orthotic footwear specialist.

It is also important to assess patients' eating patterns before providing oral care. Patients should be asked whether problems are noted with chewing, swallowing, or the fit of their dentures, if any. Patients may have changed the type of food in their diet as a result of chewing difficulties. The presence of an ulcer or irritation may impair chewing and cause patients to avoid eating. This is common in older persons with poorly fitting dentures.

Patient Expectations. As is the case in any nursing assessment, it is important to know what patients expect from nursing care. For hygiene care, patients may simply expect to have hygiene preferences and practices applied in the health care setting. Nurses can assess patients' expectations by asking questions such as "To make you most comfortable and feeling at home, how can I best perform your bath and personal care?" or "How can we help you care for your teeth, nails, and hair, now that you are at home?"

Understanding patients' expectations and applying them in practice is important in establishing a trusting relationship. Truly individualizing hygiene care shows respect for patients' needs. As the nurse learns what each patient expects, this information can be incorporated into the individual's plan of care (see "Planning" section later in this chapter).

◆ Nursing Diagnosis

Through assessment nurses determine the condition of the skin, oral cavity, and other tissues, as well as a patient's need for and ability to meet personal hygiene needs. As nurses review all data gathered, they need to think about their knowledge pertaining to pre-existing conditions and then look for clusters of data suggesting a problem trend. For example, an older person with degenerative arthritis can present with pain in the joints, weakness, mobility limitations in the dominant hand, and a generally unkempt appearance. A closer review of assessment data reveals defining characteristics of an inability to wash body parts and difficulty turning and regulating a water faucet. The nursing diagnosis of *bathing/hygiene self-care deficit* is supported and becomes part of the plan of care. The accurate selection of nursing diagnoses requires critical thinking to identify actual or potential health problems. Assessment activities must be thorough in identifying all appropriate defining characteristics so that an accurate diagnosis can be made (Box 38-5).

The focus of nursing interventions depends on whether a patient has an actual alteration (e.g., impaired tissue integrity) or is at risk for a problem (e.g., risk for impaired oral mucous membrane). The patient with an actual alteration requires extensive hygiene care, which is often more thorough than routine care. For example, if the patient has skin breakdown, the nurse must initiate care more frequently to keep intact skin surfaces clean and dry and to eliminate factors such as moisture or drainage that can worsen the condition of the skin. The nurse must also provide care to promote healing of injured skin surfaces (see Chapter 46). If the patient is at risk for a problem, the nurse must institute preventive measures. In both cases, it may be beneficial to involve the wound-ostomy nurse in care planning. In the case of risk for impaired oral mucous membranes, it is important to keep the mucosa well hydrated, minimize foods irritating to tissues, and provide cleansing that soothes and reduces tissue inflammation.

The identification of related factors guides in the selection of nursing interventions. Diagnoses of *impaired oral mucous membrane related to malnutrition* and *impaired oral mucous membrane related to chemical trauma* require very different interventions. When malnutrition is a causal factor, the nurse needs to confer with a dietitian for appropriate dietary supplements and incorporate patient education into the plan. When mucosa are injured as a result of chemical trauma from chemotherapy, techniques for cleaning and hydrating inflamed tissues and eliminating sources of irritation are the focus of nursing care. Although many nursing diagnoses associated with hygiene problems are possible, the following are a few of the more common diagnoses:

- *Impaired dentition*
- *Fatigue*
- *Ineffective health maintenance*
- *Risk for infection*
- *Deficient knowledge about hygiene practices*
- *Impaired physical mobility*
- *Impaired oral mucous membrane*
- *Self-care deficit, bathing/hygiene, dressing/grooming, toileting*
- *Chronic low self-esteem*
- *Risk for impaired skin integrity*
- *Ineffective tissue perfusion*

BOX 38-5 NURSING DIAGNOSTIC PROCESS

Assessment Activities	Defining Characteristics	Nursing Diagnosis
Observe patient's attempt to bathe self either in bed or at bathroom sink. (*Note:* Be sure positioning does not restrict potential movement.)	Unable to wash body or body parts	*Self-care deficit in bathing or hygiene related to upper extremity weakness and generalized fatigue*
Assess patient's upper extremity strength, range of motion, and coordination.	Restricted upper extremity range of motion and strength Coordination adequate	
Ask patient about level of fatigue after bathing.	Complains of fatigue and needs to rest after bathing	
Obtain vital signs before and after bathing.	Pulse elevated from 90–110 beats per minute, blood pressure stable, respirations elevated from 16–22 breaths per minute	

◆ Planning

During planning, nurses synthesize information from multiple resources (Figure 38-6). Professional nursing standards and evidence-informed clinical guidelines are especially important to consider when developing a care plan for the patient. For example, the clinical practice guidelines of the Canadian Diabetes Association (2013) offer valuable foot care guidelines for diabetic patients. Critical thinking ensures that the patient's plan of care integrates knowledge about the individual patient, including preferences, health status, equipment needed, assistance available, and previous experience in providing hygiene care. Certain patients have multiple nursing diagnoses. The concept map (Figure 38-7) shows graphically how numerous nursing diagnoses can be interrelated.

Goals and Outcomes. The nurse and the patient work together to identify goals and expected outcomes and to develop an individualized care plan based on the patient's nursing diagnoses (Box 38-6). Goals are established with the patient's self-care abilities and resources in mind and focus on maintaining or improving the condition of the skin and mucosa, oral mucosa, or dental hygiene, for example. Outcomes should be appropriate, realistic, measurable, and achievable within patient limitations.

When providing patient hygiene, nurses care for a variety of patients with different self-care abilities and needs. For example, for a patient who has hemiparesis after a cerebrovascular accident, the nurse and the patient might develop the following goal: "Patient's musculoskeletal system remains free of breakdown or contractures." A series of realistic individualized expected outcomes would then be established

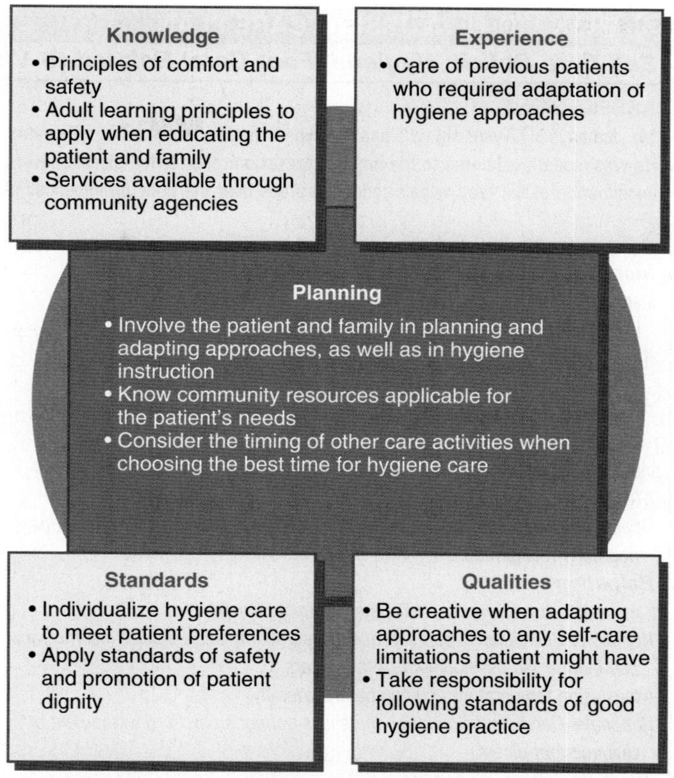

FIGURE 38-6 Critical thinking model for hygiene planning.

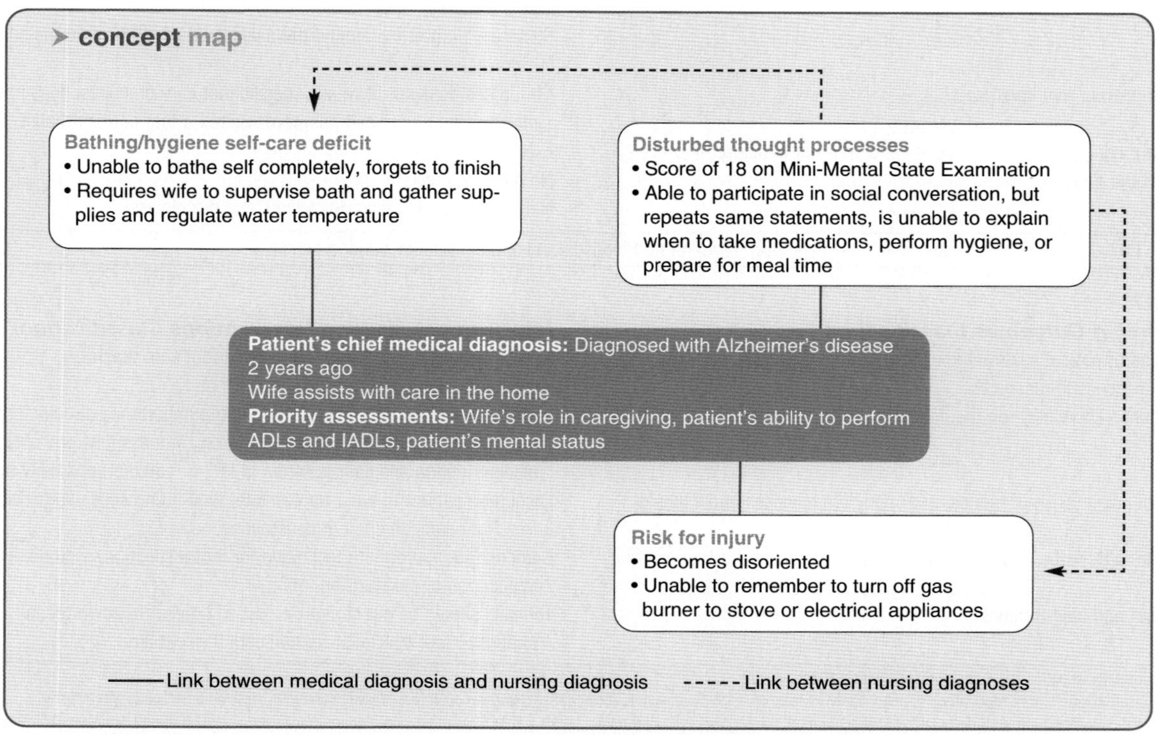

FIGURE 38-7 Concept map for a patient with Alzheimer's disease and hygiene needs. *ADLs,* Activities of daily living; *IADLs,* instrumental activities of daily living.

BOX 38-6 NURSING CARE PLAN

Self-Care Deficit: Hygiene (Foot Care) Related to Visual Impairment and Knowledge Deficit

ASSESSMENT

Mr. James is a 77-year-old who has had type 1 diabetes mellitus for 30+ years. He was recently admitted to the hospital for uncontrolled blood glucose levels. Examination of his feet reveals reddened areas over the bony prominences of the toes and calluses to the soles of the feet and to both heels. Mr. James's toenails are unkempt, yellow, and thickened. He states that he is unable to see well enough to trim his toenails because he has cataracts.

Assessment Activities	***Findings and Defining Characteristics***
Inspection	
Inspect the feet for dry, rough skin, fissures, calluses, lesions, blisters, inflammation, edema. *Rationale: Daily inspection is especially important for those patients at increased risk for developing pressure injuries.* *Prevention: Early recognition of risk factors associated with diabetic foot issues.*	Redness over bony prominences of toes Calluses on soles of feet and heels
Inspect the toenails for discoloration, thickness, and any abnormal findings (e.g., ingrown toenails). *Rationale: Monitor for signs of infections, redness, erythema for prevention and early recognition.*	Unkempt, yellow, thickened toenails
Palpation	
Palpate the dorsalis pedis and posterior tibial pulses. *Rationale: Decreased circulation due to neuropathy and vascular insufficiency can lead to the development of foot ulcers.*	Pedal pulses weak bilaterally
Assess skin temperature and compare bilaterally. *Rationale: Decreased circulation increases patient's risk for development of diabetic foot ulcers.*	Feet are cool to the touch bilaterally
Palpate for edema, tenderness. *Rationale: Bilateral dependent edema occurs with diabetic neuropathy.*	No edema or tenderness
Assess sensation. *Rationale: Neuropathy is a major risk factor for the development of foot ulcers.*	Decreased sensation bilaterally
Assess range of motion.	Range of motion is within normal limits
Protection	
Assess type and condition of footwear.	Patient wears ill-fitting shoes that are well worn, have slippery soles, and are approximately 10 years old Socks are tight fitting around the ankles and have holes on the soles
Hygiene	
Inquire about present foot care practices.	Mr. James does not have any specific foot care practices, does not use moisturizing lotion, and has never visited a foot care specialist
Inspect feet for odour, cleanliness, excessive dryness or moisture, and the condition of the nails.	Excessive dryness No odour is present Nails are unkempt, long, thickened, and discoloured

NURSING DIAGNOSIS: Self-care deficit: Hygiene (foot care) related to visual impairment and knowledge deficit.

PLANNING

Goals (Nursing Outcomes Classification)*	***Intervention (Nursing Interventions Classification)*** [†]
Attain baseline of patient's current knowledge and practices regarding foot hygiene and access to resources.	Assess patient's knowledge and current foot care practices. Assess patient's ability to perform ADLs and IADLS.
Increase patient's knowledge on the importance of foot hygiene.	Provide instruction on the need for and the importance of daily inspection of the feet for signs of skin breakdown (e.g., redness, blisters, abrasions, ulcers); friction and calluses from ill-fitting footwear; and daily hygiene.
Eliminate underlying cause of redness over bony prominences and calluses.	Encourage patient to wear appropriate, well-fitting shoes and socks that are free from damage and not constricting.
Patient is able to describe and demonstrate proper technique for foot hygiene.	Demonstrate appropriate technique for foot inspection, hygiene, and application of moisturizing lotion.
Nails are clean and well-trimmed.	Toenails should be cut straight across to prevent ingrown toenails. Refer patient to foot specialist for nail care if necessary.

ADLs, Activities of daily living; *IADLs,* instrumental activities of daily living.
*Outcome classification labels from Moorhead, S., Johnson, M., Maas, M. L., & Swanson, E. (Eds.). (2013). *Nursing outcomes classification (NOC)* (5th ed.). St. Louis, MO: Mosby.
[†]Intervention classification labels from Bulechek, G. M., Butcher, H. K., & McCloskey Dochterman, J. (Eds.). (2013). *Nursing interventions classification (NIC)* (6th ed.). St. Louis, MO: Mosby Elsevier.

EVALUATION

Patient's foot hygiene practices have improved. Feet are clean, skin integrity is maintained, feet are free from injury, and there is a decrease in dryness. Patient is seeing a foot care specialist every 3 to 4 weeks for nail care, callus removal, and foot assessment. Appropriate, well-fitting footwear is worn.

to assist the patient in meeting this goal. These outcomes may include the following:

- Patient's skin is clean, dry, and intact without signs of inflammation.
- Patient's skin remains elastic and well hydrated.
- Patient's range of joint motion remains within normal limits on both affected and unaffected sides.

Setting Priorities. The patient's condition influences the plan for delivering hygiene. A seriously ill patient usually needs a daily bath because body secretions accumulate and can lead to skin breakdown. An older patient at home may require a visit from a home care aide to assist with a tub bath. Patients who are normally inactive during the day and have skin that tends to be dry may need to bathe only twice a week. Nurses must plan for necessary assistance for patients who are weakened or possess poor coordination. For example, a patient who has hemiparesis and has difficulty getting out of the tub should have a tub chair, handrails, or extra personnel available for help.

Timing is also important in planning hygiene. Being interrupted in the middle of a bath to undergo a diagnostic procedure can frustrate and embarrass a patient. After extensive diagnostic tests (e.g., a stress test), it may be best to delay hygiene and allow a patient to rest.

Continuity of Care. It is important to plan for care throughout the hospital stay, from admission to discharge, whether to a rehabilitation facility or back home. When a patient needs assistance as a result of a self-care limitation, the family becomes a valuable resource. Family members can usually assist with hygiene measures but may need support and guidance in adapting techniques to fit patient limitations. Nurses must be aware of equipment and procedures that were used while the patient was in the hospital or facility so that the patient and family are knowledgeable about the care, have the skill needed to provide the care, and have access to necessary equipment. In addition, various community resources may be needed. For example, if the nurse is involved in the care of a homeless patient, the nurse may need to be aware of the location of clothing distribution centres for basic hygiene supplies or a shelter where bathing facilities are available. Forming partnerships with social workers or staff in local area churches and schools can assist in ensuring that patients have the resources they need to maintain hygiene.

◆ Implementation

Providing hygiene is a very basic part of a patient's care. The use of caring practices helps to alleviate the patient's anxiety and promote comfort and relaxation while the nurse performs each hygiene measure. For example, while giving a patient a bath and changing a gown, the nurse needs to use a gentle approach in turning and repositioning the patient and use a soft, gentle voice while conversing with the patient to help relieve any fears or concerns. For patients with symptoms such as pain or nausea, administering symptom relief therapies before starting hygiene care helps to prepare the patient for the procedure.

Another important part of implementation is assisting patients to administer their own hygiene. This includes educating patients on proper hygiene techniques and connecting patients with the community resources necessary to enable them to perform hygiene care. The same patients at risk for hygiene problems are those in greatest need of understanding their risks, knowing the implications, and having the information they need to make choices about when and how hygiene is performed.

Health Promotion. In primary health care settings, nurses educate and counsel patients and families on appropriate hygiene techniques. A new mother needs assistance in learning how to bathe her newborn infant. An older person needs to become informed about the importance of regular ear care to avoid hearing deficits resulting from accumulated cerumen. When assisting patients, nurses must maintain the standards for hygiene illustrated in this chapter and incorporate adaptations as needed to their patients' lifestyle, living arrangements, abilities, and preferences. Guidelines to assist nurses in providing education to patients about hygiene are presented in Box 38-7.

Acute and Restorative Care. Nursing knowledge and skills needed for performing hygiene care are consistent across all health care settings where acute and restorative care are provided. In addition, some of the skills in this section are applicable in areas of health promotion.

In health care settings where patients receive direct nursing care, a variety of scheduled hygiene measures are provided (Box 38-8). Times of providing such measures may change because of factors affecting the organization or the scheduling of care such as planned diagnostic and treatment procedures, the patient's need for more hygiene, or the nurse's work assignment.

Bathing and Skin Care

Bathing and skin care are a part of total hygiene. The extent of patients' bath and the methods used for bathing depend on their physical abilities, health problems, and the degree of hygiene required. If patients are physically dependent or cognitively impaired, nurses need to increase skin assessment and provide skin care directed toward reducing the risk for skin breakdown. When bathing cognitively impaired patients, nurses must consider these patients' special needs and challenges (Box 38-9). These patients can easily become afraid, may use physical and verbal aggressive behaviours to avoid bathing, and may also display self-injurious behaviours (Wolf & Czekanski, 2015).

A complete bed bath is used with patients who are totally dependent and require total hygiene care. It is an activity that can be

BOX 38-7 Educating Patients About Hygiene Care

- Make instructions relevant. After assessing a patient's knowledge, motivation, and health beliefs, provide information that relates to the patient's situation and will be most useful in resolving the patient's problem. For example, when offering foot care instruction to a patient with diabetes mellitus, explain how the circulation to the feet can be impaired and how that poses a risk for poor healing and infection should the skin become cut or broken.
- Adapt teaching of techniques to the patient's personal bathing facilities. Not all patients will have the ideal situation that exists in a health care setting (e.g., easily accessible shower or a bedside table to place over a bed). Use the facilities or equipment that the patient has so that personal-care items are easy to reach, the patient's safety is ensured, and the patient feels comfortable when performing hygiene. For example, a young mother may feel more comfortable bathing an infant in a baby bath chair.
- Teach the patient steps to take to avoid injury. Almost any hygiene procedure can pose risks (e.g., cutting a nail too close to the skin, failing to adjust the water temperature of a bath, or using tap water for contact lens care). Any instruction you provide must clearly outline safety risks.
- Reinforce infection control practices. Damage to the skin, mucosa, eyes, or other tissues creates an immediate risk for infection. Be sure the patient understands the relationship between healthy and intact skin and tissues, hand hygiene practices, and the prevention of infection.

exhausting for patients, even if the nurse provides all the care. Nurses must anticipate and assess whether patients are physically able to tolerate a complete bath. Observing for verbal and nonverbal cues provides a measure of their physical tolerance. A **partial bed bath** involves bathing only those body parts that would cause discomfort or odour if not cleaned, and those areas not easily reached by the patient. This includes perineal care. Aging or dependent patients in need of only partial hygiene and self-sufficient bedridden patients unable to reach all body parts receive partial bed baths. Nurses need to carefully assess patients to determine the amount of assistance required during hygiene care. Skill 38-1 outlines the procedures for bathing a bedridden client.

When administering a complete or partial bath, it is important to assess the condition of the skin to determine which type of cleaning product is necessary or whether the patient requires daily bathing. Patients with excessively dry skin are predisposed to skin impairment. The nurse may decide to skip a bath for a day or bathe only badly soiled areas. The use of a soap that contains emollients is another option. Lubricating the skin with lotion can also help reduce dryness.

The tub bath or shower can be used to give a more thorough bath than a bed bath. Safety is of primary concern because the surface of a tub or shower stall is slippery. In some settings, it is necessary to obtain a physician's or nurse practitioner's order for a shower or tub bath. In some agencies, showers are equipped with a chair for patients with weakness or poor balance. Both tubs and showers should be equipped with grab bars for patients to hold on to during their entry and exit and when manoeuvring. Patients vary in how much assistance they need. Regardless of the type of bath the patient receives, the following guidelines should be used:

- *Provide privacy.* Close the door or pull the room curtains around the bathing area. While bathing the patient, expose only the areas being bathed.
- *Maintain safety.* Keep the side rails up while away from the patient's bedside. This is critical for dependent, debilitated, and unconscious patients. (*Note:* When side rails are used as a restraint, a physician's order may be needed. Check your agency's policy.) Place the call light within the patient's reach if you are leaving the room temporarily.
- *Maintain warmth.* The room should be kept warm because the patient is partially uncovered and may become chilled. Wet skin causes an excess loss of heat through convection. Control drafts. Keep the patient covered, exposing only the body part being washed during the bath.
- *Promote independence.* Encourage the patient to participate in as many of the bathing activities as possible. Offer assistance when needed.
- *Anticipate needs.* Bring a new set of clothing and hygiene products to the bedside or bathroom.

BOX 38-8 Hygiene Care Schedule in Acute and Long-Term Care Settings

Early Morning Care

When nurses work the night shift, they may be required to provide basic hygiene to patients getting ready for breakfast, scheduled tests, or early morning surgery. Early morning care (often referred to as "A.M. care") includes offering a bedpan or urinal if the patient is not ambulatory, washing the patient's hands and face, and assisting with oral care.

Routine Morning Care

Before or after breakfast, care includes offering a bedpan or urinal to patients confined to bed; providing a bath or shower; giving perineal care; giving oral hygiene and foot, nail, and hair care; assisting with shaving, giving a back rub; changing the patient's gown or pyjamas; changing the bed linens; and straightening the patient's bedside unit and room. This is often referred to as "complete A.M. care."

Afternoon Care

Hospitalized patients often undergo many exhausting diagnostic tests or procedures in the morning. In rehabilitation centres, patients may participate in physiotherapy during the morning. Afternoon hygiene care includes washing the hands and face, assisting with oral care, offering a bedpan or urinal to those patients who are not ambulatory, and straightening bed linen.

Evening, or Hour-Before-Sleep, Care

Before bedtime, nurses can offer personal hygiene care that helps a patient relax to promote sleep. Evening care, or P.M. care, may include changing soiled bed linens, gowns, or pyjamas; assisting the patient in washing the face and hands; providing or assisting with oral hygiene; giving a back massage; and offering a bedpan or urinal to nonambulatory patients. Patients should be asked if they would like a beverage, such as juice, if permitted.

BOX 38-9 EVIDENCE-INFORMED PRACTICE

Bathing Patients Who Have Dementia or Alzheimer's Disease

Provide individualized and flexible patient-centred care:

- Obtain bathing history—what works, what doesn't work.
- Identify bathing preferences from the patient, other caregivers, or family.
- Determine the method that is least distressing to the patient (e.g., soaking feet in the bathtub; use of prepackaged commercial bath cleansing products [see Figure 38-8]; no-rinse shampoo cap—if hair washing causes the patient distress).
- If patient fears water, try using coloured water or drawing a bubble bath.
- Prepare the bath environment in advance, with adequate lighting and necessary supplies (soap, shampoo, towels, etc.).
- Minimize the time the patient is unclothed, and ensure that the bathing environment is warm.
- Use distraction and negotiation instead of demands (e.g., give the patient a washcloth to keep hands occupied).
- Minimize noise in the bathing area or play the patient's favourite music softly in the background.
- Set priorities regarding which body parts need bathing and which parts can be "skipped" (e.g., separate hair washing from bathing).
- Assess whether the patient requires glasses or a hearing aid, which can assist with communication (remove aids as required during bathing after communicating your intent to the patient).
- Praise the patient's accomplishments.

Adapted from Alzheimer Society of Canada. (2015). *Personal care.* Retrieved from http://www.alzheimer.ca/en/Living-with-dementia/Day-to-day-living/Personal-care; and Wolf, Z., & Czekanski, K. (2015). Bathing disability and bathing persons with dementia. *Medsurg Nursing, 24*(1), 9–22.

SKILL 38-1 BATHING A PATIENT

Delegation Considerations

Skills of bathing may be delegated to an unregulated care provider. Instructions about the following should be provided:

- The importance of not massaging reddened skin areas
- The clarification of early signs of impaired skin integrity
- The importance of reporting changes in the patient's skin
- Proper positioning of an in-dwelling catheter during perineal care
- The importance of reporting any perineal drainage, excoriation, or rash observed

Equipment

- Washcloths and bath towels
- Wash basin
- Bath blanket (warm, if possible)
- Cleaning solution (agency or patient specific)
- Personal hygiene items (unscented deodorant, powder, lotion)
- Clean hospital gown or patient's own pyjamas or gown
- Bed linen
- Linen bag
- Disposable gloves
- Disposable wipes
- Bedpan or urinal

PROCEDURE

STEPS	RATIONALE
General Instructions	
1. Review orders for specific safety measures concerning the patient's movement, positioning, or isolation precautions.	• Prevents accidental injury to the patient during bathing activities. • Determines level of assistance required by the patient.
2. Explain procedure, and ask patient for suggestions on how to prepare supplies. Encourage and promote independence by asking the patient how much of the bath he or she wishes to complete.	• Promotes patient's cooperation and participation. • Promotes patient's comfort and provides an opportunity to include cultural or personal hygiene preferences in hygiene care. • Patient participates in plan of care.
3. Assess patient's ability to perform self-care and allow patient to perform as much of the bath as possible.	• Determines the amount of assistance required and the need for specialized equipment or additional personnel. • Encourages and promotes independence.
4. Assess patient's tolerance for activity, comfort level, cognitive ability, and musculoskeletal function.	• Determines patient's ability to perform self-care and level of assistance required. Also, determines type of bath to administer (e.g., tub bath or partial bed bath).

CRITICAL DECISION POINT: *Patients whose level of independence and mobility change frequently may require more or less assistance during bathing.*

STEPS	RATIONALE
5. Assess patient's bathing preferences: frequency, type of hygiene products, and other factors related to patient preferences.	• Encourages and promotes patient participation.
6. Ask whether patient has noticed any problems or unusual marks on skin. Observe the skin throughout the procedure, paying particular attention to areas that were previously soiled or reddened or showed early signs of breakdown.	• Provides information to direct physical assessment of skin during bathing.
7. Begin complete or partial bed bath, or tub/whirlpool bath or shower.	
A. Complete or partial bed bath	
(1) Close room doors and draw the room divider curtain.	• Privacy ensures patient's mental and physical comfort.
(2) Prepare equipment and supplies.	• Reduces transmission of microorganisms and avoids interrupting the procedure or leaving the patient unattended to retrieve missing equipment.
(3) For nonambulatory patients, offer a bedpan or urinal. Provide a towel and washcloth for perineal care afterward.	• Patient will feel more comfortable after voiding. Prevents the interruption of bath.
(4) Perform hand hygiene. If patient's skin is soiled with drainage or body secretions, put on disposable gloves. Ensure that the patient is not allergic to latex.	• Reduces transmission of microorganisms.
(5) Place hospital bed at appropriate level, lower side rail closest to you. Assist patient in assuming a comfortable position, preferably supine. Bring or have the patient move toward side closest to you.	• Raising the height of the bed to the appropriate position facilitates proper body mechanics. Maintains patient's comfort throughout procedure. Minimizes strain on back muscles because you do not have to reach across the bed.
(6) Loosen the top covers. Place bath blanket over the top sheet. Remove top sheet from under the blanket. If possible, have patient hold bath blanket while you withdraw sheet. Optional: Use the top sheet when a bath blanket is not available.	• Removal of top linens prevents them from becoming soiled or moist during the bath. Blanket provides warmth and privacy. The patient is not exposed unnecessarily.

Continued

SKILL 38-1 BATHING A PATIENT—cont'd

STEPS	RATIONALE
(7) If top sheet is to be reused, fold it for replacement later. If not, dispose in linen bag, taking care not to allow linen to contact uniform.	• Proper disposal helps prevent transmission of microorganisms.
(8) Assist patient with oral hygiene. See Skill 38-3.	
(9) Remove patient's gown or pyjamas. If the patient has an intravenous (IV) line infusing and the gown has snaps, simply unsnap and remove the gown without disconnecting the IV tubing. If the gown does not have snaps, remove gown from the arm without IV line first; then lower the IV container or remove from the pump and slide the gown covering the affected arm over the tubing and container. Rehang IV container and check flow rate (see Step 7A[9] illustrations) or reset pump rate. Do not disconnect the tubing. If an extremity is injured or has reduced mobility, begin removal from the unaffected side. Ensure that the fresh gown has snaps.	• Provides full exposure of body parts during bathing. Undressing unaffected side first allows easier manipulation of gown over body part with reduced range of motion (ROM). • Manipulation of IV tubing and container will possibly disrupt flow rate.

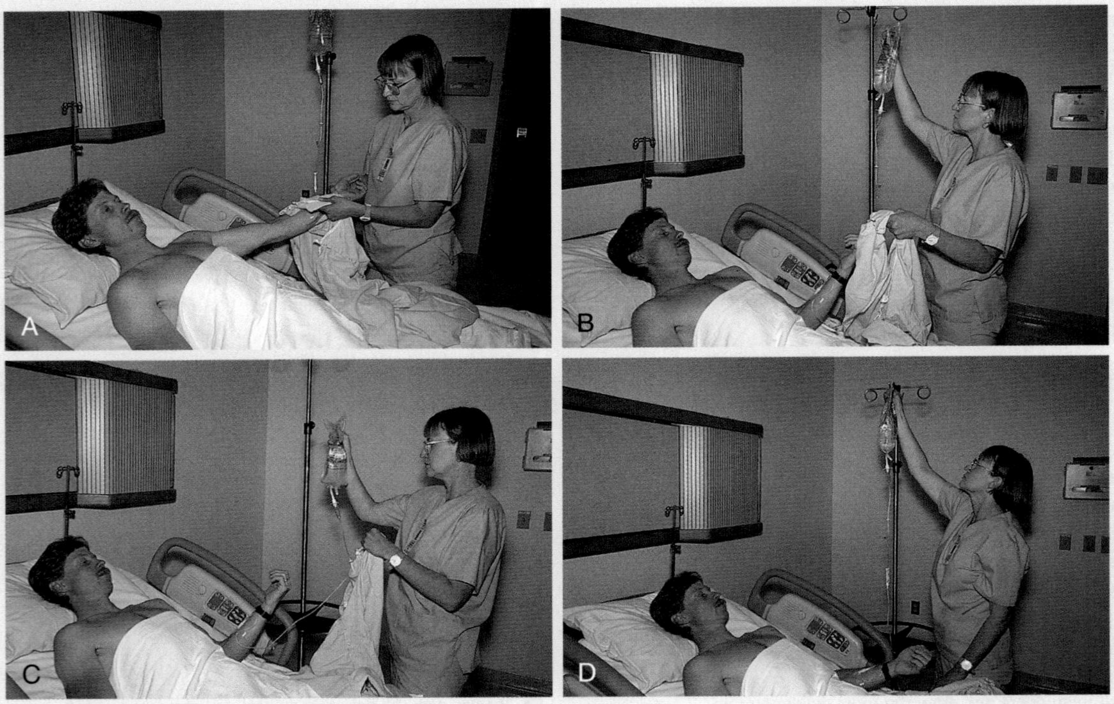

STEP 7A(9) **A,** Remove patient's gown. **B,** Remove IV bag from pole. **C,** Slide IV tubing through arm of patient's gown. **D,** Rehang IV bag and check flow rate.

CRITICAL DECISION POINT: *If available, be sure that patients with an IV line or upper extremity injury have a gown with snap or tie sleeves; this ensures easy access to the upper extremities during hygiene.*

CRITICAL DECISION POINT: *When an IV pump is used, it may be appropriate to manually adjust the IV flow rate to keep-vein-open (KVO) and remove the IV tubing from the pump (check agency policy). Once the gown has been removed, reset the pump to the prescribed IV flow rate (see Chapter 40).*

STEPS	RATIONALE
(10) Raise the side rail. Fill a wash basin two-thirds full with warm water. Have patient place fingers in water to test temperature tolerance. Change the water as necessary throughout the bath.	• Raising side rail maintains the patient's safety as you leave the bedside. Warm water promotes comfort, relaxes muscles, and prevents unnecessary chilling. Testing the temperature prevents accidental burns.
(11) Remove pillow, if allowed, and raise head of the bed 30–45 degrees. Place bath towel under the patient's head. Place a second bath towel over patient's chest.	• Removal of the pillow makes it easier to wash the patient's ears and neck. The placement of towels prevents soiling of the bed linen and bath blanket.
(12) Immerse washcloth in water and wring thoroughly. If desired, fold the washcloth around the fingers of your hand to form a mitt (see Step 7A[12] illustration).	• A mitt retains water and heat better than a loosely held washcloth and prevents splashing and cold edges from brushing against the patient.

STEPS	RATIONALE
(13) Inquire whether the patient is wearing contact lenses. Wash patient's eyes with plain warm water. Use a different section of mitt for each eye. Move mitt from inner to outer canthus (see Step 7A[13] illustration). Soak any crusts on eyelid for 2–3 minutes with damp cloth before attempting removal. Dry eyes thoroughly but gently.	• Soap irritates eyes. The use of separate sections of the mitt reduces infection transmission. Bathing the eye from inner to outer canthus prevents secretions from entering the nasolacrimal duct. Pressure can cause internal injury.

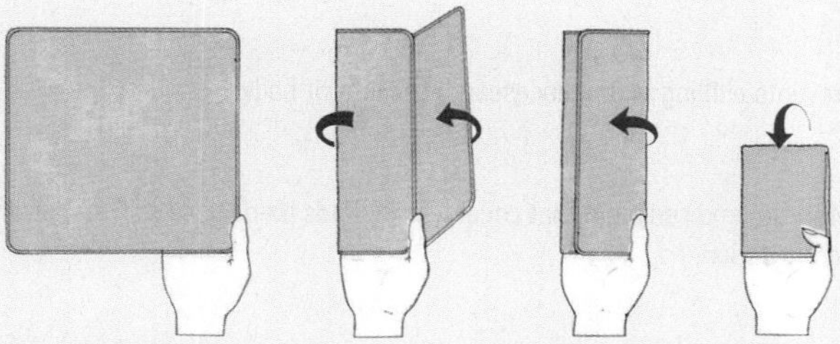

STEP 7A(12) Steps for folding washcloth to form a mitt.

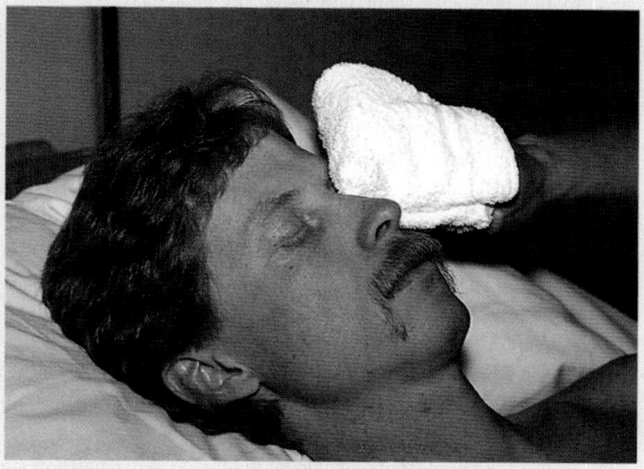

STEP 7A(13) Wash eye from inner to outer canthus.

STEPS	RATIONALE
(14) Ask whether patient prefers to use soap on his or her face. Wash, rinse, and thoroughly dry all areas of the face, neck, and ears. (Men may wish to shave at this point or after the bath.)	• Soap tends to dry the face, which is exposed to air more than other body parts.
(15) Expose patient's arm that is farthest from you and place bath towel lengthwise under the arm.	• Prevents soiling of bed. Washing far side first eliminates contaminating clean areas once they are washed.
(16) Bathe arm using long, firm strokes from distal to proximal areas (fingers to axilla). Raise and support arm as needed while thoroughly washing the axilla (see Step 7A[16] illustration).	• Soap lowers the surface tension of the skin and facilitates the removal of debris and bacteria when friction is applied during washing. Long, firm strokes stimulate circulation. Movement of the arm exposes the axilla and exercises the joint's normal ROM.

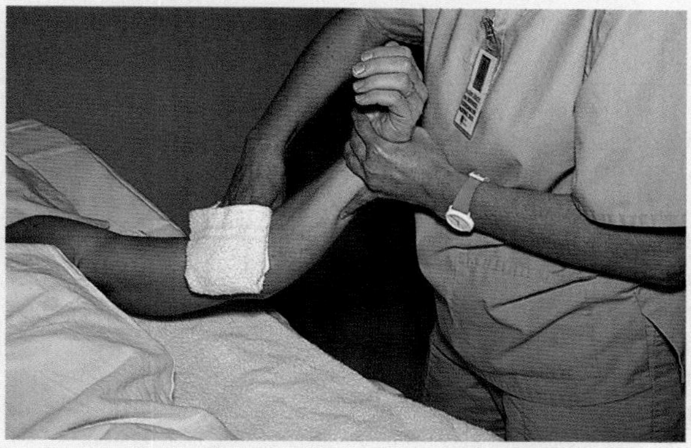

STEP 7A(16) Washing from fingers to axilla.

STEPS	RATIONALE
(17) Rinse and dry arm and axilla thoroughly. If patient uses deodorant or talcum powder, apply it. Be sure to use unscented products where possible.	• Excess moisture causes skin maceration or softening. Deodorant controls body odour.
(18) Fold bath towel in half and lay it on the bed beside the patient. Place a basin on the towel. Immerse patient's hand in water. Allow hand to soak for 3–5 minutes before washing hand and fingernails (see Skill 38-2). Remove basin and dry hand well.	• Soaking softens cuticles and calluses of the hand, loosens debris beneath nails, and enhances the feeling of cleanliness. Thorough drying removes moisture from between fingers. *Note:* Do not soak if the patient is diabetic or is cognitively impaired and unable to understand the procedure.
(19) Cover the arm with bath blanket or towel. Repeat steps 15–18 for the other arm.	

CRITICAL DECISION POINT: *If a patient is at risk for falls, be sure the two side rails are up before obtaining fresh water or other supplies. Remember, side rails cannot be used as a restraint unless ordered.*

Continued

SKILL 38-1 BATHING A PATIENT—cont'd

STEPS	RATIONALE
(20) Cover patient's chest with a bath towel, and fold bath blanket down to the umbilicus. With one hand, lift edge of towel away from patient's chest. With washcloth or mitted hand, bathe chest using long, firm strokes. Take special care to wash skinfolds under the patient's breasts. Keep patient's chest covered between wash and rinse periods. Dry well.	• Draping prevents unnecessary exposure of body parts. The towel maintains warmth and privacy. Secretions and dirt collect easily in areas of tight skinfolds. Skinfolds are susceptible to excoriation if not cleaned and dried properly.
(21) Place bath towel lengthwise over patient's chest and abdomen. (Two towels may be needed.) Fold blanket down to just above the pubic region.	• Prevents chilling and unnecessary exposure of body parts.
(22) With one hand, lift the bath towel. With mitted hand, bathe the abdomen, giving special attention to bathing the umbilicus and abdominal folds. Keep the abdomen covered between washing and rinsing. Dry well.	• Moisture and sediment that collect in skinfolds predispose skin to maceration and irritation.
(23) Cover patient's chest and abdomen with top of the bath blanket or bath towels. Expose far leg by folding blanket toward midline. Be sure other leg and perineum are covered.	• Maintains patient's warmth and comfort. Prevents chilling and unnecessary exposure.
(24) Place bath towel lengthwise under the far leg and, using firm strokes (unless contraindicated), wash, rinse, and dry thoroughly. Support the leg with one hand if patient is unable to support it.	• Promotes venous return.

CRITICAL DECISION POINT: *Patients with a history of deep vein thrombosis (DVT) or hypercoagulation disorders should not have their lower extremities washed with long, firm strokes.*

STEPS	RATIONALE
(25) Clean the foot, making sure to bathe between toes. Clean and clip nails as per physician or nurse practitioner orders (see Skill 38-2). Dry well. If skin is dry, apply lotion.	• Secretions and moisture can accumulate between the toes. Lotion helps retain moisture and soften the skin. • Patient's own nail clippers should be used to avoid the transmission of microorganisms.

CRITICAL DECISION POINT: *Do not massage any reddened area on the patient's skin as it can increase the risk of skin breakdown (Maher, Meehan, Hertz, et al., 2013).*

STEPS	RATIONALE
(26) Repeat Steps 23–25 for the other leg and foot.	
(27) Assist patient in assuming a prone or side-lying position (as applicable). Place the towel lengthwise along the patient's side. Put on disposable gloves if not done so already.	• Exposes back and buttocks for bathing. Prevents contact with microorganisms in body secretions.
(28) Wash, rinse, and dry patient's back from neck to buttocks using long, firm strokes (see Step 7A[28] illustration). Pay special attention to folds of the buttocks and the anus for redness or skin breakdown. Give a back massage (see Chapter 31). Change bath water if necessary and put on disposable gloves.	• Skinfolds near buttocks and anus may contain fecal secretions that harbour microorganisms. • Prolonged pressure on the sacral area or other bony prominences may lead to the development of pressure injuries. • Changing the water prevents the transfer of microorganisms from the anal area to genitalia.

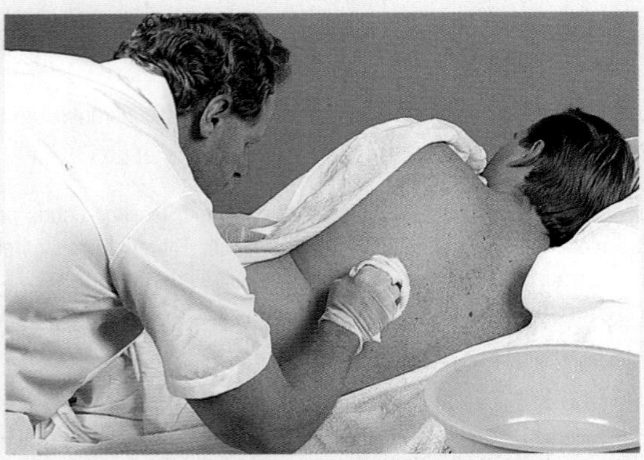

STEP 7A(28) Washing patient's back.

STEPS	RATIONALE
(a) Female perineal care	
(a1) Assist patient in assuming a dorsal recumbent position, if not contraindicated. Cover chest and upper extremities with a towel and lower extremities with a bath blanket. Expose only the genitalia. (If patient can wash, covering entire body with a bath blanket may be preferable.) Clean the perineal area. Pay special attention to skinfolds. Patients at risk for infection of the genitalia, urinary tract, or reproductive tract include those with in-dwelling catheters or fecal or urinary incontinence. If fecal material is present, enclose in a fold of underpad and remove with disposable wipes.	• Provides easy access to genitalia. • Patients capable of performing a partial bath usually prefer to wash their own genitalia. • Secretions that accumulate on surface of skin surrounding genitalia act as a reservoir for infection. • Cleaning reduces transmission of microorganisms from the anus to the urethra or genitalia.
(a2) Wash labia majora. Wipe from the perineum to the rectum. Repeat on the opposite side using a different section of the washcloth.	• Wiping from the perineum to the rectum reduces the chance of transmitting fecal organisms to the urinary meatus.
(a3) Separate the labia with your nondominant hand, exposing the urethral meatus and vaginal orifice. Wash downward from the pubic area toward the rectum in one smooth stroke (see Step 7A[28][a3] illustration). Use a separate section of cloth for each stroke. Cleanse thoroughly around the labia minora, clitoris, and vaginal orifice.	• Cleaning method reduces the risk of transferring microorganisms to the urinary meatus (cleaning from area of least contamination to most contamination, as secretions that collect around the labia minora facilitate bacterial growth). (For menstruating women or patients with in-dwelling urinary catheters, clean with disposable wipes.)
(a4) Assist patient to a comfortable position.	
(a5) Remove disposable gloves and perform hand hygiene.	• Helps prevent the transmission of infection.
(b) Male perineal care	
(b1) Lower the side rails, and assist patient to a supine position. Note restriction in mobility. Patients at risk for infection of the genitalia, urinary tract, or reproductive tract include uncircumcised males and patients with in-dwelling catheters or fecal or urinary incontinence.	• Provides full exposure of male genitalia. • Patients capable of performing a partial bath usually prefer to wash their own genitalia.
(b2) Gently raise the penis, and place a bath towel underneath. Gently grasp the shaft of penis. If the patient is uncircumcised, retract the foreskin (see Step 7A[28][b2] illustration). If the patient has an erection, perineal care can be deferred until later.	• Gentle but firm handling reduces the chance of the patient having an erection. Secretions capable of harbouring microorganisms collect underneath the foreskin. Cleaning the penis can lead to an erection, which can embarrass both the patient and you.

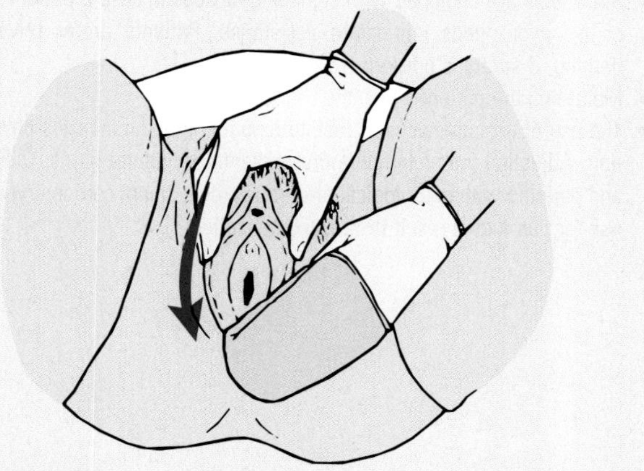

STEP 7A(28)(a3) Cleanse from perineum to rectum (front to back).

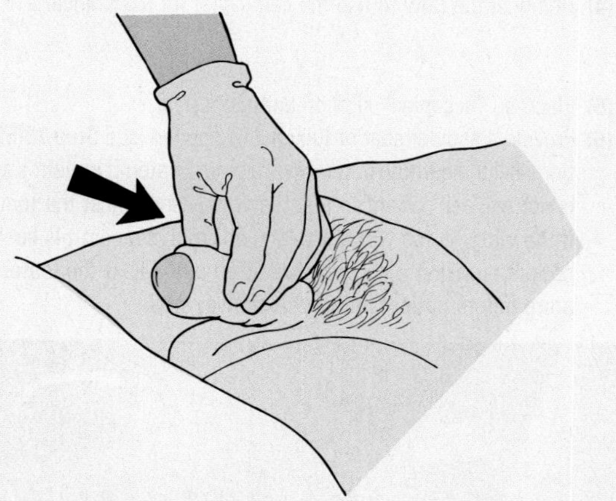

STEP 7A(28)(b2) Fully retract foreskin.

STEPS	RATIONALE
(b3) Wash tip of the penis at the urethral meatus first, using a circular motion. Clean from the meatus outward. Rinse and dry gently.	• The direction of the cleaning moves from areas of least contamination to most contamination, preventing microorganisms from entering the urethra.
(b4) Return foreskin to its natural position.	• Tightening of the foreskin around the shaft of the penis can cause local edema and discomfort.

Continued

SKILL 38-1 BATHING A PATIENT—cont'd

STEPS	RATIONALE
(b5) Wash the shaft of the penis with gentle but firm downward strokes. Pay special attention to the underlying surface of the penis. Rinse and dry thoroughly.	• The underlying surface of the penis may have a greater accumulation of secretions.
(b6) Gently clean scrotum, making sure to wash underlying skinfolds. Rinse and dry thoroughly.	• Pressure on scrotal tissue can be painful to the patient. Secretions collect between skinfolds.
(b7) Inspect the surface of external genitalia after cleaning.	• Thick secretions may cover underlying skin lesions or areas of breakdown. Evaluation determines the need for additional hygiene.
(b8) If patient has bowel or urinary incontinence, apply a thin layer of skin barrier cream to the buttock, anus, and perineal area.	• Protects skin from excess moisture and toxins from urine and stool.
(b9) Assist patient to a comfortable position and cover with bath blanket.	
(29) Assist patient in dressing. Comb patient's hair. Women may want to apply makeup, and men may wish to shave at this point. Assist patient to a chair or wheelchair.	• Promotes patient's body image.
(30) Make the patient's bed (see Skill 38-5).	• Provides a clean environment.
(31) Remove soiled linen and place it in a linen bag. Clean and replace the bathing equipment. Replace the call light and personal possessions. Leave the room as clean and comfortable as possible.	• Helps prevent the transmission of microorganisms. A clean environment promotes the patient's comfort. Keeping the call light and articles of care within reach promotes the patient's safety.
(32) Remove disposable gloves (if applied) and perform hand hygiene.	• Reduces the transmission of microorganisms.
B. Tub or whirlpool bath or shower (verify with agency policy whether a physician's or nurse practitioner's order is needed and whether you need to remain in the room during the patient's bath)	
(1) Check tub or shower for cleanliness. Use cleaning techniques outlined in agency policy. Place rubber mat on tub or shower bottom. Place disposable bath mat or towel on the floor in front of the tub or shower.	• Cleaning helps prevent the transmission of microorganisms. Mats prevent slipping and falling.
(2) Collect all hygienic aids, toiletry items, and linens requested by the patient. Place within easy reach of the tub or shower.	• Placing items close at hand prevents possible falls when patient reaches for equipment.
(3) Assist patient to the bathroom if necessary. Have patient wear a robe and slippers to bathroom.	• Assistance prevents accidental falls. Wearing a robe and slippers prevents chilling and provides for privacy and comfort.
(4) Demonstrate how to use the call signal for assistance.	• Bathrooms are equipped with signalling devices in case a patient feels faint or weak or needs immediate assistance. Patients prefer privacy during bathing, if safety is not jeopardized.
(5) Place an "occupied" sign on bathroom door.	• Maintains the patient's privacy.
(6) Provide a shower seat or tub chair if needed (see Step 7B[6] illustration). Fill the bathtub halfway with warm water. If patient's sensation is normal, ask patient to test the water, and adjust the temperature if the water is too warm. Explain which faucet controls hot water. If patient is taking a shower, turn it on and adjust the water temperature before patient enters the shower stall.	• The use of assistive devices facilitates bathing and minimizes physical exertion. Adjusting water temperature prevents accidental burns. Older persons and patients with neurological alterations (e.g., spinal cord injury) are at high risk for burns as a result of reduced sensation.

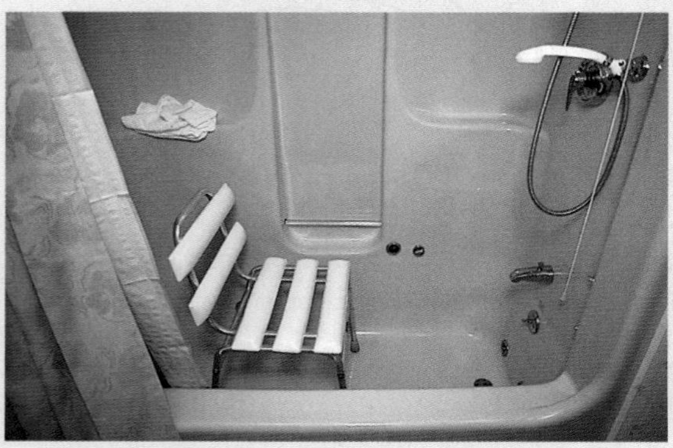

STEP 7B(6) Shower seat for patient safety.

STEPS	RATIONALE
(7) Instruct the patient to use safety bars when getting in and out of the tub or shower. Caution the patient against the use of bath oil in tub water.	• Prevents slipping and falling. Oil causes tub surfaces to become slippery.
(8) Instruct the patient not to remain in tub longer than 20 minutes. Debilitated patients should not be left alone while in the tub. Observe ROM during bath.	• Prolonged exposure to warm water may cause vasodilation and pooling of blood, leading to lightheadedness or dizziness. Measures joint mobility.
(9) Return to the bathroom when the patient signals, and knock before entering.	• Provides privacy.
(10) For the patient who is unsteady, drain the tub of water before patient attempts to get out of it. Place a bath towel over patient's shoulders. Assist patient in getting out of tub as needed, and assist with drying. If the patient is weak or unstable, have another person assist.	• Prevents accidental falls. Patient may become chilled as water drains.

CRITICAL DECISION POINT: *Weak or unstable patients need extra assistance in getting out of a tub. Planning for additional personnel is essential before attempting to assist a patient from the tub.*

STEPS	RATIONALE
(11) Observe patient's skin, paying particular attention to areas that were previously soiled or reddened or showed early signs of breakdown.	• Techniques used during bathing should leave skin clean and clear.
(12) Assist patient as needed in donning a clean gown or pyjamas, slippers, and robe. (In a home setting, the patient may don regular clothing.)	• Maintains warmth to prevent chilling.
(13) Assist patient to his or her room and a comfortable position in a bed or chair.	• Maintains relaxation gained from bathing.
(14) Clean the tub or shower according to agency policy. Whirlpool baths may require special cleaning. Remove soiled linen and place it in a linen bag. Discard disposable equipment in the proper receptacle. Place an "unoccupied" sign on the bathroom door. Return supplies to the storage area.	• Helps prevent transmission of infection through soiled linen and moisture.
(15) Perform hand hygiene.	• Reduces the transfer of microorganisms.

UNEXPECTED OUTCOMES	RELATED INTERVENTIONS
Areas of excessive dryness, rashes, or irritation, or signs of pressure injury on patient's skin	• Review agency's skin care policy regarding special cleaning and moisturizing products. • Limit the frequency of complete baths. • Complete a pressure injury assessment (see Chapter 46). • Obtain a special bed surface if patient is at risk for or has skin breakdown.
Inflammation of skin and genitalia, with localized tenderness, swelling, and presence of foul-smelling discharge	• Bathe the area frequently to keep it clean and dry. • Obtain an order for a sitz bath. • Apply a protective barrier. • Notify the physician or nurse practitioner and apply prescribed antibacterial or antifungal ointment or cream.
Patient expresses perineal discomfort	• Increase the frequency of perineal care. • Assess the perineum for signs of excoriation, swelling, irritation, or discharge.
Patient unable to perform perineal care correctly	• Review perineal care with the patient. • Position the patient and have patient observe the cleaning procedure.
Patient becomes excessively fatigued and unable to cooperate or participate in bathing	• Reschedule bathing to a time when the patient is more rested. • Patients with cardiopulmonary conditions and breathing difficulties may require a pillow or elevated head of the bed during bathing. • Notify the physician or nurse practitioner about changes in the patient's fatigue level. • Schedule rest periods.
Patient seems unusually restless or complains of discomfort	• Consider analgesia before bathing. • Schedule rest periods before bathing.

Continued

SKILL 38-1 BATHING A PATIENT—cont'd

STEPS	RATIONALE

RECORDING AND REPORTING

- Record the condition of skin and any significant findings (e.g., reddened areas, bruises, nevi, or joint or muscle pain).
- Report any evidence of alterations in skin integrity or increased wound secretions to the person in charge or the physician.
- Record the presence of any abnormal findings (e.g., the character and amount of discharge or condition of the genitalia), and record any related procedure you perform.
- Record the appearance of a suture line, if present.
- Report any break in a suture line or the presence of abnormalities to the person in charge or the physician.
- Record all procedures performed, the amount of assistance provided, the patient's reaction, and the extent of the patient's participation.

HOME CARE CONSIDERATIONS

- Assess the patient's tub and shower area for the need for safety devices (e.g., grab bars, bath mats).
- Assess the patient for the need for assistive bathing devices (e.g., shower chair, hand-held shower).
- Instruct caregivers to assess the patient's perineal area daily for signs of infection and skin breakdown.

OLDER PERSON CONSIDERATIONS

- Check the temperature of water carefully as the patient's sensitivity to temperature may be impaired.
- Continent patients may not require bathing every day, especially if dry skin is a problem.

Bag Baths. An innovative approach to the traditional bed bath was developed because of concern for patients who are predisposed to dry skin and the risk for infection. When wash basins are not cleaned and dried completely after use, contamination with Gram-negative organisms may occur. Successive uses of the basin may cause a patient's skin to harbour more Gram-negative organisms. The "bag bath" (Figure 38-8) is a specially prepared package containing 10 washcloths that are premoistened with a mixture of water and a nonrinsable cleaner. The bag bath package is warmed in a microwave before use, and a different cloth is used for each part of the patient's body. With this technique, the skin air-dries because towel drying removes the emollient that is left behind after the water–cleaner solution evaporates. Health care personnel who have used the bag bath products report shorter bathing times and increased patient satisfaction and staff productivity (Howe, 2008).

Perineal Care. Perineal care is usually part of a complete bed bath (see Skill 38-1). Patients most in need of perineal care are those at greatest risk for acquiring an infection (e.g., patients who have in-dwelling urinary catheters, patients who are recovering from rectal or genital surgery or childbirth, uncircumcised males, patients who are incontinent, or patients who are morbidly obese). In addition, women who are having a menstrual period require good perineal care. Patients who are able to perform self-care should be encouraged to do so. Sometimes nurses can feel embarrassed when providing perineal care, particularly for patients of the opposite sex. Similarly, patients may feel embarrassed, but this should not cause nurses to overlook patients' hygiene needs. A professional, dignified, and sensitive approach can reduce embarrassment and put patients at ease.

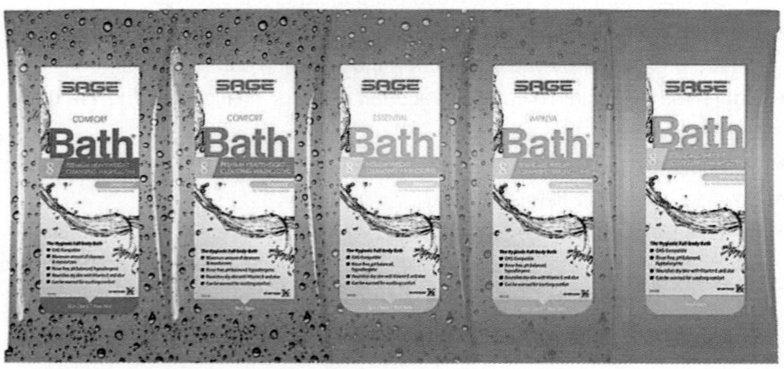

FIGURE 38-8 **Commercial bath cleansing pack.** (From Sage Products, Cary, IL. [2017]. Retrieved from http://shopsageproducts.com/no-rinse-bathing.)

If patients perform self-care, various problems such as vaginal and urethral discharge, skin irritation, and unpleasant odours may go unnoticed. Nurses must be alert for complaints of burning during urination or localized tenderness, excoriation, or pain in the perineum. Nurses should also inspect their patients' bed linen for signs of discharge.

Back Rub. A back rub or massage is often performed after a patient's bath. It promotes relaxation, relieves muscular tension, stimulates circulation, and improves sleep. Massage is associated with a reduction in blood pressure, and a reduction in pain, and it decreases anxiety and depression (Nelson, 2015). Patients generally report that they are more comfortable after a back rub or massage and find the experience pleasant, regardless of the length of the massage.

When providing a back rub, relaxation can be enhanced by reducing any noise and ensuring that the patient is comfortable. Because some individuals may dislike physical contact, it is important to ask the patient whether he or she would like a back rub and whether gentle or deep massage is preferred. The patient's medical record should be reviewed for any contraindications to massage (e.g., fractured ribs, burns of the skin, or heart surgery). Back rubs are an important strategy to reduce the incidence and prevalence of pressure injures. Box 38-10 examines this strategy along with the associated costs and nursing implications.

Foot and Nail Care. Foot and nail care should be incorporated into a person's regular hygiene routine. Routine care involves soaking to soften the cuticles, thorough cleansing, drying, and proper nail trimming. The exception involves patients with diabetes mellitus, who do not soak their feet because of the risk of infection. When providing

BOX 38-10 EVIDENCE-INFORMED PRACTICE

Reducing the Incidence and Prevalence of Pressure Injuries

According to a study by Leijon, Bergh, and Terstappen (2013), the mean prevalence rate of pressure injuries in acute care settings is 23%. Pressure injuries cause patients stress, pain, and suffering; increased length of hospital stay; and increased workload for health care staff. Estimated costs of treating a patient with an uncomplicated pressure injury are $2 400 to $3 200 per month, and treatment for a complicated injury is estimated to be $12 000, which includes supplies and nursing care (Orsted, Rosenthal, & Woodbury, et al., 2009). The goal of the Pressure Ulcer Awareness and Prevention (PUAP) program, created by the Canadian Association of Wound Care (CAWC) (2017), is to increase awareness of the high cost of pressure injuries through education and support, to improve clinical practice, and to create and improve current policies in health care facilities, to shift the focus from treatment to prevention of pressure injuries.

Nursing Implications

One of the key components of the nursing history and physical examination is the assessment of the integument for pre-existing conditions or risk assessment for potential breakdown in skin integrity. Risk assessment can be accomplished by using the Braden Scale for Assessment of Pressure Ulcer Risk (see Table 46-2) to identify those patients at risk so that strategies can be implemented to reduce their risk. Nurses are in a position to have an impact on the financial costs of pressure injuries to both the health care system and patients by completing thorough, daily skin assessment during hygiene care or independently for early recognition and early intervention.

Dibsie, L. G. (2008). Implementing evidence-based practice to prevent skin breakdown. *Critical Care Nursing Quarterly, 31*(2), 140–149; Leijon, S., Bergh, I., & Terstappen, K. (2013). Pressure ulcer prevalence, use of preventive measures, and mortality risk in an acute care population: A quality improvement project. *Journal of Wound, Ostomy and Continence Nursing, 40*(5), 469–474; Orsted, H. L., Rosenthal, S., & Woodbury, M. G. (2009). Pressure ulcer awareness and prevention program: A quality improvement program through the Canadian Association of Wound Care. *Journal of Wound, Ostomy and Continence Nurses, 36*(2), 178–183.

foot and nail care, patients may remain in bed or sit in a chair (Skill 38-2). In some settings or with specific patients, such as a person with diabetes mellitus, a physician's or nurse practitioner's order is needed to trim the toenails. Before implementing this procedure, check your agency's policy.

During the procedure, time is taken to teach the patients and family members the proper techniques for cleaning and nail trimming. Measures to prevent infection and promote good circulation should be stressed. Patients learn to protect their feet from injury, keep their feet clean and dry, and wear footwear that fits properly. Patients are instructed on the proper way to inspect all surfaces of the feet and hands for lesions, dryness, and signs of infection. It is important for patients to recognize any abnormalities and the importance of reporting these conditions to their caregiver.

Patients with diabetes mellitus and/or peripheral vascular disease are at risk for the development of foot ulcers as a result of poor peripheral blood supply to the feet and decreased sensation in the feet. These lesions are slow to heal because of compromised circulation over time and can result in amputation (Bateman, 2014). Appropriate patient teaching and daily foot care practices, along with early detection of diabetic foot ulcers, can decrease the risk of amputation (Canadian Diabetes Association, 2013).

Patients with diabetes mellitus or peripheral vascular disease should be provided information regarding how circulation directly affects the health and integrity of tissues of the feet and should be advised to use the following guidelines in a routine foot and nail care program:

- Inspect the feet daily, including the tops and soles of the feet, the heels, and the areas between the toes. Use a mirror to help inspect the feet thoroughly or ask a family member to check daily.
- If you have diabetes mellitus, you should receive a thorough foot examination at least once a year. If you have one or more high-risk foot conditions, you should be evaluated more frequently and referred to a specialist as necessary.
- Wash the feet daily using lukewarm water; *do not soak.* If you have reduced sensation, you may want to use a bath thermometer at home to test the water temperature. Thoroughly dry the feet and in between toes.
- Do not cut corns or calluses or use commercial removers. Consult a physician, podiatrist, or certified foot nurse.
- If your feet perspire excessively, apply a nonallergenic foot powder.
- If dryness is noted along the sides of the feet, rub a nonallergenic lotion gently into the skin, wiping off any excess. *Do not apply lotion between the toes, as excessive moisture can result in infection.*
- Trim the toenails straight across and square; do not use scissors. Consult a podiatrist as needed.
- Do not use over-the-counter preparations or home remedies. Consult a physician, podiatrist, or certified foot nurse.
- Constricting garments such as elastic stockings, knee-high hose, garters, and crossing the legs while sitting should be avoided as these can cause impaired circulation to the lower extremities.
- Wear clean, dry socks or stockings daily. Change socks twice a day if feet perspire heavily. Socks should be free of holes or repairs that might cause pressure on the tissue.
- Do not walk barefoot.
- Wear properly fitted shoes with porous uppers if possible. The soles of shoes should be flexible and nonslipping. Shoes should be sturdy, closed in, and not restrictive to the feet. New shoes should be worn for short periods of time over several days to break them in, to avoid the formation of blisters. Patients with increased plantar pressure (e.g., due to erythema or callus) should use footwear that cushions and redistributes pressure. Patients with bony deformity (e.g., a bunion or Charcot's joint) may need extra-wide or extra-deep shoes with cushioned insoles.
- Do not wear high-heeled, open-toed, or pointed-toe shoes.
- Exercise regularly to improve circulation to the lower extremities. Walk slowly and elevate, rotate, flex, and extend the feet at the ankles. Dangle the feet over the side of the bed for 1 minute, then extend both legs and hold them parallel to the bed while lying supine for 1 minute, and, finally, rest for 1 minute.
- Do not apply hot water bottles or heating pads directly to the feet.
- Wash minor cuts immediately and dry them thoroughly. Use only mild cleaners. Antibiotics are not generally required for wounds with no signs of infection. Contact a multidisciplinary foot-care team to treat cuts or lacerations (Canadian Diabetes Association, 2013).

Any patients who require regular, thorough foot care should have a caregiver or family member able to provide care during times when the patient is incapacitated. Patients with visual difficulties, physical constraints preventing movement, or cognitive problems that impair their ability to assess the condition of the feet need caregiver or family assistance.

SKILL 38-2 PERFORMING NAIL AND FOOT CARE

Delegation Considerations

The skill of nail and foot care for the nondiabetic patient can be delegated to a regulated or an unregulated care provider; however, this skill should not be delegated if the patient is diabetic. It is important to discuss the following:

- That nail clipping must be performed by the nurse
- Any special considerations for patient positioning

Equipment

- Wash basin
- Emesis basin
- Washcloth and bath towel
- Nail clippers (the patient's)
- Emery board or nail file
- Unscented lotion
- Disposable bath mat
- Paper towels
- Disposable gloves

PROCEDURE

STEPS	RATIONALE
1. Identify patients at risk for foot or nail problems:	• Certain conditions increase the likelihood of foot or nail problems.
A. Older person	• Poor vision, lack of coordination, or inability to bend over contributes to difficulty in performing foot and nail care. Normal physiological changes of aging also result in nail and foot problems (Bateman, 2014).
B. Diabetes mellitus	• Vascular changes associated with diabetes mellitus reduce blood flow to peripheral tissues. Breaks in skin integrity place a diabetic patient at high risk for a skin infection. Meticulous foot assessment and care reduce the diabetic patient's risk of debilitating foot problems (Bateman, 2014).
C. Heart failure or renal disease	• Both conditions can increase tissue edema, particularly in dependent areas (e.g., feet). Edema reduces blood flow to neighbouring tissues.
D. Cerebrovascular accident (stroke)	• The presence of residual foot or leg weakness or paralysis results in altered walking patterns. An altered gait pattern increases friction and pressure on feet.
2. Assess patient's knowledge of foot and nail care practices.	• Determines patient's need for health teaching.
3. Ask female patients about whether they use nail polish and polish remover frequently.	• Chemicals in these products can cause excessive dryness.
4. Assess patient's ability to care for nails or feet; consider visual alterations, fatigue, and musculoskeletal weakness.	• Demonstrates patient's knowledge of proper foot care. Determines the amount of assistance and teaching required.
5. Assess types of home remedies (e.g., aloe vera, herbal preparations) that the patient uses.	• Some preparations can cause injury to soft tissue; always consult a foot-care expert (Canadian Diabetes Association, 2013).
A. Over-the-counter chemical preparations to remove corns or calluses	• Chemical preparations can cause burns and ulcerations.
B. Cutting or shaving of corns or calluses with razor blade or scissors	• Cutting of corns or shaving calluses may result in a break in skin integrity and increases the risk for infection.
C. Use of oval corn pads	• Oval pads may exert pressure on the toes, thereby decreasing circulation to surrounding tissues.
D. Application of adhesive tape	• The skin of older persons is thin and delicate and prone to tearing when adhesive tape is removed.
6. Assess type of footwear worn by patients: Are socks worn? Are shoes tight or ill fitting? Are garters or knee-high nylons worn? Is footwear clean?	• Some types of shoes and footwear may predispose patients to foot and nail problems (e.g., infection, areas of friction, ulcerations). In patients with diabetes mellitus, nonhealing plantar ulcerations have been identified as one of the primary causes of lower limb amputation (Canadian Diabetes Association, 2013).
7. Observe patient's walking gait. Have the patient walk down a hall or in a straight line (if able).	• Structural as well as painful disorders of the feet can cause limping or an unnatural gait.
8. Assist an ambulatory patient to sit in a bedside chair. Help a bed-bound patient to a supine position with head of the bed elevated. Place disposable bath mat on the floor under patient's feet or place a towel on the mattress.	• Sitting in a chair facilitates immersing feet in the basin. The bath mat protects feet from exposure to soil or debris.
9. Obtain a physician's or nurse practitioner's order for cutting nails if agency policy requires it.	• The patient's skin may be accidentally cut. Certain patients are more at risk for infection, depending on their medical condition.
10. Explain the procedure to the patient, including the fact that proper soaking requires several minutes.	• Patient must be willing to place fingers and feet in basins for 10–20 minutes. Patient may become anxious or fatigued.

CRITICAL DECISION POINT: *Patients with diabetes do not soak hands and feet. Soaking increases their risk of infection due to maceration of the skin.*

STEPS	RATIONALE
11. Perform hand hygiene. Arrange equipment on an overbed table.	• Reduces transmission of microorganisms. Easy access to equipment prevents delays.
12. Fill wash basin with warm water. Test water temperature.	• Warm water softens nails and thickened epidermal cells, reduces inflammation of the skin, and promotes local circulation. Proper water temperature prevents burns.
13. Place basin on bath mat or towel.	• Avoids spills; this maintains safety of the care provider and the patient.
14. Fill emesis basin with warm water, and place basin on paper towels on overbed table.	• Warm water softens nails and thickened epidermal cells.
15. Pull curtain around the bed or close the room door (if desired).	• Maintaining the patient's privacy reduces anxiety.
16. Inspect all surfaces of the fingers, toes, feet, and nails. Pay particular attention to areas of dryness, inflammation, or cracking. Also inspect the areas between toes, heels, and soles of feet.	• The integrity of feet and nails determines the frequency and level of hygiene required. Heels, soles, and sides of the feet are prone to irritation from ill-fitting shoes.

CRITICAL DECISION POINT: *Patients with peripheral vascular diseases or diabetes mellitus, older persons, and patients whose immune system is suppressed may require nail care from a specialist to reduce the risk of infection.*

17. Assess colour and temperature of toes, feet, and fingers. Assess capillary refill. Palpate radial and ulnar pulses of each hand and dorsalis pedis pulses of feet (see Chapter 32).	• Assesses the adequacy of blood flow to extremities. Peripheral vascular disease can contribute to poor wound healing. Patients who are immunocompromised or who have neuropathy or peripheral vascular disease are at increased risk of foot infections (Canadian Diabetes Association, 2013).
18. Instruct patient to place his or her fingers in the emesis basin and place arms in a comfortable position. Assist patient to place feet in the basin.	• Prolonged positioning can cause discomfort unless normal anatomical alignment is maintained. • Patients with muscular weakness may have difficulty positioning their feet.
19. Allow patient's feet and fingernails to soak for 10–20 minutes (unless the patient has diabetes). Rewarm water after 10 minutes.	• Softening of corns, calluses, and cuticles ensures easy removal of dead cells and easy manipulation of cuticles.
20. Clean gently under the fingernails with an orange stick or the wooden end of a cotton-tipped swab while fingers are immersed (see Step 20 illustration). Remove fingers from the emesis basin, and dry thoroughly.	• The orange stick removes debris under nails that harbours microorganisms. Thorough drying impedes fungal growth and prevents maceration of the tissues.
21. Using nail clippers, clip fingernails straight across and even with the tops of fingers (see Step 21 illustration). Using a file, shape the nails straight across. If patient has circulatory problems, do not cut the nail; only file the nail.	• For infection-control purposes, use the patient's own nail clippers. Cutting straight across prevents splitting of the nail margins and the formation of sharp nail spikes that can irritate lateral nail margins. Filing prevents cutting the nail too close to the nail bed.

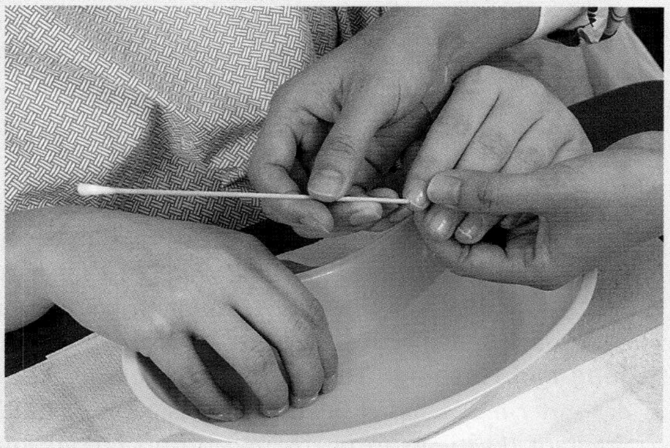

STEP 20 Clean fingernails with the end of a cotton-tipped swab or an orange stick.

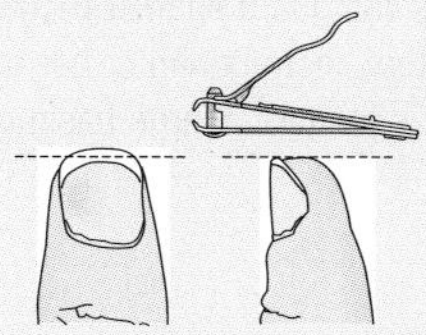

STEP 21 Using nail clippers, trim nails straight across.

22. Push cuticle back gently with a wet facecloth. Thoroughly dry the hands.	• Reduces incidence of inflamed cuticles. Thorough drying impedes fungal growth and prevents maceration of the tissues.
23. Move the overbed table away from the patient.	• Provides easier access to the feet.
24. Put on disposable gloves, and scrub callused areas of the feet with a washcloth.	• Gloves help prevent the transmission of fungal infection. Friction removes dead skin layers.
25. Clean gently under nails with an orange stick. Remove feet from basin, and dry them thoroughly.	• Removal of debris and excess moisture reduces chances of infection.
26. Clean and trim the toenails using the procedures in Steps 21 and 22. Do not file the corners of toenails.	• For infection control purposes, use the patient's own nail clippers. Shaping corners of toenails may damage tissues.
27. Apply lotion to feet and hands, and assist patient back to bed and into a comfortable position.	• Lotion lubricates dry skin by helping to retain moisture.

Continued

SKILL 38-2 PERFORMING NAIL AND FOOT CARE—cont'd

STEPS	RATIONALE
28. Remove disposable gloves and place in a receptacle. Clean and return the equipment and supplies to the proper place. Dispose of soiled linen in a hamper. Perform hand hygiene.	• Reduces the transmission of infection.
29. Inspect the nails and surrounding skin surfaces after soaking and nail trimming.	• Determines the condition of skin and nails. Allows caregiver to note any remaining rough nail edges.
30. Ask patient to explain or demonstrate nail care.	• Evaluates patient's level of learning techniques.
31. Observe patient's walk after toenail care.	• Evaluates the level of comfort and mobility achieved.

UNEXPECTED OUTCOMES	RELATED INTERVENTIONS
Inflammation and tenderness of cuticles and surrounding tissues	• Repeated soakings may be needed to relieve inflammation and loosen layers of cells from calluses or corns. • Patient with diabetes or peripheral vascular disease may require referral to a podiatrist. • Antifungal cream may be needed.
Localized areas of tenderness on feet, with calluses or corns at points of friction	• Change in footwear may be needed. • Refer to a podiatrist
Appearance of ulcer between toes or other pressure areas on foot	• Notify physician. • Refer to a podiatrist. • Increase frequency of foot assessment and hygiene.

RECORDING AND REPORTING

- Document the procedure and any observations (e.g., breaks in the skin, inflammation, ulcerations) on the patient's record sheets using the forms provided by your agency or facility.
- Report any breaks in the skin or ulcerations to the person in charge or the physician. These breaks are serious in patients with diabetes, peripheral vascular disease, and illnesses that impair circulation. Special foot care treatments may be needed.

HOME CARE CONSIDERATIONS

- If the patient has diabetes or decreased peripheral circulation, alternative therapies or foot soaking should be carried out only after consulting with a physician.
- An alternative therapy would be moleskin applied to areas of the feet that are experiencing friction—this is less likely to cause pressure than corn pads. Spot adhesive bandages can guard against friction, but they do not have padding to protect against pressure.
- If the patient is ambulatory, instruct him or her to soak feet in a bathtub.
- If the patient's mobility is limited, a large basin or pan can be used for soaking.

Oral Hygiene

Oral hygiene helps to maintain the healthy state of the mouth, teeth, gums, lips, and tongue (Canadian Dental Association, 2017). Brushing cleans the teeth of food particles, plaque, and bacteria. It also massages the gums and relieves any discomfort resulting from unpleasant odours and tastes. Flossing helps to further remove plaque and bacteria from between the teeth to reduce gum inflammation and infection. Complete oral hygiene enhances well-being and comfort and stimulates the appetite.

Patients also benefit from a diet that excludes foods that contribute to plaque formation and tooth decay and that promotes healthy periodontal structures (Canadian Dental Association, 2017). Plaque-forming foods include carbonated beverages, breads, and starches. Oral hygiene immediately after a meal further reduces plaque. Nurses can assist patients in maintaining good oral hygiene by teaching them the importance of correct techniques and a routine daily schedule.

Patients of all ages should be advised to have a dental checkup at least every 6 months. Education about common gum and tooth disorders and methods of prevention can motivate patients to follow good oral hygiene practices. Nurses need to provide assistance with oral hygiene for weakened or disabled patients. When patients have variations in oral mucosal integrity, hygiene techniques should be adapted to ensure thorough and effective care (Box 38-11).

Brushing and Flossing. Thorough tooth brushing at least four times a day (after meals and at bedtime) is basic to an effective oral hygiene program. If patients are unable to perform oral care four times per day, they should do it at least once during the day and always at night. All tooth surfaces should be brushed thoroughly with a fluoride toothpaste. A toothbrush should have a straight handle and a brush small enough to reach all areas of the mouth. A toothbrush with soft, rounded bristles should be used to stimulate gums without causing bleeding. Toothbrushes should be replaced every 3 months (Canadian Dental Association, 2017). Older patients with reduced dexterity and grip may require an enlarged handle with an easier grip or an electric toothbrush (Mitchell & Shoemaker, 2017). One simple way to make an enlarged brush handle is to pierce a soft rubber ball and push the brush handle through it or glue a short piece of plastic tubing around the handle. Commercially made foam rubber toothbrushes are useful for patients with sensitive gums. However, swabbing fails to clean teeth adequately because plaque accumulates around the base of the teeth.

BOX 38-11 FOCUS ON OLDER PERSONS

Dental Care

- Many older persons are edentulous (without teeth), and the teeth that are present are often diseased or decayed (Huang, Chan, & Young, 2013).
- The periodontal membrane weakens, making it more prone to infection; periodontal disease can predispose older persons to systemic infection.
- The presence of chronic illnesses (e.g., diabetes mellitus, renal insufficiency, and cardiovascular diseases) increases older persons' risk for periodontal disease (Marino, Albala, Sanchez, et al., 2014).
- Dentures or partial plates may not fit properly, causing pain and discomfort; this can, in turn, affect digestive processes, the enjoyment of food, and nutritional status (Marino et al., 2014).
- Weaker jaw muscles and shrinkage of the bony structure of the mouth may increase the work of chewing and lead to increased fatigue when eating (Marino et al., 2014).
- Dry mouth can be caused by an age-related decline in saliva secretion, as well as by over 400 medications that are frequently used by older persons (Marino et al., 2014).
- Poor nutritional status in some older persons can increase the risk for and severity of dental problems (e.g., caries, periodontal disease, receding gums, and tooth degeneration) (Huang et al., 2013).
- An inability or unwillingness to access dental care and the belief that tooth loss is a natural outcome of aging are reasons why some older persons do not seek dental care (Marino et al., 2014).
- Financial limitations, low income, and lack of transportation also contribute to inadequate dental care of some older persons.

Foam rubber swabs should be used in moderation. Electric toothbrushes can be used, but nurses should consult their agency's policy to ascertain whether their use is permitted. Lemon-glycerine sponges should not be used because they dry mucous membranes and erode teeth enamel. "Moi-Stir" is a common brand-name salivary supplement that improves moisture and the texture of the tongue and mucosa.

When teaching patients about mouth care, the nurse should recommend that they not share toothbrushes with family members or drink directly from a bottle of mouthwash. Cross-contamination occurs easily. The use of disclosure tablets or drops to stain the plaque that collects at the gum line can be useful for showing patients how effectively they brush.

Patients can experience conditions that threaten the integrity of the oral mucosa. For example, mucosal changes associated with aging, use of chemotherapeutic drugs, or dehydration require a change in oral hygiene. More frequent mouth care and use of anti-infective agents are examples of ways nurses can revise approaches to meet patient needs. Unconscious patients and those with artificial airways (e.g., endotracheal or tracheal tubes) need more frequent and specialized oral hygiene. These patients have an increased risk of aspiration and, subsequently, aspiration pneumonia, and they also have more problems with dry and inflamed oral mucosa.

The amount of assistance needed by the patient when brushing the teeth may vary. Many patients can perform their own oral care and should be encouraged to do so. Nurses should observe patients when they are brushing their teeth to be sure proper techniques are being used. When assisting with or providing oral hygiene, the nurse must determine the amount of assistance needed and the individual's oral hygiene preferences (Skill 38-3).

Flossing. Dental flossing removes plaque and bacteria from between teeth. Flossing involves inserting waxed or unwaxed dental floss between all tooth surfaces, one space at a time. Flossing at least once a day is sufficient (Canadian Dental Association, 2017). To prevent bleeding, patients who are receiving chemotherapy or radiation or who are on anticoagulant therapy should use unwaxed floss and avoid vigorous flossing near the gum line. Applying toothpaste to the teeth before flossing allows fluoride to come in direct contact with tooth surfaces, aiding in cavity prevention. Because it is important to clean all tooth surfaces thoroughly, the nurse should not rush flossing. Placing a mirror in front of the patient helps the nurse to demonstrate the proper method for holding the floss and cleaning between the teeth. Flossing a patient's teeth is not realistic or appropriate in all care settings. However, flossing may be done more frequently in rehabilitation and long-term care settings.

Patients With Special Needs. Some patients require special oral hygiene methods because of their level of dependence on the care provider or the presence of oral mucosa problems. Unconscious patients are susceptible to drying of mucous-thickened salivary secretions because they are unable to eat or drink, frequently breathe through the mouth, and often receive oxygen therapy. Unconscious patients also cannot swallow salivary secretions that accumulate in the mouth. These secretions often contain Gram-negative bacteria that can cause pneumonia if aspirated into the lungs. While providing hygiene to unconscious patients, nurses must protect them from choking and aspiration. While cleaning the oral cavity, the nurse should never use his or her fingers to hold the patient's mouth open, as a human bite is highly contaminated. It may be necessary to perform mouth care at least every 2 hours for the unconscious patient. Research shows that the use of chlorhexidine with oral hygiene reduces the risk of ventilator-associated pneumonia (Enwere, Elofson, Forbes, et al., 2016). The nurse needs to explain the steps of mouth care and the sensations the patient will feel, and advise the patient when the procedure is completed (Skill 38-4).

Patients who receive chemotherapy, radiation, or nasogastric tube intubation or who have an infection of the mouth can suffer from stomatitis, an inflammation of the oral mucosa that can cause burning, pain, and a change in food tolerance. Gentle brushing and flossing are important in preventing bleeding of the gums. Patients should be advised to avoid alcohol and commercial mouthwash and to stop smoking. Normal saline rinses (approximately 30 mL) used upon awaking in the morning, after each meal, and at bedtime can effectively clean the oral cavity. The rinses can be increased to every 2 hours, if necessary. The physician or nurse practitioner may order a mild oral analgesic for pain control.

Patients with diabetes mellitus frequently have periodontal disease and should have regular, yearly (or more frequently if necessary) visits to the dental professional for oral health assessment and care. All tissues should be handled gently with a minimum of trauma. Patients should learn to follow rigid cleaning schedules, at least four times a day.

Denture Care. Patients should be encouraged to clean their dentures on a regular basis to avoid gingival infection and irritation. When patients become disabled, the care provider or family caregiver can

SKILL 38-3 PROVIDING ORAL HYGIENE

Delegation Considerations

The skill of oral hygiene can be delegated to an unregulated care provider (UCP). It is important to discuss the following with the UCP:

- How to adapt the procedure for a patient who is at risk of aspiration (e.g., those with an impaired level of consciousness or impaired swallowing, and those who are confused)
- To immediately report excessive patient coughing or choking during or after oral hygiene
- To report any bleeding of the oral mucosa or gums, lesions, or patient report of pain
- To report any concerns with dentures (e.g., ill-fitting or broken dentures)

Equipment

- Soft-bristled toothbrush
- Nonabrasive fluoride toothpaste or dentifrice
- Dental floss
- Water glass with cool water
- Normal saline or an essential oil antiseptic mouthwash (optional; follow patient's preference)
- Emesis basin
- Tongue blade
- Face towel
- Paper towels
- Disposable gloves

PROCEDURE

STEPS	RATIONALE
1. Determine patient's oral hygiene practices:	• Allows caregiver to identify errors in technique, deficiencies in preventive oral hygiene, and patient's level of knowledge regarding dental care.
A. Frequency of tooth brushing and flossing	
B. Type of toothpaste or dentifrice used	
C. Last dental visit	
D. Frequency of dental visits	
E. Type of mouthwash or moistening preparation, such as over-the-counter saliva substitutes or sugar-free gum with xylitol	• Mouthwash provides a pleasant aftertaste but can dry mucosa after extended use if it has an alcohol base.
2. Assess risk for oral hygiene problems (see Table 38-5).	• Certain conditions increase the likelihood of impaired oral cavity integrity and the need for preventive care.
3. Assess patient's risk for aspiration: impaired swallowing, reduced gag reflex.	• An accumulation of secretions and dentifrice can increase the patient's risk for aspiration if the patient's ability to control oral secretions is impaired.
4. Assess patient's ability to grasp and manipulate a toothbrush. (For older persons, try a 30-second tooth brushing assessment.)	• A toothbrush test is useful in assessing dexterity and strength. Determines level of assistance required.
5. Prepare equipment at bedside.	• Avoids interrupting the procedure or leaving the patient unattended while retrieving missing equipment.
6. Perform hand hygiene and put on disposable gloves.	• Reduces the transmission of microorganisms.
7. Inspect the integrity of the lips, teeth, buccal mucosa, gums, palate, and tongue (see Chapter 32).	• Determines status of patient's oral cavity and the extent of need for oral hygiene.
8. Identify the presence of common oral problems:	• Helps determine type of hygiene patient requires and information patient needs for self-care.
A. Dental caries—chalky white discoloration of a tooth or the presence of brown or black discoloration	
B. Gingivitis—inflammation of gums	
C. Periodontitis—receding gum lines, inflammation, gaps between teeth	• Receding gums can occur with aging, and as a result, older patients require meticulous oral hygiene.
D. Halitosis—bad breath	
E. Cheilosis—cracking of the lips	
F. Stomatitis—inflammation of the oral tissues	• Patients receiving immunosuppressive chemotherapy (e.g., cancer chemotherapy) and patients with suppressed immune function are at risk for stomatitis (Gupta & West, 2016).
G. Dry, cracked, coated tongue	
9. Explain the procedure to the patient and discuss preferences regarding the use of hygiene aids.	• Some patients feel uncomfortable about having a caregiver care for their basic needs. Patient involvement with the procedure minimizes anxiety.
10. Raise the bed to a comfortable working position. Raise head of the bed (if patient's condition allows) and lower the side rail. Move the patient, or help patient move closer. A side-lying position can be used.	• Raising the bed and repositioning the patient prevents straining of muscles. A semi-Fowler position helps prevent patient from choking or aspirating.
11. Place paper towels on an overbed table, and arrange other equipment within easy reach.	• Prevents soiling of the tabletop. Equipment prepared in advance ensures a smooth, safe procedure.
12. Place a towel over patient's chest.	• Prevents soiling of bed linen and patient's clothing.
13. Apply toothpaste to brush, holding brush over the emesis basin. Pour a small amount of water over toothpaste.	• Moisture aids in the distribution of toothpaste over tooth surfaces.

STEPS	RATIONALE
14. The patient may assist by brushing. Hold toothbrush bristles at a 45-degree angle to gum line (see Step 14 illustration, part A). Be sure tips of bristles rest against and penetrate under gum line. Brush inner and outer surfaces of upper and lower teeth by brushing from gum to crown of each tooth. Clean biting surfaces of teeth by holding top of bristles parallel with teeth and brushing gently back and forth (see Step 14 illustration, part B). Brush sides of teeth by moving bristles back and forth (see Step 14 illustration, part C).	• Angle allows brush to reach all tooth surfaces and to clean under gum line where plaque and bacteria accumulate. Back-and-forth motion dislodges food particles caught between teeth and along chewing surfaces.
15. Have patient hold brush at a 45-degree angle and lightly brush over surface and sides of tongue (see Step 15 illustration). Avoid initiating gag reflex.	• Microorganisms collect and grow on the tongue's surface and contribute to bad breath. Gagging may cause aspiration of toothpaste. Evaluates patient's ability to use correct technique.

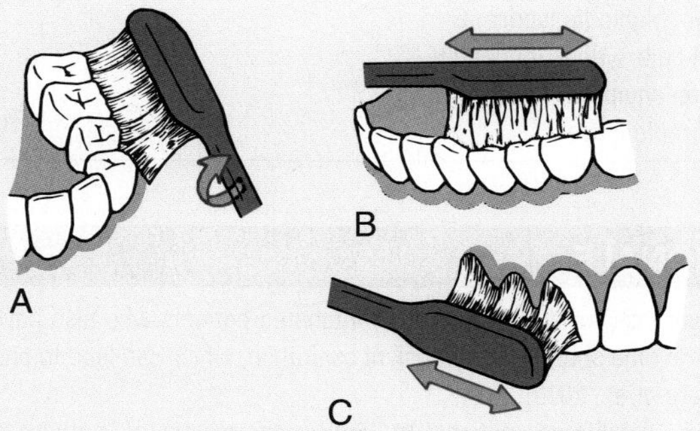

STEP 14 Directions for toothbrush placement. **A,** Gum line is brushed at a 45-degree angle. **B,** Parallel position is used for brushing biting surfaces. **C,** Lateral position is used for brushing sides of teeth.

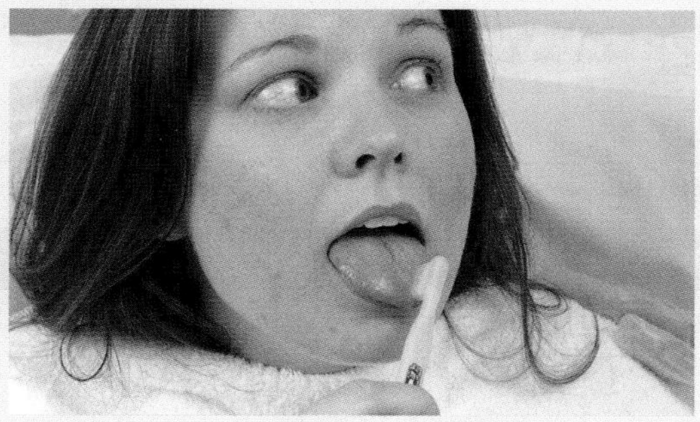

STEP 15 Assisting patient with brushing tongue.

STEPS	RATIONALE
16. Allow patient to rinse mouth thoroughly: taking several sips of water, swishing water across all tooth surfaces, and spitting into the emesis basin.	• Irrigation removes food particles.
17. Allow patient to gargle and rinse mouth with mouthwash as desired.	• Mouthwash can be effective in reducing plaque and gingivitis (Canadian Dental Association, 2017).
18. Assist in wiping patient's mouth.	• Promotes sense of comfort.
19. Allow patient to floss.	• Reduces tartar between tooth surfaces.
20. Allow patient to rinse mouth thoroughly with cool water and spit into emesis basin. Assist in wiping patient's mouth.	• Irrigation removes plaque and tartar from the oral cavity.
21. Ask patient whether any area of oral cavity feels uncomfortable or irritated. Inspect the oral cavity.	• Pain can indicate a problem.
22. Assist patient to comfortable position, remove emesis basin and bedside table, raise side rail, and lower bed to the original position.	• Provides for patient comfort and safety.
23. Wipe off overbed table, discard soiled linen and paper towels in appropriate containers, remove soiled gloves, and return equipment to the proper place.	• Proper disposal of soiled equipment helps prevent the spread of microorganisms.
24. Remove gloves, and perform hand hygiene.	• Reduces the transmission of microorganisms.
25. Ask patient to describe proper hygiene techniques.	• Evaluates patient's learning.

UNEXPECTED OUTCOMES	RELATED INTERVENTIONS
Dryness and inflammation of oral mucosa	• Increase frequency of oral hygiene. • Increase patient's hydration (if permitted). • Apply water-soluble lubricant to the patient's lips.
Retraction of gum margins from teeth, localized areas of inflammation, and bleeding around gum margins	• Determine whether patient has an underlying bleeding tendency (e.g., anti-coagulant therapy). • Report findings to the physician or person in charge. • Use a soft-bristled toothbrush. • Increase frequency of oral hygiene.
Signs of dental caries	• Refer patient to a dentist. • Teach patient oral hygiene techniques.

RECORDING AND REPORTING

- Record all procedures on a flow sheet provided by your agency or facility. Note the condition of the oral cavity in the patient care notes.
- Report any bleeding or the presence of lesions to the person in charge or the physician.

HOME CARE CONSIDERATIONS

- Teach the patient and caregiver to assess the oral cavity daily to determine any effects of medications on the oral cavity (e.g., reddened, inflamed gums).

SKILL 38-4 PERFORMING MOUTH CARE FOR AN UNCONSCIOUS OR DEBILITATED PATIENT

Delegation Considerations

Oral hygiene of an unconscious or debilitated patient can be delegated to an unregulated care provider (UCP). You must first assess the patient for the gag reflex and determine whether the person providing assistance can safely use oral suctioning for clearing the patient's oral secretions (see Chapter 39). When delegating tasks to a UCP, it is important to instruct him or her about the following:

- The proper way to position the patient for mouth care
- How to safely use oral suctioning for clearing oral secretions (see Chapter 40)
- To report to any bleeding of the mucosa or gums, any painful reaction by the patient, or excessive coughing or choking

Equipment

- Antiseptic oral rinse (e.g., chlorhexidine gluconate)
- Small soft-bristled toothbrush
- Sponge swab (e.g., Toothette swab)
- Oral airway
- Padded tongue blade
- Face towel
- Paper towels
- Emesis basin
- Water glass with cool water
- Water-soluble lip lubricant
- Small-bulb syringe (optional)
- Suction equipment
- Disposable gloves

PROCEDURE

STEPS	RATIONALE
1. Assess patient's risk for oral hygiene problems (see Table 38-5).	• Oral care is provided frequently to intubated patients who also have a nasogastric tube and who are at risk of aspiration, which can lead to pneumonia (Enwere et al., 2016).
2. Explain procedure to patient.	• Allows debilitated patient to anticipate procedure without anxiety. Unconscious patients retain the ability to hear.
3. Test for the presence of a gag reflex by touching the posterior pharyngeal wall with a tongue blade.	• Reveals whether patient is at risk for aspiration.

CRITICAL DECISION POINT: *Patients with an impaired gag reflex require oral care as well. You must determine the type of suction apparatus needed at the bedside to protect the patient's airway against aspiration.*

STEPS	RATIONALE
4. Raise bed to the appropriate height; lower head of the bed (if patient's condition permits) and then lower the side rail.	• Allows use of good body mechanics and reduces the risk of injury.
5. Pull curtain around the bed, or close the room door.	• Provides privacy.
6. Perform hand hygiene and put on disposable gloves.	• Reduces the transfer of microorganisms. Gloves prevent contact with microorganisms in blood or saliva.
7. Place paper towels on an overbed table and arrange equipment. If needed, turn on a suction machine and connect tubing to the suction catheter.	• Prevents soiling of the tabletop. Equipment prepared in advance ensures a smooth, safe procedure.
8. Position patient on side (Sims' position) with head turned well toward dependent side. Move patient close to side of the bed. Raise the side rail.	• Turning the patient's head to the side allows secretions to drain from the mouth instead of collecting in the back of the pharynx. Prevents aspiration. Moving the patient close to the side of the bed facilitates proper body mechanics.
9. Place a towel under patient's head and an emesis basin under the chin.	• Prevents soiling of bed linen and patient's gown.
10. Carefully separate upper and lower teeth with padded tongue blade by inserting blade, quickly but gently, between back molars. Insert blade when patient is relaxed, if possible. Do not use force (see Step 10 illustration).	• Prevents patient from biting down on your fingers and provides access to oral cavity.

CRITICAL DECISION POINT: *Never use fingers to separate the patient's teeth.*

STEPS	RATIONALE
11. Inspect condition of the oral cavity (see Chapter 32).	• Determines condition of the oral cavity and the need for hygiene.
12. Clean mouth using brush or sponge Toothette swabs moistened with chlorhexidine solution if patient condition can tolerate it; otherwise, moisten with water. Clean chewing and inner and outer tooth surfaces. Swab roof of mouth, gums, and inside cheeks. Gently swab or brush tongue, but avoid stimulating gag reflex (if present). Moisten clean swab or Toothette swab with water to rinse. (Bulb syringe may also be used to rinse.) Repeat rinse several times.	• Brushing action removes food particles between teeth and along chewing surfaces. Swabbing helps remove secretions and crusts from mucosa and moistens mucosa. Rinsing removes any debris and cleaning agent and provides for patient comfort.
13. Suction secretions as they accumulate, if necessary.	• Suction removes secretions and fluid that can collect in the posterior pharynx.

STEPS	RATIONALE
14. Apply a thin layer of water-soluble lubricant to lips (see Step 14 illustration).	• Lubricates lips to prevent drying and cracking.

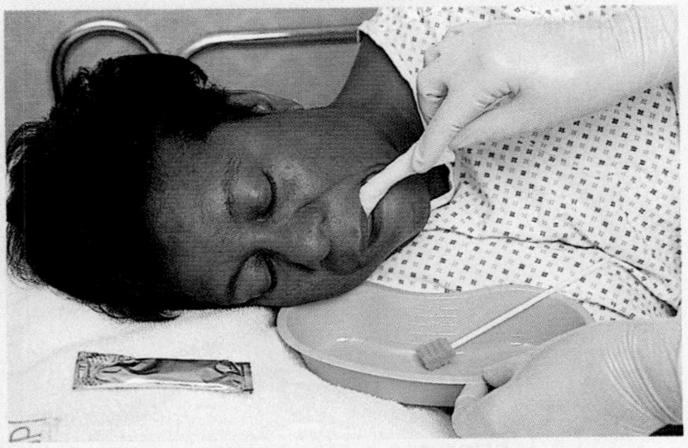

STEP 10 Separate upper and lower teeth with padded tongue blade.

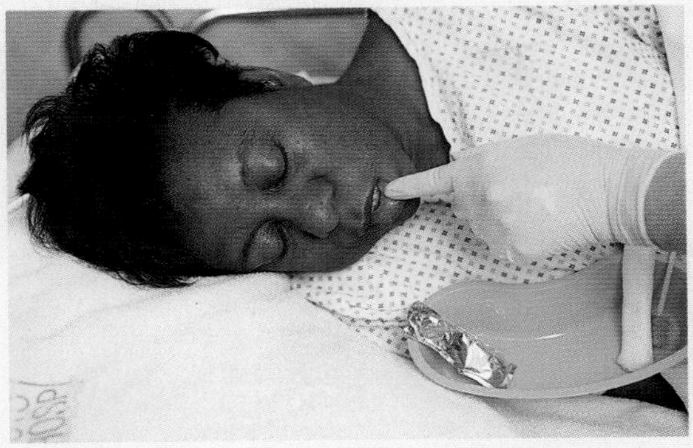

STEP 14 Application of water-soluble moisturizer to lips.

STEPS	RATIONALE
15. Inform patient that procedure is completed.	• Provides meaningful stimulation to unconscious or less responsive patient.
16. Put on clean gloves, and inspect oral cavity.	• Determines efficacy of cleaning. Once thick secretions are removed, underlying inflammation or lesions may be revealed.
17. Ask debilitated patient whether mouth feels clean.	• Evaluates level of comfort.
18. Reposition patient in a comfortable position, raise side rail as appropriate or as ordered, and return the bed to original position.	• Maintains patient's comfort and safety. Raising all four side rails may be considered a restraint, and a physician's order is needed.
19. Clean equipment and return to its proper place. Place soiled linen in the proper receptacle.	• Proper disposal of soiled equipment helps prevent the spread of microorganisms.
20. Remove and discard gloves. Perform hand hygiene.	• Reduces the transmission of microorganisms.
21. Assess patient's respirations on an ongoing basis.	• Ensures early recognition of aspiration.

UNEXPECTED OUTCOMES	RELATED INTERVENTIONS
Secretions or crusts remaining on oral mucosa, tongue, or gums	• Increase frequency of oral hygiene. • Try using a pediatric-size toothbrush—it may provide better hygiene if the oral cavity is difficult to access.
Localized inflammation of gums or mucosa	• Increase frequency of oral hygiene with a soft-bristled toothbrush. • Apply moisturizing gel on the oral mucosa. • Chemotherapy and radiation can cause stomatitis. To provide relief and promote oral hygiene, topical anti-inflammatories and anaesthetics may be prescribed (Gupta & West, 2016).
Aspiration of secretions	• Suction oral airway. • Perform tracheal bronchial suctioning. • Notify the physician.

RECORDING AND REPORTING

- Record the procedure, including pertinent observations (e.g., the presence of bleeding gums, dry mucosa, ulcerations, or crusts on the tongue).
- Report any unusual findings to the person in charge or the physician.

HOME CARE CONSIDERATIONS

- Oral cavity should be irrigated with a bulb syringe.
- Mouth care should be given at least twice a day. Caregivers can buy nonprescription oral care solutions (e.g., chlorhexidine solutions) at most pharmacies.
- Have caregivers demonstrate positioning of the patient that will prevent aspiration.

assume responsibility for denture care (Box 38-12). Dentures are patients' personal property and need to be handled with care because they can be easily broken. They must be removed at night to give the gums a rest and prevent bacterial buildup. Dentures should be kept covered in water when they are not worn to prevent warping, and they should always be stored in an enclosed, labelled cup and placed in a patient's bedside stand. Patients should be discouraged from removing dentures and placing them on a napkin or tissue because they could be easily thrown away.

Hair and Scalp Care

A person's appearance and feeling of well-being can often depend on the way his or her hair looks and feels. Illness or disability may prevent patients from maintaining daily hair care. Immobilized patients' hair soon becomes tangled. Dressings may leave sticky blood or antiseptic solutions on the hair. In the clinic and home care setting, nurses may encounter patients who have head lice. Proper hair care is important to patients' body image. Brushing, combing, and shampooing are basic hair hygiene measures for all patients.

BOX 38-12 PROCEDURAL GUIDELINE

Care of Dentures

Delegation Considerations

The skill of denture care can be delegated to an unregulated care provider (UCP). It is important to discuss the following with the UCP:

- To report any cracks found in the dentures
- To report any patient complaints of oral discomfort
- To report any signs of irritation, inflammation, or lesions

Equipment

- Soft-bristled toothbrush or denture toothbrush
- Denture cleaning agent or toothpaste
- Denture adhesive (optional)
- Glass of water
- Emesis basin or sink
- Washcloth
- Disposable gloves
- Denture cup (if dentures are to be stored after cleaning)

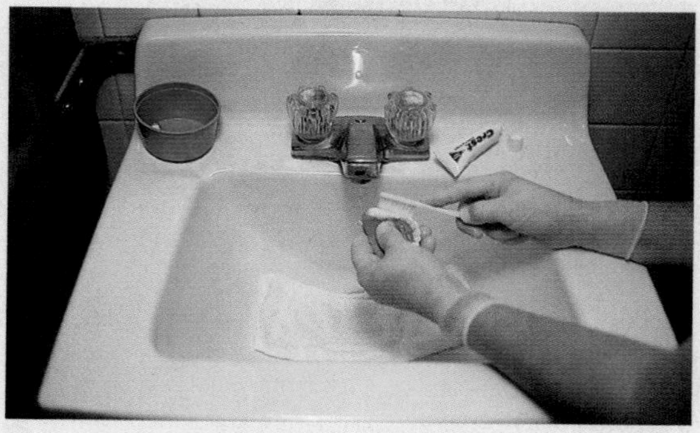

STEP 5 Brushing dentures.

Procedure

1. Ask patient whether dentures fit and whether the gums or mucous membranes are tender or irritated.
2. Ask patient about preferences for denture care and products used. If patient is unable to care for own dentures, you must provide this care. Clean dentures for the patient during routine mouth care.
3. Fill emesis basin with tepid water or, if using sink, place washcloth in bottom of sink and fill sink with 2.5 cm of water.
4. Remove dentures. If patient is unable to do this independently, perform hand hygiene and put on gloves, grasp upper plate at front with thumb and index finger wrapped in gauze, and pull downward. Gently lift lower denture from jaw, and rotate one side downward to remove from patient's mouth. Place dentures in emesis basin or sink.
5. Apply cleaning agent to brush and brush surfaces of dentures (see Step 5 illustration). Hold dentures close to water. Hold the brush horizontally, and use a back-and-forth motion to clean biting surfaces. Use short strokes from the top of the denture to biting surfaces to clean outer and inner teeth surfaces. Hold the brush vertically, and use short strokes to clean inner tooth surfaces. Hold the brush horizontally, and use a back-and-forth motion to clean the undersurface of dentures.
6. Rinse thoroughly in tepid water.
7. Some patients use an adhesive to seal dentures in place. If so, apply a thin layer to the undersurface before inserting.
8. If patient needs assistance with the insertion of dentures, moisten the upper denture and press firmly to seal it in place. Then insert moistened lower denture. Ask whether dentures feel comfortable.
9. Dentures should be removed at night and the gums cleaned gently. Dentures should be stored in a denture container that is labelled with the patient's name and placed in the bedside table to prevent loss.
10. Remove and discard gloves and perform hand hygiene.

Brushing and Combing. Frequent brushing and combing helps to keep hair clean and distributes oil evenly along hair shafts and prevents hair from tangling. Patients should be encouraged to maintain routine hair care. However, patients with limited mobility or weakness and those who are confused require assistance. Patients in a hospital or long-term care facility appreciate the opportunity to have their hair brushed and combed before being seen by others.

When caring for patients from different cultures, it is important to learn as much as possible from them or their family about their preferred hair care practices. Cultural preferences affect how hair is combed and styled. Nurses should never trim or cut a patient's hair without the patient's consent.

Long hair can easily become matted when patients are confined to bed, even for a short period. When lacerations or incisions involve the scalp, blood and topical medications can also cause tangling. Frequent brushing and combing keeps long hair neatly groomed. Braiding can help to avoid repeated tangles; however, braids should be unbraided periodically and the hair combed to ensure good hygiene. Braids made too tightly can result in bald patches. Nurses must always obtain permission from patients, if conscious, before braiding their hair.

To brush the hair, part it into two sections and separate each into two more sections. It is easier to brush smaller sections of hair. Brushing from the scalp toward the hair ends minimizes pulling. Moistening the hair with water frees tangles for easier combing.

Patients who develop head lice require special considerations in the way combing is performed. The lice are small, about the size of a sesame seed. Bright light or natural sunlight is necessary for the lice to be seen. Thorough combing is recommended and may remove nits (empty eggshells) if infestation is extensive. To remove head lice, the following steps are used:

- Put on a disposable gown and gloves.
- Use a grooming comb or hairbrush to remove any tangles.
- Divide the patient's hair in sections and fasten off the hair that is not being combed.
- Comb out from the scalp to the end of the hair (special fine-tooth combs are available in drugstores).
- Between each pass, dip the comb in a cup of water or use a paper towel to remove nits.
- After combing, look through the hair carefully for attached live lice.
- Catch live lice with tweezers or comb.
- Move to next section of hair after combing thoroughly.
- Instruct the family to clean the comb with an old toothbrush and dental floss and boil the comb (if possible). The ideal would be to discard the comb after each use, but some patients' financial situations may prevent the purchase of multiple combs.
- Instruct the family to comb and screen for lice daily.
- Instruct the family to separate the patient's clothes and then wash them in hot water.

- Instruct caregivers on how to prevent the transmission of lice:
  - Do not share bed linens.
  - Avoid placing your bare hand on the patient's head.
  - Immediately wash your hands after providing hair care.
  - Separate all hair care products.

If a pediculicidal shampoo is ordered, instruct the patient and caregiver on the proper use of shampoo. Lindane, an organochloride, can have neurological side effects. Shampoos containing lindane are contraindicated for those patients under 50 kg, neonates, those who take medications that lower seizure threshold (e.g., bupropion), and patients who have human immunodeficiency virus (HIV), owing to increased risk of seizures (Drugs.com, 2017). As with any medication preparation, it is important to review and understand the product information provided in the packaging.

Shampooing. To promote and restore hair and scalp health, patients should be instructed to keep hair clean, combed, and brushed regularly. Patients may also need to know how to check for and remove parasites, such as lice (see Table 38-4). Nurses should inform patients that they need to notify their primary caregiver of changes in the texture and distribution of hair, which may indicate a serious systemic problem.

Frequency of shampooing depends on patients' daily routines and the condition of their hair. Nurses should remind patients in hospitals or long-term care facilities that staying in bed, perspiring excessively, or undergoing treatments that leave blood or solutions in the hair may result in them needing more frequent shampooing.

For patients at home who have limited mobility, it can be challenging to find ways that they can shampoo their hair without causing injury to themselves. If patients are able to take a shower or bath, their hair can usually be shampooed without difficulty. A shower or tub chair may be used for ambulatory, weight-bearing patients who become fatigued or faint. Hand-held shower nozzles enable patients to wash their hair in the tub or shower. Patients allowed to sit in a chair may choose to be shampooed in front of a sink or over a wash basin. However, bending is limited or contraindicated in certain conditions (e.g., eye surgery or neck injury). In these situations, the nurse needs to teach the patient and family members the degree of bending allowed.

If patients are unable to sit but can be moved, the nurse may transfer the patient to a stretcher for transportation to a sink or shower equipped with a hand-held nozzle. This equipment is commonly found in long-term care facilities. Again, the nurse needs to exercise caution when positioning the patient's head and neck, particularly for patients with any form of head or neck injury.

If patients are unable to sit in a chair or be transferred to a stretcher, shampooing must be done while the patient is in bed (Box 38-13). A special shampoo trough can be positioned under the patient's head to catch water and suds. After shampooing, patients like having their hair styled and dried. Dry shampoos that reduce the need to wet the patient's hair are also available but are not highly effective. These dry shampoo preparations vary, and the application procedures, listed on the container, should be followed exactly. Also available are prepackaged shampoo cloths, which can be used to shampoo a patient in bed or in a chair. In some agencies, a physician's or nurse practitioner's order is necessary to shampoo the dependent patient.

Shaving. Shaving facial hair can be done after a bath or shampoo. Women may prefer to shave their legs or axillae while bathing. When assisting a patient, the nurse should take care to avoid cutting the patient with a razor blade. Patients prone to bleeding (e.g., those receiving anticoagulants or high doses of aspirin, those with low platelet counts) must use an electric razor. Before using an electric razor, it is good to check for frayed cords and other electrical hazards, as well as the agency's policy with respect to the use of these razors. Each razor blade or electric razor should be used on only one patient, to prevent spread of infection.

Before a razor blade is used for shaving, the skin must be softened to prevent pulling, scraping, or cuts. This is done by placing a warm washcloth over the male patient's face for a few seconds, then applying shaving cream or lathering a mild soap to soften the skin. If the patient is unable to shave, the nurse may perform the task. To avoid causing discomfort or razor cuts, the nurse gently pulls the skin taut and uses short, firm razor strokes in the direction in which the hair grows (Figure 38-9). Short downward strokes work best to remove hair over the upper lip. A patient usually can explain the best way to move the razor across the skin. In dark-skinned patients, facial hair tends to be curly and can become ingrown unless shaved close to the skin.

Moustache and Beard Care

Patients with moustaches or beards require daily grooming. Keeping these areas clean is important because food particles and mucus can easily collect in the hair. If the patient is unable to carry out self-care, the nurse must perform this care for the patient. Beards can be gently combed out. A shaggy or unkempt moustache or beard can be trimmed, only with consent from the patient or family. For cultural or religious reasons, trimming or shaving off a moustache or beard cannot be performed without the patient's or family's consent.

Care of the Eyes, Ears, and Nose

Special attention is given to cleaning the eyes, ears, and nose during a routine bath and when drainage or discharge accumulates. This aspect of hygiene not only makes patients more comfortable, it also improves sensory perception (see Chapter 47). Care focuses on preventing infection and maintaining normal sensory function and requires approaches that consider patients' special needs.

Basic Eye Care. Cleaning the eyes simply involves washing them with a clean washcloth moistened in water. Soap may cause burning and irritation (see Skill 38-1). Direct pressure should never be applied over the eyeball because it may cause serious injury. When cleaning a patient's eyes, use a clean washcloth and cleanse from the inner to outer canthus. Use a different section of the washcloth for each eye. Unconscious patients often require more frequent eye care.

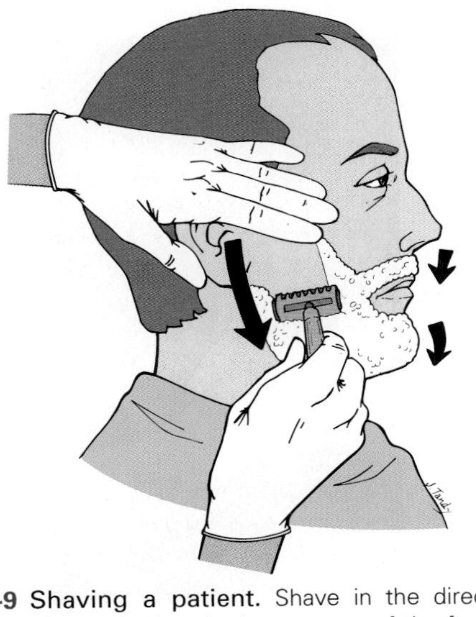

FIGURE 38-9 Shaving a patient. Shave in the direction of hair growth. Use longer strokes on the larger areas of the face. Use short strokes around the chin and lips. (From Sorrentino, S. A. [2004]. *Assisting with patient care* [2nd ed., p. 320, Fig. 17-5]. St. Louis, MO: Mosby.)

BOX 38-13 PROCEDURAL GUIDELINE

Shampooing the Hair of a Bed-Bound Patient

Delegation Considerations

The skill of shampooing hair can be delegated to an unregulated care provider (UCP). It is important to discuss the following with the UCP:

- To follow any precautions necessary in positioning the patient
- To report any patient complaints of neck pain
- To report condition of the scalp and hair

Equipment

- Bath towels
- Washcloths
- Shampoo
- Hair conditioner (if available)
- Water pitcher with warm water
- Plastic shampoo trough
- Wash basin
- Bath blanket
- Waterproof pad
- Clean comb and brush
- Hair dryer (if warranted by patient's condition)
- Disposable gloves (optional)

Procedure

1. Before washing the patient's hair, ensure that this procedure is not contraindicated for the patient. Certain medical conditions, such as head and neck injuries, spinal cord injuries, and arthritis, could place the patient at risk for injury during shampooing because of positioning and manipulation of the patient's head and neck.
2. Put on gloves if needed. Inspect the hair and scalp before initiating the procedure to determine the presence of any conditions that may require the use of special shampoos or treatments (e.g., for dandruff or the removal of dried blood).
3. Place waterproof pad under patient's shoulders, neck, and head (see Step 3 illustration). Position patient supine, with head and shoulders at top edge of the bed. Place a plastic trough under the patient's head and a wash basin at end of the trough. Be sure the trough spout extends beyond the edge of the mattress.

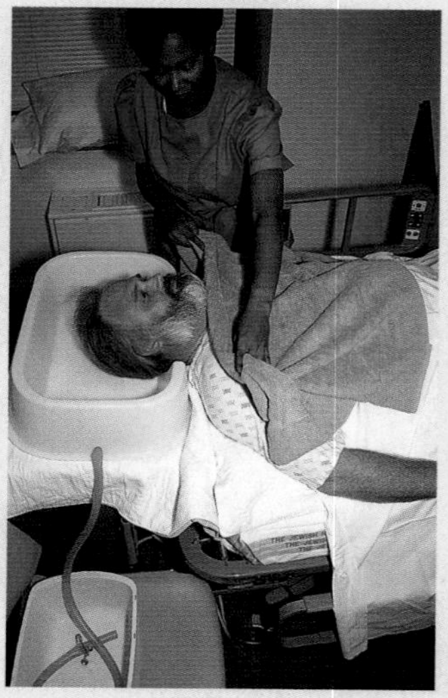

STEP 3 Pad has been placed under shoulders, neck, and head.

4. Place rolled towel under patient's neck and bath towel over patient's shoulders.
5. Brush and comb patient's hair.
6. Obtain warm water.
7. Offer patient the option of holding a face towel or washcloth over the eyes.
8. Slowly pour water from a water pitcher over hair until it is completely wet (see Step 8 illustration). If hair contains matted blood, don gloves, apply peroxide to dissolve the clots, and then rinse the hair with saline. Apply small amount of shampoo.

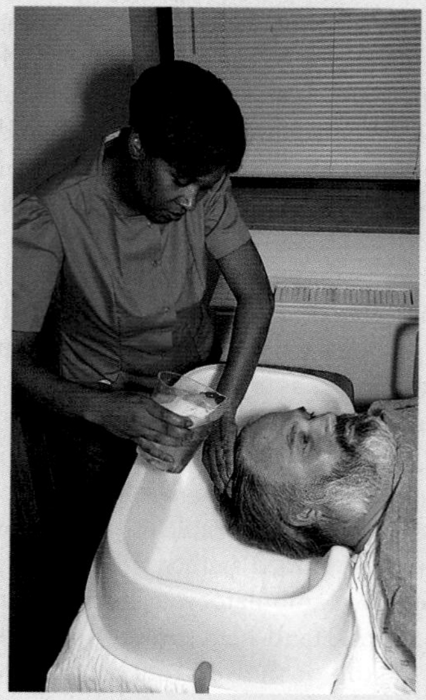

STEP 8 Pour water over hair.

9. Work up lather with both hands. Start at the hairline and work toward back of the neck. Lift head slightly with one hand to wash back of the head. Shampoo sides of the head. Massage scalp by applying pressure with fingertips, if not contraindicated.
10. Rinse hair with water. Make sure water drains into basin. Repeat rinsing until hair is free of soap.
11. Apply conditioner or cream rinse, if requested, and rinse hair thoroughly.
12. Wrap patient's head in bath towel. Dry patient's face with cloth used to protect eyes. Dry off any moisture along the neck or shoulders.
13. Dry patient's hair and scalp. Use a second towel if first becomes saturated.
14. Comb hair to remove tangles, and dry with dryer if desired (not available in all agencies or facilities).
15. Apply oil preparation or conditioning product to hair, if desired by patient.
16. Assist patient to a comfortable position, and complete styling of hair.

Secretions may collect along the lid margins and inner canthus when the blink reflex is absent or an eye does not close completely. It may be necessary to place an eye patch over the involved eye to prevent corneal drying and irritation. Lubricating eye drops may be given according to the physician's or nurse practitioner's orders.

Eyeglasses. Glasses are made of hardened glass or plastic that is impact-resistant to prevent shattering. Nevertheless, because of their cost, extra care should be taken when cleaning glasses, and they should be protected from breakage or other damage when they are not worn. Glasses should be put in a case in a drawer of the bedside table when not in use and labelled with the patient's name.

Cool water is sufficient for cleaning glass lenses. A soft cloth is best for drying to prevent scratching the lens; paper towels can scratch a lens. Plastic lenses in particular are scratched easily, and special cleansing solutions and drying cloths are available for them. It is good to use whatever the patient's eye care specialist recommends.

Contact Lenses. A contact lens is a small, round, transparent, and sometimes coloured disc that fits directly over the cornea of the eye. Contact lenses are designed specifically to correct refractive errors of the eye or abnormalities in the cornea's shape. They are relatively easy to apply and remove.

Contact lenses are available in daily-wear, extended-wear, and disposable varieties. All lenses must be removed periodically to prevent ocular infection and corneal ulcers or abrasions. Patient education must include a discussion of proper lens care techniques to avoid microbial infections (e.g., keratitis) (Cheung, Nagra, & Hammersmith, 2016) (Box 38-14).

Daily-wear lenses should be removed overnight for cleaning and disinfecting; extended-wear lenses can be worn for up to 30 days without being removed (Health Canada, 2006). Disposable lenses are available in daily-wear and extended-wear varieties. Extended-wear disposable lenses are usually replaced every 1 to 2 weeks. Pain, tearing, discomfort, and redness of the conjunctivae may be symptoms of lens overwear. The persistence of symptoms after lens removal may indicate serious ocular injury.

Contact lenses accumulate secretions and foreign matter while they are being worn. These materials deteriorate and then irritate the eye, causing distorted vision and the risk for infection. Contact lenses should be cleaned and thoroughly disinfected once removed. Patients should be cautioned to never use saliva, homemade saline, or tap water when cleaning lenses as these solutions may contain microorganisms that can cause serious infections.

Artificial Eyes. Patients with artificial eyes have had an **enucleation**, or removal, of an entire eyeball as a result of a tumour growth, severe infection, or eye trauma. Some artificial eyes are permanently implanted, whereas others can be removed for routine cleaning. Patients with an artificial eye usually prefer to care for their own eye. Nurses should respect the patient's wishes and assist by assembling needed equipment.

Patients may at times require assistance in prosthesis removal and cleaning. To remove an artificial eye, retract the lower eyelid and exert slight pressure just below the eye (Figure 38-10). This action causes the artificial eye to rise from the socket because the suction holding the eye in place has been broken. A small rubber bulb syringe or medicine dropper bulb may also be used to create a suction effect. The suction created by placing the bulb tip directly over the eye and squeezing lifts the artificial eye from the socket.

The artificial eye is usually made of glass or plastic. Warm normal saline is used to clean the prosthesis. The edges of the eye socket and surrounding tissues should also be cleaned, with soft gauze moistened in saline or clean tap water. Signs of infection should be reported immediately because bacteria can spread to the neighbouring eye, underlying sinuses, or even underlying brain tissue. To reinsert the eye, retract the upper and lower lids and gently slip the eye into the socket,

BOX 38-14 PATIENT TEACHING

Contact Lens Care

Objectives

- Patient will be able to identify warning signs of corneal irritation and eye infection.
- Patient will be able to clean and care for contact lenses correctly.

Teaching Strategies

Encourage the patient to see a vision care specialist (ophthalmologist or optometrist) regularly:

- For low-risk patients: birth to 24 months: by age 3 months; age 2–5 years: prior to attending school; age 6–19 years: annually; age 20–64 years: every 1–2 years; and over age 65 years: annually
- The vision care specialist will determine the frequency for high-risk patients (Alberta Association of Optometrists, n.d.)

Teach the patient the following facts about contact lens care:

- Special cleaning solutions should be used when cleaning and disinfecting contact lenses.
- Never use fingernail on a lens to remove dirt or debris that does not loosen during washing with cleaning solutions.
- Follow recommendations of the lens manufacturer or your eye care practitioner when cleaning and disinfecting lenses.
- Remember the mnemonic RSVP: *r*edness, *s*ensitivity, *v*ision problems, and *p*ain (Health Canada, 2006). If one of these problems occurs, remove the contact lenses immediately. If problems continue, contact a vision care specialist.
- Lenses become very slippery once cleaning solution is applied.
- If a lens is dropped on a hard surface, moisten your finger with the cleaning or wetting solution and gently touch the lens to pick it up. Then clean, rinse, and disinfect the lens.
- Lenses should be kept moist or wet when not worn.
- Use fresh solution daily when storing and disinfecting lenses.
- Do not wipe the lens with a tissue or towel.
- Thoroughly wash and rinse the lens storage case on a daily basis. Clean it periodically with soap or liquid detergent; rinse it thoroughly with warm water and air-dry it.
- To avoid a mix-up, always start with the same lens when removing or inserting lenses.
- Throw away disposable or planned replacement lenses after the prescribed wearing period.

Evaluation

- Ask the patient to identify the warning signs of corneal irritation and eye infection.
- Ask the patient to describe methods of improper contact lens handling that can lead to infection.
- Ask the patient to describe the techniques required to clean and store contact lenses.

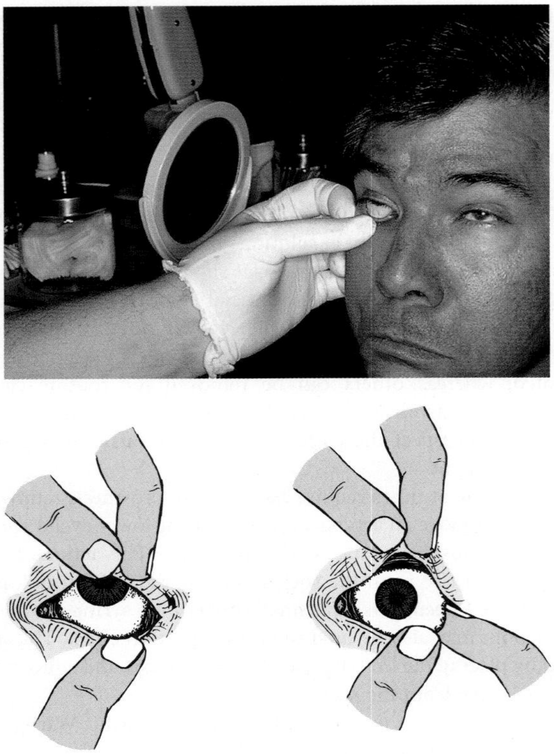

FIGURE 38-10 Removal of a prosthetic eye To remove an artificial eye, retract the lower eyelid and exert slight pressure just below the eye. This action causes the artificial eye to rise from the socket because the suction holding the eye in place has been broken. A small, rubber bulb syringe or medicine-dropper bulb can also be used to create a suction effect. Place the bulb tip directly over the eye and squeeze it to create suction needed to lift the eye from the socket. (Not pictured.)

fitting it neatly under the upper eyelid. An artificial eye may be stored in a labelled container filled with tap water or saline.

Ear Care. Routine ear care involves cleaning the ear with the end of a moistened washcloth, rotated gently into the ear canal. When cerumen is visible, a gentle, downward retraction at the entrance of the ear canal may cause the cerumen to loosen and slip out. Nurses should warn patients never to use sharp objects such as bobby pins or paper clips to remove cerumen as this can traumatize the ear canal and rupture the tympanic membrane. Use of cotton-tipped applicators should also be avoided because they can cause cerumen to become impacted within the canal.

Children and older persons commonly have impacted cerumen. Excessive or impacted cerumen can usually be removed only by irrigation, which usually requires a physician's or nurse practitioner's order. If a patient has a history of a perforated eardrum or if perforation is discovered during assessment, the procedure is contraindicated. Before irrigation, instill three drops of glycerine at bedtime to soften the cerumen and three drops of hydrogen peroxide twice a day to loosen the cerumen. Then irrigation with approximately 250 mL of warm water (at 37°C) into the ear canal mechanically washes away loosened cerumen. The use of cold or hot water can cause nausea or vomiting.

The patient may sit or lie on his or her side with the affected ear up. To irrigate the ear, place a small curved basin under the affected ear to catch the irrigating solution, and use a bulb-irrigating syringe. The tip of the syringe should not occlude the ear canal, to avoid exerting pressure against the tympanic membrane. Direct a gentle irrigation at the top of the canal to loosen the cerumen from the sides of the canal. After the canal is clear, wipe off any moisture from the ear and inspect the canal for remaining cerumen.

Hearing Aid Care. Hearing aids are instruments made up of miniature parts working together as a system to amplify sound in a controlled manner. Aids receive normal low-intensity sound inputs and deliver them to the ear as louder outputs. The new class of hearing aids can reduce background noise interference. Computer chips placed in the aids allow for fine adjustments to a specific patient's hearing needs. Hearing aids are used by both hard-of-hearing individuals (those with a slight or moderate hearing loss) and deaf individuals (those with severe or profound hearing loss). While mechanical dysfunction of the external or middle ear causes conductive hearing loss, which could be due to impacted cerumen or a foreign body that obstructs the transmission of sound, sensorineural (perceptive) hearing loss indicates a pathology in the inner ear, cranial nerve VII damage, or presbycusis (gradual nerve degeneration that occurs with aging) (Cullington, Kitterick, Debold, et al., 2016). Although cochlear implants in children with significant hearing loss are becoming more widely available, there is no statistical information available regarding the number of children in Canada who have received cochlear implants; however, Fitzpatrick and Brewster (2010) undertook a survey that examined the growing use of cochlear implantation for adults. According to their results, by 2007, 2 534 adults had received cochlear implants in Canada. Resource allocation and access were two of the major concerns affecting the number of adult cochlear implantation surgeries performed.

Three popular types of hearing aids are available. An *in-the-canal (ITC) aid* is the newest, smallest, and least visible hearing aid and fits entirely in the ear canal. It has cosmetic appeal, is easy to manipulate and place in the ear, does not interfere with wearing eyeglasses or using the telephone, and can be worn during most physical exercise. However, it requires an adequate ear diameter and depth for proper fit. It does not accommodate progressive hearing loss, and it requires manual dexterity to operate, insert, remove, and change the batteries. Also, cerumen tends to plug this model more than the other models.

An *in-the-ear (ITE, or intra-aural) aid* (Figure 38-11, *A*) fits into the external auditory canal and allows for better fine-tuning. It is more powerful and stronger than the ITC aid and therefore is useful for a wider range of hearing loss. It is easy to position and adjust and does not interfere with wearing eyeglasses. It is, however, more noticeable than the ITC aid and is not recommended for persons with moisture or skin problems in the ear canal.

A *behind-the-ear (BTE, or postaural) aid* (Figure 38-11, *B*) hooks around and behind the ear and is connected by a short, clear, hollow plastic tube to an ear mould inserted into the external auditory canal. It allows for fine-tuning. It is the largest of the three aids and is useful for patients with rapidly progressive hearing loss or manual dexterity difficulties and those who find partial ear occlusion intolerable. Disadvantages are that it is more visible, may interfere with wearing eyeglasses and using a phone, and is more difficult to keep in place during physical exercise. Box 38-15 reviews patient education guidelines for the care and use of a hearing aid.

Nasal Care. The patient can usually remove secretions from the nose by gently blowing into a soft tissue. The patient should be cautioned against harsh blowing; this can create pressure capable of injuring the eardrum, nasal mucosa, and even sensitive eye structures. Bleeding from the nares is a sign of harsh blowing.

If the patient is unable to remove nasal secretions, the nurse can assist by using a wet washcloth or a cotton-tipped applicator moistened in water or saline. The applicator should never be inserted beyond the

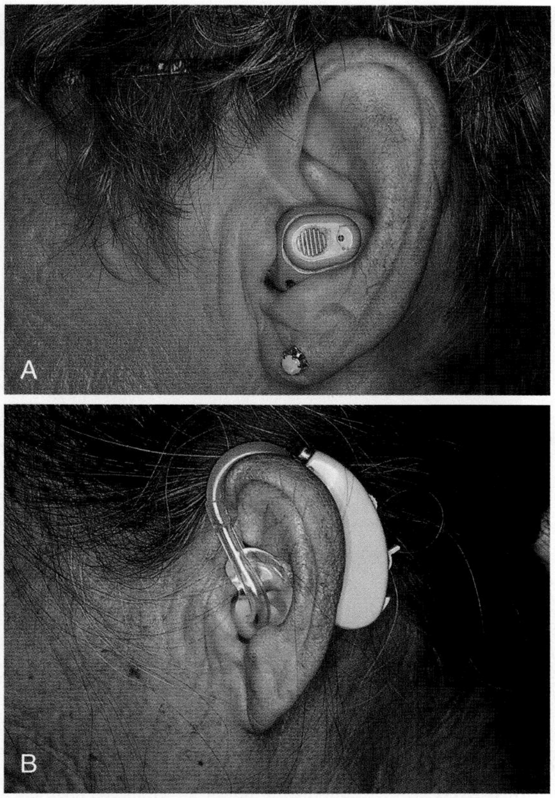

FIGURE 38-11 Two common types of hearing aids. **A,** In the ear. **B,** Behind the ear.

length of the cotton tip. Excessive nasal secretions can also be removed by gentle suctioning.

When patients have a nasogastric, feeding, or endotracheal tube inserted through the nose, the nurse should change the tape anchoring it when soiled or if it becomes loose. When tape becomes moist from nasal secretions, the skin and mucosa can easily become macerated. Friction from the tube can cause tissue sloughing. After carefully removing the tape, the nurse maintains hold of the tubing and thoroughly cleans and dries the nasal surface (see Chapter 42).

Patient's Room Environment

Attempting to make a patient's room as comfortable as possible is an important priority. The patient's room should be comfortable, safe, and large enough to allow the patient and several visitors to move about freely. Room temperature and ventilation are difficult to control; however, noise and odours can be controlled to create a more comfortable environment. Keeping the room neat and orderly also contributes to the patient's sense of well-being.

Maintaining Comfort. The nature of what constitutes a comfortable environment depends on the patient's age, severity of illness, and level of daily activity. Depending on the patient's age and physical condition, the room temperature should be maintained between 20°C and 23°C, if possible. Infants, older persons, and the acutely ill may need a warmer room. However, certain acutely ill patients (e.g., patients with head injuries) may benefit from cooler room temperatures to lower the body's metabolic demands to reduce intracranial pressure.

A good ventilation system keeps stale air and odours from lingering in the room. The acutely ill, infants, and older persons must be protected from drafts by ensuring that they are adequately dressed and covered with a lightweight blanket.

BOX 38-15 Care and Use of Hearing Aids by the Patient

- Initially, wear a hearing aid for short periods; then gradually increase the wearing time to 10–12 hours.
- Once inserted, turn the aid slowly to one-third to one-half volume.
- Remember that a whistling sound indicates too high a volume, incorrect ear mould insertion, an improper fit of the aid, or a buildup of earwax or fluid.
- Adjust the volume to a comfortable level for talking at a distance of 1 m.
- Do not wear the aid under heat lamps, while using a hair dryer, or in very wet, cold weather.
- Keep in mind that batteries can last 70–85 hours—1 week with daily wearing of 10–12 hours.
- Remove or disconnect the battery when not in use.
- Replace ear moulds every 2–3 years.
- Routinely check the battery compartment: Is it clean? Are batteries inserted properly? Is the compartment shut all the way?
- Remember that dials on the hearing aid should be clean and easy to rotate, creating no static during adjusting.
- Keep the aid clean.
- Aids are usually cleaned with a soft cloth and warm soapy water; see the manufacturer's instructions.
- Avoid the use of hairspray and perfume while wearing the hearing aid; the residue from the spray can cause the aid to become oily and greasy.
- Do not submerse the aid in water.
- Routinely check the cord or tubing (depending on type of aid) for cracking, fraying, and poor connections.
- Follow up with an audiologist routinely to evaluate the effectiveness of the current aid.
- Remember that the frequencies of newer computerized hearing aids can be easily adjusted.

Data from Eliopoulous, C. (2013). *Gerontological nursing* (8th ed.). Philadelphia, PA: Lippincott Williams & Wilkins; Miller, C. A. (2014). *Nursing for wellness in older adults* (7th ed.). Philadelphia, PA: Lippincott Williams & Wilkins; and Touhy, T. A., & Jett, K., (2016). *Toward healthy aging: Human needs and nursing response* (9th ed.). St. Louis, MO: Mosby.

Good ventilation also reduces lingering odours caused by draining wounds, vomitus, bowel movements, and unemptied urinals. Room deodorizers can help remove many unpleasant odours but should be used with discretion in consideration of the patient's possible embarrassment. Before using room deodorizers, it is important to determine that the patient is not allergic or sensitive to the deodorizer itself. Vanilla, poured onto a gauze inside a basin, and placed under the bed, can work well to discreetly mask unpleasant odours. Bedpans and urinals should be emptied and rinsed promptly. Thorough hygiene measures are the best way to control body or breath odours.

Ill patients seem to be more sensitive to common hospital noises (e.g., IV pump alarms, suction apparatus, or stretchers exiting an elevator). The nurse should explain the source of any unfamiliar noise to the patient and family members. Until the patient is familiar with hospital noises, the noise level should be controlled as much as possible. This can also help the patient sleep (see Chapter 41).

Proper lighting is necessary for everyone's safety and comfort. A brightly lit room is usually stimulating, and a darkened room is best for rest and sleep. Room lighting can be adjusted by closing or opening drapes, regulating overbed lights, and closing or opening room doors. When entering a patient's room at night, the nurse should refrain from abruptly turning on an overhead light unless necessary.

Room Equipment. Although variations in hospital rooms exist across health care settings, a typical hospital room contains the following basic pieces of furniture: an overbed table, a bedside stand, chairs, and a bed (Figure 38-12). Long-term care and rehabilitation facilities may have similar equipment. The overbed table rolls on wheels and can be adjusted to various heights over the bed or a chair. The table provides an ideal working space for performing procedures. It also provides a surface on which to place meal trays, toiletry items, and objects frequently used by the patient. The bedpan and urinal should not be placed on the overbed table. The bedside stand is used to store the patient's personal possessions and hygiene equipment. A telephone (if supplied), water pitcher, and drinking cup are commonly found on top of the bedside stand.

Most hospital rooms contain an armless straight-backed chair or an upholstered lounge chair with arms. Straight-backed chairs are convenient to use when temporarily transferring the patient from the bed, such as during bed making. Lounge chairs tend to be more comfortable when a patient is willing and able to sit for an extended period.

Each room usually has an overbed light. Additional portable lighting can be used to provide extra light during bedside procedures. Other equipment usually found in a patient's room is a call bell, a television set (not available in all agencies and facilities), a wall-mounted blood pressure gauge, oxygen and vacuum wall outlets, and personal-care items. Special equipment designed for comfort or positioning patients includes foot boots, special mattresses, and bed boards (see Chapters 45 and 46). Nurses should check their agency's policy and the manufacturers' directions before using comfort and positioning equipment.

Beds. Seriously ill patients may remain in bed for a long time. Because a bed is the piece of equipment used most by a hospitalized patient, it should be designed for comfort, safety, and adaptability for changing positions. The typical hospital bed has a firm mattress on a metal frame that can be raised and lowered horizontally. Many hospitals are converting the standard hospital bed to one in which the mattress surface can be electronically adjusted for patient comfort. Different bed positions are used to promote patient comfort, minimize symptoms, promote lung expansion, and improve access during certain procedures (Table 38-6).

The position of a bed is usually changed by electrical controls incorporated into the patient's call light and in a panel on the side or foot of the bed (Figure 38-13). However, some facilities do have hospital beds that are manually controlled. It is important to become familiar with the use of the bed controls. Ease in raising and lowering a bed and in changing the position of the bed head and foot eliminates undue musculoskeletal strain on the care provider. Instructions should be provided to the patients on the proper use of controls; they should be cautioned against raising the bed to a position that might cause harm.

TABLE 38-6 Common Bed Positions

Position	Description	Uses
Fowler's 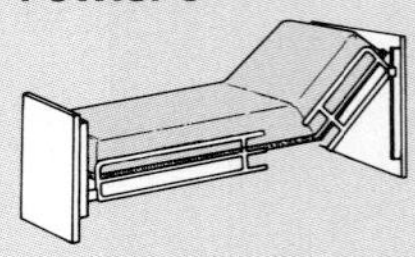	Head of bed raised to angle of 45 degrees or more; semisitting position; foot of bed may also be raised at knee	Is preferred while patient eats Is used during nasogastric tube insertion and nasotracheal suction Promotes lung expansion
Semi-Fowler's 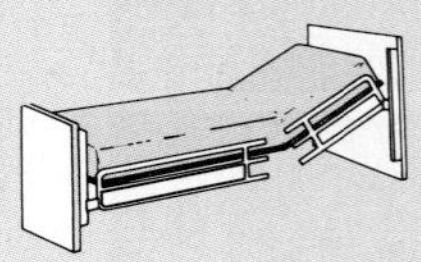	Head of bed raised approximately 30 degrees; inclination less than Fowler's position; foot of bed may also be raised at knee	Promotes lung expansion Is used when patients receive gastric feedings to reduce regurgitation and risk of aspiration
Trendelenburg's 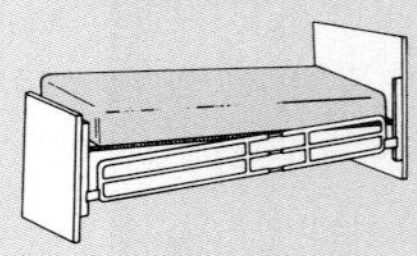	Entire bed frame tilted with head of bed down	Is used for postural drainage Facilitates venous return in patients with poor peripheral perfusion
Reverse Trendelenburg's 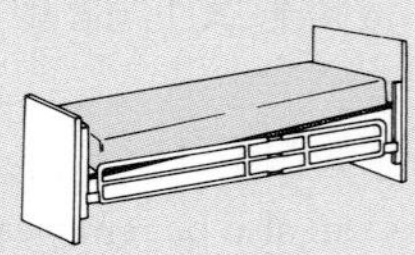	Entire bed frame tilted with foot of bed down	Is used infrequently Promotes gastric emptying Prevents esophageal reflux
Flat 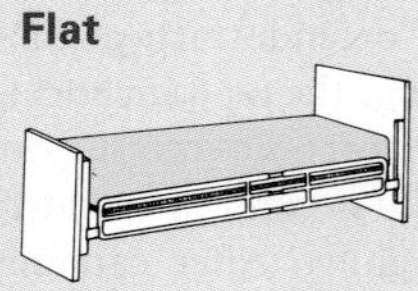	Entire bed frame horizontally parallel with floor	Is used for patients with vertebral injuries and in cervical traction Is used for patients who are hypotensive Is generally preferred by patients for sleeping

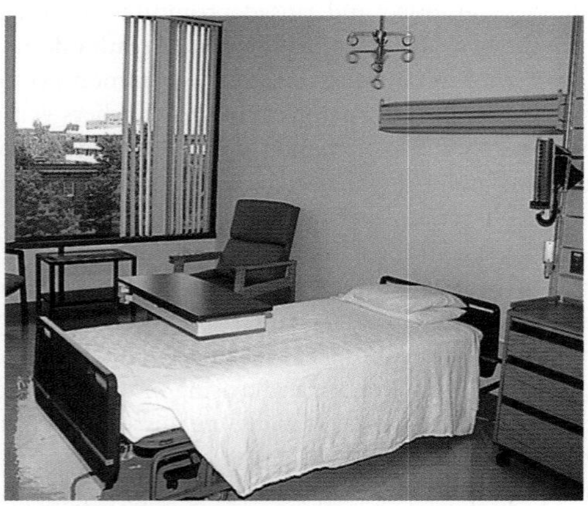

FIGURE 38-12 A typical hospital room.

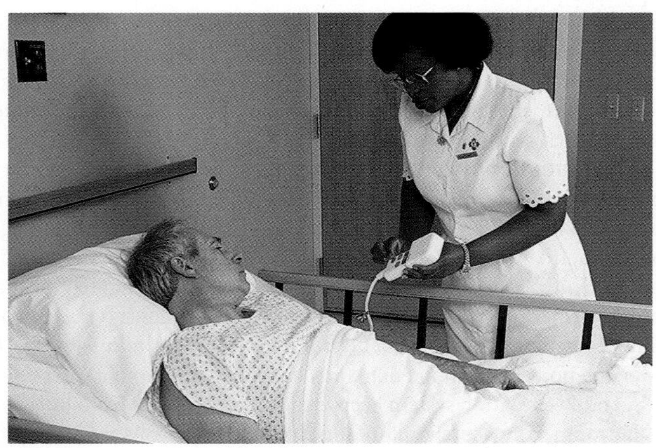

FIGURE 38-13 Instruct patient in use of call light and bed controls.

Beds contain safety features such as locks on the wheels or casters, and alarms. Wheels should be locked when the bed is stationary to prevent accidental movement. Alarms should be turned on to protect patients at risk for falls when getting out of bed without assistance. Side rails protect patients from accidental falls. The headboard can be removed from most beds. This is important when the medical team must have easy access to the patient's head, such as during cardiopulmonary resuscitation.

Bed making. A patient's bed should be kept clean and comfortable. This requires frequent inspections to be sure linen is clean, dry, and free of wrinkles. When patients are diaphoretic, have draining wounds, or are incontinent, nurses should check frequently for soiled linen.

The bed is usually made in the morning after the patient's bath or while the patient is in the shower, sitting in a chair eating, or out of the room for procedures or tests. Throughout the day, bed linens should be straightened when they become loose or wrinkled. The bed linen should also be checked for food particles after meals and for wetness or soiling. Linens that are soiled or wet should be changed.

When changing bed linen, nurses need to follow the principles of medical asepsis by keeping soiled linen away from their uniform (Figure 38-14). Soiled linen is placed in special linen bags before discarding it in a hamper. To avoid air currents, which can spread microorganisms, bed linens should never be shaken. To avoid transmitting infection, soiled linen should not be placed on the floor. If clean linen touches the floor, it should be immediately discarded.

During bed making, it is important to use proper body mechanics (see Chapter 36). The bed should always be raised to the appropriate height before changing linen so that you do not have to bend or stretch over the mattress. You should also move back and forth to opposite sides of the bed while putting on new linen. Body mechanics is also important when turning or repositioning the patient in bed.

When patients are confined to a bed, organize bed-making activities to conserve time and energy (Figure 38-15 and Skill 38-5). The patient's privacy, comfort, and safety are all important. To help promote comfort and safety, use side rails to aid positioning and turning, keep a call light within the patient's reach, and maintain the proper bed position. After making a bed, always return it to the lowest horizontal position to prevent accidental falls should the patient get in and out of the bed alone.

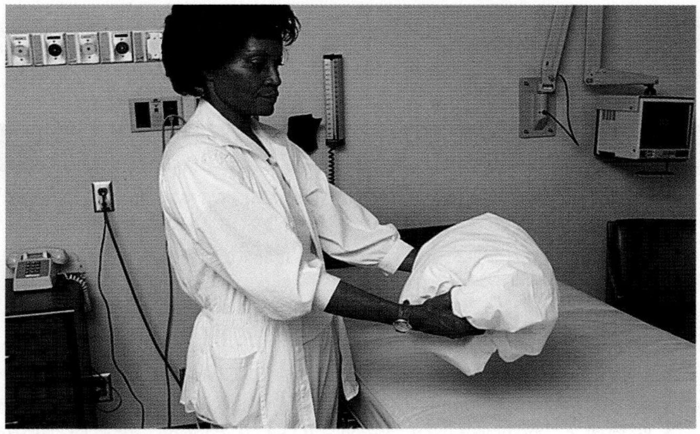

FIGURE 38-14 Holding linen away from the uniform prevents contact with microorganisms.

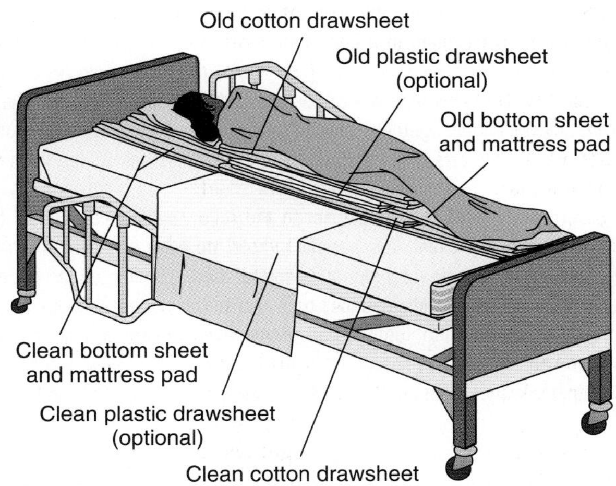

FIGURE 38-15 Equipment for making an occupied bed.

SKILL 38-5 MAKING AN OCCUPIED BED

Delegation Considerations

The skill of making an occupied bed can be delegated to an unregulated care provider (UCP). It is important to discuss the following with the UCP:

- Any precautions or activity restrictions for the patient
- What to do if wound drainage, dressing material, drainage tubes, or IV tubing becomes dislodged or is found in the linens
- What to do if the patient becomes fatigued

Equipment

See Figure 38-15.

- Linen bag(s)
- Bottom sheet (flat or fitted)
- Drawsheet (optional)
- Top sheet
- Blanket
- Bedspread
- Waterproof pads or soaker pad (optional)
- Pillowcases
- Bedside chair or table
- Disposable gloves (optional)
- Towel
- Disinfectant

Continued

SKILL 38-5 MAKING AN OCCUPIED BED—cont'd

PROCEDURE

STEPS	RATIONALE
1. Assess potential for patient incontinence or excess drainage on bed linen.	• Determines the need for protective waterproof pads or extra bath blankets on the bed.
2. Check chart for orders or specific precautions concerning movement and positioning.	• Ensures patient safety and the use of proper body mechanics.
3. Explain procedure to the patient, noting that he or she will be asked to turn on side and roll over linen.	• Minimizes anxiety and encourages cooperation.
4. Perform hand hygiene and put on gloves. (Gloves are worn only if linen is soiled or if contact with body secretions is possible.)	• Reduces the transmission of microorganisms.
5. Assemble equipment and arrange it on a bedside chair or table. Remove unnecessary equipment such as a dietary tray or items used for hygiene.	• Assembling all equipment provides for a smooth procedure and assists in increasing the patient's comfort. Placing linen on a clean surface minimizes spread of infection.
6. Draw room curtain around bed or close room door.	• Maintains patient's privacy.
7. Adjust bed height to a comfortable working position. Lower any raised side rail on one side of bed. Remove the call light.	• Minimizes strain on the back. It is easier to remove and put on linen evenly with bed in a flat position. Provides easy access to bed and linen.
8. Loosen top linen at foot of the bed.	• Makes linen easier to remove.
9. Remove bedspread and blanket separately. If bedspread and blanket are soiled, place them in a linen bag. Keep soiled linen away from your uniform.	• Reduces the transmission of microorganisms.
10. If blanket and bedspread are to be reused, fold them by bringing the top and bottom edges together. Fold the farthest side over onto nearer bottom edge. Bring top and bottom edges together again. Place folded linen over back of chair.	• Folding method facilitates replacement and minimizes wrinkles.
11. Cover patient with a bath blanket in the following manner: Unfold bath blanket over top sheet. Ask patient to hold top edge of the bath blanket. If patient is unable to help, tuck top of bath blanket under patient's shoulder. Grasp top sheet under bath blanket at patient's shoulders and bring sheet down to foot of bed. Remove the sheet and discard in a linen bag.	• Bath blanket provides warmth and keeps body parts covered during linen removal.
12. With assistance from another, slide mattress toward head of the bed.	• If mattress slides toward foot of the bed when head of the bed is raised, it is difficult to tuck in linen. In addition, it is uncomfortable for the patient because the patient's feet may be pressed against or hang over the foot of the bed.
13. Position patient on the far side of the bed, turned onto his or her side and facing away from you. Be sure side rail in front of patient is up. Adjust pillow under patient's head.	• Turning patient onto side provides space for placement of clean linen. Side rail ensures patient's safety, preventing forward falls from the bed surface, and helps patient in moving.
14. Loosen bottom linens, moving from head to foot. With seam side down (facing the mattress), fanfold bottom sheet and drawsheet toward patient—first drawsheet, then bottom sheet. Tuck edges of linen just under buttocks, back, and shoulders. Do not fanfold mattress pad if it is to be reused (see Step 14 illustration).	• Prepares for removal of all bottom linen simultaneously. Provides maximum workspace for placing clean linen. Later, when patient turns to other side, soiled linen can be removed easily.
15. Wipe off any moisture on exposed mattress with towel and appropriate disinfectant.	• Reduces the transmission of microorganisms.
16. Put clean linen on exposed half of the bed:	
A. Place clean mattress pad on bed by folding it lengthwise with centre crease in middle of bed. Fanfold top layer over mattress. (If pad is reused, simply smooth out any wrinkles.)	• Putting on linen over bed in successive layers minimizes energy and time used in bed making.

STEPS	RATIONALE

B. Unfold bottom sheet lengthwise so that centre crease is situated lengthwise along centre of bed. Fanfold sheet's top layer toward centre of bed alongside the patient. Smooth bottom layer of sheet over mattress, and bring the edge over closest side of the mattress. Pull fitted sheet smoothly over mattress ends. Allow edge of flat unfitted sheet to hang about 25 cm over mattress edge. Lower hem of bottom flat sheet should lie seam down and even with bottom edge of mattress (see Step 16B illustration).

- Proper positioning of linen on one side ensures that adequate linen will be available to cover opposite side of bed. Keeping seam edges down eliminates irritation to patient's skin.

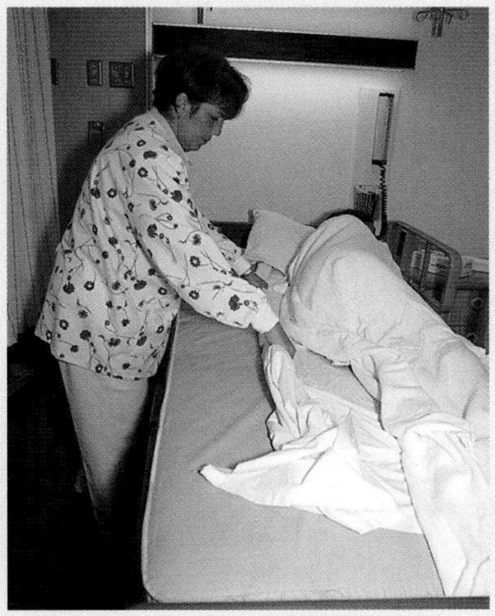

STEP 14 Old linen tucked under patient.

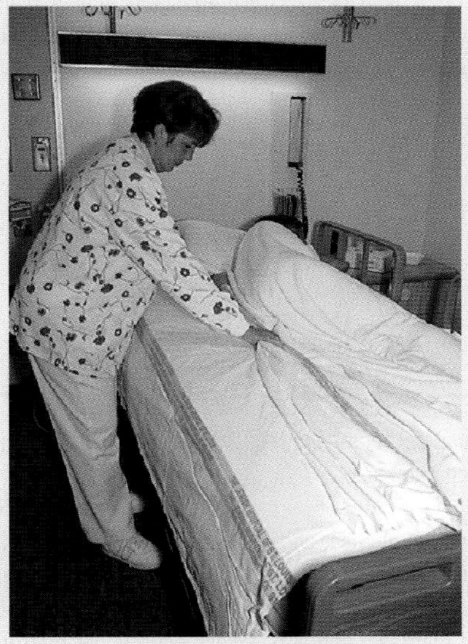

STEP 16B Clean linen applied to bed.

17. Mitre bottom flat sheet at head of bed (if fitted sheets are not in use):

- Mitred corner cannot be loosened easily even if patient moves frequently in bed.

A. Face head of bed diagonally. Place hand away from head of bed under top corner of mattress, near mattress edge, and lift.

B. With other hand, tuck top edge of bottom sheet smoothly under mattress so that side edges of sheet above and below the mattress would meet if brought together.

C. Face side of the bed and pick up top edge of sheet at approximately 45 cm from top of mattress (see Step 17C illustration).

D. Lift sheet, and lay it on top of mattress to form a neat triangular fold, with lower base of the triangle even with the mattress side edge (see Step 17D illustration).

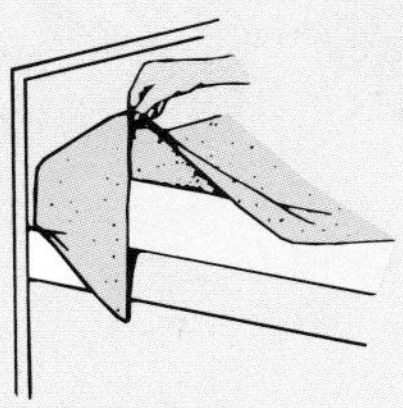

STEP 17C Pick up top edge of sheet.

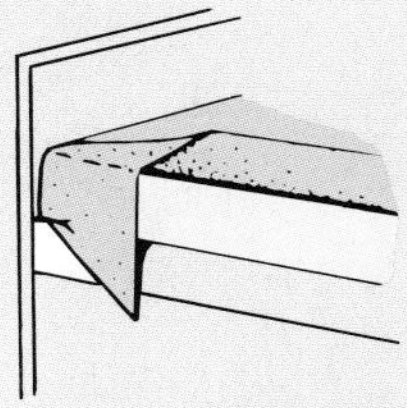

STEP 17D Sheet on top of mattress in a triangular fold.

Continued

SKILL 38-5 MAKING AN OCCUPIED BED—cont'd

STEPS	RATIONALE

E. Tuck lower edge of sheet, which is hanging free below the mattress, under the mattress. Tuck with palms down, without pulling triangular fold (see Step 17E illustration).

F. Hold portion of sheet covering side of mattress in place with one hand. With the other hand, pick up top of triangular linen fold and bring it down over side of the mattress (see Step 17F illustrations). Tuck this portion under mattress (see Step 17F illustrations).

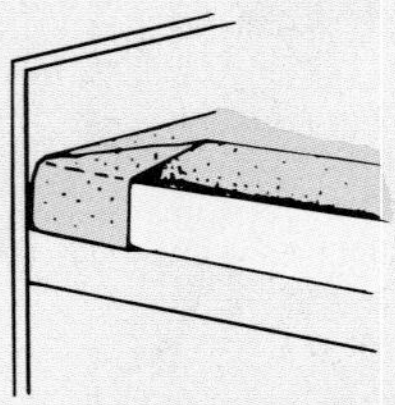

STEP 17E Lower edge of sheet tucked under mattress.

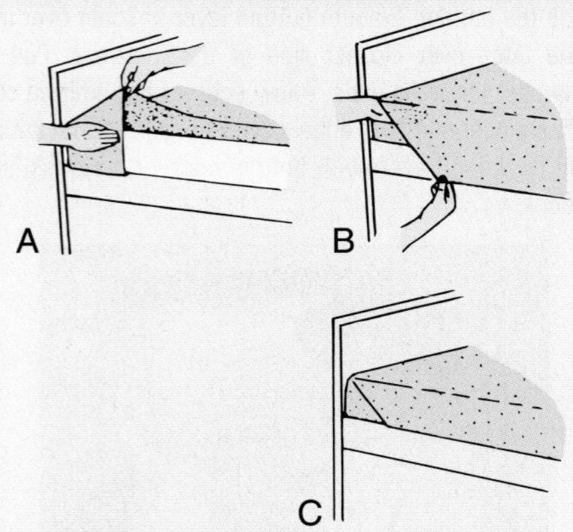

STEP 17F A and B, Triangular fold placed over side of mattress. **C**, Linen tucked under mattress.

18. Tuck remaining portion of sheet under the mattress, moving toward foot of the bed. Keep linen smooth.
- Folds of linen are source of irritation for patient.

19. *(Optional)* Open drawsheet so that it unfolds in half. Lay centrefold along middle of bed lengthwise, and position sheet so that it will be under the patient's buttocks and torso (see Step 19 illustration). Fanfold top layer toward patient, with edge along the patient's back. Smooth bottom layer out over the mattress, and tuck excess edge under mattress (keep palms down).
- Drawsheet is used to lift and reposition the patient. Placement under patient's torso distributes most of the patient's body weight over the sheet.

20. Place waterproof pad over drawsheet, with centrefold against patient's side. Fanfold top layer toward patient.
- Protects bed linen from being soiled.

21. Have patient roll slowly toward you, over the layers of linen. Raise side rail on working side, and go to other side of the bed.
- Positions patient for removal and placement of linens. Maintains patient's safety and body alignment during turning.

22. Lower side rail. Assist patient in positioning on other side, over folds of linen (see Step 22 illustration). Loosen edges of soiled linen from under mattress.
- Exposes opposite side of bed for removal of soiled linen and placement of clean linen. Makes linen easier to remove.

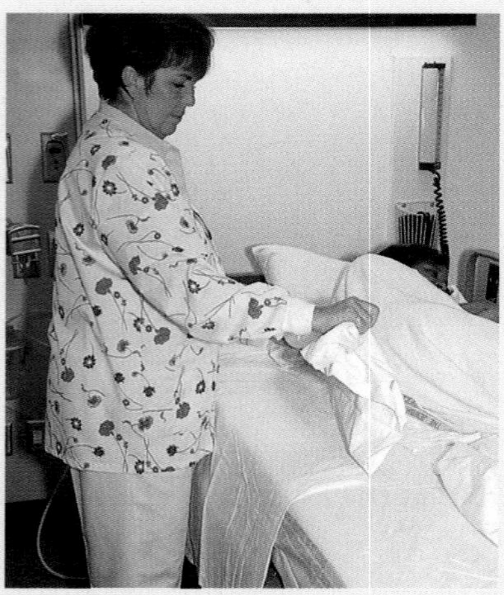

STEP 19 Optional drawsheet.

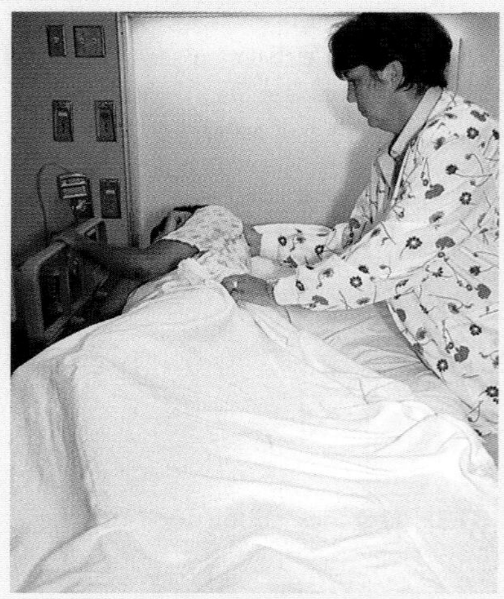

STEP 22 Assist patient to roll over folds of linen.

23. Remove soiled linen by folding it into a bundle or square, with soiled side turned in. Discard in linen bag. If necessary, wipe mattress with antiseptic solution, and dry mattress surface before putting on new linen.
- Reduces the transmission of microorganisms.

24. Pull clean, fanfolded linen smoothly over edge of mattress from head to foot of bed.
- Smooth linen will not irritate patient's skin.

25. Assist patient in rolling back into supine position. Reposition pillow.
- Maintains patient's comfort.

STEPS	RATIONALE
26. Pull fitted sheet smoothly over mattress ends. Mitre top corner of bottom sheet (see Step 17). When tucking corner, be sure that sheet is smooth and free of wrinkles.	• Wrinkles and folds can cause irritation to the skin.
27. Facing side of the bed, grasp remaining edge of bottom flat sheet. Lean back; keeping back straight, pull while tucking excess linen under mattress. Proceed from head to foot of the bed. (Avoid lifting mattress during tucking to ensure fit.)	• Proper use of body mechanics while tucking linen prevents injury.
28. Smooth fanfolded drawsheet out over bottom sheet. Grasp edge of the sheet with palms down, lean back, and tuck sheet under mattress. Tuck from middle to top and then to bottom.	• Tucking first at top or bottom may pull sheet sideways, causing poor fit.
29. Place top sheet over patient with centrefold lengthwise down middle of bed. Open sheet from head to foot, and unfold over patient.	• Sheet should be equally distributed over bed by correctly positioning centrefold.
30. Ask patient to hold clean top sheet, or tuck sheet around patient's shoulders. Remove the bath blanket and discard in linen bag.	• Sheet prevents exposure of body parts. Having patient hold sheet encourages patient participation in care.
31. Place blanket on bed, unfolding it so that crease runs lengthwise along middle of bed. Unfold blanket to cover patient. Top edge should be parallel with edge of top sheet and 15–20 cm from top sheet's edge.	• Blanket should be placed to cover patient completely and provide adequate warmth.
32. Place bedspread over bed according to Step 31. Be sure that top edge of bedspread extends about 2.5 cm above blanket's edge. Tuck top edge of bedspread over and under top edge of blanket.	• Gives bed neat appearance and provides extra warmth.
33. Make cuff by turning edge of top sheet down over top edge of the blanket and bedspread.	• Protects patient's face from rubbing against blanket or bedspread.
34. Standing on one side at foot of the bed, lift mattress corner slightly with one hand and tuck linens under mattress. Tuck top sheet and blanket under together. Be sure that linens are loose enough to allow movement of patient's feet. Making a horizontal toe pleat is an option (see Step 34 illustration).	• Makes neat-appearing bed. Pressure injuries can develop on patient's toes and heels from feet rubbing against tight-fitting bed sheets.

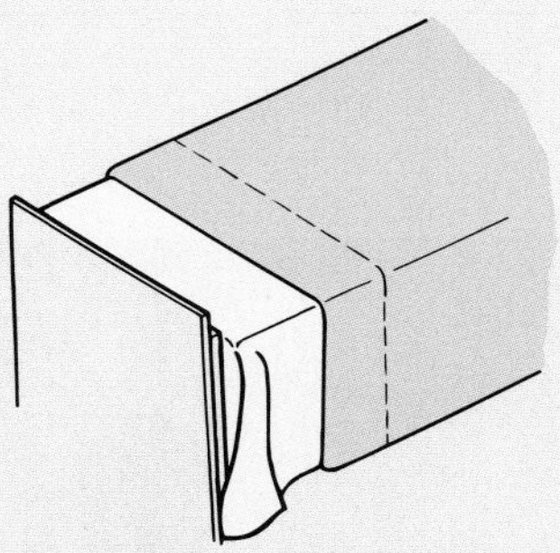

STEP 34 Optional toe pleat.

STEPS	RATIONALE
35. Make modified mitred corner with top sheet, blanket, and bedspread (see Box 38-16, Step 20 illustration):	• Ensures that top covers will not loosen easily.
A. Pick up side edge of top sheet, blanket, and bedspread approximately 45 cm from foot of the mattress. Lift linen to form triangular fold, and lay it on bed.	
B. Tuck lower edge of sheet, which is hanging free below mattress, under the mattress. Do not pull triangular fold.	
C. Pick up triangular fold, and bring it down over mattress while holding linen in place alongside of the mattress. Do not tuck tip of triangle.	• Secures top linen but keeps even edge of blanket and top sheet draped over mattress.
36. Raise side rail. Make other side of bed; spread sheet, blanket, and bedspread out evenly. Fold top edge of bedspread over the blanket and make cuff with top sheet (see Step 33); make modified mitred corner at foot of bed (see Step 35).	• Side rail protects patient from accidental falls.
37. Change pillowcase:	
A. Have patient raise his or her head. While supporting patient's neck with one hand, remove pillow. Allow patient to lower head.	• Support of neck muscles prevents injury during flexion and extension of neck.
B. Remove soiled case by grasping pillow at open end with one hand and pulling case back over pillow with the other hand. Discard case in linen bag.	• Pillows slide out easily, thus minimizing contact with soiled linen.

Continued

SKILL 38-5 MAKING AN OCCUPIED BED—cont'd

STEPS	RATIONALE
C. Grasp clean pillowcase at centre of closed end. Gather case, turning it inside out over the hand holding it. With the same hand, pick up the middle of one end of the pillow. Pull pillowcase down over pillow with the other hand.	• Eases sliding of pillowcase over pillow.
D. Be sure pillow corners fit evenly into corners of the pillowcase. Place pillow under the patient's head.	• Poorly fitting case constricts fluffing and expansion of the pillow and interferes with patient comfort.
38. Place call bell within the patient's reach, and return the bed to comfortable position.	• Ensures patient safety and comfort.
39. Open room curtains, and rearrange furniture. Place personal items within easy reach on overbed table or bedside stand. Return bed to a comfortable height.	• Promotes sense of well-being.
40. Discard dirty linen in a hamper or chute, remove gloves, and perform hand hygiene.	• Helps prevent the transmission of microorganisms.
41. Ask whether patient feels comfortable.	• Ensures that bed linens are clean and smooth.
42. While you are performing this skill, inspect the patient's skin for areas of irritation.	• Folds in linen can cause pressure on the skin.
43. Observe the patient for signs of fatigue, dyspnea, pain, or discomfort throughout the skill.	• Provides data about patient's level of activity tolerance and ability to participate in other procedures.

UNEXPECTED OUTCOMES	RELATED INTERVENTIONS
Discomfort caused by linen fold	• Tighten sheets. • Change patient's position frequently.
Signs of breakdown of patient's skin	• Institute skin care measures to reduce risk of pressure injury (see Chapter 46). • Change patient's position frequently.

RECORDING AND REPORTING

- Making an occupied bed need not be recorded.

When possible, a bed should be made while it is unoccupied (Box 38-16). Use clinical judgement regarding the best time to have the patient sit up in a chair while the bed is made. When making an unoccupied bed, follow the basic principles for making an occupied bed.

An unoccupied bed can be open or closed. In an open bed, the top covers are folded back so that a patient can easily get into bed. In a closed bed, the top sheet, blanket, and bedspread are drawn up to the head of the mattress and under the pillows. A closed bed is prepared in a hospital room before a new patient is admitted to that room.

A surgical, recovery, or postoperative bed is a modified version of the open bed. The top bed linen is arranged for easy transfer of the patient from a stretcher to the bed. The top sheets and bedspread are not tucked or mitred at the corners. Instead, the top sheets are folded to one side or to the bottom third of the bed (Figure 38-16). This makes it easier to transfer the patient into the bed.

Linens. In any health care agency, it is important to have an adequate supply of linen to care appropriately for patients. Many agencies have "nurse servers," either within or just outside a patient's room, where a daily supply of linen is stored. Because of the emphasis on cost control in health care, it is important to not bring excess linen into a patient's room. Linen brought into a patient's room, if unused, must be discarded for laundering, which can increase an agency's costs. Excess linen lying around a patient's room creates clutter and obstacles for patient care activities.

Before bed making, it is important to collect necessary bed linen and the patient's personal items. In this way, the nurse has all equipment accessible to prepare the bed and room. Linens are pressed and folded to help prevent the spread of microorganisms and to make bed making easier. When fitted sheets are not available, flat sheets usually are pressed with a centre crease to be placed down the centre of the bed. The linen unfolds easily to the sides, with creases often fitting over the mattress edge. A complete linen change is not always necessary. The sheet, blanket, and bedspread may be reused for the same patient if they are not wet or soiled.

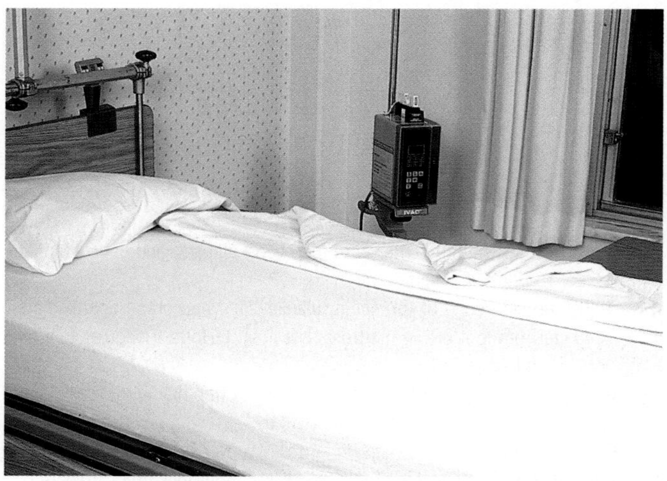

FIGURE 38-16 Surgical or recovery bed.

BOX 38-16 PROCEDURAL GUIDELINE

Making an Unoccupied Bed

Delegation Considerations

The skill of making an unoccupied bed can be delegated to an unregulated care provider (UCP).

Equipment

- Linen bag
- Bottom sheet (flat or fitted)
- Drawsheet (optional)
- Top sheet
- Blanket
- Bedspread
- Waterproof pads or soaker pad (optional)
- Pillowcases
- Bedside chair or table
- Disposable gloves (if linen is soiled)
- Washcloth
- Antiseptic cleanser

Procedure

1. Determine whether patient has been incontinent or excess drainage is on linen. Gloves will be necessary.
2. Assess activity orders or restrictions in mobility to plan whether patient can get out of bed for the procedure. If so, assist patient to bedside chair or recliner.
3. Raise bed to a comfortable working position. Lower the side rails on both sides of the bed.
4. Remove soiled linen and place in linen bag. Avoid shaking or fanning linen.
5. Reposition mattress and wipe off any moisture using a washcloth moistened in antiseptic solution. Dry thoroughly.
6. Put on all bottom linen on one side of bed before moving to opposite side.
7. Be sure fitted sheet is placed smoothly over mattress. To put on a flat unfitted sheet, allow about 25 cm to hang over mattress edge. Lower hem of the sheet should lie seam down, even with bottom edge of the mattress. Pull remaining top portion of sheet over top edge of the mattress.
8. While standing at head of the bed, mitre top corner of bottom sheet (see Skill 38-5, Step 17).
9. Tuck remaining portion of unfitted sheet under the mattress.
10. *Optional and agency or facility specific:* Put on a drawsheet, laying centre fold along middle of the bed lengthwise. Smooth drawsheet over the mattress and tuck excess edge under mattress, keeping palms down.
11. Move to opposite side of the bed, and spread bottom sheet smoothly over edge of mattress from head to foot of the bed.
12. Put on fitted sheet smoothly over each mattress corner. For an unfitted sheet, mitre the top corner of bottom sheet (see Skill 38-5, Step 17), making sure corner is taut.
13. Grasp remaining edge of unfitted bottom sheet and tuck tightly under the mattress while moving from head to foot of the bed. Smooth folded drawsheet over the bottom sheet and tuck under mattress, first at middle, then at top, and then at bottom.
14. If needed, put on a waterproof pad or soaker pad over bottom sheet.
15. Place top sheet over bed with vertical centre fold lengthwise down middle of the bed. Open sheet out from head to foot, being sure top edge of the sheet is even with top edge of the mattress.
16. Make horizontal toe pleat (optional): Stand at foot of bed and fanfold sheet 5–10 cm across bed. Pull sheet up from bottom to make fold approximately 15 cm from bottom edge of the mattress (see Skill 38-5, Step 34).
17. Tuck in remaining portion of the sheet under foot of mattress. Place blanket over the bed with top edge parallel to top edge of sheet and 15–20 cm down from edge of sheet. (*Optional:* Put on additional bedspread over bed.)
18. Make cuff by turning edge of top sheet down over top edge of the blanket and bedspread.
19. Standing on one side at foot of the bed, lift mattress corner slightly with one hand, and with the other hand tuck top sheet, blanket, and bedspread under the mattress. Be sure the pleats are not pulled out.
20. Make modified mitred corner with top sheet, blanket, and bedspread. After triangular fold is made, do not tuck tip of triangle (see Step 20 illustration).
21. Go to other side of the bed. Spread sheet, blanket, and bedspread out evenly. Make cuff with top sheet and blanket. Make modified mitred corner at foot of the bed.
22. Put on clean pillowcase.
23. Place call light within patient's reach on a bed rail or pillow and return bed to height allowing for patient transfer. Assist the patient in getting into bed.
24. Arrange patient's room. Remove and discard supplies. Perform hand hygiene.

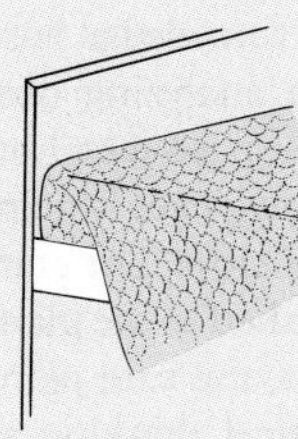

STEP 20 Modified mitred corner.

Disposal of linen must be done in such a way as to minimize the spread of infection (see Chapter 33). Agency policies provide guidelines for the proper way to bag and dispose of soiled linen. After a patient is discharged, all bed linens are sent to the laundry, the mattress and bed are cleaned by housekeeping staff, and new bed linen is applied.

◆ Evaluation

Patient Care. Evaluation of hygiene measures occurs both during and after each particular skill. For example, while bathing a patient, closely inspect the skin to determine whether drainage or other soiling has been effectively removed from the skin's surface. Once the bath is completed, ask the patient whether his or her comfort and relaxation have improved. When evaluating for the effectiveness of hygiene measures, observe for changes in the patient's behaviour. Does the patient assume a more relaxed position? Is the patient free of body odour? Is the patient able to fall asleep? Does the patient's facial expression convey a sense of comfort?

Frequently, it takes time for hygiene care to result in an improvement in a patient's condition. The presence of oral lesions, a scalp infestation, or skin excoriation often requires repeated measures and a combination of nursing interventions. Evaluate for improvement in the patient's condition over time and determine whether existing therapies are effective.

Throughout evaluation, consider the goals of care and evaluate whether expected outcomes are achieved. A critical thinking approach

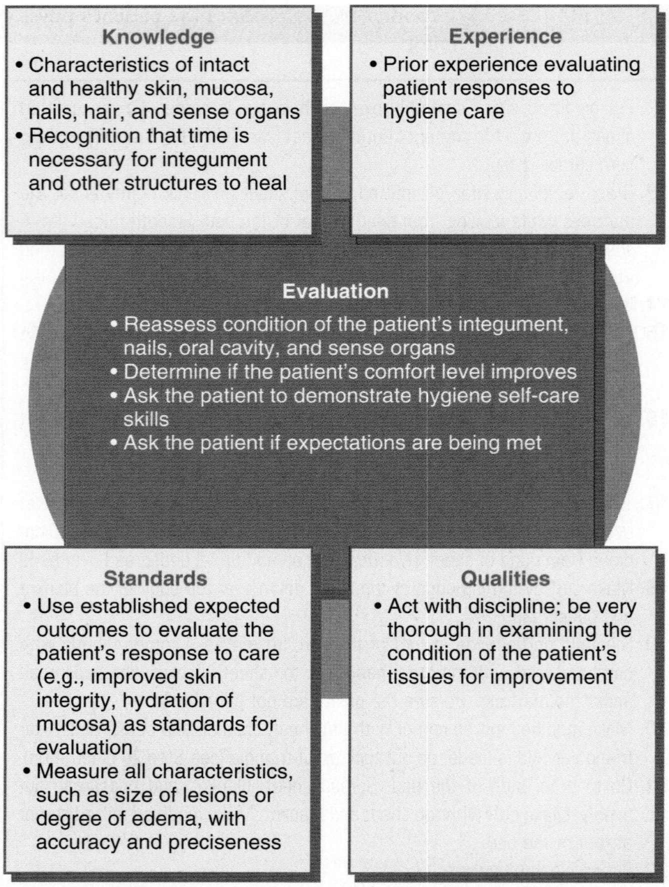

FIGURE 38-17 Critical thinking model for hygiene evaluation.

ensures that consideration is given to all factors when evaluating a patient's care (Figure 38-17). Knowledge base and experience provide important perspectives when analyzing observations made about a patient. For example, once you have seen how dehydration of the oral mucosa clears with repeated hygiene, it helps you to recognize when progress in another patient is slow. The standards for evaluation are the expected outcomes established in the planning stage of the patient's care. If outcomes are not met, the care plan may need to be revised. Continual application of critical thinking and clinical judgement is necessary when considering all evaluation findings.

Patient Expectations. The final portion of the evaluation considers whether a patient's expectations have been met through hygiene care. The nurse might ask the patient, "Do you feel your bath and back rub helped to make you comfortable?" "Can you suggest ways in which we can improve your foot care?" "What further measures do you think are necessary to keep your mouth clean and refreshed?"

Patients' expectations are important guidelines in determining patient satisfaction. As the care provider, you must feel comfortable in addressing your patients' concerns and expectations. A caring approach can facilitate a discussion of these issues.

KEY CONCEPTS

- Nurses determine a patient's ability to perform self-care and provide hygiene care according to the patient's needs and preferences.
- During hygiene care, the nurse can integrate other activities such as physical assessment, wound care, and range-of-motion exercises.
- While providing daily hygiene needs, nurses use teaching and communication skills in developing a caring relationship with the patient.
- Various personal, sociocultural, socioeconomic, and developmental factors influence patients' hygiene practices.
- Patients' health beliefs predict the likelihood of their assuming health-promoting behaviour, such as the maintenance of good hygiene.
- Nurses might not assess all body regions before administering hygiene; however, routine assessment of the patient's condition is undertaken whenever care is given.
- Patients with reduced sensation, vascular insufficiency, and immobility are at greater risk for impaired skin integrity.
- Before carrying out basic hygiene measures, nurses must perform an assessment of each patient's physical and cognitive abilities, including muscle strength, flexibility and dexterity, balance, coordination, activity tolerance, and ability to comprehend. For patients suffering symptoms such as pain or nausea, administering symptom relief therapies before performing hygiene procedures better prepares the patient.
- Patients with diabetes mellitus require special nail and foot care.
- When administering oral care to unconscious patients, measures must be taken to prevent aspiration.
- A patient's room should be comfortable, safe, and uncluttered, to provide for patient comfort and safety.
- An evaluation of hygiene care is based on the patient's sense of comfort, relaxation, well-being, and understanding of hygiene techniques.

CRITICAL THINKING EXERCISES

1. Jack Hines, a 19-year-old, remains in the hospital after a motorcycle accident in which he suffered multiple traumatic injuries. Jack has limited mobility due to casts to his left leg and arm. Discuss important factors to consider when administering hygiene care. Identify two nursing diagnoses and interventions, with rationales.
2. Marian Goyeau, a 40-year-old woman, was admitted into the hospital for treatment of a malignant breast lesion. Marian is undergoing chemotherapy along with radiation treatment. During your assessment, she complains of a loss of appetite, nausea and vomiting, and sores in her mouth. Marian is suffering from stomatitis. Identify two nursing diagnoses and interventions, with rationales.
3. Michelle Tweed, a 78-year-old woman, was transferred from an acute care hospital to a rehabilitation facility after a cerebrovascular accident. She exhibits right hemiparesis and aphasia and is incontinent of urine and stool. During the initial assessment, you discover that Mrs. Tweed has reddened areas on both heels, and her perineum and buttocks are excoriated. Identify two priority nursing diagnoses. Discuss at least three factors that contributed to Mrs. Tweed's impaired skin integrity.

REVIEW QUESTIONS

1. Mr. Mazzuca presents with an ulcer on his left foot. His diabetes mellitus is considered when planning care for him. In providing teaching on foot care, which of the following is most important to include?
   1. Daily inspection of his feet
   2. Application of lotion to his feet and between his toes daily
   3. Daily soaking of his feet in hot water
   4. Cutting his toenails in the shape of a curve

2. A 35-year-old man is interested in obtaining information about the cause of his psoriasis. Which of the following should be included in the patient teaching?
   1. Psoriasis is contagious.
   2. Psoriasis can be related to poor hygiene.
   3. Psoriasis is not contagious.
   4. Psoriasis can be cured.
3. A 75-year-old woman who has a history of diabetes and peripheral vascular disease has been trying to remove a corn from the bottom of her foot with a pair of scissors. Patient teaching should include which of the following?
   1. Increased circulation in her feet could cause severe bleeding if she were to injure her foot with the scissors.
   2. Peripheral vascular disease increases her risk of developing more corns.
   3. Diabetes mellitus places her at an increased risk for infection if she has an open wound on her foot.
   4. Her chronic disease limits her range of motion, and she may not be able to safely see or reach the corn on the bottom of her foot.
4. A thorough skin assessment is very important because the skin can provide information about which of the following?
   1. Support systems
   2. Circulatory status
   3. Psychological wellness
   4. Fundamental skills
5. A dark-skinned patient is in the Critical Care Unit after a motor vehicle collision. In assessing for cyanosis, the nurse would expect to find which characteristics in this patient's skin?
   1. Ruddy colour
   2. Generalized pallor
   3. Ashen, grey, or dull appearance
   4. Patchy areas of pallor
6. When assessing for inflammation in a darkly pigmented patient, the nurse would do which of the following?
   1. Assess the skin for swelling
   2. Palpate the skin for edema and increased warmth
   3. Assess the oral mucosa for cyanosis
   4. Palpate the skin for tenderness
7. Before providing mouth care to an unconscious patient, which of the following should be considered first?
   1. Presence of a gag reflex
   2. Condition of the skin
   3. Presence of pain
   4. Availability of equipment
8. When providing hair care for a patient, which of the following is not an important consideration?
   1. Caregiver preferences
   2. Family preferences
   3. Cultural preferences
   4. Patient preferences
9. Which of the following is the correct technique when providing eye care?
   1. Eyes should be cleaned from the outer to the inner canthus.
   2. Eyes should be cleaned from the inner to the outer canthus.
   3. Eye hygiene is not necessary.
   4. It is acceptable to clean eyes from either direction.
10. Which of the following is important to consider when providing hygiene care for patients?
    1. Use communication skills that promote a caring therapeutic relationship.
    2. Provide privacy, convey respect, and promote independence.
    3. Provide an environment that promotes the patient's physical and mental comfort.
    4. All of the above.

Answers: 1. 1; **2.** 3; **3.** 3; **4.** 2; **5.** 3; **6.** 2; **7.** 1; **8.** 1; **9.** 2; **10.** 4

Rationales for the Review Questions appear at the end of the book.

RECOMMENDED WEBSITES

Alzheimer Society of Canada: http://www.alzheimer.ca.

The Alzheimer Society of Canada website offers important information on Alzheimer's disease and other dementias, treatment, research, support, and services.

Canadian Dental Association: http://www.cda-adc.ca.

The Canadian Dental Association website offers information on maintaining optimal oral health, including oral hygiene for older persons.

Canadian Diabetes Association: http://www.diabetes.ca.

The Canadian Diabetes Association website (Diabetes Canada) offers information on the different types of diabetes, treatment, research, and services.

Public Health Agency of Canada: http://www.publichealth.gc.ca.

This website is a valuable resource offering information on healthy living, disease, and injury prevention.

REFERENCES

Alberta Association of Optometrists. (n.d.). *Eye exam frequency*. Retrieved from https://www.optometrists.ab.ca/web/AAO/Patients/Eye_Exam_Frequency.aspx.

Bateman, S. (2014). Principles of preventative foot care. *British Journal of Community Nursing, Suppl.*, S30–S38.

Canadian Dental Association. (2017). *Your oral health—Caring for your teeth*. Retrieved from http://www.cda-adc.ca/en/oral_health/cfyt/.

Canadian Diabetes Association. (2013). *Foot care*. Retrieved from http://guidelines.diabetes.ca/browse/chapter32.

Cheung, N., Nagra, P., & Hammersmith, K. (2016). Emerging trends in contact lens-related infections. *Current Opinion in Ophthalmology, 27*(4), 327–332. doi:10.1097/ICU.0000000000000280.

Cowdell, F., & Steventon, K. (2015). Skin cleansing practices for older people: A systematic review. *International Journal of Older People Nursing, 10*(1), 3–13. doi:10.1111/opn.12041.

Cullington, H., Kitterick, P., Debold, L., et al. (2016). Have cochlear implant, won't have to travel: Introducing telemedicine to people with cochlear implants. *American Journal of Audiology, 25*(3S), 299–302. doi:10.1044/2016_AJA-16-0018.

Cummings, C., Finlay, J. C., MacDonald, N. E., et al. (2016). *Head lice infestations: A clinical update*. Retrieved from http://www.cps.ca/documents/position/head-lice.

Drugs.com. (2017). *Lindane shampoo*. Retrieved from https://www.drugs.com/cdi/lindane-shampoo.html.

Dulan, A., Sheridan, D., & Laucher, M. (2016). Using transdermal drug patches for older adults. *Nursing, 46*(11), 69. doi:10.1097/01.NURSE.0000502752.25946.46.

Enwere, E., Elofson, K., Forbes, R., et al. (2016). Impact of chlorhexidine mouthwash prophylaxis on probable ventilator-associated pneumonia in a surgical intensive care unit. *International Journal of Critical Illness and Injury Science, 6*(1), 3–8. doi:10.4103/2229-5151.177368.

Fitzpatrick, E. M., & Brewster, L. (2010). Adult cochlear implantation in Canada: Results of a survey. *Canadian Journal of Speech-Language Pathology and Audiology, 34*(4), 290–296.

Gupta, A., Gupta, A., Singh, T., et al. (2016). Role of oral care to prevent VAP in mechanically ventilated intensive care unit patients. *Saudi Journal of Anaesthesia, 10*(1), 95–97.

Gupta, A., & West, H. J. (2016). Mucositis (or stomatitis). *JAMA Oncology, 2*(10), 1379.

Halloran, L. (2015). Body piercing: Avoiding complications. *Journal for Nurse Practitioners, 11*(1), 142–143. Retrieved from http://www.npjournal.org/article/S1555-4155(14)00650-3/pdf.

Health Canada. (2006). *It's your health: Contact lenses (Catalogue No. 0-662-35396-X)*. Ottawa: Author. Retrieved from http://www.hc-sc.gc.ca/hl-vs/iyh-vsv/med/lenses-lentilles-eng.php.

Howe, L. (2008). Education and empowerment of the nursing assistant: Validating their important role in skin care and pressure ulcer prevention, and demonstrating productivity enhancement and cost savings. *Advances in Skin & Wound Care, 21*(6), 275–281.

Huang, D., Chan, K., & Young, B. (2013). Poor oral health and quality of life in older US adults with diabetes mellitus. *Journal of the American Geriatrics Society, 61*(10), 1782–1788. doi:10.1111/jgs.12452.

Leijon, S., Bergh, I., & Terstappen, K. (2013). Pressure ulcer prevalence, use of preventive measures, and mortality risk in an acute care population: A quality improvement project. *Journal of Wound, Ostomy, and Continence Nursing, 40*(5), 469–474. doi:10.1097/WON.0b013e3182a22032.

Maher, A. B., Meehan, A. J., Hertz, K., et al. (2013). Acute nursing care of the older adult with fragility hip fracture: An international perspective (part 2). *International Journal of Orthopaedic and Trauma Nursing, 17*(1), 4–18. doi:10.1016/j.ijotn.2012.09.002.

Marino, R., Albala, C., Sanchez, H., et al. (2014). Prevalence of diseases and conditions which impact on oral health and oral health self-care among older Chileans. *Journal of Aging and Health, 27*(1), 3–16. doi:10.1177/0898264314533723.

Mitchell, J., & Shoemaker, A. (2017). Oral health care for nurse educators, part 1: Birth to 6 years old. *Teaching and Learning in Nursing, 12*, 69–72. Retrieved from http://www.sciencedirect.com/science/article/pii/S1557308716301524.

Nelson, N. (2015). Massage therapy: Understanding the mechanisms of action on blood pressure. A scoping review. *Journal of the American Society of Hypertension, 9*(10), 785–793. doi:10.1016/j.jash.2015.07.009.

Orsted, H. L., Rosenthal, S., & Woodbury, M. G. (2009). Pressure ulcer awareness and prevention program: A quality improvement program through the Canadian Association of Wound Care. *Journal of Wound, Ostomy, and Continence Nursing, 36*(2), 178–183.

Pemayun, T., Naibaho, R., Novitasari, D., et al. (2015). Risk factors for lower extremity amputation in patients with diabetic foot ulcers: A hospital-based case control study. *Diabetic Foot & Ankle, 6*, 29629. doi:10.3402/dfa.v6.29629.

Sardo, P., Simões, C., Alvarelhão, J., et al. (2015). Pressure ulcer risk assessment: Retrospective analysis of Braden Scale scores in Portuguese hospitalized adult patients. *Journal of Clinical Nursing, 24*(21–22), 3165–3176. doi:10.1111/jocn.12927.

Wolf, Z., & Czekanski, K. (2015). Bathing disability and bathing persons with dementia. *Medsurg Nursing, 24*(1), 9–22.

39

Cardiopulmonary Functioning and Oxygenation

Canadian content written by Giuliana Harvey, RN, MN, Heather MacLean, RN, MN
Original chapter by Erin H. McCalley, RN, BSN, MS, CCRN, CCNS

OBJECTIVES

Mastery of content in this chapter will enable you to:

- Define the key terms listed.
- Describe the structure and function of the cardiopulmonary system.
- Identify the physiological processes of cardiac output, myocardial blood flow, and coronary artery circulation.
- Diagram the electrical conduction system of the heart.
- Describe the relationship among cardiac output, preload, afterload, contractility, and heart rate.
- Identify the physiological processes involved in ventilation, perfusion, and exchange of respiratory gases.
- Describe the neural and chemical regulation of respiration.
- Describe the impact of a patient's level of health, age, lifestyle, and environment on cardiopulmonary oxygenation.
- Identify and describe clinical outcomes as a result of disturbances in conduction, altered cardiac output, impaired valvular function, myocardial ischemia, and impaired tissue perfusion.
- Identify and describe clinical outcomes of hyperventilation, hypoventilation, and hypoxemia.
- Identify nursing care interventions in the primary care, acute care, and restorative and continuing care settings that promote oxygenation.

KEY TERMS

Afterload, p. 955
Anemia, p. 959
Angina pectoris, p. 963
Asystole, p. 960
Atelectasis, p. 957
Atrial fibrillation, p. 960
Bronchoscopy, p. 968
Cardiac index (CI), p. 955
Cardiac output, p. 954
Cardiopulmonary rehabilitation, p. 1006
Cardiopulmonary resuscitation (CPR), p. 1005
Chest physiotherapy (CPT), p. 979
Chest tube, p. 998
Cor pulmonale, p. 958
Cyanosis, p. 964
Diaphragmatic breathing, p. 1009
Diffusion, p. 958
Dyspnea, p. 967
Dysrhythmias, p. 960
Electrocardiogram (ECG), p. 955
Expiration, p. 957
Hematemesis, p. 968
Hemoptysis, p. 968
Hemothorax, p. 1001
High-flow devices, p. 1002
Humidification, p. 979
Hypercapnia, p. 959
Hyperventilation, p. 964
Hypoventilation, p. 964
Hypovolemia, p. 959
Hypoxia, p. 964
Incentive spirometry, p. 997
Inspiration, p. 957
Low-flow devices, p. 1002
Mediastinal chest tube, p. 1000
Myocardial contractility, p. 955
Myocardial infarction (MI), p. 963
Myocardial ischemia, p. 962
Nasal cannula, p. 1002
Nebulization, p. 979
Normal sinus rhythm (NSR), p. 955
Orthopnea, p. 968
Pneumothorax, p. 998
Postural drainage, p. 980
Preload, p. 955
Pulse oximeter, p. 974
Pursed-lip breathing, p. 1009
Stroke volume, p. 955
Subcutaneous emphysema, p. 998
Ventilation, p. 956
Ventricular fibrillation, p. 960
Ventricular tachycardia, p. 960
Wheezing, p. 968

MEDIA RESOURCES

http://evolve.elsevier.com/Canada/Potter/fundamentals/

- Audio Chapter Summaries
- Examination Review Questions
- Concept Map Creator
- Case Study with Questions
- Audio Glossary
- Content Updates
- Video Clips

Oxygen is required to sustain life. The cardiac and respiratory systems function to supply the body's oxygen demands. Blood is oxygenated through the mechanisms of ventilation, perfusion, and transport of respiratory gases. Neural and chemical regulators control the rate and depth of respiration in response to tissues' changing oxygen demands.

SCIENTIFIC KNOWLEDGE BASE

Cardiovascular Physiology

Cardiopulmonary physiology involves delivery of (a) deoxygenated blood (blood that is high in carbon dioxide and low in oxygen) to the right side of the heart and to the pulmonary circulation and (b) oxygenated blood from the lungs to the left side of the heart and the tissues. The cardiac system delivers oxygen, nutrients, and other substances to the tissues and removes the waste products of cellular metabolism through the cardiac pump, the circulatory vascular system, and the integration of other systems (e.g., respiratory, digestive, and renal) (McCance & Huether, 2014).

Structure and Function. The right ventricle pumps blood through the pulmonary circulation. The left ventricle pumps blood to the systemic circulation (Figure 39-1). The circulatory system exchanges respiratory gases, nutrients, and waste products between the blood and the tissues.

Myocardial Pump. The pumping action of the heart is essential to maintaining oxygen delivery. Coronary artery disease and cardiomyopathic (enlarged heart) conditions result in a diminished stroke volume (i.e., the volume of blood ejected from the ventricles) and decreased pump effectiveness. Hemorrhage and dehydration decrease pump effectiveness by decreasing the amount of blood ejected from the ventricles, thereby reducing circulating blood volume. The four chambers of the heart fill with blood during diastole and empty during systole.

The myocardial (cardiac muscle) fibres have contractile properties that enable them to stretch during filling. In a healthy heart, this stretch is proportionally related to the strength of contraction. As the myocardium stretches, the strength of the subsequent contraction increases; this is known as the *Frank–Starling (Starling's) law* of the heart. In the diseased heart, Starling's law does not apply because the stretch of the myocardium is beyond the heart's physiological limits. The subsequent contractile response results in insufficient ventricular ejection (volume), and blood begins to "back up" in the pulmonary (left heart failure) or systemic circulation (right heart failure).

Myocardial Blood Flow. To maintain adequate blood flow to the pulmonary and systemic circulation, myocardial blood flow must supply sufficient oxygen and nutrients to the myocardium itself. Blood flow through the heart is unidirectional. There are four heart valves that ensure this forward blood flow (see Figure 39-1). During ventricular diastole, the atrioventricular (mitral and tricuspid) valves open and blood passively flows from the higher-pressure atria into the relaxed ventricles. Toward the end of ventricular diastole, the atria contract, sending increased blood flow through the atrioventricular valves into the ventricles; this is known as "atrial kick." Ventricular pressure will continue to rise, thus causing the atrioventricular valves to close. This represents S_1, or the first heart sound. After ventricular filling, the systolic phase begins.

During the systolic phase, semilunar (aortic and pulmonic) valves open and blood flows from the ventricles into the aorta and pulmonary artery. As the ventricles empty, ventricular pressures decrease, allowing closure of the semilunar valves. Closure of these valves represents S_2, or the second heart sound. Patients with valvular disease may have backflow or regurgitation of blood through the incompetent valve, causing a murmur that is heard on auscultation (see Chapter 32 for further information about health assessment and physical examination).

Coronary Artery Circulation. Blood in the atria and ventricles does not supply oxygen and nutrients to the myocardium itself. The coronary circulation is the branch of the systemic circulation that supplies the myocardium with oxygen and nutrients and removes waste. The coronary arteries fill during ventricular diastole (McCance & Huether, 2014). The right and left coronary arteries arise from the aorta just above and behind the aortic valve through openings called the *coronary ostia* (coronary openings). The left coronary artery, the most abundant blood supply, feeds the left ventricular myocardium, which is more muscular and does most of the heart's work (Box 39-1).

Systemic Circulation. The arteries and veins of the systemic circulation deliver nutrients and oxygen to and remove waste from the tissues. Oxygenated blood flows from the left ventricle by way of the aorta and into large systemic arteries. These arteries branch into smaller arteries, into arterioles, and finally into the smallest vessels, the capillaries. At the capillary level, the exchange of respiratory gases, nutrients, and wastes occurs, and the tissues are oxygenated. The waste products exit the capillary network by way of the venules that join to form veins. These veins form larger veins, which carry deoxygenated blood to the right side of the heart, where it is returned to pulmonary circulation.

Blood Flow Regulation. The amount of blood ejected from the left ventricle each minute is the cardiac output. The normal cardiac output is 4 to 6 L/minute in the healthy 68-kg adult at rest. The circulating volume of blood changes according to the oxygen and metabolic needs of the body. For example, during exercise, pregnancy, and fever the

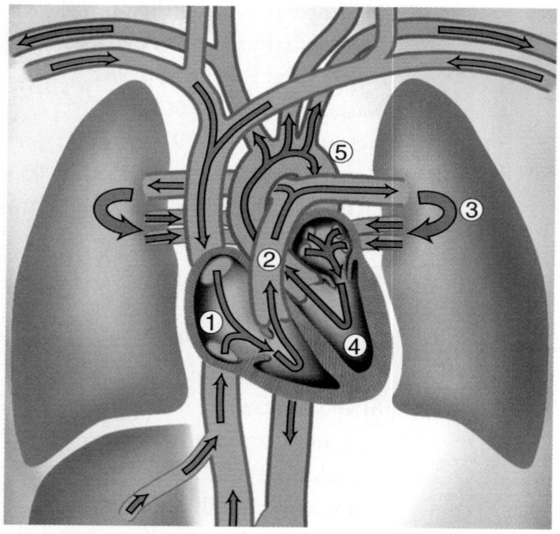

FIGURE 39-1 Schematic representation of blood flow through the heart. *Arrows* indicate direction of flow. *1,* The right atrium receives venous blood from the inferior and superior venae cavae and the coronary sinus. The blood then passes through the tricuspid valve into the right ventricle. *2,* With each contraction, the right ventricle pumps blood through the pulmonic valve into the pulmonary artery and to the lungs. *3,* Oxygenated blood flows from the lungs to the left atrium by way of the pulmonary veins. *4,* It then passes through the mitral valve and into the left ventricle. *5,* As the heart contracts, blood is ejected through the aortic valve into the aorta and thus enters the systemic circulation. (From Lewis, S. L., Heitkemper, M. M., Dirksen, S. R., Bucher, L., Camera I., Barry, M. A., Goldsworthy, S., & Goodridge, D. [Eds.]. [2014]. *Medical-surgical nursing in Canada: Assessment and management of clinical problems* [3rd Canadian ed., p. 844, Fig. 34-1]. Toronto: Elsevier Canada.)

BOX 39-1 Coronary Arteries

Right Coronary Artery

Right Atrium, Anterior Right Ventricle

Supplies

- Posterior aspect of septum (90% of population)
- Posterior papillary muscle
- Sinus and atrioventricular nodes (80–90% of population)
- Inferior aspect of left ventricle

Left Coronary Arteries

Left Anterior Descending Artery

Supplies

- Anterior left ventricular wall
- Anterior interventricular septum (septal branches supply conduction system, bundle of His, and bundle branches)
- Anterior papillary muscle
- Left ventricular apex
- Right ventricle

Circumflex Artery

Supplies

- Left atrium
- Posterior surfaces of left ventricle
- Posterior aspects of septum

cardiac output increases, but during sleep it decreases. Cardiac output is represented by the following formula:

$$\text{Cardiac output (CO)} = \text{Stroke volume (SV)} \times \text{Heart rate (HR)}$$

Cardiac output in the older person may be affected by increased arterial wall tension and moderate myocardial hypertrophy due to an increased systolic blood pressure.

Cardiac index (CI) is the adequacy of the cardiac output for an individual. It takes into account the body surface area (BSA) of the patient. The CI is determined by dividing the cardiac output by the BSA. The normal range is 2.5 to 4 L/min/m^3. Both cardiac output and the CI are measured with invasive pulmonary artery catheters.

Stroke volume is the amount of blood ejected from the left ventricle with each contraction. It can be affected by the amount of blood in the left ventricle at the end of diastole (preload), the resistance to left ventricular ejection (afterload), and myocardial contractility.

Preload is essentially the end-diastolic volume. The ventricles stretch when filling with blood. The more stretch on the ventricular muscle, the greater the contraction and the greater the stroke volume (Starling's law). In clinical situations, the preload and subsequent stroke volume can be manipulated by changing the amount of circulating blood volume. For example, in the patient with hemorrhagic shock, fluid therapy and replacement of blood increases volume, thus increasing the preload and stroke volume, which in turn increases cardiac output. If volume is not replaced, preload decreases, the cardiac output decreases, and, ultimately, the venous return to the right atrium decreases, further decreasing preload and cardiac output.

Afterload is the resistance to left ventricular ejection—the work that the heart must overcome to fully eject blood from the left ventricle. The diastolic aortic pressure is a good clinical measure of afterload. For example, in a patient with hypertension, the afterload is greater than normal, increasing the cardiac workload. Afterload in this situation can be manipulated by decreasing systemic blood pressure.

The invasive measurement and monitoring of these cardiopulmonary hemodynamics is usually performed in Critical Care Units. Some step-down or special care units may also have the capability to measure and monitor hemodynamics.

Myocardial contractility also affects stroke volume and cardiac output. Poor contraction decreases the amount of blood ejected by the ventricles during each contraction. Drugs that can increase the force of myocardial contraction include digitalis preparations, epinephrine, and sympathomimetic drugs (drugs that mimic the effects of the sympathetic nervous system). Injury to the myocardial muscle, such as an acute myocardial infarction (AMI), can cause a decrease in myocardial contractility. The myocardium of the older person is more rigid and slower in recovering its contractility (Touhy & Jett, 2014).

Heart rate affects blood flow because of the interaction between rate and diastolic filling time. With a sustained heart rate greater than 160 beats per minute, diastolic filling time decreases, decreasing stroke volume and cardiac output. The heart rate of the older person is slow to increase under stress and is likely related to lack of conditioning rather than age. Exercise remains a health promotion strategy beneficial to maintaining health and cardiac function for all ages (Heart and Stroke Foundation of Canada [HSFC], 2017a).

Conduction System. The rhythmic relaxation and contraction of the atria and ventricles depend on continuous, organized transmission of electrical impulses. These impulses are generated and transmitted by way of the cardiac conduction system (Figure 39-2).

The heart's conduction system generates the necessary action potentials that conduct the impulses required to initiate the electrical chain of events resulting in the heartbeat. The autonomic nervous system influences the rate of impulse generation, the speed of transmission through the conductive pathway, and the strength of atrial and ventricular contractions. Sympathetic nerve fibres, which increase the rate of impulse generation and the speed of impulse transmission, innervate all parts of the atria and ventricles. The parasympathetic fibres originating from the vagus nerve decrease the rate and innervate all parts of the atria and ventricles, as well as the sinoatrial (SA) and atrioventricular (AV) nodes.

The conduction system originates with the SA node, the "pacemaker" of the heart. The SA node is in the right atrium next to the entrance of the superior vena cava. Impulses are initiated at the SA node at an intrinsic rate of 60 to 100 beats per minute. The average resting adult rate is approximately 75 beats per minute (McCance & Huether, 2014).

The electrical impulses are then transmitted through the atria along intra-atrial pathways to the AV node. The AV node mediates impulses between the atria and the ventricles. The intrinsic rate of the normal AV node is 40 to 60 beats per minute. The AV node assists atrial emptying by delaying the impulse before transmitting it through the bundle of His and the ventricular Purkinje network. The intrinsic rate of the bundle of His and the ventricular Purkinje network is 20 to 40 beats per minute.

An electrocardiogram (ECG) reflects the electrical activity of the conduction system. An ECG monitors the regularity and path of the electrical impulse through the conduction system; however, it does not reflect muscular work of the heart. The normal sequence on the ECG is called normal sinus rhythm (NSR) (Figure 39-3).

NSR implies that the impulse originates at the SA node and follows the normal sequence through the conduction system. The P wave represents the electrical conduction through both atria. Atrial contraction follows the P wave. The PR interval represents the impulse travel time through the AV node, through the bundle of His, and to the Purkinje fibres. The normal length for the PR interval is 0.12

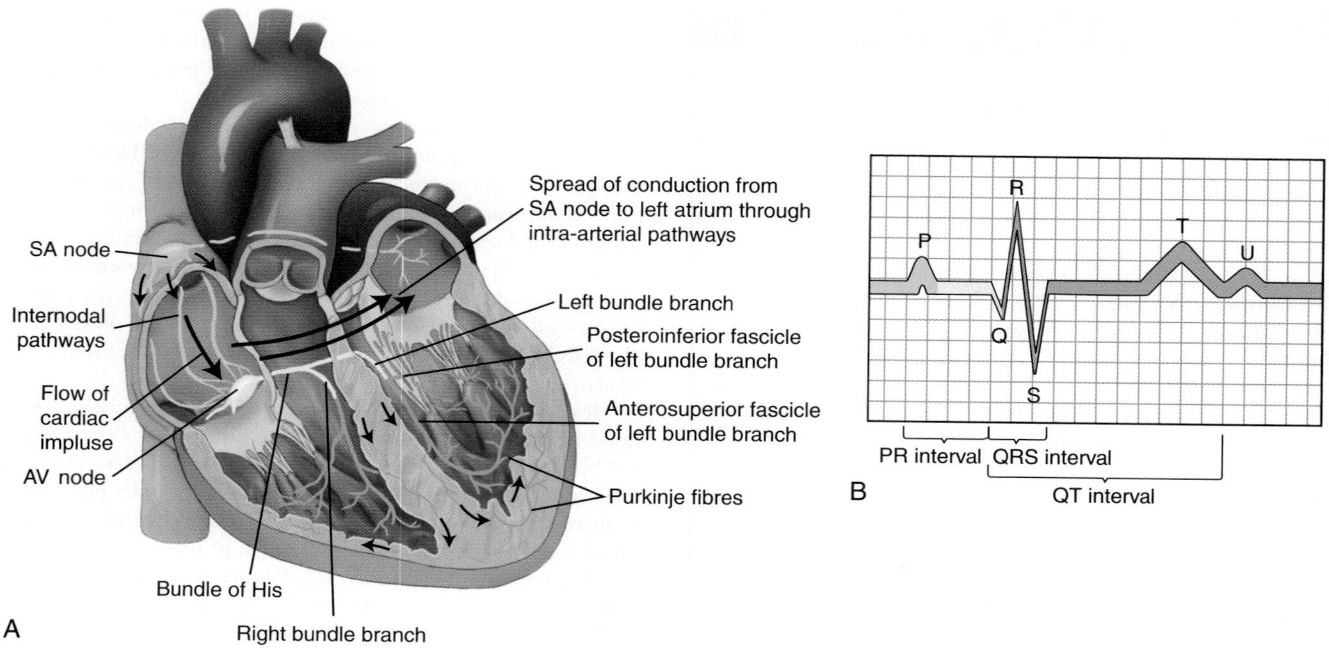

FIGURE 39-2 A, Conduction system of the heart. **B,** The normal electrocardiogram pattern. *AV,* Atrioventricular; *SA,* sinoatrial. (From Lewis, S. L., Heitkemper, M. M., Dirksen, S. R., Bucher, L., Camera I., Barry, M. A., Goldsworthy, S., & Goodridge, D. [Eds.]. [2014]. *Medical-surgical nursing in Canada: Assessment and management of clinical problems* [3rd Canadian ed., p. 845, Fig. 34-4]). Toronto: Elsevier Canada.)

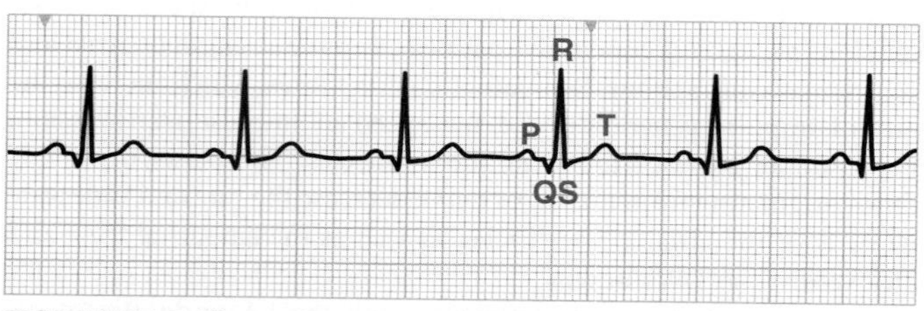

FIGURE 39-3 Normal electrocardiogram waveform. (From Lewis, S. L., Heitkemper, M. M., Dirksen, S. R., Bucher, L., Camera I., Barry, M. A., Goldsworthy, S., & Goodridge, D. [Eds.]. [2014]. *Medical-surgical nursing in Canada: Assessment and management of clinical problems* [3rd Canadian ed., p. 955, Fig. 38-8]. Toronto: Elsevier Canada.)

to 0.20 seconds (120–200 msec). An increase in the time (i.e., >0.20 seconds) indicates that there is a block in the impulse transmission through the AV node; a decrease (i.e., <0.12 seconds) indicates the initiation of the electrical impulse from a source other than the SA node.

The QRS complex indicates that the electrical impulse has travelled through the ventricles. Normal QRS duration is 0.06 to 0.10 seconds (60–100 msec). An increase in QRS duration indicates a delay in conduction time through the ventricles. Ventricular contraction usually follows the QRS complex.

The QT interval represents the time needed for ventricular depolarization and repolarization. The normal QT interval is 0.12 to 0.42 seconds (120–420 msec). Changes in electrolyte values, such as in hypocalcemia or during therapy with drugs such as disopyramide (Norpace), amiodarone (Cordarne), and sotolol (Sotacor), can increase the QT interval. Shortening of the QT interval occurs with digitalis therapy, hyperkalemia, and hypercalcemia.

Respiratory Physiology

Most cells in the body obtain their energy from chemical reactions involving oxygen and the elimination of carbon dioxide. The exchange of respiratory gases occurs between environmental air and the blood. There are three steps in the process of oxygenation: ventilation, perfusion, and diffusion.

Structure and Function. Conditions or diseases that change the structure and function of the lung can alter respiration. The respiratory muscles, pleural space, lungs, and alveoli (Figure 39-4) are essential for ventilation, perfusion, and exchange of respiratory gases. Gases are moved into and out of the lungs through pressure changes. Intrapleural pressure is either negative or less than atmospheric pressure, which is 760 mm Hg at sea level. For air to flow into the lungs, intrapleural pressure must become more negative, setting up a pressure gradient between the atmosphere and the alveoli. The diaphragm and external intercostal muscles contract to create a negative pleural pressure and increase the size of the thorax for inspiration. Together, relaxation of the diaphragm and contraction of the internal intercostal muscles allows air from the lung to escape. The coordination of the respiratory muscles is essential for effective respiration and gas exchange. The lung transfers oxygen from the atmosphere into the alveoli, where the oxygen is exchanged for carbon dioxide. The alveoli transfer oxygen and carbon dioxide to and from the blood through the alveolar membrane.

Ventilation is the process of moving gases into and out of the lungs. Ventilation requires coordination of the muscular and elastic properties of the lung and thorax, as well as intact innervation. The major inspiratory muscle of respiration is the diaphragm. It is innervated by the phrenic nerve, which exits the spinal cord at the fourth cervical vertebra. Perfusion relates to the ability of the cardiovascular system to pump oxygenated blood to the tissues and return deoxygenated blood to the lungs. Diffusion is responsible for moving the molecules

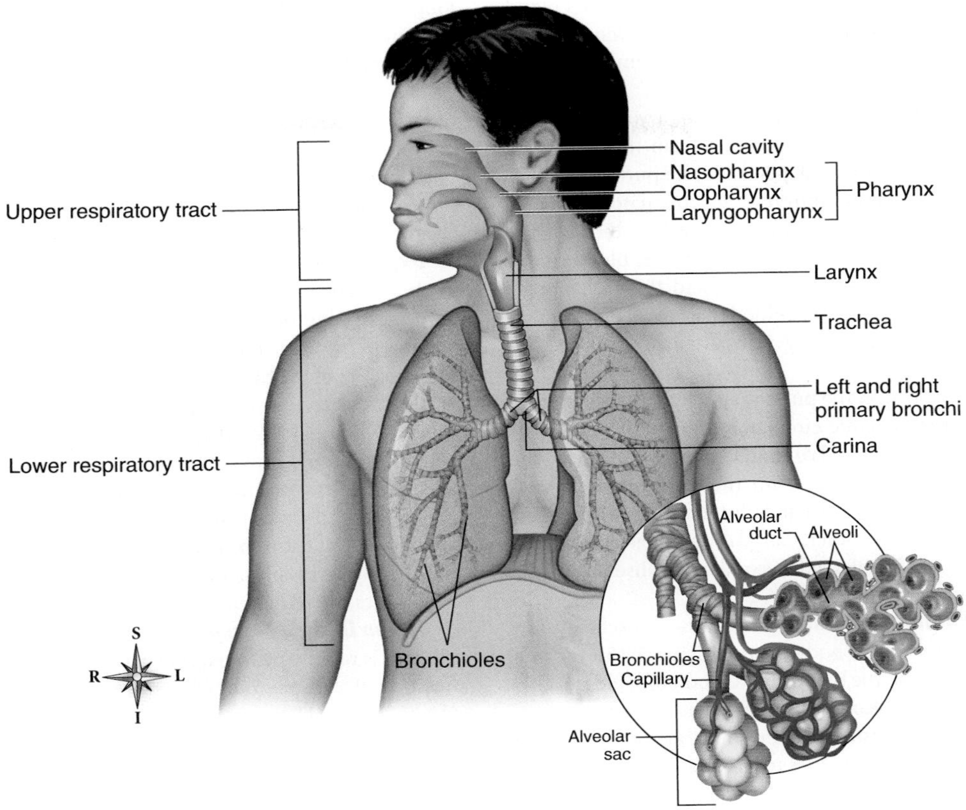

FIGURE 39-4 Structures of the pulmonary system. (From Huether, S. E., & McCance, K. L. [2017]. *Understanding pathophysiology* [6th ed. p. 671, Fig. 26-1]. St. Louis, MO: Elsevier.)

from one area to another. For the exchange of respiratory gases to occur, the organs, nerves, and muscles of respiration must be intact and the central nervous system able to regulate the respiratory cycle.

Work of Breathing. Breathing is the effort required for expanding and contracting the lungs. In the healthy individual, breathing is quiet and accomplished with minimal effort. The amount of energy expended on breathing depends on the rate and depth of breathing, the ease with which the lungs can be expanded (compliance), and airway resistance.

Inspiration is an active process, stimulated by chemical receptors in the aorta. Expiration is a passive process that depends on the elastic-recoil properties of the lungs, requiring little or no muscle work. Elastic recoil is produced by elastic fibres in lung tissue and by surface tension in the fluid film lining the alveoli. Surfactant is a chemical produced in the lungs that maintains the surface tension of the alveoli and keeps them from collapsing. Patients with advanced chronic obstructive pulmonary disease (COPD) lose the elastic recoil of the lungs and thorax. As a result, the patient's work of breathing is increased. In addition, patients with certain pulmonary diseases can have decreased surfactant production and may, in turn, develop atelectasis. Atelectasis is the collapse of the alveoli that prevents normal gas exchange between carbon dioxide and oxygen.

Accessory muscles of respiration can increase lung volume during inspiration. Patients with COPD, especially emphysema, frequently use these muscles to increase lung volume. Prolonged use of the accessory muscles of respiration does not promote effective ventilation and causes fatigue. During assessment, one observes elevation of the patient's clavicles during inspiration.

Compliance is the ability of the lungs to distend or expand in response to increased intra-alveolar pressure. Compliance is decreased in diseases such as pulmonary edema, interstitial and pleural fibrosis, and congenital or traumatic structural abnormalities such as kyphosis or fractured ribs.

Airway resistance is the pressure difference between the mouth and the alveoli in relation to the rate of flow of inspired gas. Airway resistance can be increased by an airway obstruction, a small airway disease (such as asthma), and tracheal edema. When resistance is increased, the amount of air travelling through the anatomical airways is decreased.

Decreased lung compliance, increased airway resistance, active expiration, or the use of accessory muscles increases the work of breathing, resulting in increased energy expenditure. To meet this expenditure, the body increases its metabolic rate, and the need for oxygen, as well as for the elimination of carbon dioxide, increases. This sequence is a vicious cycle for a patient with impaired ventilation, causing further deterioration of respiratory status and the ability to oxygenate adequately.

Lung Volumes and Capacities. Spirometry is used to measure the volume of air entering or leaving the lungs. Variations in lung volumes may be associated with health states such as pregnancy, exercise, obesity, or obstructive and restrictive conditions of the lungs. The amount of surfactant, degree of compliance, and strength of respiratory muscles can affect pressures and volumes within the lungs.

Pulmonary Circulation. The primary function of the pulmonary circulation is to move blood to and from the alveolocapillary membrane in order for gas exchange to occur. The pulmonary circulation serves as a reservoir for blood so that the lung can increase its blood volume without large increases in pulmonary artery or venous pressures. The pulmonary circulation also acts as a filter, removing small thrombi before they can reach vital organs.

The pulmonary circulation begins at the pulmonary artery, which receives poorly oxygenated mixed venous blood from the right ventricle. Blood flow through this system depends on the pumping ability of the right ventricle, which has an output of approximately 4 to 6 L/minute. The flow continues from the pulmonary artery through the pulmonary arterioles to the pulmonary capillaries, where blood comes in contact with the alveolocapillary membrane and the exchange of respiratory gases occurs. The oxygen-rich blood then circulates through the pulmonary venules and pulmonary veins, returning to the left atrium.

Pressure and resistance within the pulmonary circulatory system is lower than that within the systemic circulatory system. The walls of the pulmonary vessels are thinner and contain less smooth muscle. The lung accepts the total cardiac output from the right ventricle and, except in cases of alveolar hypoxia or cor pulmonale, does not direct blood flow from one region to another. **Cor pulmonale** is a condition in which the right ventricle is enlarged, secondary to diseases of the lung, thorax, or pulmonary circulation.

Respiratory Gas Exchange. Respiratory gases are exchanged in the alveoli and the capillaries of the body tissues (Figure 39-5). Oxygen is transferred from the lungs to the blood, and carbon dioxide is transferred from the blood to the alveoli to be exhaled as a waste product. At the tissue level, oxygen is transferred from the blood to tissues, and carbon dioxide is transferred from tissues to the blood to return to the alveoli and be exhaled. This transfer is dependent on the process of diffusion.

Diffusion is the movement of molecules from an area of higher concentration to an area of lower concentration. Diffusion of respiratory gases occurs at the alveolocapillary membrane, and the rate of diffusion can be affected by the thickness of the membrane. Increased thickness of the membrane impedes diffusion because gases take longer to transfer across. Patients with pulmonary edema, pulmonary infiltrates, or a pulmonary effusion have an increased thickness of the alveolocapillary membrane, resulting in slowed diffusion, slowed exchange of respiratory gases, and impaired delivery of oxygen to tissues. The surface area of the membrane can be altered as a result of chronic disease (e.g., emphysema), acute disease (e.g., pneumothorax), or a surgical process (e.g., lobectomy). The alveolocapillary membrane can be destroyed or may thicken, changing the rate of diffusion. When fewer alveoli are functioning, the surface area is decreased.

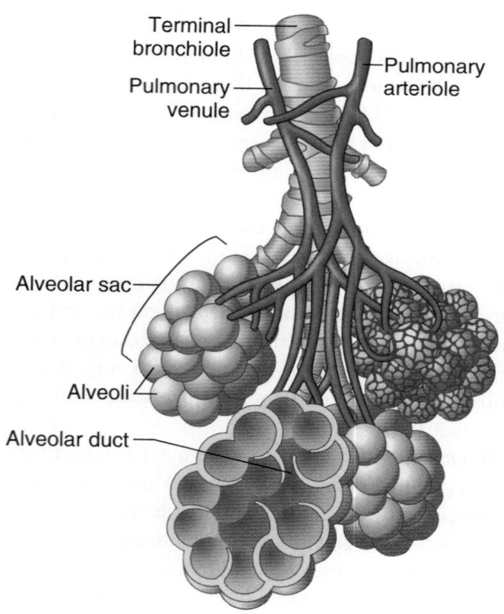

FIGURE 39-5 Alveoli. (From Huether, S.E., & McCance, K.L. [2017]. *Understanding pathophysiology* [6th ed., p. 671, Fig. 26-4]. St. Louis, MO: Elsevier.)

Oxygen Transport. The oxygen transport system consists of the lungs and cardiovascular system. Delivery depends on the amount of oxygen entering the lungs (ventilation), blood flow to the lungs and tissues (perfusion), rate of diffusion, and oxygen-carrying capacity. The capacity of the blood to carry oxygen is influenced by the amount of dissolved oxygen in the plasma, amount of hemoglobin, and tendency of hemoglobin to bind with oxygen. Only a relatively small amount of required oxygen, less than 1%, is dissolved in the plasma. Most oxygen is transported by hemoglobin, which serves as a carrier for oxygen and carbon dioxide. The hemoglobin molecule combines with oxygen to form oxyhemoglobin. The formation of oxyhemoglobin is easily reversible, allowing hemoglobin and oxygen to dissociate, which frees oxygen to enter tissues.

Carbon Dioxide Transport. Carbon dioxide diffuses into red blood cells and is rapidly hydrated into carbonic acid (H_2CO_3) because of the presence of carbonic anhydrase. The carbonic acid then dissociates into hydrogen (H^+) and bicarbonate (HCO_3^-) ions. The hydrogen ion is buffered by hemoglobin, and the HCO_3^- diffuses into the plasma (see Chapter 40). In addition, some of the carbon dioxide in red blood cells reacts with amino acid groups, forming carbamino compounds. This reaction can occur rapidly without the presence of an enzyme. Reduced hemoglobin (deoxyhemoglobin) can combine with carbon dioxide more easily than oxyhemoglobin, thus venous blood transports most of the carbon dioxide.

Regulation of Respiration. Regulation of respiration is necessary to ensure sufficient oxygen intake and carbon dioxide elimination to meet the body's demands (e.g., during exercise, infection, or pregnancy). Neural and chemical regulators control the process of respiration. Neural regulation includes the central nervous system control of respiratory rate, depth, and rhythm. Chemical regulation involves the influence of chemicals such as carbon dioxide and hydrogen ions on the rate and depth of respiration (Box 39-2).

Factors Affecting Oxygenation

Adequacy of circulation, ventilation, perfusion, and transport of respiratory gases to the tissues is influenced by four types of factors: (1) physiological, (2) developmental, (3) lifestyle, and (4) environmental. Developmental, lifestyle, and environmental factors will be presented in a later section.

Physiological Factors. Any condition that affects cardiopulmonary functioning directly affects the body's ability to meet oxygen demands. The general classifications of cardiac disorders are disturbances in conduction, impaired valvular function, myocardial hypoxia, cardiomyopathic conditions, and peripheral tissue hypoxia. Respiratory disorders include hyperventilation, hypoventilation, and hypoxia.

Other physiological processes affecting a patient's oxygenation are alterations that affect the oxygen-carrying capacity of blood, such as anemia; increases in the body's metabolic demands (e.g., pregnancy, fever, infection); and alterations that affect chest wall movement or the central nervous system (Table 39-1).

Decreased Oxygen-Carrying Capacity. Hemoglobin carries most of the oxygen to tissues. Anemia and inhalation of toxic substances

BOX 39-2 Physiological Processes of Oxygenation

Neural Regulation
Maintains rhythm and depth of respiration and balance between inspiration and expiration.

Cerebral Cortex
Voluntary control of respiration delivers impulses to the respiratory motor neurons by way of the spinal cord; accommodates speaking, eating, and swimming.

Medulla Oblongata
Automatic control of respiration occurs continuously.

Chemical Regulation
Maintains appropriate rate and depth of respirations according to changes in the blood's carbon dioxide (CO_2), oxygen (O_2), and hydrogen ion (H^+) concentration.

Chemoreceptors
Located in the medulla, aortic body, and carotid body. Changes in chemical content of O_2, CO_2, and H^+ stimulate chemoreceptors, which in turn stimulate neural regulators to adjust the rate and depth of ventilation to maintain normal arterial blood gas levels. Chemical regulation can occur during physical exercise and with some illnesses. It is a short-term adaptive mechanism.

TABLE 39-1 Physiological Processes Affecting Oxygenation

Process	Effect on Oxygenation
Anemia	Decreases oxygen-carrying capacity of blood
Toxic inhalant	Decreases oxygen-carrying capacity of blood
Airway obstruction	Limits delivery of inspired oxygen to alveoli
High altitude	Atmospheric oxygen concentration is lower and inspiratory oxygen concentration decreases
Fever	Increases metabolic rate and tissue oxygen demand
Decreased chest wall motion (e.g., from musculoskeletal impairments)	Prevents lowering of diaphragm and reduces anteroposterior diameter of thorax on inspiration, reducing volume of air inspired

decrease the oxygen-carrying capacity of blood by reducing the amount of available hemoglobin to transport oxygen. Anemia, a hemoglobin level lower than normal, is a result of decreased hemoglobin production, increased red blood cell destruction, blood loss, or a combination of these factors. Patients will have complaints of fatigue, decreased activity tolerance, and increased breathlessness, as well as pallor (especially seen in the conjunctiva of the eye) and an increased heart rate.

Carbon monoxide is the most common toxic inhalant that decreases the oxygen-carrying capacity of blood. The affinity for hemoglobin to bind with carbon monoxide is greater than 200 times its affinity to bind with oxygen, creating a functional anemia. Because of the bond's strength, carbon monoxide is not easily dissociated from hemoglobin, making the hemoglobin unavailable for oxygen transport.

Decreased Inspired Oxygen Concentration. When the concentration of inspired oxygen declines, the blood has less oxygen-carrying capacity. Decreases in the fraction of inspired oxygen concentration (FiO_2) can be caused by an upper or lower airway obstruction limiting delivery of inspired oxygen to alveoli; decreased environmental oxygen, such as at high altitudes; or decreased inspiration as a result of an incorrect oxygen concentration setting on respiratory therapy equipment.

Hypovolemia. Hypovolemia is caused by conditions such as shock and severe dehydration resulting from extracellular fluid loss and reduced circulating blood volume. With a significant fluid loss, the body tries to adapt by increasing the heart rate and peripheral vasoconstriction to increase the volume of blood returned to the heart and, in turn, increase the cardiac output.

Increased Metabolic Rate. Increased metabolic activity causes increased oxygen demand. When body systems are unable to meet this increased demand, the level of oxygenation declines. An increased metabolic rate is a normal physiological response to pregnancy, wound healing, and exercise because the body is building tissue. Most people can meet the increased oxygen demand and do not display signs of oxygen deprivation. Fever increases the tissues' need for oxygen, and as a result, carbon dioxide production also increases.

If the febrile state persists, the metabolic rate remains high and the body begins to break down protein stores, resulting in muscle wasting and decreased muscle mass. Respiratory muscles such as the diaphragm and intercostal muscles are also wasted. The body attempts to adapt to the increased carbon dioxide levels by increasing the rate and depth of respiration. The patient's work of breathing increases, and the patient will eventually display signs and symptoms of hypoxemia. Patients with pulmonary diseases are at greater risk for hypoxemia and hypercapnia (a greater than normal amount of carbon dioxide in the blood). Assessment findings include an increased rate and depth of respiration, use of the accessory muscles of respiration, pursed-lip breathing, and decreased activity tolerance.

Conditions Affecting Chest Wall Movement. Any condition that reduces chest wall movement can result in decreased ventilation. If the diaphragm cannot fully descend with breathing, the volume of inspired air decreases, and less oxygen is delivered to the alveoli and, subsequently, to tissues.

Pregnancy. As the fetus grows during pregnancy, the greater size of the uterus pushes abdominal contents upward against the diaphragm. In the last trimester of pregnancy, the inspiratory capacity declines, resulting in dyspnea on exertion and increased fatigue.

Obesity. Morbidly obese patients have reduced lung volumes as a result of the heaviness of the lower thorax and abdomen, particularly when in the recumbent and supine positions. These patients have a reduction in compliance as a result of encroachment of the abdomen into the chest, increased work of breathing, and decreased lung volumes, and they may experience fatigue and have carbon dioxide retention. In some patients, an obesity–hypoventilation syndrome develops in which oxygenation is decreased and carbon dioxide is retained, resulting in daytime sleepiness. Morbidly obese patients may also develop obstructive sleep apnea, characterized by excessive daytime somnolence and loud snoring and apneic periods during sleep. The obese patient is also susceptible to pneumonia after surgery or an upper respiratory tract infection because the lungs cannot fully expand and pulmonary secretions are not mobilized in the lower lobes.

Musculoskeletal Abnormalities. Musculoskeletal impairments in the thoracic region reduce oxygenation. Such impairments may result from abnormal structural configurations, trauma, muscular diseases, and diseases of the central nervous system. Abnormal structural configurations impairing oxygenation include those that affect the rib cage, such as pectus excavatum (an indentation of the lower sternum), and those that affect the vertebral column, such as kyphosis, lordosis, or scoliosis.

Trauma. The person with multiple rib fractures can develop a flail chest, a condition in which fractures cause instability in part of the chest wall. The unstable chest wall allows the lung underlying the injured area to contract on inspiration and bulge on expiration, resulting in hypoxia. Chest wall or upper abdominal incisions may also decrease chest wall movement as the patient uses shallow respirations to minimize chest wall movement to avoid pain. Excessive or high doses of narcotic analgesics may depress the respiratory centre, further decreasing respiratory rate and chest wall expansion.

Neuromuscular Diseases. Diseases such as muscular dystrophy affect oxygenation of tissues by decreasing the patient's ability to expand and contract the chest wall. Ventilation is impaired, and atelectasis, hypercapnia, and hypoxemia can occur. Myasthenia gravis, Guillain-Barré syndrome, and poliomyelitis affect respiratory functioning and result in hypoventilation. Myasthenia gravis interferes with normal transmission of impulses from nerves to muscles, involving the whole body, including muscles of respiration. Guillain-Barré syndrome and poliomyelitis cause inflammation and paralysis of muscle groups. Guillain-Barré syndrome usually results in an ascending pattern of paralysis. Respiratory muscles become paralyzed as paralysis ascends to the thoracic region. Poliomyelitis may lead to general or local paralysis. Both disorders may reverse, but poliomyelitis usually results in more residual paralysis.

Central Nervous System Alterations. Diseases or trauma involving the medulla oblongata and spinal cord may result in impaired respiration. When the medulla oblongata is affected, neural regulation of respiration is damaged and abnormal breathing patterns may develop. If the phrenic nerve is damaged, the diaphragm may not descend, thus reducing inspiratory lung volumes and causing hypoxemia. Cervical trauma at C3 to C5 can result in paralysis of the phrenic nerve. Spinal cord trauma below the fifth cervical vertebra usually leaves the phrenic nerve intact but damages nerves that innervate the intercostal muscles, preventing anteroposterior chest expansion.

Influences of Chronic Disease. Oxygenation can be decreased as a direct consequence of chronic disease. It can also be decreased as a secondary effect, as with anemia. The physiological response to chronic hypoxemia is the development of a secondary polycythemia (increase in red blood cells). This adaptive response is the body's attempt to increase the amount of circulating hemoglobin to increase the available oxygen-binding sites.

Alterations in Cardiac Functioning

Illnesses and conditions that affect cardiac rhythm, strength of contraction, blood flow through the chambers, myocardial blood flow, and peripheral circulation cause alterations in cardiac functioning. Older persons experience alterations in cardiac function due to calcification of the conduction pathways, thicker and stiffer heart valves from lipid accumulation and fibrosis, and a decrease in the number of pacemaker cells in the SA node (Meiner, 2011; Touhy & Jett, 2014).

Disturbances in Conduction. Some disturbances in conduction are a result of electrical impulses that do not originate from the SA node. These rhythm disturbances are called **dysrhythmias**, meaning a deviation from the normal sinus heart rhythm (Table 39-2). Dysrhythmias may occur as a primary conduction disturbance; as a response to ischemia, valvular abnormality, anxiety, or drug toxicity; as a result of caffeine, alcohol, or tobacco use; or as a complication of acid–base or electrolyte imbalance (see Chapter 40). Such disturbances may be life-threatening and require treatment with medication or defibrillation (Box 39-3).

Dysrhythmias are classified by cardiac response and site of impulse origin. Cardiac response can be tachycardiac (>100 beats/min), bradycardiac (<60 beats/min), a premature (early) beat, or a blocked (delayed or absent) beat. Tachydysrhythmias and bradydysrhythmias can lower cardiac output and blood pressure. Tachydysrhythmias reduce cardiac output by decreasing diastolic filling time. Bradydysrhythmias lower cardiac output because of the decreased heart rate.

Atrial fibrillation is a common type of dysrhythmia in older persons. The electrical impulse in the atria is chaotic and originates from multiple sites. The rhythm is irregular because of the multiple pacemaker sites and the unpredictable conduction to the ventricles. The QRS complex is normal; however, it occurs at irregular intervals. Atrial fibrillation is often described as an irregularly irregular rhythm.

Abnormal impulses originating above the ventricles are referred to as *supraventricular dysrhythmias*. The abnormality on the waveform is the configuration and placement of the P wave. Ventricular conduction usually remains normal, and a normal QRS complex is observed.

Ventricular dysrhythmias represent an ectopic site of impulse formation within the ventricles. It is ectopic in that the impulse originates in the ventricle, not the SA node. The configuration of the QRS complex is usually widened and bizarre. P waves may or may not be present; often they are buried in the QRS complex. **Ventricular tachycardia** and **ventricular fibrillation** are life-threatening rhythms that require immediate intervention. Ventricular tachycardia is considered a life-threatening dysrhythmia because of the decreased cardiac output and the potential to deteriorate into ventricular fibrillation or sudden cardiac death (HSF and American Heart Association [AHA], 2015).

Asystole is a lethal rhythm associated with no apparent electrical activity. The patient has no cardiac output and thus no palpable pulse. If the patient is on a cardiac monitor, the lack of electrical activity is noted by an absent rhythm. Asystole can occur as a primary event, it may follow ventricular fibrillation, or it can occur in patients with complete heart block. Asystole must be treated immediately.

Altered Cardiac Output. Failure of the myocardium to eject sufficient volume to the systemic and pulmonary circulations can result in heart failure. Heart failure is a growing epidemic with approximately 50 000 Canadians newly diagnosed each year (HSFC, 2016). Primary coronary artery disease, cardiomyopathic conditions, valvular disorders, and pulmonary disease lead to myocardial pump failure.

BOX 39-3 Automated External Defibrillator (AED)

- An automated external defibrillator is a device used to administer an electrical shock through the chest wall to the heart.
- Built-in computers assess the victim's heart rhythm and determine if defibrillation is needed.
- The AED delivers a shock to the victim.
- It can be used by nonmedical personnel.
- It is used to strengthen the chain of survival. Every minute of a sudden cardiac arrest without defibrillation decreases the survival rate by 7%–10%

Heart and Stroke Foundation of Canada (2016). HSFC National AED Program. Retrieved from https://resuscitation.heartandstroke.ca/programs/aed/nationalaed

Left-Sided Heart Failure. Left-sided heart failure is an abnormal condition characterized by impaired functioning of the left ventricle as a result of elevated pressures and pulmonary congestion. If left ventricular failure is significant, the amount of blood ejected from the left ventricle drops greatly, resulting in decreased cardiac output. Assessment findings may include decreased activity tolerance, breathlessness, dizziness, and confusion as a result of tissue hypoxia from the diminished cardiac output. As the left ventricle continues to fail, blood begins to pool in the pulmonary circulation, causing pulmonary congestion. Clinical findings include crackles on auscultation, hypoxia, shortness of breath on exertion and often at rest, cough, and paroxysmal nocturnal dyspnea.

Right-Sided Heart Failure. Right-sided heart failure results from impaired functioning of the right ventricle characterized by venous congestion in the systemic circulation. Right-sided heart failure more commonly results from pulmonary disease or from long-term left-sided failure. The primary pathological factor in right-sided failure is elevated pulmonary vascular resistance (PVR). As the PVR continues to

TABLE 39-2 Common Basic Cardiac Dysrhythmias

Rhythm Characteristics and Etiology	Clinical Significance and Management
Sinus Tachycardia	
Regular rhythm, rate 100–180 beats/min (higher in infants), normal P wave, normal QRS complex.	Patient with damaged heart may not be able to sustain increased myocardial oxygen consumption by increased heart rate.
Rate increase may be a normal response to exercise, emotion, or stressors such as pain, fever, pump failure, hyperthyroidism, and certain drugs (e.g., caffeine, nitrates, epinephrine, nicotine).	Correct underlying causes; discontinue drugs producing the adverse effect.
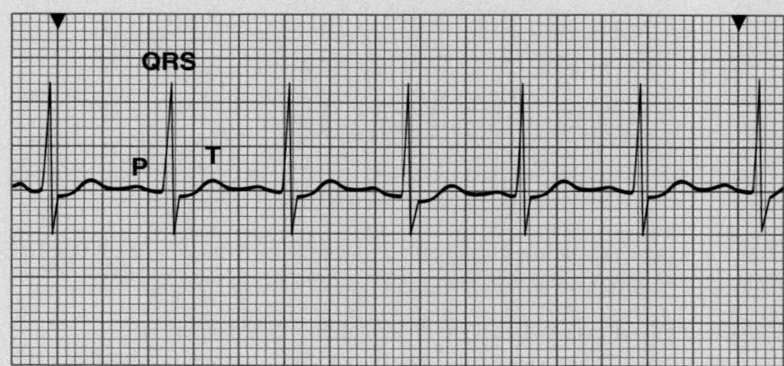 Sinus tachycardia (From Wesley, K. [2011]. *Huzar's basic dysrhythmias and acute coronary syndrome interpretation and management* [4th ed., p. 87, Fig. 5-5B]. St. Louis, MO: Mosby.)	
Sinus Bradycardia	
Regular rhythm, rate <60 beats/min, normal P wave, normal PR interval, normal QRS complex.	No clinical significance unless associated with signs and symptoms of reduced cardiac output such as dizziness or syncope or presence of chest pain.
Rate decrease may be a normal response to sleep or in well-conditioned athletes; abnormal drops in rate may be caused by diminished blood flow to the sinoatrial (SA) node, vagal stimulation, hypothyroidism, increased intracranial pressure, or pharmacological drugs (e.g., digoxin, propranolol, quinidine, procainamide).	Bradycardia with hypotension and decreased cardiac output is treated with atropine; a pacemaker may be required.
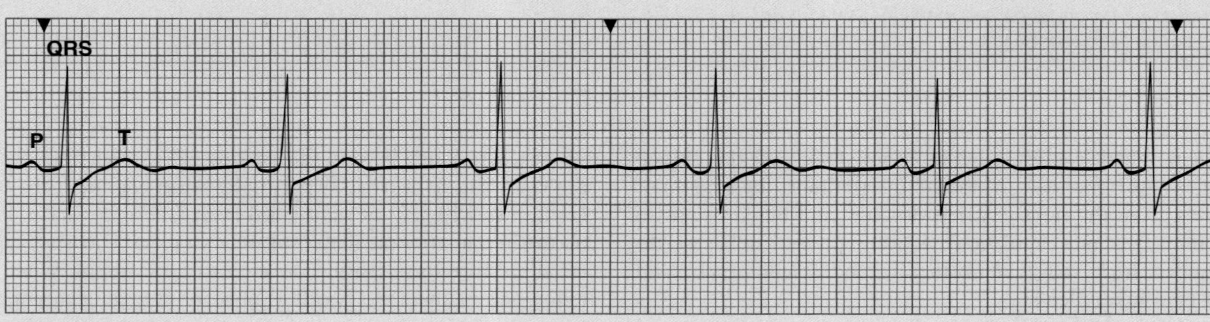 Sinus bradycardia (From Wesley, K. [2011]. *Huzar's basic dysrhythmias and acute coronary syndrome interpretation and management* [4th ed., p. 82, Fig. 5-3A]. St. Louis, MO: Mosby.)	

Continued

TABLE 39-2 Common Basic Cardiac Dysrhythmias—cont'd

Rhythm Characteristics and Etiology	Clinical Significance and Management
Atrial Fibrillation (A-fib)	
Chaotic, irregular atrial activity resulting in an irregular ventricular response. No identifiable P waves. Irregular ventricular response resulting in an irregular cardiac rate and rhythm. The rate is determined by the conduction of the multiple atrial impulses across the atrioventricular (AV) node. A-fib is caused by aging, calcification of the SA node, or changes in myocardial blood supply.	There is a loss of the atrial kick (portion of the cardiac output squeezed in the ventricles with a coordinated atrial contraction), pooling of blood in the atria, and development of microemboli. The patient may complain of fatigue, a fluttering in the chest, or shortness of breath if the ventricular response is rapid. A-fib is a commonly occurring dysrhythmia in the aging and older person. Anticoagulants such as warfarin (Coumadin) may be used to reduce the risk of stroke. Warfarin is prescribed on the basis of the international normalized ratio (INR) and thus dose adjustments are based on daily INR results.

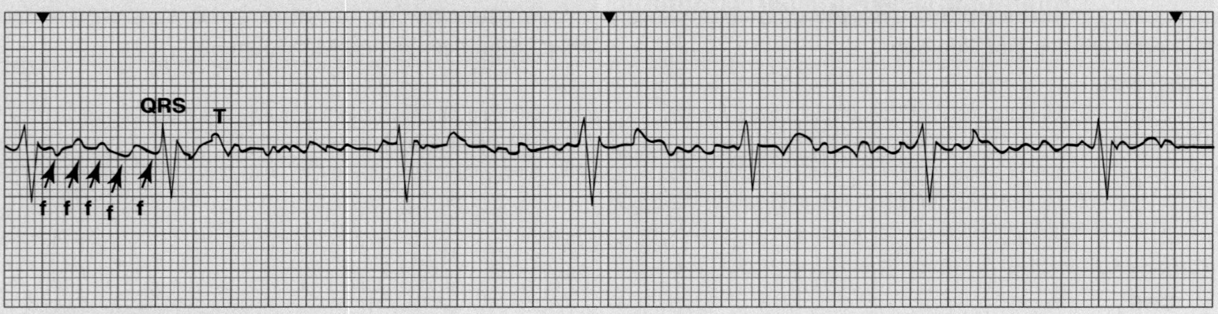

Coarse atrial fibrillation

(From Wesley, K. [2011]. *Huzar's basic dysrhythmias and acute coronary syndrome interpretation and management* [4th ed., p. 103, Fig. 6-7F]. St. Louis, MO: Mosby.)

Rhythm Characteristics and Etiology	Clinical Significance and Management
Ventricular Tachycardia	
Rhythm slightly irregular, rate 100–200 beats/min, P wave absent, PR interval absent, QRS complex wide and bizarre, >0.12 seconds.	Results in a decreased cardiac output due to decreased ventricular filling time; may lead to severe hypotension and loss of pulse and consciousness.
Caused by changes in the normal pacemaker of the heart, such as decrease in blood flow, ischemia, or embolus.	If pulseless, interventions may include defibrillation, cardiopulmonary resuscitation (CPR), and medications (Heart and Stroke Foundation [HSF] & American Heart Association [AHA], 2015).

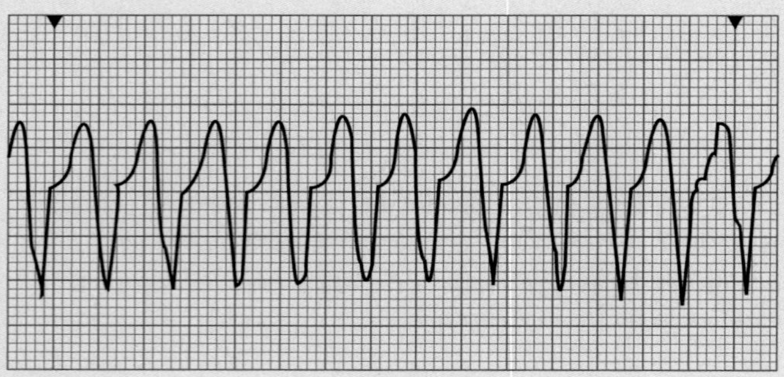

VT

(From Wesley, K. [2011]. *Huzar's basic dysrhythmias and acute coronary syndrome interpretation and management* [4th ed., p. 122, Fig. 8-2C]. St, Louis, MO: Mosby.)

rise, the right ventricle must generate more work, and the oxygen demand of the heart increases. As the failure continues, the amount of blood ejected from the right ventricle declines, and blood begins to "back up" in the systemic circulation. Clinically, the patient has weight gain, distended neck veins, hepatomegaly and splenomegaly, and dependent peripheral edema.

Impaired Valvular Function. Valvular heart disease is an acquired or congenital disorder of a cardiac valve characterized by stenosis and obstructed blood flow or valvular degeneration and regurgitation of blood. When stenosis occurs in the semilunar valves (aortic and pulmonic valves), the adjacent ventricles must work harder to move the ventricular volume beyond the stenotic valve. Over time, the stenosis can cause the ventricle to hypertrophy (enlarge), and if the condition is left untreated, left- or right-sided heart failure can occur. If stenosis occurs in the atrioventricular valves (mitral and tricuspid valves), the atrial pressure rises, causing the atria to hypertrophy. When regurgitation occurs, there is a backflow of blood into an adjacent chamber. For example, in mitral regurgitation, the mitral leaflets do not close completely. When the ventricles contract, blood escapes back into the atria, causing a murmur, or "whooshing" sound (see Chapter 32).

Myocardial Ischemia. Myocardial ischemia results when the supply of blood to the myocardium from the coronary arteries is

TABLE 39-2 Common Basic Cardiac Dysrhythmias—cont'd

Rhythm Characteristics and Etiology	Clinical Significance and Management
Ventricular Fibrillation Uncoordinated electrical activity. No identifiable P, QRS, or T wave. Causes include sudden cardiac death, electrical shock, acute myocardial infarction, drowning, or trauma. 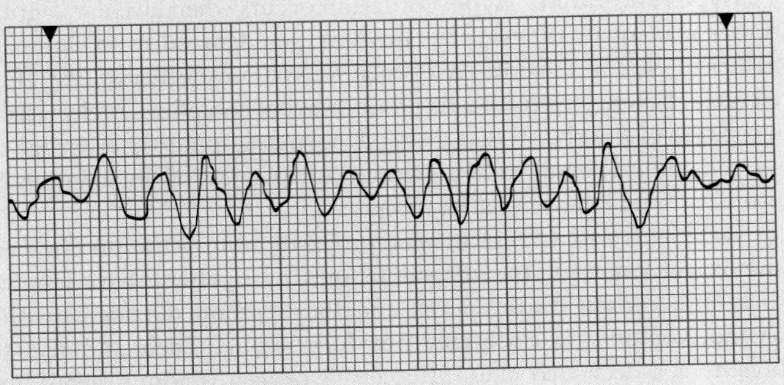 Coarse ventricular fibrillation (From Wesley, K. [2011]. *Huzar's basic dysrhythmias and acute coronary syndrome interpretation and management* [4th ed., p. 127, Fig. 8-5C]. St. Louis, MO: Mosby.)	Acute loss of pulse and respiration. Defibrillation, CPR, and medications may be used as initial interventions for ventricular fibrillation (HSF & AHA, 2015). The 2015 *American Heart Association Guidelines for CPR and Emergency Cardiovascular Care* recommend the establishment of automated external defibrillator programs in public locations where there is a relatively high likelihood of witnessed cardiac arrest (HSF & AHA, 2015; see Box 39-3).
Asystole Classically referred to as a "flat line." There are no electrical impulses and therefore no QRS complex, no contraction, and no cardiac output. Possible causes are hypoxia, hyperkalemia and hypokalemia, pre-existing acidosis, drug overdose, and hypothermia. 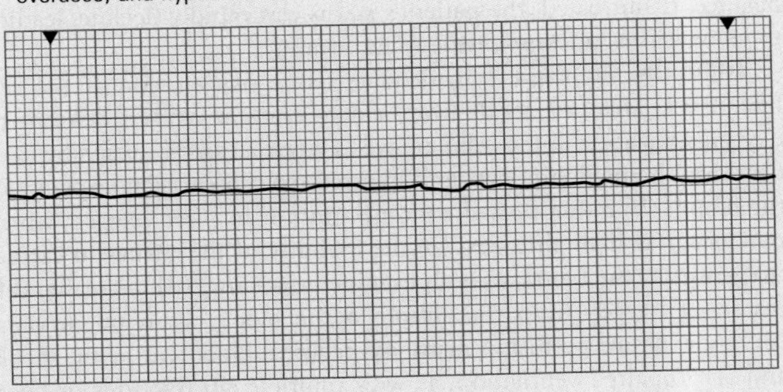 Ventricular asystole (From Wesley, K. [2011]. *Huzar's basic dysrhythmias and acute coronary syndrome interpretation and management* [4th ed., p. 132, Fig. 8-8C]. St, Louis, MO: Mosby.)	The unresponsive patient will have no pulse, blood pressure, or respirations. The management of asystole consists of CPR, medications, and correction of the underlying cause (HSF & AHA, 2015).

Adapted from Wesley, K. (2011). *Huszar's basic dysrhythmias and acute coronary syndrome interpretation and management* (4th ed.) St. Louis, MO: Mosby.

insufficient to meet the oxygen demands of the organ. Common manifestations of this ischemia include angina pectoris, myocardial infarction, and acute coronary syndrome.

Angina Pectoris. Angina pectoris is usually a transient imbalance between myocardial oxygen supply and demand. The condition results in chest pain that is aching, sharp, tingling, or burning, or that feels like pressure. The chest pain may be left-sided or substernal and may radiate to the left or both arms, and to the jaw, neck, and back. In some patients, anginal pain may not radiate. The pain can last from 3 to 5 minutes (McCance & Huether, 2014). Patients report that pain is often precipitated by activities that increase myocardial oxygen demand (e.g., exercise, anxiety, or stress). The pain is usually relieved with rest and coronary vasodilators, the most common being a nitroglycerine preparation.

Myocardial Infarction. Myocardial infarction (MI) results from sudden decreases in coronary blood flow or an increase in myocardial oxygen demand without adequate coronary perfusion. Infarction occurs because of ischemia (which is reversible) and necrosis (which is not reversible) of myocardial tissue. After 20 minutes of myocardial ischemia, cellular death occurs (McCance & Huether, 2014).

In men, chest pain associated with MI is usually described as crushing, squeezing, or stabbing. The pain may be retrosternal and left precordial, and it may radiate from down the left arm to the neck, jaws, teeth, epigastric area, and back. The pain occurs at rest or on exertion, lasts more than 20 minutes, and is unrelieved by rest, position change, or sublingual nitroglycerine administration.

Chest pain remains the most common symptom in both men and women but does not have to be present to indicate an MI (HSFC,

2017b). The language women use to describe their pain may differ as they may describe it as pressure or tightness; this may influence their diagnosis and treatment (HSFC, 2018, p. 6). It is important to note that sex and gender differences may exist in heart disease, for example, when it comes to heart disease women are "under-researched, under-diagnosed and under-treated, and under-supported during recovery" (HSFC, 2018, p. 2). Atypical symptoms such as nausea, indigestion, fatigue, and shortness of breath may be present in both men and women (HSFC, 2017b).

As women get older, the risk of heart disease increases (AHA, 2015a). In a recent report by the HSFC (2018) they state "we still struggle to untangle and apply new knowledge about women and heart disease, and why some women—Indigenous women, ethically diverse women, women living in poverty, and women in remote and rural locations—often face even greater inequities (p. 2). HSFC (2018) state "Indigenous people of Canada-First Nations, Metis and Inuit are two times more likely to develop heart disease," with indigenous women more likely to die from heart disease at a younger age compared to non-indigenous women (p. 14).

Acute Coronary Syndrome. Acute coronary syndrome (ACS) includes unstable angina, non-ST-segment elevation MI, and ST-segment elevation MI. There is an imbalance in the oxygen supply and demand to the myocardium. Causes include nonocclusive thrombus on pre-existing plaque; coronary vasospasm; arterial narrowing from atherosclerosis; inflammation or infection; and secondary unstable angina from anemia, fever, or hypoxemia. Symptoms may not be constant and may present atypically. Patients with classic AMI symptoms are more easily identified. Intermediate risk factors for ACS include smoking, hypertension, diabetes, high cholesterol, physical inactivity, obesity, and a family history of cardiac disease (AHA, 2015b).

Alterations in Respiratory Functioning

Illnesses and conditions that affect ventilation or oxygen transport cause alterations in respiratory functioning. The three primary alterations are hyperventilation, hypoventilation, and hypoxia.

The goal of ventilation is to produce a normal arterial carbon dioxide tension ($PaCO_2$) between 35 and 45 mm Hg and maintain a normal arterial oxygen tension (PaO_2) between 80 and 100 mm Hg. Hyperventilation and hypoventilation refer to alveolar ventilation and not to the patient's respiratory rate. Arterial oxygen levels can be monitored using a noninvasive oxygen saturation monitor. The normal range is 95% to 100%. Hypoxia refers to a decrease in the amount of arterial oxygen.

Hyperventilation. Hyperventilation is a state of ventilation in excess of that required to eliminate the normal venous carbon dioxide produced by cellular metabolism. Anxiety, infections, drugs, or an acid–base imbalance can induce hyperventilation, as well as hypoxia associated with pulmonary embolus or shock. Acute anxiety can lead to hyperventilation and may cause loss of consciousness from excess carbon dioxide exhalation. Fever can cause hyperventilation. As a patient's body temperature increases, there is an increase in the metabolic rate, thereby increasing carbon dioxide production. The clinical response is an increased rate and depth of respiration.

Hyperventilation may also be chemically induced. Salicylate (aspirin) poisoning causes excessive stimulation of the respiratory centre as the body attempts to compensate for excess carbon dioxide. Amphetamines also increase ventilation by raising carbon dioxide production. Hyperventilation can also occur as the body tries to compensate for metabolic acidosis by producing a respiratory alkalosis. For example, the diabetic patient who has gone into diabetic ketoacidosis is producing large amounts of metabolic acids. The respiratory system tries to correct the acid–base balance by overbreathing. Ventilation increases to reduce the amount of carbon dioxide available to form carbonic acid (see Chapter 40). Hemoglobin does not release oxygen to tissues as readily, and tissue hypoxia results. As symptoms worsen, the patient may become more agitated, which further increases the respiratory rate and can result in respiratory alkalosis.

Hypoventilation. Hypoventilation occurs when alveolar ventilation is inadequate to meet the body's oxygen demand or to eliminate sufficient carbon dioxide. As alveolar ventilation decreases, $PaCO_2$ is elevated. Severe atelectasis can produce hypoventilation. Atelectasis is a collapse of the alveoli that prevents normal respiratory exchange of oxygen and carbon dioxide. As alveoli collapse, less of the lung can be ventilated and hypoventilation occurs.

In patients with COPD, the inappropriate administration of excessive oxygen can result in hypoventilation. These patients have adapted to a high carbon dioxide level, and their carbon dioxide–sensitive chemoreceptors are essentially not functioning. Their stimulus to breathe is a decreased PaO_2. If excessive oxygen is administered, the oxygen requirement is satisfied and the stimulus to breathe is negated. High concentrations of oxygen (e.g., >24%–28% [1–3 L/min]) prevent the PaO_2 from falling and obliterate the stimulus to breathe, resulting in hypoventilation. The excessive retention of carbon dioxide may lead to respiratory arrest.

Signs and symptoms of hypoventilation include mental status changes, dysrhythmias, and potential cardiac arrest. Treatment requires improving tissue oxygenation, restoring ventilatory function, treating the underlying cause of the hypoventilation, and achieving acid–base balance. If untreated, the patient's status can rapidly decline, leading to convulsions, unconsciousness, and death.

Hypoxia. Hypoxia is inadequate tissue oxygenation at the cellular level. This can result from a deficiency in oxygen delivery or oxygen utilization at the cellular level. Hypoxia can be caused by (a) a decreased hemoglobin level and lowered oxygen-carrying capacity of the blood; (b) a diminished concentration of inspired oxygen, which may occur at high altitudes; (c) the inability of the tissues to extract oxygen from the blood, as with cyanide poisoning; (d) decreased diffusion of oxygen from the alveoli to the blood, as in pneumonia; (e) poor tissue perfusion with oxygenated blood, as with shock; and (f) impaired ventilation, as with multiple rib fractures or chest trauma.

The clinical signs and symptoms of hypoxia include apprehension, restlessness, inability to concentrate, declining level of consciousness, dizziness, and behavioural changes. The patient with hypoxia is unable to lie down and appears fatigued and agitated. Vital sign changes include an increased pulse rate and increased rate and depth of respiration. The patient with a narcotic overdose, such as a heroin overdose, may display signs of hypoventilation. During early stages of hypoxia, the blood pressure is elevated unless the condition is caused by shock. As the hypoxia worsens, the respiratory rate may decline as a result of respiratory muscle fatigue.

Cyanosis, or blue discoloration of the skin and mucous membranes caused by the presence of desaturated hemoglobin in capillaries, is a late sign of hypoxia. The presence or absence of cyanosis is not a reliable measure of oxygenation status. Central cyanosis, observed in the tongue, soft palate, and conjunctiva of the eye, where blood flow is high, indicates hypoxemia. Peripheral cyanosis, seen in the extremities, nail beds, and earlobes, is often a result of vasoconstriction and stagnant blood flow. Hypoxia is a life-threatening condition. Untreated, it can produce cardiac dysrhythmias that result in death. Hypoxia is managed by administration of oxygen and treatment of the underlying cause, such as airway obstruction.

NURSING KNOWLEDGE BASE

Developmental Factors

According to the Canadian Association of Schools of Nursing (CASN, 2015), foundational knowledge of human development expanding over the lifespan is an essential domain to consider when developing a plan of care. The developmental stage of the patient and the normal aging process can affect tissue oxygenation.

Infants and Toddlers. Infants and toddlers are at risk for upper respiratory tract infections as a result of frequent exposure to other children and exposure to second-hand smoke. In addition, during the teething process, some infants develop nasal congestion, which encourages bacterial growth and increases the potential for respiratory tract infection. Upper respiratory tract infections are usually not dangerous, and infants or toddlers recover with little difficulty.

School-Aged Children and Adolescents. School-aged children and adolescents are exposed to respiratory infections and respiratory risk factors such as second-hand smoke and cigarette smoking. A healthy child usually does not have adverse pulmonary effects from respiratory infections. A person who starts smoking in adolescence and continues to smoke into middle age, however, has an increased risk for cardiopulmonary disease and lung cancer.

Young and Middle-Aged Adults. Young and middle-aged adults are exposed to multiple cardiopulmonary risk factors: an unhealthy diet, lack of exercise, stress, over-the-counter and prescription drugs not used as intended, illegal drugs, and smoking. By reducing these modifiable factors patients may decrease their risk for cardiac or pulmonary diseases. During youth and middle age, lifelong habits and lifestyles are established. It is thus important to help these patients make good choices and informed decisions about the rest of their lives and their health care practices.

Older Persons. The cardiac and respiratory systems undergo changes throughout the aging process (Box 39-4). The changes are associated with calcification of the heart valves, SA node, and costal cartilages. The arterial system develops atherosclerotic plaques. Osteoporosis leads to changes in the size and shape of the thorax.

The trachea and large bronchi become enlarged from calcification of the airways. The alveoli enlarge, decreasing the surface area available for gas exchange. The number of functional cilia is reduced, causing a decrease in the effectiveness of the cough mechanism, putting the older person at increased risk for respiratory infections (Touhy & Jett, 2014). Ventilation and transfer of respiratory gases decline with age because the lungs are unable to expand fully, leading to lower oxygenation levels.

Lifestyle Risk Factors

Lifestyle modifications that influence cardiopulmonary functioning are frequently difficult because a patient is being asked to change a

BOX 39-4 FOCUS ON OLDER PERSONS

Changes to Cardiac and Respiratory Systems

- The tuberculin skin test is an unreliable indicator of tuberculosis in older persons. They frequently display false-positive or false-negative skin test reactions.
- Older persons are at an increased risk for reactivation of dormant organisms that have been present for decades, as a result of age-related changes in the immune system.
- The standard 5-TU Mantoux test is given and repeated or repeated with the 250-TU strength to create a booster effect.
- If the older person has a positive reaction, a complete history is necessary to determine any risk factors.
- Cardiac problems differ from other chronic conditions in that, when they become acute, symptoms worsen rapidly and necessitate hospitalization, whereas other chronic conditions can be managed in the home (Touhy & Jett, 2014).
- Regulating blood pressure in the older person results in 30% fewer strokes, 64% fewer cases of heart failure, 23% fewer fatal cardiac events, and 21% fewer cardiac-related deaths (Touhy & Jett, 2014).
- Mental status changes are often the first signs of respiratory problems and may include forgetfulness and irritability.
- Older persons may not complain of dyspnea until it affects the activities of daily living that are important to them.
- Changes in the older person's cough mechanism may lead to retention of pulmonary secretions, airway plugging, and atelectasis, if cough suppressants are not used with caution.
- Age-related changes in immune function lead to a decrease in cell-mediated and humoral immunity, causing an increased risk of respiratory infections (McCance & Huether, 2014).
- Alterations in the thorax that occur from ossification of costal cartilage, decreased space between vertebrae, and diminished respiratory muscle strength lead to impairment of chest expansion and oxygenation (Touhy & Jett, 2014).

BOX 39-5 FOCUS ON PRIMARY HEALTH CARE

Positive Lifestyle Practices for Cardiopulmonary Health Promotion

As part of a primary health care focus, it is important to educate young to older persons about the following lifestyle practices that promote cardiopulmonary health:

- Maintain ideal body weight.
- Eat a low-fat, low-salt, calorie-appropriate diet.
- Engage in regular aerobic exercise 30 to 60 minutes daily.
- Use a filter mask when exposed to occupational hazards.
- Use stress-reduction techniques.
- Reduce exposure to secondary infections.
- Do not smoke.
- Avoid second-hand smoke and other pollutants.
- Have annual visits with a health care provider.
- Monitor blood pressure.
- Monitor cholesterol and triglyceride levels.
- Request an annual influenza vaccine, especially if at risk for the development of influenza.
- Request a pneumococcal vaccine, if appropriate.

habit or behaviour that may be enjoyed, such as cigarette smoking or eating certain foods; however, these changes can be achieved with encouragement, support, and time (Box 39-5). Risk factor modification is important and includes smoking cessation, weight reduction, a low-cholesterol and low-sodium diet, management of hypertension, and moderate exercise. Although it may be difficult to change long-term behaviour, assisting patients with healthy behaviours can slow or halt the progression of cardiopulmonary diseases.

Poor Nutrition. Nutrition affects cardiopulmonary function in several ways. Severe obesity decreases lung expansion, and the increased body weight increases oxygen demands to meet metabolic needs. The malnourished patient may experience respiratory muscle wasting, resulting in decreased muscle strength and respiratory excursion. Cough efficiency is reduced secondary to respiratory muscle weakness, putting the patient at risk for retention of pulmonary secretions. Diets high in fat increase cholesterol and atherogenesis in the coronary arteries.

Patients who are morbidly obese, malnourished, or both are at risk for anemia. Diets high in carbohydrates may play a role in increasing the carbon dioxide load for patients with carbon dioxide retention. As carbohydrates are metabolized, an increased load of carbon dioxide is created and excreted via the lungs.

Hypertension affects approximately a quarter of adult Canadians (Leung et al., 2017, p. 558). Health behaviour modification, such as reduction in dietary sodium, could assist with the management of hypertension (Hypertension Canada, 2017). Diets high in potassium may prevent and help improve control over hypertension. A 2000-calorie diet high in fibre, potassium, calcium, and magnesium, with an emphasis on fruits, vegetables, and low-fat dairy foods and low in saturated and total fat, is recommended to help prevent and reduce the effects of hypertension. More recently, it has been found that adhering to a Mediterranean diet that is supplemented with extra-virgin olive oil or nuts may reduce the risk of cardiovascular events (Estruch, et al., 2013). Additionally, it has been recommended that reducing intake of concentrated sugars such as those found in ultra-processed foods and beverages be considered for those with coronary heart disease (DiNicolantonio, Lucan, & O'Keefe, 2015, p. 464). The HSFC (2017c) recommends that an individual's total intake of free sugars not exceed 10% (ideally less than 5%) of total daily calorie intake. Consumption of energy drinks by young adults should also be reduced given the increase in related emergency room visits (Kozik, Shah, Bhattacharyya, et al., 2016, p. 1205). Energy drinks have been found to increase systolic blood pressure, alter electrolytes, and cause cardiac arrhythmias (Kozik et al., 2016, p. 1205).

Inadequate Exercise. Exercise increases the body's metabolic activity and oxygen demand. The rate and depth of respiration increase, enabling the person to inhale more oxygen and exhale excess carbon dioxide. A physical exercise program has many benefits (see Chapter 36). People who exercise for 30 to 60 minutes daily have a lower pulse rate and blood pressure, decreased cholesterol level, increased blood flow, and greater oxygen extraction by working muscles. Fully conditioned people can increase oxygen consumption by 10 to 20% because of increased cardiac output and increased efficiency of the myocardial muscle (James, Oparil, Carter, et al., 2014).

Smoking. Cigarette smoking is associated with a number of diseases, including heart disease, chronic obstructive lung disease, and lung cancer. Smoking is a risk factor for heart disease, stroke, cancer, and respiratory disease (McCance & Huether, 2014). Inhaled nicotine causes vasoconstriction of peripheral and coronary blood vessels, increasing blood pressure, and decreasing blood flow to peripheral vessels. Women who take birth control pills and smoke cigarettes are at increased risk for cardiovascular problems such as thrombophlebitis and pulmonary emboli.

Cigarette smoking is the leading cause of cancer death in Canada, accounting for more than 85% of lung cancer cases in Canada (Canadian Cancer Society, 2017). Regular exposure to second-hand smoke contributes to heart disease and respiratory illnesses such as asthma and bronchitis (Statistics Canada, 2016). Lung cancer is the leading cause of cancer death for both men and women (Canadian Cancer Society, 2017). It is estimated that 1 in 11 men and 1 in 15 women will develop lung cancer in their lifetime (Canadian Cancer Society, 2017). The 5-year survival rate (2006–2008) for females with lung cancer is 20% and in males, 14% (Canadian Cancer Society, 2017). If lung cancer is detected when the disease is still localized, the survival rate is 49%. However, lung cancer is often diagnosed only when it has reached an advanced stage. If a substantial number of health care providers implement even minimal smoking cessation interventions, a decrease in related tobacco diseases will result (Registered Nurses' Association of Ontario [RNAO], 2007, p. 13). RNAO (2007) has developed Best Practice Guidelines and recommendations for nurses to assist their patients with smoking cessation (see RNAO, 2007).

Substance Abuse. Excessive use of alcohol and other drugs can impair tissue oxygenation in two ways. First, the person who chronically abuses substances often has a poor nutritional intake. With the resultant decrease in intake of iron-rich foods, hemoglobin production declines. Second, excessive use of alcohol and certain other drugs can depress the respiratory centre, reducing the rate and depth of respiration and the amount of inhaled oxygen. Substance abuse by either smoking or inhaling, such as crack cocaine or inhaling fumes from paint or glue cans, causes direct injury to lung tissue that can lead to permanent lung damage and impaired oxygenation.

Stress. A continuous state of stress or severe anxiety increases the body's metabolic rate and the oxygen demand. The body responds to anxiety and other stresses with an increased rate and depth of respiration. Most people can adapt, but some, particularly those with chronic illnesses or acute life-threatening illnesses such as an MI, cannot tolerate the oxygen demands associated with anxiety (see Chapter 29).

Environmental Factors

The environment can also influence oxygenation. The incidence of pulmonary disease is higher in smoggy, urban areas than in rural areas. In addition, the patient's workplace may increase the risk for pulmonary disease. Some occupational pollutants are asbestos, talcum powder, dust, and airborne fibres. Asbestosis is an occupational lung disease that develops after exposure to asbestos. The lung in asbestosis is characterized by diffuse interstitial fibrosis, creating a restrictive lung disease. It can also cause pleural mesotheliomas and pleural plaques. Patients at risk for developing asbestosis include those working with textiles, fireproofing, or milling or in the production of paints, plastics, or some prefabricated construction. Patients exposed to asbestos who also smoke are at increased risk of developing lung cancer.

CRITICAL THINKING

Successful critical thinking requires a synthesis of knowledge, experience, information gathered from patients, critical thinking qualities, and intellectual and professional standards. Clinical judgements require nurses to anticipate the information necessary, analyze the data, and make decisions regarding the patient's care. During the assessment, nurses need to consider all elements that build toward making an appropriate nursing diagnosis (Figure 39-6).

To understand the oxygen demands of a patient and the ability of the patient's body to meet those demands, nurses need to integrate knowledge from nursing and other disciplines, previous experiences, and information gathered from patients. Professional standards, such

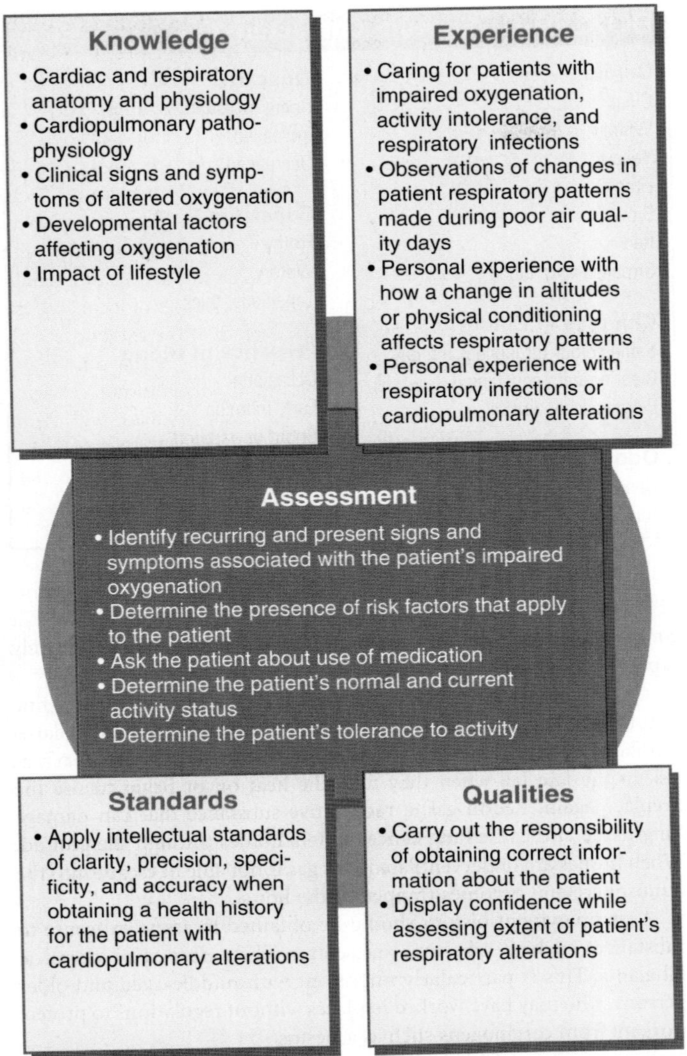

FIGURE 39-6 Critical thinking model for oxygenation assessment.

as those developed by the HSFC, the Canadian Cardiovascular Society, the Canadian Lung Association, the Canadian Thoracic Society, and the Canadian Foundation for Infectious Diseases Society, provide valuable guidelines for the care and management of patients with altered oxygenation.

❖ NURSING PROCESS

◆ Assessment

The nursing assessment of a patient's cardiopulmonary functioning includes an in-depth history of the patient's normal and present cardiopulmonary function, past impairments in circulatory or respiratory functioning, and measures that the patient uses to optimize oxygenation. The history should include a review of drug, food, and other allergies, such as pet dander, mould, and environmental triggers.

Through physical examination of the patient's cardiopulmonary status, the extent of existing signs and symptoms is determined. A review of laboratory and diagnostic test results provides valuable data on respiratory and ventilatory parameters.

Health History

The health history should focus on the patient's ability to meet oxygen needs. The health history for cardiac function includes pain and characteristics of pain, dyspnea, fatigue, peripheral circulation, cardiac risk factors, and the presence of past or concurrent cardiac conditions. The health history for respiratory function includes presence of a cough, shortness of breath, wheezing, pain, environmental exposures, frequency of respiratory tract infections, pulmonary risk factors, past respiratory problems, current medication use, and smoking history or exposure to second-hand smoke.

Pain. Chest pain needs to be thoroughly evaluated with regard to location, duration, radiation, and frequency. Cardiac pain does not occur with respiratory variations and is most often on the left side of the chest; in men, it radiates to the left arm. Chest pain in women is much less definitive and may be a sensation of choking, breathlessness, or pain that radiates through to the back. Pericardial pain resulting from an inflammation of the pericardial sac is usually nonradiating and may occur with inspiration.

Pleuritic chest pain is peripheral and may radiate to the scapular regions. It is worsened by inspiratory manoeuvres, such as coughing, yawning, and sighing. Pleuritic pain is often caused from an inflammation or infection in the pleural space and is described as knife-like, lasting from a minute to hours and always in association with inspiration.

Musculoskeletal pain may be present following exercise, rib trauma, and prolonged coughing episodes. This pain is also aggravated by inspiratory movements and may easily be confused with pleuritic chest pain.

Fatigue. Fatigue is a subjective sensation in which the patient reports a loss of endurance. Fatigue in the patient with cardiopulmonary alterations is often an early sign of worsening of the chronic underlying process. To provide an objective measure of fatigue, the patient may be asked to rate the fatigue on a scale of 0 to 10, with 10 being the worst level of fatigue and 0 representing no fatigue.

Smoking. It is important to determine patients' direct and secondary exposure to cigarette smoke. Nurses should ask patients about any history of smoking, including the number of years smoked and the number of packages smoked per day. This is recorded as pack-year history. For example, if a patient smoked two packs a day for 20 years, the patient would have a 40 pack-year history (packages per day × years smoked).

It is also important to determine if the patient is exposed to second-hand smoke from family or co-workers. Exposure to second-hand smoke increases the patient's risk for chronic lung or cardiac diseases.

Dyspnea. Dyspnea is a clinical sign of hypoxia and manifests as breathlessness. It is the subjective sensation of difficult or uncomfortable breathing. Dyspnea is shortness of breath associated with exercise or excitement, but in some patients dyspnea may be present without any relation to activity or exercise. Dyspnea is associated with many conditions, such as pulmonary diseases, cardiovascular diseases, neuromuscular conditions, and anemia. Guidelines have been developed by the Registered Nurses' Association of Ontario (RNAO) to address nursing assessment and management of patients experiencing dyspnea associated with COPD (RNAO, 2005/2010). In addition, dyspnea may occur in pregnant women in the final months of pregnancy. Environmental factors, such as pollution, cold air, and smoking, may also cause or worsen dyspnea.

Dyspnea can be associated with clinical signs such as exaggerated respiratory effort, use of the accessory muscles of respiration, nasal flaring, and marked increases in the rate and depth of respirations. The use of a visual analogue scale (VAS) can help patients make an objective assessment of their dyspnea. The VAS is a 100-mm vertical line with end points of 0 and 10. Zero is equated with no dyspnea and 10 is equated with the worst breathlessness the patient has experienced. Studies have validated the use of the VAS to evaluate a patient's dyspnea in the clinical setting (Pang, Collins, Sauser, et al., 2014). Nurses can evaluate the effectiveness of nursing interventions by monitoring a patient's assessment of his or her dyspnea.

If the patient has a history of dyspnea, it is important to determine the circumstances under which it occurred, such as with exertion, stress, or respiratory tract infection. The nurse should also determine whether the patient's perception of dyspnea affects the ability to lie flat. **Orthopnea** is an abnormal condition in which the person must use multiple pillows when lying down or must sit with the arms elevated and leaning forward to breathe. The number of pillows required for sleeping, such as two- or three-pillow orthopnea, usually quantifies the presence of orthopnea.

Cough. Cough is a sudden, audible expulsion of air from the lungs. The person breathes in, the glottis is partially closed, and the accessory muscles of expiration contract to expel the air forcibly. Coughing is a protective reflex to clear the trachea, bronchi, and lungs of irritants and secretions. The carina, the point of bifurcation of the right and left mainstem bronchus, is the most sensitive area for cough production. A cough is difficult to evaluate, and almost everyone has periods of coughing. Patients with a chronic cough tend to deny, underestimate, or minimize their coughing, often because they are so accustomed to it that they are unaware of how frequently it occurs.

Coughing is classified according to the time when the patient most frequently coughs. Patients with chronic sinusitis may cough only in the early morning or immediately after rising from sleep. This clears the airway of mucus resulting from sinus drainage. Patients with chronic bronchitis generally produce sputum all day, although greater amounts are produced after rising from a semi-recumbent or flat position. This is a result of the dependent accumulation of sputum in the airways and is associated with reduced mobility (see Chapter 45). When a patient has a cough, it is important to determine its frequency and whether it is productive or nonproductive. A productive cough results in sputum production, material coughed up from the lungs that may be swallowed or expectorated. Sputum contains mucus, cellular debris, and microorganisms, and it may contain pus or blood. When assessing a patient's cough, collect data about the type and quantity of sputum. Instruct the patient to try to produce some sputum; the patient should be careful not to simply clear the throat to produce a sample of saliva. Then inspect it for colour, consistency, odour, and amount (Box 39-6).

If **hemoptysis** (bloody sputum) is reported, determine if it is associated with coughing and bleeding from the upper respiratory tract, from sinus drainage, or from the gastrointestinal tract (**hematemesis**). In addition, the hemoptysis should be described according to amount, colour, and duration and whether it is mixed with sputum. When the patient reports bloody or blood-tinged sputum, diagnostic tests, such as examination of sputum specimens, chest X-ray examinations, **bronchoscopy**, and other X-ray studies, should be performed.

Wheezing. **Wheezing** is characterized by a high-pitched musical sound caused by high-velocity movement of air through a narrowed airway. Wheezing may be associated with asthma, acute bronchitis, or pneumonia. Wheezing can occur on inspiration, expiration, or both. It is important to determine if there are any precipitating factors, such as respiratory infection, allergens, exercise, or stress.

Environmental or Geographical Exposures. Environmental exposure to many inhaled substances is closely linked with respiratory disease. Nurses should investigate exposures in a patient's home and workplace. The most common environmental exposures in the home are cigarette smoke, carbon monoxide, and radon. In addition, it is good to determine whether a patient who is a nonsmoker is passively exposed to smoke.

BOX 39-6 Sputum Characteristics

Colour	**Quantity**
Clear	Same as usual
White	Increased
Yellow	Decreased
Green	
Brown	**Consistency**
Red	Frothy
Streaked with blood	Watery
	Tenacious, thick
Changes in Colour	
Same colour throughout the day	**Presence of Blood**
Clearing with coughing	Occasional
Progressively darker	Early morning
	Bright or dark red
Odour	Blood tinged
None	
Foul	

Carbon monoxide poisoning can result from a blocked furnace flue or fireplace. The patient may have vague complaints of general malaise, flu-like symptoms, and excessive sleepiness. Patients are particularly at risk in the late fall when they turn the heat on or begin to use the fireplace again. Radon gas, a radioactive substance that can damage lung tissue and cause lung cancer, enters homes through the ground. When homes are underventilated, this gas is not able to escape into the atmosphere and becomes trapped in the home.

An employment history should be obtained to assess exposure to substances such as asbestos, coal, cotton fibres, fumes, or chemical inhalants. This is particularly important with middle-aged and older persons, who may have worked in places without regulations to protect workers from carcinogens such as asbestos.

Exposure to pathogens may occur during travel. Schistosomiasis can be acquired in Asia, Africa, the Caribbean, and South America. This is infection of a human with a species of fluke found in fresh water that has been contaminated by human feces. Coccidioidomycosis is a fungal disease caused by inhalation of *Coccidioides immitis*, a wind-borne spore carried on dust particles.

Respiratory Infections. A health history should contain information about the patient's frequency and duration of respiratory tract infections. Although everyone occasionally experiences a cold, for some people it can result in bronchitis or pneumonia. On average, patients will have four colds per year. Nurses should determine if patients have had a pneumococcal or flu vaccine in the past. Questioning older persons about receiving these vaccines is especially important, given their increased risk for respiratory disease (Touhy & Jett, 2014). Nurses should ask about any known exposure to tuberculosis (TB) and the results of the tuberculin skin test.

Nurses also need to determine a patient's risk for human immunodeficiency virus (HIV) infection. Patients with a history of intravenous (IV) drug use and multiple unprotected sexual partners are at risk of developing HIV infection. Patients may not display any symptoms of HIV infection until they present with *Pneumocystis carinii* (PCP) or *Mycoplasma* pneumonia. Presentation with PCP or *Mycoplasma* pneumonia indicates a significant depression of the patient's immune system and progression to acquired immune deficiency syndrome (AIDS).

Allergies. When obtaining a respiratory system history, inquire about airborne allergens. The patient's allergic response may be watery eyes, sneezing, runny nose, or respiratory symptoms, such as cough or wheezing. Ask the patient specific questions about the type of allergens, response to these allergens, and successful and unsuccessful relief measures. In addition, determine the impact that environmental air quality and second-hand smoke exposure has on the patient's allergy and symptoms.

Safe nursing practice also includes obtaining information about food, drug, or insect-sting allergies. These data are usually obtained on initial history and physical examination. However, it is important to double-check this information with the patient, especially when obtaining information about respiratory allergens.

Health Risks. Familial risk factors, such as a family history of lung cancer or cardiovascular disease, need to be investigated. Documentation should include which blood relatives have had the disease and their present level of health or age at time of death. Other family risk factors include the presence of infectious diseases, particularly TB. It is important to determine who in the patient's household has been infected and the status of treatment.

Medications. The health history should also list medications the patient is using. These could include prescribed medications, over-the-counter drugs, folk medicine, herbal medicines, alternative therapies, and illicit drugs and substances. Such medications may have adverse effects by themselves or through interactions with other drugs. A person using a prescribed bronchodilator drug, for example, may decide that using an over-the-counter inhalant will also be beneficial. Many of these contain ephedrine or ma huang, a natural chemical that acts like epinephrine. This product may react with the prescribed medication by potentiating or decreasing the effect of the prescribed medication. Patients taking warfarin (Coumadin) for blood thinning will prolong the prothrombin time (international normalized ratio [INR]) results if they are taking gingko biloba, garlic, or ginseng with the anticoagulant. The drug interaction could precipitate a life-threatening bleed.

> **Safety Alert** During history taking, ask patients to list all of the over-the-counter and herbal supplements they are taking to ensure that medication interactions do not develop.

When patients are prescribed drugs for which toxic levels can be monitored by blood analyses, nurses need to review these laboratory values. Common drugs that can be monitored are digitalis preparations (digitalis levels), anticoagulants such as warfarin (Coumadin; INR level), and phenobarbital (phenobarbital levels). Toxic effects of these medications can impair cardiopulmonary functioning.

It is important to determine whether a patient uses illicit drugs. These drugs, particularly parenterally administered narcotics, which are often diluted with talcum powder, can cause pulmonary disorders resulting from the irritant effect of the powder on lung tissues.

As with all medication, nurses need to assess a patient's knowledge and ability to self-administer medications correctly (see Chapter 34). Of particular importance is the assessment of the patient's understanding of potential adverse effects of the medications. Patients should be able to recognize adverse reactions and be aware of the dangers in combining prescribed medications with over-the-counter drugs.

Physical Examination

The physical examination performed to assess the patient's level of tissue oxygenation includes evaluation of the cardiopulmonary system (see Chapter 32). Special consideration should be given when assessing the older person because changes in the cardiopulmonary system occur with the aging process (Table 39-3). These changes may result in changes in the patient's activity tolerance, level of fatigue, or transient changes in vital signs and may not be associated with a specific cardiopulmonary disease.

Inspection. Using inspection techniques, the nurse performs a head-to-toe observation of the patient for skin and mucous membrane colour, general appearance, level of consciousness, adequacy of systemic circulation, breathing patterns, and chest wall movement (Table 39-4). Any abnormalities should be investigated during palpation, percussion, and auscultation.

Inspection includes observations of the nails for clubbing. Clubbed nails, obliteration of the normal angle between the base of the nail and the skin, are seen in patients with prolonged oxygen deficiency, endocarditis, and congenital heart defects.

Chest wall movement is observed for retraction, sinking in of soft tissues of the chest between the intercostal spaces. The nurse should also observe for paradoxical breathing, asynchronous breathing, and the patient's breathing pattern (Table 39-5). In paradoxical breathing, the chest wall contracts during inspiration and expands during exhalation. Infants can experience sternal and substernal chest wall retractions with only a slight inspiratory effort because of the pliability of the chest wall. The anteroposterior diameter of the chest wall should be noted; conditions such as emphysema, advancing age, and COPD can cause the chest to assume a rounded shape.

Palpation. Palpation of the chest provides assessment data in several areas. It is used to document the type and amount of thoracic excursion, elicit any areas of tenderness, and identify tactile fremitus, thrills, heaves, and the cardiac point of maximal impulse (PMI). Palpation also aids in detecting abnormal masses or lumps in the axilla and breast tissue. Palpation of the extremities provides data about the peripheral circulation, the presence and quality of peripheral pulses, skin temperature, colour, and capillary refill (see Chapter 32).

The feet and legs should be palpated to assess for the presence or absence of peripheral edema. Patients with alterations in their cardiac function, such as those with heart failure or hypertension, often have pedal or lower extremity edema. Edema is graded from 1+ to 4+, depending on the depth of visible indentation after firm application of a finger (see Chapter 32).

Palpation of the pulses in the neck and extremities is performed to assess arterial blood flow (see Chapter 32). A scale of 0 (absent pulse) to 3+ (full, bounding pulse) is used to describe what is palpated. The normal pulse is graded at 2+, and a weak, thready pulse is graded as 1+.

Percussion. Percussion is used to detect the presence of abnormal fluid or air in the lungs. It also aids in determining diaphragmatic excursion (see Chapter 32).

Auscultation. Auscultation helps in identifying normal and abnormal heart and lung sounds (see Chapter 32). Auscultation of the cardiovascular system should include assessment for normal S_1 and S_2 sounds, the presence of abnormal S_3 and S_4 sounds (gallops), and murmurs or rubs. Auscultation is also used to identify a bruit over the carotid arteries, abdominal aorta, and femoral arteries.

Auscultation of lung sounds involves listening for movement of air throughout all lung fields—anterior, posterior, and lateral. Adventitious breath sounds occur with collapse of a lung segment, fluid in a lung segment, or narrowing or obstruction of an airway. Auscultation is also used to evaluate the patient's response to interventions for improving the respiratory status.

TABLE 39-3 Assessment Findings in the Aging Cardiopulmonary System

Function	Pathophysiological Change	Key Clinical Findings
Heart		
Muscle contraction	Thickening of the ventricular wall, increased collagen and decreased elastin in the heart muscle	Decreased cardiac output Diminished cardiac reserve
Blood flow	Heart valves become thicker and stiffer, more often in the mitral and aortic valves	Systolic ejection murmur
Conduction system	The SA node becomes fibrotic from calcification; the number of pacemaker cells in the SA node decreases	Increased PR, QRS, and Q-T intervals, decreased amplitude of the QRS complex
Arterial vessel compliance	Vessels become calcified, loss of arterial distensibility, decreased elastin in the vessel walls, more bends and twists (tortuous) in the vessels	Hypertension, with an increase in systolic blood pressure Fluctuation in blood pressure
Lungs		
Breathing mechanics	Decreased chest wall compliance, loss of elastic recoil Decreased respiratory muscle mass/strength	Prolonged exhalation phase Decreased vital capacity
Oxygenation	Increased ventilation–perfusion mismatch Decreased alveolar surface area Decreased carbon dioxide diffusion capacity	Decreased PaO_2 (arterial oxygen tension) Decreased cardiac output Slightly increased $PaCO_2$ (arterial carbon dioxide tension)
Breathing control/ breathing pattern	Decreased responsiveness of central and peripheral chemoreceptors to hypoxemia and hypercapnia	Increased respiratory rate Decreased tidal volume
Lung defence mechanisms	Decreased number of cilia Decreased IgA production and humoral and cellular immunity	Decreased airway clearance Diminished cough reflex
Sleep and breathing	Decreased respiratory drive Decreased tone of upper airway muscles	Increased risk of aspiration and infection Decreased PaO_2 Snoring, obstructive sleep apnea

TABLE 39-4 Inspection of Cardiopulmonary Status

Abnormality	Cause
Eyes	
Xanthelasma (yellow lipid lesions on eyelids)	Hyperlipidemia
Corneal arcus (whitish opaque ring around junction of cornea and sclera)	Hyperlipidemia in young to middle-aged adults, normal finding in older persons with arcus senilis
Pale conjunctivae	Anemia
Cyanotic conjunctivae	Hypoxemia
Petechiae on conjunctivae	Fat embolus or bacterial endocarditis
Mouth and Lips	
Cyanotic mucous membranes	Decreased oxygenation (hypoxia)
Pursed-lip breathing	Associated with chronic lung disease
Neck Veins	
Distension	Associated with right-sided heart failure
Nose	
Flaring nares	Air hunger, dyspnea
Chest	
Retractions	Increased work of breathing, dyspnea
Asymmetry	Chest wall injury
Skin	
Peripheral cyanosis	Vasoconstriction and diminished blood flow
Central cyanosis	Hypoxemia
Decreased skin turgor	Dehydration (normal finding in older persons, as a result of decreased skin elasticity)
Dependent edema	Associated with right-sided heart failure
Periorbital edema	Associated with kidney disease
Fingertips and Nail Beds	
Cyanosis	Decreased cardiac output or hypoxia
Splinter hemorrhages	Bacterial endocarditis
Clubbing	Chronic hypoxemia

From Ball, J. W., Dains, J. E., Flynn, J. A., Solomon, B. S., & Stewart, R. W. (2015). *Seidel's physical examination handbook* (8th ed.). St. Louis, MO: Elsevier.

TABLE 39-5 Assessment of Breathing Pattern

Pattern and Rate (Breaths/Minute)	Clinical Significance
Eupnea (12–20) 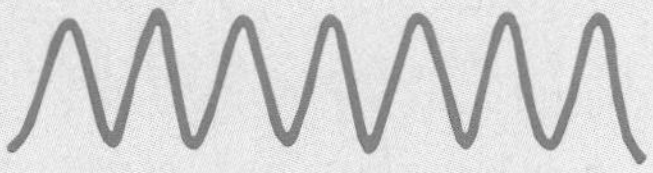	Normal rate in the adult
Tachypnea (>20) 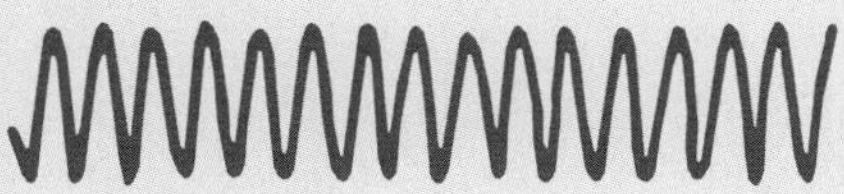	Can result from anxiety or response to pain or fever, respiratory failure, shortness of breath, or a respiratory infection. May lead to respiratory alkalosis, paresthesia, tetany, and confusion
Bradypnea (<12) 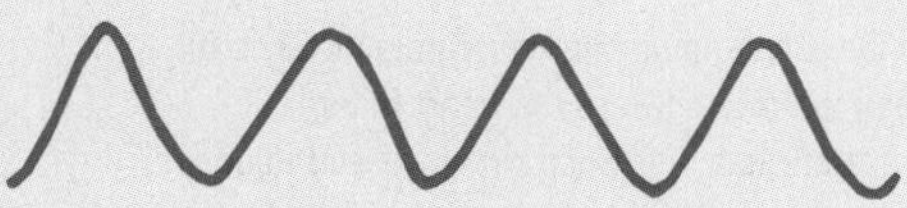	Results from sleep, respiratory depression, drug overdose, or central nervous system lesion
Apnea (absence of respiration >15 seconds) 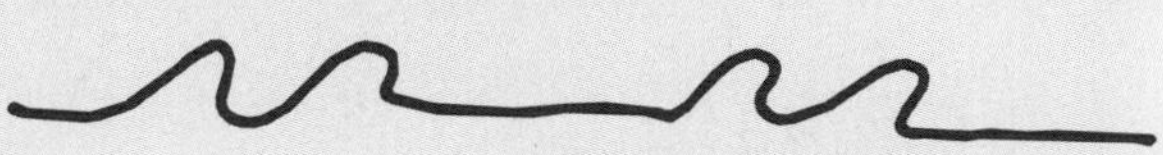	May be intermittent, such as in sleep apnea, or prolonged, as in a respiratory arrest
Kussmaul's respirations (usually >35, may be slow or normal) 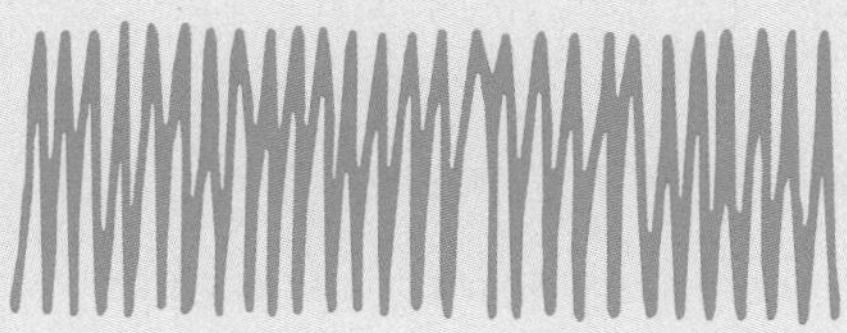	Tachypnea pattern associated with metabolic imbalance such as diabetic ketoacidosis, metabolic acidosis, or renal failure

BOX 39-7 Tuberculosis Skin Testing

- Skin testing is used to determine past exposure to *Mycobacterium* tuberculosis.
- Tuberculosis skin testing (TST) is performed by administering an intradermal injection of 0.1 mL of tuberculin-purified protein derivative on the inner surface of the forearm. The injection produces a pale elevation of the skin (a wheal) 6–10 mm in diameter. Afterward, the injection site may be circled, and the patient is instructed not to wash off the circle.
- Tuberculin skin tests are read 48–72 hours after injection. If the site is not read within 72 hours, the patient must undergo another skin test.
- Positive results are indicated by a palpable, elevated, hardened, reddened area around the injection site, caused by edema and inflammation from the antigen–antibody reaction. The site is measured in millimetres. A positive test result occurs when the site is ≥10 mm.
- Reddened flat areas are *not* positive reactions and are not measured.
- TST in older persons (see Box 39-4) and those with altered immune function (e.g., HIV, patients receiving chemotherapy) is less reliable.

Diagnostic Tests

There are a variety of diagnostic tests used to monitor cardiopulmonary functioning. Some of these tests can be obtained through screening, simple blood specimens, X-ray films, or other noninvasive means. One such screening mechanism is TB skin testing (Box 39-7). This is a simple test that is usually required annually for health care workers to monitor possible TB exposure. In contrast, invasive diagnostic tests, such as a thoracentesis, can be quite painful, depending on the patient's tolerance for pain.

Tables 39-6 and 39-7 and Box 39-8 summarize diagnostic testing used in the assessment and evaluation of patients with cardiopulmonary alterations. The nurse should explain the procedure and tell the patient what to expect, to reduce the patient's anxiety. The patient must understand the importance of following instructions, such as holding the breath as requested and not coughing during the procedure. After any procedure, the patient is monitored for signs of changes in cardiopulmonary functioning, sudden shortness of breath, pain, oxygen desaturation, and anxiety. The nurse needs to promote the patient's comfort and encourage the patient to rest after the test, because many patients find these tests to be tiring.

Patient Expectations

During assessment, nurses should ask patients what they expect from the encounter and what their priority is for management of their health. In identifying expectations, nurses involve patients in the decision-making process and allow them to participate in their care and know what will happen to them (Box 39-9). For example, if the nurse plans a smoking-cessation or weight-reduction program for a patient who is not ready for the change, both the nurse and the patient will become frustrated. It is important to establish short-term, realistic goals that build to a larger goal. For example, reducing the fat in the patient's diet might start out with replacing food such as whole milk with 2% milk and gradually introducing skim milk. A sudden change

TABLE 39-6 Cardiopulmonary Diagnostic Blood Studies

Test and Normal Values	Interpretation
Complete Blood Count (CBC)	
Normal values for a CBC vary with age and gender.	A CBC determines the number and type of red and white blood cells per cubic millimetre of blood.
Cardiac Blood Studies	
CK (creatinine kinase) MB Levels rise 3–6 hours after infarction occurs. Peaks in 12–24 hours and then returns to normal within 2 days.	Cardiac enzymes are used to diagnose acute myocardial infarcts. CK-MB is specific to the myocardial cell and may quantify myocardial damage and timing of the onset of the infarction.
Two cardiac-specific troponins released after a myocardial infarction:	Cardiac troponins become elevated as early as 3 hours after myocardial injury.
Cardiac troponin I (cTnI) <0.03 ng/mL	Often remains elevated for 7–10 days.
Cardiac troponin T (cTnT)* <0.1 ng/mL	Often remains elevated for up to 10–14 days.
B-Type Natriuretic Peptide (BNP) BNP <100 ng/L	BNP is a marker for heart failure and assists with identifying pulmonary or cardiac causes for shortness of breath. The more elevated the levels, the more severe the heart failure.
C-reactive protein <10 mg/L	C-reactive protein is used to detect inflammation if there is a high suspicion of tissue injury or infection in the body. It may also be used to assess for risk of developing coronary artery disease and stroke.
Serum Electrolytes	
Potassium (K^+) 3.5–5 mmol/L	Patients on diuretic therapy are at risk for hypokalemia (low potassium). Patients receiving angiotensin-converting enzyme inhibitors are at risk for hyperkalemia (elevated potassium).
Cholesterol	
Cholesterol <5.20 mmol/L	Contributing factors include sedentary lifestyle, intake of saturated fatty acids, and familial hypercholesterolemia.
Low-density lipoprotein (LDL)-cholesterol (bad cholesterol) <3.4 mmol/L	High LDL cholesterol (hypercholesterolemia) is caused by excessive intake of saturated fatty acids, dietary cholesterol intake, and obesity. Familial hypercholesterolemia and hyperlipidemia are also contributing factors, as are hypothyroidism, nephrotic syndrome, and diabetes mellitus.
High-density lipoprotein (HDL)-cholesterol (good cholesterol) Male: >0.75 mmol/L Female: >0.91 mmol/L	Low HDL cholesterol is caused by cigarette smoking, obesity, lack of regular exercise, β-adrenergic blocking agents, genetic disorders of HDL metabolism, hypertriglyceridemia, and type 2 diabetes.
Triglycerides Male: 0.45–1.81 mmol/L Female: 0.40–1.52 mmol/L	Obesity, excessive alcohol intake, diabetes mellitus, β-adrenergic blocking agents, and genetic predisposition cause hypertriglyceridemia.

*May see high-sensitivity (hs) cTnT for early detection of low levels related to cTnT.
Data from Pagana, K. D., Pagana, T. J., & Pagana, T. N. (2015). *Mosby's diagnostic and laboratory test reference* (12th ed.). St. Louis, MO: Mosby.

from whole to skim milk will most likely fail, because the change is too great. A plan for adding exercise to the patient's lifestyle could start with a commitment to exercise once a week for 20 minutes, or the patient could commit to a weight-reduction plan of 2 kg per month.

When addressing a patient's expectations, remember that your goals and expectations may not always coincide with those of your patient. By addressing the patient's concerns and expectations, you will establish a relationship that can address other health care goals and expected outcomes. Knowing the mindset of patients and respecting their wishes will go a long way toward helping patients make significant lifestyle changes to benefit their health.

◆ Nursing Diagnosis

Patients with an altered level of oxygenation can have nursing diagnoses that are primarily from a cardiovascular or pulmonary origin. Each nursing diagnosis is based on specific defining characteristics and the related etiology (Box 39-10). Nurses use the information gathered in the nursing assessment to identify and cluster the defining characteristics. The clustered defining characteristics support the nursing diagnosis.

Nursing diagnoses appropriate for the patient with alterations in oxygenation include, but are not limited to, the following:

- *Activity intolerance*
- *Risk for activity intolerance*
- *Ineffective airway clearance*
- *Anxiety*
- *Ineffective breathing pattern*
- *Decreased cardiac output*
- *Impaired comfort*
- *Impaired verbal communication*
- *Ineffective individual coping*
- *Fatigue*
- *Fear*
- *Risk for imbalanced fluid volume*

TABLE 39-7 Cardiac Function Diagnostic Tests

Test	Significance
12-Lead electrocardiogram (ECG)	Graphic recording of the electrical impulses generated by the heart, during the cardiac cycle. The test is used to detect abnormal electrical activity and the electrical position of the heart. The ECG includes 12 leads: I, II, III, AVR, AVL, AVF, and V1–6. It provides a 360-degree view of the heart.
Holter monitor	Portable ECG worn by the patient. The test produces a continuous ECG tracing over a period of time. Patients keep a diary of activity, noting when they experience rapid heartbeats or dizziness. Evaluation of the ECG recording along with the diary provides information about the heart's electrical activity during activities of daily living.
ECG exercise stress test	ECG is monitored while the patient walks on a treadmill at a specified speed and duration of time. Used to evaluate the cardiac response to physical stress. The test is not a valuable tool for evaluation of cardiac response in women because of increased false-positive findings among women.
Thallium stress test	An ECG stress test with the addition of thallium-201-injected IV. The test determines coronary blood flow changes with increased activity.
Electrophysiological study (EPS)	Invasive measure of intracardiac electrical pathways. Provides more specific information about difficult-to-treat dysrhythmias. EPS assesses the adequacy of antidysrhythmic medication.
Echocardiography	A transthoracic echo (TTE) is a noninvasive measure of heart structure and heart wall motion. Graphically demonstrates overall cardiac performance. Echocardiography can be performed via the esophagus and is referred to as transesophageal echocardiography or TEE.
Scintigraphy	Radionuclide angiography. Used to evaluate cardiac structure, myocardial perfusion, and contractility.
Cardiac catheterization and angiography	Used to visualize cardiac chambers, valves, the great vessels, and coronary arteries. Pressures and volumes within the four chambers of the heart can also be measured.

Data from Pagana, K. D., Pagana, T. J., & Pagana, T. N. (2015). *Mosby's diagnostic and laboratory test reference* (12th ed.). St. Louis, MO: Mosby.

- *Impaired gas exchange*
- *Ineffective health maintenance*
- *Risk for infection*
- *Deficient (specify) knowledge*
- *Risk for impaired skin integrity*
- *Disturbed sleep pattern*
- *Ineffective tissue perfusion*
- *Impaired spontaneous ventilation*

◆ Planning

During planning, nurses use critical thinking skills to synthesize information from multiple sources (Figure 39-7). Critical thinking ensures that the nurse's plan of care integrates individualized patient needs. Professional standards are especially important to consider when developing a care plan. These standards often establish scientifically proven guidelines for selecting effective nursing interventions.

Goals and Outcomes. An individualized care plan is developed for each nursing diagnosis (Box 39-11). In collaboration with the patient, the nurse sets realistic expectations for care. Goals should be individualized and realistic with measurable outcomes.

Patients with impaired oxygenation require a nursing care plan directed toward meeting the actual or potential oxygenation needs of the patient. Individual outcomes are derived from patient-centred needs. For example, the goal of maintaining a patent airway can be evaluated by specific outcomes for the patient. These might include the following expected outcomes:

- Patient's lungs are clear to auscultation.
- Patient achieves maintenance and promotion of bilateral lung expansion.
- Patient coughs productively.
- Oxygen saturation is maintained or improved.

Often a patient with cardiopulmonary disease has multiple nursing diagnoses (Figure 39-8). In this case, the nurse needs to identify when goals or outcomes apply to more than one diagnosis. The presence of multiple diagnoses also makes priority setting a critical activity.

Setting Priorities. The patient's level of health, age, lifestyle, and environmental risks affect the level of tissue oxygenation. Patients with severe impairments in oxygenation frequently require nursing interventions in multiple areas. Nurses need to consider what the most important goal is during the limited amount of time a patient is seen in the hospital or primary care setting. For example, in an acute care setting, maintaining a patent airway has a higher priority than improving the patient's exercise tolerance. The need for a patent airway is an immediate need. In a second example, when caring for a patient who has an abdominal incision, pain control may have a greater priority than coughing and deep breathing. Again, in this situation, controlling the patient's pain ultimately will facilitate coughing and deep breathing.

However, in a community-based or primary setting, the priority may focus on smoking cessation, exercise, diet modifications, or a combination of these activities. Both the nurse and the patient need to be focused on the same goal and expected outcomes to be successful. In addition to being individualized, each goal should be realistic and attainable for the patient.

Collaborative Care. The time spent with the patient in any setting is limited. Therefore, nurses need to collaborate with family members, colleagues, and other specialists to accomplish the goals and outcomes that have been determined. Some patients may need to improve their exercise and activity tolerance; for some patients, their continuity of care may involve enrolling in a community-based cardiopulmonary rehabilitation program. Another patient may have the same health care need but is unable to leave the home, and home physiotherapy is needed.

Collaboration with physiotherapists, nutritionists, and community-based nurses may be valuable for a patient with heart failure or chronic

BOX 39-8 Common Respiratory Tests and Methods

Oxygenation Tests

Pulse oximetry: A **pulse oximeter** is a device used to indirectly measure pulse rate and oxygen saturation. A sensor is attached to the patient's finger, toe, nose, earlobe, or forehead (see figure). Accuracy is directly related to the perfusion of the probe area, a systolic blood pressure >90 mm Hg, and the hemoglobin level. Decreased levels correlate well with arterial oxygen levels and are used to trend oxygenation over time. Normal peripheral capillary oxygen saturation (SpO_2) values are greater than 95%. An SpO_2 below 70% is life-threatening.

- *Arterial blood gas:* A radial or femoral artery is punctured to obtain arterial blood. Tests measure the oxygen concentration in the blood, the hydrogen ion concentration (pH), partial pressure of carbon dioxide ($PaCO_2$), and the partial pressure of oxygen (PaO_2). Normal values are as follows:
  - pH 7.35–7.45
  - $PaCO_2$ 35–45 mm Hg
  - PaO_2 80–100 mm Hg
  - SaO_2 95–100%

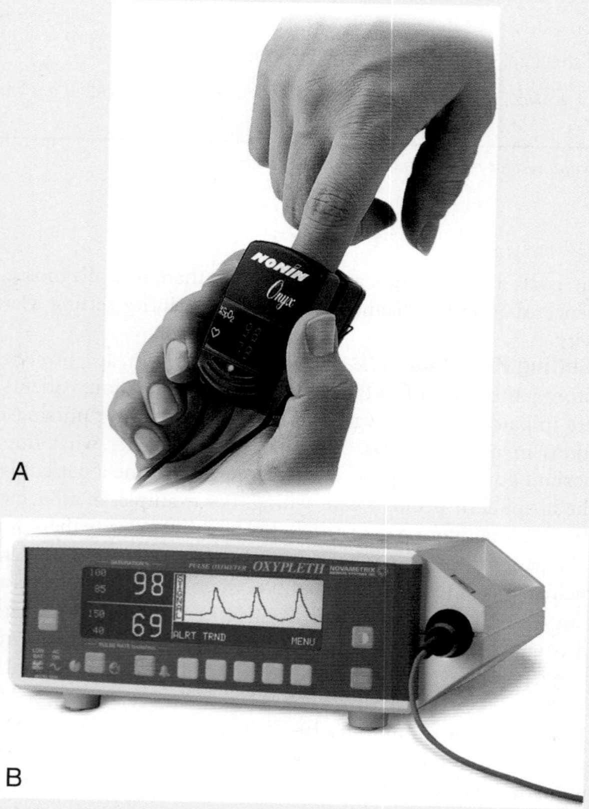

A, Portable pulse oximeter displays oxygen saturation (SpO_2) and pulse rate. **B,** A pulse oximeter displays the oxygen saturation and pulse rate as a digital reading. (From Lewis, S. L., Heitkemper, M. M., Dirksen, S. R., Bucher, L., Barry, M. A., Goldsworthy, S., & Goodridge, D. [Eds.]. [2014]. *Medical-surgical nursing in Canada: Assessment and management of clinical problems* [3rd Canadian ed., p. 614, Fig. 28-7 A]. Toronto: Elsevier Canada. [A, Courtesy Nonin Medical Inc., Plymouth, Minnesota; B, Courtesy Respironics, Inc., Murrysville, Pennsylvania.])

Pulmonary Function Tests

Pulmonary function tests measure lung volume (the amount of air moving into and out of the lungs) and capacity (how much air the lungs can hold). Respiratory therapists usually conduct these tests. The patient takes as deep a breath as possible and forcefully exhales into a mouthpiece attached to a machine. Pulmonary readings are recorded and compared with previous readings and with average normal values, which vary depending on the patient's age, gender, weight, height, and race. These tests are used to diagnose and monitor pulmonary disease and conditions (e.g., asthma, emphysema). They are also used to evaluate postoperative lung conditions.

Imaging

- *Chest X-ray examination:* Usually posteroanterior and lateral films are taken to adequately visualize all of the lung fields. A radiograph of the thorax is used to observe the lung fields for fluid, infiltrates (e.g., pneumonia), masses (e.g., lung cancer), fractures, pneumothorax, and other abnormal processes.
- *Computed tomography (CT) scan:* A CT scan provides visualization of fine detail of the lungs and other structures in the thorax. It is often used as part of the assessment of patients with pneumonia, lung masses, and suspected pulmonary emboli.
- *Ventilation/perfusion (nuclear medicine) lung scan:* This scan is used to detect pulmonary emboli. The results from two separate scans are compared: the perfusion scan uses an injected radioactive tracer to measure pulmonary blood flow, and the ventilation scan shows the pulmonary distribution of a different inhaled tracer. Mismatches (areas of ventilation without corresponding perfusion or blood flow) indicate pulmonary emboli.

Methods of Obtaining Respiratory Specimens for Analysis

Specimens are cultured so they can be used to detect the presence of blood, microbes, and abnormal cells. A variety of methods are used to obtain respiratory specimens.

- *Sputum tests:* Sputum is mucus from the respiratory system that is expectorated through the mouth. Sputum specimens are obtained when the patient coughs up sputum from the bronchi and trachea; specimens are easier to obtain in the morning when the secretions are coughed up upon awakening. Sputum tests include (a) *sputum culture and sensitivity (C and S)* test, used to identify a specific microorganism growing in the sputum and to identify drug resistance and sensitivities; (b) *sputum for acid-fast bacillus (AFB)*, a test used to screen for the presence of AFB for detection of TB by early-morning specimens on three consecutive days; and (c) *sputum for cytology*, used to identify abnormal lung cancer and differentiate the type of cancer cells (small cell, oat cell, large cell).
- *Bronchoscopy:* A narrow, flexible, fibre-optic scope is passed into the trachea and bronchi to enable visual examination of the tracheobronchial tree. The procedure is performed to obtain fluid, sputum, or biopsy samples, and to remove mucous plugs or foreign bodies.
- *Thoracentesis:* This involves surgical perforation of the chest wall and pleural space with a needle to aspirate fluid for diagnostic or therapeutic purposes or to remove a specimen for biopsy. The procedure is performed using aseptic technique and local anaesthetic. The patient usually sits upright with the anterior thorax supported by pillows or an overbed table.
- *Nasopharyngeal aspirate or swab:* This swab is used to detect respiratory viruses. Aspirates are the best specimens from young children, whereas swabs can be used for obtaining samples from older children and adults.

Data from Pagana, K. D., Pagana, T. J., & Pagana, T. N. (2015). *Mosby's diagnostic and laboratory test reference* (12th ed.). St. Louis, MO: Mosby.

BOX 39-9 CASE STUDY

Understanding Cardiac Rehabilitation: A Personal Story and Case Study

During my evening shift Mr. Evans (a pseudonym), a 48-year-old male was admitted to the cardiac medical unit with a late-presenting myocardial infarction (MI). He presented to the emergency department with mid-scapular pain. Mr. Evans did not relate the symptoms to a cardiac event. One of our initial conversations indicated he was anticipating returning to work upon discharge from the hospital. I met his wife soon afterward, who shared with me her sense of being overwhelmed with the dietary changes, new medications, and her husband's "denial" of the current diagnosis. Toward the later part of my shift I took the opportunity to inquire about their understanding of the cardiac rehabilitation program and their intention to use the resource. I used this opportunity to teach Mr. Evans and his wife about cardiac rehabilitation. They developed an understanding of this resource and began to recognize that it was more than just an exercise program. Mr. Evans and his wife understood that cardiac rehabilitation encompassed a holistic approach to wellness with members of an interdisciplinary team who have expertise in different areas of clinical practice. Cardiac rehabilitation offered this couple ongoing support and strategies for lifestyle changes to promote wellness.

1. How do nurses assess patients' and families' readiness to learn?
2. What pertinent members of the interdisciplinary team support patients and families during cardiac rehabilitation? What are key elements of the conversation with patients and families regarding cardiac rehabilitation?
3. In addition to patients who have been diagnosed with an MI, what other patients might also benefit from cardiac rehabilitation?

BOX 39-10 NURSING DIAGNOSTIC PROCESS

Assessment Activities	Defining Characteristics	Nursing Diagnosis
Ask patient or family about patient's mood, attentiveness, memory, and activity level.	Confusion Decreased activity Fatigue Irritability Restlessness Sleepiness	*Impaired gas exchange related to decreased lung expansion*
Observe patient's respirations.	Dyspnea Impaired gas exchange related to collapsed alveoli Nasal flaring Tachypnea Use of accessory muscles	
Inspect skin and mucous membranes.	Diaphoresis Pallor Moist skin	
Auscultate chest.	Decreased respiratory excursion Abnormal, distant lung sounds	

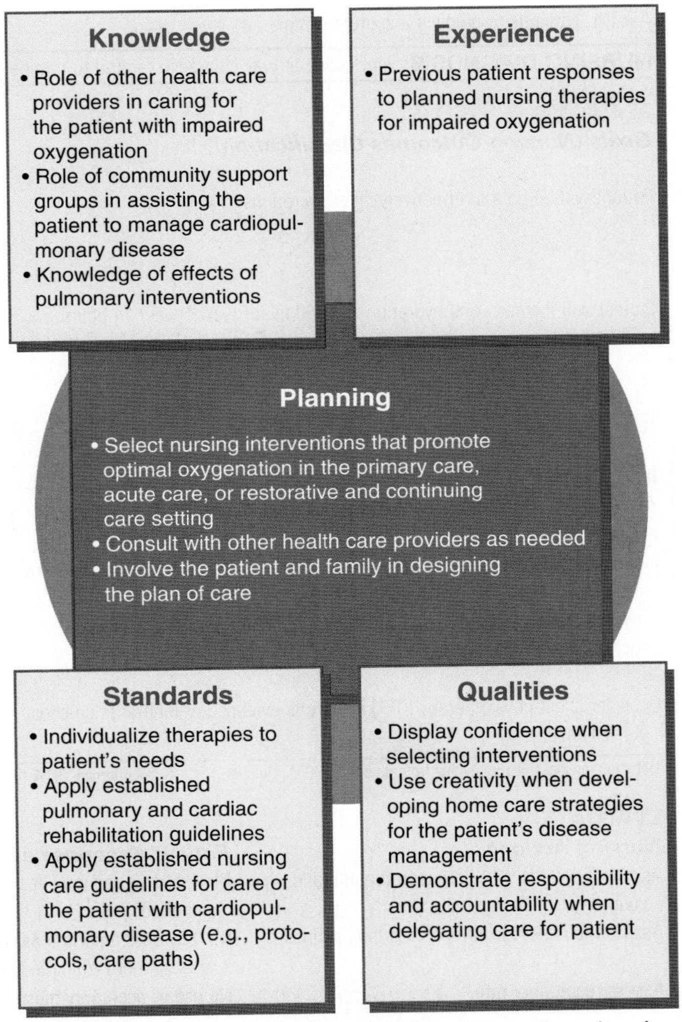

FIGURE 39-7 Critical thinking model for oxygenation planning.

lung conditions and is an essential component of primary health care. These professionals work with the patient and the community to optimize resources to assist the patient in attaining the highest level of wellness. In addition, professionals can help to identify community resources and support systems for both the patient and family in preventing and managing symptoms related to cardiopulmonary diseases.

◆ Implementation

Nursing interventions for promoting and maintaining adequate oxygenation include independent nursing actions such as health-promotion and disease-prevention behaviours, positioning, and coughing techniques. Interdependent or dependent interventions include oxygen therapy, lung inflation techniques, hydration, medication administration, and chest physiotherapy (CPT).

Health Promotion

Maintaining the patient's optimal level of health is important in reducing the number and severity of respiratory symptoms. Prevention of respiratory infections is foremost in maintaining optimal health. Providing cardiopulmonary-related health information (Box 39-12

BOX 39-11 NURSING CARE PLAN

Ineffective Airway Clearance/Retained Secretions

ASSESSMENT

Mr. Edwards, an older person with a history of chronic obstructive pulmonary disease (COPD), comes to the primary care office with complaints of continued coughing. He reports having an intermittent productive cough and occasionally produces thick yellow sputum. His vital signs are temperature 38.5°C, pulse 104 beats per minute, respirations 28 breaths per minute, and blood pressure 130/85 mm Hg, and his SpO_2 is 84% on room air. He continues to smoke 2 to 3 cigarettes a day, an improvement from his previous 10 to 15 per day. Mr. Edwards does not exercise and needs to complete his self-care activities slowly, given his shortness of breath.

Assessment Activities	*Findings and Defining Characteristics*
Ask Mr. Edwards how long he has had this cough.	He replies, "I have a morning cough every day, but this cough is different. It started about a week ago."
Ask Mr. Edwards what is different about this cough.	He replies, "My ribs are getting sore. I can't cough up anything, my mouth is dry, and I have become more fatigued over the past week."
Observe Mr. Edwards's skin and mucous membranes.	His skin and mucous membranes are dry.
Auscultate lung fields.	Abnormal lung sounds are in the upper lobes. The lower lobes are clear.
Ask Mr. Edwards how many glasses of water he drinks daily.	Over the last week he has drunk two to three glasses a day.
Ask Mr. Edwards to produce a sputum sample.	He is unable to produce a sputum sample for evaluation.

NURSING DIAGNOSIS: Ineffective airway clearance related to retained secretions and reduced fluid intake.

PLANNING

*Goals (Nursing Outcomes Classification)**	*Expected Outcomes*
	Respiratory Status: Airway Patency
Patient will be able to effectively clear secretions.	Lung sounds will be normal in 48 hours. Sputum will be thin, white, and watery. Respiratory rate will be within 20–24 breaths/min in 48 hours. Patient will be able to clear airway by coughing.
Patient will increase oral hydration to 1 000 mL of water every 24 hours.	Oral mucous membranes will be pink and moist. Patient will verbalize that his mouth is not dry. Patient will notice an increase in ease of sputum production. Patient will report that his sputum is thin, white, and watery.

*Outcome classification labels from Moorhead, S., Johnson, M., Maas, M. L., & Swanson, E. (Eds.). (2013). *Nursing outcomes classification (NOC),* (5th ed.). St. Louis, MO: Elsevier.

INTERVENTIONS

Interventions (Nursing Interventions Classification)†	*Rationale*
Airway Management	
Increase fluids to 1 000 mL in 24 hours if not contraindicated by cardiovascular disease.	Fluids help to liquefy secretions and promote ease of removal (Hong & Galvagno, 2013). Fluids will relieve oral mucosa and skin dryness.
Have patient deep-breathe and cough every 2 hours four to five times.	Retained secretions predispose patient to atelectasis and pneumonia.
Teach patient effective cough techniques.	Coughing techniques will help to clear the airway effectively and decrease fatigue from ineffective coughing (Borge, Hagen, Mengshoel, et al., 2014).
Consider chest physiotherapy (CPT) if there is evidence of infiltrates on chest X-ray film.	Standards for CPT include sputum production >30 mL/day or infiltrates on chest X-ray film.

†Intervention classification labels from Bulechek, G. M., Butcher, H. K., & Dochterman, J. M. (Eds.). (2013). *Nursing interventions classification (NIC)* (6th ed.). St. Louis, MO: Elsevier.

EVALUATION

Nursing Actions	*Patient Response and Findings*	*Achievement of Outcome*
Ask Mr. Edwards if he can deep-breathe and cough.	Mr. Edwards reports, "It is easier to cough up my secretions now."	Patient is able to clear airway by coughing.
Assess the chest for adventitious lung sounds.	Mr. Edwards reports that he has not heard any wheezing or rattling in his chest.	Lungs clear to auscultation in all fields.
Assess respiratory rate.	No use of accessory muscles of respiration. Normal breathing pattern and respiratory rate.	Respiratory rate is between 20 and 24 breaths/min.
Assess patient's level of hydration.	Mucous membranes are moist. Mr. Edwards reports, "My mouth isn't so dry anymore."	Oral mucous membranes are pink and moist.
Observe appearance of sputum.	Sputum is thin, white, and watery.	Sputum is thin, white, and watery.

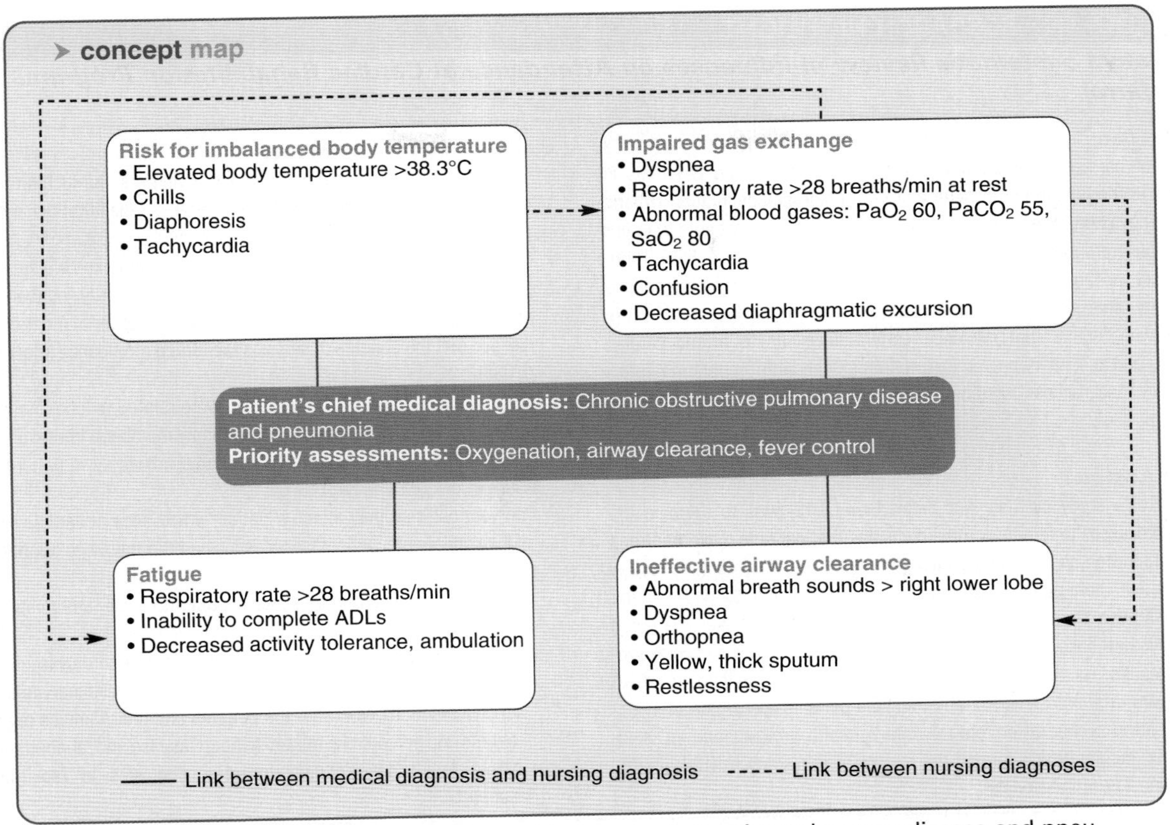

FIGURE 39-8 Concept map for a patient with chronic obstructive pulmonary disease and pneumonia. *ADLs,* Activities of daily living.

BOX 39-12 PATIENT TEACHING

Cardiovascular Disease

Objectives

- Patient will be able to describe the risk factors associated with cardiovascular disease.
- Patient will be able to demonstrate health promotion behaviours.

Teaching Strategies

- Explain to the patient about modifying risk factors, such as quitting smoking, reducing alcohol intake, being attentive to sugar intake, and modifying high-fat and high-carbohydrate diets.
- Inform the patient about other risk factors for cardiovascular disease, such as diabetes, obesity, physical inactivity, stress, and oral contraceptives.
- Discuss with the patient the importance of regular blood pressure and blood cholesterol monitoring (total cholesterol, high-density lipoprotein, low-density lipoprotein, and triglyceride levels).
- Educate the patient about low-fat, low-salt, and calorie-appropriate diets. Provide sample menus.
- Educate the patient about the benefits of exercising 30–60 minutes a day to help reduce weight and lower blood pressure. Help the patient develop an exercise program.

Evaluation

- Ask the patient to describe the modifiable and nonmodifiable risk factors for cardiovascular disease.
- Ask the patient to verbalize strategies for balanced nutrition.
- Obtain the patient's weight and blood pressure.
- Monitor the patient's serum cholesterol (total, high- and low-density lipids) and triglyceride levels.

and Box 39-13) is an important nursing responsibility and part of a primary health care model.

Vaccinations. Annual influenza vaccines are recommended for everyone 6 months and older (Centers for Disease Control [CDC], 2017a). Individuals with chronic illnesses (heart, lung, kidney, diabetes, or immunosuppressed), infants, older persons, and pregnant women should be immunized (CDC, 2017a). The vaccine is also recommended for people in close or frequent contact with anyone in the high-risk groups. Vaccination should begin as soon as the vaccine becomes available, if possible by October (CDC, 2017a). In Canada, it is estimated that, in a given year, an average of 12 200 hospitalizations and approximately 3 500 deaths occur due to influenza (Health Canada, 2016). After the vaccination, antibodies develop against the strains of the virus. When exposed to the influenza virus, the antibodies assist with preventing infection or reduce the severity of illness.

Pneumococcal vaccine is recommended for patients at increased risk of developing pneumonia, those with chronic illnesses or immunosuppression (such as HIV/AIDS), those living in special environments

BOX 39-13 RESEARCH HIGHLIGHT

A Qualitative Systematic Review of Influences on Attendance at Cardiac Rehabilitation Programs After Referral

Research Focus

Attendance at cardiac rehabilitation and secondary prevention programs is instrumental in the prevention of heart disease in high-risk populations (Clark, King-Shier, Thompson, et al., 2012, p. 835). Up to half of all patients who are referred to these programs do not participate (Clark et al., 2012, p. 835). There has been little research done to examine strategies for increasing attendance and to identify what influences attendance after referral (Clark et al., 2012, p. 835). Identifying factors that influence patient decisions to attend cardiac rehabilitation and secondary prevention programs would inform potential interventions to increase access for those requiring cardiac health services (Clark et al., 2012, p. 836).

Research Abstract

The purpose of a study by Clark and colleagues (2012) was to examine the factors and processes that influence the decisions that patients make to attend cardiac rehabilitation and secondary prevention services. A systematic review using qualitative meta-analysis was the method employed to gather data. Relevant qualitative studies that met specific identified criteria were gathered from numerous databases and a meta-ethnographic approach was used to synthesize the results. For the purpose of this study, Clark and colleagues (2012) defined the term *attendance* as "whether eligible patients participate in a secondary prevention service after referral from a health professional" (p. 836). There were 90 studies that informed the results of this study (2010 patients, 120 caregivers, 312 professionals).

Evidence-Informed Practice

- There were both personal and contextual barriers and facilitators that influenced patients' decisions to attend cardiac rehabilitation and secondary prevention services (Clark et al., 2012, p. 840).
- The personal barriers to attendance were related to knowledge of programs, perceived beliefs about heart disease, patient identity, as well as financial and occupational constraints. An increased sense of control over heart disease and the benefits of services facilitated attendance (Clark et al., 2012, p. 838).
- The contextual barriers of attendance were related to long-distance travel to programs and a lack of support from family members. Interestingly, families and health care providers were considered influential in patient attendance (Clark et al., 2012, p. 840).
- Interventions that may promote patient attendance at cardiac rehabilitation and secondary preventions services include the following (Clark et al., 2012, p. 840):
  - Providing personalized feedback to patients on the "suitability" of services (p. 840)
  - Facilitating patients' sense of control over their cardiovascular health
  - With the assistance of members from the interdisciplinary team, engaging in conversations with both the patients and their families regarding their beliefs and perceptions related to heart disease and rehabilitation services
  - Using face-to-face or web-based mechanisms to facilitate required support.

Clark, A. M., King-Shier, K. M., Thompson, D. R., Spaling, M. A., Duncan, A. S., Stone, J. A., et al. (2012). A qualitative systematic review of influences on attendance at cardiac rehabilitation programs after referral. *American Heart Journal, 164*(6), 835–845. doi:10.1016/j.ahj.2012.08.020.

such as long-term care facilities, and patients over the age of 65 years (CDC, 2017b).

Healthy Lifestyle Behaviour. Identification and elimination of risk factors for cardiopulmonary disease is an important part of primary health care. Nurses need to encourage patients to eat a healthy, low-fat, high-fibre diet; to monitor their cholesterol, triglyceride, high-density lipoprotein (HDL), and low-density lipoprotein (LDL) levels and reduce stress; to exercise; and to maintain a body weight in proportion to their height.

Elimination of use of cigarettes and other tobacco products, reduction in exposure to pollutants, monitoring of air quality, and adequate hydration are additional behaviours that promote health. Patients should be encouraged to examine their habits and to make changes to achieve their goals.

Exercise is a key factor in maintaining a healthy heart and lungs. Patients should be encouraged to exercise three to four times a week for 20 to 30 minutes. Aerobic exercise is necessary to improve lung function, strengthen muscles, and achieve better health. Walking is one of the most efficient ways of getting a good aerobic workout. Many shopping malls have programs that allow people to enter the mall before shops open and to use the enclosed area for walking. Some have measured and posted the distances to help people plan their activity and measure their progress. Patients should be taught how to take their pulse and pace themselves; it is better to walk 15 minutes every day than to walk to exhaustion to achieve a goal. Patients should plan a time interval and walk for the designated time. Gradually, they will notice that the distance increases as their endurance and fitness improve.

Patients with cardiopulmonary alterations need to minimize their risk for infection, especially during the winter months. Nurses need to teach patients to avoid large, crowded places; to keep their mouth and nose covered; and to be sure to dress warmly, including a scarf, hat, and gloves. This is especially important during the peak of the influenza season.

Patients with known cardiac disease and those with multiple risk factors should be cautioned to avoid exertion in cold weather. Shovelling snow is especially risky and in many patients can precipitate a cardiac event. Other activities, such as hanging holiday lights and decorations in the extreme cold, can precipitate chest pain and bronchospasm. Patients should be advised to avoid drinking alcohol before going out into cold weather because it blunts the respiratory drive when used in excess and may contribute to exposure to the cold by making the patient feel warm when the patient is really not protected from the cold.

Patients should also be taught to plan for the hot summer months. Activities should be limited to early in the day or late in the evening, when temperatures are lower. Patients should take care to maintain adequate hydration and sodium intake; this is especially true for those patients taking diuretics. Caffeinated and alcoholic beverages should be limited or avoided completely, because they act as diuretics and can contribute to dehydration.

Environmental Pollutants. Avoiding exposure to second-hand smoke is essential to maintaining optimal cardiopulmonary function. Most businesses and restaurants now ban smoking or have separate areas designated as smoking areas. If patients are exposed to second-hand smoke in their home environment, counselling and support may be necessary to assist the smoker in successful smoking cessation or alterations in behaviour patterns, such as smoking outside.

Exposure to chemicals and pollutants in the work environment must also be considered. Patients such as farmers, painters, carpenters, and others who are exposed to pollutants benefit from the use of particulate filter masks to reduce inhalation of particles.

Acute Care

According to the Canadian Association of Schools of Nursing (CASN, 2015), one of the key competency domains for baccalaureate nurses is to consider interventions according to their abilities to monitor and manage complex patient needs. Patients with acute pulmonary illnesses require nursing interventions directed toward halting the pathological process (e.g., respiratory tract infection), shortening the duration and severity of the illness (e.g., hospitalization with pneumonia), and preventing complications from the illness or treatments (e.g., health care–associated infection resulting from invasive procedures).

Dyspnea Management. Dyspnea is difficult to quantify and to treat. Treatment modalities need to be individualized for each patient, and more than one therapy is usually implemented. The underlying process that causes or worsens dyspnea must be treated and stabilized initially, then four additional therapies—pharmacological measures, oxygen therapy, physical techniques, and psychosocial techniques—are implemented. Pharmacological treatments may include bronchodilators, steroids, mucolytics, and low-dose anti-anxiety medications. Oxygen therapy can reduce dyspnea associated with exercise. Physical techniques, such as cardiopulmonary reconditioning through exercise, breathing techniques, and cough control, can help to reduce dyspnea. Relaxation techniques, biofeedback, and meditation are physiological measures that the patient can use to help lessen the sensation of dyspnea.

Airway Maintenance. The airway is patent when the trachea, bronchi, and large airways are free from obstructions. Airway maintenance requires adequate hydration to prevent thick, tenacious secretions. Proper coughing techniques remove secretions and keep the airway open. A variety of interventions, such as suctioning, CPT, and nebulizer therapy, assist the patient in managing alterations in airway clearance.

Mobilization of Pulmonary Secretions. The ability of a patient to mobilize pulmonary secretions may make the difference between a short-term illness and a long recovery involving complications. Nursing interventions that promote mobilization of pulmonary secretions help the patient to achieve and maintain a clear airway, and encourage lung expansion and gas exchange.

Humidification. Humidification is the process of adding water to gas. Temperature is the most important factor affecting the amount of water vapour a gas can hold. The percentage of water in the gas in relation to its capacity for water is the relative humidity. Air or oxygen with a high relative humidity keeps the airways moist and helps loosen and mobilize pulmonary secretions. Humidification is necessary for patients receiving oxygen therapy at >4 L/minute. Bubbling oxygen through water can add humidity to the oxygen delivered to the upper airways, as with a nasal cannula or face mask.

An oxygen hood is used for infants and a humidity tent is used for children with illnesses such as croup and tracheitis to liquefy secretions and assist in the reduction of fever (Hockenberry & Wilson, 2015). To prevent nonhumidified air or oxygen from entering the tent, the nebulizer at the top of the humidity tent remains filled with water. Air in the humidity tent can become cool and may fall below 20°C, thus causing the child to become chilled. Children in humidity tents require frequent changes of clothing and bed linen to remain dry and warm.

Nebulization. Nebulization is a process of adding moisture or medications to inspired air by mixing particles of varying sizes with the air. A nebulizer uses the aerosol principle to suspend a maximum number of water drops or particles of the desired size in inspired air. The moisture added to the respiratory system through nebulization improves clearance of pulmonary secretions. Nebulization is often used for administration of bronchodilators and mucolytic agents.

When the thin layer of fluid that supports the mucous layer over the cilia is allowed to dry, the cilia are damaged and cannot adequately clear the airway. Humidification through nebulization enhances mucociliary clearance, the body's natural mechanism for removing mucus and cellular debris from the respiratory tract.

Chest physiotherapy. Chest physiotherapy (CPT) is a group of therapies used in combination to mobilize pulmonary secretions. These therapies include postural drainage, chest percussion, and vibration. CPT should be followed by productive coughing and suctioning of the patient who has a decreased ability to cough. CPT is recommended for patients who produce greater than 30 mL of sputum per day or have evidence of atelectasis by chest X-ray examination. This procedure can be safely used with infants and young children; however, conditions and diseases unique to children may at times contraindicate this procedure. CPT is used for a select group of patients. Box 39-14 describes the guidelines for determining if CPT is indicated for the patient.

Chest percussion involves striking the chest wall over the area being drained. The hand is positioned so that the fingers and thumb touch and the hands are cupped (Figure 39-9). Percussion on the surface of the chest wall sends waves of varying amplitude and frequency through the chest, changing the consistency and location of the sputum. Chest percussion is performed by striking the chest wall alternately with cupped hands (Figure 39-10). Percussion is performed over a single

BOX 39-14 Guidelines for Chest Physiotherapy

Nursing care and selection of chest physiotherapy (CPT) skills are based on specific assessment findings. The following guidelines are designed to help in physical assessment and subsequent decision making:

- Know the patient's normal range of vital signs. Conditions such as atelectasis and pneumonia requiring CPT can affect vital signs. The degree of change is related to the level of hypoxia, overall cardiopulmonary status, and tolerance of activity.
- Know the patient's medications. Certain medications, particularly diuretics and antihypertensives, cause fluid and hemodynamic changes. These changes may decrease the patient's tolerance of the positional changes of postural drainage. Steroid medications increase the patient's risk of pathological rib fractures and often contraindicate rib shaking.
- Know the patient's medical history. Certain conditions, such as increased intracranial pressure, spinal cord injuries, and abdominal aneurysm resection, contraindicate the positional changes of postural drainage. Thoracic trauma or surgery may also contraindicate percussion, vibration, and rib shaking.
- Know the patient's level of cognitive function. Participation in controlled coughing techniques requires the patient to follow instructions. Congenital or acquired cognitive limitations may alter the patient's ability to learn and participate in these techniques.
- Be aware of the patient's exercise tolerance. CPT manoeuvres are fatiguing. When the patient is not used to physical activity, initial tolerance for the manoeuvres may be decreased. However, with gradual increases in activity and planned CPT, patient tolerance for the procedure will improve.

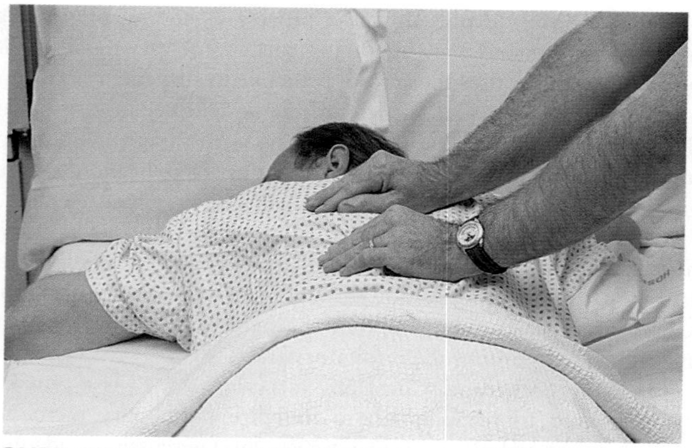

FIGURE 39-9 Hand position for chest wall percussion during chest physiotherapy.

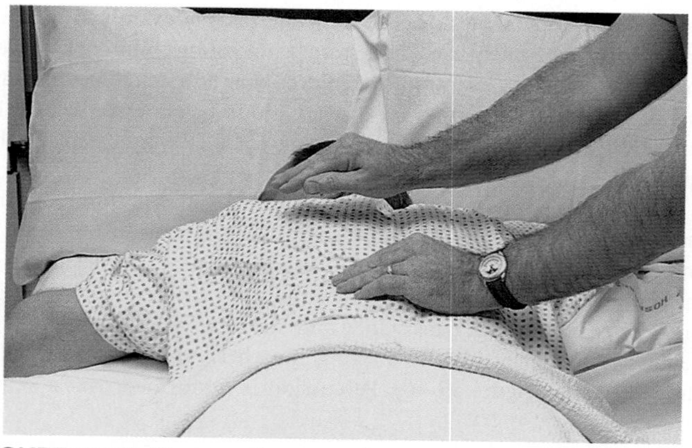

FIGURE 39-10 Chest wall percussion, alternating hand clapping against the patient's chest wall.

layer of clothing, not over buttons, snaps, or zippers. The single layer of clothing prevents slapping the patient's skin. Thicker or multiple layers of material dampen the vibrations.

Percussion is contraindicated in patients with bleeding disorders, osteoporosis, or fractured ribs. It is important to percuss the lung fields and not over the spine, abdomen, lower ribs, or breastbone to prevent injury to the spleen, liver, or kidneys (Cystic Fibrosis Foundation, 2012).

Vibration is a fine, shaking pressure applied to the chest wall only during exhalation. This technique is thought to increase the velocity and turbulence of exhaled air, facilitating secretion removal. Vibration increases the exhalation of trapped air and may shake mucus loose and induce a cough.

Postural drainage is the use of positioning techniques that draw secretions from specific segments of the lungs and bronchi into the trachea. Coughing or suctioning normally removes secretions from the trachea. The procedure for postural drainage can include most lung segments (Table 39-8). Because patients may not require postural drainage of all lung segments, the procedure is based on clinical assessment findings. For example, patients with left lower lobe atelectasis may require postural drainage of only the affected region, whereas a child with cystic fibrosis may require postural drainage of all lung segments.

Suctioning Techniques. Suctioning is necessary when a patient is unable to clear respiratory tract secretions with coughing. The suctioning techniques include oropharyngeal and nasopharyngeal suctioning, orotracheal and nasotracheal suctioning, and suctioning of an artificial airway.

These techniques are based on common principles. In most cases, sterile technique is used for suctioning because the trachea is considered sterile. The mouth is considered clean, thus the suctioning of oral secretions should be performed after suctioning of the oropharynx and trachea. Each type of suctioning requires the use of a round-tipped catheter with a number of side holes at the distal end of the catheter. Frequency of suctioning is determined by patient assessment and need. If secretions are identified by inspection or auscultation techniques, suctioning is required. Because sputum is not produced continuously or every 1 or 2 hours but occurs as a response to a pathological condition, there is no rationale for routine suctioning of all patients every 1 to 2 hours. In addition, suctioning reduces the amount of the available dead space in the oropharynx and trachea, often resulting in significant desaturation. It is important to monitor the patient to ensure adequate oxygenation. Too-frequent suctioning can put the patient at risk for development of hypoxemia, hypotension, arrhythmias, and possible trauma to the mucosa of the lungs (Lynn-McHale, 2011).

Oropharyngeal and Nasopharyngeal Suctioning. The oropharynx extends behind the mouth from the soft palate above the level of the hyoid bone and contains the tonsils. The nasopharynx is located behind the nose and extends to the level of the soft palate. Oropharyngeal or nasopharyngeal suctioning is used when the patient is able to cough effectively but is unable to clear secretions by expectorating or swallowing. The suction procedure is used after the patient has coughed (Skill 39-1). As the amount of pulmonary secretions is reduced and the patient is less fatigued, the patient may be able to expectorate or swallow the mucus, and suctioning is no longer required.

Orotracheal and Nasotracheal Suctioning. Orotracheal or nasotracheal suctioning is necessary when the patient with pulmonary secretions is unable to manage secretions by coughing and does not have an artificial airway (see Skill 39-1). A catheter is passed through the mouth or nose into the trachea. The nose is the preferred route because stimulation of the gag reflex is minimal. The procedure is similar to nasopharyngeal suctioning, but the catheter tip is moved farther into the patient's trachea. The entire procedure from catheter passage to its removal should be done quickly, lasting no longer than 10 seconds (American Association of Respiratory Care [AARC], 2010). Unless in respiratory distress, the patient should be allowed to rest between passes of the catheter. If the patient is using supplemental oxygen, the oxygen cannula or mask should be replaced during rest periods.

Tracheal Suctioning. Tracheal suctioning is accomplished through an artificial airway such as an endotracheal tube or tracheostomy tube (see Skill 39-1). The suction catheter should be no greater than one-half the size of the internal diameter of the artificial airway (AARC, 2010). Secretion removal should be as atraumatic as possible. To avoid trauma to the mucosa of the lung, never apply suction pressure while inserting the catheter, and maintain suction pressure less than 150 mm Hg in adults (AARC, 2010). Apply suction intermittently *only* as the catheter is withdrawn. Rotating the catheter will enhance removal of secretions that have adhered to the sides of the endotracheal tube. Apply a mask and goggles, and wear a barrier gown to prevent splashes with body fluids.

The practice of normal saline instillation (NSI) into artificial airways to improve secretion may be harmful and is not recommended. Clinical studies comparing suctioning after NSI with standard suctioning have not demonstrated any clinical or significant results (AARC, 2010).

The two current methods of suctioning are the open and closed methods. Open suctioning involves a sterile catheter that is opened at

TABLE 39-8 Positions for Postural Drainage

Lung Segment	Position of Patient
Adult	
Bilateral 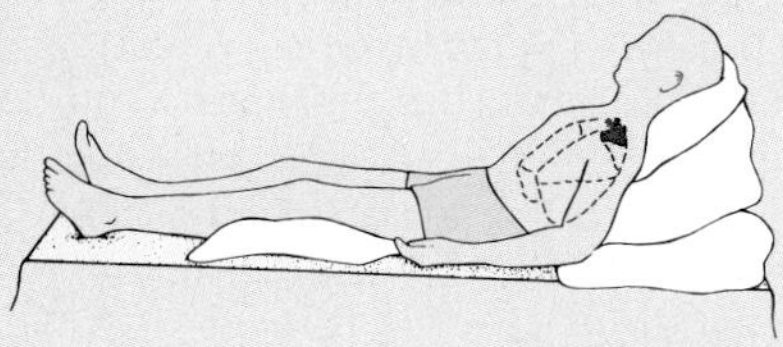	High-Fowler's position
Apical segments	
Right upper lobe—anterior segment 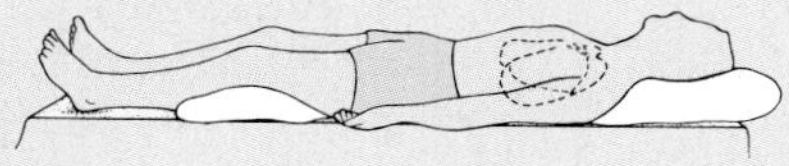	Supine with head of bed elevated 15–30 degrees
Left upper lobe—anterior segment 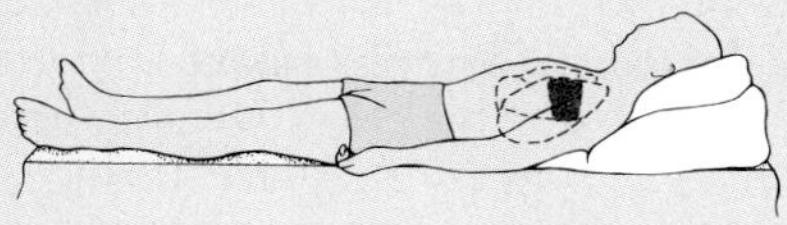	Supine with head elevated
Right upper lobe—posterior segment 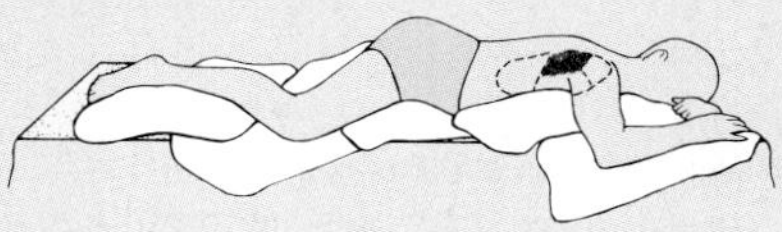	Side lying with right side of chest elevated on pillows
Left upper lobe—posterior segment 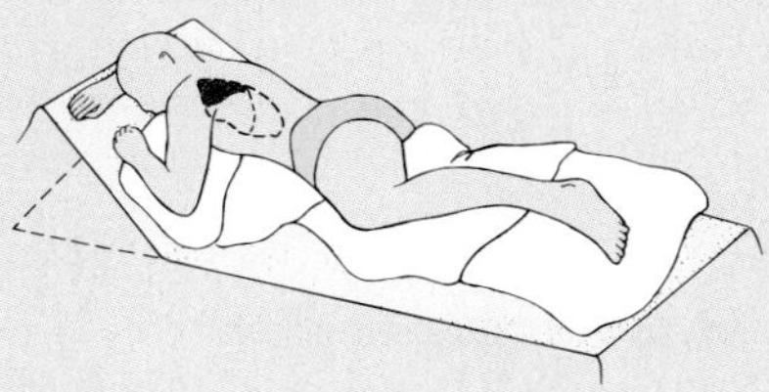	Side lying with left side of chest elevated on pillows
Right middle lobe—anterior segment 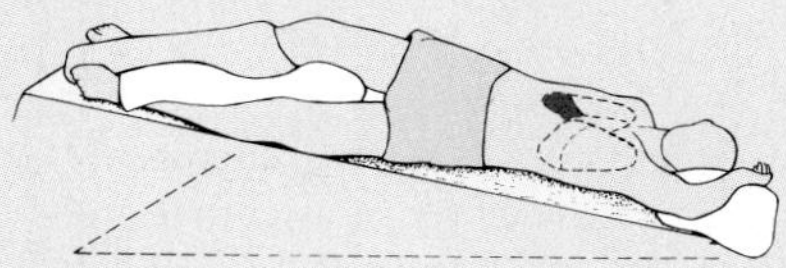	Three-fourths supine position with dependent lung in Trendelenburg's position
Right middle lobe—posterior segment 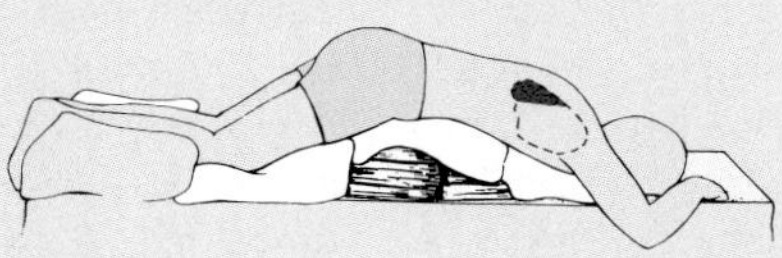	Prone with thorax and abdomen elevated
Both lower lobes—anterior segments 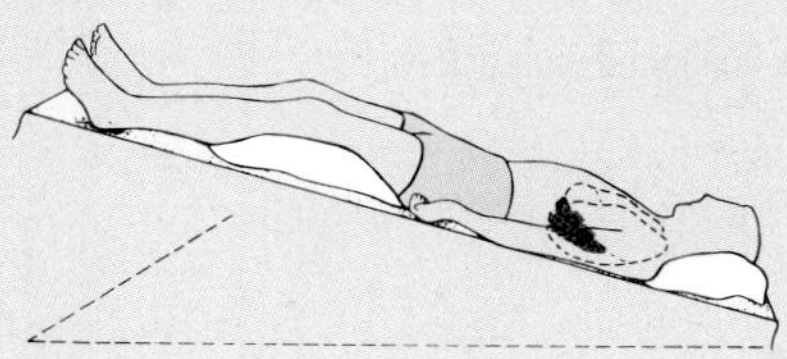	Supine in Trendelenburg's position

Continued

TABLE 39-8 Positions for Postural Drainage—cont'd

Lung Segment	Position of Patient
Left lower lobe—lateral segment 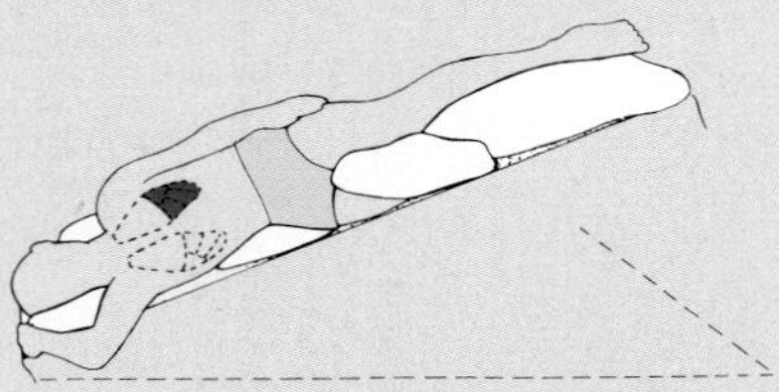	Right side lying in Trendelenburg's position
Right lower lobe—lateral segment 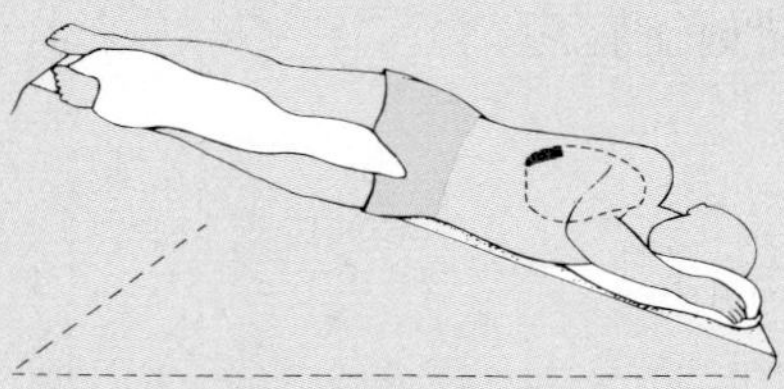	Left lateral in Trendelenburg's position
Right lower lobe—posterior segment 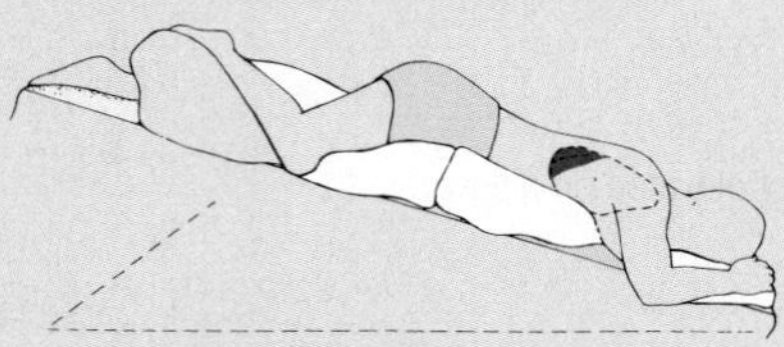	Prone in Trendelenburg's position with abdomen and thorax elevated
Both lower lobes—posterior segments 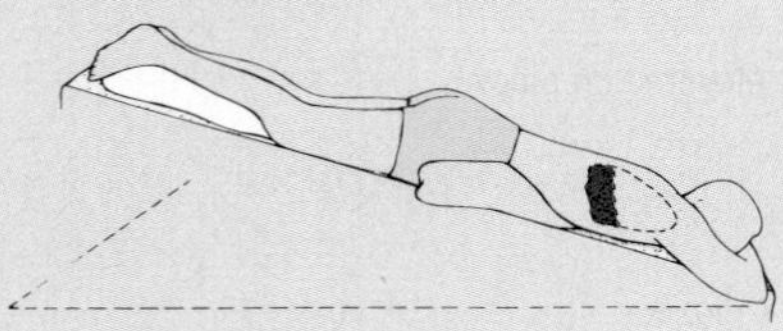	Prone in Trendelenburg's position with abdomen and thorax elevated
Child	
Bilateral—apical segments 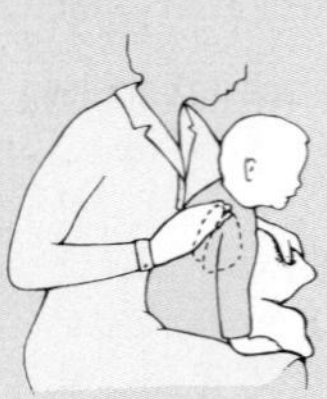	Sitting on nurse's lap, leaning slightly forward, flexed over pillow
Bilateral—middle anterior segments 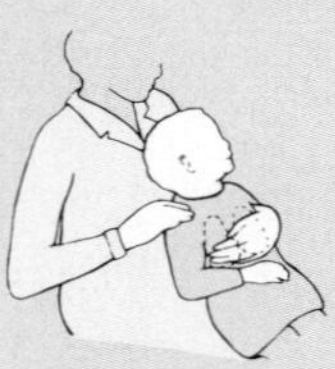	Sitting on nurse's lap, leaning against nurse
Bilateral lobes—anterior segments 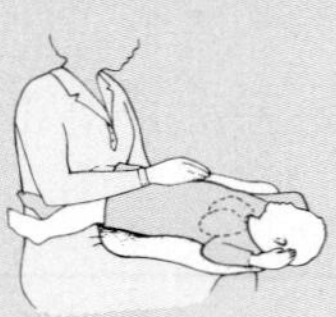	Lying supine on nurse's lap, back supported with pillow

SKILL 39-1 SUCTIONING

Delegation Considerations

If the patient has been assessed and determined to be stable, the skill of performing suctioning of an established tracheostomy can be delegated to an unregulated care provider (UCP) when the patient has a permanent tracheostomy tube or is receiving oropharyngeal suctioning. Before delegating this skill, do the following:

- Discuss with the UCP any unique modifications of the skill, such as the need to reapply any supplemental oxygen equipment following the procedure.
- Discuss appropriate suction limits.
- Instruct the UCP to report any change in the patient's respiratory status, signs and symptoms of hypoxemia, secretion colour or volume, or unresolved coughing or gagging.
- Instruct the UCP to report any change in the patient's colour, vital signs, or pain level.

Equipment

- Appropriate-size suction catheter (smallest diameter that will remove secretions effectively) or Yankauer catheter (oral suction)
- Nasal or oral airway (if indicated)
- Two sterile gloves or one sterile and one clean disposable glove (refer to technique)
- Clean towel or paper drape
- Portable or wall suction
- Mask, goggles, or face shield
- Connecting tube (1.8 metres)
- Pulse oximeter and stethoscope

Equipment for procedure without closed-suction catheter

- Small Y adapter (if catheter does not have a suction-control port)
- Water-soluble lubricant
- Sterile basin
- Sterile normal saline solution or water (approximately 100 mL)

PROCEDURE

STEPS	RATIONALE
1. Assess for signs and symptoms of upper and lower airway obstruction requiring nasotracheal or orotracheal suctioning, abnormal respiratory rate, adventitious sounds, nasal secretions, gurgling, drooling, restlessness, gastric secretions, or vomitus in mouth, and coughing without clearing secretions from airway.	• Physical signs and symptoms result from decreased oxygen to tissues, as well as pooling of secretions in upper and lower airways. A complete assessment is required before and after suction procedure (American Association of Respiratory Care [AARC], 2004).
2. Assess signs and symptoms associated with hypoxia and hypercapnia: decreased SpO_2, increased pulse and blood pressure, increased respiratory rate, apprehension, anxiety, decreased ability to concentrate, lethargy, decreased level of consciousness (especially acute), increased fatigue, dizziness, behavioural changes (especially irritability), dysrhythmias, pallor, and cyanosis.	• Physical signs and symptoms resulting from decreased oxygen to tissues indicate need for suctioning. Anxiety and pain consume oxygen and, in turn, worsen the signs of hypoxia.
3. Determine factors that normally influence upper or lower airway functioning:	
• Fluid status	• Fluid overload may increase amount of secretions. Dehydration promotes thicker secretions.
• Lack of humidity	• The environment influences secretion formation and gas exchange, necessitating airway suctioning when the patient cannot clear secretions effectively.
• Pulmonary disease, chronic obstructive pulmonary disorder, pulmonary infection	• Increases patient's risk for retaining pulmonary secretions. Patients with respiratory infections are prone to increased secretions that are thicker and sometimes more difficult to expectorate.
• Anatomy	• Abnormal anatomy can impair normal drainage of secretions. For example, nasal swelling, a deviated septum, or facial fractures may impair nasal drainage. Tumours in or around the lower airway may impair secretion removal by occluding or externally compressing the lumen of the airway.
• Changes in level of consciousness	• Impairs patient's ability to cough independently or follow instructions to cough and clear airway.
• Decreased cough or gag reflex, dysphagia, presence of a feeding tube	• Increases patient's risk for aspiration and subsequent pulmonary infection.
• Allergies, sinus drainage	• Increases volume of secretions in pharynx.
4. Identify contraindications to nasotracheal suctioning: occluded nasal passages; nasal bleeding, epiglottitis, or croup; acute head, facial, or neck injury or surgery, coagulopathy, or bleeding disorder; irritable airway or laryngospasm or bronchospasm; gastric surgery with high anastomosis; myocardial infarction (AARC, 2004).	• These conditions are contraindications to nasal suctioning because passage of the catheter through the nasal route causes trauma to existing facial trauma or surgery, increases nasal bleeding, or causes severe bleeding in the presence of bleeding disorders. With epiglottitis, croup, laryngospasm, or irritable airway, the entrance of a suction catheter via the nasal route causes intractable coughing, hypoxemia, and severe bronchospasm, necessitating emergency intubation or tracheostomy. Hypoxemia may worsen cardiac damage in myocardial infarction (AARC, 2004).

Continued

SKILL 39-1 SUCTIONING—cont'd

STEPS	RATIONALE
5. Examine sputum microbiology data.	• Certain bacteria are easier to transmit or require isolation because of virulence or antibiotic resistance.
6. Assess patient's understanding of the procedure.	• Reveals need for patient instruction and encourages cooperation.
7. Obtain prescriber's order if indicated by agency policy.	• Some institutions require a prescriber's order for tracheal suctioning.
8. Explain to patient how the procedure will help clear the airway and relieve breathing problems and that temporary coughing, sneezing, gagging, or shortness of breath is normal. Encourage patient to cough out secretions. Have patient practise coughing, if able. Splint surgical incisions, if necessary.	• Encourages cooperation and minimizes risks, anxiety, and pain.
9. Explain the importance of coughing and encourage coughing during procedure.	• Facilitates secretion removal and may reduce frequency and duration of future suctioning.
10. Help patient to assume a position comfortable for you and for the patient (usually semi-Fowler's or sitting upright with head hyperextended, unless contraindicated). Stand on patient's right if you are right-handed or on his or her left if you are left-handed.	• Reduces stimulation of gag reflex, promotes patient comfort and secretion drainage, and prevents aspiration. Hyperextension facilitates insertion of the catheter into the trachea. Position facilitates catheter insertion.
11. Place pulse oximeter on patient's finger. Take reading and leave pulse oximeter in place.	• Provides baseline oxygen level to determine patient's response to suctioning.
12. Place towel across patient's chest.	• Reduces transmission of microorganisms by protecting gown from secretions.
13. Perform hand hygiene. Apply mask, gown, goggles, or face shield if splashing is likely.	• Reduces transmission of microorganisms.
14. Connect one end of connecting tubing to suction machine and place the other end in a convenient location near patient. Turn suction device on and set vacuum regulator to appropriate negative pressure: 100 to 150 mm Hg for adults (AARC, 2010), 60 to 100 mm Hg for infants and children, 40 to 60 mm Hg for pre-term infants (Hockenberry & Wilson, 2015). ***Appropriate pressure may vary; check institutional policy.***	• Excessive negative pressure damages nasal pharyngeal and tracheal mucosa and induces greater hypoxia. Negative pressure should not exceed 150 mm Hg because high pressure increases the risk for airway trauma, hypoxemia, and atelectasis (AARC, 2010).
15. If indicated, increase supplemental oxygen therapy to 100% or as indicated by prescriber's orders. Encourage patient to deep-breathe.	• Hyperoxygenation provides some protection from suction-induced decline in oxygenation. Hyperoxygenation is most effective in the presence of hyperinflation, such as when encouraging the patient to deep-breathe or to increase ventilator tidal volume settings (Soule & Bennett, 2014).
16. Preparation for all types of suctioning:	
A. Open suction kit or catheter using aseptic technique. If a sterile drape is available, place it across the patient's chest or on the overbed table. Do not allow the suction catheter to touch any nonsterile surfaces.	• Prepares catheter and helps prevent transmission of microorganisms. A sterile drape provides a sterile surface on which to lay the suction catheter between passes, if needed.
B. Unwrap or open sterile basin and place on bedside table. Fill basin or cup with approximately 100 mL of sterile normal saline solution or water (see Step 16B illustration).	• Normal saline or water is needed to flush catheter and tubing after each suction pass.

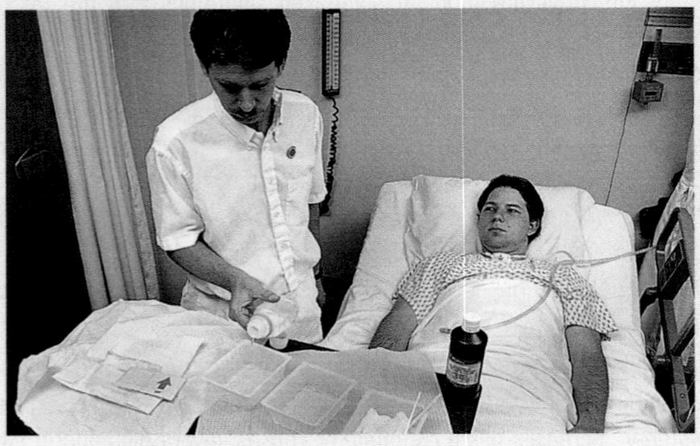

STEP 16B Pouring sterile saline into basin.

STEPS	RATIONALE
C. Turn on suction device. Set regulator to appropriate negative pressure.	
17. Suction airway.	
A. Oropharyngeal suctioning	
(1) Apply clean disposable gloves and mask or face shield (if splashing is likely).	• Suction of oral cavity does not require use of sterile gloves. Suction may cause splashing of body fluids.

STEPS	RATIONALE
(2) Attach Yankauer to connecting tubing. Check that equipment is functioning properly by suctioning a small amount of water or normal saline from the cup or basin.	
(3) Remove oxygen mask if present. Keep oxygen mask near patient's face. Nasal cannula may remain in place (if present).	• Allows access to patient's mouth. Reduces chances of hypoxia.

CRITICAL DECISION POINT: *Be prepared to quickly reapply oxygen mask if SpO_2 falls or respiratory distress develops during or at the end of suctioning.*

STEPS	RATIONALE
(4) Insert Yankauer into the patient's mouth. With suction applied, move catheter around mouth, including pharynx and gum line, until secretions are cleared.	• Movement of catheter prevents suction tip from invaginating oral mucosal surfaces, thus potentially causing trauma.
(5) Encourage patient to cough, and repeat suctioning if needed. Replace oxygen mask if used.	• Coughing moves secretions from lower to upper airways into mouth.
(6) Suction water from basin through catheter until catheter is cleared of secretions. Turn off suction.	• Clearing secretions before they dry reduces the probability of transmission of microorganisms and enhances delivery of preset suction pressures.
(7) Place catheter in a clean, dry area for reuse.	• Facilitates prompt removal of airway secretions when suctioning is needed in the future. Moist environment encourages microorganism growth.

CRITICAL DECISION POINT: *Do not store the catheter where it will come in contact with secretions or excretions, which promote bacterial growth. If the patient is capable of self-oral suctioning, place the catheter within reach.*

B. Nasopharyngeal and nasotracheal suctioning

STEPS	RATIONALE
(1) Open lubricant. Squeeze small amount onto open sterile catheter package without touching package. Lubricant is *not* necessary for artificial airway suctioning.	• Prepares lubricant while maintaining sterility. Water-soluble lubricant is used to avoid lipoid aspiration pneumonia. Excessive lubricant can occlude the catheter.
(2) Apply sterile glove to each hand, or apply nonsterile glove to nondominant hand and sterile glove to dominant hand.	• Reduces transmission of microorganisms and allows nurse to maintain sterility of suction catheter.
(3) Pick up suction catheter with dominant hand without touching nonsterile surfaces. Pick up connecting tubing with nondominant hand. Secure catheter to tubing (see Step 17B[3] illustration).	• Maintains catheter sterility. Connects catheter to suction.

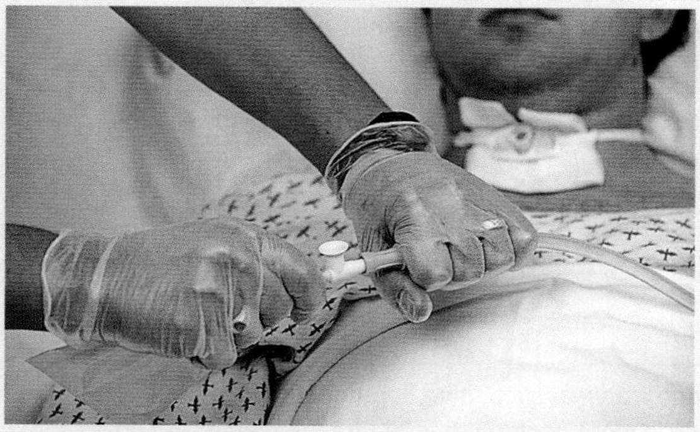

STEP 17B(3) Attaching catheter to suction.

STEPS	RATIONALE
(4) Check that the equipment is functioning properly by suctioning a small amount of normal saline solution from the basin.	• Ensures equipment function; lubricates catheter and tubing.
(5) Lightly coat distal 6–8 cm (2–3 inches) of catheter with water-soluble lubricant.	• Lubricates catheter for easier insertion.
(6) Remove oxygen delivery device, if applicable, with nondominant hand. *Without applying suction* and using dominant thumb and forefinger, gently insert catheter into naris during inhalation. ***Never apply suction during insertion.***	• Application of suction pressure while introducing catheter into nasopharyngeal tissues increases risk of damage to mucosa. When advanced into trachea, suction could damage mucosa and increase risk of hypoxia.
(7) *Nasopharyngeal:* As the patient takes a deep breath, insert catheter following natural course of naris; slightly slant catheter downward and advance to back of pharynx. Do not force through naris. In adults, insert catheter about 20 cm (6–8 inches); in older children, 16–20 cm (6–8 inches); in infants and young children, 4–14 cm (3–5½ inches) into trachea until resistance is met or patient coughs; then pull back 1–2 cm (½ inch).	• Proper placement ensures removal of pharyngeal secretions. Pulling back on catheter before initiating suctioning prevents invagination of the tracheal membrane (AARC, 2010).

Continued

SKILL 39-1 SUCTIONING—cont'd

STEPS	RATIONALE
(a) Apply intermittent suction for no more than 10 seconds by placing and releasing nondominant thumb over catheter vent (AARC, 2010). Slowly withdraw catheter while rotating it back and forth between thumb and forefinger.	• Intermittent suction safely removes pharyngeal secretions. Suction time of >10 seconds increases risk for suction-induced hypoxemia (AARC, 2010).
(8) *Nasotracheal:* As patient takes a deep breath advance catheter following natural course of naris, slightly slanted and downward to just above entrance into larynx and then the trachea. Allow patient to take a breath. Quickly insert catheter approximately 15–20 cm (6–8 inches) (in adult) into trachea (see Step 17B[8] illustration). Patient will begin to cough, then pull back catheter 1–2 cm (½ inch) before applying suction. *Note*: In older children, advance 16–20 cm (6–8 inches); in young children and infants, 8–14 cm (3–5½ inches).	• Ensures catheter will be inserted into trachea with minimal stress to patient.

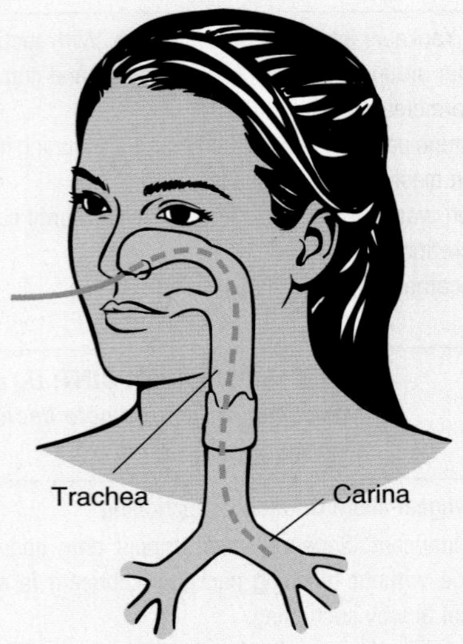

STEP 17B(8) Distance of insertion of nasotracheal catheter.

CRITICAL DECISION POINT: *Insert catheter during patient inhalation, especially if inserting catheter into trachea because epiglottis is open. If there is difficulty passing the catheter, ask the patient to cough or say "ahh."* Do not insert during swallowing *or catheter will most likely enter the esophagus.* Never *apply suction during insertion. Patient should cough. If patient gags or becomes nauseated, catheter is most likely in the esophagus and must be removed.*

STEPS	RATIONALE
(a) *Positioning option for nasotracheal suctioning:* In some instances, turning the patient's head to the right will help you suction the left mainstem bronchus; turning head to the left will help you suction the right mainstem bronchus. If resistance is felt after insertion of catheter for maximum recommended distance, the catheter has probably hit carina. Pull the catheter back 1–2 cm (½ inch) before applying suction.	• Turning the patient's head to the side elevates the bronchial passage on the opposite side and facilitates passage of the catheter.

CRITICAL DECISION POINT: *Use nasal approach and perform tracheal suctioning before pharyngeal suctioning whenever possible. The mouth and pharynx contain more bacteria than the trachea does. If copious oral secretions are present before beginning the procedure, suction the mouth with an oral suction device.*

STEPS	RATIONALE
(b) Apply intermittent suction for 10 seconds by placing and releasing nondominant thumb over vent of catheter and slowly withdrawing catheter while rotating it back and forth between dominant thumb and forefinger. Encourage patient to cough. Replace oxygen device, if applicable.	• Intermittent suction and rotation of catheter prevent injury to mucosa. If the catheter "grabs" mucosa, remove thumb to release suction. Suctioning longer than 10 seconds can cause cardiopulmonary compromise, usually from hypoxemia or vagal overload.

CRITICAL DECISION POINT: *Monitor patient's vital signs and oxygen saturation during the procedure, note if the patient's pulse drops more than 20 beats per minute or increases more than 40 beats per minute, or oxygen saturation falls below 90% or 5% from baseline, in which case cease suctioning.*

STEPS	RATIONALE
(9) Rinse catheter and connecting tubing with normal saline or water until cleared.	• Removes secretions from catheter. Secretions that remain in suction catheter or connecting tubing decrease suctioning efficiency.

STEPS	RATIONALE
(10) Assess for need to repeat suctioning procedure. Do not perform more than two passes with the catheter. Allow adequate time (at least 1 minute) between suction passes for ventilation and oxygenation (AARC, 2010). Ask patient to deep-breathe and to cough.	• Observe for alterations in cardiopulmonary status. Suctioning can induce hypoxemia, dysrhythmias, laryngospasm, and bronchospasm (AARC, 2010). Deep breathing reventilates and reoxygenates alveoli and reduces the risk for suction-induced hypoxemia. Repeated passes clear the airway of excessive secretions but can also remove oxygen and may induce laryngospasm.
C. Artificial airway (tracheostomy or endotracheal [ET] tube) suctioning	

CRITICAL DECISION POINT: *If a risk for splash is present or if patient is on respiratory precautions, gown, face shield or mask, and goggles may be required.*

STEPS	RATIONALE
(1) Apply personal protective equipment as needed.	• Reduces transmission of microorganisms.
(2) Apply one sterile glove to each hand, or apply nonsterile glove to nondominant hand and sterile glove to dominant hand.	• Reduces transmission of microorganisms and allows nurse to maintain sterility of suction catheter.
(3) Pick up suction catheter with dominant hand without touching nonsterile surfaces. Pick up connecting tubing with nondominant hand. Secure catheter to tubing.	• Maintains catheter sterility. Establishes suction.
(4) Check that equipment is functioning properly by suctioning a small amount of saline from the basin by occluding suction vent.	• Ensures equipment function; lubricates catheter and tubing.
(5) Hyperoxygenate patient before suctioning, using manual resuscitation bag-valve device and increasing FiO_2 for several minutes; or if mechanically ventilated use the ventilator to provide additional breaths without increasing tidal volume. Some mechanical ventilators have a button that, when pushed, delivers oxygen for a few minutes and then resets to the previous value.	• Hyperoxygenation for 30–60 seconds decreases suction-induced hypoxemia. Most sources recommend hyperoxygenation with 100% oxygen in the adult patient (AARC, 2010).
(6) If patient is receiving mechanical ventilation, open swivel adapter or, if necessary, remove oxygen or humidity delivery device with nondominant hand.	• Exposes artificial airway.
(7) Without applying suction, gently but quickly insert catheter using dominant thumb and forefinger into artificial airway (it is best to time catheter insertion with inspiration) until resistance is met or patient coughs, then pull back 1 cm (½ inch).	• Application of suction pressure while introducing catheter into the trachea increases risk of damage to tracheal mucosa and greater hypoxia through removal of entrained oxygen present in airways. The action of pulling back stimulates cough and removes catheter from mucosal wall so that catheter is not resting against tracheal mucosa during suctioning.

CRITICAL DECISION POINT: *If unable to insert catheter past the end of the endotracheal tube, the catheter is probably caught in the Murphy eye (i.e., side hole at the distal end of the endotracheal tube that allows for collateral airflow in the event of main stem intubation). If this happens, rotate catheter to reposition it away from the Murphy eye, or withdraw it slightly and reinsert with the next inhalation. Usually the catheter meets resistance at the carina. One indication that the catheter is at the carina is acute onset of coughing, because the carina contains many cough receptors. The catheter should be pulled back 1 cm (½ inch).*

STEPS	RATIONALE
(8) Apply intermittent suction for no longer than 10 seconds by placing and releasing nondominant thumb over vent of catheter; slowly withdraw catheter while rotating it back and forth between dominant thumb and forefinger (AARC, 2010) (see Step 17C[8] illustration). Encourage patient to cough. Watch for respiratory distress.	• Intermittent suction and rotation of catheter prevent injury to tracheal mucosal lining. If catheter "grabs" mucosa, remove thumb to release suction.

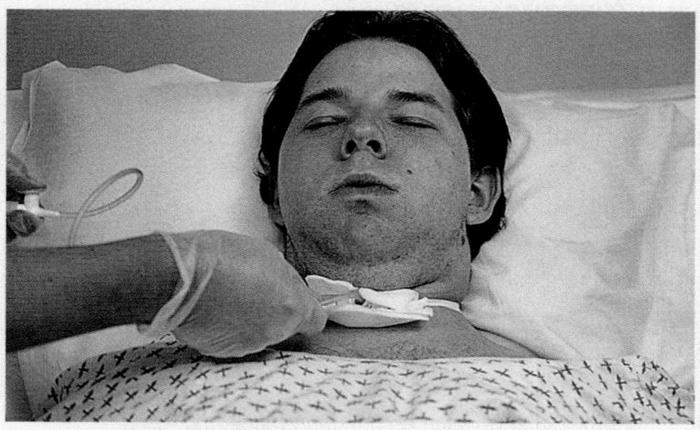

STEP 17C(8) Suctioning tracheostomy.

Continued

SKILL 39-1 SUCTIONING—cont'd

STEPS	RATIONALE
CRITICAL DECISION POINT: *If patient develops respiratory distress during suction procedure, immediately withdraw catheter and supply additional oxygen and breaths as needed. Oxygen can be administered directly through the catheter in an emergency. Disconnect suction and administer 100% oxygen through the catheter.*	
(9) If patient is receiving mechanical ventilation, close swivel adapter or replace oxygen delivery device.	• Re-establishes the artificial airway.
(10) Encourage patient to deep-breathe, if able. Some patients respond well to several manual breaths from the mechanical ventilator or bag-valve device.	• Reoxygenates and re-expands alveoli. Suctioning can cause hypoxemia and atelectasis.
(11) Rinse catheter and connecting tubing with normal saline until clear. Use continuous suction.	• Removes catheter secretions. Secretions left in tubing decrease suction and provide environment for microorganism growth. Secretions left in connecting tube decrease suctioning efficiency.
(12) Assess patient's cardiopulmonary status for secretion clearance and complications. Repeat Steps 17C(5) through 17C(11) once or twice more to clear secretions. Allow adequate time (at least 1 full minute) between suction passes for ventilation and reoxygenation. Perform oropharyngeal and nasopharyngeal (if necessary) suctioning to clear secretions (Steps 17A, 17B). Do not suction nose again after suctioning mouth.	• Suctioning can induce dysrhythmias, hypoxia, and bronchospasm and impair cerebral circulation or adversely affect hemodynamics (AARC, 2010). • The upper airway is considered clean and lower airway is considered sterile. Therefore, the same catheter can be used to suction from sterile to clean areas, but not from clean to sterile areas.
18. Complete procedure:	
A. Disconnect catheter from connecting tubing. Roll catheter around fingers of dominant hand. Pull glove off inside out so that catheter remains in glove. Pull off other glove over first glove in same way to contain contaminants. Discard into appropriate receptacle. Turn off suction.	• Reduces transmission of microorganisms. Clean equipment should not be touched with contaminated gloves.
B. Remove towel and place in laundry or remove drape and discard in appropriate receptacle.	
C. Reposition patient as indicated by condition. You may need to reapply clean gloves for patient's personal care (e.g., oral hygiene).	• Proper positioning based on patient's condition promotes comfort, encourages secretion drainage, and reduces risk of aspiration.
D. If indicated, readjust oxygen to original level.	• Helps patient's blood oxygen level return to baseline.
E. Discard remainder of normal saline into appropriate receptacle. If basin is disposable, discard into appropriate receptacle. If basin is reusable, rinse and place in soiled utility room.	• Solution is contaminated.
F. Remove goggles, mask, face-shield, and gown, and place in appropriate receptacles; perform hand hygiene.	• Reduces transmission of microorganisms.
G. Place unopened suction kit on suction machine table or at head of bed according to institution preference.	• Provides for immediate access of suction catheter and equipment in the event of an emergency or for the next suctioning procedure.
19. Compare patient's vital signs and SpO_2 saturation before and after suctioning.	• Identifies physiological effects of suction procedure to restore airway patency.
20. Ask patient if breathing is easier and if congestion is decreased. Auscultate lungs and compare respiratory assessment before and after suctioning.	• Provides subjective confirmation that airway obstruction is relieved with suctioning procedure.
21. Observe airway secretions.	• Provides data to document presence or absence of respiratory tract infection.

UNEXPECTED OUTCOMES	RELATED INTERVENTIONS
Worsening respiratory status	• Limit length of suctioning. • Determine need for more frequent suctioning, possibly of shorter duration. • Determine need for supplemental oxygen, supply oxygen between suction passes. • Notify health care provider.
Return of bloody secretions	• Determine amount of suction pressure used. It may need to be decreased. • Ensure suction completed correctly by using intermittent suction and rotation of catheter. • Evaluate suctioning frequency. • Provide more frequent oral hygiene. • Determine other factors, such as prolonged bleeding time.

STEPS	RATIONALE
Unable to pass suction catheter through first naris attempted	• Try other naris or oral route. • Insert nasal airway, especially if suctioning through patient naris frequently. • Guide catheter along naris floor to avoid turbinates. • If obstruction is mucus, apply suction to relieve obstruction, but do not apply suction to mucosa. If obstruction is thought to be a blood clot, consult physician. • Increase lubrication of catheter.
Paroxysms of coughing	• Administer supplemental oxygen. • Allow patient to rest between passes of suction catheter. • Consult health care provider regarding need for inhaled bronchodilators or topical anaesthetics.
No secretions obtained	• Evaluate patient's fluid status. • Assess for signs of infection. • Determine need for chest physiotherapy. • Assess adequacy of humidification on oxygen delivery device.

RECORDING AND REPORTING

- Record the amount, consistency, colour, and odour of secretions and patient's response to procedure; document patient's pre-suctioning and post-suctioning cardiopulmonary status.

HOME CARE CONSIDERATIONS

- Nurses need to adhere to best practices for infection control while weighing cost-effectiveness in the setting of a chronic situation. If the patient has an established tracheostomy or requires long-term nasotracheal suctioning and infection is not present, clean suction technique is appropriate.
- Instruct the patient and family in infection-control measures for emptying the secretion jar. These secretions should be emptied in the toilet but they have a splash risk. Instruct the caregiver to apply a mask (shield if available) and gloves and bring the secretion jar as close to the toilet bowel as possible to decrease the risk of splash.

the time of suctioning. Sterile gloves are worn to perform the suction procedure. Closed suctioning involves a multiple-use suction catheter encased in a plastic sheath (Figure 39-11). Closed suctioning is most often used on patients who require mechanical ventilation to support their respiratory efforts, because it permits continuous delivery of oxygen while suction is performed, thus reducing the risk of oxygen desaturation. Although sterile gloves are not required in this procedure, at least nonsterile (i.e., disposable) gloves are recommended to prevent contact with splashes from body fluids.

Artificial Airways. An artificial airway is indicated for patients with a decreased level of consciousness or an airway obstruction and to aid in the removal of tracheobronchial secretions.

Oral Airway. The oral airway, the simplest type of artificial airway, prevents obstruction of the trachea by displacement of the tongue into the oropharynx (Figure 39-12). The oral airway extends from the teeth to the oropharynx, maintaining the tongue in the normal position. The correct-size airway must be used. Proper oral airway size is determined by measuring the distance from the corner of the mouth to the angle of the jaw just below the ear. The length is equal to the distance from the flange of the airway to the tip. If the airway is too small, the tongue is not held in the anterior portion of the mouth; if the airway is too large, it may force the tongue toward the epiglottis and obstruct the airway.

The airway is inserted by turning the curve of the airway toward the cheek and placing it over the tongue. When the airway is in the

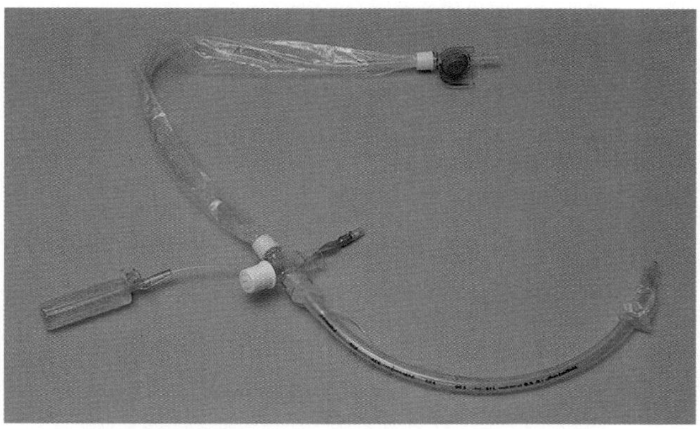

FIGURE 39-11 Ballard tracheal care, closed suction.

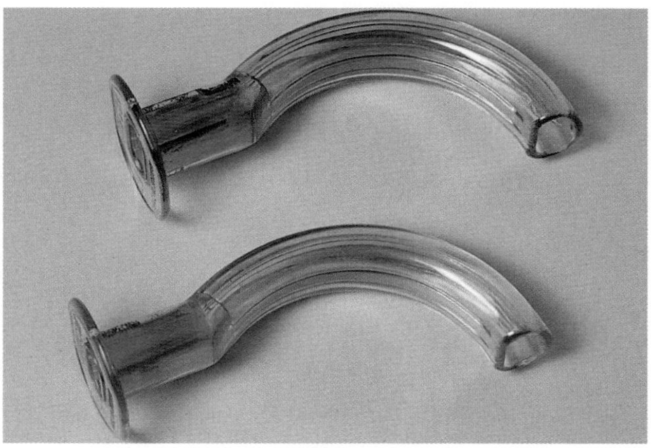

FIGURE 39-12 Artificial oral airways.

oropharynx, turn it so that the opening points downward. When correctly placed, the airway moves the tongue forward away from the oropharynx, and the flange, the flat portion of the airway, rests against the patient's teeth. Incorrect insertion merely forces the tongue back into the oropharynx.

Endotracheal and Tracheal Airway. An artificial airway is for a patient with decreased level of consciousness or airway obstruction and aids in removal of tracheal bronchial secretions. The presence of an artificial airway places the patient at high risk for infection and airway injury. Sterile technique must be used in caring for and maintaining an artificial airway to help prevent health care–associated infections. Artificial airways need to be cared for and maintained in the correct position to prevent airway damage (Skill 39-2).

Endotracheal (ET) tubes are used as short-term artificial airways to administer mechanical ventilation, relieve upper airway obstruction, protect against aspiration, or clear secretions. Only health care providers with special training may insert ET tubes. ET tubes are generally removed within 14 days; however, they may be used for a longer period of time if the patient is showing progress toward weaning from mechanical ventilation and extubation.

If the patient requires long-term assistance from an artificial airway, a tracheostomy is considered. A surgical incision is made into the trachea, and a short artificial airway (a tracheostomy tube) is inserted.

Maintenance and Promotion of Lung Expansion. Nursing interventions to maintain or promote lung expansion include noninvasive and invasive techniques. Noninvasive techniques are ambulation, positioning, and incentive spirometry. An invasive procedure is management of a chest tube.

Ambulation. Immobility is a major factor contributing to atelectasis and ventilator-associated pneumonia. Early ambulation has been correlated with increased general strength and lung expansion. Mobility programs should include input from respiratory therapists and physiotherapists (Atkins & Kautz, 2014).

Positioning. In the healthy, completely mobile person, adequate ventilation and oxygenation are maintained by frequent position changes during daily activities. Frequent changes of position are simple and cost-effective methods for reducing the risks of stasis of pulmonary secretions and decreased chest wall expansion.

The most effective position for patients with cardiopulmonary diseases is the 45-degree semi-Fowler's position, using gravity to assist in

SKILL 39-2 CARE OF AN ARTIFICIAL AIRWAY

Delegation Considerations

This skill should not be routinely delegated to an unregulated care provider (UCP). It is the nurse's responsibility to perform endotracheal care. In some settings, patients who have well-established tracheostomy tubes may have the care delegated to UCPs. It is the nurse's responsibility to assess and ensure that proper artificial airway care is provided. In addition, UCPs may perform other aspects of the patient's care. The nurse must instruct the UCPs about the following:

- To report any changes in the patient's respiratory status, level of consciousness, confusion, restlessness, irritability, changes in vital signs (range to report), decreased pulse oximetry level (values to report), or change in level of comfort
- To report abnormal colour of tracheal stoma and drainage
- Emergency procedures in case the tracheostomy tube inadvertently becomes dislodged when ties are changed

Equipment

Endotracheal (ET) tube care

- Towel
- ET and oropharyngeal suction equipment
- 2.5 to 4 cm adhesive or waterproof tape (not paper or silk tape) or commercial ET tube holder and mouthguard (follow manufacturer's instructions for securing)
- Two pairs of disposable (nonsterile) gloves
- Adhesive remover swab or acetone on a cotton ball
- Mouth care supplies (e.g., toothbrush, toothpaste, toothette for edentulous patients)
- 0.12–0.20% chlorhexidine mouthwash rinse or gel
- Face cleanser (e.g., wet washcloth, towel, soap, shaving supplies)
- Clean 2 × 2 gauze
- Tincture of benzoin, liquid adhesive, or skin prep pads
- Mask, goggles, face shield (if indicated)
- Stethoscope
- Oral airway

Tracheostomy care

- Towel
- Tracheostomy suction supplies
- Sterile tracheostomy care kit, if available, or three sterile 4 × 4 gauze pads
- Sterile cotton-tipped applicators
- Sterile tracheostomy dressing
- Sterile basin
- Small sterile brush (or disposable cannula)
- Tracheostomy ties (e.g., twill tape, manufactured tracheostomy ties, Velcro tracheostomy ties)
- Normal saline (NS)
- Scissors
- Pair of sterile and clean gloves
- Mask, goggles, face shield (if indicated)

PROCEDURE

STEPS	RATIONALE
1. Perform pulmonary assessment:	
A. Auscultate lung sounds.	• Provides baseline information.
B. Assess condition and patency of airway and surrounding tissues.	• Indicates if additional skin care to irritated areas is needed. Identifies potential pressure areas.
C. Note type and size of tube, movement of tube, and cuff size.	• Movement of tube predisposes the patient to tracheal trauma or tube dislodgement and may indicate the need for another size airway. Cuff size indicates the amount of air needed to properly inflate cuff.
2. Explain procedure to the patient and family.	• Reinforces information given to patient and family and provides an opportunity for them to ask additional questions.
3. Position patient: Usually supine or semi-Fowler's.	• Provides access to the site and facilitates completion of the procedure.
4. Place towel across patient's chest.	• Reduces transmission of microorganisms and protects linens and bedclothes.
5. Perform hand hygiene. Apply mask, goggles, or face shield (if indicated).	• Reduces transmission of microorganisms.
6. Perform airway care.	
A. Endotracheal tube care	
(1) Observe for signs and symptoms of need to perform care of the artificial airway: **(a)** Soiled or loose tape **(b)** Pressure sores on nares, lip, or corner of mouth **(c)** Unstable tube **(d)** Excessive secretions	• A patient with an artificial airway is at increased risk because of the inability to control secretions or difficulty in controlling them, and because of pressure points of the artificial airway.
(2) Identify factors that increase the risk of complications from ET tubes: **(a)** Type and size of tube **(b)** Movement of tube up and down trachea **(c)** Cuff size **(d)** Duration of placement	• A tube moving up and down the trachea predisposes the patient to tracheal trauma or dislodgement. Cuff underinflation may allow aspiration, whereas overinflation causes tracheal mucosa injury (Hess, 2005).
(3) Determine proper ET tube depth as noted by centimetres at lip or gum line. This line is marked on the tube and recorded in the patient's record at time of intubation.	• Ensures that tube is a proper depth to adequately ventilate both lungs and that tube is not too high (causing vocal cord damage) or too low (causing right main-stem intubation, thus ventilating only right lung).
(4) Suction ET tube (see Skill 39-1):	• Removes secretions. Diminishes patient's need to cough during procedure.

CRITICAL DECISION POINT: *An oral airway should be immediately accessible in the event that the patient bites down and obstructs the ET tube.*

STEPS	RATIONALE
(a) Instruct patient not to bite or move ET tube with tongue or pull on tubing; removal of tape can be uncomfortable.	• Prepares patient for procedure and what to expect.
(b) Leave Yankauer suction catheter connected to suction source.	• Prepares for oropharyngeal suctioning.
(5) Prepare method to secure endotracheal tube (check agency policy).	• Adhesive tape must be placed around the head from cheek to cheek below the ears. Avoid placing it over the ears, as this may result in a pressure sore.
(a) *Tape method:* Cut piece of tape long enough to go completely around patient's head from naris to naris plus 15 cm (6 in): for an adult, approximately 30–60 cm (1–2 ft). Lay adhesive side up on bedside table. Cut and lay 8–15 cm (3–6 in) of tape, adhesive side down, in centre of long strip to prevent tape from sticking to hair.	
(b) *Commercially available endotracheal tube holder:* Open package per manufacturer's instructions. Set device aside with the head guard in place and the Velcro strips open.	• Commercial devices are latex-free, fast, and convenient.
(6) Apply clean gloves, and instruct assistant to apply gloves and hold ET tube firmly at patient's lips. Note the number marking on the ET tube at the gum line.	• Reduces transmission of microorganisms. Maintains proper tube position and prevents accidental extubation.

CRITICAL DECISION POINT: *Do not allow helper to hold the tube away from the lips or nares. Doing so allows too much "play" in the tube and increases the risk for tube movement and accidental extubation. Never let go of the ET tube because the tube could become dislodged.*

Continued

SKILL 39-2 CARE OF AN ARTIFICIAL AIRWAY—cont'd

STEPS	RATIONALE
(7) Remove old tape or device.	
(a) *Tape:* Carefully remove tape from ET tube and patient's face. If tape is difficult to remove, moisten it with (soapy) wet washcloth, water, or adhesive tape remover. Discard tape in appropriate receptacle if nearby. If not, place soiled tape on bedside table or on distant end of towel.	• Provides access to skin under tape for assessment and hygiene. Reduces transmission of microorganisms.
(b) *Commercially available device:* Remove Velcro strips from ET tube, and remove ET tube holder from patient.	• The Velcro adhesive strips hold the ET tube in place and provide a marker to measure distance to patient's lips or gums. These devices permit access to patient's mouth and lips for ease in oropharyngeal suctioning and oral hygiene.
(8) Remove excess secretions or adhesive left on patient's face. Use adhesive remover swab to remove excess adhesive left on face after tape removal. Wash adhesive remover from face.	• Promotes hygiene. Retained adhesive can cause damage to skin and prevent adhesion of new tape.
(9) Remove oral airway or bite block if present. Keep ET tube cuff inflated.	• Provides access and complete observation of patient's oral cavity.

CRITICAL DECISION POINT: *Do not remove oral airway if patient is actively biting. Wait until tape or device is partially or completely secured to ET tube.*

STEPS	RATIONALE
(10) Clean mouth, gums, and teeth opposite ET tube with powdered tooth brush or brush with nonfoaming antiseptic paste for 3–4 minutes (Booker, Murff, Kitko, et al., 2013). Rinse carefully with sterile water, and suction orally as needed during brushing and rinsing. Moisten brush with sterile water to rinse, then use brush or a clean toothette to apply chlorhexidine rinse or gel (Booker et al., 2013; Labeau, Van de Vyver, Brusselaers, et al., 2011). Perform oral care twice daily at 12-hour intervals minimally (Booker et al., 2013). If necessary, administer oropharyngeal suctioning with Yankauer catheter.	• The use of an oral antiseptic for oral care of intubated patients has a beneficial effect in preventing ventilator-associated pneumonia (Booker et al., 2013; Labeau et al., 2011). Suctioning removes pooled secretions.
(11) Note "cm" ET tube (oral ET tube only) marking at lips or gums. With help of assistant, move ET tube to opposite side or centre of mouth. Do not change tube depth.	• Prevents formation of pressure sores at sides of patient's mouth. Ensures correct position of tube and allows for quick visual scan of displaced tube (Cooper, 2013). Measuring the tube at the lip line can be distorted because of edema, trauma, or the disease process.
(12) Repeat oral cleaning as in Step (9) on opposite side of mouth.	• Removes secretions from mouth and oropharynx.
(13) Clean face and neck with soapy washcloth; rinse and dry. Shave male patient as necessary.	• Moisture and beard growth prevent adhesive tape adherence.
(14) Use small amount of skin protectant or liquid adhesive on clean 2 × 2 gauze and dot on upper lip (oral ET tube) or across nose (nasal ET tube) and cheeks to ear. Allow to dry completely.	• Protects and makes skin more receptive to tape.
(15) Secure ET tube.	
(a) *Tape method:*	
(a1) Slip tape under patient's head and neck, adhesive side up. Do not twist tape or catch hair, or allow tape to stick to itself. It helps to stick tape gently to the tongue blade, which serves as a guide as tape is passed behind the patient's head. Centre tape so that double-faced tape extends around the back of the neck from ear to ear.	• Positions tape to secure ET tube in proper position.

STEPS	RATIONALE
(a2) On one side of face, secure tape from ear to naris (nasal ET tube) or over lip to ET tube (oral ET tube). Tear remaining tape in half lengthwise, forming two pieces that are 1–1.5 cm (¼–½ inch) wide. Secure bottom half of tape across upper lip (oral ET tube) or across top of nose (nasal ET tube; see Step 6A[15][a2] illustration, part A). Wrap top half of tape around tube (see Step 6A[15][a2] illustration, part B). Tape should encircle tube at least two times for security.	• Secures tape to face. Using top tape to wrap tube prevents downward drag on ET tube.

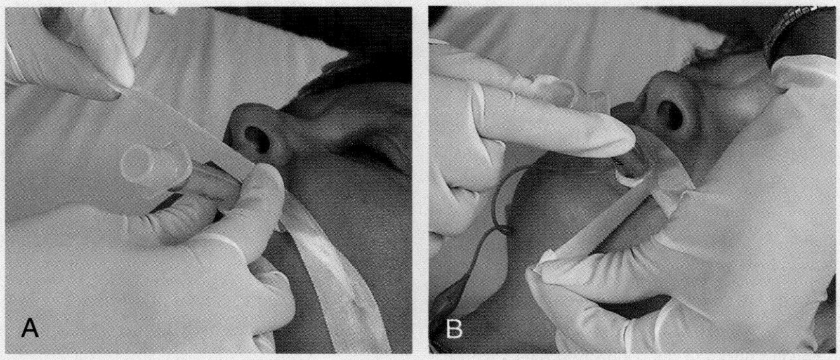

STEP 6A(15)(a2) A, Securing bottom half of tape across patient's upper lip. **B,** Securing top half of tape around tube.

(a3) Gently pull other side of tape firmly to pick up slack, and secure it to remaining side of face (see Step 6A[15][a3] illustration). Have assistant release hold when tube is secure. You may want the assistant to help reinsert the oral airway.	• Secures tape to face and ET tube. Tube should be at same depth at the lips. Check earlier assessment for verification of tube depth in centimetres.

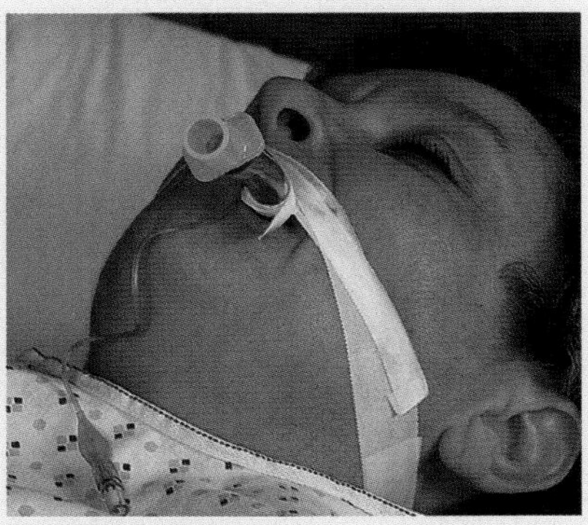

STEP 6A(15)(a3) Tape securing ET tube.

(b) *Commercially available device:*

(b1) Place ET tube through opening designed to secure ET tube. Ensure that pilot balloon to the ET tube is accessible.	• Commercially available holders have a slit in the front of the holder designed to secure the ET tube.
(b2) Place Velcro strips of ET holder under patient at occipital region of the head.	• Ensures that the ET tube remains at the correct depth as determined during assessment.
(b3) Verify that ET tube is at the established position using the lip or gum line as a guide.	• The ET tube needs to be secure so that the position of the tube remains at the correct depth.
(b4) Secure Velcro strips at base of the patient's head. Leave 1 cm (½ inch) slack in the strips.	
(b5) Verify that tube is secure, that it does not move forward from patient's mouth or backward down into patient's throat. Ensure that there are no pressure areas on oral mucosa or occipital region of the head.	• The tube must be secure so that the position of the tube remains at the correct depth. The tube can be secured without being tight and causing pressure.

Continued

SKILL 39-2 CARE OF AN ARTIFICIAL AIRWAY—cont'd

STEPS	RATIONALE
(16) Clean oral airway in warm, soapy water and rinse well. Then rinse in chlorhexidine rinse, shake excess solution from oral airway. *Option:* Insert new oral airway if secretions are difficult to remove.	• Promotes hygiene. Reduces transmission of microorganisms.
(17) For unconscious patient, reinsert oral airway without pushing tongue into oropharynx.	• Prevents patient from biting ET tube and allows access for oropharyngeal suctioning. An oral airway in a conscious, cooperative patient may cause excessive gagging and pressure injuries to the mouth and tongue.
B. Tracheostomy care	
(1) Observe for signs and symptoms of need to perform tracheostomy care:	• A patient with a tracheostomy tube is at increased risk because of loss of natural airway protection of the upper airway.
(a) Soiled or loose ties or dressing	
(b) Nonstable tube	
(c) Excessive secretions	
(2) Suction tracheostomy (see Skill 39-1). Before removing gloves, remove soiled tracheostomy dressing and discard in glove with coiled catheter.	• Removes secretions so as not to occlude outer cannula while inner cannula is removed. Reduces need for patient to cough. Prevents aspiration of retained secretions. • Disposal method helps to contain microorganisms.
(3) Prepare equipment:	
(a) Open sterile tracheostomy kit. Open two 4 × 4 inch gauze packages using aseptic technique, and pour normal saline (NS) on one package. Leave the second package dry. Open two packages of cotton-tipped swabs and pour NS on one package. Do not recap NS.	• Preparation and organization of equipment allow for efficient tracheostomy care and reconnecting of the patient to an oxygen source in a timely manner.
(b) Open sterile tracheostomy dressing package.	
(c) Unwrap sterile basin and pour approximately 2 cm (1 in) of NS into it.	
(d) Open small sterile brush package and place aseptically into sterile basin.	
(e) Prepare length of twill tape long enough to go around patient's neck two times, approximately 60–75 cm (20–25 in) for an adult. Cut ends on diagonal. Lay aside in dry area.	• Cutting ends of tie on diagonal aids in inserting tie through eyelet.
(f) If using commercially available tracheostomy tube holder, open package according to manufacturer's directions.	
(4) Remove oxygen source if present. Pre-oxygenate for a minimum of 30 seconds by asking patient to take five to six deep breaths or use a manual resuscitation bag connected to 100% oxygen. Apply oxygen source loosely over tracheostomy if patient desaturates during procedure.	• Replenishes oxygen lost during suctioning (AARC, 2010).
(5) Apply sterile gloves. Keep dominant hand sterile throughout procedure.	• Reduces transmission of microorganisms.

CRITICAL DECISION POINT: *For tracheostomy tube with no inner cannula or Kistner button, continue with Step B(8).*

STEPS	RATIONALE
(6) If a nondisposable inner cannula is used:	
(a) While touching only the outer aspect of the tube, unlock and remove inner cannula with nondominant hand. Drop inner cannula into NS basin.	• Removes inner cannula for cleaning. NS loosens secretions from inner cannula.
(b) Place tracheostomy collar or T tube and ventilator oxygen source over or near outer cannula. (*Note:* T tube and ventilator oxygen devices cannot be attached to all outer cannulas when inner cannula is removed.)	• Maintains supply of oxygen to patient.
(c) To prevent oxygen desaturation in affected patients, quickly pick up inner cannula and use small brush to remove secretions inside and outside cannula (see Step 6B[6][c] illustration).	• Tracheostomy brush provides mechanical force to remove thick or dried secretions.
(d) Hold inner cannula over basin and rinse with NS, using nondominant hand to pour NS.	• Removes secretions from inner cannula.

STEPS	RATIONALE
(e) Replace inner cannula and secure "locking" mechanism (see Step 6B[6][e] illustration). Reapply ventilator or oxygen sources.	• Secures inner cannula and re-establishes oxygen supply.

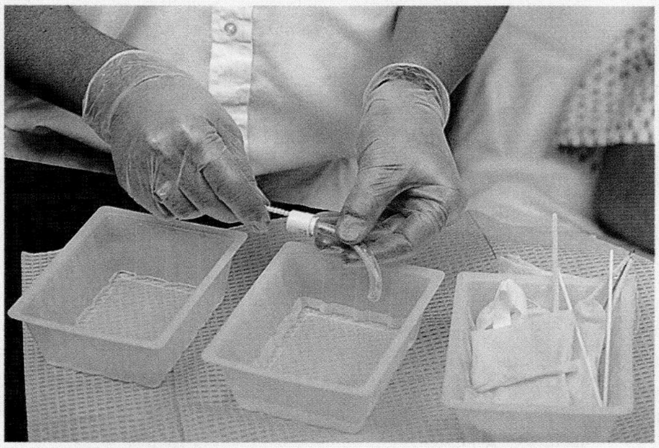

STEP 6B(6)(c) Cleaning the tracheostomy inner cannula.

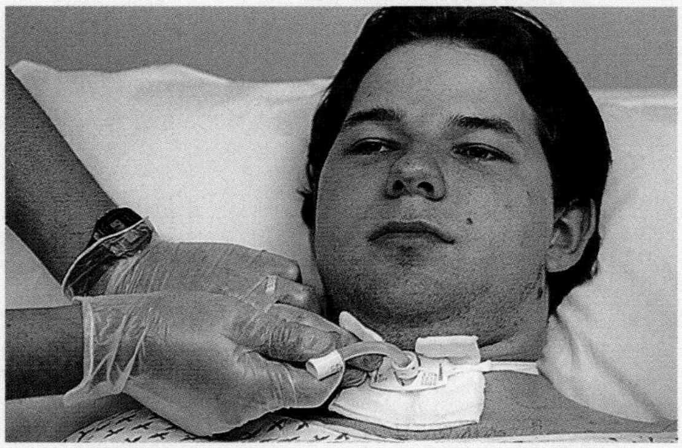

STEP 6B(6)(e) Reinserting the inner cannula.

STEPS	RATIONALE
(7) If a disposable inner cannula is used:	
(a) Remove cannula from manufacturer's packaging.	
(b) While touching only the outer aspect of the tube, withdraw inner cannula and replace with new cannula. Lock into position.	
(c) Dispose of contaminated cannula in appropriate receptacle and apply oxygen source.	• Prevents unnecessary oxygen desaturation.
(8) Using NS-saturated cotton-tipped swabs and 4 × 4 gauze, clean exposed outer cannula surfaces and stoma under faceplate, extending 5–10 cm (2–4 inches) in all directions from stoma (see Step 6B[8] illustration). Clean in circular motion from stoma site outward, using dominant hand to handle sterile supplies.	• Aseptically removes secretions from stoma site. Moving in outward circle pulls mucus and other contaminants from stoma to periphery.

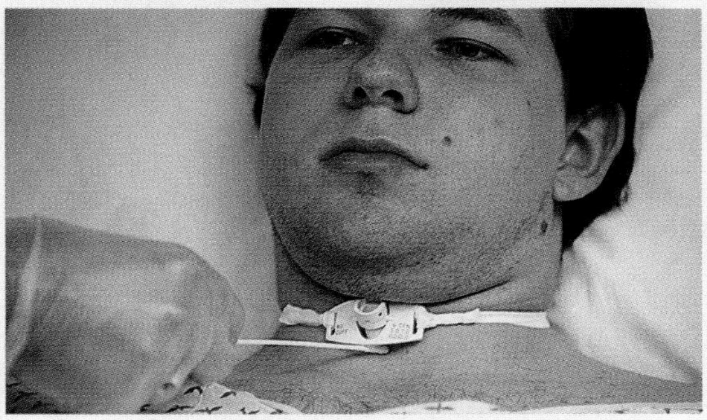

STEP 6B(8) Cleaning around stoma

STEPS	RATIONALE
(9) Using NS-prepared cotton-tipped swabs and 4 × 4 gauze, clean outer tracheostomy tube flange and skin surfaces. Using dry 4 × 4 gauze, pat lightly at skin and exposed outer cannula surfaces.	• Dry surfaces prevent formation of moist environment conducive to growth of microorganisms and prevent skin excoriation.
(10) Secure tracheostomy.	
(a) *Tracheostomy tie method:*	
(a1) Instruct assistant to apply gloves and hold tracheostomy tube securely in place while ties are cut.	• Promotes hygiene, reduces transmission of microorganisms, and secures tracheostomy tube.

CRITICAL DECISION POINT: *Assistant must not release hold on tracheostomy tube until new ties are firmly tied, to reduce risk of accidental extubation. If no assistant is present, do not cut old ties until new ties are in place and securely tied.*

Continued

SKILL 39-2 CARE OF AN ARTIFICIAL AIRWAY—cont'd

STEPS	RATIONALE
(a2) Take prepared tie and insert one end of tie through faceplate eyelet, and pull ends even (see Step 6B[10][a2] illustration).	

CRITICAL DECISION POINT: *Tracheostomy obturator should be kept at bedside with a fresh tracheostomy to facilitate reinsertion of the outer cannula, if dislodged. An additional tracheostomy tube of the same size and kind should be kept on hand for emergency replacement (Morse, Whitmer, & McIntosh, 2013).*

STEPS	RATIONALE
(a3) Slide both ends of tie behind head and around neck to other eyelet, and insert one tie through second eyelet.	
(a4) Pull snugly.	• Secures tracheostomy tube in place.
(a5) Tie ends securely in double square knot, allowing space for only one loose or two snug fingerwidths in tie.	• One-finger slack prevents ties from being too tight when tracheostomy dressing is in place and prevents movement of tracheostomy tube into lower airway.
(a6) Insert fresh tracheostomy dressing under clean ties and faceplate (see Step 6B[10][a6] illustration).	• Absorbs drainage. Dressing prevents pressure on clavicle heads.

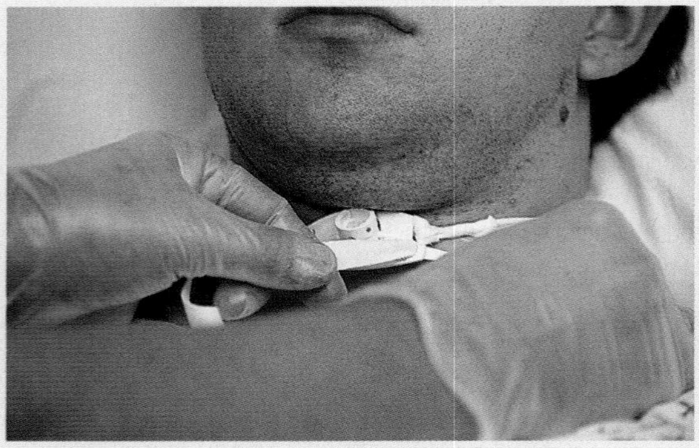

STEP 6B(10)(a2) Replacing tracheostomy ties when an assistant is not available. Do not remove old tracheostomy ties until new ones are secure.

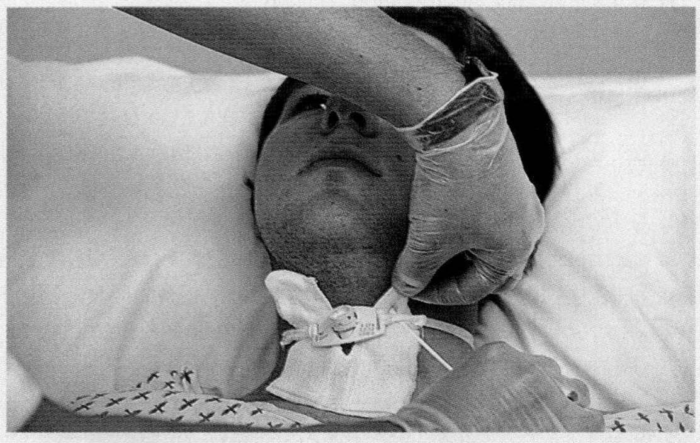

STEP 6B(10)(a6) Applying tracheostomy dressing.

STEPS	RATIONALE
(b) *Tracheostomy tube holder method:*	
(b1) While wearing gloves, maintain secure hold on tracheostomy tube. This can be done with an assistant, or, when an assistant is not available, by leaving the old tracheostomy tube holder in place until new device is secure.	• Prevents accidental displacement of tube.
(b2) Align strap under patient's neck. Ensure that Velcro attachments are positioned on either side of tracheostomy tube.	
(b3) Place narrow end of ties under and through faceplate eyelets. Pull ends even, and secure with Velcro closures.	
(b4) Verify that there is space for only one loose or two snug fingerwidth(s) under neck strap. Insert fresh tracheostomy dressing under clean ties and faceplate.	
7. Position patient comfortably and assess respiratory status.	• Promotes comfort. Some patients may require post-tracheostomy care suctioning.
8. Replace any oxygen delivery devices.	• Maintains oxygen therapy.
9. Remove and discard gloves and face shield. Replace cap on NS. Perform hand hygiene.	• Reduces transmission of infection. Once opened, NS can be considered free of bacteria for 24 hours, after which it should be discarded.
10. Compare respiratory assessments before and after procedure.	• Identifies any changes in presence and quality of breath sounds after procedure.
11. Observe depth and position of tubes.	• Verifies that position of tube is correct.
12. Assess security of tape or commercial ET or tracheostomy tube holder by tugging at tube.	• Artificial airway should not move. Patient may cough.
13. Assess skin around mouth and oral mucosa (ET tube) and tracheostomy stoma for drainage, pressure, and signs of irritation.	• Skin breakdown or irritation should not be present.

STEPS	RATIONALE

UNEXPECTED OUTCOMES	RELATED INTERVENTIONS
Accidental extubation of ET tube	• Call for assistance. • Assist respirations with bag mask as needed. • Assess patient for airway patency, spontaneous breathing, and vital signs. • Prepare for re-intubation.
Accidental decannulation of tracheostomy tube	• Call for assistance while remaining with patient. • Replace old tracheostomy tube with new spare tube of same size and kind kept at bedside. • Prepare to manually ventilate patient who develops respiratory distress.
Breath sounds not equal bilaterally with ET tube in place	• Evaluate ET tube for proper depth. If incorrect, arrange for ET tube to be repositioned as allowed by institution. • Obtain order for chest X-ray study to verify placement, if applicable.
Hard, reddened areas with or without excessive or foul-smelling secretions	• This indicates infection. Notify physician. • Increase frequency of tube care. • Remove inner cannula, if applicable, for cleaning and suctioning.
Insecure tube, artificial airway moves in or out, coughed out by patient	• Assess patient's respiratory status and observe for the presence of mucus plugs. • Adjust or apply new ties.
Breakdown, pressure areas, or stomatitis (tracheostomy tube)	• Increase frequency of tube care. • Make sure skin areas are clean and dry.

RECORDING AND REPORTING

- Record respiratory assessments before and after care.
- Record ET tube care: depth of ET tube, frequency and extent of care, patient tolerance, and any complications related to presence of the tube.
- Record tracheostomy care: type and size of tracheostomy tube, frequency and extent of care, patient tolerance, and any complications related to presence of the tube.

HOME CARE CONSIDERATIONS (TRACHEOSTOMY ONLY)

- Instruct caregivers on how to obtain supplies.
- Instruct caregivers on signs and symptoms of respiratory distress, tube dysfunction, and respiratory and stoma infections.
- At home, clean technique is used with nonsterile gloves, and routine tracheostomy care should be done at least once a day after discharge from hospital.

lung expansion and reduce pressure from the abdomen on the diaphragm. When the patient is in this position, the nurse needs to ensure that the patient does not slide down in bed, which could reduce lung expansion. A patient with unilateral lung disease (e.g., pneumothorax, atelectasis, pneumonia, thoracotomy, multiple trauma affecting one lung) should be positioned with the unaffected lung down ("good lung down"). This promotes better perfusion of the healthy lung, improving oxygenation. In the presence of pulmonary abscess or hemorrhage, the patient should be placed with the affected lung down to prevent drainage toward the unaffected (healthy) lung.

Incentive Spirometry. Incentive spirometry is a method of encouraging voluntary deep breathing by providing visual feedback to patients about inspiratory volume. Incentive spirometry is used to promote deep breathing and to prevent or treat atelectasis in the postoperative patient. The use of an incentive spirometer to promote lung expansion and thus prevent postoperative pulmonary complications following abdominal surgery is supported by research (AARC, 2011; Cassidy, Rosenkranz, McCabe, et al., 2013).

Flow-oriented incentive spirometers consist of one or more plastic chambers containing freely moving coloured balls. The patient inhales slowly and with an even flow to elevate the balls and keep them floating as long as possible to ensure a maximally sustained inhalation. Volume-oriented incentive spirometry devices have a bellows that is raised to a predetermined volume by an inhaled breath (Figure 39-13). An achievement light or counter is used to provide feedback.

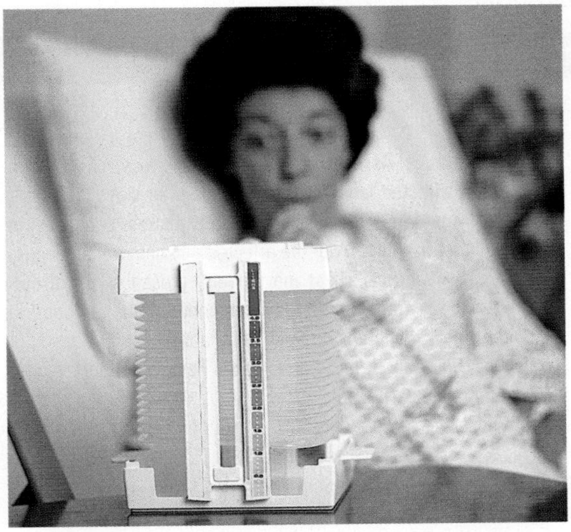

FIGURE 39-13 Volume-oriented spirometer.

The aim of incentive spirometry is to encourage patients to breathe to their normal inspiratory capacities. A postoperative inspiratory capacity one-half to three-fourths of the preoperative volume is acceptable because of postoperative pain. Administration of pain medications before incentive spirometry will help the patient achieve deep breathing by reducing pain and splinting (see Chapter 48). The AARC Guidelines (AARC, 2011) recommend 5–10 breaths per session every hour while the patient is awake.

Chest Tubes. Chest tubes are inserted to remove air and fluids from the pleural space, prevent air or fluid from re-entering the pleural space, and re-establish normal intrapleural and intrapulmonic pressures. A chest tube is a catheter inserted through the thorax to remove fluid or air. There are a variety of chest drainage systems on the market. In addition to the usual disposable waterless system, the mobile chest drain may be used. Mobile systems rely on gravity, not suction, for drainage. In specific patients, these mobile drains reduce the length of time needed for the chest tube, improve ambulation, and decrease the length of time spent in the hospital (Carroll, 2017). Mobile chest drains are lighter and smaller, thus the patient is able to move more easily, reducing the risk for deep vein thrombosis and pulmonary embolism.

Chest tubes are commonly used after chest surgery and chest trauma and for pneumothorax or hemothorax to promote lung re-expansion (Skill 39-3).

A pneumothorax is a collection of air in the pleural space. The loss of negative intrapleural pressure causes the lung to collapse. There are a variety of mechanisms that are associated with a pneumothorax. It may occur spontaneously or as a result of chest trauma, such as a stabbing or the chest striking the steering wheel in a motor vehicle accident. A pneumothorax may also result from the rupture of an emphysematous bleb on the surface of the lung (a large bulla resulting from the destruction caused by emphysema) or from an invasive procedure, such as insertion of a subclavian IV line.

A patient with a pneumothorax usually feels pain as atmospheric air irritates the parietal pleura. The pain may be sharp and pleuritic. Dyspnea is common and worsens as the size of the pneumothorax increases.

SKILL 39-3 CARE OF PATIENTS WITH CHEST TUBES

Delegation Considerations

This skill should not be delegated to an unregulated care provider (UCP). However, a UCP may assist with other aspects of the patient's care. It is important to inform the UCP of the following:

- Proper positioning of the patient with chest tubes to facilitate chest tube drainage and optimal function of the system
- How to ambulate and transfer a patient with chest drainage
- To report to the nurse any changes in vital signs, including oxygen saturation, chest pain, sudden shortness of breath, or excessive bubbling in the water-seal chamber
- To immediately report to the nurse a disconnection of the system, any change in type and amount of drainage, sudden bleeding, or sudden cessation of bubbling

Equipment

- Disposable chest drainage system (see Figure 39-14)
- Suction source and set-up (wall canister or portable)
- Disposable (nonsterile) gloves
- 5-cm tape
- Sterile gauze sponges
- Two shodded hemostats
- Stethoscope
- Pulse oximeter

PROCEDURE

STEPS	RATIONALE
1. Perform hand hygiene and assess patient.	
A. Pulmonary status: Assess for respiratory distress, chest pain, breath sounds over affected lung area, and stable vital signs (see Chapter 30). Signs and symptoms of increased respiratory distress or chest pain include decreased breath sounds over the affected and nonaffected lungs, marked cyanosis, asymmetrical chest movements, presence of **subcutaneous emphysema** (air trapped in the subcutaneous tissue) around tube insertion site or neck, hypotension, and tachycardia.	• Signs and symptoms should reflect improvement in respiratory distress and chest pain after insertion of chest tube. • Notify physician immediately.
B. Vital signs, SpO_2, and level of orientation. Review patient's current hemoglobin and hematocrit levels.	• Changes in pulse and blood pressure may indicate infection, respiratory distress, or pain. Reflects blood loss and subsequent levels of oxygenation.
C. Pain: If possible, ask patient to rate level of pain on a scale of 0 to 10.	• Chest tubes can be painful and interfere with a patient's mobility, coughing and deep breathing, and rehabilitation.
2. Observe:	
A. Chest tube dressing and site surrounding tube insertion.	• Ensures that dressing is intact and occlusive seal remains without air or fluid leaks and that area surrounding insertion site is free of drainage or skin irritation.
B. Tubing for kinks, dependent loops, or clots.	• Maintains a patent, freely draining system, preventing fluid accumulation in the chest cavity. Presence of kinks, dependent loops, or clotted drainage increases the risk for infection, atelectasis, and tension pneumothorax (Carroll, 2017).
C. Chest drainage system, which should be upright and below level of tube insertion.	• Facilitates drainage; the system must be in this position to function properly.

STEPS	RATIONALE
3. Provide two shodded hemostats or approved clamps for each chest tube, attached to the top of patient's bed with adhesive tape. Chest tubes are clamped only under specific circumstances per prescriber's order or nursing policy and procedure:	• Shodded hemostats have a covering to prevent hemostat from penetrating the chest tube once changed. The use of these shodded hemostats or other clamp prevents air from re-entering the pleural space (Bauman & Handley, 2011).
A. To assess air leak.	
B. To quickly empty or change disposable systems; performed by a nurse who has received education in the procedure.	
C. To assess if patient is ready to have the chest tube removed (which is done by prescriber's order); monitor the patient for recurrent pneumothorax.	
4. Position patient.	• Permits optimal drainage of fluid and air.
A. Semi-Fowler's to high-Fowler's position to evacuate air (pneumothorax).	• Air rises to the highest point in the chest. Pneumothorax tubes are usually placed on the anterior aspect at the midclavicular line, second or third intercostal space.
B. High-Fowler's position to drain fluid (hemothorax, effusion).	• Permits optimal drainage of fluid. Posterior tubes are placed on the midaxillary line, eighth or ninth intercostal space.
5. Maintain tube connection between chest and drainage tubes; ensure that it is intact and secured. Check patency of air vents in system:	• Secures chest tube to drainage system and reduces risk of air leak causing breaks in airtight system.
A. Water-sealed vent must be without occlusion.	• Permits displaced air to pass into atmosphere.
B. Suction-control chamber vent must be without occlusion when suction is used.	• Provides safety factor of releasing excess negative pressure into the atmosphere. Too little suction prevents lung re-expansion and increases patient risk for infection, atelectasis, and tension pneumothorax. Too much suction damages the lung tissue and perpetuates existing air leaks.
C. Confirm that valves are unobstructed. Waterless systems have relief valves without caps. For dry suction systems, the positive pressure relief valve must remain unobstructed.	• Provides safety factor of releasing excess negative pressure.
6. Coil excess drainage tubing on mattress or chair. Secure with rubber band, safety pin, or plastic clamp. Allow enough space for patient to reposition.	• The length of tubing should be tailored to each patient to avoid excessive coiling or loop formation. Fluid collection in the loop may occlude system (Carroll, 2017).
7. Adjust tubing to hang in a straight line from top of mattress to drainage chamber. If chest tube is draining fluid, indicate time (e.g., 0900) on drainage system with adhesive tape or write-on surface of disposable commercial system.	• Provides a baseline for continuous assessment of type and quality of drainage.

CRITICAL DECISION POINT: *Check institutional policy before stripping or milking chest tubes. This practice is being discontinued at most institutions because it is believed that stripping the tube greatly increases intrathoracic pressure, which damages the pleural tissue and causes or worsens an existing pneumothorax. Although the literature is contradictory, milking may be done in selected patients (e.g., fresh postoperative thoracic surgery in presence of multiple clots). There is evidence that milking is associated with a significant increase of pleural fluid drainage; however, it does not improve postoperative morbidity and mortality and therefore cannot be recommended as a* routine *postoperative procedure (Dango, Sienel, Passlick, et al., 2010).*

STEPS	RATIONALE
8. Perform hand hygiene.	• Reduces transmission of infection.
9. Evaluate:	
A. Vital signs and pulse oximetry as ordered or if patient's condition changes.	• Provides ongoing data about the patient's level of oxygenation.
B. Chest tube dressing.	• Appearance of drainage may be due to tube occlusion, causing drainage to exit around tube.

CRITICAL DECISION POINT: *Check the dressing carefully because it must remain occlusive. It can come loose from the skin, although this may not be readily apparent. Follow hospital policy as needed to maintain seal.*

STEPS	RATIONALE
C. Tubing: It should be free of kinks and dependent loops.	• Straight and coiled drainage tube positions are optimal for pleural drainage. However, when a dependent loop is unavoidable, periodic lifting and drainage of the tube will promote pleural drainage.
D. Chest drainage system: It should be upright and below level of tube insertion. Note presence of clots or debris in tubing.	• The system must be in the upright position to function and facilitate proper drainage.
E. Water seal for fluctuations with patient's inspiration and expiration.	

Continued

SKILL 39-3 CARE OF PATIENTS WITH CHEST TUBES—cont'd

STEPS	RATIONALE
(1) Waterless system: Diagnostic indicator for fluctuations for patient's inspirations and expirations.	• In a nonmechanically ventilated patient, fluid should rise in the water seal or diagnostic indicator with inspiration and fall with expiration. The opposite occurs in a patient who is mechanically ventilated. This indicates the system is properly functioning.
(2) Water-seal system: Bubbling in the water-seal chamber.	• When system is initially connected to patient, bubbles are expected from the chamber. These are from air that was present in the system and in the patient's intrapleural space. After a short time, the bubbling stops. Fluid will continue to fluctuate in the water seal on inspiration and expiration until the lung is re-expanded or the system becomes occluded.
(3) Water-seal system: Bubbling in the suction-control chamber (when using suction).	• The suction-control chamber has constant gentle bubbling. Tubing remains free of obstruction and the suction source is turned to the appropriate setting.
F. Waterless system: Bubbling in diagnostic indicator.	• Mechanism to observe for the presence of tidalling.
G. Waterless system: The suction control (float ball) indicates the amount of suction that the patient's intrapleural space is receiving.	• The suction float ball dictates the amount of suction in the system. The float ball allows no more suction than allowed by its setting. If the suction source is set too low, the suction float ball cannot reach the prescribed setting. In this case, the suction must be increased for the float ball to reach the prescribed setting.
H. Type and amount of fluid drainage: Note colour and amount of drainage, patient's vital signs, and skin colour. Assess the fluid in the collection tubing, not just the drainage in the collection chamber. The normal amount of drainage is as follows:	
(1) In the adult: <50–200 mL/hour immediately after surgery in a mediastinal chest tube; approximately 500 mL in first 24 hours.	• A **mediastinal chest tube** is commonly used following open heart surgery. It is inserted in the mediastinum (below the sternum) and is connected to a drainage system. This tube drains blood or fluid, thus preventing accumulation around the heart. Dark-red drainage is expected only in the postoperative period, turning serous with time.
(2) In the adult: Between 100 and 300 mL of fluid may drain in a pleural chest tube in an adult during the first 3 hours after insertion. The 24-hour rate is 500–1000 mL. Drainage is grossly bloody during the first several hours after surgery and then changes to serous. Remember that a sudden gush of drainage may be retained blood and not active bleeding. This increase in drainage can result from patient position changes.	• Re-expansion of lungs forces drainage into the tube. Coughing can also cause large gushes of drainage or air. Acute bleeding indicates hemorrhage.

CRITICAL DECISION POINT: *Inform the health care provider, remain with the patient, and assess vital signs and cardiopulmonary status if drainage suddenly increases, is bright red, or if there is >100 mL/hour of bloody drainage (except for the first 3 hours postoperative). This may indicate hemorrhage or perforation of the lung.*

STEPS	RATIONALE
I. Observe patient for decreased respiratory distress and chest pain, auscultate lung sounds over affected area, and monitor SpO_2.	• An increase in respiratory distress and/or chest pain, decrease in breath sounds over affected and unaffected lungs, cyanosis, asymmetrical chest movements, subcutaneous emphysema around the insertion site or neck, hypotension, tachycardia, and/or a mediastinal shift are critical and indicate a change in patient status (e.g., excessive blood loss, tension pneumothorax). This must be reported immediately to the patient's health care provider.
J. Pain: Ask patient to evaluate pain on a level of 0 to 10.	• May indicate the need for medication for pain.

UNEXPECTED OUTCOMES	RELATED INTERVENTIONS
Continuous bubbling in water-sealed chamber	• This indicates a leak between the patient and water seal. • Assess all connections between the patient and drainage system, and tighten any loose connections. • Check institution policy, and if instructed, cross-clamp chest tube close to patient's chest. If bubbling stops, air leak is inside patient's thorax or at chest tube insertion site. Unclamp tube, and notify health care provider immediately. Reinforce chest dressing. Leaving a chest tube clamped causes a tension pneumothorax and mediastinal shift.
Chest tube is dislodged	• Immediately apply pressure over chest tube insertion site. • Have assistant apply occlusive gauze dressing and tape three sides. • Notify health care provider.

STEPS	RATIONALE
Tension pneumothorax	• Determine that chest tubes are not clamped, kinked, or occluded. Obstructed chest tubes trap air in the intrapleural space when an air leak originates within the patient. • Notify health care provider immediately. • Prepare immediately for another chest tube insertion; obtain a flutter (Heimlich) valve or large-gauge needle for short-term emergency release of air in the intrapleural space. Have emergency equipment (e.g., oxygen, code cart) near patient.
Substantial increase in bright red drainage	• Obtain vital signs and monitor drainage. • Assess patient's cardiopulmonary status and notify health care provider.
Sudden cessation of chest tube drainage	• Observe for kink and possible clot in the chest drainage system. • Assess for mediastinal shift or respiratory distress (medical emergency) and notify health care provider.

RECORDING AND REPORTING

- Record in patient care record the patency of chest tube; presence, type, and amount of drainage; presence of fluctuations; patient's vital signs; chest dressing status; amount of suction and water seal; and level of comfort.

HOME CARE CONSIDERATIONS

- Patients with chronic conditions (e.g., uncomplicated pneumothorax, effusions, empyema) that require a chest tube may be discharged home with smaller mobile chest drains. These systems do not have a suction-control chamber and use a mechanical one-way valve instead of a water-seal chamber.
- Instruct patient in how to ambulate and remain active with a home chest tube drainage system.
- Provide patient with information on when to contact health care providers regarding changes in drainage system (e.g., chest pain, breathlessness, change in drainage).

A **hemothorax** is an accumulation of blood and fluid in the pleural cavity between the parietal and visceral pleurae, usually as a result of trauma. It produces a counterpressure and prevents the lung from full expansion. A hemothorax can also be caused by the rupture of small blood vessels from inflammatory processes, such as pneumonia or TB. In addition to pain and dyspnea, signs and symptoms of shock can develop if blood loss is severe.

Disposable systems, such as an Atrium or Pleur-Evac chest drainage system, are one-piece moulded plastic units that provide for a single- or multiple-chamber closed drainage system (Figure 39-14). A single-chamber system allows air from a pneumothorax to bubble out of the water seal and escape through the air outlet, preventing air from re-entering the intrapleural space (Perry, Potter, & Ostendorf, 2014). A two- or three-chamber system drains both a hemothorax and a pneumothorax. The two-chamber system allows fluid to flow into a collection chamber and air to flow into the water seal chamber (Perry et al., 2014). A three-chamber system permits the drainage of fluid and air through controlled suction (Perry et al., 2014). The two- and three-chamber systems have two compartments—one for fluid or blood and a second for a water seal or a one-way valve (Perry et al., 2014). The three-chamber system has a third compartment for suction control, which may or may not be used (Perry et al., 2014).

There are two types of commercial drainage devices: water-seal and waterless systems. Although the principles of the waterless system are similar to those of the water-seal system, there are structural differences. The waterless system does not require fluid for setup, and the water seal is replaced by a one-way valve (Perry et al., 2014). The suction chamber, which does not depend on water, contains a float ball that is set by a control dial after the suction source is initiated (Perry et al., 2014). Dry suction chest drainage systems (see Figure 39-14) provide higher suction pressure levels. A self-compensating regulator controls dry suction units, and a dial is set to the prescribed suction

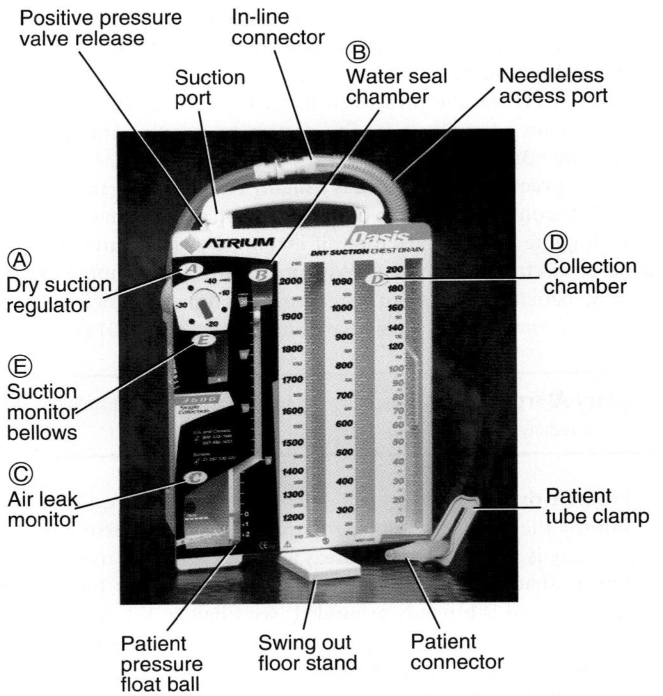

FIGURE 39-14 Dry suction chest drainage system. (Courtesy Atrium Medical Corp. From Perry, A. G., Potter, P. A., & Ostendorf, W.R. [2014]. *Clinical nursing skills & techniques* [8th ed., p. 661, Fig. 26-9]. St. Louis, MO: Mosby.)

control setting (Perry et al., 2014). Pressure is set between −10 cm H_2O and −40 cm H_2O.

Special considerations. Clamping a chest tube is only done under specific circumstances (see Skill 39-3) and is determined by a prescriber's orders or institution policy. The chest drainage unit must be handled carefully and the drainage device maintained below the patient's chest. If the tubing disconnects from the drainage unit, the patient is instructed to exhale as much as possible and to cough. This manoeuvre rids the pleural space of as much air as possible. The care provider needs to cleanse the tips of the tubing and reconnect them quickly. If the drainage unit is broken, the end of the chest tube can be quickly submerged in a container of sterile water to re-establish the seal. Clamping the chest tube may result in a tension pneumothorax. Air pressure builds in the pleural space, collapsing the lung and creating a life-threatening event.

Removal of chest tubes requires patient preparation. This includes administering pain medication 30 minutes prior to removal. Patients report various sensations during chest tube removal. The most frequent sensations include burning, pain, and a pulling sensation.

Maintenance and Promotion of Oxygenation. Promotion of lung expansion and of mobilizing secretions and maintaining a patent airway assists the patient in meeting oxygenation needs. Some patients, however, also require oxygen therapy to keep a healthy level of tissue oxygenation.

Oxygen Therapy. Oxygen therapy is widely available and used in a variety of settings to relieve or prevent tissue hypoxia. Any patient with impaired tissue oxygenation can benefit from controlled oxygen administration. Oxygen is not a substitute for other treatment, however, and should be used only when indicated. Oxygen should be treated as a drug. It has dangerous side effects, such as atelectasis or oxygen toxicity (Heuer & Scanlan, 2009). As with any drug, the dosage or concentration of oxygen should be continuously monitored. The nurse needs to routinely check the prescriber's orders to verify that the patient is receiving the prescribed oxygen concentration. The rights of medication administration also pertain to oxygen administration (see Chapter 34).

Safety precautions. Oxygen is a highly combustible gas. Although it will not spontaneously burn or cause an explosion, it can easily cause a fire to ignite in a patient's room if it contacts a spark from an open flame or electrical equipment. With increasing use of home oxygen therapy, patients and health care providers must be aware of the dangers of combustion (Kassis, Savetamal, Assis, et al., 2014).

> **Safety Alert** Oxygen in high concentrations has a great combustion potential and readily fuels fire.

Promote oxygen safety by using the following measures:

- Inform the patient, visitors, roommates, and all personnel that smoking is not permitted in areas where oxygen is in use.
- Ensure that all electrical equipment in the room is functioning correctly and is properly grounded (see Chapter 37). An electrical spark in the presence of oxygen can result in a serious fire.
- Locate the closest fire extinguisher.
- Know the fire procedures and the evacuation route for the area.
- Check the oxygen level of portable tanks before transporting a patient, to ensure that enough oxygen in the tank exists to complete the transport.

Supply of Oxygen. Oxygen is supplied to the patient's bedside either by oxygen tanks or through a permanent wall-piped system. Oxygen tanks are transported on wide-based carriers that allow the tank to be placed upright at the bedside. Regulators are used to control the amount of oxygen delivered. One common type is an upright flowmeter with a flow adjustment valve at the top. A second type is a cylinder indicator with a flow adjustment handle. In the home setting, oxygen therapy is also supplied in a variety of methods, including refillable cylinders.

In the hospital or home, oxygen tanks are delivered with the regulator in place. In the hospital, the respiratory care department usually connects the regulator to the oxygen source. Home care vendors are usually responsible for connecting the oxygen tank to the regulator for home use.

Methods of Oxygen Delivery. Oxygen delivery devices can be considered low-flow or high-flow systems. **Low-flow devices** such as nasal cannulas, simple face masks, and reservoir masks provide oxygen in concentrations that vary with the patient's respiratory pattern (Heuer & Scanlan, 2009). **High-flow devices** deliver oxygen rates above the normal inspiratory flow rate and thus provide a fixed FiO_2 (fraction of inspired oxygen) regardless of the patient's inspiratory flow and breathing pattern (Heuer & Scanlan, 2009). The Venturi mask is an example of a high-flow device.

Nasal cannula. A **nasal cannula** is a low-flow device used for oxygen delivery (Skill 39-4). The two nasal prongs, approximately 1.5 cm long, protrude from the centre of a disposable tube and are inserted into the nares (Figure 39-15). Oxygen is delivered via the cannulas with a flow rate of up to 6 L/minute. Flow rates greater than 4 L/minute are not often used because of the drying effect on the mucosa and the relatively little increase in delivered oxygen concentration. If flow rates are greater than 4L/minute, humidification is required (AARC, 2007). It is important to know what flow rate produces a given percentage of inspired oxygen concentration (FiO_2; Table 39-9). Nurses must also be alert for skin breakdown over the ears and in the nares from too tight an application of the nasal cannula.

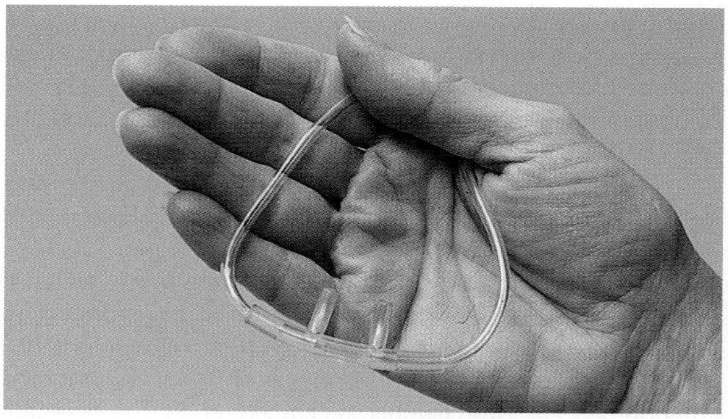

FIGURE 39-15 Nasal cannula.

TABLE 39-9 Approximate FiO_2 With Different Oxygen Delivery Devices

Oxygen Delivery Device	Required Litre Flow (L/minute)	Approximate Percent Oxygen
Nasal cannula	1–2	24–28
	3–4	32–36
	5–6	40–44
Simple face mask	5–6	40
	6–7	50
	7–8	60
Venturi mask	4	24–28
	8	35–40
	12	50–60

SKILL 39-4 APPLYING A NASAL CANNULA OR OXYGEN MASK

Delegation Considerations

This skill cannot be delegated to an unregulated care provider (UCP). The nurse is responsible for assessing the patient and providing safe and accurate oxygen therapy, including adjustment of oxygen flow rate and evaluation of patient response. It is important to instruct the UCP about the following:

- Correct placement and adjustment of delivery device
- The type of equipment and the oxygen flow rate
- Unexpected outcomes associated with the oxygen delivery device (e.g., increased rate of breathing, decreased level of consciousness, increased confusion, pain, changes in vital signs) and the need to inform the nurse if any of these outcomes occur

Equipment

- Oxygen delivery device (e.g., nasal cannula or oxygen mask)
- Oxygen tubing
- Humidifier, if indicated
- Sterile water for humidification, if indicated
- Oxygen source
- Oxygen flowmeter
- Appropriate room signs

PROCEDURE

STEPS	RATIONALE
1. Inspect patient for signs and symptoms associated with hypoxia and presence of airway secretions.	• Left untreated, hypoxia can produce cardiac dysrhythmias and death. Presence of airway secretions decreases the effectiveness of oxygen delivery.

CRITICAL DECISION POINT: *Patients with sudden changes in their vital signs, level of consciousness, or behaviour may be experiencing profound hypoxia. Patients who demonstrate subtle changes over time may have worsening of a chronic or existing condition or have a new medical condition.*

STEPS	RATIONALE
2. Obtain patient's most recent SpO_2 or arterial blood gas (ABG) values. Review patient's medical record for the medical order for oxygen, noting delivery method, flow rate, and duration of oxygen therapy.	• Provides objective baseline data to use to compare outcome of oxygen therapy. Ensures safe and accurate oxygen administration.
3. Explain to the patient and family what the procedure entails and the purpose of oxygen therapy.	• Decreases patient's anxiety, which reduces oxygen consumption and increases patient cooperation.
4. Perform hand hygiene.	• Reduces transmission of infection.
5. Attach oxygen delivery device (e.g., nasal cannula, mask) to oxygen tubing and attach to humidified oxygen source adjusted to prescribed flow rate (see Step 5 illustration).	• Humidity prevents drying of nasal and oral mucous membranes and airway secretions. Ensures correct oxygen delivery.
6. Place tips of cannula into patient's nares, and adjust elastic headband or plastic slide until cannula or face mask fits snugly and comfortably (see Step 6 illustration).	• Directs flow of oxygen into patient's upper respiratory tract. Patient is more likely to keep device in place if it fits comfortably.

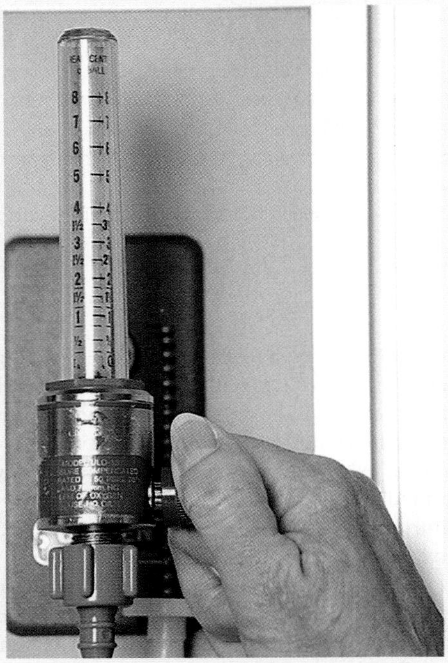

STEP 5 Adjusting flowmeter to prescribed oxygen flow rate.

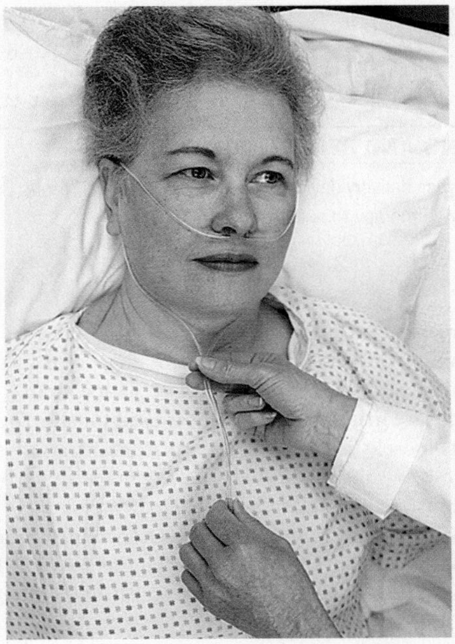

STEP 6 Adjusting nasal cannula to fit patient and ensure comfort.

Continued

SKILL 39-4 APPLYING A NASAL CANNULA OR OXYGEN MASK—cont'd

STEPS	RATIONALE
7. Maintain sufficient slack on oxygen tubing and secure to patient's clothes.	• Allows patient to turn head without dislodging nasal cannula or causing mask to shift position.
8. Observe for proper function of oxygen delivery device:	• Ensures patency of delivery device and accuracy of prescribed oxygen flow rate.
(a) Nasal cannula: Cannula is positioned properly in the nares.	• Provides prescribed oxygen rate and reduces pressure on tips of nares.
(b) Reservoir nasal cannula oxymizer: Fit as for nasal cannula. Reservoir is positioned under patient's nose or worn as a pendant.	• Oxygen-conserving cannula, indicated for long-term oxygen use.
(c) Nonrebreathing mask: Apply mask over patient's mouth and nose to form a tight seal. The valves on the mask close, so exhaled air does not enter reservoir bag.	• Does not allow exhaled air to be rebreathed. Valves on mask side ports permit exhalation but close during inhalation to prevent inhaling room air.
(d) Partial rebreathing mask: Apply mask over patient's mouth and nose to form a tight seal. Ensure that the bag remains partially inflated.	• Allows exhaled air to mix with inhaled air. Ports on the side of the mask permit most of the expired air to escape; however, the bag remains partially inflated.
(e) Venturi mask: Apply mask over patient's mouth and nose to form a tight seal. Select appropriate flow rate.	• Reduces buildup of carbon dioxide.
9. Check cannula/mask every 8 hours. Keep humidification container filled at all times.	• Ensures patency of cannula/mask and oxygen flow. Prevents inhalation of dehumidified oxygen.
10. Observe patient's nares and superior surface of both ears for skin breakdown.	• Oxygen therapy can cause drying of nasal mucosa. Pressure on ears from cannula tubing or elastic can cause skin irritation.
11. Perform hand hygiene.	• Reduces transmission of microorganisms.
12. Verify oxygen flow rate, proper setup, and prescriber's orders.	• Ensures delivery of prescribed oxygen flow rate and patency of cannula/mask.
13. Inspect patient for relief of symptoms associated with hypoxia.	• Indicates that hypoxia is corrected or reduced.

UNEXPECTED OUTCOMES	RELATED INTERVENTIONS
Worsening respiratory status	• Check that oxygen delivery device is patent, not kinked, and attached to the oxygen flowmeter. • Check oxygen level set on flowmeter; determine if delivered amount is consistent with prescriber's order. • If not using wall oxygen, determine if the oxygen source contains enough oxygen to deliver the prescribed oxygen amount. • Notify health care provider.
Dry nasal and upper airway mucosa	• If oxygen flow rate is >4 L/min, determine the need for humidification. • Assess the patient's fluid status and increase fluids if appropriate. • Provide frequent oral care. • Obtain prescriber's order for use of sterile nasal saline intermittently.
Skin breakdown over ears	• Adjust tightness of elastic strap as needed. • Use good hygiene and skin care around the ears. • Place soft, woven 4 × 4 gauze pads between elastic and ears. • Reposition elastic strap frequently.

RECORDING AND REPORTING

- Record oxygen delivery device and litre flow in medical record. Document patient and family education. Report oxygen delivery device, litre flow, and response to changes in therapy to oncoming shift.

Oxygen masks. An oxygen mask is a device used to administer oxygen, humidity, or heated humidity. It is shaped to fit snugly over the mouth and nose and is secured in place with a strap.

The simple face mask (Figure 39-16) is used for short-term oxygen therapy. It fits loosely and delivers oxygen concentrations from 40 to 60%. The mask is contraindicated for patients with carbon dioxide retention because retention can be worsened.

The partial rebreathing mask and the non-rebreathing mask are low-flow devices with a reservoir bag (Figure 39-17). The partial rebreather mask provides an oxygen concentration of 40 to 70% with a minimum flow rate of 10 L/minute (Heuer & Scanlan, 2009). The non-rebreather provides a high concentration of oxygen at 60 to 80% with a minimum flow rate of 10 L/minute (Heuer & Scanlan, 2009). Oxygen flows into the reservoir bag and mask during inhalation; one-way valves on the non-rebreather mask prevent expired air from flowing back into the bag. The nurse should frequently inspect the bag to make sure it is inflated. If it is deflated, the patient may be breathing large amounts of exhaled carbon dioxide. High-flow oxygen systems should be humidified (AARC, 2007).

The Venturi mask (Figure 39-18), a high-flow device, can be used to deliver oxygen concentrations of 24 to 60% with oxygen flow rates of 4 to 12 L/minute, depending on which flow-control meter is selected (see Table 39-9). This mask entrains room air to achieve a consistent and precise oxygen concentration. The Venturi mask is helpful for patients with COPD who require low, constant oxygen concentrations.

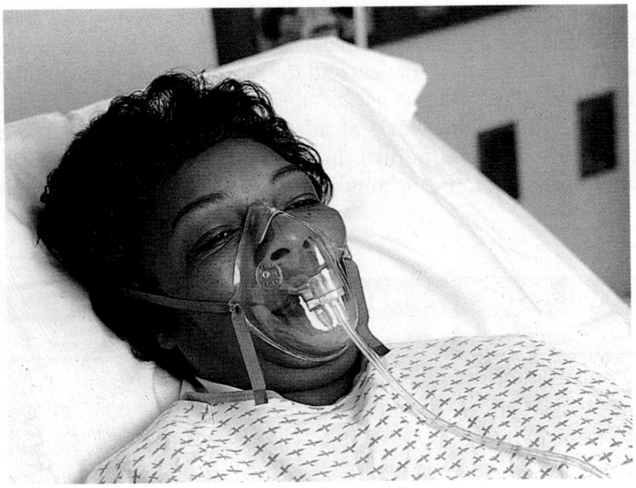

FIGURE 39-16 Simple face mask.

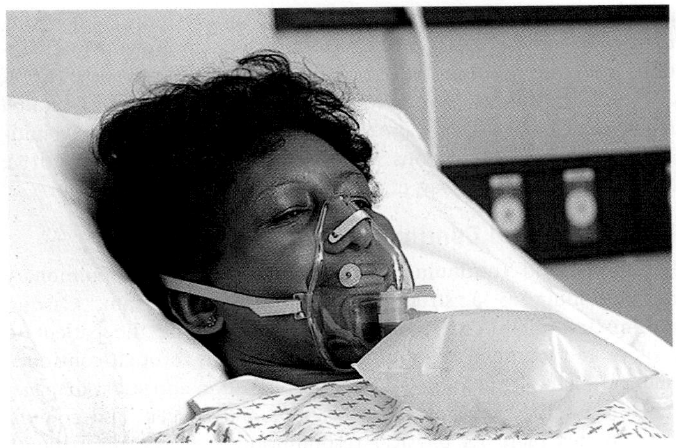

FIGURE 39-17 Plastic face mask with reservoir bag.

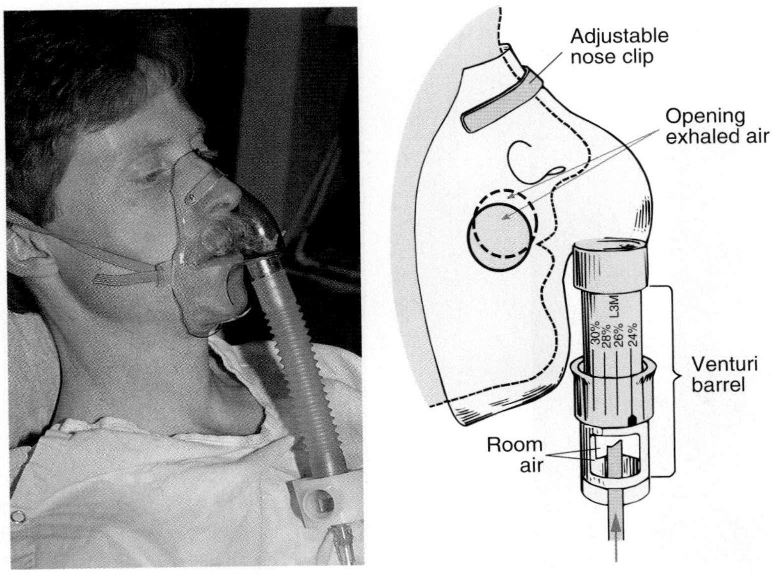

FIGURE 39-18 Venturi mask.

Home Oxygen Therapy. Indications for home oxygen therapy include a PaO_2 of 55 mm Hg or less or an SaO_2 of 88% or less on room air at rest, on exertion, or with exercise (Qaseem, Wilt, Weinberger, 2011). Home oxygen therapy has a beneficial effect for patients with chronic cardiopulmonary diseases. This therapy improves patients' exercise tolerance and fatigue levels and in some situations assists in the management of dyspnea. When home oxygen is required, it is usually delivered by nasal cannula. When a patient has a permanent tracheostomy, however, a T tube or tracheostomy collar is necessary (AARC, 2007). Three types of oxygen are used: compressed oxygen, liquid oxygen (Figure 39-19), and oxygen concentrators. The advantages and disadvantages (Table 39-10) of each type are assessed, along with the patient's needs and community resources, before placing a certain delivery system in the home. In the home, the major consideration is the oxygen delivery source.

Patients requiring home oxygen need extensive teaching to be able to continue oxygen therapy at home efficiently and safely (Skill 39-5). This includes oxygen safety, regulation of the amount of oxygen, and how to use the prescribed home oxygen delivery system. It is important to coordinate the efforts of the patient and family, home care nurse, home respiratory therapist, and home oxygen equipment vendor. The social worker usually assists with arranging for the home care nurse and oxygen vendor.

Restoration of Cardiopulmonary Functioning. If a patient's hypoxia is severe and prolonged, cardiac arrest may result. A *cardiac arrest* is a sudden cessation of cardiac output and circulation. When this occurs, oxygen is not delivered to tissues, carbon dioxide is not transported from tissues, tissue metabolism becomes anaerobic, and metabolic and respiratory acidosis occurs. Permanent heart, brain, and other tissue damage occurs within 4 to 6 minutes.

Cardiopulmonary Resuscitation. Cardiac arrest is characterized by an absence of pulse and respiration. When a patient has had a cardiac arrest, cardiopulmonary resuscitation (CPR) must be initiated. CPR is a basic emergency procedure of artificial respiration and manual external cardiac massage. Most nursing students are required to have successfully completed a CPR course before their clinical experiences.

Emphasis is placed on ensuring that high-quality CPR is performed (AHA, 2015c; 2017). Compressions must be provided at the appropriate rate and depth, the person administering CPR allowing for complete chest recoil after each compression, minimizing interruptions in compressions, and avoiding excessive ventilation (AHA, 2015c). The 2015 *American Heart Association Guidelines for CPR and Emergency Cardiovascular Care* reinforces the importance of early initiation of chest compressions and early defibrillation (AHA, 2015c; Neumar, Shuster, Callaway, et al., 2015).

Restorative and Continuing Care

Restorative and continuing care may emphasize cardiopulmonary reconditioning as a structured rehabilitation program. Cardiopulmonary rehabilitation involves actively helping the patient to achieve and maintain an optimal level of health through controlled physical exercise, nutrition counselling, relaxation and stress management techniques, prescribed medications and oxygen, and compliance to this plan. As physical reconditioning occurs, the patient's symptoms of dyspnea, chest pain, fatigue, and activity intolerance should decrease. The patient's anxiety, depression, or somatic concerns also often decrease. The patient and the rehabilitation team define the goals of rehabilitation.

Hydration. Maintenance of adequate systemic hydration keeps mucociliary clearance normal. In patients with adequate hydration, pulmonary secretions are thin, white, watery, and easily removable

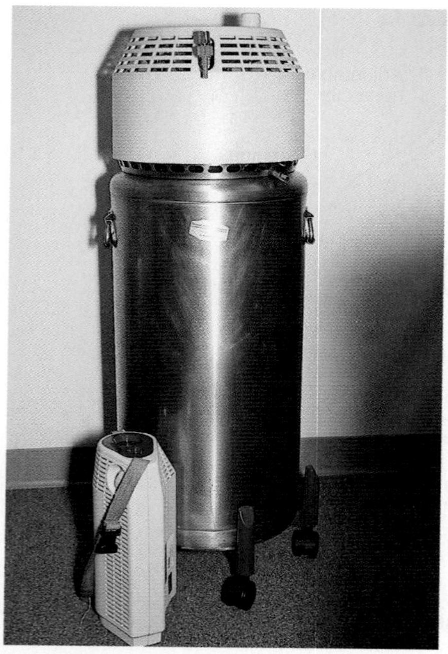

FIGURE 39-19 Primary and portable liquid oxygen source for ambulation.

TABLE 39-10 Home Oxygen Systems

Primary Use	Advantages	Disadvantages
Compressed Gas Cylinders		
Stationary and portable intermittent therapy; Used for exercise or sleep only	100% oxygen, relatively inexpensive, no loss of gas during storage, relatively portable, delivery of up to 15 L/min	Bulky, possibly unsightly, frequent refilling necessary with continuous use
Compressed Gas		
Small cylinder with compressed gas for easy portability	Allows from 1 to 5 hours of portable oxygen	Only lasts a few hours, E-cylinders not appropriate as sole source of oxygen
Liquid Oxygen Systems (see Figure 39-19)		
Used with active patients	100% oxygen, conveniently portable, portable units refilled at home, delivery of up to 6 L/min	Usually weekly delivery necessary for refill, evaporates if not used, potential for frostbite at connections and if liquid is spilled
Oxygen Concentrators		
Stationary system for patients requiring low-flow continuous oxygen and limited mobility	Provides large source of oxygen, inexpensive, delivery of 1–5 L/min, delivery up to 10 L/min with certain models	Oxygen concentration decreases as litre flow increases, power supply needed, electric bill increase, second system needed for portability

SKILL 39-5 USING HOME OXYGEN EQUIPMENT

Delegation Considerations

This skill should not be delegated to an unregulated care provider (UCP). However, once the patient is stable on home oxygen therapy, the UCP may perform certain aspects of care. The nurse is responsible for assessing the patient, checking the device setup, and providing safe and accurate oxygen therapy. The nurse must instruct the UCP about the following:

- Unique needs of the patient (e.g., home nasal cannula or mask) and any assistance needed in filling liquid canisters
- The type of equipment that the patient should have in the home and the oxygen flow rate
- Unexpected outcomes associated with the oxygen delivery device (e.g., increased rate of breathing, decreased level of consciousness, increased confusion, pain), and the need to inform the nurse if any occur

Equipment

- Nasal cannula, oxygen mask, or other prescribed delivery device (see Skill 39-4)
- Humidification device if oxygen delivery greater than 4 L/min
- Oxygen tubing
- Home oxygen delivery system with appropriate equipment
- "No Smoking/Oxygen in Use" sign for each entrance to home

PROCEDURE

STEPS	RATIONALE
1. While patient is in the hospital, determine patient's or family's ability to use oxygen equipment correctly. In the home setting, reassess for appropriate use of equipment.	• Physical or cognitive impairments of patient necessitate instructing a family member or significant other in how to operate home oxygen equipment. Ongoing assessment enables the nurse to determine specific components of skill that the patient or family easily complete.
2. Assess home environment for adequate electrical service if oxygen concentrator is used.	• Oxygen concentrators require electricity to work. Continuous oxygen therapy must not be interrupted.
3. Assess patient's and family's ability to observe for signs and symptoms of hypoxia.	• Hypoxia occurs at home despite use of oxygen therapy. Worsening of a patient's physical condition or another underlying condition, such as a change in respiratory status, can cause hypoxia.
4. Determine appropriate resources in the community for equipment and assistance, including maintenance and repair services, and medical equipment supplier.	• Ensure readily available assistance for patients with home oxygen systems.
5. In case of power failure, determine appropriate backup system when using a compressor. Have a spare oxygen tank available.	• Many municipalities require that patients with home oxygen equipment notify emergency medical services (EMS) before bringing the equipment home. When there is a power outage, EMS calls the home, and in some cases the home is on a priority list for having power restored.
6. Perform hand hygiene.	• Reduces transmission of infection.
7. Place oxygen delivery system in a clutter-free environment that is well ventilated; away from walls, drapes, bedding, combustible materials; and at least 2.4 meters (8 feet) from heat source.	• Prevents injury from improper placement of oxygen equipment.
8. Demonstrate steps for preparation and completion of oxygen therapy.	• Demonstration is a reliable technique for teaching psychomotor skills and encourages patient to ask questions.
A. Compressed oxygen system	
(1) Turn cylinder valve counterclockwise two to three turns with wrench. Store wrench with oxygen tank.	• Turns on oxygen. Keep wrench available.
(2) Check cylinders by reading amount on pressure gauge.	• Verifies adequate oxygen supply for patient use.
B. Oxygen concentrator system	
(1) Plug concentrator into appropriate outlet.	• Provides power source.
(2) Turn on power switch.	• Starts concentrator motor.
(3) Alarm will sound for a few seconds.	• Alarm turns off when desired pressure inside concentrator is reached.
C. Liquid oxygen system	
(1) Check liquid system by depressing button at lower right corner and reading the dial on the stationary oxygen reservoir or ambulatory tank.	• Verifies adequate oxygen supply.
(2) Collaborate with medical equipment provider to receive instruction on refilling ambulatory tank.	• Ambulatory tanks of liquid oxygen must be filled when empty.

CRITICAL DECISION POINT: *Fill ambulatory tanks only when they are empty. Liquid oxygen is stored at or below −183°C (−297°F) inside the reservoir, and the temperature inside the ambulatory tank is warmer. If cold oxygen from the reservoir mixes with warmer oxygen left in the ambulatory tank, the ambulatory tank may malfunction.*

STEPS	RATIONALE
(3) Refilling oxygen tank:	
(a) Wipe both filling connectors with a clean, dry, lint-free cloth.	• Removes dust and moisture from system.
(b) Turn off flow selector of ambulatory unit.	
(c) Attach ambulatory unit to stationary reservoir by inserting adapter from ambulatory tank into adapter of stationary reservoir.	• Secures connections.

Continued

SKILL 39-5 USING HOME OXYGEN EQUIPMENT—cont'd

STEPS	RATIONALE
(d) Open fill valve on ambulatory tank, and apply firm pressure to top of stationary reservoir (see Step 8C[3][d] illustration). Stay with unit while it is filling. You will hear a loud hissing noise. The tank fills in about 2 minutes.	• Prevents leaking of oxygen during filling process. If oxygen leaks during filling process, the connection between ambulatory tank and reservoir will ice up and stick together.

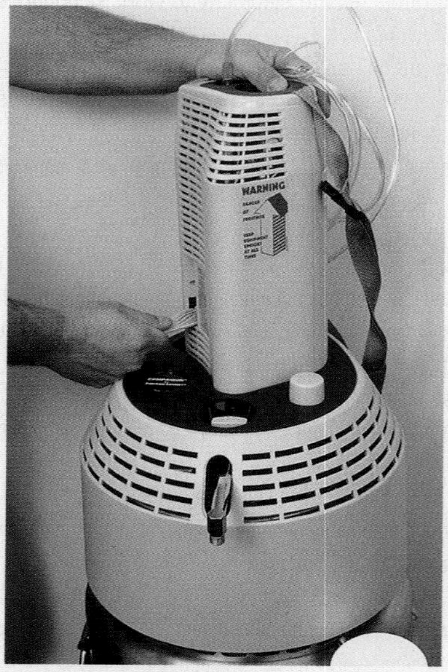

STEP 8C(3)(d) Fill valve on ambulatory tank is open while applying firm pressure to top of ambulatory unit.

STEPS	RATIONALE
(e) Disengage ambulatory unit from stationary reservoir when hissing noise changes and vapour cloud begins to form from stationary unit.	• Overfilling causes the ambulatory unit to malfunction from high pressure in the tank.
(f) Wipe both filling connectors with a clean, dry, lint-free cloth.	• Ice sometimes forms during filling. Wiping removes moisture from oxygen system.

CRITICAL DECISION POINT: *If ambulatory unit does not separate easily, valves from the reservoir and ambulatory unit may be frozen together. Wait until the valves warm to disengage (about 5–10 minutes). Do not touch any frosted areas because contact with skin may cause skin damage from frostbite.*

STEPS	RATIONALE
9. Connect oxygen delivery device to oxygen system.	• Connects oxygen source to delivery system.
10. Adjust to prescribed flow rate (L/min).	• Ensures appropriate oxygen prescription.
11. Place oxygen delivery device on patient. Ensure patient has two sets of oxygen delivery devices and tubing.	• Delivers oxygen to patient. Extra devices are used when equipment is cleaned or in case of malfunction.
12. Perform hand hygiene.	• Reduces transmission of microorganisms.
13. Instruct patient and family not to change oxygen flow rate.	• Provides prescribed amount of oxygen. Exceeding prescribed oxygen may be harmful (e.g., COPD).
14. Guide the patient and family as they perform each step. Provide written material for reinforcement and review.	• Allows nurse to correct errors in technique and discuss their implications.
15. Instruct the patient or family to notify the health care provider if signs or symptoms of hypoxia or respiratory tract infection occur.	• Respiratory tract infections increase oxygen demand and may affect oxygen transfer from lungs to blood. They may cause severe exacerbation of patient's pulmonary disease.
16. Discuss emergency plan for power loss, natural disaster, and acute respiratory distress. Have patient or family call 911 and notify health care provider and home care agency.	• Ensures appropriate response and can prevent worsening of patient's condition.
17. Instruct patient in safe home oxygen practices, including placing "No Smoking/Oxygen in Use" signs at each entrance to the home, not allowing smoking in the home, keeping oxygen tanks away from open flames, and storing tanks upright.	• Ensures safe use of oxygen in the home and prevents injury to patient and family.

STEPS	RATIONALE
18. Monitor rate of oxygen delivery. All oxygen-delivery equipment should be checked at least daily by patient or caregiver.	• Determines if patient is regulating oxygen at prescribed rate.
19. Oxygen-delivery equipment must be maintained and serviced routinely according to the manufacturer's guidelines (AARC, 2007).	

UNEXPECTED OUTCOMES	RELATED INTERVENTIONS
Patient reports no oxygen flow	• Check tank pressure gauge. If level of oxygen is low, refill tank if portable, or provide alternative source of oxygen, such as concentrator or H cylinder. • Notify home oxygen supplier of need for refill. • Reassure patient and family.
Unable to fill portable liquid oxygen from main source	• Check to see that portable tank is connected correctly. • Determine if valve is frozen. • Contact home oxygen supplier for service visit. • Provide alternative oxygen source if necessary.

RECORDING AND REPORTING

- Record the patient's and family's ability to safely use the home oxygen equipment. Report the type of home oxygen equipment to be used and the patient's and family's understanding of how to use the equipment, knowledge of safety guidelines and unexpected outcomes, and ability to demonstrate proper use of the oxygen delivery device.

with minimal coughing. Excessive coughing to clear thick, tenacious secretions is fatiguing and energy depleting. The best way to maintain thin secretions is to provide a fluid intake of 1 500 to 2 000 mL/day unless contraindicated by cardiac status. The colour, consistency, and ease of secretion expectoration can determine the adequacy of hydration.

Coughing Techniques. Coughing is effective for maintaining a patent airway. Coughing enables the patient to remove secretions from both the upper and lower airways. The normal series of events in the cough mechanism are deep inhalation, closure of the glottis, active contraction of the expiratory muscles, and glottis opening. Deep inhalation increases the lung volume and airway diameter, allowing the air to pass through partially obstructing mucous plugs or other foreign matter. Contraction of the expiratory muscles against the closed glottis causes a high intrathoracic pressure to develop. When the glottis opens, a large flow of air is expelled at a high speed, providing momentum for mucus to move to the upper airways, where it can be expectorated or swallowed.

The effectiveness of coughing is evaluated by sputum expectoration, the patient's report of swallowed sputum, or clearing of adventitious sounds by auscultation. Patients with chronic pulmonary diseases, upper respiratory tract infections, and lower respiratory tract infections should be encouraged to deep-breathe and cough at least every 2 hours while awake. Patients with a large amount of sputum should be encouraged to cough every hour while awake and every 2 to 3 hours while asleep until the acute phase of mucus production has ended. Coughing techniques include deep breathing and coughing for the postoperative patient, cascade, huff, and quad coughing.

With the *cascade cough,* the patient takes a slow, deep breath and holds it for 2 seconds while contracting expiratory muscles. Then the patient opens the mouth and performs a series of coughs throughout exhalation, thereby coughing at progressively lowered lung volumes. This technique promotes airway clearance and a patent airway in patients with large volumes of sputum.

The *huff cough* stimulates a natural cough reflex and is generally effective only for clearing central airways. While exhaling, the patient opens the glottis by saying the word "huff." With practice, the patient inhales more air and may be able to progress to the cascade cough.

The *quad cough* technique is used for patients without abdominal muscle control, such as those with spinal cord injuries. While the patient breathes out with a maximal expiratory effort, the patient or nurse pushes inward and upward on the abdominal muscles toward the diaphragm, causing the cough.

Respiratory Muscle Training. Respiratory muscle training improves muscle strength and endurance, resulting in improved activity tolerance. Respiratory muscle training may prevent respiratory failure in patients with COPD.

One method for respiratory muscle training is the incentive spirometer resistive breathing device (ISRBD). Resistive breathing is achieved by placing a resistive breathing device into a volume-dependent incentive spirometer. Muscle training is achieved when the patient uses the ISRBD on a scheduled routine (e.g., twice a day for 15 minutes or four times a day for 15 minutes).

Breathing Exercises. Breathing exercises include techniques to improve ventilation and oxygenation. The three basic techniques are deep breathing and coughing exercises, pursed-lip breathing, and diaphragmatic breathing. Deep breathing and coughing exercises are routine interventions for postoperative patients (see Chapter 48).

Pursed-Lip Breathing. Pursed-lip breathing involves deep inspiration and prolonged expiration through pursed lips to prevent alveolar collapse. The patient is instructed to take a deep breath while sitting up and to exhale slowly through pursed lips, as if blowing through a straw. The patient then blows through a straw into a glass of water to learn the technique. Patients need to gain control of the exhalation phase so that it is longer than inhalation. The patient is usually able to perfect this technique by counting the inhalation time and gradually increasing the count during exhalation. In studies using pulse oximetry as a feedback tool, patients have been able to demonstrate an increase in their arterial oxygen saturation during pursed-lip breathing.

Diaphragmatic Breathing. Diaphragmatic breathing is more difficult and requires the patient to relax intercostal and accessory respiratory muscles while taking deep inspirations. The patient

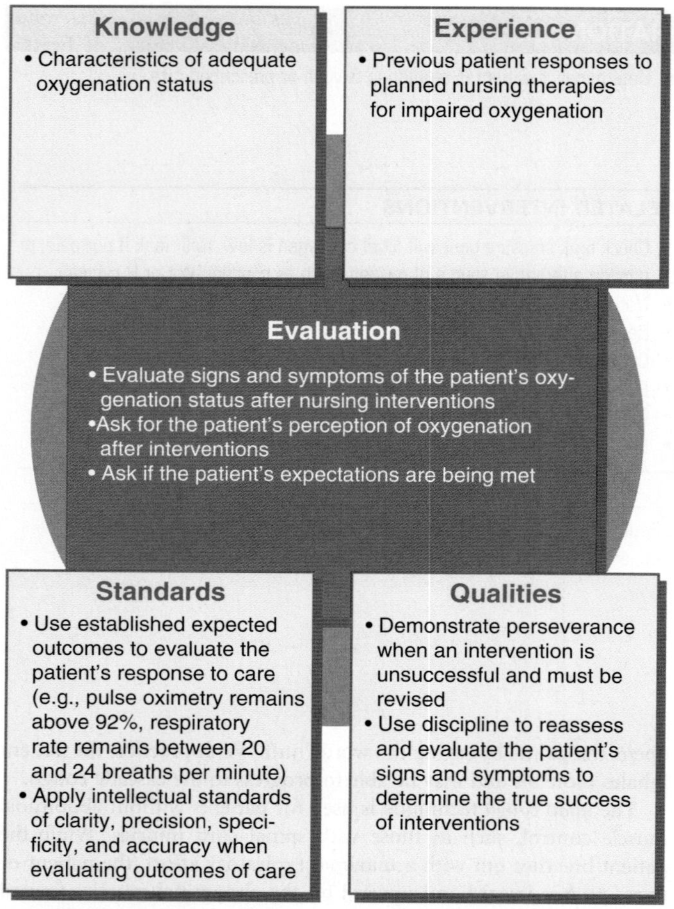

FIGURE 39-20 Critical thinking model for oxygenation evaluation.

concentrates on expanding the diaphragm during controlled inspiration and is taught to place one hand flat below the breastbone and above the waist, and the other hand 2 to 3 cm below the first hand. The patient is asked to inhale while the lower hand moves outward during inspiration. The patient observes for inward movement as the diaphragm ascends. These exercises are initially taught with the patient in the supine position and then practised while the patient sits and stands. The exercise is often used with the pursed-lip breathing technique.

Diaphragmatic breathing is also useful for patients with pulmonary disease, for postoperative patients, and for women in labour to promote relaxation and provide pain control. The exercise improves efficiency of breathing by decreasing air trapping and reducing the work of breathing.

◆ Evaluation

Nursing interventions and therapies are evaluated by comparing the patient's progress with the goals and expected outcomes of the nursing care plan. The nurse evaluates the actual care given to the patient by the health care team on the basis of the expected outcomes (Figure 39-20).

Patient Care. The patient is the only one who can evaluate his or her degree of breathlessness. The patient should be asked to rate breathlessness on a scale of 1 to 10, with 1 being no shortness of breath and 10 being severe shortness of breath. Arterial blood gas levels, pulmonary function tests, vital signs, ECG tracings, and physical assessment data provide objective measurement of the success of therapies and treatments. Outcomes are compared with expected outcomes to determine the patient's health status. Continuous evaluation helps to determine whether new or revised therapies are required and if new nursing diagnoses have developed and require a new plan of care.

When nursing measures directed toward improving oxygenation are unsuccessful, the nurse must immediately modify the nursing care plan. Nurses should not hesitate to notify the physician about a patient's deteriorating oxygenation status. Prompt notification can avoid an emergency situation, or even the need for CPR.

Patient Expectations. It is important to ask patients if their expectations of care have been met. For example, the nurse can ask the patient, "Do you feel as though you will be able to use the breathing techniques we have practised at home?" If the patient does not think this will work at home, then the patient's expectations for care management have not been met.

The nurse should ask the patient whether all questions and needs have been met. If not, the nurse needs to spend more time understanding what the patient wants and needs to meet his or her expectations. Working closely with the patient will enable the nurse to redefine those patient expectations that can be realistically met within the limitations of the patient's condition and treatment.

KEY CONCEPTS

- The primary function of the heart is to deliver deoxygenated blood to the lungs for oxygenation and to deliver oxygen and nutrients to the tissues.
- Preload, afterload, contractility, and heart rate alter cardiac output.
- Cardiac dysrhythmias are classified by cardiac activity and site of impulse origin.
- The primary function of the lungs is to transfer oxygen from the atmosphere into the alveoli and to transfer carbon dioxide out of the body as a waste product.
- Ventilation is the process of providing adequate oxygenation from the alveoli to the blood.
- Compliance, or the ability of the lungs to expand and contract, depends on the function of musculoskeletal and neurological systems and on other physiological factors.
- The process of inspiration (active process) and expiration (passive process) is caused by changes in intrapleural and intra-alveolar pressures and lung volumes.
- Respiration is controlled by the central nervous system and by chemicals within the blood.
- Decreased hemoglobin levels alter the patient's ability to transport oxygen.
- Impaired chest wall movement reduces the level of tissue oxygenation.
- Hyperventilation is a respiratory rate greater than that required to maintain normal levels of carbon dioxide.
- Hypoventilation causes carbon dioxide retention.
- Hypoxia occurs if the amount of oxygen delivered to tissues is too low.
- The health history and assessment include information about the patient's cough, dyspnea, fatigue, wheezing, chest pain, environmental exposures, respiratory infection, cardiopulmonary risk factors, and use of medications.
- Diagnostic and laboratory tests may be needed to complete the database for a patient with decreased oxygenation.

- Breathing exercises improve ventilation, oxygenation, and sensations of dyspnea.
- Nebulization delivers small drops of water or particles of medication to the airways.
- Chest physiotherapy includes postural drainage, percussion, and vibration to mobilize pulmonary secretions.
- Coughing and suctioning techniques are used to maintain a patent airway.
- Oxygen therapy is used to improve levels of tissue oxygenation and is delivered by a nasal cannula, various oxygen masks, or the use of an artificial airway.

CRITICAL THINKING EXERCISES

1. Ms. Delgado is a 56-year-old postmenopausal woman with a history of hypertension. She presents to her primary care office with complaints of nausea, indigestion, increased fatigue, and shortness of breath with increased activity for the past 16 hours. What questions would you ask Ms. Delgado in the nursing health history?
2. Mr. Kwan has recently immigrated to Canada. He comes to the clinic because he has been increasingly fatigued, has a persistent cough, has been losing weight, and awakens at night with sweats. What questions would be important to ask when completing the nursing health history?
3. Mrs. Leblanc, age 45 years, has been admitted to the hospital with community-acquired pneumonia. She has a productive cough, fever, chills, crackles and wheezes on auscultation of her chest, and a heart rate of 104 beats per minute. What nursing diagnosis would you consider for this patient? What nursing interventions would be appropriate for her? What health promotion interventions need to be initiated before discharge from the hospital?
4. Mr. Chen Lee, age 72 years, is on a medical unit for a recent diagnosis of COPD. He uses his call bell to indicate that he feels short of breath. His respiratory rate is 32 breaths per minute and oxygen saturation is 86% on room air. What immediate nursing interventions would you initiate?

REVIEW QUESTIONS

1. The nurse is completing an admission assessment of a patient who was diagnosed with anemia. Which assessment finding has the greatest implication for this patient's plan of care?
   1. Fatigued when ambulating
   2. Increased activity tolerance when ambulating
   3. Decreased breathlessness when ambulating
   4. Oxygen saturation of 95% on room air when ambulating
2. A patient on a cardiac unit who was initially in a normal sinus rhythm informs the nurse of increasing shortness of breath. Referencing Figure Q-2, which interventions are appropriate for this change in rhythm? *(Select all that apply.)*
   1. Warfarin (Coumadin)
   2. Prepare for defibrillation
   3. Lopressor (Metoprolol)
   4. Apply nasal cannulas at 2 L/min
   5. Elevate the head of the bed
   6. Preparing for transcutaneous pacing
   7. Review the current partial thromboplastin time (PTT) lab value
3. A patient returns from thoracic surgery with a chest tube. One hour after the initial physical assessment the nurse notes 750 mL in the last hour of bright red drainage in the collection chamber of the chest tube. Prioritize the list of nursing interventions.
   1. Take vital signs
   2. Prepare to administer intravenous fluids
   3. Notify most responsible health care provider
   4. Suggest a current complete blood count be collected
4. What assessment finding is consistent with a patient who has a fever?
   1. A decrease in carbon dioxide
   2. The presence of cyanosis
   3. An increase in carbon dioxide
   4. An increase in muscle mass
5. A patient is diagnosed with the dysrhythmia of normal sinus tachycardia. Referencing Figure Q-5, which anatomical structure is responsible for the tachycardia?
6. A patient is discharged after being diagnosed and treated for heart failure. What health promotion strategies are important to consider with this patient? (*Select all that apply.*)
   1. Monitor weekly weight
   2. Eat low-fat and low-sodium Mediterranean diet
   3. Engage in regular aerobic activity
   4. Take vitamin D daily
   5. Consider annual flu and pneumococcal vaccines
   6. Notify health care provider if oxygen demands decrease
7. A patient admitted to the medical unit with a pneumothorax begins to experience confusion and restlessness. The vital signs are temperature 35.8°C, pulse 110, respirations 32, and blood pressure 110/68. What is the potential diagnosis?
   1. Atelectasis
   2. Ventricular tachycardia
   3. Dementia
   4. Hypoxia

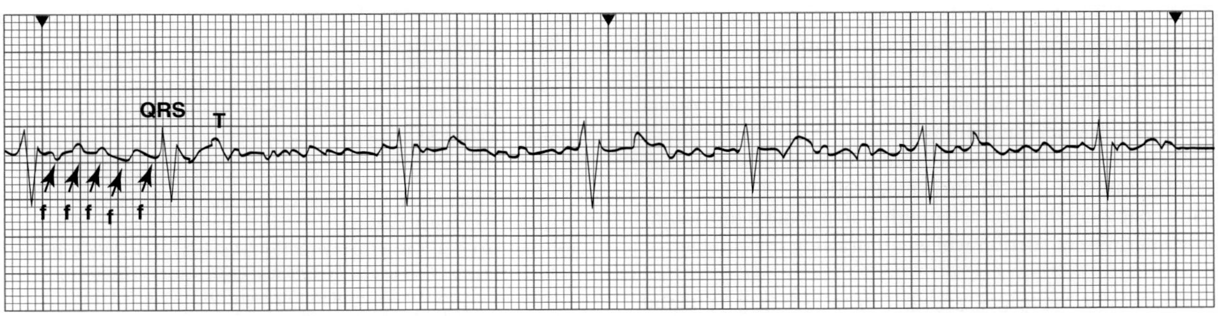

FIGURE Q-2 Coarse atrial fibrillation. (From Wesley, K. [2011]. *Huszar's basic dysrhythmias and acute coronary syndrome interpretation and management* [4th ed., p. 103, Fig. 6-7F]. St. Louis, MO: Mosby.)

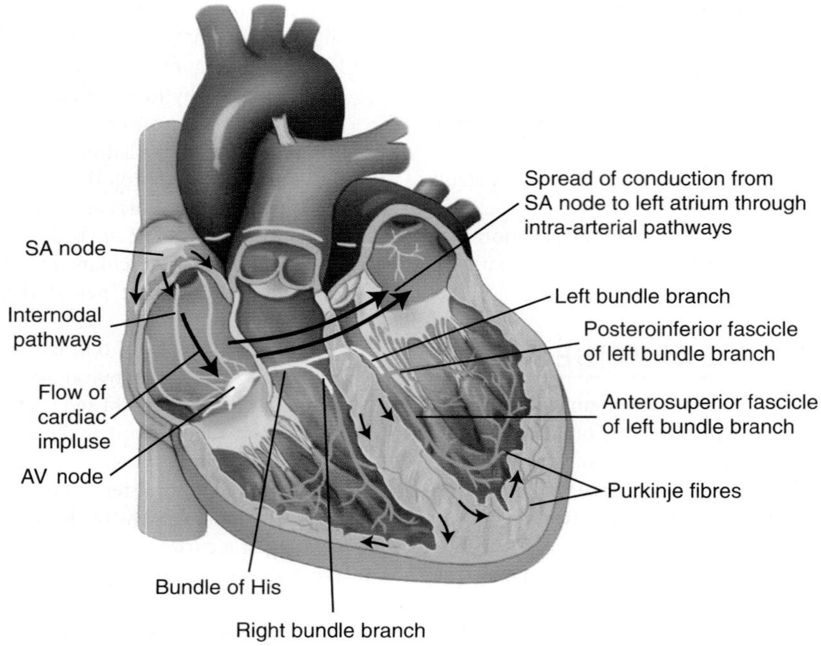

FIGURE Q-5 (From Lewis, S. L., Heitkemper, M. M., Dirksen, S. R., Bucher, L., Camera I., Barry, M. A., Goldsworthy, S., & Goodridge, D. [Eds.]. [2014]. *Medical-surgical nursing in Canada: Assessment and management of clinical problems* [3rd Canadian ed., p. 845, Fig. 34-4]. Toronto: Elsevier Canada.)

8. What is the likely long-term risk factor associated with long-term smoking?
   1. Cardiopulmonary disease and lung cancer
   2. Obesity and diabetes
   3. Stress-related illnesses and pneumothorax
   4. Hypotension and bradycardia
9. A patient with a fresh tracheostomy requires suctioning. During suctioning the patient develops respiratory distress. What is the priority sequence?
   1. Immediately withdraw catheter
   2. Supply additional oxygen as needed
   3. Take vital signs
   4. Disconnect suction
   5. Remain with the patient until oxygen returns to baseline
10. Apply intermittent suction for ______________ seconds by placing and releasing nondominant thumb over vent of catheter and slowly withdrawing while rotating it back and forth between dominant thumb and forefinger.
11. A patient has a suspected tension pneumothorax following the insertion of a chest tube. What action is considered a nursing priority?
    1. Assess the chest tube to ensure it is not clamped or occluded.
    2. Cross-clamp the chest tube close to the patient's chest.
    3. Change the dressing using nonocclusive material.
    4. Instruct the patient to deep-breathe and cough.
12. Which of the following statements best describes the correct method for nasotracheal suctioning?
    1. Use clean gloves to complete the procedure.
    2. Insert the catheter 1–2 cm during expiration.
    3. Lightly coat 2–3 cm of catheter with water-soluble lubricant.
    4. Apply intermittent suction while withdrawing the catheter.

Answers: 1. 1; **2.** 1, 3, 4, 5; **3.** 1, 3, 4, 2; **4.** 3; **5.** sinoatrial node (SA node); **6.** 2, 3, 5; **7.** 4; **8.** 1; **9.** 1, 2, 4, 3, 5; **10.** 10 seconds; **11.** 1; **12.** 4

Rationales for the Review Questions appear at the end of the book.

RECOMMENDED WEBSITES

Canadian Thoracic Society: https://cts.lung.ca/

The Canadian Thoracic Society provides evidence-informed information and resources regarding respiratory health.

Canadian Cardiovascular Society: http://www.ccs.ca/en/

The Canadian Cardiovascular Society provides evidence-informed information and resources on cardiovascular health.

Heart and Stroke Foundation of Canada: http://www.heartandstroke.ca

The Heart and Stroke Foundation is a national voluntary, nonprofit organization whose mission is to improve the health of Canadians by preventing heart disease and stroke through research, health promotion, and advocacy.

REFERENCES

American Association of Respiratory Care (AARC). (2004). Clinical practice guideline: Nasotracheal suction. *Respiratory Care, 49*, 1080–1084.

American Association of Respiratory Care (AARC). (2007). AARC Clinical practice guideline, oxygen therapy in the home or alternate site health care facility. *Respiratory Care, 52*(1), 1063.

American Association of Respiratory Care (AARC). (2010). Endotracheal suctioning of mechanically ventilated patients with artificial airways. *Respiratory Care, 55*(60), 758–764.

American Association of Respiratory Care (AARC). (2011). Clinical practice guideline: Incentive spirometry. *Respiratory Care, 56*(10), 1600.

American Heart Association (AHA). (2015a). *Heart attack symptoms in women.* Retrieved from http://www.heart.org/HEARTORG/Conditions/HeartAttack/WarningSignsofaHeartAttack/Heart-Attack-Symptoms-in-Women_UCM_436448_Article.jsp#.WApQGzL2aos.

American Heart Association (AHA). (2015b). *Acute coronary syndrome.* Retrieved from http://www.heart.org/HEARTORG/Conditions/HeartAttack/AboutHeartAttacks/Acute-Coronary-Syndrome_UCM_428752_Article.jsp#.WApUY3osAmU.

American Heart Association (AHA). (2015c). *Highlights of the 2015 American Heart Association guidelines update for CPR and ECC.* Retrieved from http://eccguidelines.heart.org/wp-content/uploads/2015/10/2015-AHA-Guidelines-Highlights-English.pdf.

American Heart Association (AHA). (2017). 2017 American Heart Association focused update on adult basic life support and cardiopulmonary resuscitation quality. *Circulation, 136*, e1–e7. doi.org/10.1161/CIR.0000000000000539.

Atkins, J. R., & Kautz, D. D. (2014). Moved to improve: Progressive mobilization in the intensive care unit. *Dimensions of Critical Care Nursing, 33*(5), 275. doi:10.1097/dcc.0000000000000063.

Bauman, M., & Handley, C. (2011). Chest tube care: The more you know, the easier it gets. *American Nurse Today, 6*(9), 27–32. Retrieved from http://www.americannursetoday.com/chest-tube-care-the-more-you-know-the-easier-it-gets.

Booker, S., Murff, S., Kitko, L., et al. (2013). Mouth care to reduce ventilator associated pneumonia. *American Journal of Nursing, 113*(10), 24. doi:10.1097/01.naj.0000435343.38287.30.

Borge, C. R., Hagen, K. B., Mengshoel, A. M., et al. (2014). Effects of controlled-breathing exercises and respiratory muscle training in people with chronic obstructive pulmonary disease: Results from evaluating the quality of evidence in systematic reviews. *BMC Pulmonary Medicine, 14*, 184. doi:10.1186/1471-2466-14-184.

Canadian Association of Schools of Nursing/Association Canadienne des Écoles de Sciences Infirmières [CASN/ACESI]. (2015). *National nursing education framework: Final report.* Retrieved from http://www.casn.ca/wp-content/uploads/2014/12/Framwork-FINAL-SB-Nov-30-20151.pdf.

Canadian Cancer Society. (2017). *Lung cancer statistics.* Retrieved from http://www.cancer.ca/en/cancer-information/cancer-type/lung/statistics/?region=on.

Carroll, P. (2017). *Chest tube and drainage management.* Retrieved from http://www.rn.org/courses/coursematerial-98.pdf.

Cassidy, M. R., Rosenkranz, P., McCabe, K., et al. (2013). I cough: Reducing post-operative complications with a multidisciplinary patient care program. *JAMA Surgery, 148*(8), 740–745. doi:10.10001/jamasurg.2013.358.

Centers for Disease Control and Prevention (CDC). (2017a). *Key facts about seasonal flu vaccine.* Retrieved from https://www.cdc.gov/flu/protect/keyfacts.htm#vaccines-available.

Centers for Disease Control and Prevention (CDC). (2017b). *Pneumococcal vaccine.* Retrieved from http://www.cdc.gov/pneumococcal/vaccination.html.

Clark, A. M., King-Shier, K. M., Thompson, D. R., et al. (2012). A qualitative systematic review of influences on attendance at cardiac rehabilitation programs after referral. *American Heart Journal, 164*(6), 835–845. doi:10.1016/j.ahj.2012.08.020.

Cooper, K. L. (2013). Evidence-based prevention of pressure ulcers in the intensive care unit. *Critical Care Nurse, 33*(6), 57. doi:10.4037/ccn2013985.

Cystic Fibrosis Foundation. (2012). *Consumer fact sheet: An introduction to postural drainage and percussion.* Retrieved from https://www.cff.org/PDF-Archive/Introduction-to-Postural-Drainage-and-Pecussion/.

Dango, S., Sienel, W., Passlick, B., et al. (2010). Impact of chest tube clearance on postoperative morbidity after thoracotomy: Results of a prospective, randomised trial. *European Journal of Cardio-thoracic Surgery, 37*(1), 51. doi:10.1016/j.ejcts.2009.06.034.

DiNicolantonio, J. J., Lucan, S. C., & O'Keefe, J. H. (2015). The evidence for saturated fat and for sugar related to coronary heart disease. *Progress in Cardiovascular Diseases, 58*, 464–472. doi:10.1016/j.pcad.2015.11.006.

Estruch, E., et al. (2013). Primary prevention of cardiovascular disease with a Mediterranean diet. *New England Journal of Medicine, 368*(14), 1279–1290. doi:10.1056/NEJMoa1200303.

Health Canada. (2016). *Canadian immunization guide chapter on influenza and statement on seasonal influenza vaccine for 2016–2017.* Retrieved from http://www.phac-aspc.gc.ca/naci-ccni/flu-2016-grippe-eng.php#ii2.

Heart & Stroke 2018 Heart Report. (2018). *Ms. Understood:* Women's hearts are victims of a system that is ill-equipped to diagnose, treat and support them. Retrieved from http://www.heartandstroke.ca/-/media/pdf-files/canada/2018-heart-month/hs_2018-heart-report_en.

Heart and Stroke Foundation (HSF) and American Heart Association (AHA). (2015). *Highlights of the 2015 American Heart Association Guidelines for CPR and ECC* (Heart and Stroke Foundation of Canada Edition). Retrieved from http://eccguidelines.heart.org/wp-content/uploads/2015/10/2015-AHA-Guidelines-Highlights-English.pdf.

Heart and Stroke Foundation of Canada (HSFC). (2016). *The burden of heart failure.* Retrieved from https://www.heartandstroke.ca/-/media/pdf-files/canada/2017-heart-month/heartandstroke-reportonhealth-2016.ashx?la=en.

Heart and Stroke Foundation of Canada (HSFC). (2017a). *The benefits of physical activity.* Retrieved from http://www.heartandstroke.ca/get-healthy/stay-active/benefits-of-physical-activity.

Heart and Stroke Foundation of Canada. (2017b). *Heart attack.* Retrieved from http://www.heartandstroke.ca/heart/conditions/heart-attack.

Heart and Stroke Foundation of Canada (HSFC). (2017c). *What is sugar?* Retrieved from http://www.heartandstroke.ca/get-healthy/healthy-eating/reduce-sugar.

Hess, D. R. (2005). Tracheostomy tubes and related appliances. *Respiratory Care, 50*(4), 497–510.

Heuer, A. J., & Scanlan, C. L. (2009). Medical gas therapy. In R. L. Wilkins, J. K. Stoller, & R. M. Kacmarek (Eds.), *Fundamentals of respiratory care* (pp. 867–901). St. Louis, MO: Mosby.

Hockenberry, M. J., & Wilson, D. (2015). *Wong's nursing care of infants and children multimedia enhanced version* (10th ed.). St. Louis, MO: Mosby.

Hong, C. M., & Galvagno, S. (2013). Patients with chronic pulmonary disease. *Medical Clinics of North America, 97*(6), 1095.

Hypertension Canada. (2017). *Health Behaviour Management.* Retrieved from http://guidelines.hypertension.ca/prevention-treatment/health-behaviour-management/.

James, P. A., Oparil, S., Carter, B., et al. (2014). 2014 Evidence-based guideline for the management of high blood pressure in adults: Report from the panel members appointed to the Eighth Joint National Committee. *JAMA: The Journal of the American Medical Association, 311*(5), 507–520. doi:10.1001/jama/2013.284427.

Kassis, A., Savetamal, A., Assis, R., et al. (2014). Characteristics of patients with injury secondary to smoking on home oxygen therapy transferred intubated to a burn center. *Journal of American College of Surgeons, 8*(6), 1182. doi:10.1016/j.jamcollsurg.2013.12.055.

Kozik, T. M., Shah, S., Bhattacharyya, M., et al. (2016). Cardiovascular responses to energy drinks in a healthy population: The C-energy study. *American Journal of Emergency Medicine, 34*, 1205–1209. doi:10.1016/j.ajem.2016.02.068.

Labeau, S. O., Van de Vyver, K., Brusselaers, N., et al. (2011). Prevention of ventilator-associated pneumonia with oral antiseptics: A systematic review and meta-analysis. *Lancet Infectious Disease, 11*(11), 845. doi:10.1016/S1473-3099(11)70127-X.

Leung, A. A., et al. (2017). Hypertension Canada's 2017 Guidelines for Diagnosis, Risk Assessment, Prevention, and Treatment of Hypertension in Adults. *Canadian Journal of Cardiology, 33*, 557–576. doi:10.1016/j.cjca.2017.03.005.

Lynn-McHale, D. J. (2011). *ACCN procedural manual for critical care* (6th ed.). St. Louis, MO: Mosby.

McCance, K. L., & Huether, S. E. (2014). *Pathophysiology: The biologic basis for disease in adults and children* (7th ed.). St. Louis, MO: Mosby.

Meiner, S. (2011). *Gerontologic nursing* (4th ed.). St. Louis, MO: Mosby.

Morse, L. L., Whitmer, E., & McIntosh, E. (2013). Tracheostomy care and complications in the intensive care unit. *Critical Care Nurse, 33*(5), 18. doi:10.4037/ccn2013518.

Neumar, R. W., Shuster, M., Callaway, C. W., et al. (2015). Part 1: Executive summary: 2015 American Heart Association Guidelines update for cardiopulmonary resuscitation and emergency cardiovascular care. *Circulation, 132*(18, Suppl. 2), S315–S367. doi:10.1161/CIR.0000000000000252.

Pang, P. S., Collins, S. P., Sauser, K., et al. (2014). Assessment of dyspnea early in acute heart failure: Patient characteristics and response differences between Likert and visual analog scales. *Academic Emergency Medicine, 21*(6), 659–666. doi:10.111/acem.12390.

Perry, A. G., Potter, P. A., & Ostendorf, W. R. (2014). *Clinical nursing skills and techniques* (8th ed.). St. Louis, MO: Mosby.

Qaseem, A., Wilt, T. J., Weinberger, S. E., et al. (2011). Diagnosis and management of stable chronic obstructive pulmonary disease: A clinical practice guideline update from the American College of Physicians, American College of Chest Physicians, American Thoracic Society, and European Respiratory Society. *Annals of Internal Medicine, 155*(3), 179–191. Retrieved from https://www.thoracic.org/statements/resources/copd/copd-guideline-acp-ats-ers-accp%20-abstract.pdf.

Registered Nurses' Association of Ontario (RNAO). (2005/2010). *Nursing care of dyspnea: The 6th vital sign in individuals with chronic obstructive pulmonary disease (COPD).* Toronto: Author. Retrieved from http://www.rnao.org/Page.asp?PageID=924&ContentID=807.

Registered Nurses' Association of Ontario (RNAO). (2007). *Integrating smoking cessation into daily nursing practice.* Toronto: Author. Retrieved from http://rnao.ca/sites/rnao-ca/files/Integrating_Smoking_Cessation_into_Daily_Nursing_Practice.pdf.

Soule, M. L., & Bennett, M. (2014). Comparison of airway management practices between registered nurses and respiratory care practitioners. *American Journal of Critical Care, 23*(3), 191. doi:10.437/ajcc2014424.

Statistics Canada. (2016). *Second-hand smoke.* Retrieved from http://www.statcan.gc.ca/pub/82-229-x/2009001/envir/shs-eng.htm.

Touhy, T. A., & Jett, K. F. (2014). *Ebersole and Hess' gerontological nursing and healthy aging* (4th ed.). St. Louis, MO: Elsevier.

40

Fluid, Electrolyte, and Acid–Base Balances

Canadian content written by Darlaine Jantzen, RN, MA, PhD
Original chapter by Linda Felver, RN, PhD

OBJECTIVES

Mastery of content in this chapter will enable you to:

- Define the key terms listed.
- Describe the distribution, composition, movement, and regulation of body fluids.
- Describe the regulation and movement of major electrolytes.
- Describe the processes involved in regulating acid–base balance.
- Describe common fluid, electrolyte, and acid–base imbalances, and identify related risk factors.
- Choose appropriate clinical assessments for fluid, electrolyte, and acid–base balances.
- Interpret basic fluid, electrolyte, and acid–base laboratory values.
- Identify and discuss nursing interventions for patients with fluid, electrolyte, and acid–base imbalances.
- Discuss the purpose of, and procedure for, initiating, maintaining, and discontinuing intravenous therapy and peripheral vascular access devices.
- Discuss the purpose and nursing care related to central vascular access devices, including preventing and recognizing associated complications.
- Discuss complications associated with intravenous therapy.
- Discuss the purpose of, and procedure for, initiating a blood transfusion and interventions to manage transfusion reaction.

KEY TERMS

Active transport, p. 1017
Aldosterone, p. 1019
Anion gap, p. 1026
Anions, p. 1016
Antidiuretic hormone (ADH), p. 1019
Arterial blood gas (ABG), p. 1024
Autologous transfusion, p. 1065
Base excess, p. 1025
Buffer, p. 1021
Cations, p. 1016
Central vascular access devices (CVADs), p. 1038
Colloid osmotic pressure, p. 1017
Colloids, p. 1038
Concentration gradient, p. 1017
Crystalloid, p. 1038
Dehydration, p. 1019
Diffusion, p. 1017
Edema, p. 1018
Electrolytes, p. 1016
Electronic infusion devices (EIDs), p. 1053
Extracellular fluid (ECF), p. 1016
Filtration, p. 1018
Fluid volume deficit (FVD), p. 1028
Fluid volume excess (FVE), p. 1038
Hemolysis, p. 1065
Homeostasis, p. 1018
Hydrostatic pressure, p. 1018
Hypercalcemia, p. 1024
Hyperchloremia, p. 1024
Hyperkalemia, p. 1024
Hypermagnesemia, p. 1024
Hypernatremia, p. 1023
Hypertonic, p. 1052
Hypocalcemia, p. 1024
Hypochloremia, p. 1024
Hypokalemia, p. 1023
Hypomagnesemia, p. 1024
Hyponatremia, p. 1023
Hypotonic, p. 1052
Hypovolemia, p. 1019
Infiltration, p. 1064
Insensible water loss, p. 1018
Interstitial fluid, p. 1016
Intracellular fluid (ICF), p. 1016
Intravascular fluid, p. 1016
Ions, p. 1016
Isotonic, p. 1052
Metabolic acidosis, p. 1026
Metabolic alkalosis, p. 1027
Obligatory water loss, p. 1018
Osmolality, p. 1017
Osmolarity, p. 1052
Osmoreceptors, p. 1019
Osmosis, p. 1017
Osmotic pressure, p. 1017
Oxygen saturation, p. 1025
Peripheral vascular access devices (PVADs), p. 1038
Peripherally inserted central catheter (PICC), p. 1038
Phlebitis, p. 1064
Respiratory acidosis, p. 1025
Respiratory alkalosis, p. 1025
Sensible water loss, p. 1018
Solutes, p. 1016
Solution, p. 1017
Solvent, p. 1017
Total parental nutrition (TPN), p. 1038
Transcellular fluid, p. 1016
Transfusion reaction, p. 1065
Vascular access devices (VADs), p. 1038

MEDIA RESOURCES

http://evolve.elsevier.com/Canada/Potter/fundamentals/

- Audio Chapter Summaries
- Examination Review Questions
- Concept Map Creator
- Case Study with Questions
- Audio Glossary
- Content Updates
- Video Clips

Fluid, electrolyte, and acid–base balances within the body are essential for normal body function (Box 40-1). These balances are maintained by ingestion, distribution, and excretion of water and electrolytes and by respiration. Within the body, these balances are maintained by the renal, pulmonary, and buffer systems. Imbalances may be caused by many factors, including altered intake, illness, or excessive losses, such as exercise-induced diaphoresis. These imbalances affect physiological processes at the cellular, tissue, and system levels of the body; therefore, understanding the mechanisms that contribute to fluid, electrolyte, and acid–base balances is essential to nursing practice.

SCIENTIFIC KNOWLEDGE BASE

This section provides a foundation for nurses' critical thinking and nursing practice. This is intended as a brief overview; anatomy and physiology textbooks expand on this information.

Water is the largest single component of the body. The average adult male weight is 60% water; however, this amount varies with age, gender, and body weight. A healthy, mobile, well-oriented adult can usually maintain normal fluid, electrolyte, and acid–base balances with renal, hormonal, and neural functions.

Distribution of Body Fluids

Body fluids are distributed in two distinct compartments, one containing intracellular fluid and the other containing extracellular fluid. **Intracellular fluid (ICF)**, or cytosol, includes all fluid within body cells, accounting for approximately 60% of the body's fluids (Amerman, 2016, p. 986).

Extracellular fluid (ECF), all the fluid outside cells, is divided into three compartments: interstitial fluid, intravascular fluid, and transcellular fluids. **Interstitial fluid**, including lymph, is the fluid between the cells and outside the blood vessels. **Intravascular fluid** is blood plasma. **Transcellular fluid**, separated from other fluid by epithelium, includes cerebrospinal, pleural, peritoneal, and synovial fluids and the fluids in the gastrointestinal tract (Figure 40-1).

Composition of Body Fluids

Electrolytes are important **solutes** in all body fluids. An electrolyte, when dissolved in an aqueous solution, separates into **ions** and is able to carry an electrical current (Amerman, 2016, p. 986). Positively charged electrolytes are **cations** (e.g., sodium [Na^+], potassium [K^+], calcium [Ca^{2+}]). Negatively charged electrolytes are **anions** (e.g., chloride [Cl^-], bicarbonate [HCO_3^-], sulphate [SO_4^-]). Electrolytes are vital to many body functions.

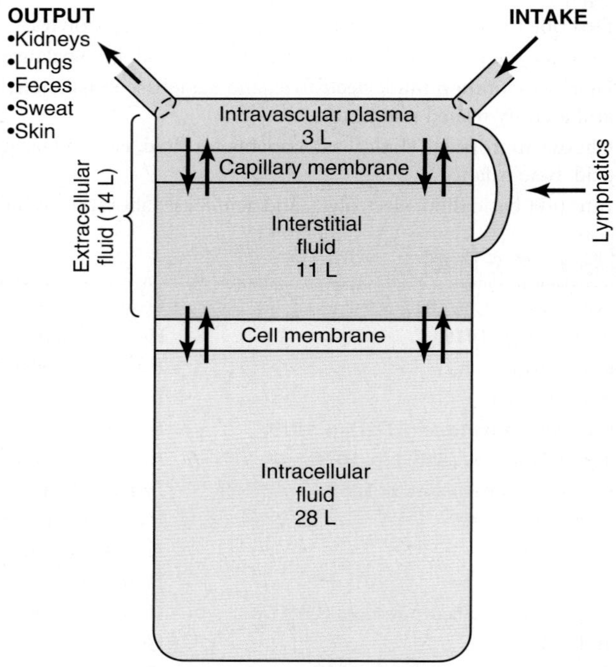

FIGURE 40-1 Body fluid distribution.

BOX 40-1 CASE STUDY

Sidney Runs

Sidney is a nursing student who is active in sports and exercise. Sidney has become aware that fluid, electrolyte, and acid–base balance is critical to healthy exercise. In the midst of studying for a biology exam, Sidney decides to go for a long run. The weather is warm, with a brisk breeze. Sidney decides to study while running. Sidney remembers that fluid, electrolyte, and acid–base balance in the human body is the result of feedback loops and concentration gradients. After a few minutes, Sidney starts to sweat, a great deal. This water needs to be replaced, either before or after the run, or both. It is possible that Sidney will need to drink an extra 3–4 litres, based on increased loss of fluid through breathing and sweating. Sodium also needs to be replaced, because sweat contains salt. Awareness that replacing water is not enough in the context of strenuous exercise, particularly when the environment is hot, has led to a market full of sports drinks. Amazingly, though, most of the time Sidney's body maintains homeostasis through normal physiology and diet, with the addition of some water. The muscles need calcium to work effectively. The exercising muscles increase the acids in the blood. Sidney remembers that acid–base balance is constantly being maintained by buffers, lungs, and kidneys. By the time Sidney returns from the run, normal physiology has responded with necessary changes, in order to provide the muscles and cardiovascular system with the fluid and electrolytes necessary, and to excrete excess hydrogen ions.

The body carefully regulates electrolyte concentration (Amerman, 2016, p. 986). The value millimoles per litre (mmol/L) represents the amount of the specific electrolyte (solute) dissolved in a litre of fluid (**solution**). The solution in which a solute is dissolved is called a **solvent**. Electrolyte concentration within fluid compartments is influenced by electrical charge. During normal physiological processes, ions are exchanged for other ions with the same electrical charge.

Electrolytes are ingested, often in the form of bulk and trace minerals or salts, and then utilized for basic physiological processes, stored for future use, or excreted. These electrolytes are important for maintaining osmotic concentrations in body fluids. They are also necessary for enzyme reactions, nerve impulses, muscle contraction, and metabolism. In addition, some minerals contribute to the regulation of hormone production and strengthening of skeletal structures.

Movement of Water and Electrolytes

Fluids and electrolytes constantly shift between compartments, often across plasma membranes, to facilitate body processes such as tissue oxygenation, acid–base balance, and urine formation. The passage of molecules across the plasma membrane occurs through passive and active transport processes. Because cell membranes separating the body fluid compartments are selectively permeable, water can pass through them easily. However, most ions and others molecules pass through them more slowly. Passive transport processes include osmosis, diffusion, and filtration.

Osmosis. **Osmosis** is the movement of water through a semipermeable membrane from an area of lesser solute concentration to an area of greater solute concentration in an attempt to equalize concentrations on both sides of the membrane (Figure 40-2). A semipermeable membrane allows water to pass through while remaining impermeable to most solutes. The rate of osmosis depends on the concentration of the solutes in the solution, temperature of the solution, electrical charges of the solutes, and differences between the osmotic pressures exerted by the solutions. The concentration of a solution is measured in osmols, which reflect the amount of a substance in solution in the form of molecules, ions, or both. Osmosis is an important concept when administering intravenous solutions, as their **osmolality** influences the potential benefits and risks. Another application of understanding osmosis is when considering the action of osmotic laxatives. These laxative salts are poorly absorbed through the intestinal lining and thus draw water into the intestinal lumen, causing an accumulation of water and softened stool. The swelling also stretches the intestine, stimulating peristalsis (Burchum & Rosenthal, 2016, p. 967).

Osmotic pressure is the pressure needed to counter the movement of water (solvent) across a semipermeable membrane from a low concentration to high concentration of solutes. A solution with a high solute concentration has a high osmotic pressure and draws water into itself. If the concentration of the solute is greater on one side of the semipermeable membrane, the rate of osmosis is faster, and solvent rapidly transfers across the membrane. This continues until equilibrium is reached.

Plasma proteins affect the blood's osmotic pressure. The three main classes of plasma proteins are albumins, globulins, and fibrinogen (Amerman, 2016, p. 725). Because albumin, produced in the liver, makes up the greatest proportion of plasma proteins, it exerts **colloid osmotic pressure** or oncotic pressure. This oncotic pressure tends to keep fluid in the intravascular compartment by pulling water from the interstitial space back into the capillaries (see Figure 40-2).

Diffusion. **Diffusion** is the movement of ions and molecules in a solution across a semipermeable membrane from an area of higher concentration to an area of lower concentration (Figure 40-3). The result is an even distribution of the solute in a solution. The rate of diffusion is affected by the molecule size, concentration, and temperature of a solution. The larger the molecule is and the cooler the solution is, the slower the rate of diffusion is. The difference between the two concentrations is known as a **concentration gradient**. Perfume permeating a room and a drop of food colouring moving through a glass of water are common examples of diffusion. A physiological example is the movement of oxygen (O_2) and carbon dioxide (CO_2) between the alveoli and blood vessels in the lungs, or the movement of lipids across the cell membrane. Some diffusion, still a passive transport process, is facilitated through a channel in the cell membrane (e.g., sodium, potassium, calcium) or with a carrier (Amerman, 2016, p. 76).

Active Transport. **Active transport** processes facilitate the movement of molecules (solutes) across the plasma membrane across a concentration gradient, using chemical energy (adenosine triphosphate [ATP]). There are two types of active transport, primary and secondary. In primary active transport, a protein binds with a solute to carry it against a concentration gradient. There are three types of pumps: uniport, symport, and antiport (Amerman, 2016, p. 79). The most commonly discussed primary active transport example, the sodium-potassium pump (Na^+/K^+ ATPase), is an antiport pump, as it transports solutes in opposite directions across the plasma membrane. Secondary active transport is more complex, as the sodium-potassium pump uses chemical energy to create a concentration gradient of sodium ions. Then, using the potential energy and a carrier protein, a

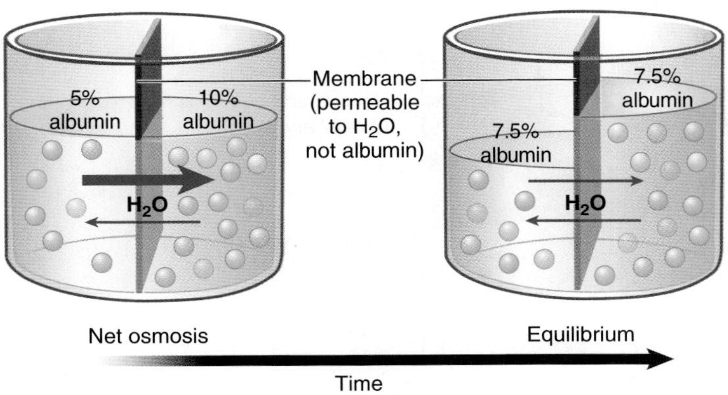

FIGURE 40-2 Osmosis.

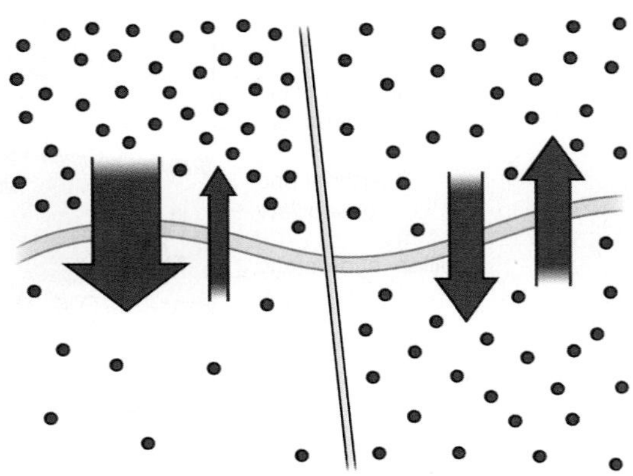
FIGURE 40-3 Diffusion.

sodium ion and a glucose molecule are transported back into the cell together (Figure 40-4).

Filtration. Filtration, the result of hydrostatic and colloid osmotic pressures, is a passive process whereby water moves into and out of the capillaries (Amerman, 2016, p. 690). Hydrostatic pressure is the force exerted by fluids within a compartment. Hydrostatic pressure in the capillaries is higher at the arteriolar end (35 mm Hg) than at the venular end (15 mm Hg). While the colloid osmotic or oncotic pressure remains stable within the capillaries, the changing hydrostatic pressures in the capillaries result in a pressure gradient. The combined pressures and the pressure gradient result in a net filtration pressure (NFP), filtering up to 2 to 4 litres of water per day into the interstitial fluid (Figure 40-5). Problems occur when hydrostatic pressure is increased on the venous side of the capillary bed, as occurs in heart failure. The normal movement of water from the interstitial space into the intravascular space by filtration is then reversed. This results in an accumulation of excess fluid in the interstitial space, known as edema. Filtration is also very important for urine formation as water and solutes are carried across the wall of the glomerular capillaries by hydrostatic or blood pressure. Falling blood pressure affects this process.

Fluid Homeostasis

Body fluids are regulated by fluid intake, hormonal controls, and fluid output in order to maintain homeostasis. Homeostasis is essential for survival. The primary hormones that regulate fluid are antidiuretic hormone, angiotensin II, aldosterone, and natriuretic peptides (Amerman, 2016, p. 992).

Fluid Output Regulation. Fluid output occurs through four organs of water loss: the kidneys, the skin, the lungs, and the gastrointestinal tract. The kidneys are the major regulatory organs of fluid balance. They receive approximately 180 L of plasma to filter each day and produce 1 200 to 1 500 mL of urine (Table 40-1). Each day an obligatory water loss of approximately 500 mL is essential, regardless of intake. This is why a person with no fluid intake will die of dehydration within a matter of days. Sensible water loss includes water loss through urine and feces.

Insensible water loss is continuous, gradual loss of water from the respiratory and skin epitheliums (Amerman, 2016, p. 990). This insensible water loss may increase in response to changes in respiratory rate and depth. Water loss from the skin is regulated by the sympathetic nervous system, which activates sweat glands. Fever may increase insensible water loss.

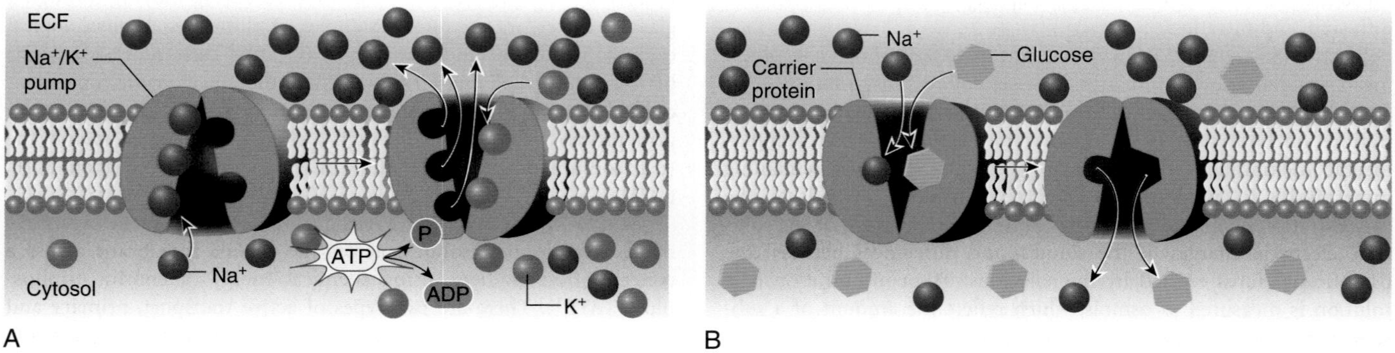

FIGURE 40-4 Secondary active transport. A, A Na^+/K^+ (sodium/potassium) pump creates a concentration gradient of sodium ions. *Left,* Na^+ ion binds to the Na^+/K^+ pump. *Right,* Adenosine triphosphate (ATP) hydrolysis fuels the transport of Na^+ into the extracellular fluid (ECF), against their concentration gradient. **B,** A carrier protein uses the potential energy of the sodium ion gradient to power the transport of glucose. *Left,* from the ECF, an Na^+ and a glucose molecule bind to another carrier protein. *Right,* The carrier protein transports the Na^+ and glucose molecule into the cell—the Na^+ with its concentration gradient, and the glucose against its concentration gradient. *ADP,* Adenosine diphosphate; *P,* protein. (Redrawn from Amerman, E. C. [2016]. *Human anatomy and physiology* [p. 81, Fig. 3.11]. Upper Saddle River, NJ: Pearson Education Inc.)

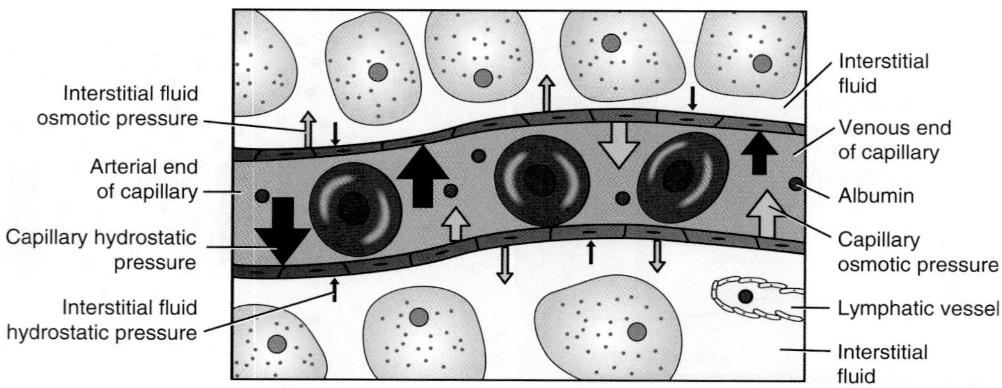

FIGURE 40-5 Capillary filtration. (From Copstead, L. C., & Banasik, J. L. [2013]. *Pathophysiology* [5th ed.]. St. Louis: Saunders.)

TABLE 40-1 Healthy Adult Average Fluid Intake and Output

	Normal (per Day)	Prolonged Heavy Exercise (per Hour)
Fluid Intake		
Fluids Ingested		
Oral	1 100–1 400 mL	280–1 100 mL/hr
Foods	800–1 000 mL	Highly variable
Metabolism	300 mL	16–50 mL/hr
TOTAL	2 200–2 700 mL	300–1 150 mL/hr
Fluid Output		
Skin (insensible and sweat)	500–600 mL	300–2 100 mL/hour
Insensible lungs	400 mL	20 mL/hr
Gastrointestinal	100–200 mL	Negligible, unless diarrhea during exercise
Urine	1 200–1 500 mL	20–1 000 mL/hr, depending on hydration status
TOTAL	2 200–2 700 mL	340–3 120 mL/hr Rehydration with Na^+-containing fluid necessary after prolonged vigorous exercise

Data from Hall, J. E. (2016). *Guyton and Hall textbook of medical physiology* (13th ed.). Philadelphia: Saunders; American College of Sports Medicine (ACSM). (2016). Position stand on exercise and fluid replacement. *Medicine & Science in Sports Exercise, 39*(2), 377.

The gastrointestinal tract plays a vital role in fluid regulation. Every day, approximately 9 L of fluid is ingested or secreted into the small intestine and then absorbed into the enterocytes of the small intestine and from the large intestine. Only approximately 100 mL is lost through the feces, under normal conditions (Amerman, 2016, p. 889). However, in the presence of a disease process, for example, diarrhea, the gastrointestinal tract may become the site of a large amount of fluid loss. This loss may have a significant impact on maintaining normal fluid homeostasis.

Fluid Intake Regulation. Fluid intake is regulated primarily through the thirst mechanism. The thirst control centre is located within the brain's hypothalamus. **Osmoreceptors** continually monitor the serum osmotic pressure, and when osmolality increases, even slightly (2% – 3%), the thirst centre is stimulated (Amerman, 2016, p. 990). An increase in plasma sodium increases the osmotic pressure and stimulates the thirst mechanism. Increased plasma osmolality can occur with any condition that interferes with the oral ingestion of fluids or with the intake of hypertonic fluids. The thirst centre will also be stimulated if plasma volume decreases, and **hypovolemia** occurs, as in excessive vomiting and hemorrhage. In addition, stimulation of the renin–angiotensin–aldosterone mechanism, potassium depletion, psychological factors, and oropharyngeal dryness initiate the sensation of thirst.

The average adult's fluid intake is about 2 200 to 2 700 mL per day; oral intake accounts for 1 100 to 1 400 mL, solid foods for about 800 to 1 000 mL, and oxidative metabolism for 300 mL daily. Patients must be in an alert state to maintain their fluid intake independently. Infants, patients with neurological or psychological problems, and some older persons who are unable to perceive or respond to the thirst mechanism are at risk for **dehydration**.

Hormonal Regulation of Fluid

Antidiuretic hormone (ADH) is stored in the posterior pituitary gland and is released in response to changes in blood osmolality. The osmoreceptors in the hypothalamus are stimulated to release ADH when the osmolality increases. ADH promotes water conservation by acting directly on the renal tubules and collecting ducts to make them more permeable to water. This, in turn, causes water to return to the systemic circulation, which dilutes the blood and decreases its osmolality. As the body attempts to compensate, the patient will experience a temporary decrease in urinary output. When the blood has been sufficiently diluted, the osmoreceptors stop the release of ADH and urinary output is restored. ADH also stimulates the thirst centre to promote fluid intake (Figure 40-6).

Aldosterone is released by the adrenal cortex in response to increased plasma potassium or falling sodium levels or as part of the renin–angiotensin–aldosterone system (RAAS) to counteract hypovolemia. To resolve hypovolemia, renin is released from the kidney in response to sympathetic nervous system stimulation and decreased renal blood flow, initiating a cascade of physiological and endocrine processes, one of which is the release of aldosterone. Aldosterone acts on the distal portion of the renal tubule to increase the reabsorption (saving) of sodium and the secretion and excretion of potassium and hydrogen.

Natriuretic peptides respond to increases in circulating blood volume. They are released from cardiac muscle cells and act on the peripheral vasculature, other hormones, and the kidney to facilitate diuresis. Natriuretic peptides increase sodium excretion and fluid loss while reducing thirst and blocking the release of ADH and aldosterone.

Regulation of Electrolytes

For normal cell function and human well-being, the body maintains a normal balance of electrolytes in the ECF and ICF, in spite of changes in intake and loss. This is accomplished primarily through electrolyte intake, absorption in the gastrointestinal tract, distribution, and excretion through the kidneys, feces, and sweat. Distribution is significant to overall electrolyte homeostasis, as some electrolytes, such as potassium, sodium, calcium, and phosphate, have very low plasma concentrations compared with cell and bone concentrations (Hall, 2016). Although fluid and electrolyte balances are inextricably linked, it is important to explore electrolyte balance separately.

Cations. Major cations within the body fluids are sodium, potassium, calcium, and magnesium (Mg^{2+}). Cations interchange when one cation leaves the cell and is replaced by another. This occurs because cells tend to maintain electrical neutrality.

Sodium Regulation. Sodium is the most abundant cation (90%) in ECF and thus exerts the greatest influence on the ECF osmotic concentration and water balance. Sodium ions are also major contributors to nerve impulse transmission, regulation of acid–base balance, and cellular chemical reactions. Normally, the intake and output of sodium is between 1.2 g and 3.3 g daily. With an increase in sodium intake and, therefore, an increase in ECF sodium content, water enters the ECF by osmosis. Therefore, increased sodium intake results in increased blood volume rather than significant changes in ECF sodium concentration.

The body continually responds to small changes in sodium content. A decrease in sodium in the ECF passing through the nephrons stimulates the RAAS to increase sodium reabsorption in the nephron. These actions indirectly increase water reabsorption as well (Amerman, 2016, 995). The normal extracellular sodium concentration is 135 to 145 mmol/L. Sustained or severe problems with sodium concentration result in high sodium, above 145 mmol/L (hypernatremia), or low sodium, below 135 mmol/L (hyponatremia).

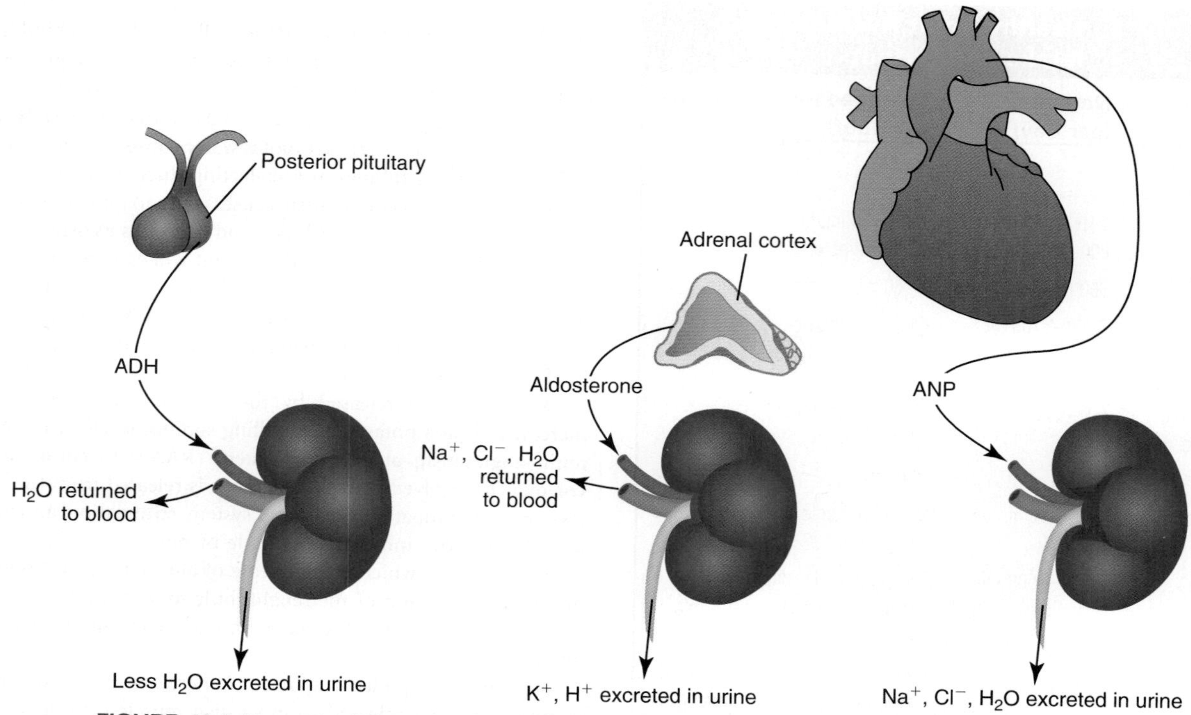

FIGURE 40-6 Hormone-influenced fluid excretion. *ADH,* Antidiuretic hormone; *ANP,* atrial natriuretic peptide; *Cl^-,* chloride; *H^+,* hydrogen ions; *H_2O,* water; *K^+,* potassium; *Na^+,* sodium.

Potassium Regulation. Potassium is the major electrolyte and principal cation in the intracellular compartment. The majority (98%) of potassium content is in the ICF. Because the potassium concentration of ECF is relatively low, the cells expend energy to maintain the potassium content of ICF. Potassium is regulated by dietary intake and strongly affected by aldosterone, insulin, and epinephrine. Extracellular potassium concentration is affected by many complex mechanisms, including those of dietary intake and renal excretion. Renal excretion is regulated by changes in potassium concentration, changes in the acidity or alkalinity of a fluid (pH measurements), sodium reabsorption, and aldosterone levels. Aldosterone secretion is triggered by many factors; therefore, potassium balance is influenced by other factors, including changes in fluid volume, blood pressure, and acidosis (Amerman, 2016, p. 997).

Potassium regulates many metabolic activities and is necessary for glycogen deposits in the liver and skeletal muscle, transmission and conduction of nerve impulses, normal cardiac conduction, and skeletal and smooth muscle contraction. The normal range for serum potassium concentrations is 3.5 to 5 mmol/L.

Calcium Regulation. Calcium is stored in bone, plasma, and body cells. Ninety-nine percent of calcium is located in bone, and only 1% is located in ECF. Approximately 50% of calcium in the plasma is bound to protein, primarily albumin, and 40% is free ionized calcium. The remaining small percentage is combined with nonprotein anions such as phosphate (PO_4^{3-}), citrate, and carbonate. Normal serum ionized calcium is 1.0 to 1.2 mmol/L. Normal total calcium is 2.25 to 2.75 mmol/L. Calcium is necessary for bone and teeth formation, blood clotting, hormone secretion, cell membrane integrity, cardiac conduction, transmission of nerve impulses, and muscle contraction.

Magnesium Regulation. Magnesium, the second most abundant intracellular cation, is essential for many intracellular activities, such as enzyme reactions. Magnesium, with a plasma concentration of 0.65 to 1.05 mmol/L, is important for bone structure and neuromuscular function, including skeletal and cardiac muscle excitability. Serum magnesium is regulated by dietary intake, renal mechanisms, and actions of the parathyroid hormone.

Anions. The three major anions of body fluids are chloride, bicarbonate, and phosphate ions.

Chloride Regulation. Chloride is the major anion in ECF. The transport of chloride follows sodium. Normal concentrations of chloride range from 97 to 107 mmol/L. Serum chloride is regulated by dietary intake and the kidneys. A person with normal renal function who has a high chloride intake will excrete a higher amount of urine chloride.

Bicarbonate Regulation. Bicarbonate is the major chemical base buffer within the body. The bicarbonate ion is found in ECF and ICF. The bicarbonate ion is an essential component of the carbonic acid–bicarbonate buffering system, which is essential to acid–base balance. The kidneys regulate bicarbonate. Normal arterial bicarbonate levels range between 22 and 26 mmol/L; venous bicarbonate is measured as carbon dioxide content, and the normal value is 24 to 30 mmol/L (Table 40-2).

Phosphate Regulation. Phosphorus is the major anion in the ICF; however, nearly all the phosphorus in the body exists in the form of phosphate. Phosphate's most important role is within the ICF, where it assists in the formation of high-energy compounds, such as ATP and nucleic acids, and in enzyme activity. Similar to magnesium and calcium, phosphate is used and stored in the skeleton. It also functions with calcium to develop and maintain teeth. Calcium and phosphate are inversely proportional; if one rises, the other falls. Phosphate also assists in acid–base regulation, promotes normal neuromuscular action, and participates in carbohydrate metabolism. Phosphate is normally absorbed through the gastrointestinal tract and is regulated by

TABLE 40-2 Laboratory Normal Values for Adults

Item Measured	Normal Value in Serum or Blood
Osmolality	280–300 mOsm/kg H_2O (SI units)
Electrolytes	
Sodium (Na^+)	136–145 mmol/L (SI units)
Potassium (K^+)	3.5–5 mmol/L (SI units)
Chloride (Cl^-)	98–106 mmol/L (SI units)
Total CO_2 (CO_2 total content)	22–30 mmol/L (SI units)
Bicarbonate (HCO_3^-)	Arterial: 22–26 mmol/L (SI units) Venous: 24–30 mmol/L (SI units)
Total calcium (Ca^{2+})	2.25–2.75 mmol/L (SI units)
Ionized calcium (Ca^{2+})	1.05–1.30 mmol/L (SI units)
Magnesium (Mg^{2+})	0.65–1.05 mmol/L (SI units)
Phosphate	0.97–1.45 mmol/L (SI units)
Anion gap	5–11 mmol/L (SI units)
Arterial Blood Gases	
pH	7.35–7.45
$Paco_2$	35–45 mm Hg (4.7–6 kPa)
PaO_2	80–100 mm Hg (10.7–133.3 kPa)
O_2 saturation	95–100% (0.95–1.00)
Base excess	−2 to +2 mmol/L (SI units)

dietary intake, renal and intestinal excretion, and parathyroid hormone. The normal serum phosphorus level is 0.9 to 1.45 mmol/L.

Regulation of Acid–Base Balance

Acid–base balance exists when the rate at which the body produces and gains acids or bases, through cellular metabolism and gastrointestinal absorption, equals the rate at which acids or bases are excreted.

This balance results in a stable concentration of hydrogen ions (H^+) in body fluids that is expressed as the pH value. Hydrogen ions are primarily excreted by the kidneys. A normal hydrogen ion level is necessary to maintain cell membrane integrity and the speed of cellular enzymatic actions.

Arterial blood pH is inversely proportional to the hydrogen ion concentration (i.e., the greater the concentration, the more acidic the solution is and the lower the pH is; the lower the concentration, the more alkaline the solution is and the higher the pH is). The pH is also a reflection of the balance between carbon dioxide, which is regulated by the lungs, and bicarbonate, a base regulated by the kidneys. Normal pH is maintained by chemical buffers, and buffer systems and regulatory mechanisms in the kidneys and lungs. A buffer is a substance or group of substances that can absorb or release hydrogen ions to stabilize pH, such as bicarbonate, phosphate, and proteins. The respiratory system, which controls the amount of carbon dioxide in the body, the hydrogen and bicarbonate ions, and therefore pH in the ECF, and the kidney are physiological buffer systems.

Buffers. Buffer systems are combinations of a weak acid and a weak base and are the short-term regulators of acid–base balance. The four main types of buffer systems are protein (amino acids, plasma proteins), hemoglobin (also a protein but unique in its buffering role), carbonic acid (H_2CO_3) and bicarbonate, and phosphate. Other types are the ammonia buffer system, a complex system that occurs in ICF, and the tubular system in the kidneys. All these buffers bind hydrogen ions until they can be permanently removed through the regulatory mechanisms in the lungs and the kidneys.

The carbonic acid–bicarbonate buffer system is used to evaluate acid–base balance, using the arterial blood gas (ABG) test. This system can be expressed as the following:

$$CO_2 + H_2O \leftrightarrow H_2CO_3 \leftrightarrow H^+ + HCO_3^-$$

$$\text{Carbon dioxide} + \text{Water} \leftrightarrow \text{Carbonic acid} \leftrightarrow \text{Hydrogen ion} + \text{Bicarbonate}$$

The carbonic acid–bicarbonate buffer system is the principal buffering system to react to change in the pH of ECF, and it reacts within seconds. Whenever carbon dioxide increases, an increase in hydrogen ions results, and whenever hydrogen ions are produced, more carbon dioxide results (Amerman, 2016, p. 1000). The lungs control the excretion of carbon dioxide, and the kidneys control the excretion of hydrogen and bicarbonate ions.

Another buffer system is the hemoglobin–oxyhemoglobin system within red blood cells (RBCs). This buffer system can have an immediate effect on pH because carbon dioxide diffuses readily into the RBCs and forms carbonic acid. The carbonic acid dissociates into hydrogen and bicarbonate ions, the latter of which diffuse into the plasma in exchange for chloride. The hydrogen ions attach to hemoglobin, whereas the carbon dioxide is carried to the lungs, where the reaction is reversed.

Regulatory Mechanisms. When the ability of buffer systems is exceeded, acid–base homeostasis is regulated by the lungs and the kidneys. The lungs adapt rapidly to an acid–base imbalance. Ordinarily, increased levels of hydrogen ions and carbon dioxide provide the stimulus for respiration. When the concentration of hydrogen ions is altered, the lungs react to correct the imbalance by altering the rate and depth of respiration. For example, when metabolic acidosis is present, respirations are increased, resulting in a greater amount of carbon dioxide being exhaled, which results in a decrease in the acidic level; when metabolic alkalosis is present, the lungs retain carbon dioxide by decreasing the respirations, thereby increasing the acidic level (Amerman, 2016, pp. 1004–1006).

The kidneys take from a few hours to several days to regulate acid–base imbalance. They regenerate or reabsorb bicarbonate in cases of acid excess and excrete it in cases of acid deficit. In addition, the kidneys use a phosphate ion to excrete hydrogen ions by forming phosphoric acid (H_3PO_4). Finally, the kidneys use the ammonia mechanism to regulate acid–base balance. In this mechanism, certain amino acids are chemically changed within the renal tubules into ammonia, which, in the presence of hydrogen ions, forms ammonium, which is excreted in the urine, thereby releasing hydrogen ions from the body (Amerman, 2016, pp. 1002–1004).

Disturbances in Electrolyte, Fluid, and Acid–Base Balances

Disturbances in electrolyte, fluid, or acid–base balance seldom occur alone and can disrupt normal body processes. For example, when body fluids are lost because of burns, illness, or trauma, the patient is also at risk for electrolyte imbalances. In addition, some untreated electrolyte imbalances (e.g., potassium loss) contribute to acid–base disturbances.

Fluid Disturbances. Fluid imbalances include volume imbalances, or disturbances in the amount of ECF, and osmolality imbalances, or disturbances in the concentration of body fluids (hyper- or hypo-osmolar imbalance). Isotonic deficit and excess exist when water and electrolytes are gained or lost in equal proportion. In contrast, osmolar imbalances are losses or excesses of only water, so the concentration (osmolality) of the serum is affected. It is important to recognize that maintaining fluid homeostasis is primarily related to circulatory volume. Hemodynamics respond quickly to changes in the intravascular compartment, followed more slowly by sodium and water balance mechanisms. Table 40-3 lists the common fluid isotonic and osmolality imbalances, the causes and signs, and related symptoms.

TABLE 40-3 Fluid Imbalances

Imbalance and Related Causes	Signs and Symptoms
Isotonic Imbalances—Water and Sodium Lost or Gained in Equal or Isotonic Proportions	
Extracellular Fluid Volume Deficit—Body Fluids Have Decreased Volume but Normal Osmolality	
Sodium and Water Intake Less Than Output, Causing Isotonic Loss: Severely decreased oral intake of water and salt Increased GI output: vomiting, diarrhea, laxative overuse, drainage from fistulas or tubes Increased renal output: use of diuretics, adrenal insufficiency (deficit of cortisol and aldosterone) Loss of blood or plasma: hemorrhage, burns Massive sweating without water and salt intake	*Physical examination:* Sudden weight loss (overnight), postural hypotension, tachycardia, thready pulse, dry mucous membranes, poor skin turgor, slow vein filling, flat neck veins when supine, dark yellow urine If severe: thirst, restlessness, confusion, hypotension; oliguria (urine output *below* 30 mL/hr); cold, clammy skin; hypovolemic shock *Laboratory findings:* Increased hematocrit; increased BUN *above* 8.9 mmol/L (hemoconcentration); urine specific gravity usually *above* 1.030, unless renal cause
Extracellular Fluid Volume Excess—Body Fluids Have Increased Volume but Normal Osmolality	
Sodium and Water Intake Greater Than Output, Causing Isotonic Gain: Excessive administration of Na^+-containing isotonic IV fluids or oral intake of salty foods and water Renal retention of Na^+ and water: heart failure, cirrhosis, aldosterone or glucocorticoid excess, acute or chronic oliguric renal disease	*Physical examination:* Sudden weight gain (overnight), edema (especially in dependent areas), full neck veins when upright or semi-upright, crackles in lungs If severe: confusion, pulmonary edema *Laboratory findings:* Decreased hematocrit, decreased BUN *below* 3.6 mmol/L (hemodilution)
Osmolality Imbalances	
Hypernatremia (Water Deficit; Hyperosmolar Imbalance)—Body Fluids Too Concentrated	
Loss of Relatively More Water Than Salt: Diabetes insipidus (ADH deficiency) Osmotic diuresis Large insensible perspiration and respiratory water output without increased water intake	*Physical examination:* Decreased level of consciousness (confusion, lethargy, coma), perhaps thirst, seizures if develops rapidly or is very severe *Laboratory findings:* Serum Na^+ level *above* 145 mmol/L, serum osmolality *above* 300 mmol/kg
Gain of Relatively More Salt Than Water: Administration of tube feedings, hypertonic parenteral fluids, or salt tablets Lack of access to water, deliberate water deprivation, inability to respond to thirst (e.g., immobility, aphasia) Dysfunction of osmoreceptor-driven thirst drive	
Hyponatremia (Water Excess; Water Intoxication; Hypo-osmolar Imbalance)—Body Fluids Too Dilute	
Gain of Relatively More Water Than Salt: Excessive ADH (SIADH) Psychogenic polydipsia or forced excessive water intake Excessive IV administration of D_5W Use of hypotonic irrigating solutions Tap-water enemas	*Physical examination:* Decreased level of consciousness (confusion, lethargy, coma), seizures if develops rapidly or is very severe *Laboratory findings:* Serum Na^+ level *below* 135 mmol/L, serum osmolality *below* 280 mmol/kg
Loss of Relatively More Salt Than Water: Replacement of large body fluid output (e.g., diarrhea, vomiting) with water but no salt	
Combined Volume and Osmolality Imbalance	
Clinical Dehydration (Extracellular Fluid Volume Deficit plus Hypernatremia)—Body Fluids Have Decreased Volume and Are Too Concentrated	
Sodium and Water Intake Less Than Output, With Loss of Relatively More Water Than Salt: All of the causes of ECV deficit (see previous causes) plus poor or no water intake, often with fever causing increased insensible water output	*Physical examination and laboratory findings:* Combination of those for ECV deficit plus those for hypernatremia (see previous signs)

ADH, Antidiuretic hormone; *BUN*, blood urea nitrogen; *ECV*, extracellular fluid volume; *GI*, gastrointestinal; D_5W, 5% dextrose in water; *IV*, intravenous; *SIADH*, syndrome of inappropriate secretion of antidiuretic hormone.

Fluid volume deficit is insufficient isotonic fluid in the extracellular compartment. Because this involves both intravascular and interstitial compartments, symptoms also relate to both compartments. Fluid volume excess is too much isotonic fluid in the extracellular compartment, and so symptoms also relate to intravascular and interstitial compartments, such as swollen fingers or ankles. Osmolar fluid imbalances involve a fluid imbalance accompanied by either elevated sodium (hypernatremia) or lower sodium (hyponatremia). Clinical dehydration, caused by reduced sodium and water intake, or loss of more water proportionately than salt, is a combined volume and osmolality imbalance. Serum sodium and osmolality values are required to diagnose hypertonic and hypotonic fluid volume deficits. Physical examination and lab values are important for diagnosing and treating these complex imbalances.

Electrolyte Imbalances. Many factors can disrupt electrolyte homeostasis, including acute infections causing diarrhea, metabolic disorders, altered electrolyte intake, sudden loss of electrolytes in the case of burns or acute vomiting, medications, and shifts in the distribution of electrolytes from cells or bones into the ECF. Table 40-4 provides a list of the causes, signs, and symptoms of electrolyte imbalances.

Sodium Imbalances. Hyponatremia is a lower-than-normal concentration of sodium in the blood (serum), which can occur with a net sodium loss or net water excess (see Table 40-3). It occurs frequently in seriously ill patients and is the most common electrolyte disturbance among older persons (El-Sharkawy, Sahota, & Lobo, 2015). Clinical indicators and treatment depend on the cause of hyponatremia and whether it is associated with a normal, decreased, or increased ECF volume. The usual situation is a loss of sodium without a loss of fluid, which results in a decrease in the osmolality of ECF. Sodium and chloride are not stored in the body; therefore, they must be consumed daily or provided through intravenous solutions in the ill.

Hypernatremia is a greater-than-normal concentration of sodium in ECF that can be caused by excess water loss or overall sodium excess (see Table 40-3). When hypernatremia occurs, the body attempts to conserve as much water as possible through renal reabsorption.

Potassium Imbalances. Hypokalemia is one of the most common electrolyte imbalances (see Table 40-4). Hypokalemia, with potassium levels less than 3.5 mmol/L, results in cardiac arrhythmias, fatigue, and altered muscle activity throughout the body (Paul, Day, & Williams, 2016, p. 301). Because the normal amount of serum potassium is so small, little tolerance for fluctuations exists. The most common cause

TABLE 40-4 Electrolyte Imbalances

Imbalance and Related Causes	Signs and Symptoms
Hypokalemia—Low Serum Potassium (K^+) Concentration	
Decreased K^+ Intake: Excessive use of K^+-free IV solutions ***Shift of K^+ Into Cells:*** Alkalosis; treatment of diabetic ketoacidosis with insulin ***Increased K^+ Output:*** Acute or chronic diarrhea; vomiting; other GI losses (e.g., nasogastric or fistula drainage); use of potassium-wasting diuretics; aldosterone excess; polyuria; glucocorticoid therapy	*Physical examination:* Bilateral muscle weakness that begins in quadriceps and may ascend to respiratory muscles, abdominal distension, decreased bowel sounds, constipation, dysrhythmias *Laboratory findings:* Serum K^+ level *below* 3.5 mmol/L; ECG abnormalities: U waves, flattened or inverted T waves; ST segment depression
Hyperkalemia—High Serum Potassium (K^+) Concentration	
Increased K^+ Intake: Iatrogenic administration of large amounts of IV K^+; rapid infusion of stored blood; excess ingestion of K^+ salt substitutes ***Shift of K^+ Out of Cells:*** Massive cellular damage (e.g., crushing trauma, cytotoxic chemotherapy); insufficient insulin (e.g., diabetic ketoacidosis); some types of acidosis ***Decreased K^+ Output:*** Acute or chronic oliguria (e.g., severe ECV deficit, end-stage renal disease); use of potassium-sparing diuretics; adrenal insufficiency (deficit of cortisol and aldosterone)	*Physical examination:* Bilateral muscle weakness in quadriceps, transient abdominal cramps, diarrhea, dysrhythmias, cardiac arrest if severe *Laboratory findings:* Serum K^+ level *above* 5 mmol/L; ECG abnormalities: peaked T waves; widened QRS complex; PR prolongation; terminal sine-wave pattern
Hypocalcemia—Low Serum Calcium (Ca^{2+}) Concentration	
Decreased Ca^{2+} Intake and Absorption: Calcium-deficient diet; vitamin D deficiency (includes end-stage renal disease); chronic diarrhea; laxative misuse; steatorrhea ***Shift of Ca^{2+} Into Bone or Inactive Form:*** Hypoparathyroidism; rapid administration of citrated blood; hypoalbuminemia; alkalosis; pancreatitis; hyperphosphatemia (includes end-stage renal disease) ***Increased Ca^{2+} Output:*** Chronic diarrhea; steatorrhea	*Physical examination:* Numbness and tingling of fingers, toes, and circumoral (around mouth) region; positive Chvostek's sign (contraction of facial muscles when facial nerve is tapped); hyperactive reflexes; muscle twitching and cramping; carpal and pedal spasms; tetany; seizures; laryngospasm; dysrhythmias *Laboratory findings:* Total serum Ca^{2+} level *below* 2.25 mmol/L or serum ionized Ca^{2+} level *below* 1.05 mmol/L; ECG abnormalities: prolonged ST segments

Continued

TABLE 40-4 Electrolyte Imbalances—cont'd

Imbalance and Related Causes	Signs and Symptoms
Hypercalcemia—High Serum Calcium (Ca^{2+}) Concentration	
Increased Ca^{2+} Intake and Absorption: Milk-alkali syndrome ***Shift of Ca^{2+} Out of Bone:*** Prolonged immobilization; hyperparathyroidism; bone tumours; nonosseous cancers that secrete bone-resorbing factors ***Decreased Ca^{2+} Output:*** Use of thiazide diuretics	*Physical examination:* Anorexia, nausea and vomiting, constipation, fatigue, diminished reflexes, lethargy, decreased level of consciousness, confusion, personality change, cardiac arrest if severe *Laboratory findings:* Total serum Ca^{2+} level *above* 2.75 mmol/L or serum ionized Ca^{2+} level *above* 1.3 mmol/L; ECG abnormalities: heart block, shortened ST segments
Hypomagnesemia—Low Serum Magnesium (Mg^{2+}) Concentration	
Decreased Mg^{2+} Intake and Absorption: Malnutrition; chronic alcoholism; chronic diarrhea; laxative misuse; steatorrhea ***Shift of Mg^{2+} Into Inactive Form:*** Rapid administration of citrated blood ***Increased Mg^{2+} Output:*** Chronic diarrhea; steatorrhea; other GI losses (e.g., vomiting, nasogastric or fistula drainage); use of thiazide or loop diuretics; aldosterone excess	*Physical examination:* Positive Chvostek's sign, hyperactive deep tendon reflexes, muscle cramps and twitching, grimacing, dysphagia, tetany, seizures, insomnia, tachycardia, hypertension, dysrhythmias *Laboratory findings:* Serum Mg^{2+} level *below* 0.65 mmol/L; ECG abnormalities: prolonged QT interval
Hypermagnesemia—High Serum Magnesium (Mg^{2+}) Concentration	
Increased Mg^{2+} Intake and Absorption: Excessive use of Mg^{2+}-containing laxatives and antacids; parenteral overload of magnesium ***Decreased Mg^{2+} Output:*** Oliguric end-stage renal disease; adrenal insufficiency	*Physical examination:* Lethargy, hypoactive deep tendon reflexes, bradycardia, hypotension Acute elevation in Mg^{2+} levels: Flushing, sensation of warmth Severe acute hypermagnesemia: Decreased rate and depth of respirations, dysrhythmias, cardiac arrest *Laboratory findings:* Serum Mg^{2+} level *above* 1.05 mmol/L; ECG abnormalities: prolonged PR interval

ECG, Electrocardiogram, *ECV*, extracellular fluid volume, *GI*, gastrointestinal, *IV*, intravenous.
Data from Felver, L. (2013). Fluid and electrolyte homeostasis and imbalances. In L. C. Copstead & J. L. Banasik (Eds.), *Pathophysiology* (5th ed.). St. Louis: Saunders.

of hypokalemia is the use of potassium-wasting diuretics such as thiazide and loop diuretics.

Hyperkalemia is a greater-than-normal amount of potassium in the blood. Lethal cardiac arrhythmias result from potassium levels over 5.0 mmol/L, as well as skeletal muscle weakness and paralysis (see Table 40-4). The primary cause of hyperkalemia is renal failure, because any decrease in renal function diminishes the amount of potassium the kidney can excrete.

Calcium Imbalances. Hypocalcemia represents a drop in serum or ionized calcium. It can result from several illnesses, some of which directly affect the thyroid and parathyroid glands (see Table 40-4). Other causes include prolonged bed rest and renal insufficiency (in which the kidneys' inability to excrete phosphorus causes the phosphorus level to rise and the calcium level to decline). Signs and symptoms can be related to diminished functioning of the neuromuscular, cardiac, and renal systems.

Hypercalcemia is an increase in the total serum concentration of calcium or ionized calcium (see Table 40-4). Hypercalcemia is frequently a symptom of an underlying disease, such as malignancy or hyperparathyroidism, resulting in excess bone reabsorption with release of calcium (McCance & Huether, 2010).

Magnesium Imbalances. Disturbances in magnesium levels are summarized in Table 40-4. Symptoms are the result of changes in neuromuscular excitability. Hypomagnesemia, a drop in serum magnesium below 0.65 mmol/L, occurs with malnutrition, malabsorption disorders, diarrhea, and alcohol withdrawal. This may cause neuromuscular symptoms, seizures, or cardiac arrhythmias. Hypermagnesemia, an increase in serum magnesium levels more than 1.05 mmol/L, depresses skeletal muscles and nerve function. Magnesium may inhibit acetylcholine, thereby causing a sedative effect.

Chloride Imbalances. Hypochloremia occurs when the serum chloride level falls below normal. Vomiting or prolonged and excessive nasogastric or fistula drainage can result in hypochloremia because of the loss of hydrochloric acid. The use of loop and thiazide diuretics also results in increased chloride loss as sodium is excreted. When serum chloride levels fall, metabolic alkalosis results as the body adapts by increasing reabsorption of the bicarbonate ion to maintain electrical neutrality.

Hyperchloremia occurs when the serum chloride level rises above normal, which usually occurs when the serum bicarbonate value falls or the sodium level rises. Hypochloremia and hyperchloremia rarely occur as single disease processes but are commonly associated with acid–base imbalance. No single set of symptoms is associated with these two alterations.

Acid–Base Balance. Arterial blood gas (ABG) analysis is the best way to evaluate acid–base balance and is based on the carbonic acid–bicarbonate buffer system. Measurement of ABGs involves analysis of six components: pH, $Paco_2$, PaO_2, oxygen saturation, base excess, and bicarbonate (see Table 40-2). Deviation from a normal value will indicate that the patient is experiencing an acid–base imbalance.

Measurements of Acidity or Alkalinity of Fluids. The pH reflects hydrogen ion concentration in the body fluids. Even a slight change can be potentially life-threatening. An increase in concentration of hydrogen ion makes a solution more acidic; a decrease makes the solution more alkaline. Normal pH value is 7.35 to 7.45; therefore, a pH value below 7.35 is acidic, and above 7.45 is alkalotic (Table 40-5).

$Paco_2$. $Paco_2$ is the partial pressure of carbon dioxide in arterial blood and is a reflection of the depth of pulmonary ventilation. The normal range is 35 to 45 mm Hg. A $Paco_2$ less than 35 mm Hg is an indication that hyperventilation has occurred. As the rate and depth of respiration increase, more carbon dioxide is exhaled, and the carbon dioxide concentration decreases. When the $Paco_2$ is more than 45 mm Hg, hypoventilation has occurred. As the rate and the depth of respiration decrease, less carbon dioxide is exhaled and more is retained, increasing the concentration of carbon dioxide.

PaO_2. PaO_2 is the partial pressure of oxygen in arterial blood. It has no primary role in acid–base regulation if it is within normal limits. A PaO_2 less than 60 mm Hg can lead to anaerobic metabolism, resulting in lactic acid production and metabolic acidosis. The normal range is 80 to 100 mm Hg.

Oxygen Saturation. Oxygen saturation is the point at which hemoglobin is saturated by oxygen. Decreasing PaO_2 causes an increase in oxygen dissociation from hemoglobin. Oxygen saturation can be affected by changes in temperature, pH, and $Paco_2$. The normal range is 95% to 99%.

Base Excess. Base excess refers to the buffering systems discussed previously, with a normal range of +2 to −2. Base excess reflects deviations from a serum pH of 7.4 (neutral). Higher values of base excess indicate alkalosis. Negative values of base excess indicate acidosis, usually the result of the elimination of too many bicarbonate ions.

Bicarbonate. Serum bicarbonate is excreted or retained by the kidneys to maintain a normal acid–base environment. It is also the principal buffer of the ECFs of the body. A normal pH is maintained with a bicarbonate ratio 20 times that of the fluid concentration of carbonic acid (McCance & Huether, 2010). The normal range is 22 to 26 mmol/L. Less than 22 mmol/L of bicarbonate usually indicates metabolic acidosis, whereas more than 26 mmol/L indicates metabolic alkalosis.

Types of Acid–Base Imbalances

The four primary types of acid–base imbalance are respiratory acidosis, respiratory alkalosis, metabolic acidosis, and metabolic alkalosis (Table 40-6).

Respiratory Acidosis. Respiratory acidosis is marked by an increased $Paco_2$, excess carbonic acid, and an increased hydrogen ion concentration (decreased pH). This occurs when respirations are not effective in excreting carbon dioxide, resulting in an increase in hydrogen concentration. With respiratory acidosis, carbon dioxide crosses the blood–brain barrier, causing neurological changes, such as headaches, irritability, and, ultimately, impaired consciousness. Hypoxemia occurs simultaneously because of respiratory depression, resulting in further neurological impairment. Electrolyte changes such as hyperkalemia and hypercalcemia may accompany the acidosis. The renal system compensates by increasing bicarbonate and eliminating hydrogen ion.

An example is the following: Mr. Butler comes to the emergency department short of breath. The first set of ABGs shows the following: pH = 7.26, $Paco_2$ = 55 mm Hg, and bicarbonate = 23 mmol/L. His body has not yet compensated for his respiratory insufficiency. A person with chronic lung disease may present with greater compensation and a pH that is closer to normal.

Respiratory Alkalosis. Respiratory alkalosis is marked by decreased $Paco_2$ and increased pH. Respiratory alkalosis can begin outside the respiratory system (e.g., anxiety with hyperventilation) or within the respiratory system (e.g., the initial phase of an asthma attack). Usually, the respiratory system corrects imbalances before compensatory changes are required.

An example is the following: Ms. Chang is hyperventilating when she comes into the emergency department. Her ABGs are as follows: pH = 7.52, $Paco_2$ = 30 mm Hg, bicarbonate = 24 mmol/L, and base

TABLE 40-5 Arterial Blood Gas Measures

Laboratory Measure	Normal Range in Adult Arterial Blood	Definition and Interpretation
pH	7.35–7.45	pH is a negative logarithm of the free H^+ concentration, a measure of how acid or alkaline the blood is. Values below 7.35 indicate abnormally acid; above 7.45 they indicate abnormally alkaline. Small changes in pH denote large changes in H^+ concentration and are clinically important.
$Paco_2$	35–45 mm Hg (4.7–6 kPa)	$Paco_2$ is partial pressure of carbon dioxide (CO_2), a measure of how well the lungs are excreting CO_2 produced by cells. Increased $Paco_2$ indicates CO_2 accumulation in blood (more carbonic acid) caused by hypoventilation; decreased $Paco_2$ indicates excessive CO_2 excretion (less carbonic acid) through hyperventilation.
HCO_3^-	22–26 mmol/L	HCO_3^- is concentration of the base (alkaline substance) bicarbonate, a measure of how well the kidneys are excreting metabolic acids. Increased HCO_3^- indicates that the blood has too few metabolic acids; decreased HCO_3^- indicates that the blood has too many metabolic acids.
PaO_2	80–100 mm Hg (10–13.3 kPa)	PaO_2 is partial pressure of oxygen (O_2), a measure of how well gas exchange is occurring in the alveoli of the lungs. Values below normal indicate poor oxygenation of the blood.
SaO_2	95%–100%	SaO_2 is oxygen saturation, the percentage of hemoglobin that is carrying as much O_2 as possible. It is influenced by pH, $Paco_2$, and body temperature. It drops rapidly when PaO_2 falls below 60 mm Hg (8 kPa).
Base excess	−2 to +2 mmol/L	Base excess is observed buffering capacity minus the normal buffering capacity, a measure of how well the blood buffers are managing metabolic acids. Values below −2 (negative base excess) indicate excessive metabolic acids; values above +2 indicate excessive amounts of bicarbonate.

TABLE 40-6 Acid–Base Imbalances

Imbalance and Related Causes	Signs and Symptoms
Respiratory Acidosis—Excessive Carbonic Acid Caused by Alveolar Hypoventilation	
Impaired Gas Exchange: Type B COPD (chronic bronchitis) or end-stage type A COPD (emphysema) Bacterial pneumonia Airway obstruction Extensive atelectasis (collapsed alveoli) Severe acute asthma episode	*Physical examination:* Headache, light-headedness, decreased level of consciousness (confusion, lethargy, coma), dysrhythmias *Laboratory findings:* Arterial blood gas alterations: pH *below* 7.35, $Paco_2$ *above* 45 mm Hg (6 kPa), HCO_3^- level normal if uncompensated or *above* 26 mmol/L if compensated
Impaired Neuromuscular Function: Respiratory muscle weakness or paralysis from hypokalemia or neurological dysfunction Respiratory muscle fatigue, respiratory failure Chest wall injury or surgery causing pain with respiration	
Dysfunction of Brainstem Respiratory Control: Drug overdose with a respiratory depressant Some types of head injury	
Respiratory Alkalosis—Deficient Carbonic Acid Caused by Alveolar Hyperventilation	
Hypoxemia from any cause (e.g., initial part of asthma episode, pneumonia) Acute pain Anxiety, psychological distress, sobbing Inappropriate mechanical ventilator settings Stimulation of brainstem respiratory control (e.g., meningitis, gram-negative sepsis, head injury, aspirin overdose)	*Physical examination:* Light-headedness, numbness and tingling of fingers, toes, and circumoral region, increased rate and depth of respirations, excitement and confusion possibly followed by decreased level of consciousness, dysrhythmias *Laboratory findings:* Arterial blood gas alterations: pH *above* 7.45, $Paco_2$ *below* 35 mm Hg (4.7 kPa), HCO_3^- level normal if short lived or uncompensated or *below* 22 mmol/L if compensated
Metabolic Acidosis—Excessive Metabolic Acids	
Increase of Metabolic Acids (High Anion Gap): Ketoacidosis (diabetes, starvation, alcoholism) Hypermetabolic state (severe hyperthyroidism, burns, severe infection) Oliguric renal disease (acute kidney injury, end-stage renal disease) Circulatory shock (lactic acidosis) Ingestion of acid or acid precursors (e.g., methanol, ethylene glycol, boric acid, aspirin overdose)	*Physical examination:* Decreased level of consciousness (lethargy, confusion, coma), abdominal pain, dysrhythmias, increased rate and depth of respirations (compensatory hyperventilation) *Laboratory findings:* Arterial blood gas alterations: pH *below* 7.35, $Paco_2$ normal if uncompensated or *below* 35 mm Hg (4.7 kPa) if compensated, HCO_3^- level *below* 22 mmol/L
Loss of Bicarbonate (Normal Anion Gap): Diarrhea Pancreatic fistula or intestinal decompression Renal tubular acidosis	
Metabolic Alkalosis—Deficient Metabolic Acids	
Increase of Bicarbonate: Excessive administration of sodium bicarbonate Massive blood transfusion (liver converts citrate to HCO_3^-) Mild or moderate ECV deficit (contraction alkalosis)	*Physical examination:* Light-headedness, numbness and tingling of fingers, toes, and circumoral region; muscle cramps; possible excitement and confusion followed by decreased level of consciousness, dysrhythmias (may be caused by concurrent hypokalemia)
Loss of Metabolic Acid: Excessive vomiting or gastric suctioning Hypokalemia Excess aldosterone	*Laboratory findings:* Arterial blood gas alterations: pH *above* 7.45, $Paco_2$ normal if uncompensated or *above* 45 mm Hg (6.0 kPa) if compensated, HCO_3^- *above* 26 mmol/L

COPD, Chronic obstructive pulmonary disease, *ECV,* extracellular fluid volume.
Data from Felver, L. (2013). Acid-base homeostasis and imbalances. In L. C. Copstead & J. L. Banasik (Eds.), *Pathophysiology* (5th ed.). St. Louis: Saunders.

excess = 2.5 mmol/L. Her kidneys have not had time to compensate and lower the bicarbonate level.

Metabolic Acidosis. Metabolic acidosis results from a decrease in serum bicarbonate or the production of organic or fixed acids. An analysis of serum electrolytes to detect an anion gap may be helpful in attempting to identify the cause of the metabolic acidosis. An anion gap reflects unmeasurable anions present in plasma and is calculated by subtracting the sum of chloride and bicarbonate from the amount of plasma sodium concentration. Compensation for metabolic acidosis initially involves an increase in respiratory rate and depth to eliminate carbon dioxide. If not quickly resolved, renal mechanisms are stimulated to increase hydrogen ion excretion, and to generate and release bicarbonate into the ECF.

An example is the following: Ms. Smith is admitted to hospital after having run her first marathon. Her electrolytes are as follows: sodium = 131 mmol/L, bicarbonate = 9 mmol/L, and chloride = 86 mmol/L. The anion gap is calculated as follows: Na – (HCO_3^- + Cl^-) = 131 – (9 + 86) = 36 mmol/L. The normal anion gap is less than 16 mmol/L (so her anion gap is high). Ms. Smith receives a diagnosis of lactic acidosis related to tissue hypoxia.

Diabetic ketoacidosis (DKA) is characterized by hyperglycemia, high ketones, and metabolic acidosis. This diabetic emergency is caused by a total lack of insulin, in type 1 diabetes, causing severely elevated glucose levels. The body responds to the glucose deficit inside the cells by mobilizing fats, a process that results in increased ketone bodies. Together, these metabolic processes cause osmotic diuresis, acidosis, and hyperkalemia. Patients with type 2 diabetes are also at risk of developing metabolic acidosis from severe hyperglycemia, although the acidosis develops more slowly and is not associated with ketosis. The clinical response to these hyperglycemic emergencies is to administer insulin and intravenous fluids. It is critical to correct water and electrolyte imbalances and restore intravascular volume, based on individual assessments and diagnostics; however, an isotonic solution such as 0.9% saline is recommended over the initial 24 to 48 hours (de Beer, Michael, Thacker, et al., 2008, p. 7; Kisiel & Marsons, 2009, p. 1097). Frequent monitoring of electrolytes, fluid balance, glucose, and ABGs is important in the treatment of DKA.

Metabolic Alkalosis. Metabolic alkalosis is marked by the heavy loss of acid from the body or by increased levels of bicarbonate. The most common causes are vomiting and gastric suction, as well as potassium deficiency, hyperaldosteronism, and diuretic therapy (Amerman, 2016, p. 1006). The body attempts to compensate by increasing the excretion of bicarbonate and decreasing the rate and the depth of respirations. Symptoms associated with metabolic alkalosis are depressed respirations and tingling of the fingers and dizziness related to secondary low calcium (Paul et al., 2016, p. 316). In serious metabolic alkalosis, cardiac arrhythmias can occur.

An example is the following: Mr. Jones comes into the clinic with persistent vomiting. His ABGs are as follows: pH = 7.63, bicarbonate = 45 mmol/L, $PaCO_2$ = 48 mm Hg, and base excess = 16 mmol/L. He is in metabolic alkalosis.

KNOWLEDGE BASE OF NURSING PRACTICE

The essential functions of fluid, electrolyte, and acid–base balances are important aspects of the scientific knowledge base of nursing practice. In all areas of nursing practice, nurses attend to the relationship between healthy water and human health (Allgood, 2009; Davidhizar, Dunn, & Hart, 2004). Regardless of the area of practice, all nurses will be involved in assessment, planning, and interventions in relation to water, electrolytes, and factors that influence acid–base balance. Identifying those most at risk for imbalances is important for promoting health and well-being (Table 40-7). Certain patients are particularly vulnerable to imbalances, including infants, older persons, and the severely ill. Patients who are disoriented or immobile are also vulnerable to imbalances because they cannot respond independently to early symptoms. If untreated, over time, the body can no longer maintain fluid and electrolyte or acid–base balances adequately, and the patient's health becomes compromised. Prolonged or severe compromises may lead to irreversible chronic health problems.

CRITICAL THINKING

Successful critical thinking requires a synthesis of knowledge, experience, information gathered from patients, critical thinking qualities, and intellectual and professional standards. Nurses must use clinical judgements to anticipate the information necessary, analyze the data, and make decisions regarding patient care.

TABLE 40-7 Risk Factors for Fluid, Electrolyte, and Acid–Base Imbalances

Age	*Very young:* ECV deficit, osmolality imbalances, clinical dehydration *Very old:* ECV excess or deficit, osmolality imbalances
Environment	*Sodium-rich diet:* ECV excess *Electrolyte-poor diet:* Electrolyte deficits *Hot weather:* Clinical dehydration
Gastrointestinal output	*Diarrhea:* ECV deficit, clinical dehydration, hypokalemia, hypocalcemia (if chronic), hypomagnesemia (if chronic), metabolic acidosis *Drainage (e.g., nasogastric suctioning, fistulas):* ECV deficit, hypokalemia; metabolic acidosis if intestinal or pancreatic drainage *Vomiting:* ECV deficit, clinical dehydration, hypokalemia, hypomagnesemia, metabolic alkalosis
Chronic diseases	*Cancer:* Hypercalcemia; with tumour lysis syndrome: hyperkalemia, hypocalcemia, hyperphosphatemia; other imbalances, depending on side effects of therapy *Chronic obstructive pulmonary disease:* Respiratory acidosis *Cirrhosis:* ECV excess, hypokalemia *Heart failure:* ECV excess; other imbalances, depending on therapy *Oliguric renal disease:* ECV excess, hyperkalemia, hypermagnesemia, hyperphosphatemia, metabolic acidosis
Trauma	*Burns:* ECV deficit, metabolic acidosis *Crush injuries:* Hyperkalemia *Head injuries:* Hyponatremia or hypernatremia, depending on ADH response *Hemorrhage:* ECV deficit, hyperkalemia if circulatory shock
Therapies	Diuretics and other medications (see Box 40-5) *IV therapy:* ECV excess, osmolality imbalances, electrolyte excesses *Parenteral nutrition:* Any fluid or electrolyte imbalance, depending on components of solution

ADH, Antidiuretic hormone; *ECV*, extracellular fluid volume; *IV*, intravenous.

NURSING PROCESS

Assessment

Patient care begins with informed assessment. This includes assessing each patient's fluid, electrolyte, and acid–base status. Using a systematic approach to collecting data and analyzing findings enables nurses to provide patient-centred care. Nurses' clinical decisions are based on the quality of their assessments and critical thinking. By gathering data through a health history and physical examination, nurses can identify patients at risk of or experiencing imbalances. During assessment (Figure 40-7), nurses must consider all elements that contribute to making appropriate nursing diagnoses.

Patient Expectations. Assessment begins with eliciting the patient's needs, values, and preferences for a patient-centred assessment. At times this may not be possible because of the severity of the patient's illness and imbalances. When able, however, it is good to begin with a focus on the patient's experience and perceptions of the illness. Has the patient experienced this before? How does the patient interpret the signs and symptoms experienced? How does the patient manage the related risks or contributing factors in his or her environment? What are the patient's concerns about the symptoms, diagnostics, or potential treatment?

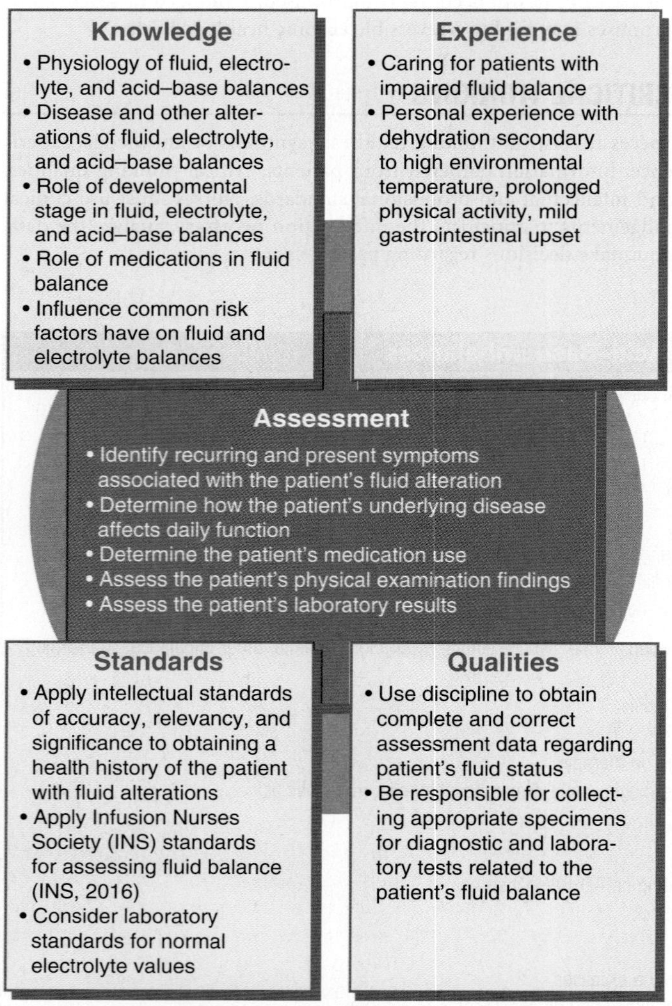

FIGURE 40-7 Critical thinking model for assessment of fluid, electrolyte, and acid–base balances.

Health History. The nursing assessment continues with a nursing health history, which is designed to reveal any risk factors or pre-existing conditions that may cause or contribute to a disturbance of fluid, electrolyte, and acid–base balances. Asking specific, focused questions will elicit the most useful data (Box 40-2).

Age. First, the patient's age is considered. An infant's proportion of total body water, approximately 75%, is greater than that of children or adults. Infants are at a greater risk for fluid volume deficit (FVD) and hyperosmolar imbalance because body water loss is proportionately greater per kilogram of weight, and therefore, they have smaller reserves.

Children ages 2 through 12 years have less stable regulatory responses to imbalance and in childhood illnesses tend to have less tolerance for large changes. Children frequently respond to illnesses with fevers of higher temperatures and longer duration than those of adults, increasing their insensible water loss. Adolescents have increased metabolic processes and water production because of the major rapid changes that occur during puberty. Adolescent girls experience changes in fluid balance with the hormonal changes associated with the menstrual cycle.

Aging has a significant impact on fluid, electrolyte, and acid–base balances and on older persons' capacity to compensate; therefore, nurses need to be able to identify the risk factors and work to prevent them (Box 40-3). With normal aging, the glomerular filtration rate is reduced, along with the number and functional capacity of nephrons. Older persons have a decreased thirst sensation. The reduction in taste may limit the amount of oral fluids consumed. Older persons have reduced aldosterone, which increases sodium excretion and may result in hyponatremia. Because older persons are more susceptible to dehydration and have a higher rate of mortality from dehydration, early detection of infection and disorders in fluid balance is very important (Shepherd, 2013). Box 40-4 outlines evidence-informed nursing practice guidelines synthesized from recent research (Arai, Butzlaff, Stotts, et al., 2014; Bunn, Jimoh, Wilsher, et al., 2015; El-Sharkawy et al., 2015; Schub & Obiamaka, 2016; Shepherd, 2013; Wotton, Crannitch, & Munt, 2008).

Reduced respiratory lung capacity impairs the ability of older persons to compensate for acid–base imbalances and maintain oxygen requirements. With increased age, patients are at risk for disorders of other body systems, including the cardiovascular, renal, and endocrine systems. In addition, older persons have a decreased ability to excrete medications.

Environmental Factors. Nurses also need to include certain environmental factors in the health history. Patients who have participated in vigorous exercise or are exposed to temperature extremes may have clinical signs of fluid and electrolyte alterations. Exposure to environmental temperatures exceeding 28°C to 30°C results in excessive sweating with weight loss. Excessive sweating with extreme exercise or exposure to high environmental temperatures can result in fluid deficits, hypernatremia, or clinical dehydration, because sweat is a hypotonic sodium-containing fluid.

Diet. The nurse should assess dietary intake (see Box 40-2) and recent changes in appetite or the ability to chew and swallow. It is good to explore if patients follow weight loss diets or gastrointestinal cleansing regimes. When nutritional intake is inadequate, the body tries to preserve its protein stores by breaking down glycogen and fat stores. When excess free fatty acids are released, metabolic acidosis can occur because the liver converts free fatty acids to ketones, which are strong acids. With high-protein diets, ketosis can also occur. After fat and carbohydrate resources are depleted, the body begins to destroy protein stores. Hypoalbuminemia occurs with lack of amino acids in the diet and with liver dysfunction. In hypoalbuminemia, the serum colloid

BOX 40-2 Nursing Assessment Questions

Nature of the Problem

- Are you currently under the care of a health care provider for management of any ongoing health problems, such as kidney or heart disease, diabetes, or blood pressure problems?
- Describe any new problems, such as vomiting, diarrhea, or a surgical procedure.

Signs and Symptoms

- In the past several weeks, have you lost or gained any weight?
- Do you feel thirsty, have a dry mouth or skin, or notice a lack of tears?
- Have you noticed a change in your urine output—decreased volume, dark colour, or concentrated appearance?
- Have you had any recent problems with vomiting or diarrhea? If so, for how long?
- Are you experiencing any problems with swelling of your hands, feet, ankles, or lower legs?
- Do you have problems breathing when you lie down at night?
- Have you noticed any dizziness, weakness, cramps, or unusual sensations, such as tingling?

Severity

- How many times a day do you urinate?
- Do you continue to feel thirsty no matter how much fluid you drink?
- Are you experiencing these symptoms more at night than in the morning?
- Are you having difficulty concentrating or do you feel confused?
- How does this compare with what is normal or usual for you?

Predisposing Factors

- Do you work or exercise in a hot environment?
- How much do you usually drink every day? What type of fluids do you drink? How much alcohol do you drink in a typical week?
- Describe your normal diet. Are you following a weight loss program? Do you use supplements for weight loss, or a salt substitute? What kind of snacks do you eat?
- Have you had any recent changes in your appetite? Have you noticed any changes in the taste of your food? Do you have any difficulty swallowing or chewing?
- Do you take any over-the-counter or prescription medications or herbal remedies?

Effect on the Patient

- How have these symptoms affected you?
- Are you losing sleep, feeling irritable, or having difficulty performing your usual daily tasks?
- What treatments or solutions have you tried to resolve these symptoms?

BOX 40-3 FOCUS ON OLDER PERSONS

Factors Affecting Fluid, Electrolyte, and Acid–Base Balance

- Body composition changes, causing a decreased percentage of body weight as water (50%), which increases risk of extracellular fluid volume (ECV) deficit and dehydration (Felver, 2013a).
- Some older people restrict fluid intake because of impaired mobility or concerns about bladder control; this increases their risk of hypernatremia and ECV deficit.
- Decreased elasticity of skin alters skin turgor even with normal fluid balance; do not rely on skin turgor to assess ECV deficit or dehydration in older persons.
- Decreased thirst sensation increases risk of hypernatremia and dehydration; do not rely on thirst to assess hypernatremia, ECV deficit, or dehydration in older persons (Touhy & Jett, 2014).
- Baroreceptors become sluggish with age, often causing brief postural hypotension; have older persons arise slowly when taking orthostatic blood pressure measurements.
- Cardiovascular changes with aging often decrease the ability to adapt to a sudden increase in vascular volume, increasing risk of pulmonary edema with rapid infusion of isotonic intravenous fluids.
- Kidneys of older persons are less able to concentrate urine, making them less able to conserve fluid when needed; this increases the risk of hypernatremia, ECV deficit, and dehydration (Touhy & Jett, 2014).
- Kidney changes of normal aging make it more difficult to excrete a large acid load, increasing the risk of metabolic acidosis.
- Increased sensitivity to anticholinergic effects of medications causes dry mouth; use several different assessments for ECV deficit and dehydration rather than relying solely on dry mouth (Burchum & Rosenthal, 2016).
- The combined effects of normal aging, chronic diseases, and multiple medications often pose challenges to maintaining fluid and electrolyte balance.

osmotic pressure is decreased, allowing fluid to shift from the circulating plasma to the interstitial fluid spaces. The nurse should also ask about complementary or alternative medicine (CAM) diet supplements or restrictions.

Lifestyle. Patients' history of smoking or alcohol consumption and of recreational drug use should be explored. These factors can alter the patient's fluid, electrolyte, and acid–base balance. Damage to the liver, kidneys, or lungs can alter compensatory mechanisms. For example, the excessive use of alcohol can ultimately cause respiratory depression, which can result in respiratory acidosis.

Medication. The nurse should obtain a complete list of current medications, including over-the-counter and herbal preparations (see Box 40-2 and Box 40-5). The nurse should evaluate the potential effects of medications to determine if specific laboratory values need to be assessed, using knowledge of physiology and pharmacology, and pharmacology references. The patient's knowledge of adverse effects and adherence to medication schedules should also be assessed.

Medical History

Acute Illness. Head and chest trauma, gastrointestinal disturbances, sepsis, shock, and second- or third-degree burns are conditions that place patients at high risk for fluid, electrolyte, and acid–base alterations. When obtaining a medical history, it is important to review any allergies. Treatment for fluid, electrolyte, and acid–base imbalances may involve exposure to latex in equipment and supplies. With neonates and infants, the nurse needs to assess the mother for known latex allergy to prevent inadvertent exposure to latex sensitization.

Burns. The burned patient can lose body fluids by many routes. The greater the body surface burned, the greater the fluid loss. Burns can result in a plasma-to-interstitial fluid shift. Plasma and interstitial

BOX 40-4 EVIDENCE-INFORMED PRACTICE

Preventing and Responding to Dehydration in Older Persons*

Evidence Summary

- Older persons are at increased risk of illness and death from dehydration, overhydration, and salt overload.
- Reduced thirst sensation and diminished appetite contribute to dehydration in older persons. Older people also have diminished capacity to correct volume losses.
- Chronic dehydration contributes to constipation in older persons.
- Adequate hydration in older persons is recommended for the prevention of falls, possibly related to hypotension or postural hypotension.
- Dehydration is a risk factor for delirium. The risk for delirium can be reduced as much as 33% with each additional glass of water consumed (El-Sharkawy et al., 2015).
- Signs and symptoms of dehydration can be easily confused with normal aging processes; therefore, assessment requires knowledge, skill, and commitment to acting on signs and symptoms.

Nursing Practice Guidelines

- Calculating fluid requirements should take into consideration individual characteristics including weight, gender, environmental factors, physical activity, and comorbidities, such as renal and cardiac disease.
- Identify risk factors for each older person from the following: age over 70 years, female, high or low body mass index, recent hospitalization, new admission to residential care, situations causing increased insensible loss (pyrexia), decreased access or ability to request fluids, and situations causing decreased intake, such as swallowing disorder (dysphagia), physical frailty, and decreased sentience. Diarrhea and vomiting are key causes of dehydration in older persons. Previous malnutrition, dehydration, polypharmacy, and having more than three medical conditions are significant risk factors.
- Establish an assessment, monitoring, and evaluation tool for identifying risk factors for older persons when initiating a caregiving relationship (e.g., on admission to residential care; with home assessment of older persons; routine health care visits)
- Assessment of hydration status should include physiological measures (urine specific gravity, urine colour, blood pressure, pulse, and respiration), as well as observed intake patterns and treatments. Recommend blood testing to determine cause and severity in suspected dehydration.
- Maintain fluid intake through documented planning using the nursing process in home, residential care, and hospital settings.
- Educate older persons and their family and friends on the importance of hydration.
- Evaluate acute losses such as diarrhea and vomiting.
- Attend more diligently to fluid balance in the context of medical issues such as diabetes, with the use of diuretics, with decreased cognitive level or functional status, and with reduced level of consciousness.
- Ensure availability of adequate fluids, including water, tea, coffee, milk, and other beverages, throughout the day and assist persons who are unable to access their own fluids. Replenish and refresh fluids through the day.
- Advocate for adequate staffing levels in residential and acute care, as inadequate staffing is closely linked to increased mortality (Shepherd, 2013).
- Promote audits of hydration practices and barriers or obstacles in health care settings and identify benchmarks for improved practice.
- Ongoing management consists of daily fluid goals, comparing current intake with physiological needs, and monitoring actual consumption of fluids and fluid-rich foods.
- Incorporate the offer of fluids, hot or cold, into regular rounds, socializing, and aspects of care using the "little and often" approach. Offer assistive devices, such as drinking straws or feeder cups, as necessary.
- Fluid status documentation should include hydration, eating habits, weight, vital signs, and fluid preferences.

*Dehydration is defined variably. Shepherd (2013) defines dehydration as equal to or greater than 1% loss of body mass through fluid loss. See text and Tables 40-3 and 40-4 for exploration of dehydration and tonicity.

fluids are also lost as burn exudate. Water vapour and heat are lost in proportion to the amount of skin that is burned away, increasing insensible losses. Blood leaks from damaged capillaries, adding to the loss of intravascular fluid volume. Sodium and water shift into the cells, further compromising ECF volume (Paul et al., 2016, p. 1844). Cell damage is accompanied by a loss of serum proteins, and a release of potassium into the intravascular fluid.

Respiratory disorders. Many alterations in respiratory function predispose the patient to respiratory acidosis. For example, pneumonia or sedative overdose interferes with the elimination of carbon dioxide due to hypoventilation. As the carbon dioxide continues to build up in the bloodstream, the body's compensatory mechanisms can no longer adapt, and the pH decreases. Likewise, hyperventilation that occurs with conditions such as fever or anxiety can cause respiratory alkalosis when too much carbon dioxide is expelled with the increased respiratory rate.

Gastrointestinal disturbances. Gastroenteritis and nasogastric suctioning result in a loss of fluid, potassium, and chloride ions. Hydrogen ions are also lost, resulting in metabolic alkalosis. In contrast, loss of bicarbonate-rich intestinal or pancreatic fluids (diarrhea, fistulas) can cause metabolic acidosis and also hypokalemia. Timely education of infant and child caregivers is necessary to prevent clinical dehydration when the infant or child is experiencing diarrhea.

Trauma. Trauma resulting in hemorrhage causes FVD or hypovolemia. In addition, crush injuries causing cellular damage bring about a massive release of potassium into the intravascular fluid, causing hyperkalemia.

Head injury. Head injury can result in cerebral edema. Occasionally, this edema creates pressure on the pituitary gland and, as a result, ADH secretion is changed. Diabetes insipidus occurs when too little ADH is secreted and the patient excretes large volumes of diluted urine with a low specific gravity. Syndrome of inappropriate antidiuretic hormone (SIADH) results in water intoxication characterized by fluid volume expansion and hyponatremia, as well as hypotonicity of fluids as a result of high urine osmolality and low serum osmolality (Amerman, 2016, p. 974).

Recent surgery. After surgery patients can exhibit many acid–base changes. The more extensive the surgery and fluid loss are during the surgical procedure, the greater the body's response is to the surgical trauma. The patient who is reluctant to breathe deeply and cough may develop respiratory acidosis as a result of retained $PaCO_2$. The patient with nasogastric suction may develop metabolic alkalosis as a result of the loss of gastric acid, fluids, and electrolytes. In addition, the stress response of surgery may cause fluid shifts postoperatively when aldosterone, glucocorticoids, and ADH are increasingly secreted, causing sodium and chloride retention, potassium excretion, and decreased urinary output.

BOX 40-5 Medications That Cause Fluid, Electrolyte, and Acid–Base Disturbances

- ACE inhibitors (e.g., captopril [Capoten]) and angiotensin II receptor blockers (e.g., Losartan [Cozaar]): Hyperkalemia
- Antidepressants, SSRIs (e.g., fluoxetine [Prozac]): Hyponatremia
- Calcium carbonate antacids: Hypercalcemia, mild metabolic alkalosis
- Corticosteroids (e.g., prednisone): Hypokalemia, metabolic alkalosis
- Diuretics, potassium-wasting (e.g., furosemide [Lasix], thiazides): ECV deficit, hyponatremia (thiazides), hypokalemia, hypomagnesemia, mild metabolic alkalosis
- Diuretics, potassium-sparing (e.g., spironolactone [Aldactone]): Hyperkalemia, mild metabolic acidosis
- Effervescent (fizzy) antacids and cold medications (high Na^+ content): ECV excess
- Laxatives: ECV deficit, hypokalemia, hypocalcemia, hypomagnesemia, metabolic acidosis
- Magnesium hydroxide (e.g., Milk of Magnesia): Hypermagnesemia
- Nonsteroidal anti-inflammatory drugs (e.g., ibuprofen [Advil]): Mild ECV excess, hyponatremia
- Penicillins, high-dose (e.g., carbenicillin): Hypokalemia, metabolic alkalosis; hyperkalemia with penicillin G (contains K^+)

ACE, Angiotensin-converting enzyme; *ECV*, extracellular fluid volume; *SSRI*, selective serotonin reuptake inhibitor.
Data from Burchum, J. R., & Rosenthal, L. D. (2016). *Lehne's pharmacology for nursing care* (9th ed.). St. Louis: Elsevier.

Chronic Illness. Chronic disease (e.g., cancer, heart failure, or renal disease) can create fluid, electrolyte, and acid–base imbalances. The normal course of the patient's chronic disease is important to know in order to anticipate how fluid, electrolyte, and acid–base status may be affected.

Cancer. The types of fluid and electrolyte imbalances that are observed in a patient with cancer depend on the type and progression of the cancer, and the related treatment. The potential electrolyte imbalances result from anatomical distortion and functional impairment from tumour growth, or tumour-related metabolic and endocrine abnormalities. Hypercalcemia can result when cancer cells secrete chemicals that prompt the release of calcium from the bone. Anorexia, stomatitis, and diarrhea, side effects of some chemotherapy or radiation, create risks for many imbalances.

Cardiovascular disease. In the patient with cardiovascular disease, diminished cardiac output reduces kidney perfusion, causing the patient to experience a decrease in urinary output. The patient will retain sodium and water, resulting in circulatory overload, and is at risk of developing pulmonary edema. Fluid and electrolyte imbalances associated with heart disease can be controlled with medications and with fluid and sodium restrictions.

Renal disorders. Kidney disease alters fluid and electrolyte balances by the abnormal retention of sodium, chloride, potassium, and water in the extracellular compartment. The plasma levels of metabolic waste products such as urea and creatinine are elevated because the kidneys are unable to filter and excrete the waste products of cellular metabolism. This elevation is toxic to cellular processes. Metabolic acidosis results when hydrogen ions are retained because of decreased renal function. Because of the renal disorder, the usual renal compensatory mechanisms, such as bicarbonate reabsorption, are not available; therefore, the body's ability to restore normal acid–base balance is limited.

The severity of fluid and electrolyte imbalance is proportional to the degree of renal failure. Acute renal failure is reversible. Although chronic kidney disease is progressive, the patient may be treated successfully with dietary control of protein and salt intake, diuretic medications, and fluid restrictions. In later stages, treatment with dialysis, transplantation, or both may be required.

Gastrointestinal disorders. Chronic gastrointestinal disorders can have a serious impact on fluid, electrolyte, and acid–base balances. Inflammatory bowel diseases, such as ulcerative colitis, regional enteritis, and celiac disease, are relatively common (Paul et al., 2016). Patients with liver failure may have a number of imbalances, including metabolic acidosis, ECF shifts in the case of ascites, and electrolyte disturbances. Key gastrointestinal assessments include the length of the illness, the presence of exacerbations in the case of inflammatory bowel disease, and the type of treatment currently being administered. It is important to determine whether the patient has a history of acute illnesses such as diarrhea or vomiting. Any condition that results in the loss of gastrointestinal fluids predisposes the patient to the development of dehydration and a variety of electrolyte disturbances.

Physical Assessment. A thorough physical examination (see Chapter 31) is necessary because fluid and electrolyte imbalances or acid–base disturbances can affect all body systems. When conducting a physical examination, nurses need to incorporate knowledge regarding the signs and symptoms of fluid, electrolyte, and acid–base imbalances; disease processes that may affect these balances; developmental considerations; and common risk factors (see Table 40-7). For example, an examination of the oral cavity may reveal signs of dehydration. Table 40-8 outlines nursing assessment findings and links these to fluid, electrolyte, and acid–base imbalances.

Assessing Fluid Intake and Output. Assessing fluid balance involves knowledge of normal fluid requirements and accurate measurement techniques and is critical to patient-centred care in the acute care setting (McGloin, 2015). Inadequate fluid management, including inaccurate calculations of fluid balance, is considered a common barrier to safety, according to many reports (McGloin, 2015). Measuring and recording fluid intake and output over a 24-hour period is a fundamental aspect of fluid balance assessment. A fluid balance chart (FBC) includes all intake (e.g., by mouth, intravenous solutions) and output (e.g., urine, nasogastric drainage) and the 24-hour balance (deficit or excess) or summary. An FBC, used in conjunction with physical assessment, is an essential component of fluid monitoring across health care settings. Recognition of trends in intake and output is also important to recognizing and responding to problems, such as fluid volume excess or clinical dehydration, promptly. Nurses can play a leadership role on the interprofessional team to promote, complete, and report accurate fluid status.

Daily weight is considered the most accurate means to evaluate fluid balance and guide the interprofessional team (Paul et al., 2016). The patient should be weighed at the same time each day with the same scale after the patient voids. The scale needs to be routinely calibrated. The patient should wear the same clothes (or clothes that weigh the same); if a bed scale is being used to weigh the patient, there should be the same number of sheets on the bed with each weighing. Patients with chronic health issues can learn to monitor their own fluid balance through weighing themselves daily, recording their weights, and reporting changes. Health care providers may direct patients with parameters and preferred action.

Intake includes all liquids taken by mouth (e.g., gelatin, ice cream, soup, juice, and water) or through nasogastric or jejunostomy feeding tubes, intravenous fluids (including both continuous and intermittent intravenous fluids), and blood or its components. A patient receiving

TABLE 40-8 Focused Nursing Assessments and Relevant Imbalances

Assessment	Imbalances
Body Weight Changes From Previous Day	
Loss of 1 kg (2.2 lbs) or more in 24 hours for adults	ECV deficit
Gain of 1 kg (2.2 lbs) or more in 24 hours for adults	ECV excess
Clinical Markers of Vascular Volume	
Blood pressure:	
Hypotension or orthostatic hypotension	ECV deficit
Light-headedness on sitting upright or standing	ECV deficit
Pulse rate and character:	
Rapid, thready	ECV deficit
Bounding	ECV excess
Fullness of neck veins:	
Flat or collapsing with inhalation when supine	ECV deficit
Full or distended when upright or semi-upright	ECV excess
Other assessments of vascular volume:	
Capillary refill: Sluggish	ECV deficit
Lung auscultation, dependent lobe: Crackles or rhonchi with progressive dyspnea	ECV excess
Urine output: Small volume of dark yellow urine	ECV deficit
Clinical Markers of Interstitial Volume	
Presence of edema: Present in dependent areas (ankles or sacrum) and possibly fingers or around eyes	ECV excess
Mucous membranes: Dry between cheek and gum, decreased or absent tearing	ECV deficit
Skin turgor: Pinched skin fails to return to normal position within 3 seconds	ECV deficit
Presence of thirst: Thirst present	Hypernatremia, severe ECV deficit
Behaviour and level of consciousness:	
Restlessness and mild confusion	Severe ECV deficit
Decreased level of consciousness (lethargy, confusion, coma)	Hyponatremia, hypernatremia, hypercalcemia, acid–base imbalances
Cardiac and Respiratory Signs of Electrolyte or Acid–Base Imbalances	
Pulse rhythm and ECG: Irregular pulse and ECG changes	K^+, Ca^{2+}, Mg^{2+}, and/or acid–base imbalances
Rate and depth of respirations:	
Increased rate and depth	Metabolic acidosis (compensatory mechanism); respiratory alkalosis (cause)
Decreased rate and depth	Metabolic alkalosis (compensatory mechanism); respiratory acidosis (cause)
Neuromuscular Markers of Electrolyte or Acid–Base Imbalances	
Muscle strength bilaterally, especially quadriceps muscles:	
Muscle weakness	Hypokalemia, hyperkalemia
Reflexes and sensations:	
Decreased deep tendon reflexes	Hypercalcemia, hypermagnesemia
Hyperactive reflexes, muscle twitching and cramps, tetany	Hypocalcemia, hypomagnesemia
Numbness, tingling in fingertips, around mouth	Hypocalcemia, hypomagnesemia, respiratory alkalosis
Muscle cramps, tetany	Hypocalcemia, hypomagnesemia, respiratory alkalosis
Tremors	Hypomagnesemia
Gastrointestinal Signs of Electrolyte Imbalances	
Inspection and auscultation:	
Abdominal distension	Hypokalemia, third-spacing of fluid
Decreased bowel sounds	Hypokalemia
Motility: Constipation	Hypokalemia, hypercalcemia

ECG, Electrocardiogram; *ECV,* extracellular fluid volume.

tube feedings may receive numerous liquid medications and water may be used to flush the tube. Over a 24-hour period, these liquids can amount to significant intake and should always be recorded on the intake and output record. Output includes urine, diarrhea, vomitus, gastric suction, and drainage from postsurgical wounds or other tubes (see Chapter 48). Daily intake should equal output plus 500 mL (to cover for insensible fluid losses).

To measure output, ambulatory patients are instructed to save their urine in a calibrated receptacle that attaches to the rim of the toilet bowl. When a patient has an in-dwelling Foley catheter, drainage tube, or suction, output is recorded at predetermined times depending on the patient's condition and prescribers' orders. Patient and family cooperation is essential for accurate intake and output measurements. The patient and the family must be taught the purpose of the measurements, including oral intake.

Recording intake and output is essential for obtaining an accurate database to evaluate hydration status. This information helps maintain an ongoing evaluation of the patient's hydration status to prevent severe imbalances. Electronic or paper forms are used to ensure consistent recording of intake and output by nurses or unregulated care providers. This recording must be accurate, and estimation is not acceptable for safe provision of care.

Laboratory Studies. Nurses need to review laboratory data, including serum and urinary electrolyte levels, hematocrit, blood creatinine level, blood urea nitrogen (BUN) levels, urine specific gravity, and ABG readings. Serum electrolyte levels are measured to determine the hydration status, the electrolyte concentration of the blood plasma, and acid–base balance. The frequency with which these electrolyte levels are measured depends on the severity of the patient's illness. Serum electrolyte tests are routinely performed on any patient entering a hospital to screen for alterations and to serve as a baseline for future comparisons. Serum and urine osmolality are also used to assess fluid balance (Arai et al., 2014, p. 464). The normal range for serum osmolality is 285 to 295 mmol/kg. With dehydration, the serum osmolality will be higher than normal.

Arterial Blood Gases. To determine ABG levels, a sample of blood from an artery is taken to assess the patient's acid–base status and the adequacy of ventilation and oxygenation. Arterial blood is drawn from a peripheral artery (usually the radial artery) or from an arterial line inserted by a physician. In some agencies, nurses are responsible for radial artery punctures. Nurses may also need to assist in the sampling process and care for the patient after the procedure. After the specimen is obtained, care is taken to prevent air from entering the syringe because this will affect the ABG analysis. The syringe should be transported to the laboratory immediately. In the event of a delay of more than 20 minutes, the syringe is submerged in crushed ice for transport to the laboratory to reduce the metabolism of cells. Pressure is applied to the puncture site for at least 5 minutes to reduce the risk of hematoma formation. The nurse can reassess the pulse after pressure has been removed.

Patient Expectations. Often the patient's fluid, electrolyte, or acid–base disturbance is so serious that it prevents a review of patient expectations. However, if a patient is alert enough to discuss care, the nurse should explore with the patient his or her short-term needs (e.g., provision of comfort from nausea) and long-term needs (e.g., understanding how to prevent alterations from occurring in the future). The nurse may also explore patient expectations with family and supportive friends. The patient's trust is strengthened through a competent response to sudden changes in condition and through clear communication with the patient, family members, or both.

◆ Nursing Diagnosis

When caring for patients with suspected fluid, electrolyte, and acid–base imbalances, it is particularly important to use critical thinking to formulate nursing diagnoses. The assessment data that establish the risk for or the actual presence of a nursing diagnosis in these areas may be subtle, and patterns and trends emerge only when nurses conscientiously assess for them. Nurses must keep in mind that many body systems may be involved. Clustering of defining characteristics will lead nurses to select the appropriate diagnoses. For example, the nursing diagnosis *deficient fluid volume* is developed to demonstrate the nursing diagnostic process in Box 40-6.

An important part of formulating nursing diagnoses is identifying the relevant causative or related factor. Nursing interventions are chosen to treat or modify the related factor. *Deficient fluid volume related to loss of gastrointestinal fluids via vomiting* requires therapies different from those needed for *deficient fluid volume related to elevated body temperature.*

Possible nursing diagnoses for patients with fluid, electrolyte, and acid–base alterations include the following:

- *Actual or risk of deficient fluid volume*
- *Actual or risk of excess fluid volume*
- *Decreased cardiac output*
- *Impaired gas exchange*
- *Acute confusion*
- *Impaired oral mucous membrane*
- *Actual or risk of impaired skin integrity*
- *Impaired mobility*
- *Ineffective therapeutic regimen management*
- *Deficient knowledge regarding disease management*

◆ Planning

During the planning process, nurses use critical thinking to synthesize information from multiple sources and to ensure that the patient's care plan integrates both scientific and nursing knowledge, the nurse's knowledge of the individual, and the patient's expectations (Figure 40-8).

Goals and Outcomes. The nurse develops an individual care plan for the nursing diagnoses (see Box 40-6 and Box 40-7). Goals or expectations for care set by the nurse and the patient should be individualized and realistic, with measurable outcomes, and developed in

BOX 40-6 NURSING DIAGNOSTIC PROCESS

Deficient Fluid Volume

Assessment Activities	Defining Characteristics
Assess blood pressure and pulse	Patient is hypotensive, with increased heart rate
Obtain daily weight measurements	Patient experiences sudden weight loss of up to 1 kg or more in 24 hours.
Observe volume of urine output and measure intake and specific gravity	Decreased volume of output in comparison to intake; increased urine specific gravity is present
Assess skin turgor	Inelastic skin turgor noted
Ask if patient is thirsty or weak	Patient verbalizes thirst and weakness
Inspect mucous membranes for degree of moisture	Dry mucous membranes are noted

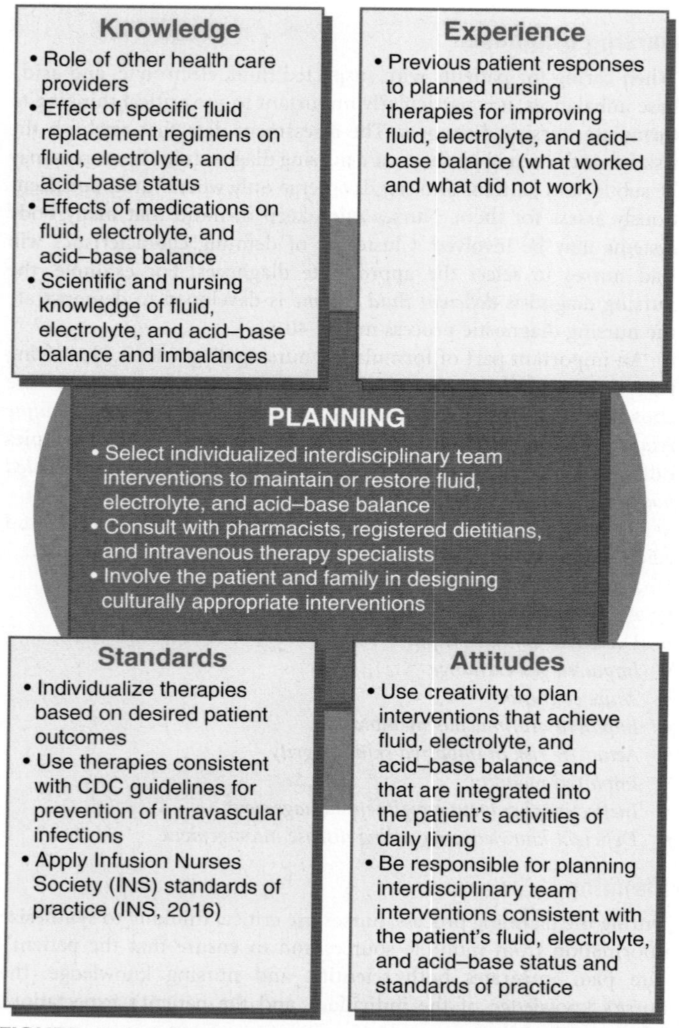

FIGURE 40-8 Critical thinking model for fluid, electrolyte, and acid–base balances planning. *CDC,* Centers for Disease Control and Prevention.

a patient-centred manner. For example, if the goal is to achieve and maintain homeostasis, the following related outcomes might be established:

- The patient will have normal fluid and electrolyte balance at discharge.
- The patient will be free of complications associated with the intravenous therapy.
- The patient will demonstrate fluid balance by moist, mucous membranes and good skin turgor.
- The patient will have serum electrolytes within the normal range within 48 hours.

Setting Priorities. The patient's clinical condition will determine which diagnosis takes priority. Many nursing diagnoses in the area of fluid, electrolyte, and acid–base balances are of highest priority because the consequences for the patient can be serious or even life-threatening. For example, in the concept map for a patient with gastroenteritis and dehydration (Figure 40-9), nausea and diarrhea caused a fluid volume deficit and electrolyte imbalances. Without treating the cause, the fluid, electrolyte, and acid–base imbalances will continue and progress.

Teamwork and Collaboration. Consultation with the patient's physician or primary health care provider may assist in setting realistic time frames for the goals of care, particularly when the patient's physiological status is unstable. During planning, it is important to collaborate as much as possible with the patient, family, and other members of the interdisciplinary health care team. Family can be particularly helpful in identifying subtle changes in a patient's behaviour associated with imbalances (e.g., anxiety, confusion, or irritability). Depending on the composition of the health care team, some therapies can be delegated, such as taking of daily weights or recording of fluid intake and output.

Infusion Therapy Team. Managing fluid, electrolyte, and acid–base imbalances often involves infusion therapy. The Infusion Nurses Society (INS) has developed standards of practice based on systematic review of the current evidence. These standards, reviewed and published regularly, are a key source for standards to inform decision making (see Figure 40-8). Vascular access device (VAD) insertion, maintenance, and surveillance for quality improvement are conducted by individuals and teams with infusion therapy education, training, and validated competency (Coram, 2015; INS, 2016, p. S17). Having a designated team for VADs, including peripheral catheters, improves patient outcomes (e.g., reduced infections), comfort (e.g., reduced number of unsuccessful attempts to initiate a VAD), and satisfaction (INS, 2016, p. S17).

For patients with acute disturbances, discharge planning must begin early. The nurse must ensure that care can continue in the home or long-term care setting with few disruptions. For example, when a patient is discharged on intravenous therapy, the nurse must determine the knowledge and skills of the person who is to assume caregiving responsibilities and make a referral for home intravenous therapy as soon as possible (Box 40-8). The nurse must also collaborate closely with other members of the health care team, such as the dietitian, pharmacist, and physician. In consultation with a dietitian, the nurse can recommend foods to increase intake of certain electrolytes or reduce intake as necessary (see Chapter 42). The pharmacist can help identify medications likely to cause electrolyte or acid–base disturbances and describe possible adverse effects of the patient's prescribed drugs. The physician directs the treatment of any fluid, electrolyte, or acid–base alteration.

◆ Implementation

Health Promotion. Health promotion activities in the area of fluid, electrolyte, and acid–base imbalances include patient education regarding fluid and electrolyte requirements, promotion of healthy environments affecting hydration, and advocating for secure access to safe water as a universal need and human right (International Council of Nurses [ICN], 2008; see also Pike-Macdonald, Best, Twomey, et al., 2007).

Patients and caregivers need to recognize risk factors for imbalances and implement appropriate preventive measures. Clear communication and use of plain language are important in health education. Parents of infants need to understand that gastrointestinal losses can quickly lead to serious imbalances. When an infant is vomiting or has diarrhea, the parent must recognize the risk and promptly seek health care to restore the infant's normal balance. Even a healthy adult is at risk for developing imbalances when subjected to high temperatures. Patients should be advised to increase water intake, maintain adequate ventilation, and refrain from excessive activity during heat waves. Box 40-4 provides guidelines for preventing dehydration in older persons. All patients with a chronic health alteration are at risk for developing changes in their fluid, electrolyte, and acid–base balances. They need to understand their own risk factors and the measures to be taken to

BOX 40-7 NURSING CARE PLAN

Fluid Volume Deficit

ASSESSMENT

Mrs. Hilda Beck is a 72-year-old seen by her health care provider this morning after falling at home and telephoning a neighbour for assistance. She lives alone in an apartment and has no chronic disease except for osteoarthritis of her hands. She has had diarrhea and vomiting for over 24 hours and has not eaten anything. Despite feeling slightly nauseated, she tried to drink a little water, because she knew she needed fluid. Mrs. Beck is admitted for intravenous (IV) fluid therapy. X-ray films indicate that she has no broken bones. Review of laboratory findings: hematocrit 55% (hemoconcentration caused by hypovolemia); sodium 148 mmol/L, and potassium 3 mmol/L. (Note: Mrs. Beck has hypokalemia in addition to extracellular fluid volume [ECV] deficit and hypernatremia [clinical dehydration].)

Assessment Activities	*Findings/Defining Characteristics**
Ask Mrs. Beck to describe when her vomiting and diarrhea began and any accompanying signs and symptoms.	She states that her gastrointestinal problems began suddenly yesterday and that she *gets weak and light-headed when she stands or sits upright*, which is why she fell. She feels *weak* and has a *dry mouth*.
Ask her about the current status of vomiting and diarrhea.	She says she was still vomiting earlier this morning. She has not done so for the past 3 hours. She feels slightly nauseated. She had three episodes of watery diarrhea this morning and more than six yesterday.
Assess Mrs. Beck's vital signs.	*Heart rate is 110 beats/min* with regular rhythm and a *weak pulse; supine blood pressure (BP) is 90/58*. Temperature and respirations are within normal limits. Postural BP measurement is not taken since patient says that she *gets light-headed when she sits upright*.
Evaluate physical signs of ECV.	Neck veins are flat when she is supine; *100 mL of dark yellow urine* in past 4 hours; dry mucous membranes between cheek and gum; prolonged capillary refill time of 5 seconds.
Weigh Mrs. Beck using a bed scale.	Weight is 55.5 kg. She states that usual weight at home is 58.5 kg (*3 kg weight loss*).

*Defining characteristics are shown in italics.

NURSING DIAGNOSIS: Deficient fluid volume related to increased output of GI fluids from vomiting and diarrhea

PLANNING

Goals (Nursing Outcomes Classification)[†] *Fluid Balance*	*Expected Outcomes*
Patient's fluid volume will return to normal by hospital discharge.	Heart rate and BP return to normal within 24 hours. Within 24 hours, Mrs. Beck does not report light-headedness when sitting or standing. Urine colour becomes light yellow within 24 hours. Daily urine output equals intake of at least 1 500 mL by discharge.
Patient will describe how to manage fluid balance at home before hospital discharge.	Mrs. Beck describes how to replace GI fluid loss with fluids that contain sodium. She describes signs and symptoms indicating need to increase fluid and sodium intake.

[†]Outcome classification labels from Moorhead, S., Johnson, M., Maas, M. L., & Swanson, E. (2012). *Nursing outcomes classification (NOC)* (5th ed.). St. Louis: Mosby.

INTERVENTIONS

Interventions (Nursing Interventions Classification)[‡] *Fluid/Electrolyte Management*	*Rationale*
Provide Mrs. Beck with her favourite fluids at her preferred temperature.	Patient-centred care takes individual preferences into account. Offer cultural preferences regarding temperature of oral fluid intake (Giger, 2013). In contrast to popular belief, moderate amounts of caffeinated beverages are not likely to have excessive diuretic effect (Shepherd, 2013).
Provide a pitcher and glass of water at Mrs. Beck's preferred temperature at her bedside; ensure that she can access and pour from it easily; provide straw if she wishes.	Weakness or chronic disease such as osteoarthritis of hands may make it difficult to manipulate a full water pitcher. Make fluid available in form that is easy for patient to access (Felver, 2013b).
Administer IV therapy as prescribed, monitoring closely for early adverse effects of complications.	IV fluid replacement augments oral replacement when ECV deficit exists. Age-appropriate care is needed because of older persons' anatomical and physiological changes that affect volume delivery (INS, 2016).
Discuss different ways to prevent and treat dehydration at home. Provide written handout of information.	Patient education is enhanced in older persons when the nurse uses multiple senses during teaching sessions (Touhy & Jett, 2014).

[‡]Intervention classification labels from Bulechek, G. M., Butcher, H. K., Dochterman, J. M., & Wagner, C. (2013). *Nursing interventions classification (NIC)* (6th ed.). St. Louis: Mosby.

Continued

BOX 40-7 NURSING CARE PLAN

Fluid Volume Deficit—cont'd

EVALUATION

Nursing Actions	*Patient Response and Finding*	*Achievement of Outcome*
Monitor vital signs, intake and output (I&O), daily weight, and postural BP when no longer light-headed. Assess neck vein fullness when supine, mucous membranes.	T 37°C, RR 10, HR 72 beats/min, BP 120/78 sitting, 122/78 standing, denies light-headedness Intake 2 000 mL, output 2 000 mL of light yellow urine Today's weight: 58.5 kg Neck veins full when supine; mucous membranes moist	Vital signs have returned to normal range. There is no postural hypotension. I&O measurements are balanced, urine is light yellow. Daily weight has returned to Mrs. Beck's normal weight. Additional markers of ECV are normal.
Evaluate effectiveness of teaching regarding maintaining fluid balance at home.	Mrs. Beck identified salty broth and commercial electrolyte replacement fluids for replacing GI fluid loss and indicated the need to increase her intake if her urine becomes dark yellow or she becomes light-headed when sitting upright.	Mrs. Beck describes effective home management of fluid balance.

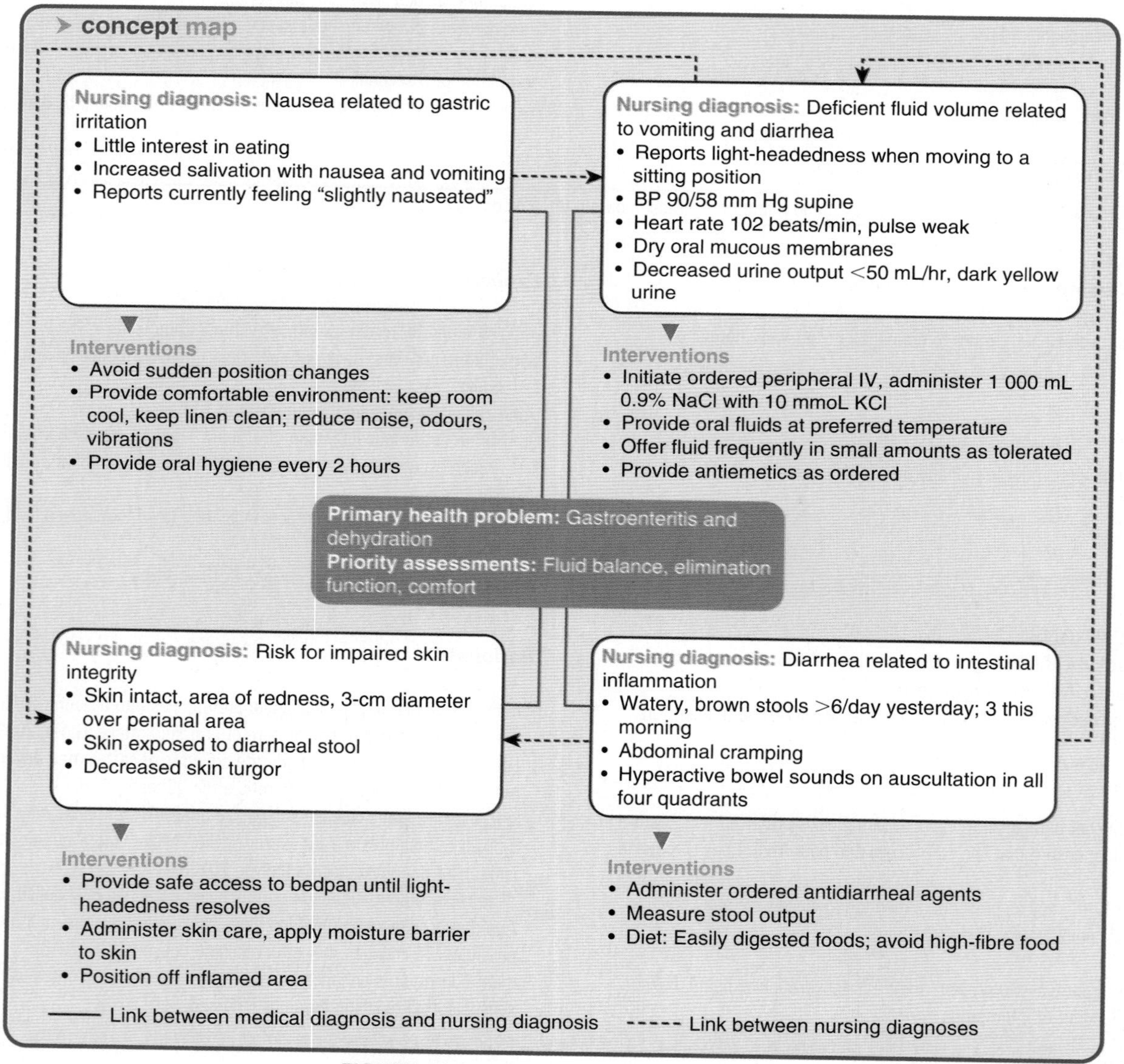

FIGURE 40-9 Concept map for Mrs. Beck.

BOX 40-8 PATIENT TEACHING

Home Intravenous Therapy

Objective

- The patient, family caregiver, or both will demonstrate competence with administering intravenous (IV) therapy safely in the home.

Teaching Strategies

- Explain the importance of IV therapy in maintaining hydration and access for the delivery of medications.
- Emphasize the risks involved when the IV system is not kept sterile.
- Be sure that the patient or family caregiver is able to manipulate the required equipment.
- Instruct them in aseptic technique and hand hygiene in the handling of all IV equipment.
- Teach them how to change IV solutions, tubing, and dressing when they become soiled or dislodged (Alexander et al., 2014). (*Note:* As the home care nurse, you may be able to visit frequently enough to perform scheduled tubing changes.)
- Teach procedures for safe disposal in appropriate containers of all sharps and IV materials exposed to blood. Keep sharps containers away from children (see Chapter 34).
- Instruct patient and caregiver to apply pressure with sterile gauze if the catheter falls out and, if the patient is on anticoagulants, to tape pieces of sterile gauze in place for at least 20 minutes with pressure or until bleeding stops.
- Instruct patient and caregiver about signs and symptoms of infiltration, phlebitis, and infection and reporting symptoms immediately.
- Instruct patient and family caregiver to report if the infusion slows or stops or if blood is seen in the tubing.
- Teach patient with family caregiver's assistance how to ambulate, perform hygiene, and participate in other activities of daily living without dislodging or disconnecting catheter and tubing:
  - For showering, protect the IV site and dressing from getting wet by covering it completely with plastic. If using an electronic infusion device, unplug around water.
  - Wear clothes that avoid pressure on the IV site and avoid trauma to the site when changing clothes.
  - Have patient avoid strenuous exercise of the arm with the IV line.

Evaluation

- Ask patient and family caregiver why it is necessary to maintain hydration and IV access for the delivery of medications.
- Ask what to do if the IV infusion stops.
- Ask patient and family caregiver to describe signs and symptoms of complications and the action they should take.
- Observe patient or family caregiver changing the IV container, tubing, and dressing.
- Observe the patient ambulating and participating in activities of daily living to see how he or she protects and manipulates the IV catheter and apparatus.

avoid imbalances. For example, patients with chronic kidney disease must avoid excess intake of fluid, sodium, potassium, magnesium, and phosphorus. Through diet education, these patients learn the types of foods to avoid and the suitable volume of fluid they are permitted daily (see Chapter 42). Patients with chronic health conditions need to be made aware of early signs and symptoms of fluid, electrolyte, and acid–base imbalances. A patient with heart disease should be instructed to obtain an accurate body weight each day at approximately the same time and to inform the health care provider of significant changes in weight from one day to another. Increase in weight, shortness of breath, orthopnea, and dependent edema are all associated with fluid retention.

Nurses engaged in health promotion can attend to environmental factors that influence the health of communities. For example, community health nurses in Newfoundland and Labrador (Pike-MacDonald et al., 2007) conducted a comprehensive community health needs study. The research was used to increase awareness of drinking water pollution, through monitoring of water quality and reporting of results to both the community and health policymakers. Globally, improved water quality and access to safe drinking water, though largely ignored, would have a significant impact on health, saving millions of lives (Allgood, 2009). While there have been successes in improving access to safe drinking water and reducing water contamination, household water treatment could bring about further advances in community health. Efforts of nurses in the developing world to provide education regarding safe drinking water and to implement safe drinking practices are saving lives. Community needs assessments and quality improvement initiatives in relation to environmental determinants of health involve attention to safe drinking and access to safe water (see Chapter 4). These efforts relate strongly to nurses' advocacy role in health promotion of healthy fluid and electrolyte levels.

Acute Care. While fluid, electrolyte, and acid–base imbalances can occur in all settings, many patients are cared for in acute care settings. Today, management of a patient's complex medical care is completed in a shorter span of time and involves expectations to perform increasingly difficult technological skills.

Enteral Replacement of Fluids. Oral replacement of fluids and electrolytes is appropriate as long as the patient is not so physiologically compromised that oral fluids cannot be replaced rapidly. Patients unable to tolerate solid foods may still be able to ingest fluids. Nurses may use strategies to encourage fluid intake, such as frequently offering small sips of fluid, ice pops, and ice chips. Ice chips should be included in the intake and output measurements, at one-half the volume of the chips (i.e., 250 mL of ice chips = 125 mL). For children with mild gastroenteritis, diluted apple juice followed by preferred fluids is an effective alternative to electrolyte maintenance fluids, with fewer treatment failures (Freedman, Willan, Boutis, et al., 2016).

Use of oral rehydration solutions (ORS) has reduced mortality related to diarrhea around the world. ORS are either glucose-electrolyte solutions or polymer-based solutions (e.g., made from rice, wheat, or maize). Evidence suggests that polymer-based solutions may be more effective in rehydration (Gregorio, Gonzales, Dans, et al., 2009). Hartling, Bellemare, Wiebe, and colleagues (2006) conducted a systematic review and concluded that oral hydration is effective and safe in treating dehydration in children with gastroenteritis, particularly with low-osmolarity solutions. A key nursing role is to encourage children and their caregivers regarding oral rehydration.

Oral replacement of fluids is contraindicated if the patient has a mechanical obstruction of the gastrointestinal tract, is at risk for aspiration, or has impaired swallowing. A feeding tube may be necessary, such as when the patient's gastrointestinal tract is healthy but the patient cannot ingest fluids (e.g., with impaired swallowing). Fluids can also be replaced through a gastrostomy or jejunostomy feeding tube or administered via a small-bore nasoenteral feeding tube. Maintaining adequate hydration for patients with enteral feeding involves an interprofessional team including dietitians, nurses, and other health care providers (Dunn, 2015). In caring for these patients, nurses need to assess for signs of dehydration and overhydration.

Restriction of Fluids. Patients who retain fluids and have fluid volume excess (FVE) require restricted fluid intake. Fluid restriction is often difficult for patients, particularly if they take medications that dry the oral mucous membranes or if they breathe through the mouth. The nurse should provide the rationale for fluid restrictions and the amount permitted. The patient and family need to understand that ice chips, gelatin, and ice cream are considered fluid. The patient should be involved in decisions regarding the amount of fluid and the distribution of fluids over the day. Patients on fluid restriction can swallow a number of pills with as little as 30 mL of liquid. Patients on fluid restriction require mouth care frequently to moisten mucous membranes, decrease the chance of mucosal drying and cracking, and maintain comfort. In experiments, patients under fluid restrictions can lose 1% to 2% body mass within 13 to 24 hours and will experience thirst strongly, except for older persons who often do not experience thirst (Arai et al., 2014; Shepherd, 2013).

Interventions for Acid–Base Imbalances. Nursing interventions to promote acid–base balance support prescribed medical therapies and are aimed at reversing the acid–base imbalance. Such imbalances can be life-threatening and require rapid correction. In collaboration with the interdisciplinary team, the nurse must maintain a functional intravenous line and provide prescribed medications, such as insulin or sodium bicarbonate, and fluid and electrolyte replacement promptly. Patients with acute acid–base disturbances often require repeated ABG analysis and close monitoring.

Parenteral Replacement of Fluids and Electrolytes. Fluid and electrolytes may be replaced through infusion directly into the circulatory system or intravenously, rather than via the digestive system. This is often referred to as *infusion therapy* (INS, 2016). Parenteral replacement includes administration of crystalloids, colloids, and total parenteral nutrition (TPN). TPN is a nutritionally adequate hypertonic solution consisting of glucose, other nutrients, and electrolytes. This solution is formulated to meet individual patient needs through interdisciplinary collaboration (e.g., dietitian, pharmacist, physician, nurse). See Chapter 42 for a full discussion of TPN and nutritional support.

The goal of intravenous fluid administration is to maintain fluid, electrolyte, and energy demands when patients are limited in their intake and to prevent or correct fluid and electrolyte disturbances from excess losses. Intravenous fluid administration enables direct access to the vascular system, permitting the continuous infusion of fluids over a period of time. Intravenous fluid therapy must be continuously regulated to assess for changes in the patient's fluid and electrolyte balances. Knowledge of the correct ordered solution, the equipment needed, the procedures required to initiate an infusion, how to regulate the infusion rate and maintain the system, how to identify and correct problems, and how to discontinue the infusion is necessary for safe and appropriate therapy. Because of the risk of transmission of infectious diseases, standard precautions must be followed when preparing to administer parenteral fluids (see Chapter 33). Patient safety and quality improvement are continuously attended to in all infusion therapy–related care (INS, 2016, p. S11). When providing infusion therapy to special populations such as infants and older persons, special competency is required. Consideration is given to anatomical and physiological differences, growth and development stage, and family preferences (INS, 2016, p. S11).

Safe administration of intravenous fluids includes an evidence-informed knowledge base related to the solution prescribed, the patient-centred rationale, equipment selection based on best practice, and potential risks and complications (Table 40-9). Safe administration of intravenous fluids also includes skills related to intravenous initiation, regulation of rate, assessment of the site and equipment, necessary techniques for maintenance of the site and prevention of infection, and, finally, discontinuation of the intravenous catheter. Consideration of the patient's unique preferences and perspectives is important throughout the intervention.

Types of solutions. The two main categories of intravenous fluids are crystalloids and colloids. Crystalloids are used most commonly and include dextrose, sodium chloride, and lactated Ringer's solutions (see Table 40-9). These solutions contain solutes that mix, dissolve, and cross semipermeable membranes. They vary in their tonicity (Figure 40-10). Colloids contain protein or starch, which does not cross semipermeable membranes and therefore remains suspended and distributed in the extracellular space, primarily the intravascular space, for up to several days. Colloids have been used to increase the osmotic pressure in the intravascular space to increase vascular volume in critical situations. Colloids are either semi-synthetic, such as dextran, pentastarch, or hetastarch, or human plasma derivatives, such as albumin, plasma proteins, or blood. Recent evidence suggests that crystalloids are as effective as colloids in many situations and are less costly (Perel & Roberts, 2012).

Vascular Access Devices. Vascular access devices (VADs) are catheters, cannulas, or infusion ports designed for repeated access to the vascular system. These devices include peripheral vascular access devices (PVADs) and central vascular access devices (CVADs) (Figure 40-11) and allow for parenteral fluid and electrolyte replacement, parenteral nutrition, and administration of medications. Peripheral cannulas are selected for short-term use, whereas central venous catheters (CVCs), peripherally inserted central catheters (PICCs), tunnelled catheters (e.g., Hickman), and implanted ports (Figure 40-12) are for long-term use or for administration of medications or solutions that

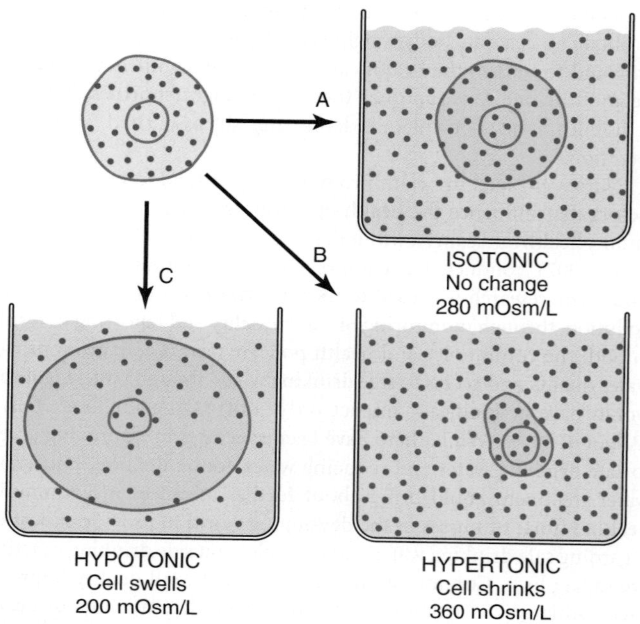

FIGURE 40-10 Effects of isotonic *(A)*, and hypertonic *(B)*, and hypotonic *(C)* solutions. (From Hall, J. E. [2016]. *Guyton and Hall textbook of medical physiology* [13th ed.]. Philadelphia: Saunders.)

TABLE 40-9 Intravenous Solutions

Solution	Concentration	Comments
Dextrose in Water Solutions		Dextrose is the name used for glucose in intravenous solutions.
Dextrose 5% in water (D_5W)	Isotonic	Isotonic when first enters vein; dextrose enters cells rapidly, leaving free water, which dilutes ECF; most of water then enters cells by osmosis.
Dextrose 10% in water ($D_{10}W$)	Hypertonic	Hypertonic when first enters vein, dextrose enters cells rapidly, leaving free water, which dilutes ECF; most of water then enters cells by osmosis.
Saline Solutions		
0.225% sodium chloride (quarter normal saline; ¼ NS; 0.225% NaCl)	Hypotonic	Saline is sodium chloride in water. Expands ECV (vascular and interstitial) and rehydrates cells.
0.45% sodium chloride (half normal saline; ½ NS; 0.45% NaCl)	Hypotonic	Expands ECV (vascular and interstitial) and rehydrates cells.
0.9% sodium chloride (normal saline; NS; 0.9% NaCl)	Isotonic	Expands ECV (vascular and interstitial); does not enter cells.
3% or 5% sodium chloride (hypertonic saline; 3% or 5% NaCl)	Hypertonic	Draws water from cells into ECF by osmosis.
Dextrose in Saline Solutions		
Dextrose 5% in 0.45% NaCl sodium chloride (D_5 ½ NS; $D_5$0.45% NaCl)	Hypertonic	Dextrose enters cells rapidly, leaving 0.45% sodium chloride.
Dextrose 5% in 0.9% sodium chloride (D_5NS; $D_5$0.9% NaCl)	Hypertonic	Dextrose enters cells rapidly, leaving 0.9% sodium chloride.
Balanced Electrolyte Solutions		
Lactated Ringer's (LR)	Isotonic	Contains Na^+, K^+, Ca^{2+}, Cl^-, and lactate, which liver metabolizes to HCO_3^-. Expands ECV (vascular and interstitial); does not enter cells.
Dextrose 5% in lactated Ringer's (D_5LR)	Hypertonic	Dextrose enters cells rapidly, leaving lactated Ringer's.

ECF, Extracellular fluid; *ECV*, extracellular fluid volume.

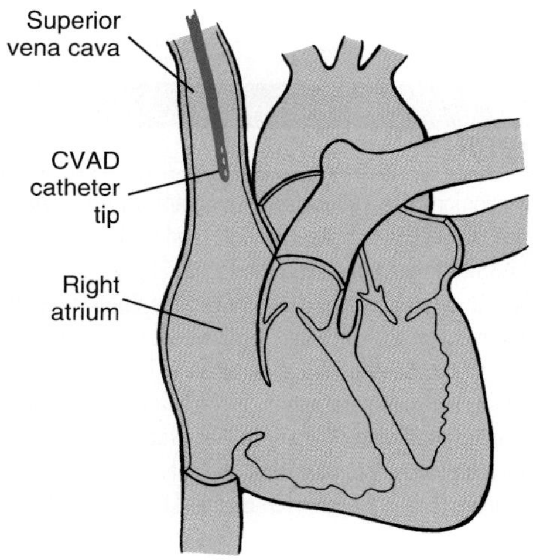

FIGURE 40-11 Central venous access devices (CVADs) deliver fluid into the superior vena cava near the heart.

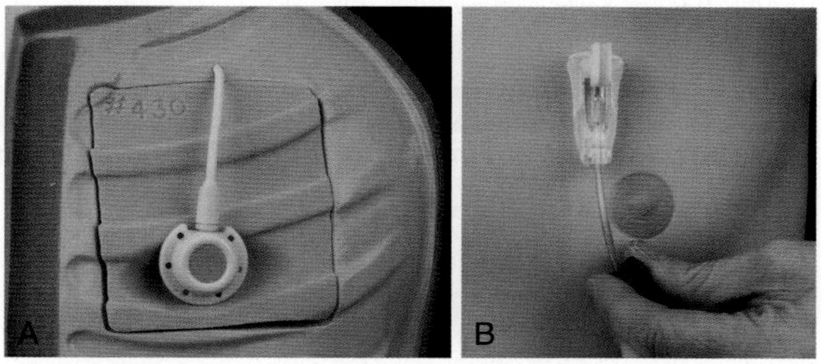

FIGURE 40-12 A, Implanted port. **B,** Accessing an implanted port. (Courtesy Darlaine Jantzen, RN, MA, PhD. Photo by Burl Jantzen.)

are irritating to veins. A midline catheter, a catheter inserted into the upper arm and terminating distal to the shoulder, is recommended for intermediate use (1–4 weeks) or when peripheral or central access is difficult or contraindicated (Ogston-Tuck, 2012, p. 476). Other reasons for using CVADs are presence of limited or poor peripheral veins, the need for good access to administer large volumes of fluid, and the need for reliable measurement of fluids. CVADs have become an essential tool in contemporary nursing practice in acute care and in community settings (INS, 2016). PICCs are quite common across settings (Figure 40-13). Correct dressing and labelling are critical to the prevention of infection and effective monitoring of the PICC site and line (Figure 40-14). Nurses play an important role in the education of patients and families regarding VADs and in decisions regarding device selection (INS, 2016; Registered Nurses' Association of Ontario [RNAO] 2004/2008). See Figure 40-15 for a comparison of midline and peripheral catheters.

Informed consent is required when providing care to patients with health challenges, and patients have the right to refuse treatment. Education regarding parenteral replacement of fluid and electrolytes or administration of treatments includes knowledge of the patient's preferred learning methods, health literacy level, and cultural preferences; organizational policy; and legislation (INS, 2016, p. S27). Nurses also play a role in the continual evaluation of the need and appropriateness of a VAD, as prompt removal of unnecessary lines is key to preventing catheter-related bloodstream infections (INS, 2016) (Box 40-9). The recommendations and discussion that follow here are general guidelines; nurses should be aware of, and follow, specific institutional and manufacturer's policy.

Peripheral vascular access devices: Nursing considerations. Comprehensive assessment is the first step in initiating any intravenous therapy (Ogston-Tuck, 2012); (Skill 40-1, Steps 2 to 6; Box 40-10). Many factors are involved in device selection, including safety concerns, treatment goals and duration, access to services such as home intravenous programs, and physical limitations. Effective communication, allowing time for questions, and education regarding the signs of complications are important to preventing and managing risks (Scales, 2011).

Text continued on p. 1050

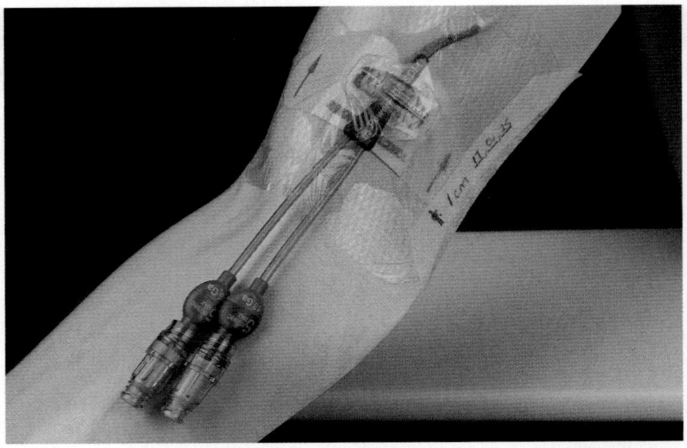

FIGURE 40-14 **Peripherally inserted central catheter (PICC) dressing and label.** (Courtesy Darlaine Jantzen, RN, MA, PhD. Photo by Burl Jantzen.)

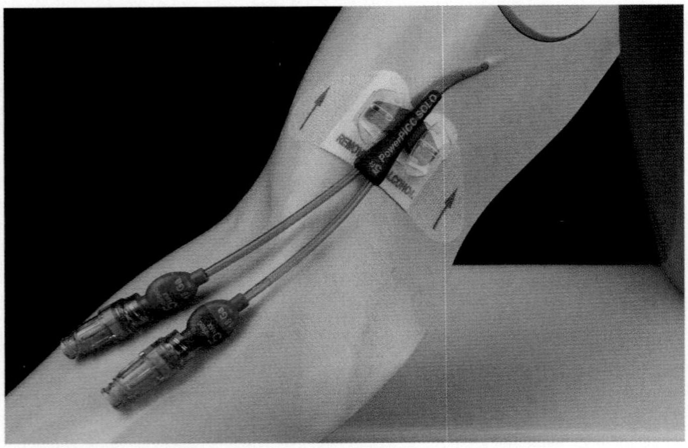

FIGURE 40-13 **Peripherally inserted central catheter (PICC) model.** (Courtesy Darlaine Jantzen, RN, MA, PhD. Photo by Burl Jantzen.)

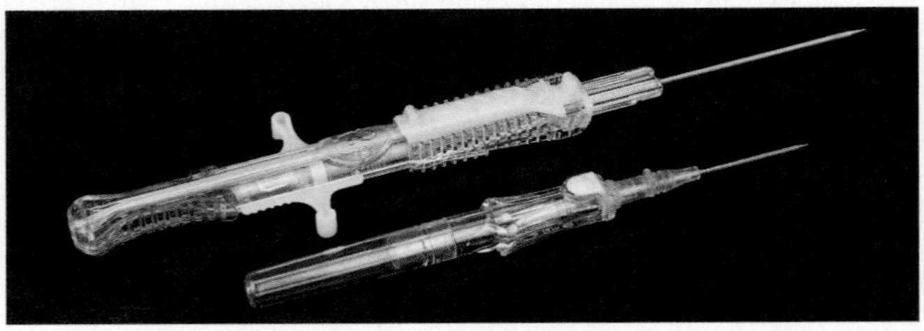

FIGURE 40-15 **Midline *(top)* and peripheral *(bottom)* intravenous catheters.** (Courtesy Darlaine Jantzen, RN, MA, PhD. Photo by Burl Jantzen.)

BOX 40-9 EVIDENCE-INFORMED PRACTICE

Preventing Central Line-Associated Bloodstream Infections (CLABSI)

PICO Question: In hospitalized adult patients, which interventions for central intravenous (IV) site care are best to prevent central line–associated bloodstream infections (CLABSI)?

Evidence Summary

CLABSI is a serious complication of IV therapy that increases morbidity, hospital length of stay, and health care costs. Research shows that effective strategies for prevention of CLABSI include the use of several evidence-informed practices together as a "bundle" or "checklist" (Chopra, Krein, Olmsted, et al., 2013). Such bundles are effective in reducing CLABSIs at the time of insertion of central lines and also during their maintenance (The Joint Commission, 2017). For example, a recommended bundle at *insertion* of a central line is hand hygiene before catheter insertion; use of maximum sterile barrier precautions on insertion; chlorhexidine skin antisepsis before insertion and during dressing changes; avoidance of the femoral vein for central venous access for adults; and daily evaluation of line necessity, with prompt removal of nonessential lines (Chopra et al., 2013). Maintenance bundles are similar, with attention to hand hygiene, catheter hub asepsis, dressing and line change, and continued daily evaluation of line necessity. For the most effective reduction in CLABSIs, research demonstrates the need for organized educational strategies and attention to institutional support and culture in addition to the use of bundled central line insertion and maintenance practices. One hospital had instituted the central line insertion bundle but still had not achieved zero CLABSI rate in the Critical Care Unit (CCU); however, with addition of a collaborative program involving staff education, daily surveillance, single-use line insertion kits, and updated policies and protocols, a zero CLABSI rate was achieved (Matocha, 2013). Dumyati, Concannon, van Wijngaarden, and colleagues (2014) reduced the CLABSI rate by 50% with a multimodal intervention that included involvement of nursing leadership and staff, education on the central line maintenance bundle components, competency evaluation, and line care audits. Zingg, Cartier, Inan, and colleagues (2014) achieved a hospital-wide clinically relevant reduction in CLABSIs with an interdisciplinary multimodal program that included educational components, single-use insertion kits, a catheter insertion checklist, and a catheter maintenance bundle.

Application to Nursing Practice

- If CLABSI prevention bundles are not used for central line insertion and maintenance at your agency, review the current research in a nursing practice committee or with your IV therapy team to influence policy and procedures and implement these bundles.
- Extend use of central line maintenance bundles to hospital units outside the CCU where patients have central lines.
- Work with infection control personnel and medical and nursing administration to establish a multidisciplinary CLABSI prevention program that includes institutional support for education, competency demonstration, use of insertion and maintenance bundles, and daily line audits.

SKILL 40-1 INITIATING A PERIPHERAL INTRAVENOUS INFUSION

Delegation Considerations

In many provinces, monitoring intravenous therapy is included within the scope of practice for licensed and registered practical nurses. In some locations, the delegating nurse is ultimately responsible for assessment and monitoring of the intravenous device. *The skill of initiating intravenous therapy should not be delegated to unregulated care providers (UCPs) or to those who have not demonstrated competence in initiating intravenous therapy* (INS, 2016, S18). Other aspects of the patient's care may be delegated to UCPs. Instruct the UCP about the following:

- To inform the nurse if the patient complains of burning sensation or appears to have discomfort, bleeding, swelling, or coolness at the catheter insertion site
- The prescribed flow rate and to report if the rate has slowed or increased
- To inform the nurse if the intravenous dressing becomes wet or compromised
- To inform the nurse if an electronic infusion device (EID) sounds or appears to be malfunctioning
- To inform the nurse if the volume of fluid in the intravenous bag is low

Equipment

- Correct intravenous solution
- Proper catheter for venipuncture (the gauge will vary with the patient's body size and the reason for intravenous fluid administration). Select the smallest gauge and shortest length possible.
- Intravenous start kit (if available): May contain a sterile drape to place under the patient's arm, a tourniquet, cleaning and antiseptic preparations, dressings, and a small roll of sterile tape
- Local anaesthetic (optional)

For intravenous fluid infusion

- Administration set (the choice depends on the type of solution and rate of administration; infants and children, patients with cardiac or renal disease, and patients taking certain medications require microdrip tubing, which provides 60 gtt/mL)
- Extension tubing (used when a longer intravenous line is necessary or to avoid manipulation of the catheter insertion site with frequent tubing changes)
- Antiseptic swabs or sticks (chlorhexidine, povidone–iodine, alcohol)
- Disposable gloves
- Tourniquet (Determine the type of tourniquet on the basis of the patient assessment, e.g., a blood pressure [BP] cuff [older person] or a rubber band [infants]. Tourniquets can be a source of contamination; use a single-use product.)
- Nonallergenic tape
- Waterproof pad (to place under patient's hand or arm)
- Intravenous pole or EID, for precise flow-control, or flow-control device, determined by patient age, patient's presenting condition, specific infusion therapy, and setting
- Special patient gown with snaps at shoulder seams, if available (makes removal with intravenous tubing easier)
- Needle disposal container (also called sharps container)
- Intravenous site protection device (optional)

For Normal Saline Lock

- Needleless connectors
- Injection cap (also called intravenous plug, adapter, CAP)
- 1 to 3 mL of sterile normal saline

Gauze Dressing Only

- 2 × 2 (5 cm × 5 cm) or 4 × 4 (10 cm × 10 cm) sterile gauze sponge
- Sterile tape

Transparent Dressing Only (Preferred)

- Transparent dressing

PROCEDURE

STEPS	RATIONALE
ASSESSMENT	
1. Review prescriber's order for type and amount of intravenous fluid, rate of fluid administration, and purpose of infusion. Follow 10 rights for administration of medications (see Chapter 34).	• An order requesting the initiation of a peripheral intravenous access and administration of an intravenous solution must be made by a physician before implementation of this procedure. Nurses assist in decision making for selection of appropriate access device.
2. Identify patient according to agency policy.	• Ensures correct patient and complies with quality and safety guidelines.

CRITICAL DECISION POINT: *Health care providers or prescribers do not write orders to "initiate peripheral access" or "perform venipuncture." "Start IV" may be written, followed by the exact intravenous therapy order. The order to perform venipuncture is implied. If the order is confusing or in question, clarify it with the health care provider before proceeding.*

Continued

SKILL 40-1 INITIATING A PERIPHERAL INTRAVENOUS INFUSION—cont'd

STEPS	RATIONALE
3. Assess for clinical variables that respond to or are affected by intravenous fluid administration. Assess for chronic illness and prescribed and over-the-counter medications.	• Provides baseline data for later evaluation of change in fluid and electrolyte status. • Analysis of data may lead to recommendations regarding slower infusion rate or contraindications to therapy.
A. Peripheral edema	• Indicates expanded interstitial fluid volume, evident in dependent body parts (e.g., feet and ankles). Excess intravenous fluids will worsen this condition.
B. Greater than 20% change in body weight	• Daily weights assist in documenting fluid retention or loss. Change in body weight of 1 kg corresponds to 1 L of fluid retention or loss.
C. Dry skin and mucous membranes	• Frequently associated with fluid volume deficit (FVD).
D. Distended neck veins	• Frequently associated with fluid volume excess (FVE) or cardiovascular alterations.
E. BP changes	• Elevations in BP may indicate volume excess, and decreased pressure may indicate FVD. These changes can be more sudden and pronounced in patients with underlying cardiopulmonary disease.
F. Irregular pulse rhythm; tachycardia	• Rate and rhythm change can occur with changes in intravascular volume, as well as changes in potassium, calcium, or magnesium. Tachycardia may indicate cardiac compensation for reduced circulating volume, whereas irregular pulse may indicate arrhythmias secondary to electrolyte imbalance.
G. Auscultation of abnormal lung sounds	• With FVE, the cardiovascular system is unable to compensate for this excess and fluid builds up in the lungs, creating abnormal lung sounds, such as crackles.
H. Decreased skin turgor. Skin fails to return to normal position in 3 seconds after pinching.	• With decreased fluid volume, the skin when pinched remains in that state for several seconds. This is called "tenting."

CRITICAL DECISION POINT: *Changes in skin turgor are a less reliable indicator for older patients because of the natural loss in skin elasticity caused by the normal aging process.*

STEPS	RATIONALE
I. Thirst	• Symptomatic of FVD. Very young, confused, and severely debilitated patients may not be able to indicate their thirst.
J. Anorexia, nausea, and vomiting	• May be present with FVE or FVD. These symptoms may also be present with the patient's underlying disease.
K. Decreased urine output	• During dehydration, the kidneys attempt to restore fluid balance by reducing urine production.
L. Behavioural changes	• May occur with FVD and acid–base imbalance. In addition, behavioural changes may be due to fever, the underlying condition, or pre-existing disease.
4. Assess patient's previous or perceived experience with intravenous therapy and arm placement preference (INS, 2016).	• Determines level of emotional support and instruction necessary for patient-centred care. If sensitive to venipunctures, a local anaesthetic may be indicated. The local anaesthetic needs to be applied 5–10 minutes prior to insertion (Burchum & Rosenthal, 2016).
5. Determine whether patient is to undergo any planned surgeries or is to receive blood infusion later.	• Allows nurse to select catheter gauge, and avoids placement in an area that will interfere with medical procedures.
6. Assess laboratory data.	• Determines priority assessments, establishes baseline, and provides information that affects insertion of devices, such as FVD, anemia.
7. Determine patient's history of allergies.	• Equipment used or medication or solution ordered may contain substances to which patient is allergic, such as iodine, adhesive, or latex.
8. Assess for the following risk factors: child or older person, presence of heart failure or renal failure, previous surgeries, or low platelet count.	• Fluid imbalances develop more rapidly in extremely young patients (infants) and older patients because such patients have proportionately larger extracellular fluid (ECF) volume, patients with heart failure may require fluid restriction and cannot adapt to sudden increases in vascular volume, and patients with renal failure cannot eliminate excess ECF. A low platelet count predisposes patients to bleeding at intravenous site. • Vascular visualization may be indicated in patients with disease-related vessel changes (e.g., diabetes), prior extended intravenous therapy, skin alterations (e.g., burns, scars), very young or advanced age, or obesity.

STEPS	RATIONALE
PLANNING	
9. Prepare patient and family by explaining the procedure, its purpose, and what is expected of the patient.	• Decreases anxiety and promotes cooperation.
10. Obtain informed consent.	• Initiation of a vascular access device (VAD) can be accepted or refused. Follow organizational policy and legislation regarding consent procedures. • Verbal consent and implied consent are types of consent in keeping with patient-centred care.
11. Assist patient to comfortable sitting or supine position.	• Enables patient to extend arm.
12. Collect and organize equipment on clean, clutter-free bedside stand or overbed table.	• Reduces risk of contamination and accidents and contributes to patient safety.
13. Change patient's gown to the more easily removed gown with snaps at the shoulder, if available.	• Use of a special intravenous gown facilitates safe removal of the gown.
14. Check intravenous solution, using the 10 rights of drug administration (see Chapter 34). Make sure prescribed additives, such as potassium and vitamins, have been added. Check solution for colour, clarity, and expiration date. Check bag for leaks, which is best if done before reaching the bedside (see Step 14 illustration).	• Intravenous solutions are medications and should be carefully checked to reduce the risk of error. • As with medication administration, use agency-approved resources (e.g., drug reference) for composition of intravenous fluids, incompatibilities, adverse effects, and special considerations. • Solutions that are discoloured, contain particles, or are expired are not to be used. (Some solutions may have slight discoloration [e.g., be pink-tinged] and still be suitable for use.) Leaky bags present an opportunity for infection and must not be used.

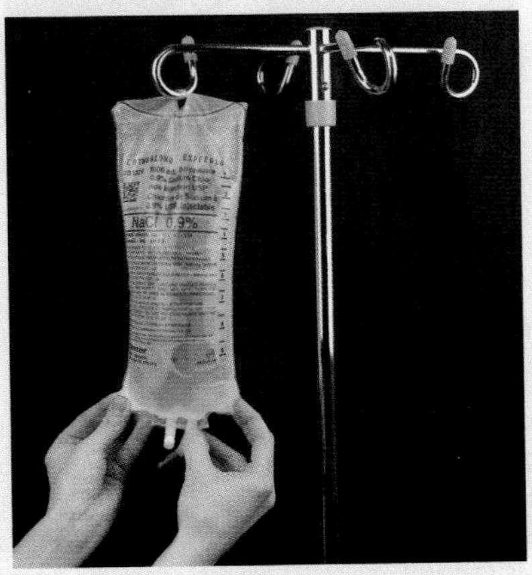

STEP 14 Check intravenous solution. (Courtesy Darlaine Jantzen, RN, MA, PhD. Photo by Burl Jantzen.)

STEPS	RATIONALE
IMPLEMENTATION	
15. Perform hand hygiene.	• Reduces spread of microorganisms, thereby helping to prevent infection.
For continuous infusion:	
16. Open the infusion set and other supplies, maintaining aseptic technique. When preparing the infusion set, do not touch point of entry for connections, and avoid removing end cap.	• Maintains sterility of equipment and reduces spread of microorganisms. Prevents bacteria from entering infusion equipment and bloodstream, and reduces transmission of infection. • EIDs may have special administration sets, in which case, follow manufacturer's instructions. • If contamination occurs, discard intravenous tubing.
17. Place roller clamp about 2 to 5 cm below drip chamber and move roller clamp to closed position. For EIDs, place roller clamp proximal to the patient.	• Close proximity of roller clamp to drip chamber allows more accurate regulation of flow rate. Moving clamp to closed position prevents accidental spillage of fluid.
18. Remove protective sheath over intravenous bag port. For bottled intravenous solution, remove metal cap and metal and rubber discs beneath cap. Use caution to avoid touching exposed opening.	• Provides access for insertion of infusion tubing into solution.
19. Insert infusion set into fluid bag or bottle by removing protector cap from tubing insertion spike (keeping spike sterile) and inserting spike into opening of intravenous bag (see Step 19 illustration). Clean rubber stopper on glass-bottled solution with antiseptic and insert spike into black rubber stopper of intravenous bottle. Hang solution container on intravenous pole at a minimum height of 90 cm above planned insertion site.	• Prevents contamination of solution from contaminated insertion spike. • Container heights of approximately 1 m are usually sufficient to overcome venous pressure and other resistance from tubing and catheter. • If contamination occurs, discard intravenous tubing and obtain a new set.

Continued

SKILL 40-1 INITIATING A PERIPHERAL INTRAVENOUS INFUSION—cont'd

STEPS	RATIONALE
20. Compress drip chamber and release, allowing it to fill one-third to one-half full. Open clamp and prime infusion tubing by filling with intravenous solution, carefully inverting valves and ports in sequence as the solution moves through the tubing (see Step 20 illustration).	• Creates vacuum effects; fluid enters drip chamber to prevent air from entering tubing. By inverting valves and ports, you allow them to fill with fluid, minimizing air bubbles.

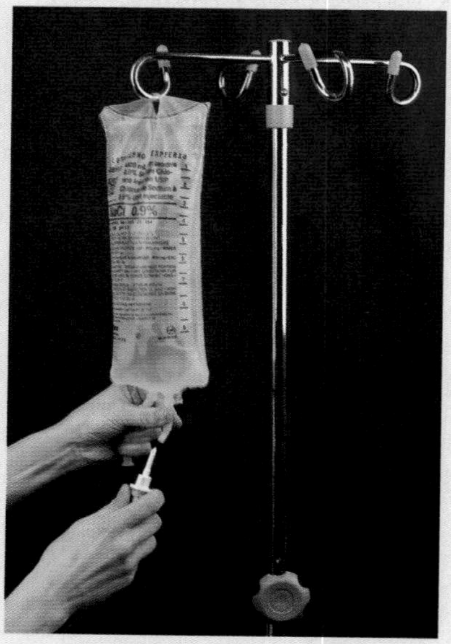

STEP 19 Inserting spike into intravenous bag. (Courtesy Darlaine Jantzen, RN, MA, PhD. Photo by Burl Jantzen.)

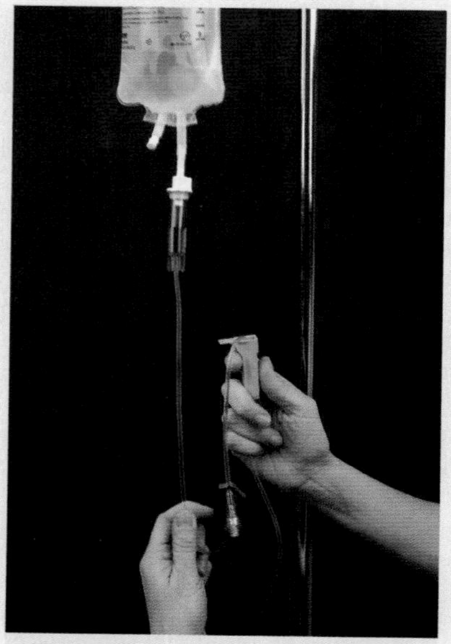

STEP 20 Priming intravenous tubing. (Courtesy Darlaine Jantzen, RN, MA, PhD. Photo by Burl Jantzen.)

STEPS	RATIONALE
21. Slowly release roller clamp to allow fluid to travel from drip chamber through tubing to needle adapter. (See Step 20, Priming intravenous tubing.) Return roller clamp to closed position after tubing is primed (filled with intravenous fluid).	• Slow filling of tubing decreases turbulence and chance of bubble formation. Removes air from tubing and permits tubing to fill with solution. Closing the clamp prevents accidental loss of fluid. • Most tubing sets can be primed without removing the end cap. If the tubing protector cap is removed, replace it promptly once the tubing is primed.
22. Be certain tubing is clear of air and air bubbles. To remove small air bubbles, firmly tap intravenous tubing where air bubbles are located. Check entire length of tubing to ensure that all air bubbles are removed. If using multiple-port tubing, turn ports upside down and tap to fill and remove air.	• Air bubbles may contribute to anxiety related to intravenous therapy and may cause EID to set off alarm, increasing anxiety further.
23. Insert primed tubing into EID set to "off" (see Step 23 illustration).	• Facilitates starting infusion as soon as intravenous site is ready.

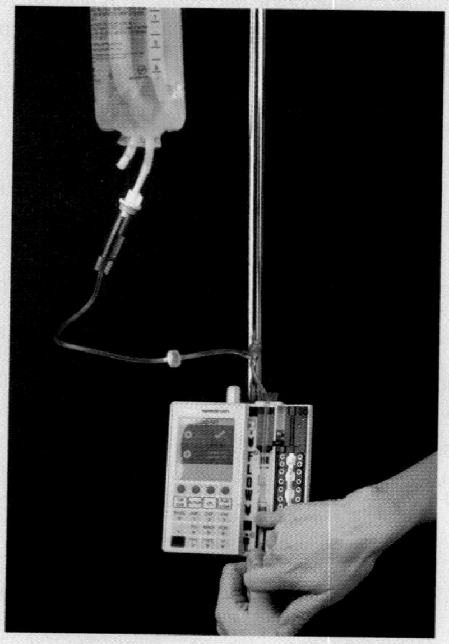

STEP 23 Primed line with EID. (Courtesy Darlaine Jantzen, RN, MA, PhD. Photo by Burl Jantzen.)

STEPS	RATIONALE
For intermittent intravenous catheter use: **24.** Prepare needleless connector and extension set. Use sterile technique to connect the needleless connector to the loop or short extension tubing. Prime with normal saline.	• Priming the extension tubing and needleless connector prevents introduction of air into the vein. • Extension sets are not recommended for continuous intravenous fluid administration, as they are potential sites of microbial contamination (INS, 2016, p. S68). • Remove needleless connector when rapid flow rates are required, or when administering red blood cells (INS, 2016, p. S68).
25. Apply disposable gloves. Eye protection and mask may be worn (see agency policy) if splash or spray of blood is possible. *Note:* Gloves can be left off to locate vein but must be applied before preparing site.	• Reduces transmission of microorganisms. Decreases exposure to bloodborne organisms (INS, 2016).

CRITICAL DECISION POINT: *Gloves can be applied before or after assessing veins. Gloves must be applied before VAD insertion. Use disposable, nonsterile gloves and no-touch technique for intravenous insertion (INS, 2016, p. S65).*

STEPS	RATIONALE
26. Apply tourniquet 10 to 15 cm above the proposed insertion site or above antecubital fossa (see Step 26 illustration) to begin vein selection. Position tourniquet so that ends are away from proposed venipuncture site. Check for presence of radial pulse. *Option:* Apply BP cuff instead of tourniquet. Inflate to a level just below patient's normal diastolic pressure. Maintain inflation at that pressure until venipuncture is completed.	• Tourniquet should be tight enough to impede venous return but not occlude arterial flow. • If patient has fragile veins, apply tourniquet loosely or not at all. • Avoid antecubital fossa for intravenous insertion, except in extreme emergencies.
27. Select the vein. Common intravenous sites for the adult include cephalic, basilic, and median cubital veins (see Figures 40-17 and 40-18).	
A. Use the most distal site in the nondominant arm, if possible.	• Venipuncture should be performed distal to proximal, which increases the availability of other sites for future intravenous therapy.
B. Avoid areas that are painful to palpation.	• May indicate inflamed vein.
C. Select a vein large enough for catheter placement.	• Prevents interruption of venous flow while allowing adequate blood flow around the catheter.
D. Choose a site that will not interfere with patient's activities of daily living or planned procedures.	• Selection of an appropriate site will minimize risk of injury and loss of the intravenous line.
E. Use the fingertips to palpate the vein by pressing downward and noting the resilient, soft, bouncy feeling as the pressure is released (see Step 27E illustration).	• Fingertips are more sensitive and are better to assess vein condition.

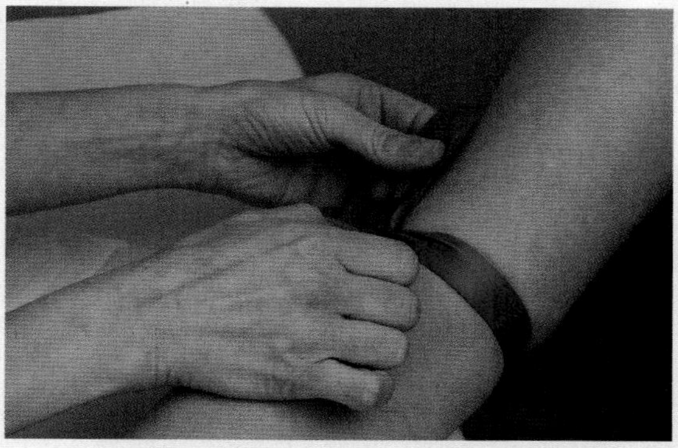

STEP 26 Apply tourniquet. (Courtesy Darlaine Jantzen, RN, MA, PhD. Photo by Burl Jantzen.)

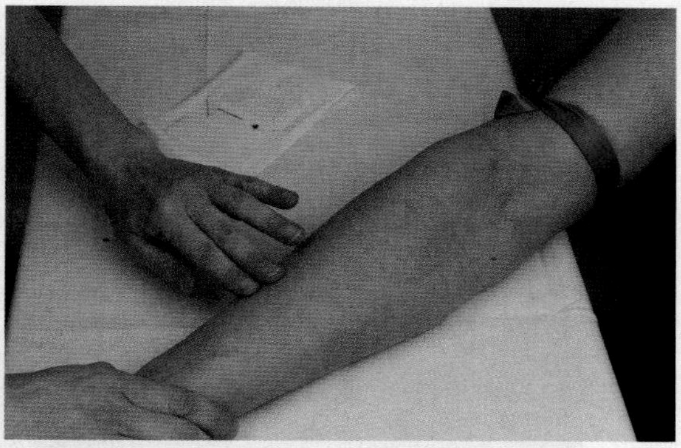

STEP 27E Palpate vein for resilience. (Courtesy Darlaine Jantzen, RN, MA, PhD. Photo by Burl Jantzen.)

STEPS	RATIONALE
F. If needed, promote venous distension by instructing the patient to open and close the fist several times, lowering the patient's arm in a dependent position, applying warmth to the arm for several minutes, and rubbing or stroking the patient's arm from distal to proximal below proposed site.	• These activities increase blood flow to the area of insertion. When these techniques are properly used, they foster venous dilation and access to the vein.

CRITICAL DECISION POINT: *Avoid vigorous rubbing and multiple tapping of patient's veins. These techniques may cause injury to the vein, such as a hematoma, or cause venous constriction.*

Continued

SKILL 40-1 INITIATING A PERIPHERAL INTRAVENOUS INFUSION—cont'd

STEPS	RATIONALE
G. Avoid sites distal to previous venipuncture site, sclerosed or hardened cordlike veins, infiltrated site or phlebotic vessels, bruised areas, and areas of venous valves or bifurcation. Avoid veins in antecubital fossa and ventral surface of the wrist.	• Such sites increase the risk of infiltration of a newly placed intravenous line and of excessive vessel damage. • Veins in the antecubital fossa are used for blood draws, and placement in this area limits mobility. The inner wrist contains numerous tendons that could be damaged.
H. Avoid fragile dorsal veins in older persons and vessels in an extremity with compromised circulation (e.g., in cases of mastectomy, dialysis graft, or paralysis).	• Venous alterations can increase risk of complications (e.g., infiltration and decreased catheter dwelling time).
28. Release tourniquet temporarily and carefully. Clip arm hair with scissors (if necessary).	• Hair impedes venipuncture and adherence of dressing. Shaving can cause microabrasions and predispose patient to infection.

CRITICAL DECISION POINT: *Do not shave area with a razor. Shaving may cause microabrasions and predispose patient to infection. Use single-patient-use scissors or disposable-head surgical clippers (INS, 2016, p. S64).*

STEPS	RATIONALE
29. (If area of insertion appears to need cleaning, use soap and water first.) Clean insertion site using firm, circular motion (centre to outward) in concentric circles 5–7.5 cm from insertion site. Use antiseptic preparation as a single agent or in combination, according to agency policy. Chlorhexidine (>0.5%) in alcohol solution is recommended. If this solution is contraindicated, povidone-iodine is a topical anti-infective agent that reduces skin surface bacteria; 70% alcohol is another antiseptic cleaning agent. Povidone-iodine must dry to be effective in reducing microbial counts. Avoid touching the cleaned site. Allow the site to dry for at least 2 minutes. If skin is touched after cleaning, repeat cleaning procedure (INS, 2016).	• Air-drying prevents chemical reactions between agents and allows time for maximum microbicidal activity of agents (INS, 2016). • Touching the cleaned area would introduce organisms from the nurse's hand to the site. • The use of chlorhexidine for insertion and with the use of ports is considered best practice (INS, 2016; Scales, 2011).
30. Reapply tourniquet or BP cuff above insertion site.	• BP cuff should be inflated <50 mm Hg, as diminished arterial flow prevents venous filling.

CRITICAL DECISION POINT: *Do not palpate the insertion site after skin antisepsis (INS, 2016, p. S65).*

STEPS	RATIONALE
31. Perform venipuncture. Anchor vein by placing thumb over vein beneath insertion site and by stretching the skin against the direction of insertion 5 to 7.5 cm distal to the site. Warn patient of a sharp stick. Puncture skin and vein, holding catheter at 10- to 30-degree angle with the bevel pointed upward slightly distal to actual site in the direction of vein (see Step 31 illustrations).	• The VAD selected should be the smallest gauge and shortest length that will accommodate the therapy (INS, 2016). • Places needle parallel to vein. When vein is punctured, risk of puncturing posterior vein wall is reduced. • Superficial veins require a smaller angle; deeper veins require a greater angle.

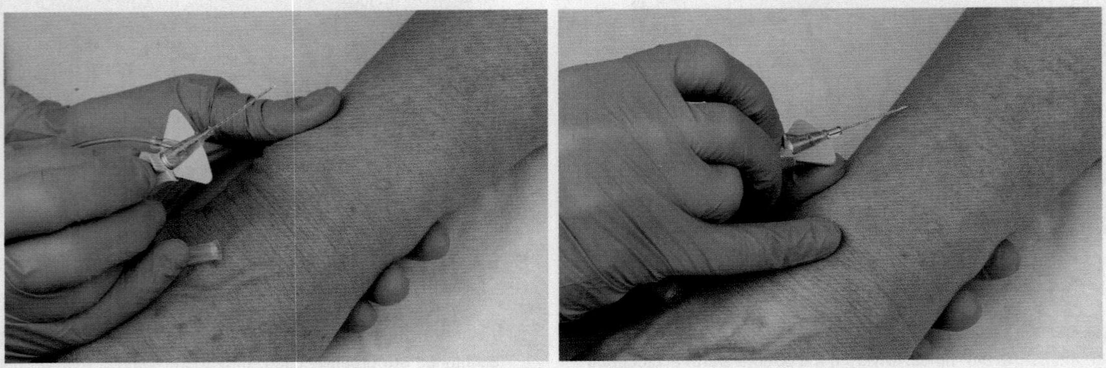

STEP 31 Stabilize vein below insertion site with skin taut and puncture vein (Courtesy Darlaine Jantzen, RN, MA, PhD. Photo by Burl Jantzen.)

CRITICAL DECISION POINT: *No more than two attempts at inserting an intravenous line should be made by a single nurse (INS, 2016, p. S64).*

STEPS	RATIONALE
32. Look for blood return through tubing of butterfly needle or flashback chamber of over-the-needle catheter, indicating that needle has entered vein (see Step 32 illustration). Lower catheter or needle until almost flush with skin. Advance until hub is near the insertion site. Do not reinsert the stylet once it is loosened. Follow manufacturer's guidelines for specific safety catheter use and for techniques for retracting stylus.	• Increased venous pressure from tourniquet increases backflow of blood into catheter or tubing. • Lowering the angle and advancing the cannula slightly allow for full penetration of vein wall, placement of catheter within vein's inner lumen, and easy advancement of catheter off stylet. • Threading catheter up to hub reduces the risk of introducing infectious organisms along the catheter length. Reinsertion of the stylet can cause catheter damage and potential catheter embolization. • Advancing stylet into vein may penetrate posterior vein wall. • Reinsertion of stylet can cause catheter shearing and potential catheter embolization.
33. Stabilize the catheter. Apply gentle but firm pressure with the index finger of nondominant hand 3 cm above insertion site. Release tourniquet or BP cuff with dominant hand. Apply gentle but firm pressure above insertion site and keep catheter stable.	• Permits venous flow, reduces backflow of blood, and prevents accidental withdrawal or dislodgement.
34. Quickly connect distal end of tubing, extension set, or needleless connector. Be sure connection is secure. Do not touch point of entry of connection. Secure connection (see Step 34 illustration).	• Prompt connection of infusion set maintains patency of vein. • Maintains sterility.

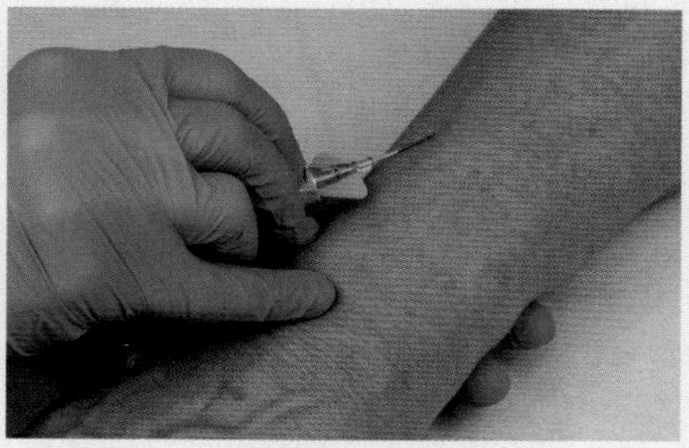

STEP 32 Blood return in flashback chamber, catheter lowered flush with skin. (Courtesy Darlaine Jantzen, RN, MA, PhD. Photo by Burl Jantzen.)

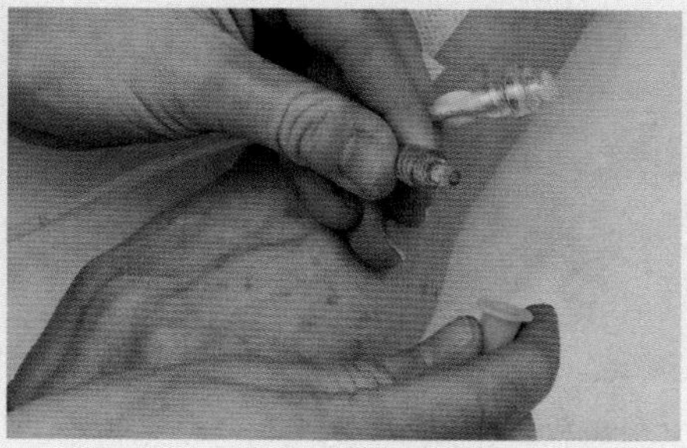

STEP 34 Secure connection, maintaining asepsis. (Courtesy Darlaine Jantzen, RN, MA, PhD. Photo by Burl Jantzen.)

STEPS	RATIONALE
For Continuous Infusion: **35A.** Release roller clamp slowly to begin infusion at a rate to maintain patency of intravenous line, or turn on EID, program it, and begin infusion at correct rate (see Skill 40-2).	• Permits venous flow and prevents clotting of vein and obstruction of flow of intravenous solution.
For intermittent infusion: **35B.** Continue to stabilize catheter with nondominant hand and attach injection cap of adapter. Insert prefilled flush solution into injection cap. Flush slowly. Maintain thumb pressure on syringe during withdrawal or close clamp on extension tubing of injection cap while still flushing last 0.2–0.4 mL of flush solution.	• Positive pressure in the catheter prevents reflux of blood into the catheter lumen. • Use volume equal to twice the internal volume of the catheter system.

CRITICAL DECISION POINT: *Be sure to calculate rate so as not to infuse intravenous solution too rapidly or too slowly.*

STEPS	RATIONALE
36. Stabilize catheter with an engineered stabilization device (ESD) (see Step 36 illustration), either alone or in combination with a securement dressing.	• Securing the catheter and tubing prevents movement and tension on the device, reducing mechanical irritation and possible phlebitis or infection (Higginson, 2015). Procedures for securing catheter vary with devices and with agency policy. Manufacturer-provided catheter stabilization devices reduce the risk of complications from peripheral VAD (INS, 2016, S73). • Joint stabilization, through use of a padded armboard, is acceptable, although sites close to joints (e.g., antecubital fossa) are not recommended (INS, 2016, S75).

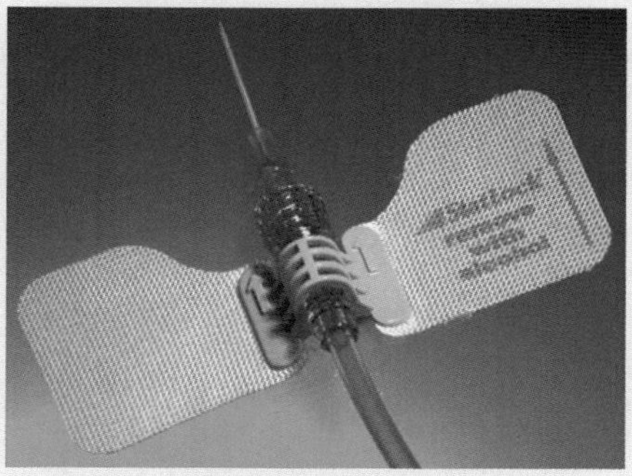

STEP 36 Catheter stabilization device. (C.R. Bard, Inc. Used with permission.)

Continued

SKILL 40-1 INITIATING A PERIPHERAL INTRAVENOUS INFUSION—cont'd

STEPS	RATIONALE
A. If applying transparent dressing, secure catheter with nondominant hand while preparing to apply dressing.	• Transparent dressings are preferred (Bernatchez, 2014) as gauze does not provide the same barrier, needs to be changed more often (every 2 days), and does not provide stabilization of the catheter, all contributing to an increased risk of infection with gauze dressings. • Additional cost of transparent dressing is offset by increased labour costs and frequency of dressing change.
37. Observe site for swelling.	• Any swelling suggests the catheter has been dislodged or was unsuccessfully inserted and must be removed.
38. Apply sterile dressing over site. **A.** Transparent dressing Carefully remove adherent backing. Apply one edge of dressing and then gently smooth remaining dressing over site (see Step 38A illustration).	• Transparent dressings are occlusive to moisture and microorganisms. Transparent dressings allow continuous inspection of the intravenous site, are more comfortable, and enable patients to bathe and shower without saturating the dressing. • Transparent dressings are occlusive to moisture and microorganisms between catheter and tubing or cap, allowing for both continuous and intermittent intravenous use.

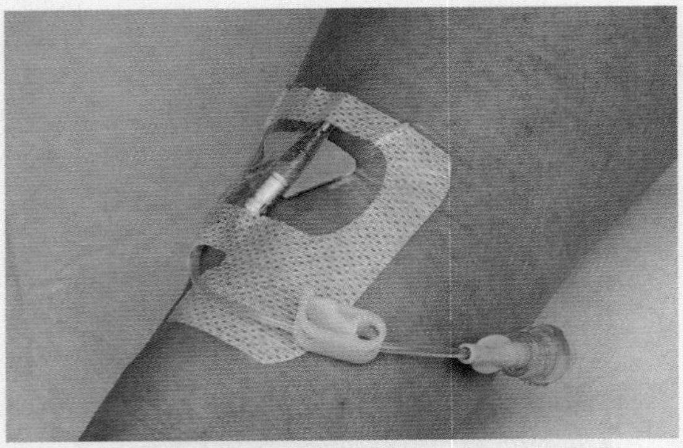

STEP 38A Apply transparent dressing. (Courtesy Darlaine Jantzen, RN, MA, PhD. Photo by Burl Jantzen.)

39. Secure tubing (see Step 39 illustration).

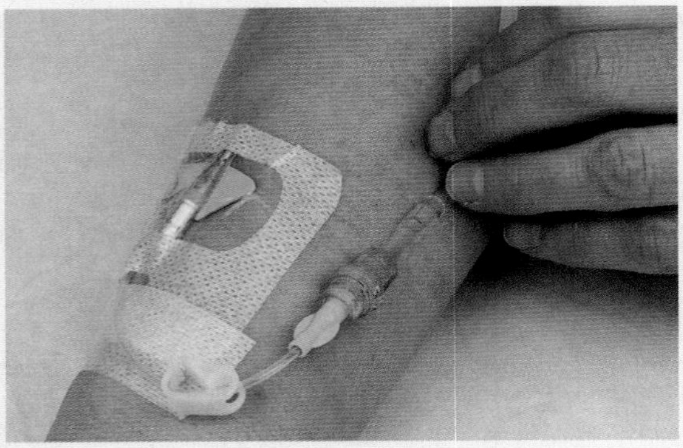

STEP 39 Secure tubing. (Courtesy Darlaine Jantzen, RN, MA, PhD. Photo by Burl Jantzen.)

STEPS	RATIONALE
40. Prepare the equipment according to expected frequency of use.	
A. *For intravenous fluid administration:* Adjust flow rate to correct drops per minute or connect to EID (see Skill 40-2, Steps 9 to 15).	• Maintains correct rate of flow for intravenous solution. Flow can fluctuate; therefore, it must be checked at intervals.
B. *For intermittent use:* Saline lock. Flush with 3 mL of sterile normal saline at prescribed frequency or according to agency policy.	• Maintains patency of intravenous catheter. While some authors recommend heparin lock, the RNAO (2004/2008) recommends use of saline for flushing and locking peripheral short catheters, after each use and daily if not in use.

STEPS	RATIONALE
41. Label dressing with date, time, gauge size and length of catheter, and your initials (see Step 41 illustration).	• Allows for easy recognition of type of device and time interval for site rotation.

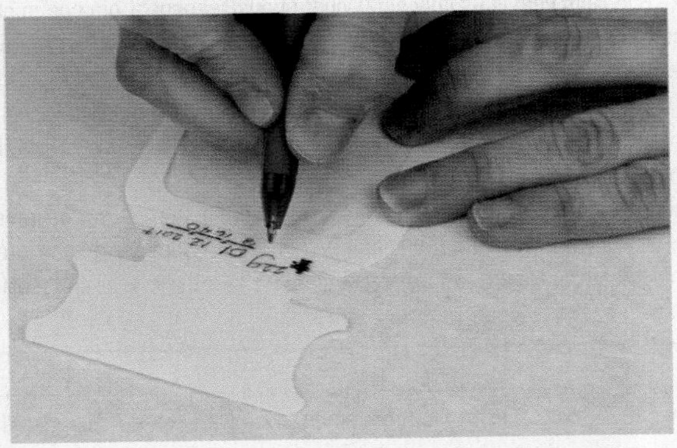

STEP 41 Label intravenous dressing. (Courtesy Darlaine Jantzen, RN, MA, PhD. Photo by Burl Jantzen.)

STEPS	RATIONALE
42. Dispose of used needles in appropriate sharps container. Discard supplies. Remove gloves and perform hand hygiene.	• Reduces transmission of microorganisms and protects staff from injury.
43. Observe patient every hour to determine whether fluid is infusing correctly:	• Correct administration of fluid volume prevents fluid imbalance.
A. Check whether correct amount of solution is infused as prescribed, by looking at time tape.	
B. Count flow rate or check rate on infusion pump.	• Accurate monitoring of rate further ensures correct volume administration.
C. Check patency of intravenous catheter or needle.	
D. Observe patient for signs of discomfort.	
E. Inspect insertion site for absence of phlebitis (see Table 40-10), infiltration (see Table 40-11), or inflammation.	
44. Document intravenous insertion, including date, time, device selected (size, type, length, brand), site, number of attempts, name of practitioner, and professional designation. A special parenteral therapy flow sheet may be used. Record patient's response to intravenous fluid, amount infused, and integrity and patency of system every 4 hours or according to agency policy.	• Precise description of insertion site is important for future consideration of sites. • Evaluation of parenteral therapy is an important part of the nursing process.
45. Observe patient every hour to determine response to therapy (i.e., measure vital signs, conduct postprocedure assessments).	• Provides continuous evaluation of type and amount of fluid delivered to patient. Hourly inspection prevents accidental fluid overload or inadequate infusion rate and identifies early incidence of vein inflammation or tissue damage. Intravenous fluids and additives are given to maintain or restore fluid and electrolyte balance. They can also cause unexpected effects, which can be serious.

UNEXPECTED OUTCOMES	RELATED INTERVENTIONS
FVD, as manifested by decreased urine output, dry mucous membranes, hypotension, and tachycardia	• Notify physician; may require readjustment of infusion rate.
FVE, as manifested by crackles in lungs, shortness of breath, and edema	• Reduce intravenous flow rate if symptoms appear and notify physician.
Electrolyte imbalances, as manifested by abnormal serum electrolyte levels; changes in mental status, neuromuscular function, and vital signs; and other signs and symptoms	• Notify physician. Additives in intravenous or type of intravenous fluid may be adjusted.
Infiltration, as indicated by swelling and possible pitting edema, pallor, coolness, pain at insertion site, and possible decrease in flow rate	• Stop infusion and discontinue intravenous therapy. Elevate affected extremity. Restart new intravenous line if continued therapy is necessary.
Phlebitis, as indicated by pain, increased skin temperature, and erythema along path of vein	• Cause of phlebitis (chemical, mechanical, bacterial, postinfusion) will inform interventions. • Stop infusion or slow infusion, depending on the determined cause. • Mechanical irritation may be treated by stabilizing catheter, elevating limb, and monitoring. • If phlebitis worsens or is causing patient distress, discontinue intravenous therapy. Restart new intravenous line if continued therapy is necessary. • Place moist, warm compress over area of phlebitis and elevate limb if possible.

Continued

SKILL 40-1 INITIATING A PERIPHERAL INTRAVENOUS INFUSION—cont'd

STEPS	RATIONALE
Bleeding at venipuncture site	• Bleeding from vein is usually slow, continuous seepage. Common in patients who have received heparin or have a bleeding disorder or if the intravenous site is over a bend in the arm or hand. • If bleeding occurs around venipuncture site and catheter is within vein, antisepsis and dressing changes are performed. Eventually, intravenous therapy may need to be discontinued. • Blood on the dressing can result when the administration set becomes disconnected from the catheter's hub. When blood appears on the dressing, verify that the system is intact and conduct site care, skin antisepsis, and dressing change.

REPORTING

- Report the following to incoming nursing staff: type of fluid, flow rate, status of venipuncture site, amount of fluid remaining in present solution, expected time to hang next intravenous bag or bottle, and any adverse effects.

HOME CARE CONSIDERATIONS

- Teach patient and family about hand hygiene and aseptic technique for all care related to the intravenous site and equipment.
- Teach caregiver to apply pressure with sterile gauze if catheter falls out and, if patient is on anticoagulant therapy, to tape several pieces of sterile gauze in place for at least 20 minutes with pressure or until bleeding stops.
- Teach patient and caregiver to perform tub bath without getting intravenous tubing wet and to unplug pump first if one is used. For showering, the patient must protect the intravenous site and dressing from getting wet by covering them completely with plastic.
- Teach patient and family to monitor intake and output using measuring devices, as necessary.
- Teach patient and family to dispose of open and sheathed needles into sharps container. All sharps containers must be stored in a safe area away from children.

BOX 40-10 Safety Guidelines for Infusion Therapy

Ensuring patient safety is an essential role of the professional nurse. To ensure patient safety, communicate clearly with members of the health care team, assess and incorporate the patient's priorities of care and preferences, and use the best evidence when making decisions about a patient's care. When performing the skills in this chapter, remember the following points to ensure safe, individualized patient care:

- Check that you have the necessary information, a prescriber's order if required, and equipment available for the procedure before beginning.
- Before initiation of therapy, check patient identification using two patient identifiers and assess the appropriate route and rate of infusion and potential incompatibilities between infusing fluids and medications (INS, 2016).
- Determine if the patient has a latex allergy or latex sensitivity and use latex-free equipment and supplies if allergy or sensitivity is present (INS, 2016, p. S35).
- Use special designated tubing for the brand of electronic infusion device (EID) and for blood transfusions and some medications.
- Review the steps of the procedure mentally before entering a patient's room (i.e., consider modifications that you may need to make for this specific patient and verify that the type of IV solution is appropriate for this patient).
- Maintain strict aseptic and sterile techniques, when required, and sterility and integrity of the IV system to prevent bloodstream infections (INS, 2016).
- If you contaminate a sterile object during the procedure, do not use it. Use a new sterile one.
- Use standard body fluid precautions during procedures and place all disposable blood-contaminated items and sharp items in designated puncture-resistant biohazard containers (INS, 2016).

Insertion and management of a PVAD are now considered a routine nursing responsibility and skill. Competency assessment and validation on an ongoing basis are required. This should be documented according to organizational policy (INS, 2016, p. S18). Vascular visualization technology is used with difficult access, in special populations, or after failed attempts to insert a PVAD and thus to avoid the need for CVAD related to successful cannulation of the PVAD (INS, 2016, p. S44). The management of PVADs requires careful monitoring of the site, patency, and dressing. The site should be assessed for phlebitis and infiltration (Table 40-10 and Table 40-11). Scales to assess for phlebitis and infiltration are important tools for nurses initiating and managing PVADs (Box 40-11) (Groll, Davies, MacDonald, et al., 2010). Although a recent systematic review of phlebitis scales recommends further study and standardization of definitions, the INS phlebitis scale is one of the most commonly used scales (see Table 40-10) (Ray-Barruel, Polit, Murfield, et al., 2014).

Central vascular access devices: Nursing considerations. A CVAD is a venous access device with a tip that terminates in a great vessel, preferably in the lower third of the superior vena cava; however, the upper right atrium is an acceptable site. The catheters are available in a variety of lengths, sizes, and numbers of lumens and are often made of silicone or polyurethane. The most common insertion sites are the internal jugular and subclavian veins; the right internal jugular vein is considered the best option (Casey & Elliot, 2010, p. 80). Skin-tunnelled catheters (STC) are tunnelled from the entry site, subcutaneously, to the preferred vein, where the catheter is inserted and advanced into the superior vena cava (Green, 2008, p. 44). PICCs are inserted through a peripheral vein, such as the basilic, median cubital, or cephalic vein, and terminate in the superior vena cava (Hamilton, 2006).

Nurses need to be able to recognize the following complications associated with CVADs: pneumothorax, arterial puncture, hemorrhage, cardiac tamponade, air embolus, hemothorax, nerve injury, hydrothorax, infection, catheter occlusion, and phlebitis. Nurses also need to be aware of strategies to prevent these complications when caring for patients with a CVAD. Evidence-informed and vigilant nursing care is important for insertion and in the maintenance of all CVADs. Nursing responsibilities for CVADs include careful monitoring, flushing, site care, and dressing changes to prevent central line–associated bloodstream infection (CLABSI). See Box 40-9 for evidence-informed practice for preventing CLABSI. Aseptic technique and diligent hand hygiene are essential for all aspects of care. Prior to insertion, chlorhexidine gluconate 2% in 70% isopropyl alcohol should be applied properly and allowed to dry. Maximal barrier precautions (including gown, mask, cap, and full drape) and ultrasound-guided procedure are key recommendations for insertion (Casey & Elliot, 2010, p. 82). Nurses must ensure that the tip placement or location has been verified and documented before the CVAD is used. Finally, the date of insertion must be documented.

Maintenance recommendations are aimed at maintaining patency and preventing complications, specifically catheter-related bloodstream infection (CR-BSI) or CLABSI. The manufacturer's stabilization device is preferred for PICCs and CVCs. Sterile, transparent, semipermeable membrane dressings are recommended (INS, 2016). Dressings are assessed daily or when they become wet, soiled, or loose. The new dressing is labelled with the site, type of CVAD, length, date, time, and nurse's initials. Transparent dressing may be left intact for

TABLE 40-10 Phlebitis Scale

Grade	Clinical Criteria
0	No symptoms
1	Erythema at access site with or without pain
2	Pain at access site with erythema and/or edema
3	Pain at access site with erythema and/or edema; streak formation; palpable venous cord
4	Pain at access site with erythema and/or edema; streak formation; palpable venous cord >2.54 cm (1 in) in length; purulent drainage

From Infusion Nurses Society. (2011). Infusion nursing standards of practice. *Journal of Infusion Nursing, 34*(1S), S1.

TABLE 40-11 Infiltration Scale

Grade	Clinical Criteria
0	No symptoms
1	Skin blanched Edema <2.54 cm (1 in) in any direction Cool to touch With or without pain
2	Skin blanched Edema 2.54–15.2 cm (1–6 in) in any direction Cool to touch With or without pain
3	Skin blanched, translucent Gross edema >15.2 cm (6 in) in any direction Cool to touch Mild–moderate pain Possible numbness
4	Skin blanched, translucent Skin tight, leaking Skin discoloured, bruised, swollen Gross edema >15.2 cm (6 in) in any direction Deep pitting tissue edema Circulatory impairment Moderate-to-severe pain Infiltration of any amount of blood product, irritant, or vesicant

From Groll, D., Davies, B., MacDonald, J., et al. (2010). Evaluation of the psychometric properties of the phlebitis and infiltration scales for the assessment of complications of peripheral vascular access devices. *Journal of Infusion Nursing, 33*(6), 385.

BOX 40-11 RESEARCH HIGHLIGHT

Using Phlebitis and Infiltration Scales for Assessing Peripheral Vascular Access Devices (PVADs)

Research Focus

Phlebitis and infiltration are common complications related to intravenous therapy. Two scales, developed by the Infusion Nurses Society (INS), are used to assess the extent of these complications. A study was done by a team of Canadian researchers to evaluate the scales' reliability, validity, and ease of use (Groll et al., 2010).

Research Abstract

The study used observation in a hospital setting and with a home nursing agency, for a total of 182 participants and 416 observations. Each participant was observed up to four times by two observers. The participants' charts were also audited. The research nurses used a data collection tool and observation form for each participant. The study evaluated the phlebitis and infiltration scales for four properties: acceptability, feasibility, reliability, and validity. The researchers concluded that the scales are easy to use and did not take long to complete. The scales were reliable and valid in both settings. The researchers also found that nurses who used the tools identified more cases of phlebitis and infiltration than were recorded in the participants' charts. These findings support the use of the INS phlebitis and infiltration scales in a variety of settings.

Evidence-Informed Practice

- Nurses in all settings are positioned to assess for complications related to PVADs.
- Scales to assess for phlebitis and infiltration are important tools for nurses initiating and managing PVADs.

Groll, D., Davies, B., Mac Donald, J., Nelson, S., & Virani, T. (2010). Evaluation of the psychometric properties of the phlebitis and infiltration scales for the assessment of complications of peripheral vascular access devices. *Journal of Infusion Nursing, 33*(6), 385–390.

up to 5 to 7 days. No dressing is required for an STC once the wound has healed, unless the patient prefers one (Green, 2008, p. 45).

The external catheter should be measured and results documented daily to ensure that the catheter remains in the correct placement. The insertion site should be inspected daily for tenderness, signs of infection, erythema, warmth, and edema, and assessment should include palpation. The chest and neck should be assessed for engorged veins and for difficulty with movement. The nurse should also assess the patient for signs of systemic infection, such as fever, chills, and hypotension (Casey & Elliot, 2010, p. 78; Scales, 2011).

Prior to accessing a CVAD, the nurse conducts a 15-second rub with 70% isopropyl alcohol, povidone-iodine, or >0.5% chlorhexidine in alcohol solution (INS, 2016). New antimicrobial devices and approaches to preventing CR-BSI are being developed and include antimicrobial catheters, needleless access devices, dressings, and lock solutions (Casey & Elliot, 2010, p. 84). To prevent occlusion of the CVAD, the device is flushed and assessed for patency according to institutional policy. The use of heparin for flushing and locking is currently an area for further study and future recommendations (e.g., Mitchell, Anderson, Williams, et al., 2009; RNAO, 2008). Totally implanted ports, used for long-term treatment such as chemotherapy, are inserted surgically and are accessed by inserting a needle through the skin into the device. They can be used up to 2 000 times (Kelly, 2009, p. s11) and have the lowest incidence of infection (Casey & Elliot, 2010, p. 80).

Patient and family education is required for all patients with a CVAD. This should include care requirements and patient restrictions.

Administration of Intravenous Therapy

Types of solutions. Many prepared intravenous solutions are available for use (Table 40-9). Solutions are classified as hypertonic, isotonic, or hypotonic (see Figure 40-10, earlier in chapter). Osmolarity, reflecting the osmolar concentration in 1 L of solution (mOsm/L), is most often used to describe fluids outside the body (Hannon, Pooler, & Porth, 2010). A solution with the same osmolarity as blood plasma is called *isotonic.* A hypertonic solution, with a higher osmotic pressure, such as 3% sodium chloride, pulls fluid from cells, causing them to shrink. An isotonic solution, with the same osmotic pressure as plasma, such as 0.9% sodium chloride, expands the body's fluid volume without causing a fluid shift from one compartment to another. A hypotonic solution, with an osmotic pressure lower than plasma, such as 0.45% sodium chloride, moves fluid into the cells, causing them to enlarge. Each of these actions occurs through osmosis.

In general, isotonic fluids are used most commonly for extracellular volume replacement (e.g., FVD after prolonged vomiting). The decision to use a hypotonic or hypertonic solution is based on the specific fluid and electrolyte imbalances. For example, the patient with a hypertonic fluid imbalance will in general receive a hypotonic intravenous solution to dilute the ECF and rehydrate the cells. All intravenous fluids should be given carefully, especially hypertonic solutions, because these pull fluid into the vascular space by osmosis, resulting in an increased vascular volume that can lead to pulmonary edema, particularly in patients with heart or renal failure. Certain additives, most commonly vitamins and potassium chloride, are frequently added to intravenous solutions.

> **Safety Alert** Under no circumstances should potassium chloride (KCl) be given by intravenous push. Direct intravenous infusion of KCl may cause death. If an intravenous fluid requires additives, a prescriber's order must specify the required additives—for example, "1 000 mL D51/2 NS with 20 mmol/L KCl at 125 mL/hour."

Patients with normal renal function who are receiving nothing by mouth should have potassium added to intravenous solutions. The body cannot conserve potassium, and even when the serum level falls, the kidneys continue to excrete potassium. Without oral or parenteral potassium intake, hypokalemia can develop quickly. Conversely, the nurse should verify that the patient has adequate renal function before administering an intravenous solution containing potassium, because hyperkalemia can develop quickly.

Equipment. Correct selection and preparation of intravenous equipment are necessary for safe and quick placement of an intravenous line (Figure 40-16). Because fluids are instilled into the bloodstream, sterile technique is necessary; the nurse should have all equipment organized for efficient insertion (see Skill 40-1). Intravenous cannulas are available in a variety of gauges. The larger the gauge, the smaller the diameter of the cannula. These cannulas are plastic tubing threaded over a needle. Once the cannula is inserted into the vein, the needle is withdrawn, leaving the cannula in place. Intravenous tubing or an intermittent infusion device, such as a needleless port, is then connected.

> **Safety Alert** Intravenous pumps or volume-control (flow-control) devices ensure a prescribed rate of infusion. A prescribed rate of infusion is vital for children, patients with renal or cardiac failure, and critically ill patients. Electronic infusion devices must be used for medications that require precise rates of administration.

Initiating an intravenous line. A venipuncture is a technique in which a vein is punctured through the skin by a sharp, rigid stylet (e.g., butterfly needle or metal needle), a partially covered plastic catheter (over-the-needle catheter), or a needle attached to a syringe. When veins are fragile or collapse, venipuncture may become extremely

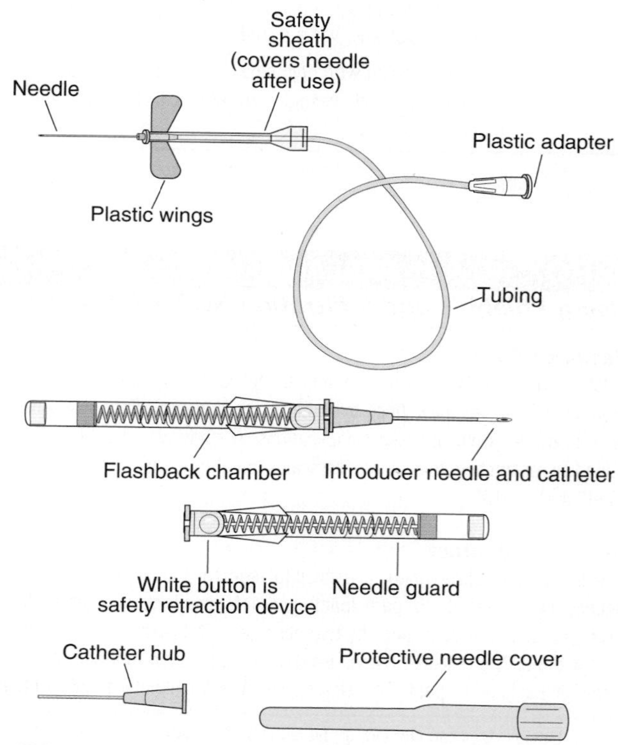

FIGURE 40-16 Options for intravenous access device.

difficult. For these difficult cases, venipuncture should be performed by an experienced, skilled practitioner. Skill 40-1 describes venipuncture for intravenous fluid infusion.

Venipuncture site. After the equipment is collected at the bedside, the nurse prepares to place the intravenous line by assessing the patient for a venipuncture site (see Skill 40-1, Step 27A). Common intravenous puncture sites are the hand and the arm (Figures 40-17 and 40-18). The use of the foot for an intravenous site is common with children but is avoided in the adult because of the danger of thrombophlebitis (INS, 2016). According to a review of the literature, replacing a PVAD every 72 hours is not supported; instead this is done when clinically indicated. However, nurses need to follow agency policy (Webster, Osborne, Rickard, et al., 2010).

When assessing the patient for potential venipuncture sites for intravenous infusion, nurses should consider conditions and contraindications that exclude certain sites. Because children and older persons have fragile veins, nurses should avoid sites that are easily moved or bumped, such as those on the dorsal surface of the hand. Venipuncture is contraindicated in a site that has signs of infection, infiltration, or thrombosis. An infected site is red, tender, swollen, and possibly warm to the touch, and exudate may be present. An infected site is not used because of the danger of introducing bacteria from the skin surface into the bloodstream. Arms on the side of a mastectomy, and extremities with an arteriovenous graft or fistula for dialysis should be avoided. It is important to place intravenous devices at the most distal point, when possible, as this allows for the use of proximal sites later if the patient needs a venipuncture site change. See Box 40-12 for guidelines concerning older persons.

Regulating the infusion flow rate. After the intravenous infusion is secured and the line is patent, the nurse must regulate the rate of infusion according to the prescriber's orders (Skill 40-2). An infusion rate that is too slow can lead to further cardiovascular and circulatory collapse in a critically ill patient. An intravenous fluid that is running too slowly can also clot more easily. An infusion rate that is too rapid can result in FVE. Fluids that run by gravity are adjusted through use of a flow control or regulator clamp. Fluids infused by an electronic infusion device or rate controller are regulated by a mechanical mechanism set at the prescribed rate. Regardless of the device in use, the patient requires close monitoring to verify the correct infusion of the intravenous solution and to detect the occurrence of any complication.

Electronic infusion devices (EIDs) or infusion pumps are necessary when administering low hourly volumes (e.g., less than 20 mL/hour) and for patients who are at risk for volume overload, such as neonatal, pediatric, and geriatric patients. In addition, when infusing high volumes of intravenous fluids (more than 150 mL/hour) to patients with impaired renal clearance, older persons, or children, or when infusing drugs or intravenous fluids that require specific hourly volumes, EIDs permit accurate infusion. EIDs deliver the infusion via positive pressure and have become standard in most settings. Recent advances in infusion technology have resulted in a variety of devices available for use to ensure accurate delivery.

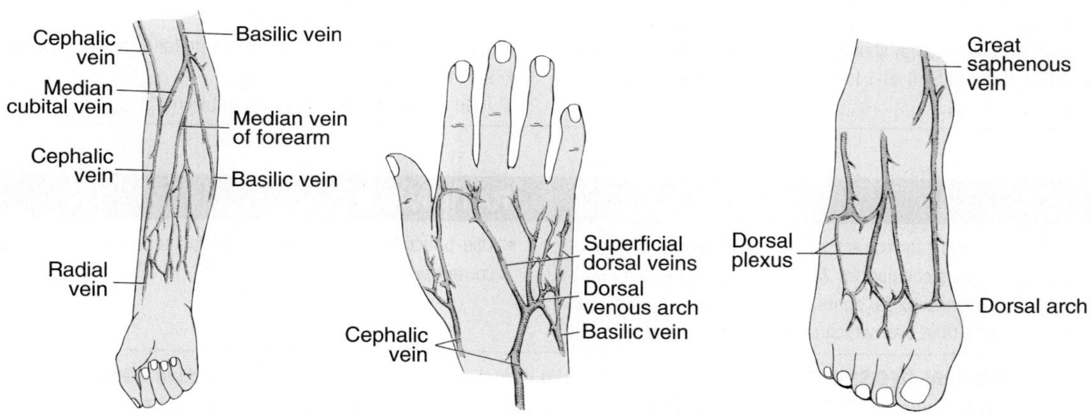

FIGURE 40-17 Common intravenous sites.

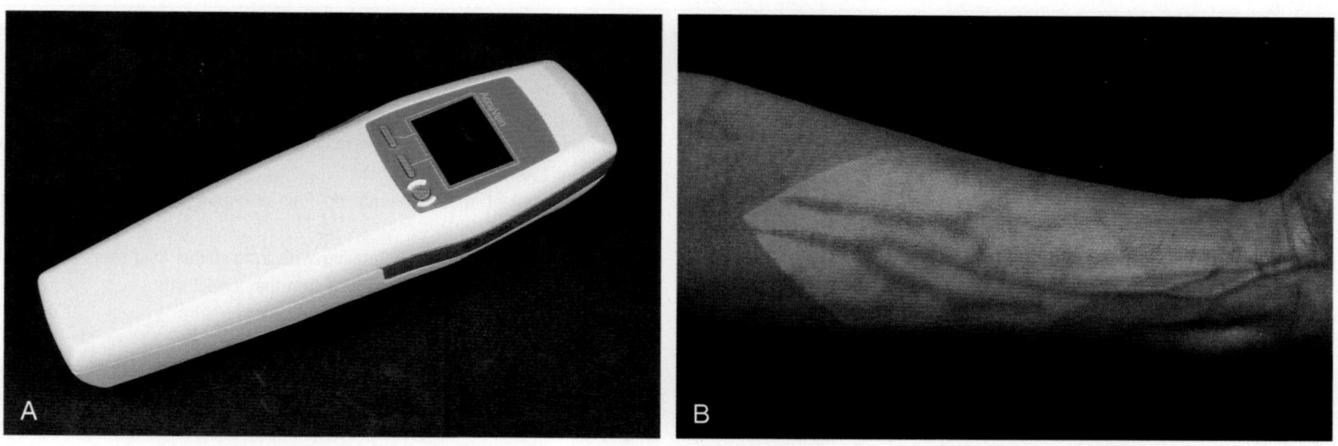

FIGURE 40-18 A, Vein finder. **B,** Veins illuminated. (Courtesy Darlaine Jantzen, RN, MA, PhD. Photo by Burl Jantzen.)

BOX 40-12 FOCUS ON OLDER PERSONS

Protection of Skin and Veins

- Use the smallest gauge cannula or needle possible (e.g., 22 to 24 gauge). Veins are very fragile, and a smaller gauge allows better blood flow to provide increased hemodilution of the intravenous fluids or medications.
- Avoid using the back of the hand for needle insertion, which may compromise the patient's need for independence and mobility.
- Impaired skin integrity may lead to susceptibility for tearing, venous sclerosis, and difficulty detecting complications.
- Avoid placement of an intravenous line in veins that are easily bumped because less subcutaneous support tissue is present.
- If the patient has fragile skin and veins, use minimal or no tourniquet pressure.
- After applying a tourniquet, venous pressure rises rapidly, the vein is overstretched, and puncture with even a thin needle can rupture the wall of the vein.
- If using a tourniquet, place it over the patient's sleeve to decrease shearing of fragile skin.
- With loss of supportive tissue, veins tend to lie more superficially; lower the insertion angle for venipuncture to 5 to 15 degrees (INS, 2016).
- If the patient has lost subcutaneous tissue, the veins lose stability and will roll away from the needle. To stabilize the vein, apply traction to the skin below the projected insertion site.
- Secure the device with a securement device for protection (Higgingson, 2015).
- Nutritional deficiencies promote fluid to migrate into tissues surrounding vessels, making intravenous access more difficult.
- Multiple medication usage (e.g., anticoagulants, antibiotics, and steroids) increases the likelihood of fragile, transparent skin that bruises and bleeds easily.
- Dehydration related to a lower percentage of body weight as water and diminished thirst mechanism contribute to difficult intravenous access.

SKILL 40-2 REGULATING INTRAVENOUS FLOW RATES

Delegation Considerations

In many provinces, regulating and monitoring intravenous therapy is included within the scope of practice for licensed and registered practical nurses. The skill of regulating intravenous therapy should not be delegated to unregulated care providers (UCPs). Refer to Skill 40-1 for important information to convey to the UCP.

Equipment

- Watch or clock with a second hand
- Paper and pencil or calculator
- Intravenous electronic infusion controller or pump (optional)
- Volume control device (optional)
- Time indicator tape for gravity infusions

PROCEDURE

STEPS	RATIONALE
1. Check patient's medical record for correct solution, additives, and time of infusion. Usual order includes solution for 24 hours, usually divided into 2 or 3 L. Occasionally, intravenous order contains only 1 L to keep vein open (KVO). Order also indicates time over which each litre is to infuse.	• Use principles of drug administration to ensure correct fluids are given to correct patient.

CRITICAL DECISION POINT: *It is common for health care providers to write an abbreviated intravenous order, such as "D5W with 20 mmol KCl 125 mL/hr continuous." This order implies that the intravenous fluid should be maintained at this rate until the order has been written for the intravenous line to be discontinued.*

STEPS	RATIONALE
2. Perform hand hygiene. Observe for patency of intravenous line and needle or catheter.	• For fluid to infuse at a proper rate, intravenous line and needle must be free of kinks, knots, and clots.
A. Open drip regulator and observe for rapid flow of fluid from solution into drip chamber and then close drip regulator to prescribed rate.	• Rapid flow of fluid into drip chamber indicates patency of intravenous line. Closing drip chamber to prescribed rate prevents fluid overload.
3. Check patient's knowledge of how positioning of the intravenous site affects flow rate.	• Fosters patient participation in maintaining most effective position of arm with intravenous equipment.
4. Verify with patient how venipuncture site feels (e.g., determine whether the patient is experiencing pain or burning sensation).	• Includes patient in decision making. Pain or burning sensation may be early indication of phlebitis.
5. Have paper and pencil or use calculator to calculate flow rate.	• The beginning student is unfamiliar with intravenous fluid rates and should use mathematical calculations to obtain the correct rate.
6. Know calibration (drop factor) in drops per millilitre (gtt/mL) of infusion set: **A. Microdrip:** 60 gtt/mL **B. Macrodrip:** 15 gtt/mL or 10 gtt/mL depending on manufacturer (will state on package)	• Microdrip tubing, also called pediatric tubing, universally delivers 60 gtt/mL and is used when small or very precise volumes are to be infused. However, different commercial parenteral administration sets for macrodrip tubing are available. Macrodrip tubing should be used when large quantities or fast rates are necessary.

STEPS	RATIONALE

CRITICAL DECISION POINT: *Know which company's infusion set your agency uses.*

STEPS	RATIONALE
7. Calculate flow rate (hourly volume) of prescribed infusion. Flow rate mL/hr = total infusion (volume in mL)/hours of infusion (time to be infused). Example: 1 000 mL/8 hr = 125 mL/1 hr	• Once hourly rate has been determined, these formulas give correct flow rate.
8. Read prescriber's orders and follow 10 rights for correct solution and proper additives.	• Intravenous fluids are medications; following 10 rights decreases chance of medication error.
9. Intravenous fluids are usually ordered by rate, such as 100 mL/hr. However, occasionally, intravenous fluids are ordered over a period of time, such as 1 000 mL D5W with 20 mmol KCl over 8 hr.	• Determines volume of fluid that should infuse hourly.
10. Place adhesive or fluid indicator tape on intravenous bottle or bag next to volume markings.	• Time taping intravenous bag gives visual cue as to whether fluids are being administered over correct period of time. Time tapes may be required for all intravenous infusions, including those on therapies infused via electronic infusion devices (EIDs). Check agency policy.

CRITICAL DECISION POINT: *Do not use felt-tipped pens or permanent markers on intravenous bags made of polyvinyl chloride because the ink could contaminate the solution (Millam & Hadaway, 2003).*

STEPS	RATIONALE
11. Select one of the following formulas to calculate minute flow rate (drops/min) on the basis of the drop factor of infusion set:	• Formulas compute correct flow rate over a minute.
A. mL/hr/60 min = mL/min and Drop factor × mL/min = drops/min	• Total volume × drop factor/infusion time in minutes. • Volume is multiplied by drop factor, and the product is divided by time (in min).
B. Alternative: mL/hr × drop factor/60 min = drops/min Using formula B above, calculate minute flow rate for bottle 1 : 1 000 mL with 20 mmol KCl *Microdrip:* 125 mL/hr × 60 gtt/mL = 7 500 gtt/hr 7 500 gtt ÷ 60 minutes = 125 gtt/min *Macrodrip:* 125 mL/hr × 15 gtt/mL = 1 875 gtt/hr 1 875 gtt ÷ 60 minutes = 31 gtt/min	• When using microdrip, mL/hr always equals gtt/min.
12. Establish flow rate by counting drops in drip chamber for 1 minute by watch; then adjust roller clamp to increase or decrease rate of infusion.	• Determines whether fluids are administered too slowly or too quickly.
13. Follow manufacturer's procedure for EIDs.	• Infusion devices are recommended for minimizing risks associated with infusion therapy.
Most pumps require the user to begin by placing the intravenous infusion tubing within ridges of control box in direction of flow (i.e., portion of tubing nearest intravenous bag at top and portion of tubing nearest patient at bottom). Required drops per minute or volume per hour and volume to be infused are selected (see Step 13 illustration). Open rate control clamp and press start button.	• Infusion pumps move fluid by compressing and milking intravenous tubing, thus propelling fluid through tubing. • Rate control clamp should be open completely while infusion controller or pump is in use.

CRITICAL DECISION POINT: *Special infusion tubing is required for some pumps (check manufacturer's directions).*

STEPS	RATIONALE
A. Monitor infusion rates and intravenous site for complications according to agency policy.	• Infusion controllers or pumps are not infallible and do not replace frequent, accurate nursing assessments. Infusion pumps may continue to infuse intravenous fluids after an infiltration has begun. All EIDs must have a free-flow protector device.
B. Assess patency and integrity of system when alarm sounds.	• Alarm indicates that electronic eye has not noted precise number of drops from drip chamber, the solution bag or bottle is empty, or flow is obstructed (e.g., kink in tubing, closed drip regulator, infiltrated or clotted needle, or air in the tubing).

Continued

SKILL 40-2 REGULATING INTRAVENOUS FLOW RATES—cont'd

STEPS	RATIONALE
14. Follow this procedure for volume control device:	
A. Place volume control device (see Step 14A illustration) between intravenous bag and insertion spike of infusion set using sterile technique.	• Reduces risk of sudden increase in fluid volume.

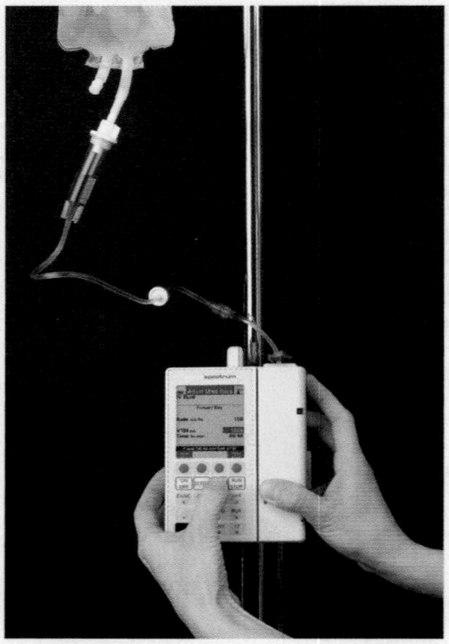

STEP 13 Program EID. (Courtesy Darlaine Jantzen, RN, MA, PhD. Photo by Burl Jantzen.)

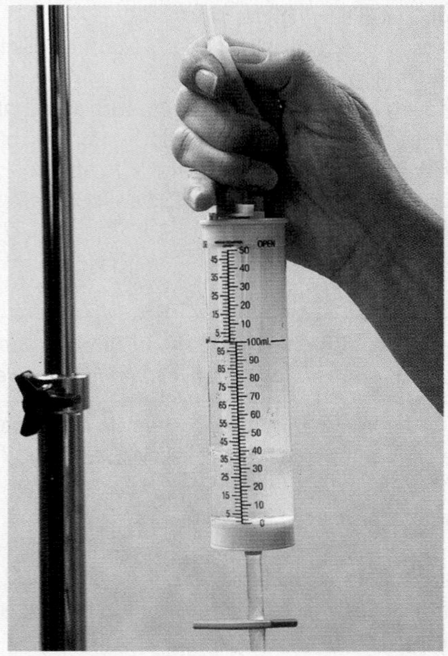

STEP 14A Volume control device. (From Perry, A. G., Potter, P. A., & Ostendorf, W. [2018]. *Clinical nursing skills and techniques* [9th ed., p. 618]. St. Louis: Mosby.)

STEPS	RATIONALE
B. Place 2 hours of fluid allotment into chamber device.	• Prevents intravenous line from running dry if nurse does not return in exactly 60 minutes. In addition, if an accidental increase in flow rate occurs, patient receives at most only a 2-hour allotment of fluid.
C. Assess system at least hourly; add fluid to volume control device. Regulate flow rate.	• Maintains patency of system.
15. Record name of solution, rate of infusion, drops/minute, and mL/hour in nurses' notes or flow sheet every 4 hours or according to patient's condition and to agency policy. Immediately record in nurses' notes or flow sheet any new intravenous fluid rates. Document use of any EID or controlling device.	• Prompt and accurate documentation informs interdisciplinary collaboration.
16. Observe patient for response to therapy. Refer to Skill 40-1, Steps 42 and 44.	• Signs and symptoms of dehydration or overhydration warrant changing rate of fluid infused.
17. Evaluate infusion site for signs of infiltration, inflammation, clot in catheter, or kink or knot in infusion tubing.	• Prevents decrease in or cessation of flow rate.

UNEXPECTED OUTCOMES	RELATED INTERVENTIONS
Sudden infusion of large volume of solution, with symptoms of dyspnea, crackles in lungs, and increased urine output, indicating fluid overload	• Slow infusion to KVO rate and notify physician immediately. New intravenous orders will be required. Patient may require diuretics.
Intravenous fluid bag runs empty, with subsequent loss of intravenous line patency	• Intravenous therapy will be restarted.
	• The intravenous infusion is slower than ordered.
	• Check patient for positional change that might affect infusion rate, height of intravenous bag, and for kinking of tubing.
	• An infiltration may be developing at intravenous site. Check condition of site.
	• If volume infused is deficient, consult physician for new order to provide necessary fluid volume.

REPORTING

- At change of shift or when leaving on break, report rate of infusion to nurse in charge or next nurse assigned to care for patient.

STEPS	RATIONALE

HOME CARE CONSIDERATIONS

- Ensure that patient is able and willing to operate the EID (if applicable) and administer intravenous therapy or that a reliable caregiver or nursing support personnel is at home to provide this intravenous therapy care.
- Teach patient and primary caregiver to time drops per minute using watch with second hand.
- Ensure proper EID function and that electrical outlets are functioning properly and grounded and infusion device has backup power, if required by type of infusate.
- Teach patient and caregiver alarms and how to troubleshoot them.
- Provide patient and caregiver with a phone number that can be accessed 24 hours a day.

Many devices have operating and programming capabilities that allow for single- and multiple-solution infusions at different rates. A variety of detectors and alarms respond to air in intravenous lines, completion of infusion, high and low pressure, low battery power, occlusion, and the inability to deliver at a preset rate.

> **Safety Alert** An anti–free-flow safeguard (preventing bolus infusion in the event of machine malfunction) is an important element of an electronic infusion device and is required. The manufacturer's recommendations for specific device features should always be checked.

Patency of the intravenous needle or catheter means that the tip of the needle or catheter has no clots and that the catheter or needle tip is not against the vein wall. A blocked catheter or needle can affect the rate of infusion of the intravenous fluids. Intravenous flow rates can also be affected by infiltration, a knot or kink in the tubing, the height of the solution, a restrictive intravenous dressing, and the position of the patient's extremity. One way to assess patency is by lowering the intravenous bag below the level of the intravenous insertion site and observing for a blood return; however, this method does not confirm patency. If no blood return occurs and fluid does not flow easily from the drip chamber when the roller clamp is opened, the nurse should assess potential causes: a clot may be occluding the cannula of the intravenous catheter, the catheter tip may be occluded against the wall of the vein, or the intravenous dressing may be too tight, thereby impeding the flow. The tubing and area around the insertion site should be inspected for anything that could obstruct the flow of intravenous fluids. A knot or kink in the tubing can decrease the flow rate. Occasionally, the tubing is kinked under a dressing; the dressing should be removed to locate the problem. The patient may also occlude the tubing by lying or sitting on it. The flow rate frequently resumes after the tubing is straightened. The height of the intravenous bag can also affect flow rates. Raising the bag usually increases the rate because of increased hydrostatic pressure.

Flexion of an extremity, particularly at the wrist or elbow, or positioning can decrease flow rates. Although VAD placement in areas of flexion is discouraged, in emergencies it may be necessary. Immobilizing with an arm board provides some protection; however, this requires vigilant assessment, and careful positioning to enable visualization and to prevent pressure. Most often it is preferred that an intravenous catheter be inserted in a new site rather than relying on a site that causes problems. However, before discontinuing the infusion hampered by an extremity position, the nurse should start the infusion in another site, to verify that the patient has other accessible veins.

Sudden increases in flow can occur accidentally. For example, a restless patient may loosen the roller clamp with a sudden movement and increase the flow rate, or the flow rate may be accidentally increased if the patient ambulates. Some intravenous catheters are positional in the patient's vein. A sudden increase in the intravenous infusion rate causes a rapid increase in vascular volume, which can make the patient critically ill or even cause death. EID and volume-control devices are designed to prevent sudden changes in infusion rate.

Maintaining the system. After the intravenous line is in place and the flow rate is regulated, the nurse must maintain the system. It is important to observe agency policy regarding maintenance of intravenous lines. Line maintenance is achieved by (1) keeping the system sterile; (2) changing solutions, tubing, and site dressings; and (3) assisting the patient with self-care activities so as not to disrupt the system.

Nurses play an important role in maintaining the integrity of both PVAD and CVAD systems to prevent infection from developing. Knowledge of potential sites for contamination informs nurses' practice (refer to Figures 40-17 and 40-18). This begins with thorough hand hygiene before and after handling any component of the intravenous system. Special training for nurses who care for patients with CVADs is the first step in preventing infections (Scales, 2011).

The integrity of the intravenous system must always be maintained. Tubing must never be disconnected because it becomes tangled or because it might be more convenient in positioning or moving a patient or applying a gown. If a patient needs more room to manoeuvre, extension tubing can be added to an intravenous line. However, the use of extension tubing should be kept to a minimum, as each connection of tubing provides an opportunity for contamination. Stopcocks for connecting more than one solution to a single intravenous site are sources of contamination and should be avoided (INS, 2016). Whenever an intravenous line is disconnected from a stopcock, the port should be plugged with a sterile cap. A port should never remain exposed to air because of the risk of contamination. A new administration set should be exchanged with the subsequent fluid change.

Intravenous tubing also contains injection ports through which adapters can be inserted for medication injections. The INS (2016) recommends intravenous tubing, when the peripheral catheter site is changed it may be used for up to 96 hours without increasing the chance of infection if it does not contain lipids, blood, or blood products. Needleless injection ports reduce the risk of needle-stick injury and reduce contamination, thereby promoting patient safety when connecting, accessing, or removing intravenous equipment (Edwards & Johnson, 2012). This risk is further minimized by using alcohol–chlorhexidine gluconate solution or povidone–iodine for cleaning the port both before and after use. Patients receiving intravenous therapy over several days will require a change of solutions. It is important to organize tasks so that this can be done in plenty of time before the solution empties and the cannula becomes clotted. Many agencies have policies regarding the "hang time" of intravenous fluids. Rickard, Vannapraseuth, McGrail, and colleagues (2009) found no need to routinely replace intravenous fluid containers and recommend further research to establish set time points for replacing intravenous fluid containers. Skill 40-3 reviews steps for changing intravenous solutions.

SKILL 40-3 MAINTENANCE OF INTRAVENOUS SYSTEM

Delegation Considerations

In many provinces, this skill is included within the scope of practice for licensed and registered practical nurses. The skill of changing intravenous solutions and tubing should not be delegated to unregulated care providers (UCPs). UCPs may be delegated the tasks of collecting supplies and assisting with comfort and safety measures. UCPs are instructed to ensure intravenous tubing is not kinked or pulled during care and ambulation. UCPs are instructed to report if intravenous solution is near empty or if there is leaking or patient experiences discomfort related to the intravenous infusion.

Equipment

Intravenous infusion

- Bottle or bag of correct type and volume of intravenous solution as ordered by physician or health care provider
- Time tape
- Infusion tubing and tubing label
- Filter (size appropriate to solution) and extension tubing (if necessary)

Intermittent Saline Lock

- Injection or disinfectant cap, loop, or short extension tubing (if necessary)
- Antiseptic swab

Normal saline flush

- Commercially available prefilled syringe filled with preservative-free normal saline (single-patient use if using multidose vial)
- Disposable gloves

Discontinuation of intravenous line

- Disposable gloves
- Sterile 2 × 2 (5 cm × 5 cm) gauze
- Tape

PROCEDURE

STEPS	RATIONALE
Changing Intravenous Solution	
1. Check prescriber's orders.	• Ensures that correct solution will be used. Intravenous therapy requires the 10 rights of medication administration.
2. If order is written for keep vein open (KVO) or to keep open (TKO), contact physician for clarification of the rate of the infusion. Note date and time when solution was last changed.	• Orders for KVO do not provide complete information and can result in fluid overload or deficit and electrolyte imbalance. A KVO order should contain a specific infusion rate (INS, 2016). Refer to agency policy. Intravenous tubing and solution should be changed at the same time.
3. Determine the compatibility of all intravenous fluids and additives by consulting appropriate literature or the pharmacy.	• Incompatibilities may lead to precipitate formation and can cause physical, chemical, and therapeutic patient changes. Precipitation may occlude patency of catheter.
4. Determine patient's understanding of need for continued intravenous therapy.	• Informs need for patient instruction.
5. Assess patency of current intravenous access site. VADs are flushed and aspirated prior to each intermittent infusion and after. VAD is locked after completed.	• If patency is occluded, a new intravenous access site may be needed. Notify physician.
6. Have next solution prepared and accessible at least 1 hour before needed. Check that solution is correct and properly labelled. Check solution expiration date and for presence of precipitate and discoloration.	• Adequate planning reduces risk of clot formation in vein caused by empty intravenous bag. Checking prevents medication error.
7. Prepare to change solution when less than 50 mL of fluid remains in bottle or bag or when a new type of solution is ordered.	• Prevents air from entering tubing and vein from clotting from lack of flow.
8. Prepare patient and family by explaining the procedure, its purpose, and what is expected of patient.	• Decreases anxiety and promotes cooperation.
9. Be sure drip chamber is at least half full.	• Provides fluid to vein while bag is changed.
10. Perform hand hygiene.	• Reduces transmission of microorganisms.
11. Prepare new solution for changing. If using plastic bag, remove protective cover from intravenous tubing port. If using glass bottle, remove metal cap and metal and rubber discs.	• Permits quick, smooth, and organized change from old to new solution.
12. Move roller clamp to stop flow rate.	• Prevents solution remaining in drip chamber from emptying while changing solutions.
13. Remove old intravenous fluid container from intravenous pole.	• Brings work to nurse's eye level.
14. Quickly remove spike from old solution bag or bottle and, without touching tip, insert spike into new bag or bottle.	• Reduces risk of solution in drip chamber running dry and maintains sterility.
CRITICAL DECISION POINT: *If spike is contaminated, a new intravenous tubing set is required.*	
15. Hang new bag or bottle of solution on intravenous pole.	• Gravity assists with delivery of fluid into drip chamber.

STEPS	RATIONALE
16. Check for air in tubing. If bubbles form, they can be removed by closing the roller clamp, stretching the tubing downward, and tapping the tubing with the finger. For larger amounts of air, swab injection port below the air with alcohol and allow to dry. Connect a syringe to this port and aspirate the air into the syringe. Reduce air in tubing by priming slowly instead of allowing a wide-open flow.	• Reduces risk of air embolus. Use of an air-eliminating filter also reduces this risk.
17. Make sure drip chamber is one-third to one-half full. If the drip chamber is too full, pinch off tubing below the drip chamber, invert the container, squeeze the drip chamber (see Step 17 illustration), hang up the bag, and release the tubing.	• Reduces risk of air entering tubing.

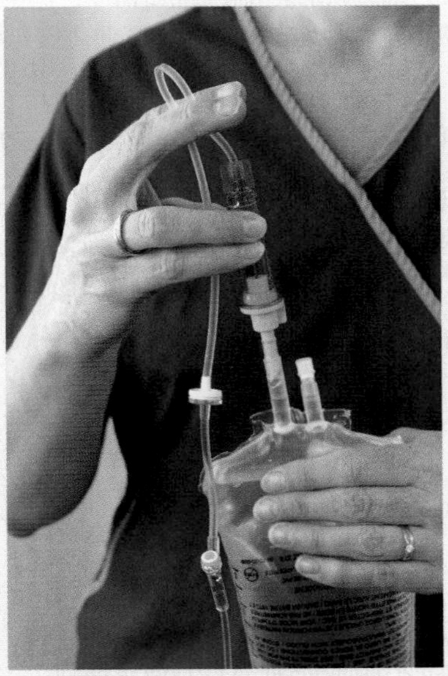

STEP 17 Pinch tubing, invert chamber, and squeeze drip chamber to remove a portion of fluid. (Courtesy Darlaine Jantzen, RN, MA, PhD. Photo by Burl Jantzen.)

STEPS	RATIONALE
18. Regulate flow to prescribed rate.	• Maintains measures to restore fluid balance and deliver intravenous fluid as ordered.
19. Mark time on label tape and place on bag. Do not use felt-tipped pens or permanent markers on intravenous bags.	• Ink from markers may leach through polyvinyl chloride containers.
20. Observe patient for signs of overhydration or dehydration to determine response to intravenous fluid therapy.	• Provides ongoing evaluation of patient's fluid and electrolyte status.
21. Observe intravenous system for patency and development of complications (e.g., infiltration or phlebitis).	• Provides ongoing evaluation of intravenous system.
Changing Intravenous Tubing	
22. Determine when new infusion set is needed:	• Note that usually the tubing and the bag, and even the site, are changed at the same time. (Refer to Steps 13–22, 33, and 34, to change bag *and* tubing.)
A. Agency policy will indicate frequency of routine change for intravenous administration sets and saline flush tubing.	• Evidence (Gillies, Wallen, Morrison, et al., 2005) recommends up to 96 hours for tubing changes.
B. Puncture of infusion tubing requires immediate change.	• Punctured tubing results in fluid leakage and bacterial contamination.
C. Contamination of tubing requires immediate change.	• Contamination of tubing allows entry of bacteria into patient's bloodstream.
D. Occlusions in existing tubing can occur after infusion of packed red blood cells, whole blood, albumin, or other blood components.	• Whole blood or blood component products can occlude or partially occlude tubing because viscous solutions adhere to walls of tubing and decrease the size of the lumen.
23. Prepare patient and family by explaining the procedure, its purpose, and what is expected of patient.	• Decreases anxiety, promotes cooperation, and prevents sudden movement of extremity, which could dislodge intravenous needle or catheter.
24. Perform hand hygiene.	• Reduces transmission of microorganisms.
25. Open new infusion set, keeping protective coverings over infusion spike and distal adapter. Secure all junctions with Luer-Locks, clasping devices, or threaded devices.	• Provides nurse with ready access to new infusion set and maintains sterility of infusion set.
26. Apply nonsterile, disposable gloves.	• Reduces risk of exposure to HIV, hepatitis, and other bloodborne pathogens.

Continued

SKILL 40-3 MAINTENANCE OF INTRAVENOUS SYSTEM—cont'd

STEPS	RATIONALE
27. If catheter hub is not visible, remove intravenous dressing while maintaining stability of catheter. If transparent dressing has to be removed, anchor catheter during disconnection.	• Hub must be accessible to provide smooth transition when removing old tubing and inserting new tubing.
28. For intravenous continuous infusion:	
A. Move roller clamp on new intravenous tubing to closed position.	• Prevents spillage of solution after bag or bottle is spiked.
B. Slow rate of infusion by regulating drip rate on old tubing. Be sure rate is at KVO rate.	• Prevents complete infusion of solution that remains in tubing, which can increase risk of occlusion of intravenous catheter or needle.
C. Compress and fill drip chamber of old tubing.	• Provides surplus of fluid in drip chamber so enough fluid is available to maintain intravenous patency while changing tubing.
D. Remove intravenous container from pole, invert container, and remove old tubing from container. Carefully hold container while hanging or taping drip chamber on intravenous pole 1 m above intravenous site.	• Fluid in drip chamber will run slowly to keep catheter patent.
E. Place insertion spike of new tubing into old solution bag opening and hang solution bag on intravenous pole.	• Permits flow of fluid from solution into new infusion tubing.
F. Compress and release drip chamber on new tubing; fill drip chamber one-third to one-half full.	• Allows drip chamber to fill and promotes rapid, smooth flow of solution through new tubing.
G. Slowly open roller clamp, remove protective cap from needle adapter (if necessary), and flush new tubing with solution. Replace cap.	• Removes air from tubing and replaces it with fluid.
H. Turn roller clamp on old tubing to closed position.	• Prevents spillage of fluid as tubing is removed from needle hub.
29. To connect to a saline lock:	
A. If a loop or short extension tubing is needed because of an awkward intravenous site placement, use sterile technique to connect the new injection cap to the loop or tubing.	
B. Swab injection cap with recommended solution for 15 seconds. Insert syringe with 1 to 3 mL saline and inject through the injection cap into the loop or short extension tubing (see Step 29B illustration). Connect tubing to injection cap.	• Removes air to prevent introduction into the vein.
30. To change (continuous or extension set) tubing at the hub, stabilize hub of catheter and apply pressure over vein just above catheter tip at least 3 cm above insertion site. Gently disconnect old tubing from catheter hub and clean cap to connect new tubing. Maintain stability of hub and quickly insert adapter of new tubing or saline lock into hub (see Step 30 illustration).	• It is important to maintain asepsis at the catheter hub. • Prevents accidental displacement of catheter or needle. • Prevents clot formation in catheter or needle and backflow of blood.

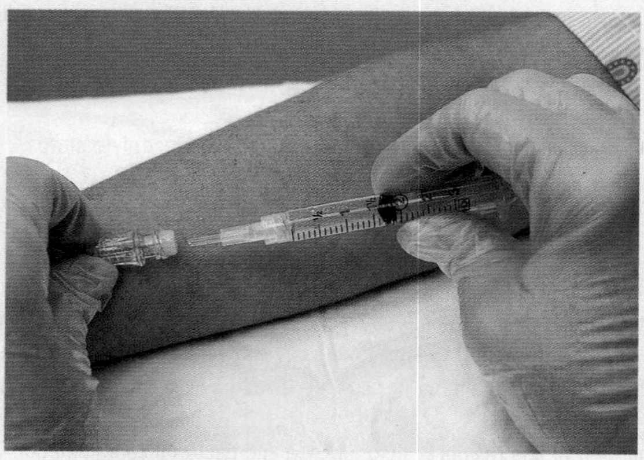

STEP 29B Inject saline into injection cap.

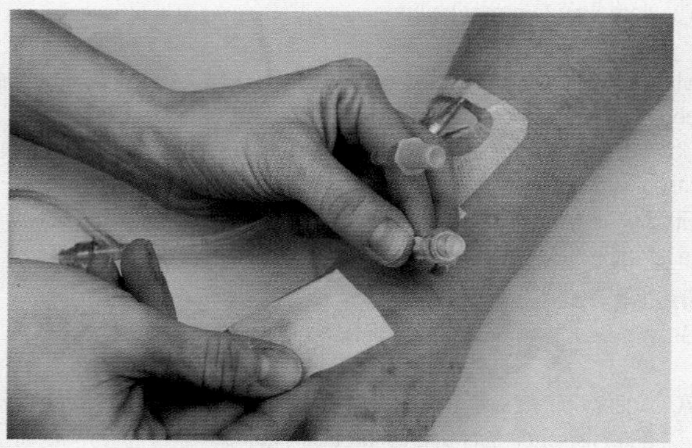

STEP 30 Clean cap to connect new tubing. (Courtesy Darlaine Jantzen, RN, MA, PhD. Photo by Burl Jantzen.)

STEPS	RATIONALE
31. Open roller clamp on new tubing. Allow solution to run rapidly for 30 to 60 seconds.	• Permits intravenous solution to enter catheter to prevent catheter occlusion.
32. Regulate intravenous drip according to prescriber's orders and monitor rate hourly.	• Maintains infusion flow at prescribed rate.
33. Apply new dressing, if needed.	• Reduces risk of bacterial infection from skin.
34. Discard old tubing in proper container.	• Reduces accidental transmission of microorganisms.
35. Remove and dispose of gloves. Perform hand hygiene.	• Reduces transmission of microorganisms.
36. Evaluate flow rate and observe connection site for leakage.	• Maintains prescribed rate of flow of intravenous fluid and determines if it is secure.

STEPS	RATIONALE
Discontinuing Peripheral Intravenous Access	
37. Check physician's order for discontinuation of intravenous therapy.	• Order is required for discontinuation of fluids or medication.
38. Explain procedure to patient. Explain that affected extremity must be held still and how long procedure will take.	• Minimizes patient's anxiety and discomfort.
39. Perform hand hygiene and apply disposable gloves.	• Reduces transmission of microorganisms.
40. Turn intravenous tubing roller clamp to closed position. Remove tape securing tubing.	
41. Remove intravenous site dressing and tape while stabilizing catheter.	• Movement of catheter will cause discomfort.
42. With dry gauze held over site, apply light pressure and withdraw the catheter, using a slow steady movement, keeping the hub parallel to the skin.	• Changing the angle of the catheter inside the vein could cause additional vein irritation, increasing the risk of postinfusion phlebitis.

CRITICAL DECISION POINT: *If patient has received anticoagulants (e.g., low-dose aspirin, warfarin sodium [Coumadin], heparin) or has a low platelet count, apply steady pressure for 5 to 10 minutes and assess bleeding.*

43. Apply pressure to the site for 2 to 3 minutes, or until no further bleeding is noted, using the dry, sterile gauze pad. Secure with tape.	• Dry pad causes less irritation to the puncture site. Subcutaneous hematoma is a common complication. When needle is removed, vein wall contracts to stop bleeding.
44. Inspect the catheter for intactness, noting tip integrity and length.	• Tips of catheter can break off, causing an embolus, an emergency situation. Notify physician if tip is broken.
45. Discard used supplies.	
46. Remove and discard gloves and perform hand hygiene.	
47. Instruct patient to report any redness, pain, drainage, or swelling that may occur after catheter removal.	• Postinfusion phlebitis may occur within 48 to 96 hours after catheter removal.

UNEXPECTED OUTCOMES	RELATED INTERVENTIONS
Incorrect flow rate; patient receives too little or too much fluid	• Readjust infusion rate to ordered rate; evaluate patient for adverse effects; notify physician.
Decreased or absent flow of intravenous fluid	• Assess intravenous infusion system for patency. • Recalibrate drip rate on new tubing. • Assess intravenous site for infiltration.

RECORDING AND REPORTING

- Record changing of tubing and solution on patient's record. A special parenteral therapy flow sheet may be used.
- Attach a piece of tape or preprinted label with the date and time of tubing change to tubing below the level of drip chamber. Labelling can ensure these items are changed at the correct intervals (Scales, 2011).

HOME CARE CONSIDERATIONS

- Emphasize to patient and family the importance of changing solutions when intravenous tubing still contains fluid.

The dressings over intravenous sites are applied to reduce the entrance of bacteria into the insertion site. The two forms of dressings are transparent and gauze. Transparent dressings reliably secure the intravenous device, allow continuous visual inspection of the intravenous site, become less easily soiled or moistened, and require less frequent changes than standard gauze. Intravenous dressings should be routinely changed as per agency policy (Skill 40-4).

To prevent the accidental disruption of an intravenous system, the nurse may need to assist the patient with hygiene, comfort measures, meals, and ambulation. Using a gown specifically made with snaps along the top sleeve seam helps facilitate changing the gown without disturbing the venipuncture site. Regular gowns are changed as follows:

1. Remove the sleeve of the gown from the arm without the intravenous line, maintaining the patient's privacy.
2. Remove the sleeve of the gown from the arm with the intravenous line.
3. Remove the intravenous solution container from its stand and pass it and the tubing through the sleeve. (If this involves removing the tubing from an intravenous electronic infusion device, use the roller clamp to slow the infusion to prevent the accidental infusion of a large volume of solution or medication.)
4. Place the intravenous solution container and tubing through the sleeve of the clean gown and hang it on its stand. (If the intravenous line is connected to an electronic infusion device, open the roller clamp. Turn on the pump.)
5. Place the arm with the intravenous line through the gown sleeve.
6. Place the arm without the intravenous line through the gown sleeve. (Breaking the integrity of an intravenous line to change a gown leads to contamination.)

SKILL 40-4 CHANGING A PERIPHERAL INTRAVENOUS DRESSING

Delegation Considerations

In many provinces, the skill of changing a peripheral intravenous dressing is included within the scope of practice for licensed and registered practical nurses. This skill should not be delegated to unregulated care providers (UCPs). UCPs may be delegated the tasks of collecting supplies, assisting with comfort measures, and distracting the patient during the procedure. UCPs are instructed to inform the nurse if the patient or UCP notes moistness on the dressing or if the dressing is no longer intact.

Equipment

- Antiseptic swab stick (chlorhexidine, povidone-iodine, or 70% alcohol, as recommended by the agency)
- Adhesive remover (if needed)
- Skin barrier
- Disposable gloves
- Sterile transparent dressing

PROCEDURE

STEPS	RATIONALE
ASSESSMENT	
1. Identify patient with two identifiers or according to agency policy. Assess site, including expiration date of dressing, dressing integrity, and cleanliness daily, or more often. Assess catheter–skin junction for signs of infection or inflammation.	• Documentation is essential for prevention of peripheral venous access catheter–related infections. • Peripheral intravenous dressings should be scheduled when intravenous system is changed; when damp, loosened, or visibly soiled; or every 5–7 days (INS, 2016, p. S82).
2. Perform hand hygiene.	• Follow principles of ANTT: Always wash hands effectively; Never contaminate key parts; Touch non-key parts with confidence; Take appropriate infective precautions (Ogston-Tuck, 2012, p. 479).
3. Observe intravenous system for proper functioning, leaking, or complications: kinks in infusion tubing or intravenous catheter. Palpate the catheter site through the intact dressing for inflammation, noting any patient complaints of pain or burning sensation.	• Moisture is a medium for bacterial growth. • Unexplained decrease in flow rate requires investigation of placement and patency of the intravenous catheter. Pain can be associated with both phlebitis and infiltration.
4. Inspect exposed catheter site for swelling or blanching and other signs of infiltration.	• Indicates fluid infusing into surrounding tissues. Will require removal of intravenous catheter.
5. Assess patient's understanding of need for continued intravenous infusion.	• Determines need for patient instruction.
PLANNING	
6. Explain procedure and purpose to patient and family. Explain that affected extremity must be held still and how long procedure will take.	• Decreases anxiety, promotes cooperation, and gives patient time frame around which personal activities can be planned.
7. Collect equipment.	• Ensures organized procedure.
8. Apply disposable gloves.	• Reduces transmission of microorganisms.
9. Remove dressing. Be cautious if catheter tubing becomes tangled or attached to dressing. When removing transparent dressing, hold catheter hub and tubing with nondominant hand.	• Prevents accidental displacement of catheter or needle. • Be aware of adhesive-related skin injury.
10. Observe insertion site for signs and symptoms of infection (redness, swelling, and exudate). If present, remove catheter and insert a new intravenous line in another site.	• Presence of infection or complication indicates need to remove vascular access device at current site.
11. If infiltration, phlebitis, or clot occurs or if ordered by prescriber, stop infusion and discontinue intravenous therapy. Restart new intravenous line if continued therapy is necessary. Place moist, warm compress over area of phlebitis.	
12. If intravenous fluid is infusing properly, gently remove any tape securing catheter. Stabilize needle or catheter with one hand. Use adhesive remover to clean skin and remove adhesive residue, if needed.	• Exposes venipuncture site. Stabilization prevents accidental displacement of catheter or needle. Adhesive residue decreases ability of new dressing to adhere tightly to skin.
13. Stabilize catheter at all times with one finger over catheter until tape or dressing is replaced.	• Prevents decannulation from vein.

STEPS	RATIONALE
14. Using circular motion, clean peripheral intravenous insertion site with antiseptic swab starting at insertion site and working outward, creating concentric circles (see Step 14 illustration). Allow swab solution to air-dry completely.	• Circular motion prevents cross-contamination from skin bacteria near venipuncture site. Antiseptics may include chlorhexidine, povidone-iodine, and alcohol. If antiseptic agents are used in combination, allow each to dry separately.

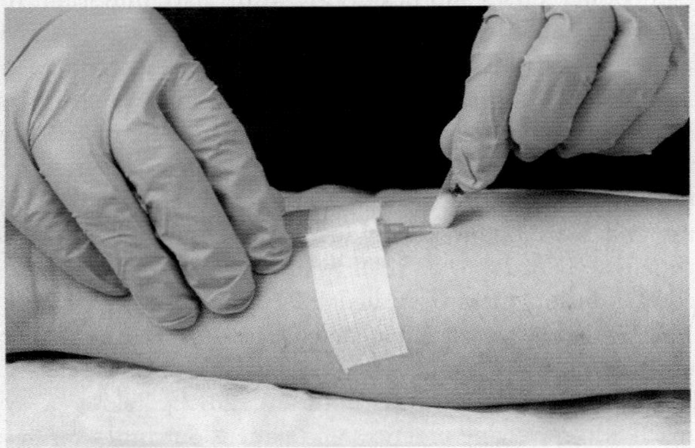

STEP 14 Clean peripheral insertion site.

CRITICAL DECISION POINT: *Do not tape over connection of access tubing or port to intravenous catheter.*

STEPS	RATIONALE
15. Apply new transparent dressing (see Skill 40-1, Step 38A).	• Ensures protection of intravenous site and reduces chance of infection.
16. Remove and discard gloves.	
17. Anchor intravenous tubing with additional pieces of tape. When using transparent polyurethane dressing, minimize the tape placed over dressing.	• Prevents accidental displacement of intravenous needle or catheter or separation of intravenous tubing from needle adapter.
18. Place insertion date, date and time of dressing change, size and gauge of catheter, and your initials directly on dressing.	• Documents dressing change.
19. Discard used equipment and perform hand hygiene.	• Reduces transmission of microorganisms.
20. Observe functioning and patency of intravenous system in response to changing dressing.	• Validates that intravenous line is patent and functioning correctly.
21. Monitor patient's body temperature.	• Elevated temperature indicates an infection that may be associated with bacterial contamination of the venipuncture site.

UNEXPECTED OUTCOMES	RELATED INTERVENTIONS
Infiltration of intravenous catheter, as evidenced by decreased flow rate or edema, pallor, or decreased temperature around insertion site	• Stop infusion and discontinue intravenous therapy. Restart new intravenous line in other extremity if continued therapy is necessary. • Elevate affected extremity.
Accidental removal of intravenous catheter or needle	• Restart intravenous infusion if continued therapy is needed.
Elevated body temperature	• Notify physician. Intravenous line may be removed and restarted. Patient will be evaluated for source of infection.
Red, edematous, or painful insertion site or presence of exudates, indicating infection at venipuncture site	• Discontinue intravenous infusion. Antibiotic therapy may begin. • Apply warm, moist compress to area of inflammation.

RECORDING AND REPORTING

- Record appearance of intravenous site, type of dressing, and status of intravenous fluid infusion.
- A special parenteral fluid flow sheet may be used for recording.

Protective devices designed to prevent accidental dislodgement of an intravenous catheter (Figure 40-19) are now available. The device fits comfortably around a patient's hand or arm and provides a plastic shield to cover the intravenous device. Protective devices extend the time a catheter remains in the vein and minimize repeated venipuncture.

The patient with an arm or a hand infusion is able to walk, unless contraindicated. A portable intravenous pole (a standard intravenous pole with wheels) is needed. Help the patient get out of bed and place the pole next to the involved arm. The patient should be instructed to hold on to the pole and push it while walking. The nurse needs to assess the equipment to make sure that the intravenous bag is at the proper height, the tubing is not tense, the flow rate is correct, and the tubing does not get contaminated. The patient should be instructed to report any blood in the tubing, a stoppage in the flow, or increased discomfort. Intravenous medications, especially antibiotics and potassium,

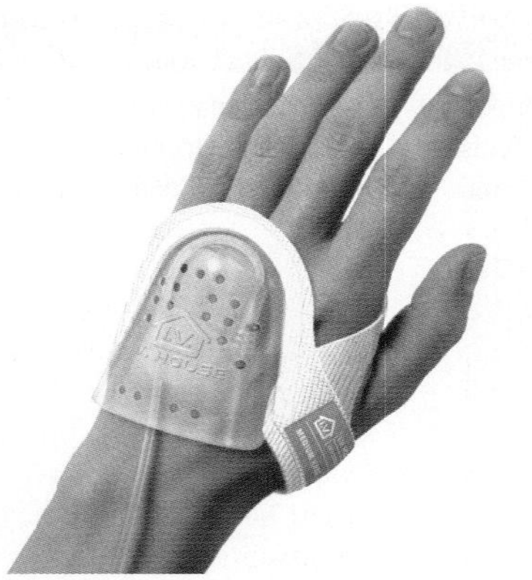

FIGURE 40-19 IV House protective device. (Courtesy IV House, St. Louis, MO.)

can cause discomfort and burning sensations at the intravenous site. Although discomfort may be relieved by repositioning the extremity, the source of discomfort must always be carefully evaluated and may necessitate starting a new intravenous line in a larger vein.

Complications of intravenous therapy. An infiltration occurs when intravenous fluids enter the surrounding space around the venipuncture site (see Table 40-11). This manifests as swelling (from increased tissue fluid) and pallor and coolness (caused by decreased circulation) around the venipuncture site. Fluid may be flowing through the intravenous line at a decreased rate or may have stopped flowing. Pain may also be present and usually results from edema. This pain increases proportionately as the infiltration continues.

When infiltration occurs, the infusion must be discontinued, and if intravenous therapy is still necessary, a new catheter is inserted into a vein in another extremity. To reduce discomfort and edema, the extremity should be raised, which promotes venous drainage. Wrapping the extremity in a warm, moist towel for 20 minutes while keeping it elevated on a pillow also promotes venous return, increases circulation, and reduces pain and edema. This can be repeated three to four times per day until resolved. Infiltration of medications that cause extravasation require specific care, outlined by institutional policy.

Phlebitis is inflammation of the vein. Selected risk factors for phlebitis include the type of catheter material, chemical irritation of additives and drugs given intravenously (e.g., antibiotics), the rate of the medication administration, the skill of the individual inserting the catheter, and the anatomical position of the catheter. Signs and symptoms may include pain, edema, erythema, increased skin temperature over the vein, and, in some instances, redness travelling along the path of the vein (INS, 2016). Dehydration may also be a contributing factor because of the increase in blood viscosity.

When phlebitis develops, the intravenous line must be discontinued and a new line inserted in another vein. Warm, moist heat on the site of phlebitis can offer some relief to the patient. Phlebitis can be dangerous because blood clots (thrombophlebitis) can occur and, in some cases, may result in emboli. Such conditions can result in permanent damage to veins and in prolonging the patient's hospitalization.

Bleeding can occur around the venipuncture site during the infusion or through the catheter needle or tubing if these become inadvertently disconnected. Bleeding is common in patients who have received heparin or who have a bleeding disorder (e.g., leukemia or thrombocytopenia). If bleeding occurs around the venipuncture site and the catheter is within the vein, a pressure dressing may be applied over the site to control the bleeding. Bleeding from a vein is usually a slow, continuous seepage and is not serious.

Discontinuing intravenous infusions. Discontinuing an infusion is necessary after the prescribed amount of fluid has been infused, when an infiltration occurs, if phlebitis is present, or if the infusion catheter or needle develops a clot at its tip. Refer to Skill 40-3 for discontinuing an intravenous infusion.

Safety and Quality Improvement. As stated throughout this text, individual nurses and health care teams have important roles in ensuring patient safety and quality improvement. For individuals administering infusion therapy, competency assessment should include psychomotor skills, such as those outlined in this chapter, as well as application of knowledge, decision making, and ethical practice. Nurses contribute to quality improvement through using standardized documentation, fostering a culture of care, demonstrating accountability, and assisting in identifying clinical quality indicators and benchmarks (INS, 2016, p. S21). Evaluating and reporting the incidence of infusion therapy–related infections is one very important example. Some nurses participate in collecting data from standardized documentation and then analyzing patient outcomes or safety for the health care team (Edwards & Johnson, 2012). Taking a systems approach and reviewing practices and patient outcomes can result in rapid implementation of changes (Coram, 2015).

In the quality and safety literature, a common approach to prevention of infection is ANTT: *A*lways wash hands effectively; *N*ever contaminate key parts; *T*ouch non-key parts with confidence; *T*ake appropriate infective precautions (Ogston-Tuck, 2012, p. 479). Bloodstream infections in both peripheral and central intravenous lines have been significantly reduced by using a disinfection cap, as a way of addressing noncompliance and variation in techniques of disinfecting the hubs of needleless connectors (DeVries, Mancos, & Valentine, 2014).

Blood Transfusion. Blood replacement or transfusion, or blood component therapy, is the intravenous administration of whole blood or a component, such as plasma, packed red blood cells (RBCs), platelets, or cryoprecipitate. Other blood products, manufactured from human plasma, include albumin (5% or 25%), intravenous immune globulin (IVIG), Rh immune globulin (RHIG), and prothrombin complex concentrate (PCC). The primary objectives for blood transfusions include the following: (1) to increase circulating blood volume after surgery, trauma, or hemorrhage; (2) to increase the number of RBCs and to maintain hemoglobin levels in patients with severe anemia; and (3) to provide selected cellular components as replacement therapy (e.g., clotting factors, platelets, albumin). Caring for patients receiving blood or blood products is a significant nursing responsibility. Thorough assessment, meticulous identification of the patient and transfusion, and careful monitoring is critical, as error could lead to dangerous and life-threatening events.

Blood Groups and Types. The most important grouping for transfusion purposes is the ABO system, which includes A, B, O, and AB blood types. The determination of blood groups is based on the presence or absence of A and B RBC antigens. Individuals with A antigens, B antigens, or no antigens belong to groups A, B, and O, respectively. The person with A and B antigens has AB blood. Individuals with type A blood naturally produce anti-B antibodies in their plasma. Similarly, individuals with type B blood naturally produce anti-A antibodies. An individual with type O blood has neither type A nor type B antigen and thus is considered a universal blood donor. Individuals with type AB blood produce neither antibody, which is why they can be universal recipients and receive any type of blood (Table 40-12). Rhesus, or Rh, factor is the second important consideration in blood typing. The Rh factor is an antigenic substance in the erythrocytes. A person with the factor is Rh positive, and a person without it is Rh negative. Blood must be matched for Rh factor as well as ABO grouping. Rh-negative people must receive only Rh-negative blood, whereas Rh-positive people can receive either Rh-negative or Rh-positive blood.

If incompatible or mismatched blood is transfused, a transfusion reactions occurs. The patient's, or recipient's, antibodies trigger RBC destruction. This response ranges from a mild response (e.g., faintness, dizziness) to severe anaphylactic shock or acute intravascular hemolysis, both of which can be life-threatening. Prompt intervention is required, including immediately stopping the transfusion, removing the tubing, and replacing the line with a normal saline infusion to maintain intravenous access.

Autologous Transfusion. Autologous transfusion, or autotransfusion, is the collection of a patient's own blood. The blood for an autologous transfusion can be obtained by preoperative donation up to 5 weeks before the planned surgery (e.g., heart, orthopedic, plastic, or gynecological). Patients can donate several units of their own blood, depending on the type of surgery and the ability of the patient to maintain an acceptable hematocrit. Another way to collect blood for an autologous transfusion is during perioperative blood salvage (e.g., during vascular and orthopedic surgery, organ transplant surgery, and traumatic injuries). The blood that has been salvaged is then reinfused during the surgery. Blood can also be salvaged postoperatively from mediastinal and chest tube drainage and after joint and spinal surgery. Autologous transfusions decrease the risk of complications such as mismatched blood and exposure to bloodborne infectious agents (Alexander, Corrigan, Gorski, et al., 2014).

Blood Transfusions. When transfusing blood or blood components, assessment is required before, during, and after the transfusion and for regulation of the transfusion, because of the risk of reactions and complications. Prior to transfusion the primary health care provider must obtain consent for transfusion, except in emergencies. The nurse then verifies that consent has been obtained, that it is current, and that the patient understands the reason for the blood transfusion. Patients with certain cultural backgrounds may abstain from blood transfusions (Box 40-13). The nurse should ask the patient if he or she has had a previous transfusion or a transfusion reaction. Before giving a transfusion, the nurse needs to explain the procedure and instruct the patient to report any side effects (e.g., chills, dizziness, or fever) once the transfusion begins. The nurse checks that the patient is properly identified, based on agency policy. This is critical to ensure that the patient is given the correct blood component, based on blood typing. Certain diagnostic tests are used to determine the need for blood component and the effectiveness of treatment, such as hemoglobin, platelet count, or tests related to clotting.

Infusion of blood components or blood products requires an order from the primary health care provider. The nurse checks patient identification, component or product to be administered, the amount or volume, the rate of administration, and any other requirements, such as premedication (e.g., intravenous diuretic). If the patient has an intravenous line in place, the nurse needs to assess the venipuncture site and determine the appropriate gauge of the intravenous catheter. A large catheter, such as 18 to 22 gauge, is recommended for adults unless rapid infusion is required (16–18 gauge). Blood administration tubing with a 70- to 260-micron filter is used, and the nurse needs to determine if the tubing is appropriate for the EID when using one. When priming blood administration tubing, 0.9% normal saline must be used to prevent hemolysis, or breakdown of RBCs. Timing of blood transfusion is extremely important. The infusion is begun within 30 minutes of accessing the blood component from the transfusion medical laboratory (TML) and is stopped after 4 hours. Bags and tubing are discarded in the biohazardous waste, according to agency policy.

Because of the danger of transfusion reactions, it is very important to use specific precautions and the ten rights of medication administration (see Chapter 34) in administering blood or blood products.

TABLE 40-12 ABO Compatibilities for Transfusion Therapy

Component	Compatibilities	
Whole Blood	**Give Type-Specific Blood Only**	
Packed red cells (stored, washed, or frozen/washed)	***Donor***	***Recipient***
	O	O, A, B, AB
	A	A, AB
	B	B, AB
	AB	AB
Fresh-frozen plasma	***Donor***	***Recipient***
	O	O
	A	A, O
	B	B, O
	AB	AB, B, A, O
Platelets	RBC: ABO and Rh compatible *preferred*	
	Donor	***Recipient***
	O	O, A, B, AB
	A	A, AB
	B	B, AB
	AB	AB

ABO, Blood group consisting of groups A, AB, B, and O.
Data from Alexander, M., Corrigan, A. M., Gorski, L. A., et al. (2014). *Core curriculum for infusion nursing* (4th ed.). Philadelphia: Lippincott.

BOX 40-13 CULTURAL ASPECTS OF CARE

Preinfusion Assessments

When a patient's natural skin contains more melanin, it becomes more difficult to identify colour changes. Intravenous complications such as phlebitis and infiltration may not be easily detected. Patients from some cultural backgrounds experience fear related to the donor process for blood. Patients with certain religious (e.g., Jehovah's Witness) or personal beliefs may abstain from receiving blood transfusions or medications.

Implications for Practice

- Establish communication. Understand the values of family elders and know whom to speak with about intravenous procedures.
- Assess patients individually to determine their acceptance of or abstinence from therapeutic regimens.
- Appreciate patients' choice related to their therapy.
- Although some patients will abstain from receiving whole blood or packed red blood cells, they will accept other blood products or alternatives.

Adapted from Rudnicke, C. (2003). Transfusion alternatives. *Journal of Infusion Nursing, 26*(3), 29.

The nurse should first obtain the patient's baseline vital signs (temperature, blood pressure, pulse, respirations, and oxygen saturation) before the transfusion begins. This allows the nurse to determine when changes in vital signs occur, which can indicate that a transfusion reaction is developing. A thorough check of the blood product, the patient, the reason for the transfusion, the volume or dose, the rate, and site ensures safe administration and that the patient is receiving the correct type of blood component or product. The rate of transfusion is usually specified in the health care provider's orders. Although the nurse is not involved in the blood labelling process, he or she is responsible for determining that the blood delivered to the patient corresponds to the blood type listed in the patient's medical record. Two registered nurses or one registered nurse and a licensed practical nurse (see agency policy) must together check the label on the blood product against the patient's identification number, blood group, and complete name. If even a minor discrepancy exists, the blood should not be given and the TML should be notified immediately. The nurse documents vital signs, time, and transfusion details on initiation, and throughout the transfusion, as the seventh right. On completion of the transfusion, the eighth right involves monitoring and documenting the patient response.

Initiation of a transfusion begins slowly, to allow for the early detection of a transfusion reaction. The nurse needs to maintain the infusion rate, monitor for side effects, assess vital signs, and promptly record all findings. The nurse continues to monitor the patient and obtain vital signs periodically during the transfusion, as directed by agency policy. The nurse should observe for hives, fever or rigors, dyspnea, cough, or back or infusion site pain and note patient complaints of unusual feelings. Upon completion, the administration tubing used for RBCs should be discarded at 4 hours or after two units; it should be discarded immediately following infusion of blood products, such as IVIG, clotting factors, and albumin. If blood components or products are contraindicated, plasma expanders may be required in cases of sudden or extreme hypovolemia.

Transfusion Reactions and Complications. Noninfectious complications from transfusions are generally more common than infectious complications. Noninfectious complications such as allergic reactions (minor to severe), hemolytic transfusion reactions, and ABO transfusion reactions are a systemic response by the body to incompatible blood or blood component (e.g., white blood cells from donor blood). Causes may also include allergic sensitivity to the potassium or citrate preservative in the blood. Several types of acute reactions can result from blood transfusions (Table 40-13). Transfusion-related acute lung injury is the most serious transfusion reaction and requires critical care. If a transfusion reaction is anticipated or suspected, vital signs must be monitored more frequently (see Table 40-13).

A second category of transfusion reactions, infectious complications, includes diseases transmitted by infected blood donors who are asymptomatic. Because all units of blood collected must undergo serological testing and screening for human immunodeficiency virus (HIV) and hepatitis B virus, the risk of acquiring bloodborne infections from blood transfusions is reduced. Bacterial sepsis is more common in platelets.

Circulatory overload, or TACO, is a risk when a patient receives large volumes of whole blood or packed RBC transfusions for massive hemorrhagic shock or when a patient with normal blood volume receives blood. Patients particularly at risk for circulatory overload are older persons and those with cardiopulmonary diseases.

> **Safety Alert** If a blood reaction is suspected, stop the transfusion immediately.

Blood transfusion reactions are life-threatening, but prompt nursing intervention can maintain the patient's physiological stability.

- Keep the intravenous line open by hanging 0.9% normal saline directly into the intravenous line and running the saline.
- Do not turn off the blood and simply turn on the 0.9% normal saline that is connected to the Y-tubing infusion set. This would cause blood remaining in the Y-tubing to infuse into the patient. Even a small amount of mismatched blood can cause a major reaction.
- Notify the primary health care provider immediately.
- Remain with the patient, observing signs and symptoms and monitoring vital signs as often as every 5 minutes.
- Prepare to administer emergency drugs such as antihistamines, vasopressors, fluids, and steroids as per physician order or protocol.
- Prepare to perform cardiopulmonary resuscitation.
- Obtain a urine specimen and send it to the laboratory to determine the presence of hemoglobin as a result of RBC hemolysis.
- Save the blood container, tubing, attached labels, and transfusion record, and return them to the laboratory.

Restorative Care

After experiencing acute alterations in fluid, electrolyte, or acid–base balance, patients often require ongoing maintenance to prevent a recurrence of health alterations. Older persons and chronically ill patients require special considerations to prevent complications from developing.

Home Intravenous Therapy. Intravenous therapy is often continued in the home setting for patients who are discharged from the hospital and have not completed their prescribed treatment or who require long-term therapy. Ideally, a family member will be available at home if the patient suddenly cannot manage the intravenous system or if a problem develops. A home care nurse will work closely with the patient and family to ensure that a sterile intravenous system is maintained and that complications are avoided or recognized promptly. Refer to Box 40-8 for a summary of patient education guidelines for home intravenous therapy.

Nutritional Support. Most patients who have had electrolyte disorders or metabolic acid–base disturbances require ongoing nutritional support. Depending on the type of disorder, fluid or food intake may be encouraged or restricted (see Chapter 42). If patients are still responsible for meal preparation, they should learn to understand the nutritional content of foods and to read the labels of commercially prepared foods.

Medication Safety. Numerous medications and over-the-counter drugs contain components or create potential adverse effects that can alter fluid and electrolyte balances. Patients with chronic disease who are receiving multiple medications and those with renal or liver disorders are at significant risk for alterations in fluid and electrolyte status (Box 40-14). Once patients return to a restorative care setting, whether in their home or in a residential care home, drug safety becomes very important. Patient and family education is essential to providing information regarding potential drug interactions and what adverse effects they can cause. It is important to review all medications with patients and encourage them to consult with their local pharmacist, especially if they try a new over-the-counter medication.

◆ Evaluation

Patient Expectations. Nurses routinely review with patients how well their concerns and expectations regarding fluid, electrolyte, or acid-base status have been addressed. Asking questions directed at

TABLE 40-13 Acute Adverse Effects of Transfusions

Adverse Effect	Cause	Clinical Manifestations	Management	Prevention
Transfusion Reactions—Caused by Immune Response to Blood Components				
Acute intravascular hemolytic	Infusion of ABO-incompatible whole blood, RBCs, or components containing 10 mL or more of RBCs Antibodies in recipient's plasma attach to antigens on transfused RBCs, causing RBC destruction	Chills, fever, low back pain, flushing, tachycardia, tachypnea, hypotension, hemoglobinuria, hemoglobinemia, sudden oliguria (acute kidney injury), circulatory shock, cardiac arrest, death	Stop transfusion and save blood bag and administration set for follow-up. Keep IV site open with normal saline infused through new tubing. Maintain BP and treat shock as ordered, if present. Obtain blood samples *slowly* to avoid hemolysis; send for serological testing. Send urine specimen to laboratory. Give diuretics as prescribed to maintain urine flow. Insert in-dwelling urinary catheter or measure each voiding to monitor hourly urine output. Dialysis may be required if acute kidney injury occurs. ***Patient safety alert:*** Do not transfuse additional RBC-containing components until transfusion service provides newly cross-matched units.	Meticulously verify and document patient identification from sample collection to component infusion.
Febrile nonhemolytic (most common)	Antibodies against donor white blood cells	Sudden shaking chills (rigors), fever (rise in temperature 0.5°C [1°F] or more from start), headache, flushing, anxiety, muscle pain	Stop transfusion. Give antipyretics as prescribed; avoid aspirin in thrombocytopenic patients. ***Patient safety alert:*** Do not restart transfusion.	Consider leukocyte-poor blood products (filtered, washed, or frozen). Pretreat with antipyretics if prior history.
Mild allergic	Antibodies against donor plasma proteins	Flushing, itching, urticaria (hives)	Stop transfusion temporarily. Give antihistamine as directed. If symptoms are mild and transient, restart transfusion slowly. ***Patient safety alert:*** Do not restart transfusion if fever, pulmonary symptoms, or hypotension develops.	Treat prophylactically with antihistamines.
Anaphylactic	Antibodies to donor plasma, especially anti-IgA	Anxiety, urticaria, dyspnea, wheezing progressing to cyanosis, severe hypotension, circulatory shock, possible cardiac arrest	Stop transfusion. Have epinephrine ready for injection (0.4 mL of 1 : 1 000 solution subcutaneously or 0.1 mL of 1 : 1 000 solution diluted to 10 mL with saline for IV use). Provide blood pressure support as ordered. Initiate CPR if indicated. ***Patient safety alert:*** Do not restart transfusion.	Transfuse extensively washed RBC products from which all plasma has been removed. Alternately use blood from IgA-deficient donor.
Other Acute Adverse Effects				
Circulatory overload	Blood administered faster than circulation can accommodate	*Dyspnea,* cough, crackles, or rales in dependent lobes of lungs; distended neck veins when upright	Turn down transfusion rate or stop transfusion. Place patient upright with feet in dependent position. Administer prescribed diuretics, oxygen, morphine. Phlebotomy may be indicated.	Adjust transfusion volume and flow rate on basis of patient size and clinical status. Have transfusion service divide unit into smaller aliquots for better spacing of fluid input.
Sepsis	Bacterial contamination of transfused blood components	Rapid onset of chills, high fever, severe hypotension, and circulatory shock *May occur:* Vomiting, diarrhea, sudden oliguria (acute kidney injury), disseminated intravascular coagulation (DIC)	Stop transfusion. Obtain culture of patient's blood and send bag with remaining blood to transfusion service for further study. Treat as ordered: antibiotics, IV fluids, vasopressors, glucocorticoids.	Collect, process, store, and transfuse blood products according to blood-banking standards and infuse within 4 hours of starting time.

ABO, Blood group consisting of groups A, AB, B, and O; *BP,* blood pressure; *CPR,* cardiopulmonary resuscitation; *IgA,* immunoglobulin A; *IV,* intravenous; *RBC,* red blood cell.

Data from Alexander, Corrigan, A. M., Gorski, L. A., et al. (2014). *Core curriculum for infusion nursing* (4th ed.). Philadelphia: Lippincott.

BOX 40-14 RESEARCH HIGHLIGHT

Managing Chronic Kidney Disease

Research Focus

Prevention of complications associated with chronic kidney disease requires attention to many biochemical parameters. In nurse-run clinics, nurses, with the guidance of physicians, are able to successfully manage these parameters through patient-centred care, health promotion, teaching, dealing with problems, taking time, use of protocols, consultations or referrals, logistics, paperwork or documentation, and nurse–physician collaboration.

Research Abstract

The purpose of the study conducted by Molzahn, Pelletier Hibbert, Gaudet, and colleagues (2008) was to describe the nature of the care provided to people with chronic kidney disease in a larger study of nurse-run, physician-monitored clinics and to describe how patients, nurses, and nephrologists described their experience with the clinics. Seven nurses, five physicians, and 22 patients participated in interviews, which were tape-recorded and transcribed. In addition to interviews, data collection involved review of 40 randomly selected charts. Themes identified related to the characteristics of the nurse, patient-centred care, health promotion, teaching, dealing with problems, time, protocols, consultations or referrals, logistics, paperwork or documentation, and nurse–physician collaboration. Challenges and outcomes were also described as part of the experience with the clinic. Patients were actively engaged in self-management and reported high levels of satisfaction with care, as well as improvements in selected outcomes. Overall, the perceptions about this model of care were positive, and the approach warrants further exploration.

Evidence-Informed Practice and Primary Health Care

- Regular assessment and management by nurses can be used to prevent cardiovascular disease and other complications of chronic kidney disease.
- Patient-centred care, teaching, and health promotion are important processes in caring for the patient with chronic kidney disease.
- Many people with chronic kidney disease are able and willing to self-manage their illness.

Molzahn, A. E., Pelletier Hibbert, M., Gaudet, D., Starzomski, R., Barrett, B., & Morgan, J. (2008). Managing chronic kidney disease in a nurse-run, physician-monitored clinic: The CanPREVENT experience. *Canadian Journal of Nursing Research, 40,* 96–112.

presenting signs and symptoms and at anticipated responses to interventions is important to the nursing process. If the patient's concerns involve having a better understanding of a chronic problem, the nurse needs to focus the evaluation on health education provided. Often the patient's level of satisfaction with care also depends on the nurse's success in involving family and friends. If the patient has concerns about returning home or to a different care setting, it will be important to evaluate if the patient feels prepared for the transition from acute care.

Patient Outcomes. The evaluation of a patient's clinical status is especially important if an acute fluid and electrolyte or acid–base imbalance exists. In some situations, the patient's condition can change very quickly, and the nurse must be able to recognize the signs and symptoms of impending problems by being aware of health alterations, the effects of medications and fluids, and the patient's presenting clinical status (see Figure 40-8). It is particularly important to evaluate the effectiveness of the interdisciplinary team interventions, review diagnoses, report outcomes, and remain open to revising the plan of care. This evaluation should include risk factors, clinical status, laboratory findings, and underlying or contributing problems.

The nurse needs to determine whether changes have occurred from the last patient assessment and analyze such changes. For example, have the physical signs and symptoms of the assessed condition begun to disappear or lessen in intensity? A patient's response to treatment of hypokalemia would be evidenced by an increasing serum potassium and a reduction in physical symptoms associated with hypokalemia.

For patients with less acute alterations, evaluation likely occurs over a longer period of time. In this situation, the nurse's evaluation may be focused more on behavioural changes (e.g., the patient's ability to follow dietary restrictions and medication schedules). The family's ability to anticipate alterations and prevent problems from recurring may also be an important element of the evaluation.

The patient's level of progress determines whether the nurse needs to continue or revise the care plan. If goals are not met, the nurse may need to consult with others on the interdisciplinary team to discuss additional methods, such as increasing the frequency of an intervention (e.g., provide more fluids to a dehydrated patient), introducing a new therapy (e.g., initiate insertion of an intravenous line), or discontinuing a particular therapy. Once outcomes have been met, the nurse can resolve the nursing diagnosis and focus on other priorities.

KEY CONCEPTS

- Body fluids are distributed in ECF and ICF compartments.
- A dynamic interplay of fluid and electrolyte intake and absorption, distribution, hormonal control, and output determines fluid and electrolyte balance.
- Volume disturbances include isotonic and osmolar deficits and excesses.
- Acid–base imbalances are buffered by chemical, biological, and physiological buffering, especially the lungs and kidneys.
- Chronic and serious illnesses increase the risk of fluid, electrolyte, and acid–base imbalances.
- Patients who are very young or very old are at greater risk for fluid, electrolyte, and acid–base imbalances.
- Assessment for fluid, electrolyte, and acid–base alterations includes the nursing health history, physical and behavioural assessments, measurements of intake and output, daily weights, and specific laboratory data.
- Osmolar imbalances and extracellular fluid volume (ECV) deficit can be corrected by enteral or parenteral administration of fluid.
- Common complications of intravenous therapy are infiltration, phlebitis, infection, ECF excess, and bleeding at the infusion site.
- Blood transfusions are given to replace fluid volume loss from hemorrhage, treat anemia, or replace coagulation factors.
- Blood transfusions can be obtained from a donor, autologously, or through perioperative salvage.
- Administration of blood or blood products requires the nurse to follow a specific procedure in order to prevent and identify transfusion reactions quickly.
- In addition to transfusion reactions, the risks of transfusion include hyperkalemia, hypocalcemia, hypervolemia or circulatory overload, and infection.
- Treatment for electrolyte disturbances includes dietary and pharmacological interventions.

- The body's chemical buffering system responds first to acid–base abnormalities.
- The goals of therapy for acid–base imbalances are to treat the underlying illness and to restore the arterial blood pH to normal.
- With new technology emerging continually, nurses need to stay current on evidence to inform practice, particularly in relation to VADs.

CRITICAL THINKING EXERCISES

1. Mrs. Emanuele is an 81-year-old woman admitted to the hospital with a 3-day history of vomiting and diarrhea. She has had only ice chips since the first episode of vomiting and is now complaining of malaise, cramping muscles, and a temperature of 39°C. Which laboratory findings would you expect to be abnormal on the basis of her complaints? What interventions would you expect the physician to order?
2. Caroline, a nurse, has just received a new patient on her unit who is to receive one unit of RBCs within the next hour. What nursing actions are necessary before administering blood? Can Caroline delegate the administration of blood to a licensed practical nurse or an unregulated care provider?
3. Carlos is caring for Mr. Rossi, a 52-year-old man who has been seen in the emergency department following a motor vehicle accident. Mr. Rossi is complaining of difficulty breathing and has a respiratory rate of 40 breaths per minute. He is transferred to the Critical Care Unit, intubated, and placed on a ventilator. A nursing student asks Carlos to interpret Mr. Rossi's last ABG results: pH = 7.30; PaO_2 = 70; $Paco_2$ = 50; bicarbonate = 24 mmol/L. What interpretation will Carlos give to the student nurse? What is the relationship between the ABG results and Mr. Rossi being intubated and ventilated?
4. Janelle is the nurse caring for Mrs. Kwan, a 59-year-old woman who has just had a total knee replacement. The physician has ordered cefazolin (Ancef) 1 g in 50 mL to run over 30 minutes intravenous three times daily. Mrs. Kwan has a continuous infusion of Ringer's lactate at 75 mL/hour in the left forearm. What type of tubing will Janelle use to administer the intravenous medication? Calculate the drops per minute for both microdriptubing (60 drops/mL) and macrodriptubing (15 drops/mL).
5. Mrs. Yoe is on a surgical unit following a total abdominal hysterectomy. She experienced postoperative bleeding and requires blood products; however, for religious and cultural reasons, she has refused blood products. What are the key principles in providing care for Mrs. Yoe? How does a health promotion perspective inform your care of Mrs. Yoe? What other options are available, and how realistic or viable are these options?
6. A 24-year-old tennis professional was admitted to the clinic with a temperature of 41°C. He has a history of playing 5-hour tennis matches in 38°C heat. His coach brought him to the clinic because he was weak and lethargic. What assessment findings would you expect to find? What interventions would be necessary? Describe a teaching plan for this patient upon discharge.

REVIEW QUESTIONS

1. One of the most common electrolyte imbalances is:
   1. Hypokalemia
   2. Hyperkalemia
   3. Hyponatremia
   4. Hypocalcemia
2. The patient most at risk for fluid volume deficits is a(n):
   1. Older person
   2. Young to middle adult
   3. Child
   4. Infant
3. One reason that older persons experience fluid and electrolyte imbalance and acid–base imbalances is that they:
   1. Eat poor-quality food
   2. Have a decreased thirst sensation
   3. Have a more severe stress response
   4. Have an overly active thirst response
4. Output recorded on an intake and output record includes:
   1. Urine, vomitus, diarrhea, and drainage from wounds
   2. Diarrhea, gastric suction, and drainage from wounds
   3. Medications, juices, and water
   4. Urine, diarrhea, vomitus, gastric suction, and drainage from wounds or tubes
5. Health promotion activities in the area of fluid and electrolyte imbalances focus primarily on:
   1. Patient teaching
   2. Dietary intake
   3. Medication regimen
   4. Physician involvement in care
6. The nurse is aware that the following medication is never given directly intravenously:
   1. Potassium chloride (KCl)
   2. Furosemide (Lasix)
   3. Dextrose
   4. Calcium gluconate
7. Many factors are initially controlled for in the intravenous insertion procedure. The nurse understands that this begins with:
   1. Hand hygiene
   2. Checking the sterility of supplies
   3. Ensuring the ten rights of medication administration
   4. Carefully checking the order for the intravenous therapy
8. Indications of intravenous fluid infiltration include:
   1. Phlebitis and coolness
   2. Edema and erythema
   3. Pallor and coolness
   4. Pain and erythema
9. A recent evidence-informed review recommends that replacing peripheral venous catheters and rotating sites should occur:
   1. Every 96 hours
   2. Every 72 hours
   3. When clinically indicated
   4. Every 48 hours
10. Fifteen minutes after blood administration, your patient develops dyspnea, a cough, and a rapid heart rate. You suspect:
    1. Sepsis
    2. Anaphylaxis
    3. Acute hemolytic reaction
    4. Circulatory overload

Answers: 1. 1; **2.** 4; **3.** 2; **4.** 4; **5.** 1; **6.** 1; **7.** 1; **8.** 3; **9.** 3; **10.** 4

Rationales for the Review Questions appear at the end of the book.

RECOMMENDED WEBSITES

Association for Vascular Access: http://www.avainfo.org

The website for the Association for Vascular Access has many links to conferences and national and international organizations regarding vascular access.

Canadian Association of Nephrology Nurses and Technologists: http://www.cannt.ca

This association exists to promote excellence in the care of patients with renal disease. They provide leadership through education, research, and dissemination of research. Nephrology nursing standards are available from the website and include standards for holistic patient care across areas of practice such as prevention, assessment, and nursing interventions.

Canadian Paediatric Society: http://cps.ca/documents/position/home-intravenoustherapy

The Canadian Paediatric Society has a position statement on home intravenous therapy for Canadian children and youth. The web resource outlines indications and summarizes research related to pediatric home intravenous therapy.

Canadian Patient Safety Institute (CPSI) (Tools and Resources): http://www.patientsafetyinstitute.ca/en/Topic/Pages/Central-Line-Infections-(CLI).aspx

CPSI focuses on a wide range of patient safety topics. Preventing central-line infections is one topic with resources for physicians and nurses. The link given here is for two sets of evidence-informed steps for insertion and care of central lines.

Canadian Vascular Access Association: http://www.cvaa.info/

The Canadian Vascular Access Association provides leadership in advocating for safe, quality vascular access by promoting education, partnerships, knowledge, and research. The mission statement highlights the role of empowering and engaging members, with a vision for optimal patient outcomes.

Infusion Nurses Society: http://www.ins1.org/default.aspxm

This society is a global leader in intravenous therapy, playing a key role in synthesizing and disseminating the best evidence and publishing standards for infusion care. The society advances best practice through their publications, professional development opportunities, and advocacy.

MedCalc: Acid–Base Calculator: http://www.medcalc.com/acidbase.html

The MedCalc acid–base program provides a calculator for acid–base status and anion gap. Other options are calculators for creatinine clearance, fractional excretion of sodium, free water deficit, and hypo- and hypernatremia.

Ontario Regional Blood Coordinating Network: http://www.transfusionontario.org/

This government-funded network provides a number of services, including an educational service for registered nurses, called Bloody Easy Blood Administration. The online learning program requires registration; however, anyone can register and complete the module and an assessment test.

Registered Nurses' Association of Ontario (RNAO) Nursing Best Practice Guidelines: http://rnao.ca/bpg/guidelines/clinical-guidelines

RNAO has developed Best Practice Guidelines for a number of aspects of nursing care, including intravenous therapy. RNAO Best Practice Guidelines address assessment, device selection, care, and maintenance of vascular access, including central vascular access devices (CVAD). RNAO guidelines can be accessed through the RNAO website (http://www.rnao.org) and clicking on Nursing Best Practice Guidelines or by going to the link above. These guidelines are based on current evidence and knowledge and constitute an excellent resource.

REFERENCES

Alexander, M., Corrigan, A. M., Gorski, L. A., et al. (Eds.), (2014). *Core curriculum for infusion nursing* (4th ed.). Philadelphia: Lippincott, Williams, and Wilkins.

Allgood, G. (2009). Safe drinking water for the most vulnerable. *International Nursing Review, 56*(3), 273–275. doi:10.1111/j.1466-7657.2009.00752.x.

Amerman, E. C. (2016). *Human anatomy and physiology*. New York: Pearson Education Inc.

Arai, S. R., Butzlaff, A., Stotts, N. A., et al. (2014). Quench the thirst: lessons from clinical thirst trials. *Biological Research for Nursing, 16*(4), 456–466. doi:10.1177/1099800413505900.

Bernatchez, S. F. (2014). Care of peripheral venous catheter sites: Advantages of transparent film dressings over tape and gauze. *Journal of the Association for Vascular Access, 19*(4), 256–261.

Bunn, D., Jimoh, F., Wilsher, S. H., et al. (2015). Increasing fluid intake and reducing dehydration risk in older people living in long-term care: A systematic review. *Journal of the American Medical Directors Association, 16*(2), 101–113. doi:10.1016/j.jamda.2014.10.016.

Burchum, J. R., & Rosenthal, L. D. (2016). *Lehne's pharmacology for nursing care* (9th ed.). St. Louis, MO: Elsevier.

Casey, A. L., & Elliott, T. S. J. (2010). Prevention of central venous catheter–related infection: Update. *The British Journal of Nursing, 19*(2), 78. doi:10.12968/bjon.2010.19.2.46289.

Chopra, V., Krein, S. L., Olmsted, R. N., et al. (2013). Prevention of central line-associated bloodstream infections: Brief update review. In P. G. Shekelle, R. M. Wachter, P. J. Pronovost, et al. (Eds.), *Making health care safer II: An updated critical analysis of the evidence for patient safety practices* (AHRQ publication no. 13-E001-EF). Rockville, MD: Agency for Healthcare Research and Quality. Retrieved from http://www.ncbi.nlm.nih.gov/books/NBK133364/.

Coram, J. (2015). A collaborative approach: Seeking excellence in vascular access. *The British Journal of Nursing, 24*(8), S16–S22. doi:10.12968/bjon.2015.24.Sup8.S16.

Davidhizar, R., Dunn, C. L., & Hart, A. N. (2004). A review of the literature on how important water is to the world's elderly population. *International Nursing Review, 51*(3), 159–166. doi:10.1111/j.1466-7657.2004.00224.x.

De Beer, K., Michael, S., Thacker, M., et al. (2008). Diabetic ketoacidosis and hyperglycaemic hyperosmolar syndrome—clinical guidelines. *Nursing in Critical Care, 13*(1), 5–11. doi:10.1111/j.1478-5153.2007.00259.x.

DeVries, M., Mancos, P. S., & Valentine, M. J. (2014). Reducing bloodstream infection risk in central and peripheral intravenous lines: Initial data on passive intravenous connector disinfection. *Journal of the Association for Vascular Access, 19*(2), 87–93. doi:10.1016/j.java.2014.02.002.

Dumyati, G., Concannon, C., van Wijngaarden, E., et al. (2014). Sustained reduction of central line-associated bloodstream infections outside the intensive care unit with a multimodal intervention focusing on central line maintenance. *American Journal of Infection Control, 42*(7), 723–730. doi:10.1016/j.ajic.2014.03.353.

Dunn, S. (2015). Maintaining adequate hydration and nutrition in adult enteral tube feeding. *The British Journal of Community Nursing, 20*(Suppl. 7), S16–S23. doi:10.12968/bjcn.2015.20.Sup6a.S16.

Edwards, C., & Johnson, C. (2012). Evaluation of a Luer-activated intravenous administration system. *Journal of the Association for Vascular Access, 17*(4), 200–207. doi:10.1016/j.java.2012.10.003.

El-Sharkawy, A. M., Sahota, O., & Lobo, D. N. (2015). Acute and chronic effects of hydration status on health. *Nutrition Reviews, 73*(Suppl. 2), 97–109. doi:10.1093/nutrit/nuv038.

Felver, L. (2013a). Fluid and electrolyte homeostasis and imbalances. In L. C. Copstead & J. L. Banasik (Eds.), *Pathophysiology* (5th ed.). St. Louis: Saunders.

Felver, L. (2013b). Fluid and electrolyte balance. In J. F. Giddens (Ed.), *Concepts for nursing practice*. St. Louis: Mosby.

Freedman, S. B., Willan, A. R., Boutis, K., et al. (2016). Effect of dilute apple juice and preferred fluids vs. electrolyte maintenance solution on treatment failure among children with mild gastroenteritis: A randomized clinical trial. *JAMA, 315*(18), 1966–1974. doi:10.1001/jama.2016.5352.

Giger, J. N. (2013). *Transcultural nursing: Assessment and intervention* (6th ed.). St. Louis: Mosby.

Gillies, D., Wallen, M. M., Morrison, A. L., et al. (2005). Optimal timing for intravenous administration set replacement. *Cochrane Database of Systematic Reviews*, (4), CD003588, doi:10.1002/14651858.CD003588.pub2.

Green, J. (2008). Care and management of patients with skin-tunnelled catheters. *Nursing Standard, 22*(42), 41–48. doi:10.7748/ns2008.06.22.42.41.c6580.

Gregorio, G. V., Gonzales, M. L. M., Dans, L. F., et al. (2009). Polymer-based oral rehydration solution for treating acute watery diarrhoea. *Cochrane Database of Systematic Reviews*, (2), CD006519, doi:10.1002/14651858.CD006519.pub2.

Groll, D., Davies, B., MacDonald, J., et al. (2010). Evaluation of the psychometric properties of the phlebitis and infiltration scales for the assessment of complications of peripheral vascular access devices. *Journal of Infusion Nursing, 33*(6), 385–390. doi:10.1097/NAN.0b013e3181f85a73.

Hall, J. E. (2016). *Guyton and Hall textbook of medical physiology* (13th ed.). Philadelphia, PA: Saunders.

Hamilton, H. (2006). Complications associated with venous access devices: Part one. *Nursing Standard, 20*(26), 43. doi:10.7748/ns2006.03.20.26.43.c4087.

Hannon, R., Pooler, C., & Porth, C. M. (2010). *Porth pathophysiology: Concepts of altered health states* (1st Cdn. ed.). Philadelphia, PA: Lippincott Williams & Wilkins.

Hartling, L., Bellemare, S., Wiebe, N., et al. (2006). Oral versus intravenous rehydration for treating dehydration due to gastroenteritis in children. *The Cochrane Database of Systematic Reviews*, (3), CD004390, doi:10.1002/14651858.CD004390.pub2.

Higgingson, R. (2015). IV cannula securement: protecting the patient from infection. *The British Journal of Nursing, 24*(8), S23–S28. doi:10.12968/bjon/2015.24.Sup8.S23.

Infusion Nurses Society (INS). (2016). Infusion nursing standards of practice. *Journal of Infusion Nursing, 39*(S1), S1–S159.

International Council of Nurses. (2008). *Universal access to clean water. International Council of Nurses position statement.* Retrieved from http://www.icn.ch/images/stories/documents/publications/position_statements/E15_Universal_Access_Clean_Water.pdf.

Kelly, L. J. (2009). The family of vascular access devices. *Journal of Infection Prevention, 10*(1), s7–s12. doi:10.1177/1757177409342156.

Kisiel, M., & Marsons, L. (2009). Recognizing and responding to hyperglycaemic emergencies. *The British Journal of Nursing, 18*(18), 1094–1098. doi:10.12968/bjon.2009.18.18.44549.

Matocha, D. (2013). Achieving near-zero and zero: Who said interventions and controls don't matter? *The Journal of Vascular Access, 18*(3), 157. doi:10.1016/j.java.2013.03.003.

McCance, K. L., & Huether, S. E. (2010). *Pathophysiology: The biologic basis for disease in adults and children* (6th ed.). Maryland Heights, MO: Mosby Elsevier.

McGloin, S. (2015). The ins and outs of fluid balance in the acutely ill patient. *The British Journal of Nursing, 24*(1), 14–18. doi:10.12968/bjon.2015.24.1.14.

Millam, D. A., & Hadaway, L. C. (2003). On the road to successful I.V. starts. *Nursing, 33*(5), 1–14.

Mitchell, M. D., Anderson, B. J., Williams, K., et al. (2009). Heparin flushing and other interventions to maintain patency of central venous catheters: A systematic review. *Journal of Advanced Nursing, 65*(10), 2007–2021.

Molzahn, A. E., Pelletier Hibbert, M., Gaudet, D., et al. (2008). Managing chronic kidney disease in a nurse-run, physician monitored clinic: The CanPREVENT experience. *The Canadian Journal of Nursing Research, 40*(3), 96–112.

Ogston-Tuck, S. (2012). Intravenous therapy: Guidance on devices, management and care. *The British Journal of Community Nursing, 17*(10), 474–484. doi:10.12968/bjcn.2012.17.10.474.

Paul, P., Day, R. A., & Williams, B. (2016). *Brunner & Suddarth's Canadian textbook of medical-surgical nursing* (3rd ed.). Philadelphia, PA: Lippincott Williams & Wilkins.

Perel, P., & Roberts, I. (2012). Colloids versus crystalloids for fluid resuscitation in critically ill patients. *Cochrane Database of Systematic Reviews,* (6), CD000567, doi:10.1002/14651858.CD000657.pub5.

Pike-MacDonald, S., Best, D. G., Twomey, C., et al. (2007). Promoting safe drinking water. *The Canadian Nurse, 103*(1), 14–19.

Ray-Barruel, G., Polit, D. F., Murfield, J. E., et al. (2014). Infusion phlebitis assessment measures: A systematic review. *Journal of Evaluation in Clinical Practice, 20*(2), 191–202. doi:10.1111/jep.12107.

Registered Nurses' Association of Ontario. (2004/2008). *Nursing Best Practice Guideline: Assessment and device selection with 2008 supplement.* Toronto: Author. Retrieved from http://rnao.ca/bpg/guidelines/assessment-and-device-selection-vascular-access.

Registered Nurses' Association of Ontario. (2008). *Care and maintenance to reduce vascular access complications: Guideline supplement.* Toronto: Author. Retrieved from http://rnao.ca/sites/rnao-ca/files/storage/related/3380_Care_and_Maintenance_to_Reduce_Vascular_Access_Complications_Supplement_FINAL.pdf.

Rickard, C. M., Vannapraseuth, B., McGrail, M. R., et al. (2009). The relationship between intravenous infusate colonisation and fluid container hang time. *Journal of Clinical Nursing, 18*(21), 3022–3028. doi:10.1111/j.1365-2702.2009.02870.x.

Scales, K. (2011). Reducing infection associated with central venous access devices. *Nursing Standard, 25*(36), 49–56. doi:10.7748/ns2011.05.25.36.49.c8517.

Schub, T., & Obiamaka, O. (2016, October 28). Hydration: Maintaining oral hydration in older adults. *CINAHL Nursing Guide.* Retrieved from http://www.cinahl.com.

Shepherd, A. B. (2013). Water, water, everywhere and not a drop to drink? *Nursing and Residential Care, 15*(8), 530–537. doi:10.12968/nrec.2013.15.8.530.

The Joint Commission (TJC). (2017). *2018 National patient safety goals.* Oakbrook Terrace, IL: Author. Retrieved from http://www.jointcommission.org/standards_information/npsgs.aspx.

Touhy, T. A., & Jett, K. F. (2014). *Ebersole and Hess' gerontological nursing & healthy aging* (4th ed.). St. Louis: Mosby.

Webster, J., Osborne, S., Rickard, C., et al. (2010). Clinically indicated replacement versus routine replacement of peripheral venous catheters. *Cochrane Database of Systematic Reviews,* (3), CD007798, doi:10.1002/14651858.CD007798.pub2.

Wotton, K., Crannitch, K., & Munt, R. (2008). Prevalence, risk factors and strategies to prevent dehydration in older adults. *Contemporary Nurse: A Journal for the Australian Nursing Profession, 31*(1), 44–56.

Zingg, W., Cartier, V., Inan, C., et al. (2014). Hospital-wide multidisciplinary multimodal intervention programme to reduce central catheter-associated bloodstream infection. *PLoS ONE, 9*(4), e93898. doi:10.1371/journal/pone.0093898.

41

Sleep

Canadian content written by Claudette Taylor, PhD, RN, NP adult
Original chapter by Patricia A. Stockert, RN, BSN, MS, PhD

OBJECTIVES

Mastery of content in this chapter will enable you to:

- Define the key terms listed.
- Compare the characteristics of rest and sleep.
- Explain the effect of the 24-hour sleep–wake cycle on biological functions.
- Discuss the mechanisms that regulate sleep.
- Describe the stages of a normal sleep cycle.
- Explain the functions of sleep and rest.
- Compare the sleep requirements of different age groups.
- Identify factors that normally promote sleep and factors that normally disrupt sleep.
- Discuss the characteristics of common sleep disorders.
- Conduct a sleep history for a patient.
- Identify nursing diagnoses appropriate for patients with sleep alterations.
- Identify nursing interventions designed to promote normal sleep cycles for individuals of all ages.
- Describe ways to evaluate sleep therapies.

KEY TERMS

Biological clocks, p. 1073
Cataplexy, p. 1078
Circadian rhythms, p. 1073
Emotional stress, p. 1081
Excessive daytime sleepiness (EDS), p. 1076
Hypersomnolence, p. 1075
Hypnotics, p. 1092
Insomnia, p. 1076
Narcolepsy, p. 1077
Nocturia, p. 1075
Nonrapid eye movement (NREM) sleep, p. 1074
Parasomnias, p. 1078
Polysomnogram, p. 1076
Rapid eye movement (REM) sleep, p. 1074
Rest, p. 1079
Sedatives, p. 1092
Sleep, p. 1073
Sleep apnea, p. 1076
Sleep architecture, p. 1080
Sleep deprivation, p. 1078
Sleep hygiene, p. 1076

MEDIA RESOURCES

http://evolve.elsevier.com/Canada/Potter/fundamentals/

- Audio Chapter Summaries
- Examination Review Questions
- Concept Map Creator
- Case Study with Questions
- Audio Glossary
- Content Updates
- Video Clips

Sleep is essential for good health. Sleep is a basic necessity of life and is as important as air, food, and water (National Sleep Foundation, 2009). Everyone requires sleep. For a variety of reasons, individuals are, on average, sleeping less. Continual sleep loss may have many, yet largely unknown, adverse outcomes for health and well-being. In the short term, insufficient sleep alters mood and decreases the ability to concentrate, make decisions, and participate in daily activities.

To help patients in identifying and treating their sleep pattern disturbances, nurses need to first understand the nature of sleep, the factors influencing sleep, and patients' sleep habits. Patients require an individualized approach that is determined on the basis of their personal habits and patterns of sleep, to address the particular problem that is disrupting their sleep. Nursing interventions are often effective in resolving short- and long-term sleep disturbances.

Sleep provides healing and restoration (Van Cauter, Spiegel, Tasali, et al., 2008). Achieving the best possible sleep quality contributes to good health and to recovery from illness. Ill patients often require more sleep and rest than healthy patients. The nature of illness, however, often prevents some patients from getting adequate rest and sleep. Sleep can also be made difficult by the environment of a hospital or extended care facility and the activities of health care providers. Some patients have pre-existing sleep disturbances, whereas other patients develop sleep problems as a result of illness or hospitalization.

SCIENTIFIC KNOWLEDGE BASE

Definition of Sleep

Sleep is a universal, dynamic, highly organized, physiological, and behavioural state required by most living organisms to maintain health and well-being (Box 41-1) (Carskadon & Dement, 2011; Collop, Salas, Delayo, et al., 2008).

Physiology of Sleep

Sleep is a cyclical, physiological, and behavioural process that alternates with longer periods of wakefulness. Sleep physiology is controlled by three distinct processes: an *ultradian* process, a *homeostatic* process (process S), and a *circadian* process (process C). The ultradian process occurs within the sleep state and is characterized by the alteration of the two sleep stages: nonrapid eye movement (NREM) sleep and rapid eye movement (REM) sleep. Process S and process C work together to regulate the timing and organization of sleep and wakefulness. Process S is dependent on the sleep–wake cycle, whereas process C functions to maintain a state of wakefulness (Achermann & Borbely, 2011; Lee-Chiong, 2008).

Circadian Rhythms. The biological functions of most living organisms are regulated by circadian rhythms. The term *circadian* is derived from the Latin words *circa*, which means "about," and *dien,* which means a day (Smith, Comella, & Hogl, 2008). People experience cyclical rhythms as part of their everyday life. The sleep–wake cycle is the most familiar of the 24-hour circadian rhythms. Numerous biological and behavioural functions are influenced by circadian rhythms. Changes in body temperature, for example, exhibit circadian rhythmicity. Normally, a person's body temperature peaks in the afternoon, decreases gradually, and then drops sharply after a person falls asleep. The initial period of a person's sleep is characterized by high levels of growth hormones and increased blood glucose concentrations, blood pressure, and heart rate. Sensory acuity and mood are also maintained by the 24-hour circadian cycle (Laposky, Bass, Kohsaka, et al., 2008).

Factors that affect circadian rhythms and daily sleep–wake cycles include light, temperature, social activities, and work routines. All individuals have biological clocks that synchronize their sleep–wake cycles, which explains why some individuals fall asleep at 9 p.m., whereas others go to bed at midnight. Different individuals also function at their best at different times of the day.

Hospitals or extended care facilities usually do not adapt care to an individual's sleep–wake cycle preferences. Typical hospital routines often interrupt sleep or prevent patients from falling asleep at their usual time. A person has poor quality of sleep if his or her sleep–wake cycle changes significantly. A serious illness is often indicated by reversals in the sleep–wake cycle, such as falling asleep during the day.

BOX 41-1 Behavioural Characteristics of Sleep

- Periodic
- Involuntary
- Reversibility
- Reduced responsiveness to environment
- Minimal movement
- Closed eyes
- Species-specific posture

Carskadon, M. A., & Dement, W. C. (2011). Normal human sleep: An overview. In M. H. Kryger, T. Roth, & W. C. Dement (Eds.), *Principles and practice of sleep medicine* (5th ed., pp. 16–41). Philadelphia, PA: Elsevier.

When the sleep–wake cycle is disrupted (e.g., by working rotating shifts), other physiological functions can also change. For example, the person may experience a decreased appetite and lose weight or may experience other common symptoms of sleep cycle disturbances, such as anxiety, restlessness, irritability, and impaired judgement. Failure to maintain the usual sleep–wake cycle can negatively influence the individual's overall health.

Sleep Regulation. Sleep involves a sequence of physiological and behavioural states maintained by highly integrated central nervous system (CNS) activity, which is associated with changes in the autonomic nervous system and endocrine, cardiovascular, respiratory, gastrointestinal, renal, and musculoskeletal systems (Lee-Chiong, 2008). Each sequence of physiological states is identified by specific physiological responses and patterns of brain activity. Special instruments provide information about the structural and physiological aspects of sleep: for example, the electroencephalogram (EEG) measures electrical activity in the cerebral cortex, the electromyogram (EMG) measures muscle tone, and the electro-oculogram (EOG) measures eye movements.

Current theory suggests that sleep is a dynamic multiphase process. The body's major sleep centre is the hypothalamus. The hypothalamus secretes hypocretins (orexins) that promote wakefulness. The anterior pituitary gland also secretes hormones (e.g., growth hormone and prolactin) that promote sleep (Lee-Chiong, 2008).

Researchers believe the ascending reticular activating system (RAS), located in the upper brain stem, contains special cells that maintain alertness and wakefulness. The RAS receives visual, auditory, pain, and tactile sensory stimuli. Activity from the cerebral cortex (e.g., emotions and thought processes) also stimulates the RAS. Arousal, wakefulness, and maintenance of consciousness result from neurons in the RAS that release serotonin and catecholamines, such as norepinephrine and dopamine (Siegel, 2011).

Whether a person remains awake or falls asleep depends on a balance of impulses received from higher centres (e.g., thoughts), peripheral sensory receptors (e.g., sound or light stimuli), and the limbic system (e.g., emotions) (Figure 41-1). As a person tries to fall asleep, the eyes close and the body assumes a relaxed position and stimuli to the RAS declines. If the room is dark and quiet, the RAS further

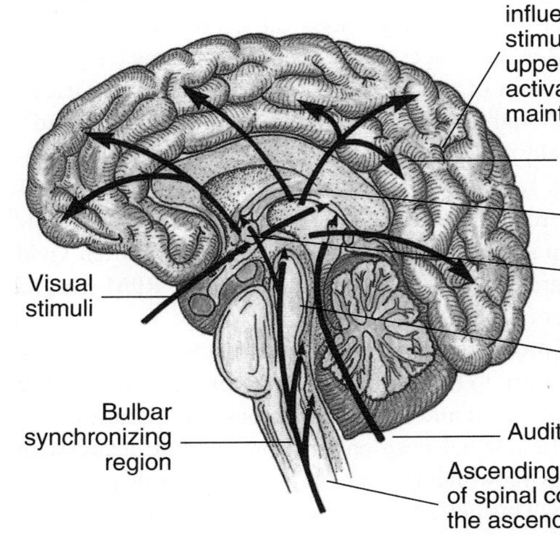

FIGURE 41-1 The reticular activating system and the bulbar synchronizing region control sensory input by intermittently activating and suppressing the brain's higher centres to control sleep and wakefulness.

BOX 41-2 Stages of the Sleep Cycle

Stage 1: Nonrapid Eye Movement

This stage represents the lightest level of sleep.
The person is unresponsive but easily aroused by sensory stimuli, such as noise.
Physiological activity begins to decrease, accompanied by a gradual fall in vital signs and metabolism.
Muscle tone is present.
When awakened from this stage, a person feels as though he or she had been daydreaming.
This stage lasts only a few minutes.
Accounts for about 2% to 5% of total sleep time in adults.

Stage 2: Nonrapid Eye Movement

This stage is a period of sound sleep.
Relaxation progresses.
Body functions continue to slow.
Muscle tone remains present.
Eye movements are absent.
Accounts for the greatest proportion (45% to 55%) of total sleep time in adults.

Stage 3: Nonrapid Eye Movement

This stage is the deepest period of sleep.
Individuals are difficult to arouse.
Muscles become completely relaxed.
Vital signs are significantly lower than during waking hours, but remain regular.
Parasomnias sometimes occur during this stage (e.g., sleepwalking, enuresis [bedwetting])
Accounts for 10% of total sleep time in adults and is more prominent during the first half of sleep.
If sleep loss has occurred previously, the sleeper will spend a considerable portion of the sleep period in this stage.

Rapid Eye Movement Sleep

Rapid eye movements are present.
Respirations are irregular and shallow.
Variable heart rate and blood pressure occur.
Vivid and elaborate dreams sometimes occur.
Dreaming occurs more frequently and is more complex than in NREM sleep.
This stage usually begins about 90 minutes after sleep has begun.
Loss of skeletal muscle tone occurs.
Gastric secretions increase.
The person is difficult to arouse.
The duration of REM sleep increases with each cycle.
Accounts for about 25% of total sleep time in adults.

Billard, M. (2008). Normal sleep. In H. R. Smith, C. L. Comella, & B. Hogl (Eds.), *Sleep medicine* (pp. 9–24). New York: Cambridge University Press; and Lee-Chiong, Jr., T. (2008). *Sleep medicine: Essentials and review.* New York: Oxford University Press.

declines. At some point, an area of the brain called the *bulbar synchronizing region (BSR)* takes over, causing sleep.

Stages of Sleep. Changes in brainwave activity, muscle tone, body temperature, and eye movements are associated with different stages of sleep (Billard, 2008). Within sleep, two separate phases have been identified: **nonrapid eye movement (NREM) sleep** and **rapid eye movement (REM) sleep** (Box 41-2). During NREM sleep, a sleeper progresses through three stages (stages 1, 2, and 3) of increasingly deeper sleep. Stage 1, a light and drowsy sleep, occurs at the beginning of sleep and is the transitional stage between wakefulness and sleeping. Stage 2 is a deeper stage of sleep, although a sleeper may be easily aroused during this stage of sleep. Stage 3 involves even deeper sleep, and this stage is known as delta sleep or slow-wave sleep (SWS). Delta sleep or SWS sleep is thought to be the most restorative of all the sleep stages. REM sleep, also known as paradoxical sleep, follows NREM sleep and is not divided into stages. REM sleep shares some characteristics of NREM sleep and of wakefulness. REM sleep is "paradoxical" in the sense that, although a person is behaviourally asleep, the individual is physiologically active—brain activity is high, rapid eye movements are occurring, twitching of the extremities occurs, and males frequently develop erections (Siegel, 2011). The most characteristic feature of REM sleep is dreaming. REM sleep dreams are often vivid and emotional (Billard, 2008; Van Cauter et al., 2008). REM sleep is the phase at the end of each sleep cycle.

Different factors promote or interfere with various stages of the sleep cycle. It is important to be aware of these factors and know about therapies that promote sleep and eliminate factors that disrupt it.

Sleep Cycle. The normal sleep pattern for an adult begins with a pre-sleep period during which the person is aware of only gradually developing sleepiness. This period normally lasts 10 to 30 minutes, but if a person has difficulty falling asleep, it can last an hour or longer. Once asleep, the person usually passes through four to five complete sleep cycles per night, each consisting of three stages of NREM sleep and a period of REM sleep (Billard, 2008). Sleep begins when adults

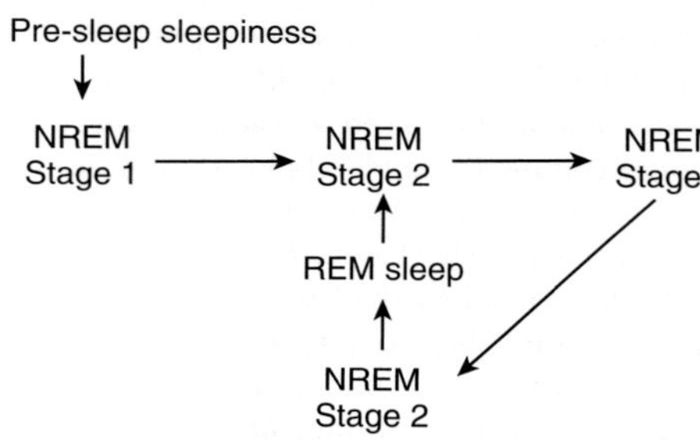

FIGURE 41-2 The stages of the adult sleep cycle. *NREM,* Nonrapid eye movement; *REM,* rapid eye movement.

enter stage 1 NREM sleep. This stage usually persists for only a few minutes, and sleep may be easily interrupted by calling the person's name or by touching them. Stage 2 NREM sleep follows and continues for approximately 10 to 25 minutes. In stage 2, a person is not so easily awakened. Stage 2 NREM sleep then goes to stage 3 NREM, back to stage 2 NREM and then to REM sleep to complete the sleep cycle (Figure 41-2). NREM sleep and REM sleep continue to alternate throughout a night in this cyclical pattern (Carskadon & Dement, 2011; Lee-Chiong, 2008). The number of sleep cycles depends on the total amount of time that a person spends sleeping.

The average length of the first cycle is 90 minutes, and subsequent cycles may last between 100 and 120 minutes. During the night, the NREM/REM sleep cycle is repeated four to five times, and with each subsequent cycle, less time is spent in stage 3 NREM sleep while the proportion of time spent in REM sleep increases. Of the total sleep time, 75% to 85% is spent in NREM sleep.

Not all people progress consistently through the stages of sleep. For example, a sleeper may move back and forth for short intervals between the NREM stages 2 and 3 before entering the REM stage. The amount of time spent in each stage varies over a person's lifespan. Newborns and children spend more time in deep sleep or SWS. This stage of sleep is highest in children, and for this reason it is often very difficult to wake young children from this particular stage of sleep. As individuals age, less time is spent in deep sleep (Carskadon & Dement, 2011; Lee-Chiong, 2008).

Functions of Sleep

Although we spend a third of our time sleeping, many of the reasons why we sleep have yet to be understood. Many theories of why we sleep have been proposed, and all of these may be partially correct. For instance, it has been proposed that sleep allows for physiological and psychological restoration (Van Cauter et al., 2008). During NREM sleep, biological functions slow. Normally, in daytime hours the heart rate of a healthy adult averages 70 to 80 beats per minute, or less, if the individual is in excellent physical condition. During sleep, the heart rate slows, beating 10 to 26 fewer times each minute, or 60 to 120 fewer beats each hour. Clearly, restful sleep is beneficial in preserving cardiac function. Other biological functions also decrease during sleep—for example, respirations, blood pressure, muscle tone, urine production, and hormone secretion (Carskadon & Dement, 2011). The body needs sleep for physiological restoration such as cell and tissue repair. Increased cell mitosis and increased protein synthesis have been observed during periods of NREM sleep (Van Cauter et al., 2008).

REM sleep is necessary for brain tissue restoration and appears to be important for cognitive restoration (Lee-Chiong, 2008). REM sleep is associated with changes in cerebral blood flow, increased cortical activity, increased oxygen consumption, and epinephrine release (Carskadon & Dement, 2011). During sleep, the brain filters stored information about the day's activities. The benefits of sleep on behaviour often go unnoticed until a problem develops as a result of sleep deprivation. A loss of REM sleep leads to feelings of confusion and suspicion.

Sleep is also believed to be important for immune function, renal function, regulation of body temperature, metabolism of glucose, and hormone secretion (Collop et al., 2008; Tibbits, 2008).

In addition to physical functioning, sleep is essential for psychological and social functioning. Without sleep, individuals are irritable and anxious and often report high levels of stress.

Dreams. *Dreaming* is defined as a mental activity that occurs while individuals are asleep. Dreams can occur during both NREM and REM sleep. The majority of dreams take place in the REM sleep stage. REM sleep–related dreams are often vivid and elaborate, whereas NREM dreams are simpler and more realistic (Lee-Chiong, 2008; Nielsen, 2011).

Studies of across-the-night changes in the characteristics of dreams suggest that dreams become more realistic as the night progresses. Dream content also appears to parallel cognitive and emotional development, as the recollection of dreams reported by children and adults is quite different (Stickgold & Wamsley, 2011).

Determinants of dreams, aside from age, include personality, physiological conditions (e.g., pregnancy), psychological conditions, pharmacological therapies, and situational factors. Personality also influences the quality of dreams; for example, a creative person has elaborate and complex dreams, whereas a depressed person dreams of helplessness (Stickgold & Wamsley, 2011). Most people dream about their immediate concerns, such as an argument with a spouse or worries over work. Sometimes a person is unaware of the fears represented in bizarre dreams. Clinical psychologists can try to analyze the symbolic nature of dreams as part of a patient's psychotherapy. The ability to describe a dream and interpret its significance sometimes helps resolve personal concerns or fears.

Numerous theories have been proposed as to why individuals dream. For centuries, dreams have been seen as messages from the gods, and this belief is upheld by many cultures today. Sigmund Freud theorized that dreams were the expression of an individual's unconscious desires and that by exploring dreams, emotional problems could be cured (Stickgold & Wamsley, 2011).

Physical Illness

Any illness that causes pain, physical discomfort, or mood problems, such as anxiety or depression, often results in sleep problems. Individuals who are ill frequently have trouble falling asleep or staying asleep. Illnesses can also force patients to sleep in unfamiliar positions. For example, when an arm or leg is in traction, patients have a difficult time finding a comfortable position for sleep.

Respiratory disease often interferes with sleep. While individuals sleep, their level of blood oxygen decreases. In healthy individuals, this decrease can be compensated for easily whereas individuals with respiratory diseases often require supportive devices, practices, or therapies to assist them while they are sleeping (Agarwal, Richardson, Krishnan, et al., 2009). Symptoms associated with respiratory diseases may require individuals to alter their position to facilitate sleeping. For example, individuals with chronic obstructive lung disease, such as emphysema, are frequently short of breath and often require two or three pillows to sleep (Lee-Chiong, 2008).

Cardiovascular disease interferes with sleep. Individuals who are obese are at greater risk for cardiovascular disease and, thus, for sleep disorders (Box 41-3). Chest pain, shortness of breath, diaphoresis, nausea, and palpitations, all symptoms associated with cardiovascular disease, frequently occur during the night and can disrupt sleep. Hypertension often causes early morning awakening and fatigue (Lee-Chiong, 2008).

The sleep of individuals with musculoskeletal disorders such as osteoarthritis and rheumatoid arthritis may be disrupted by the pain that often accompanies these conditions (Lavigne, Smith, Denis, et al., 2011).

Nocturia, or urination during the night, disrupts sleep and the sleep cycle. This condition is most common in older people with reduced bladder tone or individuals who have cardiac disease, diabetes, or problems with elimination. After a person awakens repeatedly to urinate, returning to sleep is difficult.

Sleep Disorders

Sleep disorders are conditions that interfere with nighttime sleep. Currently, more than 80 sleep disorders have been identified in the literature. The American Academy of Sleep Medicine developed the International Classification of Sleep Disorders version 2 (ICSD2), which classifies these disorders into eight major categories (Box 41-4).

Increasingly, evidence suggests sleep disorders are related to serious medical conditions. Individuals with sleep disorders are at risk for developing hypertension, diabetes, and cardiovascular and neurological diseases. Sleep disorders can affect individuals of all ages, and the prevalence of these disorders increases with advancing age (Bloom, Ahmed, Alessi, et al., 2009). Individuals with sleep disorders may complain of difficulty falling asleep or staying asleep, daytime sleepiness, **hypersomnolence**, or abruptly falling asleep during the daytime (Bae & Avidan, 2008).

The insomnias are primary disorders related to difficulty falling asleep. Individuals with sleep-related breathing disorders have disordered respirations during sleep. Hypersomnia is a group of disorders that are not due to sleep related breathing disorders, and are caused by disturbances in circadian rhythms or in nocturnal sleep. The parasomnias are undesirable behaviours that usually occur during sleep.

BOX 41-3 RESEARCH HIGHLIGHT

Sleep Duration and Obesity

Research Focus

Research has shown an association between obesity, sleep time, and the occurrence of sleep disorders. The prevalence of obesity has increased considerably over the past 25 years and is considered a global epidemic (Magee, Iverson, Huang, et al., 2008). *Obesity* refers to an excess of body fat and is a disorder that occurs when body fat excess impairs the health of individuals. Obesity is associated with an increased risk of many chronic diseases, including heart disease, diabetes, hypertension, and cancer (Anic, Titus-Ernstoff, Newcomb, et al., 2010). Prior research has shown that obesity increases morbidity and mortality.

Shorter sleep times have become increasingly more prevalent in Western countries for many reasons, including lifestyle choices, work or family requirements, or prevailing physical or psychological problems. Over the past several years, sleep duration in adults has decreased, on average, by 1.5 to 2 hours per night, and many individuals are reporting sleeping fewer than 6 hours per night. Researchers wanted to determine whether shorter sleep time increases the risk of obesity.

Research Abstract

Patel, Blackwell, Redline, and colleagues (2008) assessed the sleep pattern of 3 110 older men and 3 219 older women using wrist actigraphy, an objective method of sleep assessment. Study results demonstrated that a sleep duration of fewer than 5 hours was associated with an increased body mass index and truncal (abdominal) fat; the fat was also associated with cardiovascular disease and diabetes.

Evidence-Informed Practice

- During assessment of a patient's health problems, ask questions related to sleep quality and sleep patterns.
- If the patient indicates a problem with sleep, conduct a thorough sleep history.
- Reinforce good sleep hygiene habits.
- Encourage patients to notify their health care provider if they begin to experience sleep problems.
- Reinforce healthy eating habits.
- Encourage patients to seek the advice of other health care providers (e.g., dietitian, nutritionist).

Patel, S. R., Blackwell, T., Redline, S., Ancoli-Israel, S., Cauley, J. A., Hillier, T. A., et al. (2008). The association between sleep duration and obesity in older persons. *International Journal of Obesity, 32*(12), 1825–1834.

Circadian rhythm sleep disorders are caused by a misalignment between the timing of sleep and the societal norm or the desires of the individual. In sleep-related movement disorders, the person experiences movements such as leg cramps or teeth grinding that disturb sleep. The "other sleep disorders category" contains sleep problems that do not fit into other categories.

Sleep laboratory studies are often used to diagnose a sleep disorder (Chervin, 2011). A polysomnogram involves the use of EEG, EMG, and EOG to monitor stages of sleep and wakefulness during nighttime sleep. The Multiple Sleep Latency Test (MSLT) provides objective information about sleepiness and selected aspects of sleep structure by measuring eye movements, muscle tone changes, and brain electrical activity during at least four napping opportunities spread throughout the day. The MSLT takes 8 to 10 hours to complete. Patients wear an Actigraph device on the wrist to measure sleep–wake patterns over an extended period of time. Actigraphy data provide information such as sleep time, number and duration of awakenings, and levels of activity and rest (Chervin, 2011).

Insomnia. Patients experience insomnia when they report problems falling asleep, staying asleep, or nonrestorative sleep. Insomnia is the second most commonly expressed complaint reported in clinical practice after pain and the most common self-reported sleep-related complaint (Wyatt & Crisostomo, 2008). Insomnia is more common in women, and its incidence increases with advancing age (Doghramji, 2010). Insomnia may be transient and may indicate an underlying physical or psychological disorder (Reeve & Bailes, 2010). People experience *transient insomnia* as a result of schedule changes (shift work, travel), situational crises, particular medications, and excessive intake of alcohol or caffeine. However, transient insomnia may lead to chronic difficulty if causes are not addressed (Reeve & Bailes, 2010).

Insomnia is often associated with poor sleep hygiene, behaviours that are problematic for initiating sleep and maintaining sleep. Management of insomnia depends on whether it is transient or indicative of an underlying disorder. Treatment may include nonpharmacological therapies such as relaxation therapy, cognitive-behavioural therapy, or pharmacological agents (e.g., hypnotics).

Behavioural and cognitive therapies have few adverse effects and show evidence of sustained improvement in sleep over a 6-month period (Doghramji, 2010; Snowden, 2008).

Sleep Apnea. Sleep apnea is a disorder in which people stop breathing for a period of at least 10 seconds while asleep (Ramar & Guilleminault, 2008). There are two types of sleep apnea: obstructive sleep apnea (OSA) and central sleep apnea. Obstructive sleep apnea is the most common form of sleep apnea and results from an obstruction of the upper airway (Cao, Guilleminault, & Kushida, 2011). Central sleep apnea represents a loss of inspiratory effort due to an underlying pathological condition (Ramar & Guilleminault, 2008).

Risk factors for developing OSA include age, obesity, gender, ethnicity, smoking, alcohol, and a positive family history. OSA is more common in Asians than in Caucasians. OSA may affect middle-aged men more frequently, particularly when they are obese. OSA is also common in postmenopausal women and in younger women and children (Ramar & Guilleminault, 2008).

Excessive daytime sleepiness (EDS) and fatigue are the most common complaints of individuals who have OSA. Those who have severe OSA often report taking daytime naps and experience a disruption in their daily activities because of sleepiness. Feelings of sleepiness are usually most intense when waking up just after falling asleep and 12 hours after the mid-sleep period.

In addition to reports of excessive daytime sleepiness, other symptoms of OSA are fatigue, morning headaches, choking or gasping upon awakening, irritability, depression, difficulty concentrating, and decreased sex drive (Cao et al., 2011; Ramar & Guilleminault, 2008). Snoring is a distinguishing characteristic of OSA, as nearly all patients with this disorder snore (Cao et al., 2011).

OSA occurs when the muscles or structures of the oral cavity or throat relax during sleep. The upper airway becomes partially or completely blocked, thereby diminishing the nasal airflow (hypopnea) or

BOX 41-4 Classification of Sleep Disorders

Insomnias
Acute insomnia (duration of less than one month)
Primary insomnia (unrelated to any other disorder)
Co-morbid insomnia (due to a medical condition)
Nonrestorative sleep
Early morning awakening

Sleep-Related Breathing Disorders
Sleep apnea
- Obstructive sleep apnea syndrome
- Central sleep apnea syndromes
  - Primary central sleep apnea
  - Central sleep apnea due to a drug or substance
  - Central sleep apnea due to a medical condition

Snoring
Upper airway resistance syndrome

Excessive Sleepiness
Narcolepsy
Narcolepsy secondary to medical disorders
Hypersomnias
- Idiopathic hypersomnia (no identifiable cause)
- Recurrent hypersomnia (repeated episodes of hypersomnia)
- Post-traumatic hypersomnia (associated with head injuries)
- Menstrual-related hypersomnia

Behaviourally induced insufficient sleep syndrome

Parasomnias
Disorders of Arousal
Sleepwalking
Sleep terrors

Parasomnias Usually Associated With REM Sleep
Nightmare disorder
REM sleep behaviour disorder
Sleep paralysis

Other Parasomnias
Sleep-related groaning
Sleep-related hallucinations
Sleep-related eating disorder
Sleep-related enuresis (bedwetting)
Due to drug or substance
Due to a medical condition

Circadian Rhythm Sleep Disorders
Primary Circadian Rhythm Sleep Disorders
Delayed sleep phase type
Advanced sleep phase type

Behaviourally Induced Circadian Rhythm Sleep Disorders
Jet lag type
Shift work type
Delayed sleep phase type
Drug or substance use

Sleep-Related Movement Disorders
Restless leg syndrome
Periodic limb movements
Sleep-related leg cramps
Sleep-related bruxism (teeth grinding)

Isolated Symptoms, Apparently Normal Variants, and Unresolved Issues
Long sleeper
Short sleeper
Snoring
Sleep talking
Benign sleep myoclonus of infancy

Other Sleep Disorders
Physiological (organic) sleep disorders
Environmental sleep disorder
Sleep disorder not due to a substance or physiological condition

Adapted from American Academy of Sleep Medicine: International classes of diseases and international classification of sleep disorders, as cited in Thorpy, M. (2011). Classification of sleep disorders. In M. H. Kryger, T. Roth, & W. C. Dement (Eds.), *Principles and practice of sleep medicine* (5th ed., pp. 680–693). Philadelphia, PA: Elsevier.

stopping it (apnea) for as long as 10 to 30 seconds (Cao et al., 2011). The person still attempts to breathe; chest and abdominal movements continue and often result in loud snoring and snorting sounds. When breathing is partially or completely diminished, each successive diaphragmatic movement becomes stronger until the obstruction is relieved. Apneic episodes are normally terminated by gasps, snorting, or brief periods of awakening.

Structural abnormalities such as a deviated septum, nasal polyps, certain jaw configurations, or enlarged tonsils predispose an individual to obstructive sleep apnea. The effort to breathe during sleep results in arousals from deep sleep often to the stage 2 cycle. In severe cases, hundreds of hypopnea or apnea episodes occur every hour, resulting in severe interference with deep sleep.

OSA causes a serious decline in the saturation level of arterial oxygen. Individuals with OSA are at risk for cardiac dysrhythmias, heart failure, pulmonary hypertension, angina, stroke, hypertension, and metabolic syndrome. Sleep apnea contributes to high blood pressure and increased risk for heart attack and stroke (National Sleep Foundation, 2009).

Individuals who have OSA rarely achieve deep sleep because sleep is often fragmented. OSA may exact a heavy emotional toll on the individuals affected and their families. OSA may affect marital relationships and interactions within and outside the family, and frequently is an embarrassment to the patient (National Sleep Foundation, 2009). Treatment for OSA includes continuous positive airway pressure (CPAP). CPAP consists of a mask that fits over the nose and mouth through which air is continuously delivered into the airway to assist in keeping it open during sleep (Ramar & Guilleminault, 2008). Other treatments include addressing the underlying cardiac or respiratory complications and emotional problems that occur as a result of the symptoms of this disorder (Atwood, Strollo, & Givelber, et al., 2011).

Narcolepsy. Narcolepsy is a common complex neurological sleep disorder for which there is no known cure. Narcolepsy is known to affect men and women of any age; however, it usually appears in adolescence. The clinical manifestations of narcolepsy are highly variable. Excessive daytime sleepiness is the most common complaint associated with narcolepsy. During the day, a person who has narcolepsy may suddenly feel an overwhelming wave of sleepiness and fall asleep

(Ahmed & Thorpy, 2010). Narcolepsy is known to have a significant impact on REM sleep and is also known to intensify the emotions associated with this stage of sleep. Many individuals with narcolepsy experience hallucinations, vivid dreams, night terrors, sleepwalking, sleep paralysis, and poor memory and concentration, or the feeling of being unable to move or talk just before waking or falling asleep. **Cataplexy**, or sudden bilateral (occasionally unilateral) loss of muscle tone accompanied by an overpowering urge to sleep, can occur at any time during the day and can last from a few seconds to as long as 30 minutes. These episodes are sporadic and can occur occasionally to several times per day. A history of cataplexy may be obtained by inquiring whether the loss of muscle tone occurs during the following: upon hearing or telling a joke, while laughing, or when angry. Other triggers are embarrassment, surprise, stress, or sexual arousal (Ahmed & Thorpy, 2010; Cook, 2008a, 2008b). Some studies show a genetic link for narcolepsy (Faraco & Mignot, 2011).

Narcolepsy may also affect energy levels, metabolism, appetite, and feelings of mental well-being. Individuals with narcolepsy can have intense cravings for carbohydrates, and greater than one-third of individuals with narcolepsy suffer from obesity (Smith et al., 2008).

Most people with narcolepsy tend to be diagnosed several years after the onset of the condition, which means most of the symptoms associated with this disorder go untreated. Prior to diagnosis, individuals are frequently regarded as "different," antisocial, lacking in motivation, and uncooperative (Jennum, Knudsen, & Kjellberg, 2009).

There is no known cure for narcolepsy; therefore, treatment is targeted at symptom management. Traditionally, individuals with narcolepsy have been treated by two groups of drugs: stimulants and antidepressants. Stimulants promote wakefulness and reduce the frequency of sleeping episodes. Modafinil is a wakefulness-promoting agent and has been shown to improve symptoms of fatigue and cognitive function (memory and concentration). Antidepressants suppress cataplexy and other REM-related symptoms (Ahmed & Thorpy, 2010; Cook, 2008a, 2008b).

Nonpharmacological management should be initiated in all individuals. Education is an important component of the treatment plan for individuals with narcolepsy. Good sleep hygiene should be emphasized. The fundamental principles of sleep hygiene are listed in Box 41-5. Other management strategies include regular exercise, strategically timed daytime naps (if possible), a high-protein diet, deep breathing exercises, and chewing gum (Cook, 2008b). Patients who have narcolepsy need to avoid factors that increase drowsiness (e.g., alcohol, heavy meals, exhausting activities, long-distance driving, and extended periods of sitting in hot, stuffy rooms).

Parasomnias. **Parasomnias** are undesirable sleep problems that occur while falling asleep, between sleep phases, or during transitions from sleep to wakefulness. The word *parasomnia* is derived from the Greek word *para* combined with the Latin word *somnus* meaning event accompanying sleep (Silvestri & Arico, 2008). The parasomnia may range from abnormal sleep-related movements to emotions, perceptions, dreaming, or behaviours. Parasomnia may be the manifestation of an underlying physical or psychological disorder or may be caused by the ingestion of drugs or other substances (Lee-Chiong, 2008). Parasomnias are more common in children than in adults (Verrier & Josephson, 2011).

Parasomnias that occur among older children include somnambulism (sleepwalking), night terrors, nightmares, nocturnal enuresis (bedwetting), body rocking, and bruxism (teeth grinding). When adults experience these symptoms, more serious disorders are often indicated. Specific treatment for these disorders varies; however, in all cases patients need to be supported and their safety maintained.

BOX 41-5 Sleep Hygiene: Fundamental Principles

- Avoid late afternoon naps.
- Decrease consumption of caffeine, tobacco, and alcohol.
- Exercise regularly, but not prior to bedtime.
- Eat regular meals, do not go to bed hungry, and decrease consumption of liquids in the evening.
- Maintain a regular sleep–wake schedule, even on weekends.
- Maintain the bedroom as an environment solely for sleep.
- Ensure a sleeping environment that is comfortable and quiet.

Milner, C. E., & Belicki, K. (2010). Assessment and treatment of insomnia in adults: A guide for clinicians. *Journal of Counseling & Development, 88*, 236–244.

Shift Work. *Shift work sleep disorder (SWSD)* is a common sleep disorder experienced by individuals who work outside the traditional 9-to-5 work day. This disorder results from imposing a sleep–wake schedule that is contrary to the body's internal circadian clock. Most commonly associated with nighttime work, the health and economic consequences of this disorder are profound. Studies suggest that individuals who engage in shift work have a high risk of developing cardiovascular disease. The most common problems reported by shift workers are excessive sleepiness, fatigue, and insomnia. Not all individuals exposed to shift work develop this disorder (Drake & Wright, 2011).

Sleep Deprivation. **Sleep deprivation** refers to insufficient sleep during a specific time period. The most common causes of sleep deprivation are lifestyle factors or work-related factors. One approach to understanding the functional significance of sleep is to consider the behavioural and physiological effects of sleep deprivation. Numerous studies on animal models subjected to periods of sleep deprivation demonstrated that sleep deprivation resulted in changes in metabolism (weight loss despite increased food intake), impaired glucose metabolism, increased heart rate, skin lesions, decreased body temperature, and, with prolonged periods, death (Van Cauter et al., 2008).

There are several types of sleep deprivation. Sleep deprivation may be observed as a reduction in sleep time where sleep time does not meet the needs of the individual, prolonged wakefulness, and sleep disruption related to a pathophysiological process (e.g., cancer). The extent to which an individual experiences the effects of sleep deprivation depends on the physiological and behavioural requirements of the individual (Orezel-GryGlewska, 2009). Moreover, the effects of sleep deprivation are cumulative, meaning a mild reduction in sleep time over a prolonged period may be detrimental to the individual (Tibbits, 2008).

Sleep deprivation may be experienced by individuals for a variety of reasons. Causes include illness (e.g., fever, difficulty breathing, or pain), emotional stress, certain medications, environmental disturbances (e.g., noise, unfamiliar surroundings, frequent nursing care), and variability in the timing of sleep due to shift work and travel. Factors contributing to sleep deprivation in hospitalized patients are outlined in Box 41-6. Physicians and nurses are particularly prone to sleep deprivation because of their long work schedules and rotating shifts (Elliott, McKinley, & Cistulli, 2011; Lei, Qiongjing, Qiuli, et al., 2009). Hospitalization, especially in Critical Care Units (CCUs), makes patients particularly vulnerable to periods of sleep deprivation. Constant environmental stimuli within the CCU, such as strange noises from equipment, invasive equipment and procedures, the frequent monitoring and care given by nurses, and continuous light, lead to an inability to sleep. Numerous studies have confirmed that CCU

BOX 41-6 Causes of Sleep Deprivation in Hospitalized Patients

Environmental Factors
Noise
Uncomfortable bed and pillows
Bright lights
Pathophysiological factors
Pain and discomfort
Use of invasive equipment such as intravenous lines, nasogastric tubes

Emotional Factors
Stress, worry
Lack of control
Lack of privacy
Anxiety about procedures and outcomes of investigations

BOX 41-7 Sleep Deprivation Symptoms

Physiological Symptoms
Ptosis, visual disturbances such as blurred vision
Clumsiness in fine motor skills
Decreased reflexes
Slowed response time
Decreased reasoning and judgement
Decreased auditory and visual alertness
Cardiac arrhythmias
Increased food intake
Decreasing satiety
Weight loss

Psychological Symptoms
Easily distracted
Confusion and disorientation
Forgetfulness
Increased sensitivity to pain
Irritability, withdrawal, apathy
Excessive sleepiness
Poor concentration
Agitation
Hyperactivity
Decreased motivation

patients frequently experience sleep deprivation (Drouot, Cabello, D'Ortho, et al., 2008; Elliot, et al., 2011).

A person's response to sleep deprivation is highly variable. Patients exhibit a variety of physiological and psychological symptoms (Box 41-7). The severity of symptoms is often related to the duration of sleep deprivation. The most effective treatment for sleep deprivation is the elimination or correction of factors that disrupt the sleep pattern. Nurses play an important role in identifying individuals' treatable sleep deprivation problems.

NURSING KNOWLEDGE BASE

Sleep and Rest

When persons are at **rest**, they usually feel mentally relaxed, free from anxiety, and physically calm. Rest does not imply inactivity, although rest is often thought of as the act of settling down in a comfortable chair or lying in bed. Usually, when individuals are at rest, they are in a state of mental, physical, and spiritual activity that leaves them feeling refreshed, rejuvenated, and ready to resume the activities of the day. Individuals have their own habits for obtaining rest and can adjust to new environments or conditions that affect their ability to rest. Rest may be obtained from reading a book, practising a relaxation exercise, listening to music, taking a long walk, or sitting quietly.

Illness and unfamiliar health care routines can easily affect the usual rest and sleep patterns of individuals entering a hospital or other health care facilities. Nurses may frequently care for patients on bed rest, which confines patients to bed in order to reduce the physical and psychological demands on their body. Patients may not necessarily feel rested because they may still have emotional worries that prevent complete relaxation. For example, concern over physical limitations or a fear of being unable to return to their usual lifestyle can cause patients to feel stressed and unable to relax. Nurses must always be aware of a patient's need for rest. Long periods without rest can lead to illness or to the worsening of an existing illness.

Normal Sleep Requirements and Patterns

Individual requirements for sleep duration and quality vary among individuals of all age groups. For example, one person may feel adequately rested after 6 hours of sleep, whereas another person may require 10 hours of sleep.

Neonates. During the first few weeks of life, newborns sleep about 16 hours a day, sleeping almost constantly during the first week. Sleep occurs equally across the day and night in newborns and is more strongly influenced by hunger than by light–dark cues. The sleep cycle of newborns is generally 40 to 50 minutes, with waking occurring after one to two sleep cycles. Sleep is classified as active sleep (REM sleep equivalent) or quiet sleep (NREM sleep equivalent). A third stage has also been identified and is known as indeterminate sleep. This sleep stage cannot be defined as either quiet sleep or active sleep by polysomnography. Newborn sleep cycles begin with active sleep; newborns spend the majority of their sleep time in this stage of sleep. The primary function of active sleep is thought to allow for the continued development of neural pathways (Crabtree & Williams, 2009; Lee-Chiong, 2008).

Infants. By age 3 months, the amount of time the newborn spends in active sleep (REM sleep equivalent) diminishes, the required hours for sleep gradually decrease, and sleep–wake periods develop into a day/night cycle. By 6 months of age, infants enter sleep through NREM sleep. The ability to sleep during the night develops by 6 to 9 months of age. At this point, the infant's sleeping pattern is characterized by a nocturnal sleep period of 10 to 12 hours' duration, and two to three daytime naps, which collectively amount to 12 to 14 hours of total sleep time. Awakening commonly occurs early in the morning, although awakening during the night is not unusual (Crabtree & Williams, 2009; Lee-Chiong, 2008).

Toddlers. By 2 years of age, most children usually require 12 to 14 hours of sleep each day, which generally includes a nap in the afternoon and, for some, a morning nap as well. This amount of sleep is needed to re-energize the toddler and for continued growth and development. Lack of sleep makes a toddler feel tired and irritable. Awakening during the night is common for toddlers. A variety of factors may influence night waking, including dreams and a fear of being separated from their parents. During this period, the percentage of REM sleep continues to fall (Crabtree & Williams, 2009; Hockenberry & Wilson, 2014).

Preschoolers. A preschooler sleeps about 13 hours a night (about 20% of which is REM sleep). By 5 years of age, the preschooler rarely takes daytime naps, except in cultures where siestas are the custom (Hockenberry & Wilson, 2014). The preschooler usually has difficulty relaxing or quieting down after long, active days and may experience bedtime fears, waking during the night, or nightmares. Partial wakening, followed by a normal return to sleep, is frequent (Hockenberry & Wilson, 2014). In the waking period, the child may exhibit brief episodes of crying, walking aimlessly, unintelligible speech, sleepwalking, or bedwetting. Numerous factors may influence the sleep pattern of preschoolers, including day care and preschool schedules, family routines, and parental expectations as to the amount of sleep required for this developmental stage (Crabtree & Williams, 2009).

School-Aged Children. The amount of sleep needed varies during the school-age years. Both gender and ethnicity may explain the variability of sleep patterns in school-aged children. A longer sleep cycle has been observed in school-aged girls compared with their same-aged male counterparts. Caucasian children have more NREM stage 1 sleep and less NREM stage 2 sleep than African American children. Most school-aged children sleep between 9 and 10 hours each night. Epidemiological studies of school-aged children have shown shorter sleep times are associated with behavioural problems and symptoms of depression (Paavonen, Porkka-Heiskanen, & Lahikainen, 2009; Seo, Sung, Lee, et al., 2010).

Adolescents. The sleep pattern of adolescents is variable across a 7-day week, with shorter sleep times occurring during the school week. Consecutive nights of shorter sleep results in "sleep debt," with adolescents recovering this sleep on weekends with longer sleep times. The demands of school (e.g., schedules, assignments, exams, and extra-curricular activities), decreased parental influence, employment, and social media appear to play a significant role in the sleep patterns of adolescents (National Sleep Foundation, 2009). Physiological (circadian and homeostatic) processes that regulate sleep and wakefulness are also thought to influence the sleep habits of adolescents (Crabtree & Williams, 2009; Lee-Chiong, 2008). This shortened sleep time often results in EDS. As a result of EDS, adolescents may experience reduced performance in school, vulnerability to accidents, behaviour and mood problems, and increased use of alcohol or other substances (Crabtree & Williams, 2009; Gradisar, Gardner, & Dohnt, 2011).

Young Adults. Most young adults average 6 to 8.5 hours of sleep per night. Approximately 20% of sleep time is REM sleep, which remains consistent throughout life. The stresses of a job, family relationships, and social activities frequently lead to both insomnia and the use of medications to aid sleep. Daytime sleepiness contributes to an increased number of accidents, decreased productivity, and interpersonal problems in this age group. Pregnancy increases the need for sleep and rest. During the third trimester of pregnancy, women may experience insomnia, periodic limb movements, restless leg syndrome, and sleep-disordered breathing (Balserak & Lee, 2011).

Middle-aged Adults. During middle adulthood, the total time spent sleeping at night begins to decline. The amount of stage 3 sleep begins to fall and continues to fall with advancing age. Insomnia is particularly common, probably because of the changes and stresses experienced in middle age. Anxiety, depression, and certain physical illnesses cause sleep disturbances. Women who have menopausal symptoms often experience insomnia (Lee & Moe, 2011).

Older Persons. Aging results in several physiological and psychological changes, and alterations in sleep patterns frequently occur because of these changes. Studies suggest that poor sleep quality is a common complaint of older persons. Approximately 50% of older persons report difficulty sleeping (Espiritu, 2008; Neikrug & Ancoli-Israel, 2010; Roepke & Ancoli-Israel, 2010). Aging is associated with changes in **sleep architecture**, or sleep pattern. Greater nighttime disturbances (increased awakenings at night), less slow-wave or deep sleep, increased frequency of daytime napping, and decreased total sleep time are changes in sleep architecture that occur with aging (Lee-Chiong, 2008).

Older women are at particular risk for sleep problems due to hormonal changes that accompany menopause. In fact, problems sleeping are reported by approximately 25% to 50% of menopausal women (Roepke & Ancoli-Israel, 2010). Hot flashes (episodes of warmth in the face and chest) occurring at night can cause problems sleeping and may lead to an increase in the frequency of nighttime awakenings and, hence, less sleep time.

Numerous other factors are also related to the sleep problems reported by older men and women. These include the presence of co-morbid physiological conditions (e.g., heart disease) and psychological conditions (e.g., depression), primary sleep disorders (e.g., insomnia), chronic pain, nocturia, use of multiple medications, and alterations in circadian rhythm expressions (Neikrug & Ancoli-Israel, 2010).

Factors Affecting Sleep

Often, several factors alter the quality and quantity of sleep, such as physiological, psychological, and environmental influences.

Drugs and Substances. Many older persons take a variety of medications to control or treat chronic conditions, and these medications can seriously disrupt sleep. Daytime sleepiness, insomnia, and fatigue often result as a direct effect of commonly prescribed medications (Box 41-8). These medications may impair waking function and alter sleep patterns, which can be problematic for individuals (Cook, 2008a, 2008b; Smith et al., 2008). Antidepressants, antihistamines, and pain medications can cause daytime sleepiness or fatigue. Beta blockers have been associated with nightmares and vivid dreams. Diuretics can cause nocturia, thereby disrupting sleep. Medications prescribed for sleep can also be problematic as a result of their sedating effects during daytime hours (Mendelson, 2011).

Lifestyle. A person's daily routine influences sleep patterns. An individual working a rotating shift (e.g., 2 weeks of day shifts followed by a week of night shifts) often has difficulty adjusting to the altered sleep schedule (National Sleep Foundation, 2017a). For example, the body's internal clock for bedtime is set at 11 p.m., but the work schedule instead forces sleep at 9 a.m. The individual is able to sleep only 3 or 4 hours because the body's clock perceives that the morning is the time to be awake and active. Difficulties with maintaining alertness during work time result in decreased and even hazardous performance. After several weeks of working a night shift, a person's biological clock usually does adjust. Other alterations in routines that disrupt sleep patterns are performing unaccustomed heavy work, engaging in late-night social activities, and changing the evening mealtime (Balkin, 2011; Belenky & Akerstedt, 2011).

Usual Sleep Patterns. In the past century, the amount of sleep obtained nightly has decreased by more than 20% (National Sleep Foundation, 2017b), which indicates that many adults are sleep deprived and experience excessive sleepiness during the day. Sleepiness becomes pathological when it occurs at times when individuals need to or want to be awake. Individuals who experience temporary sleep deprivation as a result of an active social evening or a lengthened work schedule usually feel sleepy the next day. However, they are usually able to overcome these feelings despite the difficulty they experience in performing tasks and remaining attentive. Much more serious than temporary sleep deprivation is a chronic lack of sleep, which causes serious alterations in the ability to perform daily functions. Sleepiness tends to be most difficult to overcome during the performance of sedentary (inactive) tasks. For example, single-vehicle accidents related to a driver falling asleep at the wheel occur most often between 2 a.m.

BOX 41-8 Drugs and Their Effect on Sleep and Wakefulness

Hypnotics
Decrease NREM stage 3 sleep as well as REM sleep
Increase daytime sleepiness
Lead to poor memory and concentration
Depress respirations
May worsen sleep apnea in older persons

Diuretics
Nighttime awakenings caused by nocturia

Antidepressants
Cognitive impairment
Psychomotor impairment
Increase of NREM stage 1 sleep
Suppression of REM sleep
Decrease in total sleep time
Daytime sleepiness

Stimulants
Caffeine
Prevents the onset of sleep
Interrupts sleep during the night
Decreases the time spent in deep sleep
Interferes with REM sleep

Alcohol
Speeds onset of sleep
Reduces REM sleep
Interrupts sleep during the night and makes returning to sleep difficult

Beta-Adrenergic Blockers
Fatigue
Insomnia
Depression
Psychomotor impairment
Nightmares
Vivid dreams

Benzodiazepines
Alter REM sleep
Increase sleep time
Increase daytime sleepiness

Narcotics
Cause somnolence
Decrease amount of time spent in deep sleep stages
Suppress REM sleep
Depress respirations
Cause cognitive impairment
Cause psychomotor impairment

Anticonvulsants
Decrease REM sleep time
May cause daytime drowsiness
May cause insomnia
Cause impaired cognition

Anti-Parkinsonian Drugs
May cause worsening of cognitive function, especially memory
Cause fatigue
Cause somnolence

and 5 a.m., as a result of the sleepiness that occurs when individuals are awake during what is their normal period of sleep (Philip, Sagaspe, & Taillard, 2011).

Emotional Stress. Sleep is frequently disrupted by worry over personal problems or a personal situation. Emotional stress causes a person to be tense and often leads to frustration when sleep does not occur. Stress also causes a person to try too hard to fall asleep, to awaken frequently during the sleep cycle, or to oversleep. Continued stress can lead to poor sleep habits.

Older patients frequently experience personal losses, such as retirement, physical impairment, or the death of a loved one, all of which can lead to emotional stress. Older persons and other individuals who live with depressive mood problems may experience delays in falling asleep, the earlier appearance of REM sleep, frequent awakening, increased total bed time, feelings of having slept poorly, and early awakening (National Sleep Foundation, 2017a).

Environment. The physical environment in which a person sleeps can significantly influence the ability to fall asleep and remain asleep. Good ventilation is essential for restful sleep. The size, firmness, and position of the bed also affect the quality of sleep. If a person usually sleeps with another individual, sleeping alone often causes wakefulness. On the other hand, sleeping with a restless or snoring bed partner can disrupt sleep.

In hospitals and other inpatient facilities, noise creates a problem for patients. Noise in hospitals is usually new or strange and often loud, and patients wake easily. While in the hospital, the sleep of patients is often fragmented, with patients experiencing increased total wake times, increased nocturnal awakenings, and decreased REM sleep and total sleep time. Environment-induced noises (e.g., nursing activities) are sources of increased sound levels. CCUs are sources for high noise levels as the result of staff consultations, monitor alarms, and equipment sounds (Elliott, et al., 2011). The environment is unpleasant for sleeping because of the close proximity of patients, noise from confused and ill patients, the ringing of alarm systems and telephones, and disturbances caused by emergencies. Noise contributes to hearing loss, delays healing, impairs the immune function, and increases blood pressure, heart rate, and stress (Patel, Chipman, Carlin, et al., 2008).

The level of light in a room affects the ability to fall asleep. Some individuals prefer a dark room for sleep, whereas others, such as children or older persons, often prefer soft lighting during sleep. Individuals may also have trouble sleeping because of the temperature of a room. A room that is too warm or too cold often causes an individual to become restless.

Exercise and Fatigue. A person who is moderately fatigued usually achieves restful sleep, especially when the fatigue is the result of enjoyable work or exercise. Exercising that is completed at least 3 hours prior to bedtime allows the body enough time to cool down and maintains a state of fatigue that promotes relaxation (National Sleep Foundation, 2009). However, excess fatigue resulting from exhausting or stressful work makes falling asleep difficult. Excess fatigue is a common problem for grade-school children and adolescents.

Food and Caloric Intake. Following good eating habits is important for proper sleep. Eating a large, heavy meal or a spicy meal at night often leads to indigestion that interferes with sleep. Insomnia can result from caffeine, alcohol, or nicotine consumed in the evening. Coffee, tea, cola, and chocolate contain caffeine and xanthines that cause sleeplessness. Individuals who have insomnia can improve their sleep by drastically reducing or completely avoiding these substances (Reeve & Bailes, 2010). Some food allergies cause insomnia. In infants, a milk allergy sometimes causes nighttime waking and crying, or colic.

Both weight loss and weight gain influence sleep patterns (Patel, 2009; Van Cauter et al., 2008). Weight gain contributes to OSA because of the increased size of the soft tissue structures in the upper airway (Wellman & White, 2011). Weight loss causes insomnia and decreased amounts of sleep (Patel, 2009). Certain sleep disorders are the result of the semi-starvation diets popular in a weight-conscious society.

CRITICAL THINKING

Successful critical thinking requires a synthesis of knowledge, including information gathered from individuals, past experience, critical thinking qualities, and intellectual and professional standards. Clinical judgements require nurses to anticipate the required information, analyze the data, and make decisions regarding patient care. Adapting to the changing needs of a patient, based on sound decision making, constitutes critical thinking. During assessment (Figure 41-3), nurses need to consider all elements, to make appropriate nursing diagnoses.

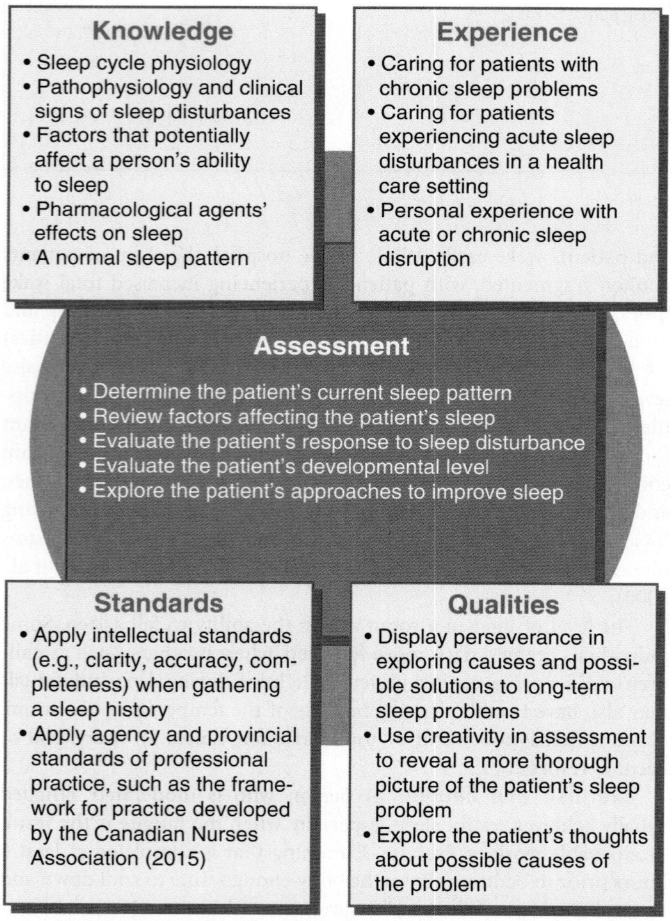

FIGURE 41-3 Critical thinking model for sleep assessment.

In the case of sleep, nurses integrate knowledge from disciplines such as nursing, pharmacology, and psychology. Nurses' experience with patients who have sleep problems, together with exploring research related to sleep, will aid in their understanding of effective forms of sleep therapies. Nurses need to use critical thinking qualities, such as perseverance, confidence, and discipline, to complete a comprehensive assessment and to develop a plan of care that can successfully manage the sleep problem. The framework for practice developed by the Canadian Nurses Association (2015) and standards of practice developed by each provincial and territorial nursing organization identify the nurse's role in patient care. In addition, evidence-informed geriatric nursing protocols for best practice, such as those in *Excessive Sleepiness* (Chasens, Williams, & Umlauf, 2008), provide specific instructions for assessing and addressing the needs of older patients with sleep disorders.

❖ NURSING PROCESS

◆ Assessment

Patients' sleep patterns are assessed by using the nursing history to gather information about factors that usually influence sleep. Because sleep is a subjective experience, only the patient is able to report whether it is sufficient and restful. If the patient is satisfied with the quantity and quality of sleep received, the nurse should consider it normal, and the nursing history is brief. If, however, a patient reports or suspects a sleep problem, the nurse needs to conduct a detailed history.

Sleep Assessment

Most individuals are able to provide a reasonably accurate estimate of their sleep patterns, particularly if any changes have occurred. In the nursing assessment, focus on understanding the characteristics of the patient's sleep problem and usual sleep habits so that your nursing care strategies to promote sleep are individualized. For example, if the nursing history reveals that a patient always reads before falling asleep, then offer reading material at bedtime.

Sources for Sleep Assessment. Usually, patients are the best resource for describing their sleep problems and how these problems differ from their usual sleep and waking patterns. The patient often knows the cause of sleep problems, such as a noisy environment or worry over a relationship. In addition, bed partners are able to provide information on the patient's sleep patterns that assists in obtaining insight regarding the nature of certain sleep disorders. For example, partners of patients with sleep apnea often complain that the patient's snoring disturbs their sleep. Often the partners must sleep in a different bed or move to another room to obtain adequate sleep. Ask bed partners whether patients have pauses of breathing during sleep and how frequently these pauses occur. Some partners mention becoming fearful when patients stop breathing during sleep.

When caring for children, seek information about sleep patterns from the parents, who are usually a reliable source of information about their child's trouble with sleeping.

An infant's difficulty in falling asleep or frequent awakenings during the night are often the result of hunger, excessive warmth, or separation anxiety. Parents of infants need to keep a 24-hour diary of their infant's waking and sleeping behaviour for several days to aid in determining the cause of the problem. Ask the parents to describe the infant's eating pattern and sleeping environment, both of which can influence sleeping behaviour. Older children often are able to verbalize the fears or worries that inhibit their ability to fall asleep. If children frequently awaken in the middle of bad dreams, parents may be able to identify the problem, although they may not be able to understand the meanings of the dreams. Ask parents to describe the typical behaviour patterns that foster or impair sleep. For example, excessive stimulation from active play or from visiting friends will predictably impair sleep. In the case of a child who experiences chronic sleep problems, ask the parents to describe provoking factors, the duration of the problem, its progression, and the child's responses.

Tools for Sleep Assessment. Although subjective reports of sleep are reliable and valid measures of sleep, some people may be inclined to exaggerate or minimize their sleeping patterns. One effective, brief method for assessing sleep quality is the use of a visual analogue scale (Chervin, 2011; Cohen, 2004). Draw a straight horizontal line 100 mm long. At the opposite ends of the line, print two opposing statements, such as "best night's sleep" and "worst night's sleep." Ask patients to mark a point on the horizontal line that corresponds to their perception of the previous night's sleep. Measure the distance of the mark along the line in millimetres; this number is a numerical value for satisfaction with sleep. Use the scale repeatedly to show change over time. Such a scale is useful to assess an individual's changes in sleep pattern over time.

Another brief subjective method to assess sleep is a numeric scale with a 0 to 10 sleep rating (Chervin, 2011; Cohen, 2004). Instruct patients to first rate their sleep quantity, then their quality of sleep on a scale of 1 to 10, with 0 being the worst sleep and 10 being the best sleep.

Sleep History

When a patient reports having received adequate sleep, a sleep history is usually brief. The information needed for nurses to plan care conducive to sleep includes the following: the usual bedtime, bedtime rituals, the preferred environment for sleeping, and the time the patient usually rises. When nurses suspect a sleep problem, they should explore the quality and characteristics of sleep in greater depth by asking patients to describe the nature of their sleep, including recent changes in their sleep pattern, sleep symptoms experienced during waking hours, use of sleep medications and other prescribed or over-the-counter medications, herbal products, diet, intake of substances such as caffeine or alcohol that influence sleep, and recent life events that may have affected the patient's mental well-being.

Description of Sleeping Problems. When a patient reports a sleep problem, the nurse needs to conduct a more detailed history. A detailed assessment ensures that the appropriate therapeutic care is provided. Open-ended questions help a patient to describe the problem more fully. After the patient provides a general description of the problem, the nurse can ask some focused questions, which will usually reveal specific characteristics that are useful in planning therapies. The nurse needs to understand the nature of the sleep problem, its signs and symptoms, its onset and duration, its severity, any predisposing factors or causes, and the overall effect on the patient. The nurse should ask specific questions related to the sleep problem (Box 41-9). Proper questioning helps to determine the type of sleep disturbance and the nature of the problem. Box 41-10 gives examples of additional questions for the nurse to ask the patient when specific sleep disorders are suspected. The questions assist in selecting specific sleep therapies and the best time for implementation.

As an adjunct to the sleep history, the patient and the patient's bed partner can keep a sleep–wake diary for 1 to 4 weeks (Lee-Chiong, 2008). The patient completes the sleep–wake diary daily to provide information on day-to-day variations in sleep–wake patterns over extended periods. Entries in the diary can include 24-hour information about various waking and sleeping health behaviours, including evening and bedtime routines, the time the patient goes to bed, the amount of time it took for the patient to fall asleep, the number of awakenings during the night, total sleep time, sleep quality (did they feel rested in the morning), the time and length of daytime napping, mealtimes, type and amount of alcohol and caffeine consumed, current medications, and daytime activities. A partner helps to record the estimated times the patient falls asleep or awakens. Although the sleep diary can provide useful information, the patient needs to be motivated to participate in recording the entries.

Usual Sleep Pattern. What constitutes "normal sleep" is difficult to define because individuals vary in their perception of the adequate quantity and quality of sleep. It is the responsibility of all health care

BOX 41-9 Nursing Assessment Questions

Nature of the Problem

What type of problem are you having with your sleep?
Why do you think your sleep is inadequate?
Describe for me a recent typical night's sleep. How is this sleep different from what you are accustomed to?

Signs and Symptoms

Do you have difficulty falling asleep, staying asleep, or waking up?
Have you been told that you snore loudly?
Have you been told you stop breathing or gasp for breath during sleep?
Do you feel drowsy or fall asleep while reading, when watching television, while driving, or when participating in other daily activities?
Do you feel excessively sleepy or irritable?
Do you have trouble concentrating during waking hours?
Do you have headaches when awakening?
Does your child awaken from nightmares?

Onset and Duration

When did you notice the problem?
How long has this problem lasted?

Severity

How long does it take you to fall asleep?
How often during the week do you have trouble falling asleep?
How many hours of sleep a night did you get this week?
How does this amount of sleep compare to what is usual for you?
What do you do when you awaken during the night or when you awaken too early in the morning?

Predisposing Factors

What do you do just before you go to bed?
Have you recently had any changes at work or at home?
Describe your mood. Have you noticed any changes in your mood recently?
What recreational drugs do you take on a regular basis?
Are you taking any new prescription or over-the-counter medications?
Do you eat food (spicy or greasy foods) or drink substances (alcohol or caffeinated beverages) that interfere with your sleep?
Do you have a physical illness that interferes with your sleep?
Does anyone in your family have a history of sleep problems?

Effect on the Patient

How has the loss of sleep affected you?

BOX 41-10 Questions to Ask to Assess for Specific Sleep Disorders

Insomnia

Do you have difficulty falling asleep?

After you fall asleep, do you have difficulty staying asleep? How many times during a night's sleep do you awaken?

When you wake up in the morning, do you feel rested? What time do you wake up in the morning? What causes you to awaken early?

What do you do to prepare for sleep? What do you do to improve your sleep?

What do you think about as you try to fall asleep?

When did you notice you had problems sleeping?

How often do you have trouble sleeping?

Do you feel excessively tired or sleepy during the day?

Do you take naps during the daytime?

Do you have any problems with performing tasks (i.e., work-related or driving) during the daytime?

Sleep Apnea

Do you snore loudly? Does anyone else in your family snore loudly?

Has anyone (e.g., spouse, bed partner, roommate) ever told you that you stop breathing for short periods during your sleep?

Do you experience headaches after awakening?

Do you have difficulty staying awake during the day?

Narcolepsy

Do you sometimes fall asleep unexpectedly? (Friends or relatives may report any occurrences.)

Do you feel excessively tired or sleepy during the day?

Do you have trouble concentrating?

Have you ever had an episode of losing muscle control or falling to the floor after a laughing episode or when angry?

Have you ever had the feeling of being unable to move or talk just before falling asleep or upon awakening?

Do you have vivid dreams when going to sleep or waking up?

providers to inquire about sleep quality of all patients. Patients need to describe their usual sleep pattern to determine the significance of the changes caused by a sleep disorder. The following questions can be asked to determine a patient's sleep pattern:

1. What time do you usually go to bed each night?
2. What time do you usually fall asleep? Do you do anything special to help you fall asleep?
3. How many times do you awaken during the night? Why?
4. What time do you typically wake in the morning?
5. What is the average number of hours you sleep each night?

The patient data are then compared with the predominant sleep pattern for other patients of the same age. On the basis of this comparison, the nurse can begin to assess for identifiable patterns, which may indicate a specific sleep disturbance, such as insomnia.

Patients with sleep problems frequently show patterns that differ drastically from their usual sleep pattern, or sometimes the change is relatively minor. Hospitalized patients usually need or want more sleep as a result of their illness; however, some patients require less sleep because they are less active. Some patients who are ill think that they need to try to sleep more than their usual amount of sleep, a perception that eventually makes sleeping difficult.

Physical and Psychological Illness. It is important to determine whether the patient has any pre-existing health problems that interfere with sleep. Poor sleep quality has been associated with numerous physiological and psychological illnesses. Chronic diseases, such as chronic obstructive pulmonary disease, and painful disorders, such as arthritis, interfere with sleep. This may occur because of the conditions themselves or because of medications taken to treat them. Several symptoms associated with these conditions, such as shortness of breath, pain, and nocturia, can potentially disrupt sleep. Psychiatric disorders can also interfere with sleep. For example, insomnia is common in individuals with schizophrenia, a chronic psychiatric disorder.

Insomnia is also common among individuals with depression. Anxiety disorders have also been associated with poor sleep (Ramsawh, Stein, & Mellman, 2011). Hence, it is very important to assess patients' sleep pattern, medical and social history (e.g., alcohol, tobacco, and caffeine consumption), and medication usage, including a description of over-the-counter and prescribed drugs. The social history can provide useful information, such as a situational crisis that may be interfering with sleep. If a patient takes medications to aid sleep, the nurse should gather information about the type and amount of medication that the patient uses, and assess the effectiveness of such medications and their effects on daytime function (Lee-Chiong, 2008).

Current Life Events. During the assessment, the nurse needs to ask whether the patient is experiencing any changes in lifestyle that could disrupt sleep. A person's occupation often offers a clue to the nature of the sleep problem (Drake & Wright, 2011). Changes in job responsibilities, rotating shifts, or long hours contribute to a sleep disturbance. The nurse can question the patient about social activities, recent travel, or mealtime schedules to help clarify the sleep assessment.

Bedtime Routines. Patients should be asked what they do to prepare for sleep. For example, the patient may drink a glass of milk, take a sleeping pill, eat a snack, or watch television. The nurse should note the habits that are beneficial compared with those that disturb sleep. For example, watching television may promote sleep for one person, whereas watching TV may stimulate another person to stay awake. Sometimes pointing out that a particular habit is interfering with sleep helps patients to find ways to change or eliminate that habit.

Special attention must be paid to a child's bedtime rituals. Parents need to report whether it is necessary, for example, to read the child a bedtime story, rock the child to sleep, or engage in quiet play. Some young children need a special blanket or stuffed animal when going to sleep.

Bedroom Environment. During the assessment, the nurse should ask the patient to describe his or her preferred bedroom conditions. These preferences may be the lighting in the room, music or television in the background, or the need to have the bedroom door open or closed. Some children require the company of a parent to fall asleep. In a health care environment, environmental distractions often interfere with sleep, such as a roommate's television, an electronic monitor in the hallway, a noisy nurses' station, or another patient who cries out at night. It is important to identify strategies that the nurse or the patient can use to reduce the effects of the distractions or to control the environment (National Sleep Foundation 2009).

Behaviours of Sleep Deprivation. Some patients are unaware of how their sleep problems affect their behaviour. The patient should be observed for behaviours such as irritability, forgetfulness, confusion, lethargy, frequent yawning, and slurred speech. If sleep deprivation has lasted a long time, psychotic behaviour, such as delusions and paranoia, sometimes develop. For example, a patient may report seeing strange objects or colours in the room, or the patient may act afraid when a nurse enters the room.

Patient Expectations

When a patient experiences a poor night's sleep, a vicious cycle of anticipatory anxiety may begin. The patient may fear that sleep will again be disturbed and will try harder and harder to sleep (Morin, 2011). When assessing a patient's sleep needs, nurses need to use a skilled, individualized, and caring approach, always asking patients what they expect regarding their sleep, the interventions they currently use, and the success of these interventions. Patients should also be asked about what other interventions they may prefer, and how they could be implemented. It is important to understand the patients' expectations regarding their sleep pattern. When patients ask for assistance because of sleep disturbances, they typically expect a nurse to respond promptly to assist them in improving their quantity and quality of sleep.

◆ Nursing Diagnosis

Nurses review their assessment to identify clusters of data that characterize a sleep pattern disturbance. When a sleep pattern disturbance is identified, it is important to be specific, as numerous factors may be the cause of these disturbances. By specifying the nature of a sleep disturbance and related factors, the nurse is able to develop with the patient interventions particular to the patient's situation. For example, interventions developed for sleep apnea will differ from those interventions developed to address sleep pattern disturbances related to psychological distress (e.g., anxiety, stress). Box 41-11 demonstrates how to use nursing assessment activities to identify and cluster defining characteristics to make an accurate nursing diagnosis related to sleep pattern disturbances.

Many factors can contribute to disturbed sleep patterns. It is important that the assessment identifies the probable cause of or factors related to the sleep disturbance, such as a noisy environment, a situational crisis, or a high intake of caffeinated beverages in the evening. These causes become the focus of interventions for minimizing or eliminating the problem. For example, if a patient is experiencing insomnia as the result of a noisy health care environment, the nurse can use strategies to promote sleep, such as controlling the noise of hospital equipment, reducing interruptions, or keeping doors closed. If the insomnia is related to worry over a threatened marital separation, the nurse can introduce coping strategies and collaborate with other health care providers regarding support groups or other services available to support the patient (Carpenito, 2016; Lei et al., 2009). If the nurse incorrectly identifies the probable cause or related factors, the patient will not benefit from the strategies to minimize or eliminate the presumed sources of disruption.

Sleep problems affect patients in other ways. For example, the nurse may find that a patient with sleep apnea is in conflict with a spouse who is tired of and frustrated over the patient's snoring. In addition, the spouse may be concerned that the patient is breathing improperly and thus is in danger. The nursing diagnosis of *compromised family coping* indicates that the nurse needs to provide support to both the patient and the patient's spouse so that they both understand sleep apnea and obtain the medical treatment needed. The following are examples of nursing diagnoses for patients with sleep problems:

- Anxiety
- Ineffective breathing pattern
- Acute confusion
- Compromised family coping
- Ineffective coping
- Ineffective health maintenance
- Fatigue
- Ineffective protection

BOX 41-11 NURSING DIAGNOSTIC PROCESS

Insomnia

Assessment Activities	Defining Characteristics
Ask the patient to describe his or her sleep pattern (past and present), the nature of the sleep problem, duration, etc.	The patient reports either a history or no history of sleep problems. The patient reports difficulty in falling asleep, staying asleep, and awakening several times during the night. Once awakened, the patient reports difficulty returning to sleep. The patient reports the need to nap during the day because of daytime sleepiness. With the use of a visual analogue scale, the patient reports feeling fatigued following a night's sleep. The patient reports no regular bedtime routine and frequently remains in bed in the morning to "catch up" on the sleep lost the previous night.
Related Factors	
Pathophysiological	The patient reports frequent awakenings during the night, for example, due to problems breathing.
Treatment	The patient reports daytime sleepiness due to medication.
Situational (personal, lifestyle)	The patient reports difficulty falling asleep and staying asleep because of a personal crisis. For example, the loss of a patient's job; the patient reports problems sleeping related to a recent diagnosis of cancer.
Observe the patient's appearance.	The patient appears pale and has dark circles under the eyes.
Observe the patient's behaviour, and ask the patient's spouse whether the patient is experiencing behavioural changes.	The patient is irritable and yawns frequently. The patient reports not feeling well-rested and having poor concentration. The spouse describes times when the patient was lethargic and distracted. The patient and the patient's spouse report napping during the day.
Determine whether the patient has experienced recent lifestyle changes.	The spouse reports that the patient recently lost his or her job and is concerned about finding a new position. The patient reports being under tremendous stress because of a family member's illness.

- Insomnia
- Disturbed sensory perception
- Sleep deprivation

◆ Planning

Goals and Outcomes. During the planning of a strategy of care, nurses again synthesize information from multiple resources to develop an individualized plan of care (Figure 41-4 and Box 41-12). Nurses must consider standards of nursing practice and clinical practice guidelines when developing a plan of care. Clinical practice guidelines are evidence-informed recommendations developed by expert practitioners and arise from a synthesis of the best evidence of a particular topic (Morin, 2011).

As the nurse plans care for the patient with sleep problems, the nurse can create a concept map to help develop a holistic approach to patient-centred care (Figure 41-5). The concept map is created after identifying the relevant nursing diagnoses from the assessment database. In this example, the nursing diagnoses are linked to the patient's anxiety related to her mother's recent cancer diagnosis.

The concept map shows the relationships between the nursing diagnoses *anxiety, disturbed sleep pattern,* and *impaired social interaction.* This approach to planning care can assist the nurse in recognizing relationships between planned interventions. For this patient, interventions and successful outcomes for one nursing diagnosis affect the resolution of another nursing diagnosis.

When developing goals and outcomes, the nurse and the patient need to collaborate. As a result, the nurse will be more likely to set realistic goals and measurable outcomes. An effective plan includes outcomes that focus on the goal of improving the quantity and quality of sleep in the home over a realistic period of time. Family members are often very helpful in contributing to the plan. A sleep promotion plan frequently requires many weeks to accomplish. The following is an example of a goal with patient outcomes:

Goal: The patient will control the environmental sources that disrupt sleep within 1 month.

Outcomes:

- The patient will identify factors in the immediate home environment that disrupt sleep within 2 weeks.
- The patient will report having a discussion with family members about environmental barriers to sleep within 2 weeks.
- The patient will report changes made in the bedroom to promote sleep within 4 weeks.
- The patient will report having fewer than two awakenings per night within 4 weeks.

Setting Priorities. The nurse needs to collaborate with the patient to establish the priority outcomes and interventions. It is important to remember that sleep problems are frequently the result of other health problems; management of these problems and their associated symptoms is the nurse's first priority. Once the symptoms are properly managed, the nurse can then focus on sleep therapies.

Collaborative Care. In collaboration with the patient and the patient's significant others, the nurse should ensure that any planned interventions, such as a change in the sleep schedule or changes to the bedroom environment, are realistic and achievable. In a health care setting, the treatments or routines should be planned so that the patient is able to rest. For example, in the Critical Care Unit, available electronic monitors can be used to track trends in vital signs without awakening the patient each hour. Other staff members should be informed of the plan of care so they can cluster activities at certain times to reduce the number of awakenings. In an extended care facility, the plan of care involves better planning of rest periods around the activities of the other residents. Often, patients' roommates have very different schedules and this must be considered.

The nature of the sleep disturbance determines whether referrals are necessary to additional health care providers. For example, if a sleep problem is related to a situational crisis or an emotional problem, the nurse may refer the patient to a psychiatric clinical nurse specialist or a clinical psychologist for counselling. When a patient has chronic insomnia, a referral to a sleep centre is beneficial. If the patient needs a referral for continued care in the community, the nurse should offer information about the sleep problem to the home care nurse. The success of sleep therapy depends on an approach that fits both the patient's lifestyle and the nature of the sleep disorder.

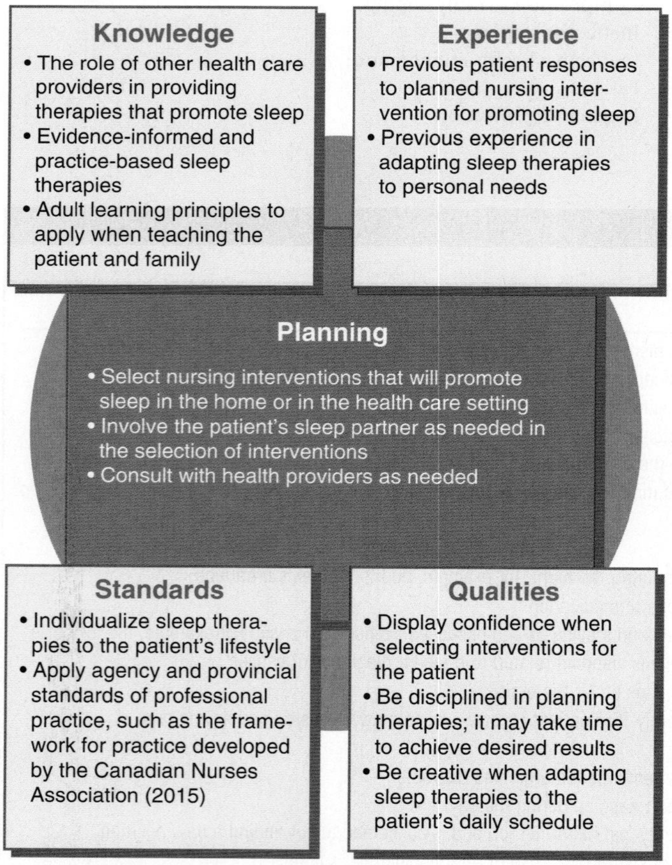

FIGURE 41-4 Critical thinking model for sleep planning.

◆ Implementation

Nursing interventions that are designed to improve the quality of a person's rest and sleep focus largely on health promotion. Patients need adequate sleep and rest to maintain active and productive lives. During times of illness, rest and sleep promotion are important for recovery. Nursing care provided in acute care, restorative care, or continuing care settings differs from nursing care in the home setting. The primary differences are in the environment and the nurse's ability to support normal rest and sleep habits. The patient's age also influences the types of therapies that are most effective. Box 41-13 provides principles for promoting sleep in older patients.

Health Promotion

Nurses can help patients in community health and home settings to develop behaviours conducive to rest and relaxation. To develop good sleep habits at home, patients and their bed partners need to learn the

BOX 41-12 NURSING CARE PLAN

Disturbed Sleep Pattern

ASSESSMENT

Andree Smith is a 36-year-old lawyer who presents to the health care centre where you are working. Andree, accompanied by her husband, has come to the clinic because she is having problems sleeping. Andree and her husband have three children, two in school and one in preschool. As you begin your assessment, Andree suddenly bursts into tears and tells you her mother has been recently diagnosed with breast cancer. Andree's assessment includes a thorough sleep history and a discussion on how this sleep problem is affecting her life. A physical examination is also conducted.

Assessment Activities	*Findings and Defining Characteristics**
Sleep pattern (present and past)	Andree reports difficulty falling asleep at night and awakening several times during the night. Andree states, *"I am so tired; I have no energy to do anything. I am irritable all of the time and I am having trouble concentrating at work."* Andree also reports that she has less patience with her children.
Relational Factors	
Pathophysiological	
Assess whether Andree has a history, a family history, or both of sleep problems.	Andree reports no personal or family history of sleep problems.
Assess whether Andree has a history of medical or psychological disorders.	Andree reports she has no history of any medical or psychiatric disorders.
Treatment	
Assess Andree's use of medications (both over-the-counter and prescription), including names, dosage, and frequency.	Andree reports she recently started taking melatonin at bedtime to help her sleep. Aside from melatonin, Andree is on no other medication.
Situational (personal, home, community)	
Ask Andree whether she has had any recent changes in her life.	Andree reports being highly anxious and states, "*Everything bothers me.*" She also reports that she has *stopped* her routine of walking 2–4 km daily because she has no energy.
Situational (personal, lifestyle)	
Ask Andree to describe her bedtime routine.	Andree reports she is going to bed between midnight and 1 a.m., which is 2 hours later than her usual bedtime. *It takes her an hour to fall asleep.* In the past, she received 7–8 hours of sleep each night, but now *it is closer to 5–6 hours.* She drinks two to three cups of coffee after dinner while surfing the Internet for information on her mother's condition. Andree also reports drinking a glass of wine before bedtime to help her relax because she has been having trouble falling asleep.
Observe Andree's appearance. Assess Andree for signs of sleep problems. Observe Andree's behaviour.	Andree appears *pale and tired.* She has *dark circles under her eyes* and is *slow to respond* to questions asked. She *yawns* frequently during the interview and appears restless.
With Andree's permission, ask her husband whether Andree has exhibited any behavioural changes.	Andree's husband reports that she is *irritable* with the children, is *forgetful,* and cries easily.

**Defining characteristics are in italic type.*

NURSING DIAGNOSIS: Insomnia related to psychological stress from mother's recent cancer diagnosis.

PLANNING

Goals (Nursing Outcomes Classification)† *Sleep*	*Expected Outcomes*
Andree will achieve an improved sense of restorative sleep within 2 weeks. Andree will report adherence to a regular bedtime routine within 1 week. Andree will achieve a more normal sleep pattern within 2 weeks. Within 2 weeks, Andree will report sleeping 7 hours nightly.	Andree will report waking less during the night and feeling rested within 2 weeks. Within 2 weeks, Andree will fall asleep within 30 minutes of going to bed.

†Outcomes from Carpenito L. J. (Ed.). (2016). Nursing diagnosis: Application to clinical practice (15th ed.). Philadelphia, PA: Lippincott Williams & Wilkins.

INTERVENTIONS

Interventions (Nursing Interventions Classification)‡ *Sleep Enhancement*	*Rationale*
Encourage Andree to establish a bedtime routine and a regular sleep pattern.	Maintaining a consistent schedule helps induce sleep (Milner & Belicki, 2010).
Instruct Andree to limit her consumption of caffeine and alcohol before bedtime.	Caffeine is a stimulant that may cause difficulty in falling asleep. Alcohol has the effect of lightening and fragmenting sleep (Milner & Belicki, 2010).

Continued

BOX 41-12 NURSING CARE PLAN

Disturbed Sleep Pattern—cont'd

Interventions (Nursing Interventions Classification)[‡]	***Rationale***
Assist Andree in identifying ways to eliminate stressful concerns about work before bedtime (e.g., taking time before actual sleep time to read a light novel).	Excess worry and intense activities before bedtime may stimulate the patient and prevent sleep (National Sleep Foundation, 2009).
Adjust the sleep environment: have Andree control the noise, temperature, and light in the bedroom.	Develop an environment conducive to sleep (Morin, 2011).
Exercise Promotion	
Encourage Andree to begin walking routinely during the day, but not 2 to 3 hours before bedtime.	Regular exercise increases activity levels and improves sleep quality. When exercise occurs just before bedtime, it can act as a stimulant that prevents sleep (National Sleep Foundation, 2009).
Simple Relaxation Therapy	
Instruct Andree on how to perform muscle relaxation before bedtime.	Relaxation therapy can help to reduce anxiety, which interferes with sleep (Lee-Chiong, 2008).

[‡]Intervention classification labels from Carpenito, L. J. (Ed.). (2016). Nursing diagnosis: Application to clinical practice (15th ed.). Philadelphia, PA: Lippincott Williams & Wilkins.

EVALUATION

Nursing Actions	***Patient Response and Finding***	***Achievement of Outcome***
Ask Andree whether she is able to fall asleep and stay asleep.	Andree responds, "It usually takes me 15 to 20 minutes to fall asleep, and I woke up once at night twice last week."	Andree reports she falls asleep within 30 minutes and wakes up less frequently during the night.
Ask Andree to describe her waking behaviours at work and home during the day.	Andree responds that she is able to concentrate on her work more. She reports she is less irritable with her children. She has restarted her walking routine.	Andree reports feeling more rested.
Observe Andree's waking nonverbal expressions and behaviour.	Andree sits in the chair without shifting position. She actively engages in conversation with you. She does not yawn during the interview. She is not as pale as she was previously and the circles under her eyes are almost gone.	Andree says she sleeps for an average of 7 hours a night.

techniques that promote sleep and the conditions that interfere with sleep (Milner & Belicki, 2010) (Box 41-14). Parents should also learn how to promote good sleep habits for their children. Patients benefit most from instructions that are formed on the basis of information about their homes and lifestyles, such as the types of activities that promote sleep for a shift worker or ways to make the home environment more conducive to sleep. Patients will be more likely to apply information that is useful and relevant to their needs.

Environmental Controls. All patients require a sleeping environment with a comfortable room temperature, proper ventilation, minimal noise, a comfortable bed, and proper lighting (Morin, 2011; National Sleep Foundation, 2009). Children and adults vary in their preferences for a comfortable room temperature. Parents should be instructed to position cribs away from open windows or drafts and to cover the infant with a light, warm blanket. Older persons often require extra blankets or covers.

Distracting noise should be eliminated so that the bedroom is as quiet as possible. In the home, the television, telephone, or the intermittent chiming of a clock can disrupt a patient's sleep. The family becomes an important part of the approach to reduce noise in the home, especially if the home is shared with several family members, all with different bedtime schedules. However, some patients are accustomed to sleeping with familiar inside noises, such as the hum of a fan. Commercial products that play soothing sounds, such as recordings of ocean waves or rainfall, can help to create a soothing environment for sleep.

The bed and mattress need to provide support and comfortable firmness. Bed boards can be placed under mattresses to provide additional support. Sometimes extra pillows can help to position a person comfortably in bed. For some patients, the position of the bed in the room also makes a difference.

Patients vary in their preference for the amount of light they can tolerate in the bedroom. Infants and older persons sleep best in softly lit rooms. Light should not shine directly on their eyes. Small table lamps can be used to prevent total darkness. For older persons, proper lighting reduces the chance of confusion and prevents falls while walking to the bathroom. Heavy shades, drapes, or slatted blinds are helpful if streetlights shine through windows, or if patients nap during the day.

Promoting Bedtime Routines. Bedtime routines help to relax patients in preparation for sleep (Milner & Belicki, 2010). Individuals should go to bed when they feel fatigued or sleepy. Going to bed while fully awake and thinking about other things often leads to insomnia and interferes with the perception of the bed as a stimulus for sleep. Newborns and infants sleep through so much of the day that a specific routine is hardly necessary. However, quiet activities, such as holding them snugly in blankets, singing or talking softly, and gentle rocking, help infants to fall asleep.

Parents need to reinforce short, predictable routines associated with preparing for bedtime (Milner & Belicki, 2010). A bedtime routine that is used consistently (e.g., the same hour for bedtime, eating a snack, or pursuing a quiet activity) helps young children to avoid delaying sleep.

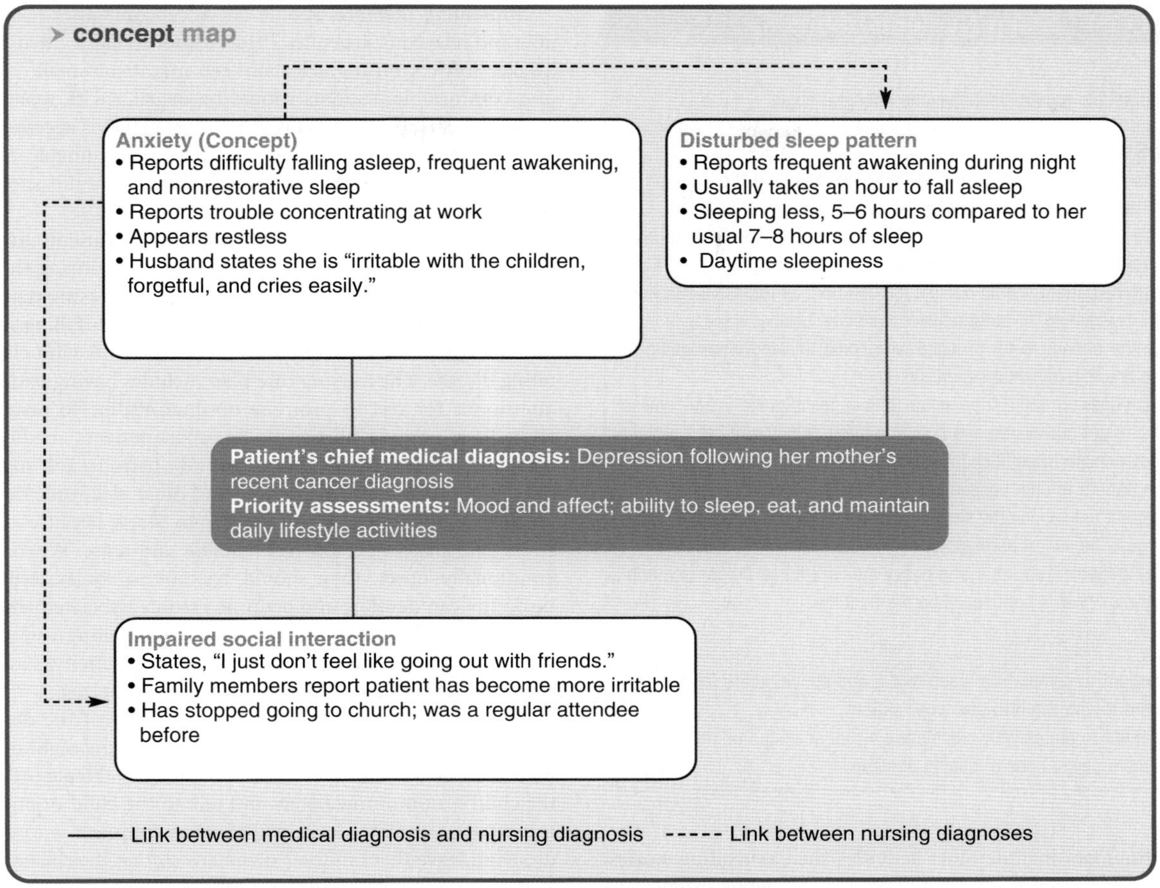

FIGURE 41-5 Concept map for a patient who has depression following the news of her mother's recent cancer diagnosis.

BOX 41-13 FOCUS ON OLDER PERSONS

Promoting Sleep

Sleep–Wake Pattern

- Maintain a regular bedtime and wake-up schedule, even on weekends or vacations (Lee-Chiong, 2008).
- Eliminate naps unless they are a routine part of the schedule.
- If naps are used, limit them to 20 minutes or less, twice a day, and avoid napping in the late afternoon or early evening.
- Go to bed when sleepy.
- Use a warm bath and relaxation techniques (reading, music, meditation, guided visual imagery) to promote sleep (Lee-Chiong, 2008).
- If unable to sleep within 15 to 30 minutes, get out of bed.
- Avoid work-related activities before bedtime (Milner & Belicki, 2010).

Environment

- Sleep where you sleep best.
- Keep noise to a minimum; use soft music to mask noise if necessary.
- Use a night light and keep the path to the bathroom free of obstacles.
- Set the room temperature to your preference; use socks to promote warmth.
- For "clock watchers" remove the clock from the bedroom
- Listen to relaxing music (Morin, 2011).

Medications

- Use sedatives and hypnotics as a last resort, and then only for the short term if absolutely necessary (Mendelson, 2011).
- Adjust medications being taken for other conditions, and assess for drug interactions that may cause insomnia or excessive daytime sleepiness (EDS).

Diet

- Limit the intake of alcohol, caffeine, and nicotine in the late afternoon and evening (Lee-Chiong, 2008; Milner & Belicki, 2010).
- Consume carbohydrates or milk as a light snack before bedtime (Milner & Belicki, 2010).
- Decrease the intake of fluids 2 to 4 hours before sleep.

Physiological and Illness Factors

- Elevate the head of the bed and provide extra pillows as preferred.
- Use analgesics 30 minutes before bed to ease aches and pains.
- Use therapeutics to control symptoms of chronic conditions as prescribed (Lavigne et al., 2011).

BOX 41-14 Sleep Hygiene Habits

Objective

- Patient will follow proper sleep hygiene habits at home.

Teaching Strategies

- Instruct the patient to try to exercise daily, preferably in the morning or afternoon, and to avoid vigorous exercise within 2 hours of bedtime.
- Caution the patient against sleeping long hours during weekends or holidays, to prevent disturbance of the normal sleep–wake cycle.
- Explain that the patient should not use the bedroom for intensive studying, snacking, TV watching, or other nonsleep activity, besides sex.
- Encourage the patient to try to avoid worrisome thinking when going to bed and to practise relaxation exercises.
- If the patient does not fall asleep within 30 minutes of going to bed, advise the patient to get out of bed and do some quiet activity until the patient feels sleepy enough to go back to bed.
- Advise the patient to limit consumption of caffeine and alcohol.
- Ask the patient to examine the sleeping environment. If noise or light is an issue, suggest the use of earplugs or eyeshades.
- Instruct the patient to avoid eating heavy meals 3 hours before bedtime; the patient may have a light snack before bedtime.

Evaluation

- Ask the patient to complete a sleep–wake and activity diary for 1 week, and compare it with the previous week's diary.
- Ask the patient to periodically complete a visual analogue or sleep rating scale to record perceptions of quality of sleep.

Bedtime routines can include quiet activities such as reading stories, colouring, allowing children to sit in a parent's lap while listening to music, or listening to a prayer.

Adults need to avoid excessive mental stimulation just before bedtime. Reading a light novel, watching an enjoyable television program, or listening to music can help a person to relax. Relaxation exercises, such as slow, deep breathing for 1 or 2 minutes, can help to relieve tension and prepare the body for rest (see Chapter 36). Guided imagery and praying also promote sleep for some patients.

At home, patients should be discouraged from trying to finish office work or to resolve family problems before bedtime. The bedroom is not a place to work, and patients need to always associate the bedroom with sleep. Working toward a consistent time for sleeping and wakening helps most patients to gain a healthy sleep pattern and to strengthen the rhythm of their sleep–wake cycle.

Promoting Safety. For any patient prone to confusion or falls, safety is critical. A small night light can assist the patient in orienting to the room environment before going to the bathroom. Beds set lower to the floor reduce the chance of a person falling when first standing. Patients should be instructed to remove clutter and small rugs from the path used to walk from the bed to the bathroom. If a patient needs assistance in ambulating from a bed to the bathroom, a small bell can be placed at the bedside to call family members. Sleepwalkers are unaware of their surroundings and are slow to react, which increases their risk of falls. Sleepwalkers should not be startled but instead gently awakened and led back to bed.

Infants' beds need to be safe. To reduce the chance of suffocation, pillows, stuffed toys, or the ends of loose blankets should not be placed in cribs. Loose-fitting plastic mattress covers are dangerous because infants can pull them over their face and suffocate. Parents should place infants on their back to prevent sudden infant death syndrome (SIDS) (National Sleep Foundation, 2009).

Promoting Comfort. People fall asleep only after feeling comfortable and relaxed (Carpenito, 2016). Minor irritants often keep patients awake. Soft cotton nightclothes keep infants or small children warm and comfortable. Patients should be instructed to wear loose-fitting nightwear. An extra blanket is sometimes all that is necessary to prevent a person from feeling chilled and thus being unable to fall asleep. Patients need to void before retiring so they are not kept awake by a full bladder.

Establishing Periods of Rest and Sleep. Patients living at home should be encouraged to stay physically active during the day so that they will be more likely to sleep at night. Increasing daytime activity reduces the likelihood of having problems with falling asleep. In the home setting, nurses frequently care for patients with chronic debilitating disease. The nursing care plan includes having patients set aside afternoons for rest to promote optimal health. To provide uninterrupted rest periods, nurses should adjust patients' medication schedules, instruct patients to void before rest periods, and suggest turning off cell phones, electronic tablets, and other electronic devices.

Stress Reduction. The inability to sleep because of emotional stress can make a person feel irritable and tense. When patients feel emotionally upset, they should try not to force sleep. Otherwise, insomnia can develop, and bedtime is soon associated with the inability to relax. A patient who has difficulty falling asleep should be encouraged to get up and pursue a relaxing activity, such as reading, rather than staying in bed and thinking about sleep.

Preschoolers have bedtime fears (e.g., fear of the dark or fear of strange noises) and frequently awaken during the night or have nightmares. When a child experiences a nightmare, the parent should enter the child's room immediately and talk to the child briefly about fears to provide a cooling-down period. One approach is to comfort children and leave them in their own beds so that their fears are not used as an excuse to delay bedtime. Keeping a light turned on in the room will also help some children. Cultural tradition can cause families to approach sleep practices differently (Box 41-15).

Bedtime Snacks. Some individuals enjoy bedtime snacks, whereas others cannot sleep after eating. A dairy product snack, such as warm milk or cocoa, contains L-tryptophan and is often helpful in promoting sleep. A full meal before bedtime often causes gastrointestinal upset and can interfere with the ability to fall asleep.

Patients should be encouraged to avoid drinking or ingesting caffeine before bedtime. Because coffee, tea, cola, and chocolate act as stimulants, they can cause a person to stay awake or to awaken throughout the night (National Sleep Foundation, 2009). Infants require special measures to minimize their nighttime awakenings for feeding. Children commonly need a middle-of-the-night bottle or to breastfeed at night. Hockenberry and Wilson (2014) recommend offering the last feeding as late as possible. Parents should be instructed not to give infants bottles in bed.

Pharmacological Approaches. Melatonin is a major hormone of the circadian system and plays an important role in promoting sleep (Buysse, 2011). Melatonin is a popular nutritional supplement to aid sleep. The recommended dosage is 0.3 to 1 mg taken 2 hours before bedtime (National Sleep Foundation, 2017a). Older persons who have decreased levels of melatonin find taking melatonin to be beneficial as a sleep aid (Lee-Chiong, 2008). Several other herbal products also assist in promoting sleep. Valerian is effective in addressing mild insomnia. It effects the release of neurotransmitters and produces a very mild sedation (Buysse, 2011). Kava helps promote sleep in patients who have sleep problems related to anxiety but needs to be used cautiously because of its potential toxic effects on the liver (Morin, 2011). Chamomile, passion flower, lemon balm, and lavender are other herbal products that have mild sedative effects. Patients should be cautioned

BOX 41-15 CULTURAL ASPECTS OF CARE

Co-Sleeping

Practices and patterns of sleep and rest vary among cultures. Culture and biology influence the development of sleep problems in children. Sleep patterns, bedtime routines, sleep aids, and sleep arrangements are a component of the cultural practices related to the use of space and the perception of comfortable distances for interactions with others. Sleep experts traditionally recommend having infants and children sleep in their own beds. Co-sleeping (i.e., the practice of infants and children sleeping with their parents) is a culturally preferred habit and is common in nonindustrialized countries. Health care providers in Canada frequently discourage this practice because of safety issues. The Canadian culture promotes independence in childhood. Because co-sleeping does not promote this independence, health care workers tend to discourage it. As a nurse, you need to be culturally sensitive when discussing co-sleeping practices with parents and developing sleeping plans for children.

Implications for Practice

- Complete a thorough sleep assessment of the child and the family.
- Discuss the risks of the child sleeping with the parents. During the discussion, remain culturally sensitive to and respectful of the parents' views.
- Co-sleeping affects the infant's normal sleep pattern by decreasing slow-wave sleep and increasing the number of nighttime arousals.
- Co-sleeping has been linked to an increased risk of sudden infant death syndrome (SIDS) under certain conditions, such as parental smoking and alcohol or drug use.
- Instruct parents who practise co-sleeping to avoid using alcohol or drugs that impair arousal. Decreased arousal prevents the parents from awakening if the child experiences problems.
- Co-sleeping should occur only with parents and not with another adult or child.
- Encourage the parents who co-sleep to use light sleeping clothes, to keep the room temperature comfortable, and to not bundle the child tightly or in too many clothes.

about the dosage and use of herbal compounds. Because some herbal compounds interact with prescribed medication, patients should avoid using these treatments together (Krystal, 2011) (see Chapter 35).

The use of nonprescription sleeping medications is not advisable. Patients need to learn the risks of such drugs. Although these drugs initially seem to be effective, over the long term, they can lead to further sleep disruption. Nurses can help patients to use behavioural and proper sleep hygiene habits to establish sleep patterns that do not require the use of drugs.

Acute Care

Patients in an acute care setting frequently have their normal rest and sleep routines disrupted, which makes them more susceptible to periods of sleep deprivation. Sleep has a restorative function; hence, in this setting, nursing interventions should focus on controlling factors in the environment that disrupt sleep, relieving physiological or psychological barriers to sleep, and providing uninterrupted rest and sleep periods for the patient. The nurse may accomplish this by organizing procedures to minimize the number of times the patient's sleep must be disrupted and by avoiding any unnecessary procedures during rest periods.

Environmental Controls. In a hospital setting, nurses can promote rest and sleep periods by reducing or eliminating environmental disturbances. When possible, the doors to patients' rooms should be closed. In semiprivate rooms, the curtains should be closed between patients. At night, the lights on a nursing unit should be dimmed. Noise levels can be reduced by conducting conversations and reports away from patient rooms and by keeping necessary conversations to a minimum, especially at night; reducing the volume of alarms, televisions, and other equipment; turning off bedside oxygen and other equipment not in use; and, when possible, avoiding noisy procedures till daytime hours (Carpenito, 2016). Patients' use of cellular telephones and laptop computers should be discouraged during rest periods, and their minimal use during the hospitalization period should be encouraged. Moreover, the nurse should limit visitors during rest periods.

Promoting Comfort. Compared with beds at home, hospital beds are often harder and of a different height, length, or width. Keeping beds clean and dry and in a comfortable position helps patients to relax. Pillows can be used for support (painful limbs, splinting of surgical incisions). Some patients who have painful illnesses require special comfort measures, such as the application of dry or moist heat, use of supportive dressings or splints, or proper positioning before retiring (Figure 41-6).

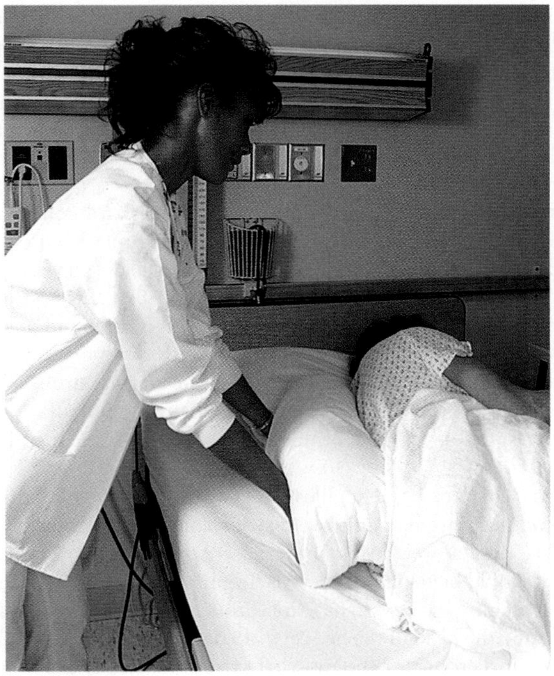

FIGURE 41-6 Positioning a patient for sleep.

Establishing Periods of Rest and Sleep. In a hospital or extended care setting, it is sometimes difficult to provide patients with the time needed to rest and sleep. However, nurses should plan their nursing care to avoid awakening patients for nonessential tasks. When possible, assessments, treatments, procedures, and routines should be scheduled for times when patients are awake. For example, if a patient's physical condition has been stable, nurses should avoid awakening the patient to check vital signs. Allowing patients to determine the timing and methods of delivery of personal care measures will promote rest. Bed baths and other routine hygiene measures should not be administered during the night simply because that timing may be most convenient for the nursing staff. Blood samples need to be drawn at a time when the patient is awake. Unless maintaining a drug's therapeutic blood level is essential, medications can be given during waking hours. Nurses need to work with the radiology department and other support services to schedule diagnostic studies and therapies at intervals that allow patients time for rest. Nurses should always try to provide patients with 2 to 3 hours of uninterrupted sleep during the night (Cmiel, Karr, & Gasser, 2004). Nurses may accomplish this by organizing procedures to minimize the number of times a patient's sleep must be disrupted and by avoiding any unnecessary procedures during rest periods.

When the patient's condition demands more frequent monitoring, activities should be scheduled to allow the patient to have extended rest periods. The nurse should plan activities in such a way both that health care personnel will avoid returning to the room every few minutes and that the patient will have up to an hour or more to rest quietly. For example, if a patient needs frequent dressing changes, is receiving intravenous therapy, and has drainage tubes from several sites, the nurse should not make a separate trip into the room to attend to each task. Instead, the nurse can use a single visit to change the dressing, regulate the intravenous system, and empty the drainage tubes. Nurses need to become patients' advocates for promoting optimal sleep, by postponing or rescheduling visits by family, asking consultants to reschedule visits, and questioning the frequency of certain procedures.

Promoting Safety. Patients with OSA are at risk for complications while in the hospital. Surgery and anaesthesia disrupt patients' normal sleep patterns. Postoperatively, these patients reach deep levels of REM sleep. This deep sleep causes muscle relaxation that can lead to OSA (Cao et al., 2011). Patients with OSA who are given opioid analgesics after surgery have an increased risk of developing airway obstruction because these medications suppress the normal arousal mechanisms (Cao et al., 2011). The nurse needs to monitor the patient's airway, respiratory rate, depth, and breath sounds frequently after surgery.

Nurses can recommend lifestyle changes to patients with OSA, including sleep hygiene improvements, alcohol moderation, smoking cessation, and a weight-loss program (Atwood et al., 2011). Such patients should be taught to prevent sleeping in the supine position by wearing a fanny pack or tight shirt with a tennis ball on the back, or by elevating the head of the bed 30 to 45 degrees (Atwood et al., 2011). As noted earlier, one of the most effective therapies is use of a nasal CPAP device at night, which requires a patient to wear a mask over the nose. The mask delivers room air at a high pressure and the air pressure prevents airway collapse. The CPAP device is portable and is effective particularly for OSA (Buchanan & Grunstein, 2011).

Another treatment option is the use of an oral appliance. These appliances advance the mandible or tongue to relieve pharyngeal obstruction (Cistulli, Ferguson, & Lowe, 2011). In cases of severe sleep apnea, the tonsils, uvula, or portions of the soft palate are surgically removed. Success with surgical procedures is variable.

Stress Reduction. Patients who are hospitalized for extensive diagnostic testing often have difficulty resting or sleeping because of uncertainty about their state of health. Giving patients control over their health care minimizes uncertainty and anxiety. Providing information about the purpose of procedures and routines and answering questions will give patients the peace of mind they need to rest or to fall asleep. During the night shift, nurses can take time to sit and talk with patients who are unable to sleep and may be able to determine the factors preventing patients from sleeping. Back rubs help patients relax more thoroughly. If a sedative is indicated, the nurse should confer with the physician to ensure the lowest dosage is used initially. A sedative should be discontinued as soon as possible, to prevent a dependence that can seriously disrupt the normal sleep cycle. Nurses should be aware that the metabolism of drugs in older persons is slower, making them more vulnerable to the adverse effects of sedatives, hypnotics, anti-anxiety drugs, and analgesics.

Restorative or Continuing Care

Nursing interventions implemented in the acute care setting are also used in the restorative or continuing care environment. Important considerations include controlling the environment, especially the noise level; establishing periods of rest and sleep; and promoting comfort. Nursing interventions related to the control of barriers to sleep are also implemented in these settings. Helping a patient achieve restful sleep in this environment sometimes takes a period of time.

Promoting Comfort. Comfort measures promote sleep and improve patients' sense of well-being. Nurses can promote comfort by offering a patient a warm bath or shower before bedtime. Other personal hygiene measures are mouth care and toileting (e.g., offering the bedpan or urinal). Back massages, soft music, and relaxation exercises also promote comfort. Proper positioning of the patient in bed is also very important. Using pillows to support limbs and other dependent body parts maintains skin integrity, thereby maintaining comfort (Milner & Belicki, 2010) (see Chapter 31).

Controlling Physiological Disturbances. Controlling the symptoms of patients with physical illnesses can promote sleep. For example, placing patients with respiratory disorders in upright bed positions and offering additional pillows may assist with their breathing. Teaching patients with chronic respiratory disorders (e.g., chronic obstructive pulmonary disease) pursed-lip breathing will decrease their respiratory rate and also promote comfort and sleep. Humidified air, the use of supplemental oxygen, if appropriate, and other pharmacological therapies (i.e., bronchodilators) are also relevant considerations.

Patients with pain, nausea, and other recurrent symptoms may require nonpharmacological and pharmacological therapies to promote sleep (Milner & Belicki, 2010; Morin, 2011). Relaxation measures (e.g., music, guided imagery) are appropriate diversional therapies. Providing pain relief with analgesics is also appropriate. To promote patients' comfort and sleep, nurses need to collaborate with physicians and other health care personnel to determine the optimal plan for relief of patients' symptoms (Milner & Belicki, 2010).

Pharmacological Approaches. Numerous pharmacological drugs, both prescription and over-the-counter, are used to manage insomnia. Conversely, polypharmacy to manage insomnia is associated with disrupted sleep patterns, including increased nocturnal awakening and decreased REM sleep and total sleep time. Therefore, CNS stimulants, such as amphetamines, caffeine, nicotine, terbutaline, theophylline, and pemoline, need to be used sparingly and only under medical management (O'Malley, Gleeson, & Weir, 2011). In addition, withdrawal from CNS depressants, such as alcohol, barbiturates, tricyclic antidepressants (amitriptyline, imipramine, and doxepin), and triazolam, can cause insomnia. Nurses need to manage these medications carefully.

Medications that induce sleep are called **hypnotics**. **Sedatives** are medications that produce a calming or soothing effect (Mendelson,

2011). Hypnotics and sedatives can be used as sleep medications and will help, if used correctly. A patient who takes sleep medications needs to understand their proper use, their risks, and their possible adverse effects. Long-term use of anti-anxiety, sedative, or hypnotic agents, however, can disrupt sleep and lead to more serious problems.

One group of drugs considered to be relatively safe is the benzodiazepines. The benzodiazepines cause relaxation, anti-anxiety, and hypnotic effects by facilitating the action of neurons in the CNS that suppress responsiveness to stimulation, thereby decreasing the levels of arousal (Mendelson, 2011). Unlike sedatives and hypnotics, benzodiazepines do not cause general CNS depression, and they also have a lower potential for abuse. These drugs are frequently prescribed because anti-anxiety effects occur at safe, nontoxic doses. In the older person, short-acting benzodiazepines, such as temazepam and triazolam, are preferred over long-acting agents (Mendelson, 2011).

Benzodiazepines need to be administered with caution in children younger than 12 years of age. These medications are contraindicated in infants younger than 6 months. Pregnant women need to avoid benzodiazepines because their use is associated with the risk of congenital anomalies. Nursing mothers do not receive these drugs because they are excreted in breast milk. Initial doses are small, and increments are added gradually, on the basis of patient response, for a limited period of time. Patients should be warned not to take more than the prescribed dose, especially if the medication seems to become less effective after the initial use. If older patients who were continent, ambulatory, and alert suddenly become incontinent, confused, or demonstrate impaired mobility, the use of benzodiazepines needs to be considered as a possible cause. Regular use of any sleep medication often leads to drug tolerance. Rebound insomnia is a problem that can be experienced after stopping the medication (Lee-Chiong, 2008). Immediately administering a sleeping medication when a hospitalized patient complains of being unable to sleep will do the patient more harm than good. Alternative approaches need to be considered for promoting sleep. Routine monitoring of the patient's response to sleeping medications is also important.

◆ Evaluation

The patient is an important source of information for evaluating outcomes related to sleep and rest. Each patient has a unique need for sleep and rest, and only the patient will know whether sleep problems have improved, and which interventions or therapies are most successful in promoting sleep (Figure 41-7). To evaluate the effectiveness of nursing interventions, the nurse makes comparisons with baseline sleep assessment data.

The nurse needs to determine whether expected outcomes have been met, using evaluative measures shortly after a therapy has been tried (e.g., by observing whether a patient falls asleep after noise has been reduced and the room has been darkened) and after a patient awakens from sleep (e.g., by asking a patient to describe the number of awakenings during the previous night). The patient and the patient's bed partner can usually provide accurate evaluative information. Over longer periods, assessment tools such as the visual analogue scale or the sleep rating scale can be used to determine whether sleep has progressively improved.

Nurses also need to evaluate the level of understanding that patients and their family members have gained after receiving instruction in sleep habits. Nurses can measure adherence to these practices during a home visit, when they are able to observe the environment. When expected outcomes are not met, the nursing measures or expected outcomes need to be revised on the basis of the patient's needs or preferences. When outcomes are not met, the nurse can ask questions

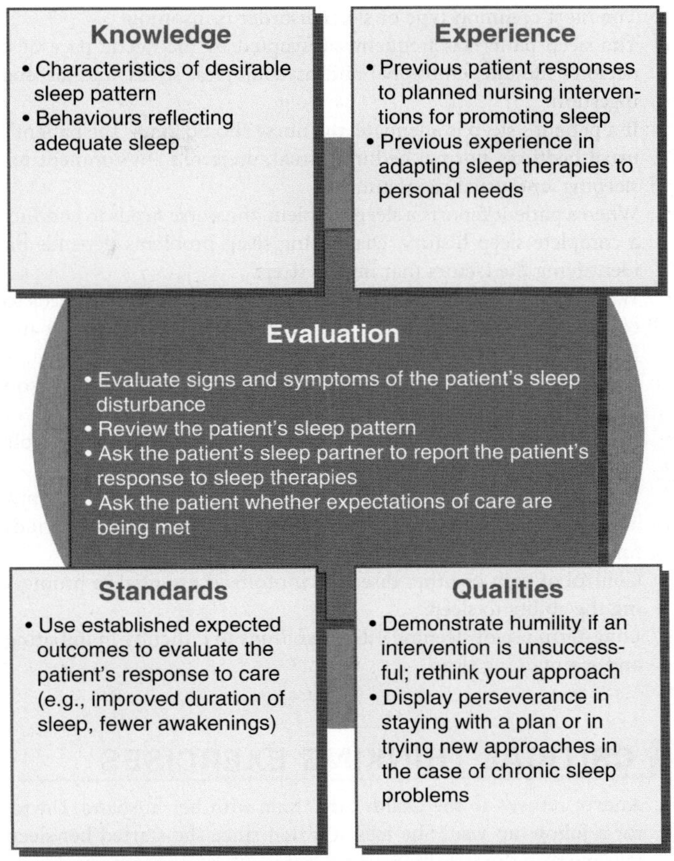

FIGURE 41-7 Critical thinking model for sleep evaluation.

such as "Do you feel as though you slept better when you exercised?" or "Do you feel rested when you wake up?"

When nurses successfully develop good relationships with patients and when they have developed therapeutic plans of care, subtle behaviours often indicate the patients' levels of satisfaction. The absence of signs of sleep problems, such as lethargy, frequent yawning, or position changes, may be noted. The nurse should ask the patient whether his or her sleep needs have been met, using such questions as "Are you feeling more rested?" or "Can you tell me if you feel we have done all we can to help improve your sleep?" If the patient's expectations have not been met, the nurse will need to spend more time trying to understand the patient's needs and preferences. Working closely with the patient and the patient's bed partner will enable the nurse to redefine the expectations that can be realistically met within the limits of the patient's condition and treatment.

KEY CONCEPTS

- Sleep provides physiological and psychological restoration.
- The 24-hour sleep–wake cycle is a circadian rhythm that influences physiological function and behaviour.
- The control and regulation of sleep depends on a balance between regulators within the central nervous system.
- During a typical night's sleep, a person passes through four to five complete sleep cycles. Each sleep cycle contains four nonrapid eye movement (NREM) stages of sleep and a period of rapid eye movement (REM) sleep.

- The most common type of sleep disorder is insomnia.
- The sleep pattern is frequently disrupted by the hectic pace of a person's lifestyle, emotional and psychological stress, and alcohol ingestion.
- If a patient's sleep is adequate, the nurse should assess the patient's usual bedtime, normal bedtime ritual, preferred environment for sleeping, and usual rising time.
- When a patient reports a sleep problem, the nurse needs to conduct a complete sleep history. Diagnosing sleep problems depends on identifying the factors that impair sleep.
- When planning interventions to promote sleep, the nurse needs to consider the characteristics of the patient's home environment and normal lifestyle.
- A regular bedtime routine of relaxing activities prepares a person physically and mentally for sleep.
- An environment with a darkened room, reduced noise, comfortable bed, and good ventilation promotes sleep.
- Important nursing interventions for promoting sleep in the hospitalized patient are controlling noise levels and establishing periods for uninterrupted sleep and rest.
- Control of pain or other disease symptoms is essential in promoting the ability to sleep.
- Long-term use of sleeping pills often leads to difficulty in initiating and maintaining sleep.

CRITICAL THINKING EXERCISES

1. Andree returns to the health care clinic with her husband, David, for a follow-up visit. She tells you that since she started her sleep hygiene plan she feels more rested but is still having some problems sleeping because of her husband's loud snoring. In addition to Andree's report of David's snoring, you note that he is overweight. On the basis of Andree's report of David's snoring, what additional assessment data should you gather from David?
2. On the basis of David's reported symptoms, what problem do you suspect he might have?
3. What action would you take at this time?
4. Andree and David also tell you that they are concerned about their 15-year-old daughter. Her grades in school are getting worse, and she says she is always tired. What do you need to know about their daughter's sleep patterns?
5. What would you recommend to Andree and David about their daughter?

REVIEW QUESTIONS

1. The nurse is gathering a sleep history from a patient who is being evaluated for obstructive sleep apnea. What symptom is the patient most likely to report?
   1. Headache
   2. Early wakening
   3. Impaired reasoning
   4. Excessive daytime sleepiness
2. When preparing a plan of care to promote sleep for a hospitalized patient, which of the following priority nursing interventions would the nurse incorporate?
   1. Ensure that the patient follows hospital routines.
   2. Avoid awakening the patient for nonessential tasks.
   3. Give prescribed sleeping medications at dinner.
   4. Turn the TV volume down for late-night programming.
3. Older persons are cautioned about the long-term use of sedatives and hypnotics because these medications are characterized by which of the following statements?
   1. They cause headaches and nausea.
   2. They are expensive and difficult to obtain.
   3. They cause severe depression and anxiety.
   4. They can lead to sleep disruption.
4. The nurse is providing health teaching for a patient using herbal compounds, such as valerian, to aid sleep. Key information about the use of herbal compounds would include the following:
   1. It can cause urinary retention.
   2. It may cause diarrhea and anxiety.
   3. It may interfere with prescribed medications.
   4. It can lead to further sleep problems over time.
5. A patient reports having vivid dreams. Through your understanding of the sleep cycle, you recognize that vivid dreaming occurs during which sleep phase?
   1. REM sleep
   2. Stage 1 NREM sleep
   3. Stage 4 NREM sleep
   4. Transition period from NREM to REM sleep
6. The nurse is providing instruction for a patient who is having difficulty falling asleep. The nurse identifies the need for further instruction when the patient says which of the following statements?
   1. I should avoid having drinks with caffeine before going to bed.
   2. If I can't get to sleep right away, I should get up and read a book.
   3. I should have an alcoholic drink before bedtime to help me relax.
   4. I should avoid exercising just before going to bed.
7. Which of the following interventions is appropriate to include in a care plan for improving sleep in the older person?
   1. Decrease fluids 2 to 4 hours before sleep.
   2. Exercise in the evening to increase fatigue.
   3. Allow the patient to sleep as late as possible.
   4. Take a nap during the day to make up for lost sleep.
8. Which statement made by a mother being discharged to home with her newborn infant indicates a need for further teaching?
   1. I won't put the baby to bed with a bottle.
   2. For the first few weeks, we are putting the cradle in our room.
   3. My grandmother told me that babies sleep better on their stomachs.
   4. I know I will have to get up during the night to feed the baby when he wakes up.
9. The nurse is developing a plan of care for a patient experiencing narcolepsy. Which of the following interventions is appropriate to include in the plan?
   1. Increase the amount of carbohydrates in the diet.
   2. Limit fluid intake 2 hours before bedtime.
   3. Preserve energy by limiting exercise to morning hours.
   4. Take one or two 20-minute naps during the day.
10. Which of the following nursing measures promotes sleep in school-aged children?
    1. Encourage evening exercise.
    2. Encourage television viewing.
    3. Ensure that the room is dark and quiet.
    4. Encourage quiet activities before bedtime.

Answers: 1. 4; **2.** 2; **3.** 4; **4.** 4; **5.** 1; **6.** 3; **7.** 1; **8.** 3; **9.** 4; **10.** 4

Rationales for the Review Questions appear at the end of the book.

RECOMMENDED WEBSITES

Canadian Lung Association: https://www.lung.ca.

This website provides information on obstructive sleep apnea (OSA), including strategies to enhance living with OSA and treatment modalities, such as continuous positive airway pressure (CPAP) devices. Sleep apnea in children is also discussed, with exploration of strategies to reduce the impact of sleep apnea, such as optimal nutrition and the use of CPAP devices.

Canadian Sleep Society: http://www.css.to.

This website provides a conduit for health care providers and researchers who are interested in sleep-related disorders, with an emphasis on sleep research performed in Canada. The site also provides information for the public on sleep-related topics and links to other sleep-related organizations, to enhance the understanding of sleep and its related disorders.

National Sleep Foundation (US): https://www.sleepfoundation.org.

This multilingual website, designed for both health care providers and the public, provides an exhaustive amount of information on a plethora of sleep-related topics—for example, restless leg syndrome, dementia, and menopause. The site provides access to sleep-related educational material and research reports, such as the 2011 annual Sleep in America poll that explores the impact of communication technology on sleep.

Public Health Agency of Canada: Sleep apnea: https://www.canada.ca/en/public-health/services/chronic-diseases/sleep-apnea.html.

This website includes publications intended for health care providers and the general public that are related to sleep apnea and other sleep disorders. It also includes a link to *Fast Facts from the 2009 Canadian Community Health Survey—Sleep Apnea Rapid Response.* This survey, conducted by Statistics Canada, estimated the prevalence of sleep apnea in the Canadian population.

Veterans Affairs Canada (VAC): http://www.veterans.gc.ca.

This website provides links to services, benefits, publications, and fact sheets relevant to Canadian veterans. Additionally, the site offers VAC information on many issues facing Canadian veterans, including the impact of post-traumatic stress disorder (PTSD) on sleep and strategies to help get a good night's sleep.

REFERENCES

Achermann, P., & Borbely, A. A. (2011). Sleep homeostasis and models of sleep regulation. In M. H. Kryger, T. Roth, & W. C. Dement (Eds.), *Principles and practice of sleep medicine* (5th ed., pp. 431–444). Philadelphia, PA: Elsevier.

Agarwal, S., Richardson, B., Krishnan, V., et al. (2009). Interstitial lung disease and sleep: What is known? *Sleep Medicine, 10*(9), 947–951. doi:10.1016/j.sleep.2009.01.004.

Ahmed, I., & Thorpy, M. (2010). Clinical features, diagnosis and treatment of narcolepsy. *Clinical Chest Medicine, 31*(2), 371–381. doi:10.1016/j.ccm.2010.02.014.

Anic, G. M., Titus-Ernstoff, L., Newcomb, P. A., et al. (2010). Sleep duration and obesity in a population-based study. *Sleep Medicine, 11*(5), 447–451. doi:10.1016/j.sleep.2009.11.013.

Atwood, C. W., Jr., Strollo, P. J., Jr., & Givelber, R. (2011). Medical therapy for obstructive sleep apnea. In M. H. Kryger, T. Roth, & W. C. Dement (Eds.), *Principles and practice of sleep medicine* (5th ed., pp. 1219–1232). Philadelphia, PA: Elsevier.

Bae, C., & Avidan, A. (2008). Sleep disorders. In H. R. Smith, C. L. Comella, & B. Hogl (Eds.), *Sleep medicine* (pp. 9–24). New York: Cambridge University Press.

Balkin, T. J. (2011). Performance deficits during sleep loss: Effects of time awake, time of day and time on task. In M. H. Kryger, T. Roth, & W. C. Dement (Eds.), *Principles and practice of sleep medicine* (5th ed., pp. 738–744). Philadelphia, PA: Elsevier.

Balserak, B. I., & Lee, K. (2011). Sleep disturbances and sleep-related disorders in pregnancy. In M. H. Kryger, T. Roth, & W. C. Dement (Eds.), *Principles and practice of sleep medicine* (5th ed., pp. 1572–1586). Philadelphia, PA: Elsevier.

Belenky, G., & Akerstedt, T. (2011). Occupational sleep medicine. In M. H. Kryger, T. Roth, & W. C. Dement (Eds.), *Principles and practice of sleep medicine* (5th ed., pp. 734–737). Philadelphia, PA: Elsevier.

Billard, M. (2008). Normal sleep. In H. R. Smith, C. L. Comella, & B. Hogl (Eds.), *Sleep medicine* (pp. 9–24). Cambridge, NY: Cambridge University Press.

Bloom, H. G., Ahmed, I., Alessi, C. A., et al. (2009). Evidence-based recommendations for the assessment and management of sleep disorders in older persons. *Journal of American Geriatrics Society, 57*(11), 761–789. doi:10.1111/j.1532-5415.2009.02549.x.

Buchanan, P., & Grunstein, R. (2011). Positive airway pressure treatment for obstructive sleep apnea-hypopnea syndrome. In M. H. Kryger, T. Roth, & W. C. Dement (Eds.), *Principles and practice of sleep medicine* (5th ed., pp. 1233–1249). Philadelphia, PA: Elsevier.

Buysse, D. J. (2011). Clinical pharmacology of other drugs used as hypnotics. In M. H. Kryger, T. Roth, & W. C. Dement (Eds.), *Principles and practice of sleep medicine* (5th ed., pp. 492–502). Philadelphia, PA: Elsevier.

Canadian Nurses Association. (2015). *Framework for the practice of registered nurses in Canada.* Ottawa: Author. Retrieved from https://www.cna-aiic.ca/~/media/cna/page-content/pdf-en/framework-for-the-pracice-of-registered-nurses-in-canada.

Cao, M. T., Guilleminault, C., & Kushida, C. A. (2011). Clinical features and evaluation of obstructive sleep apnea and upper airway resistance syndrome. In M. H. Kryger, T. Roth, & W. C. Dement (Eds.), *Principles and practice of sleep medicine* (5th ed., pp. 1206–1218). Philadelphia, PA: Elsevier.

Carpenito, L. J. (2016). *Nursing diagnosis: Application to clinical practice* (15th ed.). Philadelphia, PA: Lippincott Williams & Wilkins.

Carskadon, M. A., & Dement, W. C. (2011). Normal human sleep: An overview. In M. H. Kryger, T. Roth, & W. C. Dement (Eds.), *Principles and practice of sleep medicine* (5th ed., pp. 16–41). Philadelphia, PA: Elsevier.

Chasens, E. R., Williams, L. L., Umlauf, M. G., et al. (2008). Excessive sleepiness. In E. Capezuti, D. Zwicker, & M. Mezey (Eds.), *Evidence-based geriatric nursing protocols for best practice* (3rd ed., pp. 459–476). New York: Springer.

Chervin, R. D. (2011). Use of clinical tools and tests in sleep medicine. In M. H. Kryger, T. Roth, & W. C. Dement (Eds.), *Principles and practice of sleep medicine* (5th ed., pp. 666–679). Philadelphia, PA: Elsevier.

Cistulli, P. A., Ferguson, K. A., & Lowe, A. A. (2011). Oral appliances for sleep-disordered breathing. In M. H. Kryger, T. Roth, & W. C. Dement (Eds.), *Principles and practice of sleep medicine* (5th ed., pp. 1266–1277). Philadelphia, PA: Elsevier.

Cmiel, C. A., Karr, D. M., Gasser, D. M., et al. (2004). Noise control: A nursing team's approach to sleep promotion. *American Journal of Nursing, 104*(2), 40–48.

Cohen, F. L. (2004). Measuring sleep. In M. Frank-Stromborg & S. J. Olsen (Eds.), *Instruments for clinical-healthcare research* (3rd ed., pp. 264–285). Boston, MA: Jones & Bartlett.

Collop, N. A., Salas, R. E., Delayo, M., et al. (2008). Normal sleep and circadian processes. *Critical Care Clinics, 24*(3), 449–460. doi:10.1016/j.ccc.2008.02.002.

Cook, N. F. (2008a). Understanding narcolepsy, part 1: Epidemiology and neurophysiology. *British Journal of Neuroscience Nursing, 4*(3), 108–114.

Cook, N. F. (2008b). Understanding narcolepsy, part 2: Accurate diagnosis and effective management. *British Journal of Neuroscience Nursing, 4*(4), 170–176.

Crabtree, V., & Williams, N. A. (2009). Normal sleep in children and adolescents. *Child and Adolescent Psychiatric Clinics of North America, 18*(4), 799–811. doi:10.1016/j.chc.2009.04.013.

Doghramji, K. (2010). The evaluation and management of insomnia. *Clinics in Chest Medicine, 31*(2), 327–339. doi:10.1016/j.ccm.2010.03.001.

Drake, C. L., & Wright, K. P., Jr. (2011). Shift work, shift work disorder and jet lag. In M. H. Kryger, T. Roth, & W. C. Dement (Eds.), *Principles and practice of sleep medicine* (5th ed., pp. 784–798). Philadelphia, PA: Elsevier.

Drouot, X., Cabello, B., D'Ortho, M. P., et al. (2008). Sleep in the intensive care unit. *Sleep Medicine Reviews, 12*(5), 391–403. doi:10.1016/j.smr.2007.11.004.

Elliott, R., McKinley, S., & Cistulli, P. (2011). The quality and duration of sleep in the intensive care setting: An integrative review. *International Journal of Nursing Studies, 48*(3), 384–400. doi:10.1016/j.ijnurstu.2010.11.006.

Espiritu, J. R. D. (2008). Aging-related sleep changes. *Clinics in Geriatric Medicine, 24*(1), 1–14. doi:10.1016/j.cger.2007.08.007.

Faraco, J., & Mignot, E. (2011). Genetics of sleep and sleep disorders in humans. In M. H. Kryger, T. Roth, & W. C. Dement (Eds.), *Principles and practice of sleep medicine* (5th ed., pp. 184–198). Philadelphia, PA: Elsevier.

Gradisar, M., Gardner, G., & Dohnt, H. (2011). Recent world-wide sleep patterns and problems during adolescence: A review and meta-analysis of age, region and sleep. *Sleep Medicine, 12*(2), 110–118. doi:10.1016/j.sleep.2010.11.008.

Hockenberry, M. J., & Wilson, D. (2014). *Wong's nursing care of infants and children* (9th ed.). New York: Mosby.

Jennum, P., Knudsen, S., & Kjellberg, J. (2009). The economic consequences of narcolepsy. *Journal of Clinical Sleep Medicine, 5*(3), 240–245.

Krystal, A. D. (2011). Pharmacologic treatments: Other medications. In M. H. Kryger, T. Roth, & W. C. Dement (Eds.), *Principles and practice of sleep medicine* (5th ed., pp. 916–930). Philadelphia, PA: Elsevier.

Laposky, A. D., Bass, J., Kohsaka, A., et al. (2008). Sleep and circadian rhythms: Key components in the regulation of energy metabolism. *Federation of European Biochemical Societies, 582*(1), 142–151. doi:10.1016/j.febslet.2007.06.079.

Lavigne, G., Smith, M. T., Denis, R., et al. (2011). Pain and sleep. In M. H. Kryger, T. Roth, & W. C. Dement (Eds.), *Principles and practice of sleep medicine* (5th ed., pp. 1442–1451). Philadelphia, PA: Elsevier.

Lee, K. A., & Moe, K. E. (2011). Menopause. In M. H. Kryger, T. Roth, & W. C. Dement (Eds.), *Principles and practice of sleep medicine* (5th ed., pp. 1592–1601). Philadelphia, PA: Elsevier.

Lee-Chiong, T., Jr. (2008). *Sleep medicine: Essentials and review.* New York: Oxford University Press.

Lei, Z., Qiongjing, Y., Qiuli, W., et al. (2009). Sleep quality and sleep disturbing factors of inpatients in a Chinese hospital. *Journal of Clinical Nursing, 18*(1), 2521–2529. doi: 10.1111/j.1365-2702.2009.02846.x.

Magee, C. A., Iverson, D. C., Huang, X. F., et al. (2008). A link between chronic sleep restriction and obesity: Methodological considerations. *Public Health, 122*(12), 1373–1381. doi:10.1016/j.puhe.2008.05.010.

Mendelson, W. B. (2011). Hypnotic medications: Mechanisms of action and pharmacologic effects. In M. H. Kryger, T. Roth, & W. C. Dement (Eds.), *Principles and practice of sleep medicine* (5th ed., pp. 483–491). Philadelphia, PA: Elsevier.

Milner, C. E., & Belicki, K. (2010). Assessment and treatment of insomnia in adults: A guide for clinicians. *Journal of Counseling & Development, 88*(2), 236–244. doi:10.1002.j.1556-6678.2010.tb00015.x/full.

Morin, C. M. (2011). Psychological and behavioral treatments for insomnia I: Approaches and efficacy. In M. H. Kryger, T. Roth, & W. C. Dement (Eds.), *Principles and practice of sleep medicine* (5th ed., pp. 866–883). Philadelphia, PA: Elsevier.

National Sleep Foundation. (2009). *Diet, exercise and sleep*. Arlington, VA: Author. Retrieved from https://sleepfoundation.org/sleep-topics/diet-exercise-and-sleep.

National Sleep Foundation. (2017a). *Melatonin and sleep*. Arlington, VA: Author. Retrieved from https://sleepfoundation.org/sleep-topics/melatonin-and-sleep.

National Sleep Foundation. (2017b). *How much sleep do adults need?* Arlington, VA: Author. Retrieved from http://www.sleepfoundation.org/article/white-papers/how-much-sleep-do-adults-need.

Neikrug, A. B., & Ancoli-Israel, S. (2010). Sleep disorders in the older adult: A mini-review. *Gerontology, 56*(2), 181–189. doi:10.1159/000236900.

Nielsen, T. (2011). Dream analysis and classification: The reality simulation perspective. In M. H. Kryger, T. Roth, & W. C. Dement (Eds.), *Principles and practice of sleep medicine* (5th ed., pp. 76–91). Philadelphia, PA: Elsevier.

O'Malley, M. B., Gleeson, S. K., & Weir, I. D. (2011). Wake-promoting medications: Efficacy and adverse effects. In M. H. Kryger, T. Roth, & W. C. Dement (Eds.), *Principles and practice of sleep medicine* (5th ed., pp. 866–883). Philadelphia, PA: Elsevier.

Orezel-GryGlewska, J. (2009). Consequences of sleep deprivation. *International Journal of Occupational Medicine and Environmental Health, 23*(1), 95–114.

Paavonen, E. J., Porkka-Heiskanen, T., & Lahikainen, A. R. (2009). Sleep quality, duration and behavioral symptoms among 5–6-year-old children. *European Child & Adolescent Psychiatry, 18*(12), 747–754. doi:10.1007/s00787-009-0033-8.

Patel, M., Chipman, J., Carlin, B. W., et al. (2008). Sleep in the intensive care unit. *Critical Care Nursing, 31*(4), 309–318. doi:10.1097/01.CNQ.0000336817.89300.08.

Patel, S. R. (2009). Reduced sleep as an obesity risk factor. *Obesity Reviews, 10*(2), 61–68. doi:10.1111/j.1467-789X.2009.00664.x.

Patel, S. R., Blackwell, T., Redline, S., et al. (2008). The association between sleep duration and obesity in older adults. *International Journal of Obesity, 32*(12), 1825–1834. doi:10.1038/ijo.2008.198.

Philip, P., Sagaspe, P., & Taillard, J. (2011). Drowsy driving. In M. H. Kryger, T. Roth, & W. C. Dement (Eds.), *Principles and practice of sleep medicine* (5th ed., pp. 769–774). Philadelphia, PA: Elsevier.

Ramar, K., & Guilleminault, C. (2008). Sleep apnea (central and obstructive). In H. R. Smith, C. L. Comella, & B. Hogl (Eds.), *Sleep medicine* (pp. 129–156). New York: Cambridge University Press.

Ramsawh, H., Stein, M. B., & Mellman, T. A. (2011). Psychiatric disorders. In M. H. Kryger, T. Roth, & W. C. Dement (Eds.), *Principles and practice of sleep medicine* (5th ed., pp. 1473–1487). Philadelphia, PA: Elsevier.

Reeve, K., & Bailes, B. (2010). Insomnia in adults: Etiology and management. *Journal for Nurse Practitioners, 6*(1), 53–60. doi:10.1016/j.nurpra.2009.09.013.

Roepke, S. K., & Ancoli-Israel, S. (2010). Sleep disorders in the elderly. *Indian Journal of Medical Research, 131*, 302–310.

Seo, W. S., Sung, H. M., Lee, J. H., et al. (2010). Sleep patterns and their age-related changes in elementary school children. *Sleep Medicine, 11*(6), 569–575. doi:10.1016/j.sleep.2010.03.011.

Siegel, J. M. (2011). Sleep mechanisms and phylogeny. In M. H. Kryger, T. Roth, & W. C. Dement (Eds.), *Principles and practice of sleep medicine* (5th ed., pp. 76–91). Philadelphia, PA: Elsevier.

Silvestri, R., & Arico, I. (2008). Parasomnias. In H. R. Smith, C. L. Comella, & B. Hogl (Eds.), *Sleep medicine* (pp. 47–55). New York: Cambridge University Press.

Smith, H. R., Comella, C. L., & Hogl, B. (Eds.), (2008). *Sleep medicine*. New York: Cambridge University Press.

Snowden, A. (2008). Insomnia: Management and treatments. *Nurse Prescribing, 6*(9), 382–389.

Stickgold, R., & Wamsley, E. J. (2011). Why we dream. In M. H. Kryger, T. Roth, & W. C. Dement (Eds.), *Principles and practice of sleep medicine* (5th ed., pp. 76–91). Philadelphia, PA: Elsevier.

Tibbits, G. M. (2008). Sleep disorders: Causes, effects and solutions. *Primary Care Clinics Office Practice, 35*(4), 817–837. doi:10.1016/j.pop.2008.07.006.

Van Cauter, E., Spiegel, K., Tasali, E., et al. (2008). Metabolic consequences of sleep and sleep loss. *Sleep Medicine, 9*(S1), S23–S28. doi:10.1016/S1389-9457(08)70013-3.

Verrier, R. L., & Josephson, M. E. (2011). Cardiac arrhythmogenesis during sleep: Mechanisms, diagnosis, and therapy. In M. Kryger, T. Roth, & W. C. Dement (Eds.), *Principles and practice of sleep medicine* (5th ed., pp. 1363–1380). Philadelphia, PA: Elsevier.

Wellman, A., & White, D. P. (2011). Central sleep apnea and periodic breathing. In M. H. Kryger, T. Roth, & W. C. Dement (Eds.), *Principles and practice of sleep medicine* (5th ed., pp. 1140–1152). Philadelphia, PA: Elsevier.

Wyatt, J. K., & Crisostomo, M. I. (2008). Insomnias. In H. R. Smith, C. L. Comella, & B. Hogl (Eds.), *Sleep medicine* (pp. 97–112). New York: Cambridge University Press.

42

Nutrition

Canadian content written by Kathryn Weaver, RN, PhD
Original chapter by Kristine Rose, BSN, MSN

OBJECTIVES

Mastery of content in this chapter will enable you to:

- Define the key terms listed.
- Explain the role of each major nutrient in proper nutrition.
- Explain the importance of maintaining a balance between energy intake and expenditure.
- List the end products of carbohydrate, protein, and fat metabolism.
- Explain the significance of saturated, unsaturated, polyunsaturated, and trans fats.
- Be aware of national position statements and recommendations regarding sugar consumption.
- Describe *Eating Well With Canada's Food Guide* and its value in planning nutritious meals.
- Specify recommended dietary intake for age and sex groups in Canada to ensure that patients meet the varied essential vitamins, minerals, and nutritional requirements throughout their growth and development.
- Understand how to plan sample menus for cardiac diets, renal diets, lactose intolerance, gluten-free, and diabetes diets.
- Describe how to count calories and substitute items for diabetic patients.
- Identify the role of the dietitian, nutritionist, and speech-language pathologist in promoting healthy diets and preventing risks such as aspiration.
- Discuss the major methods of nutritional assessment.
- Identify three major nutritional problems, the patients who are at risk, and related nutrition therapy.
- Formulate a plan of care to help meet the specific nutritional needs of infants, toddlers, preschoolers, school-aged children, adolescents, adults, and older persons.
- Plan for the daily nutritional intake of pregnant women.
- Identify the potential nutritional deficits associated with vegetarian diets, giving special consideration to vegan and lacto-ovo diets.
- Identify any risks associated with genetically modified food.
- Explain how to set up a meal tray for the visually impaired patient.
- Discuss diet counselling and patient teaching in relation to patient expectations.
- State the goals of enteral and parenteral nutrition.
- Describe the procedure for initiating and maintaining tube feedings and avoiding related complications.

KEY TERMS

Amino acids, p. 1099
Anabolism, p. 1102
Anorexia, p. 1125
Anorexia nervosa, p. 1108
Anthropometry, p. 1113
Aquaporins, p. 1100
Aspiration, p. 1102
Basal metabolic rate (BMR), p. 1098
Body mass index (BMI), p. 1113
Bulimia nervosa, p. 1108
Carbohydrates, p. 1099
Catabolism, p. 1102
Cholesterol, p. 1100
Chyme, p. 1102
Complementary proteins, p. 1100
Complex carbohydrates, p. 1099
Dietary reference intakes (DRIs), p. 1103
Dysphagia, p. 1102
Elemental formulas, p. 1141
Enteral nutrition, p. 1135
Enzymes, p. 1102
Essential amino acids, p. 1099
Fat-soluble vitamins, p. 1100
Fatty acids, p. 1100
Food security, p. 1105
Fortified foods, p. 1099
Functional foods, p. 1099
Genetically modified (GM) food, p. 1099
Gluconeogenesis, p. 1103
Glycemic index, p. 1099
Glycogenesis, p. 1103
Glycogenolysis, p. 1103
Hypervitaminosis, p. 1101
Ideal body weight (IBW), p. 1113
Ketones, p. 1103
Lipid emulsions, p. 1156
Lipids, p. 1100
Macrominerals, p. 1101
Metabolism, p. 1102
Minerals, p. 1101
Modular formulas, p. 1141
Monounsaturated fatty acids, p. 1100
Nitrogen balance, p. 1100
Nonessential amino acids, p. 1099
Novel food, p. 1099
Nutrient density, p. 1099
Nutrients, p. 1099
Nutritional assessment, p. 1113
Nutritional screening, p. 1113
Organic food, p. 1099
Parenteral nutrition, p. 1149
Peristalsis, p. 1102
Polymeric formulas, p. 1141
Polyunsaturated fatty acids, p. 1100
Refeeding syndrome, p. 1149
Resting energy expenditure (REE), p. 1098
Saccharides, p. 1099

MEDIA RESOURCES

http://evolve.elsevier.com/Canada/Potter/fundamentals/

- Audio Chapter Summaries
- Examination Review Questions
- Concept Map Creator
- Case Study with Questions
- Audio Glossary
- Content Updates
- Video Clips

Proper nutrition and food safety—important to all Canadians—are a shared responsibility among government, industry, health providers, and consumers. Food supplies energy for accomplishing everyday activities, building and repairing tissues, and regulating organs and systems while helping to prevent the contraction of certain diseases and aid in the recovery from other diseases. Food also holds symbolic meaning for many cultures and communities. Since the 1930s, Health Canada has worked collaboratively with federal partners, provinces, territories, and other stakeholders to enhance nutritional health and well-being through evidence-informed nutrition policies and standards. These efforts to advise and inform about the safety and nutritional value of food have promoted environments that support Canadians in making healthy food choices (Health Canada, 2015).

As nurses, we must pay as much attention to our patients' diets as to their illnesses, treatments, and therapies. In fact, in illnesses such as type 1 diabetes mellitus, a common health concern across Western nations, diet can be a major treatment, and nurses are key professionals responsible for educating patients and families about food choices and available technology (e.g., insulin pumps) that influence the course of the disease and assist in self-management. Along with type 1 diabetes, other conditions, such as type 2 diabetes, hypertension, and inflammatory bowel disease, require highly specialized nutritional support protocols that include diets low in sugars, cholesterol, or salt (Leung, Nerenberg, Daskalopoulou, et al., 2016).

In comparison to citizens of other developed countries, the nutritional health of Canadians is good. This story may be changing, however, as Canadians face evolving demographic and economic issues that include a rising poverty rate, a decline in resources available to rural and remote communities, the aging of the population, and the social isolation or marginalization of certain groups of citizens. To illustrate, nearly one in six Canadians was at least 65 years old in 2015 (Statistics Canada, 2015); these older persons are choosing to stay in their own homes longer, placing them at risk for poor nutrition associated with mobility impairments and social isolation. Also, rates of stay-at-home spouses have dropped significantly, from 1.5 million in 1976 to 500 000 in 2014 (Statistics Canada, 2015), which leaves the majority of preschool children in day care or school while parents work. According to the *2015 National Report Card on Child and Family Poverty in Canada*, one in five Canadian children, more than 1.3 million, live below the poverty line. Poverty rates are even worse among children who are from Indigenous and racialized communities, in immigrant families, or in families affected by disability (Lloyd & Bailey, 2015). Indigenous populations increased by 232 385 people, or 20.1%, between 2006 and 2011, compared with 5.2% for the non-Indigenous population (Statistics Canada, 2016a). This increase is significant because Indigenous children account for approximately 7% of all children in Canada (Statistics Canada, 2016a), with 60% of First Nations children on reserves living below the poverty line (Kirkup, 2016). Alongside the increase in Indigenous population there is an increase in immigrant population, with nearly 56.9% of the 1 162 900 foreign-born people who immigrated to Canada between 2006 and 2011 coming from Asia and the Middle East. Together, recent immigrants comprised 17.2% of the foreign-born population and 3.5% of Canada's total population (Statistics Canada, 2016b). All these factors, along with the larger international issues arising from free trade and globalization, influence the nutritional health of Canadians.

One trend that has taken on alarming proportions is the increase in overweight and obesity. In 2014, 14 222 521 or approximately 54% of adult Canadians reported height and weight that classified them as being overweight or obese (Statistics Canada, 2017). Likewise, the prevalence of obesity has tripled over the past three decades (Government of Canada, 2016a). Close to one third (31.5%) of 5- to 17-year-olds, an estimated 1.6 million, were classified as overweight (19.8%) or obese (11.7%) in 2009 to 2011 (Roberts, Shields, de Groh, et al., 2015), with the percentage of boys aged 5 to 11 years who were obese (19.5%) being more than three times the percentage of girls who were obese (6.3%). Type 2 diabetes, an illness largely preventable through healthy eating and weight management (Canadian Diabetes Association [CDA], 2016) that in the past occurred mainly in older individuals, is now being diagnosed in Canadian children (Government of Canada, 2015). Among Indigenous people, rates of type 2 diabetes are three to five times higher than those of the general population (Health Canada, 2013a). Factors adversely affecting the nutritional health of today's Canadian society are serious, and the resultant conditions border on epidemic proportions. It is critical that nurses acquire nutritional knowledge to apply to the complexities of diseases, diverse populations, and current demographics (age, gender, income level, and culture).

SCIENTIFIC KNOWLEDGE BASE

Nutrients: the Biochemical Units of Nutrition

The body requires fuel to provide energy for the chemical reactions that enable cellular growth and repair, organ function, and body movement. The energy requirement of a person at rest is called the **basal metabolic rate (BMR)**. This is the energy needed to maintain life-sustaining activities (breathing, circulation, heart rate, and temperature) for a specific period of time. The **resting energy expenditure (REE)** is a measurement that accounts for BMR plus energy to digest meals and perform mild activity. REE is a baseline of energy requirement accounting for approximately 60% to 75% of our daily needs. Factors of age, body mass, gender, fever, environmental temperature, pregnancy, lactation, starvation, stress, illness, injury, infection, activity level, thyroid function, or the use of certain drugs may affect energy requirements or metabolism.

In general, when energy requirements are completely met by kilocalorie (kcal) intake in food, weight does not change. A kilocalorie (referred to as a "calorie" by the general public) is the unit of energy required to raise 1 kilogram of water by 1°C. When the kilocalories ingested exceed energy demands over time, a person gains weight. If the kilocalories ingested fail to meet energy requirements, a person loses weight.

Nutrients are the elements supplied by food that are necessary for body processes and function. Energy needs are met from three categories of nutrients: carbohydrates, proteins, and fats. Other nutrients are water, vitamins, and minerals, which do not provide energy but contribute to metabolic processes, including acid–base balance. A nutrient is considered essential if the body cannot manufacture it in a sufficient quantity to meet metabolic demands.

Foods are described according to **nutrient density**, the proportion of essential nutrients to the number of kilocalories. High nutrient-density foods, such as fruits and vegetables, provide a large number of nutrients in relation to kilocalories. Low nutrient-density foods, such as alcohol or refined sugar, are high in kilocalories but nutrient poor.

Foods may also be described as functional, organic, or novel. **Functional foods** (Agriculture and Agri-Food Canada, 2017) have had biologically active ingredients added that have demonstrated health benefits (e.g., probiotic yogurt, or pea fibre–fortified breads and pasta). **Fortified foods** have additional vitamins and/or minerals to provide added health benefits (e.g., fortified soy beverages and fruit juice with calcium), or are enhanced with bioactive components through plant breeding, genetic modification, processing, or special livestock feeding techniques (e.g., eggs, milk, and meat with omega-3). **Organic foods** are vegetables, fruit, eggs, milk, and meat produced without synthetic (human-made) pesticides, herbicides, and fertilizers; genetically modified organisms (GMOs); antibiotics or growth hormones; or irradiation or ionizing radiation (a way to preserve food with radiation energy). Organic farmers may use natural pesticides approved for organic food production (EatRight Ontario, 2017a). **Novel** or **genetically modified (GM) food** has undergone the practice of inserting the genes of one organism into another organism, often to resist disease and develop desired characteristics, such as a hardier texture, higher nutritional value, or faster growth (EatRight Ontario, 2017b). A review of 12 long-term studies (>90 days and up to 2 years in duration) and 12 multigenerational studies (from two to five generations) on the effects of diets containing GM corn, potato, soybean, rice, or triticale (a wheat and rye hybrid) on animal health did not suggest any health hazards and, for the most part, presented evidence to show GM plants as being nutritionally equivalent to their non-GM counterparts and as safe for use in food and feed (Snell, Bernheim, Bergé, et al., 2012). Nonetheless, Health Canada assesses the safety of all genetically modified and other novel foods proposed for sale in Canada because novel food products do not have a history of safe use as a food (Health Canada, 2017a). There is no mandatory labelling of these foods in Canada, despite intensive public campaigning and 20 years of polling that has consistently shown over 80% of Canadians want these labels (Canadian Biotechnology Action Network, 2018). According to Bawa and Anilakumar (2013), the public lacks trust in institutions and institutional activities regarding GM foods and perceives that institutions have failed to take account of the public's actual concerns. On December 13, 2016, the House of Commons Standing Committee on Agriculture and Agri-Food recommended greater transparency in the regulation of GM animals and government support for independent research into the health, environmental, and other effects of genetic modification technologies (House of Commons, Standing Committee on Agriculture and Agri-Food, 2016).

Carbohydrates. **Carbohydrates** are the recommended main source of energy in the diet. Each gram of carbohydrate produces 4 kcal and serves as the main source of fuel (glucose) for the brain, skeletal muscles during exercise, red and white blood cell production, and cell function of the renal medulla. Carbohydrates are obtained primarily from plant foods, except for lactose (milk sugar), and are classified according to their carbohydrate units, or **saccharides**.

Monosaccharides such as glucose (dextrose) or fructose (fruit sugar) are the building blocks of all other carbohydrates and cannot be broken down into a more basic carbohydrate unit. Disaccharides such as sucrose, lactose, and maltose are composed of two monosaccharides minus one unit of water. Both monosaccharides and disaccharides are classified as **simple carbohydrates** called *sugars.* Polysaccharides are composed of many carbohydrate units and are classified as **complex carbohydrates**. They include starch (stored form of glucose in plants) and glycogen (stored glucose in animals and humans). Some polysaccharides cannot be digested because humans do not have enzymes capable of breaking them down. Insoluble fibres are not digestible and include cellulose, hemicellulose, and lignin. Soluble fibres include pectin, guar gum, and mucilage. Dietary fibre is important to disease prevention, as it decreases low-density lipoprotein (LDL) cholesterol associated with the development of heart disease (Wadhera, Steen, Khan, et al., 2016).

Carbohydrate-rich foods are ranked according to their **glycemic index**, the effect on blood glucose levels and insulin response (CDA, 2018). Carbohydrates that release glucose rapidly into the bloodstream (e.g., white bread, candy) have a high glycemic index. Carbohydrates that produce only small fluctuations in blood glucose (e.g., barley, lentils) have a low glycemic index and offer long-term health benefits of sustaining weight loss, prolonging physical endurance, and reducing risks associated with heart disease and diabetes.

The Heart and Stroke Foundation of Canada (2017a) recommends consuming no more than 10% total calories per day from added sugars and ideally less than 5%; for an average 2 000 calorie-a-day diet, 10% is about 48 grams (or 12 teaspoons) of added sugars. Sugar is found in many foods, both naturally, such as in vegetables, fruit, and milk, and added. While foods containing natural sugars are an important part of a healthy diet because they also contain important nutrients, added sugars provide energy (calories) but no nutritional value on their own. Sugars are often added to processed foods to improve their flavour, colour, texture, and shelf life. Added sugar may be listed as glucose, fructose, dextrose, maltose, or sucrose on the ingredient listing on food labels. If any of these sugars are listed as the first or second ingredient on a food label, the food is likely high in sugar. One can of a soft drink contains approximately 10 teaspoons of daily added sugar. Other foods often high in added sugar include energy drinks, fruit-flavoured drinks, sports drinks, hot chocolate, specialty coffees, baked goods, and desserts. Consuming too much sugar is associated with heart disease, stroke, obesity, diabetes, high blood cholesterol, cancer, and dental cavities.

Proteins. Proteins are essential for synthesis (building) of body tissue in growth, maintenance, and repair. Collagen, hormones, enzymes, immune cells, DNA, and RNA are all composed of protein. In addition, blood clotting, fluid regulation, and acid–base balance require proteins. Nutrients and many pharmacological substances are transported in the blood by proteins.

The simplest form of protein is the amino acid. As with other nutrients, **essential amino acids** are those that the body cannot synthesize but must have provided in the diet. **Nonessential amino acids** can be synthesized by the body. **Amino acids** are linked together by peptide bonds to form larger protein molecules called *polypeptides*. Simple proteins such as albumin and insulin contain only amino acids or their derivatives. The combination of a simple protein with a nonprotein substance produces a more complex protein, such as lipoprotein, formed by a combination of a lipid (fat) and a simple protein.

Protein quality is determined by the balance of essential amino acids. Incomplete proteins lack a sufficient quantity of one or more essential amino acids and include cereals, legumes (beans, peas), and vegetables. A complete protein contains all of the nine essential amino acids in sufficient quantity to support growth and maintain nitrogen balance. Examples of foods that contain complete proteins are chicken, soybeans, fish, and cheese. Complete proteins are referred to as *high-quality proteins*. **Complementary proteins** are pairs of incomplete proteins that, when combined, supply the total amount of protein provided by complete protein sources.

Protein is the only major nutrient that contains nitrogen (it is 16% nitrogen) and is the only source of nitrogen for the body. Thus, nitrogen can be used to determine protein balance in the body. **Nitrogen balance** is achieved when the intake and output of nitrogen are equal. When the intake of nitrogen exceeds the output, the body is in positive nitrogen balance, which is required for growth, normal pregnancy, maintenance of lean muscle mass and vital organs, and wound healing. The nitrogen retained by the body is used for the building, repair, and replacement of body tissues. Negative nitrogen balance occurs when the body loses more nitrogen than it gains—for example, with severe infection, burns, fever, starvation, head injury, and trauma. The increased nitrogen loss is the result of body tissue destruction or loss of nitrogen-containing body fluids through urine, feces, sweat, and, at times, bleeding or vomiting. Nutrition during this period must provide nutrients to put patients into positive balance for healing.

Protein can be used to provide energy (4 kcal/g), but because of protein's essential role in growth, maintenance, and repair, adequate kilocalories should be provided in the diet from nonprotein sources. Protein is spared as an energy source when carbohydrate in the diet is sufficient to meet the energy needs of the body.

Fats. Fats (**lipids**) are the most calorically dense nutrient, providing 9 kcal/g. In addition to serving as fuel that supplies energy, fat cushions vital organs, lubricates body tissue, insulates, and protects cell membranes. Fats are composed of glycerol and fatty acids. **Triglycerides** circulate in the blood and are made up of three fatty acids attached to a glycerol. **Fatty acids** are composed of chains of carbon and hydrogen atoms with an acid group on one end of the chain and a methyl group at the other. Fatty acids can be **saturated,** in which each carbon in the chain has two attached hydrogen atoms, or **unsaturated,** in which an unequal number of hydrogen atoms are attached and the carbon atoms attach to each other with a double bond. **Monounsaturated fatty acids** have one double bond, whereas **polyunsaturated fatty acids** have two or more double carbon bonds. Most animal fats have high proportions of saturated fatty acids, whereas vegetable fats have higher amounts of monounsaturated and polyunsaturated fatty acids. The various types of fatty acids have significance for health and the incidence of disease, including heart disease, stroke, certain cancers, and diabetes, and are referred to in the dietary guidelines from the Heart and Stroke Foundation of Canada (2017b), the Canadian Cancer Society (2018), the Canadian Diabetes Association (2016), and the Canadian Cardiovascular Society (Anderson, Grégoire, Pearson, et al., 2016).

Trans fatty acids have received attention for their role in the development of coronary artery disease (Academy of Nutrition and Dietetics, 2014; Peterson & Zu, 2016). Formed by the partial hydrogenation of vegetable oils and mostly found in prepared foods, snack foods, and margarines, trans fats raise blood levels of so-called bad cholesterol (LDL-cholesterol) while lowering blood levels of so-called good cholesterol (high-density lipoprotein [HDL]-cholesterol), which protects against heart disease (Government of Canada, 2016b). Trans fatty acids have also been associated with diabetes (De Souza, Mente, Maroleanu, et al., 2015; Peterson & Zu, 2016), Alzheimer's disease and cognitive decline (Barnard, Bunner, & Agarwal, 2014; Morris & Tangney, 2014), infertility in men and women (Chavarro, Mínguez-Alarcón, Mendiola, et al., 2014; Sharma, Biedenharn, Fedor, et al., 2013), and prostate cancer in men (Brasky, Darke, Song, et al., 2013). The evidence, however, is inconclusive and contradictory.

Increased research and consumer awareness have led to mandatory nutrition labelling of trans fats in Canada since 2005. The acceptable macronutrient distribution range (AMDR), the range associated with reduced risk of chronic illness while providing essential intake of total fat, is 20% to 35% for adults (Academy of Nutrition and Dietetics, 2014). It is recommended that Canadians decrease their intake of the proportion of saturated and trans fatty acids. This is best accomplished by using soft margarines (liquid or tub varieties) over harder, stick forms, looking for "0 g trans fat" on the nutrition facts label, and choosing whole, natural foods and foods made with unhydrogenated oil rather than partially hydrogenated or hydrogenated vegetable oils or saturated fat.

Cholesterol is often discussed in connection with fats, although it is a sterol, not a triglyceride (Schlenker & Gilbert, 2014). It occurs naturally in animal foods but is also synthesized by the liver. Cholesterol deposits in blood vessel walls cause atherosclerosis, which is the underlying cause of coronary artery disease.

Water. Water is a critical component of the body because cell function depends on a fluid environment. Water makes up 60% to 70% of total body weight. The percentage of total body water is greater for lean people than for obese people because muscle contains more water than any other tissue except blood. Infants have the greatest percentage of total body water, and older people have the least. When deprived of water, a person cannot survive for more than a few days. Water helps regulate body temperature and acts as a solvent for nutrients and waste products. Water passes freely through membranes that separate body fluids inside (intracellular) and outside (extracellular) cells. Various water-transport proteins called **aquaporins** function as water-selective channels in many cells, altering the speed at which water crosses cell membranes and influencing conditions such as cataract formation, hypertension, and salivary gland function (Verkman, Anderson, & Papadopoulos, 2014).

Fluid needs are met by ingesting liquids and solid foods high in water content, such as fresh fruits and vegetables. Water is also produced during digestion when food is oxidized. In a healthy individual, fluid intake from all sources equals fluid output through elimination, respiration, and sweating (see Chapters 36 and 38). An ill person can have an increased need for fluid (e.g., with fever or gastrointestinal losses) and also a decreased ability to excrete fluid (e.g., with cardiopulmonary or renal disease), which may lead to the need to restrict fluid intake.

Vitamins. **Vitamins** are organic substances essential to normal metabolism. The body is unable to synthesize most vitamins in the required amounts and depends on dietary intake. The quantity of vitamins in food is affected by food processing, storage, and preparation. Vitamin content is usually highest in fresh foods used quickly after minimal exposure to heat, air, or water. Certain vitamins function as antioxidants that neutralize substances called *free radicals*, which are thought to produce oxidative damage to body cells and tissues and to increase a person's risk for various cancers. Vitamins with antioxidant properties include water-soluble vitamin C and fat-soluble beta-carotene and vitamins A and E (Schlenker & Gilbert, 2014).

Fat-Soluble Vitamins. The **fat-soluble vitamins** (A, D, E, and K) can be stored in the body. With the exception of vitamin D, these vitamins are provided only through dietary intake. Vitamin D is provided by both dietary intake and synthesis in the body with exposure to sunlight. *Canada's Food Guide* recommends that adults consume 500 mL (2 cups) of milk each day in order to receive adequate vitamin D. Yet, because vitamin D needs increase after the age of 50 and obtaining adequate vitamin D from the diet alone is very difficult, Health Canada (2012) recommends that all adults over the age of 50 take a daily vitamin D supplement of 10 micrograms (mcg; 400 IU) in addition to following *Canada's Food Guide*. The body can store fat-soluble vitamins; therefore, hypervitaminosis can result from megadoses (intentional or unintentional) of supplemental vitamins, excessive amounts of vitamins in fortified food, and excessive fish oils.

Water-Soluble Vitamins. The water-soluble vitamins are vitamins C and B complex (which consists of eight vitamins: thiamine, riboflavin, niacin, vitamin B_6, folate, vitamin B_{12}, pantothenic acid, and biotin). Another element, choline, is sometimes classified as a B vitamin. Water-soluble vitamins are easily destroyed by cooking and must be provided in the daily food intake. Although water-soluble vitamins are not stored in the body, toxicity may still occur with vitamin megadoses.

Minerals. Minerals are inorganic elements essential to the body as catalysts in biochemical reactions. Minerals become part of the structure of the body and its enzymes. For example, iron becomes attached to protein globin to form hemoglobin, which enhances oxygen-carrying capacity. Minerals are classified as macrominerals when the daily requirement is 100 mg or more and as microminerals or trace elements when less than 100 mg is needed daily. The macrominerals are calcium, sodium, potassium, phosphorus, magnesium, sulphur, and chloride. Trace minerals include iron, iodine, fluoride, zinc, selenium, chromium, copper, manganese, molybdenum, and cobalt. Other trace minerals such as aluminum, cadmium, arsenic, and boron have possible but not clearly delineated nutritional functions. Arsenic, aluminum, and cadmium have toxic effects.

Anatomy and Physiology of the Digestive System

Digestion. Digestion of food consists of mechanical breakdown that results from chewing, churning, and mixing with fluid, as well as chemical reactions by which food is reduced to its simplest form. Each part of the gastrointestinal system has an important digestive or absorptive function (Figure 42-1).

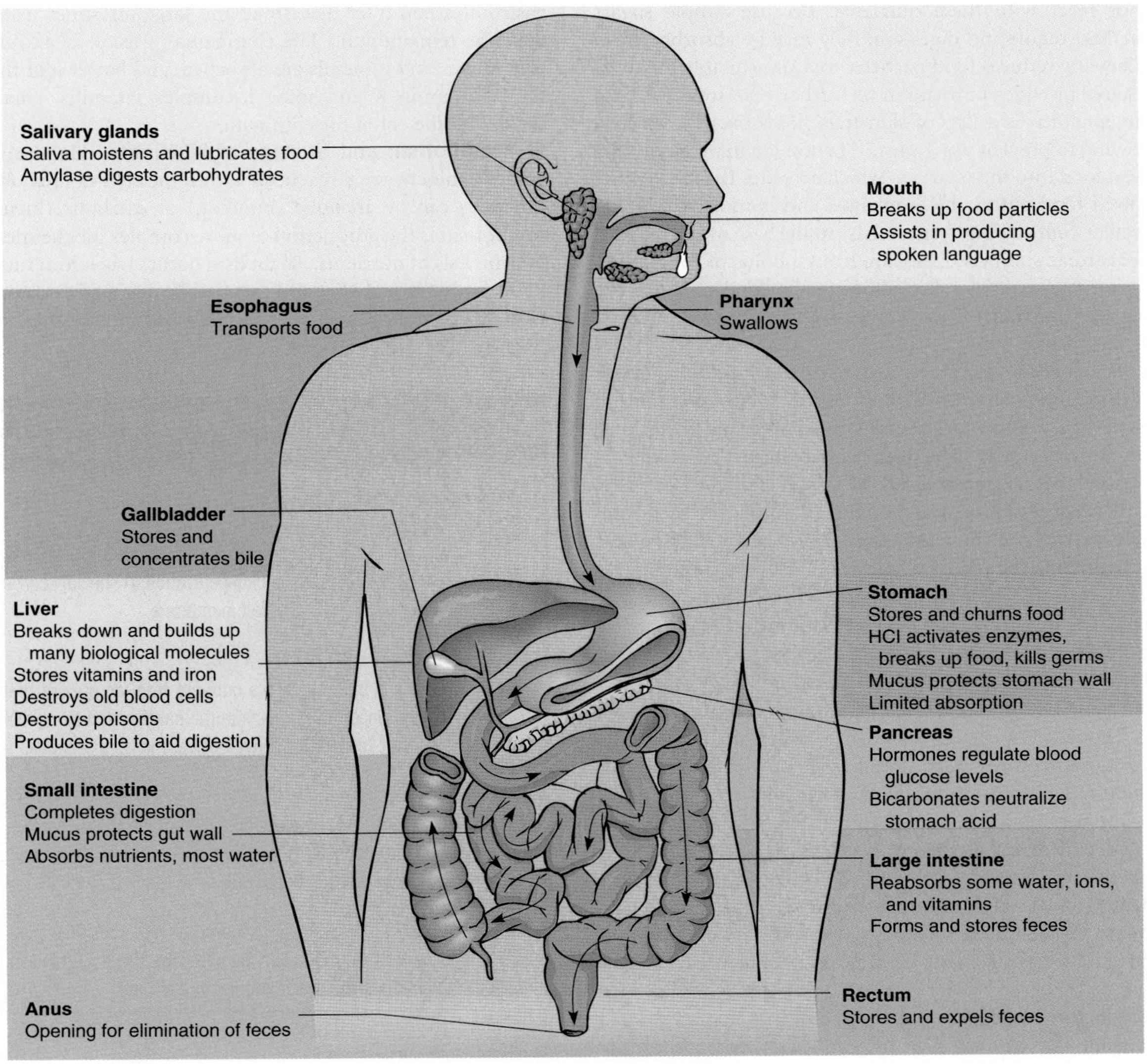

FIGURE 42-1 Summary of digestive system anatomy and organ function. *HCl,* Hydrochloric acid. (From Rolin Graphics.)

Enzymes are an essential component of the chemistry of digestion. Enzymes are protein-like substances that act as catalysts to speed up chemical reactions. Most enzymes have one specific function and function best at a specific pH. The secretions of the gastrointestinal tract have vastly different pH levels. For example, saliva is relatively neutral, gastric juice is highly acidic, and the secretions of the small intestine are alkaline.

The mechanical, chemical, and hormonal activities of digestion are interdependent. Enzyme activity depends on the mechanical breakdown of food to increase the surface area for chemical action. Hormones regulate the flow of digestive secretions needed for enzyme supply. The secretion of digestive juices and the motility of the gastrointestinal tract are also regulated by physical, chemical, and hormonal factors. Action in the gastrointestinal tract is increased by nerve stimulation from the parasympathetic nervous system (e.g., the vagus nerve).

Digestion begins in the mouth, where chewing mechanically breaks down food. The food is mixed with saliva, which contains ptyalin (salivary amylase), an enzyme that acts on cooked starch to begin its conversion to maltose. The longer food is chewed, the more starch digestion occurs in the mouth. Proteins and fats are broken down physically but remain unchanged chemically because enzymes in the mouth do not react with these nutrients. Because simple sugars (monosaccharides) require no digestion, they may be absorbed from the mouth. Chewing reduces food particles to a size suitable for swallowing, and saliva provides lubrication to further ease swallowing of the food. The epiglottis is a flap of skin that closes over the trachea during swallowing to prevent **aspiration**. The tongue manoeuvres the mass of chewed food into the pharynx, which activates the swallowing reflex. Swallowed food enters the esophagus and is moved along by wavelike muscular contractions (**peristalsis**) to the base of the esophagus, above the cardiac sphincter. Pressure from a bolus of food at the cardiac sphincter causes it to relax, allowing the food to enter the fundus (uppermost portion) of the stomach. Difficulty swallowing is referred to as **dysphagia**.

In the stomach, pepsinogen is secreted by chief cells and then converted by hydrochloric acid (HCl) to pepsin, a protein-splitting enzyme. Gastric lipase and amylase are produced to begin fat and starch digestion, respectively. The stomach's pyloric glands secrete gastrin, a hormone that triggers parietal cells to secrete intrinsic factor (IF) and HCl. IF is necessary for absorption of vitamin B_{12} in the ileum. HCl also destroys bacteria, increases the absorbability of iron and calcium, and maintains the pH of the gastric juice. The lining of the stomach is protected from autodigestion by a thick layer of mucus. Alcohol and aspirin are two substances directly absorbed through the lining of the stomach. The muscular walls of the stomach produce a churning action that continues mechanical digestion. The stomach acts as a reservoir where food remains for approximately 3 hours, within a range of 1 to 7 hours.

Food leaves the antrum, or distal stomach, via the pyloric sphincter and enters the duodenum as an acidic, liquefied mass called **chyme**. Chyme flows into the duodenum and is quickly mixed with bile, intestinal juices, and pancreatic secretions. Secretin and cholecystokinin (CCK) are hormones secreted by the mucosa of the small intestine. Secretin activates release of bicarbonate from the pancreas, raising the pH of chyme. CCK inhibits further gastrin secretion and initiates the release of additional digestive enzymes from the pancreas and gallbladder.

Bile is manufactured in the liver and stored in the gallbladder. Bile acts as a detergent, as it emulsifies fat to permit enzyme action while suspending fatty acids in solution. Pancreatic secretions contain six enzymes: amylase to digest starch; lipase to break down emulsified fats; and trypsin, elastase, chymotrypsin, and carboxypeptidase to break down proteins.

Peristalsis continues in the small intestine, mixing the secretions with the chyme. The mixture becomes increasingly alkaline, inhibiting the action of the gastric enzymes and promoting the action of the duodenal secretions. Epithelial cells in the inner walls of the small intestine secrete enzymes to facilitate digestion. These enzymes include sucrase, lactase, maltase, lipase, and peptidase. The major portion of digestion occurs in the small intestine, producing glucose, fructose, and galactose from carbohydrates; amino acids and dipeptides from proteins; and fatty acids, glycerides, and glycerol from lipids. Approximately 5 hours are required to pass food through the small intestine via peristalsis.

Absorption. The small intestine is the primary absorption site for nutrients. Its inner surface is lined with fingerlike projections called *villi*, which increase the surface area available for absorption. Nutrients are absorbed by means of passive diffusion, osmosis, active transport, and pinocytosis (Box 42-1).

The main source of water absorption is via the intestine. Approximately 7 L of gastrointestinal secretions and 1.2 L of oral intake, totalling 8.2 L of fluid, must be managed daily within the gastrointestinal tract. The small and large intestines reabsorb 8.1 L a day. The remaining 0.1 L is eliminated in feces. In addition to water, electrolytes and minerals are absorbed, and bacteria in the colon synthesize vitamin K and some B-complex vitamins. Finally, feces are formed in the colon for elimination.

Metabolism and Storage of Nutrients. **Metabolism** refers to all of the biochemical reactions within the cells of the body. Metabolic processes can be anabolic (building) or catabolic (breaking down). **Anabolism** is the production of more complex biochemical substances by synthesis of nutrients. Anabolism occurs when lean muscle is added to the body through diet and exercise. Amino acids are anabolized into tissues, hormones, and enzymes. **Catabolism** is the breakdown of

BOX 42-1 Mechanisms for Intestinal Absorption of Nutrients

Mechanism Definition

Active Transport

In this energy-dependent process, particles move from an area of greater concentration to an area of lesser concentration. A special "carrier" is needed to move the particle across the cell membrane.

Passive Diffusion

The force by which particles move outward from an area of greater concentration to lesser concentration constitutes passive diffusion. The particles do not need a special "carrier" to move outward in all directions.

Osmosis

In this process, water moves through a membrane that separates solutions of different concentrations. Water moves to equalize the concentration pressures on both sides of the membrane.

Pinocytosis

Large molecules of nutrients are engulfed by the absorbing cell when the molecule attaches to the absorbing cell membrane.

Data from Nix, S. (2013). *Williams' basic nutrition and diet therapy* (14th ed.). St. Louis, MO: Mosby; and Schlenker, E. D., & Gilbert, J. A. (2014). *Essentials of nutrition and diet therapy* (11th ed.). St. Louis, MO: Mosby.

biochemical substances into simpler substances. Starvation is an example of catabolism, when wasting of body tissues occurs. Normal metabolism and anabolism are physiologically possible when the body is in positive nitrogen balance, whereas catabolism occurs during physiological states of negative nitrogen balance.

Nutrients absorbed in the intestines are transported via the circulatory system to body tissues. Through the chemical changes of metabolism, nutrients are converted into a number of substances required by the body. Carbohydrates, protein, and fat undergo metabolism to produce chemical energy and to maintain a balance between anabolism and catabolism. To carry out the body's work, the chemical energy produced by metabolism is converted to other types of energy. For example, muscle contraction involves mechanical energy, nervous system function involves electrical energy, and the mechanisms of heat production involve thermal energy. All of these forms of energy originate in metabolism.

Nutrient metabolism consists of three main processes:

1. Catabolism of glycogen into glucose, carbon dioxide, and water (glycogenolysis)
2. Anabolism of glucose into glycogen for storage (glycogenesis)
3. Catabolism of amino acids and glycerol into glucose for energy (gluconeogenesis)

Glycogen, synthesized from glucose and stored in small reserves in liver and muscle tissue, provides energy during brief periods of fasting and maintains blood glucose levels as we sleep. Amino acids can be converted to fat and stored or catabolized into energy via gluconeogenesis. All body cells except red blood cells and neurons can oxidize fatty acids into ketones for energy in the absence of dietary carbohydrates (glucose). Some of the nutrients required by the body are stored in body tissues. The body's major form of reserve energy is fat, stored as adipose tissue.

Elimination. Chyme is moved by peristaltic action through the ileocecal valve into the large intestine, where it becomes feces. As feces move toward the rectum, water is absorbed into the intestinal mucosa. The longer the material stays in the large intestine, the more water is absorbed, causing the feces to become firmer. Exercise and fibre stimulate peristalsis. Feces contain cellulose and similar indigestible substances, sloughed epithelial cells from the gastrointestinal tract, digestive secretions, water, and microbes.

Dietary Guidelines

Dietary Reference Intakes. In 1997, the Food and Nutrition Board of the American National Institute of Medicine/National Academy of Sciences, in partnership with Health Canada, developed dietary reference intakes (DRIs) with respect to age, sex, pregnancy, and lactation (Health Canada, 2013b). The DRIs present evidenced-informed criteria for an acceptable range of minimum to maximum amounts of nutrients, vitamins, and minerals needed to avoid deficiencies or toxicities. The DRIs have four components: (1) the estimated average requirement (EAR), which is the recommended amount of a nutrient sufficient to maintain a specific body function for 50% of the population based on age and gender; (2) the recommended dietary allowance (RDA), which is the average needs of 98% of the population, not the exact needs of an individual (Murphy, Guenther, & Kretsch, 2006); (3) the upper intake level (UL), which is the highest level believed to pose no risk of adverse health events but is not a recommended level of intake; and (4) the adequate intake (AI), which is the suggested intake for individuals that is based on observed or scientifically determined estimates of nutrient intakes and is used when insufficient evidence exists to set the RDA. Because this evidence is continually evolving, clinicians should consult current resources, such as Health Canada web pages and other evidence-informed literature, when determining a patient's specific nutrition needs or supplementation.

Food Guidelines. In 1942, Health Canada developed Canada's first food guide, *Canada's Official Food Rules*. Since then, the food guide has undergone many changes in name, appearance, and content. However, its ultimate purpose—to inform daily food choices and promote optimal nutritional health—has not changed. The current guide, called *Eating Well With Canada's Food Guide*, last updated in 2007 (Figure 42-2), is based on a range of evidence resulting from focus groups, online consultations, regional meetings, and reviews of literature about the environmental context in which Canadians make food choices. Although the scientific basis for the 2007 guide is largely consistent with the latest diet and health evidence, the guide is scheduled to be revised in 2017–2018. Its review by Health Canada indicated that there are challenges in understanding and applying certain aspects (e.g., using food guide servings and healthy meals and snacks recommendations) and that the current format is not meeting the needs of all audiences (e.g., some want more detail, while others would prefer less). The revision will strengthen dietary guidance for replacing saturated fat with unsaturated fat to help decrease the risk of heart disease and reducing high intakes of sugar-sweetened beverages to help decrease the risk of obesity. Only high-quality, peer-reviewed systematic reviews and reports from leading scientific organizations and governmental agencies will be considered. As with the 2007 revision, input from health professional groups, industry, and the public will help ensure that the recommendations are scientifically sound and address those characteristics of the diet most relevant to the promotion of health and reduction of chronic disease for Canadian populations. During the revision process, the *Food Guide* can continue to be used as a trusted source of information on healthy eating (Health Canada, 2017a).

Included in the general guidelines of *Eating Well With Canada's Food Guide* are specific suggestions for food choices. Consumers are told to make at least half their grain selections whole grain; eat at least one dark green and one orange vegetable per day; and use vegetables and fruits more than juice, which contains a lower amount of fibre. Lower-fat dairy products, lean meats, and choices from the lower-fat meat group (e.g., legumes, tofu) are encouraged. The minimum intake of unsaturated fats is 30 to 45 mL. Two *Food Guide* servings of fish each week are suggested on the basis of evidence relating fish consumption and reduced risk of cardiovascular disease. The *Food Guide* lists water as a calorie-free way to quench thirst and recommends community water supplies be fluoridated to the level of 1 mg/L. No directional statements are provided to target calorie intakes (Jessri & L'Abbe, 2015).

Recommended intakes and nutritional values according to *Canada's Food Guide* are shown in Table 42-1.

Canada's Food Guide notes the importance of physical activity in maintaining energy balance and recommends that adults spend 30 to 60 minutes per day carrying out some physical activity and that children and youth spend at least 90 minutes per day. The guide provides advice on the use of vitamin and mineral supplementation when the recommended food intake pattern does not ensure adequate amounts. Although not specified in the guide, Canadians are advised to limit salt to "healthy" levels, alcohol to no more than 5% of total energy, and caffeine to no more than 400 mg for the general population, no more than 300 mg (or a little over two 8-oz [237 mL] cups of coffee per day) for women of childbearing age, and no more than 2.5 mg/kg/day for children (Health Canada, 2013c).

Eating Well With Canada's Food Guide has been adapted for First Nations, Inuit, and Métis populations (Health Canada, 2010).

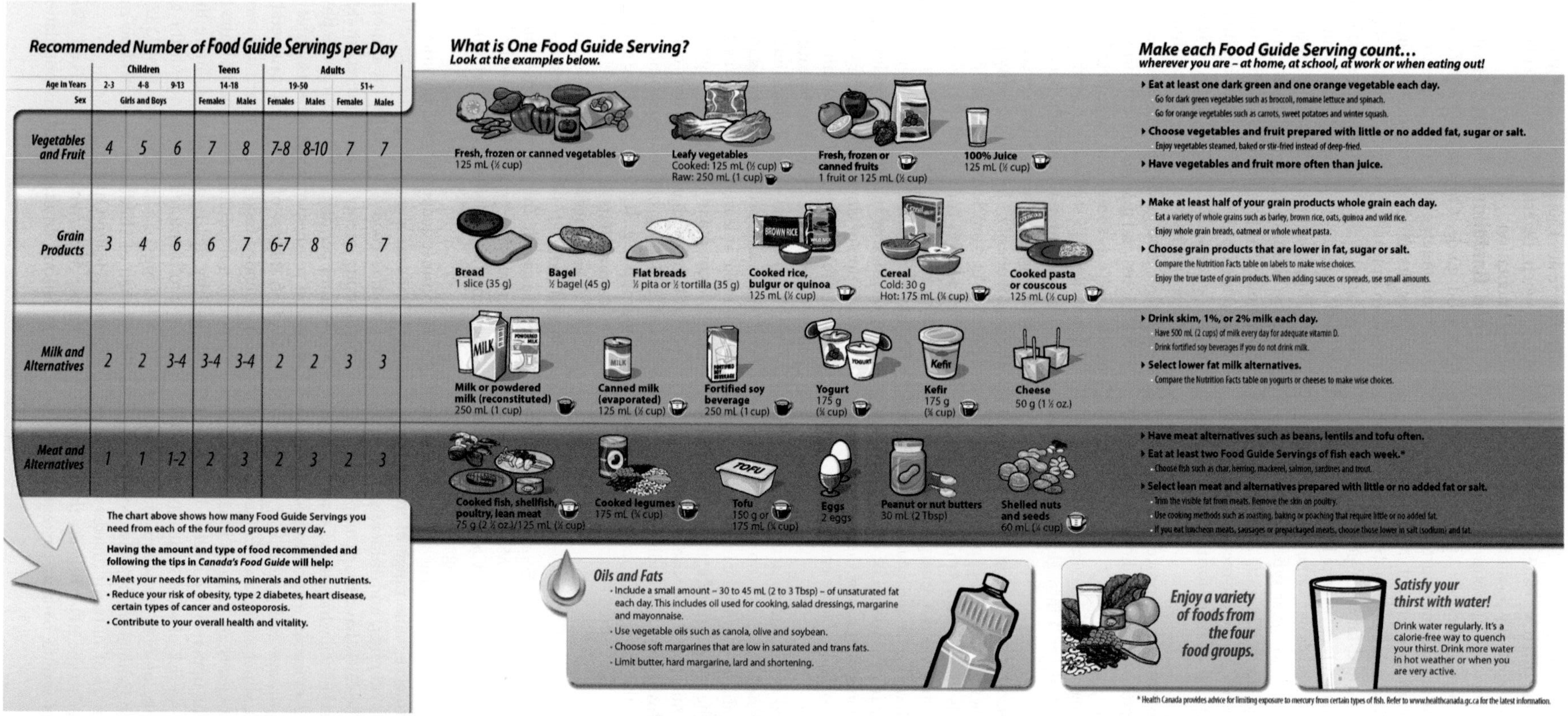

FIGURE 42-2 Extract from *Eating Well With Canada's Food Guide.* (From Health Canada. [2007]. *Eating well with Canada's food guide* [Catalogue No. H164-38/1-2007E]. Ottawa: Author. Retrieved from http://www.hc-sc.gc.ca/fn-an/food-guidealiment/index_e.html. Reproduced with permission of the Minister of Public Works and Government Services Canada.)

TABLE 42-1 Summary of Recommended Intakes and Nutritional Values According to *Eating Well With Canada's Food Guide*

VEGETABLES AND FRUIT		GRAIN PRODUCTS		MILK AND ALTERNATIVES		MEAT AND ALTERNATIVES	
Years of Age	**Servings Per Day**	**Years of Age**	**Servings Per Day**	**Years of Age**	**Servings Per Day**	**Years of Age**	**Servings Per Day**
2–3	4	2–3	3	2–3	2	2–8	1
4–8	5	4–8	4	4–8	2	9–13	1–2
9–13	6	9–13	6	9–13	3–4	Girls: 14–18	2
Girls: 14–18	7	Girls: 14–18	6	14–18	3–4	Boys: 14–18	3
Boys: 14–18	8	Boys: 14–18	7	Adults: 19–51	2	Women: 19–50	2
Women: 19–50	7–8	Women: 19–50	6–7	Adults: 51+	3	Men: 19–50	3
Men: 19–50	8–10	Men: 19–50	8			Women: 51+	2
Adults: 51+	7	Women: 51+	6			Men: 51+	3
		Men: 51+	7				

Some Important Nutrients in the Food Groups

VEGETABLES AND FRUIT	GRAIN PRODUCTS	MILK AND ALTERNATIVES	MEAT AND ALTERNATIVES
Carbohydrate	Protein	Protein	Protein
Fibre	Carbohydrate	Fat	Fat
Folate	Fibre	Carbohydrate	Thiamin
Vitamin B_6	Thiamin	Riboflavin	Riboflavin
Vitamin C	Riboflavin	Vitamin B_{12}	Niacin
Vitamin A	Niacin	Vitamin A	Vitamin B_6
Magnesium	Folate	Vitamin D	Vitamin B_{12}
Potassium	Iron	Calcium	Iron
	Zinc	Zinc	Zinc
	Magnesium	Magnesium	Magnesium
	Potassium	Potassium	Potassium

Adapted from Health Canada. (2007). *Eating well with Canada's food guide.* Ottawa, ON: Author. Retrieved from http://www.hc-sc.gc.ca/fn-an/food-guide-aliment/index_e.html. Reproduced with permission of the Minister of Public Works and Government Services Canada.

Examples of foods traditional to Canadian Indigenous populations are wild plants and seaweed in the fruit and vegetable groups, bannock as a grain product, and wild game as a meat alternative. Included in the online *Food Guide* is a link to a government website for advice on limiting exposure to mercury from eating locally caught fish. Instructions are also given for including traditional fats in the diet such as seal and whale oil, ooligan grease, and bacon fat.

In the past, Canada's Indigenous peoples subsisted on foods obtained from hunting, trapping, fishing, gathering, and agriculture. The resulting diet, high in animal protein and low in fat and carbohydrates, provided adequate energy and nutrients. In replacing traditional foods with contemporary market foods, the current diet became lower in iron, folacin, calcium, vitamins A and D, fibre, fruit, and vegetables and higher in fat and sugar intakes. Patterns of food consumption are further influenced by issues of food security (ability to acquire acceptable foods), preferences in body size, individual taste preferences, availability of particular species for food, knowledge of the nutritional deficits of store-bought food, and alteration of the natural environment. Health problems such as anemia, dental caries, heart disease, obesity, and diabetes are related to such patterns (National Collaborating Centre for Aboriginal Health, 2012).

To date, *Canada's Food Guide* has not been modified to recognize the nutritional concerns of Chinese Canadians or other immigrant groups, although it has been translated into 10 languages. In a scoping review to assess the current literature on issues pertaining to immigrant nutritional health, Sanou, O'Reilly, Ngnie-Teta, et al. (2014) reported that immigrants usually have fewer chronic conditions and tend to be healthier than the Canadian-born population when they first arrive in the country, owing to the selection effect of immigrants. However, changes due to living environment, unfamiliarity with grocery stores, availability of foods, and lifestyle factors such as urbanization and language barriers then impede the immigrants' efforts to maintain their traditional dietary practices. In attempting to acquire the ingredients necessary for replicating familiar dishes, immigrants are limited to highly processed versions that are high in fat and sodium, therefore increasing their risk for chronic conditions. Long exposure to Canadian culture is associated with increased prevalence of obesity among immigrants.

Canada's Food Guide cannot stand alone as a tool to inform certain groups, including new immigrants and some Indigenous peoples, who ostensibly face more barriers to food literacy than other groups. Consideration should be given to support health providers and other stakeholders in making nutritional information more effective, understandable, and accessible for household use (Brichta & Howard, 2013). The need for further examples of culturally appropriate foods and portions will, no doubt, be addressed through ongoing revisions to the *Food Guide*.

The Nutrition Label. Since December 12, 2007, mandatory nutrition labelling of a nutrition facts table listing energy (calories) and 13 nutrients (fat, saturated fat, trans fat, cholesterol, sodium, carbohydrate, fibre, sugars, protein, vitamin A, vitamin C, calcium, and iron) has been required on most prepackaged foods in Canada. This easy-to-read table, which appears on food labels in a consistent appearance, provides consumers with information to make informed food choices and compare products (Figure 42-3). This information includes (a) the specific amount of the food item that makes up the serving size, an amount that may differ from the *Food Guide* serving size, and (b) the percent daily value (% DV), a general guideline of how the food's nutrient content contributes to daily diet. It is important to note that the % DV is based on a 2 000-calorie/day adult diet and thus does not address recommended nutrient intake for those who are pregnant or breastfeeding. The following diet-related health claims have been established from recognized health and scientific information:

- A healthy diet low in sodium and high in potassium may reduce high blood pressure risk.
- A healthy diet adequate in calcium and vitamin D may reduce the risk of osteoporosis.
- A healthy diet low in saturated fat and trans fat may reduce the risk of heart disease.
- A healthy diet rich in vegetables and fruit may reduce the risk of some types of cancer.

Nutrition Facts
Per 1 burger (130 g)

Amount			% Daily Value
Calories 340			
Fat 27 g			42 %
Saturated Fat 12 g + Trans Fat 2 g			70 %
Cholesterol 70 mg			
Sodium 330 mg			14 %
Carbohydrate 3 g			1 %
Fibre 0 g			0 %
Sugars 3 g			
Protein 24 g			
Vitamin A	0 %	Vitamin C	0 %
Calcium	2 %	Iron	30 %

FIGURE 42-3 Example of food label. (From Health Canada. [2015]. *The nutrition facts table*. Ottawa: Author. Retrieved from http://healthycanadians.gc.ca/eating-nutrition/label-etiquetage/understanding-comprendre/nutrition-fact-valeur-nutritive-eng.php. Reproduced with the permission of the Minister of Public Works and Government Services Canada.)

Some other nutrient content claims as regulated by the Canadian government (Canadian Food Inspection Agency, 2014) are the following:

- *Free* indicates the number of calories or the amount of a nutrient is nutritionally insignificant in a specified amount of food.
- Claims for *saturated fatty acids* include a restriction on levels of both saturated and trans fatty acids.
- The claim *(naming the percent) fat-free* is allowed only if accompanied by the statement *low fat* or *low in fat*.
- The nutrient content claim *light* is restricted to foods that meet the criteria for either *reduced in energy* or *reduced in fat*.
- The only nutrient content claims permitted for foods for children under 2 years of age are *source of protein, excellent source of protein, more protein, no added sodium,* and *no added sugar*.
- A claim of *reduced in energy* or *reduced in calories* is allowed if the item has at least 25% fewer calories than the food to which it is compared.

Health Promotion and Disease Prevention: A Call to Action from Dietitians. In 2011, the United Nations recommended monitoring the trends of noncommunicable diseases, scaling up measures to reduce risk factors (including unhealthy diet), strengthening health systems and services, and improving access to health care. In response, Dietitians of Canada (2012) called for coordinated action to promote healthy eating through the highest levels of political commitment and cross-sector collaboration to provide (a) equitable access to adequate, healthy, and safe food, (b) supportive environments for healthy eating, (c) comprehensive surveillance and monitoring of food, diet, and health, and (d) access to dietitian services in all sectors. Dietitians of Canada has a sustained history of advocating for a continued leadership commitment to nutrition labelling; food fortification; food policy and regulation, including consistent nutrition information and standard serving sizes on nutrition labels; the national reduction of salt, sugar, and trans fat content in packaged and prepared foods; and using the (National) Nutritious Food Basket Protocol (e.g., http://www.health.gov.on.ca/en/pro/programs/publichealth/oph_standards/docs/nutritious_food_basket.pdf) in calculating the cost of a healthy diet to reduce poverty-related food insecurity.

Dietitians and nutritionists are highly prepared to help patients meet their nutritional needs. A dietitian must successfully complete a 4-year Bachelor of Science in Nutritional Sciences, a 1-year internship, and a nationwide exam before being registered with the Commission of Dietetic Registration and licensed to practise. Registered dietitians work in the hospital, clinic, or community or in public health, in private practice settings, and in food and nutrition industries. Their recommendations and treatment plans are informed by the evidence of scientific studies. In contrast, nutritionists are unregulated in Canada, have varying degrees of education, and complete a certificate program. Because nutritionists are not clinically trained to treat patients with diseases, they often work in private practices and deliver group nutrition and cooking classes. The term *registered nutritionist* is regulated in Alberta, New Brunswick, Nova Scotia, and Quebec and is used there interchangeably for *registered dietitian*.

NURSING KNOWLEDGE BASE

Nutrition During Human Growth and Development

Infants Through School-Aged Children. Infancy is marked by rapid growth with high protein, vitamin, mineral, and energy requirements. The average (50th percentile) birth weight of a full-term (40-week gestation) Canadian newborn boy is 3 613 g; that for a

Canadian newborn girl, 3 470 g (Kramer, Platt, Wen, et al., 2001). A healthy birth weight for newborns ranges from 2 500 to 3 999 g (Region of Waterloo Public Health, 2017). The infant usually doubles birth weight at 4 to 5 months and triples it at 1 year. An energy intake of approximately 110 kcal/kg/day is needed in the first 3 months of infancy, 100 kcal/kg/day between 3 and 6 months, 95 kcal/kg/day for 6–9 months, and 100 kcal/kg/day from 9 months to 1 year (Perry et al., 2016). Commercial formulas and human breast milk each provide approximately 20 kcal/30 mL. A full-term newborn is able to digest and absorb simple carbohydrates, proteins, and a moderate amount of emulsified fat. Spitting up is a natural consequence of the baby's anatomy because the short esophagus and small stomach allow liquid to escape from the stomach easily (Winter, 2017). Spitting up may occur during the first year until the gastroesophageal sphincter (which opens to allow food to enter the stomach and gas to escape after meals) matures and the child learns to sit independently. The average energy intake in a breastfeeding infant is 500 kcal/day (based on an average milk intake of 0.78 L/day (Perry et al., 2016). Infants need 100 or more mL/kg per day of fluid because a large portion of their total body weight is water.

Breastfeeding. Health Canada, Canadian Paediatric Society, the Dietitians of Canada, and the Breastfeeding Committee for Canada (Infant Feeding Joint Working Group, 2015) recommend breastfeeding as the optimal method of infant feeding and the exclusive use of breast milk for the first 6 months of the infant's life. Breastfeeding confers immunological and allergy protection to the infant during the period of breastfeeding, is economical and convenient (breast milk is always fresh and at the correct temperature), and provides an excellent opportunity for mother and infant to interact. Breast milk changes as a baby grows, is easier to digest than formula, helps protect against sudden infant death syndrome, and may also have a protective effect against obesity (Gionet, 2015). Breastfed infants need supplemental vitamin D because breast milk has only 1 to 10 IU/250 mL (Infant Feeding Joint Working Group, 2015), or 60% of the vitamin D needed by infants under 1 year of age. Other vitamin or mineral supplementation is not recommended for the first 6 months.

In 2011–2012, 89% of Canadian mothers breastfed their baby, a slight increase from 85% in 2003 (Gionet, 2015). Breastfeeding rates ranged from 57% in Newfoundland and Labrador to 96% in British Columbia and the Yukon. Mothers who breastfed exclusively for at least 6 months were generally older, had postsecondary qualifications, and were more often married or common-law status (91%), compared with mothers who did not breastfeed (70%). Among mothers who breastfed for less than 6 months, about 44% stopped because they perceived having insufficient breast milk, 18% had difficulty with breastfeeding technique, and 9% experienced a medical condition of the mother or baby. Canadian health practitioners are encouraged to promote exclusive breastfeeding by creating an appropriate "baby-friendly" environment of awareness and support to enable women to breastfeed throughout the continuum of care from hospitals to community health services (Pound, Unger, & Canadian Paediatric Society, Nutrition and Gastroenterology Committee, Hospital Paediatrics Section, 2012/2015).

Formula. Commercially prepared infant formulas, cow's milk–based and iron fortified, are designed to contain the approximate nutrient composition of human milk. Protein in the formula is typically supplied as whey, soy, cow's milk base, casein hydrolysate, or elemental amino acids. The composition, processing, packaging, and labelling of all infant formulas are regulated under Canadian food and drug laws. Although it is now also possible to supplement commercial infant formula with probiotics for the treatment of infantile colic, evidence is inconclusive and only a few strains have been tested (Martin, Ling, & Blackburn, 2016). Further investigations are needed to provide evidence-informed guidelines.

Specialty formulas are indicated for infants with detected or suspected pathology. Health providers caring for new mothers and their infants can address mothers' concerns about infant formulas and help them make informed choices when selecting the best substitute for human milk.

Regular cow's milk should not be used in infant formula before 9 to 12 months of age because it may cause gastrointestinal bleeding, is too concentrated for the infant's kidneys, increases the risk of milk product allergies, and is a poor source of iron and vitamins C and E (Martin et al., 2016). Honey as a potential source of botulism toxin should not be used in the infant's diet, as the toxin can be fatal in children under 1 year of age (World Health Organization [WHO], 2017).

Introduction to Solid Food. Breast milk or formula provides sufficient nutrition for the first 6 months of the infant's life. After that, iron-rich solids are introduced to meet the infant's nutrient needs (Infant Feeding Joint Working Group, 2015). Cues indicating readiness for solid foods are the appearance of fine motor skills of the hand and fingers, hand-to-mouth movement, interest in adult food and self-feeding, increased milk consumption, ability to move food to the back of the mouth, and ability to sit alone in a high chair (Infant Toddler Forum, 2014). Puréed smooth foods are typically the first semi-solid food to be introduced to an infant. The addition of foods to an infant's diet should be governed by the infant's nutrient needs and physical readiness to handle different forms of foods and by the need to detect and control allergic reactions. New foods should be introduced one at a time, at least 3 to 4 days apart, to help see if the baby is allergic to any new food. The new food should be one single type of food, not a mixture of different foods (Newfoundland Labrador Public Health, 2013). It is best to introduce new foods before milk or other foods to avoid infant rejection due to satiety (Health Canada, 2014a).

The growth rate slows during toddler years (ages 1 to 3 years). The toddler needs fewer kilocalories but an increased amount of protein in relation to body weight; consequently, appetite may decrease at about 18 months of age. Toddlers exhibit strong food preferences and become picky eaters. Small, frequent meals consisting of breakfast, lunch, and dinner, with interspersed, nutrient-dense snacks, may improve nutritional intake (Leung et al., 2012). Snacks work best mid-way between meals and should not be offered if the timing or quantity of snacking will interfere with the child's appetite for the next meal. Calcium and phosphorus are important for healthy bone growth. Whole milk should be used until the toddler reaches 2 years of age to help ensure adequate intake of fatty acids for brain and neurological development. Toddlers and preschoolers need vitamin D supplementation until their diet includes at least 10 mcg (400 IU) per day of vitamin D from other dietary sources (i.e., drinking two cups of milk daily and eating one to two servings of fish weekly). Toddlers who consume more than 720 mL of milk daily in lieu of other foods may develop milk anemia, as milk is a poor source of iron.

The oral health of infants and children needs to focus on preventing cavities. Children who sleep with a bottle are at particular risk of developing early childhood tooth decay (ECTD), a severe type of tooth decay that can affect baby teeth, especially the upper front teeth. The sugars from the milk, juice, and drinks left in the mouth combine with bacteria in plaque to create an acid that damages the enamel of a tooth. The longer and more often food is left in the mouth, the greater the chance of developing ECTD (Health Canada, 2009). Dental visits should begin within 6 months of the eruption of the first tooth or by 1 year of age at the latest. From the age of 3 years, twice-yearly dental inspections are recommended. Children under 3 years of age should have their teeth brushed by an adult, and parents need to supervise children less than 6 years of age during brushing (Canadian Dental Association, 2018).

Preschoolers' (3 to 5 years old) dietary requirements are similar to those of toddlers. They consume slightly more than toddlers, and nutrient density is more important than quantity. Encouragement of healthy eating is an important goal of parenting, and parents should try to use attractive food presentations and fun, educational initiatives rather than unhealthy food as a reward (Leung et al., 2012; Public Health Nutritionists of Saskatchewan, 2015). Because preschoolers have small stomachs, they need to eat small amounts of food more often throughout the day. One *Food Guide* serving from a food group can be divided into smaller amounts and served throughout the day. For example, half a serving of meat and alternatives may be served at two different meals, such as one egg at lunch and about 35 g (1 oz) of chicken for dinner (Health Canada, 2016a).

Safety Alert Foods such as hot dogs, candy, gum, cough drops, chewable vitamins, sunflower seeds, fish with bones, peanuts, marshmallows, grapes, raw vegetables, popcorn, and snacks on toothpicks or skewers have been implicated in choking deaths of preschoolers and toddlers and should be avoided or prepared in a safe manner (Cyr & Canadian Paediatric Society, Injury Prevention Committee, 2016).

School-aged children, 6 to 12 years old, grow at a slower and steadier rate, with a gradual decline in energy requirements per unit of body weight. The school-aged child gains 3 to 5 kg in weight and 6 cm in height per year until puberty. Despite better appetites and more varied food intake, school-aged children's diets should be carefully assessed for adequate protein and vitamins A and C. School-aged children frequently fail to eat a proper breakfast and have an unsupervised food intake at school. High amounts of fat, sugar, and salt can result from a liberal intake of commercially prepared snack foods. Recently, only 1 in 10 Canadian youth were found to meet fruit and vegetable (FV) recommendations (Minaker & Hammond, 2016). FV consumption is associated with reduced risk for chronic diseases, including some cancers, cardiovascular disease, obesity, and all-cause mortality (Wang, Ouyang, Liu, et al., 2014). Youth who meet FV recommendations are more likely to be younger (Grade 6 compared to Grades 8 to 9) and get good grades at school (Minaker & Hammond, 2016). Children who increase fruit consumption have tended to show less body mass index (BMI) gain compared to those with constantly low or decreasing fruit consumption (Bayer, Nehring, Bolte, et al., 2014).

According to the WHO cut-offs, an estimated 32.8% of 5- to 11-year-olds in Canada are overweight or obese (Roberts et al., 2015). Children living in Newfoundland and Labrador, Northwest Territories, and the Yukon in 2014 were more likely to be overweight than children in British Columbia (Statistics Canada, 2016c). Health risks associated with being overweight or obese in childhood include hypertension and high cholesterol, which are risk factors for cardiovascular disease; impaired glucose tolerance, insulin resistance, and type 2 diabetes; breathing problems, such as sleep apnea and asthma; joint problems and musculoskeletal discomfort; fatty liver disease, gallstones, and gastro-esophageal reflux (i.e., heartburn); and social and psychological problems, such as discrimination and poor self-esteem, which can continue into adulthood (Bariatric and Metabolic Institute, 2017). These diseases and disorders, traditionally limited to adults, are manifesting in Canadian youth (Public Health Agency of Canada [PHAC], 2012). The prevention and treatment of obesity in childhood and adolescence is a critical public health issue and, ultimately, an important determinant of long-term health. Strategies to reduce childhood overweight and obesity include (a) making it a collective priority by Ministers of Health to champion and encourage shared leadership and action from government departments and other sectors of Canadian society; (b) coordinating policy priorities to identify and address the risk of overweight and obesity in children early, to make children's social and physical environments more supportive of physical activity and healthy eating, and to increase the availability and accessibility of nutritious foods and decrease the marketing of foods and beverages high in fat, sugar, and/or sodium to children; and (c) monitoring progress in reducing childhood overweight and obesity (PHAC, 2012).

Adolescents. During adolescence, physiological age is a better guide to nutritional needs than chronological age. Energy needs to increase to meet the greater metabolic demands of growth. The daily requirement of protein also increases. Calcium and vitamin D are essential for the rapid bone growth that occurs during adolescence, and girls need a continuous source of iron to replace menstrual blood losses. Boys also need adequate iron for muscle development. In addition to meats and fish, greens, nuts, dried fruits, and whole grains are iron-rich foods (Marcus, 2013). Iodine supports increased thyroid activity, so adolescents' use of iodized table salt helps ensure adequate intake. B-complex vitamins are needed to support heightened metabolic activity.

The adolescent's diet is influenced by many factors other than nutritional needs, including concern about body image and appearance, desire for independence, and fad diets. Nutritional deficiencies may occur in adolescent girls as a result of dieting (Findlay, S. M., & Canadian Paediatric Society, Adolescent Health Committee, 2004/2016) and use of oral contraceptives (Dante, Vaiarelli, & Facchinetti, 2014). Adolescent girls 14 to 18 years old may have inadequate intakes of vitamin B_6, vitamin B_{12}, folate, zinc, iron, magnesium, phosphorus, and vitamin A. Their median calcium, potassium, and fibre intakes are below the AI level (Health Canada, 2012). The adolescent boy's diet may be inadequate in vitamin A and magnesium.

Snacks provide approximately 25% of teenagers' total dietary intake. The consumption of fast foods has been associated with excess weight gain, which may be related to the higher energy and fat content of most of these foods. More than 80% of Canadian adolescents report sodium intakes in excess of the UL—(Health Canada, 2017b). Fast-food restaurants also offer larger portions of food, and consumers are eating greater amounts (Benton, 2015). To counteract this trend among adolescents, health promotion initiatives (e.g., reducing the availability of junk foods in school cafeterias and vending machines) are being implemented in schools to develop supportive environments for healthier eating.

The onset of eating disorders such as **anorexia nervosa** or **bulimia nervosa** often occurs during early adolescence, when individuals are establishing independence and autonomy. Dieting and weight control are viewed as a defence for feelings of inadequacy or ineffectiveness. In later adolescence, when facing the task of separation–individualization, similar conflicts may arise (Weaver, 2015). Recognition of eating disorders is essential for early intervention (Table 42-2).

Nurses who work with adolescents experiencing eating disorders need to be aware of the many implications that such a diagnosis can have on an adolescent. The ever-present threat to physical health must be carefully monitored. Beyond the illness and treatment, these youth experience difficult emotions and face issues of identity, low self-esteem, and autonomy. The case study in Box 42-2 conveys a nurse's experiences caring for an adolescent girl with an eating disorder.

Sports and regular exercise necessitate dietary modification to meet the increased energy needs of adolescents. Carbohydrates, both simple

TABLE 42-2 Potential Assessment for Eating Disorders

Anorexia Nervosa

A. Restriction of energy intake leading to *significantly low body weight* in the context of age, sex, developmental trajectory, and physical health.
B. Intense fear of gaining weight or becoming fat, or persistent behaviour that interferes with weight gain, even though at a significantly low weight.
C. Self-evaluation based on body weight or shape; lacking recognition of the seriousness of current low body weight.

Specify severity:
Mild: BMI >17 kg/m^2
Moderate: BMI 16–16.99 kg/m^2
Severe: BMI 15–15.99 kg/m^2
Extreme: BMI <15 kg/m^2

Bulimia Nervosa

A. Recurrent episodes of binge eating (eating, in a discrete period of time [e.g., 2 hours], an amount of food larger than usual for most people) and experiencing a sense of lack of control over eating during an episode.
B. Recurrent inappropriate compensatory behaviours (e.g., self-induced vomiting, use of laxatives or diuretics, strict dieting or fasting, or vigorous exercise) in order to prevent weight gain.
C. The binge eating and inappropriate compensatory behaviours both occur, on average, at least once a week for 3 months.
D. Self-evaluation unduly influenced by body weight or shape.
E. Does not occur exclusively during episodes of anorexia nervosa.

Specify severity:
Mild: An average of 1–3 episodes of inappropriate compensatory behaviours per week
Moderate: An average of 4–7 episodes of inappropriate compensatory behaviours per week
Severe: An average of 8–13 episodes of inappropriate compensatory behaviours per week
Extreme: An average of 14 or more episodes of inappropriate compensatory behaviours per week

BMI, Body mass index.
From American Psychiatric Association. (2013). *Diagnostic and statistical manual of mental disorders* (5th ed.). Washington, DC: Author. Copyright 2013, American Psychiatric Association. Reprinted with permission.

and complex, are the main source of energy. Protein needs increase to 1.0 to 1.5 g/kg per day; fat needs do not increase. All athletes need to ingest water before and after exercise to prevent dehydration, especially in hot environments. It is not necessary to supplement the diet with vitamins and minerals, but intake of iron-rich foods is required to prevent anemia (Pasricha, Low, Thompson, et al., 2014) and of calcium with vitamin D to prevent stress fractures (Sonneville, Gordon, Kocher, et al., 2012).

Parents often have more influence over the adolescent diet than they believe they have. Effective strategies include limiting the amount of unhealthy foods kept at home and enhancing the appearance and taste of healthy foods. Making healthy foods more convenient and available and working to change social norms that determine what foods are "cool" are other ways to promote optimal nutritional health among adolescents (Krølner, Jørgensen, Aarestrup, et al., 2012).

Pregnancy occurring within 4 years of menarche may place the mother and fetus at risk because of the mother's anatomical and physiological immaturity. Malnutrition at the time of conception increases risk to the adolescent and her fetus. Most teenage girls do not want to gain weight, thus counselling adolescent girls on the nutritional needs associated with pregnancy may be difficult; suggestions are better tolerated than rigid directions. The diet of pregnant adolescents is often deficient in calcium, iron, and vitamins A and C. Prenatal vitamin and mineral supplements are recommended.

Young and Middle-Aged Adults. The demands for most nutrients are reduced as the growth period ends. Adults need nutrients for energy, maintenance, and repair, although their energy needs usually decline over the years. Obesity may become a problem as a result of decreased physical exercise, frequent dining out, and the increased ability to afford more luxury foods. Women who use oral contraceptives may need extra vitamins. Iron and calcium intake continues to be important.

Maintaining good oral health is important throughout adulthood. Poor oral hygiene and periodontal disease are potential risk factors for systemic diseases such as bacteremia, endocarditis, cardiopulmonary disease, and diabetes mellitus and for adverse outcomes in pregnancy (Arigbede, Babatope, & Bamidele, 2012; Parihar, Katoch, Rajguru, et al., 2015).

Pregnancy. Nutrition during pregnancy influences birth weight and survival chances in infants. Generally, the fetus's needs are met at the expense of the mother. If nutrient sources are not available or are unsafe (such as foods affected by the *Listeria* bacteria, which can cross through the placenta), both will suffer. Food poisoning during the first 3 months of pregnancy can cause a miscarriage. Later in the pregnancy, it can cause the baby to be born prematurely, a stillbirth, or a baby who is born very ill. Thus, it is paramount that pregnant women are careful about what they eat and how they store, prepare, and cook their food. To lower the risk of food poisoning, pregnant women should avoid eating hot dogs and non-dried deli meats straight from the package without further heating, dishes containing raw eggs or seafood, unpasteurized dairy products and fruit juices, raw sprouts, and pâtés and meat spreads that have to be refrigerated before use (Health Canada, 2016b). The nutritional status of the mother at the time of conception is important because significant aspects of fetal growth and development often occur before pregnancy is suspected.

The energy requirements associated with pregnancy are related to the mother's body weight and activity levels. Pregnant women need 100 kcal per day above the usual allowance during the first trimester and approximately 300 extra calories per day in the second and third trimesters. The additional nutrients should be obtained by including an extra two to three *Food Guide* servings from any of the four food groups daily (Health Canada, 2014b). Including these extra servings, the daily menu for pregnant women consists of seven to eight servings of vegetables and fruit, six to seven servings of grain products, two servings of milk and alternatives, and two servings of meat and alternatives. A sample weekly menu is available at "My Menu Planner": http://www.eatrightontario.ca/en/MenuPlanner.aspx. It is recommended that pregnant women have at least 150 g of cooked fish each week to ensure intake of omega-3 fats and other important nutrients and take a multivitamin containing 0.4 mg of folic acid and 16 to 20 mg of iron every day (Health Canada, 2014b). Rigid recommendations about weight gain should be avoided because the quality of nutrition during pregnancy is more important than weight gain per se or than the number of kilocalories consumed per day.

Calcium intake is especially critical during the third trimester, when fetal bones are mineralized. Iron may be supplemented to provide for increased maternal blood volume, fetal blood storage, and maternal blood loss during delivery. Iodine needs increase 15 to 17% because of increased activity of the thyroid gland. Folic acid intake is particularly important for DNA synthesis and the growth of red blood cells. Inadequate intake may lead to fetal neural tube defects, anencephaly, or maternal pre-eclampsia (Wen, Guo, Rodger, et al., 2016). Health

BOX 42-2 CASE STUDY

The Need for Understanding Nutrition in Psychiatric-Mental Health Nursing*

Sasha, a 14-year-old girl with a diagnosis of anorexia nervosa, was admitted to the hospital for refeeding and nutritional support. While brushing her hair and getting ready for the day, she reported slight chest pain and faintness. As Sasha's nurse, I performed a basic head-to-toe assessment, including postural vitals (blood pressure, pulse, and symptoms obtained with the patient in supine and standing or sitting positions). Additionally, I followed up on Sasha's most recent blood work. Findings from my assessment included a postural heart rate jump of 60 beats per minute, slight swelling or edema in her ankles, and a decrease in serum phosphate levels. These findings were indicative of refeeding syndrome, a serious and potentially life-threatening condition associated with shifts in fluids and electrolytes, most commonly seen in malnourished patients who are experiencing refeeding. I passed along this information to the rest of Sasha's treatment team so we could prevent serious complications that could include heart problems, impaired mental status, and seizures.

In making sure to introduce calories in a safe manner, as standard practice we perform calculations based on the person's age, height, and previous growth history to achieve a healthy target body weight. This may mean that if a person diagnosed with an eating disorder cannot finish a meal, we provide a calorie drink to replace the number of calories not consumed. As nurses, we may consult with a dietitian or a nutritionist; yet, in order to sufficiently support patients and families, we need to have a basic understanding of nutrition. Without application of such knowledge, there could have been serious implications to Sasha's refeeding and treatment. Thankfully, because that knowledge guided my assessment and the treatment team's response, Sasha was able to move past the barrier of refeeding syndrome, reaching her target weight upon discharge.

After reading the case study, consider the integral role that nutrition plays in the adolescent girl's growth and development as well as its influence on the illness and its treatment. What is the impact of maintaining an unhealthy low weight on the adolescent girl's bone, cardiac, and reproductive health? Given the pressing need to restore physiological status through increasing caloric intake and returning to a healthy body weight, why was the nurse cautious with refeeding and diligent with bedside assessments? What nutritional support and teaching are required in caring for adolescents affected by eating disorders and their families?

*By Sydney Ellis, RN.

BOX 42-3 FOCUS ON OLDER PERSONS

Factors Affecting Nutritional Status

- Age-related gastrointestinal changes that affect digestion of food and maintenance of nutrition include changes in the teeth and gums, decreased bite force, reduced saliva production, atrophy of oral mucosal epithelial cells, increased taste threshold, decreased thirst sensation, reduced gag reflex, and decreased esophageal and colonic peristalsis (Rémond, Shahar, Gille, et al., 2015).
- Presence of other diseases, such as diabetes and cognitive impairments related to delirium, dementia, and depression, increase risk of poor nutrition (Leslie & Hankey, 2015).
- Malnutrition in older persons has multiple causes, such as low income, low educational level, lack of physical functional level to meet activities of daily living, loss, dependency, loneliness, and lack of transportation (Ramage-Morin & Garriguet, 2015).
- Medications may have adverse effects, such as causing anorexia (loss of appetite), xerostomia (severe dryness of the mouth), early satiety, and impaired smell and taste perception. Older persons are more likely to be prescribed medications than younger individuals (Pilgrim, Robinson, Sayer, et al., 2015).
- Intake of calcium, vitamin D, and phosphorus may be deficient, increasing the risk for osteoporosis. Vitamin B_{12} may be deficient among older persons because of the high prevalence of gastrointestinal pathology and use of medications that alter vitamin B_{12} pharmacokinetics (Lachner, Steinle, & Regenold, 2012).
- Many nutrients interact with medications, and nurses should consult a drug handbook for information about specific interactions.

care providers, however, should not advise higher doses of folic acid than prescribed amounts, especially in late pregnancy, because this may slightly promote the risk of asthma in offspring (Blatter, Han, Y., Forno, et al., 2013; Brown, Reeves & Bertone-Johnson, 2014). Other supplements may also have health risks. For example, vitamin A is essential to maternal and fetal health but is teratogenic (harmful to embryo or fetal growth and development) when consumed in excess (National Institutes of Health, 2016a).

Pregnant women should drink at least eight glasses of water daily. They should also avoid artificial sweeteners, alcohol, excessive caffeine, and all drugs not specifically ordered, as these substances pass through the placenta and affect the growing baby. Adequate fluid and fibre intake and moderate exercise help prevent constipation, which is commonly associated with pregnancy in response to the growing uterus, pregnancy hormones, and iron supplementation.

Lactation. Lactating women need 500 kcal per day above the usual allowance because milk production increases energy requirements. *Eating Well With Canada's Food Guide* suggests that lactating women ingest the same nutrient levels as recommended during pregnancy. The need for calcium remains the same as during pregnancy, but lactating women require additional vitamins A and C. Daily intake of water-soluble vitamins (B and C) is needed to ensure adequate levels in breast milk. Fluid intake should be adequate but need not be excessive. Caffeine, alcohol, and drugs are excreted in breast milk and thus should be avoided (Butte & Stuebe, 2016). Alcohol passes freely into mother's milk and has been found to peak at about 30 to 60 minutes after consumption, or 60 to 90 minutes when taken with food. It takes a 55-kg woman about 2 to 3 hours to eliminate from her body the alcohol in one serving of beer or wine (La Leche League, 2015).

Older Persons. Adults aged 65 years and older have a decreased need for energy because the metabolic rate slows with age. However, vitamin and mineral requirements remain unchanged from middle adulthood.

Many factors influence the nutritional status of older persons (Box 42-3). Income is significant; for those living on a fixed income, the amount of money available to buy food may be reduced. A large number of older patients benefit from home-delivered or congregate meal services. Health status is another important factor. The older person may be following a therapeutic diet; have difficulty eating because of physical symptoms, lack of teeth, or dentures; or be at risk for drug–nutrient interactions. Thirst sensation may diminish, leading to inadequate fluid intake or dehydration (see Chapter 40). Meats may be avoided because of the cost or difficulty to chew them. Cheese, eggs, and peanut butter are useful high-protein alternatives. Cream soups and meat-based vegetable soups are nutrient-dense sources of protein; yet, commercial soups and packaged meats contain a high salt content. Milk continues to be an important food for older persons to protect against osteoporosis (a decrease of bone-mass density). Although research has shown that older men lag behind women by approximately a decade in developing osteoporosis, screening and treatment are necessary for both older men and women (National Osteoporosis Foundation, 2014). The diets of older persons should contain choices from all food groups and may require a vitamin and mineral supplement.

Alternative Food Patterns

Many people follow special patterns of food intake that are based on religion (Table 42-3), cultural background (Box 42-4) ethics, health beliefs, personal preference, or concern for the efficient use of land to produce food. Such special diets are not necessarily more or less nutritious than diets based on *Eating Well With Canada's Food Guide* or other nutritional guidelines because good nutrition depends on a balanced intake of all required nutrients.

Vegetarian Diet. Vegetarianism is the consumption of a diet predominantly of plant foods. Vegetarian diets, in general, are low in saturated fat and cholesterol and high in fibre, folate, antioxidants such as vitamin C and E, potassium, and magnesium. Because of this, vegetarian diets may lead to lower blood pressure, improved cholesterol

TABLE 42-3 Religion-Based Dietary Restrictions and Guidelines

Islam	Christianity	Hinduism	Judaism	Church of Jesus Christ of Latter-Day Saints (Mormons)	Seventh-Day Adventists
Pork	Minimal or no alcohol	All meats	Pork	Alcohol	Pork
Alcohol	Holy-day observances may restrict meat	Alcohol	Predatory fowl	Tobacco	Shellfish
Caffeine		Onions	Shellfish (eat only fish with scales)	Caffeine	Alcohol
Emulsifiers made from animal fats, especially margarines		Garlic	Rare meats	Limit meat	Vegetarian diet encouraged
Ramadan fasting sunrise to sunset for 1 month			Blood (blood sausage, etc.)		
Ritualized methods of animal slaughter required for meat ingestion			Do not mix milk or dairy products with meat dishes		
			Must adhere to kosher food preparation methods		
			24 hours of fasting on Yom Kippur, a day of atonement		
			No leavened bread eaten during Passover (8 days)		
			No cooking on the Sabbath (Saturday)		

BOX 42-4 CULTURAL ASPECTS OF CARE

Nutrition

Food patterns developed as a child, through habits and culture, interact to influence food intake. Culture also influences the meaning of food not related to nutrition. Eating is associated with sentiments and feelings such as "good" and "bad." For example, children are often rewarded for "being good" with a treat such as candy. They then associate candy with "being good." Food is also the first thing parents give to their children, usually in the moments after birth, and it is measurable. While love and advice are offered, a tall glass of milk or a second helping of homemade casserole can be immediately seen and can make parents feel they have done something positive for their child.

The incidence of lactose intolerance around the world occurs in the following ethnic or racial groups: Asian-Pacific, African and African American, Native American, Mexican American, Middle Eastern, and Whites. This condition affects nutrient absorption, and calcium deficiency results. See Table 42-7 for food lists appropriate to lactose intolerance diets.

The theory of "hot" and "cold" foods predominates in many cultures. The foundation of the theory is that to keep harmony with nature, one must balance "cold," "hot," "wet," and "dry." Some cultures believe hot characterizes warmth, strength, and reassurance, whereas cold represents menace and weakness. Classification of a food has nothing to do with spiciness but is a symbolic representation of temperature.

Implications for Practice

- Identify the meaning that certain types of food have for each patient.
- Lactose and other food intolerances unique to specific cultures require diet adaptation to meet nutrient, mineral, and vitamin daily-intake requirements.
- In some cultures, specific conditions require hot foods. Menstruation, cancer, pneumonia, earache, colds, paralysis, headache, and rheumatism are "cold" illnesses requiring hot foods (e.g., rice, grain cereals, alcohol, beef, lamb, chili peppers, chocolate, cheese, temperate-zone fruits, eggs, peas, goat's milk, corn husks, oils, peanuts, onions, pork, radishes, tamales).
- Other conditions, such as pregnancy, fever, infections, diarrhea, rashes, ulcers, liver problems, constipation, kidney problems, and sore throats, are "hot" conditions requiring cold foods (e.g., beans, citrus fruits, tropical fruits, dairy products, most fresh vegetables, honey, raisins, chicken, fish, and goat meat).

Adapted from Giger, J. N. (2016). *Transcultural nursing: Assessment and intervention* (7th ed.). St. Louis, MO: Elsevier Health Sciences.

levels, healthier weight, and less incidence of type 2 diabetes (Heart and Stroke Foundation, 2017b; Trapp & Levin, 2012).

Vegetarian diets may include the following:

1. Semi or partial-vegetarian: May eat some milk products, eggs, poultry, and fish while primarily consuming plant-based foods
2. Pesco-vegetarian: May eat fish, eggs, dairy products, grains, vegetables, fruits, legumes, seeds, and nuts while avoiding meat and poultry
3. Lacto-ovo-vegetarian: Eating eggs, dairy products, grains, vegetables, fruits, legumes, seeds, and nuts while avoiding meat, poultry, and fish
4. Lacto-vegetarian: Eating dairy products, grains, vegetables, fruits, legumes, seeds, and nuts while avoiding meat, fish, poultry, and eggs
5. Vegan: Eating grains, vegetables, fruits, legumes, seeds, and nuts while avoiding meat, fish, poultry, eggs, dairy, and honey

Appropriately planned vegetarian diets can help prevent colon cancer (Orlich, Singh, Sabate, et al., 2015). Specifically, vegan diets seem to confer lower risk for overall and for female-specific cancer, compared to other dietary patterns; lacto-ovo-vegetarian diets seem to confer protection from cancers of the gastrointestinal tract (Tantamango-Bartley, Jaceldo-Siegl, Fan, et al., 2013).

It may take planning across the lifespan to get enough protein, iron, zinc, calcium, vitamins D and B_{12}, and omega-3 fats from foods or supplements (Dietitians of Canada, 2014). As a general rule, our bodies need approximately 0.8 grams of protein for every kilogram of body weight. This means that a person weighing 60 kg requires approximately (60 kg $\times$ 0.8) 48 grams of protein daily. Children who follow a vegetarian diet are at risk for protein, iron, and vitamin deficiencies such as vitamin B_{12} (Amit & Canadian Paediatric Society, 2010/2016). Based on the lower digestibility of plant proteins, it is suggested that protein intake may need to be increased by 30 to 35% for infants up to 2 years of age, 20 to 30% for 2- to 6-year-olds, and 15% to 20% for those older than 6 years of age. A range of plant protein products are needed because particular amino acids that are abundant in some foods may be limited in other foods and vice versa. By consuming a wide variety of foods, the amino acids "complement" each other to provide the essential amino acids in proper balance. Sources of protein include soy and soy products; meat alternatives (e.g., textured vegetable protein and veggie burgers); dried beans (e.g., kidney, black, and white beans), peas (e.g., chickpeas and black-eyed peas), and lentils (e.g., red, brown, and green lentils); and grains, nuts, and seeds (Dietitians of Canada, 2014). For children under the age of 4, certain high-protein foods such as whole nuts or seeds are to be avoided, as they represent a choking risk (Cyr & Canadian Paediatric Society, Injury Prevention Committee, 2016).

Recognizing that iron deficiency is the most common nutritional deficiency in children, it is essential that food sources rich in iron are included for this population. Canadian adolescent girls and women of reproductive age who are vegetarian are at greater risk for low iron stores because diets high in plant foods contain dietary iron inhibitors (National Institutes of Health, 2016b). Vegetarian athletes need almost twice the iron of non-vegetarians and should have their iron checked periodically by their primary care provider to determine if a supplement is needed (Dietitians of Canada, 2013a). Vegan iron sources include the above protein sources, specifically firm or extra firm tofu, pinto and adzuki beans, almonds, and sesame seeds (Dietitians of Canada, 2014). Iron is additionally found in fruits such as prunes, raisins, and apricots; dark green vegetables such as collards, okra, and bok choy; and blackstrap molasses (Dietitians of Canada, 2014). The form of iron present in foods of plant origin is not well absorbed by the body; its rate of absorption can be increased by incorporating foods high in vitamin C (e.g., oranges and grapefruit and their juices, lemons, limes, kiwis, mangos, cantaloupe, potatoes, sweet peppers, broccoli, snow peas, and some green leafy vegetables).

Calcium deserves special attention in vegetarian food guidelines. A major criticism of using *Canada's Food Guide* for vegetarian diet planning is that soy milk is the only vegan milk alternative mentioned. In addition to fortified soy drinks and products (e.g., soy yogurts, tofu), good vegan sources of calcium include navy beans and white beans; nuts and nut products such as almonds and almond butter; seeds such as sesame seeds and their butter (tahini); blackstrap molasses; vegetables such as bok choy, okra, collard greens, and turnip greens; and fruits such as figs and fortified orange juice (Dietitians of Canada, 2014).

Zinc is found in soy products; dried beans, peas, and lentils; nuts such as peanuts, pecans, and cashews; seeds such as pumpkin and flax; and whole grains and fortified cereals.

Unsupplemented vegan diets do not provide vitamin B_{12}. It is recommended by Dietitians of Canada (2013b) that all people over the age of 50, regardless of type of diet, take at least 2.4 mcg of vitamin B_{12} in supplements and fortified foods (e.g., fortified nondairy milks, fortified meat alternatives, and breakfast cereals). Vitamin B_{12} is also contained in Red Star nutritional yeast, the only brand of nutritional yeast in Canada fortified with vitamin B_{12}. It has a similar flavour to cheese and can be sprinkled on top of casseroles and in soups. Vegan diets require a source of vitamin D when sun exposure is insufficient. Good sources of vitamin D include fortified soy and other fortified non-dairy drinks and soft margarines (Dietitians of Canada, 2014). It is recommended that people over the age of 50 take 400 IU of vitamin D each day from a supplement (Dietitians of Canada, 2014). There is no mention of vegetarian sources of omega-3 in *Canada's Food Guide*. Omega-3 fats are found in oils (canola, flax seed, walnut, and soybean); ground flax seed; and soybeans, tofu, and walnuts.

CRITICAL THINKING

Critical thinking requires the gathering and synthesizing of knowledge, experience, and information from patients that is gained through intellectual and professional standards. Clinical judgements involve the anticipation of required information, analysis of the data, and openness to new ideas and multiple perspectives when making decisions regarding patient care. Critical thinking is thus a dynamic process. During assessment (Figure 42-4), all elements that contribute to the rendering of appropriate nursing diagnoses are considered.

When assessing nutrition, the nurse must integrate knowledge from nursing and other disciplines, previous experiences, information gathered from patients and families about food preferences, clinical observations, and dietary history. Professional standards, such as the DRIs and *Eating Well With Canada's Food Guide* (Health Canada, 2016c), provide guidelines for assessing and maintaining patient nutritional status. Other professional standards from the Heart and Stroke Foundation of Canada, the Canadian Cancer Society, Canadian Society for Clinical Nutrition, and Diabetes Canada are available. These standards are research based and regularly updated for optimal care.

NURSING PROCESS AND NUTRITION

Nurses are in an excellent position to recognize signs of poor nutrition and take steps to initiate change. Close contact with patients and their families enables nurses to make observations about physical status, food intake, weight changes, and responses to therapy.

Assessment

Early recognition of malnourished or at-risk patients has a strong, positive influence on both short- and long-term health outcomes. A

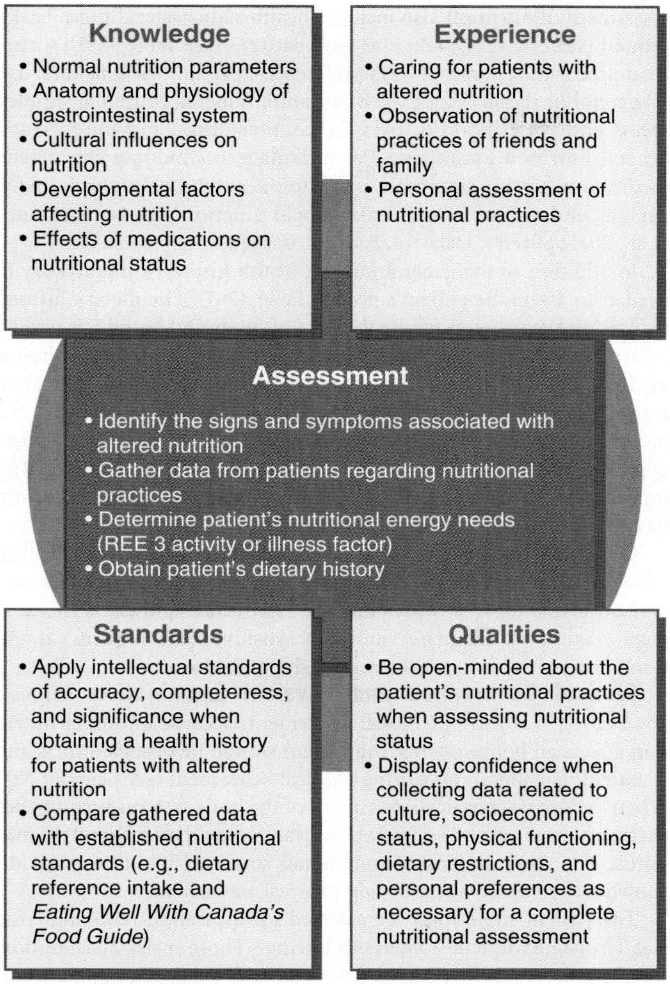

FIGURE 42-4 Critical thinking model for nutrition assessment. *REE,* Resting energy expenditure.

recent study identified that 45% of adult patients who were hospitalized for more than 2 days were nutritionally at risk upon hospital admission and that such malnutrition increases hospital stays by approximately 3 days longer than nourished patients, costing the health care system $1 500 to $2 000 per malnourished patient in 2012 dollars (Canadian Malnutrition Task Force, 2016). Other studies have found poorer quality of life, poorer physical functioning, and higher care complexity in malnourished cardiac patients (Pathirana, Lokunarangoda, Ranathunga, et al., 2014) and delayed wound healing in malnourished surgical patients (Mahakalkar, Modi, Yeola, et al., 2014). Baxter, Al-Madhaki, and Zlotkin (2014) reported the overall prevalence of malnutrition using body mass index (BMI) for age in Canadian pediatric patients as being 39.6% to 46%, of which 8.8% and 30.8% of admitted patients were under- and over-nourished, respectively. Furthermore, 6.9% to 13% were determined to be acutely malnourished and 13.4% chronically malnourished. The high prevalence of overall malnutrition suggests that initial screening using simple anthropometric measures should be conducted on hospital admission so that patients can receive appropriate nutrition-specific care.

Nutritional screening is a process of identifying characteristics known to be associated with nutrition problems to identify those who have a nutrition diagnosis and would benefit from further assessment and treatment by a dietitian (Canadian Malnutrition Task Force, 2016).

TABLE 42-4 Canadian Nutrition Screening Tool (CNST), 2014

Ask the patient the following questions	Yes	No
1. Have you lost weight in the past 6 months without trying to lose this weight? • *If the patient reports a weight loss but gained it back, consider it as a NO weight loss.*		
2. Have you been eating less than usual for more than a week?		
• *Two "YES" answers indicate nutrition risk.* • If the patient is uncertain regarding weight loss, ask if clothing is now fitting more loosely. • If the patient is unable to answer the questions, a knowledgeable informant can be asked to provide the information.		

From Laporte, M. (June 2013). *Part of a presentation given at the Canadian Nutrition Society Conference.* Retrieved from http://nutritioncareincanada.ca/sites/default/uploads/files/Comparison-of-nutrition-screening-tools-for-hospital-use.pdf.

The Canadian Nutrition Screening Tool (CNST) (Table 42-4) is a nutrition-risk screening tool that consists of two questions about weight loss and fluid intake. Two "YES" answers indicate increased nutritional risk (Laporte, Keller, Payette, et al., 2015).

If the patient was not at risk upon admission, the person should be rescreened 1 week later. As well, inadequate food intake (<50% of meals provided) should be identified and patients weighed weekly (Davidson, 2014).

Nutritional assessment goes beyond nutritional screening and involves five major areas: anthropometry, laboratory tests, dietary and health history, clinical observation and physical examination, and patient expectations. It is important to assess nutritional status when a condition exists that interferes with the patient's ability to ingest, digest, or absorb adequate nutrition. No single area or measurement accurately determines nutritional status, and a patient's personal and social health context needs to be considered.

Anthropometry. Anthropometry is a measurement system of the size and makeup of the body. Height and weight are obtained for each patient admission to any health care setting. If height cannot be measured with the patient standing, the patient should be positioned lying flat in bed as straight as possible with arms folded on the chest and measured lengthwise. If possible, the patient should be weighed at the same time each day, on the same scale, and with the same apparel. Serial measures over time provide more useful information than one-time measurement. An ideal body weight (IBW) provides an estimate of what a person should weigh. Rapid weight gain usually reflects fluid shifts. Five hundred mL of fluid equals 0.45 kg. For example, for a patient with renal failure or heart failure, a weight increase of 0.9 kg is significant, as it may indicate that the patient has retained a litre of fluid. Recent weight changes should be documented.

Body mass index (BMI) measures weight corrected for height and serves as an alternative to traditional height–weight relationships.

Calculation of BMI is achieved by dividing the patient's weight in kilograms by height in metres squared: Weight (kg)/Height^2 (m^2). The BMI nomogram is available on Health Canada's website, at http://www.hc-sc.gc.ca/fn-an/nutrition/weights-poids/guide-ld-adult/bmi_chart_java-graph_imc_java-eng.php. A BMI measuring between 25 and 30 indicates overweight, and greater than 30 defines obesity (Health Canada, 2016d). The BMI is a valid measurement of weight in relation to health; however, it is not recommended for use as the sole measurement of body composition or level of fitness because it does not differentiate between excess fat and muscle or bone and does not consider age, gender, or ethnicity (Al Dokhi & Shahid Habib, 2013; Gutterman, 2014). Care must be taken when interpreting overweight and obesity results for Canadian child obesity, as cutoff points different from adult cutoffs have been used. In 2015, the Canadian Task Force on Preventive Care recommended the use of the 2014 WHO growth charts; this recommendation was also endorsed by the College of Family Physicians of Canada (Canadian Task Force on Preventive Care, 2015).

Heart and Stroke Foundation research indicates that for most people, the waist circumference (WC) measurement may be used to determine health risk. Overweight people who carry excess pounds around the waist are at greater risk of heart disease and stroke than those who carry it on their hips, thighs, and buttocks. The WC is measured at the part of the trunk located midway between the lower costal margin (bottom of lower rib) and the iliac crest (top of pelvic bone) while the person is standing, with feet somewhat apart. The person doing the measuring should stand beside the individual and fit the tape snugly, without compressing any underlying soft tissues. The circumference should be measured to the nearest 0.5 cm, at the end of a normal expiration. In men, a WC of 102 cm (40 inches) or greater places them at significant increased risk for heart disease and stroke. In women, this measurement is 88 cm (35 inches) or more (Health Canada, 2016d; Heart and Stroke Foundation, 2017c).

Laboratory and Biochemical Tests. No single laboratory or biochemical test can be used to diagnose malnutrition. Factors that may alter test results include fluid balance, liver function, kidney function, and the presence of disease. Common laboratory tests used to study nutritional status include measures of plasma proteins such as albumin, transferrin, prealbumin, retinol-binding protein, total iron-binding capacity, and hemoglobin. After feeding, the response time for changes in these proteins ranges from hours to weeks. The metabolic half-life of albumin is 21 days; transferrin, 7 days; prealbumin, 2 days; and retinol-binding protein, 12 hours. A meta-analysis of 63 studies, which included 2 125 patients, investigated the effects of starvation on serum albumin levels in otherwise healthy individuals and reported that the levels remained normal until the patients reached extreme states of starvation (BMI <12 or greater than 6 weeks of starvation) when the malnutrition was already physically evident (Lee, Oh, Lee, et al., 2015). From this finding, it is evident that albumin cannot be reliably used as a marker for diagnosing protein-calorie malnutrition. Serum albumin levels are affected by hydration; hemorrhage; renal or hepatic disease; AIDS; high-output drainage of wounds, drains, burns, or the gut; steroid administration; albumin infusions; age; pregnancy; and trauma, burns, stress, or surgery. Albumin level is a better indicator of chronic illnesses, whereas prealbumin level is a preferred indicator of acute conditions.

Nitrogen balance is important to establish serum protein status (see "Proteins" section). Nitrogen balance is calculated as nitrogen intake minus nitrogen loss from the body and is useful for evaluating protein metabolism because nitrogen is an essential part of protein building blocks—amino acids. Nitrogen output can be measured through laboratory analysis of a 24-hour urinary urea nitrogen level (Bharadwaj, Ginoya, Tandon, et al., 2016). For patients with diarrhea or fistula drainage, a further addition of 2 to 4 g of nitrogen output is estimated. A positive (more nitrogen taken in than put out) 2- to 3-g nitrogen balance is ideal for anabolism. In contrast, negative (more nitrogen put out than taken in) nitrogen balance is present in catabolic states, such as starvation or physiological stress.

Dietary History and Health History. The nurse needs to gather information about the patient's illness or activity level to determine energy needs and compare that information with food intake. Nursing assessment of nutrition also includes health status; age; cultural background (see Box 42-4); religious food patterns (see Table 42-3); socioeconomic status; personal food preferences; psychological factors; use of alcohol or illegal drugs; use of vitamin, mineral, or herbal supplements and prescription or over-the-counter drugs; and the patient's general nutrition knowledge. Polypharmacy, or multiple concurrent medication use, is a significant predictor of nutritional status in older persons and requires careful assessment (Illario, Maione, Rusciano, et al., 2016; Silveira, Dalastra, & Pagotto, 2014).

In addition to the general nursing health history, a diet history is needed to assess the patient's needs (Table 42-5). The dietary history focuses on the patient's habitual intake of foods and liquids, as well as information about preferences, ability to obtain food, and allergies. Eliciting the diet and health history requires careful and respectful exploration of the patient's perceived health status to identify any hidden areas of concern, such as high use of alcoholic beverages, which Quintero-Platt, González-Reimers, Martín-González, et al. (2015) found to be associated with vitamin D deficiency, low lean mass, liver dysfunction, and greater long-term mortality.

Outpatients may keep a food diary spanning several days, which will enable more accurate calculation of nutritional intake and comparison to *Eating Well With Canada's Food Guide* and DRIs to see if dietary habits are adequate. Culturally sensitive food-frequency questionnaires may also be used to establish patterns over time.

Clinical Observation and Physical Examination. Clinical observation is key to nutritional assessment. Because improper nutrition affects all body systems, the patient should be observed for signs of nutritional alterations during physical assessment (see Chapter 32). When the general physical assessment of the body systems is complete, pertinent areas can be rechecked to evaluate the patient's nutritional status. The clinical signs of nutritional status (Table 42-6) provide guidelines for observation during physical assessment.

The patient should also be assessed for aspiration (choking) risk and dysphagia (difficulty when swallowing). Those at risk of aspiration may have decreased levels of alertness, decreased gag or cough reflexes, difficulty managing saliva, or a wet, gurgling voice. The warning signs of dysphagia include coughing during eating; change in voice tone or quality after swallowing; abnormal movements of the mouth, tongue, or lips; slow, weak, imprecise, inconsistent, or uncoordinated speech; abnormal gag reflex; delayed swallowing; incomplete oral clearance or pocketing of food or medications; and regurgitation. In Canada, approximately half of all new stroke patients older than 65 years of age live with dysphagia for months after the stroke. Patients with dysphagia often do not show overt signs such as coughing when food enters the airway. Aspiration may be silent; this absence of any outward sign or distress is known as "silent aspiration," reported as occurring in over 40% of patients (Cohen, Roffe, Beavan, et al., 2016) but unsuspected as the cause of death by clinicians in one third of these patients (Hu, Yi, & Ryu, 2014). Early detection of dysphagia improves outcomes such as malnutrition, dehydration, pulmonary compromise, mortality, length of hospital stay, and overall health care expenditures (Hebert, Lindsay, McIntyre, et al., 2016; Wirth, Dziewas, Beck, et al., 2016).

The 2015 Canadian Stroke Rehabilitation Best Practice Guidelines (Hebert et al., 2016) recommend early assessment of all stroke patients by rehabilitation professionals with specialized training in stroke care and recovery. Along with nurses, the core rehabilitation interprofessional team includes physiatrists, other physicians with expertise in stroke rehabilitation, occupational therapists, physiotherapists, speech-language pathologists, social workers, and dietitians. Nurses should implement aspiration precautions (Skill 42-1) and refer patients at risk of malnutrition, including those with dysphagia, to a dietitian for nutrition assessment and ongoing management.

TABLE 42-5 Obtaining a Dietary History (Acronym: FASTCHECK)	
Components of a Dietary History	**Areas to Assess and Questions to Ask**
***F*ood Practices**	
Number, type, and location of meals eaten per day	How many meals do you eat? At what times do you usually eat? Are these scheduled meals or snacks? Where do you usually eat meals and snacks? With whom?
Food preferences	What types of food do you like?
Food-preparation practices	Who prepares the food?
Food-purchasing practices	Who purchases the food?
***A*llergies**	
	Are you allergic to any foods? Specify these foods. What happens when you eat these foods? Specify the type of allergic response (e.g., hives, itching, anaphylaxis). What is done to treat allergies (e.g., EpiPen, oral antihistamines)?
***S*ymptoms**	
Indigestion, heartburn, gas, alterations in taste	What foods cause indigestion, gas, or heartburn? Does this occur each time you eat the food? Have you noticed any changes in taste? Did these changes occur with medications or following an illness?
Relief practices	What relieves the symptoms?
***T*wenty-Four Hour Recall**	
To conduct the 24-hour diet recall (National Cancer Institute, 2017), ask the patient to describe every item of food and drink ingested in a 24-hour period. The easiest time period to recall is from the time one awakens to the time one goes to bed again. a. Using open-ended questions and systematic repetition, ask, "When you first woke up yesterday, what was the first thing you put in your mouth?" "How much of it did you have?" "What time was that?" "What did you eat or drink next?" Do not ask about specific meals. Do ask for foods and drinks between any meals and at bedtime. b. Ask for specific types of foods and drinks: for example, "What kind of milk—whole, fat-free?" What kind of rice—brown, white?" c. Record time and amounts of all food eaten. d. Find out about methods of preparation (e.g., salt, fat) and ingredients in mixed dishes. e. Record intake of drinks to assess the adequacy of fluid intake. f. Determine if this intake is typical of most days. g. Record type and amount of alcoholic beverages and nonfood items consumed. Document servings consumed under "Other foods and beverages." After all the information for the diet history is collected, evaluate the 24-hour recall by a. Counting and recording the number of servings eaten for each food group b. Comparing servings eaten to recommended daily servings appropriate for the age and sex of the patient Be aware that an individual may have difficulty estimating portion sizes and remembering everything, that 24 hours may not be representative of diet, and that the individual may feel pressure to say what is perceived as desired.	
***C*hewing and Swallowing**	Do you wear dentures? Full or partial? Orthodontic devices? Are the dentures or devices comfortable? Assess the condition of the patient's teeth. Do you experience mouth pain or sores (e.g., cold sores, canker sores)? Do you have difficulty swallowing? Do you cough or gag when you swallow?
***H*unger**	
Appetite	Have you had a change in appetite? Have you noticed a change in weight? Was this change an anticipated change (e.g., were you following a weight-reduction diet)?
Satiety	Do you stop eating when feeling full? Do you pick at food between meals or eat substantially before bedtime?
***E*limination Patterns**	
	How often do you have bowel movements? Do you experience diarrhea with meals or specific foods? If yes, how do you manage the diarrhea? Do you experience constipation? If yes, how do you manage it?
***C*hemical Substances**	
Medication use	What medications do you take?
Over-the-counter substances	Do you take any over-the-counter medications that your doctor does not prescribe? If yes, specify them.
Alcohol	How many servings of alcoholic beverages do you drink each day—one, two, three, five, ten, or more?
Supplements	Describe any nutritional or herbal supplements you use.
***K*nowledge**	
	Do you believe your current diet is adequate for meeting your energy needs? If not, what would you like to change?

TABLE 42-6 Clinical Signs of Nutritional Status

Body Area	Signs of Good Nutrition	Signs of Poor Nutrition
General appearance	Alert; responsive	Listless, apathetic, cachectic appearance
Weight	Weight appropriate for height, age, body build	Obese or underweight appearance (special concern for underweight)
Posture	Erect posture; straight arms and legs	Sagging shoulders; sunken chest; humped back
Muscles	Well-developed, firm muscles; good tone; some fat under skin	Flaccid appearance, poor tone, underdeveloped tone; tenderness; edema; wasted appearance; inability to walk properly
Nervous system control	Good attention span; lack of irritability or restlessness; normal reflexes; psychological stability	Inattention; irritability; confusion; burning and tingling of hands and feet (paresthesia); loss of position and vibratory sense; weakness and tenderness of muscles (may result in inability to walk); decrease or loss of ankle and knee reflexes
Gastrointestinal function	Good appetite and digestion; normal regular elimination; no palpable organs or masses	Anorexia; indigestion; constipation or diarrhea; liver or spleen enlargement
Cardiovascular function	Normal heart rate and rhythm; lack of murmurs; normal blood pressure for age	Rapid heart rate (above 100 beats/minute), enlarged heart; abnormal rhythm; elevated blood pressure
General vitality	Endurance; energy; good sleep habits; vigorous appearance	Easily fatigued; lack of energy; falling asleep easily; tired and apathetic appearance
Hair	Shiny, lustrous appearance; firmness; strands not easily plucked; healthy scalp	Stringy, dull, brittle, dry, thin, and sparse, depigmented appearance; strands that can be easily plucked
Skin (general)	Smooth and slightly moist skin with good colour	Rough, dry, scaly, pale, pigmented, irritated appearance; bruises; petechiae; subcutaneous fat loss
Face and neck	Uniform colour; smooth, pink, healthy appearance; lack of swelling	Greasy, discoloured, scaly, swollen appearance; dark skin over cheeks and under eyes; lumpiness or flakiness of skin around nose and mouth
Lips	Smoothness; good colour; moist (not chapped or swollen) appearance	Dry, scaly, swollen appearance; redness and swelling (cheilosis); angular lesions at corners of mouth; fissures or scars (stomatitis)
Mouth, oral membranes	Reddish pink, intact mucous membranes in oral cavity	Swollen, boggy oral mucous membranes
Gums	Pink; healthy appearance; lack of swelling or bleeding	Spongy gums that bleed easily; marginal redness, inflammation; receding gums
Tongue	Pink or deep reddish colour; lack of swelling; smoothness, presence of surface papillae; lack of lesions	Swelling, scarlet, and raw appearance; magenta colour, beefiness (glossitis); hyperemic and hypertrophic papillae; atrophic papillae
Teeth	Lack of cavities and pain; bright, straight appearance; lack of crowding; well-shaped jaw; clean appearance with no discoloration	Unfilled caries; absent teeth; worn surfaces; mottling (fluorosis); malpositioned appearance
Eyes	Bright, clear, shiny appearance; lack of sores at corner of membranes; eyelids moist and healthy pink colour; prominent blood vessels or lack of mound of tissue or sclera; lack of fatigue circles beneath eyes	Pale eye membranes (pale conjunctivae); redness of membrane (conjunctival infection); dryness; signs of infection; buildup of keratin debris in the conjunctiva (Bitot's spots), redness and fissuring of eyelid corners (angular palpebritis); dryness of eye membrane (conjunctival xerosis); dull appearance of cornea (corneal xerosis); soft cornea (keratomalacia)
Neck (glands)	Lack of enlargement	Thyroid enlargement
Nails	Firm, pink appearance	Spoon shape (koilonychia); brittleness; ridges
Legs, feet	Lack of tenderness, weakness, or swelling; good colour	Edema; tender calves; tingling; weakness
Skeleton	Lack of malformation	Bowlegs; knock knees; chest deformity at diaphragm; prominent scapulae and ribs

From Hood, W. A. (2015). Nutritional status assessment in adults technique. *Medscape*. Retrieved from http://emedicine.medscape.com/article/2141861-technique; Kirkpatrick, K. (2014, February 18). 9 ways your body is trying to tell you that your diet stinks. *Huffington Post*. Retrieved from http://www.huffingtonpost.com/kristin-kirkpatrick-ms-rd-ld/diet-problems_b_4456679.html.

SKILL 42-1 ASPIRATION PRECAUTIONS

Delegation Considerations

The assessment of aspiration risk and determination of positioning cannot be delegated to unregulated care providers (UCPs). However, UCPs may feed patients after receiving instructions about aspiration precautions. It is important to instruct UCPs about the following:

- Appropriate patient positioning to decrease aspiration risk
- Reporting of any onset of coughing, gagging, or pocketing of food

Equipment

- Chair or electric bed (to allow patient to sit upright)
- Thickening agents as needed (commercial prethickened products or commercial thickening agent)
- Tongue blade
- Penlight

PROCEDURE

STEPS	RATIONALE
1. Give patients who are not alert within the first 24 hours post-stroke nothing by mouth (NPO) and monitor closely.	• Risk of aspiration is high (Hebert et al., 2016).
2. Patients should be screened for swallowing deficits as soon as they are alert and ready for trialling oral intake using a valid screening tool by an expert in dysphagia.	• An individualized management plan should be developed to address dysphagia, dietary needs, and specialized nutrition plans (Hebert et al., 2016).
3. Assess patients for signs and symptoms of dysphagia (e.g., cough, change in voice after swallowing). Video fluoroscopic swallow study or fibre-optic endoscopic examination of swallowing should be performed on all patients considered at risk for pharyngeal dysphagia or poor airway protection, based on results from the bedside swallowing assessment (Hebert et al., 2016).	• Patients at risk include those who have chronic obstructive pulmonary disease or neurological or neuromuscular diseases and those who have had trauma to or surgical procedures of the oral cavity or throat.
4. Ask patient about any difficulties with chewing or swallowing foods with different textures.	• Certain types of food are more easily aspirated.
5. Ensure that the clinical bedside screening trial is conducted by a speech language pathologist (SLP) or appropriately trained specialist.	• The SLP is qualified to assess and to advise on the safety of the patient's swallowing ability and the consistency of diet and fluids.
6. Elevate head of patient's bed so that hips are flexed at a 90-degree angle and head is flexed slightly forward, or help patient to the same position in a chair.	• Reduces risk of aspiration (Metheny, 2016).
7. The clinical bedside screening trial involves giving 3 to 10 mL of water, and if that is well tolerated, it is followed by a small cup (50–90 mL) of water.	• The Water Swallow Test is a useful bedside screening tool for aspiration in stroke patients, especially for its convenience and cost-effectiveness in clinical practice. The test accuracy is related to the water volume; water volumes of 3 mL (Hayashi, Yahiro, Sakuragi, et al., 2016), 50 mL (Martino, Maki, & Diamant, 2014), and 90 mL (Chen, Chuang, Leong, et al., 2016) have been tested and recommended for screening aspiration in stroke patients. There is no consensus among studies of the method of screening for dysphagia in the adult stroke population (Almeida, Cola, Pernambuco, et al., 2015; Hayashi et al., 2016).
8. For a patient who may feed self, explain that you are initially observing while the patient eats:	• Self-feeding may reduce the risk of pneumonia (Hebert et al., 2016) and increases patient cooperation.
A. Observe patient consume various consistencies of food and liquids, watching for signs of dysphagia.	• Referral to a dietitian and SLP is appropriate if patient has difficulty with a particular consistency.
B. Note at the end of the meal if patient becomes tired.	• Fatigue increases risk of aspiration.
C. Report signs and symptoms of dysphagia.	• Signs or symptoms indicate the need for further evaluation of swallowing by an SLP in collaboration with the radiology department, such as a fluoroscopic swallow study (Hebert et al., 2016; Koidou, Kollias, Sdravou, et al., 2013). A significant number of individuals who aspirate do not exhibit signs and symptoms of dysphagia (Teasell, Foley, Martino, et al., 2016).
D. Place identification on patient's record indicating that dysphagia is present.	• Alerts the health care team to the problem and helps the team to develop and implement an individualized plan of care.
9. For patients who require supervision or assistance with eating because dysphagia and risk of aspiration have been identified, explain that you will assist them with their meal:	• Increases patient comfort.
A. Perform hand hygiene.	• Reduces transmission of microorganisms.

Continued

SKILL 42-1 ASPIRATION PRECAUTIONS—cont'd

STEPS	RATIONALE
B. As ordered or recommended by the feeding/swallowing team, add thickener to thin liquids to create the consistency of nectar, honey, or pudding.	• Thin liquids such as water and fruit juice are difficult to control in the mouth and are more easily aspirated (Leder, Judson, Sliwinski, et al., 2013). It is essential to follow the team's determination for consistency because best practices have not yet been established (Steele, Alsanei, Ayanikalath, et al., 2015). It was shown that in a specific subset of individuals who swallowed puree consistency without aspiration but exhibited pharyngeal dysphagia and aspiration with thin liquid consistency, both nectar-like and honey-like thickened liquids were swallowed without aspiration, with 100% success (Leder et al., 2013).
C. Place 1/2 (2.5 g) to 1 teaspoon (5 g) of food on unaffected side of the mouth, allowing utensil to touch the mouth or tongue.	• Provides patient with tactile cues to begin eating.
D. Place hand on throat to gently palpate swallowing event as it occurs. Swallowing twice is often necessary to clear the pharynx.	• Helps evaluate swallowing effort.
E. Provide verbal coaching and positive reinforcement while feeding patient. • Feel the food in your mouth. • Chew and taste the food. • Raise your tongue to the roof of your mouth. • Think about swallowing. • Close your mouth and swallow. • Swallow again. • Cough to clear the airway.	• Verbal cueing keeps patient focused on swallowing. Positive reinforcement enhances patient's confidence in ability to swallow.
F. Observe for coughing, choking, gagging, and drooling of food; suction airway as necessary.	• These are indications that suggest dysphagia and risk for aspiration.
G. Provide rest periods as necessary during meal to avoid rushed or forced feeding.	• Avoiding fatigue decreases the risk of aspiration.
H. Using a penlight and tongue blade, gently inspect patient's oral cavity during and after the meal to detect pockets of food.	• Pockets of food in the mouth often indicate difficulty swallowing.
I. Ask patient to remain sitting upright for at least 30 minutes after the meal.	• Reduces the risk of gastroesophageal reflux, which causes aspiration (Teasell et al., 2016).
J. Help patient to perform hand hygiene and mouth care. Provide education and support to enable patient to meet his or her oral hygiene needs, be able to select and use appropriate oral hygiene equipment, and recognize and manage difficulty of swallowing.	• Mouth care after meals helps control dental plaque and maintain patient's oral hygiene (Teasell et al., 2016).
K. Record intake and report any observations indicative of feeding and swallowing difficulties.	
L. Ensure return of patient's tray to appropriate place, and perform hand hygiene.	• Reduces spread of microorganisms.
10. Weigh patient weekly at the same time on the same scale.	• Determines if weight is stable and reflects adequate caloric level.

UNEXPECTED OUTCOMES	RELATED INTERVENTIONS
Coughs, gags, food "stuck in throat," or left in mouth	• Patient may require a swallowing evaluation. • Initiate consultation with an SLP for swallowing exercises and techniques to improve swallowing and reduce risk of aspiration. • Notify the nurse in charge, health care provider, and SLP of any symptoms that occurred during meal and which foods caused the symptoms.
Avoidance of certain textures of food	• Change consistency and texture of food.
Weight loss	• Discuss findings with the nurse in charge, health care provider, SLP, or registered dietitian.

RECORDING AND REPORTING

- Document the following in the patient's chart: patient's tolerance of various food textures, amount of assistance required, position during meal, absence or presence of any symptoms of dysphagia, and amount eaten.
- Report any coughing, gagging, choking, or swallowing difficulties to the nurse in charge or the health care provider.

Safety Alert The importance of safety considerations (i.e., checking consistency of fluid, correct drinking utensil and volume of fluid, 90-degree head-of-bed elevation, supervision) for patients with impaired swallowing cannot be overstressed. Healthy people can tolerate the dynamic and often fast flow of liquids during swallowing to cleanly direct liquids past the airway and into the esophagus. However, individuals with dysphagia find the flow of liquids difficult to control during passage through the pharynx. This can result in impaired airway protection. One method of managing this challenge is to thicken liquids so that they flow more slowly, thus allowing the individual time to coordinate safe swallowing. Liquids are thickened to various levels of viscosity with a range of starches and gums, including commercially prepared products, and typically range from the least viscous liquid (akin to the thickness of nectar) for mild dysphagia to increasingly thicker liquids (honey-like and spoon-thick or pudding consistency) for more severe dysphagia (Cichero, 2013). Prescription of fluid thickness is patient specific.

Patients who have dysphagia are not to drink with a straw unless specifically advised by their therapist. When deemed safe to use, drinking straws reduce the volumes of discrete sips. Narrower straw diameters are associated with smaller bolus volumes (Clark, Anderson, & Hietpas, 2014). A straw may make it easier to get the liquid into the mouth and to take sequential sips without liquid spilling out of the mouth; however, healthy adult participants who drank from a cup ingested significantly more than those who used a straw (Veiga, Fonseca, & Bianchini, 2014). Additional study is needed to determine whether individuals with dysphagia demonstrate similar patterns of bolus size associated with straws (Cichero, 2013; Clark et al., 2014; Clark & Shelton, 2014).

Patient Expectations. Because patients rely on nurses and other health care providers to identify problems, nurses must be knowledgeable about nutrition, nutritional screening, assessment, and referral to meet patient expectations and needs.

◆ Nursing Diagnosis

Assessment enables determination of any actual or potential nutrition problems. Assessment data are clustered together to inform a clinical judgement about individual, family, or community responses to problems and life processes. A problem may occur when overall intake is significantly decreased or increased, or when one or more nutrients are not ingested or absorbed. For example, a man is seen at the community health clinic with a diagnosis of dysthymia (a chronic form of depression that is milder in severity than major depression) and with the profile shown in Box 42-5. Specific diagnoses are related to the actual nutritional problem (e.g., excessive intake) but may also involve problems that place the patient at risk for nutritional or health difficulties, such as physical inactivity.

The nursing diagnostic statement is based on defining characteristics present in the assessment database. The suspected health problem related to the nursing diagnosis is stated. The following are examples of nursing diagnoses relevant to nutritional problems that may pertain to the 52-year-old man with dysthymia being seen at the community health clinic (see Box 42-5):

- *Excess fluid volume*
- *Health maintenance, ineffective*
- *Imbalanced nutrition: more than body requirements*
- *Fatigue*
- *Hopelessness*
- *Activity intolerance*
- *Risk for impaired cardiovascular function*
- *Social isolation*

BOX 42-5 NURSING DIAGNOSTIC PROCESS

Imbalanced Nutrition: More Than Body Requirements

Assessment Activities	Data and Defining Characteristics
Obtain height and weight	52-year-old man Height: 180 cm Weight: 122 kg Body mass index (BMI) = 37.7
Obtain 24-hour food history	Lack of satiety High fat and carbohydrate intake, three meals plus a large evening snack/day, three to four beers per day
Fluid	Fluid intake is cola, beer, and juice, all high caloric and lacking nutrient density
Physical assessment	Short of breath on walking Large abdomen Blood pressure: 158/88 mm Hg Pulse: 102 beats/minute Respirations: 32 breaths/minute Reports low energy, fatigue, and intermittent feelings of hopelessness since his partner left him last year
Laboratory values	Cholesterol and triglycerides elevated. All others within normal limits
Medication	None
Social	Eats out with his 12- and 14-year-old sons two times a week. Says, "My sons are the only thing I have to look forward to. Without them, I would just be sitting behind my desk at work all day or else laid back in front of the TV at night."

◆ Planning

The planning for enhanced, optimal nutritional status requires a higher level of care than simply correcting problems. Information from multiple sources must be synthesized to devise an individualized approach to care that is responsive to the patient's needs (Figure 42-5). All data sources need to be considered when developing a nursing care plan (Box 42-6). It is crucial to refer to published standards that are based on scientific findings.

In clinical situations, patients have multiple related problems. The concept map in Figure 42-6 shows the relationship of nursing diagnoses for a patient with diabetes.

Goals and Outcomes. Goals and outcomes and priorities of care reflect the patient's physiological, therapeutic, and individualized needs. Mutually planned goals negotiated between the patient, nurse, and dietitian help ensure success. An overall goal for an obese patient might be "to achieve appropriate BMI height–weight range or be within 10% of ideal body weight." To accomplish this, it is important to establish regular, attainable goals, such as moderate weight loss, rather than one large, overwhelming goal (Weinberg, 2013). These smaller goals or outcomes can help the patient achieve the goal:

- Daily nutritional intake meets the minimal DRIs.
- Daily nutritional fat intake is less than 30%.
- Sugared beverages are removed from diet.
- Patient refrains from eating between meals and after dinner.
- Patient loses 0.5 to 1 kg per week.

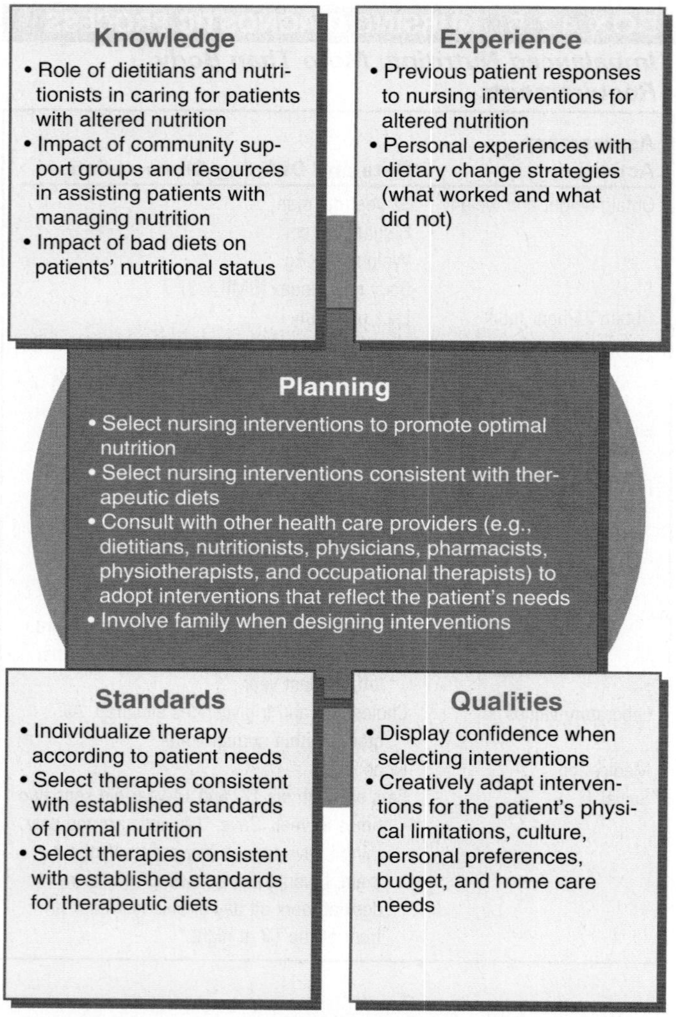

FIGURE 42-5 Critical thinking model for nutrition planning.

The setting of goals and outcomes requires interdisciplinary input. A satisfactory care plan requires accurate exchange of information between disciplines.

Setting Priorities. By identifying patients at risk for nutritional problems, health providers can help prevent or minimize these problems through timely interventions. Although changes in the patient's weight are often gradual, improving nutritional intake is a priority. With acute illness or surgery, food intake is often altered. The priority of care may be to provide optimal preoperative nutrition support for patients with malnutrition. Resumption of food intake postoperatively depends on the return of bowel function, the extent of the surgical procedure, and presence of complications (see Chapter 48).

Sometimes other priorities take precedence. For example, patients who have had throat surgery must be out of pain and comfortable before nutritional priorities can be addressed. It is also important to collaborate with the patient and family when setting care priorities so that all persons involved in the patient's care understand and support these priorities. Food purchase and preparation may involve the family, and the care plan may not succeed without their commitment, involvement, and understanding.

Continuity of Care. In any health care setting, continuity of care is essential, including continuity of nutritional interventions. Hospital discharge planning should extend nutritional interventions to the home or long-term care facility. In extended settings, the dietitian monitors the patient's nutritional status and intake and makes recommendations for changes.

When patients require long-term care or care at home, occupational therapists can help them to choose assistive devices, such as large-handled utensils and cups with a space for the nose. Food preparation areas can be rearranged to maximize the patient's function. Speech language pathologists (SLPs) recommend appropriate dietary textures and feeding strategies and assist patients with swallowing exercises and techniques to reduce aspiration risk.

Diet Planning. Diet planning to manage specific illnesses such as diabetes, cardiac or renal disease, and conditions of lactose and gluten intolerance usually requires the patient to consult with a dietitian, nurse, and other interdisciplinary team members to develop relevant knowledge and skills (Table 42-7).

Example of Diabetic Meal Planning. Patients who are diagnosed with diabetes cannot properly use and store glucose for energy. Glucose comes from foods such as fruit, milk, some vegetables, starchy foods, and sugar. To control blood glucose, patients need to eat a diet of healthy foods with a controlled amount of glucose, be active, and may need to take insulin or oral antihyperglycemic agents.

Meal planning to control blood glucose levels is structured around eating three meals per day at regular times and spacing meals no more than 6 hours apart. Healthy snacks may be needed. Sugars and sweets such as sugar, regular soft drinks, desserts, candies, jam, and honey are limited. High-fat food such as fried foods, chips, and pastries are limited because they may cause weight gain, which lessens blood glucose control and decreases heart health (Diabetes Canada, 2018). Eating more high-fibre foods is recommended for satiety and to lower blood glucose and cholesterol levels. Persons living with diabetes are instructed to drink water rather than regular soft drinks and fruit juice, which raise blood glucose. Regular physical activity improves blood glucose control.

Diabetes Canada recommends the plate method (Figure 42-7) to control portion sizes.

Persons living with diabetes should have at each meal at least three out of the four key food groups from *Eating Well with Canada's Food Guide*: vegetables and fruit, grain products, milk and alternatives, and meat and alternatives (Diabetes Canada, 2018). Fats are added in small amounts to help control weight and blood cholesterol. Carbohydrate counting, which focuses on foods that contain carbohydrate, as these raise blood glucose the most, is used to plan meals. The goal for grams of carbohydrate at each meal and snack is chosen in consultation with the registered dietitian and diabetic nurse educator to help reach or maintain a healthy weight. For accuracy in determining the carbohydrate content of food portions, patients are taught to use measuring cups and food scales and to check the nutrition label on food packages, food composition books, restaurant fact sheets, and pertinent websites. They are to write down what they eat and drink throughout the day (Diabetes Canada, 2018).

◆ Implementation

Chronic Disease, Nutrition, and Prevention. Chronic diseases are long term and not contagious. They include diseases such as obesity, diabetes, cardiovascular diseases, cancers, chronic respiratory diseases, osteoporosis, mental illnesses, and dental diseases. Half of Canadians (52%) over the age of 20 live with a chronic disease. This includes the 62% of adults and 32% of children and youth who have excess weight or obesity; the more than one in four who live with diabetes (which is expected to rise to one in three by 2020); the 1.3 million people who live with heart disease, the leading cause of death

BOX 42-6 NURSING CARE PLAN

Imbalanced Nutrition: Less Than Body Requirements

ASSESSMENT

Belinda Wong, a nurse practitioner in a community health centre, is seeing 68-year-old Mrs. Cooper, who has a history of heart failure. Recently, Mrs. Cooper noticed a weight loss (15%). She has been taking an antidepressant (sertraline) for 3 months for an initial episode of depression related to the loss of her husband 6 months ago. Mrs. Cooper was referred for counselling 3 months ago to help with grief and depression. When Belinda inquired about Mrs. Cooper's financial situation, Mrs. Cooper responded that it was difficult living on an income from the Canada Pension Plan, but she was able to manage.

Assessment Activities	***Data and Defining Characteristics***
Ask Mrs. Cooper about her food intake during the last 2 days.	She says she drinks one glass of juice in the morning and two or three cups of coffee. She may eat a sandwich in the late afternoon. "I'm just not interested in food. It has no taste."
Assess Mrs. Cooper's knowledge base by asking her what she sees as strengths of her diet, about areas in which her diet is ineffective, and what resources she uses in guiding her meal planning.	She says she does not need to worry about being overweight and believes her diet is adequate for her needs, as she does not feel hungry. She says she thinks she should be eating more vegetables and drinking more milk. Her meal preparation is "quick and easy," which pleases her. She says she is "too tired to fuss over food."
Assess her use of medication.	She takes the following prescribed medications as instructed on a daily basis: sertraline, digoxin (cardiac glycoside), chlorothiazide (diuretic), and captopril (antihypertensive).
Ask Mrs. Cooper about social interaction.	Mrs. Cooper says she is lonely and does not get out much, although her psychologist recommended more socializing. Her friends at church call to ask her to come to meetings, but she is not ready. She says she tires easily.
Weigh Mrs. Cooper and assess her posture.	This weight loss occurred over 6 months, down 11 kg. She has stooped posture. She has a low body mass index (BMI) of 17.
Observe Mrs. Cooper for signs of poor nutrition.	Dull, thinning hair Dry, scaling skin Pale conjunctivae and mucous membranes
Palpate her muscles and extremities.	2+ bilateral pitting ankle edema Generalized poor muscle tone

NURSING DIAGNOSIS: *Imbalanced nutrition:* less than body requirements related to a decreased ability to ingest food as a result of depression and loss of appetite associated with antidepressant use.

PLANNING

Goals (Nursing Outcomes Classification)*	***Expected Outcomes***
	Weight Control
Mrs. Cooper will progressively gain weight.	Patient will gain 0.5 to 1 kg/month until goal of 59 kg is reached.
	Nutritional Status: Nutrient Intake
Mrs. Cooper will consume adequate nourishment each day.	Patient will ingest 1 900 kcal/day, including 50 g of protein per day.
Mrs. Cooper will exhibit no signs of malnutrition.	Physical assessment and laboratory values will be within normal limits.

*Outcome classification labels are adapted from Moorhead, S., Johnson, M., Maas, M. L., & Swanson, E. (2013). *Nursing outcomes classification* (NOC) (5th ed.). St. Louis: Elsevier.

INTERVENTIONS

Interventions (Nursing Interventions Classification)†	***Rationale***
Nutritional Counselling	
Coordinate a plan of care with Mrs. Cooper, her family doctor, therapist, and dietitian.	Successful nutrition care planning involves an interdisciplinary approach (Tappenden Quatrara, Parkhurst, et al., 2013).
Individualize menu plans.	Encourages intake by incorporating food preferences (Weaver, Dwyer, Fulgoni, et al., 2014).
Teach Mrs. Cooper about the value associated with consulting *Eating Well With Canada's Food Guide.*	Health Canada (2016c) recommendations for food selections provide optimal nutrition.
Nutritional Monitoring	
Monitor Mrs. Cooper monthly for weight gain, anemia, serum albumin level, and total lymphocyte count (TLC).	Weight gain should be slow and progressive. Serum albumin of 40 g/L and TLC of 1 500/mm^3 are within normal limits (Robinson, 2015).
Perform physical assessment of hair, eyes, mouth, skin, and muscle tone.	To monitor for improved nutritional status.
Nutritional Management	
Encourage Mrs. Cooper to eat small meals and increase dietary intake to help offset anorexia secondary to use of sertraline.	Sertraline is a selective serotonin reuptake inhibitor (SSRI) medication; diminished taste and anorexia are common effects of SSRIs. Frequent small meals help to reduce anorexia-associated weight loss.

Continued

BOX 42-6 NURSING CARE PLAN

Imbalanced Nutrition: Less Than Body Requirements—cont'd

Interventions (Nursing Interventions Classification)†	*Rationale*
Encourage fluid intake early in the day.	Older persons need eight 250-mL glasses per day of fluid from beverage and food sources. Concentrating intake in the morning and early afternoon prevents nocturia.
Encourage fibre intake.	Fibre helps prevent constipation.
Encourage Mrs. Cooper to have congregate meals (lunch at senior centre) five times per week.	Eating with others encourages good nutrition and promotes socialization with peers. Overcoming social isolation is helpful for older persons who do not exercise and eat nutritiously (Government of Canada, 2014).

†Intervention classification labels adapted from Bulechek, G. M., Butcher, H. K., Dochterman, J. M., & Wagner, C. (Eds.). (2012). *Nursing interventions classification (NIC)* (6th ed.). St. Louis: Elsevier.

EVALUATION

Nursing Actions	*Patient Response and Finding*	*Achievement of Outcome*
Ask Mrs. Cooper to keep a food diary for 3 days.	Her diary reflects that she ate her main meal at the senior centre at noon, had fruit and grain products for breakfast, and had a sandwich with fruit and milk in the evening.	Mrs. Cooper is selecting more nutritionally rich foods, consistent with current guidelines.
Observe Mrs. Cooper's appearance.	Her skin is less pale, hair appears to be in better condition and styled. Ankle edema is present, but less than 1+.	Mrs. Cooper has improved physical parameters of nutrition; still needs follow-up.
Weigh Mrs. Cooper.	Weight gain of 2 kg in 4 weeks.	Weight gain is steady; she is still below ideal body weight.
Ask Mrs. Cooper about appetite and energy level.	Mrs. Cooper responds that on days when she eats at the senior centre, her appetite seems better and she "wants to do more things." She notes that weekends are very lonely.	Weekday support for nutritional status appears effective. Mrs. Cooper needs to increase activity status and nutritional intake during weekends.

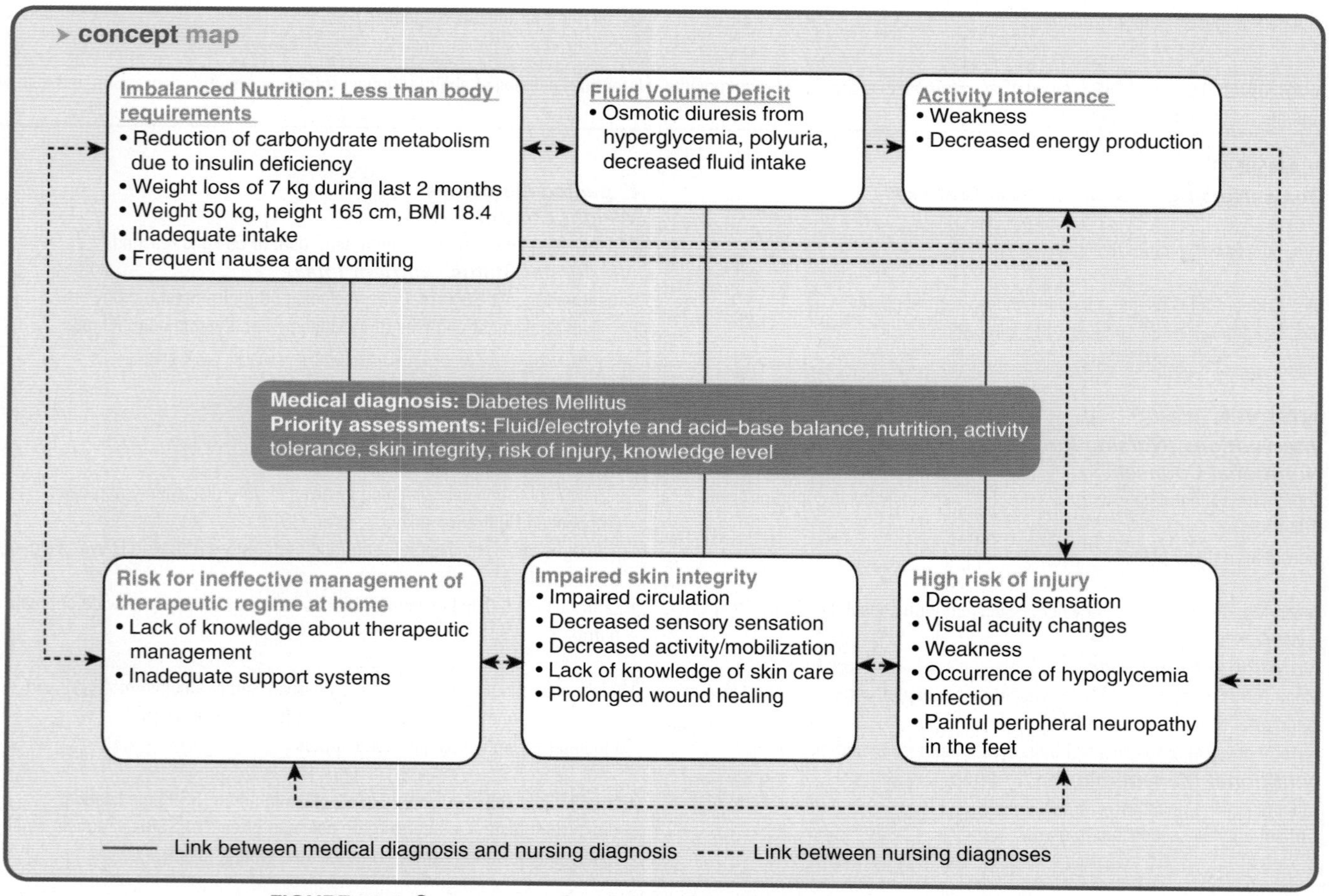

FIGURE 42-6 Concept map for patient with diabetes. *BMI,* Body mass index.

TABLE 42-7 Sample Menu Planning for Cardiac and Renal Diets and for Lactose-Intolerant and Gluten-Free Diets

Health Concern	Menu Planning With Daily Servings and Examples
Cardiac Goal is to reduce hypertension and overweight to prevent risk of stroke and heart attack	The **DASH diet**, similar to *Canada's Food Guide*, recommends a higher level of vegetable and fruit intake. DASH food groups: vegetables; fruit; grains (mainly whole grains); low-fat or no-fat dairy foods; lean meats, poultry and fish; nuts, seeds and dry beans; and fats and oils. DASH daily servings and examples: • Vegetables: 4–5 servings 250 mL (1 cup) raw leafy vegetables 125 mL (½ cup) cooked vegetables 170 mL (6 oz) juice • Fruit: 4–5 servings 1 medium piece of fruit 63 mL (¼ cup) dried fruit 125 mL (½ cup) fresh, frozen, or canned fruit • Grains (mainly whole grains): 7–8 servings 1 slice bread 250 mL (1 cup) ready-to-eat cereal 125 mL (½ cup) cooked rice, pasta, or cereal • Low-fat or no-fat dairy foods: 2–3 servings 250 mL (1 cup) milk 250 mL (1 cup) yogurt 50 g (1½ oz) cheese • Lean meats, poultry and fish: 2 servings or less 85 g (3 oz) cooked lean meats, skinless poultry, or fish • Nuts, seeds, and dry beans: 4–5 servings per week 1/3 cup (1.5 oz) nuts 30 mL (2 tbsp) peanut butter 2 tbsp (½ oz) seeds 1/2 cup cooked dry beans or peas • Fats and oils: 2–3 servings 5 mL (1 tsp) soft margarine 15 mL (1 tbsp) low-fat mayonnaise 30 mL (2 tbsp) light salad dressing 5 mL (1 tsp) vegetable oil
Renal Goal is to meet nutritional needs, reduce workload on the kidneys, preserve kidney function that is left (before starting dialysis), and control buildup of food wastes like urea	There is no "special kidney diet" for everyone. Each person has individual nutritional needs depending on his or her age, medical history, amount of kidney function, activity level, and other factors. • **Fats**—Use monounsaturated and polyunsaturated fats such as olive oil, canola oil, and safflower oil. • **Protein**—Prior to starting dialysis, a low-protein diet (2 servings of 75–90 g protein foods per day) may be helpful. Once dialysis starts, the person needs to eat more protein (about 3 servings of 75–90 g protein foods per day) to replace muscle and tissue loss. Egg whites, egg white powder, or protein powder are good protein sources. • **Calcium and phosphorus**—Limit foods that contain large amounts of phosphorus, which can cause itchy skin or painful joints and loss of calcium from bones. High- and moderate-phosphorus foods include milk, cheese, and other milk products, and protein foods such as seeds, nuts, dried peas, beans, and bran cereals. Colas and soft drinks also contain phosphorus. When dairy products cannot be incorporated in the daily diet, calcium supplements help prevent bone problems and vitamin D controls the balance of calcium and phosphorous. The provider or dietitian can discuss how best to get these nutrients. • **Sodium**—Do not add salt to food. Reducing sodium helps control high blood pressure and prevents fluid retention. Read food labels to find hidden salt and avoid foods that contain a lot of salt, sodium, or MSG. Avoid salt substitutes, as they are high in potassium. • **Potassium**—Cardiac arrhythmias may result from a buildup of potassium. It is best to choose low-potassium fruits such as apples, pears, plums, and blueberries. Vegetables such as bean sprouts, cabbage, green beans, and lettuce are also low in potassium. • **Fluids**—As kidney disease gets worse, fluid intake may need to be limited as too much fluid will lead to shortness of breath, an emergency that needs immediate medical attention. Soups, gelatin desserts, and ice cream are considered fluids. The provider and dialysis nurse will let the patient know how much to drink every day. Tips to keep from becoming thirsty include avoiding salty foods, freezing juice in an ice cube tray and eating it like a popsicle (these ice cubes are counted in the daily amount of fluids), and staying cool on hot days. • **Carbohydrates**—As a good source of energy, calories from carbohydrates may replace the calories from protein if a low-protein diet is recommended. Most fruits, breads, grains, and vegetables provide energy, as well as fibre, minerals, and vitamins. Fruits and vegetables that contain large amounts of potassium may be limited. High-potassium oranges and orange juice, nectarines, kiwis, raisins or other dried fruit, bananas, cantaloupe, honeydew melon, prunes, and nectarines should be limited. Also limit or avoid asparagus, avocado, potatoes, tomatoes or tomato sauce, winter squash, pumpkin, avocado, and cooked spinach. • **Fats** –Monounsaturated and polyunsaturated fats (olive oil, canola oil, safflower oil) can be a good source of calories that help protect heart health. • **Iron** –People with advanced kidney failure also have anemia and usually need extra iron. Foods that contain extra iron are liver, beef, pork, chicken, lima and kidney beans, and iron-fortified cereals. The provider or dietitian will determine which foods with iron can be eaten because of the kidney disease.

Continued

TABLE 42-7 Sample Menu Planning for Cardiac and Renal Diets and for Lactose-Intolerant and Gluten-Free Diets—cont'd

Health Concern	Menu Planning With Daily Servings and Examples
Lactose Intolerance	Lactose is a sugar found in milk and milk products. Lactose intolerance happens when the body does not have enough lactase (enzyme needed to digest lactose). Without lactase, undigested lactose passes into the large intestine where it is fermented by bacteria, causing bloating, gas, cramping, nausea, diarrhea, and weight loss (in children). Most people with lactose intolerance can tolerate some lactose in their diet. They are encouraged to eat small amounts of foods or beverages that have lactose with their meals. Lower lactose-containing foods eaten in small amounts (60–125 mL) can include cottage cheese, hard, aged cheese (cheddar, Swiss, Parmesan), yogurt, chocolate milk, and sour cream. If these amounts cause discomfort, persons can try eating less or using lactose-free products or foods low in lactose, preferably fortified with calcium, such as lactose-hydrolyzed milk (e.g., Lactaid, Lacteeze) and soy and rice beverages. Lactase enzyme drops or tablets reduce the lactose in milk or dairy products. Many foods that contain lactose are also important sources of calcium and vitamin D. Other sources of these nutrients are needed if lactose-containing foods are avoided. Examples of alternate sources of calcium are canned salmon (with the bones) and sardines, fortified soy and rice beverages, and calcium-fortified fruit juices. Lactose-free sources of vitamin D include fish, liver, and egg yolks. Lactose-free soy and rice beverages and non-hydrogenated margarine have been fortified with vitamin D. Persons are advised to talk to a registered dietitian if concerned they are not getting enough calcium from food and if they should take a calcium supplement.
Gluten-Free Goal is to treat celiac disease by avoiding foods that contain gluten	Gluten is a protein found in grains such as wheat, barley, rye, and triticale. Gluten causes inflammation in the small intestines of people with celiac disease. Foods that are naturally gluten-free include beans, seeds, and nuts in their natural, unprocessed form; fresh eggs; fresh meats, fish, and poultry (not breaded, batter-coated or marinated); fruits and vegetables; and most dairy products. Various gluten-free products, such as bread and pasta, are available in grocery stores. Grains and starches that are gluten-free include arrowroot, buckwheat, corn and cornmeal, flax, quinoa, rice, and gluten-free flours (rice, soy, corn, potato, and bean). It is critical to avoid wheat and other products unless labelled "gluten-free." Health Canada's regulatory requirement for "gluten-free" foods does not refer to any specific threshold for gluten in products represented as "gluten-free"; however, Health Canada considers levels of gluten protein below 20 parts per million generally not representing health risks to consumers with celiac disease. The Canadian Food Inspection Agency (2016) published a position on the Compliance and Enforcement of Gluten-Free Claims that reflects the Health Canada position. Persons living with celiac disease must be alert to hidden sources of gluten. The list of ingredients on all labels must be read every time.

Cardiac diet: Heart and Stroke Foundation of Canada. (2016). *The DASH diet to lower high blood pressure.* Retrieved from http://www.heartandstroke.ca/get-healthy/healthy-eating/dash-diet.
Renal diet: U.S. National Library of Medicine. (2015). *Diet—chronic kidney disease.* Retrieved from https://medlineplus.gov/ency/article/002442.htm.
Lactose diet: Dietitians of Canada. (2013). *Healthy eating guidelines for managing lactose intolerance.* Retrieved from http://www.dietitians.ca/Your-Health/Nutrition-A-Z/Lactose/Managing-Lactose-Intolerance.aspx.
Gluten-free diet: Canadian Celiac Association. (2016). *About celiac disease.* Retrieved from http://www.celiac.ca/?page_id=882; Canadian Food Inspection Agency. (2012). *Compliance and Enforcement of Gluten-Free Claims.* Retrieved from http://www.inspection.gc.ca/food/labelling/food-labelling-for-industry/allergens-and-gluten/gluten-free-claims/eng/1340194596012/1340194681961; Canadian Food Inspection Agency. (2016). *Gluten-free claims.* Retrieved from http://www.inspection.gc.ca/food/labelling/food-labelling-for-industry/allergens-and-gluten/eng/1388152325341/1388152326591?chap=2.

and hospitalizations in Canada; and the two in five Canadians with high blood pressure or considered prehypertensive (Dietitians of Canada, 2015).

The main focus of the WHO's 2013–2020 Global Action Plan is on the prevention and control of four types of chronic diseases—cardiovascular diseases, cancer, chronic respiratory diseases, and diabetes—which make the largest contribution to morbidity and mortality and which share behavioural risk factors of tobacco use, unhealthy diet, physical inactivity, and harmful use of alcohol. WHO (2013) recommends (a) provision of sufficient, safe, and varied food supplies to prevent malnutrition and reduce the risk of chronic diseases and (b) tackling root causes of malnutrition (i.e., genetic factors, poverty, and inequity) via political and social action, of which nutritional programs can be one aspect.

Health Promotion/Illness Prevention. Nurses are in a key position to educate patients about proper nutritional habits that may promote health and prevent the development of many diseases. Early identification of potential or actual problems is the best way to avoid more serious problems. Outpatient and community-based settings are key locations for nursing assessment of nutritional practices and status. Frequently, nurses are in a position to educate families about nutrition, inform them of community resources, and provide contact information so that families can direct questions to a dietitian or other professional nurse.

Insufficient income is the most significant barrier to healthy eating (Track, 2015). Food selection and quantity are positively associated with income. Across Canada, approximately 8.3% of households experience food insecurity; however, in Nunavut, nearly half (48.7%) of families with children lack access to basic food because of their low income (Mehler Paperny, 2015). Elsewhere in the world, low-income preschoolers and toddlers had the lowest mean intake of fruits and milk and dairy products compared to middle- and high-income groups (Mohd Shariff, Lin, Sariman, et al., 2015). Higher fruit and vegetable intake among children has been associated with better education of mothers (Van Ansem, Schrijvers, Rodenburg, et al., 2014) and food availability at home (Lehto, Ray, Te Velde, et al., 2014), both of which relate to income status. At the same time, lower socioeconomic status and issues of cost, accessibility, and parental time commitment are

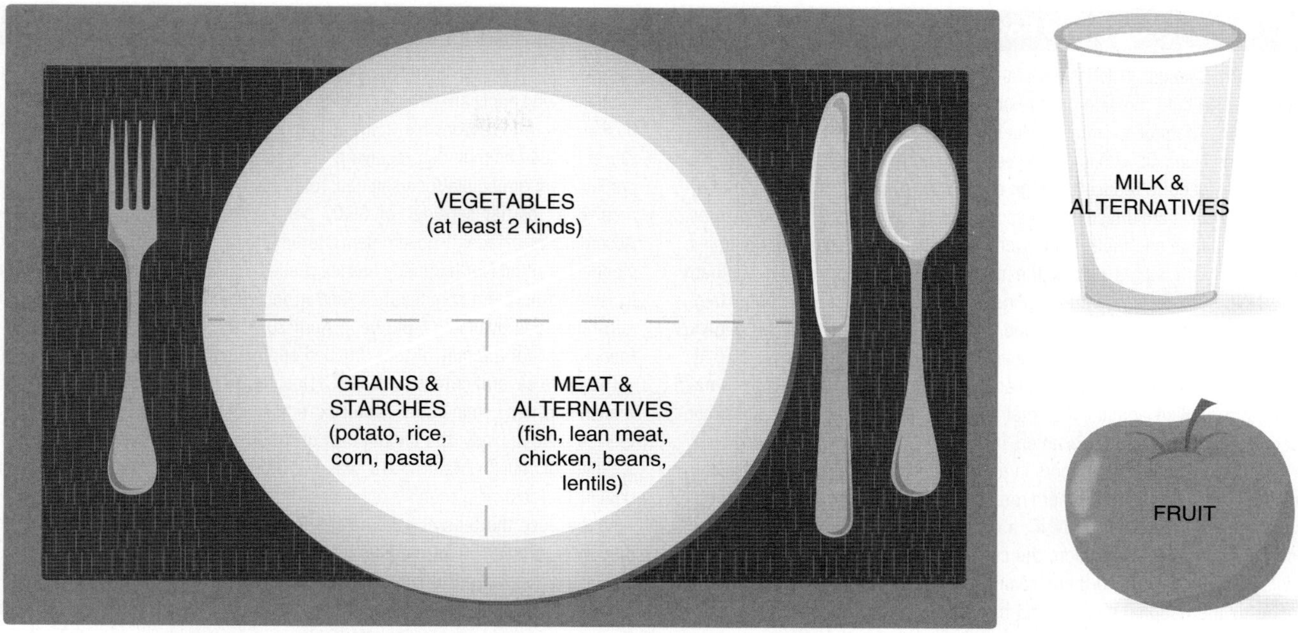

FIGURE 42-7. Plate method for meal planning. (Based on Diabetes Canada. [2017]. *Basic meal planning.* Retrieved from https://www.diabetes.ca/diabetes-and-you/healthy-living-resources/diet-nutrition/basic-meal-planning.)

associated with physical inactivity in Canadian children (Lipnowski & Canadian Paediatric Society, Healthy Active Living and Sports Medicine Committee, 2012).

In March 2016, 863 492 people received food from a food bank in Canada, an increase of 1.3% from the same time the previous year, and of 28% from March 2008; food banks assisted 2.4% of the Canadian population, with 35.6% of those helped under the age of 18 years (Food Banks Canada, 2016). The problem is worsened when children cannot access nutritional programs at schools: Canada is the only G8 country without a national school-based feeding program (Howard & Edge, 2013). Besides children, members of at-risk population groups for food insecurity also include Indigenous peoples, lone-parent families, women, immigrants, and older persons.

Although mandatory fortification of staple foods with micronutrients has helped to reduce income-related disparities (Dwyer, Wiemer, Dary, et al., 2015), other interventions are also needed to counter the threat to good nutrition and health from lack of purchasing power at individual and collective levels. For those on limited budgets, food preparation can be modified for substances that need to be used sparingly; for example, bean or cheese dishes can often replace meat. Menu planning a week in advance helps patients adhere to a specific diet, eat nutritiously, and stay within their budget. A nurse or dietitian may check menus for content. Often, simple tips can help, such as baking rather than frying to reduce fat intake, using lemon juice or spices to add flavour to low-sodium diets, and avoiding grocery shopping when hungry because it can lead to spontaneous purchases of foods not included in meal plans. Strategies to help financially disadvantaged groups improve their nutrition include collective kitchens and gardens (Loopstra & Tarasuk, 2013), coalitions with community-based organizations, antipoverty advocacy, and political commitment to policies of full employment (Wells, 2016). Also important are public-awareness forums (Food Secure Canada, 2015) and a rights-based approach to food security at federal and provincial levels (Blay-Palmer, 2016) with support to families that have inadequate resources to meet their daily nutritional needs (Food Banks Canada, 2016). See Box 42-7 for an example of an innovative program that aims to increase food security for individuals, families, and communities.

> **Safety Alert** Food safety is also an important public health issue. Food-borne illnesses can occur from poor hygiene practices and improper food storage or preparation. Nurses should educate patients about reducing the risks of food-borne illnesses (Table 42-8 and Box 42-8).

Acute Care. Many factors influence nutritional intake in acute care settings. Ill or debilitated patients often have loss of appetite (**anorexia**). The ketosis that accompanies starvation can further suppress appetite, as can the pain that results from surgical procedures and trauma. During hospitalizations, mealtimes are often interrupted or the patient is too fatigued or uncomfortable to eat. Worry about families, finances, employment, or illness often interferes with getting an adequate diet. Medications may impair taste, cause nausea, interfere with absorption, or affect metabolism. Diagnostic testing may disrupt mealtimes or require a nothing by mouth (NPO) status. Patients who are NPO and receive only standard intravenous (IV) fluids for more than 7 days are at nutritional risk.

Nurses must continuously assess patient nutritional status and plan interventions that promote normal dietary intake, digestion, and metabolism of nutrients. Patients may have a gradual progression of dietary intake or need therapeutic diets to manage their illnesses (Box 42-9).

Promoting Appetite. In providing an environment that promotes a patient's appetite, it is important to eliminate unpleasant odours, provide oral hygiene as needed to remove disagreeable tastes, and maintain patient comfort. Certain medications can affect dietary and nutrient intake; for example, insulin, glucocorticoids, and thyroid hormones affect metabolism. Other medications, such as antifungal

BOX 42-7 Focus on Food Security

Nutrition North Canada (NNC) is a federal government subsidy program launched on April 1, 2011 to provide northerners in 103 isolated communities in Saskatchewan, Manitoba, Ontario, Quebec, Labrador, Yukon, the Northwest Territories, and Nunavut with improved access to perishable nutritious food. The program is designed to reduce the high cost to consumers of food in the north where grocery costs are driven by transportation, the cost of maintaining stores, staff costs, spoilage and theft, high inventory costs, and retailer profit margins.

NNC works with stores across the north and food suppliers in southern Canada. NNC subsidizes (a) various perishable and nutritious food items (e.g., fruit, vegetables, milk, eggs, meat, and cheese) shipped by air to an eligible community and (b) traditional food commercially processed in the North (e.g., Arctic char, musk-ox, and caribou) shipped by air to an eligible community. Retail subsidies are applied against the total cost of an eligible product (including product purchasing cost, transportation, insurance, and overhead) shipped by air to an eligible community. Customers in eligible communities can purchase subsidized food from registered northern retailers or directly from registered southern suppliers. To be eligible for NNC, a community must lack year-round road, rail, or marine access. In addition, the community must meet the territorial or provincial definition of a northern community, have a year-round population according to the national census, and have an airport, post office, or grocery store.

Based on a market-driven model, the subsidy is provided to retailers and suppliers who apply and are selected to register with the program. In turn, these businesses are responsible for passing on the full subsidy to consumers. Currently, 84 communities receive a "full subsidy" of between $1.20 and $16 per kilogram of eligible food shipped; retailers in the remaining 19 communities receive a "partial subsidy" of $0.05 per kilogram of eligible food shipped. According to a federal government statement in early 2015, "the results are clear—Nutrition North Canada has succeeded in reducing prices of eligible food in isolated northern communities, and in increasing the amount of perishable nutritious food available." Between April 2011 and March 2015, the cost of a food basket for a family of four dropped approximately 5%, or $94 per month.

There are several criticisms of NNC. Despite its reported success, the cost of food in northern communities is still extremely high. In communities that receive the full NNC subsidy, the annual cost of the Revised Northern Food Basket for a family of four in March 2013 was $21 372, or $411 per week—more than double the cost of a roughly equivalent basket of food purchased in Toronto. Also, because the federal government does not currently have access to information on retailer profit margins, it cannot be verified that the NNC subsidy is being fully passed on to consumers. In sum, NNC is an innovative attempt to reduce food insecurity to remote regions of Canada's north; however, further review is needed to gauge its effectiveness.

From Pegg, S. (2016). *Food Banks Canada: Is Nutrition North Canada on shifting ground?* Retrieved from https://www.foodbankscanada.ca/getmedia/b9aa8a8f-b66b-4efc-b7d6-03f54dc77427/Is-Nutrition-North-Canada-on-Shifting-Ground.pdf.aspx

TABLE 42-8 Food Safety

Food-Borne Disease	Organism	Food Source	Symptoms*
Botulism	*Clostridium botulinum*	Improperly home-canned foods, smoked and salted fish, ham, sausage, shellfish	Symptoms vary from mild discomfort to death in 24 hours, initial nausea and dizziness progressing to motor (respiratory) paralysis
Escherichia coli	*Escherichia coli 0157:H7*	Undercooked meat (ground beef)	Severe cramps, nausea, vomiting, diarrhea (may be bloody), renal failure. Appears 1–8 days after eating, lasts 1–7 days
Listeriosis	*Listeria* species *L. monocytogenes*	Soft cheese, meat (hot dogs, pâté, lunch meats), unpasteurized milk, poultry, seafood	Severe diarrhea, fever, headache, pneumonia, meningitis, endocarditis, appears 3–21 days after infection
Perfringens enteritis	*Clostridium* species *C. perfringens*	Cooked meats, meat dishes held at room or warm temperature	Mild diarrhea, vomiting. Appears 8–24 hours after eating, lasts 1–2 days
Salmonellosis	*Salmonella* species *S. typhi* *S. paratyphi*	Milk, custards, egg dishes, salad dressing, sandwich fillings, polluted shellfish	Mild to severe diarrhea, cramps, vomiting. Appears 12–24 hours after ingestion, lasts 1–7 days
Shigellosis	*Shigella* species *S. dysenteriae*	Milk, milk products, seafood, salads	Mild diarrhea to fatal dysentery. Appears 7–36 hours after ingestion, lasts 3–14 days
Staphylococcus	*Staphylococcus* species *S. aureus*	Custards, cream fillings, processed meats, ham, cheese, ice cream, potato salad, sauces, casseroles	Severe abdominal cramps, pain, vomiting, diarrhea, perspiration, headache, fever, prostration. Appears 1–6 hours after ingestion, lasts 1–2 days

*Symptoms are generally more severe for youngest and oldest age groups.
From Nix, S. (2013). *Williams' basic nutrition and diet therapy* (14th ed.). St. Louis, MO: Mosby.

agents, can affect taste. Some psychotropic medications affect appetite, cause nausea, and alter taste. At times the nurse and dietitian can help the patient select foods to reduce the altered taste sensations or nausea. In other situations, medication may need to be changed. Physicians may order pharmacological agents to stimulate appetite (e.g., cyproheptadine [Periactin], megestrol [Megace]) or to manage symptoms that interfere with nutrition.

Assisting Patients With Feeding

Many conditions, including cancer, stroke, and neuromuscular disorders, can cause feeding difficulties. The task of feeding requires nursing knowledge and skilled intervention to protect patient safety, independence, and dignity.

Before Feeding. The nurse should assess the patient's risk of aspiration (see "Assessment" in this chapter and Skill 42-1). The patient

BOX 42-8 PATIENT TEACHING

Food Safety

Objectives

- Patient will verbalize measures to prevent food-borne illness.
- Patient will understand the primary types of illness and how they are transmitted.
- Patient will not experience food-borne illness.

Teaching Strategies

Populations particularly at risk are older and younger people and immunosuppressed individuals. Instruct patients on the following:

- Wash hands with warm, soapy water for at least 20 seconds before touching or eating food.
- Separate cutting boards. Use one board for produce and another for raw meat, poultry, fish, and seafood.
- Wash fresh fruits and vegetables thoroughly.
- Do not eat raw meats or drink unpasteurized milk.
- Do not buy or consume food that has passed the expiration date.
- Keep foods properly refrigerated at 4°C and frozen at −18°C.
- Wash dishes and cutting boards with hot, soapy water or use a bleach sanitizer of 5 mL bleach in 750 mL water.
- Thaw food, especially raw meat, poultry, fish, or seafood, in the refrigerator.
- Cook food completely, using a clean thermometer to measure the temperature of meat, poultry, and fish. Keep a temperature chart that gives the safe cooking temperatures of foods handy to always know at what temperature each food is fully cooked. Insert the thermometer probe into the thickest part of the food to ensure accuracy.
- Refrigerate leftovers within 2 hours. Do not save for more than 4 days in the refrigerator.
- Wash dishcloths and towels regularly, or use paper towels.
- Clean the inside of the refrigerator and microwave regularly to prevent microbial growth.
- Wash reusable grocery bags frequently.

Evaluation

- Ask patient to describe measures to prevent food-borne illnesses.
- Observe the patient at home for safe practices, if making a home visit.

From EatRight Ontario. (2016). *Test the temperature—Use a thermometer for food safety.* Retrieved from https://www.eatrightontario.ca/en/Articles/Food-safety/Test-the-temperature-%E2%80%93-Use-a-thermometer-for-food.aspx; Government of Canada. (2014). *Food safety and you.* Retrieved from https://www.canada.ca/en/health-canada/services/general-food-safety-tips/food-safety-you.html

BOX 42-9 Diet Progression and Therapeutic Diets

Clear Liquid

This diet is limited to broth, bouillon, coffee, tea, carbonated beverages, clear fruit juices, gelatin, or Popsicles.

Thickened Liquid

All liquids (e.g., juice, tea, coffee, water, etc.) must be thickened to the appropriate consistency (nectar, honey, or pudding) as recommended by the speech language pathologist/feeding team when thin fluids cannot be safely swallowed and may be aspirated.

Full Liquid

To a clear- or thickened-liquid diet can be added smooth-textured dairy products, custards, refined cooked cereals, vegetable juice, puréed vegetables, or any fruit juices.

Puréed

This diet includes all of the above with the addition of scrambled eggs, puréed meats, vegetables, fruits, or mashed potatoes and gravy.

Mechanical Soft

This diet includes all of the above with the addition of ground or finely diced meats, flaked fish, cottage cheese, cheese, rice, potatoes, pancakes, light breads, cooked vegetables, cooked or canned fruits, bananas, soups, or peanut butter.

Soft or Low Residue

Low-fibre, easily digested foods, such as pastas, casseroles, moist tender meats, canned cooked fruits and vegetables, desserts, cakes, and cookies without nuts or coconut, can be added.

High Fibre

This diet includes fresh uncooked fruits, steamed vegetables, bran, oatmeal, and dried fruits.

Low Sodium

A low-sodium diet is limited to 4 g (no added salt), 2 g, 1 g, or 500 mg sodium (severe sodium restriction), requiring selective food purchases.

Low Cholesterol

This diet is restricted to <200 mg/day cholesterol, in keeping with the National Cholesterol Education Program (NCEP) recommendations (Heimburger, 2016) and the Heart and Stroke Foundation of Canada (2017c).

Diabetic

In general, people with diabetes should follow a healthy diet recommended for the general population in *Eating Well With Canada's Food Guide* (Diabetes Canada, 2018; Dietitians of Canada, 2017). This includes consuming a variety of foods from the four food groups (grain products, vegetables and fruits, milk products, meat and alternatives), attaining and maintaining a healthy body weight, decreasing total fat intake to <30% of calories, and ensuring an adequate intake of carbohydrate, protein, essential fatty acids, vitamins, and minerals.

Regular

Dietary restrictions are not necessary unless specified.

should sit as upright as possible with head tilted slightly forward and may be supported by pillows, foam wedges, or rolled towels. A patient who is lying back or has the neck arched or hyperextended should not be fed because these positions create an open airway susceptible to aspiration. Glasses, hearing aids, and dentures should be functioning and in place. Clothing and bedding should be protected with napkins, towels, or aprons, and these items should not be called "bibs." The nurse needs to ensure that the suction apparatus at the bedside has been checked.

During Feeding. The patient should be kept upright. To feed the patient the nurse uses a rocking motion of the utensil on the patient's tongue. When the patient has hemiplegia (one-sided weakness), the head should be tilted slightly toward the stronger side to avoid pouching (Lampert, 2015) and small bites of food placed on the stronger side of the patient's mouth. If indicated by the feeding/swallowing team, the patient can take a drink between each mouthful of food to ease the process of eating. The patient should be observed for pouching of food. A metal teaspoon is usually the best utensil to use for feeding patients with bite reflexes.

The nurse needs to assess swallowing during feeding and give patients with dysphagia enough time to chew, allowing at least 5 to 10 seconds or longer for each bite or sip. Two completed swallows should be observed between mouthfuls. The patient's Adam's apple should move up and down. If the food is still present, the nurse can offer an empty spoonful to stimulate swallowing.

The nurse who is helping the patient to eat should sit in the patient's line of vision and provide prompting, encouragement, and direction, both verbally and nonverbally, when appropriate. The nurse avoids hovering with the next spoonful of food as this may cause a patient to hurry and worsen any swallowing difficulties. Patience, attention, and time are essential. When possible, the nurse should try to heed special requests, such as for the food to be warmed up. Nurses can promote comfort and a sense of independence by providing opportunities for patients to direct the order and speed at which they want to eat. The nurse should give the patient as much choice as possible, for instance, by asking if the patient wants peas and potatoes together or separate on the spoon. The family can be asked about the patient's favourite foods. Because mealtime is usually a social activity, it is important that nurses and other health providers talk to patients during meals. Nurses can use this opportunity to educate patients about therapeutic diets, medications, or adaptive devices.

Patients with visual deficits also need special assistance. If possible, the nurse should read aloud menu items and let the patient choose the meal. The patient should be told when the meal has arrived and where the tray is placed. Food needs to be positioned within the patient's visual field. If the patient wears glasses or contact lenses, they should be clean and in place. A dark tray or cloth can be placed under a light plate to define the plate edges, making it easier to locate the food. Patients with poor vision or blindness may be able to feed themselves if adequate care and information is given. The nurse can describe where certain foods are located on a plate (Figure 42-8) using either the clock-face method (e.g. "The meat is at 6 o'clock, mashed potatoes are at 9 o'clock, and the peas at 12 o'clock") or by saying items are at the top, bottom, or right or left side of the plate (Vision Australia, 2012). Meat should be placed at 6 o'clock, or at the bottom of the plate, as this is easiest for cutting. The patient should be told where the beverage is located in relation to the plate (e.g., "The glass of water is to the right or above 2 o'clock"). The nurse should ask the patient if he or she would like assistance with removing packaging from items. Hot drinks should be in non-spill containers; the nurse needs to tell the patient where they are placed.

When food intake is less than usual because of illness or fatigue, nutrient-dense items should be provided first. Small frequent meals, five to six per day, may be required. Patients with decreased motor skills may retain more independence by using large-handled adaptive utensils, which are easier to grip and manipulate.

After Feeding. The patient should remain upright for 30 minutes after eating. The nurse should check again for pocketing of food. If the patient needs to lie down because of fatigue, the head of the bed can be raised to sitting-up level. Intake should be noted and documented. The nurse needs to identify if any particular food was eaten faster (e.g., a preference) or with difficulty (e.g., soft meat may need to be replaced with ground), and report and document any instances of choking and fatigue. After each meal, the patient should perform oral hygiene.

Restorative and Continuing Care

Patients discharged from a hospital with dietary prescriptions often need dietary education to plan meals that meet specific therapeutic

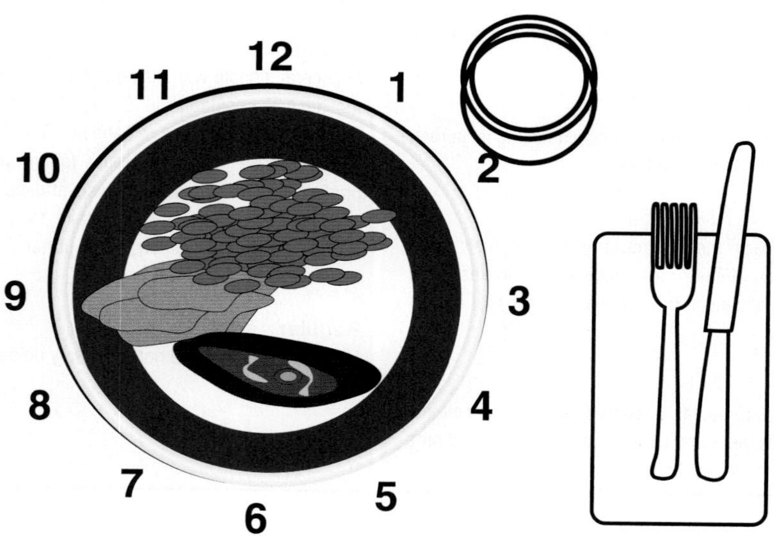

FIGURE 42-8 Using the clock-face method to identify contents and location of food on a plate.

requirements. Restorative care includes immediate postsurgical care and routine medical care pertinent to hospitalized and home care patients. The case study in Box 42-10 illustrates the need for nurses to educate visitors about a patient's nutritional status in order to avoid complications and enhance the patient's recovery following abdominal surgery.

After surgical intervention, particularly bowel resections and colon surgery, coordinated bowel motility temporarily ceases. This lack of coordinated propulsive action prevents effective transit of intestinal contents or tolerance of oral intake and leads to the accumulation of gas and fluids within the bowel. Motility typically returns within 1–3 days (Cagir, 2017).

◆ Evaluation

Care plans should reflect achievable goals and outcomes. Nurses need to evaluate outcomes of nursing actions and be alert for signs that goals are being met. They also need to allow adequate time for testing each nursing approach to a problem.

Patient Care. The effectiveness of nutritional interventions is best measured by meeting the expected patient outcomes and goals of care (Figure 42-9). Nutrition therapy does not always produce rapid results. Ongoing comparisons may be made with baseline measures of weight, serum albumin or prealbumin, and protein and kilocalorie intake. Medications may produce unwanted adverse effects. If gradual weight gain is not observed, or if weight loss continues, the prescription may need to be adjusted. Changes in health condition may indicate a need to change the nutritional care plan. Interdisciplinary team members should be consulted, and the patient should be an active participant whenever possible. The patient's ability to incorporate dietary lifestyle changes with the least amount of stress or disruption will ensure success. When expected outcomes are not met, the interventions or outcomes need to be revised on the basis of the patients' needs and preferences.

Patient Expectations. Patients expect competent and accurate care. They expect nurses to alter the care plan if outcomes of nutritional therapies are unsuccessful. Nurses' expectations and health values may differ from those held by patients. By working closely with patients, nurses can understand their expectations and try to meet them within the limits of their conditions and treatments.

SELF-MONITORING OF BLOOD GLUCOSE

Self-monitoring of blood glucose (SMBG) is a cornerstone of diabetes management. By providing a real-time blood glucose reading, SMBG enables the patient to make decisions regarding diet, exercise, and medication management.

Portable blood glucose meters are used at the hospital bedside and by patients who perform SMBG independently (Figure 42-10). In Canada, the only continuous glucose monitoring system (CGMS) available is the Medtronic MiniMed Paradigm REAL-Time System. A sensor is inserted under the skin, and data are sent from the sensor to a transmitter, which displays the glucose value on an insulin pump continuously; values are updated every 5 minutes (Figure 42-11). This system assists the patient and health care provider to identify trends and track patterns. Thus, it is particularly useful for managing insulin therapy, alerting the patient during episodes of hypoglycemia and hyperglycemia, and allowing prompt, immediate, and corrective action.

The blood glucose level reported by a laboratory is sometimes higher than the measurement by the patient's home glucose monitor or the hospital's portable meter. This is because some meters measure capillary blood glucose from whole blood (via finger stick), whereas laboratory venous samples yield plasma readings. Plasma samples, or venous samples, are 15–20% higher because plasma has a higher water content than that of whole blood, so there is more dissolved glucose in plasma than in whole blood (Austin, 2013). Most blood

BOX 42-10 CASE STUDY

*Not a Textbook Recovery**

My 46-year-old patient had come back to the floor after undergoing a total bowel resection. The protocol that we follow for reintroducing oral fluids, food, and medications is very strict because of the large surgical interruption in the body's natural state. The patient was NPO and on intravenous (IV) fluids until he produced flatus and bowel sounds in all four quadrants.

During my initial postoperative assessment of this patient, he had no bowel sounds in any quadrant. I explained to him the protocol for nutritional supplementation following surgery. For 24 to 48 hours, he would be placed on a clear fluid diet that would be advanced as he progressed through his recovery. My patient, unfortunately, told his family that he was starving. Because they were not fully aware of the protocol, they gave him something to eat. His body was not ready to handle food, and he became nauseated and vomited the food he had eaten, as well as coffee ground emesis. The coffee ground emesis indicated that he required abdominal decompression. I placed a nasogastric (NG) tube, which for several days was connected to low intermittent suction to alleviate his abdominal distension. I replaced NG tube losses 1 : 1 with an additional IV solution to maintain electrolyte balance. Blood work was done at least once a day to monitor electrolyte levels, hemoglobin, and any dehydration. When it was apparent that his recovery was taking longer than planned, we closely monitored his lab results for any signs of decreased nutritional status. We also began the process of determining whether total parental nutrition (TPN) would be appropriate. However, before needing to progress to TPN, we began to see improved laboratory results and were able to stop and remove the NG tube and suction, as he had regained faint bowel sounds in all four quadrants. We started him on a clear fluid diet, which he tolerated well, so we advanced him to a full fluid diet, which he also tolerated well. He regained full bowel sounds and had flatus the following day. We were able to advance him all the way to a regular diet. His lab work showed no nutritional deficits, and he continued on to make a full recovery.

What I hope undergraduate nurses will take away from this case is that meeting nutritional needs in patients following surgery is always different—rarely does a patient follow a "textbook" recovery. Decisions must be based on not only the nurse's past experiences and expertise but also on the unique combination of the patient's past medical history, symptoms, and family support. Nurses need to follow their patients in providing appropriate person-led interventions that promote the best outcomes for a particular care situation.

In this case study, how and why did the nurse evaluate her patient's bowel motility? What nutritional teaching is required for patients who have undergone bowel resection surgery and their families?

*By Ashley Kay, RN, BN; MN student.

glucose meters (BGMs) for home use now report blood glucose only in terms of plasma glucose to be more readily compared with laboratory values.

Instructions for using a BGM accompany each product. Because errors in monitoring technique can cause errors in management strategies, thorough patient education is crucial. Once initial education has occurred, follow-up educational sessions should take place at each subsequent patient contact and also be timed to coincide with regular appointments for reassessment. In addition, patients must be taught to calibrate their BGM and use control solutions. In Canada, the control solutions are not included in the BGM kits and are not stocked by most pharmacies. A person with diabetes must call the company to ask for the control solution, and it will be sent to them at no charge. The control solution has a very narrow expiry date and once opened lasts only 3 months. The person must run the control test every week.

The chief advantage of SMBG is that it supplies immediate information about blood glucose levels that can be used to make adjustments in food intake, activity patterns, and medication dosages. It also produces accurate records of daily glucose fluctuations and trends, as well as alerting the patient to acute episodes of hyperglycemia and hypoglycemia. SMBG is recommended as an essential part of daily diabetes management for all people using insulin or oral hypoglycemic agents (OHAs). The frequency of monitoring depends on several factors, including the patient's glycemic goals, type of diabetes, ability and willingness to perform the test independently, and treatment regimen. It is recommended that patients with type 1 diabetes test their blood glucose at least three times per day and include both preprandial and postprandial testing. Those using an insulin pump may test more

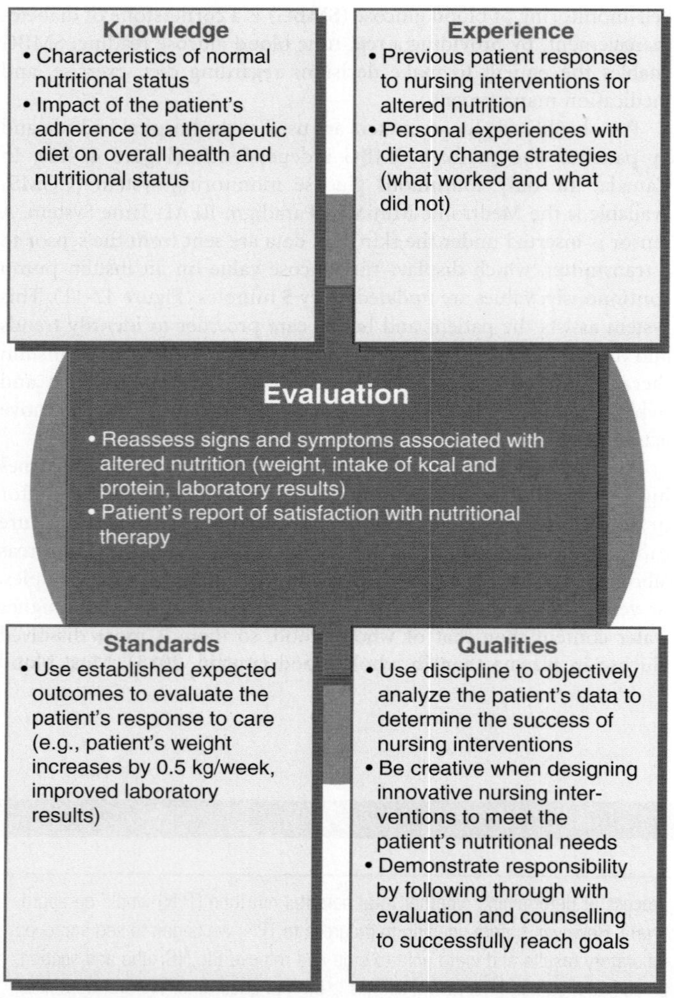

FIGURE 42-9 Critical thinking model for nutritional evaluation.

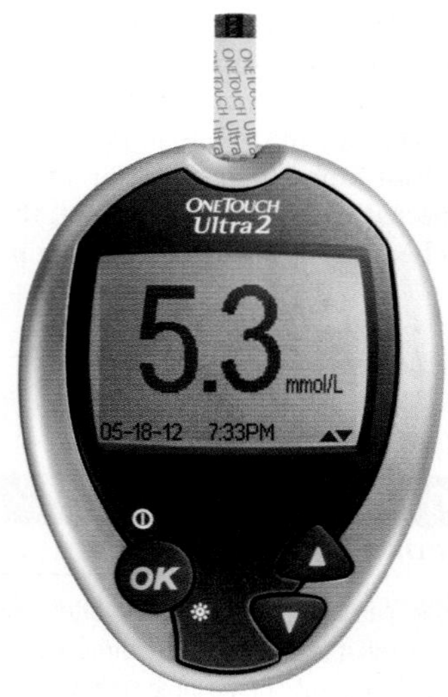

FIGURE 42-10 Blood glucose monitor. (Courtesy LifeScan, Inc., Milpitas, CA.)

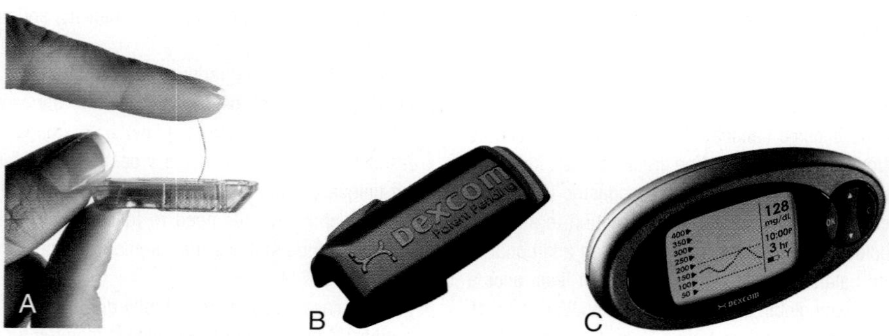

FIGURE 42-11 A tiny sensor **(A)** implanted under skin transmits continuous reading to receiver **(B)**, to alert wearer of any deviation from desired glucose target range. Readings are displayed and stored on the monitor **(C)**. (Courtesy DexCom, Inc.)

frequently. People with type 2 diabetes treated with OHAs or through lifestyle changes alone have more variable and individualized testing regimens. For patients with type 2 diabetes treated with once-daily insulin and OHAs, monitoring at least once daily is recommended (CDA, 2013).

Blood glucose testing should also be performed whenever hypoglycemia is suspected so that immediate action can be taken if necessary. When the person with diabetes is ill, the blood glucose should be tested every 2 to 4 hours to determine the effects of this stressor on blood glucose level (CDA, 2013). If a patient is visually or cognitively impaired or has limited manual dexterity, the degree to which SMBG can be performed independently must be evaluated carefully. (See Skill 42-2 for a description of how to monitor blood glucose.)

SKILL 42-2 BLOOD GLUCOSE MONITORING

When venipuncture cannot be performed to obtain capillary blood, skin puncture is an alternative method to reduce the frequency of needle sticks and for self-management of diabetes mellitus. The procedure is less painful than venipuncture, and patients can perform this procedure.

There are two methods for self-testing of blood glucose level. Both methods require obtaining a large drop of blood by skin puncture. A hand-held single-use lancet or an automatic lancet-holder device can be used. The drop of blood is then applied on the specially prepared testing strip.

The first self-testing method involves visually reading the reagent strip by comparing it with the colour chart on the container. Examples of such strips are Chemstrip bG, Glucostix, and TrendStrips. If the colour on the strip appears between two reference blocks on the chart, the user may need to estimate the results. Consequently, results of blood glucose measurement using this method may not always be accurate.

The second type of blood glucose monitoring entails the use of reflectance meters (see Figure 42-10). A variety of meters are on the market, such as the Glucometer II (Ames), Accu-Chek III (Boehringer Mannheim), Glucoscan 3000 (LifeScan), and OneTouch (LifeScan). After a drop of blood from the skin puncture is placed on the testing strip, the meter provides an accurate measurement of blood glucose level in less than 60 seconds.

For these meters, a wet-wash or dry-wipe method of testing is used. To perform a wet wash, the user flushes the blood-coated testing strip with water before inserting the strip into the glucose meter. The dry-wipe method requires the user to wipe off the blood-coated testing strip with a dry cotton ball before making a reading. Some products do not require blood to be flushed or wiped before a reading. The various methods enable measurement of blood glucose between 1.1 and 44.4 mmol/L, which is a sensitive measurement of blood glucose level.

These meters differ in the amount of blood needed for each test, testing speed, overall size, ability to store test results in memory, cost of the meter, and cost of test strips (Tsai, 2015). Some larger meters are voice activated, which is helpful for older persons with visual impairments. The amount of time to complete the glucose testing with the current glucose meters varies from 5 seconds to 50 seconds. Some meters can be programmed to monitor glucose levels for a continuous 72 hours.

Most meters allow for alternative sites, such as the forearm, palm, and thigh. Two new methods of obtaining glucose measurement are available on the market. Minimally invasive glucose meters have a very small, fine plastic sensor inserted through the abdomen, and they provide continuous readings of blood glucose levels. A biosensor is taped on the external abdomen (Figure 42-11). Using a hand-held wireless meter, the patient activates the biosensor to transmit the blood glucose level at any time without puncturing the skin. Another model, the noninvasive glucose meter, punctures the skin not with a needle but with laser technology.

Delegation Considerations

The task of measuring blood glucose level after skin puncture (capillary puncture) can be delegated to an unregulated care provider (UCP) who is specifically instructed in performing the skill. The nurse must first assess the patient to determine that it is appropriate to delegate blood glucose monitoring. If the patient's condition changes frequently, this task should not be delegated. The nurse directs the UCP by

- Explaining appropriate sites to use for puncture and when to obtain glucose levels
- Reviewing expected levels and when to report to the nurse unexpected glucose levels

Equipment

- Antiseptic swab
- Cotton ball or tissue
- Sterile lancet or blood-letting device
- Heel-warming device (*optional*)
- Paper towel
- Blood glucose meter (e.g., OneTouch)
- Blood glucose test strips (brand determined by meter used)
- Disposable gloves

PROCEDURE

STEPS	RATIONALE
1. Assess understanding of procedure and purpose. Determine whether patient with diabetes mellitus understands how to perform test and realizes importance of glucose monitoring.	• Data set guidelines for nurse to develop teaching plan.
2. Determine whether specific conditions need to be met before or after sample collection (e.g., with fasting, after meals, after certain medications, before insulin doses).	• Dietary intake of carbohydrates and ingestion of concentrated glucose preparations alter blood glucose levels.
3. Determine whether risks exist for performing skin puncture (e.g., low platelet count, anticoagulant therapy, bleeding disorders).	• Abnormal clotting mechanisms increase risk for local ecchymosis and bleeding.

Continued

SKILL 42-2 BLOOD GLUCOSE MONITORING—cont'd

STEPS	RATIONALE
4. Assess area of skin to use as puncture site. Inspect the patient's fingers, toes, and heel. Alternative sites are the palm, arm, and thigh. Avoid areas that have bruises and open lesions.	• Sides of fingers, toes, and heels are commonly selected because they have fewer nerve endings. Measurements at alternative sites are meter specific and may be different from measurements at traditional sites (McCulloch, 2017). As an alternative to the traditional fingertip site, periungual puncture sites are associated with less pain, good reproducibility, and no significant difference in the values of blood glucose obtained (Cristiano, Catanuso, Di Gregorio, et al., 2015). • The puncture site should not be edematous, inflamed, or recently punctured because these factors cause increased interstitial fluid and blood to mix and also increase the risk for infection.
5. Review health care provider's order for times and frequency of measurement.	• Health care provider determines test schedule on the basis of patient's physiological status and risk for glucose imbalance.
6. If diabetic patient performs test at home, assess patient's ability to handle skin-puncturing device. The patient may choose to continue self-testing while in hospital.	• Patient's physical health may change (e.g., vision disturbance, fatigue, pain, disease process), preventing patient from performing test.
7. Expected outcomes after completion of procedure:	
• Puncture site shows no evidence of bleeding or tissue damage.	• Hemostasis achieved. Lancet or needle did not puncture skin too deeply.
• Blood glucose level is normal.	• Normal fasting glucose level is 4 to 6 mmol/L, indicating good metabolic control.
• Patient demonstrates procedure.	• Patient demonstrates psychomotor learning.
• Patient explains test results.	• Patient validates knowledge.
8. Explain procedure and purpose to patient or family, or both. Offer patient and family opportunity to practise testing procedures. Provide resources and teaching aids for patient.	• Such explanations promote understanding and cooperation.
9. Perform hand hygiene before procedures.	• Hand hygiene reduces transfer of microorganisms.
10. Instruct patient to perform hand hygiene with soap and warm water, if patient is able.	• Handwashing promotes skin cleaning and vasodilation at selected puncture site. It establishes practice for patient when test is performed at home. Because of its ability to remove food residue from the hands and fingers, handwashing is superior to using alcohol pads to cleane the test site.
11. Position patient comfortably in chair or in semi-Fowler's position in bed.	• This position ensures easy accessibility to puncture site. Patient will assume position when self-testing.
12. Remove test strip from container, then tightly seal cap. Check code on the test strip vial.	• Sealing cap protects unused strips from accidental discoloration caused by exposure to air or light. Code on test strip vial must match code entered into the glucose meter.
13. Turn on glucose meter, if necessary.	• Turning on activates meter.

CRITICAL DECISION POINT: *Some monitors are activated when the test strip is inserted and therefore do not have a specific on-off switch.*

STEPS	RATIONALE
14. Insert strip into glucose meter (refer to manufacturer's directions), and make necessary adjustments (see Step 14 illustration).	• Some machines must be calibrated; others require zeroing of timer. Each meter is adjusted differently.

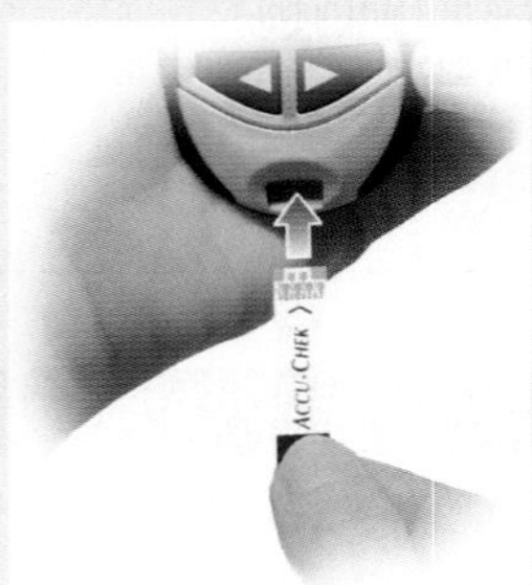

STEP 14 Load test strip into meter. (Courtesy Accu-Chek Glucometer.)

STEPS	RATIONALE
15. Remove unused glucose test strip from meter and place on paper towel or clean, dry surface with test pad facing up (see manufacturer's directions).	• Moisture on strip can alter accuracy of final test results.
16. Apply disposable gloves.	• Wearing gloves reduces risk for contamination by blood.

STEPS	RATIONALE
17. Choose puncture site. Puncture site should be vascular. In adults, select lateral side of finger; be sure to avoid central tip of finger, which has more dense nerve supply.	• Vascularity ensures free flow of blood after puncture.
18. Hold the finger that you will puncture in dependent position while gently massaging finger toward puncture site.	• Massage increases blood flow to area before puncture.
19. Clean site with antiseptic swab, and allow it to dry completely.	• The site must be allowed to dry because alcohol can cause blood to hemolyze.
20. Remove cover of lancet or blood-letting device. Hold lancet perpendicular to puncture site, and pierce finger or heel quickly in one continuous motion (do not force lancet).	• Cover keeps tip of lancet or needle sterile.
21. Some employers use lancet devices with an automatic blade retraction system. This reduces the possibility of self-sticks, preventing exposure to blood-borne pathogens. Place blood-letting device firmly against side of finger and push release button, causing needle to pierce skin (see Step 21 illustration).	• Blood-letting devices are designed to pierce skin to a specific depth, ensuring adequate blood flow. Perpendicular position ensures proper skin penetration.
22. Wipe away first droplet of blood with cotton ball. (See manufacturer's directions for meter used.)	• First drop of blood may contain more serous fluid than blood cells.
23. Lightly squeeze puncture site (without touching) until a second large droplet of blood has formed (see Step 23 illustration). Repuncturing is necessary if a large enough drop does not form to ensure accurate test results. (See manufacturer's direction regarding how blood is applied.)	• Adequate-sized droplet is needed to activate monitor and obtain accurate results. Excessive squeezing of tissues during blood sample collection may contribute to pain, bruising, scarring, hemolysis, and contamination of the blood with interstitial and intracellular fluid, leading to inaccurate results (Krleza, Dorotic, Grzunov, et al., 2015).

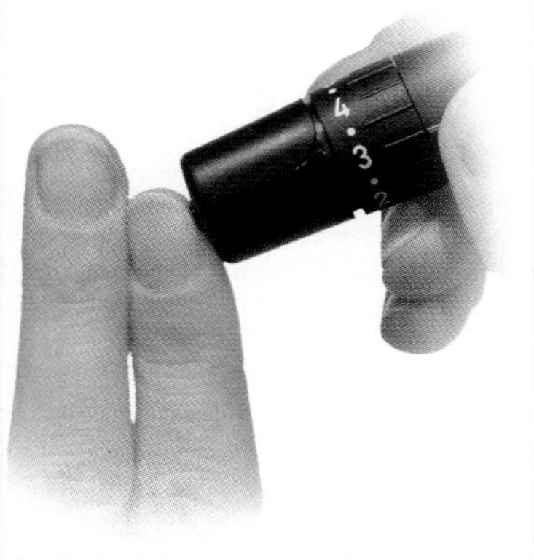

STEP 21 Prick side of patient's finger with lancet. (Courtesy Accu-Chek Glucometer.)

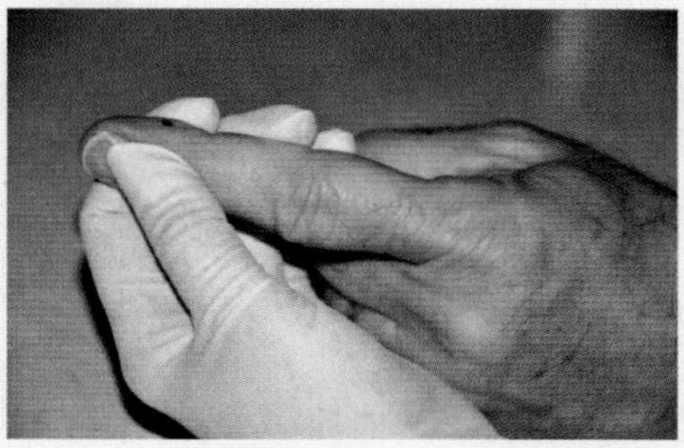

STEP 23 Squeeze puncture site until a large droplet of blood is expressed.

CRITICAL DECISION POINT: *Diabetic patients frequently have peripheral vascular disease. This makes it difficult to produce a large drop of blood after a fingerstick. To improve blood flow, be sure to hold patient's finger in dependent position before puncturing.*

STEPS	RATIONALE
24. Obtain test results.	• Exposure of blood to test strip for prescribed time ensures proper results.

CRITICAL DECISION POINT: *Some meters (such as OneTouch [LifeScan]) require blood sample to be applied to test strip already in the meter. Once the drop of blood is applied, the meter automatically calculates the reading.*

STEPS	RATIONALE
A. Be sure meter is still on. Bring test strip in the meter (in this example, an Accu-Check) to the drop of blood (see Step 24A illustration). The blood will be absorbed into the test strip (see manufacturer's instructions).	• Blood is absorbed into strip, and glucose device will show message on screen to signal that enough blood is obtained.

CRITICAL DECISION POINT: *Do not scrape blood onto the test strips or apply blood to wrong side of test strip. This prevents accurate glucose measurement. Ensure enough blood is applied to completely fill the test window. Otherwise a false reading or error message will be displayed.*

Continued

SKILL 42-2 BLOOD GLUCOSE MONITORING—cont'd

STEPS	RATIONALE
B. The blood glucose test result will appear on the screen (see Step 24B illustration). Some devices beep when measurement is completed.	

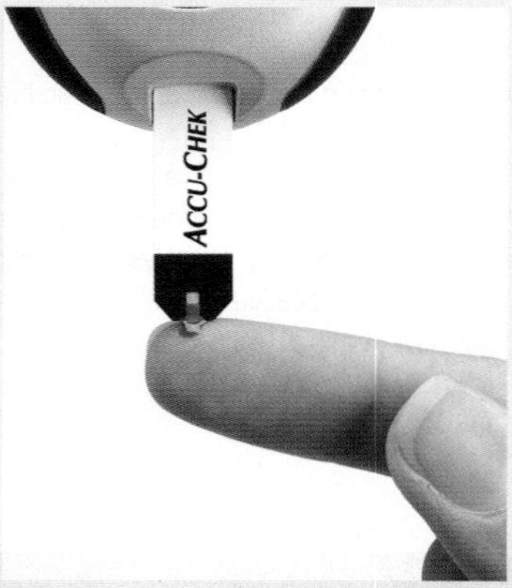

STEP 24A Touch the test strip to the blood drop. Blood is absorbed into the test strip. (Courtesy Accu-Chek Glucometer.)

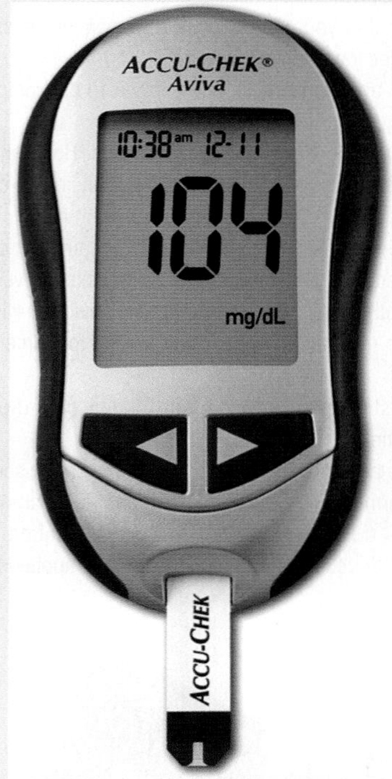

STEP 24B Results appear on meter screen. (Courtesy Accu-Chek Glucometer.)

STEPS	RATIONALE
25. Turn meter off. Dispose of test strip, lancet, and gloves in proper receptacle.	• Meter is battery powered. Proper disposal reduces risk for needlestick injury and spread of infection.
26. Discuss test results with patient.	• Discussion promotes participation and provides a perfect teaching opportunity for continued self-monitoring of blood glucose testing.
27. Reinspect puncture site for bleeding or tissue injury.	• Site is possibly a source of discomfort and infection.
28. Compare glucose meter reading with normal blood glucose levels and previous test results.	• Comparison helps determine whether glucose level is normal.
29. Ask patient to discuss procedure.	• Discussion validates patient's level of learning.
30. Ask patient to explain test and results.	• Results of test may cause anxiety. Patient may misunderstand specific step of procedure.

UNEXPECTED OUTCOMES	RELATED INTERVENTIONS
Puncture site bruised and continues to bleed	• Apply pressure. • Elevate hand above level of heart • Notify health care provider.
Blood glucose level above or below target range	• Continue to monitor patient. • Check for medication orders regarding deviations in glucose level. • Administer insulin or carbohydrate source as ordered, depending on glucose level. • Notify health care provider.
Glucose meter malfunction	• Review instructions for troubleshooting glucose meter. • Repeat test. • Call the 1-800 company phone number found at the back of every blood glucose testing meter.
Patient misunderstanding of procedure and results	• Repeat instructions to patient. • Have patient demonstrate procedure.

STEPS	RATIONALE

RECORDING AND REPORTING

- In nurses' notes or special flow sheet, record procedure, glucose level, and action taken for abnormal range.
- Describe response, including appearance of puncture site, in nurses' notes.
- Record and report abnormal blood glucose levels.
- Stress importance of timing the testing of blood glucose levels, particularly in patients with diabetes mellitus.

TEACHING CONSIDERATIONS

- Provide information on where a patient with diabetes mellitus can obtain testing samples, if applicable. When possible, teach with the same meter that the patient will use at home.
- Provide patient with information on where to obtain assistance if glucose meter has malfunctioned.
- Instruct patient in what to do and whom to contact if glucose meter malfunctions.

PEDIATRIC CONSIDERATIONS

- Young children should be allowed to choose puncture site.
- Heel and great toe are common puncture sites in infants.
- It is necessary to assess for localized complications in heels of premature infants who must have blood drawn repeatedly.
- Heel warming facilitates obtaining a specimen from a neonate.
- Infection or abscess of the heel and necrotizing osteochondritis are the most serious complications of heelstick puncture in infants.
- To avoid osteochondritis, the puncture should not be deeper than 0.85 mm for premature neonates up to 3 kg, or 2.0 mm for infants under 6 months of age, and is made at the outer aspect of the heel (Krleza et al., 2015).
- The earlobe has been used to obtain blood and to estimate arterial blood gas content, based on the hypothesis that blood from dilated capillaries of the earlobe contains a higher proportion of arterial than venous blood. However, studies have shown contradictory results on the accuracy of this technique for blood gas measurement (Vaquer, Masip, Gili, et al., 2014).
- Young children should be allowed with parent to demonstrate technique; technique can be incorporated in play activity for further understanding.

AGE-RELATED CONSIDERATIONS

- Warming fingertips may facilitate obtaining specimen.
- Some older persons have vision or dexterity problems that interfere with performing self-fingersticks.

HOME CARE CONSIDERATIONS

- Patients can use glucose meters routinely in their homes.
- Patients should be encouraged to attend a diabetic support group if it is needed.
- As visual acuity may affect a patient's ability to perform self-testing at home, there are new blood glucose testing meters that have talking ability (Tsai, 2015).

Reproduced from Perry, A. G., & Potter, P. A. (2010). *Clinical nursing skills and techniques* (7th ed., pp. 1153–1158). St. Louis, MO: Elsevier/Mosby.

ENTERAL TUBE FEEDING

Enteral nutrition refers to nutrients given via the gastrointestinal tract. When the patient cannot ingest food but is still able to digest and absorb nutrients, enteral tube feeding is indicated. Feeding tubes can be inserted through the nose (or orally if necessary) into the stomach or intestines (nasogastric-orogastric or nasointestinal-orointestinal tubes), surgically through a stoma (a surgically created opening) into the stomach or jejunum (gastrostomy or jejunostomy tubes), or endoscopically (percutaneous endoscopic gastrostomy [PEG] or jejunostomy [PEJ] tubes).

A registered nurse may insert nasogastric or orogastric tubes for abdominal decompression and for enteral feedings with an order from a physician (Saskatoon Health Region, 2017). Large-diameter (large-bore) sump tubing nasogastric tubes are most often used for both decompression and short-term enteral feeding, whereas small-bore, silastic tubing with insertion stylet is used for longer-term feeding needs. The small-bore nasogastric or nasojejunal tube is preferred over large-bore tubes as they reduce patient discomfort and gastric erosion (Holmes, 2012) and can be used for longer periods (Silk & Quinn, 2015). All other tubes must be inserted by a physician. In some settings (e.g., the Critical Care Unit), a large tube is used to start the tube feed and if the patient tolerates it for the first 24 to 48 hours, a small-bore tube is then inserted. As well, if the patient has a small-bore tube placed in the duodenum, the physician may elect to leave the sump tube in the stomach for gastric decompression and prevent vomiting or aspiration. If enteral nutrition therapy is to be administered for less than 4 weeks, nasoenteral tubes may be used. Surgical or endoscopically placed tubes are preferred for long-term feeding (>4 weeks) to reduce the discomfort of a nasal tube and to provide a more secure, reliable access (Villela, Sakai, Almeida, et al, 2014). Box 42-11 conveys the everyday experiences of a child and his family with long-term tube feeding. Patients with gastroparesis (decreased or absent innervation to the stomach causing delayed gastric emptying) or esophageal reflux, those at risk for aspiration, and those with a history of aspiration pneumonia require placement of tubes beyond the stomach into the intestine (Blumenstein, Shastri, & Stein, 2014).

Box 42-12 lists indications for enteral nutrition. The nurse inserts the nasoenteral tube (Skill 42-3), and the nurse or others, including

BOX 42-11 CASE STUDY

*Working With Riley and His Family**

I had the opportunity to look after Riley, an active 3-year-old who loved being read to and playing with super-hero action figures. Riley was meeting all of his developmental milestones except one: He had never learned to eat enough to sustain himself and appropriately gain weight. Although Riley ate a small amount of food (potato chips and hot dogs), no physical, psychosocial, or emotional cause for his reluctance to eat was found. Eventually it was decided to put in a G-tube, which Riley simply called a "button" after hearing nurses use this term. Riley often played with the G-tube and occasionally pulled it out. He seemed to think the G-tube was an extension of his body and was surprised to find out that not everyone had a G-tube.

I became involved in Riley's care once he was discharged home. As a community care nurse, my primary roles were to provide emotional support to Riley's parents while providing age-appropriate care for Riley. My family-centred approach included recognizing the parents as the decision makers in their child's life and focusing on the family's abilities and challenges. I reinforced the teaching that had occurred within the hospital related to Riley's G-tube and nutritional needs. In addition, I helped Riley's family navigate various health and social systems to ensure that adequate supports were in place.

Despite numerous attempts to decrease the nighttime feedings, Riley was not able to maintain sufficient intake for the G-tube to be removed or for the feedings to be completely discontinued. From my perspective, most health care providers were completely supportive; however, a few contravened family-oriented care by negatively judging Riley's family and suggesting that his parents were somehow responsible for Riley's nutritional challenges. For example, one health care provider suggested that Riley's parents preferred the G-tube as it took less time than convincing Riley to try to eat enough nutritious food to maintain his weight.

Riley is now 12 years old and still has a G-tube in place; he receives a tube feeding every second night. He does well in school and actively participates in sports, although he is sometimes self-conscious about his "button." Riley's mother continues to worry that he will dislodge the G-tube while playing sports. From this situation of caring for Riley and his parents over time, I have learned that children are incredibly resilient, even when faced with a significant health challenge, and that both children and their families thrive when family-centered care is provided.

In reading the case study of the young boy living with a G-tube, what are the advantages of the family-centred approach to care that the community nurse used to help meet the child's nutritional needs? What teachings about the G-tube and children's nutrition are critical? How might you engage Riley in discussing the meaning that G-tube feeding holds for him?

*By Donna Bulman, RN, PhD, University of New Brunswick.

BOX 42-12 Indications for Enteral Nutrition

Cancer

- Head and neck
- Upper gastrointestinal tract

Critical Illness or Trauma

- Respiratory failure with prolonged intubation/inadequate oral intake
- Patients in critical care with suspected/evidence of catabolism
- Trauma patients, especially those in a hypermetabolic state (e.g., burns)

Neurological and Muscular Disorders

- Brain neoplasm
- Stroke
- Cerebrovascular accident
- Neuromuscular disorders (e.g., amyotrophic lateral sclerosis, multiple sclerosis, Parkinson's disease)
- Dementia:

Patients with advanced dementia are offered quality-of-life diets; they risk injury with multiple insertions related to self-extubation of feeding tubes. Enteral feeding for end-stage dementia is controversial. Common reasons to initiate enteral feedings in these patients include prolonging survival, improving quality of life, preventing pressure injuries, and palliative care. However, the evidence to support artificial nutrition in people with advanced dementia is limited. Expert consensus is that artificial hydration and nutrition in people with advanced dementia are not appropriate when swallowing problems or disinclination to eat is a result of advancing disease, and that they should not be used solely to prolong life (Parker & Power, 2013). Decisions about artificial nutrition in people with dementia should be made on an individual basis after conducting a comprehensive, multidisciplinary assessment that includes confirmation of advanced dementia and the absence of an acute, potentially reversible cause of the swallowing difficulty. It is paramount to involve the person's family or caregivers to manage their expectations and to ensure that the wishes of the person with dementia are taken into account.

- Myopathy
- Parkinson's disease

Gastrointestinal Disorders

- Enterocutaneous fistula
- Inflammatory bowel disease
- Mild pancreatitis

Other Situations

- Respiratory failure with prolonged intubation
- Inadequate oral intake
- Continuous feedings
- Supine positioning:
  A 45-degree elevation is recommended when possible for supine patients to reduce their risk of aspiration and, if intubated, prevent ventilator-associated pneumonia (Dhaliwal, Cahill, Lemieux, et al., 2014).

Supine position is an indication for enteral feeding. Enteral feedings may be provided at the same rate as in the prone position, since they are likely to have the same residual in either position (Saez de la Fuente, Saez de la Fuente, Estelles, et al., 2014).

- Cerebral vascular accident
- Local trauma
- Anorexia nervosa
- Difficulty chewing and swallowing
- Severe depression

SKILL 42-3 INSERTING A SMALL-BORE NASOENTERIC OR ORAL TUBE FOR ENTERAL FEEDING

Delegation Considerations

At most Canadian institutions, the insertion of a sump naso/orogastric tube without stylet is an advanced nursing competency, requiring one-time certification. The insertion of a silastic feeding tube with stylet is considered a delegated medical function requiring yearly recertification. For this reason, this skill should not be delegated to unregulated care providers or those without a certified competency.

Equipment

- Nasogastric or nasointestinal (orogastric or orointestinal) tube (8 to 12 Fr) with guide wire or stylet
- Stethoscope
- 60-mL or larger Luer-Lok or catheter-tip syringe
- Entriflex nasogastric feeding tubes with safe enteral connections. (This weighted polyurethane feeding tube is designed for nasogastric and nasoduodenal feeding with a slimmer, lighter weighted tip for easier insertion. The feeding port is incompatible with Luer-Lok or intravenous [IV] connections, reducing the risk of accidental connection or inadvertent administration of IV-intended medications through the feeding tube, a practice started in Great Britain and the United States to address the JCAHO [2014] Tubing Misconnections Sentinel Alert.)
- Hypoallergenic tape and tincture of benzoin or tube fixation device
- Scissors
- pH indicator strip (scale 0.0 to 11.0)
- Medication cup or container for aspirated fluid
- Glass of water and straw (not required for intubated patients)
- Water-soluble lubricant
- Emesis basin
- Absorbent pad
- Facial tissues
- Disposable gloves (multiple pairs needed)
- Suction equipment in case of aspiration
- Penlight to check placement of nasopharynx
- Tongue blade
- Disposable tape measure
- Felt-tip marker

PROCEDURE

STEPS	RATIONALE
1. Assess patient's need for enteral tube feeding: NPO (nothing by mouth) status, functional gastrointestinal tract, inability to ingest sufficient nutrients.	• Identifying patients who need tube feedings before they become nutritionally depleted may help to prevent complications related to malnutrition.
A. Review physician's order for insertion of tube and enteral feeding schedule.	• Procedures and tube feedings require a physician's order.
2. Explain procedure to patient.	• Patient can cooperate with the process.
3. Assess patency of nares. Have patient close each nostril alternately and breathe. Examine each naris for patency and skin breakdown.	• Nares may be obstructed or irritated, or a septal defect may be present.
4. Assess the gag reflex by placing a tongue blade in patient's mouth, touching uvula to induce a gag response.	• This activity assesses ability to swallow and determines whether the patient is at risk for aspiration.

CRITICAL DECISION POINT: *Patients with impaired level of consciousness, or who are intubated and sedated, may also have impaired gag reflex, and their risk of aspiration is increased during this type of procedure and subsequent tube feedings. For patients who are intubated, sedated, or too ill to participate in the procedure, ensure that the patient's head is tilted toward the chest for enteral feeding tube insertion.*

STEPS	RATIONALE
5. Review patient's medical history for nasal problems (e.g., nosebleeds, oral or facial surgery, anticoagulation therapy, history of aspiration).	• Nasoenteral tubes are contraindicated in patients with recent nasal surgery, facial traumas, nosebleeds, or surgical procedures requiring a transsphenoid approach (e.g., to remove pituitary tumours) or who are receiving anticoagulation therapy (Metheny, 2016).
6. Perform hand hygiene.	• Hand hygiene reduces transfer of microorganisms.
7. Auscultate abdomen for bowel sounds.	• Absence of bowel sounds may indicate decreased or absent peristalsis and increased risk for aspiration or abdominal distension.
8. Explain procedure to patient and how to communicate during insertion by raising index finger to indicate gagging or discomfort.	• Explanations reduce anxiety and help patient assist in insertion.

Continued

SKILL 42-3 INSERTING A SMALL-BORE NASOENTERIC OR ORAL TUBE FOR ENTERAL FEEDING—cont'd

STEPS	RATIONALE
9. Stand on same side of bed as naris for insertion, and assist patient to high Fowler's position unless contraindicated. Place pillow behind patient's head and shoulders.	• These actions facilitate manipulation of tube. Fowler's position reduces risk of aspiration and promotes effective swallowing.
10. Place absorbent pad over patient's chest. Keep facial tissues within reach.	• Pad prevents soiling of gown. Insertion of tube may cause patient's eyes to tear.
11. Determine length of tube to be inserted and mark with tape: Traditional method for placing the tube to the stomach: Measure distance from tip of nose to earlobe and then to xiphoid process of sternum (see Step 11 illustration).	• Length approximates distance from nose to stomach for 98% of patients. For duodenal or jejunal placement, an additional 20 to 30 cm is required.

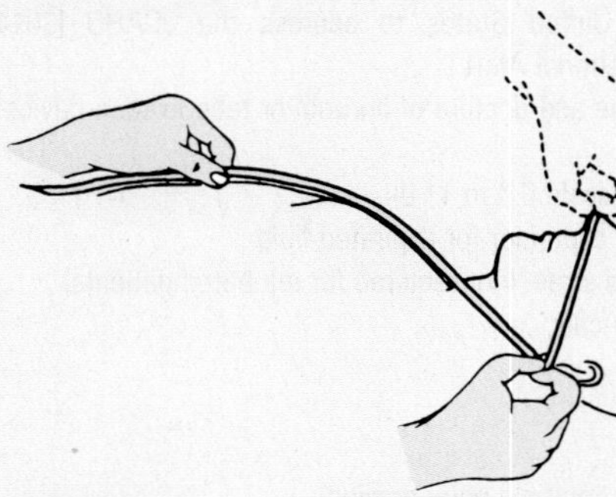

STEP 11 Length of tube to be inserted is equal to distance from tip of nose to earlobe to xiphoid process.

If placing the tube to small bowel (duodenum), follow agency-specific protocol; for example, the administration of 10 mg metoclopramide as a bowel motility agent, turning patient on right side, and injecting 200 cc of air to inflate the stomach.

STEPS	RATIONALE
12. Prepare nasogastric or nasointestinal tube for insertion according to manufacturer recommendation: **A.** Plastic tubes should *not* be iced.	• Tubes that are iced become stiff and inflexible, causing trauma to mucous membranes.
13. Perform hand hygiene and put on gloves.	• Hygiene and gloves reduce transmission of microorganisms.
A. If long-term tube, inject 10 mL of water from 30 mL or larger catheter-tip syringe into the tube and insert stylet/guide wire.	• Water releases a mechanism in the tip of the tube holding the guide wire in place to enable the guide wire to be removed following tube insertion.
B. Make certain that guide wire is securely positioned against weighted tip and that connections are snugly fitted together.	• Secure positioning and snug-fitting connections promote smooth passage of tube into gastrointestinal tract. Improperly positioned stylet can induce serious trauma (i.e., tracheal perforation, pneumothorax).
14. Cut tape 10 cm long or prepare tube fixation device. Split one end of tape lengthwise 5 cm.	• Tape is used to anchor tubing after insertion.
15. Dip tube with surface lubricant into glass of water. If tube is not prelubricated, use water-soluble lubricant.	• Activates lubricant to facilitate passage of tube into naris to gastrointestinal tract.
16. Insert tube through nostril to back of throat (posterior nasopharynx). Aim back and down toward ear.	• Natural contour facilitates passage of tube into gastrointestinal tract and reduces gagging by patient.
17. Have patient tilt head toward chest after tube has passed through nasopharynx.	• Tilting head forward closes off glottis and reduces risk of tube entering trachea. This technique is also used in patients who are intubated and sedated.

CRITICAL DECISION POINT: *Encourage a patient who is alert and communicating to swallow by giving small sips of water or ice chips when possible. For patients who are intubated and sedated, or are not able to participate in the procedure, tilt patient's head toward the chest. Advance tube as patient swallows or as patient's head is tilted toward chest. Rotate tube 180 degrees while inserting.*

STEPS	RATIONALE
18. Emphasize the need to mouth-breathe and swallow during the procedure (when possible).	• Mouth-breathing and swallowing facilitate passage of tube and alleviate patient's fear during the procedure.
19. When tip of tube reaches the carina (about 25 cm in an adult), stop insertion, hold end of tube near your ear, and listen for air exchange from the distal portion of the tube.	• **If air is heard, the tube could be in the respiratory tract; remove tube and start over. This listening step should never be used to verify tube placement** (Metheny, 2016).
20. Advance tube each time patient swallows until desired length has been passed.	• Advancing tube while patient swallows reduces discomfort and trauma to patient.

STEPS	RATIONALE

CRITICAL DECISION POINT: *Do not force tube insertion. If resistance is met or patient starts to cough, choke, or become cyanotic, stop advancing the tube and pull tube back. It is important to note that heavily sedated, comatose, or paralyzed patients may not exhibit a cough or gag reflex during insertion and so this should not be used as the sole method of determining improper tube placement. It is also possible to slip a small-bore feeding tube into the trachea down past an endotracheal tube without loss of oxygenation; therefore, X-ray examination is the definitive step in determining tube placement.*

21. Check for position of tube in back of patient's throat with penlight and tongue blade.

- Tube may be coiled, kinked, or entering trachea. (Withdraw tube immediately if tube is coiled, respiratory status of patient changes, or patient begins to cough and skin colour changes. If distress is not present, withdraw tube fully and retry. Note whether tube was kinked; if so, it is likely to kink again in the same place.)

22. Perform measures to verify placement of tube, once desired length has been passed. Secure tube before X-ray examination, because it may become dislodged during procedure.

- Tube placement must be verified by X-ray examination before enteral feedings are initiated. Other tests that can be done at the bedside to ensure ongoing placement are as follows:
  - Observe for a change in length of the external portion of the feeding tube, as indicated by movement of the marked portion of the tube.
  - Review routine chest and abdominal radiography reports to look for notations about tube location.
  - Observe changes in volume of aspirate from the feeding tube—a large increase in volume may signal the upward dislocation of a small-bowel feeding tube in the stomach; persistent inability to withdraw fluid (or only a few drops of fluid) from the tube may signal upward displacement of a gastric tube into the esophagus.
  - Measure the pH of feeding tube aspirates.
  - Encourage obtaining of a radiograph to confirm tube position if the tube's position is in doubt (Metheny, 2016).

CRITICAL DECISION POINT: *Auscultation is not a reliable method for verification of tube placement because a tube inadvertently placed in the lungs, pharynx, or esophagus can transmit a sound similar to that of air entering the stomach (Boeykens et al., 2014; National Association of Children's Hospitals, 2012).*

23. After gastric aspirates are obtained (see Box 42-16), anchor tube to patient's nose and avoid pressure on nares. Mark exit site with indelible ink. Select one of the following options:

- A properly secured tube allows the patient more mobility and prevents trauma to nasal mucosa. Mark tube at tip of naris; measure from line to end of tube; tape and secure to maintain position.

A. Apply tape.

(1) Apply tincture of benzoin or other skin adhesive on tip of patient's nose and tube and allow it to become "tacky."

- Skin adhesive helps tape adhere better and protects patient's skin.

(2) Place the intact end of tape over bridge of patient's nose. Wrap each of the 5-cm strips around tube as it exits nose. Change position of tube at naris every 8 hours (q8h) (see Step 23A(2) illustration).

- Securing tape to nares prevents tissue necrosis. Changing tube position avoids erosion of naris.

B. Apply tube fixation device, using shaped adhesive patch.

- Fixation device secures tube and reduces friction on nares (Ambutas, Staffileno, & Fogg, 2014).

(1) Apply wide end of patch to bridge of nose.

(2) Slip connector around tube as it exits nose (see Step 23B(2) illustration).

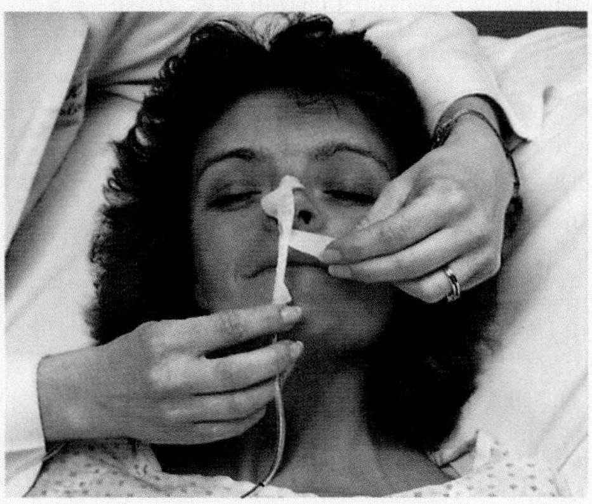

STEP 23A(2) Wrapping tape to anchor nasoenteral tube.

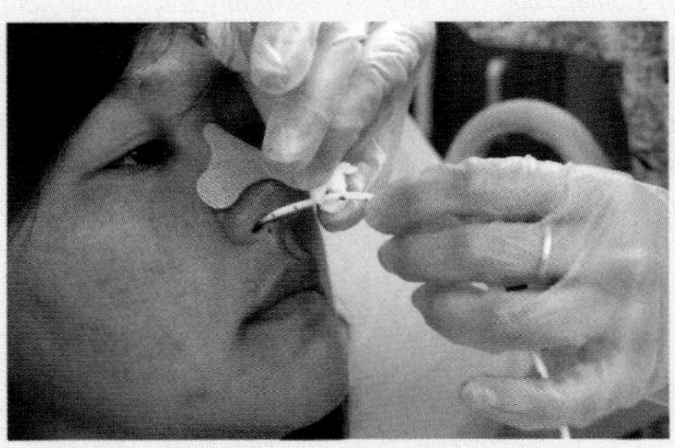

STEP 23B(2) Slipping connector around feeding tube.

Continued

SKILL 42-3 INSERTING A SMALL-BORE NASOENTERIC OR ORAL TUBE FOR ENTERAL FEEDING—cont'd

STEPS	RATIONALE
24. A second anchoring of tube against cheek with gauze and transparent dressing may be advised, so that tube does not rest over bony points.	• Fastening the tube this way may help prevent the tube from being pulled by confused patients and avoids pressure points. However, the available evidence on interventions to reduce nasogastric tube dislodgement and adverse events is of limited quantity and validity (Brugnolli, Ambrosi, Canzan, et al., 2014).
25. For intestinal placement, position patient on right side, when possible, until correct placement has been verified radiologically. Remove gloves. Perform hand hygiene, and assist patient to a comfortable position.	• Positioning patient on right side promotes passage of the tube into the small intestine (duodenum or jejunum).

CRITICAL DECISION POINT: *Leave stylet/guide wire in place until correct position is ensured by X-ray film or check agency policy that states how long you can leave the wire or stylet in place if the X-ray or interpretation is delayed. Never attempt to reinsert partially or fully remove stylet/guide wire while feeding tube is in place.*

Clinically sound judgement is always required for nasogastric insertion and placement verification. Cortrak is a device used to place small-bore tubes, in an effort to improve efficiency and reduce patient discomfort by checking placement as the tube is inserted at bedside. This reduces the need to verify placement. Cortrak involves computer technology to guide clinicians in the placement of nasoenteric feeding tubes. The device aids feeding tube placement by showing the relative location of the feeding tube tip as it descends into the tract. The tip of the feeding tube stylet has an electromagnetic transmitter. A receiver unit is placed on the patient's xiphoid during the procedure, to acquire the signal (Smithard, Barrett, Hargroves, et al., 2015).

STEPS	RATIONALE
26. Obtain X-ray film of abdomen.	• Placement of tube is verified by X-ray examination (Dhaliwal et al., 2014; Metheny, 2016).
27. Perform hand hygiene, apply clean gloves, and administer oral hygiene (see Chapter 38). Clean tubing at nostril.	• Oral hygiene promotes patient comfort and integrity of oral mucous membranes.
28. Remove gloves, dispose of equipment, and perform hand hygiene.	• These actions reduce transmission of microorganisms.
29. Inspect patient's naris and oropharynx for any irritation after insertion.	• If tube insertion was difficult, irritation of naris or oropharynx may have occurred.
30. Ask patient whether he or she feels comfortable.	• Patient's level of comfort is evaluated. (This may be a challenge if a language barrier exists or if the patient has dementia or is confused.)
31. Observe patient for any difficulty breathing or for coughing or gagging.	• Improper position of the tube may cause these symptoms or increase symptoms in patients who have heart failure, pneumonia, asthma, and other cardiac or respiratory conditions.
32. Auscultate lung sounds.	• Abnormal lung sounds can be an early sign of aspiration.
33. Assess for feeding tube placement at 4-hour intervals to ensure that the tube has remained in the desired location.	To repeat from Step 22: • Observe for a change in length of the external portion of the feeding tube. • Observe changes in volume of aspirate from the feeding tube. • Measure the pH of feeding tube aspirates. • Encourage obtaining of a radiograph to confirm tube position if the tube's position is in doubt.
34. Assess for intolerance to feedings every 4 hours.	• Monitor gastric residual volumes, abdominal discomfort, nausea/vomiting, and abdominal girth/distension (Dhaliwal et al., 2014).

UNEXPECTED OUTCOMES	RELATED INTERVENTIONS
Aspiration of stomach contents into the respiratory tract (immediate response), evidenced by coughing, dyspnea, cyanosis, auscultation of crackles or wheezes	• Position patient on side. • Suction nasotracheally and orotracheally. • Consult physician immediately to order chest X-ray examination.
Aspiration of stomach contents into respiratory tract (delayed response), evidenced by dyspnea, fever, auscultation of crackles or wheezes	• Consult physician to obtain order for chest X-ray film. • Prepare for possible initiation of antibiotics.
Development of bacterial aspiration pneumonia from contaminated saliva for patients NPO or being fed enterally.	• Limited oral hydration leads to dry mouth and increased concentration of oral bacteria. It is imperative that scrupulous oral hygiene be maintained for these individuals, which includes using a soft toothbrush to clean teeth, gums, roof of mouth, and cheeks. Patients and their families must be counselled regarding this risk for those who are discharged home or maintain self-care (Casaubon, Suddes, Acute Stroke Best Practices Working Group, 2013; Maeda & Akagi, 2014).

UNEXPECTED OUTCOMES	RELATED INTERVENTIONS
Displacement of feeding tube to another site (e.g., from duodenum to stomach, which may occur when patient coughs or vomits)	• Confirm that mark on tube (made at initial insertion) is at exit site (if tube is moved, mark at new exit site). • Remeasure distance from naris to tip of xyphoid process, and compare with baseline measurement from insertion. • Aspirate gastrointestinal contents and measure pH (Boeykens et al., 2014). • Discuss findings with physician. • Reconfirm placement by X-ray film (optional). • If tube is displaced, prepare to remove displaced tube, and insert and verify placement of new tube. • If there is a question of aspiration, obtain chest X-ray film.
CRITICAL DECISION POINT: *To prevent clogging of feeding tube in relation to feedings, flush feeding tube with tap water (Fisher & Blalock, 2014) after checking residual volume, after intermittent feeding, every 4 hours during continuous feedings, and before and after administration of medications. On average, use 15 to 30 mL or more of water for flushing. The amount of water required varies with the individual length of tube. Try to find an alternative route for medication administration when small-bore tubes (especially the temporary nasogastric silastic tubes) are used because they frequently clog.*	
Clogging of feeding tube	• To prevent feeding-tube clogging that results from medication, use liquid forms of medication whenever possible. When the solid form of dosage is used, make sure tablets can be crushed and that there is no contraindication to crushing them (i.e., sustained-release cardiac medications should *not* be crushed as they will adversely affect the patient's hemodynamic status [heart rate and blood pressure]) and that capsules can be opened; dissolve tablets or capsules well, and administer each medication separately (Lohmann, Gartner, Kurze, et al., 2015). • Aspirate gastric contents with 60-mL syringe to assess patency of tube. • Irrigate tube with water. Research clearly supports water as the best choice for initial declogging efforts (Fisher & Blalock, 2014). • Notify physician and prepare to administer pancrelipase or other enzymatic declogging agent upon physician order or standing protocol. Pancrelipase dissolves foodstuff but is ineffective in dissolving pill particles. • Attempt to clear tube with pancrelipase using a 50- to 60-mL syringe. Do *not* use a small-barrel syringe (i.e., 20 cm or less) because smaller syringes have greater psi (pounds per square inch) and injection of air or liquid under high pressure (above 40 psi) may cause tube rupture (Fisher & Blalock, 2014).
Irritation of naris and nasal mucosa	• Provide hygiene, and remove and replace tube. (*Note:* This action requires a physician's order.) • Consider removing tube and inserting it into the other naris (physician order required).

RECORDING AND REPORTING

- Record and report type and size of tube placed, location of distal tip of tube (mark and measure), patient's tolerance of procedure, pH value, and confirmation of tube position by X-ray examination.

family in the home setting, can administer enteral tube feedings. It is highly recommended that tube placement be verified by X-ray examination before the patient receives the first enteral feeding.

Enteral nutrition has been used successfully after surgery or trauma to provide fluids, electrolytes, and nutritional support. Gastric ileus may prevent nasogastric feedings, while nasointestinal or jejunostomy tubes allow successful postpyloric feeding of formula directly into the small intestine or jejunum or beyond the pyloric sphincter of the stomach (Blumenstein et al., 2014). Enteral feedings can be administered through a nasoenteric tube (Skill 42-4) or via a gastrostomy or jejunostomy tube (Skill 42-5).

Initiating Enteral Tube Feedings

Enteral formulas are usually one of four types. **Polymeric formulas** (1.0 to 2.0 kcal/mL) include milk-based blenderized foods prepared by hospital dietary staff or in the patient's home. The polymeric classification also includes commercially prepared whole-nutrient formulas. For this type of formula to be effective, the patient's gastrointestinal tract must be able to absorb whole nutrients. **Modular formulas** (3.8 to 4.0 kcal/mL) are single-macronutrient (e.g., protein, glucose, polymers, or lipids) preparations and are not nutritionally complete. This type of formula is added to other foods for meeting the patient's individual nutritional needs. **Elemental formulas** (1.0 to 3.0 kcal/mL)

SKILL 42-4 ADMINISTERING ENTERAL FEEDINGS VIA NASOENTERIC TUBE

Delegation Considerations

Administration of enteral tube feeding via nasoenteric tube is an institution-specific procedure that may or may *not* be delegated to unregulated care providers (UCPs) after the nurse verifies tube placement. The nurse is responsible for patient assessment. Depending on the institution's protocol, the nurse directs the UCPs to

- Ensure that the patient is sitting upright in a chair or in bed
- Infuse the feeding slowly
- Report any difficulty infusing the feeding or any discomfort voiced by the patient

Equipment

- Disposable feeding bag and tubing or ready-to-hang system
- 30-mL or larger Luer-Lok or catheter-tip syringe
- Stethoscope
- pH indicator strip (scale 0 to 14)
- Infusion pump (required for intestinal feedings): use pump designed for tube feedings
- Prescribed enteral feedings
- Disposable gloves
- Equipment to obtain blood glucose by fingerstick

PROCEDURE

STEPS	RATIONALE
1. Assess patient's need for enteral tube feedings: impaired swallowing, tracheostomy, decreased level of consciousness, head or neck surgery, facial trauma, surgical procedures involving upper alimentary canal.	• Identify patients who need tube feedings before they become nutritionally depleted.
2. Evaluate patient's nutritional status (see Table 42-4). Obtain baseline weight and laboratory values (e.g., albumin, transferrin, prealbumin). Assess patient for fluid volume excess or deficit, electrolyte abnormalities, and metabolic abnormalities, such as hyperglycemia.	• Enteral feedings are intended to restore or maintain a patient's nutritional status. Fluid volume assessment provides objective data to measure effectiveness of feedings.
3. Verify physician's order for formula, rate, route, and frequency and for laboratory data and bedside assessments, such as fingerstick blood glucose measurement.	• Tube feedings, laboratory tests, and bedside tests must be ordered by the physician.
4. Explain procedure to patient.	• Well-informed patients tend to be cooperative and comfortable.
5. Perform hand hygiene.	• Hand hygiene reduces transmission of microorganisms.
6. Auscultate for bowel sounds before feeding.	• Absence of bowel sounds may indicate decreased ability of gastrointestinal tract to digest or absorb nutrients.
7. Prepare feeding container to administer formula:	
A. Check expiration date on formula and integrity of container.	• Tube feedings administered within the designated shelf life from a container without cracks or breaks reduces the patient's risk of acquiring tube feeding–borne gastrointestinal infections.
B. Have tube feeding formula at room temperature.	• Cold formula may cause gastric cramping and discomfort because the liquid is not warmed by the mouth and esophagus.
C. Perform hand hygiene and apply gloves.	
D. Shake formula container well, and fill feeding container with formula (see Step 7D illustration). Open stopcock on tubing and fill with formula to remove air.	• Filling the tubing with formula prevents excess air from entering. • Tubing must be free of contamination, to prevent bacterial growth.

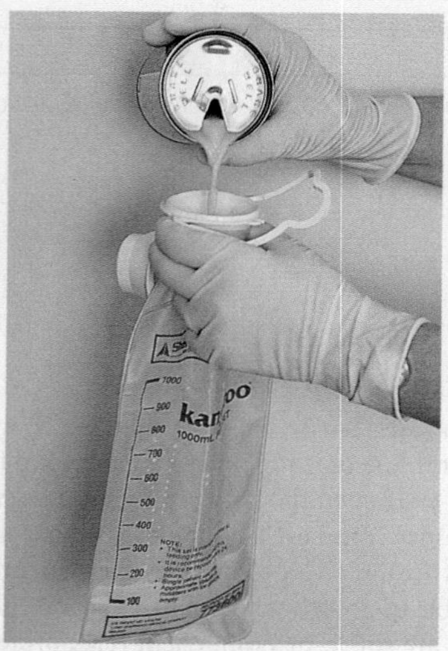

STEP 7D Pouring formula into feeding container.

STEPS	RATIONALE
E. Connect tubing to container as needed, or prepare ready-to-hang container.	

CRITICAL DECISION POINT: *Tube feedings are infused by feeding pumps and the tubes do not fit intravenous (IV) pump.*

STEPS	RATIONALE
8. For intermittent feeding, have syringe ready, and ensure formula is at room temperature.	• Cold formula may cause gastric cramping.
9. Place patient in high Fowler's position, or elevate head of bed to at least 45 degrees.	• Elevating the patient's head helps prevent aspiration.
10. Verify tube placement (see Box 42-15). Consider the results from pH testing together with the aspirate's appearance.	• On occasion, colour alone may differentiate gastric from intestinal placement. Because most intestinal aspirates are stained by bile to a distinct yellow colour and most gastric aspirates are not so stained, the difference may be distinguished. However, colour differences among the stomach and intestine are often difficult to discern, and the aspirate's colour must be considered in combination with other assessment data (Ellett et al., 2014).
11. Check pH of aspirate; confirm measurement of length of tube from naris to tip of connection port; ensure original mark is in the same position.	• Aspirates from initially placed nasogastric tubes with a pH of ≤5.5 are reliable to differentiate if the tube is in or outside the stomach, but this does not completely rule out esophageal placement (Boeykins et al., 2014; Meert, Caverly, Kelm, et al., 2015).
12. When available, check CO_2 at the distal end of naso- or orogastric (NG/OG) tubes.	• The detection of CO_2 at the distal end of NG/OG tubes (capnography) to ascertain unsuspected respiratory placement was 100% accurate in 10 critically ill adults (Ellett et al., 2014). Based on available research, more than one method of monitoring the placement of NG/OG tubes at the bedside should be used; an abdominal radiograph should be obtained if there is any doubt that the tube ends in the stomach.

CRITICAL DECISION POINT: *Auscultation is not considered a reliable method for verification of placement of tube because a tube inadvertently placed in lungs, pharynx, or esophagus can transmit sound similar to that of air entering stomach (Ellett et al., 2014; Metheny, 2016).*

13. Check for gastric residual.

A. Draw 30 mL of air with syringe. Connect to end of feeding tube. Flush tube with air.

B. Pull back evenly to aspirate gastric contents (see Step 13B illustration).

• Residual volume indicates whether gastric emptying is delayed. The Canadian Critical Care Nutrition guideline recommends a range of 250 to 500 mL (Dhaliwal et al., 2014). For pediatric patients, the amount of residual volume will be less. What constitutes a high gastric residual volume is debated. Volumes greater than 200 are considered high in critically ill patients who have airways in place. Depending on agency policy and physician or dietitian decision, if residual volume exceeds 500 mL, feedings may be withheld. However, because secretion of saliva and gastric fluids alone may total 188 mL/hour, a gastric residual volume of 200 may be too low a criterion for stopping the feeding (Flynn Makic, Rauen, & VonRueden, 2013). Further research is needed to recommend the frequency of the need to monitor gastric residual volumes. One event of elevated residual volume should not prompt cessation of enteral tube feeding but instead should prompt the nurse to monitor for signs and symptoms of intolerance (Flynn Makic et al., 2013).

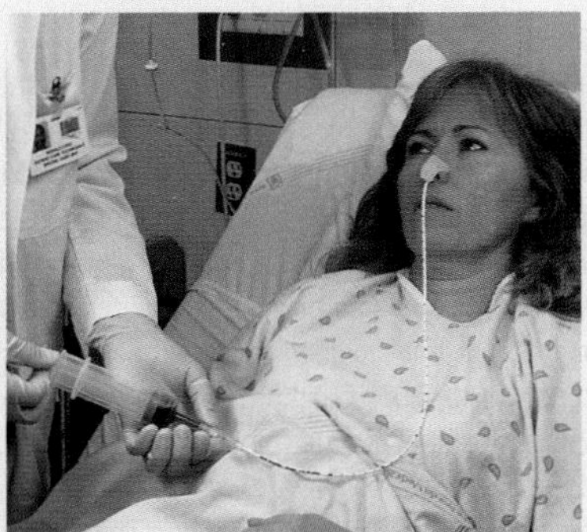

STEP 13B Check for gastric residual (small-bore tube).

Please note that if checking for gastric residual when a small-bore tube is in place, consult agency policy. Soft, small-bore tubes may collapse when GRV is checked, making assessment of residuals falsely low (Rollins & Boggs, 2013).

Remember that tube location is important. A tube in the small bowel would have ongoing secretions and much more residual and, therefore, checking residuals would not be necessary.

C. Return aspirated contents to stomach if specified by agency policy.

• Return of aspirate is also a controversial topic that requires further research (Parker, Torrazza, Li, et al., 2015).

Continued

SKILL 42-4 ADMINISTERING ENTERAL FEEDINGS VIA NASOENTERIC TUBE—cont'd

STEPS	RATIONALE
14. Flush tubing with 30 to 50 mL of tap water at room temperature (Rice, 2016).	• Ensure tube is clear and patent.
15. Label feeding tube bag. Complete and post nutrition label on bag to indicate type of formula, rate, time, and date.	
16. Initiate feeding:	
A. Syringe or intermittent feeding:	
(1) Pinch proximal end of the feeding tube.	• Pinching prevents air from entering patient's stomach.
(2) Remove plunger from syringe and attach barrel of syringe to end of tube.	
(3) Fill syringe with measured amount of formula (see Step 16A[3] illustration). Release tube and hold syringe high enough to allow it to empty gradually by gravity, and refill; repeat until prescribed amount has been delivered to the patient.	• Gradual emptying of tube feeding by gravity from syringe or feeding bag reduces risk of abdominal discomfort, vomiting, or diarrhea induced by bolus or too-rapid infusion of tube feedings.
(4) If feeding bag is used, hang feeding bag on an IV pole (see Step 16A[4] illustration). Fill bag with prescribed amount of formula, and allow bag to empty gradually over at least 30 minutes, depending on the amount of feeding.	• A feeding pump is used to infuse the formula. An IV pump must not be used for enteral feedings.

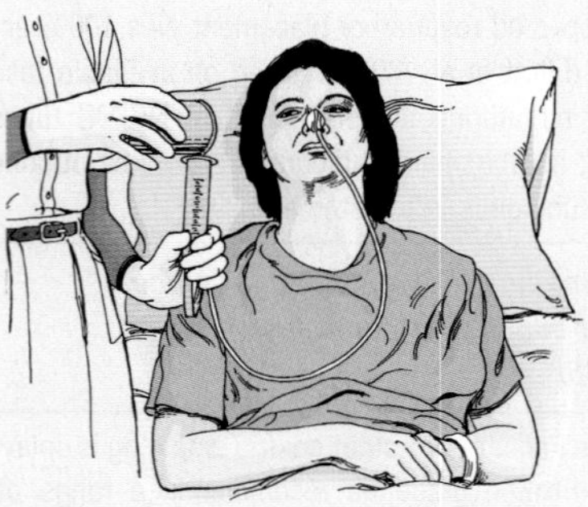

STEP 16A(3) Fill syringe with formula.

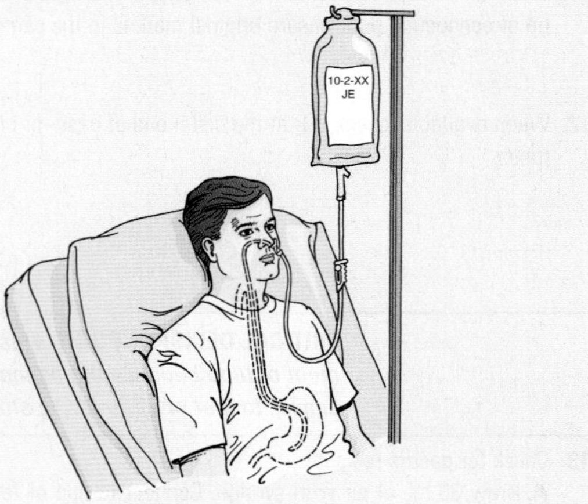

STEP 16A(4) Administration via feeding bag.

STEPS	RATIONALE
(5) Document tube assessment for placement, formula infusing, and infusion rate; elevate head of bed to at least 45 degrees.	
B. Continuous-drip method (see Step 16B illustration):	• Continuous feeding method is designed to deliver a prescribed hourly rate of feeding. This method reduces risk of abdominal discomfort. **Patients who receive continuous-drip feedings should have residuals checked as per agency policy.** Frequency of checking gastric residuals varies, and research has not clearly determined the need. A protocol of enteral nutrition management without residual gastric volume monitoring was found not inferior to a similar protocol that included residual gastric volume monitoring as protection against ventilator-assisted pneumonia (Reignier, Mercier, Le Gouge, et al., 2013). Residual gastric volume monitoring leads to unnecessary interruptions of enteral nutrition delivery with subsequent inadequate feeding and, arguably, should be removed from the standard care of critically ill patients receiving invasive mechanical ventilation and early enteral nutrition (Reignier et al., 2013). In nursing practice, however, gastric residual volumes are usually checked every 4 hours × 48 hours post-initiation of new continuous feed. For established gastric feeds (greater than 48 hours), residuals are checked when patients exhibit signs of gastric intolerance (abdominal distension, nausea, and vomiting). Measurement of gastric residuals every 4 hours is prudent in critically ill patients (Saskatoon Health Region, 2017).
(1) Prime and hang feeding bag and tubing.	
(2) Connect distal end of tubing to the proximal end of the feeding tube.	
(3) Connect tubing through infusion pump and set rate (see illustration).	
(4) Do *not* hang any longer than a 4-hour supply, to decrease risk of food spoilage potentially resulting in gastrointestinal irritation or infection.	• Tube placement verification is difficult with continuous feeding because pH of formula affects the stomach pH.

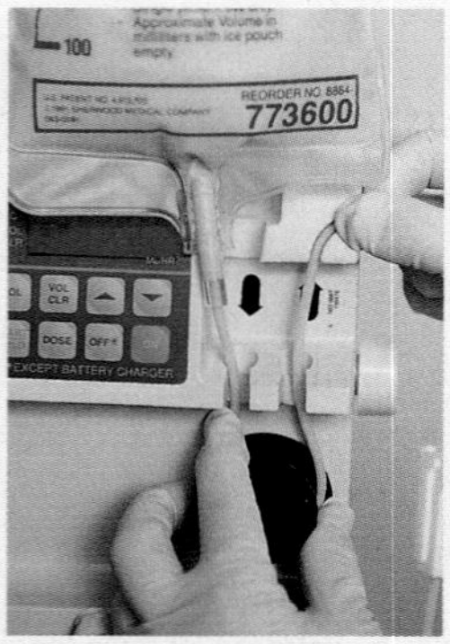

STEP 16B Prime and connect tubing through infusion pump.

STEPS	RATIONALE
17. Advance the rate of tube feeding gradually (see Box 42-13).	• Tube feedings should be advanced gradually to prevent diarrhea and gastric intolerance to formula.
18. After intermittent infusion or at end of continuous infusion, flush nasoenteral tubing with water. On average, 30 mL of water is used, but the amount can vary from 10 mL to over 30 mL. Repeat every 4 to 6 hours. Remove gloves and perform hand hygiene.	• Flushing maintains patency of feeding tube and provides patient with a source of water to help maintain fluid and electrolyte balance.

CRITICAL DECISION POINT: *It may be necessary to consult with a dietitian to recommend a total free water requirement per day. This avoids the potential of fluid overload.*

STEPS	RATIONALE
19. When tube feedings are not being administered (e.g., they may be held prior to tests or procedures such as extubation), cap or clamp the proximal end of the feeding tube.	• Closing the end of the tube prevents air from entering stomach between feedings and prevents contamination.
20. Rinse bag and tubing with water whenever feedings are interrupted or every 8 hours.	• Rinsing bag and tubing clears old tube formula and reduces bacterial growth.
21. Change bag and tubing every 24 hours.	• Changing bag and tubing reduces patient's exposure to bacterial growth occurring in those items.
22. Measure amount of aspirate (residual) every 8 to 12 hours.	• These measurements help evaluate tolerance of tube feeding.
23. Monitor fingerstick blood glucose level every 6 hours until maximum administration rate is reached and maintained for 24 hours.	• These levels alert the nurse to patient's tolerance of glucose. Remember that if feedings are stopped, monitor for any drop in glucose level—especially if patient is on insulin therapy.
24. Monitor intake and output every 8 hours and compute 24-hour totals.	• Intake and output are indications of fluid balance or fluid volume excess or deficit.
25. Weigh patient daily until maximum administration rate is reached and maintained for 24 hours; then weigh patient three times per week.	• Weight gain is an indicator of improved nutritional status; however, sudden gain of more than 1 kg in 24 hours usually indicates fluid retention.
26. Observe patient's respiratory status.	• Increased respiratory rate may indicate aspiration of tube feeding.
27. Observe return of normal laboratory values.	• Improving laboratory values (e.g., albumin, transferrin, and prealbumin) indicate an improved nutritional status.

UNEXPECTED OUTCOMES (IN ADDITION TO THOSE IDENTIFIED IN SKILL 42-1)	RELATED INTERVENTIONS
Gastric residual exceeding 200 to 500 mL (see agency policy) For example, according to Saskatoon Health Region (2017): • If the residual is less than or equal to 350 mL, refeed the aspirated volume and continue feeding as before. • If the residual is greater than or equal to 350 mL, refeed 350 mL, discard remaining aspirated volume, and hold feed × 4 hours. Restart the feed at 10 mL/hr and increase by 10 mL/hr every 1 hour back to the previous tolerated rate. • If the residual is greater than or equal to 350 mL a second time, refeed 350 mL, discard remaining aspirated volume, and hold feed × 6 hours.	• See Step 13 for further information about residual volumes. If established by agency policy, withhold feeding and notify physician. • Maintain patient in semi-Fowler's position, or have head of bed elevated at least 30 to 45 degrees. • Perform physical assessment. • Assess glycemic control.
Diarrhea three times or more in 24 hours	• Notify physician. • Confer with dietitian. • Institute skin-care measures. • Diarrhea could indicate formula is being administered too rapidly (Saskatoon Health Region, 2017). • Look for other causes of the diarrhea (e.g., antibiotics; consider change in antibiotics only for patients receiving antibiotics).
Nausea and vomiting	• Notify physician. • Check patency of tube. • Aspirate for residual. • Auscultate for bowel sounds.

RECORDING AND REPORTING

- Record amount and type of feeding and patient's response to tube feeding, patency of tube, and any side effects.
- Report patient's tolerance and adverse effects.

HOME CARE CONSIDERATIONS

- Teach patient or primary caregiver how to determine correct placement of feeding tube using pH strips.
- Inform patient or primary caregiver of signs associated with pulmonary aspiration and delayed gastric emptying.
- Describe signs and symptoms associated with feeding tube complications, and advise when to call physician.

SKILL 42-5 ADMINISTERING ENTERAL FEEDINGS VIA GASTROSTOMY OR JEJUNOSTOMY TUBE

Delegation Considerations

Administration of enteral tube feeding via a gastrostomy or jejunostomy tube is a procedure that—depending on agency policy—can be delegated to an unregulated care provider (UCP) after the nurse verifies tube placement. UCPs should never test the position of the tube or give the first dose of a tube feeding.

- Ensure that the patient is sitting upright in a chair or in bed, and instruct the UCP to infuse the feeding slowly.
- Instruct the UCP to report any difficulty infusing the feeding or any discomfort voiced by the patient.

Equipment

- Disposable feeding container or ready-to-hang bag.
- 30-mL or larger Luer-Lok or catheter-tip syringe
- Formula
- Infusion pump: Use pump designed for tube feedings
- pH indicator strips (scale 0 to 14)
- Medication cup or container for aspirated fluid
- Stethoscope
- Disposable gloves
- Equipment to obtain blood glucose by fingerstick

PROCEDURE

STEPS	RATIONALE
1. Assess patient's need for enteral tube feedings (see Skill 42-3 and Skill 42-4): impaired swallowing, decreased level of consciousness, surgical procedures involving upper alimentary tract, need for long-term enteral nutrition.	• This assessment identifies patients who need tube feedings before they become nutritionally depleted. Enteral feeding preserves the function and mass of the gut, promotes wound healing, diminishes hypermetabolism in burn injuries, and may decrease infection in critically ill patients (Blumenstein et al., 2014; Rahnemai-Azar, Rahnemaiazar, Naghshizadian, et al., 2014).
2. Obtain baseline weight and laboratory values (blood glucose, albumin, transferrin, prealbumin).	• Enteral feedings are intended to restore or maintain nutritional status. Baseline weight and laboratory values provide objective data to measure effectiveness of feedings.
3. Verify physician's order for formula, rate, route, and frequency.	• Tube feedings must be ordered by a physician.
4. Perform hand hygiene.	• Hygiene reduces transmission of microorganisms.
5. Explain procedure to patient.	• Well-informed patients are more cooperative and more at ease than patients who are ill-informed.
6. Auscultate for bowel sounds before feeding. Consult physician if bowel sounds are absent.	• Absence of bowel sounds may indicate decrease in or absence of peristalsis and increased risk of aspiration or abdominal distension.
7. Assess gastrostomy or jejunostomy site for breakdown, irritation, or drainage.	• Infection, pressure from tube, or drainage of gastric secretions can cause skin breakdown.
8. Perform hand hygiene and apply gloves.	
9. Prepare feeding container to administer formula:	
A. Have tube feeding formula at room temperature.	• Cold formula may cause gastric cramping and discomfort because the liquid is not warmed by mouth and esophagus.
B. Connect tubing to container as needed, or prepare ready-to-hang bag.	• Tubing must be free of contamination, to prevent bacterial growth.
C. Shake formula well. Fill container and tubing with formula.	• Placement of formula through tubing prevents excess air from entering gastrointestinal tract.
10. For intermittent feeding, have syringe ready and ensure formula is at room temperature.	• Cold formula may cause gastric cramping.
11. Elevate head of bed to 45 degrees.	• Elevating patient's head helps prevent chance of aspiration.
12. Apply gloves and verify tube placement.	
A. Gastrostomy tube: Attach syringe and aspirate gastric secretions; observe their appearance and check pH. Return aspirated contents to stomach unless the volume exceeds 100 mL or specified amount based on patient's age. If the volume is greater than 100 mL or the specified amount on several consecutive occasions, check agency policy regarding stopping the feeding and notifying the physician.	• Fluid from gastric tube of patient who has fasted for at least 4 hours usually has a pH of 1 to 4, especially when patient is not receiving a gastric-acid inhibitor. Continuous administration of tube feedings may elevate pH (Temblett & George, 2013). Gastric residual may indicate whether gastric emptying is delayed.
B. Jejunostomy tube: Aspirate intestinal secretions, observe their appearance, and check pH.	• Presence of intestinal fluid indicates that end of the tube is in the small intestine (i.e., the duodenum or jejunum). In general, the intestinal residual is very small (10 mL or less). If fluid appears acidic on pH test, if fluid looks like gastric fluid, or if the residual volume is large (more than 10 mL), displacement of the tube into the stomach may have occurred.
13. Flush with 30 mL of room temperature tap water.	

STEPS	RATIONALE
14. Initiate feedings:	• Gastrostomy and jejunostomy feedings are usually given continuously to ensure proper absorption. However, initial feedings may be given by bolus to assess patient's tolerance to formula. See Box 42-13 for guidelines to advance enteral feedings.
A. Syringe feedings:	
(1) Pinch proximal end of gastrostomy or jejunostomy tube.	• Pinching prevents excess air from entering the patient's stomach and prevents the leaking of gastric contents.
(2) Remove plunger and attach barrel of syringe to end of tube; then fill syringe with formula.	
(3) Release tube and elevate syringe. Allow syringe to empty gradually by gravity. Refill until prescribed amount has been delivered to patient.	• Gradual administration of tube feedings by gravity reduces the risk of diarrhea induced by bolus tube feedings.
B. Continuous drip method:	• Continuous-feeding method is designed to deliver a prescribed hourly rate of feeding. This method reduces the risk of diarrhea and risk of abdominal discomfort. Patients who receive continuous-drip feedings should have residuals checked as per agency policy and tube placement verified every 4 hours. It is usual to measure gastric residuals every 4 hours in critically ill patients (Saskatoon Health Region, 2017). • Gastric residual volumes can be reduced in noncritically ill patients after the first 48 hours of being fed.
(1) Verify that volume in container is sufficient for length of feeding (4 to 8 hours, check manufacturer's recommendations).	
(2) Hang container on IV pole, and clear tubing of air.	• Hanging the container allows for gravity-based flow of formula, which prevents accumulation of air in the patient's stomach.
(3) Thread tubing into pump according to manufacturer's directions.	
(4) Connect tubing to end of gastrostomy or jejunostomy tube.	
(5) Begin infusion at prescribed rate.	
15. Administer water via feeding tube as ordered with or between feedings.	• Water helps patients maintain fluid and electrolyte balance.
16. Flush tube with 30 mL of water every 4 to 6 hours and before and after administering medications via feeding tube.	• Flushing maintains patency of tube and provides patient with some free water. Small jejunal tubes are prone to clogging and are difficult to replace (Fisher & Blalock, 2014).
17. When tube feedings are not being administered, cap or clamp the proximal end of the gastrostomy or jejunostomy tube.	• Closing the end of the tube prevents excess air from entering the gastrointestinal tract between feedings and prevents leakage of gastric contents.
18. Rinse container and tubing with water after all intermittent feedings.	• Rinsing clears formula from tubing and reduces bacterial growth in container and tubing. The container and tubing should be changed every 24 hours.
19. Assess skin around tube exit site. Before site has healed, clean with normal saline. A small precut gauze dressing may be applied to exit site and secured with tape. The dressing is assessed for drainage and changed daily and as needed. Once site has healed, clean the skin around the tube daily with warm water and mild soap. A fully healed tubing exit site is left open to air. If patient received nasogastric feedings before tube insertion and then undergoes a procedure, tube is not used for first 4 to 6 hours after procedure. (Patient will be NPO status the night before the procedure. Postprocedure documentation—as per agency policy—will indicate when to use tube.) Feeding will resume at previous nasogastric rates once it is safe to begin feeding.	• Report any drainage, redness, swelling, or displacement of the tube to the physician. Leakage of gastric drainage may cause skin irritation. • Postprocedure monitoring is performed to check for bleeding.
20. Dispose of supplies, and perform hand hygiene.	• Hygiene helps prevent transmission of microorganisms.
21. Evaluate patient's tolerance to tube feeding. Measure the amount of aspirate every 8 to 12 hours.	• Measurements help in evaluation of tolerance of tube feeding.
22. Monitor fingerstick blood glucose level every 6 hours until maximum administration rate is reached and maintained for 24 hours.	• Alerts nurse to patient's tolerance of glucose.
23. Monitor intake and output every 24 hours.	• Intake and output are indications of fluid balance or fluid volume excess.
24. Weigh patient daily until maximum administration rate is reached and maintained for 24 hours; then weigh patient three times per week.	• Weight gain indicates improved nutritional status; however, a sudden gain of more than 1 kg in 24 hours usually indicates fluid retention.
25. Observe return of normal laboratory values.	• Improved laboratory values (albumin, transferrin, prealbumin) indicate improving nutritional status.
26. Inspect stoma site for impaired skin integrity.	• Enteral tubes can cause pressure and excoriation at the stoma site. In addition, gastric secretions irritate patient's skin.

Continued

SKILL 42-5 ADMINISTERING ENTERAL FEEDINGS VIA GASTROSTOMY OR JEJUNOSTOMY TUBE—cont'd

STEPS	RATIONALE

UNEXPECTED OUTCOMES	RELATED INTERVENTIONS
Aspiration of formula when gastric emptying is delayed or formula is administered too rapidly and produces vomiting	• Position patient in side-lying position. • Suction airway. • Notify physician. • Obtain chest X-ray film.
Skin breakdown around gastrostomy or jejunostomy site	• Institute skin care practices. • Use pressure relief measures around tube. • Provide appropriate wound care (see Chapter 46).

RECORDING AND REPORTING

- Record amount and type of feeding and patient's response to tube feeding, patency of tube, stoma site, and skin integrity, and document any side effects.
- Report to incoming nursing staff type of feeding, status of feeding tube, patient's tolerance, and adverse effects.

HOME CARE CONSIDERATIONS

Teaching patient or primary caregiver how to determine correct placement of feeding tube

- Aspirate and check pH.
- Measure tube length.

Signs associated with pulmonary aspiration and delayed gastric emptying

- Advise patient or primary caregiver to be alert for increased or laboured breathing.
- Instruct patient or caregiver to report shortness of breath.
- Instruct patient or caregiver to report enlarged or tender abdomen.
- Instruct patient or caregiver to be alert for residuals exceeding 200 mL (increased residuals may be related to aspiration) (Metheny, 2016).

Reinforcing signs and symptoms associated with feeding tube complications and when to call physician

- Shortness of breath
- Laboured breathing
- Cramping, vomiting
- Diarrhea two to three times per day
- Constipation
- Tube occlusion
- Tube length increase of 3 to 5 cm or dislodgement

contain predigested nutrients that are easier for a partially dysfunctional gastrointestinal tract to absorb. Finally, **specialty formulas** (1.0 to 2.0 kcal/mL) are designed to meet specific nutritional needs in certain illnesses (e.g., liver failure, pulmonary disease, or human immunodeficiency virus [HIV] infection).

Tube feedings are typically started at full strength at slow rates (Box 42-13). The hourly rate is increased every 12 to 24 hours if no signs of intolerance (nausea, cramping, vomiting, diarrhea) appear.

Studies have demonstrated a beneficial effect of enteral feedings in comparison with parenteral (intravenously administered) nutrition. Feeding by the enteral route may reduce sepsis, blunt the hypermetabolic response to trauma, and maintain intestinal structure and function (Silk & Quinn, 2015). To remove the tube, the procedure outlined in Box 42-14 is used.

Preventing Complications

A serious complication associated with enteral feeding is aspiration of enteral formula into the tracheobronchial tree. Aspiration of enteral formula into the lungs irritates the bronchial mucosa, resulting in decreased blood supply to affected pulmonary tissue (Blumenstein et al., 2014). This leads to necrotizing infection, pneumonia, and potential abscess formation. The high glucose content serves as a bacterial growth medium, thereby promoting infection. Adult respiratory distress syndrome is also frequently associated with pulmonary aspiration. Common conditions that increase the risk of aspiration include coughing, nasotracheal suctioning, an artificial airway, decreased level of consciousness, and lying flat during and after feeding.

Researchers have investigated the problems associated with nasoenteral tube placement, type of feeding instilled, rate of feeding, and complications associated with tube feeding. Small-bore feeding tubes create less discomfort for patients and are currently most often used (Figure 42-12). For adults, most of these tubes are 8 to 12 Fr and 91 to 109 cm long. A stylet is often used during insertion of a small-bore tube to stiffen it. The stylet is removed when the correct position of the feeding tube is confirmed.

At present, the most reliable method for verification of placement of small-bore feeding tubes is X-ray examination (Box 42-15). Measuring the pH of secretions withdrawn from the feeding tube may also help differentiate the location of the tube (Box 42-16). Patients who take acid inhibitor medications usually have an acidic pH value ranging from 4.0 (after 4 hours of fasting) to 6.0 (with continuous enteral nutrition infusion). In contrast, intestinal aspirate has a pH of

7.8 to 8.0. More precise indicators are needed to help differentiate the source of tube feeding aspirate (Boeykens, Steeman, & Duysburgh, 2014; Ellett, Cohen, Croffie, et al., 2014).

Major complications of enteral nutrition are outlined in Table 42-9. Of special note, severely malnourished patients are at risk for electrolyte disturbances from refeeding syndrome (metabolic disturbances that occur as a result of reinstituting nutrition) because cations such as potassium, magnesium, and phosphate move intracellularly during enteral nutrition or parenteral nutrition therapy. Recall also the appearance of refeeding syndrome in the case study of the adolescent living with anorexia nervosa (see Box 42-2). There can be situations where enteral nutrition is not effective in nourishing the body and your role as a nurse is to support a patient in a different way. Box 42-17 tells the story of a nurse who learned the importance of nourishing a person's soul.

BOX 42-13 Advancing the Rate of Tube Feeding

Intermittent

1. Start formula at ordered concentration.
2. If based on physician order and agency policy, infuse bolus of formula over at least 20 to 30 minutes via syringe or feeding container.
3. Begin feedings with no more than 150 to 250 mL at one time. Increase incrementally by 50 mL per feeding per day for adults to achieve needed volume and calories in six to eight feedings. Rates for pediatric patients may be increased by 5 to 10 mL per 8 to 24 hours. (*Note:* Concentrated formulas at full strength may be infused at slower rates until tolerance is achieved.)

Continuous

1. Start formula at ordered concentration full strength for isotonic formulas (concentration of all nutrients in the formula is the same as the concentration of plasma—the fluid component of blood—at approximately 300 mOsm/kg water) or at ordered concentration. Usually hypertonic formulas are also started at full strength but at a slower rate because hypertonic formulas create a pressure gradient that draws water into the intestine and may cause diarrhea and cramping.
2. Begin infusion rate at designated rate.
3. Advance rate slowly (e.g., 10 to 20 mL/hour per day, depending on patient's age) to target rate if tolerated (tolerance indicated by absence of nausea and diarrhea and by low gastric residuals).

LARGE-BORE TUBE AND NASOGASTRIC OR OROGASTRIC SUCTIONING

Gastric decompression is the use of suction to drain the stomach to relieve blockage of the intestinal tract, to wash out stomach contents when a person has taken poisonous material or after surgery (Gastric suction, 2017).

After surgery, the objectives for drainage are as follows:

- Reduce abdominal distension
- Speed the return of bowel function
- Reduce the chance of wound dehiscence and hernia

The two types of tubes most commonly used for gastric decompression are the Levine and Salem sump tube. The tubes are large: 16 to 18 Fr may be inserted through nares or orally (Silk & Quinn, 2015). (See Skill 42-6 and Box 42-18.)

Medication

It is recommended that medications *not* be administered via large-bore tube while suctioning is required. If a large-bore tube must be used, then suctioning should be withheld for at least 30 minutes after medication is administered. Nurses need to consult with the pharmacist and refer to institutional or agency policy.

PARENTERAL NUTRITION

Parenteral nutrition is a form of specialized nutrition support in which nutrients are provided intravenously. Safe administration of this form of nutrition depends on appropriate assessment of nutrition needs, meticulous management of the central venous catheter (CVC) or central venous access device (CVAD), and careful monitoring to

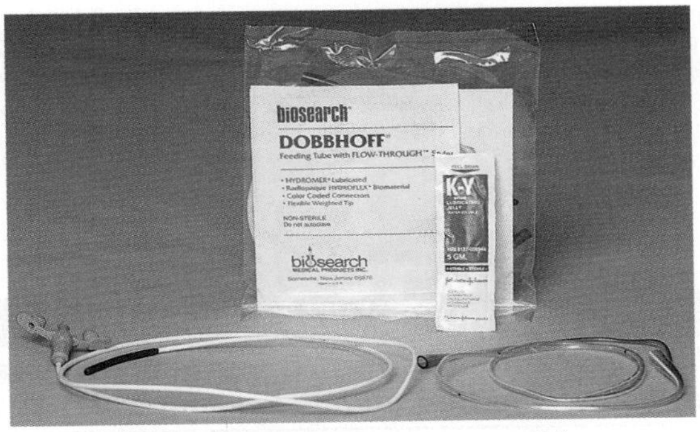

FIGURE 42-12 Enteral tubes, small bore.

BOX 42-14 PROCEDURAL GUIDELINE
Discontinuing Enteral Feedings via Nasogastric Tube

Equipment:

- Clean gloves, facial tissues, towel or absorbent pad, disposable bag

Procedure:

1. Check the physician's order to discontinue nasogastric tube.
2. Educate patient about what to expect during procedure:
   A. Patient may experience irritation of nose and throat, as well as watering of the eyes.
   B. Encourage patient to breathe out as the tube is being removed, to promote comfort and ease of removal.
3. Perform hand hygiene and apply gloves.
4. Assist patient to sit up in high Fowler's position, if possible (to protect patient from drainage). Encourage patient participation.
   A. Place towel over patient's chest.
   B. Provide tissues to patient.
5. Disconnect tube from pump and from patient's gown.
6. Ask patient to take a deep breath and exhale slowly; pinch tube and withdraw it slowly.
7. Provide oral care to patient; provide skin care around patient's nares.
8. Document procedure and total fluid balances.

BOX 42-15 RESEARCH HIGHLIGHT

Accuracy in Determining Placement of Feeding Tubes

Research Focus

Two possible adverse outcomes of enteral nutrition are (1) accidental placement of a nasoenteral feeding tube into the lung and (2) pulmonary aspiration of gastric contents.

Research Abstract

The precise incidence of accidental tube misplacements into the lung is unknown, but estimates of close to 5% have been cited. Patients at highest risk are those with a decreased level of consciousness; those who are confused, uncooperative, or agitated; those who have an endotracheal tube; those who have undergone recent extubation; and those with poor gag reflex. A feeding tube accidentally inserted into the lung may end in the tracheobronchial tree or may perforate into the pleural space. In either event, efforts are made to detect the misplacement before the introduction of tube feedings because inadvertent infusion of formula into the lung promotes tissue consolidation, pneumonia, and respiratory failure. The most accurate method for checking feeding tube placement is X-ray examination; the most effective nonradiological method is aspirating fluid from the feeding tube, measuring its pH, and describing its appearance. Although observing for respiratory distress is helpful in alert patients (especially when firm large-diameter tubes are used), it is of little benefit in those who have a decreased level of consciousness and when small-bore tubes are used. Risk factors for pulmonary aspiration in tube-fed patients include feeding into the stomach in the presence of gastric atony (which results in high gastric residual volumes), poor gag reflexes, mechanical ventilation, and flat positioning in bed. Bedside methods used to detect pulmonary aspiration are not well defined.

Evidence-Informed Practice

- Radiography is the most reliable method available to confirm correct feeding tube location, and radiographic verification is required in most acute care facilities when small-bore tubes are initially inserted.
- When the radiographic method is not feasible, measurement of CO_2 levels at the distal end of the tube have been found to be accurate in critically ill adults (Ellett et al., 2014).
- A less reliable method involves testing the feeding tube aspirate's pH and observing its appearance. A properly obtained pH of 0 to 5.5 is a good indication of gastric placement; a pH of 6 or higher could indicate placement in the lung, intestine, or stomach, in which gastric pH is usually high. Intestinal fluid is usually bile-stained (dark golden yellow); in contrast, gastric fluid is usually grassy green, off-white to tan, or clear and colourless.
- A supplementary method to confirm placement consists of marking the feeding tube with indelible ink at the exit site from the naris or lip at the time of radiography. The nurse must confirm this mark before feeding or administering medication through the tube. The measurement from naris to tip of tube must also be recorded. The exit-point mark is not a foolproof indication of correct tube placement, inasmuch as the tube's distal tip can move from its original position while the external portion remains intact.
- The auscultatory method should *not* be used to determine tube location.
- The dye method (adding Blue No. 1 food colouring to enteral formula to assist with the detection of formula aspirated into the lung) is no longer used because of its association with patient deaths.

Blumenstein, I., Shastri, Y. M., & Stein, J. (2014). Gastroenteric tube feeding: Techniques, problems and solutions. *World Journal of Gastroenterology, 20*(26), 8505–8524. doi:10.3748/wjg.v20.i26.8505; Boeykens, K., Steeman, E., & Duysburgh, I. (2014). Reliability of pH measurement and the auscultatory method to confirm the position of a nasogastric tube. *International Journal of Nursing Studies, 51*(11), 1427–1433. doi:10.1016/j.ijnurstu.2014.03.004; Dhaliwal, R., Cahill, N., Lemieux, M., & Heyland, D. K. (2014). The Canadian critical care nutrition guidelines in 2013: An update on current recommendations and implementation strategies. *Nutrition in Clinical Practice, 29*(1), 29-43; Ellett, M. L. C., Cohen, M. D., Croffie, J. M. B., Lane, K. A., Austin, J. K., & Perkins, S. M. (2014). Comparing bedside methods of determining placement of gastric tubes in children. *Journal for Specialists in Pediatric Nursing , 19*(1), 68–79. doi:10.1111/jspn.12054; Food and Drug Administration. (2003; updated 2015). FDA public health advisory: Subject: Reports of blue discoloration and death in patients receiving enteral feedings tinted with the dye FD&C Blue No. 1. Retrieved from http://www.fda.gov/ForIndustry/ColorAdditives/ColorAdditivesinSpecificProducts/InMedicalDevices/ucm142395.htm; Metheny, N. A. (2016). Prevention of aspiration in adults. *Critical Care Nurse, 36*(1), e20–e24. doi:10.4037/ccn2016831; Saskatoon Health Region. (2013). Nasogastric/orogastric tube: Insertion, care of, and removal. Retrieved from https://www.saskatoonhealthregion.ca/about/NursingManual/1040.pdf.

BOX 42-16 PROCEDURAL GUIDELINE

Obtaining Gastrointestinal Aspirate for pH Measurement, Large- and Small-Bore Feeding Tubes: Intermittent and Continuous Feeding

Critical Decision Point: Obtaining gastrointestinal aspirate for pH measurement to verify placement is crucial, whether a large- or small-bore tube is used and whether the tube will be used for decompression or feeding. *Note:* An X-ray examination to verify tube placement must be completed before enteral feedings are initiated.

Delegation Considerations:

The skill of measuring pH in gastrointestinal aspirate should *not* be delegated to unregulated care providers.

Equipment:

- 60 mL syringe
- pH test paper (scale of 0 to 11)
- Absorbent pad
- Small medication cup
- Disposable gloves

Procedure:

1. Perform hand hygiene. Perform measures to verify placement of tube:
   A. For intermittently fed patients, test placement immediately before feeding (usually a period of at least 4 hours will have elapsed since previous feeding). More frequent checking has been associated with increased clogging of small-bore tubes. To avoid clogging, flush tube with 30 mL of water after aspirating for the residual volume (Fisher & Blalock, 2014).
   B. For continuously tube-fed patients, check agency policy. If the patient is tolerating the feedings without incident and other indicators of correct location are present (the mark on the tube at the exit site has remained in its original position, and the most recent X-ray films confirm correct position of tube), it is reasonable to continue feedings. **If risk of tube displacement is high and the tube has moved, consider the need for an X-ray film to verify placement** (Ellett et al., 2014; Metheny, 2016). Plan to test pH at times when feeding may be withheld (e.g., during

BOX 42-16 PROCEDURAL GUIDELINE

Obtaining Gastrointestinal Aspirate for pH Measurement, Large- and Small-Bore Feeding Tubes: Intermittent and Continuous Feeding—cont'd

diagnostic testing, during chest physiotherapy, or to avoid medication interaction).

C. Wait at least 1 hour after medication administration by tube or mouth.

2. Apply disposable gloves.
3. Draw 30 mL of air, or an equivalent amount for infants and children, into syringe, then attach syringe to end of feeding tube. Flush tube with the 30 mL of air to clear out formula or medications before attempting to aspirate fluid. It will probably be more difficult to aspirate fluid from the small intestine than from the stomach. Repositioning the patient from side to side may be helpful. More than one bolus of air through the tube may be needed.
4. Draw back on syringe and obtain 5 to 10 mL of gastric aspirate. Observe appearance of aspirate (see illustration Step 4A). Gently mix aspirate in syringe. Then expel a few drops into a clean medicine cup. Dip the pH strip into the fluid or apply a few drops of the fluid to the strip (see illustration Step 4B). Compare the colour of the strip with the colour on the chart provided by the manufacturer.

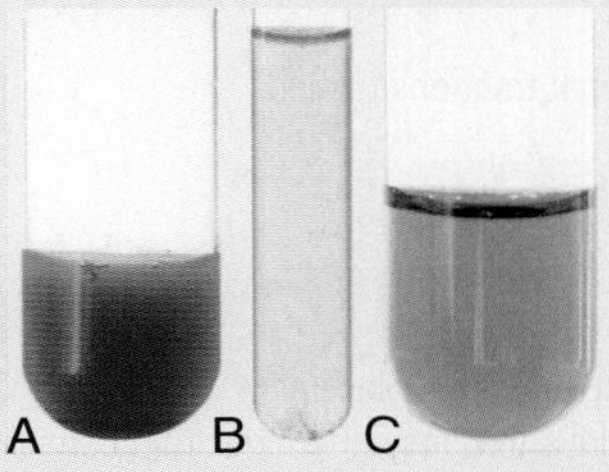

STEP 4A Gastrointestinal contents. **A,** Stomach. **B,** Stomach. **C,** Intestinal. (Courtesy Dr. Norma A. Metheny, Professor, St. Louis University School of Nursing.)

A. The pH of gastric fluid usually ranges from 1–2 up to 4–5 (Helmenstine, 2017).

B. The pH of intestinal fluid is usually higher than 6.

C. Patients with continuous tube feeding may have a pH of 5 or higher.

D. The pH of pleural fluid from the tracheobronchial tree is generally higher than 6.

5. Remove gloves and discard supplies. Perform hand hygiene.

Critical Decision Point: If after repeated attempts it is not possible to aspirate fluid from a tube that was originally confirmed by X-ray examination to be in the desired position, the tube is considered correctly placed if (1) no risk factors for tube dislocation exist, (2) the tube has remained in the original taped position and the tube's measurement remains constant, and (3) the patient is not experiencing difficulty (Irving, Lyman, Northington, et al., 2014). If in doubt, repeat radiographic examination of patient to confirm placement.

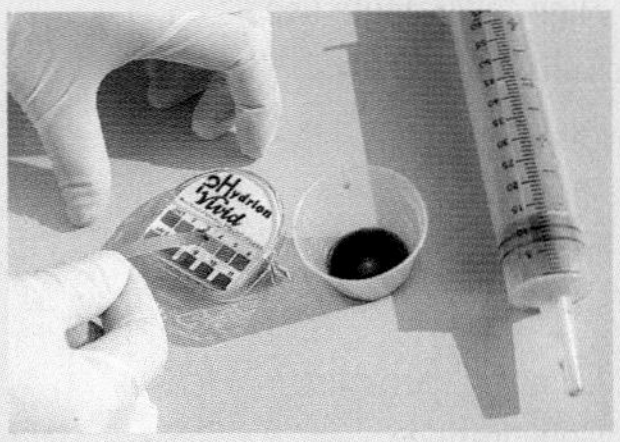

STEP 4B Comparing pH strip with colour chart.

TABLE 42-9 Complications of Enteral Tube Feeding

Problem	Possible Cause	Intervention
Pulmonary aspiration	Regurgitation of formula	Verify tube placement
	Feeding tube displaced	Reposition tube and verify tube placement
	Patient in supine position	Elevate head of bed 45 degrees during feedings and for 2 hours afterward
	Deficient gag reflex	Reassess for return of normal gag reflex; until then, place patient on aspiration precautions and place patient in supine position
	Gastroesophageal reflux disease	Verify tube placement
	Delayed gastric emptying	Lower rate of delivery to increase tolerance
Diarrhea	Hyperosmolar formula or medications	Deliver formula continuously, deliver at lower rate, dilute formula, or change to isotonic enteral nutrition (physician order required and may consult with dietitian)
	Allergy to elixir ingredients (sorbitol)	Liquid medications are often sweetened with sorbitol; consider this as possible cause of diarrhea
	Antibiotic therapy	Antibiotics may destroy normal intestinal flora; physician may change medication; treat symptoms with antidiarrheal agents
	Bacterial contamination	Do not hang formula longer than 4–8 hours in bag; wash bag out well when refilling; change tube feeding bags every 24 hours; use aseptic practices Check expiration dates
	Malabsorption	Check for pancreatic insufficiency; use low-fat, lactose-free formula and continuous feedings
Constipation	Lack of fibre	Select a formula containing fibre
	Lack of free water	Add water as needed as flushes*
	Medications	Evaluate adverse effects; suggest stool softener or bulk-forming laxative
	Inactivity	Monitor patient's ability to ambulate; collaborate with physician for activity order or physiotherapy

Continued

TABLE 42-9 Complications of Enteral Tube Feeding—cont'd

Problem	Possible Cause	Intervention
Tube occlusion	Pulverized medications given per tube	Irrigate with 30 mL water before and after each medication per tube*
		Ideally, each medication should be given separately
	Insufficient tube irrigation	Dilute crushed medications if not liquid
	Sedimentation of formula	Shake cans well before administering (read label)
	Reaction of incompatible medications or formula	Read pharmacological information on compatibility of drugs and formula
Tube displacement	Coughing, vomiting	Replace tube and confirm placement before restarting tube feeding
	Tube not taped securely	With placement verification, check that tape is secure (nasoenteral)
Abdominal cramping, nausea, or vomiting	High osmolality of formula	Suggest an isotonic formula, or dilute current formula
		Suggest use of lactose-free formula
		Stop feeding if there is a risk of gastrointestinal tract obstruction
		Use greater proportion of carbohydrate
		Warm formula to room temperature
	Rapid increase in rate or volume	Lower rate of delivery to increase tolerance
	Delayed gastric emptying	If the gastric residual is >250 mL after a second gastric residual check, a promotility agent should be considered
		A full assessment should be conducted to find out reason for high level
	Lactose intolerance	Suggest use of lactose-free formula
	Intestinal obstruction	Stop feeding if there is a risk of gastrointestinal tract obstruction
	High-fat formula used	Use greater proportion of carbohydrate
	Cold formula used	Warm formula to room temperature
Delayed gastric emptying	Diabetic gastroparesis	Consult with physician regarding medication for increasing gastric motility
	Prematurity	Check for residual (see agency policy)
	Inactivity	Consult physician regarding advancing tube to intestinal placement
		Monitor medications and pathological conditions that may affect gastrointestinal motility
Serum electrolyte imbalance	Excess gastrointestinal losses	Monitor serum electrolyte levels daily
	Dehydration	Provide free water as per dietitian's recommendation
	Cirrhosis	Know of links with specific pathological condition
	Heart failure, edema	Monitor patient's weight
	Diabetes mellitus	Monitor glucose tolerance and type of feedings
Increased respiratory quotient	Overfeeding of carbohydrates	Balance kilocalorie needs provided from fat, protein, and carbohydrate with greater proportion of fat in formula (to decrease CO_2 production)
Fluid overload	Refeeding syndrome in malnutrition	Restrict fluids if necessary, and use either a specialized formula or a diluted enteral formula at first
	Excess free water or diluted (hypotonic) formula	Monitor levels of serum proteins and electrolytes
		Use a more concentrated formula with fluid volume excess that does not carry a risk of refeeding syndrome
Hyperosmolar dehydration	Hypertonic formula with insufficient free water	Slow rate of delivery, dilute, or change to isotonic formula

*Check first for fluid restrictions that would affect volume of water given. A physician's order is required to add free H_2O; this will be patient-specific.

BOX 42-17 CASE STUDY

*Nourishing the Mind and Soul**

Phoebe, a 62-year-old woman with end-stage cancer, was admitted to palliative care for management of symptoms including anxiety, pain, and anorexia. Daily nursing interventions involved assessing and maintaining Phoebe's overall comfort in mind, body, and soul. Although Phoebe was experiencing less pain and anxiety, she continued to have little interest in food or eating. As a nursing instructor, I guided a student nurse to explore Phoebe's loss of appetite. Phoebe expectedly denied any interest in eating, stating, "I'm just not hungry." A loss of appetite is not unusual at the end of life. As one's body begins to "turn off," energy from food is no longer required; and yet, when the student nurse asked Phoebe if there was anything she was craving, Phoebe responded, surprisingly, "a roast chicken dinner with all the fixings!" Although Phoebe was not hungry in the traditional sense, she was hungry for a roast chicken dinner experience. Excited about helping Phoebe, the student nurse connected with Phoebe's daughter to grant Phoebe's wish to have a chicken dinner with her closest family members. Thankfully, the palliative care unit had a full kitchen for patients and their families. When the day arrived, Phoebe's family set to work in the kitchen. Soon the unit was filled with the nostalgic smell of a roasting chicken. Phoebe was delighted! This was the first meal she had looked forward to in quite some time. When dinnertime arrived, Phoebe, in her finest clothes, was wheeled to the family kitchen. She moved her fork through her plate of dinner, but did not

BOX 42-17 CASE STUDY

Nourishing the Mind and Soul—cont'd*

eat any of it. Still, she laughed and told stories with her loved ones. When their meal was finished, although exhausted, Phoebe was glowing! Although her physical body no longer required food for energy, the experience of a sentimental meal and close family members to share it with was required to nourish Phoebe's mind and soul.

Exploring Phoebe's loss of appetite was based on principles of dignity, hope, comfort, and quality of life for people facing the end of life. We focused on Phoebe's needs and health care wishes in order to reinforce her personal autonomy, right to be actively involved in her own care, and greater sense of control. The student and I played a key role in the palliative approach to care by initiating communication that honoured Phoebe's values and preferences and supported her family. Critically reflecting on the need for compassionate and holistic family-oriented care helped us provide a therapeutic presence and maximize quality of life (and death) to Phoebe and her family.

In the situation of caring for Phoebe, the instructor and student strove to satisfy the craving of the palliative care patient through a chicken dinner experience. Knowing that food holds symbolic meaning for people, how might this same goal be accomplished if the physical setting did not have a full kitchen? In what other ways might nurses nurture their patients' soul at the end of life?

*By Amy Carrier Fanjoy, BN, RN; MN student, University of New Brunswick.

SKILL 42-6 INSERTING A LARGE-BORE NASOENTERIC OR OROGASTRIC TUBE FOR GASTRIC SUCTIONING

Delegation Considerations

This skill requires problem-solving and knowledge application unique to a professional nurse. For this reason, this skill should *not* be delegated to unregulated care providers.

Equipment

- Nasogastric or nasointestinal (orogastric or orointestinal) tube (12 to 18 Fr)
- Stethoscope
- 60-mL or larger Luer-Lok or catheter-tip syringe
- Hypoallergenic tape and tincture of benzoin or tube fixation device
- Scissors
- pH indicator strip (scale of 0 to 14)
- Glass of water and straw (not required for intubated patients)
- Water-soluble lubricant
- Emesis basin
- Absorbent pad
- Facial tissues
- Disposable gloves (multiple pairs needed)
- Suction equipment in case of aspiration
- Penlight to check placement in nasopharynx
- Tongue blade
- Disposable tape measure
- Felt-tip marker
- Suction device for continuous or intermittent suctioning

PROCEDURE

STEPS	RATIONALE
1. Assess the need for large-bore tube (i.e., for gastric suctioning or lavage).	• Identify patients who require gastric drainage or flushing.
A. Review physician's order for type of tube and enteral feeding schedule.	• **Procedure and tube feedings require a physician's order.**
2. Perform hand hygiene. Assess patency of nares. Have patient close each nostril alternately and breathe. Examine each naris for patency and skin breakdown.	• Nares may be obstructed or irritated, or septal defect may be present.
3. Assess the gag reflex. Place tongue blade in patient's mouth, touching uvula to induce a gag response.	• Assessing gag reflex identifies patient's ability to swallow and determines risk for aspiration.

CRITICAL DECISION POINT: *Patients with impaired level of consciousness or who are intubated and sedated may also have impaired gag reflex, and their risk of aspiration is increased during this type of procedure and subsequent tube feedings. For a patient who is intubated, sedated, or too ill to participate, ensure that the patient's head is tilted toward the chest for enteral feeding tube insertion.*

Continued

SKILL 42-6 INSERTING A LARGE-BORE NASOENTERIC OR OROGASTRIC TUBE FOR GASTRIC SUCTIONING—cont'd

STEPS	RATIONALE
4. Review patient's medical history for nasal problems (e.g., nosebleeds, oral or facial surgery, anticoagulation therapy, history of aspiration).	• Nasoenteral tubes are contraindicated in patients who have undergone recent nasal surgery, have sustained facial traumas, have nosebleeds, or are receiving anticoagulation therapy. Recently, a Foley catheter placed emergently in the left naris of an injured cyclist for nasopharyngeal hemorrhage was shown on follow-up imaging to be positioned in the frontal lobe (Veeravagu, Joseph, Jiang, et al., 2013). Because of such risk for improper tube placement, caution must be exercised while performing any endonasal procedure in the settings of trauma where disruption of the anterior cranial base is possible.
5. Perform hand hygiene (before auscultating abdomen).	• Hygiene reduces transfer of microorganisms.
6. Auscultate patient's abdomen for bowel sounds.	• Absence of bowel sounds may indicate decrease in or absence of peristalsis and increased risk for aspiration or abdominal distension.
7. Explain procedure to patient and how to communicate during intubation, by raising index finger to indicate gagging or discomfort.	• Information reduces anxiety and helps patient assist in insertion. Patients who are alert and communicating tolerate the procedure better than other patients.
8. Stand on same side of bed as naris for insertion, and assist patient to high Fowler's position unless that position is contraindicated. Place pillow behind patient's head and shoulders.	• Fowler's position allows easier manipulation of tube, reduces risk of aspiration, and promotes effective swallowing.
9. Place absorbent pad over patient's chest. Keep facial tissues within reach.	• Pad prevents soiling of gown. Insertion of tube may cause patient's eyes to tear.
10. Determine length of tube to be inserted, and mark with tape. Traditional method: Measure distance from tip of nose to earlobe to xiphoid process of sternum (see Step 10 illustration).	• Length approximates distance from nose to stomach in 98% of patients. For duodenal or jejunal placement, an additional 20 to 30 cm is required.

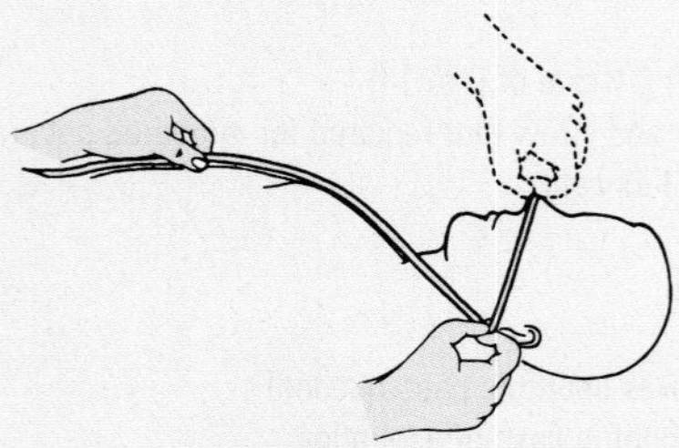

STEP 10 Length of tube to be inserted is equal to distance from tip of nose to earlobe to xiphoid process.

STEPS	RATIONALE
11. Prepare nasogastric or nasointestinal tube for intubation.	
12. Perform hand hygiene, and put on gloves.	• Hygiene and gloves reduce transmission of microorganisms.
13. Cut tape 10 cm long or prepare tube fixation device. Split one end of tape lengthwise 5 cm.	• To be used to anchor tubing after insertion.
14. Dip tube with surface lubricant into glass of water. If tube is not self-lubricating, then water-soluble lubricant should be used.	• Activates lubricant to facilitate passage of tube into naris to gastrointestinal tract. Do not use petroleum-based products because of the risk of aspiration into the lung and resultant chemical pneumonitis.
15. Insert tube through nostril to back of throat (posterior nasopharynx). Aim back and down toward ear.	• Natural contour facilitates passage of tube into gastrointestinal tract and reduces gagging by patient.
16. Have patient tilt head toward chest after tube has passed through nasopharynx.	• Tilting head forward closes off glottis and reduces risk of tube's entering trachea. This technique is also used in patients who are intubated and sedated.

CRITICAL DECISION POINT: *Encourage patients who are alert and communicating to swallow by giving small sips of water or ice chips when possible. For patients who are intubated and sedated or not able to participate, tilt head toward chest. Advance the tube as patient swallows or as head is tilted toward chest. Rotate tube 180 degrees while inserting.*

STEPS	RATIONALE
17. Emphasize the need to mouth-breathe and swallow during the procedure (when possible).	• Mouth-breathing and swallowing facilitate passage of tube and alleviate patient's fears during the procedure.
18. When tip of tube reaches the carina (about 25 cm in an adult), stop insertion, hold end of tube near your ear, and listen for air exchange from the distal portion of the tube.	• **If air is heard, the tube could be in the respiratory tract; remove tube and start over. This listening step should never be used to verify tube placement** (Metheny, 2016).

STEPS	RATIONALE
CRITICAL DECISION POINT: *Do not force tube insertion. If resistance is met or patient starts to cough, choke, or become cyanotic, stop advancing the tube and pull tube back.*	
19. Check for position of tube in back of throat with penlight and tongue blade.	• Tube may be coiled, kinked, or entering trachea. (Withdraw tube immediately if tube is coiled, if respiratory status of patient changes, or if patient begins to cough and skin colour changes; if distress is not present, withdraw tube fully and retry. Note whether tube was kinked; if so, it is likely to kink again in the same place.)
20. Perform measures to verify placement of tube, by measuring pH.	• *Note:* Tube placement must be verified by X-ray examination before enteral feeds are initiated. Another test that can be done at the bedside to ensure ongoing placement is to measure pH of aspirated gastric fluids.
A. Examine gastric contents and yield.	• Respiratory and gastric contents may look similar, but aspirating gastric contents yields a greater amount, whereas aspirating respiratory contents may yield only a few millilitres.
CRITICAL DECISION POINT: *Auscultation is no longer considered a reliable method for verification of tube placement because a tube inadvertently placed in the lungs, pharynx, or esophagus can transmit a sound similar to that of air entering the stomach (Boeykens et al. , 2014; National Association of Children's Hospitals, 2012).*	
21. After gastric aspirates are obtained, anchor tube to patient's nose and avoid pressure on nares. Mark exit site on tube with indelible ink. Select one of the following options to secure tube:	• A properly secured tube allows the patient more mobility and prevents trauma to nasal mucosa. Mark tube at tip of naris; measure from line to end of tube; tape and secure to maintain position.
A. Apply tape	
(1) Apply tincture of benzoin or other skin adhesive on tip of patient's nose and tube and allow it to become "tacky."	• Skin adhesive helps tape adhere better and protects skin.
(2) Place intact end of tape over bridge of patient's nose. Wrap each of the 5-cm strips around tube as it exits nose.	• Securing tape to nares prevents tissue necrosis.
B. Apply tube fixation device, using shaped adhesive patch.	• Device secures tube and reduces friction on nares.
(1) Apply wide end of patch to bridge of patient's nose.	
22. Fasten end of nasogastric tube to patient's gown with a piece of tape (not safety pin).	• Fastening tape to gown reduces traction on the naris if tube moves. Tape is recommended because safety pins may become unfastened and possibly cause injury to the patient.
23. Remove gloves. Perform hand hygiene and apply clean gloves, and administer oral hygiene (see Chapter 38). Clean tubing at nostril.	• Oral hygiene promotes patient comfort and integrity of oral mucous membranes.
24. Remove gloves, dispose of equipment, and perform hand hygiene.	• Hygiene reduces transmission of microorganisms.
25. Inspect naris and oropharynx for any irritation after insertion.	• If tube insertion was difficult, irritation of naris or oropharynx may have occurred.
26. Ask patient whether he or she feels comfortable.	• Patients' level of comfort is evaluated. (This may be a challenge if a language barrier exists or if the patient has dementia or is confused.)
27. Observe patient for any difficulty breathing, for coughing, or for gagging.	• Improper position of the tube may cause these symptoms or increase symptoms in patients who have heart failure, pneumonia, asthma, and other cardiac or respiratory conditions.
28. Auscultate lung sounds.	• Abnormal lung sounds can be an early sign of aspiration.
29. Connect tube to suction device as ordered.	• May be ordered as a continuous or intermittent suction and at various pressures (e.g., 80 mm Hg). In some circumstances, tubes are placed by surgeon but contraindicated or strict protocols for flush or suction (i.e., post-esophagectomy).

BOX 42-18 PROCEDURAL GUIDELINE

Providing Suction

Equipment:

- Suction device, connecting tubing (connector as required)

Procedure:

1. Check the physician's order for type and amount of suction. Suctioning may be ordered as continuous or intermittent. The amount must be ordered by the physician.
2. To reduce the patient's anxiety, educate the patient about the procedure.
3. Wash hands thoroughly to limit spread of microorganisms.
4. Set up suction device as per institution or agency policy.
5. Set type and amount of suction as ordered.
6. Monitor patient and suction system regularly. Provide data for overall care. Monitor for bleeding or blockage:
   Patient: Note abdominal distension, nausea, feeling of discomfort, bowel sounds, electrolyte levels.
   Device: Note kinks, blockages, flow, and settings.
   Drainage: Note amount, colour, and consistency.
7. Secure tubing as described in Skill Box 42-3, Step 23A(2). Keep tubing higher than stomach to facilitate drainage. Secure tubing to prevent inadvertent pulling or removal.
8. Measure output at least every 8 hours or as per institutional or agency policy.
9. Document as per institution or agency protocol.

BOX 42-19 Indications for Parenteral Nutrition

Nonfunctional Gastrointestinal Tract

Massive small bowel resection or gastrointestinal surgery
Paralytic ileus
Intestinal obstruction
Trauma to abdomen, head, or neck
Severe malabsorption
Intolerance of enteral feeding (established by trial)
Chemotherapy, radiation therapy, bone marrow transplantation

Extended Bowel Rest

Enterocutaneous fistula
Inflammatory bowel disease exacerbation
Severe diarrhea
Moderate to severe pancreatitis

Preoperative Total Parenteral Nutrition

Preoperative bowel rest
Treatment for comorbid severe malnutrition in patients with nonfunctional gastrointestinal tracts
Severely catabolic patients when gastrointestinal tract is nonusable for more than 4 to 7 days

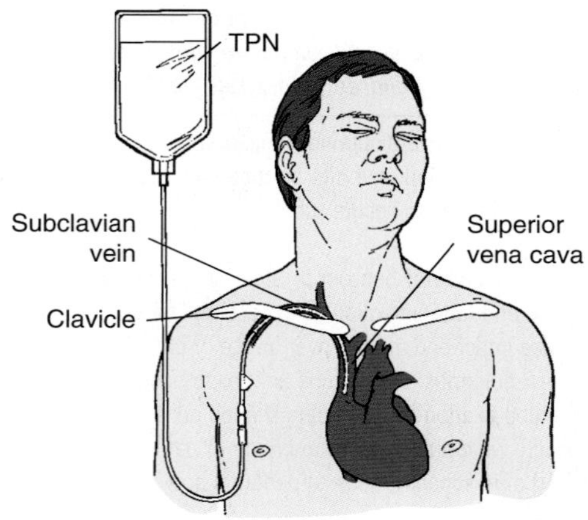

FIGURE 42-13 Parenteral nutrition via central venous catheter (CVC). *TPN,* Total parenteral nutrition. (From Mosby's dictionary of medicine, nursing, and health professionals [10th ed.], 2017. St. Louis, MO: Mosby.)

prevent or treat metabolic complications. Parenteral nutrition is administered in a variety of settings, including the patient's home. Regardless of the setting, the nurse adheres to the same principles of asepsis and infusion management to ensure safe nutrition support.

Patients who are unable to digest or absorb enteral nutrition benefit from parenteral nutrition. Patients in highly stressed physiological states, such as sepsis, head injury, or burns, are also candidates for parenteral nutrition therapy. Box 42-19 lists other indications for parenteral nutrition. Clinical and laboratory monitoring by a multidisciplinary team is required throughout parenteral nutrition therapy. The need for continued parenteral nutrition is re-evaluated regularly, with the goal of eventually using the gastrointestinal tract. Disuse of the gastrointestinal tract has been associated with villus atrophy and generalized cell shrinkage. Translocation of bacteria from the local gut to systemic regions has been noted in relation to gastrointestinal cell shrinkage; such translocation can result in gram-negative septicemia.

Lipid emulsions provide supplemental kilocalories and prevent deficiencies of essential fatty acids. These emulsions can be administered through a separate peripheral catheter, through the CVC by Y-connector tubing (see Chapter 40), or as an admixture to the parenteral nutrition solution. The addition of lipid emulsion to the parenteral nutrition solution is called a *3-in-1 admixture* and is administered over a 24-hour period. The admixture should not be used if oil droplets are observed or if an oil or creamy layer is observed on the surface of the admixture. This observation indicates that the emulsion has broken into large lipid droplets that can cause fat emboli if administered. Lipid emulsions are white and opaque; thus, care should be taken to avoid confusing enteral formula with parenteral lipids.

Contraindications to giving lipids are hyperlipidemia, lipid nephrosis, severe liver failure, and egg allergy.

Initiating Parenteral Nutrition

Patients with short-term nutritional needs often receive intravenous solutions of less than 10% dextrose in a peripheral vein in combination with amino acids and lipids. Peripheral solutions are not as calorically dense and therefore are less irritating to the peripheral veins, and their use is usually temporary. Administering parenteral nutrition with greater than 10% dextrose requires a CVC (Figure 42-13) that is placed into a high-flow central vein (such as the superior vena cava) by a physician using sterile technique (see Chapter 40).

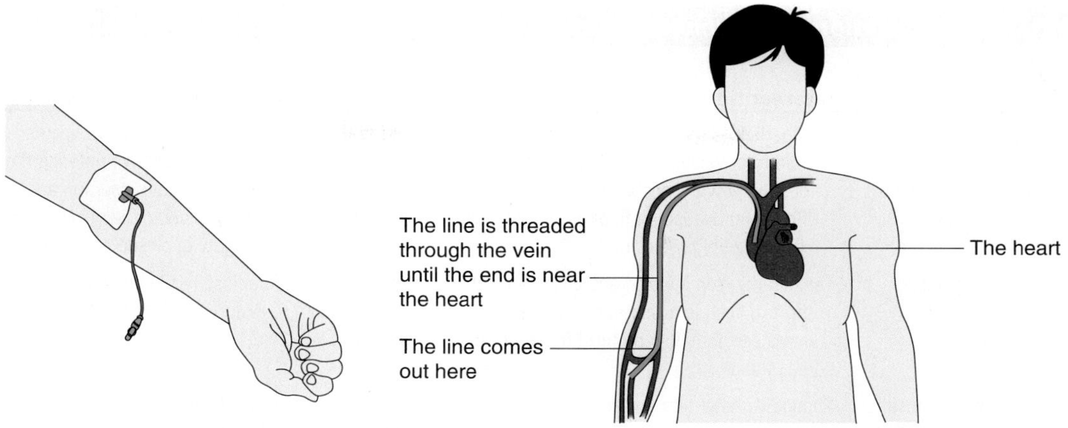

FIGURE 42-14 Peripherally inserted central catheter (PICC) line insertion.

Nurses who have special training insert peripherally inserted central catheters (PICCs) that are started in a vein of the forearm or upper arm and threaded into the subclavian vein or the superior vena cava (Figure 42-14).

After central catheter or PICC placement is verified by chest X-ray examination or radiographically confirmed and documented, the catheter is flushed with saline or heparin. The physician may suture the CVC in place. A PICC is usually stabilized with sterile strips of tape and a sterile dressing. The types of dressings to be applied vary between institutions and a variety of policies and protocols are adhered to. The nurse who is new to the nursing unit can check the appropriate dressing protocol and policy before proceeding. Wing-to-tip of the PICC should be measured and documented daily. With a tube suspected of migrating 2 cm or more, all fluids should be stopped and radiography should be repeated for placement verification. Also to verify placement, the PICC line may be flushed by specially trained nurses and, if noted to be occluded, special procedures (e.g., alteplase) are carried out to ensure line patency.

Before beginning any parenteral infusion, the nurse verifies the physician's order and inspects the solution for particulate matter or a break in the lipid emulsion. An infusion pump is always used. An initial rate of 40 to 60 mL/hour may be recommended. In some institutions, the solutions are infused separately at a specified rate until the therapy is no longer required. In this instance, each solution would have a separate infusion pump. Parenteral nutrition in the hospital is infused 24 hours a day. The parenteral infusion is refrigerated until needed, whereas the lipids are stored at room temperature.

The rate is gradually increased until the patient's complete nutritional needs are supplied. Patients who receive parenteral nutrition at home frequently administer the entire daily solution over 12 hours at night. This allows the patient to disconnect from the infusion each morning, flush the central catheter, and have independent mobility during the day.

Preventing Complications

Complications of parenteral nutrition include mechanical complications from insertion of the CVC, infection, and metabolic alterations (Table 42-10). Pneumothorax occurs when a puncture in the pulmonary system results in accumulation of air in the pleural cavity and subsequent impairment in breathing. Pneumothorax is usually accompanied by symptoms of sudden sharp chest pain, dyspnea, and coughing. In relation to parenteral nutrition, pneumothorax most often occurs during CVC placement.

Electrolyte abnormalities should be corrected before starting parenteral nutrition. Calorie goals should be reached gradually. It is very important to base the caloric and protein needs on the patient's current weight to avoid overfeeding.

The goal is for patients to switch from parenteral nutrition to enteral nutrition and/or oral feeding. Specified weights and intakes are recorded. Once patients are meeting one-third to one-half of their kilocalorie needs per day, parenteral nutrition is usually decreased to half the original volume. Enteral nutrition feedings should then be increased to meet needs. When 75% of daily energy needs are consistently met with tube feeding, parenteral nutrition may be discontinued. Patients who make the transition from parenteral nutrition to oral feedings typically have early satiety and decreased appetite. Calorie and protein counts are recommended when patients begin taking soft foods. Parenteral nutrition should be gradually decreased in response to increased oral intake. If oral intake is inadequate, small, frequent meals may prove helpful. Some institutions will discontinue lipid emulsion first, then parenteral infusion is continued until requirements are met.

KEY CONCEPTS

- Nurses must have current, culturally sensitive nutritional knowledge to apply to the complexities of health care and illness and to the changing needs of diverse populations and demographics.
- A balanced diet featuring carbohydrates, fats, proteins, vitamins, and minerals provides the essential nutrients to carry out the body's normal physiological functioning throughout the lifespan.
- Through digestion, food is broken down into its simplest form for absorption. Digestion and absorption occur mainly in the small intestine.
- Dietary reference intakes (DRIs) provide a range of values that address the needs of groups (estimated average requirement) and individuals (adequate intakes, recommended dietary allowances, and tolerable upper intake level).
- Guidelines for dietary change advocate reduced saturated and trans fats, reduced sodium, and reduced refined sugars, as well as an increased intake of complex carbohydrates and fibre.
- Nutritional screening helps in identifying patients at risk of malnourishment. Because improper nutrition can affect all body systems, nutritional assessment includes total physical assessment.

TABLE 42-10 Complications of Parenteral Nutrition (PN)

Problem	Signs and Symptoms	Intervention	Rationale
Air embolism	Tachypnea, apnea, wheezing, hypotension, cyanosis	Turn patient to left lateral decubitus position, instruct patient to perform Valsalva manoeuvre (holding one's breath and "bearing down"), and lower head of bed. Cap the open end of catheter or tape perforation in catheter wall. Administer oxygen; notify physician.	The Valsalva manoeuvre increases venous pressure to prevent air from entering the bloodstream during catheter insertion and when catheter is disconnected or cap is changed. Maintaining integrity of closed system prevents air emboli.
Catheter occlusion	No flow or sluggish flow through the catheter	Temporarily stop infusion and flush with saline or heparin. If effort to flush is unsuccessful, attempt to aspirate clot; if still unsuccessful, follow protocol for use of thrombolytic agent (e.g., alteplase).	Alteplase has been shown to be effective in restoring catheter patency.
Catheter sepsis	Fever, chills, glucose intolerance, positive blood culture	Change catheter site dressing if it becomes wet or contaminated, use sterile mask and gloves when changing dressing or tubing, catheter caps, or parenteral nutrition containers. Change infusion tubing regularly (usually every 24 hours). Assess insertion sites for signs and symptoms of infection (see Chapter 33). Do not hang a single container of parenteral nutrition for more than 24 hours or a container of lipids more than 12 hours; use an inline 0.22 mcg filter when possible.	Filtered tubing is required to remove bacteria. With 3-in-1-admixture TPN, filtration is not possible because of large lipid molecules.
Electrolyte imbalance	Monitor Na, Ca, K, Cl, PO_4, Mg, and CO_2 levels	See Chapter 40 for signs of deficiency or toxicity. Monitor intake, output, and electrolytes, especially potassium, magnesium, and phosphorous levels during the first week of parenteral therapy. Check total parenteral nutrition (TPN) for supplemental electrolyte levels at regular intervals—often weekly. Notify physician of imbalances. Supplemental vitamin K must be given as ordered throughout therapy.	Adequate hydration and balance of electrolytes is essential for normal function of cells and organs. Vitamin K can be synthesized by microflora found in the jejunum and ileum with normal use of the gastrointestinal tract; however, because parenteral nutrition circumvents gastrointestinal use, exogenous vitamin K must be administered.
Hypercapnia	Increased O_2 consumption, increased CO_2, respiratory quotient >1.0, minute ventilation	Ventilator-dependent patients are at risk; to prevent, monitor parameters, provide 30% —60% of energy requirements as fat per physician's order.	Because the combustion of fat yields less carbon dioxide than either carbohydrate or protein combustion, a higher fat diet may be preferable for reducing hypercapnia.
Hypoglycemia	Diaphoresis, shakiness, confusion, loss of consciousness	To prevent, do not discontinue PN abruptly but taper rate down to within 10% of infusion rate 1 to 2 hours before stopping. If hypoglycemia is suspected, test blood glucose level, and administer IV bolus of 10% dextrose per physician order if necessary.	Sudden discontinuation of the solution can cause hypoglycemia. Patients with diabetes are especially at risk.
Hyperglycemia	Thirst, headache, lethargy, increased urination	Monitor blood glucose level daily until it is stable and then as ordered or as needed. PN is initiated slowly and tapered up to maximal infusion rate. Additional insulin may be required during therapy if problem persists (or if patient has diabetes mellitus).	Prevent and correct hyperglycemia because its development during PN has been independently associated with higher rates of mortality and hospital complications (Gosmanov & Umpierrez, 2013).
Hyperglycemic hyperosmolar nonketonic dehydration or coma	Hyperglycemia (>500 mg/dL), glycosuria, serum osmolarity >350 mOsm/L, confusion, azotemia, headache, severe signs of dehydration (see Chapter 40), hypernatremia, metabolic acidosis, convulsions, coma	To prevent, monitor blood glucose, blood urea nitrogen, serum osmolarity, glucose in urine, and fluid losses; administer insulin as ordered; replace fluids as needed; maintain consistent infusion rate; and provide 30% of daily energy needs as fat. Patients at risk are those who are hypermetabolic, those receiving steroids, older persons, diabetic patients, those who have impaired renal or pancreatic function, and those who are septic.	Too-rapid administration of hypertonic dextrose can result in an osmotic diuresis and dehydration (see Chapter 40). Thus, if an infusion falls behind schedule, the nurse should not increase the rate in an attempt to catch up.

TABLE 42-10 Complications of Parenteral Nutrition (PN)—cont'd

Problem	Signs and Symptoms	Intervention	Rationale
Refeeding syndrome	Cardiac dysrhythmias, heart failure, respiratory distress, convulsions, coma, or death	Watch malnourished or cachectic patients for low serum (extracellular) levels of electrolytes and edema.	Ingestion of concentrated glucose increases the basal metabolic rate and is accompanied by increases in endogenous insulin production, which causes cations (potassium, magnesium, and phosphorus) to move intracellularly. The shifting of electrolytes and fluid balance increases cardiac workload and heart rate as well as increased oxygen consumption, which strains the respiratory system.
Pneumothorax	Severe dyspnea, cyanosis, radiographic confirmation	Complication that occurs upon catheter insertion may evolve slowly afterward. Monitor patient for first 24 hours for pulmonary distress.	Enables pneumothorax to be detected early and monitors for enlargement.
Thrombosis of central vein	Unilateral edema of neck, shoulder, and arm; pain	Notify physician. Prevention of catheter-related thromboses includes proper positioning of the catheter and prevention of infections. Thromboprophylaxis for patients with a central venous catheter is not recommended.	Thromboprophylaxis is not recommended, based on the results of randomized controlled trials, in which there was no statistically significant difference (Roila, 2012). Confirmatory research and cost-effectiveness analysis of this approach are needed before it is recommended.

- Interdisciplinary collaboration is essential to helping a patient achieve optimal nutrition.
- Special diets alter the composition, texture, digestibility, and residue of foods to suit the patient's particular needs.

CRITICAL THINKING EXERCISES

1. Charlene MacDonald, a 63-year-old accountant, is overweight with a sedentary lifestyle, uses alcohol infrequently, consumes restaurant food for most meals, and takes 400 IU of vitamin D daily. She wants to undergo cataract surgery to improve her vision; however, the surgeon has advised her to take off at least 10 kg of weight before the operation. Ms. MacDonald weighs 90 kg and has a height of 156 cm. Her waist circumference is 100 cm. What indications would lead you to believe Ms. MacDonald is adequately caring for her health? What additional laboratory tests and dietary and health history information are needed to perform a comprehensive nutritional assessment? What conclusions can you draw from the information available about Ms. MacDonald's weight status? Using *Eating Well With Canada's Food Guide*, what suggestions would you make to Ms. MacDonald to help her achieve weight loss?
2. Corey Green, a 32-year-old mother, is considering switching her entire family to a vegan diet because she believes it will make her 3-year-old twin daughters healthier. What nutritional concerns should you watch for? How would you assess the family's nutritional needs and monitor for such concerns? What advice would you offer to Corey to enhance her family's health while following a vegan diet? Plan one day of meals for this family, indicating food servings for the twins that would meet their protein needs and respect the vegan food diet.
3. Daniele, a middle-school student, is unhappy with her shape and weight. Using an Internet site, she calculated her BMI as 29 one month ago. "I am the smallest person in my family, but I am too fat!" she thought. During the past 4 months, she has skipped breakfast and lunch and exercised for 2 hours a day to "tone up." Her skin, lips, and hair are becoming dry. Daniele denies having lost weight even though her clothes look loose and baggy. Her friends told the homeroom teacher that Daniele goes to the bathroom immediately after eating any food. The teacher requests that you plan a session with Daniele to increase her understanding of her daily nutritional requirements and of healthy eating patterns. What will you discuss with Daniele?

REVIEW QUESTIONS

1. A function of carbohydrates in the diet is to:
   1. Enable chemical reactions
   2. Promote growth and repair of tissues
   3. Supply energy
   4. Maintain water balance
2. A patient asks if he should take vitamin pills to get the nutrients his body needs. You tell him that essential nutrients:
   1. Are made by the body
   2. Generally must be supplied by food
   3. Include herbal teas and alcohol
   4. Are best obtained through taking vitamin pills
3. Which patient would usually exhibit positive nitrogen balance?
   1. Patient with HIV/AIDS infection
   2. Patient admitted with anorexia nervosa
   3. Patient with 30% burn injury
   4. Patient in third trimester of pregnancy
4. What are the determinants of healthy eating? *(Select all that apply.)*
   1. Educational level
   2. Income
   3. Food preferences
   4. Vitamin supplementation
   5. Availability and accessibility of fresh produce
   6. Policies that increase taxation of high-energy, low-nutrient dense foods

5. When a patient is unable to take fluid or food by eating normally over an extended period of time, what is the best alternative?
    1. Liquid nutrients through a tube leading from the mouth or nose to the stomach or intestine
    2. Giving solutions through a tubing in a peripheral vein
    3. Giving continuous tube feedings regulated via an electric feeding pump
    4. Giving feedings through a tube inserted through the skin and tissue of the abdomen
6. A nutrient content claim of *light* means:
    1. The food may be light in colour
    2. The food has no added sugar or salt
    3. The food is reduced in calories or fat by 10%
    4. The levels of saturated and trans fatty acids are restricted
7. When a mother tells you that she would like to switch her 15-month-old toddler from whole to skim milk so the child will not get "too fat," you encourage her to continue with the whole milk because:
    1. Whole milk has more calcium than skim
    2. Whole milk has a longer refrigerated storage life
    3. Whole milk costs the same as skim milk
    4. Whole milk contains fatty acids needed for the toddler's brain development
8. Which intervention is appropriate for the patient experiencing dysphagia?
    1. Encourage the patient to rest lying down for at least 30 minutes after a meal.
    2. Offer thin liquids to make swallowing easier.
    3. Place the food on the strong side of the patient's mouth.
    4. Leave the patient with all food items within easy reach and tell the patient when you will come back to take away the tray.
9. The nurse cares for a patient with dysphagia. Which action(s) by the nurse reflect appropriate care for the patient?
    1. The nurse assesses the client's ability to swallow.
    2. The nurse positions the client at a 45-degree angle.
    3. The nurse offers the client clear fluids.
    4. The nurse instructs the client to place food on the left side of the mouth.
    5. The nurse consults with the physical therapist for feeding positioning.
10. Older persons at risk for malnutrition:
    1. Have the security of living on a fixed income
    2. Know about the amounts of fat, sodium, and cholesterol in the foods they eat
    3. Experience age-related gastrointestinal changes such as reduced saliva production, increased taste threshold, and decreased peristalsis
    4. Have diseases such as diabetes and depression well controlled
11. The nursing activity most likely to prevent the clogging of a nasogastric feeding tube is:
    1. Attaching the tubing to suction after each feeding
    2. Filling the tube with water and clamping it after each feeding
    3. Clamping the tube before all of the nourishment has drained
    4. Giving the patient ice chips to suck after each feeding

Answers: 1. 3; **2.** 2; **3.** 4; **4.** 1, 2, 3, 5, 6; **5.** 1; **6.** 4; **7.** 4; **8.** 3; **9.** 1; **10.** 3; **11.** 2

Rationales for the Review Questions appear at the end of the book.

RECOMMENDED WEBSITES

Diabetes Canada: https://www.diabetes.ca.
This website provides information about signs and symptoms of various types of diabetes, tips for living with diabetes, and useful clinical practice guidelines.

Dietitians of Canada: http://www.dietitians.ca/.
Dietitians of Canada is an association of food and nutrition professionals committed to the health and well-being of Canadians. This website contains numerous resources about nutrition and links to other resources and research abstracts.

Health Canada: Eating Well with Canada's Food Guide: http://www.hc-sc.gc.ca/fn-an/food-guide-aliment/index-eng.php.
This web page provides information about using and ordering *Eating Well With Canada's Food Guide*, now available in 10 languages other than English: Arabic, Chinese, Farsi (Persian), Korean, Punjabi, Russian, Spanish, Tagalog, Tamil, and Urdu.

Health Canada Food and Nutrition: http://www.hc-sc.gc.ca/fn-an/index-eng.php.
This web page provides information for the public about food, nutrition, food safety issues, allergy alerts, food policy and legislation, and other nutrition issues.

Heart and Stroke Canada: www.heartandstroke.ca.
Public education about heart and stroke warning signs and prevention strategies for healthy eating, increasing physical activity, and reducing stress are found on this site.

National Eating Disorder Information Centre (NEDIC): http://www.nedic.ca.
This website provides information, resources, and support for individuals, families, and professionals regarding eating disorders and weight preoccupation.

National Heart, Lung, and Blood Institute: The DASH Eating Plan: https://www.nhlbi.nih.gov/health-topics/dash-eating-plan/.
The Dietary Approaches to Stop Hypertension (DASH) is an eating plan low in total fat, saturated fat, and cholesterol, and rich in fruits, vegetables, and low-fat dairy products. The DASH eating plan is developed for patients with hypertension and is based on clinical studies that showed how elevated blood pressure levels can be reduced with specific eating habits.

Office of Nutrition Policy and Promotion (ONPP): http://www.hc-sc.gc.ca/ahc-asc/branch-dirgen/hpfb-dgpsa/onpp-bppn/index-eng.php.
The Office of Nutrition Policy and Promotion promotes the nutritional health and well-being of Canadians. This web page contains current information about nutrition and Canadian nutrition policy.

Ontario Public Health Association (OPHA): http://opha.on.ca/Nutrition-Resource-Centre/Home.aspx.
The Ontario Public Health Association has created the Nutrition Resource Centre, which provides support and resources to support healthy eating.

REFERENCES

Academy of Nutrition and Dietetics. (2014). Position of the academy of nutrition and dietetics: dietary fatty acids for healthy adults. *Journal of the Academy of Nutrition and Dietetics, 114*(1), 136–153. doi:10.1016/j.jand.2013.11.001.

Agriculture and Agri-Food Canada. (2017). *Functional foods and natural health products.* Retrieved from http://www.agr.gc.ca/eng/industry-markets-and-trade/statistics-and-market-information/by-product-sector/functional-foods-and-natural-health-products/?id=1170856376710.

Al Dokhi, L., & Shahid Habib, S. (2013). Composition and physical fitness scoring in Saudi adults by bioelectrical impedance analysis. *Acta Clinica Croatic, 52,* 189–194.

Almeida, T. M., Cola, P. C., Pernambuco, L. A., et al. (2015). Screening tools for oropharyngeal dysphagia in stroke. *Audiology—Communication Research, 20*(4), 361–370. doi:10.1590/2317-6431-2015-1571.

Ambutas, S., Staffileno, B. A., & Fogg, L. (2014). Reducing nasal pressure ulcers with an alternative taping device. *Medsurg Nursing, 23*(2), 96–100.

Amit, M., & Canadian Paediatric Society, Community Paediatrics Committee. (2010 reaffirmed 2016). Position statement on vegetarian diets in children and adolescents. *Paediatric and Child Health, 15*(5), 303–314. Retrieved from http://www.cps.ca/documents/position/vegetarian-diets.

Anderson, T. J., Grégoire, J., Pearson, G. J., et al. (2016). 2016 Canadian Cardiovascular Society guidelines for the management of dyslipidemia for the prevention of cardiovascular disease in the adult. *Canadian Journal of Cardiology, 32*(11), 1263–1282. doi:10.1016/j.cjca.2016.07.510.

Arigbede, A. O., Babatope, B. O., & Bamidele, M. K. (2012). Periodontitis and systemic diseases: A literature review. *Journal of Indian Society of Periodontology, 16*(4), 487–491. doi:10.4103/0972-124X.106878.

Austin, R. P. (2013). Is plasma glucose a better measure? *Diabetes Forecast*. Retrieved from http://www.diabetesforecast.org/2013/jun/is-plasma-glucose-a-better-measure.html.

Bariatric and Metabolic Institute. (2017). *Health risks of childhood obesity*. UC San Diego Health. Retrieved from https://health.ucsd.edu/specialties/surgery/bariatric/weight-loss-surgery/adolescent-weight-loss/Pages/health-risks.aspx.

Barnard, N. D., Bunner, A. E., & Agarwal, U. (2014). Saturated and trans fats and dementia: A systematic review. *Neurobiology of Aging, 35*(Suppl. 2), S65–S73. doi:10.1016/j.neurobiolaging.2014.02.030.

Bawa, A. S., & Anilakumar, K. R. (2013). Genetically modified foods: Safety, risks and public concerns—a review. *Journal of Food Science and Technology, 50*(6), 1035–1046. doi:10.1007/s13197-012-0899-1.

Baxter, J.-A. B., Al-Madhaki, F. I., & Zlotkin, S. H. (2014). Prevalence of malnutrition at the time of admission among patients admitted to a Canadian tertiary-care paediatric hospital. *Paediatrics & Child Health, 19*(8), 413–417.

Bayer, O., Nehring, I., Bolte, G., et al. (2014). Fruit and vegetable consumption and BMI change in primary school-age children: a cohort study. *European Journal of Clinical Nutrition, 68*(2), 265–270. doi:10.1038/ejcn.2013.139.

Benton, D. (2015). Portion size: What we know and what we need to know. *Critical Reviews in Food Science and Nutrition, 55*(7), 988–1004. doi:10.1080/10408398.2012.679980.

Bharadwaj, S., Ginoya, S., Tandon, P., et al. (2016). Malnutrition: Laboratory markers vs nutritional assessment. *Gastroenterology Report, 4*(4), 272–280. doi:10.1093/gastro/gow013.

Blatter, J., Han, Y., Forno, E., et al. (2013). Folate and asthma. *American Journal of Respiratory & Critical Care Medicine, 188*(1), 12–17. doi:10.1164/rccm.201302-0317PP.

Blay-Palmer, A. (2016). Power imbalances, food insecurity, and children's rights in Canada. *Frontiers in Public Health, 4*, 117. doi:10.3389/fpubh.2016.00117.

Blumenstein, I., Shastri, Y. M., & Stein, J. (2014). Gastroenteric tube feeding: Techniques, problems and solutions. *World Journal of Gastroenterology, 20*(26), 8505–8524. doi:10.3748/wjg.v20.i26.8505.

Boeykens, K., Steeman, E., & Duysburgh, I. (2014). Reliability of pH measurement and the auscultatory method to confirm the position of a nasogastric tube. *International Journal of Nursing Studies, 51*(11), 1427–1433. doi:10.1016/j.ijnurstu.2014.03.004.

Brasky, T. M., Darke, A. K., Song, X., et al. (2013). Plasma phospholipid fatty acids and prostate cancer risk in the select trial. *Journal of the National Cancer Institute, 105*(15), 1132–1141. doi:10.1093/jnci/djt174.

Brichta, J., & Howard, A. (2013). *What's to eat? Improving food literacy in Canada*. The Conference Board of Canada, October 28, 2013. Retrieved from http://www.conferenceboard.ca/e-library/abstract.aspx?did=5727.

Brown, S. B., Reeves, K. W., & Bertone-Johnson, E. R. (2014). Maternal folate exposure in pregnancy and childhood asthma and allergy: a systematic review. *Nutrition Reviews, 72*(1), 55–64. doi:10.1111/nure.12080.

Brugnolli, A., Ambrosi, E., Canzan, F., et al. (2014). Securing of naso-gastric tubes in adult patients: A review. *International Journal of Nursing Studies, 51*(6), 943–950. doi:10.1016/j.ijnurstu.2013.12.002.

Butte, N. F., & Stuebe, A. (2016). Patient education: Maternal health and nutrition during breastfeeding (Beyond the Basics). *UpToDate*. Retrieved from http://www.uptodate.com/contents/maternal-health-and-nutrition-during-breastfeeding-beyond-the-basics.

Cagir, B. (2017). Postoperative ileus. *Medscape*. Retrieved from http://emedicine.medscape.com/article/2242141-overview.

Canadian Biotechnology Action Network. (2018). *Polls on GM food labelling in Canada. 1994–present*. Retrieved from https://cban.ca/gmos/issues/labeling/polls-on-gm-food-labelling-canada/.

Canadian Cancer Society. (2018). *Eat well*. Retrieved from http://www.cancer.ca/en/prevention-and-screening/reduce-cancer-risk/make-healthy-choices/eat-well/?region=on.

Canadian Dental Association. (2018). *Cleaning teeth*. Retrieved from http://www.cda-adc.ca/en/oral_health/cfyt/dental_care_children/cleaning.asp.

Canadian Diabetes Association (CDA). (2013). *Monitoring glycemic control*. Retrieved from http://guidelines.diabetes.ca/executivesummary/ch9.

Canadian Diabetes Association (CDA) (2016). *Clinical practice guidelines*. Toronto: Author. Retrieved from http://guidelines.diabetes.ca/fullguidelines.

Canadian Diabetes Association (CDA) (2018). *The glycemic index*. Toronto: Author. Retrieved from http://www.diabetes.ca/diabetes-and-you/healthy-living-resources/diet-nutrition/the-glycemic-index.

Canadian Food Inspection Agency. (2014). *Nutrient content claims*. Retrieved from http://www.inspection.gc.ca/food/labelling/food-labelling-for-industry/nutrient-content/eng/1389905941652/1389905991605.

Canadian Food Inspection Agency. (2016). *Gluten-free claims*. Retrieved from http://www.inspection.gc.ca/food/labelling/food-labelling-for-industry/allergens-and-gluten/eng/1388152325341/1388152326591?chap=2.

Canadian Malnutrition Task Force. (2016). *Costs of hospital malnutrition*. Retrieved from http://nutritioncareincanada.ca/sites/default/uploads/files/Precis%20of%20Costs%20of%20Hospital%20Malnutrition.pdf.

Canadian Task Force on Preventive Care. (2015). *Obesity in children (2015)*. Retrieved from https://canadiantaskforce.ca/guidelines/published-guidelines/obesity-in-children/.

Casaubon, L. K., Suddes, M., & Acute Stroke Best Practices Working Group 2013. (2013). Acute inpatient stroke care. In M. P. Lindsay, G. Gubitz, M. Bayley, et al. (Eds.), *Canadian best practice recommendations for stroke care*. Ottawa, ON: Heart and Stroke Foundation of Canada. Retrieved from http://strokebestpractices.ca/wp-content/uploads/2013/05/Ch4_SBP2013_Acute-Inpatient-Care_22MAY13_EN_FINAL4.pdf.

Chavarro, J. E., Mínguez-Alarcón, L., Mendiola, J., et al. (2014). Trans fatty acid intake is inversely related to total sperm count in young healthy men. *Human Reproduction, 29*(3), 429–440. doi:10.1093/humrep/det464.

Chen, P.-C., Chuang, C.-H., Leong, C.-P., et al. (2016). Systematic review and meta-analysis of the diagnostic accuracy of the water swallow test for screening aspiration in stroke patients. *Journal of Advanced Nursing, 72*(11), 2575–2586. doi:10.1111/jan.13013.

Cichero, J. A. (2013). Thickening agents used for dysphagia management: Effect on bioavailability of water, medication and feelings of satiety. *Nutrition Journal, 12*, 54. doi:10.1186/1475-2891-12-54.

Clark, H. M., Anderson, C. C., & Hietpas, F. (2014). Volumes of discrete sips from straws of varying internal diameters. *American Journal of Speech-language Pathology, 23*(1), 84–89. doi:10.1044/1058-0360(2013/13-0032).

Clark, H. M., & Shelton, S. (2014). Training effects of the effortful swallow under three exercise conditions. *Dysphagia, 29*(5), 553–563. doi:10.1007/s00455-014-9544-7.

Cohen, D. L., Roffe, C., Beavan, J., et al. (2016). Post-stroke dysphagia: A review and design considerations for future trials. *International Journal of Stroke, 11*(4), 399–411. doi:10.1177/1747493016639057.

Cristiano, C., Catanuso, M., Di Gregorio, C., et al. (2015). Comparing the use of traditional sites and alternative sites puncture for determination of blood glucose by glucometer. *British Journal of Medical Practitioners, 8*(4), a835. Retrieved from http://www.bjmp.org/files/2015-8-4/bjmp-2015-8-4-a835.pdf.

Cyr, C., & Canadian Paediatric Society, Injury Prevention Committee. (2016). Position statement on preventing choking and suffocation in children. *Paediatrics, Children and Health, 17*(2), 91–92. Retrieved from http://www.cps.ca/documents/position/preventing-choking-suffocation-children#ref50.

Dante, G., Vaiarelli, A., & Facchinetti, F. (2014). Vitamin and mineral needs during the oral contraceptive therapy: a systematic review. *International Journal of Reproduction, Contraceptives. Obstetrics and Gynecology, 3*, 1–10. doi:10.5455/2320-1770.ijrcog20140301. Retrieved from http://jeffreydachmd.com/wp-content/uploads/2013/03/Vitamin_mineral_contraceptive_Giulia_Dante_Reprod_Contracept_Obstet_Gynecol_2014.pdf.

Davidson, B. (2014). *Nurses are pivotal in the care of malnourished hospital patients*. CSGNA Conference. Niagara Falls, Ontario. October 2, 2014. Retrieved from https://www.eiseverywhere.com/file_uploads/6d14c3dd1b95f25812772487730e33f6_SS4NursesarepivotalBridgetDavidson.pdf.

De Souza, R. J., Mente, A., Maroleanu, A., et al. (2015). Intake of saturated and trans unsaturated fatty acids and risk of all cause mortality, cardiovascular disease, and type 2 diabetes: Systematic review and meta-analysis of observational studies. *British Medical Journal, 351*, h3978. doi:10.1136/bmj.h3978.

Dhaliwal, R., Cahill, N., Lemieux, M., et al. (2014). The Canadian critical care nutrition guidelines in 2013: an update on current recommendations and implementation strategies. *Nutrition in Clinical Practice, 29*(1), 29–43.

Diabetes Canada. (2018). *Basic meal planning*. Retrieved from https://www.diabetes.ca/diabetes-and-you/healthy-living-resources/diet-nutrition/basic-meal-planning.

Dietitians of Canada. (2012). *Health promotion and disease prevention: A call to action from dietitians. Submission to the House of Commons Standing Committee on Health*. Retrieved from http://www.dietitians.ca/Downloads/Public/2012-01-30-Standing-Comm-Health-HESA-Health-Pr-(1).aspx.

Dietitians of Canada. (2013a). *Eating well for vegetarian athletes*. Retrieved from http://www.dietitians.ca/Your-Health/Nutrition-A-Z/Sports-Nutrition-(Adult)/Eating-Well-for-Vegetarian-Athletes.aspx.

Dietitians of Canada. (2013b). *Do I need a vitamin or mineral supplement?* Retrieved from http://www.dietitians.ca/Your-Health/Nutrition-A-Z/Supplements/Do-I-Need-a-Supplement-.aspx.

Dietitians of Canada. (2014). *Healthy eating guidelines for vegans*. Retrieved from http://www.dietitians.ca/Your-Health/Nutrition-A-Z/Vegetarian-Diets/Eating-Guidelines-for-Vegans.aspx.

Dietitians of Canada. (2015). *Dietitians and chronic disease management: The impact of diet counselling*. Retrieved from http://www.dietitians.ca/Downloads/Public/Chronic-Disease-2-pager.aspx.

Dietitians of Canada. (2017). *Planning meals using Eating Well with Canada's Food Guide*. Retrieved from http://www.dietitians.ca/Downloads/Public/Senior-Friendly-collection.aspx.

Dwyer, J. T., Wiemer, K. L., Dary, O., et al. (2015). Fortification and health: Challenges and opportunities. *Advances in Nutrition, 6*, 124–131. doi:10.3945/an.114.007443.

EatRight Ontario. (2017a). *Understanding organic foods*. Retrieved from http://www.eatrightontario.ca/en/Articles/Farming-Food-production/Organic-Foods-and-Growing-Methods-FAQ.aspx#.VTF1tBPF9lB.

EatRight Ontario. (2017b). *Understanding genetically modified foods. EatRight Ontario*. Retrieved from https://www.eatrightontario.ca/en/Articles/Food-technology/Biotechnology/Novel-foods/Understanding-Genetically-Modified-Foods.aspx.

Ellett, M. L. C., Cohen, M. D., Croffie, J. M. B., et al. (2014). Comparing bedside methods of determining placement of gastric tubes in children. *Journal for Specialists in Pediatric Nursing: JSPN, 19*(1), 68–79. doi:10.1111/jspn.12054.

Findlay, S. M., & Canadian Paediatric Society, Adolescent Health Committee. (2004 reaffirmed 2016). Position statement: Dieting in adolescence. *Pediatrics & Child Health, 9*, 487–491. Retrieved from http://www.cps.ca/documents/position/dieting-adolescence.

Fisher, C., & Blalock, B. (2014). Clogged feeding tubes: A clinician's thorn. *Practical Gastroenterology, 127*, 16–22. Retrieved from https://med.virginia.edu/ginutrition/wp-content/uploads/sites/199/2014/06/Parrish-March-14.pdf.

Flynn Makic, M. B., Rauen, C. A., & VonRueden, K. T. (2013). Questioning common nursing practices. What does the evidence show? Assessing gastric residual volume. *American Nurse Today, 8*(3).

Food Banks Canada (2016). *HungerCount 2016*. Toronto: Author. Retrieved from https://www.foodbankscanada.ca/getmedia/6173994f-8a25-40d9-acdf-660a28e40f37/HungerCount_2016_final_singlepage.pdf.

Food Secure Canada. (2015). *Resetting the table: A people's food policy for Canada* (2nd ed.). Retrieved from https://foodsecurecanada.org/sites/foodsecurecanada.org/files/fsc-resetting-2015_web.pdf.

Gastric suction. (2017). *MedlinePlus*. Retrieved from https://medlineplus.gov/ency/article/003882.htm.

Gionet, L. (2015). *Statistics Canada: Health at a glance. Breastfeeding trends in Canada*. (Statistics Canada Catalogue no. 82-624-X.) Retrieved from http://www.statcan.gc.ca/pub/82-624-x/2013001/article/11879-eng.htm.

Gosmanov, A. R., & Umpierrez, G. E. (2013). Management of hyperglycemia during enteral and parenteral nutrition therapy. *Current Diabetes Reports, 13*(1), 155–162. http://doi.org/10.1007/s11892-012-0335-y.

Government of Canada. (2014). *National Seniors Council report on the social isolation of seniors* (Cat. No.: Em12-6/2014E-PDF.) Retrieved from https://www.canada.ca/content/dam/nsc-cna/documents/pdf/policy-and-program-development/publications-reports/2014/Report_on_the_Social_Isolation_of_Seniors.pdf.

Government of Canada. (2015). *Type 2 diabetes*. Retrieved from http://healthycanadians.gc.ca/diseases-conditions-maladies-affections/disease-maladie/diabete-eng.php.

Government of Canada. (2016a). *Childhood obesity*. Retrieved from http://healthycanadians.gc.ca/healthy-living-vie-saine/obesity-obesite/risks-risques-eng.php.

Government of Canada. (2016b). *Trans and saturated fats*. Retrieved from http://healthycanadians.gc.ca/eating-nutrition/healthy-eating-saine-alimentation/nutrients-nutriments/fats-lipides-eng.php.

Gutterman, S. (2014). *Obesity and mortality*. Presented at the Living to 100 Symposium. Orlando, FL. Society of Actuaries. January 8–10, 2014.

Hayashi, M., Yahiro, A., Sakuragi, Y., et al. (2016). Impaired swallowing in hospitalized patients: An observational study in a community hospital in Japan (2012–2014). *Nursing Research, 65*(5), 389–396. doi:10.1097/NNR.0000000000000178.

Health Canada. (2009). *Early childhood tooth decay*. Ottawa: Author. Retrieved from http://www.hc-sc.gc.ca/hl-vs/oral-bucco/care-soin/child-enfant-eng.php.

Health Canada. (2010). *Eating well with Canada's food guide—First Nations, Métis, and Inuit*. Ottawa: Author. Retrieved from https://www.canada.ca/en/health-canada/services/food-nutrition/reports-publications/eating-well-canada-food-guide-first-nations-inuit-metis.html.

Health Canada. (2012). *Do Canadian adolescents meet their nutrient requirements through food intake alone?* Ottawa: Author. Retrieved from http://www.hc-sc.gc.ca/fn-an/surveill/nutrition/commun/art-nutr-adol-eng.php.

Health Canada. (2013a). *First Nations and Inuit health: Diabetes*. Ottawa: Author. Retrieved from http://www.hc-sc.gc.ca/fniah-spnia/diseases-maladies/diabete/index-eng.php.

Health Canada. (2013b). *Dietary reference intakes*. Ottawa: Author. Retrieved from http://www.hc-sc.gc.ca/fn-an/nutrition/reference/index-eng.php.

Health Canada. (2013c). *Health Canada reminds Canadians to manage their caffeine consumption*. Ottawa: Author. Retrieved from http://healthycanadians.gc.ca/recall-alert-rappel-avis/hc-sc/2013/34021a-eng.php.

Health Canada. (2014a). *Infant nutrition*. Ottawa: Author. Retrieved from http://healthycanadians.gc.ca/healthy-living-vie-saine/infant-care-soins-bebe/nutrition-alimentation-eng.php.

Health Canada. (2014b). *Healthy eating and pregnancy*. Ottawa: Author. Retrieved from http://healthycanadians.gc.ca/healthy-living-vie-saine/pregnancy-grossesse/general-information-renseignements-generaux/eating-alimentation-eng.php.

Health Canada. (2015). *Food and nutrition*. Ottawa: Author. Retrieved from http://www.hc-sc.gc.ca/fn-an/index-eng.php.

Health Canada. (2016a). *Healthy eating for children*. Ottawa: Author. Retrieved from https://www.canada.ca/en/health-canada/services/tips-healthy-eating-tips-families/healthy-eating-children.html.

Health Canada. (2016b). *Food safety*. Retrieved from https://www.canada.ca/en/health-canada/services/food-safety-vulnerable-populations/food-safety-pregnant-women.html.

Health Canada. (2016c). *Eating well with Canada's food guide*. Ottawa: Author. Retrieved from http://www.hc-sc.gc.ca/fn-an/food-guide-aliment/index-eng.php.

Health Canada. (2016d). *Canadian guidelines for body weight classification in adults—Quick reference tool for professionals*. Ottawa: Author. Retrieved from http://www.hc-sc.gc.ca/fn-an/nutrition/weights-poids/guide-ld-adult/cg_quick_ref-ldc_rapide_ref-eng.php.

Health Canada. (2017a). *Revision process for Canada's food guide*. Ottawa: Author. Retrieved from http://healthycanadians.gc.ca/eating-nutrition/healthy-eating-saine-alimentation/food-guide-aliment/revision-process-procedure-de-revision-eng.php.

Health Canada. (2017b). *Sodium in Canada*. Ottawa: Author. Retrieved from http://www.hc-sc.gc.ca/fn-an/nutrition/sodium/index-eng.php.

Heart and Stroke Foundation of Canada. (2017a). *What is sugar?* Retrieved from http://www.heartandstroke.ca/get-healthy/healthy-eating/reduce-sugar.

Heart and Stroke Foundation of Canada. (2017b). *For vegetarians*. Retrieved from https://www.heartandstroke.ca/get-healthy/healthy-eating/specific-diets/for-vegetarians.

Heart and Stroke Foundation of Canada. (2017c). *Blood cholesterol [Including How to manage your cholesterol]*. Retrieved from http://www.heartandstroke.ca/heart/risk-and-prevention/condition-risk-factors/high-cholesterol.

Hebert, D., Lindsay, P., McIntyre, A., et al. (2016). Canadian stroke best practice recommendations: Stroke rehabilitation practice guidelines, update 2015. *International Journal of Stroke, 11*(4), 459–484. doi:10.1177/1747493016643553. Retrieved from http://journals.sagepub.com/doi/pdf/10.1177/1747493016643553.

Heimburger, D. C. (2016). Nutrition's interface with health and disease. In L. Goldman & A. L. Schafer (Eds.), *Goldman-Cecil medicine* (25th ed., Vol. 1, pp. 1426–1430). Philadelphia, PA: Elsevier Saunders.

Helmenstine, A. M. (2017). *pH and acidity of the stomach*. Retrieved from http://chemistry.about.com/od/lecturenoteslab1/a/Stomach-Ph.htm.

Holmes, S. (2012). Enteral nutrition: An overview. *Nursing Standard, 26*(39), 41–46.

House of Commons, Standing Committee on Agriculture and Agri-Food. (2016). *Genetically modified animals for human consumption. Report of the Standing Committee on Agriculture and Agri-Food*. Retrieved from https://www.ourcommons.ca/Content/Committee/421/AGRI/Reports/RP8674228/agrirp04/agrirp04-e.pdf.

Howard, A., & Edge, J. (2013). *Enough for all: Household food security in Canada*. Ottawa: The Conference Board of Canada. Publication 14-058.

Hu, X., Yi, E. S., & Ryu, J. H. (2014). Aspiration-related deaths in 57 consecutive patients: Autopsy study. *PLoS ONE, 9*(7), e103795. doi:10.1371/journal.pone.0103795.

Illario, M., Maione, A. S., Rusciano, M. R., et al. (2016). NutriLive: An integrated nutritional approach as a sustainable tool to prevent malnutrition in older people and promote active and healthy ageing—The EIP-AHA Nutrition Action Group. *Advances in Public Health, 2016*, doi:10.1155/2016/5678782. 5678782.

Infant Feeding Joint Working Group. (2015) *Nutrition for healthy term infants: Recommendations from six to 24 months*. Retrieved from https://www.canada.ca/en/health-canada/services/food-nutrition/healthy-eating/infant-feeding/nutrition-healthy-term-infants-recommendations-birth-six-months/6-24-months.html.

Infant Todller Forum. (2014). *Developmental stages in infant and toddler feeding*. Retrieved from https://www.infantandtoddlerforum.org/media/upload/pdf-downloads/3.5_Developmental_Stages_in_Infant_and_Toddler_Feeding_NEW.pdf.

Irving, S. Y., Lyman, B., Northington, L., et al. (2014). Nasogastric tube placement and verification in children: Review of the current literature. *Critical Care Nurse, 34*(3), 67–78. doi:10.4037/ccn2014606.

Jessri, M., & L'Abbe, M. R. (2015). The time for an updated Canadian Food Guide has arrived. *Applied Physiology, Nutrition, and Metabolism, 40*, 854–857. doi:10.1139/apnm-2015-0046.

Joint Commision: Accreditation, Health Care, Certification. (2014). Managing risk during transition to new ISO tubing connector standards. *Sentinel Event Alert, 53*, Retrieved from https://www.jointcommission.org/assets/1/6/SEA_53_Connectors_8_19_14_final.pdf.

Kirkup, K. (May 17, 2016). 60% of First Nation children on reserve live in poverty, institute says. *The Canadian Press*. Retrieved from http://www.cbc.ca/news/

indigenous/institute-says-60-percent-fn-children-on-reserve-live-in-poverty-1.3585105.

Koidou, I., Kollias, N., Sdravou, K., et al. (2013). Dysphagia: A short review of the current state. *Educational Gerontology, 39*(11), 812–827. doi:10.1080/03601277.2013.766518.

Kramer, M. S., Platt, R. W., Wen, S. W., et al. for the Fetal/Infant Health Study Group of the Canadian Perinatal Surveillance System. (2001). A new and improved population-based Canadian reference for birth weight for gestational age. *Pediatrics, 108*(2), e35. Retrieved from http://www.pediatrics.org/cgi/content/full/108/2/e35.

Krleza, J. L., Dorotic, A., Grzunov, A., et al. (2015). Capillary blood sampling: National recommendations on behalf of the Croatian Society of Medical Biochemistry and Laboratory Medicine. *Biochemia Medica, 25*(3), 335–358. doi:10.11613/BM.2015.034.

Krølner, R., Jørgensen, T. S., Aarestrup, A. K., et al. (2012). The Boost study: Design of a school- and community-based randomised trial to promote fruit and vegetable consumption among teenagers. *BioMed Central Public Health, 12*, 191. doi:10.1186/1471-2458-12-191.

Lachner, C., Steinle, N. I., & Regenold, W. T. (2012). The neuropsychiatry of vitamin B12 deficiency in elderly patients. *Journal of Neuropsychiatry and Clinical Neurosciences, 24*, 5–15. doi:10.1176/appi.neuropsych.11020052.

La Leche League. (2015). *What about drinking alcohol and breastfeeding?* Retrieved from http://www.llli.org/faq/alcohol.html.

Lampert, L. (2015). *How to feed a patient with dysphagia.* Retrieved from https://www.ausmed.com/articles/how-to-feed-a-patient-with-dysphagia/.

Laporte, M., Keller, H., Payette, H., et al. (2015). Validity and reliability of the new Canadian Nutrition Screening Tool in the "real-world" hospital setting. *European Journal of Clinical Nutrition, 69*(5), 558–564. doi:10.1038/ejcn.2014.270.

Leder, S. B., Judson, B. L., Sliwinski, E., et al. (2013). Promoting safe swallowing when puree is swallowed without aspiration but thin liquid is aspirated: Nectar is enough. *Dysphagia, 28*(1), 58–62. doi:10.1007/s00455-012-9412-2.

Lee, J. L., Oh, E. S., Lee, R. W., et al. (2015). Serum albumin and prealbumin in calorically restricted, non-diseased individuals: A systematic review. *American Journal of Medicine, 128*(9), 1023-e1.

Lehto, E., Ray, C., Te Velde, S. J., et al. (2014). Mediation of parental educational level on fruit and vegetable intake among schoolchildren in ten European countries. *Public Health Nutrition, 18*(01), 1–11. doi:10.1017/S136898001300339X.

Leslie, W., & Hankey, C. (2015). Aging, nutritional status and health. *Healthcare, 3*, 648–658. doi:10.3390/healthcare3030648.

Leung, A. A., Nerenberg, K., Daskalopoulou, S. S., CHEP Guidelines Task Force, et al. (2016). Hypertension Canada's 2016 Canadian hypertension education program guidelines for blood pressure measurement, diagnosis, assessment of risk, prevention, and treatment of hypertension. *Canadian Journal of Cardiology, 32*(5), 569–688. doi:10.1016/j.cjca.2016.02.066.

Leung, A. K., Marchand, V., Sauve, R. S., et al. (2012). The "picky eater": The toddler or preschooler who does not eat. *Paediatrics & Child Health, 17*(8), 455–457.

Lipnowski, S., & Canadian Paediatric Society, Healthy Active Living and Sports Medicine Committee. (2012). Healthy active living: Physical activity guidelines for children and adolescents. *Paediatric Child Health, 17*(4), 209–210. Retrieved from http://www.cps.ca/documents/position/physical-activity-guidelines#ref4.

Lloyd, M., & Bailey, A. (2015, November 24). *One in five Canadian children lives in poverty.* News 1130. Retrieved from http://www.news1130.com/2015/11/24/canadian-children-poverty/.

Lohmann, K., Gartner, D., Kurze, R., et al. (2015). More than just crushing: a prospective pre-post intervention study to reduce drug preparation errors in patients with feeding tubes. *Journal of Clinical Pharmacy & Therapeutics, 40*(2), 220–225. doi:10.1111/jcpt.12250.

Loopstra, R., & Tarasuk, V. (2013). Perspectives on community gardens, community kitchens and the Good Food Box program in a community-based sample of low-income families. *Canadian Journal of Public Health, 104*(1), e55–e59. Retrieved from http://journal.cpha.ca/index.php/cjph/article/viewFile/3528/2746.

Maeda, K., & Akagi, J. (2014). Oral care may reduce pneumonia in the tube-fed elderly: A preliminary study. *Dysphagia, 29*(5), 616–621. doi:10.1007/s00455-014-9553-6.

Mahakalkar, C. C., Modi, S., Yeola, M., et al. (2014). Malnutrition in hospitalised patients; a real concern in surgical outcomes. *International Journal of Research in Medical Science, 2*, 250–257. doi:10.5455/2320-6012.ijrms20140248.

Marcus, J. (2013). Lifecycle nutrition: Healthy eating throughout the ages. In *Culinary nutrition: The science and practice of healthy cooking* (p. 475–543). Waltham, MA: Elsevier.

Martin, C. R., Ling, P.-R., & Blackburn, G. L. (2016). Review of infant feeding: Key features of breast milk and infant formula. *Nutrients, 8*(5), 279. doi:10.3390/nu8050279. Retrieved from http://www.mdpi.com/2072-6643/8/5/279/htm.

Martino, R., Maki, E., & Diamant, N. (2014). Identification of dysphagia using the Toronto Bedside Swallowing Screening Test (TOR-BSST©): Are 10 teaspoons of water necessary? *International Journal of Speech-Language Pathology, 16*(3), 193–198. doi:10.3109/17549507.2014.902995.

McCulloch, D. K. (2017). Patient education: Self-blood glucose monitoring in diabetes mellitus (Beyond the Basics). *UpToDate.*, Retrieved from https://www.uptodate.com/contents/self-monitoring-of-blood-glucose-in-diabetes-mellitus-beyond-the-basics.

Meert, K. L., Caverly, M., Kelm, L. M., et al. (2015). The PH of feeding tube aspirates from critically ill infants. *American Journal of Critical Care, 24*(5), e72–e77. doi:10.4037/ajcc2015971.

Mehler Paperny, A. (2015, March 25). *Going hungry: 12% of NB families can't afford healthy food.* Global News New Brunswick. Retrieved from http://globalnews.ca/news/1903255/going-hungry-why-millions-of-canadians-cant-afford-healthy-food/.

Metheny, N. A. (2016). Prevention of aspiration in adults. *Critical Care Nurse, 36*(1), e20–e24. doi:10.4037/ccn2016831.

Minaker, L., & Hammond, D. (2016). Low frequency of fruit and vegetable consumption among Canadian youth: Findings from the 2012/2013 Youth Smoking Survey. *Journal of School Health, 86*(2), 135–142. doi:10.1111/josh.12359.

Mohd Shariff, Z., Lin, K. G., Sariman, S., et al. (2015). The relationship between household income and dietary intakes of 1-10 year old urban Malaysian. *Nutrition Research and Practice, 9*(3), 278–287. doi:10.4162/nrp.2015.9.3.278.

Morris, M. C., & Tangney, C. C. (2014). Dietary fat composition and dementia risk. *Neurobiology of Aging, 35*(Suppl. 2), S59–S64. doi:10.1016/j.neurobiolaging.2014.03.038.

Murphy, S. P., Guenther, P. M., & Kretsch, M. J. (2006). Using the dietary reference intakes to assess intakes of groups: Pitfalls to avoid. *Journal of the American Dietetic Association, 106*, 1550–1553.

National Association of Children's Hospitals (NACH), ECRI Institute (2012). *Blind pediatric NG tube placements continue to cause harm.* Overland Park, KS: Child Health Patient Safety Organization, Inc.

National Cancer Institute. (2017). *Dietary assessment primer.* Retrieved from https://dietassessmentprimer.cancer.gov/.

National Collaborating Centre for Aboriginal Health (2012). *The state of knowledge of Aboriginal health: A review of Aboriginal public health in Canada.* Prince George, BC: Author. Retrieved from https://www.ccnsa-nccah.ca/docs/context/RPT-StateKnowledgeReview-EN.pdf.

National Institutes of Health. (2016a). *Vitamin A: fact sheet for health professionals.* Retrieved from https://ods.od.nih.gov/factsheets/VitaminA-HealthProfessional/.

National Institutes of Health. (2016b). *Iron: Dietary supplement fact sheet.* Retrieved from https://ods.od.nih.gov/factsheets/Iron-HealthProfessional/.

National Osteoporosis Foundation. (2014). *Clinician's guide to prevention and treatment of osteoporosis: 2014 Issue, Version 1.* Retrieved from https://my.nof.org/bone-source/education/clinicians-guide-to-the-prevention-and-treatment-of-osteoporosis.

Newfoundland Labrador Public Health. (2013). *Feeding your baby: 6-12 months.* Retrieved from http://www.cssd.gov.nl.ca/publications/pdf/healthyliving/Feeding_Your_Baby.pdf.

Orlich, M. J., Singh, P. N., Sabate, J., et al. (2015). Vegetarian dietary patterns and the risk of colorectal cancers. *Journal of the American Medical Association, 175*(5), 767–776. doi:10.1001/jamainternmed.2015.59.

Parihar, A. S., Katoch, V., Rajguru, S. A., et al. (2015). Periodontal disease: A possible risk-factor for adverse pregnancy outcome. *Journal of International Oral Health: JIOH, 7*(7), 137–142.

Parker, L., Torrazza, R. M., Li, Y., et al. (2015). Aspiration and evaluation of gastric residuals in the NICU: State of the science. *Journal of Perinatal & Neonatal Nursing, 29*(1), 51–59. doi:10.1097/JPN.0000000000000080.

Parker, M., & Power, D. (2013). Management of swallowing difficulties in people with advanced dementia. *Nursing Older People, 25*(2), 26–31.

Pasricha, S.-J., Low, M., Thompson, J., et al. (2014). Iron supplementation benefits physical performance in women of reproductive age: A systematic review and meta-analysis. *Journal of Nutrition*, doi:10.3945/jn.113.189589.

Pathirana, A. K., Lokunarangoda, N., Ranathunga, I., et al. (2014). Prevalence of hospital malnutrition among cardiac patients: Results from six nutrition screening tools. *SpringerPlus, 3*, 412. doi:10.1186/2193-1801-3-412.

Perry, S. E., Hockenberry, M. J., Lowdermilk, D. L., et al. (Eds.), (2016). Chapter 26: Newborn nutrition and feeding. In *Maternal Child Nursing Care in Canada* (2nd ed.). Toronto: Elsevier.

Peterson, M. K., & Zu, K. (2016, February/March). Trans fats: Current scientific update. *Food Safety Magazine.* Retrieved from http://www.foodsafetymagazine.com/magazine-archive1/februarymarch-2016/trans-fats-current-scientific-update/.

Pilgrim, A., Robinson, S., Sayer, A. A., et al. (2015). An overview of appetite decline in older people. *Nursing Older People, 27*(5), 29–35. doi:10.7748/nop.27.5.29.e697.

Pound, C. M., Unger, S. L., & Canadian Paediatric Society, Nutrition and Gastroenterology Committee, Hospital Paediatrics Section. (2012 updated 2015). The Baby-Friendly Initiative: Protecting, promoting and supporting breastfeeding. *Paediatrics & Child Health, 17*(6), 317–321. Retrieved from http://www.cps.ca/documents/position/baby-friendly-initiative-breastfeeding.

Public Health Agency of Canada. (2012). *Curbing childhood obesity: A federal, provincial and territorial framework for action to promote healthy weights.* Retrieved from http://www.phac-aspc.gc.ca/hp-ps/hl-mvs/framework-cadre/index-eng.php.

Public Health Nutritionists of Saskatchewan. (2015). *Helping children to be competent eaters.* Retrieved from http://www.fhhr.ca/Documents/NUN2015SchoolAgeEditionfinal_000.pdf.

Quintero-Platt, G., González-Reimers, E., Martín-González, M. C., et al. (2015). Vitamin D, vascular calcification and mortality among alcoholics. *Alcohol and Alcoholism, 50*(1), 18–23.

Rahnemai-Azar, A. A., Rahnemaiazar, A. A., Naghshizadian, R., et al. (2014). Percutaneous endoscopic gastrostomy: Indications, technique, complications and management. *World Journal of Gastroenterology, 20*(24), 7739–7751. doi:10.3748/wjg.v20.i24.7739.

Ramage-Morin, P. L., & Garriguet, D. (2015). *Nutritional risk among older Canadians.* Ottawa: Statistics Canada. Retrieved from http://www.statcan.gc.ca/pub/82-003-x/2013003/article/11773-eng.htm.

Region of Waterloo Public Health. (2017). *Quick stats. Birth weight and birth weight for gestational age, Waterloo Region, 2013, 2014 & 2015.* Retrieved from http://chd.region.waterloo.on.ca/en/researchResourcesPublications/resources/BIRTH_WEIGHT_GESTATIONAL_AGE.pdf.

Reignier, J., Mercier, E., Le Gouge, A., Clinical Research in Intensive Care and Sepsis (CRICS) Group, et al. (2013). Effect of not monitoring residual gastric volume on risk of ventilator-associated pneumonia in adults receiving mechanical ventilation and early enteral feeding: A randomized controlled trial. *Journal of the American Medical Association, 309*(3), 249–256. doi:10.1001/jama.2012.196377.

Rémond, D., Shahar, D. R., Gille, D., et al. (2015). Understanding the gastrointestinal tract of the elderly to develop dietary solutions that prevent malnutrition. *Oncotarget, 6*(16), 13858–13898.

Rice, T. W. (2016). Sterile water and enteral feeding: Fear over logic. *Practical Gastroenterology, 156*, 34–40. Retrieved from https://med.virginia.edu/ginutrition/wp-content/uploads/sites/199/2014/06/Parrish-October-16-2.pdf.

Roberts, K., Shields, M., de Groh, M., et al. (2015). *Overweight and obesity in children and adolescents: Results from the 2009 to 2011 Canadian Health Measures Survey.* Ottawa: Statistics Canada. Retrieved from http://www.statcan.gc.ca/pub/82-003-x/2012003/article/11706-eng.htm.

Robinson, R. (2015). Low serum albumin and total lymphocyte count as predictors of 30-day hospital readmission in patients 65 years of age or older. *PeerJ, 3*, e1181. doi:10.7717/peerj.1181.

Roila, F. (2012). *Expert point of view* [In response to Lavau-Denes, 2012, Does prophylaxis prevent catheter-related thrombosis?]. Retrieved from http://www.ascopost.com/issues/november-15-2012/expert-point-of-view-fausto-roila-md/.

Rollins, C. J., & Boggs, J. H. (2013). Adult enteral nutrition. In B. K. Aldredge, R. Coreli, M. E. Ernst, et al. (Eds.), *Koda-Kimble & Young's applied therapeutics* (10th ed., pp. 884–907). Philadelphia: Wolters, Lippincott, Williams & Wilkins.

Saez de la Fuente, I., Saez de la Fuente, J., Estelles, M. D. Q., et al. (2014). Enteral nutrition in patients receiving mechanical ventilation in a prone position. *Journal of Parenteral and Enteral Nutrition, 40*(2), 250–255. doi:10.1177/0148607114553232.

Sanou, D., O'Reilly, E., Ngnie-Teta, I., et al. (2014). Acculturation and nutritional health of immigrants in Canada: A scoping review. *Journal of Immigrant and Minority Health, 16*(1), 24–34. doi:10.1007/s10903-013-9823-7.

Saskatoon Health Region. (2017). *Nasogastric/orogastric tube: Insertion, care of, and removal.* Retrieved from https://www.saskatoonhealthregion.ca/about/NursingManual/1040.pdf.

Schlenker, E. D., & Gilbert, J. A. (2014). *Williams' essentials of nutrition and diet therapy* (11th ed.). St. Louis, MO: Mosby Elsevier.

Sharma, R., Biedenharn, K. R., Fedor, J. M., et al. (2013). Lifestyle factors and reproductive health: Taking control of your fertility. *Reproductive Biology and Endocrinology, 11*, 66. doi:10.1186/1477-7827-11-66.

Silk, D. B. A., & Quinn, D. G. (2015). Dual-purpose gastric decompression and enteral feeding tubes rationale and design of novel nasogastric and nasogastrojejunal tubes. *Journal of Parenteral and Enteral Nutrition, 39*(5), 531–543. doi:10.1177/0148607114551966.

Silveira, E. A., Dalastra, L., & Pagotto, V. (2014). Polypharmacy, chronic diseases and nutritional markers in community-dwelling older. *Revista Brasileira de Epidemiologia, 17*(4), 818–829. doi:10.1590/1809-4503201400040002.

Smithard, D., Barrett, N. A., Hargroves, D., et al. (2015). Electromagnetic sensor-guided enteral access systems: A literature review. *Dysphagia, 30*, 275. doi:10.1007/s00455-015-9607-4.

Snell, C., Bernheim, A., Bergé, J.-B., et al. (2012). Assessment of the health impact of GM plant diets in long-term and multigenerational animal feeding trials: A literature review. *Food and Chemical Toxicology, 50*, 1134–1148. doi:10.1016/j.fct.2011.11.048.

Sonneville, K. R., Gordon, C. M., Kocher, M. S., et al. (2012). Vitamin D, calcium, and dairy intakes and stress fractures among female adolescents. *Archives of Pediatrics & Adolescent Medicine, 166*(7), 595–600. doi:10.1001/archpediatrics.2012.5.

Statistics Canada (2015). *Canada's population estimates: Age and sex, July 1, 2015.* Ottawa: Author. Retrieved from http://www.statcan.gc.ca/daily-quotidien/150929/dq150929b-eng.htm.

Statistics Canada. (2016a). *Aboriginal peoples in Canada: First Nations People, Métis and Inuit.* Ottawa: Author. Retrieved from https://www12.statcan.gc.ca/nhs-enm/2011/as-sa/99-011-x/99-011-x2011001-eng.cfm.

Statistics Canada. (2016b). *Immigration and ethnocultural diversity in Canada.* Ottawa: Author. Retrieved from https://www12.statcan.gc.ca/nhs-enm/2011/as-sa/99-010-x/99-010-x2011001-eng.cfm.

Statistics Canada. (2016c). *Body mass index, overweight or obese, self-reported, youth, by sex, provinces and territories (Percent).* Retrieved from http://www.statcan.gc.ca/tables-tableaux/sum-som/l01/cst01/health84b-eng.htm.

Statistics Canada. (2017). *Obesity.* Ottawa: Author. Retrieved from http://www.statcan.gc.ca/eng/help/bb/info/obesity.

Steele, C. M., Alsanei, A. W., Ayanikalath, S., et al. (2015). The influence of food texture and liquid consistency modification on swallowing physiology and function: A systematic review. *Dysphagia, 30*(1), 2–26. doi:10.1007/s00455-014-9578-x.

Tantamango-Bartley, Y., Jaceldo-Siegl, K., Fan, J., et al. (2013). Vegetarian diets and the incidence of cancer in a low-risk population. *Cancer Epidemiology, Biomarkers & Prevention, 22*(2), 286–294. doi:10.1158/1055-9965.EPI-12-1060.

Tappenden, K. A., Quatrara, B., Parkhurst, M. L., et al. (2013). Critical role of nutrition in improving quality of care: An interdisciplinary call to action to address adult hospital malnutrition. *Journal of the Academy of Nutrition and Dietetics, 13*, 1219–1237. doi:10.1016/j.jand.2013.05.015.

Teasell, R., Foley, N., Martino, R., et al. (2016). *Dysphagia and aspiration following stroke.* Retrieved from http://www.ebrsr.com/sites/default/files/Chapter%2015_Dysphagia%20and%20Aspiration%20Following%20Stroke_with%20appendix.pdf.

Temblett, P., & George, G. (2013). pH testing to confirm nasogastric tube position on the ICU: Are we wasting our time? *Critical Care, 17*(Suppl. 2), 245. doi:10.1186/cc12183.

Track, L. (2015). *Hungry for justice: Advancing a right to food for children in BC.* BC Civil Liberties Association. Retrieved from https://bccla.org/wp-content/uploads/2015/06/20150501-Hungry-For-Justice-Advancing-a-Right-to-Food-for-Children-in-BC.pdf.

Trapp, C., & Levin, S. (2012). Preparing to prescribe plant-based diets for diabetes prevention and treatment. *Diabetes Spectrum, 25*(1), 38–44. doi:10.2337/diaspect.25.1.38.

Tsai, A. (2015, March). Meters: Does your device measure up? What to look for when buying a blood glucose meter. *Diabetes Forecast,* Retrieved from http://www.diabetesforecast.org/2015/mar-apr/meters-does-your-device-measure-up.html.

United Nations (2011, May 19). *Prevention and control of non-communicable diseases—Report of the Secretary General. A/66/83.* Retrieved from http://www.un.org/ga/search/view_doc.asp?symbol=A/66/83&Lang=E.

Van Ansem, W. J., Schrijvers, C. T., Rodenburg, G., et al. (2014). Maternal educational level and children's healthy eating behaviour: Role of the home food environment (cross-sectional results from the INPACT study). *International Journal of Behavioral Nutrition and Physical Activity, 11*, 113. doi:10.1186/s12966-014-0113-0.

Vaquer, S., Masip, J., Gili, G., et al. (2014). Earlobe arterialized capillary blood gas analysis in the intensive care unit: A pilot study. *Annals of Intensive Care, 4*, 11. doi:10.1186/2110-5820-4-11.

Veeravagu, A., Joseph, R., Jiang, B., et al. (2013). Traumatic epistaxis: Skull base defects, intracranial complications and neurosurgical considerations. *International Journal of Surgery Case Reports, 4*(8), 656–661. doi:10.1016/j.ijscr.2013.04.033.

Veiga, H. P., Fonseca, H. V., & Bianchini, E. M. (2014). Sequential swallowing of liquid in elderly adults: Cup or straw? *Dysphagia, 29*(2), 249–255. doi:10.1007/s00455-013-9503-8.

Verkman, A. S., Anderson, M. O., & Papadopoulos, M. C. (2014). Aquaporins: Important but elusive drug targets. *Nature Reviews Drug Discovery, 13*, 259–277. doi:10.1038/nrd4226.

Villela, E. L., Sakai, P., Almeida, M. R., et al. (2014). Endoscopic gastrostomy replacement tubes: Long-term randomized trial with five silicone commercial models. *Clinical Nutrition, 33*, 221–225. doi:10.1016/j.clnu.2013.04.015.

Vision Australia. (2012). *Caring for patients who are blind or have low vision.* Retrieved from http://www.visionaustralia.org/living-with-low-vision/family-friends-and-carers/caring-for-patients-who-are-blind-or-have-low-vision.

Wadhera, R. K., Steen, D. L., Khan, I., et al. (2016). A review of low-density lipoprotein cholesterol, treatment strategies, and its impact on cardiovascular disease morbidity and mortality. *Journal of Clinical Lipidology, 10*(3), 472–489. doi:10.1016/j.jacl.2015.11.010.

Wang, X., Ouyang, Y., Liu, J., et al. (2014). Fruit and vegetable consumption and mortality from all causes, cardiovascular disease, and cancer: Systematic review and dose–response meta-analysis of prospective cohort studies. *British Medical Journal, 349*(g4490). doi:10.1136/bmj.g4490.

Weaver, C. M., Dwyer, J., Fulgoni, V. L., III, et al. (2014). Processed foods: Contributions to nutrition. *American Journal of Clinical Nutrition, 99*(6), 1525–1542. doi:10.3945/ajcn.114.089284.

Weaver, K. (2015). Feeding and eating disorders. In W. Austin & M. A. Boyd (Eds.), *Psychiatric nursing for Canadian practice* (3rd ed., pp. 523–571). Philadelphia: Lippincott Williams & Wilkins.

Weinberg, R. S. (2013). Goal setting in sport and exercise: Research and practical applications. *Revista da Educação Física / UEM, 24*(2), 171–179. doi:10.4025/reveducfis.v24.2.17524.

Wells, D. (2016). Living wage campaigns and building communities. *Alternate Routes: A Journal of Critical Social Research, 27*, 235–246. Retrieved from http://www.alternateroutes.ca/index.php/ar/article/viewFile/22400/18182.

Wen, S. W., Guo, Y., Rodger, M., et al. (2016). Folic acid supplementation in pregnancy and the risk of pre-eclampsia—A cohort study. *PLoS ONE, 11*(2), e0149818. doi:10.1371/journal.pone.0149818.

Winter, H. S. (2017). Patient education: Acid reflux (gastroesophageal reflux) in infants (beyond the basics). *UpToDate*. Retrieved from http://www.uptodate.com/contents/acid-reflux-gastroesophageal-reflux-in-infants-beyond-the-basics.

Wirth, R., Dziewas, R., Beck, A. M., et al. (2016). Oropharyngeal dysphagia in older persons—From pathophysiology to adequate intervention: A review and summary of an international expert meeting. *Clinical Interventions in Aging, 11*, 189–208. doi:10.2147/CIA.S97481.

World Health Organization. (2013). *Global action plan for the prevention and control of noncommunicable diseases 2013–2020*. WHO Document Production Services, Geneva, Switzerland. Retrieved from http://apps.who.int/iris/bitstream/10665/94384/1/9789241506236_eng.pdf?ua=1.

World Health Organization. (2017). *Botulism fact sheet*. Retrieved from http://www.who.int/mediacentre/factsheets/fs270/en/.

43

Urinary Elimination

Canadian content written by Kathleen F. Hunter, RN, NP, PhD, GNC(C), NCA
Original chapter by Donna L. Thompson, MSN, CRNP, RNP-BC, CCCN-AP

OBJECTIVES

Mastery of content in this chapter will enable you to:

- Define the key terms listed.
- Describe the process of urination.
- Identify factors that commonly influence urinary elimination.
- Compare common alterations in urinary elimination.
- Identify two modalities of renal replacement therapy.
- Obtain a nursing health history for a patient with urinary elimination problems.
- Identify nursing diagnoses appropriate for patients with alterations in urinary elimination.
- Obtain urine specimens.
- Describe characteristics of normal and abnormal urine.
- Describe the nursing implications of common diagnostic tests of the urinary system.
- Discuss nursing measures to promote normal micturition and to reduce episodes of incontinence.
- Insert a urinary catheter.
- Discuss nursing measures to reduce urinary tract infection.
- Irrigate a urinary catheter.

KEY TERMS

Bacteremia, p. 1168
Bacteriuria, p. 1168
Catheter-associated UTI (CAUTI), p. 1169
Catheterization, p. 1188
Cystitis, p. 1168
Dysuria, p. 1168
Hematuria, p. 1167
Micturition, p. 1166
Nephrostomy, p. 1171
Pelvic floor muscle exercises (PFMEs), p. 1206
Postvoid residual (PVR), p. 1172
Pyelonephritis, p. 1168
Renin, p. 1167
Suprapubic catheterization, p. 1203
Ureterostomy, p. 1171
Urinary incontinence (UI), p. 1169
Urinary retention, p. 1169

MEDIA RESOURCES

http://evolve.elsevier.com/Canada/Potter/fundamentals/

- Audio Chapter Summaries
- Examination Review Questions
- Concept Map Creator
- Case Study With Questions
- Audio Glossary
- Content Updates
- Video Clips

Normal elimination of urinary wastes is a basic function. Many illnesses and conditions, both acute and chronic, can affect the urinary function. Nurses play a key role in assessment of urinary tract function, promotion of continence and management of incontinence and optimal bladder emptying. Understanding the reasons for urinary elimination problems and finding evidence-informed solutions acceptable to patients are essential nursing functions.

SCIENTIFIC KNOWLEDGE BASE

Urinary elimination depends on the coordinated function of the kidneys, ureters, bladder, and urethra. Kidneys remove wastes (excess water and by-products of metabolism) from the blood to form urine. Ureters transport urine from the kidneys to the bladder. The bladder stores urine until the urge to urinate develops. Micturition (urination) occurs when a complex neural response allows the bladder to contract, the urethral sphincter to relax, and urine to leave the body through the urethra (Figure 43-1).

Upper Urinary Tract

Kidneys. The kidneys lie on either side of the vertebral column behind the peritoneum and against deep muscles of the back. The kidneys extend from the twelfth thoracic vertebra to the third lumbar vertebra. Normally, the left kidney is higher than the right one because of the anatomical position of the liver.

Waste products of metabolism that collect in the blood are filtered in the kidneys. Blood reaches each kidney by a renal (kidney) artery that branches from the abdominal aorta. The *nephron* is the functional unit of the kidney, where waste products are removed and urine is formed. Nephrons also play a key role in fluid and electrolyte balance (Doig & Huether, 2014).

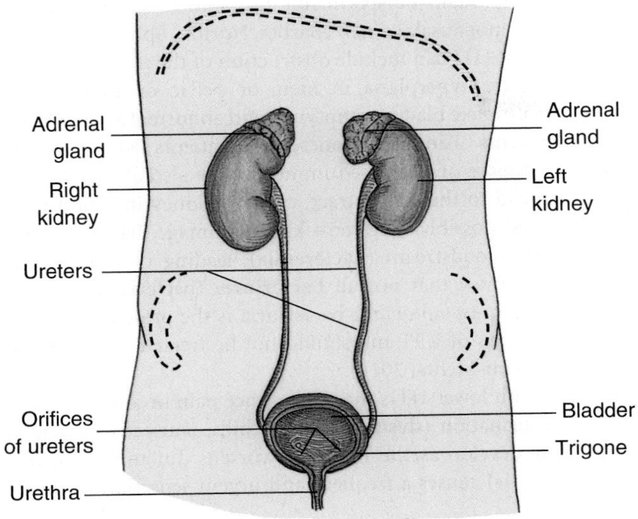

FIGURE 43-1 Organs of the urinary system.

A cluster of blood vessels forms the capillary network of the *glomerulus* of the nephron, which is the initial site of filtration of the blood and the beginning of urine formation. The glomerular capillaries permit filtration of water, glucose, amino acids, urea, creatinine, and major electrolytes. Large proteins and blood cells normally do not filter through the glomerulus. The presence of proteins (proteinuria) or blood (hematuria) in urine is a sign of glomerular injury.

The glomerulus filters approximately 125 millilitres (mL) of plasma per minute (180 litres [L] per day). Most (99%) of the filtrate is reabsorbed into the plasma, with the remaining 1% excreted as urine. The reabsorption process maintains fluid and electrolyte balance (Doig & Huether, 2014). Normal urine production ranges from 1 to 2 L per day and is affected by many factors, including fluid intake and body temperature (Doig & Huether, 2014). An output of less than 30 mL per hour may indicate renal alterations.

The kidneys play a role in other functions including the production of red blood cells (RBCs), blood pressure regulation, and bone mineralization. Erythropoietin stimulates RBC production and maturation in the bone marrow (Doig & Huether, 2014). Patients with chronic alterations in kidney function cannot produce sufficient quantities of this hormone and are therefore prone to anemia.

Renin, another hormone produced by the kidneys, plays a role in blood pressure control by regulating renal blood flow via the renin–angiotensin–aldosterone system (RAAS). Renin is released from the juxtaglomerular cells when blood pressure decreases, converting angiotensinogen (a substance synthesized by the liver) into angiotensin I. Angiotensin I is converted to angiotensin II in the lungs. Angiotensin II causes vasoconstriction and stimulates aldosterone release from the adrenal cortex. Aldosterone causes retention of water, which increases blood volume. The kidneys also produce prostaglandin E2 and prostacyclin, which are important in maintaining renal blood flow through vasodilation. These mechanisms increase arterial blood pressure and renal blood flow (Doig & Huether, 2014).

The kidneys play a role in calcium and phosphate regulation by producing a substance that converts vitamin D into its active form. The disruption of these other regulatory functions in patients with kidney impairment can lead to bone disease from impaired calcium resorption, hypertension, and anemia.

Ureters. Urine enters the renal pelvis from the collecting ducts and travels to the bladder through the ureters. The *ureters* are tubular structures that enter the urinary bladder obliquely through the posterior wall, at the ureterovesical junction (the juncture of the ureters and the bladder). Peristaltic waves cause urine to enter the bladder in spurts rather than steadily. Contraction of the bladder compresses the ureters at the junction during micturition to prevent the reflux of urine.

An obstruction within a ureter, such as a kidney stone (renal calculus), can result in distension of the ureter (hydroureter) and backup of urine to the pelvis of the kidney (hydronephrosis), potentially causing long-term renal impairment.

Lower Urinary Tract

Bladder. The urinary *bladder* is a hollow, distensible muscular organ lined with uroepithelium that stores and excretes urine. It is composed of the lower trigone base, lying between the ureter and urethral openings, and the upper dome of the detrusor muscle. When empty, the bladder lies behind the symphysis pubis in the pelvic cavity. It rests against the anterior wall of the rectum in men and against the anterior walls of the cervix and vagina in women.

The bladder expands as it becomes filled with urine. During filling, pressure remains low as the relaxed bladder is normally highly compliant. When the bladder is full, it expands and extends above the symphysis pubis. Contraction of the detrusor expels urine from the body. In a pregnant woman, the developing fetus pushes against the bladder, reducing its capacity and causing a feeling of fullness.

Urethra. Urine travels from the bladder through the *urethra* (a fibromuscular tube) and passes outside of the body through the urethral meatus. The urethra transverses the pelvic floor muscles, a layer of skeletal muscle that stabilizes the urethra and forms part of the continence mechanism. Circular smooth muscle and striated sphincter muscle (also known as the *external sphincter*, or *rhabdosphincter*) in the urethra also contribute to closure between voids and aid in continence. In women, the urethra is approximately 3–4 cm long. This short length predisposes females to infection. The male urethra is about 18–20 cm long (Doig & Huether, 2014).

Act of Urination

Urination, also known as *micturition* or *voiding*, is the process of bladder emptying. Micturition requires simultaneous contraction of the bladder and relaxation of the outlet. Neural control of voiding and continence is dependent on a complex flow of information between the bladder, spinal cord, and brain (Birder, Chai, Griffiths, et al., 2013), involving both autonomic and somatic nerves. Infants void reflexively, with activation of the pontine micturition centre in the pons of the brainstem from signals of fullness from the bladder. Sensory nerves from the bladder and urethra carry efferent signals through the spinal reflex arc and up the spinal cord to the pontine micturition centre in the brainstem. Afferent signals move back down, inhibiting sympathetic fibres of the hypogastric nerve innervating the bladder and Onuf's nucleus in the sacral spinal cord where motor neurons innervating the rhabdosphincter are located, resulting in relaxation of the sphincter and contraction of the detrusor muscle. As the child matures, voluntary control over bladder emptying develops with involvement of higher-level brain structures including the forebrain, allowing for suppression of the voiding reflex. Forebrain circuits for safety, emotions, and societal propriety play a role in voluntary micturition. Voluntary contraction of the pelvic floor muscles also plays a role in maintaining continence. In adults, the first urge to void is usually felt when there is 250 to 300 mL of urine accumulated in the bladder (Doig & Huether, 2014), with a strong urge at 500 mL. Structural damage to connecting pathways can result in loss of the ability to suppress the voiding reflex, resulting in urinary urgency incontinence (Birder et al., 2013).

Factors Influencing Urination

Many factors influence the volume and quality of urine and a person's ability to urinate (Box 43-1), including sociocultural, psychological, and pathophysiological conditions.

Common Alterations in Urinary Elimination

Most patients with urinary problems have disturbances in the act of micturition that involve a failure to store urine, a failure to empty urine, or both. Disturbances may be acute or chronic and result from infection, an overactive bladder, impaired contractility, obstruction to urine outflow, or inability to control micturition voluntarily due to mechanical or neural dysfunction.

Urinary Tract Infections. Urinary tract infection (UTI) can involve the lower urinary tract, causing cystitis, urethritis, and, in males, prostatitis. Women are more susceptible to infection because of the short urethra and the proximity of the rectum to the urethral meatus. Risk factors for UTI in women include sexual activity, pregnancy, diaphragm or spermicide use, and low vaginal estrogen level in postmenopausal women (Barber, Norton, Spivak, et al., 2013). Other causes of UTI can include obstruction of the urinary tract (e.g., benign prostatic hyperplasia in men, or pelvic organ prolapse in women), incomplete bladder emptying, and abnormal anatomy. Older persons, patients using antibiotics, and patients with progressive underlying disease or decreased immunity are also at increased risk. UTI can spread to the upper tract, causing kidney infection (**pyelonephritis**) and possibly long-term kidney damage. Bacteria can also spread to the bloodstream (**bacteremia**), leading to urosepsis. It is important to know that not all **bacteriuria** (bacteria in the urine) causes infection. *Asymptomatic* bacteriuria is the presence of bacteria but no symptoms of UTI and should not be treated with antibiotics (Mody & Juthani-Mehta, 2014).

Patients with lower UTIs may experience pain or a burning sensation during urination (**dysuria**). Fever, chills, nausea, vomiting, and malaise may develop as the infection worsens. Inflammation of the bladder (**cystitis**) causes a frequent and urgent sensation of the need

BOX 43-1 Factors Influencing Urinary Elimination

Psychological Factors

- Anxiety and emotional stress may cause a sense of urgency and increased frequency of urination.
- Anxiety also may prevent a person from being able to urinate because of inhibited relaxation of perineal muscles and urinary sphincter. Attempting to void in a public restroom also may result in a temporary inability to urinate.
- Privacy and adequate time to urinate are important to most people.

Sociocultural Factors

- Cultural, gender and religious practices vary and can influence voiding habits.
- Transportation, cost, and language barriers may limit access to services for chronic conditions, including urinary incontinence, for newcomers to Canada (Harrington, Wilson, Rosenberg et al., 2013, p. 6) and those in rural and remote communities, including some Indigenous groups.
- Cultural practices such as female genital cutting, practised in sub-Saharan Africa and Egypt, can lead to obstetrical complications as well as difficulty voiding, urinary tract infections, and chronic pain (Perron, Senikas, Burnett, et al., 2013, p. 1029), and health care providers need to avoid stigmatizing these women.

Fluid Balance

- If fluids and the concentration of electrolytes and solutes are in equilibrium, an increase in fluid intake causes an increase in urine production.
- Drinks that contain caffeine promote increased urine formation (diuresis).
- Alcohol inhibits the release of antidiuretic hormone (ADH), resulting in increased urine production.

Diagnostic Examination

- Diagnostic examinations (i.e., cystoscopy) that involve instrumentation of the bladder may cause short-term urethra trauma and hematuria.
- Instrumentation (e.g., catheterization) of the urinary tract increases risk of infection.

Surgical Procedures

- Postoperative urinary retention (POUR) can occur after receiving anaesthetic. Increasing age and female gender are also risk factors for POUR (Wu, Auerbach, & Aaronson, 2012).
- Some modes of postoperative pain control, such as nurse- or patient-controlled epidural analgesia, are associated with higher rates of POUR than are newer approaches, including continuous local anaesthetic wound infiltration (Ventham, Hughes, O'Neill, et al., 2013).
- Surgery involving lower abdominal and pelvic structures can impair urination because of local trauma to surrounding tissues.

Pathological Conditions

- Conditions affecting the central nervous system (stroke, multiple sclerosis, Parkinson's disease, dementia) can result in the inability to suppress the voiding reflex, resulting in urgency and urgency incontinence.
- Neurological disease, including diabetes and multiple sclerosis, may also affect peripheral nerve function and result in impaired contractility and poor bladder emptying.
- Spinal cord injury above the lumbar region can result in detrusor sphincter dyssynergia (poor emptying as the sphincter contracts with the bladder). Persons with injury at or above the sixth thoracic vertebrae are at risk for life-threatening hypertension (autonomic dysreflexia), which can be triggered by bladder distension (Boss & Huether, 2014, p. 593).
- People with advanced dementia often experience difficulties with object recognition (agnosia), task performance (apraxia), and wayfinding (visuospatial challenges), which can affect independent toileting and continence.
- Conditions that slow or hinder mobility (e.g., arthritis, Parkinson's disease) also interfere with being able to get to the toilet or remove clothing.
- Urine volume and quality are affected by prerenal (e.g., dehydration, hemorrhage), renal (e.g., diabetes-related kidney disease), and postrenal (e.g., obstructed urine flow from renal calculi or benign prostatic hyperplasia) factors.

Medications

- Diuretics prevent reabsorption of water and certain electrolytes, increasing urine output.
- Many drugs (e.g., bladder antimuscarinics, antidepressants) have anticholinergic adverse effects which can inhibit contractility, resulting in urinary retention.
- Other drugs (amlodipine) can cause peripheral edema, resulting in increased nocturia (nighttime voids).
- Hypnotics, sedatives, and opioids may decrease alertness and the ability to recognize the need to void.

to void and may cause incontinence. Irritation to bladder and urethral mucosa results in blood-tinged urine (hematuria). Cloudy, foul-smelling urine, or a change in urine colour, in the absence of other symptoms, does not indicate infection. Some foods (e.g., beets, blackberries) and medications (e.g., rifampin, phenazopyridine, and senna) can darken or discolour urine or cause an odour (e.g., from asparagus) (Pagana & Pagana, 2013). If infection spreads to the upper urinary tract (i.e., to the kidneys, causing pyelonephritis), rapid onset of flank or lower back pain, tenderness, fever, and chills can occur.

In Canada, UTIs are among the most common health care–associated infections, with the majority of these UTIs attributed to in-dwelling urinary catheters (Canadian Patient Safety Institute, 2016). Catheter-associated UTI (CAUTI) results in additional hospital days, morbidity, and mortality for patients. The trend in Canada is to reduce unnecessary use of in-dwelling catheters in all settings and remove them as soon as clinically indicated. Common accepted indications for insertion of a urinary catheter are in Table 43-1. Catheters should never be inserted for nursing convenience. The most common organism associated with CAUTI is *Escherichia coli*, although other bacteria can lead to infection (Nicolle, 2014). Bacteria ascend the catheter tubing, and shortly after a catheter is inserted a biofilm starts to form as organisms adhere to the catheter surface. As long as the catheter remains in the bladder, the biofilm remains and matures. Urease-producing bacteria can cause encrustation with a crystalline biofilm. The chance of CAUTI occurring increases each day that the catheter remains in place (Cottenden, Bliss, Buckley, et al., 2013), hence the focus on avoiding unnecessary catheterization and timely removal.

TABLE 43-1 Indications for Insertion of an In-Dwelling Urinary Catheter

Length of Catheterization	Indications
Short-term catheter (fewer than 14 days)	• Select surgical procedures/postoperative care (e.g., urological surgery, prolonged surgery) • Accurate monitoring of urine output every 1–2 hours in critically ill patients • Prolonged immobilization due to trauma • Acute urinary retention or bladder outlet obstruction • Instillation of medications into the bladder • End-of-life care *only if* required for comfort
Long-term catheter (more than 14 days)	• Bladder outlet obstruction pending surgery or if the patient is not suitable for surgical intervention • Chronic retention related to neurological disease if intermittent catheterization is not feasible • Stage 3 or 4 sacral pressure injury or perineal skin breakdown in incontinent patients • Intractable urinary incontinence if alternate approaches have been tried but not successful

Adapted from Lo, E., Nicolle, L. E., Coffin, S. E., Gould, C., Maragakis, L. L., Meddings. J., et al. (2014). Strategies to prevent catheter-associated urinary tract infections in acute care hospitals: 2014 Update. *Infection Control and Hospital Epidemiology, 35*(5), 464–479. doi:10.1086/675718; Gould, C. V., Umscheid, C. A., Agarwal, R. K., Kuntz, G., Pegues, D. A., & the Healthcare Infection Control Practices Advisory Committee. (2010). Guideline for prevention of catheter-associated urinary tract infections 2009. *Infection Control and Hospital Epidemiology, 31*, 319–326.

Urinary Incontinence and Other Lower Urinary Tract Symptoms. Urinary incontinence (UI) is "any involuntary loss of urine" (Staskin, Kelleher, Bosch, et al., 2013, p. 363) and often occurs along with other lower urinary tract symptoms including storage (e.g., daytime frequency, nocturia, urgency), voiding (e.g., intermittent or slow stream, hesitancy), and postmicturition symptoms (e.g., postmicturition dribble). There are many types of UI (Table 43-2), including urgency, stress, mixed (urgency and stress), UI associated with chronic retention (previously called *overflow UI*), functional, and multifactorial. Stress UI is more common in women than in men but changes to mixed UI with aging. Men also experience more UI with aging, usually the urgency type. Overactive bladder (OAB) syndrome includes bladder urgency, often with increased frequency and nocturia, and may or may not include urgency UI. OAB occurs in the absence of obvious pathology or UTI (Staskin et al., 2013, p. 364). Urgency UI has been identified as one of the most bothersome symptoms for individuals (Agarwal, Eryuzlu, Cartwright, et al., 2014). In Canada, at least 7% of women and 3.5% of men have daily moderate-to-severe incontinence, with an estimated cost of $8.5 billion dollars to individuals, employers, and the health care system (Canadian Continence Foundation, 2014). Psychosocial impact ranges from minor lifestyle changes to stigma, embarrassment, and self-imposed social isolation.

> **Safety Alert** Continued episodes of incontinence create the potential for skin breakdown. The immobilized patient who experiences frequent incontinence is especially at risk for pressure injuries (see Chapter 46). Timely and meticulous skin care is essential.

Nocturia. Nocturia is a prevalent and bothersome lower urinary tract symptom defined as waking from sleep one or more times to void and has been associated with increased mortality (Bergman, Sih, & Weiss, 2015). Prevalence of nocturia increases with age and is seen in multiple conditions, including OAB, prostate enlargement (men), excess urine production at night (nocturnal polyuria) associated with peripheral edema in heart failure, obstructive sleep apnea, and loss of arginine vasopressin (antidiuretic hormone) circadian rhythm. Polyuria can also occur in metabolic imbalances such as hyperglycemia and hypercalcemia.

Regardless of the cause, it is important to learn whether a patient wakes at night to void, or voids because he or she is awake. Assessment includes evaluation of lower urinary tract symptoms, post-void residual urine, and a bladder diary with 24-hour urine output (time and volume of each void). Treatment options may include reducing fluid intake in the evening, elevating the feet for 1 to 2 hours before bedtime to encourage return of fluid from the lower extremities, medication to reduce the volume of urine produced overnight, or medication to relax the bladder muscle.

> **Safety Alert** Micturition syncope is a type of situational syncope that is reflex mediated and triggered by micturition and defecation, leading to a slow heart rate and hypotension resulting in transient loss of consciousness. Dehydration, fatigue, and medical illness are thought to play a role. To avoid injury, at-risk patients should be cautioned to sit when voiding and not to stand up suddenly.

Urinary Retention. Urinary retention is the marked accumulation of urine in the bladder as a result of the bladder's inability to empty. Normally, urine production slowly fills the bladder and prevents activation of stretch receptors until the bladder distends to a certain extent. The micturition reflex then occurs, and the bladder

TABLE 43-2 Types of Urinary Incontinence

Definition	Causes/Risk Factors	Common Interventions
Transient Urinary Incontinence (UI): Urine loss resulting from causes outside of or affecting the urinary system, that resolves when the underlying causes are treated	DISAPPEAR (Northwood & Whytock, 2014) • *D*elirium • *I*ntake of fluids • *S*tool impaction • *A*trophic vaginitis • *P*sychological problems (depression) • *P*harmaceuticals • *E*xcess urine output • *A*bnormal lab values (e.g., hyperglycemia) • *R*estricted mobility	Identify and treat the underlying cause. Conservative: supportive measures such as fluid and bowel management, toileting assistance, containment pads if required Pharmacological: medication review and appropriate adjustment by prescriber. Women with atrophic vaginitis may benefit from low-dose vaginal estrogen.
Urgency UI: Urine loss associated with or immediately preceded by a sudden and urgent need to void that cannot be postponed. Can be part of overactive bladder (OAB) syndrome	Central nervous system disorders (dementia, cerebrovascular accident, Parkinson's disease, multiple sclerosis) and outflow obstruction, particularly in men with an enlarged prostate	Conservative: fluid and bowel management, caffeine reduction, pelvic floor muscles exercises (PFMEs), scheduled voiding regimes, urgency suppression and bladder retraining Pharmacological: bladder antimuscarinic agents (e.g., oxybutynin, tolterodine, solifenacin, fesoterodine) or β-3 adrenoreceptor agonist agent (mirabegron) Surgical/Invasive: injection of botulinum toxin into bladder, sacral nerve stimulation
Stress UI: Urine loss resulting from increased intra-abdominal pressure (e.g., coughing, sneezing, laughing, lifting)	Most common in women (poor sphincter closure), but can occur in men after radical prostatectomy. Risk factors in women include obesity, number of deliveries, ethnicity (White women are at greater risk), weakness of the pelvic floor, heavy lifting, and prior hysterectomy.	Conservative: lifestyle strategies (weight loss, fluid and bowel management, smoking cessation, caffeine reduction), PFMEs, pessary Pharmaceutical: serotonin-norepinephrine reuptake inhibitor in women (duloxetine) Surgical: in women, urethral bulking, tapes and slings, colposuspension; artificial sphincter in men
Mixed UI: Urine loss that has features of both stress and urge incontinence		Combinations of urgency and stress UI interventions
UI associated with chronic retention of urine (previously overflow UI): Involuntary loss of urine when the bladder does not completely empty with a high residual urine volume or a palpable nonpainful bladder remaining after voiding	Bladder outlet obstruction from prostate enlargement, or pelvic organ prolapse (POP) or fecal impaction Poor contractility of the bladder (detrusor) muscles seen in neurological conditions (e.g. diabetes, spinal cord injury). Spinal lesions C2–T12 can result in a hyperreflexive bladder with loss of coordination between bladder contraction (dyssenergia). Lesions below S1 can lead to an areflexive bladder and poor emptying (Doig & Huether, 2014, p. 1345).	Conservative: fluid and bowel management, scheduled voiding regimes (e.g., timed voiding), double voiding, intermittent catheterization, in-dwelling urinary catheter (last resort) Pharmaceutical: outlet obstruction in men: α-antagonists (tamsulosin, terazosin), 5-α reductase inhibitors (dutasteride, finasteride) Surgical: prostate surgery, intraurethral stent, botulinum toxin to detrusor
Functional UI: Urine loss due to inability to reach the toilet	Cognitive, physical function or mobility impairments	Conservative: timed toileting (scheduled or prompted voiding), containment products (e.g., pads, condom catheter)—supplementary but not a substitute for toileting assistance
Multifactorial UI: Urine loss due to multiple interacting factors both inside and outside the urinary tract	Comorbid conditions, medications, age-related changes, and environmental factors (e.g., bathroom access)	Treatment of comorbid conditions, assessment of environment and provision of equipment (e.g., commode), containment products (e.g., pads, condom catheter)

empties. With urinary retention, the bladder becomes unable to respond to the micturition reflex and thus is unable to empty. Urine continues to collect in the bladder, causing feelings of pressure, discomfort, tenderness over the symphysis pubis, restlessness, and diaphoresis. As retention progresses, overflow incontinence may occur. Pressure in the bladder builds to a point at which the urethral sphincter is unable to hold back urine and a small volume escapes. Urinary retention results from an underactive or acontractile detrusor muscle or urethral obstruction. Acute urinary retention can occur postpartum or following urogenital surgery, as a result of medication adverse effects (e.g., anticholinergic adverse effects), or from fecal impaction. Postoperative urinary retention (POUR), a type of acute urinary retention, occurs most frequently following orthopedic, genitourinary, and rectal surgery (Steggall, 2013), with risk factors including older age, prolonged surgery, type of anaesthesia, and sedating medications. Chronic urinary retention can occur in men with prostate enlargement and in women with pelvic organ prolapse, urethral stricture, or in conditions that alter motor and sensory innervation of the bladder.

Key signs of acute urinary retention are absence of urine output over several hours, bladder distension, restlessness, diaphoresis, and moderate-to-extreme abdominal discomfort. A patient under the influence of anaesthetics or analgesics may feel only pressure, but an alert patient experiences severe pain as the bladder distends beyond its normal capacity. A person with chronic urinary retention may not be aware of the overfull bladder. In severe urinary retention, the bladder may hold a litre or more of urine, well over the normal capacity of 400–600 mL. Intermittent catheterization may be needed to empty the bladder and reduce the risk of overflow incontinence and UTI.

> **Safety Alert** In individuals with spinal cord injury at the T5–T6 level or above, bladder distension can be a cause of autonomic dysreflexia. The intact sympathetic nervous system below the spinal lesion triggers a sympathetic response resulting in vasoconstriction and hypertension that can be life threatening (Boss & Huether, 2014, p. 593).

Urinary Diversions. A urinary stoma to divert the flow of urine from the kidneys directly to the abdominal surface is created for several reasons, including cancer of the bladder, trauma, radiation injury to the bladder, fistulas, and chronic cystitis. A urinary diversion may be temporary or permanent. The patient with an incontinent urinary diversion must wear an ostomy appliance continuously because no sphincter control exists to regulate urine flow. Local irritation and skin breakdown occur when urine comes in contact with the skin for long periods. Figure 43-2 illustrates two approaches to urinary diversion.

The ileal loop or conduit involves separating a loop of intestinal ileum with its blood supply intact. The ureters are implanted into the isolated segment of ileum, with the remaining ileum reconnected. The isolated ileal segment can then be used as a conduit for continuous urine drainage or fashioned into a continent reservoir (Konety, Barbour, & Carroll, 2013). The continent pouch provides urinary storage in a leak-proof pouch. A portion connected to the abdominal wall acts as a continent nipple, and intermittent catheterization is therefore needed for emptying. The disadvantage of an ileal conduit or reservoir is that if urine outflow becomes obstructed, irreversible damage to the kidneys can occur secondary to chronic infections or hydronephrosis.

A **ureterostomy** involves bringing the end of one or both ureters to the abdominal surface. To avoid the need for two collecting devices, a transureteroureterostomy connects the ureters and brings one out through the abdominal wall. In some cases, a tube may need to be placed directly into the renal pelvis to provide urinary drainage. This procedure is called a **nephrostomy** (Figure 43-3).

It is essential that stoma appliances fit correctly, that the patient (or caregiver) is capable of changing the appliance easily, and that skin around the stoma remains protected and intact. Unprotected skin that comes in contact with urine will quickly become macerated and break down, causing pain, infection, increased hospital stays, and potential breakdown of the stoma. All patients must be referred to an enterostomal nurse for preoperative stoma fitting and assessment and should be followed closely for several months postoperatively. The patient should also be referred to the United Ostomy Association of Canada, an invaluable source of advice and networking.

A urinary diversion poses threats to a patient's body image, and adjustment to it takes time. Although a normal lifestyle is possible with a stoma, adjustment can be difficult and each person will cope differently.

Renal Failure. Irreversible damage to the glomeruli or renal tubules causes decline in kidney function and leads to end-stage renal disease. In end-stage disease, there is severely reduced or absent urine output from the bladder, and metabolic disturbances result

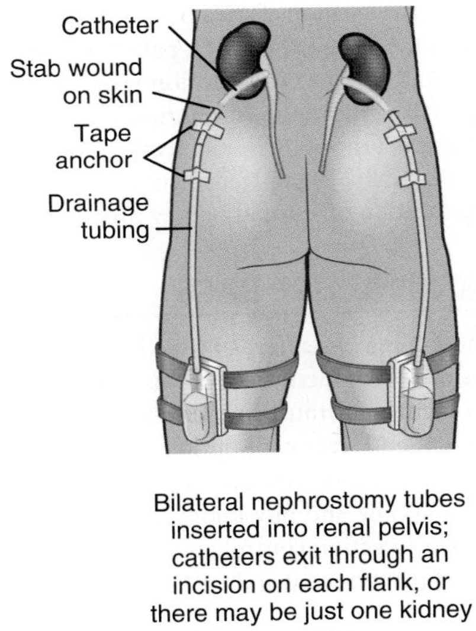

FIGURE 43-3 Nephrostomy tubes.

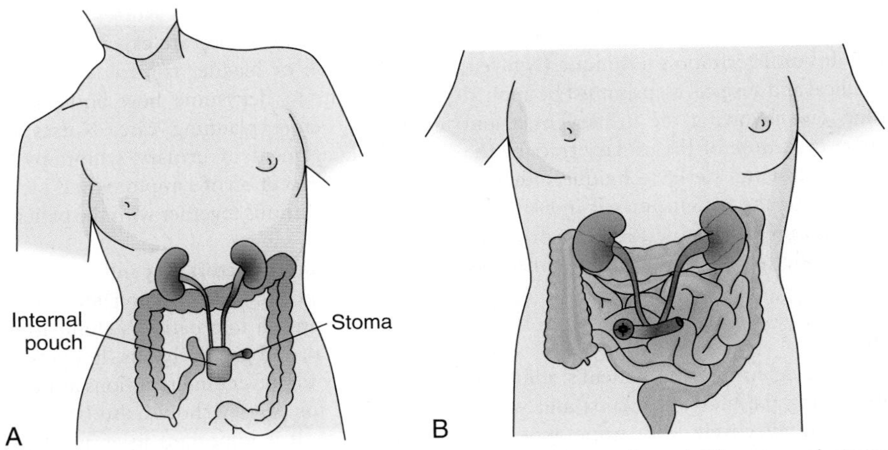

FIGURE 43-2 Types of urinary diversions: (A) Internal pouch and (B) external stoma.

in uremic syndrome, including increased nitrogenous wastes in the blood, altered regulatory functions causing marked fluid and electrolyte abnormalities, nausea, vomiting, headache, coma, and risk of convulsions. The condition may be managed conservatively with medications and a regimen of dietary and fluid restrictions. Severe disease requires renal replacement therapy, either dialysis or organ transplantation. Dialysis may take one of two forms: peritoneal or hemodialysis. Both dialysis modalities can be applied for a short or long time, but specialized equipment and nurses with specific training must be available.

Peritoneal dialysis is an indirect method of cleaning the blood of waste products and excess fluid using osmosis and diffusion. The peritoneum functions as a semipermeable membrane for the procedure. A sterile electrolyte solution (dialysate) is instilled into the peritoneal cavity by gravity via a surgically placed catheter. The dialysate is left in the cavity for a prescribed time interval and then drained out by gravity. Hemodialysis involves using a machine equipped with a semipermeable filtering membrane (artificial kidney) that removes accumulated waste products and excess fluids from the blood. Dialysate fluid is pumped through one side of the filter membrane (artificial kidney) while the patient's blood passes through the other side. The processes of diffusion, osmosis, and ultrafiltration clean the patient's blood, which is returned through a specially placed vascular access device such as an arteriovenous fistula or hemodialysis catheter. Organ transplantation is the replacement of a patient's diseased kidney with a healthy one from a living or cadaver donor of compatible blood and tissue type. Special medications (immunosuppressives) are administered for life to prevent the body from rejecting the transplanted organ. Unlike dialysis, successful organ transplantation offers the patient the potential for restoration of normal kidney function.

NURSING KNOWLEDGE BASE

Urinary elimination is a basic human function that is usually a private process. Nurses are often the first to become aware that a patient has elimination problems and must be alert to cues, prepared to discuss relevant assessment and treatment options, and able to provide counselling and support. These skills require a sound base of scientific knowledge related to anatomy and physiology, as well as an understanding of concepts such as infection control and hygiene, normal growth and development, and psychosocial and cultural considerations.

Infection Control and Hygiene

The urinary tract is considered to be sterile. Nurses must use infection-control principles to help prevent the development and spread of UTIs, as well as to treat existing infections (see Chapter 33). Hospital-acquired UTIs are often related to poor hand hygiene, improper catheter care, or faulty catheterization technique (Nguyen, 2013). Knowledge of both medical and surgical asepsis must be applied meticulously when providing care involving the urinary tract and external genitalia. Any invasive procedure of the urinary tract by the nurse, such as catheterization, necessitates sterile technique, although clean technique may be practised by the patient for self-intermittent catheterization in the home. Procedures such as perineal care or examination of the genitalia must be undertaken with care to minimize risk of infection.

Growth and Development

Growth and development factors determine the patient's ability to control the act of urination during the lifespan. Infants and young children cannot concentrate urine effectively, with urine appearing light yellow and clear.

Relative to their body size, infants and children excrete large volumes of urine. For example, a 6-month-old infant who weighs 6 to 8 kg excretes 400 to 500 mL of urine daily. As the neurological system matures, a toddler of 2 to 3 years of age is able to associate the sensations of bladder filling and urination. A child must be able to recognize the feeling of bladder fullness, hold urine for 1 to 2 hours, and communicate the sense of urgency to an adult. Many toddlers may then be able to control the urethral sphincter, and toilet training can begin. Young children need their parents' understanding, patience, and consistency. A child may not gain full control of micturition until 4 or 5 years of age. Daytime control of micturition is easier to accomplish than nighttime control and occurs earlier in the child's development, usually by 2 years of age. Occasional daytime accidents or nocturnal enuresis (bedwetting) may continue until 5 years of age.

The adult normally voids 1 500 to 1 600 mL of urine daily, or approximately 500 mL every 4 hours. During pregnancy, urinary frequency is common and susceptibility to UTIs is increased. In women, child-bearing and hormonal changes during menopause may contribute to urinary difficulties. In men, prostate enlargement can begin in the 40s and continue throughout the lifespan, resulting in urinary frequency and possibly retention.

Changes in kidney and bladder function also occur with aging. The kidney's ability to concentrate urine or reabsorb water and sodium declines. Alterations in kidney function include a reduction in glomerular filtration rate, from 125 mL per minute in younger adults to 60 to 70 mL per minute in adults 80 years of age. The older person often experiences nocturia, due in part to age-related changes in vasopressin secretion (Wagg, Chen, Kirschner-Hermanns, et al., 2013). The functional capacity of the bladder decreases, resulting in increased urinary frequency. Detrusor contractility also decreases, contributing to less effective emptying, elevated **postvoid residuals (PVRs)** (the volume remaining in the bladder after a void), and increased susceptibility to UTI. A decrease in urethral closure pressure in women, which is generally associated with a decline in estrogen levels, can contribute to an increase in incontinence (Wagg et al., 2013). Older men commonly experience incomplete bladder emptying associated with prostatic enlargement.

Psychosocial and Cultural Considerations

Nurses must consider that urinary elimination problems may result in alterations of sexuality and self-concept (which includes body image, self-esteem, roles, and identity). The embarrassment associated with elimination problems may delay or prevent seeking help. Individuals with incontinence often blame themselves for their condition and go to great lengths, including self-imposed social isolation, to keep others from finding out about it. Nurses must therefore initiate discussion by asking patients if they are experiencing any issues related to urinary elimination or bladder control, as a routine part of care. It is also important to determine how bothersome symptoms are for each patient before planning care. Nurses have a role in promoting self-management of urinary symptoms through understanding the patient's perception of symptoms and identifying effective and acceptable interventions together with the patient (Wilde, Bliss, Booth, et al., 2014).

Sociocultural factors may influence the patient's expectation of the degree of privacy and location for attending to urinary needs. The nurse's approach to a patient's elimination needs must consider cultural, social, and gender habits. If a patient prefers privacy, the nurse should try to prevent interruptions as the patient voids. A patient with less need for privacy should also be treated with understanding and acceptance. It is important to ensure that the patient is comfortable when he or she is trying to void. In some cultures, people prefer to squat over a receptacle rather than sit on one. Culture dictates when and where it is appropriate to urinate. In some cultures, a woman with urinary needs should be assisted only by another woman.

CRITICAL THINKING

Critical thinking during assessment of urinary elimination requires the integration of evidence-informed knowledge from nursing and other disciplines, experiential knowledge, and an understanding of the patient's perceptions of the alterations in elimination and their impact. Critical thinking also involves an understanding of relevant cultural, environmental, and personal factors, including the unique goals of every patient. Empathy, teaching, and ongoing support are needed to assist the patient in meeting these goals and maintaining improvement. In Canada, little research has been undertaken to understand urinary symptoms and problems among Indigenous groups, in spite of the prevalence of risk factors such as diabetes in these populations. Moving forward, partnerships with Indigenous people need to be formed, in order to gain better understanding and address urinary health needs.

Professional standards provide valuable directions for treatment and management of elimination problems. When planning and implementing care for patients with alterations in urinary elimination, nurses need to use standards developed by professional organizations, such as the Canadian Nurse Continence Advisors Association, the Canadian Continence Foundation, the United Ostomy Association of Canada, and the Urology Nurses of Canada.

❖ NURSING PROCESS AND ALTERATIONS IN URINARY FUNCTION

◆ Assessment

In order to identify a urinary elimination problem and gather data for a care plan, nurses obtain information by collecting a health history, performing a focused physical assessment, assessing the patient's urine, and reviewing information from diagnostic tests and examinations. Nurses use critical thinking to synthesize this information as assessment proceeds (Figure 43-4). Adequate assessment should result in the formulation of nursing diagnoses appropriate for alterations in urinary elimination. Nurses should be alert to individual needs related to normal aging that predispose older persons to certain elimination problems (Box 43-2).

Health History. The nursing health history includes a review of the patient's urinary elimination pattern and lower urinary tract

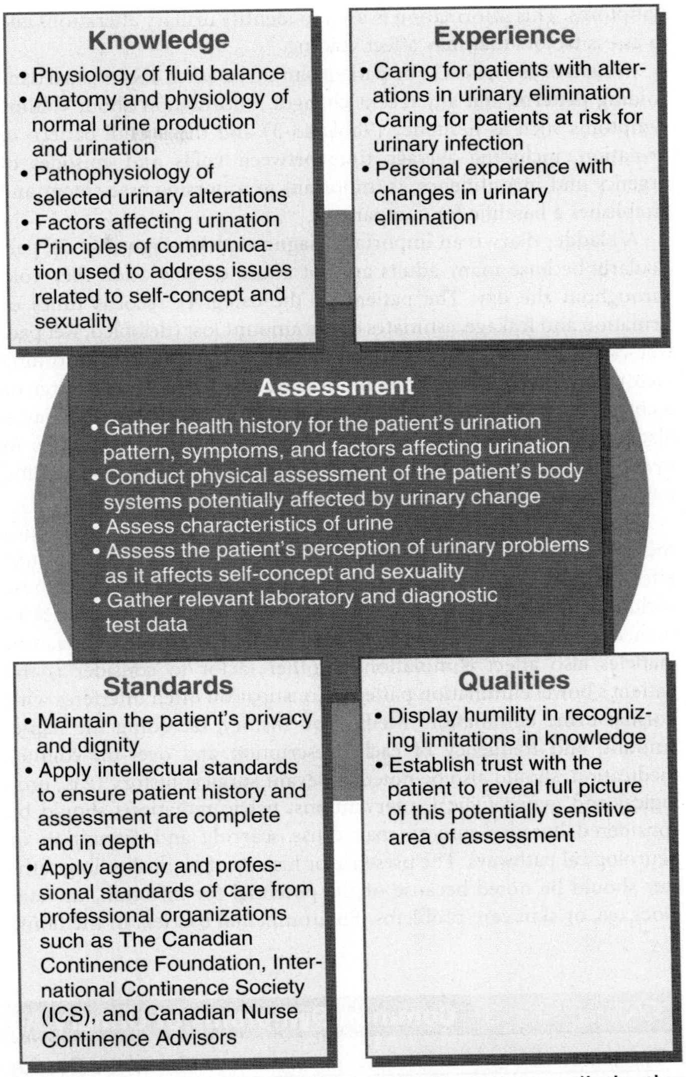

FIGURE 43-4 Critical thinking model for urinary elimination assessment.

BOX 43-2 FOCUS ON OLDER PERSONS

Physiological Changes Associated With Urinary Problems

- Physiological changes in the lower urinary tract occur in continent as well as incontinent older persons.
- Dilute urine discourages bacterial growth; therefore, older persons should be encouraged to increase their fluid intake to at least six glasses a day, unless medically contraindicated (Wagg et al., 2013).
- Cranberries can prevent bacteria from adhering to the bladder wall, and cranberry products may help reduce recurrent urinary tract infections in women, although a systematic review found the effect smaller than previously identified. Many people stop using the juice as they do not like the taste, and cranberry extract tablets and capsules were found ineffective (Jepson, Williams, & Craig, 2012).
- Restriction of fluids 2 hours before sleep, combined with elevating the legs to allow for venous return and bladder emptying before bedtime (leg elevation for at least 1 hour), may decrease the incidence of nocturia (Wagg et al., 2013).
- In-dwelling catheters should not be used routinely in older persons unless other options have been tried. The risk of infection increases dramatically for catheterized patients (Wagg et al., 2013).
- Treating asymptomatic bacteriuria in older persons is not recommended.
- Incontinence is not a normal part of aging, and efforts should be made to assess incontinence and provide interventions to promote return to continence.

symptoms. This information is used to identify urinary alterations and to assess factors that may affect voiding.

Pattern of Urination. The patient should be asked about usual daily voiding patterns and any recent changes. Information about voiding symptoms such as hesitancy (Table 43-3) and the overall pattern of urination, including average time between voids and episodes of urgency and incontinence, is important to a nursing assessment and establishes a baseline for comparison.

A bladder diary is an important diagnostic tool (Figure 43-5), particularly because many adults are not aware of how often they void throughout the day. The patient or the caregiver records times of urination and leakage, estimates of the amount lost (dribbled, wet pad, wet clothing), and types and amount of fluids ingested. Recording factors that precipitated urination or leakage, such as a strong urge or a cough, is particularly helpful. The number of pad changes per day is also useful information. A 3-day (72-hour) voiding diary helps in evaluating lifestyle habits (e.g., fluid intake) in relation to the voiding pattern and symptoms (Canadian Continence Foundation, 2014).

Factors Affecting Urination. The nurse must consider the patient's medical history, surgical history, and current environment that may affect urination. Many medical conditions can affect voiding. These include acute conditions such as infection or trauma. Chronic diseases such as multiple sclerosis, spinal cord injury, stroke, dementia, and diabetes also affect elimination. Another factor to consider is the patient's bowel elimination pattern. Constipation often interferes with normal urine elimination. Medication history, including the name, amount, and frequency of each prescription and over-the-counter medication, should also be noted. Relevant surgical history (e.g., urological and gynecological interventions, pelvic radiation) should be considered because surgery may cause scarring and disruption of neurological pathways. The presence or history of an in-dwelling catheter should be noted because of the potential for infection, catheter blockage, or skin care problems. Environmental barriers in the home or health care setting also should be evaluated. The nurse needs to assess the patient's mobility and ability to dress or undress and use the toilet independently. Such aids as elevated toilet seats, grab bars, or a portable commode may be needed.

One of the most important parts of the assessment is the impact of alterations in elimination on the patient's lifestyle and quality of life. The impact of urinary incontinence in particular can be substantial; it is important to discuss changes the patient has made to cope with the condition. It is also important to note whether the patient has previously seen a health care provider for help with or advice on urination.

Physical Assessment. A physical examination (see Chapter 32) provides nurses with data with which they can determine the presence and severity of urinary elimination problems. The primary structures reviewed are the skin and mucosal membranes of the perineum, urethral and vaginal orifices, bladder (by palpation), and rectum.

Skin and Mucosal Membranes. The nurse assesses the condition of the skin and mucosal membranes. Problems with urinary elimination are often associated with fluid and electrolyte disturbances. By assessing skin turgor and the oral mucosa, the nurse is assessing the patient's hydration status. Urinary incontinence increases the risk of skin breakdown (see Chapter 46).

Kidneys. Flank pain usually develops if the kidneys become infected or inflamed. The nurse can assess for flank tenderness early in the disease by percussing the costovertebral angle (the angle formed by the spine and the twelfth rib). Auscultation is also performed to detect the presence of a renal artery bruit (sound resulting from turbulent blood flow through a narrowed artery).

Nurses with advanced examination skills learn to palpate the kidneys during abdominal examination. The kidneys' position, shape, and size can reveal renal swelling.

Bladder. In adults, the bladder rests below the symphysis pubis and is difficult to palpate. When distended, the bladder rises above the

TABLE 43-3 Common Symptoms of Urinary Alterations

Symptom	Common Causes or Associated Factors
Incontinence: Involuntary loss of urine	See Table 43-2
Urgency: Sudden and compelling urge to void that cannot be postponed	Overactive bladder syndrome that is neurogenic, sensory, or idiopathic; calculi or tumour; urinary tract infection (UTI)
Dysuria: Painful or difficult urination	Bladder inflammation; urethral trauma; UTI; inflammation of urethra, sphincter, or both
Frequency: Voiding more than eight times in 24 hours	Increased fluid intake, bladder infection or inflammation, increased pressure on bladder (pregnancy, psychological stress), incomplete emptying, small bladder capacity, overactive bladder syndrome, polyuria
Hesitancy: Difficulty initiating urination	Hypotonic bladder, anxiety, urethral stricture, obstruction associated with prostate enlargement
Polyuria: Voiding large amounts of urine	Excess fluid intake, diabetes mellitus or diabetes insipidus (hyperglycemia), diuretic use, nocturnal polyuria, postobstructive diuresis
Oliguria: Diminished urinary output relative to intake (usually 400 mL/24 hours)	Dehydration, renal failure, increased antidiuretic hormone (ADH) secretion
Nocturia: Getting up at night to void one or more times	Excessive fluid intake before bed (especially coffee or alcohol), renal disease, overactive bladder, heart failure with peripheral edema, prostate enlargement, sleep apnea
Dribbling: Leakage of urine despite voluntary control of urination	Stress incontinence, overflow from urinary retention, postvoid pooling of urine in the urethra (men)
Hematuria: Blood in the urine	Kidney or bladder neoplasms, renal disease, infection of kidney or bladder, trauma, calculi, bleeding disorders, UTI
Elevated postvoid residual urine	Neurogenic bladder, prostate enlargement, trauma, pelvic organ prolapse, inflammation or stricture of urethra

Bladder Diary DAY 1

TIME	AMOUNT URINATED		URGENCY?		LEAKAGE		DRINKS	
	How many times	How much	Yes	No	How many times	How much	Which drink	How much
EXAMPLE:	3 times		✓		once		water	1 cup
6-8 am								
8-10 am								
10-12 pm								
12-2 pm								
2-4 pm								
4-6 pm								
6-8 pm								
8-10 pm								
10-12 pm								
12-2 am								
2-4 am								
4-6 am								

A little Some A lot

Bladder Diary DAY 2

TIME	AMOUNT URINATED		URGENCY?		LEAKAGE		DRINKS	
	How many times	How much	Yes	No	How many times	How much	Which drink	How much
EXAMPLE:	3 times		✓		once		water	1 cup
6-8 am								
8-10 am								
10-12 pm								
12-2 pm								
2-4 pm								
4-6 pm								
6-8 pm								
8-10 pm								
10-12 pm								
12-2 am								
2-4 am								
4-6 am								

A little Some A lot

FIGURE 43-5 Sample urinary diary. (From Canadian Continence Foundation. [2016]. Retrieved from http://www.canadiancontinence.ca/pdfs/Bladder-Diary.pdf.)

symphysis pubis at the midline of the abdomen and may extend to just below the umbilicus. On inspection, a swelling or convex curvature of the lower abdomen may be noted. The nurse should lightly palpate the lower abdomen. The partially filled bladder normally feels smooth and rounded. As light pressure is applied to the bladder, the patient may feel the urge to urinate, tenderness, or even pain. Percussion of a full bladder yields a dull note.

The Female Perineum. When examining the female patient, the nurse requests that she assume a dorsal recumbent position to provide full exposure of the genitalia. The perineum is inspected for skin integrity and for the presence of a rash associated with incontinence and the use of containment pads. The rash may be monilial (maculopapular, red rash) or an ammonia contact perineal dermatitis (papular with macerated skin). The nurse needs to inspect the vaginal orifice carefully for signs of inflammation and describe any drainage.

Also, the urethral meatus should be assessed and the presence of any discharge, inflammation, or lesions noted. Normally, the meatus is pink and appears as a small, slitlike opening below the clitoris and above the vaginal orifice. It may recede well into the vaginal vault with aging, making catheterization difficult. Discharge from the meatus is normally not present. If it is present, specimens of urethral discharge should be obtained before the patient voids.

Speculum examination and assessment of pelvic floor strength in females are advanced skills. On speculum examination, the vagina can be assessed for pelvic organ prolapse, vaginal atrophy, and atrophic vaginitis, a common result of estrogen depletion after menopause. Signs of atrophy include dry, thin, pale mucosa with loss of rugae; a urethral caruncle (red urethral meatus) or red labia and vaginal walls indicate inflammation associated with vaginitis (Weber, Limpens, & Roovers, 2015). Pelvic floor muscle strength can be digitally assessed in women by gently inserting a gloved finger into the vagina. The examiner asks the patient to squeeze around the finger as firmly as possible, and then hold the contraction for up to 10 seconds. Digital assessment is very useful in helping the patient to identify the pelvic floor muscles correctly.

The Male Perineum. The male urethral meatus normally appears as a small opening at the tip of the penis. The nurse should inspect the meatus for any discharge, inflammation, or lesions. If the foreskin needs to be retracted in uncircumcised men to see the meatus, it must be replaced to avoid constriction of the glans. Disposable gloves should be worn when retracting the foreskin. Pelvic floor muscle strength can be digitally assessed in men by gently inserting a gloved finger into the rectum and asking the patient to squeeze around it.

Assessment of Urine. Assessment of urine involves measuring the patient's fluid intake and urine output and observing characteristics of the urine.

Intake and Output. It is important to assess the patient's average daily fluid intake. If an accurate measurement of fluid intake is needed from the patient who is at home, the nurse can ask him or her to show a commonly used glass or cup on which the intake estimate is based. In a health care setting, a patient's fluid intake is measured either when the prescriber orders intake and output measurements or when nursing judgement warrants a more precise measurement (see Chapter 40). A change in urine volume is a significant indicator of fluid alterations or kidney disease. While caring for the patient, the nurse assesses urine volume by measuring output with each voiding (using a urine hat, bedpans, or urinals) (Figure 43-6). Special receptacles (urometers) are attached between in-dwelling catheters and drainage bags and are a convenient means of accurately measuring urine volume (Figure 43-7). A urometer holds 100 to 200 mL of urine. After measuring urine with a urometer, the nurse drains the cylinder into the urinary drainage bag or into a receptacle for disposal. Urometers are indicated when precise hourly measurements of urine are needed.

When urine from a drainage bag is measured, the urine should be drained into a plastic graduated receptacle for more precise measurement of output (Figure 43-8). Each patient should have a graduated receptacle for his or her exclusive use to prevent potential cross-contamination.

Nurses should report any extreme increase or decrease in urine volume. An hourly output of less than 30 mL for more than 2 hours is cause for concern. Similarly, consistently high volumes of urine (polyuria), over 2 000 to 2 500 mL daily, should be reported to a physician.

Characteristics of Urine. During assessment the patient's urine is also inspected for colour, clarity, and odour.

Colour. Normal urine ranges from a pale, straw colour to amber, depending on its concentration. Urine is usually more concentrated in the morning or with fluid-volume deficits. As a person drinks more fluids, urine becomes less concentrated.

Bleeding from the kidneys or ureters causes dark red urine; bleeding from the bladder or urethra causes urine to become bright red. Various medications and foods also change urine colour and will cause a false positive on a urinalysis. For example, phenazopyridine, a urinary analgesic, colours the urine bright orange. Eating beets, rhubarb, or blackberries may cause red urine. Special dyes used in intravenous diagnostic studies also discolour urine. Dark amber urine may result from high concentrations of bilirubin caused by liver dysfunction or vitamin B. The nurse should document and report any abnormal colour or sediment, especially if the cause is unknown.

Clarity. Normal urine appears transparent at voiding, but may become cloudy if left standing. In patients with renal disease, urine may appear cloudy or foamy because of high protein concentrations. Urine also will appear thick and cloudy as a result of bacteria.

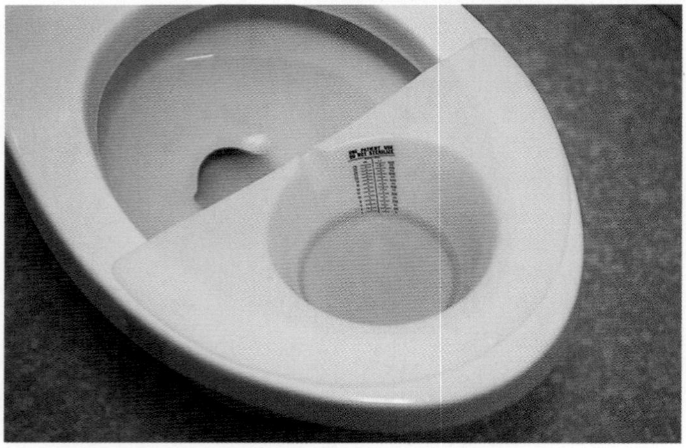

FIGURE 43-6 Urine hat.

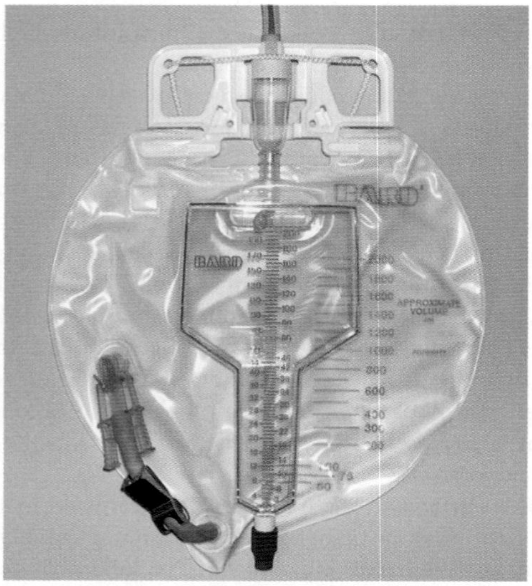

FIGURE 43-7 Urometer. (Courtesy Michael Gallagher, RN, BSN, OSF, Saint Francis Medical Center, Peoria, IL.)

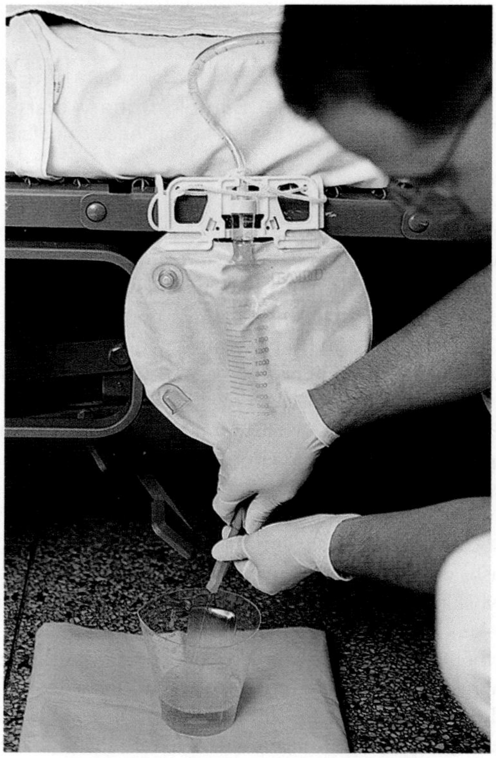

FIGURE 43-8 Urine drainage bag.

TABLE 43-4 Urine Testing

Collection Type (Use of Specimen)	Nursing Considerations
Random specimen (routine urinalysis or collection for other tests such as urine electrolytes)	Can be collected during normal voiding, from an in-dwelling catheter or a urinary diversion collection bag. Collected in a clean specimen cup.
Clean-voided or midstream specimen (culture and sensitivity)	See Skill 43-1. Collected in a sterile specimen cup.
Catheter specimen (culture and sensitivity and other tests)	If the patient has an in-dwelling catheter, a specimen can be collected using the aseptic technique through the special port (see Figure 43-9) found on the side of the catheter. When symptomatic CAUTI is suspected and the specimen is for culture and sensitivity, the catheter should be changed prior to specimen collection and initiation of antibiotics, as biofilm has likely formed on the old catheter (Nicolle, 2014). Clamp the tubing below the port, allowing fresh, uncontaminated urine to collect in the tube. After wiping the port with an antimicrobial swab, insert a sterile syringe tip and withdraw at least 3 to 5 mL of urine.
	Using the sterile aseptic technique, transfer the urine to a sterile container (see Chapter 33).
Timed urine specimens (for measuring levels of adrenal cortical steroids or hormones, creatinine clearance, or protein quantity tests)	Time required between collections may be 2, 12, or 24 hours. The timed period begins after the patient urinates and ends with a final voiding at the end of the time period. The patient voids into a clean receptacle, and the urine is transferred to the special collection container, which may contain special preservatives. Each specimen must be free of feces and toilet tissue. Missed specimens make the entire collection inaccurate. Check agency policy and with the laboratory for specific instructions.

CAUTI, Catheter-associated urinary tract infection.

Odour. Urine has a characteristic odour. The more concentrated the urine, the stronger the odour. Stagnant urine has an ammonia odour, which is common in patients who are repeatedly incontinent. A sweet or fruity odour occurs from acetone or acetoacetic acid (by-products of incomplete fat metabolism) seen with diabetes mellitus or starvation.

Urine Testing. It is common to collect urine specimens for laboratory testing (Table 43-4). The type of test being done determines the method of collection. All specimens are labelled with the patient's name, the date, and the time of collection. Specimens should be transported to the laboratory quickly to ensure accuracy of test results. Agency infection control policies require adherence to standard precautions or routine practices by all personnel during the handling of specimens (see Chapter 33).

Specimen collection. For specimen collection, the nurse collects random, clean-voided or midstream (Skill 43-1), sterile (Figure 43-9), and timed specimens.

Urine collection in children. Collecting specimens from infants and children is often difficult. School-aged children and adolescents are usually able to cooperate, although they may be embarrassed. Preschool children and toddlers have difficulty voiding on request. Offering a young child fluids 30 minutes before requesting a specimen may help. The nurse must use terms for urination that the child can understand. A young child may be reluctant to void in unfamiliar receptacles. A potty-chair or specimen hat placed under the toilet seat is usually effective. Special collection devices must be used for infants and toddlers who are not toilet trained. Clear plastic, single-use bags with self-adhering material can be attached over the child's urethral meatus. Specimens should not be obtained by squeezing urine from the diaper material because test results may be inaccurate.

Common Urine Tests

Urinalysis. The laboratory performs a urinalysis on a specimen obtained through any of the previously described methods. Table 43-5 lists normal values for a urinalysis. The specimen should be examined as soon as possible after it is collected, preferably within 2 hours. For

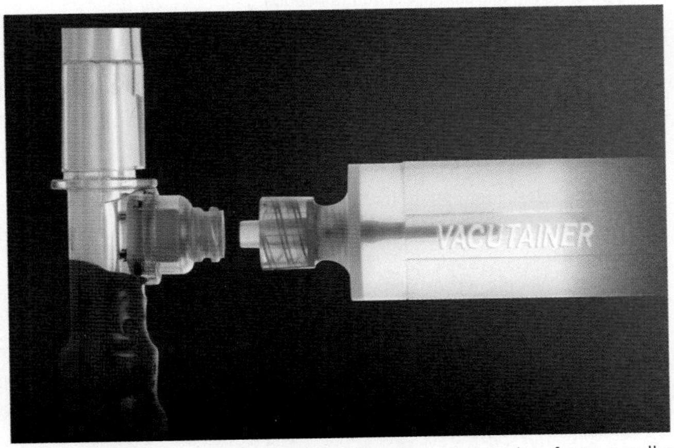

FIGURE 43-9 Urine specimen collection. Aspiration from a collection port in drainage tubing on an in-dwelling catheter (needleless technique). (Courtesy and © Becton, Dickinson and Company.)

protein, the first voided specimen in the morning is preferred, to ensure a uniform concentration of constituents (Pagana & Pagana, 2013). For a quick screening, the nurse can perform certain portions of the urinalysis with special reagent strips. The strip is dipped into the urine and observed for a colour change in the time interval designated on the package.

Specific gravity. The *specific gravity* is the weight or degree of concentration of a substance compared with an equal amount of water. A urine specimen is poured into a special dry, clean cylinder. The weighted urinometer is suspended in the cylinder of urine. The concentration of dissolved substances in the urine aids in the determination of a patient's fluid balance. This measurement is always done as part of a complete urinalysis. Nurses working in a Critical Care Unit may be responsible for doing periodic measurement of specific gravity of urine as part of a complete assessment of specific patients.

SKILL 43-1 COLLECTING A MIDSTREAM (CLEAN-VOIDED) URINE SPECIMEN

Delegation Considerations

Collecting a midstream (clean-voided) urine specimen may be delegated to unregulated care providers (UCPs). If appropriate, an alert patient who is physically able may be instructed to collect the specimen. It is the nurse's responsibility to ensure that this specimen is obtained correctly and in a timely manner. Be aware of agency policy regarding specimen collection.

Instruct the UCP to inform you of the following:

- When the specimen was obtained
- Whether the patient was unable to initiate a stream or had pain or burning on urination
- Whether the collected specimen is dark, bloody, or cloudy; is odorous; or contains mucus

Equipment

- Soap or cleaning solution, washcloth, towel, and handwashing basin
- Commercial kit for clean-voided specimen or individual supplies as listed
- Sterile cotton balls or sterile gauze pads
- Antiseptic solution (e.g., clorhexidine or providone-iodine) or sterile normal saline or water, as approved by agency; check for patient allergy, and if allergy exists, provide an alternative
- Sterile water
- Sterile specimen collection cup or jar
- Sterile and nonsterile (disposable) gloves
- Bedpan, bedside commode, or specimen hat
- Completed specimen label
- Completed laboratory requisition form

PROCEDURE

STEPS	RATIONALE
1. Assess voiding status of patient:	
A. When patient last voided	• May indicate readiness to void.
B. Level of awareness or developmental stage	• Reveals patient's ability to cooperate during procedure.
C. Mobility, balance, and physical limitations	• Determines level of assistance needed in acquiring specimen.
2. Assess patient's understanding of purpose of test and method of collection.	• Information allows for clarification and promotes patient cooperation.
3. Explain procedure to patient:	
A. Reason midstream specimen is needed	
B. Ways patient and family can assist	• Helps patient understand the procedure.
C. Ways to obtain specimen free of feces	• Feces change characteristics of urine and may cause abnormal values.
4. Provide fluids to drink a half-hour before collection unless contraindicated (i.e., fluid restriction) if patient does not feel urge to void.	• Improves likelihood of patient being able to void.
5. Identify patient and perform hand hygiene.	• Ensures accuracy of specimen collection. Decreases likelihood of transfer of microorganisms.
6. Provide privacy for patient by closing door or bed curtain.	• Privacy allows patient to relax and produce specimen more quickly.
7. Give patient or family members soap, washcloth, and towel to clean perineal area.	• Patient may prefer to wash own perineal area. Cleaning prevents contamination of specimen as urine passes from urethra.
8. Apply nonsterile gloves and assist nonambulatory patients with perineal care. Assist female patient onto bedpan. Raise head of bed.	• Provides easy access to perineal area to collect specimen. Semi-sitting position may ease voiding.
9. Using surgical asepsis, open sterile kit (see Step 9 illustration) if using one or prepare sterile supplies. Apply sterile gloves after opening sterile cup, placing cap with sterile inside surface up; do not touch inside of container or cap (see Chapter 33).	• The sterile technique is essential to maintain sterility of equipment and specimen. Sterile gloves prevent the transmission of microorganisms. A contaminated specimen is the most frequent reason for inaccurate reporting of urine cultures and sensitivities.

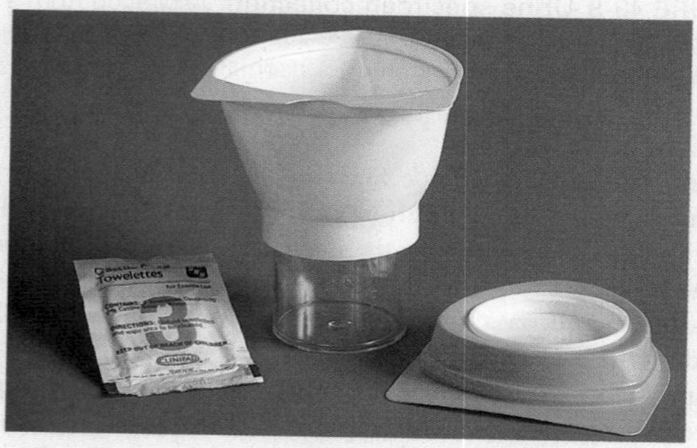

STEP 9 Commercial midstream urine collection kit.

STEPS	RATIONALE
10. Pour antiseptic solution over cotton balls or gauze pads unless kit contains prepared gauze pads in antiseptic solution.	• Cotton balls or gauze pads will be used to further clean the perineum.

STEPS	RATIONALE
11. Assist or allow patient to independently clean perineum and collect specimen:	
A. Female patient	
(1) Spread labia with thumb and forefinger of nondominant hand.	• Provides access to urethral meatus.
(2) Clean area with cotton ball or gauze and approved solution, moving from front (above urethral orifice) to back (toward anus; see Step 11A[2] illustration). Using a fresh swab each time, repeat front-to-back motion three times (begin left side, then right side, then centre).	• Clean from area of least contamination to area of greatest contamination to decrease bacterial levels.
(3) If agency policy indicates, rinse area with sterile water, and dry with cotton ball or gauze.	• Prevents contamination of specimen with antiseptic solution.
(4) While you or the patient continue holding labia apart, patient should initiate stream; after stream is achieved, pass container into stream and collect 30 to 60 mL (see Step 11A[4] illustration).	• Initial stream flushes out microorganisms that accumulate at the urethral meatus and prevents transfer into specimen.

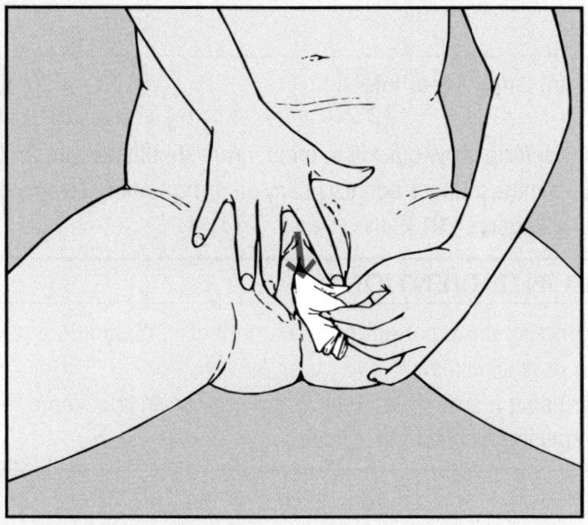

STEP 11A(2) Cleaning technique (female).

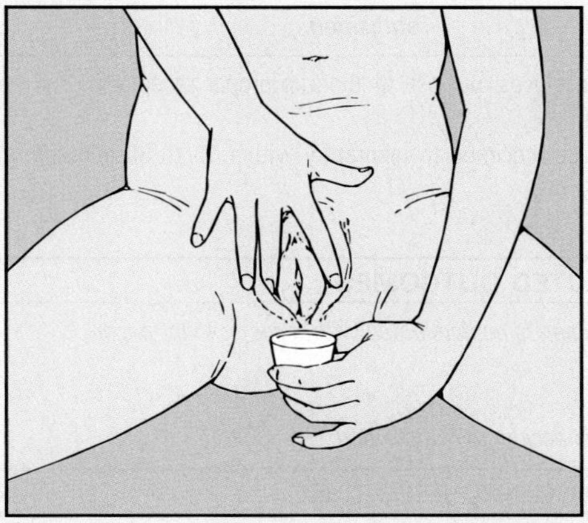

STEP 11A(4) Specimen collection (female).

STEPS	RATIONALE
B. Male patient	
(1) Hold patient's penis with one hand or have the patient hold his penis; using circular motion and antiseptic swab or cotton ball with approved solution, clean end of penis, moving from centre to outside (see Step 11B[1] illustration). In uncircumcised men, the foreskin should be retracted before cleaning.	• Clean from area of least contamination to area of greatest contamination to decrease bacterial levels.
(2) If agency procedure indicates, rinse area with sterile water, and dry with cotton ball or gauze.	• Prevents contamination of specimen with antiseptic solution.
(3) After patient has initiated urine stream, pass specimen collection container into stream and collect 30 to 60 mL (see Step 11B[3] illustration).	• Initial stream flushes out microorganisms that accumulate at the urethral meatus and prevents transfer into specimen. • The amount required to be collected may vary from agency to agency, depending on collection equipment and laboratory procedures.

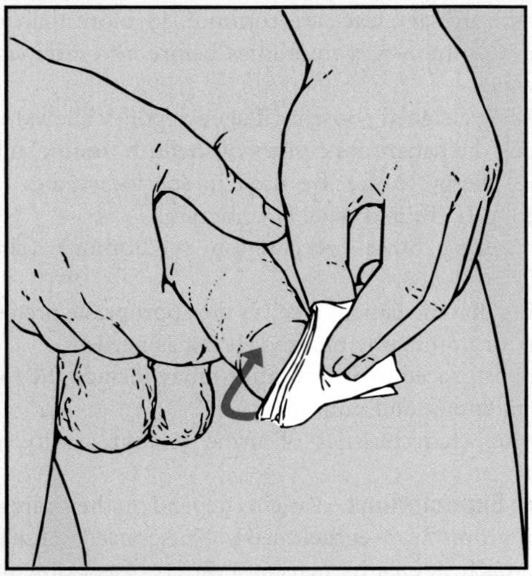

STEP 11B(1) Cleaning technique (male).

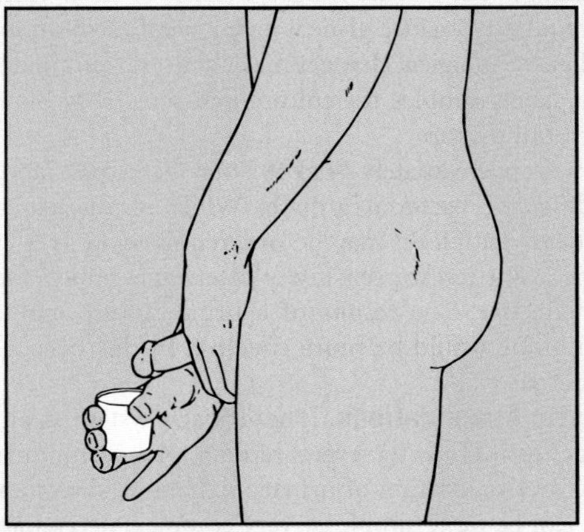

STEP 11B(3) Specimen collection (male).

Continued

SKILL 43-1 COLLECTING A MIDSTREAM (CLEAN-VOIDED) URINE SPECIMEN—cont'd

STEPS	RATIONALE
12. Remove specimen container before flow of urine stops and before releasing labia or penis. Patient finishes voiding in bedpan or toilet. If foreskin was retracted for specimen collection, it must be replaced over the glans.	• Prevents contamination of specimen with skin flora. If foreskin is not replaced, swelling and constriction may occur, causing pain and possible obstruction of urine flow.
13. Replace cap securely on specimen container (touch outside only).	• Retains sterility of inside of container and prevents spillage of urine.
14. Clean any urine from exterior surface of container, and place in a plastic specimen bag.	• Prevents transfer of microorganisms to others.
15. Remove bedpan (if applicable), assist patient to comfortable position, and provide handwashing basin if needed.	• Promotes relaxing environment.
16. Label specimen, and attach laboratory requisition.	• Prevents inaccurate identification that could lead to errors in diagnosis or treatment.

CRITICAL DECISION POINT: *If patient is menstruating, indicate this information on the laboratory requisition.*

STEPS	RATIONALE
17. Remove gloves, dispose of them in proper receptacle, and perform hand hygiene.	• Reduces transmission of infection.
18. Transport specimen to laboratory within 15 to 30 minutes or refrigerate immediately.	• Because bacteria grow quickly in urine, urine should be sent to the laboratory within 30 minutes. Check agency policy on refrigeration if transport is delayed. (Pagana & Pagana, 2013).

UNEXPECTED OUTCOMES	RELATED INTERVENTIONS
Urine specimen is contaminated with feces or toilet paper	• Repeat instruction to patient or assist patient in obtaining a new specimen. • Obtain a new specimen. • Consider using a straight catheterization to obtain specimen.
Specimen is accidentally discarded	• Repeat specimen collection.

RECORDING AND REPORTING

- Record date and time urine specimen was obtained in nurses' notes.
- Notify physician or nurse practitioner of any significant abnormalities.

HOME CARE CONSIDERATIONS

- If patient is required to collect specimen as an outpatient, a clean technique may be used. Provide proper instruction for collection.
- Appropriate equipment must be given to the patient and family.
- Information on storing the specimen until time of delivery to doctor's office or hospital laboratory must be provided.

If questions regarding the accuracy of specific gravity measurements arise, a urine osmolality test should be obtained. Although both tests measure urine concentration, the osmolality test is more accurate because it measures the total number of particles in a solution (see Chapter 40).

Urine culture. For a urine culture, a sterile or clean-voided sample of urine is required. Because urine is an excellent medium for bacterial growth and bacteriological changes may alter test results, facilities may require that urine samples for culture and sensitivity be stored in a refrigerator until pickup.

Usually it is approximately 24 to 48 hours before the laboratory can report findings of bacterial growth. While results are awaited, a broad-spectrum antibiotic may be ordered as soon as a culture has been obtained. The test for sensitivity determines which specific antibiotics are effective. The results of a urine culture may show that another antibiotic would be more effective. In this case, a new antibiotic is ordered.

Diagnostic Examinations. The urinary system is amenable to accurate diagnostic study by several radiographic techniques. The two approaches for visualization of urinary structures, direct and indirect techniques, can be quite simple or very complex, necessitating extensive nursing intervention. These procedures are further subdivided into invasive or noninvasive categories (Table 43-6). One noninvasive procedure involves computed tomography (CT).

Many of the nursing responsibilities related to diagnostic examinations of the urinary tract are common to more than one type of procedure. Common responsibilities before an examination include the following:

- Witnessing a signed consent (if agency policy allows)
- Assessing the patient for history of shellfish (iodine) allergy, which predicts allergy to the dye used in specific studies (intravenous pyelogram [IVP] and renal arteriogram)
- Administering bowel preparation medications (check agency policy)
- Ensuring that the patient receives the appropriate pretest diet (clear liquids) or nothing by mouth (NPO), as needed

Common postprocedure interventions may include the following:

- Assessing intake and output
- Observing characteristics of urine (colour, clarity, presence of blood)

Patient Expectations. Patients depend on their caregivers to recognize and promptly meet their needs. Nurses need to use a skilled and caring approach, be creative in using a variety of assessment techniques, and serve as patient advocates. A caring nurse will meet the patient's

TABLE 43-5 Routine Urinalysis

Measurement (Normal Value)	Interpretation
Routine Laboratory Value	
pH (4.6–8.0, average 6.0)	pH indicates acid–base balance. Urine that stands for several hours becomes alkaline. An acid pH helps protect against bacterial growth.
Protein (none or up to 8 mg/100 mL)	Protein is not normally present in urine. It is seen in renal disease because damage to glomeruli or tubules allows protein to enter urine.
Glucose (none)	Diabetic patients have glucose in their urine as a result of the inability of tubules to reabsorb high glucose concentrations (180 mg/100 mL). Ingestion of high concentrations of glucose may cause some glucose to appear in the urine of healthy people.
Ketones (none)	Patients whose diabetes mellitus is poorly controlled experience breakdown of fatty acids. Ketones are end products of fat metabolism. Patients with dehydration, starvation, or excessive aspirin usage also may have ketonuria.
Blood (up to two red blood cells [RBCs])	Damage to glomeruli or tubules may allow RBCs to enter the urine. Trauma, disease, or surgery of the lower urinary tract also may cause blood to be present. In women, blood in a routine urine specimen may indicate contamination with menstrual fluid.
Specific gravity (1.010–1.025)	Specific gravity measures concentration of particles in urine. High specific gravity reflects concentrated urine, and low specific gravity reflects diluted urine. Dehydration, reduced renal blood flow, and increased antidiuretic hormone (ADH) secretion elevate specific gravity. Overhydration, early renal disease, and inadequate ADH secretion reduce specific gravity.
Microscopic Examination	
White blood cells (WBCs) (0–4 per low-power field)	Greater numbers may indicate urinary tract infection (UTI).
Bacteria (none)	Bacteria indicate UTI. (Patient may or may not have symptoms.)
Casts (none)	Casts are cylindrical bodies whose shapes take on the likeness of objects within the renal tubule. Types include hyaline, WBCs, RBCs, granular cells, and epithelial cells. Their presence is always an abnormal finding and indicates renal alterations.

Data from Pagana, K. D., & Pagana, T. J. (2013). *Mosby's diagnostic and laboratory test reference* (11th ed.). St. Louis, MO: Mosby.

needs in a way that is acceptable and individualized to the patient and the family situation. Patients with alterations in urinary elimination expect nurses to be respectful of privacy needs and sensitive to the impact of urinary impairments on sexuality and self-concept. The nurse and patient should develop the care plan together whenever possible and establish goals that are mutually acceptable. Cultural practices and personal preferences also must be considered.

◆ Nursing Diagnosis

A thorough assessment of the patient's urinary elimination function reveals patterns of data that allow the nurse to make relevant and accurate nursing diagnoses. The diagnosis may focus on a specific alteration or an associated problem, such as impaired skin integrity related to urinary incontinence. Identification of defining characteristics leads the nurse to select an appropriate diagnosis. Specifying related factors for each diagnosis enables selection of individualized nursing interventions (see Chapter 14). A sample of diagnostic reasoning is found in Box 43-3. Nursing diagnoses common to patients with alterations in urine elimination include the following:

- *Disturbed body image*
- *Pain (acute, chronic)*
- *Self-care deficit, toileting*
- *Impaired skin integrity*
- *Impaired urinary elimination*
- *Urinary incontinence (transient, urge, stress, mixed, functional, UI associated with chronic retention of urine (formerly overflow)*
- *Urinary retention*

BOX 43-3 NURSING DIAGNOSTIC PROCESS

Assessment Activities	Defining Characteristics	Nursing Diagnosis
Have patient describe situations that accompany urine leakage.	Patient states that she "loses a little urine" whenever she sneezes, coughs, or laughs. Patient states that she has been having problems for several years.	*Stress urinary incontinence related to decreased pelvic muscle tone and urethral sphincter trauma*
Observe patient behaviour.	Patient is wearing a menstrual minipad continuously. Patient is reluctant to interact with others and tries not to cough or laugh.	
Review medical history.	Patient is menopausal and has had three vaginal births.	

TABLE 43-6 Diagnostic Examinations

Name of Procedure	Purpose and Method of Procedure	Special Nursing Considerations
Noninvasive Procedures		
Abdominal roentgenogram (plain film; kidney, ureter, bladder [KUB], or flat plate)	To determine the size, shape, symmetry, and location of the kidneys; diagnose urinary calculi; preliminary X-ray imaging before intravenous pyelogram (IVP).	No special preparation or precautions; bowel preparation is required if preliminary X-ray imaging is before IVP.
Computerized axial tomographic (CT) scan	A computerized X-ray procedure used to obtain detailed images of structures within a selected plane of the body. The computer reconstructs a cross-sectional image and thus allows the physician to view pathological conditions such as tumours and obstructions.	Bowel preparation as per agency or physician preference. Assess patient for shellfish (iodine) allergy if a CT scan with contrast material is ordered. Prepare patient for the procedure (e.g., patient will be placed into a large machine and need to lie still, feelings of claustrophobia occur in some patients).
Intravenous pyelogram (IVP)	To view the collecting ducts and renal pelvis and outline the ureters, bladder, and urethra with the use of dye, which is excreted through the urine. A special dye is injected intravenously. The patient's ability to empty the bladder is assessed through a postvoiding X-ray film.	Bowel preparatrion will be completed as per agency or physician preference. Only clear liquids are permitted until after test is completed. Assess patient for shellfish (iodine) allergy before test. After test, fluid intake is encouraged to dilute and flush dye from patient. Observe for late symptoms of allergic reaction (rash, throat tightness, difficulty breathing, etc.).
Retrograde pyelogram	Series of X-ray films that provide detailed anatomical views of the ureter, ureteropelvic junction, renal pelvis, and calyces. A ureteral catheter is placed in the lower ureteral segment, and contrast material is injected or infused into the upper urinary tract.	Same as for IVP.
Retrograde urethrogram (RUG)	To obtain oblique X-ray films of the male urethra by instilling a small volume of iodine-bound contrast material into the urethra from a retrograde direction.	Assess patient for shellfish (iodine) allergy before test.
Renal (kidney) scan	To determine renal blood flow, anatomical structure of the kidneys, and excretory function using a radioisotope.	Usually no bowel preparation is needed, but check agency policy. After test, only precaution is rinsing bedpan or urinal after use and flushing the urine, as urine will contain a minute amount of radioisotope. Rinse fluid carefully using a double flush.
Renal ultrasonography	To identify gross renal structures and structural abnormalities in the kidney using high-frequency, inaudible sound waves.	No bowel preparation is needed.
Bladder ultrasonography	To identify structural abnormalities of bladder or lower urinary tract. Also used to estimate the volume of urine in the bladder and to measure postvoid residual volume.	Patient may be asked to drink fluids before the ultrasonography to cause bladder distension for better results. To measure postvoid residual volume, ultrasonography should be performed within 15 minutes of void. No special care is necessary after either study.
Invasive Procedures		
Endoscopy	Use of an endoscope allows for direct visualization, specimen collection, or treatment of the interior of the kidney (nephroscopy), ureter (ureteroscopy), bladder (cystoscopy), and urethra (cystourethroscopy). Although this procedure may be accomplished using local anaesthesia, it is more commonly performed using general anaesthesia or conscious sedation to avoid unnecessary anxiety and trauma for the patient.	Signed consent is obtained. If ordered, a bowel preparation is completed. Follow agency policy for preoperative preparation and checklist (see Chapter 48). After patient's return, assess the vital signs and the characteristics of urine, monitor intake and output, encourage ingestion of fluids, and observe for fever, dysuria, and pain in the suprapubic region.

TABLE 43-6 Diagnostic Examinations—cont'd

Name of Procedure	Purpose and Method of Procedure	Special Nursing Considerations
Arteriogram (angiography)	Used primarily to visualize the renal arteries or their branches to detect narrowing or occlusion. A catheter is placed in one of the femoral arteries and introduced up to the level of the renal arteries. Radiopaque contrast is injected through the catheter while X-ray images are taken in rapid succession.	Signed consent is required. Assess for shellfish (iodine) allergy. Follow agency preprocedure checklist. After the procedure, monitor vital signs frequently until patient is stable; bed rest is maintained for prescribed time interval; fluids are encouraged to flush the contrast from the system. Also monitor the affected extremity for neurocirculatory function (pulse, skin temperature, sensation, and movement), and observe catheter site for bleeding, swelling, increased tenderness, or hematoma formation. Physician must be notified immediately of any postprocedure abnormality.
Uroflometry and Urodynamic testing	Uroflometry measures rate of urine expelled and is noninvasive. The patient voids into a urine flowmeter. Complete urodynamics determines bladder and sphincter function in the case of urinary obstruction or urinary incontinence. A catheter is inserted, the urine is drained, and sterile water or contrast liquid is used to fill the bladder. Pressure readings are taken and compared with the patient's reported sensations.	Explain the need for the patient to report all sensations during the test. After the test, assess the patient for sensations of sweating, pain, nausea, bladder fullness, or a strong urge to void.

Data from Pagana, K. D., & Pagana, T. J. (2013). *Mosby's diagnostic and laboratory test reference* (11th ed.). St. Louis, MO: Mosby.

Common symptoms that contribute to a nursing diagnosis of impaired urinary elimination, such as frequency, urgency, and nocturia, were described in Table 43-3. Each of these symptoms is associated with multiple underlying disorders. Nurses need to assimilate what has been learned from personal history-taking, physical assessment, and diagnostic tests to determine a nursing diagnosis and an appropriate care plan.

◆ Planning

During planning, nurses integrate the knowledge gained from assessment and the knowledge related to resources and available therapies to develop an individualized care plan (Box 43-4). The patient's needs should be matched with clinical and professional standards recommended in the literature (Figure 43-10). Building a relationship of trust with the patient is important because implementing the care plan involves interaction of a very personal nature.

Goals and Outcomes. The care plan for alterations in urinary elimination must include realistic and individualized goals along with relevant outcomes. The nurse and patient must collaborate in setting goals and outcomes. A general goal might be normal urinary elimination, but the individual goal may differ depending on the problem. The goals may be short term or long term. For example, for a patient with urinary retention after surgery, the short-term goal may be "Patient will have normal voiding with complete bladder emptying within 24 hours." Relevant expected outcomes for this goal may include the following:

- Patient will void within 8 hours.
- Urinary output of 300 mL or greater will occur with each voiding.
- Patient's bladder will not be distended on palpation.
- Patient will not continually feel an urge to void.

Conversely, the patient with stress incontinence may have a long-term goal that involves weeks of pelvic floor muscle exercises (PFMEs; also known as *Kegel exercises*) to achieve urinary control: "Patient will achieve improved urinary continence within 12 weeks after start of pelvic floor muscle exercise program." Goals must be reasonably achievable for the patient and be relevant to the patient's situation.

Setting Priorities. Urinary elimination is a personal and intimate activity. The nurse must establish a relationship with the patient that promotes open discussion. A supportive and collaborative environment helps to make the patient's priorities apparent and fosters mutual understanding of realistic goals.

When a patient has multiple nursing diagnoses (Figure 43-11), the nurse must recognize the primary health problem and its influence on other problems. In the example of the patient with cognitive impairment, the resultant incontinence creates several risks. Focusing on management of incontinence will often help to resolve more than one nursing diagnosis. Although physical care needs may appear to have higher priority, psychological needs related to self-esteem or sexuality may be of higher priority to the patient. Attention to the patient's perceived needs may be the most satisfactory and successful approach to accomplishing all of the goals. Reinforcement and praise of good health habits can improve adherence to the care plan.

Continuity of Care. The care plan incorporates health promotion activities and therapeutic interventions for patients. Preventive interventions may be required for patients at risk for urinary problems. It is important to consider the patient's home environment and normal elimination routines when planning therapies. Consultation with other health care providers and with the patient's family is often necessary. For example, the physiotherapist can design an exercise plan to increase strength and endurance so that the patient will be able to ambulate to the bathroom. The need for home care services should be explored and appropriate referrals made. The family may need to alter the home environment to make it easier and safer for the patient to use the bathroom.

◆ Implementation

Implementation is the action phase of the nursing process. Nurses carry out the independent and collaborative activities needed to assist the patient in achieving the desired outcomes and goals. Independent

BOX 43-4 NURSING CARE PLAN

Mixed Urinary Incontinence

ASSESSMENT

Kay, a home care nurse, is seeing Mrs. Grayson, a 75-year-old widow, at her home. Mrs. Grayson was referred by her physician because of arthritis and early dementia. She has had three urinary tract infections in the past year. She lives alone, but her daughter lives less than a 10-minute drive away. Kay's assessment included a discussion of Mrs. Grayson's current health problems.

Assessment Activities	**Findings and Defining Characteristics**
Ask Mrs. Grayson about how she is coping with her arthritis.	She responds, "It slows me down. The pain medication is helping, but it takes me longer to get out of my chair and get anywhere." Mrs. Grayson begins to cry and states, "You can see the plastic cover on my chair. I'm so embarrassed; sometimes I can't get out of the chair fast enough and I lose my water. I've been wearing those diapers lately."
Ask Mrs. Grayson to describe how long she has had trouble controlling her urine and whether she has ever sought help.	Mrs. Grayson says that she has had trouble with dribbling for more than 10 years, but she didn't think anything could be done because of her age. Over the past few years, it has gotten worse. With little warning, she has to rush to the bathroom and is often wet on the way. She also leaks when she coughs.
Ask Mrs. Grayson about any changes, such as new medication, that may have contributed to her worsening symptoms.	Mrs. Grayson says that she has not started any new medications.
Ask Mrs. Grayson to complete a bladder diary for 3 days when she is likely to be at home most of the time, and provide a receptacle so that she can measure several of her voids. Establish a diary format she understands and can work with.	Mrs. Grayson completes the diary for only 2 days because she finds it difficult to write everything down and often forgets to do this task.
Assess bladder diary findings and discuss patterns with Mrs. Grayson so she becomes aware of her usual bladder routines and is more able to participate in her care planning.	The diary findings discussed are as follows: 1. Largest volume void is 200 mL and longest interval between voids is 1.25 hours. Mrs. Grayson is up two times at night to void. 2. Two episodes of incontinence occur on the way to the bathroom. Mrs. Grayson records that she gets a sudden urge to void but is "very wet" on the way to the bathroom. 3. Mrs. Grayson also records that she can feel herself dribbling while coughing. 4. Fluid intake is low, averaging 800 mL per 24 hours.

NURSING DIAGNOSIS: *Mixed incontinence.* Mrs. Grayson has symptoms of urge incontinence: frequency, incontinence associated with severe urgency, and nocturia. She also describes episodes of stress incontinence. Her impaired mobility makes it more difficult to get to the bathroom in time. Mrs. Grayson also may be at risk for a urinary tract infection (UTI) due to reduced fluid intake.

PLANNING

Goals (Nursing Outcomes Classification)*	**Expected Outcomes**
Patient will review bladder diary and think about aspects of her elimination pattern that may be amenable to change.	Enhanced understanding of bladder function
Patient will report reduced episodes of incontinence within 1 month and longer intervals between voids.	Reduced episodes of urinary incontinence
Patient will increase fluid intake to help ensure adequate hydration and prevent urinary tract infection.	Adequate hydration

*Outcome classification labels from Moorhead, S., Johnson, M., Maas, M. L., & Swanson, E. (Eds.). (2013). *Nursing outcomes classification (NOC)* (5th ed.). St. Louis, MO: Mosby.

INTERVENTIONS

Interventions (Nursing Interventions Classification)	**Rationale**
Urinary Incontinence Care	
Discuss "normal" bladder habits with patient as well as her actual patterns of intake and output, based on the bladder diary.	The success of conservative therapies for urinary incontinence (UI) such as pelvic floor muscle exercises (PFMEs) requires motivation and ongoing commitment and self-care, meaning that the patient must be an active part of assessment and care planning. Provide written reminders for individuals with memory issues. Toileting education and prompted voiding with support of caregivers may be of help (Drennan, Greenwood, Cole, et al., 2012).

BOX 43-4 NURSING CARE PLAN

Mixed Urinary Incontinence—cont'd

Interventions (Nursing Interventions Classification)	***Rationale***
Refer for continence specialist to assess pelvic floor strength, to establish baseline and to teach patient appropriate muscle to tighten. Instruct patient to practise PFMEs at least twice a day. The continence specialist will also assess for urogenital atrophy.	Cognitively intact and motivated older persons can learn PFMEs when able to identify the correct musculature. Growing evidence supports the positive impact of PFMEs in women with stress UI and overactive bladder (OAB) syndrome, including the reflex inhibition of involuntary detrusor contractions (Moore et al., 2013). Persons with early dementia may be helped with written instructions and reminders from caregivers. Urogenital atrophy is a contributor to UTI in older women that can be treated with low-dose vaginal estrogen.
Work with patient to establish a manageable program of bladder training, asking the patient to void at regular, prespecified intervals throughout the day based on maximum intervals in bladder diary (1.25 hours). Gradually increase the interval by 15 to 30 minutes per week as tolerated, until an acceptable pattern is achieved. Patient will need prompting and support from caregivers to undertake this.	Bladder training reduces frequency and urgency in women with OAB syndrome (Milne, 2008) but may be more successful when pelvic floor muscle strength has improved.
Discuss safety issues related to the patient's nocturia and the possibility of acquiring a bedside commode.	Older persons who get up at night to urinate are more likely to experience a fall. Because older persons are also at increased risk for bone fractures, it is important to identify persons with nocturia and to ensure that appropriate safety precautions are taken.
Encourage patient to increase noncaffeinated fluid intake gradually to approximately 1 500 mL during the day, with fluid intake restricted after suppertime.	Adequate hydration will help prevent UTI and maintain dilute urine. Avoiding fluids before bedtime may reduce nocturia.

EVALUATION

Nursing Action	***Patient Response and Finding***	***Achievement of Outcome***
Ask Mrs. Grayson to complete a bladder diary at regular intervals (monthly or every 2 months) to compare to the baseline diary. Provide written instructions.	Three months after initiating conservative treatment, patient responds, "I'm dry most of the time now."	Mrs. Grayson has reduced her episodes of incontinence and increased the interval between voids. She is now voiding every 3 hours on average and is up one or two times at night. She reports that she feels better because she is getting more sleep.

activities are those determined by nurses using their own judgement, for example, teaching self-care activities to the patient. Collaborative activities are those prescribed by the physician that nurses carry out, such as medication administration.

Health Promotion. The focus of health promotion is to assist the patient in understanding and participating in self-care practices that will preserve and protect healthy urinary system function. People with urinary incontinence and other lower urinary tract symptoms may think that these are normal, or they may lack awareness of treatment options. Such negative attitudes prevent them from reporting symptoms and seeking help (Seshan & Muliira, 2013). Targeted health promotion and education can improve how people perceive bladder problems and help-seeking. Nurses must maintain an open, caring attitude and provide bladder health education to those seeking information. Key aspects of continence promotion and education, based on international recommendations (Newman, Buckley, Gordon, et al., 2013), are summarized in Box 43-5.

Patient Education. Success of therapies aimed at solving or minimizing urinary elimination problems depends in part on successful patient education. Although many patients may need to learn about all aspects of urinary elimination, the nurse should first focus the teaching on the patient's specific elimination problems. For example, patients who practise poor hygiene benefit most from learning about the normal sterility of the urinary tract and ways to prevent infection. Patients also learn the significance of symptoms of urinary alterations so that early preventive health care can be initiated.

BOX 43-5 Continence Promotion and Education

- To eliminate stigma and increase awareness of strategies that can improve quality of life, continence awareness should be a part of health education and advocacy.
- Health care and community service providers should be a part of continence awareness programs.
- Care delivery for continence services should be based on a chronic disease model.
- Professional and patient education is needed to improve knowledge and practice.

Nurses can easily incorporate teaching while providing nursing care. For example, when attempting to increase a patient's fluid intake, a good time to discuss the benefits of this action is while giving fluids with medications or meals. Teaching about perineal hygiene may be appropriate while giving a bath or performing catheter care.

Promoting Regular Micturition. Maintaining regular patterns of urinary elimination can help prevent many urination problems. Patients with urinary incontinence commonly void frequently throughout the day to avoid accidental urine loss. However, frequent voiding (e.g., at hourly intervals) may contribute to creating a small-capacity bladder. Conversely, patients who hold their urine for long periods

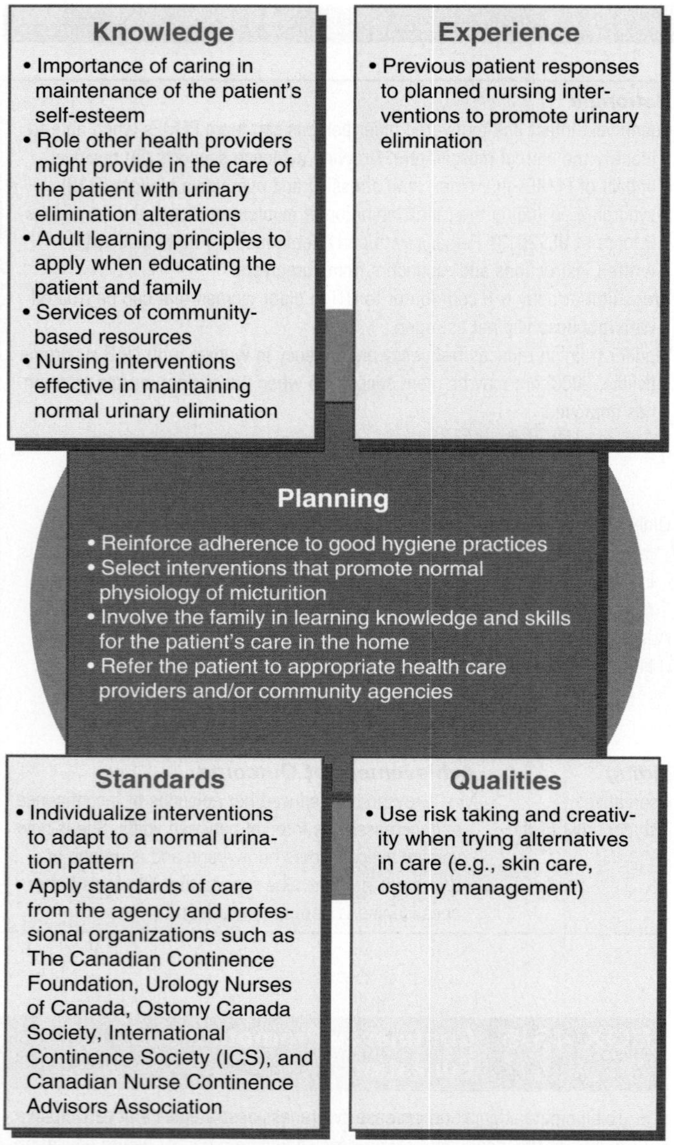

FIGURE 43-10 Critical thinking model for urinary elimination planning.

(more than 8 hours) may develop a hypotonic bladder with incomplete emptying. Nurses should reinforce the importance of voiding regularly (approximately every 3 to 4 hours) to help maintain a normal bladder capacity (400 to 500 mL). Because constipated stool in the rectum may compress the urethra and impede emptying, nurses should emphasize the importance of regular bowel movements and encourage measures to enhance regularity, including diets rich in fibre (see Chapter 44).

Many nursing measures have been designed to promote normal voiding in patients at risk for urination difficulties and in patients with established urination problems. Nurses can initiate many of these measures independently.

Stimulating micturition reflex. The patient's ability to void depends on feeling the urge to urinate, being able to control the urethral sphincter, and being able to relax during voiding. Nurses can help a patient learn to relax and stimulate the micturition reflex by enabling the patient to assume the normal position for voiding. A woman is better able to void in a squatting or sitting position. If the woman is unable to use toilet facilities, the nurse can help her into a sitting position on a bedpan or bedside commode. A smaller slipper bed pan may be easier for the patient to use. A man voids more easily in a standing position. If the man cannot reach toilet facilities, he may stand at the bedside and void into a urinal (a metal or plastic receptacle for urine). A female urinal, with an elongated spout, may be helpful to women with limited mobility (Figure 43-12).

Providing certain sensory stimuli also may promote relaxation and voiding. The sound of running water helps many patients void. Stroking the inner thigh may stimulate sensory nerves and promote the micturition reflex. The nurse can also pour warm water over the patient's perineum to create the urge to urinate. If urine output is being measured, the nurse must first measure the volume of water that will be poured over the perineal area.

Maintaining elimination habits. Many patients follow routines to promote normal voiding. In a hospital or long-term care facility, nursing routines may conflict with those of patients. When a patient is admitted to hospital or other care setting, the nurse should obtain information on usual voiding patterns when taking the nursing history. Integrating patients' habits into the care plan fosters normal voiding and will assist in preventing problems related to urination.

Maintaining adequate fluid intake. Patients with urinary incontinence often reduce fluid intake because they believe that this will help keep them dry. In reality, maintaining an adequate fluid intake of 1 500 to 2 000 mL promotes continence because concentrated urine can irritate the bladder mucosa. Fluid intake should not include caffeinated beverages, which have a diuretic effect. The patient should be reminded that many vegetables and fruits have a high fluid content and can contribute to daily fluid intake. At the patient's home, it may be helpful to establish a schedule for drinking fluids (e.g., with meals or medications). Fluids should be minimized after supper to minimize nocturia.

The nurse can teach the patient to avoid foods and fluids that may cause worsening of lower urinary tract symptoms:

- Tobacco (smoker's cough aggravates stress urinary incontinence)
- Alcohol (acts as a diuretic)
- Substances containing caffeine, such as coffee, tea, and chocolate (may worsen urgency and urgency incontinence, increases frequency) (Northwood & Hunter, 2014)
- Carbonated beverages
- Artificial sweeteners (e.g., Aspartame)

Promoting Complete Bladder Emptying. Under normal circumstances, a small amount of urine (50 mL) remains in the bladder after voiding (residual urine) because the urinary sphincters close. Thus, people normally remain continent and dry. People with residual urine are able to remain dry when their urethral closure pressure is sufficient to prevent leakage. However, urinary incontinence may occur when too much residual urine is in the bladder or when the urinary sphincters are too weak to maintain closure pressure. As well as contributing to incontinence, residual urine can be a medium for bacterial growth.

Patients should be encouraged to take their time while voiding and to try again when they feel they have not emptied their bladders fully (double voiding). Those with consistently elevated PVRs (>100 mL) may require intermittent catheterization. Portable bladder scanners offer a noninvasive means of assessing PVRs. Box 43-6 describes the procedure for using a bladder scanner.

Preventing Infection. One of the most important considerations for a patient with alterations in urinary elimination is the need to prevent infection of the urinary system. Good perineal hygiene that includes cleaning the urethral meatus after each voiding or bowel movement is essential. Patients with limited dexterity due to conditions such as

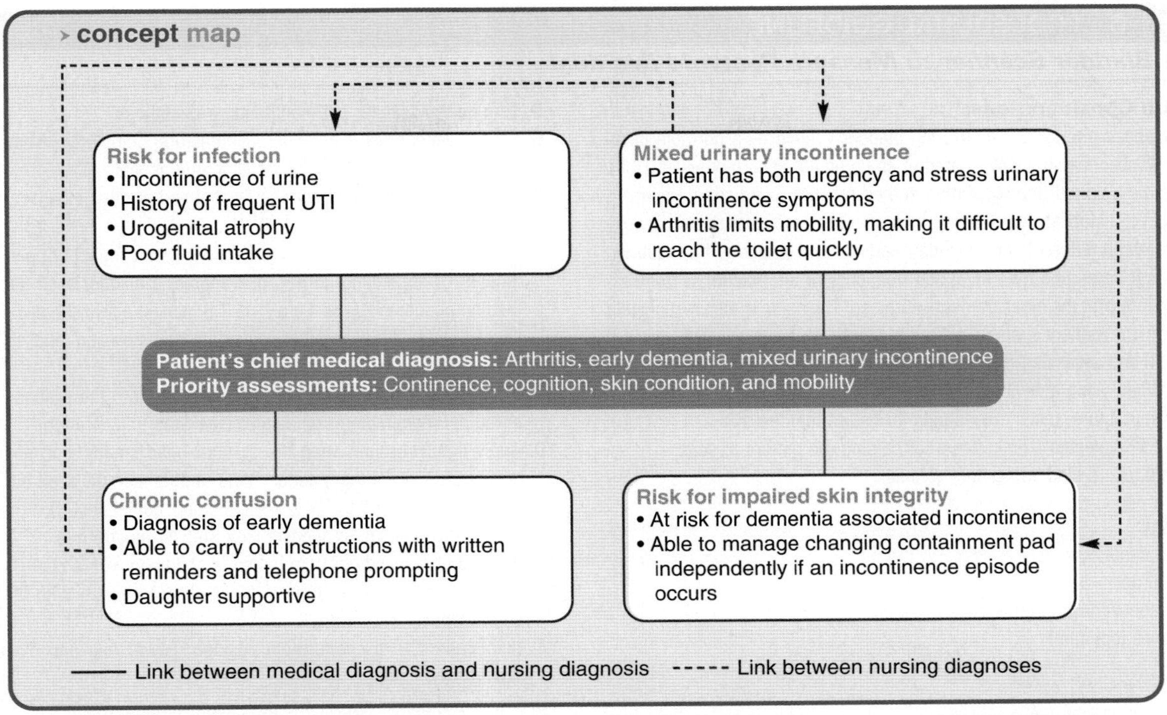

FIGURE 43-11 Concept map for patient with mixed urinary incontinence, early dementia, and recurrent urinary tract infection (UTI).

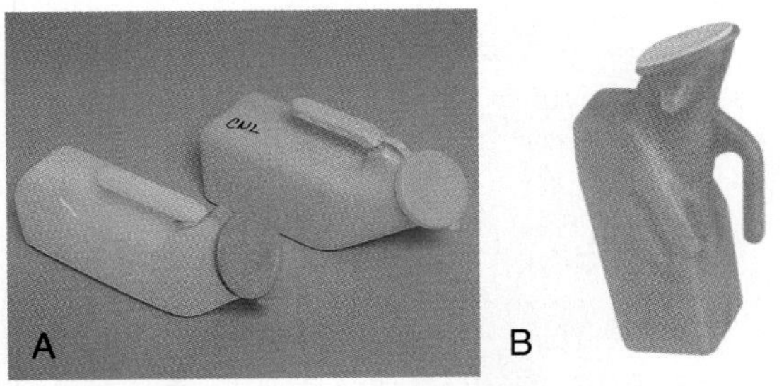

FIGURE 43-12 Types of male **(A)** and female **(B)** urinals. (**B,** Courtesy Briggs Medical Service Co.)

arthritis or stroke can benefit from the use of a squirt bottle filled with warm water to rinse the perineum after defecation.

Maintaining an adequate daily intake of fluids (1 500 to 2 000 mL) maintains renal function and promotes regular micturition. Dehydration can contribute to urinary incontinence, as concentrated urine can irritate the bladder (Northwood & Hunter, 2014). Urine is normally acidic and tends to inhibit growth of microorganisms.

Catheters and Incontinence Products. Many measures can be used in health care settings to decrease the incidence of urinary alterations. Use of a urinary catheter requires a prescriber order and should only be implemented when the criteria for insertion of an in-dwelling urinary catheter (see Table 43-1) have been met. Incontinence alone is not a reason to insert a urinary catheter. Patients experiencing incontinence should be managed with an individualized combination of incontinence products and conservative and pharmacological interventions prior to any consideration of catheterization.

Special Considerations in Acute Care. Conservative interventions listed in Table 43-2 are discussed in detail in the next section. Many are appropriate to implement in acute care. In particular, toileting strategies should be implemented and continence aids, such as urinals, should be used first to avoid unnecessary use of containment products (pads) or in-dwelling urinary catheters. In-dwelling catheters should only be inserted when absolutely indicated, and in acute care, continued use of an in-dwelling catheter should be reassessed daily (Leis & Soong, 2017). Nurses have a key role to play in reassessment and reminders to remove catheters that are no longer needed.

Maintaining Elimination Habits. Patients usually require time to void. Requesting a urine specimen on demand does not contribute to relaxation and normal voiding habits. Patients should be given at least 30 minutes to provide a specimen. Patients normally void upon awakening or before meals; therefore, the nurse should offer them the opportunity to use toilet facilities then. Also important is the need to respond promptly to patients' urges to urinate. Delays in assisting patients to the bathroom may interfere with normal micturition and contribute to incontinence. This is particularly the case with patients who have OAB syndrome.

> **Safety Alert** Many falls by older persons are related to the urge to urinate. Anticipate an older person's need to urinate and provide scheduled bathroom visits. Make sure that the pathway between the bed and the toilet facility is clear of any barriers.

Privacy is essential to normal voiding. If the patient cannot reach the bathroom, the bedside curtain should be closed. The debilitated patient at home may prefer to use a bedside commode screened by a partition or room divider. Young children are often unable to void in the presence of people other than their parents.

BOX 43-6 PROCEDURAL GUIDELINE

Using a Bladder Scanner to Measure Postvoid Residual

Delegation Considerations:

In some provinces, the skill of measuring bladder volume by a portable ultrasound bladder scanner can be delegated to an unregulated care provider (UCP). Nurses must be aware of the legislation in their practice jurisdiction. However, it is important to establish competency in bladder scan measurements because reliability between different care provider readings can be poor. The regulated nurse must first determine the timing and frequency of the bladder scan measurement and interpret the measurements obtained. The nurse is also responsible for assessing the patient's ability to toilet before measurement of postvoid residual (PVR) and assessing the abdomen for distension if urinary retention is suspected. When using a device:

- Follow manufacturer recommendations for use of the device.
- Measure PVR volumes 10 minutes after helping the patient to void.
- Report and record bladder scanner volumes.

Equipment:

- Bladder scanner
- Ultrasound gel
- Cleaning agent for scanner head, such as an alcohol pad
- Clean gloves (optional)

Steps:

1. Identify patient, using two identifiers (e.g., name and birthday or name and medical record number) according to agency policy.
2. Perform hand hygiene. Discuss procedure with patient. If the measurement is for PVR, ask him or her to void and measure and record voided urine volume. (Apply gloves if patient requires assistance with voiding). The scan measurement should be within 10 minutes of voiding.
3. Help patient to the supine position with the head slightly elevated. Raise bed to appropriate working height. If side rails are raised, lower side rail on working side.
4. Expose patient's lower abdomen.
5. Turn on the scanner per manufacturer guidelines.
6. Set the gender designation per manufacturer guidelines. Women who have had a hysterectomy should be designated as male.
7. Wipe the scanner head with an alcohol pad or other cleanser and allow to air-dry.
8. Palpate the patient's symphysis pubis (pubic bone). Apply a generous amount of ultrasound gel (or, if available, a bladder scan gel pad) to the midline abdomen 2.5 to 4 cm (1 to 1.5 inches) above the symphysis pubis. The ultrasound gel ensures adequate transmission and thus accurate measurement.
9. Place the scanner head on the gel, ensuring that the scanner head is oriented per manufacturer guidelines (see Step 9 illustration).
10. Apply light pressure, keep the scanner head steady, and point it slightly downward toward the bladder. Press and release the scan button.
11. Verify accurate aim (refer to manufacturer guidelines). Complete the scan and print the image (if needed) (see Step 11 illustration).
12. Remove ultrasound gel from patient's abdomen with a paper towel.
13. Remove ultrasound gel from scanner head and wipe with alcohol pad or other cleanser; let air-dry.
14. Help patient to a comfortable position. Lower bed and place side rails accordingly.
15. Dispose of soiled towels and pad. Perform hand hygiene.

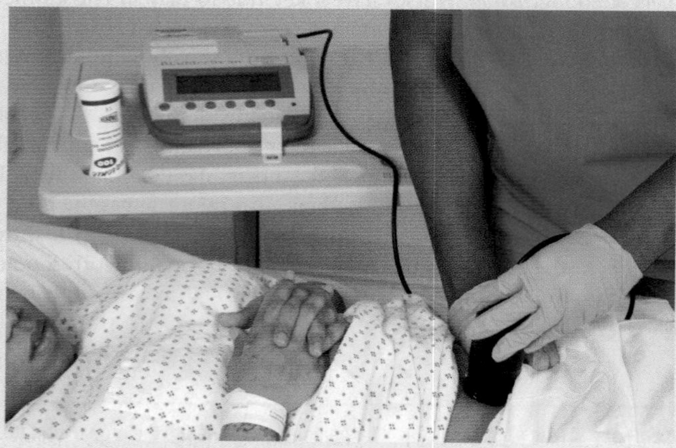

STEP 9 Point scanner head slightly downward toward bladder.

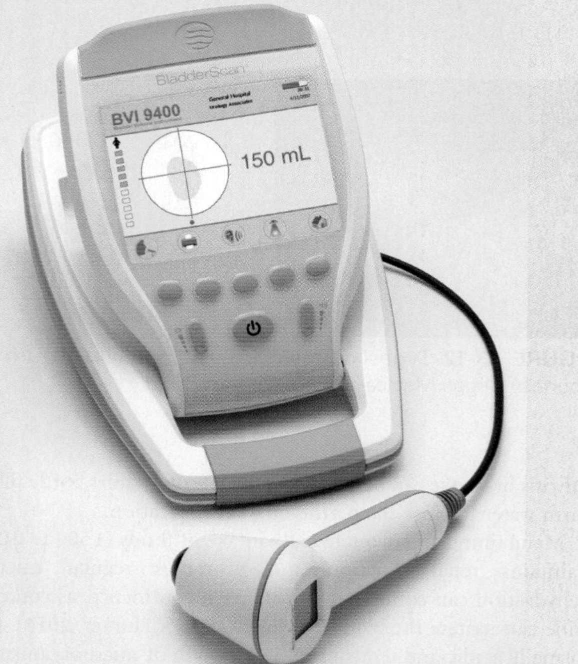

STEP 11 Bladder scan image (Courtesy Verathon, Inc.)

When possible, nurses should encourage the continued use of special measures that a patient uses to void. The patient may be able to relax and void more easily while reading or listening to music. Having a cup or glass of fluids also may promote urination.

Catheterization. Catheterization of the bladder involves introducing a narrow tube through the urethra and into the bladder to allow a continuous flow of urine into a drainage receptacle. Indications for in-dwelling urethral catheterization, which is to be avoided if possible, were provided earlier in the chapter, in Table 43-1, along with discussion about CAUTI prevention. Intermittent catheterization is used to empty the bladder in people with poorly contractile bladder or bladder sphincter dyssenergia, and it is commonly used long term in persons with spinal cord injury or spinal bifida. Intermittent catheterization can be used to collect a sterile urine specimen, but only in patients who are unable to provide a midstream specimen. Bladder catheterization carries the risk of CAUTI, blockage, and trauma to the urethra, so it is preferable to rely on other measures for either specimen collection or the management of incontinence (Cottenden et al., 2013).

Types of catheterization. Catheters may be intermittent or in-dwelling (retention). With the intermittent technique, a single-use straight catheter (Figure 43-13, *A*) is introduced urethrally for 5 to 10 minutes, just long enough to drain the bladder. The straight catheter has a single lumen with a small opening about 1.3 cm from the tip. Urine drains from the tip, through the lumen, and into a receptacle. Intermittent catheterization is performed by the patient or by a nurse and is common in patients who have incomplete bladder emptying due to neurogenic conditions (e.g., spinal cord injury). In the hospital, intermittent catheterization is sterile to reduce the risk of health care–associated infections. In the community, patients use the clean intermittent catheterization technique and reuse their catheters many times. Catheters are washed with soap and water and left to air-dry until the next use. Clean intermittent self-catheterization is felt to be a safe technique for those self-managing bladder emptying in the home (Cottenden et al., 2013).

The coude catheter is a type of catheter that has a curved tip and is used for male patients who have an enlarged prostate that partly obstructs the urethra. It is less traumatic during insertion because it is stiffer and easier to control than the straight-tip catheter. However, use of this type of catheter requires special education.

An in-dwelling or Foley catheter (Figure 43-13, *B*) is retained for longer periods in the bladder by means of a small balloon that anchors it against the bladder neck. In acute care, the catheter remains in place until daily review of necessity indicates it should be removed. Some acute care settings have catheter-removal prompt systems to remind the nurse to assess if the catheter is still needed and to get a physicians' order to remove it if no longer appropriate. Patients with long-term catheters need to have an individualized routine for changing established on the basis of agency policy and pattern of blockage. A blocked catheter should be changed as soon as possible. In-dwelling catheters are either two lumen (the most common type; one lumen drains urine and the other carries sterile water to inflate or deflate the balloon) or three lumen (the third lumen allows for irrigation). The triple-lumen catheter (Figure 43-13, *C*) is used for continuous bladder irrigation. They can be used on a short-term or long-term basis.

Catheters are manufactured in many different materials (latex, silicone, Teflon) and come in many different diameters. Guidelines on how to make appropriate decisions regarding catheter selection are provided in Box 43-7.

Catheter insertion. For urethral catheterization of any type, a physician's order is required. The nurse must use strict aseptic technique (see Chapter 33). Organizing equipment before beginning the procedure prevents interruptions. The steps for inserting in-dwelling and single-use straight catheters are basically the same. The difference lies in the procedure taken to inflate the in-dwelling catheter balloon and secure the catheter. Skill 43-2 lists the steps for inserting in-dwelling and single-use straight catheters in both men and women.

Closed drainage systems. After inserting an in-dwelling catheter, the nurse needs to maintain a closed urinary drainage system to minimize the risk of infection. Urinary drainage bags are plastic and can hold about 1 000 to 1 500 mL of urine. The drainage bag should never be raised above the level of the patient's bladder. The bag should hang on the bed frame or wheelchair, without touching the floor. Urine in the bag and tubing can become a medium for bacteria, and infection is likely to develop if urine flows back into the bladder. Therefore, the bag should not be hung on the bed's side rails because from there it can be raised above the level of the bladder accidentally. When the patient ambulates, the drainage bag must be held below the patient's waist.

Text continued on p. 1198

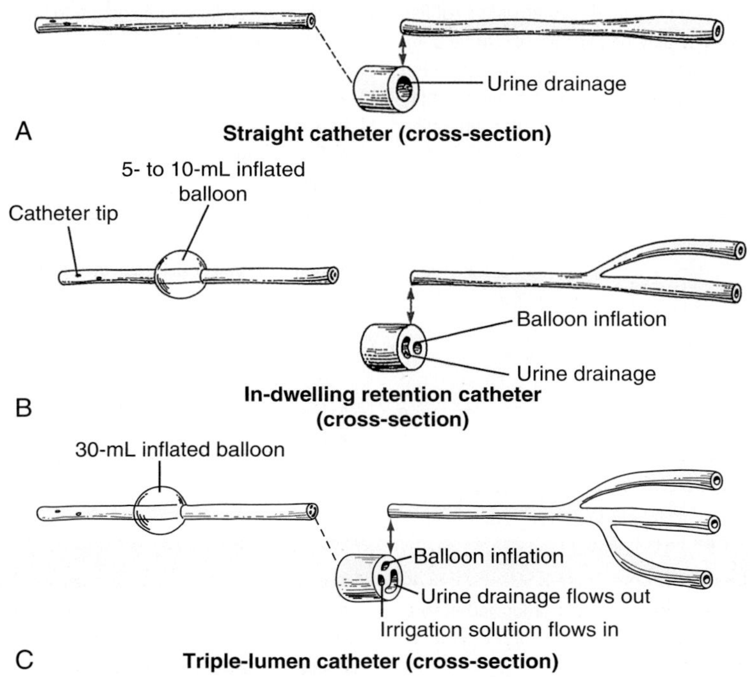

FIGURE 43-13 **A,** Straight catheter (cross-section), **B,** In-dwelling (Foley) retention catheter (cross-section). **C,** Triple-lumen catheter (cross-section).

BOX 43-7 Guidelines for Appropriate Catheter Selection

- The catheter size should be determined according to the size of the patient's urethral canal. When the French system is used, the larger the gauge number, the larger the catheter size. In general, an 8 to 10 Fr gauge is required for children, 10 to 12 for adult females, and 12 to 16 for adult males (Cottenden et al., 2013). The smallest effective catheter size is preferred in order to prevent trauma.
- After urological procedures (prostatectomy), a 20 to 24 Fr three-lumen catheter may be used to allow clot drainage and irrigation.
- The expected time required for catheterization will determine the catheter material selection (Teflon- or silicone-coated latex, 100% silicone, hydrophilic-coated latex).
- Plastic catheters are suitable only for intermittent use because of their inflexibility. Some intermittent catheters are hydrophilic (add water to make lubricious) or prelubricated to decrease friction and discomfort on insertion.
- Latex catheters come with or without a coating (silicone, Teflon, or silver). Be aware of patient allergies to any of these materials. Latex catheters may become encrusted more quickly than other materials (Cottenden et al., 2013).
- Pure silicone or hydrophilic polymer-coated catheters are best suited for long-term use (2 to 3 months) because they cause less encrustation at the urethral meatus and cause less friction and irritation to tissues (Cottenden et al., 2013).
- Silicone catheters have larger interior lumens than those of other catheters of the same size and may allow for more efficient urine drainage.
- For patients who develop encrustations and blockages frequently, the use of an inexpensive catheter changed every 7 to 10 days (depending on their pattern of blockage) may be more economical. Monitor patient's pattern of blocking and change prior to usual blockage time.
- For short-term use, silver-hydrogel catheters may delay the onset of bacteriuria.
- Balloon size is also important to consider when selecting an in-dwelling catheter. Balloon sizes range from 3 mL (pediatric) to large postoperative volumes (30 mL). In adults, the 10-mL size allows for optimal drainage, whereas the 30-mL size is used after prostatectomy to provide hemostasis of the prostatic bed (Cottenden et al., 2013).
- Only sterile water should be used to inflate the balloon because saline may crystallize, resulting in incomplete deflation of the balloon at the time of removal.
- Urine leakage around the catheter may be due to bladder spasms secondary to constipation or fecal impaction, the use of a large catheter balloon (30 mL) or a large catheter (>18 Fr) that causes irritation, the presence of a urinary tract infection, kinking of the catheter, or trauma at the bladder neck from traction on the balloon. A change in lumen size, the use of anticholinergic medication, or a referral to a urologist may be warranted.

SKILL 43-2 INSERTING AND REMOVING A STRAIGHT (INTERMITTENT) OR IN-DWELLING CATHETER

Delegation Considerations

Catheterization is usually not delegated to unregulated care providers (UCPs). However, in some settings, agency policy may permit this skill to be delegated to UCPs who have been properly instructed. UCPs routinely assist with positioning the patient and maintaining patient privacy and comfort, empty urine from the collection bag, and provide perineal care. If a UCP is performing the skill, instruct him or her to inform a nurse of the following:

- Patient discomfort or fever
- Abnormal colour, odour, or amount of urine in drainage bag

Equipment

Catheterization kit containing the following sterile items:

- Gloves (extra pair optional)
- Drapes, one fenestrated
- Lubricant
- Antiseptic cleaning solution
- Cotton balls
- Forceps
- Prefilled syringe with sterile water to inflate the balloon of an in-dwelling catheter
- Catheter of correct size and type for procedure (i.e., intermittent or in-dwelling)
- Sterile drainage tubing with collection bag and multipurpose tube holder or tape, safety pin, and elastic band for securing tubing to bed if patient is bed bound (for an in-dwelling catheter)
- Receptacle or basin (usually bottom of catheterization tray)
- Specimen container
- Blanket

PROCEDURE

STEPS	RATIONALE
1. Review patient's medical record, including prescriber's order and nurses' notes.	• Determines purpose of inserting catheter: preparation for surgery, urinary irrigations, collection of sterile specimens, measurement of residual urine, and size and style of catheter. Assess for previous catheterization, including catheter size, response of patient, and time of last catheterization.

STEPS	RATIONALE
2. Close bedside curtain or door.	• Offers privacy, reduces embarrassment, and aids in relaxation during procedure.
3. Assess status of patient:	
A. Ask patient when he or she last voided, or check intake and output flow sheet, or palpate bladder.	• Determines time of last voiding or potential for bladder fullness.
B. Level of awareness or developmental stage	• Reveals the patient's ability to cooperate and the level of explanation needed.
C. Mobility and physical limitations of patient	• Affects the way that the patient is positioned.
D. Patient's gender and age	• Determines catheter size: 8 to 10 Fr is generally used for children, 10 to 12 for adult females, 12 to 16 for adult males.
E. Distended bladder	• Causes pain. Can indicate need to insert catheter if patient is unable to void independently.
F. Perform hand hygiene. Apply clean gloves. Inspect perineum for erythema, drainage, and odour.	• Reduces infection. Determines condition of the perineum.
G. Note any pathological condition that may impair passage of catheter (e.g., enlarged prostate in men, pelvic organ prolapse in women).	• Obstruction prevents passage of catheter through urethra into the bladder. Use of coude catheter may be required for men.
H. Allergies	• Procedure risks exposure to antiseptic, tape, latex, and lubricant. Betadine allergies are common; if the patient is unaware of allergy, ask if allergic to shellfish.
4. Assess patient's knowledge of the purpose for catheterization.	• Reveals need for patient instruction.
5. Explain procedure to patient.	• Promotes cooperation.
6. Arrange for extra nursing personnel to assist as necessary.	• Patient may be unable to assume positioning for procedure.
7. Perform hand hygiene.	• Reduces transmission of microorganisms.
8. Raise bed to appropriate working height.	• Promotes use of proper body mechanics.
9. Facing patient, stand on left side of bed if right-handed (on right side of bed if left-handed). Clear the bedside table and arrange equipment.	• To insert catheter successfully, you must assume a comfortable position with all equipment easily accessible.
10. Raise side rail on opposite side of bed, and lower side rail on working side.	• Promotes patient safety.
11. Place waterproof pad under patient.	• Prevents soiling of bed linens.
12. Position patient:	
A. Female patient	
(1) Assist to dorsal recumbent position (supine with knees flexed). Ask patient to relax thighs so that the hips can be rotated externally.	• Provides good visualization of perineal structures. Support legs with pillows to reduce muscle tension and promote comfort.
(2) Assist to side-lying (Sims') position with upper leg flexed at hip if unable to assume dorsal recumbent position. If this position is used, you must take extra precautions to cover rectal area with drape to reduce chance of cross-contamination.	• This alternative position is used if patient cannot abduct legs at hip joint (e.g., if patient has arthritic joints). Support patient with pillows if necessary to maintain position.
B. Male patient	
(1) Assist to supine position with thighs slightly abducted.	• Comfortable position for patient that aids in visualization.
13. Drape patient:	• Avoids unnecessary exposure of body parts and maintains patient's comfort.
A. Female patient (see Step 13A illustration)	
(1) Drape with bath blanket. Place blanket in diamond fashion over patient, with one corner at patient's midsection, side corners over each thigh and abdomen, and last corner over perineum.	

Continued

SKILL 43-2 INSERTING AND REMOVING A STRAIGHT (INTERMITTENT) OR IN-DWELLING CATHETER—cont'd

STEPS	RATIONALE
B. Male patient (see Step 13B illustration)	
(1) Drape upper trunk with bath blanket and cover lower extremities with bed sheets, exposing only genitalia.	

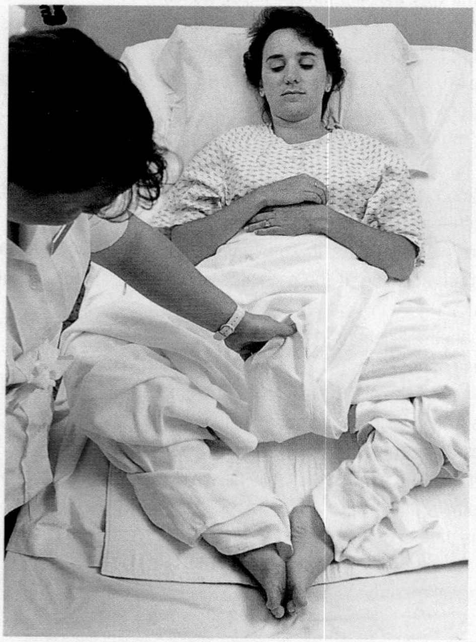

STEP 13A Draping technique (female).

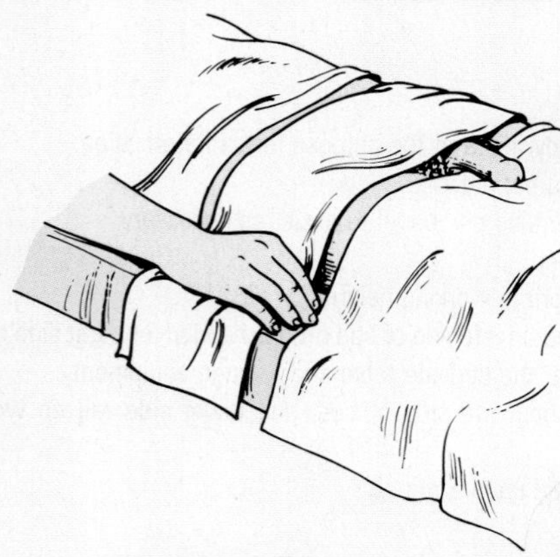

STEP 13B Draping technique (male).

STEPS	RATIONALE
14. Wearing disposable gloves, wash perineal area with soap and water as needed; dry thoroughly. Remove and discard gloves; perform hand hygiene.	• Reduces microorganisms near urethral meatus and allows further opportunity to visualize perineum and landmarks.
15. Position lamp to illuminate perineal area (have an assistant hold flashlight, if necessary).	• Permits accurate identification and good visualization of urethral meatus.
16. Open package containing drainage system; place drainage bag over edge of bottom bed frame, and bring drainage tube up between side rails and mattress.	• Prepares system for eventual connection with catheter.

CRITICAL DECISION POINT: *This step is necessary only when an in-dwelling catheter is being inserted and a drainage system is not part of the catheterization kit.*

STEPS	RATIONALE
17. Open catheterization kit according to directions, keeping bottom of container sterile.	• Prevents transmission of microorganisms from table or work area to sterile supplies. The materials in the kit are arranged in sequence of use.
18. Place plastic bag that contained kit within reach of work area to use as a waterproof bag to dispose of used supplies.	• Allows you to handle sterile supplies without contamination.
19. Apply sterile gloves (see Chapter 33).	

CRITICAL DECISION POINT: *If underpad is the first item in the catheterization kit, place pad plastic side down under patient, touching only the edges so as to maintain sterility. Then apply sterile gloves.*

STEPS	RATIONALE
20. Organize supplies on sterile field. Open inner sterile package containing catheter. Pour sterile antiseptic solution into correct compartment containing sterile cotton balls. Open packet containing lubricant. Remove specimen container (lid should be placed loosely on top) and prefilled syringe from collection compartment of tray, and set them aside on sterile field.	• Maintains principles of surgical asepsis and organizes work area. • *Note:* Pretesting of balloon is no longer recommended because catheters are pretested during manufacturing and inflation may distort the balloon, leading to increased trauma.
21. Lubricate 2.5 to 5 cm of catheter for women and 12.5 to 17.7 cm for men.	• Makes insertion of the catheter easier by decreasing friction.

CRITICAL DECISION POINT: *Some catheters have plastic sheaths over them that must be removed before lubrication. In some cases, the prescriber may order local anaesthetic lubricant.*

STEPS	RATIONALE
22. Apply sterile drape:	
A. Female patient	
(1) Allow top edge of drape to form a cuff over both gloved hands. Place drape on bed between patient's thighs. Slip cuffed edge just under buttocks, taking care not to touch contaminated surface with gloves.	• Outer surface of drape covering hands remains sterile. Sterile drape against sterile gloves is sterile.
(2) Pick up fenestrated sterile drape and allow it to unfold without touching any unsterile objects. Apply drape over perineum, exposing labia and being sure not to touch contaminated surface (see Step 22A illustration).	• Maintains sterility of work surface.
B. Male patient	
(1) Two methods are used for draping, depending on preference. *First method:* Apply drape over thighs and under penis without completely opening fenestrated drape. *Second method:* Apply drape over thighs just below penis. Pick up fenestrated sterile drape, allow it to unfold without touching any unsterile objects, and drape it over penis with fenestrated slit resting over penis (see Step 22B[1] illustration).	• Maintains sterility of work surface.

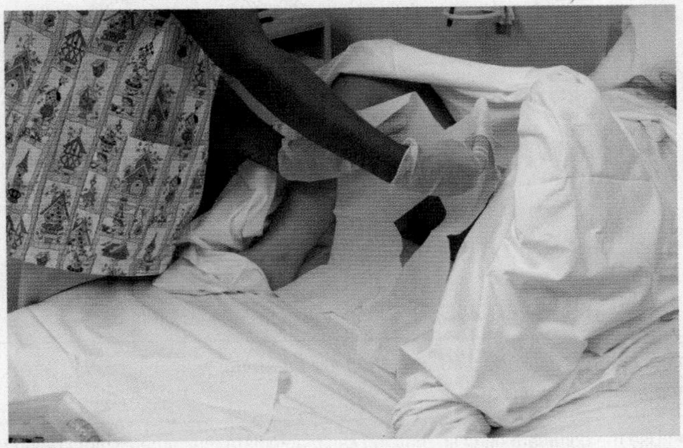

STEP 22A(2) Place sterile fenestrated drape (with opening in centre) over perineum with labia exposed.

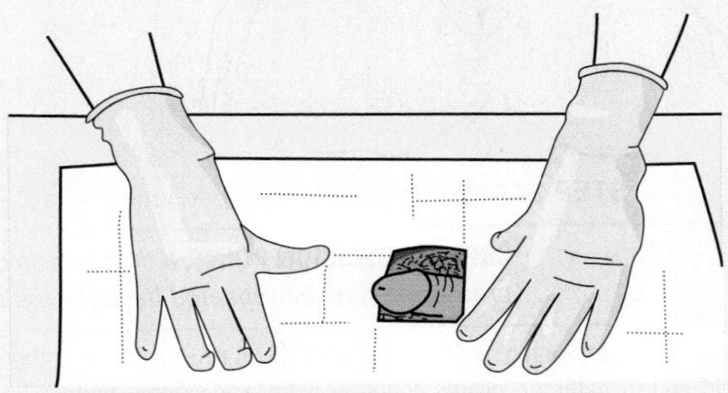

STEP 22B(1) Draping male with fenestrated drape.

23. Place sterile tray and contents on sterile drape. Open specimen container.	• Provides easy access to supplies during catheter insertion. Maintains aseptic technique during procedure.
24. Clean urethral meatus:	
A. Female patient	
(1) With nondominant hand, carefully retract labia to fully expose urethral meatus. Maintain position of nondominant hand throughout procedure.	• Full visualization of urethral meatus is provided. Full retraction prevents contamination of urethral meatus during cleaning.
(2) Using forceps held in sterile dominant hand, pick up cotton ball saturated with antiseptic solution, and clean perineal area, microwiping from clitoris toward anus (front to back). Using a new cotton ball for each area, wipe along the far labial fold, near labial fold, and directly over centre of urethral meatus (see Step 24A[2] illustration).	• Cleaning reduces number of microorganisms at urethral meatus. Use of a single cotton ball for each wipe prevents transfer of microorganisms. Cleaning for each of the three areas proceeds from area of least contamination to that of most contamination. Dominant hand remains sterile.

CRITICAL DECISION POINT: *If the labia close during cleaning, then the cleaning procedure must be repeated because the area has become contaminated.*

Continued

SKILL 43-2 INSERTING AND REMOVING A STRAIGHT (INTERMITTENT) OR IN-DWELLING CATHETER—cont'd

STEPS	RATIONALE
B. Male patient	
(1) If patient is not circumcised, retract foreskin with nondominant hand. Grasp penis at shaft just below glans. Retract urethral meatus between thumb and forefinger. Maintain nondominant hand in this position throughout procedure.	• If foreskin is accidentally released or if penis is dropped during cleaning, the process must be repeated because the area has become contaminated.
(2) With sterile dominant hand, pick up cotton ball with forceps and clean penis. Move in a circular motion from urethral meatus down to base of glans. Repeat cleaning three more times, using a clean cotton ball each time (see Step 24B[2] illustration).	• Cleaning reduces number of microorganisms at urethral meatus and proceeds from area of least contamination to that of most contamination. Dominant hand remains sterile.

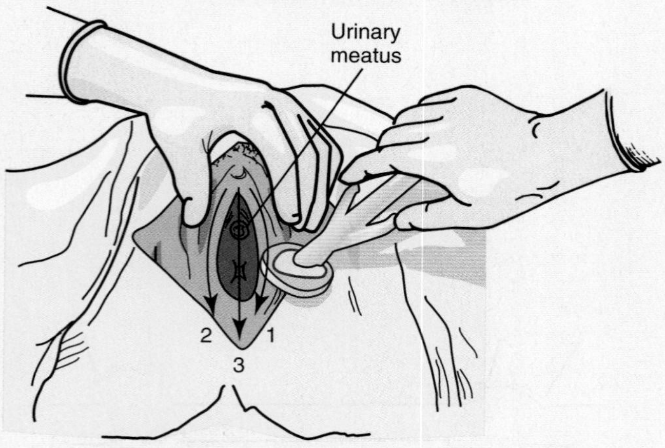

STEP 24A(2) Cleaning female perineum.

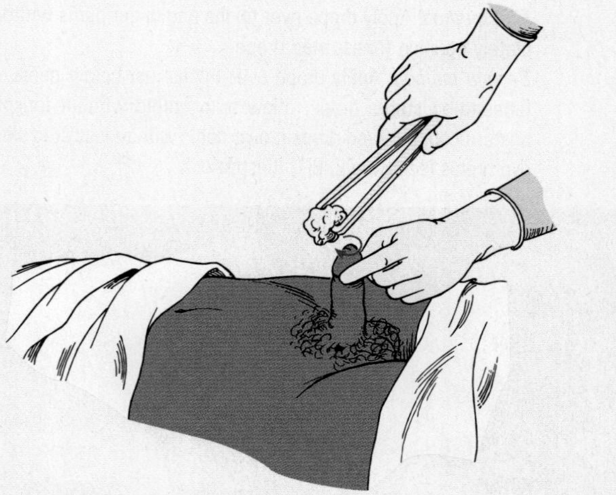

STEP 24B(2) Cleaning technique (male).

CRITICAL DECISION POINT: *If the foreskin does not remain retracted during cleaning, then the cleaning procedure must be repeated because the area has become contaminated.*

STEPS	RATIONALE
25. Pick up catheter with gloved dominant hand, 7.5 to 10 cm from catheter tip. Hold end of catheter loosely coiled in palm of dominant hand. (Optional: May grasp catheter with forceps.)	• Use the dominant hand so that you can manipulate the catheter more readily. Place distal end of catheter in urine tray receptacle if straight catheterization is ordered.
26. Insert catheter:	
A. Female patient	
(1) Ask patient to bear down gently as if voiding, and slowly insert catheter through urethral meatus (see Step 26A[1] illustration).	• Relaxation of urethral sphincter and pelvic floor muscle aids in insertion of catheter.

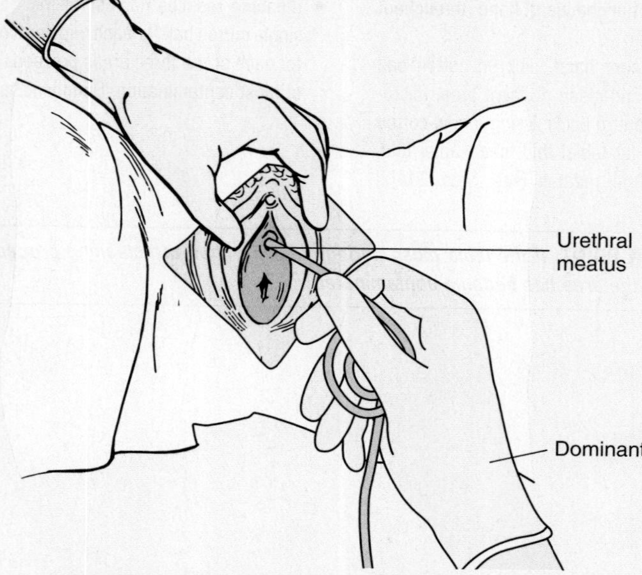

STEP 26A(1) Inserting catheter into female urinary meatus.

STEPS	RATIONALE
(2) Advance catheter a total of 5 to 7.5 cm in adult female or **until urine flows out of catheter's end.** When urine appears, advance catheter another 2.5 to 5 cm. *Do not force against resistance.*	• Female urethra is short. Appearance of urine indicates that the catheter tip is in bladder or lower urethra. Further advancement of catheter ensures bladder placement.
(3) Release labia and hold catheter securely with nondominant hand. Slowly inflate balloon if in-dwelling catheter is being used (see Step 26A[3] illustrations; see Step 29).	• Catheter may be expelled accidentally by bladder or sphincter contraction.

CRITICAL DECISION POINT: *If no urine appears, check whether catheter is in vagina. If misplaced, leave catheter in vagina as landmark indicating where not to insert, and insert another through urethral meatus.*

STEPS	RATIONALE
B. Male patient	
(1) Lift penis to position perpendicular to patient's body and apply light traction (see Step 26B[1] illustration).	• Straightens urethral canal to ease catheter insertion.

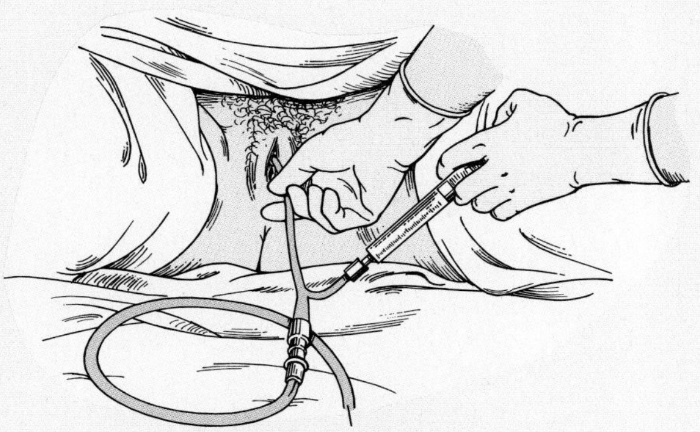

STEP 26A(3) Inflating balloon (in-dwelling catheter)

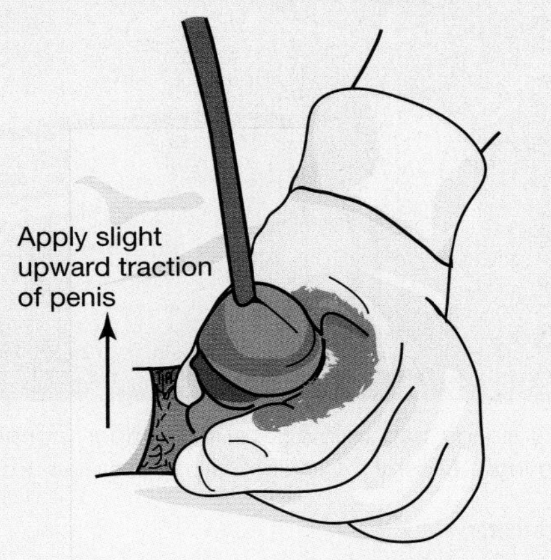

STEP 26B(1) Position penis perpendicular to body for catheter insertion.

STEPS	RATIONALE
(2) Ask patient to bear down as if voiding, and slowly insert catheter through urethral meatus.	• Relaxation of urethral sphincter and pelvic floor muscle aids in insertion of catheter.
(3) Advance catheter 17 to 22.5 cm in adult male or **until urine flows out of catheter's end**. If resistance is felt, withdraw catheter; do not force it through urethra. When urine appears, advance catheter another 2.5 to 5 cm. *Do not use force against resistance.*	• The adult male urethra is long. It is normal to meet resistance at the prostate. When resistance is felt, you should hold the catheter firmly without forcing it. After a few seconds, the muscle relaxes and the catheter is advanced. Appearance of urine indicates that the catheter tip is in bladder or urethra. Advancement of the catheter to the bifurcation ensures proper placement.
(4) Lower penis and hold catheter securely in nondominant hand. Place end of catheter in urine tray. Inflate balloon if in-dwelling catheter is being used (see Step 29).	• Catheter may be expelled accidentally by bladder or urethral contraction. Collection of urine prevents soiling and provides output measurement.
(5) Reduce (or reposition) the foreskin.	• Paraphimosis (retraction and constriction of the foreskin behind the glans penis) secondary to catheterization may occur if foreskin is not reduced.
27. Collect urine specimen as needed. Fill specimen cup or jar to desired level (20 to 30 mL) by holding end of catheter over cup with your dominant hand.	• Allows sterile specimen to be obtained for culture analysis.
28. Allow bladder to empty fully (about 800 to 1 000 mL) unless institution policy restricts maximal volume of urine to drain with each catheterization. Check institution policy before beginning catheterization.	• As always, you should monitor the patient's condition; if the vital signs change or bleeding occurs, temporarily stop the flow of urine and continue when the patient's condition warrants. Retained urine may serve as a reservoir for growth of microorganisms.

CRITICAL DECISION POINT: *If a single-use straight catheter was inserted, withdraw it slowly but smoothly until it is removed.*

STEPS	RATIONALE
29. Inflate balloon fully per manufacturer's recommendation and then release catheter with nondominant hand and pull gently.	• Inflation of balloon anchors the catheter tip in place above the bladder outlet to prevent the catheter's removal. Note size of balloon on catheter. Most commonly, a 5-mL balloon is used, but a 30-mL balloon may be ordered in some cases. A prefilled syringe may be included with the kit. Use only the amount included. Do not overinflate the balloon. A 5-mL balloon should be inflated with the supplied amount (10 mL) to allow symmetrical expansion.

Continued

SKILL 43-2 INSERTING AND REMOVING A STRAIGHT (INTERMITTENT) OR IN-DWELLING CATHETER—cont'd

STEPS	RATIONALE
CRITICAL DECISION POINT: *If resistance to inflation is noted or if patient complains of pain, the balloon may not be entirely within the bladder. Stop inflation, aspirate the fluid injected into the balloon, and advance the catheter a little more before attempting to inflate the balloon again.*	
30. Attach end of in-dwelling catheter to collecting tube of drainage system. Drainage bag must be below level of bladder. Attach bag to bed frame; do not place bag on bed's side rails (see Step 30 illustration).	• In-dwelling catheters drain the bladder by gravity. Attaching to the bed frame prevents accidental pulling of the catheter when a bed rail is lowered.

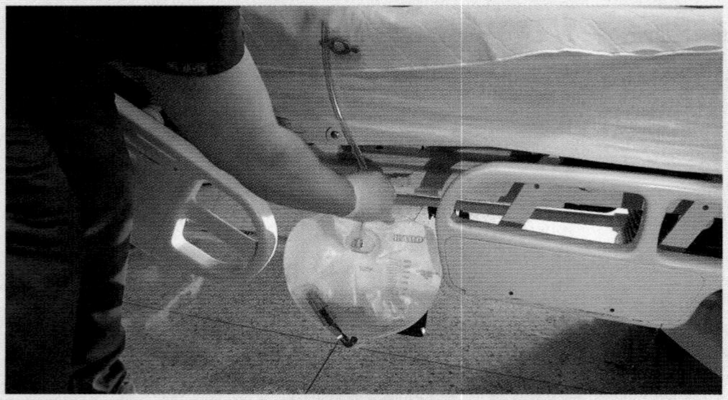

STEP 30 Drainage bag below level of bladder, connected to bed-frame. (Copyright Mosby's Clinical Skills: Essentials Collection.)

STEPS	RATIONALE
31. Anchor catheter:	
A. Female patient	
(1) Secure catheter tubing to inner thigh or abdomen with a strip of nonallergenic tape (or multipurpose tube holders with a Velcro strap). Allow for slack so that movement of thigh does not create tension on catheter (see Step 31A[1] illustration).	• Anchoring catheter to inner thigh reduces pressure on urethra, thus reducing possibility of tissue injury (Cottenden et al., 2013).
B. Male patient	
(1) Secure catheter tubing to top of thigh or lower abdomen (with penis directed toward chest). Allow for slack so that movement does not create tension on catheter (see Step 31B[1] illustration).	• Anchoring catheter to lower abdomen reduces pressure on urethra at junction of penis and scrotum, thus reducing possibility of tissue injury. Unsecured catheters may cause traction and pressure that leads to severe tissue erosion and damage to the urethral sphincter and urethra, particularly in males (Getliffe & Fader, 2007).

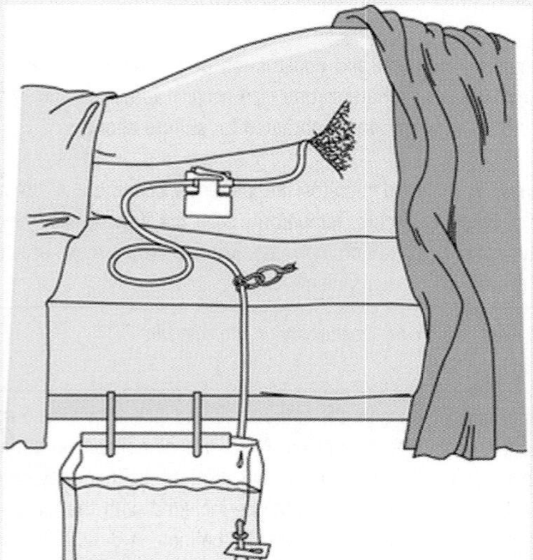

STEP 31A(1) Tape catheter to inner thigh (female) and coil extra tubing on bed and attach to sheet. (From Sorrentino, S. A., Remmert, L.N., & Wilk, M.J. [2018]. *Mosby's Canadian textbook for the support worker* [4th ed., Figure 31-11A]. Toronto: Elsevier.)

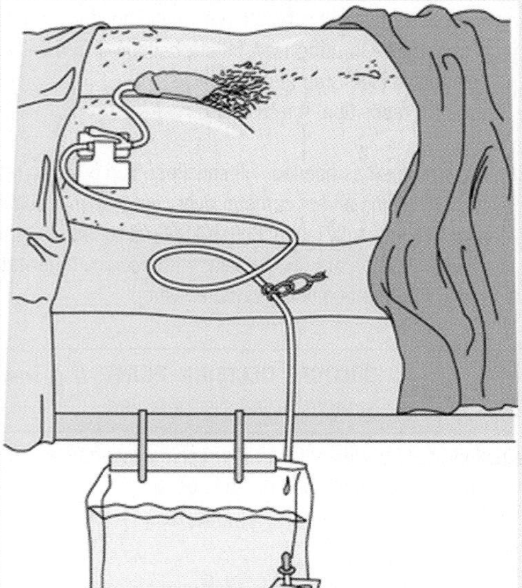

STEP 31B(1) Tape catheter to lower thigh (male) and coil extra tubing on bed and attach to sheet. (From Sorrentino, S. A., Remmert, L.N., & Wilk, M.J. [2018]. *Mosby's Canadian textbook for the support worker* [4th ed., Figure 31-11B]. Toronto: Elsevier.)

STEPS	RATIONALE
32. Assist patient to comfortable position. Wash and dry perineal area as needed.	• Maintains comfort and security.
33. Remove gloves and dispose of equipment, drapes, and urine in proper receptacles.	• Reduces transmission of microorganisms.
34. Perform hand hygiene.	• Reduces transmission of microorganisms.
35. Palpate bladder.	• Determines whether distension has been relieved.
36. Ask about patient's comfort.	• Determines whether patient's sensation of discomfort or fullness has been relieved.
37. Observe character and amount of urine in drainage system.	• Determines whether urine is flowing adequately.
38. Ensure that no urine is leaking from catheter or tubing connections.	• Prevents injury to patient's skin.
39. Removal of in-dwelling Foley catheter:	
A. Review medical order for removal of catheter. In cases of genitourinary surgery, it is especially important to obtain an order.	• Premature removal of catheter in patients who have undergone genitourinary surgery could injure the patient.
B. Perform hand hygiene, put on clean gloves, and provide privacy.	• Procedure requires use of medical asepsis.
C. Prepare the patient:	• Prepares patient, to minimize anxiety.
(1) Provide an explanation of procedure.	
(2) Position patient with waterproof pad under buttocks and cover with bath blanket, exposing only genital area and catheter. Position females in dorsal recumbent position and male patients in supine position.	• Shows respect for patient dignity by only exposing genital area and catheter.
(3) Remove catheter securement device and free drainage tubing.	
D. If needed, provide hygiene of genital area with soap and water.	• Antiseptic cleaners have not been proven to decrease risk for catheter-associated UTI (Gould, Umscheid, Agarwal, et al., 2010; Lo et al., 2014).
E. Move syringe plunger up and down to loosen, and then withdraw plunger to 0.5 mL. Insert hub of syringe into inflation valve (balloon port). Allow balloon fluid to drain into syringe by gravity. Make sure that entire amount of fluid is removed by comparing removed amount to volume needed for inflation.	• Partially inflated balloon can traumatize urethral wall during removal. Passive drainage of catheter balloon will prevent formation of ridges in balloon. These ridges can cause discomfort or trauma during removal.
F. Pull catheter out smoothly and slowly. Examine it to ensure that it is whole. Catheter should slide out easily. Do not use force. If you note any resistance, repeat Step 39E to remove remaining water. Notify health care provider if balloon does not deflate completely.	• Promotes patient comfort and safety.
G. Wrap contaminated catheter in waterproof pad. Unhook collection bag and drainage tubing from bed.	• Reduces transmission of microorganisms.
H. Reposition patient as necessary. Provide hygiene as needed. Lower level of bed and position side rails accordingly.	
I. Empty, measure, and record urine present in drainage bag. Discard in appropriate receptacle. Remove and discard gloves. Perform hand hygiene.	• Records urinary output. Reduces transmission of microorganisms.
J. Encourage patient to maintain or increase fluid intake (unless contraindicated).	• Maintains normal urine output.
K. Initiate voiding record or bladder diary. Instruct patient to report when urge to void occurs and that all urine needs to be measured. Make sure that patient understands how to use collection container.	• Evaluates bladder function.
L. Ensure easy access to toilet, commode, bedpan, or urinal. Place urine "hat" on toilet seat if patient is using toilet. Place call bell within easy reach.	

UNEXPECTED OUTCOMES	RELATED INTERVENTIONS
Urethral or perineal irritation or discomfort	• Observe for leaking catheter; replace if necessary. • Assess whether in-dwelling catheter is anchored properly. • Perform perineal hygiene and catheter care more frequently.
Fever or odour, or small, frequent voidings, burning sensations, or bleeding on voiding	• Obtain a new sterile specimen from the catheter port. • Notify prescriber.
Urinary retention and inability to void after catheter is removed	• Provide adequate fluid intake and ensure patient privacy. • If patient is unable to void 6 to 8 hours after catheter removal, notify prescriber.

Continued

SKILL 43-2 INSERTING AND REMOVING A STRAIGHT (INTERMITTENT) OR IN-DWELLING CATHETER—cont'd

STEPS	RATIONALE

RECORDING AND REPORTING

- Report and record type and size of catheter inserted, amount of fluid used to inflate the balloon, characteristics of urine, amount of urine, reasons for catheterization, specimen collection if appropriate, and patient's response to procedure and teaching concepts.
- Initiate intake and output record.
- If catheter is definitely in bladder and no urine is produced within 1 hour, absence of urine should be reported to prescriber immediately.

HOME CARE CONSIDERATIONS

- Patients who are at home may use a leg bag during the day and switch to a large-volume bag at night so that sleep can be uninterrupted. Attach the large-volume bag to the spigot at the bottom of the leg bag.
- Patients may catheterize themselves at home, using a clean technique.

If the catheter must be disconnected from the drainage tubing, both tips should be cleaned with an alcohol swab before being reconnected, to minimize the transfer of microorganisms into the tubing.

Most drainage bags contain an antireflux valve to prevent urine in the bag from re-entering the drainage tubing and contaminating the patient's bladder. A spigot at the base of the bag is used to empty the bag. The spigot should always be clamped, except during emptying, and tucked into the protective pouch on the side of the bag (see agency policy). To ensure that the drainage system remains unobstructed, the nurse should check for kinks or bends in the tubing, avoid positioning the patient on the drainage tubing, and observe for clots or sediment that may occlude the collecting tubing.

Routine catheter care. Patients with in-dwelling catheters have a number of special care needs. Nursing measures are directed at maintaining patient comfort, preventing infection, and maintaining an unobstructed flow of urine.

Perineal hygiene. Buildup of secretions or encrustation at the catheter insertion site is a source of irritation and potential infection. Nurses should provide perineal hygiene (see Chapter 38) at least twice daily, after a bowel movement, or as needed for a patient with an in-dwelling catheter. Soap and water or skin cleansers are effective in reducing the number of microorganisms around the urethra and help to maintain skin health and patient comfort. The nurse should take care not to accidentally advance the catheter upward into the bladder during cleaning as this action risks introducing bacteria into the bladder.

Catheter care. In addition to routine perineal hygiene, many institutions recommend that patients with catheters receive special care three times a day and after defecation or bowel incontinence to help minimize discomfort and infection (Skill 43-3).

Fluid intake. All patients with catheters should have a daily fluid intake of at least 2 000 to 2 500 mL. Encouraging self-management in patients with a long-term catheter can improve their fluid intake (Wilde, Crean, McMahon, et al., 2016), which can be met through oral intake or intravenous infusion. A high fluid intake produces a large volume of urine that flushes the bladder and keeps the catheter tubing free of sediment.

Preventing infection. The most important strategy in preventing the onset of infection is performing hand hygiene between patients. Maintaining a closed urinary drainage system is also important (Lo, Nicolle, Coffin, et al., 2014). A break in the system can lead to the introduction of microorganisms. Locations at risk are the site of catheter insertion, the drainage bag, the spigot, the tube junction, and the junction of the tube and the bag (Figure 43-14).

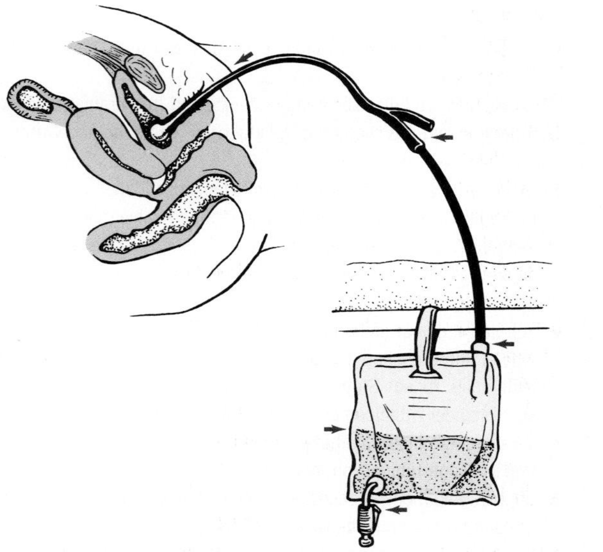

FIGURE 43-14 Potential sites for introduction of infectious organisms into a urinary drainage system.

In addition, the nurse should monitor the patency of the system to prevent pooling of urine within the tubing. Bacteria can travel up drainage tubing to grow in pools of urine. If this urine flows back into the patient's bladder, an infection will likely develop. The patient should be observed for symptoms of UTI, and any changes in his or her condition need to be documented. Suggested methods to prevent infections in catheterized patients are provided in Box 43-8.

Catheter irrigations and instillations. Sometimes it may be necessary to irrigate an in-dwelling urinary catheter using a triple-lumen catheter and sterile solution to maintain patency after urogenital surgery or to prevent blood clots from occluding the catheter. This is usually done by a continuous closed-bladder irrigation. Occasionally, an intermittent closed irrigation may be ordered if the catheter is occluded and it is deemed harmful to remove the catheter (e.g., after urological surgery). A prescriber may order bladder instillations for select bladder medications, with instruction as to how long the medication stays in the bladder. Unnecessary catheter irrigation should be avoided (Lo et al., 2014). If a catheter becomes occluded by sediment and encrustation, it should be changed to avoid flushing debris

SKILL 43-3 IN-DWELLING CATHETER CARE

Delegation Considerations

Perineal care is often part of routine hygiene care that is delegated to unregulated care providers (UCPs). Proper assessment and care of the perineal area requires professional clinical judgement. If the patient has had trauma or surgical procedures that involve the perineal area, care of this area should not be delegated.

- Instruct the UCP to report any patient discomfort, perineal pain, perineal discharge, or odour to a nurse. The UCP should also report on the condition of the catheter and drainage tubing (e.g., leaks, encrustations, or any discoloured or foul-smelling urine).

Equipment

- Catheter care kit or individual supplies
- Disposable gloves
- Cotton balls or large swabs
- Clean washcloth and towel
- Warm water and soap
- Antiseptic swab or cloth (if agency policy directs)
- Bath blanket
- Waterproof absorbent pad

PROCEDURE

STEPS	RATIONALE
1. Assess for episode of bowel incontinence or patient discomfort or provide care as per agency routine regarding hygiene measures (see Chapter 38).	• Accumulation of secretions or feces causes irritation to perineal tissues and acts as a source of bacterial growth.
2. Explain procedure to patient. Offer the able patient an opportunity to perform self-care.	• Reduces anxiety and promotes cooperation. Embarrassment may motivate patient to perform own hygiene.
3. Close door or bedside curtain.	• Maintains patient privacy.
4. Perform hand hygiene.	• Reduces transmission of infection.
5. Position patient.	
A. Female patient	• Ensures easy access to perineal tissues.
(1) Dorsal recumbent position	
B. Male patient	
(1) Supine or Fowler's position	
6. Place waterproof pad under patient.	• Prevents soiling of bed linens.
7. Drape bath blanket over patient so that only perineal area is exposed.	• Prevents unnecessary exposure of body parts.
8. Apply gloves.	
9. Remove anchor device to free catheter tubing.	
10. With nondominant hand:	
A. Female patient	
(1) Gently retract labia to expose urethral meatus and catheter insertion site fully, maintaining position of hand throughout procedure.	• Provides full visualization of urethral meatus. Full retraction prevents contamination of urethral meatus during cleaning.
B. Male patient	• If foreskin is accidentally released or penis is dropped during cleaning, the process must be repeated because the area has become contaminated.
(1) Retract foreskin if not circumcised, and hold penis at shaft just below glans, maintaining position throughout procedure.	
11. Assess urethral meatus and surrounding tissue for inflammation, swelling, and discharge. Note amount, colour, odour, and consistency of discharge. Ask patient if any burning or discomfort has been experienced.	• Determines presence of local infection and status of hygiene.
12. Clean perineal tissue:	
A. Female patient	
(1) Use clean cloth and perineal cleanser. Clean around urethral meatus and catheter. Moving from pubis toward anus, clean labia minora. Use a clean side of the cloth for each wipe. Finally, clean around anus. Dry each area well.	• Reduces the number of microorganisms at the urethral meatus. Use of a clean cloth prevents transfer of microorganisms.
B. Male patient	• Cleaning moves from area of least contamination to that of most contamination.
(1) While spreading urethral meatus, clean around catheter first, and then wipe in circular motion around meatus and glans.	
13. Reassess urethral meatus for discharge.	• Determines whether cleaning is complete.

Continued

SKILL 43-3 IN-DWELLING CATHETER CARE—cont'd

STEPS	RATIONALE
14. While stabilizing the catheter with the nondominant hand, use a towel and perineal cleanser to wipe in a circular motion along length of catheter for 10 cm (see Step 14 illustration).	• Reduces presence of secretions or drainage on exterior surface of catheter. • Some agencies may use antiseptic swab or cloth to wipe off tubing. Check policy.

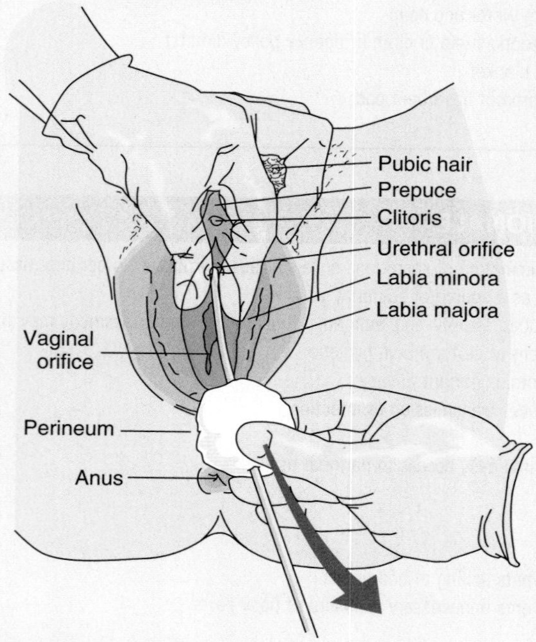

STEP 14 Cleaning catheter during catheter care (From Sorrentino, S. [2007]. *Mosby's textbook for nursing assistants.* St. Louis: Mosby.)

STEPS	RATIONALE
15. In male patient, reduce (or reposition) the foreskin.	• Prevents trauma to the head of the penis.
16. Re-anchor catheter tubing.	• Prevents trauma to the urethra.
17. Place patient in a safe, comfortable position.	• Promotes comfort.
18. Dispose of contaminated supplies, remove gloves, and perform hand hygiene.	• Reduces spread of infection.

UNEXPECTED OUTCOMES	RELATED INTERVENTIONS
Urethral discharge	• Increase frequency of in-dwelling catheter care. • Notify prescriber. • Assess for urethral trauma. • Monitor urine output.

RECORDING AND REPORTING

- Report and record the presence and characteristics of drainage, the condition of the perineal tissue, and any discomfort reported by the patient.
- If infection is suspected, report findings to prescriber.

HOME CARE CONSIDERATIONS

- If patient is discharged with an in-dwelling catheter in place, the patient and family should be taught catheter care as well as educated about the signs and symptoms that should be reported to a nurse or prescriber. A referral for home care may be needed.

containing bacteria into the bladder. Bladder irrigations or washouts to "unblock" such catheters that break the closed urinary drainage system increase risk of UTI.

Maintenance of a closed system is essential during continuous or intermittent irrigations (see Skill 43-4) and instillations. An order from a prescriber is needed for all irrigations and instillations.

Removal of in-dwelling catheter. When removing an in-dwelling catheter, the nurse needs to promote normal bladder function and prevent trauma to the urethra. Timely removal of in-dwelling catheters that are no longer required is a key intervention in reducing the incidence of CAUTI (Lo et al., 2014).

The patient may experience some discomfort when voiding after initial removal of the catheter. Until the bladder regains full tone, the patient may experience urinary frequency or retention. Ongoing complaints of dysuria and frequency may indicate an infection. The patient's urinary function is assessed by noting the first voiding after

BOX 43-8 Preventing Catheter-Associated Urinary Tract Infection (CAUTI)

- In acute care, urinary catheters should be inserted using aseptic technique with sterile equipment.
- Securing in-dwelling catheters prevents movement and pulling on the catheter, reducing urethral trauma.
- Maintain a closed urinary drainage system.
- Maintain unobstructed flow of urine through the catheter, drainage tubing, and drainage bag.
- Keep the urinary drainage bag below the level of the bladder at all times.
- Avoid dependent loops in urinary drainage tubing.
- Prevent the urinary drainage bag from touching or dragging on the floor.
- Use a separate measuring receptacle for each patient when emptying the urinary drainage bag. Do not allow the drainage spigot to touch the receptacle.
- Drain all urine from the tubing into bag and empty the drainage bag before patient transfer or activity.
- Empty the drainage bag when half-full.
- Perform routine perineal hygiene daily and after soiling. Be sure to use a wipe to clean the length of the exposed catheter.
- Obtain urine samples using the sampling port. Clean the port with disinfectant and use a sterile syringe or cannula.
- Quality improvement programs should be in place that alert providers that a catheter is in place and, in acute care, trigger daily review of need.

From Gould, C. V., Umscheid, C. A., Agarwal, R. K., Kuntz, G., Pegues, D. A., & the Healthcare Infection Control Practices Advisory Committee. (2010). Guideline for prevention of catheter-associated urinary tract infections 2009. *Infection Control and Hospital Epidemiology, 31,* 319–326. doi:10.1086/651091; Lo, E., Nicolle, L. E., Coffin, S. E., Gould, C., Maragakis, L. L., Meddings J., et al. (2014). Strategies to prevent catheter-associated urinary tract infections in acute care hospitals: 2014 update. *Infection Control and Hospital Epidemiology, 35*(5), 464–479. doi:10.1086/675718.

SKILL 43-4 CLOSED CATHETER IRRIGATION

Delegation Considerations

Closed catheter irrigation is usually not delegated to unregulated care providers (UCPs). Closed catheter irrigation is usually done in patients with complications such as gross hematuria or after a urological surgery.

- UCPs may assist with other aspects of patient care, such as positioning the patient and measuring intake and output.
- Instruct the UCP to report any complaints of pain, discomfort, or fever to a nurse.
- Instruct the UCP to report the presence of clots in the output or a change in output to a nurse.

Equipment

- Closed intermittent method:
  - Antiseptic swab
  - Sterile irrigation solution at room temperature
  - Sterile container
  - Luerlock needleless syringe to access port (check manufacturer requirements)
  - Clamp to temporarily occlude catheter as irrigant is instilled
- Closed continuous method:
  - Sterile irrigation solution at room temperature
  - Irrigation tubing and clamp
  - IV pole
  - Antiseptic swab
  - Bath blanket

PROCEDURE

STEPS	RATIONALE
1. Assess prescriber's order for type of irrigation (continuous or intermittent) and irrigation solution to use.	• Ensures proper selection of equipment.
2. Assess colour of urine and presence of mucus or sediment.	• Determines whether patient is bleeding, has infection, or is sloughing tissue.
3. Determine type of catheter in place:	
A. Triple lumen (one lumen to inflate balloon, one to instill irrigation solution, one to allow outflow of urine).	• Triple lumen is for closed continuous irrigation.
B. Double lumen (one lumen to inflate balloon, one to allow outflow of urine).	• Double lumen may be in place for closed intermittent irrigation/instillation.
4. Determine patency of drainage tubing.	• Ensures that drainage tubing is not kinked, clamped incorrectly, or looped.
5. Assess amount of urine in drainage bag (may want to empty drainage bag before irrigation).	• If drainage bag is not empty, you will need to subtract urine volume from the amount drained to determine whether all irrigant has returned.
6. Explain procedure and purpose to patient.	• Helps patient relax and cooperate during procedure.
7. Perform hand hygiene and apply disposable gloves for closed methods.	• Prevents transmission of microorganisms.
8. Provide privacy by pulling bed curtains closed. Fold back covers so that the catheter is exposed. Cover patient's upper torso with bath blanket.	• Promotes patient comfort.
9. Assess lower abdomen for bladder distension.	• Detects whether catheter is malfunctioning or blocking urinary drainage.
10. Position patient in dorsal recumbent or supine position.	• Promotes patient comfort and provides easy access to catheter.

Continued

SKILL 43-4 CLOSED CATHETER IRRIGATION—cont'd

STEPS	RATIONALE
11. *Closed intermittent irrigation (with double-lumen catheter):*	
A. Prepare prescribed sterile solution in sterile graduated cup.	• Ensures that irrigating fluid remains sterile.
B. Draw sterile solution into syringe by using aseptic technique.	

CRITICAL DECISION POINT: ***Avoid cold solution as irrigant because it may cause bladder spasm and discomfort.***

STEPS	RATIONALE
C. Clamp in-dwelling catheter just distal to injection (specimen) port.	• Occlusion of catheter allows irrigant to be instilled into catheter.
D. Clean injection port with antiseptic swab (same port used for specimen collection).	• Reduces transmission of infection.
E. Insert needless syringe tip through port.	
F. Slowly inject fluid into catheter and bladder.	• Slow, continuous pressure reduces trauma to the bladder wall.

CRITICAL DECISION POINT: ***If catheter does not irrigate easily, stop the irrigation. The catheter may be occluded or tip may be placed in the urethra and not in the bladder. Contact prescriber, as the catheter may need to be removed or replaced.***

STEPS	RATIONALE
G. Withdraw syringe, remove clamp, and allow solution to drain into drainage bag. If instillation was ordered by prescriber, keep clamped to allow solution to remain in bladder for ordered time.	• Allows drainage by gravity. Some medications stay in the bladder for a specific time. Do not leave unattended.

CRITICAL DECISION POINT: ***If solution is to remain in bladder, do not forget to unclamp tubing at the end of the instillation period.***

12. Closed continuous irrigation (with triple-lumen catheter) (see Step 12 illustration).

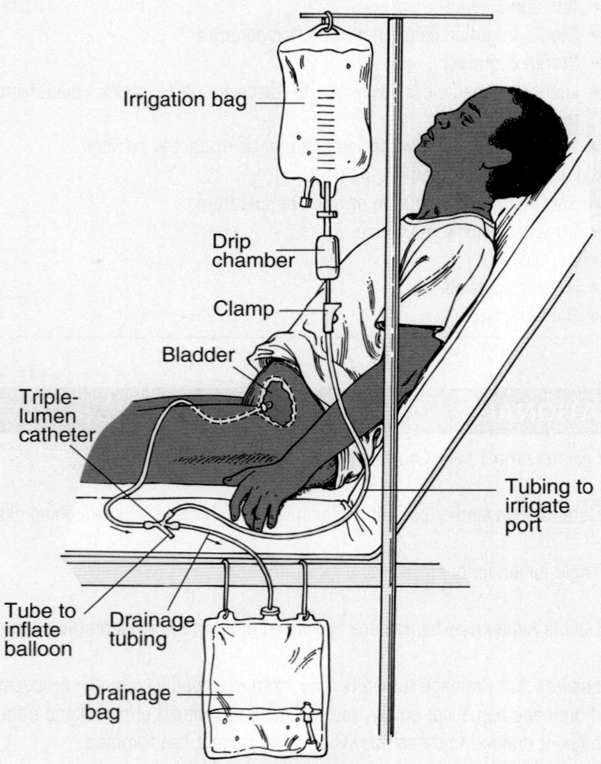

STEP 12 Closed continuous bladder irrigation.

STEPS	RATIONALE
A. Using the aseptic technique, insert tip of sterile irrigation tubing into bag of sterile irrigating solution.	• Prevents entrance of microorganisms.
B. Close clamp on tubing and hang bag of solution on IV pole.	
C. Open clamp and allow solution to flow through (prime) tubing, keeping end of tubing sterile. Close clamp.	• Removes air from tubing.

STEPS	RATIONALE
D. Wipe off irrigation port of triple-lumen catheter with antiseptic swab, and then attach to irrigation tubing.	• Third lumen provides means for irrigation solution to enter bladder. System must remain sterile.
E. Be sure that drainage bag and tubing are securely connected to the drainage port of triple-lumen catheter.	• Ensures that urine and irrigation solution will drain from bladder.
F. For intermittent flow, clamp tubing on drainage system, open clamp on irrigation tubing, and allow prescribed amount of fluid to enter bladder (100 mL is normal for adults). Close irrigation clamp and then open drainage tubing clamp. (Optional: Leave clamp closed for time ordered. See previous Critical Decision Point.)	• Fluid instills through catheter into bladder, flushing system. Fluid drains out after irrigation is completed.
G. For continuous drainage, calculate drip rate and adjust clamp on irrigation tubing accordingly. Be sure that clamp on drainage tubing is open and check volume of drainage in drainage bag. Ensure that drainage tubing is patent, and avoid kinks.	• Ensures continuous, even irrigation of catheter system. • Prevents accumulation of solution in bladder, which may cause bladder distension and possible injury.
13. When irrigation is complete, dispose of contaminated supplies, remove gloves, and perform hand hygiene.	• Prevents spread of infection.
14. Calculate fluid used to irrigate bladder and catheter and subtract from total output.	• Determines accurate urinary output.
15. Assess characteristics of output: viscosity, colour, and presence of matter (e.g., sediment, clots, blood).	• Evaluates results of irrigation.

UNEXPECTED OUTCOMES	RELATED INTERVENTIONS
Irrigating solution does not return or is not flowing at prescribed rate, possible occlusion of catheter	• Examine tubing for kinks, clots, or urine sediment. • Evaluate for bladder distension. • Notify prescriber if irrigant is retained, if patient complains of pain, or if bladder is distended.
Bright red bleeding with irrigation	• Assess for shock (check vital signs, skin colour, and moisture). • Closed intermittent—stop irrigation • Closed continuous—leave flowing • Notify prescriber immediately.
Increased cloudiness of urine, fever	• Monitor fever. • Notify prescriber. • Obtain sterile urine specimen if ordered by prescriber.
Increase in pain	• Examine tubing for kinks, clots, or urine sediment. • Evaluate for bladder distension. • Notify prescriber.

RECORDING AND REPORTING

- Record type and amount of irrigation solution used, amount returned as drainage, and the character of drainage.
- Record and report any findings such as complaints of fever, pain, sudden bleeding, inability to instill fluid into bladder, or presence of blood clots.

HOME CARE CONSIDERATIONS

- If patient is discharged with an in-dwelling catheter and requires bladder irrigations, either the patient or the patient's family must be properly instructed on how to perform this task or a referral made to home care.
- Teach patient and family to observe urine colour, clarity, odour, amount, and signs of obstruction or urinary tract infection.

catheter removal and by documenting the time and amount of voiding during the next 24 to 48 hours. The nurse should record the time and amount of voids, including incontinence, on a bladder record. An ultrasound bladder scanner can assist with monitoring PVR urine. If amounts are small, frequent assessment for bladder distension, abdominal pain, dribbling, incontinence, and any sensation of incomplete empting is necessary. If 8 hours elapse without voiding or if the patient experiences discomfort, it may become necessary to reinsert the catheter. The prescriber should be notified.

Alternatives to Urethral Catheterization. Absorbent pads can be an aid to containing urine loss. Two alternatives for urinary drainage can be used to avoid the risks associated with catheters inserted through the urethra: suprapubic catheterization and condom catheters.

Absorbent pads. Both disposable and washable absorbent pads are available in many absorbencies and styles. These include insert pads designed for women and men to wear with underwear, all-in-one briefs, pull-ups, and underpads (Cottenden et al., 2013). Absorbent pads for urine are designed with multiple layers to absorb urine. Some people may need a combination of products to manage incontinence. Incontinence pads are helpful to contain urine leakage but not a replacement for assisting patients to the toilet.

Suprapubic catheterization. Suprapubic catheterization involves surgical placement of a catheter through the abdominal wall above the symphysis pubis and into the urinary bladder (Figure 43-15). For those needing long-term catheterization, a suprapubic rather than urethrally inserted catheter may be an option for comfort, although CAUTI can still occur (Hunter, Bharmal, & Moore, 2013). A physician performs the procedure under local or general anaesthesia. The catheter is anchored in place with sutures, a commercially prepared body seal, or both. Long-term suprapubic catheter users may have a Foley catheter, and once the track is healed, nurses may be authorized to change this type of device. Urine drains into a urinary drainage bag. Maintenance of the tubing and drainage bag is the same as for an in-dwelling catheter. The suprapubic catheter is relatively painless and reduces the incidence of infection commonly seen with in-dwelling catheters. Studies comparing the use of this method of urinary drainage have shown mixed results. While infection rates may be slightly lower, the long-term complications are similar (Hunter et al., 2013). Sediment, clots, encrustations, or the abdominal wall itself can block the suprapubic catheter. Adequate fluid intake will help minimize the risk of blockage by sediment or infection due to stagnation. The suprapubic catheter must remain patent at all times. Nurses must monitor the patient's intake and output carefully, monitor the appearance of urine, and observe for signs of infection (e.g., fever and chills). Nurses also should administer skin care around the insertion site.

Condom catheters. The second alternative to catheterization is the condom catheter (external urinary catheter; Box 43-9), which may be suitable for incontinent or comatose men who still have complete and spontaneous bladder emptying. The condom is a soft, pliable sheath that slips over the penis. It may be worn at night only or continuously, depending on the patient's needs. The most common is the self-adhesive silicone condom sheath or sheath with brush-on adhesive, although some are still secured with a strip of elastic tape (European Association of Urology Nurses, 2016). Latex products are also still available; the nurse needs to ensure that the patient does not have a latex allergy if one is used. Care must be taken to ensure that whatever type or size of condom is used, blood supply to the penis is not impaired. Standard adhesive tape should never be used to secure a condom catheter because this tape does not expand with changes in penis size and is painful to remove.

Condom catheters are associated with less risk of UTI, but infections may result from buildup of secretions around the urethra, trauma to the urethral meatus, or buildup of pressure in the outflow tubing. Condom catheters must be applied and changed according to the manufacturers' directions to prevent abrasion, dermatitis, ischemia, necrosis, edema, and maceration of the penis. Frequent skin assessment is vital.

For a man with a retracted penis, maintaining a conventional condom catheter may prove difficult. To help alleviate this problem, special externally applied devices are available that are secured by hydrocolloid strips (Figure 43-16), or specially designed underwear can be used. The manufacturer's guidelines for product application should be consulted.

Maintenance of Skin Integrity. Prolonged exposure of skin to urine and stool can lead to inflammation and maceration, resulting in incontinence-associated dermatitis (IAD) (Gray, McNichol, & Nix, 2016). Continuous exposure of the perineal area or skin around an ostomy can also lead to gradual maceration and excoriation (see

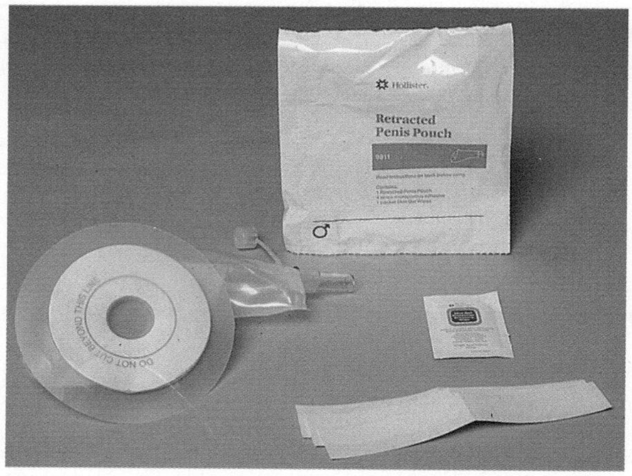

FIGURE 43-16 Retracted penis pouch external urinary device.

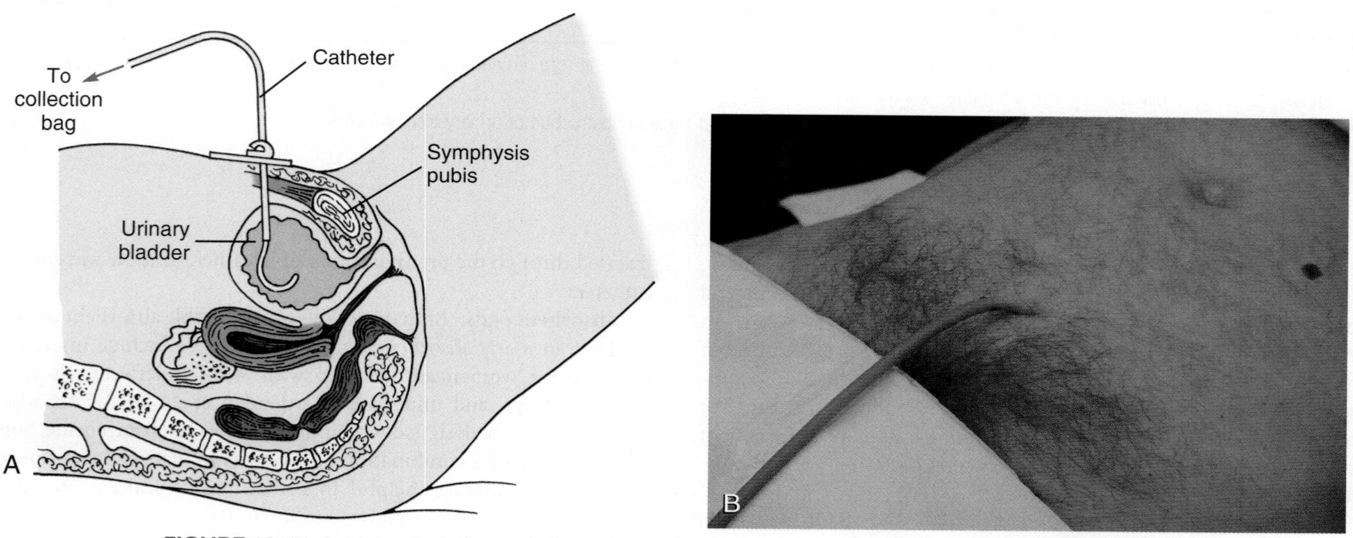

FIGURE 43-15 **A,** Placement of suprapubic catheter above symphysis pubis. **B,** Suprapubic catheter without a dressing.

BOX 43-9 PROCEDURAL GUIDELINE

Applying a Condom Catheter

Delegation Considerations:

The application of a condom catheter can be delegated to unregulated care providers (UCPs). The registered nurse is responsible for assessing the condition of the penis over time and should inform the UCP to notify the registered nurse of any signs of skin irritation or tissue swelling.

Equipment:

- Condom catheter (may be self-adhesive or provided with elastic adhesive tape)
- Collection bag
- Basin with warm water
- Towel and washcloth
- Disposable gloves
- Scissors

Procedure:

1. Check prescriber's order.
2. Perform hand hygiene.
3. Assess urinary elimination patterns, the patient's ability to urinate voluntarily, and continence.
4. Assess the patient's mental status to determine appropriate teaching related to condom catheter care.
5. Assess condition of penis and scrotum. Ensure that the foreskin of the uncircumcised male is not retracted.
6. Assess the patient's knowledge of the purpose of the condom catheter.
7. Explain procedure to patient.
8. Raise bed to working height and raise far upper side rail.
9. Using sheet, drape patient so that only genitals are exposed.
10. Prepare condom catheter and drainage system (see manufacturer's directions).
11. Apply gloves and provide perineal care.
    A. If necessary, clip hair at base of penile shaft.
12. Apply skin preparation to penile shaft and allow to dry.
13. Holding penis in nondominant hand, apply condom by rolling smoothly onto penis. *Note:* Leave a 2.5-cm to 5-cm space between tip of penis and end of catheter (see Step 13 illustration).
14. Secure condom catheter:
    A. If self-adhesive catheter is used, follow the manufacturer's directions.
    B. If elastic adhesive is used, wrap the strip of adhesive over the condom catheter to secure it in place, using a spiral technique (see Step 14A illustration). *Note:* Adhesive tape must never be used.

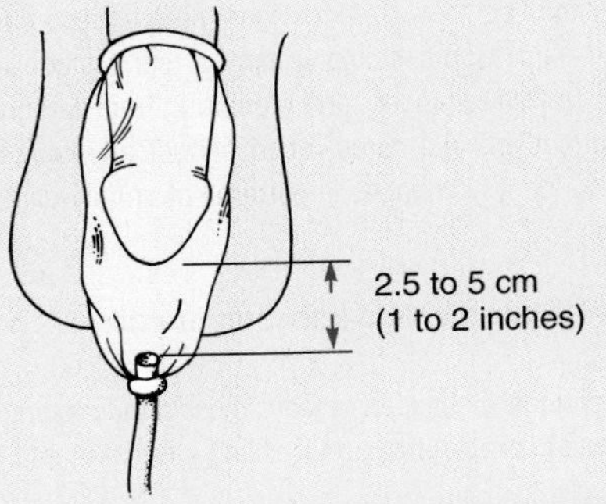

STEP 13 Distance between end of penis and tip of catheter.

15. Attach catheter to leg drainage bag. If using large drainage bag, attach to lower bed frame.
16. Make patient comfortable.
17. Observe urinary drainage, drainage tube patency, condition of penis, and tape placement.

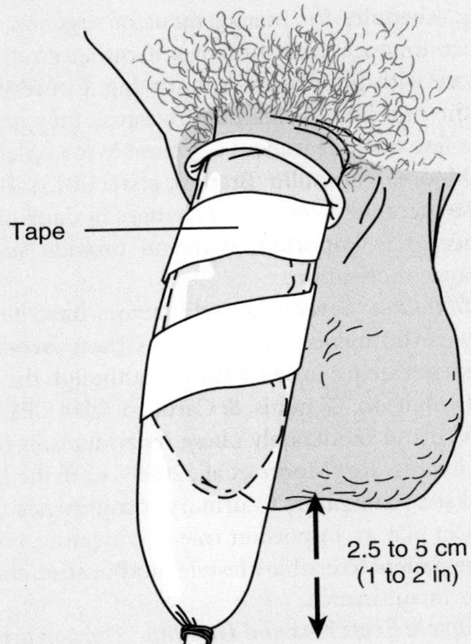

STEP 14B Elastic tape is applied in spiral fashion to secure the condom catheter to the penis.

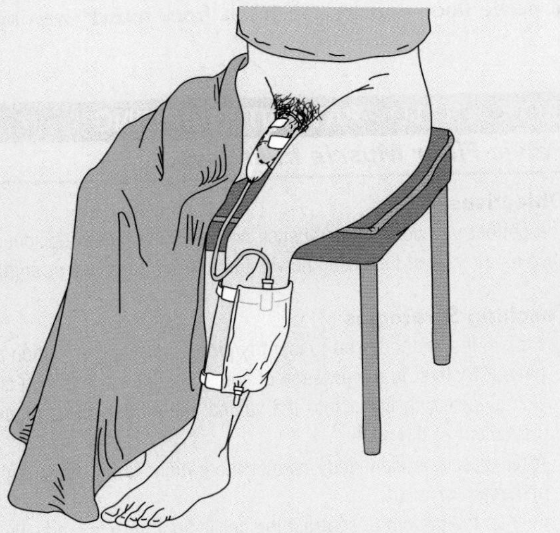

STEP 15 Attach condom catheter to leg bag.

Chapter 46). Washing with pH-balanced soap and warm water or no rinse cleanser is the best way to remove urine. Body lotion keeps skin moisturized and barrier cream products help protect the skin. Patients who soil their clothing should receive partial baths and dry clothing and bed linens immediately after voiding. If fungal growth develops, a steroid or antifungal ointment may be prescribed.

Conservative Management to Promote Continence. In acute, rehabilitation, restorative, and continuing care settings, a number of approaches have shown success in improving bladder control. They include lifestyle changes, pelvic floor muscle exercises, bladder retraining, and toileting schedules for management of urgency, stress, and mixed urinary incontinence. Intermittent self-catheterization may be an option for those with poor bladder emptying. Conservative therapies should be the first line of treatment because they generally are noninvasive, have few side effects, and are feasible for older as well as younger adults (Moore, Dumoulin, Bradley, et al., 2013). Because the success of all these therapies necessitates changes in daily lifestyle and ongoing adherence, it is important that you provide support and follow-up to enhance motivation.

Lifestyle Modification. Several lifestyle factors have been associated with urinary incontinence. Smoking has been associated with increased risk of incontinence in some studies, although the link is not completely clear (Robinson, Giarenis, & Cardozo, 2014). Extra weight, particularly in obese and moderately obese individuals, is believed to increase intrapelvic pressure (Moore et al., 2013). Caffeine has a weak diuretic effect and may contribute to urinary incontinence (Robinson et al., 2014). You can play an important role in educating, counselling, and supporting the patient to enable lifestyle modification that reduces the risk factors for incontinence.

Pelvic Floor Muscle Exercises and Training. The pelvic floor musculature (PFM) spans the opening in the bony pelvis and combines with connective tissue to provide structural support for the pelvic organs. A well-toned PFM maintains the bladder neck in position to ensure that any increase in intra-abdominal pressure, as occurs with coughing, is transmitted not only to the bladder but also to the bladder neck to maintain closure. Contraction of the PFM results in urethral compression as the urethra is pulled forward toward the symphysis pubis (Dumoulin, Hay-Smith, & Habée-Séguin, 2014). Poor tone in the pelvic floor muscles can result from muscle wasting caused by prolonged immobility, frequent straining in association with urinary or fecal elimination, stretching of muscles during childbirth, menopausal muscle atrophy, or traumatic damage.

Pelvic floor muscle exercises (PFMEs), formerly known as *Kegel exercises*, improve the strength of pelvic floor muscles through hypertrophy and recruitment of additional muscle fibres associated with repetitive contractions (Dumoulin et al., 2014). These exercises are an evidence-informed treatment for stress incontinence, overactive bladders, and mixed causes of urinary incontinence (Moore et al., 2013). They are often taught to women prenatally and to men undergoing prostatectomy. Patients begin these exercises by trying to suppress passing flatus rectally to teach them the correct muscles to contract. The exercises are then practised at nonvoiding times (Box 43-10). Patients should be alert and motivated to perform the exercises. They also should be aware that it may take 12 to 16 weeks to notice appreciable change, but that maintaining the exercises is important in order to obtain a positive outcome. Pelvic floor muscle training (PFMT) involves a systematic program, led by a specialist physiotherapist or specialized continence nurse, for patients with poor pelvic floor tone who need additional coaching and biofeedback.

Bladder Training. The goal of bladder training is to increase gradually the interval between voids and to decrease voiding frequency (Wagg et al., 2013). The overall purpose is to restore a normal pattern of voiding. For bladder training to be successful, patients must be alert, motivated, and physically able to follow a training program. The program includes education, scheduled voiding, and positive reinforcement.

The first step in bladder training is establishing a baseline. The patient or caregiver completes a urinary diary to assess maximum voiding intervals. It is not uncommon for the patient with frequency or an overactive bladder to void small amounts hourly or more often. An initial training schedule for such a patient might involve a voiding schedule of every 75 minutes while awake, increasing every 1 to 3 weeks by 15-minute increments toward a 3-hour schedule. The rate of incremental changes will depend on the patient's progress and on his or her ability to adhere to a rigid schedule. Urge suppression techniques, such as counting backward from 100 when the urge to void is felt and performing pelvic floor muscle contractions, are helpful. The nurse must be aware that the patient who has experienced an episode of

BOX 43-10 PATIENT TEACHING
Pelvic Floor Muscle Exercises

Objectives

The patient will achieve continence or experience fewer episodes of incontinence as a result of increased pelvic floor muscle tone and strength.

Teaching Strategies

- Explain the method used to identify proper muscle contraction by having the patient try to stop the passage of flatus. Female patients can check contraction by inserting finger into the vagina; male patients can look for a slight movement of the penis.
- After muscle is identified, instruct the patient to lie down with knees bent and apart, or to sit.
- Instruct the patient to contract the pelvic floor muscle gradually and hold the contraction for up to 10 seconds without tensing the muscles of the legs, buttocks, back, or abdomen. Remind the patient to breathe during the exercise.
- Instruct the patient to relax the muscle gradually for an equal time period between each contraction.
- The patient should perform 10 repetitions three times a day.
- Patients with mild cognitive impairment or early stage dementia can be supported by written reminders and prompting from caregivers.
- Teach the patient and the caregiver to periodically keep a 24- to 72-hour urinary diary to identify changes in patterns of urinary elimination.

Evaluation

- Ask the patient if he or she has practised the exercises and how often practice occurs.
- Specialized continence clinicians assess muscle tone during vaginal (female) or rectal (male) examination by asking the patient to perform the contraction.
- Monitor the patient's urinary diary.
- Ask the patient and the caregiver about degree of satisfaction related to the control achieved over urinary elimination.

incontinence in public will be particularly hesitant to deter voiding for even brief periods.

Prompted Voiding, Timed Toileting, and Habit Retraining. Timed toileting, habit retraining, and prompted voiding are potentially useful strategies for patients with cognitive or physical impairment, or both, who rely on caregiver assistance. Timed toileting and habit retraining involve assessment of a patient's normal pattern of voiding to establish a toileting schedule that preempts incontinence or reduces the number of incontinence episodes (Wagg et al., 2013). Such interventions are labour intensive, which may limit their feasibility. When combined with positive reinforcement, this approach is also called *prompted voiding*. This is best suited for daytime use in settings where caregivers are able to follow the protocol and with patients who do not require more than one person to assist with transfer and show improvement in an initial 3-day trial.

Intermittent Self-Catheterization. Some patients with chronic disorders such as spinal cord injury learn to perform self-catheterization. The patient must be physically able to manipulate equipment and assume a position for successful catheterization. The nurse must teach the patient the structure of the urinary tract, the clean versus sterile technique, the importance of adequate fluid intake, and the frequency of self-catheterization. In general, the goal is to have patients perform self-catheterization every 6 to 8 hours, although the schedule should be individualized.

Pharmacological Strategies. Drug therapy, either alone or in combination with other therapies, can help problems of urinary incontinence and retention. The major categories of medication are presented in Table 43-7.

Safety Alert α-Adrenergic blockers may cause postural hypotension and increase the patient's risk of falling and injury. Instruct patients taking these medications to plan their nighttime toileting and to get out of bed slowly.

TABLE 43-7 Medications Used to Treat Urinary Incontinence and Retention

Classification	Action	Generic Name	Adverse Effects	Contraindications, Effects, or Alerts/ Comments
Urgency incontinence: Antimuscarinics (anticholinergics)	• Anticholinergic/antimuscarinic • Inhibits effect of acetylcholine on smooth muscle antispasmodic	Oxybutynin tolterodine trospium fesoterodine solifenacin	Constipation Dry mouth Blurred vision Confusion and decreased cognition in older persons Urinary retention	Narrow-angle glaucoma Gastrointestinal obstruction Ulcerative colitis Myasthenia gravis Retention elevated residual
β-3 Adrenoreceptor agonist	Stimulates β-3 adrenoreceptors to promote detrusor (bladder) relaxation	Mirabegron	May increase blood pressure	Not for use in those with systolic BP >180 mm Hg or diastolic BP >110 mm Hg
Urinary incontinence (UI) associated with chronic retention of urine (previously from prostatic hyperplasia): α-Adrenergic blockers	Block α receptors to relax bladder neck or proximal urethra and reduce symptoms of obstructive voiding	Terazosin doxazosin tamsulosin	Postural hypotension Syncope fainting	Patients taking antihypertensives will require dosage titration
UI associated with chronic retention of urine (previously overflow UI) related to poor bladder contraction: Cholinergic agents	Thought to stimulate detrusor contraction	Bethanechol	May cause urethral resistance	Little effect in chronic urinary retention. Research limited to postsurgical retention, but little efficacy has been shown.
Stress or urge incontinence in women: Low-dose, topical hormone replacement therapy	Reduces irritation and atrophic vaginitis. Can reduce symptoms of overactive bladder and stress incontinence as well as reducing frequency of urinary tract infections	Low-dose estrogen creams, tablets, or rings	Sore breasts Spotting (rare with very low dose)	History of endometrial, ovarian, or breast cancer
Nocturia: Antidiuretic hormone analogues	To treat primary nocturnal enuresis (bedwetting) in children and nocturnal polyuria in adults by decreasing urine output through replacing arginine vasopressin (antidiuretic hormone)	Desmopressin	Hyponatremia	Caution required for use in frail older persons

From Gorodzinsky, F. P. (2014). Therapeutic choices: Urinary incontinence in children. In *Compendium of Therapeutic Choices: RxTx database*. Canadian Pharmacists Association. Retrieved from https://www.e-therapeutics.ca; Sadowski, C. A. (2015). Therapeutic choices: Urinary incontinence in adults. In *Compendium of Therapeutic Choices: RxTx database*. Canadian Pharmacists Association. Retrieved from https://www.e-therapeutics.ca; Wagg, A. W., Chen, L. K., Kirschner-Hermanns, R., Kuchel, G. A., Johnson, T., Ostaszkiewicz, J, et al. (2013). Incontinence in the frail elderly. In P. Abrams, L. Cardozo, S. Khoury, & A. Wein (eds.), *Incontinence* (5th ed., pp. 1001–1100). Paris: ICUD-EAU.

◆ Evaluation

Patient Care. The patient is the best source of evaluation of outcomes and responses to nursing care (Figure 43-17). However, nurses will also evaluate the effectiveness of nursing interventions through comparisons with baseline data. The nurse should evaluate for changes in the patient's voiding pattern, the presence of urinary tract alteration, and the patient's physical condition. Actual outcomes are compared with expected outcomes to determine the patient's health status. Continuous evaluation enables the nurse to determine whether new or revised therapies are required or if any new nursing diagnoses have developed.

Patient Expectations. If, as a nurse, you have developed a trusting relationship with a patient, indications of the patient's degree of satisfaction with his or her care will be evident. The patient may smile or nod in appreciation. However, you need to confirm whether the patient's expectations have been met to full satisfaction. You may need to ask specifically about the patient's degree of urinary control and comfort. If simply asked, "How are you feeling today?" the patient may reply with a noncommittal "Okay." However, you need specific information about how well an intervention has met the patient's need in order to continue or revise the care plan. You can also assist the patient in redefining unrealistic expectations when impairment in function is not likely to be altered as completely as he or she might like.

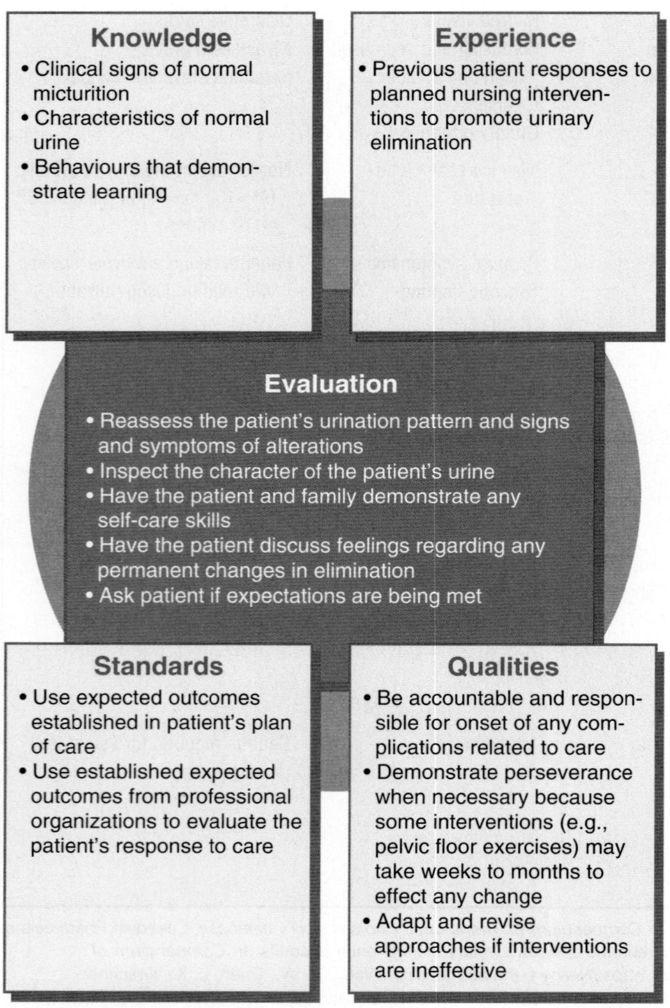

FIGURE 43-17 Critical thinking model for urinary elimination evaluation.

KEY CONCEPTS

- The act of micturition, or voiding, is influenced by complex interactions between the bladder, spinal cord, and brain, involving both autonomic (involuntary) and somatic (voluntary) nerves. Symptoms common to urinary disturbances include urgency, frequency, dysuria, polyuria, oliguria, and difficulty in starting the urinary stream.
- When collected properly, a clean-voided urine specimen does not contain bacteria from the urethral meatus.
- Methods of promoting the micturition reflex assist patients in sensing the urge to urinate and urethral sphincter relaxation.
- An increased fluid intake results in increased urine formation, which reduces the risk of urinary tract infections.
- An in-dwelling urinary catheter remains in the bladder for an extended period and has potential for biofilm formation, making the risk of infection greater than with intermittent catheterization.
- Closed catheter irrigation may be needed to maintain catheter patency and prevent blood clots, especially after urological surgery.
- A catheter drainage system should be a closed system positioned to allow free drainage of urine by gravity.
- Incontinence is classified as transient, urge, stress, mixed, and functional. Each type can be addressed through a variety of nursing interventions and prescribed treatments.
- Nurses need to follow specific guidelines for in-dwelling catheter insertion, to reduce the occurrence of catheter-associated urinary tract infection. In acute care, nurses have an important role in advocating for removal of in-dwelling catheters if these are no longer needed.

CRITICAL THINKING EXERCISES

1. Mrs. Rodriguez is 77 years old and has had problems with urgency for the past 2 years. The episodes are becoming increasingly frequent. She has been attempting to deal with the problem by using an absorbent pad in her underwear, but she feels as though everyone knows about her incontinence. The embarrassment of urinary odours often keeps her at home. She has given up attending daily mass at church.
   a. How can you help Mrs. Rodriguez regain control of her urinary elimination?
   b. What nursing diagnoses apply to Mrs. Rodriguez?
   c. For one of the diagnoses, provide one goal or outcome and two nursing interventions.
2. Mrs. Brownell is 37 years old and has been admitted with back pain radiating downward into her groin. She has also noticed blood in her urine for a week, but she was hoping it would go away. She is scheduled to undergo an intravenous pyelogram (IVP) in 4 hours.
   a. What is the purpose of the IVP?
   b. What nursing care is needed before Mrs. Brownell goes to the radiography department?
   c. Provide at least two nursing responsibilities for care of a patient who has undergone an IVP.
3. Mrs. Fenton is 70 years old and has physical limitations related to rheumatoid arthritis. Her daughter, with whom she lives, has brought her to her family practitioner's office. You are the family nurse practitioner in the practice. As you assess Mrs. Fenton, you ask her how she is coping. She begins to answer but then starts to cry and says, "I know when I have to go to the bathroom, but I often don't make it in time." Her daughter asks you for suggestions on how to manage, as she has noticed that her mother's perineal skin is reddened and sore. What assessments need to be completed before planning interventions for Mrs. Fenton's care?

REVIEW QUESTIONS

1. The normal adult urine output is:
   1. 1 000 mL/day
   2. 1 500 to 1 600 mL/day
   3. 3 000 to 3 200 mL/day
   4. 4 000 mL/day
2. In addition to removal of waste products of metabolism, which of the following describes the role of the kidneys?
   1. Secretion of antidiuretic hormone
   2. Regulation of growth hormone
   3. Fluid and electrolyte balance
   4. Albumin manufacturing
3. Postrenal alterations result from obstruction to the flow of urine in the urinary collecting system caused by:
   1. Dehydration
   2. Calculi
   3. Hemorrhage
   4. Diabetes mellitus
4. Which of the following is *not* a risk factor for urinary tract infection (UTI)?
   1. Catheterization
   2. Antibiotic use
   3. Acidic urine
   4. Spermicide use
5. Hospital-acquired UTIs are often related to poor hand hygiene and:
   1. Urinary drainage bags
   2. Poor perineal hygiene
   3. Poor catheterization technique
   4. Poor urinary output
6. The urine may appear cloudy because of the presence of white blood cells (WBCs) or:
   1. Bacteria
   2. Urinary drainage bags
   3. Blood clots
   4. Poor perineal hygiene
7. Prompted voiding is most appropriate for:
   1. Patients with cognitive disorders
   2. Patients with small-capacity bladders
   3. Patients with urinary obstruction
   4. Male patients after prostatectomy
8. A patient with stress incontinence:
   1. Is incontinent after a strong urge to void
   2. Is unaware of the need to void
   3. Loses small amounts of urine with increased intra-abdominal pressure (e.g., coughing)
   4. Exhibits a small-capacity bladder
9. Ensuring that an in-dwelling catheter drainage bag is lower than the bladder prevents:
   1. Urine flowing back into the bladder, which will likely cause an infection
   2. Urinary retention
   3. Reflex incontinence
   4. Urinary incontinence
10. When applying a condom catheter requiring an elastic adhesive tape, it is important to secure the catheter on the penile shaft in such a manner that the catheter is:
    1. Tight and draining well
    2. Dependent and draining well
    3. Secured with adhesive tape applied in a circular pattern
    4. Snug and secure, but does not cause constriction to blood flow
11. The nurse can provide support to the patient with incontinence by:
    1. Discussing long-term care placement
    2. Recommending long-term catheterization
    3. Referring to local continence services and websites
    4. Informing the patient that nothing can be done
12. Lifestyle choices to improve incontinence include:
    1. Immunization
    2. Weight loss
    3. Cholesterol management
    4. Regular medical examination

Answers: 1. 2; **2.** 3; **3.** 2; **4.** 3; **5.** 3; **6.** 1; **7.** 1; **8.** 3; **9.** 1; **10.** 4; **11.** 3; **12.** 2

Rationales for the Review Questions appear at the end of the book.

RECOMMENDED WEBSITES

Canadian Association for Enterostomal Therapy: http://www.caet.ca
The Canadian Association for Enterostomal Therapy (CAET) is a professional organization that represents enterostomal therapy nurses, who provide services for patients with abdominal stomas (openings), fistulas, draining wounds, or selected skin, gastrointestinal, and genitourinary disorders. CAET promotes education, standards, and research for enterostomal practice.

Canadian Continence Foundation: http://www.continence-fdn.ca
The Canadian Continence Foundation is a national, nonprofit organization that serves the education needs of people experiencing incontinence. The foundation implements and promotes professional education and research to advanced treatment and management of incontinence.

Canadian Nurse Continence Advisors Association (CNCA): http://www.cnca.ca/
This national association is mandated to enhance the specialty of nurse continence advisors (NCA) in Canada by promoting education, research, and clinical practice.

Continence Products Advisor: https://www.continenceproductadvisor.org/
This website provides noncommercial, evidence-informed information for consumers and health care providers on continence products, including a wide variety of devices and equipment to support continence.

International Continence Society (ICS): https://www.ics.org/
This organization is an international society with a global focus to improve quality of life for those affected by urinary, bowel, and pelvic floor disorders. ICS addresses education, research, and advocacy regarding incontinence.

Kidney Foundation of Canada: http://www.kidney.ca
This national volunteer organization is committed to reducing the burden of kidney disease through funding research, providing education and support, promoting access to health care, and increasing public awareness about kidney health and organ donation.

Ostomy Canada Society: http://www.ostomycanada.ca
This voluntary organization is dedicated to assisting people with bowel or bladder diversions by providing support and information.

Urology Nurses of Canada: http://www.unc.org
Urology Nurses of Canada (UNC) is the professional organization for urological nurses in Canada. Its website offers links to urological-related information, including UNC's professional standards.

REFERENCES

Agarwal, A., Eryuzlu, L. N., Cartwright, R., et al. (2014). What is the most bothersome lower urinary tract symptom? Individual- and population-level perspectives for both men and women. *European Urology*, *65*(6), 1211–1217. doi:10.1016/j.eururo.2014.01.019.

Barber, A. E., Norton, J. P., Spivak, A. M., et al. (2013). Urinary tract infections: Current and emerging management strategies. *Clinical Infectious Diseases*, *57*(5), 719–724. doi:10.1093/cid/cit284.

Bergman, A. M., Sih, A. M., & Weiss, J. P. (2015). Nocturia: An overview of evaluation and treatment. *Bladder, 2*(2), e13. doi:10.14440/bladder.2015.42.

Birder, L., Chai, T., Griffiths, D., et al. (2013). Neural control. In P. Abrams, L. Cardozo, S. Khoury, et al. (Eds.), *Incontinence* (5th ed., pp. 181–259). Paris: ICUD-EAU.

Boss, B. J., & Huether, S. E. (2014). Chapter 18: Disorders of the central and peripheral nervous systems and the neuromuscular junction. In K. L. McCance, S. E. Huether, V. L. Brashers, et al. (Eds.), *Pathophysiology: The biological basis for disease in adults and children* (7th ed., pp. 581–640). St. Louis: Mosby.

Canadian Continence Foundation. (2014). *The impact of incontinence in Canada: A briefing document for policy makers*. Retrieved from http://www.canadiancontinence.ca/pdfs/en-impact-of-incontinence-in-canada-2014.pdf.

Canadian Patient Safety Institute. (2016). *Hospital harm improvement resource: Urinary tract infection*. Retrieved from http://www.patientsafetyinstitute.ca/en/toolsResources/Hospital-Harm-Measure/Documents/Resource-Library/HHIR%20UTI.pdf.

Cottenden, A., Bliss, D., Buckley, B., et al. (2013). Management using continence products. In P. Abrams, L. Cardozo, S. Khoury, et al. (Eds.), *Incontinence* (5th ed., pp. 1653–1786). Paris: ICUD-EAU.

Doig, A. K., & Huether, S. E. (2014). Chapter 37: Structure and function of the renal and urologic systems. In K. L. McCance, S. E. Huether, V. L. Brashers, et al. (Eds.), *Pathophysiology: The biological basis for disease in adults and children* (7th ed., pp. 1319–1339). St. Louis: Mosby.

Drennan, V. M., Greenwood, N., Cole, L., et al. (2012). Conservative interventions for incontinence in people with dementia or cognitive impairment living at home: A systematic review. *BMC Geriatrics, 12*, 77. Retrieved from http://www.biomedcentral.com/1471-2318/12/77.

Dumoulin, C., Hay-Smith, E. J. C., & Habée-Séguin, G. M. (2014). Pelvic floor muscle training versus no treatment, or inactive control treatments, for urinary incontinence in women. *Cochrane Database of Systematic Reviews*, (5), CD005654, doi:10.1002/14651858.CD005654.pub3.

European Association of Urology Nurses (2016). *Evidence-based guidelines for best practice in urological health care: Male external catheters in adults*. Arnhem, The Netherlands: European Association of Urology Nurses. Retrieved from http://patients.uroweb.org/wp-content/uploads/Male-External-Catheters-in-Adults_LR.pdf.

Getliffe, K., & Fader, M. (2007). Catheters and containment products. In K. Getliffe & M. Dolman (Eds.), *Promoting continence: A clinical and research resource* (3rd ed., pp. 259–308). Edinburgh, Scotland: Bailliere-Tindall/Elsevier.

Gould, C. V., Umscheid, C. A., Agarwal, R. K., et al., the Healthcare Infection Control Practices Advisory Committee. (2010). Guideline for prevention of catheter-associated urinary tract infections 2009. *Infection Control and Hospital Epidemiology, 31*, 319–326. doi:10.1086/651091.

Gray, M., McNichol, L., & Nix, D. (2016). Incontinence-associated dermatitis: Progress, promises and ongoing challenges. *Journal of Wound, Ostomy, and Continence Nursing, 43*(2), 188–192. doi:10.1097/WON.0000000000000217.

Harrington, D. W., Wilson, K., Rosenberg, M., et al. (2013). Access granted! Barriers endure: Determinants of difficulties accessing specialist care when required in Ontario, Canada. *BMC Health Services Research, 13*, 146. doi:10.1186/1472-6963-13-146.

Hunter, K. F., Bharmal, A., & Moore, K. N. (2013). Long-term bladder drainage: Suprapubic catheter versus other methods: A scoping review. *Neurourology and Urodynamics, 32*(7), 944–951. doi:10.1002/nau.22356.

Jepson, R. G., Williams, G., & Craig, J. C. (2012). Cranberries for preventing urinary tract infections. *Cochrane Database of Systematic Reviews*, (10), Art.No.:CD001321, doi:10.1002/14651858.CD001321.pub5.

Konety, B. R., Barbour, S., & Carroll, P. R. (2013). Urinary diversion and bladder substitutions. In J. McAninch & T. F. Lue (Eds.), *Smith and Tanagho's general urology* (18th ed.). New York: McGraw-Hill.

Leis, J., & Soong, C. (2017). *Lose the tube: A toolkit for early removal of urinary catheters on inpatient wards*. Choosing Wisely Canada. Retrieved from https://choosingwiselycanada.org/wp-content/uploads/2017/07/CWC_Urinary-Catheter_Toolkit_All_v1.2_2017-07-12.pdf.

Lo, E., Nicolle, L. E., Coffin, S. E., et al. (2014). Strategies to prevent catheter-associated urinary tract infections in acute care hospitals: 2014 update. *Infection Control and Hospital Epidemiology, 35*(5), 464–479. doi:10.1086/675718.

Milne, J. L. (2008). Behavioral therapies for overactive bladder: Making sense of the evidence. *Journal of Wound, Ostomy & Continence Nursing, 35*, 93–1011.

Mody, L., & Juthani-Mehta, M. (2014). Urinary tract infections in older women: A clinical review. *JAMA: Journal of the American Medical Association, 311*(8), 844–854. doi:10.1001/jama.2014.303.

Moore, K., Dumoulin, C., Bradley, C., et al. (2013). Adult conservative management. In P. Abrams, L. Cardozo, S. Khoury, et al. (Eds.), *Incontinence* (5th ed., pp. 1101–1227). Paris: ICUD-EAU.

Newman, D. K., Buckley, B., Gordon, D., et al. (2013). Continence promotion, education and primary prevention. In P. Abrams, L. Cardozo, S. Khoury, et al. (Eds.), *Incontinence* (5th ed., pp. 1789–1827). Paris: ICUD-EAU.

Nguyen, H. T. (2013). Bacterial infections of the genitourinary tract. In J. McAninch & T. F. Lue (Eds.), *Smith and Tanagho's general urology* (18th ed.). New York: McGraw Hill.

Nicolle, L. E. (2014). Catheter-associated urinary tract infections. *Antimicrobial Resistance and Infection Control, 3*(23), 2–8. doi:10.1186/2047-2994-3-23.

Northwood, M., & Hunter, K. F. (2014). Treatment of urinary incontinence. In P. Eyles (Ed.), *Promoting continence care: A bladder and bowel handbook for care providers.* Canadian Nurse Continence Advisor Association (2nd ed., pp. 44–52). Hamilton ON: McMaster University Press.

Northwood, M., & Whytock, S. (2014). Transient causes of urinary incontinence. In P. Eyles (Ed.), *Promoting continence care: A bladder and bowel handbook for care providers.* Canadian Nurse Continence Advisor Association (2nd ed., pp. 26–34). Hamilton, ON: McMaster University Press.

Pagana, K. D., & Pagana, T. J. (2013). *Mosby's diagnostic and laboratory test reference* (11th ed.). St. Louis, MO: Mosby.

Perron, L., Senikas, V., Burnett, M., et al. (2013). Female genital cutting. *Journal of Obstetrics and Gynecology Canada, 35*(11), 1028–1045.

Robinson, D., Giarenis, I., & Cardozo, L. (2014). You are what you eat: The impact of diet on overactive bladder and lower urinary tract symptoms. *Maturitas, 79*(1), 8–13. doi:10.1016/j.maturitas.2014.06.009.

Seshan, V., & Muliira, J. K. (2013). Self-reported urinary incontinence and factors associated with symptom severity in community dwelling adult women: Implications for women's health promotion. *BMC Women's Health, 13*, 16. doi:10.1186/1472-6874-13-16.

Staskin, D., Kelleher, C., Bosch, R., et al. (2013). Initial assessment of urinary incontinence in adult male and female patients. In P. Abrams, L. Cardozo, S. Khoury, et al. (Eds.), *Incontinence* (5th ed., pp. 361–388). Paris: ICUD-EAU.

Steggall, M. (2013). Post-operative urinary retention. *Nursing Standard, 28*(5), 43–48.

Ventham, N. T., Hughes, M., O'Neill, S., et al. (2013). Systematic review and meta-analysis of continuous local anaesthetic wound infiltration versus epidural analgesia for postoperative pain following abdominal surgery. *British Journal of Surgery, 100*(10), 1280–1289. doi:10.1002/bjs.9204.

Wagg, A. W., Chen, L. K., Kirschner-Hermanns, R., et al. (2013). Incontinence in the frail elderly. In P. Abrams, L. Cardozo, S. Khoury, et al. (Eds.), *Incontinence* (5th ed., pp. 1001–1100). Paris: ICUD-EAU.

Weber, M. A., Limpens, J., & Roovers, J. P. (2015). Assessment of vaginal atrophy: A review. *International Urogynecology Journal, 26*, 15–28. doi:10.1007/s00192-014-2464-0.

Wilde, M. H., Bliss, D. Z., Booth, J., et al. (2014). Self-management of urinary and fecal incontinence. *American Journal of Nursing, 114*(1), 38–45.

Wilde, M. H., Crean, H. F., McMahon, J. M., et al. (2016). Testing a model of self-management of fluid intake in community-residing long-term indwelling catheter users. *Nursing Research, 65*(2), 97–106. doi:10.1097/NNR.0000000000000140.

Wu, A. K., Auerbach, A. D., & Aaronson, D. S. (2012). National incidence and outcomes of postoperative urinary retention in the Surgical Care Improvement Project. *American Journal of Surgery, 204*(2), 167–171. doi:10.1016/j.amjsurg.2011.11.012.

44

Bowel Elimination

Canadian content written by Jennifer Skelly, RN, PhD
Original chapter by Jane Fellows, MSN, CWOCN

OBJECTIVES

Mastery of content in this chapter will enable you to:

- Define the key terms listed.
- Discuss the role of gastrointestinal organs in digestion and elimination.
- Describe the integrated processes of oral pharyngeal swallowing and breathing.
- Describe the functions of the large intestine.
- Explain the physiological aspects of normal defecation.
- Discuss the psychological and physiological factors that influence the elimination process.
- Describe the common physiological alterations in elimination.
- Assess a patient's pattern of elimination.
- List the nursing diagnoses related to alterations in elimination.
- Describe the nursing implications for common diagnostic examinations of the gastrointestinal tract.
- List the nursing measures that promote normal elimination.
- List the nursing measures included in bowel training.
- Discuss the nursing measures required for patients with a bowel diversion.
- Use critical thinking in the provision of care to patients with alterations in bowel elimination.

KEY TERMS

MEDIA RESOURCES

http://evolve.elsevier.com/Canada/Potter/fundamentals/

- Audio Chapter Summaries
- Examination Review Questions
- Concept Map Creator
- Case Study With Questions
- Audio Glossary
- Content Updates
- Video Clips

Bowel elimination is crucial to human function and hence critical for nurses to understand in the care of their patients. The gastrointestinal (GI) system is a remarkable structure that allows the ingestion of food and absorption of nutrients and, ultimately, the elimination of waste.

Regular elimination of bowel waste is essential for normal body functioning. Alterations in bowel elimination are often early indications of problems within either the GI tract or another body system.

To manage the bowel elimination problems of patients, as a nurse, you must understand the normal elimination process and the factors that promote, impede, or cause alterations in elimination. Of particular concern in managing bowel elimination is supportive nursing care that is respectful of the patient's privacy and emotional needs.

SCIENTIFIC KNOWLEDGE BASE

The purposes of the GI tract are to ingest food, break down the ingested food into absorbable forms (digestion), absorb fluid and nutrients, prepare food for both absorption and use by the body's cells, and

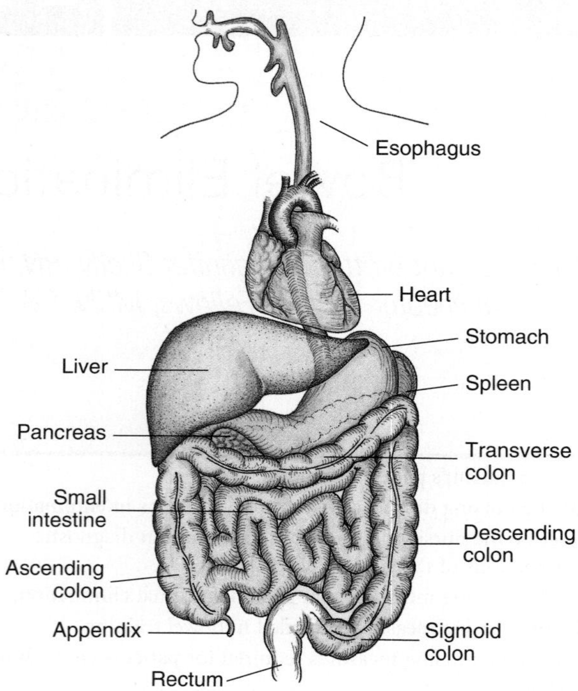

FIGURE 44-1 Organs of the gastrointestinal tract (with the heart as a reference point).

provide temporary storage of feces. The GI tract is a series of hollow, multilayered, muscular organs that are lined with mucous membranes (Figure 44-1). The mucosal and muscle layers are innervated by the intrinsic enteric nervous system comprising sensory, interneuronal, and motor fibres. The rate of rhythmic contractions is specific to each organ and is controlled by the pacemaker cells in the muscle layers. The central nervous system receives input from the GI tract through sensory fibres, which travel in the vagus and sympathetic nerves. Extrinsic sympathetic and parasympathetic motor nerves terminate on the enteric nervous system and act to modulate the activity of the intrinsic enteric nervous system. The GI tract begins at the mouth and continues through to the anus. The mouth, esophagus, and stomach receive food, and initial digestion occurs. The duodenum, jejunum, and ileum are where most digestion and absorption occurs. Finally, the cecum, colon, and rectum store and then eliminate waste. The salivary glands, liver, and pancreas are accessory organs that aid digestion. The GI tract also functions as a specialized immune system, preventing bacteria and viruses of the nonsterile lumen from entering the bloodstream (Hannon & Porth, 2017).

Mouth

The mouth is the point of entry into the GI tract. The mouth mechanically and chemically breaks down nutrients into usable sizes and forms. The teeth **masticate** food, breaking it down into a soft, moist ball (a **bolus**) suitable for swallowing. Saliva, which is produced by the salivary glands in the mouth, dilutes and softens the food in the mouth for easier swallowing and commences digestion of carbohydrates. In addition, mucus from the salivary glands lubricates the passage of the bolus through the pharynx and down the esophagus during swallowing.

Swallowing begins with the lips closing and the tongue curling with its tip and then the back being pressed to the roof of the mouth (Figure 44-2). The action of swallowing tips the bolus into the pharynx. The pharyngeal cavity is common to both the GI tract and the respiratory tract. The swallowed bolus must cross the nasopharynx, and the soft palate must elevate toward the nasopharynx to prevent material from entering the back of the nose. To prevent aspiration, the vocal cords in the glottis close, the epiglottis moves downward to seal off the trachea, and breathing is inhibited in the central nervous system. The bolus enters the esophagus through the relaxed upper esophageal sphincter. This complex process is under striated muscle control and requires an intact nervous system (Hannon & Porth, 2017).

Esophagus

The esophagus provides a conduit to the stomach through the chest cavity. The esophagus is a straight tube about 25 cm in length. Smooth muscle layers of the esophagus provide the peristaltic contractions to move food along its length. Its mucous membranes secrete mucus that aids in the lubrication of food. Sphincters on either end of the esophagus prevent air from entering the esophagus and stomach during breathing and reflux of stomach contents into the esophagus (Hannon & Porth, 2017).

The bolus travels down the relaxed esophagus mainly by gravity to the lower esophageal sphincter, which is opened by the initiation of swallowing in the pharynx and upper esophageal sphincter. A wave of **peristaltic contractions** propels the bolus into the stomach. Peristaltic contractions relax over the bolus and contract behind the bolus, thus moving contents through the length of the GI tract. If the bolus moves slowly or is stuck, a local reflex will relax the area ahead of the bolus and produce a powerful contraction behind the bolus. In the esophagus, this action is known as *secondary peristalsis*. Tertiary contractions of the esophagus are frequently simultaneous and are produced by irritation of the mucosa by gastric contents. These contractions can be extremely painful and may mimic cardiac chest pain (Hannon & Porth, 2017).

Stomach

The stomach performs several tasks: storage of swallowed food and liquid, mixing of food with liquid and gastric digestive juices, and the controlled emptying of its contents through the pyloric sphincter into the small intestine. The stomach is a baglike structure located in the upper quadrant of the abdomen.

Peristaltic and mixing contractions of the stomach are controlled by the intrinsic pacemaker activity of the smooth muscle cells. Similar to other sections of the GI tract, the stomach is innervated by the enteric nervous system and connections to the parasympathetic and sympathetic nervous systems. The emptying of the stomach is regulated by neural and hormonal mechanisms.

The stomach produces two key GI hormones: gastrin and ghrelin. Gastrin stimulates gastric acid secretion. Ghrelin is newly discovered and has growth hormone–releasing activity and stimulates food intake and digestion while reducing energy expenditures. Gastrin and somatostatin regulate the secretion of acid and pepsin in the stomach.

The stomach also secretes hydrochloric acid (HCl) and the intrinsic factor. HCl facilitates the digestion of protein and is antibacterial. The intrinsic factor is essential in the absorption of vitamin B_{12}. Mucus protects the stomach mucosa from acidity and enzyme activity (Hannon & Porth, 2017). The rate at which the stomach empties depends on the content of the dissolved and partially digested bolus (**chyme**). Water diffuses from both the stomach and the small intestine and is emptied rapidly. Carbohydrates are emptied only slightly more slowly, particularly if they are not strongly acidic. Proteins empty even more slowly and in smaller amounts as determined by the acidity of the chyme. Fats are emptied the slowest of all. The controlled emptying

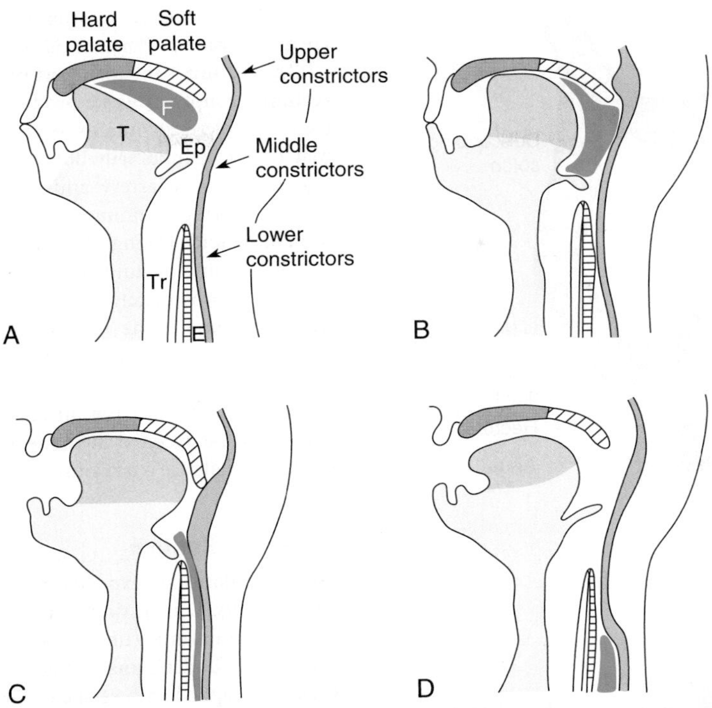

FIGURE 44-2 Oral and pharyngeal events during swallowing. A, The bolus (*F*) is propelled into the pharynx by placement of the tongue (*T*) on the hard palate. **B,** Further propulsion is caused by movement of the more distal regions of the tongue against the palate. Contraction of the upper constrictors of the pharynx and the soft palate separates the oropharynx from the nasopharynx. **C,** Contraction of the pharynx and relaxation of the cricopharyngeal muscle propel the bolus through the upper esophageal sphincter. Upward movement of the glottis and downward movement of the epiglottis (*Ep*) seal off the trachea (*Tr*), and the respiratory drive is inhibited in the central nervous system. **D,** The bolus is now in the esophagus (*E*) and is propelled into the stomach by a peristaltic contraction. (From Johnson, L. R. [2013]. *Gastrointestinal physiology* [7th ed., p. 28, Fig. 3-1]. St. Louis, MO: Mosby.)

allows the pancreatic secretions and bile to neutralize the chyme and secrete enzymes for luminal digestion (Hannon & Porth, 2017).

Small Intestine

The small intestine consists of the duodenum, jejunum, and ileum. The duodenum is about 22 cm long and connects the stomach to the jejunum. The duodenum also contains the opening for the common bile duct and main pancreatic duct. The jejunum and ileum are over 7 m long and are folded closely to fit in the abdomen (Hannon & Porth, 2017).

The duodenum continues to process the chyme from the stomach. The chyme that enters the duodenum is acidic and contains partially digested protein, carbohydrates, and unemulsified fats. The presence of these substances stimulates the release of the hormones secretin and cholecystokinin from the duodenal mucosa. Secretin stimulates the pancreas to secrete bicarbonate to neutralize the acid. Cholecystokinin stimulates the pancreas to secrete the following enzymes: (1) amylases, which convert carbohydrates to disaccharides; (2) proteases, which further hydrolyze proteins into smaller peptides; and (3) lipases, which hydrolyze triglycerides into fatty acids and monoglycerides. The presence of fats in the duodenum further stimulates cholecystokinin release, which causes the gallbladder to contract, which in turn releases bile to emulsify the fats. Any blockage of the release of these enzymes prevents the digestion of fats and proteins and results in large, fatty, and foul-smelling stools. Undigested fats and proteins reach the colon and are responsible for the changes in fecal appearance (Hannon & Porth, 2017).

The second section of the small intestine, the jejunum, is approximately 2.7 m long. Its primary function is the absorption of carbohydrates and proteins. The ileum, which is approximately 3.7 m long, specializes in the absorption of water, certain vitamins, iron, fats, and bile salts. Most nutrients and electrolytes are absorbed in the small intestine, specifically by the duodenum and the jejunum.

If the small intestine function is impaired, the digestive process is greatly altered. For example, conditions such as inflammation, surgical resection, or obstruction can disrupt contractile activity, reduce the area of absorption, or block the passage of chyme. As a result, electrolyte and nutrient deficiencies can develop (Hannon & Porth, 2017).

Large Intestine

The lower GI tract is called the large intestine because it is larger in diameter than the small intestine; however, at 1.5 to 1.8 m in length, it is much shorter. The large intestine is the primary organ of bowel elimination and is divided into the cecum, the colon, and the rectum (Figure 44-3).

Chyme from the terminal ileum enters the cecum of the large intestine, propelled by waves of peristalsis through the ileocecal sphincter, a circular muscle layer that regulates ileal emptying and prevents regurgitation of fecal contents. After a meal, the gastroileal

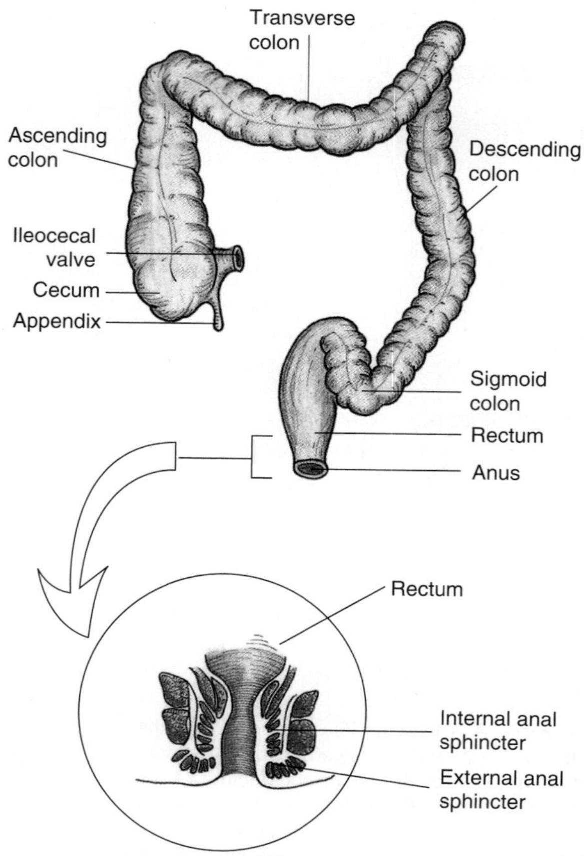

FIGURE 44-3 Divisions of the large intestine.

reflex causes the terminal ileum to contract regularly, and the sphincter opens with each contraction, thereby pushing the ileal contents into the colon.

The colon is divided into the ascending, transverse, descending, and sigmoid colons. The colon's muscular tissue allows it to accommodate and eliminate large quantities of waste and gas (**flatus**). The colon has three functions: absorption, secretion, and elimination. Each day, a large volume of water and significant amounts of sodium and chloride are absorbed by the colon (Doughty, 2006).

Two types of muscle contractions occur in the colon: slow-mixing contractions and mass **peristalsis** (or mass movement). Slow-mixing contractions move contents through the colon and expose the chyme to the mucosa, where active absorption of sodium and chloride causes water absorption and dries the chyme to feces. Intestinal content is the main stimulus for the slow-mixing contractions. Mass peristalsis movements then push the feces toward the rectum. The ingestion of food is the main stimulus for mass peristalsis, which is known as the **gastrocolic reflex**. In adults, these mass movements occur only three or four times each day (Hannon & Porth, 2017).

When the slow-mixing contractions increase and the mass peristalsis diminishes, water continues to be absorbed and the feces dry out, resulting in constipation. Conversely, when the mixing movements are decreased and the mass peristalsis is increased, the water has less time to be absorbed, and the stool will be watery (diarrhea) (Hannon & Porth, 2017).

The secretory function of the colon aids in electrolyte balance. Bicarbonate is secreted in exchange for chloride. Approximately 4 to 9 mmol of potassium is also excreted daily. Extreme alterations in colon function (e.g., diarrhea) can cause severe electrolyte disturbances (Hannon & Porth, 2017).

The rectum is the final portion of the large intestine. Normally, the rectum is empty of waste products, or **feces**, until just before defecation. The rectum contains vertical and transverse folds of tissue that may help to temporarily hold fecal contents during **defecation**. Each fold contains an artery and vein that can become distended from pressure during straining. This distension can result in the formation of hemorrhoids (Doughty, 2006).

The volume of fluids absorbed by the GI tract is high. Oral fluid intake is approximately 1.2 L per day; an additional 7 L of fluid enters from the blood as the result of the secretion of digestive enzymes by the mucosa, liver, gallbladder, and pancreas, and by osmosis as the numbers of molecules in the lumen increase by digestion. Absorption from the small and large intestine amounts to 8.1 L per day, leaving 100 mL to be excreted in the feces. Therefore, maintaining fluid and electrolyte balance is a key function of the GI system (Hannon & Porth, 2017).

Anus and Rectum

Feces and flatus are expelled from the rectum through the anal canal and the anus. Contraction and relaxation of the internal anal sphincter is under autonomic (unconscious) control, whereas the external anal sphincter is under somatic neural (conscious) control. The anal canal is richly supplied with sensory and motor nerve fibres to help control continence. Additionally, the maintenance of the acute anorectal angle formed by the puborectalis and levator ani (pelvic floor) muscles plays a key role in continence (Doughty, 2006).

When feces enter the rectum, the internal anal sphincter relaxes and this enables the anal canal to determine if the contents are solid or liquid. This action occurs concurrently with the reflexive contraction of the external sphincter. Additionally, this contraction can be accompanied by a voluntary squeeze of the sphincter muscles. The rectum is able to hold feces until their presence stimulates stretch receptors in the mucosa, producing an urge to defecate. The patient then seeks out an appropriate place to defecate, assumes a squatting position to straighten the anorectal angle, and voluntarily relaxes the external sphincter. Bearing down tenses abdominal muscles. The pelvic floor muscles relax and the feces enter the lower rectum. Involuntary propulsive contractions continue until the rectum is emptied. When the last of the feces passes, the external anal sphincter reflexively closes (Bliss & Norton, 2010).

NURSING KNOWLEDGE BASE

Process of Defecation

The physiological factors critical to bowel function and defecation include the acute anorectal angle; reflexes that cause the external anal sphincter to contract when the internal anal sphincter relaxes; pressure in the anal canal at rest facilitated by the internal anal sphincter and voluntary action of the external anal sphincter; sensory response of the rectum to filling with feces; absorption of fluid from the intestine to create formed stool consistency; complete evacuation of the rectum; and physical and cognitive abilities to get to the bathroom when needed (Bliss & Norton, 2010). Normal defecation should be painless, resulting in the passage of a soft, formed stool.

Defecation begins with contractions in the left colon, moving the stool toward the anus. When a stool reaches the rectum, the distension causes relaxation of the internal anal sphincter and signals an awareness of the need to defecate. At the time of defecation, the external sphincter relaxes and abdominal muscles contract to increase intrarectal pressure and force the stool out (Doughty, 2006). Pressure can be exerted to expel feces through a voluntary contraction of the abdominal muscles and the diaphragm while maintaining forced expiration against a closed airway. This action is termed the Valsalva manoeuvre. This action should be avoided by patients, particularly those with heart disease, as the increased intrathoracic pressure, immediate tachycardia, and reflex bradycardia can cause cardiac arrest (Marsh, 2005).

Position During Defecation. Instead of straining, patients should be taught about the optimal position to facilitate defecation. Squatting is the normal position during defecation. Toilets are designed to facilitate this posture, by allowing the person to lean forward, exert intra-abdominal pressure, and contract the thigh muscles. Bulging out the abdomen—rather than contracting the abdominal muscles—more effectively opens the bowels (Figure 44-4) (Doughty, 2006). For patients who are immobilized in bed, defecation is often difficult. In a supine position, it is impossible to contract the muscles used during defecation. If the patient's condition permits, the head of the bed should be raised; this action assists the patient to a more normal sitting position on a bedpan, enhancing the ability to defecate (Ostaszkiewicz, Hornby, Millar, et al., 2010).

Promotion of Normal Defecation. Several interventions can stimulate the defecation reflex, affect the character of feces, or increase peristalsis to help patients evacuate bowel contents normally and without discomfort.

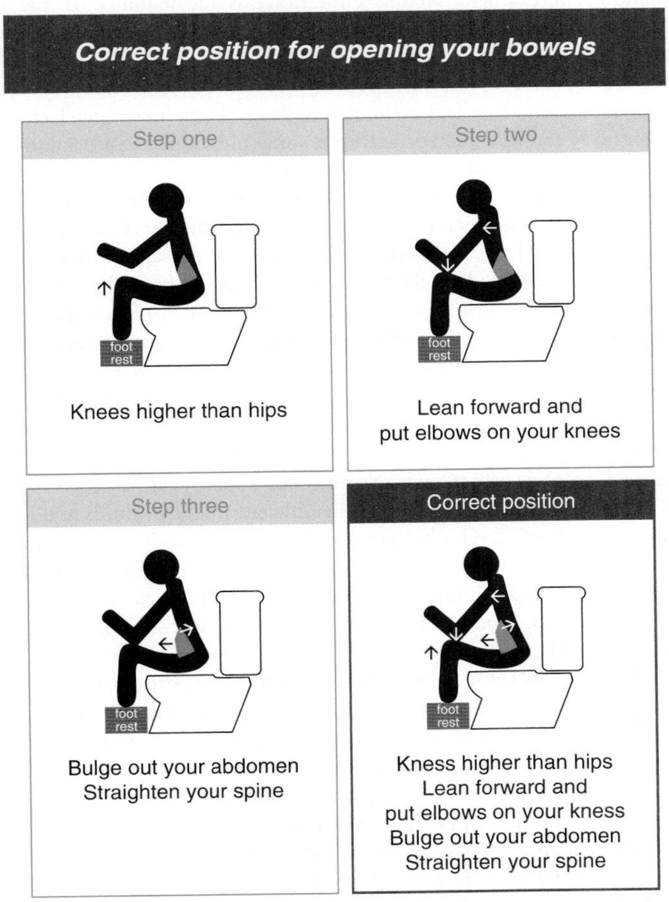

FIGURE 44-4 Correct position for opening the bowels during defecation. (Redrawn by permission of Ray Addison, Nurse Consultant in Bladder and Bowel Dysfunction, and Wendy Ness, Colorectal Nurse Specialist. Produced by Norgine Pharmaceuticals Limited, 2003.)

Sitting Position. Nurses might need to assist patients who have difficulty sitting because of muscular weakness and mobility problems. Regular toilets are too low for patients who are unable to lower themselves to a sitting position because of joint- or muscle-wasting diseases. Elevated toilet seats require less effort to sit or stand; however, they can create difficulties in achieving a squat position. In many provinces and territories, elevated toilet seats can be acquired through a service agency for minimal or no cost. The community nurse must assess the patient's capabilities in the home and the requirement for any additional equipment to facilitate daily living (Ostaszkiewicz et al., 2010).

Positioning on Bedpan. Patients restricted to bed must use bedpans for defecation. Women use bedpans to pass both urine and feces, whereas men use bedpans only for defecation. Sitting on a bedpan can be extremely uncomfortable. Nurses need to help patients to position themselves comfortably. Two types of bedpans are available (Figure 44-5). The regular bedpan, made of metal or hard plastic, has a curved, smooth upper end, a sharp-edged lower end, and is approximately 5 cm deep. A fracture pan, designed for patients with body or leg casts, has a shallow upper end and is approximately 1.3 cm deep. The upper end of the pan fits under the buttocks toward the sacrum, and the lower end fits just under the upper thighs. The pan should be high enough so that feces enter the pan. A metal bedpan should be warmed with water first, then dried.

Nurses need to ensure that the patient's privacy is maintained during bowel elimination. The call light and a supply of toilet paper should be within easy reach. When the patient finishes, the nurse should respond to the call signal immediately and remove the pan. The patient likely will require assistance with wiping. To remove the pan, the nurse can ask the patient to roll off to the side or to raise the hips. The pan should be held steady to avoid spilling. It is important to avoid pulling or shoving the pan from under the patient's hips; these actions can pull the patient's skin and cause tissue injury, such as shearing (see Chapter 46). After the pan is removed, while wearing gloves, the nurse cleans the anal and perineal areas and assists the patient with hand hygiene.

After assessing the stool, the nurse should immediately empty the bedpan's contents into the toilet or in a special receptacle in the utility room. The bedpan should be rinsed thoroughly. Care must be taken to avoid splashing the contents or the rinse. Avoiding spillage is of critical importance when using universal infection control precautions. The patient uses the same bedpan each time. The nurse charts the characteristics of the feces.

When positioning a patient on a bedpan, the nurse needs to use the proper method to prevent muscle strain and discomfort. This means never trying to lift a patient onto a bedpan. A patient should never be placed on a bedpan and then left with the bed flat unless demanded

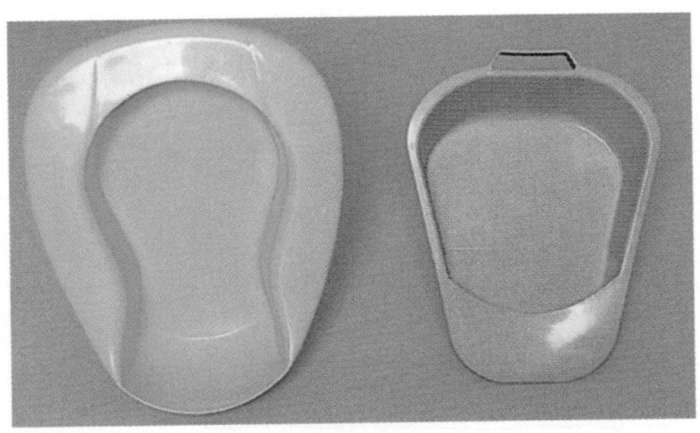

FIGURE 44-5 Types of bedpans. **Left,** regular bedpan. **Right,** fracture bedpan.

by activity restrictions. When the bed is flat, the hips remain hyperextended.

Figure 44-6 shows proper and improper positions on a bedpan. The best method is to ensure that the patient is positioned high in bed. The patient's head is raised about 30 degrees to prevent hyperextension of the back and to provide support to the upper torso. The patient then raises the hips by bending the knees and lifting the hips upward. The nurse places his or her hand, palm up, under the patient's sacrum, resting the elbow on the mattress and using it as a lever to help in lifting, while slipping the pan under the patient. Patients who have had abdominal surgery are hesitant to exert strain on suture lines and may have difficulty positioning themselves on a bedpan. To prevent abrasions, the nurse should not force the pan along the patient's skin. Nurses must always wear gloves when handling a bedpan.

If the patient is immobile or if it is unsafe to allow the patient to exert such effort, as the patient's nurse you can assist the patient to roll onto the bedpan by using the following steps:

1. Lower the head of the bed flat and assist the patient to roll onto one side, backside toward you.
2. Place the bedpan firmly against the buttocks, down into the mattress with the open rim toward the patient's feet (Figure 44-7).
3. Keeping one hand against the bedpan, place your other hand around the patient's far hip. Ask the patient to roll back onto the pan, flat in bed. Do not shove the pan under the patient.
4. When the patient is positioned comfortably, raise the head of the bed 30 degrees.
5. Place a rolled towel or small pillow under the lumbar curve of the patient's back for added comfort.

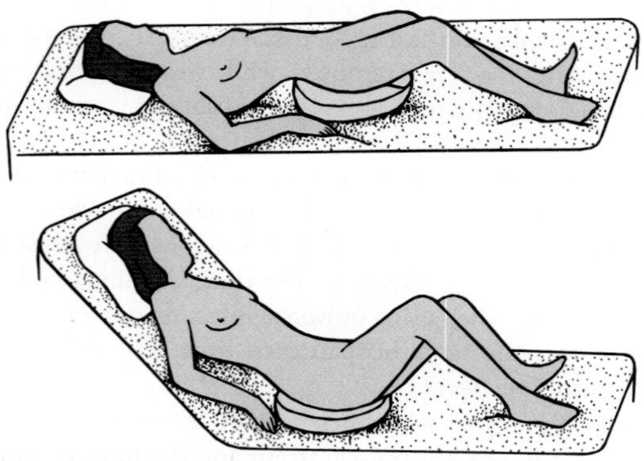

FIGURE 44-6 Positions on a bedpan. **Top,** Improper positioning of patient. **Bottom,** Proper positioning of the patient reduces back strain.

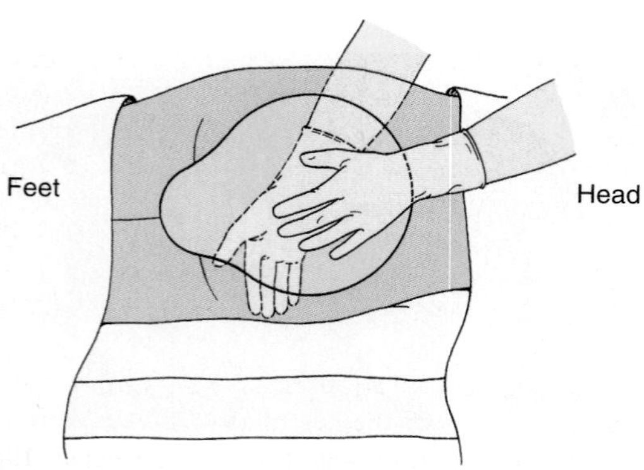

FIGURE 44-7 Positioning an immobilized patient on a bedpan.

6. Raise the knee gatch or ask the patient to bend the knees to assume a squatting position. Do not raise the knee gatch if contraindicated (Doughty, 2006).

Factors Affecting Normal Bowel Elimination

Many factors influence the process of bowel elimination. Knowledge of these factors enables nurses to anticipate measures required to maintain a normal pattern of bowel elimination.

Diet. The food a person eats influences bowel elimination. Regular daily food intake helps to maintain a routine pattern of peristalsis in the colon. **Fibre,** the indigestible residue in the diet, provides the bulk of fecal material. Dietary fibre is classified as insoluble and soluble fibre. Insoluble fibre is found in whole grains, wheat bran, and vegetables and does not dissolve in water. It is effective in preventing constipation. Soluble fibres are found in some beans, certain fruits and vegetables, and wheat bran. Soluble fibre forms a gel when mixed with water and is not as effective in preventing constipation. When a patient's dietary fibre level is low, the stool becomes dry, hard, and difficult to pass (Registered Nurses' Association of Ontario [RNAO], 2011).

Ingestion of a high-fibre diet or taking a fibre supplement can improve the likelihood of a regular bowel elimination pattern if other factors are normal. However, because fibre retains fluid in the GI tract, when additional fibre is ingested, adequate fluid intake is essential; inadequate fluid intake can lead to serious constipation or impaction. Recommended daily fluid intake for adults is at minimum 1.5 L.

Intolerance to certain foods can cause problems with bowel elimination. For example, **lactose intolerance** is the inability to digest lactose, the predominant sugar in milk. When lactose cannot be absorbed, it acts as an osmotic laxative, resulting in diarrhea, gaseous distension, and cramping (Lomer, Parkes, & Sanderson, 2008). Individuals who have lactose intolerance must learn how much lactose their body can tolerate. For example, some individuals can drink one glass of milk without effect, but not two.

Fluid Intake. An inadequate fluid intake or disturbances that result in fluid loss (such as vomiting) can affect the character of feces. Fluid liquefies intestinal contents to ease their passage through the colon. Reduced fluid intake slows the passage of food through the intestine and can result in hardening of the stool. Unless a medical contraindication exists, an adult should drink six to eight glasses (1 400 to 2 000 mL) of noncaffeinated fluid daily (RNAO, 2011). Equally important is to avoid consuming large amounts of caffeinated beverages, such as tea and coffee, as they can be irritating to the bowel and dehydrating. Some patients find that artificial sweeteners can be a bowel irritant as well (Cowie, Northwood, Robbs, et al., 2014).

Older persons tend to have an insufficient intake of fluids and are more at risk of developing constipation. Sometimes, older persons reduce their fluid intake in an attempt to reduce micturition (see Chapter 43). In addition, in some individuals an increased ingestion of milk or milk products may slow peristalsis and cause constipation (RNAO, 2011).

Physical Activity. Physical activity promotes peristalsis, whereas immobilization depresses peristalsis. Thus, early ambulation is encouraged as a patient's illness begins to resolve or as soon as possible after surgery, to promote maintenance of peristalsis and thereby normal bowel elimination. Maintaining the tone of skeletal muscles used during defecation is important. Weakened abdominal and pelvic floor muscles impair the ability to increase intra-abdominal pressure and to control the external sphincter. Muscle tone may be weakened or lost as a result of long-term illness or neurological disease that impairs nerve transmission. Patients who experience these changes in the abdominal and pelvic floor muscles are at increased risk for constipation (Doughty, 2006; Schnelle, Leung, Rao, et al., 2010).

Personal Bowel Elimination Habits. Personal bowel elimination habits can affect bowel function. Most individuals benefit from being able to use their own toilet facilities at a time that, for them, is both most effective and most convenient. A busy work schedule may prevent a person from going to the bathroom in response to the urge to defecate, thus disrupting regular habits and possibly causing constipation. A person should establish a regular time for bowel elimination (Doughty, 2006). In an institution, the nurse can facilitate this process by establishing toileting times (RNAO, 2011).

As discussed earlier, the ingestion of food is the main stimulus for mass peristalsis, which is known as the *gastrocolic reflex*. This reflex frequently leads to the need to defecate after a meal. The reflex is strongest when the stomach is empty, and this is why breakfast is referred to as the "triggering meal" for a bowel movement for most people. The nurse can capitalize on this by offering the patient assistance to toilet 15 to 20 minutes after the patient's breakfast.

Privacy. The patient's privacy must be maintained during bowel elimination. In hospital or long-term care settings, where patients may be in ward accommodation, maintaining visual, auditory, and olfactory privacy is important. Ignoring the call to stool because the patient is embarrassed can begin a cycle of constipation (RNAO, 2011).

Privacy and sensitivity must also be attended to when discussing bowel elimination with patients. Patients are cautious about discussing bowel elimination because they are embarrassed to broach the subject. It is the nurse's responsibility to ask about bowel elimination problems and to create a therapeutic climate for the patient to voice his or her concerns (Bliss & Norton, 2010).

CRITICAL THINKING

Successful critical thinking requires a synthesis of knowledge, experience, information gathered from patients, critical thinking attitudes, and intellectual and professional standards. Clinical judgements require nurses to anticipate the information necessary, analyze the data, and make decisions regarding patient care. During the assessment (Figure 44-8), nurses must consider all elements that build toward making appropriate diagnoses and determining the contributing factors to a patient's issues.

To assess a patient's bowel elimination, nurses must integrate their knowledge from nursing and other disciplines to better understand a patient's response to bowel elimination interruptions. As emphasized earlier, patients often respond to disruptions in bowel elimination with embarrassment. Sensitivity on the nurse's part is essential.

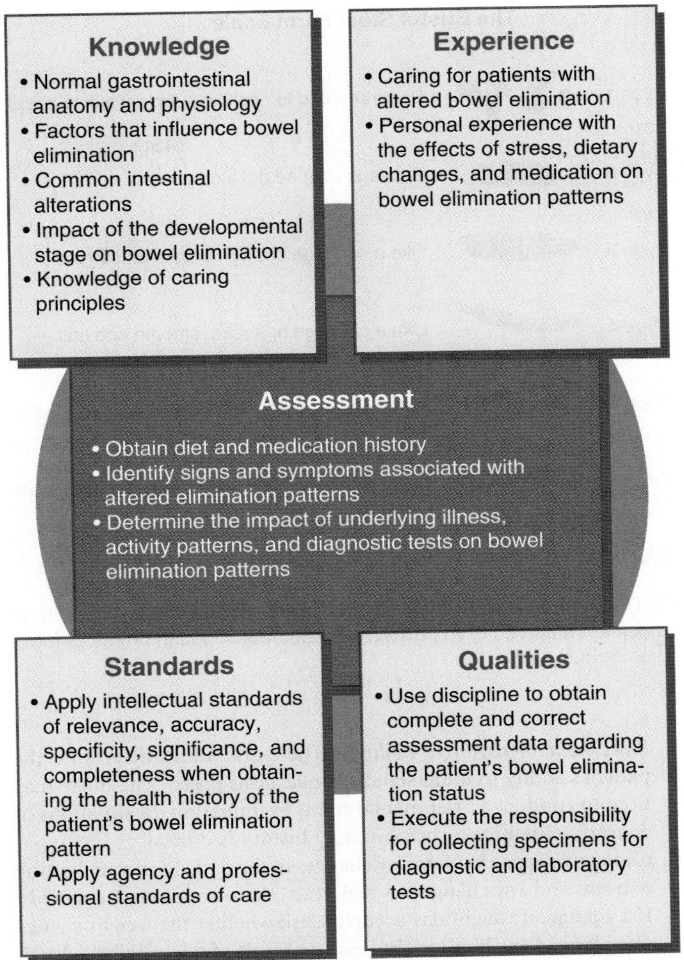

FIGURE 44-8 Critical thinking model for bowel elimination assessment.

❖ NURSING PROCESS AND BOWEL ELIMINATION

◆ Assessment

Assessment for bowel elimination patterns and abnormalities includes a nursing health history, a physical assessment of the abdomen, inspection of fecal characteristics, and a review of relevant test results. In addition, the nurse needs to determine the patient's perception of the problem and goals for treatment, medical history, pattern and types of fluid and food intake, chewing ability, medications, and recent illnesses and stressors.

Health History. The nursing health history provides a review of the patient's usual bowel patterns and habits. What a patient defines as "normal" may differ from factors and conditions that typically promote normal bowel elimination. The nurse can determine the patient's problems by first identifying the normal and abnormal patterns and habits and then understanding the patient's perception of what is normal and abnormal regarding bowel elimination. Much of the nursing health history can be organized around the factors that affect bowel elimination:

- *Determination of the patient's usual bowel elimination pattern:* The frequency and time of day of the patient's bowel eliminations should be noted. Have the patient or caregiver complete a bowel elimination diary for a week to enable an accurate assessment of the typical bowel elimination pattern.
- *The patient's description of the usual stool characteristics:* The patient's description should indicate whether the stool is normally watery or formed, soft or hard; the typical colour; whether the stool floats or sinks; and whether blood is present. Ask the patient to describe the usual shape of the stool and the number of stools per day. The Bristol Stool Chart is a handy figure to show patients to determine the nature of their usual stools (Figure 44-9).
- *Identification of routines followed to promote normal bowel elimination:* Examples of routines to promote bowel elimination are drinking hot liquids, eating specific foods, or taking time to defecate at a certain time of the day.
- *Assessment of the use of laxatives, suppositories, or enemas:* It is important to assess whether the patient uses enemas, laxatives, suppositories, or bulk-forming food additives in order to have a bowel movement. Ask the patient how often such an aid is used.

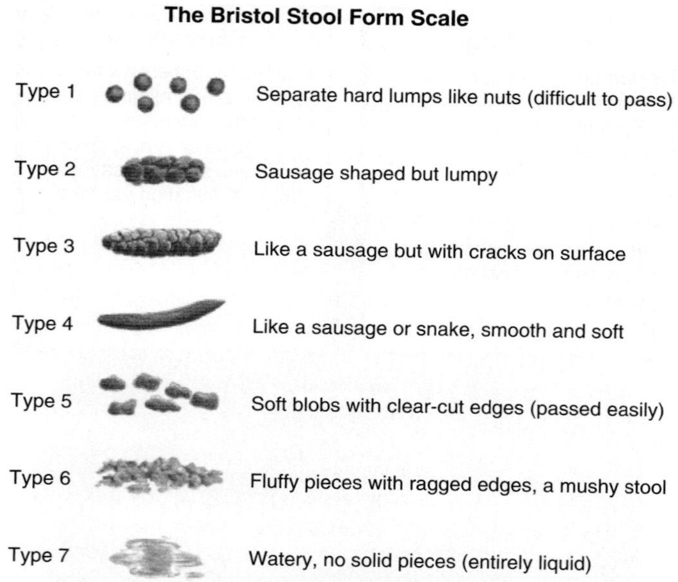

FIGURE 44-9 The Bristol Stool Chart. (From *Bristol stool form guideline.* Retrieved from http://www.aboutconstipation.org/stool-form-guide.html.)

- *Assessment of cognitive abilities:* The nurse must determine the patient's ability to understand the questions posed. The nurse may need to conduct a brief mental status examination. In situations of concern, obtaining a corroborating history is critical.
- *Changes in appetite:* Note any changes in the patient's normal eating patterns and any change in weight (i.e., the amount lost or gained). If a change of weight has occurred, ask whether the weight change was planned, such as weight loss as a result of a low-calorie diet.
- *Diet history:* Determine the patient's dietary preferences. Assess the intake of fruits, vegetables, cereals, and breads and whether mealtimes are regular or irregular. In the case of the patient who is frail and living alone, determine whether acquiring food requires assistance (e.g., financial help, food preparation assistance, or transportation to a grocery store with a full selection of fresh fruits and vegetables).
- *Description of daily fluid intake:* Determine the type and amount of fluid consumed in a typical day. The patient might need to estimate the amount by using common household measurements.
- *History of surgery or illnesses affecting the GI tract:* This information can help to explain symptoms and to assess the patient's potential for maintaining or restoring a normal bowel elimination pattern. A patient's family history of GI cancer is also relevant to the nursing assessment.
- *Medication history:* Ask for a list of the patient's current medications. The medication history must include both prescribed and over-the-counter medications (e.g., laxatives, antacids, iron supplements, and analgesics) that might alter defecation or fecal characteristics. The community nurse should ask to see the medications.
- *Emotional state:* The patient's emotional state can significantly alter the frequency of defecation. During assessment, observe and ask directly about the patient's emotions and the presence of stress.
- *History of exercise:* Ask the patient to describe the type and amount of daily exercise and if there have been any recent changes to this activity level.
- *History of pain or discomfort:* Ask whether the patient has a history of abdominal or anal pain or pain with defecation. The quality, radiation, triggers, and location of pain may help to identify the source of the problem.
- *Environment and adaptive aids:* Patients have many different living arrangements. Where patients live may affect their toileting habits. If the patient is sharing living quarters, how many bathrooms are available? Does the patient have his or her own bathroom, or does the patient need to share the facilities and thus adjust the time the bathroom is used to accommodate other persons? If the patient lives alone, is he or she capable of ambulating to the toilet safely? If the patient is not independent in bowel management, who assists the patient and how? Does the patient use a bedpan, commode, or urinal? Does the patient wear incontinence products? Does the patient use a raised toilet seat or require grab bars?
- *Mobility and dexterity:* The patient's mobility and dexterity need to be evaluated to determine whether the patient needs assistive devices or personal assistance.
- *Presence and status of bowel diversions:* If the patient has an ostomy, assess the frequency of fecal drainage, the character of the feces, the appearance and condition of the stoma (e.g., the colour, the presence of swelling, and signs of irritation), the type of fecal collection device used, and the methods used to maintain the ostomy's function.

Physical Assessment. The physical assessment (see Chapter 32) is used to evaluate a patient's body systems and functions that are likely to be affected by the presence of bowel elimination problems.

Mouth. The nurse's inspection of the mouth includes examining the patient's teeth, tongue, and gums. Poor dentition or poorly fitting dentures influence the ability to chew (see Chapter 42). Sores in the mouth can make eating not only difficult but also painful. A dry mouth may indicate dehydration (Jarvis, Browne, MacDonald-Jenkins, et al., 2014).

Abdomen. All four abdominal quadrants should be inspected for contour, shape, symmetry, and skin colour. Masses, peristaltic waves, scars, venous patterns, stomas, and lesions should be noted. Normally, peristaltic waves are not visible; however, observable peristalsis can be a sign of intestinal obstruction.

Abdominal distension appears as an overall outward protuberance of the abdomen. Distension may be caused by intestinal gas, large tumours, or fluid in the peritoneal cavity. A distended abdomen feels tight, like a drum, and the skin appears taut, as if stretched (Jarvis et al., 2014).

Percussion is used to detect lesions, fluid, or gas in the abdomen. Familiarity with the five percussion notes (see Chapter 32) enables identification of the underlying abdominal structures. Gas or flatulence creates a tympanic note. Masses, tumours, and fluid are dull to percussion.

The abdomen is auscultated with the stethoscope to assess bowel sounds in each quadrant (see Chapter 32). Normal bowel sounds occur every 5 to 15 seconds and last from 1 second to several seconds. While auscultating, the nurse should note the character and frequency of the bowel sounds. An increase in pitch or a tinkling sound may be heard when the abdomen is distended. The lack of bowel sounds or the presence of hypoactive sounds (fewer than five sounds per minute) occurs when the patient has a paralytic ileus, such as after abdominal surgery. High-pitched and hyperactive bowel sounds (35 or more sounds per minute) occur when the small intestine is obstructed or when inflammatory disorders are present (Jarvis et al., 2014).

The nurse should gently palpate the abdomen for masses or areas of tenderness (see Chapter 32). During this procedure, the nurse needs to encourage the patient to relax. Tensing of the abdominal muscles interferes with palpating underlying organs or masses (Jarvis et al., 2014).

Rectum. The area around the anus is inspected for lesions, discolorations, inflammation, and hemorrhoids. Abnormalities should be carefully recorded (see Chapter 32) (Jarvis et al., 2014).

Factors Related to Altered Patterns of Bowel Elimination

Age-Related Changes. Normal age-related changes affect bowel elimination (Table 44-1). In addition, many issues associated with aging can significantly alter bowel elimination, including polypharmacy, poor nutrition, life stressors, and comorbidities (Meiner, 2011).

Older persons also lose muscle tone in the perineal floor and the anal sphincter. Although the integrity of the external sphincter may remain intact, older persons may have difficulty controlling bowel evacuation and are at risk for incontinence. In addition, older persons may have a slowing of the nerve impulses to the anal region: some individuals are less aware of the need to defecate and, as a result, develop irregular bowel movements and are at risk for constipation (Meiner, 2011).

Infectious Disease. Microbial agents, including viruses, bacteria, and protozoa, can infect the GI tract. These infections can cause diarrhea and inflammatory or ulcerative changes in the small or large intestine. Most infections are spread by the oral–fecal route, through contaminated food or water.

The rotavirus is an example of a viral infection and is responsible for most nonbacterial food-borne epidemic gastroenteritis in all age groups. The virus is shed before and for days after clinical illness. Very few infectious virons are actually needed to cause disease. Rotavirus infection begins after about 24 hours' incubation and presents with mild to moderate fever and vomiting, followed by watery stools. Treatment is focused on preventing dehydration (Hannon & Porth, 2017).

Clostridium difficile (*C. difficile*) colitis is a bacterial infection associated with antibiotic therapy. Treatment with broad-spectrum antibiotics can lead to the disruption of the normal flora of the colon, creating colonization by *C. difficile* and the release of toxins that damage the mucosa and cause inflammation. The infection manifests with mild to moderate diarrhea and lower abdominal cramping. It is the most frequent cause of health care–associated infectious diarrhea in Canada and other developed countries (Dubberke, Butler, Yokoe, et al., 2010). Stool specimen collection for the testing of *C. difficile* or its toxins should be done as soon as possible after onset of diarrhea. Treatment includes immediate discontinuation of the antibiotic and in cases where symptoms are severe, treatment is aimed at eradication of *C. difficile* (Hannon & Porth, 2017).

The primary mode of transmission for *C. difficile* within health care facilities is by person-to-person spread. Contact precautions should be implemented for patients with acute diarrhea suspected or confirmed to be caused by *C. difficile* infection. Patients should be placed on contact precautions, preferably in a single room, until the diarrhea is resolved or its cause is determined not to be infectious. Hand hygiene should be performed frequently after patient care, contact with the patient's environment, and removing gloves at point of care; just prior to leaving the patient's room; after handling fecal matter; and after handling bedpans and commodes (Public Health Agency of Canada, 2013).

Outbreaks of the highly contagious Norwalk virus are common in Canadian schools, hospitals, day care centres, and nursing homes. The Norwalk virus has been described as "the winter vomiting disease" and rapidly spreads to staff, students, and patients. When the Norwalk virus is detected, standard infection control procedures need to be implemented rapidly, accompanied by further precautions, such as isolation of the affected units, strict handwashing protocols, the wearing of gloves and gowns, and a thorough washing down of the affected units. When an outbreak occurs, the institution is frequently closed to visitors, and infected staff are required to remain off duty until they are symptom-free for 48 hours. In healthy individuals, symptoms last from 12 to 60 hours. The very young, older persons, and ill patients are at danger from dehydration and electrolyte imbalance (Conly & Johnston, 2003).

Irritable Bowel Syndrome. Irritable bowel syndrome (IBS) is a functional GI disorder with chronic intestinal symptoms that cannot be explained by structural or biochemical abnormalities. The symptoms of IBS can include abdominal pain, altered bowel function, flatulence, bloating, nausea, anorexia, and diarrhea. The hallmark symptom is abdominal pain that is relieved by defecation and accompanied by a change in the frequency or consistency of stools (Hannon & Porth, 2017).

TABLE 44-1 Normal Age-Related Changes in the Gastrointestinal Tract

Portion of Gastrointestinal Tract	Functional or Physiological Change	Age-Related Causes
Mouth	Difficulty chewing and oral dryness	Medications can decrease saliva production Taste buds atrophy
Esophagus	Increased incidence of acid reflux	Reduced motility Loss of muscle and ligament tone Decreased esophageal contractions
Stomach	Decrease in acid secretions Not able to accommodate large amounts of food Increased risk of peptic ulcer disease, anemia, and stomach cancer	Degeneration of gastric mucosa
	Decrease in mucosal thickness	Loss of parietal cells also leads to loss of the intrinsic factor, which is needed for vitamin B_{12}, iron, calcium, and folic acid absorption.
Small intestine	Decreased nutrient absorption	Atrophy of muscle and mucosal surfaces
Large intestine	Increased risk of diverticuli Increased occurrence of constipation Missed defecation signal	Atrophy of mucosa Atherosclerotic vascular changes Decrease in tone of internal and external sphincters

Data from Meiner, S. (2011). *Gerontologic nursing* (4th ed.). St. Louis, MO: Mosby.

IBS is related to diet, stress, and psychological factors and its onset may be triggered by a GI infection. The precise pathophysiology of IBS is not understood. Management is multimodal, based on the patient's most troublesome symptoms and includes counselling, dietary modifications, and medications (such as bulking agents, antispasmodics, and antidepressants) (Quartero, Meiniche-Schmidt, Muris, et al., 2005). The nurse can support the patient with IBS by offering coaching on stress management and on maintaining a high-fibre diet (Hannon & Porth, 2017).

Inflammatory Bowel Disease. Inflammatory bowel disease (IBD) is thought to be an autoimmune disease. There are two main types of IBD, ulcerative colitis (UC) and Crohn's disease (CD). UC typically affects only the large intestine, while CD can affect any part of the GI tract from the mouth to anus. The cause of UC and CD is thought to be multifactorial; these factors are just now starting to be understood. Patients experience a range of symptoms associated with inflammation of the gut, including abdominal pain, fever, vomiting, diarrhea, rectal bleeding, anemia, and weight loss. There is currently no known cure, but symptoms can be managed through use of anti-inflammatory steroids or immunosuppressants to reduce inflammation, dietary changes to try and remove environmental triggers, and (in severe cases) surgery to remove damaged portions of the bowel (de Lang, & Barrett, 2015).

Diabetes. Patients with diabetes frequently report problems with constipation, diarrhea, or both that are due to GI autonomic neuropathy. Hyperglycemia can directly reduce or slow gastric contractions and the GI emptying rate. GI symptoms are more prevalent in patients with poor glycemic control. Symptoms can be improved with dietary changes, including reducing fats and increasing daily fibre intake (Bharucha, Low, Camilleri, et al., 2008; Duby, Campbell, Setter, et al., 2004).

Pain. Normally, the act of defecation is painless. However, several conditions can result in discomfort, including hemorrhoids, rectal surgery, rectal fistulas, and abdominal surgery. In these instances, to avoid pain, the patient often suppresses the urge to defecate. As a result, constipation and impaction may develop.

Pelvic Floor Trauma. Trauma to the pelvic floor muscles from pregnancy, labour and delivery, and aging can affect bowel elimination in women.

As pregnancy advances, the size of the fetus increases and pressure is exerted on the rectum. A temporary obstruction created by the fetus impairs the passage of feces. Slowing of peristalsis during the third trimester often leads to constipation. A pregnant woman's frequent straining during defecation or delivery can result in the formation of permanent hemorrhoids. Damage to the perineum extending to the anal sphincters during labour can also alter sphincter integrity (Doughty, 2006).

Older women, particularly those who have borne children, frequently develop loss of tone and weakening of the ligaments and muscles of the anterior and posterior vaginal walls. This condition can lead to cystocele (the dropping of the bladder into the vagina), rectocele (the pouching of the feces-filled rectum into the vagina), and sometimes complete prolapse of the uterus out of the vagina. All of these conditions alter the anorectal angle and can inhibit complete evacuation (Doughty, 2006). Nurse continence advisors (i.e., registered nurses who are specially educated in continence care) treat these problems by educating patients about high-fibre diets and teaching pelvic floor muscle exercises, often referred to as *Kegel exercises* (Cowie et al., 2014).

Acute Illness, Surgery, and Anaesthesia. The GI system may be affected by any acute illness. Changes in the patient's fluid status, mobility patterns, nutrition, and sleep cycle can affect regular bowel habits. Surgical interventions on the GI tract affect bowel elimination, as will surgery on other systems, such as the musculoskeletal and cardiovascular systems.

The general anaesthetic agents used during surgery cause temporary cessation of peristalsis (see Chapter 48). Inhaled anaesthetic agents block the parasympathetic impulses to the enteric nervous system, and the stress of surgery stimulates the sympathetic nervous system. The anaesthetic's action slows or stops the integrated contractions. Pain control medication that contains opioids has the adverse effects of slowing mass peristalsis (or mass movement) and increasing the slow-mixing contractions and fluid absorption from the colon. Thus, following surgery, abdominal discomfort from intraluminal gas and constipation are frequent, and the surgeon's postoperative orders typically include bowel routine with laxatives and enemas if bowel movements do not occur within 2 to 3 days. Thus, nurses need to note whether and when the first bowel movement postsurgery occurs, because the patient may require treatment for constipation. Early postoperative ambulation stimulates the evacuation of flatus, stimulates peristalsis, and alleviates abdominal pain (Lewis et al., 2014).

The patient who receives local or regional anaesthesia is less at risk for bowel elimination alterations because bowel activity may be affected minimally or not at all. Any surgery that involves direct manipulation of the bowel temporarily stops peristalsis. This condition, called paralytic ileus, usually lasts 24 to 48 hours. If the patient remains inactive or is unable to eat after surgery, return of normal bowel function may be further delayed (Lewis, Heitkemper, O'Brien, et al., 2014).

Enteral Feeding. Patients receiving enteral feeding will experience changes in bowel elimination. When the absorptive area of the small intestine is reduced, patients may receive nutrition through enteral feeding administered by tube into the GI tract. Enteral feeding contains nutrients that do not need further digestion to be rapidly absorbed by the diminished area of the intestine.

Patients receiving their nutrition through enteral feeding may experience diarrhea. This can be due to the feed running too quickly, medications, or an active infection (Lewis et al., 2014). Conversely, a patient could experience problems with constipation. This is usually related to the type of formula used, and a change to a high-fibre formula may resolve the constipation (Lewis et al., 2014). Again, medications the patient is taking must be examined for their effects on the GI system (Lewis et al., 2014).

Medications That Affect Elimination. Medication may have certain expected actions on the bowel; for example, some medications promote defecation, and others control diarrhea. In addition, medications prescribed for acute and chronic conditions may have secondary effects on the patient's bowel elimination patterns (Table 44-2).

Laboratory Tests. Laboratory and diagnostic examinations yield useful information concerning bowel elimination problems (Table 44-3). Laboratory analysis of fecal contents can detect pathological conditions, such as tumours, bleeding, and infection.

Fecal Specimens. Nurses are directly responsible for ensuring that fecal specimens are accurately obtained, properly labelled in appropriate containers, and transported to the laboratory on time. Institutions provide special containers for fecal specimens. Some tests require specimens to be placed in chemical preservatives.

Medical aseptic technique should be used during collection of stool specimens (see Chapter 33). Because approximately 25% of the solid portion of a stool is bacteria from the colon, disposable gloves should be worn when handling fecal specimens.

Hand hygiene is necessary for anyone who might come in contact with the specimen. The patient can often obtain the specimen if

TABLE 44-2 Medications and the Gastrointestinal System

Medication	Action
Opioids	Increase the mixing action of segmentation contractions and slow the propulsive contractions, often resulting in constipation, nausea, vomiting, or anorexia (Lilley, Rainforth Collins, Snyder, et al., 2016).
Anticholinergics (such as atropine)	Inhibit gastric acid secretion and depress gastrointestinal motility. Although anticholinergics are useful in treating hyperactive bowel disorders, they can cause constipation (Lilley et al., 2016).
Antibiotics	Frequently produce diarrhea by disrupting the normal bacterial flora in the gastrointestinal tract. Antibiotic use has been shown to promote infection with the highly contagious *C. difficile,* which has a high mortality rate in older persons. Concurrently taking a probiotic acidophilus supplement has been shown to reduce the incidence of diarrhea and to reduce the risk of *C. difficile* infections (McFarland, 2006).
Nonsteroidal anti-inflammatory drugs (such as acetylsalicylic acid)	Prostaglandin inhibitors are used to treat arthritis pain but can also promote gastrointestinal irritation that can range from dyspepsia to life-threatening hemorrhage (Lilley et al., 2016).
Histamine$_2$ (H_2) antagonists (such as ranitidine) Proton pump inhibitors (such as omeprazole)	Reduce the secretion of hydrochloric acid and are commonly used to treat many acid-related disorders. These drugs suppress gastric acid secretion and may also predispose patients to GI infections (Lilley et al., 2016).
Iron	Can cause blackening of the stool and can lead to constipation (Lilley et al., 2016).
Calcium carbonate	Adverse gastrointestinal effects include constipation, obstruction, nausea, vomiting, and flatulence (Lilley et al., 2016).

TABLE 44-3 Laboratory and Diagnostic Tests for Bowel Function

Measurement	Interpretation
Laboratory Tests	
Total bilirubin	Increased levels of bilirubin may result from hepatobiliary diseases, obstructions in the bile duct, certain anemias, and reactions to blood transfusions.
Alkaline phosphatase	Elevated levels of alkaline phosphatase may indicate obstructive hepatobiliary diseases, hepatobiliary carcinomas, bone tumours, or healing fractures.
Amylase	Elevated levels of amylase may indicate abnormalities of the pancreas, such as inflammation, tumours, cholecystitis, necrotic bowel, and diabetic ketoacidosis.
Carcinoembryonic antigen (CEA)	The carcinoembryonic antigen is elevated in the presence of cancer, inflammation of the gastrointestinal (GI) tract, or hepatobiliary organs.
Direct Visualization	
Endoscopy	A colonoscopy is a routine examination for persons 50 years of age and older. Normally, the GI tract is free of polyps, tumours, inflammation, ulcers, hernias, obstruction, and ulcerations. If a lesion, such as a polyp, is identified, the prescriber removes the growth or a portion of the growth and sends it to pathology for analysis. If bleeding is present, the prescriber may attempt to coagulate the source. In some cases, the identification of an abnormality may indicate the need for follow-up surgery for the patient.
Indirect Visualization	
X-ray with contrast medium	An X-ray may show the presence of acute abnormalities in the GI tract. A series of X-rays will allow for indirect visualization of the entire tract. The presence of tumours, ulcerations, inflammation, or other abnormalities may indicate the need for further diagnostic testing and medical or surgical intervention.

From Chernecky, C. C., & Berger, B. (2008). *Laboratory tests and diagnostic procedures.* St. Louis, MO: Saunders Elsevier.

properly instructed. The nurse should explain to the patient that feces cannot be mixed with urine or water. For this reason, the patient must defecate into a clean, dry bedpan or a special container placed under the toilet seat (Dubberke et al., 2010).

Tests performed by the laboratory for occult (microscopic) blood in the stool and stool cultures require only a small sample. About 2.5 cm of formed stool or 15 to 30 mL of liquid diarrhea stool is collected. Tests for measuring the output of fecal fat require a 3- to 5-day collection of stool. All fecal material must be saved throughout the test period.

After obtaining a fecal specimen, the nurse needs to label and tightly seal the container, complete the laboratory requisition forms, and record the specimen collections in the patient's medical record. The nurse should avoid delays in sending specimens to the laboratory because some tests, such as measurements for ova and parasites, require the stool to be warm. When stool specimens are allowed to stand at room temperature, bacteriological changes occur that can alter the test results.

A common laboratory test that can be done at home or at the patient's bedside is the **fecal occult blood test (FOBT)**, or guaiac test,

BOX 44-1 PROCEDURAL GUIDELINE
Measuring Fecal Occult Blood

Delegation Considerations:
This skill can be delegated to unregulated care providers (UCPs). The nurse directs the UCP to report immediately if blood is detected. The nurse also assesses the significance of the findings.

Equipment:
- Hemoccult test paper
- Wooden applicator
- Clean gloves
- Clean, dry container to collect sample

Procedure:
1. Explain to the patient the purpose of the test and how the patient can assist. Patients can collect their own specimens if possible. Specimen must be free of urine and toilet paper.
2. Perform hand hygiene.
3. Apply clean disposable gloves.
4. Obtain uncontaminated stool specimen.
5. Use the tip of the wooden applicator to obtain a small portion of a stool specimen. Ensure that the specimen is free of toilet paper.
6. Open the flap of the hemoccult slide. Using the wooden applicator, thinly smear the stool in the first box of the guaiac paper. Apply a second fecal specimen from a different portion of the stool to the slide's second box (see Step 6 illustration).
7. Close the slide cover and send the sample to the laboratory per the institution's policies and procedures.
8. Wrap the wooden applicator in a paper towel. Remove gloves and discard in the proper receptacle.
9. Perform hand hygiene.
10. Record any unusual fecal characteristics.

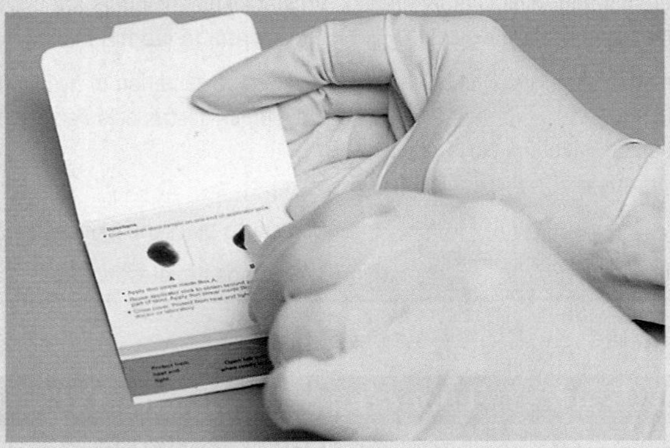

STEP 6 Application of the fecal specimen on guaiac paper.

BOX 44-2 Screening for Colon Cancer

Risk Factors
- Older than 50 years of age
- Family history of colorectal cancer (particularly parent, child, or sibling)
- History of inflammatory bowel disease (e.g., ulcerative colitis or Crohn's disease)
- High-fat and low-fibre diet
- Obesity
- Excessive alcohol consumption
- Smoking
- Physically inactive

Warning Signs
- Unexplained change in bowel patterns
- Rectal bleeding
- Unexplained weight loss
- Urgent need to empty bowel
- Unexplained stool incontinence

Screening Tests
- Fecal occult blood test (FOBT) at least every 2 years after age 50
- If patient has family history of colorectal cancer in first-degree relative or has symptoms, colonoscopy

From Ontario Ministry of Long-Term Care. (2016). *Colon cancer check.* Retrieved from http://www.health.gov.on.ca/en/pro/programs/coloncancercheck/fobt_multilingual.aspx.

which measures microscopic amounts of blood in the feces (Box 44-1). This test is useful as a diagnostic screening for colon cancer (Box 44-2). A single positive result does not confirm GI bleeding. The test should be repeated at least three times while the patient refrains from ingesting foods and medications that can cause false-positive results. For example, during the test period, the patient should avoid ingesting red meat, poultry, fish, some raw vegetables, vitamin C, aspirin, or other nonsteroidal anti-inflammatory drugs (NSAIDs) that can cause false-positive results (Ontario Ministry of Long-Term Care, 2016). Patients who receive anticoagulants or who have a bleeding disorder or a GI disorder known to cause bleeding (e.g., intestinal tumours, bowel inflammation, or ulcerations) should be regularly screened for fecal occult blood.

Fecal characteristics. Inspection of fecal characteristics (Table 44-4) reveals information about the nature of bowel elimination alterations. Several factors can influence each characteristic. A key to assessment is knowing whether any recent changes have occurred. The patient can best provide this information during the health history assessment.

Diagnostic Examinations. A variety of radiological and diagnostic tests may be ordered for the patient who experiences altered bowel elimination (Box 44-3). GI structures may be visualized using either a direct or indirect approach. Each test has a prescribed preparation routine for emptying the GI area under study to facilitate visualization. Many facilities use conscious sedation during these procedures. Nurses need to be sure they understand the safety precautions involved in the use of this form of anaesthesia. In many institutions, special training is required. A crash cart must be present at the bedside, and the patient must be monitored continuously with pulse oximetry and frequent vital signs, usually every 15 minutes during and immediately following the procedure. Nurses need to check agency policy regarding the use of sedation for these examinations (Pagana, Pagana, & Pike-MacDonald, 2013).

Diagnostic Tests. Diagnostic examinations that involve visualization of GI structures often require that portions of the bowel be empty. The patient receives a prescribed bowel preparation before the test. Usually, the patient is asked to drink a large volume (4 L) of a solution containing a nonabsorbable inert molecule, such as polyethylene

TABLE 44-4 Characteristics of Feces

Characteristic	Normal	Abnormal	Cause of Abnormality
Colour	Brown	White or clay	Absence of bile pigment, such as in obstructive jaundice
		Black or tarry (i.e., melena)	Iron ingestion or upper gastrointestinal bleeding
		Red	Lower gastrointestinal bleeding, hemorrhoids
		Pale with fat or frothy	Malabsorption of fat
		Mucus or pus	Spastic constipation, colitis, excessive straining
		Bloody mucus	Blood in feces, inflammation, infection, hemorrhoids
Odour	Pungent; affected by food type	Noxious change	Blood in feces or infection
Consistency	Soft, formed	Liquid	Diarrhea, reduced absorption
		Hard	Constipation
Frequency	Daily or two to three times weekly	More than three times a day or less than once a week	Hypomotility or hypermotility (multifactorial)
Shape	Resembles diameter of rectum	Narrow, pencil shaped	Anal or distal rectal carcinoma
Constituents	Undigested food, dead bacteria, fat, bile pigment, cells lining intestinal mucosa, water	Blood, pus, foreign bodies, mucus, worms	Internal bleeding, infection, swallowed objects, irritation, inflammation
		Excess fat	Malabsorption syndrome, enteritis, pancreatic disease, surgical resection of intestine

From Jarvis, C., Browne, A., MacDonald-Jenkins, J., & Luctkar-Flude, M. (Eds.). (2014). *Physical examination and health assessment* (2nd Canadian ed.). Toronto: Elsevier Canada; and Swartz, M. H. (2009). *Textbook of physical diagnosis history and examination* (6th ed.). Philadelphia, PA: Saunders Elsevier.

BOX 44-3 Radiological and Diagnostic Tests

Flat Plate Radiography
- A simple X-ray film of the abdomen that requires no preparation.

Computerized Tomography Scan
- An X-ray examination of the body from many angles uses a scanner and is analyzed by a computer.
- The preparation may be either nothing by mouth (NPO) or no preparation.
- The patient must be informed of the need to lie very still. If claustrophobia is a problem, light sedation may be used.

Ultrasound Imaging
- Technique used to visualize the abdomen and organs within.
- High-frequency sound waves echo off body organs to create a picture.
- The preparation depends on the organ to be visualized and may include either fasting or no preparation.

Upper Gastrointestinal Barium Swallow Esophagram
- An X-ray examination uses an opaque contrast medium (e.g., barium) to visualize the structure and motility of the upper gastrointestinal tract, including the pharynx, esophagus, and stomach.
- The patient must be restricted to NPO after midnight the night before the examination.
- The patient must remove all jewellery and other metallic objects.
- After the test, the patient must increase fluids to facilitate passage and elimination of the barium.

Lower Gastrointestinal Barium Enema
- An X-ray examination uses an opaque contrast medium to visualize the lower gastrointestinal tract.
- The preparation includes a bowel preparation or cathartic to empty any remaining stool particles.

Upper Gastrointestinal Endoscopy
- An endoscopic examination of the upper gastrointestinal tract allows a more direct visualization via a lighted fibre-optic tube.
- The preparation is similar to that of the upper gastrointestinal barium swallow.
- A light sedation is required.

Colonoscopy
- An endoscopic examination of the rectum and colon that uses a long, flexible tube (i.e., a colonoscope) inserted into the rectum.
- Bowel must be clean and free of fecal material.
- Light sedation is required.

Sigmoidoscopy
- An examination of the interior of the sigmoid colon.
- Preparation is similar to that of a colonoscopy.
- Light sedation is required.

Magnetic Resonance Imaging
- A noninvasive examination uses magnetic and radio waves to produce a picture of the inside of the body.
- Provides better contrast between normal and pathological tissue than an ultrasound.
- The preparation is NPO 4 to 6 hours before examination.
- No metallic objects are allowed in the room, including metal objects on clothes.

From Pagana, K. D., Pagana, T. J., & Pike-MacDonald, S. A. (2013). *Mosby's Canadian manual of diagnostic and laboratory tests* (1st Canadian ed.). Toronto: Elsevier.

glycol. Other medications, cathartics, or enemas may also be used. In addition, the patient is not allowed to eat or drink after midnight of the day preceding examinations such as a colonoscopy, endoscopy, or other testing that requires visualization of the lower GI tract. Following the diagnostic procedure, the patient may experience changes in bowel elimination, such as increased gas or loose stools. These changes will stop when the patient resumes a normal eating pattern (Pagana et al., 2013).

◆ Nursing Diagnosis

Nursing assessment of the patient's bowel function reveals data that may indicate an actual or potential bowel elimination problem or a problem resulting from bowel elimination alterations. The concept map in Figure 44-10 depicts how the nursing diagnosis of constipation may be related to other diagnoses. In this example, a patient with cancer has developed constipation as a result of activity intolerance and imbalanced nutrition. Both conditions are a result of the patient's pain. Diagnoses that may apply to patients with bowel elimination problems include the following:

- *Bowel incontinence*
- *Constipation*
- *Risk for constipation*
- *Perceived constipation*
- *Diarrhea*

A patient's associated problems, such as body-image changes or skin breakdown, require interventions unrelated to bowel function impairment. In some instances, however, nurses need to direct as much attention to the associated problem as to the bowel elimination problem.

Nurses' ability to identify the correct nursing diagnosis depends not only on the thoroughness of assessment but also on recognition of defining characteristics and factors that can impair bowel elimination (Box 44-4). The nurse needs to determine the patient's risk and then institute measures to ensure maintenance of normal bowel function.

Common Bowel Elimination Problems. Nurses may care for patients who have or are at risk for bowel elimination problems because of emotional stress (anxiety or depression), inflammatory diseases, prescribed therapy, disorders impairing defecation, or physiological changes in the GI tract, such as surgical alteration of intestinal structures.

Constipation. Constipation is a symptom, not a disease (Box 44-5). The signs of constipation vary among patients but usually include infrequent bowel movements (fewer than three per week), difficult evacuation of feces, inability to defecate at will, and hard feces (Ginsberg, Phillips, Wallace, et al., 2007). Common signs are abdominal pain and distension and a sensation of fullness and pressure in the rectum. Straining during defecation is also an associated sign. When intestinal motility slows, the fecal mass becomes exposed over time to the intestinal walls and most of the fecal water is absorbed. Little water is left to soften and lubricate the stool. Passage of a dry, hard stool may cause rectal pain (Ginsberg et al., 2007). Constipation is a common concern during acute hospital admissions for older persons (Box 44-6).

Constipation can be a significant hazard to health. Straining during defecation may cause problems to the patient who has recently

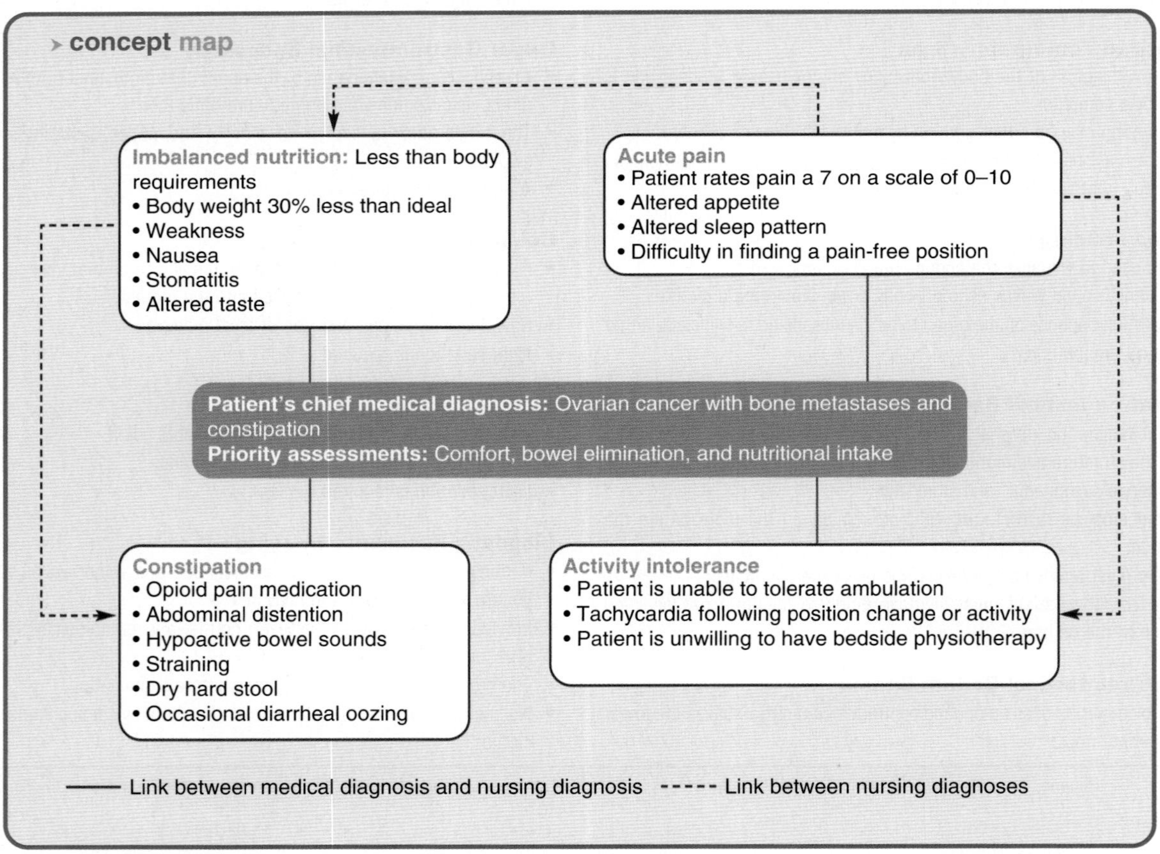

FIGURE 44-10 Concept map for a patient who has ovarian cancer with bone metastases and constipation.

undergone abdominal, gynecological, or rectal surgery. The effort to pass a stool can cause sutures to separate, thereby reopening the wound. Patients who have a history of cardiovascular disease, diseases causing elevated intraocular pressure (glaucoma), and increased intracranial pressure should prevent constipation and avoid using the Valsalva manoeuvre. The Valsalva manoeuvre can be avoided by exhaling through the mouth during straining. Constipation also affects a person's quality of life (Bliss & Norton, 2010).

Patients may experience constipation as a result of medications they are taking. Medications that cause constipation include anticholinergics, antidepressants, antiemetics, antihistamines, antihypertensives, anti-Parkinson agents, antipsychotics, antacids containing aluminum, analgesics, NSAIDs, histamine-2 blockers, hypnotics, diuretics, sedatives, iron supplements, and opioids (RNAO, 2011).

Constipation can also occur in conjunction with the treatment of urinary conditions, as an adverse effect of the medication but also because individuals with urinary incontinence may reduce their fluid intake to reduce the frequency of their need to urinate (Ginsberg et al., 2007).

Impaction. Fecal **impaction** results from unrelieved constipation and can lead to overflow incontinence. Fecal impaction is a collection of hardened feces that are wedged in the rectum and cannot be expelled.

BOX 44-4 NURSING DIAGNOSTIC PROCESS

Assessment Activities	Defining Characteristics	Nursing Diagnosis
Inspect the abdomen for shape, symmetry.	Distended abdomen	*Diarrhea related to gastrointestinal disorder*
Auscultate for bowel sounds.	Bowel sounds are hyperactive and audible without a stethoscope.	
Percuss for general tympany.	Hyperresonance is present with gaseous distension.	
Assess frequency of stools.	Patient reports having more than three loose bowel movements a day, accompanied by muscle cramps.	
Assess hydration status.	Loss of skin turgor and dry mucous membranes.	
Have patient describe the pain, cramping, or any associated factors.	Pain is colicky in nature and spasmodic.	
Evaluate the perianal area for redness and irritation.	Breakdown of perianal tissues	

From Ackley, B., & Ladwig, G. (Eds.). (2011). *An evidence-based guide to planning care* (9th ed.). St. Louis, MO: Mosby Elsevier; and Jarvis, C., Browne, A., MacDonald-Jenkins, J., & Luctkar-Flude, M. (Eds.). (2014). *Physical examination and health assessment* (2nd Canadian ed.). Toronto: Elsevier Canada.

BOX 44-5 Common Causes of Constipation

- Ignoring the urge to defecate
- Sedentary lifestyle, including lengthy bed rest or lack of regular exercise
- A low-fibre diet high in animal fats (e.g., meats, dairy products, eggs) and refined sugars (e.g., rich desserts)
- A low noncaffeinated fluid intake
- Prolonged and overuse of laxatives
- Polypharmacy
- Comorbidities such as Parkinson's disease, multiple sclerosis, rheumatoid arthritis, chronic bowel diseases, depression, eating disorders, hypothyroidism, hypocalcemia, or hypokalemia
- Neurological conditions that block the nerve impulse to the colon (e.g., spinal cord injuries, tumours)

From Ginsberg, D. A., Phillips, S. F., Wallace, J., & Josephson, K. L. (2007). Evaluating and managing constipation in the elderly. *Urologic Nursing, 27,* 191–200; and Registered Nurses' Association of Ontario. (2011). *Prevention of constipation in the older adult population.* Toronto: Registered Nurses' Association of Ontario.

BOX 44-6 RESEARCH HIGHLIGHT

Constipation in Older Persons During an Acute Hospital Stay

Research Focus

Bowel problems during hospitalization can be common and distressing in older persons. In some cases, hospital stays can be lengthened if constipation is not addressed. The majority of guidelines and research done on constipation in older persons focus on patients in a long-stay hospital or in long-term care. Very few studies have been done on factors that predict the onset of constipation in the acutely hospitalized older person. Identifying factors that precipitate constipation during an acute hospital stay would facilitate starting a specific, preventative care plan for constipation early in an older person's hospital stay.

Research Abstract

The purpose of the study by Cardin, Minicuci, Droghi, and colleagues (2009) was to identify any factors predicting the onset of constipation in acutely hospitalized older patients. The goal was to create an evidence-informed identification of which patients need early preventative measures. The study involved 192 patients over the age of 67 who were consecutively admitted for various medical conditions to an acute care ward in an Italian hospital. All patients were interviewed upon arrival, and detailed information was collected about their physical health, mental status, dietary problems, medication use, and consistency of feces. Information on constipation and medication use during their hospital stay was also collected.

Evidence-Informed Practice

- Use of laxatives at home was a factor in constipation during the hospital stay.
- Satisfaction with bowel movements is reduced in patients who must stay in bed for lengthy periods of time during their hospitalization.
- Patients who have had cerebrovascular accidents are also more unsatisfied with their bowel movements during their hospital stay.
- Nurses working in acute care should assess their patients for at-home laxative use upon admission and put in place a plan to prevent constipation for patients who used laxatives at home, are likely to remain in bed for longer than 2 weeks, or who have had a cerebrovascular accident.

Cardin, F., Minicuci, N., Droghi, A. T., Inelmen, E. M., Sergi, G., & Terranova, O. (2009). Constipation in acutely hospitalized older patients. *Archives of Gerontology and Geriatrics, 50,* 277–281. doi:10.1016/j.archger.2009.04.007.

In cases of severe impaction, the mass can extend into the sigmoid colon. Patients who are immobile, dehydrated, have impaired rectal sensation, depression, delirium, and dementia are most at risk for impaction.

An obvious sign of impaction is the inability to pass a stool for several days, despite the repeated urge to defecate. A continuous oozing of diarrhea stool may develop when the liquid portion of feces located higher in the colon seeps around the impacted mass. Loss of appetite (anorexia), nausea or vomiting, abdominal distension and cramping, and rectal pain may accompany the condition. If nurses suspect an impaction, they can gently perform a digital examination of the rectum and palpate for the impacted mass (Cowie et al., 2014).

Diarrhea. Diarrhea is an increase in the number of stools (several bowel movements per day) and the passage of liquid, unformed feces. Diarrhea can be acute or chronic. Diarrhea can be caused by infectious organisms (as discussed earlier), food intolerances, medications (including chemotherapy), or intestinal disease. Intestinal contents pass through the small and large intestine too quickly to allow the usual absorption of fluid and nutrients. Irritation within the colon can result in an increased mucus secretion. As a result, feces become watery and the patient may be unable to control the urge to defecate (Hannon & Porth, 2017).

Excess loss of colonic fluid can result in serious fluid, electrolyte, or acid–base imbalances. Older persons are particularly susceptible to complications associated with diarrhea (see Chapter 40). Repeated passage of diarrhea stools exposes the skin of the perineum and the buttocks to irritating intestinal contents; therefore, meticulous skin care and containment of fecal drainage is needed to prevent skin breakdown (see Chapter 38) (Hannon & Porth, 2017).

The aims of treatment are to remove the precipitating conditions and to slow peristalsis. Drugs that are opiumlike (such as loperamide) are used to decrease GI motility and stimulate water and electrolyte absorption. Antidiarrheal medications should not be used with patients who have blood in their stool or a high fever, because they could risk worsening the disease. Antibiotics are used only when enteric pathogens have been identified (Hannon & Porth, 2017).

Communicable food-borne pathogens can also cause diarrhea. The risk of food-borne illnesses can be greatly reduced by thorough hand washing after using the bathroom and before and after preparing foods, and by properly storing and preparing fresh produce and meats. When diarrhea is the result of a food-borne virus, the goal is usually to rid the system of the pathogen, not to slow peristalsis.

Incontinence. Bowel incontinence is the inability to control the passage of feces and gas from the anus. Bowel incontinence is devastating to patients and has a significant effect on functional, social, and psychological well-being (Bliss, Fischer, Savik, et al., 2004). The possible embarrassment of soiling clothes can lead to self-imposed social isolation (Cowie et al., 2014). Contributing factors to bowel incontinence include diet, fluid intake (in particular, caffeine), alcohol, and nicotine (Cowie et al., 2014). Physical conditions that impair anal sphincter function, compliance, or control can cause incontinence. Additionally, patients without the cognitive awareness of the urge to defecate are at risk for incontinence (Cowie et al., 2014). Conditions that create frequent, loose, large-volume, watery stools are predispositions for bowel incontinence (Bliss, Johnson, Savik, et al., 2000). Bowel incontinence can be successfully managed and treated with nursing intervention (Box 44-7).

Flatulence. In most healthy individuals, 100 to 200 mL of gas is present in the GI tract. Gas in the upper GI tract may increase from the swallowing of air. Gas production in the colon occurs from bacteria digesting cellulose in the colon.

As gas accumulates in the lumen of the intestines, the bowel wall stretches and distends, resulting in flatulence. Flatulence is a common cause of abdominal fullness, pain, and cramping. Normally, intestinal gas escapes through the mouth (belching) or the anus (passing of flatus). For a person eating a normal diet, 50 to 500 mL of gas is passed 10 to 15 times a day. However, if intestinal motility is reduced as a result of the effects of opiates, general anaesthetics, abdominal surgery, or immobilization, flatulence can become severe enough to cause abdominal distension and severe, sharp pain (Lewis et al., 2014).

Hemorrhoids. Hemorrhoids are dilated, engorged veins in the lining of the rectum. They are either external or internal. External hemorrhoids are clearly visible as protrusions of skin. If the underlying vein is hardened, a purplish discoloration (i.e., thrombosis) may be visible. This condition causes increased pain, and the hemorrhoid may need to be excised. Internal hemorrhoids have an outer mucous membrane. Increased venous pressure as a result of pregnancy, heart failure, chronic liver disease, or straining at defecation can cause hemorrhoids. The presence of hemorrhoids is frequently accompanied by fecal soiling of undergarments and irritation of the distended veins by

BOX 44-7 CASE STUDY

Bowel Incontinence

Miranda is 58-year-old woman with diabetes who has come to the continence program about her problem with bowel incontinence. She tells the nurse continence advisor that she has been trying to manage her incontinence on her own for the past 6 months. She reports that she has two to three bowel accidents a day. The stools are soft and she has no warning and no control when the urge to defecate occurs. It is so unpredictable that she is no longer comfortable leaving home, which is limiting her activity. She has been a diabetic for 10 years, taking Metformin, but struggles to keep her blood sugar within normal range. She has gained 23 kg (50 lbs) in the last year so she has switched to diet cola, consuming four to six cans a day. She has reduced her dietary fibre intake because she felt it was making her bowel incontinence worse.

A careful assessment identified the following factors potentially contributing to her bowel incontinence:

- Restricting her diet/fibre intake can have an impact on the consistency of her stools. Many individuals manipulate their diets, thinking it is the way to manage their bowels.
- Her fluid intake of diet cola contains both caffeine and artificial sweetener, which have the potential to increase peristalsis, resulting in loose stools (Cowie et al., 2014).

Miranda agreed to begin to reduce her diet cola intake and replace it with water, and to drink at least four to five 237-mL (8-ounce) glasses of water over the course of the day. A consultation with a dietitian was arranged to review her diabetic diet and to begin gradually increasing her dietary fibre with the goal over time to achieve about 25 mg of fibre per day. A regular toileting time after her breakfast was established, to promote regular bowel movements (Cowie et al., 2014).

Gradually, over the next 3 months, with support and coaching, Miranda successfully regained her bowel control. She was so relieved to be able to go about her daily activities once again without worrying about whether she would have an embarrassing accident.

overly vigorous cleaning of the anus. Meticulous cleaning following a bowel movement may reduce the possibility of irritation (Lewis et al., 2014).

◆ Planning

During the planning of care, the nurse synthesizes information from multiple resources (Figure 44-11). Critical thinking ensures that the plan of care integrates all the nurse knows about the patient and the clinical problem. Nurses must rely on professional standards. The guidelines on incontinence (see Chapter 43) can assist nurses in protecting the patient's skin, promoting continence, and reducing the embarrassment associated with incontinence. In addition, the Agency for Health Care Policy and Research (AHCPR), the Registered Nurses' Association of Ontario (RNAO), and the Canadian Association of Wound Care (CAWC) have guidelines on the reduction of pressure injuries; these guidelines can assist the nurse in developing care plans for patients with bowel incontinence (see Chapter 46).

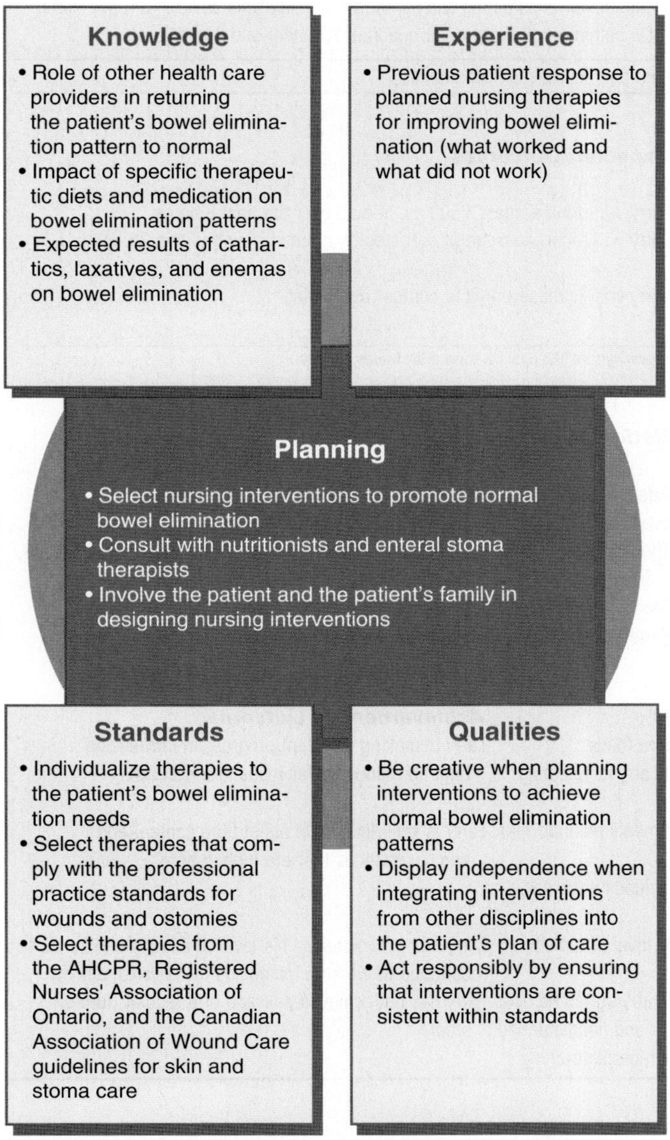

FIGURE 44-11 Critical thinking model for bowel elimination planning. *AHCPR,* Agency for Health Care Policy and Research.

Goals and Outcomes. The nurse and the patient establish goals and outcomes by incorporating the patient's bowel elimination habits or routines as much as possible and by reinforcing routines that promote health. The nurse must also consider pre-existing health concerns. For example, if the patient is at risk for the worsening of heart failure, an outcome of increased fluid intake must be tailored to the patient's cardiac function and ability to safely handle the increased fluid. For another example, if the patient's bowel habits caused the elimination problem, the nurse can help the patient learn new bowel habits. The overall goal of returning the patient to a normal bowel elimination pattern may include the following outcomes:

- The patient practises regular defecation habits.
- The patient lists the proper fluid and food intake needed to achieve regular bowel elimination.
- The patient implements a regular exercise program.
- The patient reports daily passage of soft, formed brown stool.
- The patient does not report any discomfort associated with defecation.

Setting Priorities. Defecation patterns vary among individuals. For this reason, the nurse and the patient must work together closely to plan effective interventions (Box 44-8). A realistic time frame to establish a normal defecation pattern for one patient might differ from that for another patient. For the patient who has a new ostomy as the result of newly diagnosed cancer, the priority of coping with cancer and its treatment may precede the patient's need to independently manage the bowel diversion. For another patient, however, when a bowel diversion is necessary, coping with the changes in body image may become a high priority for both the patient and the patient's family.

Continuity of Care. When patients are disabled or debilitated by illness, nurses need to include the patient's family in the plan of care. Family members often have the same bowel elimination habits as the patient. Thus, teaching both the patient and the patient's family is an important part of the care plan. Other health team members, such as dietitians and enterostomal therapist (ET) nurses, can be valuable resources. When patients require surgical intervention, a critical pathway may be used to coordinate the activities of the multidisciplinary health care team.

The patient who has alterations in bowel elimination will require intervention from many members of the health care team. Certain tasks, such as assisting patients onto the bedpan or bedside commode, are appropriate to delegate to unregulated care providers (UCPs). The nurse needs to remind the UCP to report any abnormal findings or difficulties encountered during the bowel elimination process. Non-nursing personnel perform many of the diagnostic tests used to evaluate the GI system. Nurses must maintain ongoing communication with these caregivers to ensure that the patient's safety, needs, wants, and concerns are addressed.

◆ Implementation

The success of nursing interventions depends on improving the patient's and the family members' understanding of bowel elimination. In the home, hospital, or long-term care facility, patients capable of learning can be taught effective bowel habits.

The patient and the patient's family need to be taught about proper diet, adequate fluid intake, and factors that stimulate or slow peristalsis, such as emotional stress. The patient should also learn the importance of establishing regular bowel routines, participating in regular exercise, and taking appropriate measures when bowel elimination problems develop.

Patient Expectations. Patients expect nurses to answer all their questions regarding diagnostic tests and the preparation for those tests.

BOX 44-8 NURSING CARE PLAN

Constipation

ASSESSMENT

Javier is a nurse who visits Larry at his home on a cattle ranch. Larry lives 40 km from town. He is 22 years old and had surgery 6 days ago for repair of a broken right leg. Larry tells Javier, "I just don't feel good."

Assessment Activities	***Findings and Defining Characteristics***
Ask Larry about his recent bowel elimination patterns over the last 5 days.	Larry has not had a bowel movement since he left the hospital 4 days ago and he feels like his abdomen is tight and sore.
Review Larry's medication.	Larry has been prescribed opioids for pain. He is taking them regularly, as prescribed.
Review Larry's dietary intake over the past day.	Larry has eaten eggs, bacon, and toast for breakfast and soup for lunch. For supper, Larry had chicken, rice, and corn. He drinks about six cups of coffee each day, no water, but will drink a cola.
Ask about any nausea or vomiting.	Larry has not felt nauseated.
Auscultate the abdomen.	Decreased bowel sounds are auscultated throughout all four abdominal quadrants.
Palpate the abdomen.	While Javier is palpating Larry's abdomen, Larry tells Javier, "It really hurts." On palpation, the left lower quadrant is tender and firm.

NURSING DIAGNOSIS: Constipation related to opiate-containing pain medication and decreased fibre intake.

PLANNING

Goals (Nursing Outcomes Classification)*	***Expected Outcomes***
Bowel Elimination	
Larry will establish normal defecation.	Larry will drink at least 1 500 mL of fluid over the next 8 hours.
Larry will voice relief from constipation.	Larry will report passage of soft stool without straining within 24 hours.
Nutritional Status: Food and Fluid Intake	
Larry will identify measures to prevent constipation.	Larry will increase the fibre content of his diet.
Larry will increase the amount of daily exercise.	

*Outcome classification labels from Ackley, B., & Ladwig, G. (Eds.). (2011). *An evidence-based guide to planning care* (9th ed.). St. Louis, MO: Mosby Elsevier.

INTERVENTIONS

Interventions	***Rationale***
Constipation or Impaction Management	
Encourage fluid intake of fruit juice, water, and other appropriate fluids.	Adequate fluid intake is necessary to prevent hard, dry stool.
Encourage activity within the limits of Larry's mobility regimen.	Even minimal activity (such as leg lifts) increases peristalsis.
Add bran flakes or bran to the diet.	The number of bowel movements is increased with consumption of bran (Bliss, Jung, Savik, et al., 2001).
Provide laxative or stool softeners as ordered.	Medications can soften the stool and prevent straining (Lilley et al., 2016).
Provide a private atmosphere for bowel elimination.	Patients should feel relaxed when moving their bowels.

EVALUATION

Nursing Actions	***Patient Response and Findings***	***Achievement of Outcome***
Ask Larry to identify foods high in fibre.	Larry is able to correctly identify high-fibre foods. Review of the 24-hour diet diary shows Larry is selecting high-fibre, low-fat foods.	Larry is making excellent progress in introducing high-fibre and low-fat foods into his diet.
Ask Larry to plan menus to increase fibre.	Review of the 24-hour diet diary shows meals planned that have high-fibre content. Larry reviews his shopping list, which includes bran, oat, and fruit products.	Larry is knowledgeable about fibre content and purchases foods that are high in fibre.
Ask Larry about increased activity.	Larry states that he has not changed his level of activity.	Larry has not increased his level of activity and needs to continue to work on increasing his physical activity.
Observe Larry's subsequent stool for characteristics such as consistency and colour.	Stools occur now every 24 to 48 hours. Larry states he does not "feel regular." The abdomen is soft and nondistended. Stools are formed and hard, and Larry reports straining.	Larry has not achieved passage of a regular, formed stool.

Patients will be concerned about discomfort and exposure. Fear of losing control of their bowel elimination is especially worrisome. Patients need reassurance that their needs will be met and that nurses are supportive. Patients expect a knowledgeable nurse who can teach them methods of promoting and maintaining a normal bowel elimination pattern.

Management of Bowel Elimination. One of the most important habits nurses can encourage patients to establish is a daily bowel routine that includes adequate fluid and food intake as well as regular exercise. The urge to defecate usually occurs within an hour following a meal, after breakfast being the most common time for most individuals. Having access to a bathroom, privacy, and a comfortable seated position are all factors in the routine. Many patients have their established routines for defecation at home, which can become disrupted if they are ill. In a hospital or long-term care facility, nurses need to ensure that treatment routines do not interfere with a patient's bowel elimination routine. The provision of privacy is important to maintain. When a patient shares the room with other patients, the curtain should be pulled around the area so the patient can relax, with the knowledge that interruptions will not occur. The call light should always be placed within the patient's reach. Bathroom doors should be closed, although the nurse may stand close by in case the patient needs assistance.

Maintenance of Proper Fluid and Food Intake. Daily fluid intake should be between 1 500 and 2 000 mL per day of noncaffeinated beverages. Dietary fibre intake should be from 25 to 30 g per day. In choosing a diet to promote normal bowel elimination, nurses need to consider the frequency of defecation, the characteristics of the feces, and the types of foods that impair or promote defecation. The patient with frequent constipation or impaction requires an increased intake of high-fibre foods and more fluids. The patient needs to understand that diet therapy is only one factor to consider and may not give immediate relief from problems such as constipation.

Many evidence-informed interventions are available to reduce the risk of constipation (Box 44-9) (RNAO, 2011).

If diarrhea is a problem, the patient can eat foods with a low-fibre content, such as applesauce, bananas, and rice, to reduce gastric upset or abdominal cramping. Diarrhea caused by illness can be debilitating. If the patient cannot tolerate foods or liquids orally, intravenous therapy (with potassium supplements) is necessary. The patient then returns to a normal diet slowly, often beginning with fluids. Excessively hot or cold fluids stimulate peristalsis, thereby causing abdominal cramps and further diarrhea. As the tolerance to liquids improves, solid foods are ordered. Following a severe diarrheal episode, milk products may need to be withheld until the enterocyte population has matured. Milk products may have the effect of perpetuating the diarrhea.

Promotion of Regular Exercise. A daily exercise program helps prevent bowel elimination problems. Walking, riding a stationary bicycle, or swimming stimulates peristalsis. Patients who are sedentary at work are most in need of regular exercise. For patients with mobility problems, such as arthritis, a passive exercise program may be helpful.

For a patient who is temporarily immobilized, the nurse should attempt ambulation of the patient as soon as possible. If the condition permits, the nurse can assist a postoperative patient in walking to a chair on the evening of the day of surgery. The patient should walk farther each day.

Exercises can help bedridden patients to more comfortably use a bedpan. The patient can practise the following exercises:

- Lie supine; tighten the abdominal muscles as though pushing them to the floor. Hold them tight to the count of three; relax. Repeat 5 to 10 times as tolerated.
- Flex and contract the thigh muscles by raising one knee slowly toward the chest. Repeat for each leg at least five times and increase the frequency as tolerated.

Bowel Retraining. The patient with incontinence is unable to maintain bowel control. A bowel retraining program can help some patients achieve normal defecation, especially those who still have some neuromuscular control.

The training program involves setting up a daily routine. By attempting to defecate at the same time each day and by using measures that promote defecation, the patient gains control of the bowel reflexes. The program requires time, patience, and consistency. The patient's physical readiness and ability to benefit from bowel training needs to be determined before undertaking such a program. A successful program includes the following:

- Assessing the patient's normal bowel elimination pattern and recording times when the patient is incontinent
- Choosing a time based on the patient's pattern to initiate defecation-control measures by assisting the patient to the toilet at the designated time
- Offering a hot drink (e.g., tea), fruit juice (e.g., prune juice), or another fluid that normally stimulates peristalsis for the patient before the selected defecation time
- Instructing the patient to avoid medications such as analgesics, which may increase constipation
- Providing privacy and setting a time limit for the defecation (15 to 20 minutes)

BOX 44-9 EVIDENCE-INFORMED PRACTICE

Prevention of Constipation in the Older Person Population

- Fluid intake of at least 1 500 to 2 000 mL per day is recommended. The preferred fluid is water because it is sodium-free and calorie-free. The patient may also benefit from drinking one to two glasses of fruit juice.
- Coffee, tea, and alcohol should be avoided because of their diuretic properties.
- A high-fibre diet (25 to 30 g/day) reduces constipation; fibre that passes though the colon acts as a sponge. As a result, bulkier and softer stools develop. In addition, the waste moves through the body more easily and results in more regular bowel movements. A high-fibre diet is not recommended for individuals who are immobile or who do not consume at least 1.5 L of fluid per day.
- The most beneficial means to prevent constipation is a combination of insoluble and soluble fibre (e.g., bran, fruits, and vegetables).
- Physical activity in combination with adequate fluid intake and a high-fibre diet is beneficial in the management of constipation. For patients who are fully mobile, walking once or twice a day for 15 to 20 minutes is sufficient.
- For individuals who are unable to walk, chair or bed exercises are recommended, such as the pelvic tilt, low trunk rotation, and single leg lifts.
- Laxatives should be used with caution. If laxatives are necessary, a stepwise progression is recommended: first bulk-forming laxatives, followed by stool softeners, osmotics, stimulants, suppositories, and enemas as a last resort.

Adapted from Registered Nurses' Association of Ontario. (2011). *Prevention of constipation in the older adult population.* Toronto: Registered Nurses' Association of Ontario.

- Instructing the patient to lean forward at the hips while sitting on the toilet, to apply manual pressure with the hands over the abdomen, and to bear down but not to strain to stimulate the colon to empty
- Refraining from making critical remarks or conveying frustration if the patient is unable to defecate
- Providing regular meals with adequate fluids and fibre (Bliss and Norton, 2010)
- Maintaining normal exercise within the patient's physical ability

Hemorrhoids. Many patients experience discomfort from alterations in their bowel elimination. Pain results when hemorrhoid tissues are directly irritated. The primary goal for the patient with hemorrhoids is to have soft-formed, painless bowel movements. Proper diet, fluids, and regular exercise improve the likelihood of the stools being soft. If the patient becomes constipated, passage of hard stools may cause bleeding and irritation. Local heat provides temporary relief to swollen hemorrhoids. A sitz bath is the most effective means of heat application.

Maintenance of Skin Integrity. The patient with diarrhea or bowel incontinence is at risk for skin breakdown when fecal contents remain on the skin. Liquid stool is usually acidic and contains digestive enzymes. Irritation from repeated wiping with toilet tissue aggravates the breakdown of skin. Bathing the skin after soiling helps but may result in more breakdown unless the skin is thoroughly dried.

When caring for an incontinent patient who is unable to ask for assistance, the nurse should check often for defecation. The anal areas can be protected with barrier cream that holds moisture in the skin to prevent drying and cracking. Yeast infections of the skin can develop easily. Several powdered antifungal agents are effective against yeast. Baby powder or cornstarch should not be used because they have no medicinal properties and they frequently cake on the skin, which makes them difficult to remove.

Medications. Medications may be used to initiate and facilitate bowel elimination. Cathartics, laxatives, and occasionally an enema are used to control constipation, whereas antidiarrheal preparations assist the patient in resolving diarrhea. All of these medications are available over the counter; stronger preparations are available through prescriptions. Patients must be cautioned not to use these over-the-counter medications on a prolonged basis without consulting their health care provider.

Laxatives are defined as products that stimulate evacuation of the formed stool from the rectum, whereas cathartics are defined as products that evacuate unformed and usually watery fecal material from the entire colon. Laxatives are thus milder in action than cathartics. When used correctly, laxatives and cathartics safely maintain normal bowel elimination patterns; however, chronic use of cathartics causes the large intestine to lose muscle tone and to become less responsive to stimulation by laxatives. Laxative overuse can also cause serious diarrhea that can lead to dehydration and electrolyte depletion. Mineral oil, a common laxative, decreases fat-soluble vitamin absorption. Laxatives can influence the efficacy of other medications by altering the transit time (i.e., the time the medication remains in the GI tract and is available for absorption).

> **Safety Alert** Excessive use of laxatives, enemas, or bulk-forming agents increases the patient's risk for diarrhea and abnormal bowel elimination and destroys the patient's normal defecation reflex. In addition, the patient may develop an altered absorption of nutrients, fluid and electrolyte imbalances, and generalized weakness. When these symptoms occur in chronically ill or older patients, they may result in an increased risk for falls and other injuries.

Cathartics and laxatives. A patient is often unable to defecate normally because of pain, constipation, or impaction. Cathartics and laxatives provide the short-term action of emptying the bowel. They are also used in bowel evacuation for patients undergoing GI tests and abdominal surgery. Although the terms *cathartic* and *laxative* are often used interchangeably, cathartics have a stronger effect on the intestines. Five types of laxatives and cathartics are available (Table 44-5).

Cathartics and laxatives are available in oral, tablet, and powder suppository dosage forms (see Chapter 34). Although the oral route is most commonly used, cathartics that are prepared as suppositories are more effective because of their stimulant effect on the rectal mucosa. Cathartic suppositories such as bisacodyl (Dulcolax) can act within 30 minutes. Older persons who use Dulcolax often have a strong, sudden urge to defecate.

Electrolyte Balance and Antidiarrheal Agents. For patients with diarrhea, frequent passage of liquid stools becomes a problem. When a person has secretory diarrhea, cells at the base of the villi secrete massive amounts of fluid into the lumen of the small intestine. However, the tip of the villi can still absorb sugars and fluids. Therefore, diarrhea can quickly lead to serious electrolyte imbalances, particularly in infants and children (see Chapter 40). Therefore, the first course of action is to immediately replace fluids by mouth. Fluids with adequate electrolyte content (e.g., Pedialyte and Gastrolyte) are a wise choice. In developing countries without a safe water supply or during epidemics of infectious diarrhea (e.g., cholera), millions of lives have been saved by using a cheap, safe, and simple method of replacing water and salts lost through diarrhea. This method, known as *oral rehydration therapy (ORT)*, involves mixing a very low-cost package of salts (sodium, potassium chloride, citrate or bicarbonate, and glucose) with boiled water.

Many patients will use over-the-counter agents, such as Imodium, to relieve common diarrhea. However, the most effective antidiarrheal agents are prescriptive opiates, such as codeine phosphate, opium tincture (Paregoric), and diphenoxylate (Lomotil). Opiates inhibit the peristaltic waves that move feces forward but also increase the segmental contractions that mix intestinal contents and expose the contents to the mucosal absorbing surface. The further effect of opiates on increasing the absorption of sodium and water also dries out the feces. As a result, more water is absorbed by the colonic mucosa. These antidiarrheal agents should be used with caution because opiates may be addictive.

Rectal Suppositories. A rectal suppository may be used to stimulate defecation for a patient having difficulty initiating a bowel movement. Rectal suppositories are solid, bullet-shaped preparations designed for easy insertion into the rectum. The suppository dissolves at body temperature and gradually spreads over the lining of the lower bowel (rectum). Glycerin suppositories are used to lubricate the stool in the rectum, facilitating evacuation. Stimulant suppositories like Dulcolax contain medication that is absorbed into the bloodstream from the rectum and stimulates the mucosa, increasing peristalsis.

Enemas. An enema is the instillation of a solution into the rectum and sigmoid colon. The primary reason for using an enema is to promote defecation by stimulating peristalsis. The volume of fluid instilled breaks up the fecal mass, stretches the rectal wall, and initiates the defecation reflex. Enemas are also used as a vehicle for administering medications that exert a local effect on rectal mucosa.

The most common use for an enema is temporary relief of constipation. Other indications include removing impacted feces; beginning a program of bowel training; and emptying the bowel before diagnostic tests, surgery, or childbirth.

Cleansing enemas. Cleansing enemas promote the complete evacuation of feces from the colon. They act by stimulating peristalsis

TABLE 44-5 Common Types of Laxatives and Cathartics

Agents and Brand Names	Action	Indications	Risks
Bulk Forming			
Methylcellulose (Benefibre)	The high-fibre content absorbs water and increases solid intestinal bulk.	These agents are the least irritating, most natural, and safest cathartics. These agents are the drugs of choice for treating chronic constipation (e.g., during pregnancy or as the result of a low-residue diet).	These agents can cause obstruction if not mixed with at least 240 mL of water or juice and swallowed quickly.
Psyllium (Metamucil)	These agents stretch the intestinal wall to stimulate peristalsis.	These agents may also be used to relieve mild, watery diarrhea.	Use caution with bulk-forming laxatives that also contain stimulants. These agents are not used in patients for whom large fluid intake is contraindicated.
Emollient or Wetting			
Docusate sodium (Colace) Docusate calcium (Surfak)	Stool softeners are detergents that lower the surface tension of feces, allowing water and fat to penetrate. They may increase the secretion of water by the intestines.	These agents are used for short-term therapy to relieve straining on defecation. These agents would be beneficial for patients who have hemorrhoids, have undergone perianal surgery, are pregnant, or are recovering from myocardial infarction.	These agents are of little value for treatment of chronic constipation.
Saline			
Magnesium citrate or citrate of magnesia (Citromag)	These agents contain a salt preparation that is not absorbed by the intestines.	These agents are used only for acute emptying of the bowel (e.g., as a preparation for endoscopic examination, in cases of suspected poisoning, or to treat acute constipation).	These agents are not used for long-term management of constipation.
Magnesium hydroxide (Milk of Magnesia)	The osmotic effect increases pressure in the bowel to act as stimulant for peristalsis.		These agents are contraindicated for patients with kidney dysfunction (to avoid a toxic buildup of magnesium).
Sodium phosphate (Fleet Enema)	Sodium phosphate		Phosphate salts are not used for patients on fluid restriction.
Stimulant Cathartics			
Bisacodyl (Dulcolax)	These agents irritate the intestinal mucosa to increase motility.	These agents may be used to prepare the bowel for diagnostic procedures.	These agents may cause severe cramping.
Castor oil (Neoloid, Purge)	These agents decrease absorption in the small bowel and colon.		These agents are not for long-term use.
Phenolphthalein (Doxidan, Correctol, Ex-Lax)	Phenolphthalein and danthron may cause pink or red urine.		
Lubricants			
Mineral oil (Haley's M-O, Petrogalar Plain)	These agents coat the fecal contents, which allows for easier passage of the stool. These agents reduce water absorption in the colon.	These agents are used to prevent straining on defecation (e.g., for patients who have hemorrhoids and for those who are recovering from perianal surgery).	These agents decrease the absorption of fat-soluble vitamins (A, D, E, and K). These agents can cause a dangerous form of pneumonia if aspirated into the lungs. Mineral oil, when taken with emollients, can increase the risk for fat emboli.

From Lilley, L. L., Harrington, S., Snyder, J. S., & Swart, B. (2011). *Pharmacology for Canadian health care practice* (2nd Canadian ed.). Toronto: Elsevier Canada.

through the infusion of a large volume of solution or through local irritation of the colon's mucosa. Solutions used in cleansing enemas include tap water, normal saline, low-volume hypertonic saline, and soapsuds solution. Each solution exerts a different osmotic effect to move fluids between the colon and the interstitial spaces beyond the intestinal wall. Infants and children should receive only normal saline because they are at risk for fluid imbalance.

A prescriber may order a high- or low-cleansing enema. The terms *high* and *low* refer to the height from which, and hence the pressure with which, the fluid is delivered. High enemas are given to cleanse the entire colon. After the enema is infused, the patient is asked to turn from the left lateral position to the dorsal recumbent position and to the right lateral position. The position change ensures that fluid reaches all of the large intestine. A low enema cleanses only the rectum and the sigmoid colon.

Tap water. Tap water is hypotonic and exerts a lower osmotic pressure than that of fluid in interstitial spaces. After infusion into the colon, tap water escapes from the bowel lumen into the interstitial spaces. The net movement of water is low. The infused volume stimulates defecation before large amounts of water leave the bowel. Tap water enemas should not be repeated because water toxicity or circulatory overload can develop if large amounts of water are absorbed.

Normal saline. Physiologically, normal saline is the safest solution to use because it exerts the same osmotic pressure as that of fluids in the interstitial spaces surrounding the bowel. The volume of infused saline stimulates peristalsis. Unlike tap water enemas, saline enemas do not create the danger of excess fluid absorption.

Hypertonic solutions. Hypertonic solutions infused into the bowel exert osmotic pressure that pulls fluids out of the interstitial spaces. The colon fills with fluid, and the resultant distension promotes defecation. Patients unable to tolerate large volumes of fluid benefit most from this type of enema, which is, by design, low volume. Patients with contraindications for this type of enema are patients who are dehydrated and young infants. A hypertonic solution of 120 to 180 mL is usually effective. The commercially prepared Fleet Enema is the most commonly used hypertonic solution.

Soapsuds. Soapsuds may be added to tap water or saline to create the effect of intestinal irritation to stimulate peristalsis. Only pure castile soap is safe to use. A liquid form of castile soap is included in most soapsuds enema kits. Harsh soaps or detergents can cause serious bowel inflammation.

Oil-Retention Enemas. Oil-retention enemas lubricate the rectum and colon. The feces absorb the oil and become softer and easier to pass. To enhance the action of the oil, the patient retains the enema for several hours, if possible.

Other Types of Enemas. Carminative enemas provide relief from gaseous distension. Use of a carminative enema improves the ability to pass flatus. An example of a carminative enema is MGW solution, which contains 30 mL of magnesium, 60 mL of glycerine, and 90 mL of water.

Medicated enemas contain drugs. An example is sodium polystyrene sulphonate (Kayexalate), which is used to treat patients with dangerously high serum potassium levels. This drug contains a resin that exchanges sodium ions for potassium ions in the large intestine. Another medicated enema is neomycin solution, which is an antibiotic used to reduce bacteria in the colon before bowel surgery.

Enema Administration. Enemas are administered in either commercially packaged, disposable units or with reusable equipment prepared before use. Sterile technique is unnecessary because the colon normally contains bacteria; however, gloves should be worn to prevent the transmission of fecal microorganisms.

The nurse should explain the procedure to the patient, including the position to assume, precautions to take to avoid discomfort, and the length of time necessary to retain the solution before defecation. If the patient is to receive the enema at home, the procedure must be explained to a family member.

Often the prescriber orders "enemas until clear." This order means that the enema is to be repeated until the patient passes fluid that is clear and contains no fecal material. As many as three enemas may be necessary, but the nurse should caution the patient against using more than three enemas. Excess enema use seriously depletes fluids and electrolytes. If the enema fails to return a clear solution after three times (check agency policy on the maximum number of enemas permitted) or if the patient seems to not tolerate the rigours of repeated enemas, the prescriber should be notified.

Giving an enema to a patient who is unable to contract the external sphincter can pose difficulties. In these cases, the enema should be given with the patient positioned on the bedpan. Giving the enema with the patient sitting on the toilet is unsafe because the curved rectal tubing can abrade the rectal wall. Skill 44-1 outlines the steps for enema administration.

Safety Alert For patients with an impaction, the fecal mass may be too large to be passed voluntarily. If enemas fail, the nurse may consider breaking up the fecal mass with his or her finger and removing it in sections (Box 44-10). The procedure will be very uncomfortable for the patient. Excess rectal manipulation may cause irritation to the mucosa, bleeding, perforation of the bowel wall, and stimulation of the vagus nerve, which results in a reflex slowing of the heart rate. Because of the procedure's potential complications, a prescriber's order is necessary for a nurse to remove a fecal impaction.

Surgical Management of Bowel Elimination

Inserting and Maintaining a Nasogastric Tube. A patient's condition or situation may warrant special interventions to decompress the GI tract. Such conditions include surgery, infections of the GI tract, trauma to the GI tract, and the absence of peristalsis.

A nasogastric (NG) tube is a pliable tube that is inserted through the patient's nasopharynx into the stomach. The tube has a hollow lumen that allows removal of gastric secretions and introduction of solutions into the stomach. NG intubation has several purposes (Table 44-6).

The Levin and Salem sump tubes are the most common tubes used for stomach decompression. The Levin tube is a single-lumen tube with holes near the tip. A sump tube may be connected to either a drainage bag or an intermittent suction device to drain stomach secretions.

TABLE 44-6 Purposes of Nasogastric Intubation

Purpose	Description	Type of Tube
Decompression	Removal of secretions and gaseous substances from the gastrointestinal tract to prevent or relieve abdominal distension	Salem sump, Levin, Miller-Abbott
Feeding (i.e., gavage; see Chapter 42)	Instillation of liquid nutritional supplements or feedings into the stomach for patients unable to swallow fluid	Duo, Dobhoff, Levin
Compression	Internal application of pressure by means of an inflated balloon to prevent internal esophageal or gastrointestinal hemorrhage	Sengstaken-Blakemore
Lavage	Irrigation of the stomach in cases of active bleeding, poisoning, or gastric dilation	Levin, Ewald, Salem sump

SKILL 44-1 ADMINISTERING A CLEANSING ENEMA

Delegation Considerations

The skill of administering an enema can be delegated to unregulated care providers (UCPs). Nurses have the responsibility to assess the patient for specific considerations, such as his or her safety, the need for alternative positioning and comfort, and the presence of stable vital signs prior to the procedure. In addition, nurses have the responsibility to determine the patient's response to the enema. If delegating this task to a UCP:

- Inform and assist the UCP in the proper way to position patients who have mobility restrictions, such as patients with arthritis or severe fatigue.
- Instruct the UCP how to position patients who have therapeutic equipment present, such as drains, intravenous catheters, or traction.
- Instruct the UCP about the specific signs and symptoms that will appear in patients not tolerating the procedure and about when the procedure must be stopped. For example, these signs and symptoms may include abdominal pain more than a pressure sensation, abdominal cramping, abdominal distension, or rectal bleeding.

Equipment

- Clean gloves
- Water-soluble lubricant
- Waterproof, absorbent pads
- Bath blanket
- Toilet tissue
- Bedpan, bedside commode, or access
- Washbasin, washcloths, towel
- Intravenous (IV) pole
- Enema bag administration
- Enema container
- Tubing and clamp (if not already attached to the enema container)
- Appropriate size rectal tube: 22 to 30 Fr
- Correct volume of warmed solution: 750 to 1 000 mL
- Prepackaged enema
- Prepackaged enema container with rectal tip

PROCEDURE

STEPS	RATIONALE
1. Assess the status of the patient: last bowel movement, normal bowel patterns, presence of hemorrhoids, mobility, external sphincter control, and abdominal pain.	• Assessment is used to determine the factors indicating a need for an enema and influences the type of enema used.
2. Assess the patient for presence of increased intracranial pressure, glaucoma, or recent rectal or prostate surgery.	• These conditions contraindicate the use of an enema.
3. Check the patient's medical record to clarify the rationale for the enema.	• The nurse needs to determine the purpose of the enema administration, either as a preparation for a special procedure or for relief of constipation.
4. Review the prescriber's order for the enema.	• A prescriber's order is required. The order determines the number and type of enemas to be given.
5. Determine the patient's level of understanding of the purpose of the enema.	• The patient's current level of understanding allows the nurse to plan for appropriate teaching measures.
6. Perform hand hygiene. Collect appropriate equipment.	• Proper hand hygiene reduces the transmission of microorganisms.
7. Correctly identify the patient and explain the procedure.	• Explaining the procedure promotes patient cooperation and reduces anxiety.
8. Assemble the enema bag with the appropriate solution and rectal tube.	
9. Perform hand hygiene and apply gloves.	• Proper hand hygiene reduces the transmission of microorganisms.
10. Provide privacy by closing the curtains around the bed or by closing the door.	• Privacy reduces the embarrassment for the patient.
11. Raise the bed to an appropriate working height; raise the side rail on the patient's left side.	• Raising the bed and use of the side rail promote good body mechanics and patient safety.
12. Assist the patient into a position lying on the left side with right knee flexed (i.e., Sims' position).	• The Sims' position allows the enema solution to flow downward by gravity along the natural curve of the sigmoid colon and rectum, thus improving retention of the solution.

CRITICAL DECISION POINT: *Patients who have poor sphincter control will have difficulty retaining the enema solution. If the patient is suspected of having poor sphincter control, position the patient on a bedpan.*

STEPS	RATIONALE
13. Place a waterproof pad under the hips and buttocks.	• A waterproof pad prevents soiling of the bed linen.
14. Cover the patient with a bath blanket, exposing only the rectal area, with the anus clearly visible.	• The bath blanket provides warmth, reduces exposure of body parts, and allows the patient to feel more relaxed and comfortable.
15. Place the bedpan or commode in an easily accessible position. If the patient will be expelling contents in toilet, ensure the toilet is available. (If the patient will be walking to the bathroom to expel the enema, place the patient's slippers and bathrobe in an easily accessible position.)	• A bedpan or commode should be nearby in case the patient is unable to retain the enema solution.
16. Administer the enema:	
A. Enema bag	
(1) Add warmed solution to the enema bag: warm the tap water as it flows from faucet, place the saline container in a basin of hot water before adding saline to the enema bag, check the temperature of the solution with a bath thermometer or by pouring a small amount of solution over your inner wrist.	• Hot water can burn intestinal mucosa. Cold water can cause abdominal cramping and is difficult to retain.

Continued

SKILL 44-1 ADMINISTERING A CLEANSING ENEMA—cont'd

STEPS	RATIONALE
(2) Raise the container, release the clamp, and allow the solution to flow long enough to fill the tubing.	• Raising the container removes air from the tubing.
(3) Reclamp the tubing.	• Reclamping prevents further loss of the solution.
(4) Lubricate 6 to 8 cm of the tip of the rectal tube with lubricating jelly.	• The lubricating jelly allows smooth insertion of the rectal tube without risk of irritation or trauma to the mucosa.
(5) Gently separate the buttocks and locate the anus. Instruct the patient to relax by breathing out slowly through the mouth.	• Exhaling promotes relaxation of the external anal sphincter.
(6) Insert the tip of the rectal tube slowly by pointing the tip in the direction of the patient's umbilicus (see Step 16A[6] illustration) for about 7 to 10 cm.	• Careful insertion prevents trauma to the rectal mucosa from an accidental lodging of the tube against the rectal wall. Insertion beyond the proper limit can cause bowel perforation.

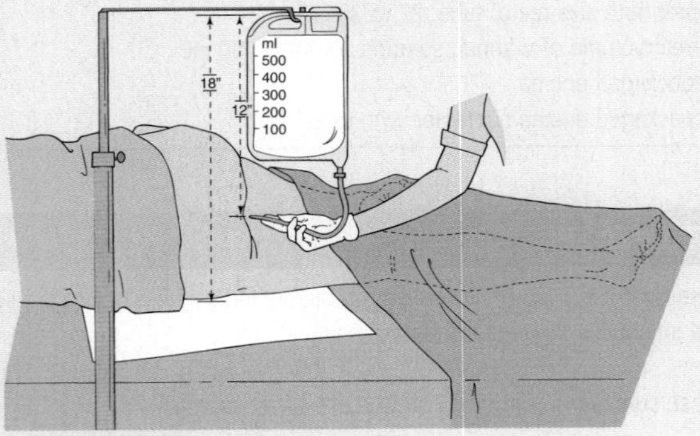

STEP 16A(6) Insertion of a rectal tube into the rectum.

CRITICAL DECISION POINT: ***If the tube does not pass easily, do not force it. Consider allowing a small amount of fluid to infuse and then try reinserting the tube slowly.***

STEPS	RATIONALE
(7) Hold the tubing in the rectum constantly until the end of the fluid instillation.	• Bowel contractions can cause expulsion of the rectal tube.
(8) Open the regulating clamp and allow the solution to enter slowly with the enema container at the patient's hip level.	• Rapid instillation can stimulate evacuation of the rectal tube.
(9) Raise the height of the enema container slowly to the appropriate level above the anus: 30 to 45 cm for a high enema, 30 cm for a regular enema, 7.5 cm for a low enema (see Step 16A[6] illustration). Instillation time varies depending on the volume of solution administered.	• Raising the height slowly allows for continuous, slow instillation of the solution. Raising the container too high causes rapid instillation and possible painful distension of the colon.
(10) Lower the container or clamp tubing if the patient complains of cramping or if fluid escapes around the rectal tube.	• Temporary cessation of instillation prevents cramping, but may prevent the patient from retaining all the fluid, thus altering the effectiveness of the enema.
(11) Clamp the tubing after all solution is instilled.	• Clamping prevents entrance of air into the rectum.
B. Prepackaged disposable container	
(1) Remove the plastic cap from the rectal tip. The tip is already lubricated, but more jelly can be applied as needed.	• Lubrication provides for smooth insertion of rectal tube while avoiding rectal irritation or trauma.
(2) Gently separate the buttocks and locate the anus. Instruct the patient to relax by breathing out slowly through the mouth.	• Breathing out promotes relaxation of the external rectal sphincter.
(3) Insert the tip of the bottle gently into the rectum about 7 to 10 cm.	• Gentle insertion prevents trauma to the rectal mucosa.
(4) Squeeze the bottle until all the solution has entered the rectum and colon. Instruct the patient to retain the solution until the urge to defecate occurs, usually within 2 to 5 minutes.	• Hypertonic solutions require only small volumes to stimulate defecation.
17. Place layers of toilet tissue around the tube at the anus and gently withdraw the rectal tube.	• The use of toilet paper provides the patient with comfort and cleanliness.
18. Explain to the patient that the feeling of distension is normal. Ask the patient to retain the solution for as long as possible while lying quietly in bed.	• The enema solution distends the bowel. The length of retention varies depending on the type of enema and the patient's ability to contract the rectal sphincter. Longer retention promotes more effective stimulation of peristalsis and defecation.
19. Discard the enema container and tubing in the proper receptacle, or rinse thoroughly with warm soap and water if the container is to be reused.	• Proper handling of the used enema container and tubing reduces the transmission and growth of microorganisms.

STEPS	RATIONALE
20. Assist the patient to the bathroom or help to position the patient on a bedpan.	• The normal squatting position promotes defecation.
21. Observe the character of the feces and solution (caution the patient against flushing the toilet until you can inspect the feces).	• The character of the expelled feces determines the efficacy of the enema.

CRITICAL DECISION POINT: *When enemas are ordered "until clear," observe the contents of the solution passed. Return is "clear" when no solid fecal material exists, but solution may be coloured.*

STEPS	RATIONALE
22. Assist patient as needed to wash the anal area with warm soap and water (if providing perineal care, use gloves).	• Fecal contents can irritate the skin. Proper hygiene promotes the patient's comfort.
23. Remove and discard gloves and perform hand hygiene.	• Proper hand hygiene reduces the transmission of microorganisms.
24. Inspect the colour, consistency, and amount of stool and fluid passed.	• The colour, consistency, and amount of stool determine whether the stool is evacuated or fluid is retained. Note any abnormalities, such as the presence of blood or mucus.
25. Assess the condition of the abdomen; cramping, rigidity, or distension can indicate a serious problem.	• The condition of the abdomen determines whether distension is relieved. Excess volume can distend or perforate the bowel.

UNEXPECTED OUTCOMES	RELATED INTERVENTIONS
Rigidity and distension of the abdomen	• Stop the enema administration if fluid is still being instilled. • Notify the prescriber and obtain vital signs.
Abdominal pain or cramping	• Slow the rate of instillation.
Bleeding	• Stop the enema administration. • Notify the prescriber and obtain vital signs.

RECORDING AND REPORTING

- Record the type and volume of the enema given and the characteristics of the results.
- Report to the prescriber if the patient failed to defecate.

HOME CARE CONSIDERATIONS

- For patients who require enemas for bowel preparation at home, instruct the patient's family not to exceed the recommended fluid volume levels or the recommended number of enemas. Emphasize to the family members the need for slow administration of warmed fluid.

BOX 44-10 PROCEDURAL GUIDELINE

Digital Removal of Stool

Delegation Considerations:

The digital removal of stool should not be delegated to unregulated care providers (UCPs).

Equipment:

- Bath blanket
- Waterproof pad
- Clean gloves
- Lubricant
- Towel
- Washcloth
- Soap and water
- Bedpan

Procedure:

1. Check the patient record for a prescriber's order for manual disimpaction.
2. Explain the procedure to the patient.
3. Perform hand hygiene. Take baseline vital signs prior to the procedure. Help the patient to lie on the left side with knees flexed and back toward you.
4. Drape the trunk and lower extremities with a bath blanket and place a waterproof pad under the buttocks. Keep a bedpan next to the patient.
5. Apply disposable gloves and lubricate the index finger of your dominant hand with lubricating jelly.
6. Gently insert the gloved index finger into the rectum and advance the finger slowly along the rectal wall toward the umbilicus.
7. Gently loosen the fecal mass by massaging around it. Work the finger into the hardened mass.
8. Work the feces downward toward the end of the rectum. Remove small pieces at a time and discard into the bedpan.
9. Reassess the patient's vital signs and look for signs of fatigue. Stop the procedure if the heart rate drops significantly or if the heart rhythm changes. Monitor for 1 hour postprocedure.
10. Continue to remove feces and allow the patient to rest at intervals.
11. After completion, wash and dry the buttocks and anal area.
12. Remove the bedpan and dispose of the feces. Remove gloves by turning them inside out, and then discard.
13. Assist the patient to the toilet or position the patient on a clean bedpan if the urge to defecate develops.
14. Perform hand hygiene. Record results of the removal of the impaction by describing the fecal characteristics.
15. Follow the procedure with enemas or cathartics as ordered by prescriber.
16. Reassess the patient's vital signs and level of comfort.

The Salem sump tube is preferable for stomach decompression. This tube has two lumina: one for removal of gastric contents (Figure 44-12) and one to provide an air vent. A blue "pigtail" is the air vent that connects with the second lumen. When the sump tube's main lumen is connected to suction, the air vent permits free, continuous drainage of secretions. The air vent should never be clamped off, connected to suction, or used for irrigation.

Bowel Diversions. Certain diseases cause conditions that prevent the normal passage of feces through the rectum. The treatment for these disorders may result in the need for a **stoma**, which is a temporary or permanent artificial opening in the abdominal wall. The opening may be either an **ileostomy**, a surgical opening in the ileum, or a **colostomy**, a surgical opening in the colon. The ends of the intestine are brought through the abdominal wall to create the stoma (RNAO, 2009).

The standard bowel diversion creates a stoma, or the patient can undergo reconstructive surgery that uses the native sphincter for bowel continence. The reconstructive surgery includes either a continent stoma procedure, which is now rarely done, or the ileoanal pouch anastomosis, which is described later (Canadian Association for Enterostomal Therapy [CAET], 2007a).

Ostomies. The location of the ostomy determines the consistency of the stool. An ileostomy bypasses the entire large intestine. As a result, stools are frequent and liquid. The same is true for a colostomy of the ascending colon (Figure 44-13). A colostomy of the transverse colon, in general, results in a more solid, formed stool (see Figure 44-13). The descending colostomy and sigmoid colostomy emit a near-normal stool (see Figure 44-13). The location of a colostomy is determined by the patient's medical problem and general condition. Colostomies have three types of construction: loop colostomy, end colostomy, and double-barrel colostomy (CAET, 2007b)

Loop colostomy. A loop colostomy is usually performed in a medical emergency when closure of the colostomy is anticipated. Loop colostomies are usually temporary large stomas constructed in the transverse colon. The surgeon pulls a loop of bowel onto the abdomen. The loop ostomy has two openings through the one stoma (see Figure 44-13). The proximal end drains stool, whereas the distal portion drains mucus (Monahan, Neighbors, Sands, et al., 2007).

End colostomy. The end colostomy consists of one stoma formed from one end of the bowel with the distal portion of the GI tract either removed or sewn closed (known as *Hartmann's pouch*) and left in the abdominal cavity. For many patients, end colostomies are a result of surgical treatment for colorectal cancer. In such cases, the rectum might also be removed. Patients with diverticulitis who are treated surgically often have a temporary end colostomy with a Hartmann's pouch (Figure 44-14).

Double-barrel colostomy. In a double-barrel colostomy (as opposed to the loop colostomy), the bowel is surgically severed and the two ends are brought out onto the abdomen (see Figure 44-13). The double-barrel colostomy consists of two distinct stomas: the proximal functioning stoma and the distal nonfunctioning stoma.

Kock continent ileostomy. The Kock continent ileostomy is created using the patient's small intestine to create a pouch. This procedure is occasionally used in the treatment of ulcerative colitis. The pouch has a continent stoma, which is a nipple-type valve that is drained with an external catheter. The patient places the external catheter intermittently in the stoma and empties the pouch several times

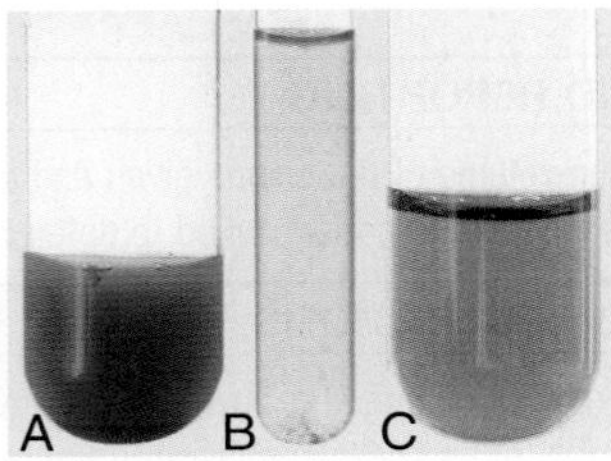

FIGURE 44-12 Gastric contents. **A,** Stomach. **B,** Stomach. **C,** Intestinal. (Courtesy Dr. Norma Metheny, St. Louis University, School of Nursing. St. Louis, MO.)

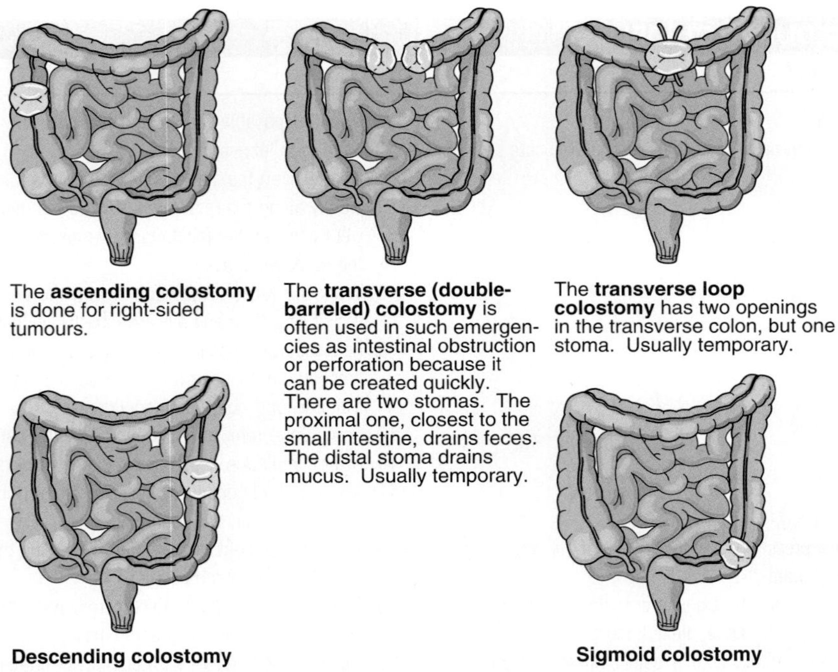

FIGURE 44-13 Different types of colostomies. (From Monahan, F. D., Neighbors, M., Sands, J. K., Marek, J. F., & Green, C. J. [2007]. *Phipps' medical-surgical nursing: Health and illness perspectives* [8th ed., p. 1262, Fig. 43-10]. St. Louis, MO: Mosby Elsevier.)

a day. The stoma is covered with a protective dressing or a stoma cap (RNAO, 2009).

Psychological Considerations. A stoma can cause serious body-image changes, particularly when it is permanent. A classic study reported by Walsh et al. (1995) measured the perception of body image in patients who had a stoma. Patients who had a long-standing history of chronic bowel disease, such as Crohn's disease or ulcerative colitis, reported an improved quality of life but a lower body image. Conversely, patients who needed an ostomy because of cancer reported a higher body image but a reduced quality of life. Patients often perceive a stoma as invasive and disfiguring; however, a well-placed stoma should not interfere with the patient's activities and can be concealed by clothing (Banks & Razor, 2003). Although clothing may conceal the ostomy, the patient feels different. Many patients have difficulty maintaining or initiating normal sexual relations. An important factor in the patient's reactions is the character of the fecal secretions and the ability to control them. The patient's self-esteem can be impaired by foul odours, spillage, or leakage of liquid stools and the inability to regulate bowel movements.

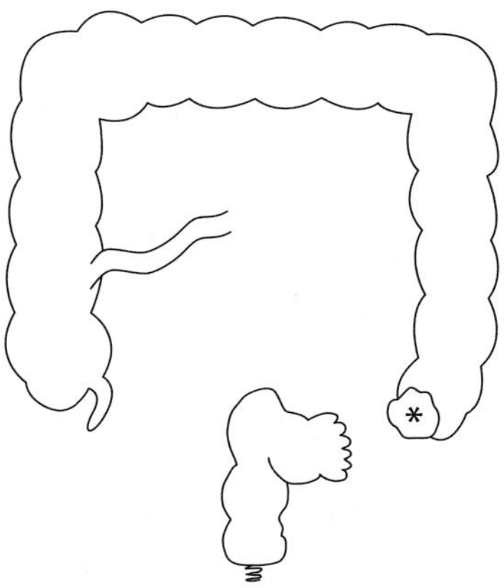

FIGURE 44-14 Hartmann's pouch procedure. (Redrawn from Registered Nurses' Association of Ontario. [2009]. *Ostomy care and management* [p. 67]. Toronto: Registered Nurses' Association of Ontario. Retrieved from http://rnao.ca/bpg/guidelines/ostomy-care-management. Illustration by Nancy Bauer, HBA, HB Admin, RN, ETN. Published with permission.)

Care of Ostomies. Patients with temporary or permanent bowel diversions have unique bowel elimination needs. Individuals with an ostomy wear a pouch or appliance to collect the **effluent** (the stool discharged from an ostomy) from the stomas (RNAO, 2009). These patients must use meticulous skin care to prevent liquid stool from irritating the skin around the stoma (Figure 44-15).

Irrigating a Colostomy. Although this practice is not as common as it once was, some patients may be instructed to irrigate their left-sided colostomies in order to regulate colon emptying. Other patients do not want to spend the additional 60 to 90 minutes in the bathroom every day, and they empty their pouch only as necessary (CAET, 2007b).

Appendix E: Sample Ostomy Teaching Record

OSTOMY TEACHING RECORD

Client: ______________________

Address: ______________________

Before Surgery: Teaching Completed	Date & Initial
Date of surgery	
Type of surgery/ostomy	
Reason for surgery	
E.T. Nurse visit	
Stoma site selection and marking	
Stoma location and appearance	
Given teaching booklets about surgery	
Given samples of pouching system	
Purpose of pouch and skin barrier	
Knowledge of others with an ostomy	
Viewed ostomy video	

After Surgery: While in Hospital Teaching Completed	Date & Initial
Stoma (size, swelling, shrinkage and appearance)	
Type of drainage while in hospital	
Observe/assist with pouch emptying	
Independent with pouch emptying	
Observe/assist with release of gas from pouch	
Independent with release of gas from pouch	
Observe/assist with pouch and skin barrier change	
Discuss odour control options	
Signs of pouch leakage (prevention and treatment)	
Viewed ostomy video and given teaching booklet (if not done pre-op)	
Who to call if problems occur after discharge from hospital	

After Surgery: Discharged Home Teaching Completed	Date & Initial
Type of drainage at home	
Stoma (size, swelling, shrinkage and appearance)	
Independent with pouch emptying	
Observe/assist with pouch and skin barrier change	
Independent with pouch and skin barrier change	
Signs of pouch leakage (prevention and treatment)	
Skin breakdown (prevention and treatment)	
Application instructions	
Supply list/where to buy	
Care of supplies/emergency kit	
Discuss odour control options	
Nutrition/dietary instructions	
Bathing	
Activity/travel	
Clothing modifications	
Sexual function concerns	
Financial Assistance (A.D.P., Private Insurance, Social Assistance, Disability)	
United Ostomy Association of Canada Support Group	
Ostomy visitor	
Discharge instructions	

Colostomy: Teaching Completed	Date & Initial
Care of perineal wound (if present)	
Mucous drainage per rectum (if rectum left in place)	
Care of a mucous fistula (if present)	
Colostomy irrigation information	
Trial of a colostomy irrigation (optional)	
Constipation/diarrhea/gas	

Ileostomy: Teaching Completed	Date & Initial
Care of perineal wound (if present)	
Mucous drainage per rectum (if rectum left in place)	
Sodium loss and replacement	
Potassium loss and replacement	
Obstruction and management	
Fluid imbalance and treatment	
Medication	

FIGURE 44-15 Sample ostomy teaching record. *A.D.P.*, Assistive Devices Program; *E.T.*, Enterostomal therapist. (From ET NOW, Red Cross Care Partners, Waterloo, Ontario.)

Specific equipment for irrigating a colostomy should be used. An enema set should never be used to irrigate a colostomy. A special cone-tipped irrigator (Figure 44-16) is used. This device prevents both bowel penetration and backflow of the irrigating solution. Patients usually sit on the toilet and place an irrigating sleeve over the stoma. The end of this sleeve extends into the bowl of the toilet. The prescriber orders the amount and type of solution. For adults, the amount ranges from 500 to 700 mL of tap water. The solution is instilled slowly through the lubricated cone tip. Irrigation should take 5 to 10 minutes. The patient then removes the cone tip and waits 30 to 45 minutes for the solution and feces to drain out of the irrigation sleeve. Once the drainage stops, the patient applies a stoma cap or a pouch. If a patient chooses to irrigate the colostomy, the timing of the irrigation can be individualized to the patient's lifestyle.

Pouching Ostomies. Ostomies require a pouch to collect fecal material. An effective pouching system protects the skin, contains fecal material, remains odour-free, and is comfortable and inconspicuous. A person wearing a pouch should feel secure in participating in any activity.

Many pouching systems are available. To ensure that a pouch fits well and meets the patient's needs, a number of factors need to be considered: the location of the ostomy; the type and size of the stoma; the amount and consistency of the effluent; the size and contour of the abdomen; the condition of the skin around the stoma; skin sensitivities or allergies; the physical activities of the patient; cognitive abilities for learning; the patient's personal preference, age, and dexterity; and the cost of the equipment. An **enterostomal therapist (ET)** is a nurse trained to care for wound and ostomy management. The staff nurse collaborates with the ET to ensure that the correct pouching system is used. For example, a referral to an ET nurse would be appropriate to plan the care of a patient who has a high-output ostomy that requires a pouch modification.

A pouching system consists of a pouch and a skin barrier (Figure 44-17). Pouches come in one- and two-piece systems that are disposable or reusable. Some pouches have the opening precut by the manufacturer; others require the stoma opening to be custom cut to the patient's specific stoma size.

Skin barriers include wafers, pastes, powders, and liquid film that are applied to the skin around the stoma. Wafer skin barriers, which are permanently attached to the ostomy pouch, are called *one-piece pouch systems*. In a *two-piece system*, the pouch can be detached from the skin barrier for emptying or changing. This system allows the skin barrier to remain around the patient's stoma for several days, thus minimizing the chance of skin damage from too-frequent removal of the skin barrier from the peristomal skin (Figure 44-18). When using a two-piece pouching system, the skin barrier and pouch must be the same corresponding size and from the same manufacturer. The pouch from one manufacturer will not fit correctly on the skin barrier from another manufacturer. The nurse needs to ensure the patient understands that an ostomy pouch made for collecting fecal matter (i.e., a pouch specifically for a colostomy or ileostomy) must be used and not a pouch for collecting urine.

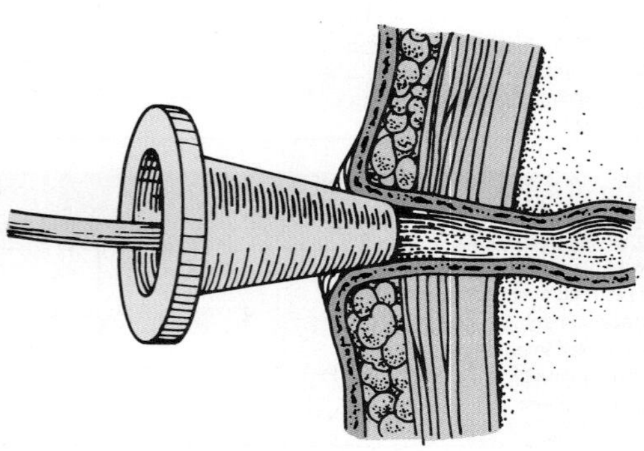

FIGURE 44-16 Ostomy irrigation cone inserted into the stoma.

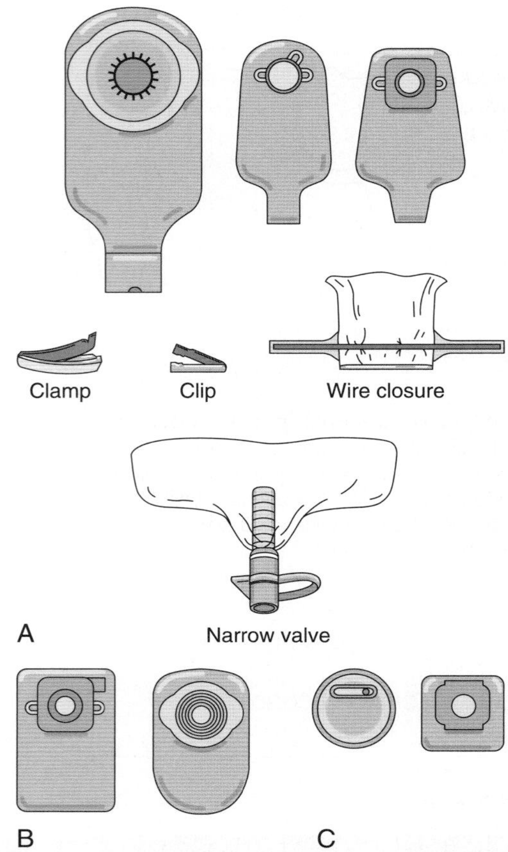

FIGURE 44-17 Common ostomy pouch products, closures, and patches. A, Drainable pouches and pouch closures. **B,** Nondrainable pouches. **C,** Patches for regulated colostomies. (From Monahan, F. D., Neighbors, M., Sands, J. K., Marek, J. F., & Green, C. J. [2007]. *Phipps' medical-surgical nursing: Health and illness perspectives* [8th ed., p. 1264, Fig. 43-11]. St. Louis, MO: Mosby Elsevier.)

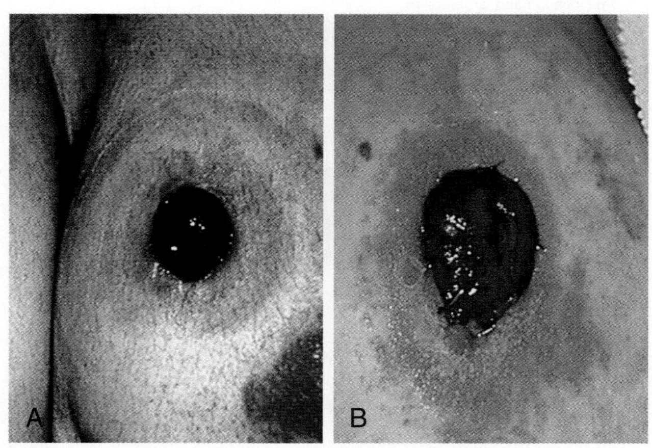

FIGURE 44-18 A, Mechanical injury to the peristomal skin. **B,** Candidiasis damage to the peristomal skin. (Permission to use these copyrighted photos has been granted by the owner, Hollister Incorporated.)

Patients need to be instructed to measure the stoma size carefully when selecting and cutting out the opening on the wafer skin barrier. A good skin barrier protects the skin, prevents irritation from repeated removal of the pouch, and is comfortable for the patient to wear. Skill 44-2 describes the steps for applying one type of pouch system.

Nutritional Considerations for Patients With Ostomies. Nutritional therapy is important for patients with ostomies. During the first weeks after surgery, many prescribers recommend low-fibre diets, particularly for ileostomy patients, because the small bowel requires time to adapt to the diversion. Low-fibre foods include bread, noodles, rice, cream cheese, eggs (not fried), strained fruit juices, lean meats, fish, and poultry. As ostomies heal, patients can eat almost any food. High-fibre foods, such as fresh fruits and vegetables, help to ensure a more solid stool, which is needed to achieve success at irrigation. Blockage must be avoided. The stoma's surgical construction can affect the likelihood of blockage.

Patients with an ileostomy should eat slowly and chew their food completely. Drinking 10 to 12 glasses of water daily also helps to prevent blockage. High-fibre foods that may cause problems include stringy meats; mushrooms; popcorn; some fruits, such as cherries; and some seafood, such as shrimp and crab. Ostomy patients may benefit

SKILL 44-2 POUCHING AN OSTOMY

Delegation Considerations

The skill of pouching a newly established ostomy should not be delegated to unregulated care providers (UCPs). Pouching of a well-established ostomy can be delegated to a UCP. The nurse must do the following:

- Assist the caregiver in selecting the appropriate pouch and skin barrier.
- Inform the caregiver of the signs of stomal and peristomal skin changes that should be reported to a nurse.
- Ask the caregiver to monitor and report the characteristics and volume of the ostomy output and report changes in volume or consistency to a nurse for further assessment.

Equipment

- Clear drainable colostomy (or ileostomy) pouch in the correct size for a two-piece system or custom cut to fit a one-piece system with an attached skin barrier
- Pouch closure device, such as a clamp or clip if needed
- Clean gloves
- Gauze pads and washcloths
- Towel or disposable waterproof barrier
- Basin with warm tap water
- Scissors and pen
- Adhesive remover (optional)

PROCEDURE

STEPS	RATIONALE
1. Perform hand hygiene.	
2. Apply gloves. Observe the skin barrier and pouch for leakage and the length of time in place. Depending on the type of pouching system used (e.g., an opaque pouch), you may need to remove the pouch to fully observe the stoma. Clear pouches permit the viewing of the stoma without their removal.	• Leakage may indicate the need for a different type of pouch or sealant.

CRITICAL DECISION POINT: *Intact skin barriers with no evidence of leakage do not need to be changed daily and can remain in place for 3 to 5 days (depending on manufacturer's guidelines).*

STEPS	RATIONALE
3. Observe the stoma for colour, swelling, trauma, and healing; the stoma should be moist and reddish-pink. Assess the type of stoma. Stomas can be flush with the skin or can be a bud-like protrusion on the abdomen.	• Stoma characteristics are one factor to consider when selecting an appropriate pouching system.
4. Measure the stoma at each pouching change. Follow the pouch manufacturer's directions and measuring guide to determine which pouch to use on the basis of the patient's stoma size. The opening around the appliance should be no greater than 2 mm larger than the stoma (Perry & Potter, 2014).	• The size of the stoma determines the correct size of equipment, which prevents trauma to the stoma. Too large an opening can permit fecal drainage to ooze from under the appliance, causing skin irritation. Too small an opening can cause the appliance to cut into the stoma (Perry & Potter, 2014).
5. Observe the abdominal incision (if present).	• The relationship of the abdominal incision to the stoma determines proper placement of the pouch.
6. Observe the effluent from the stoma and record the intake and output. Empty the pouch if it is more than one-third to one-half full. Ask the patient about skin tenderness. Remove gloves and perform hand hygiene.	• Effluent from the stoma is caustic. If effluent comes in contact with the sensitive peristomal skin, the risk of skin breakdown increases. Pouches must be emptied because the weight of the pouch may disrupt the seal of adhesive on the skin (Perry & Potter, 2014).
7. Assess the abdomen for the best type of pouching system to use. Consider the following: **A.** Contour and peristomal plane **B.** Presence of scars, incisions **C.** Location and type of stoma	• The characteristics of the abdomen determine the pouching system selection and the need for additional equipment. For a stoma to have an adequate seal with an ostomy appliance, the stoma must be placed within the abdominal rectus muscle, away from abdominal creases and folds, away from the bony understructures, and surrounded by at least 5 cm of smooth surface on all sides (Perry & Potter, 2014).
8. Assess the patient's self-care ability to determine the best type of pouching system to use.	• Patients who have difficulty using their hands or who have limited vision may find a one-piece system or a precut pouch and skin barrier more desirable to use; others prefer being able to keep the skin barrier in place for several days, changing just the pouch, and therefore prefer the two-piece system.

Continued

SKILL 44-2 POUCHING AN OSTOMY—cont'd

STEPS	RATIONALE
9. After removing the skin barrier and pouch, assess the skin around the stoma, noting scars, folds, skin breakdown, and the peristomal suture line, if present. Keep the pouch loosely attached to the stoma to collect any drainage while the system is being changed.	• Assessing the skin around the stoma determines the need for barrier paste to increase adherence of the pouch to the skin or to fill in irregularities.

CRITICAL DECISION POINT: *If the skin around the stoma is discoloured, weeping, itchy, or sore, refer the patient to an ostomy specialist (Perry & Potter, 2014).*

STEPS	RATIONALE
10. Determine the patient's emotional response, knowledge, and understanding of an ostomy and its care.	• Understanding the patient's perspective assists in determining both the extent to which the patient is able to participate in care and the patient's need for teaching and the clarification of information.
11. Explain the procedure to the patient; encourage the patient's interaction and questions.	• Explaining the procedure reduces the patient's anxiety and encourages the patient's participation.
12. Perform hand hygiene. Assemble the equipment and close the room curtains or door.	• Proper hand hygiene reduces the transmission of infection. Organizing the equipment optimizes the use of time and conserves the patient's and nurse's energy. Privacy reduces the embarrassment for the patient.
13. Position the patient either standing or in a semi-reclining position and draped. If seated, position the patient either on or in front of the toilet.	• When the patient is semi-reclined, fewer wrinkles ease the application of the pouching system; draping maintains the patient's dignity.
14. Perform hand hygiene and apply disposable gloves.	• Proper hand hygiene reduces the transmission of microorganisms.
15. Place the towel or disposable waterproof barrier under the patient.	• The towel or waterproof barrier protects the bed linen.
16. Completely remove the used pouch and skin barrier by gently pushing the skin away from the barrier. An adhesive remover may be used to facilitate removal of the skin barrier.	• Working gently reduces trauma; jerking irritates the skin and can cause tears.
17. Clean the peristomal skin gently with warm tap water using gauze pads or a clean washcloth; do not scrub the skin; dry completely by patting the skin with gauze or a towel.	• Avoid the use of soap because it leaves a residue on the skin that interferes with pouch adhesion to the skin. Skin must be as dry as the skin barrier; the pouch does not adhere to wet skin. If blood appears on the gauze pad, do not be alarmed; the stoma, if rubbed, may ooze some blood from the cleaning process. The stoma's surface is a highly vascular mucous membrane. Bleeding into the pouch is abnormal.
18. Measure the stoma for the correct size of pouching system needed, using the manufacturer's measuring guide (see Step 18 illustration).	• Measuring the stoma ensures accuracy in determining the correct pouch size needed. The stoma shrinks and does not reach its usual size for 6 to 8 weeks.
19. Select the appropriate pouch for the patient on the basis of your patient assessment. For a custom cut-to-fit pouch, use an ostomy guide to cut an opening on the pouch 2 mm larger than the stoma before removing the backing (Perry & Potter, 2014). Prepare the pouch by removing the backing from the barrier and adhesive (see Step 19 illustration). For an ileostomy, apply a thin circle of barrier paste around the opening in the pouch; allow to dry.	• The barrier paste facilitates the seal and protects the skin. The size of the pouch opening keeps drainage off the skin and reduces the risk of damage to the stoma during peristalsis or physical activity. The pouch and skin barrier are changed whenever leaking occurs. They can also be changed before or after a tub bath or shower. The stool is alkaline, which is an irritant on the skin; fecal bacteria can colonize on the skin and increase the risk of infection. Change the pouch and skin barrier when the patient is comfortable; before a meal is better because this timing avoids increased peristalsis and the chance of evacuation during the pouch change.

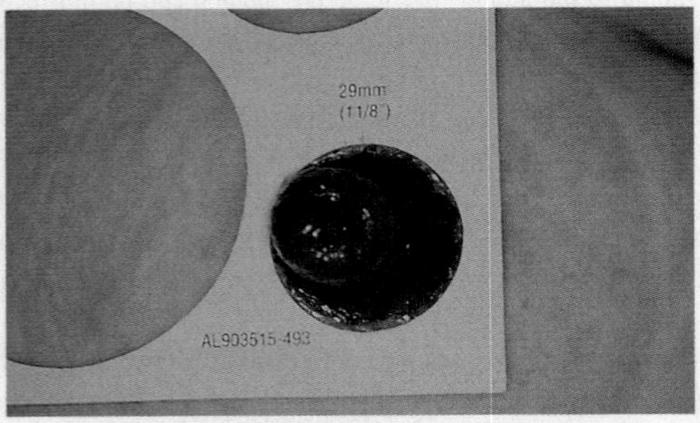

STEP 18 Measuring a stoma.

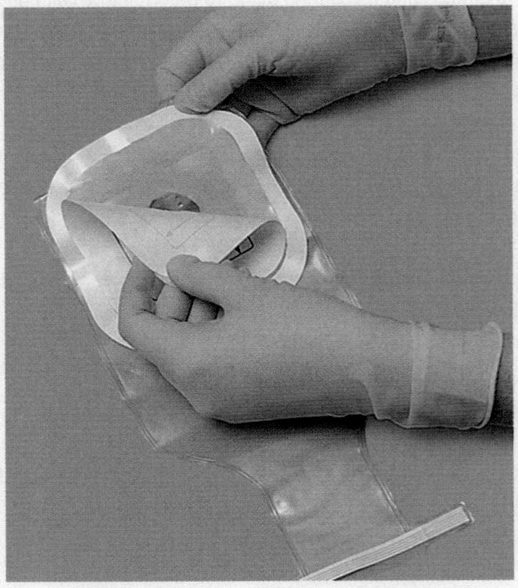

STEP 19 Preparing an ostomy pouch.

STEPS	RATIONALE

CRITICAL DECISION POINT: *If the patient has a large volume of liquid stool from an ileostomy, consider using a high-output pouch that will contain the volume of effluent and reduce the frequency of pouch emptying.*

20. Apply the skin barrier and pouch. If creases occur next to the stoma, use a barrier paste to fill in; let dry 1 to 2 minutes.

CRITICAL DECISION POINT: *If the patient has a surgical incision near the stoma, the skin barrier may need to be trimmed to fit.*

A. For a one-piece pouching system:

(1) Use skin sealant wipes on the skin directly under the adhesive skin barrier or pouch; allow to dry. Press the adhesive backing of the pouch or skin barrier smoothly against the skin, starting from the bottom and working up and around the sides.

(2) Hold the pouch by the barrier, centre it over the stoma, and press down gently on the barrier; the bottom of the pouch should point toward the patient's knees (see Step 20A[2] illustration).

(3) Maintain gentle finger pressure around the barrier for 1 to 2 minutes.

B. For a two-piece pouching system:

(1) Apply the flange (the barrier with adhesive) as in steps above for a one-piece system (see Step 20B[1] illustration). Then snap on the pouch and maintain finger pressure.

- The flange creates a wrinkle-free, secure seal and decreases irritation from the adhesive on skin.

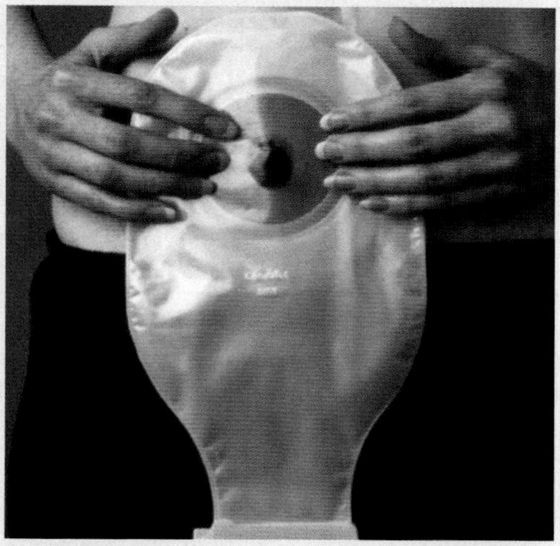

STEP 20A(2) Applying a one-piece pouch. (Courtesy ConvaTec, Princeton, NJ.)

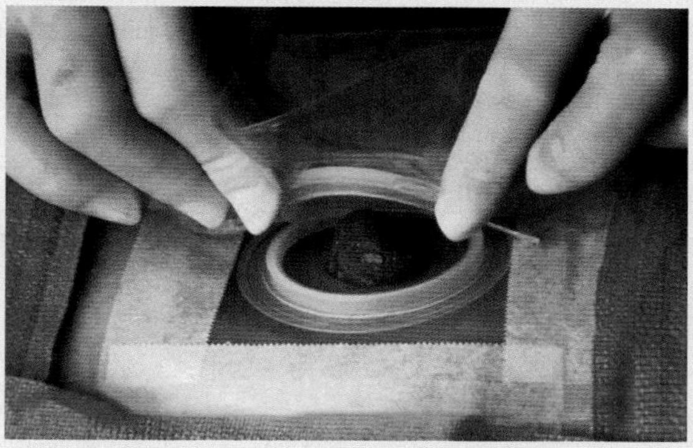

STEP 20B(1) Application of a barrier-paste flange; separate inner surface and position. Courtesy ConvaTec, Princeton, NJ.)

C. For both pouching systems, gently tug on the pouch in a downward direction.

- Tugging on the pouch determines whether the pouch is securely attached.

21. Apply a nonallergenic paper tape around the pectin skin barrier in a "picture frame" method. Half of the tape should be on the skin barrier and half on the patient's skin. Some patients prefer a belt attached to the pouch for extra security in place of the tape.

- "Picture framing" the pectin skin barrier adds to the security of keeping the pouch system attached securely.

CRITICAL DECISION POINT: *If the patient chooses to wear a belt, ensure that it is not fastened too tightly, by placing two fingers between the belt and the patient's skin.*

22. Fold the bottom of drainable open-ended pouches up once and close using a closure device such as a clamp (or follow the manufacturer's instructions for closure).

- Proper closure maintains a secure seal to prevent leaking.

23. Properly dispose of the old pouch and the soiled equipment.

24. Remove gloves and perform hand hygiene.

- Proper hand hygiene reduces the transmission of microorganisms.

25. Change a one- or two-piece pouch every 3 to 7 days unless it is leaking; a pouch can remain in place for tub bath or shower; after a bath or shower, pat the adhesive dry.

- Avoid unnecessary trauma to the skin from too-frequent changes. Drying the adhesive ensures the adhesion of the pouch.

Continued

SKILL 44-2 POUCHING AN OSTOMY—cont'd

STEPS	RATIONALE
26. Ask whether the patient feels discomfort around the stoma.	• The patient's perception of discomfort determines the presence of skin irritation.
27. While the pouch is removed and the skin is being cleaned, note the appearance of the skin around the stoma and the existing incision (if present). Re-inspect the condition of the skin barrier and adhesive.	• Assessing the skin and existing incision determines the condition of the tissues and the progress of healing. The condition of the skin barrier and adhesive can indicate the presence of leaks.
28. Observe the patient's nonverbal behaviours as the pouch is applied. Ask whether the patient has any questions about the pouching.	• Nonverbal behaviours indicate the patient's emotional response to the stoma and his or her readiness for learning. The patient's questions determine the level of understanding of the procedure.

UNEXPECTED OUTCOMES	RELATED INTERVENTIONS
Damage of the peristomal skin	Assess for the following conditions and report their occurrence to the prescriber for treatment: • Mechanical damage (see Figure 44-18, *A*) due to inappropriate skin care or incorrect tape removal) • Chemical damage due to the effluent coming into contact with the peristomal skin or a skin reaction to the adhesive • Damage due to a fungus (e.g., candidiasis; see Figure 44-18, *B*), usually caused by excessive skin moisture
Necrosis of stoma (purple or black discoloration, dryness, failure to bleed, or sloughing of tissue)	• Assess the circulation to the stoma. • Observe for excessive edema or tension on the bowel suture line (if present). • Immediately report this finding to the prescriber.

RECORDING AND REPORTING

- Chart the type of pouch and skin barrier applied.
- Record the amount, appearance, and texture of the stool; the condition of the peristomal skin; and the condition of any sutures.
- Report any of the following to the charge nurse or the prescriber, or both:
  - Any abnormal appearance of the stoma, the suture line, the peristomal skin, the character of output, or the absence of bowel sounds.
  - No flatus in 24 to 36 hours and no stool by the third day.
- Document abdominal distension, excessive tenderness, and the nature of bowel sounds.
- Record the patient's level of participation and need for instruction.

HOME CARE CONSIDERATIONS

- Evaluate the patient's home toileting facilities. Note the presence of adequate toileting facilities.
- Caution the patient that most ostomy pouches and barriers cannot be flushed down the toilet; they clog the plumbing system. Dispose of used ostomy pouch according to agency policy and local sanitation regulations.

from avoiding foods that cause gas and odour, such as broccoli, cauliflower, dried beans, and Brussels sprouts.

◆ Evaluation

Patient Care. The effectiveness of care depends on success in meeting the goals and expected outcomes of care. Optimally, the patient will be able to have regular, pain-free defecation of soft, formed stools. The patient is the only person who is able to determine whether the bowel elimination problems have been relieved and which therapies were most effective (Figure 44-19). The patient will also be able to demonstrate information learned regarding establishment of a normal bowel elimination pattern. The patient will be able to demonstrate any skills learned, such as ostomy protocols and skin protection. The patient will be able to accomplish normal defecation by manipulating components of daily living, such as diet, fluid intake, and exercise. The patient will have minimal reliance on artificial means of defecation, such as enemas and laxative use.

Patient Expectations. If the nurse has been successful in establishing a therapeutic relationship with the patient, the patient will feel more comfortable in discussing the intimate details often associated with bowel elimination. The patient will also not be as fearful of embarrassment as the nurse assists the patient with his or her bowel elimination needs. The patient will relate a feeling of comfort and freedom from pain as bowel elimination needs are met within the limits of the patient's condition and treatment.

KEY CONCEPTS

- The mechanical breakdown of food elements, gastrointestinal motility, and selective absorption and secretion of substances by the large intestine influence the character of feces.
- Food high in fibre content and an increased fluid intake keep feces soft.
- Ongoing use of cathartics, laxatives, and enemas affects and delays the reflexes of normal defecation.
- Vagal stimulation, which slows the heart rate, may occur during straining while defecating, receiving enemas, and during digital removal of an impacted stool.
- The greatest danger from diarrhea is developing an imbalance of fluids and electrolytes.

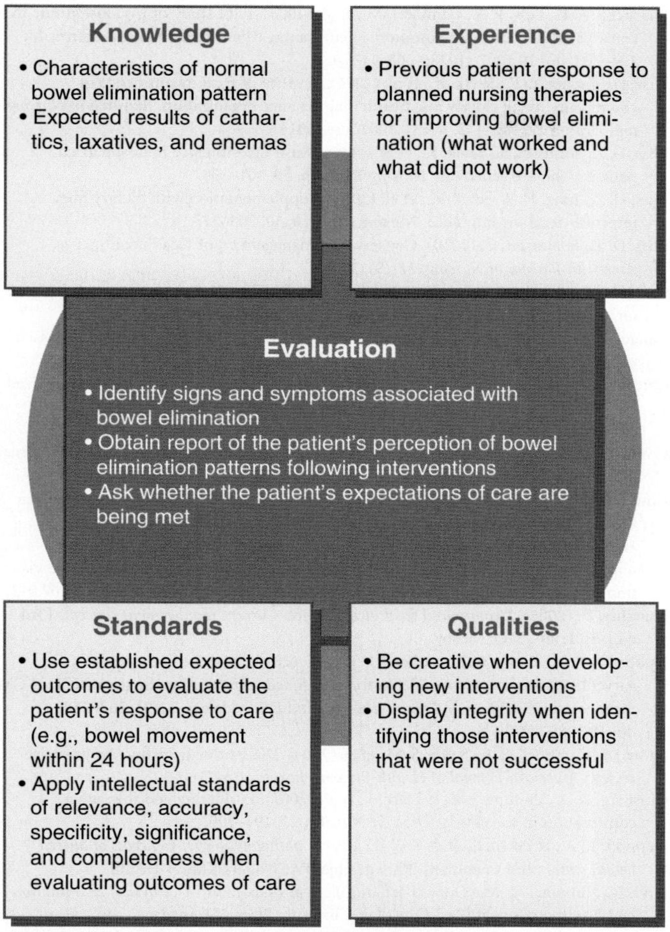

FIGURE 44-19 Critical thinking model for bowel elimination evaluation.

- The location of an ostomy influences the consistency of the stool.
- Assessment of bowel elimination patterns should focus on bowel habits, factors that normally influence defecation, recent changes in bowel elimination, and a physical examination.
- Indirect and direct visualization of the lower gastrointestinal tract requires cleansing of the bowel before the procedure.
- When selecting a diet to promote normal bowel elimination, the nurse needs to consider the frequency of defecation, the fecal characteristics, and the effect of foods on the gastrointestinal function.
- Proper positioning on a bedpan allows the patient to assume a position similar to squatting without experiencing muscle strain.
- Nasogastric intubation decompresses the gastric contents by removing secretions and gaseous products from the gastrointestinal tract.
- The purposes of gastric decompression are to keep the gastrointestinal tract free of secretions, to reduce nausea and gas, and to decrease the risk of vomiting and aspiration.
- Proper selection and use of an ostomy pouching system are necessary to prevent damage to the skin around the stoma.
- Dangers during digital removal of stool include traumatizing the rectal mucosa and promoting vagal stimulation.
- Skin breakdown can occur after repeated exposure to liquid stool.

CRITICAL THINKING EXERCISES

1. A 19-year-old man with a history of good health and regular exercise is your patient at the university health service facility where you work. He complains of increasing diarrhea and abdominal cramping; he has no weight loss. He states that on rare occasions he noticed blood on the toilet paper he used. What additional pieces of assessment data do you need?
2. A long-term care facility has invited you to present a talk on preventing bowel incontinence in their residents. What points of information do you include in your presentation?
3. A 22-year-old man is to undergo surgery for Crohn's disease. He will have a new pouching ileostomy. He and his mother need to learn what the ileostomy means for his future bowel elimination needs. What do you tell them?
4. Mrs. Pidpahora is 82 years old and a resident in a long-term care facility. She has just been assessed for acute confusion in the emergency department and admitted to your ward. In her documentation, you see that she has become more confused and forgetful since she moved into long-term care 4 months ago. She spends most of her time in bed or sitting in a chair in her room. She is occasionally incontinent of urine and has not had a bowel movement in 5 days. She is taking the following medications and supplements: levothyroxine (Synthroid), calcium carbonate, vitamin D, chlorothiazide, risperidone, chloral hydrate. What steps would you take to understand and address her apparent constipation (Neil, Curran, & Wattis, 2003; Robson, Kiely, & Lembo, 2000; Spina & Scordo, 2002)?

REVIEW QUESTIONS

1. Most nutrients and electrolytes are absorbed in which of the following areas?
   1. Colon
   2. Stomach
   3. Esophagus
   4. Small intestine
2. During the nursing assessment, the patient reveals that he has diarrhea and cramping every time he eats ice cream. He attributes this reaction to the cold nature of the food. These symptoms might be associated with which of the following?
   1. Food allergy
   2. Irritable bowel syndrome
   3. Lactose intolerance
   4. Increased peristalsis
3. The nurse is assessing a 55-year-old patient who is in the clinic for a routine physical examination. Under which of the following scenarios would the nurse instruct the patient to obtain fecal occult blood testing (FOBT)?
   1. The patient has a family history of polyps.
   2. The patient reports rectal bleeding.
   3. A palpable mass is detected on digital examination.
   4. The patient is due for a routine examination for colon cancer.
4. Which of the following agents decreases colonic propulsive contractions while increasing the mixing of contractions?
   1. Antidiarrheal opiate agents
   2. Hypertonics
   3. Cathartics
   4. Laxatives
5. Which of the following situations results in diarrhea that occurs with a fecal impaction?
   1. A clear liquid diet
   2. Irritation of the intestinal mucosa

3. Seepage of stool around the impaction
4. Inability of the patient to form a stool

6. A cleansing enema is ordered for a 55-year-old patient before intestinal surgery. What amount of solution should be instilled?
   1. 150 to 200 mL
   2. 200 to 400 mL
   3. 400 to 750 mL
   4. 750 to 1 000 mL
7. During the enema, the patient complains of pain. You note rectal bleeding and blood in the return fluid. What action do you take?
   1. Stop the instillation.
   2. Slow the rate of instillation.
   3. Stop the instillation, notify the prescriber, and obtain vital signs.
   4. Tell the patient to breathe slowly and relax.
8. What is one of the greatest problems in caring for a patient with a nasogastric tube?
   1. Dehydration
   2. Maintaining comfort
   3. Constipation
   4. Nutritional therapy
9. What term is given to the stool discharged from an ostomy?
   1. Effluent
   2. Cathartics
   3. Colonic fluid
   4. Mucosa
10. What term describes a nurse trained to care for ostomy patients?
    1. Enterostomal therapist
    2. Nurse practitioner
    3. Ostomy practitioner
    4. GI therapist

Answers: 1. 4; 2. 3; 3. 4; 4. 1; 5. 3; 6. 4; 7. 3; 8. 2; 9. 1; 10. 1

Rationales for the Review Questions appear at the end of the book.

RECOMMENDED WEBSITES

Canadian Cancer Society: http://www.cancer.ca
This website is a source for general information about all types of cancers, as well as Canadian statistics of the prevalence, mortality, and survival rates for specific cancers.

Canadian Digestive Health Foundation: http://www.cdhf.ca/
The Canadian Digestive Health Foundation (CDHF) supports research and education in the management and cure of digestive diseases and disorders.

Canadian Nurse Continence Advisors: www.cnca.ca
This website has both professional and patient resources on education and research about urinary and bowel incontinence.

Colorectal Cancer Association of Canada: http://www.colorectal-cancer.ca
Colorectal cancer is the second most common cause of cancer deaths in Canada. The Colorectal Cancer Association of Canada is a nonprofit organization that supports individuals with colorectal cancer, their families, and caregivers.

Registered Nurses' Association of Ontario, BPG Ostomy Care and Management: http://rnao.ca/bpg/guidelines/ostomy-care-management

Registered Nurses' Association of Ontario, BPG Prevention of Constipation in the Older Adult Population: http://rnao.ca/bpg/guidelines/prevention-constipation-older-adult-population

REFERENCES

Banks, N., & Razor, B. (2003). Preoperative stoma site assessment and marking: Trained RNs can improve ostomy outcomes. *American Journal of Nursing, 103*(3), 64A–64D.

Bharucha, A. E., Low, P. A., Camilleri, M., et al. (2008). Pilot study of pyridostigmine in constipated patients with autonomic neuropathy. *Clinical Autonomic Research, 18*, 194–202. doi:10.1007/s10286-008-0476-x.

Bliss, D., Fischer, L. R., Savik, K., et al. (2004). Severity of fecal incontinence in community living elderly in a health maintenance organization. *Research in Nursing and Health, 27*, 162–173. doi:10.1002/nur.20014.

Bliss, D. Z., Johnson, S., Savik, K., et al. (2000). Fecal incontinence in hospitalized patients who are acutely ill. *Nursing Research, 49*, 101–108.

Bliss, D. Z., Jung, H.-J., Savik, K., et al. (2001). Supplementation with dietary fiber improves fecal incontinence. *Nursing Research, 50*, 203–213.

Bliss, D. Z., & Norton, C. (2010). Conservative management of fecal incontinence. *American Journal of Nursing, 111*(9), 30–38.

Canadian Association for Enterostomal Therapy (CAET). (2007a). *A guide to living with an ileostomy.* Retrieved from https://caet.ca/ileostomy-guide/.

Canadian Association for Enterostomal Therapy (CAET). (2007b). *A guide to living with a colostomy.* Retrieved from https://caet.ca/colostomy-guide/.

Cardin, F., Minicuci, N., Droghi, A. T., et al. (2009). Constipation in acutely hospitalized older patients. *Archives of Gerontology and Geriatrics, 50*, 277–281. doi:10.1016/j.archger.2009.04.007.

Conly, J. M., & Johnston, B. L. (2003). Norwalk virus: Off and running. *Canadian Journal of Infectious Diseases, 14*, 11–13.

Cowie, B., Northwood, M., Robbs, L., et al. (2014). P. Eyles (Ed.), *Promoting continence care: A bladder and bowel handbook for care providers.* [Custom courseware] Hamilton, ON: McMaster University Press.

de Lang, K. M., & Barrett, J. C. (2015). Understanding inflammatory bowel disease via immunogenetics. *Journal of Autoimmunity, 64*, 91–100. doi:10.1016/j.aut.2015.07.013.

Doughty, D. (2006). *Urinary and fecal incontinence: Current management concepts* (3rd ed.). St. Louis, MO: Mosby.

Dubberke, E. R., Butler, A. M., Yokoe, D. S., et al. (2010). Multicenter study of surveillance for hospital-onset *Clostridium difficile* infection by the use of ICD-9-CM diagnosis codes. *Infection Control and Hospital Epidemiology, 31*(3), 262–268. doi:10.1086/650447.

Duby, J. J., Campbell, R. K., Setter, S. M., et al. (2004). Diabetic neuropathy: An intensive review. *American Journal of Health-System Pharmacy, 61*, 160–173.

Ginsberg, D. A., Phillips, S. F., Wallace, J., et al. (2007). Evaluating and managing constipation in the elderly. *Urologic Nursing, 27*, 191–200.

Hannon, R. A., & Porth, C. (Eds.), (2017). *Porth pathophysiology: Concepts of altered health states* (2nd Canadian). Philadelphia, PA: Wolters Kluwer Health.

Jarvis, C., Browne, A., MacDonald-Jenkins, J., et al. (Eds.), (2014). *Physical examination and health assessment* (2nd Canadian). Toronto: Elsevier Canada.

Lewis, S., Heitkemper, M., O'Brien, P., et al. (2014). *Medical-surgical nursing in Canada: Assessment and management of clinical problems* (3rd Canadian). Toronto: Elsevier Canada.

Lilley, L. L., Rainforth Collins, S., Snyder, J. S., et al. (2016). *Pharmacology for Canadian health care practice* (3rd Canadian). Toronto: Elsevier Canada.

Lomer, M. C. E., Parkes, G. C., & Sanderson, J. D. (2008). Review article: Lactose intolerance in clinical practice—Myths and realities. *Alimentary Pharmacology and Therapeutics, 27*, 93–103.

Marsh, G. B. (2005). *Miller-Keane encyclopedia and dictionary of medicine, nursing and allied health* (7th ed.). St. Louis, MO: Saunders.

McFarland, L. V. (2006). Meta-analysis of probiotics for the prevention of antibiotic associated diarrhea and the treatment of *Clostridium difficile* disease. *American Journal of Gastroenterology, 101*, 812–822.

Meiner, S. E. (2011). *Gerontologic nursing* (4th ed.). St. Louis, MO: Elsevier Mosby.

Monahan, F. D., Neighbors, M., Sands, J. K., et al. (2007). *Phipps' medical-surgical nursing: Health and illness perspectives* (8th ed.). St. Louis, MO: Mosby Elsevier.

Neil, W., Curran, S., & Wattis, J. (2003). Antipsychotic prescribing in older people. *Age and Aging, 32*, 475–483.

Ontario Ministry of Long-Term Care. (2016). *Colon cancer check.* Retrieved from http://www.health.gov.on.ca/en/pro/programs/coloncancercheck/fobt_multilingual.aspx.

Ostaszkiewicz, J., Hornby, L., Millar, L., et al. (2010). The effects of conservative treatment for constipation on symptom severity and quality of life in community-dwelling adults. *Journal of Wound, Ostomy Continence Nursing, 37*(2), 193–198. doi:10.1097/WON.0b013e3181cf7206.

Perry, A. G., & Potter, P. A. (2014). *Clinical nursing skills and techniques* (8th ed.). St. Louis, MO: Mosby Elsevier.

Public Health Agency of Canada. (2013). Clostridium Difficile *infection: Prevention and control guidance for management in acute care settings.* Retrieved from http://www.phac-aspc.gc.ca/nois-sinp/guide/c-dif-acs-esa/index-eng.php.

Quartero, A. O., Meiniche-Schmidt, V., Muris, J., et al. (2005). Bulking agents, antispasmodic and antidepressant medication for the treatment of irritable bowel syndrome. *Cochrane Database of Systematic Reviews*, (2), CD003460, doi:10.1002/14651858.CD003460.pub2.

Registered Nurses' Association of Ontario (RNAO). (2009). *Ostomy care and management.* Toronto: Author. Retrieved from http://rnao.ca/bpg/guidelines/ostomy-care-management.

Registered Nurses' Association of Ontario (RNAO). (2011). *Prevention of constipation in the older adult population*. Toronto: Author. Retrieved from http://rnao.ca/bpg/guidelines/prevention-constipation-older-adult-population.
Robson, K. M., Kiely, D. K., & Lembo, T. (2000). Development of constipation in nursing home residents. *Diseases of the Colon and Rectum, 45*, 940–945.
Schnelle, J. F., Leung, F. W., Rao, S. S. C., et al. (2010). A controlled trial of an intervention to improve urinary and fecal incontinence and constipation. *Journal of the American Geriatrics Society, 58*, 1504–1511. doi:10.1111/j.1532-5415.2010.02978.x.
Spina, E., & Scordo, M. G. (2002). Clinically significant drug interactions with antidepressants in the elderly. *Drugs and Aging, 19*, 299–320.
Walsh, B. A., et al. (1995). *Psychometric evaluation of body image and quality of life following ostomy surgery*. Oral abstract presented at the Wound, Ostomy Continence Nurses (WOCN) Society 27th Annual Conference, Denver, CO.

45

Mobility and Immobility

Canadian content written by Jill Vihos, RN, BScN, MN, PhD
Original chapter by Judith A. McCutchan, RN, ASN, BSN, MSN, PhD

OBJECTIVES

Mastery of content in this chapter will enable you to:

- Define the key terms listed.
- Discuss physiological and pathological influences on body alignment and joint mobility.
- Identify changes in physiological and psychosocial function that are associated with immobility.
- Assess for correct and impaired body alignment and mobility.
- Formulate appropriate nursing diagnoses for impaired mobility.
- Develop individualized nursing care plans for patients with impaired mobility.
- Compare and contrast active and passive range-of-motion (ROM) exercises.
- Describe essential techniques when assisting with active and passive ROM exercises, assisting a patient to move up in bed, repositioning a patient, assisting a patient to a sitting position, and transferring a patient from a bed to a chair or from a bed to a stretcher.
- Describe interventions for improving or maintaining patients' mobility.
- Evaluate the nursing care plan for maintaining body alignment and mobility.

KEY TERMS

Activity tolerance, p. 1259
Anthropometric measurements, p. 1260
Atelectasis, p. 1250
Bed rest, p. 1249
Body alignment, p. 1247
Body mechanics, p. 1247
Chest physiotherapy (CPT), p. 1267
Disease atrophy, p. 1249
Disuse osteoporosis, p. 1251
Embolus, p. 1250
Exercise, p. 1258
Footdrop, p. 1251
Friction, p. 1247
Gait, p. 1254
Hemiparesis, p. 1247
Hemiplegia, p. 1247
Hypostatic pneumonia, p. 1250
Immobility, p. 1249
Instrumental activities of daily living (IADLs), p. 1282
Joints, p. 1247
Joint contracture, p. 1251
Ligaments, p. 1247
Mobility, p. 1246
Muscle atrophy, p. 1249
Negative nitrogen balance, p. 1250
Orthostatic hypotension, p. 1250
Osteoporosis, p. 1251
Paraplegia, p. 1248
Pathological fractures, p. 1248
Posture, p. 1247
Pressure injury, p. 1252
Pressure ulcers, p. 1247
Quadriplegia, p. 1248
Tendons, p. 1247
Thrombus, p. 1250
Trochanter roll, p. 1271
Urinary stasis, p. 1252

MEDIA RESOURCES

http://evolve.elsevier.com/Canada/Potter/fundamentals/

- Audio Chapter Summaries
- Examination Review Questions
- Concept Map Creator
- Case Study With Questions
- Audio Glossary
- Content Updates
- Video Clips

Mobility refers to the ability to move easily and independently. To maintain optimal physical mobility, the musculoskeletal and nervous systems of the body must be intact and functioning. Illnesses, surgery, injuries, pain, and aging can temporarily or permanently impair mobility. Nurses need to know the many hazards created by immobility and how to prevent them. Nurses also need to know how to care for patients who are immobile. This care includes positioning the patient who is immobile so that optimal body alignment is attained, and moving and transferring patients when they cannot do so independently. Clinical nursing practices related to mobility require the incorporation of scientific and nursing and skills to provide comprehensive care.

SCIENTIFIC KNOWLEDGE BASE

Nature of Movement

Movement is a complex process that requires coordination between the musculoskeletal and nervous system. As a nurse, you will assess how a patient's physical and psychological condition affects body movement. Body mechanics are the coordinated efforts of the musculoskeletal and nervous systems to maintain balance, posture, and body alignment during lifting, bending, moving, and performing activities of daily living (ADLs). Knowing how patients initiate movement and understanding your own movements requires a basic understanding of body mechanics. Lifting techniques historically used in nursing practice can cause debilitating injuries to nurses and other health care providers (Burnfield, McCrory, Shu, et al., 2013; Griffis, 2012). In Canada, government legislation and institution policy require nurses to use evidence-informed guidelines regarding body alignment, balance, gravity, and friction when implementing nursing interventions such as positioning patients, determining the risk of patient falls, and selecting the safest way to move or transfer patients (Healey & Darowski, 2012) (see Chapter 36).

Alignment and Balance. The terms body alignment and posture are analogous and refer to the positioning of the joints, tendons, ligaments, and muscles while standing, sitting, and lying. Being in correct body alignment means that the individual's centre of gravity is stable. Correct body alignment reduces strain on musculoskeletal structures, minimizes the risk of injuries and falls, aids in maintaining adequate muscle tone, and contributes to balance. Balance is enhanced with a wide base of support and correct body posture and when the body's centre of gravity is kept low and within the base of support (see Chapter 36).

Balance is required for maintaining a static position (e.g., sitting), moving (e.g., walking), and performing ADLs. Disease, injury, pain, physical development (e.g., age), life changes (e.g., pregnancy), medications (e.g., in which dizziness or drowsiness is an adverse effect), and deconditioning (as a result of prolonged immobility) can compromise the ability to remain balanced. Impaired balance is a major threat to mobility and physical safety and contributes to a fear of falling and self-imposed activity restrictions (McMahon & Fleury, 2012) (see Chapter 36).

Gravity and Friction. *Weight* is the force exerted on a body by gravity. The force of weight is always directed downward, which is why an unbalanced object falls. Unsteady patients fall when their centre of gravity becomes unbalanced; the gravitational pull of their weight moves outside their base of support.

To lift an object or person safely, the lifter has to overcome the weight of the object and know its centre of gravity. In symmetrical objects the centre of gravity is at the exact centre of the object. However, people are not geometrically perfect; their centre of gravity is usually at 55 to 57% of standing height and is located in the midline. This is why only using the principles of body mechanics in lifting patients is not sufficient, as this can lead to injury of a nurse or other health care provider (see Chapter 36).

Friction is a force that occurs in a direction opposing movement. The greater the surface area of the object to be moved, the greater the friction. A larger object produces greater resistance to movement. The force exerted against the skin while the skin remains stationary and the bony structures move is called *shear*. An example of shear is when the head of a hospital bed is elevated beyond 60 degrees and gravity pulls a patient so that the bony skeleton moves toward the foot of the bed while the skin remains against the sheets. The blood vessels in the underlying tissue are stretched and damaged, resulting in impeded blood flow to the deep tissues. Ultimately, pressure ulcers often develop within the undermined tissue; the surface tissue appears less affected. To decrease surface area and reduce friction when a patient is unable to assist in moving up in bed, nurses use ergonomic assistive devices such as friction-reducing transfer sheets and full-body slings. Full-body slings are used to mechanically lift a patient off the surface of a bed, thereby preventing friction, tearing, or shearing the patient's skin and protecting the nurse and other staff from injury (Burnfield et al., 2013).

Whenever possible, nurses should use some of the patient's strength when lifting, transferring, or moving the patient. The procedure should be explained to the patient and the patient told when and what body parts to move. The result should be a synchronized movement in which the patient can participate and in which friction is decreased. By involving the patient, the nurse may have the added benefit of increasing the patient's participation in self-care, thus promoting his or her sense of accomplishment.

Pathological Influences on Mobility

Many pathological conditions affect mobility, including both congenital and acquired impairments, degenerative and episodic conditions, and diseases affecting virtually every body system. Although a complete description of each is beyond the scope of this chapter, an overview of four categories of pathological influences is presented here: postural abnormalities, impaired muscle development, damage to the central nervous system, and direct trauma to the musculoskeletal system.

Postural Abnormalities. Congenital or acquired postural abnormalities affect the efficiency of the musculoskeletal system, as well as body alignment, balance, and appearance. During assessment, the nurse observes body alignment and range of motion (ROM; see Chapter 36). Postural abnormalities can cause pain, impair alignment or mobility, or both. Knowledge about the characteristics, causes, and treatment of common postural abnormalities (Table 45-1) is necessary for lifting, transferring, and positioning a patient. Some postural abnormalities may limit ROM. Nurses intervene to maintain a patient's maximum ROM in unaffected joints and then often collaborate with physiotherapists to design interventions to strengthen affected muscles and joints, improve the patient's posture, and adequately use affected and unaffected muscle groups. Referral to or collaboration with a physiotherapist and occupational therapist may enhance nursing interventions for a patient with a postural abnormality.

Impaired Muscle Development. Injury and disease can lead to numerous alterations in musculoskeletal function. For example, the muscular dystrophies are a group of familial disorders that cause degeneration of skeletal muscle fibres. They are the most prevalent of the muscle diseases in childhood. Patients with muscular dystrophies experience progressive, symmetrical weakness and wasting of skeletal muscle groups, with increasing disability and deformity (McCance & Huether, 2014).

Damage to the Central Nervous System. Damage to any component of the central nervous system that regulates voluntary movement results in impaired body mobility. Trauma from a head injury, ischemia from a stroke or cerebrovascular accident (CVA), hemorrhage, tumour, or bacterial infection such as meningitis can damage the cerebellum or the motor strip in the cerebral cortex. Damage to the cerebellum causes problems with balance, and motor impairment is directly related to the amount of destruction of the motor strip. For example, a person with a right-sided cerebral hemorrhage with necrosis has destruction of the right motor strip that results in left-sided hemiplegia (muscle paralysis) or hemiparesis (muscle weakness). Trauma to the spinal cord also impairs mobility. For example, a complete transection of the spinal cord results in a bilateral loss of

TABLE 45-1 Postural Abnormalities

Abnormality	Description	Cause	Possible Treatments*
Torticollis	Inclining of head to the affected side, in which the sternocleidomastoid muscle is contracted	Congenital or acquired condition	Surgery, heat, support, or immobilization, depending on cause and severity, gentle range of motion
Lordosis	Exaggeration of anterior convex curve of lumbar spine	Congenital condition Temporary condition (e.g., pregnancy)	Spine-stretching exercises (based on cause)
Kyphosis	Increased convexity in curvature of thoracic spine	Congenital condition Rickets, osteoporosis Tuberculosis of the spine	Spine-stretching exercises, sleeping without pillows, use of bed board, bracing, spinal fusion (based on cause and severity)
Kypholordosis	Combination of kyphosis and lordosis	Congenital condition	Similar to methods used in kyphosis or lordosis (based on cause) Immobilization and surgery (based on cause and severity)
Scoliosis	Lateral "S" or "C"-shaped curvature of spinal column with vertebral rotation, unequal heights of hips and shoulders	Sometimes a consequence of numerous congenital, connective tissue, and neuromuscular disorders. Poliomyelitis Spastic paralysis Unequal leg length	Approximately half of children with scoliosis require surgery. Nonsurgical treatment is with braces and exercises.
Kyphoscoliosis	Abnormal anteroposterior and lateral curvature of spine	Congenital condition Poliomyelitis Cor pulmonale	Immobilization and surgery (based on cause and severity)
Congenital hip dysplasia	Hip instability with limited abduction of hips and, occasionally, adduction contractures (head of femur does not articulate with acetabulum because of abnormal shallowness of acetabulum)	Congenital condition (more common with breech deliveries)	Maintenance of continuous abduction of the thigh so that head of femur presses into the centre of acetabulum Abduction splints, casting, surgery
Knock-knee (genu valgum)	Legs curved inward so that knees come together as person walks	Congenital condition Rickets	Knee braces, surgery if not corrected by growth
Bowlegs (genu varum)	One or both legs bent outward at knee, which is normal until two to three years of age	Congenital condition Rickets	Slowing rate of curving if not corrected by growth With rickets, increase of vitamin D, calcium, and phosphorus intake to normal ranges
Clubfoot	95%: medial deviation and plantar flexion of foot (equinovarus) 5%: lateral deviation and dorsiflexion (calcaneovalgus)	Congenital condition	Casts, splints such as Denis–Browne splint, and surgery (based on degree and rigidity of deformity)
Footdrop	Inability to dorsiflex and evert foot because of peroneal nerve damage	Congenital condition Trauma Improper position of a patient who is immobilized	None (cannot be corrected) Prevention through physiotherapy Bracing with ankle–foot orthotic
Pigeon-toes (metatarsus adductus or metatarsus varus)	Internal rotation of forefoot or entire foot, common in infants, often accompanied by development dysplasia of the hip	Congenital condition Habit	Growth, wearing reversed shoes, casting, bracing

*Severity of the condition and its cause will dictate treatment, which must be individualized.
Based on McCance, K. L., & Huether, S. E. (2014). *Pathophysiology: The biologic basis for disease in adults and children* (7th ed.). St. Louis, MO: Mosby.

voluntary motor control below the level of the trauma because motor fibres are cut. Injury above the first thoracic vertebra results in **quadriplegia** (also known as *tetraplegia*) (four-limb paralysis) and injury below that level results in **paraplegia** (two-limb paralysis).

Direct Trauma to the Musculoskeletal System. Direct trauma to the musculoskeletal system can result in bruises, contusions, sprains, and fractures. A *fracture* is a disruption of bone tissue continuity. Fractures most commonly result from direct external trauma but can also occur as a consequence of some deformity of the bone (e.g., **pathological fractures** of osteoporosis, Paget's disease, metastatic cancer, or osteogenesis imperfecta). Young children are usually able to form new bone more easily than adults and, as a result, have few complications after a fracture. Treatment often includes positioning the fractured bone in proper alignment and immobilizing it to promote healing and restore function. Even this temporary immobilization can result in some muscle atrophy, loss of tone, and joint stiffness. After the fracture has healed, physiotherapy may be required to regain functional losses.

NURSING KNOWLEDGE BASE

Mobility–Immobility

Fully understanding mobility requires more than an overview of the physiology and regulation of movement by the musculoskeletal and nervous systems. Nurses must also know how to apply these scientific principles in the clinical setting to determine the safest way to move patients and to understand the effect of immobility on the physiological, psychological, and developmental aspects of patient care.

Factors Influencing Mobility–Immobility. To determine how to move patients safely, nurses need to assess a patient's ability to move. As stated earlier, *mobility* refers to a person's ability to move about freely. Immobility refers to the inability to move about freely. Mobility and immobility are best understood as the end points of a continuum, with many degrees of partial mobility in between. Some patients move back and forth on this continuum, but for other patients, immobility is absolute and continues indefinitely. The terms *bed rest* and *impaired physical mobility* are frequently used when discussing patients on the mobility–immobility continuum.

Bed rest is an intervention that restricts patients to bed for therapeutic reasons. Although it is much less commonly used, health care providers often prescribe this intervention. Patients with a wide variety of conditions are placed on bed rest. The general objectives of bed rest are as follows:

- To reduce physical activity and the oxygen needs of the body
- To reduce pain, including postoperative pain, and the need for large doses of analgesics
- To promote safety for patients recovering from the effects of anaesthetics or who are sedated
- To allow patients who are ill or debilitated to rest
- To allow patients who are exhausted the opportunity for uninterrupted rest

The duration of bed rest depends on the illness or injury and the patient's prior state of health.

The effects of muscular deconditioning associated with lack of physical activity are often apparent in a matter of days. The individual of average weight and height without a chronic illness on bed rest loses muscle strength from baseline levels at a rate of 3% a day. Deconditioning can occur to any individual regardless of age. Immobility is also associated with cardiovascular, skeletal, and other organ changes. The term disease atrophy describes the tendency of cells and issue to reduce in size and function in response to prolonged inactivity resulting from bed rest, trauma, casting of a body part, or local nerve damage (McCance & Huether, 2014). *Impaired physical mobility* is defined by the North American Nursing Diagnosis Association as a state in which the individual experiences or is at risk of experiencing limitation of physical movement (Ackley & Ladwig, 2014).

Periods of immobility due to disability or injury or prolonged bed rest can cause major physiological, psychological, and social effects. These effects can be gradual or immediate and vary from patient to patient. The greater the extent and the longer the duration of immobility, the more pronounced are the consequences. The patient with complete mobility restrictions is continually at risk for adverse effects of immobility. When possible, it is imperative that patients, especially older persons, have limited bed rest and that their activity is more than movement from bed to chair. Loss of walking independence increases hospital stays, need for rehabilitation services, or nursing home placement. In addition, the deconditioning related to reduced walking increases the risk for patient falls (Gillis, MacDonald, & MacIssac, 2008; Pashikanti & Von Ah, 2012).

Systemic Effects of Immobility. All body systems work more efficiently with some form of movement. Exercise has positive outcomes for all major systems of the body (see Chapter 36). When there is an alteration in mobility, each body system is at risk for impairment. The severity of the impairment depends on the patient's overall health, degree and length of immobility, and age. For example, persons with chronic illness develop pronounced effects of immobility. (See case study of person with Multiple Sclerosis Box 45-1.)

Metabolic Changes. Changes in mobility alter endocrine metabolism, calcium resorption, and functioning of the gastrointestinal system. The endocrine system, made up of hormone-secreting glands, maintains and regulates vital functions such as (1) response to stress and injury; (2) growth and development; (3) reproduction; (4) maintenance of the internal environment; and (5) energy production, use, and storage.

When injury or stress occurs, the endocrine system triggers a series of responses aimed at maintaining blood pressure and preserving life. The endocrine system is important in maintaining homeostasis. Tissues and cells live in an internal environment that the endocrine system helps regulate through maintenance of sodium, potassium,

BOX 45-1 CASE STUDY

Immobility

Kate is a 36-year-old female who has multiple sclerosis and was admitted to the neurology unit 3 days ago for exacerbation of symptoms. She came to the emergency department with a chief concern of weakness, difficulty balancing, and extreme pain, with loss of muscle function in her legs. Kate was diagnosed with multiple sclerosis 3 years ago. She is married and has two children, ages 7 years and 4 years. Prior to admission, she adhered closely to her medication regime and continued her very active lifestyle, enjoying outdoor activities with her family. Since hospital admission 3 days ago, Kate's muscle function in her lower extremities has deteriorated significantly and she is unable to leave her bed and cannot walk.

1. Describe the physiological risks of immobility and the assessments that need to be performed to ensure Kate's safety and well-being.
2. Identify a potential nursing diagnosis for Kate as related to her immobility.
3. Develop a plan of care with a focus on mobility for Kate. Identify and describe interventions to be implemented to prevent and reduce the adverse effects of immobility. Explain how you would evaluate your plan of care (include how you would appraise the effectiveness of interventions implemented and health outcomes).
4. Identify psychological implications of immobility. How does Kate's hospitalization affect her role as a mother and caregiver? Explore how Kate's acute hospitalization affects her family as a unit of care.

water, and acid–base balance. The endocrine system also helps regulate energy metabolism. Thyroid hormone increases the basal metabolic rate (BMR), and energy becomes available to cells through the integrated action of gastrointestinal and pancreatic hormones (McCance & Huether, 2014).

Immobility disrupts normal metabolic functioning, decreasing the metabolic rate; altering the metabolism of carbohydrates, fats, and proteins; causing fluid, electrolyte, and calcium imbalances; and causing gastrointestinal disturbances such as decreased appetite and slowing of peristalsis. However, in the presence of an infectious process, patients who are immobilized may have an increased BMR as a result of fever or wound healing because these increase cellular oxygen requirements (McCance & Huether, 2014).

A deficiency in calories and protein is characteristic of patients with a decreased appetite secondary to immobility. The body is constantly synthesizing proteins and breaking them down into amino acids to form other proteins. When the patient is immobile, the body excretes more nitrogen (the end product of amino acid breakdown) than it ingests in proteins, resulting in **negative nitrogen balance**. Weight loss, decreased muscle mass, and weakness result from tissue catabolism (tissue breakdown) (McCance & Huether, 2014). Another metabolic change associated with immobility is calcium resorption (loss) from bones. Immobility causes the release of calcium into circulation. Normally, the kidneys can excrete the excess calcium. However, if the kidneys are unable to respond appropriately, hypercalcemia results. Pathological fractures occur if calcium resorption continues as a patient remains on bed rest or continues to be immobile (McCance & Huether, 2014).

Impairments of gastrointestinal functioning caused by decreased mobility vary. Difficulty in passing stools (constipation) is a common symptom, although pseudodiarrhea may result from a fecal impaction (accumulation of hardened feces). This finding is not normal diarrhea, but rather liquid stool passing around the area of impaction. Left untreated, fecal impaction can result in a mechanical bowel obstruction that may partially or completely occlude the intestinal lumen, blocking normal propulsion of liquid and gas. The resulting fluid in the intestine produces distension and increases intraluminal pressure. Over time, intestinal function becomes depressed, dehydration occurs, absorption ceases, and fluid and electrolyte disturbances worsen.

Respiratory Changes. Regular aerobic exercise is known to enhance respiratory functioning. In contrast, lack of movement and exercise places patients at higher risk for respiratory complications. Patients who are immobile are at a high risk of developing pulmonary complications such as **atelectasis** (collapse of alveoli) and **hypostatic pneumonia** (inflammation of the lung from stasis or pooling of secretions). Both conditions decrease oxygenation, prolong recovery, and add to the patient's discomfort (Lewis, Dirksen, Heitkemper, et al., 2013). In atelectasis, secretions block a bronchiole or a bronchus, and the distal lung tissue (alveoli) collapses as the existing air is absorbed, producing hypoventilation. The site of the blockage determines the severity of atelectasis. A lung lobe or even a whole lung may collapse. At some point in the development of these complications, there is a proportional decline in the patient's ability to cough productively. Ultimately, the distribution of mucus in the bronchi increases, particularly when the patient is in the supine, prone, or lateral position. Mucus accumulates in the dependent regions of the airways. Hypostatic pneumonia frequently results because mucus is an excellent medium for bacterial growth.

Cardiovascular Changes. Immobilization also affects the cardiovascular system, frequently resulting in orthostatic hypotension, increased cardiac workload, and thrombus formation.

Orthostatic hypotension is a drop of blood pressure greater than 20 mm Hg in systolic blood pressure and of 10 mm Hg in diastolic blood pressure. Symptoms include dizziness, light-headedness, nausea, tachycardia, pallor, or fainting when the patient changes from a lying or sitting position to a standing position (Ball, Dains, Flynn, et al., 2015). In the immobilized patient, decreased circulating fluid volume, pooling of blood in the lower extremities, and decreased autonomic response occur. These responses are especially evident in older persons.

As the workload of the heart increases, its oxygen consumption does as well. Therefore, the heart works harder and less efficiently during periods of prolonged rest. As immobilization increases, cardiac output falls, further decreasing cardiac efficiency and increasing workload.

Patients who are immobile are also at risk for thrombus formation. A **thrombus** is an accumulation of platelets, fibrin, clotting factors, and the cellular elements of the blood attached to the interior wall of a vein or artery, sometimes occluding the lumen of the vessel (Figure 45-1). Three factors contribute to venous thrombus formation: (1) loss of integrity of the vessel wall (e.g., injury during surgical procedures), (2) alterations in blood flow (e.g., slow blood flow in calf veins associated with bed rest), and (3) alterations in blood constituents (e.g., a change in clotting factors or increased platelet activity). These three factors are sometimes referred to as *Virchow's triad* (McCance & Huether, 2014). A dislodged venous thrombus, called an **embolus**, may travel through the circulatory system to the lungs and impair circulation and oxygenation. Venous emboli that travel to the lungs are called *pulmonary emboli* and may be life-threatening. More than 90% of all pulmonary emboli begin in the legs or pelvis (Copstead-Kirkhorn & Banasik, 2011). As a nurse, you will practise in numerous situations when deep vein thrombosis must be prevented, especially during perioperative care.

Musculoskeletal Changes. Immobility affects the musculoskeletal system by causing temporary or permanent impairment or permanent disability. Restricted mobility may result in loss of endurance, strength, and muscle mass as well as decreased stability and balance. Other effects of restricted mobility affecting the skeletal system are impaired calcium metabolism and impaired joint mobility.

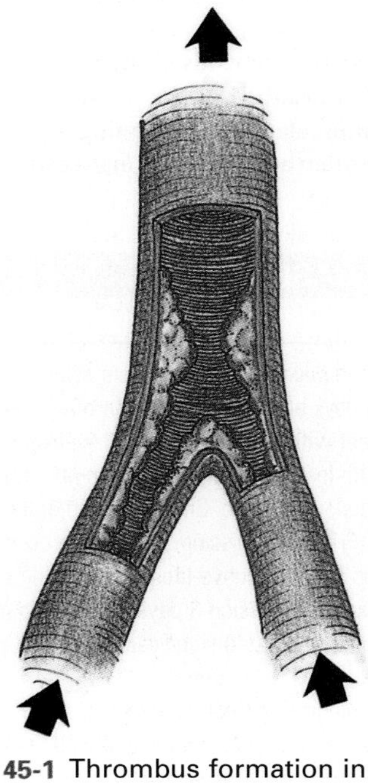

FIGURE 45-1 Thrombus formation in a vessel.

BOX 45-2 PATIENT TEACHING

Patients With Osteoporosis

Objective

- Patient will identify strategies to prevent or limit the severity of osteoporosis.

Teaching Strategies

- Instruct patient (and caregiver, if present) on common risk factors and how to modify lifestyle (e.g., eliminating smoking, caffeine, alcohol).
- Teach patient and caregiver the current recommended dietary allowances for calcium and vitamin D, and review foods high in calcium and vitamin D.
- Instruct patient and caregiver to do appropriate types of weight-bearing exercises as recommended by the physician or physiotherapist to prevent injury or fractures.
- Teach patient and caregiver about safety, fall prevention, and strategies to create a safe home environment.
- Instruct patient and caregiver in self-administration of appropriate medication as ordered by the physician.
- Foster a positive self-image in the patient by providing realistic yet optimistic and positive feedback about changes in the patient's appearance and mobility.

Evaluation

- Patient and caregiver identify strategies to modify the patient's lifestyle, such as stopping smoking, reducing caffeine or alcohol intake, or increasing dietary calcium.
- Patient and caregiver identify foods high in calcium and vitamin D.
- Patient and caregiver demonstrate appropriate weight-bearing exercises.
- Patient and caregiver identify safety strategies to prevent falls.
- Patient and caregiver demonstrate appropriate knowledge about medications.
- Patient and caregiver express positive but realistic feedback regarding the effects of disease.

Muscle effects. Because of protein breakdown, a patient loses lean body mass during immobility. The reduced muscle mass makes it difficult for patients to sustain activity without increased fatigue. If immobility continues and the patient does not exercise, there is further loss of muscle mass.

Prolonged immobility often leads to *disuse atrophy*, the pathological reduction in normal size of muscle fibres after prolonged inactivity from bed rest, trauma, casting, or local nerve damage. Loss of endurance, decreased muscle mass and strength, and joint instability (see "Skeletal Effects" section) put patients at risk for falls.

Skeletal effects. Immobilization causes two skeletal changes: impaired calcium metabolism and joint abnormalities. Because immobilization results in bone resorption, the bone tissue is less dense, or is atrophied, and disuse osteoporosis results, putting the patient at risk for pathological fractures. Bone resorption also causes calcium to be released in the blood, and hypercalcemia results.

Osteoporosis is a major health concern in Canada. Eighty percent of all fractures in women over 50 are related to osteoporosis. Fragility fractures are responsible for excess mortality and morbidity (Papaioannou, Morin, Cheung, et al., 2010). Although primary osteoporosis is different in origin from the osteoporosis that results from immobility, it is imperative that nurses recognize that immobilized patients are at high risk for accelerated bone loss if they have primary osteoporosis. Important interventions for preventing disability in patients with primary osteoporosis who become immobilized include early patient evaluation, and consultation with and referral to physicians, dietitians, occupational therapists, and physiotherapists. Patient teaching should focus on limiting the severity of the disease through diet and activity (Box 45-2).

Immobility can also lead to joint contractures. A joint contracture is an abnormal and possibly permanent condition characterized by fixation of a joint. Flexor muscles for joints are stronger than extensor muscles and therefore contribute to the formation of contractures. Disuse, atrophy, and shortening of the muscle fibres cause joint contraction. When a contracture occurs, the joint cannot obtain full ROM. Contractures may leave a joint or joints in a nonfunctional position (Figure 45-2) and can be permanent. Early prevention of contractures is essential (Clavet, Hebert, Fergusson, et al., 2011).

One common and debilitating contracture is footdrop (Figures 45-3 and 45-4). When footdrop occurs, the foot is permanently fixed in plantar flexion. Ambulation is difficult with the foot in this position

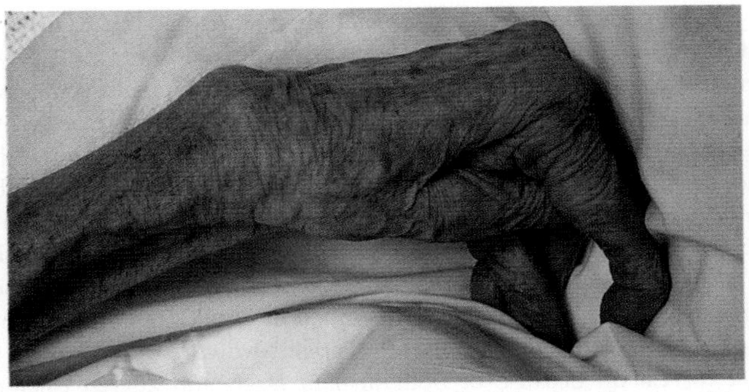

FIGURE 45-2 A contracture of the joints in the fingers. (From Sorrentino, S. A., Wilk, M. J., & Newmaster, R. [2009]. *Mosby's Canadian textbook for the support worker* [2nd ed., p. 429, Fig. 24-1]. Toronto: Elsevier.)

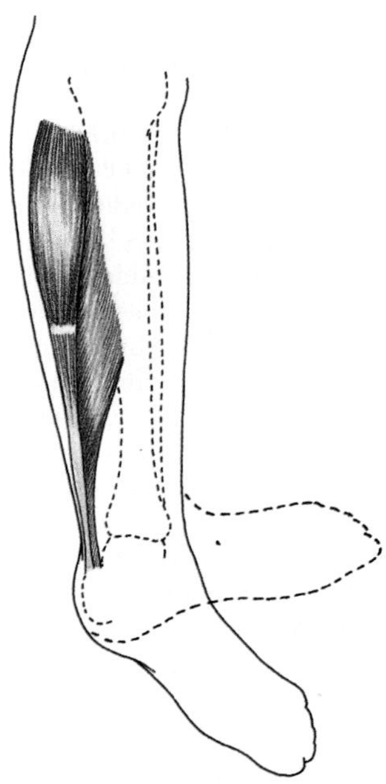

FIGURE 45-3 Footdrop. The ankle is fixed in plantar flexion. Normally, the ankle is able to flex (*dotted line*), which eases walking.

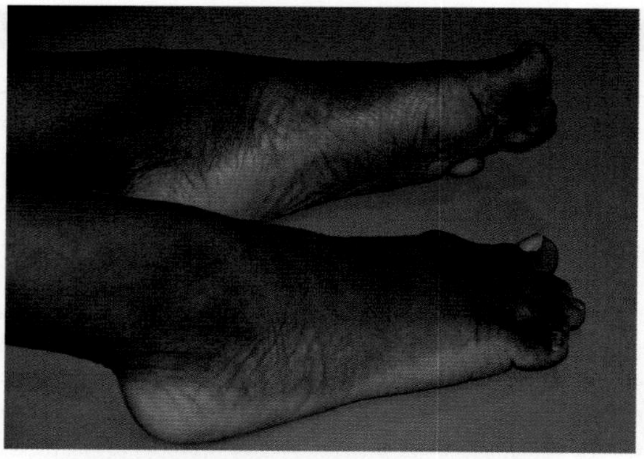

FIGURE 45-4 Patient with bilateral footdrop.

because the patient cannot dorsiflex the foot. A patient with footdrop is unable to lift the toes off the ground. Footdrop can be associated with a variety of etiologies, including prolonged bed rest, peroneal nerve damage, peripheral neuropathy, and CVAs (strokes).

Urinary Elimination Changes. Immobility alters a patient's urinary elimination. In the upright position, urine flows out of the renal pelvis and into the ureters and bladder because of gravitational forces. When the patient is recumbent or flat, the kidneys and the ureters move toward a more level plane. Urine formed by the kidney must enter the bladder unaided by gravity. Because the peristaltic contractions of the ureters are insufficient to overcome gravity, the renal pelvis may fill before urine enters the ureters. This condition, called **urinary stasis**, increases the risk of urinary tract infection and renal calculi (see Chapter 43). *Renal calculi* are calcium stones that lodge in the renal pelvis and pass through the ureters. Patients who are immobile are at risk for calculi because of both urinary stasis and altered calcium metabolism leading to hypercalcemia.

As the period of immobility continues, fluid intake can diminish, and this increases the risk for dehydration. As a result, urinary output may decline around the fifth or sixth day after immobilization and the urine is often highly concentrated. This concentrated urine increases the risk for calculi formation and infection. Patients who are immobile may have limited access to bathing equipment and be unable to perform adequate perineal hygiene, which may also increase the risk of urinary tract contamination by *Escherichia coli* bacteria.

Patients who are immobile may not be getting up to use the bathroom or even a bedside commode. Voiding on a bedpan or using a urinal does not provide the usual sensory stimulation to void and does not allow gravity to act on the bladder sphincter. Consequently, patients may be unable to void or completely empty their bladder. This leads to residual urine in the bladder, which increases the risk of infection. Complete urinary retention requires catheterization. Both intermittent catheterization and in-dwelling catheters increase the risk of developing urinary tract infection.

Integumentary Changes. The changes in metabolism that accompany immobility add to the harmful effect of pressure on the skin in immobilized patients. This makes immobility a major risk factor for pressure injuries. Preventing a pressure injury is much less expensive than treating one; therefore, preventative nursing interventions are imperative (Registered Nurses' Association of Ontario [RNAO], 2011a).

A **pressure injury** is localized damage to the skin and/or underlying soft tissue as a result of prolonged ischemia (decreased blood supply in the tissues). The injury can present as intact skin or an open ulcer (pressure ulcer) and may be painful. A pressure injury is characterized initially by inflammation and usually forms over a bony prominence. Ischemia develops when the pressure on the skin is greater than the pressure inside the small peripheral blood vessels supplying blood to the skin. Adequate blood flow is necessary to supply oxygen and nutrients for tissue metabolism and the elimination of metabolic wastes. Pressure affects cellular metabolism by decreasing or totally eliminating tissue circulation.

People who are conscious and have voluntary muscle control and normal perception of pressure perceive decreased circulation to tissue. They change positions regularly to increase circulation to tissue and thus prevent the formation of pressure injuries. Individuals with impaired sensation or mobility may require assistance to regularly reposition themselves, to avoid the development of pressure injuries. The location of bony prominences, involving the skin most at risk for breakdown, varies depending on patient positioning. Individuals require frequent position changes, whether they are lying down or sitting.

> **Safety Alert** Implement a comprehensive skin care program to prevent skin breakdown in all patients, from neonates to older persons. Effective skin care programs include accurate and consistent assessment and documentation as well as interventions to protect the skin (e.g., turning the patient every 2 hours and using mechanical devices such as lifts when you need to move the patient; RNAO, 2011a).

Psychosocial Effects of Immobility. Immobilization can contribute to decreased social interaction, social isolation, sensory deprivation, loss of independence, and role changes (Parker, 2012). These in turn may lead to emotional reactions, behavioural responses, sensory alterations, and changes in coping. Every patient responds to immobility differently.

Patients who are immobilized can become depressed because of changes in role, self-concept, and other factors. *Depression* is an affective disorder characterized by exaggerated feelings of sadness, melancholy, dejection, worthlessness, emptiness, and hopelessness out of proportion to reality. Depression can result from worrying about present and future levels of health, finances, and family needs. Because immobilization removes the patient from a daily routine, he or she has more time to worry about disability. Worrying can quickly increase the patient's depression, causing withdrawal. By assessing behavioural changes throughout a patient's restricted mobility, nurses are better equipped to identify changes in self-concept, recognize early signs of depression, and develop nursing interventions.

Developmental Changes. Immobility often leads to developmental changes in very young children and in older persons. The immobilized young or middle-aged adult who has been healthy may experience few, if any, developmental changes. However, exceptions exist, and patients must be fully assessed for developmental implications. For example, when a mother has complications at childbirth and as a result cannot interact with the newborn infant as expected, both the mother and infant need to be assessed for sufficient maternal–infant attachment.

Infants, Toddlers, and Preschoolers. The newborn infant's spine is flexed and lacks the anteroposterior curves of the adult. As the baby grows, musculoskeletal development permits support of weight for standing and walking. Posture is awkward because the head and upper trunk are carried forward. Because body weight is not evenly distributed along a line of gravity, posture is off balance, and falls occur often. When the infant, toddler, or preschooler is immobilized, it is usually because of trauma or the need to correct a congenital skeletal abnormality. Prolonged immobilization can delay the child's gross motor skills, intellectual development, or musculoskeletal development. Nurses caring for immobilized children should plan activities that provide physical and psychosocial stimuli.

Adolescents. The adolescence stage is usually initiated by a tremendous growth spurt (see Chapter 23). Growth is frequently uneven. Prolonged immobilization may alter adolescent growth patterns. When the activity level is reduced because of trauma, illness, or surgery, the adolescent may lag behind peers in gaining independence. Social isolation is a concern for this age group when immobilization occurs.

Adults. An adult who has correct posture and body alignment feels good, looks good, and generally appears self-confident. The healthy adult also has the necessary musculoskeletal development and coordination to carry out ADLs. When periods of prolonged immobility occur, however, all physiological systems are at risk. In addition, the role of the adult may change with regard to the family or social structure. The adult may lose identity and self-concept associated with a job.

Older Persons. A progressive loss of total bone mass (strength), muscle strength, and aerobic capacity occurs in older persons. Some of the possible causes of this loss are decreased physical activity, hormonal changes, and bone resorption. Older persons may walk more slowly, take smaller steps, and appear less coordinated. Adverse effects of prescribed medications can include altering of a sense of balance or changes in blood pressure, which increase older persons' risks for falls and injuries (see Chapter 24). The outcomes of a fall include possible injury, hospitalization, loss of independence, and psychological effects (McMahon & Fleury, 2012).

Older persons may experience functional-status changes secondary to hospitalization and altered mobility status (Box 45-3). Immobilization of older persons increases their physical dependence on others and accelerates functional losses (Padula, Hughes, & Baumhover, 2009). Immobilization of some older persons results from a degenerative disease, neurological trauma, or chronic illness. In others, immobilization can occur suddenly, such as after a stroke. When providing nursing care for an older person, nurses should develop a care plan that encourages the patient to perform as many self-care activities as possible, thereby maintaining the highest level of mobility and functionality. Nurses may inadvertently contribute to a patient's immobility by providing unnecessary help with activities such as bathing and transferring.

BOX 45-3 Functional Decline in Hospitalized Immobile Older Persons

For many older persons, admission to the hospital often results in functional decline despite the treatment for which they were admitted. Some older persons have problems with mobility and can quickly regress to a dependent state. Rapid intervention of an interdisciplinary health team is required to maintain the patient's functional capacity.

- Usual aging is associated with decreased muscle strength and aerobic capacity, which becomes exacerbated if a patient's nutritional state is poor.
- A nutritional assessment needs to be included in the plan of care for the older person experiencing immobility.
- Anorexia and insufficient assistance with eating food lead to malnutrition, which contributes to the known problems associated with immobility.
- Improved nutrition increases the patient's ability to perform physical reconditioning exercises (Padula et al., 2009).
- There is a direct relationship between the success of older persons' rehabilitation and their nutritional status.

Adapted from Touhy, T., Jett, K., Boscart, V., & McCleary, L. (2012). *Ebersole & Hess' gerontological nursing and healthy aging* (1st Canadian ed.). Toronto: Elsevier Canada.

CRITICAL THINKING

Critical thinking requires nurses to combine knowledge, experience, patient data, and professional standards. Each of these sources must be integrated into the nurse's diagnosis and care plan for the patient with impaired mobility (Figure 45-5). A creative approach can also be helpful. Best Practice Guidelines such as those developed by the Registered Nurses' Association of Ontario (RNAO) provide valuable guides for managing complications associated with immobility. In addition, many health care facilities have standards of practice related to the lifting and transferring of patients and the prevention of falls and pressure sores.

NURSING PROCESS

Nurses must apply the nursing process and use a critical thinking approach to develop individualized care plans for patients with mobility impairments or risk for immobility. The aim of the care plan is to improve the patient's functional status, promote self-care, maintain psychological well-being, and reduce the hazards of immobility.

Assessment

Nursing assessment must incorporate a patient's normal mobility status, the effects, if any, of diseases or conditions on mobility, and the

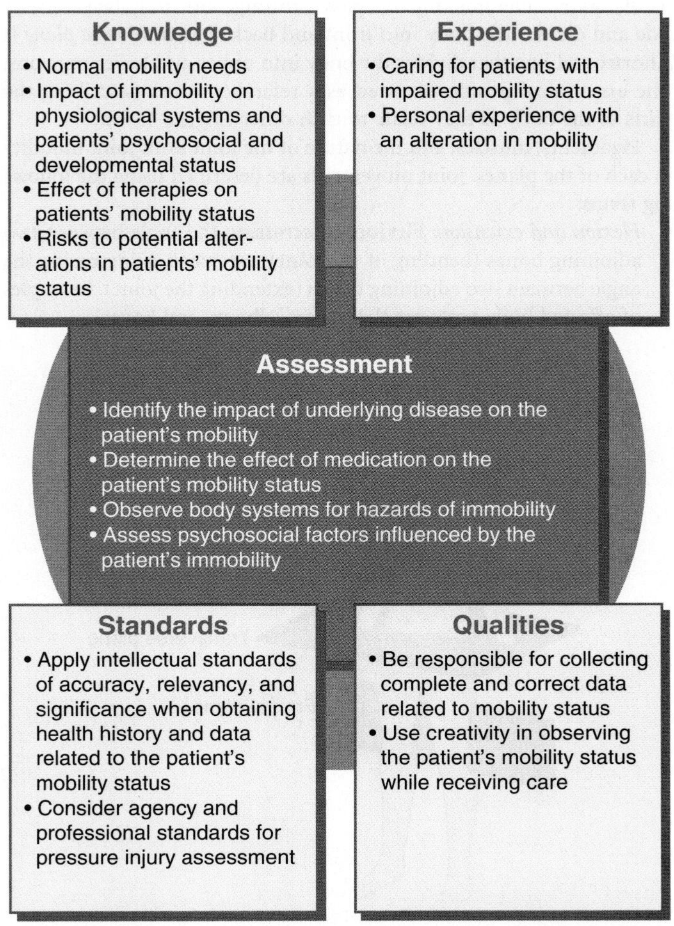

FIGURE 45-5 Critical thinking model for mobility assessment.

patient's risk for mobility alterations as a result of treatments. During assessment, nurses critically analyze findings to ensure that they make patient-centred clinical decisions required for safe nursing care.

Patient Expectations. Usually, the nurse will assess a patient's degree of mobility and immobility during the health history interview and physical examination. It is important to remember that the patient is a partner in providing information and designing the plan of care, and to understand how the patient perceives any limitations in mobility. Has the patient had a disability for an extended period of time, or is the patient well adapted to the use of an assist device or even a wheelchair? Is the limitation in mobility sudden and unexpected, causing the patient to be fearful or full of questions? Nurses must always convey respect for the patient's preferences, values, and needs during assessment and when designing a plan of care (Ackley & Ladwig, 2014).

Mobility. Assessment of patient mobility focuses on ROM, gait, exercise and activity tolerance, and body alignment. When unsure of the patient's abilities, the nurse begins assessment of mobility with the patient in the most supportive position and moves to higher levels of mobility according to the patient's tolerance. Generally, the nurse starts assessing movement while the patient is lying, then proceeds to assessing sitting positions in bed, transfers to chair, and, finally, gait. This sequence of assessment helps to protect the patient's safety.

Range of Motion. *Range of motion (ROM)* is the maximum amount of movement available at a joint in one of the four planes of the body: medial, sagittal, frontal, or transverse. The *medial plane* is a line through the axis of the body, separating the body into equal halves, a left side and a right side. The *sagittal plane* is any plane parallel to the medial plane. The *frontal plane* passes through the body from side to side and divides the body into front and back. The *transverse plane* is a horizontal line that divides the body into upper and lower portions. The anatomical position is used as a reference when describing the parts of the body as they relate to each other (Figure 45-6).

Ligaments, muscles, and the nature of the joint limit joint mobility in each of the planes. Joint movements are described using the following terms:

- *Flexion and extension:* Flexion is decreasing the angle between two adjoining bones (bending of the joint); extension is increasing the angle between two adjoining bones (extending the joint). Examples of affected body parts are the fingers, elbows, and knees.

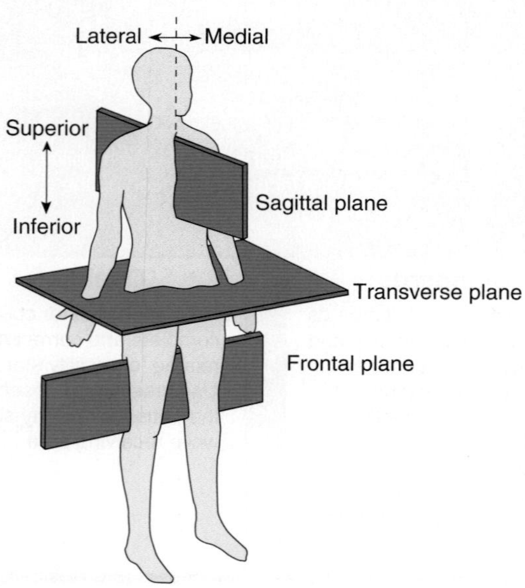

FIGURE 45-6 Planes of the body.

- *Hyperextension:* This is movement of a body part beyond its normal resting extended position.
- *Dorsiflexion and plantar flexion:* Dorsiflexion is the flexion of toes and foot upward; plantar flexion is the bending of toes and foot downward.
- *Abduction and adduction:* Abduction is movement of an extremity away from the midline of the body; adduction is movement of an extremity toward the midline of body (e.g., arms, fingers, and legs).
- *Eversion and inversion:* Eversion is the turning of a body part away from the midline; inversion is the turning of a body part toward the midline (e.g., feet).
- *Pronation and supination:* Pronation is movement of a body part so that the front or ventral surface faces downward; supination is movement of a body part so that the front or ventral surface faces upward (e.g., hands, forearm).
- *Internal and external rotation:* Internal rotation is rotation of the joint inward; external rotation is rotation of the joint outward (e.g., hip).
- *Circumduction:* This is the circular movement of a limb in a cone-shaped manner (e.g., shoulder).

Assessment of ROM is important as a baseline measure to determine a patient's mobility status and to later compare and evaluate whether loss in joint mobility has occurred as a result of clinical changes or treatments. When assessing ROM, the nurse needs to physically examine the patient for stiffness, swelling, pain, limited movement, and unequal movement, and ask the patient whether any of these features are present. Patients whose mobility is restricted require ROM exercises to reduce the hazards of immobility, such as contractures. Limited ROM often indicates inflammation such as arthritis, fluid in the joint, or altered nerve supply. Increased mobility (beyond normal ROM) of a joint sometimes indicates connective tissues disorders, ligament tears, or possible joint fractures.

The nurse needs to assess the type of ROM exercise a patient can perform. First, the medical plan of care is considered and if active ROM exercises are appropriate; then the patient's ability to engage in active ROM exercise is assessed. ROM exercises may be active (the patient is able to move all joints through his or her ROM unassisted), passive (the patient is unable to move independently, and the nurse moves each joint through its ROM), or somewhere in between (Table 45-2). Passive ROM exercises are prescribed for patients who are unable to move because of paralysis, sedation, or generalized weakness. Passive ROM exercises improve joint mobility, prevent contractures, and help prepare the patient for ongoing rehabilitation exercises (Smith, Caple, & Pravikoff, 2016). With a patient who is weak, the nurse may provide support while the patient performs most of the movement, or the patient may be able to move some joints actively while the nurse passively moves others (Box 45-4). The nurse's assessment will help to determine the patient's need for assistance, teaching, or reinforcement. In general, exercises should be as active as health and mobility allow. Assessment data from patients with limited joint movements vary on the basis of the area affected.

Gait. The term **gait** is used to describe a particular manner or style of walking. It is a coordinated action that requires the integration of sensory function, muscle strength, proprioception, balance, and a properly functioning central nervous system (vestibular system and cerebellum). The gait cycle begins with the heel strike of one leg and continues to the heel strike of the other leg. Assessing a patient's gait helps nurses to draw conclusions about balance, posture, safety, and ability to walk without assistance, all of which affect the risk of falling. Here are a few ways to assess a patient's gait:

1. Observe the patent entering the room, and note speed, stride, and balance.

TABLE 45-2 Range-of-Motion Exercises

Body Part	Type of Joint	Type of Movement	Range (Degrees)	Primary Muscles
Neck, cervical spine	Pivotal	Flexion: Bring chin to rest on chest.	45	Sternocleidomastoid
		Extension: Return head to erect position.	45	Trapezius
	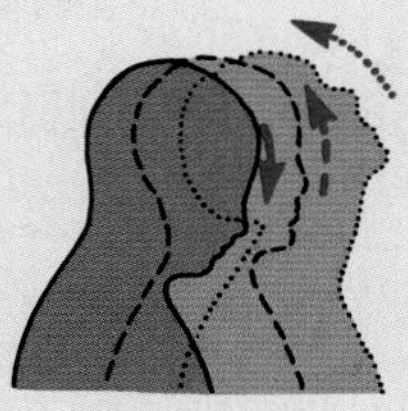	Hyperextension: Bend head back as far as possible.	10	Trapezius
	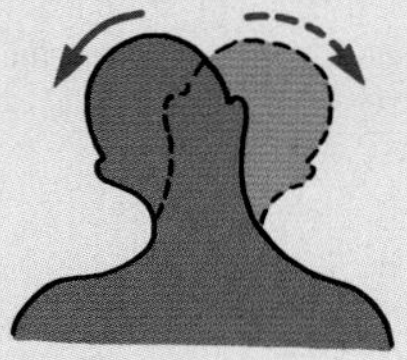	Lateral flexion: Tilt head as far as possible toward each shoulder.	40–45	Sternocleidomastoid
	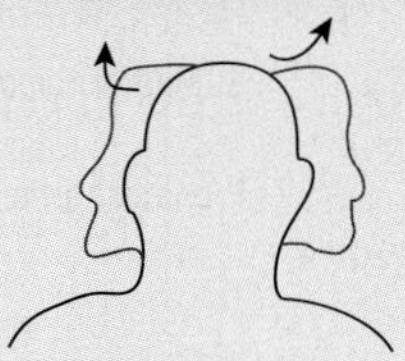	Rotation: Turn head as far as possible along transverse plane to look to each side.	180	Sternocleidomastoid, trapezius
Shoulder	Ball and socket	Flexion: Raise arm from side position forward to position above the head.	180	Coracobrachialis, biceps brachii, deltoid, pectoralis major
	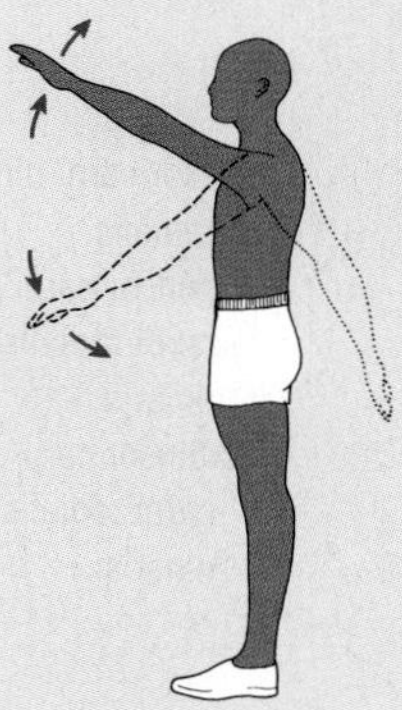	Extension: Return arm to position at side of the body.	180	Latissimus dorsi, teres major, triceps brachii
		Hyperextension: Move arm behind body, keeping elbow straight.	45–60	Latissimus dorsi, teres major, deltoid
	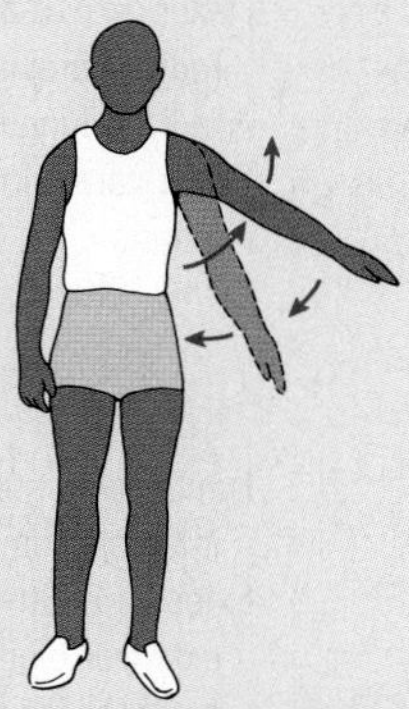	Abduction: Raise arm to side to position above head with palm away from head.	180	Deltoid, supraspinatus
		Adduction: Lower arm sideways and across body as far as possible.	320	Pectoralis major
	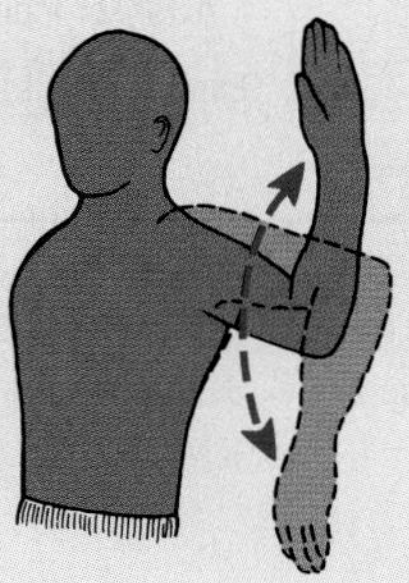	Internal rotation: With elbow flexed, rotate shoulder by moving arm until thumb is turned inward and toward back.	90	Pectoralis major, latissimus dorsi, teres major, subscapularis
		External rotation: With elbow flexed, move arm until thumb is upward and lateral to head.	90	Infraspinatus, teres major, deltoid

Continued

TABLE 45-2 Range-of-Motion Exercises—cont'd

Body Part	Type of Joint	Type of Movement	Range (Degrees)	Primary Muscles
	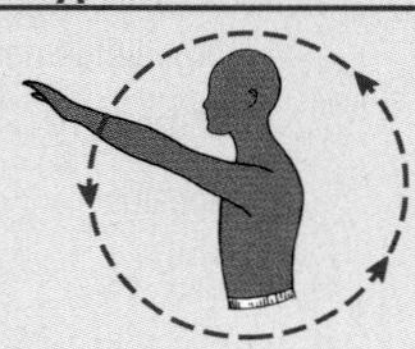	Circumduction: Move arm in full circle. (Circumduction is a combination of all movements of the ball-and-socket joint.)	360	Deltoid, coracobrachialis, latissimus dorsi, teres major
Elbow	Hinge 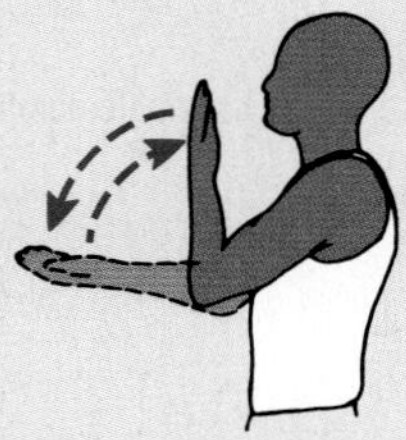	Flexion: Bend elbow so that lower arm moves toward its shoulder joint and the hand is level with the shoulder.	150	Biceps brachii, brachialis, brachioradialis
		Extension: Straighten elbow by lowering hand.	150	Triceps brachii
Forearm	Pivotal 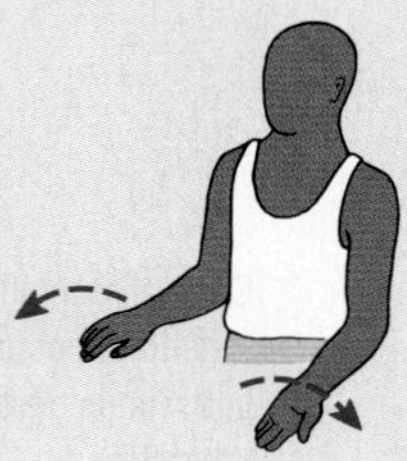	Supination: Turn lower arm and hand so that the palm is up.	70–90	Supinator, biceps brachii
		Pronation: Turn lower arm so that the palm is down.	70–90	Pronator teres, pronator quadratus
Wrist	Condyloid 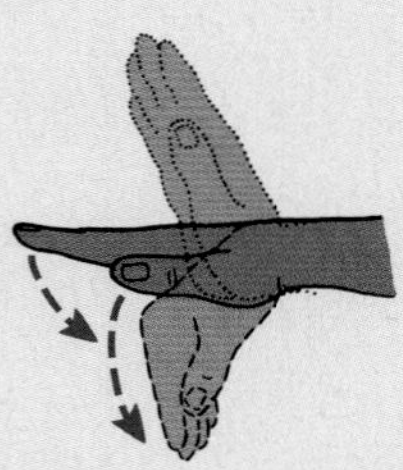	Flexion: Move palm toward inner aspect of forearm.	80–90	Flexor carpi ulnaris, flexor carpi radialis
		Extension: Move fingers and hand posterior to midline.	80–90	Extensor carpi radialis brevis, extensor carpi radialis longus, extensor carpi ulnaris
		Hyperextension: Bring dorsal surface of hand back as far as possible.	80–90	Extensor carpi radialis brevis, extensor carpi radialis longus, extensor carpi ulnaris
	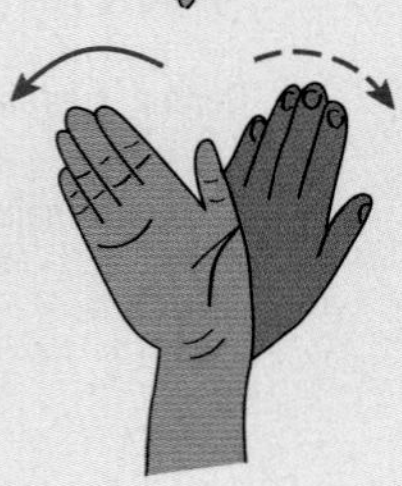	Abduction (radial deviation): Place hand with palm up and extend wrist laterally toward the thumb.	Up to 30	Flexor carpi radialis, extensor carpi radialis brevis, extensor carpi radialis longus
		Adduction (ulnar deviation): Place hand with palm up and extend wrist medially toward the fifth finger.	30–50	Flexor carpi ulnaris, extensor carpi ulnaris
Fingers	Condyloid hinge 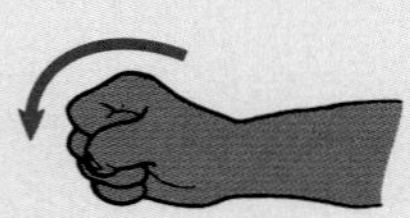	Flexion: Make a fist.	90	Lumbricals, interosseous volaris, interosseous dorsalis
		Extension: Straighten fingers.	90	Extensor digiti quinti proprius, extensor digitorum communis, extensor indicis proprius
	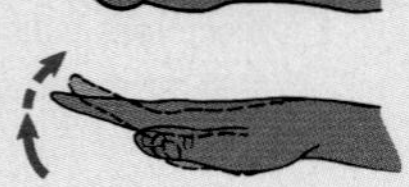	Hyperextension: Bend fingers back as far as possible.	30–60	Extensor digitorum

TABLE 45-2 Range-of-Motion Exercises—cont'd

Body Part	Type of Joint	Type of Movement	Range (Degrees)	Primary Muscles
	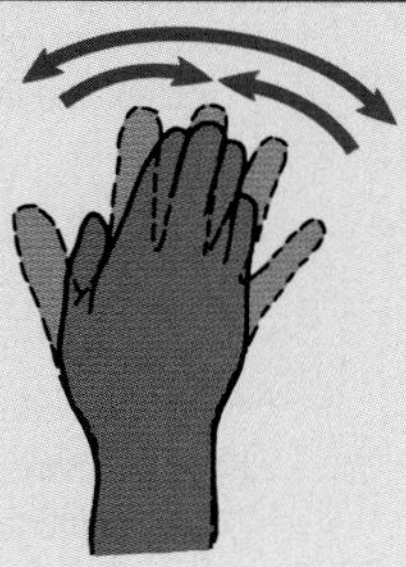	Abduction: Spread fingers apart.	30	Interosseous dorsalis
		Adduction: Bring fingers together.	30	Interosseous volaris
Thumb	Saddle 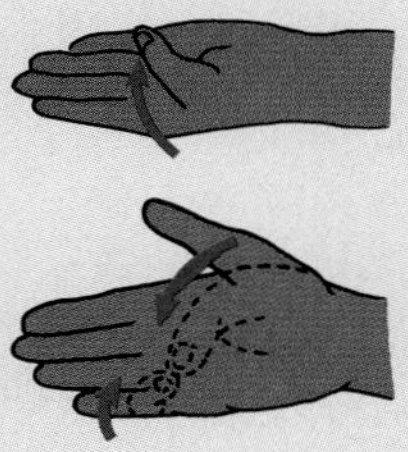	Flexion: Move thumb across palmar surface of hand.	90	Flexor pollicis brevis
		Extension: Move thumb straight away from hand.	90	Extensor pollicis longus, extensor pollicis brevis
		Abduction: Extend thumb laterally (usually done when placing fingers in abduction and adduction).	30	Abductor pollicis brevis
		Adduction: Move thumb back toward hand.	30	Adductor pollicis obliquus, adductor pollicis transversus
		Opposition: Touch thumb to each finger of the same hand.		Opponeus pollicis, opponeus digiti minimi
Hip	Ball and socket 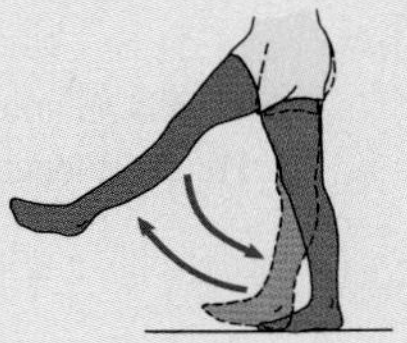	Flexion: Move leg forward and up.	90–120	Psoas major, iliacus, sartorius
		Extension: Move leg back beside other leg.	90–120	Gluteus maximus, semitendinosus, semimembranosus
	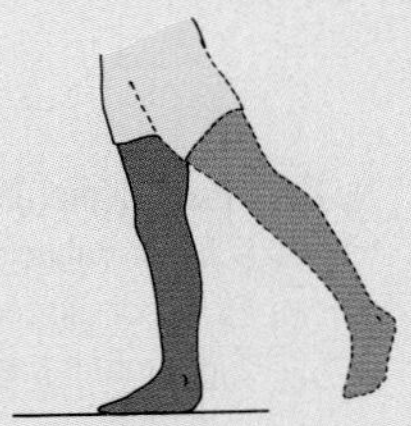	Hyperextension: Move leg behind the body.	30–50	Gluteus maximus, semitendinosus, semimembranosus
	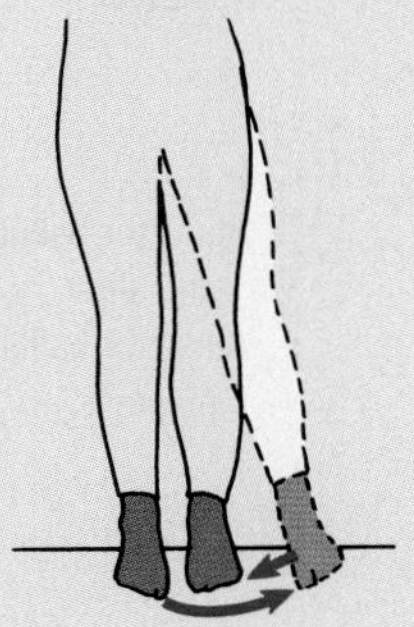	Abduction: Move leg laterally away from the body.	30–50	Gluteus medius, gluteus minimus
		Adduction: Move leg back toward medial position and beyond, if possible.	30–50	Adductor longus, adductor brevis, adductor magnus
	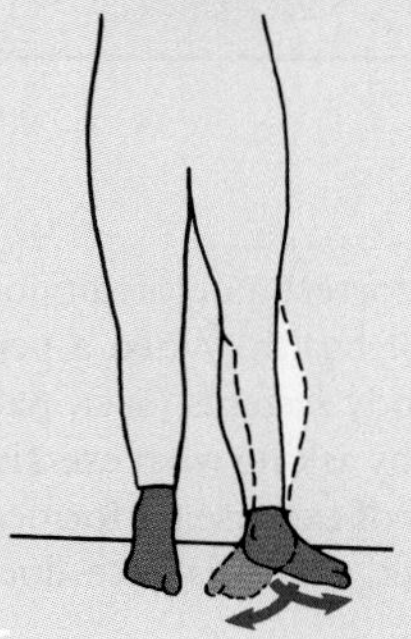	Internal rotation: Turn foot and leg toward other leg.	90	Gluteus medius, gluteus minimus, tensor fasciae latae
		External rotation: Turn foot and leg away from other leg.	90	Obturatorius internus, obturatorius externus

Continued

TABLE 45-2 Range-of-Motion Exercises—cont'd

Body Part	Type of Joint	Type of Movement	Range (Degrees)	Primary Muscles
	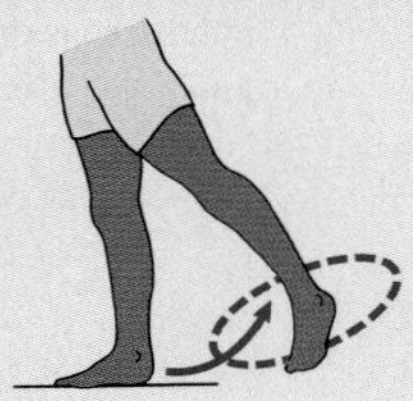	Circumduction: Move leg in a circle.		Psoas major, gluteus maximus, gluteus medius, adductor magnus
Knee	Hinge 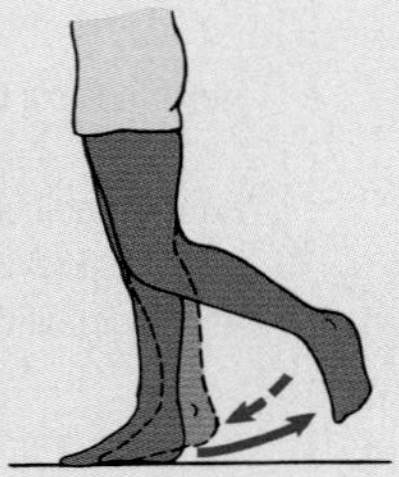	Flexion: Bring heel back toward back of thigh.	120–130	Biceps femoris, semitendinosus, semimembranosus, sartorius
		Extension: Return leg to the floor.	120–130	Rectus femoris, vastus lateralis, vastus medialis, vastus intermedius
Ankle	Hinge 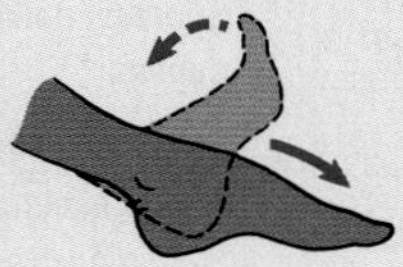	Dorsiflexion: Move foot so that toes are pointed upward.	20–30	Tibialis anterior
		Plantar flexion: Move foot so that toes are pointed downward.	45–50	Gastrocnemius, soleus
Foot	Gliding 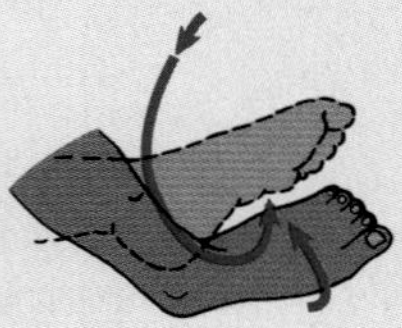	Inversion: Turn sole of foot medially.	10 or less	Tibialis anterior, tibialis posterior
		Eversion: Turn sole of foot laterally.	10 or less	Peroneus longus, peroneus brevis
Toes	Condyloid 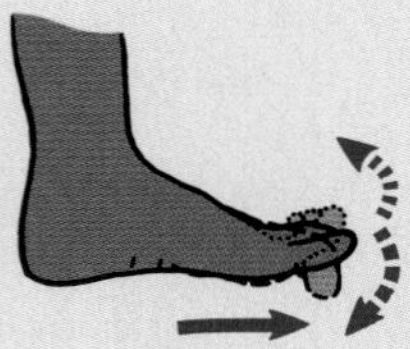	Flexion: Curl toes downward.	30–60	Flexor digitorum, lumbricalis pedis, flexor hallucis brevis
		Extension: Straighten toes.	30–60	Extensor digitorum longus, extensor digitorum brevis, extensor hallucis longus
	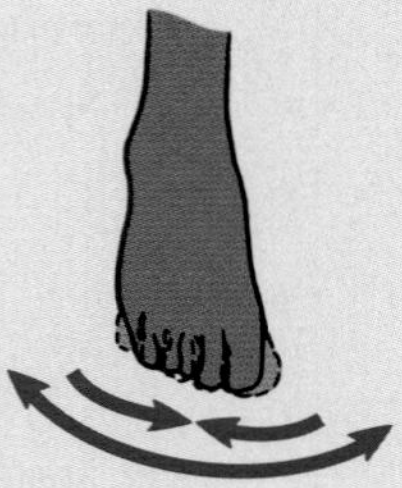	Abduction: Spread toes apart.	15 or less	Abductor hallucis, interosseous dorsalis
		Adduction: Bring toes together.	15 or less	Adductor hallucis, interosseous plantaris

2. Ask the patient to walk across the room, turn, and come back.
3. Ask the patient to walk heel-to-toe in a straight line. This may be difficult for older patients, even in the absence of disease, so stay at the patient's side during the walk.

Exercise and Activity Tolerance. Exercise is physical activity for conditioning the body, improving health, and maintaining fitness. It can be used as therapy to correct a deformity or to restore the overall body to a maximal state of health. When a person exercises, physiological changes occur in body systems (see Chapter 36). Nurses assess a patient's exercise history by asking what exercise the patient normally engages in and the amount of exercise performed daily and weekly. For example, if a patient walks, what distance does the person typically

BOX 45-4 How to Perform Passive Range-of-Motion Exercises

1. Perform hand hygiene.
2. Identify the patient using two unique identifiers (e.g., chart, wrist band).
3. Explain the procedure and its purpose to the patient. Provide additional information, as needed.
4. Assess the patient's health status, including pain, to determine the patient's activity tolerance and need for analgesia.
5. Assist the patient into a comfortable position in a bed or chair.
6. Perform range-of-motion exercises, working from head to toe:
   a. Head and neck: flexion, extension, rotation, lateral flexion
   b. Shoulder: flexion, extension, abduction, adduction, internal rotation, external rotation
   c. Elbow: flexion, extension, supination, pronation
   d. Wrist: flexion, extension, adduction, abduction, rotation
   e. Hand, fingers, and thumb: flexion, extension, adduction, abduction, opposition, circumduction of thumb
   f. Hip: flexion, extension, abduction, adduction, internal rotation, external rotation*
   g. Knee: flexion, extension
   h. Ankle: plantar flexion, dorsiflexion, inversion, eversion
   i. Feet and toes: flexion, extension

*Contraindicated in patients who have had total hip arthroplasties.
Adapted from Smith, N., Caple, C., & Pravikoff, D. (2016). Range-of-motion exercises, passive. CINAHL Nursing Guide, EBSCO Publishing. *Nursing Practice and Skill-CEU*. CINAHL AN: T703878.

walk, and how often? If a patient does not exercise regularly, the nurse will want to focus on their activity tolerance.

Activity tolerance is the type and amount of exercise or work that a person is able to perform without undue exertion or possible injury. Assessment of a patient's activity tolerance is necessary when planning activities for the patient, such as walking, ROM exercises, or ADLs. Activity tolerance assessment includes data from physiological, emotional, and developmental domains (see Chapter 36).

When a patient's activity begins after a period of inactivity, the nurse should monitor the patient for symptoms such as dyspnea, fatigue, or chest pain. If these symptoms develop, the nurse must assess for a change in vital signs (heart rate and blood pressure). A weak or debilitated patient is unable to sustain even slight changes in activity because of the increased demand for energy. Simple tasks such as eating or moving in bed often result in extreme fatigue. When the patient experiences decreased activity tolerance, the nurse must carefully assess the time needed by the patient to recover. Decreasing recovery time indicates improved activity tolerance.

People who are depressed, worried, or anxious are frequently unable to tolerate exercise. Patients who are depressed tend to withdraw from activity rather than participate in it. Patients who worry or are anxious expend a great amount of mental energy and often report feeling fatigued. Because of this, they may experience physical and emotional exhaustion.

Developmental changes also affect activity tolerance. As the infant enters the toddler stage, the activity level increases and the need for sleep declines. The child entering preschool or primary grades expends mental energy in learning and may require more rest after school or before strenuous play. The adolescent going through puberty may require more rest because much of the body's energy is expended for growth and hormone changes (see Chapter 23).

Changes may still occur through the adult years, but many of these changes are related to work and lifestyle choices. Pregnancy causes fluctuations in a woman's energy tolerance, especially during the first and third trimesters. Hormonal changes and fetal development use body energy, and the woman may be unable or unmotivated to carry out physical activities. During the last trimester, fetal development consumes a great deal of the mother's energy, and the size and location of the fetus may limit the mother's ability to take a deep breath, resulting in less oxygen being available for physical activities.

As the person grows older, activity tolerance changes. Muscle mass is reduced, posture changes, and bone composition changes. Changes in the cardiopulmonary system, such as decreased maximum heart rate and decreased lung compliance, affect the intensity of exercise. With progressing age, some older persons still exercise but do so at a reduced intensity. The more inactive a patient becomes, the more pronounced these activity changes are.

Body Alignment. Nursing assessment of body alignment is done with the patient lying, sitting, or standing. This assessment has the following objectives:

- Determining normal physiological changes in body alignment resulting from growth and development for each individual patient
- Identifying deviations in body alignment caused by incorrect posture
- Providing opportunities for patients to observe their posture
- Identifying learning needs of patients for maintaining correct body alignment
- Identifying trauma, muscle damage, or nerve dysfunction
- Obtaining information about other factors contributing to poor alignment, such as fatigue, malnutrition, and psychological problems

The first step in assessing body alignment is to put the patient at ease so the person does not assume unnatural or rigid positions. When assessing the body alignment of a patient who is immobilized or unconscious, pillows and positioning supports should be removed from the bed and the patient placed in the supine position.

Standing. When the patient is standing, it is good to check for the following signs of correct body alignment:

- The head is erect and midline.
- When observed posteriorly, the shoulders and hips are straight and parallel.
- When observed posteriorly, the vertebral column is straight.
- When observed laterally, the head is erect and the spinal curves are aligned in a reversed "S" pattern. The cervical vertebrae are anteriorly convex, the thoracic vertebrae are posteriorly convex, and the lumbar vertebrae are anteriorly convex.
- When observed laterally, the abdomen is comfortably tucked in and the knees and ankles are slightly flexed. The person appears comfortable and does not seem conscious of the flexion of knees or ankles.
- The arms hang comfortably at the sides.
- The feet are placed slightly apart to achieve a base of support, and the toes are pointed forward.
- When viewing the patient from behind, the centre of gravity is in the midline, and the line of gravity is from the middle of the forehead to a midpoint between the feet. Laterally, the line of gravity runs vertically from the middle of the skull to the posterior third of the foot (Figure 45-7).

Sitting. Characteristics of correct alignment of the sitting patient include the following (Figure 45-8):

- The head is erect, and the neck and vertebral column are in straight alignment.
- The body weight is evenly distributed on the buttocks and thighs.
- The thighs are parallel and in a horizontal plane.

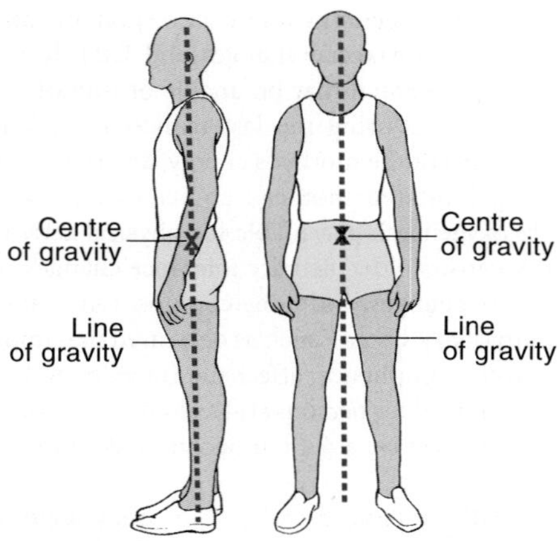

FIGURE 45-7 Correct body alignment when standing.

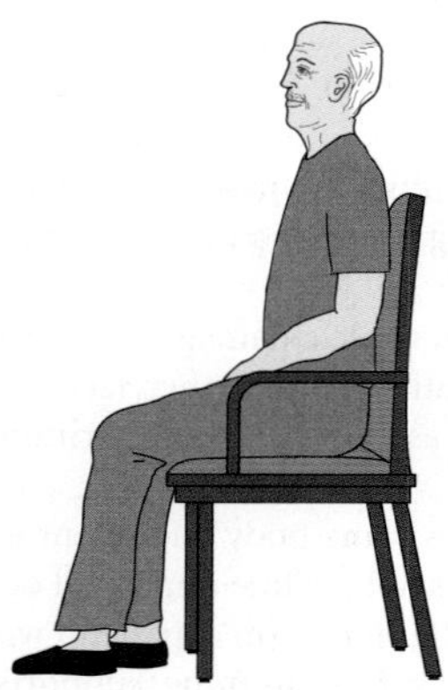

FIGURE 45-8 Correct body alignment when sitting. The patient's feet are flat on the floor, the calves do not touch the chair, and the back is straight and against the back of the chair. (From Sorrentino, S. A., Wilk, M.J. & Newmaster, R. [2009]. *Mosby's Canadian textbook for the support worker* [2nd ed., p. 412, Fig. 23-20]. Toronto: Elsevier.)

- Both feet are supported on the floor or on wheelchair footrests. With patients of short stature, a footstool can be used to ensure ankles are comfortably flexed.
- A 2.5- to 5-cm space is maintained between the edge of the seat and the popliteal space on the posterior surface of the knee. This space ensures that no pressure is on the popliteal artery or nerve to decrease circulation or impair nerve function.
- The patient's forearms are supported on the armrest, in the lap, or on a table in front of the chair.

It is particularly important to assess alignment when the patient is sitting if the patient has muscle weakness, muscle paralysis, or nerve damage. Patients who have these problems have diminished sensation in the affected area and are unable to perceive pressure or decreased circulation. Proper alignment while sitting reduces the risk of musculoskeletal system damage. The patient with severe respiratory disease may assume a posture of leaning on a table in front of the chair in an attempt to breathe more easily. This is called *orthopnea*.

Lying. People who are conscious have voluntary muscle control and normal perception of pressure. As a result, they usually assume a position of comfort when lying down. Because their ROM, sensation, and circulation are within normal limits, they change positions when they perceive muscle strain and decreased circulation.

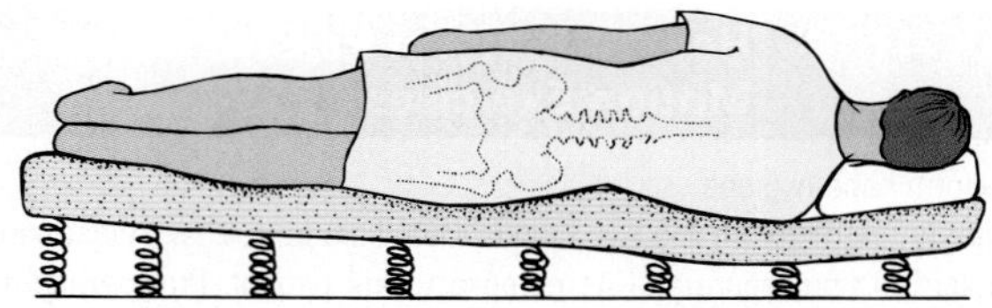

FIGURE 45-9 Lateral lying position for assessment of body alignment.

Assessment of body alignment for a patient who is immobilized or bedridden is done with the patient in the lateral position. All positioning supports should be removed from the bed except for the pillow under the head, and the body is supported with an adequate mattress (Figure 45-9). This position allows for full view of the spine and back and provides other baseline body alignment data, such as whether the patient can remain positioned without aid. The vertebrae should be aligned, and the position should not cause discomfort. Patients with impaired mobility (e.g., traction or arthritis), decreased sensation (e.g., hemiparesis following a CVA), impaired circulation (e.g., diabetes), or lack of voluntary muscle control (e.g., spinal cord injury) are at risk for damage when lying down.

Immobility

Physiological Assessment. Assessment of the patient for physiological hazards of immobility is done while performing a head-to-toe physical assessment (see Chapter 32). Additionally, the examiner should focus on the patient's psychosocial and developmental dimensions. The physiological hazards of immobility that may be identified during a nursing assessment are summarized below and in Table 45-3.

Metabolic system. When assessing metabolic functioning, nurses use anthropometric measurements (measures of height, weight, and skin fold thickness) to evaluate muscle atrophy. In addition, the nurse may need to analyze intake and output records to determine whether a fluid imbalance exists (see Chapter 40). Does intake equal output? Dehydration and edema can increase the rate of skin breakdown in a patient who is immobilized. Monitoring laboratory data such as electrolytes, serum protein (albumin and total protein) levels, and blood urea nitrogen can help in determining metabolic functioning.

Assessment of wound healing and monitoring of food intake and elimination patterns will help to determine altered gastrointestinal functioning and potential metabolic problems. If a patient who is immobile has a wound, the rate of healing indicates how well nutrients are being delivered to tissues. Normal progression of healing indicates that metabolic needs of injured tissues are being met. Anorexia occurs commonly in patients who are immobilized. The patient's food intake should be assessed before the meal tray is removed to determine the amount eaten. The patient's dietary patterns and food preferences are assessed at the onset of immobilization, to help prevent nutritional imbalances.

Respiratory system. A respiratory assessment is performed at least every 2 hours for patients with restricted activity. The nurse needs to inspect chest wall movements during the full inspiratory–expiratory cycle. If a patient has an atelectatic area, chest movement may be asymmetrical. The entire lung region should be auscultated to identify diminished breath sounds, crackles, or wheezes. Auscultation is focused on the dependent lung fields because pulmonary secretions tend to collect in these lower regions. The nurse needs to perform a complete respiratory assessment to identify the presence of secretions and to determine nursing interventions necessary for optimal respiratory function.

TABLE 45-3 Physiological Hazards of Immobility

System	Assessment Techniques	Abnormal Findings
Metabolic	Inspection	Slowed wound healing, abnormal laboratory data
	Inspection	Muscle atrophy
	Anthropometric measurements (mid-upper arm circumference, triceps skinfold measurement)	Decreased amount of subcutaneous fat
	Palpation	Generalized edema
Respiratory	Inspection	Asymmetrical chest wall movement, dyspnea, increased respiratory rate
	Auscultation	Crackles, wheezes, decreased air entry
Cardiovascular	Auscultation	Orthostatic hypotension
	Auscultation, palpation	Increased heart rate, third heart sound, weak peripheral pulses
	Inspection	Dependent edema in feet and legs (if seated) and in sacrum (if lying)
Musculoskeletal	Inspection, palpation	Decreased range of motion, erythema, increased diameter in calf or thigh
	Palpation	Joint contracture
	Inspection	Activity intolerance, muscle atrophy, joint contracture
Elimination	Inspection	Decreased urine output, cloudy or concentrated urine, decreased frequency of bowel movements
	Palpation	Distended bladder and abdomen
	Auscultation	Decreased bowel sounds
Skin	Inspection, palpation	Break in skin integrity

Cardiovascular system. Cardiovascular assessment of the patient who is immobile includes blood pressure monitoring, evaluation of apical and peripheral pulses, and observation for signs of venous stasis (e.g., edema and poor wound healing). All patients should have their vital signs monitored during the first few attempts at sitting or standing.

The nurse needs to move the patient gradually during position changes from supine to sitting or standing and assess for dizziness when monitoring orthostatic blood pressures. When performing this procedure, the nurse assesses and documents orthostatic changes. First, the nurse obtains baseline blood pressure and pulse measurements with the patient in the supine position, and then assists the patient to a position sitting at the side of the bed. The patient should remain sitting for 3 minutes before the blood pressure and pulse are taken. The nurse should remain with the patient in a sitting position and continually monitor the patient for dizziness or lightheadedness. If the patient has no dizziness or drop in blood pressure (≥20 mm Hg systolic or 10 mm Hg diastolic), the nurse assists the patient to a standing position and retakes the blood pressure and pulse immediately when the patient stands and again after 3 minutes of standing. The patient should be monitored closely for dizziness throughout this procedure. The longer the period of immobility, the greater the risk of hypotension when the patient stands (McCance & Huether, 2014).

The nurse also needs to assess the apical and peripheral pulses. Recumbent positions increase cardiac workload and result in an increased pulse rate. In some patients, particularly older persons, the heart may not tolerate the increased workload, and a form of cardiac failure may develop. A third heart sound, heard at the apex with the bell of the stethoscope, can be an early indication of heart failure. Monitoring of peripheral pulses will enable the nurse to evaluate the heart's ability to pump blood. Absence of a peripheral pulse in the lower extremities should be documented and reported immediately to the patient's health care provider, especially if the pulse was present previously.

Edema may develop in patients who have had injury or whose heart is unable to handle the increased workload of bed rest. Because edema moves to dependent body regions, assessment of the patient who is immobile includes inspection of the sacrum, legs, and feet. If the heart is unable to tolerate the increased workload, peripheral body regions, such as the hands, feet, nose, and earlobes, will be colder than central body regions. Edema can be caused by other means, such as renal impairment, and by certain medications, such as steroids. The nurse must look for other sources of edema beyond heart failure and immobility. Deep vein thrombosis (DVT) is a hazard of restricted mobility. To assess for a DVT, the patient's elastic stockings or sequential compression devices (SCDs) are removed every 8 hours (or according to agency policy) and the calves observed for redness, warmth, and tenderness. Homans' sign, or calf pain on dorsiflexion of the foot, is contraindicated in patients when a DVT is suspected as vigorous dorsiflexion may dislodge the thrombus.

Measurement of bilateral calf circumference and recording it daily can serve as an alternative assessment for DVT. To do this, the nurse marks a point on each calf 10 cm from the midpatella. The circumference is measured each day, using the mark for placement of the tape measure. Unilateral increases in calf diameter can be an early indication of thrombosis. Because DVTs can also occur in the thigh, daily thigh measurements should be taken if the patient is prone to thrombosis. In many patients, DVTs can be prevented by their taking part in active exercise and wearing compression devices, in conjunction with prescribed anticoagulant treatment.

If a patient has a DVT, an embolus can dislodge and travel through the circulatory system to the lung, causing a pulmonary embolism (PE). The signs and symptoms of PE vary depending on the size of the embolus and, hence, the extent of occlusion of the pulmonary vasculature. A massive PE can cause sudden and profound shock, including hypotension, tachycardia, tachypnea, hypoxia, and chest pain. Individuals can die within hours if the PE is not identified and treated quickly (McCance & Huether, 2014).

Musculoskeletal system. Major musculoskeletal abnormalities to identify during nursing assessment include decreased muscle tone and strength, loss of muscle mass, reduced ROM, and contractures. The anthropometric measurements described previously may indicate loss of muscle mass.

During assessment of ROM, the nurse can detect muscle tone by asking the patient to relax and then passively moving each limb at several joints to get a feeling for any resistance or rigidity that may be present. Muscle strength is assessed by having the patient assume a stable position and then performing manoeuvres to demonstrate strength of the major muscle groups (see Chapter 36). Assessment of ROM is important as a baseline against which later measurements can be compared to evaluate whether a loss in joint mobility has occurred. ROM can be measured with a goniometer.

Disuse osteoporosis cannot be identified by physical assessment. However, patients on prolonged bed rest, postmenopausal women, patients taking steroids, and people with increased serum and urine calcium levels have a greater risk for bone demineralization. The nurse should consider the risk of disuse osteoporosis when planning nursing interventions. Although some falls result in injury, others occur because of pathological fractures secondary to osteoporosis. Patients who are at risk for osteoporosis should have their diet assessed for calcium intake (Papaioannou et al., 2010).

Integumentary system. Early identification of high-risk patients and of their risk factors can aid in preventing pressure injuries. The patient's skin must be continually assessed for breakdown and colour changes, such as pallor or redness. The nurse must consistently use a standardized tool, such as the Braden Scale. This screening tool is used to identify patients with high risk for impaired skin integrity or early changes in the condition of their skin. Early identification allows for early intervention. The skin should be observed often during routine care (e.g., when the patient is turned, during hygiene measures, and when providing for elimination needs). Skin assessment should occur every 2 hours (RNAO, 2011a) and is based on patients' mobility, hydration, and physiological status. It is essential to promptly identify changes in the skin and underlying tissues.

Elimination system. To determine the effects of immobility on elimination, the patient's total intake and output needs to be assessed each shift and every 24 hours. The amounts should be compared over time. The nurse needs to determine that the patient is receiving the correct amount and type of fluids orally or parenterally (see Chapter 40). Inadequate intake and output or fluid and electrolyte imbalances increase the risk for renal system impairment, ranging from recurrent infections to kidney failure. Dehydration also increases the risk for skin breakdown, thrombus formation, respiratory infections, and constipation.

Immobility impairs gastrointestinal peristalsis. Assessment of bowel elimination status includes an analysis of a patient's dietary choices and fluid intake, review of medications, monitoring of the frequency and consistency of bowel movements, and an abdominal examination (RNAO, 2011b). With accurate assessment, the nurse will be able to intervene before constipation and fecal impaction occur.

Psychosocial Assessment. Many alterations in psychological, sociocultural, cognitive, and developmental functioning are related to immobility. Often these problems are interrelated. Nursing care must focus on all of these dimensions, not just on physical problems (Box 45-5). Often the focus of immobility is on the early visible physical problems, such as skin impairment, but the psychosocial and developmental aspects of immobility should not be overlooked.

Abrupt changes in cognition may have a physiological cause, such as surgery, a medication reaction, a PE, or an acute infection. For example, the primary symptom of compromised older persons with an acute urinary tract infection or fever is confusion. Identifying confusion is an important component of the nurse's assessment. Acute confusion in older persons is not normal and should be thoroughly examined (RNAO, 2016; Touhy, Jett, Boscart, et al., 2012).

Common reactions to immobilization are boredom, feelings of isolation, depression, and anger. The patient's history should be explored and mental health concerns or disorders identified. The nurse needs to observe for changes in a patient's emotional status and listen carefully to family if they report emotional changes. The nurse must identify patients who are at greater risk for social isolation and their available resources. Examples of change that may indicate psychosocial concerns are a cooperative patient who becomes less cooperative, or an independent patient who asks for more help than is necessary. The nurse should investigate reasons for such alterations. Identifying how the patient usually copes with loss is vital (see Chapter 25). A change in mobility status, whether permanent or not, may cause a grief reaction. Families are a key resource for information about behaviour changes.

Unexplained changes in the sleep–wake cycle should be identified and corrected. Nurses can prevent or minimize most stimuli that interrupt the sleep–wake cycle (e.g., nursing activities, a noisy environment, or discomfort). However, the effects of some medications such as analgesics, sleeping pills, or cardiovascular drugs can also cause sleep disturbances (see Chapter 41).

Because psychosocial changes usually occur gradually, it is important to observe the patient's behaviour on a daily basis. If behavioural changes occur, the cause(s) should be determined and the changes evaluated as short or long term. Identifying the cause helps the nurse to design appropriate nursing interventions. For example, a fear of falling often limits the bariatric or older person's mobility; fear may be related to past experiences of falling and not being able to get up (RNAO, 2011c). Interventions include encouraging the patient to lean

BOX 45-5 RESEARCH HIGHLIGHT

The Meaning of Mobility

Research Focus

It is widely known that decreased mobility contributes to physical and psychological impairment. Little is known, however, about the significance of mobility to other residents and to nurses in long-term care facilities. The purpose of this study was to determine nurses' and residents' perceptions of mobility in order to develop strategies that would support mobility in the institutionalized adult.

Research Abstract

In this exploratory, qualitative study by Bourret, Bernick, Cott, and colleagues (2002), residents and nursing staff made up focus groups in three long-term care facilities. A total of 20 residents and 15 nurses participated in the study. When asked about the importance of mobility, both groups identified it as key to quality of life. Older persons equated mobility with freedom, choice, and independence. Nurses valued mobility and associated it with freedom and autonomy. Both nurses and residents viewed having to wait for assistance as an impediment to mobility. Nurses identified further obstacles such as heavy workload and lack of time. Residents focused on physical barriers such as steep ramps, crowded elevators, and the negative attitudes of staff.

Evidence-Informed Practice

- Mobility is central to patients' quality of life and well-being.
- Nurses play a key role in assessing and assisting patients with their mobility needs.
- Nurses should focus on minimizing obstacles to mobility.
- Nurses should coordinate with other health care providers to meet patients' mobility needs.
- Nurses need to use creative strategies to encourage mobility in older persons.

Bourret, E., Bernick, L., Cott, C., & Kontos, P. (2002). The meaning of mobility for residents and staff in long-term care facilities. *Journal of Advanced Nursing, 37*(4), 338–345.

forward before standing, rather than standing straight up, and teaching the patient how to get up and down from the floor, with assistance if needed.

Developmental Assessment. Nurse need to include a developmental assessment of patients who are immobilized, to ensure that their patients' holistic needs are met. When caring for a young child, it is good to determine whether the child can meet developmental tasks and is progressing normally. The child's development may regress or be slowed because of immobilization. After identifying a child's developmental needs, the nurse should design nursing interventions that maintain normal development and provide physical and psychological stimuli, and assure the parents that developmental delays are usually temporary (see Chapter 22).

Immobilization of a family member changes the family's functioning. The family's response to this change may lead to problems, stress, and anxieties. When children see parents who are immobile, they may have difficulty understanding what is occurring and coping.

Immobility can have a significant effect on the older person's levels of health, independence, and functional status. Nursing assessment enables the nurse to determine the older person's ability to meet needs independently and to adapt to developmental changes such as declining physical functioning and altered family and peer relationships. A decline in developmental functioning needs prompt investigation to determine why the change occurred and what can be done to return the patient to an optimal level of functioning as soon as possible. Activities that reduce immobility and promote participation in ADLs are vital to prevent functional decline (Nagarkar, Swapnil, & Shruti, 2014). Assessment should also include the patient's home and community, to identify factors that are risks to the patient's mobility and safety (see Chapter 37).

Patient Expectations

Patients may have unrealistic expectations of themselves or of their caregivers. They may agree with the staff and understand their own limitations, or they may set their expectations of themselves too high or too low. Some patients may expect caregivers to complete all activities, and other patients may want to do as much as possible. It is important to explore patient expectations by asking patients to explain what they know about their mobility status, what questions they and their families have, and how the immobility is affecting their goals.

◆ Nursing Diagnosis

A patient who is partially or completely immobilized may have one or more nursing diagnoses. The two diagnoses most directly related to mobility problems are *impaired physical mobility* and *risk for disuse syndrome*. The diagnosis of *impaired physical mobility* is used for the patient who has some limitation but is not completely immobile. The diagnosis of *risk for disuse syndrome* should be considered for the patient who is immobile and at risk for multisystem pathophysiology because of inactivity. The list of potential diagnoses is extensive, because immobility affects multiple body systems:

- *Activity intolerance*
- *Ineffective airway clearance*
- *Ineffective breathing pattern*
- *Ineffective individual coping*
- *Risk for disuse syndrome*
- *Risk for fluid volume deficit*
- *Impaired gas exchange*
- *Risk for infection*
- *Risk for injury*
- *Impaired physical mobility*
- *Impaired skin integrity*
- *Risk for impaired skin integrity*
- *Disturbed sleep pattern*
- *Social isolation*
- *Ineffective (peripheral) tissue perfusion*
- *Impaired urinary elimination*

Assessment reveals clusters of data indicating whether a patient is at risk or if an actual problem-focused diagnosis exists. The clusters of data can indicate at-risk factors or defining characteristics that are observable assessment cues to support a problem-focused diagnostic label. In the case of a problem-focused diagnosis, the assessment data will reveal a related factor or causative factor for the diagnosis. Identifying the related factor allows nurses to identify the most appropriate interventions to manage or eliminate the related factor. Accurate identification of nursing diagnosis (on the basis of assessment data) is important to planning patient-centred goals and subsequent nursing interventions that will best help the patient. For example, *impaired physical mobility related to bed rest* requires different interventions than those for *impaired physical mobility related to pain in the left shoulder*. Nurses need to identify and cluster defining characteristics that support the nursing diagnosis selected (Box 45-6). The diagnosis related to reluctance to initiate movement requires slightly different interventions aimed at keeping the patient as mobile as possible and encouraging the patient to perform self-care and ROM. The diagnosis related to pain requires the nurse to assist the patient with comfort measures so the patient is then willing and more able to move. In both situations, the nurse explains how activity enhances healthy body functioning.

Immobility may also lead to complications such as PEs or pneumonia. If these conditions develop, the nurse will need to collaborate with the physician or nurse practitioner for prescribed therapy to intervene.

◆ Planning

During planning, nurses synthesize information from resources such as knowledge of the roles of respiratory therapy, occupational therapy, and physiotherapy; professional standards such as the RNAO (2011a, 2011b, 2011c) guidelines for prevention of falls and pressure injuries;

BOX 45-6 NURSING DIAGNOSTIC PROCESS

Assessment Activities	Defining Characteristics	Nursing Diagnosis
Measure range of motion (ROM) during exercises of extremities.	Patient has limited ROM with left shoulder. Patient has impaired coordination while attempting to perform ROM with left shoulder.	*Impaired physical mobility related to left shoulder pain*
Observe patient use left shoulder in activities of daily living.	Patient is reluctant to attempt movement with left shoulder.	
Ask patient about perception of pain.	Patient complains of sharp pain in shoulder.	
Ask patient about endurance and activity tolerance.	Patient reports decreased muscle strength in left shoulder.	

qualities involving creativity and perseverance; and past experience with similar patients (Figure 45-10). Professional standards are especially important to consider when developing a plan of care. These standards often establish scientifically proven guidelines for selecting effective nursing interventions. As previously stated, the patient is a full partner in designing the plan of care, and this input must be reflected when establishing the goals and outcomes of care.

Goals and Outcomes. Nurses develop an individualized care plan for each nursing diagnosis (Box 45-7). It is important to set realistic expectations for care and include the patient and his or her family. Goals should be individualized, realistic, and measurable, focusing on prevention of problems or risks to body alignment and mobility.

Nurses develop goals and expected outcomes to help patients achieve their highest level of mobility and reduce the hazards of immobility. For example, a patient who has left-sided paralysis after a stroke may have two long-term goals. The first, directed toward improved mobility, is "Patient uses walker to ambulate safely around the home and grocery store." A parallel goal, directed toward the hazards of immobility, is "Patient's skin will remain intact." Both of these goals are essential to restoring the patient's maximum mobility. Because sensation is impaired, both the patient and caregivers must be aware of the patient's need to have the skin free of pressure. Expected outcomes for the goal of maintaining skin integrity include:

- Patient's skin colour and temperature return to normal baseline within 20 minutes of position change.
- Patient's skin remains dry and intact.

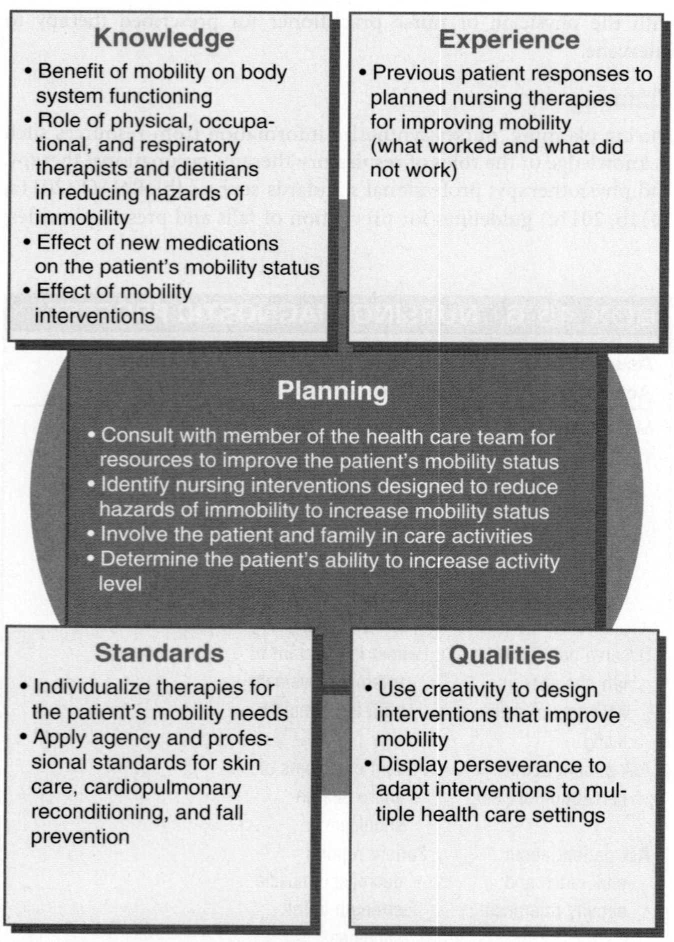

FIGURE 45-10 Critical thinking model for immobility planning.

Setting Priorities. The impact that a problem has on a patient's mental and physical health determines the immediacy of any problem. Nurses need to set priorities when planning care to ensure that immediate needs are met first. This is particularly important when patients have multiple diagnoses (Figure 45-11). Therapies should be planned according to the severity of risks to the patient. The plan should be individualized according to the patient's developmental stage, level of health, and lifestyle.

Potential complications should not be overlooked. Many times, actual problems such as pressure injuries and disuse osteoporosis get addressed only after they develop. Therefore, nurses must be vigilant in monitoring the patient, reinforcing prevention techniques to both the patient and other caregivers, and supervising unregulated care providers (UCPs) in carrying out activities aimed at preventing complications of impaired mobility.

Teamwork and Collaboration. Care of the patient experiencing alterations in mobility requires a team approach. The interventions planned for the patient may be done directly by the nurse or delegated to UCPs. UCPs can reinforce leg exercises, use of the incentive spirometer, and coughing and deep breathing. They may also turn and position patients, apply elastic stockings, and assess leg circumferences and height and weight.

Because many of the skills associated with care of the patient who is immobile can be delegated, nurses need to be vigilant in performing routine assessments to identify any developing complications early. It is also the nurse's responsibility to inform the UCP when patients are at risk for immobility hazards so that complications can be prevented. For example, although turning and positioning of a patient who is comatose may be delegated, the nurse must ensure that it is done correctly and that the position is changed frequently enough to reduce the risk of poor alignment and future injury to the skin and musculoskeletal system. The frequency of turning is based on patient assessment for risk of developing pressure injuries (see Chapter 46).

Nurses collaborate with other health team members such as physiotherapists or occupational therapists when considering a patient's mobility needs. For example, physiotherapists are a resource for planning ROM or strengthening exercises, and occupational therapists are a resource for planning ADLs that patients need to modify or relearn. Wound care specialists and respiratory therapists are often involved in patient care, especially with patients who are experiencing complications related to their immobility. The nurse can consult with a registered dietitian when the patient is experiencing nutritional problems, and consult a social worker or psychologist to assist with coping or other psychosocial issues.

Discharge planning begins when a patient enters the health care system. In anticipation of the patient's discharge from an institution, it is important to make appropriate referrals or consult a case manager to ensure that the patient's needs are met at home. The patient's home environment should be considered when setting goals and planning therapies to maintain or improve body alignment and mobility. Referrals should be made early in the care process for ongoing care and therapy at home to help the patient remain mobile or further regain mobility at home.

◆ Implementation

Health Promotion. Health promotion activities are an essential part of primary health care and include a variety of interventions that can be divided into education, prevention, and early detection. Examples of health promotion activities that address mobility and immobility include prevention of work-related injury, fall prevention measures, exercise, and early detection of bone or joint abnormalities.

BOX 45-7 NURSING CARE PLAN

Impaired Physical Mobility

ASSESSMENT

Ms. Barbara Adams, an 84-year-old patient, has been admitted for rehabilitation after a total hip replacement for osteoarthritis 5 days ago. The wound is clean, dry, and intact. Staples are to be removed in 9 days. She is weight bearing as tolerated (WBAT). She is not able to safely transfer independently from a chair to the bed. She states that she is "afraid of falling" and frequently refuses to get out of bed. She rates her pain as a 2 on a scale of 0 to 10. Ms. Adams has a history of smoking. She states that she needs pain medication to help her sleep during the night but does not need any during the day.

Assessment Activities	*Findings and Defining Characteristics*
Assess Ms. Adams's pain level. Ask her to rate her pain on a scale from 0 to 10.	She rates her pain as a 2 on a scale of 0 to 10. She states that she needs pain medication at night to help her sleep, but does not need any during the day.
Assess Ms. Adams's ability to transfer.	She is not able to transfer without assistance from chair to bed.
Ask Ms. Adams how her surgery has affected her mobility.	She responds that she is "afraid of falling," and she frequently refuses to get out of bed.
Assess Ms. Adams's wound status.	Wound is clean, dry, and intact.

NURSING DIAGNOSIS: Impaired physical mobility related to musculoskeletal impairment from surgery and a fear of falling.

PLANNING

*Goals (Nursing Outcomes Classification)**	*Expected Outcomes*
Ms. Adams will be free from skin breakdown by discharge.	***Tissue Integrity: Skin*** Patient's skin will remain intact. Patient's skin will be free of erythema.
Ms. Adams will exhibit no evidence of deep vein thrombosis (DVT) by discharge.	***Tissue Perfusion: Peripheral*** Patient's calf diameters will remain within 1 cm of baseline through discharge. Patient's lower extremity pulses will remain equal. Patient will have no complaints of calf pain.
Ms. Adams will be able to safely transfer with assistive device by discharge.	***Mobility Level*** Ms. Adams will be able to move from her bed to her chair and back again using her walker with one-person assistance within 5 days. Ms. Adams will be able to transfer from her chair to her bedside commode using her walker within 5 days. Patient will state fear of falling during transfer is less within 2 days.

*Outcome classification labels from Moorhead, S., Johnson, M., Maas, M. L., & Swanson, E. (Eds.). (2013). *Nursing outcomes classification (NOC)* (5th ed.). St. Louis, MO: Mosby.

INTERVENTIONS

Interventions (Nursing Interventions Classification)†	*Rationale*
Circulatory Care	
Administer low-dose heparin as ordered.	Administration of low-dose heparin has been shown to reduce risk for vein thrombosis.
Apply graduated compression stockings as ordered and remove them each shift for hygiene.	Application increases venous tone, improving venous return and reducing venous stasis.
Reinforce antiembolic exercises while awake.	Exercises promote venous return.
Assist patient out of bed slowly.	Moving slowly will decrease the likelihood of orthostatic hypotension. Moving the patient slowly will also avoid the perception by the patient of being rushed, which may cause the patient to become fearful.
Skin Surveillance	
Instruct patient to shift position every 1 to 1.5 hours while awake.	Position changes should occur every 1 to 1.5 hours or more frequently if needed. This reduces the risk of pressure injury development.
When patient is recumbent, place patient in 30-degree lateral position.	The 30-degree lateral position reduces pressure from the sacral area and reduces the risk of skin breakdown (RNAO, 2011a).
Keep patient's heels off bed by placing a pad under the lower legs.	Use of a thin pad under the lower legs raises the heels just enough so that a paper can slide between the heels and the bed, thereby reducing the pressure on the heels so that tissue blood flow is maintained (RNAO, 2011a).
Positioning	
Explain positioning procedure to patient.	Reduces anxiety
Refer patient to physiotherapy for transfer training.	Helps to strengthen muscles used in transfer
Encourage patient to assist in transfer and positioning.	Promotes independence
Teach patient safe positioning after total hip replacement—for example, no hip flexion >90 degrees, do not cross legs, do not lie on affected side, and when in bed use a pillow between the knees.	Minimizes risk of dislocation of hip. Patient education is important for continued rehabilitation and healing.

†Intervention classification labels from Bulechek, G. M., Butcher, H. K., & Dochterman, J. M. (Eds.). (2013). *Nursing interventions classification (NIC)* (6th ed.). St. Louis, MO: Mosby.

Continued

BOX 45-7 NURSING CARE PLAN

Impaired Physical Mobility—cont'd

EVALUATION

Nursing Actions	*Patient Response and Finding*	*Achievement of Outcome*
Ask Ms. Adams if her mobility has improved postoperatively. Observe patient transfer from bed to chair.	Patient is able to transfer from the chair to the bed with assistance.	Patient has achieved goal of transferring with assistance.
Observe Ms. Adams's skin integrity at each shift.	Patient's wound remains clean, dry, and intact. No breakdown is noted on extremities or the sacral area.	Patient has achieved outcome that skin will remain intact.
Perform circulatory assessment of extremities at every shift.	Patient's calf diameters remain within 1 cm of baseline. Swelling, pain, redness, and warmth are not evident.	DVT is not evident.
Ask Ms. Adams to rate her fear of falling on a scale of 0 to 10.	Patient rates fear of falling a 7 on a scale of 0 to 10. Patient is getting out of bed every shift.	Outcome of decrease in fear of falling has not been totally achieved. Continue to encourage patient.

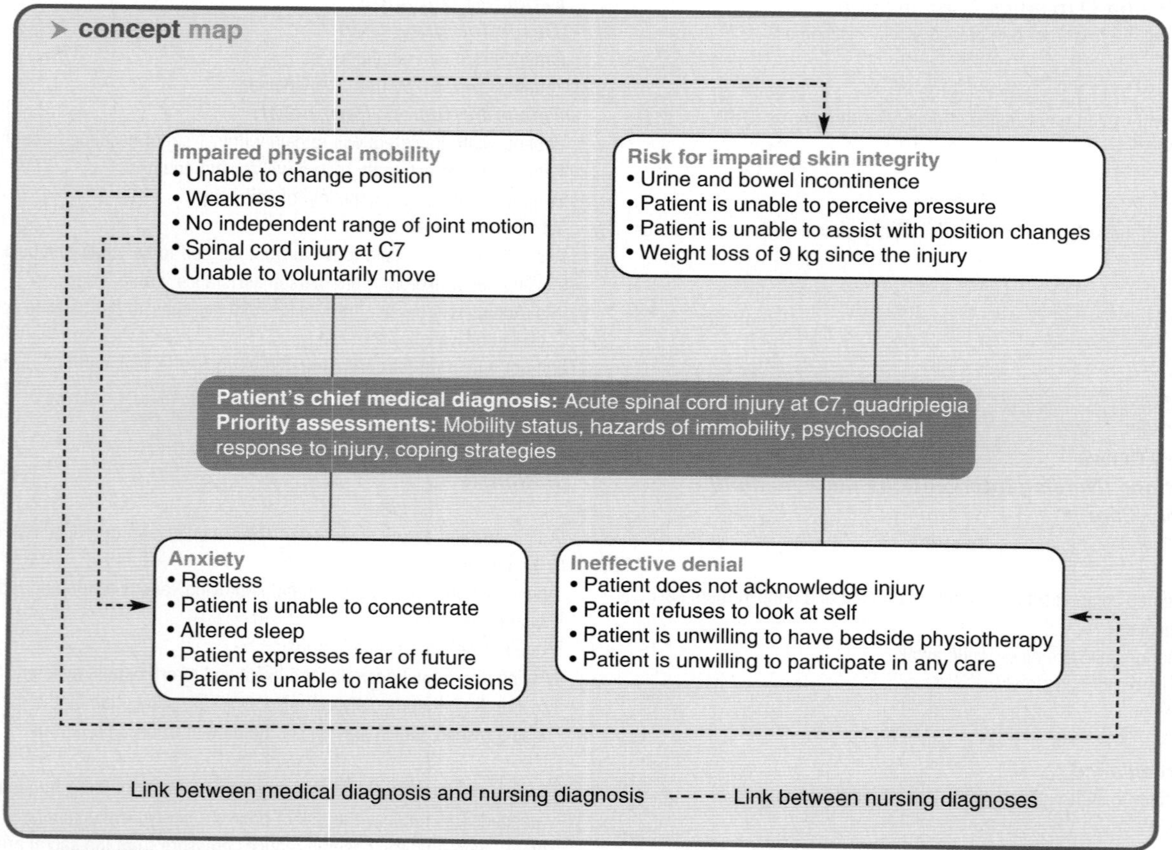

FIGURE 45-11 Concept map for patient with quadriplegia related to an acute spinal cord injury at C7.

Prevention of Work-Related Musculoskeletal Injuries. Injuries occur as a result of overexertion, which can result in back injuries and other musculoskeletal problems. Back injuries are often the direct result of improper lifting and bending. The most common back injury is strain on the lumbar muscle group, which includes the muscles around the lumbar vertebrae. Injury to these areas affects the ability to bend forward, backward, and from side to side and limits the ability to rotate the hips and lower back. Staff use of ergonomic programs in health care facilities can reduce costs, injuries to employees, and missed work days (Hunter, Branson, & Davenport, 2010).

Nurses and other health care staff are especially at risk for injury to lumbar muscles when lifting, transferring, or positioning immobilized patients. Nurses need to be aware of agency policies and protocols that protect staff and patients from injury. When transferring a patient, the nurse must always perform a functional assessment of the patient to determine the assistance the nurse will need (see Chapter 36).

Current evidence supports use of mechanical or other ergonomic assistive devices as the safest way to reposition patients who are unable to do these activities themselves. Many agencies have instituted no-lift policies (see Chapter 36).

Exercise. Although many diseases and physical problems cause or contribute to immobility, it is important to remember that exercise programs enhance feelings of well-being and improve endurance, strength, and health (see Chapter 36). Exercise reduces the risk of many health problems, such as cardiovascular disease, diabetes, and osteoporosis. The Self-Management Resource Center (2015) chronic disease self-management program encourages appropriate exercise for maintaining and improving strength, flexibility, and endurance. All patients should be encouraged to find a type of exercise that meets their lifestyle and particular health-related needs. Nurse can collaborate with a physiotherapist to design individualized exercise programs for patients who have challenges with mobility.

Acute Care

In the acute care setting, interventions are used to reduce the hazards of immobility. Nurses should know proper positioning and transferring techniques to safely move patients (see Chapter 36).

Patients in acute care settings who experience altered physical mobility may demonstrate problems associated with adverse effects of immobility, such as impaired respiratory status, orthostatic hypotension, and impaired skin integrity. Nurses need to design interventions to reduce the impact of immobility on body systems and prepare the patient for the restorative phase of care.

Metabolic System. Because the body needs protein to repair injured tissue and rebuild depleted protein stores, the patient who is immobilized should be on a high-protein, high-calorie diet. A high-calorie intake provides sufficient fuel to meet metabolic demands and replace subcutaneous tissue. The nurse should ensure that the patient is taking vitamin B and C and supplements when necessary. Supplementation with vitamin C is needed for skin integrity and wound healing; vitamin B complex assists in energy metabolism.

If the patient is unable to eat, nutrition must be provided parenterally or enterally. Enteral feedings include delivery through a nasogastric, gastrostomy, or jejunostomy tube of high-protein, high-calorie solutions with complete requirements of vitamins, minerals, and electrolytes (see Chapter 42). *Total parenteral nutrition* refers to delivery of nutritional supplements through a central or peripheral intravenous catheter.

Respiratory System. Patients who are immobilized and have reduced ventilation can benefit from a variety of nursing interventions that promote expansion of the chest and lungs, prevent stasis of pulmonary secretions, maintain a patent airway, and promote adequate exchange of respiratory gases. These patients need to frequently fully expand their lungs to maintain their elastic recoil property. In addition, secretions accumulate in the dependent areas of the lungs. Often patients with restricted mobility experience weakness; as this progresses the cough reflex gradually becomes inefficient. All of these factors put the patient at risk of developing pneumonia. The stasis of secretions in the lungs is life-threatening for an immobilized patient.

Promoting Expansion of the Chest and Lungs. To promote re-expansion of dependent lung regions, the nurse should assist the patient with repositioning at least every 2 hours. As stated earlier, re-expansion maintains the elastic recoil property of the lungs and clears the dependent lung regions of pulmonary secretions.

Deep-breathing exercises, incentive spirometry, controlled coughing, and chest physiotherapy are nursing interventions available to promote lung expansion. The patient should be encouraged to deep breathe and cough every 1 to 2 hours. Alert patients can be taught to deep breathe or yawn every hour or to use an incentive spirometer (see Chapter 39). The nurse can instruct the patient to take in three deep breaths and cough with the third exhalation. This technique produces a more forceful, productive cough without excessive fatigue. These respiratory interventions will aid alveolar expansion and prevent atelectasis. Coughing also reduces the stasis of pulmonary secretions.

Preventing Stasis of Pulmonary Secretions. Stagnant secretions accumulating in the bronchi and lungs may lead to growth of bacteria and subsequent development of pneumonia. Changing the patient's position every 2 hours can reduce stagnation of secretions. This change rotates the dependent lung, mobilizing secretions.

Patients who are immobile need to have an adequate fluid intake. Unless there is a medical contraindication, an adult needs to drink at least 1 100 to 1 400 mL of noncaffeinated fluids daily. This helps keep mucociliary clearance normal. In patients free from infection and with adequate hydration, pulmonary secretions will appear thin, watery, and clear. The patient can easily remove the secretions by coughing. Without adequate hydration, the secretions are thick and difficult to remove. Offering fluids that patients prefer on a regularly timed schedule also helps bowel and urine elimination and aids in maintaining circulation and skin integrity.

Chest physiotherapy (CPT) (percussion and positioning) is an effective method for preventing stasis of pulmonary secretions. CPT techniques help the patient to drain secretions from specific segments of the bronchi and lungs into the trachea so that the patient can cough and expel the secretions. Respiratory assessment findings can be used to identify areas of the lungs requiring CPT (see Chapter 39).

Maintaining a Patent Airway. Patients who are immobilized are generally weakened. If weakness progresses, the cough reflex gradually becomes inefficient. The stasis of secretions in the lungs may be life-threatening because hypostatic pneumonia can easily develop. The dislodging and mobilizing of the stagnant secretions reduce the risk of pneumonia. Assessment findings that indicate pneumonia include productive cough with greenish-yellow sputum; fever; pain on breathing; crackles and wheezes; and dyspnea. Nurses should actively work with patients to deep breathe and cough every 1 to 2 hours as described earlier, in the section "Promoting Expansion of the Chest and Lungs."

In the patient who is immobilized, an obstructed airway is usually the result of a mucous plug. Nurses can implement several therapies (e.g., CPT) to reduce the risk of mucous plugs and to maintain a patent airway. Nasotracheal or orotracheal suction techniques may be used to remove secretions in the upper airways of a patient who is unable to cough productively. This procedure must be performed aseptically. Nurses can also suction secretions when patients have artificial airways such as an endotracheal or tracheal tube. A catheter is inserted into the artificial airway using sterile technique. This can be used to remove pulmonary secretions from the upper and lower airways (see Chapter 39).

Cardiovascular System. The effects of bed rest or immobilization on the cardiovascular system include orthostatic hypotension, increased cardiac workload, and thrombus formation. Nursing therapies should be designed to minimize or prevent these alterations.

Reducing Orthostatic Hypotension. Patients who are immobile usually have increased pulse rate and decreased pulse pressure and blood pressure. A large decrease in blood pressure when rising to a sitting or standing position (orthostatic hypotension) can result in lightheadedness and fainting (McCance & Huether, 2014). When patients who are on bed rest or have been immobile are able to move to a sitting or standing position, they often experience orthostatic hypotension.

Interventions should be directed toward reducing or eliminating the effects of orthostatic hypotension. The nurse should attempt to get the patient moving as soon as the physical condition allows, even if this only involves sitting at the side of the bed (dangling) or moving to a chair. Changing position slowly and gradually aids in preventing orthostatic hypotension. The patient should be helped to sit on the side of the bed for a few minutes as this activity helps maintain muscle tone and increase venous return. When mobilizing a patient for the first time, the nurse should always perform a functional assessment using a safe patient handling algorithm (see Chapter 36). This is a precautionary step that prevents the nurse and patient from injury and allows the patient to do as much of the transfer as possible.

Reducing Cardiac Workload. Cardiac workload is increased by immobility. A nursing intervention that reduces cardiac workload involves instructing patients to avoid using a Valsalva manoeuvre when moving up in bed, defecating, or lifting household objects. During a Valsalva manoeuvre a patient holds the breath and strains, which increases intrathoracic pressure, thus decreasing venous return and cardiac output. When the strain is released, venous return and cardiac output immediately increase and systolic blood pressure and pulse pressure rise. These pressure changes produce a reflex bradycardia and a possible decrease in blood pressure that may cause sudden cardiac death in patients with heart disease. The patient should be reminded to breathe out while defecating, lifting, or moving side to side or moving up in bed.

Preventing Thrombus Formation. The most cost-effective way to address the problem of DVT is through prevention (prophylaxis). It begins with identifying patients at risk and continues throughout the time patients are immobile or otherwise at risk. This requires collaboration between nurses and health care providers. Using frequent patient assessment, nurses can identify risk factors. Interventions to reduce the risk of thrombus formation in patients who are immobilized include leg exercises, encouraging fluids intake, position changes, and patient teaching of preventive measures. Intervention begins when the patient becomes immobile. Preoperative patients should be given this information before surgery (see Chapter 48).

Prophylaxis also includes anticoagulation, mechanical prevention with graduated compression stockings, and intermittent pneumatic compression devices. These interventions require a prescriber's order. Anticoagulants most often prescribed include unfractionated heparin (UFH) (usually given as 5 000 units two or three times daily), low-molecular-weight heparins (LMWH) (e.g., tinzaparin, enoxaparin, and dalteparin), and vitamin K antagonists (e.g., warfarin).

Bleeding is a potential adverse effect of anticoagulant medications because anticoagulants suppress clot formation. The nurse must continually assess the patient for signs of bleeding, such as bruising, hematuria, coffee ground–like vomitus or gastrointestinal aspirate, guaiac-positive stools, and bleeding gums. Although most patients receiving prophylactic doses of anticoagulants do not experience adverse effects, the risk of bleeding is present.

SCDs and intermittent pneumatic compression (IPC) devices are used to prevent blood clots in the lower extremities. These consist of sleeves or stockings made of fabric or plastic that are wrapped around the leg and secured with Velcro (Box 45-8). The sleeves are then connected to a pump that alternately inflates and deflates the stocking around the leg. A typical cycle is inflation for 10 to 15 seconds and deflation for 45 to 60 seconds. Inflation pressures average 40 mm Hg. Use of SCDs or IPCs on the legs decreases venous stasis by increasing venous return through the deep veins of the legs. For optimal results, use of SCD or IPC devices is begun as soon as possible and maintained until the patient becomes fully ambulatory. Graduated compression stockings can help prevent DVT, but patients must receive the right size, and the SCD or IPC must be used correctly. Comprehensive nursing care includes removing the SCD or IPC every shift to verify skin integrity and assess skin for pressure points. Additionally, peripheral neurovascular assessment of the extremity including extremity colour, sensation, movement, temperature, palpation of distal pulses, and assessment for edema must be performed by the nurse every shift.

Elastic stockings (sometimes called *thromboembolic device [TED] hose* or thigh-high antiembolic stockings) aid in maintaining external

BOX 45-8 PROCEDURAL GUIDELINE

Application of Sequential Compression Stockings

Delegation Considerations

The skill of applying sequential compression stockings (SCSs) can be delegated to unregulated care providers (UCPs). The nurse is responsible for assessing circulation in the extremities; therefore, when application of the SCSs is delegated, it is important to instruct the UCP to do the following:

- Notify the nurse if the patient complains of pain in the leg.
- Notify the nurse if discoloration develops in the extremities.

Equipment

- Tape measure, sequential compression stockings, stockinette, hygiene supplies

Procedure

1. Assess the patient for the need for sequential compression stockings.
2. Obtain baseline assessment data about the status of circulation, pulse, and skin integrity on the patient's lower extremities before initiating application of sequential compression stockings.
3. Measure the patient for proper-size stocking by measuring around the largest part of the patient's thigh. Review the manufacturer's directions regarding measuring for proper fit.
4. Perform hand hygiene. Provide hygiene to lower extremities if needed.
5. Place a protective stockinette over the patient's leg.
6. Wrap the stocking around the leg, starting at the ankle, with the opening over the patella (see Step 6 illustration).
   A. Attach the stockings to the insufflator and verify that the intermittent pressure is between 35 and 45 mm Hg.
7. Record date and time of stocking application, and stocking length and size in nurses' notes.
8. Record condition of skin and circulatory assessment.
9. Monitor skin integrity and circulation to the patient's lower extremities as ordered or according to the manufacturer's guidelines.

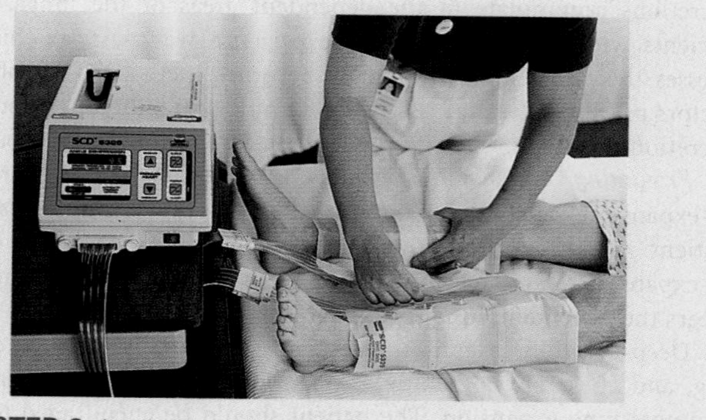

STEP 6 Application of sequential compression stocking.

pressure on the muscles of the lower extremities and thus promote venous return (Box 45-9). When considering applying elastic stockings, the nurse must first assess the patient's suitability for wearing them. Stockings should not be applied if any local condition affects the leg (e.g., any skin lesion, gangrenous condition, or recent vein ligation) because application may compromise circulation. The nurse will need to measure the patient's legs with a tape measure to determine proper stocking size. The stockings must be applied properly, and must be removed and reapplied at least once per shift. The nurse must assess circulation at the toes to ensure that the hose are not too tight. The stockings should always be clean and dry; it may be useful for the patient to have two pairs.

Proper positioning used with other therapies (e.g., heparin or elastic stockings) reduces a patient's risk of thrombus formation because compression of the leg veins is minimized. When positioning patients, the nurse must use caution to prevent pressure on the posterior knee and deep veins in the lower extremities. Patients should be taught to avoid the following: crossing the legs, sitting for prolonged periods of time, wearing clothing that constricts the legs or waist, putting pillows under the knees, and massaging the legs.

ROM exercises can reduce the risk of contractures and aid in preventing thrombi. Activity causes contraction of the skeletal muscles, which in turn exerts pressure on the veins to promote venous return, thereby reducing venous stasis. Specific exercises that help prevent thrombophlebitis are ankle pumps, foot circles, and knee flexion. Ankle pumps, sometimes called *calf pumps*, include alternating plantar flexion and dorsiflexion. To perform foot circles, the patient rotates the ankle. Encourage patients to make letters of the alphabet with their feet every 1 to 2 hours. Knee flexion involves alternately extending and flexing the knee. These exercises are sometimes referred to as antiembolic exercises and should be done hourly while the patient is awake.

Suspected DVT should be reported immediately to the patient's health care provider. The nurse needs to elevate the leg but avoid pressure on the suspected thrombus area. The family, patient, and all health care personnel should be instructed to not massage the area because of the danger of dislodging the thrombus.

Musculoskeletal System. Exercise to prevent excessive muscle atrophy and joint contractures helps maintain musculoskeletal function. If a patient is unable to move part or all of the body, the nurse can perform passive ROM exercises for all immobilized joints while bathing the patient and at least two or three more times a day (see "Restorative Care" section). If one extremity is paralyzed, the patient can be taught to put each joint independently through its ROM.

BOX 45-9 PROCEDURAL GUIDELINE

Application of Elastic Stockings

Delegation Considerations

The skill of applying elastic stockings can be performed by unregulated care providers (UCPs). The nurse is responsible for assessing circulation to the lower extremities; therefore, when application of the stockings is delegated, it is important to instruct the UCP to report if the patient develops leg pain or discoloration.

Equipment

- Tape measure, elastic stockings, hygiene supplies

Procedure

1. Assess the need for elastic stockings and condition of the patient's skin.
2. Observe for conditions that might contraindicate use of stockings.
3. Perform hand hygiene. Provide hygiene to lower extremities if needed.
4. Use tape measure to measure the patient's legs to determine proper stocking size (measure according to manufacturer's directions). Elastic stockings come in two lengths: knee length and thigh length.
5. Apply stockings:
   A. Turn elastic stocking inside out up to the heel. Place one hand into the sock, holding heel. Pull top of sock with the other hand inside out over foot of sock.
   B. Place patient's toes into the foot of the elastic stocking, making sure that sock is smooth (see Step 5B illustration).

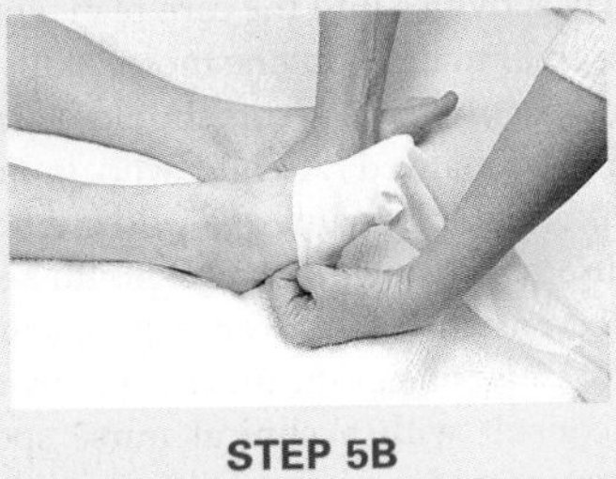

STEP 5B

   C. Slide remaining portion of sock over the patient's foot, being sure that the toes are covered. Make sure the foot fits into the toe and heel position of the sock (see Step 5C illustration).
   D. Slide top of sock up over patient's calf until sock is completely extended. Be sure sock is smooth and no ridges or wrinkles are present, particularly behind the knee (see Step 5D illustration).
6. Instruct patient not to roll socks partially down.
7. Record date and time of stocking application, and stocking length and size in nurses' notes.
8. Record condition of skin and circulatory assessment.

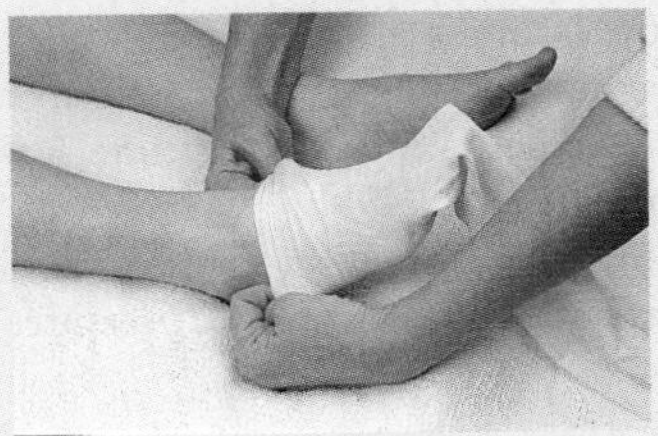

STEP 5C

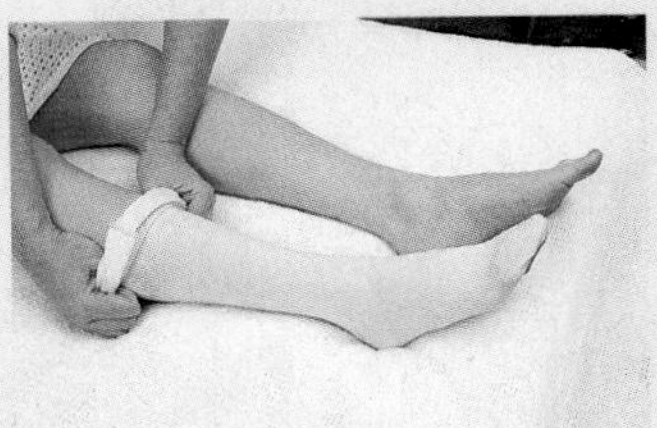

STEP 5D

Patients on bed rest should have active ROM exercises incorporated into their daily schedules. Nurses teach patients to integrate exercises during ADLs.

Some orthopedic conditions require frequent passive ROM exercises to restore the injured joint's function after surgery, such as a total knee arthroplasty. This is beneficial when the patient must gradually increase the degree and duration of flexion and extension. Patients with such conditions may use automatic equipment (continuous passive motion [CPM]) for passive ROM exercises (Figure 45-12). The CPM machine moves an extremity to a prescribed angle for a prescribed period. A multiprofessional approach is used when CPM therapy is prescribed. In most institutions, physiotherapists are responsible for first-time administration and adjustment of CPM machines. It is important to assess the patient's pain level and administer analgesia as needed before using CPM.

Elimination System. The nursing interventions for maintaining optimal urinary functioning are directed at keeping the patient well hydrated and preventing urinary stasis, calculi, and infections without causing bladder distension.

Adequate hydration (i.e., at least 1 100 to 1 400 mL of noncaffeinated fluids per day) helps prevent renal calculi and urinary tract infections. The patient who is well hydrated should void large amounts of dilute urine that are approximately equal to fluid intake. If the patient is incontinent, the care plan can be modified to include toileting aids and a hygiene schedule so that the increased urinary output does not cause skin breakdown.

To prevent bladder distension, the nurse needs to assess the frequency and amount of urinary output. A patient who continually dribbles urine and whose bladder is distended may have overflow incontinence. If the patient does not have voluntary control of bladder elimination, bladder training may be necessary. If the patient experiences bladder distension, the nurse may be required to insert a straight catheter or an in-dwelling Foley catheter (see Chapter 43).

The frequency and consistency of bowel movements must be recorded. A diet rich in fluids, fruits, vegetables, and fibre can facilitate normal peristalsis. If a patient is unable to maintain regular bowel patterns, stool softeners, cathartics, or enemas may be needed (see Chapter 44).

Integumentary System. The major risk to the skin from restricted mobility is the formation of pressure injuries. Early identification of high-risk patients helps prevent pressure injuries. As stated earlier, preventing a pressure injury is much less expensive than treating one, and thus preventive nursing interventions are imperative, as outlined in the RNAO (2011a) Best Practice Guideline *Risk Assessment and Prevention of Pressure Ulcers.*

Interventions aimed at prevention include positioning, skin care, and the use of therapeutic devices to relieve pressure. The immobilized patient's position should be changed according to the patient's activity level, perceptual ability, treatment protocols, and daily routines. Although turning the patient every 1 to 2 hours is recommended for preventing pressure injuries, it may also be necessary to use devices for relieving pressure on the skin. The amount of time that a patient sits uninterrupted in a chair should be limited to 1 hour or less, although this time interval is individualized. Patients need to be repositioned frequently because uninterrupted pressure leads to skin breakdown. Nurses need to teach patients who are able to shift their weight in a chair to do so every 15 minutes. Patients who are chair-bound should have a device for the chair that reduces pressure; however, doughnut-shaped devices should not be used (RNAO, 2011a). If a pressure injury does develop, treatment should commence immediately based on RNAO's (2007) Best Practice Guideline *Assessment and Management of Stage I–IV Pressure Ulcers.*

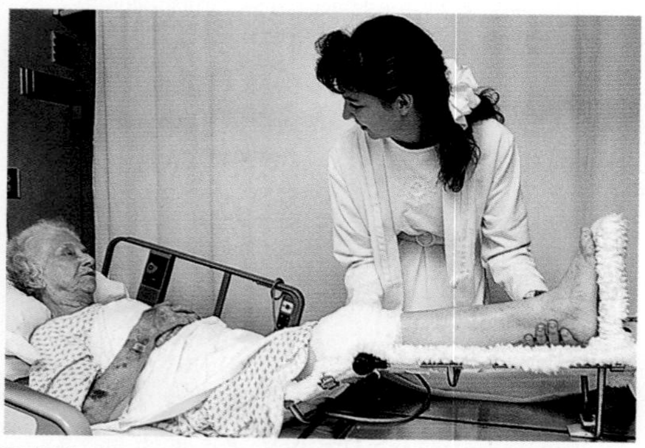

FIGURE 45-12 Continuous passive motion machine.

Psychosocial Changes. Nurse can use assessment data to identify the psychosocial effects of prolonged immobilization. People who have a tendency toward depression or mood swings are at greater risk for developing psychosocial changes during bed rest or immobilization.

The nurse should anticipate changes in the patient's psychosocial status and provide routine and informal socialization. The nurse needs to observe the patient's ability to cope with restricted mobility. If the nursing care plan is not improving coping patterns, a clinical nurse specialist, counsellor, social worker, spiritual advisor, or other consultant may be needed. Their recommendations should be incorporated into the care plan.

Nursing activities should be planned to enable a patient to talk and interact with staff. If possible, the patient should be placed in a room with others who are mobile and interactive. If a private room is required, staff members and family should be asked to visit throughout the shift to provide meaningful interaction.

Nurses can provide stimuli to maintain a patient's orientation. Maintaining a calendar and clock; providing a newspaper, books, radio, or television; and encouraging visits from significant others may reduce the risk of social isolation and delirium (RNAO, 2016). Spending time in the room talking and listening to the patient also helps reduce isolation.

Nurses can involve patients in their care by encouraging them to perform as many ADLs as independently as possible. Patients should continue to perform personal grooming if they did so before their mobility was restricted. This type of activity preserves the patient's dignity and gives the patient a sense of accomplishment.

In institutional health care settings, nursing care activities should not be scheduled between 2200 hours and 0700 hours to minimize interruptions of sleep. For example, the nurse may administer medications and assess vital signs at the time when the patient is turned or receives special skin care.

Developmental Changes in Children. Ideally, patients with mobility challenges continue normal development; nursing interventions can help with this. Nursing care needs to provide mental and physical stimulation, particularly for a young child. Nurses need to incorporate play activities into the care plan. For example, completing puzzles helps a child to develop fine motor skills, and reading helps the child to develop cognitively. Parents should be encouraged to stay with a child who is hospitalized. A child who is immobilized should be placed with children of the same age who are not immobilized, unless a contagious disease is present. A child should be allowed to participate in nursing interventions such as dressing changes and cast care. The nurse needs to assess for significant changes from normal behavioural patterns and consult with a clinical nurse specialist, counsellor, or other health care provider who specializes in children when needed.

Positioning Devices and Techniques. Patients with impaired function of the nervous, skeletal, or muscular system and with general weakness often require help to attain proper body alignment while in bed or sitting. Skin integrity should be assessed regularly for pressure points or skin breakdown when using positioning devices.

Several positioning devices are available for maintaining good body alignment for patients:

- *Pillows:* Provide support, elevate body parts, and can splint incisional areas, reducing postoperative pain during activity or coughing and deep breathing. Before using a pillow, determine whether it is the proper size. A thick pillow under the patient's head increases cervical flexion, leading to strain on joints and muscles of the neck and upper back, and compression of blood vessels and nerves that supply the neck. A thin pillow under body prominences may be inadequate to protect skin and tissue from damage caused by pressure. When additional pillows are unavailable, or if they are an improper size, use folded sheets, blankets, or towels as positioning aids.
- *Wedge (or abductor) pillow:* This is a triangular-shaped pillow made of heavy foam used to maintain the legs in abduction after total hip replacement surgery.
- *Foot boot:* Prevents footdrop by maintaining the feet in dorsiflexion. Foot boots are made of rigid plastic or heavy foam (Figure 45-13). They keep the foot flexed at the proper angle and the weight of the bed sheets off the toes. Remove the foot boots two or three times a day to assess skin integrity and joint mobility.
- *Trochanter roll:* Prevents external rotation of the hips when the patient is in a supine position. A trochanter roll is formed by folding a cotton bath blanket lengthwise to a width that will extend from the greater trochanter of the femur to the lower border of the popliteal space (Figure 45-14). The blanket is placed under the buttocks and then rolled counterclockwise until the thigh is in neutral position or in inward rotation. When correct alignment of the hip is achieved, the patella faces directly upward.
- *Sandbags:* These are sand-filled plastic tubes or bags that can be shaped to body contours. Sandbags can be used in place of or in addition to trochanter rolls. They immobilize an extremity or maintain body alignment.
- *Hand rolls:* These maintain the thumb in slight adduction and in opposition to the fingers. A hand roll maintains the hand, thumb, and fingers in a functional position, thus preventing contractures (Figure 45-15). Evaluate the hand roll to make sure that the hand is indeed in a functional position. Hand rolls are most often used for patients whose arms are paralyzed or who are unconscious. Do not use rolled washcloths as hand rolls, because they do not keep the thumb well abducted, especially in patients who have a spastic paralysis.
- *Hand–wrist splints:* These are individually moulded for the patient to maintain proper alignment of the thumb (slight adduction) and the wrist (slight extension). Use splints only on the patient for whom the splint was made (Figure 45-16) and follow the splint schedule (e.g., wear for 2 hours, remove for 2 hours).
- *Trapeze bar:* This is a triangular device that descends from a securely fastened overhead bar attached to the bed frame. A trapeze bar allows the patient to use his or her upper extremities to raise the trunk off the bed, to assist in transfer from the bed to a wheelchair, or to perform arm exercises (Figure 45-17). It is a useful device for increasing independence, maintaining upper body strength, and decreasing the shearing action from sliding across or up and down in bed.

Although each procedure for positioning has specific guidelines, there are universal steps to follow for patients who require positioning

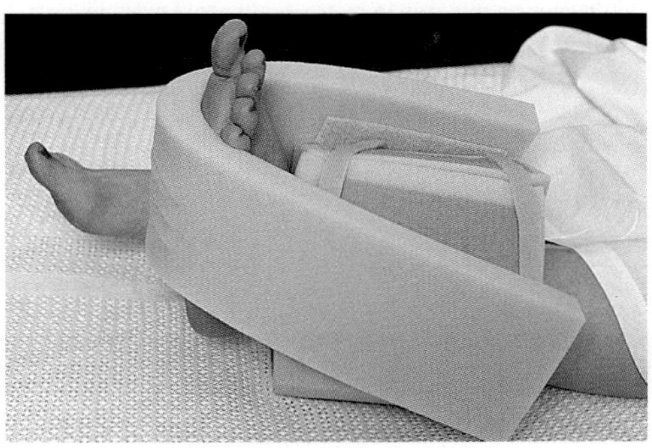

FIGURE 45-13 Foot boot.

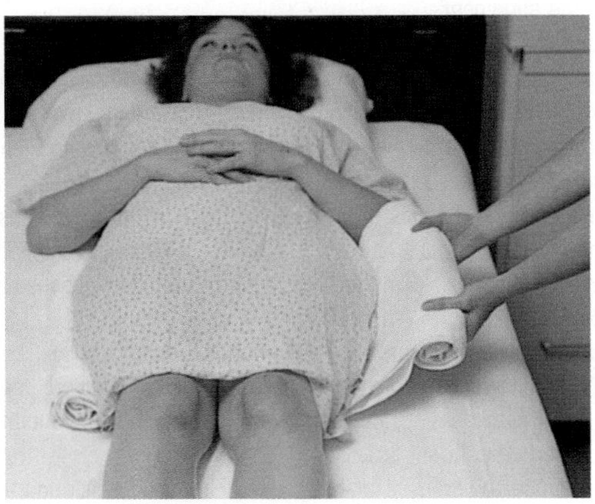

FIGURE 45-14 Trochanter roll.

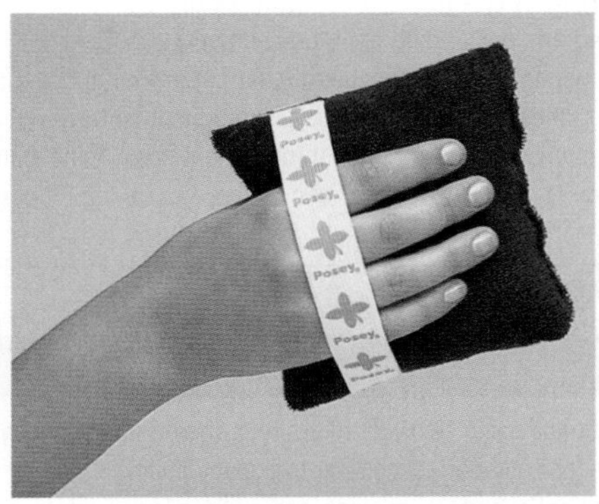

FIGURE 45-15 Hand roll. (Courtesy J. T. Posey, Arcadia, CA.)

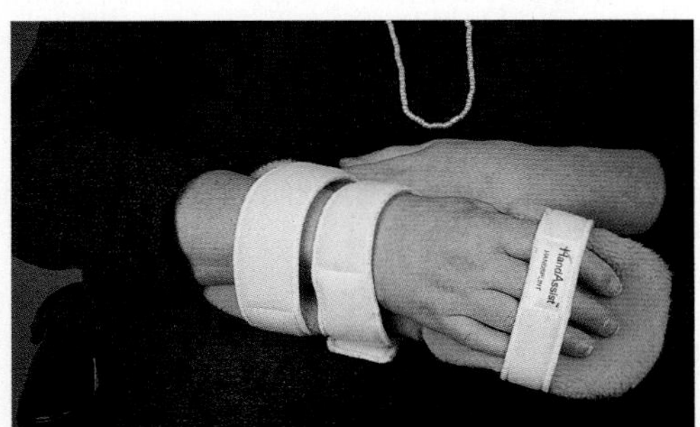

FIGURE 45-16 Hand–wrist splint. (From Sorrentino, S. A., Wilk, M. J., & Newmaster, R. [2009]. *Mosby's Canadian textbook for the support worker* [2nd ed., p. 431, Fig. 24-8]. Toronto: Elsevier.)

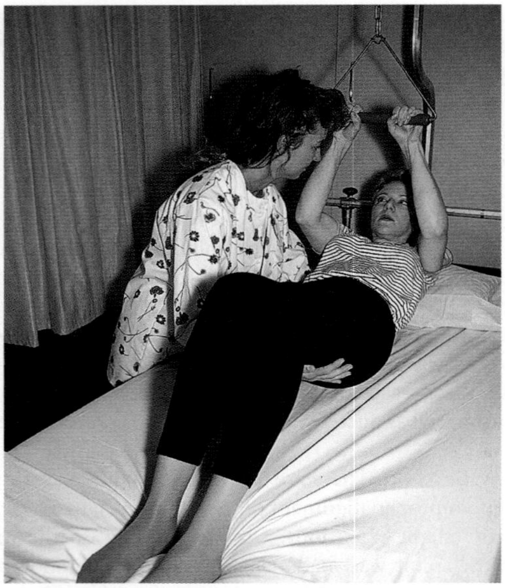

FIGURE 45-17 Patient using a trapeze bar.

assistance (Skill 45-1). Following the guidelines reduces the risk of injury to the musculoskeletal system when a patient is lying or sitting. When joints are unsupported, their alignment is impaired. Joints must be positioned in a slightly flexed position or their mobility is decreased. During positioning, the nurse must also assess bony prominences (pressure points; see Figure 46-2). When actual or potential pressure areas exist, nursing interventions involve removal of the pressure, thus decreasing the risk for development of pressure injuries and further trauma to the musculoskeletal system. For these patients the 30-degree lateral position is used.

Supported Fowler's Position. In the supported Fowler's position, the head of the bed is elevated 45 to 60 degrees and the patient's knees are slightly elevated without pressure to restrict circulation in the lower legs; the patient is sitting up in bed. The head of the bed should not be elevated more than 60 degrees because this would increase shearing force on the patient's back and heels. The patient's illness and overall condition influence the angle of head and knee elevation and the length of time that the patient should remain in the supported Fowler's position. Supports must permit flexion of the hips and knees and proper alignment of the normal curves in the cervical, thoracic, and lumbar vertebrae. The following are common trouble areas for the

SKILL 45-1 MOVING AND POSITIONING PATIENTS IN BED

Delegation Considerations

The skills of moving and positioning patients in bed can be delegated to unregulated care providers (UCPs). The nurse is responsible for assessing the patient's level of comfort and for any potential hazards. Instruct the UCP about:

- Any moving and positioning limitations unique to patient
- Individual needs for body alignment (e.g., patient with spinal cord injury)
- Scheduled times to reposition patient throughout shift
- When to request assistance (e.g., if the patient has a spinal cord injury, when the patient is unable to assist the nurse, has a lot of equipment, or is confused)

Equipment

- Pillows
- Appropriate safe patient-handling assistive device (e.g., friction-reducing transfer sheet)
- Positioning devices as required (e.g., trochanter roll, extra pillows, hand rolls)
- Side rails

ASSESSMENT

STEPS	RATIONALE
1. Identify patient using two identifiers (e.g., name and birthday or name and medical record number), according to agency policy.	• Ensures correct patient. Complies with the Joint Commission (2018) standards and improves patient safety.
2. Assess patient's body alignment and comfort level while patient is lying down.	• Provides baseline data for later comparisons. Determines ways to improve position and alignment.
3. Assess for risk factors that may contribute to complications of immobility:	• Increased risk factors require more frequent repositioning.
• Paralysis: Hemiparesis resulting from cerebrovascular accident (CVA); decreased sensation	• Paralysis impairs movement and causes muscle tone changes; sensation is often affected. Because of difficulty in moving and poor awareness of the involved body part, the patient is unable to protect and position the affected body part (Lewis et al., 2013).
• Impaired mobility: Traction or arthritis or other contributing disease processes	• Traction or arthritic changes of affected extremity result in decreased range of motion (ROM).
• Impaired circulation	• Decreased circulation to skin and underlying tissues predisposes the patient to pressure sores.
• Age: Very young, older persons	• Premature and young infants require frequent turning because their skin is fragile. Normal physiological changes associated with aging predispose older persons to greater risks for developing complications of immobility (Drake, Redfern, Sherburne, et al., 2012).
• Sensation: Decreased from CVA, paralysis, neuropathy	• Because of poor awareness of body part or reduced sensation, patient is unable to protect and position body part from pressure.

STEPS	RATIONALE
• Level of consciousness and mental status	• Determines need for special aids or devices. Patients with altered levels of consciousness may not understand instructions or be able to help during positioning.
• Assess condition of patient's skin.	• Provides a baseline to determine effects of positioning.
4. Assess patient's physical ability to help with moving and positioning:	• Enables nurse to use patient's mobility, coordination, and strength. Determines need for additional help. Ensures patient's and nurse's safety (VISN8, 2015).
• Age	• Some older persons may move more slowly and with less strength.
• Disease process	• Cardiopulmonary disease may require the patient to have the head of the bed elevated.
• Strength, coordination	• Determines amount of assistance provided by patient during position change.
• ROM	• Limited ROM may contraindicate certain positions.
5. Assess health care provider's orders before positioning. Clarify whether any positions are contraindicated because of the patient's condition (e.g., spinal cord injury; respiratory difficulties; certain neurological conditions; presence of incisions, drain, or tubing).	• Placing patient in an inappropriate position could cause injury.
6. Perform hand hygiene.	• Reduces transfer of microorganisms.
7. Assess for the presence of tubes, incisions, and equipment (e.g., traction).	• Alters positioning procedure and affects patient's ability to independently change positions.
8. Assess the ability and motivation of the patient, family members, and primary caregiver to participate in moving and positioning the patient in bed in anticipation of discharge to home.	• Determines ability of the patient and caregivers to assist with positioning.
PLANNING	
1. Collect appropriate equipment. Based on functional assessment of the patient, get assistance as needed. Close door to room or bedside curtains.	• Having appropriate number of people to position patient prevents patient and nurse injury. Provides for patient privacy.
2. Perform hand hygiene.	• Reduces transfer of microorganisms.
3. Adjust level of bed to a comfortable working height. If two or multiple nurses are involved in positioning, raise height of the bed to the comfort zone of the tallest nurse.	• Raises level of work to centre of gravity and provides for patient's and nurse's safety. • For the tallest nurse, adjusting bed to his or her working height prevents exaggerated bending at the waist, which can lead to injury when repositioning.
4. Remove all pillows and devices used for positioning.	• Reduces interference with positioning.
5. Explain procedure to patient.	• Decreases anxiety and increases patient cooperation.
IMPLEMENTATION	
1. Assist patient in moving up in bed.	• Determines degree of risk in repositioning patient and technique required to safely assist patient.
A. Can patient assist?	
(1) Fully able to assist, nurse assistance not needed; nurse stands by to assist.	
(2) Partially able to assist; patient can assist with nurse using positioning cues or aids (e.g., friction-reducing transfer sheet).	

CRITICAL DECISION POINT: *Before lowering head of bed to flatten bed, account for all tubing, drains, and equipment to prevent dislodgement or tipping if caught in the mattress or bed frame as bed is lowered.*

STEPS	RATIONALE
B. Assist patient in moving up in bed using friction-reducing transfer sheets (two or more nurses).	• This is not a one-person task. Helping a patient move up in bed without help from other co-workers or without the aid of assistive devices is not recommended or considered safe for the patient or the nurse. If the patient is unable to fully assist, refer to Step C.
(1) Position patient supine with head or bed flat or in Trendelenburg position in bed if this is tolerated. A nurse stands on each side of bed.	• Enables nurse to assess body alignment. Reduces pull of gravity, friction, and possible shear on patient's skin. With the bed in Trendelenburg position, gravity helps with moving patient proximally in bed.
(2) Lower side rails. Remove pillow from under the head and shoulders, and place pillow at head of bed.	• Prevents striking of patient's head against head of the bed.
(3) Turn patient side to side to place repositioning device under patient. Ensure patient's shoulders and hips are on the repositioning device being used.	• Reduces surface area and friction. • Supports patient's body weight and reduces friction during movement.

Continued

SKILL 45-1 MOVING AND POSITIONING PATIENTS IN BED—cont'd

STEPS	RATIONALE
(4) Return patient to supine position. Instruct patient to lie flat on back, cross arms on chest, and bend the knees. If the patient is unable to bend knees, place a pillow under lower legs to decrease friction during repositioning.	• Even distribution of the patient's weight makes lifting and positioning easier.
(5) Fanfold repositioning device (e.g., friction-reducing transfer sheet) on both sides, with each nurse grasping firmly (palms up) near the patient.	• Provides strong handles to grip transfer sheet without slipping. Palms-up grip is safe and effective as it promotes use of the more powerful biceps muscles.
(6) Nurses or workers assume a six-checkpoint position (Alberta Health Services, 2010): **(a)** "3 for the top"—ears over shoulders and shoulders over hips **(b)** "3 for the bottom"—tighten stomach and push buttocks back while keeping body weight over the heels. Reposition trunk forward by bending at the hips and not at the waist. **(c)** Elbows tucked in **(d)** Safe effective grip (palms up) **(e)** Comfort zone (bend elbows and tuck elbows into sides, move hands to shoulders and to hips) **(f)** Weight transfer—stable base, transfer side to side and front to back	• Promotes optimal body mechanics. • Maintains three natural curves of the spine. • Stable and flexible base helps maintain balance and centre of gravity during transfer. • Keeps load close. • Facilitates use of more powerful quadriceps and biceps muscle groups.
(7) Grasp top sheet at the patient's shoulder and hip level (palms up). Place feet shoulder-width apart and point foot nearest the head of the bed in the direction of the move (forward–backward stance; see Step 1B[7] illustration).	• Facing the direction of movement prevents twisting of nurse's body while moving the patient. • A stable base of support increases balance. This stance enables the nurse to shift body weight as the patient is repositioned up in bed, thereby reducing force needed to move load.
(8) Instruct patient to flex neck, tilting chin toward chest.	• Prevents hyperextension of neck when moving patient up in bed.
(9) Instruct patient to assist moving by bending knees and pushing with feet on bed surface.	• Reduces friction. Increases patient mobility. Decreases workload.
(9) The primary nurse counts, "1-2-3 slide." Instruct patient to push with heels and elevate trunk while breathing out on the command word "slide" thus moving toward head of bed.	• Prepares patient for repositioning. Reinforces assistance in moving up in bed. Increases patient cooperation. Breathing out avoids Valsalva manoeuvre.
(10) On command "slide," rock and shift weight from back to front leg. At the same time, the patient pushes with heels and elevates trunk.	• Rocking enables the nurse to improve balance and overcome inertia. Shifting weight counteracts the patient's weight and reduces the force needed to move load. The patient's assistance reduces friction and workload.
(11) Tuck in top sheet of friction-reducing transfer sheet after repositioning. If using transitory slider sheet, remove from under patient.	• Patient will slide if slider set remains under patient.

2. Position patient in one of the following positions using correct body alignment to protect pressure areas. Begin with patient lying supine and reposition in bed following Step 1B.

A. Position patient in supported Fowler's position (see Step 2A illustration).

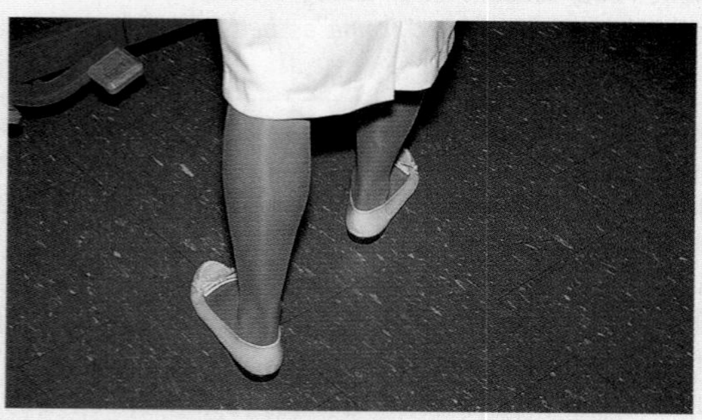

STEP 1B(7) Position of feet: feet placed apart in a forward-to-backward stance.

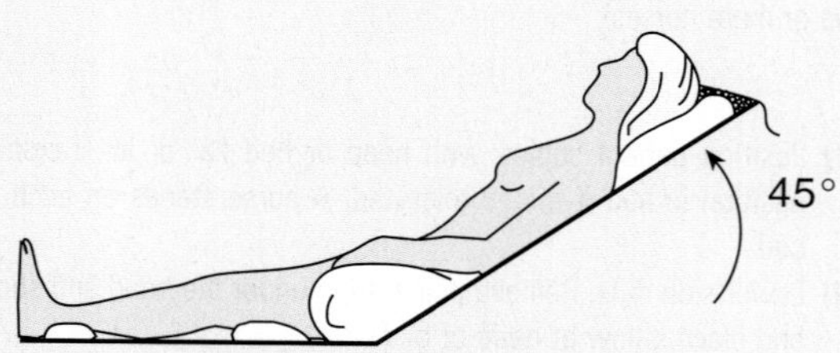

STEP 2A Supported Fowler's position.

STEPS	RATIONALE
(1) With patient supine, elevate head of bed 45 to 60 degrees if not contraindicated.	• Increases comfort, improves ventilation, and increases patient's opportunity to socialize or relax.
(2) Rest patient's head against mattress or on a small pillow.	• Prevents flexion contractures of cervical vertebrae.
(3) Use pillows to support arms and hands if the patient does not have voluntary control or use of hands and arms.	• Prevents shoulder subluxation from effect of downward pull of unsupported arms, promotes circulation by preventing venous pooling, and prevents flexion contractures of arms and wrists.

STEPS	RATIONALE
(4) Position pillow at lower back.	• Supports lumbar vertebrae and decreases flexion of vertebrae.
(5) Place a small pillow under thigh.	• Prevents hyperextension of knee and occlusion of popliteal artery caused by pressure from body weight.
(6) Position patient's heel in heel boots or other heel pressure relief devices.	• Heel pressure relief devices are more effective than pillows for consistently reducing pressure from the mattress on the heels. When pillows are used, they must be repositioned each time the patient moves or is repositioned (Bangova, 2013).

CRITICAL DECISION POINT: *To keep feet in proper alignment and prevent footdrop, use foot support devices. A foot cradle may also be used in patients with poor peripheral circulation as a means of reducing pressure on the tips of a patient's toes.*

STEPS	RATIONALE
B. Position patient with hemiplegia in supported Fowler's position.	
(1) Elevate head of bed 45 to 60 degrees. Adjust head of bed according to patient's condition. For example, those with increased risk of pressure injuries remain at a 30-degree angle (semi-Fowler's).	• Increases comfort, improves ventilation, and increases patient's opportunity to relax.
(2) Position patient in sitting position as straight as possible.	• Counteracts tendency to slump toward affected side. Improves ventilation and cardiac output, and decreases intracranial pressure. Improves patient's ability to swallow and helps to prevent aspiration of food, liquids, and gastric secretions.
(3) Position head on a small pillow with the chin slightly forward. If patient is totally unable to control head movement, avoid hyperextension of the neck.	• Prevents hyperextension of neck. Too many pillows under the head may cause or worsen neck flexion contracture.
(4) Provide support for involved arm and hand on overbed table in front of patient. Place arm away from patient's side and support elbow with pillow. • Position *flaccid* hand in a normal resting position with the wrist slightly extended, arches of hand maintained, and fingers partially flexed. You may use a hand grip or section of rubber ball cut in half; clasp patient's hands together. • Position *spastic* hand with wrist in neutral position or slightly extended; fingers should be extended with palm down. It may be difficult to position spastic hands without the use of specially made splints for the patient (discuss with occupational therapist).	• Paralyzed muscles do not automatically resist pull of gravity as they do normally. As a result, shoulder subluxation, pain, and edema may occur.
(5) Flex patient's knees and hips by using a pillow or folded blanket under the knees.	• Ensures proper alignment. Flexion prevents prolonged hyperextension, which could impair joint mobility.
(6) Support feet in dorsiflexion with firm pillow or therapeutic boots or splints.	• Prevents footdrop. Stimulation of ball of the foot by a hard surface has a tendency to increase muscle tone in a patient with extensor spasticity of lower extremity. Therapeutic boots or splints are manufactured with thick padding to cushion the heel and prevent pressure injuries.
C. Position patient in supported supine position.	
(1) Be sure patient is comfortable on back with head of bed flat.	• Some patients' physical conditions will not tolerate a supine position.
(2) Place a small rolled towel under the lumbar area of the back.	• Provides support for lumbar spine.
(3) Place a pillow under upper shoulders, neck, or head.	• Maintains correct alignment and prevents flexion contractures of cervical vertebrae.
(4) Place trochanter rolls or sandbags parallel to lateral surface of the patient's thighs if patient is immobile.	• Reduces external rotation of hip.
(5) Position patient's heels in heel boots or other heel pressure relief device (check agency policy).	• Heel pressure relief devices are more effective than pillows for consistently reducing pressure from the mattress on the heels. Reducing pressure on heels prevents possible pressure sores.
(6) If needed, support feet in dorsiflexion with foot support devices (check agency policy).	• Maintains dorsiflexion and prevents footdrop.

Continued

SKILL 45-1 MOVING AND POSITIONING PATIENTS IN BED—cont'd

STEPS	RATIONALE
(7) Place pillows under pronated forearms, keeping upper arms parallel to patient's body (see Step 2C[7] illustrations).	• Reduces internal rotation of shoulder and prevents extension of elbows. Maintains correct body alignment.

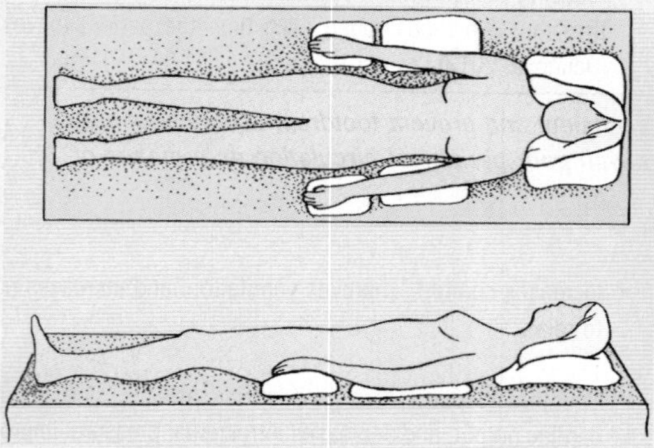

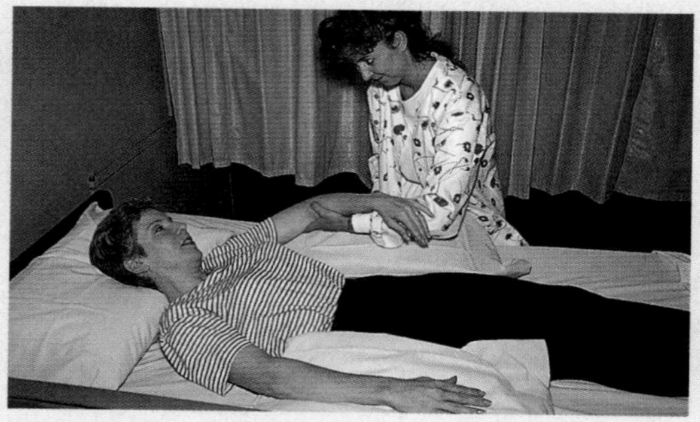

STEP 2C(7) Supine position with pillows in place.

STEPS	RATIONALE
(8) Place hand rolls in patient's hands. Consider occupational therapy referral for use of hand splints, if necessary.	• Reduces extension of fingers and abduction of thumb. Maintains thumb slightly adducted and in opposition to fingers.
D. Position hemiplegic patient in supine position.	
(1) Assess patient to determine that the person is comfortable on his or her back with the head of bed flat.	• Some patients' physical conditions do not tolerate supine position.
(2) Place folded towel or small pillow under shoulder of affected side.	• Decreases possibility of pain, joint contracture, and subluxation. Maintains mobility in muscles around shoulder to permit normal movement patterns.
(3) Keep affected arm away from body with elbow extended and palm up. (An alternative is to place arm out to side, with elbow bent and hand toward head of the bed.)	• Maintains mobility in arm, joints, and shoulder to permit normal movement patterns. (Alternative position counteracts limitation of ability of arm to rotate outward at shoulder [external rotation]. External rotation must be present to raise arm overhead without pain.)

CRITICAL DECISION POINT: *Position the affected hand in one of the recommended positions for flaccid or spastic hand.*

STEPS	RATIONALE
(4) Place a folded towel under the hip of patient's involved side.	• Diminishes effect of spasticity in entire leg by controlling hip position.
(5) Flex affected knee 30 degrees by supporting it on a pillow or folded blanket.	• Slight flexion breaks up abnormal extension pattern of leg. Extensor spasticity is most severe when the patient is supine.
(6) If needed, support feet in dorsiflexion with foot support devices (check agency policy).	• Maintains foot in dorsiflexion and prevents footdrop. Foot support devices prevent stimulation to ball of foot by hard surface, which has a tendency to increase muscle tone in a patient with extensor spasticity of lower extremity.
E. Position patient in prone position. This requires two staff members to safely position patient.	• In certain patients with pulmonary conditions such as acute respiratory distress syndrome, the use of a prone position can help improve oxygenation.
(1) With a repositioning device under patient and one nurse standing on each side of the bed, reposition patient toward one side of the bed. Ensure that side rail on opposite side is up for safety.	• Prepares patient for positioning.
(2) With patient supine, the primary nurse grasps the top sheet at the patient's shoulder and hip level using a safe effective grip (palms up, elbows tucked in to sides) and assumes a position to use a front-to-back weight transfer.	• Promotes use of stronger biceps muscles. Front-to-back weight transfer promotes nurses' safety by preventing rotation of spine that can lead to injury.
(3) The secondary nurse positions to perform a back-to-front weight transfer and places hands on the patient's shoulder and hip to provide directional guidance only.	
(4) Primary nurse counts "1-2-3 slide," and on command word "slide" primary worker performs a front-to-back weight transfer while the secondary worker uses a back-to-front weight transfer. Nurses use a combined slide-and-turn motion so the patient first slides toward the primary worker and is then turned onto his or her side. At the end of the move, the patient will be facing the secondary nurse.	

STEPS	RATIONALE
(5) Roll patient over arm positioned close to body, with elbow straight and hand under hip. Position on abdomen in centre of the bed.	• Positions patient correctly so that alignment can be maintained. • Diminishes effects of spasticity in entire leg by controlling hip position. Slight hip flexion breaks up abnormal extension pattern of leg; extensor spasticity is most severe when the patient is supine.
(6) Turn patient's head to one side and support head with a small pillow (see Step 2E[6] illustration).	• Reduces flexion or hyperextension of cervical vertebrae.
(7) Place small pillow under patient's abdomen below level of diaphragm (see Step 2E[7] illustration).	• Reduces pressure on breasts of some female patients and decreases hyperextension of lumbar vertebrae and strain on lower back. Improves breathing by reducing mattress pressure on diaphragm.
(8) Support arms in flexed position, level at shoulders.	• Maintains proper body alignment. Support reduces risk of joint dislocation.
(9) Support lower legs with pillows to elevate toes (see Step 2E[9] illustration).	• Prevents footdrop. Reduces external rotation of hips. Reduces mattress pressure on toes.

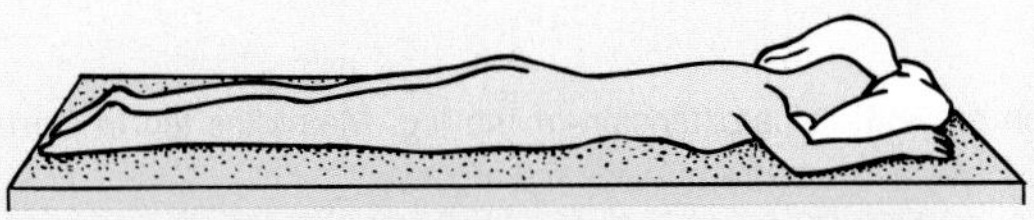

STEP 2E(6) Prone position, head supported with pillow.

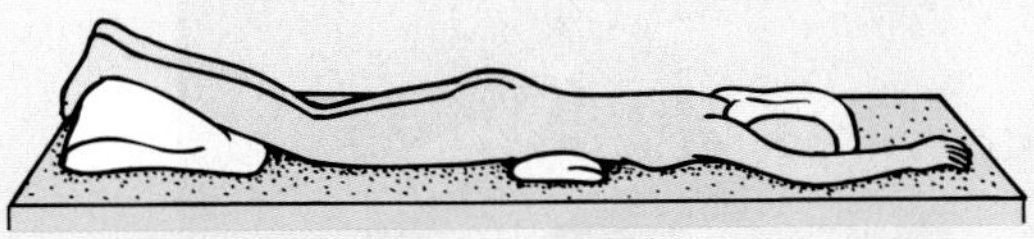

STEP 2E(7) Prone position, pillow under patient's abdomen and feet.

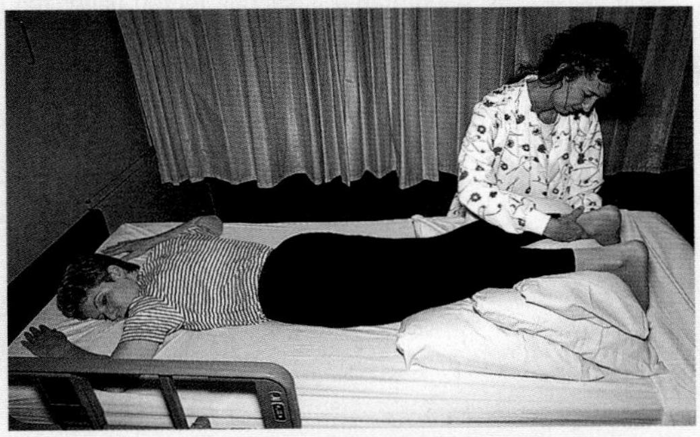

STEP 2E(9) Prone position with pillows supporting lower legs.

F. Position patient with hemiplegia in prone position.

CRITICAL DECISION POINT: *Increase frequency of position changes if pressure areas begin to appear, joint mobility becomes impaired or worsened, or patient complains of discomfort. Consult with physiotherapist and occupational therapist as needed. Use 30-degree lateral position to help prevent pressure injuries.*

STEPS	RATIONALE
(1) Move patient toward unaffected side.	• Creates room for proper patient alignment in centre of bed when patient is rolled onto abdomen.
(2) Roll patient onto side.	
(3) Place pillow on patient's abdomen.	• Prevents sagging of abdomen when patient is rolled over; decreases hyperextension of lumbar vertebrae and strain on lower back.
(4) Roll patient onto abdomen by positioning involved arm close to patient's body, with elbow straight and hand under hip. Roll patient carefully over arm.	• Prevents injury to affected side.
(5) Turn head toward involved side.	• Promotes development of neck and trunk extension, which is necessary for standing and walking.
(6) Position involved arm out to side, with elbow bent, hand toward head of bed, and fingers extended (if possible).	• Counteracts limitation of the arm's ability to rotate outward at the shoulder (external rotation). External rotation must be present to raise arm over head without pain.
(7) Flex knees slightly by placing pillow under legs from knees to ankles.	• Flexion prevents prolonged hyperextension, which could impair joint mobility.
(8) Keep feet at right angle to legs by using a pillow high enough to keep toes off mattress.	• Maintains feet in dorsiflexion.
G. Position patient in 30-degree lateral (side-lying) position.	
(1) Lower head of bed completely or as low as the patient can tolerate.	• Provides position of comfort for patient and removes pressure from bony prominences on back and buttocks.
(2) Position patient in supine position at side of bed opposite direction toward which patient is to be turned. Reposition upper trunk, supporting shoulders first, followed by repositioning of lower trunk, supporting hips. Raise side rails and move to opposite side of bed.	• Provides room for patient to turn to side.
(3) Prepare to turn patient onto side. Flex patient's knee that will not be next to mattress. Place one hand on the patient's hip and one hand on the patient's shoulder.	• Positioning will set up leverage for easy turning.
(4) Roll patient onto side toward you.	• Rolling decreases trauma to tissues. In addition, patient is positioned so that leverage on hip makes turning easy.

Continued

SKILL 45-1 MOVING AND POSITIONING PATIENTS IN BED—cont'd

STEPS	RATIONALE
(5) Place pillow under patient's head and neck.	• Maintains alignment. Reduces lateral neck flexion. Decreases strain on sternocleidomastoid muscle.
(6) Bring shoulder blade forward.	• Prevents patient's weight from resting directly on shoulder joint.
(7) Position both arms in a slightly flexed position. The upper arm is supported by a pillow level with the shoulder; the other arm, by the mattress.	• Decreases internal rotation and adduction of the shoulder. Supporting both arms in a slightly flexed position protects joint and improves ventilation because chest is able to expand more easily.
(8) Place your hands under patient's hips and bring dependent hip slightly forward so angle from hip to mattress is approximately 30 degrees.	• The 30-degree lateral position reduces pressure on trochanter.
(9) Place tuck-back pillow behind patient's back. (Make by folding pillow lengthwise. The smooth area is slightly tucked under the patient's back.)	• Provides support to maintain patient on side.
(10) Place pillow under semiflexed upper leg level at hip from groin to foot (see Step 2G[10] illustrations).	• Flexion prevents hyperextension of the leg. Maintains leg in correct alignment. Prevents pressure on bony prominence.

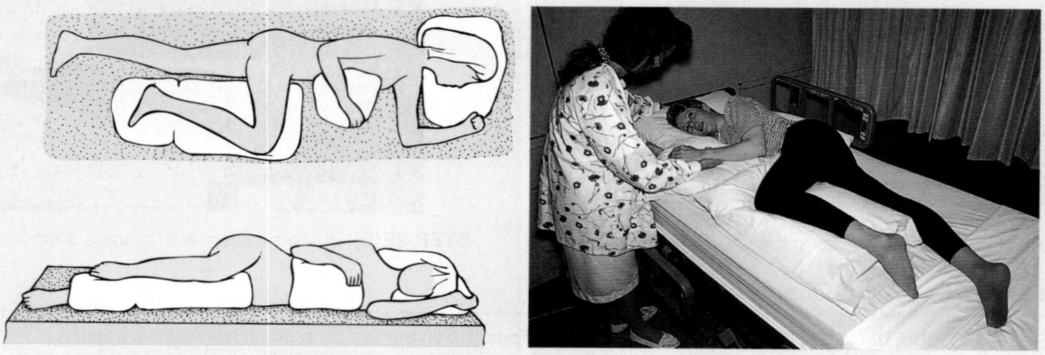

STEP 2G(10) Side-lying position with pillows in place.

STEPS	RATIONALE
(11) Support feet in dorsiflexion with foot support devices (check agency policy).	• Maintains dorsiflexion of foot. Prevents footdrop. Foot support devices prevent stimulation to ball of foot by hard surface, which has tendency to increase muscle tone in patient with extensor spasticity of lower extremity.
H. Position patient in Sims' (semiprone) position (one nurse).	
(1) Lower head of bed completely.	• Provides for proper body alignment while patient is lying down.
(2) Assess patient's level of comfort in the supine position.	• Some patient's physical conditions do not tolerate supine position.
(3) Position patient in supine position on side of bed opposite direction the patient is to be turned. Reposition upper trunk, supporting the shoulders first; reposition lower trunk, supporting hips. Raise side rails and move to opposite side of bed.	• Prepares patient for positioning.
(4) Move to other side of bed and roll patient on side. Position patient in lateral position and lying partially on abdomen, with dependent shoulder lifted out and arm placed at patient's side.	• Patient is rolled only partially onto abdomen.
(5) Place a small pillow under patient's head.	• Patient is rolled only partially onto abdomen.
(6) Place pillow under flexed upper arm, supporting arm level with shoulder.	• Maintains proper alignment and prevents lateral neck flexion. Prevents internal rotation of shoulder.
(7) Place pillow under flexed upper leg, supporting leg level with hip.	• Prevents internal rotation of hip and adduction of leg. Flexion prevents hyperextension of leg. Reduces mattress pressure on knees and ankles.
(8) Support feet in dorsiflexion with foot support devices (check agency policy) (see Step 2H[8] illustration).	• Maintains foot in dorsiflexion. Prevents footdrop. Foot support devices prevent stimulation to ball of foot by hard surface, which has tendency to increase muscle tone in patient with extensor spasticity of lower extremity.

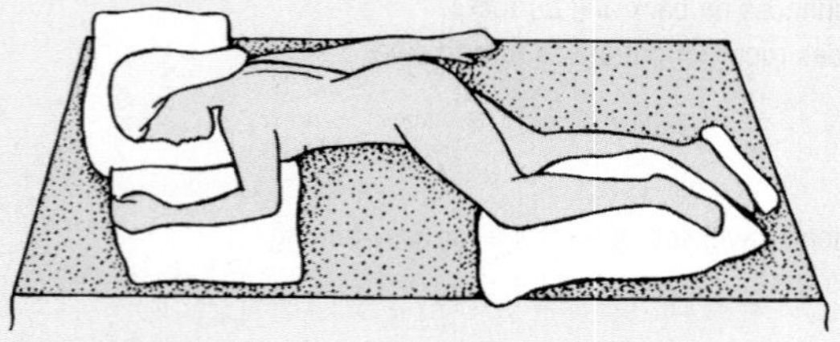

STEP 2H(8) Sims' (semiprone) position with pillows in place.

STEPS	RATIONALE
I. Logrolling patient (three to five nurses).	

CRITICAL DECISION POINT: *Supervise and aid UCPs when a prescriber's order is to logroll a patient. In patients who have suffered a spinal cord injury or are recovering from neck, back, or vertebral column surgery the spinal column must be maintained in straight alignment to prevent further injury.*

STEPS	RATIONALE
(1) Place patient in supine position on side of bed opposite direction to be turned.	• Prepares patient for turning onto side.
(2) Place small pillow between patient's knees.	• Prevents tension on the spinal column and adduction of the hip.
(3) Cross patient's arms on chest and bend knee on the opposite side the patient will be turned toward.	• Prevents injury to arms. • Facilitates weight transfer when logrolling.
(4) Position two nurses on side of bed to which the patient will be turned. Position third nurse on the other side of bed (see Step 2I[4] illustration).	• Distributes weight equally among nurses. • For patients with spinal cord injury or vertebral column trauma, stabilizing the patient's head and neck facilitates synchronous movement of the vertebral column when logrolling and prevents injury to the patient.

SAFETY ALERT: *If a patient has a spinal cord injury, or actual or suspected vertebral column fracture, a fourth nurse must be positioned at the head of the bed to stabilize the patient's head and neck to ensure synchronous movement of the entire vertebral column when logrolling. If needed, use a fifth nurse on the same side as the third nurse.*

STEPS	RATIONALE
(5) The nurse on the opposite side of the bed passes the edge of the transfer sheet to the nurses on the side of the bed to which patient is to be turned. These nurses fan fold or roll the sheet and then grasp the sheet using a safe effective grip (palms up, elbows at sides) and position themselves to do a front-to-back weight transfer.	• Provides strong handles to grip the transfer sheet or pull sheet without slipping. • Palms up, elbows at sides facilitates maximum use of the stronger biceps muscles. • Safety of the nurse is facilitated by using a front-to-back weight transfer, as this action prevents rotation of the spine that can lead to injury.
(6) The nurse on the opposite side of the bed positions open palmed hands on the patient's shoulder and hip to provide directional guidance only. For the nurses on the side that the patient is to be turned: the first nurse grasps the transfer sheet at the patient's shoulders and lower back, and the second nurse grasps the transfer sheet at the patient's hips and lower thighs.	
(7) The nurse on the opposite side of the bed counts "1-2-3 roll," and on the command word "roll" the two nurses perform a front-to-back weight transfer, while the nurse on the opposite side of the bed gently guides the patient using a back-to-front weight transfer. At the completion of the move, the patient will be facing the two nurses (see Step 2I[7] illustration).	• Maintains proper alignment in the patient by moving all body parts at the same time, preventing tension or twisting of the spinal column.

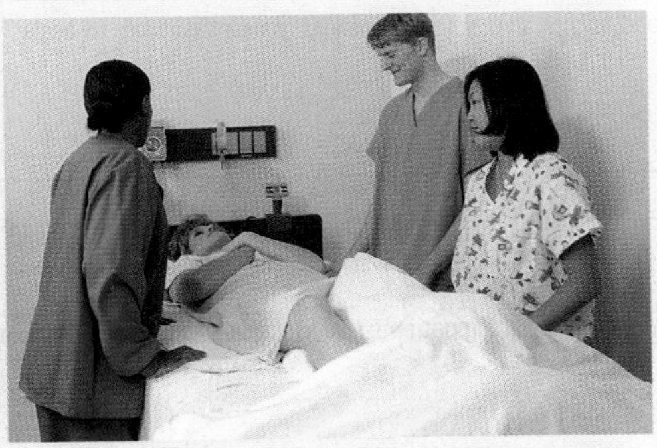

STEP 2I(4) Position nurses on each side of patient.

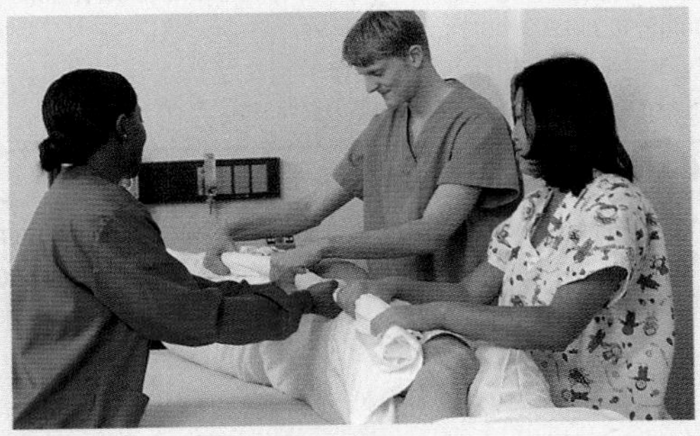

STEP 2I(7) Move patient as a unit, maintaining proper alignment.

STEPS	RATIONALE
(8) The nurse on the opposite side of the bed places pillows along the length of the patient (see Step 2I[8] illustration).	• Pillows keep the patient aligned.

Continued

SKILL 45-1 MOVING AND POSITIONING PATIENTS IN BED—cont'd

STEPS	RATIONALE
(9) Gently lean the patient as a unit back toward the pillows for support (see Step 2I[9] illustration).	• Ensures continued straight alignment of spinal column, preventing injury.

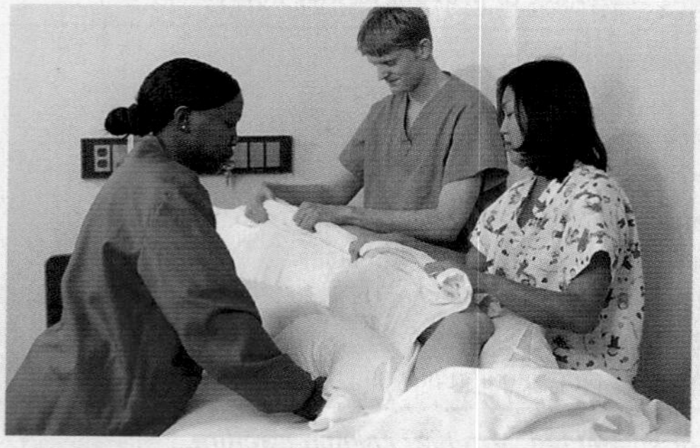

STEP 2I(8) Place pillows along patient's back for support.

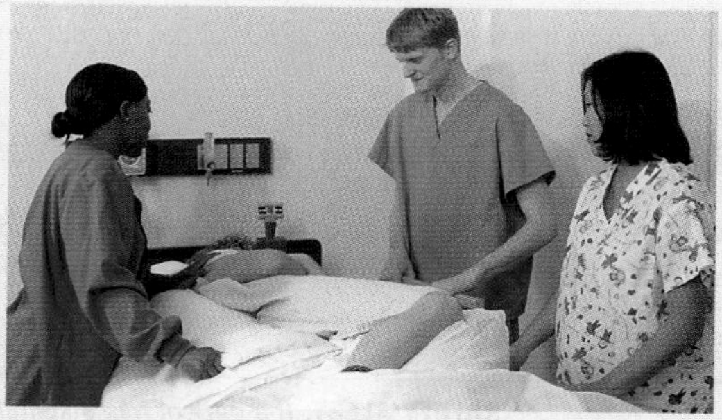

STEP 2I(9) Gently lean patient as a unit against pillows.

STEPS	RATIONALE
3. Perform hand hygiene.	• Reduces transmission of microorganisms.

EVALUATION

1. Evaluate patient's level of comfort and ability to assist in position change.	• Patients with reduced activity tolerance and increased levels of pain may find position changes very tiring and will need post-position change interventions to restore their level of comfort.
2. After each position change, evaluate patient's body alignment and assess pressure areas. Observe for areas of erythema or breakdown involving skin.	• Prompt identification of poor alignment reduces risks to the patient's skin and musculoskeletal systems.

UNEXPECTED OUTCOMES	RELATED INTERVENTIONS
Joint contractures develop or worsen (Cause: Improper positioning results in shortening of muscles)	• Consult physiotherapy and/or occupational therapy. • Ensure that activity and ROM orders are implemented consistently.
Skin erythema and breakdown (Cause: Inadequate frequency of repositioning)	• Increase frequency of turning and repositioning. • Place turning schedule above patient's bed. • Implement other activities per agency skin care policy or protocol (e.g., assess more frequently, consult dietitian, place patient on pressure-relieving mattress).
Patient avoids moving	• Administer analgesia as ordered by health care provider to ensure patient's comfort before moving if patient is in pain. • Allow pain medication to take effect before positioning. • Provide patient education about benefits of moving.

RECORDING AND REPORTING

- Document repositioning or turning and any relevant observations during procedure (e.g., condition of skin, joint movement, patient's ability to assist with positioning) in nurses' notes.
- Report observations at change of shift.
- Document your evaluation of patient learning.

HOME CARE CONSIDERATIONS

- Teach the family about the importance of body mechanics for themselves and the patient.
- Teach family how to use safe patient-handling equipment, if necessary.
- Teach the patient and family about the signs of skin breakdown and the importance of safety during positioning patients with decreased sensation or mobility.

patient in the supported Fowler's position (see Skill 45-1 for preventive measures):

- Increased cervical flexion because the pillow at the head is too thick and the head thrusts forward
- Hyperextension of the knees, allowing the patient to slide to the foot of the bed
- Pressure on the posterior aspect of the knees, decreasing circulation to the feet
- External rotation of the hips
- Arms hanging unsupported at the patient's sides
- Unsupported feet or pressure on the heels
- Unprotected pressure points at the sacrum and heels
- Increased shearing force on the back and heels when the head of bed is raised greater than 60 degrees

Supine Position. The supine position is a back-lying position. In the supine position, the relationship of body parts is essentially the same as in good standing alignment except that the body is in the horizontal plane. Pillows, trochanter rolls, and hand rolls or arm splints are used to increase comfort and reduce injury to the skin or musculoskeletal system. The mattress should be firm enough to support the cervical, thoracic, and lumbar vertebrae. Shoulders are supported, and the elbows are slightly flexed to control shoulder rotation. A foot support is used to prevent footdrop and maintain proper alignment. The following are some common trouble areas for patients in the supine position (see Skill 45-1 for preventive measures):

- Increased cervical flexion because the pillow at the head is too thick and the head thrusts forward
- Head flat on the mattress
- Shoulders unsupported and internally rotated
- Elbows extended
- Thumb not in opposition to the fingers
- Hips externally rotated
- Unsupported feet
- Unprotected pressure points at the occipital region of the head, vertebrae, coccyx, elbows, and heels

Prone Position. The patient in the prone position is lying chest down. Often the head is turned to the side. If a pillow is under the head, it should be thin enough to prevent cervical flexion or extension and maintain alignment of the lumbar spine. Placing a pillow under the lower leg permits dorsiflexion of the ankles and some knee flexion, which promotes relaxation. If a pillow is unavailable, the ankles should be in dorsiflexion over the end of the mattress. Although the prone position is seldom used in practice, nurses should consider this as an alternative, especially in patients who normally sleep in this position. The prone position may also have some benefits for patients with acute respiratory distress syndrome and acute lung injury (Barbas, Faissol, Matos, et al., 2012). Specialty beds that safely position acutely ill patients in the prone position are available.

Nurses should assess for and correct any of the following potential trouble points for patients in the prone position (see Skill 45-1 for preventive measures):

- Neck hyperextension
- Hyperextension of the lumbar spine
- Plantar flexion of the ankles
- Unprotected pressure points at the chin, elbows, hips, knees, and toes

Side-Lying Position. In the side-lying (or lateral) position, the patient is resting on the side with the major portion of body weight on the dependent hip and shoulder. A 30-degree lateral position is recommended for patients at risk for pressure injuries. Trunk alignment should be the same as in standing. For example, the structural curves of the spine should be maintained, the head should be supported in line with the midline of the trunk, and rotation of the spine needs to be avoided. The following trouble points are common in the side-lying position (see Skill 45-1 for preventive measures):

- Lateral flexion of the neck
- Spinal curves out of normal alignment
- Shoulder and hip joints internally rotated, adducted, or unsupported
- Lack of support for the feet
- Lack of protection for pressure points at the ear, shoulder, anterior iliac spine, trochanter, and ankles
- Excessive lateral flexion of the spine if the patient has large hips and a pillow is not placed superior to the hips at the waist

Sims' Position. Sims' position differs from the lateral position in the distribution of the patient's weight. In Sims' position, the weight is placed on the anterior ilium, humerus, and clavicle. Trouble points common in Sims' position include the following (see Skill 45-1 for preventive measures):

- Lateral flexion of the neck
- Internal rotation, adduction, or lack of support to the shoulders and hips
- Lack of support for the feet
- Lack of protection for pressure points at the ilium, humerus, clavicle, knees, and ankles

Transfer Techniques. Nurses often provide care for patients who must be assisted to change positions, who must be moved up in bed, or who must be transferred from a bed to a chair or from a bed to a stretcher. Use of proper body mechanics will enable you as a nurse to position, move, or transfer patients safely and also protect you from injury to the musculoskeletal system (see Chapter 36). Although many transfer techniques are used, the following general guidelines should be followed in any transfer procedure:

- Raise the side rail on the side of the bed opposite you to prevent the patient from falling out of bed.
- Elevate the level of the bed to a comfortable working height.
- Assess the patient's mobility and strength to determine what assistance the patient can offer during transfer.
- Determine the need for assistance from other care providers or mechanical lifts.
- Explain the procedure to the patient and describe what is expected of the patient.
- Assess for correct body alignment and pressure areas after each transfer.

> **Safety Alert** Recognition of your own personal strengths and limits is crucial. Moving a patient who is completely immobilized by yourself is dangerous and not allowed in many agencies. If you are attempting transfer or moving techniques for the first time, you should request help to reduce the risk of injury to yourself and to the patient.

Repositioning Patients. When repositioning a patient, a safe transfer is the first priority. Patients require various levels of assistance to move up in bed, move to the side-lying position, or sit up at the side of the bed. For example, a young, healthy woman may need only a little support as she sits at the side of the bed for the first time after childbirth, whereas an older person may need help from one or more nurses to do the same task 1 day after abdominal surgery.

The nurse must always enlist the patient's help to the fullest extent possible. To determine what the patient is able to do alone and how many people are needed to help move the patient in bed, the nurse needs to assess the patient to determine whether the illness, injury, or treatment contradicts exertion (e.g., cardiovascular disease, spinal cord injury, vertebral column surgery).

Next, the nurse must perform a functional assessment of the patient (Table 45-4). A functional assessment includes the following;

- Determine whether the patient is able to communicate his or her needs and comprehend and follow directions.
- Assess the patient's vision and hearing.
- Assess the patient's medical status, including conditions and limitations that will affect the move, attachments or appliances, pain and fatigue, and medications that will affect the move.
- Assess the patient's hand grip strength.
- Assess the patient's ability to raise the hips when knees are bent and feet are on the bed (bridging).
- Assess the patient's ability to roll side to side in bed.

If the patient is deficient in any of these assessments, at least two nurses are required to safely transfer and reposition the patient in bed. As the patient's nurse, you must then determine the comfort level of

TABLE 45-4 Safe Patient Handling Functional Assessment Record

Question	Yes/No/Not Applicable	Comments
Patient Health Information		
Communication		
Is patient able to communicate needs?		
Is vision and hearing adequate? List aides if used.		
Cognitive Status		
Is patient able to recall instructions?		
Is patient able to judge capabilities in moving?		
Emotional/Behaviour Status		
Is patient cooperative and predictable in behaviour?		
Is patient mood stable?		
Medical Status		
Conditions/limitations that will affect move		
Does the patient have attachments/appliances?		
Does the patient have pain/fatigue?		
Is the patient on medication that will affect move?		
Functional Assessment		
Can patient grip, push, and pull hands? Right / Left		
In supine position, can the patient raise hips with knees bent and feet on bed?		
Can the patient roll side to side in bed? Right / Left		
Can the patient get into a sitting position at the side of the bed and maintain sitting position for 15 seconds?		
Can the patient straighten at least one leg and hold for 3 seconds? Right / Left		
Can the patient get into a standing position?		If "no" a mechanical lift is required.
Is patient able to bear body weight for 15 seconds?		If "no" a mechanical lift is required.
Is patient predictable and reliable in physical and mental performance?		If "no" a mechanical lift is required.
Are all caregivers able to perform the task?		

From Alberta Health Services. (2010). *It's your move.* Retrieved from http://ahamms01.http.internapcdn.net/ahamms01/Content/AHS_Website/modules/iym/presentation.html.

the patient and evaluate personal strength and knowledge of the procedure.

Finally, determine whether the patient is too heavy or immobile for you to complete the procedure alone (see Skill 45-1). Use of mechanical transfer devices may be warranted (Figure 45-18), and agency lifting and transferring policies must be followed.

Assessment criteria and tools have been developed to help nurses gather data and to assess and plan for the safe transfer of patients. An example of a safe patient handling functional assessment record form is shown in Table 45-4.

Restorative Care

The goal of restorative care for the patient who is immobile is to maximize functional mobility and independence and reduce residual functional deficits such as impaired gait and decreased endurance. The focus in restorative care is on not only ADLs that relate to physical self-care but also **instrumental activities of daily living (IADLs)**. IADLs are activities that are necessary to be independent in society beyond eating, grooming, transferring, and toileting. They include such skills as shopping, preparing meals, banking, and taking medications.

In restorative care, nurses use many of the interventions described in the "Health Promotion" and "Acute Care" sections in this chapter, but the emphasis is on working collaboratively with patients and their significant others and with other health care providers. The goal is to enhance the patient's quality of life by helping the patient return to maximal functional ability in both ADLs and IADLs.

Intensive specialized rehabilitation such as occupational or physiotherapy is common. If the patient is in an institution, he or she will likely go to the therapy department two to three times a day. Your role as a nurse is to work collaboratively with these professionals and reinforce exercises and teaching. For example, after a stroke, a patient will likely receive gait training from a physiotherapist, speech rehabilitation from a speech therapist, and training from an occupational therapist on getting dressed and preparing food. Working with allied health providers on an interdisciplinary plan of care, you can reinforce and further enhance the patient's mobilization. The therapy may not be able to restore total functional health, but it may help the patient adapt to limited mobility and related complications.

Restorative interventions are focused on the regaining of mobility. According to evidenced-informed protocols, common restorative interventions used by nurses include promotion of exercises for maintaining or regaining joint mobility and teaching of the use of assistive devices for walking (Box 45-10). Items frequently used to help a patient adapt to mobility limitations include walkers, canes, wheelchairs, and assistive devices such as raised toilet seats, reaching sticks, special silverware, and adaptive clothing with Velcro closures.

Range-of-Motion (ROM) Exercises. To ensure adequate joint mobility, the nurse needs to teach the patient about ROM exercises. When the patient does not have voluntary motor control, the patient should start with passive ROM exercises. Walking also increases joint mobility. Occasionally, patients need to use assistive devices such as crutches or walkers to help them walk.

Patients with restricted mobility are unable to perform some or all ROM exercises independently. Such patients include those with limited movement in one extremity and those who are completely immobilized. ROM exercises should be provided to maintain maximum joint mobility.

To ensure that patients routinely receive ROM exercises, the nurse should schedule them at specific times, perhaps with another nursing activity, such as during the patient's bath. This will enable the nurse to systematically reassess mobility while improving the patient's ROM. In

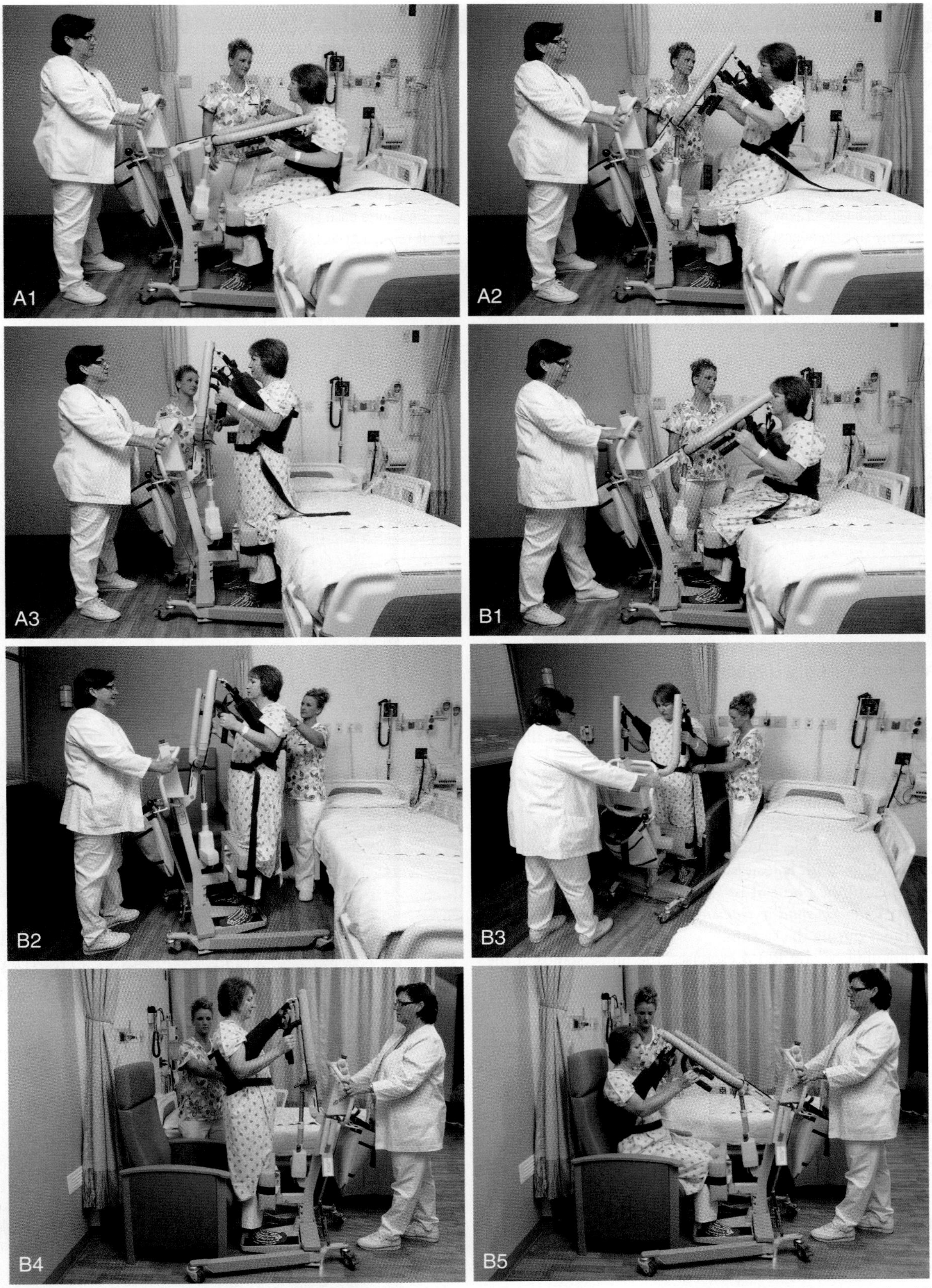

FIGURE 45-18 Using a motorized lift for patient transfer. A1, Safety straps are secured appropriately when using a motorized lift to help a patient move to standing position. **A2,** Patient grasps handles as the nurse enables motorized lift. **A3,** Patient is in standing position with feet on the floor and is ready to ambulate to a chair with nurses' help. **B1,** When the patient is unable to walk, the nurse secures safety straps, and platform of the motorized lift is used. **B2,** Patient in upright position. **B3,** Positioning patient in front of chair. **B4,** Explaining to patient the need to hold on to the handles as motorized lift begins to lower patient into chair. **B5,** Guiding patient into chair.

BOX 45-10 EVIDENCE-INFORMED PRACTICE

Exercise Promotion in Older Persons and Individuals at Risk for Inadequate Activity

- Increase patient's awareness of current activity levels.
- Encourage patient to contemplate change in activity level.
- Provide information about the benefits of exercise.
- Determine any impediments to exercise.
- Provide choices of physical activities.
- Assist patient in preparing for an activity program.
- Provide information about how to safely carry out the exercise (e.g., proper walking, safety considerations).
- Assist patient in strengthening exercise tolerance and activity levels.
- Emphasize patient's ability to become more active.
- Provide resources for social exercise groups (e.g., fitness groups, community walking programs, walking in local shopping malls).
- Assist patient in establishing an activity program.
- Provide positive, constructive feedback.
- Increase physical activity as appropriate for patient's mobility status.
- Assist patient in developing a long-term exercise plan.
- Visit the patient while he or she is participating in an exercise program.
- Assist patient in maintaining an activity program.
- Recognize each success.
- If relapse occurs, remind patient that it is okay and to continue with the exercise program.
- Maintain a supportive environment.
- Encourage family and friends to participate in the exercise program.

Adapted from Jitramontree, N. (2010). Evidence-Based Practice Guideline: Exercise promotion: Walking in elders. *Journal of Gerontological Nursing 36*(11), 10-18.

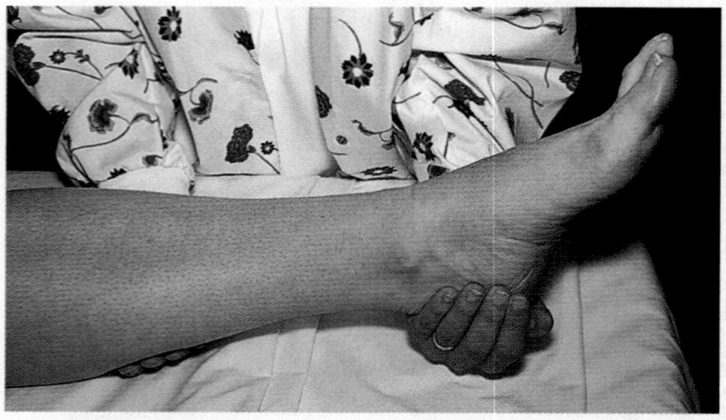

FIGURE 45-19 Using a cupped hand to support a joint.

addition, during bathing, the extremities and joints are usually put through complete ROM.

Unless contraindicated, the care plan should include movement of the patient's extremities through the fullest ROM possible. ROM exercises may be active, passive, or somewhere in between (active assisted). Passive ROM exercises should begin as soon as the patient's ability to move the extremity or joint is lost. Movements are carried out slowly and smoothly, just to the point of resistance; ROM should not cause pain. *Never force a joint beyond its capacity.* Each movement should be repeated five times during the session.

When performing passive ROM exercises, the nurse stands at the side of the bed closest to the joint being exercised. Passive ROM exercises are performed using a head-to-toe sequence and moving from larger to smaller joints. If an extremity is to be moved or lifted, the nurse can place a cupped hand under the joint to support it (Figure 45-19), support the joint by holding the adjacent distal and proximal areas (Figure 45-20), or support the joint with one hand and cradle the distal portion of the extremity with the remaining arm (Figure 45-21). See Table 45-2 for detailed ROM exercises and illustrated motion for each joint.

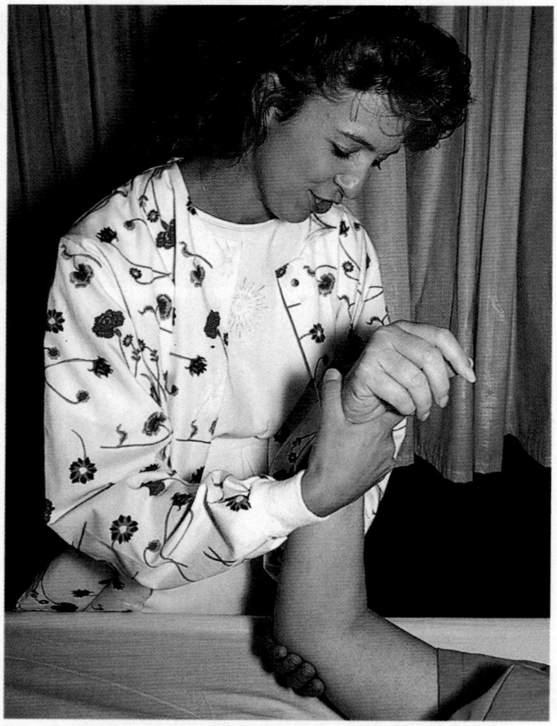

FIGURE 45-20 Supporting the joint by holding the distal and proximal areas adjacent to the joint.

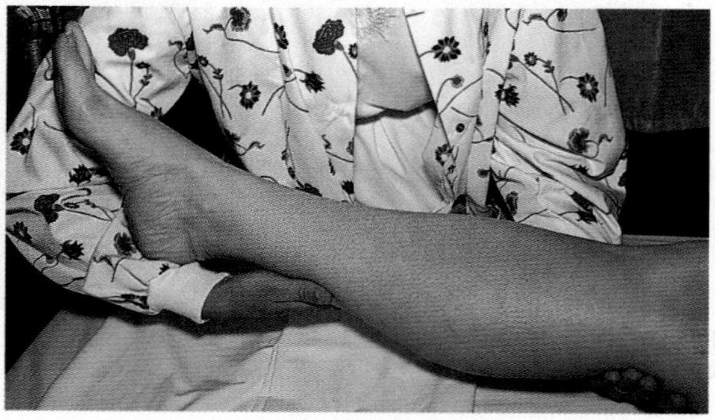

FIGURE 45-21 Cradling the distal portion of an extremity.

◆ Evaluation

Patient Care. To evaluate outcomes and response to nursing care, the effectiveness of all interventions needs to be measured. The actual outcomes are compared with the outcomes selected during planning. The nurse needs to evaluate specific interventions designed to promote body alignment, improve mobility, and protect the patient from the hazards of immobility. The nurse also evaluates patient and family instruction to prevent future risks to body alignment and hazards of

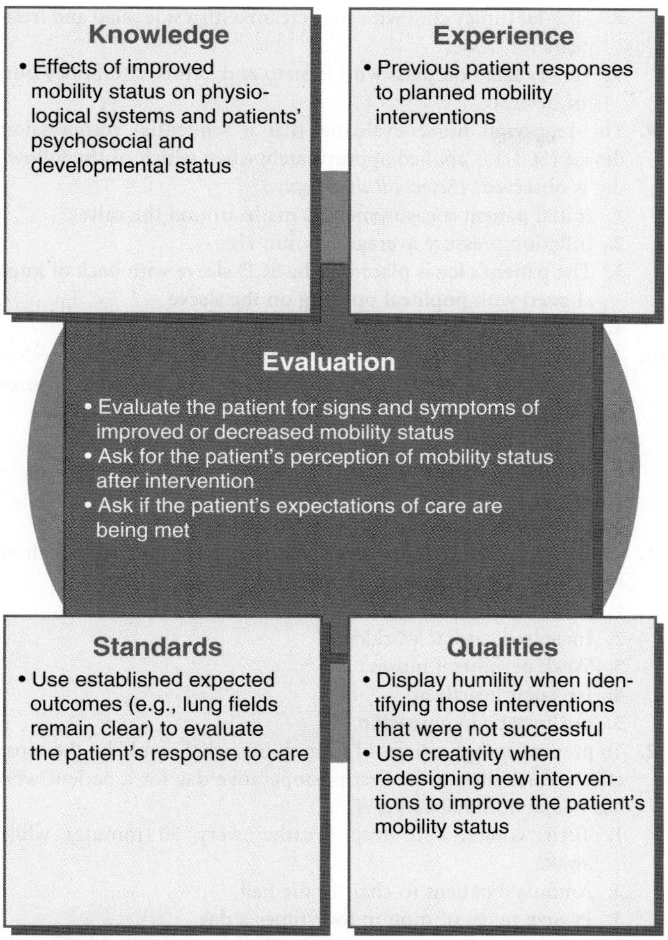

FIGURE 45-22 Critical thinking model for immobility evaluation.

immobility (Figure 45-22). The evaluation enables the nurse to determine whether new or revised therapies are required and if new nursing diagnoses have developed.

Patient Expectations. Patients who are immobile and dependent on others for some or all of their needs can become overly dependent or try to do too much themselves too early. Finding the balance between independence and dependence is a difficult task. Patients will want control over mobility that is personally satisfactory. For the patient who is completely dependent on others for care, control over how and when things are done may be very important. Do patients feel they are treated with dignity? Do caregivers treat them as adults? Are they given opportunities to make meaningful choices? These are important questions nurses need to consider regarding patient expectations.

KEY CONCEPTS

- Body mechanics are the coordinated efforts of the musculoskeletal and nervous systems as the person moves, lifts, bends, stands, sits, lies down, and completes daily activities.
- Balance is assisted through nervous system control by the cerebellum and inner ear.
- Range-of-motion (ROM) exercises include one or all of the body joints and can be active or passive.
- Body alignment is the condition of joints, tendons, ligaments, and muscles in various body positions.
- Balance is achieved when a wide base of support is present, the centre of gravity falls within the base of support, and a vertical line falls from the centre of gravity through the base of support.
- Developmental stages influence body alignment and mobility; the greatest impact of physiological changes on the musculoskeletal system is observed in children and older persons.
- The risk of disabilities related to immobilization depends on the extent and duration of immobilization and the patient's overall level of health.
- Immobility may result from illness or trauma or may be prescribed for therapeutic reasons (bed rest).
- Immobility presents hazards in the physiological, psychological, and developmental dimensions.
- The nursing process and critical thinking synthesis are used to provide care for patients who are experiencing or are at risk for the adverse effects of impaired body alignment and immobility.
- After identifying nursing diagnoses, nurses plan and implement interventions to prevent or minimize the hazards and complications of impaired body alignment and immobilization.
- Patients with weakness and impaired function of the nervous, skeletal, or muscular system often require nursing assistance to attain proper body alignment while in bed or sitting and to transfer from a bed to a chair.
- Positioning devices help patients maintain good body alignment while lying or sitting.
- Assistive devices to promote walking include canes, walkers, and crutches.

CRITICAL THINKING EXERCISES

1. You are caring for a 57-year-old man who had bilateral total knee replacements for osteoarthritis 2 days ago. He is beginning to transfer to a chair with help. He is 45 kg overweight and has a history of deep vein thrombosis. He has compression stockings, continuous passive range of motion, and a saline lock. Make a list of potential nursing diagnoses.
2. When you are conducting a home visit for a 75-year-old woman, the patient's granddaughter runs in and says, "Did you show the nurse the sore on your leg that you got from falling yesterday?" What questions about mobility are important to ask the patient? How do you begin your assessment?
3. You are caring for a 68-year-old man who is immobilized after spinal cord trauma from a motor vehicle accident. What potential complications would you assess for in this patient?

REVIEW QUESTIONS

1. An older person has limited mobility as a result of a total knee replacement. During assessment, the nurse notes that the patient has difficulty breathing while lying flat. Which of the following assessment data support a possible pulmonary problem related to impaired mobility? *(Select all that apply.)*
   1. BP is 128/84
   2. Respirations are 26/min on room air
   3. HR is 114 beats/min
   4. Crackles over lower lobes heard on auscultation
   5. Pain reported as 3 on scale of 0 to 10 after medication

2. A patient has been on bed rest for over 4 days. On assessment, the nurse identifies the following as a sign associated with immobility:
   1. Decreased peristalsis
   2. Decreased heart rate
   3. Increased blood pressure
   4. Increased urinary output
3. The nurse puts elastic stockings on a patient following major abdominal surgery. The nurse teaches the patient that the stockings are used after a surgical procedure to ________________.
   1. Increase blood pressure
   2. Promote venous return to the heart
   3. Prevent pressure injuries
   4. Assist with range of motion exercises
4. A nurse is teaching a community group about ways to minimize the risk of developing osteoporosis. Which of the following statements reflect understanding of what was taught? *(Select all that apply.)*
   1. "I usually go swimming with my family at the YMCA three times a week."
   2. "I need to ask my doctor if I should have a bone mineral density check this year."
   3. "I don't drink milk at dinner. I'll eat my broccoli or cabbage to get the calcium I need in my diet."
   4. "I'll check the label of my multivitamin. If it has calcium, I can save money by not taking another pill."
   5. "My lactose intolerance should not be a concern when considering my calcium intake."
5. A nurse is caring for an older person who has had a fractured hip repaired. In the first few postoperative days, which of the following nursing measures will best facilitate the resumption of activities of daily living for this patient?
   1. Encouraging use of an overhead trapeze for positioning and transfer
   2. Frequent family visits
   3. Assisting the patient to a wheelchair once per day
   4. Ensuring that there is an order for physiotherapy
6. An older person has been bedridden for 2 weeks. Which of the following complaints by the patient indicates to the nurse that he or she is developing a complication of immobility?
   1. Loss of appetite
   2. Gum soreness
   3. Difficult swallowing
   4. Left ankle joint stiffness
7. A patient is receiving 5 000 units of heparin subcutaneously every 12 hours while on prolonged bed rest to prevent thrombophlebitis. Because bleeding is a potential adverse effect of this medication, the nurse should continually assess the patient for the following signs of bleeding: *(Select all that apply.)*
   1. Bruising
   2. Pale yellow urine
   3. Bleeding gums
   4. Coffee ground–like vomitus
   5. Light brown stool
8. The nurse is caring for a patient whose calcium intake must increase because of high-risk factors for osteoporosis. Which of the following menus should the nurse recommend?
   1. Cream of broccoli soup with whole-wheat crackers, cheese, and tapioca for dessert
   2. Hot dog on a whole-wheat bun with a side salad and an apple for dessert
   3. Low-fat turkey chili with sour cream with a side salad and fresh pears for dessert
   4. Turkey salad on toast with tomato and lettuce and honey bun for dessert
9. The registered nurse evaluates that a sequential compression device (SCD) is applied appropriately when which of the following is observed? *(Select all that apply.)*
   1. Initial patient measurement is made around the calves.
   2. Inflation pressure averages 40 mm Hg.
   3. The patient's leg is placed in the SCD sleeve with back of knee aligned with popliteal opening on the sleeve.
   4. Yellow light indicates SCD device is functioning.
10. A patient on prolonged bed rest is at an increased risk to develop this common complication of immobility if preventive measures are not taken:
    1. Myoclonus
    2. Pathological fractures
    3. Pressure injuries
    4. Pruritis
11. The effects of immobility on the cardiac system include which of the following? *(Select all that apply.)*
    1. Thrombus formation
    2. Increased cardiac workload
    3. Weak peripheral pulses
    4. Irregular heartbeat
    5. Orthostatic hypotension
12. To prevent complications of immobility, what would be the most effective activity on the first postoperative day for a patient who has had abdominal surgery?
    1. Turn, cough, and deep breathe every 30 minutes while awake
    2. Ambulate patient to chair in the hall
    3. Passive range of motion four times a day
    4. Immobility is not a concern the first postoperative day
13. Which of the following nursing interventions should be implemented to maintain a patent airway in a patient on bed rest?
    1. Isometric exercises
    2. Administration of low-dose heparin
    3. Suctioning every 4 hours
    4. Use of incentive spirometer every 2 hours while awake
14. Place the following options in the order in which elastic stockings should be applied.
    1. Identify patient using two identifiers.
    2. Smooth any creases or wrinkles.
    3. Slide the remainder of the stocking over the patient's heel and up the leg.
    4. Turn the stocking inside out until the heel is reached.
    5. Assess the condition of the patient's skin and circulation of the legs.
    6. Place toes into foot of the stocking.
    7. Measure patient's legs to determine proper stocking size.
15. Which of the following are physiological outcomes of immobility?
    1. Increased metabolism
    2. Reduced cardiac workload
    3. Decreased lung expansion
    4. Decreased oxygen demand

Answers: 1. 2, 3, 4; **2.** 1; **3.** 2; **4.** 1, 2, 3; **5.** 1; **6.** 4; **7.** 1, 3, 4; **8.** 1; **9.** 2, 3; **10.** 3; **11.** 1, 2, 5; **12.** 2; **13.** 4; **14.** 1, 5, 7, 4, 6, 3, 2; **15.** 3

Rationales for the Review Questions appear at the end of the book.

RECOMMENDED WEBSITES

(American) Association of Rehabilitation Nurses: http://www.rehabnurse.org/
This website provides an extensive list of links to resources for nurses working with patients with actual or potential impairments or disabilities. It provides information about both prevention and treatment. Although the content has an American orientation, it is also useful to Canadian nurses.

Canadian Association of Rehabilitation Nurses (CARN): http://www.carn.ca
This website provides access to CARN and includes information about membership, education events, and Canadian certification in rehabilitation nursing.

Canadian Physical Activity Guidelines: http://www.csep.ca/en/guidelines/links-to-csep-guidelines
The Canadian Society of Exercise Physiologists provides guides to physical activity for all age groups and has developed guidelines specific to persons with spinal cord injuries. The guidelines provided through this website are a good source of consumer education on the benefits of activity.

Osteoporosis Canada: http://www.osteoporosis.ca
Osteoporosis Canada is a national organization that works toward educating and supporting individuals and communities in the prevention and treatment of osteoporosis. This website provides numerous links to evidence-informed resources on osteoporosis.

The Registered Nurses' Association of Ontario (RNAO) Best Practice Guidelines: Prevention of Falls and Injury in the Older Adult: http://rnao.ca/bpg/guidelines/prevention-falls-and-fall-injuries-older-adult
The RNAO has developed a series of practice guidelines based on the consensus of nurse experts across a variety of practice, academic, and research agencies. This site provides information on patient participation in ADLs, cognition, continence, strength, gait, and balance in relation to the risk for falls.

REFERENCES

Ackley, B., & Ladwig, G. (2014). *Nursing diagnosis handbook: An evidence-based guide to planning care* (10th ed.). St. Louis, MO: Mosby.

Alberta Health Services (AHS). (2010). *It's your move.* Retrieved from http://ahamms01.http.internapcdn.net/ahamms01/Content/AHS_Website/modules/iym/presentation.html.

Ball, J. W., Dains, J. E., Flynn, J. A., et al. (2015). *Seidel's guide to physical examination* (8th ed.). St. Louis, MO: Mosby.

Bangova, A. (2013). Prevention of pressure ulcers in nursing home residents. *Nursing Standard, 27*(24), 54–61.

Barbas, C., Faissol, G., Matos, J., et al. (2012). Goal-oriented respiratory management for critically ill patients with acute respiratory distress syndrome. *Critical Care Research Practice*, Article 952168. doi:10.1155/2012/952168.

Bourret, E., Bernick, L., Cott, C., et al. (2002). The meaning of mobility for residents and staff in long-term care facilities. *Journal of Advanced Nursing, 37*(4), 338–345.

Burnfield, J. M., McCrory, B., Shu, Y., et al. (2013). Comparative kinematic and electromyographic assessment of clinician- and device-assisted sit-to-stand transfers in patients. *Journal of the American Physical Therapy Association, 93*(10), 1331–1341. doi:10.2522/ptj.20120500.

Clavet, H., Hebert, P. C., Fergusson, D. A., et al. (2011). Joint contractures in the intensive care unit: Association with resource utilization and ambulatory status at discharge. *Disability and Rehabilitation, 33*(2), 105–112. doi:10.3109/09638288.2010.486468.

Copstead-Kirkhorn, L., & Banasik, J. (2011). *Pathophysiology* (4th ed.). Philadelphia, PA: Saunders.

Drake, J., Redfern, W. S., Sherburne, E., et al. (2012). Pediatric skin care: What do nurses really know? *Journal for Specialists in Pediatric Nursing, 17*(4), 329–338. doi:10.1111/j.1744-6155.2012.00342.x.

Gillis, A., MacDonald, B., & MacIsaac, A. (2008). Nurses' knowledge, attitudes, and confidence regarding preventing and treating deconditioning in older adults. *Journal of Continuing Education in Nursing, 39*(12), 547–554.

Griffis, H. (2012). Adverse risk: A dynamic interaction model of patient moving and handling. *Journal of Nursing Management, 20*(6), 713–736. doi:10.1111/j.13652834.2011.01276.x.

Healey, F., & Darowski, A. (2012). Older patients and falls in hospitals. *Clinical Risk, 18*(5), 170–176. doi:10.1258/cr.2012.012020.

Hunter, B., Branson, M., & Davenport, D. (2010). Saving costs, saving health care providers' backs, and creating a safe patient environment. *Nursing Economics, 28*(2), 130–134.

Joint Commission. (2018). *2018 National patient safety goals.* Retrieved from https://www.jointcommission.org/standards_information/npsgs.aspx.

Lewis, S. L., Dirksen, S. R., Heitkemper, M. M., et al. (2013). *Medical-surgical nursing: Assessment and management of clinical problems* (9th ed.). St. Louis: Mosby.

McCance, K. L., & Huether, S. E. (2014). *Pathophysiology: The biologic basis for disease in adults and children* (7th ed.). St. Louis, MO: Mosby.

McMahon, S., & Fleury, J. (2012). External validity of physical activity interventions for community-dwelling older adults with fall risk: A quantitative systematic literature review. *Journal of Advanced Nursing, 68*(10), 2140–2154. doi:10.1111/j.1365-2648.2012.05974.x.

Nagarkar, A. K., Swapnil, G., & Shruti, K. (2014). Chronic diseases and functional decline: A cross sectional study among older adults in India. *Indian Journal of Gerontology, 28*(1), 37–50.

Padula, C. A., Hughes, C., & Baumhover, L. (2009). Impact of a nurse-driven mobility protocol on functional decline in hospitalized older adults. *Journal of Nursing Care Quality, 24*(4), 325–331. doi:10.1097/NCQ.0b013e3181a4f79b.

Papaioannou, A., Morin, S., Cheung, A. M., et al. (2010). 2010 clinical practice guidelines for the diagnosis and management of osteoporosis in Canada: Summary. *Canadian Medical Association Journal, 182*, 1864–1873. doi:10.1503/cmaj.100771.

Parker, K. (2012). Psychosocial effects of living with a leg ulcer. *Nursing Standard, 26*(45), 52–62.

Pashikanti, L., & Von Ah, D. (2012). Impact of early mobilization protocol on the medical surgical inpatient population: An integrated review of literature. *Clinical Nurse Specialist, 26*(2), 87–94. doi:10.1097/NUR.0b013e31824590e6.

Registered Nurses' Association of Ontario (RNAO). (2007). *Assessment and management of stage I to IV pressure ulcers (revised).* Toronto: Author. Retrieved from http://rnao.ca/sites/rnao-ca/files/Assessment__Management_of_Stage_I_to_IV_Pressure_Ulcers.pdf.

Registered Nurses' Association of Ontario (RNAO). (2011a). *Prevention of falls and fall injuries in the older adult.* Toronto: Author. Retrieved from http://rnao.ca/sites/rnao-ca/files/Prevention_of_Falls_and_Fall_Injuries_in_the_Older_Adult.pdf.

Registered Nurses' Association of Ontario (RNAO). (2011b). *Risk assessment and prevention of pressure ulcers.* Toronto: Author. Retrieved from http://rnao.ca/sites/rnao-ca/files/Risk_Assessment_and_Prevention_of_Pressure_Ulcers.pdf.

Registered Nurses' Association of Ontario (RNAO). (2011c). *Prevention of constipation in the older adult population.* Toronto: Author. Retrieved from http://rnao.ca/sites/rnao-ca/files/Prevention_of_Constipation_in_the_Older_Adult_Population.pdf.

Registered Nurses' Association of Ontario (RNAO). (2016). *Delirium, dementia and depression in older adults: Assessment and care.* Retrieved from http://rnao.ca/bpg/guidelines/assessment-and-care-older-adults-delirium-dementia-and-depression.

Smith, N., Caple, C., & Pravikoff, D. (2016). *Range-of-motion exercises, passive. CINAHL Nursing Guide.* EBSCO Publishing. Nursing Practice and Skill-CEU. CINAHL AN: T703878.

Self-Management Resource Center. (2015). *Patient education: Chronic disease self-management program.* Retrieved from http://patienteducation.stanford.edu/programs/cdsmp. https://www.selfmanagementresource.com/programs/small-group/chronic-disease-self-management/.

Touhy, T., Jett, K., Boscart, V., et al. (2012). *Ebersole & Hess' gerontological nursing and healthy aging* (1st Canadian ed.). Toronto: Elsevier Canada.

VISN8 Patient Safety Center. (2015). *Algorithms for safe patient handling and movement.* Retrieved from https://www.publichealth.va.gov/employeehealth/patient-handling/.

46

Skin Integrity and Wound Care

Canadian content written by Rosemary Kohr, RN, BA, BScN, MScN, PhD, Tertiary Care Nurse Practitioner Certificate

Original chapter by Janice C. Colwell, RN, MS, CWOCN, FAAN

OBJECTIVES

Mastery of content in this chapter will enable you to:

- Describe the key terms listed.
- Discuss the risk factors that contribute to pressure injury formation.
- Recognize the stages of pressure injury.
- Describe the etiology and key components of venous, arterial, diabetic, and malignant wounds.
- Discuss the normal process of wound healing.
- Describe the differences between wounds that heal by primary and secondary intention.
- Describe the complications of wound healing.
- Explain the factors that impede or promote wound healing.
- Describe the differences in nursing care for acute and chronic wounds.
- Describe the types of dressings appropriate for moist wound healing.
- Complete an assessment for a patient with impaired skin integrity.
- List nursing diagnoses associated with impaired skin integrity.
- Develop a nursing care plan for a patient with impaired skin integrity.
- List appropriate nursing interventions for a patient with impaired skin integrity.
- State evaluation criteria for a patient with impaired skin integrity.

KEY TERMS

Abrasion, p. 1306
Approximated, p. 1301
Blanching, p. 1290
Collagen, p. 1292
Darkly pigmented skin, p. 1290
Debridement, p. 1317
Dehiscence, p. 1309
Drainage evacuators, p. 1330
Epithelialization, p. 1303
Eschar, p. 1301
Evisceration, p. 1309
Exudate, p. 1301
Fibrin, p. 1303
Fistula, p. 1309
Friction, p. 1292
Granulation tissue, p. 1301
Hematoma, p. 1308
Hemorrhage, p. 1308
Hemostasis, p. 1303
Hyperemia, p. 1290
Induration, p. 1293
Laceration, p. 1306
Nonviable tissue, p. 1299
Pressure injury, p. 1289
Primary intention, p. 1301
Puncture, p. 1306
Purulent, p. 1307
Sanguineous, p. 1307
Secondary intention, p. 1302
Serosanguineous, p. 1307
Serous, p. 1307
Shear, p. 1292
Slough, p. 1301
Sutures, p. 1329
Tissue ischemia, p. 1290
Wound, p. 1301
Wound contraction, p. 1303

MEDIA RESOURCES

http://evolve.elsevier.com/Canada/Potter/fundamentals/

- Audio Chapter Summaries
- Examination Review Questions
- Concept Map Creator
- Case Study With Questions
- Audio Glossary
- Content Updates
- Video Clips

Skin, the body's largest organ, constitutes 15% of the total adult body weight (Wysocki, 2016). It protects against disease-causing organisms; senses pain, temperature, and touch; and synthesizes vitamin D. Injury to the skin poses risks to safety and triggers a complex healing response.

As a nurse, one of your most important responsibilities is to monitor skin integrity and prevent skin breakdown. Understanding normal wound healing helps in planning, implementing, and assessing interventions that maintain skin integrity and optimize wound healing.

SCIENTIFIC KNOWLEDGE BASE

Skin

The skin has two layers: the epidermis and the dermis (Figure 46-1). These two layers are separated by a membrane, often referred to as the dermal–epidermal junction. The epidermis, or top layer, also consists of several layers. The stratum corneum is the thin, outermost layer of the epidermis, consisting of flattened, keratinized cells. The cells originate from the innermost epidermal (or basal) layer. These cells divide, proliferate, and migrate toward the epidermal surface.

After cells reach the stratum corneum, they flatten and die. This constant movement ensures replacement of surface cells sloughed during normal desquamation or shedding. The stratum corneum protects underlying cells and tissues from dehydration and prevents the entrance of certain chemical agents. The stratum corneum allows the evaporation of water from the skin and permits the absorption of certain topical medications.

The dermis, the inner layer of the skin, provides tensile strength, mechanical support, and protection to the underlying muscles, bones, and organs. It differs from the epidermis in that it contains mostly connective tissue and few skin cells. Collagen (a tough, fibrous protein), blood vessels, and nerves are in the dermal layer. Fibroblasts, which are responsible for collagen formation, are the only distinctive cell type within the dermis.

Understanding skin structure helps nurses to maintain skin integrity and promote wound healing. Intact skin protects the patient from chemical and mechanical injuries. When the skin is injured, the epidermis functions to resurface the wound and restore the barrier against invading organisms while the dermis responds to restore the structural integrity (collagen) and the physical properties of the skin. Age alters skin characteristics and makes skin more vulnerable to damage. Box 46-1 provides a summary of the changes in aging skin.

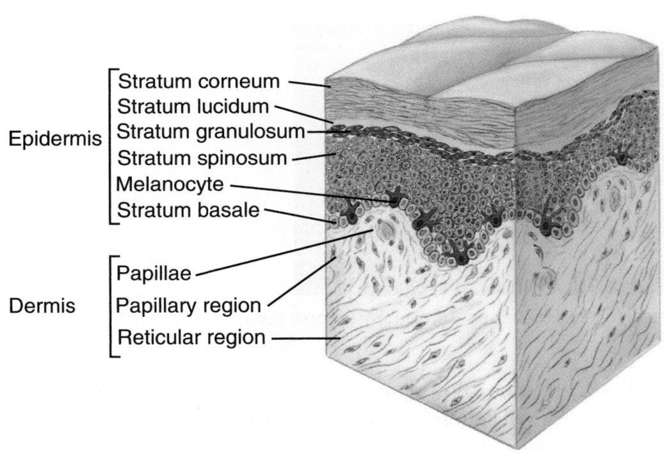

FIGURE 46-1 Layers of skin. (From Applegate, E. [2006]. *The anatomy and physiology learning system* [3rd ed.]. St. Louis: Saunders.)

Pressure Injury

Pressure ulcer, pressure sore, decubitus ulcer, and *bedsore* have long been used as terms describing impaired skin integrity related to unrelieved, prolonged pressure. However, this terminology has been changed to *pressure injury*, and staging now uses numbers rather than Roman numerals (National Pressure Ulcer Advisory Panel [NPUAP], 2017). This change reflects the fact that not all impaired skin integrity results in a pressure injury. Deep tissue injury and stage 1 are injury to the tissue without breaking the skin, although at high risk of further damage. The pressure injury guidelines developed by the Registered Nurses' Association of Ontario (RNAO) (RNAO, 2016) provide consistency with the NPUAP standards. A **pressure injury** is localized to skin and underlying tissue, usually over a bony prominence, as a result of pressure, shear, or friction, or a combination of these factors and is affected by moisture, nutrition, perfusion, and comorbidities (Figure 46-2).

Pressure injuries have a high prevalence rate in all health care settings. While it is a challenge to arrive at accurate figures, the classic study by Woodbury and Houghton (2004) estimates that one in four individuals within the Canadian health care system—including acute care, complex continuing care, home care, and long-term care—has some issue with skin integrity, and reflects current clinician observation. The consistent "take-home" message is that many chronic wounds are preventable and, with appropriate management, healable.

The impact of pressure injury and other chronic wounds on quality of life is significant, as normal activities may be restricted because of pain, odour, or treatments. Costs associated with chronic wound care can substantially increase the burden on the health care system. It has been estimated that chronic wounds' cost to the Canadian health care system is approximately $3.9 billion annually—approximately 3% of total health care expenditures (Wounds National Stakeholder Roundtable Report, 2012).

Thus, it is essential that attention be paid to the causes of pressure injury as well as to the healing process of wounds. The focus of this chapter is on pressure injury prevention and treatment options, but other chronic wounds, such as diabetic, arterial, venous, and malignant wounds, will also be briefly discussed and are important for nurses to recognize and treat. Additional resources are readily available on websites for the Canadian Association of Wound Care (CAWC), the Canadian Association of Enterostomal Therapists (CAET), and RNAO,

BOX 46-1 FOCUS ON OLDER PERSONS

Skin-Associated Issues

- Age-related changes, such as reduced skin elasticity, decreased collagen, and thinning of underlying muscle and tissues, cause the older person's skin to be easily torn via mechanical trauma, especially shearing forces (Wysocki, 2016).
- Concomitant medical conditions and polypharmacy, common in the older person, interfere with wound healing.
- The attachment between the epidermis and dermis becomes flattened in older persons, allowing skin to be easily torn from mechanical trauma (e.g., tape removal).
- Aging causes a diminished inflammatory response, resulting in slow epithelialization and wound healing (Doughty & Sparks-Defriese, 2016).
- The hypodermis decreases in size with age. Older patients have little subcutaneous padding over bony prominences, so they are more prone to skin breakdown (Wysocki, 2016).
- Reduced nutritional intake, commonly seen in older persons, increases the risk of pressure injury development and impaired wound healing (Gould et al., 2015).

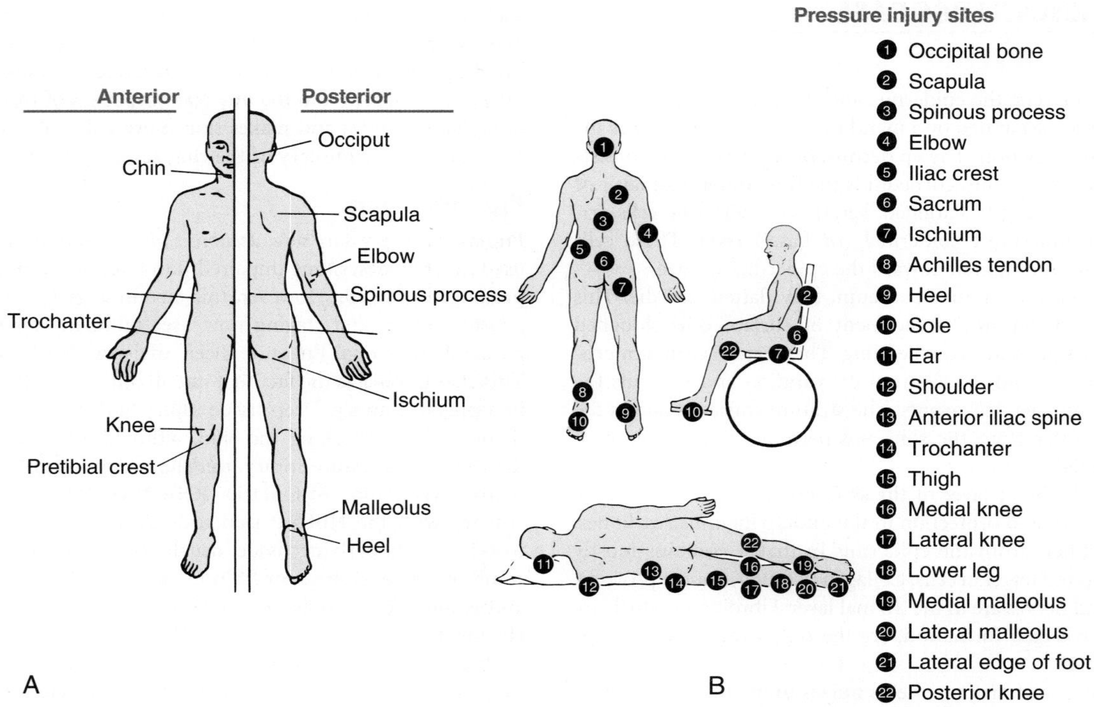

FIGURE 46-2 **A,** Bony prominences most frequently underlying pressure injury. **B,** Common pressure injury sites. (Adapted from Trelease, C. C. [1988]. Developing standards for wound care. *Ostomy/Wound Management, 20,* 46.)

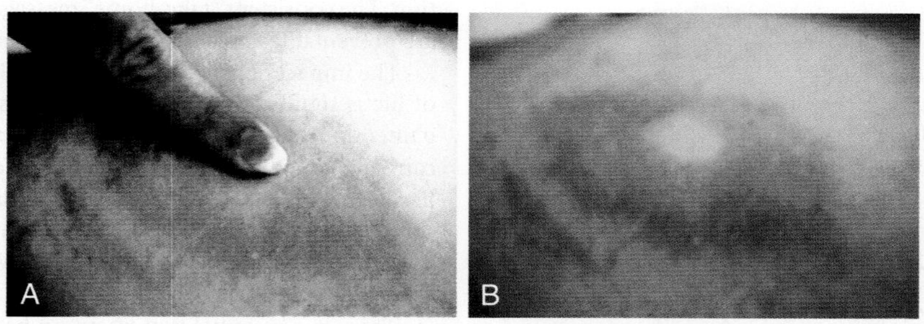

FIGURE 46-3 **A,** Reactive hyperemia. **B,** Blanching erythema: blanches with fingertip pressure.

which has produced a large number of evidence-informed Best Practice Guidelines for pressure injuries, venous leg ulcers, diabetic foot ulcers, continence, and constipation, among others. These and other resources are provided in the "Recommended Websites" section at the end of this chapter.

Pathogenesis of Pressure Injury. Pressure is the major element in the cause of pressure injury. Three pressure-related factors contribute to the development of pressure injuries: (1) pressure intensity, (2) pressure duration, and (3) tissue tolerance.

Pressure Intensity. A classic research study identified capillary closing pressure as the minimal amount of pressure required to collapse a capillary (e.g., when the pressure exceeds the normal capillary pressure range of 15 to 32 mm Hg) (Burton & Yamada, 1951). Therefore, if pressure applied over a capillary exceeds the normal capillary pressure and the vessel is occluded for a prolonged period of time, tissue ischemia, or reduction in blood flow, can occur. If the patient has decreased sensation and thus does not have the cue of discomfort to prompt shifting (off-loading) pressure, tissue death may result. The clinical presentation of obstructed blood flow occurs when the nurse evaluates areas of pressure. After a period of tissue ischemia, if pressure is relieved and blood flow returns, the skin turns red. The effect of this redness is vasodilatation (blood vessel expansion), called hyperemia (redness) (Figure 46-3, *A*). The area of hyperemia is evaluated by pressing a finger over the affected area. If the area blanches (turns lighter in colour) (Figure 46-3, *B*) and the redness returns when you remove your finger, hyperemia is transient and is an attempt to overcome the ischemic episode; thus, it is called *blanching hyperemia* (Pieper, 2016). If, however, the erythematous area does not blanch *(nonblanching erythema)* (Figure 46-4) when you apply pressure, deep tissue damage is probable.

Blanching occurs when the normal red tones of light-skinned patients are absent. Blanching does not occur in patients with darkly pigmented skin. The definition derived by The Task Force on the Implications for Darkly Pigmented Intact Skin in the Prediction and Prevention of Pressure Ulcers (Bennett, 1995) still stands today (Edsberg, Black, Goldberg, et al, 2016). Darkly pigmented skin is defined as skin that "remains unchanged (does not blanch) when pressure is applied over a bony prominence, irrespective of the patient's race or ethnicity." Characteristics of intact dark skin that will alert nurses to the potential for pressure injuries are found in Box 46-2.

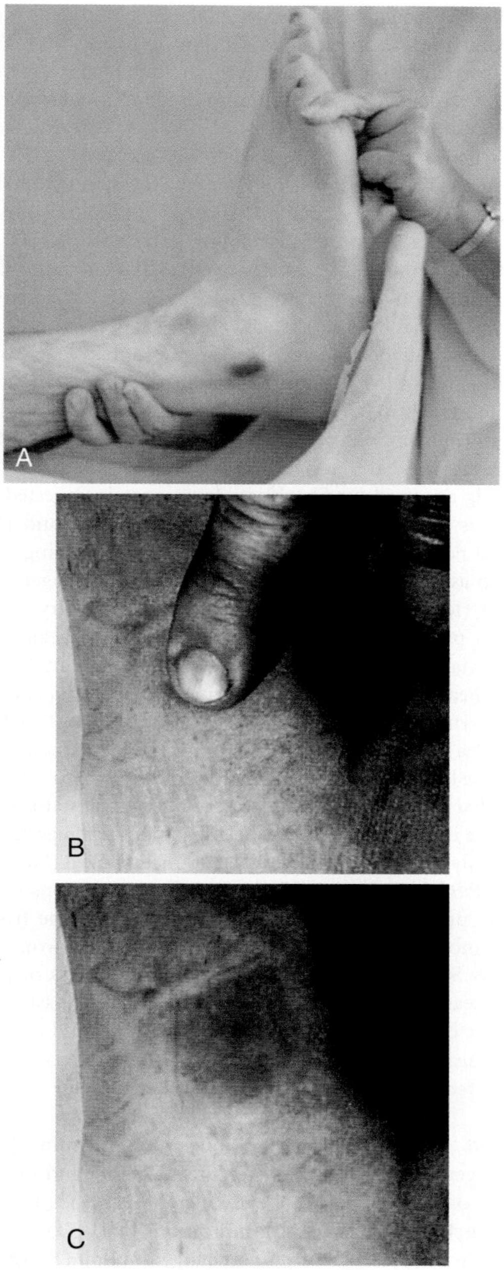

FIGURE 46-4 A, Reactive hyperemia. **B** and **C,** In nonblanching erythema, the area is much darker than the surrounding skin and does not blanch with fingertip pressure. (Pires, M., & Muller, A. [1991]. Detection and management of early tissue pressure indicators: A pictorial essay. *Progressions, 3*[3], 3.)

Pressure Duration. Two considerations are related to duration of pressure. Low pressures over a prolonged time period and high-intensity pressure over a short period of time both cause tissue damage. Extended pressure occludes blood flow and nutrients and contributes to cell death (Pieper, 2016). Clinical implications of pressure duration include evaluating the amount of pressure (check the skin for reactive hyperemia) and the amount of time that a patient tolerates pressure (check to be sure that after removing pressure, the affected area blanches).

Tissue Tolerance. The ability of tissue to endure pressure depends on the integrity of both the tissue and supporting structures. The extrinsic factors of shear, friction, and moisture affect the ability of the skin to tolerate pressure: the greater the degree to which these factors are present, the more susceptible the skin will be to damage from pressure. Another factor related to tissue tolerance pertains to the ability of the underlying skin structures (blood vessels, collagen) to assist in redistributing pressure. Systemic factors such as poor nutrition, age, and low blood pressure affect tissue tolerance to externally applied pressure.

BOX 46-2 Characteristics of Dark Skin at Risk of Skin Breakdown

Dark skin tones, especially darkly pigmented skin, may not demonstrate change in colour with a pressure injury. To assess a dark-skinned patient for the presence of a stage 1 pressure injury, the following should be considered:

Assess the skin in a well-lit environment.
Use natural light or halogen light.
Avoid florescent light.
Assess the following (assess noninjured skin areas first):

Colour

- Colour remains unchanged and does not blanch when pressure is applied.
- If patient previously had a pressure injury, that area of skin might be lighter than the original colour.
- Localized areas of inflammation may take on an eggplant (purplish-blue or violet) colour rather than appearing reddened.

Temperature

- Circumscribed area of intact skin may be warm to touch. As tissue changes colour, intact skin feels cool to touch.
- Inflammation is detected by making comparisons to surrounding skin.

Appearance

- Edema may occur with induration and appear taut and shiny.
- Injured skin with a stage 1 pressure injury might show low resilience. Document tissue resilience: tissue on palpation is boggy or mushy when compared to surrounding skin.

Palpation

- Surrounding area may be sensitive or tender to touch or may be hard or lumpy on palpation.

Adapted from Nix, D. P. (2016). Skin and wound inspection and assessment. In R. A. Bryant & D. P. Nix (Eds.), *Acute and chronic wounds: Current management concepts* (5th ed.). St. Louis: Elsevier.

NURSING KNOWLEDGE BASE

Prediction and Prevention of Pressure Injury

A major aspect of nursing care is the maintenance of skin integrity. Consistent, planned skin care interventions are critical to ensuring high-quality care. Nurses need to take every opportunity to observe and assess their patients' skin for impaired skin integrity.

Risk Factors for Pressure Injury Development. A variety of factors predisposes a patient to pressure injury. These factors are often directly related to disease, such as a decreased level of consciousness, the after-effects of trauma, or the presence of a cast, or are secondary to an illness, such as decreased sensation after a cerebrovascular accident.

The use of a pressure injury risk assessment tool, such as the Braden Scale (Braden & Bergstrom, 1988; discussed later), provides an initial assessment to determine appropriate interventions and ongoing regular assessment to evaluate skin status and treatment efficacy.

Impaired Sensory Perception. Patients with altered sensory perception of pain and pressure are at more risk of impaired skin integrity than are patients with normal sensation. Patients with impaired sensory perception of pain and pressure may not feel increased, prolonged pressure or pain and are at high risk of developing a pressure injury.

Impaired Mobility. Patients unable to independently change positions are at risk of pressure injury development. For example, patients with spinal cord injuries have decreased or absent motor and sensory perception and are unable to reposition themselves.

Alteration in Level of Consciousness. Patients who are confused or disoriented or with changing levels of consciousness may not be able to understand the sensation of pressure and respond by repositioning independently. As well, they may not be able to communicate discomfort or pain. Patients in a coma cannot perceive pressure and are unable to move voluntarily to relieve pressure.

Shear. **Shear** is the force exerted parallel to the skin and results from both gravity pushing down on the body and resistance (friction) between the patient and a surface (Pieper, 2016). For example, shear force occurs when the head of the bed is elevated and the skeleton starts to slide but the skin is fixed because of friction with the bed (Figure 46-5). In addition, shear force occurs when a patient is transferred from the bed to a stretcher and the patient's skin is pulled across the bed. When shear is present, the skin and subcutaneous layers adhere to the surface of the bed, while layers of muscle and the bones slide in the direction of body movement. The underlying tissue capillaries are stretched and angulated by the shear force. As a result, necrosis occurs deep within the tissue layers, causing undermining of the dermis. Heels are particularly vulnerable to injury from shear as patients are often repositioned in bed without the heels being supported.

Friction. The force of two surfaces moving across one another, such as the mechanical force exerted when skin is dragged across a coarse surface such as bed linens, is called **friction** (Wound, Ostomy and Continence Nurses [WOCN], 2010). Unlike shear injuries, friction injuries affect the epidermis, or top layer of the skin. The denuded skin appears red and painful and is sometimes referred to as a "sheet burn." A friction injury occurs in a patient who is dragged over the bed surface instead of being lifted slightly during position changes.

Moisture. The presence and duration of moisture on the skin increases the risk of ulcer formation. Moisture reduces the skin's resistance to other physical factors such as pressure and shear force. Prolonged moisture softens skin, which makes it more susceptible to damage. Immobilized patients, who are unable to take care of their own hygiene needs, depend on nurses to keep their skin dry and intact. Skin moisture originates from wound drainage, excessive perspiration, and fecal or urinary incontinence.

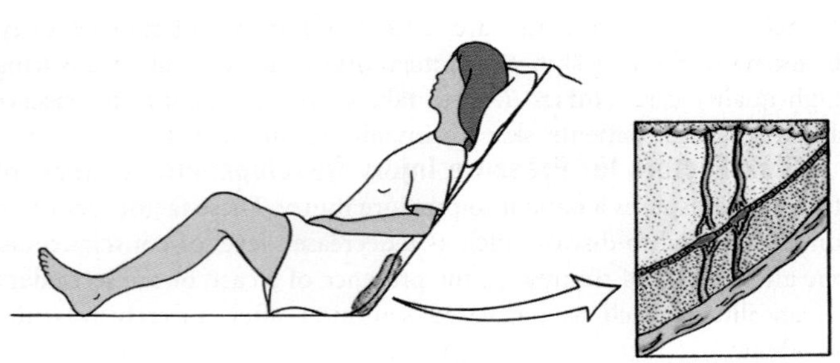

FIGURE 46-5 Sketch of shear force exerted against the sacral area.

Nutrition. Adequate nutritional intake is essential for not only wound healing but also wound prevention (Kennerly, Boss, Yap, et al., 2015). In particular, high-protein oral nutritional supplementation is necessary in patients whose prealbumin or albumin, hemoglobin, and serum zinc stores are low (Litchford, Dorner, & Posthauer, 2014; Posthauer, Banks, Dorner, et al., 2015; RNAO, 2016).

For patients weakened or debilitated by illness, nutritional therapy is especially important. A patient who has undergone surgery (see Chapter 48) and is well nourished still requires at least 1 500 kcal/day for nutritional maintenance. Alternatives such as enteral feedings and parenteral nutrition (see Chapter 42) are available for patients unable to maintain normal food intake.

Normal wound healing requires proper nutrition (Table 46-1). Deficiencies in any of the nutrients result in impaired or delayed healing (Stotts, 2016a). Physiological processes of wound healing depend on availability of protein, vitamins (especially A and C), and trace minerals: zinc and copper. **Collagen** is a protein formed from amino acids acquired by fibroblasts from protein ingested in food. Vitamin C is necessary for the synthesis of collagen, and vitamin A reduces the negative effects of steroids on wound healing. Trace elements such as zinc (used for epithelialization and collagen synthesis) and copper (for collagen fibre linking) are also necessary.

Calories provide the energy to support wound healing. Protein needs, especially, are increased. A balanced nutrient intake is critical for wound healing, including protein, fat, carbohydrates, vitamins, and minerals. Serum proteins are biochemical indicators of malnutrition (Stotts, 2016a). Although serum albumin is the most frequently measured of these laboratory parameters, it is not sensitive to rapid changes in nutritional status. The best measure of nutritional status is prealbumin because it reflects not only what the patient has ingested but also what the body has absorbed, digested, and metabolized (Stotts, 2016a).

Tissue Perfusion. Oxygen fuels the cellular functions essential to the healing process; therefore, the ability to perfuse the tissues with adequate amounts of oxygenated blood is critical to wound healing (Doughty & Sparks-Defriese, 2016). Patients with shock or peripheral vascular diseases, such as diabetes, are at risk of poor tissue perfusion due to poor circulation. Oxygen requirements depend on the phase of wound healing; for instance, chronic tissue hypoxia is associated with impaired collagen synthesis and reduced tissue resistance to infection.

Infection. Wound infection prolongs the inflammatory phase, delays collagen synthesis, prevents epithelialization, and increases the production of proinflammatory cytokines, which leads to additional tissue destruction (Stotts, 2016b). Indications that a wound infection is present are the presence of pus; a change in odour, volume, or the character of wound drainage; redness in the surrounding tissue; fever; or pain (Box 46-3).

Pain. Uncontrolled pain can affect the patient's ability to tolerate movement and can decrease tissue perfusion because of rapid, shallow breathing and tensed muscles. In addition, the patient's appetite may be diminished because of nausea from pain, and if the restorative powers of sleep are not accessible, the individual may feel hopeless and depressed from the unrelenting nature of both the wound and the persistent pain (Kohr & Gibson, 2008; Upton, Solowiej, & Woo, 2014).

Age. Physiological changes occur with aging. These changes will affect the healing trajectory of a wound. For example, decrease in the functioning of macrophages leads to a delayed inflammatory response, delayed collagen synthesis, and slower epithelialization.

Psychosocial Impact of Wounds. The patient's psychological response to any wound is part of the nursing assessment. Body-image changes often impose a great stress on the patient's adaptive mechanisms. In addition, body-image changes influence self-concept (see

TABLE 46-1 Role of Selected Nutrients in Wound Healing

Nutrient	Role in Healing	Recommendations	Sources
Calories	Fuel for cell energy "protein protection"	35–40 kcal/kg/day, or enough to maintain positive nitrogen balance	
Protein	Fibroplasia, angiogenesis, collagen formation, and wound remodelling, immune function	1.0–1.5 g/kg/day, or enough to maintain positive nitrogen balance	Poultry, fish, eggs, beef
Vitamin C (ascorbic acid)	Collagen synthesis, capillary wall integrity, fibroblast function, immunological function, antioxidant	100–1 000 mg/day Need long time before clinical scurvy from vitamin C deficiency develops Low toxicity	Citrus fruits, tomatoes, potatoes, fortified fruit juices
Vitamin A	Epithelialization, wound closure, inflammatory response, angiogenesis, collagen formation Can reverse steroid effects on skin and delayed healing	1 600–2 000 retinol equivalents per day Supplement if deficient 20 000 units × 10 days	Green leafy vegetables (spinach), broccoli, carrots, sweet potatoes, liver
Vitamin E	No known role in wound healing, antioxidant	None	Fish, oysters, liver, dark meat, eggs, legumes
Zinc	Collagen formation, protein synthesis, cell membrane and host defences	15–30 mg Correct deficiencies No improvement in wound healing with supplementation unless zinc deficient Use with caution: large doses can be toxic May inhibit copper metabolism and impair immune function	Vegetables, meats, legumes
Fluid	Essential fluid environment for all cell functions	30–35 mL/kg/day Increase by another 10–15 mL/kg if patient is on an air-fluidized bed	Use noncaffeine, nonalcoholic fluids without sugar Water is best: 6–8 glasses/day

Adapted from Ayello, E. A., Thomas, D. R., & Litchford, M. A. (1999). Nutritional aspects of wound healing. *Home Health Nurse, 17*(11), 719; and Stotts, N. A. (2016). Nutritional assessment and support. In R. A. Bryant & D. P. Nix (Eds.), *Acute and chronic wounds: Current management concepts* (5th ed.). St. Louis, MO: Mosby.

BOX 46-3 Classic Signs of Wound Infection

- Pain and tenderness at the wound site
- Erythema (reddening of the surrounding tissue)
- Edema (swelling), **induration** (increased firmness of the tissue)
- Inflammation of wound edges
- Purulent discharge
- Warmth in surrounding tissue
- Fever, chills
- Foul odour
- Elevated white blood cell count
- Delayed healing

Chronic Wounds

These show the above signs and symptoms as well as the following:

- Increased exudates
- Bright red discoloration of granulation tissue
- New areas of slough or breakdown on the wound surface
- Undermining (dead space under the edges of the wound)

Chapter 26) and sexuality (see Chapter 27). Nurses must ensure that the patient's personal and social resources for adaptation are a part of the assessment. Factors that affect the patient's perception of the wound include the presence of scars, drains (drains are often necessary for weeks or even months after certain procedures), odour from drainage, and temporary or permanent prosthetic devices.

CRITICAL THINKING

Successful critical thinking requires a synthesis of knowledge, experience, information gathered from patients, critical thinking attitudes, and intellectual and professional standards. Clinical judgement involves anticipating the information necessary, analyzing the data, and making decisions regarding patient care. Critical thinking is always changing. During assessment, it is important to consider all elements that build toward making appropriate nursing diagnoses (Figure 46-6).

When caring for patients who have impaired skin integrity and chronic wounds, nurses must integrate knowledge from nursing and other disciplines, previous experiences, and information gathered from patients to understand the risks to skin integrity and wound healing. Knowledge of normal musculoskeletal physiology, the pathogenesis of pressure injuries, normal wound healing, and the pathophysiology of underlying diseases provides nurses with a scientific basis for care. Wounds Canada (formerly Canadian Association of Wound Care) (Orsted, Keast, Foret-Lalande, et al., 2017) and the RNAO (2016) provide evidence-derived guidelines for assessment of the risk of impaired skin integrity, prevention measures, and interventions to promote wound healing, as well as other standards of practice that nurses should use in planning care. Past experience with patients at risk of impaired skin integrity or with patients with wounds increases the experiential knowledge base helping nurses to identify interventions.

Finally, as a nurse, you need to ensure that you remain attentive during assessment to obtain comprehensive and correct assessment data. As identified previously, a *continuum* exists to wound healing that

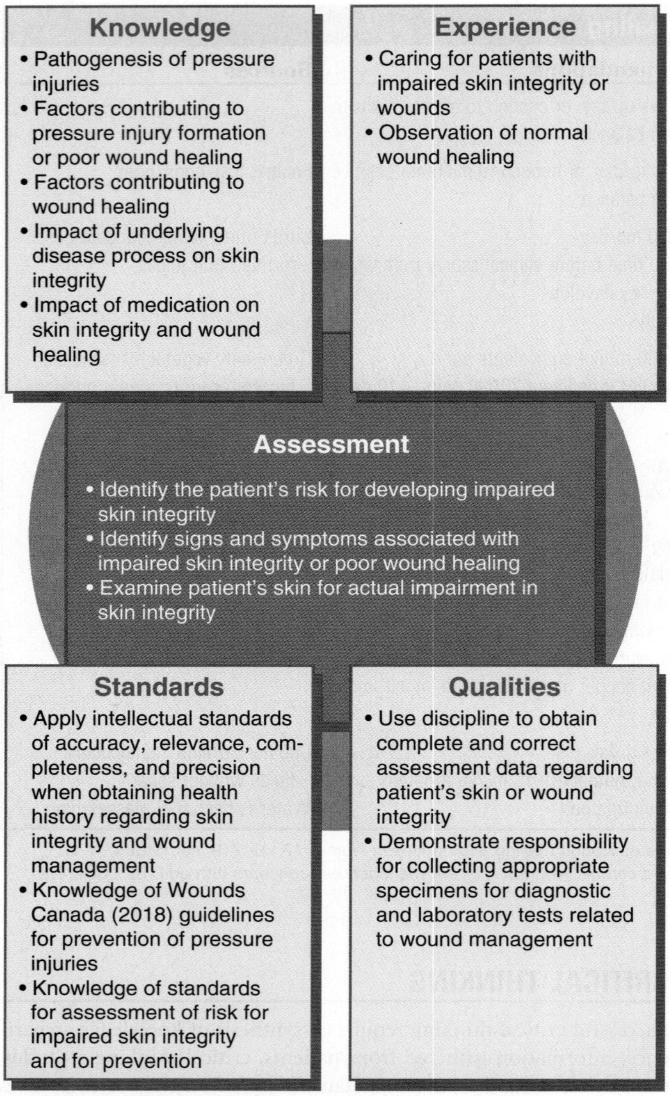

FIGURE 46-6 Critical thinking for skin integrity and wound care assessment.

implies change over time. You need to be aware that the patient and the skin or wound condition will not remain static, so you should reassess on a regular basis and adjust your plan of care accordingly. Knowledge and experience regarding wound healing will assist you in taking advantage of all the available and appropriate treatment options.

Assessment for tissue pressure damage involves visual and tactile inspection of the skin. The nurse's baseline assessment will determine the patient's normal skin characteristics and any potential or actual areas of breakdown (see Figure 46-2) . Nurses need to take into account the specific characteristics of a patient's skin, including pigmentation and effects of aging or medication (Bennett, 1995; Gould, Abadir, Brem, et al., 2015). Assessment characteristics of darkly pigmented skin appear in Boxes 46-2 and 46-4.

Particular attention must be paid to areas located over bony prominences or under casts, traction, splints, braces, collars, or other orthopedic devices. Oxygen tubing around noses and ears should be inspected. The frequency of pressure checks depends on the schedule of appliance application and the skin's response to the external pressure (Figure 46-7).

When hyperemia is noted, the nurse must document the location, size, and colour and reassess the area after 1 hour (Figure 46-8, *A*).

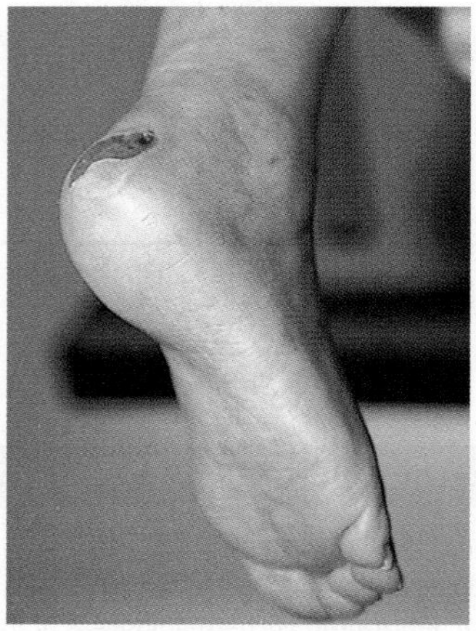

FIGURE 46-7 A pressure injury on the heel caused by pressure exerted by the mattress.

BOX 46-4 CULTURAL ASPECTS OF CARE

Skin Colour Impact

As a nurse, your ability to detect cyanosis and other changes in skin colour in patients is an important clinical skill. However, this detection becomes a challenge in dark-skinned patients. Cyanosis is a slightly bluish greyish slate-like or dark purple discoloration of the skin due to tissues near the skin surface having low oxygen saturation. Colour differentiation of cyanosis varies according to skin pigmentation. In dark-skinned patients, you need to know the individual's baseline skin tone. You should not confuse the normal hyperpigmentation of Mongolian spots that are seen on the sacrum of African, Indigenous, and Asian individuals as cyanosis. Observe the patient's skin in non-glare daylight. The Gaskin's Nursing Assessment of Skin Color (GNASC) is a useful assessment tool for identifying changes in skin colour that increase the patient's risk of pressure injuries.

Implications for Practice

- Cyanosis is difficult but possible to detect in the dark-skinned patient.
- Be aware of situations that produce changes in skin tone, such as inadequate lighting.
- Examine body sites with the least melanin, such as under the arm, for underlying colour identification.
- Evaluate pigmented skin for colour-specific changes in skin tone.

Adapted from Gaskin, F. C. (1986). Detection of cyanosis in the person with dark skin. *Journal of National Black Nurses' Association, 1,* 52; Myers, J. (2015). Challenges of identifying eczema in darkly pigmented skin. *Nursing Children and Young People, 27*(6), 24–28; National Pressure Ulcer Advisory Panel (NPUAP). (2016). *Pressure injury stages.* Retrieved from http://www.npuap.org/resources/educational-and-clinical-resources/npuap-pressure-injury-stages/; and Henderson, C. T., Ayello, E. A., Sussman, C., Leiby, D. M., Bennett, M. A., Dungog, E. F., et al. (1997). Draft definition of stage I pressure ulcers: Inclusion of persons with darkly pigmented skin. *Advances in Wound Care, 10*(5), 16–19.

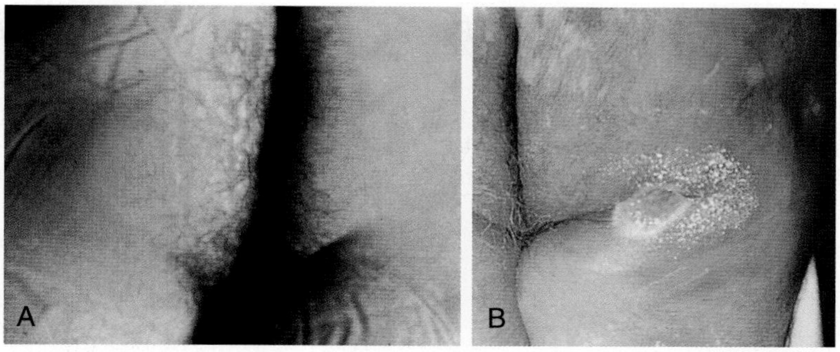

FIGURE 46-8 A, Hyperemia on ischial tuberosity. **B,** Ulcer. (Pires, M., & Muller, A. [1991]. Decision and management of early tissue pressure indicators: A pictorial essay. *Progressions, 3*[3], 3.)

When abnormal reactive hyperemia is suspected, the nurse needs to outline the affected area with a marker to make reassessment easier. These signs are early indicators of impaired skin integrity, but damage to the underlying tissue is sometimes more progressive (Figure 46-8, *B*). Palpation with the fingertips will help the nurse assess and identify induration or other damage to skin and underlying tissues.

The nurse should gently palpate the reddened tissue, observing for blanching as normal skin tones return in patients with light-toned skin. In addition, the nurse needs to palpate for induration, noting size in millimetres or centimetres of the induration around the injured area. Changes in the temperature of the surrounding skin and tissues should also be noted.

❖ NURSING PROCESS

◆ Assessment

Skin integrity is subject to change over time. Baseline and continual assessment data support critical information about the patient's skin integrity and the increased risk of developing pressure injuries. The specific factors, such as continence status or mobility, help focus the nurse's assessment (Box 46-5).

Skin

Nurses should ensure that ongoing assessment occurs to guard against skin breakdown, and nurses should treat any tears or wounds promptly. The neurologically impaired patient, the chronically ill patient in long-term care, the patient with diminished mental status, and patients in the Critical Care Unit (CCU) or oncology, hospice, or orthopedic departments all have an increased potential of developing pressure injuries.

Risk Assessment

By identifying and promptly treating at-risk patients, nurses can spare patients with little risk of pressure injury development the unnecessary and sometimes costly preventive treatments and related risks of complications (Skill 46-1). Prevention and treatment of pressure injuries are *major* nursing priorities, no matter what the health care setting. Evidence exists that a program of prevention guided by consistent risk assessment simultaneously reduces the institutional incidence of pressure injuries by as much as 60% and decreases the costs of prevention at the same time (Braden, 2001). The Braden Pressure Ulcer Risk Assessment Scale has been identified by Wounds Canada and the RNAO Best Practice Guidelines as a reliable and valid risk assessment tool across all health care sectors and is the most commonly used (Orsted et al., 2017; RNAO, 2016). However, an assessment tool is exactly that, a tool to assist nurses in planning intervention strategies and evaluation of a patient's skin on an ongoing basis. No assessment tool can replace your clinical judgement as a nurse (RNAO, 2016).

BOX 46-5 Nursing Assessment Questions

Skin Integrity

Sensation

- Do you have any loss of feeling in your feet or legs or anywhere else?
- Do you feel more (or less) sensitive to heat or cold?

Mobility

- Do you have any physical conditions, injury, or paralysis that limits your mobility?
- Can you easily change your position?
- Is it painful to move?

Continence

- Do you have any problems with urine or bowel continence?
- Do you need help when you use the toilet?
- How often do you need to use the toilet? During the day? During the night?

Presence of a Wound

- How did this wound happen?
- When did the wound occur?
- When did you last receive a tetanus shot?
- What happened to this wound since it occurred? Is it getting better? Or worse?
- What treatments, activities, or care have slowed or helped the wound healing process? Are there other things we could be doing to improve things?
- Is the wound painful? If so, can you describe the pain (burning, stabbing, sharp, dull, etc.) or is it itchy? What have you been doing to manage this? Is it working?
- What would you like, in terms of the goal for yourself, in relation to this wound and its healing?

Braden Scale

The Braden Scale (Table 46-2) was developed on the basis of risk factors in a nursing home population (Bergstrom, Braden, Laguzza, et al., 1987). It is the most widely used risk assessment tool in North America to assess patients for risk of skin breakdown. What is important to note is that the Braden Scale comprises six subscales: sensory perception, moisture, activity, mobility, nutrition, and friction and

SKILL 46-1 ASSESSMENT FOR RISK OF PRESSURE INJURY DEVELOPMENT

Delegation Considerations

Assessment of patients for risk of pressure injury should not be delegated to unregulated care providers (UCPs); however, prevention strategies should be included in their work plan. Check with your institution's policy in this regard.

Prevention

- Document changes to patient's skin, such as redness, blistering, abrasions, or cuts.
- Keep patient's skin dry: clean well after incontinence (urine or stool) or exposure to other body fluids.
- Reposition patient according to frequency established in nursing care plan or agency policy.
- Avoid trauma to patient's skin from tape, pressure, friction, or shear.

Equipment

- Use a risk assessment tool: Braden Scale (used in this skill) or other tool, according to agency policy.
- Documentation record

PROCEDURE

STEPS	RATIONALE
1. Identify at-risk individuals needing prevention and specific risk factors.	• Identification determines factors that increase the patient's risk of developing pressure injuries (Braden, 2014; RNAO, 2016).
A. Use a validated risk assessment tool (e.g., the Braden Scale).	• Consistent, reliable, comparable assessments are ensured (Gadd & Morris, 2014; NPUAP, 2016; RNAO, 2016).
B. Assess the patient on admission to the hospital, long-term care facility, home care program, or other health care facility.	• A baseline assessment is provided.
C. Inspect the condition of the patient's skin at least once a day (see Box 46-5) and examine all bony prominences, noting skin integrity. (Check agency policy for reassessment and reassess at periodic intervals.) If redness or discoloration is noted, palpate area of redness for blanchable erythema.	• Routine skin assessments will identify changes in patient's risk of pressure injuries. • Nonblanchable erythema or discoloration in the patient's skin may be an early indicator of skin injury (Pieper, 2016).

CRITICAL DECISION POINT: *In dark-skinned patients, the discoloration appears as a deepening of the normal colour (see Box 46-2). Darkly pigmented skin does not always show direct changes in colour (Bennett, 1995; NPUAP, 2016).*

STEPS	RATIONALE
D. Observe all assistive devices, such as braces or casts, and medical equipment, such as nasogastric and enteral tubes and catheters, for pressure points.	• Presence of medical equipment may cause pressure and skin breakdown in sensitive regions, such as nostrils, ears, or other bony prominences.
2. Determine patient's ability to respond meaningfully to pressure-related discomfort (sensory perception).	• Patients with completely, very, or slightly limited ability to respond to pressure-related discomfort cannot communicate discomfort, will have a limited ability to feel pain, and, thus, risk developing pressure injuries.
3. Assess the degree to which patient's skin is exposed to moisture.	• Exposure to excessive moisture increases the risk of skin breakdown due to changes in skin pH and maceration of skin.
4. Evaluate the patient's activity level.	• The patient who is bedfast, chairfast, or only walks occasionally limits repositioning and pressure off-loading due to physical inactivity.
A. Determine patient's ability to change and control body position (mobility).	• Potential for friction and shear injury increases when the patient is completely dependent on others for position change.
B. Determine patient's preferred positions.	• Habitual positioning (e.g., lying on one side or the other) may result in skin breakdown as the patient may resist repositioning to different areas.
5. Assess patient's usual food and fluid intake pattern (nutrition and hydration).	• A patient who never eats a complete meal, rarely eats a complete meal, or has limited fluid intake is at risk of skin breakdown.
A. Review weight pattern and nutritional laboratory values.	• Decreased nutritional status is linked with pressure ulcer formation and poor wound healing (Kennerly et al., 2015; RNAO, 2016).
B. Complete a fluid intake assessment.	• Fluid imbalance, either dehydration or edema, can increase the patient's risk of pressure injuries.
6. Evaluate the presence of friction and shear.	• The patient who has spastic limbs, requires maximum assistance in moving, or slides against sheets when moved is at an increased risk of skin damage.

STEPS	RATIONALE
7. Document the risk assessment on admission, on a regular basis according to institutional policy, and if any change in status occurs (Sibbald, Orsted, et al., 2006).	• The documentation provides a baseline to track risk of development of pressure injuries and allow planning of interventions.
A. Observe the Braden Scale scores: as they become lower, predicted risk becomes higher. Existing skin breakdown increases the risk by one level.	• Scores: 15–16, mild risk 13–14, moderate risk 10–12, high risk <10, very high risk • Existing skin breakdown indicates risk factors are already present and require attention.
B. Link the risk assessment to preventive protocols.	• Prevention protocols will target problem areas to assist in prevention of skin breakdown (Gadd & Morris, 2014).
C. Institute mild-risk interventions (score of 15–16). Plan of care should include frequent turning; maximum remobilization; off-load heel pressure; use of pressure-reducing support surface; managing moisture, nutrition, and friction and shear.	• The risk of skin breakdown is decreased.
D. Institute moderate-risk interventions (score of 13–14). Plan of care should include interventions for mild risk (Step 7C), as well as use of foam wedges to position the patient in the 30-degree lateral position.	• The increased risk of skin breakdown is decreased with appropriate interventions.
E. Institute high-risk interventions (score of 10–12). Plan of care should include interventions for moderate risk (Step 7D), as well as instructions to turn the patient with small shifts in weight.	• The factors that contribute to skin breakdown are identified, and appropriate interventions are planned.
F. Institute very high-risk interventions (score of <10). Plan of care should include interventions for high risk (Step 7E) as well as use of a pressure-relieving surface, which still requires frequent repositioning of patient.	• Plan interventions to decrease the effects of immobility, decreased sensory perception, moisture, friction, shear, decreased activity, and nutritional issues in a high-risk individual.
8. Provide education to patient and family regarding pressure injury risk.	• Patient and family understand and participate as much as possible in the interventions designed to reduce pressure injury risk.
9. Evaluate measures to reduce pressure injury development.	• Evaluation on a regular basis provides opportunity to assess and adjust interventions.
A. Observe patient's skin for areas at risk.	• Patient's response to risk-reduction interventions is determined over time.
B. Observe tolerance of patient for positioning.	• Frequent change in position further reduces patient's risk of developing pressure injuries.
C. Monitor the success of a toileting program or other measures to reduce the frequency of incontinence of urine or stool.	• Avoiding moisture from urine or stool on patient's skin reduces risk of skin breakdown.
D. Evaluate laboratory nutrition values.	• Value of nutritional supplements in improving nutritional status is determined.

UNEXPECTED OUTCOMES	RELATED INTERVENTIONS
No blanching when skin is firmly pressed, purple discoloration, or significant colour change	• Reassess frequency of turning schedule. • Implement agency's skin care protocols. • Consider support surface to reduce pressure injury risk.

RECORDING AND REPORTING

- Record patient's risk score and subscores.
- Record appearance of skin (at pressure points, etc.).
- Describe position, turning intervals, pressure-relieving devices, and other prevention strategies.
- Report any need for additional consultations (e.g., wound care specialist or dietitian) for the high-risk patient.

HOME CARE CONSIDERATIONS

- Instruct caregiver to use the 30-degree lateral position. This position reduces pressure over the trochanter.
- Pressure-relief manoeuvres need to be individualized for patient needs and the home environment. Provide the family with resources to access equipment.

TABLE 46-2 Braden Scale for Predicting Pressure Sore Risk

Patient's Name ________________________ Evaluator's Name ________________________ Date of Assessment ________________

Characteristic	Score: 1	Score: 2	Score: 3	Score: 4
Sensory Perception				
Ability to respond meaningfully to pressure-related discomfort	1. Completely limited Unresponsive (does not moan, flinch, or gasp) to painful stimuli due to diminished level of consciousness or sedation. OR Limited ability to feel pain over most of body surface.	2. Very limited Responds only to painful stimuli. Cannot communicate discomfort except by moaning or restlessness. OR Has a sensory impairment that limits the ability to feel pain or discomfort over half of body.	3. Slightly limited Responds to verbal commands but cannot always communicate discomfort or need to be turned. OR Has some sensory impairment that limits ability to feel pain or discomfort in one or two extremities.	4. No impairment Responds to verbal commands. Has no sensory deficit that would limit ability to feel or voice pain or discomfort.
Moisture				
Degree to which skin is exposed to moisture	1. Constantly moist Skin is kept moist almost constantly by perspiration, urine, etc. Dampness is detected every time patient is moved or turned.	2. Moist Skin is often, but not always, moist. Linen must be changed at least once a shift.	3. Occasionally moist Skin is occasionally moist, requiring an extra linen change approximately once a day.	4. Rarely moist Skin is usually dry. Linen only requires changing at routine intervals.
Activity				
Degree of physical activity	1. Bedfast Confined to bed.	2. Chairfast Ability to walk severely limited or nonexistent. Cannot bear own weight or must be assisted into chair or wheelchair.	3. Walks occasionally Walks occasionally during day but for very short distances, with or without assistance. Spends majority of each shift in bed or chair.	4. Walks frequently Walks outside the room at least twice a day and inside room at least once every 2 hours during waking hours.
Mobility				
Ability to change and control body position	1. Completely immobile Does not make even slight changes in body or extremity position without assistance.	2. Very limited Makes occasional slight changes in body or extremity position but unable to make frequent or significant changes independently.	3. Slightly limited Makes frequent though slight changes in body or extremity position independently.	4. No limitations Makes major and frequent changes in position without assistance.
Nutrition				
Usual food intake pattern	1. Very poor Never eats a complete meal. Rarely eats more than one-third of any food offered. Eats two servings or less of protein (meat or dairy products) per day. Takes fluids poorly. Does not take a liquid dietary supplement. OR Is NPO or maintained on clear liquids or IVs for more than 5 days.	2. Probably inadequate Rarely eats a complete meal and generally eats only about half of any food offered. Protein intake includes only three servings of meat or dairy products per day. Occasionally will take a dietary supplement. OR Receives less than optimum amount of liquid diet or tube feeding.	3. Adequate Eats over half of most meals. Eats a total of four servings of protein (meat, dairy products) each day. Occasionally will refuse a meal but will usually take a supplement if offered. OR Is on a tube feeding or total parenteral nutrition regimen that probably meets most nutritional needs.	4. Excellent Eats most of every meal. Never refuses a meal. Usually eats a total of four or more servings of meat and dairy products. Occasionally eats between meals. Does not require supplementation.

TABLE 46-2 Braden Scale for Predicting Pressure Sore Risk—cont'd

Friction and Shear	1. Problem Requires moderate to maximum assistance in moving. Complete lifting without sliding against sheets is impossible. Frequently slides down in bed or chair, requiring frequent repositioning with maximum assistance. Spasticity, contractures, or agitation leads to almost constant friction.	2. Potential problem Moves feebly or requires minimum assistance. During a move, skin probably slides to some extent against sheets, chair, restraints, or other devices. Maintains relatively good position in chair or bed most of the time but occasionally slides down.	3. No apparent problem Moves in bed and in chair independently and has sufficient muscle strength to lift up completely during move. Maintains good position in bed or chair at all times.
TOTAL SCORE			

NPO, Nothing by mouth.

shear. While the total score provides a prediction of risk of skin breakdown, nurses must pay attention to the subscales. When a subscale result is low, interventions should be initiated, relevant to that indicator (Gadd & Morris, 2014). Remember, the *lower* the score, the *higher* the risk; the total score ranges from 6 to 23, and a lower total score indicates a higher risk of pressure injury development (Braden & Bergstrom, 1989). The cutoff score for onset of pressure injury risk with the Braden Scale in the general adult population is 18 (Ayello & Braden, 2002). The Braden Scale is highly reliable and has been widely used to identify patients at greatest risk of pressure injuries (Bergstrom et al., 1987; Braden & Bergstrom, 1994; Orsted et al., 2017).

Case Example. Your patient is Mrs. Hetje Lamont, an 85-year-old widow with a recent left-sided stroke who lives alone and who has been admitted to your acute care medical floor. She has obvious slurred speech and some facial drooping; her left arm is flaccid and she tells you she "can't feel it at all." She has been incontinent of urine since the stroke and is wearing an adult continence product. She seems alert (oriented to time, place, person) but has been noted to be "a bit confused and weepy at times." Her status has been nothing by mouth (NPO) for the past 48 hours, in preparation for a swallowing assessment. (She is currently receiving only IV normal saline.) Her daughter tells you that Mrs. Lamont "has been eating like a bird" for the past few weeks.

When you come to the bedside, she is lying on her right side and has difficulty moving without help. She is too weak to ambulate and needs assistance to sit in a chair.

Questions:

- What is her score on the Braden Scale?
- From the subscore results, what interventions would be appropriate?
- How often would you reassess your patient for risk of skin breakdown?

Classification of Pressure Injury

Nurses need to assess pressure injury at regular intervals using systematic variables to evaluate wound healing, plan appropriate interventions, and evaluate progress. One method nurses can use for assessment of a pressure injury is a staging system. Staging systems for pressure injury are based on the description of the depth of tissue destroyed. Accurate staging requires knowledge of the skin layers. A major drawback of a staging system is that a wound covered with necrotic tissue cannot be staged because the necrotic tissue is covering the depth of the wound (Figure 46-9). The necrotic tissue must be debrided or removed to expose the wound base to allow for assessment.

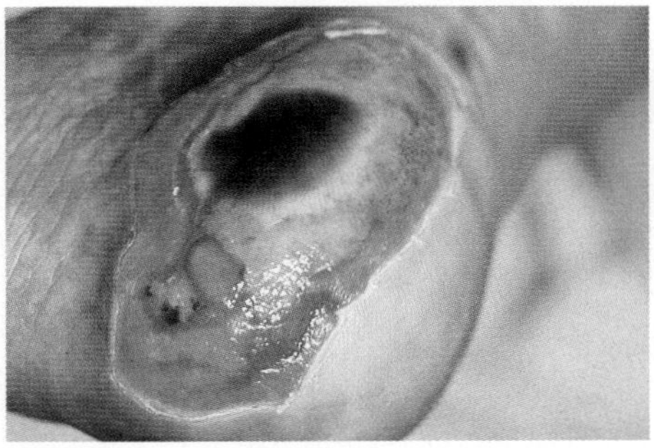

FIGURE 46-9 Pressure injury with tissue necrosis.

The National Pressure Ulcer Advisory Panel (NPUAP) (2007) proposed a four-stage classification system with an additional deep tissue injury descriptor (Table 46-3). In 2016, the NPUAP revised the staging definitions, including changing the terminology from *pressure ulcer* to *pressure injury*. While this may seem confusing, it addresses the problem of deep tissue injury and stage 1, which appear as intact skin, not as an ulcer. In addition, the use of Roman numerals (I, II, II, IV) has been changed to numbers (1, 2, 3, 4) for simpler documentation. Where pressure injury is observed, documentation needs to occur. Staging describes the pressure injury depth at the point of assessment. Thus, once staged, the wound as it heals (or deteriorates) is identified as (for example) a healing stage 3 pressure injury (Nix, 2016). While this is a very recent change in documentation naming, it does not change the descriptions of the actual pressure injury (Box 46-6).

In addition, Bennett (1995) suggested that when nurses assess patients with darkly pigmented skin, proper lighting is important to accurately assess the skin (see Box 46-2). Either natural light or a halogen light is recommended. This prevents the blue tones that fluorescent light sources produce on darkly pigmented skin, which interfere with accurate assessment.

For a wound with **nonviable tissue**, the nurse needs to include the amount (percentage) and appearance (colour) of viable and nonviable

TABLE 46-3 Guidelines for Staging Pressure Injury

The following criteria can be used as a visual aid to help identify and appropriately stage pressure injury. The definitions were derived from work done by the National Pressure Ulcer Advisory Panel and published in February 2007; revision April 2016.

Suspected Deep Tissue Injury

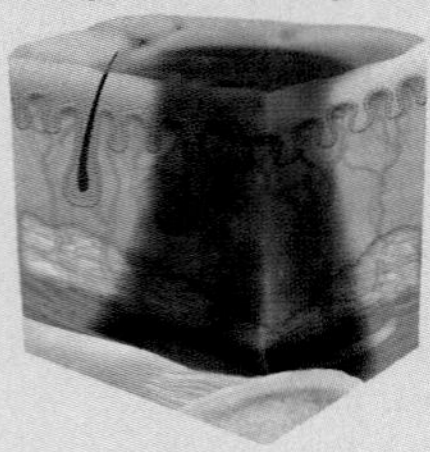

Intact or nonintact skin with localized area of persistent nonblanchable deep red, maroon, purple discoloration or epidermal separation revealing a dark wound bed or blood-filled blister. Pain and temperature change often precede skin colour changes. Discoloration may appear differently in darkly pigmented skin. This injury results from intense or prolonged pressure and shear forces at the bone–muscle interface. The wound may evolve rapidly to reveal the actual extent of tissue injury, or it may resolve without tissue loss.

Stage 1

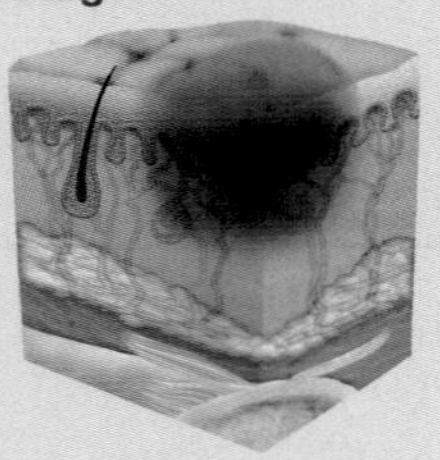

Intact skin with a localized area of nonblanchable erythema, which may appear differently in darkly pigmented skin. Presence of blanchable erythema or changes in sensation, temperature, or firmness may precede visual changes. Colour changes do not include purple or maroon discoloration; these may indicate deep tissue pressure injury.

Stage 2

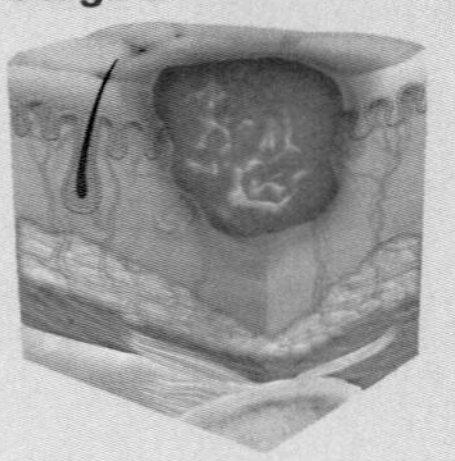

Partial-thickness loss of skin with exposed dermis. The wound bed is viable, pink or red, and moist and may also present as an intact or ruptured serum-filled blister. Adipose (fat) is not visible and deeper tissues are not visible. Granulation tissue, slough, and eschar are not present. These injuries commonly result from adverse microclimate and shear in the skin over the pelvis and shear in the heel. This stage should not be used to describe moisture-associated skin damage (MASD), including incontinence-associated dermatitis (IAD), intertriginous dermatitis (ITD), medical adhesive–related skin injury (MARSI), or traumatic wounds (skin tears, burns, abrasions).

Stage 3

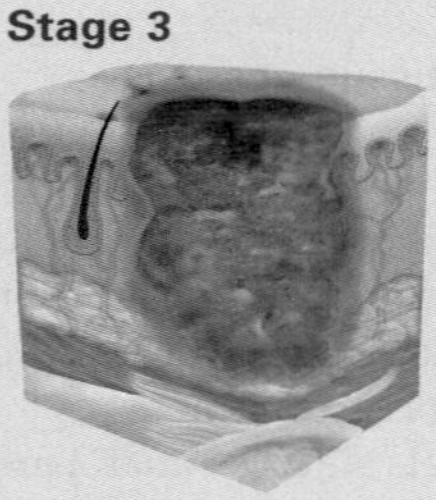

Full-thickness loss of skin, in which adipose (fat) is visible in the ulcer and granulation tissue and epibole (rolled wound edges) are often present. Slough, eschar, or both may be visible. The depth of tissue damage varies by anatomical location; areas of significant adiposity can develop deep wounds. Undermining and tunnelling may occur. Fascia, muscle, tendon, ligament, cartilage, and bone are not exposed.

Stage 4

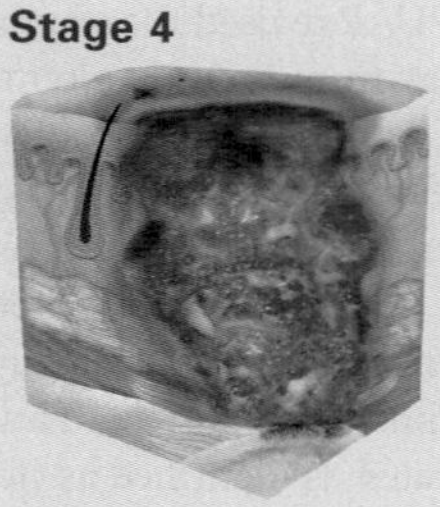

Full-thickness skin and tissue loss with exposed or directly palpable fascia, muscle, tendon, ligament, cartilage, or bone in the ulcer. Slough, eschar, or both may be visible. Epibole (rolled edges), undermining, tunneling, or a combination of these often occur. Depth varies by anatomical location.

Unstageable

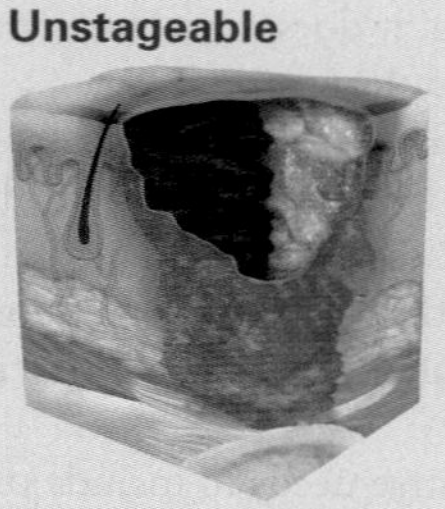

Full-thickness skin and tissue loss in which the extent of tissue damage within the ulcer cannot be confirmed because it is obscured by slough or eschar. If slough or eschar is removed, a stage 3 or stage 4 pressure injury will be revealed. Stable eschar (i.e., dry, adherent, intact without erythema or fluctuance) on the heel or ischemic limb should not be softened or removed.

From National Pressure Ulcer Advisory Panel. (2016). *Pressure injury stages*. Retrieved from http://www.npuap.org/resources/educational-and-clinical-resources/npuap-pressure-injury-stages/.

BOX 46-6 National Pressure Ulcer Advisory Panel Staging Guidelines

Suspected Deep Tissue Injury
Please refer to Table 46-3 for a description of a suspected deep tissue injury.

Further Description
Deep tissue injury may be difficult to detect in individuals with dark skin tones. Evolution may include a thin blister over a dark wound bed. The wound may further evolve and become covered by thin eschar. Evolution may be rapid, exposing additional layers of tissue, even with optimal treatment.

Stage 1
Please refer to Table 46-3 for a description of a stage 1 pressure injury.

Further Description
The area may be painful, firm, soft, warmer, or cooler as compared with adjacent tissue. Stage I may be difficult to detect in individuals with dark skin tones. The stage may indicate at-risk persons (a heralding sign of risk).

Stage 2
Please refer to Table 46-3 for a description of a stage 2 pressure injury.

Further Description
The stage presents as a shiny or dry, shallow ulcer without slough or bruising. (Bruising indicates suspected deep tissue injury.) This stage should not be used to describe skin tears, tape burns, perineal dermatitis, maceration, or excoriation.

Stage 3
Please refer to Table 46-3 for a description of a stage 3 pressure injury.

Further Description
The depth of a stage 3 pressure injury varies by anatomical location. The bridge of the nose, ear, occiput, and malleolus do not have subcutaneous tissue, and stage 3 pressure injury can be shallow. In contrast, areas of significant adiposity can develop extremely deep stage 3 pressure injury. The bone or tendon is not visible or directly palpable.

Stage 4
Please see Table 46-3 for a description of a stage 4 pressure injury.

Further Description
The depth of a stage 4 pressure injury varies by anatomical location. The bridge of the nose, ear, occiput, and malleolus do not have subcutaneous tissue and these ulcers can be shallow. Stage 4 injuries can extend into muscle or supporting structures (e.g., fascia, tendon, or joint capsule) or both, making osteomyelitis possible. Exposed bone or tendon is visible or directly palpable.

Unstageable
Please refer to Table 46-3 for a description of an unstageable pressure injury.

Further Description
Until enough slough or eschar is removed to expose the base of the wound, the true depth and, therefore, stage cannot be determined. Stable (dry, adherent, intact without erythema or fluctuance) eschar on the heels serves as "the body's natural (biological) cover" and should not be removed. The staging system was defined by Shea in 1975 and provides a name to the amount of anatomical tissue loss. The original definitions were confusing to many clinicians and led to inaccurate staging of wounds associated with or due to perineal dermatitis and those due to deep tissue injury.

From National Pressure Ulcer Advisory Panel. (2007). Pressure ulcer definitions. Retrieved from http://www.npuap.org/documents/NPUAP2007_PU_Def_and_Descriptions.pdf. Revised 2016.

tissue. This will assist the nurse in developing the appropriate plan of care based on the healing ability of the wound.

Granulation tissue is red, moist tissue composed of new blood vessels, the presence of which indicates progression toward healing. Soft yellow or white tissue is characteristic of **slough** (a stringy substance attached to the wound bed), which will need to be removed before the wound is able to heal. Black or brown necrotic tissue is **eschar**, which usually needs to be removed before healing can proceed. Sharp debridement of a wound, to remove nonviable tissue, can be performed only by a nurse who has the appropriate knowledge, skill, and clinical judgement and agency or institution policy and procedure in place.

The measurement of the size of the wound provides overall changes in size, which is an indicator for wound healing progress (Nix, 2016). Consistent measurement of length × width is appropriate to track progress. While a disposable ruler is likely most readily available, mobile technology has developed automated and accurate wound measurement tools, which are becoming more accessible (Bills, Berriman, Noble, et al., 2016). Depth is obtained by using a sterile cotton-tipped applicator to gently probe for tunnelling and undermining in the wound bed.

Wound **exudate** describes the amount, colour, consistency, and odour of wound drainage and is part of the wound assessment. Excessive exudate usually indicates presence of an infection. Nurses should also evaluate the condition of the skin surrounding the wound for redness, warmth, maceration, or edema (swelling). The presence of any of these factors on the periwound skin indicates wound deterioration.

Wound Classifications

A **wound** is a disruption of the integrity and function of tissues in the body (Bryant & Clark, 2016). It is imperative that nurses understand that *all wounds are not created equal.* Understanding the etiology of a wound is important because the treatment for the wound varies, depending on the underlying disease process. Some treatments are even harmful to certain wounds, so nurses always need to obtain a complete history, including the etiology of the wound.

Wounds can be classified in many ways. Wound classification systems describe the status of skin integrity, cause of the wound, severity or extent of tissue injury or damage, cleanliness of the wound (Table 46-4), or descriptive qualities of wound tissue, such as colour (Figure 46-10). Wound classifications enable nurses to understand the risks associated with a wound and implications for healing.

Process of Wound Healing

Wound healing comprises integrated physiological processes. The tissue layers involved and their capacity for regeneration determine the mechanism for repair of any wound (Doughty & Sparks-Defriese, 2016). Two types of wounds are those with loss of tissue and those without. A clean surgical incision is an example of a wound with little tissue loss. The surgical wound heals by **primary intention**. The skin edges are **approximated**, or closed, and the risk of infection is low.

TABLE 46-4 Wound Classification

Description	Causes	Implications for Healing
Onset and Duration		
Acute		
A wound that proceeds through an orderly and timely reparative process that results in sustained restoration of anatomical and functional integrity.	Trauma, a surgical incision	Wounds are usually easily cleaned and repaired. Wound edges are clean and intact.
Chronic		
Wound that fails to proceed through an orderly and timely process to produce anatomical and functional integrity.	Vascular compromise, chronic inflammation, or repetitive insults to the tissue (Doughty & Sparks-Defriese, 2016)	Continued exposure to insult impedes wound healing.
Healing Process		
Primary Intention		
Wound that is closed.	Surgical incision, wound that is sutured or stapled	Healing occurs by epithelialization; heals quickly with minimal scar formation.
Secondary Intention		
Wound edges are not approximated.	Pressure wounds, surgical wounds that have tissue loss	Wound heals by granulation tissue formation, wound contraction, and epithelialization.
Tertiary Intention		
Wound is left open for several days, then wound edges are approximated.	Wounds that are contaminated and require observation for signs of inflammation	Closure of wound is delayed until risk of infection is resolved (Doughty & Sparks-Defriese, 2016).

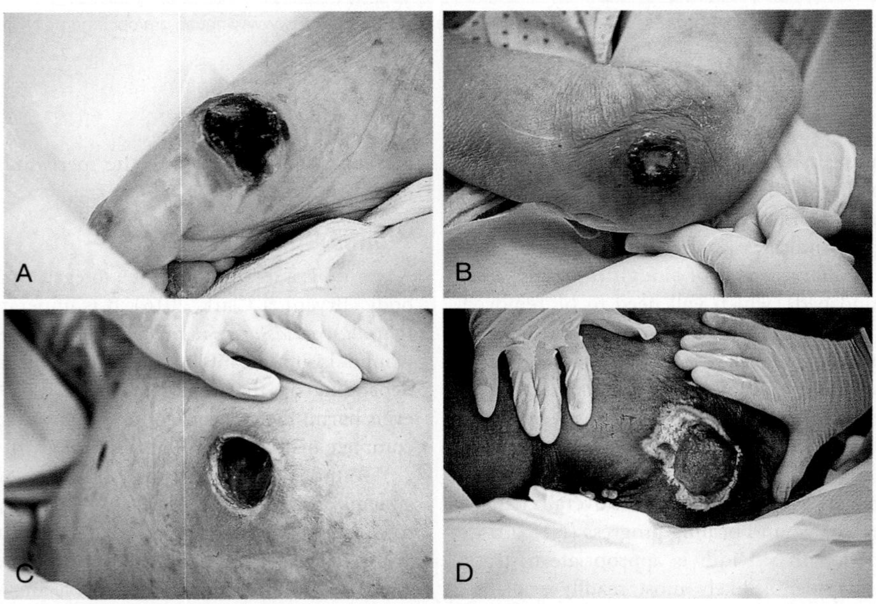

FIGURE 46-10 Wounds classified by colour assessment. A, Black wound. **B,** Yellow wound. **C,** Red wound. **D,** Mixed-colour wound. (Courtesy Scott Health Care—A Molnlycke Company. Philadelphia, PA.)

Healing occurs quickly, with minimal scar formation, as long as infection and secondary breakdown are prevented (Doughty & Sparks-Defriese, 2016). In contrast, a wound involving loss of tissue, such as a burn, pressure injury, or severe laceration, heals by **secondary intention.** The wound is left open until it becomes filled by scar tissue. It takes longer for a wound to heal by secondary intention; thus, the chance of infection is greater. If scarring from secondary intention is severe, loss of tissue function is often permanent (Figure 46-11).

Wound Repair

Partial-thickness wounds are shallow wounds involving loss of the epidermis (top layer) and possibly partial loss of the dermis. Epidermal

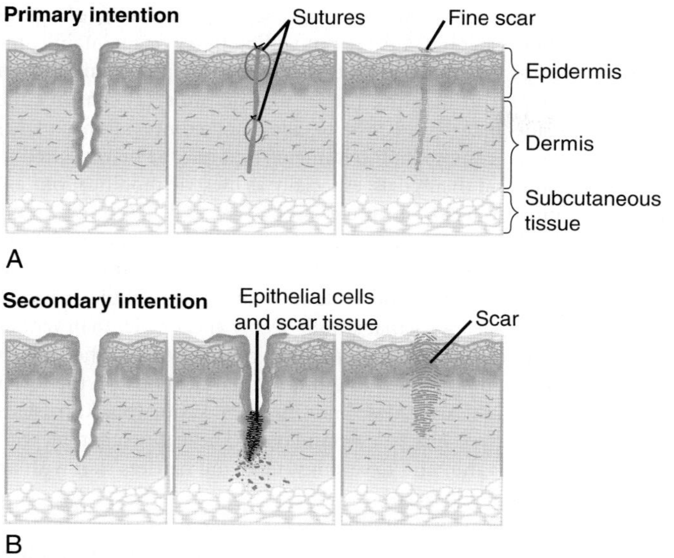

FIGURE 46-11 A, Wound healing by primary intention such as a surgical incision. Wound healing edges are pulled together and approximated with sutures or staples, and healing occurs by connective tissue deposition. **B,** Wound healing by secondary intention. Wound edges are not approximated, and healing occurs by granulation tissue formation and contraction of the wound edges. (Bryant, R. A., & Nix, D. P. [Eds.]. [2016]. *Acute and chronic wounds: Nursing management* [5th ed.]. St. Louis, MO: Elsevier. Used with permission.)

wounds, such as a clean surgical wound or an abrasion, heal by regeneration. However, full-thickness wounds extending into the dermis (involving both layers of tissue) heal by scar formation because deeper structures do not regenerate. Pressure injuries are an example of full-thickness wounds.

Partial-Thickness Wound Repair. Three components make up the healing process of a partial-thickness wound: inflammatory response, epithelial proliferation (reproduction) and migration, and re-establishment of the epidermal layers. Tissue trauma causes the *inflammatory response,* which, in turn, causes redness and swelling to the area, as well as a moderate amount of serous exudate. Normally, this response is limited to the first 24 hours after wounding. Epithelial cells begin to regenerate, providing new replacement cells. This *epithelial proliferation and migration* starts at the wound edges and the epidermal cells lining the epidermal appendages, allowing for quick resurfacing. Epithelial cells begin migrating across the wound bed soon after wounding. A wound left open to air can resurface within 6 to 7 days, whereas a wound that is kept moist can resurface in 4 days. The difference in the healing rate is related to the fact that epidermal cells only migrate across a moist surface. In a dry wound, the cells migrate down into a moist level before migration can occur (Doughty & Sparks-Defriese, 2016). New epithelium is only a few cells thick and must undergo *re-establishment of the epidermal layers.* The cells slowly re-establish normal thickness and appear as dry pink tissue.

Full-Thickness Wound Repair. Inflammatory, proliferative, and remodelling phases are involved in the healing process of a full-thickness wound. Note the differences between partial- and full-thickness wounds.

Inflammatory Phase. The *inflammation stage* is the body's reaction to wounding, beginning within minutes of injury and, in full-thickness wounds, lasting approximately 3 days. During **hemostasis**, injured blood vessels constrict, and platelets gather to stop bleeding. Clots form a **fibrin** matrix that later provides a framework for cellular repair. Damaged tissue and mast cells secrete histamine, resulting in vasodilation of surrounding capillaries and exudation of serum and white blood cells into damaged tissues. This results in localized redness, edema, warmth, and throbbing. The inflammatory response is beneficial, and attempting to cool the area or reduce the swelling has no value unless the swelling occurs within a closed compartment (e.g., ankle or neck).

Leukocytes (white blood cells) reach the wound within a few hours. The primary white blood cell is the neutrophil, which begins to ingest bacteria and small debris. The second important leukocyte is the monocyte, which transforms into macrophages.

The macrophages are the "garbage cells" that clean a wound of bacteria, dead cells, and debris by phagocytosis. Macrophages continue the process of clearing the wound of debris and release growth factors that attract fibroblasts, the cells that synthesize collagen (connective tissue). Collagen appears as early as the second day and is the main component of scar tissue.

In a clean wound, the inflammatory phase accomplishes control of bleeding and establishes a clean wound bed. The inflammatory phase is prolonged if too little inflammation occurs, as in debilitating diseases such as cancer or after the administration of steroids. Too much inflammation also decreases the speed of healing, as arriving cells compete for available nutrients.

Proliferative Phase. The *proliferative phase,* in which new blood vessels appear as reconstruction progresses, lasts from 3 to 24 days. The main activities during this phase are filling of the wound with granulation tissue, contraction of the wound, and resurfacing of the wound by epithelialization. Fibroblasts, which synthesize collagen, are present in this phase, providing the matrix for granulation, in turn supporting re-epithelialization. Collagen provides strength and structural integrity to a wound. During this period, the wound contracts to reduce the area that requires healing (**wound contraction**). Lastly, epithelial cells migrate from the wound edges to resurface. In a clean wound, when the proliferative phase is complete, the vascular bed has been re-established and the area filled with replacement tissue (collagen/granulation tissue), and the surface has been repaired (**epithelialization**). Impairment of healing during this stage usually results from systemic factors such as age, anemia, hypoproteinemia, and zinc deficiency.

Remodelling. *Maturation,* the final stage of healing, can take up to 2 years to occur, depending on the depth and extent of the wound. The collagen scar continues to reorganize and gain strength for several months. Usually, scar tissue contains fewer pigmented cells (melanocytes) and has a lighter colour than normal skin. Healed wounds are at risk for pressure injury as they usually do not have the tensile strength of the tissue they replace.

All chronic wounds described in this chapter are discussed in detail in the RNAO Best Practice Guidelines, which are readily available online at http://www.rnao.org.

Skin Tears

Aging skin is at a greater risk of developing skin tears because of the thinning of the epidermis. Dehydration, poor nutrition, prolonged use of corticosteroids, impaired sensory perception, and cognitive impairment are all risk factors for skin breakdown. When moving older person patients in bed or transferring them from bed to gurney for tests, for example, nurses need to be careful in their handling of these patients. Skin tears and bruising are common problems in this population (Figure 46-12). Any open area on the skin creates the potential for infection (portal of entry for bacteria). Using tape or adhesive dressings on fragile skin can also precipitate skin tears. The use of simple, high-quality gauze pads held in place with a woven cotton wrapped bandage (e.g., Kling wrap) or a soft silicone dressing that will not adhere to the skin is effective in protecting the area from further damage and supporting wound healing.

Venous and Arterial Wounds

Venous and arterial wounds are the result of poor circulation and occur in the lower extremities. Venous ulcers are the most common type of lower extremity wound and account for approximately 80% of leg wounds. In addition, these wounds have a recurrence rate of 70% (Gould, Dosi, Couch, et al., 2016).

Venous Ulcers. Venous ulcers are superficial and irregular in shape (Figure 46-13, *A*). These wounds usually have a large amount of exudate caused by edema in the surrounding tissue. Venous insufficiency is related to weak vein walls in the legs; furthermore, limited range of motion in the ankle decreases the ability of the calf muscle to pump. Serum and red blood cells leak into the surrounding tissue, which causes the characteristic brownish hemosiderin staining of tissue and skin. In chronic venous insufficiency, the edema in the tissue becomes firm and the lower legs develop a wooden-like appearance, called *lipodermatosclerosis*.

Treatment of Venous Leg Ulcers. It is important that nurses assess the ankle-brachial pressure index before using compression therapy to prevent, treat, or diminish edema in the lower legs (RNAO, 2004). Because venous leg ulcers are often hard-to-heal wounds, patients may have tried a variety of products, such as lanolin in topical moisturizers, topical antibiotics, or others. These products may create allergic contact dermatitis, and it is best to avoid anything but the simplest, natural products to clean, debride, moisten, and cover. Normal saline, autolytic debriding agents, preservative-free hydrogels, and soft silicone dressings can be used. Products to avoid are those with preservatives, chemicals in the dressing, and fragrances. Edema control is essential, but many patients are not willing to try or maintain compression therapy. A wound care specialist with training in compression therapy is helpful in assisting nurses to determine (1) whether the patient has adequate blood flow to allow for compression and (2) different types of compression treatments that may be better suited to certain patients and their goals, especially as lifestyle modifications are usually required to heal venous ulcers.

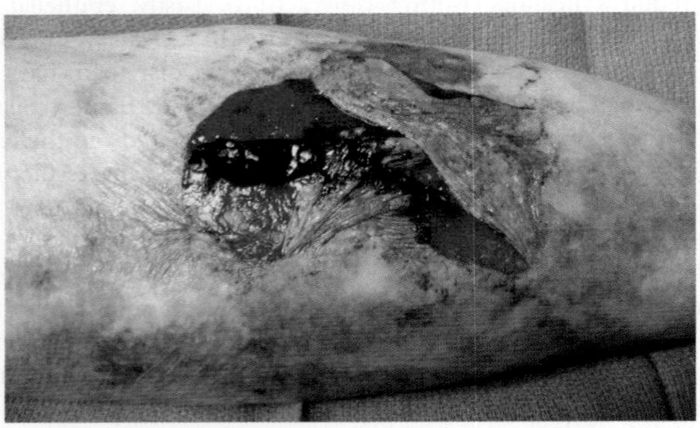

FIGURE 46-12 Skin tear. (Courtesy Rose Hamm. Cain, J. E. [2009]. *Mosby's PDQ for wound care* [p. 18]. St. Louis, MO: Mosby.)

Arterial Ulcers. Arterial ulcers (also called *ischemic ulcers*) are caused by inadequate blood flow to the lower extremity (unlike venous ulcers, which are caused by poor blood return). Arterial ulcers have a "punched-out" appearance that is both deeper and smaller than venous ulcers. They are often located on the feet, over the tips of the toes, or on the toe joints, but are also found on other locations on the lower leg (Figure 46-13, *B*). Arterial wounds may be necrotic (black, crusted) in appearance or have very pale wound beds. The legs of a patient with arterial disease are thin and have shiny, taut, and hairless skin with an almost translucent appearance.

Because of the nature of this disease, arterial wounds are quite resistant to healing and could be considered "maintenance" wounds, where the goal is to provide comfort and protection from infection. These wounds are not good candidates for debridement because poor blood flow will limit ability to heal. The best option for treatment is to keep these wounds clean and dry. Often, a solution of povidone (Betadine) (10% in a 1% solution) can be made using 0.25 povidone to 0.75 normal saline. When gauze pads soaked in the solution are used, they should be placed in or on the wound and changed once daily; this will decrease bacteria in the wound and promote drying of the tissue. Both of these results are useful in nonhealing wounds such as arterial ulcers.

Diabetic Ulcers

In Canada, more than 11 million people are living with diabetes or prediabetes (where blood sugar is higher than normal range), according to the Canadian Diabetes Association (2016). The Indigenous population has much higher percentages of individuals with diabetes (25% of Indigenous individuals older than 65 years have diabetes). Diabetes is a disease that requires major lifestyle changes, including careful monitoring of blood glucose. Complications related to poorly controlled diabetes have serious results: renal failure, which may require dialysis; diabetic neuropathy, which may lead to limb amputation (Figure 46-14); and retinal neuropathy, which leads to blindness. People with diabetes have compromised healing potential. Any break in the skin can cause long-term problems because these wounds resist healing. Forty-five percent of lower-extremity amputations occur in individuals with diabetes. One lower-limb amputation of a nontraumatic nature (e.g., diabetes-related) will result in a second limb

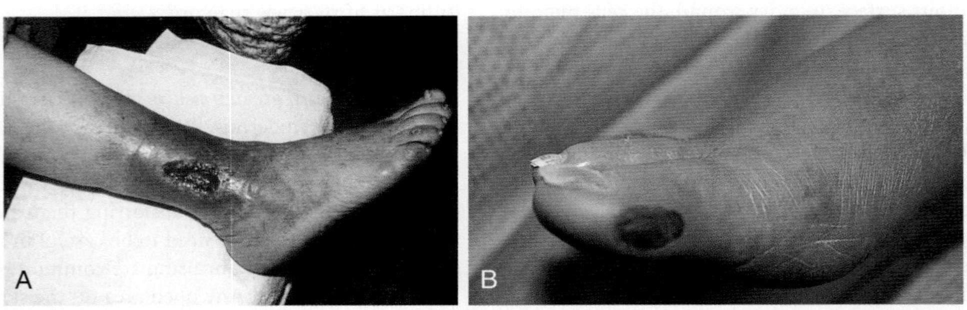

FIGURE 46-13 A, Venous leg ulcer. **B,** Arterial lower limb wound. (Bryant, R., & Nix, D. [2016]. *Acute and chronic wounds: Current management concepts* [5th ed., Plates 34 and 35]. St. Louis, MO: Elsevier.)

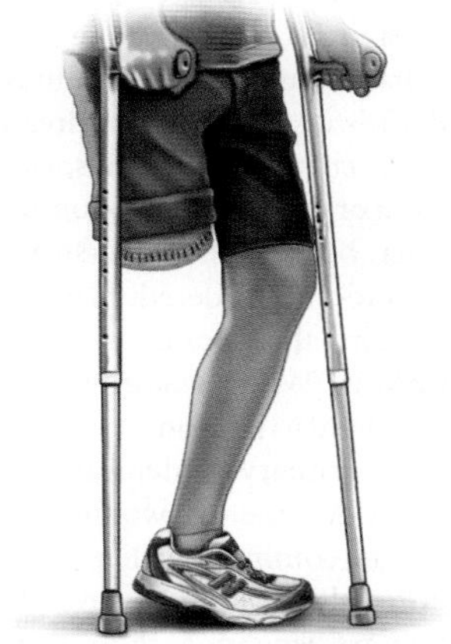

FIGURE 46-14 Person with above-knee amputation.

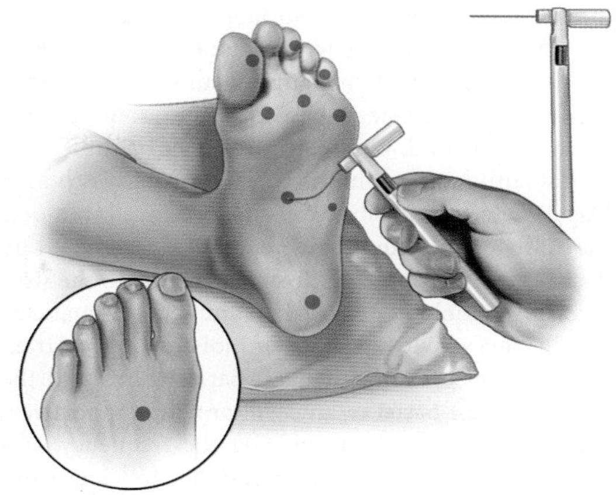

FIGURE 46-16 Monofilament test.

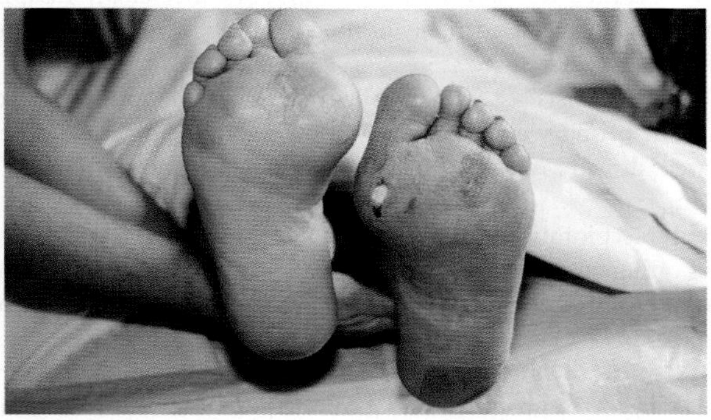

FIGURE 46-15 Diabetic foot with callus and packing in wound. (Bryant, R., & Nix, D. [2016]. *Acute and chronic wounds: Current management concepts* [3rd ed., Plate 38]. St. Louis MO: Elsevier. Reprinted with permission.)

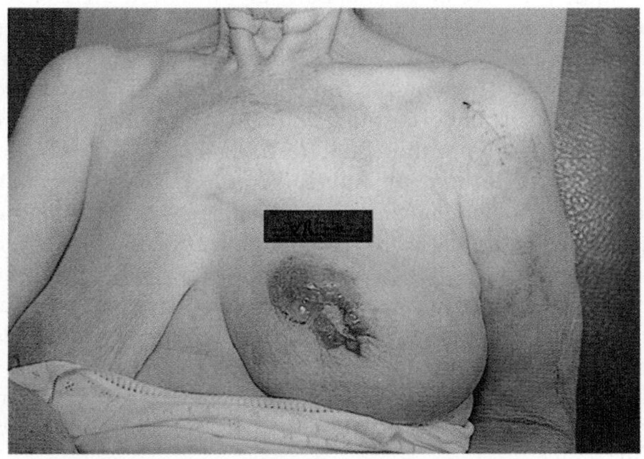

FIGURE 46-17 Malignant breast tumour. (Bale, S., & Jones, V. [2005]. *Wound care nursing: A patient-centred approach* [2nd ed., p. 195, Fig. 9-16]. St. Louis, MO: Mosby. Reprinted with permission.)

amputation within 3 years and death within 5 years (Tentolouris, Al-Sabbagh, Walker, et al., 2004). These are sobering statistics and reinforce how important it is for nurses to provide education, as well as careful assessment and early intervention, to patients with diabetes.

Diabetic ulcers occur because of neuropathic changes related to diabetes. They most commonly are found over bony prominences located on the plantar surface of the foot, over the metatarsal heads, and beneath the heels. These changes include sensory neuropathy, loss of protective sensation (e.g., a decrease in the ability to feel pain or temperature change); autonomic neuropathy, or absence of sweating leading to dry skin with fissures, cracks, and calluses over pressure points (heels and ball of the foot); and motor neuropathy, resulting in changes in muscle contractions leading to high arches and cocked-up "hammer" toes. These contribute to pressure points, creating calluses (Figure 46-15).

Assessment. Assessment of the feet in patients with diabetes with a monofilament test (Pop-Busui, Bolton, Feldman, et al., 2017) determines the extent of neuropathy (Figure 46-16). However, in patients with diabetes, it can be assumed that peripheral neuropathy is a risk; nurses should provide education and conduct close inspection and palpation of the feet and lower legs. Prevention starts with patient teaching regarding appropriate footwear, including wearing hard-soled shoes at home; testing water temperature before bathing or showering; and good foot care, available from a certified foot-care specialist such as a chiropodist.

Diabetic Wound Treatment. If the diabetic wound can heal, then necrotic tissue and callus buildup must be debrided to establish a clean wound bed and diminish pressure. Sharp or surgical debridement should be performed only by a qualified health care provider (RN or MD) with appropriate skills and knowledge and supported by agency or institution policy regarding sharp and surgical debridement. Incorrect sharp or surgical debridement can significantly harm the patient. Diabetic wounds may be prophylactically treated with some form of topical antimicrobial dressing. If the patient complains of pain at the wound site, particularly persistent pain, osteomyelitis (bone infection) should be suspected. The nurse needs to ensure that the physician or advanced practice nurse primarily responsible for the patient is aware of this so that appropriate action can be taken.

Malignant or Fungating Wounds

Cancer tumours may extrude through the skin as swollen masses with numerous fissures that drain purulent, often very malodorous exudate, that sometimes bleed when cleaned or touched. Typical sites for fungating wounds are the side of the face or neck and the breast or groin area (Figure 46-17). These wounds are not only painful at dressing change but also often embarrass the patient because of their odour and unsightliness. They are malignant wounds that will not heal, but the tumours may be reduced in size with radiation or chemotherapy.

Care of the malignant or fungating wound requires attention to environmental and extrinsic issues such as odour, drainage, and appearance of the wound. Odour control may be difficult and may require topical antifungal or antimicrobial dressings such as metronidazole (Flagyl) or a topical silver dressing. Various types of charcoal dressings are also available to provide odour management but are not always effective once they are wet. To avoid trauma to the wound bed, adhesive dressings should not be used, but rather atraumatic dressings, such as soft silicone, which will allow for moisture vapour transfer and will decrease pain at dressing changes. Barrier films and the use of silicone (dimethicone)-based creams will provide supportive care and protect the periwound skin. Minimizing the frequency of dressing changes as well as using "low-profile," nonbulky dressings will enhance quality of life.

Acute and Surgical Wounds

As a nurse, you may be in situations in which you are assessing a wound, either at the time of injury before treatment, or after therapy, when the wound is relatively stable. Each situation requires you to make different observations and to take different actions. Regardless of the setting, it is important that you obtain information regarding the cause and history of the wound (see Box 46-5).

Emergency Setting, or Acute, Wounds. Nurses see wounds in any setting, including the clinic, emergency department, youth camps, or their own backyard. When a patient's condition is judged to be stable because of the presence of spontaneous breathing, a clear airway, and a strong carotid pulse (see Chapter 39), the nurse should inspect the wound for bleeding. The type of wound determines criteria for inspection. For example, a patient presenting with an abrasion would not likely require the nurse to inspect for signs of internal bleeding, but the nurse should do so in the event of a puncture wound.

An **abrasion** is superficial with little bleeding and is considered a partial-thickness wound. The wound often appears "weepy" because of plasma leakage from damaged capillaries. A **laceration**, which is a jagged, unintentional (i.e., nonsurgical) wound, sometimes bleeds more profusely, depending on the wound's depth and location. For example, minor scalp lacerations tend to bleed profusely because of the rich blood supply to the scalp. Lacerations greater than 5 cm long or 2.5 cm deep cause serious bleeding. Puncture wounds bleed in relation to the depth and size of the wound; for example, a nail puncture does not cause as much bleeding as a knife wound. The primary dangers of puncture wounds are internal bleeding and infection.

The wound should be inspected for contaminate material. Most traumatic wounds are dirty. Soil, broken glass, shreds of cloth, and foreign substances clinging to penetrating objects sometimes become embedded in the wound.

The next step is to assess the size (including depth) of the wound. A deep laceration requires suturing. A large open wound may expose bone or tissue that needs to be protected.

When the injury is a result of trauma from a dirty penetrating object, the nurse needs to determine when the patient last received a tetanus toxoid injection. Tetanus bacteria reside in soil and in the gut of humans and animals. A tetanus antitoxin injection is necessary if the patient's last one was more than 5 years ago.

Stable Setting, or Surgical Wounds. When the patient's condition is stabilized (e.g., after surgery or treatment), the wound is assessed to determine its healing progress. If the wound is covered by a dressing and the dressing is intact and not saturated with drainage, the nurse should not directly inspect the wound unless serious complications are suspected. Here, the nurse only needs to inspect the dressing and external drains.

Dressings contaminated with external drainage (e.g., feces or urine) need to be changed, as well as saturated dressings with leakage to periwound tissue. When changing dressings, care should be taken to avoid accidental removal or displacement of underlying drains. Because removal of dressings may be painful, the nurse must assess the patient's need for an analgesic, and once ordered, make sure it is given at least 30 minutes before exposing the wound.

Wound Appearance. When assessing wound appearance the nurse needs to check whether the wound edges are closed. A surgical incision healing by primary intention should have clean, well-approximated edges. A **puncture** wound is usually a small, circular wound with the edges coming together toward the centre. Crusts from exudate often form along wound edges.

If the wound edges are separated, the nurse needs to inspect the condition of tissue at the wound base, looking for complications such as dehiscence and evisceration. The outer edges of a wound normally appear inflamed for the first 2 to 3 days, but this slowly disappears. Within 7 to 10 days, a normally healing wound resurfaces with epithelial cells, and edges close.

Table 46-5 lists assessment characteristics for abnormal wound healing in primary and secondary wounds. If an infection develops, the area directly surrounding the wound becomes inflamed and swollen.

Skin discoloration usually results from bruising of interstitial tissues or hematoma formation. Blood collecting beneath the skin first takes on a bluish or purplish appearance. Gradually, as clotted blood is broken down, shades of brown and yellow appear.

Character of Wound Drainage. The amount, colour, odour, and consistency of drainage should be noted. The amount of drainage depends on the location and extent of the wound. For example, drainage is minimal after a simple appendectomy. In contrast, a large abscess may drain a moderate amount for several days. When an accurate measurement of the amount of drainage within a dressing is needed, the nurse can weigh the dressing and compare it with the weight of the

TABLE 46-5 Assessment of Abnormal Healing in Primary and Secondary Intention Wounds

Primary Intention Wounds	Secondary Intention Wounds
Wounds' incision line poorly approximated	Pale or fragile granulation tissue; granulation tissue bed is excessively dry or moist
Drainage present more than 3 days after closure	Exudate present
Inflammation decreased in first 3 to 5 days after injury	Necrotic or sloughy tissue present in wound base
No epithelialization of wound edges by day 4	Epithelialization not continuous
No healing ridge by day 9	Fruity, earthy, or putrid odour present Presence of fistula(s), tunnelling, undermining

Adapted from Stotts, N. A., & Cavanaugh, C. E. (1999). Assessing the patient with a wound. *Home Healthcare Nurse, 17*(1), 27.

same dressing when clean and dry. The general rule is that 1 g of drainage equals 1 mL of drainage volume. Another method of quantifying wound drainage is to chart the number of dressings used and frequency of changes. An increase or decrease in number or frequency of dressings will indicate a relative increase or decrease in wound drainage.

The colour and consistency of drainage vary depending on the type of drainage, including **serous**, **sanguineous**, **serosanguineous**, and **purulent** (Table 46-6). If drainage has a pungent or strong odour, infection should be suspected.

The wound's appearance is described according to the characteristics observed. An example of accurate recording follows:

Abdominal incision is 5 cm in width, in RLQ (right lower quadrant); wound edges well approximated without inflammation or exudate. 1.2 cm diameter circle of serous drainage present on one 4 × 4 gauze changed every 8 hours.

TABLE 46-6 Types of Wound Drainage

Type	Appearance
Serous	Clear, watery plasma 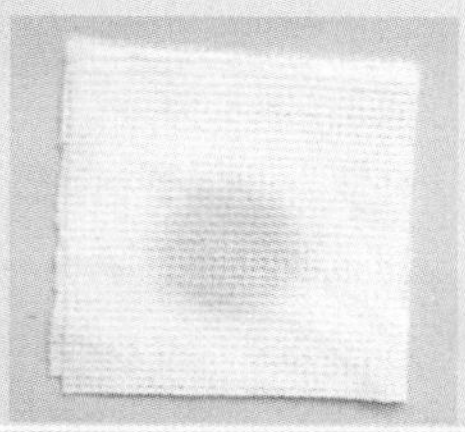
Purulent	Thick, yellow, green, tan, or brown 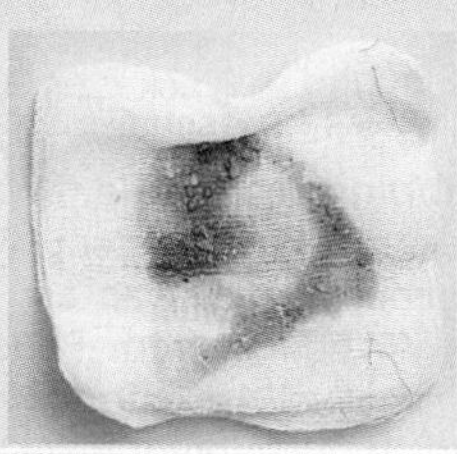
Serosanguineous	Pale, red, watery: mixture of clear and red fluid 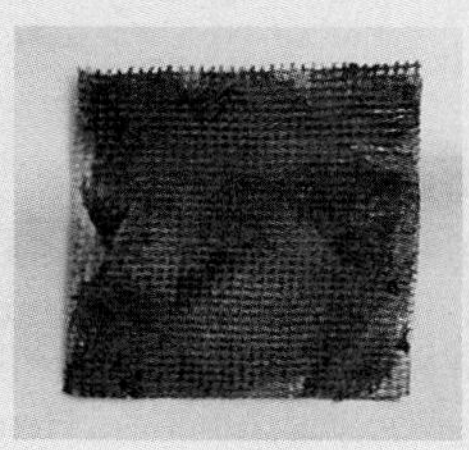
Sanguineous	Bright red: indicates active bleeding 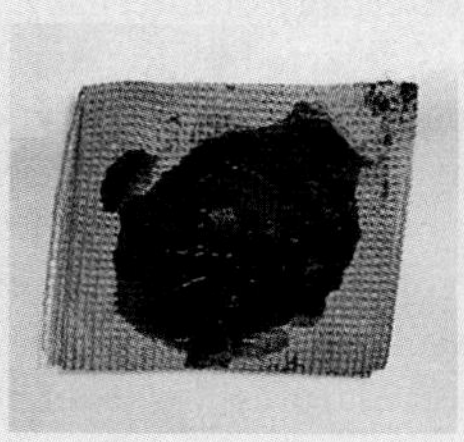

Drains. If a large amount of drainage is anticipated, a drain is often inserted in or near a surgical wound. Some drains are sutured in place. *Exercise caution when changing the dressing around drains, regardless of whether they are sutured, to prevent accidental removal.* A Penrose drain lies under a dressing; at the time of placement, a pin or clip is placed through the drain to prevent it from slipping farther into a wound (Figure 46-18). It is usually the nurse's responsibility to pull or advance the drain as drainage decreases to permit healing deep within the wound site.

When assessing the number of drains, drain placement, character of drainage, and condition of collecting equipment, the nurse must first observe the security of the drain and its location with respect to the wound. Next to note is the character of drainage. If a collecting device is available, the drainage volume should be measured. Because a drainage system needs to be patent, the nurse must look for drainage flow through the tubing, as well as around the tubing. *A sudden decrease in drainage through the tubing may indicate a blocked drain, which may require surgical revision. Contact the physician in this case.* When a drain is connected to suction, the system needs to be assessed to ensure that the pressure ordered is being exerted. Evacuator units such as a Hemovac or Jackson-Pratt (Figure 46-19) exert a constant low pressure as long as the suction device (bladder or bag) is fully compressed.

These types of drainage devices are often referred to as self-suction. If the evacuator device is unable to maintain a vacuum on its own, the nurse must notify the surgeon, who will then order a secondary vacuum system (such as wall suction). If fluid accumulates within the tissues, wound healing will not progress at an optimal rate, increasing risk of infection.

Wound Closures. Surgical wounds are closed with staples, sutures, or wound closures. A frequent skin closure is the stainless steel staple. The staple provides more strength than nylon or silk sutures and causes less irritation to tissue. However, the nurse should look for irritation around staple or suture sites and note whether closures are intact. Normally, for the first 2 to 3 days after surgery, skin around sutures or staples is edematous. Continued swelling indicates that closures are too tight. Overly tight suture material may cut into the skin, which can lead to wound separation or wound dehiscence. Early suture removal reduces formation of defects along the suture line and minimizes chances of unattractive scar formation.

Tissue adhesive such as Dermabond forms a strong bond across apposed wound edges, which allows normal healing to occur below. It can be used to replace small sutures for incisional repair. The product is applied across the approximated wound edges, which are then held together until the solution dries, providing an adhesive closure. Although surgeons generally use it for small superficial lacerations, some may use it on larger wounds, where subcutaneous sutures are needed (Januchowski & Ferguson, 2014).

Palpation of the Wound. When inspecting a wound, it is important to observe for swelling or separation of wound edges. Wearing sterile gloves, the nurse lightly presses the wound edges to detect localized areas of tenderness or drainage collection. If pressure causes fluid

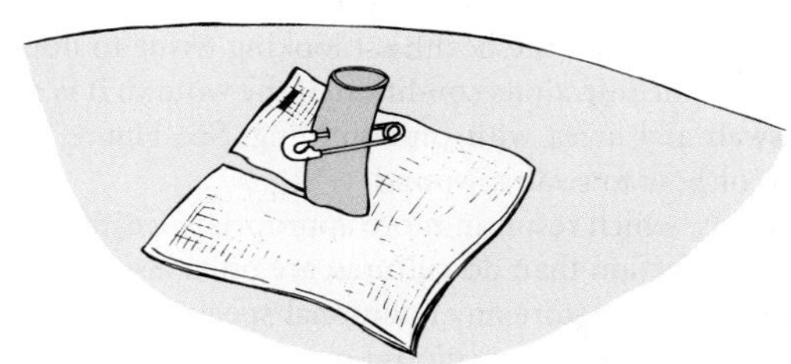

FIGURE 46-18 Penrose drain.

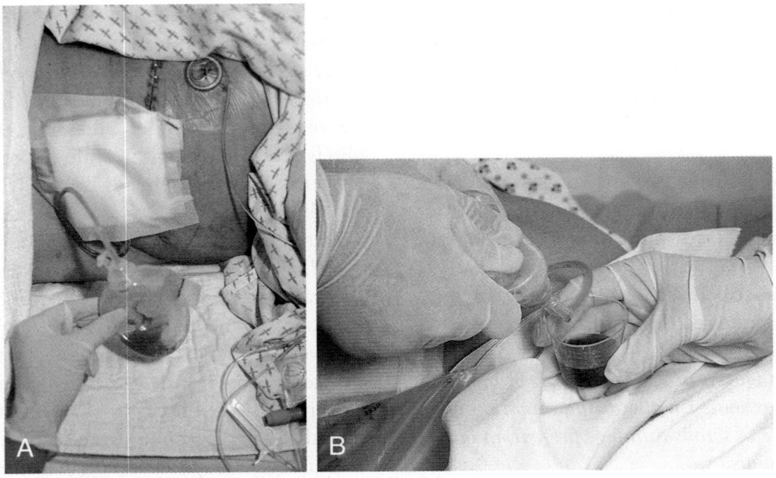

FIGURE 46-19 **Jackson-Pratt drainage device.** **A,** Drainage tubes and reservoir. **B,** Emptying drainage reservoir.

BOX 46-7 Recommendations for Standardized Techniques for Wound Cultures*

Quantitative Swab Procedure

- Clean the wound surface with a *nonantiseptic* (i.e., sterile water or normal saline) solution.
- Use a sterile swab from a culturette tube.
- Rotate the swab in 1 cm^2 of clean tissue in the open wound (see Figure 46-20). Apply pressure to the swab to elicit tissue fluid (Stotts, 2016b). Insert the tip of the swab into the appropriate sterile container, and transport to the laboratory.

*Check agency policy to determine whether you need to obtain an order from a health care provider.

Adapted from Stotts, N. A. (2016). Wound infection: Diagnosis and management. In R. A. Bryant & D. P. Nix (Eds.), *Acute and chronic wounds: Current management concepts* (5th ed.). St. Louis, MO: Elsevier.

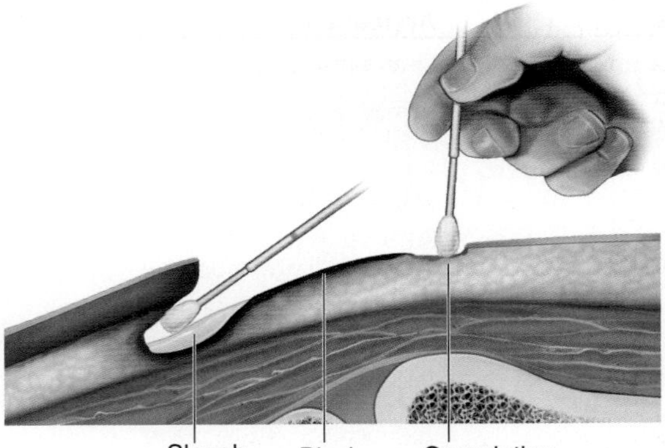

FIGURE 46-20 **Swabbing technique.** Swab wound from healthiest looking tissue to obtain results consistent with infectious condition of wound. It is also appropriate to swab any areas with undermining. (Illustration by Nancy A. Bauer. From Bauer, N. A. [2007, revised]. *RNAO best practice guideline: Assessment and management of stage I–IV pressure ulcers* [p. 100]. Toronto: RNAO.)

to be expressed, the character of the drainage should be noted. The patient is normally sensitive to palpation of wound edges; however, extreme tenderness may be indicative of infection.

Wound Cultures. If purulent or suspicious-looking drainage is detected, a specimen of the drainage may need to be obtained for culture (see Chapter 33). A wound culture sample should never be collected from old drainage. Resident colonies of bacteria from the skin grow within exudate and are not always the true causative organisms of a wound infection. First the wound is cleaned with normal saline to remove skin flora. Aerobic organisms grow in superficial wounds exposed to the air, and anaerobic organisms tend to grow within body cavities. The nurse should use a different method of specimen collection for each type of organism as per agency policy (Box 46-7). A wound is swabbed from the healthiest looking tissue to obtain results consistent with the infectious condition of the wound. It is also appropriate to swab any areas with undermining. See Figure 46-20 for a description of how to swab a wound.

Gram stains, which result in more appropriate treatment earlier in the course of infection than do cultures, are often also performed, but they do not usually require any additional specimens. The gold standard of wound culture is tissue biopsy, obtained by a physician or nurse with specialized training (Stotts, 2016b).

Complications of Wound Healing

Hemorrhage. Hemorrhage, or bleeding from a wound site, is normal during and immediately after initial trauma. Hemostasis occurs within several minutes unless large blood vessels are involved or the patient has poor clotting function. Hemorrhages that occur after hemostasis indicate a slipped surgical suture, a dislodged clot, infection, or erosion of a blood vessel by a foreign object (e.g., a drain). Hemorrhage occurs externally or internally.

Internal bleeding is detected by looking for distention or swelling of the affected body part, a change in the type and amount of drainage from a surgical drain, or signs of hypovolemic shock. A hematoma is a localized collection of blood underneath the tissues. It appears as a swelling, a change in colour, sensation, or warmth, or a mass that often takes on a bluish discoloration. A hematoma near a major artery or vein is dangerous because pressure from the expanding hematoma obstructs blood flow.

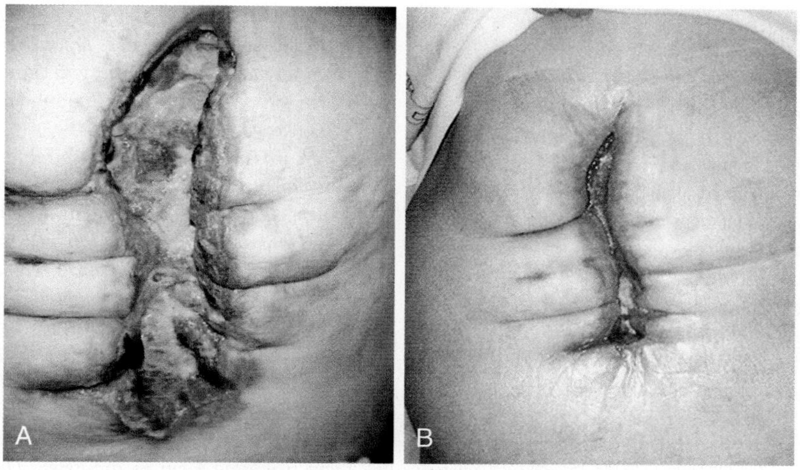

FIGURE 46-21 A, Dehisced wound before wound V.A.C. therapy. **B,** Dehisced wound after wound V.A.C. therapy. (Courtesy Kinetic Concepts, Inc. San Antonio, TX.)

External hemorrhaging is obvious. The dressings covering the wound need to be observed for bloody drainage. If bleeding is extensive, the dressing soon becomes saturated, and frequently blood drains from under the dressing and pools beneath the patient. *Observe all wounds closely, particularly surgical wounds, in which the risk of hemorrhage is greatest during the first 24 to 48 hours after surgery or injury.*

Infection. Wound infection is the second most common health care–associated infection (see Chapter 33). However, infection may not be revealed through a lab culture due to poor culture technique or administration of antibiotics. In fact, all chronic wounds are considered contaminated with bacteria. What differentiates contaminated wounds from infected wounds is the amount of bacteria present. It is generally agreed that infected wounds have more than 100 000 (10^5) organisms per gram of tissue (Stotts, 2016b). The chances of wound infection are greater when the wound contains necrotic tissue, when contaminants are in or near the wound, and when blood supply and local tissue defences are reduced.

Bacterial infection inhibits wound healing. Some contaminated or traumatic wounds show signs of infection early, within 2 to 3 days. A surgical wound infection may not develop until day 4 or 5. The patient has a fever, tenderness and pain at the wound site, and an elevated white blood cell count. The edges of the wound appear inflamed. If drainage is present, it is odorous and purulent and is a yellow, green, or brown colour, depending on the causative organism.

Dehiscence. When a wound fails to heal properly, the layers of skin and tissue separate. This most commonly occurs before collagen formation (3 to 11 days after injury). Dehiscence is the partial or total separation of wound layers. A patient at risk of poor wound healing (e.g., poor nutritional status, infection, or obesity) is at risk of dehiscence. However, obese patients have a higher risk because of the constant strain placed on their wounds and the poor healing qualities of fat tissue (Pierpont, Dinh, Salas, et al., 2014). Dehiscence involves abdominal surgical wounds and may occur after a sudden strain, such as coughing, vomiting, or sitting up (Figure 46-21). Patients often report feeling as though something has given way. *When an increased amount of serosanguineous drainage from a wound occurs, be alert for the potential for dehiscence.* A strategy to prevent dehiscence is to provide support to the area, using a folded thin blanket or pillow placed over an abdominal wound when the patient is coughing. This splints and supports healing tissue when coughing increases intra-abdominal pressure.

BOX 46-8 Risk of Skin Breakdown From Body Fluids

Low Risk	Urine
Saliva	Ascitic fluid
Serosanguineous drainage	Purulent exudate
Moderate Risk	**High Risk**
Bile	Gastric drainage
Stool	Pancreatic drainage

Evisceration. With total separation of wound layers, evisceration (protrusion of visceral organs through a wound opening) sometimes occurs. It is an emergent condition that requires surgical repair. *When evisceration occurs, quickly place sterile towels soaked in sterile saline over the extruding tissues to reduce the chance of bacterial invasion and drying of the tissues and contact the physician.* If the organs protrude through the wound, blood supply to the tissues is compromised. The patient should not receive anything by mouth (NPO), and the nurse needs to observe for signs and symptoms of shock, and prepare the patient for emergency surgery.

Fistulas. A fistula is an abnormal passage between two organs or between an organ and the outside of the body. Most fistulas form as a result of poor wound healing or complication of disease, such as Crohn's disease. Trauma, infection, radiation exposure, and diseases such as cancer will prevent tissue layers from closing properly and will allow the fistula tract to form. Fistulas increase the risk of infection and fluid and electrolyte imbalances from fluid loss. Chronic drainage of fluids through a fistula also predisposes a patient to skin breakdown (Box 46-8).

◆ Nursing Diagnosis

Through assessment, clusters of data reveal whether an actual or a risk of *impaired skin integrity* exists. Assessment data may support more than one diagnostic label. For example, a postoperative patient has purulent drainage from a surgical wound and reports tenderness around the area of the wound. These data support a nursing diagnosis of *impaired skin integrity related to a contaminated wound* (Box 46-9). After completing an assessment of the patient's wound, the nurse

BOX 46-9 Impaired Skin Integrity Related to a Contaminated Wound

Assessment Activities That Define Characteristics

Inspect surface of skin: presence of wound, break in skin integrity.

Yellow, foul-smelling drainage comes from wound.

Edges of wound are red and warm, not approximated.

Sutures remain in place. Inspect wound for signs of healing.

Brown-red drainage occurs 5 days after surgery.

Edges of wound are not approximated.

Obtain patient's temperature, heart rate, white blood cell count, and serum albumin level.

Patient is febrile, heart rate is 125 beats per minute, leukocyte (white blood cell) count is 12 000/mm^3, and serum albumin level is less than 3.5 mg/100 mL.

identifies nursing diagnoses that will direct supportive and preventive care. Multiple nursing diagnoses are associated with impaired skin integrity and wounds:

- *Risk of infection*
- *Imbalanced nutrition: less than body requirements*
- *Acute or chronic pain*
- *Impaired physical mobility*
- *Impaired skin integrity*
- *Risk of impaired skin integrity*
- *Ineffective tissue perfusion*
- *Impaired tissue integrity*

Some patients are at risk of poor wound healing because of previously defined factors that impair healing. Thus, even though the patient's wound appears normal, the nurse would identify nursing diagnoses, such as *impaired nutrition* or *ineffective tissue perfusion,* that direct nursing care toward support of wound repair.

The nature of a wound can cause problems unrelated to wound healing. *Alteration in comfort* and *impaired mobility* are problems that have implications for the patient's eventual recovery. For example, a large abdominal incision can cause enough pain to interfere with the patient's ability to turn in bed effectively.

◆ Planning

After identifying nursing diagnoses, the nurse develops a plan of care for the patient who is at risk or who has actual impaired skin integrity. During planning, the nurse synthesizes information from multiple resources (see Figure 46-6). Critical thinking ensures that the patient's plan of care integrates all that the nurse knows about the individual, as well as key critical thinking elements. Professional standards of practice are especially important to consider when developing a plan of care. As the patient's nurse, ask yourself what aspects of care you are able to perform without medical orders, what aspects of care you can delegate to other regulated health care providers, and what are the patient goals.

For many patients, the wound is only a part of the story. For example, consider the following scenario:

You are caring for Mrs. Kathy Crane, a 65-year-old woman who lives with her recently retired husband and who has a 30-year history of diabetes mellitus. She currently takes insulin, but her diabetes is poorly controlled because of her inability to adhere to a 1 200-calorie diabetic diet and her "hit or miss" approach to testing her serum glucose on a regular basis. She is 32 kg overweight.

For the last 10 years, she has reported decreased sensation in her lower extremities. She does not practise good foot care; she cuts her own toenails and, at home, goes barefoot or wears socks. She regularly soaks her feet in an Epsom-salt footbath because she "read this was good for your feet."

She was admitted to the hospital for elective repair of an abdominal aneurysm. The surgery went well, but postoperatively Mrs. Crane had difficulty ambulating and performing coughing and deep breathing exercises. On her second postoperative day, she developed pneumonia, which required intravenous antibiotics. During the course of her pneumonia, Mrs. Crane stated she was "too tired" to walk or get up to use the commode or toilet. She required an adult continence product as she was now incontinent of urine and stool. She complained of pain when repositioned and would generally reposition herself on her back. Two weeks after her surgery, Mrs. Crane developed a large draining sacral wound, which is now 6 cm in diameter. The base of the wound can be visualized down to bone (stage 4). In addition, she has a smaller, stage 3 ulcer on her left heel. Skin assessment also reveals areas of prolonged redness over pressure points, especially on the right heel and over both hips.

When planning care for Mrs. Crane, you can use a concept map to individualize care for her, as she has multiple health problems and related nursing diagnoses (Figure 46-22). This map assists you in using critical thinking skills to organize complex patient assessment data and related nursing diagnoses with the patient's chief medical diagnosis. As you identify linkages between nursing diagnoses and medical diagnosis, the concept map also links potential interventions with the patient's health care needs and goals in mind.

Goals and Outcomes

Nursing care is based on the patient's identified needs and priorities. The nurse's first job is to ensure being on the same path with the patient, regarding the establishment of goals and expected outcomes. In addition, the nurse needs to determine whether the wound is likely to heal. For example, a pressure injury with unrelieved pressure, along with the patient's possible poor nutritional intake, is unlikely to heal. In addition, patients in terminal stages of illness may not have the physiological resources to heal, despite optimal environmental supports. Thus, it is important to plan interventions according to risk of skin breakdown, type and severity of the wound, and complications, such as infection, poor nutrition, and peripheral vascular diseases, which affect wound healing.

A goal frequently identified is to see wound improvement within a 2-week period. The outcomes of this goal could include the following:

- Higher percentage of granulation tissue in the wound base
- No further skin breakdown in any body location
- An increase in caloric intake of 10%

These outcomes are reasonable if the overall goal for the patient is to heal the injury. Other goals of care for patients with wounds include preventing infection, maintaining skin integrity, comfort, and health promotion.

Setting Priorities

Nurses establish nursing care priorities in wound care based on the comprehensive patient assessment goal expectations and established outcomes. These priorities also depend on whether the patient's condition is stable or acute (emergent). An acute wound needs immediate intervention, whereas in the presence of a chronic, stable wound, other factors, such as mobilization, may have greater priority. No matter

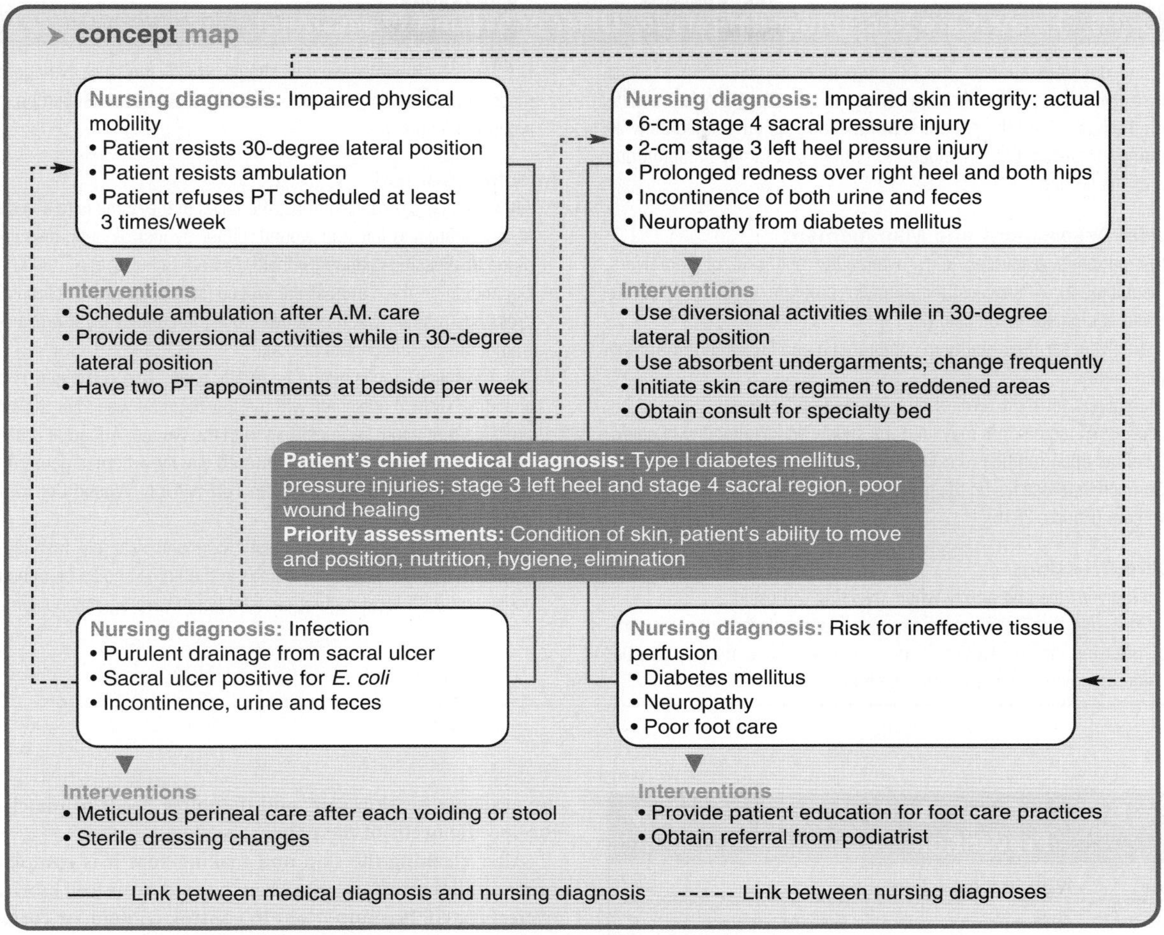

FIGURE 46-22 Concept map for a patient with a chronic wound. *PT,* Physiotherapy.

what the risk is of developing pressure injuries, preventive interventions such as skin care practices, appropriate positioning, and elimination of friction and shear are priorities. Promotion of skin health is also essential. Existing skin breakdown, from skin tears to large chronic wounds, requires ongoing attention because it is frequently the reason for both hospitalization and decrease in quality of life for patients, no matter what the setting. Patient and family preferences, daily activities, and the healing potential of the wound need to be included in the collaborative setting of priorities.

Collaborative Care

Wound care is not just a nursing responsibility; it is a team effort, including a physiotherapist, occupational therapist, dietitian, pharmacist, and physician, as well as the patient, family, and nurse. With early discharge from health care settings, it is important to consider what resources are required to plan for the patient's ongoing care. Anticipating wound care needs and related equipment and resources, such as referral to a home care agency or outpatient wound care clinic, supports not only wound healing but also the patient's independence.

Patients and their families often need to continue the objectives of wound management after discharge (Box 46-10). Nurses need to consider caregiver ability, as well as time needed to change a particular dressing when selecting the treatment to use after discharge. In particular, in the community, frequency of home visits is a key factor in resource management. Patients, families, and caregivers need to be provided with education and knowledge so that they understand the importance of good nutrition, pressure off-loading (particularly when sitting in a recliner chair for long periods of time), and how different wound dressings are used. The nurse's role, no matter the health care setting, is to work with the patient and family to develop and support their understanding and involvement to optimize wound healing as much as possible.

◆ Implementation: Preventing Skin Breakdown

Health Promotion. The most effective intervention for problems with skin integrity and wound care is prevention. Prompt, early identification of patient risk factors aids in the prevention of pressure injuries. Use of a risk assessment tool, such as the Braden Scale (see Table 46-2), is a first step in identifying a patient's risk of skin breakdown. Table 46-7 provides nursing interventions based on risk factors identified in the Braden Scale. If risk factors are identified, the nurse must follow up with interventions. The three major areas of nursing interventions for prevention of skin breakdown are (1) skin care, including hygiene and moisture management; (2) mechanical loading and support devices, including positioning and use of therapeutic surfaces; and (3) education (RNAO, 2016).

Topical Skin Care. Nurses need to perform frequent skin assessments (see Box 46-5), at a minimum of once a day; however, high-risk patients may require more frequent skin assessments, such as every

BOX 46-10 Home Care Recommendations for Ulcer or Wound Assessment

Assessment and documentation of the pressure ulcer should occur at least weekly, unless evidence of deterioration exists, in which case you need to reassess both the wound and the patient's overall management immediately. In the home setting, it is essential to include the patient and family in monitoring the progress of the wound.

Psychosocial Assessment and Management

- Assess the patient's resources (e.g., availability and skill of caregivers, finances, equipment). A successful treatment program requires adequate caregiver and equipment resources.
- Evaluate caregivers for their ability to comprehend and implement the treatment requirements.
- Evaluate caregivers for their level of strength and endurance.
- Consider economic factors that may limit the supply and availability of equipment, as well as opportunities to relieve caregivers.
- Use an approach that focuses on the psychosocial and physical factors affecting wound care (House, 2015).

Wound Care Dressings

- Consider caregiver time and ability when selecting a dressing.
- Consider a dressing that, while more expensive per unit, may decrease frequency of dressing change (which is more cost-effective than a cheaper dressing requiring more frequent dressing change).
- Dressings for healable wounds should provide moisture management without macerating or drying out the wound bed, decrease bioburden, and support wound debridement.

Infection Control

- All wounds are colonized; thus, the focus in the home is to avoid introduction of contamination into the wound, either by instruments, dressings, or technique at dressing change (Sibbald, Orsted, Schultz, et al., 2003).
- Depending on the status of the wound (surgical/acute or chronic), secondary dressings may be clean or sterile, but the contact layer dressing should be from a sterile (unopened) package.
- The "no-touch" technique is generally used. This technique is a method of changing surface dressings without touching the wound or the surface of any dressing that might be in contact with the wound. Adherent dressings should be grasped by the corner and removed slowly, whereas gauze dressings can be pinched in the centre and lifted off (WOCN Wound Committee & APIC, 2012).
- Place soiled dressings in a plastic bag and securely fasten bag closure. Disposal of contaminated dressings in the home should be done in a manner consistent with local regulations and home care agency policies.

TABLE 46-7 A Quick Guide to Pressure Injury Prevention

Risk Factor	Nursing Interventions
Decreased sensory perception	Assess pressure points for signs of nonblanching reactive hyperemia. Provide a pressure-redistribution surface.
Moisture	Assess need for incontinence management. After each incontinent episode, clean area with no-rinse perineal cleaner and protect skin with a moisture-barrier ointment.
Friction and shear	Reposition patient by using a drawsheet to lift the patient off the surface. Ensure heels are also supported. Provide a trapeze to facilitate movement. Position patient at a 30-degree lateral turn and limit head elevation to 30 degrees.
Decreased activity or mobility	Establish and post an individualized turning schedule. Ensure functionality of pressure off-loading devices for wheelchair, bed.
Poor nutrition	Assess teeth or dentures; ensure good mouth care. Provide adequate nutritional and fluid intake; assist with intake, as necessary. Consult dietitian for nutritional evaluation.

shift. In addition, the patient's skin must be kept clean and dry. Assessment and skin hygiene are two initial defences for preventing skin breakdown. To clean the skin, soaps and hot water should be avoided. Instead, use cleaners with nonionic surfactants that are gentle to the skin (Orsted et al., 2017; RNAO, 2016). Many types of products are available for skin care, and the nurse needs to match their use to the specific needs of the patient.

After cleaning the skin and making sure it is completely dry, the nurse applies moisturizer to keep the epidermis well lubricated but not oversaturated. It is important to control, contain, or correct incontinence, perspiration, and wound drainage (Bryant & Clark, 2016).

To aid in preventing and managing incontinence, clinicians find the RNAO *Best Practice Guidelines on Promoting Continence Using Prompted Voiding* (2002) helpful, although the Canadian Urological Association (CUA) has also developed Canadian guidelines, accessible on the CUA website. Patients who have fecal incontinence and who are also receiving enteral tube feeding provide a management challenge. When patients have an incontinent episode, the affected area should be gently cleaned and dried, and a thick layer of moisture barrier applied to the exposed area. A moisture barrier protects skin from excessive moisture and bacteria found in the urine or stool. The barrier should not interfere with the function of the adult continence brief. It is helpful to use the expertise of an advanced practice nurse with a focus on wound care or management of incontinence while caring for at-risk patients. Methods for controlling or containing incontinence vary. While medication and surgery are available treatments, the nurse can explore behavioural techniques with the patient, such as prompted or timed voiding. The guidelines mentioned earlier (RNAO and CUA) provide excellent information to assist nurses in developing appropriate treatment plans for patients.

Before initiating use of absorbent pads and adult continence briefs, the nurse should explore the use of the behavioural techniques mentioned earlier. These absorptive products are used only as part of the treatment plan for an incontinent patient. Only products that wick moisture away from the patient's skin should be used (Bryant & Clark, 2016; Wounds Canada, 2017a). Underpads need to be used with caution, because some of these pads do not wick the drainage away from the patient's skin and will cause skin damage. In addition, patients who are provided with low air loss or other specialty pressure-relief bed surfaces require continence pads designed specifically for the bed surface.

Positioning. Positioning interventions reduce pressure and shearing force to the skin. Elevating the head of the bed to 30 degrees or less will decrease the chance of pressure injuries developing from shearing forces (RNAO, 2016). A *Cochrane Review* of studies examining repositioning related to pressure injury prevention (Gillespie, Chaboyer, McInnes, et al., 2014) indicated that there were limited reliable results as to timed repositioning (e.g., 2, 3, 4 or 6 hours). However, the authors did state that repositioning of the individual with decreased mobility function is important. Nurses should be aware of their patient's activity level, perceptual ability, and daily routines (Braden, 2001; RNAO, 2016) when determining a repositioning approach that will be of benefit to the individual. When repositioning a patient, the nurse should use positioning devices to protect bony prominences (RNAO, 2016). The RNAO guidelines also recommend a 30-degree lateral position, which should prevent positioning directly over a bony prominence. To prevent shear and friction injuries, the nurse should use a sheet to lift, rather than drag, the patient when changing positions, and ensure the heels are supported as well. It is helpful to use the expertise of physiotherapists and occupational therapists who are skilled at assessment and treatment modalities for both seating and positioning for beds, chairs, and wheelchairs.

> **Safety Alert**
> Incorrect positioning of an immobile patient may create a shearing injury. When repositioning the patient, obtain assistance. With at least one other caregiver, place a drawsheet under the patient, and then, grasping the sides of the sheet, use it to lift the patient up and toward the new position. Remember to ensure the heels are not dragging on the bed, as this may contribute to shearing and friction injuries.

If the patient can sit in a chair, the duration of sitting should be limited. For example, if it was determined that the patient should be repositioned every 2 hours, then the duration of sitting should be less than 2 hours. In the sitting position, the pressure on the ischial tuberosities is greater than in the supine position. In addition, patients with some independent mobility should be encouraged to shift weight every 15 minutes when sitting (RNAO, 2016). Shifting weight provides short-term relief on the ischial tuberosities. In addition, patients should sit on a foam, gel, or air cushion to redistribute weight away from the ischial areas. The nurse can engage assistance of the physiotherapist or occupational therapist to ensure that cushions are correctly inflated and positioned. Rigid and doughnut-shaped cushions are contraindicated because they reduce blood supply to the area, which results in wider areas of ischemia (RNAO, 2016).

After repositioning the patient, the nurse should reassess the skin. See Box 46-2 for identifying characteristics that indicate early signs of tissue ischemia in darkly pigmented skin. For patients who have light-toned skin, the nurse should check for normal reactive hyperemia and blanching.

Reddened areas should never be massaged. Massaging reddened areas increases breaks in the capillaries in the underlying tissues and increases the risk of injury to those tissues and of pressure injury formation (RNAO, 2016).

Support Surfaces (Therapeutic Beds and Mattresses). A *support surface* is a specialized device for pressure redistribution designed for management of tissue loads, microclimate, and other therapeutic functions (i.e., mattresses, integrated bed system, mattress replacement, overlay or seat cushion, or seat cushion overlay) (NPUAP, 2007). A variety of support surfaces exist, including specialty beds and mattresses that reduce the hazards of immobility to the skin and musculoskeletal system. However, none of them eliminates the need for meticulous nursing care, and no single device eliminates the effects of pressure on the skin.

When selecting support surfaces, the nurse must thoroughly assess the patient's needs. Knowledge about support surface characteristics (Table 46-8) will assist the nurse in clinical decision making, along with consultations with the physiotherapist and occupational therapist.

The nurse must fully explain to patients and families why and how these specialty surfaces need to be used (Box 46-11). Some common errors when support surfaces are used are placing the wrong side of the support surface toward the patient, not plugging in or turning on powered support surfaces, using inappropriate absorbent underlay or bedding, failing to do "hand checks," and improper inflation (too much or too little) for some support surfaces. Hand checks are done by placing the hand under the support surface (or, if an overlay, between it and the standard mattress or cushion), at the pressure point, with the palm facing up and fingers flat. There should be at least 2.5 cm of support surface between the patient's pressure point and the caregiver's hand. If not, the support cushion or bed surface does not provide adequate support.

Education. Education of the patient and caregivers is an important nursing function (Orsted et al., 2017). What is important is that nurses individualize teaching to meet the language, educational level, and learning needs for each patient, especially older patients or those for whom English is not their first language. Nurses can use a variety of educational tools, including web-based learning, YouTube videos, and written materials, when teaching patients and caregivers or family members how to prevent and treat skin breakdown. Materials can be accessed from reputable government, educational, and national organizations such as the Canadian Association of Wound Care (renamed Wounds Canada) and the Canadian Association of Enterostomal Therapists (see "Recommended Websites" section). The wound care industry also provides excellent educational materials, although some may be product specific. Nurses can readily access any of these sites through an Internet search engine.

BOX 46-11 PATIENT TEACHING

Pressure-Redistribution Surfaces

Objectives

- Patient and family will describe their understanding of the purposes and basic operations of the pressure-redistribution surfaces.

Teaching Strategies

- Explain reasons for the pressure-redistribution surface.
- Explain proper body mechanics while using the pressure-redistribution surface.
- Educate patient and family about the use and care of the pressure-redistribution surface.
- Explain additional pressure-redistribution measures.

Evaluation

- Patient and family will state the basic purposes for the pressure-redistribution surface.
- Patient and family will describe the function of the pressure-redistribution surface.
- Patient and family will demonstrate proper use of the pressure-redistribution surface.

TABLE 46-8 Support Surfaces

Categories and Definitions	Mechanism of Action	Indications	Examples of Manufacturers in Canada*
Low-Air-Loss			
Available in a mattress placed directly on the existing bed frame or an overlay placed directly on top of an existing surface	Pressure redistribution Provides a flow of air to assist in managing the heat and humidity of the skin	Prevention or treatment of skin breakdown	Arjo-Huntleigh EHOB Hill-Rom Quart Healthcare
Nonpowered			
Any support surface not requiring or using external sources of energy for operation. Examples: foam, interconnected air-filled cells	Pressure redistribution Air moves to and from cells as body position changes	Prevention or treatment of skin breakdown	Arjo-Huntleigh EHOB Hill-Rom Quart Healthcare
Air-Fluidized Beds			
Surfaces that change load distribution properties when powered and when patient is in contact with the surface	Provides pressure redistribution via a fluidlike medium created by forcing air through beads, as characterized by immersion and envelopment	Prevention or treatment of skin breakdown May also be used to protect newly flapped or grafted surgical sites and for patients with excessive moisture	Arjo-Huntleigh Hill-Rom
Lateral Rotation			
Provides passive motion to promote mobilization of respiratory secretions and provides low-air-loss therapy	Features a support surface that provides rotation about a longitudinal axis, as characterized by degree of patient turn, duration, and frequency	Treatment and prevention of pulmonary complications associated with immobility	Arjo-Huntleigh Hill-Rom Quart Healthcare

*Refer to company website for specific product information.

In addition, nurses need to be aware of the meaning of the experience of a chronic wound for patients and their caregivers (Orsted et al., 2017; RNAO, 2016). Through research, clinicians are beginning to explore the concerns and issues faced by patients and their frail older spouses caring for their loved ones with pressure injuries (Goldberg & Beltz, 2010; Koschwanez, Kerse, Darragh, et al., 2013). Nurses need to plan interventions to meet the identified psychosocial needs of patients and their caregivers (Orsted et al., 2017; RNAO, 2016).

Management of Pressure Injury. Treatment of patients with pressure injury requires a holistic, team approach (RNAO, 2016). Aspects of pressure injury treatment include local care of the wound and supportive measures such as adequate nutrients and redistribution of pressure (Skill 46-2), which may call for the expertise of other members of the interdisciplinary health care team, including the physician, physiotherapist, occupational therapist, dietitian, pharmacist, and social worker.

Optimizing wound healing requires monitoring of the wound, but unless infection is suspected or present, the wound will heal best when undisturbed. Many current wound dressings are designed to remain in place for up to a week or even longer, and this approach supports healing in chronic, noninfected wounds (Orsted et al., 2017; RNAO, 2016). However, this does not diminish the need to regularly assess and document the wound: its location, stage, size, tissue type and amount, exudate, and the surrounding skin condition (Nix, 2016).

The use and documentation of a systematic approach to assessment of pressure injury leads to better decision making and optimum outcomes (Padula, Mishra, Makic, et al., 2014). Several healing and documentation tools are available for nurses to use to document wound assessments over time. Using a tool helps link the assessment to outcomes so that an evaluation of the plan of care follows objective criteria (Padula et al., 2014). For example, the Bates-Jensen Wound Assessment Tool (BWAT) contains 13 items that can be used to assess wound characteristics, which are then rated by the nurse, using a Likert-type scale (score of 1 indicates the healthiest and 5 indicates the least healthy attribute for each characteristic). The scoring assists in evaluating whether the goals of the wound management plan are effective. Tools such as the BWAT may seem overly detailed and time consuming, but when used accurately and regularly, they provide a method of ensuring reliable documentation of nursing actions.

Many organizations are turning to electronic documentation systems, including wound care documentation. These approaches are rapidly taking the place of "paper and pen" versions of documentation and assessment, and often provide options for wound photography and automated wound measurement as well as embedded best practice recommendations (Florczak, Scheurich, Croghan, et al., 2012; Geller, 2014).

Wound Management. Maintenance of a physiological local wound environment is the goal of effective wound management (Bryant & Nix 2016). To maintain a healthy wound environment, nurses need to address the following directives: prevent and manage infection, clean the wound, remove nonviable tissue, manage exudate, maintain the wound in a moist environment, and protect the wound. A wound will not move through the phases of wound healing if the wound is infected. Prevention of wound infection includes wound irrigation, cleaning, and removal of nonviable tissue.

Cleaning a Wound. Only noncytotoxic wound cleaners, such as normal saline or commercial wound cleaners, should be used to clean wounds. Noncytotoxic cleaners will not damage or kill

SKILL 46-2 TREATING PRESSURE INJURIES

Delegation Considerations

The skill of treating pressure injuries cannot be delegated to unregulated care providers (UCPs). In some practice settings, nurses can delegate *nonsterile* dressing application for chronic, established wounds when a nurse has evaluated and designated the protocol. The *assessment* of the wound remains within the scope of the nurse, however, even if the dressing change is delegated. Instruct nursing assistive personnel to do the following:

- Report changes in skin integrity to a nurse immediately.
- Report pain, fever, or wound drainage to a nurse immediately.
- Report any potential contamination to the existing dressing (e.g., patient incontinence or other bodily fluids; dressing becomes dislodged).

Equipment

- Disposable gloves (clean)
- Plastic bag for dressing disposal
- Disposable measuring tape
- Cotton-tipped applicators (sterile)
- Topical cleaning agent
- Dressing of choice (see Table 46-9)
- Hypoallergenic tape (if needed)
- Documentation record
- Measurement tool to record ongoing wound progress

PROCEDURE

STEPS	RATIONALE
1. Assess patient's level of comfort using a scale of 1 to 10 and the need for pain medication.	• Pain management enables better tolerance for dressing change.
2. Determine if patient has allergies to topical agents.	• Topical agents cause localized skin reactions.
3. Review order for topical agent or dressing.	• Administration of proper medication and treatment is ensured.
4. Close room door or bedside curtains. Position patient to allow dressing removal.	• Privacy is provided; area is accessible for dressing change.
5. Perform hand hygiene, and apply clean gloves. Remove dressing, and place in plastic bag.	• Transmission of microorganisms is reduced; accidental exposure to body fluids is prevented.
6. Assess pressure injury or wound. All pressure wounds need individual assessments (see Step 6 illustration).	• Consistent assessment will provide the basis for evaluating wound progress (RNAO, 2016).
A. Note colour, type, and percentage of tissue present in the wound base.	• Determining tissue type assists in dressing selection.
B. Measure width and length of the wound(s). Determine width by measuring the dimension from left to right and the length from top to bottom.	• Wound size will change as healing progresses; therefore, longest and widest areas of the wound will change over time. Measuring width and length by measuring the same area will provide a consistent measurement (Nix, 2016).
C. Measure depth of wound using sterile cotton-tipped applicator (see Step 6 illustration).	• Depth is important to determine wound volume. Although surface area adequately represents tissue loss in stage 2 wounds, volume more adequately represents tissue loss in stage 3 and 4 wounds (RNAO, 2016).
D. Measure depth of undermining using sterile cotton-tipped applicator to gently probe under skin edges (see Step 6 illustration).	• Undermining represents loss of underlying tissue (subcutaneous and muscle) to a greater extent than the skin. Undermining indicates progressive tissue loss.

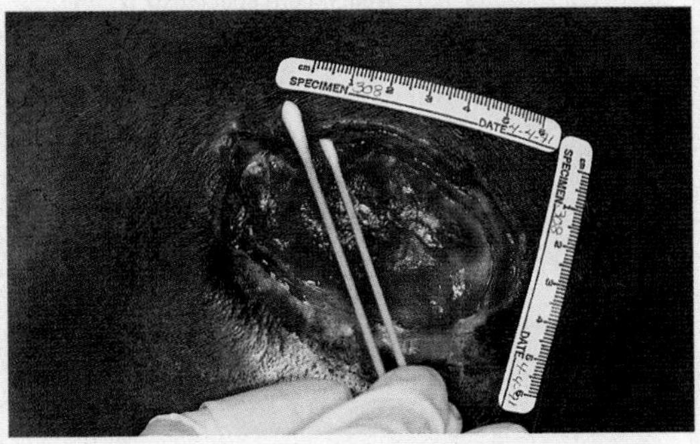

STEP 6 Measuring wound depth (Steps B, C, and D.)

STEPS	RATIONALE
7. Assess periwound skin for maceration, redness, and denuded areas.	• Deterioration of skin around a wound indicates infection, excessive wound exudate, or skin stripping from adhesive removal.
8. Change to sterile gloves, if needed (check agency policy).	• Avoid potential contamination of wound from external source. Refer to institutional policy regarding use of clean or sterile gloves.
9. Clean wound thoroughly with warmed normal saline, tap water, or cleaning agent.	• Wound debris must be removed to support healing tissue (RNAO, 2016).
10. Apply topical agents, as prescribed.	
A. Enzymatic debridement, as prescribed Carefully read instructions.	
(1) Apply thin, even layer of ointment over necrotic areas of ulcer only, where eschar has been scored if required. Protect periwound skin.	• A thick layer of ointment is not necessary; a thin layer absorbs and is more effective (Bryant & Niix, 2016). Check manufacturer's directions for frequency of application.

Continued

SKILL 46-2 TREATING PRESSURE INJURIES—cont'd

STEPS	RATIONALE
(2) Apply secondary nonadherent gauze dressing directly over wound.	• Wound is protected. Bacteria are prevented from entering wound.
(3) Tape securely in place.	• Dressing is kept in place. Use tape or adhesive that will not irritate skin.
B. Hydrogel	
(1) Cover surface of ulcer with thin layer of hydrogel using applicator or gloved hand.	• A moist wound environment is maintained.
(2) Apply secondary nonadherent gauze dressing or transparent dressing over wound, and adhere to intact skin.	• Wound base is covered and hydrogel–wound interface is maintained.
C. Calcium alginate or hydrofibre	
(1) Lightly pack wound with alginate or hydrofibre using applicator or gloved fingers.	• Wound moisture is maintained while excess drainage is absorbed.
(2) Apply secondary dressing of nonadherent gauze, absorbent pad, or foam over alginate. Tape in place.	• Alginate is held against wound surface.
11. Remove gloves, dispose of soiled supplies. Perform hand hygiene.	• Transmission of microorganisms is reduced.
12. Assess wound at each dressing change or sooner if the wound or patient's condition deteriorates (Nix, 2016). Utilize agency's tool for wound assessment.	• Not all patients with wounds will follow a healing trajectory, due to comorbidities. Consistent assessment provides a record of healing progress, deterioration, or stalled wound.
13. Compare wound assessment to identified plan of care, and discuss with health care team if there is increase in size of wound, increased presence of pain, foul-smelling drainage, or increase in devitalized tissue.	• Wound care is an interdisciplinary activity and requires involvement of the team of health care providers as well as the patient and family.

CRITICAL DECISION POINT: *A clean pressure wound should show evidence of approximately 30% healing within 2 to 4 weeks. Do not use the pressure injury staging system to measure healing. The system measures depth of wound, not healing (WOCN, 2010).*

14. Complete wound documentation required for one of the wound assessment instruments per agency's protocol.	• Assessments compared over time will determine progress toward wound healing.

UNEXPECTED OUTCOMES	RELATED INTERVENTIONS
Maceration of skin surrounding wound	• Reduce exposure of surrounding skin to topical agents and moisture. • Consider use of a skin barrier on periwound skin. • Use a dressing that will wick exudate away from periwound skin.
Deepening of wound and increased drainage	• Notify health care team regarding possible wound infection • Obtain necessary wound cultures as required • Obtain additional consults (e.g., wound care specialist).

RECORDING AND REPORTING

- Record assessment of wound (including measurement) in patient's record.
- Describe type of topical agent used, dressing applied, and patient's response.
- Report any deterioration in wound appearance (including odour).

HOME CARE CONSIDERATIONS

- Assess ability of patient or family to manage dressing changes and provide education (demonstrate and ensure that family, patient, or both can show or describe how to manage dressings and support).
- Patients need to dispose of contaminated dressings in the home in a manner consistent with local regulations (WOCN, 2010).
- Discuss need for a home pressure-redistribution surface or bed.

fibroblasts and healing tissue (Bryant & Nix, 2016). Cytotoxic solutions to absolutely avoid are sodium hypochlorite solution (Dakin's solution—essentially bleach), acetic acid, povidone-iodine, and hydrogen peroxide. These are *not* to be used in clean granulating wounds because they inhibit wound healing (Orsted et al., 2017; RNAO, 2016).

Recently, there has been significant interest in determining the relative safety of tap water in cleaning and irrigating wounds. From the research literature, there appears to be no particular risk related to using tap water from safe (municipal) water sources (Queirós, Santos, Apóstolo, et al., 2014). However, when using tap water in rural areas or from unknown sources, or if there could be potential contamination from the delivery system (e.g., rusted faucet or pipes), it is good to err on the side of caution and use sterile water or normal saline as the cleaner of choice.

Irrigation. Irrigation is a common method of delivering the wound cleaning solution to the wound. Studies have shown that an optimal effective range of irrigation pressures exists that ensure adequate removal of bacteria (RNAO, 2016; Rodeheaver, 2012). To ensure an irrigation pressure within the correct range, nurses should use a 35-mL syringe with a 19-gauge angiocatheter or a single 100-mL saline squeeze bottle. Both methods will enhance wound cleaning, but by delivering saline at a pressure between 4 and 15 psi (Bryant & Nix2016), trauma to the wound bed is avoided.

Debridement. Debridement is the removal of nonviable, necrotic tissue and is necessary to rid the injury of a source of infection, to enable visualization of the wound bed, and to provide a clean base for healing. However, a dry necrotic heel ulcer is an exception. According to the RNAO (2016) guidelines, stable, dry, black eschar on heels should not be debrided if no evidence of infection (e.g., pain, purulence, or erythema) appears. The method of debridement—mechanical, autolytic, chemical, or sharp or surgical—will depend on which is most appropriate to the patient's condition and care goals (Orsted et al., 2017; RNAO, 2016). During the debridement process, it is important to remember that increases in wound exudate, odour, and size are likely to be observed. Nurses need to assess and effectively manage pain that may occur with debridement (Orsted et al., 2017; RNAO, 2016).

Mechanical debridement, or a "wet-to-dry" saline gauze dressing, is *not* considered appropriate, as it is nonselective in its removal of both devitalized and viable tissue (Orsted et al., 2017). Biological debridement is the use of maggot therapy. Sterile maggots are used in a wound because they ingest the dead tissue and do not impede granulation (Sun, Chen, Zhang, et al., 2016). Chemical or enzymatic debridement is another option. Topical enzymes induce changes in the substrate, resulting in the breakdown of necrotic tissue (Carter, Gilligan, Waycaster, et al., 2016). Depending on the type of enzyme used, the preparation either digests or dissolves tissue. Care must be taken to apply only to the wound bed, never periwound tissue.

Current best practice treatment options are autolytic and sharp or surgical debridement (the gold standard). In autolytic debridement synthetic dressings are used over a wound to allow the eschar and fibrinous slough within the wound to be self-digested by the action of enzymes that are present in wound fluids (Orsted et al., 2017). Dressings that support moisture at the wound surface (e.g., hydrogel or hydrocolloid) maintain a moist wound bed ("moist like your eyeball"), which allows the movement of epithelial cells and facilitates wound closure; however, a wound that has excessive exudate (drainage) provides an environment that supports bacterial growth, macerates the periwound skin, and slows the healing process (Orsted et al., 2017). If exudate is excessive, an absorptive dressing (e.g., calcium alginate, hydrofibre, or foam) should be used, and volume, consistency, and odour of drainage evaluated to determine whether infection may be present.

Sharp or surgical debridement is the most efficient way to reach vitalized tissue at the base of a wound and is also used when sepsis can be localized and excised. Surgical debridement with a scalpel, scissors, or other sharp instrument should be performed only by health care providers with knowledge, skill, and competence to perform the procedure, usually physicians and advanced practice nurses (e.g., nurse practitioners). As a nurse, your regulating authority (e.g., College of Nurses) and your agency or institution policy mandates whether you are able to perform sharp or surgical debridement.

It is important to remember that the wound will not heal, regardless of the use of topical therapy (Bryant & Nix, 2016), unless the causative factors (e.g., malnourishment, shear, friction, pressure, and moisture) are controlled or eliminated. In addition, as the wound goes through the phases of healing, the treatment plan will need to be altered. For example, in the management of a wound with slough and necrotic tissue, the nurse may initially use a hydrocolloid dressing to autolytically debride the wound. Because the hydrocolloid dressing interacts with the wound to gradually liquefy and debride the slough/necrotic tissue, it should be left intact—up to 1 week if possible. Once the wound is free of necrotic, sloughy tissue, the nurse would discontinue the hydrocolloid dressing and choose a different type of dressing after assessing the wound base characteristics. Continued reassessment is key to supporting the wound as it moves through the phases of wound healing. It cannot be stressed enough how important it is for nurses to explain the process of wound healing to the patient and family.

Growth Factors. Growth factors regulate most of the key actions of cells during wound healing, and topical growth factors regulate the healing of chronic wounds (Schultz, 2016). Through extensive studies of the molecular regulation of healing, researchers now better understand the role of various growth factors involved in wound healing, including epidermal growth factor, platelet-derived growth factor, fibroblast growth factor, and transforming growth factor. Depending on the setting, nurses may be responsible for the use of this treatment modality.

Nutritional Status. Nutritional assessment and support of the patient with a wound is a vital component in normal cellular integrity and tissue repair (Molnar, Vlad, & Gumus, 2016; Stotts, 2016a; Weiss, Fingar, Barrett, et al., 2016). Nurses need to correct inadequate nutrition and support healing through early intervention. The Canadian Malnutrition Task Force (2017) recommends nutritional assessment within 24 hours of admission. The patient's mouth and skin should be assessed for signs of nutritional deficiencies (see Chapter 42). Reassessments reflect changes in status and effects of interventions (Litchford et al., 2014). Box 46-12 defines parameters for clinically significant malnutrition (Agency for Health Care Policy and Research [AHCPR], 1994; Cederholm, Bosaeus, Barazzoni, et al., 2015).

Protein Status. Patients with a potential for or actual decreased serum albumin levels or poor protein intake need a nutritional evaluation to ensure proper caloric intake (Laporte, Keller, Payette, et al., 2015; Orsted et al., 2017). A patient can lose as much as 50 g of protein per day from an open, weeping pressure injury. Although the recommended intake of protein for adults is 0.8 g/kg/day, a higher intake of

BOX 46-12 AHCPR* Recommendations for Nutritional Assessment and Management of Pressure Injury

Assessment of Clinically Significant Malnutrition

Serum albumin is less than 3.5 mg/100 mL.
Total lymphocyte count is less than 1 800/mm^3.
Body weight has decreased more than 15%.

Interventions

- Involve dietitian to prevent malnutrition and ensure adequate dietary intake.
- Maintain serum albumin level greater than 3.5 mg/100 mL.
- Maintain total lymphocyte count greater than 1 800/mm^3.
- Perform an abbreviated nutritional assessment, according to institutional policy and as defined by the Subjective Global Assessment at least every 3 months for patients who are unable to take food by mouth or who experience an involuntary change in weight.
- Encourage dietary intake or supplementation if a patient with a pressure injury is malnourished. If dietary intake continues to be inadequate, impractical, or impossible, use nutritional support (usually tube feeding) to place the patient into positive nitrogen balance (approximately 30 to 35 calories/kg/day and 1.25 to 1.50 g of protein/kg/day) according to the goals of care.
- Give vitamin and mineral supplements if you suspect or confirm deficiencies.

**AHCPR,* Agency for Health Care Policy and Research.
Adapted from Agency for Health Care Policy and Research, Panel for Treatment of Pressure Ulcers in Adults. (1994). *Treatment of pressure ulcers: Clinical practice guideline no. 15.* (AHCPR Pub No. 95-0653). Rockville, MD: Agency for Health Care Policy and Research, Public Health Service, U.S. Department of Health and Human Services.

protein up to 1.8 g/kg/day is necessary for healing. Increased protein intake helps rebuild epidermal tissue. Increased caloric intake helps replace subcutaneous tissue. Vitamin C promotes collagen synthesis, capillary wall integrity, fibroblast function, and immunological function.

Hemoglobin. A low hemoglobin level decreases delivery of oxygen to the tissues and leads to further ischemia. When possible, hemoglobin should be maintained at 12 g/100 mL.

Dressings

For surgical wounds that heal by primary intention, it is common to remove dressings as soon as drainage stops. In contrast, when a wound is healing by secondary intention, the dressing material becomes a means for providing an optimal healing environment.

Purposes of Dressings. A dressing serves several purposes:

- Protects wound from microorganism contamination
- Aids in hemostasis
- Promotes healing by absorbing drainage and supports autolytic debridement
- Supports or splints the wound site
- Protects the patient from seeing the wound (if perceived as unpleasant)
- Promotes thermal insulation of the wound surface
- Provides a moist environment for the wound bed

In a normally healing wound, when wound drainage is minimal, the healing process forms a natural fibrin seal that eliminates the need for a dressing. Wounds with extensive tissue loss always need a dressing.

A pressure dressing is applied with elastic bandages, exerts localized downward pressure over an actual or potential bleeding site, and eliminates dead space in underlying tissues so that wound healing progresses normally. Pressure dressings need to be checked to be sure that they do not interfere with circulation to a body part. Skin colour, pulses in distal extremities, the patient's comfort, and changes in sensation should be assessed. Pressure dressings are not routinely removed.

Specific dressings cover and protect certain types of wounds, such as large wounds, wounds with drainage tubes or suction catheters in the wound, wounds that need frequent changing, and fistulas. For these wounds, pouches or special wound collection systems cover the wound and collect wound drainage. Some of these devices have a plastic flange on the front of the wound pouch, which allows the nurse to change wound packing without removing the wound pouch from the skin.

Understanding the method of action and purpose of the dressing selection facilitates wound healing (Bryant & Nix 2016). When the nurse identifies the objectives for care of the wound, the dressing choice becomes clear. For example, a wound requiring exudate management requires a different type of dressing than one that requires debridement.

A primary function of a dressing on a healing wound is to protect the fragile wound bed. Most traditional surgical dressings have three layers: a contact or primary layer, an absorbent layer, and an outer protective or secondary layer. The contact dressing covers the incision and part of the adjacent skin. Fibrin, blood products, and debris adhere to the contact dressing's surface. A dressing that does not adhere to the wound bed, such as soft silicone, will not cause the dressing to stick to the suture line. Use of dry gauze or improper removal of the dressing will disrupt the healing epidermal surface. If a dressing sticks to the surgical incision, the dressing needs to be saturated with saline solution or water to release it from the incisional area and prevent trauma to the wound bed.

Types of Dressings. Wet-to-dry and wet-to-moist dressings are still often ordered, despite extensive research literature over the past 40 years that has clearly identified *moist wound healing* dressings as the optimal dressing choice to manage and support healing within the wound. As clinical researchers develop more appropriate dressings, it is essential to understand the reason why wet-to-dry and wet-to-moist dressings are neither current best practice nor supported in the research literature.

The basic premise behind the wet-to-dry dressing is to put a wet dressing (gauze and normal saline) on a wound, allow it to dry out, and then pull off the now-dry dressing, thereby mechanically debriding the wound. This is not effective, however, since the action is nonselective, so healthy granulating tissue is removed along with any necrotic or sloughy tissue. In addition, this type of action is inevitably painful to the patient; given the current availability of nontraumatic dressings, this seems an unnecessary condition for patient care.

Wet-to-moist dressings involve the use of a saline-soaked gauze that is not left to dry out on the wound, but rather kept moist on the wound through frequent dressing changes. Research has shown that frequency of dressing changes has a negative impact on wound healing (the disruption of fragile granulation tissue, cooling down the wound bed). As well, the dressing that is moistened with normal saline becomes a hypertonic environment that pulls fluid out of the wound bed in a way that leaves a slurry of blood and proteins on the surface of the wound, which, if not kept constantly moist, dries out (becoming a wet-to-dry dressing).

However, since these approaches are still used in some situations, as a nurse, you need to know the steps to follow when applying this type of dressing to a wound. It is strongly recommended that you consider alternatives (and there are many) to this approach, since it is not effective in promoting wound healing. You are encouraged to discuss the rationale for moist wound healing for the patient in question with the other care providers, in order to support evidence-informed best practices (Ovington, 2001).

Dressings vary by type of material and mode of application (wet or dry) (Skill 46-3). They need to be easy to apply, comfortable, and made of materials that promote wound healing. Wounds Canada has "Product Picker" guidelines (2017b) that nurses can use in selecting dressings that respond to the need of the wound, based on the goal for the wound: to heal, to protect from infection, to provide comfort, or to maintain current status (e.g., nonhealing wound). As with an unfamiliar medication, if, as a nurse, you are using a dressing you are not familiar with, you should look it up to learn its properties and how to use it correctly. A dressing designed to wick away exudate and avoid skin stripping from adhesives will protect the periwound skin. Protecting the wound bed requires a dressing that will maintain a moist wound bed (not too dry, not too wet), prevent contamination from external sources such as feces or urine, and be conformable to the wound and surrounding tissue (Box 46-13; see also Table 46-9). In addition, if the wound is deep, undermining, or has tunnelling or sinus tracts, ensure that the "packing" is actually not jammed into the wound: it should be packed lightly to prevent abscess development but to support the healthy closure of the wound (from the inside outward). In this situation, lightly pack the wound with appropriate dressing material— for example, in a dry base wound, a nonwoven gauze moistened with hydrogel; in a wet/contaminated base wound, hypertonic sodium ribbon (goes in dry); and in an infected wound bed, cadexomer iodine/silver/honey dressing (Orsted et al., 2017; Sibbald, Orsted, Coutts, et al., 2006).

Woven Gauze Dressings. In the past, woven gauze dressings were commonly used to provide coverage for wounds; however, research has demonstrated that their efficacy in wound healing is limited (Orsted et al., 2017). Nonwoven gauze nonetheless remains useful as packing material (e.g., Nu-gauze), and is available in different textures and in

SKILL 46-3 APPLYING DRY AND MOIST DRESSINGS

Delegation Considerations

The skill of applying dry and moist dressings to the new acute wound (generally a surgical wound) cannot be delegated to unregulated care providers (UCPs). In some settings, nurses can delegate aspects of wound care, such as changing of dressings using *clean* techniques for chronic wounds. The *assessment* of the wound remains within the scope of the nurse, however, even if the dressing change is delegated. Instruct nursing assistive personnel to do the following:

- Report pain, fever, bleeding, or wound drainage to a nurse immediately.
- Report any potential contamination to the existing dressing (e.g., patient incontinence or other bodily fluids; dressing becomes dislodged).

While surgeons often have specific orders for postsurgical (acute) wounds, it is important to support wound healing using best practice. Ensuring the wound is protected from potential contamination, observing for signs of infection, and attention to the patient's need for analgesic prior to dressing change are all important considerations.

Equipment

- Sterile gloves
- Variety of gauze dressings and pads
- Irrigation kit
- Cleaning solution
- Sterile solution
- Clean, disposable gloves
- Tape, ties, or bandages, as needed
- Waterproof bag
- Extra gauze dressings, or abdominal pads

PROCEDURE

STEPS	RATIONALE
1. Perform hand hygiene. Obtain information about wound characteristics (e.g., size, location, history of wound progress or management).	• Transmission of microorganisms is reduced. Plan for proper type and amount of supplies needed. Know when assistance ("an extra pair of hands") is needed to apply and affix dressing.
2. Assess patient's level of comfort. If analgesic has been ordered, assess need and provide if required.	• Removal of a dry dressing is painful; some patients require pain medication.
3. Review orders for dressing change procedure. Be prepared to adjust dressing depending on wound progress.	• Orders indicate type of dressing or applications to use; wounds change over time, so previous dressing may not be appropriate to current state of wound.
4. Explain procedure to patient, respond to questions. Instruct patient not to touch wound area or opened dressing supplies.	• Explanation decreases anxiety. Sudden, unexpected movement on patient's part may result in contamination of wound and supplies.
5. Close room or cubicle curtains and windows.	• Privacy is provided; airborne microorganisms are reduced.
6. Position patient comfortably, drape with bath blanket to expose only wound site.	• Wound is accessible; unnecessary exposure is minimized.
7. Place disposable bag within reach of work area. Fold top of bag to make cuff (see Step 7 illustration).	• Soiled dressings can easily be disposed of. Bag's outer surface is not soiled.

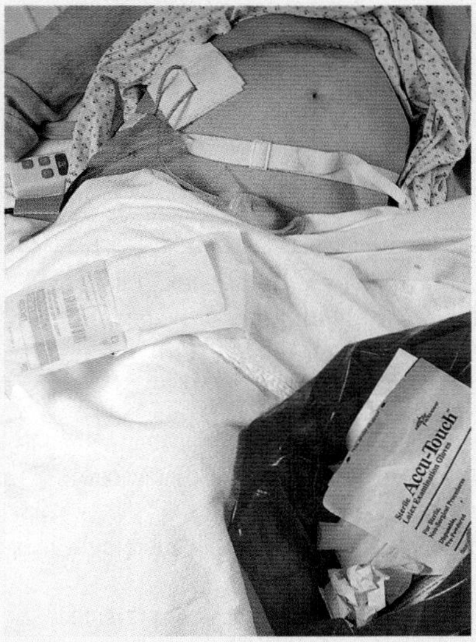

STEP 7 Disposable waterproof bag placed near the dressing site.

STEPS	RATIONALE
8. Apply face mask and protective eyewear, if needed.	• Transmission of pathogens to exposed tissues is reduced. Mask and eyewear protect from splashes.
9. Put on clean, disposable gloves; remove tape, bandage, or ties.	• Transmission of infectious organisms from soiled dressings to hands is prevented.

Continued

SKILL 46-3 APPLYING DRY AND MOIST DRESSINGS—cont'd

STEPS	RATIONALE
10. Remove tape: pull parallel to skin toward dressing; remove remaining adhesive from skin.	• Pulling tape toward dressing reduces stress on suture line or periwound skin.
11. With gloved hand, carefully remove gauze dressings one layer at a time, taking care not to dislodge drains or tubes.	• Appearance of drainage is sometimes upsetting to patient. Removal of one layer at a time reduces the chance of accidental removal of underlying drains.
A. If dressing sticks on a wet-to-dry dressing, do not moisten it; instead, gently free dressing, and alert patient of potential discomfort.	• Wet-to-dry dressing should debride wound (Ramundo, 2016). Do not wet the dressing to remove it. However, reassess and select other method of debridement.

CRITICAL DECISION POINT: *Never use a wet-to-dry dressing in a clean granulating wound. Use only for debridement and only if other debridement options are unavailable (Ramundo, 2016).*

STEPS	RATIONALE
12. Observe character and amount of drainage on dressing and appearance of wound.	• Estimate of drainage amount and appearance of wound assist in determining progress.
13. Fold dressings with drainage contained inside, and remove gloves inside out. With small dressings, remove gloves inside out over dressing (see Step 13 illustration). Dispose of gloves and soiled dressings in disposable bag. Perform hand hygiene.	• Transmission of microorganisms is reduced. Hands do not come into contact with material on gloves.
14. Open sterile dressing tray or individually wrapped sterile supplies. Place on bedside table (see Step 14 illustration).	• Sterile dressings remain sterile while on or within sterile surface. Preparation of supplies prevents break in technique during dressing change.

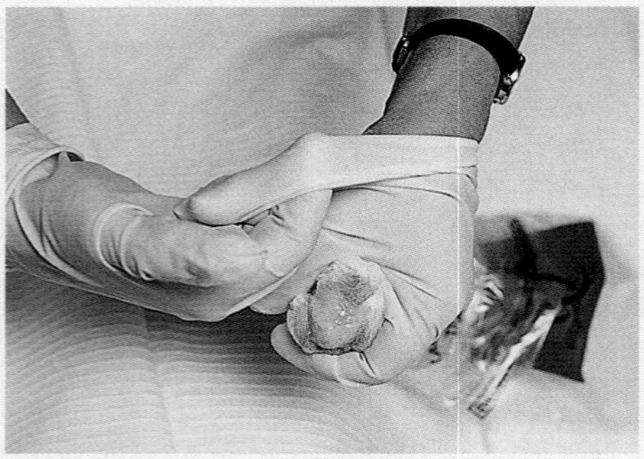

STEP 13 Removal of disposable gloves over contaminated dressing.

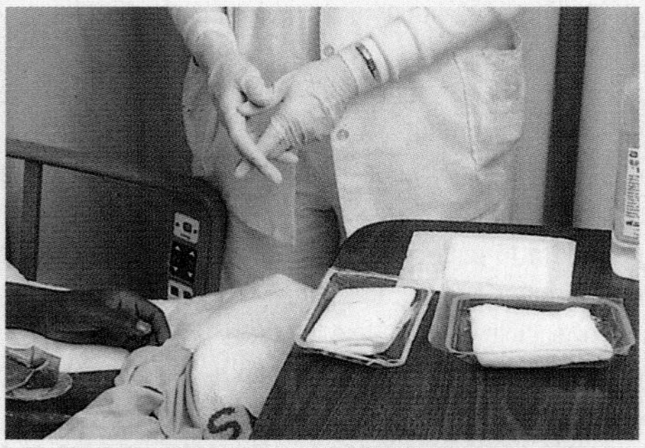

STEP 14 Sterile dressing equipment.

STEPS	RATIONALE
15. If required, clean or irrigate wound:	
A. Pour ordered solution into sterile irrigation container or use single-use bottle of normal saline.	
B. Using syringe or single-use bottle, irrigate wound at 10–15 psi	• 10–15 psi will effectively remove loose debris without damage to the granulating tissue of the wound bed.
C. Continue until the irrigation flow is clear.	• Use patient positioning to assist in irrigation (e.g., side-lying).
D. Dry surrounding skin.	

CRITICAL DECISION POINT: *Some wound cleaners are available in spray bottles with "stream." Use "spray" setting to loosen debris and stream function to irrigate. Do not irrigate sinus tracks or wounds where the base of the wound cannot be determined.*

STEPS	RATIONALE
16. Apply dressing:	
A. Dry dressing	
(1) Perform hand hygiene. Apply sterile gloves.	• Sterile supplies can be handled without contamination.
(2) Inspect wound for appearance, drains, drainage, and integrity.	• Wound healing status is indicated.
(3) Clean wound with solution: Use warmed (body temperature) solution when possible	• Cold or room temperature solution can affect growth factor and impede healing.
(a) Clean from least contaminated area to most contaminated area.	• Contamination of previously cleaned area is prevented.
(4) Gently pat periwound area to dry.	• Protection and absorption of wound drainage is provided.
(5) Apply appropriate type of dressing to cover the wound.	• Wound is protected from external environment.
(6) Apply topper (cover) dressing if required.	• Topper dressing prevents strikethrough of wound drainage and provides a surface to tape the dressing in place.
B. Moist dressing	
(1) Perform hand hygiene. Apply clean gloves.	
(2) Remove old dressings, discard in secure garbage container.	

STEPS	RATIONALE

(3) Assess surrounding skin (see Step 16B[3] illustration). Discard gloves.

- Surrounding skin assessment provides an evaluation of wound management.

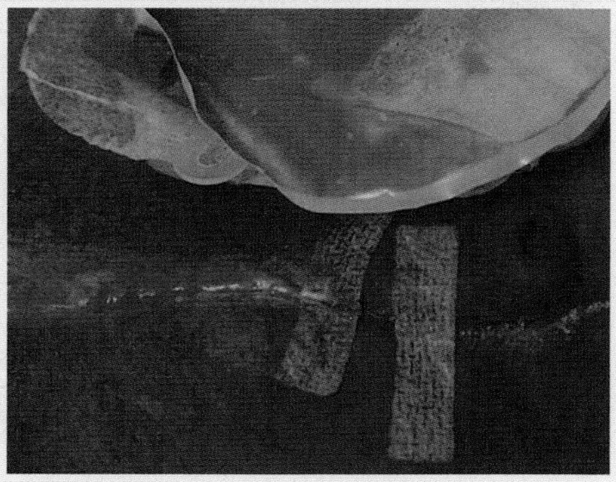

STEP 16B(3) Exposure of wound facilitates assessment of wound and surrounding skin.

(4) Perform hand hygiene. Apply sterile gloves as required.

- Handling of sterile supplies can occur without contamination.

(5) Clean wound base with warmed-to-body-temperature (if possible) normal saline or commercially prepared wound cleaner. Assess wound base.

- Cleaning removes wound debris for adequate assessment.

(6) Moisten gauze with prescribed solution. Gently wring out excess solution. Unfold.

- Gauze needs to be moist to allow for absorption of wound debris.

(7) Apply gauze as a single layer (see Step 16B[7] illustration) directly onto the wound surface. If wound is deep, gently and lightly "pack" dressing into wound base by hand or with forceps until all wound surfaces are in contact with the gauze. If tunnelling is present, use a cotton-tipped applicator to place gauze into tunnelled area. Be sure gauze does not touch the surrounding skin (see Step 16B[7] illustration).

- Inner gauze needs to be moist, not dripping wet, to absorb drainage and adhere to debris. Excessively moist dressings result in moisture-associated skin damage (maceration) in the periwound skin (Gray & Weir, 2007). The wound needs to be loosely packed to facilitate wicking of drainage into absorbent outer layer of dressing.

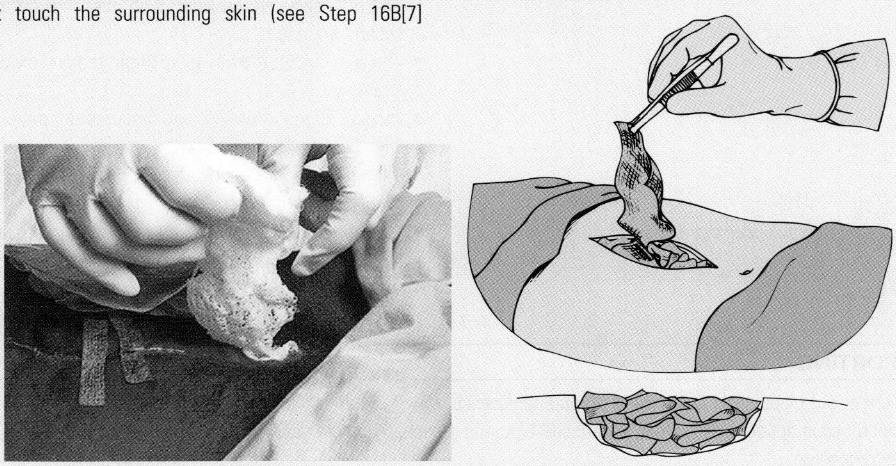

STEP 16B(7) Packing wound with single layer of gauze.

(8) Cover with sterile dry gauze and topper dressing.

- Topper dressing prevents strikethrough of wound drainage and provides a surface to tape the dressing in place.

17. Secure dressing.

A. Tape: Apply nonallergenic tape to secure dressing in place.

- The goal for securing a dressing is to keep the dressing in place and intact without causing damage to underlying and surrounding skin.

B. Montgomery ties (see Figure 46-23)

- Protect periwound skin from breakdown through frequent dressing changes.

(1) Expose adhesive surface of tape on end of each tie.

(2) Place ties on opposite sides of dressing.

(3) Place adhesive directly on skin, or use skin barrier.

- Skin barrier (Stomahesive) protects intact skin from stretch and tension of adhesive tape.

Continued

SKILL 46-3 APPLYING DRY AND MOIST DRESSINGS—cont'd

STEPS	RATIONALE
C. For dressings on an extremity, secure dressing with rolled gauze or an elastic net (see Step 17C illustration)	

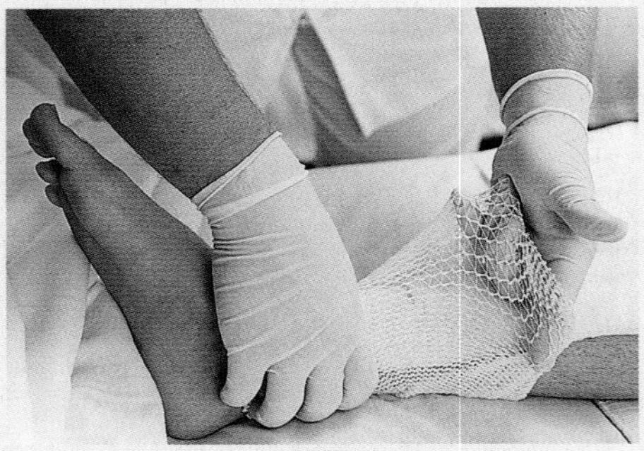

STEP 17C Elastic net securing a lower extremity dressing.

STEPS	RATIONALE
18. Remove gloves, and dispose of in bag. Remove any mask or eyewear.	• Transmission of infection is reduced.
19. Dispose of supplies, and perform hand hygiene.	• Transmission of infection is reduced.
20. Assist patient to comfortable position.	• Patient's sense of well-being is promoted. Comfort is enhanced.

UNEXPECTED OUTCOMES	RELATED INTERVENTIONS
Wound appears inflamed, tender, with or without drainage	• Monitor patient for signs of infection (e.g., increased temperature or white blood cell count). • Obtain wound culture. • Notify health care provider.
Wound drainage increases	• Increase frequency of dressing changes. • Notify health care provider, who may consider drain placement to facilitate wound drainage.
Wound bleeds during dressing change	• Observe colour. If drainage is bright red and excessive, you will need to apply pressure. • Inspect along dressing and underneath patient to determine amount of bleeding. • Obtain vital signs, as needed. • Notify health care provider.
Sensation that "something has given way under the dressing"	• Observe wound for increased drainage or separation of sutures. • Protect wound. Cover with sterile moist dressing. • Instruct patient to lie still. • Notify health care provider.

RECORDING AND REPORTING

- Immediately report brisk, bright-red bleeding or evidence of wound dehiscence or evisceration to health care provider.
- Report wound and periwound tissue appearance, colour, and tissue type and presence and characteristics of exudate, type and amount of dressings used, and tolerance of patient to procedure.
- Record patient's level of comfort and effective analgesic and comfort measures.
- Write date and time dressing applied on tape in ink (not marker).

HOME CARE CONSIDERATIONS

- More expensive specialty dressings are sometimes used because they have longer wear-time and often have antimicrobial properties.
- Assess ability of patient and family to manage dressing changes independently, and teach as possible.
- Patients need to dispose of contaminated dressings in the home in a manner consistent with local regulations.

various lengths and sizes; the 4 × 4 and ribbon dressings are the most common. Gauze can be saturated with solutions and used to clean and pack a wound. When used to lightly pack a dry wound, the gauze should be moistened with hydrogel, which will hydrate a dry wound bed. A simple gauze "island" dressing can be used over clean wounds with little or no drainage. The "island" refers to the gauze pad surrounded by a lightly adhesive fabric. Acute surgical wounds are most likely to be packed with saline-moistened nonwoven gauze and the dressing changed at frequent intervals, usually determined by the surgeon.

Transparent Film Dressings. Self-adhesive, transparent film dressings are occlusive and trap the wound's moisture over the wound,

BOX 46-13 WOCN* Dressing Recommendations

- Use a dressing that will continuously provide a moist ("like your eyeball") environment. Wet-to-dry dressings should be avoided.
- Perform wound care using topical dressings as determined by a thorough assessment. No specific studies have proven an optimal dressing type for pressure wounds.
- Choose a dressing that keeps the surrounding intact (periwound) skin dry while keeping the wound bed moist.
- Choose a dressing that controls exudate but does not desiccate the wound bed.
- Consider caregiver time, ease of use, availability, and cost when selecting a dressing.
- Eliminate wound dead space by loosely filling all cavities with dressing material.

**WOCN*, Wound, ostomy, and continence nurses.
Adapted from Wound, Ostomy and Continence Nurses Society. (2003, 2010). *Guideline for prevention and management of pressure ulcers.* WOCN Clinical Practice Guidelines Series. Glenview, IL: Author.

providing a moist environment. The transparent film dressing has been used for small, superficial wounds such as skin tears or for protection of high-risk skin. However, transparent film dressings can be difficult to remove and can cause unnecessary trauma to fragile periwound tissue. The transparent film must be removed with a "lateral pull" technique, in which the nurse supports the dressing with one hand while lifting (and breaking the adhesive seal) with the other, instead of just pulling off the dressing. Bearing these factors in mind, nurses can use transparent film dressing to affix gauze, and it can also function as a secondary dressing or provide autolysis for small wounds.

Transparent film is particularly useful in securing intravenous (IV) lines and other tubing since these dressings tend to provide an occlusive barrier, which does not allow significant moisture–vapour transfer and can potentially create macerated periwound skin.

Transparent film does permit a view of the wound, but some newer dressings, such as clear acrylic absorbent dressings, offer more moisture–vapour transfer capability and longer wear time.

Nonadherent Contact Layer Dressings. A variety of nonadherent dressings are available and provide protection to the fragile granulating tissue while allowing the interstitial fluid and moisture from the wound to evaporate. This provides a moist "like your eyeball" environment

TABLE 46-9 Wound Care Dressings

CLASS		LOCAL WOUND CARE*			CARE CONSIDERATIONS
	Description	Tissue Debridement	Infection	Moisture Balance	Indications and Contraindications
1. Films and membranes	Semipermeable adhesive sheet. Impermeable to H_2O molecules and bacteria	+	–	–	Moisture vapour transmission rate varies from film to film. Should not be used on draining or infected wounds.* Create occlusive barrier against infection.
2. Nonadherent contact layer	Sheets of low adherence to tissue. Nonmedicated tulles, silicone, and petrolatum-based woven dressings	–	–	–	Allows drainage to seep through pores to secondary dressing and evaporate off the wound. Requires a cover (absorbent) dressing.
3. Hydrogels	Polymers with high H_2O content. Available in gels, solid sheets, or impregnated gauze	++	–	+	Should not be used on draining wounds. Solid sheets should not be used on infected wounds.
4. Hydrocolloids	May contain gelatin, sodium, carboxymethylcellulose, polysaccharides, or pectin, or a combination of these. Sheet dressings are occlusive and have polyurethane film outer layer	+++	+/–	++	Should be used with care on fragile skin. Should not be used on heavily draining or infected wounds.* Create occlusive barrier to protect the wound from outside contamination. Characteristic odour may accompany dressing change and should not be confused with infection.
5. Calcium alginates	Sheets or fibrous ropes of calcium sodium alginate (seaweed derivative). Have hemostatic capabilities	++	+	+++	Should not be used on dry wounds. Avoid packing into narrow deep sinuses because of low tensile strength. Bioreabsorbable.
6. Composite dressings	Multilayered, combination dressings to increase absorbency and autolysis	+	–	+++	Use on wounds on which dressing may stay in place for several days.*
7. Foams	Nonadhesive or adhesive polyurethane foam. May have occlusive backing. Sheets or cavity packing. Some have fluid lock.	–	–	+++	Use on moderate to heavily draining wounds. Occlusive foams should not be used on heavily draining or infected wounds.*
8. Charcoal	Contains odour-absorbent charcoal within product	–	–	+	Some charcoal products are inactivated by moisture. Ensure that dressing edges are sealed.

Continued

TABLE 46-9 Wound Care Dressings—cont'd

CLASS		LOCAL WOUND CARE*			CARE CONSIDERATIONS
	Description	Tissue Debridement	Infection	Moisture Balance	Indications and Contraindications
9. Hypertonic	Sheet, ribbon, or gel impregnated with sodium concentrate.	+	+	++	Gauze ribbon should not be used on dry wounds. May be painful on sensitive tissue. Gel may be used on dry wounds.
10. Hydrophilic fibres	Sheet or packing strip of sodium carboxymethylcellulose. Converts to a solid gel when activated by moisture (fluid lock).	+	–	+++	Best for moderate amount of exudate. Should not be used on dry wounds. Avoid packing into narrow deep sinuses because of low tensile strength.
11. Antimicrobials	Medical-grade honey, silver, cadexomer iodine, gentian violet/methylene blue—with vehicle for delivery: sheets, gels, alginates, foams, or paste	+	+++	+	Broad spectrum against bacteria. Not to be used on patients with known hypersensitivities to any product components.
12. Other devices	NPWT applies localized negative pressure to surface and margins of wound. Dressings consist of polyurethane or polyvinyl alcohol materials.	–	+	+++	Pressure-distributing wound dressing actively removes fluid from the wound and promotes wound edge approximation. Advanced skill required for patient selection for this therapy.
13. Biological	Living human fibroblasts provided in sheets at ambient or frozen temperatures. Extracellular matrix. Collagen-containing preparations. Hyaluronic acid. Platelet-derived growth factor.	–	–	–	Should not be used on wounds with infection, sinus tracts, excessive exudate, or on patients known to have hypersensitivity to any of the product components. Cultural issues related to source. Advanced skill required for patient selection for this therapy.

*"+" Indicates the appropriateness of the dressing for tissue debridement, infection, and moisture balance. "–" Indicates the dressing is not considered beneficial in these areas. Use with caution if critical colonization is suspected.
NPWT, Negative pressure wound therapy.
From Registered Nurses' Association of Ontario. (2011, revised 2016). *RNAO best practice guideline: Assessment and management of stage I–IV pressure ulcers* (pp. 102–103). Toronto: Author.

that promotes healing. As well, the contact layer can remain undisturbed while a secondary cover dressing can be changed as needed (when saturated or soiled). Early forms of contact layer dressings were tulle (paraffin) or petrolatum jelly, which may decrease the effectiveness of moisture–vapour transfer. Some of the newer petrolatum-based or silicone contact layers are more effective in this regard. These dressings are designed to be placed over the open wound and draped across the intact periwound skin. It is important for wound healing to allow these contact layer dressings to remain in place for a number of days and change the secondary dressing only as needed.

Soft Silicone Dressings. Soft silicone dressings are composed of silicone that functions as an atraumatic wound contact layer. A main advantage of soft silicone is its removal without causing trauma to the wound bed or the periwound skin. Different types of soft silicone dressings are wound contact layers (useful for skin tears) and absorbent dressings for exudating wounds. Soft silicone dressings are particularly relevant in decreasing pain during dressing change and are especially useful in dealing with fungating wounds or any wound where the periwound skin is fragile, such as in pediatric patients.

Hydrocolloid Dressings. Hydrocolloid dressings have complex formulations of colloidal, elastomeric, and adhesive components. These dressings are adhesive and occlusive. The wound contact layer of the dressing forms a gel as fluid is absorbed and maintains a moist healing environment. Hydrocolloids support healing in clean granulating wounds, autolytically debride necrotic wounds, and are available in a variety of sizes and shapes.

A hydrocolloid dressing has the following characteristics:

- Has minimal absorption capabilities and is best for autolytically debriding a dry or slightly moist wound with fibrinous or necrotic debris
- Maintains wound bed moisture
- Slowly liquefies necrotic debris
- Is impermeable to external bacteria and other contaminants
- Is self-adhesive and conforms to the body well
- Acts as a preventive dressing for high-risk friction areas
- May be left in place for 5 to 7 days

This type of dressing is most useful on shallow to moderately deep wounds. Hydrocolloid dressings should not be used in heavily draining wounds or in full-thickness or infected wounds. Because of the manner in which hydrocolloids interact with the wound bed matter, when the dressing is removed, residue in the wound bed may be confused with pus (colour, odour) until the wound is cleaned. Hydrocolloids are quite adherent to the periwound skin and should be used with caution where the periwound tissue is fragile or friable.

Hydrogel Dressings. Hydrogel dressings donate moisture to the wound bed (hence, the term *hydro,* indicating "water") and are gauze or sheet dressings impregnated with water- or glycerin-based amorphous gel. This type of dressing hydrates wounds and absorbs some smaller amounts of exudate. Hydrogel dressings are for partial-thickness and full-thickness wounds, deep wounds with minimal drainage, necrotic wounds, burns, and radiation-damaged skin. They are very useful with painful wounds because they are soothing to the patient, do not adhere to the wound bed, and cause minimal trauma during dressing removal. Hydrogels should not be used on draining wounds; sheets should not be used on infected wounds. Hydrogels come in a sheet dressing or in a tube. When using hydrogel from a tube, the gel should not be squirted directly into the wound; rather, use a sterile gauze dressing or sterile implement (e.g., tongue depressor) to apply the gel so that potential contamination of the tube from matter in the wound is avoided.

Hydrogel has the following characteristics:

- Is soothing and reduces pain in the wound
- Provides a moist environment
- Debrides the wound (by softening the necrotic tissue)
- Does not adhere to the wound base and is easy to remove

Foam Dressings. Foam dressings are composed of nonadhesive or adhesive polyurethane foam, are provided as sheets or packing, and come in a variety of sizes and shapes. They are useful for wounds with large amounts of drainage or for autolytic debridement because they can be left intact for up to 7 days. Some foam dressings have a "fluid lock" to wick drainage off the wound and periwound skin, which prevents maceration. Furthermore, nonborder foam dressings can be cut to fit around drainage tubes.

Calcium Alginate Dressings. Calcium alginate dressings are manufactured from seaweed and are available in sheet and rope form. The alginate forms a thickened, stronger surface when it comes in contact with wound fluid. These highly absorbent dressings are useful in highly draining wounds and also provide hemostasis in friable tissue. Calcium alginate dressings are bioreabsorbable but should be removed from the wound.

Another type of dressing very useful for highly exudative wounds is hydrofibres, composed of sodium carboxymethylcellulose. These are available in sheets or ribbon and are used in similar situations to the calcium alginates. The main advantage of the hydrofibre dressing is that when exposed to fluid, it becomes a solid gel. This is particularly useful when the wound bed or wound edge is friable, for example, in malignant fungating wounds.

Neither of these dressings should be used on or in dry wounds. Secondary dressing (usually some form of absorbent pad) is required.

Composite Dressings. Composite dressings are a combination of two different dressing types. These multilayered dressings are designed to provide both absorption and autolysis. Composite dressings can remain in place for up to 3 days.

Topical Treatment for Infected Wounds. Superficially infected wounds require topical dressings to deal with the bacteria within the wound and surrounding tissue. Deep tissue infection requires the addition of antibiotic therapy, which can be determined from wound swab cultures (Sibbald, Woo, & Ayello, 2006). Topical dressings include hypertonic sodium solutions, slow-release iodine, gentian violet/methylene blue, medical-grade honey, and silver antimicrobials. The manufacturer's directions need to be followed for use.

Hypertonic Dressings. Hypertonic dressings go on dry and are of benefit to draining or wet wounds. They contain a high concentration of sodium, which pulls out interstitial fluid, decreases edema to improve blood flow to the tissue surrounding the wound, and establishes a negative environment for bacterial growth. These dressings are available in ribbon, sheet, or gel form and are designed to be changed every 24–48 hours. Some patients find that the hypertonic dressings sting. Effectiveness and patient comfort should be reassessed on a daily basis and use of these dressings stopped when the wound is no longer wet.

Cadexomer Iodine. Cadexomer iodine dressings are available in sheets or a tube and provide the toxicity of iodine in a starch matrix. The iodine downloads into the wound bed in a controlled fashion, targeting only bacteria. The colour change of the dressing indicates its efficacy: it is brownish-orange when applied and gradually changes to cream-coloured as the iodine is absorbed. This process usually takes 72 hours, so the dressing should be left intact for 3 days. Changing the dressing more frequently will interfere with the effectiveness of the product. Large amounts of cadexomer iodine should be used with caution (see product monograph for limits). Cadexomer iodine should not be used in breastfeeding women or patients with thyroid conditions or shellfish allergy.

Silver Dressings. Silver dressings have antimicrobial effects similar to cadexomer iodine, against approximately 150 different pathogens, including fungal infections, methicillin-resistant *Staphylococcus aureus* (MRSA), and vancomycin-resistant enterococci (VRE). Silver dressings come in sheet, ribbon, rope, woven, and foam formats in a variety of sizes. The amount of silver in the dressing, which affects the kill rate (speed and sustainability), varies, and silver dressings require moisture to become activated—either from the wound bed exudate or with the use of a scant amount of hydrogel laid down in the base of the wound first. In addition, some silver dressings require a secondary dressing, and their efficacy ranges from 3 to 7 days, depending on the product. No sensitivity to silver dressings has been reported, but patients do occasionally complain of stinging as the silver is activated. Some forms of silver dressings may leave a dark stain on the periwound skin.

Honey (Medical-Grade Leptosperum Honey). Honey has long been known to have antimicrobial properties. As a treatment option for infected or suspected infection in wounds, it is particularly effective as it changes the pH in the wound bed, creating a negative environment for bacterial proliferation and produces a low concentration of hydrogen peroxide, which does not damage the healing tissue. As well as killing bacteria (e.g., MRSA and VRE), it has a significant impact on decreasing wound odour. The medical-grade format of Manuka honey is available in colloid, alginate, gel, and paste. It is particularly useful in pilonidal cysts as it can be applied in a warmed liquefied format directly into the wound, with a hydrofibre and simple cover dressing. The wound can be irrigated and more of the medical-grade honey introduced to the wound. Often wounds treated with honey will have an increase in drainage initially and may require more frequent dressing changes.

Gentian Violet/Methylene Blue. Gentian violet/methylene blue–impregnated dressing provides bacteriostatic coverage to help manage wound bioburden and protect against infection. It has exhibited a broad spectrum of activity against microorganisms such as MRSA, VRE, and *Candida*. The available dressings are in a foam-type format in squares and tubes, which are useful for deeper, narrow wounds. Effectiveness of the dressing is indicated by the change in colour and moisture in the dressing. The dressing will absorb drainage and become white. The first application is assessed at 24 hours; subsequent dressings can remain intact (and re-moistened if needed) for up to 72 hours. As with every dressing you are not familiar with, check the product monograph or website for complete information on use.

Negative Pressure Wound Therapy. Negative pressure wound therapy (NPWT) is another modality for dressings. The approach uses a machine that applies localized negative pressure to the surface and margins of the wound, pulling up the base of the wound and enhancing healing rates. It can be very effective, particularly for wounds in which rapid healing is viable, and will enhance patients' quality of life. Over the past few years, smaller, mobile versions of NPWT have become available for many different types of wounds. NPWT is a relatively expensive method, but in the appropriate situation, it can significantly increase wound healing, thus decreasing the requirement for health care resources, including hospitalization. Usually these dressings are changed three times a week.

NPWT is also used to enhance the viability of split-thickness skin grafts. Placing it over the graft intraoperatively decreases the ability of the graft to shift and evacuates fluids that build up under the graft (Frantz, Broussard, Mendez-Eastman, et al., 2016).

Changing Dressings. When changing a dressing, it is important to keep in mind that the characteristics of the wound may have changed since the previous dressing change. The nurse can still have similar dressings as previously used within close proximity—in hospital settings, where any unused dressing in a patient room may be discarded, it is best to leave the dressings nearby, but outside the patient's room. As well, nurses should be familiar with the location and type of underlying drains or tubing and any specific supplies that may be required. Poor preparation can result in a break in aseptic technique (see Chapter 33), accidental dislodging of a drain, unnecessary discomfort to the patient, or time wasted in searching for supplies.

As a nurse, your judgement in modifying a dressing change procedure is important during wound care. If the character of a wound changes, notify the wound care specialist or physician. Ensure open and clear communication with the physician or wound specialist or nurse who documents your interventions, even though you do not require a medical order to change a dressing. However, if a specific order is written, it is the nurse's responsibility to assess the current status of the wound in relation to the order. Has the wound changed? Would a different dressing be more effective? Nurses need to communicate this to the physician or wound specialist on the team.

An order to "reinforce dressing prn" (add dressings without removing the original one) is common immediately after surgery, when the surgeon does not want accidental disruption of the suture line or bleeding. The medical or operating room record usually indicates whether drains are present and from what body cavity they drain. After the first dressing change, nurses need to document in the patient care plan the location of drains, type (and number) of dressing materials, and other pertinent information related to care of the wound.

Clean or Sterile Technique. The body of literature about sterile versus clean dressing techniques is growing. The RNAO guidelines (2011, 2016) recommend sterile dressings, good handwashing, and clean gloves changed between each of the patient's wounds or when soiled. For surgical wounds, preliminary research indicates no difference in the healing rate of wounds when a clean rather than a sterile dressing change technique is used. Although aseptic or sterile technique is often used for surgical wound care, the most important aspects of this approach are to ensure as clean a field as possible with the use of sterile dressing packs, sterile scissors and forceps, and sterile dressings and gloves.

Preparing for Dressing Change (in Any Care Setting). To prepare a patient for a dressing change, nurses must do the following:

- Administer required analgesics so that peak effects occur during the dressing change
- Describe steps of the procedure to lessen patient anxiety
- Gather all supplies required for the dressing change
- Recognize normal signs of healing
- Answer questions about the procedure or the wound

Nurses must always consider teaching the patient and family how to change the dressing, particularly in the home care setting. The nurse needs to demonstrate dressing changes to the patient and family and then provide an opportunity for them to practise changing a dressing when the nurse is present. In acute care, by the time the patient is ready to be discharged, wound healing has usually progressed past the point when complications such as dehiscence or evisceration might occur.

Packing a Wound. When packing a wound, the nurse must first assess the size, depth, and shape of the wound, then assess for tunneling and undermining of the wound. These wound characteristics will help determine the size and type of dressing material needed to pack the wound. Many dressing materials, such as alginates, are used to pack wounds. If nonwoven gauze is the appropriate dressing material, saturate the gauze with the ordered solution, wring it out, unfold it, and lightly pack it into the wound. The entire wound surface needs to be in contact with part of the moist gauze dressing (see Skill 46-3). As stated in the RNAO guidelines (2011, 2016), "keeping the wound moist and the surrounding intact skin dry" (p. 43) will prevent maceration and help maintain a moist wound environment, and when using a dressing "*loosely* pack any sinus tract or cavity to eliminate dead space" (p. 77).

The wound should not be packed too tightly; use a light touch. Over-packing the wound causes pressure on the tissue in the wound bed, decreasing blood flow to the area and preventing healing and wound closure. The amount of packing placed in the wound should be documented to ensure there is no chance for any packing material to be left in the wound when the dressing is changed.

Securing Dressings. Tape, ties, a secondary dressing, or gauze net is used to secure a dressing over a wound site. The choice of anchoring depends on the wound size and location, the presence of drainage, frequency of dressing changes, and patient's level of activity. Of equal importance is the potential for skin stripping as tape is applied and removed frequently from the same area of skin. Patients with chronic wounds tend to have skin that is fragile and prone to breakdown. Thus, it is important to pay attention to the method used in affixing dressings.

If tape must be used, ensure that the periwound skin is not excoriated or at risk of breakdown, and that the patient does not have an allergy or sensitivity to tape. Nonallergenic paper and silicone tapes are available to minimize skin reactions. Common adhesive tape adheres strongly to the skin's surface, whereas elastic adhesive tape compresses closely around pressure bandages and permits more movement of a body part. Skin sensitive to adhesive tape becomes severely inflamed and denuded and, in some cases, even sloughs when the tape is removed. A barrier wipe is used to protect the periwound skin and provide additional "tack" to help tape adhere but not damage the underlying skin. The skin under the tape should be assessed at each dressing change. If the skin does not remain intact or is irritated, an alternative solution (e.g., paper or silicone tapes or Montgomery ties) is used.

Tape is available in various widths. Choose the size that sufficiently secures the dressing. Strips of 7.6-cm adhesive tape will likely ensure that a large dressing does not continually slip off. Other options, such as gauze wrap or burn-net dressings, may also be used.

When applying tape, ensure that the skin is dry so that the tape will adhere to several centimetres of skin on both sides of the dressing in a "window-pane" fashion. If needed, place tape across the middle of the dressing. When securing the dressing, press the tape gently, exerting pressure away from the wound. With tension occurring in both directions away from the wound, skin distortion and irritation is minimized. Never apply tape over irritated or broken skin. Barrier film or spray can assist with adherence of the tape and protect the periwound skin from breakdown due to tape adhesives.

To remove tape safely, loosen the tape ends and gently pull the outer end parallel with the skin surface toward the wound. Apply light traction to the skin away from the wound as the tape is loosened and removed. The traction minimizes pulling on the skin. If tape covers an area of hair growth, the patient experiences less discomfort if the tape is pulled in the direction of hair growth. Adhesive remover can also be used to release the tape from the skin, but is not recommended as it can dry out the skin.

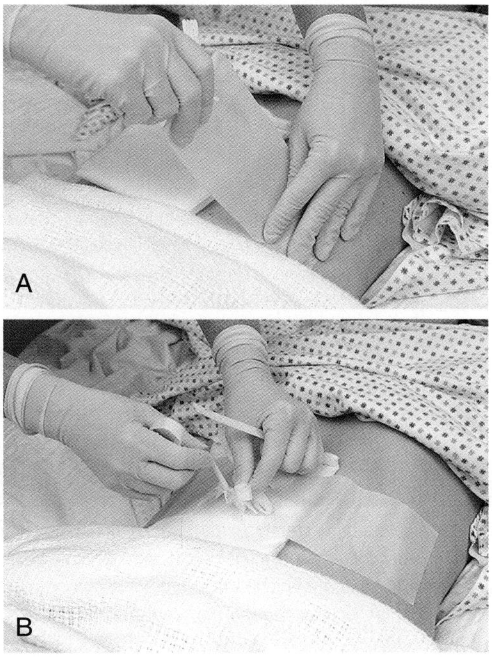

FIGURE 46-23 Montgomery ties. **A,** Each tie is placed at side of dressing. **B,** Securing ties encloses dressing.

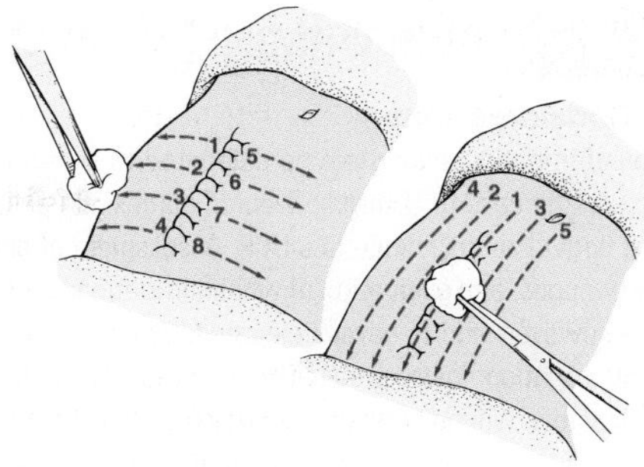

FIGURE 46-24 Methods for cleaning a wound site.

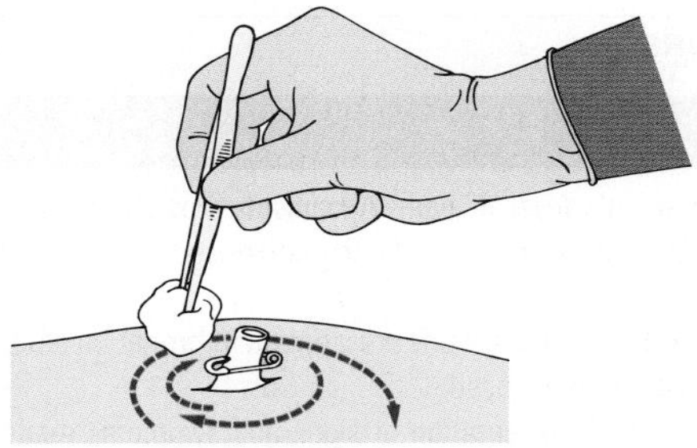

FIGURE 46-25 Cleaning a drain site.

When frequent dressing changes are required, particularly for large abdominal or chest wounds, avoid repeated removal of tape from sensitive skin by using dressings secured with pairs of reusable Montgomery ties (Figure 46-23). Each section consists of a long strip; half contains an adhesive backing to apply to the skin, and the other half folds back and contains a cloth tie to fasten across a dressing and untie at dressing changes.

Comfort Measures. A wound is often painful, depending on the extent of tissue injury and the patient's other medical health issues. Several techniques can be used to minimize discomfort during wound care. Administration of analgesic medications 30 to 45 minutes before dressing changes (depending on a drug's time of peak action) reduces discomfort. Careful removal of tape, gentle cleaning of wound edges, and careful manipulation of dressings and drains minimize stress on sensitive tissues. Often, propping and positioning the patient with pillows or foam wedges can decrease positioning pain or discomfort, particularly in complex, time-consuming dressing changes.

Surgical or Traumatic Wound Considerations

Basic Skin Cleaning for Surgical or Traumatic Wounds. Surgical or traumatic wounds are cleaned by applying noncytotoxic solutions with sterile gauze or by irrigating. The following three principles are important when cleaning an incision or the area surrounding a drain:

1. Clean in a direction from the least contaminated area, such as from the wound or incision to the surrounding skin (Figure 46-24) or from an isolated drain site to the surrounding skin (Figure 46-25).
2. Use gentle friction when applying solutions locally to the skin.
3. When irrigating, allow the solution to flow from the least to most contaminated area (Skill 46-4).

Never use the same piece of gauze to clean across an incision or wound twice. Use gauze to clean the periwound skin, not the open wound. Open wound beds are damaged by the abrasive contact of gauze.

Cleaning Skin and Drain Sites. In cases in which the open drain leaks onto surrounding skin, ensure that the drainage is removed from the skin to avoid maceration or excoriation of the tissue from possibly caustic drainage. The drain itself may also need to be cleaned on a regular basis to avoid a buildup of potentially contaminated material.

Drain sites are a source of contamination because moist drainage harbours microorganisms. If a wound has a dry incisional area and a moist drain site, use two separate swabs or gauze pads, one to clean from the top of the incision toward the drain and one to clean from the bottom of the incision toward the drain. To clean the area of an isolated drain site, clean around the drain, moving in circular rotations outward from a point closest to the drain. In this situation, the skin near the site is more contaminated than the site itself. To clean circular wounds, use the same technique as in cleaning around a drain.

Irrigation. Irrigation is a special way of cleaning wounds. An irrigating syringe is used to flush the area with a constant low-pressure flow of noncytotoxic solution (usually saline). The gentle washing action of the irrigation cleans a wound of exudate and debris. Irrigations are particularly useful for open, deep wounds. A common refrain regarding irrigation is *Irrigate, irrigate, irrigate . . . and then irrigate some more.* However, it is important to check that the irrigant is not left pooled in the wound bed (usually by repositioning the patient to allow gravity to assist in drainage).

Wound Irrigation. Irrigation of an open wound requires sterile technique. A 35-mL syringe with a 19-gauge angiocatheter (Bryant & Nix, 2016) or a single-use bottle of normal saline is used to deliver the solution, so as not to damage healing wound tissue. A wound opening should never be occluded with a syringe, because this results in the introduction of irrigating fluid into a closed space. In this case, the pressure of the fluid causes tissue damage and discomfort. Always irrigate a wound with the syringe tip over but not in the drainage site.

SKILL 46-4 PERFORMING WOUND IRRIGATION

Delegation Considerations

The skill of wound irrigation should not be delegated to unregulated care providers (UCPs). In the case of a chronic wound, nurses can delegate cleaning of the wound with clean technique to a UCP. Assessment of any wound, care of acute new wounds, and evaluation of wound irrigation is the responsibility of the nurse, however, and is never delegated. When a wound is stable or requires clean irrigation, instruct the UCP to do the following:

- Report any change in wound appearance or increased wound drainage to the nurse.
- Use proper clean technique to avoid cross-contamination from irrigation syringes and equipment.

Equipment

- Irrigant or cleaning solution (volume 1.2 to 2 times the estimated wound volume)
- Irrigation delivery system, depending on amount of pressure desired:
  - Sterile 35-mL irrigation syringe with sterile soft angiocatheter or 19-gauge needle (WOCN, 2010) or whirlpool or hand-held shower, if appropriate.
- Disposable gloves and sterile gloves (check agency policy)
- Waterproof underpad, if needed
- Dressing supplies
- Disposable waterproof bag
- Gown, if risk of spray
- Goggles, mask, or both if risk of spray

PROCEDURE

STEPS	RATIONALE
1. Assess patient's level of pain. Administer prescribed analgesic 30 to 45 minutes before starting wound irrigation procedure.	• Discomfort may be related directly to the wound or indirectly to muscle tension or immobility. Increased comfort permits patient to move more easily and be positioned to facilitate wound irrigation.
2. Review medical record for any prescription for irrigation of open wound and type of solution to be used.	• Open wound irrigation requires medical order, including type of solution to use.
3. Assess recent documentation of signs and symptoms related to patient's open wound.	• Data are used as baseline to indicate change in condition of wound (Orsted, et al., 2017).
A. Condition of skin and wound	
B. Elevation of body temperature	• Elevated temperature may indicate response to infection.
C. Drainage from wound (amount, colour)	• Amount will decrease as healing takes place.
D. Odour	• Strong odour may indicate infection.
E. Consistency of drainage	• Leukocytes produce thick drainage.
4. Explain procedure of wound irrigation and cleaning.	• Information will reduce patient's anxiety.
5. Perform hand hygiene.	• Transmission of microorganisms is reduced.
6. Position patient comfortably to permit gravitational flow of irrigating solution through wound and into collection receptacle. Position patient so that wound is vertical to collection basin.	• Directing solution from top to bottom of wound and from clean to contaminated area prevents further infection. Positioning patient during planning stage provides bed surfaces for later preparation of equipment.
7. Warm irrigation solution to approximate body temperature.	• Warmed solution increases comfort and reduces vascular constriction response in tissues.
8. Form cuff on waterproof bag and place it near bed.	• Cuffing helps to maintain large opening, thereby permitting placement of contaminated dressing without touching refuse bag itself.
9. Close room door or bed curtains.	• Privacy is maintained.
10. Apply gown, goggles, or mask, if needed.	• Gown, goggles, and mask protect from splashes or sprays of blood and body fluids.
11. Put on disposable gloves, remove soiled dressing, and discard in waterproof bag. Discard gloves.	• Transmission of microorganisms is reduced.
12. Prepare equipment; open sterile supplies.	
13. Put on sterile gloves (check agency policy).	
14. Irrigate wound with wide opening:	
A. Fill 35-mL syringe with irrigation solution.	• Flushing wound helps remove debris and facilitates healing by secondary intention.
B. Attach 19-gauge needle or angiocatheter.	• Angiocatheter provides ideal pressure for cleaning and removal of debris.
C. Hold syringe tip 2.5 cm above upper end of wound and over area being cleaned.	• Holding the tip above the wound prevents syringe contamination. Careful placement of the syringe prevents unsafe pressure of the flowing solution.
D. Using continuous pressure, flush wound; repeat Steps 14A, 14B, and 14C until solution draining into basin is clear.	• Clear solution indicates that all debris has been removed.
15. Irrigate deep wound with very small opening:	
A. Attach soft angiocatheter to filled irrigating syringe.	• Catheter permits direct flow of irrigant into wound. Expect wound to take longer to empty when opening is small.
B. Lubricate tip of catheter with irrigating solution; then gently insert tip of catheter and pull out about 1 cm.	• Tip is not in fragile inner wall of wound.
C. Using slow, continuous pressure, flush wound.	

CRITICAL DECISION POINT: ***Caution:*** *Splashing may occur during this step.*

STEPS	RATIONALE
D. Pinch off catheter just below syringe while keeping catheter in place.	• Sterile solution will not be contaminated.
E. Remove and refill syringe. Reconnect to catheter and repeat until solution draining into basin is clear.	
16. Clean wound with hand-held shower:	• Method is useful for patients able to shower with assistance or independently. Shower may be accomplished at home. A shower table is helpful for bed-bound or acutely ill patients.
A. With patient seated comfortably in shower chair, adjust spray to gentle flow; water temperature should be warm.	
B. Cover showerhead with clean washcloth, if needed.	
C. Shower for 5 to 10 minutes with showerhead 30 cm from wound.	

CRITICAL DECISION POINT: *Consider culturing a wound if it has a foul and purulent odour, if inflammation surrounds the wound, if a nondraining wound begins to drain, or if the patient is febrile.*

STEPS	RATIONALE
17. Obtain cultures, if needed, after cleaning with nonbacteriostatic saline.	• Routine culturing of open wounds is not recommended (Orsted et al., 2017; RNAO, 2016). If required, quantitative bacterial cultures (tissue biopsy or wound fluid by needle aspiration) should be performed rather than swab cultures, which often detect only surface bacterial contaminants.
18. Dry wound edges with gauze; dry patient, if shower or whirlpool is used.	• Maceration of surrounding tissue is prevented if excess moisture is dried.
19. Apply appropriate dressing (see Skill 46-3 and Box 46-13).	• Protective barrier and healing environment for wound are maintained.
20. Remove gloves and, if worn, mask, goggles, and gown.	• Transfer of microorganisms is prevented.
21. Dispose of equipment and soiled supplies. Perform hand hygiene.	• Transmission of microorganisms is reduced.
22. Assist patient to comfortable position.	
23. Assess type of tissue in the wound bed.	• Wound healing progress is identified and type of wound cleaning needed is determined.
24. Inspect dressing periodically.	• Patient's response to wound irrigation and need to modify plan of care are determined.
25. Evaluate skin integrity.	• Whether extension of wound has occurred is determined.
26. Observe patient for signs of discomfort.	• Patient's pain should not increase as a result of wound irrigation.
27. Observe for presence of retained irrigant.	• Retained irrigant is a medium for bacterial growth, and subsequent infection may occur.

UNEXPECTED OUTCOMES	RELATED INTERVENTIONS
Wound does not appear to heal	• Obtain wound culture. • Notify physician, who may change frequency of dressing, irrigation, or both.
Wound drainage increases	• Apply more absorbent gauze. • Increase the frequency of irrigation.

RECORDING AND REPORTING

- Record wound irrigation and patient response on progress notes.
- Immediately report to attending physician any evidence of fresh bleeding, sharp increase in pain, retention of irrigant, or signs of shock.
- At change of shift, report expected and unexpected outcomes that have occurred.

HOME CARE CONSIDERATIONS

- Determine if tap water is potable (e.g., treated municipal water supply) and home is adequately clean. If patient or caregiver is to irrigate wound, change dressing, or both, explain method, demonstrate it, and have them explain and show you.
- You can teach the patient or caregiver how to make normal saline, if conditions warrant and cost is an issue. Determine safety (of handling boiling water). Normal saline can be made by using 10 mL of salt in 1 L of boiling water and should be discarded after 24–48 hours (Barr, 1995).

Fluid needs to flow directly into the wound and not over a contaminated area before entering the wound. Skill 46-4 lists steps for wound irrigation. Avoid irrigating wounds when the base cannot be determined (e.g., tunnelling sinus) or into a body cavity.

Sutures. A surgeon closes a wound by bringing the wound edges as close together as possible to reduce scar formation. Proper wound closure involves control of bleeding and minimal trauma and tension to tissues.

Sutures are threads or metal used to sew body tissues together. The patient's history of wound healing, the site of surgery, the tissues involved, and the purpose of the sutures determine choice of suture material. For example, if the patient has had repeated surgery for an abdominal hernia, wire sutures may be used to provide greater strength for wound closure. In contrast, a small laceration of the face calls for use of very fine polyester sutures to minimize scar formation.

Sutures are available in a variety of materials, including silk, steel, cotton, linen, wire, nylon, and polyester. Steel staples are a common type of outer skin closure that cause less trauma to tissues than do sutures, while providing extra strength. Tape closures such as Steri-Strips applied over the wound to keep the edges closed are also used, although adhesive glue is now commonly used as well.

Sutures are placed within tissue layers in deep wounds as well as superficially, as the final means for wound closure. Deep sutures are usually an absorbable material that will disappear over time; however, sutures are foreign bodies and, thus, are capable of causing local inflammation. The surgeon tries to minimize tissue injury by using the finest suture possible and the smallest number necessary.

Suture Removal. Policies vary within institutions as to who is able to remove sutures. If it is appropriate for the nurse to remove them, an order is required. Special scissors with curved cutting tips or special staple removers slide under the skin closures for suture removal (Figure 46-26). If the suture line appears to be healing better in certain locations than in others, the surgeon may choose to have only some sutures removed (e.g., every other one).

To remove staples, simply insert the tips of the staple remover under each wire staple. While slowly closing the ends of the staple remover together, squeeze the centre of the staple with the tips, freeing the staple from the skin (see Figure 46-26).

To remove sutures, first check the type of suturing used (Figure 46-27). With intermittent suturing, the surgeon ties each individual suture made in the skin. Continuous suturing, as the name implies, is a series of sutures with only two knots, one at the beginning and one at the end of the suture line. Retention sutures are placed more deeply than skin sutures, and nurses may or may not remove them, depending on agency policy.

The manner in which the suture crosses and penetrates the skin determines the method for removal. Never pull the visible portion of a suture through underlying tissue. Sutures on the skin's surface harbour microorganisms and debris, but the portion of the suture beneath the skin is sterile. Pulling the contaminated portion of the suture through tissues may lead to infection. Suture materials should be clipped as close to the skin edge on one side as possible and the suture pulled through from the other side (Figure 46-28).

Drainage Evacuation. When drainage interferes with healing, drainage evacuation is achieved by using either a drain alone or a drainage tube with continuous suction. Special skin barriers need to be applied, including hydrocolloid dressings, similar to those used with ostomies (see Chapter 44), around drain sites. The skin barriers are soft material applied to the skin with adhesive. Drainage flows on the barrier but not directly on the skin.

Drainage evacuators (Figure 46-29) are convenient, portable units that connect to tubular drains lying within a wound bed and exert a safe, constant, low-pressure vacuum to remove and collect drainage. To set the suction on a drainage evacuator with the drainage port open, the lever on the diaphragm is raised. Push straight down on the lever to lower the diaphragm. Closure of the port prevents escape of air and creates vacuum pressure. The nurse needs to ensure that suction is exerted and connection points between the evacuator and tubing are intact. After the evacuator collects drainage, its volume and character should be assessed every shift and as needed. When the evacuator fills, the nurse measures output by emptying the contents into a graduated cylinder and immediately resets the evacuator to apply suction.

Bandages and Binders. A simple gauze dressing is often not enough to immobilize or provide support to a wound. Binders and

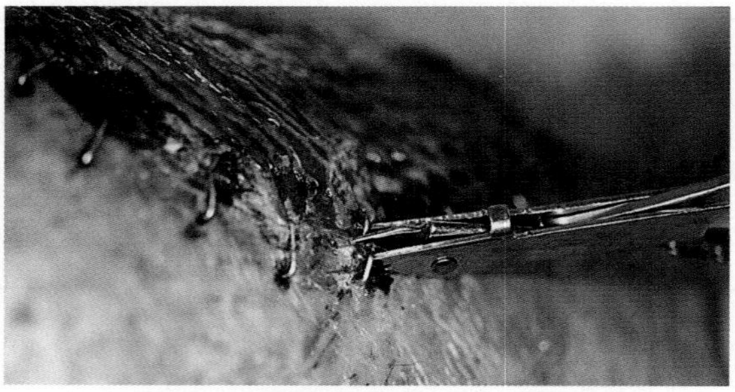

FIGURE 46-26 Staple remover.

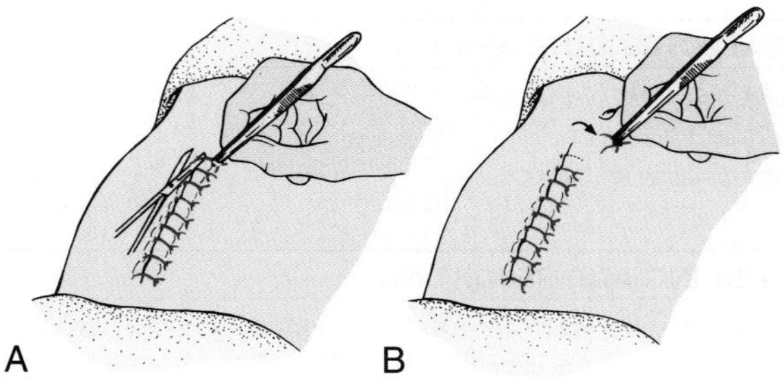

FIGURE 46-28 Removal of intermittent suture. **A,** Cut the suture as close to the skin as possible, away from the knot. **B,** Remove the suture and never pull the contaminated stitch through the tissues.

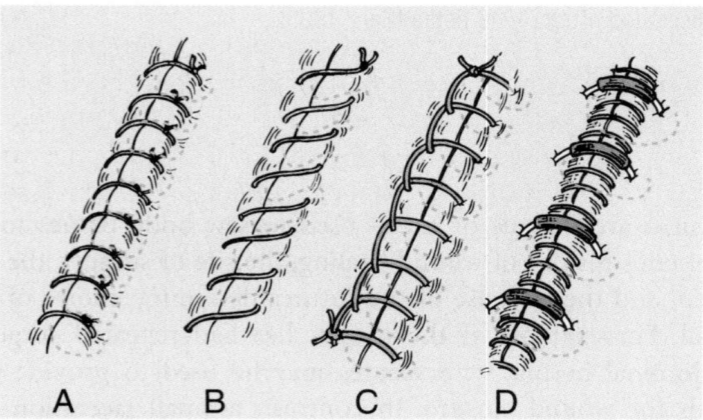

FIGURE 46-27 Examples of suturing methods. **A,** Intermittent. **B,** Continuous. **C,** Blanket continuous. **D,** Retention.

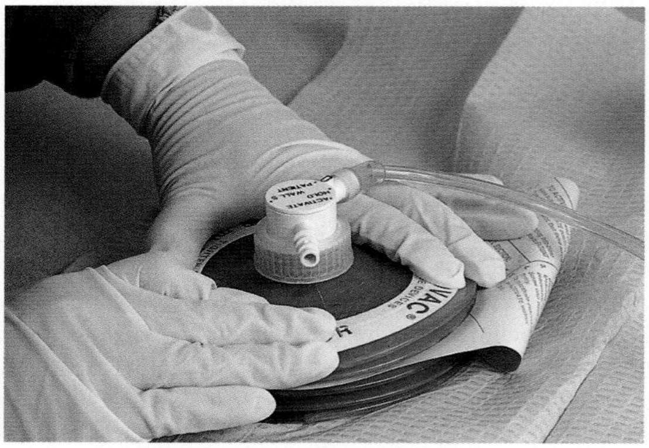

FIGURE 46-29 Drainage evacuator.

bandages applied over or around dressings provide extra protection and therapeutic benefits by doing the following:

- Creating pressure over a body part (e.g., an elastic pressure bandage applied over an arterial puncture site)
- Immobilizing a body part (e.g., an elastic bandage applied around a sprained ankle)
- Supporting a wound (e.g., an abdominal binder applied over a large abdominal incision and dressing)
- Reducing or preventing edema (e.g., a well-supporting bra to minimize breast discomfort after delivery of a baby)
- Securing a splint (e.g., a bandage applied around hand splints for correction of deformities)
- Securing dressings (e.g., elastic webbing applied around leg dressings after a vein stripping)

Bandages are available in rolls of various widths and materials, including gauze, elasticized knit, elastic webbing, flannel, and muslin. Gauze bandages are lightweight and inexpensive, conform easily to the contours of the body, and permit air circulation to prevent skin maceration. Elastic bandages conform well to body parts but also exert pressure.

Principles for Applying Bandages and Binders. Correctly applied bandages and binders do not cause injury to underlying and nearby body parts or create discomfort for the patient. For example, a chest binder should not be so tight as to restrict chest wall expansion. Before applying a bandage or binder, the following are nursing responsibilities:

- Inspecting the skin for abrasions, edema, discoloration, or exposed wound edges
- Covering exposed wounds or open abrasions with a sterile dressing
- Assessing the condition of underlying dressings and changing them, if soiled
- Assessing the skin of underlying areas that will be distal to the bandage for signs of circulatory impairment (coolness, pallor or cyanosis, diminished or absent pulses, swelling, numbness, and tingling) to provide a means for comparing changes in circulation after bandage application

After applying a bandage, the nurse needs to assess, document, and immediately report changes in circulation, skin integrity, comfort level, and body function (e.g., ventilation, movement). When applying the bandage, the nurse should readjust it, as necessary. The nurse should also explain to the patient that the binder may feel relatively firm or tight. The nurse needs to carefully assess a bandage to be sure that it is properly applied (according to the written order) and is providing therapeutic benefit. Any soiled bandages need to be replaced.

Binder application. Binders are especially designed for the body part to be supported. Most binders are made of elastic or cotton. The most common types of binders are the abdominal binder and breast binder (Skill 46-5). Well-fitting bras are more common now than breast binders, although both methods provide support after breast surgery or exert pressure to reduce lactation in a woman after childbirth.

Abdominal binders. An abdominal binder supports large abdominal incisions that are vulnerable to tension or stress as the patient moves or coughs. An abdominal binder is secured with safety pins, Velcro strips, or metal stays.

Bandage application. Rolls of bandage secure or support dressings over irregularly shaped body parts. Each roll has a free outer end and a terminal end at the centre of the roll. The rolled portion of the bandage is its body, and its outer surface is placed against the patient's skin or dressing. Skill 46-6 describes the steps for applying an elastic bandage.

The Whole Person, the Whole Team

Skin management and wound care require the involvement of the health care team because the factors that create skin breakdown, such as pressure and nutrition, are assessed and treated by experts within the health care team: physiotherapist, occupational therapist, dietitian, nurse, physician, social worker, and pharmacist. In addition, the wound belongs to the patient and you need to recognize the impact of the individual on both the development and healing potential of a wound.

Case Study. Mr. John Purata is an 84-year-old man who has returned to his home in a long-term care facility where you are looking after the ulcer on his sacrum, developed during his stay in acute care after hip replacement surgery. Mr. Purata has been too tired to get up for meals, and you have noticed that his nutritional status is declining. Although he is on a pressure-relief surface, Mr. Purata tends to lie on his back. You have mentioned to him the importance of repositioning to assist in healing the wound, but he merely closes his eyes and tells you he is fine the way he is. When you and the other staff in the long-term care facility try to get him up to walk, Mr. Purata is hesitant and requires a great deal of coaching and encouragement to walk even a few steps. He then says he is too tired to go further and asks to go back to bed. He is frequently lying in bed, with eyes closed and the lights dim. His daughter and son are concerned that he seems to have lost his "get up and go" attitude. The wound is not improving, and you are concerned.

- What are the key issues that need to be addressed?
- What members of the health care team need to be involved?
- What would be realistic goals for Mr. Purata?
- How would you develop a plan of care for this patient?

◆ Evaluation

Nursing interventions for reducing and treating pressure injuries are evaluated by determining the patient's response to nursing therapies and whether the patient achieved each goal (Figure 46-30). To evaluate outcomes and responses to care, nurses measure the effectiveness of interventions. The optimal outcomes are to prevent injury to the skin and tissues, reduce injury to the skin and underlying tissues, and restore skin integrity.

Because each patient has different risk factors for impaired skin integrity, nurses need to individualize nursing interventions. Patients with minimal mobility impairments or relatively stable health status need only a few measures.

Patients with impaired skin integrity need assessment on an ongoing basis for factors that contribute to skin breakdown. This includes a comprehensive skin assessment and a wound assessment using a validated risk assessment tool. Assessment provides the foundation for the plan of care and is critical for monitoring the effectiveness of the plan (Nix, 2016).

Nurses need to include the patient and the caregiver in the assessment process. It is important to determine what they know about impaired skin integrity and develop a plan of care to provide education. Chronic wounds such as pressure injuries take time to heal, and it is likely that the patient will be in the home or long-term care setting with the pressure injury.

If the identified outcomes are not met for a patient with impaired skin integrity, questions to ask include the following:

- Was the etiology of the skin impairment addressed? Were pressure, friction, shear, and moisture components identified; did the plan of care decrease the contribution of each of these components?
- Was wound healing supported by providing the wound base with a moist protected environment?

SKILL 46-5 APPLYING AN ABDOMINAL OR BREAST BINDER

Delegation Considerations

The skills of applying a binder (abdominal or breast) can be delegated to unregulated care providers (UCPs). The nurse is responsible for wound assessment and the evaluation of wound care interventions. You need to complete an assessment of the patient's ability to breathe deeply, cough effectively, and move independently; assess skin for irritation or abrasion; assess the incision or wound and dressing; and assess the patient's comfort level before a binder or sling is applied for the first time. When delegating the skill of applying a binder, instruct the UCP to do the following:

- Immediately report any change in the patient's respiratory status.
- Report an increase in wound drainage.
- Report changes in skin integrity under or adjacent to the binder.
- Remove the binder at prescribed intervals.

Equipment

- Disposable gloves, if wound drainage is present
- Abdominal binder:
  - Correct size cloth or elastic straight binder
  - Safety pins (6 to 8), unless Velcro closure or metal fasteners are attached
- Breast binder:
  - Correct size binder
  - Safety pins (approximately 12), unless Velcro closure is attached

PROCEDURE

STEPS	RATIONALE
1. Observe patient with need for support of chest or abdomen. Observe ability to breathe deeply and cough effectively.	• Baseline assessment determines patient's ability to breathe and cough. Impaired ventilation of lungs can lead to alveolar atelectasis and inadequate arterial oxygenation.
2. Review medical record, if medical prescription for particular binder is required, and reasons for application.	• Application of supportive binders may be used on nursing judgement. In some situations, physician input is required.
3. Inspect skin for actual or potential alterations in integrity. Observe for irritation, abrasion, skin surfaces that rub against each other, or allergic response to adhesive tape used to secure dressing.	• Actual impairments in skin integrity can be worsened with application of a binder. Binder can cause pressure and excoriation.
4. Inspect any surgical dressing.	• Dressing replacement or reinforcement precedes application of any binder.
CRITICAL DECISION POINT: *Dressing should be clean and dry, and incision or wound should be entirely covered by dressing.*	
5. Assess patient's comfort level, using analogue scale of 0 to 10 (see Chapter 31), noting any objective signs and symptoms of pain.	• Data will determine effectiveness of binder placement.
CRITICAL DECISION POINT: *Expect patient in moderate to severe pain to have diaphoresis, tachycardia, and elevated blood pressure.*	
6. Gather necessary data regarding size of patient and appropriate binder.	• Proper fit of binder will be ensured.
7. Explain procedure to patient.	• Patient will understand and be more cooperative.
8. Teach skill to patient or significant other.	• Anxiety is reduced and continuity of care after discharge is ensured.
9. Perform hand hygiene and apply gloves (if likely to contact wound drainage).	• Transmission of microorganisms is reduced.
10. Close curtains or room door.	• Patient's comfort and dignity are maintained.
11. Apply binder.	
A. Abdominal binder:	
(1) Position patient in supine position with head slightly elevated and knees slightly flexed.	• Muscular tension on abdominal organs is minimized.
(2) Fanfold far side of binder toward midline of binder.	• Patient's time in uncomfortable position is reduced.
(3) Instruct and help patient to roll away from you toward raised side rail while firmly supporting abdominal incision and dressing with hands.	• Pain and discomfort are reduced.
(4) Place fanfolded ends of binder under patient.	• Placement and centring of binder are accomplished with minimal discomfort.
(5) Instruct or assist patient to roll over folded ends.	
(6) Unfold and stretch ends out smoothly on far side of bed.	• Skin integrity and comfort are maintained.
(7) Instruct patient to roll back into supine position.	• Chest expansion and adequate wound support are facilitated when binder is closed.
(8) Adjust binder so that supine patient is centred over binder using symphysis pubis and costal margins as lower and upper landmarks.	• Support from binder is centred over abdominal structures, which reduces incidence of decreased lung expansion.

STEPS	RATIONALE
CRITICAL DECISION POINT: *Cover any exposed areas of an incision or wound with sterile dressing.*	
(9) Close binder. Pull one end of binder over centre of patient's abdomen. While maintaining tension on that end of binder, pull opposite end of binder over centre and secure with Velcro closure tabs, metal fasteners, or horizontally placed safety pins.	• Continuous wound support and comfort are provided.
B. Breast binder:	
(1) Assist patient in placing arms through binder's armholes.	• Binder placement process is made easier for patient.
(2) Assist patient to supine position in bed.	• Supine positioning facilitates normal anatomical position of breasts; facilitates healing and comfort.
(3) Pad area under breasts, if necessary.	• Skin contact with undersurface is prevented.
(4) Using Velcro closure tabs or horizontally placed safety pins, secure binder at nipple level first. Continue closure process above and then below nipple line until entire binder is closed.	• Horizontal placement of pins may reduce risk of uneven pressure or localized irritation.
(5) Make appropriate adjustments, including individualizing fit of shoulder straps and pinning waistline darts to reduce binder size.	• Support to patient's breasts is maintained.
(6) Instruct and observe skill development in self-care related to reapplying breast binder.	• Self-care is an integral aspect of discharge planning. Skin integrity and comfort level goals are ensured.
12. Remove gloves and perform hand hygiene.	• Cross-infections are prevented.
13. Assess patient's comfort level, using analogue scale of 0 to 10, noting any objective signs and symptoms.	• Effectiveness of binder placement is determined. Binders should not increase discomfort.
14. Adjust binder, as necessary.	• Comfort and chest expansion are promoted.
15. Observe site for skin integrity, circulation, and characteristics of the wound. (Periodically remove binder and surgical dressing to assess wound characteristics.)	• Binder should not result in complication to skin, wound, or underlying organs.
16. Assess patient's ability to breathe properly.	• Any impaired ventilation and potential pulmonary complications are identified.
17. Identify patient's need for assistance with activities such as combing hair.	• Mobility of upper extremities may be limited, depending on severity and location of incision.

UNEXPECTED OUTCOMES	RELATED INTERVENTIONS
Patient's pain increases	• Remove binder and assess wound. • Reapply binder using less pressure.
Patient develops impaired skin integrity under the binder	• Remove binder. • Initiate skin care measures to heal affected site.

RECORDING AND REPORTING

- Report any skin irritation at between-shift report.
- Record application of binder, condition of skin, circulation, integrity of dressing, and patient's comfort level.
- Report ineffective lung expansion to physician immediately.

HOME CARE CONSIDERATIONS

- Abdominal and breast binders can be washed and air-dried.
- Instruct caregiver to avoid excessive pressure with binder application.

SKILL 46-6 APPLYING AN ELASTIC BANDAGE

Delegation Considerations

The application of an elastic bandage can be delegated to unregulated care providers (UCPs). The nurse is responsible for wound assessment and the evaluation of the wound. In addition, the nurse should assess for adequate circulation to the extremity distal to the elastic bandage (e.g., pulse, skin temperature, capillary refill). When delegating this skill to a UCP, instruct about any restrictions that the patient might have (e.g., unable to independently raise leg or independently roll over). Also instruct the UCP to report the following:

- Any change in the skin colour of the patient's injured extremity
- Any increases in the patient's pain

Equipment

- Correct width and number of bandages
- Safety pins, clips, or adhesive tape
- Disposable gloves, if wound drainage is present

PROCEDURE

STEPS	RATIONALE
1. Perform hand hygiene and apply gloves, if needed. Inspect skin for alterations in integrity as indicated by abrasions, discoloration, chafing, or edema. (Look carefully at bony prominences.)	• Altered skin integrity contraindicates the use of elastic bandages.
2. Inspect surgical dressing. Remove gloves and perform hand hygiene.	• Surgical dressing replacement or reinforcement precedes application.
3. Observe adequacy of circulation (distal to bandage) by noting surface temperature, skin colour, and sensation of body parts to be wrapped.	• Comparison of area before and after application of bandage is necessary to ensure continued adequate circulation. Impairment of circulation may result in coolness to touch when compared with opposite side of body, cyanosis or pallor of skin, diminished or absent pulses, edema or localized pooling, and numbness or tingling of part.
4. Review medical record for specific orders related to application of elastic bandage. Note area to be covered, type of bandage required, frequency of change, and previous response to treatment.	• Specific prescription may direct procedure, including factors such as extent of application (e.g., toe to knee, toe to groin) and duration of treatment.
5. Identify patient's and primary caregiver's present knowledge level of skill, if bandaging will be continued at home.	• Planning and teaching should be individualized.
6. Explain procedure to patient.	• Increased knowledge promotes cooperation and reduces anxiety.
7. Teach skill to patient or primary caregiver.	• Anxiety is reduced and continuity of care after discharge is ensured.
8. Perform hand hygiene and apply gloves if drainage is present.	• Transmission of microorganisms is reduced.
9. Close room door or curtains.	• Patient's comfort and dignity are maintained.
10. Help patient to assume comfortable, anatomically correct position.	• Alignment is maintained, and musculoskeletal deformity is prevented.

CRITICAL DECISION POINT: *Bandages applied to lower extremities are applied before patient sits or stands. Elevation of dependent extremities for 20 minutes before bandage application will enhance venous return.*

STEPS	RATIONALE
11. Hold roll of elastic bandage in dominant hand and use other hand to lightly hold beginning of bandage at distal body part. Continue transferring roll to dominant hand as bandage is wrapped.	• Appropriate and consistent bandage tension is maintained.

CRITICAL DECISION POINT: *Toes or fingertips should be visible for follow-up circulatory assessment.*

STEPS	RATIONALE
12. Apply bandage from distal point toward proximal boundary using variety of turns to cover various shapes of body parts.	• Bandage is applied in a manner that conforms evenly to body part and promotes venous return.
13. Unroll and very slightly stretch bandage.	• Uniform bandage tension is maintained.
14. Overlap turns by one-half to two-thirds width of bandage roll.	• Uneven bandage tension and circulatory impairment are prevented.
15. Secure first bandage with clip or tape before applying additional rolls.	
16. Apply additional rolls without leaving any uncovered skin surface. Secure last bandage applied.	• Wrinkling and loose ends are prevented.
17. Remove gloves, if worn, and perform hand hygiene.	• Transmission of microorganisms is reduced.
A. Assess distal circulation when bandage application is complete and at least twice during 8-hour period.	• Early detection and management of circulatory impairment ensure healthy neurovascular status.
B. Observe skin colour for pallor or cyanosis.	
C. Palpate skin for warmth.	
D. Palpate pulses and compare bilaterally.	
E. Ask if patient is aware of pain, numbness, tingling, or other discomfort.	• Neurovascular changes indicate impaired venous return.
F. Observe mobility of extremity.	• Joint immobility is determined; if bandage is too tight, movement will be restricted.
18. Have patient demonstrate bandage application.	• Return demonstration documents learning.

STEPS	RATIONALE

UNEXPECTED OUTCOMES	RELATED INTERVENTIONS
Impaired circulation distal to elastic bandage	• Release bandage. • Palpate extremity and assess pulse, temperature, and capillary refill. • Reapply dressing with less pressure.
Break in skin under elastic bandage	• Remove bandage. • Reapply bandage with less pressure.
Inability of patient to change dressing	• Determine barriers to applying bandage. • Explore options (e.g., different type of dressing).

RECORDING AND REPORTING

- Document condition of the wound, integrity of dressing, application of bandage, circulation, and patient's comfort level.
- Report any changes in neurological or circulatory status to the nurse in charge or physician.

HOME CARE CONSIDERATIONS

- Instruct patient or caregiver not to secure bandages too tightly, which interferes with circulation.
- Elastic bandages that are used to reduce swelling are best applied to the feet in the morning, before getting out of bed.
- Always remove an elastic bandage daily and inspect the area.

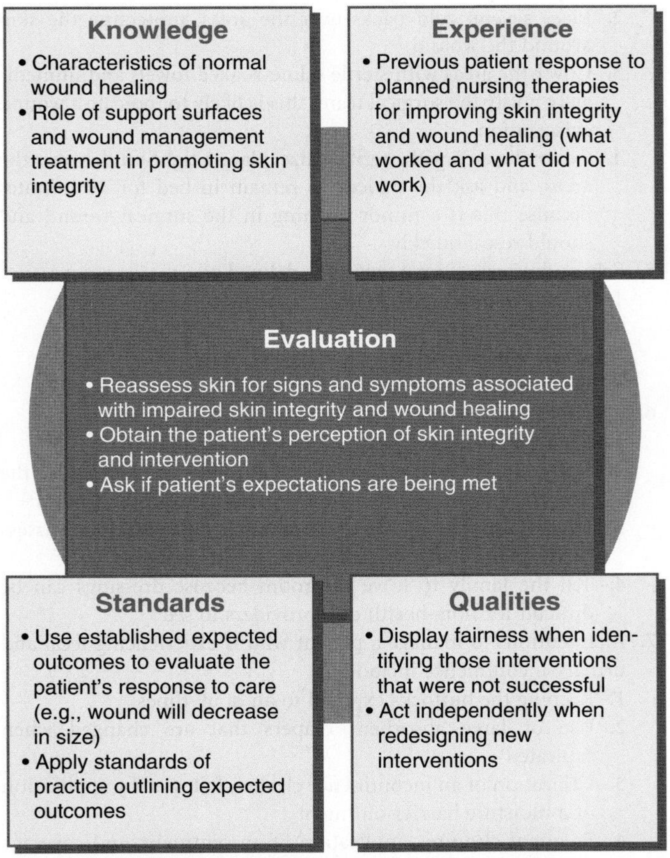

FIGURE 46-30 Critical thinking model for skin integrity and wound care evaluation.

- Were issues such as nutrition assessed and a plan of care developed that provided the patient with the calories to support healing?

Finally, nurses must evaluate the need for additional referrals to other experts in wound management, such as occupational therapists, dietitians, and wound care specialists. Care of the patient with a pressure injury requires a multidisciplinary team approach.

KEY CONCEPTS

- Prevention of skin breakdown is a major nursing focus for all patients, irrespective of their age or the health care setting.
- Patients should be assessed for risk of skin breakdown with the use of a validated risk assessment tool, such as the Braden Scale, on admission to care and at regularly scheduled intervals—unless health status changes (then more frequently).
- Low score in any subscale of the assessment tool should be addressed and monitored.
- Alterations in mobility, sensory perception, level of consciousness, and nutrition, as well as the presence of moisture, increase the risk of developing pressure injuries.
- Preventive skin care is aimed at controlling external pressure on bony prominences and keeping the skin clean, well lubricated, hydrated, and free of excess moisture.
- Proper positioning (the 30-degree rule) reduces the effects of pressure and guards against shearing force.
- Wound assessment requires a description of the appearance of the wound base, size (length × width × depth), presence of exudate, and the periwound skin condition.
- Moist wound-healing approaches are based on evidence and support the healing cycle of wounds.
- Wounds require pressure off-loading, adequate nutrition and hydration, blood flow, and an absence of infection to heal.
- Arterial, venous, and diabetic wounds are often the result of impaired peripheral circulation to the extremities.

- Wound irrigation should be at room or body temperature and provide 4 to 15 psi of pressure to avoid damaging fragile granulating tissue.
- Therapeutic beds and mattresses redistribute the effects of pressure; selection is based on assessment data to identify the best bed for individual needs.
- Cleaning and topical agents used to treat pressure injuries vary according to the stage of the pressure injury and condition of the wound bed. Assessment of the ulcer enables nurses to select proper skin care agents.
- Nutritional interventions are directed at improving wound healing through increasing protein and calorie levels, as required.
- When extensive tissue loss occurs, a wound heals by secondary intention.
- The chances of wound infection are greater when the wound contains dead or necrotic tissue, when foreign bodies lie on or near the wound, and when the blood supply and tissue defences are reduced.
- The principles of wound first aid include control of bleeding, cleaning, and protection.
- The layers of a dry dressing absorb drainage and prevent the entrance of bacteria.
- A moist environment supports wound healing.
- When cleaning wounds or drain sites, the nurse cleans from the least to most contaminated area, away from wound edges.
- A bandage or binder should be applied in a manner that does not impair circulation or irritate the skin.

CRITICAL THINKING EXERCISES

Mrs. Stein, who is 76 years of age, is at postoperative day 7 after a total hip replacement. She developed redness and oozing of foul-smelling, tan-coloured drainage from the hip incision on postoperative day 4. Significant medical history includes arthritis and mild hypertension. Because of surgical pain at the incision site, she did not easily transfer from her bed to the chair. Now on day 7, she notes some pain at the incision and complains of a painful, burning sensation in the sacral region. She is continent of urine and stool but continues to "scoot" over to the side of the bed when preparing for bed-to-chair transfers.

1. The staples from the surgical incision were removed and an order was written for a moist saline gauze dressing to be applied to the area three times a day. Would this be the approach that best supports wound healing? Provide a rationale and suggest alternative approaches. When the dressing is removed, what are the critical factors to assess?
2. A head-to-toe skin assessment is done per institutional policy on a daily basis. At the most recent assessment, redness was noted over the sacral area, and on direct examination, a small area of denuded tissue was noted. The involved area has minimal depth and a red, moist base. How would you describe the impairment in skin integrity in your charting?
3. What will you include in your plan of care to address the impairment in skin integrity in the sacral area?
4. Mrs. Stein will be discharged tomorrow. What issues must be assessed regarding her care before discharge? Explain why those issues are of importance.

REVIEW QUESTIONS

1. When repositioning an immobile patient, the nurse notices redness over a bony prominence. When the area is assessed, the red spot blanches with a fingertip touch, indicating:
   1. A local skin infection requiring antibiotics
   2. This patient has sensitive skin and requires special bed linen
   3. A stage 3 pressure injury needing the appropriate dressing
   4. Reactive hyperemia, a reaction that causes the blood vessels to dilate in the injured area
2. This type of pressure injury is an observable, pressure-related alteration of intact skin, whose indicators, compared with an adjacent or opposite area on the body, may include changes in one or more of the following: skin temperature (warmth or coolness), tissue consistency (firm or beefy feel), and sensation (pain or itching).
   1. Stage 1
   2. Stage 2
   3. Stage 3
   4. Stage 4
3. When obtaining a wound culture to determine the presence of a wound infection, the specimen should to be taken from the:
   1. Necrotic tissue
   2. Wound drainage
   3. Drainage on the dressing
   4. Wound after it has first been cleaned with appropriate cleaner
4. Postoperatively, the patient with a closed abdominal wound reports a sudden "pop" after coughing. When you examine the surgical wound site, the sutures are open and pieces of small bowel are noted at the bottom of the now opened wound. The correct intervention would be to:
   1. Allow the area to be exposed to air until all drainage has stopped
   2. Place several cold packs over the areas, protecting the skin around the wound
   3. Cover the areas with sterile saline-soaked towels and immediately notify the surgical team; this is likely to indicate a wound evisceration
   4. Cover the area with sterile gauze, place a tight binder over the areas, and ask the patient to remain in bed for 30 minutes because this is a minor opening in the surgical wound and should reseal quickly
5. Serous drainage from a wound is defined as:
   1. Fresh bleeding
   2. Thick and yellow
   3. Clear, watery plasma
   4. Beige to brown and foul-smelling
6. Before changing a dressing, the nurse should:
   1. Read the medical orders and follow them exactly
   2. Gather together all the supplies that might be required for the dressing change and remove the dressing from the wound
   3. Discuss the plan to change the dressing with the patient, assess the need for analgesia, and provide it, if necessary
   4. Tell the family to leave the room because dressings can be difficult for non–health care providers to see
7. Interventions to manage a patient who is experiencing fecal and urinary incontinence include:
   1. Keeping the buttocks exposed to air at all times
   2. Use of large absorbent diapers that are changed when saturated
   3. Utilization of an incontinence cleaner, followed by application of a moisture barrier ointment
   4. Frequent cleaning, application of an ointment, and coverage of the areas with a thick, absorbent towel
8. The best description of a hydrocolloid dressing is:
   1. A seaweed derivative that is highly absorptive
   2. Premoistened gauze placed over a granulating wound
   3. A debriding enzyme that is used to remove necrotic tissue

4. A dressing that forms a gel that interacts with the wound surface

9. A binder placed around a surgical patient with a new abdominal wound is indicated for:
   1. Collection of wound drainage
   2. Reduction of abdominal swelling
   3. Reduction of stress on the abdominal incision
   4. Stimulation of peristalsis (return of bowel function) by direct pressure

10. Patients with pressure injuries require:
    1. Repositioning every 4 to 6 hours
    2. Bed rest and a quiet environment
    3. Frequent dressing changes
    4. Nutritional assessment from a dietitian

Answers: 1. 4; 2. 1; 3. 4; 4. 3; 5. 3; 6. 3; 7. 3; 8. 4; 9. 3; 10. 4

Rationales for the Review Questions appear at the end of the book.

RECOMMENDED WEBSITES

Canadian Association for Enterostomal Therapy (CAET): http://www.caet.ca.

CAET is an association of health care providers (ET nurses) promoting education, research, and standards for enterostomal nursing practice. Nurses with the ET designation have obtained additional post-baccalaureate level certification to offer care to patients with the following conditions: abdominal stomata (openings), fistulae, draining wounds, and selected disorders of the integumentary (skin), gastrointestinal, and genitourinary systems.

Connecting Learners with Knowledge: Skin & Wound Community Practice: https://www.clwk.ca/communities-of-practice/skin-wound-community-of-practice/.

This website provides a number of useful tools and educational videos for clinicians with a role in wound care. It was developed and is supported by the British Columbia Provincial Nursing Skin & Wound Care Committee.

European Pressure Ulcer Advisory Panel: http://www.epuap.org.

Created in 1996, this group of health care providers and wound care experts works to lead and support all European countries in the efforts to prevent and treat pressure injuries. The mission statement is "to provide the relief of persons suffering from or at risk of pressure ulcers, in particular through research and the education of the public." Numerous links to European wound care organizations appear on the website.

National Pressure Ulcer Advisory Panel (NPUAP): http://www.npuap.org.

The NPUAP provides multidisciplinary leadership for improved patient outcomes in pressure injury prevention and management through education, public policy, and research.

Registered Nurses' Association of Ontario (RNAO) Best Practice Guidelines: http://rnao.ca/bpg.

This website provides links to the RNAO Best Practice Guidelines, including the revised version of *Risk Assessment and Prevention of Pressure Ulcers and Assessment and Management of Stage I to IV Pressure Ulcers*, now called *Assessment and Management of Pressure Injuries for the Interprofessional Team* (3rd edition), which can be downloaded for no cost as a pdf file or purchased through RNAO.

The South West Regional Wound Care Program: http://swrwoundcareprogram.ca.

This website, also known as "The Toolkit" contains skin, wound, and ostomy care–related resources for health care providers and members of the public, primarily intended for those within the Southwest catchment of Ontario. Similar to the other sites provided here, this website is open access and provides a wealth of information on best practices in wound care, including information for patients.

World Wide Wounds: http://www.worldwidewounds.com.

World Wide Wounds is an online, peer-reviewed journal with a focus on current research and evidence-informed practice issues related to wound care.

Wound Care Management: http://www.lhsc.on.ca/wound.

This website is a clinical resource, based on evidence-informed best practices for wound care. The site includes numerous links to online resources, including those for typical wounds and dressing options.

Wound, Ostomy and Continence Nurses (WOCN) Society: http://www.wocn.org.

The WOCN Society is a professional nursing society that supports the practice and delivery of expert health care to patients with wounds, ostomies, and incontinence.

Wounds Canada (formerly Canadian Association of Wound Care (CAWC): https://www.woundscanada.ca.

Wounds Canada is the new name for the Canadian Association of Wound Care, an interprofessional national organization dedicated to prevention, treatment, evaluation, and scholarship regarding wound care across the continuum of care. This website has quick reference guides and best practice articles available for downloading on all aspects of wound care practice, as well as information on upcoming seminars, conferences, and scholarship funding opportunities.

REFERENCES

Agency for Health Care Policy and Research (AHCPR), Panel for Treatment of Pressure Ulcers in Adults. (1994). *Treatment of pressure ulcers: Clinical practice guideline no. 15 (Pub No. 95-0653)*. Rockville, MD: Agency for Health Care Policy and Research, Public Health Service, U.S. Department of Health and Human Services.

Ayello, E. A., & Braden, B. (2002). How and why to do pressure ulcer risk assessment. *Advances in Skin & Wound Care, 15*(13), 125. doi:10.1097/00129334-200205000-00008.

Barr, J. E. (1995). Principles of wound cleansing. *Ostomy/Wound Management, 41*(Suppl. 7A), 15S–21S, discussion 22S.

Bennett, M. A. (1995). Report of the task force on the implications for darkly pigmented intact skin in the prediction and prevention of pressure ulcers. *Advances in Wound Care, 8*(6), 34.

Bergstrom, N., Braden, B. J., Laguzza, A., et al. (1987). The Braden Scale for Predicting Pressure Sore Risk. *Nursing Research, 36*, 205–210.

Bills, J. D., Berriman, S. J., Noble, D. L., et al. (2016). Pilot study to evaluate a novel three-dimensional wound measurement device. *International Wound Journal, 13*(6), 1372–1377. doi:10.1111/iwj.12534.

Braden, B. J. (2001). Risk assessment in pressure ulcer prevention. In D. L. Krasner, G. Rodeheaver, & R. G. Sibbald (Eds.), *Chronic wound care: A clinical source book for healthcare professionals*. Wayne, PA: HMP Communications.

Braden, B., & Bergstrom, N. (1988). *Braden Scale for Predicting Pressure Sore Risk*. Retrieved from http://www.bradenscale.com/images/bradenscale.pdf.

Braden, B. J., & Bergstrom, N. (1989). Clinical utility of the Braden Scale for Predicting Pressure Sore Risk. *Decubitus, 2*(3), 50.

Braden, B. J., & Bergstrom, N. (1994). Predictive validity of the Braden Scale for pressure sore risk in a nursing home population. *Research in Nursing & Health, 17*, 459.

Bryant, R. A., & Clark, R. A. F. (2016). Skin pathology and types of damage. In R. A. Bryant & D. P. Nix (Eds.), *Acute and chronic wounds: Current management concepts* (5th ed.). St. Louis, MO: Elsevier.

Bryant, R. A., & Nix, D. P. (2016). Principles of woundhealing. In R. A. Bryant & D. P. Nix (Eds.), *Acute and chronic wounds: Current management concepts* (5th ed.). St. Louis, MO: Elsevier.

Burton, A. C., & Yamada, S. (1951). Relation between blood pressure and flow in the human forearm. *Journal of Applied Physiology, 4*, 329.

Canadian Association of Wound Care (Wounds Canada, 2018). *Best practice recommendations for the prevention and management of pressure injuries*. Retrieved from https://www.woundscanada.ca/docman/public/health-care-professional/bpr-workshop/172-bpr-prevention-and-management-of-pressure-injuries-2/file.

Canadian Diabetes Association. (2016). *Clinical practice guidelines 2016: Interim update*. Toronto: Author. Retrieved from http://guidelines.diabetes.ca/update.

Canadian Malnutrition Task Force. (2017). *Subjective global assessment form*. http://nutritioncareincanada.ca/tools/assessment-sga.

Carter, M. J., Gilligan, A. M., Waycaster, C. R., et al. (2016). Treating pressure ulcers with clostridial collagenase ointment: Results from the US Wound Registry. *Wound Repair and Regeneration, 24*(5), 904–912. doi:10.1111/wrr.12548.

Cederholm, T., Bosaeus, I., Barazzoni, R., et al. (2015). Diagnostic criteria for malnutrition—An ESPEN consensus statement. *Clinical Nutrition, 34*, 335e40.

Doughty, D. B., & Sparks-Defriese, B. (2016). Wound-healing physiology. In R. A. Bryant & D. P. Nix (Eds.), *Acute and chronic wounds: Current management concepts* (5th ed.). St. Louis, MO: Elsevier.

Edsberg, L. E., Black, J. M., Goldberg, M., et al. (2016). Revised National Pressure Ulcer Advisory Panel Pressure Injury Staging System: Revised Pressure Injury Staging System. *Journal of Wound, Ostomy and Continence Nursing, 43*(6), 585–597.

Florczak, B., Scheurich, A., Croghan, J., et al. (2012). An observational study to assess an electronic point-of-care wound documentation and reporting system regarding user satisfaction and potential for improved care. *Ostomy/Wound Management, 58*(3), 46–51.

Frantz, R. A., Broussard, C. L., Mendez-Eastman, S., et al. (2016). Devices and technology in wound care. In R. A. Bryant & D. P. Nix (Eds.), *Acute and chronic wounds: Current management concepts* (5th ed.). St. Louis, MO: Elsevier.

Gadd, M. M., & Morris, S. M. (2014). Use of the Braden Scale for pressure ulcer risk assessment in a community hospital setting: The role of total score and individual subscale scores in triggering preventive interventions. *Journal of Wound, Ostomy & Continence Nursing, 41*(6), 535–538.

Geller, L. (2014). Leading change in wound care. *Canadian Nurse*, May, 2014.

Gillespie, B. M., Chaboyer, W. P., McInnes, E., et al. (2014). Repositioning for pressure ulcer prevention in adults. *Cochrane Database of Systemic Reviews*, (4), CD009958.

Goldberg, E., & Beltz, J. (2010). The lived experience of diverse elders with chronic wounds. *Ostomy/Wound Management, 56*(11), 36–46.

Gould, L., Abadir, P., Brem, H., et al. (2015). Chronic wound repair and healing in older persons: Current status and future research. *Wound Repair and Regeneration, 23*(1), 1–13.

Gould, L. J., Dosi, G., Couch, K., et al. (2016). Modalities to treat venous ulcers: Compression, surgery, and bioengineered tissue. *Plastic and Reconstructive Surgery, 138*(3S), 199S–208S.

Gray, M., & Weir, D. (2007). Prevention and treatment of moisture-associated skin damage (maceration) in the periwound skin. *Journal of Wound, Ostomy and Continence Nursing, 34*(2), 153. doi:10.1097/01.WON.0000264827.80613.05.

House, S. L. (2015). Psychological distress and its impact on wound healing: An integrative review. *Journal of Wound, Ostomy & Continence Nursing, 42*(1), 38–41. doi:10.1097/WON.0000000000000080.

Januchowski, R., & Ferguson, W. J. (2014). The clinical use of tissue adhesives: A review of the literature. *Osteopathic Family Physician, 6*(2), 25–29.

The Joint Commission (TJC). (2018). *Pain management*. Retrieved from http://www.jointcommission.org/topics/pain_management.aspx.

Kennerly, S., Boss, L., Yap, T. L., et al. (2015). Utility of Braden Scale nutrition subscale ratings as an indicator of dietary intake and weight outcomes among nursing home residents at risk for pressure ulcers. *Healthcare, 3*(4), 879–897.

Kohr, R., & Gibson, M. (2008). Doing the right thing: Using hermeneutic phenomenology to understand management of wound pain. *Ostomy/Wound Management, 54*(4), 52–60.

Koschwanez, H. E., Kerse, N., Darragh, M., et al. (2013). Expressive writing and wound healing in older persons: A randomized controlled trial. *Psychosomatic Medicine, 75*(6), 581–590.

Laporte, M., Keller, H. H., Payette, H., et al. (2015). Validity and reliability of the new Canadian Nutrition Screening Tool in the 'real-world' hospital setting. *European Journal of Clinical Nutrition, 69*(5), 558–564. doi:10.1038/ejcn.2014.270.

Litchford, M. D., Dorner, B., & Posthauer, M. E. (2014). Malnutrition as a precursor of pressure ulcers. *Advances in Wound Care, 3*(1), 54–63.

Molnar, J. A., Vlad, L. G., & Gumus, T. (2016). Nutrition and chronic wounds: Improving clinical outcomes. *Plastic and Reconstructive Surgery, 138*(3S), 71S–81S.

National Pressure Ulcer Advisory Panel (NPUAP). (2007). *Terms and definitions related to support surfaces*. Retrieved from http://www.npuap.org/wp-content/uploads/2012/03/NPUAP_S3I_TD.pdf.

National Pressure Ulcer Advisory Panel (NPUAP). (2016). *Pressure injury stages*. Retrieved from http://www.npuap.org/resources/educational-and-clinical-resources/npuap-pressure-injury-stages/.

National Pressure Ulcer Advisory Panel (NPUAP). (2017). *Position statement on staging—2017 clarifications*. Retrieved from http://www.npuap.org/wp-content/uploads/2012/01/NPUAP-Position-Statement-on-Staging-Jan-2017.pdf.

Nix, D. (2016). Patient assessment and evaluation of healing. In R. A. Bryant & D. P. Nix (Eds.), *Acute and chronic wounds: Current management concepts* (5th ed.). St. Louis, MO: Elsevier.

Orsted, H., Keast, D., Foret-Lalande, L., et al. (2017). *Best practice recommendations for the prevention and management of wounds*. Wounds Canada. Retrieved from https://www.woundscanada.ca/docman/public/health-care-professional/165-wc-bpr-prevention-and-management-of-wounds/file.

Ovington, L. (2001). Hanging wet-to-dry dressings out to dry. *Home Healthcare Nurse, 19*(8), 477–483.

Padula, W. V., Mishra, M. K., Makic, M. B. F., et al. (2014). A framework of quality improvement interventions to implement evidence-based practices for pressure ulcer prevention. *Advances in Skin & Wound Care, 27*(6), 280–284.

Pieper, B. (2016). Mechanical forces: Pressure, shear and friction. In R. A. Bryant & D. P. Nix (Eds.), *Acute and chronic wounds: Current management concepts* (5th ed.). St. Louis, MO: Elsevier.

Pierpont, V. N., Dinh, T. P., Salas, R. E., et al. (2014). Obesity and surgical wound healing: A current review. *ISRN Obesity*, doi:10.1155/2014/638936. Article ID 638936.

Pop-Busui, R., Boulton, A. J., Feldman, E. L., et al. (2017). Diabetic neuropathy: A position statement by the American Diabetes Association. *Diabetes Care, 40*(1), 136–154.

Posthauer, M. E., Banks, M., Dorner, B., et al. (2015). The role of nutrition for pressure ulcer management: National Pressure Ulcer Advisory Panel, European Pressure Ulcer Advisory Panel, and Pan Pacific Pressure Injury Alliance white paper. *Advances in Skin & Wound Care, 28*(4), 175–188.

Queirós, P., Santos, E., Apóstolo, J., et al. (2014). The effectiveness of cleansing solutions for wound treatment: A systematic review. *JBI Database of Systematic Reviews and Implementation Reports, 12*(10), 121–151.

Ramundo, J. M. (2016). Wound debridement. In R. A. Bryant & D. P. Nix (Eds.), *Acute and chronic wounds: Current management concepts* (5th ed.). St. Louis, MO: Mosby.

Registered Nurses' Association of Ontario (RNAO). (2002). *Promoting continence using prompted voiding*. Toronto: Author. Retrieved from http://rnao.ca/bpg/guidelines/promoting-continence-using-prompted-voiding.

Registered Nurses' Association of Ontario (RNAO). (2004). *Assessment and management of venous leg ulcers*. Toronto: Author. Retrieved from http://rnao.ca/bpg/guidelines/assessment-and-management-venous-leg-ulcers.

Registered Nurses' Association of Ontario (RNAO). (2011). *Best Practice Guideline: Assessment and management of stage I to IV pressure ulcers*. Toronto: Author.

Registered Nurses' Association of Ontario (RNAO). (2016). *Assessment and management of pressure injuries for the interprofessional team, third edition*. Retrieved from http://rnao.ca/bpg/guidelines/pressure-injuries.

Rodeheaver, G. T. (2012). Wound cleansing, wound irrigation, wound disinfection. In D. L. Krasner, G. T. Rodeheaver, & R. G. Sibbald (Eds.), *Chronic wound care: A clinical source book for healthcare professionals* (5th ed.). Wayne, PA: HMP Communications.

Schultz, G. (2016). Molecular regulation of wound healing. In R. A. Bryant & D. P. Nix (Eds.), *Acute and chronic wounds: Current management concepts* (5th ed.). St. Louis, MO: Elsevier.

Sibbald, R. G., Orsted, H. L., Coutts, P. M., et al. (2006). Best practice recommendations for preparing the wound bed: Update 2006. *Wound Care Canada, 4*, 15–29.

Sibbald, R. G., Orsted, H., Schultz, G. S., et al. (2003). Preparing the wound bed 2003: Focus on infection and inflammation. *Ostomy/Wound Management, 49*(11), 24–51.

Sibbald, R. G., Woo, K., & Ayello, E. A. (2006). Increased bacterial burden and infection: The story of NERDS and STONES. *Advances in Skin & Wound Care, 19*, 447–461.

Stotts, N. A. (2016a). Nutritional assessment and support. In R. A. Bryant & D. P. Nix (Eds.), *Acute and chronic wounds: Current management concepts* (5th ed.). St. Louis, MO: Elsevier.

Stotts, N. A. (2016b). Wound infection: Diagnosis and management. In R. A. Bryant & D. P. Nix (Eds.), *Acute and chronic wounds: Current management concepts* (5th ed.). St. Louis, MO: Elsevier.

Sun, X., Chen, J. A., Zhang, J., et al. (2016). Maggot debridement therapy promotes diabetic foot wound healing by up-regulating endothelial cell activity. *Journal of Diabetes and Its Complications, 30*(2), 318–322.

Tentolouris, N., Al-Sabbagh, S., Walker, M., et al. (2004). Mortality in diabetic and nondiabetic patients after amputations performed from 1990 to 1995: A 5-year follow-up study. *Diabetes Care, 27*, 1598–1604.

Upton, D., Solowiej, K., & Woo, K. Y. (2014). A multinational health professional perspective of the prevalence of mood disorders in patients with acute and chronic wounds. *International Wound Journal, 11*(6), 627–635.

Weiss, A. J., Fingar, K. R., Barrett, M. L., et al. (2016). *Characteristics of hospital stays involving malnutrition, 2013*. Healthcare Cost and Utilization Project. Statistical brief #210. Rockville, MD: Agency for Healthcare Research and Quality (AHRQ). Retrieved from https://www.hcup-us.ahrq.gov/reports/statbriefs/sb210-Malnutrition-Hospital-Stays-2013.pdf.

Woodbury, M. G., & Houghton, P. E. (2004). Prevalence of pressure ulcers in Canadian healthcare settings. *Ostomy/Wound Management, 50*(10), 22–38.

Wound, Ostomy and Continence Nurses Society (WOCN). (2010). *Guideline for prevention and management of pressure ulcers (WOCN clinical practice guidelines series)*. Glenview, IL: Author.

Wound, Ostomy and Continence Nurses Society (WOCN) Wound Committee, & Association for Professionals in Infection Control and Epidemiology (APIC) 2000 Guidelines Committee. (2012). Clean vs. sterile dressing techniques for management of chronic wounds: A fact sheet. *Journal of Wound, Ostomy & Continence Nursing, 39*(Suppl. 2), S30–S34. doi:10.1097/WON.0b013e3182478e06.

Wounds Canada. (2017a). *Foundations of best practice for skin and wound management*. Retrieved from https://www.woundscanada.ca/health-care-professional/education-health-care-professional/advanced-education/12-healthcare-professional/110-supplements.

Wounds Canada. (2017b). *Product pickers*. Retrieved from https://www.woundscanada.ca/health-care-professional/183-resources-industry-partner/288-product-picker.

Wounds National Stakeholder Round-Table Report. (2012, June). Retrieved from https://www.scribd.com/doc/108577300/WOUNDS-National-Stakeholder-Round-Table-Report.

Wysocki, A. B. (2016). Anatomy and physiology of skin and soft tissue. In R. A. Bryant & D. P. Nix (Eds.), *Acute and chronic wounds: Current management concepts* (5th ed.). St. Louis, MO: Elsevier.

47

Sensory Alterations

Canadian content written by Pamela G. Hawranik, RN, MN, PhD
Original chapter by Jill Parsons, RN, PhD

OBJECTIVES

Mastery of content in this chapter will enable you to:

- Describe the key terms listed.
- Differentiate among the processes of reception, perception, and reaction to sensory stimuli.
- Discuss the relationship of sensory function to an individual's level of wellness.
- Discuss common causes and effects of sensory alterations.
- Discuss common sensory changes that normally take place as individuals age.
- Conduct an assessment of an individual's sensory status.
- Develop a plan of care for individuals with sensory alterations.
- Identify interventions for preventing sensory deprivation and controlling sensory overload.
- Describe conditions in the health care setting or patient's home that nurses can adjust to promote meaningful sensory stimulation.
- Discuss ways to maintain a safe environment for patients with sensory deficits.
- Identify the benefits of working with an interdisciplinary team.
- Evaluate the effects of the nursing process when caring for patients with sensory alterations.

KEY TERMS

Age-related macular degeneration (AMD), p. 1342
Aphasia, p. 1347
Audiologist, p. 1357
Auditory, p. 1339
Carpal tunnel syndrome, p. 1346
Cataracts, p. 1342
Central auditory processing disorders, p. 1343
Cerumen, p. 1343
Conductive hearing loss, p. 1343
Delirium, p. 1344
Diabetic retinopathy, p. 1342
Expressive aphasia, p. 1347
Glaucoma, p. 1343
Global aphasia, p. 1347
Gustatory, p. 1339
Health promotion, p. 1353
Hyperesthesia, p. 1357
Kinesthetic, p. 1339
Myopia, p. 1343
Olfactory, p. 1339
Otitis media, p. 1343
Otolaryngologist, p. 1357
Ototoxic, p. 1349
Perception, p. 1341
Presbycusis, p. 1343
Presbyopia, p. 1343
Proprioceptive, p. 1345
Receptive aphasia, p. 1347
Refractive error, p. 1343
Retinal detachment, p. 1343
Sensorineural hearing loss, p. 1343
Sensory deficit, p. 1341
Sensory deprivation, p. 1343
Sensory overload, p. 1344
Stereognosis, p. 1339
Strabismus, p. 1344
Tactile, p. 1339
Tinnitus, p. 1343
Tympanic membrane, p. 1340
Vertigo, p. 1343
Visual, p. 1339
Xerostomia, p. 1343

MEDIA RESOURCES

http://evolve.elsevier.com/Canada/Potter/fundamentals/

- Audio Chapter Summaries
- Examination Review Questions
- Concept Map Creator
- Case Study With Questions
- Audio Glossary
- Content Updates
- Video Clips

People rely on a variety of sensory stimuli to give meaning and order to events occurring in their environment. The senses help form the perceptual base of our world (Touhy, Jett, Boscart, et al., 2012). Stimulation comes from many sources inside and outside the body, particularly through the senses of sight (**visual**), hearing (**auditory**), touch (**tactile**), smell (**olfactory**), and taste (**gustatory**). The body also has a **kinesthetic** sense that enables a person to be aware of the position and movement of body parts without seeing them. **Stereognosis** is a sense that allows a person to recognize an object's size, shape, and texture. Meaningful stimuli allow a person to learn about the environment and are necessary for healthy functioning and normal development.

Sensory alterations have been perceived by many as inevitable with aging and, therefore, are overlooked and not treated (Cacchione, 2014; Crews & Campbell, 2004). However, sensory alterations can occur at any age and can have multiple causations. They can also have a substantial detrimental effect on the individual's ability to care for themselves in their home, maintain independence, and learn and adopt necessary self-care practices (Cacchione, 2014). Individually, hearing and vision loss are associated with depression, cognitive decline, delirium, functional decline, and falls (Robinson, Feng, Woods, et al., 2013). More serious is dual sensory impairment, such as both vision and hearing loss. This can be associated with depression, delirium, falls, cognitive decline, and mortality (Karpa, Gopinath, Beath, et al., 2010). Olfactory, tactile, and gustatory impairments, such as swallowing difficulties, may result in nutritional problems with resultant weight loss, dehydration, cognitive changes, and skin breakdown (Franks, Chuah, King, et al., 2015; Mueller, 2015).

Many patients seeking health care have pre-existing sensory alterations (e.g., cataracts) or more than one sensory alteration (e.g., both hearing and visual deficits). Others may develop sensory alterations because of medical treatment (e.g., hearing loss from antibiotic use). In other cases, there can be environmental causes resulting in sensory deficits, such as hearing loss due to frequent exposure to occupational noise. The health care environment itself can cause sensory alterations. For example, a hospital unit is often a place of unfamiliar sights, sounds, and smells that can lead to sensory overload resulting in delirium. In contrast, being hospitalized can also lead to sensory deprivation in some individuals due to the lack of meaningful contact with familiar supports, such as family and friends.

As a nurse, you must be able to recognize the factors that can lead to sensory alterations, know how those factors can be prevented or minimized, understand the implications of sensory alterations, and work with the patient in facilitating his or her independence and self-care needs.

SCIENTIFIC KNOWLEDGE BASE

Normal Sensation

The nervous system continuously receives thousands of bits of information from sensory nerve receptors, relays the information through appropriate channels, and integrates the information into a meaningful response. Sensory stimuli reach the sensory receptors and can elicit an immediate reaction or present information to the brain to be stored for future use. The nervous system must be intact for sensory stimuli to reach appropriate brain centres and for the individual to perceive the sensation. After interpreting the significance of a sensation, the person can then react to the stimulus (Tables 47-1 and 47-2).

Reception, perception, and reaction are the three components of any sensory experience. Reception begins with stimulation of a receptor nerve cell, which is usually designed for only one type of stimulus, such as light, touch, or sound. In the case of special senses, the

TABLE 47-1 Normal Hearing

Function	Anatomy and Physiology
The Ear	
Transmits to the brain an accurate pattern of all sounds received from the environment, the relative intensity of these sounds, and the direction from which they originate.	The auditory system is composed of three major parts: external or outer ear, middle ear, and inner ear (see Figure 47-1, *B*).
External Ear	
The purpose of the hair follicles and the cerumen is to protect against the entry of foreign matter into the canal and lubricate the canal to inhibit growth of bacteria and fungi. The external auditory canal shelters the tympanic membrane and maintains the elasticity of the tympanic membrane by maintaining a relatively constant temperature and humidity.	The external ear is composed of the auricle (or pinna) and the external auditory canal. The pinnae direct and funnel sound waves into the external auditory canal and then to the eardrum (**tympanic membrane**). The outer one-third of the canal is lined with hair follicles and glands that secrete cerumen or ear wax.
Middle Ear	
The function of the middle ear is to transmit sound from the external auditory canal to the inner ear. The functions of the tympanic membrane are to cause the ossicles to vibrate in order to transmit sound waves to the inner ear and to protect the middle ear.	The middle ear consists of the tympanic membrane, the ossicles, and the oval window. The tympanic membrane is located at an oblique angle at the end of the auditory canal. The ossicles are three small bones (malleus, incus, and stapes). They are often nicknamed hammer, anvil, and stirrup, respectively. Movement of the stapes in the oval window creates vibrations in the fluid of the inner ear.
Inner Ear	
When vibrations at the oval window are transmitted to the inner ear they distort and move the fluid and hair cells in the labyrinth. The inner ear converts sound waves for the transmission and interpretation by the brain regarding body position, sound, and movement. The impulses are then transmitted along the eighth cranial nerve to the brain.	The inner ear contains three interconnected bony structures: cochlea, vestibule, and semicircular canals. They are often called the labyrinth because of their winding canal system. They contain fluid and tiny hair cells.

TABLE 47-2 Normal Vision

Function	Anatomy and Physiology
The Eye	
Transmits to the brain an accurate pattern of light reflected from solid objects in the environment and transformed into colour and hue.	The external parts of the eye include the eyebrows, eyelids, eyelashes, conjunctiva, cornea, sclera, and tear ducts. The internal structures include the sclera, cornea, choroid, ciliary body, iris, pupil, lens, and retina (see Figure 47-1, *A*). Light rays enter the convex cornea and begin to converge. Fine adjustment of light rays occurs as they pass through the pupil and through the lens. The ciliary muscles change the shape of the lens to focus the light on the retina. The retina has a pigmented layer of cells to enhance visual acuity. The sensory retina contains the rods and cones—photoreceptor cells sensitive to stimulation from light. Photoreceptor cells send electrical impulses by way of the optic nerve to the brain.

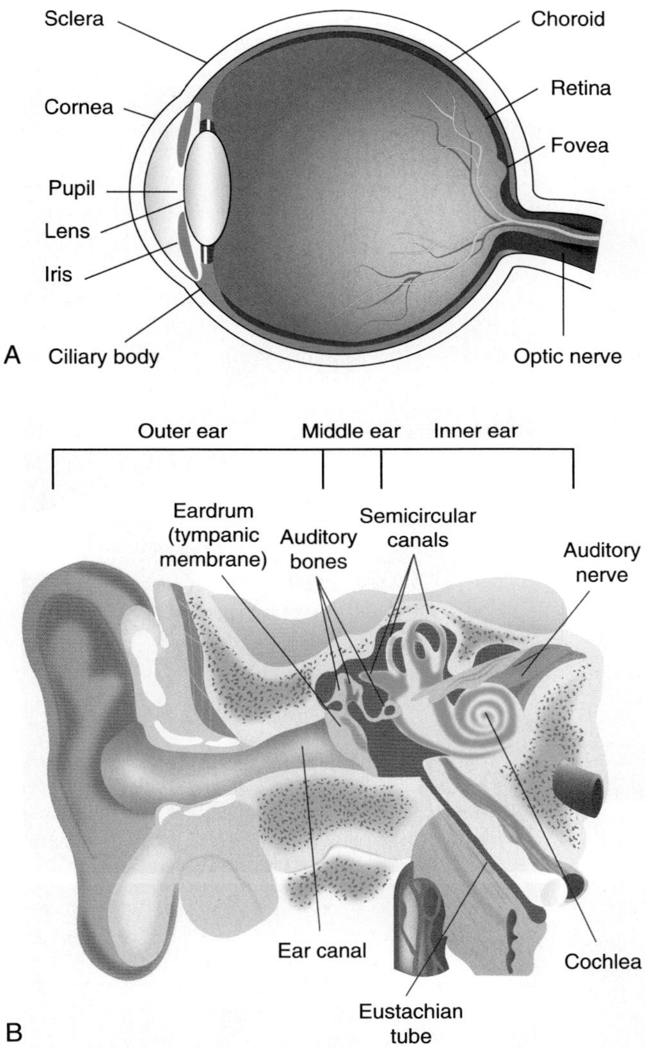

FIGURE 47-1 Anatomy of the eye and ear. A, Anatomy of the eye. **B,** Anatomy of the ear. (**A,** National Eye Institute, https://nei.nih.gov/photo; **B,** https://www.allamericanhearing.com/i-wonder-if-i-have-a-hearing-loss/anatomy-of-the-ear/.)

receptors are grouped close together or located in specialized organs (McCance & Huether, 2014), such as the taste buds of the tongue or the retina of the eye (Figure 47-1, *A*). When a nerve impulse is created, it travels along pathways to the spinal cord or directly to the brain. For example, sound waves stimulate hair cell receptors within the organ of Corti (located in the inner ear), which causes impulses to travel along the eighth cranial nerve to the acoustic area of the temporal lobe (Figure 47-1, *B*). Sensory nerve pathways usually cross over to send stimuli to opposite sides of the brain.

The actual **perception** or awareness of unique sensations depends on the receiving region of the cerebral cortex, where specialized brain cells interpret the quality and nature of sensory stimuli. When the person becomes conscious of the stimuli and receives the information, perception takes place. Perception includes integration and interpretation of the stimuli on the basis of the person's experiences. A person's level of consciousness influences how well stimuli are perceived and interpreted. Any factors lowering consciousness impair sensory perception.

If sensation is incomplete, such as blurred vision, or if the person has a cognitive impairment, he or she may misinterpret the stimuli and may react inappropriately (e.g., become aggressive). It is impossible to react to all the multiple stimuli entering the nervous system. The brain prevents sensory bombardment by discarding or storing sensory information. A person will usually react to stimuli that are most meaningful or significant at the time. After continued reception of the same stimulus, however, a person stops responding, and the sensory experience goes unnoticed. For example, a person concentrating on reading a good book may not be aware of music in the background. This adaptability phenomenon occurs with most sensory stimuli, except for those of pain.

Sensory Deficits

A loss in the normal function of sensory reception and perception is a **sensory deficit**. The prevalence of sensory deficits is of concern, particularly with the increase in the number of people reaching 65 years and over.

When senses are impaired, the sense of self is affected. Initially, a person may withdraw by avoiding communication or socialization with others in an attempt to cope with the sensory loss. It becomes difficult for the person to interact safely with the environment until new skills are learned. When a deficit develops gradually or when considerable time has passed since the onset of an acute sensory loss, the person may learn to rely on unaffected senses. When one sense is impaired, people depend on their other intact senses. However, individuals with dual sensory impairments, for example, vision and hearing loss, have increased difficulty compensating (Perlmutter, Bhorade, Gordon, et al., 2010).

Patients with sensory deficits may change behaviour in effective or ineffective ways. For example, one patient with a hearing impairment may turn the unaffected ear toward the speaker to hear better, whereas another patient may avoid people to avoid the embarrassment of not being able to understand their speech.

Visual Deficits. Most vision loss in Canada is caused by one of five eye conditions: age-related macular degeneration (AMD), cataract, diabetic retinopathy, glaucoma, and refractive errors.

Age-Related Macular Degeneration. Age-related macular degeneration (AMD) is the leading eye disease causing vision loss in Canada. It is incurable. It usually affects people over 50 years of age. It is a condition in which the macula (located in the centre of the retina) results in a gradual or sudden loss of central vision. First signs may include blurring of reading matter, distortion or loss of central vision, and distortion of vertical lines (see Figure 47-2, *B*).

Cataract. Every individual will develop cataracts if they live long enough. Cataracts usually develop gradually and without pain, resulting in blurring, decreased vision, and glare. Cloudy or opaque areas in part of or the entire lens interfere with passage of light through the lens (see Figure 47-2, *C*). Although associated with aging, cataracts can also be caused by diabetes, injury, or medications, especially steroids.

Diabetic Retinopathy. Diabetic retinopathy is the result of pathological changes that occur in the blood vessels of the retina, resulting in decreased vision or vision loss caused by hemorrhage and macular edema. It is the leading cause of vision loss in Canadians under 50 years of age. Long-term or poorly managed diabetes can lead to progressive damage to the blood vessels that feed the retina. These blood vessels leak into the retina, resulting in severe vision loss or blindness (see Figure 47-2, *D*).

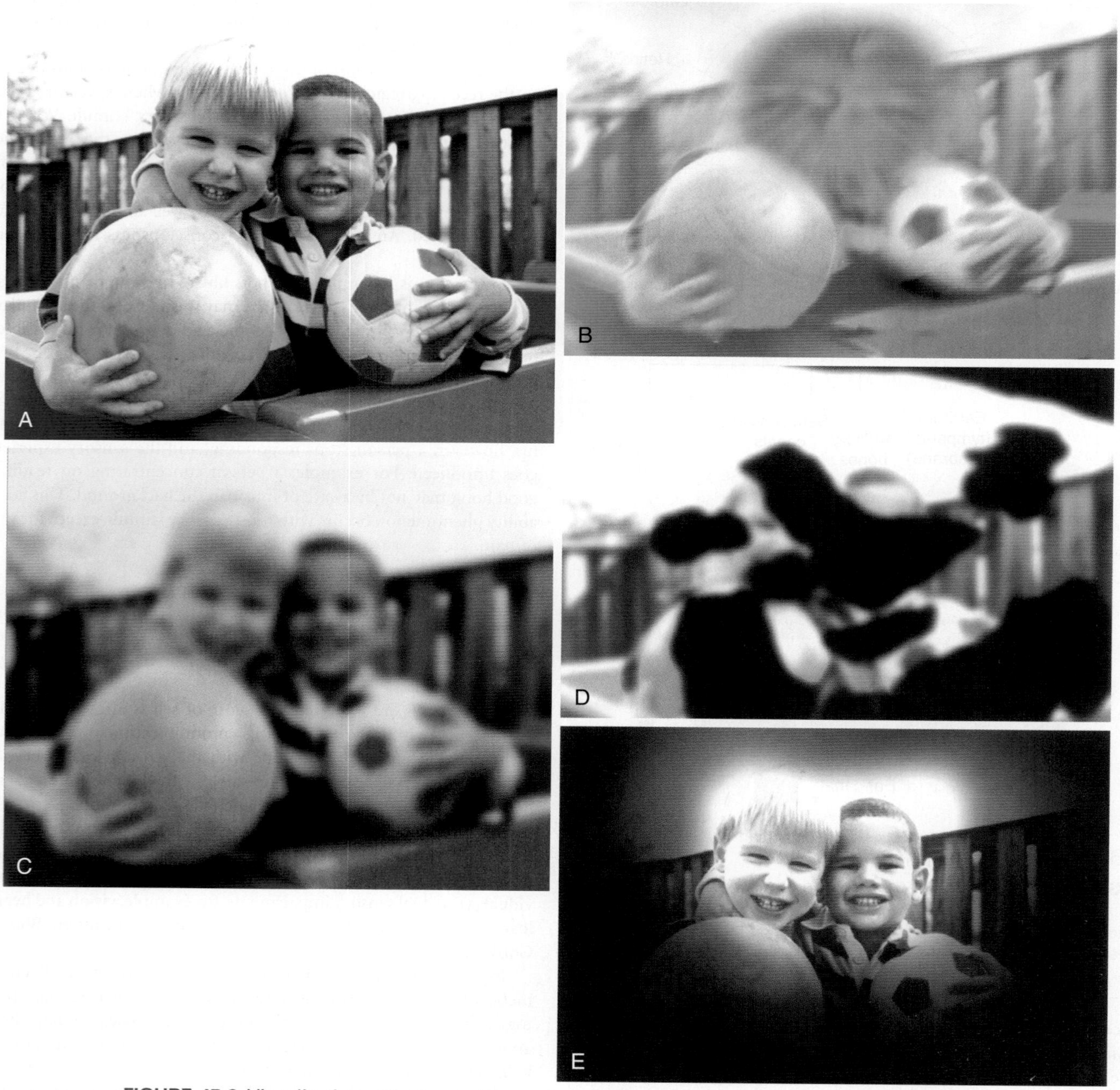

FIGURE 47-2 Visualizations when eye disease is present. **A,** Normal vision. **B,** Age-related macular degeneration. **C,** Cataract. **D,** Diabetic retinopathy. **E,** Glaucoma. (National Eye Institute, https://nei.nih.gov/photo.)

Glaucoma. Glaucoma is the second most common cause of vision loss in Canadians over 65 years of age. One of the most common causes of blindness, it can develop at any age, but affects 1 in 100 Canadians over 40 years of age (Muzychka, 2009). It results in increased fluid pressure inside the eye that can eventually damage the optic nerve. Left untreated, it can result in visual field loss, decreased visual acuity, a halo effect seen around objects, and blindness (see Figure 47-2, *E*). Glaucoma can be idiopathic in origin or may be caused by eye injury, inflammation, tumours, diabetes, or medications such as steroids.

Dry Eyes. Dry eyes occur more frequently with aging. This condition results in a gritty feeling, pain, itching, blurred vision, light sensitivity, redness, and sometimes excessive tears as a compensatory response.

Refractive Errors. Refractive errors are the most frequent yet most easily correctible source of vision loss. They occur when a person's vision is reduced and corrective lenses are used to correct the error. There are three types of refractive error: myopia (nearsightedness), hyperopia (farsightedness), and presbyopia (difficulty reading small print).

Retinal Detachment. Retinal detachment occurs when the retina develops small holes or tears. This may occur with thinning of the retina with aging or from separation of the vitreous from the retina and is more common in persons with a family history of retinal detachment. Nearsightedness, infection, or injury, such as trauma to the eye, are other causes (Canadian Ophthalmological Society, 2007).

Hearing Deficits

Conductive Hearing Loss. Conductive hearing loss results when sound waves are not effectively transmitted through the outer and middle ear to the inner ear. Common causes are partial or total blockage of the ear canal, such as blockage caused by colds, allergies, and ear infections.

Presbycusis. Presbycusis is a common progressive hearing disorder in older persons that results in the inability to hear high-pitched sounds, making speech seem more muffled and unclear (Public Health Agency of Canada, 2006).

Central Auditory Processing Disorders. Central auditory processing disorders involve damage to the auditory centres and pathways in the central cortex. Some causes include traumatic brain injury, tumours, and heredity.

Cerumen Accumulation. Buildup of cerumen (earwax) can occur in the external auditory canal. Hard cerumen causes conduction deafness. This is more common in older people.

Ménière's Disease. Ménière's disease is a disorder of the inner ear characterized by hearing loss, tinnitus, and vertigo (sudden loss of balance). It likely is caused by increased fluid in the inner ear. This disorder usually begins in people between the ages of 20 and 50 years.

Otitis Media. Otitis media is an infection of the middle ear that is common in infants and children. Recurrent or chronic otitis media can cause damage to the eardrum or middle ear, resulting in permanent hearing loss.

Otosclerosis. Otosclerosis is a hereditary condition, resulting in hardening of the ossicles in the middle ear and gradual and progressive hearing loss that is usually accompanied by tinnitus (background noises in the ear, hissing or ringing sounds, or discrete tones or pulses).

Sensorineural Hearing Loss. Sensorineural hearing loss results from damage to the inner ear (cochlea) or hearing nerve in the brain, or the hair cells in the cochlea or of the nerve cells between the inner ear and central auditory cortex. Adult sensorineural hearing loss can be caused by excessive noise levels; certain medications; viruses; and metabolic, vascular, and other systemic alterations. Metabolic changes, however, appear to be the most significant factor affecting age-related hearing loss (Sprinzl & Riechelman, 2010).

Tinnitus. Tinnitus affects about 10 to 15% of the population. It is often described as a ringing, buzzing, or pulsating sound in the ear. It can be intermittent or constant, have one or more tones, and vary in volume. It does not always include hearing loss (Canadian Hearing Society, 2018a,b,).

Balance Deficit. Benign positional vertigo is a common condition among older persons, usually resulting from vestibular dysfunction. Frequent episodes of vertigo or disequilibrium are precipitated by a change in the position of the head.

Taste Deficits. Xerostomia is a decrease in salivary production that leads to thicker mucus and dry mouth. It may result from the adverse effects of medications such as antihistamines. This condition can interfere with the ability to eat and leads to appetite and nutritional problems.

Taste alterations are manifested by food aversions and decreased caloric intake. These can occur frequently in patients with cancer and as people age.

Neurological Deficits. Peripheral neuropathy is a common disorder that is very common in people with diabetes and in older persons. Sensations such as tingling or pins and needles, numbness, weakness, and pain are felt, often starting in the lower legs and feet. Onset is insidious and difficult to diagnose early on. It is estimated that up to 47% of diabetics have peripheral neuropathy (Dworkin, Malone, Panarites, et al., 2010; Hanewinckel, Ikram, & van Doorn, 2016).

Sensory processing disorder is a condition in which the brain has trouble receiving and responding to information that comes from the senses. Common sounds may be painful or overwhelming for the individual or light touch may be considered painful. This condition tends to be found in children but can be diagnosed in adults. This disorder is often seen in conditions such as autism spectrum disorder (Howe & Stagg, 2016).

Sensory Alterations

The most common types of sensory alterations are sensory deficits, sensory deprivation, and sensory overload. When a patient has more than one sensory alteration, the ability to function and relate effectively within the environment can be seriously impaired.

Sensory Deprivation. The reticular activating system in the brain stem mediates all sensory stimuli to the cerebral cortex. Even in deep sleep, individuals are able to receive stimuli. Sensory stimulation must be of sufficient quality and quantity to maintain a person's awareness. When a person experiences an inadequate quality or quantity of stimulation, sensory deprivation occurs. Three types of sensory deprivation include (1) reduced sensory input (e.g., caused by sensory deficit from visual or hearing loss), (2) elimination of pattern or meaning from input (e.g., exposure to strange environments), and (3) restriction of the environment (e.g., bed rest or reduced environmental variation) that produces monotony and boredom (Touhy & Jett, 2014).

A decrease in stimuli can occur when patients are placed in isolation. Isolation precautions are used for patients who test positive for transmissible organisms such as *Clostridium difficile* (*C. diff.*), which causes an inflammation of the colon and deadly diarrhea. There has been an almost four-fold increase in the *C. difficile* infection attributable mortality rate in Canadian hospitals from 1997 to 2005 (1.5% of cases to 5.7%, respectively, $p < .001$) (Gravel, Miller, Simor, et al., 2009). When placed in isolation, the person is confined to his or her room, and the number of people entering the room, as well as the person's contact with the outside world, is reduced. Nurses are required to follow transmission-based precautions, which include frequent hand hygiene and the use of masks and gloves. Most organisms are transmitted via the hands of caregivers. Masks may prevent visualization of caregivers' faces, and gloves will alter the sense of touch. Patients who are moved into isolation are at risk of developing delirium. **Delirium** is a serious, potentially preventable complication (Wofford & Vacchiano, 2011). It is an acute, short-term disturbance of consciousness that may last a few hours or become permanent if not detected and treated. Delirium is characterized by acute onset of inattention, disorganized thinking, hallucinations, and agitation (Baker, Taggart, Nivens, et al., 2015).

Sensory deprivation has many serious effects (Box 47-1). The symptoms can easily cause nurses and physicians to believe that a patient is psychologically ill and confused, is suffering from severe electrolyte imbalance, or is under the influence of psychotropic drugs. Nurses can help prevent sensory deprivation by being aware of the contributing factors and identifying patients who are at risk. Prompt action to reduce or eliminate the risk factors and treat the resultant behavioural changes is important (Baker et al., 2015).

Sensory Overload. When a person receives multiple sensory stimuli and cannot perceptually disregard or selectively ignore some stimuli, **sensory overload** occurs. Excessive sensory stimulation prevents the brain from appropriately responding to or ignoring certain stimuli. Because of the multitude of stimuli leading to overload, the person no longer perceives his or her environment in a way that makes sense. Overload prevents meaningful response by the brain; the person's thoughts race, attention moves in many directions, and anxiety and restlessness may occur. As a result, overload causes a state similar to that produced by sensory deprivation. However, in contrast to deprivation, overload is individualized. The amount of stimuli necessary for healthy function varies with each individual. A person's tolerance to sensory overload may vary by level of fatigue, attitude, and emotional and physical well-being.

BOX 47-1 Effects of Sensory Deprivation

Cognitive
- Reduced capacity to learn
- Inability to think or to problem solve
- Poor task performance
- Disorientation/confusion
- Bizarre thinking
- Increased need for socialization, altered mechanisms of attention

Affective
- Boredom
- Restlessness
- Increased anxiety
- Emotional lability (e.g., rapid mood swings)
- Panic
- Increased need for physical stimulation

Perceptual
- Alterations in
  - Visual/motor coordination
  - Reduced colour perception
  - Less tactile accuracy
  - Changes in ability to perceive size and shape
  - Changes in spatial and time judgement

From Potter, P., Perry, A., Stockert, P., & Hall, A. (2017). *Fundamentals of nursing* (9th ed.). St. Louis, MO: Elsevier.

The acutely ill patient may easily be affected by sensory overload. The patient in constant pain or who undergoes frequent monitoring of vital signs or lack of sleep is at risk. Multiple stimuli can combine to cause overload even if the patient is receiving a comforting word or a gentle back rub. Admission to a Critical Care Unit (CCU) can be a precipitating factor for sensory overload and delirium (Sendelbach & Guthrie, 2009). Lights are always on; sounds can be heard from monitoring equipment, staff conversations, equipment alarms, and the activities of people in the unit.

The behavioural changes associated with sensory overload can easily be confused with mood swings or simple disorientation. Symptoms such as racing thoughts, scattered attention, restlessness, and anxiety need to be observed. Gestures such as pulling at the sheets or tubing or plucking at unseen things in the air are often exhibited. Constant reorientation, control of excessive stimuli, and, if possible, providing care in blocks of time become an important part of the patient's care. Providing clocks and calendars, dimming lights, family support, and clear communication can help prevent sensory overload and delirium in patients (Robinson, Rich, Weitzel, et al., 2008).

NURSING KNOWLEDGE BASE

Factors Influencing Sensory Function

Many factors influence sensory function, including the patient's age, the quantity and quality of stimuli, family support, environment, medications, culture and ethnicity, and various chronic illnesses. While each of these factors is described here separately, there is rarely one factor responsible for sensory alteration. Most often there are multiple factors present that interact, causing changes in sensory functioning, such as in a newborn baby in the CCU. Not only does the environment influence the senses, but the medical condition of the infant and his or her developmental level or physical maturity may impair the child's sensory functioning. Sensory alternation also affects the child's medical condition.

Age. Infants and children are at risk for visual and hearing impairment because of a number of genetic, prenatal, and postnatal conditions. A concern with high-risk neonates is that early intense visual and auditory stimulation can adversely affect visual and auditory pathways and alter the developmental course of other sensory organs (Hockenberry & Wilson, 2015).

Six out of 10 children experience reading difficulties due to uncorrected or undetected vision problems, and nearly 25% of school-age children have vision problems (National Coalition for Vision Health, 2015). Certain eye conditions can lead to visual impairment. **Strabismus** (crossed eyes) usually begins in infancy or childhood. School children with significant strabismus have self-image problems. It is often treated by surgically adjusting the tension on the eye muscles. Amblyopia (lazy eye) is poor vision in an eye that did not develop normal sight during early childhood. The main causes of amblyopia are strabismus, refractive errors, or cloudiness of the eye tissues (Canadian Ophthalmological Society, 2007).

With aging comes an increase in the incidence of sensory loss. A study by Humes (2015) reported that middle-aged adults experience declines in both sensory and cognitive processing. The changes that were observed were between that of young and older persons. This finding suggests that age-related decline in sensory processing is continuous rather than abruptly beginning in old age.

The incidence of vision loss is also more prevalent with aging. The four most common causes of blindness increase with age. After age 40, the number of cases of vision loss doubles every decade, and it triples at age 75. Individuals who have vision loss are more likely than those without vision problems to

- Be admitted to a nursing home, 3 years earlier
- Experience twice the number of falls
- Experience three times the incidence of depression
- Have four times as many hip fractures
- Have double the mortality rate (National Coalition for Vision Health, 2015)

Presbyopia is a normal visual change that occurs in individuals over 40 years of age. It is caused by age-related stiffening of the lens of the eye, resulting in an inability of the lens to change shape to allow focusing (accommodation) clearly on close objects, such as reading a newspaper (Barnes & Sewell, 2014). Other visual difficulties normally associated with aging include reduced visual fields, increased glare sensitivity, impaired night vision, reduced accommodation and depth perception, and reduced colour discrimination (Speros, 2009) (Box 47-2). Colours with short wavelengths, such as blues, pinks, beiges, and greens, become more difficult to distinguish, while colours with long wavelengths, such as reds, oranges, and yellows, are easier to discriminate. The visual changes can occur gradually, and in many cases older people may not notice their vision deteriorating until it significantly interferes with their ability to engage in regular or everyday activities, or when they realize that the vision loss is taking place (Gold, Zuvela, & Hodge, 2007).

Every year in Canada, more than 1 000 children are born with a permanent hearing loss (Canadian Infant Hearing Task Force, 2016). It has many causes and each hearing loss is unique to the individual (Canadian Hard of Hearing Association, 2010). Aging is the number one cause of hearing loss. Hearing changes include decreased hearing acuity, speech intelligibility, pitch discrimination, and hearing threshold (Box 47-3). Older persons hear low-pitched sounds best but have difficulty hearing conversation over background noise. Speech sounds are garbled, and reception of and reaction to speech are delayed. Older people have difficulty discriminating particular consonants (*z, t, f, g*) and high-frequency sounds (e.g., *s, sh, ph, k*) (presbycusis). A problem with age-related hearing loss is that some individuals may not even be aware of their deficit, or what they may have considered age-related changes are, in fact, abnormal changes. A serious concern for persons with a hearing deficit is that they may be inappropriately labelled as confused (Touhy & Jett, 2014).

The olfactory system, which gives us the ability to detect odours in the environment, declines with age, owing to normal physiological aging changes (Masurkar & Devanand, 2014). Diminished sense of smell results from a reduction in the number of olfactory sensory neurons and bulb cells. Changes include a reduction in olfactory nerve fibres by the age of 50 years, reduced taste discrimination, and reduced sensitivity to odours. More than half of people 65 years of age and older report a change in sense of smell. This can result in decreased enjoyment of eating and drinking, as well as pose a safety risk for detecting harmful odours in the environment.

Diminished sense of taste with aging likely results from a reduction in the function or number of taste buds, along with decreased saliva production. Smoking, poor oral hygiene, nasal polyps, and radiation therapy may also contribute to diminished taste sensation (Capezuti, Siegler, & Mezey, 2008). Changes in sensory perception can affect the enjoyment of food and dietary choices and can lead to malnutrition in older people (Methven, Jimenez-Pranteda, & Lawlor, 2016).

Proprioceptive changes after the age of 60 years include increased difficulty with balance, spatial orientation, and coordination. Proprioceptive dysfunction can be caused by vestibular dysfunction and neuropathy, or any factor that affects the reception, transmission, perception, or interpretation of proprioceptive stimuli (McCance & Huether, 2014). Older persons experience tactile changes, including declining sensitivity to pain, pressure, and temperature. Factors affecting tactile changes are numerous and include trauma, infection, metabolic or vascular changes, degenerative diseases, and drugs such as sedatives (McCance & Huether, 2014).

Nurses must be careful not to assume automatically that a patient's sensory problem is related to advancing age. Nurses must conduct a careful assessment to determine the true cause(s).

Stimuli. As mentioned earlier, the presence or absence and the quantity of stimuli can affect the individual's cognitive and mental status. Sensory deprivation and sensory overload can occur. Meaningful stimuli reduce the incidence of sensory deprivation and may help to alleviate sensory overload. In a patient's home or a long-term care facility, meaningful stimuli may include pets, music, television, family photographs, a calendar, and a clock. The presence of others can offer positive stimulation.

Family Support. The amount and quality of contact with family members and significant others can influence the degree of isolation a patient feels. The absence of visitors during hospitalization or residency in a long-term care facility can also affect sensory status. This is a common problem in hospital settings where visitation is restricted. The ability to discuss fears or concerns with loved ones is an important coping mechanism for most people. Therefore, the absence of meaningful conversation can cause a person to become sensorially deprived, and nurses may not be alerted to this problem until behavioural changes occur.

Environment. A person's work environment can increase the risk for sensory alterations. Individuals who are exposed to loud noises at work or who have occupations that involve the risk of exposure to chemicals or flying particles should be screened for hearing and visual problems. Approximately 9 000 Canadians experience some form of hearing impairment due to occupational exposure each year (Health Canada, 2010). Noise exposure over time, coupled with the loss of blood supply to the cochlea with aging, will result in hearing loss. Harmful noise levels occur in the workplace and in recreational environments. Poor noise control, inadequate hearing protection, and lack of education about the risks of hearing loss are contributing factors. Military personnel, farmers, lawn care workers, and people

BOX 47-2 Aging Changes to Vision That Affect Visual Ability

Peripheral vision decreases
Pupils shrink in size
Ciliary muscles that change the shape of the lens become less flexible
Cornea becomes more opaque and yellowed
Tear production decreases
Lens becomes thickened and cloudy

BOX 47-3 Aging Changes to Hearing That Affect Hearing Ability

Increased rigidity of the ossicles
Decreased elasticity of the tympanic membrane
Increased cerumen production
Decreased number of neurons and blood vessels
Loss of hair cells in inner ear

who work around power tools and loud music are at risk for occupation-related hearing loss (Fausti, Wimington, Helt, et al., 2005).

Occupations that require repetitive manual work involving flexion and extension at the wrist, forceful grip with the hand, or vibrations of the hand and arm can cause pressure on the median nerve, resulting in carpal tunnel syndrome (Giersiepen & Spallek, 2011), a condition characterized by swelling or inflammation of the wrists. This inflammation creates pressure on the nerve as it passes through the narrow area (the carpal tunnel) in the wrist. The patient can experience numbness, tingling, pain, and a reduction of the grip strength and function of the affected hand (Ibrahim, Khan, Goddard, et al., 2012).

Older farmers and ranchers and other outdoor workers must deal with the effects of aging as well as the hazards in their work environment. They are subject to noise injury from the equipment, leading to hearing loss. Fatigue, reduced vision, arthritis, and slower reaction time that occur with aging can increase these workers' risk for injury. Older agricultural workers dealing with toxins (pesticides and herbicides) may experience loss of vision or sense of touch.

As discussed earlier, the hospital environment can place a patient at risk for sensory alterations from exposure to environmental stimuli or a change in sensory input, due to immobility because of bed rest, disability, or physical circumstances (e.g., casts or traction), or when placed in isolation. Infants in neonatal intensive care units experience an overload of sensory stimuli from the bright lights, excessive noise, and painful procedures. This sensory overload alters their physiological responses and can lead to decreased social interaction, altered rest and sleep patterns, restlessness, irritability and crying, as well as overall reduction in auditory response and motor development (Cabral, da Silva, Tudella, et al., 2015; Darcy, Hancock, & Ware, 2008) (Box 47-4).

Children have unique developmental, biological, and behavioural characteristics that make them particularly vulnerable to environmental hazards, including toxins such as mercury, lead, pesticides, second-hand smoke, and moulds. Their metabolism is rapid, they drink more water per body volume than adults, and breathe more rapidly, taking in more air per body volume than adults. Exposure to such toxins can result in learning disabilities, impaired hearing, numbness or pain, impaired sensation, impaired coordination, and other symptoms, depending on the toxin and the nature of the exposure (Dunn, Burns, & Sattler, 2003).

Medications. Aging changes and the high prevalence of chronic disease in older persons increase the likelihood of this population taking multiple medications, either those prescribed by a health care practitioner or taken by self-medication. Multiple medications can have considerable risks for the individual (Hubbard, O'Mahony, & Woodhouse, 2013; Oyarzun-Gonzalez, Myers, Muldoon, et al., 2015). *Self-medication* is defined as self-administration of medicine, without a prescription from a licensed professional (Jerez-Roig, Medeiros, Silva, et al., 2014). Generally, the medicine is suggested or shared by a relative or friend. Hearing loss may occur as an adverse effect of prescription medications, such as thiazide diuretics and certain antibiotics.

Medications can contribute to numerous adverse effects and combination toxicity. Overuse of laxatives, which are available over the counter, can lead to bowel dependency.

Ethnicity. Certain sensory deficits have been found to occur at higher rates with certain genders and ethnicities. Regarding vision loss, some findings that are based on ethnicity include the following:

- Whites have somewhat higher rates of overall vision loss in Canada compared to visible minorities.
- Older (aged 60+) visible minority women have the highest rates of cataract, while older visible minority males have the lowest rates.
- Men from visible minority populations have high rates of glaucoma.
- White Canadians are more likely to have vision loss from AMD than Black Canadians; the reverse is true for refractive errors.
- Chinese-Canadians have double the rate of AMD compared to White Canadians and may have twice the rate of diabetic retinopathy.
- Chinese-Canadian children are more likely to experience nearsightedness than children who are White.
- Indigenous Canadians have higher rates of diabetic retinopathy. Inuit populations have much higher rates of primary open-angle glaucoma (Access Economics Pty Limited, 2008).

Vision loss affects women slightly more than men; however, this may reflect the greater longevity of women (Access Economics Pty Limited, 2008). More research needs to be conducted to identify whether gender and ethnicity are the causative factors or whether other factors such as lifestyle, poverty, inadequate nutrition, genetics, access to treatment, or environment are the causative or associative factors.

BOX 47-4 RESEARCH HIGHLIGHT

The Neonatal Intensive Care Unit and Sensory Processing in Preterm Infants

While a neonatal intensive care unit can increase the survival rate of preterm infants, it also exposes infants to sensory stimuli that can be harmful to their immature systems. A descriptive cross-sectional study of 30 infants, with 15 preterm infants and a control group of 15 full-term infants, examined their sensory processing. The authors of the study found a significant difference between the two groups of infants in their reactions to deep tactile pressure. Early childhood experience is a crucial factor in the health and well-being of the infant and also at a later age. It is important for the nurse to detect changes in sensory development, plan strategies to decrease the sensory overload, and refer the infant for intervention that continues until the child reaches school age.

Cabral, T., da Silva, L., Martinez, C., & Tudella, E. (2016). Analysis of sensory processing in preterm infants. *Early Human Development, 103*, 77–81.

CRITICAL THINKING

Critical thinking involves synthesizing knowledge and information gathered from patients, experience, and intellectual and professional standards. During assessment (Figure 47-3), nurses consider all critical thinking elements that help them make appropriate nursing diagnoses. Rowles and Russo (2009) discuss how nurses need critical thinking skills to provide individualized, evidence-informed care to meet patients' complex needs. Critical thinking requires interpreting and synthesizing information to make decisions in planning and delivering nursing care.

Care for patients with sensory alterations requires integration of knowledge from several areas: normal anatomy and physiology of the sensory and nervous systems, the pathophysiology of sensory deficits and factors that affect sensory function, therapeutic communication principles, and normal aging changes. This information enables nurses to conduct appropriate assessments, anticipate what to recognize when a patient describes a sensory problem, and recognize abnormalities. For example, knowing that someone with glaucoma will have tunnel vision (i.e., they can see clearly at the centre of their visual field but cannot see the periphery) will help the nurse recognize that when the person is sitting down for a meal he or she may not see the location of the cup or other dining utensils that would be outside the centre of their vision.

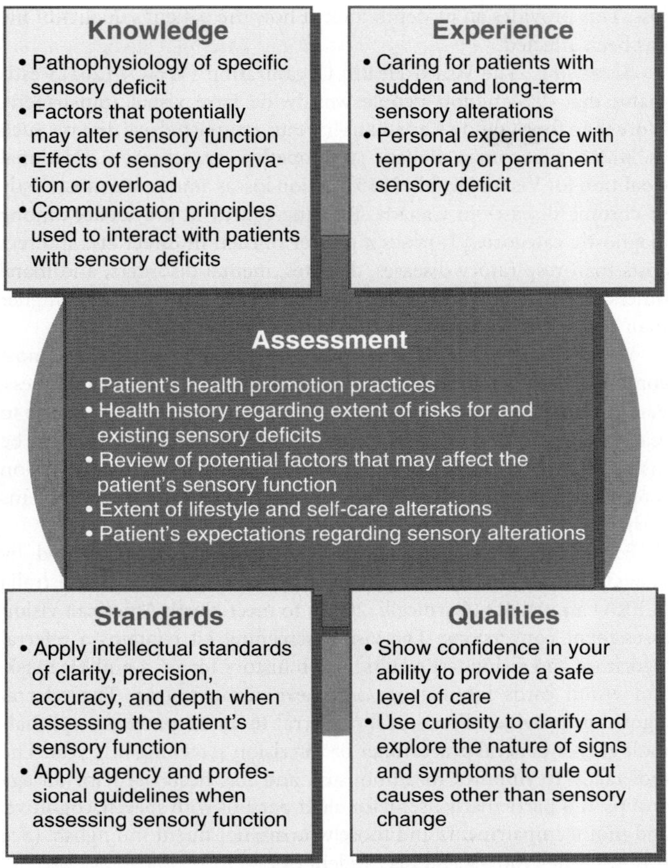

FIGURE 47-3 Critical thinking model for sensory alterations assessment.

Previous experience in caring for patients with sensory deficits enables you as a nurse to recognize limitations in function in each new patient and how those limitations might affect the patient's ability to carry out daily activities. For example, after caring for a patient with a hearing impairment, you will be able to conduct a more effective assessment of the next patient.

Standards of care and practice, such as those from the Canadian Ophthalmological Society, the Registered Nurses' Association of Ontario (RNAO), the Canadian Gerontological Nursing Association, and the Canadian National Institute for the Blind (CNIB), provide criteria for screening sensory problems and for establishing standards for competent, safe, and effective care and practice. Using critical thinking, nurses can conduct a thorough assessment and then plan, implement, and evaluate care that will enable the patient to function safely and effectively.

❖ NURSING PROCESS

◆ Assessment

When assessing patients with or at risk for sensory alterations, nurses must consider how the patient's particular illness may lead or has led to sensory changes. As well, all the factors that may influence sensory function must be considered. For example, if the patient has a hearing impairment, the nurse's communication style needs to be adjusted and assessment is focused on relevant criteria related to hearing deficits. Nurses collect a history that assesses the patient's current sensory status and the degree to which a sensory deficit affects the patient's lifestyle, psychosocial adjustment, developmental status, self-care ability, and safety. The assessment must also focus on the quality and quantity of environmental stimuli.

The location of the patient assessment is important. There should be privacy with no distractions. The nurse should sit at the same eye level as the patient, to create a supportive atmosphere and reduce the power differential between the nurse and the patient. To understand the nature of a communication problem, the nurse must know whether a patient has trouble speaking, understanding, naming, reading, or writing. Patients who have existing sensory deficits often develop alternative ways of communicating.

A deaf or hearing-impaired patient may read lips, use sign language, listen with the help of a hearing aid, or read and write notes. Visually impaired patients may be unable to observe facial expressions and other nonverbal behaviours that clarify the content of spoken communication. Instead, they rely on voice tones and inflections to detect the emotional tone of communication. Nurses need to face such patients, allowing them to see the nurse's face and mouth movements clearly. If the person has a visual impairment, the nurse should speak clearly with a moderate rate of speech and pause to determine understanding. Lighting should be sufficient. If the patient cannot hear the nurse well, the patient will watch the nurse's mouth movements in order to understand the nurse's questions. The nurse should not sit with a window behind him or her as this creates glare for the patient, who then cannot see facial features and mouth movements.

Patients with **aphasia** have varied degrees of inability to speak, interpret, or understand language. **Expressive aphasia**, a motor type of aphasia, is the inability to name common objects or express simple ideas in words or writing. For example, a patient understands a question but is unable to express an answer. Sensory or **receptive aphasia** is the inability to understand written or spoken language; a patient is able to express words but is unable to understand questions or comments of others. **Global aphasia** is the inability to understand language or communicate orally.

The temporary or permanent loss of the ability to speak is extremely traumatic to an individual. The nurse should assess for alternate communication methods and whether they cause anxiety. The nurse needs to determine whether the patient has developed a sign-language system or symbols to communicate his or her needs.

A family member who is identified as a caregiver or a support person to the patient should be included in the nurse's interview, either at the same time as the interview with the patient or in a separate interview. If it is suspected that the patient is not providing accurate information about his or her health or cannot provide adequate information, a separate interview with a family member should be held. The nurse may need to clarify the patient's health problems or medications or the family member's perception of how the patient is coping or managing daily activities. If the family member is a caregiver to the patient, the nurse may need to interview him or her to discover the person's coping ability and stress level as caregiver.

Use of Assistive Devices. Nurses need to assess for the use of assistive devices (e.g., hearing aids or glasses) and the sensory effects for patients. This includes learning how often the devices are used daily, the patient's or family caregiver's method for cleaning devices, and the patient's knowledge of what to do when a problem develops. However, just because the patient has an assistive device, the nurse should not assume that it works or that the patient uses it or benefits from it.

Many people are reluctant to wear a hearing aid (Adams-Wendling & Pimple, 2008). Several factors may determine a person's likelihood of wearing a hearing aid: perceived need for improved hearing, attitude toward the hearing problem, and motivation to seek solutions. Cost may also be a concern for having hearing assessed and for purchasing a hearing aid if the patient is not covered by a provincial health plan. In some provinces, hearing aids must be purchased from an approved dispenser or dealer for the cost to be covered by the provincial health programs (Canadian Hard of Hearing Association, 2015).

Sensory Alterations History. The nursing health history includes assessment of the nature and characteristics of sensory alterations or any problem related to an alteration. The history begins with asking the patient to describe the sensory deficit, as in the examples provided in Box 47-5. The patient's ethnic or cultural background needs to be considered because certain sensory deficits are more common in certain groups. It is also important to ensure that patients are able to communicate in the examiner's language, in order to be able to answer questions and describe their condition accurately.

Knowledge about the onset and duration of the sensory alteration can be helpful. The nurse can then learn how long the patient has taken measures to adjust to the alteration. It is also useful to assess the patient's self-rating for a sensory deficit, by simply saying, "Rate your hearing as excellent, good, fair, poor, or bad." Then, from the patient's self-rating, the nurse can explore the patient's perception of a sensory loss. This provides an in-depth look at how the patient's quality of life has been affected.

Screening. The World Health Organization (WHO) (2012) estimates that 285 million people worldwide have visual impairment. More than four million Canadians have an age-related eye disease, such as AMD, glaucoma, diabetic retinopathy, or cataracts (National Coalition for Vision Health, 2015). Vision loss is among the most costly of chronic diseases in Canada. Ranking fourth in prevalence among diagnostic categories, it poses a greater burden in direct and indirect costs than respiratory diseases, diabetes, mental disorders, and many others. Measured in direct health-related costs, vision loss ranks higher than any disease category in Canada (Muzychka, 2009).

Visual impairment is common during childhood. The most common visual problem is a refractive error such as nearsightedness. Parents must know signs suggesting visual impairment (e.g., failure to react to light and reduced eye contact from the infant) and should be instructed to report these signs to a physician immediately. Vision screening of school-aged children and adolescents can detect problems early.

For vision assessment, a vision screening kit was adapted by Hawranik and Bell (2007), from the Centre of Eye Research Australia (CERA) and WHO (Carnicelli, 2001), to meet North American vision assessment conversions. The vision screening kit contains a referral algorithm and vision test results, vision history forms, a pinhole mask, and vision cards for distance and near vision testing. The referral algorithm provides direction for referral to an optometrist, ophthalmologist, or general practitioner or for vision screening in 1 year. The tool takes 10 minutes to administer, and has been used for all age groups. It is particularly useful for older persons with speech, cognitive, and motor impairments and those who are not fluent in English. (See Box 47-6 for vision screening guidelines.)

Children at risk for hearing impairment include those with a family history of childhood hearing impairment, perinatal infection (rubella, herpes, cytomegalovirus), low birth weight, chronic ear infection, and Down syndrome. Nurses should advise pregnant women of the

BOX 47-5 Nursing Assessment Questions

Nature of the Problem

- What problem are you having with your vision/hearing?
- What have you tried to correct the vision/hearing difficulty?
- Do you use any devices to improve your vision/hearing?
- How effective are your glasses or hearing aids?

Signs and Symptoms

- Ask a patient with visual alterations: Do you require books with large print or on audiotape? Are you able to prepare a meal or write a cheque? Do you notice any eye irritation or drainage?
- Ask a patient with hearing alterations: Which types of sounds or tones do you have difficulty hearing? Do people tell you that they have to "shout" for you to hear them? Do people ask you not to talk so loud? Do you have a ringing, crackling, or buzzing in your ears? Is there pain—sharp, dull, burning, itching? Have you noticed any redness, swelling, or drainage? Any signs of infection?

Onset and Duration

- When did you notice the problem? How long has it lasted?
- Does it come and go, or is it constant?
- What makes the problem better or worse?

Predisposing Factors

- Do you work or participate in any activities that have the potential for vision/hearing injury? If so, how do you protect your hearing and vision?
- Do you have a family history of cataracts, glaucoma, macular degeneration, or hearing loss?
- When was your last vision/hearing examination?

Effect on Patient

- What effect has your vision/hearing problem had on your work, family, or social life?
- Have changes in your vision/hearing affected your feelings of independence?
- How does your vision/hearing problem make you feel about yourself?
- Do you have problems with routine care of glasses, contact lenses, or hearing aids?

BOX 47-6 Recommended Vision Screening Guidelines for Infants, Children, Youth, and Adults

- Newborns to 3 months of age should undergo a complete examination of the skin and external eye structures and inspection of the red reflex to assess for lenticular opacities or posterior eye disease. Abnormal exams should warrant an urgent referral to an ophthalmologist. Any newborns at risk for retinopathy of prematurity or family histories of hereditary ocular disease should be referred to an ophthalmologist.
- From 6 to 12 months of age, the above examinations should also be done, as well as assessments of ocular alignment, corneal light reflexes, and fixation and following.
- From 3 to 5 years of age, the above examinations should be done, as well as visual acuity testing with an age-appropriate tool.
- For children and youth aged 6 to 18, routine screenings and examinations with any visual complaints are indicated (Amit & Canadian Paediatric Society Community Paediatrics Committee, 2009/2016).
- Patients between the ages of 40 and 64 years should have an eye examination every 2 to four years. Examinations should occur every 1 to 2 years if the patient's family has a history of glaucoma, or if the patient has had a serious eye injury in the past, is taking steroid medications, or is over 65 years of age (Smith & Neely, 2007).

importance of early prenatal care, avoidance of ototoxic drugs, and testing for syphilis or rubella.

Children with chronic middle ear infections, a common cause of impaired hearing, should receive periodic auditory testing. Parents must be warned of the risks (e.g., exposure to smoke, previous history of ear infections, siblings with otitis media, attending day care) and should seek medical care when their child has symptoms of earache or respiratory infection (Kerschner, Lindstrom, Pomeranz, et al., 2005).

Many teenagers and young adults already have permanent hearing loss caused by exposure to excessive noise from electronic listening devices, automobile stereo systems, and concerts. According to Vogel and colleagues (2008), electronic players may be the most significant risk factor for music-induced hearing loss in adolescents. Parents and children need to take precautions when involved in activities associated with high-intensity noise. If someone has to shout in a person's ear to be understood in a noisy environment, the person is at risk for permanent hearing loss if exposed to this level of noise for just 5 minutes per day (Health Canada, 2005).

The guidelines for hearing screening for adults are less prescriptive. In general, if a patient works or lives in an environment where the noise level is high, routine screening is highly recommended and may be mandated by occupational health and safety measures in the workplace. Nurses in occupational settings can assess for symptoms of tinnitus and make prompt referrals. Early detection may prevent hearing disabilities. Barnett (2007) recommends that, since aging is associated with degenerative changes, patients over 40 have a routine hearing assessment. Adults must not accept hearing loss as a natural part of aging. If a hearing loss does occur, it is important to have regular hearing testing. Nurses should encourage patients to follow through with recommendations for hearing aids.

There are a number of bedside assessment tools that can be used to assess hearing impairment. The screening version of the Hearing Handicap Inventory for the Elderly (HHIE-S) is a 5-minute, 10-item questionnaire designed to assess how a patient perceives the emotional and social effects of hearing loss. The greater the handicapping effect from the hearing loss, the higher the score (Stark & Hickson, 2004). The Minimum Data Set (MDS) assessment can be used at admission and on a regular basis to detect conductive, sensorineural, or mixed hearing loss (Adams-Wendling & Pimple, 2008).

A health history can also reveal any recent changes in a patient's behaviour. Often friends or family are the best resources for this information because the patient may be unaware of any change. Details will be revealed by asking the following questions:

- Have you noticed any change in their hearing (e.g., television being turned louder)?
- Has your family member or friend shown any recent mood swings (e.g., outbursts of anger, nervousness, fear, or irritability)?
- Have you noticed him or her avoiding social activities?
- Has your mother fallen recently?

It is important to remember that many adults are sensitive about admitting losses and may hesitate to share information.

The nurse should also rely on personal observation of the patient to detect sensory alterations. Some useful observations indicating hearing loss are the following: the patient seems inattentive to others, responds to questions inappropriately, believes people are talking about him or her, has trouble following clear directions, asks to have something repeated, has monotonous voice quality and speaks unusually loudly or softly, has the television unusually loud, and leans head to one side when being spoken to (Touhy et al., 2012).

Acknowledging a need to improve hearing is a person's first step. Nurses can give patients useful information on the benefits of wearing a hearing aid. A wide variety of aids are available that may not only successfully enhance a person's hearing but can also be cosmetically acceptable. It is also important to have a significant other available to assist with hearing aid adjustment (Box 47-7).

BOX 47-7 Troubleshooting Hearing Aid Malfunction

Objectives

- Patient and family member will identify source of malfunction in hearing aid.
- Patient and family member will demonstrate hearing aid care.

Teaching Strategies

- Show patient and family member locations on hearing aid device where damage (e.g., cracks, fraying) is likely to occur: ear mould or case, earphone, dials, cord, and connection plugs.
- Demonstrate battery replacement and stress the importance of having an extra set of unused batteries available.
- Review method to check volume: turn dial to maximum gain and then check. Is voice clear?
- Consult manufacturer's directions for specific care measures for cleaning battery case and ear mould.
- Review factors to report to hearing aid laboratory: static, distortion of sound, poor volume quality.

Nurses are often consulted for guidance when changes in vision and hearing occur. Consequently, a nurse's knowledge of screening techniques is important. It is also important that nurses are familiar with the normal aging process, as well as the signs and symptoms of common diseases so that appropriate suggestions for referral can be made.

Factors other than sensory deprivation or overload may cause impaired perception (e.g., medications or pain). The patient's medication history should be assessed, which includes prescribed and over-the-counter medications, as well as herbal products and caffeine. This history includes gaining information regarding the frequency, dose, method of administration, and last time these medications were taken. Nurses should conduct a thorough pain assessment when pain is suspected to be causing perceptual problems.

Mental Status. Mental status assessment is an important component of any evaluation of sensory function. This is particularly important as visual impairment is a risk factor for cognitive decline (Whitson, Cousins, Burchett, et al., 2007). Visual impairment can be associated with hallucinations. Approximately 14 to 20% of individuals with AMD will develop Charles Bonnet syndrome (Crumbliss, Taussig, & Jay, 2009). This syndrome is characterized by visual hallucinations, ocular pathology causing visual deterioration, and preserved cognitive status. Affected individuals are fully aware that the hallucinations are not real. They are reluctant to report these experiences, fearing that they may be diagnosed with a dementia (Boxerman, Wittich, & Overbury, 2015; Menon, 2005; Nair, Nair, Shah, et al., 2014).

Observing the patient during history-taking, physical examination, and nursing care provides valuable data for evaluation of a patient's mental status. An assessment of mental status is valuable particularly if sensory deprivation or overload is suspected. The nurse should observe the patient's physical appearance and behaviour, measure the patient's cognitive ability, and assess the patient's emotional status. The Mini-Mental State Examination (MMSE) is an example of a tool that can be used to measure disorientation, altered conceptualization and abstract thinking, and change in problem-solving abilities (Folstein, Folstein, & McHugh, 1975) (see Chapter 32). For example, a patient with severe sensory deprivation may not be able to carry on a conversation, remain attentive, or display recent or past memory.

If the patient resides in his or her own home, it is good to check for cleanliness in the home, spoiled food on the counter or in the fridge, misplaced items, inappropriate dress, and losing the way to the store or other locations he or she used to frequent.

Physical Assessment. To identify sensory deficits and their severity, nurses need to assess vision, hearing, olfaction, taste, and the ability to discriminate light touch, temperature, pain, and position. Chapter 32 describes assessment techniques in detail. Table 47-3 summarizes assessment techniques for identifying sensory deficits. The data will be more accurate if the examination room is private, quiet, and comfortable for the patient.

Ability to Perform Self-Care. Patients' functional abilities in their home environment or health care setting, including feeding, dressing, grooming, and toileting, should be assessed. For example, the nurse can assess whether a patient with altered vision can find items on a meal tray and can read directions on a prescription. Vision loss

TABLE 47-3 Assessment of Sensory Function

Assessment	Behaviour Indicating Deficit (Children)	Behaviour Indicating Deficit (Adults)
Vision		
Ask patient to read newspaper, magazine, or lettering on menu. Measure visual acuity with Snellen chart (see Chapter 32) or the Vision Screening Tool. Assess visual fields and depth perception. Assess pupil size and accommodation to light. Ask patient to identify colours on colour chart or crayons. Observe patient conducting activities of daily living (ADLs).	Self-stimulation, including eye rubbing, body rocking, sniffing or smelling, arm twirling; hitching (using legs to propel while in sitting position) instead of crawling	Poor coordination, squinting, underreaching or overreaching for objects, persistent repositioning of objects, impaired night vision, accidental falls
Hearing		
Perform conventional assessment, including whisper and tuning fork (see Chapter 32). Perform audiometry, if indicated. Observe patient conversing with others. Assess patient's perception of hearing ability and history of tinnitus. Inspect ear canal for hardened cerumen.	Frightened when unfamiliar people approach, no reflex or purposeful response to sounds, failure to be awakened by loud noise, slow or absent development of speech, greater response to movement than to sound, avoidance of social interaction with other children	Blank looks, decreased attention span, lack of reaction to loud noises, increased volume of speech, positioning of head toward sound, smiling and nodding of head in approval when someone speaks, use of other means of communication such as lip-reading or writing, complaints of ringing in ears
Touch		
Assess patient for sensitivity to light touch (see Chapter 32) and temperature. Check patient's ability to discriminate between sharp and dull stimuli. Assess whether patient can distinguish objects (coin or safety pin) in the hand with eyes closed. Ask whether patient feels unusual sensations.	Inability to perform developmental tasks related to grasping objects or drawing, repeated injury from handling of harmful objects (e.g., hot stove, sharp knife)	Clumsiness, overreaction or underreaction to painful stimulus, failure to respond when touched, avoidance of touch, sensation of pins and needles, numbness
Smell		
Ask patient to close eyes and identify several nonirritating odours (e.g., coffee, vanilla).	Difficult to assess until child is 6 or 7 years old, difficulty discriminating noxious odours	Failure to react to noxious or strong odour, increased body odour, decreased sensitivity to odours
Taste		
Ask patient to sample and distinguish different tastes (e.g., lemon, sugar, salt). Have patient drink or sip water and wait 1 minute between each taste. Ask patient if recent weight change has occurred.	Inability to tell whether food is salty or sweet, possible ingestion of strange-tasting things	Change in appetite, excessive use of seasoning and sugar, complaints about taste of food, weight change
Position Sense		
Perform conventional tests for balance and position sense (see Chapter 32).	Clumsiness, extraneous movement, excessive arm swinging in children with hyperactivity or learning difficulty Inability to sit or stand as per expected milestones	Poor balance and spatial orientation, shuffling gait, reduced response to brace self when falling, slow and deliberate movements, a history that includes falls

contributes to an increase in self-administered medication errors and increased rates of hospitalization (Pelletier, Thomas, & Shaw, 2009). The nurse should determine a visually impaired patient's ability to perform daily routines such as reading bills, writing cheques, or driving a vehicle at night. Does a patient's loss of balance prevent rising from a toilet seat safely? Any impairment in the ability to perform self-care has implications for planning discharge from a health care setting and for providing resources within the home. Vision loss with older people increases the risk of falls and the likelihood of being institutionalized (Pelletier et al., 2009).

Health Promotion Habits. Nurses must assess the daily routines that patients follow to maintain sensory function. What type of eye and ear care is incorporated into daily hygiene? For those individuals who participate in sports or recreational activities or who work in a setting where ear or eye injury is a possibility (e.g., chemical exposure or constant exposure to loud noise), it is good to determine if safety glasses or hearing protective devices (HPDs) are worn. Do patients who use assistive devices such as eyeglasses, contact lenses, or hearing aids know how to care for them (see Chapter 38)? Are the devices used? Are they in proper working order?

Hazards. A patient with sensory alterations is at risk for injury if the living environment is unsafe. For example, a patient with visual impairment cannot see potential hazards clearly. A patient with proprioceptive problems may lose balance easily and fall. The condition of the home, the rooms, and the front and back entrances can be problematic for the patient with sensory alterations. Some of the more common hazards are the following:

- Uneven, cracked walkways leading to front or back door
- Doormats with slippery backing
- Extension and telephone cords in the main route of walking traffic
- Loose area rugs on hardwood floors or tiles; runners placed over carpeting
- Bathrooms without shower or tub grab bars
- Water faucets unmarked to designate hot and cold
- Bathroom floor with slippery surface
- Absence of smoke detectors in rooms
- Unlit stairways, lack of handrails
- Floors cluttered with material and excessive furniture, including footstools
- Kitchen equipment (e.g., ranges, irons, toasters) with hard-to-read settings

Patients living with visual impairment may also be unable to read medication labels and syringe gauges. Therefore, the nurse should ask the patient to read a label to determine whether he or she can adequately see the instructions. If a patient has a hearing impairment, the nurse should check to see whether the sounds of a doorbell, telephone, smoke alarm, and alarm clock are easy to discriminate.

In the hospital environment, caregivers often forget to rearrange furniture and equipment to keep paths from the bed and chair to the bathroom and entrance clear. Walking into a patient's room and looking for safety hazards must be a routine part of nursing care. Check frequently for the following:

- Is the call light within easy, safe reach?
- Are intravenous (IV) poles on wheels and easy to move?
- Are footstools against the bed?
- Are suction machines, IV pumps, or drainage bags positioned so that a patient can rise from a bed or chair easily?

◆ Nursing Diagnosis

After assessment, nurses review all available data and look for patterns and trends suggestive of a health problem relating to sensory alterations (Box 47-8). For example, a patient's advanced age, inattentiveness during conversations, and self-rating of hearing as "poor" are all defining characteristics for the nursing diagnosis of *disturbed sensory perception (auditory)*. Nurses need to validate their findings to ensure the accuracy of the diagnosis. For example, the diagnosis of disturbed thought processes could mistakenly be made if the nurse does not confirm the patient's hearing deficit and perception of poor hearing.

As well, the factor that likely causes the patient's health problem must be determined. In the previous example, impacted cerumen is the cause of the patient's hearing alteration. The etiology or related factor of a nursing diagnosis is a condition that can be affected by nursing interventions. The etiology must be accurate; otherwise, nursing therapies will be ineffective. For a patient with impacted cerumen, regular irrigation of the ear canal has the potential to improve auditory perception (Armstrong, 2009). In contrast, if the patient's auditory alteration were related to hearing loss from nerve deafness, nursing interventions for alternative communication methods would be necessary.

The patient may also have health care problems for which sensory alteration is the etiology, such as with the diagnosis of risk for injury. People with vision loss have double the incidence of falls and double the incidence of difficulties in daily living compared with those without vision loss (National Coalition for Vision Health, 2015). Nurses may also select nursing diagnoses by recognizing the way that sensory alterations affect a patient's ability to function (e.g., self-care deficit). In addition, most patients present themselves to health care providers with multiple diagnoses. In the example of the concept map in Figure 47-4, a patient with retinal detachment has the nursing diagnosis of disturbed sensory perception, which can lead to risk for falls and fear. Nurses must recognize patterns of data that reveal health problems created by the patient's sensory alteration. Examples of nursing diagnoses that might apply to patients with sensory alterations are the following:

- *Impaired adjustment*
- *Impaired verbal communication*
- *Risk for injury*

BOX 47-8 NURSING DIAGNOSTIC PROCESS

Assessment Activities	Defining Characteristics	Nursing Diagnosis
Assess patient's visual acuity.	Has reduced ability to see objects clearly. Needs brighter light to read. Has trouble distinguishing edges of stairs. May have fallen or have had a recent fracture.	*Risk for injury related to visual impairment from cataract formation*
Visit home setting and inspect for any hazards that may pose risks to patient.	Lighting in rooms, hallways, and stairwells is very dim. Carpet in living room is old, and edges are curled up. Steps lead up to front entrance of home.	
Review medical record from clinic visit.	Bilateral cataracts	

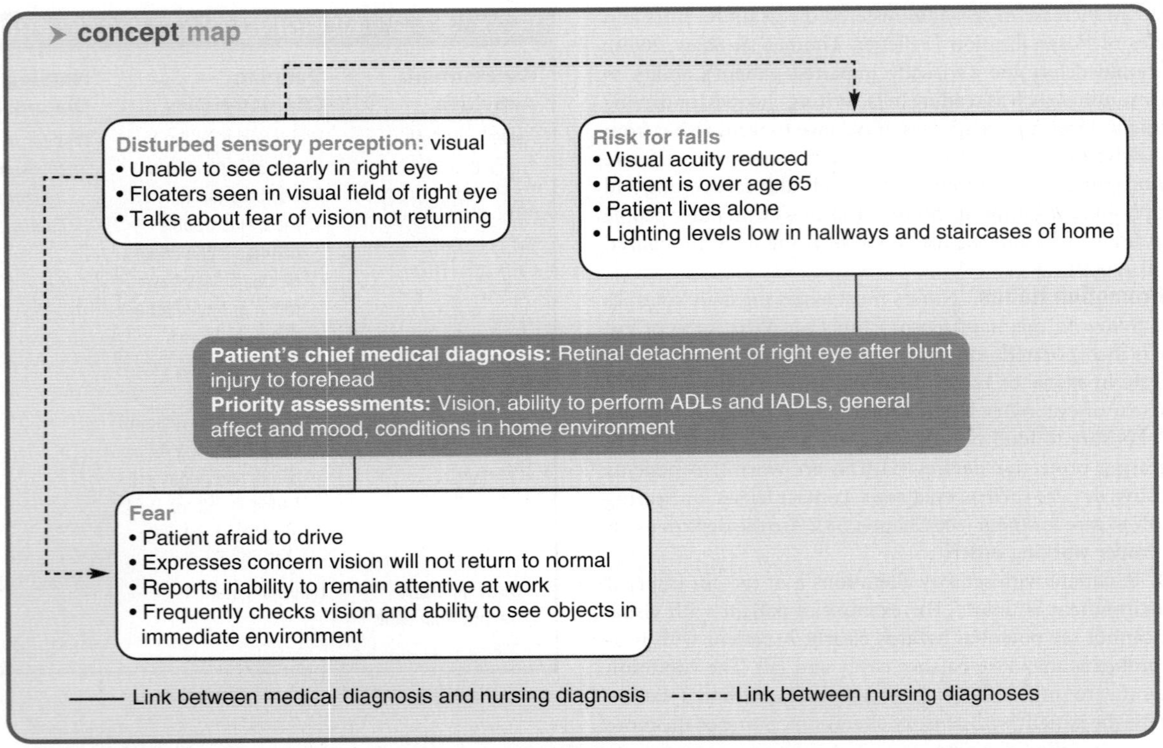

FIGURE 47-4 **Concept map for patient with retinal detachment.** *ADLs,* Activities of daily living; *IADLs,* instrumental activities of daily living.

- *Impaired physical mobility*
- *Self-care deficit—for example, bathing, oral hygiene*
- *Situational low self-esteem*
- *Risk for falls*
- *Social isolation*

◆ Planning

During planning, nurses use critical thinking skills to synthesize information from multiple sources (Figure 47-5), including knowledge gained from the assessment and knowledge of how sensory deficits affect normal functioning. In this way, nurses can recognize the extent of a patient's deficit and know the type of interventions most likely to be helpful. Also to consider are the role that other health care providers can play in planning care and the available community resources (e.g., CNIB) that may be useful. These resources and the nurse's previous experience in caring for patients with sensory alterations can be invaluable when planning nursing approaches.

When applying critical thinking to planning care, professional standards can be particularly useful. These standards, in the form of clinical pathways or clinical practice guidelines, often recommend interventions based on research evidence for the patient's condition. For example, patients who have visual deficits and are hospitalized may be placed on a fall prevention protocol that will incorporate research-based precautions to ensure patient safety.

Goals and Outcomes. During planning, as a nurse you will develop an individualized plan of care for each nursing diagnosis (Box 47-9). With the patient, develop a realistic plan that incorporates what you know about the patient's sensory problems and the extent to which sensory function can be maintained or improved. If maintenance or improvement is not realistic, preventing injury and learning alternative ways of maintaining independence are key. Goals and outcomes should be realistic and measurable. A goal of care for a patient with an actual or potential sensory alteration may be this: "The patient will regain improvement in hearing acuity within 2 weeks." Associated outcomes for this goal might be the following:

- The patient will report using communication techniques for improved reception of messages within 2 weeks.
- The patient will successfully demonstrate the technique for cleaning the hearing aid within 1 week.
- The patient will self-report improved hearing acuity.

Setting Priorities. Priorities of care must be set with regard to the type and extent of sensory alteration that affects a patient. For example, a patient who enters the emergency department after experiencing eye trauma may have priorities of reducing anxiety and preventing further injury to the eye. In contrast, a patient who is being discharged from an outpatient surgery department following cataract removal may have the priority of learning about any self-care requirements. In both cases, however, safety is always a top priority. The patient can also help prioritize aspects of care. For example, patients may wish to learn ways to communicate more effectively or to participate in favourite hobbies, given their sensory limitation.

Some sensory alterations are short term (e.g., a patient suffering sensory or perceptual alterations as a result of sensory overload in a Critical Care Unit) (Box 47-10). Appropriate interventions are thus likely to be temporary (e.g., frequent reorientation or introduction of intimate and pleasant stimuli, such as a back rub). Sensory alterations such as permanent visual loss require long-term goals of care for patients to adapt. Sometimes it becomes necessary for the patient to make major changes in self-care activities, communication, or socialization. Patients who have sensory alterations at the time of entering a health care setting often already have strategies they developed to adapt their lifestyle to their sensory limitations. Nurses need to allow persons with sensory impairment to control whatever part of their care they can.

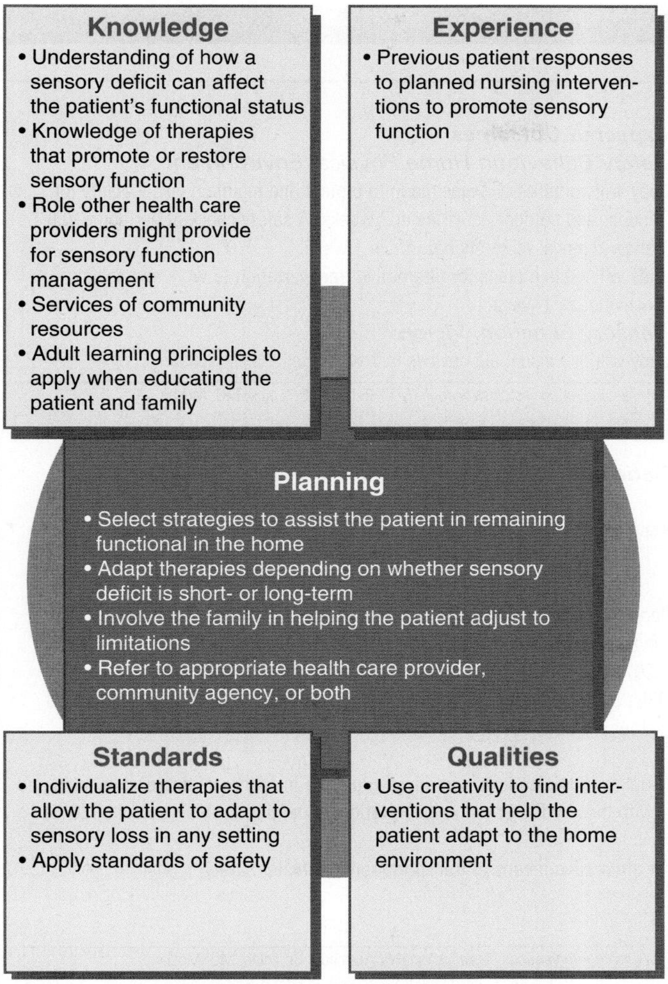

FIGURE 47-5 Critical thinking model for sensory alterations planning.

◆ Implementation

Nursing interventions involve the patient and family. The most effective interventions enable the patient with sensory alterations to function safely with existing deficits and to continue a normal lifestyle. Learning to adjust to sensory impairments can occur at any age with proper support and resources.

When developing a plan of care, it is important to consider all resources available to patients. The family can play a key role in providing meaningful stimulation and learning ways to help the patient adjust to any limitations. Family members should understand how a patient's sensory impairment affects normal daily activities. Family and friends can be more supportive when they understand sensory deficits and the types of elements that worsen or lessen sensory problems. Resources are available within a community that provide information that assists patients with personal management needs and can also provide practical tips and emotional support for family members who are caregivers. For example, the CNIB, Canadian Hearing Society, and the Canadian Association of the Deaf offer resource materials and product information (see "Recommended Websites" section). Nurses need to help family members to focus on the person's abilities rather than on his or her disability.

As part of a multidisciplinary health care team, the nurse may also refer the patient to other health care providers. Early referrals to occupational or speech therapists, for example, can speed a patient's recovery. If a patient has experienced a major loss of sensory function and is also unable to manage medical needs, such as medication self-administration or dressing changes, referral to home care may be an option. Numerous community-based resources (e.g., CNIB, Canadian Association of Independent Living Centres, or the Canadian Hearing Society) are also available. The nurse may be able to arrange for a volunteer to visit the patient or have printed materials made available that describe ways to help cope with sensory problems.

In the community, **health promotion** related to sensory alterations is delivered in doctors' offices, homes, community centres, schools, and industry. Public health nurses, for example, conduct newborn hearing

BOX 47-9 NURSING CARE PLAN

Disturbed Sensory Perception

ASSESSMENT

Judy Long is a 70-year-old widow who lives alone. She tells the community health nurse that her vision has become progressively blurred over the last several years. She comments that she is having her neighbour drive her places.

Assessment Activities	***Findings and Defining Characteristics***
Ask Judy to describe her vision changes.	Judy states, "My left eye seems to have a film over it that makes my vision blurred. I am having difficulty reading. I also have difficulty with night driving; the headlights are large and blurred."
Ask Judy to describe any life changes that have occurred since the change in vision.	Judy indicates that she has always managed her home and done volunteering. She says she is losing her independence because she has to have someone drive her, and she is now hesitant to use stairs at home.
Assess Judy's visual acuity.	Judy cannot read the Snellen chart with the left eye.
Ask Judy the results of the visit to the ophthalmologist.	Judy states that she was told she has a cataract in the left eye and a cataract beginning in her right eye; surgery is planned on her left eye.
Conduct a home hazard assessment.	The home is cluttered, the lighting is dim, and the stairs going into the house have no handrails.

NURSING DIAGNOSIS: Risk for injury.

Continued

BOX 47-9 NURSING CARE PLAN

Disturbed Sensory Perception—cont'd

PLANNING

Goals (Nursing Outcomes Classification)*	***Expected Outcomes***
	Safety Behaviour: Home Physical Environment
Judy will maintain independence in a safe home environment.	Judy will verbalize changes made to protect and maintain visual acuity for indoor and outdoor activities in 2 weeks. A safety check of her home will show removal of safety hazards in 1 week. Judy will explain plans for alternative transportation to work and social activities in 1 week.
	Sensory Function: Vision
Judy will make the best use of existing visual function.	Judy will use visual aid devices in 1 week.

*Outcome classification labels from Moorhead, S., Johnson, M., Maas, M. L., & Swanson, E. (Eds.). (2013). *Nursing outcomes classification (NOC)* (5th ed.). St. Louis, MO: Mosby.

INTERVENTIONS

Interventions (Nursing Interventions Classification)[†]	***Rationale***
Environmental Management	
Teach Judy how to improve the safety of her environment, such as making sure her home is free of clutter, footstools, and electrical cords, and to avoid rearranging furniture.	Keeping the area clutter free reduces the risk of injury (Lim & Sung, 2012).
Teach Judy to use a light over the shoulder for reading and writing.	People with cataracts see better with wider illumination (Perlmutter, 2013).
Encourage use of a magnifier for Judy to use to read the newspaper and mail and advise her on where to purchase it.	Devices will provide magnification to improve visual acuity (Touhy & Jett, 2014).
Encourage her to make an appointment with an ophthalmologist within the next 4 weeks.	Older persons need a routine eye examination annually or as recommended (Touhy & Jett, 2014).
Emotional Support	
Encourage Judy to express feelings regarding loss of vision and lifestyle changes.	People with vision loss experience triple the incidence of depression compared with those without vision loss (National Coalition for Vision Health, 2015).
Family Involvement	
Confer with Judy on selecting a family member, friend, or community resource person who can provide transportation until after the eye condition has been corrected.	An alternative means of transportation will foster safety.

[†]Intervention classification labels are from Bulechek, G. M., Butcher, H. K., & Docherterman, J. M. (2013). *Nursing interventions classification (NIC)* (6th ed.). St. Louis, MO: Mosby.

EVALUATION

Nursing Actions	***Patient Response and Finding***	***Achievement of Outcome***
Ask Judy to describe the changes that have made the home environment safer.	Judy responds that the family has removed the clutter, and handrails have been placed at the entryway. Lighting has been placed behind her chair, and 100-watt lights are in the living room.	Judy reports feeling safer walking up and down the stairs and moving about in her home. The home hazards have been reduced.
During a home visit, observe the home environment for safety hazards.		
Observe Judy's verbal and nonverbal responses to the lifestyle adaptations.	Judy says, "I feel safer when walking in my home."	
As Judy uses a magnifier, have her read a medication label.	Judy is able to read the name of her medication and dosage correctly.	Better use is made of current vision.
Ask Judy if she is able to maintain a degree of independence with the environmental and lifestyle modifications.	Judy states, "I am more independent at home, and until surgery, I do not mind someone driving for me."	Judy has attained some degree of independence.
Ask Judy to identify source of transportation.	Judy says a family member has agreed to drive her for shopping and to her surgery.	Judy has transportation through the weeks required for the surgical experience.

screenings during well-baby clinics and reinforce the importance of parents following the Canadian Ophthalmological Society eye examination guidelines. In long-term care facilities, the nurse can use the Vision Screening Tool at admission to provide a baseline and then annually to assess for changes in vision. In school health programs, the nurse can stress the importance of maintaining the health of eyes and ears. Occupational health nurses play a key role in preventing injury, such as ensuring that safety standards are followed.

Preventive Safety. Trauma is a common cause of blindness in children. Penetrating injuries from propulsive objects such as firecrackers, slingshots, rubber bands, or rocks, and penetrating wounds from sticks, scissors, or toys are just a few examples. Parents and

BOX 47-10 Health Promotion in Practice

Ms. T is in the coronary care unit recovering from coronary artery bypass surgery. Although she is alert and comfortable and her physical needs have been met, she seems anxious. You ask her if she is worried about anything and she says, "I am feeling closed in with all these tubes and the sound of machines all around; it feels like there's not enough air here." You take a minute to demonstrate a simple deep breathing exercise, you do it with her, and encourage her to do this frequently. This intervention alleviates her anxiety and provides her with a tool for self-care.

From Miller, C. (2013). *Fast facts. Health promotion in nursing: Promoting wellness in a nutshell.* New York: Springer Publishing (p. 6).

children require education about ways to avoid eye trauma. Safety equipment can easily be found in most sports shops and large department stores and online. In some Canadian jurisdictions, legislation or association bylaws mandate the wearing of protective equipment (e.g., visors in minor hockey) (CNIB, 2015a).

Since the required use of hockey visors in amateur sport, there has been a steady decline in the incidence of eye injuries from hockey. The biggest barrier that remains today is the stigma associated with using visors and face masks. Parents should play an active role in encouraging their children to wear eye protection on the ice (CNIB, 2015a).

Adults are at risk for eye injury while working in jobs involving exposure to chemicals or flying objects. The Canadian Centre for Occupational Health and Safety has guidelines for safety in the workplace. Employers are required to have employees wear eye goggles or use equipment such as HPDs to reduce the risk of injury. Eyewash stations should be provided where a worker is exposed to potential contact with a biological or chemical substance (Canadian Centre for Occupational Health and Safety, 2017). Nurses in occupational health settings can reinforce use of protective devices and ensure that features such as eyewash stations are in close proximity to the risk for injury.

Preventing hearing loss requires individuals to avoid exposure to continuously high noise levels and brief, loud impulse noise. The potential for hearing loss increases as the decibel level rises. Various provincial jurisdictions mandate occupational noise exposure limits (e.g., Government of Alberta, 2009). HPDs should be worn by patients who must work around noise. Earplugs and earphones are useful in blocking high-decibel sounds.

Another means of hearing-loss prevention involves regular immunization of children against diseases capable of causing hearing loss (e.g., rubella, mumps, and measles). Public health nurses, nurse practitioners, and nurses who work in physicians' offices, schools, and community clinics should reinforce the importance of early and timely immunization. When a child or an adult develops any type of health problem, caution should be used in prescribing drugs that are ototoxic.

Adaptations for Visual Loss. When a patient experiences changes in visual acuity, peripheral vision, adaptation to the dark, or depth perception, safety becomes a concern. With reduced peripheral vision, a patient cannot see panoramically because the outer visual field is less discrete. This creates a special hazard for driving or walking in crowded areas. Adults with reduced adaptation to the dark require three times as much light to see objects as they did as young adults. With reduced depth perception, a person cannot see how far away objects are located, making walking down stairs or over uneven surfaces dangerous.

Driving can also be a safety hazard. Reduced peripheral vision may prevent a driver from seeing a car in an adjacent lane. Reduced adaptation to the dark and sensitivity to glare make driving at night a significant risk. Although vision is a primary consideration for safety, other factors exist as well. In the case of older persons, decreased reaction time, reduced hearing, and decreased strength in the legs and arms may further compromise driving skills. Safety tips for those who continue to drive include driving in familiar areas, not driving during rush hour, avoiding major highways for local drives, using rear-view and side-view mirrors when changing lanes, and avoiding driving at dusk or at night. Older drivers with visual impairment are 40% more likely to have caused a collision than those without visual impairment. Auto collisions are the number one cause of accidental death in 65- to 74-year-olds (Alberta Transportation, 2014).

In Ontario, drivers over the age of 80 are required to renew their licences every 2 years. The renewal process involves a vision test, a written test, a group educational session, and a driving test for some applicants (Ontario Ministry of Transportation, 2014). British Columbia requires a driver's retest for individuals approaching their eightieth birthday. Drivers need to complete a medical examination, vision test, and road test (BCAA Traffic Safety Foundation, 2007).

Visual alterations can make conducting normal activities of daily living more difficult. Because of reduced depth perception, patients can trip on throw rugs, runners, or stairs. Flooring or carpeting should be kept in good repair. The patient should be advised to use low-pile carpeting. Thresholds between rooms should be level with the floor. Clutter should be removed to ensure clear pathways for walking. Furniture should be arranged so that the patient can move about easily without fear of tripping or running into objects. Any stairwell should have a securely fastened handrail extending the full length of the stairs.

Front and back entrances to homes, work areas, and stairwells need to be properly lit. Light fixtures need higher-wattage bulbs with wider illumination. Although less energy efficient, incandescent lighting may be preferred over fluorescent lighting because of the flickering of fluorescent lights. The CNIB website offers suggestions for lighting and other modifications for the visually impaired. A light switch should be located at the top and bottom of stairwells. It is also important that lighting on the stairs does not cast shadows. The nurse should ensure that the patient is able to see the edge of each step clearly, especially the first and last steps. When possible, steps inside and outside the home should be replaced with ramps.

When a patient is unable to see visual contrasts, a number of interventions can be helpful. Sometimes settings on electrical appliances and equipment are only highlighted in black and white or shades of grey. Coloured tape, paint, nail polish, or raised label dots can be used to colour-code appliance dials. Colour can also be useful to highlight the edge of stairs. Applying a broad strip of coloured tape at the stair edge can help a person better see the edges. The nurse can tour the home with the patient to find opportunities for colour-coding. Telephones with large numbers or "picture phones" may be helpful to connect with significant others.

The nurse should also ensure that the patient is able to self-administer medications safely. Labels on medication containers should be in large print. A friend or spouse should always be familiar with dosage schedules. Using a magnifying glass or having family members read prescription medication labels for the patient may be helpful. Audible prescription labelling may become more common in the future (McMahon & Curtis, 2009). People who are visually impaired may have some difficulty manipulating eyedroppers. Eye-drop dispensers are available and often allow older or people with vision loss to independently administer their drops.

The pupil's ability to adjust to light diminishes with age, resulting in the older person becoming more sensitive to glare. Nurses can suggest ways for the patient to minimize glare, such as selecting satin and nonglossy finishes for walls and countertops in the home, selecting a tile pattern for flooring, and choosing sheer curtains, tinted windows, or adjustable shades to reduce outdoor light. Wearing sunglasses outside can reduce the glare of direct sunlight.

The ability to read is important to everyone. Therefore, patients should be encouraged to use their glasses whenever possible (e.g., during procedures and patient instruction), which helps patients remain oriented, maintain some control, and retain their dignity. Patients with reduced visual acuity may need more than corrective lenses. A pocket magnifier can help a patient read most printed material. Telescopic lens eyeglasses are smaller, are easier to focus, and have a greater range. Books and other publications are also available in larger print. If a patient has a legal or other important document he or she wishes to read, standard copying machines have enlarging capabilities. Closed-circuit television magnifying units or portable or desktop video magnifiers using solid-state digital technology enlarge written characters. Minimum and maximum magnification varies from 12 to 60 times the original, depending on the screen size. As well, many word-processing programs allow print to be enlarged, as do e-reader tablets. Audio-recorded books are available and can be readily purchased in bookstores or online or borrowed from public libraries or CNIB.

With aging, a person experiences a change in colour perception. Nurses can offer suggestions of ways the patient may decorate a room and paint hallways or stairwells so that differentiations can be made in surfaces and objects in a room.

The patient with recent visual impairment often requires help with walking. The presence of an eye patch, frequently instilled eye drops, and the swelling of eyelid structures following surgery are just a few factors that can cause a patient to need more assistance than usual. A sighted guide can give confidence to the visually impaired person and ensure safe mobility. The CNIB has published a manual for assisting someone with vision loss (CNIB, 2012). Touhy et al. (2012) list four suggestions for a sighted guide:

- Ask the patient if he or she wants a "sighted guide."
- If assistance is accepted, offer an elbow or arm. Instruct the patient to grasp your arm just above the elbow. If necessary, physically assist the person by guiding his or her hand to your arm or elbow.
- Go one half-step ahead and slightly to the side of the person. The shoulder of the person should be directly behind your shoulder. If the person is frail, place his or her hand on your forearm.
- Relax and walk at a comfortable pace. Warn the patient when you approach doorways or narrow spaces.

While walking the patient, describe the course of movement and ensure that obstacles have been removed. A patient with visual impairment should never be left standing alone in an unfamiliar area. For patients who undergo eye surgery, it is important to teach family members techniques for assisting with ambulation. For those patients who are blind, mobility training is available from CNIB. Guide dogs may also prove useful (CNIB, 2015b). A patient who spends considerable time in bed should have a call light nearby. Necessary objects should be placed in front of the patient to prevent falls caused by reaching over the bedside. Side rails may also be useful to provide added security. At night, a night-light reduces the time required for the eyes to adapt to the dark and enables the patient to see well enough to function without keeping the regular light on.

The nurse should face the patient when speaking, use simple sentences, and speak more slowly and at a normal volume. It is wise to note on the intercom button and the patient's chart if the patient is deaf or blind. A patient lacking the ability to speak cannot call out for assistance. Patients should have message boards or the call light easily available.

Adaptations for Reduced Hearing. To maximize residual hearing function, the nurse works closely with the patient to suggest ways to modify the environment. Telephones and televisions can be amplified. Alarm clocks that shake the bed or activate a flashing light are useful devices. An innovative way to enrich the lives of those with a hearing impairment is recorded music. Some patients with severe hearing loss can hear music recorded in the low-frequency sound cycles. Closed captioning, in which audio content and non-speech information, such as the identity of speakers and sound effects, are described using words or symbols, is available for many television programs.

Important environmental sounds may best be heard if amplified or changed to a lower-pitched, buzzer-like sound. Lamps are available that respond with light to sounds such as doorbells, burglar alarms, smoke detectors, and babies crying. These lamps can be purchased from hearing aid dealers, telephone companies, and appliance stores. Signalling devices allow the person with hearing loss to have greater independence. Family members or anyone who calls the patient regularly should learn to let the telephone ring for longer periods. Amplified receivers for telephones and telephone communications devices use a computer and a printer to transfer words over the telephone for people who are hearing impaired. Both sender and receiver must have the special device to complete a call. Telecommunication relay services (TRS) are available from most telephone companies. A telephone operator service translates voice to text and vice versa. Video relay services (VRS) are also available. VRS enables individuals with hearing disabilities who use American Sign Language to communicate with voice telephone users through video equipment rather than through typed text. Video equipment links the VRS user with an operator so that they can see and communicate with each other in signed conversation (Government of Canada, Canadian Radio-Television and Telecommunications Commission, 2017). The Canadian Hard of Hearing Association (2009) document entitled *Keys to the Communication Revolution* provides a list of key technological breakthroughs for the hearing impaired; however, some of these technologies are not readily available in Canada at this time.

When beginning a conversation with a patient who has a hearing deficit, it helps to reduce any background noise by turning off or lowering the volume of any television, appliance, or radio (Box 47-11). It is also helpful to have conversations in settings where the acoustics are better, which aids in controlling and muffling extraneous background noises. In a group setting, forming a semicircle in front of the patient helps him or her see who is speaking next, thereby fostering group involvement. The patient with a hearing impairment may be able to speak normally. However, the deaf patient's inability to hear self-spoken words may cause serious speech alterations. Patients may use sign language (American or Quebec Sign Language), lip-read, write with a pad and pencil, or learn to use a computer, electronic tablet, or smartphone for communication. Special communication boards that contain common terms used in nursing care (e.g., pain, bathroom, dizzy, or walk) help patients express their needs.

Patient instruction is one aspect of communication. Patients can learn by listening to audiotapes or the sound portion of a televised teaching session. Patients with hearing impairment may benefit from written instructional materials and visual teaching aids (e.g., posters and graphs).

If a patient has any of the following ear conditions, a hearing aid cannot be used: visible congenital or traumatic deformity of the ear, active drainage in the last 90 days, sudden or progressive hearing loss within the last 90 days, acute or chronic dizziness, unilateral sudden hearing loss within the last 90 days, visible cerumen accumulation or a foreign body in the ear canal, pain or discomfort in the ear, or an

BOX 47-11 Communication Methods for Patients With Hearing Impairment

- Get the patient's attention. Do not startle the patient when entering the room. Do not approach a patient from behind. Be sure the patient knows you wish to speak.
- Face the patient and stand or sit on the same level. Be sure your face and lips are illuminated to promote lip-reading. Keep hands away from the mouth.
- If the patient wears glasses, be sure they are clean so that your gestures and face can be seen.
- If the patient wears a hearing aid, make sure it is in place and working.
- Speak slowly and articulate clearly. Older persons may take longer to process verbal messages.
- Use a normal tone of voice and inflections of speech. Do not speak with something in your mouth.
- When you are not understood, rephrase rather than repeat the conversation.
- Use visible expressions. Speak with your hands, your face, and your eyes.
- Do not shout. Loud sounds are usually higher pitched and may impede hearing by accentuating vowel sounds and concealing consonants. If it is necessary to raise your voice, speak in lower tones.
- Speak toward the patient's best or unaffected ear. Use written information to enhance the spoken word.
- Do not restrict a deaf patient's hands. Ensure that IV lines are not secured to both of the patient's hands if the preferred method of communication is sign language.
- Avoid speaking from another room or while walking away.
- Record a hearing impairment in the medical record.

audiometric air–bone gap of 15 decibels or greater. All but the last of these can be detected on physical examination. Referrals to or recommendations that the patient see an otolaryngologist or audiologist for further counselling should be made (Ebersole et al., 2011).

Another option for those with severe to profound hearing loss is a cochlear implant. This is a small, complex electronic device that can help provide a sense of sound to a person who is profoundly deaf or severely hard of hearing. The implant consists of an external portion that sits behind the ear and a second portion that is surgically placed under the skin. An implant does not restore normal hearing. Instead, it can give a deaf person a useful representation of sounds in the environment and help him or her understand speech. A Pocket Talker can also be used to augment spoken volume.

Adaptations for Reduced Taste and Olfaction. Nurses can easily promote the sense of taste by using measures to enhance remaining taste perception.

Good oral hygiene keeps the taste buds well hydrated. Taste perception is heightened if foods are well seasoned, differently textured, and eaten separately. Flavoured vinegar or lemon juice can add tartness to food. The nurse can ask the patient what foods appeal most to taste. If taste perception is improved, food intake and appetite will also improve. A patient can learn to check dates on food packages and the colour and texture of food. Leftovers should be kept in labelled containers with the preparation date.

A reduced sensitivity to odours means that the patient may be unable to smell leaking gas, a smouldering cigarette or fire, or spoiled food. The patient should use smoke and carbon monoxide detectors and other alternative precautions, such as checking ashtrays or placing cigarette butts in water. Pilot gas flames should be checked visually or professionally on a regular basis.

Stimulation of the sense of smell with aromas such as brewing coffee, cooking garlic, and baking bread can heighten taste sensation. Blending or mixing foods should be avoided because these actions make it difficult to identify tastes. Smell can be improved by strengthening pleasant olfactory stimulation. A patient's environment can be made more pleasant with smells such as cologne, mild room deodorizers, fragrant flowers, and sachets, although the patient must be assessed for allergies or sensitivities before using these items. Certain aromas may actually cause patients to lose their appetite.

Removal of unpleasant odours improves the quality of a person's environment. Nurses should keep a patient's room clean, empty bedpans or urinals after use, remove and dispose of soiled dressings, and keep bathroom doors closed.

Adaptations for Reduced Tactile Sensation. Patients with reduced tactile sensation usually have the impairment over a limited portion of their bodies. Nurses can stimulate existing function by using touch therapeutically. If the patient is willing to be touched, hair brushing, a back rub, and touching of the arms or shoulders are ways of increasing tactile contact. When sensation is reduced, firm pressure may be necessary for the patient to feel the nurse's hand. Turning and repositioning can also improve the quality of tactile sensation. When invasive procedures are being performed, it is important to use touch by holding the patient's hands and keeping them warm and dry.

If a patient is overly sensitive to tactile stimuli (hyperesthesia), nurses must minimize irritating stimuli. Keeping bed linens loose to minimize direct contact with the patient and protecting the skin from exposure to irritants are helpful measures. If the patient has numbness and tingling or pain in the hands, as with carpal tunnel syndrome, special wrist splints may be worn to dorsiflex the wrist to relieve the nerve pressure. For those patients who use computers, special keyboards and wrist pads are available to decrease the pressure on the median nerve, aid in relief of pain, and promote healing.

Patients with reduced tactile sensation risk injury because they are unable to sense pressure on bony prominences or the need to change position. These patients rely on nurses for timely repositioning, moving tubes or devices they may be lying on, and turning them to avoid skin breakdown. When the patient is less able to sense temperature variations, nurses should be extra cautious when applying heat and cold therapies and preparing bathwater. Nurses must check the condition of the patient's skin frequently.

The Braden Scale (see Chapter 46) (Braden & Bergstrom, 1988) is a validated tool for assessing pressure injury risk for patients in acute or long-term care and community settings (Registered Nurses' Association of Ontario [RNAO], 2015; Stevenson, 2009). Those identified as at risk are monitored closely to implement preventive and treatment strategies as indicated.

When patients have reduced sensation in their extremities, they are also at risk for injury from exposure to temperature extremes. Nurses should caution them on the use of water bottles or heating pads (see Chapter 46). The temperature of bathwater should always be checked before stepping into the tub.

Safety Alert To create a safe environment, the nurse begins by looking at the results of the home and therapeutic environment assessment (see Chapter 37).

Adaptations to the Environment. The patient with recent sensory impairment requires a complete orientation to the immediate environment. Reorientation to the institutional environment may be provided by ensuring that name tags on uniforms are visible, addressing the patient by name, explaining where the patient is (especially if patients are transported to different areas for treatment), and using conversational cues to time or location. Nurses can reduce the tendency for patients to become confused by offering short, simple, repeated explanations and reassurance. Family members and visitors can also help orient patients to the hospital surroundings.

Patients with serious visual impairment must feel comfortable in knowing the boundaries of the immediate environment. They may want to touch the boundaries of a room or objects to gain a sense of their surroundings. The patient may need to walk through a room and feel the walls to establish a sense of direction. Nurses can help by describing furniture or equipment within the room. As it takes time to absorb a room's arrangement, the patient may need further reorientation, with the nurse explaining the location of key items (e.g., call light, telephone, and chair).

It is important to keep all objects in the same position and place. Simply moving a chair aside may create a dangerous safety hazard. The nurse needs to ask the patient if any item should be arranged to make ambulation easier. Traffic patterns should be kept clear, and use of furniture with sharp edges should be avoided. The patient who is blind needs extra time to perform tasks and a detailed description of how to perform an activity.

Patients confined to bed are at risk for sensory deprivation. Normally, movement gives an integrated awareness of the self through vestibular and tactile stimulation. A person's sensory perception is influenced by movement patterns. The limited movement of bed rest changes how a person interprets the environment; surroundings seem different, and objects seem to assume shapes different from normal. A person who is on bed rest requires routine stimulation through range-of-motion exercises, positioning, and participation in self-care activities (as appropriate). Comfort measures such as washing the patient's face and hands and providing back rubs can help improve the quality of stimulation and lessen the chance of sensory deprivation. Planning time to talk with patients is also essential. The nurse should explain unfamiliar environmental noises and sensations. As well, a calm, unhurried approach during contact with a patient gives the nurse quality time to help reorient and familiarize the patient with care activities. The patient who is well enough to read will benefit from a variety of reading materials.

Promoting Self-Care. The ability to perform self-care is essential for self-esteem. People with chronic conditions who are supported to perform self-care report a higher quality of life, independence, and self-esteem, along with lower levels of depression, anxiety, and fatigue (Robinson, 2010). Frequently, family members and nurses believe that patients with sensory impairments require assistance when, in fact, they can help themselves. Useful guidelines are available to assist patients with visual or tactile impairment so that they can help themselves with daily living activities. For example, a meal tray can be set up as though food on the tray and condiments and drinks around the tray are numbers on the face of a clock. The visually impaired patient can easily become oriented to the items after the nurse or family member explains each item's location.

The patient with visual problems may need assistance in reaching toilet facilities safely. Safety bars should be installed near the toilet. It may be helpful to have the bar a different colour than the wall for easier visibility. Towels should never be placed on safety bars because they may interfere with a person's grasp. Toilet paper should be within easy reach. The use of sharply contrasting colours, especially red, on drawers and other places helps promote functional independence. Choosing clothes that match can be an issue, but techniques such as hanging clothes together on a hanger or marking them with similar labels often overcome this difficulty. The patient's preference must always be considered when helping to arrange or buy clothes.

If tactile sense is diminished, the patient can dress more easily with zippers or Velcro strips, pullover sweaters or blouses, and elasticized waists. If a patient has partial paralysis and reduced sensation, the affected side should be dressed first.

Patients with proprioceptive problems may lose balance easily. Floor mats should have rubberized, skid-proof bottoms. They should be checked and replaced as needed. Bathrooms should have nonskid surfaces in the tub and shower. Grab bars should be installed either vertically or horizontally in tubs and showers, depending on how the patient is able to grasp or hold on to the bar. Nurses can instruct family members to supervise ambulation and sitting, make frequent checks to prevent falls, and help caution the patient against leaning forward.

Any sensory impairment has a significant influence on body image, and it is important for the patient to feel well-groomed and attractive. Some patients may need assistance with basic grooming. Others may need assistance with medication selection, clothing identification, and learning to manage routine procedures, such as blood pressure and glucose monitoring. A variety of aids are available to help individuals with varying types of sensory deficits. It is important to assist patients in maintaining a degree of independence and in having as much control over the management of their care and lifestyle as possible.

◆ Evaluation

Evaluation of Patient Care. It is essential to determine whether care measures maintain or improve patients' ability to interact and function within their environment. Only patients themselves will know if their sensory abilities are improved and which interventions or therapies are most successful in facilitating a change in their performance (Figure 47-6). Nurses can collaborate with family members to determine if a patient's ability to function within the home has improved. To evaluate the effectiveness of nursing interventions, nurses use critical thinking and make comparisons with the baseline sensory assessment data to evaluate if sensory alterations have changed.

If, as a nurse, you have developed a good relationship with a patient and have a therapeutic plan of care, subtle behaviours often indicate the level of the patient's satisfaction. Note whether the patient responds appropriately, such as by smiling. As well, observe whether the patient interacts more and is not asking to have information repeated. Ask the patient, "Can you tell me if you feel we have done all we can do to help improve your ability to hear?" If the patient's expectations have not been met, then you need to spend more time understanding the patient's needs and specific preferences. Ask the patient, "What else can the health care team do to meet your needs?" Working closely with the patient and family will enable you to redefine expectations that can be realistically met within the limits of the patient's condition and therapies. Interventions are effective when goals and expectations have been met.

Patient Outcomes. As the nurse, you determine if expected outcomes have been met. The nature of the sensory alteration influences the way you evaluate the outcome of care. Look back on the goals and interventions for nursing care. Discuss goals and interventions with the patient, family, and multidisciplinary team members and reflect on their perspectives of meeting these goals. What went well? What could have been improved? What still needs to be done? What is the patient's perception of the nursing care? For example, you use proper communication techniques with a patient with a hearing deficit and then evaluate whether the patient has gained the ability to hear or interact more effectively. When expected outcomes have not been achieved, it may

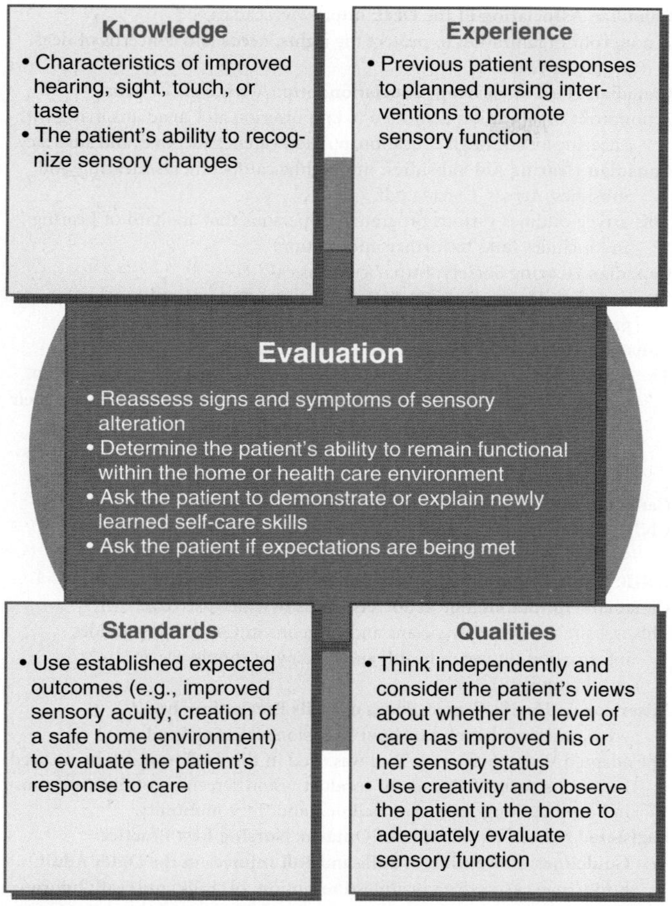

FIGURE 47-6 Critical thinking model for sensory alterations evaluation.

be necessary to change interventions or alter the patient's environment. Family members may need to be involved in support of the patient. You may also consult with the multidisciplinary team (e.g., physician, occupational therapist, audiologist) for suggestions to achieve unmet needs. The patient must be involved in all evaluation and planning activities.

If nursing care has been directed at improving sensory acuity, evaluate the integrity of the sensory organs and the patient's ability to perceive stimuli. Any interventions designed to relieve problems associated with sensory alterations are evaluated on the basis of the patient's ability to function normally without injury. When you attempt to directly or indirectly (through education) alter the patient's environment, evaluation is directed at observing whether the patient makes environmental changes. When patient teaching is designed to improve a patient's sensory function, it is important to determine whether the patient is following recommended therapies. Asking the patient to explain or demonstrate self-care skills aids in evaluating the level of learning that has occurred. It is often necessary to reinforce previous instruction if learning has not taken place. The results of your evaluation will determine whether to continue the existing plan of care, make modifications, or end the use of certain interventions.

Acknowledgment

The chapter author gratefully acknowledges Donnie McIntosh, BN, MEd, for her contributions in the revisions of this chapter.

KEY CONCEPTS

- When sensory function is impaired, the sense of self is impaired and can affect one's ability to socialize.
- Multiple factors can result in sensory alterations, which are sometimes difficult to identify separately.
- Uncorrected vision impairment can lead to falls, fractures, depression, social isolation, behavioural changes, and cognitive impairment.
- Aging usually results in a gradual decline of acuity in all senses.
- It is important to differentiate between medical conditions or disease symptoms and normal aging changes.
- Patients who are older, immobilized, or confined in isolated environments are at risk for sensory alterations.
- Assessment of a patient's health promotion habits helps reveal risks for sensory impairment.
- An individual may not admit to a sensory loss.
- The plan of care for patients with sensory alterations needs to include participation from family members in the assessment and in the intervention plan.

CRITICAL THINKING EXERCISES

1. Mr. Kalinski is a 54-year-old farmer who is having a physical examination. Overall, his health is good. His wife reports that over the past year she has noticed bruising on his arms and legs and burns on his arms. He says he has no idea how they got there and that they do not hurt. What assessment data are needed? What is your nursing diagnosis? Are there several? What specific interventions may be needed?
2. Mrs. Martell, 79 years old, is visiting the nurse practitioner clinic for a routine checkup for the first time. You notice that she needed help reading the paper forms requesting information on her health history. She also told you she is having increased difficulty driving at night. What questions would you ask and what screening would you do regarding her visual difficulties, in addition to your full assessment?
3. You have an opportunity to speak with a group of parents and students regarding prevention of hearing problems. What information would you share with this varied age group to promote healthy hearing?
4. You are a nurse in a long-term care facility. It is suspected that Mrs. Donovan may have *C. diff.* As a precaution, you place her in isolation in her room until the test results arrive. She has been in isolation for 4 days now. She has been displaying angry behaviour, not recognizing staff, and asking when she can return home. What would your assessment include? Identify your nursing diagnosis or diagnoses. What type of interventions can you and your staff carry out for Mrs. Donovan?

REVIEW QUESTIONS

1. Select the sense that enables a person to be aware of the position and movement of body parts without seeing them:
   1. Tactile
   2. Auditory
   3. Gustatory
   4. Kinesthetic
2. A sense that allows a person to recognize an object's size, shape, and texture is:
   1. Tactile
   2. Gustatory

3. Kinesthetic
4. Stereognostic

3. A patient who is in constant pain and undergoes frequent monitoring of vital signs is at risk for experiencing sensory:
   1. Deficits
   2. Stimuli
   3. Overload
   4. Deprivation
4. Proprioceptive changes after 60 years of age include increased:
   1. Hearing and vision impairment
   2. Vision impairment and difficulty with spatial orientation
   3. Difficulty with balance, spatial orientation, and coordination
   4. Hearing impairment and difficulty with balance and coordination
5. For a patient who has a hearing impairment, the nurse should
   1. Approach a patient quietly from behind
   2. Select a public area to have a spoken conversation
   3. Face the patient when speaking and speak slower and at a normal volume
   4. Face the patient when speaking and use a louder-than-normal tone of voice
6. When obtaining a history of the patient's hearing loss, the nurse should ask,
   1. "How long have you been deaf?"
   2. "Do you also have vision problems?"
   3. "Why don't you pay attention to me while I speak?"
   4. "How does your hearing now compare with your hearing a year ago?"
7. A realistic goal for an older patient who drives is to:
   1. Drive very slowly all of the time
   2. Always drive at night to prevent sun glare
   3. Drive during rush hour when others are on the road
   4. Use rear-view and side-view mirrors when changing lanes
8. To prevent hearing impairment among children, a nursing intervention is to teach parents, schoolteachers, and children to:
   1. Administer antibiotics to reduce the risk of infections
   2. Avoid activities in which crowds and loud noises occur
   3. Delay childhood immunizations until hearing can be verified
   4. Take precautions when involved in activities associated with high-intensity noises
9. A high priority in a home assessment for a patient with diminished olfaction is the inclusion of:
   1. Extra lighting in hallways
   2. Smoke detectors on all levels
   3. Amplified telephone receivers
   4. A low-temperature water setting
10. Sensory deficits happen when a problem with sensory reception or perception occurs. As a result, patients may:
    1. Rely solely on one sense
    2. Respond normally to stimuli
    3. Withdraw socially to cope with the loss
    4. Function safely within their environment

Answers: 1. 4; **2.** 4; **3.** 3; **4.** 3; **5.** 3; **6.** 4; **7.** 4; **8.** 4; **9.** 2; **10.** 3

Rationales for the Review Questions appear at the end of the book.

RECOMMENDED WEBSITES

Accessible Media Inc.: http://www.ami.ca/about-ami.
Accessible Media Inc. is a nonprofit audio newsstand that broadcasts international, national, regional, and local stories from over 600 Canadian newspapers and magazines.

Canadian Association of the Deaf: http://www.cad.ca.
A nonprofit organization to protect the rights, needs and concerns of deaf people in Canada.

Canadian Hard of Hearing Association: http://www.chha.ca/chha/.
A nonprofit organization dedicated to empowering all Canadians living with a hearing loss through education, public awareness, services and advocacy.

Canadian Hearing Aid Subsidies: http://chha.ca/documents/Hearing_Aid_Subsidies_Across_Canada.pdf.
This article outlines various programs for persons that are hard of hearing and includes links to further information.

Canadian Hearing Society: http://www.chs.ca/.
The Canadian Hearing Society provides services that prevent hearing loss and promote the independence of deaf and hearing-impaired people.

Canadian Helen Keller Centre: http://www.chkc.org/.
The Canadian Helen Keller Centre (CHKC) provides training programs to individuals who are deaf-blind to help them increase and maintain their independence and autonomy, access services in the community, and decrease isolation. The website provides links relevant to deaf-blindness and communicating with people who are deaf-blind.

Canadian National Institute for the Blind (CNIB): http://www.cnib.ca/.
CNIB is a national, voluntary organization that offers information and support to people with vision loss.

CNIB: Guide Dogs: http://www.cnib.ca/en/living/guide-dog/.

Canadian Ophthalmological Society: http://www.cos-sco.ca/.
This website is for eye physicians and surgeons in Canada. It provides information on vision health and when you should see an ophthalmologist.

Misericordia Health Centre, Focus on Falls Prevention: http://www.misericordia.mb.ca/AboutUs/VisionScreening.html.
The adapted Vision Screening Tool was used in this facility and is being used in various parts of Canada to conduct vision screening of older persons in hospitals, long-term care facilities, and the community.

Registered Nurses' Association of Ontario, Nursing Best Practice Guidelines: Prevention of Falls and Fall Injuries in the Older Adult: http://rnao.ca/sites/rnao-ca/files/Prevention_of_Falls_and_Fall_Injuries_in_the_Older_Adult.pdf.
These guidelines outline evidence-based approaches for preventing falls and reducing fall injuries for older adults.

SeeHear Canada: http://see-hear.ca/.
SeeHear screens hearing and vision for both elementary-aged children in their schools and adults in their workplaces.

Voice for Deaf and Hard of Hearing Children: http://www.voicefordeafkids.com/.
A nonprofit organization that provides support and education for the general public on deaf and hard of hearing children.

REFERENCES

Access Economics Pty Limited. (2008). *Cost of vision loss in Canada.* Toronto: Canadian Ophthalmological Society & Canadian National Institute for the Blind. Retrieved from http://www.cnib.ca/eng/cnib%20document%20library/research/covl_full_report.pdf.

Adams-Wendling, L., & Pimple, C. (2008). Nursing management of hearing impairment in nursing facility residents. *Journal of Gerontological Nursing, 34*(11), 9–17.

Alberta Transportation. (2014). *Information for mature drivers.* Retrieved from https://www.transportation.alberta.ca/content/docType45/Production/SeniorsPamphlet.pdf.

Amit, M., & Canadian Paediatric Society, Community Paediatrics Committee. (2009/2016). Vision screening in infants, children and youth. *Paediatrics & Child Health, 14*(4), 246–248. Retrieved from https://www.cps.ca/en/documents/position/children-vision-screening.

Armstrong, C. (2009). Diagnosis and management of cerumen impaction. *American Family Physician, 80*(9), 1011–1013.

Baker, N., Taggart, H., Nivens, A., et al. (2015). Delirium: Why are nurses confused? *Medsurg Nursing, 24*(1), 15–22.

Barnes, S., & Sewell, D. (2014). The value and underutilization of simple reading glasses in geropsychiatry inpatient settings. *American Journal of Alzheimer's Disease & Other Dementias, 29*(8), 657–659. doi:10.1177/1533317514539034.

Barnett, T. O. (2007). Problems of the ear. In F. Monahan, J. Sands, M. Neighbors, et al. (Eds.), *Phipps' medical-surgical nursing: Health and illness perspectives* (8th ed.). St. Louis, MO: Mosby.

BCAA Traffic Safety Foundation. (2007). *Mature Drivers Program: Driver's re-test.* Retrieved from http://www.tsf-bcaa.com/pdf/Driver_Re_test.pdf.

Boxerman, H., Wittich, W., & Overbury, O. (2015). Charles Bonnet syndrome in older adults with age-related macular degeneration: Its relationship to depression and mild cognitive impairment. *British Journal of Visual Impairment, 33*(1), 19–30. doi:10.1177/0264619614557529.

Braden, B., & Bergstrom, N. (1988). *Braden Scale for Predicting Pressure Sore Risk.* Retrieved from http://www.bradenscale.com/images/bradenscale.pdf.

Cabral, T., da Silva, L., Tudella, E., et al. (2015). Motor development and sensory processing: A comparative study between preterm and term infants. *Research in Developmental Disabilities, 36*, 102–107.

Cacchione, P. (2014). Sensory impairment: A new research imperative. *Journal of Gerontological Nursing, 40*(4), 3–5. doi:10.3928/00989134-20140306-01.

Canadian Centre for Occupational Health and Safety. (2017). *Emergency showers and eyewash stations.* Retrieved from http://www.ccohs.ca/oshanswers/safety_haz/emer_showers.html.

Canadian Hard of Hearing Association. (2009). *Hearing Awareness Project: Keys to the communication revolution.* Retrieved from http://chha.ca/chha/projects-keys.php.

Canadian Hard of Hearing Association. (2015). *Canadian hearing aid subsidies and workers compensation.* Retrieved from http://chha.ca/documents/Hearing_Aid_Subsidies_Across_Canada.pdf.

Canadian Hearing Society. (2018a). *Facts and figures.* Retrieved from http://www.chs.ca/facts-and-figures.

Canadian Hearing Society. (2018b). *Tinnitus and sound sensitivity consultation.* Retrieved from http://www.chs.ca/services/tinnitus-and-hyperacusis-consultations.

Canadian Infant Hearing Task Force. (2016). *Position statement on early hearing detection and intervention (EHDI): Canadian Infant Hearing Task Force.* Retrieved from http://www.infanthearingcanada.ca/wp-content/uploads/2016/01/2016-EHDI-CIHTF-Position-Statement.pdf.

Canadian National Institute for the Blind (CNIB). (2012). Step-by-step: *A how-to manual for guiding someone who is blind or partially sighted.* Retrieved from http://www.cnib.ca/en/about/Publications/vision-health/Documents/CNIB_STEP_BY_STEP_2012_ENG%20FINAL-s.pdf.

Canadian National Institute for the Blind (CNIB). (2015a). *Eye safety in hockey.* Retrieved from http://www.cnib.ca/en/your-eyes/safety/at-play/Pages/hockey.aspx.

Canadian National Institute for the Blind (CNIB). (2015b). *Guide dogs.* Retrieved from http://www.cnib.ca/en/living/guide-dog/.

Canadian Ophthalmological Society. (2007). *Retinal detachment: A serious problem.* Retrieved from http://www.eyesite.ca/english/public-information/eye-conditions/pdfs/RetinalDetach_e.pdf.

Capezuti, E. A., Siegler, E. L., & Mezey, M. D. (2008). *Encyclopedia of elder care. The comprehensive resource on geriatric and social care* (2nd ed.). New York: Springer Publishing.

Carnicelli, A. (2001). *Vision screening for older people: A joint initiative between the Royal Victoria Eye and Ear Hospital and the Centre for Eye Research Australia.* East Melbourne, Australia: Royal Victoria Eye and Ear Hospital and the Centre for Eye Research Australia.

Crews, J., & Campbell, V. (2004). Vision impairment and hearing loss among community-dwelling older Americans: Implications for health and functioning. *American Journal of Public Health, 94*, 823–829.

Crumbliss, K., Taussig, M., & Jay, W. (2009). Vision rehabilitation and Charles Bonnet syndrome. *Seminars in Ophthalmology, 23*, 121–126.

Darcy, A., Hancock, L., & Ware, E. (2008). A descriptive study of noise in the neonatal intensive care unit: Ambient levels and perceptions of contributing factors. *Advances in Neonatal Care, 8*(3), 165–175. Republished in *Advances in Neonatal Care, 8*(5 Suppl.), S16–S26.

Dunn, A., Burns, C., & Sattler, B. (2003). Environmental health of children. *Journal of Pediatric Health Care, 17*(5), 223–231.

Dworkin, R., Malone, D., Panarites, C., et al. (2010). Impact of postherpetic neuralgia and painful diabetic peripheral neuropathy on health care costs. *Journal of Pain, 11*(4), 360–368. doi:10.1016/j.jpain.2009.08.005.

Ebersole, P., Touhy, T., Hess, P., et al. (2011). *Toward healthy aging: Human needs and nursing response* (8th ed.). St. Louis, MO: Mosby/Elsevier.

Fausti, S. A., Wimington, D. J., Helt, P. V., et al. (2005). Hearing health and care: The need for improved hearing loss prevention and hearing conservation practices. *Journal of Rehabilitation Research and Development, 42*(4), 45–61. doi:10.1682/JRRD.2005.002.0039.

Folstein, M., Folstein, S., & McHugh, P. (1975). "Mini-Mental State": A practical method for grading the cognitive state of patients for the clinician. *Journal of Psychiatric Research, 12*(3), 189–198. doi:10.1016/0022-3956(75)90026-6.

Franks, K., Chuah, M., King, A., et al. (2015). Connectivity of pathology: The olfactory system as a model for network-driven mechanisms of Alzheimer's disease pathogenesis. *Frontiers in Aging Neuroscience, 7*, 1–12. doi:10.3389/fnagi.2015.00234.

Giersiepen, K., & Spallek, M. (2011). Carpal tunnel syndrome as an occupational disease. *Deutsches Arzteblatt International, 108*(4), 238–242. doi:10.3238/arztebl.2011.0238.

Gold, D., Zuvela, B., & Hodge, W. (2007). Perspectives on low vision service in Canada: A pilot study. *Canadian Journal of Ophthalmology, 41*(3), 348–354.

Government of Canada. Canadian Radio-television and Telecommunications Commission. (2017). *Video Relay Services.* Retrieved from https://crtc.gc.ca/eng/phone/acces/rela.htm.

Government of Alberta. (2009). *Occupational Health and Safety Act. Noise exposure.* Retrieved from https://work.alberta.ca/documents/WHS-LEG_ohsc_2009.pdf.

Gravel, D., Miller, M., Simor, A., et al. (2009). Health care-associated Clostridium difficile infection in adults admitted to acute care hospitals in Canada: A Canadian nosocomial infection surveillance program study. *Clinical Infectious Diseases, 48*, 568–576.

Hanewinckel, R., Ikram, M., & van Doorn, P. (2016). Assessment scales for the diagnosis of polyneuropathy. *Journal of the Peripheral Nervous System, 21*(2), 61–73. doi:10.1111/jns.12170.

Hawranik, P., & Bell, S. (2007). Vision care in long-term care facilities: An overlooked need. *Canadian Journal of Geriatrics, 10*(3, Suppl. 1), 15–18.

Health Canada. (2005). *It's your health: Hearing loss and leisure noise.* Ottawa: Author. Retrieved from http://publications.gc.ca/collections/collection_2008/hc-sc/H50-3-166-2005E.pdf.

Health Canada. (2010). *Noise from machinery intended for the workplace.* Ottawa: Author. Retrieved from http://www.hc-sc.gc.ca/ewh-semt/noise-bruit/machinery-machines-eng.php.

Hockenberry, M. J., & Wilson, D. (2015). *Wong's nursing care of infants and children* (8th ed.). St. Louis, MO: Mosby.

Howe, F., & Stagg, S. (2016). How sensory experiences affect adolescents with an autistic spectrum condition within the classroom. *Journal of Autism and Developmental Disorders, 46*(5), 1656–1668. doi:10.1007/s10803-015-2693-1.

Hubbard, R. E., O'Mahony, M. S., & Woodhouse, K. W. (2013). Medication prescribing in frail older people. *European Journal of Clinical Pharmacology, 69*(3), 319–326. doi:10.1007/s00228-012-1387-2.

Humes, L. (2015). Age-related changes in cognitive and sensory processing: Focus on middle-aged adults. *American Journal of Audiology, 24*(2), 94–97. doi:10.1044/2015_AJA-14-0063.

Ibrahim, I., Khan, W., Goddard, N., et al. (2012). Carpal tunnel syndrome: A review of the recent literature. *Open Orthopedic Journal, 6*, 69–76. doi:10.2174/1874325001206010069.

Jerez-Roig, J., Medeiros, L., Silva, V., et al. (2014). Prevalence of self-medication and associated factors in an elderly population: A systematic review. *Drugs and Aging, 31*(2), 883–896. doi:10.1007/s40266-014-0217-x.

Karpa, M., Gopinath, B., Beath, K., et al. (2010). Associations between hearing impairment and mortality risk in older persons: The Blue Mountains Hearing Study. *Annals of Epidemiology, 20*(6), 452–459. doi:10.1016/j.annepidem.2010.03.011.

Kerschner, J. E., Lindstrom, D. R., Pomeranz, A., et al. (2005). Comparison of caregiver otitis media risk factor knowledge in suburban and urban primary care environments. *International Journal of Pediatric Otorhinolaryngology, 69*, 49–56.

Lim, Y., & Sung, M. (2012). Home environmental and health-related factors among home fallers and recurrent fallers in community dwelling older Korean women. *International Journal of Nursing Practice, 18*(5), 481–488. doi:10.1111/j.1440-172X.2012.02060.x.

Masurkar, A., & Devanand, D. (2014). Olfactory dysfunction in the elderly: Basic circuitry and alterations with normal aging and Alzheimer's disease. *Current Geriatric Reports, 3*(2), 91–100. doi:10.1007/s13670-014-0080-y.

McCance, K. L., & Huether, S. E. (2014). *Pathophysiology: The biologic basis for disease in adults and children* (7th ed.). St. Louis, MO: Elsevier Mosby.

McMahon, J., & Curtis, A. (2009). Methods of reading information on labels of prescription medications by persons who are visually impaired. *Journal of Visual Impairment & Blindness, 103*(5), 303–308.

Menon, G. (2005). Complex visual hallucinations in the visually impaired: A structured history-taking approach. *Archives of Ophthalmology, 123*(3), 349–355.

Methven, L., Jimenez-Pranteda, M., & Lawlor, J. (2016). Sensory and consumer science methods used with older adults: A review of current methods and recommendations for the future. *Food Quality and Preferences, 48*(Pt. B), 333–344. doi:10.1016/j.foodqual.2015.07.001.

Mueller, C. (2015). Nutrition assessment and older adults. *Topics in Clinical Nutrition, 30*(1), 94–102. doi:10.1097/TIN.0000000000000022.

Muzychka, M. (2009). *Environmental scan of vision health and vision loss in the provinces and territories of Canada.* Toronto: National Coalition for Vision Health.

Nair, A., Nair, A., Shah, B., et al. (2014). Seeing the unseen: Charles Bonnet syndrome revisited. *Psychogeriatrics, 15*(3), 204–208. doi:10.1111/psyg.12091.

National Coalition for Vision Health. (2015). *Vision loss in Canada.* Toronto: Author. Retrieved from http://www.canadianjournalofophthalmology.ca/article/S0008-4182(07)80039-1/abstract.

Ontario Ministry of Transportation. (2014). *Aging and driving: Ontario's licence renewal program for drivers age 80 and above.* Retrieved from http://www.mto.gov.on.ca/english/driver/pdfs/ges-booklet-english.pdf.

Oyarzun-Gonzalez, X., Myers, S., Muldoon, S., et al. (2015). Cognitive decline and polypharmacy in an elderly population. *Journal of the American Geriatrics Society, 63*(1), 397–399. doi:10.1111/jgs.13283.

Pelletier, A., Thomas, J., & Shaw, F. (2009). Vision loss in older persons. *American Family Physician, 79*(11), 963–970.

Perlmutter, M. (2013). Home lighting assessment for clients with low vision. *American Journal of Occupational Therapy, 67*(6), 674–682. doi:10.5014/ajot.2013.006692.

Perlmutter, M., Bhorade, A., Gordon, M., et al. (2010). Cognitive, visual, auditory, and emotional factors that affect participation in older adults. *American Journal of Occupational Therapy, 64*(4), 570–579. doi:10.5014/ajot.2010.09089.

Public Health Agency of Canada. (2006). *Hearing loss info sheet for seniors.* Retrieved from http://seniorspolicylens.ca/Root/Materials/Adobe%20Acrobat%20Materials/Hearing_Loss_Info-Sheet.pdf.

Registered Nurses' Association of Ontario (RNAO). (2015). *Nursing best practice guidelines: Risk assessment and prevention of pressure ulcers. Summary of recommendations.* Toronto: Author. Retrieved from http://rnao.ca/bpg/guidelines/risk-assessment-and-prevention-pressure-ulcers.

Robinson, B., Feng, Y., Woods, C., et al. (2013). Prevalence of visual impairment and uncorrected refractive error—Report from a Canadian urban population-based study. *Ophthalmic Epidemiology, 20*(3), 123–130. doi:10.3109/09286586.2013.789915.

Robinson, F. (2010). Self-care for people with long-term conditions. *Practice Nurse, 40*(8), 9–10.

Robinson, S., Rich, C., Weitzel, T., et al. (2008). Delirium prevention for cognitive, sensory, and mobility impairments. *Research and Theory for Nursing Practice, 22*(2), 103–113. doi:10.1891/0889-7182.22.2.103.

Rowles, C. J., & Russo, B. L. (2009). Strategies to promote critical thinking and active learning. In D. M. Billings & J. A. Halstead (Eds.), *Teaching in nursing: A guide for faculty* (3rd ed., pp. 238–261). St. Louis, MO: Saunders Elsevier.

Sendelbach, S., & Guthrie, P. (2009). Evidence-based guideline: Acute confusion/delirium identification, assessment, treatment, and prevention. *Journal of Gerontological Nursing, 35*(11), 11–18.

Smith, S. C., & Neely, S. (2007). Nursing management: Visual and auditory problems. In S. L. Lewis, M. Heitkemper, S. Dirksen, et al. (Eds.), *Medical-surgical nursing: Assessment and management of clinical problems* (7th ed.). St. Louis, MO: Mosby Elsevier.

Speros, C. I. (2009). More than words: Promoting health literacy in older adults. *Online Journal of Issues in Nursing, 14*(3), K1.

Sprinzl, G., & Riechelmann, H. (2010). Current trends in treating hearing loss in elderly people: A review of the technology and treatment options—A mini-review. *Gerontology, 56*(3), 351–358. doi:10.1159/000275062.

Stark, P., & Hickson, L. (2004). Outcomes of hearing aid fitting for older people with hearing impairment and their significant others. *International Journal of Audiology, 43*, 390–398.

Stevenson, K. (2009). Pressure ulcer prevention: When are we negligent? *Wound Care Canada, 7*(2), 30–32.

Touhy, T., & Jett, P. (2014). *Ebersole and Hess' gerontological nursing & healthy aging* (4th ed.). St. Louis: Mosby.

Touhy, T., Jett, A., Boscart, V., et al. (2012). *Ebersole & Hess's gerontological nursing and healthy aging* (Canadian ed.). Toronto: Elsevier Canada.

Vogel, I., Brug, J., Hosli, E. J., et al. (2008). MP3 players and hearing loss: Adolescents' perceptions of loud music and hearing conversation. *Journal of Pediatrics, 152*(3), 400–404. doi:10.1016/j.jpeds.2007.07.009.

Whitson, H. E., Cousins, S. W., Burchett, B. M., et al. (2007). The combined effect of visual impairment and cognitive impairment on disability in older people. *Journal of the American Geriatrics Society, 55*, 885–891.

Wofford, K., & Vacchiano, C. (2011). Sorting through the confusion: Adverse cognitive change after surgery in adults. *American Association of Nurse Anesthetists, 79*(4), 335–342.

World Health Organization (WHO). (2012). *WHO releases the new global estimates on visual impairment.* Retrieved from http://www.who.int/blindness/en/.

48

Care of Surgical Patients

Canadian content written by Frances Fothergill-Bourbonnais, RN, PhD
Original chapter by Antoinette Falker, DNP, RN, CMSRN, CBN, GCNS-BC

OBJECTIVES

Mastery of content in this chapter will enable you to:

- Define the key terms listed.
- Understand the aspects of perioperative nursing care.
- Differentiate between classifications of surgery and types of anaesthesia.
- List factors to include in the preoperative, intraoperative, and postoperative assessment of a surgical patient.
- Demonstrate postoperative exercises: diaphragmatic breathing, coughing, turning, and leg exercises.
- Design a preoperative teaching plan.
- Prepare a patient for surgery.
- Explain the nurse's role in the operating room.
- Describe the rationales for nursing interventions designed to prevent postoperative complications.
- Explain the differences and similarities in caring for ambulatory (day) surgical patients and caring for inpatient surgical patients.

KEY TERMS

Abdominal gas, p. 1406
Antiembolism stockings, p. 1396
Atelectasis, p. 1368
Bariatric, p. 1368
Cholecystectomy, p. 1365
Circulating nurse, p. 1395
Clinical pathways, p. 1378
Convalescence, p. 1398
Dehiscence, p. 1370
Dermatomes, p. 1401
General anaesthesia, p. 1396
Informed consent, p. 1378
Latex sensitivity, p. 1394
Local anaesthesia, p. 1397
Malignant hyperthermia, p. 1401
Paralytic ileus, p. 1402
Perioperative nursing, p. 1363
Postanesthesia Recovery Score (PARS), p. 1398
Postanesthesia Recovery Score for Ambulatory Patients (PARSAP), p. 1399
Preoperative teaching plan, p. 1375
Procedural sedation, p. 1397
Regional anaesthesia, p. 1396
Same-day surgery, p. 1364
Scrub nurse, p. 1395
Sequential compression device, p. 1396

MEDIA RESOURCES

http://evolve.elsevier.com/Canada/Potter/fundamentals/

- Audio Chapter Summaries
- Examination Review Questions
- Concept Map Creator
- Case Study With Questions
- Audio Glossary
- Content Updates
- Video Clips

Perioperative nursing care includes care given before (preoperative), during (intraoperative), and after (postoperative) surgery. Surgical procedures generally take place in a hospital, although some minor surgical procedures can be conducted in a physician's office. Perioperative nursing is based on nurses' understanding of several important principles, including the following:

- Excellence in perioperative practice
- Interprofessional teamwork
- Effective and therapeutic communication and collaboration with the patient, the patient's family, and the surgical team
- Effective and efficient patient assessment and intervention in all phases
- Advocacy on behalf of the patient and the patient's family
- Understanding of cost containment
- Understanding of patient safety

As a nurse, you must act as an advocate for your patient, communicate with compassion, thoroughly document care, and emphasize patient safety in all phases of care. The nursing process provides a basis for perioperative nursing, with the nurse individualizing strategies so that the patient receives continuity of care from admission into the health care system through convalescence. By using the nursing process, nurses can help to anticipate patient needs and minimize complications. The World Health Organization (WHO) has produced the Surgical Safety Checklist (WHO, 2008) to facilitate patient safety throughout the operative procedure.

The continuing care of the surgical patient has shifted from hospital-based to home-based convalescence, with the patient and family assuming increased responsibility. As the length of hospital stays decreases, the educational needs of the patients and their families increase. Patients are sent home often with complex medical or surgical conditions that require education and follow-up. Effective teaching and early discharge planning by the nurse are essential to ensure positive surgical outcomes (Suhonen & Leino-Kilpi, 2006).

HISTORY OF SURGICAL NURSING

Surgery gave physicians the means to treat conditions that were difficult or impossible to manage solely through medicinal applications. Early surgeons had little knowledge of the principles of asepsis, and anaesthesia techniques were primitive and unsafe. Indeed, the early surgeon's success was based on speed. The discovery of anaesthesia, in the 1840s, revolutionized surgery. Anaesthesia provided a combination of analgesia, muscle relaxation, and amnesia, which allowed the time for surgical procedures to be extended. The value of handwashing and the development of germ theory in the 1860s (Pasteur) and 1870s (Koch) triggered the study of aseptic technique, which reduced postoperative infections and mortality. Joseph Lister (1827–1912) was associated with antisepsis, or listerism. Initially, antisepsis was one way to protect patients from pathogens in the environment. After experimenting with carbolic acid dressings and continuous carbolic acid sprays during surgical operations, Lister, in 1867, described a reduced incidence of gangrene and mortality. He eventually abandoned carbolic acid by 1890, when Koch demonstrated heat to be more effective than chemicals for sterilizing instruments (Porter, 1997). Therefore, Pasteur, Lister, and Koch helped provide a scientific basis to help prevent infection in hospitals.

Asepsis and the techniques associated with it ensured that the patient did not acquire in-hospital infections. Germ theory influenced nursing practice through the creation of carefully delineated procedures designed to preserve asepsis (McPherson, 1996). Nurses working in the first operating rooms (ORs) cleaned the rooms and equipment, prepared the solutions and dressings, performed technical tasks such as obtaining supplies, administered anaesthetics as graduates, and occasionally accompanied patients to the surgical ward to deliver nursing care.

In Canada, OR nursing became part of training at the Montreal General Hospital in 1890 ("Nurses life in the Montreal General Hospital," 1892). Toronto General Hospital, St. Michael's Hospital in Toronto, and Winnipeg General Hospital quickly followed suit. OR nursing in the early twentieth century became organized around the technology of surgery. Nurses ensured that the aseptic conditions of the surgical environment were maintained by all personnel and, along with physicians, became the first specialists in anaesthesia. As sterile ORs developed, OR nursing became a specialty separate from anaesthesia and surgical nursing. Two roles emerged: the sterile scrub nurse, who handled the instruments and passed them to the surgeon, and the circulating nurse, who ensured that all sponges used in operations were accounted for outside the patient's body and that aseptic conditions were maintained. OR nursing was confined to activities in and around the OR and was a well-established field of practice by the 1920s.

During the Second World War, a proliferation of courses that focused on OR nursing developed. These post-diploma courses subsequently enabled nurses to join the military, where they were highly valued as working with trauma patients (Toman, Heap, & Frize, 2006). During the Second World War, the expertise of nurses in caring for soldiers with traumatic injuries accelerated. "The primary purpose of dressings shifted from one of limiting blood loss in the field to one of preventing infection and accelerating healing—while also shifting the level of knowledge and expertise to perform dressing changes and treat the underlying wounds" (Toman, 2007, p. 135).

The trend of including OR experience in training continued into the 1960s. However, during the 1970s, a change occurred in nursing education, whereby nurses were expected to acquire a broad knowledge base. As a result, many schools eliminated OR experience from the curriculum, believing that it focused only on manual skills (Sandelowski, 2000). What was not recognized was the role that OR nurses play in ensuring patients' comfort and safety and continuity of care before, during, and after their surgical journey.

In 1956 in the United States, the Association of Operating Room Nurses (AORN) was formed. The organization developed standards of nursing practice that outlined the perioperative nurse's scope of responsibility. AORN was the first nursing organization to develop structure, process, and outcome standards as defined by the American Nurses Association. AORN has since changed its name to the Association of periOperative Registered Nurses; however, AORN is still used as its acronym. The organization continues to be a driving force for the practice of perioperative nursing and works closely with Canadian associations. Perioperative nurses care for patients during preoperative, intraoperative, and postoperative periods. They work collaboratively with surgeons, anaesthetists, registered nurse first assistants, nurses and other health care providers.

In Canada, the Operating Room Nurses Association of Canada (ORNAC) was founded in 1983. The mission of this professional organization is the promotion and advancement of excellence in the provision of perioperative care to patients and the professional growth and personal enhancement of perioperative registered nurses. It sets the standards for Canadian perioperative nursing practice. Specifically, ORNAC values are (1) knowledge—education and research are essential components that guide practice; (2) collaboration—with nurses within the specialty, organizations, agencies, and other disciplines; (3) respect—for worth, quality, diversity, and importance of patients and each other; (4) professionalism—to advance the specialty; and (5) continuous quality improvement—to achieve excellence. Opportunities exist in conjunction with the Canadian Nurses Association (CNA) for registered nurses to obtain perioperative nursing certification. To advance nursing standards in the field, the National Association of Perianesthesia Nurses of Canada (NAPANc, 2014) has published the third edition of its standards. Areas covered include, for example, nursing process, ethics, continuing competence, and research. In addition to NAPANc, there are provincial associations for perioperative nursing. For example, the Ontario PeriAnesthesia Nurses Association (OPANA) was founded in 1985 to represent all nurses in Ontario who are involved in the care of patients pre- and postanaesthesia. These nursing environments are usually same-day (ambulatory) care, postanaesthetic care units, and preadmission units. The vision of OPANA is that of a respected nursing practice that promotes high-quality patient care throughout the perianaesthesia road to recovery. Perianaesthesia nursing is considered a specialty area of nursing practice.

Same-Day (Ambulatory) Surgery

A more recent change in the surgical field is the advent of same-day surgery, also referred to as *ambulatory surgery* or *short-stay surgery*. In **same-day surgery**, the patient is admitted on the day of surgery, has the surgery, and then goes home the same day. These services are provided within a hospital setting. More than half of all surgical procedures are conducted on an outpatient basis, including ophthalmic, gastroenterological, gynaecological, otorhinolaryngological, orthopaedic, cosmetic and restorative, and general procedures, and the incidence of same-day surgery has greatly increased. The process of admitting patients and then observing them overnight (23-hour admission) can also occur.

There are distinct benefits for the patient who has same-day surgery. Anaesthesia drugs that metabolize rapidly with few after-effects allow for shorter operative times. Nurses recognize the benefit of early postoperative ambulation and encourage patients to assume an active role in recovery. Same-day surgery also results in shorter hospital stays, as patients are usually discharged the day of surgery. This reduces the possibility of developing hospital-acquired infections, which occur when patients become colonized with bacteria found in the hospital setting. Procedures such as tumour biopsies and gallbladder removal (cholecystectomy) can now be done using laparoscopic procedures. Because of the small incision required, a laparoscopic cholecystectomy involves a hospital stay of only a few to 24 hours and a recovery period of a week. In contrast, a traditional open cholecystectomy requires a larger abdominal incision and involves a hospital stay of 3 to 5 days and a recovery period of at least 4 weeks. Thus, many surgeons use laparoscopic procedures for a variety of surgical interventions, thereby decreasing the length of surgery, hospitalization, and associated costs. Laparoscopic approaches are just one form of the increasingly used minimally invasive surgical (MIS) techniques. For example, specialized instruments and cameras as well as medical imaging equipment can be used for procedures such as pyeloplasty (Francis & Winfield, 2006), total hip arthroscopy (Burden, 2007), vascular surgery, or minimally invasive brain surgery. There is also robotic–laparoendoscopic single-site surgery with instruments dedicated to this approach, such as the da Vinci SI surgical system (Autorino, Kaouk, Stolzenburg, et al., 2013). Construction of new OR suites is increasingly providing dedicated rooms for MIS, and thus OR nurses are being educated about their role related to the techniques as well as intraoperative patient care.

Same-day surgery requires that nurses provide extensive preoperative and postoperative teaching and assess the patient's available support systems and readiness for self-care. For example, discharge education should include potential complications and what to do about them, instructions on care of incision sites, any drains, diet and activity, pain management, and telephone numbers to contact. Surgical day care nurses frequently call patients at home on the day after surgery to inquire about how recovery is progressing. As well, home care nurses must refer the patient to appropriate community agencies for services such as physiotherapy. Currently, apps are being developed for the web and for cell phone use. These apps are being used to help prepare patients mentally for surgery as well as provide education regarding the surgical procedure and postoperative care.

Role of Registered Nurse First Assistant (RNFA). The RNFA is an experienced perioperative nurse who has completed advanced education that provides additional knowledge along with advanced technical skills. The RNFA works collaboratively with surgeons and other members of the surgical team (Registered Nurses' Association of Ontario [RNAO], 2017). ORNAC has been advocating for the RNFA role since late 1980s, and the role was formally recognized in Canada in 1994.

Introduction of Anaesthetist's Assistant (AA). Recently, AAs have been introduced into the OR environment. The AAs set up equipment used for anaesthesia and assist with all aspects of the anaesthetic care plan, such as assisting with intubation and regional anaesthesia as well as satellite procedures like diagnostic imaging. AAs work under the direct supervision of an anaesthetist. Admission requirements, for example, to the Michener Institute, for an AA credentialing program are to have a respiratory therapist diploma or BScN with a minimum of 2 years' critical care experience.

SCIENTIFIC KNOWLEDGE BASE

Classification of Surgery

Surgical procedures are classified according to seriousness, urgency, and purpose (Table 48-1). A procedure may fall into more than one classification. For example, surgical removal of a disfiguring scar is minor in seriousness, elective in urgency, and reconstructive in purpose. Frequently, the classes overlap. An urgent procedure is also considered major in seriousness. As well, the same operation may be performed for different reasons on different patients. For example, a gastrectomy may be performed as an emergency procedure to resect a bleeding ulcer or as an urgent procedure to remove a cancerous growth. The classification indicates to nurses the level of care a patient might require. Hospitals have a system for prioritizing the booking of surgeries based on their classification.

The American Society of Anesthesiologists (ASA) assigns classification on the basis of a patient's physical status (PS) independent of the proposed surgical procedure (Table 48-2). In a Canadian study, Sankar, Johnson, Beattie, and colleagues (2014) found that the ASA-PS scale has moderate interrater reliability and is a valid marker of a patient's preoperative health status. ASA-PS class I and class II patients are acceptable for ambulatory surgery. Patients in classes IV and V require inpatient surgery because they are at higher risk for complications (e.g., cardiac or pulmonary complications). The ASA classification system is used in Canadian hospitals.

NURSING KNOWLEDGE BASE

Nursing knowledge offers important contributions for the care of the perioperative patient. For example, nursing research has shown the benefit of preoperative education in promoting positive patient outcomes after surgery. Structured preoperative teaching that includes, for example, the ORNAC (2015) standards as well as a return demonstration of postoperative exercises has been shown to improve outcomes such as pain severity, pulmonary function, length of stay, and patients' levels of anxiety.

Significant evidence-informed knowledge is also available for proper wound care interventions. Nursing research has contributed to what is known about the characteristics of wound healing and the types of applications most likely to be beneficial (see Chapter 46).

Within the OR setting, knowledge has improved the standards for infection control and patient safety. For example, surgical hand scrubs (see Chapter 33) can now be performed without the use of brushes, as a result of research that has shown the efficacy of alcohol-based hand rubs (Suchomel, Koller, Kundi, et al., 2009). Evidence-informed practice changes within the OR improve the quality of care for surgical patients and, ultimately, improve patient outcomes.

CRITICAL THINKING

Successful critical thinking requires a synthesis of knowledge, information gathered from patients, nursing experience, critical thinking qualities, and intellectual and professional standards. Clinical judgements require nurses to anticipate the information necessary, analyze the data, and make decisions regarding patient care. A patient's condition is always changing. During assessment (Figure 48-1), nurses must consider all of the elements that contribute to making appropriate nursing diagnoses.

When caring for the perioperative patient, nurses make clinical care decisions by integrating knowledge of anatomy, physiology, pathophysiology, and the surgical stress response with previous experiences in caring for surgical patients and information gathered from the

TABLE 48-1 Classification of Surgical Procedures

Type	Description	Examples
Seriousness		
Major	Involves extensive reconstruction or alteration in body parts; poses great risks to well-being	Coronary artery bypass, colon resection, removal of larynx, resection of lung lobe
Minor	Involves minimal alteration in body parts; often designed to correct deformities; involves minimal risks compared with major procedures	Cataract extraction, facial plastic surgery, tooth extraction
Urgency		
Elective	Usually is optional and may not be necessary for health	Bunionectomy, facial plastic surgery, breast reconstruction, removal of wart
Urgent	Is necessary for patient's health; may prevent additional problems from developing (e.g., tissue destruction or impaired organ function); not necessarily emergency	Excision of cancerous tumour, removal of gallbladder for stones, vascular repair for obstructed artery (e.g., coronary artery bypass)
Emergency	Must be done immediately to save life or preserve function of body part	Repair of perforated appendix, repair of traumatic amputation, control of internal hemorrhaging
Purpose		
Diagnostic	Surgical exploration that allows physician to confirm diagnosis; may involve removal of tissue for further diagnostic testing	Exploratory laparotomy (incision into peritoneal cavity to inspect abdominal organs), breast biopsy
Ablative	Excision or removal of diseased body part	Amputation, removal of appendix, cholecystectomy
Palliative	Relieves or reduces intensity of disease symptoms; will not produce cure	Colostomy, debridement of necrotic tissue, removal of brain tumour
Reconstructive or restorative	Restores function or appearance to traumatized or malfunctioning tissues	Internal fixation of fractures, scar revision
Procurement for transplant	Removal of organs, tissues, or both from a person pronounced dead for purpose of transplantation into another person. Sometimes there are living donors such as one person donating a kidney to another.	Kidney, heart, or liver transplant
Constructive	Restores function lost or reduced as a result of congenital anomalies	Repair of cleft palate, closure of atrial septal defect in heart
Cosmetic	Performed to improve personal appearance	Blepharoplasty to correct eyelid deformities; rhinoplasty to reshape nose

TABLE 48-2 Physical Status (PS) Classification of the American Society of Anesthesiologists (ASA)

Class	Description	Characteristics and Examples
PS-I	A normal, healthy patient	No physiological, biological, or organic disturbance
PS-II	A patient with a mild systemic disease	Disease imposes minimal restriction on activity; e.g., hypertension (HTN), obesity, diabetes mellitus
PS-III	A patient with a severe systemic disease that limits activity but is not incapacitating	Disease limits activity (e.g., severe diabetes with systemic complications); history of myocardial infarction, angina pectoris, or poorly controlled HTN
PS-IV	A patient with a severe systemic disease that is a constant threat to life	Severe cardiac, pulmonary, renal, hepatic, or endocrine dysfunction
PS-V	A moribund patient who is not expected to survive without the operation	Surgery is done as a last recourse or as a resuscitative effort; e.g., major multisystem or cerebral trauma, ruptured aneurysm, or large pulmonary embolus
PS-VI	A patient declared brain dead whose organs could be considered for donor purposes	

NOTE: The addition of an "E" to the physical status class indicates emergency surgery, such as PS-IE, PS-IIE, and so on.

Adapted from *Physical status (PS) classification.* (2008). Reprinted with permission of the American Society of Anesthesiologists, 520 N. Northwest Highway, Park Ridge, IL, 60068-2573, http://asahq.org/clinical/physicalstatus.htm.

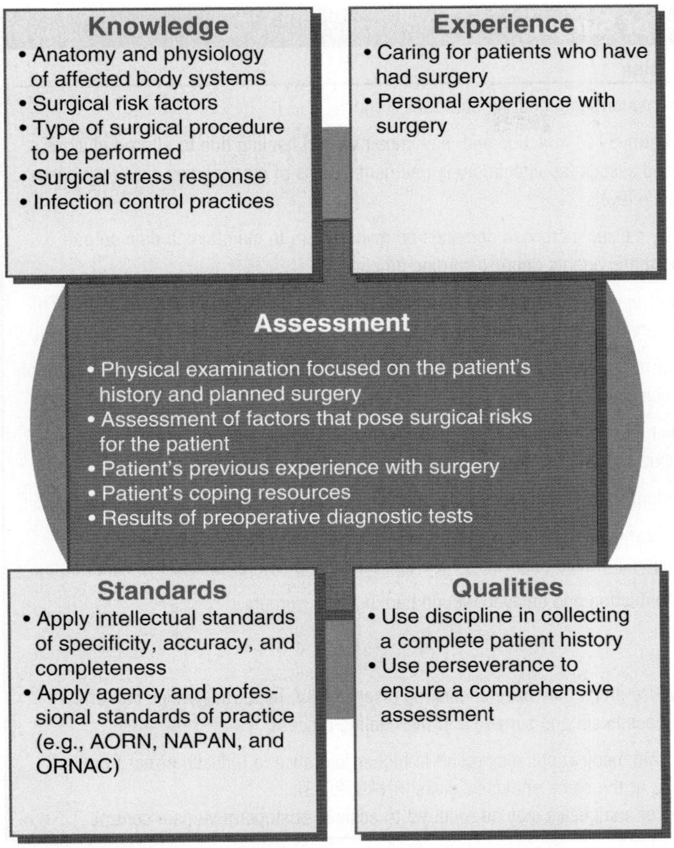

FIGURE 48-1 **Critical thinking model for surgical patient assessment.** *AORN,* Association of periOperative Registered Nurses; *NAPAN,* National Association of Perianesthesia Nurses; *ORNAC,* Operating Room Nurses Association of Canada.

patient, such as medical and surgical history, potential for surgical risk, and coping resources. Nurses' use of critical thinking qualities, such as perseverance, is needed to develop a plan of care that provides successful perioperative care (e.g., airway management, infection control, pain management, and discharge planning). Professional standards and guidelines developed by, for example, AORN (2004), NAPANc, OPANA, and ORNAC, as well as agency policies, provide valuable information for perioperative management and evaluation of processes and outcomes.

❖ NURSING PROCESS IN THE PREOPERATIVE SURGICAL PHASE

Surgical patients enter the health care setting in different stages of health. A patient may enter the hospital on a predetermined day feeling relatively healthy and prepared to face elective surgery. In contrast, a victim of a motor vehicle collision may face emergency surgery with no time to prepare. The ability to establish rapport and maintain a professional relationship with the patient is an essential component of the preoperative phase. Nurses must do this quickly but compassionately and effectively.

The surgical patient may undergo tests and procedures to confirm or rule out problems requiring surgery. Usually patients scheduled for same-day surgery have tests done several days before surgery. Testing done the day of surgery is usually limited to such tests as glucose monitoring for the patient with diabetes. Nurses must be familiar with the tests, their purpose, and how to monitor results.

The patient meets many members of the interprofessional team, including surgeons, anaesthesiologists, physiotherapists, and nurses. All play a role in the patient's care and recovery. Family members attempt to provide support through their presence but face many of the same stressors as the patient. Nurses must communicate effectively with the patient and family because *the nurse–patient relationship is the foundation of care* (see Chapter 17). Nurses need to assess the patient's physical, emotional, and spiritual well-being and cultural heritage; recognize the degree of surgical risk; coordinate diagnostic tests; identify nursing diagnoses and nursing interventions; and establish outcomes in collaboration with the patient and his or her family. Pertinent data and the care plan are communicated among the members of the surgical team.

◆ Assessment

The assessment of the surgical patient is intended to establish the patient's baseline preoperative function to assist in preventing and recognizing possible postoperative complications. Assessment of the surgical patient can be extensive. Ambulatory surgical programs require that patient data be completed several days in advance. Since patients are admitted only hours before the surgical event, nurses must organize and verify data obtained preoperatively to implement a perioperative care plan. This occurs not only with the ambulatory care patient but also with the patient who will require a more prolonged hospital stay. Increasingly, patients are admitted on the day of surgery, even for such major procedures as open heart surgery and bowel surgery.

Most assessments begin in a preadmission clinic before admission for surgery. The purpose of the preadmission is to prepare the patient physically and emotionally for surgery (OPANA, 2009a). Patients may answer a self-report inventory and the nurse may complete an initial physical examination, draw blood or complete other laboratory tests, begin teaching, identify potential risks, and answer questions. This streamlines the care required for the patient on the day of surgery. In the immediate preoperative period, nurses assess the patient's understanding of previous teaching and individualize patient and family care.

The physician usually performs a comprehensive history and physical examination with follow-up by the preadmission nurse. In this case, the nurse needs to review assessments and testing already completed and to highlight significant information (e.g., the patient being on diuretics). The focus is on key measurements for all body systems to ensure that no obvious problems are overlooked and that the patient has understood education previously provided. Even though the surgeon will screen the patient before scheduling surgery, preoperative assessment occasionally reveals an abnormality that delays or cancels surgery. For example, the patient may have a cough and low-grade fever on admission. This may indicate the onset of infection, and the surgeon will need to be notified immediately.

Nursing Health History. The nurse should conduct an initial interview to collect a patient history similar to that described in Chapter 32. If a patient is unable to relate all the necessary information, the nurse should rely on family members as resources.

Medical History. A review of the patient's medical history should include past illnesses and the primary reason for currently seeking medical care. The patient's current medical record and medical records from past hospitalizations are excellent sources of data.

Pre-existing illnesses can influence the choice of anaesthetic agents used and the patient's ability to tolerate surgery and reach full recovery (Table 48-3). Patients must be carefully screened for medical

TABLE 48-3 Medical Conditions That Increase Risks of Surgery

Type of Condition	Reason for Risk
Bleeding disorders (thrombocytopenia, hemophilia)	Increase risk of hemorrhaging during and after surgery.
Diabetes mellitus	Increases susceptibility to infection and may impair wound healing due to altered glucose metabolism and associated circulatory impairment. Stress of surgery may cause increases in blood glucose levels.
Heart disease (recent myocardial infarction, dysrhythmias, heart failure) and peripheral vascular disease	Stress of surgery causes increased demands on myocardium to maintain cardiac output. General anaesthetic agents depress cardiac function.
Obstructive sleep apnea	Administration of opioids increases risk of airway obstruction postoperatively. Patients will desaturate as revealed by drop in oxygen saturation by pulse oximetry.
Upper respiratory infection	Increases risk of respiratory complications during anaesthesia (e.g., pneumonia and spasm of laryngeal muscles).
Liver disease	Alters metabolism and elimination of drugs administered during surgery and impairs wound healing and clotting time because of alterations in protein metabolism.
Fever	Predisposes patient to fluid and electrolyte imbalances and may indicate underlying infection.
Chronic respiratory disease (emphysema, bronchitis, asthma)	Reduces patient's means to compensate for acid–base alterations (see Chapter 40). Anaesthetic agents reduce respiratory function, increasing risk for severe hypoventilation.
Immunological disorders (leukemia, HIV, bone marrow depression, and use of chemotherapeutic drugs or immunosuppressive agents)	Increase risk of infection and delayed wound healing after surgery.
Abuse of street drugs	Patients who abuse drugs may have underlying disease (HIV, hepatitis), which can affect response to anaesthesia and surgery and the healing process.
Chronic pain	Regular use of pain medications may result in higher tolerance, a reduced effect from repeated doses of the same analgesic class (RNAO, 2013). Increased doses of analgesics may be required to achieve postoperative pain control.

conditions that may increase the risk for complications during or after surgery. For example, a patient who has a history of heart failure may experience a further decline in cardiac function both intraoperatively and postoperatively. Intravenous (IV) fluids may need to be administered at a slower rate, or a diuretic may need to be given if blood transfusions are required.

Risk Factors. Various conditions and factors increase a person's risk when undergoing surgery. Knowledge of risk factors enables nurses to take necessary precautions in planning care.

Age. Infants are at risk during surgery because of their immature physiological status. During surgery, nurses and physicians are especially concerned with maintaining an infant's normal body temperature. The infant's shivering reflex is underdeveloped, and often wide temperature variations occur. Anaesthesia adds to the risk because anaesthetics can cause vasodilation and heat loss.

During surgery, an infant has difficulty maintaining a normal circulatory blood volume. The total blood volume of an infant is considerably less than that of an older child or an adult. Therefore, even a small amount of blood loss can be serious. A reduced circulatory volume makes it difficult for the infant to respond to increased oxygen demands during surgery. In addition, the infant is highly susceptible to complications associated with dehydration. However, if blood or fluids are replaced too quickly, overhydration may occur. Other important and unique aspects of a child's surgical care are airway management, treatment of seizures, management of temperature alterations, identification and treatment of emergence delirium and delayed emergence from anaesthesia, treatment of pain and agitation, and availability of age-appropriate emergency equipment and medications.

Older patients are also at risk for complications. With advancing age, a patient's physical capacity to adapt to the stress of surgery is hampered. A recent Canadian study examined 257 older patients who underwent emergency general surgery. More than 50% experienced an in-hospital complication following surgery, the most common being cardiac events, surgical infection or sepsis, and postoperative bleeding (Lees, Merani, Tauh, et al., 2015). Despite the risk, the majority of patients undergoing surgery are older persons. Table 48-4 summarizes the physiological factors that place older patients at risk during surgery.

Nutrition. Normal tissue repair and resistance to infection depend on adequate nutrients. Surgery intensifies this need. After surgery, a patient requires at least 1 500 kcal/day to maintain energy reserves. Increased protein, vitamins A and C, and zinc facilitate wound healing (see Chapters 42 and 46). A malnourished patient is prone to poor tolerance of anaesthesia, negative nitrogen balance, delayed blood clotting mechanisms, infection, poor wound healing, and the potential for multiple organ failure. If a patient is having elective surgery, attempts to correct nutritional imbalances should be made before the surgery. However, if a malnourished patient must undergo an emergency procedure, efforts to restore nutrients will occur after surgery.

Obesity. Obesity increases surgical risk by reducing respiratory and cardiac functions. Hypertension, coronary artery disease, diabetes mellitus, and heart failure are common in the bariatric (obese) population. Embolus, atelectasis (partial or total collapse of the alveoli), and pneumonia are also more frequent postoperative complications in the obese patient. The patient may have difficulty resuming normal physical activity after surgery. The obese patient is susceptible to poor wound healing and wound infection because of the structure of fatty tissue, which contains a poor blood supply. This slows delivery of essential nutrients, antibodies, and enzymes needed for wound healing (see Chapter 46). It is often difficult to close the surgical wound of an

TABLE 48-4 Physiological Factors That Place the Older Person at Risk During Surgery

Alterations	Risks	Nursing Implications
Cardiovascular System		
Degenerative change in myocardium and valves	Reduced cardiac reserve and arrhythmias	Assess baseline vital signs. Recognize the longer time period required for heart rate to return to normal after stress on the heart and evaluate the occurrence of tachycardia accordingly.
Rigidity of arterial walls and reduction in sympathetic and parasympathetic innervation to heart	Alterations may predispose patient to postoperative hemorrhage or an increase in systolic and diastolic blood pressure	Maintain adequate fluid balance to minimize either dehydration or circulatory overload.
Increase in calcium and cholesterol deposits within small arteries; thickened arterial walls	Predispose patient to clot formation in lower extremities	Instruct patient on techniques for performing leg exercises and proper turning. Apply elastic stockings, sequential compression devices.
Integumentary System		
Decreased subcutaneous tissue and increased fragility of skin	Prone to pressure injuries and skin tears	Assess skin at least every 4 hours; pad all bony prominences during surgery. Turn or reposition at least every 2 hours (see Chapter 46).
Pulmonary System		
Stiffening and reduction in size of the rib cage	Reduced vital capacity. Could retain secretions	Instruct patient on proper technique for coughing and deep breathing.
Reduced range of movement in diaphragm	Residual capacity (volume of air left in lung after normal breath) increases, reducing amount of new air brought into lungs with each inspiration	When possible, have patient ambulate and sit in chair frequently.
Stiffened lung tissue and enlarged air spaces	Alteration reduces blood oxygenation	Obtain baseline oxygen saturation; measure as indicated throughout perioperative period.
Renal System		
Reduced blood flow to kidneys	Increased risk of shock when blood loss occurs	For patients hospitalized before surgery, determine baseline urinary output for 24 hours.
Reduced glomerular filtration rate and excretory times	Limits ability to eliminate drugs or toxic substances	Assess for adverse response to drugs.
Reduced bladder capacity	Voiding frequency increases, and larger amount of urine stays in bladder after voiding. Sensation of need to void may not occur until bladder is filled.	Instruct patient to notify nurse immediately when sensation of bladder fullness develops. Keep call light and bedpan within easy reach. Toilet every 2 hours, or more frequently if indicated.
Neurological System		
Sensory losses, including reduced tactile sense	Decreased ability to respond to early warning signs of surgical complications such as delirium	Inspect bony prominences for signs of pressure that patient may not sense. Orient patient to surrounding environment. Observe for nonverbal signs of pain.
Decreased reaction time	Confusion after anaesthesia. Delirium is a disturbance of attention and awareness that develops over a short period of time (Adamis, Rooney, Meagher, et al., 2015). Delirium manifests in three subtypes: hyperactive, hypoactive, and mixed (Page & Ely, 2011). Older patients undergoing surgery are at high risk for delirium. Delirium can be caused by medications such as narcotics, or by physiological reasons such as infection or dehydration.	Allow adequate time for patient to respond, process information, and perform activities. Use Best Practice Guidelines (BPGs) on screening for and caregiving strategies for older persons with delirium, dementia, and depression (RNAO, 2010a, 2010b). Institute fall precautions (RNAO, 2005/2011).

Continued

TABLE 48-4 Physiological Factors That Place the Older Person at Risk During Surgery—cont'd

Alterations	Risks	Nursing Implications
Metabolic System		
Lower basal metabolic rate	Reduced total oxygen consumption	Ensure adequate nutritional intake when diet is resumed, but avoid intake of excess calories.
Reduced number of red blood cells and hemoglobin levels	Ability to carry adequate oxygen to tissues is reduced	Administer blood products if required. Monitor blood test results.
Change in total amounts of body potassium and water volume	Greater risk for fluid or electrolyte imbalance occurs	Monitor electrolyte levels and supplement as necessary.
Impaired thermoregulatory mechanisms	Cold operating rooms; exposure of body parts during procedure, intravenous (IV) fluids, medications	Ensure careful, close monitoring of patient temperature; provide warm blankets; monitor cardiac function; warm IV fluids.

obese patient because of the thick adipose layer. An obese patient is also at risk for dehiscence (opening of the suture line).

Immunocompetence. For the patient with cancer, radiation therapy may be given preoperatively to reduce the size of the cancerous tumour so that it can be removed surgically. Radiation has some unavoidable effects on normal tissue, such as excess thinning of skin layers, destruction of collagen, and impaired vascularization of tissue. Ideally, the surgeon waits 4 to 6 weeks after completion of radiation treatments to perform surgery. Otherwise, the patient may face serious problems with wound healing. In addition, chemotherapeutic drugs used for cancer treatment, immunosuppressive medications used to prevent rejection after organ transplantation, and steroids used to treat a variety of inflammatory conditions increase the risk for infection.

Fluid and Electrolyte Imbalances. The body responds to surgery as if it is a form of trauma. As a result of the adrenocortical stress response, sodium and water are retained and potassium is lost within the first 2 to 5 days after surgery. The severity of the stress response influences the degree of fluid and electrolyte imbalances. The more extensive the surgery, the greater is the stress response. A patient who is hypovolemic or who has serious preoperative electrolyte alterations is at significant risk during and after surgery. For example, an excess or depletion of potassium increases the chance of dysrhythmia. If the patient has pre-existing renal, gastrointestinal, or cardiovascular abnormalities, the risk for fluid and electrolyte alterations is even greater.

Pregnancy. The perioperative care plan must address the needs of both the mother and the developing fetus. Surgery is performed on a pregnant patient only on an emergency basis. All the mother's major systems are affected during pregnancy. For example, cardiac output significantly increases, as does respiratory tidal volume to accommodate the increase in metabolic rate. Gastrointestinal motility decreases, hormone levels increase, and energy levels decrease with advancing pregnancy. Laboratory and hemodynamic values change. Fibrinogen levels increase, making pregnant patients more susceptible to the development of deep vein thrombosis because of increased coagulability. Hemoglobin and hematocrit levels decrease, mostly as a result of the effects of hemodilution (increased circulating volume). The white blood cell (WBC) count is elevated when the woman is near term and postpartum without the presence of infection. However, infection always must be ruled out in the presence of an elevated WBC count. General anaesthesia is administered with caution because of the increased risk for fetal death and preterm labour. Psychological considerations for the mother and family are essential.

Previous Surgeries. Although previous surgery does not necessarily present as a risk factor, a patient's past experience with surgery can highlight many potential issues. The nurse should ask the patient to recall the previous type of surgery, level of discomfort, extent of disability, and overall level of care provided. Any complications that the patient experienced must be addressed. It is also important to assess patients for nausea and vomiting with previous surgeries, as research has shown they can be troublesome symptoms that are not always adequately medicated (Wilson, Watt-Watson, Hodnett, et al., 2016) and can increase the risk for aspiration. Prior anaesthesia records may be a useful source of information if previous problems such as malignant hyperthermia occurred. This information helps nurses to anticipate the patient's preoperative and postoperative needs. Previous surgery also may influence the level of physical care required after a surgical procedure. For example, a patient who has had a previous thoracotomy for resection of a lung lobe has a greater risk for postoperative pulmonary complications than does a patient with intact, normal lungs.

Perceptions and Understanding of Surgery. The surgical experience affects not only the patient, but also the entire family. The nurse must therefore prepare both the patient and the family. Identifying a patient's and family's knowledge, expectations, and perceptions allows the nurse to plan teaching and to provide individualized emotional support measures.

Each patient feels fearful when entering the surgical setting. Some fears are due to past hospital experiences, warnings received from friends and family, or lack of knowledge. The nurse must assess the patient's understanding of the planned surgery and its implications. For example, the nurse needs to determine whether the patient undergoing a breast biopsy recognizes that she will have a biopsy performed, not a mastectomy. The nurse might ask questions such as "Tell me what you think will happen before and after surgery," or "Explain what you know about your surgery." If a patient is misinformed or unaware of the reason for surgery, the nurse must confer with the physician before the patient is sent to the surgical suite. It is also good to determine whether further explanations are needed related to routine preoperative and postoperative procedures. When a patient is well prepared and knows what to expect, the patient's knowledge is reinforced and accuracy and consistency are maintained.

Medication History. If a patient regularly uses prescription or over-the-counter medications, the surgeon or anaesthesiologist may temporarily discontinue the drugs before surgery or adjust the dosages. Certain medications have special implications for the surgical patient, creating greater risks for complications or interacting negatively with anaesthetic agents (Table 48-5). For example, nurses must instruct patients in a preadmission unit to ask the physician whether usual medications should be taken on the morning of surgery. Patients also

TABLE 48-5 Medications With Special Implications for the Surgical Patient

Drug Class	Effects During Surgery
Antibiotics	Antibiotics can potentiate action of anaesthetic agents. For example, if taken within 2 weeks before surgery, aminoglycosides (gentamicin, tobramycin, neomycin) may cause mild respiratory depression due to depressed neuromuscular transmission.
Antidysrhythmics	Antidysrhythmics can reduce cardiac contractility and impair cardiac conduction during anaesthesia.
Anticoagulants	Anticoagulants alter normal clotting factors and thus increase risk of hemorrhaging. They should be discontinued before surgery. Aspirin (ASA) is a commonly used medication that can alter clotting mechanisms. Many older patients take ASA, and the nurse should be alert as to whether they have discontinued use presurgery. Most surgeons will have the patient stop taking ASA 4 to 5 days before the surgery.
Anticonvulsants	Long-term use of certain anticonvulsants (e.g., phenytoin [Dilantin] and phenobarbital) can alter the metabolism of anaesthetic agents.
Antihypertensives	Antihypertensives may interact with anaesthetic agents to cause bradycardia, hypotension, and impaired circulation. Some may inhibit synthesis and storage of norepinephrine in sympathetic nerve endings.
Corticosteroids	With prolonged use, corticosteroids cause adrenal atrophy, which reduces the body's ability to withstand stress. Before and during surgery, dosages may be temporarily altered.
Insulin	Diabetic patients' need for insulin after surgery is altered. Stress response and intravenous administration of glucose solutions can increase dosage requirements after surgery. Decreased nutritional intake can decrease dosage requirements.
Diuretics	Diuretics potentiate electrolyte imbalances (particularly potassium) after surgery.
Nonsteroidal anti-inflammatory drugs (NSAIDs)	NSAIDs inhibit platelet aggregation and may prolong bleeding time, increasing susceptibility to postoperative bleeding.
Herbal therapies: ginger, gingko, ginseng	Some herbal therapies have the ability to affect platelet activity and increase susceptibility to postoperative bleeding. Ginseng may increase hypoglycemia with insulin therapy.

should be asked whether any herbal preparations are used, because many patients do not view herbs as medications and may omit them from their medication history (see Chapter 35). Certain herbs may interfere with the action of other medications (a pharmacist must be consulted). For hospitalized patients, prescription drugs taken preoperatively are automatically discontinued postoperatively unless the physician reorders them. It is important for the nurse to be aware of the patient's previous medications that likely will need to be resumed postoperatively (e.g., antihypertensives).

Allergies. Nurses must assess for allergies to drugs that may be given during a phase of the surgical experience. In addition, it is critical to assess for latex, food, and contact allergies (e.g., allergies to tape, ointments, or solutions). A patient may be too young or have too few exposures to drugs to know whether he or she has any allergies. The type of allergic response is also very important to assess. Allergies need to be delineated from unpleasant adverse effects. For example, the patient may state that codeine causes nausea (an adverse effect), or that it causes hypotension and confusion (an allergy). When asking a patient about allergies, the nurse needs to realize that the term *allergy* can be confusing for some patients. Asking a patient whether he or she has ever "had a problem with a medication or substance" may be a helpful approach.

It is critical that the patient be asked specifically about latex allergies because a latex-free environment must be provided for patients with latex allergies. Nurses ensure that a list of the patient's allergies is noted appropriately in his or her medical record or the electronic chart, as well as in any other places designated by institutional policy, such as an allergy band.

Smoking Habits. The patient who smokes is at greater risk for postoperative pulmonary complications than one who does not. The chronic smoker already has an increased amount and thickness of mucous secretions in the lungs. General anaesthetics increase airway irritation and stimulate pulmonary secretions, which are retained as a result of reduction in ciliary activity during anaesthesia. After surgery, the patient who smokes has greater difficulty clearing the airways of mucous secretions and needs education on the importance of postoperative deep breathing and coughing (see Chapter 39). In addition, smoking can compromise blood flow to the heart, which can affect the response to surgery. Nurses play a key role in reducing smoking and can refer to nursing Best Practice Guidelines (BPGs) on smoking cessation (RNAO, 2007), when appropriate. During the postoperative period, nicotine replacement therapy may be required to support the patient who smokes.

Alcohol Ingestion and Substance Use and Abuse. Habitual use of alcohol and illegal drugs predisposes the patient to adverse reactions to anaesthetic agents. The patient also may experience a cross-tolerance to anaesthetic agents, necessitating higher-than-normal amounts. In addition, the physician may need to increase postoperative dosages of analgesics. Patients with a history of excessive alcohol ingestion also may be malnourished, which may contribute to delayed wound healing. These patients are at risk for liver disease, portal hypertension, and esophageal varices (predisposing the patient to bleeding disorders). The patient who habitually uses alcohol and is required to remain in the hospital for longer than 24 hours is also at risk for acute alcohol withdrawal and its more severe form, delirium tremens.

Family Support. It is important for nurses to determine the extent of the patient's support from family members or friends. Because blood relations do not always define family, it is best to have the patient identify his or her sources of support (see Chapter 19). Surgery can result in temporary or permanent disability that requires added assistance during recovery. The patient usually cannot immediately assume the same level of physical activity enjoyed before surgery. Often a patient returns home with dressings to change or exercises to perform. With same-day surgery, patients and families assume responsibility for postoperative care. The family is an important resource for the patient with physical limitations and provides the emotional support needed to motivate the patient to return to a previous state of health. In addition, the family may better remember preoperative and postoperative teaching.

The nurse should ask whether family members or friends could provide support. The patient may want someone present when the nurse provides instructions or explanations. Family presence should be encouraged when feasible, especially for patients having ambulatory surgery. Often a family member can become the patient's coach, offering valuable support during the postoperative period, when the patient's participation in care is vital.

Occupation. The nurse should assess the patient's occupational history to anticipate the possible effects of surgery on recovery and eventual work performance. Any restrictions should be explained before a patient returns to work, such as lifting, use of the extremities, or climbing stairs. When a patient is unable to return to his or her job, the nurse should confer with a social worker or occupational therapist to refer the patient to job-training programs or to help the patient seek economic assistance.

Preoperative Preparation for Pain Assessment and Management. Surgical manipulation of tissues, treatments, and positioning on the OR table may result in postoperative pain for the patient. Pain is a very personal experience and requires an individualized care plan. Preoperatively, the nurse should prepare the patient and family for the assessment and management of pain (see Chapter 31), including the patient's and the family's expectations for pain management after surgery. The nurse should begin education regarding pain management as soon as possible (Box 48-1). The preoperative assessment should introduce to the patient the use of a pain instrument to rate the presence and severity of pain postoperatively (see Chapter 31). Several instruments for both pediatric and adult patients are available. Frequent pain assessments with the patient are necessary to alert the nurse to treat the pain and assess the adequacy (outcome) of pain interventions.

Review of Emotional Health. Surgery is psychologically stressful. The patient may be anxious about the surgery and its implications. Patients often feel that they are powerless over their situation. Family members may perceive the patient's surgery as a disruption of their lifestyle. Hospitalization and the recovery period at home may be lengthy. The family is usually concerned about the patient returning to a normal, productive life. When the patient has chronic illness, the family may be fearful that surgery will result in further disability or may be hopeful that the patient will improve. To understand the impact of surgery on a patient's and a family's emotional health, the nurse should assess the patient's feelings about surgery, self-concept, body image, and coping resources.

It is often difficult to assess feelings thoroughly when ambulatory surgery is scheduled; nurses usually have less time to establish a relationship with patients. In some day surgical programs, the nurse may visit with a patient in the home or on the telephone before surgery. If visiting in a hospital room, the nurse should choose a time for discussion after admitting procedures or diagnostic tests have been completed. The nurse should explain to the patient that it is normal to have fears and concerns. The patient's ability to share feelings partially depends on the nurse's willingness to listen, be supportive, and clarify misconceptions.

If the patient feels powerless, the nurse should attempt to determine the reason. The medical diagnosis may generate apprehension of increased dependence and loss of physical or mental function. The thought of being "put to sleep" under anaesthesia may create concern about loss of control. Most patients want to retain the power to make decisions about treatment. Nurses must assure patients of their right to ask questions and seek information.

A patient may be angry about the need for surgery. For example, a young person may feel that it is unfair to have a disorder that typically affects older people. Surgery may occur at a time when it is inconvenient or potentially disruptive. The patient occasionally may express anger verbally at the nurse or the physician. Being argumentative or overly demanding, refusing to cooperate, and criticizing the health care team's efforts to provide care are manifestations of the patient's anger and anxiety.

Body Image. Surgical removal of any diseased body part may leave permanent disfigurement or alteration in body function. Loss of certain body functions (e.g., with a colostomy or ureterostomy) may compound patients' fears. Nurses should assess for the body-image alterations that patients perceive will result from surgery. Patients will respond differently depending on their culture, self-concept, and degree of self-esteem (see Chapter 26). Excision of breast tissue, colostomy, ureterostomy, hysterectomy, or removal of the prostate gland may affect patients' perceptions of their sexuality.

Nurses should encourage patients to express their concerns about sexuality. The patient facing even temporary sexual dysfunction

BOX 48-1 RESEARCH HIGHLIGHT

A Randomized Controlled Trial of an Individualized Preoperative Education Intervention for Symptom Management After Total Knee Arthroplasty

Research Focus

The aim of this study was to determine the effect of preoperative educational intervention on postsurgical pain and nausea.

Research Abstract

Total knee replacement is a common surgical procedure performed to reduce pain and immobility usually caused by osteoarthritis. Pain and nausea are common symptoms for patients after this procedure. Although previous research studies have examined educational interventions for pain prevention and treatment in this population, none of the studies focused on analgesic pain management and antiemetic therapy. This Canadian study aimed to determine the effect of an individualized preoperative educational intervention on interference, due to pain, with activities on postoperative day 3, and the effect of this educational intervention on nausea, pain, and analgesic and antiemetic administration on postoperative days 1, 2, and 3. Topics covered in the intervention included the importance of pain management to promote activity, communicating with health professionals, asking for analgesics and antiemetics, misbeliefs about taking medications, and nonpharmacological measures. The sample of 143 participants was randomized to the intervention group or to standard care. Those in the standard group got the usual teaching. Those in the intervention group received the usual teaching plus a booklet on symptom management, an individual teaching session, and a follow-up support call. The results revealed that there were no differences between the two groups. Participants had severe nausea and pain and yet received antiemetics and analgesics in insufficient doses. The authors concluded that more than individualized teaching is required to reflect a change in symptom management. They suggested further research is needed on modifying factors in the hospital system to bring about change in symptom management.

Wilson, R., Watt-Watson, J., Hodnett, E., & Tranmer, J. (2016). A randomized controlled trial of an individualized preoperative education intervention for symptom management after total knee arthroplasty. *Orthopaedic Nursing, 35*(1), 20–28.

requires understanding and support. Discussions about the patient's sexuality should be held with the patient's sexual partner so that both individuals can gain a shared understanding of how to cope with limitations in sexual function.

Coping Resources. When reviewing the patient's coping resources, it is important to ask him or her about specific family members and friends who may provide support. Once they are identified, these individuals should be included in any patient teaching and interventions aimed at managing stress and anxiety. If the patient has had previous surgery, the nurse should determine what behaviours helped to resolve any tension or nervousness. The nurse may instruct the patient on relaxation exercises that can help control anxiety.

Culture. Patients come from diverse cultural and religious backgrounds that affect the way they perceive and react to their surgical experience. If cultural, ethnic, and religious differences are not acknowledged and incorporated into the perioperative care plan, desired surgical outcomes may not be achieved. Therefore, learning about a patient's cultural and ethnic heritage helps nurses provide effective perioperative care. Although it is important to recognize and plan for differences based on culture, nurses also must recognize that members of the same culture are individuals and may not hold these shared beliefs. Box 48-2 highlights some cultural care aspects in the perioperative period.

BOX 48-2 CULTURAL ASPECTS OF CARE

Providing Culturally Sensitive Care to Patients Undergoing Surgery

Providing individualized education and perioperative nursing care to patients of various cultural, religious, and ethnic groups can be challenging. Using a variety of resources available within a health care agency, whether in written from or from the Internet, will help nurses to provide culturally sensitive care.

Implications for Practice

- Preoperative assessment should include a cultural assessment with questions regarding such topics as primary language spoken, feelings about surgery and pain, pain management, expectations, support system, and feelings toward self-care with postoperative implications (e.g., Does patient relate to concept of pain? Does patient follow custom that gives family members control over decisions?).
- Use the services of a professional interpreter if necessary to communicate with a patient. Use pictures or phrase cards with various languages to communicate with a patient whose language is different than yours; these cards can be used to assess pain, comfort, temperature, and so forth.
- Provide preoperative and postoperative educational materials in a variety of languages.

Resources

A document from Nova Scotia provides a guide for cultural competence (Marshall, 2005): *A Cultural Competence Guide for Primary Health Care Professionals in Nova Scotia.* Retrieved from http://healthteamnovascotia.ca/cultural_competence/Cultural_Competence_guide_for_Primary_Health_Care_Professionals.pdf.

The Canadian Nurses Association (CNA, 2010) has a relevant position statement, *Promoting Cultural Competence in Nursing.* Retrieved from https://www.cna-aiic.ca/~/media/cna/page-content/pdf-en/ps114_cultural_competence_2010_e.pdf?la=en.

The College of Nurses of Ontario (CNO, 2009) has a practice guideline, *Culturally sensitive care.* Retrieved from http://www.cno.org/globalassets/docs/prac/41040_culturallysens.pdf.

Patient Expectations. Patients rely on their caregivers for information, comfort, pain control, adequate monitoring, and performance of interventions that ensure their safety throughout the surgical experience. Thus nurses need to have a caring attitude, advocate for the patient, be skilled in surgical assessment and interventions, and anticipate the patient's needs throughout the perioperative period. Nurses must understand the patient's expectations in order to develop an individualized care plan. Does the patient expect full pain relief or simply to have pain reduced? Does the patient expect to be independent immediately after surgery, or does he or she expect to be fully dependent on nursing staff or on family members? These are only a few of the questions that need to be asked of the surgical patient to establish a care plan congruent with his or her needs and expectations.

Physical Examination. Nurses should conduct a partial or complete physical examination, depending on the patient's preoperative condition (see Chapter 32). Assessment focuses on findings related to the patient's medical history and on body systems that likely will be affected by the surgery.

General Survey. The nurse should first observe the patient's general appearance. Gestures and body movements may reflect weakness caused by illness. The patient may appear malnourished. Height, body weight, and history of recent weight loss are important indicators of nutritional status.

Preoperative vital signs, including blood pressure while sitting and standing, provide important baseline data with which alterations that occur during and after surgery can be compared. Some institutions request that blood pressure be obtained in both arms for comparison. Anxiety and fear commonly cause elevations in heart rate and blood pressure. As the effects of the anaesthesia diminish after surgery, vital sign findings are compared with the preoperative baseline. Preoperative assessment of vital signs is also important to rule out fluid and electrolyte abnormalities (see Chapter 30).

An elevated temperature before surgery is a cause for concern. If the patient has an underlying infection, the surgeon may choose to postpone surgery until the infection has been treated. An elevated body temperature increases the risk for fluid and electrolyte imbalances after surgery.

Head and Neck. The condition of oral mucous membranes is one indicator of the patient's level of hydration. A dehydrated patient is at risk for developing serious fluid and electrolyte imbalances during surgery. Inspection of the soft palate and nasal sinuses can reveal sinus drainage, indicative of respiratory or sinus infection. Cervical lymph node enlargement may reveal local or systemic infection.

The jugular veins should be inspected for distension. Excess fluid within the circulatory system or failure of the heart to contract efficiently may lead to jugular vein distension and reveal a risk for cardiovascular complications during surgery.

During the examination of the oral mucosa, loose or capped teeth must be identified because they could become dislodged during endotracheal intubation. Dentures must be noted so that they can be removed before surgery, especially if general anaesthesia is required.

Integument. The nurse should carefully inspect the skin, especially over bony prominences, such as the heels, elbows, sacrum, and scapula. During surgery, a patient must lie in a fixed position, often for several hours. As a result, the patient may have an increased risk for pressure injuries (see Chapter 46), especially if the patient is older and skin is thin and dry and has poor turgor. Chronic use of steroids also increases the patient's susceptibility to skin tears. In addition, the overall condition of the skin reveals the patient's level of hydration.

Thorax and Lungs. Assessment of the patient's breathing pattern and chest excursion aids in assessing ventilatory capacity. A decline in ventilatory function places the patient at risk for respiratory complications. For example, a patient who has high abdominal surgery will have difficulty breathing deeply because of a painful abdominal incision. Auscultation of breath sounds will indicate whether the patient has pulmonary congestion or narrowing of airways.

Existing atelectasis or moisture in the airways will be aggravated during surgery. Serious pulmonary congestion may cause postponement of the surgery. Certain anaesthetics can cause laryngeal muscle spasm; thus, if wheezing in the airways is heard on auscultation preoperatively, the patient is at risk for further airway narrowing during surgery and after extubation (removal of the endotracheal tube). The physician should be made aware of these findings.

Heart and Vascular System. The nurse should assess the character of the apical, radial, and peripheral pulses; the capillary refill; and the colour and temperature of the patient's extremities. If peripheral pulses are not palpable, a Doppler instrument should be used to assess their presence. Acceptable capillary refill occurs in less than 3 seconds. Measurement of capillary refill and assessment of peripheral pulses are particularly important for the patient having vascular surgery or orthopaedic surgery (see Chapter 32).

Abdomen. The abdomen should be assessed for size, shape, symmetry, and presence of distension. Assessment of preoperative bowel sounds is useful as a baseline. The nurse also should ask the patient whether he or she has regular bowel movements and inquire about the colour and consistency of stools.

Neurological Status. Preoperative assessment of neurological status is imperative for all patients who will be receiving general anaesthesia. The baseline neurological status assists with the assessment of ascent from anaesthesia. During the health history and physical assessment, the nurse observes the patient's level of orientation, alertness, and mood, noting whether the patient answers questions appropriately and can recall recent and past events. A patient who will have surgery for neurological disease (e.g., brain tumour or aneurysm) may demonstrate an impaired level of consciousness or altered behaviour.

If the patient is scheduled for spinal anaesthesia, preoperative assessment of gross motor function and strength is important. Spinal anaesthesia causes temporary paralysis of the lower extremities. The nurse should be aware if a patient enters surgery with weakness or impaired mobility of the lower extremities so that, when the spinal anaesthetic wears off, full motor function is not expected to return.

Diagnostic Screening. Before a patient has surgery, the surgeon may order diagnostic tests as determined by the patient's history and physical assessment. Table 48-6 lists common diagnostic tests performed preoperatively based on the patient's medical history. The tests ordered are also determined by the procedure itself. For procedures where blood loss is expected (e.g., hip and knee replacements), a type and cross-match would be indicated preoperatively. The surgeon will designate the number of blood units to have available during surgery. Table 48-7 outlines the purpose and normal values for the more common blood tests. If diagnostic tests reveal severe problems, the surgeon may cancel surgery until the condition stabilizes. Nurses are responsible for the preparation of patients for diagnostic studies and for coordinating completion of the tests. Nurses also review diagnostic results as they become available, not only to alert physicians to these findings and to assist with planning appropriate therapy, but also to integrate these findings into nursing decisions related to patient care.

If a patient has a history of heart disease, an electrocardiogram (ECG) is usually ordered. The ECG measures the electrical activity of the heart to assess the heart rate, rhythm, and other factors. A chest X-ray (an examination of the condition of the heart and lungs) is usually required for thoracic surgery or if the patient has certain medical conditions.

Pulmonary function testing and arterial blood gas analysis may be performed on patients with pre-existing lung disease. Blood glucose levels and glycosylated hemoglobin (HbA1c) are measured on patients with diabetes. HbA1c measures the amount of hemoglobin A1c in the blood, which reflects the patient's average blood glucose level over the long term (Pagana, Pagana, & Pike-MacDonald, 2013).

TABLE 48-6 Common Diagnostic Tests Performed Preoperatively Based on Patient History

History	Tests
Hepatic disease	International normalized ratio (INR); activated partial thromboplastin time (aPTT); liver enzymes, such as serum aspartate aminotransferase; alkaline phosphatase
Cardiovascular disease	blood urea nitrogen (BUN), creatinine, complete blood count (CBC), chest X-ray, electrocardiogram (ECG)
Pulmonary disease	CBC, chest X-ray, ECG, blood gases
Central nervous system disease	White blood cell (WBC) count, electrolytes, BUN, creatinine, glucose, electroencephalography (EEG)
Medications	
Diuretics	Electrolytes, and perhaps BUN and creatinine
Steroids	Electrolytes, glucose
Anticoagulants	INR, aPTT

Autologous infusions are an option for some patients who choose to donate their own blood before surgery. Although Canadian Blood Services screens all blood donors and blood products for infections such as human immunodeficiency virus (HIV) and hepatitis, some patients are more comfortable donating their own blood. The donation usually must be made several weeks before the scheduled surgery. Because of the short time frame now from preadmission to day of surgery, autologous infusions may not always be possible as there may not be enough time to complete the process. Autotransfusion via the use of a cell-saver device during surgery may be possible if physicians anticipate large blood loss (e.g., open heart surgery).

◆ Nursing Diagnosis

Nurses cluster patterns of defining characteristics gathered during assessment to identify nursing diagnoses for the surgical patient (Box 48-3). The patient with pre-existing health problems is likely to have a variety of risk diagnoses. For example, a patient with pre-existing bronchitis who has abnormal breath sounds and a productive cough will be at risk for ineffective airway clearance. In addition, a patient who undergoes a surgical procedure is at risk for developing infection at the surgical site, the IV site, or in the bloodstream (sepsis). A diagnosis of risk for infection will require the nurse's attention from admission through convalescence.

The related factors for each diagnosis establish directions for nursing care that will be provided during one or all of the surgical phases. For example, the diagnosis of risk for infection related to an invasive procedure will require different interventions from those if the related factor is inadequate immune response. Preoperative nursing diagnoses enable the nurse to take precautions and actions ensuring that the care provided during the intraoperative and postoperative phases is consistent with the patient's needs.

Nursing diagnoses made preoperatively will also focus on the potential risks a patient may face after surgery. Preventive care is essential so

TABLE 48-7 Diagnostic Screening for Surgical Patients

Measurement and Normal Values	Interpretation
Complete Blood Count (CBC) *Red blood cells (RBCs):* Men: 4.7–6.1 × 10^{12}/L; Women: 4.2–5.4 × 10^{12}/L *Hemoglobin (Hgb):* Men: 140–180 mmol/L; Women: 120–160 mmol/L *Hematocrit (Hct):* Men: 0.42–0.52; Women: 0.37–0.47 *White blood cells (WBCs):* Adults and children >2 years: 5–10 × 10^9/L	Peripheral venous sample of blood measures RBCs, WBCs, Hgb, and Hct. May reveal infection, low blood volume, and potential for oxygenation problems. Surgeon may order blood replacement.
Serum Electrolytes *Sodium (Na):* 136–145 mmol/L *Potassium (K):* 3.5–5.0 mmol/L *Chloride (Cl):* 98–106 mmol/L *Bicarbonate (HCO_3):* 22–26 mmol/L	Peripheral venous sample of blood reveals significant fluid and electrolyte imbalances preoperatively. Attention is given to Na, K, and Cl levels. Intravenous (IV) fluid replacement may be indicated preoperatively.
Coagulation Studies *International normalized ratio (INR):* 0.8–1.20 *Activated partial thromboplastin time (APTT):* 30–40 seconds *Platelets:* 150–400 × 10^9/L	INR, aPTT, and platelet counts reveal clotting ability of blood. These studies are used to indicate patients at risk for bleeding tendencies or thrombus formation.
Serum Creatinine *Men:* 53–106 mcmol/L *Women:* 44–97 mcmol/L	Ability of kidneys to excrete creatinine, a by-product of muscle metabolism, indicates renal function. Elevated level can indicate renal failure.
Blood Urea Nitrogen (BUN) 3.6–7.1 mmol/L	Ability of kidneys to excrete urea and nitrogen indicates renal function. BUN becomes elevated if patient is dehydrated. Preoperative IV fluid replacement may be needed.
Glucose *Fasting:* 4.0–6.0 mmol/L	Finger stick or peripheral blood sample. Patients may require treatment of low or high levels preoperatively and postoperatively. Elevated blood sugar levels are usually the result of a deficiency in insulin secretion (type 1 diabetes), insulin action, or combination of both (type 2 diabetes).

Adapted from Pagana, K. D., Pagana, T. J., & Pike-MacDonald, S. A. (2013). *Mosby's Canadian manual of diagnostic and laboratory tests* (1st Canadian ed.). Toronto: Elsevier.

that the surgical patient can be managed effectively. The following are common nursing diagnoses relevant to the surgical patient:

- *Ineffective airway clearance*
- *Risk for allergy response to latex*
- *Anxiety*
- *Disturbed body image*
- *Risk for ineffective thermoregulation*
- *Ineffective breathing pattern*
- *Ineffective coping*
- *Fear*
- *Risk for deficient fluid volume*
- *Risk for infection*
- *Risk for perioperative positioning injury*
- *Deficient knowledge (specify)*
- *Impaired physical mobility*
- *Acute pain*
- *Powerlessness*
- *Impaired skin integrity*
- *Disturbed sleep pattern*
- *Delayed surgical recovery*

◆ Planning

During planning, nurses once again synthesize information from multiple resources (Figure 48-2). For example, knowledge pertaining to adult learning principles, coupled with the patient's unique needs, will ensure a well-designed **preoperative teaching plan**. Critical thinking ensures that the patient's care plan integrates the nurse's knowledge, previous experience, and established standards of care. Previous experience in caring for surgical patients helps nurses anticipate how to approach patient care (e.g., complications to prevent and anticipate, and methods to reduce anxiety). Professional standards and evidence-informed practices are especially important to consider when developing a care plan, as they provide a scientific basis for selecting effective nursing interventions. Nurses need

BOX 48-3 NURSING DIAGNOSTIC PROCESS

Assessment Activities	Defining Characteristics	Nursing Diagnosis
Ask patient to describe previous surgical experiences.	Patient mentions a traumatic prior experience with surgery	*Fear related to knowledge deficit and previous surgical experience*
Ask patient about preoperative education and preparation before admission.	Unaware of preoperative testing	
Observe patient's nonverbal behaviour.	Patient's behaviour indicates fear and tension	
Assess vital signs.	Increased heart rate	

Ackley, B. J., & Ladwig, G. B. (2011). *Nursing diagnosis handbook: An evidenced based guide to planning care* (9th ed.). St. Louis, MO: Elsevier.

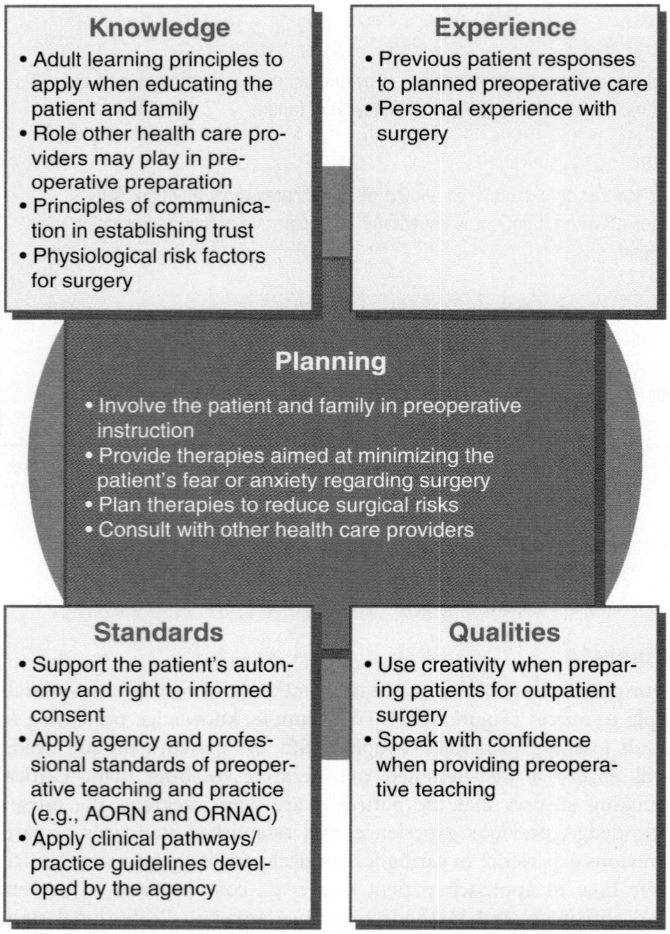

FIGURE 48-2 Critical thinking model for surgical patient planning. *AORN,* Association of periOperative Registered Nurses; *ORNAC,* Operating Room Nurses Association of Canada.

to develop an individualized care plan for each nursing diagnosis (Box 48-4). The nurse and the patient together can set realistic expectations for care.

Successful planning requires the involvement of both the surgical patient and the family in establishing the care plan. Early patient involvement minimizes surgical risks and postoperative complications. A patient who is well informed about the surgical experience is less likely to be fearful and can prepare to participate in the postoperative recovery phase so that outcomes can be met. Diagnosis, interventions, and outcomes are established to ensure recovery or maintenance of the preoperative state.

Goals and Outcomes. The preoperative care plan is based on individualized nursing diagnoses. This plan is reviewed and modified during the intraoperative and postoperative periods. Outcomes established for each goal of care provide measurable behavioural evidence to gauge the patient's progress toward meeting the stated goals.

The following example provides a goal of care and expected outcomes relevant for the preoperative surgical patient:

- Patient is able to verbalize the significance of postoperative exercises.
- Patient verbalizes prevention of lung congestion and pneumonia as reasons for deep breathing and coughing exercises.
- Patient verbalizes promotion of blood flow to prevent leg clots as reason for postoperative leg exercises.
- Patient verbalizes rationale for early ambulation, as it improves lung function, assists with return of bowel function, and promotes recovery.

Note: Incentive spirometry as a treatment is used much less now or not at all in the hospital setting. Agostini and Singh (2009) conducted a review of the literature examining the use of incentive spirometry following thoracic surgery. Postoperative physiotherapy regimes with or without incentive spirometry appeared to be effective following thoracic surgery, compared to no physiotherapy. In Restrepo, Wettstein, Wittnebel and colleagues' (2011) update on the American Association of Respiratory Care Clinical Practice Guidelines related to incentive spirometry, the authors made several recommendations, one of which is that incentive spirometry alone is not recommended for routine use in pre- and postoperative care. The guideline also suggests that deep breathing exercises provide the same benefit as incentive spirometry in the pre- and postoperative setting. In addition, incentive spirometry is not recommended for prevention of atelectasis in patients who have undergone upper abdominal surgery or coronary artery bypass graft surgery. Strickland, Rubin, Drescher, et al. (2013) also reported that routine use of incentive spirometry cannot be supported as a therapy to prevent postoperative complications.

Setting Priorities. Using clinical judgement, nurses should prioritize nursing diagnoses and interventions based on the assessed unique needs of each patient. Patients who need emergency surgery may experience changes in their physiological status that require the nurse to reprioritize quickly. For example, if a patient's blood pressure begins to drop, hemodynamic stabilization becomes a priority over education. Generally, when the preoperative situation is more controlled, the approach to each patient needs to reflect an understanding of the implications of the patient's age, physical and psychological health, educational level, and cultural and religious practices. Increasingly, patients are preparing advanced medical directives to indicate their wishes regarding any unexpected aggressive medical treatment that might arise.

◆ Implementation

Preoperative nursing interventions provide the patient with an understanding of the surgery and prepare the patient not only physically and

BOX 48-4 NURSING CARE PLAN

Deficient Knowledge Regarding Preoperative and Postoperative Care Requirements

ASSESSMENT

Mrs. Campana is an 80-year-old woman scheduled to be admitted in 5 days for elective bowel resection. Joe Marrero is the nurse in the clinic surgery service assigned to prepare Mrs. Campana for surgery. During his initial discussion with Mrs. Campana, Joe observes her to be alert and oriented. Mrs. Campana has severely reduced visual acuity but is able to hear Joe's questions clearly.

Assessment Activities	*Findings and Defining Characteristics*
Ask Mrs. Campana about previous surgeries and her experience with them.	She responds, "I had surgery over 20 years ago, and I was in the hospital for 10 days."
Ask Mrs. Campana what she has been told regarding her surgery.	She states that her surgeon explained the procedure using a picture of the bowel and indicating the location of the part to be removed.
Ask Mrs. Campana what she has been told regarding preoperative preparation and what to expect postoperatively.	She states that she received information from the surgeon's office regarding medicines to stop taking and those she should take on the morning of surgery, her diet before surgery and when to stop eating, and whom to call with questions. She does not recall receiving information regarding what to expect postoperatively.
Assess Mrs. Campana's ability to read typical font type.	She is unable to read the text font on the newspaper; she can read the headlines with her glasses.
Assess Mrs. Campana's family and support system for preoperative and postoperative assistance.	She states that her daughter will be coming into town on the day of surgery to help her after surgery.

NURSING DIAGNOSIS: Deficient knowledge regarding preoperative and postoperative care requirements related to lack of exposure to information.

PLANNING

*Goals (Nursing Outcomes Classification)**	*Expected Outcomes*
	Knowledge of Treatment Procedures
Patient will understand the postoperative routines of surgical care by day before surgery.	Patient will discuss monitoring routines after surgery by morning of surgery in the preoperative period. Patient will be able to describe importance of postoperative exercises by morning of surgery, including turn, cough, and deep breathing; incentive spirometer; and leg exercises. Patient will be able to describe schedule for activity and nutritional management postoperatively by day 1 after surgery.
Patient will participate actively in postoperative recovery activities by day 1 after surgery.	Patient will successfully perform postoperative exercises by morning of surgery in the preoperative period.

*Outcome classification labels from Moorhead, S., Johnson, M., & Maas, M. L. (Eds.). (2013). *Nursing outcomes classification (NOC)* (5th ed.). St. Louis, MO: Mosby.

INTERVENTIONS

Interventions (Nursing Interventions Classification)†	*Rationale*
Teaching in the Preoperative Period	
Provide patient and her daughter with hospital website and YouTube instructions that explain preoperative and postoperative routines. Supply instruction booklet designed for the visually impaired. Make a follow-up call to patient and to her daughter to give them an opportunity to ask questions and voice concerns. Document all phases of education—preoperative before admission, day of surgery, and postoperative—provided to patient in her record.	Preadmission education can require less teaching time and better performance of exercises on admission. Knowing what to expect can help to reduce anxiety in patients who are undergoing surgery. Carr, Thomas, and Wilson-Barnett (2005) conducted a study with women undergoing major gynecological surgery to explore the impact of anxiety and depression on pain experience over time following surgery. The results revealed that preoperative anxiety was predictive of postoperative anxiety as well as higher pain scores and that nurses need to identify these patients so that interventions can be implemented. In addition, the authors suggested that patients may benefit from specific information, such as length of stay or what the pain will be like.
On admission to hospital, demonstrate to patient and daughter the performance of postoperative exercises and how to get out of bed.	Demonstration is an effective method to reinforce didactic instruction.
Explain sensations to be expected postoperatively (e.g., incisional pain that will be controlled with medications, intravenous [IV], nasogastric tube, wound care, frequent vital signs assessments).	Teaching about sensory aspects (what the patient sees, feels, smells) should be structured.
Give patient opportunity to demonstrate postoperative exercises before surgery.	Return demonstration measures patient learning and provides an opportunity to reinforce instruction.

Continued

BOX 48-4 NURSING CARE PLAN

Deficient Knowledge Regarding Preoperative and Postoperative Care Requirements—cont'd

Interventions (Nursing Interventions Classification)[†]	*Rationale*
Correct any unrealistic expectations the patient or daughter may have regarding surgery.	Unrealistic expectations, when unmet, can contribute to patient's anxiety. Psychological preparation for surgery reduces anxiety.

[†]Intervention classification labels from Dochterman, J. M., Bulecheck, G. M., & Butcher, H. K. (Eds.). (2013). *Nursing interventions classification (NIC)* (6th ed.). St. Louis, MO: Mosby.

EVALUATION

Nursing Actions	*Patient Response and Finding*	*Achievement of Outcome*
Ask patient to describe typical monitoring and care activities after surgery. Document evaluation of patient's understanding and demonstration of learned activities in patient's record.	She is able to verbalize typical monitoring and care after surgery. She states that the instruction booklet and YouTube instructions were both helpful.	Mrs. Campana has a good understanding of the typical postoperative course.
Observe patient's demonstration of postoperative exercises.	She is able to demonstrate leg exercises and deep breathing and coughing exercises.	Mrs. Campana is able to demonstrate the postoperative exercises her daughter showed her.
Explore with patient and daughter if they have any remaining fears or concerns.	Both Mrs. Campana and her daughter deny any fears or concerns at the present time.	Informational and psychological needs of Mrs. Campana and her daughter have been met.

psychologically for surgical intervention but also to be an active participant in the recovery process.

Informed Consent. Surgery cannot be legally or ethically performed until a patient understands the need for a procedure, the steps involved, the risks, the expected results, and alternative treatments. The surgeon is responsible for explaining the procedure and obtaining the informed consent. Often today, the consent is signed in the physician's office or in the preadmission unit. If, as a nurse, you are involved in obtaining the signature, you must ensure before signing that the patient understands the procedure. If the patient is unclear about the procedure, the consent should not be signed and the physician should be notified (see Chapter 8).

Preoperative Teaching. Education is an important aspect of the patient's surgical experience. Preoperative teaching reflects a patient's expected postoperative course of events and has a positive influence on the patient's recovery.

Nurses in preadmission clinics may contact patients up to 1 week before surgery to answer the patient's questions and reinforce explanations. Preoperative information and instructions may include telephone calls, mailings from the physician's office or hospital, preoperative teaching guidelines and checklists, and the use of hospital websites or clinical pathways (Figure 48-3).

Pritchard (2011) has discussed the importance of giving appropriate information to patients preoperatively. Information needs to be tailored to address patients' individual needs; this targeted information, then, is meaningful to the patient. Establishing a relationship with patients facilitates understanding of their specific situation so that information given addresses their concerns. Pritchard (2011) suggests that the use of standard information sheets, such as preoperative information sheets, is not sufficient to address patients' information needs or to reduce their preoperative anxiety.

Including family members in preoperative preparation is advised. Family members need to be aware of the normal expectations after discharge from the hospital. They also may recognize untoward events that may unfold once the patient is home. If anxious relatives do not understand routine postoperative events, their anxiety will likely heighten the patient's fears and concerns. Preoperative preparation of family members can help to minimize anxiety and misunderstanding.

Nurses should provide patients with information about sensations typically experienced after surgery. Preparatory information helps patients anticipate the steps of a procedure and thus helps them form realistic images of the surgical experience. When events occur as predicted, patients are better able to cope and attend to them. For example, in the OR, the anaesthesiologist may apply ointment to patients' eyes to prevent corneal damage. Warning patients about sensations of blurred vision will reduce their anxiety on awakening from surgery. Sensations that may be described include expected pain at the surgical site, tightness of dressings, dryness of the mouth, or a sore throat resulting from an endotracheal tube.

Anxiety and fear are barriers to learning, and both emotions are heightened as surgery approaches. The nurse should assess the surgical patient's readiness and ability to learn. If the patient is capable of and receptive to learning, information should be presented in a logical sequence, beginning with preoperative events and advancing to intraoperative and postoperative routines. The following discussion addresses aspects of patient knowledge that demonstrate a patient's understanding of the surgical experience.

Patient Cites Reasons for Preoperative Instructions and Exercises. If given a rationale for preoperative and postoperative procedures, the patient is better prepared to participate in his or her care. Every preoperative teaching program includes explanation and demonstration of postoperative exercises: diaphragmatic breathing, coughing, turning, and leg exercises. These exercises are designed to prevent postoperative complications (Skill 48-1). Physiotherapists, as part of the interprofessional team, can facilitate patient mobility postoperatively.

If the patient is measured for elastic stockings or sequential compression devices, the nurse must teach about the purpose of these devices and the nursing care that will be required after their application (see Chapter 45).

After explaining each exercise, the nurse should demonstrate it. Nurses act as a coach, guiding the patient through each exercise. For example, as a nurse, you assess whether the patient is sitting properly and help the patient place his or her hands in the proper position during breathing. You then allow the patient time for independent practice.

Patient States the Time of Surgery. The patient and family should be told the approximate time that surgery will begin. If the hospital has a busy OR schedule, it is best to let them know whether other procedures are scheduled before the patient's. The surgeon usually informs the patient and family of the anticipated length of surgery. Unanticipated delays may occur for many reasons. The family needs to be aware that delays do not necessarily indicate a problem.

Text continued on p. 1389

The Ottawa Hospital | L'Hôpital d'Ottawa

☐ Civic ☐ General

CLINICAL PATHWAY

Total Hip Arthroplasty, Primary/Revision and Hip Resurfacing

IN PATIENT 5 FLOW SHEET

Pre-Admission Unit (PAU)	Day of Surgery Pre-op — Same Day Admission / Surgical Day Care Unit (SDA/SDCU)
Date: yyaa ________ mm ______ dj ______	Date: yyaa ________ mm ______ dj ______
Critical Path	**Critical Path**
Assessment and teaching per Pre-Admission Unit (PAU) standards of care and procedure specific education material. Pre-operative diagnostic testing as per Medical Directive for Pre-Admission Diagnostic Testing for Elective Surgery. **Additional Orders** • X-ray if ordered on Pre-op orders (SPO 297 ORT) **Discharge Planning** • Discuss expected length of stay of 1 day for hip resurfacing and total hip replacement and 1 to 3 days for total hip arthroplasty revision • As per patient history, identify issues that could cause delay of discharge and discuss discharge preparation. • Ensure patient has Total Hip Arthroplasty patient education booklet order # CP 04 B	**Assessment and teaching per Same Day Admission standards of care and procedure specific education material. Pre-operative diagnostic testing as per Medical Directive for Pre-Admission Diagnostic Testing for Elective Surgery.**
Patient Outcomes	**Patient Outcomes**
Patient Teaching • Understands pre-op instructions and events • Understands usual post-op course, plan for pain management, and usual self care measures to prevent post-op complications – per patient education booklet **Discharge Planning** • Understands usual length of stay and expected discharge time of 10 a.m. post-op day 1, 2 or 3 • Appropriate discharge plan in place or if no suitable discharge plan in place – consult required health-care provider as appropriate	**Patient Teaching** • Adherence with pre-op instructions • Understands usual events/expectations of operative day • Understands usual post-op course, plan for pain management, and usual self care measures to prevent post-op complications – per patient information booklet
Patient progress corresponds with clinical pathway	**Patient progress corresponds with clinical pathway**
Nursing: ☐ Yes ☐ No Signature: ____________ Time: ______ NTV – circle above, VC ______	**Nursing:** ☐ Yes ☐ No Signature: ____________ Time: ______ NTV – circle above, VC ______

Variance Codes (VC)

186	Activity variance	NTV	Non-Tracked Variance
492	Not discharged by end of pathway – continued need for acute care	OFF	Ordered off clinical pathway
510	Not discharged by end of pathway – non-medical reason		

CP 04 A (REV 11/2016) CHART – DOSSIER

FIGURE 48-3 Preoperative patient instructions for a clinical pathway for a total hip arthroplasty. The first day of a 6-day pathway highlights what the patient can expect before surgery. *DVT*, Deep venous thrombosis; *NVS*, neuro vital signs; *PVA*, peripheral vascular assessment. (Courtesy The Ottawa Hospital, Ottawa, ON.)

Continued

Patient ______________________ Chart No. ______________

Day of Surgery Post-op / Post Anesthetic Care Unit (PACU)	
Date: yyaa ________ mm ______ dj ______	
Critical Path	**Patient Outcomes**
Oxygen saturation monitoring (SpO_2) and oxygen administration per oxygen titration protocol. **Vital signs (VS), assessment, treatment, and teaching per PACU standards of care.** **Additional Orders** • Bedrest • NPO to clear fluids prn • Pillow between knees • In/out catheterization as ordered • May transfer to ward when PACU discharge criteria is achieved	**Pain Control** • Indicates adequate pain control. Pain equal or less than 3 at rest, equal or less than 5 with activity; pain not preventing movement; patient satisfied with pain control. • Achieves PACU discharge criteria for transfer to ward

Patient progress corresponds with clinical pathway

☐ Yes ☐ No Signature: ______________________, Initial ________ Time: ________ NTV – circle above, VC ________

D = 8-12 h day shift **E** = evening shift, if applicable **N** = 8-12 h night shift

Variance Codes (VC)

186	Activity variance	**NTV**	Non-Tracked Variance
492	Not discharged by end of pathway – continued need for acute care	**OFF**	Ordered off clinical pathway
510	Not discharged by end of pathway – non-medical reason		

CP 04 A (2 – 6) **CHART**

FIGURE 48-3, cont'd

Patient ______________________________ Chart No. ______________

Day of Surgery Post-op Ward	
Date: yyaa ________ mm ______ dj ______	
Critical Path	**Patient Outcomes**
Assessments/Treatments • VS, PVA/NVS, SpO_2, pain q4h × 24 hrs • Monitor dressing q4 hours • Pillow between legs at all times • Pain management per Acute Pain Service (APS) or Orthopedic orders as applicable • Oxygen per Oxygen Titration Protocol	**Assessments/Treatments** • Minimal oozing on dressing **Pain Control** • Indicates adequate pain control. Pain equal or less than 3 at rest, equal or less than 5 with activity; pain not preventing movement; patient satisfied with pain control.
Activity • Deep breathing and coughing (DB & C) • Up in chair × 1 ______ initial if able • Mobilize if able • Activity as tolerated • **Verify orders for Weight bearing status and hip precautions**	**Activity** • Completes transfer with assistance • Demonstrates understanding of positioning while in bed
Nutrition • Diet as ordered	**Nutrition** • Able to tolerate diet as ordered
Elimination • Monitor bowel sounds and elimination	**Elimination** • Patient has bowel sounds • Patient able to void **Prevention of DVT** • Performs ankle pumping exercises • Prophylaxis medication started
Patient Teaching • Reinforce: – DB & C – Ankle pumping exercises – Pillow positioning to maintain good alignment • Pain management • Hip precautions • Weight bearing status • Bowel management • Ensure patient has Total Hip Arthroplasty booklet	**Patient Teaching** • Demonstrates: – DB & C – Pillow positioning and leg alignment – Ankle pumping exercises – Understanding of hip precautions – Understanding of pain management – Understanding of weight bearing status – Use of mobility aids
Discharge Planning • Review discharge plan and consult appropriate health-care provider if potential problems identified – Possible discharge tomorrow if discharge criteria met	

Patient progress corresponds with clinical pathway

D ☐ Yes ☐ No Signature: ______________________, Initial ________ Time: ________ NTV – circle above, VC ________

E ☐ Yes ☐ No Signature: ______________________, Initial ________ Time: ________ NTV – circle above, VC ________

N ☐ Yes ☐ No Signature: ______________________, Initial ________ Time: ________ NTV – circle above, VC ________

D = 8-12 h day shift **E** = evening shift, if applicable **N** = 8-12 h night shift

Variance Codes (VC)

186	Activity variance	**NTV**	Non-Tracked Variance
492	Not discharged by end of pathway – continued need for acute care	**OFF**	Ordered off clinical pathway
510	Not discharged by end of pathway – non-medical reason		

CP 04 A (3 – 6) **CHART**

FIGURE 48-3, cont'd

Continued

Patient ______________________ **Chart No.** ______________

Post-op Day 1

Date: yyaa ______ mm ______ dj ______

Critical Path	Patient Outcomes
Assessments/Treatments • VS with SpO_2, PVA/NVS q shift • Pain assessment q4h • Discontinue saline lock if IV access no longer required • Monitor dressing q4h • Discontinue bulky dressing and change to strip dressing • Pillow between legs at all times • Pain management as per APS or Orthopedic orders as applicable • Wean off APS pain modality if applicable • Oxygen per Oxygen Titration Protocol. Wean if possible. **Activity** • **Verify orders for Weight bearing status and hip precautions** • DB & C • Exercise program with Physiotherapy • Up in chair × 3: at ______ initial ______ at ______ initial ______ at ______ initial ______ • Ambulate • Gait training on stairs if applicable **Nutrition** • Diet as ordered **Elimination** • Monitor bowel sounds and elimination **Patient Teaching** • Reinforce: – DB & C – Ankle pumping exercises – Pillow positioning to maintain good alignment • Pain management • Hip precautions • Weight bearing status • Bowel management • Ensure patient has Total Hip Arthroplasty booklet **Discharge Planning** • Review discharge plan **Discharge** • Consider for possible discharge today if discharge criteria met • If unable to discharge today, discuss discharge plan with patient	**Assessments/Treatments** • Minimal oozing on dressing **Pain Control** • Indicates adequate pain control. Pain equal or less than 3 at rest, equal or less than 5 with activity; pain not preventing movement; patient satisfied with pain control. **Wound** • Minimal oozing • Incision dry and intact • Edges well approximated **Activity** • Completes transfer with assistance progressing to independent • Ambulates with assistance progressing to independent • Performs exercises according to self-directed exercise program • Ambulates in stairs as needed **Nutrition** • Able to tolerate diet as ordered **Elimination** • Voiding well • Patient has bowel sounds **Patient Teaching** • Demonstrates: – DB & C – Pillow position and leg alignment – Ankle pumping exercises – Understanding of hip precautions – Understanding of pain management – Understanding of weight bearing status – Use of mobility aids **Discharge Criteria for Early Discharge Pathway** • Post-op x-ray arranged • No evidence of DVT • No discharge/redness/swelling from incision • Ambulates independently/safely with mobility devices • Manages stairs as needed • Time to Up and Go Test score less than or equal to 30 seconds • **Patient and family verbalizes/understands:** – Post discharge care – Signs and symptoms of DVT – Emergency resources – Wound care – Equipment recommendations for home safety – Pain management – Bowel management – Hip precautions – Exercise program

Patient progress corresponds with clinical pathway **D** = 8-12 h day shift **E** = evening shift, if applicable **N** = 8-12 h night shift

D ☐ Yes ☐ No Signature: ______________, Initial ______ Time: ______ NTV – circle above, VC ______

E ☐ Yes ☐ No Signature: ______________, Initial ______ Time: ______ NTV – circle above, VC ______

N ☐ Yes ☐ No Signature: ______________, Initial ______ Time: ______ NTV – circle above, VC ______

Variance Codes (VC)

186	Activity variance	**NTV**	Non-Tracked Variance
492	Not discharged by end of pathway – continued need for acute care	**OFF**	Ordered off clinical pathway
510	Not discharged by end of pathway – non-medical reason		

CP 04 A (4 – 6) **CHART**

FIGURE 48-3, cont'd

Patient ______________________ **Chart No.** ______________________

Post-op Day 2

Date: yyaa ________ mm ______ dj ______

Critical Path	**Patient Outcomes**
Assessments/Treatments • VS, PVA/NVS q shift • Pain assessment q4h • Discontinue saline lock if IV access no longer required • Pain management as per Orthopedic orders • Discontinue Oxygen Titration Protocol	**Assessments/Treatments** • Patient hemodynamically stable **Pain Control** • Indicates adequate pain control. Pain equal or less than 3 at rest, equal or less than 5 with activity; pain not preventing movement; patient satisfied with pain control. **Wound** • Minimal oozing
Activity • **Verify orders for Weight bearing status and hip precautions** • Continue exercise program • Up in chair × 3 minimum: at ______ initial ______ at ______ initial ______ at ______ initial ______ • Ambulate • Gait training on stairs if applicable	**Activity** • Ambulates independently using assistive devices • Ambulates on stairs as needed • Transfers independently using appropriate mobility devices
Nutrition • Diet as ordered	**Nutrition** • Able to tolerate diet as ordered
Elimination • Monitor bowel sounds and elimination	**Elimination** • Patient has bowel sounds • Patient able to void
Patient Teaching • Reinforce: – DB & C – Ankle pumping exercises – Pillow positioning to maintain good alignment • Pain management • Hip precautions • Weight bearing status • Bowel management • Ensure patient has Total Hip Arthroplasty booklet	**Patient Teaching** • Demonstrates: – DB & C – Pillow position and leg alignment – Understanding of hip precautions – Understanding of weight bearing status – Use of mobility aids – Ankle pumping exercises – Understanding of pain management
Discharge • Consider for possible discharge today if discharge criteria met • If unable to discharge today, discuss discharge plan with patient	**Discharge Criteria** • Post-op x-ray done • No evidence of DVT • No discharge/redness/swelling from incision • Ambulates independently/safely with mobility devices • Manages stairs as needed • Time to Up and Go Test score less than or equal to 30 seconds • **Patient and family verbalizes/understands:** – Post discharge care – Signs and symptoms of DVT – Emergency resources – Wound care – Equipment recommendations for home safety – Pain management – Bowel management – Hip precautions – Exercise program

Patient progress corresponds with clinical pathway **D** = 8-12 h day shift **E** = evening shift, if applicable **N** = 8-12 h night shift

D ☐ Yes ☐ No Signature: ______________________, Initial ______ Time: ______ NTV – circle above, VC ______

E ☐ Yes ☐ No Signature: ______________________, Initial ______ Time: ______ NTV – circle above, VC ______

N ☐ Yes ☐ No Signature: ______________________, Initial ______ Time: ______ NTV – circle above, VC ______

Variance Codes (VC)

186	Activity variance	**NTV**	Non-Tracked Variance
492	Not discharged by end of pathway – continued need for acute care	**OFF**	Ordered off clinical pathway
510	Not discharged by end of pathway – non-medical reason		

FIGURE 48-3, cont'd

Continued

Patient ______________________________ Chart No. ______________________________

Post-op Day 3

Date: yyaa __________ mm ________ dj ________

Critical Path	Patient Outcomes
Assessments/Treatments • VS with PVA/NVS q shift • Pain assessment q4h • Discontinue saline lock • If incisional drainage notify physician • Pain management as per Orthopedic orders **Activity** • **Verify orders for Weight bearing status and hip precautions** • Continue exercise program • Up in chair × 3 minimum: at ________ initial ________ at ________ initial ________ at ________ initial ________ • Ambulate • Gait training on stairs if applicable **Nutrition** • Diet as ordered **Elimination** • Monitor bowel sounds and elimination **Patient Teaching** • Reinforce: – DB & C – Ankle pumping exercises – Pillow positioning to maintain good alignment • Pain management • Hip precautions • Weight bearing status • Bowel management • Ensure patient has Total Hip Arthroplasty booklet **Discharge Planning** • If unable to discharge today, continue care as per post-op day 3 pathway until discharged **Discharge** • Discharge by 10 a.m. once discharge criteria met unless otherwise indicated by physician	**Pain Control** • Indicates adequate pain control. Pain equal or less than 3 at rest, equal or less than 5 with activity; pain not preventing movement; patient satisfied with pain control. **Activity** • Ambulates independently using assistive devices • Transfers independently using appropriate mobility devices • Ambulates on stairs as needed **Nutrition** • Able to tolerate diet as ordered **Elimination** • Patient has bowel sounds • Patient is voiding **Patient Teaching** • Demonstrates: – DB & C – Pillow position and leg alignment – Ankle pumping exercises – Understanding of hip precautions – Understanding of pain management – Understanding of weight bearing status – Use of mobility aids **Discharge Criteria** • Post-op x-ray done • No evidence of DVT • No discharge/redness/swelling from incision • Ambulates independently/safely with mobility devices • Manages stairs as needed • Time to Up and Go Test score less than or equal to 30 seconds • **Patient and family verbalizes/understands:** – Post discharge care – Signs and symptoms of DVT – Emergency resources – Wound care – Equipment recommendations for home safety – Pain management – Bowel management – Hip precautions – Exercise program

Patient progress corresponds with clinical pathway **D** = 8-12 h day shift **E** = evening shift, if applicable **N** = 8-12 h night shift

D ☐ Yes ☐ No Signature: ______________________________, Initial ________ Time: ________ NTV – circle above, VC ________

E ☐ Yes ☐ No Signature: ______________________________, Initial ________ Time: ________ NTV – circle above, VC ________

N ☐ Yes ☐ No Signature: ______________________________, Initial ________ Time: ________ NTV – circle above, VC ________

Variance Codes (VC)

186	Activity variance	**NTV**	Non-Tracked Variance
492	Not discharged by end of pathway – continued need for acute care	**OFF**	Ordered off clinical pathway
510	Not discharged by end of pathway – non-medical reason		

FIGURE 48-3, cont'd

SKILL 48-1 DEMONSTRATING POSTOPERATIVE EXERCISES

Delegation Considerations

The skill of demonstrating postoperative exercises should not be delegated to unregulated care providers (UCPs). However, other aspects of patient care may be delegated. When using UCPs be sure to do the following:

- Educate the UCP to encourage patients to practise exercises regularly, following instruction.
- Instruct the UCP to inform the nurse if patients are unwilling to perform these exercises.

Equipment

- Pillow or wrapped blanket (used to splint surgical incision during coughing)
- Positive expiratory pressure (PEP) device might be used

PROCEDURE

STEPS	RATIONALE
1. Assess the patient's risk for postoperative respiratory complications. Review the medical history to identify presence of chronic pulmonary conditions (e.g., emphysema, chronic bronchitis, asthma), any condition that affects chest wall movement, history of smoking, and presence of reduced hemoglobin.	• General anaesthesia predisposes the patient to respiratory problems because the lungs are not fully inflated during surgery and the cough reflex is suppressed, so that mucus collects within airway passages. After surgery, the patient may have reduced lung volume and require greater efforts to cough and breathe deeply; inadequate lung expansion can lead to atelectasis and pneumonia. The patient is at greater risk for developing respiratory complications if other chronic lung conditions are present. Smoking damages ciliary clearance and increases mucous secretion. Reduced hemoglobin level can lead to inadequate oxygenation.
2. Assess patient's ability to cough and breathe deeply by having the patient take a deep breath and observing movement of shoulders and chest wall. Measure chest excursion during deep breath. Ask patient to cough after taking a deep breath.	• Reveals maximum potential for chest expansion and ability to cough forcefully; serves as baseline to measure ability to perform exercises after surgery.
3. Assess risk for postoperative thrombus formation. (Older patients, those with active cancer, and those immobilized for more than 3 days are most at risk.) Observe for localized tenderness along the distribution of the venous system, swollen calf or thigh, calf swelling more than 3 cm compared with asymptomatic leg, pitting edema in symptomatic leg, and collateral superficial veins. If any of these signs are present, notify the physician. The most common test for diagnosing deep venous thrombosis (DVT) is ultrasound. A D-dimer test may also be done (National Heart Lung and Blood Institute [NHLBI], 2011).	• Venous stasis, decreased perfusion, and vein trauma exist simultaneously for thrombus formation to occur (Lewis, Dirksen, Heitkemper, et al., 2014). After general anaesthesia, circulation is slowed, thus increasing the risk for clot formation. Immobilization results in decreased muscular contraction in the lower extremities, which promotes venous stasis.
4. Assess the patient's ability to move independently while in bed.	• Determines existence of any mobility restrictions.
5. Explain postoperative exercises to the patient, including their importance to recovery and physiological benefits.	• Information allows the patient to understand the significance of exercises and can motivate learning. People tend to learn new skills when benefits can be gained.
6. Demonstrate exercises.	
A. Diaphragmatic breathing	
(1) Assist the patient to a comfortable sitting position on side of bed or in chair or to standing position.	• Upright position facilitates diaphragmatic excursion.
(2) Stand or sit facing the patient.	• Allows the patient to observe the breathing exercise.

Continued

SKILL 48-1 DEMONSTRATING POSTOPERATIVE EXERCISES—cont'd

STEPS	RATIONALE
(3) Instruct the patient to place palms of hands across from each other, down and along lower borders of anterior rib cage. Place tips of third fingers lightly together (see Step 6A[3] illustration). Demonstrate for the patient.	• Position of hands allows the patient to feel movement of the chest and abdomen as the diaphragm descends and lungs expand.

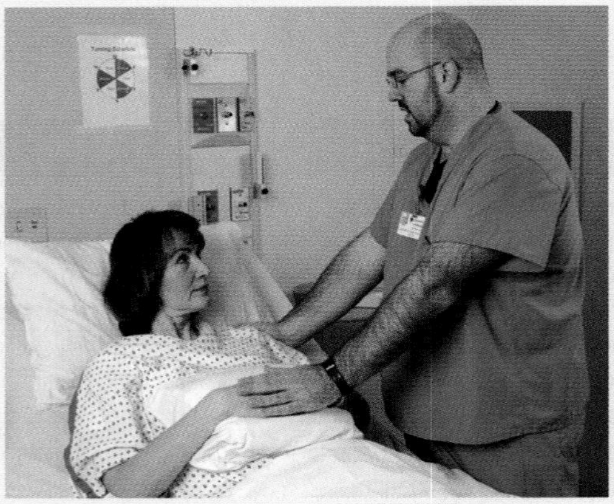

STEP 6A(3) Deep breathing exercise—placement of hands on upper abdomen during inhalation.

STEPS	RATIONALE
(4) Have the patient take slow, deep breaths, inhaling through the nose and pushing abdomen against hands. Tell the patient to feel the middle fingers separate during inhalation. Demonstrate.	• Taking slow, deep breaths prevents panting or hyperventilation. Inhaling through the nose warms, humidifies, and filters air.
(5) Explain that the patient will feel normal downward movement of the diaphragm during inspiration. Explain that abdominal organs descend and the chest wall expands.	• Explanation and demonstration focus on normal ventilatory movement of the chest wall. The patient develops understanding of how diaphragmatic breathing feels.
(6) Avoid using auxiliary chest and shoulder muscles while inhaling and instruct the patient in same manner.	• Using auxiliary chest and shoulder muscles increases useless energy expenditure.
(7) Have the patient hold a slow, deep breath for a count of three and then slowly exhale through the mouth as if blowing out a candle (with pursed lips). Tell the patient that middle fingertips will touch as the chest wall contracts.	• Allows for gradual expulsion of all air and helps prevent airway collapse by facilitating the maintenance of positive airway pressure.
(8) Repeat breathing exercise three to five times.	• Allows the patient to observe a slow, rhythmic breathing pattern.
(9) Have the patient practise the exercise. Instruct the patient to take 10 slow, deep breaths every hour while awake during the postoperative period until mobile.	• Repetition of the exercise reinforces learning. Regular deep breathing prevents postoperative complications.
B. Positive expiratory pressure (PEP) device.	• The PEP device creates pressure in the lungs and keeps airways from closing. It helps move mucus up.
(1) Perform hand hygiene.	• Reduces transmission of microorganisms.
(2) Set PEP device to the setting ordered. PEP allows exhalation against resistance, therefore increasing airway pressure (Strickland et al., 2013). There is no high-level evidence to support the routine use of PEP, except in patients with cystic fibrosis (Strickland et al., 2013).	• The higher the setting, the more effort will be required by the patient. Ideally, it should deliver 10–20 cm H_2O during passive expiration (American Association for Respiratory Care [AARC], 1993; Cincinnati Children's Hospital Medical Center, 2018).
(3) Instruct the patient to assume semi-Fowler's or high-Fowler's position, and place nose clip on the patient's nose.	• Promotes optimal lung expansion and expectoration of mucus (AARC, 1993).
(4) Have the patient place lips around the mouthpiece. The patient should take a full breath and then exhale two to three times longer than inhalation. Pattern should be repeated for 10 to 20 breaths.	• Ensures that all breathing is done through the mouth and that the device is used properly.
(5) Remove device from the mouth and have the patient take a slow, deep breath and hold for 3 seconds.	• Promotes lung expansion before coughing.
(6) Instruct the patient to exhale in quick, short, forced exhalations or "huffs."	• "Huff" coughing, or forced expiratory technique, promotes bronchial hygiene through increased expectoration of secretions.

STEPS	RATIONALE
C. Controlled coughing	
(1) Explain the importance of maintaining an upright position.	• Position facilitates diaphragm excursion and enhances thorax expansion.
(2) Demonstrate coughing. Take two slow, deep breaths, inhaling through the nose and exhaling through the mouth.	• Deep breaths expand the lungs fully so that air moves behind mucus and facilitates the effects of coughing.
(3) Inhale deeply a third time and hold breath to count of three. Cough fully for two or three consecutive coughs without inhaling between coughs. (Tell the patient to push all air out of lungs.)	• Consecutive coughs help remove mucus more effectively and completely than one forceful cough.

CRITICAL DECISION POINT: *Coughing may be contraindicated after brain or eye surgery.*

(4) Caution the patient against simply clearing the throat instead of coughing. Explain that coughing will not cause injury to incision when done correctly.	• Clearing the throat does not remove mucus from deep in airways. Postoperative incisional pain makes it harder for the patient to cough effectively.
(5) If surgical incision will be abdominal or thoracic, teach the patient to place one hand over the incisional area and the other hand on top of it. During breathing and coughing exercises, the patient presses gently against the incisional area to splint or support it. A pillow over the incision is optional (see Step 6C[5] illustration).	• Surgical incision cuts through muscles, tissues, and nerve endings. Deep breathing and coughing exercises place additional stress on the suture line and cause discomfort. • Splinting the incision with hands provides firm support and reduces incisional pulling. (Some patients prefer to have a pillow to place over the incision.)

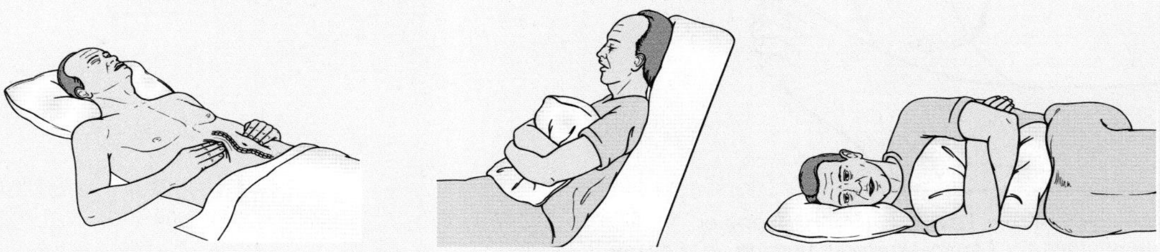

STEP 6C(5) Techniques for splinting incision. (From Lewis, S. L., Dirksen, S. R., Heitkemper, M. M., et al. [2014]. *Medical-surgical nursing in Canada: Assessment and management of clinical problems* [3rd Canadian ed.]. Toronto: Elsevier.)

(6) The patient continues to practise coughing exercises, splinting imaginary incision. Instruct the patient to cough two to three times every 2 hours while awake.	• Value of deep coughing with splinting is stressed to expectorate mucus effectively with minimal discomfort.
(7) Instruct the patient to examine sputum for consistency, odour, amount, and colour changes.	• Sputum consistency, odour, amount, and colour changes may indicate presence of pulmonary complication, such as pneumonia.
D. Turning (Note that turning properly applies when patient is in hospital, as well as once patient returns home.)	
(1) Instruct the patient to assume supine position and move to side of bed if permitted by surgery. Have the patient move by bending knees and pressing heels against the mattress to raise and move buttocks (see Step 6D[1] illustration). Top side rails on both sides of the bed should be raised.	• Positioning begins on side of the bed so that turning to other side will not cause the patient to roll toward the bed's edge.
(2) Instruct the patient to place right hand over the incisional area to splint it.	• Supports and minimizes pulling on the suture line during turning.
(3) Instruct the patient to keep right leg straight and flex left knee up (see Step 6D[3] illustration). If back or vascular surgery was performed, patient will need to logroll or will require assistance with turning.	• Straight leg stabilizes the patient's position. Flexed left leg shifts weight for easier turning.

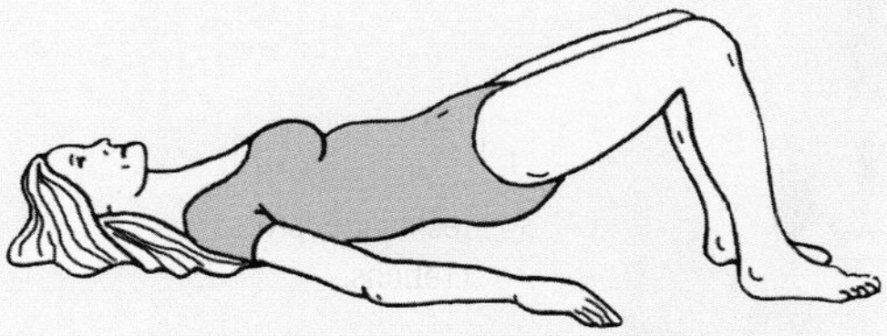

STEP 6D(1) Buttocks lift.

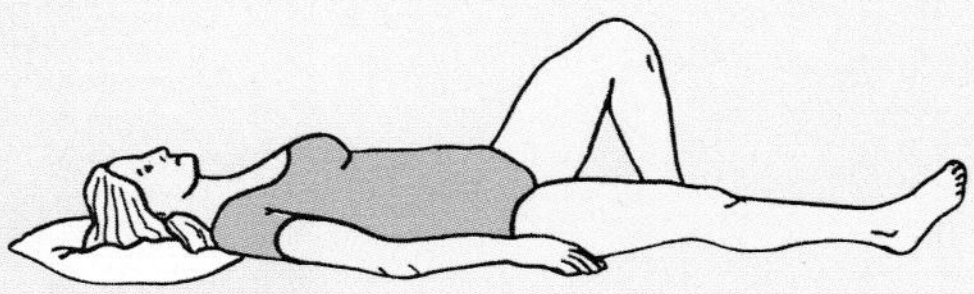

STEP 6D(3) Leg position for turning.

Continued

SKILL 48-1 DEMONSTRATING POSTOPERATIVE EXERCISES—cont'd

STEPS	RATIONALE
(4) Have the patient grab the right side rail with left hand, pull toward right, and roll onto right side.	• Pulling toward side rail reduces effort needed for turning.
(5) Instruct the patient to turn every 2 hours while awake.	• Reduces risk of vascular and pulmonary complications.
E. Leg exercises Patients do these in hospital and once at home	
(1) Have the patient assume supine position in bed. Demonstrate leg exercises by performing passive range-of-motion exercises and simultaneously explaining exercise.	• Provides normal anatomical position of lower extremities.
(2) Rotate each ankle in complete circle. Instruct the patient to draw imaginary circles with big toe (see Step 6E[2] illustration). Repeat five times.	• Leg exercises maintain joint mobility and promote venous return to prevent thrombi.

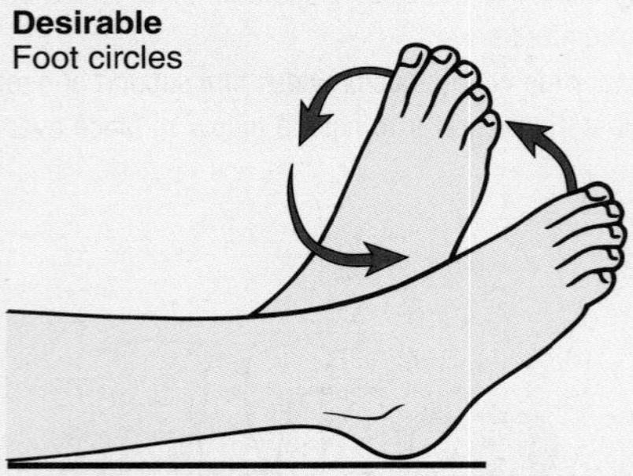

STEP 6E(2) Foot circles. (From Lewis, S. M., Heitkemper, M. M., Dirksen, S. R., et al. [2014]. *Medical-surgical nursing in Canada: Assessment and management of clinical problems* [3rd Canadian ed.]. Toronto: Elsevier.)

(3) Alternate dorsiflexion and plantar flexion of both feet. Direct the patient to feel calf muscles contract and relax alternately (see Step 6E[3] illustrations, parts A and B). Repeat five times.	• Stretches and contracts gastrocnemius muscles.

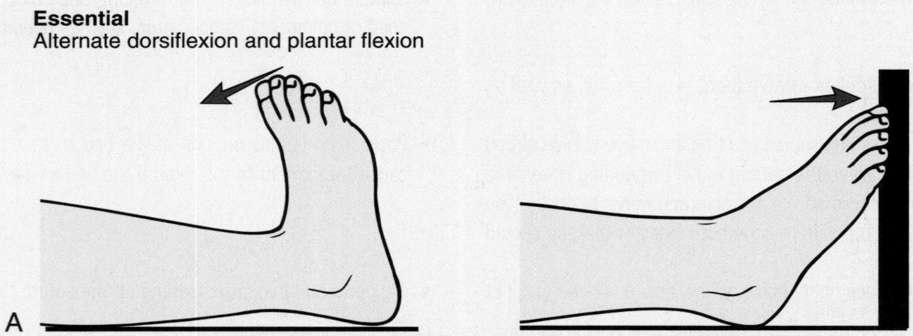

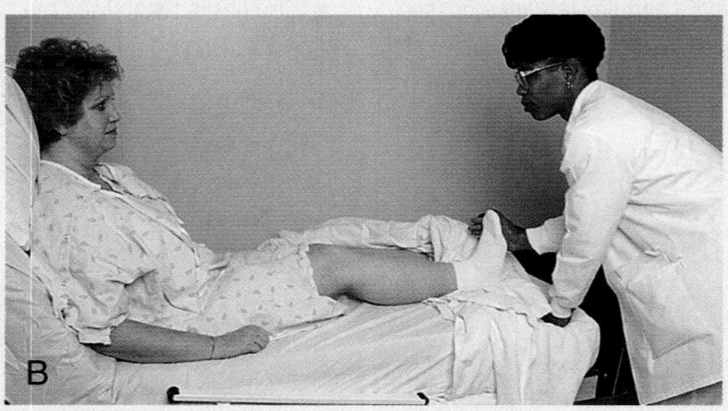

STEP 6E(3) A, Alternate dorsiflexion and plantar flexion. **B,** Patient pushes feet to perform plantar flexion. (From Lewis, S. M., Heitkemper, M. M., Dirksen, S. R., et al. [2014]. *Medical-surgical nursing in Canada: Assessment and management of clinical problems* [3rd Canadian ed.]. Toronto: Elsevier.)

STEPS	RATIONALE
(4) Perform quadriceps setting by tightening thigh and bringing knee down toward mattress, then relaxing (see Step 6E[4] illustration). Repeat five times.	• Contracts muscles of upper legs, maintains knee mobility, and enhances venous return.
(5) Have the patient alternately raise each leg straight up from the bed surface, keeping legs straight, and then have the patient bend leg at hip and knee (see Step 6E[5] illustration). Repeat five times.	• Promotes contraction and relaxation of quadriceps muscles.

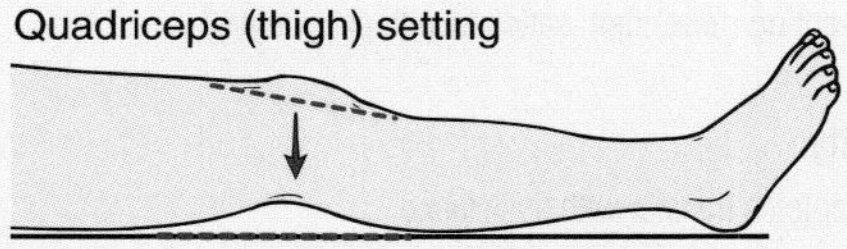

STEP 6E(4) Quadriceps (thigh) setting. (From Lewis, S. M., Heitkemper, M. M., Dirksen, S. R., et al. [2014]. *Medical-surgical nursing in Canada: Assessment and management of clinical problems* [3rd Canadian ed.]. Toronto: Elsevier.)

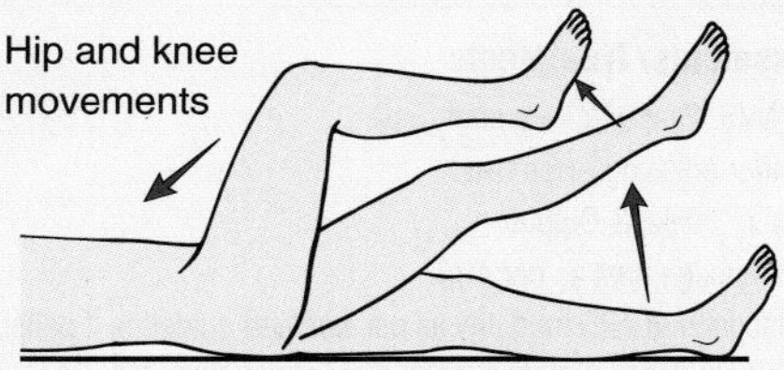

STEP 6E(5) Hip and knee movements. (From Lewis, S. L., Heitkemper, M. M., Dirksen, S. R., et al. [2014]. *Medical-surgical nursing in Canada: Assessment and management of clinical problems* [3rd Canadian ed.]. Toronto: Elsevier.)

STEPS	RATIONALE
7. Have the patient practise exercises at least every 2 hours while awake. Instruct the patient to coordinate turning and leg exercises with diaphragmatic breathing and coughing exercises.	• Repetition of sequence reinforces learning. Establishes routine for exercises that develops habit for performance. Sequence of exercises should be leg exercises, turning, breathing, and coughing.
8. Observe the patient's ability to perform all exercises independently.	• Ensures that the patient has learned correct techniques. Documents the patient's education and provides data for instructional follow-up.

UNEXPECTED OUTCOMES	RELATED INTERVENTIONS
Inability to perform exercises correctly after surgery	• Assess for the presence of anxiety, pain, and fatigue. • Teach the patient stress reduction techniques, pain management strategies, or both. • Repeat the teaching, using additional demonstration or repeat demonstration at a time when family members or friends are present.
Unwillingness to perform exercises postoperatively because of incisional pain of thorax or abdomen (deep breathing, coughing, and turning) or because of surgery involving lower abdomen, groin, buttocks, or legs (leg exercises, turning)	• Instruct the patient to ask for pain medication 30 minutes before performing postoperative exercises or to use patient-controlled analgesia (PCA) immediately before exercising. • Report to the surgeon inadequate pain relief and the need to change analgesic or increase dose.

RECORDING AND REPORTING

- Record the exercises demonstrated and whether the patient can perform them independently.
- Report any problems the patient has in practising exercises to the nurse assigned to the patient on the next shift for follow-up.

Patient Knows Where the Postoperative Unit Is and Where the Family Will Be During Surgery and Recovery. The unit to which the patient is admitted before surgery may be different from the postoperative unit. The family needs to know where the patient will be taken after surgery. The nurse also should explain where the family can wait and where the surgeon will attempt to find family members after surgery. Many institutions have implemented programs in which the circulating nurse gives periodic reports to the family in the waiting room when prolonged surgeries are involved. If the patient will be taken to a special unit postoperatively, it helps to orient the patient and family members to the unit's environment before surgery. Programs designed to connect with the family also have been developed in day-surgery areas (Andrews, 2009).

Patient Discusses Anticipated Postoperative Monitoring and Therapies. The patient and family need to know about postoperative events. If they understand the frequency of postoperative vital sign monitoring before surgery occurs, they will be less apprehensive when nurses do this. Nurses can also explain whether the patient is likely to have IV lines, monitoring lines, dressings, or drainage tubes or whether he or she will require ventilator support.

Patient Describes Surgical Procedures and Postoperative Treatment. After the surgeon has explained the basic purpose of the surgical procedure, the patient may ask the nurse additional questions to clarify any misunderstandings. Pre-established teaching standards, such as those integrated in clinical pathways for preoperative and postoperative care (Figure 48-4), give nurses an excellent guide for instruction. A good starting point is to ask what the patient has been told. If the patient has limited understanding about the surgery, the nurse can provide additional explanations. If necessary, the surgeon can be asked to re-inform the patient.

Patient Describes Postoperative Activity Resumption. The type of surgery a patient undergoes affects the speed with which normal physical activity and regular eating habits can be resumed. Nurses should explain that it is normal to progress gradually in both activity and eating. If the patient tolerates activity and diet well, activity levels will progress more quickly.

Patient(e) ______________________ Chart No. – N° du dossier ______________________

Post-op Day 1 — Jour 1 post-opératoire

Date: yyaa ________ mm ______ dj ______

Critical Path	Patient Outcomes
Assessments/Treatments • VS, NVS, Pain q4h → q shift, SpO_2 • Monitor dressing / Hemovac • Monitor Intake & Output • Pain management as per APS – Discontinue APS modality as per weaning guideline if patient meets criteria – If single dose intrathecal only: discontinue from APS 24 hours following time of injection **Activity** • DB&C • Exercise program • Pivot transfer with walker • Confirm weight bearing status • Up in chair x 2 ________ initial, ________ initial • Ambulate x 1 with assistance: ________ initial • Assistive devices, specify: ________________ **Nutrition** • Diet as ordered **Elimination** • Catheter as ordered **Patient Teaching** • Reinforce exercise program • Proper pillow positioning • Hip precautions • If on Low Molecular Weight Heparin – start self injection teaching and provide booklet • Ensure patient has Total Hip Arthroplasty patient information booklet • Pain management	**Pain Control** • Adequate pain control achieved: Pain ≤ 3 rest, ≤ 5 activity; pain not preventing movement; satisfied with pain control **Activity** • Completes transfer with assistance • Performs exercises according to self directed exercise program **Prevention of DVT** • Demonstrates appropriate exercises & positioning for prevention of DVT • Verbalizes understanding of anticoagulant therapy **Patient Teaching** • Verbalizes understanding of "Total Hip Arthroplasty" instructions and exercise program • Understands basics of self injection if applicable • Demonstrates: – Proper positioning – Understanding of weight-bearing status

Patient progress corresponds with clinical pathway

Physiotherapy:

☐ Yes ☐ No Signature: ____________________ Time: ________ NTV – circle above, VC ________

Nursing:

D ☐ Yes ☐ No Signature: ____________________, Initial ________ Time: ________ NTV – circle above, VC ________

E ☐ Yes ☐ No Signature: ____________________, Initial ________ Time: ________ NTV – circle above, VC ________

N ☐ Yes ☐ No Signature: ____________________, Initial ________ Time: ________ NTV – circle above, VC ________

D = 8-12 h day shift **E** = evening shift, if applicable **N** = 8-12 h night shift

Variance Codes (VC)

186	Activity variance	**510**	Not discharged by end of pathway – non-medical reason
653	Consult not sent by Day 3	**NTV**	Non-Tracked Variance
492	Not discharged by end of pathway – continued need for acute care	**OFF**	Ordered off clinical pathway

 CHART – DOSSIER CP 4A (3 – 7)

FIGURE 48-4 Clinical pathway for a total hip arthroplasty, primary/revision and hip resurfacing. Highlights what the patient can expect on the first day after surgery. (Courtesy The Ottawa Hospital, Ottawa, ON.)

Patient Describes Pain-Relief Measures. Typically, one of the patient's fears is pain. The family is also concerned for the patient's comfort. Pain after surgery is to be expected. The nurse should inform the patient and family of interventions available for pain relief (e.g., analgesics, positioning, splinting, and relaxation exercises; see Chapter 31). The patient needs to know the schedule for analgesic drugs, their route of administration, and their effects.

Patients having surgery may avoid taking pain-relief drugs for fear of becoming dependent on them. Nurses should encourage the patient to use analgesics as needed and explain to the patient that the risks of becoming dependent are minimal. The patient needs to understand that unless the pain is controlled, it will be difficult to participate in postoperative therapy such as mobilization. The patient should be encouraged to inform a nurse before the pain becomes a constant discomfort. If a patient waits until pain becomes excruciating, an analgesic may not provide relief at the dose prescribed. Patients who will have patient-controlled analgesia (PCA) after surgery should be taught how to push the button when they begin to feel discomfort and should understand that use of PCA will not cause overmedication (see Chapter 31). The patient should also understand the length of time that it takes for the drug to begin working. Information from preoperative assessment will be helpful to the nurse when teaching about pain-relief measures. Pain reporting and expectations regarding pain management based on a patient's cultural beliefs are areas that need to be explored both individually and systematically through research (Douglas, 1999; Ramer, Richardson, Cohen, et al., 1999). For example, Lovering (2006) conducted a collaborative inquiry project in Saudi Arabia to examine cultural attitudes and beliefs in patients and staff about the causes, treatment, and experiences of pain.

Patient Expresses Feelings Regarding Surgery. If the patient is admitted to the hospital during the preoperative surgical phase, frequent visits by staff, diagnostic testing, and physical preparation for surgery consume a lot of time; as a result, the patient has few opportunities to reflect on the upcoming surgical experience. Nurses must recognize the patient as a unique individual. The patient and family need time to express their feelings about the surgery. The patient's level of anxiety influences the frequency of discussions. While delivering bedside care, the nurse can encourage expression of concerns. Family members may wish to discuss their concerns without the patient present so that their fears will not frighten the patient and vice versa. Establishing a trusting and therapeutic relationship with the patient and family allows this to happen.

Acute Care. Activities in the acute care setting during the preoperative phase focus on interventions to prepare the patient physically for surgery. This occurs less frequently now, as many patients enter hospital on the day of surgery.

Physical Preparation. The degree of preoperative physical preparation depends on the patient's health status and on the surgery to be performed. A seriously ill patient receives more supportive care in the form of medications, IV fluid therapy, and monitoring than does a patient facing a minor elective procedure. Nurses should explain the purpose of all procedures.

Maintenance of normal fluid and electrolyte balances. The patient requiring surgery is vulnerable to fluid and electrolyte imbalances as a result of inadequate preoperative intake, excessive fluid losses during surgery, and the physiological effect of third spacing (redistribution of intravascular fluid into interstitial space) in the initial postoperative period (see Chapter 40). A patient traditionally took nothing by mouth (NPO) after midnight on the morning of surgery to keep the stomach empty and thus reduce the risk of vomiting and aspiration. Recommendations for preoperative fasting have been published by the Canadian Anesthesiologists' Society (2005/2018) and by the American Society of Anesthesiologists (ASA, 2011). They recommended fasting from clear liquids at least 2 hours before elective procedures requiring general anaesthesia, regional anaesthesia, or sedation/analgesia. The nurse should remove fluids and solid foods from the patient's bedside and post a sign over the patient's bed to alert hospital personnel and family members about fasting restrictions. The patient may be instructed to take specific medications (e.g., cardiovascular medications, anticonvulsants, or antibiotics) with a sip of water. A patient who is at home on the evening before surgery must understand the importance of the specific fasting period that has been ordered. Patients can rinse their mouths with water or mouthwash and brush their teeth immediately before surgery as long as they do not swallow water. The nurse must notify the surgeon and anaesthesiologist if the patient has eaten or consumed fluids during the fasting period.

During surgery, normal mechanisms for controlling fluid and electrolyte balances, including respiration, digestion, circulation, and elimination, are disturbed. The surgical procedure may cause extensive losses of blood and other body fluids. The surgical stress response aggravates any fluid and electrolyte imbalances. The patient's preoperative diet should include foods high in protein, with sufficient carbohydrates, fat, and vitamins. If a patient cannot eat because of gastrointestinal alterations or impairments in consciousness, an IV route for fluid replacement is started. The physician assesses serum electrolyte levels to determine the type of IV fluids and electrolyte additives to administer. Patients with severe nutritional imbalances may require supplements containing concentrated protein and glucose (see Chapter 42).

Reduction of risk of surgical wound infection. The risk of developing a surgical wound infection is determined by the amount and type of microorganisms contaminating a wound, the susceptibility of the host, and the surgical wound itself. All three factors interact to cause infection. Antibiotics may be ordered in the preoperative period and may be administered prophylactically. For example, prior to colorectal surgery, antibiotics are given orally or intravenously which cover aerobic and anaerobic bacteria and reduce the risk of surgical wound infection (Nelson, Gladman, & Barbateskovic, 2014).

Microorganisms grow and multiply on the skin. Without proper skin preparation, the risk of postoperative wound infection is high. Many surgeons instruct patients to bathe or shower the evening before surgery. Some physicians may request that patients bathe or shower more than once, whereas others may ask patients to give special attention to cleaning the proposed operative site. This attention could include the use of an antibacterial soap. Depending on the surgical procedure, a patient may also shower on the morning of surgery. If the surgical procedure involves the head, neck, or upper chest area, the patient may be required to shampoo his or her hair. Cleaning and trimming of fingernails and toenails also may be necessary.

The need for hair removal is less common now and depends on the amount of hair, the location of the incision, and the surgical procedure planned. Hair removal can damage and cause breaks in the patient's skin, which may allow for the entry of microorganisms. If required, hair is removed with a clipper or shaver as close to the time of surgery as possible. Tanner, Norrie, and Melen (2011) conducted a review of studies examining hair removal to reduce surgical site infection. They found no significant difference in infections between patients with hair removal and those without. However, the number of patients studied was small and further research is suggested.

Short hospital stays can reduce the chance of a hospital-acquired infection. Respiratory, urinary tract, and wound infections can all be acquired during hospitalization. This is one advantage of ambulatory surgical procedures, because the patient usually returns home once the surgery has been completed.

Precautions for patient requiring infection-control procedures. If a patient requires surgery but also has an infectious process, the OR must be notified in advance to ensure appropriate preparation. For example, patients with tuberculosis would be placed in a reverse airflow OR suite and subsequently in a reverse airflow room in the postanaesthesia care unit (PACU). Patients with methicillin-resistant *Staphylococcus aureus* (MRSA) may have their surgery performed at the end of the day so that the surgical suite can be cleaned afterward. These patients on transfer to the PACU are placed in an isolation room. Many hospitals now require that all "same-day admit" patients be screened for MRSA and vancomycin-resistant enterococci (VRE).

Prevention of bowel incontinence. The patient may receive a bowel preparation (e.g., a cathartic or enema) if the surgery involves the lower gastrointestinal system or lower abdominal organs. Manipulation of portions of the gastrointestinal tract during surgery results in absence of peristalsis for 24 hours or longer. Enemas and cathartics, such as GoLYTELY, cleane the gastrointestinal tract to prevent intraoperative incontinence and postoperative constipation. An empty bowel reduces the risk for injury to the intestines and minimizes contamination of the operative wound if a portion of the bowel is incised or opened accidentally, or if colon surgery is planned (see Chapter 44).

Promotion of rest and comfort. Rest is essential for normal healing. Anxiety about the impending surgery can easily interfere with the patient's ability to relax or sleep. As well, the underlying condition requiring surgery may be painful, further impairing rest.

If the patient is admitted to the hospital before the day of surgery, the nurse should attempt to make the patient's environment quiet and comfortable. Sometimes the patient is ordered an anxiolytic agent for the night before surgery. Anxiolytic agents such as benzodiazepines (e.g., alprazolam [Xanax]) act on the cerebral cortex and limbic system to relieve anxiety and promote sleep (Lehne, 2007).

An advantage of ambulatory surgery or same-day surgical admissions is that the patient is able to sleep at home the night before surgery. He or she is likely to get more rest in a familiar environment. The nonhospitalized patient also may have medication ordered by the physician if apprehension about surgery interferes with a good night's rest.

Preparation on the Day of Surgery. Nurses must complete a number of interventions before releasing the patient for surgery.

Hygiene. Basic hygiene measures provide additional comfort before surgery. The patient may want to bathe before surgery. Because the patient cannot wear personal nightwear to the OR, the nurse must provide a clean hospital gown. If the patient has been NPO for the last several hours, his or her mouth may be very dry. The nurse may offer the patient mouthwash and toothpaste, again with the caution not to swallow any water.

Hair and cosmetics. During surgery with general anaesthesia, the patient's head is positioned to introduce an endotracheal tube into the airway (see Chapter 39). This procedure may involve manipulation of the patient's hair and scalp. To avoid injury, the patient should be asked to remove hairpins or clips before leaving for surgery. Hairpieces or wigs also should be removed. Long hair can be braided. The patient will wear a disposable hat before entering the OR.

During and after surgery, the anaesthesiologist and nurses will assess skin and mucous membranes to determine the patient's level of oxygenation and circulation. Therefore, all makeup (lipstick, powder, blush, nail polish) should be removed to expose normal skin and nail colouring. Pulse oximetry is capable of recording accurate measurements through most nail polish colours, but removal is still considered good practice. Contact lenses, false eyelashes, and eye makeup also must be removed. The patient's glasses can be stored or given to the family immediately before the patient enters the OR.

Removal of prostheses. It is easy for any type of prosthetic device to become lost or damaged during surgery. The patient must remove all prostheses, including partial or complete dentures, artificial limbs, artificial eyes, and hearing aids. If a patient has a brace or a splint, the nurse may need to determine whether it should remain with the patient.

Many patients are embarrassed at having to remove dentures, wigs, or other devices that enhance their personal appearance. Privacy should be offered as these personal items are removed. Patients may be allowed to keep personal items until they reach the preoperative area. For safekeeping, dentures must be placed in special containers labelled with the patient's name and other identification required by the agency. In many institutions, nurses must make an inventory of all prosthetic devices or personal items and lock them away according to agency policy. It is also common practice for nurses to give prostheses to family members or to keep items like dentures at the patient's bedside. Documentation in the nursing notes, the surgical checklist, or per agency policy should reflect these actions.

Safeguarding valuables. If a patient has any valuables, the nurse should give them to family members or secure them for safekeeping. Many hospitals require patients to sign a release form that frees the institution of responsibility for any lost valuables. Valuables usually can be stored and locked in a designated location. Often patients are reluctant to remove wedding rings or religious medals. A wedding band can be taped in place. However, if there is a risk that the patient will experience swelling of the hand or fingers (related to mastectomy, hand surgery, or fluid shifts), the wedding band should be removed. For safety, metal items, such as for pierced areas, should also be removed. The location of valuables is documented per hospital policy.

Preparing the bowel and bladder. The patient may require an enema or cathartic on the morning of surgery to ensure that the colon is empty. If so, it should be given at least 1 hour before the patient is scheduled to leave for surgery, allowing time for the patient to defecate without rushing. The nurse should instruct the patient to void just before leaving for the OR and before giving preoperative medications. An empty bladder prevents a patient from becoming incontinent during surgery. This is important during abdominal surgery, when it may be necessary for the surgeon to manipulate the bladder. An empty bladder also makes abdominal organs more accessible during surgery. The last time of voiding is charted. If the patient is unable to void, this should be noted on the preoperative (preprocedure) checklist. An in-dwelling urinary catheter may be placed if the surgery is long or the incision will be in the lower abdomen.

Vital signs. The nurse must measure a final preoperative set of vital signs. The anaesthesiologist uses these values as a baseline during surgery. If preoperative vital signs are abnormal, surgery may need to be postponed. The physician should be notified of any abnormalities before sending the patient to surgery.

Documentation. Before the patient goes to the OR, the nurse needs to check the contents of the medical record to ensure that pertinent laboratory results are present. Any abnormal findings in laboratory results, such as low potassium, should be reported. Consent forms need to be checked for accuracy of information. A preoperative or preprocedure checklist (Figure 48-5) provides nurses with guidelines to ensure that nursing interventions are completed. Nurses should also check the nursing notes to ensure that documentation of care is current. This is especially important if the hospitalized patient experienced unexpected problems on the night before surgery. The OR should be alerted through notation of any positioning challenges for the patient, such as difficulty flexing knees, or of any sensory impairment.

Performing special procedures. A patient's condition may warrant special interventions before surgery. The patient may need IV infusions

The Ottawa Hospital | L'Hôpital d'Ottawa

PRE PROCEDURE CHECKLIST
FEUILLE DE VÉRIFICATION PRÉ-INTERVENTION

Nurse to initial each column – L'infirmière doit parapher chaque colonne	Yes Oui	No Non	N/A S/O
Addressograph plate – Plaque d'adressographe			
Precautions if yes, check – Précautions si oui, cochez : ❑ contact(es) ❑ airborne – aériennes ❑ droplet – gouttelettes ❑ other – autre :			
Identity bracelet verified – Bracelet d'identité vérifié			
Allergies status confirmed, bracelet on prn-Statut d'allergies confirmé, bracelet mis prn			
Weight – Poids : ❑ kg ❑ lbs			
Consent CON 17 completed as per policy Admin. no. (00291) – Consentement CON 17 rempli selon la politique Admin n° (00291)			
Blood and blood products consent CON 66 completed as per policy Admin. no. (00045) Consentement à recevoir du sang ou des produits sanguins CON 66 rempli selon la politique Admin n° (00045)			
Consult notes/Medical history – Notes de consultation/Antécédents médicaux ❑ on chart – au dossier ❑ on – sur OACIS			
Patient Admission History – Antécédents du patient à l'admission (NUR 71 A) ❑ on chart – au dossier ❑ on – sur OACIS			
Medication Administration Records (MAR) – Fiches d'administration des médicaments (FAM)			
Teeth – Dents : ❑ capped – couronne ❑ loose – branlante Removed – Enlevé(s) : ❑ dentures dentiers ❑ bridge pont ❑ glasses lunettes ❑ contacts verres de contacts ❑ makeup/nail polish maquillage/vernis à ongles ❑ jewellery/body piercing bijoux/perçage corporel Hearing aid – Appareil auditif : ❑ removed – enlevé ❑ in ear – dans l'oreille (case must be labelled and sent to OR – L'étui doit être étiquetté et envoyé au bloc opératoire)			
Communication barrier – Conflit de communication If yes, Interpreter to accompany patient to OR – Si oui, l'interprète doit accompagner le patient au bloc opératoire			
Skin integrity problem – Problème de l'intégrité de la peau Site :			
Surgical implants – Implants chirurgicaux Site :			
Pacemaker/Internal defibrillator – Stimulateur cardiaque/Défibrillateur interne			
Antibiotics ordered – Antibiotiques ordonnés ❑ Sent to OR with patient – Envoyés au bloc avec le patient ❑ Given/started on unit – Administré/débuté à l'unité			
Diagnostic testing completed as per orders or pathway – Examens diagnostiques complets selon ordonnances ou plan			
Blood glucose by point of care testing (POCT) – Glycémie par tests aux points de service			
Pregnancy test – Examen de grossesse Done prn – Fait prn : ❑ + ❑ -			
CPR & Plan of Treatment – RCR et plan de traitement (SPO 238 on front of chart – au devant du dossier)			
NPO since – À jeun depuis :			
Family/SDM have been notified of procedure time ❑ Patient refused ❑ No family available Person Notified (name) Telephone number Date/Time notified			

PRINTED NAME-NOM EN LETTRES MOULÉES	SIGNATURE	INIT	DATE (yyaa-mm-dj)	TIME HEURE

ORA 06 (04/2015) Cat.: 412550 CHART-DOSSIER

FIGURE 48-5 Preprocedure checklist. (Courtesy The Ottawa Hospital, Ottawa, ON.)

started or a nasogastric tube inserted before leaving the patient unit for surgery. These procedures also may be done once the patient is in the preoperative area or in the OR.

Administering preoperative medications. The advent of ambulatory surgery has reduced the use of preoperative medications. However, the anaesthesiologist or surgeon may order preanaesthetic drugs ("on-call medications," "pre-ops") to reduce the patient's anxiety, the amount of general anaesthesia required, the risk of nausea and vomiting and resultant aspiration, and respiratory tract secretions.

The nurse should provide all nursing care measures before giving the patient preoperative medications at the prescribed time. The consent form needs to be signed before the administration of these medications. In addition, the patient should be helped to void. Because the drugs cause sedation, the patient should not be allowed to leave the bed or stretcher until personnel arrive to transport him or her to the OR. The patient should be warned to expect drowsiness and a dry mouth.

> **Safety Alert** Explain to the patient the effects of any preoperative medications. Remind the patient to remain in bed or on the stretcher. Raise the side rails and keep the bed or stretcher in the low position. Place the call light within easy reach of the patient.

Latex sensitivity or allergy. As the incidence and prevalence of latex sensitivity and allergy has increased, the need to recognize potential sources of latex is critical. Guidelines developed through Canadian and American health care organizations are also available for the management of latex allergies and safe latex use in health care facilities (Sussman & Gold, 2004). For example, the Canadian Allergy, Asthma, and Immunology Foundation (1994) has a fact sheet on latex allergy.

The OR and PACU can contain innumerable products that have latex in them. Some common sources are gloves, IV tubing, syringes, and rubber stoppers on bottles and vials. Latex is also present in objects that may be overlooked, such as adhesive tape, disposable electrodes, endotracheal tube cuffs, protection sheets, and ventilator equipment. However, many hospitals have moved to latex-free products. Persons most at risk are people with a previous sensitivity to latex or rubber products, people with neural tube defects such as spina bifida, patients with a history of multiple surgeries, health care providers, and those with a history of contact dermatitis or atopic immunological reactions (OPANA, 2009b). Symptoms of a latex reaction can include local effects ranging from urticaria and flat or raised red patches to vesicular, scaling, or bleeding eruptions. Acute dermatitis also may be present. Rhinitis and rhinorrhea are other common symptoms in both mild and severe latex reactions. Immediate hypersensitivity reactions can be life-threatening, with the patient exhibiting focal or generalized urticaria, edema, bronchospasm, and mucous hypersecretion, which can compromise respiratory status. Vasodilatation compounded by increased capillary permeability can lead to circulatory collapse and eventual death.

Protocols exist for patients with a latex allergy or sensitivity. Patients with this allergy are identified preoperatively. Latex-free kits are available; they include latex-free equipment (e.g., a latex-free ambu bag) and follow the patients throughout their hospitalization. Although latex kits are available, the move to latex-free products has decreased their use. It is recommended that the patient with a latex allergy be scheduled as the first case of the day in the OR (OPANA, 2009b). The patient can then be safely accommodated by using appropriate latex-free items during the perioperative period and recovery. Box 48-5 lists precautions for patients with latex sensitivity or allergy.

BOX 48-5 EVIDENCE-INFORMED PRACTICE

Latex Precautions

1. Survey the patient care area and remove any products containing latex (e.g., examination gloves, rubber sheets, or blood pressure cuff).
2. Place a latex precautions label on the patient's chart and latex precautions signs on the door to the patient's room and on the transport cart.
3. Use only nonlatex gloves. Order an adequate supply.
4. Review the supplies to be used for the patient and substitute with latex-free supplies as necessary.
5. Review the medications to be administered and verify that they are latex-free. Include the following steps:
   a. Notify the pharmacy of the need for latex precautions.
   b. Verify that all prescribed medications are latex-free.
   c. Place a sign in the area where medications (including mixing solutions) are kept, indicating that the patient is on latex precautions.
   d. Use latex-free syringes.
6. Review the intravenous supplies to be used and verify that they are latex-free. Include the following steps:
   a. Use latex-free solutions.
   b. Use latex-free tubing.
   c. Use latex-free syringes, including those for patient-controlled analgesia.
   d. Use latex-free tape.
7. Verify that bedding and support garments are latex-free (e.g., mattress protectors, anti-embolism stockings, and binders).
8. Verify that dressings and tape are latex-free.
9. Notify the family and visitors of the use of latex precautions.
10. Routinely survey the patient care area to verify that latex products are not present (e.g., examination gloves, balloons).
11. Before transfer to another area or agency, notify care providers of the need for latex precautions.
12. Provide education programs about latex allergy to health care providers, patients, and family or caregivers. This education should include the following:
    a. Definition of latex allergy
    b. Exposures to latex
    c. Latex avoidance
    d. Signs and symptoms of a reaction to latex
    e. Emergency treatment of a reaction to latex

Adapted from Sussman, G., & Gold, M. (2004). *Guidelines for the management of latex allergies and safe latex use in health care facilities.* Retrieved from http://www.accai.org/public/physicians/latex.htm; and Ontario Perianesthesia Nurses Association (OPANA). (2009). *Management of patients with latex allergies* (pp. 121–123). Dundas, ON: Author.

Surgical safety checklist. The World Health Organization (WHO, 2008) has a surgical safety checklist, a tool designed by experts in surgery, anaesthesia, and nursing, that can be used to foster communication between surgeons and nurses about a patient's condition and risk factors at critical time points: during sign in, time out (surgical phase), and sign out. This checklist is endorsed by the Canadian Patient Safety Institute (2009).

Eliminating wrong site and wrong procedure surgery. Whenever an invasive surgical procedure is to be performed, the nurse and the surgeon must ensure that the site has been marked by the surgeon (see agency policy). Indelible ink may be used to mark left and right distinction, multiple structures (e.g., fingers), and levels of the spine. The nurse also must verify the patient and the procedure to be performed. In addition, once the patient reaches the OR, he or she is introduced to the surgical team. The patient is asked to describe what procedure is being performed and to indicate the site for the surgery. The consent form is verified.

◆ Evaluation

Patient Care. The nurse in the preoperative area will be the source for evaluating outcomes during the preoperative period (Figure 48-6). With regard to the preoperative patient's care plan, limited time is available to evaluate the outcomes. The patient's current status is compared with expected outcomes to determine whether new or revised interventions or nursing diagnoses need to be implemented.

Because interventions continue during and after surgery, evaluation of many goals and outcomes do not occur until after surgery. For example, the nurse will not be able to evaluate the success in preventing postoperative wound infection or promoting return of normal physiological function until a few days after surgery. If the patient is having ambulatory surgery, he or she will return home; therefore, the effectiveness of certain interventions is evaluated at follow-up appointments.

Patient Expectations. Determining whether the patient's expectations have been met regarding preoperative teaching may be difficult. Nurses are evaluating patients in a hurried atmosphere because there are many things that need to be accomplished in a short amount of time. The patient's surgery may be an emergency, or performance of various procedures may make it difficult for nurses to find time for evaluation. It is important that nurses remember to attend to the patient's emotional needs (privacy, fear, anxiety), as well as to his or her physical needs. The patient should be given an opportunity to state whether expectations have been met. If expectations have not been met, the nurse needs to work closely with the patient to redefine expectations that can be realistically met within the time limits imposed by the particular setting.

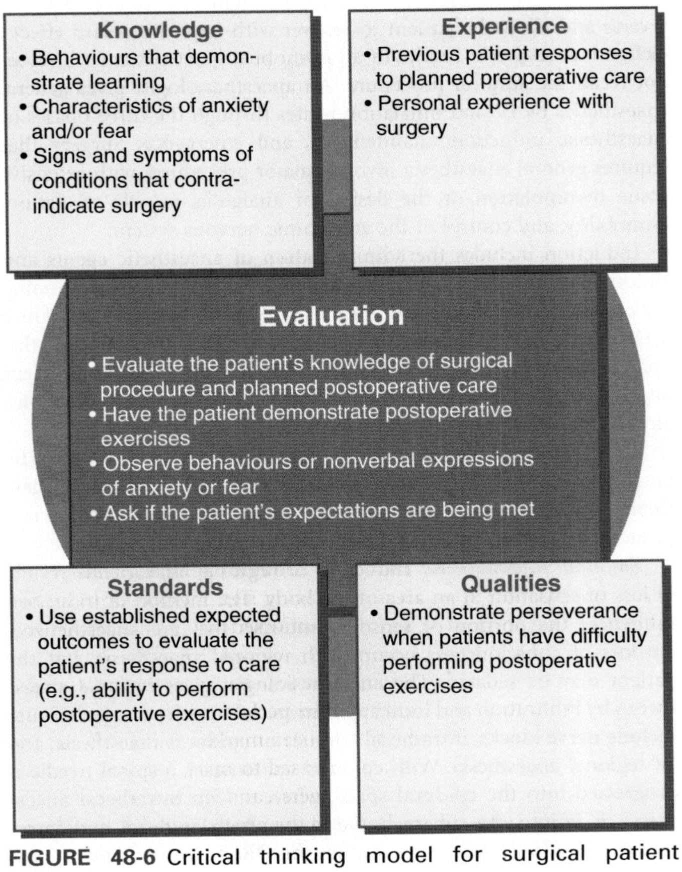

FIGURE 48-6 Critical thinking model for surgical patient evaluation.

TRANSPORT TO THE OPERATING ROOM

Personnel in the OR notify the nursing division or ambulatory surgery area when it is time for the patient's surgery. In many hospitals, an orderly or transporter brings a stretcher for transporting the patient. The transporter checks the patient's identification bracelet against the patient's chart to ensure that the right person is going to surgery. Because the patient may have received preoperative drugs, the nurses and transporter assist the patient when transferring from bed to stretcher to prevent falls. The ambulatory surgery patient may ambulate to the OR if able to do so and not medicated. The nurse should provide the family with an opportunity to visit before the patient is transported to the OR, then direct the family to a waiting area. In some hospitals, the family may be allowed to wait with the patient in the OR holding area until he or she is transported into the OR.

After the patient leaves the nursing unit, the bed and the room are prepared if the patient is returning to the same nursing unit. For recording vital signs, many institutions now have automated blood pressure machines. In addition, with bedside monitoring equipment, patient information can be scanned at the bedside and entered into the electronic chart. Other materials required at the bedside include the following:

- Emesis basin
- Clean gown
- Washcloth, towel, and facial tissues
- IV pole and, often, IV pump
- Suction equipment (if needed)
- Oxygen equipment (if needed)
- Extra pillows for positioning the patient comfortably
- Bed pads to protect bed linens from drainage
- Bed raised to stretcher height with bed linens pulled back and furniture moved to accommodate the stretcher and equipment (such as IV lines)

INTRAOPERATIVE SURGICAL PHASE

Care of the patient during surgery requires careful preparation and knowledge of the events that occur during the surgical procedure. The nurse usually functions in one of two roles in the OR: circulating nurse or scrub nurse. The **circulating nurse** must be a registered nurse. Responsibilities of this nurse include reviewing the preoperative assessment, establishing and implementing the intraoperative care plan, evaluating the care, and providing for continuity of care postoperatively. The circulating nurse assists with procedures, such as endotracheal intubation as needed. In addition, this nurse monitors sterile technique and a safe OR environment, assists the surgeon and surgical team by providing additional supplies, verifying sponge and instrument counts, and maintaining accurate and complete written records.

The **scrub nurse** may be a registered nurse or a registered practical nurse. This nurse maintains a sterile field during the surgical procedure, assists with applying sterile drapes, hands the surgeons instruments and other sterile supplies, and completes sponge and instrument counts.

Preoperative (Holding) Area

In most hospitals, the patient enters a holding area outside the OR. The nurse in the holding area validates the patient's identification and the location of the surgery. The nurse also verifies that appropriate data have been obtained, assesses a patient's readiness both physically and emotionally, and reinforces teaching. Nurses in the holding area are members of the OR staff and wear surgical scrub suits, hats, and footwear in accordance with infection control policies. In some ambulatory surgical settings, a perioperative primary nurse admits the patient, circulates for the operative procedure, and manages the patient's recovery and discharge.

In the preoperative area, the nurse or the anaesthesiologist may insert an IV catheter into the patient's arm to establish a route for fluid replacement and IV drugs. A large-bore (18-gauge) IV catheter is used for easy infusion of fluids and blood products if necessary. The nurse also applies a blood pressure cuff. The cuff will remain in place throughout the surgery so that the anaesthesiologist can assess blood pressure readings. The nurse usually reviews the preoperative checklist, and the anaesthesiologist may perform a patient assessment at this time.

If any preoperative medications have been given, the patient begins to feel drowsy. The temperature in the holding area and adjacent OR suites is usually cool, and the patient should be offered an extra blanket. The patient's stay in the holding area is usually brief.

Admission to the Operating Room

Nurses transfer the patient to the OR via a stretcher. Usually the patient is still awake and will notice nurses and physicians wearing surgical masks, gowns, and eyewear. The staff carefully transfer the patient to the OR table, after ensuring that the stretcher and table are locked in place. After the patient is on the table, a safety strap is fastened around the patient. The nurse supports the patient by explaining procedures and encouraging the patient to ask questions. Sights and sounds in the surgical suite can seem frightening to patients.

NURSING PROCESS IN THE INTRAOPERATIVE SURGICAL PHASE

Assessment

In the holding area, the nurse conducts a focused preoperative assessment to verify that the patient is ready for surgery and to plan intraoperative care. Because patients will not be able to speak for themselves while under general anaesthesia, this preoperative assessment in the OR is important for the patient's safety.

> **Safety Alert** Verification of the patient's name by patient response compared with chart and ID bracelet is completed before sedation. The chart is reviewed for consent forms, allergies, medical history, physical assessment findings, test results, and verification of preoperative medications. The nurse verifies with the patient the planned surgical procedure and the surgical site before anaesthesia is administered. Some agencies ask the patient to mark the surgical site. The nurse ensures that the patient's prosthetic devices and valuables have been removed.

Nurses review the preoperative care plan to establish an intraoperative care plan and assess the patient's psychological comfort.

Nursing Diagnosis

Nurses review preoperative nursing diagnoses and modify them to individualize the care plan in the OR.

Planning

Goals and Outcomes. Patient-centred outcomes of preoperative care extend into the intraoperative phase. For example, one goal would be to maintain skin integrity. An expected outcome would be that the patient will have intact skin and show no signs of redness.

Implementation

A primary focus of intraoperative care is to prevent injury and complications related to anaesthesia, surgery, positioning, and equipment used. The perioperative nurse serves as an advocate for the patient during surgery and protects the patient's dignity and rights at all times.

Physical Preparation. After safely securing the patient on the OR table, the nurse applies monitoring devices to the patient before surgery. Patients receiving general and regional anaesthesia undergo continuous ECG monitoring during surgery. Small plastic electrodes are placed on the chest and extremities to record electrical activity of the heart. A monitor in the OR displays the heart's electrical activity. Pulse oximetry will be used to monitor oxygen saturation. An electrical cautery grounding pad is applied to the skin. Antiembolism stockings or sequential compression devices may be applied intraoperatively (especially during long surgeries) or postoperatively according to agency policy (see Chapter 45). The nurse documents device application and patient tolerance to procedures.

Introduction of Anaesthesia. Patients undergoing surgical procedures receive one of four types of anaesthesia: general, regional, local, or procedural sedation.

General Anaesthesia. General anaesthesia is a state of total unconsciousness resulting from anaesthetic drugs (Merchant, Chartrand, Dain, et al., 2016). Modern anaesthetic agents are much easier to reverse and allow the patient to recover with fewer untoward effects. General anaesthesia results in an immobile, quiet patient who does not recall the surgical procedure. An anaesthesiologist gives general anaesthetics by IV and inhalation routes through the three phases of anaesthesia: induction, maintenance, and emergence. Surgery that requires general anaesthesia involves major procedures with extensive tissue manipulation or the desire for analgesia, muscle relaxation, immobility, and control of the autonomic nervous system.

Induction includes the administration of anaesthetic agents and endotracheal intubation. The maintenance phase includes positioning the patient, preparing the skin for incision, and the surgical procedure itself. Appropriate levels of anaesthesia are maintained during this phase. During emergence, anaesthetics are decreased and the patient begins to awaken. Because of the short half-life of current medications, emergence often begins to occur in the OR.

The duration of anaesthesia depends on the length of surgery. The greatest risks from general anaesthesia are the adverse effects of anaesthetic agents, including cardiovascular depression or irritability, respiratory depression, and hepatic and renal damage.

Regional Anaesthesia. Induction of regional anaesthesia results in loss of sensation in an area of the body. The method of induction influences the portion of sensory pathways that are anaesthetized. No loss of consciousness occurs with regional anaesthesia, but the patient may be sedated. The anaesthesiologist gives regional anaesthetics by infiltration and local application. Administration techniques include nerve blocks, intrathecal (spinal) or epidural anaesthesia, and IV regional anaesthesia. With epidural anaesthesia, a spinal needle is progressed into the epidural space, whereas with intrathecal anaesthesia, it is into the subarachnoid space. Both epidural and intrathecal anaesthesia affect motor, sensory, and sympathetic nerves. With intrathecal anaesthesia, the onset of anaesthesia is faster and the amount of medication required is much less than with epidural anaesthesia.

Infiltrative anaesthetics do involve risks, particularly in the case of intrathecal (spinal) anaesthesia. Because the level of anaesthesia may rise, which means that the anaesthetic agent moves upward in the spinal cord, breathing may be affected. This migration of the anaesthetic agent depends on the drug type, amount, and patient position. If the level of anaesthesia rises, respiratory paralysis may develop, requiring resuscitation. Elevation of the upper body prevents respiratory paralysis. The patient may experience a sudden fall in blood pressure, which results from extensive vasodilation caused by the anaesthetic block to sympathetic vasomotor nerves and pain and motor nerve fibres. The patient requires careful monitoring during and immediately after surgery.

Because the patient is responsive and capable of breathing voluntarily, it is not necessary for the anaesthesiologist to use an endotracheal tube. OR personnel can gain a false sense of security because of the patient's relative alertness. Nurses must remember that burns and other trauma can occur on the anaesthetized part of the body without the patient's being aware of these injuries. Therefore, nurses must observe the position of the extremities and the condition of the skin frequently.

Local Anaesthesia. Local anaesthesia involves loss of sensation at the desired site (e.g., a growth on the skin or the cornea of the eye). The anaesthetic agent (e.g., lidocaine) inhibits nerve conduction until the drug diffuses into the body's circulation. It may be injected locally or applied topically. The patient experiences a loss in pain and touch sensation at the site. Local anaesthesia is commonly used for minor procedures performed in ambulatory surgery. Physicians may infiltrate the operative area with local anaesthetics to promote postoperative pain relief. For example, peripheral nerve blocks produce anaesthetic effect both at and distal to the site of injection (Turjanica, 2007).

Procedural sedation. Procedural sedation (sometimes referred to as conscious sedation) is routinely used for procedures that do not require complete anaesthesia but rather a depressed level of consciousness. Sedation is a state of reduced excitement achieved by the administration of a sedative agent (Merchant et al., 2016). The Ramsay Sedation Scale (RSS modified) can be used as a guide to levels of sedation (van Dishoeck, van der Hooft, Simoons, et al., 2009). With this sedation, procedures that need to be performed can be more acceptable to the patient. The patient must independently retain a patent airway and airway reflexes and must be able to respond appropriately to physical and verbal stimuli (Merchant et al., 2016). Ketamine has become popular for procedural sedation.

Advantages of procedural sedation include adequate sedation and reduction of fear and anxiety with less risk than general anaesthesia and a more rapid recovery. Sedation does not reduce sensation of pain; therefore, other treatments may be required to reduce pain. A variety of diagnostic and therapeutic procedures are appropriate for procedural sedation (burn dressing changes, some cosmetic surgery, pulmonary biopsy and bronchoscopy, colonoscopy, and many others). Nurses assisting with the administration of local anaesthesia and procedural sedation must demonstrate competency in the care of these patients. Knowledge of anatomy, physiology, cardiac dysrhythmias, procedural complications, and pharmacological principles related to the administration of individual agents is essential. Nurses also must be able to assess, diagnose, and intervene in the event of untoward reactions and demonstrate skill in airway management and oxygen delivery. Resuscitation equipment must be readily available when local anaesthesia or procedural sedation is used. AORN (2018) has guidelines on care of the patient receiving anaesthesia and care of patients receiving moderate sedation or analgesia.

Positioning the Patient for Surgery. When general anaesthesia is being used, the nursing personnel and surgeon often do not position the patient until the stage of complete relaxation is achieved. The choice of position is usually determined by the surgical approach. Ideally, the patient's position provides good access to the operative site and sustains adequate circulatory and respiratory function. It should not impair neuromuscular structures. The patient's comfort and safety must be considered.

Normal range of joint motion is maintained in an alert person by pain and pressure receptors. If a joint is extended too far, pain stimuli provide a warning that muscle and joint strain is too great. In a patient who is anaesthetized, normal defence mechanisms cannot guard against joint damage, muscle stretch, and strain. The muscles are so relaxed that it is relatively easy to place the patient in a position that the individual normally could not assume while awake. The patient then remains in a given position, often for several hours. Although it may be necessary to place a patient in an unusual position, attempts should be made to maintain correct alignment and protect the patient from pressure, abrasion, and other injuries. Attachments to the operating table allow protection and padding of extremities and bony prominences. Positioning should not impede normal movement of the diaphragm or interfere with circulation to body parts. If restraints are necessary, the area to be restrained should be padded to prevent skin trauma.

Documentation of Intraoperative Care. During the intraoperative phase, the nursing staff continues the preoperative care plan. Strict asepsis must be followed to minimize the risk of surgical wound infection. IV fluid infusion and monitoring of urinary and nasogastric output are examples of actions nurses will take to maintain the patient's fluid balance. Throughout the surgical procedure, an accurate record is kept of patient care activities and procedures performed by OR personnel. Documentation of intraoperative care provides useful data for the nurse who will care for the patient postoperatively.

◆ Evaluation

Interventions implemented during the intraoperative phase are evaluated throughout the surgical procedure.

Patient Care. Nurses perform intraoperative evaluation of the patient. Blood pressure, heart rate and rhythm, and oxygen saturation are monitored continuously. Temperature is measured during and upon completion of the surgical procedure. Intake and output is carefully recorded. The skin is inspected under the grounding pad and at areas where pressure from positioning may have been exerted.

Patient Expectations. Nurses should frequently question patients not undergoing general anaesthesia regarding pain, numbness, perceived room temperature, and overall comfort. The circulating nurse provides updates to family members in the waiting room.

POSTOPERATIVE SURGICAL PHASE

After surgery, a patient's care can become complex as a result of physiological changes that may occur. Patients who have undergone general anaesthesia are more likely to face complications than those who have had only local anaesthesia or procedural sedation. The patient who has had general anaesthesia usually has undergone extensive surgery as well. In contrast, an ambulatory surgical patient who has had local anaesthesia with no sedation and has stable vital signs may be discharged immediately. A patient who has undergone regional or general anaesthesia usually is transferred to the PACU to be stabilized before discharge to the nursing unit or back to the ambulatory surgery area.

To assess a patient's postoperative condition, nurses must apply critical thinking while relying on information from the preoperative nursing assessment, knowledge regarding the surgical procedure performed, and events occurring during surgery. This information helps nurses detect any changes and make decisions about the patient's care. A variation from the patient's norm may indicate the onset of surgery-related complications. Along with the anaesthesiologist or anaesthetist assistant, the circulating nurse may accompany the patient to the PACU and report to the nurse to provide continuity of care.

A patient's postoperative course involves two phases: the immediate recovery period and postoperative convalescence. For an ambulatory surgical patient, recovery normally lasts only 1 to 2 hours, and convalescence occurs at home. For a hospitalized patient, recovery may last a few hours, and convalescence occurs in the hospital over one or more days, depending on the extent of the surgery and the patient's response to it.

Immediate Postoperative Recovery

Before the patient arrives in the PACU, the PACU nurse obtains data from the surgical team in the OR regarding the patient's general status and the need for special equipment and nursing care. Careful planning allows the nursing staff to consider placement of patients in the PACU. For example, patients who have undergone spinal anaesthesia are aware of their surroundings and may benefit from being in a quieter part of the PACU, away from patients who need frequent monitoring. The patient with a serious infection such as tuberculosis should be isolated from other patients. Standard precautions or routine practices for infection control are used for all patients (see Chapter 33). Nurses must be familiar with agency and professional protocols related to preventing respiratory infection transmission (Public Health Ontario, 2012).

When the patient is admitted to the PACU, the nursing staff can inform family members. Usually, nurses would advise family members to remain in the designated waiting area so that they can be found when the surgeon arrives to explain the patient's condition. The surgeon is responsible for describing the patient's status, the results of surgery, and any complications that may have been encountered. Nurses can be a valuable resource to the family if complications arose during the operative phase.

When the patient enters the PACU (Figure 48-7), nurses and members of the surgical team confer about the patient's status. The surgical team's report includes a review of anaesthetic agents administered so that nurses can anticipate both how quickly a patient should regain consciousness and his or her analgesic needs. A report on IV fluids or blood products administered during surgery alerts nurses to the patient's fluid and electrolyte balances. The surgeon often reports any special concerns (e.g., whether the patient is at risk for hemorrhaging or infection). The anaesthesiologist discusses whether there were complications during surgery, such as excessive blood loss or cardiac irregularities. Frequently, this report takes place while PACU nurses are admitting the patient. A nurse will attach the patient to monitoring equipment such as the noninvasive blood pressure monitor, ECG monitor, and pulse oximeter. Patients usually receive some form of oxygen in this immediate recovery period. The nurse takes vital signs when the patient arrives and confirms these with the surgical team.

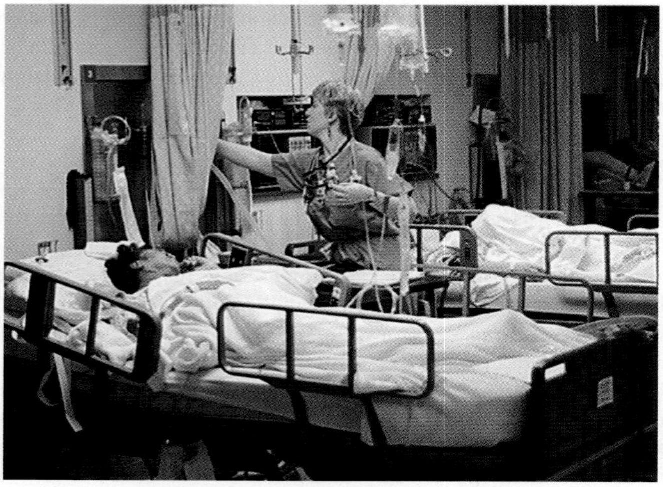

FIGURE 48-7 Postanaesthesia care unit.

After reviewing events in the OR, the PACU nurse conducts a complete assessment of the patient's status. This assessment should be performed rapidly and thoroughly and be targeted to the needs of the postsurgical patient. Standards of perianaesthetic nursing practice, such as those of NAPANc (2014), which are used by OPANA, function as a guide for agencies in outlining the urgent nature and components of the admission assessment as well as ongoing monitoring of patient status. A systems approach to assessment is discussed in a later section outlining the nursing process in postoperative care. Nursing care in the PACU focuses on monitoring and maintaining respiratory, circulatory, neurological, and fluid and electrolyte status; assessing wound status; and assessing and managing pain (see "Nursing Process in Postoperative Care").

Discharge From the Postanaesthesia Care Unit

Nurses evaluate readiness for discharge from the PACU by comparing vital sign stability with the preoperative data. Other outcomes for discharge are body temperature control, good ventilatory function, orientation to surroundings, absence of complications, minimal pain and nausea, controlled wound drainage, adequate urine output, and fluid and electrolyte balances. Patients who had more extensive surgery that required anaesthesia of longer duration usually recover more slowly. Many PACU staff use an objective scoring system that helps to delineate when patients may be discharged. The Aldrete score, or the Postanesthesia Recovery Score (PARS), is the most widely used scoring tool (Table 48-8). The patient must receive a composite score of 8 to 10 before discharge from the PACU. Some agencies have modified this scoring system; for example, some remove movement of extremities and add presence of pain, and some agencies require that the patient have a composite score of 10 before discharge from the PACU. If the patient's condition is still poor after 2 to 3 hours, the stay in the PACU lengthens or the surgeon may transfer the patient to a Critical Care Unit (CCU). More recently, some agencies have been using the Post-Anesthesic Discharge Scoring System (PADSS).

When the patient is ready to be discharged from the PACU, the PACU nurse may call the nursing unit to report the patient's status, including vital signs, respiratory status, the type of surgery and anaesthesia performed, any complications that occurred during surgery or in the PACU, blood loss, level of consciousness, general physical condition, type and amount of fluids received, and presence of IV lines, drainage tubes, and dressings. The nurse also should review physician orders that require attention. The PACU nurse's report helps the nurse in the acute patient care area to anticipate special patient needs and obtain necessary equipment. Any outstanding family issues are also addressed.

Orderlies or other personnel, who might include nurses, transport the patient on a stretcher. Usually the PACU nurse does not accompany the patient to the surgical unit, but a verbal report will be given to the acute care nurse reviewing the patient's condition and course of care. Some institutions have policies related to which patients must be

TABLE 48-8 Postanaesthetic Recovery Score or Modified Aldrete Score

Parameter	Task	Score
Activity	Able to move four extremities voluntarily or on command	2
	Able to move two extremities voluntarily or on command	1
	Unable to move extremities voluntarily or on command	0
Respiration	Able to breathe deeply and cough freely	2
	Dyspnea or limited breathing	1
	Apneic	0
Blood pressure	± 20% of preanaesthetic level	2
	± 20–49% of preanaesthetic level	1
	± 50% of preanaesthetic level	0
Consciousness	Fully awake	2
	Arousable on calling	1
	Not responding	0
Oxygen saturation	SpO_2 >94% on room air	2
	Needs O_2 inhalation to maintain SpO_2 >94%	1
	SpO_2 <94% even with extra O_2	0
Total		

Adapted from Aldrete, J. A., & Kroulik, D. (1970). A post-anesthetic recovery score. *Anesthesia and Analgesia, 49,* 924–934; and Aldrete, J. A. (1998). Modifications to the post-anesthesia score for use in ambulatory surgery. *Journal of PeriAnesthesia Nursing, 13*(3), 148.

accompanied by a nurse, such as those who have experienced recent seizure activity or who have had upper airway surgery. Staff members assist in safely transferring the patient to a bed (see Chapter 36).

Recovery in Ambulatory Surgery

The thoroughness and extent of postoperative recovery care depend on the ambulatory patient's condition, type of surgery, and anaesthesia. There are two phases of postanaesthesia recovery. During phase I, nurses focus on helping the patient safely transition from a totally anaesthetized state to one requiring less acute interventions. After patients become stable and no longer require such intensive monitoring, nurses transfer them to phase II recovery. During phase II, nurses focus on continuing the recovery process, addressing the patient's needs, and preparing the patient and family for discharge from phase II (NAPANc, 2014).

With new anaesthetic agents and techniques, patients experience a more rapid awakening in the OR (Apfelbaum, Walawander, Grasela, et al., 2002; Fredman, Sheffer, Zohar, et al., 2002; Saar, 2001). Therefore, some ambulatory surgery patients may bypass phase I. This is known as *fast tracking* (Rice, Muckler, Miller, et al., 2015; White, Rawal, Nguyen, et al., 2003). Phase II recovery may consist of a room equipped with medical recliner chairs, side tables, and footrests. Kitchen facilities for preparing light snacks and beverages are usually located in the area, along with bathrooms. Aldrete (1998) has added five more areas of functional assessment for the ambulatory surgery patient, which constitute the Postanesthesia Recovery Score for Ambulatory Patients (PARSAP) (Table 48-9). The phase II environment is designed to promote both the patient's and the family's comfort and well-being until discharge. Nurses continue to monitor patients but not at the same intensity as during phase I. In phase II recovery, nurses initiate postoperative teaching with patients and family members (Box 48-6).

TABLE 48-9 Expanded Postanaesthesia Recovery Score for Ambulatory Patients

Parameter	Task	Score
Activity	Able to move four extremities voluntarily or on command	2
	Able to move two extremities voluntarily or on command	1
	Unable to move extremities voluntarily or on command	0
Respiration	Able to breathe deeply and cough freely	2
	Dyspnea or limited breathing	1
	Apneic	0
Blood pressure	± 20% of preanaesthetic level	2
	± 20–49% of preanaesthetic level	1
	± 50% of preanaesthetic level	0
Consciousness	Fully awake	2
	Arousable on calling	1
	Not responding	0
Oxygen saturation	SpO_2 >94% on room air	2
	Needs O_2 inhalation to maintain SpO_2 >94%	1
	SpO_2 <94% even with extra O_2	0
Dressing	Dry and clean	2
	Wet but marked and not increasing	1
	Growing area of wetness	0
Pain	Pain-free	2
	Mild pain handled by oral medication	1
	Severe pain requiring parenteral medication	0
Ambulation	Able to stand up and walk straight*	2
	Vertigo when erect	1
	Dizziness when supine	0
Fasting or feeding	Able to drink fluids	2
	Nauseated	1
	Nausea and vomiting	0
Urine output	Has voided	2
	Unable to void but comfortable	1
	Unable to void and uncomfortable	0
Total		

NOTE: Total score must be at least 18 for patient to be discharged to home.
*May be substituted by Romberg's test, or by picking up 12 clips in one hand.
Adapted from Aldrete, J. A., & Kroulik, D. (1970). A post-anesthetic recovery score. *Anesthesia and Analgesia, 49,* 924–934; and Aldrete, J. A. (1998). Modifications to the post-anesthesia score for use in ambulatory surgery. *Journal of PeriAnesthesia Nursing, 13,* 148.

Ambulatory surgical patients are discharged to home when they meet certain criteria. A patient being monitored by PARSAP must achieve a score of 18 or higher before being discharged. An exception may be allowed if the patient was unable to walk or move his or her extremities before surgery (Aldrete, 1998). Postoperative nausea and vomiting may occur once the patient is home even if the symptoms were not present at the time of discharge. Attention must be paid to these symptoms, because they affect patient recovery, whether in the hospital or at home for ambulatory surgical patients (Lichtor & Chang, 2012). An option for therapy includes the prophylactic use of the drug ondansetron (Lehne, 2007).

BOX 48-6 PATIENT TEACHING

Postoperative Instructions for Ambulatory Surgical Patients

Objectives

- Patient will verbalize resources to contact for assistance.
- Patient will describe signs and symptoms of postoperative problems.
- Patient will list the name and dose of medications to self-administer.
- Patient will describe guidelines related to specific surgery.

Teaching Strategies

- Provide instruction sheet with physician's or nurse's telephone number, surgery centre's number, and follow-up appointment date and time. Allow patient and family to ask questions.
- Explain to family members the signs and symptoms of infection for which to observe.
- Explain name, dose, schedule, and purpose of medications. Provide drug information leaflets.
- Explain activity restrictions, diet progression, and any special wound care related to specific surgery. Provide instruction sheet with clear, focused explanations.

Evaluation

- Ask patient to describe signs indicating potential problems and normal convalescence.
- Ask patient to explain when and how to call health care providers such as the home care nurse.
- Make sure patient records follow-up appointment in diary or on an electronic device.
- Ask patient and family members to describe the signs and symptoms of infection.
- Ask patient to verbalize name of drug, dose, and when to take.
- Ask patient to demonstrate proper activity or movement and wound care.

Written postoperative instructions and prescriptions are reviewed with the patient and the family, and the nurse should ensure that they verbalize understanding of these instructions. The patient is discharged to the care of a responsible adult.

Postoperative Convalescence

Inpatients are kept in the PACU until their condition stabilizes; they are then transported to the postoperative nursing unit. Ambulatory surgery patients will return home. Nursing care focuses on returning the patient to a relatively functional level of wellness as soon as possible. The speed of convalescence depends on the presurgical general state of health, the type or extent of surgery, the risk factors involved, and any postoperative complications.

NURSING PROCESS IN POSTOPERATIVE CARE

Nursing care in the PACU is focused on managing pain and monitoring and maintaining respiratory, circulatory, fluid and electrolyte, and neurological status. Other important assessments include temperature, skin and incision or wound status, and genitourinary and gastrointestinal function. Nurses in the surgical unit continue to assess these critical factors until the patient's discharge from the acute care facility.

Assessment

After patient assessment upon arrival to the PACU, the nurse repeats evaluation of vital signs and other key observations at least every 15 minutes or more frequently, depending on the patient's condition and unit policy. This assessment usually continues until discharge from the PACU. Once the patient is returned to the surgical unit, the nurse admitting the patient takes vital signs immediately in order to compare them with the PACU findings. Vital sign monitoring in the surgical nursing unit initially should be at least hourly for 4 hours and then every 4 hours, unless complications develop. Frequency of assessment should always be based on the patient's current condition, which can change rapidly, especially during the postoperative period.

Nurses need to thoroughly document their assessment, including circulatory and respiratory status, level of consciousness, temperature, condition of dressings and drains, pain and comfort level, skin warmth and colour, ability to move extremities, IV fluid status, and urinary output measurements. Patient data can be entered on flow sheets, by electronic documentation, or as written progress notes. The initial findings are a baseline for comparing any postoperative changes.

Once the patient returns to the acute care area, the nurse's focus is on completing the assessment, meeting the patient's immediate needs, and providing an opportunity for the family to be with the patient. The call light and emesis basin should be within the patient's reach. The nurse can explain the purpose of postoperative procedures or equipment and the patient's status. The family should know that the patient will fall in and out of sleep for most of the rest of the day, owing to the effects of general anaesthesia and pain medication. The family also should be reminded that frequent assessments are to be expected and that limited sensation and movement in the patient's extremities may remain for a few hours if he or she had intrathecal (spinal) or epidural anaesthesia.

Respiration. Major concerns for the nurse caring for patients postanaesthesia and after surgery are hypoventilation, hypoxemia, and airway obstruction. Certain anaesthetic agents may cause respiratory depression. Thus, nurses must be especially alert for shallow, slow breathing and a weak cough. Airway patency, respiratory rate, rhythm, depth of ventilation, symmetry of chest wall movement, breath sounds, and colour of mucous membranes must all be assessed. If breathing is unusually shallow, placing a hand near the patient's nose or mouth allows the nurse to feel exhaled air. Pulse oximetry should reflect 92 to 100% saturation. Some agencies now have directives that allow nurses to administer oxygen at 3 L/minute via nasal prongs if the patient has a saturation of less than 92%.

The patient often has an oral or nasal airway (see Chapter 39) inserted in the OR after removal of the endotracheal tube to maintain a patent airway until the patient can protect his or her airway. As the patient awakens in the PACU, he or she will spit out the airway or the nurse will ask him or her to spit it out. The patient's ability to do so signifies the return of a normal gag reflex.

One of the nurse's greatest concerns is airway obstruction. A number of factors can contribute to obstruction, including weak pharyngeal or laryngeal muscle tone from anaesthetics; secretions in the pharynx, bronchial tree, or trachea; and laryngeal or subglottic edema (Litwack, 1999). Signs of airway obstruction include snoring, nasal flaring, and use of accessory muscles to breathe (Barone, Pablo, & Barone, 2004). In the postanaesthetic patient, the tongue causes the majority of airway obstructions. Ongoing assessment of airway patency is crucial. Patients are often kept in a side-lying position until airways are clear.

In the acute care area, nurses continue to assess respiratory status and breath sounds. Older patients, smokers, and patients with a history of respiratory disease are prone to developing complications such as atelectasis or pneumonia. The patient is also assessed for any signs of shortness of breath with activity.

Circulation. The patient is at risk for cardiovascular complications resulting from actual or potential blood loss from the surgical site, adverse effects of anaesthesia, electrolyte imbalances, and depression of normal circulatory regulating mechanisms. Careful assessment of heart rate and rhythm, along with blood pressure, reveals the patient's cardiovascular status. A rhythm strip is usually obtained postoperatively, compared with any preoperative ECG tracings, and mounted on the PACU record. The vital signs are monitored at least every 15 minutes throughout the PACU recovery phase. Preoperative vital signs are compared with postoperative values. The physician should be notified if the patient's blood pressure drops progressively with each check or if the heart rate changes or becomes irregular.

The nurse assesses circulatory perfusion by noting capillary refill, pulses, and the colour and temperature of the nail beds and skin. If the patient has had vascular surgery or has casts or constricting devices that may impair circulation, the nurse should assess peripheral pulses and capillary refill distal to the site of surgery. For example, after surgery to the femoral artery, the posterior tibial and dorsalis pedis pulses are assessed. The nurse should also compare pulses in the affected extremity with those in the nonaffected extremity.

A common early circulatory problem is hemorrhage. Blood loss may occur externally through a drain or incision, or internally. Either type of hemorrhage may result in a fall in blood pressure; elevated heart and respiratory rates; thready pulse; cool, clammy, pale skin; and restlessness. Often, the first sign of hemorrhage is restlessness. Signs such as thready pulse and clammy skin are noted much later, after significant blood loss has occurred. To prevent deterioration of the patient, the surgeon must be notified of significant changes, from baseline, of heart rate, blood pressure, and respirations. The nurse must maintain IV fluid infusion and may need to increase IV replacement fluids. The patient's vital signs are monitored every 15 minutes or more frequently until his or her condition stabilizes. Oxygen may need to be continued. Volume replacement and medications to promote perfusion to vital organs such as the brain may be considered. Crystalloids such as Ringer's lactate are commonly used (Diepenbrock, 2012). Plasma expanders (colloids) may be used instead of blood transfusions. Colloids may be made from blood products (i.e., albumin), but artificial colloids, such as hetastarch, may also be used (Diepenbrock, 2012). Colloids may be used in hypovolemic shock (Annane, Siami, Jaber, et al., 2013). Blood counts and coagulation studies are drawn and sent to the laboratory. The potential for cardiovascular complications remains when the patient is transferred to the acute care area. In that area, nurses continue to assess the same factors that were identified in the PACU.

Temperature Control. The OR and recovery room environments are kept extremely cool. The patient's anaesthetically depressed level of body function results in a lowering of metabolism and a fall in body temperature. When patients begin to awaken, they usually complain of feeling cold and uncomfortable. The length of time spent in the OR and laminar flow rooms contributes to heat loss. Surgeries that require an open body cavity also contribute to heat loss. Older persons and pediatric patients are at higher risk for developing problems associated with hypothermia. Hypothermia can cause cardiac irregularities, hypotension, and coagulopathy (Barone et al., 2004).

In rare instances, **malignant hyperthermia**, a genetically determined condition and a life-threatening complication of anaesthesia, develops. Due to the release of intracellular calcium, muscle contractions occur throughout the body. Other symptoms can be tachypnea, cardiac arrhythmias, unstable blood pressure, cyanosis, and skin mottling. An elevated temperature, a sign of the condition, occurs late. It is often seen during the induction phase of anaesthesia and is managed by discontinuing the anaesthetic agent causing the condition, administering oxygen, and starting dantrolene (Barone et al., 2004). Fluid resuscitation is required. Without prompt detection and treatment, it can be fatal.

For all patients, temperature is monitored closely in the acute care area. Because an elevated temperature may be the first indication of an infection, nurses need to evaluate the patient for a potential source of infection, including the IV site (if present), the surgical incision or wound, and the respiratory and urinary tracts. The physician must be notified, because further evaluation, including blood, sputum, and urinary cultures, likely will be needed. In older patients, fever may not be seen with infection (Litwack, 2006).

Fluid and Electrolyte Balances. Because of the surgical patient's risk for fluid and electrolyte abnormalities, nurses need to assess the patient's hydration status and monitor cardiac and neurological function for signs of electrolyte alterations (see Chapter 40). Laboratory values will be monitored and compared with the patient's baseline values.

One of the nurse's important responsibilities is monitoring the rate and maintaining the patency of IV infusions. The patient's only source of fluid intake immediately after surgery is through IV catheters. Nurses must inspect the catheter insertion site to ensure that the catheter is properly positioned within a vein so that fluid flows freely. Nurses need to record the intravenous infusions received as well as any sources of oral intake once peristalsis returns. All sources of output are measured, including urine, surgically placed drains, gastric drainage, and drainage from wounds, and any insensible loss from diaphoresis is noted. Daily weights may be assessed postoperatively if the patient has a known cardiac or renal history (e.g., heart failure). It is important to compare preoperative and postoperative weights and to be consistent in the scale used, the amount of clothing worn by the patient, and the time of day to obtain accurate weight measurement. *Accurate recording of intake and output is crucial.* It is also important to be aware of the amount of fluids received in the intraoperative and immediate postoperative period. For example, if large amounts of fluid were received during surgery, the patient may exhibit signs of fluid retention, such as pedal edema or abnormal breath sounds.

Neurological Functions. The patient is often drowsy in the PACU. As anaesthetic agents are metabolized, the patient's reflexes return, muscle strength is regained, and a normal level of orientation returns. A patient should at least be oriented to self and to the hospital before discharge from the PACU. Gag reflexes (see Chapter 32), hand grips, and movement of the patient's extremities are assessed. If the patient has had surgery involving a portion of the neurological system, a more thorough neurological assessment needs to be conducted, including assessing pupil size and reaction.

Patients who had regional anaesthesia begin to experience a return in motor function before tactile sensation. The patient's sensation is checked along **dermatomes** (segmental skin areas innervated by specific segments of the spinal cord). Knowing where anaesthesia was introduced, the nurse is able to check the distribution of the spinal nerves affected (see Chapter 32). Typically, the nurse assesses the dermatome level by touching the patient bilaterally and documenting where he or she feels touch. The sense of touch can be tested using a paper clip, for example. Assessment of extremity strength, movement, and sensation continues to be important if spinal or epidural anaesthesia has been given, although the patient should remain in the PACU until sensation and voluntary movement of the lower extremities have been re-established.

Skin Integrity and Condition of the Wound. In the PACU, nurses assess the condition of the patient's skin, noting rashes, petechiae, abrasions, or burns. A rash may indicate a drug sensitivity or allergy. Abrasions or petechiae may result from a clotting disorder or from inappropriate positioning that injures skin layers. Burns may indicate that an electrical cautery grounding pad was incorrectly placed on the patient's skin. Burns or serious injury to the skin should be documented in an incident report (see Chapter 15). The nurse should also make a note if the patient complains of any burning or pain in the eye that could indicate a corneal abrasion.

After surgery, most wounds are covered with a dressing that protects the site and collects drainage. Nurses need to observe the amount, colour, odour, and consistency of drainage on dressings. Serosanguinous drainage is the most common type of drainage occurring immediately after surgery. The amount of drainage is estimated by noting the number of saturated gauze sponges. If drainage appears on the outer surface of a dressing, another way to assess drainage is by drawing a circle around the outer perimeter of the drainage on the dressing and dating it with the time noted. This way, nurses can easily note if drainage is increasing (see Chapter 46).

The nurse on the surgical nursing unit usually will have the first opportunity to view and thoroughly assess and document the status of the incision or wound. Initially, it is important to note if wound edges are approximated and no active bleeding or drainage is present. The wound needs to be assessed for redness, swelling, signs of infection, and slipped sutures or staples. Wound assessment is especially important because it forms the baseline for continued monitoring during the patient's hospital stay.

Pressure injuries can occur in the patient undergoing surgery. Older patients may have several risk factors, such as nutritional or cardiovascular deficiencies or diabetes that predispose them to these injuries (Walton-Geer, 2009). It is important to assess the patient's mobility level. If the patient is unable or unwilling to turn, pressure injuries can occur. Nurses should use the Braden Scale to determine the patient's risk of developing pressure injuries (RNAO, 2016). Preventive measures such as a turning schedule and pressure-reduction devices can be instituted (see Chapter 46).

Genitourinary Function. Depending on the surgery, a patient may not regain voluntary control over urinary function for 6 to 8 hours after anaesthesia. An epidural or spinal anaesthetic may prevent the patient from feeling bladder fullness. The nurse should palpate the lower abdomen just above the symphysis pubis for bladder distension or use a bladder scanner to identify the amount of urine in the bladder. If the patient has a urinary catheter, there should be a continuous flow of urine—30 to 50 mL/hour in adults. The colour and the odour of the urine should be observed. Surgery involving portions of the urinary tract normally causes bloody urine for at least 12 to 24 hours, depending on the type of surgery. The nurse needs to conduct ongoing assessment of genitourinary function.

Gastrointestinal Function. Anaesthetics slow gastrointestinal motility and may cause nausea. Normally during the immediate recovery phase, faint or absent bowel sounds are auscultated in all four quadrants. The abdomen is inspected for distension that may be caused by an accumulation of gas. In a patient who has had abdominal surgery, distension will develop if internal bleeding occurs; however, this is a late sign of bleeding. Distension also may occur in the patient who develops a paralytic ileus as a result of handling of the bowel in surgery.

Nurses need to closely monitor the patient's initial oral intake for potential aspiration or the presence of nausea and vomiting. Assessment also includes checking every 4 to 8 hours for return of peristalsis. Routinely, nurses auscultate the abdomen to detect return of normal bowel sounds; 5 to 30 loud gurgles per minute over each quadrant indicates that peristalsis has returned. High-pitched tinkling sounds accompanied by abdominal distension suggest that the bowel is not functioning properly. The nurse should ask the patient if he or she is passing gas (flatus). This is an important sign indicating normal bowel function. If a nasogastric tube is in place, the nurse needs to assess the patency of the tube (see Chapter 44), the colour and amount of any drainage, and (if ordered) the level of suction required.

Pain and Comfort. Pain management is included in the overall aim of ensuring patient comfort. Comfort is also achieved through nursing measures such as bathing and providing clean bedding. As patients awaken from general anaesthesia, the sensation of pain becomes prominent. Pain can be perceived before full consciousness is regained. Acute incisional pain causes patients to become restless and may be responsible for temporary changes in vital signs. It is difficult for patients to begin coughing and undertaking deep breathing exercises when they experience pain. The patient who had regional or local anaesthesia may not experience pain initially because the incisional area is still anaesthetized.

Assessment of the patient's discomfort and evaluation of pain-relief therapies are essential nursing functions. Pain scales are an effective method for nurses to assess postoperative pain, evaluate response to analgesics, and objectively document pain severity (see Chapter 31). In addition, best practice guidelines provide guidance for decision making (RNAO, 2013). By frequently assessing pain, nurses can evaluate the effectiveness of interventions (e.g., positioning, analgesics) throughout the patient's recovery. The nurse's caring presence at the bedside fosters communication between the nurse and the patient, which in turn enables effective pain management.

Patient Expectations. The nurse assesses the patient's and family's expectations and perceived progress in the recovery and convalescence phases. Ongoing assessment of expectations regarding pain control, comfort level, dietary intake, activity level, and readiness for discharge are also performed. The nurse determines the patient's and the family's expectations regarding needs at home and incorporates these into the care plan.

◆ Nursing Diagnosis

Nurses determine the status of problems identified from preoperative nursing diagnoses and cluster new relevant data to identify new diagnoses. Previously defined diagnoses, such as *impaired skin integrity*, may continue as a postoperative problem. The nurse may identify new risk factors leading to identification of nursing diagnoses. For example, an older patient who has undergone major abdominal surgery and who has a pre-existing problem of reduced hip mobility resulting from arthritis will likely have the diagnosis of *impaired physical mobility*. The surgery itself may add risk factors for the patient. Nurses also consider the needs of a patient's family when making diagnoses. For example, difficulties of the family coping with the patient's condition require nursing intervention. Early dialogue with the family can aid in identifying any challenges.

◆ Planning

Because of the critical nature of the immediate postoperative period, the nursing care in the PACU involves close monitoring of the patient and frequent assessments to ensure a return to stable physiological function. During the convalescent phase, the nurse uses current physical assessment data and analysis of the preoperative nursing health history for planning the patient's care. The surgeon's postoperative plan and the institution's clinical pathways are also guidelines. Typical postoperative plans include the following:

- Frequency of vital sign monitoring and other assessments such as oxygen saturation
- Types of IV fluids and rates of infusion
- Postoperative medications (especially those for pain and nausea)
- Resumption of preoperative medications as condition allows (some oral medications will be converted to the IV route with

appropriate dose adjustment). Some institutions have a medication reconciliation and orders form to be used in the postoperative period.

- Fluids and food allowed by mouth
- Level of activity that the patient is allowed to resume
- Position that the patient is to maintain while in bed
- Intake and output
- Laboratory tests and diagnostic studies
- Special directions (e.g., surgical drains to suction, tube irrigations, dressing changes)
- Patient teaching and discharge planning

Goals and Outcomes. Nurses consider the effects of the stress of surgery and the limitations it produces when establishing goals, patient outcomes, and nursing interventions for the patient. Measurable outcomes with indicators help to ensure timely and appropriate recovery from surgery. For example, the patient at risk for impaired physical mobility should have specific outcomes that include targeted ambulation (e.g., steps to take and distance down hallway) and range of joint movement. After each outcome is met, the patient ultimately will achieve the goal of independent mobility at a preoperative level or better. The nurse carefully considers all goals of care established during the preoperative surgical phase. The following is an example of goals and outcomes for the postoperative period:

- Patient achieves a return of normal physiological function after surgery.
- Patient's vital signs return to preoperative baseline.
- Patient's airway is patent and respirations are even and unlaboured.
- Patient's temperature returns to baseline. Patient's fluid and electrolyte levels remain balanced.
- Patient verbalizes feeling of increased strength and ability to move.

Setting Priorities. In the PACU, priorities of care include the assessment and stability of the patient's airway; interventions for an impaired airway; assessment of the patient's respiratory, circulatory, neurological, and fluid and electrolyte status; and pain control. As the patient progresses on the acute care unit, priorities should focus on advancement of patient activity. The patient generally will have multiple nursing diagnoses. Nurses may re-establish priorities several times as the patient's health status changes.

Continuity of Care. In the recovery phase, nurses collaborate on the care plan with staff from respiratory therapy, physiotherapy, occupational therapy, dietary, social work, home care, and other areas to meet the patient's needs. The goal of all these disciplines is to assist the patient to return to the best possible level of functioning with a smooth transition to home. The family's role in the care plan to foster recovery is also essential.

BOX 48-7 FOCUS ON OLDER PERSONS

Risks of Surgery

- Advances in medical technology and therapies allow patients to live longer, but often with chronic illness such as heart disease, and these chronic diseases account for about 70% of all deaths in Canada (Canadian Hospice Palliative Care Association, 2014). Therefore, nurses are caring for many more surgical patients of advanced age and are required to know the age-related factors that affect the outcomes of a surgical procedure. Hypothermia and postoperative embolism may be seen in older persons (Clayton, 2008).
- A smaller margin of physiological reserve makes the older person less able to compensate during the perioperative period for changes that can occur due to infection, hemorrhage, alterations in blood pressure, and fluid and electrolyte abnormalities.
- Older patients are at greater risk for postoperative delirium after procedures such as hip replacement and cardiac surgery (Brooks, 2012; OPANA, 2009a). A rapid decline in cognitive function, fluctuations in awareness and orientation, disturbed sleep–wake cycle, and personality and mood changes characterize the typical presentation. Delirium may be the first indicator of infection, fluid or electrolyte imbalances, or deteriorating respiratory or hemodynamic status. Postoperative delirium is associated with extended lengths of hospital stay, loss of independence, increased morbidity and mortality, and increased health care costs (Ansaloni, Catena, Chattat, et al., 2010; Inouye, 2006). Delirium may present as hyperactive, hypoactive, or mixed (Barr, Fraser, Puntillo, et al., 2013).
- Altered and unexpected drug responses are often related to different pharmacokinetics in the older person. Thus, when caring for the perioperative older patient, nurses must be alert to the possibility of a high risk for adverse medication events with the administration of anaesthetic agents and postoperative analgesics, especially narcotics. "Start lower and go slow" should be the guiding principle when medicating older persons, because of their slower drug-clearance capability (RNAO, 2007).

Data from Brooks, P.B. (2012). Postoperative delirium in elderly patients. *American Journal of Nursing, 112*(9), 38-49; Canadian Hospice Palliative Care Association. (2014). *Fact sheet: Hospice Palliative Care in Canada.* Retrieved from http://www.chpca.net/media/330558/Fact_Sheet_HPC_in_Canada%20Spring%202014%20Final.pdf; Clayton, J. L. (2008). Special needs of older adults undergoing surgery. *AORN Journal, 87*(3), 557–570; Registered Nurses' Association of Ontario (RNAO). (2007). *Assessment and management of pain in the elderly.* Retrieved from http://rnao.ca/sites/rnao-ca/files/Assessment_and_Management_of_Pain_in_the_Elderly_-_Learning_Package_for_LTC.pdf; Registered Nurses' Association of Ontario (RNAO). (2013). *Assessment and management of pain* (3rd. ed.). Retrieved from http://www.rnao.org/Page.asp?PageID=924&ContentID=720.

◆ Implementation

Health Promotion. Primary causes of postoperative complications include the surgical wound, the effects of prolonged immobilization during surgery and convalescence, preoperative risks such as age (Box 48-7), and the influence of anaesthesia and analgesics. Nursing interventions in the postoperative period are directed at preventing complications so that the patient returns to the highest level of functioning possible. Failure of the patient to become actively involved in recovery adds to the risk for complications (Table 48-10). Virtually any body system can be affected. Nurses must consider the interrelationship of all systems and therapies provided.

Maintaining Respiratory Function. To prevent respiratory complications, pulmonary interventions should be started early. The benefits of thorough preoperative teaching are realized when patients are able to participate actively. When the patient awakens from anaesthesia, the nurse may need to assist him or her in maintaining a patent airway. The following measures maintain airway patency:

- Position the patient on one side with the face downward and the neck slightly extended to facilitate a forward movement of the tongue and the flow of mucous secretions out of the mouth. A small folded towel supports the head. Another positioning technique to promote a patent airway involves slightly elevating the head of the bed and slightly extending the patient's neck, with the head turned to the side. The PACU nurse may need to perform a jaw thrust manoeuvre or chin lift continuously to maintain the airway in some patients. The patient should never be positioned with arms over or across the chest because this reduces maximum chest expansion.
- Suction artificial airways and the oral cavity for mucous secretions (see Chapter 39). Care must be taken to avoid eliciting the gag reflex, which could cause vomiting.

TABLE 48-10 Postoperative Complications

Complication	Cause
Respiratory System	
Atelectasis: Collapse of alveoli with retained mucous secretions. Signs and symptoms include elevated respiratory rate, dyspnea, fever, crackles auscultated over involved lobes of lungs, productive cough, decreased oxygen saturation.	Inadequate lung expansion. Anaesthesia, analgesia, and immobilized position prevent full lung expansion. There is greater risk in patients with upper abdominal surgery who have pain during inspiration and repress deep breathing.
Pneumonia: Inflammation of alveoli. It may involve one or several lobes of lung. Development in lower dependent lobes of lung is common in immobilized surgical patient. Signs and symptoms include fever, chills, productive cough, chest pain, purulent mucus, and dyspnea as well as decreased oxygen saturation.	Poor lung expansion with retained secretions or aspirated secretions.
Hypoxemia: Inadequate concentration of oxygen in arterial blood. Signs and symptoms include restlessness, decreased mental alertness, dyspnea, high or low blood pressure, tachycardia or bradycardia, diaphoresis, and cyanosis.	Respirations are depressed by anaesthetics or analgesics. Increased retention of mucus with impaired ventilation occurs because of pain or poor positioning.
Pulmonary embolism: Embolus blocking pulmonary arterial blood flow to one or more lobes of lung. Signs and symptoms include dyspnea, sudden chest pain, cyanosis, tachycardia, and drop in blood pressure.	Same factors lead to formation of thrombus or embolus. Immobilized surgical patient with pre-existing circulatory or coagulation disorders is at risk.
Circulatory System	
Hemorrhage: Loss of large amount of blood externally or internally in short period of time. Signs and symptoms include hypotension, weak and rapid pulse, cool and clammy skin, rapid breathing, restlessness, and reduced urine output.	Slipping of suture or dislodged clot at incisional site. Patients with coagulation disorders are at greater risk. Blood loss with fractures can also occur.
Hypovolemic shock: Inadequate perfusion of tissues and cells from loss of circulatory fluid volume. Signs and symptoms are same as for hemorrhage.	In surgical patient, hypovolemic shock is usually caused by hemorrhage.
Thrombophlebitis: Inflammation of vein often accompanied by clot formation. Veins in legs are most commonly affected. Signs and symptoms include swelling and inflammation of involved site and aching or cramping pain. Vein feels hard, cordlike, and sensitive to touch.	Venous stasis is aggravated by prolonged sitting or immobilization. Trauma to vessel wall and hypercoagulability of blood increase risk of vessel inflammation.
Thrombus: Formation of clot attached to interior wall of a vein or artery, which can occlude the vessel lumen. Signs and symptoms include localized tenderness along distribution of the venous system, swollen calf or thigh, calf swelling more than 3 cm compared with asymptomatic leg, pitting edema in symptomatic leg, collateral superficial veins, and decrease in pulse below location of thrombus (if arterial).	Venous stasis (see discussion of thrombophlebitis) and vessel trauma. Venous injury is common after surgery of legs, abdomen, pelvis, and major vessels. Patients with pelvic and abdominal cancer or traumatic injuries to the pelvis or lower extremities are at high risk for thrombus formation.
Embolus: Piece of thrombus that has dislodged and circulates in bloodstream until it lodges in another vessel, commonly in the lungs, heart, brain, or mesentery.	Thrombi form with increased coagulability of blood (e.g., polycythemia).
Gastrointestinal System	
Paralytic ileus: Nonmechanical obstruction of the bowel caused by physiological, neurogenic, or chemical imbalance associated with decreased peristalsis.	Handling of intestines during surgery can lead to loss of peristalsis for a few hours to several days.
Abdominal distension: Retention of air within intestines and abdominal cavity during gastrointestinal surgery. Signs and symptoms include increased abdominal girth, tympanic percussion over abdominal quadrants, and patient complaints of fullness, "gas pains," and referred shoulder pain.	Slowed peristalsis from anaesthesia, bowel manipulation, or immobilization. During laparoscopic surgeries, influx of air for procedure causes distension.
Nausea and vomiting: Symptoms of improper gastric emptying or chemical stimulation of vomiting centre. Patient complains of gagging or feeling full or sick to stomach.	Abdominal distension, fear, severe pain, medications, eating or drinking before peristalsis returns.
Genitourinary System	
Urinary retention: Involuntary accumulation of urine in bladder as a result of loss of muscle tone. Signs and symptoms include inability to void, restlessness, and bladder distension. It appears 6 to 8 hours after surgery.	Effects of anaesthesia and narcotic analgesics. Local manipulation of tissues surrounding bladder as well as edema interfere with bladder tone. Poor positioning of patient impairs voiding reflexes.
Urinary tract infection: An infection of the urinary tract as a result of bacterial or yeast contamination. Signs and symptoms include dysuria, itching, abdominal pain, possible fever, cloudy urine, white blood cells, and leukocyte esterase positive on urinalysis.	Most frequently a result of catheterization of the bladder.

TABLE 48-10 Postoperative Complications—cont'd

Complication	Cause
Integumentary System	
Wound infection: An invasion of deep or superficial wound tissues by pathogenic microorganisms. Signs and symptoms include warm, red, and tender skin around incision; fever and chills; and purulent material exiting from drains or from separated wound edges. Infection usually appears 3 to 6 days after surgery.	Infection is caused by poor aseptic technique or contaminated wound or surgical site before surgical exploration. For example, with a bowel perforation, the patient is at increased risk for a wound infection because of bacterial contamination from the large intestine.
Wound dehiscence: Separation of wound edges at suture line. Signs and symptoms include increased drainage and appearance of underlying tissues. This usually occurs 6 to 8 days after surgery.	Malnutrition, obesity, preoperative radiation to surgical site, old age, poor circulation to tissues, and unusual strain on suture line from coughing or positioning cause dehiscence.
Wound evisceration: Protrusion of internal organs and tissues through incision. Usually occurs 6 to 8 days after surgery.	See discussion of wound dehiscence. Patient with dehiscence is at risk for developing evisceration.
Skin breakdown: Result of pressure or shearing forces. Surgical patients are at increased risk if alterations in nutrition and circulation are present, resulting in edema and delayed healing.	Prolonged periods on the operating room (OR) table and in the bed postoperatively can lead to pressure breakdown. Skin breakdown results from shearing during positioning on the OR table and improper pulling of the patient up in bed.
Nervous System	
Complex pain situations: These might include situations in which pain is unresponsive to standard treatment or where there are multiple sources of pain.	The source may be related to, for example, surgical site or concomitant injuries or pathology.

The following measures promote expansion of the lungs:

- Encourage diaphragmatic breathing exercises every hour while patients are awake. Maximal inspirations lasting 3 to 5 seconds open up alveoli.
- Encourage early ambulation. Walking causes patients to assume a position that does not restrict chest wall expansion and stimulates an increased respiratory rate.
- Help patients who are restricted to bed to turn on their side every 1 to 2 hours while awake and to sit when possible. Turning permits expansion of the lungs. Sitting causes lowering of abdominal organs, thus facilitating diaphragmatic movement and lung expansion.
- Keep the patient comfortable. A patient who is comfortable will be able to participate in the postoperative regimen. Assess, document, treat, and evaluate the patient's pain on a regular basis.

The following measures promote removal of pulmonary secretions if they are present:

- Encourage coughing exercises every 2 hours while patients are awake, and maintain pain control to promote a deep, productive cough. Coughing may be contraindicated for patients who have had eye or intracranial surgery because of the potential increase in intraocular or intracranial pressure.
- Provide oral hygiene to facilitate expectoration of mucus. The oral mucosa becomes dry when patients are NPO or are placed on limited fluid intake.
- Initiate orotracheal or nasotracheal suction for patients who are too weak or unable to cough (see Chapter 39).
- Administer oxygen as ordered and monitor oxygen saturation with a pulse oximeter.

Preventing Circulatory Complications. Measures directed at preventing circulatory complications avert circulatory stasis. Some patients are at greater risk of venous stasis because of the nature of their surgery or medical history. The following measures promote normal venous return and circulatory blood flow:

- Encourage patients to perform leg exercises at least every hour while awake. Exercise may be limited in an affected extremity involving vascular repair or realignment of fractured bones and torn cartilage.
- Apply elastic antiembolism stockings or sequential compression stockings as ordered by the physician (see Chapter 45). The antiembolism stockings should be removed at least once per shift. Perform a thorough assessment of the skin of the lower extremities at this time.
- Encourage early ambulation. Some patients are expected to ambulate on the evening of surgery, depending on the severity of the surgery and their condition. Even if a patient has an epidural catheter or a PCA device, ambulation should be encouraged. The degree of activity allowed progresses as the condition improves. Before ambulation, assess the patient's vital signs. Abnormalities may contraindicate ambulation. If vital signs are at baseline, first help the patient to sit on the side of the bed. Patient complaints of dizziness are a sign of postural hypotension. Rechecking the patient's blood pressure will help to determine whether ambulation is safe. Assist with ambulation by standing at the patient's side and ensuring that he or she can stand safely and walk steadily. The first few times out of bed, patients may be able to walk only a few metres. This should improve each time. Evaluate tolerance to activity by periodically assessing the pulse rate as the patient ambulates.
- Avoid positioning patients in a manner that interrupts blood flow to their extremities. While in bed, patients should not have pillows or rolled blankets placed under their knees. Compression of the popliteal vessels can cause thrombi. When patients sit in chairs, their legs should be elevated on footstools. A patient should never be allowed to sit with one leg crossed over the other.
- Administer anticoagulant drugs as required. Physicians often order prophylactic doses of anticoagulants, such as heparin or Fragmin (dalteparin), for patients at greatest risk for thrombus formation.
- Promote adequate fluid intake. Adequate hydration prevents concentrated buildup of formed blood elements, such as platelets and red blood cells. When the plasma volume is low, these elements may gather and form small clots within blood vessels.

Achieving Rest and Comfort. A surgical patient's pain increases as the effects of anaesthesia diminish. The patient becomes more aware of the surroundings and more perceptive of discomfort. The incisional area may be only one source of pain. Irritation from abdominal gas, drainage tubes, tight dressings or casts, and the muscular strains caused from positioning on the OR table can cause discomfort.

It is common to administer narcotic analgesics immediately after surgery. Initial analgesic doses are usually given by IV infusion in the PACU and titrated to patient comfort. After an anaesthetized patient is awake and aware, PCA may be used. This is given by IV or subcutaneous infusion or via an epidural, often with Dilaudid or morphine. The PCA system allows patients to administer their own analgesics from a specially prepared pump (see Chapter 31). If patients are able to gain a sense of control over their pain, they usually have fewer postoperative problems. Currently, the Ambit pump is being used at some institutions for ambulatory patients who have had, for example, shoulder or knee surgery. Patients can administer a bolus and they are usually operating them at home for 1–2 days. Some patients receive epidural analgesia that may be continued during the recovery period (see Chapter 31). Increasingly, patients are being prescribed a combination of opioid and nonopioid analgesics in an effort to decrease opioid-related adverse effects (White, 2008) in the postoperative period. For example, as soon as peristalsis returns, patients may be given a combination of acetaminophen and a nonsteroidal anti-inflammatory drug.

In the acute care area, nurses continue pain assessment and determine the effectiveness of interventions. Patients who will have PCA after surgery should be taught how to push the button when they begin to feel pain, and they should understand that use of PCA will not cause them to overmedicate. Patients should be taught to administer PCA prior to activities that may increase pain, such as mobilization. If the patient has a PCA system and is trying to use it more frequently than the amount programmed, the nurse should investigate his or her pain further and contact the physician or the advanced practice nurse on the acute pain service to increase, for example, the amount of medication received. PCA provides a useful monitor of the effectiveness of pain medication. As oral intake is tolerated, the nurse facilitates changing the patient's pain medication from IV to oral administration. It is important to ensure adequate pain coverage when the patient is switched from an IV to an oral route (Snell, Fothergill Bourbonnais, & Durocher-Hendricks, 1997). Sometimes patients are given a subcutaneous injection of analgesia before transfer to the acute care area to ensure pain control over this time period. Intramuscular injections of analgesics are seldom used now. The importance of nonpharmacological interventions should not be overlooked. The nurse should assess which care measures may contribute to pain and use nonpharmacological measures to treat it. An example would be to lower the head of the bed and use a pillow for incisional splinting while turning a patient with recent abdominal surgery. Nurses can also use other methods of promoting pain relief, such as positioning, back rubs, distraction, or imagery. Ice packs may be ordered for patients undergoing joint replacement.

Pain can slow recovery significantly. The patient becomes reluctant to cough, breathe deeply, turn, ambulate, or perform necessary exercises. Nurses should assess the patient's pain thoroughly (see Chapter 31). It should not be assumed that the pain is from the surgery. When the patient asks for pain medication, it is important to determine the location, intensity, and character of the pain. During the first 24 to 48 hours after surgery, the nurse should provide analgesics on a regular basis around the clock to improve pain control (RNAO, 2013). If pain medications are not relieving discomfort, the nurse should notify the physician or the acute pain service after completing a thorough assessment. In addition, recognizing the potential complications of analgesics and knowing what to do if they occur is an important role of the postoperative nurse.

Acute Care

Temperature Regulation. Temperature regulation is important in the postoperative period. Patients are often cool after surgery, so the PACU nurse should provide warmed blankets in the immediate postoperative period. If the patient's temperature is 35.6°C or below, a warming device such as the Bair Hugger may be used. Increasing body warmth causes the patient's metabolism to rise and circulatory and respiratory functions to improve.

Shivering may not be a sign of hypothermia but rather a side effect of certain anaesthetic agents. Meperidine (Demerol) may be given in small increments to decrease shivering. Deep breathing and coughing help to expel retained anaesthetic gases.

Malignant hyperthermia is a potentially lethal condition that can occur in patients who receive general anaesthesia (OPANA, 2009a). It should be suspected when there is unexpected tachycardia and tachypnea; jaw muscle rigidity; body rigidity of limbs, abdomen, and chest; or hyperkalemia. Temperature elevation is a late sign. The PACU nurse will immediately administer dantrolene sodium ordered by the physician.

Infection is another possible cause of temperature elevation. The following interventions decrease the risk of postoperative infections: encouraging deep breathing and coughing, assisting with early ambulation, removing in-dwelling urinary catheters and IV catheters once the patient is voiding and drinking, and providing aseptic care of the surgical wound. Cultures are obtained from patients suspected of having infections (see Chapter 46).

Maintaining Neurological Function. Orientation to the environment is important in maintaining the patient's mental status. The nurse needs to reorient the patient, explain that surgery has been completed, and describe procedures and nursing measures. The patient who was properly prepared before surgery is less likely to be anxious when nurses provide care. Any change in level of consciousness should be promptly reported to a physician.

Maintaining Fluid and Electrolyte Balances. An important nursing responsibility is maintaining patency and prescribed rate of IV infusions and monitoring fluid and electrolyte balances in the postoperative period. As the patient begins to take and tolerate oral fluids, the IV rate will be decreased. When an ambulatory surgical patient awakens and is able to tolerate fluids by mouth without gastrointestinal upset, the IV catheter is removed. When the patient no longer needs a continuous IV infusion, the IV line may be saline locked to preserve the site for antibiotics or other use (see Chapter 40). The patient also may receive blood products or artificial volume expanders, depending on blood loss during and after surgery.

Promoting Normal Bowel Elimination and Adequate Nutrition. Normally a patient who has had general anaesthesia does not receive fluids to drink in the PACU because of bowel sluggishness, the risk of nausea and vomiting, and grogginess from general anaesthesia. To minimize nausea, the patient should avoid sudden movement. For patients identified as being at high risk for the development of nausea and vomiting or patients who must not vomit (e.g., eye surgery), a combination of antiemetics may be recommended (Lichtor & Chang, 2012). If the patient has a nasogastric tube, it is important to note the position of the tube and observe for drainage. If suction is required, the nurse needs to verify that it is maintained at the required level (see Chapter 44). Occlusion of a nasogastric tube results in accumulation of gastric contents within the stomach.

The patient likely will begin taking ice chips or sips of fluids once he or she is returned to the acute care unit. If these are tolerated, a clear liquid meal usually will be ordered. Interventions to prevent gastrointestinal complications will promote return of normal elimination and faster return of normal nutritional intake. It takes several days for a patient who has had surgery on gastrointestinal structures (e.g., a colon resection) to resume a normal diet. Normal peristalsis may not return for 2 to 3 days. In contrast, the patient whose gastrointestinal tract is unaffected directly by surgery can resume dietary intake after recovering from the effects of anaesthesia. The following measures promote return of normal elimination:

- Maintain a gradual progression in dietary intake. For the first few hours after surgery, a patient receives only IV fluids. If bowel sounds are active and the physician orders a normal diet for the first evening after surgery, begin by providing clear liquids, such as water, ginger ale, broth, or tea, after nausea subsides. Overloading the patient with large amounts of fluids may lead to distension and vomiting. If the patient tolerates liquids without nausea, advance the diet as ordered. Patients who have had abdominal surgery are usually NPO for the first 24 to 48 hours after the procedure. As peristalsis returns, provide clear liquids, followed by full liquids, a light diet of solid foods, and, finally, the patient's usual diet. Encourage intake of foods high in protein and vitamin C.
- Promote ambulation and exercise. Physical activity stimulates a return of peristalsis. The patient who suffers abdominal distension and "gas pain" may obtain relief while walking.
- Maintain an adequate fluid intake. Fluids keep fecal material soft for easy passage. Fruit juices and warm liquids are especially effective.
- Administer fibre supplements, stool softeners, and rectal suppositories such as Dulcolax (bisacodyl) as ordered. If constipation or distension develops, the physician may attempt to stimulate peristalsis with cathartics or enemas, but caution must be exercised.

It is also important to promote adequate food intake by stimulating the patient's appetite:

- Remove sources of noxious odours and provide small servings of nonspicy foods.
- Assist the patient to a comfortable position during mealtime. The patient should sit, if possible, to minimize pressure on the abdomen.
- Provide desired servings of food. For example, a patient may be more willing to face his or her first meal when servings are not large.
- Provide frequent oral hygiene. Adequate hydration and cleaning of the oral cavity eliminate dryness and bad tastes.
- Provide meals when the patient is rested and free from pain. Often a patient loses interest in eating if mealtime has been preceded by exhausting activities, such as ambulation, coughing and deep breathing exercises, or extensive dressing changes. When a patient has pain, the associated nausea often causes a loss of appetite.

Promoting Urinary Elimination. The depressant effects of anaesthetics and analgesics impair the sensation of bladder fullness. If bladder tone is reduced, the patient has difficulty starting urination. However, patients should void within 8 to 12 hours after surgery. Because a full bladder can be painful and often causes restlessness in recovery, it may become necessary to insert a catheter. If the patient has an in-dwelling urinary catheter, the goal should be to have it removed as soon as possible because of the high risk for development of a health care–associated infection.

Patients who undergo surgery of the urinary system frequently have an in-dwelling urinary catheter inserted to maintain free urinary flow until voluntary control of urination returns. The following measures promote normal urinary elimination (see Chapter 43):

- Help the patient to assume normal positions during voiding. The male patient may need assistance to stand to void. Bedpans make voiding difficult. A female patient will have better results if she is able to use a toilet or a bedside commode.
- Check the patient frequently for the need to void. A patient restricted to bed needs assistance in handling and using bedpans or urinals. Often the patient acquires a sudden feeling of bladder fullness and urgency to void and will need help quickly.
- Assess for bladder distension. If a patient does not void within 8 hours of surgery or if bladder distension is present, it may be necessary to insert a straight in-and-out urinary catheter. A physician's order is needed for this. Continued difficulty in voiding may necessitate an in-dwelling catheter, although the risk for a urinary tract infection increases.
- Monitor intake and output. Urine output should be at least 30 mL/hour for adults. If the urine is dark, concentrated, and low in volume, the physician should be notified. A patient can easily become dehydrated as a result of fluid loss from the surgical wound. Measure intake and output for several days after surgery until normal fluid intake and urinary output are achieved.

Promoting Wound Healing. A surgical wound undergoes considerable stress during convalescence. Inadequate nutrition, impaired circulation, and metabolic alterations increase the risk for delayed healing (see Chapter 46). Strain on sutures from coughing, vomiting, distension, and movement of body parts can disrupt the wound layers. Nurses need to protect the wound and promote healing. A critical time for wound healing is 24 to 72 hours after surgery, after which time a seal is established. If a wound becomes infected, it usually occurs 3 to 6 days after surgery. Nurses must use the aseptic technique during dressing changes and wound care (see Chapters 33 and 46). Surgical drains must remain patent so that accumulated secretions can escape from the wound bed. Ongoing observation of the wound aids in identifying early signs and symptoms of infection.

Maintaining and Enhancing Self-Concept. The appearance of wounds, bulky dressings, and extruding drains and tubes threaten a patient's self-concept. The effects of surgery, such as disfiguring scars, may create permanent changes in the patient's body image. If surgery leads to impairment in body function, the patient's role within the family can change significantly.

Nurses should observe patients for alterations in self-concept. Patients may show revulsion toward their appearance by refusing to look at incisions, carefully covering dressings with bedclothes, or refusing to get out of bed because of tubes and devices. The fear of not being able to return to a functional role in the family may cause patients to avoid participating in the care plan.

The family becomes an important part of efforts to improve the patient's self-concept. The nurse can explain the patient's appearance and encourage the family to be accepting of the patient's concerns and promote the patient's independence. If the condition is permanent, the family and patient will go through a grieving process. The nurse can be very supportive throughout this process. The following measures help to maintain the patient's self-concept:

- Provide privacy during dressing changes or inspection of the wound. Keep room curtains closed around the bed when changing and applying dressings, and drape the patient so that only the dressing or incisional area is exposed.
- Maintain the patient's hygiene. Wound drainage and antiseptic solutions from the surgical skin preparation dry on the patient's skin surface and cause irritation. When patients return to the unit, they should be given a postoperative bath and provided oral hygiene. In addition, a complete bath on the first day after surgery can make the patient feel renewed. When the patient's gown becomes soiled by wound drainage, offer a clean gown and washcloth. Keep the patient's hair clean and neatly combed. Offer frequent oral hygiene. Room deodorizers may be useful if the odour from drainage seems particularly troublesome to the patient and the family.

- Prevent drainage devices from overflowing. Contents of drainage collections are measured every 8 hours or 12 hours for output recording and are emptied as they become full. Maintain a pleasant environment. Self-concept is heightened by the patient being in pleasant, comfortable surroundings. Store or remove unused supplies and keep the patient's bedside orderly and clean.
- Offer opportunities for the patient to discuss feelings about his or her appearance. A patient who avoids looking at an incision may need to discuss fears or concerns. A patient having surgery for the first time is often more anxious than one who has had multiple surgeries. When the patient chooses to look at an incision for the first time, the area should be clean. Eventually, the patient should be able to care for the incision site by applying simple dressings or cleaning the affected area.
- Provide the family with opportunities to discuss ways to promote the patient's self-concept. Encouraging independence can be difficult for a family member who has a strong desire to assist the patient in any way. By knowing about the appearance of a wound or incision, family members can be supportive during dressing changes. The topic or tone of a conversation can also help family members support a patient who is dwelling on fears and concerns. Family members should not avoid discussing the future. However, they need help to know when it is appropriate to discuss future plans. Then the patient and family can work together to discuss realistic plans for the patient's return home.

Restorative and Continuing Care. The nurse, the patient, and the family work to prepare the patient for discharge. Education regarding wound care, activity level, diet, medications, and specifics related to the type of surgery is an ongoing process throughout hospitalization. After discharge, some patients will need assistance from home care services with tasks such as wound care (Box 48-8). For patients with ambulatory surgery, focused education within the limited time in care is essential. Including the family or a significant person provides a resource for the patient once he or she is at home (see Box 48-6). With both ambulatory and hospitalized patients, nurses make patients aware of a wide variety of educational materials, including those from the hospital website. For example, educational materials with many pictures should be used with patients who have limited reading ability. Materials should be sensitive to various cultures and religions. However, the provision of materials does not ensure understanding. Verification, return demonstration, and ongoing clarification are required.

◆ Evaluation

Patient Care. Nurses evaluate the effectiveness of care provided to the surgical patient on the basis of expected outcomes after nursing interventions. In all surgical settings, nurses consult with the patient and family to gather evaluation data. The nurse can evaluate the outcomes of the patient who had ambulatory surgery by telephoning the patient's home, asking specific questions to determine whether complications have developed and whether the patient understands restrictions or medications. This call is usually placed 24 hours after surgery, which allows the nurse to evaluate the progress of recovery.

In an acute care setting, evaluation of the patient is ongoing. If a patient fails to progress as expected, the nurse revises the patient's care plan according to the priorities of the patient's needs. Every effort is made to assist the patient in returning to as healthy and functional a state as possible. Nursing evaluation also includes determining the extent to which the patient and the family have learned self-care measures.

Patient Expectations. With shorter hospital stays and ambulatory surgery, it is especially important to evaluate patient expectations early in the postoperative process. Pain relief is usually a priority. Asking the patient if everything possible has been done to alleviate pain, including nonpharmacological measures, can determine whether the patient's needs have been met. Timeliness of response to the patient's needs, such as scheduled times for pain medication and prompt answering of a call light, may increase satisfaction. The patient usually wants to be discharged from acute care as soon as possible and when indicated by the physician. In some institutions, for continuity of care, the electronic chart is started in the preadmission unit, then follows the patient to day surgery unit, then to the OR, then the PACU.

Good communication among members of the interprofessional team ensures that patient needs are met and that discharge plans are in place, and enhances the patient's satisfaction with care.

BOX 48-8 FOCUS ON PRIMARY HEALTH CARE

Recovery at Home

Regardless of the length of time the patient spends in the hospital, it is essential that nurses ensure that the patient and family have the appropriate information and skills needed to continue a successful recovery at home. However, time is often very limited, especially with the move toward preadmission units and short hospital stays. A comprehensive approach is needed to ensure continuity of care from hospital to home. A patient is often expected to continue dressing care, follow any activity restrictions, continue medication therapy, and observe for signs and symptoms of complications upon returning home. In addition, the patient needs someone to be present for the first 24 hours to ensure that no delayed reaction from the anaesthesia occurs, such as difficulty breathing. A referral to home care assists patients who are unable to perform self-care activities. Close association with home care services is required for some patients if dressing changes or physiotherapy is needed. It is useful to have a case management nurse in attendance at discharge to convey what tasks a patient can perform effectively. Berg, Arestedt, and Kjellgren (2013) conducted a qualitative study of 31 patients in Sweden recovering from day surgery. The results indicated that patients need knowledge regarding what is considered a normal recovery and how to care for themselves after surgery.

KEY CONCEPTS

- Perioperative nursing is nursing care provided to the surgical patient before, during, and after surgery.
- Surgery is classified by level of severity, urgency, and purpose.
- The preoperative period may be several days or only a few hours long.
- Preoperative assessment of vital signs and physical findings provides an important baseline with which to compare postoperative assessment data.
- Nursing diagnoses of the surgical patient may pose implications for nursing care during one or all phases of surgery.
- Primary responsibility for obtaining informed consent rests with the patient's surgeon.
- Structured preoperative teaching has a positive influence on a patient's postoperative recovery.
- Basic to preoperative teaching is an explanation of all preoperative and postoperative activities and demonstration of postoperative exercises.
- In ambulatory surgery, nurses must use the limited time available to educate patients, assess their health status, and prepare them for surgery.

- A routine preoperative (preprocedure) checklist can be used as a guide for final preparation of the patient before surgery.
- Many responsibilities of nurses within the OR focus on protecting the patient from potential harm.
- All medications taken before surgery are automatically discontinued after surgery unless a physician reorders the drugs.
- Family members or other supportive networks are important in assisting patients with any physical limitations and in providing emotional support during postoperative recovery and ongoing care at home.
- Assessment of the postoperative patient centres on the body systems most likely to be affected by anaesthesia, immobilization, and surgical trauma.
- Accurate pain assessment and intervention are necessary for healing.
- Nurses in the postoperative surgical unit provide the discharge education required so that the patient and the family can manage at home.

CRITICAL THINKING EXERCISES

1. An 82-year-old patient is admitted for surgery on a fractured hip caused by a fall. What postoperative complications are typical in the older patient undergoing this type of surgery?
2. Mr. B. is a 52-year-old patient who will undergo thoracic surgery. He has smoked one pack of cigarettes per day for 30 years. What type of pulmonary preventive measures would you expect Mr. B to need postoperatively?
3. Mrs. C. was admitted for same-day surgery for an inguinal hernia repair. What discharge criteria would be used for Mrs. C., and what discharge instructions would she require?
4. Your patient is scheduled for abdominal hysterectomy at 2:00 p.m. Based on NPO guidelines, what fasting schedule should you implement in collaboration with the surgeon and the anaesthesiologist?
5. You are doing preoperative teaching for a patient undergoing a minimally invasive surgical technique. Identify one advantage of this type of surgery.

REVIEW QUESTIONS

1. An obese patient is at risk for poor wound healing and for wound infection postoperatively because:
   1. Ventilatory capacity is reduced
   2. Fatty tissue has a poor blood supply
   3. Risk for dehiscence is increased
   4. Resuming normal physical activity is delayed
2. The nurse should ask each patient preoperatively for the name and dose of all prescription and over-the-counter medications taken before surgery because they:
   1. May cause allergies to develop
   2. Are automatically ordered postoperatively
   3. May create greater risks for complications or interact with anaesthetic agents
   4. Should be taken on the morning of surgery with sips of water
3. A patient who smokes two packs of cigarettes per day is most at risk postoperatively for which of the following?
   1. Infection
   2. Pneumonia
   3. Hypotension
   4. Cardiac dysrhythmias
4. Family members should be included when the nurse teaches the patient preoperative exercises so that they can:
   1. Supervise the patient at home
   2. Coach the patient postoperatively
   3. Practise with the patient while waiting to be taken to the operating room
   4. Relieve the nurse by getting the patient to do his or her exercises every 2 hours
5. In the postoperative period, measuring input and output helps assess which of the following?
   1. Renal and circulatory function
   2. Patient comfort
   3. Neurological function
   4. Gastrointestinal function
6. In the PACU, one measure taken to maintain airway patency is to:
   1. Suction the pharynx and bronchial tree
   2. Give oxygen through a mask at 10 L/minute
   3. Position the patient so that the tongue falls forward
   4. Sit patient in high-Fowler's position
7. Which one of the following measures promotes normal venous return and circulatory blood flow?
   1. Suctioning artificial airways and the oral cavity
   2. Monitoring fluid and electrolyte status during every shift
   3. Having the patient deep-breathe and cough
   4. Encouraging the patient to perform leg exercises at least once an hour while awake
8. A patient with an international normalized ratio (INR) or an activated partial thromboplastin time (APTT) greater than normal is at risk postoperatively for:
   1. Anemia
   2. Bleeding
   3. Infection
   4. Cardiac dysrhythmias
9. When the patient is engaging in deep breathing and coughing exercises, it is important to have the patient sitting because this position:
   1. Is more comfortable
   2. Facilitates expansion of the thorax
   3. Increases the patient's view of the room and is more relaxing
   4. Helps the patient to splint with a pillow
10. In the postoperative period, if a patient has unexpected tachycardia and tachypnea; jaw muscle rigidity; body rigidity of limbs, abdomen, and chest; or hyperkalemia, the nurse should suspect which of the following?
    1. Infection
    2. Hypertension
    3. Pneumonia
    4. Malignant hyperthermia

Answers: 1. 2; 2. 3; 3. 2; 4. 2; 5. 1; 6. 3; 7. 4; 8. 2; 9. 2; 10. 4

Rationales for the Review Questions appear at the end of the book.

RECOMMENDED WEBSITES

Canadian Anesthesiologists' Society: http://www.cas.ca.
This website offers patient information about anaesthesia and provides guidelines for using anaesthesia.

National Association of PeriAnesthesia Nurses of Canada: http://www.napanc.org.
Perianaesthesia nurses are registered nurses with advanced knowledge in the care of patients during all phases of perianaesthesia, including, for

example, nurses in postanaesthetic care units, same-day surgery, and diagnostic imaging. The aim of this organization is to advance education for perianaesthesia nurses across Canada.

Ontario PeriAnesthesia Nurses Association: http://www.opana.org.

This website provides position statements on and standards of perianaesthesia nursing practice.

Operating Room Nurses Association of Canada: http://www.ornac.ca.

This website provides practice standards for Canadian operating room nurses, as well as information on certification with the Canadian Nurses Association (CNA).

REFERENCES

Adamis, D., Rooney, S., Meagher, D., et al. (2015). A comparison of delirium diagnosis in elderly medical inpatients using the CAM, DRS-R98, DSM-IV and DSM-5 criteria. *International Psychogeriatrics, 27*(6), 883–889.

Agostini, P., & Singh, S. (2009). Incentive spirometry following thoracic surgery: What should we be doing? *Physiotherapy, 95*, 76–82.

Aldrete, J. A. (1998). Modifications to the post anesthesia score for use in ambulatory surgery. *Journal of PeriAnesthesia Nursing, 13*, 148–155.

American Association for Respiratory Care (AARC). (1993). AARC clinical practice guideline: Use of positive airway pressure adjuncts to bronchial hygiene therapy. *Respiratory Care, 38*(5), 516–521. Retrieved from http://www.rcjournal.com/cpgs/papcpg.html.

American Society of Anesthesiologists (ASA). (2011). Practice guidelines for the preoperative fasting and the use of pharmacologic agents to reduce the risk of pulmonary aspiration: Application to healthy patients undergoing elective procedures. Updated report by the American Society of Anesthesiologists Committee on Standards and Practice Parameters. *Anesthesiology, 114*(3), 495–511. doi:10.1097/ALN.0b013e3181fcbfd9.

Andrews, S. M. (2009). Patient family-centered care in the ambulatory surgery setting. *Journal of PeriAnesthesia Nursing, 24*(4), 244–246. doi:10.1016/j.jopan.2009.05.100.

Annane, D., Siami, S., Jaber, S., et al. (2013). Effects of fluid resuscitation with colloids versus crystalloids on mortality in critically ill patients presenting with hypovolemic shock. The CRISTAL randomized trial. *Journal of the American Medical Association, 310*(17), 180–187. doi:10.1001/jama.2013.280502.

Ansaloni, L., Catena, F., Chattat, R., et al. (2010). Risk factors and incidence of postoperative delirium in elderly patients after elective and emergency surgery. *The British Journal of Surgery, 97*, 273–280. doi:10.1002/bjs.6843.

Apfelbaum, J. L., Walawander, C. A., Grasela, T. H., et al. (2002). Eliminating intensive postoperative care in same-day surgery patients using short-acting anesthetics. *Anesthesiology, 97*(1), 66–74.

Association of periOperative Registered Nurses (AORN). (2004). *Standards, recommended practices, and guidelines*. Denver, CO: Author.

Association of periOperative Registered Nurses (AORN). (2018). *Guidelines for perioperative practice*. http://www.aornstandards.org/content/current.

Autorino, R., Kaouk, J. H., Stolzenburg, J.-U., et al. (2013). Current status and future directions of robotic single site surgery: A systematic review. *European Urology, 63*(2), 266–280. doi:10.1016/j.eururo.2012.08.028.

Barone, C. P., Pablo, C. S., & Barone, G. W. (2004). Postanesthetic care in the critical care unit. *Critical Care Nurse, 24*(1), 38–46.

Barr, J., Fraser, G. L., Puntillo, K., et al. (2013). Clinical practice guidelines for the management of pain, agitation, and delirium in adult patients in the intensive care unit. *Critical Care Medicine, 41*(1), 263–306. doi:10.1097/CCM.0b013e3182783b72.

Berg, K., Arestedt, K., & Kjellgren, K. (2013). Postoperative recovery from the perspective of day surgery patients: A phenomenographic study. *International Journal of Nursing Studies, 50*, 1630–1638.

Brooks, P. B. (2012). Postoperative delirium in elderly patients. *American Journal of Nursing, 112*(9), 38–49.

Burden, N. (2007). Care of the orthopedic patient in the ambulatory surgery setting. *Journal of PeriAnesthesia Nursing, 22*(3), 207–210.

Canadian Allergy Asthma and Immunology Foundation. (1994). *Natural rubber latex allergy*. Orleans, ON: Author. Retrieved from http://www.allergyfoundation.ca/index.php?page=64.

Canadian Anesthesiologists' Society. (2005/2018). *Guidelines to the practice of anesthesia. The pre-anesthetic checklist*. Retrieved from http://www.cas.ca/English/Page/Files/97_Appendix%203.pdf.

Canadian Hospice Palliative Care Association (CHPCA). (2014). *Fact sheet: Hospice palliative care in Canada*. Retrieved from http://www.chpca.net/media/330558/Fact_Sheet_HPC_in_Canada%20Spring%202014%20Final.pdf.

Canadian Nurses Association (CNA). (2010). *Promoting cultural competence in nursing*. Ottawa: Author. Retrieved from https://www.cna-aiic.ca/~/media/cna/page-content/pdf-en/ps114_cultural_competence_2010_e.pdf?la=en.

Canadian Patient Safety Institute. (2009). *Surgical safety checklist*. Retrieved from http://www.patientsafetyinstitute.ca/en/toolsResources/Documents/Interventions/Surgical%20Safety%20Checklist/Detailed%20Explanation%20of%20the%20Checklist.pdf.

Carr, E. J., Thomas, V. N., & Wilson-Barnet, J. (2005). Patient experiences of anxiety, depression and acute pain after surgery: A longitudinal perspective. *International Journal of Nursing Studies, 42*, 521–530.

Cincinnati Children's Hospital Medical Center. (2018). *Positive expiratory pressure*. Retrieved from cincinnatichildrens.org/health/p/positive-expiratory-pressure.

Clayton, J. L. (2008). Special needs of older adults undergoing surgery. *AORN Journal, 87*, 557–570. doi:10.1016/j.aorn.2008.02.006.

College of Nurses of Ontario (CNO). (2009). *Culturally sensitive care*. Retrieved from http://www.cno.org/globalassets/docs/prac/41040_culturallysens.pdf.

Diepenbrock, N. H. (2012). *Quick reference to critical care* (4th ed.). Philadelphia, PA: Lippincott Williams & Wilkins.

Douglas, M. (1999). Pain as the fifth vital sign: Will cultural variations be considered? *Journal of Transcultural Nursing, 10*, 285.

Francis, P., & Winfield, H. N. (2006). Care of the patient undergoing robotic assisted laparoscopic pyeloplasty. *Urologic Nursing, 26*, 110–115.

Fredman, B., Sheffer, O., Zohar, E., et al. (2002). Fast-track eligibility of geriatric patients undergoing short urologic procedures. *Anesthesia and Analgesia, 94*, 560–564.

Inouye, S. K. (2006). Delirium in older persons. *New England Journal of Medicine, 354*, 1157. doi:10.1056/NEJMra052321.

Lees, M. C., Merani, S., Tauh, K., et al. (2015). Perioperative factors predicting poor outcome in elderly patients following emergency general surgery: a multivariate regression analysis. *Canadian Journal of Surgery, 58*(5), 312–317. doi:10.1503/cjs.011614.

Lehne, R. (2007). *Pharmacology for nursing care* (6th ed.). St. Louis: Elsevier.

Lewis, S. L., Dirksen, S. R., Heitkemper, M. M., et al. (2014). *Medical-surgical nursing in Canada: Assessment and management of clinical problems* (3rd Canadian ed.). Toronto: Elsevier Canada.

Lichtor, J. L., & Chang, F. (2012). Nausea and vomiting treatment after surgery: We can still do better. *Anesthesiology, 117*(3), 454–455. doi:10.1097/ALN.0b013e318267ef54.

Litwack, K. (1999). *Core curriculum for perianesthesia nursing practice* (4th ed.). Philadelphia, PA: Saunders.

Litwack, K. (2006). Adjusting postsurgical care for older patients. *Nursing, 36*(1), 66–67.

Lovering, S. (2006). Cultural attitudes and beliefs about pain. *Journal of Transcultural Nursing, 17*(4), 389–395.

Marshal, M. (2005). *A cultural competence guide for primary health care professionals in Nova Scotia*. Halifax: Government of Nova Scotia. Retrieved from http://www.multiculturalmentalhealth.ca/wp-content/uploads/2013/10/Cultural_Competence_guide_for_Primary_Health_Care_Professionals-Nova-Scotia-.pdf.

McPherson, K. (1996). *Bedside matters: The transformation of Canadian nursing, 1900–1990*. Toronto: Oxford University Press.

Merchant, R., Chartrand, D., Dain, S., et al. (2016). Guidelines to the practice of anesthesia—Revised edition. *Canadian Journal of Anesthesia, 63*, 86–112. doi:10.1007/s12630-015-0470-4.

National Association of PeriAnesthesia Nurses in Canada (NAPAN). (2014). *Standards for practice*. New Bandon, NB: Author. Retrieved from http://napanc.ca/index.php/standards.

National Heart, Lung and Blood Institute (NHLBI). (2011). *What is deep vein thrombosis?* Retrieved from https://www.nhlbi.nih.gov/health/health-topics/topics/dvt.

Nelson, R. L., Gladman, E., & Barbateskovic, M. (2014). Antimicrobial prophylaxis for colorectal surgery. *Cochrane Database of Systematic Reviews*, (5), article no. CD001181.

Nurse's life in the Montreal General Hospital. (1892, October). *Dominion Monthly Magazine*, 541–550.

Operating Room Nurses Association of Canada (ORNAC). (2015). *The ORNAC standards, guidelines, and position statements for perioperative Registered Nurses*. https://www.ornac.ca/en/standards.

Ontario PeriAnesthesia Nurses Association (OPANA). (2009a). *Standards of perianesthetic nursing practice*. Dundas, ON: Author.

Ontario PeriAnesthesia Nurses Association (OPANA). (2009b). *Management of patients with latex allergies* (pp. 121–123). Dundas, ON: Author.

Pagana, K. D., Pagana, T. J., & Pike-Macdonald, S. A. (2013). *Mosby's Canadian manual of diagnostic and laboratory tests* (1st Canadian ed.). Toronto: Elsevier.

Page, V., & Ely, E. W. (2011). *Delirium in critical care*. Cambridge, UK: Cambridge University Press.

Porter, R. (1997). *The greatest benefit to mankind: A medical history of humanity*. New York: W. W. Norton.

Pritchard, M. J. (2011). Using targeted information to meet the needs of surgical patients. *Nursing Standard, 25*(51), 35–39.

Public Health Ontario. (2012). *Best practices for infection prevention and control programs in Ontario in all health care settings* (3rd ed.). Toronto: Queen's Printer for Ontario.

Retrieved from https://www.publichealthontario.ca/en/eRepository/BP_IPAC_Ontario_HCSettings_2012.pdf.

Ramer, L., Richardson, J. L., Cohen, M. Z., et al. (1999). Multimeasure pain assessment in an ethnically diverse group of patients with cancer. *Journal of Transcultural Nursing, 10*, 94–101.

Registered Nurses' Association of Ontario (RNAO). (2005/2011). *Prevention of falls and fall injuries in the older adult*. Retrieved from http://rnao.ca/sites/rnao-ca/files/Prevention_of_Falls_and_Fall_Injuries_in_the_Older_Adult.pdf.

Registered Nurses' Association of Ontario (RNAO). (2007). *Assessment and management of pain in the elderly*. Toronto: Author. Retrieved from http://rnao.ca/sites/rnao-ca/files/Assessment_and_Management_of_Pain_in_the_Elderly_-_Learning_Package_for_LTC.pdf.

Registered Nurses' Association of Ontario (RNAO). (2010a). *Caregiving strategies for older adults with delirium, dementia and depression* (Guideline Supplement). Toronto: Author. Retrieved from http://rnao.ca/sites/rnao-ca/files/Caregiving_Strategies_for_Older_Adults_with_Delirium_Dementia_and_Depression.pdf.

Registered Nurses' Association of Ontario (RNAO). (2010b). *Screening for delirium, dementia and depression in older adults* (Guideline Supplement). Toronto: Author. Retrieved from http://rnao.ca/sites/rnao-ca/files/Screening_for_Delirium_Dementia_and_Depression_in_the_Older_Adult.pdf.

Registered Nurses' Association of Ontario (RNAO). (2013). *Assessment and management of pain* (3rd ed.). Toronto: Author. Retrieved from http://rnao.ca/sites/rnao-ca/files/AssessAndManagementOfPain2014.pdf.

Registered Nurses' Association of Ontario (RNAO). (2016). *Assessment and management of pressure injuries for the interprofessional team* (3rd ed.). Toronto: Author. Retrieved from http://rnao.ca/bpg/guidelines/pressure-injuries.

Registered Nurses' Association of Ontario (RNAO). (2017). *Registered Nurse First Assistant Interest Group*. Toronto: Author. Retrieved from http://rnao.ca/connect/interest-groups/rnfa.

Restrepo, R. D., Wettstein, R., Wittnebel, L., et al. (2011). Incentive spirometry 2011. *Respiratory Care, 56*(10), 1600–1604. doi:10.4187/respcare.01471.

Rice, A. N., Muckler, V. C., Miller, W. R., et al. (2015). Fast-tracking ambulatory surgery patients following anesthesia. *Journal of PeriAnesthesia Nursing, 30*(2), 124–133.

Saar, L. (2001). Use of a modified postanesthesia recovery score in phase II perianesthesia period of ambulatory surgery patients. *Journal of PeriAnesthesia Nursing, 16*(2), 82–89.

Sandelowski, M. (2000). *Devices and desires: Gender, technology and American nursing*. Chapel Hill, NC: University of North Carolina Press.

Sankar, A., Johnson, S. R., Beattie, W. S., et al. (2014). Reliability of the American Society of Anesthesiologists physical status scale in clinical practice. *British Journal of Anaesthesia, 113*(3), 424–432. doi:10.1093/bja/aeu100.

Snell, C. C., Fothergill-Bourbonnais, F., & Durocher-Hendriks, S. (1997). Patient controlled analgesia and intramuscular injections: A comparison of patient pain experiences and postoperative outcomes. *Journal of Advanced Nursing, 25*, 681–690.

Strickland, S. L., Rubin, B. K., Drescher, G. S., et al. (2013). AARC clinical practice guideline: Effectiveness of nonpharmacologic airway clearance therapies in hospitalized patients. *Respiratory Care, 58*(12), 2187–2193. doi:10.4187/respcare.02925.

Suchomel, M., Koller, W., Kundi, M., et al. (2009). Surgical hand rub: Influence of duration of application on the immediate and three-hours effects of n-propanol and isopropanol. *American Journal of Infection Control, 37*(4), 289–293.

Suhonen, R., & Leino-Kilpi, H. (2006). Adult surgical patients and the information provided to them by nurses: A literature review. *Patient Education and Counseling, 61*, 5–15.

Sussman, G., & Gold, M. (2004). *Guidelines for the management of latex allergies and safe latex use in health care facilities*. Retrieved from http://www.acaai.org/public/physicians/latex.htm.

Tanner, J., Norrie, P., & Melen, K. (2011). Preoperative hair removal to reduce surgical site infection (Review). *The Cochrane Database of Systematic Reviews*, (11), CD004122, doi:10.1002/14651858.CD004122.pub4.

Toman, C. (2007). *An officer and a lady*. Vancouver: UBC Press.

Toman, C., Heap, R., & Frize, M. (2006). Canadian women in engineering and science: Historical and contemporary perspectives. *Scientia Canadensis, 29*, 155–175.

Turjanica, M. A. (2007). Postoperative continuous peripheral nerve blockade in the lower extremity total joint arthroplasty population. *Medsurg Nursing, 16*, 151–154.

van Dishoeck, A. M., van der Hooft, T., Simoons, M. L., et al. (2009). Reliable assessment of sedation level in routine clinical practice by adding an instruction to the Ramsay Scale. *European Journal of Cardiovascular Nursing, 8*(2), 125–128.

Walton-Geer, P. S. (2009). Prevention of pressure ulcers in the surgical patient. *AORN Journal, 89*(3), 538–548.

White, P. (2008). Pain management after ambulatory surgery—Where is the disconnect? *Canadian Journal of Anesthesia, 55*(4), 201–207.

White, P. F., Rawal, S., Nguyen, J., et al. (2003). PACU fast-tracking: An alternative to "bypassing" the PACU for facilitating the recovery process after ambulatory surgery. *Journal of PeriAnesthesia Nursing, 18*, 247–253.

Wilson, R., Watt-Watson, J., Hodnett, E., et al. (2016). A randomized controlled trial of an individualized preoperative education intervention for symptom management after total knee arthroplasty. *Orthopaedic Nursing, 35*(1), 20–28.

World Health Organization. (2008). *Safe surgery checklist*. Retrieved from who.int/patientsafety/safesurgery/ss_checklist/en/.

A APPENDIX

Practical Nursing in Canada

Written by Joyce Engel, RN, PhD

OBJECTIVES

Mastery of content in this appendix will enable you to:

- Define the key terms listed.
- Explain how practical nursing has evolved as a regulated nursing group in Canada.
- Discuss the current issues and trends that affect practical nurses in Canada.
- Differentiate the scope of practice of the practical nurse from that of the registered nurse and unregulated health care provider.
- Explain how legislation, regulatory bodies, and professional associations govern the practice of practical nurses.
- Predict the future role of practical nurses within the Canadian health care system.

KEY TERMS

acuity, p. 1413
authorized act, p. 1415
competence, p. 1420
controlled act (restricted act), p. 1415
credentialling, p. 1415
creeping credentialism, p. 1412
delegation, p. 1421
educational laddering, p. 1417
entry-to-practice competencies, p. 1415
epidemiology, p. 1424
hybridization, p. 1414
jurisprudence, p. 1416
licensed practical nurse (LPN), p. 1412
practical nursing, p. 1412
proactive, p. 1424
protected title, p. 1412
registered nurse (RN), p. 1413
registered practical nurse, p. 1413
registration, p. 1412
specialization, p. 1415
speciation, p. 1414
standards of practice, p. 1419
supervision, p. 1421
unregulated care provider (UCP), p. 1419

HISTORY OF PRACTICAL NURSING IN CANADA

Practical nursing became a profession in the late 1930s. Initially it began as a hospital-based program with few common standards and hardly any legislative control. Beginning in the 1970s, practical nursing has been recognized as a distinct profession that necessitates formal education. Up until the mid-1970s, minimal high school preparation was necessary for admission to a practical nursing program and the program was likely a short apprenticeship in a hospital setting. No licensure examination was required and no official **registration**, **protected title**, or professional body existed.

Between 2006 and 2015, the supply of **licensed practical nurses (LPNs)** grew by over 50%, with the proportion of LPNs working in community settings increasing from 9% to 12.8% over the same period (Canadian Institute for Health Information [CIHI], 2016a), suggesting the growing recognition of the value of LPNs in all health care settings.

The Evolution of Practical Nursing

Practical nursing has evolved in a similar way in most provinces. It has also followed a pattern similar to that which other occupations have followed when established as professions. Abbott (1988) studied 130 occupations and noted that as they develop into professions, a number of common characteristics are evident:

- National professional association
- Government-sponsored licensing legislation
- Professional examinations
- A professional school separate from schools for other professions
- A university-based professional education
- A code of ethics
- A national-level journal
- Accreditation (e.g., United States) and certification (e.g., United Kingdom) programs

Practical nursing evidences most of these characteristics, except for university education requirements and a national-level journal. In addition, licensed practical nursing has undergone a series of name and designation changes and has experienced, in particular, a phenomenon known as **creeping credentialism**, or the requirement for increasing levels of education.

Canada. As early as 1914, the Canadian National Association for Trained Nurses (called the Canadian Nurses Association [CNA] since 1924) recognized the value of practical nursing, especially in the provision of care to patients in the home (College of Licensed Practical Nurses of British Columbia [CLPNBC], 2011). The first practical nurses were usually called either nursing aides (if female) or orderlies (if male).

In 1931, practical nurses in Canada numbered 4 700. By 1947, this number had increased to more than 7 900, largely because of increased hospital service needed after the Second World War. The first formal education program specifically for practical nurses (as opposed to for nursing aides or orderlies) began in Manitoba in 1945 (CIHI, 2010; CLPNBC, 2011). The first legislative acts were introduced in the 1940s and controlled the education, testing, licensing, regulation, and practice of practical nursing.

Many of the changes in the education of the practical nurse reflect the same changes that occurred earlier in the education of the registered nurse (RN). Education programs have become longer and more complex and have moved from hospital schools to postsecondary institutions, such as colleges. Rather than continuing to emphasize tasks and procedures, education programs have begun to focus more on holistic principles of nursing.

In the 1980s, most provinces developed regulations to govern practical nursing and required graduates to write a national licensing examination provided by the Canadian Nurses Association Testing Service (CNATS). In 2016, the national licensing examination moved to a computer-based format and is available in all provinces except the Yukon and Newfoundland and Labrador (which continue to offer a paper-based format) and in Quebec (Assessment Strategies Inc. [ASI], 2017). Table A-1 presents historical highlights in the evolution of practical nursing in selected provinces.

United States. In the United States, the first official practical nurse program was started by the Ballard School in New York in 1893, with a 3-month course to train women in simple nursing care, home care, and cooking (Knecht, 2017).

Nurses in the United States were the first to use the term *licensed practical nurse (LPN)*, which set a precedent that many Canadian jurisdictions have since followed.

United Kingdom. Before the early 1990s, nursing education in the United Kingdom was provided in nursing schools that were attached to hospitals. Project 2000, started in the early 1990s in the United Kingdom, aimed to increase the professional stature of nursing by removing nursing education from its hospital service base and placing it in postsecondary educational institutions. Today, nursing education in the United Kingdom takes place in the postsecondary school system at the college or technical school level (NursingNetUK, n.d.). Courses in enrolled nursing (the closest equivalent to practical nursing) no longer officially exist. Therefore, practical nurses from other countries cannot be certified in nursing in the United Kingdom unless they undergo upgrading in their training.

The Demand for Practical Nursing

In the late 1940s and early 1950s, demand for practical nurses increased significantly in most jurisdictions. A number of factors were responsible for this increased demand, which included political and economic pressures, changes within the nursing profession, and ecological and sociological factors.

Political and Economic Pressures. As roles for women expanded after the Second World War and more opportunities were available in a range of occupations and professions, the number of nurses decreased. This shortage of RNs came at a time when patients' acuity (i.e., level of sickness) was increasing in institutions. In addition, the increasing age of the population required more supportive care in communities and long-term care facilities, and private enterprise began exerting a greater economic influence on health care.

Because this public demand for safe and competent practice increased at the same time as economic and personnel challenges, practical nursing became more important within the health care system. Practical nursing offered an economical but highly competent workforce to meet the needs of patients in hospitals and of those requiring long-term care.

Changes Within Nursing

Nursing Education. The changing methods of educating nurses also contributed to the personnel and economic challenges in the health care sector. For many years, hospitals and other health care agencies depended on nursing students for free staffing of their institutions. When nursing education moved from a hospital base to a postsecondary base (beginning in the early 1970s), the number of staff who were available on hospital units decreased suddenly. Institutions responded by employing greater numbers of less trained health care assistants and aides to provide basic care. This reliance on a less prepared workforce was a concern for the public, who expected accountability and professionalism in health care. These expectations have resulted in higher standards and mandatory registration requirements for all categories of nurse, including the practical nurse.

Registration Laws. In the early twentieth century, beginning legislation was secured by RNs that outlined aspects of practice and preparation for practice such as nursing curricula and admission criteria. In addition, permissive registration protected the title of registered nurse but not who could use it. As long as health care providers did not claim to be registered, they could practise many nursing activities and claim to be a nurse.

After the Second World War, the public began demanding more qualified practitioners. As a result, mandatory registration was established, which laid out scopes of practice and protected not only titles but also who could use the title of registered nurse. Nurse registration laws were also amended to allow the creation of another level within nursing practice. Most provinces now have two categories of nurses: RNs (including nurse practitioners) and practical nurses. A nurse in the practical nurse category can use the title *licensed practical nurse (LPN)* or, in Ontario, *registered practical nurse*. In the four Western provinces, registered psychiatric nurses, a third category of nursing, also exists.

Development of Categories Within the Nursing Profession. The evolution of at least two categories of Canadian nurses and, in the Western provinces, three categories, distinguishes nursing from some other professions. The medical profession, for example, essentially has one level of practitioner (a medical doctor) and many subspecialties (e.g., pediatrics, ophthalmology, orthopedics, and so on). Because medical practice involves many responsibilities, some are ceded to practitioners such as optometrists, who have a unique, limited scope of practice and make no claims to be medical doctors.

Even though medical doctors cede limited activities to nonmedical professionals, they maintain their own professional position, which involves the central tasks of diagnosis and treatment of disorders, functions that are clear to the public. Nursing, however, has developed a much less definitive practice, and divisions between the professional knowledge base and functions of the categories of nurses are somewhat unclear to employers, the public, and even to nurses. Basic theory and practice are common to both categories of nurses and are divided only by depth of knowledge and complexity of care required. Patient complexity, predictability, and stability, however, are hardly absolute and can be difficult to define. As a result, there is sometimes confusion about the boundaries between registered and practical nurses. Ecological and sociological theories applied to nursing provide possible insights into the development and confusion around the categories of nurse in Canada because they articulate reaction to change and the competition that occurs among groups for power, reward, roles and functions, and even professional survival.

Ecological and Sociological Factors

Ecology Theory Applied to Nursing. Ecology theory in general describes changes in populations, such as companies and professions, that result from environment and evolution (Wilson, 1992).

To survive, groups compete for niches (places or functions in any system) and evolve to cope effectively with environmental changes.

TABLE A-1 History of Practical Nursing in Selected Provinces

Province	Year	Significant Developments and Comments
British Columbia	1951	*Practical Nurse Act* passed
	1965	*Practical Nurses Act* legally approved
		Council of LPNs established as the licensing body
	1991	Council of LPNs becomes an independent regulatory body of the Ministry of Health
	1996	The Council of LPNs in BC becomes the College of LPNs of British Columbia under the *Health Professions Act*
Alberta	1945	The School for Nursing Aides established in Calgary, sponsored by Department of Veterans Affairs and Canadian Vocational Training
	1947	*The Provincial Nursing Aides Act* passed, which allowed licensing of the Certified Nursing Aide
	1961	Alberta Certified Nursing Aide Association (ACNAA) incorporated
	1972	Alberta Certified Nursing Aide Association, along with eight other practical nursing associations, becomes a founding member of the Canadian Association of Practical Nurses and Nursing Assistants
	1978	*Nursing Assistant Registration Act* combines aide and orderly in one category of RNA (registered nursing assistant)
	1987	Professional Council of RNAs (PCRNA) becomes first health care discipline under *Health Disciplines Act.* Registered nursing assistants become self-regulatory with a distinct scope of practice.
		Nursing assistant graduates required to write Canadian Practical Nurse Registration Examination (national licensing examination)
	1990	RNAs change title to LPNs
		Professional Council of RNAs becomes Professional Council of LPNs
	1995	Mandatory educational upgrading instituted as a result of LPN devaluation and membership decline
	1998	Council changes its name to College of Licensed Practical Nurses of Alberta
	1999	*Health Disciplines Act* becomes *Health Professions Act,* which will eventually include all regulated health care professions under their separate provincial colleges
	2003	The College of Licensed Practical Nurses of Alberta is formally proclaimed
	2004	LPNs in specialized practice are recognized by the *Health Professions Act*
	2006	Diploma is approved as the entry-to-practice requirement
Manitoba	1945	First official practical nurse education program in Canada
Ontario	1938	Centres begin offering 6-month courses for nursing assistants
	1941–1945	With approval of Ontario Department of Health, Registered Nurses' Association of Ontario (RNAO) sponsors eight 6-month training programs for nursing assistants
	1947	*Nurses Act* is amended to allow title of Certified Nursing Assistant (CNA)
	1963	CNA title is changed to Registered Nursing Assistant (RNA)
	1990	RNA training programs moved to community colleges
	1993	RNA title is changed to Registered Practical Nurse (RPN)
	2001	College of Nurses of Ontario passes a regulation to require all RPNs to obtain their basic diploma through an enhanced 2-year program in a provincial college as an entry-to-practice requirement beginning January 2005
	2002	All practical nursing programs are offered in colleges
New Brunswick	1977	Legislature established an act of incorporation, giving the Association of New Brunswick Registered Nursing Assistants the responsibility of education, registration, and discipline of registered practical nurses
	1987 and 2000	Unsuccessful attempts to change the RNA title to Licensed Practical Nurse through the New Brunswick Legislature
	2002	The *Licensed Practical Nurses Act* recognizes the new LPN title
		The Association of New Brunswick Licensed Practical Nurses becomes the name of the provincial association

Data from Association of New Brunswick Licensed Practical Nurses (2012), *About ANBLPN.* Retrieved from https://www.anblpn.ca/; Canadian Institute for Health Information (CIHI). (2010). *Regulated nurses: Canadian trends, 2005 to 2009* (p. 81). Retrieved from https://secure.cihi.ca/free_products/nursing_report_2005-2009_en.pdf; College of Licensed Practical Nurses of Alberta. (2016). *History of Alberta's licensed practical nurses.* Retrieved from https://www.clpna.com/about-clpna/history-alberta-lpns/; College of Licensed Practical Nurses of British Columbia. (2011). *History of LPNs in BC and Canada.* Retrieved from https://www.clpnbc.org/What-is-an-LPN/History-of-LPNs-in-B-C-and-Canada; and Registered Practical Nurses Association of Ontario. (2013). *History of practical nursing and RPNAO.* Retrieved from https://www.rpnao.org/about/history.

Groups that have too narrow a function or that fail to compete successfully lose their niche to other groups. Niches may change, which requires successful adaptation through either competing for a new niche or acquiring the niche first and establishing a solid place in it.

Two concepts in biological evolution that can be applied to practical nursing are the concepts of *speciation* and *hybridization.* In **speciation**, the species divides into one or more subspecies, each with its own particular function or niche. In **hybridization**, the new species adopts characteristics of one or more of the ancestor species (Van House & Sutton, 2000).

Out of the single species in nursing, two "subspecies" have arisen: the RN and the LPN. As discussed earlier, some provinces also have a third "subspecies," the registered psychiatric nurse, who has a college education and is educated to provide care to patients with mental illness. The niche for the RN is wider than that of the LPN, and the niche for the registered psychiatric nurse is the narrowest of all. Hybridization can also be applied to nursing. Nursing has adopted characteristics of other "species," such as use of ideas and technology that were previously exclusively medical functions. For example, taking blood pressure, starting intravenous infusions, and making certain types of diagnoses are now nursing functions that used to be medical functions.

It is interesting that whereas nursing has developed speciation, medicine has avoided speciation and instead developed specialization. Whereas nurses share functions, doctors cede specific unwanted functions to different professionals. The sharing of functions among practical and registered nurses is what contributes to the public and professional confusion about the roles of the two levels of nurses.

Sociology Applied to Nursing. Sociology is the study of group roles, functions, and interactions. Abbott's (1988) unique theory about professions can be melded with ecology theory to provide additional insight into the development of professions. According to Abbott, a profession attempts to keep certain tasks or problems for itself and shares them with others only if it can do so without endangering its own niche.

Abbott (1988) also believed that a profession protects itself and its niche position by possessing a sound knowledge base. In other words, acquiring knowledge is central to developing a strong professional identity. Abbott believed that knowledge sets a true profession apart from a mere occupation and helps to "redefine its problems and tasks, defend them from interlopers, and seize new problems…", which enables "survival in the competitive system of professions" (p. 8).

Professional tasks are either objective (knowledge and technology based) or subjective (culturally or legally based) in nature. Some objective tasks unique to nursing have been the development of the nursing process and nursing diagnoses. Subjective tasks are most clearly seen in the legal criteria for nursing defined in each province. Authorized acts or controlled acts (e.g., in Ontario) or restricted acts (e.g., in British Columbia) are acts that are harmful unless performed by qualified persons. The *Ontario Nursing Act 1991* defines which of the 13 authorized acts specified in the *Regulated Health Professions Act* nurses are allowed to perform. These include four acts that nurses in Ontario are allowed to perform: (1) performing a procedure below the dermis or mucous membrane; (2) placing an instrument, hand, or finger into a body opening; (3) administering a substance by injection or inhalation; and (4) dispensing a drug (College of Nurses of Ontario [CNO], 2018a). In order to perform controlled acts authorized to nurses through legislation, nurses must have the skills and knowledge necessary to perform the acts. It is also important to note that while nurses may be allowed to perform controlled acts under legislation, organizational policies may restrict or limit their performance.

Objective tasks are more resistant to change than are subjective tasks. Change in environment often brings in new tasks, new knowledge, and new technology. Failure to adapt to changes in the environment can result in a loss of niche, role, and position for a profession (Van House & Sutton, 2000). A successful profession is supported in its adaptation to changes by changes in laws and regulations, public opinion, and workplace practices and rules, all of which reflect culture and society.

Practical nursing has had mixed success in adapting to environmental forces. Jurisdictions have enacted definitive legal supports (such as registration, licensing, and protected title) for the particular knowledge base and specified range of tasks that characterize practical nursing. Despite this, LPNs still strive to clarify their role for both the public and the government. Their knowledge and practice are similar to that of RNs, but workplaces continue to be challenged to maximize and make appropriate use of LPNs, thus underusing or exploiting skills and knowledge of LPNs. Therefore,

> *Abbott's [1988] analysis also casts light on the debate raging in most professional schools—what is the perfect balance between theory and practice? A student focusing solely on theory (or the abstract knowledge base) lacks the skills and tools to practice the profession; however, Abbott [warned] that practice-based knowledge lacks abstraction…a thorough understanding of the knowledge base, not simply the tools and skills, is most likely to provide safe passage to the new environment (Van House & Sutton, 2000, p. 60).*

In order to adapt to changing needs and practices in health care and to optimize their professional roles, practical nurses in Canada continue to work toward balance in both theory and practice. Basic education is increasing in complexity and in the promotion of the concept of lifelong learning. In addition to basic education, many practical nurses complete credentialling in specialty areas after graduation, which enhances the individual's basic knowledge base and skills and increases professional credibility.

PRACTICAL NURSING TODAY: ISSUES AND TRENDS

Educational Preparation and Entry-to-Practice Competencies

Patients' needs are more complex than ever. Practical nurses must respond to increased acuity, multiple comorbidities among patients experiencing chronic disorders, wide cultural and social variations among patients, and a continuing trend toward home and community care. In response, national entry-to-practice competencies are reviewed with key stakeholder groups and revised by the Canadian Council for Practical Nurse Regulators (CCPNR), which includes representatives from all jurisdictions in Canada who license and regulate practical nurses, with the assistance of Assessment Strategies Inc. (CCPNR, 2013). These competencies, which are adopted by provincial and territorial jurisdictions, change with varying needs of the practice environment. The competencies serve to outline what the public can expect of practical nurses and guide educational preparation of practical nurses. Entry-to-practice competencies reflect minimum standards of knowledge, skills, attitudes, and judgement expected of beginning practical nurses and include competencies related to:

- Therapeutic relationships
- Interprofessional and collaborative relationships with patients and members of the health care team
- Clinical decision making
- Comprehensive assessments of patients
- Evaluation of care
- Promotion of patients' rights and responsibilities
- Facilitation of health education and health promotion
- Adherence to legal requirements of practical nursing practice, including documentation
- Professional and ethical conduct
- Leadership

Thus, as the practice environment changes, the education of practical nurses is guided by entry-to-practice competencies that also change to respond to the environment's needs. This results in educational programs that are increasingly demanding in scope and depth and that include strong theory and hands-on preparation.

Entry to a Practical Nurse Program. Entry requirements for practical nursing programs have become more vigorous. Canadian practical nursing programs require that applicants have a high school diploma. Most require that applicants have high marks in language and in one or two sciences. Mature students without a high school diploma may be admitted to many postsecondary institutions if applicants can demonstrate equivalent learning through other forms of education or can successfully complete pre-entrance student testing.

Location and Length of Program. In most Canadian jurisdictions, practical nursing programs are 2-year (approximately four semesters) diploma programs and are offered in postsecondary institutions. In order to facilitate student access to nursing education, some educational institutions offer practical nursing programs through nontraditional delivery methods such as distance education and online learning. The trend toward longer and more complex education for practical nurses is fuelled by the increased complexity of the patient base, new and rapid developments in technology, increased public expectations, professional competitiveness, and expanded opportunities for practice.

These increases in the educational requirements for entry to practice have both positive and negative aspects for the individual professional, the profession, the workplace, the government, and society in general. Positive effects include increases in employment opportunities, national and international mobility, and quality of service to the public. Negative effects may include increases in educational costs for the individual and society, delay of the professional's entry into the job market, problems in workplace collective agreements, exacerbation of job shortages, and creation of economic burdens for employers when increased education results in expectations of higher compensation.

Instructors in Practical Nursing Programs. Canadian nursing instructors are usually required to have clinical experience and educational preparation that is at least one level beyond that of their students. At one time, this meant that RNs taught aides and practical nurses. Today, almost without exception, RNs with baccalaureate degrees teach in practical nursing programs. Many have master's degrees or doctorates in nursing, education, or other related areas. LPNs may be hired as course instructors or as assistants under the direction of a lead course instructor. RNs and LPNs are most often involved with teaching students in clinical areas. These clinical teachers may be hired directly by a postsecondary institution or may be employees of the agency in which clinical practice takes place. Importantly, practising LPNs serve as role models and support students educationally during preceptorship experiences.

Student Clinical Practice. In order to prepare students for practice as LPNs, it is important to secure clinical settings that provide opportunity for solid practice of knowledge and skills gained in the classroom and laboratory settings, reflect the diverse settings in which LPNs practise, and enable students to work to the full scope of practice of LPNs. Securing appropriate clinical placements for students can be a challenge, for two main reasons:

1. Some acute care areas (e.g., surgery, acute medicine, pediatrics) either do not use LPNs or restrict what LPNs are able to do, perhaps because of unit or institutional mandates or unfamiliarity with the competency levels of LPNs.
2. Clinical areas are frequently inundated with requests for clinical placements of students from various health care fields, which is an especially prominent problem in large urban centres. As a result, practical nursing programs are incorporating innovative approaches to prepare students for clinical placements. These include use of computerized human patient simulators and clinical simulations in order to increase student confidence and enhance readiness to practise before clinical practicum experiences. In addition, scheduling of clinical learning has extended to weekends and a variety of other shifts. Program delivery models have also been adjusted to allow for clinical placements during summer months, when clinical settings may be more readily available.

Requirements for Practice as a Licensed Practical Nurse

In order to practise, practical nurses must become registered in the provincial or territorial jurisdiction in which they intend to practise. The professional regulatory colleges in the provinces and territories are mandated to set requirements for registration or licensing.

Educational Preparation. Applicants for registration must demonstrate successful and recent completion of a nursing education program that prepares them to safely and capably perform the entry-to-practice competencies expected of practical nurses in the jurisdiction to which they are applying. For students who are applying for registration in the province or territory where they have taken an approved educational program, this requirement will be satisfied when the educational program provides documentation to the regulatory college that the students have successfully completed their program. If an applicant is applying from outside the province or territory, then the regulatory college evaluates documentation from the applicant to determine if the educational background of the applicant is equivalent to that received by applicants from provincial or territorial programs. Recent graduates of programs may be able to practise with a temporary license until they write and pass the national licensing exams.

Evidence of Practice. Applicants for registration must also present evidence of recent practice as a practical nurse. For most applicants, this requirement is met through the recent completion of an approved educational program. Applicants who have already been in practice must provide evidence of recent employment as an LPN or RPN, including details about the settings in which practice occurred, job descriptions, and patient population served.

Registration Examinations. When the regulatory college is satisfied that recent graduates of programs (or internationally prepared nurses) have met educational, experience, and other requirements, the final step in registration is applying to write the Canadian Practical Nurse Registration Examination after submitting application and administration fees. As stated earlier, as of 2016, the national licensing examination is offered in a computer-based format in all provinces except the Yukon and Newfoundland and Labrador, which offer a paper-based format, and in Quebec. This examination, which is based on the national entry-to-practice competencies, includes approximately 170 multiple-choice questions and is provided by Assessment Strategies Inc. (ASI), in partnership with Pearson VUE. In addition to flexibility in testing sites and testing dates, computer-based testing enables access to an interactive examination database and study resources (ASI, 2017). Applicants for registration may also need to pass jurisprudence examinations that test knowledge and comprehension of laws and regulations, by-laws, and standards that govern provincial nursing practice (CNO, 2018b). In some provinces (e.g., British Columbia), LPNs are required to write the jurisprudence examination not only upon first application for registration but also periodically thereafter (CLPNBC, n.d.)

Once the registration examination is written, applicants are notified of the results of their examination by email. If unsuccessful, they are provided with a breakdown of the examination results to assist in further preparation. Unsuccessful examination writers will not be allowed to register as nurses until they pass the examination. The number of times that the exam can be repeated is directed by the regulatory body of the province or territory in which registration is sought.

Usually, the school receives a summary of the passing and failing marks in that class and information about the school's success in relation to other programs in its jurisdiction and in Canada. Privacy of examination marks is an issue in many areas. In Ontario, for instance, students must sign a waiver that allows their examination results to be sent to their educational institution. When the examination results are sent to the school, the student names are obscured.

Other Requirements. Because professionals have a position of power, concerns inevitably arise that they could take advantage of vulnerable persons, especially young children and older persons. Thus, applicants are required to provide evidence of good character and fitness to practise, which includes completion of a criminal record check and disclosure of mental or physical health problems that would have an impact on the ability to practise safely, competently, and ethically. Safe care involves the ability to communicate clearly and accurately; therefore, applicants must also provide information as to fluency in the use of the English language and, possibly, in the French language (depending on the province or territory).

Continuing Education Issues

Laddering. Should health care aides be given the opportunity to become practical nurses? Should practical nurses be given the opportunity to become degree nurses? The concept of educational laddering, or *bridging,* recognizes prior learning and acknowledges that knowledge and expertise are acquired in various ways. It provides a means by which individuals can progress in their careers with reasonable access to other levels or categories of education and nursing. Institutions across Canada offer academic pathways that bridge health care aide (or personal support worker) and practical nursing programs, as well as practical nursing and registered nursing programs.

Postgraduate Certification. Practical nurses can further their education and their contribution to the profession by specializing in specific fields. Practical nurses have plentiful opportunities to obtain certification in specialty areas after graduation from a basic program. These certificates may be offered to LPNs or to both registered and practical nurses. Examples of specialty areas are certification in operating room technique and management, foot care, gerontology and geriatric nursing, dialysis, women's health, specialized mental health, and occupational nursing.

The Role of the Practical Nurse

Most jurisdictions recognize that practical nursing is a separate category within the wider field of professional nursing. There is also recognition that LPNs and RNs study from the same body of nursing knowledge. Registered nurses study this content in greater detail and over a longer period of time, which allows for a deeper base in clinical practice, as well as in decision making, leadership, and research utilization. Practical nurses study for a shorter period, which results in a more focused knowledge and skills base (CNO, 2014).

While 31.5% of LPNs work in long-term and chronic care and this remains a key setting for their practice, the proportion of LPNs in community and hospital settings is increasing. In 2015, the number of LPNs in hospital care (48.5%) was greater than that in long-term care, and 12.2% were in community settings (CIHI, 2016a). Additionally, LPNs were being hired into acute care areas that may not have been previously available to them, such as operating rooms, emergency rooms, maternal child nursing, and mental health, where they work independently or collaboratively with RNs. LPNs also work in community settings, such as community health centres, home care, nursing stations, and public health units, as well as in physician's offices, educational institutions, government agencies, occupational health, and industrial settings. LPNs may also be self-employed. LPNs in these settings, in addition to direct client or patient care, can occupy a variety of diverse roles, such as educators and administrators (CIHI, 2010). Consequently, practical nurse programs are providing instruction in skills and knowledge needed to care for stable patients in acute care settings (e.g., intravenous therapy, oxygen therapy) and long-term care settings, as well as in community and mental health.

Table A-2 lists the percentages of practical nurses in Canada employed in different areas of responsibility in 2015.

Workplace Issues

Recent declines in the number of nurses in health care have prompted concerns about the adequacy of the nursing workforce of the future. While data on the workforce suggest that this decline is related to retirements, fewer students graduating, and unique occurrences such as the introduction of Ontario's Declaration of Practice in 2014 (CIHI, 2015a, 2015b), declines or nearly parallel inflows and outflows in some categories of nurses prompt close attention to additional factors that may be causing nurses to relocate, leave the profession, or decide not

TABLE A-2 Number and Percentage Distribution of Licensed Practical Nurses Employed in Practical Nursing by Area of Responsibility (2015)

	Count	Percentage
Total direct care	97 923	100
Geriatric/Long-term care	40 623	41.5
Medical/Surgical	14 857	15.2
Nursing in several clinical areas	7 594	7.8
Psychiatric/Mental health	4 464	4.6
Rehabilitation	3 344	3.4
Home care	2 778	2.8
Community health	2 340	2.4
Operating room	2 222	2.3
Palliative care	1 892	1.9
Emergency room	1 826	1.9
Maternal/Newborn	1 428	1.5
Ambulatory care	1 061	1.1
Pediatric	1 033	1.1
Public health	541	0.6
Oncology	205	0.2
Occupational health	191	0.2
Critical care (burn)	145	0.1
Other patient care	11 379	11.6
Total	76 240	100.0%

Modified from Canadian Institute for Health Information (CIHI). (2016). *Regulated nurses, 2015: Report: LPN data tables: Table 19.* Retrieved from https://www.cihi.ca/en/lpn_2015_data_tables_en_xlsx.

to renew their registration. A large study by Nowrouzi, Giddens, Gohar, and colleagues (2016) that reviewed the literature on workplace issues and workplace satisfaction among both RNs and LPNs suggested a number of factors thought to contribute to nurses' stress, burnout, and, potentially, absenteeism, poor-quality care or productivity, or decision to leave the profession and health care:

- Overtime
- Long hours, especially 12-hour shifts
- Short staffing
- Situations of ethical distress
- Working for several employers
- Violence in the workplace
- Conflicted or noncollaborative relationships with other nurses or with physicians
- Lack of institutional support or commitment for nursing activities
- Feelings of powerlessness
- Amount of compensation

Workforce Trends

Despite recent declines in the numbers of nurses in the health workforce, the supply of practical nurses continues to grow overall in Canada (CIHI, 2016b). As evidence of this trend, CIHI (2016b) data suggest that the inflow of LPNs to the profession as a result of new graduates, migration from other countries, and nurses returning to the workforce is more than double the outflow from the profession resulting from retirement, family responsibilities, returning to school, or choosing another occupation. This suggests a growing supply of LPNs, as evidenced in employment data. In 2006, 67 300 LPNs (including Ontario registered practical nurses) were employed, and 101 319 were employed in 2015 (CIHI, 2016c), which suggests not only that there are more LPNs available to the workforce but also that more LPNs are being employed (Table A-3 summarizes the distribution of the Canadian LPN workforce by jurisdiction). This growth is particularly dramatic in British Columbia and Alberta, where the supply of LPNs from 2006 to 2015 has more than doubled, as well as in provinces such as Quebec and Ontario (CIHI, 2016d).

In addition to the growing supply and employment of LPNs, this workforce is becoming younger, with over one-third of LPNs being younger than 35 years of age. Full-time employment tends to occur less among younger nurses, however, which may be related to factors such as less availability of full-time positions, continuation of education, gaining experience through employment in multiple positions, and the desire for greater work–life balance (CIHI, 2016b). Employment trends also indicate that there is increased decline in the numbers of regulated nurses who work in rural and remote areas, which points to greater potential difficulties for patients accessing high-quality care in these areas.

Internationally prepared LPNs in Canada comprise less than 3% of the practical nurse workforce, which represents a slight increase from 2007 to 2011. Most of these nurses have attended programs in the Philippines or the United Kingdom (CIHI, 2012). Nurses from international jurisdictions must meet regulatory requirements of the province or territory in which they wish to practise, which include writing the registration examination and meeting standards of educational preparation. A number of bridge training programs are available to help qualified immigrants meet the Canadian regulatory requirements (Government of Ontario [Immigration], 2016). The trends in supply and employment of LPNs suggest that there may be more hiring of LPNs in diverse health care settings and perhaps even wider acceptance of the significant roles that LPNs can play in contemporary health care in Canada. Data also suggest, however, that the number of regulated nurses who are middle-aged (i.e., ages 34 to 54 years) is declining, which is troubling, because this group is important in the support of older regulated nurses and in mentorship to younger nurses who are entering the nursing workforce (CIHI, 2016e). Additionally, the growing inflow of LPNs, which is partially related to migration of nurses, may mean that LPNs are becoming somewhat more mobile, which can affect the stability of health care settings. Conversely, this trend may also mean that LPNs have more opportunities than in the

TABLE A-3 Licensed Practical Nursing Workforce, by Jurisdiction and Canada, 2005 to 2015

	2005	2006	2007	2008	2009	2010	2011	2012	2013	2014	2015
NL	2698	2639	2598	2530	2521	2495	2480	2230	2223	2221	2245
PEI	606	599	623	631	665	590	621	639	609	527	548
NS	3127	3174	3160	3250	3357	3530	3710	3652	3707	3664	3774
NB	2633	2646	2734	2731	2729	2802	2905	2927	2995	2996	3061
QUE	16293	17104	17492	19581	19184	20244	21394	22633	23873	24852	24867
ONT	24458	25084	26126	27435	28804	30423	31446	32839	35260	37248	39069
MAN	2590	2652	2671	2615	2651	2732	2836	2935	2952	2968	3032
SASK	2194	2224	2381	2514	2629	2723	2806	2816	2842	3134	3230
ALTA	5313	5614	5986	6232	6669	7301	7720	8342	8948	10080	10801
BC	4884	5412	5791	6705	7577	8235	8501	9015	9985	10264	10483
YT	56	60	59	62	64	63	76	92	100	105	110
NWT	101	92	88	94	94	86	92	91	91	95	99
Canada	64953	67300	69709	74380	76944	81224	84587	88211	93585	98124	101 319

NOTE: Totals may not sum to 100% due to rounding. Data released by the Canadian Institute for Health Information (CIHI) may differ from data from other sources due to CIHI's nationally standardized methodology.

From Canadian Institute for Health Information (CIHI) (2016). *Regulated nurses, 2015: LPN data tables: Table 1.* Retrieved from https://www.cihi.ca/en/lpn_2015_data_tables_en_xlsx.

past, which can be of interest to persons who are considering becoming a LPN. The declining numbers of regulated nurses in remote and rural areas (CIHI, 2016b) may present a challenging but interesting area of employment and opportunity for LPNs, particularly those with some experience.

STANDARDS AND SCOPE OF PRACTICE

Standards of Practice

As a regulated profession, practical nursing is responsible for establishing its own **standards of practice**. The professional regulatory body for LPNs in each jurisdiction (e.g., the provincial college of practical nurses) has the authority to set standards of practice for its members. It also has the authority to ensure that members meet these standards.

Standards of practice are written statements that detail the level of performance expected of nurses in a particular jurisdiction. They provide general guidelines about several aspects of professional practice and performance. The practice of any nurse can be continually measured against these standards. They also demonstrate to the public that the profession of practical nursing is dedicated to protecting public safety and providing high-quality care.

Although they differ in details, most standards of practice for practical nurses in Canada offer performance guidelines for the following areas (among others): nursing process (i.e., assessment, participation in nursing diagnoses, planning, implementation, evaluation), ethics, education, leadership, research, and collaboration with other professionals.

Each individual nurse and the regulatory body are responsible for standards—the individual nurse for knowing and using them and the regulatory body for publishing and enforcing them. In addition, the professional association and employers must support these standards in practice and in theory. Finally, members of the public are responsible for being good consumers of the professional health care they receive.

Ethics in Nursing

Ethics refers to the moral principles or values that guide people when they decide what is right and what is wrong. Ethics influences behaviour and relationships with other people. Providing ethical nursing care means that the nurse forms a dynamic, caring, helping relationship with the patient in order to help the patient achieve and maintain optimal health.

Regulatory bodies for practical nursing are responsible for establishing and promoting codes of ethics or statements of values that are agreed upon by members of a profession and guide ethical decision making. The following values are promoted in most codes of ethics for LPNs:

- Being accountable for one's actions
- Upholding the patient's rights to privacy and confidentiality
- Providing care that maintains the patient's dignity
- Demonstrating respect for the patient at all times
- Promoting integrity by providing safe, competent, and ethical nursing care
- Evaluating one's work and maintaining competency

Scope of Practice

Scope of practice refers to the legal limits of a professional role. Four categories of regulated nurses provide patient care. In addition, **unregulated care providers (UCPs)** (e.g., nurse's aides, health care aides, personal support workers) work alongside nurses to provide patient care. Each category of regulated nurse has its own scope of practice. These scopes of practice are each different because each category of regulated nurse has different education, legal authority, and performance requirements.

In Table A-4, the educational preparation and decision making related to patients and context of practical and registered nurses are compared. While specific scopes of practice may differ among jurisdictions, it is common to find that as the complexity and unpredictability of the patient's condition and risk of negative outcomes increase, practical nurses will need more collaboration and support from RNs. This support initially may involve consultation with the RN and may lead to sharing the patient assignment with the RN or the RN's taking responsibility for the patient (CNO, 2014; Licensed Practical Nurses Association of Prince Edward Island, 2011) (Figure A-1). It may be within an LPN's scope of practice to care for a stable postoperative patient; however, if the patient's vital signs become unstable and urine output decreases below normal limits, the condition of the patient may require care that exceeds that scope of practice. When the LPN recognizes that the patient's condition has become more complex and unpredictable, the LPN needs to consult with the RN and may determine that the patient is experiencing signs of shock that require physician attention. It is essential that LPNs and RNs are aware of each other's scopes of practice because this awareness enhances their ability to work collaboratively to determine and deliver the most appropriate plan of care.

It is important to note that boundaries between scopes of practice of LPNs and RNs vary because of shifts in the health needs of patients and because of ongoing development of competencies beyond basic preparation for practice. Such boundaries may shift when the health needs of a patient change, necessitating reconsideration of the scopes of practice of the LPN and RN. The boundaries between scopes of practice of LPNs and UCPs are more definite because little of the basic knowledge and few competencies are shared between the two roles.

Challenges to Working to Full Scope of Practice. Although graduates of practical nursing programs are prepared to perform skills that are considered entry-to-practice competencies and consistent with their scope of practice, many factors can influence their ability to do so in the workplace. Additionally, practical nurses can and do acquire skills and knowledge consistent with the scope of practice for practical nurses beyond those needed for entry to practice, such as operating room techniques, special foot care, orthopedic care, dialysis care, and specialized gerontological care.

Theoretically, any health care skill that a family member or lay person can be taught can be performed by a nurse, as long as the nurse has the appropriate knowledge base and has demonstrated initial and continued competency and judgement in the application of the skill. LPNs need to be aware, however, that family members are not bound by the same legal restrictions that may apply to the role of LPNs.

Even if a health care skill is considered part of the scope of practice, LPNs may be restricted from performing such activities as the administration of injections or initiation of intravenous therapy by institutional or regional policies or practices and variations in what LPNs are allowed to do across jurisdictions, across institutions, and even across units. In order to determine what can be included in the LPN's role, the LPN needs to continuously update his or her knowledge base from the professional association, the regulatory body, agency policies, and evidence bases such as research and other relevant sources.

While regulatory bodies and employers place parameters on what LPNs are able to do, it is important for LPNs to recognize the

TABLE A-4 Educational Preparation and Decision Making Related to Care Provision for Practical and Registered Nurses

	Practical Nurse	Registered Nurse
Entry-level education	Completion of a recognized practical nursing education program and successful completion of the Canadian Practical Nurse Registration Examination	Completion of a recognized baccalaureate program and successful completion of the NCLEX
Patient	Educated to work collaboratively with patients (individuals, families, groups, and communities) and with members of the health care team across the continuum of health	Educated to work collaboratively with patients (individuals, families, groups, populations, and communities) and with members of the health care team across the continuum of health
Context of practice	Works as a team member in all settings and provides leadership (e.g., directs unregulated care providers [UCPs], mentors students, represents nursing and nursing care issues)	Works as an independent practitioner or team member, and provides leadership (e.g., leads interprofessional teams, directs UCPs, makes decisions about resource allocation) in all settings
Implementation	Coordinates care of less acute, less complex, less variable patients with more predicable outcomes Provides elements of care for highly complex patients in close consultation with the RN Initiates certain restricted or controlled activities, providing the LPN has the knowledge and **competence** (or ability) to do so, without an order from an authorized health professional	Coordinates care of patients regardless of acuity, complexity, variability, or predictability Directs plans of care for highly complex patients Initiates restricted or controlled activities that are common to and different from those authorized to the practical nurse, providing the RN has the knowledge and competence to do so, without an order from an authorized health professional

From College of Licensed Practical Nurses of British Columbia (CLPNBC). (2016). *Scope of practice for licensed practical nurses.* Retrieved from https://www.clpnbc.org/Documents/Practice-Support-Documents/Scope-of-Practice-ONLINE.aspx; College of Nurses of Ontario (CNO). (2014). *RN and registered practical nurse practice: The client, the nurse, and the environment.* Retrieved from http://www.cno.org/globalassets/docs/prac/41062.pdf; and Nurses Association of New Brunswick and Association of New Brunswick Licensed Practical Nurses. (2015). *Guidelines for intraprofessional collaboration: Registered nurses and licensed practical nurses working together.* Retrieved from http://www.anblpn.ca/downloads/working_together.pdf.

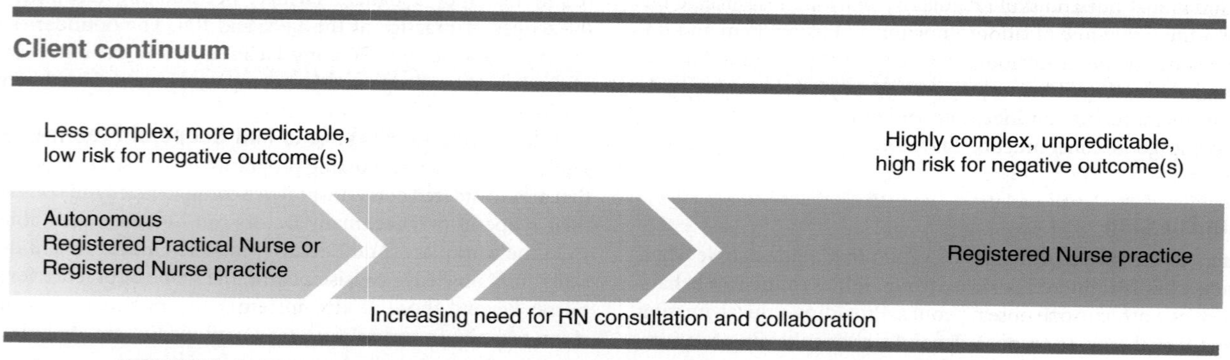

FIGURE A-1 Client continuum. (From College of Nurses of Ontario [CNO]. [2014]. *RN and Registered Practical Nurse practice: The client, the nurse and the environment [Practice Guideline].* Toronto: Author [p. 5]. Retrieved from http://www.cno.org/globalassets/docs/prac/41062.pdf.)

responsibility that they assume for their individual practice through licensure. What this means is that LPNs are obligated to ensure that they have the necessary knowledge and skills to perform safe care, as well as to determine when safe care of a patient is beyond their scope of practice and level of competence and requires consultation with other health care providers or RNs.

Inevitably, LPNs in various areas develop different competencies as their knowledge and skills develop, through experience and taking post-basic courses. Once they have acquired additional skills and knowledge, LPNs must be employed in areas where these expanded capabilities can be continuously practised and where LPNs are allowed to work to their full scope of practice. As individual competencies are enhanced and scopes of practice are expanded, nurses and employers must continuously seek clarification of their roles so that employers, for example, are fully aware of new competencies of LPNs, at the entry level and beyond. Employers must also develop clear policies to address the expanded practices of all nursing staff. Unfortunately, this does not always occur, resulting in a mismatch between the "scope of employment" and the "scope of practice" for which LPNs are prepared.

In response to the changing health care system, however, which includes employer demand, rising patient acuity levels, nursing shortages, and professional organizational efforts, progress has been made in the effort to allow LPNs to apply their full scope of practice. This trend shifts LPNs from a task orientation to a competency base and, in the process, improves patient care and professional job satisfaction.

Optimizing and clearly defining roles for both LPNs and RNs can also lead to more cost-effective nursing care.

Interprofessional and Intraprofessional Collaborative Practice

The LPN is a team member and thus should always work in a collaborative manner with other health care personnel. Interprofessional collaboration includes communicating with the patient, the family, and other health care workers to define, implement, and evaluate the plan of care. Good working relationships and intraprofessional collaboration between LPNs and RNs in the team are essential in the delivery of quality patient care. The LPN also makes suggestions and referrals to individual members of the health care team and in team meetings in which patient care and concerns are discussed. Full understanding of all roles and clear and appropriate communication are integral to effective collaboration within a team.

Leadership: Supervising and Delegating

The LPN is often in a position to supervise or to delegate, as well as to be the recipient of **supervision** and **delegation**. In order to supervise and delegate, the LPN must have sufficient knowledge, skill, attitude, and judgement. Both supervision and delegation, although different skills, serve to protect the public and the profession by ensuring that a task is performed safely and competently.

Supervision. Supervision is usually required by individuals who are new to a skill or role, such as students of a profession, new members of a profession, and professionals or nonprofessionals (such as family members or UCPs). The person who is supervising usually has experience in that knowledge and skill and may or may not be a member of the same profession or occupational group.

Supervision is an intervention and usually part of an ongoing and developing relationship. The purposes of supervision are to enhance competent functioning of an inexperienced person and to protect the public and the professional practice. Because supervision requires continual observation, monitoring, and evaluation, the supervisor must have a positive, collaborative relationship with the person being supervised. Both parties in the relationship must understand the roles that each must play. People receiving instruction should be supervised until they can safely perform the task alone. Supervision may occur in many forms, such as a one-on-one observation, an interview with the patient who has received care, or an analysis of the written report of a task. The supervisor provides evaluative information about the task performed as soon as is feasible.

If supervision of a skill occurs in a more isolated instance, the development of a relationship and the analysis of progress are more difficult.

Delegation. In delegation, authority to perform a restricted task or function is transferred to another person or group. The nurse must make this decision carefully. Professional standards are quite clear in this matter. Before delegating a task to another person, the nurse must ensure that the person to whom delegation is being made has the required knowledge, skill, and judgement to perform that function. The nurse must consider numerous other factors before a function is delegated to someone else:

- The associated risks and benefits for the patient
- The need for another person to perform the task
- The ability of the person to maintain competence in the procedure over time
- The ability to provide adequate supervision once the skill has been learned

The Commonwealth of Massachusetts (2016) has identified "five rights of delegation" for nurses, which are applicable to nurses working at all levels:

- The right task,
- The right circumstances,
- The right person,
- The right direction or communication, and
- The right supervision and evaluation.

In addition, the nurse must know institutional policies and procedures about delegation and whether the particular function may be legally delegated. This is particularly crucial because of increasing numbers of UCPs with varied skill sets and functions within the health care system. Responsibility does not stop once a task is delegated to another person. The delegating nurse retains ultimate responsibility for the correct completion of the task. The College of Nurses of Ontario (2013) developed a useful decision tree to help the nurse decide whether a function can be delegated to another person (Figure A-2).

Continuing Education and Expanded Competencies

The LPN is expected to continue professional growth and acquire a range of knowledge, skills, and judgement beyond that of the minimal entry-to-practice standards. Many educational opportunities are available to the nurse from postsecondary institutions, professional organizations, employers, and charitable agencies (e.g., Diabetes Canada). Increasingly, nurses are encouraged to attend educational events offered by other health care providers, such as respiratory therapists, pharmacists, physiotherapists, and gerontologists. This cross-professional education is also immensely valuable in encouraging greater understanding and collaboration among members of the health care team.

LEGISLATION, REGULATORY BODIES, AND PROFESSIONAL ASSOCIATIONS

Legislation, regulatory bodies, and professional associations govern the practice of nursing. These have been created to protect public safety and promote ethical practice.

Legislation

In most provinces and territories, nursing practice has similar legal regulatory requirements (education, registration, and complaints and disciplinary processes) and professional standards (scope and standards of practice, and competency issues). Laws that govern regulated health care professions serve to protect the best interests of the public by regulating health care practitioners and determining how, what, and where they practise.

Acts That Govern Specific Health Care Professions. In most provinces and territories, each profession has its own governing law, called an *act.* For example, medical doctors, registered nurses, practical nurses, chiropractors, and so forth are each governed by a professional act. These acts list specific tasks that these professionals are allowed to perform because they have the required skills, which may overlap with those of other professions.

Acts That Govern Multiple Health Care Professions. Some provinces have removed separate acts for individual health care professions and are replacing them with a single, generic act that applies to all health care professions. In Ontario, this act is called the *Regulated Health Professions Act,* and in British Columbia, it is called the *Health Professions Act.* This trend is occurring for several reasons:

- The public is demanding safe and accountable practice.
- New technology, which is increasingly complex and invasive, is potentially dangerous if improperly used. Professionals must, with

Nurse considers teaching/delegating* a procedure.

Am I competent to perform the procedure?

YES — **NO** Do not teach/delegate.

Am I competent to teach/delegate the procedure?

YES — **NO** Do not teach/delegate.

Consider:

- risks and benefits of performing procedure;
- predictability of outcomes;
- safeguards and resources available; and
- other factors in situation.

Can I safely teach/delegate the procedure, considering the factors?

YES — **NO** Do not teach/delegate.

Is care provider available with potential to perform procedure?

YES — **NO** Do not teach/delegate.

- Teach care provider.
- Determine competence.
- Identify conditions for performing and indicators for seeking assistance.

Is there a mechanism to determine ongoing competence?

YES — **NO** Do not teach/delegate.

Ensure that a monitoring mechanism is in place.

* Delegating refers to controlled act procedures.

FIGURE A-2 Decision tree for teaching or delegating performance of a procedure. (From College of Nurses of Ontario. [2013]. *Working with unregulated care providers* [p. 8]. Retrieved from http://www.cno.org/globalassets/docs/prac/41014_workingucp.pdf.)

great care, administer treatments such as radiation therapy, drugs for cancer, surgery, and injections.

- People requiring health care have increasingly complex physical, emotional, and social needs.
- As many professions expand their scope of practice and acquire new knowledge and skill sets, significant overlap in knowledge and skills occurs between various groups. These general health care acts attempt to apply a regulatory structure common to all groups.
- Health care professionals are more mobile today (i.e., they move between jurisdictions) and may have wide variations in knowledge and competence.
- The number and variety of health care professions have increased.

These generic health care acts list professions that are regulated by the law and activities that only members of certain professions are authorized to perform. All the laws governing the actions of health care providers, whether they are profession-specific acts or generic health care acts, include statements about the type of educational background necessary to enter a professional school and the type and length of education the professional schools must offer. The laws also require the profession to set up a governing body to monitor and regulate professional practice in the public interest.

Regulatory Bodies

According to the professional and health care acts, each profession must have a regulatory body that governs it. As the health care environment changes, regulatory bodies adapt by modifying practice standards and guidelines accordingly. Depending on the province or territory, this regulatory body may be called a *college,* a *council,* an *association,* or a *board.* Its primary mandate is to protect the public by controlling the activities of the professionals. In order to practise or use their professional title, all professionals must be members of their regulatory body.

Functions of the Regulatory Body. Each regulatory body uses many methods to protect the public, including the following:

- Ensure that professionals have the necessary credentials to practise in the specific province or territory
- Determine whether qualifying examinations are necessary
- Register the professional as a member of the profession once all criteria for membership have been met
- Keep a public register of the names, registration numbers, and business addresses of all members
- Define scope of practice and competency standards, according to professional standards and the existing laws
- Ensure that members renew or update registration and maintain competency criteria on a regular basis
- Receive and investigate complaints from the public or other professionals about member practices, and discipline members as necessary
- Publish disciplinary results regularly (i.e., name, registration number, offence, and disciplinary decision)
- Approve practical nursing programs in their jurisdiction

Some people have expressed concern that members' right to privacy is compromised by the publication of names, registration numbers, and business addresses of registered health care providers, as well as of disciplinary actions. Because of public safety, regulatory bodies and most provincial and territorial governments believe that publishing this information supersedes the provider's right to privacy.

Protecting or Reserving Titles. Usually, regulatory bodies are also responsible for ensuring that the members' professional title (e.g., LPN, medical doctor) is protected, or reserved. This means that only registered members are authorized to call themselves by the professional title. The protected title is usually related to the terms used in the jurisdiction, but protection is usually also extended to other, synonymous terms. For example, in Ontario, all of the following related terms and abbreviations are protected: *nurse, registered practical nurse, LPN, PN,* and their variants.

The colleges of LPNs are the regulatory bodies responsible for superintending the profession of licensed practical nursing in the public interest. As such, the college sets the requirements for the privilege of using the professional titles related to LPN. The professional title assures the public and other care providers that the individual has been evaluated and found capable of practising within the established standards.

Self-Regulation. Public good must be balanced with individuality, as must government laws with professional input. Professional self-regulation in nursing means that each nurse is expected to assume personal responsibility for maintaining competence and personal, physical, social, and emotional fitness to practise. Self-regulation also means that nurses establish standards of practice and an ethical framework for the nursing profession as a whole.

Self-regulation is a privilege that is entrusted to a regulating college in order to serve and protect the public interest.

The Registration Process for the Practical Nurse (Credentialling). In all territories and provinces of Canada, registration with the local regulatory body must proceed through a specific process. The regulatory body (also called a *registering body*) in each jurisdiction determines whether the applicant has sufficient educational background and competency for registration in the particular area. To be registered as practical nurses, applicants must prove that their education meets requirements for theoretical and clinical hours in specified topics and clinical areas. They also must provide evidence of competent practice by passing the Canadian licensing examination. The requirement for evidence of successful, current practice is satisfied if an applicant is a recent graduate of a program in the province where registration is sought. Applicants from out of province or territory, and out of country, or those who are returning to work must provide evidence of recent competent work (usually within the past 3 to 5 years) in the practical nursing field, as well as successful completion of the Canadian licensing examinations or their equivalent. If the certification examination, educational preparation, or evidence of competent practice are not accepted by the regulatory body, then applicants may need to write the Canadian licensing examination, or take theoretical or clinical courses in order to meet current Canadian standards. As already noted, in many jurisdictions, applicants must also pass a criminal record check before registering to practise.

Professional Associations

In Prince Edward Island and Ontario, the professional association is separate from the regulatory body (e.g., the College of Nurses of Ontario is the regulatory body and the Registered Practical Nurses Association of Ontario is the professional association). In all other provinces and territories, however, they are the same body. The purpose of most professional associations is to advocate for and promote the particular profession they serve. The objectives of the Registered Practical Nurses Association of Ontario (2013) include the following:

- Advocating for registered practical nurses in diverse settings, resulting in optimum patient health services through policy, legislation, and regulation
- Advocating for quality, respectful working environments for registered practical nurses
- Enhancing the professional competencies of registered practical nurses by ensuring the research, development, and delivery of quality educational programs
- Promoting the benefits of membership to registered practical nurses in order to ensure a strong and unified professional voice
- Promoting a closer working relationship with other health and related organizations

There are fundamental differences between a regulatory body and a professional association. Protection of the public is the distinct mandate of the regulatory body, whereas promoting professional development is the mandate of the professional association. Many nurse leaders and politicians believe that regulatory bodies and professional associations should not be combined because doing so may lead to public confusion and conflicts of interest. In the interests of both professional issues and public accountability, the professional association and regulatory body must remain in continuous, effective communication.

Practical nurses in provinces and territories that do not have a professional association separate from the regulatory body can access the Canadian Practical Nurses Association (CPNA) for professional advocacy and promotion issues. Unlike membership in the regulatory body, membership in the professional association is usually voluntary.

The Canadian Association of Practical Nurse Educators, an affinity group of the nationwide Association of Canadian Community Colleges, offers educational and networking opportunities and holds yearly conferences for educators throughout Canada.

Benefits of Membership in the Professional Association. Members of professional associations enjoy the following benefits:

- Emotional support from other professionals by sharing thoughts, feelings, and ideas
- Enhancement of a personal and collective knowledge base, thus contributing to individual and group growth
- Belonging to a strong force for change (groups often lobby for change more effectively than do individuals)
- Achievement of economic advantages (e.g., better insurance rates through a group plan)
- Opportunities to network

In summary, nursing is a complex profession that exists in a challenging environment under constant legal and professional changes. No nurse works alone; an LPN is always in an environment with the public and other health care providers. Each nurse must understand how legislation, regulatory bodies, and professional associations work together to inform safe and competent practice.

THE FUTURE OF PRACTICAL NURSING IN CANADA

The health care system in Canada is continually changing, and these changes have an effect on practical nursing. Both Abbot (1988) and Wilson (1992) believed that organisms and professions that do not respond to change lose their niche positions and either fade to unimportant entities controlled by others or die out completely. According to Wilson, "Homogeneity means vulnerability" (p. 301). In order to cope effectively, nurses must be proactive and view change as a challenge and an opportunity rather than a threat. By doing so, nursing will maintain or advance its niche position in health care.

General Health Care Trends

A number of current and projected changes have the potential to affect practical nursing. Various sources (Engel, Prentice, & Larsen, 2014; Public Health Agency of Canada [PHAC], 2015) have outlined the issues that will impact the delivery of health care services in Canada, some of which include the following:

- Enhanced use of technology for health records, robotics in treatment, and teaching
- Increased public demands for access and transparency in information and health care provision
- Sustainability of the current public funding model for health care
- Strong public interest in having a voice in health services
- Growing population of older persons
- Increased acuity of patients in institutional care
- Emergence of new infectious diseases (e.g., Zika virus)
- Continued gaps in access to services and in quality in rural, remote, and Indigenous communities
- Health of Indigenous people
- Increased prevalence of chronic disorders and multiple comorbidities

These trends within the Canadian health care system and in the health of Canadians drive discussions around appropriate staffing mixes, alternative delivery models, and alternative funding models. For example, as costs increase in health care, there is strong interest in leveraging wider partnerships among public, nonprofit, and business sources (PHAC, 2015). With over half of the Canadian population over 20 years of age experiencing at least two or more chronic disorders, there is impetus toward having a better understanding of chronic disease, as well as a shift toward considering how health education and promotion can be helpful in preventing chronic disorders and promoting good quality of life. Prevention efforts are also focussed on reducing the frequency of falls among older persons at home and of nonintentional injuries, which can have devastating and long-term effects for those who experience these events. Concern with access to services and care has led to a heightened focus on community, rehabilitation, and home-based services, the need for a national pharmaceutical strategy, and an emphasis on exploration of innovations that may lead to increased access to quality services in rural and remote regions of Canada, as well as among Indigenous people (PHAC, 2015). As Villeneuve and MacDonald (2006) predicted, interprofessional care has assumed significance in the current health care environment, where complex patient needs and evolving technology and care strategies require the expertise of professionals working together and with patients to leverage the expertise that each can bring to health care. Although there is emphasis on the value of interprofessional teams, there continues to be concern about optimal staffing and skill mixes needed to achieve health outcomes, even within intraprofessional teams such as nursing, which raises the need for a national human resources plan for health care.

General concerns about the prevalence of mental health issues in Canada have also highlighted the need to address the mental health of the health care workforce, whose members face the challenges of violence from patients and other health care providers. They also are needing to adjust to ongoing changes brought about by technology, complex health needs, and continual emergence of new research and innovations.

Implications for Practical Nursing

Continuous rapid change requires professionals to respond appropriately in order to cope effectively. Practical nurses need to be lifelong learners and develop increasingly broad-based competencies to adapt to changing occupational demands. This is not the time to focus solely on one narrow skill set or to cling stubbornly only to the knowledge base acquired in undergraduate school.

Modern technological treatment is increasingly expensive and time intensive. Practical nurses have the knowledge, abilities, attitudes, and skills to contribute significantly to newly evolving primary health care models. Practical nurses of the future will likely need to have increased knowledge of epidemiology and play a greater role in illness prevention, health promotion, and health teaching for patients throughout the lifespan. For instance, nurses will likely be required to provide information to reduce infectious and chronic lifestyle-related diseases such as cancer, diabetes, obesity, and heart–lung disorders. Health teaching for individuals and groups will involve teaching about healthy lifestyles, collaboration with the patient and others, and empowerment of patients to make their own health care decisions.

Because health care problems are often too complex to be addressed by any one person, practical nurses will need to focus more on working collaboratively in teams and networks of health care providers. The trend toward interprofessional health care models will require nurses to be increasingly aware of current scopes of practice among all workers. Care maps and critical pathways may be emphasized over narrow frameworks unique to one profession and facilitate collaboration, as well as reduce chances of error.

Nurses may need to be more aware of conflicts of interest if health care moves into corporate models. If professional values clash with corporate values, professional colleagues and the professional association will become increasingly important sources of information and support.

Computer use has become the norm rather than the exception in most health care institutions. Practical nurses will need computer literacy to use technology in direct patient care and to pursue their education.

Nurses work with an increasingly diverse and multicultural population base. Practical nurses of the future will thus have to develop more knowledge and skill in applying concepts from the humanities and social sciences such as psychology, sociology, and anthropology.

Possible Evolution of the Practical Nurse Role

Changes in Educational Standards for Entry to Practice. In view of the likely expanding roles for the practical nurse, a high school diploma will continue to be the minimum requirement for entry into a practical nursing program. Some knowledge of or fluency in a second language would be useful in our increasingly multicultural society.

Practical nurse education programs need to be at least 2 academic years in length and must occur in a postsecondary institution that meets general program standards for preparing professionals to meet entry-to-practice requirements. These programs must be academically sound and include components of pure science, social science, and humanities, as well as interprofessional education. Beyond the basic program, there will need to be more opportunities for LPNs to gain partial or full transfer credit into baccalaureate nursing programs. Additionally, many other opportunities will need to exist for nurses to gain expertise in specific health care areas while retaining a practical nursing identity. Should a university degree in practical nursing be available? Some places in the United States offer degrees in practical nursing, but this would need to be explored further to understand its benefits and challenges in Canada. These challenges include the potential blurring of roles between LPNs and RNs and questions about how a baccalaureate would change employment opportunities for LPNs.

Scope of Practice and New Competencies. The practical nursing profession faces an exciting future. The practical nursing scope of practice will continue to evolve in response to changes in the Canadian health care system. Villeneuve and MacDonald (2006) proposed that the structure of the health care system and the delivery of nursing by regulated nursing professions will be very different in the future. They predicted that, by 2020, registered nurses would undertake more of the primary care that is currently provided by general practitioners. If this becomes reality, how will it affect the role of practical nurses? They also predicted that, by 2020, the proportion of practical nurses would increase and that most nurses would work in community settings and in interprofessional teams. Practical nurses would also likely play a greater role in preoperative and perioperative settings and assume primary responsibility for rehabilitation and long-term care; this trend is already occurring. Villeneuve and MacDonald (2006) envisioned acute care in 2020 as a combination of all categories of nurses. Despite changes in roles, collaborative practice between RNs and practical nurses is viewed as important in health care delivery.

Practical nurses of the future will continue to acquire separate postgraduate competencies in specific areas through postbasic education and on-the-job training and experience, making them well positioned to work with patients with diverse needs and illness and diverse cultural experiences. This will mean ongoing dialogue with RNs to plan for future roles and scopes of practice that serve all stakeholders in the Canadian health care system.

If professionals in acute care increase their use of the critical pathway (care map) system, practical nurses will likely have expanded roles in areas such as Critical Care Units. They would be able to work with more unstable patients because the critical pathway system allows for more interdependence and collaboration, technological and personnel help, and distinct instructions for care and consultation. The RN would continue with the role of case manager.

What Is the Final Answer?

What will happen to practical nursing in the future? No one knows for certain, but ecological and sociological studies of professions indicate that individuals and groups—both animal and human—grow, develop, change, flourish, fade out, and disappear. According to Wilson (1992), "Environment is the theatre and evolution is the play" (p. 80).

Practical nurses and registered nurses may always maintain separate scopes of practice for survival reasons. Practical nursing will position its significance for health care of the future by developing more diverse and specialized competencies in our changing society. It must develop competencies that address the needs of the environment. It must change to meet health care demands. Health care, more specifically, nursing, is the theatre, and constant change is the play. If practical nurses wish to maintain their particular niche in the health care system, it is essential that they respond effectively in this environment of continued rapid change.

KEY CONCEPTS

- Nursing is the largest single group of health care providers in Canada.
- After the Second World War, nursing registration laws were amended to create two levels of nursing practice.
- Practical nursing was recognized in the 1970s as a distinct profession that necessitates formal education.
- Education programs for practical nurses have become longer and more complex and have moved from hospital settings to postsecondary institutions.
- Ecology theory describes the need for a group to compete for niches and evolve to cope effectively with environmental changes.
- In most Canadian jurisdictions, practical nursing programs are diploma programs that run for 2 academic years and are offered at postsecondary institutions.
- The main difference between registered nurses and practical nurses is the depth and breadth of their knowledge base.
- Licensed practical nurses have a strong foundation in clinical practice, decision making, and critical thinking.
- Practical nurses work in a range of settings, including direct care, administration, and education.
- As a regulated profession, practical nursing is responsible for establishing its own standards of practice.
- Practical nurses are expected to continue professional growth and acquire a range of knowledge, skill, and judgement beyond that of minimal entry-to-practice standards.
- Delivery of cost-effective nursing care involves optimizing the scope of practice and clearly defining roles for both categories of nurses.
- Self-regulation is a privilege that is entrusted to a regulating body in order to serve and protect the public interest.
- Continuous change in the health care system requires the practical nursing profession to adapt in regard to entry to practice and scope of practice.

CRITICAL THINKING EXERCISES

1. The delivery of health care will be different in the future. If registered nurses begin to play a larger role in primary health care, how will that affect the future roles of practical nurses and personal support workers? How would you design the human resources structure of the Canadian health care system of the future?
2. Noreen, the manager of a surgical unit, is reviewing her tight budget and staffing complement. One-quarter of her staff consists of practical nurses and the remainder consists of RNs. The responsibilities of the practical nurses have not changed on her unit for the last 10 years. Based on what you know about scope of practice and delegation, what suggestions would you have for Noreen? What resources would you suggest that she access?
3. A newly graduated practical nurse is caring for a patient after a total knee replacement. Eight hours after the patient's return to the unit, he begins to complain of shortness of breath and chest pain on

inhalation. The nurse identifies that oxygen saturation levels are falling and air entry is decreased to the patient's left lower lobe. The nurse has never encountered this type of situation before. Describe how the practical nurse and RN can partake in consultation and collaboration in this situation.

REVIEW QUESTIONS

1. A practical nurse identifies as an LPN. In order to use the title of LPN, the nurse must have done which of the following?
   1. Completed an accredited practical nursing program
   2. Become registered with a regulatory body
   3. Passed the NCLEX national licensing examination
   4. Procured employment as a practical nurse
2. Which of the following applies to the scope of practice for LPNs?
   1. Only those with medical backgrounds have a scope of practice.
   2. A scope of practice is not required for practical nurses unless they are working in acute care settings.
   3. A scope of practice cannot be altered once it has been established through legislation.
   4. A scope of practice will vary among jurisdictions across Canada.
3. The movement toward wider competencies, registration, scopes of practice, and laddering by LPNs in Canada is consistent with which aspect of ecological theory?
   1. Successful groups establish niches that are not shared with other groups.
   2. Surviving groups are successful in coping with the influences and changes in their environment.
   3. Professional groups must establish a unique knowledge and skill base.
   4. Survival is based on the development of many subgroups that subsume responsibilities of other professions.
4. Which of the following depicts the concept of laddering in the continued knowledge and skill development of LPNs?
   1. An LPN takes an intravenous (IV) course because IV initiation is required in the clinical setting.
   2. An LPN receives prior learning recognition toward an RN program.
   3. An LPN takes a business course to become team leader.
   4. An LPN obtains certification as a wound care specialist.
5. In Canada, practical nursing was established in which decade as a distinct profession that required a formal education?
   1. 1930s
   2. 1970s
   3. 1980s
   4. 1990s
6. Which of the following individuals is not licensed under law to practise as a nurse in Canada?
   1. A health care provider who has taken a short training program to provide personal care to older persons in a nursing home.
   2. A graduate of a nursing program who has completed studies but not applied to the regulatory college to practise.
   3. A graduate of a nursing program who has successfully written licensing exams and whose application for licensing has been granted.
   4. A graduate of a nurse practitioner program who has satisfied all requirements for licensing as a registered nurse in another category.
   5. A nurse who has moved to Canada from another country.
7. A high-school student wonders about employment opportunities as an LPN. Which of the following would provide an accurate profile of what the student could expect as an LPN?
   1. Opportunities for LPN practice are very limited in Canada due to rising acuity levels in patients.
   2. The student could expect to work exclusively with older persons as an LPN.
   3. Employers are reluctant to hire LPNs who do not have degree preparation.
   4. Full-time employment for new graduates may be limited.
8. In most Canadian jurisdictions, entry-level LPNs (registered practical nurses) graduate from which of the following?
   1. Certificate programs
   2. Two-year college diploma programs
   3. Baccalaureate degree programs
   4. Hospital-based programs
9. The activities that practical nurses are authorized to perform are outlined in which of the following?
   1. Entry-to-practice competencies
   2. Scope of practice
   3. Terminal outcomes
   4. National law
10. Which of the following situations would be guided by codes of ethics for practical nurses? *(Select all that apply.)*
    1. An LPN needs information on how to add specific medications to an IV line.
    2. An informal caregiver and friend of an older person is curious and asks for details about the person's past history and current treatment plan.
    3. An employer refuses to allow LPNs to work to their full scope of practice.
    4. A practical nurse is unsure of how to delegate tasks to UCPs.
    5. An LPN asks to retake an IV course because the LPN recognizes that his or her IV skills have lapsed.

Answers: 1. 2; **2.** 4; **3.** 2; **4.** 2; **5.** 3; **6.** 1; **7.** 4; **8.** 2; **9.** 2; **10.** 2, 5

Rationales for the Review Questions appear at the end of the book.

REFERENCES

Abbott, A. D. (1988). *The system of professions: An essay on the division of expert labor.* Chicago, IL: University of Chicago Press.

Assessment Strategies Inc. (2017). *Canadian Practical Nurse Examination: Computer based testing.* Retrieved from http://cpnre.ca/abouttheexam_computer-based_testing_e.asp.

Canadian Council for Practical Nurse Regulators (CCPNC). (2013). *Entry-to-practice competencies for licensed practical nurses.* Retrieved from https://www.clpnbc.org/Documents/Practice-Support-Documents/Entry-to-Practice-Competencies-(EPTC)-LPNs.aspx.

Canadian Institute for Health Information (CIHI). (2010). *Regulated nurses: Canadian trends, 2005 to 2009.* Retrieved from https://secure.cihi.ca/free_products/nursing_report_2005-2009_en.pdf.

Canadian Institute for Health Information (CIHI). (2012). *Regulated nurses: Canadian trends 2007–2011.* Retrieved from https://secure.cihi.ca/free_products/Regulated_Nurses_EN.pdf.

Canadian Institute for Health Information (CIHI). (2015a). *Regulated nurses, 2014.* Retrieved from https://secure.cihi.ca/free_products/RegulatedNurses2014_Report_EN.pdf.

Canadian Institute for Health Information (CIHI). (2015b). *Supply of nurses declines for the first time in 2 decades.* Retrieved from https://www.cihi.ca/en/nurses_2014_pubsum_en.pdf.

Canadian Institute for Health Information (CIHI). (2016a). *Regulated nurses, 2015: Canada and jurisdictional highlights.* Ottawa: Author. Retrieved from https://www.cihi.ca/en/pt_highlights_final_en.pdf.

Canadian Institute for Health Information (CIHI). (2016b). *Regulated nurses, 2015: Report.* Retrieved from https://secure.cihi.ca/free_products/Nursing_Report_2015_en.pdf.

Canadian Institute for Health Information (CIHI). (2016c). *Regulated nurses, 2015: LPN data tables: Table 15.* Retrieved from https://www.cihi.ca/en/lpn_2015_data_tables_en_xlsx.

Canadian Institute for Health Information (CIHI). (2016d). *Regulated nurses, 2015: LPN data tables: Table 1.* Retrieved from https://www.cihi.ca/en/lpn_2015_data_tables_en_xlsx.

Canadian Institute for Health Information (CIHI). (2016e). *Regulated nurses, 2015: LPN data tables: Table 19.* Retrieved from https://www.cihi.ca/en/lpn_2015_data_tables_en_xlsx.

College of Licensed Practical Nurses of British Columbia (CLPNBC). (n.d.). *About CLPNBC: Frequently asked questions: Jurisprudence.* Retrieved from https://www.clpnbc.org/FAQs#JPexpand.

College of Licensed Practical Nurses of British Columbia (CLPNBC). (2011). *History of LPNs in BC and Canada.* Retrieved from https://www.clpnbc.org/What-is-an-LPN/History-of-LPNs-in-B-C-and-Canada.

College of Nurses of Ontario (CNO). (2013). *Working with unregulated care providers.* Retrieved from https://www.cno.org/globalassets/docs/prac/41014_workingucp.pdf.

College of Nurses of Ontario (CNO). (2014). *RN and RPN practice: The client, the nurse, and the environment.* Retrieved from http://www.cno.org/globalassets/docs/prac/41062.pdf.

College of Nurses of Ontario (CNO). (2018a). *Legislation and regulation. RHPA: scope of practice, controlled acts model.* Retrieved from http://www.cno.org/globalassets/docs/policy/41052_rhpascope.pdf.

College of Nurses of Ontario (CNO). (2018b). *Jurisprudence examination.* Retrieved from http://www.cno.org/en/become-a-nurse/entry-to-practice-examinations/jurisprudence-examination/.

Commonwealth of Massachusetts. (2016). *Five rights of delegation.* Retrieved from http://www.mass.gov/eohhs/gov/departments/dph/programs/hcq/dhpl/nursing/nursing-practice/advisory-rulings/unlicensed-assistive-personnel/five-rights-of-delegation.html.

Engel, J., Prentice, D., & Larsen, P. (2014). Introduction to chronicity in Canada. In M. Kramer-Kile, J. Osuiji, P. Larsen, et al. (Eds.), *Chronic illness in Canada: Impact and intervention* (pp. 3–28). Burlington, MA: Jones & Bartlett Learning.

Government of Ontario [Immigration]. (2016). *Working in Ontario: Nursing.* Retrieved from http://www.ontarioimmigration.ca/en/working/OI_HOW_WORK_NURSE_CM.html.

Knecht, P. (2017). *Success in practical/vocational nursing, from student to leader.* St. Louis, MO: Elsevier.

Licensed Practical Nurses Association of Prince Edward Island. (2011). *Exemplary care: Registered nurses and licensed practical nurses working together.* Retrieved from https://www.arnpei.ca/data/RNsandLPNsWorkingTogether.pdf.

Nowrouzi, B., Giddens, E., Gohar, B., et al. (2016). The quality of work life of registered nurses in Canada and the United States: A comprehensive literature review. *International Journal of Occupational and Environmental Health, 22*(4), 341–358. doi: 10.1080/10773525.2016.1241920.

NursingNet.UK. (n.d.). *Training: A brief history.* Retrieved from http://nursingnetuk.com/about/?_ts=2725.

Public Health Agency of Canada. (2015). *Centre for Chronic Disease Prevention: Strategic plan 2016–2019: Improving health outcomes—a paradigm shift.* Retrieved from http://www.phac-aspc.gc.ca/cd-mc/assets/pdf/ccdp-strategic-plan-2016-2019-plan-strategique-cpmc-eng.pdf.

Registered Practical Nurses Association of Ontario. (2013). *Mission and objectives.* Retrieved from https://www.rpnao.org/content/mission-vision.

Van House, N. A., & Sutton, S. A. (2000). The panda syndrome: An ecology of LIS education [Electronic version]. *Journal of Education for Library and Information Science, 41*(1), 52–68. doi:10.2307/40324088.

Villeneuve, M., & MacDonald, J. (2006). *Toward 2020: Visions for nursing.* Ottawa, ON: Canadian Nurses Association.

Wilson, E. O. (1992). *The diversity of life.* Cambridge, MA: Harvard University Press.

B APPENDIX

Laboratory Values

Adapted by Jana Lok

The tables in this appendix list some of the most common tests, their normal values, and possible etiologies of abnormal values. Laboratory values are expressed in the Système International d'Unités (SI) units, which are used in Canada. Conventional units, used in the United States, are presented after the SI units in parentheses. Laboratory values may vary with different techniques and in different laboratories. Possible etiologies are presented in alphabetical order. SI abbreviations and other symbols appearing in the tables are defined as follows:

<	=	less than
>	=	greater than
≥	=	greater than or equal to
≤	=	less than or equal to
AU	=	arbitrary unit
cm H_2O	=	centimetres of water
dL	=	decilitre
EU	=	Ehrlich unit
fL	=	femtolitre
g	=	gram
IU	=	international unit
kPa	=	kilopascal
kU	=	kilounit
L	=	litre
mcg	=	microgram (one millionth [10^{-6}] of a gram)
mcIU	=	micro–international unit (one millionth [10^{-6}] of an international unit)
mcL	=	microlitre
mcmol	=	micromole
mEq	=	milliequivalent
mg	=	milligram (one thousandth [10^{-3}] of a gram)
microkat	=	microkatal
microU	=	microunit
mL	=	millilitre
mm	=	millimetre
mm Hg	=	millimetre of mercury
mmol	=	millimole
mOsm	=	milliosmole
mU	=	milliunit (one hundredth [10^{-2}] of a unit)
nmol	=	nanomole (one billionth [10^{-9}] of a mole)
ng	=	nanogram (one billionth [10^{-9}] of a gram)
pg	=	picogram (one trillionth [10^{-12}] of a gram)
pmol	=	picomole (one trillionth [10^{-12}] of a mole)
U	=	unit

TABLE B-1 Serum, Plasma, and Whole Blood Chemistries

Test	Normal Values: SI Units (Conventional Units)	POSSIBLE ETIOLOGY: Higher Values	POSSIBLE ETIOLOGY: Lower Values
Acetone		Diabetic ketoacidosis, high-fat diet, low-carbohydrate diet, starvation	—
• Quantitative	<200 mcmol/L (<1.16 mg/dL)		
• Qualitative	Negative (negative)		
Alanine aminotransferase (ALT; formerly known as serum glutamate pyruvate transferase [SGPT])	4–36 U/L (same as in SI units)	Liver disease, shock	—
Albumin	35–50 g/L (3.5–5 g/dL)	Dehydration	Burns, chronic liver disease, malabsorption, malnutrition, nephrotic syndrome, pregnancy, inflammatory disease
Aldolase	<8.0 mU/L (3–8.2 Sibley-Lehninger U/dL)	Infection, muscle trauma, skeletal muscle disease, hepatocellular disease, MI	Late muscular dystrophy, renal disease, hereditary fructose intolerance
α_1-Antitrypsin	0.85–2.13 g/L (85–213 mg/dL)	Acute and chronic inflammation and infection, arthritis, malignancy, stress, syndrome, thyroid infections	Chronic lung disease (early onset of emphysema), malnutrition, nephrotic syndrome, end-stage cancer

TABLE B-1 Serum, Plasma, and Whole Blood Chemistries—cont'd

Test	Normal Values: SI Units (Conventional Units)	POSSIBLE ETIOLOGY Higher Values	Lower Values
Alpha-fetoprotein	0–40 mcg/L (<40 ng/mL)	Cancers of testes, lymphoma, stomach, colon, breasts and ovaries, carcinoma of liver, neural tube defects or multiple pregnancies in pregnant women, fetal distress or congenital abnormalities, fetal death	In pregnant women, fetal trisomy 21 or fetal wastage
Ammonia	6–47 mcmol/L (10–80 mcg/dL)	GI bleeding, hepatic encephalopathy, portal hypertension, severe liver disease, Reye syndrome, severe heart failure or congestive hepatomegaly	Hyperornithinemia, essential or malignant hypertension
Amylase	100–300 U/L (60–120 Somogyi units/dL)	Acute and chronic pancreatitis, mumps (salivary gland disease), perforated ulcers	Acute alcoholism, cirrhosis of liver, extensive destruction of pancreas
Ascorbic acid	23–85 mcmol/L (0.4–1.5 mg/dL)	Excessive ingestion of vitamin C	Connective tissue disorders, hepatic disease, renal disease, rheumatic fever, vitamin C deficiency
Aspartate aminotransferase (AST) (formerly known as serum glutamic oxaloacetic transferase [SGOT])	0–35 U/L (same as SI units)	Acute hepatitis, liver disease, MI, pulmonary infarction, skeletal muscle disease	Chronic renal dialysis, acute renal disease, pregnancy, diabetic ketoacidosis
B-type (brain-type) natriuretic peptide	<100 mcg/L (<100 ng/mL)	Heart failure, MI, hypertension, cor pulmonale	—
Bicarbonate	21–28 mmol/L (21–28 mEq/L)	Chronic use of loop diuretics, compensated respiratory acidosis, metabolic alkalosis	Acute renal failure, compensated respiratory alkalosis, diarrhea, metabolic acidosis
Bilirubin • Total • Indirect • Direct	 5.1–17 mcmol/L (0.3–1.0 mg/dL) 3.4–12 mcmol/L (0.2–0.8 mg/dL) 1.7–5.1 mcmol/L (0.1–0.3 mg/dL)	Biliary obstruction, hemolytic anemia, impaired liver function, pernicious anemia, prolonged fasting, Dubin-Johnson syndrome, sickle cell anemia, sepsis, hepatitis	—
Blood gases*			
• Arterial pH	7.35–7.45 (same as SI units)	Alkalosis	Acidosis
• Venous pH	7.31–7.41 (same as SI units)	Alkalosis	Acidosis
• Partial pressure of carbon dioxide in arterial blood ($PaCO_2$)	35–45 mm Hg (same as SI units)	Compensated metabolic alkalosis, respiratory acidosis	Compensated metabolic acidosis, respiratory alkalosis
• Partial pressure of oxygen in arterial blood (PaO_2)	80–100 mm Hg (same as SI units)	Administration of high concentration of oxygen	Chronic lung disease, decreased cardiac output
• Partial pressure of oxygen in venous blood (PvO_2)	40–50 mm Hg (same as SI units)		
Calcium	2.25–2.75 mmol/L (9–10.5 mg/dL)	Acute osteoporosis, hyperparathyroidism, multiple myeloma, vitamin D intoxication	Acute pancreatitis, hypoparathyroidism, liver disease, malabsorption syndrome, renal failure, vitamin D deficiency
Calcium, ionized	1.05–1.30 mmol/L (4.5–5.6 mg/dL)	—	—
Carbon dioxide (CO_2 content)	21–28 mmol/L (21–28 mEq/L)	Severe vomiting, COPD, metabolic alkalosis	Chronic use of loop diuretics, renal failure, DKA, starvation, metabolic acidosis, shock
Beta-carotene	1.4–4.7 mcmol/L (75–253 mcg/dL)	Cystic fibrosis, hypothyroidism, pancreatic insufficiency	Dietary deficiency, malabsorption disorders
Chloride	98–106 mmol/L (98–106 mEq/L)	Corticosteroid therapy, dehydration, excessive infusion of normal saline, metabolic acidosis, respiratory alkalosis, uremia	Addison's disease, heart failure, diarrhea, metabolic alkalosis, overhydration, respiratory acidosis, SIADH, vomiting

Continued

TABLE B-1 Serum, Plasma, and Whole Blood Chemistries—cont'd

Test	Normal Values: SI Units (Conventional Units)	POSSIBLE ETIOLOGY Higher Values	Lower Values
Cholesterol	<5 mmol/L (<200 mg/dL) age dependent	Biliary obstruction, cirrhosis, hypothyroidism, hyperlipidemia, idiopathic hypercholesterolemia, renal disease, uncontrolled diabetes	Corticosteroid therapy, extensive liver disease, hyperthyroidism, malnutrition
• High-density lipoproteins (HDL)	>1.55 mmol/L (>60 mg/dL)		
• Low-density lipoproteins (LDL)	<2.59 mmol/L (<100 mg/dL)		
Cholinesterase (RBC)	5–10 U/L (same as SI units)	Exercise, sickle cell disease	Acute infections, insecticide intoxication, liver disease, muscular dystrophy
Copper	11–22 mcmol/L (70–140 mcg/dL)	Cirrhosis, contraceptive use by female patient	Wilson's disease
Cortisol		Adrenal adenoma, Cushing's syndrome, hyperthyroidism, pancreatitis, stress	Addison's disease, adrenal insufficiency, hypopituitary states, hypothyroidism, liver disease
• 0800 Hours	138–635 nmol/L (5–23 mcg/dL)		
• 1600 Hours	<83–359 nmol/L (3–13 mcg/dL)		
Creatine	15.3–76.3 mcmol/L (0.2–1.0 mg/dL)	Active rheumatoid arthritis, biliary obstruction, hyperthyroidism, renal disease, severe muscle disease	Diabetes mellitus
Creatine kinase (CK)		Brain damage, exercise, musculoskeletal injury or disease, MI, numerous intramuscular injections, severe myocarditis	—
• Male	55–170 U/L (same as SI units)		
• Female	30–135 U/L (same as SI units)		
Creatine kinase isozyme of heart (CK-MB [CK-2])		Acute MI	—
• Male	2–6 mcg/L (2–6 ng/mL)		
• Female	2–5 mcg/L (2–5 ng/mL)		
Creatine kinase mass fraction	<5% fraction of total CK	—	—
Creatinine		Severe renal disease	Diseases with decreased muscle mass (e.g. muscular dystrophy, myasthenia gravis)
• Male	53–106 mcmol/L (0.6–1.2 mg/dL)		
• Female	44–97 mcmol/L (0.5–1.1 mg/dL)		
Ferritin (serum)		Anemia of chronic disease (infection, inflammation, liver disease), sideroblastic anemia	Iron-deficiency anemia, severe protein deficiency
• Male	26–674 pmol/L (12–300 ng/mL)		
• Female	22–337 pmol/L (10–150 ng/mL)		
Folic acid (folate)	11–57 mmol/L (5–25 ng/mL)	Hypothyroidism, pernicious anemia	Alcoholism, hemolytic anemia, inadequate diet, malabsorption syndrome, malnutrition, megaloblastic anemia
Gamma-glutamyltranspeptidase (GGT)		Cholestasis, cytomegalovirus infection, Epstein-Barr, liver disease, MI, pancreatitis	—
• Male	8–38 U/L (same as SI units)		
• Female	5–27 U/L (same as SI units)		
Glucose, fasting	4–6 mmol/L (70–110 mg/dL)	Acute stress, cerebral lesions, Cushing's syndrome, diabetes mellitus, hyperthyroidism, pancreatic insufficiency	Addison's disease, hepatic disease, hypothyroidism, insulin overdosage, pancreatic tumour, pituitary hypofunction, postdumping syndrome
Glucose, 2-hr oral glucose tolerance testing (OGTT)		Diabetes mellitus	Hyperinsulinism
• Fasting	4–6 mmol/L (70–110 mg/dL)		
• 1 hr	<11.1 mmol/L (<200 mg/dL)		
• 2 hr	<7.8 mmol/L (<140 mg/dL)		
Haptoglobin	0.5–2.2 g/L (50–220 mg/dL)	Acute MI, infectious and inflammatory processes, malignant neoplasms	Chronic liver disease, hemolytic anemia, mononucleosis, systemic lupus erythematosus, toxoplasmosis, transfusion reactions

TABLE B-1 Serum, Plasma, and Whole Blood Chemistries—cont'd

Test	Normal Values: SI Units (Conventional Units)	POSSIBLE ETIOLOGY Higher Values	POSSIBLE ETIOLOGY Lower Values
Homocysteine		Cardiovascular disease, cerebrovascular disease, peripheral vascular disease, cystinuria, vitamin B_6 or B_{12} deficiency, folate deficiency, malnutrition	—
• 0–30 years	4.6–8.1 mcmol/L (same as SI units)		
• 30–59 years			
• Male	6.13–11.2 mcmol/L (same as SI units)		
• Female	4.5–7.9 mcmol/L (same as SI units)		
• >59 years	5.8–11.9 mcmol/L (same as SI units)		
Insulin	43–186 pmol/L (6–26 microU/mL)	Acromegaly, adenoma of islet cells, obesity, untreated mild case of type 2 diabetes mellitus	Diabetes mellitus, obesity
Iron		Excessive RBC destruction, hemochromatosis, massive transfusion	Anemia of chronic disease, iron-deficiency anemia
• Male	14–32 mcmol/L (80–180 mcg/dL)		
• Female	11–29 mcmol/L (60–160 mcg/dL)		
Total iron-binding capacity (TIBC)	45–82 mcmol/L (250–460 mcg/dL)	Iron-deficiency state, oral contraceptive use, polycythemia	Cancer, chronic infections, pernicious anemia, uremia
Lactic acid (venous blood)	0.6–2.2 mmol/L (5–20 mg/dL)	Acidosis, heart failure, severe liver disease, shock, tissue ischemia	—
Lactic dehydrogenase (LDH)	100–190 U/L (same as SI units)	Heart failure, hemolytic disorders, hepatitis, metastatic cancer of liver, MI, pernicious anemia, pulmonary embolus and infarction, skeletal muscle damage	—
Lactic dehydrogenase isoenzymes			
• LDH_1	0.17–0.27 (17%–27%)	MI, pernicious anemia, strenuous exercise	—
• LDH_2	0.27–0.37 (27%–37%)	Exercise, pulmonary embolus, sickle cell crisis	—
• LDH_3	0.18–0.25 (18%–25%)	Malignant lymphoma, pulmonary embolus	—
• LDH_4	0.03–0.08 (3%–8%)	Systemic lupus erythematosus, pancreatitis, pulmonary infarction, renal disease	—
• LDH_5	0.0–0.05 (0%–5%)	Heart failure, hepatitis, pulmonary embolus and infarction, skeletal muscle damage, strenuous exercise	—
Lipase	0–160 U/L (same as SI units)	Acute and chronic pancreatitis, hepatic disorders, pancreatic disorder (cancer, pseudocyst), perforated peptic ulcer, salivary gland inflammation or tumour	—
Magnesium	0.74–1.07 mmol/L (1.8–2.6 mEq/L)	Addison's disease, hypothyroidism, renal failure	Chronic alcoholism, hyperparathyroidism, hyperthyroidism, hypoparathyroidism, malnutrition, severe malabsorption
Myoglobin	1.0–5.3 nmol/L (<90 ng/mL)	MI, myositis, malignant hyperthermia, muscular dystrophy, skeletal muscle ischemia or trauma, rhabdomyolysis, seizures	Polymyositis
Osmolality	280–300 mmol/kg (280–300 mOsm/kg)	Chronic renal disease, dehydration, diabetes mellitus, hypernatremia, shock	Addison's disease, diuretic therapy, hyponatremia, overhydration
Oxygen saturation		Increased inspired oxygen, polycythemia vera	Anemia, cardiac decompensation, decreased inspired oxygen, respiratory disorders
• Arterial	95%–100% (same as SI units)		
• Venous	60%–80% (same as SI units)		

Continued

TABLE B-1 **Serum, Plasma, and Whole Blood Chemistries—cont'd**

Test	Normal Values: SI Units (Conventional Units)	POSSIBLE ETIOLOGY Higher Values	POSSIBLE ETIOLOGY Lower Values
pH	*See* Blood gases		
Phenylalanine	0–121 mcmol/L (0–2 mg/dL)	Phenylketonuria	—
Phosphatase, acid	2.2–10.5 U/L (0.13–0.63 U/L)	Advanced Paget's disease, cancer of prostate, hyperparathyroidism	—
Phosphatase, alkaline (ALP)	35–120 U/L (0.5–2.0 mckat/L)	Bone diseases, cirrhosis, malignancy of liver/ bone, marked hyperparathyroidism, obstruction of biliary system, rickets	Excessive vitamin D ingestion, hypothyroidism, milk-alkali syndrome
Phosphorus, phosphate	0.97–1.45 mmol/L (3.0–4.5 mg/dL)†	Bone metastasis, healing fractures, hypoparathyroidism, hypocalcemia, renal disease, vitamin D intoxication	Chronic alcoholism, diabetes mellitus, hypercalcemia, hyperparathyroidism, vitamin D deficiency
Potassium	3.5–5.0 mmol/L (3.5–5.0 mEq/L)	Acute or chronic renal failure, Addison's disease, dehydration, diabetic ketosis, excessive dietary or IV intake, massive tissue destruction, metabolic acidosis	Burns, Cushing's syndrome, deficient dietary or IV intake, diarrhea (severe), diuretic therapy, GI fistula, insulin administration, pyloric obstruction, starvation, vomiting
Prostate-specific antigen (PSA)	<4 mcg/L (<4 ng/mL)	Benign prostatic hypertrophy, prostate cancer, prostatitis	—
Proteins		Burns, cirrhosis (globulin fraction), dehydration	Congenital agammaglobulinemia, increased capillary permeability, inflammatory disease, liver disease, malabsorption, malnutrition
• Total	64–83 g/L (6.4–8.3 g/dL)		
• Albumin	35–50 g/L (3.5–5 g/dL)		
• Globulin	23–34 g/L (2.3–3.4 g/dL)		
• Albumin/globulin ratio	1.5:1–2.5:1 (same as SI units)	Multiple myeloma (globulin fraction), shock, vomiting	Malnutrition, nephrotic syndrome, proteinuria, renal disease, severe burns
Pseudocholinesterase (serum)	8–18 U/mL (same as SI units)	—	—
Renin		Renal hypertension, salt-losing GI disease (vomiting/diarrhea), volume decrease (e.g., hemorrhage)	Increased salt intake, primary aldosteronism
• Upright position	0.03–1.2 ng/L/sec (0.1–4.3 mg/mL/hr)		
Sodium	135–145 mmol/L (135–145 mEq/L)	Corticosteroid therapy, dehydration, impaired renal function, increased dietary or IV intake, primary aldosteronism	Addison's disease, decreased dietary or IV intake, diabetic ketoacidosis, diuretic therapy, excessive loss from GI tract, excessive perspiration, water intoxication
Testosterone		Adrenal hyperplasia, adrenal or pituitary tumours, testicular tumours	Hypofunction of testes
• Male	174–729 pmol/L (50–120 pg/mL)		
• Female	3.5–29.5 pmol/L (1.0–8.5 pg/mL)	Polycystic ovary, virilizing tumours	—
Thyroxine (T_4), total	64–154 nmol/L (5–12 mcg/dL)	Hyperthyroidism, thyroiditis	Cretinism, hypothyroidism, myxedema
Thyroxine (T_4), free	10–36 pmol/L (0.8–2.8 ng/dL)	Hyperthyroidism, metastatic neoplasms	Hypothyroidism, pregnancy
Triiodothyronine (T_3) uptake	24–34 AU (24%–34%)	—	—
Triiodothyronine (T_3)	1.7–5.2 pmol/L (110.4–337.7 ng/dL)	Hyperthyroidism	Hypothyroidism
Thyroid-stimulating hormone (TSH)	2–10 mIU/L (2–10 mcIU/mL)	Graves' disease, myxedema, primary hypothyroidism	Secondary hypothyroidism
Triglycerides		Diabetes mellitus, hyperlipidemia, hypothyroidism, liver disease	Hyperthyroidism, malabsorption syndrome, malnutrition
• Male	0.45–1.81 mmol/L (40–160 mg/dL)		
• Female	0.40–1.52 mmol/L (35–135 mg/dL)		
Troponin T (cTnT)	<0.1 mcg/L (<0.1 ng/mL)	Cardiac muscle damage (resulting from MI, myocarditis, or pericarditis), chronic renal failure, multiorgan failure, severe heart failure	—
Troponin I (cTnI)	<0.35 mcg/L (<0.35 ng/mL)		—

TABLE B-1 Serum, Plasma, and Whole Blood Chemistries—cont'd

Test	Normal Values: SI Units (Conventional Units)	POSSIBLE ETIOLOGY Higher Values	POSSIBLE ETIOLOGY Lower Values
Urea nitrogen, blood (blood urea nitrogen [BUN], serum urea nitrogen)	3.6–7.1 mmol/L (10–20 mg/dL)	Burns, dehydration, GI bleeding, increase in protein catabolism (fever, stress), renal disease, shock, urinary tract infection	Fluid overload, malnutrition, severe liver damage, SIADH
Uric acid • Male • Female	 240–501 mcmol/L (4.0–8.5 mg/dL) 160–430 mcmol/L (2.7–7.3 mg/dL)	Alcoholism, eclampsia, gout, gross tissue destruction, high-protein weight reduction diet, leukemia, multiple myeloma, renal failure	Administration of uricosuric drugs
Vitamin A	0.52–2.09 mcmol/L (15–60 mcg/dL)	Excess ingestion of vitamin A	Vitamin A deficiency
Vitamin B_{12}	118–701 pmol/L (160–950 pg/mL)	Chronic myeloid leukemia	Malabsorption syndrome, pernicious anemia, strict vegetarianism, total or partial gastrectomy
Zinc	11.5–18.5 mcmol/L (75–120 mcg/dL)	—	Alcoholic cirrhosis

*Because arterial blood gases are influenced by altitude, the values for $PaCO_2$, PaO_2, and PvO_2 decrease as altitude increases. The lower values are normal for an altitude of 1.6 km (1 mile).

†Values for older adults are significantly lower than those for younger adults.

COPD, chronic obstructive pulmonary disease; *DKA,* diabetic ketoacidosis; *GI,* gastrointestinal; *IV,* intravenous; *MI,* myocardial infarction; *RBC,* red blood cell; *SIADH,* syndrome of inappropriate antidiuretic hormone.

TABLE B-2 Hematology

Test	Normal Values: SI Units (Conventional Units)	POSSIBLE ETIOLOGY Higher Values	POSSIBLE ETIOLOGY Lower Values
Bleeding time (Ivy method)	1–9 min	Aspirin ingestion, clotting factor deficiency, defective platelet function, thrombocytopenia, vascular disease, von Willebrand's disease	—
Activated partial thromboplastin time (aPTT)	30–40 sec* (same as SI units)	Deficiency of one or more of the following: factor I, II, V, or VIII; factors IX and X; factor XI; and factor XII Hemophilia; heparin therapy; liver disease	—
Partial thromboplastin time (PTT)	60–70 sec (same as SI units)	Same as for aPTT	—
Activated coagulation time or automated clotting time (ACT)	70–120 sec (same as SI units)	Same as for aPTT	—
Prothrombin time (PT; Protime)	11–12.5 sec* (same as SI units)	Deficiency of one or more of the following: factor I, II, V, VII, or X Liver disease; vitamin K deficiency; warfarin therapy	—
International normalized ratio (INR)	0.81–1.20 (same as SI units)	Same as for PT	—
Thrombin time	8–12 sec (same as SI units)	DIC, increased tendency to bleed	—
Fibrinogen	2.0–5.0 g/L (60–100 mg/dL)	Burns (after first 36 hr), inflammatory disease	Burns (during first 36 hr), DIC, severe liver disease
Fibrin split (degradation) products	<10 mg/L (<10 mcg/mL)	Acute DIC, massive hemorrhage, massive trauma, primary fibrinolysis	—
D-dimer	<3.0 mmol/L (<50 ng/mL)	Deep-vein thrombosis, DIC, myocardial infarction, unstable angina	—
Erythrocyte count† (RBC count] [altitude dependent]) • Male • Female	 $4.7–6.1 \times 10^{12}/L$ $4.2–5.4 \times 10^{12}/L$	Dehydration, high altitudes, polycythemia vera, severe diarrhea	Anemia, leukemia, post hemorrhage

Continued

TABLE B-2 Hematology—cont'd

Test	Normal Values: SI Units (Conventional Units)	POSSIBLE ETIOLOGY Higher Values	Lower Values
Mean corpuscular volume (MCV) [Hct/RBC]	80–95 fL (80–95 mm³)	Folic acid and vitamin B_{12} deficiency, liver disease, macrocytic anemia	Microcytic anemia
Mean corpuscular hemoglobin (MCH) [Hb/RBC]	27–31 pg (same as SI units)	Macrocytic anemia	Microcytic anemia
Mean corpuscular hemoglobin concentration (MCHC) [Hb/Hct]	32–36 g/dL (32%–36%)	Intravascular hemolysis, spherocytosis	Hypochromic anemia
Erythrocyte sedimentation rate (ESR), Westergren Method • Male • Female	 ≤15 mm/hr (same as SI units) ≤20 mm/hr (same as SI units)	*Moderate increase:* acute hepatitis, myocardial infarction, rheumatoid arthritis *Marked increase:* acute and severe bacterial infections, malignancies, pelvic inflammatory disease	Malaria, severe liver disease, sickle cell anemia
Hematocrit (altitude dependent)† • Male • Female	 0.42–0.52 volume fraction (42%–52%) 0.37–0.47 volume fraction (37%–47%)	Dehydration, high altitudes, polycythemia	Anemia, bone marrow failure, hemorrhage, leukemia, overhydration
Hemoglobin (altitude dependent)† • Male • Female	 140–180 g/L (14–18 g/dL) 120–160 g/L (12–16 g/dL)	Chronic obstructive pulmonary disease, high altitudes, polycythemia	Anemia, hemorrhage
Hemoglobin, glycosylated or glycated (hemoglobin A_{1c} [HbA_{1c}])	<6% (adult without diabetes)	Nondiabetic hyperglycemia, poorly controlled diabetes mellitus	Chronic blood loss, chronic renal failure, pregnancy, sickle cell anemia
Red cell distribution width (RDW)	11%–14.5% (same as SI units)	—	Anisocytosis, macrocytic anemia, microcytic anemia
Platelet count (thrombocytes)	150–400 × 10^9/L (150,000–400,000/mm³)	Acute infections, chronic granulocytic leukemia, chronic pancreatitis, cirrhosis, collagen disorders, polycythemia, post splenectomy	Acute leukemia, cancer chemotherapy, DIC, hemorrhage, infection, systemic lupus erythematosus, thrombocytopenic purpura
Reticulocyte count (manual)	0.5%–2% total number of RBC	Hemolytic anemia, polycythemia vera	Hypoproliferative anemia, macrocytic anemia, microcytic anemia
WBC count†	5–10 × 10^9/L (5000–10,000/mm³)	Inflammatory and infectious processes, leukemia	Aplastic anemia, autoimmune diseases, overwhelming infection, side effects of chemotherapy and irradiation
WBC differential			
• Segmented neutrophils	2.5–7.5 × 10^9/L (62%–68%)	Bacterial infections, collagen diseases, Hodgkin's disease	Aplastic anemia, viral infections
• Band neutrophils	0–1 × 10^9/L (0%–9%)	Acute infections	—
• Lymphocytes	1.0–4.0 × 10^9/L (1000–4000/mm³; 20%–40%)	Chronic infections, lymphocytic leukemia, mononucleosis, viral infections	Corticosteroid therapy, whole body irradiation
• Monocytes	0.1–0.7 × 10^9/L (100–700/mm³; 2%–8%)	Acute infections, chronic inflammatory disorders, Hodgkin's disease, malaria, monocytic leukemia	—
• Eosinophils	0.00–0.5 × 10^9/L (50–500/mm³; 1%–4%)	Allergic reactions, eosinophilic and chronic granulocytic leukemia, Hodgkin's disease, parasitic disorders	Corticosteroid therapy
• Basophils	0.02–0.05 × 10^9/L (15–50/mm³; 0.5%–1%)	Hypothyroidism, myeloproliferative diseases, ulcerative colitis	Hyperthyroidism, stress
Sickle cell solubility	Negative (negative)	Sickle cell anemia	—

*For patients receiving anticoagulant therapy, aPTT is 1.5–2.5 times the control value in seconds; PT is 1.5–2.0 times the control value in seconds.
†Components of complete blood count (CBC).
DIC, disseminated intravascular coagulation; *RBC,* red blood cell; *WBC,* white blood cell.

TABLE B-3 **Serology–Immunology**

Test	Normal Values: SI Units (Conventional Units)	POSSIBLE ETIOLOGY Higher Values	Lower Values
Antinuclear antibody (ANA)	Negative at 1 : 40 dilution (same as SI units)	Chronic hepatitis, rheumatoid arthritis, scleroderma, systemic lupus erythematosus (SLE)	—
Anti-DNA antibody	Negative <70 U/mL (same as SI units)	SLE	—
Anti-RNP (ribonucleoprotein)	Negative (negative)	Mixed connective tissue disease, scleroderma, rheumatoid arthritis, Sjögren's syndrome, SLE	—
Anti-Sm (Smith)	Negative (Negative)	SLE	—
Antistreptolysin-O (ASO)	≤160 Todd units/mL (same as SI units)	Acute glomerulonephritis, rheumatic fever, streptococcal infection	—
C-reactive protein (CRP)	<10 mg/L (<1.0 mg/dL)	Acute infections, any inflammatory condition (e.g., acute rheumatic fever/arthritis), widespread malignancy	—
Carcinoembryonic antigen (CEA)	<5 mcg/L (5 ng/mL)	Carcinomas of colon, liver, pancreas; chronic cigarette smoking; inflammatory bowel disease; other cancers	—
Complement assay components • Total • C3 • C4	 75–160 kU/L (75–160 U/mL) 0.55–1.2 g/L (55–120 mg/dL) 0.2–0.5 g/L (20–50 mg/dL)	—	Acute glomerulonephritis, rheumatoid arthritis, serum sickness, subacute bacterial endocarditis, SLE
Direct antihuman globulin test (DAT) or direct Coombs' test	Negative (negative) (no agglutination)	Acquired hemolytic anemia, drug reactions, hemolytic disease of the newborn, transfusion reactions	—
Fluorescent treponemal antibody absorption (FTAAbs)	Negative (nonreactive)	Syphilis	—
Hepatitis A antibody	Negative (negative)	Hepatitis A	—
Hepatitis B surface antigen (HBsAg)	Negative (negative)	Hepatitis B	—
Hepatitis C antibody	Negative (negative)	Hepatitis C	—
Immunoglobulins			
• IgA	0.85–3.85 g/L (85–385 mg/dL)	Autoimmune disorders, chronic infection, chronic liver disease, IgA myeloma, rheumatoid arthritis	Burns, hereditary telangiectasia, malabsorption syndromes
• IgD	Minimal	Chronic infection, connective tissue disease	—
• IgE	24–400 mcg/L	Anaphylactic shock, atopic disease (allergies), parasite infections	—
• IgG	5.65–17.65 g/L (565–1765 mg/dL)	Hepatitis, IgG monoclonal gammopathy, infections—acute and chronic, SLE	Acquired deficiencies, burns, congenital deficiencies, immunosuppression, nephrotic syndromes
• IgM	0.55–3.75 g/L (55–375 mg/dL)	Acute infections, liver disease, rheumatoid arthritis	Congenital and acquired antibody deficiencies, lymphocytic leukemia, protein-losing enteropathies
Monospot or Mono-Test	Negative (<1 : 28 titre)	Infectious mononucleosis	—
Rheumatoid factor (RA factor)	Negative or <60 IU/mL by nephelometric method	Rheumatoid arthritis, Sjögren's syndrome, SLE	—
RPR (rapid plasma reagin) test	Negative or nonreactive (same as SI units)	Febrile diseases, IV drug abuse, leprosy, malaria, rheumatoid arthritis, syphilis, SLE	—
VDRL (Venereal Disease Research Laboratory) test	Negative or nonreactive (same as SI units)	Syphilis	—
Thyroid antibodies	Titre <1 : 100 (same as SI units)	Early hypothyroidism, Graves' disease, Hashimoto's thyroiditis, pernicious anemia, SLE, thyroid carcinoma	—

IV, intravenous.

TABLE B-4 Urine Chemistry

Test	Specimen	Normal Values: SI Units (Conventional Units)	POSSIBLE ETIOLOGY Higher Values	Lower Values
Acetone (ketones)	Random	Negative (negative)	Diabetes mellitus, high-fat and low-carbohydrate diets, starvation states	—
Aldosterone	24 hr	17–70 nmol/24 hr (2–26 mcg/24 hr)	*Primary aldosteronism:* Adrenocortical tumours *Secondary aldosteronism:* Cardiac failure, cirrhosis, large dose of ACTH, salt depletion	Adrenocorticotropic hormone (ACTH) deficiency, Addison's disease, corticosteroid therapy
Amylase	24 hr	100–300 U/L (60–120 Somogyi units/dL)	Acute pancreatitis	—
Bence Jones protein	Random	Negative (negative)	Biliary duct obstruction, multiple myeloma	—
Bilirubin	Random	5.1–16 mcmol/L (0.3–1.0 mg/dL)	Gallstones Dubin-Johnson Syndrome Rotor Syndrome	—
Calcium	24 hr	2.25–2.75 mmol/day (9.0–10.5 mg/dL)	Bone tumour, hyperparathyroidism, milk-alkali syndrome, lymphoma, Addison's Disease	Hypoparathyroidism, malabsorption of calcium and vitamin D, renal failure, pancreatitis
Catecholamines	24 hr		Heart failure, pheochromocytoma, progressive muscular dystrophy	
• Epinephrine		<109 nmol/day (<20 mcg/24 hr)		
• Norepinephrine		<590 nmol/day (<100 mcg/24 hr)		
Chloride	24 hr	110–250 mmol/day (110–250 mEq/day)	Dehydration, Cushing's syndrome, eclampsia, kidney dysfunction	Burns, diarrhea, excess perspiration, menstruation, vomiting, Addison's disease, heart failure
Copper	24 hr	0.6 mcmol/day (<40 mcg/day)	Cirrhosis, Wilson's disease	—
Coproporphyrin	24 hr	<300 nmol/day (<200 mcg/day)	Lead poisoning, oral contraceptive use, poliomyelitis	—
Creatine	24 hr		Acromegaly, disease affecting renal function, diabetic nephropathy	Decreased muscle mass (e.g., muscular dystrophy, myasthenia gravis)
• Male		53–106 mcmol/day (0.6–1.2 mg/dL)		
• Female		44–97 mcmol/L (0.6–1.2 mg/dL)		
Creatinine	24 hr		Anemia, leukemia, muscular atrophy, salmonellosis	Renal disease
• Male		53–106 mcmol/L (0.6–1.2 mg/dL)		
• Female		44–97 mcmol/L (0.5–1.1. mg/dL)		
Creatinine clearance	24 hr	1.42–2.25 mL/sec (85–135 mL/min)	—	Renal disease
• Male		1.78–2.32 mL/sec (107–139 mL/min)		
• Female		1.45–1.78 mL/sec (87–107 mL/min)		
Estriol	24 hr		Gonadal or adrenal tumour	Agenesis of ovaries, endocrine disturbance, menopause, ovarian dysfunction
• Female				
• Ovulatory phase		28–100 mcg/24 hr (104–370 nmol/L)		
• Luteal phase		22–80 mcg/24 hr (81–296 nmol/L)		
• Pregnancy		≤166,455 nmol/day (≤45,000 mcg/day)		
• Menopause		1.4–19.6 mcg/24 hr (5.2–72.5 nmol/L)		
• Male		5–18 mcg/24 hr (18–67 nmol/L)	—	—

TABLE B-4 Urine Chemistry—cont'd

Test	Specimen	Normal Values: SI Units (Conventional Units)	POSSIBLE ETIOLOGY Higher Values	Lower Values
Glucose	Random	Random: negative; 24-hour: <2.78 mmol/24 hr (<0.5 g/24 hr)	Diabetes mellitus, low renal threshold for glucose resorption, physiological stress, pituitary disorders	—
Hemoglobin	Random		Extensive burns, glomerulonephritis, hemolytic anemias, hemolytic transfusion reaction	—
• Male		140–180 mmol/L (14–18 g/dL)		
• Female		120–160 (12–16 g/dL)		
5-Hydroxyindole-acetic acid (5-HIAA)	24 hr	10–40 mcmol/day (2–8 mg/24 hr)	Malignant carcinoid syndrome	—
Ketone bodies	Random	Negative (negative)	Alcoholism, fasting, high-protein diets, marked ketonuria, poorly controlled diabetes mellitus, starvation	—
Lead	24 hr	<0.40 mcmol/day (<80 mcg/day)	Lead poisoning	—
Metanephrine	24 hr	12–60 pg/mL	Pheochromocytoma	—
Myoglobin	Random	1.0–5.3 nmol/L (<90 ng/mL)	Crushing injuries, electric injuries, extreme physical exertion	—
pH	Random	4.6–8.0 (average, 6.0)	Chronic renal failure, compensatory phase of alkalosis, salicylate intoxication, vegetarian diet	Compensatory phase of acidosis, dehydration, emphysema
Phenylpyruvic acid	Random	Negative (negative)	Phenylketonuria	—
Phosphorus, inorganic	24 hr	0.97–1.45 mmol/L (3.0–4.5 mg/dL)	Fever, hypoparathyroidism, nervous exhaustion, rickets, tuberculosis	Acute infections, nephritis
Porphobilinogen	Random	Negative (negative)	Acute intermittent porphyria, liver disorders	—
	24 hr	0–6.6 mg/24 hr (0–2 mg/24 hr)		
Potassium	24 hr	25–100 mmol/day (25–100 mEq/L/day)	Chronic renal failure, starvation, Cushing's syndrome, hyperaldosteronism, alkalosis, diuretic therapy	Reduced intake, dehydration, Addison's disease, malnutrition, vomiting, diarrhea, acute renal failure
Protein (dipstick)	Random	Negative (negative)	Heart failure, nephritis, nephrosis, physiological stress	—
Protein (quantitative)	24 hr	<0.15 g/day (<150 mg/day)	Cardiac failure, inflammatory processes of urinary tract, nephritis, nephrosis, toxemia of pregnancy	—
• At rest		0.05–0.08 g/day (<50–80 mg/day)		
• During exercise		<0.25 g/day (<250 mg/day)		
Sodium	24 hr	40–250 mmol/day (40–250 mEq/day)	Acute tubular necrosis	Hyponatremia
Specific gravity	Random	1.005–1.030 (usually, 1.010–1.025)*	Albuminuria, dehydration, fever, GI losses (vomiting/diarrhea), glycosuria, SIADH	Diabetes insipidus, diuresis, overhydration
Titratable acidity	24 hr	20–50 mEq/day (same as SI units)	Metabolic acidosis	Metabolic alkalosis
Uric acid	24 hr	1.48–4.43 mmol/day (250–750 mg/24 hr)	Gout, leukemia	Nephritis
Urobilinogen	24 hr	0.5–4.0 mg/24 hr (0.5–4.0 Ehrlich units/24 hr)	Hemolytic disease, hepatic parenchymal cell damage, liver disease	Complete obstruction of bile duct
Uroporphyrins	24 hr		Lead poisoning, liver disease, porphyria	—
• Male		10–53 nmol/24 hr (8–44 mcg/24 hr)		
• Female		10–26 nmol/24 hr (4–22 mcg/24 hr)		
Vanillylmandelic acid	24 hr	<35 mcmol/day (<6.8 mg/24 hr)	Pheochromocytoma, neuroblastomas	—

*Values decrease with age.
GI, gastrointestinal; *SIADH,* syndrome of inappropriate antidiuretic hormone.

TABLE B-5 Gastric Analysis

Test	Normal Values: SI Units (Conventional Units)	POSSIBLE ETIOLOGY Higher Values	Lower Values
Basal			
Free hydrochloric acid	0.3 mmol/L (0.3 mEq/L)	Hypermotility of stomach	Pernicious anemia
Total acidity	15–45 mmol/L (15–45 mEq/L)	Gastric and duodenal ulcers, Zollinger-Ellison syndrome	Gastric carcinoma, severe gastritis
Poststimulation			
Free hydrochloric acid	10–130 mmol/L (10–130 mEq/L)	—	—
Total acidity	20–150 mmol/L (20–150 mEq/L)	—	—

TABLE B-6 Fecal Analysis

Test	Normal Values: SI Units (Conventional Units)	POSSIBLE ETIOLOGY Higher Values	Lower Values
Fecal fat	7–21 mmol/day (2–6 g/24 hr)	Chronic pancreatic disease, cystic fibrosis, malabsorption syndrome, obstruction of common bile duct, short gut syndrome	—
Urobilinogen	51–372 mcmol/100 g of stool (30–220 mg/100 g of stool)	Hemolytic anemias	Complete biliary obstruction
Mucus	Negative (negative)	Mucous colitis, spastic constipation	—
Pus	Negative (negative)	Chronic bacillary dysentery, chronic ulcerative colitis, localized abscesses	—
Blood*	Negative (negative)	Anal fissures, hemorrhoids, inflammatory bowel disease, malignant tumour, peptic ulcer	—
Colour			
• Brown		Various shades, depending on diet	—
• Clay		Biliary obstruction or presence of barium sulphate	—
• Tarry		More than 100 mL of blood in GI tract	—
• Red		Blood in large intestine	—
• Black		Blood in upper GI tract, or iron medication	—

*Ingestion of meat may produce false-positive results. Patient may be placed on a meat-free diet for 3 days before the test.
GI, gastrointestinal.

TABLE B-7 Cerebrospinal Fluid Analysis

Test	Normal Values: SI Units (Conventional Units)	POSSIBLE ETIOLOGY Higher Values	Lower Values
Pressure	<20 cm H_2O (same as SI units)	Hemorrhage, intracranial tumour, meningitis	Head injury, spinal tumour, subdural hematoma
Blood	Negative (negative)	Intracranial hemorrhage	—
Cell count (age dependent)			
• White blood cells (WBCs)	0–5 × 10^6 WBCs/L (1–5 WBCs/mcL)	Inflammation or infections of CNS	—
• Red blood cells (RBCs)	Negative (negative)		—
Chloride	116–122 mmol/L of CSF (116–122 mEq/L of CSF)	Uremia	Bacterial infections of CNS (meningitis, encephalitis)
Glucose	2.8–4.2 mmol/L (50–75 mg/dL)	Diabetes mellitus, viral infections of CNS	Bacterial infections and tuberculosis of CNS
Protein			
• Lumbar	0.15–0.45 g/L (15–45 mg/dL)	Guillain-Barré syndrome, poliomyelitis, traumatic tap	—
• Cisternal	0.15–0.25 g/L (15–25 mg/dL)	Syphilis of CNS	—
• Ventricular	0.05–0.15 g/L (5–15 mg/dL)	Acute meningitis, brain tumour, chronic CNS infections, multiple sclerosis	—

NB: All of the changes are based on the values presented in the Pagana & Pagana textbook.
CNS, central nervous system; *CSF,* cerebrospinal fluid.

REVIEW QUESTION RATIONALES

CHAPTER 1

1. **The correct answer is 1.** The *Lalonde Report* shifted emphasis from a medical to a behavioural approach to health. It concluded that the traditional medical approach to health care was inadequate and that "further improvements in the environment, reductions in self-imposed risks, and a greater knowledge of human biology" are necessary to improve the health status of Canadians.
2. **The correct answer is 4.** The *Ottawa Charter for Health Promotion* supported a socioenvironmental approach to health. It identified prerequisites for health: peace, shelter, education, food, income, a stable ecosystem, sustainable resources, social justice, and equity.
3. **The correct answer is 1.** Labonte (1993) categorized the major determinants of health in a socioenvironmental approach as psychosocial risk factors and socioenvironmental risk conditions. Political, social, and cultural forces affect health and well-being directly and indirectly through their influence on personal health behaviours. Socioenvironmental risk conditions can contribute to psychosocial risk factors, which can then result in unhealthy behaviours.
4. **The correct answer is 1.** Given that the determinants of health are broad, healthy public policy must extend beyond traditional health care agencies and government health care departments to other sectors such as agriculture, education, transportation, labour, social services, energy, and housing. Therefore, policymakers in all government sectors and organizations should know the health consequences of their policies.
5. **The correct answer is 2.** Primary prevention includes activities that protect against a disease before signs and symptoms occur. Examples are immunization (to prevent infectious diseases) and reduction of risk factors (such as inactivity, smoking, and exposure to air pollution).
6. **The correct answer is 3.** Rather than focusing only on helping people develop healthy behaviours, the aim of health promotion is to create healthy public policy, supportive environments, community action, and personal skill. Health promotion is committed to empowerment and community-based health planning and addresses health issues within the context of the social, economic, and political environment. It therefore is political.
7. **The correct answer is 2.** The belief that health is primarily an *individual* responsibility is most congruent with the behavioural approach to health. The behavioural approach places responsibility for health on the individual, thereby favouring health promotion strategies such as education. Strategies are often based on the assumption that if people know the risk factors of disease, they will engage in healthy behaviours.
8. **The correct answer is 3.** Rather than focusing primarily on interventions at the societal level, the population health promotion model advocates that interventions be implemented toward individuals and families, communities, individual sectors of society (such as health care or environmental sectors), and society as a whole.
9. **The correct answer is 2.** Income and social status are the greatest determinants of health. Canadians who live in poverty have poorer health and are more likely to die earlier and to suffer more illnesses than those with higher incomes, regardless of age, sex, race, culture, and place of residence.
10. **The correct answer is 2.** Health promotion is directed toward increasing the level of well-being and self-actualization.

CHAPTER 2

1. **The correct answers are 2, 3, and 4.** The CIHI, CHI, and CIHR are all involved in monitoring, innovating, researching, and reporting on these critical measures of the health care delivery. Canada e-Health does not exist. The Consumer Association of Canada is an advocacy group.
2. **The correct answers are 1 and 2.** Both Indigenous and RCMP are federal responsibility according to the legislation. Some newcomers and immigrants and military members are given inclusion and some are not, so answers 3 and 4 are not correct. Individuals in transit remain covered by their province of origin for 3 months.
3. **The correct answer is 2.** The mentor recognizes that health promotion is a major component in the PHC model. Answers 1, 3, and 5 are about interventions, procedures, and duties, which are a function but not a focus. Institutionalization is not a focus in public health, although there are situations that may incite such actions (e.g., nonadherence to taking medication for tuberculosis).
4. **The correct answer is 4.** These principles are stated in the *Canada Health Act.* Other answers include values, and approaches to health delivery and sustainability, but not the principles that are officially articulated.
5. **The correct answer is 5.** Adult day supports are respite and relief settings in the community rather than in the home or institution. Home care may not meet the needs of this family in the short term as it is obvious that the woman needs a break from caregiving. Palliative care would be inappropriate as there is no indication of a terminal condition. Both hospital and ambulatory care would be inappropriate for this patient.
6. **The correct answers are 2, 4, and 5.** The skills of the nurse practitioner, dietician, and social worker bring a holistic approach to the patient, and with the assistance of the translator, there is a greater chance of ensuring clear communication and understanding of issues, challenges, and opportunities. The physician and the pharmacist have roles in the care of pregnant women but bring little to the dialogue of how to select and prepare healthier foods and how to use food as part of the health care plan.
7. **The correct answer is 3.** Only answer 3 recognizes the community and cultural aspects of this issue. Answers 1 and 4 are heavily weighted toward the medical model. Answer 2 may actually occur but should be based on local input and reflect local beliefs and preferred ways.
8. **The correct answer is 1.** Each of the answers has elements of truth. Answer 1 recognizes the need for succession planning that is compassionate and respectful of the career of aging nurses and their potential contributions to the new nursing cadre. Answer 2 is somewhat blaming, implying that the nurses are not self-regulating their work behaviors and risks. Answer 3

acknowledges the potential for technology to alleviate certain aspects of the work environment, but there is no "replacement" motive. Answer 4 does not reflect efforts to increase enrollments and to ensure ethical recruitment internationally. Answer 5 acknowledges the complexity of the nursing workforce but is not innovative or progressive.

9. **The correct answer is 2.** Screening programs, such as mammography or cervical screening, are significant secondary prevention programs offered in many locations and countries. An example of primary prevention would be an awareness campaign on hypertension. Tertiary care might include a stroke protocol for emergency (ambulance) services. Rehabilitation could include an aphasia support group for improving communication.
10. **The correct answer is 2.** Primary care has historically been the domain of physicians, but nurse practitioners and doctors of nursing practice, among others, are now offering primary care services, often in a partnership model with a physician.

CHAPTER 3

1. **The correct answer is 2.** Florence Nightingale, considered to be the founder of modern nursing, spearheaded the movement to improve standards of nursing care in the mid-nineteenth century.
2. **The correct answer is 2.** The earliest nursing care was provided by Indigenous nurses, followed by the Grey Nuns. Both groups used herbal remedies to relieve symptoms. Nuns cared for the sick at home and, later, in hospitals. Formal nurses' education started later, in the 1870s.
3. **The correct answer is 3.** Simone Roach was a Catholic sister. Religious sisters are committed to living a life according to religious counsels. One of the underlying values she identified in 1979 was rooted in religious belief: the sanctity of human life.
4. **The correct answer is 4.** Throughout her career, Nightingale promoted the status of nursing. She also believed that only women should be nurses. There is a low percentage of men in nursing (6.4%). The apprenticeship model is no longer used in Canada. The field of public health nursing started after Nightingale's death.
5. **The correct answer is 2.** Education standards are monitored by provincial regulators and associations.

CHAPTER 4

1. **The correct answer is 1.** The overall goals of a population health approach are to maintain and improve the health of the entire population and to eliminate health disparities. The population health approach provides a framework for thinking about health and for taking action to improve the health of populations. Action is directed primarily at community levels.
2. **The correct answer is 2.** Public health nursing merges knowledge from the public health sciences with professional nursing theories to safeguard and improve the health of populations in the community.
3. **The correct answer is 3.** Community-based nursing involves acute, chronic, and palliative care of patients and families that enhances their capacity for self-care and promotes autonomy in decision making.
4. **The correct answer is 4.** Vulnerable populations of patients are those who are likely to develop health problems as a result of excess risks, who experience barriers when trying to access to health care services, or who are dependent on others for care.
5. **The correct answer is 4.** Competent care of vulnerable populations does not include offering financial or legal advice.
6. **The correct answer is 2.** Physical, emotional, and sexual abuse, as well as neglect, are major public health problems affecting older persons, women, and children.
7. **The correct answer is 2.** A successful community health nursing practice requires an ability to build relationships with the community and to be responsive to changes within the community.
8. **The correct answer is 3.** Perinatal classes, infant care, child safety, and cancer screening are just some of the health education programs in which a nurse in community practice may participate as a nurse educator.
9. **The correct answer is 1.** The nurse as consultant provides information and supports participation in health activities. In this role, the nurse responds to inquiries about and makes referrals to community resources.
10. **The correct answer is 1.** The community can be viewed as having three components: locale or structure, the social systems, and the people.

CHAPTER 5

1. **The correct answer is 4.** A theory is a purposeful set of assumptions or propositions that show relationships between concepts. Theories are useful because they provide a systematic view of explaining, predicting, and prescribing phenomena.
2. **The correct answer is 3.** The drive for early theorizing about nursing practice came from nursing educators, who noted that traditional ways of preparing professional nurses were becoming outdated.
3. **The correct answer is 1.** The nursing process originally involved four steps: assessment, planning, intervention, and evaluation.
4. **The correct answer is 1.** Each conceptual framework attempted to define nursing by creating a theoretical definition for the substance and structure of the key bodies of knowledge needed to understand clinical situations. This knowledge was called the *metaparadigm concepts* and included person, environment, health care, and nursing care.
5. **The correct answer is 3.** The central question confronting early theorists about nursing practice remained as follows: How does a nurse organize and make sense of all available knowledge and apply it intelligently to the challenges that arise in an individual clinical case?
6. **The correct answer is 1.** Kuhn challenged the traditional notion of science as a logical progression of discoveries. He argued that major scientific developments occurred when scientists thought about problems in radically new and different ways.
7. **The correct answer is 1.** The main features of the McGill model were "a focus on health rather than illness and treatment, on all family members rather than the patient alone, on family goals rather than on the nurse's, and on family strengths rather than their deficits."
8. **The correct answer is 4.** Peplau defined the essence of nursing as the interpersonal relationship between the nurse and the patient. She viewed this relationship as interactive and therapeutic, in which the goal was to investigate the meaning of a patient's behavior and support that patient to achieve independent living.
9. **The correct answer is 2.** Canadian theorist Evelyn Adam articulated the essence of nursing as a helping process. From her perspective, the nurse played a complementary–supplementary role in supporting the patient's strength, knowledge, and will.

10. **The correct answer is 2.** Systems theory accounted for the whole of an entity (the system) and its component parts (subsystems), as well as the interactions between the parts and the whole.
11. **The correct answer is 2.** Parse's nursing model does not articulate goals for nursing in the traditional sense of defining health; instead, it relies on the notion of people in a continuous process of making choices and changing health care priorities.

CHAPTER 6

1. **The correct answer is 2.** Using evidence-informed decision making has been found to improve the quality of patient care.
2. **The correct answer is 4.** Quasi-experimental studies are considered to be quantitative; the other answers are qualitative designs. Quasi-experimental designs are an adaptation of the experimental design. Measurement of outcome variables occurs before and after an intervention (treatment) is given to research subjects. As the design incorporates measurement in a structured way, it is a quantitative design.
3. **The correct answer is 3.** Naming other participants is not required for informed consent. The consent form must describe the purpose of the study, the role of the subjects, types of data that are to be obtained, how the data are obtained, the duration of the study, subject selection, procedures, risks to the subject, potential benefits, alternatives to participation, and contact information.
4. **The correct answer is 3.** A quasi-experimental research design is one in which groups are formed and the conditions are controlled, but the subjects are not randomly assigned to a control group or treatment conditions.
5. **The correct answer is 4.** As well as using knowledge based on systematic research studies, evidence-informed practice also takes into account a nurse's clinical experience, practice trends, and patient preferences.

CHAPTER 7

1. **The correct answer is 3.** By understanding their personal values, nurses better understand their patients' and colleagues' values. In "value conflict," personal values are at odds with those of a patient, a colleague, or an institution. Values clarification plays a major role in resolving these dilemmas.
2. **The correct answer is 4.** *Justice* refers to fairness. The term is often used during discussions about resources. The question in this situation is how to determine the just distribution of resources. What constitutes a fair distribution of resources may not always be clear.
3. **The correct answer is 3.** *Maleficence* refers to harm or hurt; thus, *nonmaleficence* is the avoidance of harm or hurt. In health care ethics, ethical practice involves not only the will to do good but also the equal commitment to do no harm.
4. **The correct answer is 4.** The nurse is attempting to understand the patient's fears so that the nurse can advocate on his or her behalf through understanding and articulating this knowledge to others.
5. **The correct answer is 4.** *Autonomy* refers to a person's independence. Autonomy represents an agreement to respect another person's right to determine a course of action. Respect for a patient's autonomy is fundamental to the practice of health care and is why patients are included in all aspects of decision making regarding their care.
6. **The correct answer is 2.** The value of autonomy is to respect a patient's choice or self-determination.
7. **The correct answer is 3.** Advocacy calls for the nurse to allow patients' opinions to be heard (give patients a voice) and to speak out for those who cannot speak.
8. **The correct answer is 3.** The nurse does not make decisions for the patient. Advocating for the patient includes protecting the patient's right to choice by providing information, obtaining informed consent for all nursing care, and respecting the patient's decisions.
9. **The correct answer is 4.** Relational ethics explores the notion of relationships as a central activity of human behaviour. Scholars who write about relational ethics maintain that relationship is central to everything that nurses do and reflects a way of "being," displayed in everyday interactions rather than a mode of decision making.
10. **The correct answer is 2.** Each step in the processing of an ethical dilemma resembles steps in critical thinking. The nurse begins by gathering information and moves through assessment and identification of the problem, planning of a solution, implementation of a solution, and evaluation of the results.

CHAPTER 8

1. **The correct answer is 1.** Statute law is created by elective legislative bodies such as Parliament and provincial or territorial legislatures. Examples of provincial statutes are the nursing practice acts throughout the country, which describe and define nursing practice within each province.
2. **The correct answer is 1.** Any intentional physical contact such as treating a patient without the patient's consent is considered battery.
3. **The correct answers are 2, 3, and 4.** The essential elements of negligence are having a duty of care, breaching the duty by providing substandard care, and harm or an injury that results from the nurse's actions or inaction.
4. **The correct answer is 4.** Negligence in nursing is conduct that falls below a standard of care established by law. No intent is needed for negligence to occur. It is characterized chiefly by inadvertence, thoughtlessness, or inattention. Therefore, failing to raise the side rails when they are ordered is negligence.
5. **The correct answer is 2.** Obtaining informed consent is part of the physician–patient relationship. If a nurse suspects that a patient does not understand a procedure for which he or she is being asked to give consent or has consented to, the nurse must notify the physician or nursing supervisor.
6. **The correct answer is 4.** If a patient is harmed as a direct result of a nursing student's actions or lack of action, the liability is generally shared by the student, the instructor, the hospital or health care facility, and the university or educational institution.
7. **The correct answer is 4.** A nurse providing emergency assistance at an accident scene would not be covered by homeowners or an employer's insurance policy because the care given would not be the responsibility of the employer. However, some provinces have passed "Good Samaritan" laws (e.g., *Alberta's Emergency Medical Act*, 1988) that prevent voluntary rescuers from being sued for wrongdoing unless it can be proved that they displayed gross negligence.
8. **The correct answer is 4.** The physician is responsible for directing medical treatment. Nurses are obligated to follow physicians' orders unless they believe the orders are in error, violate hospital policy, or would harm patients.

9. **The correct answer is 4.** Patients can still be identified even if their name is not provided. Individuals can be identified even if a posting is done anonymously or by using a pseudonym. There is a mistaken belief that privacy controls allow the communication to be viewed only by the intended recipient. It is the nurses' role to safeguard all patient information learned in the course of treatment. It is to be shared only on a need-to-know basis with members of the health care team directly involved in the patient's care, when legally required, or where failure to disclose may lead to significant harm.

CHAPTER 9

1. **The correct answers are 1, 2, 3, and 4.** The environmental risks include all of the factors listed, which could lead to various diseases and injuries.
2. **The correct answer is 2.** The nurse would analyze the DALY indicator to assist with understanding the GBD of a country.
3. **The correct answers are 1, 2, and 3.** The SDGs align with a planetary perspective that focuses on poverty; they address the health of all persons of all ages; and they target health risks of low-, middle-, and high-income countries.
4. **The correct answer is 2.** In Canada, rather than assimilation, the preferred outcome is multiculturalism, in which immigrants and other people maintain their culture and different people of diverse cultures interact peacefully within the nation. Canadians believe, as stated in the multiculturalism policy, that citizens should be able to retain their traditions within a Canadian context.
5. **The correct answer is 1.**
6. **The correct answer is 2.** Cultural safety is the outcome of nursing education that enables safe care to be defined by those who receive the care. When a person acts on his or her prejudices, discrimination—treating people unfairly on the basis of their group membership—occurs.
7. **The correct answer is 1.** Ethnocentrism is the root of stereotypes, biases, and prejudices against other people who are perceived to be different from the valued group.
8. **The correct answer is 3.** Disparities in health outcomes between rich and poor patients illustrate the influence of socioeconomic factors on morbidity and mortality. Social factors such as poverty and lack of access to health resources compromise the health status of poor and unemployed patients.
9. **The correct answer is 3.** Global health focuses on issues that directly or indirectly affect health but that can transcend national boundaries.

CHAPTER 10

1. **The correct answer is 1.** Indigenous people who went to residential schools had problems with showing affection to their children, as they were not shown affection at residential schools and thus did not know how to parent their children in a warm manner. This pattern of parenting was passed down from generation to generation. Therefore, children of residential school survivors may not have had affection shown to them as children and consequently do not know to show affection to their own children.
2. **The correct answer is 2.** The federal government pays for health care for First Nations people who live on reserve and are Treaty Indians. This is according to the treaties and the *Indian Act*, a colonial policy.
3. **The correct answer is 3.** When the man asks for a sweet grass ceremony and to see the hospital Indigenous Elder, he is attending to his spirituality. Also, the Indigenous view of health is holistic, which takes into account the spiritual, physical, emotional, and mental aspects of a person. Answer 1 is incorrect because while historical trauma must be taken into account, *cultural genocide* rather than spiritual genocide would be important. Answers 2 and 4 are incorrect because the Indigenous world view focuses on community as a whole, rather than on individualism.
4. **The correct answer is 2.** Not all Indigenous people have traditional beliefs. Because of exposure to Western religions during colonialism, Indigenous peoples have a variety of beliefs, including Christianity, Catholicism, and other faiths. Some Indigenous people have no religious faith, and some have no knowledge of their traditions.
5. **The correct answer is 1.** Personal health practices and coping skills include smoking habits, which contribute to COPD. Physical environments can contribute to COPD and asthma among Indigenous people because they may live in poor housing with mould and other contaminants as well as poor ventilation and in areas that are overcrowded. Finally, level of education affects rates of respiratory illness in that higher levels of income are linked with better housing, the ability to connect with medical services, and better health literacy.
6. **The correct answer is 2.** Indigenous families have decreased access to health care for a variety of reasons, including lack of transportation, living in remote and rural locations without health care services, language barriers, poverty, and racism.
7. **The correct answer is 1.** Studies have shown that the most effective deterrent to suicide in Indigenous communities is self-determination and taking back culture and language (e.g., creating art). Communities that have these aspects have much lower rates of suicides than do communities who do not have these aspects.
8. **The correct answer is 2.** This would be the most impactful use of time, as well as the most appropriate, because the nurse would be helping the community work toward self-determination and would be helping to increase the cultural capacity of the community, which has been shown to decrease suicide rates and increase mental health. It would be long-acting and could have an impact on the entire community as families could learn their language and pass it down to generations. Learning one's Indigenous language is part of reconnecting with Indigenous knowledge systems.
9. **The correct answer is 3.** Asking an Indigenous patient where he or she is from demonstrates cultural humility on the part of the nurse and shows the patient that the nurse is interested in who the person is. The other three answers demonstrate a nurse making assumptions about the patient, which is not culturally safe.
10. **The correct answer is 4.** In asking the patient to tell the nurse more about the medicine, the nurse is demonstrating cultural safety and humility. By expressing concern, the nurse is being honest, educating the patient, and collaborating with the patient to work out the best outcome for her, thus demonstrating respect.
11. **The correct answer is 3.** A Métis person must have recent connections to the Métis community and self-identify as Métis. It is not enough to have ancestry from several generations ago. Also, Métis people are not defined solely through ethnicity.

CHAPTER 11

1. **The correct answers are 2, 3, and 4.** Transformational leadership is most fundamentally relational and inclusive of others in inspiring a shared vision for change and innovation. There is not a focus on the attributes of one leader.

2. **The correct answer is 3.** Collaborative models ensure that the needs of patients and populations determine the practice model (team composition) that is best situated to provide the best care. Persons (individuals, families, communities) are considered core members of teams making decisions about care.
3. **The correct answers are 3 and 4.** RNs do not delegate care to LPNs who have autonomous scopes of practice; RNs delegate to UCPs but remain accountable for the care delegated. RNs must understand team members' scopes of practice in order to ensure safe and appropriate delegation.
4. **The correct answer is 4.** Decentralized structures allow for shared decision making. Answers 1, 2, and 3 are not management structures.
5. **The correct answer is 3.** *Accountability* refers to answering for one's actions. One is required to come forward with full transparency and information about a decision or error.
6. **The correct answer is 1, 2, and 4.** Systems should focus on preventing mistakes and not just detection of them, thus shifting frames of accountability to view mistakes as opportunities for learning and affirming values of safety and quality. Staffing models and ratios have been shown to be associated with safety and quality care outcomes.
7. **The correct answer is 1.** A first step in providing leadership and supporting collaborative practice is to understand the UCP's role, scope of practice, and perspective; the need for educational sessions should be collaboratively determined.
8. **The correct answers are 1, 2, 3, and 4.** All apply to leadership for the promotion of primary health care.
9. **The correct answer is 4.** This patient is acutely ill and requires ongoing assessment and care by the RN; a bed bath may be safely delegated within the UCP scope of practice, with the RN remaining accountable for the patient and assuming all other aspects of care.
10. **The correct answers are 1 and 3.** A nurse-sensitive outcome is directly related to the care that nurses provide to patients; nurses oversee patient mobility in long-term care, and they are the primary providers of wound care.

CHAPTER 12

1. **The correct answer is 2.** The nurse seeks information to enhance his or her own knowledge base and uses information literacy skills to determine the scientific merit of the information retrieved.
2. **The correct answers are** 1. Assessment: **e**—collecting data about the patient's hoped-for health outcomes; 2. Nursing diagnosis: **d**—identifying the concern or problem to be resolved; 3. Planning: **a**—deciding what to do; 4. Implementation: **c**—taking action to intervene; 5. Evaluation: **b**—identifying the criteria to be used to determine if the patient's goals were attained.
3. **The correct answer is 3.** At the basic level of critical thinking, thinking is concrete and based on a set of rules or principles. In this case, the nurse uses the institution's procedures manual to confirm how to complete a specific procedure.
4. **The correct answer is 2.** The nursing process consists of five steps: assessment, nursing diagnosis, planning, implementation, and evaluation. During the assessment phase, the nurse engages in systematic observation to discern the patient's current health status—for example, the nurse gathers data (amount of drainage) to determine what action should be taken (notify physician or not).
5. **The correct answer is 3.** The nurse's knowledge base is an important component of critical thinking. The nurse demonstrates inquisitiveness in reading the nursing literature and preparing to apply what he learned in interacting with his patient.
6. **The correct answer is 3.** The nurse seeks information to solve a particular problem. The nurse notices that the intravenous infusion is not functioning correctly and uses her knowledge to solve the problem.
7. **The correct answer is 3.** Based on an assessment and analysis of the physical signs and symptoms, the nurse diagnoses the patient's health status. The nurse conducts both physical and behavioural observations, consults other sources of information, and draws conclusions about the health status of the infant based on the patterns observed.
8. **The correct answer is 1.** Reflection involves recalling a situation purposefully to evaluate performance and improve nursing practice. The nurse here purposefully recalls a situation to determine how he can work toward improving his clinical competency.
9. **The correct answers are 1, 2, and 3.** All three actions are needed to develop a sound, evidence-informed position of your own. Taking a side prematurely and assuming that the authorities are well informed about the information needed are not evident of critical thinking. The nurse utilizes critical thinking skills and dispositions to seek information and acquire a deeper understanding of the issue and the assumptions underlying the opposing points of view. The nurse remains open-minded and uses evidence to develop an informed position.
10. **The correct answers are** 1. Inference: **a**; 2. Evaluation: **d**; 3. Explanation: **e**; 4. Self-regulation: **b**; 5. Open-mindedness: **c**.
11. **The correct answer is 1.** On the basis of patient's descriptions the nurse draws a conclusion based on behaviour patterns indicative of ineffective coping.

CHAPTER 13

1. **The correct answer is 3.** Analyzing and interpreting data, documentation, and sharing of data with other health care providers cannot be done until data are validated and determined accurate.
2. **The correct answer is 4.** Documenting nursing care and reviewing data with other health care providers are part of intervention, not assessment. Making inferences is the step after data clustering.
3. **The correct answer is 3.** Diagnosis and treatment of clients' responses describes the entire nursing process; a common nursing language refers to the process of developing nursing diagnoses; identification of a disease refers to evaluation. A nursing diagnosis for an individual client is the clinical judgement about responses to actual and potential health problems or life processes.
4. **The correct answer is 4.** Evaluating nursing care is evaluation, gathering client information is assessment, and helping nurses focus on their role refers to the entire nursing process.
5. **The correct answer is 4.** A wellness nursing diagnosis describes levels of wellness in an individual, family, or community that can be enhanced. A risk nursing diagnosis describes human responses to health conditions or life processes that may develop in a vulnerable individual. An actual nursing diagnosis describes responses to health conditions or life processes that exist in an individual, family, or community. A potential nursing diagnosis is one under consideration during data interpretation.
6. **The correct answer is 2.** An actual nursing diagnosis describes responses to health conditions or life processes that exist in an individual, family, or community. A potential nursing diagnosis is one under consideration during data interpretation. A wellness

nursing diagnosis describes levels of wellness in an individual, family, or community that can be enhanced. A risk nursing diagnosis describes human responses to health conditions or life processes that may develop in a vulnerable individual.

7. **The correct answer is 1.** Risk factors are evidence considered during assessment; related factors are those contributing to the diagnosis; the complete statement is the nursing diagnosis.
8. **The correct answer is 2.** The client is the best source of information.
9. **The correct answers are 1 and 2.** The other answers are related factors but do not define the primary diagnosis.

CHAPTER 14

1. **The correct answer is 1.** Maintaining proper drainage of the wound is a high priority for this client immediately after surgery. The condition of the intravenous dressing, the client's comfort, and obtaining more intravenous fluids are important, but they do not have the highest priority in this situation.
2. **The correct answers are 1 and 2.** The descriptions "afebrile until discharge" and "without phlebitis by the third postoperative day" reflect the actual condition or state of the client.
3. **The correct answer is 4.** Rating pain acuity on a scale is the only report of the expected outcome in measurable terms.
4. **The correct answer is 4.** *Collaboration* means that a number of health care providers are involved in care.
5. **The correct answer is 3.** Successful planning requires that nurses collaborate with the client and family, consult with other members of the health care team, and review relevant literature. Critical pathways are care plans that detail the essential steps in the care of clients with a specific clinical problem and describe the expected progress of the client. Concept mapping provides a visual representation showing the connections between many problems. The purpose is not quality assurance in the health care facility. Multidisciplinary communication is enhanced through the use of critical pathways. Standardized care plans, not concept maps, provide a standardized format for client problems.
6. **The correct answer is 2.** Cardiopulmonary resuscitation is an example of a life-saving measure to protect the client. Administering analgesics is a physical care technique; it is not a life-saving measure. Stress-reduction therapy is an example of a counselling technique. Teaching the client how to take his or her pulse is an example of the nursing intervention of teaching.
7. **The correct answer is 3.** Auscultation of lung sounds is an evaluation of the effectiveness of suctioning, which is the nursing intervention being evaluated.
8. **The correct answer is 1.** Goals and expected outcomes are objective criteria developed in the plan of care used to judge a client's response to care. Answers 2 and 4 are both subjective observations of the nurse based on client feedback.
9. **The correct answer is 3.** Determining adherence to the medical regime is the priority. Antibiotics must be taken routinely and consistently to maintain adequate blood levels. Additional data are required as related to the plan of care prior to pursuing other nursing interventions.

CHAPTER 15

1. **The correct answer is 1.** This information about a fellow nursing student is confidential. Another nursing student cannot share it with classmates or visit that ill student because the student learned of the ill student's admission accidentally in the course of his work. The student has no right to access the record of the ill student, because that student is not caring for the ill student.
2. **The correct answer is 4.** Enter only objective descriptions of the patient's behaviour, not opinions or judgements. Do not write retaliatory or critical comments about a patient; in a court of law, such comments can be used as evidence of nonprofessional behaviour or poor quality of care.
3. **The correct answer is 3.** Subjective data are what the patient says, and this is often in his or her own words, between quotation marks.
4. **The correct answer is 4.** Enter only objective descriptions of the patient's behaviour, not opinions or judgements. Do not write retaliatory or critical comments about a patient; in a court of law, such comments can be used as evidence of nonprofessional behaviour or poor quality of care.
5. **The correct answer is 1.** Patients frequently request copies of their health records, and they have the right to do so. Each institution has policies for controlling the manner in which records are shared. In most situations, patients are required to give written permission for release of medical information.
6. **The correct answer is 4.** Use complete, concise descriptions of care so that documentation is objective and factual. Avoid using empty phrases such as "well tolerated," which is too generalized and has no meaning.
7. **The correct answer is 3.** Acuity ratings or records provide a method of determining the hours of care and staff required for a given group of patients. A patient's acuity level is based on the type and number of nursing interventions required for providing care in a 24-hour period.
8. **The correct answers are:** 1. P, 2. S, 3. A, 4. O. **S** (*subjective:* "The pain increases every time I try to turn on my left side.") **O** (*objective:* Left lower abdominal surgical incision, 3 inches in length, closed, sutures intact, no drainage. Pain noted on mild palpation.) **A** (*assessment:* Acute pain related to tissue injury from surgical incision.) **P** (*plan:* Repositioned patient on right side. Encouraged patient to use patient-controlled analgesia.)
9. **The correct answers are 1, 2, 4, and 5.**
10. **The correct answers are 1 and 4.**
11. **The correct answer is 1.** The direct entry of orders eliminates issues related to illegible handwriting and transcription errors.
12. **The correct answer is 3.** Clinical decision support systems (CDSSs) are computerized programs used within the health care setting to aid and support clinical decision making. The knowledge base within a CDSS contains rules and logic statements that link information required for clinical decisions to generate tailored recommendations for individual patients, which are presented to nurses as alerts or warnings.
13. **The correct answer is 3.** Nurses need to make sure that patient-identifiable information (e.g., files, stickers, information in notebooks, worksheets) is not taken home and is disposed of correctly in a secure bin for shredding.

CHAPTER 16

1. **The correct answer is 3.** Changes in the health care system have led to an increased need for high-quality, comparable, aggregated data to support effective decision making—whether decisions are at the clinical level, the local or regional level, or the system level. Nurses recognize the value of adopting technology to support evidence-informed professional practice, innovation, and nursing data collection and representation.

2. **The correct answer is 4.** Nursing needs standardized documentation to facilitate aggregation of nursing data, to support comparison and analysis, to enhance communication among nurses, and to improve representation regarding nursing contributions.
3. **The correct answer is 2.** The CNA formally adopted ICNP as the terminology of choice for professional nursing practice. Standardized nursing terminology using ICNP® is being implemented via the C-HOBIC project. This project will examine nursing-sensitive outcomes and compare these measures across various clinical settings. Because all outcomes are coded using ICNP, this comparison will have a stronger impact and allow for greater analysis.
4. **The correct answer is 1.** Although all nurses must practise using both the Standards of Care (provincial legislation) and the national *Code of Ethics*, all nurses must be aware of both pieces of federal legislation governing the privacy of health information in Canada. The *Privacy Act* and the *Personal Information Protection and Electronic Documents Act* (PIPEDA) prohibit nurses from disclosing personal health information about any patient, with very limited exceptions.
5. **The correct answer is 3.** Nurses can enact the *e-Nursing Strategy* by engaging in advocacy for access and participation and engaging in developing their competencies. Additionally, as a nurse you should work toward the seven key outcomes as identified by the CNA. These include the following:
   a. Integrating ICT into your practice to achieve good patient outcomes
   b. Having the required information and knowledge to support your practice
   c. Facilitating human resources planning
   d. Support for new models of nursing practice and health services delivery
   e. Improved connections between nursing groups
   f. Improved quality of nurses' work environments
   g. Contributing to the global community of nursing
6. **The correct answer is 1.** Many professional and informal nursing communities are available to foster nurses' engagement in the informatics communities. Canada Health Infoway solicits clinician engagement in support of development of the pan-Canadian EHR. One can be a voluntary member of any (or several) Standards Collaborative Working Groups (SCWG) and contribute to specific aspects of EHR development. The Canadian Nursing Informatics Association (CNIA) is the national group that all nurses are welcome to join. Additionally, many provinces have special-interest groups that are dedicated to nursing informatics. COACH is another choice for nurses to join a national Canadian group. International opportunities include AMIA, IMIA-SIGNI, and HISA. Nurses may also consider other informal communities, such as listservs, wikis, and blogs, and other social networks, such as Facebook. It is critical, however, to remember that most informal communities are not held to the professional content standards like those of more formal organizations, and content should be considered with caution.

CHAPTER 17

1. **The correct answer is 4.** Assessment of a patient's ability to communicate includes gathering data about the many contextual factors that influence communication. These include the participants' internal factors and characteristics, the nature of their relationship, the situation prompting communication, the environment, and the sociocultural elements present. Assessing these contextual factors helps the nurse make sound decisions during the communication process.
2. **The correct answer is 3.** Active listening means being attentive to what the patient is saying both verbally and nonverbally. The acronym *SOLER* represents facilitative skills for attentive listening: **S** (*sit* facing the patient); **O** (observe an *open posture*—that is, keep arms and legs uncrossed); **L** (*lean* toward the patient); **E** (establish and maintain intermittent *eye contact*); **R** (*relax*).
3. **The correct answer is 1.** A helping relationship between nurse and patient does not just happen; it is created with care and skill and is built on the patient's trust in the nurse. During the orientation phase of a relationship, the nurse sets the tone for the relationship by adopting a warm, empathic, and caring demeanour. During this phase, the relationship is often superficial, uncertain, and of a social nature. The phase is a period of getting to know each other and establishing trust.
4. **The correct answer is 3.** Interacting with patients who have conditions that impair communication requires sensitivity and creativity. Communication techniques must be adapted to the patient's unique circumstances and sensory, motor, and cognitive needs. The nurse must be patient, ask simple questions, encourage the patient to converse, and allow sufficient time for the patient to understand and respond. Visual cues and communication aids may be useful in communicating with aphasic patients.
5. **The correct answer is 1.** Nurses function in roles that require interaction with multiple members of the health care team. Many elements of the nurse–patient relationship are also applied in these interprofessional relationships, which are focused on accomplishing the work and goals at the point of care. It is especially important to involve the patient and family in decisions about the plan of care, to determine whether suggested methods are acceptable.
6. **The correct answer is 3.** *Clarifying* means checking whether understanding is accurate, as in restating an unclear or ambiguous message to elicit the sender's meaning. Instead of restating the message, you can also ask the other person to rephrase it, explain further, or give an example of what he or she means.
7. **The correct answer is 4.** Focusing is used to centre on key elements or concepts of a message. If conversation is vague or rambling, or if patients begin to repeat themselves, focusing is a useful technique.
8. **The correct answer is 2.** Intrapersonal communication, or self-talk, is a powerful communication tool. It strongly influences perceptions, feelings, self-concept, and behaviour and can replace negative thoughts with positive assertions.
9. **The correct answer is 2.** A tip for improved communication with older persons is to stick to one topic at a time.
10. **The correct answer is 2.** In the zones of personal space and touch, the personal zone (45 cm to 1 m) includes nursing activities such as sitting at a patient's bedside and documenting the patient's health history.

CHAPTER 18

1. **The correct answers are 1 and 2.** Personal knowing is related to Sally's response to Mrs. Brandt's crying. This made her respond to find out what emotion the crying was related to so that Sally would know what intervention she might need to provide. Aesthetic knowing is related to Sally's approach to Mrs. Brandt and her crying. Sally was ready to provide comfort if her crying was a negative emotional reaction to something.
2. **The correct answers are 2, 3, and 5.** Jordan was promoting and respecting informed decision making by trying to determine the situation that brought the youth to live on the street. Jordan also

was preserving the youth's dignity by treating him for a coffee and being open to listening to him and gaining an understanding of the youth's lived experience. Jordan chose to not ignore the youth who was asking for money for coffee. But he did not just give him money, he also provided a connection by taking the youth with him for a coffee and treating him with respect. Jordan was demonstrating his ability of being accountable to this ethical value of nursing.

3. **The correct answers are 2, 3, and 4.** Jordan demonstrated *interpreting*: While Jordan did not initially notice the homeless youth, he was reminded about his growing knowledge from nursing classes about social justice issues in society. Therefore, he was using analytic reasoning, which caused him to focus on his intuitive reasoning to want to reach out to the youth. Jordan chose to gain more understanding by using his narrative reasoning by first offering to take the youth to coffee with him and then to further respond by listening to the youth and suspending his own judgement about circumstances that might have led to the youth's situation. Thus, he created an interaction with the youth that provided a social connection between the two of them and provided the potential space for openness that might allow further interactions and potential other forms of nursing interventions. Jordan demonstrated *responding* in that his response to the youth's request for money for coffee enabled Jordan to exercise his nursing skills in creating a therapeutic interaction with the youth. Jordan not only granted the youth's request but also realized the need to ensure that the youth was provided a connection through a social encounter in which he was open to the youth without demonstrating judgement about the youth's circumstances that led to his homelessness. Jordan's approach to learning from the youth over coffee was a means of learning about the lived experience of a person living on the street and of being open to seeking out what the youth might have as a goal for himself. With such information Jordan might be able to facilitate community-based supports for the youth and in this way reinforce the value he saw in the youth as a member of society. Jordan demonstrated *reflection-in-action* in that he became alerted to the youth's situation and connected this to his learning. He was able to integrate the learning into his community-based practice learning and, in doing so, likely would experience reflection-on-action following the interaction with the youth.
4. **The correct answers are 1, 3 and 4.** *Affinity* is at play in this scenario. Jasmine is a student nurse and does not know the doctor. He, in turn, has not worked with Jasmine and does not know what her competence level is. So without knowing her competence the doctor lashes out in his frustration at not having the test done for his patient, without checking why it wasn't done. This interaction shows limited *respect* by the doctor to Jasmine in her situation. She is viewed as likely not competent to know the answer to the question, so the doctor does not explore the reason with Jasmine. Jasmine then feels very intimidated and is reluctant to share the correct information with the doctor, for fear of his further retribution. In terms of *control*, Jasmine will naturally see herself in a limited power position in the situation. The doctor is in control, and he has demonstrated his power over not just her but the situation itself. This further reinforces Jasmine's decision to keep quiet and let someone else tell him why the MRI was not done.

CHAPTER 19

1. **The correct answer is 4.** The nurse must think of family as defined by each individual. In other words, the nurse can think of the family as a set of relationships that the patient identifies as family or as a network of individuals who influence each other's lives, whether the ties are biological or legal.
2. **The correct answer is 2.** The blended family is formed when both parents bring children from previous relationships into a new, joint living situation or when children from the current union and children from previous unions are living together.
3. **The correct answer is 4.** The family is the primary social context in which health promotion and disease prevention take place. The family's beliefs, values, and practices also strongly influence health-promoting behaviours of its members.
4. **The correct answer is 3.** Health promotion researchers have focused on the stress-moderating effect of hardiness and resiliency as factors that contribute to long-term health. Family hardiness comprises the internal strengths and durability of the family unit. Family resiliency is the ability to cope with expected and unexpected stressors.
5. **The correct answer is 2.** When the family as patient is the approach, the nurse focuses on the entire family, its processes, and relationships (e.g., parenting or family caregiving).
6. **The correct answer is 1.** *Internal structure* refers to the people who are included in the family and how they are connected to each other. Specifically, this question assesses family composition, a subcategory of internal structure. *Family composition* refers to the individual members who form the family. The family composition is not limited to the traditional nuclear family; instead, it may include any of the various family forms.
7. **The correct answer is 3.** In considering family nursing from a relational inquiry perspective, there is an explicit focus on understanding the family in context (sociocultural, geo-political, and economic contexts).
8. **The correct answer is 3.** Letting be and change, as well as emancipatory action, are two of the assessing and intervening approaches described by Hartrick Doane and Varcoe (2005) in *Family nursing as relational inquiry: Developing health promoting practice.*
9. **The correct answer is 4.** *Expressive functioning* refers to the ways in which people communicate. Emotional communication is a subcategory of expressive functioning and encompasses the range and types of feelings that are expressed by the family.
10. **The correct answer is 1.** Circular questions facilitate change by inviting the family to discover their own answers; they help explain a problem.
11. **The correct answer is 3.** In an effective family interview, the nurse can engage a family to assess, explore, and identify strengths and problems. The nurse can also decide to intervene or to refer the family to another health care provider.

CHAPTER 20

1. **The correct answer is 3.** Psychomotor learning involves acquiring skills that require the integration of mental and muscular activity; therefore, teaching a patient to use an inhaler requires the use of the psychomotor domain. The patient masters skills by manipulating equipment and practicing manual skills. The cognitive domain involves intellectual behaviour and thinking. The affective domain involves emotions and feelings. *Attentional* refers to the act of careful observing or listening.
2. **The correct answer is 2.** If a patient's learning ability is impaired or if distractions are present, the nurse should modify or postpone teaching activities. Any physical condition (e.g., pain, fatigue, or hunger) that depletes energy also impairs the ability to learn.

Therefore, the nurse should teach the patient when pain medications are working. When visitors are in the room they may be distracting. While awake and alert just before lunch, the patient may be hungry, and there is a risk of being interrupted by meals arriving. When patients focus on the stressors in their lives, part of patient-centred care is to respect this; such stressors will distract them from learning.

3. **The correct answer is 3.** Readiness to learn is related to the grieving stage. Patients cannot learn when they are unwilling or unable to accept the reality of illness. However, properly timed teaching can help a patient to adjust to illness or disability. When a patient is in denial or disbelief, the nurse should teach in the present tense (e.g., explain what the patient needs to know to be discharged). Teaching the spouse is not patient centred, does not replace patient involvement, and may be counterproductive. If the patient is not open to education, providing information about what she needs to know in a few weeks is less important than what the patient needs to know at present. Answer 4 is incorrect; it is important to respect where the patient is at this point in time and understand that the patient needs time to process the diagnosis.
4. **The correct answers are 4 and 5.** As a child matures, intellectual growth moves from the concrete to the abstract. By developing topics that require activities and problem solving, the nurse is considering the adolescents' level of development and will engage the students in learning about nutrition. By exploring the students' current understanding, the nurse is assessing learning needs. Lectures do not provide the interaction preferable for this age group. Language should be appropriate to the age and education level of the group, and for this group everyday language would be appropriate. The focus of the teaching is nutrition, not eating disorders.
5. **The correct answers are 2, 4, and 6.** To plan a patient-centred education activity with a specific cultural group, it is essential to involve members of the group in the assessment and planning of the activity. This way the nurse can incorporate cultural values, beliefs, and practice into the plan. By assessing the community in general, the nurse may fail to identity the needs and expectations of this particular group. There is nothing to indicate the need for special cognitive considerations for this group that would require simplistic material. Focusing on Western concepts would not be a patient-centred approach, would dismiss the cultural experience of health and illness by this cultural group, and may limit their ability to self-manage their health.
6. **The correct answer is 1.** The telling approach is useful when limited information must be taught over a short period of time (e.g., preparing a patient for an emergency diagnostic procedure). Selling, entrusting, and participation activities take place over time and with interaction and negotiation that is usually not possible in emergency situations.
7. **The correct answer is 3.** Role play is used to help teach new ideas and attitudes. During role play, patients play themselves or someone else and rehearse a desired behaviour. Simulations help the learner to problem solve in a scenario. Analogies are used to translate complex concepts into simpler, more familiar language and ideas. Demonstrations are used to teach specific psychomotor skills.
8. **The correct answers are 1 and 3.** Learning disabilities are disorders that may impair the ability to acquire, organize, remember, understand, or apply information. When teaching patients with learning disabilities or other barriers to learning, a recommended technique is to demonstrate procedures, such as measuring dosages, and then ask for return demonstrations, thus providing the opportunity to clarify instructions and time to review procedures. Patients should be given information on multiple occasions to reinforce knowledge and understanding. Written material is often difficult for individuals with learning disabilities to understand or use. Individuals with learning disabilities often require *more time* to understand material.
9. **The correct answer is 2.** In general, teaching and learning begin when a person identifies a need for knowing or acquiring an ability to do something. Receiving written instructions, being able to understand the markings on the syringe, or having the dexterity to do the task are important but do not indicate a readiness to learn.
10. **The correct answers are 1, 4, and 5.** Demonstrations help teach psychomotor skills, such as preparing a syringe. The patient can observe a skill before practicing it. Simulation gives the patient the opportunity to practise understanding of the skill, and video or computer instructions can be used to reinforce learning. Group instruction and one-to-one discussion are useful for providing information and answering questions but are not the best teaching methods to use in this scenario.
11. **The correct answer is 1.** Understanding how to self-manage an acute episode is a priority and needs to be addressed first. While teaching about environmental factors such as cigarette smoke, purchasing of medical alert bracelets, and healthy diet and lifestyle are all aspects of teaching for an asthmatic patient, the management of an acute episode takes priority.
12. **The correct answer is "application."** This demonstrates the patient's ability to apply knowledge in a different context.

CHAPTER 21

1. **The correct answer is 4.** Growth is the quantitative, or measurable, aspect of an individual's increase in physical measurements. Measurable growth indicators include changes in height, weight, teeth, skeletal structures, and sexual characteristics.
2. **The correct answer is 1.** Moral development is the ability of an individual to distinguish right from wrong and to develop ethical values on which to base his or her actions.
3. **The correct answer is 1.** Organicism is a theoretical focus on the organism itself. According to theories in this tradition, development is a result of biologically driven behaviour and the person's adaptation to the environment.
4. **The correct answer is 1.** Three major categories of factors influence human growth and development: genetics, environment, and the interaction between these two. The family is an example of an environmental factor. Family influences through its values, beliefs, customs, and specific patterns of interaction and communication.
5. **The correct answer is 4.** Psychiatrist Robert Havighurst believed his findings described a sequential process that takes place between the internal life (personality) of adults and their outer world (culture, lifestyle).
6. **The correct answer is 4.** The zone of proximal development, described by Vygotsky, is the difference between a child's current developmental achievement and a child's capabilities, given the child's physical and emotional maturation level. For example, a 12-month-old child may be walking by holding on to furniture but be developmentally able to walk independently. A sensitive caregiver could help the child achieve independent walking by encouraging activities that help the child gain confidence to walk alone.
7. **The correct answer is 1.** During formal operations, the individual's thinking moves to abstract and theoretical subjects. Thinking

can venture into such subjects as achieving world peace, finding justice, and seeking meaning in life. Adolescents can organize their thoughts in their minds. New cognitive powers allow the adolescent to achieve more far-reaching problem solving.

8. **The correct answer is 2.** The microsystem consists of the immediate settings, activities, and personal relationships of the individual. Examples of microsystems are family, classroom, workplace, and recreation group.
9. **The correct answer is 3.** According to Keating and Hertzman's (1999) population health approach, human development is a population phenomenon. They referred to the strong association between the health of a population, developmental outcomes, and the social and economic forces affecting the larger society. Therefore, improving community housing would be an attempt to improve the health of the population.
10. **The correct answer is 4.** According to resilience theory, protective processes shield people from adversity and include social supports, such as high-quality day care.

CHAPTER 22

1. **The correct answers are 2, 3, and 4.** Infants with low birth weight have an increased risk for learning disorders, temperament problems, neurological and motor impairment, and developmental delays.
2. **The correct answer is 1.** Up to 10% of birth weight is lost in the first few days after birth, primarily through fluid losses by respiration, urination, defecation, and low fluid intake. Supplementation with formula is not needed because breastfeeding is considered the most complete nutritional source until the infant is about 6 months of age.
3. **The correct answer is 2.** Hepatitis B vaccine can be administered at months 0, 1, and 6, with at least 4 weeks between the first and second dose, at least 2 months between the second and third dose, and at least 4 months between the first and third dose. Alternatively, it can be administered as DTaP-HB-IPV-Hib vaccine, with the first dose at 2 months of age.
4. **The correct answer is 4.** According to Piaget (1952), during the preoperational thought stage of cognitive development, toddlers recognize that they are separate beings from their mothers, but they are unable to assume another person's viewpoint. They use symbols to represent objects, places, and people. This function is demonstrated when children imitate the behaviour of another person that they viewed earlier (e.g., pretend to shave like their daddy).
5. **The correct answers are 1 and 4.** The preschool period encompasses the years between 3 and 5 years of age. The play of preschool children becomes more social after the third birthday as it shifts from parallel to associative play. Most 3-year-old children are able to play with one other child in a cooperative manner in which they make something or play designated roles, such as mother and baby. By the age of 4 years, children play in groups of two or three, and by 5 years, the group has a temporary leader for each activity.
6. **The correct answers are 1, 3, 4, 5, and 6.** Warning signs of suicide, which often occur for at least a month before suicide is attempted, are deterioration in school performance; social withdrawal; loss of initiative; loneliness, sadness, and crying; appetite and sleep disturbances; and verbalization of suicidal thought.
7. **The correct answer is 4.** The nurse is legally required to report all cases of suspected child abuse or neglect to authorities.
8. **The correct answer is 3.** "Administration of the seasonal influenza vaccine should usually be postponed in persons with serious acute illnesses until their symptoms have abated. Immunization should not be delayed because of minor acute illness, with or without fever. If significant nasal congestion is present that might impede delivery of...[live attenuated influenza vaccine (LAIV)] to the nasopharyngeal mucosa, inactivated vaccines can be administered or LAIV can be deferred until resolution of the illness" (Public Health Agency of Canada, 2016c, Key Information: How section, para. 5).
9. **The correct answer is 4.** Being like their peers is extremely important for adolescents. However, the range of age at menarche is 10 to 18, with an average of 12.25. The beginning of breast development ranges from age 8 to 13. As with increases in height and weight, the pattern of sexual changes is more significant than their time of onset. Large deviations from normal patterns necessitate investigation.
10. **The correct answers are 1, 3, and 4.** Injuries, including self-inflicted injuries and injuries caused by motor vehicle accidents and poisoning, are the leading cause of death in adolescents. Eating disorders are thought to be more common among girls, but boys may also suffer from these disorders. Tobacco use, although decreasing, continues to be a problem among adolescents.

CHAPTER 23

1. **The correct answers are 1, 3, and 6.** The nurse recognizes that patients with obesity are more likely to have elevated blood glucose associated with type 2 (non-insulin-dependent) diabetes mellitus, body mass index (BMI) above 30 kg/m^2, and high blood pressure. A fasting blood glucose level of 5 mmol/L is within the normal range. A BMI of 28 kg/m^2 is indicative of a patient being overweight, but is not considered obesity. A blood pressure of 125/85 mmHg is moderately elevated, but is still considered within the normal range for a middle-aged adult patient.
2. **The correct answer is 1.** The patient is generally in good health, and promotion of good health practices are indicated among young adults. Primary, secondary, and tertiary prevention efforts may be indicated for specific conditions that the young adult may be at risk of acquiring. However, these are not necessarily indicated for all young adults.
3. **The correct answers are 1, 2, 4, 5, and 6.** Each of these elements determines health outcomes among young and middle adult patients. Sexuality is an incorrect response because differences between sexual desire, sexual behaviour, and sexual identity typically do not affect a prescribed course of therapy.
4. **The correct answer is 4.** Quickening is the sensation of movement or of abdominal gas caused by fetal movement. Morning sickness is usually associated with the first trimester of pregnancy and is the result of increased serum hormone levels. Amenorrhea is associated with fertilization and implantation of the egg and increased hormone levels during the first trimester of pregnancy. Increased colostrum is the result of hormone influences that prepare the breasts for lactation and occurs during the third trimester of pregnancy.
5. **The correct answer is 2.** Although firearm injuries occur as a result of criminal activities, they do not represent 80% of the firearm injuries in Canada. Approximately 80% of suicides in Canada are firearm related, therefore 20% of suicides are the result of firearms and 50% of suicides are the result of firearms are incorrect answers.

6. **The correct answer is 1.** HIV-positive gay men should be included in intervention development to overcome stigma and power imbalances experienced by these men in the health care system. Collaborating with the Medical Health Officer provides a good way to engage additional stakeholders in intervention development but does not include the perspectives of the patients and may actually decrease the likelihood of cultural safety, especially if the Medical Health Officer is perceived as part of the institutional barriers limiting access to care for HIV-positive gay men. Engaging family members in smoking reduction and cessation intervention development may strengthen family support systems for HIV-positive gay men and may improve intervention success, but this does not demonstrate cultural safety. Acknowledging the cultural traditions of HIV-positive gay men demonstrates cultural awareness, but implementing a standardized smoking reduction and cessation intervention demonstrates lack of cultural competence. Neither of these actions are consistent with a cultural safety approach to intervention development.
7. **The correct answer is 3.** The nurse is assessing potential health risks, not the presence of an actual disease state. There is limited to no evidence to suggest that poor personal hygiene contributes to myocardial infarction. Lifestyle is a less important consideration in this case than family history is. Hereditary disease is incorrect because there is not sufficient evidence to determine that the patient actually has a disease state that could contribute to a myocardial infarction.
8. **The correct answer is 1.** When parents teach back what they have learned, describe how to access additional information, and report when to contact health care providers, they are demonstrating that they have increased health literacy. The parents who listen to the nurse and thank the nurse for sharing knowledge with them are not providing sufficient evidence that they have increased health literacy about care for their newborn. Parents who are able to teach back what they have learned and were actively engaged in the learning process meet some of the criteria for increased health literacy, but there is insufficient evidence that the parents are able to implement what they have learned. Parents who listen and are able to describe how to care for their newborn but report that they do not understand what was taught have self-identified learning deficit and require further teaching with the nurse to increase health literacy.
9. **The correct answer is 1.** The nurse is using gender-neutral terminology and seeking clarification from the patient about how to address the patient in conversation. It is incorrect to call the patient by their name and use gender-specific language when addressing them; this discounts them and can contribute to erasure. It is incorrect to refuse care to a transmasculine patient on the basis of philosophical and religious beliefs. Although the nurse does have the right to have his or her own philosophical and religious beliefs, this needs to be addressed in a way that does not limit the health care options of the patient. In some situations the nurse may be required to provide safe and ethical care to the patient until an appropriate replacement for the nurse can be found. This is an ethical issue that you need to contemplate and reflect on to determine how you will respond when you encounter patients with beliefs that are different from your own. Encouraging a patient to formula feed takes away the patient's autonomy to make their own choice in how to care for their health and the health of their newborn.
10. **The correct answers are 1, 2, and 5.** Biofeedback, imagery, and relaxation are all effective stress management techniques. Medication has the potential for medication overuse and abuse. Additionally, nonpharmacological approaches are more effective at overcoming stress and have less potential for adverse effects. Time management strategies are not specific for stress management; however, they may be beneficial for helping to reduce stress. Assertiveness training is not specific for the management of stress and is more appropriate for situations that may contribute to stress for a patient.

CHAPTER 24

1. **The correct answer is 4.** Two factors contribute to the projected increase in the number of older persons: the aging of the baby-boom generation and the growth of the population segment older than 85 years. The baby boomers are the adults born between 1946 and 1964.
2. **The correct answer is 3.** The three common conditions affecting cognition are delirium, dementia, and depression. The nurse may find that distinguishing among these three conditions is challenging, but it is essential.
3. **The correct answer is 2.** Sexuality is increasingly recognized as an important factor in the lives of older persons. All older persons, whether healthy or frail, need to express sexual feelings. Sexuality involves love, warmth, sharing, and touching, not just the act of intercourse.
4. **The correct answer is 1.** The libido does not decrease in older persons, although frequency of sexual activity may decline. An older woman who does not understand physical changes affecting sexual activity may be concerned that her sex life is nearly over. The older man may feel the same when he discovers a change in the firmness of his erection, a decreased need for ejaculation with each orgasm, or a longer recovery period between episodes of intercourse.
5. **The correct answer is 3.** Presbyopia (the gradual decline in the ability to focus on near objects) is common in older persons.
6. **The correct answer is 1.** Presbycusis, common in older persons, is a decrease in the ability to hear high-pitched sounds and sibilant consonants such as "s," "sh," and "ch".
7. **The correct answer is 1.** Taste buds atrophy and lose sensitivity. Older persons are less able to discern among salty, sweet, sour, and bitter tastes.
8. **The correct answer is 4.** The anteroposterior diameter of the thorax increases. The incidence of osteoporosis is increased in older persons; vertebral changes caused by osteoporosis lead to dorsal kyphosis, the curvature of the thoracic spine sometimes called "dowager's hump."
9. **The correct answer is 1.** Frontotemporal dementia has an insidious onset and progresses slowly. Early symptoms include poor hygiene, lack of social tact, hyperorality, and sexual disinhibition. Incontinence is an early symptom in frontotemporal dementia, whereas it is a late symptom in the more common Alzheimer's disease.
10. **The correct answer is 2.** A palliative approach includes care for persons with life–limiting illnesses, which may be noncancer or cancer. It is an approach that focuses on generalist care, not specialized palliative care services.

CHAPTER 25

1. **The correct answer is 1.** An actual loss is any loss of a person or object that can no longer be felt, heard, known, or experienced by the individual. Lost objects that have been valued by a patient

include any possession that is worn out, misplaced, stolen, or ruined.

2. **The correct answer is 2.** A perceived loss is any loss that is uniquely defined by the grieving patient. It may be less obvious to others.
3. **The correct answer is 3.** Situational loss includes any sudden, unpredictable external event.
4. **The correct answer is 4.** During Bowlby's phase of disorganization and despair, an individual may constantly examine how and why the loss occurred.
5. **The correct answer is 4.** During Kübler-Ross's stage of depression, the person finally realizes the full impact and significance of the loss and may feel overwhelmingly lonely and withdraw from interpersonal interaction.
6. **The correct answer is 2.** Worden's task 3 is to adjust to the environment in which the deceased is missing. According to Worden, a person does not realize the full impact of a loss for at least 3 months. At this point, many friends and associates make less frequent contact, and the person is left to ponder the full impact of loneliness.
7. **The correct answer is 3.** Loneliness and problems associated with completing the tasks of daily living are two of the most common and difficult adjustments for older bereaved spouses.
8. **The correct answer is 4.** Expression of hopefulness is an expected outcome for patients experiencing a loss.
9. **The correct answer is 2.** For transplantation of organs, ventilatory and circulatory support must be maintained until the organs are harvested. The family must clearly understand that the patient is "brain dead" and that the equipment (i.e., ventilator and vasopressor medications) is not keeping the patient alive but keeping the physical body in a state so that the organs will not be damaged before being harvested.
10. **The correct answer is 3.** Palliative care allows patients to make more informed choices, achieve better alleviation of symptoms, and have more opportunity to manage unfinished business.

CHAPTER 26

1. **The correct answer is 2.** Self-concept is how a person thinks about himself or herself. It is a subjective sense of the self and a complex mixture of unconscious and conscious thoughts, attitudes, and perceptions. Mastectomy is a surgical procedure that alters the appearance and function of the body. Although the changes may not be apparent to other people when the individual is dressed, these bodily changes have a significant impact on the individual.
2. **The correct answer is 3.** Body image depends only partly on the reality of the body. Body image involves attitudes related to the body, including physical appearance, structure, or function. Feelings about body image include those related to sexuality, femininity and masculinity, youthfulness, health, and vitality. These mental images are not always consistent with a person's actual physical structure or appearance.
3. **The correct answer is 3.** An individual's identity is affected by stressors throughout life but is particularly vulnerable during adolescence, a time characterized by many changes.
4. **The correct answer is 1.** Identity confusion results when a person does not maintain a clear, consistent, and continuous consciousness of personal identity.
5. **The correct answer is 3.** By asking clients how they feel about themselves, the nurse is seeking information about their self-esteem.
6. **The correct answer is 1.** Increasing the client's self-awareness is achieved through establishing a trusting nurse–client relationship that allows the client to openly explore thoughts and feelings.
7. **The correct answers are 1, 2, and 4.** A client with poor self-esteem often avoids eye contact, has a stooped or slumped posture, and/or an untidy, unkempt appearance.
8. **The correct answer is 4.** *Role performance* refers to the way in which individuals perceive their ability to carry out significant roles. The patient is worried about his ability to work and provide for his family as a result of his surgery on his back. This is part of his role as a husband and father.
9. **The correct answer is 2.** Risk-taking behaviours such as early involvement with intercourse, having unprotected sex, substance abuse, and reckless driving are often associated with poor self-esteem and self-concept.
10. **The correct answers are 2 and 4.** Inquiring about the client's family responsibilities and relationships with his or her relatives is appropriate when assessing the client's roles responsibilities and relationships. Question 1 is more appropriate for assessing self-esteem, and questions 3 and 5 are more appropriate when inquiring about body image.

CHAPTER 27

1. **The correct answer is 3.** *Gender identity* refers to the degree to which a person identifies as male, female, or some combination thereof. It begins in early childhood as the child becomes aware of the differences of the sexes and perceives that he or she is male or female.
2. **The correct answer is 2.** *Sexual health* means that a person has freedom from physical and psychological impairment, awareness of and positive attitudes toward sexual functioning, and accurate knowledge about sexuality.
3. **The correct answer is 4.** Sexual dysfunction is the absence of complete sexual functioning.
4. **The correct answer is 1.** A major problem in dealing with STIs is that symptoms are absent or go unnoticed. Finding and treating the people who have them can be difficult. Some people who are infected may not even know that they are.
5. **The correct answer is 2.** The most common bacterial STI is genital chlamydia. (HIV infection, AIDS, and HPV are viral STIs.) A chlamydial infection may cause an abnormal genital discharge and burning with urination. There are many serious complications of genital chlamydia in women, including chronic pelvic pain, infertility, and ectopic pregnancy.
6. **The correct answer is 1.** Contraceptive methods that require a health care provider's intervention include hormonal contraception, intrauterine devices (IUDs), the diaphragm, the vaginal contraceptive ring, the cervical cap, and surgical procedures (vasectomy and tubal ligation).
7. **The correct answer is 2.** Effectiveness rates are as follows: for birth control pills, 91 to 99%; for the contraceptive sponge, 68 to 80% for women who have had children, and 84 to 91% for women who have not had children; for vaginal spermicides, 72 to 82%; and for the female condom, 79 to 95%.
8. **The correct answer is 2.** The most valuable tool that you can use when providing care in areas of sexuality is effective, nonjudgemental communication. A perceptive and educated approach to talking about sexuality can offer the support that many patients require. Effective communication about sexuality requires caring, sensitivity, tact, compassion, the use of appropriate language, and nondiscriminatory attitudes.

9. **The correct answer is 3.** When caring for older persons, you may need to adjust your assessment approach. When gathering a sexual history from an older person, it is important to keep in mind that the patient may have difficulty discussing intimate details with health care providers. You are responsible for helping maintain the sexuality of older persons by offering the opportunity to discuss any concerns. Often, asking questions on the topic of sexuality in a comfortable, relaxed manner facilitates older persons' discussion of their sexual needs.
10. **The correct answer is 1.** A useful framework to guide planning is the PLISSIT model, developed by Annon (1976). **P** stands for "permission giving." During assessment, the nurse can bring up the topic of sexuality and can give the individual permission to talk about sexual concerns. **LI** stands for "limited information," which is basic information regarding sexuality and sexual functioning. **SS** stands for "specific suggestions," whereby the nurse provides specific suggestions regarding a sexual concern or issue. If the nurse is not equipped to address a particular concern, he or she should refer the patient to another health care provider. **IT** stands for "intensive therapy." At this level of intervention, the nurse's role is to refer the patient to a qualified practitioner, such as a social worker or a sex counsellor, for individualized therapy.

CHAPTER 28

1. **The correct answer is 3.** Caring for a patient's spiritual needs means caring for the whole person, accepting his or her beliefs and experiences, and helping the patient with issues surrounding meaning and hope. Praying for the patient and calling for a religious leader may be appropriate in some situations, but those situations must be directed by the patient and considered carefully.
2. **The correct answer is 2.** Atheists do not believe in the existence of God. Agnostics believe that any ultimate reality is unknown. This does not mean that spirituality is not an important concept for the atheist or agnostic. Atheists search for meaning in life through their work and their relationships with other individuals. However, it is important not to assume that *spirituality* would be an acceptable term to describe this search for meaning because of its long relationship to religion.
3. **The correct answers are 2 and 4.** Research has indicated that spiritual practices provide structure and support for patients. There are also many different types of spiritual practices that will look different for each individual. Spiritual practices are not always assigned a high priority by nurses because they may not see it as an important part of modern medicine. However, it is important to note that it is often a critical part of a patient's personal medicine.
4. **The correct answer is 1.** Presence is an important way of being with patients that facilitates spiritual care.
5. **The correct answers are 2 and 3.** Those from the Hindu tradition may observe important days of fasting and they are more comfortable with same-sex care providers. Removal of religious symbols can cause distress, and prayer is preferred in private. It is important to understand and facilitate these practices.
6. **The correct answer is 4.** Reviews of spirituality in the literature have indicated that it is associated with meaning, purpose, and connectedness. Although spirituality is closely affiliated with religion for some individuals, individuals on a spiritual journey may or may not describe themselves as religious.
7. **The correct answers are 2, 3, and 4.** Research has indicated that patients prefer support for their own spiritual practices rather than the more intimate interventions that may be implemented by nurses. Adopting an attitude of open curiosity allows patients to share their spiritual beliefs. Patients also want nurses to know about their personal beliefs and spiritual practices.
8. **The correct answer is 4.** Values are an important part of religion and spirituality. Times of grief and suffering may lead to changes in those values.
9. **The correct answer is 3.** Spiritual assessment requires a great deal of sensitivity and should be adapted to the circumstances.
10. **The correct answers are 1 and 5.** Relational practice is respectful, compassionate, and authentic inquiry into the experience of another and is foundational for all of nursing care. Therefore, it helps to create an environment for sensitive spiritual care.

CHAPTER 29

1. **The correct answer is 1.** The medulla oblongata controls vital functions necessary for survival, including heart rate, blood pressure, and respiration.
2. **The correct answer is 4.** The general adaptation syndrome is a three-stage reaction to stress. During the alarm reaction, rising hormone levels result in increases in blood volume, blood glucose levels, epinephrine and norepinephrine levels, heart rate, blood flow to muscles, oxygen intake, and mental alertness.
3. **The correct answer is 3.** Post-traumatic stress disorder (PTSD) can develop after a traumatic injury or event.
4. **The correct answer is 3.** Situational stress can arise from the person's current circumstances, such as moving, changing jobs, and adjusting to a chronic illness or condition.
5. **The correct answer is 2.** The nurse uses the interview to determine the patient's perception of the stressor by asking the patient what is of most concern at this time.
6. **The correct answer is 4.** Three primary modes of coping with stress are to decrease exposure to stress-producing situations, increase resistance to stress by increasing action-oriented coping strategies, and learn skills that reduce physiological response to stress. A support group can provide information about a wide range of coping strategies, guidance about reducing exposure to stressful situations, and shared training sessions on techniques to reduce physiological responsiveness.
7. **The correct answer is 2.** In the presence of anxiety-provoking thoughts and events, a common physiological symptom is muscle tension. Physiological tension will be diminished through a systematic approach of relaxing major muscle groups.
8. **The correct answer is 4.** Rapid changes in health care technology, diversity in the workforce, organizational restructuring, and changing work systems can place stress on nurses.
9. **The correct answer is 1.** A crisis creates a turning point in a person's life because it changes the direction of a person's life in some way. The precipitating event usually occurs from 1 to 2 weeks before the individual seeks help, but it may have occurred within the past 24 hours. In general, a crisis is resolved in some way within approximately 6 weeks.

CHAPTER 30

1. **The correct answer is 3.** Bradycardia is a slow heart rate, slower than 60 beats per minute in adults. Bradypnea is an abnormally slow rate of breathing, slower than 12 breaths per minute.
2. **The correct answer is 1.** An inefficient contraction of the heart that fails to transmit a pulse wave to the peripheral pulse site

creates a pulse deficit. To assess a pulse deficit, the nurse and a colleague assess radial and apical rates simultaneously and then compare rates. The difference between the apical and radial pulse rates is the pulse deficit.

3. **The correct answer is 1.** The normal temperature range gradually drops as individuals approach older adulthood. Older persons have a narrower range of body temperatures than do younger adults. Oral temperatures of 35°C are not unusual for older persons in cold weather. However, the average body temperature of older persons is approximately 36°C.
4. **The correct answer is 3.** The blood pressure measurement is high at 140/96 and the heart rate is within normal range at 70 beats per minute; therefore, the nurse would administer the scheduled metoprolol.
5. **The correct answer is 3.** The respiratory rate measurement and shortness of breath indicate that the patient has tachypnea. A stooped or slumped position impairs ventilatory movement and lying flat prevents full chest expansion; in comparison, a straight, erect posture promotes full chest expansion, which can sometimes decrease shortness of breath, thereby improving the respiratory rate.
6. **The correct answers are 1, 2, and 4.** Patients should never alter the prescribed antihypertensive medication unless otherwise directed by their ordering health care provider as this could lead to unstable blood pressure management. It is important to teach patients about measures they can take to modify their diet (e.g., sodium and fat reduction, alcohol limitations) and reduce stress. Additionally, many will require instruction on how to measure their blood pressure at home, on acceptable values, and when to notify health care providers when values are out of range.
7. **The correct answer is 1.** The blood pressure measurements indicate that the patient has orthostatic hypotension. If orthostatic hypotension is assessed, the patient is assisted to a supine position, and the physician or nurse in charge is then notified. While obtaining orthostatic measurements, the nurse observes for other symptoms of hypotension, such as fainting, weakness, or light-headedness.
8. **The correct answer is 2.** If the nurse detects an abnormal rate while palpating a radial pulse, the next step is to assess the apical rate. The apical rate requires auscultation of heart sounds, which provides a more accurate assessment of cardiac contraction.
9. **The correct answer is 3.** Diseases causing poor oxygenation, such as asthma or chronic obstructive pulmonary disease (COPD), cause an increase in pulse rate.
10. **The correct answer is 3.** A reduction in respiratory rate and depth will not reflect inaccuracies in measurement as this is the purpose of obtaining oxygen saturation levels. Reduced circulation to extremities due to disease or hypothermia can cause poor transmittal of information to the oximeter's probe. Bright light near the measuring probe can cause inaccurate readings as the oximeter obtains saturation readings through the measurement of light through a photo detector, and if there is too much ambient light, results could be influenced. Covering the measuring site with a blanket while taking the reading would help to improve readings.
11. **The correct answer is 3.** The patient has a diagnosis of heart failure, and if there is an existing cardiac or respiratory problem, the stress of a fever can be great because cellular metabolism increases and oxygen consumption rises. The heart and respiratory rates then increase to meet the greater metabolic needs of the body for nutrients. This increased metabolism requires additional oxygen. If the demand for additional oxygen cannot be met, cellular hypoxia (inadequate oxygenation) occurs, sometimes causing angina (chest pain), as this patient is noting. Water loss through increased respiration and diaphoresis can also be excessive, placing a patient at risk for fluid volume deficit. Interventions during a fever may include oxygen therapy and maintaining optimum fluid volume status; this is why the order of normal saline 100 mL/hour is reasonable, along with the order of supplemental oxygen. The patient is complaining of chest pain, thus an electrocardiogram could be ordered to rule out a possible myocardial infarction. The order to question would be the metoprolol, as the blood pressure is low and metoprolol is an antihypertensive medication; giving it would only make the blood pressure drop more.

CHAPTER 31

1. **The correct answer is 3.** Imagery is a visualization technique used by the patient to decrease pain sensation by focusing on pleasurable images. Distraction involves directing the patient's attention to something within the immediate environment to reduce pain awareness. Relaxation exercises involve techniques that lessen physical and mental tension through focus on consciously releasing muscle tension. Recall is not a nonpharmacological pain strategy.
2. **The correct answer is 4.** Referred pain is perceived in an area distant from its point of origin. Transient pain is brief and passes quickly and may be at its point of origin. Superficial pain originates in the skin or subcutaneous tissue. Phantom pain may reflect injury to the peripheral nervous system and may occur in a person who has lost part of a limb.
3. **The correct answer is 3.** The Northern Pain Scale is a self-report scale for developmentally age-appropriate young Inuit children experiencing acute pain episodes. The FLACC tool is most appropriate for children who are nonverbal. The Numerical Rating Scale is indicated for children (older than 9 years) and adults experiencing acute pain who are able to use numbers to rate the intensity of their pain. The Wong-Baker Scale, although a self-report scale specific for this age group, is not as culturally appropriate.
4. **The correct answer is 3.** Increased blood pressure is an involuntary sympathetic nervous system response to moderate pain. Heart rate would increase because of activation of the sympathetic nervous system. Restlessness and protection of the painful area are behavioural responses.
5. **The correct answer is 4.** The nurse can only make an accurate diagnosis of pain after having performed a complete patient assessment. The patient's withdrawal from communication, grimacing, moaning, and verbalizations of discomfort will need to be considered.
6. **The correct answer is 3.** Descriptive scales are used both to assess pain severity and to evaluate changes in a patient's condition. A rating of 7 or more on a 0–10 scale requires immediate attention. The dose was insufficient.
7. **The correct answer is 3.** Teaching patients about pain reduces anxiety and helps them to achieve a sense of control. When a patient is anticipating pain, the nurse needs to explain procedures and any associated discomfort. A confident explanation of the procedure helps nurses gain a patient's trust. When patients are informed about an upcoming painful experience, they often perceive the actual experience as less unpleasant.
8. **The correct answer is 4.** Relaxation and guided imagery are examples of mind–body interactions to decrease pain sensation, whereas physical interventions are techniques that focus solely

on the body. Adjuvants are drugs used to enhance the effect of opioids, whereas patient-controlled analgesia is a drug delivery system.

9. **The correct answer is 3.** OPQRSTUV is the acronym that can be used to remember the components of a pain assessment.
10. **The correct answer is 2.** PCA is a drug delivery by which the patient, not the nurse or family, is in control of the delivery of the pain management program. Although the patient may use less medication because it is self-administered, before the pain becomes too severe, the primary goal of this delivery system is not to minimize the quantity of analgesia needed to control pain.

CHAPTER 32

1. **The correct answer is 1.** Appearance and behaviour are assessed during a general survey. Measurement of vital signs and observing specific body systems are separate components of the physical assessment process and are usually done after the general survey. Conducting a detailed health history usually occurs before the physical examination. Data from the health history guide the physical exam.
2. **The correct answer is 3.** Compared to the fingertips, palmar surface, and base of the hands, the dorsal surface has comparatively less superficial blood supply and less muscle mass. Therefore, it remains slightly cooler to touch and so offers a better contrast by which to detect warm skin during physical examination. Rectal temperature reflects core body temperature rather than skin temperature. Rectal temperature is not the preferred option for temperature measurement in a child 7 years old if other options are available (i.e., tympanic, oral).
3. **The correct answers are 1, 3, 4, and 5.** Skin lesions that are symmetrical, uniform in colour, and less than 6 mm in diameter are less likely to be dangerous. The warning signs of dangerous skin lesions include asymmetry or irregular borders, more than one colour, changes in size or colour, bleeding, and tenderness.
4. **The correct answer is 3.** Rhonchi are loud, low-pitched, rumbling, coarse sounds heard most often during inspiration or expiration. Crackles are moist sounding, most often heard during inspiration and clearing with coughing. Wheezes are high-pitched, musical sounds that are usually louder on expiration than inspiration. Normal breath sounds are clear.
5. **The correct answer is 3.** S_2 correlates with the closure of the aortic and pulmonic valves. S_1 correlates with the closure of the mitral and tricuspid valves.
6. **The correct answer is 2.** When bones are fractured, it is important to assess pulses in the region of fracture to ensure circulation is not compromised. The scaphoid bone is in the wrist; therefore, assessing the radial pulse helps ensure circulation in the scaphoid region. The dorsalis pedis pulse is on the top of the foot, the posterior tibialis pulse on the inner ankle, and the apical pulse at the apex of the heart, making assessment of these pulses less important given the presenting concern.
7. **The correct answer is 2, 4, 3, 1.** The order of an abdominal examination is inspection, auscultation, percussion, palpation. The order of an abdominal examination differs slightly from assessments in the other systems. The examiner begins with inspection and follows with auscultation. By using auscultation before palpation, there is less chance of altering the frequency and character of bowel sounds.
8. **The correct answer is 2.** A painless, pea-sized lump is an abnormal finding that needs to be reported to the patient's health care provider. The testes are normally round, movable, and smooth, rather than lumpy. The nurse should advise the patient to do a testicular self-examination monthly. The best time is after a warm bath or shower, when the scrotal skin is less thick.
9. **The correct answers are 1 and 2.** The knee is a hinge joint capable of the movement of flexion and extension. Flexion is the movement of decreasing the angle between two adjoining bones. Extension is the movement of increasing the angle between two adjoining bones. Abduction is the moving away from the midlines of the body. Adduction is moving toward midline of the body. Internal rotation is rotation of a joint inward. External rotation is rotation of a joint outward.
10. **The correct answer is 4.** Interpreting abstract ideas or concepts reflects the capacity for abstract thinking. For an individual to explain common phrases such as "A stitch in time saves nine" or "Don't count your chickens before they're hatched" requires a higher level of intellectual function. The examiner should note whether the patient's explanations are relevant and concrete. The patient with altered mental status will probably interpret the phrase literally or merely rephrase the words. Judgement requires a comparison and evaluation of facts and ideas to understand their relationships and to form appropriate conclusions. Asking how much the patient knows about his or her illness or the reason for seeking health care can assess a patient's knowledge. Association involves finding similarities or associations between concepts.
11. **The correct answers are 2, 3, and 4.** Cranial nerves (CN) III (oculomotor), IV (trochlear), and VI (abducens) are responsible for motor function of the eye muscles and can be assessed by observing a patient's directions of gaze. CN II (optic) is responsible for visual acuity. CN VII (facial) is responsible for facial expressions. CN XI (spinal accessory) is responsible for movement of the head and shoulders
12. **The correct answers are 1, 2, and 4.** Elevated blood pressure is not a normal physical finding in any patient, whereas each of the three other choices is a common variation of normal findings based on the individual's biocultural background.

CHAPTER 33

1. **The correct answer is 1.** If an infection can be transmitted from one person to another either directly or indirectly, it is a communicable (infectious, contagious) disease.
2. **The correct answer is 1.** MRSA is transmitted by direct and indirect contact. It is spread by physical contact between an infected or colonized individual and a susceptible host. It can also be spread by contact between a susceptible host and a contaminated intermediate object.
3. **The correct answer is 4.** The interval when a patient manifests signs and symptom specific to the type of infection (e.g., common cold manifested by sore throat, sinus congestion, or rhinitis) is the illness stage.
4. **The correct answer is 2.** Hand hygiene is the most important and most basic technique in preventing the transmission of infections. Hand hygiene includes using an alcohol hand rub before and after providing patient care, or handwashing with soap and water when hands are visibly soiled, and performing a surgical scrub when necessary. The components of good handwashing are using an adequate amount of soap, rubbing the hands together to lather the soap and create friction, and rinsing under a stream of water.
5. **The correct answer is 3.** Washing with soap and water takes a minimum of 40 to 60 seconds when all components are considered (including drying time).

6. **The correct answer is 2.** Before isolation measures are instituted, the patient must understand the nature of the disease or condition, the purposes of isolation, and the steps for carrying out specific precautions. The nurse also take measures to improve the patient's sensory stimulation during isolation.
7. **The correct answer is 4.** The primary reason for gowning is to prevent the contamination of clothes during contact with the patient. Gowns protect health care workers and visitors from coming in contact with infected material, blood, or body fluid.
8. **The correct answer is 2.** Hand hygiene must be performed before and after direct patient contact; before and after contact with the patient's environment; after contact with blood, body fluids, and the patient's secretions and excretions and after contact with equipment or articles contaminated by them; and before gloves are put on and removed.
9. **The correct answer is 2.** Contact precautions are needed when standard precautions or routine practices are not sufficient to prevent transmission. *C. difficile* spores have a high potential for environmental contamination and can be spread to other patients via health care workers' hands and contaminated equipment.
10. **The correct answer is 1.** During surgical handwashing the hands need to be above the elbows at all times. Water runs by gravity from fingertips to elbows, flowing from the least contaminated areas.

CHAPTER 34

1. **The correct answer is 1.** Right to refuse has been added to the rights of medication administration. It is important to remember that a patient has the right to refuse a medication. Ensuring that patients know that they have the right to refuse is important to maintain person-centred care. Patients need to be informed that they have this right, but at the same time, they also need to be fully informed about the potential consequences of their refusal.
2. **The correct answer is 2.** A medication order is required for any medication to be administered. To protect patient safety, nurses should ensure the medication order contains all the elements (e.g., medication name, dose, route). If the medication order is incomplete, the nurse should inform the prescriber and ensure completeness before carrying out the medication order. Incomplete transcriptions are a source of medication errors.
3. **The correct answer is 1.** The primary contraindications to administering oral medications include the presence of gastrointestinal alterations, the inability of a patient to swallow foods or fluids, the risk of aspiration in patients with impaired ability to swallow, and the use of gastric suction.
4. **The correct answer is 1.** A medication error is any event that could cause or lead to a patient either receiving inappropriate medication therapy or failing to receive appropriate medication therapy. Most medication errors occur when nurses fail to follow routine procedures, such as checking dose calculations, deciphering illegible handwriting, and recording the names of or administering medications with which they are unfamiliar.
5. **The correct answer is 4.** Apply the following formula for solid dose forms of medications: Dose ordered/Dose on hand × Amount on hand = Amount to administer

$$500\ \text{mg}/250\ \text{mg} \times 1\ \text{tablet} = 2\ \text{tablets}$$

Therefore, if the physician orders 500 mg orally (PO) of Keflex and the medication is only available in tablets containing 250 mg, 2 tablets should be administered.

6. **The correct answer is 3.** Subcutaneous injections involve placing medications into the loose connective tissue under the dermis. Because subcutaneous tissue is not as richly supplied with blood as the muscles, absorption is commonly slower than intramuscular injections.
7. **The correct answer is 1.** Nurses are responsible for following legal provisions when administering controlled substances (drugs that alter the mind or behaviour patterns), which can be dispensed only with a prescription. Violations of the *Narcotic Control Act* are punishable by fines, imprisonment, and loss of nurse licensure or registration.
8. **The correct answer is 2.** Pharmacokinetics is the study of how medications enter the body, reach their site of action, are metabolized, and exit the body. Nurses must use their knowledge of pharmacokinetics when timing medication administration, judging the patient's risk for alterations in medication action, and observing the patient's response.
9. **The correct answer is 4.** Official publications, such as the *British Pharmacopoeia* and the *Canadian Formulary*, set standards for drug strength, quality, purity, packaging, safety, labelling, and dosage form. Physicians, nurses, and pharmacists depend on these standards to ensure that patients receive pure drugs in safe and effective dosages.
10. **The correct answer is 1.** Administration of the *Food and Drugs Act* and the *Controlled Drugs and Substances Act* is carried out by the Health Protection Branch (HPB) of the federal government. Before a new drug can be marketed in Canada, an application for approval must be made to the HPB. After intensive testing, the HPB reviews the application. When sufficient information has been accumulated to ensure its safety, the drug is released for general use.

CHAPTER 35

1. **The correct answer is 3.** Despite the success of allopathic medicine (traditional Western medicine), many health conditions are difficult to treat. Patients with health conditions such as arthritis, chronic back pain, gastrointestinal problems, allergies, headaches, and insomnia choose to explore alternative methods to relieve their symptoms. Answers 1, 2, and 4 are incorrect, as these are complex health problems requiring consultation and treatment from a medical physician before seeking assistance from complementary approaches.
2. **The correct answer is 4.** Many complementary approaches, such as acupuncture and massage therapy, require diagnostic and therapeutic methods specific to their field, whereas other complementary approaches, such as guided imagery and breath work, are, in general, easily learned and applied.
3. **The correct answer is 1.** Most Canadians have used complementary and alternative medicine therapy to prevent illness or maintain wellness. One study reported that 74% of Canadians had used some form of complementary and alternative medicine in their lifetime with the purpose of preventing illness, maintaining wellness, or both.
4. **The correct answer is 1.** Holistic nursing encompasses and treats the mind, body, and spirit of the patient. Nurses can use holistic interventions such as relaxation therapy, guided imagery, music therapy, simple touch, massage, and prayer. Such interventions affect the whole person (mind–body–spirit) and are economical, noninvasive, nonpharmacological complements to traditional medical care.

5. **The correct answer is 2.** Some complementary and alternative medicine approaches and techniques involve natural processes, such as breathing, concentration, and simple touch, to help patients feel better and cope with chronic conditions. These techniques can be learned with minimum preparation, and many of these procedures can be used with patients as part of the nurse's independent nursing practice (Dossey & Keegan, 2013). Adequate assessment and the patient's permission are prerequisites for implementing a complementary medicine therapy.
6. **The correct answer is 1.** According to one of the principles of complementary and alternative medicine approaches, the individual must be actively involved in the treatment. Patients achieve better responses if they are involved in decision making and are able to practise the techniques or exercises daily. The patient must commit to implementing and maintaining the therapy until a desired outcome is achieved.
7. **The correct answer is 3.** St. John's wort is effective as a mild antidepressant and sedative.
8. **The correct answer is 1.** Meditation can augment the effects of certain drugs. For example, individuals taking antihypertensive, antidepressant, or antianxiety medications should be monitored. Prolonged practice of meditation techniques may, in some cases, lead to less need for certain medications, and some doses of medications may need to be adjusted.
9. **The correct answer is 2.** Acupuncture techniques are used to stimulate and activate the body's self-healing abilities. Bringing the patient's body back into balance through the transfer of energy refers to therapeutic touch. Chiropractic therapy involves treatment of diseases of the spine and joints, and in meditation a state of relaxation is created through reducing neural impulses sent to the brain.
10. **The correct answer is 4.** Therapeutic touch is a training-specific therapy that was developed in the 1970s by a nurse, Dr. Dolores Krieger. Although the philosophical and religious assumptions of therapeutic touch differ from those of other Eastern healing modalities, both practices involve trained practitioners who attempt to direct their own balanced energies in an intentional and motivated manner toward the patient.

CHAPTER 36

1. **The correct answer is 3.** Two points of support on the floor maintain a safe balance.
2. **The correct answers are 1, 2, and 3.** This position improves the patient's balance by providing a wider base of support.
3. **The correct answer is 1.** Three points of support maintain a safe balance.
4. **The correct answer is 2.** Patients are more open to developing an exercise program when they are at a stage of readiness to change their behaviour.
5. **The correct answers are 3 and 5.** Patient assistance promotes independence and strength while minimizing workload. A broad base of support increases stability.
6. **The correct answer is 1.** Physical inactivity, hormonal changes, and increased osteoclastic activity contribute to progressive loss of total bone mass in older persons. This increases the patient's risk of falls and injuries.
7. **The correct answer is 3.** It is increasingly evident that children are less active, resulting in an increase in childhood obesity and type 2 diabetes. Strategies for physical activity incorporated early into a child's daily routine may provide a foundation for lifetime commitment to exercise and physical fitness.
8. **The correct answer is 3.** Body mechanics alone are not sufficient to prevent musculoskeletal injuries when positioning or transferring patients. Teaching the use of patient-handling equipment or a lift team in combination with proper body mechanics is more effective.
9. **The correct answer is 2.** Patient understanding is confirmed when the patient is able to explain information or demonstrate it back. Inability to explain or demonstrate indicates the need for repeat instruction or trying a new approach. Teach Back is a way to confirm that a nurse has explained to a patient what he or she needs to know in a manner that the patient understands.
10. **The correct answer is 2.** When ascending stairs on crutches, the patient usually uses a modified three-point gait.
11. **The correct answers are 1, 2, 3, and 4.** By assessing the patient thoroughly, the nurse makes the correct decision concerning his or her ability to manage the patient safely, the need for additional personnel, the patient's ability or inability to help the nurse with the transfer, and the proper equipment to use for the transfer.
12. **The correct answer is 2.** Three-point alternating, or three-point gait requires the patient to bear all of the weight on one foot. In a three-point gait, the patient bears weight on both crutches and then on the uninvolved leg, repeating the sequence.
13. **The correct answer is 3.** Although the patient was discharged from the procedure recovery room, the patient did have some conscious sedation. This sedation may affect the patient's ability to safely follow directions and participate in the transfer; therefore, additional help would be needed to safely transfer the patient from the bed to the stretcher.
14. **The correct answer is 4.** In persons with type 2 diabetes, regular exercise can improve the body's use of glucose and fatty acids, thereby decreasing blood glucose level.
15. **The correct answer is 3.** Musculoskeletal disorders are the most prevalent and debilitating occupational health hazards for nurses. Preventive interventions are needed to avoid the hazards and economic burdens associated with patient-handling tasks. The Canadian Patient Safety Institute calls for the use of assistive equipment and devices to promote a safe health care environment for nurses and their patients.

CHAPTER 37

1. **The correct answer is 2.** In Canada, accidental injuries are the leading cause of death for individuals between the ages of 1 and 34 years.
2. **The correct answer is 2.** Adolescents are at greatest risk for injury from motor vehicle accidents, suicide, and substance abuse.
3. **The correct answer is 1.** Advancing age and the concurrent physiological changes in vision, hearing, mobility, reflexes, circulation, and the ability to make quick judgements predispose older persons to falls.
4. **The correct answer is 2.** WHMIS consists of three main elements: worker education programs, cautionary labelling of products, and the provision of MSDSs.
5. **The correct answer is 2.** Procedure-related accidents occur during therapy. They include medication and fluid administration errors, the improper application of external devices, and accidents related to the improper performance of procedures (e.g., improper Foley catheter insertion).
6. **The correct answer is 4.** A patient who cannot weight bear needs to be moved using a mechanical lift, to protect the nurse from injury and in turn maintain the safety of the patient.

7. **The correct answer is 3.** Restraints are *not* considered a long-term intervention. Restraints are used only after other alternatives have been tried, and the least restrictive method of restraint is used. The use of restraints must be part of the patient's medical treatment. Restraints are considered a short-term intervention; once they have been applied, regular assessments are needed to determine whether they should be continued.
8. **The correct answer is 3.** The poison control centre phone number should be visible on the telephone in homes with young children and in their parents' cell phone. In all cases of suspected poisoning, this number should be called immediately, before any intervention.
9. **The correct answer is 4.** Having a family member with the patient at all times is an unrealistic expectation; a trained sitter may be used if constant observation is required. Attending to personal needs, offering diversionary activities, and camouflaging IV lines may help to avoid the need for a restraint.

CHAPTER 38

1. **The correct answer is 1.** As patients with diabetes often have decreased sensation in their feet, feet should be inspected daily for signs of skin breakdown or infection; changes in colour, temperature, and sensation; and any discoloration or thickening of toenails. Daily inspection can help decrease the development of foot ulcers and subsequent complications.
2. **The correct answer is 3.** Psoriasis is a chronic inflammatory skin condition, the exact cause of which is unknown, and there is currently no cure. It is thought to be an immune-mediated disease whereby the person's immune system reacts against its own cells. It is not contagious and cannot be passed from one person to another. It is not related to poor hygiene.
3. **The correct answer is 3.** With her chronic disease, she may have decreased sensation and circulation, and an increased healing time. She is at a higher risk of developing infection and foot ulcers, which are difficult to treat and slow to heal.
4. **The correct answer is 2.** The skin holds information about the body's circulation, nutritional status, and signs of systemic disease.
5. **The correct answer is 3.** Pallor in a patient with dark skin appears ashen, grey, or dull.
6. **The correct answer is 2.** Inflammation is not easily recognized, and it is often necessary to palpate the skin for increased warmth, taut surfaces that may indicate edema, and induration (hardening of the tissue) as redness at the site of the inflammation is not able to be seen in a dark-skinned patient.
7. **The correct answer is 1.** Gag reflex should be tested in order to avoid aspiration of oral contents during oral hygiene care.
8. **The correct answer is 1.** The patient should always be included in the care plan. Cultural preferences should always be considered. If the patient is unconscious, the family can provide information on hair care preferences.
9. **The correct answer is 2.** This action prevents secretions from entering the nasolacrimal duct.
10. **The correct answer is 4.** It is important to do all of these actions.

CHAPTER 39

1. **The correct answer is 1.** Anemia, a lower than normal hemoglobin level, is a result of decreased hemoglobin production, increased red blood cell destruction, blood loss, or a combination of these factors. Patients will have complaints of fatigue, decreased activity tolerance, and increased breathlessness, as well as pallor (especially seen in the conjunctiva of the eye) and an increased heart rate.
2. **The correct answers are 1, 3, 4, and 5.** The appropriate interventions for a patient with a new onset of atrial fibrillation are to be anticoagulated, control the ventricular response, apply oxygen, and elevate the head of the bed. These interventions reduce the cardiac workload and maximize cardiac output. The anticoagulant reduces the risk of stroke, and an INR is the most appropriate lab value for patients taking Coumadin.
3. **The correct answer is 1, 3, 4, 2.** Hypovolemia is caused by conditions such as shock and severe dehydration resulting from extracellular fluid loss and reduced circulating blood volume. The nurse begins with a set of vital signs to inform the health care provider of the patient's current health status. The nurse can suggest that the health care provider order current blood work, including a complete blood count. The nurse then prepares for intravenous infusion, remains with the patient, and continues to assess vital signs as well as cardiopulmonary status. There is the possibility that this patient will return to the operating room, thus the patient should not receive food or drink.
4. **The correct answer is 3.** Fever increases the tissues' need for oxygen, and as a result, carbon dioxide production also increases. If the febrile state persists, the metabolic rate remains high and the body begins to break down protein stores, resulting in muscle wasting and decreased muscle mass. Respiratory muscles such as the diaphragm and intercostal muscles are also wasted.
5. **The correct answer is sinoatrial node (SA node).** The SA node is the pacemaker of the heart with an intrinsic rate of 60–100 beats per minute. The heart rate increase may be a normal response to exercise, caffeine, emotion, and pain.
6. **The correct answers are 2, 3, and 5.** Health promotion for patients with heart failure should address the importance of a low-sodium and low-fat Mediterranean diet, routine exercise, and annual vaccines (including pneumococcal). Taking daily weight and recognizing symptoms of increased oxygen demand are important. Vitamin D intake is not related to symptoms or treatment of heart failure.
7. **The correct answer is 4.** Hypoxia is inadequate tissue oxygenation at the cellular level. The clinical signs and symptoms of hypoxia include apprehension, restlessness, inability to concentrate, a decreased level of consciousness, dizziness, and behavioural changes. Vital sign changes include an increased pulse rate and increased rate and depth of respirations. During the early stages of hypoxia the blood pressure is elevated.
8. **The correct answer is 1.** A person who starts smoking in adolescence and continues to smoke into middle age has an increased risk for cardiopulmonary disease and lung cancer.
9. **The correct answer is 1, 2, 4, 3, 5.** The immediate actions include the removal of the source of obstruction before administering oxygen.
10. **The correct answer is 10 seconds.** Suctioning longer than 10 seconds can cause cardiopulmonary compromise.
11. **The correct answer is 1.** If an unexpected outcome resulting from a chest tube is a tension pneumothorax, it is important to determine if the cause is related to the chest tube being clamped, kinked, or occluded.
12. **The correct answer is 4.** Applying intermittent suction while withdrawing the catheter prevents injury to the tracheal mucosal lining. Sterile gloves should be used for this procedure; lightly coat 6–8 cm of the catheter, and, in adults, insert catheter approximately 15–20 cm during inspiration.

CHAPTER 40

1. **The correct answer is 1.** Hypokalemia is one of the most common electrolyte imbalances, in which an inadequate amount of potassium circulates in extracellular fluid (ECF). When severe, hypokalemia can affect cardiac conduction and function. Because the normal amount of serum potassium is so small, fluctuations are poorly tolerated. The most common cause of hypokalemia is the use of potassium-wasting diuretics such as thiazide and loop diuretics.
2. **The correct answer is 4.** An infant's proportion of total body water (70 to 80% total body weight) is greater than that of children or adults. Infants are not protected from fluid loss because they ingest and excrete a relatively greater daily water volume than do adults. Therefore, they are at a greater risk for fluid volume deficit and hyperosmolar imbalance because body water loss is proportionately greater per kilogram of weight. In addition, infants are dependent on others for fluid intake.
3. **The correct answer is 2.** Older persons experience a number of age-related changes that can affect fluid, electrolyte, and acid–base balances. They have a decreased thirst sensation, which may affect their oral intake of fluids. The kidneys have a decrease in the glomerular filtration rate and in the number of filtering nephrons. These changes can mean that in the presence of sodium depletion or overload, the older person may be unable to maintain homeostasis, and the imbalance is instead worsened.
4. **The correct answer is 4.** For patients in health care settings, measurement of intake and output is a nursing intervention routinely used for patients after a procedure, patients who are febrile, patients with restricted fluids, or patients who receive diuretic or intravenous therapy. Output includes urine, diarrhea, vomitus, gastric suction, and drainage from postsurgical wounds or other tubes.
5. **The correct answer is 1.** Health promotion activities in the area of fluid, electrolyte, and acid–base imbalances focus primarily on patient teaching. Patients and caregivers need to recognize risk factors for these imbalances and implement appropriate preventive measures.
6. **The correct answer is 1.** Under no circumstances should potassium chloride (KCl) be given by intravenous push. A direct intravenous infusion of KCl can be fatal. If an intravenous fluid is to have additives, a physician's order must be obtained that includes the required additives.
7. **The correct answer is 1.** The patient's microflora and contamination by insertion are initially controlled for in the procedure for intravenous insertion. However, the other factors are controlled through conscientious use of infection control principles. This begins with thorough hand hygiene before and after the nurse handles any component of the intravenous system.
8. **The correct answer is 3.** An infiltration occurs when intravenous fluids enter the surrounding space around the venipuncture site. This is manifested as swelling (from increased tissue fluid) and pallor and coolness (caused by decreased circulation) around the venipuncture site.
9. **The correct answer is 3.** Although many policies recommend replacing peripheral venous access devices and rotating sites to prevent phlebitis, the most recent evidence-informed review suggests that this is unnecessary, is costly, and may increase patient discomfort unnecessarily; therefore, current recommendations are to rotate sites on the basis of clinical indications, including painful site, redness, swelling, or hardness at the site.
10. **The correct answer is 4.** Although tachycardia and possibly some dyspnea with acute hemolytic and anaphylactic reactions will occur, the most common symptoms of circulatory overload related to blood administration are cough, dyspnea, and tachycardia. In other reactions, fever, chills, or both also occur.

CHAPTER 41

1. **The correct answer is 4.** Excessive daytime sleepiness (EDS) is the most common complaint of people with obstructive sleep apnea (OSA). People with severe OSA may report experiencing a disruption in their daily activities because of sleepiness.
2. **The correct answer is 2.** In hospitals and long-term care facilities, patients may have difficulty finding the time they need to rest and sleep. The nurse should plan care to avoid awakening patients for nonessential tasks. The nurse should schedule assessments, treatments, procedures, and routines for times when patients are awake. For example, the nurse should not wake a stable patient to check vital signs.
3. **The correct answer is 4.** The use of nonprescription sleeping medications is not advisable. Patients should learn the risks of such drugs. Over the long term, these drugs can lead to further sleep disruption even when they initially seemed to be effective. Older persons should be cautioned about using over-the-counter antihistamines because of their long duration of action that can cause confusion, constipation, urinary retention, and increased risk of falls.
4. **The correct answer is 4.** Patients should be cautioned about the dosage and use of herbal compounds because active ingredients can vary from product to product. Herbal compounds may interact with prescribed medication, and concurrent use should be avoided.
5. **The correct answer is 1.** Although dreams occur during both nonrapid eye movement (NREM) and rapid eye movement (REM) sleep, the dreams of REM sleep are more vivid and elaborate and are believed to be functionally important to learning, memory processing, and adaptation to stress.
6. **The correct answer is 3.** Alcohol can initially make a person feel drowsy; however, it can also cause a person to awaken during the night and can cause difficulty returning to sleep.
7. **The correct answer is 1.** Limiting alcohol, caffeine, and nicotine and decreasing fluids 2 to 4 hours before sleep may promote sleep for older persons.
8. **The correct answer is 3.** The Canadian Paediatric Society recommends that apparently healthy infants be placed in the supine position during sleep because of an association between the prone position and the occurrence of sudden infant death syndrome (SIDS).
9. **The correct answer is 4.** Narcolepsy is a dysfunction of mechanisms that regulate the sleep and wake states. Excessive daytime sleepiness (EDS) is the most common complaint associated with this disorder. Brief daytime naps no longer than 20 minutes help reduce subjective feelings of sleepiness. During the day, the person may suddenly feel an overwhelming wave of sleepiness and fall asleep; REM sleep can occur within 15 minutes of falling asleep.
10. **The correct answer is 4.** Sleep needed during the school years is individualized because of varying activity and health levels. Six-year-olds average 11 to 12 hours of sleep nightly, whereas 11-year-olds sleep 9 to 10 hours. Six- or seven-year-olds can usually be persuaded to go to bed by encouraging quiet activities.

CHAPTER 42

1. **The correct answer is 3.** Carbohydrates are the main source of energy in the diet.
2. **The correct answer is 2.** Essential nutrients are generally supplied by food.
3. **The correct answer is 4.** When the intake of nitrogen exceeds the output, the body is in positive nitrogen balance, which is required for growth, normal pregnancy, maintenance of lean muscle mass and vital organs, and wound healing.
4. **The correct answers are 1, 2, 3, 5, and 6.** Individual income, education, and food preferences combine with collective factors such as geographic proximity to nutritious food and taxation of certain categories of foodstuffs, for example, carbonated beverages, candies and confectionery, and snack food products at a higher rate that influences food selection and quantity.
5. **The correct answer is 1.** When a patient is unable to take fluid or food by eating normally over an extended period of time, nutrients are needed, and giving liquid nutrients through a nasal or oral enteral feeding tube will ensure adequate nutrition.
6. **The correct answer is 4.** The nutrient content claim *light* is permitted only on foods reduced in fat or reduced in calories. The percent of reduction in calories or fat has not been established for the claim *light*.
7. **The correct answer is 4.** Whole milk helps ensure adequate intake of fatty acids necessary for brain and neurological development.
8. **The correct answer is 3.** The stronger side can do the work of chewing and swallowing.
9. **The correct answer is 1.** The nurse must assess the patient's ability to swallow before attempting feeding. Patients are to be positioned in sitting position or as upright as tolerable. Patients with dysphagia may require thickened fluids to reduce choking risk. As permitted, food is placed in the stronger side of the mouth (see Question 8 above). The speech-language pathologist and the dietician are the most qualified allied health providers to plan for feeding of dysphasic patients.
10. **The correct answer is 3.** Age-related factors affect appetite, comfort, and digestion of food.
11. **The correct answer is 2.** Filling the tube with water and clamping it after each feeding will *most* likely prevent clogging of a nasogastric feeding tube.

CHAPTER 43

1. **The correct answer is 2.** The normal adult urine output is 1 500 to 1 600 mL/day.
2. **The correct answer is 3.** In addition to removal of waste products of metabolism, the kidneys have a role in fluid and electrolyte balance through filtration and reabsorption of water, glucose, and major electrolytes. Antidiuretic hormone is secreted from the posterior pituitary gland, growth hormone is regulated by hormones from the hypothalamus, and albumin is produced in the liver.
3. **The correct answer is 2.** Postrenal alterations result from obstruction to the flow of urine in the urinary collecting system anywhere between the renal pelvis and the urethral meatus. Urine is formed by the urinary system but cannot be eliminated by normal means. Urinary obstruction can be caused by calculi (stones), blood clots, or tumours.
4. **The correct answer is 3.** The urine is normally acidic, which inhibits bacterial growth and may prevent UTIs. Residual urine left in the bladder becomes alkaline and is an ideal medium for microbial growth.
5. **The correct answer is 3.** Hospital-acquired UTIs are often related to poor hand hygiene and urinary catheterization. The introduction of a catheter through the urethra provides a direct route for microorganisms to enter the bladder.
6. **The correct answer is 1.** The urine appears cloudy because of the presence of white blood cells (WBCs) or bacteria. Having the urine stand for a long time after collecting may also cause cloudiness.
7. **The correct answer is 1.** Prompted voiding is a useful strategy for patients with cognitive or physical impairment, or both, who rely on caregiver assistance.
8. **The correct answer is 3.** With stress incontinence, urine loss results from increased intra-abdominal pressure (e.g., coughing, sneezing, laughing, lifting). It usually involves a small volume of urine loss (less than 50 mL) and usually occurs in women or in men following radical prostatectomy. Pregnancy and delivery, weak pelvic floor muscles, heavy lifting, and obesity are sometimes contributing factors.
9. **The correct answer is 1.** The drainage bag should never be raised above the level of the patient's bladder. It should hang on the bed frame or wheelchair without touching the floor. Urine in the bag and tubing can become a medium for bacteria, and infection is likely to develop if urine flows back into the bladder.
10. **The correct answer is 4.** Care must be taken to ensure that, whatever type or size of condom is used, blood supply to the penis is not impaired. Therefore, the condom catheter should be snug and secure but should not cause constriction of blood flow.
11. **The correct answer is 3.** In many cases, incontinence can be reduced through careful assessment, determination of possible causes and contributors, and implementation of management strategies. Referral to a local continence service that can provide this expertise and reliable web-based resources can be sources of information for the patient.
12. **The correct answer is 2.** Research has demonstrated that weight loss in the overweight individual can be an effective strategy in improving incontinence, particularly in women with stress incontinence.

CHAPTER 44

1. **The correct answer is 4.** Most nutrients and electrolytes are absorbed in the small intestine, specifically in the duodenum and jejunum.
2. **The correct answer is 3.** Lactose intolerance is the inability to digest lactose, which is the predominant sugar in milk and milk products. Lactose intolerance is caused by a shortage of the enzyme lactase. Lactase is normally produced by the cells that line the small intestine and is needed to digest lactose; however, lactase is genetically programmed to disappear in adulthood in everyone except in individuals of northern European ancestry. As a result, many adults cannot digest lactose, which results in diarrhea, gaseous distension, and cramping.
3. **The correct answer is 4.** Fecal occult blood testing (FOBT), or the guaiac test, is a common laboratory test that can be done at home or at the patient's bedside. This test measures microscopic amounts of blood in the feces. FOBT is useful as a diagnostic screening test for colon cancer.
4. **The correct answer is 1.** Antidiarrheal opiate agents decrease intestinal muscle tone to slow the passage of feces. Opiates inhibit the peristaltic waves that move feces forward, but they also increase segmental contractions that mix the intestinal contents and expose them to the mucosal-absorbing surface.

5. **The correct answer is 3.** An obvious sign of impaction is the inability to pass a stool for several days, despite the repeated urge to defecate. When a continuous oozing of diarrhea stool develops, impaction should be suspected. The diarrhea is the result of the liquid portion of feces, located higher in the colon, seeping around the impacted mass.
6. **The correct answer is 4.** Cleansing enemas promote the complete evacuation of feces from the colon. The amount of solution to be instilled in an adult is 750 to 1 000 mL.
7. **The correct answer is 3.** The specific signs and symptoms of intolerance to an enema include abdominal pain that is greater than a pressure sensation, abdominal cramping, abdominal distension, or rectal bleeding. The enema must be stopped. Notify the prescriber and obtain vital signs.
8. **The correct answer is 2.** One of the greatest problems in caring for a patient with a nasogastric tube is maintaining comfort. The tube is a constant irritation to nasal mucosa. The nurse must assess the condition of both nares and mucosa for inflammation and excoriation.
9. **The correct answer is 1.** The stool discharged from an ostomy is called *effluent.*
10. **The correct answer is 1.** A nurse trained to care for ostomy patients is an enterostomal therapist (ET).

CHAPTER 45

1. **The correct answers are 2, 3, and 4.** Patients who are immobile are at high risk for developing pulmonary complications. The most common respiratory complications are atelectasis (collapse of alveoli) and hypostatic pneumonia (inflammation of the lung from stasis or pooling of secretions). Ultimately, the distribution of mucus in the bronchi increases, particularly when the patient is in the supine, prone, or lateral position.
2. **The correct answer is 1.** Immobility disrupts normal metabolic functioning: decreasing the metabolic rate; altering the metabolism of carbohydrates, fats, and proteins; causing fluid, electrolyte, and calcium imbalances; and causing gastrointestinal disturbances such as decreased appetite and slowing of peristalsis.
3. **The correct answer is 2.** Wearing of elastic stockings promotes venous return to the heart. Elastic stockings (sometimes called *antiembolic stockings*) aid in maintaining external pressure on the muscles of the lower extremities and thus promote venous return. Increase in venous return helps reduce the stasis of blood, thereby reducing the risk for deep vein thrombosis in the lower extremities.
4. **The correct answers are 1, 2, and 3.** Patients at risk for or diagnosed with osteoporosis have special health promotion needs. Patients who are at risk should be encouraged to get screened for osteoporosis. Nurses also need to assess these patients' diets for calcium and vitamin D intake. Multivitamins do not always have the needed amount of calcium for every individual. A patient needs to know his or her requirement and make a decision based on that.
5. **The correct answer is 1.** The trapeze bar enables the patient to pull with the upper extremities to raise the trunk off the bed, aid in transfer from bed to wheelchair, or perform upper-arm exercises. It increases independence and maintains upper-body strength to aid in performing activities of daily living.
6. **The correct answer is 4.** Patients whose mobility is restricted require range-of-motion (ROM) exercises daily to reduce the hazards of immobility. Temporary immobilization results in some muscle atrophy, loss of muscle tone, and joint stiffness. Two weeks of joint immobilization without ROM can quickly result in contractures.
7. **The correct answers are 1, 3, and 4.** Because bleeding is a potential adverse effect of these medications, the nurse needs to continually assess the patient for signs of bleeding such as hematuria, bruising, coffee ground–like vomitus or gastrointestinal aspirate, guaiac-positive stools, and bleeding gums.
8. **The correct answer is 1.** The nurse needs to teach the patient, caregiver, or both the current recommended dietary allowances for calcium and review foods high in calcium (e.g., milk fortified with vitamin D, leafy green vegetables, yogurt, and cheese).
9. **The correct answers are 2 and 3.** The most effective way to prevent deep vein thrombosis is through an aggressive program of prophylaxis. A properly functioning SCD inflates with a pressure around 40 mm Hg. Inflation pressure averages 40 mm Hg, and the patient's leg should be placed in the SCD sleeve with the back of the knee aligned with the popliteal opening on the sleeve. Measurement involves length of leg, not calf. A green light indicates that the SCD device is functioning.
10. **The correct answer is 3.** Immobility is a major risk factor for pressure injuries. Any break in the integrity of the skin is difficult to heal. Preventing a pressure injury is much less expensive than treating one; therefore, preventive nursing interventions are imperative.
11. **The correct answers are 1, 2, and 5.** The three major changes in the cardiac system with immobility are orthostatic hypotension, increased cardiac workload, and thrombus formation.
12. **The correct answer is 2.** Prevention of complications of immobility begins when the patient becomes immobilized. Ambulating every 30 minutes is not necessary and disruptive to the healing process. Active patient participation in exercise is more beneficial to preventing venous stasis.
13. **The correct answer is 4.** Incentive spirometry opens the airway, preventing atelectasis.
14. **The correct answer order is 1, 5, 7, 4, 6, 3, 2.**
15. **The correct answer is 3.** Physiological outcomes of immobility include decreased metabolism, increased cardiac workload, decreased lung expansion, and increased oxygen demand.

CHAPTER 46

1. **The correct answer is 4.** When the skin is being compressed, blood flow is slowed and the skin becomes pale. After the pressure is relieved, the skin in the affected area turns red (erythema), which is a result of the blood vessels expanding (vasodilation) to allow more blood into the area to overcome the ischemic episode. This process is called *normal reactive hyperemia.* The reddened area is assessed by pressing a fingertip over it. If the area blanches (turns white or a pale colour) and the erythema returns when the finger is removed, the reactive hyperemia is likely transient. If, however, the reddened area does not blanch when finger pressure is applied (abnormal reactive hyperemia), suspect deep tissue damage.
2. **The correct answer is 1.** A stage 1 pressure injury is an observable pressure-related alteration of intact skin, whose indicators, as compared with an adjacent or opposite area on the body, may include changes in skin temperature (warmth or coolness), tissue consistency (firm or beefy feel), and sensation (pain or itching).
3. **The correct answer is 4.** If purulent or suspicious-looking wound drainage is present or there is a change in a previously healing chronic wound, obtaining a specimen of the drainage for culture may be necessary. The wound culture sample should never be

collected from old drainage. Resident colonies of bacteria from the skin grow within exudate and may not be the true causative organisms of a wound infection. Before culturing a wound, clean the base of the wound with normal saline to remove superficial slough and debris. Select the cleanest part of the wound bed (granulating tissue is optimal), press the swab into a 1-cm square area of this cleanest part of the wound, and rotate fully, pressing to express fluid beneath the surface of the wound bed.

4. **The correct answer is 3.** When evisceration occurs, place sterile towels soaked in sterile saline over the extruding tissues to reduce chances of bacterial invasion and drying of the tissues. If the organs protrude through the wound, blood supply to the tissues is compromised. The patient should be allowed nothing by mouth (NPO), observed for signs and symptoms of shock, and prepared for emergency surgery.
5. **The correct answer is 3.** Serous drainage is clear, watery plasma.
6. **The correct answer is 3.** Ensuring that the patient understands the plan of care will decrease anxiety and increase the patient's feeling of control. Pain can also have a negative impact on wound healing; thus, assessing the need for analgesia and providing it before the dressing change supports optimal healing and patient comfort and control.
7. **The correct answer is 3.** Exposure to fecal and urinary incontinence creates a caustic environment on the skin that leads to excoriation and further breakdown, once the skin is no longer intact. An incontinence cleanser and a moisture barrier ointment will remove urine and feces from the skin, leaving a protective (usually silicone-based) barrier that repels moisture.
8. **The correct answer is 4.** Hydrocolloid dressings are dressings with complex formulations of colloidal, elastomeric, and adhesive components that are both adhesive and occlusive. The wound contact layer of this dressing forms a gel as fluid is absorbed and maintains a moist healing environment.
9. **The correct answer is 3.** An abdominal binder will support the wound and reduce stress on large abdominal incisions that are vulnerable to tension or stress as the patient moves or coughs.
10. **The correct answer is 4.** The body requires additional energy to heal pressure injury. Dietitians are trained in thorough assessment of caloric requirements and intake for effective wound healing and, thus, are essential members of the health care team looking after patients with skin breakdown. In addition, dietitians are knowledgeable about different sources of nutrition, including supplements or tube feeding, if required.

CHAPTER 47

1. **The correct answer is 4.** A kinesthetic sense enables a person to be aware of the position and movement of body parts without seeing them.
2. **The correct answer is 4.** Stereognosis is a sense that allows a person to recognize an object's size, shape, and texture.
3. **The correct answer is 3.** When a person receives multiple sensory stimuli and cannot perceptually disregard or selectively ignore some stimuli, sensory overload occurs. The patient in constant pain or who undergoes frequent monitoring of vital signs is at risk. Multiple stimuli can combine to cause overload.
4. **The correct answer is 3.** Proprioceptive changes after the age of 60 years include increased difficulty with balance, spatial orientation, and coordination.
5. **The correct answer is 3.** For a patient with hearing impairment, the nurse should face the patient when speaking, use simple sentences, and speak more slowly and at a normal volume.
6. **The correct answer is 4.** The nursing health history includes assessment of the nature and characteristics of sensory alterations or any problem related to an alteration. The nurse begins by asking the patient to describe the sensory deficit; for example, "How does your hearing now compare with your hearing a year ago?"
7. **The correct answer is 4.** Older persons who drive should be advised as follows: Do not drive during rush hour. Use rear-view and side-view mirrors when changing lanes. Avoid driving at dusk or at night. Drive slowly, but not too slowly. Keep your car in good working condition.
8. **The correct answer is 4.** Hearing loss caused by noisy environments was once thought to affect primarily older individuals; however, recent research has observed this loss in youth. Nurses should routinely teach parents and children to take precautions when involved in activities associated with high-intensity noise. Nurses should assess patients for noise exposure and participate in providing hearing conservation classes for teachers, students, and patients.
9. **The correct answer is 2.** Olfaction is the sense of smell. A patient who cannot smell smoke may not know that something is burning. A smoke detector would be essential.
10. **The correct answer is 3.** When senses are impaired, the sense of self is impaired. Initially, a person may withdraw by avoiding communication or socialization with others in an attempt to cope with the sensory loss.

CHAPTER 48

1. **The correct answer is 2.** The obese patient is susceptible to poor wound healing and to wound infection because of the structure of fatty tissue, which contains a poor blood supply. This slows delivery of essential nutrients and enzymes needed for wound healing.
2. **The correct answer is 3.** If a patient regularly uses prescription or over-the-counter medications, the surgeon or anaesthesiologist may temporarily discontinue the drugs before surgery or adjust the dosages. Certain medications have special implications for the surgical patient, creating greater risks for complications or interacting negatively with anaesthetic agents.
3. **The correct answer is 2.** The patient who smokes is at greater risk for postoperative pulmonary complications than a patient who does not smoke.
4. **The correct answer is 2.** The family is an important resource for a patient with physical limitations and can provide the emotional support needed to motivate the patient to return to a previous state of health. Often, a family member can become the patient's coach, offering valuable support during the postoperative period.
5. **The correct answer is 1.** Accurate recording of intake and output helps in assessing renal and circulatory function. For example, nurses measure all sources of output, including urine, surgically placed drains, gastric drainage, and drainage from wounds, and note any insensible loss from diaphoresis.
6. **The correct answer is 3.** The patient is positioned on one side with the face downward and the neck slightly extended to facilitate a forward movement of the tongue and the flow of mucous secretions out of the mouth.
7. **The correct answer is 4.** To promote normal venous return and circulatory blood flow, patients should be encouraged to perform leg exercises at least every hour while awake. Other measures include applying elastic stockings or sequential compression device as ordered, encouraging early ambulation, positioning

the patient so that blood flow is not interrupted, administering anticoagulant drugs as ordered, and promoting adequate fluid intake.

8. **The correct answer is 2.** International normalized ratio (INR) and activated partial thromboplastin time (APTT) indicate the clotting ability of blood, which if greater than normal reveal patients at risk for bleeding tendencies.
9. **The correct answer is 2.** Maintaining an upright position facilitates diaphragm excursion and enhances expansion of the thorax.
10. **The correct answer is 4.** Malignant hyperthermia is a potentially lethal condition that can occur in patients who received general anaesthesia. It should be suspected when there is unexpected tachycardia and tachypnea; jaw muscle rigidity; body rigidity of limbs, abdomen, and chest; or hyperkalemia. Temperature elevation is a late sign.

APPENDIX A

1. **The correct answer is 2.** The requirements to become registered include completion of an approved practical nurse program and providing evidence of recent practice. Practical nurses write the Canadian Practical Nurse Registration Examination, not the NCLEX. In order to use the protected title of LPN, the LPN must be registered.
2. **The correct answer is 4.** In order to practise as an LPN, practical nurses must be licensed within their jurisdiction, regardless of the setting in which they intend to practise. Through legislation, scopes of practice are determined for all regulated professionals, regardless of whether they are a medical practitioner (i.e., physician) or from another category. Scopes of practice reflect social and professional advances and will vary by jurisdiction because each province is responsible for its own legislation regarding regulated professions.
3. **The correct answer is 2.** Without adaptation or successful responses to change, the creation of specialized knowledge and skills and niches in practice can result in being squeezed out when the environment changes or losing the support of government and other power groups. The formation of subgroups is known as *speciation,* and the subsumption of characteristics of another profession is known as *hybridization*, neither of which may result in survival.
4. **The correct answer is 2.** *Laddering* refers to the recognition of prior learning and experience in order to achieve a higher credential (such as a baccalaureate in nursing). While certifications, skills-based learning, and continuing education advance the skills and career of the LPN, they are not part of laddering to a different level of credential.
5. **The correct answer is 3.** In the 1940s, the first formal education program for practical nursing was established in Manitoba and the first legislative act that laid out education requirements was passed. It was not until the 1970s that practical nursing was recognized as a distinct profession that required formal education. Practical nursing moved to colleges in Ontario, in the 1990s.
6. **The correct answer is 1.** Only those who are able to satisfy all requirements (e.g., evidence of satisfactory practice, completion of an approved nursing program, criminal record check, success on licensing examinations) for licensure and have applied and been approved for licensure by their regulatory body can practise as a nurse in the category to which they apply (the NP graduate could practise as an LPN or general class RN but not as an NP). Unregulated health care providers are not regulated and, therefore, cannot practise as a nurse.
7. **The correct answer is 4.** While historically, LPNs have been hired into long-term care areas where there is a predominance of older persons, the numbers hired in acute care and other areas is increasing. New graduates are more likely to secure part-time employment in multiple settings. Baccalaureate education is not required for LPNs.
8. **The correct answer is 2.** Requirements to register as an LPN or RPN include graduation from a formal, approved education program, which is a 2-year college diploma program. Certificate and hospital-based training programs were the initial approaches to LPN education. Baccalaureate education is not an entry-level requirement.
9. **The correct answer is 2.** A scope of practice is determined through provincial law and governs what LPNs can legally do. Terminal outcomes outline the competencies expected of practical nurse graduates at the end of an educational program and are based on entry-to-practice competencies, as well as scopes of practice.
10. **The correct answers are 2 and 5.** Codes of ethics provide general guidelines about practice and behaviour and would not include specific details as to how to administer medication. A code of ethics would include self-evaluation in order to maintain competency. Confidentiality and privacy are part of ethical behaviour. Negotiation related to use of skills is a workplace and regulatory responsibility.

Page numbers followed by "*f*" indicate figures, "*t*" indicate tables, and "*b*" indicate boxes.

Q

R

SPECIAL FEATURES

PATIENT TEACHING

CONCEPT MAPS

RESEARCH HIGHLIGHTS